Quick Table of Contents

D1159513

PORTH PATHOPHYSIOLOGY

Concepts of Altered Health States

PORTH PATHOPHYSIOLOGY
Concepts of Altered Health States

SECOND CANADIAN EDITION

RUTH A. HANNON, NP-PHC, MHA, MSFNP-BC, DNP(C)

Assistant Professor
School of Nursing
McMaster University
Hamilton, Ontario

CAROL M. PORTH, RN, MSN, PhD (Physiology)

Professor Emeritus
College of Nursing
University of Wisconsin—Milwaukee
Milwaukee, Wisconsin

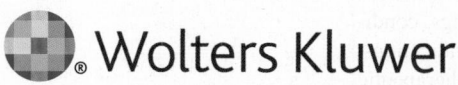 Wolters Kluwer

Philadelphia • Baltimore • New York • London
Buenos Aires • Hong Kong • Sydney • Tokyo

Executive Editor: Sherry Dickinson
Product Development Editor: Katherine Burland
Editorial Assistant: Dan Reilly
Marketing Manager: Dean Karampelas
Production Project Manager: Marian Bellus
Design Coordinator: Joan Wendt
Manufacturing Coordinator: Karin Duffield
Prepress Vendor: Aptara, Inc.

9 8 7 6 5 4 3 2 1

Printed in China

Library of Congress Cataloging-in-Publication Data
Porth pathophysiology : concepts of altered health states / [edited by] Ruth A. Hannon, Carol M. Porth.
– Second Canadian edition.
    p. ; cm.
    Pathophysiology
    Based on: Porth's Pathophysiology : concepts of altered health states / [edited by] Sheila C. Grossman, Carol M. Porth. Ninth edition. [2014].
    Includes bibliographical references and index.
    ISBN 978-1-4511-9289-6
    I. Hannon, Ruth A., editor. II. Porth, Carol, editor. III. Pathophysiology (Porth). Based on (work):
IV. Title: Pathophysiology.
    [DNLM: 1. Disease–Nurses' Instruction. 2. Pathology–Nurses' Instruction.
3. Physiology–Nurses' Instruction. QZ 4]
    RB113
    616.07–dc23
                                                            2015032546

While there have been so many people regularly encouraging me, I want to specifically thank Andrew and Narelle, who in their own way are my biggest supporters.

—RUTH A. HANNON

Contributors to the Second Canadian Edition

Jonathan Barrios, NP-PHC, MScN, PhD(c)
Nursing Instructor
Ryerson University
Toronto, Ontario
CHAPTER 44: DISORDERS OF THE MALE GENITOURINARY
  SYSTEM

Jason R. Faulhaber, MD
Assistant Program Director
Infectious Diseases Fellowship Training Program
Carilion Medical Center
Roanoke, Virginia
CHAPTER 20: ACQUIRED IMMUNODEFICIENCY SYNDROME

Ellen Gretsinger, RN(EC), BSc, MSFNP, DNP(c)
Primary Health Care Nurse Practitioner
Smithville Medical Centre Family Health Team
Smithville, Ontario
Primary Health Care Nurse Practitioner Instructor
McMaster University
Hamilton, Ontario
CHAPTER 46: DISORDERS OF THE FEMALE
  REPRODUCTIVE SYSTEM

Kim Litwack, RN, PhD, FAAN, APNP
Associate Dean for Academic Affairs
University of Wisconsin—Milwaukee
Milwaukee, Wisconsin
Family Nurse Practitioner
Advanced Pain Management
Madison, Wisconsin
CHAPTER 49: SOMATOSENSORY FUNCTION, PAIN,
  AND HEADACHE

Peter Margetts, MD, PhD
Professor of Medicine
Division of Nephrology
McMaster University
Hamilton, Ontario
CHAPTER 34: ACUTE RENAL INJURY AND CHRONIC
  KIDNEY DISEASE

Christopher McLaughlin, MD, PhD
Chief Ophthalmology Resident
Hamilton Regional Eye Institute
McMaster University
Hamilton, Ontario
CHAPTER 54: DISORDERS OF VISUAL FUNCTION

Lesley L. Moisey, RD, MSc, PhD(c)
PhD Candidate and Consulting Dietitian
University of Waterloo
Waterloo, Ontario
CHAPTER 39: ALTERATIONS IN NUTRITIONAL STATUS

Joanna Pierazzo, RN, MScN, PhD
Assistant Professor
School of Nursing, McMaster University
Hamilton, Ontario
CHAPTER 50: DISORDERS OF MOTOR FUNCTION
CHAPTER 51: DISORDERS OF BRAIN FUNCTION

Charlotte Pooler, RN, MN, PhD
Clinician Scientist
Palliative/End of Life Care & Community Programs
Alberta Health Services, Edmonton Zone
Faculty of Nursing, University of Alberta
Edmonton, Alberta
CHAPTER 26: HEART FAILURE AND CIRCULATORY
  SHOCK
CHAPTER 27: STRUCTURE AND FUNCTION OF THE
  RESPIRATORY SYSTEM
CHAPTER 28: RESPIRATORY TRACT INFECTIONS, NEOPLASMS,
  AND CHILDHOOD DISORDERS

Carol M. Porth, RN, MSN, PhD
Professor Emerita
University of Wisconsin—Milwaukee
Milwaukee, Wisconsin
CHAPTER 18: INFLAMMATION, TISSUE REPAIR, AND
  WOUND HEALING

Otto Sanchez, MD, PhD
Professor
Faculty of Health Sciences
University of Ontario Institute of Technology
Oshawa, Ontario
CHAPTER 8: NEOPLASIA

Diana Sherifali, RN, PhD, CDE
Associate Professor
School of Nursing, McMaster University
Hamilton, Ontario
CHAPTER 42: DIABETES MELLITUS AND THE
  METABOLIC SYNDROME

Contributors to the First Canadian Edition

Anna Barkman, RN, BN, MN
Instructor
School of Nursing
Faculty of Health and Community Studies
Mount Royal College
Calgary, Alberta
(Chapters 22, 23, 24, 25, 26)

Lynn Miles, RN, BScN, MSc, PhD
Professor
Mohawk College
Hamilton, Ontario
(Chapter 59)

Lesley L. Moisey, MSc, RD, PhD(c)
PhD Candidate and Consulting Dietitian
University of Waterloo
Waterloo, Ontario
(Chapter 39)

Joanna Pierazzo, RN, BEd, MScN, PhD
Assistant Professor
School of Nursing, McMaster University
Hamilton, Ontario
(Chapters 50, 51)

Otto Sanchez, MD, PhD
Professor
Faculty of Health Sciences
University of Ontario Institute of Technology
Oshawa, Ontario
(Chapter 8)

Linda Slater-MacLean, RN, BScN, MN, CNCC(C)
Clinical Nurse Specialist, Critical Care
University of Alberta Hospital
Edmonton, Alberta
(Chapters 30, 31, 32, 33, 34)

Contributors to the Ninth U.S. Edition

Cynthia Bautista, PhD, RN, CNRN, CCNS, ACNS-BC
Neuroscience Clinical Nurse Specialist
Yale New Haven Hospital
New Haven, Connecticut
(Chapters 48, 49, 50, 51)

Jaclyn Conelius, PhD, APRN, FNP-BC
Assistant Professor
School of Nursing, Fairfield University
Fairfield, Connecticut
(Chapters 21, 22, 23, 24, 25, 26)

Sally O. Gerard, DNP, RN, CDE
Assistant Professor of Nursing and Coordinator,
  Nursing Leadership Track
School of Nursing
Fairfield University
Fairfield, Connecticut
(Chapters 40, 41)

Lisa Grossman, MD, MPH
Administrative Chief Resident
Obstetrics/Gynecology
Columbia University Medical Center
New York, New York
(Chapters 6, 7, 45, 46, 47)

Theresa Kessler, PhD, RN, ACNS-BC, CNE
Professor
Valparaiso University
Valparaiso, Indiana
(Chapters 32, 52)

Melissa Kramps, DNP, APRN
Nurse Practitioner
Memory Disorders Center
New York, New York
(Chapter 3)

Zachary Krom, MSN, RN, CCRN
Service Line Educator: Adult Surgery
Yale New Haven Hospital
New Haven, Connecticut
(Chapters 36, 37, 38)

Christine Kurtz, DNP, PMHCNS-BC
Adjunct Assistant Professor
College of Nursing
Valparaiso University
Valparaiso, Indiana
(Chapter 52)

Jessie Moore, MS, APRN
Program Coordinator, Weight Loss Surgery
Yale New Haven Hospital—Saint Raphael Campus
New Haven, Connecticut
(Chapter 39)

Nancy Moriber, PhD, CRNA, APRN
Visiting Assistant Professor and Director, Nurse
  Anesthesia Track
School of Nursing
Fairfield University
Fairfield, Connecticut
(Chapters 17, 19)

Martha Burke O'Brien, MS, ANP-BC, APRN
Director of Student Health Services
Trinity College
Hartford, Connecticut
(Chapter 54)

Eileen O'Shea, DNP, RN
Assistant Professor
School of Nursing
Fairfield University
Fairfield, Connecticut
(Chapter 2)

Kathleen Wheeler, PhD, APRN, PMHNP-BC, FAAN
Professor
School of Nursing
Fairfield University
Fairfield, Connecticut
(Chapter 53)

The preparation of this second Canadian edition has only been made possible by the extensive work of previous editions of *Pathophysiology: Concepts of Altered Health States*. Carol M. Porth's major emphasis, as a nurse-physiologist, has always been "to relate normal body functioning to the physiologic changes that participate in disease production and occur as a result of disease, as well as the body's remarkable ability to compensate for these changes." She believes that "the beauty of physiology is that it integrates all of the aspects of human genetics, molecular and cellular biology, and organ anatomy and physiology into a functional whole that can be used to explain both the physical and psychological aspects of altered health." It has been her philosophy "to share the beauty of the human body and to emphasize that in disease as in health, there is more 'going right' in the body than is 'going wrong'." It is based on this perspective that we hope all our readers "will learn to appreciate the marvellous potential of the body."

This Canadian edition is adapted from the ninth edition of *Porth's Pathophysiology: Concepts of Altered Health States*. In the process of writing a Canadian perspective, the commonalities were far more extensive than the differences. Of course, the underlying pathophysiology that contributes to alterations in health is not unique to individual countries; however, minor differences do occur with regard to units of measurement, predominant etiologies, epidemiology, and management. This Canadian edition maintains all the features of the ninth edition and, while maintaining an international focus, gives supplementary attention to Canadian specific content.

FEATURES

A variety of features appear throughout the book to enhance learning.

Illustrations

Over 800 illustrations appear throughout this book and have been carefully developed or chosen to support the concepts that are presented in the text. There is a balance between line drawings of anatomic structures and pathophysiologic processes, flow charts, and photographic illustrations of disease states to enhance conceptual learning, linking text content to illustration content. Clinical illustrations depict the clinical manifestations of selected disease states.

Understanding

The Understanding feature focuses on key physiologic processes and phenomena that form a basis for understanding the disorders presented in the text. This feature, which is illustrated in full colour, breaks a process or phenomenon down into its consecutive parts and presents them in a sequential manner, providing an insight into the many opportunities for disease processes to disrupt the sequence.

Reading and Learning Aids

Objectives, appearing at the beginning of each major section in a chapter, provide a focus of study, while *Summary* boxes appearing at the end of each major section provide a review and reinforcement of the main content. *Key concept boxes* are intended to help the reader retain and use text information by identifying major ideas or concepts. *Tables* and *charts* are designed to present complex information in a format that is meaningful and easy to remember. *Review Exercises* appear at the end of each chapter and assist the reader in using a conceptual approach to solving problems related to chapter content. This edition also includes a glossary, and a table of normal laboratory values. The table of laboratory values includes Standard International (SI) and conventional units, as well as Internet addresses for conversion resources.

STUDENT AND INSTRUCTOR RESOURCES

A variety of ancillary materials are available to support students and instructors alike.

Resources for Students

Student Resources on thePoint include:

- Review Questions
- Animations
- Activities
- And more!

Resources for Instructors

Instructor Resources on thePoint include:

- A **Test Generator**, containing more than 1,000 multiple choice questions
- **PowerPoint** presentations
- Pre-lecture Quizzes
- An **Image Bank**, containing over 500 images from the text in formats suitable for printing, projecting, and incorporating into websites
- And more!

Acknowledgements

This second Canadian edition of *Porth Pathophysiology: Concepts of Altered Health States* continues to build on the high standards set out by Carol M. Porth. Carol and her team provided a solid foundation and I am indebted to her for this. While many of the foundational authors from the first edition have moved on, the chapters were refined with the help of equally talented Canadian contacts.

I would like to thank my many colleagues from work including the Science Team—Kirsten, Terry, and Peter, plus others from across Canada who have helped to enrich the content with their constructive comments.

It has been a pleasure to work with the team at Wolters Kluwer as they provided significant patience and guidance though this process. The editorial and production staff included Executive Editor Sherry Dickinson, Product Development Editor Katherine Burland, Editorial Assistant Dan Reilly, and Production Project Manager Marian Bellus, among others.

Contents

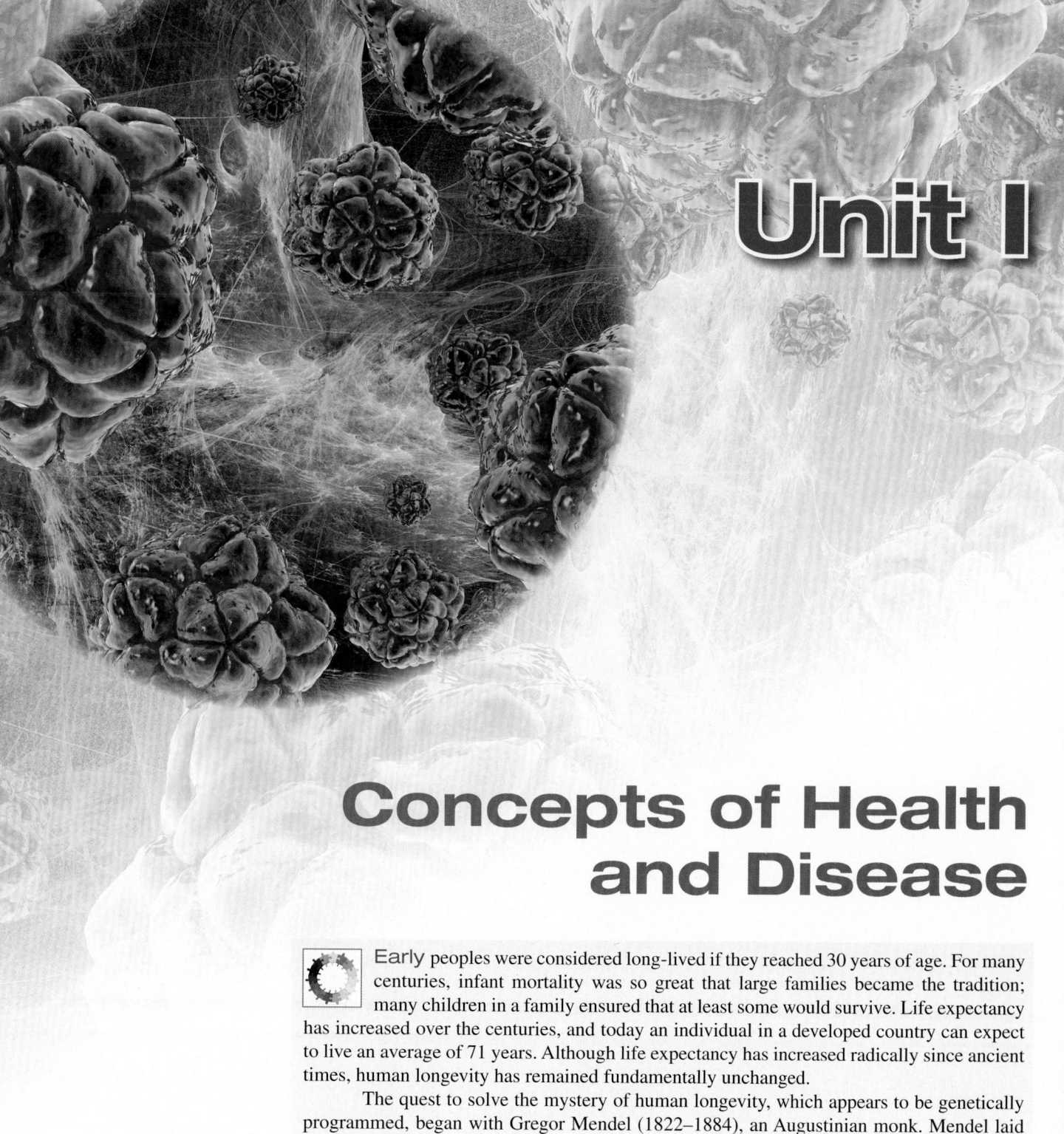

Unit I

Concepts of Health and Disease

Early peoples were considered long-lived if they reached 30 years of age. For many centuries, infant mortality was so great that large families became the tradition; many children in a family ensured that at least some would survive. Life expectancy has increased over the centuries, and today an individual in a developed country can expect to live an average of 71 years. Although life expectancy has increased radically since ancient times, human longevity has remained fundamentally unchanged.

The quest to solve the mystery of human longevity, which appears to be genetically programmed, began with Gregor Mendel (1822–1884), an Augustinian monk. Mendel laid the foundation of modern genetics with the pea experiments he performed in a monastery garden. Today, geneticists search for the determinant, or determinants, of the human life span. Up to this time, scientists have failed to identify an aging gene that would account for a limited life span. However, they have found that cells have a finite reproductive capacity. As they age, genes are increasingly unable to perform their functions. The cells become poorer and poorer at making the substances they need for their own special tasks or even for their own maintenance. Free radicals, mutation in a cell's DNA, and the process of programmed cell death are some of the factors that work together to affect a cell's functioning.

Concepts of Health and Disease

The term *pathophysiology,* which is the focus of this book, may be defined as the physiology of altered health. The term combines the words *pathology* and *physiology.* Pathology (from the Greek *pathos,* meaning "disease") deals with the study of the structural and functional changes in cells, tissues, and organs of the body that cause or are caused by disease. Physiology deals with the functions of the human body. Thus, pathophysiology deals not only with the cellular and organ changes that occur with disease, but with the effects that these changes have on total body function. Pathophysiology also focuses on the mechanisms of the underlying disease and provides the background for preventive as well as therapeutic health care measures and practices. This chapter is intended to orient the reader to the concepts of health and disease, various terms that are used throughout the book, the sources of data and what they mean, and the broader aspects of pathophysiology in terms of the health and well-being of populations.

CONCEPTS OF HEALTH AND DISEASE

After completing this section of the chapter, you should be able to meet the following objectives:

- State the World Health Organization definition of health.
- State a definition of pathophysiology.
- Characterize the disease process in terms of etiology, pathogenesis, morphology, clinical manifestations, and prognosis.
- Explain the meanings of reliability, validity, sensitivity, specificity, and predictive value as they relate to observations and tests used in the diagnosis of disease.

What constitutes health and disease often is difficult to determine because of the way different people view the topic. What is defined as health is determined by many factors, including heredity, age and sex, cultural and ethnic differences, as well as individual, group, and societal perspectives.

Health

In 1948, the Preamble to the Constitution of the World Health Organization (WHO) defined health as a "state of complete physical, mental, and social well-being and not merely the absence of disease and infirmity," a definition that has not been amended since that time.[1] Although ideal for many people, it also has been criticized for being too vague. In the 1980s the WHO shifted towards health promotion namely targeting public and population health including disease prevention while protecting health.[2] The Public Health Agency of Canada, when discussing the complexity of health for Canadians, recognizes that health is determined by multiple interactions between social and economic factors, the physical environment, an individual's biology and behaviour, plus governmental policies all within Canada's unique universal access to health care.[3]

Disease

A disease is considered an acute or chronic illness that one acquires or is born with that causes physiologic dysfunction in one or more body system. Each disease generally has specific signs and symptoms that characterize its pathology and identifiable etiology. The aspects of the disease process include etiology, pathogenesis, morphologic changes, clinical manifestations, diagnosis, and clinical course.

Etiology

The causes of disease are known as *etiologic factors*. Among the recognized etiologic agents are biologic agents (*e.g.,* bacteria, viruses), physical forces (*e.g.,* trauma, burns, radiation), chemical agents (*e.g.,* poisons, alcohol), and nutritional excesses or deficits. At the molecular level, it is important to distinguish between abnormal molecules and molecules that cause disease.[4] This is true of diseases such as cystic fibrosis, sickle cell disease and familial hypercholesterolemia, in which the genetic abnormality of a single amino acid, transporter molecule, or receptor protein produces widespread effects on health.

Most disease-causing agents are nonspecific, and many different agents can cause disease of a single organ. On the other hand, a single agent or traumatic event can lead to disease of a number of organs or systems. Although a disease agent can affect more than a single organ and a number of disease agents can affect the same organ, most disease states do not have a single cause. Instead, the majority of diseases are multifactorial in origin. This is particularly true of diseases such as cancer, heart disease, and diabetes. The multiple factors that may predispose an individual to a particular disease often are referred to as *risk factors.*

One way to view the factors that increase the risk for disease is to group them into categories according to whether they were present at birth or acquired later in life. *Congenital conditions* are defects that are present at birth, although they may not be evident until later in life. Congenital conditions may be caused by genetic influences, environmental factors (*e.g.,* viral infections in the mother, maternal drug use, irradiation, or intrauterine crowding), or a combination of genetic and environmental factors. *Acquired conditions* are those that are caused by events that occur after birth. These include injury, exposure to infectious agents, inadequate or improper nutrition, lack of oxygen, inappropriate immune responses, and neoplasia. Many diseases are thought to be the result of a genetic predisposition and an environmental event or events that serve as a trigger to initiate disease development. Significant advances in molecular biology linked with further genomic knowledge is helping to identify disease etiology with the potential for personalized medicine including individual interventions.[5]

Pathogenesis

While etiology describes what sets the disease process in motion, *pathogenesis* explains how the disease process evolves. In other words, pathogenesis is the sequence of cellular and tissue events that take place from the time of initial contact with an etiologic agent until the ultimate expression of a disease. Although etiology and pathogenesis are two terms often used interchangeably, their meanings are quite different. For example, atherosclerosis often is cited as the etiology (or cause) of coronary artery disease. In reality, the progression of the inflammatory process from a fatty streak to the occlusive vessel lesion seen in people with coronary artery disease represents the pathogenesis of the disorder. The true etiology of atherosclerosis remains largely uncertain.

Morphology

Morphology refers to the fundamental structure or form of cells or tissues. *Morphologic changes* are concerned with both the gross anatomic and microscopic changes that are characteristic of a disease. *Histology* deals with the study of the cells and extracellular matrix of body tissues. The most common method used in the study of tissues is the preparation of histologic sections—thin, translucent sections of human tissues and organs—that can be examined with the aid of a microscope. Histologic sections play an important role in the diagnosis of many types of cancer. A *lesion* represents a pathologic or traumatic discontinuity of a body organ or tissue. Descriptions of lesion size and characteristics often can be obtained through the use of radiographs, ultrasonography, and other imaging methods. Lesions also may be sampled by biopsy and tissue samples subjected to histologic study.

Clinical Manifestations

Diseases can manifest in a number of ways. Sometimes the condition produces manifestations, such as fever, that make it evident that the person is ill. In other cases, the condition is silent at the onset and is detected during examination for other purposes or after the disease is far advanced.

Signs and *symptoms* are terms used to describe the structural and functional changes that accompany a disease. A *symptom* is a subjective sensation that is noted by the person with a disorder, whereas a *sign* is a manifestation that is noted by an external observer. Pain, difficulty in breathing, and dizziness are symptoms that may occur with a disease. An elevated temperature, a swollen extremity, or changes in pupil size are objective signs that can be observed by someone other than the person with the disease. Signs and symptoms may be related to the primary disorder or they may represent the body's attempt to compensate for the altered function caused by the pathologic condition. Many pathologic states are not observed directly—one cannot see that a person is hemorrhaging or that he or she has decreased pulmonary gas exchange. Instead, what can be observed is the body's attempt to compensate for changes in function brought about by the disease, such as the tachycardia that accompanies blood loss or the increased respiratory rate that occurs with pneumonia.

A *syndrome* is a compilation of signs and symptoms (*e.g.,* chronic fatigue syndrome) that are characteristic of a specific disease state. *Complications* are possible adverse extensions of a disease or outcomes from treatment. *Sequelae* are lesions or impairments that follow or are caused by a disease.

Diagnosis

A *diagnosis* is the designation as to the nature or cause of a health problem (*e.g.,* bacterial pneumonia or hemorrhagic stroke). The diagnostic process usually requires a careful history and physical examination. The history is used to obtain a person's account of his or her symptoms and their progression, and the factors that contribute to a diagnosis. The physical examination is done to observe for signs of altered body structure or function.

The development of a diagnosis involves weighing competing possibilities and selecting the most likely one from among the conditions that might be responsible for the person's clinical presentation. The clinical probability of a given disease in a person of a given age, sex, race, lifestyle, and locality often is influential in arrival at a presumptive diagnosis. Laboratory tests, radiologic studies, computed tomography (CT) scans, and other tests often are used to determine or confirm a diagnosis.

An important factor when interpreting diagnostic test results is the determination of whether they are normal or abnormal. For example, it must be determined whether a particular blood count is above normal, within the normal range, or below normal. What is termed a *normal* value for a laboratory test is established statistically from test results obtained from a selected sample of people. The normal values refer to the 95% distribution (mean plus or minus two standard deviations [mean ± 2 SD]) of test results for the reference population.[6] Thus, the normal levels for serum sodium (135 to 145 mmol/L) represent the mean serum level for the reference population ± 2 SD. The normal values for some laboratory tests are adjusted for gender, other comorbidities, or age. For example, the normal hemoglobin range for women is 120 to 160 g/L, and for men, 140 to 174 g/L.[7] Serum creatinine level often is adjusted for age in the elderly, and normal values for serum phosphate differ between adults and children.

Laboratory parameters are interpreted based on validity, reliability, sensitivity, and specificity of the measurement.[8] *Validity* refers to the extent to which a measurement tool measures what it is intended to measure. This often is assessed by comparing a measurement method with the best possible method of measure that is available. For example, the validity of blood pressure measurements obtained by a sphygmomanometer might be compared with those obtained by intra-arterial measurements. *Reliability* refers to the extent to which an observation, if repeated, gives the same result. A poorly calibrated blood pressure machine may give inconsistent measurements of blood pressure, particularly of pressures in either the high or low range. Reliability also depends on the persons making the measurements. For example, blood pressure measurements may vary from one observer to another because of the technique that is used (*e.g.,* different observers may deflate the cuff at a different rate, thus obtaining different values), the way the numbers on the manometer are read, or differences in hearing acuity.

In the field of clinical laboratory measurements, *standardization* is aimed at increasing the trueness and reliability of measured values. Standardization relies on the use of written standards, reference measurement procedures, and reference materials.[9] In Canada, the Health Products and Food Branch of Health Canada regulates in vitro diagnostic devices, including clinical laboratory instruments, test kits, and reagents. Manufacturers who propose to market new diagnostic devices must submit information on their instrument, test kit, or reagent to Health Canada, as required by existing statutes and regulations. Health Canada reviews this information to decide whether the product may be marketed in Canada.

Measures of sensitivity and specificity are concerned with determining how likely or how accurately the test or observation will identify people with and without the disease[10] (Fig. 1.1). *Sensitivity* refers to the proportion of people with a disease who are positive for that disease on a given test or observation (called a *true-positive* result). If the result of a

FIGURE 1.1 • The relationship between a diagnostic test result and the occurrence of disease. There are two possibilities for the test result to be correct (true positive and true negative) and two possibilities for the result to be incorrect (false positive and false negative). (From Fletcher R. H., Fletcher S. W. (2005). *Clinical epidemiology: The essentials* (4th ed., p. 36). Philadelphia, PA: Lippincott Williams & Wilkins.)

very sensitive test is negative, it tells us the person does not have the disease and that the disease has been excluded or "ruled out." *Specificity* refers to the proportion of people without the disease who are negative on a given test or observation (called a *true-negative* result). Specificity can be calculated only from among people who do not have the disease. A test that is 95% specific correctly identifies 95 of 100 normal people. The other 5% are *false-positive* results. A false-positive test result can be unduly stressful for the person being tested, whereas a *false-negative* test result can delay diagnosis and jeopardize the outcome of treatment.

Predictive value is the extent to which an observation or test result is able to predict the presence of a given disease or condition.[9–12] A *positive predictive value* refers to the proportion of true-positive results that occurs in a given population. In a group of women found to have "suspect breast nodules" in a cancer screening program, the proportion later determined to have breast cancer would constitute the positive predictive value. A *negative predictive value* refers to the true-negative observations in a population. In a screening test for breast cancer, the negative predictive value represents the proportion of women without suspect nodules who do not have breast cancer. Although predictive values rely in part on sensitivity and specificity, they depend more heavily on the prevalence of the condition in the population. Despite unchanging sensitivity and specificity, the positive predictive value of an observation rises with prevalence, whereas the negative predictive value falls.

Clinical Course

The clinical course describes the evolution of a disease. A disease can have an acute, subacute, or chronic course. An *acute disorder* is one that is relatively severe, but self-limiting. *A chronic disease* implies a continuous, long-term process. A chronic disease can run a continuous course or can present with exacerbations (aggravation of symptoms and severity of the disease) and remissions (a period during which there is a decrease in severity and symptoms). *A subacute disease* is intermediate or between acute and chronic: it is not as severe as an acute disease and not as prolonged as a chronic disease.

The spectrum of disease severity for infectious diseases, such as hepatitis B, can range from preclinical to persistent chronic infection. During the *preclinical stage,* the disease is not clinically evident but is destined to progress to clinical disease. As with hepatitis B, it may be possible to transmit a virus during the preclinical stage. *Subclinical disease* is not clinically apparent and is not destined to become clinically apparent. It is diagnosed with antibody or culture tests. Most cases of tuberculosis are not clinically apparent, and evidence of their presence is established by skin tests. *Clinical disease* is manifested by signs and symptoms. A persistent chronic infectious disease persists for years, sometimes for life. *Carrier status* refers to an individual who harbours an organism but is not infected, as evidenced by antibody response or clinical manifestations. This person still can infect others. Carrier status may be of limited duration or it may be chronic, lasting for months or years.

IN SUMMARY

The term pathophysiology, which is the focus of this book, may be defined as the physiology of altered health. A disease has been defined as any deviation from or interruption of the normal structure or function of any part, organ, or system of the body that is manifested by a characteristic set of symptoms or signs and whose etiology, pathology, and prognosis may be known or unknown. The causes of disease are known as etiologic factors. Pathogenesis describes how the disease process evolves. Morphology refers to the structure or form of cells or tissues; morphologic changes are changes in structure or form that are characteristic of a disease.

A disease can manifest in a number ways. A symptom is a subjective complaint, such as pain or dizziness, whereas a sign is an observable manifestation, such as an elevated temperature or a reddened throat. A syndrome is a compilation of signs and symptoms that are characteristic of a specific disease state.

A diagnosis is the designation as to the nature and cause of a health problem. The diagnostic process requires a careful history and physical examination. Laboratory tests, radiologic studies (e.g., CT scans), and other tests are used to confirm a diagnosis. The value of many tests is based on their reliability and validity, as well as their sensitivity and specificity.

The clinical course of a disease describes its evolution. It can be acute (relatively severe, but self-limiting), chronic (continuous or episodic, but occurring over a long period of time), or subacute (not as severe as acute or as prolonged as chronic). Within the disease spectrum, a disease can be designated preclinical, or not clinically evident; subclinical, not clinically apparent, and not destined to become clinically apparent; or clinical, characterized by signs and symptoms.

HEALTH AND DISEASE IN POPULATIONS

After completing this section of the chapter, you should be able to meet the following objectives:

- Define the term epidemiology.
- Compare the meaning of the terms incidence and prevalence as they relate to measures of disease frequency.
- Compare the sources of information for and limitations of mortality and morbidity statistics.
- Differentiate primary, secondary, and tertiary levels of prevention.

The health of individuals is closely linked to the health of the community and to the population it encompasses. The ability to traverse continents in a matter of hours has opened the world to disease issues of populations at a global level. Diseases that once were confined to local areas of the world now pose a threat to populations throughout the world.

As we move through the 21st century, we are continually reminded that the health care system and the services it delivers are targeted to particular populations. Managed care systems are focused on a population-based approach to planning, delivering, providing, and evaluating health care. The focus of health care also has begun to emerge as a partnership in which individuals are asked to assume greater responsibility for their own health.

Epidemiology and Patterns of Disease

Epidemiology is the study of disease occurrence in human populations.[10] It was initially developed to explain the spread of infectious diseases during epidemics and has emerged as a science to study risk factors for multifactorial diseases, such as heart disease and cancer. Epidemiology looks for patterns of persons affected with a particular disorder, such as age, race, dietary habits, lifestyle, or geographic location. In contrast to biomedical researchers, who seek to elucidate the mechanisms of disease production, epidemiologists are more concerned with whether something happens than how it happens. For example, the epidemiologist is more concerned with whether smoking itself is related to cardiovascular disease and whether the risk of heart disease decreases when smoking ceases. On the other hand, the biomedical researcher is more concerned about the causative agent in cigarette smoke and the pathway by which it contributes to heart disease.

Much of our knowledge about disease comes from epidemiologic studies. Epidemiologic methods are used to determine how a disease is spread, how to control it, how to prevent it, and how to eliminate it. Epidemiologic methods also are used to study the natural history of disease, to evaluate new preventative and treatment strategies, to explore the impact of different patterns of health care delivery, and to predict future health care needs. As such, epidemiologic studies serve as a basis for clinical decision making, allocation of health care dollars, and development of policies related to public health issues.

Prevalence and Incidence

Measures of disease frequency are an important aspect of epidemiology. They establish a means for predicting what diseases are present in a population and provide an indication of the rate at which they are increasing or decreasing. A *disease case* can be either an existing case or the number of new episodes of a particular illness that are diagnosed within a given period. *Incidence* reflects the number of new cases arising in a population at risk during a specified time. The population at risk is considered to be persons without the disease but who are at risk for developing it. It is determined by dividing the number of new cases of a disease by the population at risk for development of the disease during the same period (*e.g.,* new cases per 1,000 or 100,000 persons in the population who

are at risk). The cumulative incidence estimates the risk of developing the disease during that period of time. *Prevalence* is a measure of an existing disease in a population at a given point in time (*e.g.,* number of existing cases divided by the current population).[10] Prevalence is not an estimate of the risk of developing a disease because it is a function of both new cases and how long the cases remain in the population. Incidence and prevalence are always reported as rates (*e.g.,* cases per 100 or cases per 100,000).

Mortality and Morbidity

Morbidity and mortality statistics provide information about the functional effects (morbidity) and death-producing (mortality) characteristics of a disease. These statistics are useful in terms of anticipating health care needs, planning of public education programs, directing health research efforts, and allocating health care dollars.

Morbidity describes the effects an illness has on a person's life. Many diseases, such as arthritis, have low death rates but make a significant impact on a person's life. Morbidity is concerned not only with the occurrence or incidence of a disease but with the persistence and long-term consequences of the disease.

Mortality statistics provide information about the causes of death in a given population. In most countries, people are legally required to record certain facts such as age, sex, and cause of death on a death certificate. Internationally agreed-upon classification procedures (the International Classification of Diseases [ICD] by the WHO) are used for coding the cause of death, and the data are expressed as death rates.[1] Crude mortality rates (*i.e.,* number of deaths in a given period) do not account for age, sex, race, socioeconomic status, and other factors. For this reason, mortality often is expressed as death rates for a specific population or age group, such as the infant mortality rate. Mortality also can be described in terms of the leading causes of death according to age, sex, race, and ethnicity. Among 15- to 24-year-olds, the three leading causes of death are injuries, suicide, and cancer, whereas the three leading causes of death for persons 65 years of age and older are circulatory system diseases (including cardiovascular and cerebral events), cancer, and then respiratory system diseases (including acute and chronic causes).[11]

Determination of Risk Factors

Conditions suspected of contributing to the development of a disease are called *risk factors*. They may be inherent to the person (high blood pressure or obesity) or external (smoking or drinking alcohol). There are different types of studies used to determine risk factors, including cross-sectional studies, case-control studies, and cohort studies.

Cross-Sectional and Case-Control Studies

Cross-sectional studies use the simultaneous collection of information necessary for classification of exposure and outcome status. They can be used to compare the prevalence of a disease in those with the factor (or exposure) with the prevalence of a disease in those who are unexposed to the factor, such as the prevalence of coronary heart disease in smokers and non-smokers. *Case-control studies* are designed to compare persons known to have the outcome of interest (*cases*) and those known not to have the outcome of interest (*controls*).[10] Information on exposures or characteristics of interest is then collected from persons in both groups. For example, the characteristics of maternal alcohol consumption in infants born with fetal alcohol syndrome (cases) can be compared with those in infants born without the syndrome (controls).

Cohort Studies

A *cohort* is a group of persons who were born at approximately the same time or share some characteristics of interest.[10] Persons enrolled in a cohort study (also called a *longitudinal study*) are followed over a period of time to observe one or more specific health outcomes. A cohort may consist of a single group of persons chosen because they have or have not been exposed to suspected risk factors; two groups specifically selected because one has been exposed and the other has not; or a single exposed group in which the results are compared with the general population.

Framingham Study. One of the best-known examples of a cohort study is the American Framingham Study, which was carried out in Framingham, Massachusetts.[12] Framingham was selected because of the size of the population, the relative ease with which the people could be contacted, and the stability of the population in terms of moving into and out of the area. This longitudinal study, which began in 1948, was set up by the United States Public Health Service to study the characteristics of people who would later develop coronary heart disease. The study consisted of 5,000 persons, aged 30 to 62 years, selected at random and followed for an initial period of 20 years, during which time it was predicted that 1,500 of them would develop coronary heart disease. The advantages of such studies are that they can explore a number of risk factors at the same time and determine the relative importance of each, and that the risk factors can be related later to other diseases such as stroke. Canada and other international communities have utilized the data collected from the original and subsequent cohorts for developing evidence-based strategies. Chart 1.1 describes some of the significant milestones from the Framingham Study.

Nurses' Health Study. Another well-known cohort study is the Nurses' Health Study, which was developed by Harvard University and Brigham and Women's Hospital. The study began in 1976 with a cohort of 121,700 female nurses, 30 to 55 years of age, living in the United States. The study expanded in 1989 to include a group of 116,000 female nurse participants.[13] Initially designed to explore the relationship between oral contraceptives and breast cancer, nurses in the study have provided answers to detailed questions about their menstrual cycles, smoking habits, diet, weight and waist measurements, activity patterns, health problems, and medication use. They have collected urine and blood samples, and even provided

---

CHART 1.1   FRAMINGHAM STUDY: SIGNIFICANT MILESTONES

- 1960—Cigarette smoking found to increase risk of heart disease
- 1961—Cholesterol level, blood pressure, and electrocardiogram abnormalities found to increase risk of heart disease
- 1967—Physical activity found to reduce risk of heart disease; obesity found to increase risk of heart disease
- 1970—High blood pressure found to increase risk of stroke
- 1976—Menopause found to increase risk of heart disease
- 1978—Psychosocial factors found to affect heart disease
- 1988—High levels of HDL cholesterol found to reduce risk of death
- 1996—Progression from hypertension to heart failure described
- 1999—Lifetime risk of developing heart disease at age 40 is one in two for men and one in three for women
- 2002—Obesity established as a risk factor for heart failure
- 2009—High leptin levels found to protect against Alzheimer's disease and dementia
- 2010—Sleep apnea tied to increased risk of stroke
- 2010—Familial risk directly associated with atrial fibrillation and stroke

(Abstracted from Framingham Heart Study (2013). Research milestones. Available online at: http://www.framinghamheartstudy.org/about/milestones.html.)

---

researchers with their toenail clippings. In selecting the cohort, it was reasoned that nurses would be well organized, accurate, and observant in their responses, and that physiologically they would be no different from other groups of women. It also was anticipated that their childbearing, eating, and smoking patterns would be similar to those of other working women.

National Longitudinal Survey of Children and Youth (NLSCY). This Canadian example of a cohort study was developed in 1994 to collect data on Canadian children from all provinces with ages initially ranging from newborn to 11 years of age. Key information about education, health, child care arrangements, and relationships is collected from both the children and the caregivers to monitor the impact these factors have over time. Subsequent biennial cycles follow the original children and with each data collection cycle new cohorts are added.[14]

Natural History

The *natural history* of a disease refers to the progression and projected outcome of the disease without medical intervention. By studying the patterns of a disease over time in populations, epidemiologists can better understand its natural history. Knowledge of the natural history can be used to determine disease outcome, establish priorities for health care services, determine the effects of screening and early detection programs on disease outcome, and compare the results of new treatments with the expected outcome without treatment.

There are some diseases for which there are no effective treatment methods available, or for which the current treatment measures are effective only in certain people. In this case, the natural history of the disease can be used as a predictor of outcome. For example, the natural history of hepatitis C indicates that 75% of people who become infected with the virus fail to clear the virus and progress to chronic infection.[15] Information about the natural history of a disease and the availability of effective treatment methods provides directions for preventive measures. In the case of hepatitis C, careful screening of blood donations and education of intravenous drug abusers can be used to prevent transfer of the virus. At the same time, scientists are striving to develop a vaccine that will prevent infection in persons exposed to the virus. The development of vaccines to prevent the spread of infectious diseases such as polio and hepatitis B undoubtedly has been motivated by knowledge about the natural history of these diseases and the lack of effective intervention measures. With other diseases, such as breast cancer, early detection through use of mammography and clinical examination increases the chances for a cure.

Prognosis refers to the probable outcome and prospect of recovery from a disease. It can be designated as chances for full recovery, possibility of complications, or anticipated survival time. Prognosis often is presented in relation to treatment options—that is, the expected outcomes or chances for survival with or without a certain type of treatment. The prognosis associated with a given type of treatment usually is presented along with the risk associated with the treatment.

Levels of Prevention

Basic healthy lifestyle choices contribute to the prevention of disease, as they may help to reduce known risk factors. There are three fundamental types of prevention: primary prevention, secondary prevention, and tertiary prevention[10] (Fig. 1.2). It is important to note that all three levels are aimed at prevention.

Primary prevention is directed at keeping disease from occurring by removing all risk factors. Examples of primary prevention include the administration of folic acid to pregnant women and women who may become pregnant to prevent fetal neural tube defects, giving immunizations to children to prevent communicable disease, and counselling people to adopt healthy lifestyles as a means of preventing heart disease.[10] Primary prevention is often accomplished outside the health care system at the community level. Some primary prevention measures are mandated by law (*e.g.,* wearing seat belts in automobiles and helmet use on motorcycles). Other primary prevention activities (*e.g.,* use of ear plugs or dust masks) occur in specific occupations.

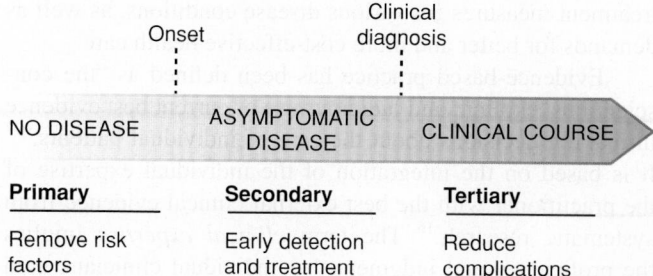

FIGURE 1.2 • Levels of prevention. Primary prevention prevents disease from occurring. Secondary prevention detects and cures disease in the asymptomatic phase. Tertiary prevention reduces complications of disease. (From Fletcher R. H., Fletcher S. W. (2005). *Clinical epidemiology: The essentials* (4th ed., p. 149). Philadelphia, PA: Lippincott Williams & Wilkins.)

Secondary prevention detects disease early when it is still asymptomatic and treatment measures can effect a cure or stop it from progressing. The use of a Papanicolaou (Pap) smear for early detection of cervical cancer is an example of secondary prevention. Screening also includes history taking (asking if a person smokes), physical examination (blood pressure measurement), laboratory tests (cholesterol level determination), and other procedures (colonoscopy) that can be "applied reasonably rapidly to asymptomatic people."[10] Most secondary prevention is done in clinical settings. All types of health care professionals (*e.g.,* physicians, nurses, dentists, audiologists, optometrists) participate in secondary prevention.

Tertiary prevention is directed at clinical interventions that prevent further deterioration or reduce the complications of a disease once it has been diagnosed. An example is the use of β-blocking adrenergic drugs to reduce the risk of death in persons who have had a myocardial infarction (heart attack). The boundaries of tertiary prevention go beyond treating the problem with which the person presents. In persons with diabetes, for example, tertiary prevention requires more than good glucose control—it includes provision for regular ophthalmologic examinations for early detection of retinopathy, education for good foot care, and treatment for other cardiovascular risk factors such as hyperlipidemia.[10] Tertiary prevention measures also include measures to limit physical impairment and the social consequences of an illness. Most tertiary prevention programs are located within health care systems and involve the services of a number of different types of health care professionals.

Evidence-Based Practice and Practice Guidelines

Evidence-based practice and evidence-based practice guidelines are used to inform clinicians, public health practitioners, health care organizations, and the public as a means of improving the quality and efficiency of health care.[16] Their development has been prompted, at least in part, by the enormous amount of published information about diagnostic and treatment measures for various disease conditions, as well as demands for better and more cost-effective health care.

Evidence-based practice has been defined as "the conscientious, explicit, and judicious use of current best evidence in making decisions about the care of individual patients."[17] It is based on the integration of the individual expertise of the practitioner with the best external clinical evidence from systematic research.[16] The term *clinical expertise* implies the proficiency and judgment that individual clinicians gain through clinical experience and clinical practice. The best external clinical evidence for disease management relies on the identification of clinically relevant research, often from the basic sciences, but especially from patient-centred clinical studies that focus on the accuracy and precision of diagnostic tests and methods, the power of prognostic indicators, and the effectiveness and safety of therapeutic, rehabilitative, and preventive regimens. Other types of evidence, such as qualitative studies, are better suited to understanding human perceptions and behaviours to enable reduction of risk factors, promotion of screening, and management of disease symptoms.

Clinical practice guidelines are systematically developed statements intended to inform practitioners and clients in making decisions about health care for specific clinical circumstances.[16,18] Guidelines differ from systematic reviews, which focus on a review of the current literature and contribute to the knowledge base for guidelines. Clinical practice guidelines should not only review but also weigh various outcomes, both positive and negative, and make recommendations. They can take the form of algorithms (step-by-step methods for solving a problem), written directives for care, or a combination thereof.

The development of evidence-based practice guidelines often uses methods such as meta-analysis to combine evidence from different studies to produce a more precise estimate of the accuracy of a diagnostic method or the effects of an intervention method. It also requires review: by practitioners with expertise in clinical content, who can verify the completeness of the literature review and ensure clinical sensibility; by experts in guideline development who can examine the method by which the guideline was developed; and by potential users of the guideline.[16]

Once developed, practice guidelines must be continually reviewed and changed to keep pace with new research findings and new diagnostic and treatment methods. For example, the National Advisory Committee on Immunizations (NACI) has been reporting to Health Canada since 1964 and recommending guidelines for all Canadians. The NACI developed and now provides regular updates for the online Canadian Immunization Guide.[18] Another example is the Canadian Hypertension Society's expert panel, which first developed evidence-based recommendations in 1977 that eventually led to the development of the annual updates for hypertension by the Canadian Hypertension Education Program (CHEP) (see Chapter 23).[19]

Evidence-based practice guidelines, which are intended to direct client care, are also important in directing research into the best methods of diagnosing and treating specific health problems. This is because health care providers use the same criteria for diagnosing the extent and severity of a particular condition such as hypertension, and because they use the same protocols for treatment.

IN SUMMARY

Epidemiology refers to the study of disease in populations. It looks for patterns such as age, race, and dietary habits of persons who are affected with a particular disorder to determine under what circumstances the particular disorder will occur. Incidence is the number of new cases arising in a given population during a specified time. Prevalence is the number of people in a population who have a particular disease at a given point in time or period. Incidence and prevalence are reported as proportions or rates (e.g., cases per 100 or 100,000 population). Mortality or death statistics provide information about the trends in the health of a population, whereas morbidity describes the effects an illness has on a person's life. It is concerned with the incidence of disease as well as its persistence and long-term consequences.

Conditions suspected of contributing to the development of a disease are called risk factors. Studies used to determine risk factors include cross-sectional studies, case-control studies, and cohort studies. The natural history refers to the progression and projected outcome of a disease without medical intervention. Prognosis is the term used to designate the probable outcome and prospect of recovery from a disease.

The three fundamental types of prevention are primary prevention, secondary prevention, and tertiary prevention. Primary prevention, such as immunization, is directed at removing risk factors so that disease does not occur. Secondary prevention, such as a Pap smear, detects disease when it still is asymptomatic and curable with treatment. Tertiary prevention, such as use of β-adrenergic drugs to reduce the risk of death in persons who have had a heart attack, focuses on clinical interventions that prevent further deterioration or reduce the complications of a disease.

Evidence-based practice and evidence-based practice guidelines are mechanisms that use the current best evidence to make decisions about the health care of individuals. They are based on the expertise of the individual practitioner integrated with the best clinical evidence from systematic review of credible research studies. Practice guidelines may take the form of algorithms (step-by-step methods for solving a problem), written directives, or a combination thereof.

References

1. World Health Organization. (2013). About WHO. Available online at: www.who.int/about/en/. Accessed September 2, 2013.
2. The Association of Faculties of Medicine of Canada. (2009). AFMC Primer on Population Health. Available online at: http://phprimer.afmc.ca/inner/primer_contents. Accessed September 2, 2013.

3. Public Health Agency of Canada. (2011). Population health. Available online at: http://www.phac-aspc.gc.ca/ph-sp. Accessed September 2, 2013.

4. Waldenstrom J. (1989). Sick molecules and our concepts of illness. *Journal of Internal Medicine 225*, 221–227.

5. Naylor S., Chen J. (2010). Unraveling human complexity and disease with systems biology and personalized medicine. *Personalized Medicine. 7*(3), 275–289.

6. Mayer D. (2010). *Essentials of Evidence-based Medicine* (2nd ed.). New York: Cambridge University Press.

7. Fischbach F., Dunning M. B. (2009). *A Manual of Laboratory and Diagnostic Tests* (8th ed., p. 68, 1008). Philadelphia, PA: Lippincott Williams & Wilkins.

8. Bickley L. (2013). *Bates' Guide to Physical Assessment and History Taking* (11th ed., pp. 43–51). Philadelphia, PA: J.B. Lippincott.

9. Wians F. H. (2009). Clinical laboratory tests: Which, why, and what do the results mean? *LabMedicine. 40*(2),105–113.

10. Fletcher R. H., Fletcher S. W. (2005). *Clinical Epidemiology: The Essentials* (4th ed.). Philadelphia, PA: Lippincott Williams & Wilkins.

11. Public Health Agency of Canada. (2008). Leading causes of death and hospitalization in Canada. Available online at: http://www.phac-aspc.gc.ca/publicat/lcd-pcd97/table1-eng.php. Accessed September 2, 2013.

12. Framingham Heart Study. (2013). Framingham Heart Study. Available online at: http://www.framinghamheartstudy.org/about/index.html. Accessed September 2, 2013.

13. Channing Laboratory. (2013). Nurses' Health Study. Available online at: www.channing.harvard.edu/nhs/. Accessed September 2, 2013.

14. Statistics Canada. (2010). National longitudinal survey of children and youth. Available online at: http://www23.statcan.gc.ca/imdb/p2SV.pl?Function=getSurvey&SDDS=4450&Item_Id=25609&lang=en. Access September 2, 2013.

15. Canadian Liver Foundation. (2012). Viral hepatitis A, B, C. Available online at: http://www.liver.ca/liver-disease/types/viral-hepatitis-a-b-c.aspx. Accessed September 2, 2013.

16. Sukhmeet S. P., Philippon M. J., Bhandari M. (2010). Principles of evidence-based medicine. *Orthop Clin North Am. 41*(2),131–138.

17. Sackett D. L. (1996). Evidence based medicine: What it is and what it isn't. *British Medical Journal 312*, 71–72.

18. Public Health Agency of Canada. (2013). National Advisory Committee on Immunization (NACI). Available online at: http://www.phac-aspc.gc.ca/naci-ccni/. Accessed September 2, 2013.

19. Hypertension Canada. (2013). Canadian hypertension education program (CHEP). Available online at: http://www.hypertension.ca/chep. Accessed September 2, 2013.

Concepts of Altered Health in Children

2

Children are not miniature adults. Physical and psychological maturation and development strongly influence the types of illnesses children experience and their responses to these illnesses. Although many signs and symptoms are the same in persons of all ages, some diseases and complications are more likely to occur in the child. In addition, there may be differences in the severity of their symptoms, expected outcomes, and types of interventions. This chapter provides an overview of the developmental stages of childhood and the related health care needs of children. Considerations for children, including specific diseases and symptoms, are presented in the different chapters throughout the book.

In the late 1800s the infant mortality rate was between 200 and 400 deaths per 1,000 live births.[1] Infectious diseases were rampant, and children, with their immature and inexperienced immune systems and their frequent exposure to other infected children, were especially vulnerable. With the introduction of sanitation and hygiene protocols, antimicrobial agents, infectious disease control, nutritional and technologic advances, and collaborative prevention initiatives (federal, provincial, local, and community levels), infant mortality decreased dramatically. Since 1979, Canada's infant mortality rate has decreased more than half. In 2009, Canada's infant mortality rate was 4.9 per 1,000 live births but the rates are higher in the prairie provinces and the Northwest Territories has the highest rate (15.5). Japan continues to have the lowest infant mortality rate of 2.4 per 1,000 live births, whereas the United States has a relatively high rate, when compared to other industrialized countries, of 6.4 per 1,000 live births. However, statistics for both Canada and the United States include very premature babies who negatively affect the results as they have lower chances of survival.[2]

One of the more perplexing causes of infant mortality is the incidence of preterm birth among women of all races and classes. Despite continued, gradual declines in the overall infant mortality rate during the latter part of the 20th century, the incidence of premature births continues to present a challenge to reducing the racial disparities in infant mortality rates, as well as the overall incidence of infant mortality. The percentage of infants born with very low birth weight (<1,500 g) has increased gradually in recent years. One reason for the increase in children born with low birth weight is that the number of twin, triplet, and higher-order multiple births has increased.[3]

GROWTH AND DEVELOPMENT

After completing this section of the chapter, you should be able to meet the following objectives:

- Characterize the use of percentiles to describe growth and development during infancy and childhood.
- Describe the major events that occur during prenatal development from fertilization to birth.
- Define the terms low birth weight, small for gestational age, and large for gestational age.
- Identify reasons for abnormal intrauterine growth.
- Describe assessment methods for determination of gestational age.

The terms *growth* and *development* describe an ongoing dynamic process that begins with a fertilized ovum and continues throughout the infant, childhood, and adolescent periods until adulthood is achieved. *Physical growth* describes changes in the body as a whole or in its individual parts. *Development,* on the other hand, embraces other aspects of growth, such as changes in capabilities, acquisitions of skills and psychosocial behaviours. Skill acquisition occurs in a standard fashion—from simple to complex and from general to the specific.[4] In addition, pediatric development progresses in a predictable sequence—from head-to-toe (cephalocaudal) and from midline to the periphery (proximodistal)[4] (Fig. 2.1). Each phase of development builds upon previous successes in order to achieve a higher-level skill. For example, the infant must first learn to roll over before he or she is able to sit up. Likewise, the toddler must learn to stand before he or she can walk.

Growth and development encompass a complex interaction between genetic and environmental influences, such as nutrition and sensory stimulation.[4] The experience of each child is unique, and the patterns of growth and development may be profoundly different for individual children within the context of what is considered *normal.* Because of the wide variability, these norms often can be expressed only in statistical terms.

Evaluation of growth and development requires comparison of an individual's growth and development with a standard. Statistics are calculations derived from measurements that are used to describe the sample measured or to make predictions about the rest of the population represented by the sample. Because all individuals grow and develop at different rates, the standard must somehow take this individual variation into account. The standard typically is derived from measurements made on a sample of individuals deemed representative of the total population. When multiple measurements of biologic variables such as height, weight, head circumference, and blood pressure are made, most values fall around the centre or middle of all the values. Plotting the data on a graph yields a bell-shaped curve, which depicts the normal distribution of these continuously variable values.

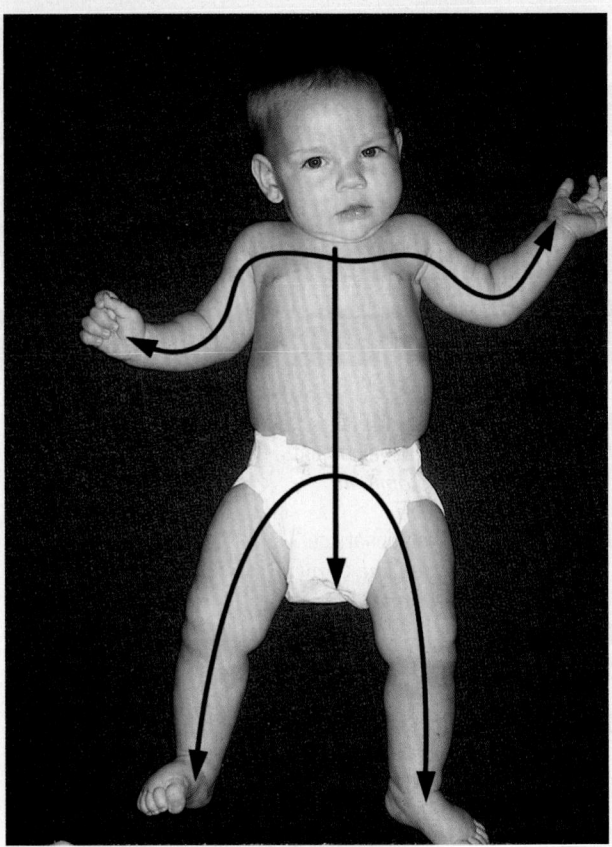

FIGURE 2.1 • The child's pattern of growth is in a head-to-toe direction, or cephalocaudal, and in an inward-to-outward pattern called proximodistal. (From Bowden V. R., Greenberg C. S. (2010). *Children and their families: The continuum of care* (2nd ed., p. 77). Philadelphia, PA: Lippincott Williams & Wilkins.)

The mean and standard deviation are common statistics used in describing the characteristics of a population. The mean represents the average of the measurements; it is the sum of the values divided by the number of values. A normal bell-shaped curve is symmetric, with the mean falling in the centre of the curve and one half of the values falling on either side of the mean. The standard deviation determines how far a value varies or deviates from the mean. The points one standard deviation above and below the mean include 68% of all values, two standard deviations 95% of all values, and three standard deviations 99.7% of all values.[5] If a child's height is within one standard deviation of the mean, he or she is as tall as 68% of children in the population. If a child's height is greater than three standard deviations above the mean, he or she is taller than 99.7% of children in the population.

The bell-shaped curve can also be marked by percentiles, which are useful for comparison of an individual's values with other values. When quantitative data are arranged in ascending and descending order, a middle value called the *median* can be described, with one half (50%) of the values falling on either side. The values can be further divided into percentiles. A percentile is a number that indicates the percentage of values for the population that are equal to or below the number. Percentiles are used most often to compare an individual's value with a set of norms. They are used extensively to develop and interpret physical growth charts and measurements of ability and intelligence.

Utilizing standardized growth charts can provide health professionals with a means to measure what is a normal growth trajectory of children, or alert them to what is an atypical pattern. The American Center for Disease Control and Prevention (CDC) charts are configured for Caucasian norms, which may not be representative of diverse ethnic cultures and new immigrants. Currently it is recommended that the newer World Health Organization (WHO) (2006) growth chart be used to measure children ages 0 to 2 years, and either the CDC (2000) growth chart or the WHO chart be utilized for all children older than two.[6] The WHO (2006) charts differ from previously used CDC growth charts in that the WHO charts were developed as the outcome of a rigorous longitudinal study, in which an international sample of children from diverse ethnic groups was sampled.[7,8] Because the WHO charts were developed based on a global sample of children, they can be applied to children regardless of ethnicity, socioeconomic status, and type of feeding.[8] Findings from recent studies support that the WHO growth charts provide a more sensitive indicator, which allows for earlier intervention in the very young age groups.[9,10] Growth charts for children can be accessed via the Canadian Paediatric Society website: http://www.cps.ca/tools-outils/who-growth-charts.

Prenatal Growth and Development

Human development is considered to begin with fertilization, the union of sperm and ovum resulting in a zygote (Fig. 2.2). The process begins with the intermingling of a haploid number of paternal (23, X or Y) and maternal (23, X) chromosomes in the ampulla of the oviduct that fuse to form a zygote.[11,12] Within 24 hours, the unicellular organism becomes a two-cell organism and, within 72 hours, a 16-cell organism called a

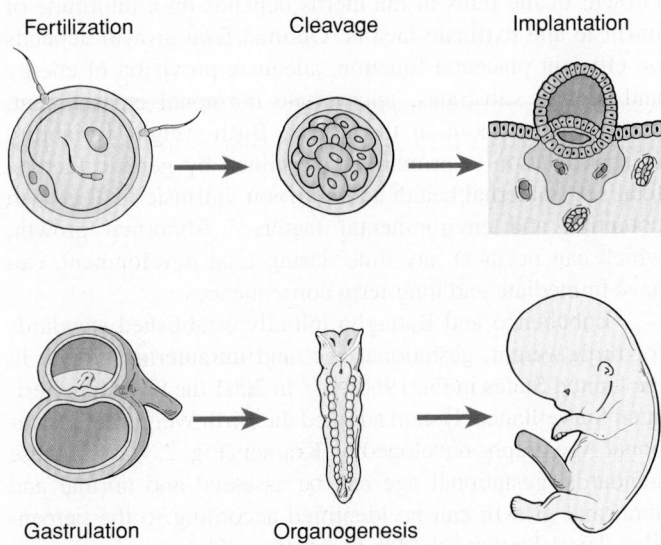

Fertilization   Cleavage   Implantation

Gastrulation   Organogenesis

FIGURE 2.2 • Milestones in embryonic development.

morula. This series of mitotic divisions is called *cleavage.* During cleavage, the rapidly developing cell mass travels down the oviduct to the uterus by a series of peristaltic movements. Shortly after entering the uterus (about 4 days after fertilization), the morula is separated into two parts by fluid from the uterus. The outer layer gives rise to the placenta (trophoblast), and the inner layer gives rise to the embryo (embryoblast). The structure is now called a *blastocyst.* By the sixth day the blastocyst attaches to the endometrium. This is the beginning of *implantation,* and it is completed during the second week of development.[11,13]

Prenatal development is divided into two main periods. The first, or *embryonic period,* begins during the second week and continues through the eighth week after fertilization.[11,12] During the embryonic period, the main organ systems are developed and many function at a minimal level. The second, or *fetal period,* begins during the ninth week. During the fetal period, the growth and differentiation of the body and organ systems occur.

Embryonic Development

Embryonic development progresses through three stages.[11] During the first stage, growth occurs through an increase in cell numbers and the elaboration of cell products. The second stage is one of morphogenesis (development of form), which includes massive cell movement. During this stage, the movement of cells allows them to interact with each other in the formation of tissues and organs. The third stage is the stage of differentiation or maturation of physiologic processes. Completion of differentiation results in organs that are capable of performing specialized functions.

Embryonic development begins during the second week of gestation with implantation of the blastocyst. As implantation of the blastocyst progresses, a small space appears in the embryoblast, which is the primordium of the amniotic cavity. Concurrently, morphologic changes occur in the embryoblast that result in formation of a flat, almost circular bilaminar plate of cells called the *embryonic disk.* The embryonic disk, which forms the embryo proper, gives rise to all three germ layers of the embryo (*i.e.,* ectoderm, mesoderm, endoderm). The third week is a period of rapid development, noted for the conversion of the bilaminar embryonic disk into a trilaminar embryonic disk through a process called *gastrulation*[11–13] (Fig. 2.2). The ectoderm differentiates into the epidermis and nervous system, and the endoderm gives rise to the epithelial linings of the respiratory passages, digestive tract, and glandular cells of organs such as the liver and pancreas. The mesoderm becomes smooth muscle tissue, connective tissue, blood vessels, blood cells, bone marrow, skeletal tissue, striated muscle tissue, and reproductive and excretory organs.

The notochord, which is the primitive axis about which the axial skeleton forms, is also formed during the third week. The neurologic system begins its development during this period. *Neurulation,* a process that involves formation of the neural plate, neural folds, and their closure, is completed by the fourth week.[11,12] Disturbances during this period can result in brain and spinal defects such as spina bifida. The cardiovascular system is the first functional organ system to develop. The primitive heart, which beats and circulates blood, develops during this period.[4]

By the fourth week, the neural tube is formed. The embryo begins to curve and fold into a characteristic "C"-shaped structure. The limb buds are visible, as are the otic pits (*i.e.,* primordia of the internal ears) and the lens placodes (primordia of the crystalline lenses). The fifth week is notable for the rapid growth of the head secondary to brain growth.

During the sixth week, the upper limbs are formed by fusion of the swellings around the branchial groove. In the seventh week, there is the beginning of the digits, and the intestines enter the umbilical cord (umbilical herniation). By the eighth week, the embryo is human-like in appearance—eyes are open, and eyelids and ear auricles are easily identified.

Fetal Development

The fetal period extends from the ninth week to birth.[11-13] During the 9th to 12th weeks, fetal head growth slows, whereas body length growth is greatly accelerated. By the 11th week, the intestines in the proximal portion of the cord have returned to the abdomen. The primary ossification centres are present in the skull and long bones, and maturation of the fetal external genitalia is established by the 12th week. During the fetal period, the liver is the major site of red blood cell formation (*i.e.,* erythropoiesis); at 12 weeks, this activity has decreased and erythropoiesis begins in the spleen. The kidney becomes functional around the 12th week, at which time urine is passed into the amniotic fluid.[13]

The 13th through 16th weeks are notable for ossification of the skeleton, scalp hair patterning, and differentiation of the ovaries in female fetuses.[11] By the 17th through 20th weeks, growth has slowed. The fetal skin is covered with a fine hair called *lanugo* and a white, cheeselike material called *vernix caseosa.* Eyebrows and head hair are visible. In male fetuses, the testes begin to descend, and in female fetuses, the uterus is formed. Brown fat, which is a specialized type of adipose tissue that produces heat by oxidizing fatty acids, also forms during this period.[11] It is found near the heart and blood vessels that supply the brain and kidneys and is thought to play a role in maintaining the temperature of these organs during exposure to environmental changes that occur after birth.

During the 21st through 25th weeks, significant fetal weight gain occurs. At 21 weeks rapid eye movements begin, and blink-startle reflexes have been reported at 22 to 23 weeks after application of a vibroacoustic noise source to the mother's abdomen.[11] The type II alveolar cells of the lung begin to secrete surfactant. The pulmonary system becomes more mature and able to support respiration during the 26th through 29th weeks. Breathing movements are present as a result of central nervous system (CNS) maturation. At this age a fetus can survive if born prematurely and given intensive care. There is substantial weight gain during this time. Although still somewhat lean, the fetus is better proportioned.

The 30th through 34th weeks are significant for an increasing amount of white fat (8% of body weight), which

gives the fetal limbs an almost chubby appearance.[11] During the 35th week, grasp and the pupillary light reflex are present. If a normal-weight fetus is born during this period, it is premature by "date" as opposed to premature by "weight."[12]

Expected time of birth is 266 days, or 38 weeks after fertilization, or 40 weeks after the last menstrual period (LMP).[11] At this time, the neurologic, cardiovascular, and pulmonary systems are developed enough for the infant to make the transition to extrauterine life. The survival of the newborn depends on this adaptation after the placenta is removed.

Birth Weight and Gestational Age

Development during the fetal period is primarily concerned with rapid growth and differentiation of tissues, organs, and systems. Fetal weight gain is linear from 20 weeks' gestation through 38 weeks' gestation. In the last half of pregnancy, the fetus gains 85% of birth weight. After 38 weeks of gestation, the rate of growth declines, probably related to the constraint of uterine size and decreased placental function.[11] After birth, weight gain resumes at a rate similar to intrauterine rates.

At birth, the average weight of the full-term newborn is 3,000 to 4,000 g. Infants weighing 2,500 g or less at birth are classified as low birth weight (LBW). LBW is further broken down into very low birth weight (VLBW) and extremely low birth weight (ELBW). VLBW is defined as a birth weight less than 1,500 g, and ELBW as a birth weight less than 1,000 g.[14]

An infant is considered term when born between the beginning of the 38th week and completion of the 41st week. An infant is considered premature when born before the end of the 37th week and postmature when born after the end of the 41st week. The lowest mortality rates occur among newborns with weights between 3,000 and 4,000 g and gestational ages of 38 to 42 weeks.[15]

Abnormal Intrauterine Growth

Growth of the fetus in the uterus depends on a multitude of intrinsic and extrinsic factors. Optimal fetal growth depends on efficient placental function, adequate provision of energy and growth substrates, appropriate hormonal environment, and adequate room in the uterus. Birth weight variability in a population is primarily determined by genetic factors, fetal sex, maternal health and nutrition, intrinsic fetal growth potential, and environmental factors.[16] Abnormal growth, which can occur at any time during fetal development, can have immediate and long-term consequences.

Lubchenco and Battaglia initially established standards for birth weight, gestational age, and intrauterine growth in the United States in the 1960s.[17,18] In 2001 the Canadian Perinatal Surveillance System adopted the Birth Weight for Gestational Age graphs developed by Kramer (Fig. 2.3). With these standards, gestational age can be assessed and normal and abnormal growth can be identified according to the percentiles. The 10th through 90th percentiles of intrauterine growth encompass 80% of births. Growth is considered abnormal

Canadian Female Singletons

FIGURE 2.3 • Classification of newborn girls by birth weight and gestational age. Similar chart is available for boys. (Source: Canadian Perinatal Surveillance System, Public Health Agency of Canada (2004) © Adapted and Reproduced with the permission of the Minister of Public Works and Government Services Canada, 2009.)

when a newborn falls above or below the 90th and 10th percentiles, respectively.[18]

Small for Gestational Age. *Small for gestational age* (SGA) is a term that denotes fetal undergrowth. SGA is defined as a birth weight less than two standard deviations below the mean for gestational age, or below the 10th percentile. The terms *small for gestational age* and *intrauterine growth retardation* (IUGR) are used interchangeably, but are not synonymous.[11,16,19] IUGR refers to a process that causes a reduction in an expected pattern of growth. SGA refers to an infant with a birth weight lower than the predetermined cut-off point.[19]

Moderate IUGR (between 3rd and 10th percentiles) and severe IUGR (below the 3rd percentile) can occur at any time during fetal development. Depending on the time of insult, the infant can have symmetric or proportional growth retardation or asymmetric or disproportional growth retardation.[14,19] Impaired growth that occurs early in pregnancy during the hyperplastic phase of growth results in a symmetric growth retardation, and there is a proportionate decrease in length, weight, and head size for gestational age.[14,19] This is irreversible postnatally. Causes of proportional IUGR include chromosomal abnormalities, congenital infections, and exposure to environmental toxins. Impaired growth that occurs later in pregnancy during the hypertrophic phase of growth results in asymmetric growth retardation.[11] Infants with IUGR due to intrauterine malnutrition often have weight reduction out

of proportion to length or head circumference but are spared impairment of head and brain growth. Tissues and organs are small because of decreased cell size, not decreased cell numbers. Postnatally, the impairment may be partially corrected with good nutrition.

Gestational growth can be affected by maternal, placental, and fetal factors. The maternal environment can have a drastic effect on birth weight and size. Underweight mothers are more likely to give birth to small-weight infants.[19] Maternal nutrition and weight gain are influenced by many factors. Women at risk for poor nutrition and poor fetal growth include adolescents, women of low economic status, women with short interpregnancy intervals, women with unusual or stringent diet restrictions, and women who do heavy physical work during pregnancy.[19] Various maternal diseases have been associated with restricted fetal growth, including prepregnancy hypertension, diabetes mellitus, and chronic maternal illnesses and infections. Growth retardation in the fetus may be related to maternal exposure to environmental agents such as recreational drugs (drugs of abuse), therapeutic drugs, and environmental hazards. Tobacco in the form of cigarette smoking during pregnancy reduces birth weight; and the reduction is related to the number of cigarettes smoked.[11,19] Occupational exposure to agents such as industrial solvents used as thinners in paint, glue, and varnishes can pose a threat to the pregnant mother and fetus.[19] Abnormal placentation comprises a broad range of pathologic processes that compromise uteroplacental blood flow and fetal growth. Fetal factors include chromosomal aberrations and gene abnormalities. There is also a progressive decrease in placental and fetal weight as the number of fetuses increases in multiple-fetus gestations. Infants of twin and triplet gestations tend to weigh less than those of singlet gestations.[15,19]

The perinatal mortality rate among infants with IUGR is 10 to 20 times that among infants whose size and weight are appropriate for gestational age.[19] The causes of this mortality are primarily hypoxia and congenital anomalies. Other complications include polycythemia, hyperbilirubinemia, and hypoglycemia. SGA infants have a larger plasma volume and circulating red cell mass, most likely the result of fetal hypoxia and subsequent erythropoietin production. Many of the SGA infants also experience fasting hypoglycemia during the first days of life, probably as the result of depleted hepatic glycogen stores.[19]

The long-term effects of growth retardation depend on the timing and severity of the insult. Many of these infants have developmental disabilities on follow-up examination, especially if the growth retardation is symmetric.[11] They may remain small, especially if the insult occurred early. If the insult occurred later because of placental insufficiency or uterine restraint, with good nutrition catch-up growth can occur and the infant may attain appropriate growth goals.

Large for Gestational Age. *Large for gestational age* (LGA) is a term that denotes fetal overgrowth and a birth weight above the 90th percentile.[15,19] The excessive growth may result from maternal or fetal factors. Maternal factors include maternal obesity and diabetes. Fetal factors consist primarily of gene and chromosome abnormalities. Maternal size has long been recognized as a factor that influences birth weight—heavy women tend to have LGA infants. Women with diabetes also tend to have LGA infants, especially if the diabetes was poorly controlled during pregnancy.[19]

Complications when an infant is LGA include birth asphyxia and trauma due to mechanical difficulties during the birth process, hypoglycemia, polycythemia, and hyperbilirubinemia.[19] Maternal hyperglycemia exposes the fetus to increased levels of glucose, which stimulate fetal pancreatic islet hyperplasia and increased insulin secretion. Insulin increases fat deposition and the result is a macrosomic (large body size) infant. Infants with macrosomia have enlarged viscera and are large and plump because of an increase in body fat. Fetal hyperinsulinemia is associated with fetal hypoxia and erythropoietin-induced polycythemia. Infants with polycythemia are at direct risk for hyperbilirubinemia.[19] LGA infants and infants of diabetic mothers are also at risk for hypoglycemia (to be discussed). Other potential long-term effects of LGA include insulin resistance, metabolic syndrome, overweight or obesity, diabetes, and early cardiovascular disease. In addition, there is increasing evidence that links high birth weight with overall leukemia risk.[20]

Assessing Gestational Age

Gestational age assessment can be divided into two categories: prenatal assessment and postnatal assessment. *Prenatal assessment* of gestational age most commonly includes careful menstrual history, physical milestones during pregnancy (*e.g.*, uterine size, detection of fetal heart rate and movements), and prenatal tests for maturity (*e.g.*, ultrasonography, amniotic fluid studies). The Nägele rule uses the first day of the LMP to calculate the day of labour by adding 7 days to the LMP and counting back 3 months.[11,21] This method may be inaccurate if the mother is not a good historian or has a history of irregular menses, which interferes with identification of a normal cycle.

Postnatal assessment of gestational age is done by examination of external physical and neuromuscular characteristics, alone or in combination. Assessment of gestational age should be a part of every initial newborn examination. Accurate assessment of gestational age facilitates risk assessment and identification of abnormalities and allows for earlier interventions. Dubowitz and Ballard developed the most common methods used in nurseries today. The Dubowitz method is comprehensive and includes 21 criteria using external physical (11) and neuromuscular (10) signs.[22] The estimate of gestational age is best done within 12 hours of birth and is accurate within 1 week. The method is less accurate for infants born at less than 30 weeks' gestational age. The Ballard method is an abbreviated Dubowitz method that includes 12 criteria, using 6 external physical and 6 neuromuscular signs[21] (Fig. 2.4). The New Ballard Score (NBS) was updated and modified to include newborns at gestational ages of 20 to 44 weeks and is the most commonly used method.[15,23]

IN SUMMARY

Growth and development begin with union of ovum and sperm and are ongoing throughout a child's life to adulthood. Abnormalities during this process can have profound effects on the individual. Prenatal development is composed of two periods, the embryonic period and the fetal period. During these periods, the zygote becomes the newborn with the organ maturity to make the adjustments necessary for extrauterine life. An infant is considered term when born between the beginning of the 38th week and completion of the 41st week. An infant is considered premature when born before the end of the 37th week and postmature when born after the end of the 41st week.

At birth, the average weight of the full-term newborn is 3,000 to 4,000 g. Infants weighing 2,500 g or less at birth are classified as being low birth weight. Low birth weight is further broken down into very low birth weight (<1,500 g) and extremely low birth weight (<1,000 g). Infants with a birth weight above the 90th percentile are considered large for gestational age. The lowest mortality rates occur among newborns with weights between 3,000 and 4,000 g and gestational ages of 38 to 42 weeks.

INFANCY

After completing this section of the chapter, you should be able to meet the following objectives:

- Describe the use of the Apgar score in evaluating infant well-being at birth.
- Describe the causes and manifestations of neonatal hypoglycemia.
- List three injuries that can occur during the birth process.
- Describe physical growth and organ development during the first year of life.
- Explain how the common health care needs of the premature infant differ from the health care needs of the term newborn or infant.
- Differentiate between organic and nonorganic failure to thrive syndrome.

Infancy is defined as the time from birth to approximately 12 months of age, the first 4 weeks of which are designated as the *newborn* or *neonatal* period. This is a period of rapid physical growth and maturation. The infant begins life as a relatively helpless organism and, through a process of progressive development, gains the skills to interact and cope with the environment. The infant begins life with a number of primitive reflexes and little body control. By 12 months, a child is able to stand alone, hold a cup and spoon, say several words, and play with toys.

Neuromuscular maturity

	−1	0	1	2	3	4	5
Posture							
Square window (wrist)	>90°	90°	60°	45°	30°	0°	
Arm recoil		180°	140–180°	110–140°	90–110°	<90°	
Popliteal angle	180°	160°	140°	120°	100°	90°	<90°
Scarf sign							
Heel to ear							

Physical maturity

Skin	Sticky, friable, transparent	Gelatinous, red, translucent	Smooth, pink; visible veins	Superficial peeling and/or rash, few veins	Cracking pale areas, rare veins	Parchment, deep cracking, no vessels	Leathery, cracked, wrinkled
Lanugo	None	Sparse	Abundant	Thinning	Bald areas	Mostly bald	
Plantar surface	Heel–toe 40–50 mm:−1 <40 mm:−2	>50 mm No crease	Faint red marks	Anterior transverse crease only	Creases anterior 2/3	Creases over entire sole	
Breast	Imperceptible	Barely perceptible	Flat areola, no bud	Stippled areola 1–2 mm bud	Raised areola 3–4 mm bud	Full areola 5–10 mm bud	
Eye/ear	Lids fused loosely:−1 tightly:−2	Lids open; pinna flat, stays folded	Slightly curved pinna; soft; slow recoil	Well-curved pinna; soft but ready recoil	Formed and firm, instant recoil	Thick cartilage, ear stiff	
Genitals: male	Scrotum flat, smooth	Scrotum empty, faint rugae	Testes in upper canal, rare rugae	Testes descending, few rugae	Testes down, good rugae	Testes pendulous, deep rugae	
Genitals: female	Clitoris prominent, labia flat	Prominent clitoris, small labia minora	Prominent clitoris, enlarging minora	Majora and minora equally prominent	Majora large, minora small	Majora cover clitoris and minora	

Maturity rating

Score	Weeks
−10	20
−5	22
0	24
5	26
10	28
15	30
20	32
25	34
30	36
35	38
40	40
45	42
50	44

FIGURE 2.4 • Ballard scoring system for determining gestational age in weeks. (From Ballard J. L., Khoury J. C., Wedig K., et al. (1991). New Ballard Score, expanded to include extremely premature infants. *Journal of Pediatrics*, 119, 417.)

Growth and Development

The average length of a full-term infant is 50 cm, with a range of 48 to 53 cm.[11,15] During the first 6 months, length increases by 2.5 cm per month. By 1 year, the increase in length is approximately 50% of the birth length. This increase is primarily in trunk growth. Typically, infants double their birth weight by 6 months and triple their birth weight by age 1.

The skull bones of newborn infants are incomplete and are connected by bands of connective tissue called *sutures*. At the junction of the sutures are wider spaces of unossified membranous tissue called *fontanelles*. The larger anterior fontanelle is palpable until about 18 months to 2 years of age; the smaller ones are replaced by bone by the end of the first year.[4] The softness of the cranial bones and loose connections of the sutures and fontanelles enable the shape of an infant's head to change (mold) during the birth process. The fibrous sutures of the infant's skull also permit the cranium to enlarge during infancy and childhood. The increase in head size is greatest during the first 2 years, the period of most rapid brain development. Premature closure of any suture in the skull is called *craniosynostosis*.[4] The cause of primary craniosynostosis is unknown, but genetic factors appear to be important. These malformations vary between genders depending on which suture is involved and are often associated with other skeletal abnormalities. The closed suture prevents growth from occurring in the affected area, but growth continues in the unaffected sutures, resulting in an abnormally shaped head. The clinical consequences of premature suture closure depend on which suture is affected[24] (Fig. 2.5).

Chest circumference at birth is smaller than head circumference. By 1 year, the head and chest are approximately equal in circumference; after 1 year, chest circumference exceeds

A

B

FIGURE 2.5 • Craniosynostosis. **A:** Scaphocephaly due to closure of the sagittal suture, in which the anterior fontanelle is small or absent, results in a long, narrow, wedge-shaped cranium. **B:** Oxycephaly due to premature closure of the coronal suture results in a high, tower-like cranium. (Adapted from Moore K. L., Dalley A. F. (2006). *Clinically oriented anatomy* (5th ed., p. 905). Philadelphia, PA: Lippincott Williams & Wilkins.)

head circumference.[4] After birth, most organ systems continue to grow and mature in an orderly fashion. Variations in growth and development are responsible for the differences in body proportions. For example, during the fetal period, the head is the predominant part because of the rapidly growing brain, whereas during infancy the trunk predominates, and in childhood the legs predominate.

Organ Systems

Organ systems must continue to grow and mature after delivery. Many are at a minimal level of functioning at birth. This often places the infant at risk for health problems.

Respiratory System. The respiratory system must make the transition from an intrauterine to an extrauterine existence. Onset of respiration must begin at birth for survival. The first breaths expand the alveoli and initiate gas exchange. The infant's respiratory rate initially is rapid and primarily abdominal, but with maturation, respiratory rate gradually slows. Maturation of the respiratory system includes an increase in the number of alveoli and growth of the airways. Infants are obligatory nose breathers until 3 to 4 months of age; any upper airway obstruction may cause respiratory distress.[4] The trachea

is small and close to the bronchi, and the bronchi's branching structures enable infectious agents to be easily transmitted throughout the lungs. The softness of the supporting cartilage in the trachea, along with its small diameter, places the infant at risk for airway obstruction. The auditory (eustachian) tube is short and straight and closely communicates with the ear, putting the infant at risk for middle ear infections.

Cardiovascular System. Birth initiates major changes in the cardiovascular system. Fetal circulation ends as the umbilical cord is clamped and the neonate begins to breathe. At birth, three fetal shunts (foramen ovale, ductus venosus, and ductus arteriosus) undergo a functional closure due to the directional change in blood flow[4,25] (Fig. 2.5). Full anatomic closure of the three shunts may take weeks to months for the healthy term newborn, and may take longer in preterm neonates.[25] At birth, the size of the heart is large in relation to the chest cavity. The size and weight of the heart doubles in the first year. Initially, the right ventricle is more muscular than the left ventricle, but this reverses in infancy. As the infant grows, the heart rate gradually slows, and systolic blood pressure rises.

Thermoregulation. Maintaining a stable body temperature is a function of heat production and conservation coupled with heat loss. Heat production in response to cold stress can occur through peripheral vascular constriction, inhibition of sweat, voluntary muscle activity, involuntary muscle activity (shivering), and nonshivering thermogenesis. However, many of these responses occur rarely in the neonate. The main source of heat production is through nonshivering thermogenesis.[26] Nonshivering thermogenesis is a physiologic process that relies heavily on heat liberated from brown fat stores.[25,26] Brown fat is found in full term newborns. Thus, thermal regulation is a greater challenge for preterm and low birth weight infants.[21] Heat loss to the environment can occur through the following mechanisms: (1) radiation, or transfer of heat from a warmer to a cooler area that is not in contact with the body; (2) convection, transfer of heat to the surrounding environment, influenced by air currents; (3) conduction, transfer of heat to a cooler surface that is in direct contact with the body; and (4) evaporation, cooling secondary to water loss from the skin.[21,27] Heat loss in the preterm infant is accelerated because of the higher ratio of surface area to body mass, reduced insulation of subcutaneous tissue, and water loss through immature skin.

INFANCY

- Infancy, which is the time from birth to 12 months of age, is a period of rapid physical growth and maturation.
- From an average birth weight of 3,000 to 4,000 g, in the full-term infant manages to triple its weight and increase its length by 50% at 1 year of age.
- Physiologic changes at birth and immature organ systems place the neonate and infant at risk for a variety of health problems.

The thermal environment of the preterm infant must be regulated carefully. Ideally, the infant should be kept in a neutral environment to maintain a stable core body temperature with minimal need for metabolic heat production through oxygen consumption. The neutral thermal environment for a given infant depends on size, gestational age, and postnatal age. In general, when infants reach a weight of 1,700 to 1,800 g, they can maintain temperature when bundled in an open crib.[27]

Gastrointestinal System. The infant's gastrointestinal system is immature, and most digestive processes are poorly functioning until approximately 3 months of age. Solid food may pass incompletely digested and be evident in the stool. The newborn's first stool is called *meconium* and is composed of amniotic fluid, intestinal secretions, shed mucosal cells, and sometimes blood from ingested maternal blood or minor bleeding of intestinal tract vessels. Passage of the dark black-green meconium should occur within the first 24 to 48 hours in healthy term newborns, but may be delayed for up to 7 days in preterm newborns or in newborns who do not receive enteral nutrition because of illness.[21]

At birth, sucking may be poor and require several days to become effective. The tongue thrust reflex is present and aids in sucking, but it disappears at approximately 6 months of age. Stomach capacity for the newborn is approximately 60 to 90 ml, but because of the limited capacity and rapid emptying, infants require frequent feeding.[21]

Genitourinary System. The infant's genitourinary system is functionally immature at birth. The kidneys do not concentrate urine well until approximately 6 weeks of age. The first void should occur within 24 hours of birth, and is typically small in amount; the urine is light in colour and odourless.[21] Small bladder capacity causes frequent voiding. Total daily volume of urine output increases during the first week, from 30 to 300 ml. Newborns who do not void or who experience a projectile stream of urine, may need further evaluation for suspected congenital anomalies or obstructions within the urinary system.[21]

Nervous System. The nervous system undergoes rapid maturation and growth during infancy. In contrast to other systems that grow rapidly after birth, the nervous system grows proportionately more rapidly before birth. The most rapid period of fetal brain growth is between 15 and 20 weeks of gestation, at which time there is a significant increase in neurons. A second increase occurs between 30 weeks' gestation and 1 year of age. Around 12 months, the weight of the infant brain is two times heavier than it was at birth and is about 2/3 that of the adult size.[4]

At birth, the nervous system is incompletely integrated, but sufficiently developed to sustain extrauterine life. Most of the neurologic reflexes are primitive reflexes. Normal newborn reflexes, which include the palmar (grasp), Moro (startle), rooting (sucking), and stepping (placing) reflexes, can be used to evaluate the newborn's and infant's developing CNS.

The maturation of the nervous system includes an increase in the size of neurons, size and number of glial cells, and number of interneuron connections and branching of axons and dendrites. As this maturation progresses, the level of infant functioning increases from simple to complex and from primitive reflexes to purposeful movement. Cortical control of motor functions is closely associated with myelination of nerve fibres. Myelination of the various nerve tracts progresses rapidly after birth and follows a cephalocaudad and proximodistal direction sequence, beginning with myelination of the spinal cord and cranial nerves and followed by the brain stem and corticospinal tracts.[4] In general, sensory pathways become myelinated before motor pathways. The acquisition of fine and gross motor skills depends on this myelination and maturation.[28]

The first year of life also is filled with psychosocial developmental milestones for the infant. Basic needs must be met before the infant can accomplish these developmental tasks. Erikson described the development of a sense of trust as the task of the first stage.[29] If trust is not acquired, the infant becomes mistrustful of others and frustrated with his or her inability to control the surrounding environment.

Health Problems of the Neonate

The most profound physiologic changes required of the newborn occur at the time of transition from intrauterine to extrauterine life. Onset of respiration must begin at birth for survival. The fetal shunts (*i.e.,* foramen ovale and ductus arteriosus) begin to close and the circulation of blood changes from a serial to parallel circuitry. Heat regulation is a response critical to the infant's survival. The newborn's large surface area and lack of subcutaneous fat predispose to excessive heat loss. Blood glucose concentration in the fetus is approximately 0.8 mmol/L less than maternal glucose concentrations and can drop to hypoglycemic levels in certain high-risk groups.

Distress at Birth and the Apgar Score

The Apgar score, devised by Dr. Virginia Apgar, is a scoring system that evaluates infant well-being at birth.[30] The system addresses five categories (*i.e.,* heart rate, respiratory effort, muscle tone, reflex irritability, and colour) with a total score ranging from 0 to 10, depending on the degree to which these functions are presented (Table 2.1). Evaluations are performed at 1 minute and 5 minutes after delivery. A score of 0 to 3 is indicative of severe distress, 4 to 6 of moderate distress, and 7 to 10 of mild to no distress. Most infants score 6 to 7 at 1 minute and 8 to 9 at 5 minutes. If the score is 7 or less, the evaluation should be repeated every 5 minutes until a score of 7 or greater is obtained. An abnormal score at 5 minutes is more predictive of problems with survival and neurologic outcome than at 1 minute.[15,21]

Neonatal Hypoglycemia

Glucose concentration normally decreases in the immediate postnatal period, with levels below 2.0 to 2.5 mmol/L considered indicative of hypoglycemia.[27] By 2 hours, the glucose

TABLE 2.1 APGAR SCORE ASSESSMENT

CRITERION	SCORE[a]		
	0	1	2
Heart rate	Absent	<100	>100
Respiratory effort	Absent	Weak, irregular	Crying
Muscle tone	Limp	Some flexion	Well flexed
Reflex irritability	No response	Grimace	Cry, gag
Colour	Pale	Cyanotic	Pink
Total	0	5	10

[a]The Apgar score should be assigned at 1 minute and 5 minutes after birth, using a timer. Each criterion is assessed and assigned a 0, 1, or 2. The total score is the assigned Apgar score. If resuscitation is required beyond the 5 minutes, additional Apgar scores also may be assigned as a method to document the response of the newborn to the resuscitation.[21]

concentration in normal-term infants stabilizes between 2.6 and 4.4 mmol/L. After the first 2 and up to 36 hours of life, concentrations below 2.6 should be considered abnormal. In neonates, classic symptoms of hypoglycemia are not always present when there is a low blood glucose level; the lack of symptoms can be misleading and may jeopardize brain metabolism.[31] Furthermore, if the neonate were to experience hypoxemia or ischemia, in addition to hypoglycemia then the newborn is at risk for permanent brain damage.[31] Thus, all infants should be screened for hypoglycemia before 6 hours of age. Blood glucose can be easily measured by heel stick using a glucometer. Signs and symptoms of neonatal hypoglycemia include: cyanosis, apnea, hypothermia, hypotonia, poor feeding, lethargy, and seizures.[31] Newborns who are at particular risk for neonatal hypoglycemia are infants of diabetic mothers (IDMs) and premature and SGA newborns. The factors related to hypoglycemia in IDMs are hyperinsulinemia and diminished glucagon secretion.[31] Glucose readily crosses the placenta, and consequently IDMs are exposed to elevated blood glucose levels, a condition that stimulates islet cell hypertrophy and hyperplasia. Several other physiologic processes occur during the transition to extrauterine life for IDMs. The combined physiologic changes result in an abnormal plasma hormonal pattern of: high insulin, low glucagon, and low epinephrine; the hormonal changes inhibit the neonate's endogenous glucose production, causing a state of hypoglycemia.[31] Newborns with high insulin blood levels or hyperinsulinemia are often large for gestational age (LGA); however, if the diabetes was well controlled during the mother's pregnancy, labour, and delivery, then the newborn may be near normal size and may be less likely to have hypoglycemia.[31] Premature and SGA infants are two more populations at risk for developing hypoglycemia. Factors related to hypoglycemia for these infants include inadequate liver glycogen stores, muscle protein, and body fat, which is needed to meet energy needs.[31] Because these infants are small in size, their enzyme systems for gluconeogenesis may not have developed fully. In addition, infants with perinatal asphyxia and some

SGA newborns may have transient hyperinsulinemia, which promotes hypoglycemia.[31]

Neonatal Jaundice/Hyperbilirubinemia

Hyperbilirubinemia in neonates pertains to an elevated serum level of bilirubin. With this condition, the infant's skin appears yellow or jaundiced in colour due to the excessive accumulation of unconjugated, lipid-soluble bilirubin[32,33] (Fig. 2-6). A newborn infant's metabolism of bilirubin is in transition from the fetal stage, during which the placenta is the principal route of elimination of lipid-soluble bilirubin, to the postnatal stage, during which the water-soluble conjugated form is excreted

FIGURE 2.6 • A newborn infant with jaundice.

from hepatic cells into the biliary system and then into the gastrointestinal tract. This transitional process takes time and more than 50% of all full-term and most preterm infants develop hyperbilirubinemia. Bilirubin is formed from the breakdown of hemoglobin in red blood cells. Red blood cells live only for 70 to 90 days in the newborn, unlike the older child, in whom red blood cells live for 120 days.[32] Normally, about two thirds of the unconjugated bilirubin produced by a term newborn can be effectively cleared by the liver. However, the relative immaturity of the newborn liver and the shortened life span of the fetal red blood cells may predispose the term newborn to hyperbilirubinemia. Delayed umbilical cord clamping may also increase the risk for developing jaundice but with the establishment of sufficient enteral nutrition, regular bowel elimination, and normal fluid volume, the liver is usually able to clear any excess bilirubin.

There are several types of neonatal jaundice: physiologic, kernicterus, and breast milk jaundice. *Physiologic jaundice* refers to jaundice in the immediate neonatal period without signs of illness. Under normal circumstances, the level of unconjugated or indirect-reacting bilirubin in umbilical cord blood is 17 to 50 μmol/L.[32,33] This level rises to less than 85 μmol/L per 24 hours, usually peaking between the third and fifth days of life and decreasing to below 34 μmol/L between 5 and 7 days of life.[32,33]

Jaundice and its underlying hyperbilirubinemia are considered pathologic if their time of appearance, duration, and pattern of appearance vary significantly from those of *physiologic jaundice*. The development of *kernicterus* or bilirubin encephalopathy is a neurologic syndrome resulting from extremely high levels of serum bilirubin (>425 μmol/L), in which bilirubin crosses the blood brain barrier and deposits unconjugated bilirubin in the basal ganglia and brain stem nuclei.[32,33] Kernicterus develops at lower bilirubin levels in preterm infants. The exact level at which bilirubin levels are harmful to infants with LBW is unclear.

Although uncommon, jaundice and elevated unconjugated bilirubin levels can also occur in breast-fed infants (*breast milk jaundice*). It occurs after the seventh day of life, with maximal concentrations as high as 170 to 205 μmol/L reached during the second to third week.[34] The current recommendation is not to stop breast-feeding but rather add supplementation of extra fluids either oral (formula) or intravenous to help decrease the serum bilirubin.

Regardless of the cause, the goal of therapy is to prevent the concentration of bilirubin in the blood from reaching neurotoxic levels.[32–34] All newborns should be screened at discharge. Treatment measures include frequent breast-feeding to prevent dehydration, phototherapy using overhead or fibre-optic pads, and, in severe cases, exchange blood transfusions. Phototherapy uses a special artificial blue light to alter bilirubin so it may be more readily excreted in the urine and stool. The need for exchange transfusion is infrequent, but is indicated when bilirubin levels reach 375 to 420 μmol/L, or if anemia is present as a result of the hemolytic process.[32]

Birth Injuries

Injuries sustained during the birth process are responsible for less than 2% of neonatal mortality and morbidity.[35] Predisposing factors for birth injuries include: maternal age (less than 16 or greater than 35), primagravida, cephalopelvic disproportion, prolonged or rapid labour, deep transverse arrest of descent of presenting part of the fetus, oligohydramnios, abnormal presentation, use of midcavity forceps or vacuum extraction, VLBW infant, extreme prematurity, large fetal head (*e.g.*, hydrocephalus), fetal anomalies, and fetal weight.[35]

Cranial Injuries. The contour of the head of the newborn often reflects the effects of the delivery presentation. The softness of the cranial bones in infants and their loose connections at the sutures and fontanelles allow the shape of the head to mold during birth. In a vertex (head-first) delivery, the head is usually flattened at the forehead with the apex rising and forming a plane at the end of the parietal bones and the posterior skull or occiput dropping abruptly (Fig. 2.7). By 1 to 2 days of age, the head has taken on a more oval shape.[21] Such molding does not occur in infants born by breech presentation or caesarean section.

Caput succedaneum is a localized area of scalp edema caused by sustained pressure of the presenting part against the cervix. The caput succedaneum may extend across suture lines and have overlying petechiae, purpura, or ecchymosis. No treatment is needed, and it usually resolves over the first week of life. *Cephalohematoma* is a subperiosteal collection of blood from ruptured blood vessels.[36] The margins are sharply delineated and do not cross suture lines. It usually is unilateral, but it may be bilateral, and it usually occurs over the parietal area. The subperiosteal bleeding may be slow and

FIGURE 2.7 • Molding of the calvaria or posterior portion of the skull in a newborn infant. (From Moore K. L., Dalley A. F. (2006). *Clinically oriented anatomy* (5th ed., p. 903). Philadelphia, PA: Lippincott Williams & Wilkins.)

therefore not apparent for 24 to 48 hours. The overlying skin is not discoloured. Skull fractures may be present. If present, usually the fractures are linear, nondepressed, and do not require treatment. Infants with cephalohematomas are usually asymptomatic. Management includes monitoring for hyperbilirubinemia. Resolution usually occurs over a period of 2 weeks to 3 months. Rarely, a cephalohematoma may develop complications. Large cephalohematomas may result in significant blood loss, causing anemia and hyperbilirubinemia. In rare cases, an infant may develop a subdural or subarachnoid hemorrhage. Calcium deposits occasionally develop, and the swelling may remain for the first year.

Fractures. Skull fractures are uncommon because the infant's compressible skull is able to mold to fit the contours of the birth canal. However, fractures can occur and more often follow a forceps delivery or severe contraction of the pelvis associated with prolonged, difficult labour. Skull fractures may be linear or depressed. Uncomplicated linear fractures often are asymptomatic and do not require treatment. Depressed skull fractures are observable by the palpable indentation of the infant's head. They require surgical intervention if there is compression of underlying brain tissue. A simple linear fracture usually heals within several months.[35,36]

The clavicle is the most frequently fractured bone during the birth process.[36] It is more common in LGA infants and occurs when delivery of the shoulders is difficult in vertex (*i.e.,* head-first) or breech presentations. The infant may or may not demonstrate restricted motion of the upper extremities, but passive motion elicits pain. There may be discolouration or deformity and, on palpation, crepitus (*i.e.,* a crackling sound from bones rubbing together), and irregularity may be found. Treatment of complete fractures consists of immobilizing the arm and shoulder and providing pain relief.[36]

Peripheral Nerve Injuries. The brachial plexuses are situated above the clavicles in the anterolateral bases of the neck. They are composed of the ventral rami of the fifth cervical (C-5) through the first thoracic (T-1) nerves. During vertex deliveries, excessive lateral traction of the head and neck away from the shoulders may cause a stretch injury to the brachial plexus on that side. In a breech presentation, excessive lateral traction on the trunk before delivery of the head may tear the lower roots of the cervical cord. If the breech presentation includes delivery with the arms overhead, an injury to the fifth and sixth cervical roots may result. When injury to the brachial plexus occurs, it causes paralysis of the upper extremity. The paralysis often is incomplete.[37]

Brachial plexus injuries include three types: Erb palsy (*i.e.,* upper arm), Klumpke palsy (*i.e.,* lower arm), and paralysis of the entire arm. Risk factors include an LGA infant and a difficult, traumatic delivery. Erb palsy or upper plexus injury involving C-5 to C-7 accounts for approximately 90% of plexus injuries.[37] It manifests with variable degrees of paralysis of the shoulder and arm. The affected arm is held in the "waiter's tip position," with adduction and internal rotation of shoulder,

FIGURE 2.8 • Position of the right arm in an infant with Erb palsy. After partial upper arm paralysis, the upper arm is held in a "waiter's tip" position with adduction and internal rotation of the shoulder, extension of the elbow with pronation of the forearm, and flexion of the wrist and fingers.

extension at the elbow, pronation of the forearm, and flexion of the wrist and fingers (Fig. 2.8). When the infant is lifted, the affected extremity is limp. The Moro reflex is impaired or absent, but the grasp reflex is present. Klumpke palsy or lower plexus injury at C-5 to T-1 is rare and presents with paralysis of the hand.[37,38] The infant has wrist drop, the fingers are relaxed, and the grasp reflex is absent. The Moro reflex is impaired, with the upper extremity extending and abducting normally while the wrist and fingers remain flaccid.[37]

Treatment of brachial plexus injuries includes immobilization, appropriate positioning, and an exercise program. Most infants recover in 3 to 6 months. If paralysis persists beyond this time, surgical repair (*i.e.,* neuroplasty, end-to-end anastomosis, nerve grafting) may be done.[37]

Health Problems of the Premature Infant

Infants born before 37 weeks gestation are considered premature. They often fall into the LBW category, with most weighing less than 2,500 g, and many weighing less than 1,500 g. Mortality and morbidity are increased in the premature population, with their rates inversely proportional to the length of gestation. Despite the advances in obstetric management since the late 1960s, the rate of premature delivery has not significantly changed, and the overall rate in Canada is 7.8%. The percentage of infants born with VLBW (<1,500 g) has increased in recent years. In 2009, 1.9% of infants born in Canada were VLBW, compared with 0.9% in 1975.[2] Recent increases have been attributed to the rise in the number of twin, triplet, and higher-order multiple births, as well as advancing maternal ages.[2]

Late preterm infants are born after 34 weeks but before 37 weeks and account for 70% to 75% of all preterm births. While these infants appear more mature and their body weight can exceed 2,500 g, they are at significant risk of developing complications and commonly require specialized care or prolonged admissions.[27]

The premature infant is poorly equipped to withstand the rigours of extrauterine transition. The organ systems are immature and may not be able to sustain life. The respiratory system may not be able to support gas exchange; the skin may be thin and gelatinous and easily damaged; the immune system is compromised and may not effectively fight infection; and the lack of subcutaneous fat puts the infant at risk for temperature instability. Complications of prematurity include respiratory distress syndrome, pulmonary hemorrhage, transient tachypnea, congenital pneumonia, pulmonary air leaks, bronchopulmonary dysplasia, recurrent apnea, glucose instability, hypocalcemia, hyperbilirubinemia, anemia, intraventricular hemorrhage, periventricular leukomalacia, necrotizing enterocolitis, circulatory instability, hypothermia, bacterial or viral infection, retinopathy of prematurity, and disseminated intravascular coagulopathies.

Respiratory Problems. The *respiratory distress syndrome* (RDS) is the most common complication of prematurity. The primary cause of RDS is the lack of surfactant in the lungs. At 24 weeks' gestation, there are small amounts of surfactant and few terminal air sacs (*i.e.,* primitive alveoli), with underdeveloped pulmonary vascularity. If an infant is born at this time, there is a poor chance of survival. By 26 to 28 weeks, there usually is sufficient surfactant and lung development to permit survival. Surfactant deficiency leads to decreased lung compliance, reduced alveolar ventilation, and atelectasis. Clinical manifestations include grunting, rapid shallow respirations, retractions, nasal flaring, and cyanosis.

The availability of exogenous surfactant replacement therapy has greatly improved the outcome of RDS. The administration of corticosteroids to women in preterm labour has been shown to accelerate lung maturation in their infants. Antenatal steroids are now the standard of care for women in preterm labour of up to 34 weeks. However, because the survival rate of the sickest infants has improved and because their management is more complex, the incidence of other complications has increased. These include air leak syndromes, bronchopulmonary dysplasia, and intracranial hemorrhage.[21,37]

Periodic breathing and *apnea of prematurity* are other common respiratory problems in premature infants. Brief apneic pauses lasting 5 to 10 seconds (*periodic breathing*) is a common finding and most often resolves without any obvious cause. In contrast, *apnea of prematurity* is defined as failure to breathe for 15 to 20 seconds or more, and often is accompanied by bradycardia or cyanosis. Apnea of prematurity may be the result of either lack of respiratory effort (central apnea) or due to an obstruction in the upper airway (obstructive apnea).[39]

Management of periodic breathing and apnea includes use of cardiorespiratory monitors and multiple other treatments depending on the cause of the apnea. Prompt tactile stimulation is often sufficient to abort mild episodes of apnea. Suctioning, repositioning, ventilator support and oxygen may be necessary for recurrent or prolonged apnea. In addition, methylxanthines (*e.g.,* caffeine, theophylline) may be used to increase central respiratory effort in recurrent apnea of prematurity. Infants with obstructive apnea may respond to nasal continuous positive airway pressure (CPAP) or bi-level positive airway pressure.[39]

Brain Injuries. Premature infants are particularly vulnerable to *intraventricular hemorrhage* (IVH) and *periventricular leukomalacia* (PVL). IVH or bleeding into the germinal matrix tissues, with possible rupture of the ventricular septum and tissue of the developing brain, is a major problem almost exclusive to preterm infants[40] (Fig. 2.9). Bleeding is thought to result from alterations in cerebral blood flow to damaged vessels in the germinal matrix, an early developmental structure that contains a fragile vascular bed that is poorly supported by connective tissue. Also with the decrease in blood flow to brain tissue, PVL, a form of ischemic white-matter brain injury adjacent to the lateral ventricles, can occur affecting motor nerve pathways leading to disabilities such as cerebral palsy. Because the germinal matrix begins to involute after 34 weeks of gestation, PVL and IVH are lesions linked to preterm infants. The incidence of these brain injuries increases with decreasing birth weight and gestational age.

Risk factors for IVH/PVL include prematurity, respiratory distress syndrome, hypoxic-ischemic injury, hypotension or hypertension, increased or decreased cerebral blood flow, pneumothorax, and hypervolemia.[40] Cranial ultrasonography

FIGURE 2.9 • Intraventricular hemorrhage in a premature infant. (From Rubin R., Strayer D. S. (Eds.). (2008). *Rubin's pathophysiology: Clinicopathologic foundations of medicine* (5th ed., p. 223). Philadelphia, PA: Lippincott Williams & Wilkins.)

is the method of choice for diagnosis, and standard grading systems (I–IV) are used to classify the extent and severity of any hemorrhage. Clinical manifestations are determined by the level (grade) of involvement. In some cases (grades I and II), no clinical manifestations may be seen. Most injuries resolve, but the more severe hemorrhages may obstruct the flow of cerebrospinal fluid, potentially causing a progressive hydrocephalus or, with white-matter damage, can lead to permanent destruction of neuronal connections.[40]

Necrotizing Enterocolitis.

Necrotizing enterocolitis (NEC) is an acquired life-threatening emergency of the gastrointestinal system in the newborn period. The disorder is characterized by various degrees of mucosal and transmural necrosis of the intestine. The incidence is 1% to 7% of admissions to the neonatal intensive care unit. This disorder is rarely seen in term infants, and incidence and fatality increase with decreasing birth weight and gestational age.[37,41]

Although the exact causes of NEC are unknown, it is suspected that three factors contribute to the disease: intestinal ischemia, oral effect of enteral feedings (metabolic substrate), and bacterial flora of the intestine have been linked to NEC pathogenic organisms. NEC most likely develops from an interaction between loss of mucosal damage caused by a variety of factors (*i.e.,* intestinal ischemia, infection) and the infant's response to the injury (circulatory, immunologic, inflammatory).[37,41] Any portion of the bowel may be affected, but the distal part of the ileum and proximal segment of the colon are involved most frequently. The necrosis of the intestine may be superficial, affecting only the mucosa or submucosa, or may extend through the entire intestinal wall (Fig. 2.10). If the full thickness of the intestinal wall is damaged, perforation can result. NEC usually has its onset in the second week, but it may occur as late as the third month in VLBW infants.[34] Age of onset is inversely related to gestational age.

FIGURE 2.10 • Neonatal necrotizing enterocolitis. Autopsy photograph of the intestine of an infant who died of necrotizing enterocolitis shows necrosis and pneumatosis of the intestine. (From Centers for Disease Control and Prevention. (2008). Public Health Image Library. ID #857 Available online at: http://phil.cdc.gov/phil/home.asp.)

Clinical manifestations of NEC are variable. However, the classic initial symptoms are usually feeding intolerance, abdominal distension, and bloody stools shortly after the first week of life. Severity of the disease ranges from mild to severe, in which bowel perforation occurs and a deteriorating clinical picture typically leads to shock. Clinical diagnosis is primarily radiographic. The radiographic hallmark of NEC is pneumatosis intestinalis or intramural air. Pneumoperitoneum is indicative of intestinal perforation.[37,41]

Treatment includes cessation of feedings, stomach decompression, broad-spectrum antibiotic coverage, fluid and electrolyte replacement, and total parenteral nutrition. Surgical intervention to excise necrotic bowel and create a stoma is necessary in approximately 25% to 50% of infants with NEC. Prevention strategies include: promotion of breast-feeding as there is decreased incidence of NEC in infants who receive human milk, and administration of probiotic preparations to increase mucosal barrier function, enhance nutrition, and reduce mucosal colonization by potential pathogens.[37,41]

Infection and Sepsis.

Sepsis is a major cause of neonatal morbidity and mortality in the neonate. Preterm infants are particularly at risk, having a 3- to 10-fold higher incidence of infection than full-term infants with normal birth weight and up to 20% of infants in neonatal intensive care units have positive blood cultures.[42] Preterm infants have a higher risk of becoming infected than full term infants (1:250 in preterm compared to 1:1,500 in full term) because of the immaturity and relative inexperience of their immune system. The majority of maternal antibodies (immunoglobulin [Ig] G) are transferred during the later weeks of gestation; in preterm infants, cord immunoglobulin levels are directly proportional to gestational age.[33] In addition, preterm infants often require invasive treatments that further increase their susceptibility to microbial invasion.[37]

The terms *early onset* and *late onset* are often used to describe two different categories related to the onset of infection. Early-onset infections are typically defined as those acquired during delivery or up to 7 days after birth. Late-onset sepsis typically occurs after the first week of life. Typically, early-onset infection results from bacteria that was acquired during the infant's passage through the birth canal or from the mother's genitourinary tract. There may be a history of obstetric complications, such as prolonged rupture of membranes, prolonged second stage of labour, or leaking membranes. The infant's health is severely impacted by early onset infections and progressive multi-organ system illness occurs. Infants with this type of sepsis frequently present with respiratory failure, shock, meningitis, disseminated intravascular coagulation, acute tubular necrosis and symmetrical peripheral gangrene.[42] The two organisms that may cause up to 80% of early onset infections are: group B beta hemolytic *Streptococcus* (GBS) and *Escherichia coli* (*E. coli*).[42,43] GBS remains the most frequent pathogen in term infants, and *E. coli* the most significant pathogen in preterm infants. Although other bacteria are less commonly found, organisms such as *Listeria monocytogenes,* enterococci, and gram-negative enteric bacilli (other than *E. coli*) must be considered.[42]

Late-onset infection is commonly acquired via person-to-person transmission or from contaminated equipment. It may be caused by the same pathogens as early onset sepsis, or by viral agents. Infants with late onset sepsis will have bacteremia and usually a focal site, such as meningitis, osteomyelitis, arthritis, and urinary tract infection. Meningitis is seen more often with late-onset infection than early-onset. Clinical signs and symptoms of late onset infection include lethargy, poor feeding, hypotonia, apathy, seizures, bulging fontanelle, fever, and hyperbilirubinemia.[37]

The manifestations of bacterial infection in the newborn result from two sources: the effects of the bacterial invasion of the microorganism and the response of the infant's immune system to the invasion.[42] Bacteria release endotoxins and other vasoactive substances, causing central vasodilation, peripheral vasoconstriction, and systemic hypovolemia. The immune response to the endotoxins leads to hemodynamic, metabolic, respiratory, CNS, gastrointestinal, and dermatologic changes. The signs of bacterial sepsis in a newborn, which can occur in all body systems, are generally nonspecific and are not easily distinguished from other causes. Therefore, it is important to have a high index of suspicion for sepsis in the newborn, especially the preterm newborn. The observation that there has been a subtle change in an infant's general condition, often marked by the nursing or maternal assessment that the infant "is not doing well," may be the first indication of infection. However, as the septicemia progresses, the signs become more severe and more specific.

Optimal prognosis depends on early diagnosis and implementation of appropriate therapy; thus, frequent and careful assessment and evaluation of the infant's physical condition can have a significant impact on outcome. Administration of antimicrobial agents to mothers during the intrapartal period or to newborns immediately postpartum has been shown to reduce the risk of early-onset GBS infection. In 2013, the Society of Obstetricians and Gynaecologists in Canada (SOGC) in collaboration with the Canadian Paediatric Society (CPS) updated the prevention of neonatal GBS disease guidelines.[44] GBS disease continues to be a threat to the newborn because of the high mortality and morbidity rates associated with the disease and the increased survival of smaller and more preterm newborns with a higher risk for GBS disease.

Health Problems of the Infant

Infants are prone to numerous health problems during the first year of life, which may become serious if not recognized and treated appropriately. Many of them may be precipitated by the relative immaturity of the organ systems. Infants are prone to nutritional disturbances, feeding difficulties, irritable infant syndrome or colic, and failure to thrive. Injuries, the major cause of death during infancy, are caused by events such as aspiration of foreign objects, suffocation, motor vehicle collisions, falls, and poisoning. Childhood diseases may be a

problem if the infant is not adequately immunized. Thus, injury and illness prevention is vital during infancy.

Nutritional Disturbances

Good nutrition is important during infancy because of rapid growth. Human milk or commercial infant formulas form the basis for the early nutritional needs of the newborn and young infant. Health Canada and the CPS recommend exclusive breast-feeding for the first 6 months of life. Human milk from a well-nourished mother is easily digested, provides sufficient nutrients and calories for normal growth and development, and has the added benefit of offering some immune protection. Vitamin D is recommended for breast-fed infants, fluoride for those receiving formula made with unfluorinated water, and dietary or supplemental iron should be added at approximately 6 months of age, when the fetal iron stores become depleted.[45]

Mothers who do not choose to breast-feed their child or who are unable to breast-feed may choose from a variety of commercial formulas designed to closely match the nutrition of human milk. Several companies produce infant formulas that contain the essential nutrients for infants. Although there are some minor differences, most infant formulas are similar, regardless of which company produces the formula.

Some infants may experience difficulties in consuming mother's milk or infant formulas that are based on cow's milk because of lactase deficiency. Lactase is an enzyme that breaks down lactose, the carbohydrate found in human milk and cow's milk. Some infant formulas contain carbohydrates other than lactose. These formulas are made from soybeans. Other feeding intolerances also may occur. Treatment of any milk or formula intolerance depends on identification of the specific offender and elimination of it from the diet. Newborns and infants frequently exhibit "spitting up" or regurgitation of formula, despite the absence of a formula intolerance. In general, cow's milk-based formulas are preferable to soy-based formulas, and changing to a soy-based formula should be undertaken only when there is a proven case of galactosemia or who cannot consume dairy based products for religious or cultural reasons. Education of the parents about the signs and symptoms of intolerance plus the reassurance that spitting up formula is normal may be all that is required. An infant that is gaining weight, appears alert and well nourished, has adequate stools, and demonstrates normal hunger is unlikely to have a formula intolerance.[45]

One area of infant nutrition that is still the subject of much controversy is the introduction of solid foods. There is great variation in advice regarding when to start solid foods and what solid foods to introduce. In general, human milk or iron-fortified infant formulas should supply most infant nutrition during the first year of life. However, solid foods usually are introduced between 4 to 6 months. When solid foods are being introduced, they should be considered as supplemental to the total nutrition and not as the main component of nutrition. The recommendation is to introduce meat, meat alternative and iron-fortified cereals as the first complementary foods.[45] Slow progression to the addition of individual foods (*e.g.*, vegetables, fruits) and textures (*e.g.*, puree, soft solids) occurs as the infant learns to chew and swallow food. Infants also become able to drink from a cup rather than a bottle during this time.

Irritable Infant Syndrome or Colic

Colic is usually defined as paroxysmal abdominal pain or cramping in an infant and usually is manifested by loud crying, drawing up of the legs to the abdomen, and extreme irritability.[46] Episodes of colic may last from several minutes to several hours a day. During this time, most efforts to soothe the infant or relieve the distress are unsuccessful. Colic is a temporary problem that resolves for the majority (up to 90%) of infants by 3 to 4 months of age. "Colic has often been described by the *rule of three:* crying for more than three hours a day, for more than 3 days a week, and for longer than three weeks in well-fed and healthy infants."[46] When parents seek advice about a colicky baby, their concerns should be substantiated by their health care provider. Because there may be an underlying organic cause, a careful history and physical examination should be performed. A history of apnea, cyanosis, or struggling to breathe may suggest previously undiagnosed pulmonary or cardiac conditions.[46] Tilting of the head and arching of the back may be indicative of gastroesophageal reflux.

There is no single etiologic factor that causes colic. Some reasons for the crying are related to feeding problems including: hunger, air swallowing, gastroesophageal reflux, and food intolerance. Therefore, the treatment of colic is not precise. Many nonmedical techniques and pharmacologic preparations have been tried. However, medications have not proven to be effective and should be avoided. Nonpharmacologic interventions include: soothing voices or singing, swaddling, slow rhythmic rocking, walking, white noise, and gentle vibration, such as car rides.[46] Support of the parents is probably the single most important factor in the treatment of colic. Many times the mother (or primary care provider) may be afraid to state just how frustrating it can be to be unable to console the infant. An open discussion of this frustration can help the mothers or care providers recognize that their feelings of frustration are normal; frequently, this gives them the added support needed to deal with their infant. Because the incidence of colic in breast-fed and bottle-fed infants is similar, mothers should be encouraged to continue breast-feeding so that the infant will continue to receive the many beneficial effects of breast-feeding.

Failure to Thrive

Failure to thrive (FTT) is a term that refers to the failure to meet expected standards of growth for infants and young children due to the inability to obtain or use essential nutrients. FTT may be organic or nonorganic.[47,48] Organic failure to thrive is the result of a physiologic cause that prevents the infant from obtaining or using nutrients appropriately. An example of organic failure to thrive is inadequate growth of an infant with deficient energy reserve because of a congenital defect that makes sucking and feeding difficult. Nonorganic failure to thrive is the result of psychological factors that prevent adequate intake of nutrition, such as poverty or poor child-parent interaction.[48]

Diagnosis of the type of FTT depends on careful examination and history of the infant and serial follow-up evaluations. Cases of organic failure to thrive usually are easier to diagnose than cases of nonorganic failure to thrive. Diagnosis of nonorganic failure to thrive requires extensive investigation of history, family situation, relationship of the care provider to the infant, and evaluation of feeding practices. The nonorganic basis should be considered early in every case of FTT in order to prevent potential developmental delays, social and emotional problems.[48]

Therapy for FTT depends on the cause. Because long-term nutritional deficiencies can result in impaired physical and intellectual growth, provision of optimal nutrition is essential. Methods to increase nutritional intake by adjusting caloric density of the formula or by parenteral nutrition may be required in cases of organic FTT.

Sudden Infant Death

Sudden unexpected infant death (SUID) is defined as the unexpected death of an infant, which after autopsy and investigation, may be attributed to metabolic disorders, hypothermia or hyperthermia, neglect or homicide, poisoning or accidental suffocation.[49] Sudden infant death syndrome (SIDS) is similar in definition, except that the cause of death is inconclusive and remains unexplained after autopsy, investigation of the death scene, and review of the child's medical and family history.[49,50] SIDS is rare during the first month of life, increases to a peak between 2 and 4 months of life, and then declines. Although its incidence has decreased since the "back to sleep" campaign was initiated in Canada in 1993, which advocated that infants be laid down to sleep in the supine position, SIDS continues to account for more infant deaths beyond the neonatal period than any other cause.[51]

Factors identified in the United States associated an increased risk of SIDS with sleeping in the prone position, prematurity and LBW, African American or Native American race, and exposure to environmental cigarette smoke; as well as young age of the mother, lack of or inadequate prenatal care, and smoking or substance use during pregnancy.[39,50] Sleeping prone has consistently been shown to increase the risk of SIDS. Originally, the CPS identified any nonprone position (*i.e.,* side or back) as being optimum for reducing the risk of SIDS. In 2013 the CPS reaffirmed that placing infants on their backs confers the lowest risk and is the preferred position.[51] Soft sleep surfaces on beds, such as comforters and pillows, also increase the risk of SIDS, as does bed sharing between infants and adults.

The exact cause of SIDS is unknown. Theories focus on brain stem abnormality, which prevents effective cardiorespiratory control. Features of SIDS include prolonged sleep apnea, increased frequency of brief inspiratory pauses, excessive periodic breathing, and impaired response to increased carbon dioxide or decreased oxygen. A diagnosis of SIDS can be made only if an autopsy is performed to exclude other causes of death. Differentiation of child abuse from SIDS is an important consideration, and each case of SIDS must be subjected to careful examination.[50]

Support of family members of an infant who dies of SIDS is crucial. Parents frequently feel guilty or inadequate as parents. The fact that there must be close scrutiny to differentiate a SIDS death from a death by child abuse adds to the guilt and disappointment felt by the family. After a diagnosis of SIDS is made, it is important that the parents and other family members receive information about SIDS. Health care providers need to be fully aware of resources available to families with a SIDS death. The siblings of the child who died of SIDS also need information and support to get through the grief process.

Injuries

Injuries are the major cause of death in infants 6 to 12 months of age. Aspiration of foreign objects, suffocation, falls, poisonings, drowning, burns, and other bodily damage may occur because of the infant's increasing ability to investigate the environment. Childproofing the environment can be an important precaution to prevent injuries. No home or environment can be completely childproofed, and close supervision of the child by a competent care provider is essential to prevent injury.

Motor vehicle collisions are responsible for a significant number of infant deaths. After 1 year of age, motor vehicle collisions become the number one cause of injuries resulting in death in children.[52] All Canadian provinces have legislation that requires infants be placed in an approved infant safety restraint while riding in a vehicle.[4] The middle of the back seat is considered the safest place for the infant to ride. Many hospitals do not discharge an infant unless there is a safety restraint system in the car. If a family cannot afford a restraint system, programs are available that donate or loan the family a restraint. Health care providers must be involved in educating the public about the dangers of carrying infants in vehicles without taking proper precautions to protect them.

Infectious Diseases

One of the most dramatic improvements in infant health has been related to widespread immunization for the major childhood communicable diseases, including diphtheria, pertussis, tetanus, polio, *Haemophilus influenzae* type B, rotavirus, pneumococcal serotypes, measles, mumps, rubella, and hepatitis B infections. Immunizations against these infectious diseases have greatly reduced morbidity and mortality in infants and young children. These immunizations are given at standard times as part of health promotion in infants and children. However, although they have lowered their prevalence, immunization programs have not completely eradicated these diseases. Immunization programs are effective only if all children receive the immunizations. Although most immunizations can be received through local health departments at no or low cost, some infants or young children do not routinely receive immunizations or do not receive the full regimen of immunizations. Methods to improve compliance and access

to immunizations are needed. Immunization recommendations are subject to change as research leads to development of improved vaccines or greater understanding of the microorganisms.

IN SUMMARY

Infancy is defined as that period from birth to 12 months of age. During this time, growth and development are ongoing. The relative immaturity of many of the organ systems places the infant at risk for a variety of illnesses. Birth initiates many changes in the organ systems as a means of adjusting to postnatal life. The birth process is a critical event, and maladjustments and injuries during the birth process are a major cause of death or disability. Premature delivery remains a significant health problem in Canada. The premature infant is at risk for numerous health problems because of the interruption of intrauterine growth and immaturity of organ systems.

EARLY CHILDHOOD

After completing this section of the chapter, you should be able to meet the following objectives:

- Define early childhood.
- Describe the growth and development of early childhood.
- Discuss the common health problems of early childhood.

Early childhood is considered to be the period of 12 months through 5 years of age. During this time, the child passes through the stages of toddler (*i.e.,* 12 months to 3 years) and preschooler (*i.e.,* 3 to 5 years). Many changes occur as the child moves from infancy through the toddler and preschool years. The major achievements are the development and refinement of locomotion and language, which take place as children progress from dependence to independence.

Growth and Development

Early childhood is a period of continued physical growth and maturation. Compared with infancy, physical growth is not as dramatic. The average child gains approximately 2 kg in weight and 7 cm in height each year.[4] The toddler's abdomen flattens, and the body becomes leaner. Physical energy peaks and the need for sleep declines to 8 to 13 hours a day, usually including one nap. By 3 years of age, visual acuity reaches 20/30 and all 20 primary teeth have erupted.[4]

The maturation of organ systems is ongoing during early childhood. The respiratory system continues its growth and maturation, but because of the relative immaturity of the airway structures, otitis media and respiratory infections are common. Infants and toddlers have barrel-shaped chests and underdeveloped intercostal muscles, which are ineffective in managing periods of respiratory distress.[4] The respiratory rate of infancy has slowed and averages 20 to 30 breaths per minute. Respirations remain abdominal until 7 years of age.[4]

EARLY CHILDHOOD

- Early childhood, which encompasses the period from 12 months through 5 years of age, is a period of continued growth and development.
- During this time, the child passes through the stages of toddler (*i.e.,* 12 months to 3 years) and preschooler (*i.e.,* 3 years through 5 years).
- The major achievements are the development and refinement of locomotion and language, which take place as children progress from dependence to independence.
- Learning is ongoing and progressive and includes interactions with others, appropriate social behaviour, and sex role functions.

Neural growth remains rapid during early childhood. By 12 months of age, the child's brain is nearly 2/3 of the adult size and has doubled in weight since birth.[4] The cephalocaudad, proximodistal principle is followed as myelinization of the cortex, brain stem, and spinal cord is completed. The spinal cord is usually completely myelinated by 2 years of age. At that time, control of anal and urethral sphincters and the motor skills of locomotion can be achieved and mastered. The continuing maturation of the neuromuscular system is increasingly evident as complex gross and fine motor skills are acquired throughout early childhood.

Growth and maturation in the musculoskeletal system continue with ossification of the skeletal system, growth of the legs, and changes in muscle and fat proportions. Legs grow faster than the trunk in early childhood; after the first year of life, approximately two thirds of the increase in height is leg growth. Muscle growth is balanced by a corresponding decrease in adipose tissue accumulation.

During early childhood, many important psychosocial tasks are mastered by the child. Independence begins to develop, and the child is on the way to becoming a social being in control of the environment. Development and refinement of gross and fine motor abilities allow involvement with a potentially infinite number of tasks and activities. Learning is ongoing and progressive and includes interactions with others, appropriate social behaviour, and sex role functions. Psychoanalytist theorist Eric Erikson described the tasks that must be accomplished in early childhood. According to Erickson, the toddler must acquire a sense of autonomy while overcoming a sense of doubt and shame and the preschooler must acquire a sense of initiative and develop a conscience.[29]

Common Health Problems

The early childhood years can pose significant health risks to the growing and maturing child. Injuries are the leading cause of death in children between the ages of 1 and 4 years; only 20- to 24-year-olds experience more injuries.[52] Locomotion and curiosity, together combined with a lack of awareness of danger, place toddlers and preschoolers at special risk for injuries. Motor vehicle collisions are responsible for almost 50% of all injuries and deaths in this group. Many injuries and deaths can be prevented by the use of appropriate seat belts and restraints. Other major causes of injuries include drowning, burns, poisoning, falls, aspiration and suffocation, and bodily damage. Infectious diseases can be a problem for children during early childhood owing to the immaturity of their immune system. This also may be the time when children first enter day care, which increases their exposure to other children and infectious diseases. The major disorders include the communicable childhood diseases (*e.g.,* common cold, influenza, varicella [chicken pox], gastrointestinal tract infections, and otitis media).[4]

Child maltreatment is an increasing problem in Canada. Although the statistics on rates of child abuse are limited, the best estimates range from one in 5 to one in 8 children in Canada undergo some form of abuse. Children at the greatest risk for maltreatment are younger than 4 years of age, female, or having a disability.[53] Child maltreatment includes physical and emotional neglect, physical abuse, and sexual abuse. Neglect is the most common type of maltreatment and can take the form of deprivation of basic necessities or failure to meet the child's emotional needs. It is often attributed to poor parenting skills. Physical abuse is the deliberate infliction of injury. The cause is probably multifactorial, with predisposing factors that include the parent, child, and environment. Sexual abuse is on the rise and includes a spectrum of types. The typical abuser is male. Children often do not report the abuse because they are afraid of not being believed but all types of child maltreatment can lead to lasting effects related to the traumatic experiences.[53]

IN SUMMARY

Early childhood is defined as the period from 12 months to 5 years of age—the toddler and preschool years. Growth and development continue but are not as dramatic as during the prenatal and infancy periods. Early childhood is a time when most organ systems reach maturity and the child becomes an independent, mobile being. There continue to be significant health risks during this period, especially from infectious diseases and injuries. Injuries are the leading cause of death during this period. Child abuse is rapidly increasing as a major health problem.

MIDDLE-TO-LATE CHILDHOOD

After completing this section of the chapter, you should be able to meet the following objectives:

- Characterize the growth and development that occur during the early school years.
- Discuss the common health problems of middle-to-late childhood.

In this text, middle-to-late childhood is defined as the period in which a child begins school through the beginning of adolescence. These 6 years, from 6 to 12 years of age, involve a great deal of change; when one recollects "childhood," these are the years most often remembered. The experiences of this period have a profound effect on the physical, cognitive, and psychosocial development of the child and contribute greatly to the adult that the child will become.

Growth and Development

Although physical growth is steady throughout middle childhood, it is slower than in the previous periods and the adolescent period to follow. During late childhood, children typically gain approximately 3 to 3.5 kg and grow an average of 6 cm per year.[4] Growth occurs discontinuously, in three to six irregularly timed spurts each year.[5]

During late childhood, a child's legs grow longer, posture improves, and his or her centre of gravity descends to a lower point. These changes make children more graceful and help them to be successful at climbing, bike riding, roller skating, and other physical activities. Body fat distribution decreases and, in combination with the lengthening skeleton, gives the child a thinner appearance. As body fat decreases, lean muscle mass increases. By 12 years of age, boys and girls have doubled their body strength and physical capabilities. Although muscular strength increases, the muscles are still relatively immature and injury from overly strenuous activities, such as difficult sports, can occur. With the gains in length, the head circumference decreases in relation to height, waist circumference decreases in relation to height, and leg length increases in relation to height.

The head grows only 2 to 3 cm during this period, indicating slower brain growth; myelination is complete by 7 years of age. Facial proportions change as the face grows faster in relation to the rest of the cranium. Primary teeth are lost and replaced by permanent teeth. When the permanent teeth first appear, they may appear to be too big for the mouth and face. This is a temporary imbalance that is alleviated as the face grows.[4]

Caloric requirements for the younger school-age child (*i.e.,* 5 to 7 years old) are usually lower compared with previous periods and with the adolescent period to follow. Cardiac growth is slow. Heart rate and respiratory rates continue to decrease, and blood pressure gradually rises. Growth of the eye continues, and the normal farsightedness of the preschool child is gradually converted to 20/20 vision by approximately 6 to 7 years.[5] Bone ossification and mineralization continue with noticeable acceleration of long bone growth. Children's bones cannot resist muscle pressure and pulling forces as well as mature bones. Precautions should be taken to prevent alterations in bone structure, such as providing properly fitting shoes and adequate desks to prevent poor posture. Children should receive routine health care screenings during this period so that common childhood conditions, such as vision and hearing deficits, obesity, and scoliosis may be addressed.[4]

MIDDLE-TO-LATE CHILDHOOD

- Middle-to-late childhood years (6 to 12 years) are those during which the child begins school through the beginning of adolescence.
- Growth during this period averages 3 to 3.5 kg and 6 cm per year, and occurs in approximately three to four bursts per year that last for approximately 8 weeks.
- Muscular strength, coordination, and stamina increase progressively, as does the ability to perform complex movements such as shooting basketballs, playing the piano, and dancing.
- During this stage, the child develops the cognitive skills that are needed to consider several factors simultaneously and to evaluate oneself and perceive others' evaluations.

Toward the end of late childhood, the physical differences between the two sexes become apparent. Girls usually enter pubescence approximately 2 years before boys, resulting in noticeable differences in height, weight, and development of secondary sex characteristics. There is much individual variation among children of the same sex. These differences can be extremely difficult for children to cope with.

Entry into the school setting has a major impact on the psychosocial development of the child at this age. The child begins to develop relationships with other children, forming groups. Peers become more important as the child moves out of the security of the family and into the bigger world. Usually during this period, children begin to form closer bonds with individual "best friends." However, the best friend relationships may frequently change. In addition, the personality of the child begins to appear. Although the personality is still developing, the basic temperament and approach to life become apparent. Although changes in personality occur with maturity, the basic elements may not change. The major task of this stage, as identified by Erikson, is the development of industry or accomplishment.[29] Failure to meet this task results in a sense of inferiority or incompetence, which can impede further progress.[4]

Common Health Problems

Common health problems seen during middle-to-late childhood include tooth decay, injury and illness, and overweight and obesity.

Tooth Decay

The incidence of dental caries has decreased since the addition of fluoride to most water systems in Canada yet the most prominent dental issue in middle childhood is tooth decay.[4] The high incidence of dental caries during late childhood is related to inadequate dental care and a high amount of dietary sugar. Children at the early part of this stage may not be as effective in brushing their teeth and may require adult assistance, but they may be reluctant to allow parental help. Therefore, health promotion includes teaching about reducing the amount of dietary sugar, proper tooth brushing, and appropriate dental care.

Injury and Illness

The chief cause of mortality in this age group is unintentional injury, primarily due to motor vehicle accidents. Specifically, most injury deaths for Canadian children between 5 and 19 years of age were due to motor vehicle traffic crash (6%) but for indigenous children and youth these injuries occur at a disproportionally higher rate compared to the national average (26%).[53,54] Falls are the leading cause for *nonfatal* injuries in children of all age groups less than 19 years of age. Establishing consistent rules for safe behaviour and reinforcing the need to wear protective sports equipment are two essential measures for injury prevention in this age group.

Although childhood cancer is rare, it is the second cause of death for children ages up to 14 years of age.[52] The most common types of cancer in these children between 0 and 14 years of age are leukemia (33%), brain and nervous system cancers (20%) and lymphomas (11%).[55]

Because of the high level of immune system competence in late childhood, these children have an immunologic advantage over earlier years. Immunization against the major communicable diseases of childhood has greatly improved the health of children in their middle childhood years. Yet, children in this age group do experience infections (*i.e.*, viral, bacterial, or fungal) from being in close contact with other children. These infections commonly occur as respiratory, gastrointestinal, or skin diseases. Other acute or chronic health problems may surface for the first time, including epilepsy and developmental or special learning disabilities. In Canada, asthma is the most common chronic disease in children less than 18 years of age.

Overweight and Obesity

Overweight and obesity is a national concern for all children in Canada, as well as a global epidemic. Overweight and obesity in children and adolescents is defined by body mass index (weight in kilograms divided by the square of height in meters) and since 2007 the recommendations are to use the World Health Organization (WHO) growth to monitor Canadian

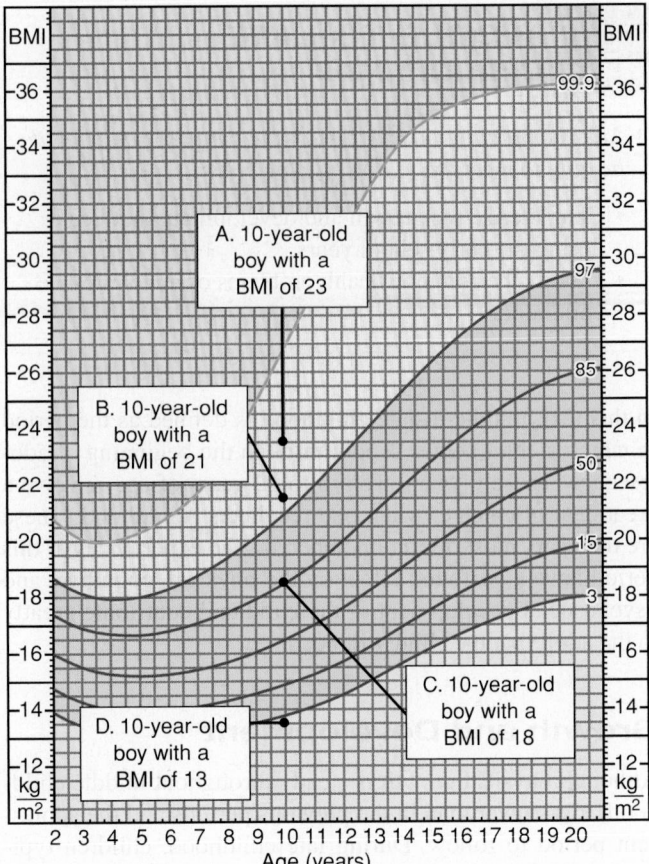

FIGURE 2.11 • Body mass index-for-age percentiles for boys 2 to 20 years of age. Overweight in children and adolescents is defined by body mass index (weight in kilograms divided by the square of height in metres) at or above the 95th percentile for children of the same age and sex. (From Centers for Disease Control and Prevention. (2007). About BMI in children and teens. Available online at: www.cdc.gov/nccdphp/dnpa/obesity/defining.htm. Calculator for determining BMI available at: http://apps.nccd.cdc.gov/dnpabmi/Calculator.aspx.)

children rather than the International Obesity Task Force (IOTF) classifications[6] (Fig. 2.11). A comparison of raw data from 1978 to the Canadian Health Measures Survey, 2009 to 2011, shows that the prevalence of overweight in children is increasing: for children 6 to 11 years of age, the prevalence increased from 13% to 20%, and for those 12 to 17 years, the prevalence increased from 11% to 20%.[56] When identifying the ethnic origin, it is noted that both black and native aboriginal children and adolescents are disproportionately affected.

There are several factors that contribute to childhood overweight/obesity including genetics, amount of calories consumed in food and drinks, and the amount of energy expended with metabolism, growth, and physical exercise. Evidence is limited regarding specific foods or dietary patterns that contribute to excessive caloric intake in children; however, large portion sizes for food and beverages, eating meals away from home, frequent snacking, consumption of energy-dense foods, and consuming beverages with added calories are often hypothesized as contributing to excessive energy intake.[4] Participating in physical activity is important for children because of its beneficial effects not only on weight, but also on blood pressure and bone strength. Media use, and specifically television viewing, may displace time children spend in physical activity. It may also contribute to increased energy consumption through excessive snacking and eating meals in front of the television. Genetic factors may increase a child's susceptibility to becoming overweight. However, this genetic susceptibility may need to exist in conjunction with other contributing factors such as a high-calorie food intake and minimal physical activity.[57]

Pediatric obesity is not just a cosmetic issue, but is associated with a significant burden of illnesses. Obesity in childhood is linked to obesity in adulthood, and does run in families; this places individuals at increased risk for developing diabetes and cardiac disease in later life. Thus, families should be encouraged to: plan meal times, provide age appropriate and healthy food portions, participate in routine physical activity, and limit sedentary behaviours.[57]

IN SUMMARY

Middle-to-late childhood is defined as that period from beginning school through adolescence. During these 6 years, growth is steady but much slower than in the infancy period. Entry into school begins the formation of relationships with peers and has a major impact on psychological development. This is a wonderful period of relatively good health secondary to an immunologic advantage, but respiratory disease poses a leading cause of illness, and motor vehicle collisions are the major cause of death. Several chronic health problems such as asthma, epilepsy, and childhood cancers may surface during this time.

Overweight and obesity, is becoming an increasingly common problem that begins in childhood. The causes of childhood overweight are undoubtedly multifactorial, but ultimately reflect an imbalance between the amount of calories the child consumes in food and beverages and the calories that the child uses to support growth and development, metabolism, and physical activity.

ADOLESCENCE

After completing this section of the chapter, you should be able to meet the following objectives:

- Characterize the physical and psychosocial changes that occur during adolescence.
- Cite the developmental tasks that adolescents need to fulfill.
- Describe common concerns of parents regarding their adolescent child.
- Discuss how the changes that occur during adolescence can influence the health care needs of the adolescent.

Adolescence is a transitional period between childhood and adulthood. It is a period of physical, emotional, cognitive growth, along with reproductive maturation. The changes of adolescence do not occur on a strict timeline; instead, they occur at different times according to a unique internal calendar. For definition's sake, adolescence is considered to begin with the development of secondary sex characteristics, around 11 or 12 years of age, and to end with the completion of somatic growth from approximately 18 to 21 years of age. Girls usually begin and end adolescence earlier than boys. The adolescent period is conveniently referred to as the *teenaged years.*[58]

ADOLESCENT PERIOD

- The adolescent period, which extends from 13 through 19 years of age, is a time of rapid changes in body size and shape, and physical, psychological, and social functioning.
- Adolescence is a time when hormones and sexual maturation interact with social structures in fostering the transition from childhood to adulthood.
- The developmental tasks of adolescence include achieving independence from parents, adopting peer codes and making personal lifestyle choices, forming or revising individual body image, and coming to terms with one's body image.

Several "tasks" that adolescents need to fulfill have been identified. These tasks include achieving independence from parents, adopting peer codes and making personal lifestyle choices, forming or revising individual body image and coming to terms with one's body image if it is not "perfect," and establishing sexual, ego, vocational, and moral identities.[4]

Growth and Development

Adolescence is influenced by attainment of developmental milestones related to puberty and influences form family, school, and peers. Physical growth occurs simultaneously with sexual maturation.[4,5] Adolescents typically experience gains of 20% to 25% in linear growth. Most of the physical growth occurs in the truncal area. The age at onset, duration, and extent of the growth vary between boys and girls and among individuals. In girls, the growth spurt usually begins around 10 to 14 years of age. It begins earlier in girls than in boys and ends earlier, with less dramatic changes in weight and height. Girls usually gain approximately 5 to 20 cm in height and 7 to 25 kg in weight. Most girls have completed their growth spurt by 16 or 17 years of age. Boys begin their growth spurt later, but it usually is more pronounced, with an increase in height of 10 to 30 cm and an increase in weight of 7 to 30 kg. Most boys continue to gain in height until 18 to 20 years of age but increases in height are possible until approximately 25 years of age.[4,5]

The changes in physical body size have a characteristic pattern. Growth in arms, legs, hands, feet, and neck is followed by increases in hip and chest size and several months later by increases in shoulder width and depth and trunk length.[4] The period of these rapid and dramatic changes may be difficult for the adolescent and parents. Shoe size may change several times over several months. Although brain size is not significantly increased during adolescence, the size and shape of the skull and facial bones change, making the features of the face appear to be out of proportion until full adult growth is attained.[4,5,59] Muscle mass and strength also increase during adolescence. Sometimes, there may be a discrepancy between the growth of bone and muscle mass, creating a temporary dysfunction with slower or less smooth movements resulting from the mismatch of bone and muscle. Body proportions undergo typical changes during adolescence. In boys, the thorax becomes broader, and the pelvis remains narrow. In girls, the opposite occurs: the thorax remains narrow, and the pelvis widens.

Organ systems also undergo changes in function, and some have changes in structure. The heart increases in size as the result of increased muscle cell size. Heart rate decreases to normal adult rates, whereas blood pressure increases rapidly to adult rates. Circulating blood volume and hemoglobin concentration increase. Boys demonstrate greater changes in blood volume and higher hemoglobin concentrations because of the influence of testosterone and their relatively greater muscle mass.[58]

Skin becomes thicker and additional hair growth occurs in both sexes. Sebaceous and sweat gland activity increases. Adrenal androgens stimulate the sebaceous glands, promoting the development of acne. Increased sweat gland activity results in perspiration and body odour. Voice changes are of significant importance during adolescence for both sexes; however, the change is more pronounced in boys.[58] The voice change results from growth of the larynx, pharynx, and lungs.[5] Greater growth occurs in the larynx of boys than in girls. The paranasal sinuses reach adult proportions, which increases the resonance of the voice, adding to the adult sound of the voice.[5,59] Dental changes include jaw growth, loss of the final deciduous teeth, and eruption of the permanent cuspids, premolars, and molars.[4] Orthodontic appliances may be needed.

The endocrine system plays a primary role in the changes throughout adolescence. Triggers that initiate the process are not completely understood. However, the result of adrenal maturation reveals physical changes in the adolescent body, such as the development of pubic and axillary hair, increased oils in the skin and hair, acne, and body odours. Another physiologic process that occurs is maturation of the hypothalamic–pituitary–gonadal axis, which is responsible for increases in circulating gonadal sex steroids.[60] Once gonadal steroid hormones are secreted at an elevated rate, overt signs of puberty are easily identified. In girls, initial signs of puberty can be seen with breast development, followed by pubic hair, and then menses approximately 2 to 2.5 years later, and in conjunction with attainment of peak height. Puberty begins later for boys, with testicular enlargement, followed by penile growth, and then the development of pubic hair.[4] Boys may also experience spontaneous erections or nocturnal seminal emissions, as a normal development of puberty. During this period, both genders will grow 3 to 4 inches over a 2-year period.[4]

In addition to reproduction maturation, changes also occur within the cortical and limbic circuits of the brain. The link between these two processes is that the brain is a target organ for steroid hormones. Essentially, neuroscientists have hypothesized that there exists a "coupling" in adolescent development between the brain and puberty hormones. As cortical and limbic circuits remodel, cognition and decision making processes are further developed, along with social behaviours. Although more research is necessary in order to enhance knowledge regarding this relationship, scientists have raised questions as to what variables and interactions occur between pubertal hormones, brain development, cognition, and behavioural maturation during the adolescent period.[61]

The behavioural and psychosocial changes that occur during adolescence are comparable to the physical changes. It is not possible to develop one guide that adequately describes and explains the tremendous changes that occur during adolescence because the experience is unique for each adolescent. There are, fortunately, some commonalities within the process that can be used to facilitate understanding of these changes. The transition from child to adult is not a smooth, continuous, or uniform process. There are frequent periods of rapid change, followed by brief plateaus. These periods can change with little or no warning, which makes living with an adolescent difficult at times.

There is one thing that persons who deal with adolescents must remember: no matter how rocky the transition from child to adult, adolescence is not a permanent disability. Health care professionals who care for adolescents may need to offer support to worried parents that the difficulties their adolescent is experiencing, and that the entire family is experiencing as a result, may be normal. The adolescent also may need reassurance that his or her feelings are not abnormal.[4,59]

Common concerns of adolescents include conflicts with parents, conflicts with siblings, concerns about school, and concerns about peers and peer relationships. Personal identity is an overwhelming concern expressed by adolescents.

Parents of adolescents also may have concerns about their child. Common concerns related to the adolescent's behaviour include rebelliousness, wasting time, risk-taking behaviours, mood swings, drug experimentation, school problems, psychosomatic complaints, and sexual activity.[4] Adolescence is a period of transition from childhood to adulthood and it is often filled with conflicts as the adolescent attempts to take on an adult role. Open communication between the adolescent and family can help make the transition less stressful; however, communication between parents and adolescents can be difficult.

Common Health Problems

Adolescence is considered to be a relatively healthy period; however, significant morbidity and mortality do occur. Common health problems experienced by adolescents include headaches, eating disorders, weight loss/weight gain and insomnia.[4] These disorders may be psychosomatic in origin. The health care worker may need to refer adolescents for specialized counselling or medical care if any of these health care concerns are exaggerated.

Additional health problems during the adolescent years (discussed below) include injury, suicide, cancer, risky sexual behaviours, adolescent pregnancy, substance abuse, including drug and alcohol abuse, and tobacco use. Health promotion is of extreme importance during the adolescent period.

There are fewer actual physical health problems during the adolescent period, but there is a greater risk of morbidity and mortality from unintentional injuries.[52,54] While the leading cause of adolescent mortality is due to unintentional injuries, the incidence of nonfatal injuries is also prevalent. Nonfatal injuries most often result from being struck by or against an object or person, due to violence, sports-related activities, or motor vehicle accidents.[52,54] Many of the injuries could be prevented with the use of simple safety measures, including automobile seat belts and bicycle and motorcycle helmets.[4]

Several factors contribute to the risk of injury during adolescence. The adolescent often is unable to recognize potentially dangerous situations, possibly because of a discrepancy between physical maturity and cognitive and emotional development. Certain behavioural and developmental characteristics of the adolescent exaggerate this problem. Adolescents typically feel the need to challenge parental or other authority. They also have a strong desire to "fit in" with the peer group. Adolescents exhibit a type of magical thinking and have a need to experiment with potentially dangerous situations or behaviours. They may have a sense of invulnerability, and believe that bad things will not happen to them, despite engaging in risky behaviours.

Another major cause of death in this age group is suicide. Although the number of adolescents reporting suicidal thoughts has decreased in the past decade, the number of suicide attempts has remained constant. Risk factors for suicide in adolescents include substance abuse, personal or family history of depression, problems at school, problems communicating with parents, current legal problems, and family ownership of a handgun. Suicide attempts are often associated with drug or alcohol abuse.

Cancer is the fourth leading cause of death in adolescents, but it is the leading cause of death from nonviolent sources. There is an increased incidence of certain types of cancer during adolescence, including lymphomas (29%), germ cell tumours including testicular or thyroid carcinomas (13%) and leukemias (12%).[55]

The increasing prevalence of sexual activity among adolescents has created unique health problems. These include adolescent pregnancy, sexually transmitted infections, and human immunodeficiency virus (HIV) transmission.[4] Associated problems include substance abuse, such as alcohol, tobacco, inhalants, and other illicit drugs. Health care providers must not neglect discussing sexual activity with the adolescent. Nonjudgmental, open, factual communication is essential for dealing with an adolescent's sexual practices. Discussion of sexual activity frequently is difficult for the adolescent and the adolescent's family. If a relationship exists between the adolescent and the health care provider, this may provide a valuable forum for the adolescent to get accurate information about safe sex, including contraception and avoidance of high-risk behaviours

for acquiring sexually transmitted infections or acquired immunodeficiency syndrome (AIDS).[58]

The number of adolescent pregnancies for Canadian females under the age of 20 was approximately 30,500 in 2005 and since 1996 the trend shows that the more common outcome for these pregnancies is abortion rather than live births. For these pregnancies approximately 45% delivered, 53% had therapeutic abortions and 2% had spontaneous abortions.[62] One fifth of all pregnancies occur within the first month after beginning sexual activity.

Risks for single teenage mothers are associated with lack of supportive networks and cognitive stimulation, socioeconomic difficulties, and decreased rates of high school graduation. Additionally, risks for infants born to young mothers include increased incidence of low birth weight and infant mortality. The topic of adolescent pregnancy involves issues related to physical and biologic maturity of the adolescent, growth requirements of the adolescent and the fetus, and unique prenatal care requirements of the pregnant adolescent. Emotional responses and psychological issues regarding relationships of the adolescent in her family and with the father of the infant, as well as how the pregnancy will affect the adolescent's future, must be considered.

Substance abuse among adolescents increased rapidly during the 1960s and 1970s but has declined since that time. However, substance abuse still is prevalent in the adolescent age group. Health care workers must be knowledgeable about the symptoms of drug abuse, the consequences of drug abuse, and the appropriate management of adolescents with substance abuse problems. Substance abuse among adolescents includes the use of tobacco products, particularly cigarettes and "smokeless" tobacco (*e.g.,* snuff, chewing tobacco, alcohol, marijuana, stimulants, inhalants, cocaine, hallucinogens, tranquilizers, and sedatives.)[4] Adolescents are at high risk for succumbing to the peer pressure to participate in substance abuse. They have a strong desire to fit in and be accepted by their peer group. It is difficult for them to "just say no." Risk-taking behaviours lead adolescents to believe that they will not get "hooked," or that the bad consequences will not happen to them. It is important that adolescents be provided with "the rest of the story" through education and constant communication with parents, teachers, role models, health care providers, and others who may have a positive influence on the adolescent.[4,5]

IN SUMMARY

Adolescence is a transitional period between childhood and adulthood. It begins with development of secondary sex characteristics (11 to 12 years) and ends with cessation of somatic growth (18 to 21 years). This is the period of a major growth spurt, which is more pronounced in boys. The endocrine system is of great importance, with its numerous hormonal changes and their initiation and continuation of the growth spurt. Psychosocial changes are equally dramatic during this period and often place tremendous pressure on relationships between adults and the adolescent. Adolescence is a relatively healthy period, but significant morbidity and mortality exist as a result of injuries, suicide, and homicide. The prevalence of sexual activity and substance abuse places the adolescent at risk for HIV infection; alcohol, tobacco, and other drug abuse; and adolescent pregnancy.

REVIEW EXERCISES

1. The vital signs of a full-term, 1-day-old newborn are temperature 38.5°C (axillary), heart rate 188 beats/minute, respirations 70 breaths/minute, blood pressure 56/36 mm Hg.

   A. *What laboratory test(s) should be performed?*

   B. *What information could be obtained from review of the maternal record that may be helpful in establishing a differential diagnosis for this infant?*

   C. *What other clinical signs should be assessed?*

2. A preterm newborn, approximately 30 weeks' gestation, is admitted to the neonatal intensive care unit. The infant exhibits respiratory distress, including tachypnea, retractions, and expiratory grunting.

   A. *Identify the two most common causes for respiratory distress in such an infant.*

   B. *Explain the etiology for the two causes identified.*

3. A 10-year-old boy is seen in the clinic for a routine physical examination. His weight is 50 kg and his height is 149 cm. His mother complains that he is constantly watching television or playing video games and seems to have no interest in riding his bike or participating in physical sports. Furthermore, he is constantly snacking and drinking sugar-sweetened cola drinks.

   A. *After calculating his BMI, use the World Health Organization (WHO) BMI chart to determine whether or not he is overweight (both the calculator and WHO's BMI charts for children are available online at: http://www.dietitians.ca/ your-health/assess-yourself/assess-your-bmi/ bmi-children.aspx).*

   B. *What suggestions might you provide for this boy and his mother?*

4. An adolescent boy is seen in the health clinic for a routine sports examination. The nurse practitioner notes that the adolescent has a mild to moderate case of facial acne. The nurse practitioner discusses the causes, prevention, and treatment of acne with the young man.

   A. *What physiologic changes contribute to the development of acne in adolescents?*

   B. *What other physical changes also occur during adolescence?*

   C. *What are common health problems in adolescents?*

References

1. Dominion of Canada. (1893). The statistical year-book of Canada for 1892. Available online at: http://www66.statcan.gc.ca/acyb_000-eng.htm. Accessed October 19, 2013.

2. Human Resources and Social Development Canada. (2013). Family life – Infant mortality. Available online at: http://www4.hrsdc.gc.ca/.3ndic.1t.4r@-eng.jsp?iid=2#M_4. Accessed October 19, 2013.

3. Statistics Canada. (2008/2013). Vital statistics: Birth database. Available online at: http://www.statscan.gc.ca. Accessed October 19, 2013.

4. Bowden V. R., Greenberg C. S. (2010). *Children and their families: The continuum of care* (2nd ed.). Philadelphia, PA: Wolters Kluwer Health/ Lippincott Williams & Wilkins.

5. Feigelman S. (2011). Growth, development and behaviour. In Kliegman R. M., Stanton B. F., St. Geme J. W., et al. (Eds.), *Nelson textbook of pediatrics* (19th ed., pp. 26–55). Philadelphia, PA: Elsevier Saunders.

6. Canadian Paediatric Society. (2010). Promoting optimal monitoring of child growth in Canada: Using the new World Health Organization growth charts. Available online at: http://www.cps.ca/en/documents/position/child-growth-charts. Accessed October 24, 2013.

7. WHO Multicentre Growth Reference Study Group. (2009). *WHO Child Growth Standards: Growth velocity based on weight, length and head circumference: Methods and development.* Geneva: World Health Organization. http://www.who.int/childgrowth/standards/velocity/tr3_velocity_report. pdf. Accessed October 19, 2013.

8. World Health Organization. (2011). Child growth standards. Available online at: http://www.who.int/childgrowth/faqs/en. Accessed October 21, 2013.

9. Maalouf-Manasseh Z., Metallinos-Katsaras E., Dewey K. G. (2011). Obesity in preschool children is more prevalent and identified at a younger age when WHO growth charts are used compared with CDC charts. *The Journal of Nutrition, 141*(6), 1154–1158.

10. Mei Z, Grummer-Strawn L. M. (2011). Comparison of changes in growth percentiles of US children on CDC 2000 growth charts with corresponding changes on WHO 2006 growth charts. *Clinical Pediatrics, 50,* 402–407.

11. Moore K. L., Persaud T. V. N. (2008). *The developing human: Clinically oriented embryology* (8th ed.). Philadelphia, PA: W.B. Saunders.

12. Lott J. W. (2007). Fetal development: Environmental influences and critical periods. In Kerner C., Lott J. W. (Eds.), *Comprehensive neonatal care: An interdisciplinary approach* (4th ed., pp. 625–647). Philadelphia, PA: Elsevier Saunders.

13. Sadler T. (2010). *Langman's medical embryology* (11th ed.). Philadelphia, PA: Lippincott Williams & Wilkins.

14. Bowers B. (2007). Prenatal, antenatal, and postnatal risk factors. In Kenner C., Lott J. W. (Eds.), *Comprehensive neonatal nursing: A physiologic perspective* (4th ed., pp. 648–665). Philadelphia, PA: Elsevier Saunders.

15. Sansoucie D. A., Calvaliere T. A. (2007). Newborn and infant assessment. In Kenner C., Lott J. W. (Eds.), *Comprehensive neonatal nursing: A physiologic perspective* (4th ed., pp. 677–718). Philadelphia, PA: Elsevier Saunders.

16. Zhang J., Merialdi M., Platt L. D., Kramer M. S. (2010). Defining normal and abnormal fetal growth: Promises and challenges. *American Journal of Obstetrics and Gynecology, 202*(6), 522–528.

17. Lubchenco L. O., Hansman C., Dressler M., Boyd E. (1963). Intrauterine growth as estimated from liveborn birthweight data at 24 to 42 weeks of gestation. *Pediatrics 32,* 793–800.

18. Kramer M. S., Platt R. W., Wen S. W., et al.; Fetal/Infant Health Study Group of the Canadian Perinatal Surveillance System. (2001). A new improved population-based Canadian reference for birth weight for gestational age. *Pediatrics. 108*(2), E35.

19. Das U. G., Sysyn G. D. (2004). Abnormal fetal growth: Intrauterine growth retardation, small for gestational age, large for gestational age. *Pediatric Clinics of North America, 51,* 639–654.

20. Caughey R. W., Michels K. B. (2009). Birth weight and childhood leukemia: A meta-analysis and review of the current evidence. *Int. J. Cancer, 124,* 2658–2670.

21. Pillitteri A. (2010). *Maternal & child health nursing: Care of the childbearing & child rearing family* (6th ed). Philadelphia, PA: Lippincott Williams & Wilkins.

22. Dubowitz L. M., Dubowitz V., Goldberg C. (1970). Clinical assessment of gestational age in the newborn infant. *Journal of Pediatrics, 77,* 1–10.

23. Ballard J. L., Khoury J. C., Wedig K., et al. (1991). New Ballard score, expanded to include extremely premature infants. *Journal of Pediatrics, 119*, 417–423.

24. Moore K. L., Dalley A. (2006). *Clinically oriented anatomy* (5th ed., pp. 904–905). Philadelphia, PA: Lippincott Williams & Wilkins.

25. Blackburn S. (2006). Placental, fetal, and transitional circulation revisited. *Journal of Perinatal & Neonatal Nursing, 20*(4), 290–294.

26. Soll R. (2008). Heat loss prevention neonates. *Journal of Perinatology, 28*, S57–S59.

27. Thilo E. H., Rosenberg A. A. (2011). The newborn infant. In Hay W. W., Hayward A. R., Levin M., et al., (Eds.), *Current pediatric diagnosis and treatment* (21st ed., pp. 9–72) New York: McGraw-Hill Medical.

28. Deoni S. C., Mercure E., Blasi A., et al. (2011). Mapping infant brain myelination with magnetic resonance imaging. *The Journal of Neuroscience, 31*(2), 784–791.

29. Erikson E. (1963). *Childhood and society.* New York: W.W. Norton.

30. Apgar V. (1953). A proposal for a new method of evaluation of the newborn infant. *Current Research in Anesthesia and Analgesia 32*, 260–267.

31. Sperling M. A. (2011). Hypoglycemia. In Kliegman R. M., Stanton B. F., St. Geme J. W., et al., (Eds.), *Nelson textbook of pediatrics* (19th ed., pp. 517–531). Philadelphia, PA: Saunders Elsevier.

32. Cohen S. M. (2006). Jaundice in the full-term newborn. *Pediatric Nursing, 32*, 202–208.

33. Canadian Paediatric Society. (2007). Guidelines for detection, management and prevention of hyperbilirubinemia in term and late preterm newborn infants (35 or more weeks' gestation). *Paediatric and Child Health, 12*(Suppl B), 1B–10B.

34. Maheshwari A., Carlo W. A. (2011). Digestive systems disorders. In Kliegman R. M., Stanton B. F., St. Geme J. W., et al. (Eds.), *Nelson textbook of pediatrics* (19th ed., pp. 600–611). Philadelphia, PA: Saunders Elsevier.

35. Pressler J. L. (2008). Classification of major newborn birth injuries. *Journal of Perinatal & Neonatal Nursing, 22*(1), 60–67.

36. Carlo W. A. (2011). The fetus and neonatal infant. In Kliegman R. M., Stanton B. F., St. Geme J. W., et al. (Eds.), *Nelson textbook of pediatrics* (19th ed., pp. 532–648). Philadelphia, PA: Elsevier Saunders.

37. Gowen C. W. (2011). Fetal and neonatal medicine. In Marcdante K. J., Kliegman R. M., Jenson H. B., et al. (Eds.), *Nelson essentials of pediatrics* (6th ed., pp. 213–263). Philadelphia, PA: Elsevier Saunders.

38. Blackburn S. T., Ditzenberger G. R. (2003). Neurologic system. In Kenner C., Lott J. W. (Eds.), *Comprehensive neonatal nursing: A multidisciplinary approach* (4th ed., pp. 624–660). Philadelphia, PA: Elsevier Saunders.

39. Carlo W. A. (2011). Respiratory tract disorders. In Kliegman R. M., Stanton B. F., St. Geme J. W. et al. (Eds.), *Nelson textbook of pediatrics* (19th ed., pp. 579–599). Philadelphia, PA: Elsevier Saunders.

40. Carlo W. A. (2011). Nervous system disorders. In Kliegman R. M., Stanton B. F., St. Geme J. W. et al., (Eds.), *Nelson textbook of pediatrics* (19th ed., pp. 565–574). Philadelphia, PA: Elsevier Saunders.

41. Neu. J., Walker W. A. (2011). Necrotizing enterocolitis. *The New England Journal of Medicine, 364*(3), 255–264.

42. Stoll B. J. (2011). Infections of the neonatal infant. In Kliegman R. M., Stanton B. F., St. Geme J. W., et al. (Eds.), *Nelson textbook of pediatrics* (19th ed., pp. 629–648). Philadelphia, PA: Elsevier Saunders.

43. Stoll B. J., Hansen N. I., Sánchez P. J., et al. (2011). Early onset neonatal sepsis: The burden of group B streptococcal and E. coli disease continues. *Pediatrics, 127*(5), 817–826.

44. Money D., Allen V. M. (2013). The prevention of early-onset neonatal group B streptococcal disease. *Journal of obstetrics and gynaecology Canada, 35*, 939–948.

45. Critch J. N. (2013). Nutrition for healthy term infants, birth to six months: An overview. *Paediatrics and Child Health, 18*(4), 206–207.

46. Goldson E., Reynolds A. (2012). Child development and behavior. In Hay W., Levin M., Deterding R. R., et al. (Eds.), *Current Diagnosis and Treatment Pediatrics* (21st ed., pp. 73–112).New York: McGraw Hill.

47. Gahagan S. (2011). Behavioral disorders. In Marcdante K. J., Kliegman R. M., Jenson H. B., et al. (Eds.), *Nelson essentials of pediatrics* (6th ed., pp. 45–61). Philadelphia, PA: Elsevier Saunders.

48. McLean H. S., Price D. T. (2011). Failure to thrive. In Kliegman R. M., Stanton B. F., St. Geme J. W., et al. (Eds.), *Nelson textbook of pediatrics* (19th ed., pp. 147–149). Philadelphia, PA: Elsevier Saunders.

49. Centers for Disease Control and Prevention (CDC). (2012). Sudden Unexpected Infant Death and Sudden Infant Death Syndrome. Available online at: http://www.cdc.gov/sids/index.htm. Accessed October 24, 2013.

50. Hunt C. F., Hauck F. R. (2011). Sudden infant death syndrome. In Kliegman R. M., Stanton B. F., St. Geme J. W., et al. (Eds.), *Nelson textbook of pediatrics* (19th ed., pp. 1421–1428). Philadelphia, PA: Elsevier Saunders.

51. Canadian Paediatric Society. (2004). Recommendations for safe sleeping environments for infants and children: Reaffirmed 2013. *Paediatric and Child Health, 9*(9), 659–663.

52. Statistics Canada. (2013). Ranking and number of deaths for the 10 leading causes of death by age group, Canada, 2009.Available online at: http://www.statcan.gc.ca/pub/84-215-x/2012001/table-tableau/tbl003-eng.htm. Accessed October 24, 2013.

53. Sinha M. (2012). Family violence in Canada: A statistical profile, 2010. Statistics Canada, No. 85-002-X.

54. Yanchar N. L., Wards L. J., Fuselli P., et al. (2012). Child and youth injury prevention: A public health approach. Available online at: http://www.cps.ca/documents/position/child-and-youth-injury-prevention. Accessed October 24, 2013.

55. Public Health Agency of Canada (PHAC). (2013). The cancer in young people in Canada program. Available online at: http://www.phac-aspc.gc.ca/cd-mc/cancer/fs-fi/cancer-adol. Accessed October 24, 2013.

56. Roberts K. C., Sheilds M., de Groh M., et al. (2012). *Overweight and obesity in children and adolescents: Results from the 2009 to 2011 Canadian Health Measure Survey.* Statistics Canada, No. 82-003-X Health Reports.

57. Krebs N. F., Primak L. E. (2011). Pediatric nutrition and nutritional disorders. In Marcdante K. J., Kliegman R. M., Jenson H. B., et al. (Eds.), *Nelson essentials of pediatrics* (6th ed, pp. 109–111). Philadelphia, PA: Elsevier Saunders.

58. Blake K., Davis V. (2011). Adolescent medicine. In Marcdante K. J., Kliegman R. M., Jenson H. B., et al. (Eds.), *Nelson essentials of pediatrics* (6th ed, pp. 265–283). Philadephia, PA: Elsevier Saunders.

59. Ball J. W., Bindler R. C., Cowen K. J. (2012). *Principles of pediatric nursing: Caring for children.* Upper Saddle River, NJ: Pearson.

60. Jospe N. (2011). Endocrinology. In Marcdante K. J., Kliegman R. M., Jenson H. B., et al. (Eds.)., *Nelson essentials of pediatrics* (6th ed, pp. 625–669). Philadelphia, PA: Elsevier Saunders.

61. Sisk C. L., Zehr J. L. (2005). Pubertal hormones organize the adolescent brain and behavior. *Frontiers in Neuroendocrinology, 26*, 163–174.

62. Statistics Canada. (2008). Pregnancy outcomes, 2005. No. 82-224-X.

Concepts of Altered Health in Older Adults

Old age is not a disease—it is strength and survivorship, triumph over all kinds of vicissitudes and disappointments, trials and illnesses.

—MAGGIE KUHN

Aging is a natural, lifelong process that brings with it unique biopsychosocial changes. For many older adults there are changes in bodily function, physical appearance, cognitive abilities, family structure, and social environment. *Gerontology* is the discipline that studies aging and the aged from biologic, psychological, and sociologic perspectives. It explores the dynamic processes of complex physical changes, adjustments in psychological functioning, and alterations in social identities.

An important first distinction is that aging and disease are not synonymous. Unfortunately, a common assumption is that growing older is inevitably accompanied by illness, disability, and overall decline in function. The fact is that the aging body can accomplish most, if not all, of the functions of its youth; the difference is that they may take longer, require greater motivation, and be less precise. But as in youth, maintenance of physiologic function is facilitated through continued use.

THE OLDER ADULT AND THEORIES OF AGING

After completing this section of the chapter, you should be able to meet the following objectives:

* State a definition for young-old, middle-old, and old-old, and characterize the changing trend in the elderly population.
* Discuss theories of biologic aging.

Who Are Older Adults?

The older adult population is typically defined in chronologic terms and includes individuals 65 years of age and older. This age was chosen somewhat arbitrarily. In the initial rudimentary legislation of 1927 some funds were provided to persons over the age of 70, but real change was initiated by the Report on Social Security for Canada in 1943 (the Marsh Report) that designated 65 years as the pensionable age. Ultimately most of Dr. Marsh's recommendations were law by 1966, and since then, the expression *old age* has been understood to apply to anyone older than 65 years. Because there is considerable heterogeneity among this group, older adults often are subgrouped into young-old (65 to 74 years), middle-old (75 to 84 years), and old-old (85+ years) to reflect more accurately the changes in function that occur. Age parameters, however, are somewhat irrelevant because chronologic age is a poor predictor of biologic function. However, chronologic age does help to quantify the number of individuals in a group and allows predictions to be made for the future.

In 2011, nearly 14.8% of the total Canadian population (4.94 million) was 65 years of age or older. In addition, the older adult population itself is getting older with the number of centenarians up 25.7% in the last 5 years. Average life expectancy has increased as a result of overall advances in health care technology, improved nutrition, and improved sanitation. The entire population of older adults is expected to grow to about 9.2 million or 23% of the total population by the year 2041 (Fig. 3.1). Women who are now 65 years of age can expect to live an additional 18.5 years (83.3 years of age), and men an additional 18.5 years (78.8 years of age).[1-4]

Women tend to outlive men throughout the aging process and make up the majority of the senior population. In 2010, 56% of the Canadian seniors over the age of 65 were women, and their proportion increases with age to account for 63% of the over 80 years group and to 80% for centenarians. Marital status also changes with advancing age. Almost one third of all older women living in the community are widowed, and there are up to four times as many widows as widowers.[3]

Among Canadian seniors 12.0% had active employment but most were retired.[4] Retirement represents a significant role change for older adults. Attitudes and adjustment to retirement are influenced by preretirement lifestyles and values. Individuals with leisure pursuits during their work life seem to adjust better to retirement than those whose lives were dominated by work. For many of today's cohort of older adults, especially the old-old, the work ethic of the Great Depression remains profoundly ingrained as the central purpose in life. When work is gone, a significant loss is felt, and something must be substituted in its place. Because leisure has not always been a highly valued activity, older adults may have difficulty learning to engage in meaningful leisure pursuits.

Loss of productive work is just one of many losses that can accompany the aging process. Loss of a spouse is a highly significant life event that commonly has negative implications for the survivor. Experts cite an increased mortality rate among recently bereaved older adults (especially men); an increased incidence of depression, psychological distress, and loneliness; and higher rates of chronic illness. Loss of physical health and loss of independence are other changes that can affect the psychosocial aspects of aging, as can relocation, loss of friends and relatives, and changes in the family structure.

Poverty is common among the elderly population and the rates vary among elderly subgroups. In 2006, 5.4% of those 65 years of age and older lived below the low income cut-off (LICO) line. The main sources of income for older persons were universal Old Age Security program, Canada/Quebec Pension Plans, income from assets, public and private pensions (30%), and earnings (23%).[1,2]

Contrary to popular belief, the majority of older adults live in community settings. Most live in some type of family setting, with a spouse, their children, or other relatives, and

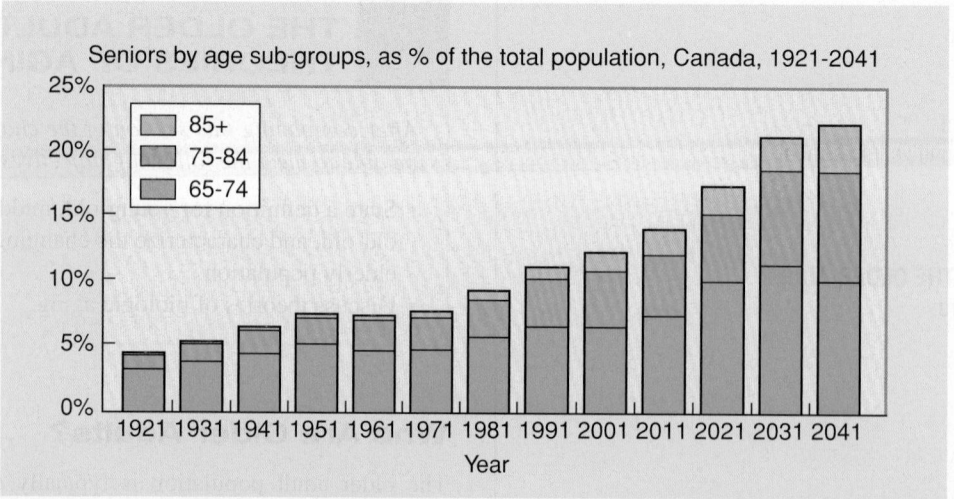

FIGURE 3.1 • Percentage of seniors in Canada comparing 1921 to the anticipated growth in 2041. Projections of people 65–74, 75–84 and 85 years of age and older as a percentage of the total Canadian population. (Source: Canada's Aging Population, Public Health Agency of Canada (2002) © Adapted and Reproduced with the permission of the Minister of Public Works and Government Services Canada, 2009.)

approximately 30% live alone. Only 2.4% of all individuals 65 years of age and older reside in health care facilities. However, this number increases close to 10% for persons 80 years of age or older.[1–3]

Older adults are the largest consumers of health care in 2010. Eighty percent of older adults reported having at least one long-term health condition. Mobility related disabilities account for 33% and approximately one sixth had difficulties with activities of daily living (ADLs). Almost half of all adult hospital beds are filled with patients 65 years of age and older.[3,4]

Theories of Aging

Multiple theories have attempted to explain the biology of aging through a variety of scientific observations at the molecular, cellular, organ, and system levels. In general, these theories can be divided into either intrinsic (developmental-genetic) or extrinsic (stochastic) theories. *Developmental-genetic theories* propose that the changes that occur with aging are genetically programmed, whereas *stochastic theories* maintain that the changes result from an accumulation of random events or damage from environmental agents or influences.[5] In reality, evidence suggests that the process of aging and longevity is multifaceted, with both genetics and environmental factors playing a role. In humans, a very long life, to beyond 90 years of age, appears to have a stronger genetic basis, which explains why centenarians and near-centenarians tend to cluster in families.[6]

OLDER ADULT

- The older population, which is subgrouped into the young-old (65 to 74 years), the middle-old (75 to 84 years), and the old-old (85+ years), has increased during the past century and is expected to continue to grow as the result of overall advances in health care technology, improved nutrition, and improved sanitation.
- As the result of increased years, many older adults are confronted with retirement, changes in lifestyle, loss of significant others, and a decline in physical functioning, but despite that a vast majority live in the community with only 4% residing in health care facilities.
- Older adults are the largest consumers of health care, requiring ongoing chronic disease management.

Developmental-Genetic Theories

The developmental-genetic theories focus on the genetic influences that determine physical condition, occurrence of disease, age of death, cause of death, and other factors contributing to longevity.[5,6] The Hayflick limit theory is based on the cellular biology work of Hayflick and Moorhead who observed more than 40 years ago that cultured human fibroblasts had a limited ability to replicate (approximately 50 population doublings) and then died.[7] Before achieving this maximum, these cells slowed their rate of division and manifested identifiable and predictable morphologic changes characteristic of senescent cells.

Another explanation of cellular aging resides with an enzyme called *telomerase* that is believed to govern chromosomal aging through its action on telomeres, the outermost extremities of the chromosome arms. With each cell division, a small segment of telomeric deoxyribonucleic acid (DNA) is lost, unless a cell has a constant supply of telomerase. In the absence of telomerase, the telomeres shorten, resulting in senescence-associated gene expression and inhibition of cell replication. It is thought that in certain cells, such as cancer cells, telomerase maintains telomere length, thereby enhancing cell replication.[8]

However, many genes that are associated with human life span are not "longevity genes," per se. For example, because mutations in the tumour suppressor genes *BRAC1* and *BRAC2* increase mortality rates associated with breast and ovarian cancer, they are rare among long-lived women.[9] Conversely, genes that reduce the risk of atherosclerosis may be more common in long-lived individuals. Genetic studies of biologic aging have explored the involvement of allelic variants in genes encoding apolipoproteins, in particular, that of apolipoprotein E (apoE). The presence of apoE4 is associated with an increased incidence of cardiovascular diseases and neurodegenerative diseases, thereby shortening life span through disease processes.[10]

Stochastic Theories

The stochastic theories propose that aging is caused by random damage to vital cell molecules (*e.g.,* mitochondrial DNA damage, oxygen radical accumulation, nuclear DNA cross-linking). The damage eventually accumulates to a level sufficient to result in the physiologic decline associated with aging.

The somatic mutation theory of aging states that the longevity and function of cells in various tissues of the body are determined by the double-stranded DNA molecule and its specific repair enzymes. DNA undergoes continuous change in response both to exogenous agents and intrinsic processes. Aging may result from conditions that produce mutations in DNA or deficits in DNA repair mechanisms.[11]

The oxidative free radical theory is another stochastic idea in which aging is thought to result partially from oxidative metabolism and the effects of free radical damage (see Chapter 5). The major byproducts of oxidative metabolism include superoxides that react with DNA, ribonucleic acid, proteins, and lipids, leading to cellular damage and aging.[5]

Another damage theory, the wear-and-tear theory, proposes that accumulated damage to vital parts of the cell leads to aging and death. Cellular DNA is cited as an example. If repair to damaged DNA is incomplete or defective, as is thought to be the case with aging, declines in cellular function might occur.[5,6]

IN SUMMARY

Aging is a natural, lifelong process that brings with it unique biopsychosocial changes. Aging is not synonymous with disease or ill health. The aging body can accomplish most or all of the functions of its youth, although they may take longer, require greater motivation, and be less precise.

The older adult population is typically defined in chronologic terms as individuals 65 years of age and older, and can be further defined as young-old (65 to 74 years), middle-old (75 to 84 years), and old-old (85+ years). The number of older persons has increased and is expected to continue to grow in the future, with an anticipated 9.2 million Canadians—23% of the population—older than 65 years of age by the year 2041.

There are two main types of theories used to explain the biologic changes that occur with aging: developmental-genetic theories, which propose that aging changes are genetically programmed, and stochastic theories, which maintain that aging changes result from an accumulation of random events or damage from environmental hazards.

PHYSIOLOGIC CHANGES OF AGING

After completing this section of the chapter, you should be able to meet the following objectives:

- Describe common skin changes that occur with aging.
- Explain how muscle changes that occur with aging affect high-speed performance and endurance.
- Describe the process of bone loss that occurs with aging.
- State the common changes in blood pressure regulation that occur with aging.
- List the changes in respiratory function that occur with aging.
- Relate aging changes in neural function to the overall function of the body.
- Briefly discuss the effects of aging on vision, hearing, taste, and smell.
- Describe changes that occur in the gastrointestinal tract with aging.
- State the significance of decreased lean body mass on interpretation of the glomerular filtration rate using serum creatinine levels.

The physiologic changes seen in the elderly reflect not only the aging process, but also the effects of years of exposure to environmental agents such as sunlight and cigarette smoke, and disease processes such as diabetes mellitus or arthritis. Overall, there is a general decline in the structure and function of the body with advancing age (Fig. 3.2). The decline results in a decreased reserve capacity of the various organ systems that consequently produce reduced homeostatic capabilities, making the older adult more vulnerable to stressors such as illness, trauma, surgery, medications, and environmental changes.

Research to identify true age-related changes as opposed to disease states is difficult. Studies using cross-sectional methodologies are the easiest to perform; however, mortality can confound the results. Although longitudinal studies tend to be more precise, they require years to perform and may not be able to account for numerous variables that enter into the aging equation, such as environment, occupation, and diet. However, it is important to differentiate, as much as possible, those changes that occur in the body as a result of aging from those that occur due to disease. This distinction allows for more accurate diagnosis and treatment of disease conditions and helps to avoid inappropriate labelling of aging changes.

Regardless of the difficulty in defining normal aging as it relates to the various organ systems, there is a pattern of gradual loss that occurs. Many of these losses begin in early adulthood, but because of the large physiologic reserve of most organ systems, the decrement does not become functionally significant until the loss reaches a certain level. Some changes, such as those that affect the skin and posture, are more visible, whereas others, such as those affecting the kidney, may go unnoticed until the person is challenged with situations such as eliminating medications.

Integumentary Changes

Changes in the skin more obviously reflect the aging process than do changes in other organ systems (see Chapter 61). Aging can impinge on the primary functions of the skin: protection from the environment, temperature regulation, fluid and electrolyte balance, sensory function, and excretion of metabolic wastes. Exposure to sunlight and harsh weather accelerates aging of the skin.

With aging, the skin becomes wrinkled and dry and develops uneven pigmentation. The thickness of the dermis, or middle layer of skin, decreases by approximately 20%, which gives the skin an overall thin and transparent quality. This is especially true for areas exposed to sunlight. Dermal collagen fibres rearrange and degenerate, resulting in decreased skin strength and elasticity.[11,12] Cellularity and vascularity of the dermis decrease with advancing age and can cause vascular fragility, leading to senile purpura (*i.e.*, skin hemorrhages) and slow skin healing. Delayed wound healing may be influenced by other factors such as poor nutrition and circulation and by changes in immune function.[13] The function of the sebaceous glands diminishes with age and leads to a decrease in sebum secretion. The decrease in size, number, and activity of the eccrine sweat glands causes a decrease in their capacity to produce sweat. Fingernails and toenails become dull, brittle, and thick, mostly as a result of decreased vascularity of the nail beds.[11–13]

Neuromuscular function
- Loss of neurons, atrophy of neuronal dendrites, impaired synaptic connections
- Declined motor strength, slowed reaction time, diminished reflexes
- Decrease in proprioceptor function that controls balance

Cardiovascular function
- Increased stiffness of blood vessels
- Decreased responsiveness to catecholamines
- Decrease in exercise heart rate
- Decrease in diastolic ventricular relaxation

Immune function
- Altered function of helper T cells
- Diminished immune response

Stature and musculoskeletal changes
- Decrease in height
- Loss of bone mass
- Decrease in muscle strength
- Skeletal bone loss

Integumentary function
- Thin, dry skin
- Decreased sebum and sweat
- Thick and brittle nails
- Sparse, grey hair

Special senses
- Decline in visual acuity
- Hearing loss
- Decline in smell

Respiratory function
- Decrease in $\dot{V}O_2$max
- Progressive loss of elastic recoil in lungs and chest wall
- Decrease in PO_2

Gastrointestinal function
- Dental problems
- Dry mouth
- Mucosal atrophy
- Constipation

Renal function
- Decrease in functional glomeruli
- Decline in renal blood flow
- Decreased glomerular filtration rate
- Decreased urine concentration ability

Genitourinary function
- Decreased bladder capacity, incomplete emptying
- Increased incidence of incontinence
- Decreased serum testosterone levels in men
- Increased vaginal dryness in women
- Decreased sexual response

FIGURE 3.2 • Clinical manifestations of aging.

Age-related changes in hair occur as well. Owing to a decline in melanin production by the hair follicle, approximately one half of the population older than 50 years of age has at least 50% grey hair, regardless of sex or original hair colour. Changes in hair growth and distribution also are seen.[12,14] Hair on the scalp, axillae, and pubis becomes more sparse, and the hairs of the ears and nostril coarsen. Skin disorders are common among the older adult population and can include skin cancers, keratoses (*i.e.,* warty lesions), xerosis (*i.e.,* excessive dryness), dermatitis, and pruritus (*i.e.,* generalized itching).[15]

Stature and Musculoskeletal Function

Aging is accompanied by a progressive decline in height, especially among older women. This decline in height is attributed mainly to compression of the vertebral column.[16] Body composition changes as well. The amount of fat increases, and lean body mass and total body water decrease with advancing age.

With aging, there is a reduction in muscle size and strength that is related to a loss of muscle fibres and a reduction in the size of the existing fibres. Although the decline in strength that occurs with aging cannot be halted, its progress can be slowed with exercise. There is a decline in high-speed performance and reaction time because of a decrease in type II muscle fibres.[17] Impairments in the nervous system also can cause movements to slow. However, type I muscle fibres, which offer endurance, are thought to remain consistent with age (see Chapter 11).

Numerous studies have reported a loss of bone mass with aging, regardless of sex, race, or body size (see Chapter 58). With aging, the process of bone formation (*i.e.,* renewal) is slowed in relation to bone resorption (*i.e.,* breakdown), resulting in a loss of bone mass and weakened bone structure. Between 30 and 35 years of age both men and women start to lose bone mass at the same rate but following menopause women accelerate this bone loss due to the decrease in estrogen production.[18] This process becomes pathologic (*i.e.,* osteoporosis) when it significantly increases the predisposition to fracture and associated complications (see Chapter 58).

The prevalence of joint disease is increased among the elderly. By age 65 years, 80% of the population has some articular disease. Osteoarthritis is so common among the elderly that it is often incorrectly assumed to be a normal age-related change rather than a disease. The synovial joints ultimately are affected by osteoarthritis, most commonly the joints of the hands, feet, knees, hips, and shoulders. It is characterized by cartilage loss and new bone formation, accounting for a distortion in articulation, limited range of motion, and joint instability (see Chapter 59).[17,18] Age is the single greatest risk factor for development of osteoarthritis, in part because of the mechanical impact on joints over time, but it also is related to injury, altered physical condition of the articular cartilage, obesity (*e.g.,* knee), congenital deformity (*e.g.,* hip), crystal deposition in articular cartilage (*e.g.,* knee), and heredity. Pain, immobility, and joint inflammation often ensue. Treatment is aimed at minimizing risk factors, weight loss if indicated, exercise to increase muscle strength, and pain relief measures.

Cardiovascular Function

Cardiovascular disease remains the leading cause of morbidity and mortality in older adults. It often is difficult to separate true age-related changes in the cardiovascular system from disease processes. The aorta and arteries tend to become stiffer and less distensible with age, the heart becomes less responsive to the catecholamines, the maximal exercise heart rate declines, and there is a decreased rate of left ventricular diastolic relaxation.

Blood Pressure

The relationship between blood pressure and risk of cardiovascular disease is continuous, consistent, and independent of other risk factors. Numerous studies have shown that systolic blood pressure progressively increases with age, whereas increases in diastolic blood pressure tend to plateau and even

decline after age 50.[11,19] As a result, there is a sharp increase in what is known as *systolic hypertension* among older adults, which occurs as a consequence of increased arterial stiffness (see Chapter 23).[20]

An elevation in systolic blood pressure accompanied by a normotensive diastolic pressure causes a dramatic increase in pulse pressure. This is a known prognostic indicator for future coronary events. Thus aggressive treatment of systolic hypertension is recommended and has been shown to demonstrate a reduction in stroke, heart failure, kidney disease, and other complications.[20,21] Individuals who are normotensive at 55 years of age have a 90% lifetime risk for development of hypertension. There is now a push to intervene when individuals are prehypertensive (*i.e.,* systolic blood pressure of 120 to 139 mm Hg or diastolic blood pressure of 80 to 89 mm Hg) with lifestyle modification strategies to prevent hypertension.[22]

Orthostatic hypotension, or a significant drop in systolic pressure on assumption of the upright position, is more common among the elderly (see Chapter 23). Compensatory cardiovascular mechanisms often are delayed or insufficient, so that a drop in blood pressure due to position change or consumption of a meal is also common. Even in the absence of orthostatic hypotension, the elderly respond to postural stress with diminished changes in heart rate and diastolic pressure. This altered response to orthostatic stress is thought to result from changes in autonomic nervous system function, inadequate functioning of the circulatory system, or both.[23]

Cardiac Function

Multiple factors determine the effect of aging on cardiac function in healthy older adults. With aging, there is an increase in left ventricular wall thickness; a delay in early left ventricular filling; a decrease in responsiveness to β-adrenergic stimulation and circulating catecholamines; a decrease in the maximal heart rate and maximal cardiac output; and an increase in systemic vascular resistance and left ventricular afterload. The afterload (*i.e.,* opposition to left ventricular ejection) rises steadily with age as the ascending aorta becomes more rigid and the resistance in peripheral arterial vessels increases.[19] Although the overall size of the heart does not increase, the thickness of the left ventricular wall may increase with age, in part responding to the increased afterload that develops because of blood vessel changes.[20]

Both left ventricular diastolic and systolic function are affected by aging. Although early diastolic filling decreases by approximately 50% between 20 and 80 years of age, more filling occurs in late diastole, in part because of more vigorous atrial contraction.[19] The augmented atrial contraction is accompanied by atrial hypertrophy and enlargement. Despite a decrease in the age-associated changes in the diastolic filling pattern in older persons, their left ventricular end-diastolic volume in the supine position does not substantially differ from that of younger persons.[19] However, it is reduced to a lesser extent in older persons than in younger persons during postural change (moving from the supine to seated position) and during graded upright exercise. Furthermore, the maximum left ventricular ejection fraction (*i.e.,* percentage of the left ventricular end-diastolic volume that is ejected during systole) that can be achieved during maximal exercise decreases with age—in this case because of a lesser decrease in left ventricular end-systolic volume. An age-associated decline in myocardial contractility is thought to contribute to this defect in end-systolic volume regulation.

The supine resting heart rate remains unchanged or decreases only slightly with age; however, the maximum heart rate that can be achieved during maximal exercise is decreased.[19] The reduction in heart rate contributes to the decrease in maximum cardiac output reserve in healthy older adults. Also the changes with the conduction system such as fibrosis of the sinoatrial node, reduction in number of sinus node pacemaker cells, or calcification of surrounding cardiac muscle or vessels can lead to conduction abnormalities.[24]

Despite aging changes and cardiovascular disease, overall cardiovascular function at rest in most healthy elderly persons is considered adequate to meet the body's needs. Cardiac output is essentially maintained in healthy older adults (men more than women) during exercise despite the decreased heart rate response, apparently because of a greater stroke volume resulting from increased end-diastolic volume during exercise.[24,25]

Respiratory Function

As lung function changes with age, it often is difficult to differentiate the effects of age from those of environmental and disease factors. Maximal oxygen consumption ($\dot{V}O_2$ max), a measure used to determine overall cardiopulmonary function, declines with age. Numerous studies have indicated that $\dot{V}O_2$ max can improve significantly with exercise and that the $\dot{V}O_2$ max of older adult master athletes can match that of their younger counterparts.

A progressive loss of elastic recoil in the lung is not caused by changes in the amount of elastin and changes in the composition of collagen fibres; rather, the decrease in surface tension increases the size of alveoli creating the loss of elastic recoil. Calcification of the soft tissues of the chest wall causes increased stiffness and thus increases the workload of the respiratory muscles. There is a loss of alveolar structure that decreases the surface area for gas exchange. Although the total lung capacity remains constant, the consequences of these changes result in an increased residual lung volume, increased functional reserve capacity, and a decline in vital capacity. There is a linear decrease in arterial oxygen tension (PO_2) of approximately 20 mm Hg from 20 to 70 years of age. This is thought to result primarily from the decrease in diffusion and the ventilation-perfusion mismatching of the aging lung.[26]

Neurologic Function

Changes at the structural, chemical, and functional levels of the nervous system occur with normal aging, but overall they do not interfere with day-to-day activities unless specific neurologic diseases come into play. The weight of the brain decreases with age, and there is a loss of neurons in the brain and spinal cord. Neuron loss is most pronounced in the cerebral cortex, especially in the superior temporal area. Additional changes take place in the neurons and supporting cells. Atrophy of the neuronal dendrites results in impaired synaptic connections, diminished electrochemical reactions, and neural dysfunction. Synaptic transmissions also are affected by changes in the chemical neurotransmitters dopamine, acetylcholine, and serotonin. As a result, many neural processes slow. Lipofuscin deposits (*i.e.,* yellow, insoluble intracellular material) are found in greater amounts in the aged brain.[25,27]

Sensorimotor changes show a decline in motor strength, slowed reaction time, diminished reflexes (especially in the ankles), and proprioception changes. These changes can cause the balance problems and slower, more deliberate movements that are frequently seen in older individuals.[28]

Even though changes in the brain are associated with aging, overall cognitive abilities remain intact. Although language skills and attention are not altered with advanced age, performance and constructional task abilities can decline, as can short-term memory and immediate recall. A change in personality or significant cognitive deficits is considered unusual with normal aging, and if either occurs, evaluation is in order. Dementia or depression can frequently be the cause.

Special Sensory Function

Sensory changes with aging can greatly affect the older adult's level of functioning and quality of life. Vision and hearing impairments due to disease states, for example, can interfere with communication and may lead to social isolation and depression.

Vision

There is a general decline in visual acuity with age, and nearly all individuals older than 55 years of age require vision correction for reading or distance. The decline occurs as a result of a smaller pupil diameter, loss of refractive power of the lens, and an increase in the scattering of light. The most common visual problem among older adults is presbyopia, or difficulty focusing on near objects. It is caused mainly by decreased elasticity of the lens and atrophy of the ciliary muscle (see Chapter 54).

Glare and abrupt changes in light pose particular problems for older adults. Both are reasons why the elderly frequently give up night driving; they also increase the risk of falls and injury. Colour discrimination changes also take place with aging. In particular, older adults have more difficulty identifying blues and greens. This is thought to be related to problems associated with filtering short wavelengths of light (*i.e.,* violet, blue, green) through a yellowed, opaque lens. Corneal sensitivity also may diminish with age, so that older adults may be less aware of injury or infection.[29]

Ophthalmologic diseases and disorders are common in the elderly. Cataracts, glaucoma, and macular degeneration are frequently seen and can greatly impair vision and function.

Both medical and surgical interventions can restore or improve vision problems that occur as a result of disease states of the eye. Low-vision aids, such as special magnifiers and high-intensity lighting that mimics sunlight, can assist in optimizing vision in otherwise uncorrectable ophthalmologic problems.

Hearing

Hearing loss is common among older adults, and some degree of impairment is almost inevitable with advancing age. It has been reported that up to 40% of independent individuals older than 65 and about half of those older than 75 years of age have a hearing impairment.[3,4]

Presbycusis, or the hearing loss of old age, is largely considered multifactorial in etiology. It occurs as a result of aging combined with auditory stressors, trauma, environmental influences, and otologic diseases, as well as genetic factors. It is characterized by a gradual, progressive onset of bilateral and symmetric sensorineural hearing loss of high-frequency tones (see Chapter 55). The hearing deficit often has both a peripheral and a central component. Speech discrimination or the ability to distinguish among words that are near-homonyms or distinguish words spoken by several different speakers, often is impaired. Accelerated speech and shouting can increase distortion and further compound the problem. When speaking to hearing-impaired older adults, it is helpful to face them directly so they can observe lip movements and facial expressions. Speech should be slow and direct. Loudness can be irritating. Rephrasing misunderstood messages also can improve understanding of the spoken word. Hearing deficits with age are not always limited to an increased detection threshold, but can include other aspects of hearing, such as sound, comprehension of speech, and noise discrimination, as noted previously.

Hearing aids can be effective for various levels of hearing loss and may greatly improve the ability to hear and communicate. Cochlear implants may be indicated for individuals with severe hearing loss not helped by hearing aids. Research in the area of hearing restoration by regeneration of cochlear hair cells as well as gene therapy holds promise.[30]

Cerumen (i.e., earwax) impaction in the external auditory canal also is commonly seen in older adults and can impair hearing. The cerumen glands, which are modified apocrine sweat glands, atrophy and produce drier cerumen. This may be partially responsible for more frequent cerumen impactions in the older adult population.[30]

Taste and Smell

Olfaction, or the sense of smell, declines with aging, possibly as a result of generalized atrophy of the olfactory bulbs and a moderate loss of olfactory neurons. Smell is a protective mechanism, and persons who cannot smell may be at risk for exposure to environmental hazards. For example, people who cannot smell smoke would be at particular risk if a fire broke out.

The sense of taste decreases with aging, but it is believed to be less affected than olfaction. In fact, in many cases what is perceived to be a decline in ability to taste is actually a defect in olfaction. Because taste and smell are necessary for the enjoyment of food flavour, older adults may not enjoy eating as much as in their youth.[29] Drugs and disease also may affect taste. Alterations in taste and smell, along with other factors such as eating alone, decreased ability to purchase and prepare food, and the high cost of some foods, may account for poor nutritional intake in some older adults. Conversely, the lack of sensory feedback may lead the person to eat more and gain weight. A decline in taste is more pronounced among older adults with Alzheimer disease, presumably because of the neuropathologic changes in the brain.[28]

Immune Function

A functional immune system is a vital component in surviving microorganism infection and damage caused by other pathogens. Immunosenescence, or age-related changes in the immune system, can pose an increased risk for some infections in the elderly. Involution of the thymus gland is complete by approximately 45 to 50 years of age, and although the total number of T cells remains unchanged, there are changes in the function of helper T cells that alter the cellular immune response of older adults. There also is evidence of an increase in various autoantibodies (e.g., rheumatoid factor) as a person ages, increasing the risk of autoimmune disorders.

Extensive studies show that although changes in immunity occur with aging, it is the compounding effects of age-related diseases and external conditions that result in an overall state of dysfunctional immunity that are responsible for the increased risk and severity of common infections in older adults. Hence, immunosenescence is a predisposing condition, but its contribution to infection risk likely is small until immunity is impaired further as a result of chronic disease, external circumstances, or repeated or chronic infections.[14] This is different from the changes related to immunosuppression resulting from certain conditions such as human immunodeficiency virus infection or immunosuppressive medications that result in unusual opportunistic infections. However, older adults are more susceptible to urinary tract infections, respiratory tract infections, wound infections, and nosocomial infections. The mortality rate from influenza and bronchopneumonia is increased in this population.[31]

Early detection of infections is more difficult in older adults because the typical symptoms, such as fever and elevated white blood cell count, often are absent or minimized. A change in mental status or decline in function often is the only presenting sign. It has been reported that frank delirium occurs in 50% of older adults with infections. Thus, infections in the elderly may be far advanced at the time of diagnosis.[14–31]

Gastrointestinal Function

The gastrointestinal tract shows less age-associated change in function than many other organ systems. Although tooth loss is common and approximately 40% to 50% of the older adult population is edentulous, it is not considered part of the normal aging process. Poor dental hygiene with associated caries and periodontal disease is the main reason for the loss. *Edentia,* or toothlessness, can lead to dietary changes and can be associated with malnutrition. Use of dentures can enhance mastication; however, taste sensation is inhibited. Because of improved dental technology and the fluoridated water supply, more persons are able to keep their teeth into their later years. *Xerostomia,* or dry mouth, also is common, but it is not universal among older adults and typically occurs as a result of decreased salivary secretions. Other causes of dry mouth can include medications, such as anticholinergics and tranquilizers, radiation therapy, and obstructive nasal diseases that induce mouth breathing.

The term *presbyesophagus* is used to denote changes in esophageal function, such as decreased motility and inadequate relaxation of the lower esophageal sphincter, that occur with aging. However, in studies that controlled for disease states such as diabetes mellitus and neuropathies, no increase in abnormal motility was observed. In general, the physiologic function of the esophagus appears to remain intact with advancing age.[25]

Atrophy of the gastric mucosa and a decrease in gastric secretions can occur in older adults. *Achlorhydria (i.e.,* decrease in hydrochloric acid secretion) occurs, probably as a result of a loss of parietal cells. Although not universal, achlorhydria is more prevalent among older adults and can cause impaired gastric absorption of substances requiring an acidic environment. *Helicobacter pylori* colonization, which is common in older adults, is thought to play a role in gastric atrophy and subsequent decline in gastric acid secretions.[32]

Atrophic gastritis and decreased secretion of intrinsic factor are more common with aging and can result in a malabsorption of vitamin B_{12}. Because vitamin B_{12} is necessary for the maturation of red blood cells, a deficiency can lead to a type of macrocytic anemia called *pernicious anemia.* Vitamin B_{12} deficiency also can cause neurologic abnormalities such as peripheral neuropathy, ataxia, and even dementia. Treatment consists of regular periodic vitamin B_{12} replacement therapy through injection or the oral form, both have shown to be as effective.[33]

The small intestine shows some age-related morphologic changes, such as mucosal atrophy; however, absorption of most nutrients and other functions appear to remain intact. Absorption of calcium, however, decreases with aging and may reflect decreased intestinal absorption along with other factors, such as reduced intake of vitamin D, decreased formation of vitamin D_3 by the skin because of reduced sun exposure, and decreased activation of vitamin D_3 by the liver and kidney.

Diverticula of the colon are common among older adults, with more than 50% of individuals older than 80 years having diverticular disease. The high incidence appears to result mainly from a low-fibre diet.[34] Constipation, or infrequent passage of hard stool, is another frequently occurring phenomenon. It often is attributed to immobility and decreased physical activity, a low-fibre diet, decreased fluid intake, and medications; malignancies and other disease states also can be responsible. Complications of constipation can include fecal impaction or obstruction, megacolon, rectal prolapse, hemorrhoids, and laxative abuse.[35]

Renal Function

Although age-related anatomic and physiologic changes occur, the aging kidney remains capable of maintaining fluid and electrolyte balance remarkably well. Aging changes result in a decreased reserve capacity, which may alter the kidney's ability to maintain homeostasis in the face of illnesses or stressors. Overall, there is a general decline in kidney mass with aging, predominantly in the renal cortex. The number of functional glomeruli decreases by 30%, with an increased percentage of sclerotic or abnormal glomeruli.[36]

Numerous cross-sectional and longitudinal studies have documented a steady, age-related decline in total renal blood flow of approximately 10% per decade after 20 years of age, so that the renal blood flow of an 80-year-old person averages approximately 300 ml/minute, compared with 600 ml/minute in a younger adult. The major decline in blood flow occurs in the cortical area of the kidney, causing a progressive, age-related decrease in the glomerular filtration rate (GFR). Serum creatinine, a byproduct of muscle metabolism, often is used as a measure of GFR. The decline in GFR that occurs with aging is not accompanied by an equivalent increase in serum creatinine levels because the production of creatinine is reduced as muscle mass declines with age.[36,37] Serum creatinine levels often are used as an index of kidney function when prescribing and calculating drug doses for medications that are eliminated through the kidneys; this has important implications for older adults. If not carefully addressed, improper drug dosing can lead to an excess accumulation of circulating drugs and result in toxicity. A formula that adjusts for age-related changes in serum creatinine for individuals 40 through 80 years of age is available (see Chapter 34).

Renal tubular function declines with advancing age, and the ability to concentrate and dilute urine in response to fluid and electrolyte impairments is diminished. The aging kidney's ability to conserve sodium in response to sodium depletion is impaired and can result in hyponatremia. A decreased ability to concentrate urine, an age-related decrease in responsiveness to antidiuretic hormone, and an impaired thirst mechanism may account for the older adult's greater predisposition to dehydration during periods of stress and illness. Older adults also are more prone to hyperkalemia and hypokalemia when stressed than are younger individuals. An elevated serum potassium may result from a decreased GFR, lower renin and aldosterone levels, and changes in tubular function. Low potassium levels, on the other hand, are more commonly caused by gastrointestinal disorders or diuretic use. Neither is the result of aging.[38]

Genitourinary Function

Both men and women undergo changes in genitourinary function as a result of the aging process. There are changes in bladder structure and function, decreases in steroid sex hormones, and changes in genital structures.

Changes in the bladder structure that occur because of the aging process can result in a decline in function. Overall, the smooth muscle and supportive elastic tissue are replaced with fibrous connective tissue. This can cause incomplete bladder emptying and a diminished force of urine stream. Bladder capacity also decreases with age, whereas the frequency of urination increases. As elastic tissue and muscles weaken, stress incontinence becomes more prevalent.

In aging women, atrophy of perineal structures can cause the urethral meatus to recede along the vaginal wall. Atrophy of other pelvic organs occurs in the aging woman because of diminished estrogen production after menopause: vaginal secretions diminish; the vaginal lining is thinner, drier, less elastic, and more easily traumatized; and normal flora are altered. These changes can result in vaginal infections, pruritus, and painful intercourse.[39]

In aging men, benign prostatic hyperplasia (BPH) is very common (see Chapter 44). The incidence progressively increases to approximately 75% of men by 80 years of age. The condition often is asymptomatic until approximately 50 years of age. Thereafter, the incidence and severity of symptoms increase with age. BPH can cause obstructive symptoms such as urinary hesitancy, diminished force of stream, retention, and postvoid dribbling; it also can cause irritative symptoms such as frequency, nocturia, urgency, and even urge incontinence.[40]

Serum testosterone levels are known to decline as men age, although the definition of and treatment for hypogonadism remain somewhat controversial. Symptoms associated with androgen deficiency in the aging man can include diminished muscle strength, stamina, and energy; loss of muscle mass; low libido (with or without erectile dysfunction); irritable mood; osteoporosis; and testicular atrophy (see Chapter 43). Although some guidelines for androgen replacement therapy for older men have been developed by several groups, there is a general lack of consensus on whether to treat.[41]

Sexual activity remains possible into late life for men and women. In general, the duration and intensity of the sexual response cycle are diminished in both sexes.[42] Women take longer to experience the physiologic changes of vaginal expansion and lubrication during the excitement phase. Penile erection in aging men takes longer to develop because of changes in neural innervation and vascular supply. Social factors affecting sexual behaviour include the desire to remain sexually active, access to a sexually functioning partner, and availability of a conducive environment.[43,44]

IN SUMMARY

There is a general decline in the structure and function of the body with advancing age, resulting in a decreased reserve capacity of the various organ systems, including the integumentary, musculoskeletal, cardiorespiratory, nervous, sensory, immune, gastrointestinal, and genitourinary systems (see Fig. 3.2). This results in a reduction of homeostatic capabilities, making the older adult more vulnerable to stressors such as illness, trauma, surgery, medication administration, and environmental changes.

FUNCTIONAL PROBLEMS ASSOCIATED WITH AGING

After completing this section of the chapter, you should be able to meet the following objectives:

- Compare information obtained from functional assessment with that obtained from a physical examination used to arrive at a medical diagnosis.
- Cite the differences between chronic and transient urinary incontinence.
- State four risk factors for falls in older individuals.
- List five symptoms of depression in older adults.
- Name a tool that can be used for assessing cognitive function.
- State the difference between delirium and dementia.

Although aging is not synonymous with disease, the aging process does lend itself to an increased incidence of illness. As chronologic age increases, so does the probability of having multiple chronic diseases. The vast majority of older adults have at least one chronic condition, and most actually have more than one.[1-3] The extent of these problems is described in Table 3.1. Older adults are more likely to experience a decline in overall health and function because of the increased incidence of chronic illness that occurs with advancing age. Because aging also brings with it a decreased ability to maintain homeostasis, illnesses often manifest in an atypical manner. For example, myocardial infarction may occur without chest pain or other presenting symptoms. Sepsis without fever is common, and pneumonia may present with acute confusion but lack the prodromal symptom of cough.

TABLE 3.1 COMMON HEALTH PROBLEMS IN OLDER ADULTS

HEALTH PROBLEMS IN OLDER ADULTS	PERCENTAGE	
	WOMEN	MEN
Hypertension	52.2	44.9
Arthritis	49.6	32.3
Diabetes	14.8	22.1
Heart disease	14.8	19.5
Urinary incontinence	12.3	9.0
At least one chronic health condition	82.9	78.6

Data from Milan, A, Vezina, M. Seniors Women, Table 10. 2011. Available online at: http://www.statcan.gc.ca/pub/89–503-x/2010001/article/11441-eng.pdf. Accessed October 17, 2013.

In addition to chronic illnesses, older adults suffer disproportionately from functional disabilities, or the inability to perform the necessary activities of daily living (ADLs). It is most likely that the decrements in health that can accompany the aging process are responsible for these functional disabilities. Among the more common functional problems of the older adult are urinary incontinence, instability and falls, sensory impairment, and depression and cognitive impairment.

Functional Assessment

Evaluation of the older adult's functional abilities is a key component of gerontologic health care. Medical diagnoses alone are incomplete without an assessment of function. Two older adults with similar medical diagnoses of arthritis, hypertension, and osteoporosis, for example, can be at opposite ends of the spectrum of functional abilities.

Assessing functional status can be done in many different ways, using a variety of methods. Measures of function should attempt, systematically and objectively, to evaluate the level at which an individual is functioning in a variety of areas, including biologic, psychological, and social health.

Selection of a screening tool to measure function depends on the purpose of data collection, the individual or target population to be assessed, availability and applicability of the instruments, reliability and validity of the screening tools, and the setting or environment. An issue that arises when assessing function is the question of capability versus performance. For example, an older adult may be able to bathe without supervision; however, the long-term care facility where the person resides may discourage it for safety reasons. Among the more commonly used assessment tools are those that measure the ability to perform ADLs and the patient's cognitive function.

When evaluating levels of function, determination of the older adult's ability to perform ADLs and instrumental ADLs (IADLs) should be included. ADLs are basic self-care tasks, such as bathing, dressing, grooming, ambulating, transferring (*e.g.,* from a chair to bed), feeding, and communicating. IADLs are more complex tasks that are necessary to function in society, such as writing, reading, cooking, cleaning, shopping, laundering, climbing stairs, using the telephone, managing money, managing medications, and using transportation. The IADL tasks indirectly examine cognitive abilities as well because they require a certain level of cognitive skill to complete.

Several tools are available for measuring functional status. One of the more commonly used tools is the Index of Activities of Daily Living. Developed by Katz in 1963 and revised in 1970, it summarizes performance in six functions: bathing, dressing, toileting, transferring, continence, and feeding. It is used as an assessment tool to determine the need for care and the appropriateness of treatment, and as a teaching aid in rehabilitation settings. Through questioning and observation, the rater forms a mental picture of the older adult's functional status as it existed during a 2-week period preceding the evaluation, using the most dependent degree of performance.[44,45] Numerous studies using the Katz Index tool show significant validity and reliability. The advantage of the tool is that it is easy to administer and provides a "snapshot" of the older adult's level of physical functioning. The disadvantage is that it does not include IADL categories that are of equal importance, especially for older adults living in the community. The Lawton Instrumental Activities of Daily Living (IADL) Scale evaluates eight domains of function necessary to assess independent living, namely ability to use the telephone, shopping, food preparation, housekeeping, laundry, mode of transportation, medication administration and ability to handle finances. It reflects how the person is functioning currently and can be used to identify new disabilities and prompt further assessment of vulnerable older adults.[46]

Urinary Incontinence

Urinary incontinence, or involuntary loss of urine, plagues over 30% of community-living individuals older than 60 years of age, 50% of hospitalized older adults, and 60% of residents in long-term care facilities.[11,40] It is estimated that 3.5 million (10%) of Canadians have some form of incontinence but these estimates may be low because individuals often fail to report symptoms of urinary incontinence, perhaps owing to the attached social stigma. Health care professionals often neglect to elicit such information as well.[47]

Incontinence is an expensive problem. A conservative estimate of cost for direct care of all Canadian adults with incontinence is over $1.9 billion annually, noting that the tendency for urinary incontinence is more prevalent with increasing age.[48] Urinary incontinence can have deleterious consequences, such as social isolation and embarrassment, depression and dependency, skin rashes and pressure sores, and financial hardship. Although urinary incontinence is a common disorder, it is not considered a normal aspect of aging. Adults with urinary incontinence can be successfully treated and even cured.[40,47]

Etiology and Pathogenesis

Changes in the micturition cycle that accompany the aging process make the older adult prone to urinary incontinence. A decrease in bladder capacity, in bladder and sphincter tone, and in the ability to inhibit detrusor (*i.e.,* bladder muscle) contractions, combined with the nervous system's increased variability in interpreting bladder signals, can cause incontinence (see Chapter 35). Impaired mobility and a slower reaction time also can aggravate incontinence.[11]

The causes of incontinence can be divided into two categories: transient and chronic. Of particular importance is the role of pharmaceuticals as a cause of transient urinary incontinence. Numerous medications, such as long-acting sedatives and hypnotics, psychotropics, and diuretics, can induce incontinence. Treatment of transient urinary incontinence is aimed at ameliorating or relieving the cause on the assumption that the incontinence will resolve.[11]

Chronic, or established, urinary incontinence occurs as a failure of the bladder to store urine or a failure to empty urine. Failure to store urine can occur as a result of detrusor muscle overactivity with inappropriate bladder contractions (*i.e.,* urge incontinence). There is an inability to delay voiding after the sensation of bladder fullness is perceived. Urge incontinence is typically characterized by large-volume leakage episodes occurring at various times of day. Urethral incompetence (*i.e.,* stress incontinence) also causes a bladder storage problem. The bladder pressure overcomes the resistance of the urethra and results in urine leakage. Stress incontinence causes an involuntary loss of small amounts of urine with activities that increase intra-abdominal pressure, such as coughing, sneezing, laughing, or exercising.[11,40,49]

Failure of the bladder to empty urine can occur because of detrusor instability, resulting in urine retention and overflow incontinence. Also called *neurogenic incontinence,* this type of incontinence can be seen with neurologic damage from conditions such as diabetes mellitus and spinal cord injury. Outlet obstruction, as with prostate enlargement and urethral stricture, also can cause urinary retention with overflow incontinence. Functional incontinence, or urine leakage due to toileting problems, occurs because cognitive, physical, or environmental barriers impair appropriate use of the toilet.[11]

Treatment

After a specific diagnosis of urinary incontinence is established, treatment is aimed at correcting or ameliorating the problem. Probably the most effective interventions for older adults with incontinence are behavioural techniques. These strategies involve educating the individual and providing reinforcement for effort and progress. Techniques include bladder training, timed voiding or habit training, prompted voiding, pelvic floor muscle (*i.e.,* Kegel) exercises, and dietary modifications.[11,49] Biofeedback, a training technique to teach pelvic floor muscle exercises, uses computerized instruments to relay information to individuals about their physiologic functions. Biofeedback can be helpful when used with other behavioural treatment techniques.[11] Use of pads or other absorbent products should be seen as a temporary measure and not as a cure. Numerous types of products are available to meet many different consumer needs.

Pharmacologic intervention may be helpful for some individuals. Oral estrogen replacement therapy in postmenopausal women is no longer recommended as a treatment approach in light of newer information about the cardiovascular side effects and increased cancer risks that estrogen can pose. However, topical estrogen in low doses is effective in decreasing urge incontinence, and to a lesser extent, stress incontinence.[11,49] Antimuscarinic drugs (*e.g.,* oxybutynin, tolterodine, darifenacin) may help with an overactive bladder and urge incontinence. Their anticholinergic side effects such as dry mouth, constipation and potential for central nervous system side effects make it necessary to weigh the risks against the benefits, which are limited at best. Newer drugs are targeting more specific muscarinic receptors and other drugs such as duloxetine and botox are currently not approved in Canada for these conditions.[11,40,49]

Surgical intervention may help to relieve urinary incontinence symptoms in appropriate patients. Bladder neck suspension or slings may assist with stress incontinence unrelieved by other interventions, and prostatectomy may be appropriate for men with overflow incontinence due to enlarged prostate. However, older adults may have medical conditions that preclude surgery. Other treatments include intermittent self-catheterization for some types of overflow incontinence, and insertable pessary devices or urethral bulking agents for stress incontinence.[11,49]

Instability and Falls

Unstable gait and falls are a common source of concern for the older adult population. The literature reveals that in Canada one in three persons over the age of 65 falls at least once per year with up to 50% sustaining a minor injury but between 5% to 20% of these falls resulting in serious injury.[50] Unintentional injuries are the sixth leading cause of death among older adults, with falls accounting for 40% of all injury deaths.[51]

The way in which a person falls can often determine the type of injury that occurs. Wrist fractures are common and frequently sustained from forward or backward falls onto an outstretched hand. Hip fractures can result from a sideways fall and are one of the most feared complications from a fall. Hip fractures predominate in the 75 years and older age group. Significant morbidity ensues from a hip fracture. The literature varies, but as much as 50% of older adults who sustain a hip fracture never regain their ability to walk independently, and up to 20% die in the year after a hip fracture.[52] The problem of falls in the older adult population is an issue of high incidence combined with a high potential for injury, owing to the high prevalence of medical problems along with physiologic changes that occur with advancing age. In addition, recovery from a fall-related injury can be lengthy and result in deconditioning, weakness and abnormality of gait, further potentiating the risk of subsequent falls.[52] An individual's activity may be restricted because of fear on the individual's or caregiver's part about possible falling. These anxieties may lead to unnecessary restrictions in independence and mobility and commonly are mentioned as a reason for institutionalization.[50,51]

Risk Factors

Although some falls have a single, obvious cause, such as a slip on a wet or icy surface, most are the result of several factors. Risk factors that predispose to falling include a combination of age-related biopsychosocial changes, chronic illnesses, and situational and environmental hazards. Table 3.2 summarizes the possible causes of falls.

Gait and stability require the integration of information from the special senses, the nervous system, and the musculoskeletal system. Changes in gait and posture that occur in healthy aged individuals also contribute to the problem of falls. The older person's stride shortens; the elbows, trunk, and knees become more flexed; toe and heel lift decrease while walking; and sway while standing increases. Muscle strength

TABLE 3.2 RISK FACTORS FOR FALLS

CATEGORY OF RISK FACTORS	EXAMPLES
Environmental hazards	Slips, trips
Age-related functional changes	Decreased muscle strength, slowed reaction time, decreased proprioception, impaired righting reflexes, increased postural sway, altered gait, impaired visual and hearing function
Cardiovascular disorders	Aortic stenosis, cardiac arrhythmias, autonomic nervous system dysfunction, hypovolemia, orthostatic hypotension, carotid sinus syncope, vertebrobasilar insufficiency
Gastrointestinal disorders	Diarrhea, postprandial syncope, vasovagal response
Genitourinary disorders	Urinary incontinence, urinary urgency/frequency, nocturia
Medication use	Alcohol, antihypertensives, cardiac medications, diuretics, narcotics, oral hypoglycemic agents, psychotropic medications, drug–drug interactions, polypharmacy
Metabolic disorders	Anemia, dehydration, electrolyte imbalance, hypothyroidism
Musculoskeletal disorders	Osteoarthritis, rheumatoid arthritis, myopathy
Neurologic disorders	Balance/gait disorders, cerebellar dysfunction, stroke with residual effects, cervical spondylosis, central nervous system lesions, delirium, dementia, normal-pressure hydrocephalus, peripheral neuropathy, Parkinson disease, seizure disorders, transient ischemic attack
Prolonged bed rest	Hypovolemia, muscle weakness from disuse and deconditioning
Respiratory disorders	Hypoxia, pneumonia
Sensory impairments	Decreased visual acuity, cataract, glaucoma, macular degeneration, hearing impairment, vestibular disorders

and postural control of balance decrease, proprioception input diminishes, and righting reflexes slow.[11,53] Because the central nervous system integrates sensory input and sends signals to the effector components of the musculoskeletal system, any alteration in neural function can predispose to falls. For this reason, falls have been associated with strokes, Parkinson disease, and normal-pressure hydrocephalus. Similarly, diseases or disabilities that affect the musculoskeletal system, such as arthritis, muscle weakness, or foot deformities, are associated with an increase in the incidence of falls.[11,53]

Age- and disease-related alterations in vision and hearing can impair sensory input, increasing the risk for falls.[54,55] Vestibular system alterations such as benign positional vertigo or Ménière disease cause balance problems that can result in falls (see Chapter 55). Input from the cardiovascular and respiratory systems influences function and ambulation. Syncope, a type of dizziness, is a transient global cerebral hypoperfusion stemming from cardiovascular symptoms. Syncope occurs fairly rapidly and usually results in falling. Syncope is common among older adults, with higher incidences among those aged 80 years and older.[23] Cognitive impairments such as dementia have been associated with an increased risk of falling, most likely because of impaired judgment and problem-solving abilities.[42,53,54]

Medications are an important and potentially correctable cause of instability and falls. Central acting medications, such as sedatives and hypnotics, have been associated with an increase in the risk of falling and injury. Diuretics can cause volume depletion, electrolyte disturbances, and fatigue, predisposing to falls. Antihypertensive drugs can cause fatigue, orthostatic hypotension, and impaired alertness, contributing to the risk of falls.[11,53]

Environmental hazards play a significant role in falling. Most falls occur in the home and often involve objects that are tripped over, such as cords, scatter rugs, and small items left on the floor. Poor lighting, ill-fitting shoes, surfaces with glare, and improper use of ambulatory devices such as canes or walkers also contribute to the problem.[53]

Prevention

Preventing falls is now recognized at the provincial and national levels as the key to controlling the potential complications that can result. Because multiple factors usually contribute to falling, the aim of the clinical evaluation is to identify risk factors that can be modified. Assessment of sensory, neurologic, and musculoskeletal systems; direct observation of gait and balance; and a careful medication inventory can help identify possible causes. Preventive measures can include a variety of interventions, such as surgery for cataracts or cerumen removal for hearing impairment related to excessive earwax accumulation.[11] Other interventions may include podiatric care, discontinuation or alteration of the medication regimen, exercise programs, physical therapy, and appropriate adaptive devices. The home also should be assessed by an appropriate health care professional (*e.g.,* occupational therapist) and recommendations made regarding modifications to promote safety. Simple changes such as removing scatter rugs, improving the lighting, and installing grab bars in the bathtub can help prevent falling.[53]

Use of specially designed external hip protector pads in high-risk older adults has demonstrated a dramatic reduction in hip fractures occurring after a fall. The impacting force and energy caused by the fall are weakened and diverted away from the greater trochanteric region by use of the pad.

Compliance is somewhat problematic, however, because individuals may be reluctant to wear the pads.[53] Vitamin D supplementation has also shown promising results and may have an independent role in the prevention of falls. Use of vitamin D is credited with improvement in functional strength and dynamic muscle performance, thereby reducing fall risk. A recent examination of systematic reviews and meta-analyses of vitamin D supplementation for prevention of hip fractures revealed a beneficial effect to high dose vitamin D supplementation combined with calcium.[56,57]

Sensory Impairment

Although sensory impairments are not imminently life-threatening, their impact on health can be substantial. Hearing impairment is associated with decreased quality of life, depression, isolation, and dementia. Visual impairment is related to increased risk of falls, hip fractures, physical disability, and depression. Nursing home residents with visual impairment are more likely to require assistance with ADLs and can be at risk for falls and hip fractures. Visual impairment also appears to increase mortality rates.[29,30,54,57]

Sensory impairment results not only from deficits in peripheral sensory structures but also from the central processing of sensory information. The older person's difficulty in processing multisensory information is seen most strikingly when there is a rapid fluctuation in the nature of the information that is received from the environment.[55]

Lack of sensory information can predispose to psychological symptoms. Charles Bonnet syndrome is an organic disorder occurring in the elderly that is characterized by complex visual hallucinations. It is associated with ocular disease and, strictly speaking, is seen in older adults with preserved intellectual functions.[58,59] Those who obtain insight into the problem generally only need reassurance that their hallucinations do not represent mental illness. For those who have limited insight and are distressed by the symptom, antipsychotics may afford some relief.[59] Both auditory and visual impairment can have important psychological effects in association with dementia. Delusions have long been associated with hearing impairment.[60] However, a recent systematic review of cohort studies that focused on late-onset psychosis determined that visual impairment was a greater risk factor.[58]

Depression and Cognitive Impairment

Depression

Depression is a significant health problem affecting the older adult population and is one of the most common geriatric psychiatric disorders. Estimates of the prevalence of depression in the elderly vary widely; however, there is a consensus that the size of the problem is underestimated owing to misdiagnosis and mistreatment. Up to 25% of community-dwelling older adults are thought to have depressive symptoms. The estimate drops to approximately 1% to 2% when diagnosis is restricted to major depression. Depressive symptoms are even more common in nursing home residents.[61]

The term *depression* is used to describe a symptom, syndrome, or disease. As listed in the fifth edition of the American Psychiatric Association's *Diagnostic and Statistical Manual of Mental Disorders* (*DSM-5*), the criteria for the diagnosis and treatment of a major depression include at least five of the following symptoms during the same 2-week period, with at least one of the symptoms being depressed mood or anhedonia (*i.e.,* loss of interest or pleasure): depressed or irritable mood; loss of interest or pleasure in usual activities; appetite and weight changes; sleep disturbance; psychomotor agitation or retardation; fatigue and loss of energy; feelings of worthlessness or excessive guilt; diminished ability to think or concentrate; and suicidal ideation, plan, or attempt.[62] Depressive symptomatology can be incorrectly attributed to the aging process, making recognition and diagnosis difficult. Depressed mood, the signature symptom of depression, may be less prominent in the older adult, and more somatic complaints and increased anxiety are reported, confusing the diagnosis. Symptoms of cognitive impairment can be seen in the depressed older adult. Although a thorough investigation is necessary to discern whether the symptoms are a result of depression versus dementia, evidence now shows that depression can be a prodromal symptom of dementia.[63]

Physical illnesses can complicate the diagnosis as well. Depression can be a symptom of a medical condition, such as pancreatic cancer, hypothyroidism or hyperthyroidism, pneumonia and other infections, congestive heart failure, dementia, and stroke.[63,64] In fact, major depression is a common consequence of stroke and occurs in about one third of all patients with ischemic stroke.[63,65] Medications such as sedatives, hypnotics, steroids, antihypertensives, and analgesics also can induce a depressive state.[63] Numerous confounding social problems, such as bereavement, loss of job or income, and loss of social support, can contribute to the diagnosis.[63]

The course of depression in older adults is similar to that in younger persons. As many as 40% experience recurrences. Suicide rates are highest among the elderly. There is a linear increase in suicide with age, most notably among white men older than 65 years of age. The exact reasons are unclear. Predictors include depression, physical illness and disability, loss of a spouse, and social isolation.[63–67]

Because diagnosis of depression can be difficult, use of a screening tool may help to measure affective functioning objectively. The Geriatric Depression Scale, an instrument of known reliability and validity, was developed to measure depression specifically in the non-institutionalized older adult population. The 30-item dichotomous scale elicits information on topics relevant to symptoms of depression among older adults, such as memory loss and anxiety.[68] Many other screening tools, each with its own advantages and disadvantages, exist to evaluate the older adult's level of psychological functioning, in its entirety or as specific, separate components of function.

Treatment. Treatment goals for older adults with depression are to decrease the symptoms of depression, improve the quality of life, reduce the risk of recurrences, improve health status, decrease health care costs, and decrease mortality. Pharmacotherapy (*i.e.,* use of antidepressants) is an effective treatment approach for the depressed older adult. The selection of a particular medication depends on a variety of factors, such as a prior positive or negative response, history of first-degree relatives responding to medication, concurrent medical illnesses that may interfere with medication use, concomitant use of non-psychotropic medications that may alter the metabolism or increase the side effect profile, likelihood of adherence, patient preference, and cost. Selective serotonin reuptake inhibitors (SSRIs), a class of antidepressants (*e.g.,* sertraline, citalopram, escitalopram), provide high specificity by blocking or slowing serotonin reuptake without the antagonism of neurotransmitter receptors or direct cardiac effects. Because of this, they are an attractive first choice for pharmacotherapy. Dosing is usually once per day, creating ease of administration. They also are less lethal in overdose than other types of antidepressants, such as the tricyclics, an important consideration because of the high suicide rate among older adults. The anticholinergic and cardiovascular side effects that can be problematic with tricyclic antidepressants (*e.g.,* nortriptyline, desipramine, amitriptyline) are minimal with SSRIs. Atypical antidepressants (*e.g.,* bupropion, mirtazapine) and serotonin and noradrenaline reuptake inhibitors (SNRIs; *e.g.,* venlafaxine, duloxetine) have begun to have a role in late-life depression. Similar in efficacy to SSRIs, clinicians may select one of these drugs for both its antidepressant and side effect properties. For example, mirtazapine is an antidepressant with associated sedation and increased appetite; it would be appropriate for a depressed elder with poor appetite and insomnia. Regardless of the classification, psychotropic medications should be given in low doses initially and gradually titrated according to response and side effects. Response to antidepressants usually requires 4 to 6 weeks at therapeutic dose levels. For a single episode of major depression, drug therapy usually should continue for a minimum of 6 months to 1 year, and 2 to 5 years for recurrent depression, to prevent relapse.[69,70]

Electroconvulsive therapy (ECT) may be the treatment of choice for older adults with severe, pharmacologically resistant major depressive episodes. Studies indicate that individuals older than 60 years of age are the largest group of patients who receive ECT. Despite the negative publicity that has been associated with ECT, the evidence for its efficacy in the treatment of depression is strong. Unfortunately, relapse after ECT is common, and alternative treatment strategies, including maintenance ECT or maintenance antidepressants after ECT, are being used.[71]

"Talking therapy," such as supportive counselling or psychotherapy, is considered to be an important part of the treatment regimen, alone or in combination with pharmacotherapy or ECT. Alterations in life roles, lack of social support, and chronic medical illnesses are just a few examples of life event changes that may require psychosocial support and new coping skills. Counselling in the older adult population requires special considerations. Individuals with significant vision, hearing, or cognitive impairments may require special approaches. Many elderly persons do not see themselves as depressed and reject referrals to mental health professionals. Special efforts are needed to engage these individuals in treatment. Cognitive behavioural therapy teaches older adults how to identify and challenge distressing thoughts, and then to reframe how they perceive or react to a situation. Some older adults may prefer this type of therapy as it is briefer and time-limited as compared to other therapies such as psychoanalysis.[72] Although depression can impose great risks for older adults, it is thought to be the most treatable psychiatric disorder in late life and therefore warrants aggressive case finding and intervention.

Dementia

Dementia is a complex and devastating problem that is a major cause of disability in the older adult population. Estimates vary, but the prevalence of cognitive impairment including dementia includes approximately 747,000 Canadians with 14.9% of these people over the age of 65. The economic costs (approximately $33 billion per year) and the pressures for caregivers for both the Canadian and worldwide populations are expected to increase significantly over the next 10 to 20 years.[73]

Although there can be a decline in intellectual function with aging, dementia, formally called *senility,* is not a normal aging process. Dementia is a syndrome of acquired, persistent impairment in several domains of intellectual function, including memory, language, visuospatial ability, and cognition (*i.e.,* abstraction, calculation, judgment, and problem solving). The cognitive changes are sufficient to impair social and occupational function. Mood disturbances and changes in personality and behaviour often accompany the intellectual deterioration.[62]

Etiology and Pathogenesis. Dementia or cognitive dysfunction can result from a wide variety of conditions, including degenerative, vascular, neoplastic, demyelinating, infectious, inflammatory, toxic, metabolic, and psychiatric disorders. Up to 70% of older adults with dementia (15 million people worldwide) are thought to have Alzheimer disease (AD), a chronic, progressive neurologic disorder of unknown cause. Two microscopic changes occur in the brain of people with AD: senile plaques that develop between neurons, and neurofibrillary tangles that develop within neurons. Researchers have speculated that inflammation around plaques destroys neighbouring neurons. Involvement of cholinergic neurons causes levels of acetylcholine in synapses to decline. Levels of acetyl cholinesterase also drop, perhaps to compensate for the loss of acetylcholine.[74,75] Vascular dementia is the second most common disorder and risk factors include ischemic stroke, hemorrhagic stroke, hypertension, hyperlipidemia, heart disease, tobacco use, and diabetes mellitus (see Chapter 53).[76–78]

Diagnosis. Currently there are no specific diagnostic tests to determine the presence of AD, and the diagnosis is made by excluding other possible causes of the dementia symptoms. The only confirmatory test for AD is examination of brain tissue on autopsy. More recently, use of positron emission tomography (PET) scans of the brain using a newer imaging molecule has proved to be of value in diagnosis. Research has shown that it can help differentiate the diagnosis by determining regional cerebral patterns of amyloid plaques and the tau neurofibrillary tangles.[79]

A commonly used tool to detect mild cognitive impairment is the Montreal Cognitive Assessment (MoCA©). It is available in 22 languages complete with details for correct scoring.[80] To detect moderate cognitive impairment the Mini-Mental State Examination (MMSE), developed by Folstein and colleagues in 1975 can be used.[81] This tool provides a brief, objective measure of cognitive functioning and has been widely used. The MMSE, which can be administered in 5 to 10 minutes, consists of a variety of questions that cover memory, orientation, attention, and constructional abilities. Both tests have been studied and found to fulfill the goal of providing a brief screening tool that quantifies cognitive impairments and documents cognitive changes over time. However, it has been cautioned that these examinations should not be used by themselves as a diagnostic tool to identify dementia.[80,81]

Treatment. Several medications have become available over the past decade to help halt further cognitive decline in Alzheimer disease. At present, three drugs (donepezil, rivastigmine, and galantamine) are available in the therapeutic category of cognitive-enhancing agents.[73,82] All three medications are acetylcholinesterase inhibitors whose action elevates acetylcholine concentrations in the cerebral cortex by slowing degradation of acetylcholine released by still-intact neurons. Donepezil has been shown to be a specific inhibitor of acetylcholinesterase with minimal side effects. The newer agents, rivastigmine and galantamine, are thought to be more selective in the binding and inactivation of acetylcholinesterase; however, adverse reactions, especially gastrointestinal symptoms, can impede therapeutic dosing. Although there still is no cure for dementia, acetylcholinesterase inhibitors are considered efficacious as antidementia drugs on the basis of improvements seen on standardized cognitive tests, as well as a slower decline in loss of function due to the disease process. There is research to suggest that there is an advantage to starting a cholinesterase inhibitor as early as possible after the diagnosis of mild AD.[73,83] There is no strong evidence to suggest that the cognitive-enhancing drugs are beneficial in people with vascular dementia. However, it would be appropriate to use them in a case of mixed AD and vascular dementia.[83]

Memantine, a moderate-affinity, uncompetitive *N*-methyl-D-aspartate (NMDA) receptor antagonist, is a newer agent that has consistently demonstrated safe and efficacious use in dementia. Glutamate is a neurotransmitter that potentially overexcites NMDA receptors, and excessive release of glutamate is believed to contribute to the neurodegeneration associated with AD. Memantine has known clinical efficacy in treating patients with moderate to severe AD but has not been proven efficacious in mild AD.[84]

There has also been interest in other neuroprotective drugs that may delay the onset or progression of AD. Nonsteroidal anti-inflammatory drugs (NSAIDs) are thought to decrease the inflammatory response to inflammatory mediators released from injured or degenerating nerve cells, although study results are somewhat inconclusive. Because of these general concerns about lack of efficacy, combined with potential side effects, NSAIDs are not considered a standard treatment for AD.[85] Cholesterol promotes beta-amyloid production. Lipid-lowering agents, such as the statin drugs, decrease cholesterol and reduce inflammation. However, thus far, studies have been disappointing in their outcomes in that they have shown no protective effect against cognitive decline.[85]

Dietary and nutritional supplements are thought to have beneficial effects in either the prevention of AD or slowing the progression of the disease. Vitamin E, an antioxidant, may play a role in AD prevention. Vitamin E, a fat-soluble vitamin, interacts with cell membranes, traps free radicals, and may interrupt chain reactions that damage cells. Although earlier studies were promising, more recent investigation of the long-term use of vitamin E did not demonstrate cognitive benefits, although the dose was markedly diminished.[85] Ginkgo biloba, another antioxidant, has unclear clinical benefits. A Cochrane review determined that the evidence supporting ginkgo biloba was not consistent or reliable.[86] Elevated plasma homocysteine concentrations have been linked as a vascular risk factor in the development of dementia and can be lowered by folic acid supplementation. A recent systematic review that studied the use of B-vitamins in the prevention and treatment of AD and dementia determined that there was insufficient evidence to support the theory that increased dietary intake or supplementation of folic acid impacted cognitive decline.[87]

Nonpharmacologic Treatment. Studies have also shown that certain mental exercises can offset some of the expected cognitive changes that can occur with aging. Cognitive training utilizes strategies to enhance cognitive functions such as memory, attention or problem solving. The goal is to maintain or improve cognitive function and compensate for deficits. This can be accomplished through both memory training approaches and computer-assisted cognitive interventions.[88] Likewise, physical exercise, such as aerobics or weight training, may have the potential for delaying functional decline in individuals with Alzheimer disease and may even help to delay the onset of dementing disorders.[89]

In more advanced cases of dementia, ensuring that the individual's physical needs, such as hygiene, bowel and bladder elimination, safety, and nutrition are met can help prevent catastrophic reactions. Providing a consistent routine in familiar surroundings also helps to alleviate stress. Matching the cognitive needs of the older adult by avoiding understimulation and overstimulation often helps in preventing behaviour problems.

The work of Hall has shown positive results in the care of older adults with AD.[90] Hall's conceptual model, progressively lowered stress threshold (PLST), proposes that the demented individual's ability to tolerate any type of stress progressively declines as the disease advances. Interventions for the older adult with dementia therefore centre on eliminating and avoiding stressors as a way to prevent dysfunctional behaviours. These stressors include fatigue, change of routine, excessive demands, overwhelming stimuli, and physical stressors. Hall's work with the PLST model has shown that individuals tend to awaken less at night, use fewer sedatives and hypnotics, eat better, socialize more, function at a higher level, and experience reduced episodes of anxiety, agitation, and other dysfunctional behaviours. Further work has shown that family caregivers trained using the PLST model improved their abilities to provide care to loved ones with dementia and lowered their own stress levels.[90]

Management of older adults with Alzheimer disease and other dementias usually involves assuming increasing responsibility for and supplying increasing care to individuals as the illness renders them incapable. Impaired judgment and cognition can prevent the older adult from making reasonable decisions and choices and eventually threatens their overall well-being. Family members often assume the monumental task of caring for older adults with dementia until the burden becomes too great, at which time many older adults may be relocated to long-term care facilities.

Delirium

It is important to differentiate dementia from delirium, also referred to as *acute confusional state*. Delirium can occur in any age group however, older adults, especially demented older adults, are far more likely to become delirious. The onset of delirium in the demented individual may be mistaken as an exacerbation of the dementia and consequently not treated as up to 70% of delirium cases go undetected.[91–93]

Delirium is an acute disorder developing over a period of hours to days and is seen frequently in hospitalized elderly patients. Prevalence rates range from 6% to 56% of hospitalized older adults, up to 53% of older adults after surgery, and up to 87% of those in intensive care.[93] Delirium is defined by the *DSM-V* as a neurocognitive disorder featuring disturbances of attention, changes in baseline cognition, and disorganized sleep–wake cycle, and which develops over a short period of time and cannot be explained by other neurocognitive disorders.[62] The severity of the symptoms tends to fluctuate unpredictably, but often is more pronounced at night.[93]

Delirium can be a presenting feature of a physical illness and may be seen with disorders such as myocardial infarction, pneumonia and other infections, cancer, and hypothyroidism. Patients with drug toxicities may present with delirium. Malnutrition, use of physical restraints, and iatrogenic events also can precipitate delirium. Delirium is associated with increased length of hospital stay and poor clinical outcomes.[91–93]

Etiology and Pathogenesis. The exact reason why delirium occurs is unclear. It is speculated that the mechanism involves the reversible impairment of multiple neurotransmitters.[91] Other possible contributing factors include vision and hearing impairments, psychological stress, and diseases of other organ systems. Delirium has a high mortality rate, ranging between 20% and 40%. Agitation, disorientation, and fearfulness—the key symptoms of delirium—place the individual at high risk for injuries such as fracture from a fall.[50]

Management. Diagnosis of delirium involves recognition of the syndrome and identification of its causes. The Confusion Assessment Method (CAM) is a validated screening tool developed to quickly and accurately identify delirium. The evaluator assesses the person for the presence of an acute onset or fluctuating course, inattention, disorganized thinking, and altered level of consciousness.[94] Management involves treatment of the underlying disease condition and symptomatic relief through supportive therapy, including removal of any type of restraint (*e.g.*, wrist restraint, Foley catheter), good nutrition and hydration, rest, comfort measures, and emotional support. Prevention of delirium is the overall goal. Avoidance of the devastating and life-threatening acute confusional state is often the key to successful management and treatment.[92,93,95]

IN SUMMARY

Health care for older adults requires unique considerations, taking into account age-related physiologic changes and specific disease states common in this population. Although aging is not synonymous with disease, the aging process does lend itself to an increased incidence of illness. The overall goal is to assist the older adult in maximizing independence and functional capabilities and minimizing disabilities that can result from various acute and chronic illnesses.

The evaluation of the older adult's functional abilities is a key component in gerontologic health care. Medical diagnoses alone are incomplete without an assessment of function. When evaluating levels of function, determination of the older adult's ability to perform ADLs and IADLs should be included.

Among the functional disorders that are common in the older population are urinary incontinence, instability and falls, sensory impairment, and depression, dementia, and delirium. The older adult is especially prone to urinary incontinence because of changes in the micturition cycle that accompany the aging process. Behavioural techniques can be an effective way to treat incontinence problems in the older adult population. Falls are a common source of concern for the older adult population. Although most fa[l]~~ do not result in serious injury, the potential for seriou~ plications and even death is real. Most falls are th~ several risk factors, including age-related bi~ changes, chronic illness, and situational ？ hazards. Both hearing and visual imp~

common in the elderly, contribute to communication problems, depression, and social isolation.

Depression is a significant but treatable health problem that often is misdiagnosed and mistreated in the older adult population. Dementia is a syndrome of acquired, persistent impairment in several domains of intellectual function, including memory, language, visuospatial ability, and cognition (*i.e.,* abstraction, calculation, judgment, and problem solving). Although there can be a slight decline in intellectual function with aging, dementia is not a normal aging process. Delirium is an acute confusional disorder developing over a period of hours to days and often is seen as a presenting feature of a physical illness or drug toxicity.

DRUG THERAPY IN THE OLDER ADULT

After completing this section of the chapter, you should be able to meet the following objectives:

- Characterize drug therapy in the older adult population.
- List five factors that contribute to adverse drug reactions in the elderly.
- Cite cautions to be used in prescribing medications for the elderly.

Drug therapy in the older adult population is a complex phenomenon influenced by numerous biopsychosocial factors. The elderly are the largest group of consumers of prescription and over-the-counter drugs. Although the older adult population comprises only about 14.8% of the Canadian population, they consume one third of all prescription drugs and 50% of all over-the-counter medications. The incidence of adverse drug reactions in the elderly is two to three times that found in young adults. This is considered to be a conservative estimate, because drug reactions are less well recognized in older adults and reactions often can mimic symptoms of specific disease states.[1,2]

Contributory Factors

Errors in the administration of medications and compliance are common among the community-dwelling older adult population. Reasons for this high rate of errors are numerous. Poor manual dexterity, failing eyesight, lack of understanding about the treatment regimen, attitudes and beliefs about medication use, mistrust of health care providers, and forgetfulness or confusion are but a few factors that can affect the adherence to medication regimens.

The role of the health care provider also can contribute improper medication use. There can be a tendency to treat symptoms with drugs rather than fully investigate the cause of those symptoms. To compound matters, accurate diagnosis of specific disease states can be difficult because older adults tend to underreport symptoms and because presenting symptoms are often atypical.[11]

Age-related physiologic changes also account for adverse effects of medications. In general, the absorption of orally ingested drugs remains essentially unchanged with age, even though the gastric pH is known to rise and gastric emptying time can be delayed. Changes in drug distribution, however, are clinically significant. Because lean body mass and total body water decrease with advancing age, water-soluble drugs such as digoxin and propranolol tend to have a smaller volume of distribution, resulting in higher plasma concentrations for a given dose and increased likelihood of a toxic reaction. Conversely, fat-soluble drugs such as diazepam are more widely distributed and accumulate in fatty tissue owing to an increase in adipose tissue with aging. This can cause a delay in elimination and accumulation of the drug over time (*i.e.,* prolonged half-life) with multiple doses of the same drug. Drug metabolism through the liver is thought to be altered owing to the decrease in hepatic blood flow seen in the older adult. Renal excretion controls the elimination of drugs from the body, and because kidney function declines with age, the rate of drug excretion decreases. This can result in an increased half-life of drugs and is why estimates of creatinine clearance are recommended to determine drug dosing.[11,96,97]

Drug use for older adults warrants a cautious approach. "Start low and go slow" is the adage governing drug prescription in geriatric pharmacology. Older adults often can achieve therapeutic results on small doses of medications. If necessary, dosing can then be titrated slowly according to response.

Further complicating matters is the issue of polypharmacy in older adults, who often have multiple disorders that may require multiple drug therapies. Polypharmacy increases the risk of drug interactions and adverse drug reactions, and decreases compliance. Drugs and disease states also can interact, causing adverse effects. For example, psychotropic drugs administered to older adults with dementia may cause a worsening of confusion; β-adrenergic blocking agents administered to an individual with chronic obstructive pulmonary disease may induce bronchoconstriction; and NSAIDs given to an older adult with hypertension can raise blood pressure further.[11,96]

The use of certain types of medications carries a high risk for older adults and should be avoided if possible. In general, long-acting drugs or drugs with prolonged half-lives can be problematic. Many sedatives and hypnotics fit into this category, and drugs such as diazepam and flurazepam should be avoided. Other classes of drugs, such as antidepressants and anxiolytics, may provide the necessary symptomatic relief and may be more appropriate for older adults than sedatives and hypnotics. Use of these agents warrants caution, however, with consideration for the unique pharmacokinetic changes that accompany aging. Drugs that possess anticholinergic properties should also be used with caution.

Anticholinergics are used for a variety of conditions; however, side effects such as dry mouth and eyes, blurred vision, and constipation are common. These drugs can also cause more serious side effects, such as confusion, urinary retention, and orthostatic hypotension. Agents that enter the central nervous system, including narcotics and alcohol, can cause a variety of problems, most notably delirium. These problems most likely occur as a result of a decreased central nervous system reserve capacity.[11,98]

Strategies

Because of the serious implications of medication use in the elderly, strategies need to be used to enhance therapeutic effects and prevent harm. Careful evaluation of the need for the medication by the health care provider is the first step. This can prove problematic as many clinical trials do not include older adults with multiple co-morbidities, forcing the practitioner to use extrapolated data from clinical trials that only included younger adult participants. Once decided, analysis of the individual's current medication regimen and disease state is necessary to prevent drug–drug interactions, drug–disease interactions, and adverse responses. Screening tools, such as the well-known Beer's Criteria or the newer Screening Tool of Older Person Prescriptions (STOPP), have been developed to avoid potentially inappropriate medications usage or prevent avoidable adverse drug events.[98,99]

Dosing should be at the low end, and frequency of drug administration should be kept to a minimum to simplify the routine and enhance compliance. Care must be taken to avoid under-prescribing as well. Subtherapeutic doses or omitting important medications due to potential fear of harm may exacerbate problems also. Timing the dose to a specific activity (*e.g.,* "take with breakfast") can also improve compliance, as can special packaging devices such as pill boxes and blister packs.

The cost of medications is another important factor for older adults on reduced, fixed incomes, as most provincial drug coverage benefits require co-payments with medications for adults over the age of 65 years. Choosing less expensive products of equal efficacy can increase compliance. The importance of educating the individual about the medication cannot be overemphasized. Health care professionals need to provide verbal and written information on the principles of medication use and on the specific medications being used. This facilitates active, involved participation by the older adult and enhances the individual's ability to make informed decisions.[11,98]

IN SUMMARY

Drug therapy in the older adult population is a complex phenomenon influenced by numerous biopsychosocial factors. Alterations in pharmacokinetics occur with advancing age and increase the likelihood of toxic reactions. "Start low and go slow" is the adage governing geriatric pharmacology. Centrally acting drugs and drugs with long half-lives should be avoided when possible. Drug–drug interactions, drug–disease interactions, and adverse reactions are increased in the elderly population. Educating the older adult about drug use is an important factor in ensuring compliance and accurate medication administration.

REVIEW EXERCISES

1. It is said that the aging body can accomplish most, if not all, of the functions of its youth; the difference is that they may take longer, require greater motivation, and be less precise.
   A. *Explain how this concept might contribute to falls in the elderly.*
2. Dementia, delirium, and depression are three conditions that commonly occur in the older adult population.
   A. *What are the defining characteristics of each condition? How are they similar? How are they different?*
3. Errors of administration and adverse drug reactions are a continual threat for the elderly.
   A. *Explain common causes of inappropriate medication use in the elderly.*

References

1. Statistics Canada. (2012). The Canadian population in 2011: Age and Sex Catalogue No. 98–311-X2011001. Available online at: http://www12.statcan.gc.ca/census-recensement/2011/as-sa/98–311-x/98–311-x2011001-eng.pdf. Accessed October 16, 2013.
2. Health Canada. (2002). Canada's aging population. Available online at: http://publications.gc.ca/collections/Collection/H39–608–2002E.pdf. Accessed October 16, 2013.
3. Milan A., Vezina M. (2011). Senior women Catalogue NO. 89–503-X. Available online at: http://www.statcan.gc.ca/pub/89–503-x/2010001/article/11441-eng.pdf. Accessed October 16, 2013.
4. Statistics Canada. (2012). Life expectancy, at birth and at age 65. Available online at: http://www.statcan.gc.ca/tables-tableaux/sum-som/l01/cst01/health72a-eng.htm. Accessed September 4, 2013.
5. Lange J., Grossman S. (2010). Theories of aging. In Mauk K. L. (Ed.), *Gerontological nursing competencies for care* (2nd ed.), pp. 50–73). Sudbury, MA: Jones and Bartlett Publishers.
6. Wheeler H. E., Kim S. K. (2011). Genetics and genomics of human ageing. *Philosophical Transactions of the Royal Society, 2011, 366,* 43–50.
7. Hayflick L., Moorehead P. S. (1965). The limited in vitro lifetime of human diploid cell strains. *Experimental Cell Research, 37,* 614–636.
8. Zanni G. R., Wick J. Y. (2011). Telomeres: Unlocking the mystery of cell division and aging. *The Consultant Pharmacist, 26,* 78–90.
9. Mai P. L., Nilanjan C., Hartge P., et al. (2009). Potential excess mortality in *BRCA1/2* mutation carriers beyond breast, ovarian, prostate, and pancreatic cancers, and melanoma. *PLoS ONE, 4,* e4812. doi:10.1371/journal.pone.0004812.
10. Vasunilashorn S., Crimmins E. M. (2009). Biodemography: Integrating disciplines to explain aging. In Bengston V. L, Gans D, Putney N. M, et al. (Eds.), *Handbook of theories of aging* (2nd ed., pp. 63–85). New York: Springer Publishing Company.
11. Kane R. L., Ouslander J. G., Abrass I. B., et al. (2009). *Essentials of clinical geriatrics* (6th ed.). New York: McGraw-Hill.

12. Veysey E., Finlay A. Y. (2010). Aging and the skin. In Fillit H. M., Rockwood K., Woodhouse K. (Eds.), *Brocklehurst's textbook of geriatric medicine and gerontology.* (7th ed., pp. 133–137). Philadelphia, PA: Saunders.

13. Zouboulis C. C., Makrantonaki E. (2011). Clinical aspects and molecular diagnostics of skin aging. *Clinics in Dermatology, 29,* 3–14.

14. Eliopoulos C. (2010). *Gerontological nursing* (7th ed.). Philadelphia, PA: Walters Kluwer Health/Lippincott Williams & Wilkins.

15. Patel G. A., Gangaram R., Lambert W. C., et al. (2010). Skin disease and old age. In Fillit H. M., Rockwood K., Woodhouse K. (Eds.), *Brocklehurst's textbook of geriatric medicine and gerontology* (7th ed., pp. 801–809). Philadelphia, PA: Saunders.

16. Gregson C. L. (2010). Bone and joint aging. In Fillit H. M., Rockwood K., Woodhouse K. (Eds.), *Brocklehurst's textbook of geriatric medicine and gerontology* (7th ed., pp. 117–122). Philadelphia, PA: Saunders.

17. Bello-Haas V. D. (2009). Neuromusculoskeletal and movement function. In Bonder B. R., Bello-Haas V. (Eds.), *Functional performance in older adults* (3rd ed., pp. 130–176). Philadelphia, PA: F.A. Davis Company.

18. Osteoporosis Canada. (2013). Osteoporosis facts and statistics. Available online at: http://www.osteoporosis.ca. Accessed October 16, 2013.

19. Howlett S. E. (2010). Effects of aging on the cardiovascular system. In Fillit H. M., Rockwood K., Woodhouse K. (Eds.), *Brocklehurst's textbook of geriatric medicine and gerontology* (7th ed., pp. 91–96). Philadelphia, PA: Saunders.

20. Lee H. Y., Oh B. H. (2010). Aging and arterial stiffness. *Circulation Journal, 74,* 2257–2262.

21. Potter J. F. (2010). Hypertension. In Fillit H. M., Rockwood K., Woodhouse K. (Eds.), *Brocklehurst's textbook of geriatric medicine and gerontology.* (7th ed., pp. 300–311). Philadelphia, PA: Saunders.

22. Kim S. J., Lee J., Jee S. H., et al. (2010). Cardiovascular risk factors for incident hypertension in the prehypertensive population. *Epidemiology and Health, 32,* e2010003. doi:10.4178/epih/e2010003.

23. Kenny R. A. (2010). Syncope. In Fillit H. M., Rockwood K., Woodhouse K. (Eds.), *Brocklehurst's textbook of geriatric medicine and gerontology* (7th ed., pp. 338–347). Philadelphia, PA: Saunders.

24. Rich, M. W. (2013). Chapter 48: Cardiovascular disease and disorders. In Durso, S. C., Sullivan, G. M. (Eds), *Geriatric review syllabus.* (8th ed.) New York, NY: American Geriatric Society.

25. Heineman J. M., Hamrick-King J., Sewell B. S. (2010). Review of the aging of physiological systems. In Mauk K. L., (Ed.). *Gerontological nursing competencies for care* (2nd ed., pp. 128–231). Sudbury, MA: Jones and Bartlett Publishers.

26. Miller M. R. (2010). Structural and physiological age-associated changes in aging lungs. *Seminars in Respiratory and Critical Care Medicine, 31,* 521–527.

27. Shankar S. K. (2010). Biology of aging brain. *Indian Journal of Pathology & Microbiology, 53,* 595–604.

28. Tarawneh R., Galvin J. E. (2010). Neurologic signs in the elderly. In Fillit H. M., Rockwood K., Woodhouse K. (Eds.), *Brocklehurst's textbook of geriatric medicine and gerontology* (7th ed., pp. 101–105). Philadelphia, PA: Saunders.

29. Hooper C. R., Bello-Haas V. D. (2009). Sensory function. In Bonder B. R., Bello-Haas V. (Eds.), *Functional performance in older adults* (3rd ed., pp. 101–129). Philadelphia, PA: F.A. Davis Company.

30. Weinstein B. E. (2010). Disorders of hearing. In Fillit H. M., Rockwood K., Woodhouse K. (Eds.), *Brocklehurst's textbook of geriatric medicine and gerontology* (7th ed., pp. 822–834). Philadelphia, PA: Saunders.

31. Tummala M. K., Taub D. D., Ershler W. B. (2010). Clinical immunology: Immune senescence and the acquired immune deficiency of aging. In Fillit H. M., Rockwood K., Woodhouse K. (Eds.), *Brocklehurst's textbook of geriatric medicine and gerontology* (7th ed., pp. 82–90). Philadelphia, PA: Saunders.

32. Feldstein R. C., Tepper R. E., Katz S. (2010). Geriatric gastroenterology: Overview. In Fillit H. M., Rockwood K., Woodhouse K. (Eds.), *Brocklehurst's textbook of geriatric medicine and gerontology* (7th ed., pp. 106–110). Philadelphia, PA: Saunders.

33. Videl-Alaball J., Butler C. C., Cannings-John R., et al. (2009). Oral vitamin B12 versus intramuscular vitamin B12 for vitamin B12 deficiency (Review). *Cochrane Database of Systematic Reviews,* (31):CD004655.

34. Wald A. (2010). The large bowel. In Fillit H. M., Rockwood K., Woodhouse K. (Eds.), *Brocklehurst's textbook of geriatric medicine and gerontology* (7th ed., pp. 661–677). Philadelphia, PA: Saunders.

35. Harari D. (2010). Constipation and fecal incontinence in old age. In Fillit H. M., Rockwood K., Woodhouse K. (Eds.), *Brocklehurst's textbook of geriatric medicine and gerontology.* (7th ed., pp. 909–925). Philadelphia, PA: Saunders.

36. Weinstein J. R., Anderson S. (2010). The aging kidney: Physiological changes. *Advances in Chronic Kidney Disease, 17,* 302–307.

37. Munang L. A, Starr J. M. (2010). Diseases of the aging kidney. In Fillit H. M., Rockwood K., Woodhouse K. (Eds.), *Brocklehurst's textbook of geriatric medicine and gerontology* (7th ed., pp. 690–696). Philadelphia, PA: Saunders.

38. Razzaque M. S. (2010). Disorders of water, electrolyte, and mineral ion metabolism. In Fillit H. M., Rockwood K., Woodhouse K. (Eds.), *Brocklehurst's textbook of geriatric medicine and gerontology* (7th ed., 697–700). Philadelphia, PA: Saunders.

39. Cooper T. K., Smith O. M. (2010). Gynecologic disorders in the elderly. In Fillit H. M, Rockwood K., Woodhouse K. (Eds.), *Brocklehurst's textbook of geriatric medicine and gerontology.* (7th ed., pp. 716–725). Philadelphia, PA: Saunders.

40. Bettez M., Tu L. M., Carlson K., et al. (2012). 2012 Update: Guidelines for adult urinary incontinence. *Canadian Urological Association journal, 6*(5), 354–363.

41. Cunningham G. R., Toma S. M. (2011). Why is androgen replacement in males controversial? *Journal of Clinical Endocrinology & Metabolism, 96,* 38–52.

42. Katz S., Downs T. D., Cash H. R., Grotz R. C. (1970). Progress in development of the Index of ADL. *Gerontologist, 10,* 20–30.

43. Chervenak J. L. (2010). Reproductive aging, sexuality and symptoms. *Seminars in Reproductive Medicine, 28,* 380–387.

44. Butler R. N., Lewis M. I. (2010). Sexuality in old age. In Fillit H. M., Rockwood K., Woodhouse K. (Eds.), *Brocklehurst's textbook of geriatric medicine and gerontology.* (7th ed., pp. 854–858). Philadelphia, PA: Saunders.

45. Katz S., Ford A. B., Jackson B. A., et al. (1963). Studies of illness in the aged: The Index of ADL. *Journal of the American Medical Association, 185*:914–919.

46. Lawton M. P., Brody E. M. (1969). Assessment of older people: Self-maintaining and instrumental activities of daily living. *Gerontologist, 9,* 179–186.

47. The Canadian Continence Foundation. (2009). Impacts of incontinence in Canada.. Available online at: http://www.canadiancontinence.ca/pdf/impacts-of-incontinence.pdf. Accessed October 16, 2013.

48. Aguzzi G., Simona B., Rosanna T. (2010). Systematic review of urinary incontinence and overactive bladder cost-of-illness studies. *The Open Pharmacoeconomic & Health Economics Journal, 2*:11–24.

49. Markland A. D., Vaughan C. P., Johnson T. M., et al. (2011). Incontinence. *Medical Clinics of North America, 95,* 539–554.

50. Scott V., Gallagher E., Higginson A., et al. (2011). Evaluation of an evidence-based education program for health professionals. *Journal of Safety Research, 42,* 501–507.

51. Statistics Canada. (2009). Leading causes of death in Canada, Table 3 [Online]. Available online at: http://www.statcan.gc.ca/pub/84-215-x/2012001/table-tableau/tbl003-eng.htm. Accessed October 17, 2013.

52. Diebold C., Fanning-Harding F., Hanson P. (2010). Management of common problems. In Mauk K. L. (Ed.). *Gerontological nursing competencies for care.* (2nd ed., pp. 454–528.). Sudbury, MA: Jones and Bartlett Publishers.

53. Studenski S. A. (2010). Falls. In Fillit H. M., Rockwood K., Woodhouse K. (Eds.), *Brocklehurst's textbook of geriatric medicine and gerontology.* (7th ed., pp. 894–902.) Philadelphia, PA: Saunders.

54. Dhital A., Pey T., Stanford M. R. (2010). Visual loss and falls: A review. *Eye, 24,* 1437–1446.

55. Setti A., Burke K. E., Kenny R. A., Newell F. N. (2011). Is inefficient multisensory processing associated with falls in older people? *Experimental Brain Research, 209,* 375–384.

56. Annweiler C., Montero-Odasso M., Schott A. M., et al. (2010). Fall prevention and vitamin D in the elderly: An overview of the key role of the non-bone effects. *Journal of Neuroengineering and Rehabilitation, 5,* 50. doi:10.1186/1743-0003-7-50.

57. Schneider J. M., Gopinath B., McMahon C. M., et al. (2011). Dual sensory impairment in older age. *Journal of Aging and Health, 23*(8), 1309–1324.

58. Brunelle S., Cole M. G., Elie M. (2011). Risk factors for the late-onset psychoses: A systematic review of cohort studies. *International journal of geriatric psychiatry, 27*(3), 240–252.

59. Schadlu A. P., Schadlu R., Shepard III J. B. (2009). Charles Bonnet Syndrome: A review. *Current Opinion in Ophthalmology, 10*, 219–222.

60. Katona C., Livingston G., Cooper C. (2010). Functional psychiatric illness in old age. In Fillit H. M., Rockwood K., Woodhouse K. (Eds.), *Brocklehurst's textbook of geriatric medicine and gerontology.* (7th ed., pp. 433–444.). Philadelphia, PA: Saunders.

61. Chen R., Copeland J. (2011). Epidemiology of depression: Prevalence and incidence. In Abou-Saleh M. T., Katona C., Kumar A. (Eds.), *Principles and practice of geriatric psychiatry* (3rd ed., pp. 479–488). West Sussex: Wiley.

62. American Psychiatric Association. (2013). *Diagnostic and statistical manual of mental disorders* (5th ed.). Arlington, VA: American Psychiatric Publishing; 2013.

63. Hermida A. P., McDonald W. M. (2011). The assessment of depressive symptoms. In Abou-Saleh M. T., Katona C., Kumar A. (Eds.), *Principles and practice of geriatric psychiatry* (3rd ed., pp. 565–572). West Sussex: Wiley.

64. Evans, M. (2011). Physical illness and depression. In Abou-Saleh M. T., Katona C., Kumar A. (Eds.), *Principles and practice of geriatric psychiatry* (3rd ed., pp. 508–514). West Sussex: Wiley.

65. Knapp P., House A. (2011). Depression after stroke. In Abou-Saleh M. T., Katona C., Kumar A. (Eds.), *Principles and practice of geriatric psychiatry* (3rd ed., pp. 515–517). West Sussex: Wiley.

66. Draper B. (2011). Suicidal behavior. In Abou-Saleh M. T., Katona C., Kumar A. (Eds.), *Principles and practice of geriatric psychiatry* (3rd ed., pp. 559–564). West Sussex: Wiley.

67. Lapierre S., Erlangsen A., Waern M., et al.; International Research Group for Suicide among the Elderly. (2011). A systematic review of elderly suicide prevention programs. *Crisis, 32*, 88–98.

68. Debruyne H., Van Buggenhout M., Le Bastard N., et al. (2009). Is the geriatric depression scale a reliable screening tool for depressive symptoms in elderly patients with cognitive impairment? *International Journal of Geriatric Psychiatry, 24*, 556–562.

69. Abou-Saleh M. T., Katona C. (2011). Pharmacological treatment of depression. In Abou-Saleh M. T., Katona C., Kumar A. (Eds.), *Principles and practice of geriatric psychiatry* (3rd ed., pp. 537–542). West Sussex: Wiley.

70. Mukai Y., Tampi R. R. (2009). Treatment of depression in the elderly: A review of the recent literature on the efficacy of single- versus dual-action antidepressants. *Clinical Therapeutics, 31*, 945–961.

71. Wilkinson D. G. (2011). Electroconvulsive therapy (ECT). In Abou-Saleh M. T., Katona C., Kumar A. (Eds.), *Principles and practice of geriatric psychiatry* (3rd ed., pp. 529–536). West Sussex: Wiley.

72. Wilkinson P. (2011). Psychotherapy of depression and dysthymia. In Abou-Saleh M. T., Katona C., Kumar A. (Eds.), *Principles and practice of geriatric psychiatry* (3rd ed., pp. 543–551). West Sussex: Wiley.

73. Alzheimer Society of Canada. (2012). Facts about dementia. Available online at: http://www.alzheimer.ca/en/About-dementia/Dementias/What-is-dementia/Facts-about-dementia. Accessed October 17, 2013.

74. Rossini P. M., Parisi L. (2011). Neurophysiology of the aging brain. In Abou-Saleh M. T., Katona C., Kumar A. (Eds.), *Principles and practice of geriatric psychiatry* (3rd ed., pp. 36–41). West Sussex: Wiley.

75. Dickstein D. L., Morrison J. H., Hof P. R. (2009). Neuropathology of aging. In Jagust W., D'Esposito M. (Eds.), *Imaging the aging brain* (pp. 27–40). New York: Oxford University Press.

76. Monsuez J. J., Gesquière-Dando A., Rivera S. (2011). Cardiovascular prevention of cognitive decline. *Cardiology Research and Practice, 2011*, 250970. doi: 10.4061/2011/250970.

77. Sharp S., Aarsland D., Day S., et al. Alzheimer's Society Vascular Dementia Systematic Review Group. (2010). Hypertension is a powerful risk factor for vascular dementia: Systematic review. *International Journal of Geriatric Psychiatry, 26*, 661–669.

78. Skoog I. (2011). Vascular dementia. In Abou-Saleh M. T., Katona C., Kumar A. (Eds.), *Principles and practice of geriatric psychiatry* (3rd ed., pp. 342–347). West Sussex: Wiley.

79. Donix M., Bookheimer S. Y., Small G. W. (2011). Physiological neuro-imaging in ageing and dementia: Metabolic and molecular scanning. In Abou-Saleh M. T., Katona C., Kumar A. (Eds.), *Principles and practice of geriatric psychiatry* (3rd ed., pp. 256–261). West Sussex: Wiley.

80. Nasreddine Z. S., Phillips N. A., Bédirian V., et al. (2005). The Montreal Cognitive Assessment. Available online at: http://www.mocatest.org/. Accessed December 10, 2008.

81. Folstein M. F., Folstein B. E., McHugh P. R. (1975). "Mini-Mental State": A practical method for grading the cognitive state of patients for the clinician. *Journal of Psychiatric Research, 12*:189–198.

82. Steinberg M., Lyketsos C. G. (2011). Pharmacological therapies in Alzheimer's disease. In Abou-Saleh M. T., Katona C., Kumar A. (Eds.), *Principles and practice of geriatric psychiatry* (3rd ed., pp. 304–311). West Sussex: Wiley.

83. Jones R. W. (2011). Drug treatment for people with dementia. *Clinical Medicine, 11*, 67–71.

84. Schneider L. S., Dagerman K. S., Higgins J. P. T., McShane R. (2011). Lack of evidence for the efficacy of memantine in mild Alzheimer disease. *Archives of Neurology, 68*, 991–998.

85. Tschanz J. T., Breitner J. C. S. (2011). Alzheimer's disease: Risk factors and preventive strategies. In Abou-Saleh M. T., Katona C., Kumar A. (Eds.), *Principles and practice of geriatric psychiatry* (3rd ed., pp. 271–280). West Sussex: Wiley.

86. Birks J., Grimley Evans J. (2009). Ginkgo biloba for cognitive impairment and dementia. *Cochrane Database of Systematic Reviews*, (1), CD003120.

87. Dangour A. D., Whitehouse P. J., Rafferty K., et al. (2010). B-Vitamins and fatty acids in the prevention and treatment of Alzheimer's disease and dementia: A systematic review. *Journal of Alzheimer's Disease, 22*, 205–224.

88. Miller K., Ercoli L., Kim J., et al. (2011). Memory training for older adults. In Abou-Saleh M. T., Katona C., Kumar A. (Eds.), *Principles and practice of geriatric psychiatry* (3rd ed., pp. 397–402.). West Sussex: Wiley.

89. Tseng C. N., Gau B. S., Lou M. F. (2011). The effectiveness of exercise on improving cognitive function in older people: A systematic review. *Journal of Nursing Research, 19*, 119–130.

90. Smith M., Gerdner L. A., Hall G. R., Buckwalter K. C. (2004). History, development and future of the progressively lowered stress threshold: A conceptual model for dementia care. *Journal of the American Geriatrics Society, 52*, 1755–1760.

91. Flaherty J. H. (2011). The evaluation and management of delirium among older persons. *Medical Clinics of North America, 95*, 555–577.

92. Ouldred E., Bryant C. (2011). Delirium: Prevention, clinical features and management. *Nursing Standard, 25*, 47–56.

93. Mittal V., Muralee S., Williamson D., et al. (2011). Delirium in the elderly: A comprehensive review. *American Journal of Alzheimer's Disease & Other Dementias, 26*, 97–109.

94. Inouye S. K., Van Dyck C. H., Alessi C. A., et al. (1990). Clarifying confusion: The confusion assessment method. *Annals of Internal Medicine, 113*, 941–948.

95. Kamholz B. (2011). Delirium. In Abou-Saleh M. T., Katona C., Kumar A. (Eds.), *Principles and practice of geriatric psychiatry* (3rd ed., pp. 195–200.). West Sussex: Wiley.

96. Corsonello A., Pedone C., Incalzi R. A. (2010). Age-related pharmacokinetic and pharmacodynamic changes and related risk of adverse drug reactions. *Current Medicinal Chemistry, 17*, 571–584.

97. Klotz U. (2009). Pharmacokinetics and drug metabolism in the elderly. *Drug Metabolism Reviews, 41*, 67–76.

98. Page R. L., Linnebur S. A., Bryant L. L., Ruscin J. M. (2010). Inappropriate prescribing in the hospitalized elderly patient: Defining the problem, evaluation tools, and possible solutions. *Clinical Interventions in Aging, 5*, 75–87.

99. Levy H. B., Marcus E. L., Christen C. (2010). Beyond the beers criteria: A comparative overview of explicit criteria. *The Annals of Pharmacotherapy, 44*, 1968–1975.

Visit thePoint **http://thePoint.lww.com for animations, journal articles, and more!**

Unit II

Cell Function and Growth

With its elegant structure and astonishing range of functions, the living cell is an object of wonder. It is the basic unit of all living organisms. There are more than 300 trillion cells in the human body, and every second of every day, more than 10 million die and are replaced.

In 1665, these impressive structures were named. While examining a thin slice of cork, Robert Hooke (1635 to 1703), an English scientist and pioneer microscopist, noted that it was made up of tiny boxlike units. The units reminded him of the small enclosures in which monks lived, and he named the microscopic spaces "cells," from the Latin word cells, meaning "small enclosures."

Although Hooke, as well as other scientists, intently studied microscopic life, few guessed the significance of the cells. That would be delayed until microscopes were advanced enough to yield more detailed information. It was with the work of Anton van Leeuwenhoek (1632 to 1723), a Dutch biologist and microscopist, that the mysteries and importance of the cell were revealed. He ground a single lens to such perfection that he was able to produce a microscope with great resolving power—one that was capable of magnifying a specimen from approximately 50 to 300 times in diameter. Van Leeuwenhoek's work, which included constructing an aquatic microscope that he used to study red blood cells and their flow through the body, was responsible for helping scientists investigate human tissue in ways that once they only dreamed of.

Cell and Tissue Characteristics

4

In most organisms, the *cell* is the smallest functional unit that can retain the characteristics necessary for life. Cells are organized into larger functional units called *tissues,* based on their embryonic origin. These tissues, in turn, combine to form the various body structures and organs. Although the cells of different tissues and organs vary in structure and function, certain characteristics are common to all cells. Cells are remarkably similar in their ability to exchange materials with their immediate environment, obtain energy from organic nutrients, synthesize complex molecules, and replicate themselves. Because most disease processes are initiated at the cellular level, an understanding of cell function is crucial to understanding the disease process. Some diseases affect the cells of a single organ, while others affect the cells of a particular tissue type, and still others affect the cells of the entire organism. This chapter discusses the structural and functional components of the cell, integration of cell function and growth, movement of molecules such as ions across the cell membrane, and parenchymal tissue types.

FUNCTIONAL COMPONENTS OF THE CELL

After completing this section of the chapter, you should be able to meet the following objectives:

- State why the nucleus is called the "control centre" of the cell.
- State the functions of the cellular organelles.
- State four functions of the cell membrane.

Although diverse in their organization, all eukaryotic cells have in common structures that perform unique functions. Eukaryotic cells are larger and have more specific parts in compartments divided by membranes called organelles. The prokaryotic cells do not have compartments and they do not possess a demarcated nucleus as the eukaryotes do. When seen under a light microscope, three major components of the cell become evident: the nucleus, the cytoplasm, and the cell membrane in the eukaryotic cells (Fig. 4.1).

Nucleus
Nuclear pore
Nucleoplasm
Chromatin
Nucleolus
Nuclear envelope

Ribosome
Rough endoplasmic reticulum
Peroxisome
Smooth endoplasmic reticulum
Cytoskeleton
Centriole (2 centrosomes)
Protein

Golgi apparatus
Cytosol
Cell membrane
Mitochondrion
Lysosome
Vesicle

FIGURE 4.1 • Composite cell designed to show in one cell all of the various components of the nucleus and cytoplasm. (From McConnell T. H., Hull K. L. (2011). *Human form human function: Essentials of anatomy and physiology* (p. 70). Philadelphia, PA: Lippincott Williams & Wilkins.)

Protoplasm

Biologists call the internal matrix of the cell *protoplasm.* Protoplasm is composed of water, proteins, lipids, carbohydrates, and electrolytes. Two distinct regions of protoplasm exist in the cell: the *cytoplasm,* which lies outside the nucleus, and the *karyoplasm* or *nucleoplasm,* which lies inside the nucleus.

Water makes up 70% to 85% of the cell's protoplasm. The second most abundant constituent (10% to 20%) of protoplasm are the cell proteins, which form cell structures and the enzymes necessary for cellular reactions. Proteins can be bound to other compounds to form nucleoproteins, glycoproteins, and lipoproteins. Lipids comprise 2% to 3% of most

cells. The most important lipids are the phospholipids and cholesterol, which are mainly insoluble in water; they combine with proteins to form the cell membrane and the membranous barriers that separate different cell compartments. Some cells also contain large quantities of triglycerides. In fat cells, triglycerides can comprise up to 95% of the total cell mass. This fat represents stored energy, which can be mobilized and used wherever it is needed in the body. Only a few carbohydrates (~1%) are found in the cell and these serve primarily as a rapid source of energy.[1] Potassium, magnesium, phosphate, sulphate, and bicarbonate ions are the major intracellular electrolytes. Small quantities of sodium, chloride, and calcium ions are also present in the cell. These electrolytes participate in reactions that are necessary for the cell's metabolism and assist in the generation and transmission of electrochemical impulses in nerve and muscle cells.

THE FUNCTIONAL ORGANIZATION OF THE CELL

- Cells are the smallest functional unit of the body.
- The nucleus is the control centre for the cell. It also contains most of the hereditary material.
- The organelles, which are analogous to the organs of the body, are contained in the cytoplasm. They include the mitochondria, which supply the energy needs of the cell; the ribosomes, which synthesize proteins and other materials needed for cell function; and the lysosomes and proteosomes, which function as the cell's digestive system.
- The cell membrane encloses the cell and provides for intracellular and intercellular communication, transport of materials into and out of the cell, and maintenance of the electrical activities that power cell function.

The Nucleus

The nucleus of the cell appears as a rounded or elongated structure situated near the centre of the cell (Fig. 4.1). All human cells are eukaryotic cells, which have at least one nucleus (prokaryotic cells, such as bacteria, lack a nucleus and nuclear membrane). Some cells contain more than one nucleus; for example, osteoclasts (a type of bone cell) typically contain 12 or more nuclei. The platelet-producing cell, the megakaryocyte, has only 1 nucleus but usually contains 16 times the normal chromatin amount.

The nucleus can be regarded as the control centre for the cell.[1] It contains the deoxyribonucleic acid (DNA) that is essential to the cell because its genes encode the information necessary for the synthesis of proteins that the cell must produce to stay alive. These proteins include structural proteins and enzymes used to synthesize other substances, including carbohydrates and lipids. Genes also represent the individual units of inheritance that transmit information from one generation to another. The nucleus is the site for the synthesis of the three types of ribonucleic acid (messenger RNA, ribosomal RNA, and transfer RNA) that move to the cytoplasm and carry out the actual synthesis of proteins. Messenger RNA (mRNA) copies and carries the DNA instructions for protein synthesis to the cytoplasm; ribosomal RNA (rRNA) is the site of protein synthesis; and transfer RNA (tRNA) transports amino acids to the site of proteins synthesis for incorporation into the protein being synthesized.[1]

Chromatin is the term denoting the complex structure of DNA and DNA-associated proteins dispersed in the nuclear matrix. Depending on its transcriptional activity, chromatin may be condensed as an inactive form of chromatin called *heterochromatin* or extended as a more active form called *euchromatin.* Because heterochromatic regions of the nucleus stain more intensely than regions consisting of euchromatin, nuclear staining can be a guide to cell activity. Evidence suggests a relationship between alterations in the chromatin, along with DNA hypermethylation, that occurs during neoplastic progression. It seems both of these processes work symbiotically not separately in their role regarding cancer.[2]

The nucleus also contains the darkly stained round body called the *nucleolus.*[1] Although nucleoli were first described in 1781, their function was unknown until the early 1960s, when it was determined that the processing of rRNA and its assembly into ribosomes occurs exclusively in the nucleolus. Nucleoli are structures composed of regions from five different chromosomes, each with a part of the genetic code needed for the synthesis of rRNA. Euchromatic nuclei and prominent nucleoli are characteristic of cells that are actively synthesizing proteins.

Surrounding the nucleus is the *nuclear envelope,* formed by two (outer and inner) nuclear membranes containing a perinuclear cisternal space between them.[1] The inner nuclear membrane is supported by a rigid network of protein filaments that bind to chromosomes and secure their position in the nucleus. The outer nuclear membrane resembles the membrane of the endoplasmic reticulum (ER) and is continuous with it. The nuclear envelope contains many structurally complex circular pores where the two membranes fuse to form a gap filled with a thin protein diaphragm.[1] Many classes of molecules, including fluids, electrolytes, RNA, some proteins, and hormones, can move in both directions through the nuclear pores. Nuclear pores apparently regulate the bidirectional exchange of molecules between the cytoplasm and the nucleus.[1]

The Cytoplasm and Its Organelles

The cytoplasm surrounds the nucleus, and it is in the cytoplasm that cellular work and function occur. Cytoplasm is essentially a colloidal solution that contains water, electrolytes, suspended proteins, neutral fats, and glycogen molecules.[1] Although not contributing to the cell's function, pigments may also accumulate in the cytoplasm. Some pigments, such as melanin, which gives skin its colour, are normal constituents of the cell. Bilirubin is a normal major pigment of bile; its excess accumulation in cells is evidenced clinically by a yellowish discolouration of the skin and sclera, a condition called *jaundice.*

Embedded within the cytoplasm are various *organelles,* which function as the organs of the cell. These organelles are separated from the cytoplasm by their own membrane. They include the ribosomes, ER, Golgi complex, mitochondria, and lysosomes.[1]

Ribosomes

The ribosomes serve as sites of protein synthesis in the cell. They are small particles of nucleoproteins (rRNA and

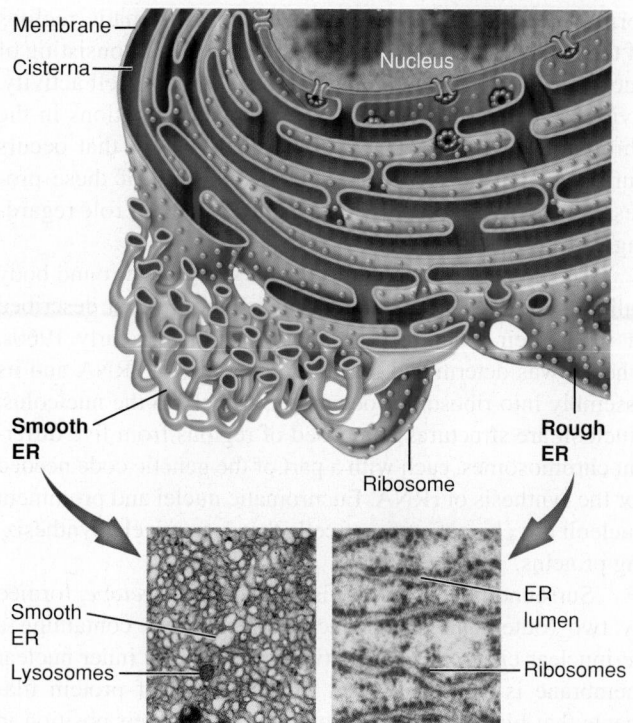

Membrane

Cisterna

Nucleus

Smooth ER

Rough ER

Ribosome

Smooth ER

Lysosomes

ER lumen

Ribosomes

FIGURE 4.2 • Types of endoplasmic reticulum and ribosomes. The rough ER consists of intricately folded membranes studded with ribosomes. Ribosomes are made of protein and rRNA organized together. (From McConnell T. H., Hull K. L. (2011). *Human form human function: Essentials of anatomy & physiology* (p. 72). Philadelphia, PA: Lippincott Williams & Wilkins.)

proteins) that are held together by a strand of mRNA to form polyribosomes (also called *polysomes*). Polyribosomes exist as isolated clusters of free ribosomes within the cytoplasm (Fig. 4.2) or attached to the membrane of the ER. Free ribosomes are involved in the synthesis of proteins, mainly enzymes that aid in the control of cell function, whereas those attached to the ER translate mRNAs that code for proteins secreted from the cell or stored within the cell (*e.g.,* granules in white blood cells).[1]

Endoplasmic Reticulum

The ER is an extensive system of paired membranes and flat vesicles that connect various parts of the inner cell (Fig. 4.2). Between the paired ER membranes is a fluid-filled space called the *matrix*.[1] The matrix connects the space between the two membranes of the nuclear envelope, the cell membrane, and various cytoplasmic organelles. It functions as a tubular communication system for transporting various substances from one part of the cell to another. A large surface area and multiple enzyme systems attached to the ER membranes also provide the machinery for a major share of the cell's metabolic functions.

Two forms of ER exist in cells: rough and smooth. *Rough ER* is studded with ribosomes attached to specific binding sites on the membrane. Proteins produced by the rough ER are usually destined to become components of lysosomes or other

organelles, be incorporated into cell membranes, or leave the cell as a secretory protein. The rough ER segregates these proteins from other components of the cytoplasm and modifies their structure for a specific function. For example, the synthesis of both digestive enzymes by pancreatic acinar cells and plasma proteins by liver cells takes place in the rough ER. All cells require a rough ER for the synthesis of lysosomal enzymes.

The *smooth ER* is free of ribosomes and is continuous with nuclear envelope. It does not participate in protein synthesis; instead, its enzymes are involved in the synthesis of lipid molecules, regulation of intracellular calcium, and metabolism and detoxification of certain hormones and drugs. It is the site of lipid, lipoprotein, and steroid hormone synthesis. The sarcoplasmic reticulum of skeletal and cardiac muscle cells is a form of smooth ER. Calcium ions needed for muscle contraction are stored and released from cisternae of the sarcoplasmic reticulum. The smooth ER of the liver is involved in glycogen storage and metabolism of lipid-soluble drugs.

Researchers are determining links between the ER and various disease processes. For example, ER stress in the gastrointestinal system has been found to be related to intestinal inflammation such as that occurs with inflammatory bowel disease.[3] Diabetes has also been linked to ER stress, which may be related to loss of pancreatic beta cell mass.[4] With myositis there is evidence that immune and nonimmune factors are the etiology of the muscle weakness.[5] The ER is being studied to determine if the dysregulation of calcium from the ER causes an increase or a decrease in the muscle weakness.[5]

Golgi Complex

The Golgi apparatus, sometimes called the *Golgi complex,* consists of stacks of thin, flattened vesicles or sacs (Fig. 4.2).[1] These Golgi bodies are found near the nucleus and function in association with the ER. Substances produced in the ER are carried to the Golgi complex in small, membrane-covered transfer vesicles. Many cells synthesize proteins that are larger than the active product. The Golgi complex modifies these substances and packages them into secretory granules or vesicles. Insulin, for example, is synthesized as a large, inactive proinsulin molecule that is cut apart to produce a smaller, active insulin molecule within the Golgi complex of the beta cells in the pancreas. In addition to producing secretory granules, the Golgi complex is thought to produce large carbohydrate molecules that combine with proteins produced in the rough ER to form glycoproteins. Recent data suggest that the Golgi apparatus complex has yet another function: it can receive proteins and other substances from the cell surface by a retrograde transport mechanism. This retrograde pathway has been exploited by several bacterial toxins, such as Shiga and cholera toxins, and plant toxins, such as ricin, that have cytoplasmic targets.

Lysosomes and Peroxisomes

Lysosomes can be viewed as the digestive system of the cell. These small, membrane-enclosed sacs contain powerful

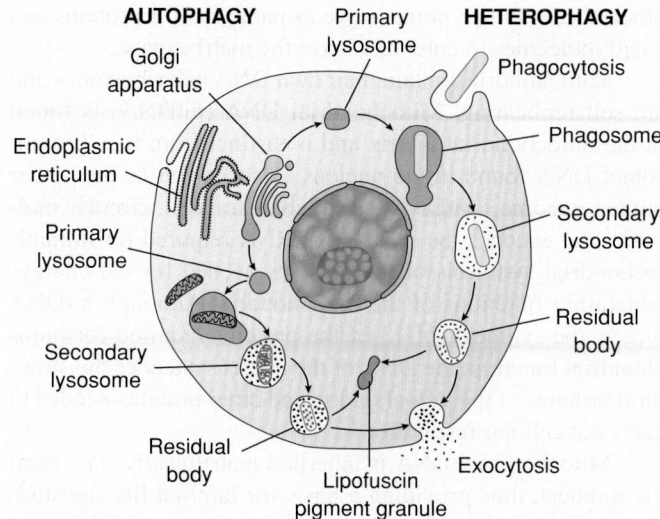

FIGURE 4.3 • The processes of autophagy and heterophagy, showing the primary and secondary lysosomes, residual bodies, extrusion of residual body contents from the cell, and lipofuscin-containing residual bodies.

hydrolytic enzymes. These enzymes can break down excess and worn-out cell parts as well as foreign substances that are taken into the cell. All of the lysosomal enzymes are acid hydrolases, which means they require an acidic environment. The lysosomes provide this environment by maintaining a pH of approximately 5 in their interior. The pH of the cytoplasm, which is approximately 7.2, serves to protect other cellular structures from this acidity. *Primary lysosomes* are membrane-bound intracellular organelles that contain a variety of hydrolytic enzymes that have not yet entered the digestive process. They receive their enzymes as well as their membranes from the Golgi apparatus. Primary lysosomes become *secondary lysosomes* after they fuse with membrane-bound vacuoles that contain material to be digested. Lysosomes breakdown phagocytosed material by either heterophagy or autophagy (Fig. 4.3).

Heterophagy refers to digestion of an exogenous substance phagocytosed from the cell's external environment.[6] An infolding of the cell membrane takes external materials into the cell to form a surrounding phagocytic vesicle, or *phagosome*. Primary lysosomes then fuse with phagosomes to form secondary lysosomes. Heterophagocytosis is most common in phagocytic white blood cells such as neutrophils and macrophages. *Autophagy* involves the segregation and disposal of damaged cellular organelles, such as mitochondria or ER, which the lysosomes must remove if the cell's normal function is to continue.[6] Autophagocytosis is most pronounced in cells undergoing atrophy. Although enzymes in the secondary lysosomes can break down most proteins, carbohydrates, and lipids to their basic constituents, some materials remain undigested. These undigested materials may remain in the cytoplasm as *residual bodies* or are extruded from the cell by exocytosis. In some long-lived cells, such as neurons and heart muscle cells, large quantities of residual bodies accumulate as lipofuscin granules or age pigment. Other indigestible pigments, such as inhaled carbon particles and tattoo pigments, also accumulate and may persist in residual bodies for decades.

Lysosomes play an important role in the normal metabolism of certain substances in the body. In some inherited diseases known as *lysosomal storage diseases,* a specific lysosomal enzyme is absent or inactive, in which case the digestion of certain cellular substances (*e.g.,* glucocerebrosides, gangliosides, sphingomyelin) does not occur.[7] As a result, these substances accumulate in the cell. There are multiple lysosome storage diseases and an example is Tay–Sachs disease, an autosomal recessive disorder, in which hexosaminidase A, which is the lysosomal enzyme needed for degrading the GM_2 ganglioside found in nerve cell membranes, is deficient. Although GM_2 ganglioside accumulates in many tissues, such as the heart, liver, and spleen, its accumulation in the nervous system and retina of the eye causes the most damage.[7,8]

Smaller than lysosomes, spherical membrane-bound organelles called *peroxisomes* contain a special enzyme that degrades peroxides (*e.g.,* hydrogen peroxide). Unlike lysosomes, peroxisomes are not formed by the Golgi apparatus. Peroxisomes are self-replicating, like mitochondria, and are initially formed by proteins produced by free ribosomes. Peroxisomes function in the control of free radicals.[6] Unless degraded, these highly unstable chemical compounds would otherwise damage other cytoplasmic molecules. For example, catalase degrades toxic hydrogen peroxide molecules to water. Peroxisomes also contain the enzymes needed for breaking down very-long-chain fatty acids, which mitochondrial enzymes ineffectively degrade. In liver cells, peroxisomal enzymes are involved in the formation of the bile acids.[6]

Proteasomes

Three major cellular mechanisms are involved in the breakdown of proteins, or *proteolysis.* One of these is by the previously mentioned endosomal–lysosomal degradation. Another cytoplasmic degradation mechanism is the *caspase pathway* that is involved in apoptotic cell death. The third method of *proteolysis* occurs within an organelle called the *proteasome.* Proteasomes are small organelles composed of protein complexes that are thought to be present in both the cytoplasm and the nucleus. This organelle recognizes misformed and misfolded proteins including transcription factors and the cyclins that are important in controlling the cell cycle that have been tagged for degradation by a small protein ubiquitin. It has been suggested that as much as one third of the newly formed polypeptide chains are selected for proteasome degradation because of quality-control mechanisms in the cell.

Mitochondria

The mitochondria are literally the "power plants" of the cell because they transform organic compounds into energy that is easily accessible to the cell. They do not make energy, but extract it from organic compounds. Mitochondria contain the enzymes needed for converting energy from sugars, lipids, and proteins into cellular energy. This multi-step process within the mitochondria is often referred to as oxidative metabolism or *cellular respiration* because it requires oxygen.[1] Cells store most of this energy as high-energy phosphate bonds in compounds such as adenosine triphosphate (ATP), using it to power the various cellular activities. Mitochondria are found close to the site of energy consumption in the cell (*e.g.,* near the myofibrils in muscle cells). The number of mitochondria in a given cell type varies by the type of activity the cell performs and the energy needed to undertake this activity.[1] For example, skeletal muscle cells have an increased number of mitochondria due to their extensive demand for energy.

Mitochondria are composed of two membranes: an outer membrane that encloses the periphery of the mitochondrion and an inner membrane that forms shelflike projections, called *cristae* (Fig. 4.4). The narrow space between the outer and inner membranes is called the *intermembrane space,* whereas the large space enclosed by the inner membrane is termed the *matrix space.*[9] The outer mitochondrial membrane contains a large number of transmembrane porins, through which water-soluble molecules may pass. Because this membrane is relatively permeable to small molecules and proteins, the contents of the intermembrane space resembles that of the cytoplasm. The inner membrane contains the respiratory chain enzymes and transport proteins needed for the synthesis of ATP. In certain regions, the outer and inner membranes contact each

other; these contact points serve as pathways for proteins and small molecules to enter and leave the matrix space.

Mitochondria contain their own DNA and ribosomes and are self-replicating. Mitochondrial DNA (mtDNA) is found in the mitochondrial matrix and is distinct from the chromosomal DNA found in the nucleus. Also known as the "other human genome," mtDNA is a double-stranded, circular molecule that encodes the rRNA and tRNA required for intramitochondrial synthesis of the proteins needed for the energy-generating functions of the mitochondria. Although mtDNA directs the synthesis of 13 of the proteins required for mitochondrial function, the DNA of the nucleus encodes the structural proteins of the mitochondria and other proteins needed to carry out cellular respiration.[6,9]

Mitochondrial DNA is inherited matrilineally (*i.e.,* from the mother), thus providing a basis for familial lineage studies. Mutations have been found in each of the mitochondrial genes, and an understanding of the role of mtDNA in certain diseases is beginning to emerge (see Chapter 7). Most tissues in the body depend, to some extent, on oxidative metabolism and can therefore be affected by mtDNA mutations.[6]

Mitochondria also function as key regulators of apoptosis or programmed cell death (see Chapter 5). The initiation of the mitochondrial pathway for apoptosis results from an increase in mitochondrial permeability and the subsequent release of proapoptotic molecules into the cytoplasm. One of

Ribosome:
protein synthesis

DNA:
encodes some
mitochondrial
proteins

Matrix

Outer membrane

Inner membrane

Enzymes:
ATP generation

FIGURE 4.4 • Mitochondrion. The inner membrane forms transverse folds called *cristae,* where the enzymes needed for the final step in adenosine triphosphate (ATP) production (*i.e.,* oxidative phosphorylation) are located. (From McConnell T. H., Hull K. L. (2011). *Human form human function: Essentials of anatomy & physiology* (p. 74). Philadelphia, PA: Lippincott Williams & Wilkins.)

these proapoptotic molecules is cytochrome c, well known for its role in mitochondrial respiration. In the cytosol, cytochrome c binds to a protein called *apoptosis activating factor-1*, initiating the molecular events involved in the apoptosis cascade. Other apoptotic proteins also enter the cytoplasm, where they bind to and neutralize the various apoptotic inhibitors, whose normal function is to block the apoptotic cascade. Both the formation of reactive oxygen species (ROS) (*e.g.*, peroxide) and the activation of the *p53* tumour suppressor gene by DNA damage or other means initiate apoptotic signalling through the mitochondria. ROS has been determined to be the etiology of cell injury to multiple diseases.[10] Dysregulated apoptosis (too little or too much) has been implicated in a wide range of diseases, including cancer, in which there is an inappropriately low rate of apoptosis, and neurodegenerative diseases, in which there is an increased or excessive rate of apoptosis.

The Cytoskeleton

Besides its organelles, the cytoplasm contains a network of microtubules, microfilaments, intermediate filaments, and thick filaments (Fig. 4.5).[6] Because they control cell shape and movement, these structures are a major component of the

FIGURE 4.5 • Microtubules and microfilaments of the cell. The microfilaments are associated with the inner surface of the cell and aid in cell motility. The microtubules form the cytoskeleton and maintain the position of the organelles.

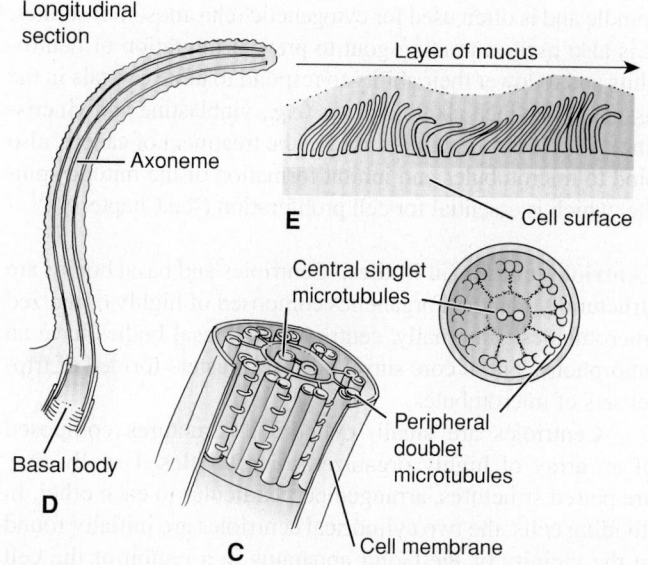

FIGURE 4.6 • **A:** The formation of a microtubule from tubulin dimers is indicated, showing the faster-growing end (+) and the slower-growing end (−). **B:** A cross-sectional view of a microtubule showing the 13 columns of spherical protofilaments. **C:** Structure of cilium, showing the nine sets of doublet microtubules surrounding a central pair of singlet microtubules. **D:** All of the microtubules are anchored to a basal body that is responsible for the formation of a core structure called the *axoneme*. **E:** The sweeping movements of cilia move the mucous layer of the respiratory tract. (**A** and **B** courtesy of Edward W. Carroll.)

structural elements called the *cytoskeleton*. The cytoskeleton also participates in the movement of entire cells.

Microtubules

Microtubules are formed from protein subunits called *tubulin*. They are long, stiff, hollow, cylindrical structures, 25 nm in outer diameter with a lumen 15 nm in diameter (Fig. 4.6). Each microtubule consists of parallel protofilaments, each composed of α- and β-tubulin dimers.[9] Microtubules are dynamic structures that can rapidly disassemble in one location and reassemble in another. During the reassembly process, the tubulin dimers polymerize in an end-to-end fashion to form protofilaments. As a result of the polymerization process, each microtubule possesses a nongrowing "minus" end and a rapidly growing "plus" end. During the disassembly process, the tubulin dimers dissociate from the protofilaments and form a pool of free tubulin in the cytoplasm. This pool is used in the polymerization process for reassembly of the protofilaments.[9]

Microtubules function in many ways, including the development and maintenance of cell form. They participate in intracellular transport mechanisms, including axoplasmic transport in neurons and melanin dispersion in pigment cells of the skin. Other functions include formation of the basic structure for several complex cytoplasmic organelles, including the centrioles, basal bodies, cilia, and flagella.[9]

The plant alkaloid *colchicine* binds to tubulin molecules and prevents the assembly of microtubules. This compound stops cell mitosis by interfering with formation of the mitotic spindle and is often used for cytogenetic (chromosome) studies. It is also used in treating gout to prevent migration of neutrophils and to lower their ability to respond to urate crystals in the tissues. The vinca alkaloid drugs (*e.g.,* vinblastine and vincristine), which are sometimes used in the treatment of cancer, also bind to microtubules and inhibit formation of the mitotic spindle, which is essential for cell proliferation (see Chapter 8).[11]

Centrioles and Basal Bodies. Centrioles and basal bodies are structurally identical organelles composed of highly organized microtubules.[9] Internally, centrioles and basal bodies have an amorphous central core surrounded by clusters formed of triplet sets of microtubules.

Centrioles are small, cylindrical structures composed of an array of highly organized microtubules. Usually they are paired structures, arranged perpendicular to each other. In dividing cells, the two cylindrical centrioles are initially found in the vicinity of the Golgi apparatus in a region of the cell called the *centrosome.* During cell division, centrioles form the mitotic spindle that aids in the separation and movement of the chromosomes.

Basal bodies are more numerous than centrioles and are found near the cell membrane in association with cilia and flagella (Fig. 4.6). They are responsible for the formation of the highly organized core of microtubules found in cilia and flagella.[9]

Cilia and Flagella. Cilia and flagella are microtubule-filled cellular extensions whose enclosing membrane is continuous with the cell membrane. Ciliated cells typically possess a large number of cilia, whereas flagellated cells have only one flagellum. In humans, the spermatozoa are the only cell type with flagella. Cilia are found on the apical (luminal) surfaces of many epithelial linings, including the nasal sinuses and passages such as the upper respiratory system. They also play a prominent role in sensory tissues such as the photoreceptor proteins in the eye (see Chapter 54), the odorant receptors of the olfactory epithelium, and the kinocilium on the hair cells in the inner ear (see Chapter 55). Cilia also act in sensory roles at critical stages of embryonic development, and they are essential for the normal functioning of many tissues,

including the kidney, during postnatal life. Recent research has linked the pathogenesis of a condition called *polycystic kidney disease* to a genetic defect in the cilia of the renal tubular cells (see Chapter 33).

A motile cilium contains nine sets of doublet microtubules that form a hollow cylinder surrounding a central pair of singlet microtubules (Fig. 4.6C). The outer doublet microtubules contain ATP motor-driven complexes that cause the adjacent microtubule doublets to slide past each other. All of these microtubules and their associated proteins are anchored to a *basal body* that is responsible for the formation of a core structure called the *axoneme* (Fig. 4.6D).[9] The axoneme serves as the internal framework that supports the cilium and provides a structure on which mechanical movement is generated. Recent evidence suggests that not all cilia contain this internal structure, and some may be missing the central pair of microtubules. Cilia lacking the central core of microtubules are often called *primary cilia,* and are immotile.

Cilia and flagella are assembled through a process called *intraflagellar transport,* during which large protein complexes are transported along the ciliary microtubules from the basal body to the ciliary tip and then back to the basal body. These protein complexes are thought to carry ciliary precursors from their site of synthesis in the cytoplasm to their site of assembly at the tip of the cilium. Genetic defects can result in improper ciliary assembly and, as a result, the cilia may be nonfunctional.[9] One of these disorders, *immobile cilia syndrome,* impairs sperm motility, causing male sterility while also immobilizing the cilia of the respiratory tract, thus interfering with clearance of inhaled bacteria, leading to a chronic lung disease called *bronchiectasis* (see Chapter 29).[9,12] Kartagener syndrome is an example of immotile cilia syndrome and involves diffuse bronchiolitis, sinus aplasia, and situs inversus totalis, which is a reversal of the thorax and abdomen organs.[12]

Microfilaments

Microfilaments are thin, threadlike cytoplasmic structures. Three classes of microfilaments exist: thin microfilaments, which are equivalent to the thin actin filaments in muscle; intermediate filaments, which are a heterogeneous group of filaments with diameter sizes between those of the thick and thin filaments; and thick myosin filaments, which are present in muscle cells, but may also exist temporarily in other cells.[6]

Muscle contraction depends on the interaction between the thin actin filaments and thick myosin filaments. Microfilaments are present in the superficial zone of the cytoplasm in most cells. Contractile activities involving the microfilaments and associated thick myosin filaments contribute to the movement of the cytoplasm and cell membrane during endocytosis and exocytosis. Microfilaments are also present in the microvilli of the intestine. The intermediate filaments assist in supporting and maintaining the asymmetric shape of cells. Examples of intermediate filaments are the keratin filaments that are found anchored to the cell membrane of epidermal keratinocytes of the skin, and the glial filaments that are found in astrocytes and other glial cells of the nervous system.[6] The *neurofibrillary tangle* found in the brain in Alzheimer disease contains microtubule-associated proteins and neurofilaments, evidence of a disrupted neuronal cytoskeleton (see Chapter 53).

The Cell (Plasma) Membrane

The cell is enclosed in a thin membrane that separates the intracellular contents from the extracellular environment. To differentiate it from the other cell membranes, such as the mitochondrial or nuclear membranes, the cell membrane is often called the *plasma membrane*. In many respects, the plasma membrane is one of the most important parts of the cell. It acts as a semipermeable structure that separates the intracellular and extracellular environments, but allows necessary substances to move across the membrane. It provides receptors for hormones and other biologically active substances, participates in the electrical events that occur in nerve and muscle cells, and aids in the regulation of cell growth and proliferation.

The cell membrane is a dynamic and fluid structure consisting of an organized arrangement of lipids, carbohydrates, and proteins (Fig. 4.7). A main structural component of the membrane is its lipid bilayer. It is a bimolecular layer that consists primarily of phospholipids, glycolipids, and cholesterol.[9] This lipid bilayer provides the basic fluid structure of the membrane and serves as a relatively impermeable barrier to all but lipid-soluble substances. Approximately 75% of the lipids are phospholipids, each with a hydrophilic (water-soluble) head and a hydrophobic (water-insoluble) tail.[9] Phospholipid molecules, along with the glycolipids, are aligned such that their hydrophilic heads face outward on each side of the membrane and their hydrophobic tails project toward the middle of the membrane. The hydrophilic heads retain water and help cells stick to each other. At normal body temperature, the viscosity of the lipid component of the membrane is equivalent to that of olive oil. The presence of cholesterol stiffens the membrane.

Although the lipid bilayer provides the basic structure of the cell membrane, proteins carry out most of the specific functions. The *integral proteins* span the entire lipid bilayer and are essentially part of the membrane. Because most of the integral proteins pass directly through the membrane, they are also referred to as *transmembrane proteins*. A second type of protein, the *peripheral proteins,* is bound to one or the other side of the membrane and does not pass into the lipid bilayer. Removal of peripheral proteins from the membrane surface usually causes damage to the membrane.[9]

The manner in which proteins are associated with the cell membrane often determines their function. Thus, peripheral proteins are associated with functions involving the inner or outer side of the membrane where they are found. Several peripheral proteins serve as receptors or are involved in intracellular signalling systems. By contrast, only the transmembrane proteins can function on both sides of the membrane or transport molecules across it.

Many integral transmembrane proteins form the ion channels found on the cell surface. These channel proteins have a complex morphology and are selective with respect to the substances they transmit. Mutations in these channel proteins, often called *channelopathies,* are responsible for a host of genetic disorders.[13] For example, in *cystic fibrosis,* the primary defect resides in an abnormal chloride channel, which results in increased sodium and water reabsorption that causes respiratory tract secretions to thicken and occlude the airways (see Chapter 29).

FIGURE 4.7 • Structure of the cell membrane showing the hydrophilic (polar) heads and the hydrophobic (fatty acid) tails. (From McConnell T. H., Hull K. L. (2011). *Human form human function: Essentials of anatomy & physiology* (p. 67). Philadelphia, PA: Lippincott Williams & Wilkins.)

The plasma membrane also contains specific water channels or pores called *aquaporins*. It is now known that aquaporin disorders are responsible for a number of diseases, including nephrogenic diabetes insipidus (see Chapter 31).

A fuzzy-looking layer surrounding the cell surface is called the *cell coat,* or *glycocalyx.* The structure of the glycocalyx consists of long, complex carbohydrate chains attached to protein molecules that penetrate the outside portion of the membrane (*i.e.,* glycoproteins); outward-facing membrane lipids (*i.e.,* glycolipids); and carbohydrate-binding proteins called *lectins.* These proteins (lectins) are responsible for a variety of activities and have anti-tumour, immunomodulatory, antifungal, and HIV-1 reverse transcriptase inhibitory processes.[14] The cell coat participates in cell-to-cell recognition and adhesion. It contains tissue transplant antigens that label cells as self or nonself. The cell coat of a red blood cell contains the ABO blood group antigens. An intimate relationship exists between the cell membrane and the cell coat. If the cell coat is enzymatically removed, the cell remains viable and can generate a new cell coat, but damage to the cell membrane usually results in cell death.

IN SUMMARY

The cell is a remarkably autonomous structure that functions in a strikingly similar manner to that of the total organism. In most cells, a single nucleus controls cell function and is the mastermind of the cell. It contains DNA, which provides the information necessary for the synthesis of the various proteins that the cell must produce to stay alive and to transmit information from one generation to another. The nucleus also is the site for the synthesis of the three types of RNA (mRNA, rRNA, tRNA) that move to the cytoplasm and carry out the actual synthesis of proteins.

The cytoplasm contains the cell's organelles and cytoskeleton. Ribosomes serve as sites for protein synthesis in the cell. The ER functions as a tubular communication system that transports substances from one part of the cell to another and as the site of protein (rough ER), carbohydrate, and lipid (smooth ER) synthesis. Golgi bodies modify materials synthesized in the ER and package them into secretory granules for transport within the cell or for export from the cell. Lysosomes, which are viewed as the digestive system of the cell, contain hydrolytic enzymes that digest worn-out cell parts and foreign materials. They are membranous structures formed in the Golgi complex from hydrolytic enzymes synthesized in the rough ER. Another organelle, the proteasome, digests misformed and misfolded proteins. The mitochondria serve as power plants for the cell because they transform food energy into ATP, to power cell activities. Mitochondria contain their own extrachromosomal DNA, important in the synthesis of mitochondrial RNAs and proteins used in oxidative metabolism. Besides its organelles, the cytoplasm contains a network of microtubules, microfilaments, intermediate filaments, and thick filaments. Microtubules are slender, stiff tubular structures that influence cell shape, provide a means of moving organelles through the cytoplasm, and effect movement of the cilia and of chromosomes during cell division. Microfilaments, which are thin, threadlike cytoplasmic structures, include the actin and myosin filaments that participate in muscle contraction.

The plasma membrane is a lipid bilayer that surrounds the cell and separates it from its surrounding external environment. Although the lipid bilayer provides the basic structure of the cell membrane, proteins carry out most of the specific functions. Transmembrane proteins frequently form transport channels for ions and other substances, whereas peripheral proteins often function as receptor sites for signalling molecules. A fuzzy-looking layer, the cell coat or glycocalyx, surrounds the cell surface. It contains tissue antigens and participates in cell-to-cell recognition and adhesion.

CONCEPTSin action**ANIMATION**

INTEGRATION OF CELL FUNCTION AND REPLICATION

After completing this section of the chapter, you should be able to meet the following objectives:

- Trace the pathway for cell communication, beginning at the receptor and ending with the effector response, and explain why the process is often referred to as signal transduction.
- Describe the phases of mitotic cell division.
- Relate the function of ATP to cell metabolism.
- Compare the processes involved in anaerobic and aerobic metabolism.

Cell Communication

Cells in multicellular organisms need to communicate with one another to coordinate their function and control their growth. The human body has several means of transmitting information between cells. These mechanisms include direct communication between adjacent cells through gap junctions, autocrine and paracrine signalling, and endocrine or synaptic signalling.[9] *Autocrine signalling* occurs when a cell releases a chemical into the extracellular fluid that affects its own activity (Fig. 4.8). With *paracrine signalling,* enzymes rapidly metabolize the chemical mediators, and therefore they act mainly on nearby cells. *Endocrine signalling* relies on hormones carried in the bloodstream to cells throughout the body. *Synaptic signalling* occurs in the nervous system, where neurotransmitters act only on adjacent nerve cells through special contact areas called *synapses.* In some parts of the body, the same chemical messenger can function as a neurotransmitter, a paracrine mediator, and a hormone secreted by neurons into the bloodstream.

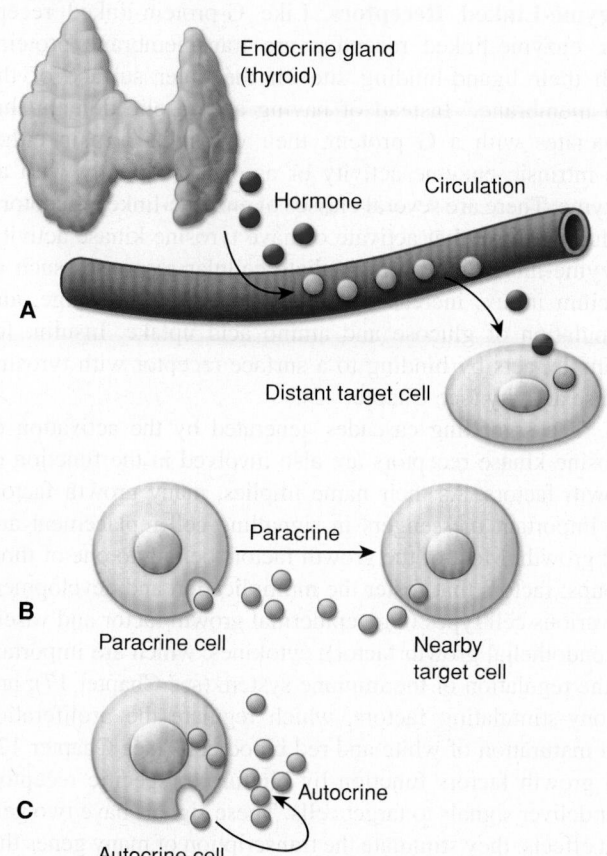

A

Endocrine gland
(thyroid)

Hormone   Circulation

Distant target cell

B

Paracrine

Paracrine cell   Nearby
target cell

C

Autocrine

Autocrine cell

FIGURE 4.8 • Examples of autocrine (**A**), paracrine (**B**), and endocrine (**C**) signalling.

CELL COMMUNICATION

- Cells communicate with each other and with the internal and external environments by a number of mechanisms, including electrical and chemical signalling systems that control electrical potentials, the overall function of a cell, and gene activity needed for cell division and cell replication.
- Chemical messengers exert their effects by binding to cell membrane proteins or receptors that convert the chemical signal into signals within the cell, in a process called *signal transduction.*
- Cells can regulate their responses to chemical messengers by increasing or decreasing the number of active receptors on their surface.

Cell Receptors

Signalling systems consist of receptors that reside either in the cell membrane (surface receptors) or within the cells (intracellular receptors). Receptors are activated by a variety of extracellular signals or *first messengers,* including neurotransmitters, protein hormones and growth factors, steroids, and other chemical messengers. Some lipid-soluble chemical messengers move through the membrane and bind to cytoplasmic or

nuclear receptors to exert their physiologic effects. Signalling systems also include transducers and effectors that are involved in conversion of the signal into a physiologic response. The pathway may include additional intracellular mechanisms, called *second messengers.* Many molecules involved in signal transduction are proteins. A unique property of proteins that allows them to function in this way is their ability to change their shape or conformation, thereby changing their function and consequently the functions of the cell. Proteins often accomplish these conformational changes through enzymes called *protein kinases* that catalyze the phosphorylation of amino acids in the protein structure.[9]

Cell Surface Receptors

Each cell type in the body contains a distinctive set of surface receptors that enable it to respond to a complementary set of signalling molecules in a specific, pre-programmed way. These proteins are not static components of the cell membrane; they increase or decrease in number according to the needs and stimulation of the cell. When excess chemical messengers are present, the number of active receptors decreases in a process called *down-regulation;* when there is a deficiency of the messenger, the number of active receptors increases through *up-regulation.* Three known classes of cell surface receptor proteins exist: G-protein-linked receptors, ion-channel-linked receptors, and enzyme-linked receptors.[6]

G-Protein-Linked Receptors. With more than 1,000 members, G-protein-linked receptors are the largest family of cell surface receptors.[6] Although many intercellular messengers exist, they rely on the intermediary activity of a separate class of membrane-bound regulatory proteins to convert external signals (first messengers) into internal signals (second messengers). Because these regulatory proteins bind to guanine nucleotides such as guanine diphosphate (GDP) and guanine triphosphate (GTP), they are called *G proteins.* G-protein-linked receptors mediate cellular responses for numerous types of first messengers, including proteins, small peptides, amino acids, and fatty acid derivatives such as the prostaglandins.[6]

Although there are differences among the G-protein-linked receptors, all share a number of features. They all have a ligand-binding extracellular receptor component, which functions as a signal discriminator by recognizing a specific first messenger, and they all undergo conformational changes with receptor binding that activates the G protein (Fig. 4.9). All G proteins are found on the cytoplasmic side of the cell membrane, and all incorporate the *GTPase cycle,* which functions as a molecular switch that exists in two states. In its activated (on) state, the G protein has a high affinity for GTP, and in its inactivated (off) state, it binds GDP.[6]

At the molecular level, G proteins are heterotrimeric (*i.e.,* they have three subunits) proteins (Fig. 4.10). The three subunits are designated alpha (α), beta (β), and gamma (γ). The α subunit can bind either GDP or GTP and contains the GTPase activity. GTPase is an enzyme that converts GTP with its three phosphate groups to GDP with its two phosphate groups.

FIGURE 4.9 • Activation of a G-protein-linked receptor and production of cyclic adenosine monophosphate (cAMP). Binding of a hormone (the first messenger) causes the activated receptor to interact with the inactive, guanine diphosphate (GDP)–bound G protein. This results in activation of the G protein and dissociation of the G protein α, β, and γ subunits. The activated α subunit of the G protein can then interact with and activate the membrane protein adenyl cyclase to catalyze the conversion of adenosine triphosphate (ATP) to the second messenger cAMP. The second messenger then activates an internal effector, which leads to the cell response.

When GDP is bound to the α subunit, the G protein is inactive; when GTP is bound, it is active. The activated G protein has GTPase activity, so eventually the bound GTP is hydrolyzed to GDP, and the G protein reverts to its inactive state. Receptor activation causes the α subunit to dissociate from the receptor and the β and γ subunits and transmit the signal from the first messenger to its effector protein. Often, the effector is an enzyme that converts an inactive precursor molecule into a second messenger, which diffuses into the cytoplasm and carries the signal beyond the cell membrane. A common second messenger is cyclic adenosine monophosphate (cAMP). It is activated by the enzyme *adenylyl cyclase,* which generates cAMP by transferring phosphate groups from ATP to other proteins.[7] This transfer changes the conformation and function of these proteins. Such changes eventually produce the cell response to the first messenger, whether it is a secretion, muscle contraction or relaxation, or a change in metabolism. Sometimes it is the opening of membrane channels involved in calcium or potassium influx.

Certain bacterial toxins can bind to the G proteins, causing inhibition or stimulation of their signal function. For example, the toxin of *Vibrio cholerae* binds and activates the stimulatory G protein linked to the cAMP system that controls the secretion of fluid into the intestine. In response to the cholera toxin, these cells overproduce fluid, leading to severe diarrhea and life-threatening depletion of extracellular fluid volume.

Enzyme-Linked Receptors. Like G-protein-linked receptors, enzyme-linked receptors are transmembrane proteins with their ligand-binding site on the outer surface of the cell membrane.[9] Instead of having a cytosolic domain that associates with a G protein, their cytosolic domain either has intrinsic enzyme activity or associates directly with an enzyme. There are several classes of enzyme-linked receptors, including those that activate or have tyrosine kinase activity. Enzyme-linked receptors mediate cellular responses such as calcium influx, increased sodium–potassium exchange, and stimulation of glucose and amino acid uptake. Insulin, for example, acts by binding to a surface receptor with tyrosine kinase activity (see Chapter 42).

The signalling cascades generated by the activation of tyrosine kinase receptors are also involved in the function of growth factors. As their name implies, many growth factors are important messengers in signalling cell replacement and cell growth. Most of the growth factors belong to one of three groups: factors that foster the multiplication and development of various cell types (*e.g.,* epidermal growth factor and vascular endothelial growth factor); cytokines, which are important in the regulation of the immune system (see Chapter 17); and colony-stimulating factors, which regulate the proliferation and maturation of white and red blood cells (see Chapter 12). All growth factors function by binding to specific receptors that deliver signals to target cells. These signals have two general effects: they stimulate the transcription of many genes that were silent in resting cells, and they regulate the entry of cells into the cell cycle and their passage through the cell cycle.

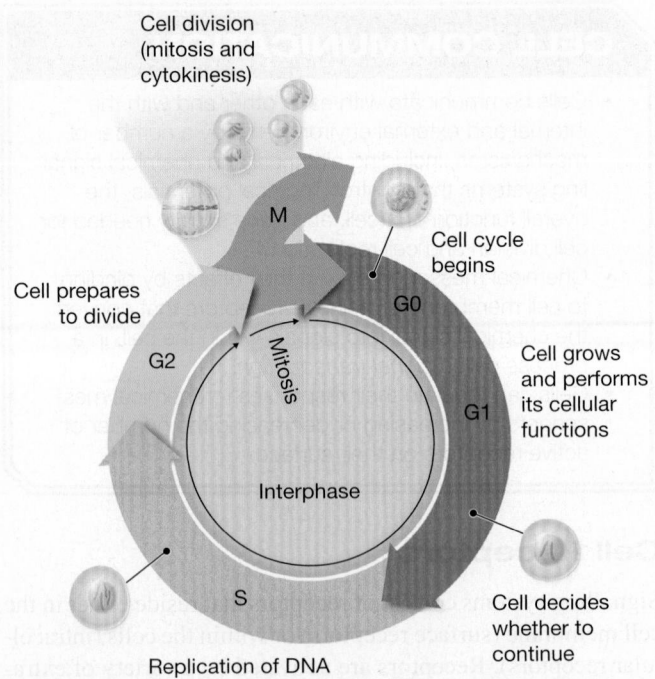

FIGURE 4.10 • The cell cycle. G_0, nondividing cell; G_1, cell growth; S, DNA replication; G_2, protein synthesis; and mitosis.) (From Wingerd B. (2014). *The human body concepts of anatomy and physiology* (3rd ed.). Philadelphia, PA: Lippincott Williams & Wilkins.)

Ion-Channel-Linked Receptors. Ion-channel-linked receptors are involved in the rapid synaptic signalling between electrically excitable cells.[6] Many neurotransmitters mediate this type of signalling by transiently opening or closing ion channels formed by integral proteins in the cell membrane. This type of signalling is involved in the transmission of impulses in nerve and muscle cells.

Intracellular Receptors

Some messengers, such as thyroid hormone and steroid hormones, do not bind to membrane receptors but move directly across the lipid layer of the cell membrane and are carried to the cell nucleus, where they influence DNA activity. Many of these hormones bind to a cytoplasmic receptor, and the receptor–hormone complex is carried to the nucleus. In the nucleus, the receptor–hormone complex binds to DNA, thereby increasing transcription of mRNA (see Chapter 6). The mRNAs are translated in the ribosomes, with the production of increased amounts of proteins that alter cell function.[7]

The Cell Cycle and Cell Division

The life cycle of a cell is called the *cell cycle.* It is usually divided into five phases: G_0, G_1, S, G_2, and M (Fig. 4.10). G_0 is the stage when the cell may leave the cell cycle and either remain in a state of inactivity or re-enter the cell cycle at another time. G_1 is the stage during which the cell begins to prepare for mitosis through DNA and protein synthesis and an increase in organelle and cytoskeletal elements. The S phase is the synthesis phase, during which DNA replication occurs and the centrioles begin to replicate. G_2 is the premitotic phase and is similar to G_1 in terms of RNA activity and protein synthesis. The M phase is the phase during which cell mitosis occurs.[9] Tissues may be composed primarily of quiescent cells in G_0, but most tissues contain a combination of cells that are continuously moving through the cell cycle and quiescent cells that occasionally enter the cell cycle. Nondividing cells, such as neurons and skeletal and cardiac muscle cells, have left the cell cycle and are not capable of mitotic division in postnatal life.[9]

Cell division, or *mitosis,* is the process during which a parent cell divides and each daughter cell receives a chromosomal karyotype identical to the parent cell.[9] Cell division gives the body a means of replacing cells that have a limited life span, such as skin and blood cells, increasing tissue mass during periods of growth and providing for tissue repair and wound healing.

Mitosis is a dynamic and continuous process. It is divided into four stages: prophase, metaphase, anaphase, and telophase (Fig. 4.11). The phase during which the cell is not undergoing division is called *interphase.* During *prophase,* the chromosomes become visible because of increased coiling of the DNA, the two centrioles replicate, and a pair moves to each side of the cell. Simultaneously, the microtubules of the mitotic spindle appear between the two pairs of centrioles. Later in prophase, the nuclear envelope and nucleolus disappear. *Metaphase* involves the organization of the chromosome pairs in the midline of the cell and the formation of a mitotic

PARENT CELL AT INTERPHASE

— Cell membrane
Nuclear envelope —
— Centriole
Cytoplasm —
Chromatin —
— Nucleolus

MITOSIS

— Centriole
— Set of chromatids

PROPHASE

— Spindle pole
— Spindle fibres

METAPHASE

ANAPHASE

CYTOKINESIS

— Microfilaments
— Cleavage furrow

TELOPHASE

Offspring cells at interphase

FIGURE 4.11 • Cell mitosis. (From McConnell T. H., Hull K. L. (2011). *Human form human function: Essentials of anatomy & physiology* (p. 79). Philadelphia, PA: Lippincott Williams & Wilkins.)

spindle composed of microtubules. *Anaphase* is the period during which separation of the chromosome pairs occurs, with the microtubules pulling one member of each pair of 46 chromosomes toward the opposite cell pole. Cell division or *cytokinesis* is completed after *telophase,* the stage during which the mitotic spindle vanishes and a new nuclear membrane develops and encloses each complete set of chromosomes.[9]

Cell division is controlled by changes in the concentrations and activity of three major groups of intracellular proteins: (1) cyclins, (2) cyclin-dependent kinases (CDKs), and (3) anaphase-promoting complex (see Chapter 8).[9] The central components of the cell cycle control system are the CDKs, whose activity depends on their association with the regulatory units called *cyclins.* Oscillations in the activity of the various CDKs lead to initiation of the different phases of the cell cycle. Cell division is also controlled by several external factors, including the presence of cytokines, various growth factors, or even adhesion factors when the cell is associated with other cells in a tissue.[9]

Cell Metabolism and Energy Sources

Energy is the ability to do work. Cells use oxygen to transform the breakdown products of the foods we eat into the energy needed for muscle contraction, transport of ions and other molecules across cell membranes, and synthesis of enzymes, hormones, and other macromolecules. *Energy metabolism* refers to the processes by which fats, proteins, and carbohydrates from the foods we eat are converted into energy or complex energy sources in the cell. Catabolism and anabolism are the two phases of metabolism. *Catabolism* consists of breaking down stored nutrients and body tissues to produce energy. *Anabolism* is a constructive process in which more complex molecules are formed from simpler ones.

The special carrier for cellular energy is ATP. ATP molecules consist of adenosine, a nitrogenous base; ribose, a five-carbon sugar; and three phosphate groups (Fig. 4.12). The phosphate groups are attached by two high-energy bonds.[9] Large amounts of free energy are released when ATP is hydrolyzed to form adenosine diphosphate (ADP), an adenosine molecule that contains two phosphate groups. The free energy liberated from the hydrolysis of ATP is used to drive reactions that require free energy. Energy from foodstuffs is used to convert ADP back to ATP. Because energy can be "saved or spent" using ATP, ATP is often called the *energy currency* of the cell.

Energy transformation takes place within the cell through two types of energy production: the *anaerobic (i.e.,* without oxygen) glycolytic pathway, which occurs within the cytoplasm, and the *aerobic (i.e.,* with oxygen) pathway, which occurs within the mitochondria. The anaerobic glycolytic pathway serves as an important prelude to the aerobic pathway. Both pathways involve oxidation–reduction reactions involving an electron donor, which is oxidized in the reaction, and an electron acceptor, which is reduced in the reaction. In energy metabolism, the breakdown products of carbohydrate, fat, or protein metabolism donate electrons and are oxidized, and the coenzymes nicotinamide adenine dinucleotide (NAD+)

FIGURE 4.12 • Adenosine triphosphate (ATP) is the major source of cellular energy. **A:** Each molecule of ATP contains two high-energy bonds, each containing about 12 kcal of potential energy. **B:** The high-energy ATP bonds are in constant flux. They are generated by substrate (glucose, amino acid, and fat) metabolism and are consumed as the energy is expended.

and flavin adenine dinucleotide (FAD) accept electrons and are reduced.[9]

Anaerobic Metabolism

Glycolysis is the process by which energy is liberated from glucose. It is an important energy provider for cells that lack mitochondria, the cell organelle in which aerobic metabolism occurs. This process also provides energy in situations when delivery of oxygen to the cell is delayed or impaired. Glycolysis involves a sequence of reactions that convert glucose to pyruvate, with the concomitant production of ATP from ADP. The net gain of energy from the glycolysis of one molecule of glucose is two ATP molecules. Although comparatively inefficient as to energy yield, the glycolytic pathway is important during periods of decreased oxygen delivery, as occurs in skeletal muscle during the first few minutes of exercise.

Glycolysis requires the presence of NAD+. Important end products of glycolysis are pyruvate and NADH (the reduced form of NAD+) plus H+. When oxygen is present, pyruvate moves into the aerobic mitochondrial pathway, and NADH + H+ delivers its electron and proton (H+) to the oxidative electron transport system.[9] Transfer of electrons from NADH + H+ to the electron transport system allows the glycolytic process to continue by facilitating the regeneration of NAD+. Under anaerobic conditions, such as cardiac arrest or circulatory shock, pyruvate is converted to lactic acid, which diffuses out of the cells into the extracellular fluid. Conversion of pyruvate to lactic acid is reversible, and after the oxygen supply has been restored, lactic acid is converted back to pyruvate and used directly for energy or to synthesize glucose.

Much of the conversion of lactic acid occurs in the liver, but a small amount can occur in other tissues. The liver removes lactic acid from the bloodstream and converts it back to glucose in a process called *gluconeogenesis*. This glucose is released into the bloodstream to be used again by the muscles or by the central nervous system (CNS). Heart muscle is also efficient in converting lactic acid to pyruvic acid and then using the pyruvic acid for fuel. Pyruvic acid is a particularly important source of fuel for the heart during heavy exercise when the skeletal muscles are producing large amounts of lactic acid and releasing it into the bloodstream.

Aerobic Metabolism

Aerobic metabolism occurs in the cell's mitochondria and involves the citric acid cycle and the electron transport chain. It is here that the carbon compounds from the carbohydrates, fats, and proteins in our diet are broken down and their electrons combined with molecular oxygen to form carbon dioxide and water as energy is released. Unlike lactic acid, which is an end product of anaerobic metabolism, the end products of aerobic metabolism (carbon dioxide and water) are generally harmless and easily eliminated from the body if necessary. In a 24-hour period, oxidative metabolism produces 300 to 500 mL of water.[9]

The citric acid cycle, sometimes called the *tricarboxylic acid* (TCA) or *Krebs cycle,* provides the final common pathway for the metabolism of nutrients. In the citric acid cycle, which takes place in the matrix of the mitochondria, an activated two-carbon molecule of acetyl-coenzyme A (acetyl-CoA) condenses with a four-carbon molecule of oxaloacetic acid and moves through a series of enzyme-mediated steps.[7] This process produces hydrogen atoms and carbon dioxide. As hydrogen is generated, it combines with NAD^+ or FAD for transfer to the electron transport system. In the citric acid cycle, each of the two pyruvate molecules formed in the cytoplasm from one molecule of glucose yields another molecule of ATP, along with two molecules of carbon dioxide and eight electrons that end up in three molecules of $NADH + H^+$ and one of $FADH_2$. Besides pyruvate from the glycolysis of glucose, products of amino acid and fatty acid degradation enter the citric acid cycle and contribute to the generation of ATP.[7]

Oxidative metabolism, which supplies 90% of the body's energy needs, takes place in the electron transport chain in the mitochondria. The electron transport chain oxidizes $NADH + H^+$ and $FADH_2$ and donates the electrons to oxygen, which is reduced to water. Energy from reduction of oxygen is used for phosphorylation of ADP to ATP. Because the formation of ATP involves the addition of a high-energy phosphate bond to ADP, the process is sometimes called *oxidative phosphorylation*.[7]

Among the members of the electron transport chain are several iron-containing molecules called *cytochromes*. Each cytochrome is a protein that contains a heme structure similar to that of hemoglobin. The last cytochrome complex is cytochrome oxidase, which passes electrons from cytochrome c to oxygen. Cytochrome oxidase has a lower binding affinity for oxygen than myoglobin (the intracellular heme-containing oxygen carrier) or hemoglobin (the heme-containing oxygen transporter in erythrocytes in the blood). Thus, oxygen is pulled from erythrocytes to myoglobin and from myoglobin to cytochrome oxidase, where it is reduced to H_2O.[7] Although iron-deficiency anemia (see Chapter 14) is characterized by decreased levels of hemoglobin, the iron-containing cytochromes in the electron transport chain in tissues such as skeletal muscle are affected as well. Thus, the fatigue that develops in iron-deficiency anemia results, in part, from impaired function of the electron transport chain.

IN SUMMARY

Cells communicate with each other by chemical messenger systems. In some tissues, chemical messengers move from cell to cell through gap junctions without entering the extracellular fluid. Other types of chemical messengers bind to receptors on or near the cell surface. Three classes of cell surface receptor proteins are known: G-protein-linked receptors, ion-channel–linked receptors, and enzyme-linked receptors. G-protein-linked receptors rely on a class of molecules called G proteins that function as an on–off switch to convert external signals (first messengers) into internal signals (second messengers). Ion-channel-linked signalling is mediated by neurotransmitters that transiently open or close ion channels formed by integral proteins in the cell membrane. Enzyme-linked receptors interact with certain peptide hormones, such as insulin and growth factors, and directly initiate the activity of the intracellular protein–tyrosine kinase enzyme.

The life cycle of a cell is called the cell cycle. It is usually divided into five phases: G_0, or the resting phase; G_1, during which the cell begins to prepare for division through DNA and protein synthesis; the S or synthetic phase, during which DNA replication occurs; G_2, which is the premitotic phase and is similar to G_1 regarding RNA and protein synthesis; and the M phase, during which cell division occurs. Cell division, or mitosis, is the process during which a parent cell divides into two daughter cells, each receiving an identical pair of chromosomes. The process of mitosis is dynamic and continuous and is divided into four stages: prophase, metaphase, anaphase, and telophase.

Metabolism is the process whereby carbohydrates, fats, and proteins from the foods we eat are broken down and subsequently converted into the energy needed for cell function. Energy is converted to ATP, the energy currency of the cell. Two sites of energy conversion are present in cells: the anaerobic glycolytic pathway in the cytoplasm and the aerobic pathway in the mitochondria. The most efficient of these pathways is the aerobic citric acid cycle and electron transport chain in the mitochondria. This pathway requires oxygen and produces carbon dioxide and water as end products. The glycolytic pathway in the cytoplasm involves the breakdown of glucose to form ATP. This pathway can function without oxygen and results in the production of lactic acid.

MOVEMENT ACROSS THE CELL MEMBRANE AND MEMBRANE POTENTIALS

After completing this section of the chapter, you should be able to meet the following objectives:

• Discuss the mechanisms of membrane transport associated with diffusion, osmosis, endocytosis, and exocytosis and compare them with active transport mechanisms.

• Describe the basis for membrane potentials.

The cell membrane serves as a barrier that controls which substances enter and leave the cell. This barrier function allows materials that are essential for cellular function to enter the cell, while excluding those that are harmful. It is responsible for differences in the composition of intracellular and extracellular fluids.

Movement of Substances Across the Cell Membrane

Movement through the cell membrane occurs in essentially two ways: passively, without an expenditure of energy, or actively, using energy-consuming processes. The cell membrane can

Understanding ▶ Cell Metabolism

Cell metabolism is the process that converts dietary fuels from carbohydrates, proteins, and fats into adenosine triphosphate (ATP), which provides for the energy needs of the cell. ATP is formed through three major pathways: (1) the glycolytic pathway, (2) the citric acid cycle, and (3) the electron transport chain. In fuel metabolism, which is an oxidation–reduction reaction, the fuel donates electrons and is oxidized, and the coenzymes nicotinamide adenine dinucleotide (NAD) and flavin adenine dinucleotide (FAD) accept electrons and are reduced.

1. Glycolytic Pathway

Glycolysis, which occurs in the cytoplasm of the cell, involves the splitting of the six-carbon glucose molecule into two three-carbon molecules of pyruvic acid. Because the reaction that splits glucose requires two molecules of ATP, there is a net gain of only two molecules of ATP from each molecule of glucose that is metabolized. The process is anaerobic and does not require oxygen (O_2) or produce carbon dioxide (CO_2). When O_2 is present, pyruvic acid moves into the mitochondria, where it enters the aerobic citric acid cycle. Under anaerobic conditions, pyruvate is converted to lactic acid, allowing glycolysis to continue as a means of supplying cells with ATP when O_2 is lacking.

2. Citric Acid Cycle

Under aerobic conditions, both of the pyruvic acid molecules formed by the glycolytic pathway enter the mitochondria, where each combines with acetyl-coenzyme to form acetyl-coenzyme A (acetyl-CoA). The formation of acetyl-CoA begins the reactions that occur in the citric acid cycle. Some reactions release CO_2 and some transfer electrons from the hydrogen atom to NADH or FADH. In addition to pyruvic acid from the glycolysis of glucose, fatty acid and amino acid breakdown products can also enter the citric acid cycle. Fatty acids, which are the major source of fuel in the body, are oxidized by a process called *beta oxidation* to acetyl-CoA for entry into the citric acid cycle.

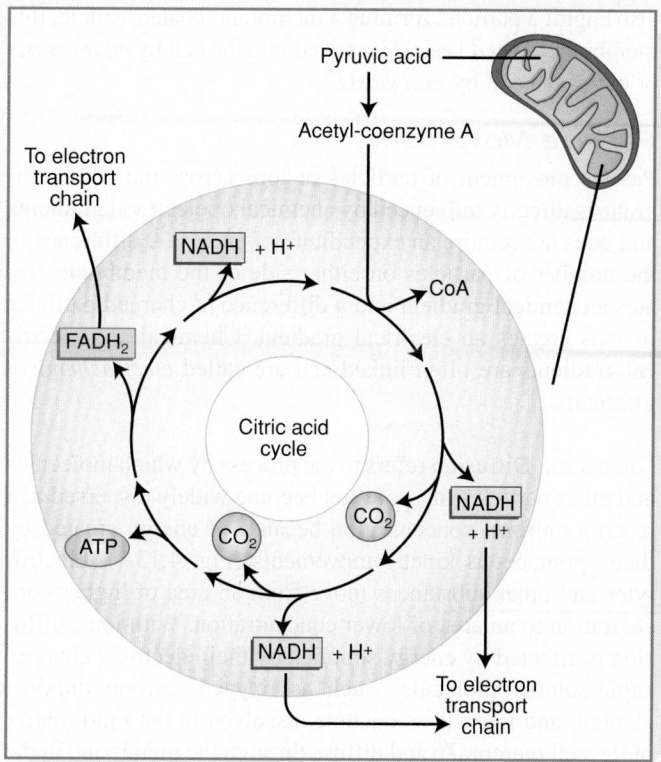

3. Electron Transport Chain

At the completion of the citric acid cycle, each glucose molecule has yielded only four new molecules of ATP (two from glycolysis and two from the citric acid cycle). In fact, the principal function of these earlier stages is to make the electrons (e^-) from glucose and other food substrates available for oxidation. Oxidation of the electrons carried by NADH and $FADH_2$ is accomplished through a series of enzymatically catalyzed reactions in the mitochondrial electron transport chain. During these reactions, protons (H^+) combine with O_2 to form water (H_2O), and large amounts of energy are released and used to add a high-energy phosphate bond to adenosine diphosphate (ADP), converting it to ATP. There is a net yield of 36 molecules of ATP from 1 molecule of glucose (2 from glycolysis, 2 from the citric acid cycle, and 32 from the electron transport chain). In general, the net amount of ATP formed from each gram of protein that is metabolized is less than for glucose, whereas that obtained from fat is greater (*e.g.*, each 16-carbon fatty acid molecule yields about 129 molecules of ATP).

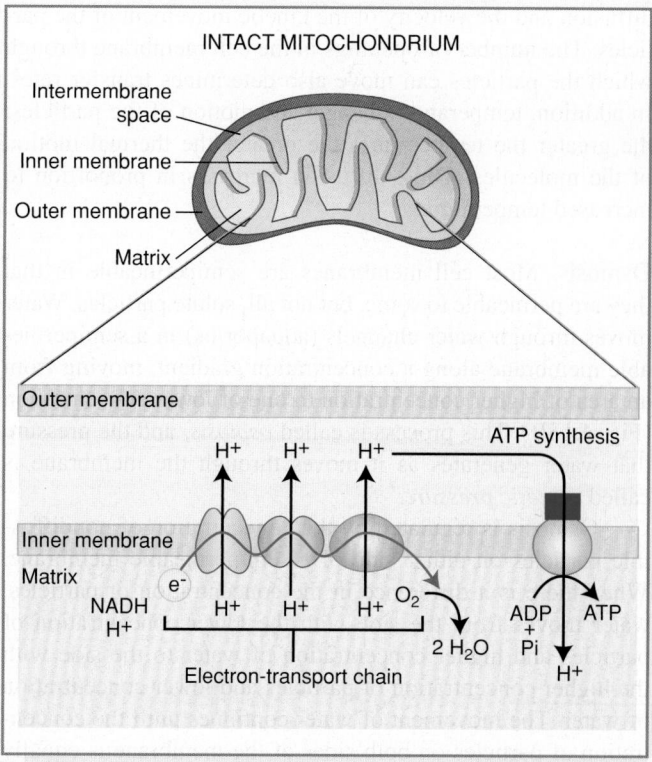

also engulf a particle, forming a membrane-coated vesicle; this membrane-coated vesicle is moved into the cell by *endocytosis* or out of the cell by *exocytosis.*[6]

Passive Movement

Passive movement of particles or ions across the cell membrane is directly influenced by chemical or electrical gradients and does not require an expenditure of energy. A difference in the number of particles on either side of the membrane creates a chemical gradient and a difference in charged particles or ions creates an electrical gradient. Chemical and electrical gradients are often linked and are called *electrochemical gradients.*[7]

Diffusion. Diffusion refers to the process by which molecules and other particles in a solution become widely dispersed and reach a uniform concentration because of energy created by their spontaneous kinetic movements (Fig. 4.13A). Electrolytes and other substances move from an area of higher concentration to an area of lower concentration. With ions, diffusion is affected by energy supplied by their electrical charge.[7] Lipid-soluble molecules such as oxygen, carbon dioxide, alcohol, and fatty acids become dissolved in the lipid matrix of the cell membrane and diffuse through the membrane in the same manner that diffusion occurs in water. Other substances diffuse through minute pores of the cell membrane. The rate of movement depends on how many particles are available for diffusion and the velocity of the kinetic movement of the particles. The number of openings in the cell membrane through which the particles can move also determines transfer rates. In addition, temperature changes the motion of the particles: the greater the temperature, the greater the thermal motion of the molecules. Thus, diffusion increases in proportion to increased temperature.

Osmosis. Most cell membranes are semipermeable in that they are permeable to some, but not all, solute particles. Water moves through water channels (aquaporins) in a semipermeable membrane along a concentration gradient, moving from an area of higher concentration to one of lower concentration (Fig. 4.13B). This process is called *osmosis,* and the pressure that water generates as it moves through the membrane is called *osmotic pressure.*[7]

Osmosis is regulated by the concentration of nondiffusible particles on either side of a semipermeable membrane. When there is a difference in the concentration of particles, water moves from the side with the lower concentration of particles and higher concentration of water to the side with the higher concentration of particles and lower concentration of water. The movement of water continues until the concentration of particles on both sides of the membrane is equally diluted or until the hydrostatic (osmotic) pressure created by the movement of water opposes its flow.

Facilitated Diffusion. Facilitated diffusion occurs through a transport protein that is not linked to metabolic energy

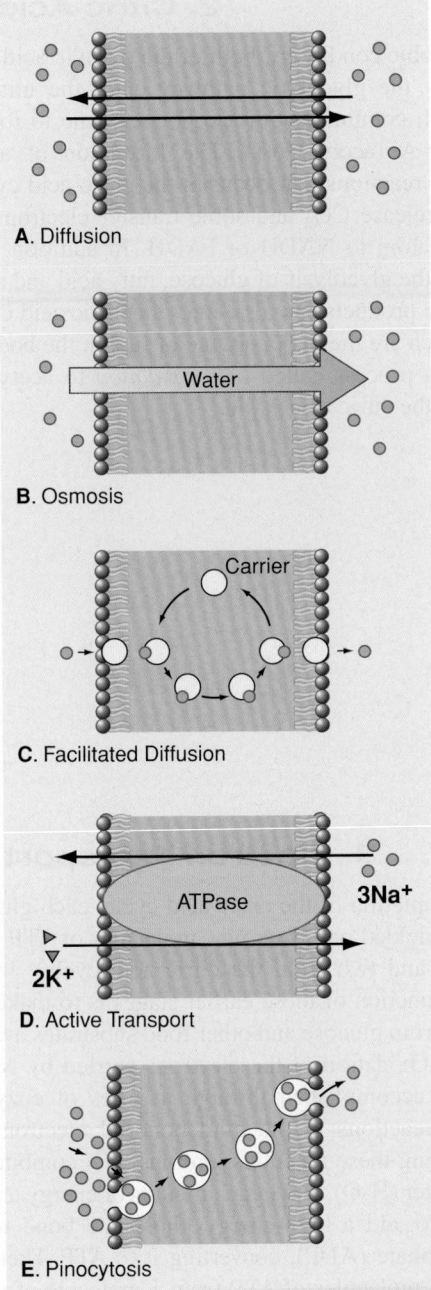

A. Diffusion

B. Osmosis

C. Facilitated Diffusion

D. Active Transport

E. Pinocytosis

FIGURE 4.13 • Mechanisms of membrane transport. **A:** In diffusion, particles move freely to become equally distributed across the membrane. **B:** In osmosis, osmotically active particles regulate the flow of water. **C:** Facilitated diffusion uses a carrier system. **D:** In active transport, selected molecules are transported across the membrane using the energy-driven (Na$^+$/K$^+$ ATPase) pump. **E:** In pinocytosis, the membrane forms a vesicle that engulfs the particle and transports it across the membrane, where it is released.

(Fig. 4.13C). Some substances, such as glucose, cannot pass unassisted through the cell membrane because they are not lipid soluble or are too large to pass through the membrane's pores. These substances combine with special transport proteins at the membrane's outer surface, are carried across the membrane attached to the transporter, and then released on the inside of the membrane. In facilitated diffusion, a substance can move only from an area of higher concentration to one of lower concentration. The rate at which a substance moves across the membrane because of facilitated diffusion depends on the difference in concentration between the two sides of the membrane. Also important are the availability of transport proteins and the rapidity with which they can bind and release the substance being transported. It is thought that insulin, which facilitates the movement of glucose into cells, acts by increasing the availability of glucose transporters in the cell membrane (see Chapter 42).[7]

Active Transport and Cotransport

Active transport mechanisms involve the expenditure of energy. The process of diffusion describes particle movement from an area of higher concentration to one of lower concentration, resulting in an equal distribution across the cell membrane. Sometimes, however, different concentrations of a substance are needed in the intracellular and extracellular fluids. For example, to function, a cell requires a much higher intracellular concentration of potassium ions than is present in the extracellular fluid, while maintaining a much lower intracellular concentration of sodium ions than the extracellular fluid. In these situations, energy is required to pump the ions "uphill" or against their concentration gradient. When cells use energy to move ions against an electrical or chemical gradient, the process is called *active transport*.[7]

The active transport system studied in the greatest detail is the sodium–potassium (Na^+/K^+)-ATPase pump (Fig. 4.13D). This pump moves sodium from inside the cell to the extracellular region, where its concentration is approximately 14 times greater than inside; the pump also returns potassium to the inside, where its concentration is approximately 35 times greater than it is outside the cell. Energy used to pump sodium out of the cell and potassium into the cell is obtained by splitting and releasing energy from the high-energy phosphate bond in ATP by the enzyme ATPase. Were it not for the activity of the Na^+/K^+-ATPase pump, the osmotically active sodium particles would accumulate in the cell, causing cellular swelling because of an accompanying influx of water (see Chapter 5).

Two types of active transport systems exist: primary active transport and secondary active transport. In *primary active transport*, the source of energy (*e.g.*, ATP) is used directly in the transport of a substance. *Secondary active transport* mechanisms harness the energy derived from the primary active transport of one substance, usually sodium, for the cotransport of a second substance. For example, when sodium ions are actively transported out of a cell by primary active transport, a large concentration gradient develops (*i.e.*, high concentration on the outside and low concentration on the inside). This concentration gradient represents a large storehouse of energy because sodium ions are always attempting to diffuse into the cell. Similar to facilitated diffusion, secondary transport mechanisms use membrane transport proteins. These proteins have two binding sites, one for sodium and the other

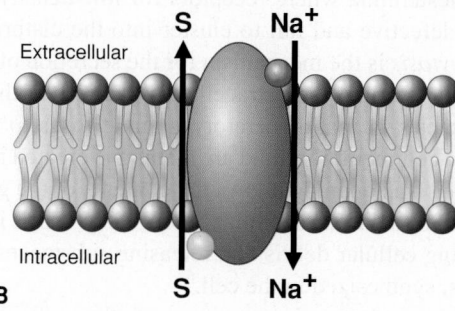

FIGURE 4.14 • Secondary active transport systems. **A:** Symport or cotransport carries the transported solute (S) in the same direction as the sodium (Na^+) ion. **B:** Antiport or countertransport carries the solute and Na^+ in the opposite direction.

for the substance undergoing secondary transport. Secondary transport systems are classified into two groups: *cotransport* or *symport* systems, in which the sodium ion and the solute are transported in the same direction, and *countertransport* or *antiport* systems, in which the sodium ion and the solute are transported in the opposite direction (Fig. 4.14).[9] An example of cotransport occurs in the intestine, where the absorption of glucose and amino acids is coupled with sodium transport.

Endocytosis and Exocytosis

Endocytosis is the process by which cells engulf materials from their surroundings. It includes pinocytosis and phagocytosis. *Pinocytosis* involves the ingestion of small solid or fluid particles. The particles are engulfed into small, membrane-surrounded vesicles for movement into the cytoplasm. The process of pinocytosis is important in the transport of proteins and strong solutions of electrolytes (Fig. 4.13E).[6]

Phagocytosis literally means "cell eating" and can be compared with pinocytosis, which means "cell drinking." It involves the engulfment and subsequent killing or degradation of microorganisms or other particulate matter. During phagocytosis, a particle contacts the cell surface and is surrounded on all sides by the cell membrane, forming a phagocytic vesicle or phagosome. Once formed, the phagosome breaks away from the cell membrane and moves into the cytoplasm, where it eventually fuses with a lysosome, allowing the ingested material to be degraded by lysosomal enzymes. Certain cells, such as macrophages and polymorphonuclear leukocytes (neutrophils), are adept at engulfing and disposing of invading organisms, damaged cells, and unneeded extracellular constituents.[6]

Receptor-mediated endocytosis involves the binding of substances such as low-density lipoproteins to a receptor on the cell surface. Binding of a ligand (*i.e.,* a substance with a high affinity for a receptor) to its receptor normally causes widely distributed receptors to accumulate in clathrin-coated pits. An aggregation of special proteins on the cytoplasmic side of the pit causes the coated pit to invaginate and pinch off, forming a clathrin-coated vesicle that carries the ligand and its receptor into the cell.[6,9] A well-studied example is familial hypercholesteremia where receptors for low-density lipoproteins are defective and fail to cluster into the clathrin-coated pits. *Exocytosis* is the mechanism for the secretion of intracellular substances into the extracellular spaces. It is the reverse of endocytosis in that a secretory granule fuses to the inner side of the cell membrane and an opening is created in the cell membrane. This opening allows the contents of the granule to be released into the extracellular fluid. Exocytosis is important in removing cellular debris and releasing substances, such as hormones, synthesized in the cell.[6]

During endocytosis, portions of the cell membrane become an endocytotic vesicle. During exocytosis, the vesicular membrane is incorporated into the plasma membrane. In this way, cell membranes can be conserved and reused.[6]

Ion Channels

The electrical charge on small ions such as sodium and potassium makes it difficult for these ions to move across the lipid layer of the cell membrane. However, rapid movement of these ions is required for many types of cell functions, such as nerve activity. This is accomplished by facilitated diffusion through selective ion channels. Ion channels are integral proteins that span the width of the cell membrane and are normally composed of several polypeptides or protein subunits that form a gating system. Specific stimuli cause the protein subunits to undergo conformational changes to form an open channel or gate through which the ions can move (Fig. 4.15). In this way, ions do not need to cross the lipid-soluble portion of the membrane but can remain in the aqueous solution that fills the ion channel. Ion channels are highly selective; some channels allow only for passage of sodium ions, and others are selective for potassium, calcium, or chloride ions. Specific interactions between the ions and the sides of the channel can produce an extremely rapid rate of ion movement. For example, ion channels can become negatively charged, promoting the rapid movement of positively charged ions.[9]

FIGURE 4.15 • Gated ion channels that open in response to a specific stimuli. **A:** Voltage-gated channels are controlled by a change in membrane potential. **B:** Ligand-gated channels are controlled by binding of a ligand to a receptor. **C:** Mechanically gated channels, which are controlled by mechanical stimuli such as stretching, often have links that connect to the cytoskeleton.

The plasma membrane contains two basic groups of ion channels: leakage channels and gated channels. Leakage channels are partially open even in the unstimulated state, whereas gated channels open and close in response to specific stimuli. Three main types of gated channels are present in the plasma membrane: *voltage-gated channels,* which have electrically operated channels that open when the membrane potential changes beyond a certain point; *ligand-gated channels,* which are chemically operated and respond to specific receptor-bound ligands, such as the neurotransmitter acetylcholine; and *mechanically gated channels,* which open or close in response to such mechanical stimulations as vibrations, tissue stretching, or pressure (Fig. 4.15).

Movement Across Capillary Membranes

An endothelial layer of cells lines the entire cardiovascular system and various types of capillary membranes allow the exchange of substances in a passive process. Simple diffusion is an important method of exchange for various substances such as oxygen and other nutrients. Another significant method of transporting ions, molecules, or particles is the movement across the capillary beds using pressure. This net movement or *filtration* is the fluid forced through the membrane due to pressure. Filtration is a balance of hydrostatic and oncotic pressures and this is discussed in detail in Chapters 21 and 30.

Membrane Potentials

Electrical potentials exist across the membranes of most cells in the body. Because these potentials occur at the level of the cell membrane, they are called *membrane potentials.*[6] In excitable tissues, such as nerve or muscle cells, changes in the membrane potential are necessary for generation and conduction of nerve impulses and muscle contraction. In other types of cells, such as glandular cells, changes in the membrane potential contribute to hormone secretion and other functions.

Electrical potentials, measured in volts (V), describe the ability of separated electrical charges of opposite polarity (+ and −) to do work. The potential difference is the difference between the separated charges. The terms *potential difference* and *voltage* are synonymous.[6] Voltage is always measured with respect to two points in a system. For example, the voltage in a car battery (6-V or 12-V) is the potential difference between the two battery terminals. Because the total amount of charge that can be separated by a biologic membrane is small, the potential differences are small and are measured in millivolts (mV), or 1/1,000 of a volt. Potential differences across the cell membrane can be measured by inserting a very fine electrode into the cell and another into the extracellular fluid surrounding the cell and connecting the two electrodes to a voltmeter. The movement of charge between two points is called *current.* It occurs when a potential difference has been established and a connection is made such that the charged particles can move between the two points.

Extracellular and intracellular fluids are electrolyte solutions containing approximately 150 to 160 mmol/L of positively charged ions and an equal concentration of negatively charged ions. These current-carrying ions are responsible for generating and conducting membrane potentials. Usually, a small excess of charged ions exists at the outer surface of the cell membrane. This is represented as positive charges on the outside of the membrane and is balanced by an equal number of negative charges on the inside of the membrane. Because of the extreme thinness of the cell membrane, the accumulation of these ions at the surfaces of the membrane contributes to the establishment of a *resting membrane potential.*

A *diffusion potential* describes the voltage generated by ions that diffuse across the cell membrane. Two conditions are necessary for a membrane potential to occur by diffusion: the membrane must be selectively permeable, allowing a single type of ion to diffuse through membrane pores, and the concentration of the diffusible ion must be greater on one side of the membrane than on the other. An *equilibrium potential* is one in which no net movement of ions occurs because the diffusion and electrical forces are exactly balanced. The equilibrium potential (or electromotive force [EMF]) for a particular ion, also known as the *Nernst potential,* can be calculated (see Clinical Application).

CLINICAL APPLICATION

The Nernst Equation for Calculating an Equilibrium Potential

The following equation, known as the *Nernst equation,* can be used to calculate the equilibrium potential (electromotive force [EMF] in millivolts [mV] of a univalent ion at body temperature of 37°C).

$$EMF\ (mV) = -61 \times \log_{10} \text{(ion concentration inside/ ion concentration outside)}$$

For example, if the concentration of an ion inside the membrane is 100 mmol/L and the concentration outside the membrane is 10 mmol/L, the EMF (mV) for that ion would be $-61 \times \log_{10}$ (100/10 [$\log_{10}$ of 10 is 1]). Therefore, it would take 61 mV of charge inside the membrane to balance the diffusion potential created by the concentration difference across the membrane for the ion.

The EMF for potassium ions using a normal estimated intracellular concentration of 140 mmol/L and a normal extracellular concentration of 4 mmol/L results in −94 mV:

$$-94\ mV = -61 \times \log_{10} \text{(140 mmol inside/4 mmol outside)}$$

This value assumes the membrane is permeable only to potassium. This value approximates the −70 to −90 mV *resting membrane potential* for nerve fibres measured in laboratory studies.

When a membrane is permeable to several different ions, the diffusion potential reflects the sum of the equilibrium potentials for each of the ions.

Understanding Membrane Potentials

Electrochemical potentials are present across the membranes of virtually all cells in the body. Some cells, such as nerve and muscle cells, are capable of generating rapidly changing electrical impulses, and these impulses are used to transmit signals along their membranes. In other cells, such as glandular cells, membrane potentials are used to signal the release of hormones or activate other functions of the cell. Generation of membrane potentials relies on (1) diffusion of current-carrying ions, (2) development of an electrochemical equilibrium, and (3) establishment of a resting membrane potential, and (4) triggering of action potentials.

1. Diffusion Potentials

A diffusion potential is a potential difference generated across a membrane when a current-carrying ion, such as the potassium (K^+) ion, diffuses down its concentration gradient. Two conditions are necessary for this to occur: (1) the membrane must be selectively permeable to a particular ion, and (2) the concentration of the diffusible ion must be greater on one side of the membrane than the other.

The magnitude of the diffusion potential, measured in millivolts, depends on the size of the concentration gradient. The sign (+ or −) or polarity of the potential depends on the diffusing ion. It is negative on the inside when a positively charged ion such as K^+ diffuses from the inside to the outside of the membrane, carrying its charge with it.

When using the Nernst equation, it is generally assumed that the potential in the extracellular fluid outside the membrane remains at zero potential and the Nernst potential is inside the membrane. The sign of the potential is negative (−) if a positive ion diffuses from the inside of the membrane to the outside and it is positive (+) if a positively charged ion diffuses from the outside to the inside of the membrane.[7]

In the resting or unexcited state, when the membrane is highly permeable to potassium, the concentration of potassium ions inside the cell is approximately 35 times greater than outside. Because of the large concentration gradient existing across the cell membrane, potassium ions tend to diffuse outward across leakage channels. As they do so, they carry their positive charges with them, causing the inside to become negative in relation to the outside. This new potential difference repels further outward movement of the positively charged potassium ion.[7] The membrane is said to be *polarized* during this stage because of the negative membrane potential that is present. The same phenomenon occurs during an *action potential* (see Chapter 49), when the membrane

2. Equilibrium Potentials

An equilibrium potential is the membrane potential that exactly balances and opposes the net diffusion of an ion down its concentration gradient. As a cation diffuses down its concentration gradient, it carries its positive charge across the membrane, thereby generating an electrical force that will eventually retard and stop its diffusion. An electrochemical equilibrium is one in which the *chemical forces driving* diffusion and the *repelling electrical forces* are exactly balanced so that no further diffusion occurs. The equilibrium potential (EMF) can be calculated by inserting the inside and outside ion concentrations into the Nernst equation.

Nernst equation

EMF (mV) = $-61 \times \log_{10}$ (ion concentration inside/ion concentration outside)

3. Resting Membrane Potential (RMP)

The RMP, which is necessary for electrical excitability, is present when the cell is not transmitting impulses. Because the resting membrane is permeable to K^+, it is essentially a K^+ equilibrium potential. This can be explained in terms of the large K^+ concentration gradient (*e.g.,* 140 mmol/L inside and 4 mmol/L outside), which causes the positively charged K^+ to diffuse outward, leaving the nondiffusible, negatively charged intracellular anions (A^-) behind. This causes the membrane to become polarized, with negative charges aligned along the inside and positive charges along the outside. The Na^+/K^+ membrane pump, which removes three Na^+ from inside while returning only two K^+ to the inside, contributes to the maintenance of the RMP.

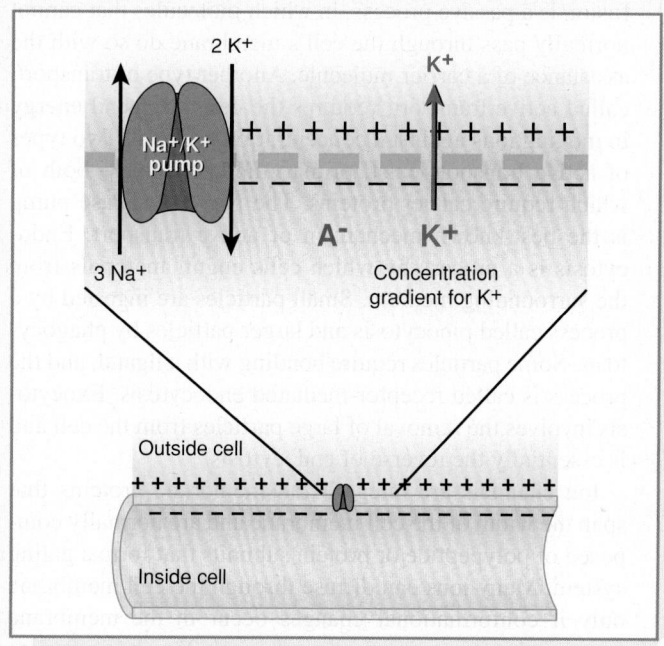

4. Action Potentials

Action potentials involve rapid changes in the membrane potential. Each action potential begins with a sudden change from the negative RMP to a positive threshold potential, causing an opening of the membrane channels for Na^+ (or other ions of the action potential). Opening of the Na^+ channels allows large amounts of the positively charged Na^+ ions to diffuse to the interior of the cell, causing the membrane potential to undergo depolarization or a rapid change to positive on the inside and negative on the outside. This is rapidly followed by closing of Na^+ channels and opening of the K^+ channels, which leads to a rapid efflux of K^+ from the cell and reestablishment of the RMP.

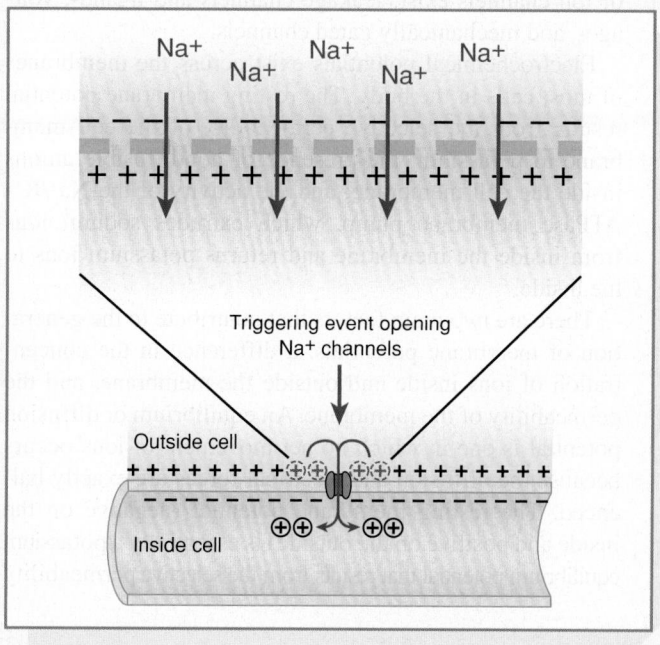

becomes highly permeable to sodium, allowing the positively charged ion to diffuse to the interior of the cell. The inflowing sodium ions produce a reversal in the normal resting membrane potential to one of the opposite polarity (positive on the inside and negative on the outside). This is called *depolarization.*

> ## IN SUMMARY
>
> Movement of materials across the cell's membrane is essential for survival of the cell. Diffusion is a process by which substances such as ions move from an area of greater concentration to one of lesser concentration. Osmosis refers to the diffusion of water molecules through a semipermeable membrane along a concentration gradient. Facilitated diffusion is a passive process, in which molecules that cannot normally pass through the cell's membrane do so with the assistance of a carrier molecule. Another type of transport, called active transport, requires the cell to expend energy in moving ions against a concentration gradient. Two types of active transport exist, primary and secondary, both of which require carrier proteins. The Na^+/K^+-ATPase pump is the best-known mechanism of active transport. Endocytosis is a process by which cells engulf materials from the surrounding medium. Small particles are ingested by a process called pinocytosis and larger particles by phagocytosis. Some particles require bonding with a ligand, and the process is called receptor-mediated endocytosis. Exocytosis involves the removal of large particles from the cell and is essentially the reverse of endocytosis.
>
> Ion channels are integral transmembrane proteins that span the width of the cell membrane and are normally composed of polypeptide or protein subunits that form a gating system. Many ions can diffuse through the cell membrane only if conformational changes occur in the membrane proteins that comprise the ion channel. Two basic groups of ion channels exist: leakage channels and ligand-, voltage-, and mechanically gated channels.
>
> Electrochemical potentials exist across the membranes of most cells in the body. The resting membrane potential results from the selective permeability of the cell membrane to potassium; the presence of nondiffusible anions inside the cell membrane; and the activity of the Na^+/K^+-ATPase membrane pump, which extrudes sodium ions from inside the membrane and returns potassium ions to the inside.
>
> There are two main factors that contribute to the generation of membrane potentials: a difference in the concentration of ions inside and outside the membrane, and the permeability of the membrane. An equilibrium or diffusion potential is one in which no net movement of ions occurs because the diffusion and electrical forces are exactly balanced. The resting membrane potential (negative on the inside and positive on the outside) is essentially a potassium equilibrium potential that results from the selective permeability

of the membrane to potassium and the large difference in potassium ion concentration that exists between the intracellular and extracellular compartments. During an action potential, the cell membrane becomes highly permeable to sodium, causing it to depolarize and reverse its polarity, becoming positive on the inside and negative on the outside.

CONCEPTS in action **ANIMATION**

BODY TISSUES

After completing this section of the chapter, you should be able to meet the following objectives:

- Explain the process of cell differentiation in terms of development of organ systems in the embryo and the continued regeneration of tissues in postnatal life.
- Describe the characteristics of the four different tissue types.
- Characterize the composition and functions of the extracellular components of tissue.

In the preceding sections, we discussed the individual cell, its metabolic processes, and mechanisms of communication and replication. Although cells are similar, their structure and function vary according to the special needs of the body. For example, muscle cells perform different functions than those of skin cells or nerve cells. Groups of cells that are closely associated in structure and have common or similar functions are called *tissues.* Four categories of tissue exist: (1) epithelium, (2) connective (supportive), (3) muscle, and (4) nerve. These tissues do not exist in isolated units, but in association with each other and in variable proportions, forming different structures and organs of the body. This section provides a brief overview of the cells in each of these four tissue types, the structures that hold these cells together, and the extracellular matrix in which they live.

Cell Differentiation

After conception, the fertilized ovum undergoes a series of divisions, ultimately forming approximately 200 different cell types. The formation of different types of cells and the disposition of these cells into tissue types is called *cell differentiation,* a process controlled by a system that switches genes on and off. Embryonic cells must become different to develop into all of the various organ systems, and they must remain different after the signal that initiated cell diversification has disappeared. The process of cell differentiation is controlled by cell memory, which is maintained through regulatory proteins contained in the individual members of a particular cell type. Cell differentiation also involves the sequential activation of multiple genes and their protein products. This means that after differentiation has occurred, the tissue type does not revert to an earlier stage of differentiation. The process of cell differentiation normally moves forward, producing cells that are more specialized than their predecessors.[1] Usually, highly differentiated cell types, such as skeletal muscle and nervous tissue, lose their ability to undergo cell division in postnatal life.

ORGANIZATION OF CELLS INTO TISSUES

- Cells with a similar embryonic origin or function are often organized into larger functional units called *tissues,* and these tissues in turn associate with other, dissimilar tissues to form the various organs of the body.
- Epithelial tissue forms sheets that cover the body's outer surface, line internal surfaces, and form glandular tissue. It is supported by a basement membrane, is avascular, and must receive nourishment from capillaries in supporting connective tissues.
- Connective tissue is the most abundant tissue of the body. It is found in a variety of forms, ranging from solid bone to blood cells that circulate in the vascular system.
- Muscle tissue contains actin and myosin filaments that allow it to contract and provide locomotion and movement of skeletal structures (skeletal muscle), pumping of blood through the heart (cardiac muscle), and contraction of blood vessels and visceral organs (smooth muscle).
- Nervous tissue, which consists of two cell types, nerve cells or neurons and glial or supporting cells, is distributed throughout the body, and serves as the body's communication system. The nervous system is divided anatomically into the CNS, which consists of the brain and spinal cord, and the peripheral nervous system (PNS), which is composed of nerve tissue outside the CNS.

Although most cells differentiate into specialized cell types, many tissues contain a few *stem cells* that apparently are only partially differentiated.[1] These stem cells are still capable of cell division and serve as a reserve source for specialized cells throughout the life of the organism. They are the major source of cells that make regeneration possible in some tissues. Stem cells have varying abilities to differentiate. Some tissues, such as skeletal muscle tissue, lack sufficient numbers of undifferentiated cells and have limited regenerative capacity. Stem cells of the hematopoietic (blood) system have the greatest potential for differentiation. These cells can potentially reconstitute the entire blood-producing and immune systems. They are the major ingredient in bone marrow transplants. Other stem cells, such as those that replenish the mucosal surface of the gastrointestinal tract, are less general but can still differentiate.

Embryonic Origin of Tissue Types

All of the approximately 200 different types of body cells can be classified into four basic or primary tissue types: epithelial, connective, muscle, and nervous (Table 4.1). These basic tissue types are often described by their embryonic origin. The embryo is essentially a three-layered tubular structure (Fig. 4.16). The outer layer of the tube is called the *ectoderm;* the middle layer, the *mesoderm;* and the inner layer, the *endoderm.* All of the adult body tissues originate from these three cellular layers. Epithelium has its origin in all three embryonic layers, connective tissue and muscle develop mainly from the mesoderm, and nervous tissue develops from the ectoderm.

Epithelial Tissue

Epithelial tissue covers the body's outer surface and lines the internal closed cavities (including blood vessels and the chambers of the heart) and body tubes that communicate with the exterior (gastrointestinal, respiratory, and genitourinary tracts). Epithelium also forms the secretory portion of glands and their ducts, and the receptors for the special senses (taste, touch, hearing, and vision).

Origin and Characteristics

Epithelial tissue is derived from all three embryonic layers.[6] Most epithelia of the skin, mouth, nose, and anus are derived from the ectoderm. Linings of the respiratory tract, gastrointestinal tract, and glands of the digestive system are of endodermal origin. The endothelial lining of blood vessels originates from the mesoderm. Many types of epithelial tissue retain the ability to differentiate and undergo rapid proliferation for replacing injured cells.

The cells that make up epithelium have three general characteristics: (1) they are characterized by three distinct surfaces: a free surface or apical surface, a lateral surface, and a basal surface; (2) they are closely apposed and joined by cell-to-cell adhesion molecules, which form specialized cell junctions; and (3) their basal surface is attached to an underlying basement membrane (Fig. 4.17). The characteristics and geometric arrangement of the cells in the epithelium determine their function. The free or apical surface is always directed toward the exterior surface or lumen of an enclosed cavity or tube, the lateral surface communicates with adjacent cells and is characterized by specialized attachment areas, and the basal surface rests on the basement membrane anchoring the cell to the surrounding connective tissue.

Epithelial tissue is avascular (*i.e.,* without blood vessels) and must therefore receive oxygen and nutrients from the capillaries of the connective tissue on which the epithelial tissue rests (Fig. 4.17). To survive, epithelial tissue must be kept moist. Even the seemingly dry skin epithelium is kept moist by a nonvitalized, waterproof layer of superficial skin cells called *keratin,* which prevents evaporation of moisture from the deeper living cells.

TABLE 4.1 CLASSIFICATION OF TISSUE TYPES

TISSUE TYPE	LOCATION
Epithelial Tissue	
Covering and lining of body surfaces	
Simple epithelium	
Squamous	Lining of blood vessels, body cavities, alveoli of lungs
Cuboidal	Collecting tubules of kidney; covering of ovaries
Columnar	Lining of intestine and gallbladder
Stratified epithelium	
Squamous keratinized	Skin
Squamous nonkeratinized	Mucous membranes of mouth, oesophagus, and vagina
Cuboidal	Ducts of sweat glands
Columnar	Large ducts of salivary and mammary glands; also found in conjunctiva
Transitional	Bladder, ureters, renal pelvis
Pseudostratified	Tracheal and respiratory passages
Glandular	
Endocrine	Pituitary gland, thyroid gland, adrenal and other glands
Exocrine	Sweat glands and glands in gastrointestinal tract
Neuroepithelium	Olfactory mucosa, retina, tongue
Reproductive epithelium	Seminiferous tubules of testis; cortical portion of ovary
Connective Tissue	
Embryonic connective tissue	
Mesenchymal	Embryonic mesoderm
Mucous	Umbilical cord (Wharton jelly)
Adult connective tissue	
Loose or areolar	Subcutaneous areas
Dense regular	Tendons and ligaments
Dense irregular	Dermis of skin
Adipose	Fat pads, subcutaneous layers
Reticular	Framework of lymphoid organs, bone marrow, liver
Specialized connective tissue	
Bone	Long bones, flat bones
Cartilage	Tracheal rings, external ear, articular surfaces
Hematopoietic	Blood cells, myeloid tissue (bone marrow)
Muscle Tissue	
Skeletal	Skeletal muscles
Cardiac	Heart muscles
Smooth	Gastrointestinal tract, blood vessels, bronchi, bladder, and others
Nervous Tissue	
Neurons	Central and peripheral neurons and nerve fibres
Supporting cells	Glial and ependymal cells in central nervous system; Schwann and satellite cells in peripheral nervous system

Basement Membrane. Underneath all types of epithelial tissue is an extracellular matrix, called the *basement membrane.* A basement membrane consists of the basal lamina and an underlying reticular layer. The terms *basal lamina* and *basement membrane* are often used interchangeably. Epithelial cells have strong intracellular protein filaments (*i.e.,* cytoskeleton) that are important in transmitting mechanical stresses from one cell to another.[6]

Cell Junctions and Cell-to-Cell Adhesions. Cells of epithelial tissue are tightly bound together by specialized junctions. These specialized junctions enable the cells to form barriers to the movement of water, solutes, and cells from one body compartment to the next. Three basic types of intercellular junctions are observed in epithelial tissues: continuous tight junctions, adhering junctions, and gap junctions (Fig. 4.18).

Continuous tight or *occluding junctions* (*i.e.,* zonula occludens), which are found only in epithelial tissue, seal the surface membranes of adjacent cells together. This type of intercellular junction prevents materials such as macromolecules in the intestinal contents from entering the intercellular space.[6]

Adhering junctions represent sites of strong adhesion between cells. The primary role of adhering junctions may be

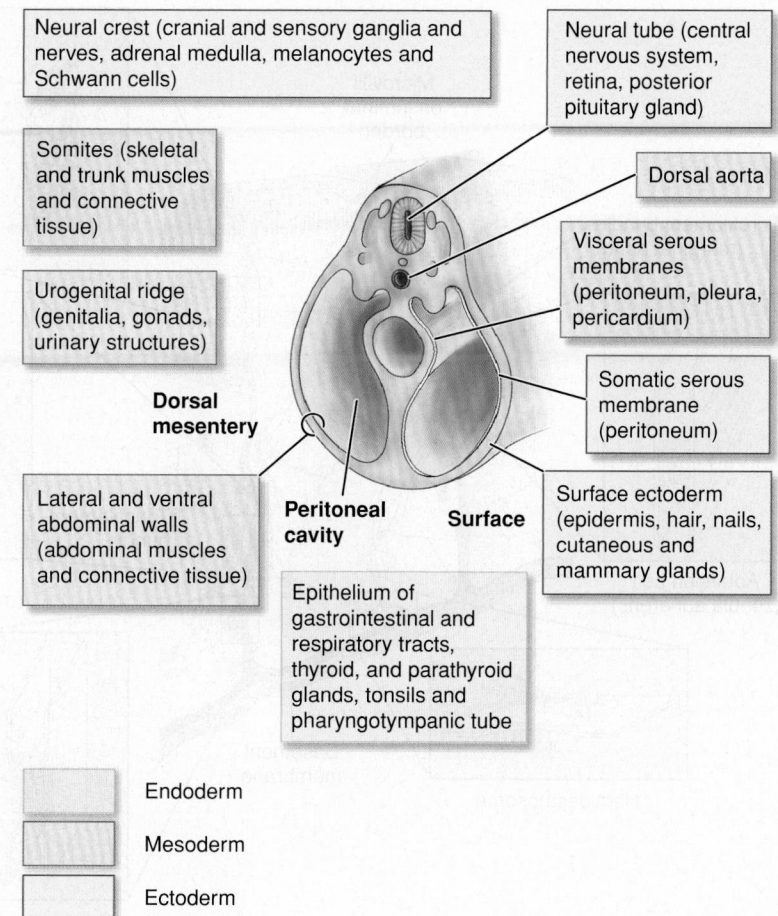

FIGURE 4.16 • Cross-section of human embryo illustrating the development of the somatic and visceral structures.

that of preventing cell separation. Adhering junctions are not restricted to epithelial tissue; they provide adherence between adjacent cardiac muscle cells as well. Adhering junctions are found as continuous, beltlike adhesive junctions (*i.e.,* zonula adherens) or scattered, spotlike adhesive junctions, called *desmosomes* (*i.e.,* macula adherens). A special feature of the

FIGURE 4.17 • Typical arrangement of epithelial cells in relation to underlying tissues and blood supply. Epithelial tissue has no blood supply of its own but relies on the blood vessels in the underlying connective tissue for nutrition (N) and elimination of wastes (W).

adhesion belt junction is that it provides an anchoring site to the cell membrane for microfilaments.[6] In epithelial desmosomes, bundles of keratin-containing intermediate filaments (*i.e.,* tonofilaments) are anchored to the junction on the cytoplasmic area of the cell membrane. A primary disease of desmosomes is *pemphigus,* which is caused by a buildup of antibodies to desmosome proteins.[10] Affected persons have skin and mucous membrane blistering. *Hemidesmosomes,* which resemble a half-desmosome, are another type of junction. They are found at the base of epithelial cells and help attach the epithelial cell to the underlying connective tissue.

Gap or *nexus junctions* involve the close adherence of adjoining cell membranes with the formation of channels that link the cytoplasm of the two cells. Gap junctions are not unique to epithelial tissue; they play an essential role in many types of cell-to-cell communication. Because they are low-resistance channels, gap junctions are important in cell-to-cell conduction of electrical signals (*e.g.,* between cells in sheets of smooth muscle or between adjacent cardiac muscle cells, where they function as electrical synapses). These multiple communication channels also enable ions and small molecules to pass directly from one cell to another.[6,9]

Types of Epithelium

Epithelial tissues are classified according to the shape of the cells and the number of layers that are present: *simple,*

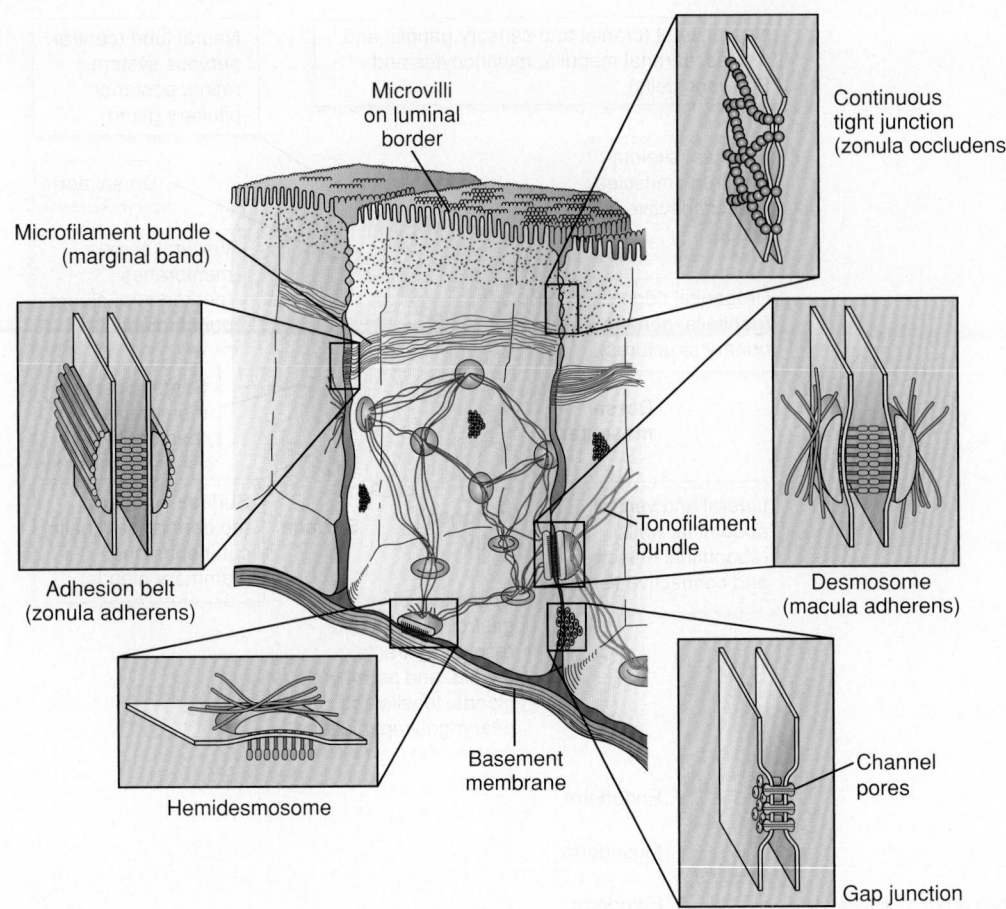

Microvilli on luminal border

Microfilament bundle (marginal band)

Adhesion belt (zonula adherens)

Hemidesmosome

Basement membrane

Continuous tight junction (zonula occludens)

Tonofilament bundle

Desmosome (macula adherens)

Channel pores

Gap junction

FIGURE 4.18 • Three types of intercellular junctions found in epithelial tissue: the continuous tight junction (zonula occludens); the adhering junction, which includes the adhesion belt (zonula adherens), desmosomes (macula adherens), and hemidesmosomes; and the gap junction.

stratified, and *pseudostratified.* The terms *squamous* (thin and flat), *cuboidal* (cube shaped), and *columnar* (resembling a column) refer to the cells' shape (Fig. 4.19).

Simple Epithelium. Simple epithelium contains a single layer of cells, all of which rest on the basement membrane. Simple squamous epithelium is adapted for filtration; it is found lining the blood vessels, lymph nodes, and alveoli of the lungs. The single layer of squamous epithelium lining the heart and blood vessels is known as the *endothelium.* A similar type of layer, called the *mesothelium,* forms the serous membranes that line the pleural, pericardial, and peritoneal cavities and cover the organs of these cavities. A *simple cuboidal epithelium* is found on the surface of the ovary and in the thyroid. *Simple columnar epithelium* lines the intestine. One form of a simple columnar epithelium has hairlike projections called *cilia,* often with specialized mucous-secreting cells called *goblet cells.* This form of simple columnar epithelium lines the airways of the respiratory tract.[6]

Stratified and Pseudostratified Epithelia. Stratified epithelium contains more than one layer of cells, with only the deepest layer resting on the basement membrane. It is designed to protect the body surface. *Stratified squamous keratinized* epithelium makes up the epidermis of the skin. *Keratin* is a tough, fibrous protein found as filaments in the outer cells of

skin. A stratified squamous keratinized epithelium is made up of many layers. The layers closest to the underlying tissues are cuboidal or columnar. The cells become more irregular and thinner as they move closer to the surface. Surface cells become totally filled with keratin and die, are sloughed off, and then replaced by the deeper cells. A stratified squamous nonkeratinized epithelium is found on moist surfaces such as the mouth and tongue. Stratified cuboidal and columnar epithelia are found in the ducts of salivary glands and the larger ducts of the mammary glands.[6] In smokers, the normal columnar ciliated epithelial cells of the trachea and bronchi are often replaced with stratified squamous epithelium cells that are better able to withstand the irritating effects of cigarette smoke.

Pseudostratified epithelium is a type of epithelium in which all of the cells are in contact with the underlying intercellular matrix, but some do not extend to the surface. A pseudostratified ciliated columnar epithelium with goblet cells forms the lining of most of the upper respiratory tract. All of the tall cells reaching the surface of this type of epithelium are either ciliated cells or mucous-producing goblet cells. The basal cells that do not reach the surface serve as stem cells for ciliated and goblet cells. *Transitional epithelium* is a stratified epithelium characterized by cells that can change shape and become thinner when the tissue is stretched. Such tissue can be stretched without pulling the superficial cells apart. Transitional epithelium is well adapted for the lining of organs

Simple squamous

Simple cuboidal

Simple columnar

Pseudostratified columnar ciliated

Transitional

Stratified squamous

FIGURE 4.19 • The various epithelial tissue types.

that are constantly changing their volume, such as the urinary bladder.

Glandular Epithelium. Glandular epithelial tissue is formed by cells specialized to produce a fluid secretion.[6] This process is usually accompanied by the intracellular synthesis of macromolecules. The chemical nature of these macromolecules is variable. The macromolecules typically are stored in the cells in small, membrane-bound vesicles called *secretory granules.* For example, glandular epithelia can synthesize, store, and secrete proteins (*e.g.,* insulin), lipids (*e.g.,* adrenocortical hormones, secretions of the sebaceous glands), and complexes of carbohydrates and proteins (*e.g.,* saliva). Less common are secretions that require minimal synthetic activity, such as those produced by the sweat glands.

All glandular cells arise from surface epithelia by means of cell proliferation and invasion of the underlying connective tissue, and all release their contents or secretions into the extracellular compartment. *Exocrine glands,* such as the sweat glands and lactating mammary glands, retain their connection with the surface epithelium from which they originated. This connection takes the form of epithelium-lined tubular ducts through which the secretions pass to reach the surface. Exocrine glands are often classified according to the way secretory products are released by their cells. In *holocrine*-type cells (*e.g.,* sebaceous glands), the glandular cell ruptures, releasing its entire content into the duct system. New generations of cells are replaced by mitosis of basal cells. *Merocrine-* or *eccrine*-type glands (*e.g.,* salivary glands, exocrine glands of the pancreas) release their glandular products by exocytosis. In *apocrine* secretions (*e.g.,* mammary glands, certain sweat glands), the apical portion of the cell, along with small portions of the cytoplasm, is pinched off the glandular cell. *Endocrine glands* are epithelial structures that have had their connection with the surface obliterated during development. These glands are ductless and produce secretions (*i.e.,* hormones) that move directly into the bloodstream.

Connective or Supportive Tissue

Connective or supportive tissue is the most abundant tissue in the body. As its name suggests, it connects and binds or supports the various tissues.[6] Connective tissue is unique in that its cells produce the extracellular matrix that supports and holds tissues together. The capsules that surround organs of the body are composed of connective tissue. Bone, adipose tissue, and cartilage are specialized types of connective tissue that function to support the soft tissues of the body and store fat. The proximity of the extracellular matrix to blood vessels allows it to function as an exchange medium through which nutrients and metabolic wastes pass.

Origin and Characteristics

Most connective tissue is derived from the embryonic mesoderm, but some is derived from the neural crest, a derivative of the ectoderm. During embryonic development, mesodermal cells migrate from their site of origin and then surround and penetrate the developing organ. These cells are called *mesenchymal cells,* and the tissue they form is called *mesenchyme.* Tissues derived from embryonic mesenchymal cells include bone, cartilage, and adipose (fat) cells. Besides providing the source or origin of most connective tissues, mesenchyme develops into other structures such as blood cells and blood vessels. Connective tissue cells include fibroblasts, chondroblasts, osteoblasts, hematopoietic stem cells, blood cells, macrophages, mast cells, and adipocytes.[6,9] The matrix of the umbilical cord is composed of a second type of embryonic mesoderm called *mucous connective tissue* or *Wharton jelly*.

Types of Connective Tissue

Adult connective tissue can be divided into two types: connective tissue proper, which is the focus of the discussion in this chapter, and specialized connective tissue (cartilage, bone, and blood cells), which is discussed in other chapters. There are four recognized types of connective tissue proper: loose (areolar), adipose, reticular, and dense connective tissue.[6,9]

Loose Connective Tissue. Loose connective tissue, also known as *areolar tissue,* is soft and pliable. It fills spaces between muscle sheaths and forms a layer that encases blood and lymphatic vessels (Fig. 4.20). Areolar connective tissue supports the epithelial tissues and provides the means by which these tissues are nourished. In an organ containing functioning epithelial tissue and supporting connective tissue, the term *parenchymal tissue* is used to describe the functioning epithelium as opposed to the connective tissue framework, or stroma.

Loose connective tissue is characterized by an abundance of ground substance and tissue fluid housing the fixed connective tissue cells: fibroblasts, mast cells, adipose or fat cells, macrophages, and leukocytes. Loose connective tissue cells secrete substances that form the extracellular matrix that supports and connects body cells. Fibroblasts are the most abundant of these cells. They are responsible for the synthesis of the fibrous and gel-like substance that fills the intercellular spaces of the body and for the production of collagen, elastic, and reticular fibres.

The *basal lamina* is a special type of intercellular matrix that is present where connective tissue contacts the tissue it supports. It is visible only with an electron microscope and is produced by the epithelial cells. In many locations, reticular fibres, produced by the connective tissue cells, are associated with the basal lamina.[6] Together the basal lamina and the reticular layer form the basement membrane seen by light microscopy. A basement membrane is found along the interface between connective tissue and muscle fibres, on Schwann cells of the PNS, on the basal surface of endothelial cells, and on fat cells. These basement membranes bond cells to the underlying or surrounding connective tissues, serve as selective filters for particles that pass between connective tissue and other cells, and contribute to cell regeneration and repair.

Adipose Tissue. Adipose tissue is a special form of connective tissue in which adipocytes predominate. Adipocytes do not generate an extracellular matrix but maintain a large intracellular space.[6] These cells store large quantities of triglycerides and are the largest repository of energy in the body. Adipose tissue helps fill spaces between tissues and helps to keep organs in place. The subcutaneous fat helps to shape the body. Because fat is a poor conductor of heat, adipose tissue serves as thermal insulation for the body. Adipose tissue exists in two forms: unilocular and multilocular. Unilocular (white) adipose tissue is composed of cells in which the fat is contained in a single, large droplet in the cytoplasm. Multilocular (brown) adipose tissue is composed of cells that contain multiple droplets of fat and numerous mitochondria (see Chapter 39).

Reticular Connective Tissue. *Reticular tissue* is characterized by a network of fibres interspersed with fibroblasts and macrophages. The fibroblasts synthesize type III collagen fibres. Reticular tissue forms the architecture of liver sinusoids, adipose tissue, bone marrow, and lymphoid tissues such as the spleen.

Dense Connective Tissue. Dense connective tissue exists in two forms: dense irregular and dense regular. Dense irregular connective tissue consists of the same components found in loose connective tissue, but exhibits a predominance of collagen fibres and fewer cells. This type of tissue can be found in the dermis of the skin (*i.e.,* reticular layer), the fibrous capsules of many organs, and the fibrous sheaths of cartilage (*i.e.,* perichondrium) and bone (*i.e.,* periosteum). It also forms the fascia that invests muscles and organs. Dense regular connective tissues are rich in collagen fibres and form the tendons and aponeuroses that join muscles to bone or other muscles and the ligaments that join bone to bone.

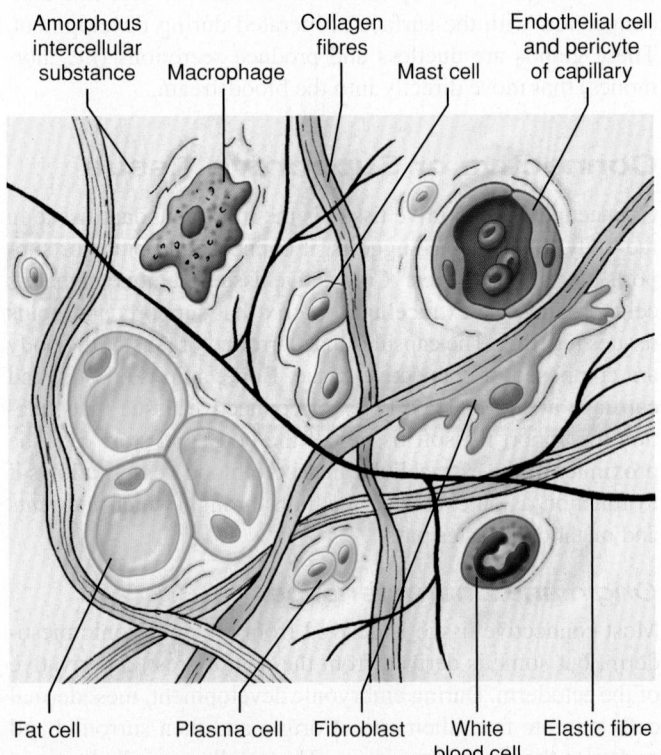

Amorphous intercellular substance · Macrophage · Collagen fibres · Mast cell · Endothelial cell and pericyte of capillary

Fat cell · Plasma cell · Fibroblast · White blood cell · Elastic fibre

FIGURE 4.20 • Diagrammatic representation of cells that may be seen in loose connective tissue. The cells lie in the extracellular matrix, which is bathed in tissue fluid that originates in the capillaries.

Muscle Tissue

Muscle tissue, whose primary function is contraction, is responsible for movement of the body and its parts and for changes in the size and shape of internal organs. Muscle tissue contains two types of fibres that are responsible for contraction: thin and thick filaments. The thin filaments are composed primarily of actin, whereas the thick filaments are composed of myosin. The two types of myofilaments occupy the bulk of the cytoplasm, which in muscle cells is called the *sarcoplasm*.[9]

There are three types of muscle tissues: *skeletal, cardiac,* and *smooth.* Skeletal and cardiac muscles are striated muscles, in which the actin and myosin filaments are arranged in large, parallel arrays in bundles, giving the muscle fibres a striped or striated appearance when observed with a microscope. *Smooth muscle* lacks striations and is found in the iris of the eye, the walls of blood vessels, hollow organs such as the stomach and urinary bladder, and hollow tubes, such as the ureters and common bile duct, that connect internal organs.[9]

Neither skeletal nor cardiac muscle can undergo the mitotic activity needed to replace injured cells. Smooth muscle, however, may proliferate and undergo mitotic activity. Some increases in smooth muscle are physiologic, as occurs in the uterus during pregnancy. Other increases, such as the increase in smooth muscle that occurs in the arteries of persons with chronic hypertension, are pathologic.

Although the three types of muscle tissue differ significantly in structure, contractile properties, and control mechanisms, they have many similarities. In the following section, the structural properties of skeletal muscle are presented as the prototype of striated muscle tissue. Smooth muscle and the ways in which it differs from skeletal muscle are also discussed. Cardiac muscle is described in Chapter 21.

Skeletal Muscle

Skeletal muscle is the most abundant tissue in the body, accounting for 40% to 45% of the total body weight.[9] Most skeletal muscles are attached to bones, and their contractions are responsible for movements of the skeleton. Each skeletal muscle is a discrete organ made up of hundreds or thousands of muscle fibres. At the periphery of skeletal muscle fibres, randomly scattered satellite cells are found. They represent a source of undifferentiated myoblast cells that may be involved in the limited regeneration capabilities of skeletal muscle. Although muscle fibres predominate, substantial amounts of connective tissue, blood vessels, and nerve fibres are also present.

Organization and Structure. In an intact muscle, the individual muscle fibres are held together by several different layers of connective tissue. Skeletal muscles such as the biceps brachii are surrounded by a dense, irregular connective tissue covering called the *epimysium* (Fig. 4.21A). Each muscle is subdivided into smaller bundles called *fascicles,* which are surrounded by a connective tissue covering called the *perimysium.* The number of fascicles and their size vary among muscles. Fascicles consist of many elongated structures called *muscle fibres,* each of which is surrounded by connective tissue called the *endomysium.* Skeletal muscles are syncytial or multinucleated structures, meaning there are no true cell boundaries within a skeletal muscle fibre.[9]

The sarcoplasm of the muscle fibre is contained within the sarcolemma, which represents the cell membrane. Embedded

FIGURE 4.21 • **A:** Connective tissue components of a skeletal muscle. **B:** Striations of the myofibril showing the overlap of contractile proteins and the A and I bands, the H zone, and the Z and M lines. **C:** The relaxed and contracted states of the myofibril showing the position of actin filaments (blue) between the myosin filaments (pink) in the relaxed muscle (top) and pulling of the Z membranes toward each other (bottom) as the muscle contracts. **D:** The sarcoplasmic reticulum with T tubules.

throughout the sarcoplasm are the contractile elements actin and myosin, which are arranged in parallel bundles called *myofibrils.* The thin, lighter-staining myofilaments are composed of actin, and the thicker, darker-staining myofilaments are composed of myosin. Each myofibril consists of regularly repeating units along the length of the myofibril, called *sarcomeres* (Fig. 4.21B).[9]

Sarcomeres are the structural and functional units of cardiac and skeletal muscle. A sarcomere extends from one Z-line to another Z-line. Within the sarcomere are alternating light and dark bands. The central portion of the sarcomere contains the dark band (A-band) consisting mainly of myosin filaments, with some overlap with actin filaments. Straddling the Z-line, the lighter I-band contains only actin filaments; therefore, it takes two sarcomeres to complete an I-band. An H-zone is found in the middle of the A-band and represents the region where only myosin filaments are found. In the centre of the H-zone is a thin, dark band, the M-band or M-line, produced by linkages between the myosin filaments. Z-lines consist of short elements that interconnect and provide the thin actin filaments from two adjoining sarcomeres with an anchoring point.

The *sarcoplasmic reticulum,* which is comparable to the smooth ER, is composed of longitudinal tubules that run parallel to the muscle fibre and surround each myofibril (Fig. 4–21D). This network ends in enlarged, saclike regions called the *lateral sacs* or *terminal cisternae.* These sacs store calcium that is released during muscle contraction. A binding protein called *calsequestrin* found in the terminal cisternae enables a high concentration of calcium ions to be sequestered in the cisternae, and only a portion are released when necessary.[9] Concentration levels of calcium ions in the cisternae are 10,000 times higher than in the sarcoplasm.

A second system of tubules consists of the *transverse* or *T tubules,* which are extensions of the plasma membrane and run perpendicular to the muscle fibre. The hollow portion or lumen of the transverse tubule is continuous with the extracellular fluid compartment. Action potentials, which are rapidly conducted over the surface of the muscle fibre, are in turn propagated by the T tubules into the sarcoplasmic reticulum. As the action potential moves through the lateral sacs, the sacs release calcium, initiating muscle contraction. The membrane of the sarcoplasmic reticulum also has an active transport mechanism for pumping calcium back into the reticulum. This prevents interactions between calcium ions and the actin and myosin myofilaments after cessation of a muscle contraction.

Skeletal Muscle Contraction. During muscle contraction, the thick myosin and thin actin filaments slide over each other, causing shortening of the muscle fibre, although the length of the individual thick and thin filaments remains unchanged (Fig. 4.21B and C). The structures that produce the sliding of the filaments are the myosin heads that form cross-bridges with the thin actin filaments (Fig. 4.22). When activated by ATP, the cross-bridges swivel in a fixed arc, much like the oars of a boat, as they become attached to the actin filament. During contraction, each cross-bridge undergoes its own cycle of movement, forming a bridge attachment and releasing it, and moving to another site where the same sequence of movement occurs. This pulls the thin and thick filaments past each other.

FIGURE 4.22 • Molecular structure of the thin actin filament (**A**) and the thicker myosin filament (**B**) of striated muscle. The thin filament is a double-stranded helix of actin molecules with tropomyosin and troponin molecules lying along the grooves of the actin strands (**C**). Sequence of events involved in sliding of adjacent actin and myosin filaments: *(1)* cocking of the myosin head occurs as ATP is split to ADP; *(2)* cross-bridge attachment; *(3)* power stroke during which the myosin head bends as it moves the actin forward; and *(4)* cross-bridge detachment occurs as a new ATP attaches to the myosin head.

Myosin is the chief constituent of the thick filament. It consists of a thin tail, which provides the structural backbone for the filament, and a globular head. Each globular head contains a binding site able to bind to a complementary site on the actin molecule. Besides the binding site for actin, each myosin head has a separate active site that catalyzes the breakdown of ATP to provide the energy needed to activate the myosin head so that it can form a cross-bridge with actin. After contraction, myosin also binds ATP, thus breaking the linkage between actin and myosin. Myosin molecules are bundled together side by side in the thick filaments such that one half have their heads toward one end of the filament and their tails toward the other end; the other half are arranged in the opposite manner.

The thin filaments are composed mainly of actin, a globular protein lined up in two rows that coil around each other to form a long helical strand. Associated with each actin filament are two regulatory proteins, tropomyosin and troponin (Fig. 4.22). *Tropomyosin,* which lies in grooves of the actin strand, provides the site for attachment of the globular heads of the myosin filament. In the noncontracted state, *troponin* covers the tropomyosin binding sites and prevents formation of cross-bridges between the actin and myosin. During an action potential, calcium ions released from the sarcoplasmic reticulum diffuse to the adjacent myofibrils, where they bind to troponin. Binding of calcium to troponin uncovers the tropomyosin binding sites such that the myosin heads can attach and form cross-bridges.[6] Energy from ATP is used to break the actin and myosin cross-bridges, stopping the muscle contraction. After the linkage between actin and myosin is broken, the concentration of calcium around the myofibrils decreases as calcium is actively transported into the sarcoplasmic reticulum by a membrane pump that uses energy derived from ATP.

The basis of *rigor mortis* can be explained by the binding of actin and myosin. As the muscle begins to degenerate after death, the sarcoplasmic cisternae release their calcium ions, which enable the myosin heads to combine with their sites on the actin molecule. Without ATP the myosin heads cannot detach from binding sites on actin and the muscle remain in a contracted state or a state of rigor until further degeneration destroys the cross-bridges between actin and myosin.

Smooth Muscle

Smooth muscle is often called *involuntary muscle* because its activity arises spontaneously or through activity of the autonomic nervous system. Smooth muscle contractions are slower and more sustained than skeletal or cardiac muscle contractions.

Organization and Structure. Smooth muscle cells are spindle shaped and smaller than skeletal muscle fibres. Each smooth muscle cell has one centrally positioned nucleus. Z-lines and M-lines are not present in smooth muscle fibres, and cross-striations are absent because the bundles of filaments are not parallel but crisscross obliquely through the cell. Instead, the actin filaments are attached to structures called *dense bodies* (Fig. 4.23). Some dense bodies are attached to

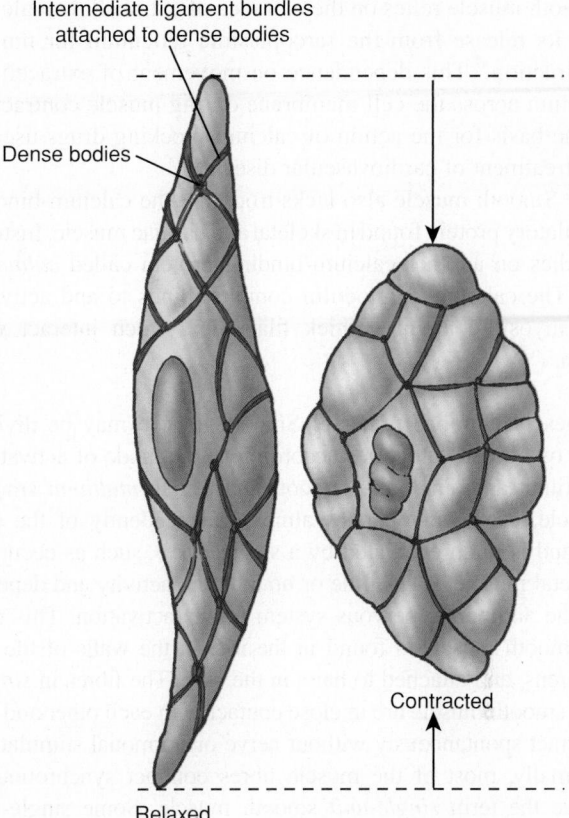

FIGURE 4.23 • Structure of smooth muscle showing the dense bodies. In smooth muscle, the force of contraction is transmitted to the cell membrane by bundles of intermediate fibres.

the cell membrane, and others are dispersed in the cell and linked together by structural proteins.[6,9]

The lack of Z-lines and the regular overlapping of contractile elements provide a greater range of tension development. This is important in hollow organs that undergo changes in volume, with consequent changes in the length of the smooth muscle fibres in their walls. Even with the distension of a hollow organ, the smooth muscle fibre retains some ability to develop tension, whereas such distension would stretch skeletal muscle beyond the area where the thick and thin filaments overlap.

Smooth muscle is usually arranged in sheets or bundles. In hollow organs, such as the intestines, the bundles are organized into the two-layered muscularis externa consisting of an outer, longitudinal layer and an inner, circular layer. A thinner muscularis mucosae often lies between the muscularis externa and the endothelium. In blood vessels, the bundles are arranged circularly or helically around the vessel wall.

Smooth Muscle Contraction. As with cardiac and skeletal muscle, smooth muscle contraction is initiated by an increase in intracellular calcium. However, smooth muscle differs from skeletal muscle in the way its cross-bridges are formed. The sarcoplasmic reticulum of smooth muscle is less developed than in skeletal muscle, and no transverse tubules are present.

Smooth muscle relies on the entrance of extracellular calcium and its release from the sarcoplasmic reticulum for muscle contraction.[6] This dependence on movement of extracellular calcium across the cell membrane during muscle contraction is the basis for the action of calcium-blocking drugs used in the treatment of cardiovascular disease.

Smooth muscle also lacks troponin, the calcium-binding regulatory protein found in skeletal and cardiac muscle. Instead, it relies on another calcium-binding protein called *calmodulin*. The calcium–calmodulin complex binds to and activates the myosin-containing thick filaments, which interact with actin.

Types of Smooth Muscle. Smooth muscle may be divided into two broad categories according to the mode of activation: multiunit and single-unit smooth muscle. In *multiunit* smooth muscle, each unit operates almost independently of the others and is often enervated by a single nerve, such as occurs in skeletal muscle. It has little or no inherent activity and depends on the autonomic nervous system for its activation. This type of smooth muscle is found in the iris, in the walls of the vas deferens, and attached to hairs in the skin. The fibres in *single-unit* smooth muscle are in close contact with each other and can contract spontaneously without nerve or hormonal stimulation. Normally, most of the muscle fibres contract synchronously, hence the term *single-unit* smooth muscle. Some single-unit smooth muscle, such as that found in the gastrointestinal tract, is self-excitable. This is usually associated with a basic slow-wave rhythm transmitted from cell to cell by nexuses (*i.e.,* gap junctions) formed by the fusion of adjacent cell membranes. The cause of this slow-wave activity is unknown. The intensity of contraction increases with the frequency of the action potential. Certain hormones, other agents, and local factors can modify smooth muscle activity by depolarizing or hyperpolarizing the membrane. Smooth muscle cells found in the uterus and small-diameter blood vessels are also single-unit smooth muscle.

Nervous Tissue

Nervous tissue is distributed throughout the body as an integrated communication system. Anatomically, the nervous system is divided into the CNS, which consists of the brain and spinal cord, and the PNS, which consists of nerve fibres and ganglia that exist outside the CNS. Nerve cells develop from the embryonic ectoderm. Nerve cells are highly differentiated and therefore incapable of regeneration in postnatal life.

Structurally, nervous tissue consists of two cell types: nerve cells or neurons, and glial or supporting cells. Most nerve cells consist of three parts: the soma or cell body, dendrites, and the axon. The cytoplasm-filled dendrites, which are multiple elongated processes, receive and carry stimuli from the environment, from sensory epithelial cells, and from other neurons to the cell. The axon, which is a single cytoplasm-filled process, is specialized for generating and conducting nerve impulses away from the cell body to other nerve cells, muscle cells, and glandular cells.

Neurons can be classified as afferent and efferent neurons according to their function. Afferent or sensory neurons carry information toward the CNS; they are involved in the reception of sensory information from the external environment and from within the body. Efferent or motor neurons carry information away from the CNS; they are needed for control of muscle fibres and endocrine and exocrine glands.

Communication between neurons and effector organs, such as muscle cells, occurs at specialized structures called *synapses*. At the synapse, chemical messengers (*i.e.,* neurotransmitters) alter the membrane potential to conduct impulses from one nerve to another or from a neuron to an effector cell. In addition, electrical synapses exist in which nerve cells are linked through gap junctions that permit the passage of ions from one cell to another.

Neuroglia (*glia* means "glue") are the cells that support neurons, form myelin, and have trophic and phagocytic functions (see Chapter 48). Four types of neuroglia are found in the CNS: astrocytes, oligodendrocytes, microglia, and ependymal cells. Astrocytes are the most abundant of the neuroglia. They have many long processes that surround blood vessels in the CNS. They provide structural support for the neurons, and their extensions form a sealed barrier that protects the CNS. The oligodendrocytes provide myelination of neuronal processes in the CNS. The microglia are phagocytic cells that represent the mononuclear phagocytic system in the nervous system. Ependymal cells line the cavities of the brain and spinal cord and are in contact with the cerebrospinal fluid. In the PNS, supporting cells consist of the Schwann and satellite cells. The Schwann cells provide myelination of the axons and dendrites, and the satellite cells enclose and protect the dorsal root ganglia and autonomic ganglion cells.

Extracellular Tissue Components

The discussion thus far has focused on the cellular components of the different tissue types. Within tissues, cells are held together by cell junctions; the space between cells is filled with an extracellular matrix; and adhesion molecules form intercellular contacts.

Extracellular Matrix

Tissues are not made up solely of cells. A large part of their volume is made up of an extracellular matrix. This matrix is composed of a variety of proteins and polysaccharides (*i.e.,* a molecule made up of many sugars).[6] These proteins and polysaccharides are secreted locally and are organized into a supporting meshwork in close association with the cells that produced them. The amount and composition of the matrix vary with the different tissues and their function. In bone, for example, the matrix is more plentiful than the cells that surround it; in the brain, the cells are much more abundant and the matrix is only a minor constituent.

Two main classes of extracellular macromolecules make up the extracellular matrix. The first is composed of polysaccharide chains of a class called *glycosaminoglycans* (GAGs), which are usually found linked to protein as proteoglycans.[10]

The second type consists of the fibrous proteins (*i.e.,* collagen and elastin) and the fibrous adhesive proteins (*i.e.,* fibronectin and laminin) that are found in the basement membrane. Members of each of these two classes of extracellular macromolecules come in a variety of shapes and sizes.

The proteoglycan and GAG molecules in connective tissue form a highly hydrated, gel-like substance, or tissue gel, in which the fibrous proteins are embedded.[10] The polysaccharide gel resists compressive forces, the collagen fibres strengthen and help organize the matrix, the rubber-like elastin adds resilience, and the adhesive proteins help cells attach to the appropriate part of the matrix. Polysaccharides in the tissue gel are highly hydrophilic, and they form gels even at low concentrations. They also accumulate a negative charge that attracts cations such as sodium, which are osmotically active, causing large amounts of water to be sucked into the matrix. This creates a swelling pressure, or turgor, that enables the matrix to withstand extensive compressive forces. This is in contrast to collagen, which resists stretching forces. For example, the cartilage matrix that lines the knee joint can support pressures of hundreds of atmospheres by this mechanism.

Glycosaminoglycan and proteoglycan molecules in connective tissue usually constitute less than 10% by weight of fibrous tissue. Because they form a hydrated gel, the molecules fill most of the extracellular space, providing mechanical support to the tissues while ensuring rapid diffusion of water and electrolytes and the migration of cells. One GAG, hyaluronan or hyaluronic acid, is thought to play an important role as a space-filler during embryonic development. It creates a cell-free space into which cells subsequently migrate When cell migration and organ development are complete, the excess hyaluronan is degraded by the enzyme hyaluronidase. Hyaluronan is also important in directing the cell replacement that occurs during wound repair (see Chapter 18).[10]

Three types of fibres are found in the extracellular space: collagen, elastin, and reticular fibres. *Collagen* is the most common protein in the body. It is a tough, nonliving, white fibre that serves as the structural framework for skin, ligaments, tendons, and many other structures. *Elastin* acts like a rubber band; it can be stretched and then returns to its original form. Elastin fibres are abundant in structures subjected to frequent stretching, such as the aorta and some ligaments. *Reticular fibres* are extremely thin fibres that create a flexible network in organs subjected to changes in form or volume, such as the spleen, liver, uterus, or intestinal muscle layer.

Adhesion Molecules

Important classes of extracellular macromolecules are the cell adhesion molecules (CAMs). CAMs can be cell-to-cell or cell-to-matrix adhesion molecules. There are four main classes of CAMs: cadherins, selectins, integrins, and the immunoglobulin (Ig) superfamily of proteins.[10] Cadherins, selectins, and integrins all depend on extracellular calcium ions (or magnesium for some integrins) to function. The calcium-independent cell-to-cell adhesion molecules belong to the Ig superfamily of proteins.

FIGURE 4.24 • Examples of homophilic and heterophilic intercellular adhesion. **A:** Homophilic adhesion can be accomplished by two identical cadherin dimer molecules joined at their N-terminal domains. **B:** Binding of the lectin domain of an integrin with the carbohydrate portions of a ligand is an example of heterophilic binding. (Courtesy of Edward W. Carroll.)

Cadherins. Cadherins link parts of the internal cytoskeleton (actin and structures called *catenins*) with extracellular cadherins of an adjacent cell. This type of linkage is called *homophilic,* meaning that molecules on one cell bind to other molecules of the same type on adjacent cells (Fig. 4.24A). More than 40 different types of cadherins are known, and they are found in such intercellular junctions as the zonula and macula adherens.[10]

Selectins. Selectins bind carbohydrates present on the ligands of an adjacent cell in a *heterophilic* type of interaction (Fig. 4.24B). In heterophilic interactions, the molecules on one cell bind to molecules of a different type on adjacent cells. Selectins are found on activated endothelial cells of blood vessels, on leukocytes, and on platelets. They, together with integrins and immunoglobulins, participate in leukocyte movement through the endothelial lining of blood vessels during inflammation.[10]

Integrins. Integrins usually assist in attaching epithelial cells to the underlying basement membrane.[10] Unlike other CAMs, they are heterodimers consisting of α and β subunits. Extracellularly, they are attached to fibronectin and laminin, the two major components of the basement membrane. Like the cadherins, their intracellular portion is linked to actin (Fig. 4.24). One group of integrins is associated with hemidesmosomes, whereas others are associated with the surface of white blood cells, macrophages, and platelets. Integrins usually have a weak affinity for their ligands unless they are associated with cellular focal contacts and hemidesmosomes. This allows some movement between cells except where a firm attachment is required to attach epithelial cells to the underlying connective tissue.

Certain integrins play an important role in allowing white blood cells to pass through the vessel wall, a process called *transmigration*. Persons affected with leukocyte adhesion deficiency are unable to synthesize appropriate integrin molecules.[10] As a result, they experience repeated bacterial infections because their white blood cells are unable to transmigrate through vessel walls.

Immunoglobulin Superfamily. The Ig superfamily proteins consist of groups of one or more Ig-like adhesion proteins that are structurally similar to antibody molecules. The best-studied example of Ig superfamily proteins are the neural cell adhesion molecules (NCAMs), which are expressed in a variety of cells, including most nerve cells. All are calcium ion independent but, unlike other CAMs, they may participate in homophilic or heterophilic interactions. Heterophilic attachments are to other members of the superfamily such as intracellular adhesion molecules (ICAMs). During early development of the CNS, cells at the roof of the neural tube express high levels of NCAM on their cell surface and are unable to move because of intercellular adhesions. Future neural crest cells lose their NCAM and begin migrating to various areas of the body. Members of the Ig superfamily also play a role in the homing process of leukocytes during inflammation.

IN SUMMARY

Body cells are organized into four basic tissue types: epithelial, connective, muscle, and nervous. The epithelium covers and lines the body surfaces and forms the functional components of glandular structures. Epithelial tissue is classified into three types according to the shape of the cells and the number of layers that are present: simple, stratified, and pseudostratified. The cells in epithelial tissue are held together by three types of intercellular junctions: tight, adhering, and gap. They are attached to the underlying tissue by hemidesmosomes.

Connective tissue supports and connects body structures; it forms the bones and skeletal system, joint structures, blood cells, and intercellular substances. Connective tissue proper can be divided into four types: loose or areolar, which fills body spaces and is characterized by an abundance of ground substance; adipose, which stores fat; reticular, which forms the architectural framework in many structures of the body; and dense, regular and irregular, which forms structures such as tendons and ligaments (regular) and the dermis of the skin (irregular).

Muscle tissue is a specialized tissue designed for contractility. Three types of muscle tissue exist: skeletal, cardiac, and smooth. Actin and myosin filaments interact to produce muscle shortening, a process activated by the presence of calcium. In skeletal muscle, calcium is released from the sarcoplasmic reticulum in response to an action potential. Smooth muscle is often called involuntary muscle because it contracts spontaneously or through activity of the autonomic nervous system. It differs from skeletal muscle in that its sarcoplasmic reticulum is less defined and it depends on the entry of extracellular calcium ions for muscle contraction.

Nervous tissue is designed for communication purposes and includes the neurons, the supporting neural structures, and the ependymal cells that line the ventricles of the brain and the spinal canal.

The extracellular matrix is made up of a variety of proteins and polysaccharides. These proteins and polysaccharides are secreted locally and are organized into a supporting meshwork in close association with the cells that produced them. The amount and composition of matrix vary with the different tissues and their function. Extracellular fibres include collagen fibres, which comprise tendons and ligaments; elastic fibres, found in large arteries and some ligaments; and thin reticular fibres, which are plentiful in organs that are subject to a change in volume (e.g., spleen and liver). Important classes of extracellular macromolecules are the adhesion molecules that maintain intercellular contacts. There are three classes of adhesion molecules that depend on extracellular calcium to function in cell adhesion: cadherins, which link parts of the internal cytoskeleton with the extracellular cadherins of an adjacent cell; selectins, which bind carbohydrates present on the ligands of adjacent cells; and integrins (some of which are magnesium dependent), which assist in attaching epithelial cells to the underlying basement membrane. The Ig superfamily of proteins are calcium-independent adhesion molecules that bind cells, such as those of the nervous system, together.

REVIEW EXERCISES

1. Tattoos consist of pigments that have been injected into the skin.
   A. *Explain what happens to the dye once it has been injected and why it does not eventually wash away.*
2. Persons who drink sufficient amounts of alcohol display rapid changes in central nervous system function, including both motor and behavioural changes, and the odour of alcohol can be detected on their breath.
   A. *Use the concepts related to the lipid bilayer structure of the cell membrane to explain these observations.*
3. The absorption of glucose from the intestine involves a cotransport mechanism in which the active primary transport of sodium ions is used to provide for the secondary transport of glucose.
   A. *Hypothesize how this information might be used to design an oral rehydration solution for someone who is suffering from diarrhea.*

References

1. Hall J. E. (2011). *Guyton and Hall Textbook of Medical Physiology.* (12th ed.). Philadelphia, PA: Saunders.

2. Brock M. V., Herman J. G., Baylin S. B. (2007). Cancer as a manifestation of aberrant chromatin structure. *Cancer Journal, 13*(1), 3–8.

3. Kaser A., Martinez-Naves E., Blumberg R. S. (2010). Endoplasmic reticulum stress: Implications for inflammatory bowel disease pathogenesis. *Current Opinion in Gastroenterology, 26*(4), 318–326.

4. Thomas S. E., Dalton L. E., Daly M. L., et al. (2010). Diabetes as a disease of endoplasmic reticulum stress. *Diabetes Metabolism Research & Reviews, 16*(8) 611–621.

5. Zong E. M., Lundberg I. (2011). Pathogenesis, classification, & treatment of inflammatory myopathies. *Nature Reviews Rheumatology, 7*(5), 297–306.

6. McConnell T. H., Hull K. L. (2011). *Human form human function: Essentials of anatomy & physiology.* Philadelphia, PA: Lippincott.

7. Boron W. F., Boulpaep E. L. (2009). *Medical physiology* (2nd ed.). Philadelphia, PA: Saunders.

8. Wang R. Y., Bodemer O. A., Watson M. S., et al. (2011). Lysosomal storage diseases: Diagnosis confirmation and management of presymptomatic individuals. *Genetics in Medicine, 13*(5), 457–484.

9. Ross M. H., Pawina W. (2011). *Histology: A text and atlas* (6th ed.). Philadelphia, PA: Lippincott.

10. Rubin R., Strayer D. (2012). *Rubin's Pathology: Clinicopathologic foundations of medicine* (6th ed.). Philadelphia, PA: Lippincott.

11. Lehne R. (2009). *Pharmacology for nursing care* (7th ed.). Philadelphia, PA: W. B. Saunders.

12. Ozkaya S., Sahin U., Gurrus A., et al. (2011). Bronchiolitis as a feature of Kartagener syndrome: A case report. *Journal of Bronchology & Interventional Pulmonology, 18*(1), 88–90.

13. Priori S. G. (2010). The fifteen years of discoveries that shaped molecular electrophysiology: Time for appraisal. *Circulation Research, 107*(4), 451–456.

14. Lam S. K., Ng T. B. (2011). Lectins: Production & practical applications. *Appl Microbiol Biotechnol, 89*(1), 45–55.

Visit thePoint **http://thePoint.lww.com for animations, journal articles, and more!**

Cellular Adaptation, Injury, and Death

5

When confronted with stresses that endanger its normal structure and function, the cell undergoes adaptive changes that permit survival and maintenance of function. It is only when the stress is overwhelming or adaptation is ineffective that cell injury, dysfunction, and eventual death occur. This chapter focuses on cellular adaptation, injury, and death.

CELLULAR ADAPTATION

After completing this section of the chapter, you should be able to meet the following objectives:

- Cite the general purpose of changes in cell structure and function that occur as the result of normal adaptive processes.
- Describe cell changes that occur with atrophy, hypertrophy, hyperplasia, metaplasia, and dysplasia and state general conditions under which the changes occur.
- Compare the pathogenesis and effects of dystrophic and metastatic calcifications.

Cells adapt to changes in the internal environment, just as the total organism adapts to changes in the external environment. Cells may adapt by undergoing changes in size, number, and type. These changes, occurring singly or in combination, may lead to atrophy, hypertrophy, hyperplasia, metaplasia, and dysplasia (Fig. 5.1). Adaptive cellular responses also include intracellular accumulations and storage of products in abnormal amounts.[1,2]

There are numerous molecular mechanisms mediating cellular adaptation, including factors produced by other cells or by the cells themselves. These mechanisms depend largely on signals transmitted by chemical messengers that exert their effects by altering gene function. In general, the genes expressed in all cells fall into two categories: operating genes that are necessary for normal function of a cell, and genes that determine the differentiating characteristics of a particular cell type. In many adaptive cellular responses, the expression of the differentiation genes is altered, whereas that of the operating genes remains unaffected. Thus, a cell is able to change size

Normal cells

Atrophy

Hypertrophy

Hyperplasia

Metaplasia

Dysplasia

— Nucleus

— Basement membrane

FIGURE 5.1 • Adaptive cell and tissue responses involving a change in cell size (atrophy and hypertrophy), number (hyperplasia), cell type (metaplasia), or size, shape, and organization (dysplasia). (From Anatomical Chart Company. (2010). *Atlas of pathophysiology* (p. 4). Springhouse, PA: Springhouse.)

or form without compromising its normal function. Once the stimulus for adaptation is removed, the effect on expression of the differentiating genes is removed and the cell resumes its previous state of specialized function. Whether adaptive cellular changes are normal or abnormal depends on whether the response was mediated by an appropriate stimulus. Normal adaptive responses occur in response to need and an appropriate stimulus. After the need has been removed, the adaptive response ceases.

CELLULAR ADAPTATION

- Cells are able to adapt to increased work demands or threats to survival by changing their size (atrophy and hypertrophy), number (hyperplasia), and form (metaplasia).
- Normal cellular adaptation occurs in response to an appropriate stimulus and ceases once the need for adaptation has ceased.

Atrophy

When confronted with a decrease in work demands or adverse environmental conditions, most cells are able to revert to a smaller size and a lower and more efficient level of functioning that is compatible with survival. This decrease in cell size is called *atrophy*. Cells that are atrophied reduce their oxygen consumption and other cellular functions by decreasing the number and size of their organelles and other structures. There are fewer mitochondria, myofilaments, and endoplasmic reticulum structures. When a sufficient number of cells are involved, the entire tissue or muscle atrophies.

Cell size, particularly in muscle tissue, is related to workload. As the workload of a cell declines, oxygen consumption and protein synthesis decrease. Furthermore, proper muscle mass is maintained by sufficient levels of insulin and insulin-like growth factor-1 (IGF-1).[3] When insulin and IGF-1 levels are low or catabolic signals are present, muscle atrophy occurs by mechanisms that include reduced synthetic processes, increased proteolysis by the ubiquitin-proteasome system, and apoptosis or programmed cell death.[4] In the ubiquitin-proteasome system, intracellular proteins destined for destruction are covalently bonded to a small protein called *ubiquitin* and then degraded by small cytoplasmic organelles called *proteasomes* (discussed in Chapter 4).[4]

The general causes of atrophy can be grouped into five categories: (1) disuse, (2) denervation, (3) loss of endocrine stimulation, (4) inadequate nutrition, and (5) ischemia or decreased blood flow. Disuse atrophy occurs when there is a reduction in skeletal muscle use. An example of disuse atrophy is seen in the muscles of extremities that have been encased in plaster casts. Because atrophy is adaptive and reversible, muscle size is restored after the cast is removed and muscle use is resumed. Denervation atrophy is a form of disuse atrophy that occurs in the muscles of paralyzed limbs. Lack of endocrine stimulation produces a form of disuse atrophy. In women, the loss of estrogen stimulation during menopause results in atrophic changes in the reproductive organs. With malnutrition and decreased blood flow, cells decrease their size and energy requirements as a means of survival.

FIGURE 5.2 • Myocardial hypertrophy. Cross-section of the heart in a patient with long-standing hypertension. (From Rubin R., Strayer D. S. (2012). *Rubin's pathology: Clinicopathologic foundations of medicine* (6th ed., p. 4). Philadelphia, PA: Lippincott Williams & Wilkins.)

Hypertrophy

Hypertrophy represents an increase in cell size, and with it an increase in the amount of functioning tissue mass. It results from an increased workload imposed on an organ or body part and is commonly seen in cardiac and skeletal muscle tissue, which cannot adapt to an increase in workload through mitotic division and formation of more cells (Fig. 5.2). Hypertrophy involves an increase in the functional components of the cell that allows it to achieve equilibrium between demand and functional capacity. For example, as muscle cells hypertrophy, additional actin and myosin filaments, cell enzymes, and adenosine triphosphate (ATP) are synthesized.[1]

Hypertrophy may occur as the result of normal physiologic or abnormal pathologic conditions. The increase in muscle mass associated with exercise is an example of physiologic hypertrophy. Pathologic hypertrophy occurs as the result of disease conditions and may be adaptive or compensatory. Examples of adaptive hypertrophy are the thickening of the urinary bladder from long-continued obstruction of urinary outflow and the myocardial hypertrophy that results from valvular heart disease or hypertension. Compensatory hypertrophy is the enlargement of a remaining organ or tissue after a portion has been surgically removed or rendered inactive. For instance, if one kidney is removed, the remaining kidney enlarges to compensate for the loss.

The initiating signals for hypertrophy appear to be complex and related to ATP depletion, mechanical forces such as stretching of the muscle fibres, activation of cell degradation products, and hormonal factors. In the case of the heart, initiating signals can be divided into two broad categories: (1) biomechanical and stretch-sensitive mechanisms; and (2) neurohumoral mechanisms that are associated with the release of hormones, growth factors, cytokines, and chemokines.[4] Internal stretch-sensitive receptors for the biochemical signals and an array of membrane-bound receptors for the

specific neurohumoral ligands, such as IGF-1 and epidermal growth factor (EGF), activate specific signal transduction pathways.[5] These pathways control myocardial growth by altering gene expression to increase protein synthesis and reduce protein degradation, thereby causing hypertrophic enlargement of the heart. A limit is eventually reached beyond which further enlargement of the tissue mass can no longer compensate for the increased work demands. The limiting factors for continued hypertrophy might be related to limitations in blood flow. In hypertension, for example, the increased workload required to pump blood against an elevated arterial pressure results in a progressive increase in left ventricular muscle mass and need for coronary blood flow.

There continues to be interest in the signalling pathways that control the arrangement of contractile elements in myocardial hypertrophy. Research suggests that certain signal molecules can alter gene expression controlling the size and assembly of the contractile proteins in hypertrophied myocardial cells. For example, the hypertrophied myocardial cells of well-trained athletes have proportional increases in width and length. This is in contrast to the hypertrophy that develops in dilated cardiomyopathy, in which the hypertrophied cells have a relatively greater increase in length than width. In pressure overload, as occurs with hypertension, the hypertrophied cells have greater width than length.[6] It is anticipated that further elucidation of the signal pathways that determine the adaptive and nonadaptive features of cardiac hypertrophy will lead to new targets for treatment.

Hyperplasia

Hyperplasia refers to an increase in the number of cells in an organ or tissue. It occurs in tissues with cells that are capable of mitotic division, such as the epidermis, intestinal epithelium, and glandular tissue.[1] Certain cells, such as neurons, rarely divide and therefore have little capacity, if any, for hyperplastic growth. There is evidence that hyperplasia involves activation of genes controlling cell proliferation and the presence of intracellular messengers that control cell replication and growth. As with other normal adaptive cellular responses, hyperplasia is a controlled process that occurs in response to an appropriate stimulus and ceases after the stimulus has been removed.

The stimuli that induce hyperplasia may be physiologic or nonphysiologic. There are two common types of physiologic hyperplasia: hormonal and compensatory. Breast and uterine enlargement during pregnancy are examples of a physiologic hyperplasia that results from estrogen stimulation. The regeneration of the liver that occurs after partial hepatectomy (*i.e.*, partial removal of the liver) is an example of compensatory hyperplasia. Hyperplasia is also an important response of connective tissue in wound healing, during which proliferating fibroblasts and blood vessels contribute to wound repair. Although hypertrophy and hyperplasia are two distinct processes, they may occur together and are often triggered by the same mechanism.[1] For example, the pregnant uterus undergoes both hypertrophy and hyperplasia as the result of estrogen stimulation.

Most forms of nonphysiologic hyperplasia are due to excessive hormonal stimulation or the effects of growth factors on target tissues.[2] Excessive estrogen production can cause endometrial hyperplasia and abnormal menstrual bleeding. Benign prostatic hyperplasia, which is a common disorder of men older than 50 years of age, is thought to be related to the action of androgens. Skin warts are an example of hyperplasia caused by growth factors produced by certain viruses, such as the papillomaviruses.

Metaplasia

Metaplasia represents a reversible change in which one adult cell type (epithelial or mesenchymal) is replaced by another adult cell type. Metaplasia is thought to involve the reprogramming of undifferentiated stem cells that are present in the tissue undergoing the metaplastic changes.[1]

Metaplasia usually occurs in response to chronic irritation and inflammation and allows for substitution of cells that are better able to survive under circumstances in which a more fragile cell type might succumb. However, the conversion of cell types never oversteps the boundaries of the primary tissue type (*e.g.,* one type of epithelial cell may be converted to another type of epithelial cell, but not to a connective tissue cell). An example of metaplasia is the adaptive substitution of stratified squamous epithelial cells for the ciliated columnar epithelial cells in the trachea and large airways of a habitual cigarette smoker. Although the squamous epithelium is better able to survive in these situations, the protective function that the ciliated epithelium provides for the respiratory tract is lost. Another example is the premalignant condition of Barrett esophagus associated with chronic gastroesophageal reflux disease (GERD) when the lower esophageal cells transform into columnar epithelium.[7] Also, continued exposure to the influences that cause metaplasia may predispose to cancerous transformation of the metaplastic epithelium.

Dysplasia

Dysplasia is characterized by deranged cell growth of a specific tissue that results in cells that vary in size, shape, and organization. Minor degrees of dysplasia are associated with chronic irritation or inflammation. The pattern is most frequently encountered in areas of metaplastic squamous epithelium of the respiratory tract and uterine cervix. Although dysplasia is abnormal, it is adaptive in that it is potentially reversible after the irritating cause has been removed. Dysplasia is strongly implicated as a precursor of cancer.[1] In cancers of the respiratory tract and the uterine cervix, dysplastic changes have been found adjacent to the foci of cancerous transformation. Through the use of the Papanicolaou (Pap) smear, it has been documented that cancer of the uterine cervix develops in a series of incremental epithelial changes ranging from severe dysplasia to invasive cancer. However,

dysplasia is an adaptive process and as such does not necessarily lead to cancer. In many cases, the dysplastic cells revert to their former structure and function.

Preterm babies who are ventilated for long periods of time due to their prematurity and lack of surfactant, and term infants who require intubation and ventilated oxygen in the first month of life, often develop bronchopulmonary dysplasia (BPD).[8] Approximately 20% of infants born at less than 30 weeks gestation and weighing less than 1,500 grams develop BPD. Although there has been some excellent therapy that has decreased some of the negative lung disease experienced by infants with BPD, many infants who develop BPD experience the long-term effects of alveolar destruction the rest of their lives.[1,8]

Intracellular Accumulations

Intracellular accumulations represent the buildup of substances that cells cannot immediately use or eliminate. The substances may accumulate in the cytoplasm (frequently in the lysosomes) or in the nucleus. In some cases the accumulation may be an abnormal substance that the cell has produced, and in other cases the cell may be storing exogenous materials or products of pathologic processes occurring elsewhere in the body. These substances can be grouped into three categories: (1) normal body substances, such as lipids, proteins, carbohydrates, melanin, and bilirubin, that are present in abnormally large amounts; (2) abnormal endogenous products, such as those resulting from inborn errors of metabolism; and (3) exogenous products, such as environmental agents and pigments that cannot be broken down by the cell.[2] These substances may accumulate transiently or permanently, and they may be either harmless or toxic.

The accumulation of normal cellular constituents occurs when a substance is produced at a rate that exceeds its metabolism or removal. An example of this type of process is fatty changes in the liver due to intracellular accumulation of triglycerides. Liver cells normally contain some fat, which is either oxidized and used for energy or converted to triglycerides. This fat is derived from free fatty acids released from adipose tissue. Abnormal accumulation occurs when the delivery of free fatty acids to the liver is increased, as in starvation and diabetes mellitus, or when the intrahepatic metabolism of lipids is disturbed, as in alcoholism.

Intracellular accumulation can result from genetic disorders that disrupt the metabolism of selected substances. A normal enzyme may be replaced with an abnormal one, resulting in the formation of a substance that cannot be used or eliminated from the cell, or an enzyme may be missing, so that an intermediate product accumulates in the cell. For example, there are at least 10 genetic disorders that affect glycogen metabolism, most of which lead to the accumulation of intracellular glycogen stores. In the most common form of this disorder, von Gierke disease, large amounts of glycogen accumulate in the liver and kidneys because of a deficiency of the enzyme glucose-6-phosphatase. Without this enzyme,

FIGURE 5.3 • Accumulation of intracellular lipofuscin. A photomicrograph of the liver of an 80-year-old man shows golden cytoplasmic granules, which represent lysosomal storage of lipofuscin. (From Rubin R., Strayer D. S. (2012). *Rubin's pathology: Clinicopathologic foundations of medicine* (6th ed., pp. 121). Philadelphia, PA: Lippincott Williams & Wilkins.)

glycogen cannot be broken down to form glucose. The disorder leads not only to an accumulation of glycogen but to a reduction in blood glucose levels. In Tay–Sachs disease, another genetic disorder, abnormal lipids accumulate in the brain and other tissues, causing motor and mental deterioration beginning at approximately 6 months of age, followed by death at 2 to 5 years of age. In a similar manner, other enzyme defects lead to the accumulation of other substances.

Pigments are coloured substances that may accumulate in cells. They can be endogenous (*i.e.,* arising from within the body) or exogenous (*i.e.,* arising from outside the body). Icterus, also called *jaundice,* is characterized by a yellow discolouration of tissue due to the retention of bilirubin, an endogenous bile pigment. This condition may result from increased bilirubin production from red blood cell destruction, obstruction of bile passage into the intestine, or toxic diseases that affect the liver's ability to remove bilirubin from the blood. Lipofuscin is a yellow-brown pigment that results from the accumulation of the indigestible residues produced during normal turnover of cell structures (Fig. 5.3). The accumulation of lipofuscin increases with age and is sometimes referred to as the *wear-and-tear pigment.* It is more common in heart, nerve, and liver cells than in other tissues and is seen more often in conditions associated with atrophy of an organ.

One of the most common exogenous pigments is carbon in the form of coal dust. In coal miners or persons exposed to heavily polluted environments, the accumulation of carbon dust blackens the lung tissue and may cause serious lung disease. The formation of a blue lead line along the margins of the gum is one of the diagnostic features of lead poisoning. Tattoos are the result of insoluble pigments introduced into the skin, where they are engulfed by macrophages and persist for a lifetime.

The significance of intracellular accumulations depends on the cause and severity of the condition. Many accumulations, such as lipofuscin and mild fatty change, have no effect on cell function. Some conditions, such as the hyperbilirubinemia that causes jaundice, are reversible. Other disorders, such as glycogen storage diseases, produce accumulations that result in organ dysfunction and other alterations in physiologic function.

Pathologic Calcifications

Pathologic calcification involves the abnormal tissue deposition of calcium salts, together with smaller amounts of iron, magnesium, and other minerals. It is known as *dystrophic calcification* when it occurs in dead or dying tissue and as *metastatic calcification* when it occurs in normal tissue.[1,2]

Dystrophic Calcification

Dystrophic calcification represents the macroscopic deposition of calcium salts in injured tissue. It is often visible to the naked eye as deposits that range from gritty, sand-like grains to firm, rock-hard material. The pathogenesis of dystrophic calcification involves the intracellular or extracellular formation of crystalline calcium phosphate. The components of the calcium deposits are derived from the bodies of dead or dying cells as well as from the circulation and interstitial fluid.

Dystrophic calcification is commonly seen in atheromatous lesions of advanced atherosclerosis, areas of injury in the aorta and large blood vessels, and damaged heart valves. Although the presence of calcification may only indicate the presence of previous cell injury, as in healed tuberculosis lesions, it is also a frequent cause of organ dysfunction. For example, calcification of the aortic valve is a frequent cause of aortic stenosis in the elderly (Fig. 5.4).

FIGURE 5.4 • Calcific aortic stenosis. Large deposits of calcium salts are evident in the cusps and free margins of the thickened aortic valve as viewed from above. (From Rubin R., Strayer D. S. (2008). *Rubin's pathology: Clinicopathologic foundations of medicine* (5th ed., p. 8). Philadelphia, PA: Lippincott Williams & Wilkins.)

Metastatic Calcification

In contrast to dystrophic calcification, which occurs in injured tissues, metastatic calcification occurs in normal tissues as the result of increased serum calcium levels (hypercalcemia). Almost any condition that increases the serum calcium level can lead to calcification in inappropriate sites such as the lung, renal tubules, and blood vessels. The major causes of hypercalcemia are hyperparathyroidism, either primary or secondary to phosphate retention in renal failure; increased mobilization of calcium from bone as in Paget disease, cancer with metastatic bone lesions, or immobilization; and vitamin D intoxication.[1]

IN SUMMARY

Cells adapt to changes in their environment and in their work demands by changing their size, number, and characteristics. These adaptive changes are consistent with the needs of the cell and occur in response to an appropriate stimulus. The changes are usually reversed after the stimulus has been withdrawn.

When confronted with a decrease in work demands or adverse environmental conditions, cells atrophy or reduce their size and revert to a lower and more efficient level of functioning. Hypertrophy results from an increase in work demands and is characterized by an increase in tissue size brought about by an increase in cell size and functional intracellular components. An increase in the number of cells in an organ or tissue that is still capable of mitotic division is called hyperplasia. Metaplasia occurs in response to chronic irritation and represents the substitution of cells of a type that is better able to survive under circumstances in which a more fragile cell type might succumb. Dysplasia is characterized by deranged cell growth of a specific tissue that results in cells that vary in size, shape, and appearance. It is often a precursor of cancer.

Under some circumstances, cells may accumulate abnormal amounts of various substances. If the accumulation reflects a correctable systemic disorder, such as the hyperbilirubinemia that causes jaundice, the accumulation is reversible. If the disorder cannot be corrected, as often occurs in many inborn errors of metabolism, the cells become overloaded, causing cell injury and death.

Pathologic calcification involves the abnormal tissue deposition of calcium salts. Dystrophic calcification occurs in dead or dying tissue. Although the presence of dystrophic calcification may only indicate the presence of previous cell injury, it is also a frequent cause of organ dysfunction (*e.g.*, when it affects the heart valves). Metastatic calcification occurs in normal tissues as the result of elevated serum calcium levels. Almost any condition that increases the serum calcium level can lead to calcification in inappropriate sites such as the lung, renal tubules, and blood vessels.

CELL INJURY AND DEATH

After completing this section of the chapter, you should be able to meet the following objectives:

- Describe the mechanisms whereby physical agents such as blunt trauma, electrical forces, and extremes of temperature produce cell injury.
- Differentiate between the effects of ionizing and nonionizing radiation in terms of their ability to cause cell injury.
- State the mechanisms and manifestations of cell injury associated with lead poisoning.
- Relate free radical formation and oxidative stress to cell injury and death.

Cells can be injured in many ways. The extent to which any injurious agent can cause cell injury and death depends in large measure on the intensity and duration of the injury and the type of cell that is involved. Cell injury is usually reversible up to a certain point, after which irreversible cell injury and death occur. Whether a specific stress causes irreversible or reversible cell injury depends on the severity of the insult and on variables such as blood supply, nutritional status, and regenerative capacity. Cell injury and death are ongoing processes, and in the healthy state, they are balanced by cell renewal.

CELL INJURY

- Cells can be damaged in a number of ways, including physical trauma, extremes of temperature, electrical injury, exposure to damaging chemicals, radiation damage, injury from biologic agents, and nutritional factors.
- Most injurious agents exert their damaging effects through uncontrolled free radical production, impaired oxygen delivery or utilization, or the destructive effects of uncontrolled intracellular calcium release.
- Cell injury can be reversible, allowing the cell to recover, or it can be irreversible, causing cell death and necrosis.
- In contrast to necrosis, which results from tissue injury, apoptosis is a normal physiologic process designed to remove injured or worn-out cells.

Causes of Cell Injury

Cell damage can occur in many ways. For purposes of discussion, the ways by which cells are injured have been grouped into five categories: (1) injury from physical agents, (2) radiation injury, (3) chemical injury, (4) injury from biologic agents, and (5) injury from nutritional imbalances.

Injury From Physical Agents

Physical agents responsible for cell and tissue injury include mechanical forces, extremes of temperature, and electrical forces. They are common causes of injuries due to environmental exposure, occupational and transportation accidents, and physical violence and assault.

Mechanical Forces. Injury or trauma due to mechanical forces occurs as the result of body impact with another object. The body or the mass can be in motion or, as sometimes happens, both can be in motion at the time of impact. These types of injuries split and tear tissue, fracture bones, injure blood vessels, and disrupt blood flow.

Extremes of Temperature. Extremes of heat and cold damage the cell, its organelles, and its enzyme systems. Exposure to low-intensity heat (43° to 46°C), such as occurs with partial-thickness burns and severe heat stroke, causes cell injury by inducing vascular injury, accelerating cell metabolism, inactivating temperature-sensitive enzymes, and disrupting the cell membrane. With more intense heat, coagulation of blood vessels and tissue proteins occurs. Exposure to cold increases blood viscosity and induces vasoconstriction by direct action on blood vessels and through reflex activity of the sympathetic nervous system. The resultant decrease in blood flow may lead to hypoxic tissue injury, depending on the degree and duration of cold exposure. Injury from freezing probably results from a combination of ice crystal formation and vasoconstriction. The decreased blood flow leads to capillary stasis and arteriolar and capillary thrombosis. Edema results from increased capillary permeability.

Electrical Injuries. Electrical injuries can affect the body through extensive tissue injury and disruption of neural and cardiac impulses. The effect of electricity on the body is mainly determined by its voltage, the type of current (*i.e.,* direct or alternating), its amperage, the resistance of the intervening tissue, the pathway of the current, and the duration of exposure.[9]

Lightning and high-voltage wires that carry several thousand volts produce the most severe damage.[2] Alternating current (AC) is usually more dangerous than direct current (DC) because it causes violent muscle contractions, preventing the person from releasing the electrical source and sometimes resulting in fractures and dislocations. In electrical injuries, the body acts as a conductor of the electrical current. The current enters the body from an electrical source, such as an exposed wire, and passes through the body and exits to another conductor, such as the moisture on the ground or a piece of metal the person is holding. The pathway that a current takes is critical because the electrical energy disrupts impulses in excitable tissues. Current flow through the brain may interrupt impulses from respiratory centres in the brain stem, and current flow through the chest may cause fatal cardiac arrhythmias.

The resistance to the flow of current in electrical circuits transforms electrical energy into heat. This is why the

FIGURE 5.5 • Electrical burn of the skin. The victim was electrocuted after attempting to stop a fall from a ladder by grasping a high-voltage line. (From Strayer D. S., Rubin E. (2008). Environmental and nutritional pathology. In Rubin E., Strayer D. S. [Eds.], *Rubin's pathology: Clinicopathologic foundations of medicine* (5th ed., p. 272). Philadelphia: Lippincott Williams & Wilkins)

elements in electrical heating devices are made of highly resistive metals. Much of the tissue damage produced by electrical injuries is caused by heat production in tissues that have the highest electrical resistance. Resistance to electrical current varies from the greatest to the least in bone, fat, tendons, skin, muscles, blood, and nerves. The most severe tissue injury usually occurs at the skin sites where the current enters and leaves the body (Fig. 5.5). After electricity has penetrated the skin, it passes rapidly through the body along the lines of least resistance—through body fluids and nerves. Degeneration of vessel walls may occur, and thrombi may form as current flows along the blood vessels. This can cause extensive muscle and deep tissue injury. Thick, dry skin is more resistant to the flow of electricity than thin, wet skin. It is generally believed that the greater the skin resistance, the greater is the amount of local skin burn, and the less the resistance, the greater are the deep and systemic effects.

Radiation Injury

Electromagnetic radiation comprises a wide spectrum of wave-propagated energy, ranging from ionizing gamma rays to radiofrequency waves (Fig. 5.6). A photon is a particle of radiation energy. Radiation energy above the ultraviolet (UV) range is called *ionizing radiation* because the photons have enough energy to knock electrons off atoms and molecules. *Nonionizing radiation* refers to radiation energy at frequencies below those of visible light. *UV radiation* represents the portion of the spectrum of electromagnetic radiation just above the visible range. It contains increasingly energetic rays that are powerful enough to disrupt intracellular bonds and cause sunburn.

Ionizing Radiation. Ionizing radiation affects cells by causing ionization of molecules and atoms in the cell, by directly hitting the target molecules in the cell, or by producing free

Wavelengths (m)

Ionizing radiation   Visible spectrum

FIGURE 5.6 • Spectrum of electromagnetic radiation.

radicals that interact with critical cell components.[1,2,10] It can immediately kill cells, interrupt cell replication, or cause a variety of genetic mutations, which may or may not be lethal. Most radiation injury is caused by localized irradiation that is used in the treatment of cancer (see Chapter 8). Except for unusual circumstances, such as the use of high-dose irradiation that precedes bone marrow transplantation, exposure to whole-body irradiation is rare.

The injurious effects of ionizing radiation vary with the dose, dose rate (a single dose can cause greater injury than divided or fractionated doses), and the differential sensitivity of the exposed tissue to radiation injury. Because of the effect on deoxyribonucleic acid (DNA) synthesis and interference with mitosis, rapidly dividing cells of the bone marrow and intestine are much more vulnerable to radiation injury than tissues such as bone and skeletal muscle. Over time, occupational and accidental exposure to ionizing radiation can result in increased risk for the development of various types of cancers, including skin cancers, leukemia, osteogenic sarcomas, and lung cancer.

Many of the clinical manifestations of radiation injury result from acute cell injury, dose-dependent changes in the blood vessels that supply the irradiated tissues, and fibrotic tissue replacement. The cell's initial response to radiation injury involves swelling, disruption of the mitochondria and other organelles, alterations in the cell membrane, and marked changes in the nucleus. The endothelial cells in blood vessels are particularly sensitive to irradiation. During the immediate post-irradiation period, only vessel dilation is apparent (e.g., the initial erythema of the skin after radiation therapy). Later or with higher levels of radiation, destructive changes occur in small blood vessels such as the capillaries and venules. Acute reversible necrosis is represented by such disorders as radiation cystitis, dermatitis, and diarrhea from enteritis. More persistent damage can be attributed to acute necrosis of tissue cells that are not capable of regeneration, and to chronic ischemia. Chronic effects of radiation damage are characterized by fibrosis and scarring of tissues and organs in the irradiated area (e.g., interstitial fibrosis of the heart and lungs after irradiation of the chest). Because

the radiation delivered in radiation therapy inevitably travels through the skin, radiation dermatitis is common. There may be necrosis of the skin, impaired wound healing, and chronic radiation dermatitis.

Ultraviolet Radiation. Ultraviolet radiation potentially causes sunburn and increases the risk of skin cancers (see Chapter 61). The degree of risk for cancer depends on the type of UV rays, the intensity of exposure, and the amount of protective melanin pigment in the skin. Skin damage produced by UV radiation is thought to be caused by reactive oxygen species and by damage to melanin-producing processes in the skin.[10] UV radiation also damages DNA, resulting in the formation of pyrimidine dimers (i.e., the insertion of two identical pyrimidine bases into replicating DNA instead of one). Other forms of DNA damage include the production of single-stranded breaks and formation of DNA–protein cross-links. Normally, errors that occur during DNA replication are repaired by enzymes that remove the faulty section of DNA and repair the damage. The importance of DNA repair in protecting against UV radiation injury is evidenced by the vulnerability of persons who lack the enzymes needed to repair UV-induced DNA damage. In a genetic disorder called *xeroderma pigmentosum,* an enzyme needed to repair sunlight-induced DNA damage is lacking. This autosomal recessive disorder is characterized by extreme photosensitivity and an increased risk of skin cancer in sun-exposed skin.[2]

Nonionizing Radiation. Nonionizing radiation includes infrared light, ultrasound, microwaves, and laser energy. Unlike ionizing radiation, which can directly break chemical bonds, nonionizing radiation exerts its effects by causing vibration and rotation of atoms and molecules. All of this vibrational and rotational energy is eventually converted to thermal energy. Low-frequency nonionizing radiation is used widely in radar, television, mobile networks (e.g., cell phones), industrial operations (e.g., heating, welding, melting of metals, processing of wood and plastic), household appliances (e.g., microwave ovens), and medical applications (e.g., diathermy). Isolated cases of skin burns and thermal injury to deeper tissues have occurred in industrial settings and from improperly used household microwave ovens. Injury from these sources is mainly thermal and, because of the deep penetration of the infrared or microwave rays, tends to involve dermal and subcutaneous tissue injury.

Chemical Injury

Chemicals capable of damaging cells are everywhere around us. Air and water pollution contain chemicals capable of tissue injury, as do tobacco smoke and some processed or preserved foods. Some of the most damaging chemicals exist in our environment, including gases such as carbon monoxide, insecticides, and trace metals such as lead.

Chemical agents can injure the cell membrane and other cell structures, block enzymatic pathways, coagulate cell proteins, and disrupt the osmotic and ionic balance of the cell. Corrosive substances such as strong acids and bases destroy cells as the substances come into contact with the body. Other chemicals may injure cells in the process of metabolism or elimination. Carbon tetrachloride (CCl_4), for example, causes little damage until it is metabolized by liver enzymes to a highly reactive free radical ($CCl_3\bullet$). Carbon tetrachloride is extremely toxic to liver cells.[1,2]

Drugs. Many drugs—alcohol, prescription drugs, over-the-counter drugs, and street drugs—are capable of directly or indirectly damaging tissues. Ethyl alcohol can harm the gastric mucosa, developing fetus (see Chapter 7), liver (see Chapter 38), and other organs. Antineoplastic (anticancer) and immunosuppressant drugs can directly injure cells. Other drugs produce metabolic end-products that are toxic to cells. Acetaminophen, a commonly used over-the-counter analgesic drug, is detoxified in the liver, where small amounts of the drug are converted to a highly toxic metabolite. This metabolite is detoxified by a metabolic pathway that uses a substance (*i.e.,* glutathione) normally present in the liver. When large amounts of the drug are ingested, this pathway becomes overwhelmed and toxic metabolites accumulate, causing massive liver necrosis.

Lead Toxicity. Lead is a particularly toxic metal. Small amounts accumulate to reach toxic levels. There are innumerable sources of lead in the environment, including flaking paint, lead-contaminated dust and soil, lead-contaminated root vegetables, lead water pipes or soldered joints, pottery glazes, newsprint, and toys made in foreign countries. Adults often encounter lead through occupational exposure. Lead and other metal smelters, miners, welders, storage battery workers, and pottery makers are particularly at risk.[1,11,12] Children may be exposed to lead through ingestion of peeling lead paint, by breathing dust from lead paint (*e.g.,* during remodelling), or from playing in contaminated soil. There has been a decline in blood lead levels of both adults and children since the removal of lead from gasoline and from soldered food cans.[11–13] Although no data for Canadian children under the age of 6 exists, it is estimated that less than 1% of adults in Canada have an increased blood lead level.[12] However

immigrant and adopted children may be at higher risk for lead toxicity if they originate from countries with higher endemic lead exposures.[11]

Lead is absorbed through the gastrointestinal tract or the lungs into the blood. A deficiency in calcium, iron, or zinc increases lead absorption. In children, most lead is absorbed through the lungs. Although children may have the same or a lower intake of lead, the absorption in infants and children is 5 to 10 times greater; thus, they are more vulnerable to lead toxicity.[2,13] Lead crosses the placenta, exposing the fetus to levels of lead that are comparable with those of the mother. Lead is stored in bone and eliminated by the kidneys. Approximately 90% of absorbed lead is stored in bone (and in the teeth of young children) compared to 70% of adults, and the remainder remains in the blood or accumulates in soft tissue deposits. Although the half-life of lead is just hours to days, bone deposits serve as a repository from which blood levels are maintained. In a sense, bone protects other tissues, but the slow turnover maintains blood levels for months to years.[13]

The toxicity of lead is related to its multiple biochemical effects.[2] It has the ability to inactivate enzymes, compete with calcium for incorporation into bone, and interfere with nerve transmission and brain development. The major targets of lead toxicity are the red blood cells, the gastrointestinal tract, the kidneys, and the nervous system.

Anemia is a cardinal sign of lead toxicity. Lead competes with the enzymes required for hemoglobin synthesis and with the membrane-associated enzymes that prevent hemolysis of red blood cells. The resulting red cells are coarsely stippled and hypochromic, resembling those seen in iron-deficiency anemia. The life span of the red cell is also decreased. The gastrointestinal tract is the main source of symptoms in the adult. This is characterized by "lead colic," a severe and poorly localized form of acute abdominal pain. A lead line formed by precipitated lead sulphite may appear along the gingival margins. The lead line is seldom seen in children. The kidneys are the major route for excretion of lead. Lead can cause diffuse kidney damage, eventually leading to renal failure. Even without overt signs of kidney damage, lead toxicity leads to hypertension.

In the nervous system, lead toxicity is characterized by demyelination of cerebral and cerebellar white matter and death of cortical cells. When this occurs in early childhood, it can affect neurobehavioural development and result in lower IQ levels and poor classroom performance.[12,13] Peripheral demyelinating neuropathy may occur in adults. The most serious manifestation of lead poisoning is acute encephalopathy. It is manifested by persistent vomiting, ataxia, seizures, papilledema, impaired consciousness, and coma. Acute encephalopathy may manifest suddenly, or it may be preceded by other signs of lead toxicity such as behavioural changes or abdominal complaints.

Because of the long-term neurobehavioural and cognitive deficits that occur in children with even moderately elevated lead levels, in the United States, the Centers for Disease

Control and Prevention and the American Academy of Pediatrics have issued recommendations for childhood lead screening.[12,13] In Canada there has never been any universal screening for lead exposure; rather, screening is done based on risk factors. A safe blood level of lead is still uncertain. At one time, 1.2 µmol/L was considered safe. Studies have clearly shown adverse health effects in children with levels as low as 0.24 to 0.48 µmol/L.[10,14] Health Canada now recommends target blood lead levels should be below 0.24 µmol/L.[12,13]

Screening for lead toxicity involves use of capillary blood obtained from a finger stick to measure free erythrocyte protoporphyrin (EP). Elevated levels of EP result from the inhibition by lead of the enzymes required for heme synthesis in red blood cells. Although the EP test is useful in detecting high lead levels, the results poorly correlate with venous blood levels and may give a false positive result if accompanied by iron deficiency anemia. The preferred venous blood sample reflects the effects of iron deficiency, a condition that increases lead absorption.[15]

Because the symptoms of lead toxicity usually are vague, diagnosis is often delayed. Anemia may provide the first clues to the disorder. Laboratory tests are necessary to establish a diagnosis. Measurement of lead levels in venous blood is usually used. Treatment involves removal of the lead source and, in cases of severe toxicity, administration of a chelating agent. Asymptomatic children with blood levels of >2.16 µmol/L usually are treated. A public health team should evaluate the source of lead because meticulous removal is needed.

Mercury Toxicity. Mercury has been used for industrial and medical purposes for hundreds of years. Mercury is toxic, and the hazards of mercury-associated occupational and accidental exposures are well known. In recent times, the primary concern of the general public with regard to the potential hazards of mercury has focused on exposure from eating certain fish, amalgams used in dentistry, and vaccines. Mercury is toxic in four primary forms: mercury vapour, inorganic divalent mercury, methyl mercury, and ethyl mercury.[16] Depending on the form of mercury exposure, toxicity involving the central nervous system and kidney can occur.

In the case of dental fillings, the concern involves mercury vapour being released into the mouth. However, the amount of mercury vapour released from fillings is very small. There is no clear evidence supporting health risk from this type of exposure, and removal of amalgams may temporarily increase blood levels of mercury.[16] The main source of methyl mercury exposure is from consumption of long-lived fish, such as tuna and swordfish. Fish concentrate mercury from sediment in the water. Only certain types of fish pose potential risk, however, and types such as salmon have miniscule amounts or no mercury. Because the developing brain is more susceptible to mercury-induced damage, it is recommended that young children and pregnant and nursing women avoid consumption of fish known to have high mercury content. Thimerosal is an ethyl mercury-containing preservative that helps prevent microorganism growth in vaccines. Concerns about

potential adverse effects have led to the making of single-dose vials that eliminate the need for thimerosal.[16] In Canada, most vaccines are either free of thimerosal or contain only trace amounts.[14]

Injury From Biologic Agents

Biologic agents differ from other injurious agents in that they are able to replicate and can continue to produce their injurious effects. These agents range from submicroscopic viruses to the larger parasites. Biologic agents injure cells by diverse mechanisms. Viruses enter the cell and become incorporated into its DNA synthetic machinery. Certain bacteria elaborate exotoxins that interfere with cellular production of ATP. Other bacteria, such as the gram-negative bacilli, release endotoxins that cause cell injury and increased capillary permeability.

Injury From Nutritional Imbalances

Nutritional excesses and nutritional deficiencies predispose cells to injury. Obesity and diets high in saturated fats are thought to predispose persons to atherosclerosis. The body requires more than 60 organic and inorganic substances in amounts ranging from micrograms to grams. These nutrients include minerals, vitamins, certain fatty acids, and specific amino acids. Dietary deficiencies can occur in the form of starvation, in which there is a deficiency of all nutrients and vitamins, or because of a selective deficiency of a single nutrient or vitamin. Iron-deficiency anemia, scurvy, beriberi, and pellagra are examples of cell injury due to lack of specific vitamins or minerals. The protein and calorie deficiencies that occur with starvation cause widespread tissue damage.

Mechanisms of Cell Injury

The mechanisms by which injurious agents cause cell injury and death are complex. Some agents, such as heat, produce direct cell injury; other factors, such as genetic derangements, produce their effects indirectly through metabolic disturbances and altered immune responses. There seem to be at least three major mechanisms whereby most injurious agents exert their effects: free radical formation, hypoxia and ATP depletion, and disruption of intracellular calcium homeostasis (Fig. 5.7).

Free Radical Injury

Many injurious agents exert damaging effects through reactive chemical species known as *free radicals*.[1,2,17,18] Free radicals are highly reactive chemical species with an unpaired electron in the outer orbit (valence shell) of the molecule. In the literature, the unpaired electron is denoted by a dot, for example •NO. The unpaired electron causes free radicals to be unstable and highly reactive, so that they react nonspecifically with molecules in the vicinity. Moreover, free radicals can establish chain reactions consisting of many events that generate new free radicals. In cells and tissues, free radicals react with proteins, lipids, and carbohydrates, thereby damaging cell membranes; inactivate enzymes; and damage nucleic acids

Injurious agents

Hypoxia/ischemia

O_2^-, H_2O_2, OH•

Free radical formation

Oxidation of cell structures and nuclear and mitchondrial DNA

Mitochondrion

↑ Intracellular Ca

Inappropriate activation of enzymes that damage cell organelles, cytoskeleton, and cell membranes; hasten ATP depletion; and fragment chromatin

ATP depletion

↓ Na⁺/K⁺-ATPase pump

↑ Anaerobic metabolism

Other effects

↑ Influx Na and H_2O

↓ Glycogen stores and intracellular pH

Detachment of ribosomes, decreased protein synthesis, and lipid deposition

Accumulation of intracellular fluids, dilation of endoplasmic reticulum, increased membrane permeability, decreased mitochondrial function

FIGURE 5.7 • Mechanisms of cell injury. The injurious agents tend to cause hypoxia/ischemia (see *middle arrow* that illustrates the manifestations that trigger anaerobic metabolism to develop leading to cellular injury). The free radical formation (left side) causes oxidation of cell structures leading to decreased ATP, and increased intracellular calcium (right side) damages many aspects of the cell also causing ATP depletion. Individually and together these three paths illustrate how injurious agents cause cell injury and death.

that make up DNA. The actions of free radicals may disrupt and damage cells and tissues.

Reactive oxygen species (ROS), also referred to as oxygen free radicals, are oxygen-containing molecules that include free radicals such as superoxide (O_2^-) and hydroxyl radical (OH•), and nonradicals such as hydrogen peroxide (H_2O_2). These molecules are produced endogenously by normal metabolic processes or cell activities, such as the metabolic burst that accompanies phagocytosis. Exogenous causes, including ionizing and UV radiation, can also cause ROS production in the body. The body neutralizes oxygen free radicals either by production of scavengers (*e.g.,* superoxide dismutase, catalase, glutathione) or intake of antioxidants (*e.g.,* selenium, carotenoids, flavonoids, ubiquinols, and vitamins C and E). *Oxidative stress* is a condition that occurs when the generation of ROS exceeds the ability of the body to neutralize and eliminate ROS.[17,18] Oxidative stress can lead to cell injury due to oxidation of cell components, activation of signal transduction pathways, and changes in gene and protein expression. DNA modification and damage can also occur as a result of oxidative stress. Although ROS and oxidative stress are clearly associated with cell and tissue damage, recent evidence shows that ROS do not always act in a random and damaging manner. Current studies have found that ROS are also important signalling molecules that are

used in healthy cells to regulate and maintain normal activities and functions such as vascular tone, insulin and vascular endothelial growth factor signalling.[17] Oxidative damage has been implicated in many diseases. Mutations in the gene for SOD are linked with amyotrophic lateral sclerosis (ALS or Lou Genrig disease).[17] Oxidative stress is thought to play an important role in the development of cancer, whereas oxidative injury is associated with vital organs and the reestablishment of blood flow after a loss of perfusion (*i.e.,* Heart attack or stroke), as occur during heart attack and stroke.[17] In addition to the many diseases and altered health conditions associated with oxidative damage, oxidative stress has been linked with the age-related functional declines that underlie the process of aging.[18]

Antioxidants are natural and synthetic molecules that inhibit the reactions of ROS with biologic structures or prevent the uncontrolled formation of ROS. Antioxidants include enzymatic and nonenzymatic compounds. Enzymes known to function as antioxidants include superoxide dismutase (SOD), catalase, glutathione peroxidase, and thioreductase. SOD forms hydrogen peroxide from superoxide. Catalase can catalyze the reaction that forms water from hydrogen peroxide.[1,2] Nonenzymatic antioxidants include carotenes (*e.g.,* vitamin A), tocopherols (*e.g.,* vitamin E), ascorbate (vitamin C), glutathione, and flavonoids, as well as micronutrients such as selenium and zinc.[19]

Nonenzymatic antioxidants often directly react with oxidants to "disarm" them. For example, vitamin C directly scavenges superoxide and hydroxyl radicals.[20]

Hypoxic Cell Injury

Hypoxia deprives the cell of oxygen and interrupts oxidative metabolism and the generation of ATP. The actual time necessary to produce irreversible cell damage depends on the degree of oxygen deprivation and the metabolic needs of the cell. Some cells, such as those in the heart, brain, and kidney, require large amounts of oxygen to provide energy to perform their functions. Brain cells, for example, begin to undergo permanent damage after 4 to 6 minutes of oxygen deprivation. A thin margin can exist between the time involved in reversible and irreversible cell damage. A classic study found that the epithelial cells of the proximal tubule of the kidney in the rat could survive 20 but not 30 minutes of ischemia.[21] During hypoxic conditions, *hypoxia-inducible factors* (HIFs) cause the expression of genes that stimulate red blood cell formation, manufacture glycolytic enzymes that produce ATP in the absence of oxygen, and increase angiogenesis[22] (*i.e.*, the formation of new blood vessels).

Cellular hypoxia can result from an inadequate amount of oxygen in the air, respiratory disease, ischemia (*i.e.*, decreased blood flow due to vasoconstriction or vascular obstruction), anemia, edema, or inability of the cells to use oxygen. In some cases of edema, the distance for diffusion of oxygen may become a limiting factor in the availability of oxygen. Hypoxemia is characterized by an insufficient amount of oxygen in the blood, resulting in decreased oxygen availability. Ischemia is characterized by impaired oxygen delivery due to decreased perfusion, with impaired removal of metabolic end products such as lactic acid. In contrast to pure hypoxemia, which depends on the oxygen content of the blood and affects all cells in the body, ischemia commonly affects blood flow through limited numbers of blood vessels and produces local tissue injury. In hypermetabolic states, cells may require more oxygen than can be supplied by normal respiratory function and oxygen transport. In shock states, cells may be injured and unable to use the oxygen available. Cellular hypoxia also serves as the ultimate cause of cell death in other injuries. For example, a physical agent such as cold temperature can cause severe vasoconstriction and impair blood flow.

Hypoxia causes a power failure in the cell, with widespread effects on the cell's structural and functional components. As oxygen pressure and availability in the cell falls, oxidative metabolism ceases and the cell reverts to anaerobic metabolism, using its limited glycogen stores in an attempt to maintain vital cell functions. Cellular pH falls as lactic acid is produced and accumulates in the cell. This reduction in pH can have adverse effects on intracellular structures and biochemical reactions. Low pH can alter cell membranes and cause chromatin clumping and cell shrinkage, and further alter oxidative metabolism within the mitochondria.

One important effect of reduced ATP is acute cellular edema caused by failure of the energy-dependent sodium/potassium (Na^+/K^+)-ATPase membrane pump, which extrudes sodium from and returns potassium to the cell. With impaired function of this pump, intracellular potassium levels decrease and sodium and water accumulate in the cell, resulting in cellular edema. The movement of water and ions into the cell is associated multiple changes including widening of the endoplasmic reticulum, increased membrane permeability, and decreased mitochondrial function.[2] To a point, the cellular changes due to ischemia are reversible if oxygenation is restored. If the oxygen supply is not restored, however, there is a continued loss of enzymes, proteins, and ribonucleic acid through the hyperpermeable cell membrane. Injury to the lysosomal membranes results in the leakage of destructive lysosomal enzymes into the cytoplasm and enzymatic digestion of cell components. Leakage of intracellular enzymes through the permeable cell membrane into the extracellular fluid provides an important clinical indicator of cell injury and death. These enzymes enter the blood and can be measured by laboratory tests.

Impaired Calcium Homeostasis

Calcium functions as an important second messenger and cytosolic signal for many cell responses. Various calcium-binding proteins, such as troponin and calmodulin, act as transducers for the cytosolic calcium signal. Calcium/calmodulin-dependent kinases indirectly mediate the effects of calcium on responses such as smooth muscle contraction and glycogen breakdown. Normally, intracellular calcium ion levels are kept extremely low compared with extracellular levels. These low intracellular levels are maintained by energy-dependent membrane-associated calcium/magnesium (Ca^{2+}/Mg^{2+})-ATPase exchange systems and sequestration of calcium ions within organelles such as the mitochondria and smooth endoplasmic reticulum.[2] Ischemia and certain toxins lead to an increase in cytosolic calcium because of increased influx across the cell membrane and the release of calcium from intracellular stores. The increased calcium level may inappropriately activate a number of enzymes with potentially damaging effects. These enzymes include the phospholipases, responsible for damaging the cell membrane; proteases that damage the cytoskeleton and membrane proteins; ATPases that break down ATP and hasten its depletion; and endonucleases that fragment chromatin. Although it is known that injured cells accumulate calcium, it is unknown whether this is the ultimate cause of irreversible cell injury.

Reversible Cell Injury and Cell Death

The mechanisms of cell injury can produce sublethal and reversible cellular damage or lead to irreversible injury with cell destruction or death (Fig. 5.8). Cell destruction and removal can involve one of two mechanisms: apoptosis, which is designed to remove injured or worn-out cells; or cell death or necrosis, which occurs in irreversibly damaged cells.

Reversible Cell Injury

Reversible cell injury impairs cell function, but does not result in cell death. Two patterns of reversible cell injury can be

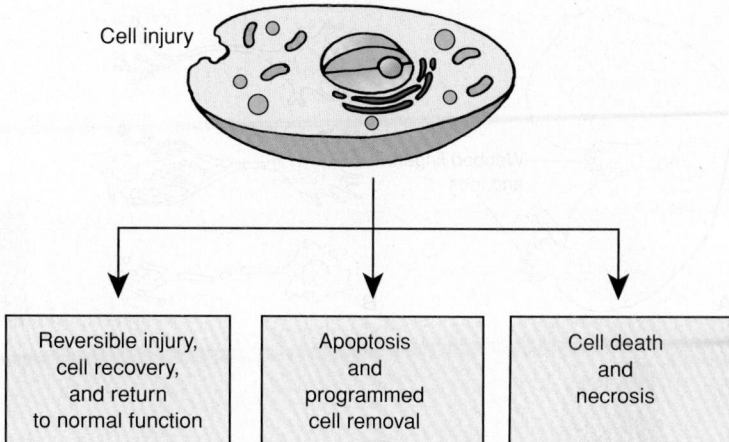

Cell injury

| Reversible injury, cell recovery, and return to normal function | Apoptosis and programmed cell removal | Cell death and necrosis |

FIGURE 5.8 • Outcomes of cell injury: reversible cell injury, apoptosis and programmed cell removal, cell death and necrosis.

observed under the microscope: cellular edema or swelling and fatty change. Cellular edema occurs with impairment of the energy-dependent Na^+/K^+-ATPase membrane pump, usually as the result of hypoxic cell injury.

Fatty changes are linked to intracellular accumulation of fat. When fatty changes occur, small vacuoles of fat disperse throughout the cytoplasm. The process is usually more ominous than cellular edema, and although it is reversible, it usually indicates severe injury. These fatty changes may occur because normal cells are presented with an increased fat load or because injured cells are unable to metabolize the fat properly. In obese persons, fatty infiltrates often occur within and between the cells of the liver and heart because of an increased fat load. Pathways for fat metabolism may be impaired during cell injury, and fat may accumulate in the cell as production exceeds use and export. The liver, where most fats are synthesized and metabolized, is particularly susceptible to fatty change, but fatty changes may also occur in the kidney, the heart, and other organs.

Programmed Cell Death

In most normal nontumour cells, the number of cells in tissues is regulated by balancing cell proliferation and cell death. Cell death occurs by necrosis or a form of programmed cell death called *apoptosis*.[1]

Apoptosis is a highly selective process that eliminates injured and aged cells, thereby controlling tissue regeneration. Cells undergoing apoptosis have characteristic morphologic features as well as biochemical changes. As shown in Figure 5.9, shrinking and condensation of the nucleus and cytoplasm occur. The chromatin aggregates at the nuclear envelope, and DNA fragmentation occurs. Then, the cell becomes fragmented into multiple apoptotic bodies in a manner that maintains the integrity of the plasma membrane and does not initiate inflammation. Changes in the plasma membrane induce phagocytosis of the apoptotic bodies by macrophages and other cells, thereby completing the degradation process.

Apoptosis is thought to be responsible for several normal physiologic processes, including the programmed destruction of cells during embryonic development, hormone-dependent

involution of tissues, death of immune cells, cell death by cytotoxic T cells, and cell death in proliferating cell populations. During embryogenesis, in the development of a number of organs such as the heart, which begins as a pulsating tube and is gradually modified to become a four-chambered pump, apoptotic cell death allows for the next stage of organ development. It also separates the webbed fingers and toes of the developing embryo (Fig. 5.10). Apoptotic cell death occurs in the hormone-dependent involution of endometrial cells during the menstrual cycle and in the regression of breast tissue after weaning from breast-feeding. The control of immune cell numbers and destruction of autoreactive T cells in the thymus have been credited to apoptosis. Cytotoxic T cells and natural killer cells are thought to destroy target cells by inducing apoptotic cell death.

Apoptosis is linked to many pathologic processes and diseases. For example, interference with apoptosis is known to be a mechanism that contributes to carcinogenesis.[23] Apoptosis is also known to be involved in the cell death associated with viral infections, such as hepatitis B and C.[24,25] Apoptosis

Phagocytic cell

FIGURE 5.9 • Apoptotic cell removal: shrinking of the cell structures (**A**), condensation and fragmentation of the nuclear chromatin (**B** and **C**), separation of nuclear fragments and cytoplasmic organelles into apoptotic bodies (**D** and **E**), and engulfment of apoptotic fragments by phagocytic cell (**F**).

FIGURE 5.10 • Examples of apoptosis: (**A**) separation of webbed fingers and toes in embryo; (**B**) development of neural connections; neurons that do not establish synaptic connections and receive survival factors may be induced to undergo apoptosis; (**C**) removal of cells from intestinal villi; new epithelial cells continuously form in the crypt, migrate to the villus tip as they age, and undergo apoptosis at the tip at the end of their life span; and (**D**) removal of senescent blood cells.

may also be implicated in neurodegenerative disorders such as Alzheimer disease, Parkinson disease, and Amyotrophic Lateral Sclerosis (ALS). However, the exact mechanisms involved in these diseases remain under investigation.

Two basic pathways for apoptosis have been described (Fig. 5.11). These are the extrinsic pathway, which is death receptor dependent, and the intrinsic pathway, which is death receptor independent. The execution phase of both pathways is carried out by proteolytic enzymes called *caspases,* which are present in the cell as *procaspases* and are activated by cleavage of an inhibitory portion of their polypeptide chain.

The *extrinsic pathway* involves the activation of receptors such as tumour necrosis factor (TNF) receptors and the Fas ligand receptor.[26] Fas ligand may be expressed on the surface of certain cells such as cytotoxic T cells, or appear in a soluble form. When Fas ligand binds to its receptor, proteins congregate at the cytoplasmic end of the Fas receptor to form a death-initiating complex. The complex then converts procaspase-8 to caspase-8. Caspase-8, in turn, activates a cascade of caspases that execute the process of apoptosis.[26] The end result includes activation of endonucleases that cause fragmentation of DNA and cell death. In addition to TNF and Fas ligand, primary signalling molecules known to activate the extrinsic pathway include TNF-related apoptosis-inducing ligand (TRAIL); the cytokine interleukin-1 (IL-1); and lipopolysaccharide (LPS), the endotoxin found in the outer cell membrane of gram-negative bacteria.

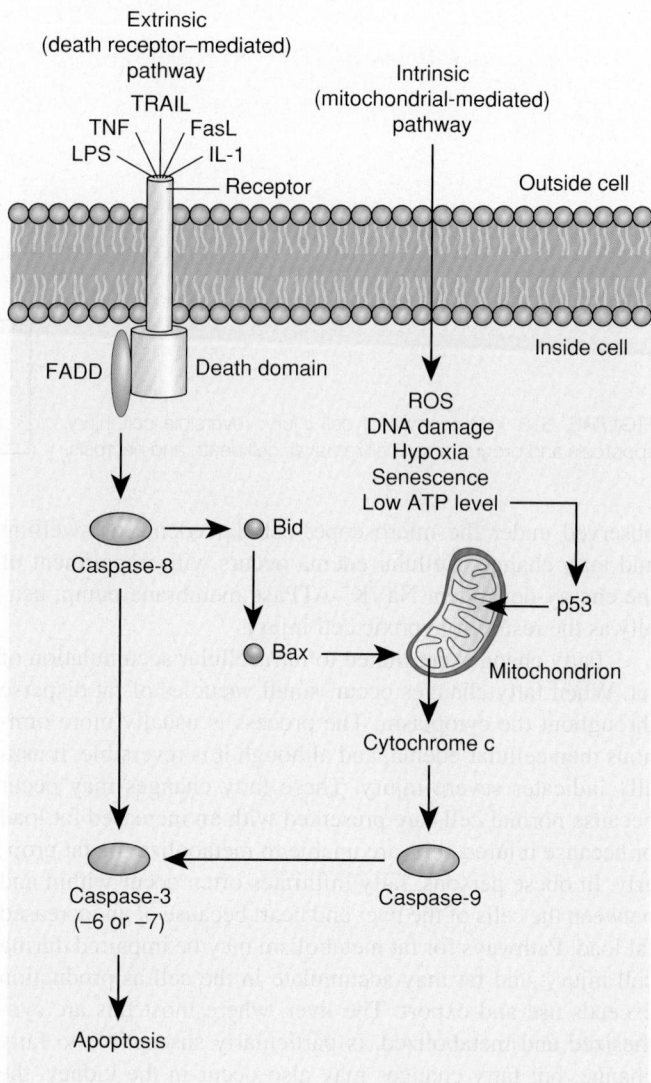

FIGURE 5.11 • Extrinsic and intrinsic pathways of apoptosis. The extrinsic pathway is activated by signals such as Fas ligand (FasL) that, on binding to the Fas receptor, form a death-inducing complex by joining the Fas-associated death domain (FADD) to the death domain of the Fas receptor. The intrinsic pathway is activated by signals, such as reactive oxygen species (ROS) and DNA damage, that induce the release of cytochrome c from mitochondria into the cytoplasm. Both pathways activate caspases to execute apoptosis.

The *intrinsic pathway,* or *mitochondrion-induced pathway,* of apoptosis is activated by conditions such as DNA damage, ROS, hypoxia, decreased ATP levels, cellular senescence, and activation of the p53 protein by DNA damage. It involves the opening of mitochondrial membrane permeability pores with release of cytochrome c from the mitochondria into the cytoplasm. Cytoplasmic cytochrome c activates caspases, including caspase-3. Caspase-3 activation is a common step to both the extrinsic and intrinsic pathways. Furthermore, activation or increased levels of proapoptotic proteins, such as Bid and Bax, after caspase-8 activation in the extrinsic pathway can lead to mitochondrial release of cytochrome c, thereby bridging the two pathways for apoptosis. Many inhibitors of apoptosis within cells are known and thought to contribute to cancer and autoimmune diseases.[27] The therapeutic actions of certain medications may induce or facilitate apoptosis. Apoptosis continues to be an active area of investigation to better understand and treat a variety of diseases.

Necrosis

Necrosis refers to cell death in an organ or tissue that is still part of a living organism.[28] Necrosis differs from apoptosis since it causes loss of cell membrane integrity and enzymatic breakdown of cell parts and triggers the inflammatory process.[1] In contrast to apoptosis, which functions in removing cells so new cells can replace them, necrosis often interferes with cell replacement and tissue regeneration.

With necrotic cell death, there are marked changes in the appearance of the cytoplasmic contents and the nucleus. These changes often are not visible, even under the microscope, for hours after cell death. The dissolution of the necrotic cell or tissue can follow several paths. The cell can undergo liquefaction (*i.e.,* liquefaction necrosis); it can be transformed to a grey, firm mass (*i.e.,* coagulation necrosis); or it can be converted to a cheesy material by infiltration of fatlike substances (*i.e.,* caseous necrosis). *Liquefaction necrosis* occurs when some of the cells die but their catalytic enzymes are not destroyed. An example of liquefaction necrosis is the softening of the centre of an abscess with the discharge of its contents. During *coagulation necrosis,* acidosis develops and denatures the enzymatic and structural proteins of the cell. This type of necrosis is characteristic of hypoxic injury and is seen in infarcted areas.[1] *Infarction (i.e.,* tissue death) occurs when an artery supplying an organ or part of the body becomes occluded and no other source of blood supply exists. As a rule, the shape of the infarction is conical and corresponds to the distribution of the artery and its branches. An artery may be occluded by an embolus, a thrombus, disease of the arterial wall, or pressure from outside the vessel.

Caseous necrosis is a distinctive form of coagulation necrosis in which the dead cells persist indefinitely as soft, cheese-like debris. It is most commonly found in the centre of tuberculosis granulomas, or tubercles, and is thought to result from immune mechanisms.[1]

Gangrene. The term *gangrene* is applied when a considerable mass of tissue undergoes necrosis. Gangrene may be classified as dry or moist. In dry gangrene, the area becomes dry and shrinks, the skin wrinkles, and its colour changes to dark brown or black. The spread of dry gangrene is slow, and its symptoms are not as marked as those of wet gangrene. The irritation caused by the dead tissue produces a line of inflammatory reaction (*i.e.,* line of demarcation) between the dead tissue of the gangrenous area and the healthy tissue (Fig. 5.12). Dry gangrene usually results from interference with the arterial blood supply to a part or area without interference in venous return, and is a form of coagulation necrosis.

In moist or wet gangrene, the area is cold, swollen, and pulseless. The skin is moist, black, and under tension. Blebs

FIGURE 5.12 • Gangrenous toes. (Biomedical Communications Group, Southern Illinois University School of Medicine, Springfield, IL.)

form on the surface, liquefaction occurs, and a foul odour is caused by bacterial action. There is no line of demarcation between the normal and diseased tissues, and the spread of tissue damage is rapid. Systemic symptoms are usually severe, and death may occur unless the condition can be arrested. Moist or wet gangrene primarily results from interference with venous return from the part. Bacterial invasion plays an important role in the development of wet gangrene and is responsible for many of its prominent symptoms. Dry gangrene is confined almost exclusively to the extremities, but moist gangrene may affect the internal organs or the extremities. If bacteria invade the necrotic tissue, dry gangrene may be converted to wet gangrene.

Gas gangrene is a special type of gangrene that results from infection of devitalized tissues by one of several *Clostridium* bacteria, most commonly *Clostridium perfringens.*[1] These anaerobic and spore-forming organisms are widespread in nature, particularly in soil; gas gangrene is prone to occur in trauma and compound fractures in which dirt and debris are embedded. Some species have been isolated in the stomach, gallbladder, intestine, vagina, and skin of healthy persons. The bacteria produce toxins that dissolve cell membranes, causing death of muscle cells, massive spreading edema, hemolysis of red blood cells, hemolytic anemia, hemoglobinuria, and renal failure.[29] Characteristic of this disorder are the bubbles of hydrogen sulphide gas that form in the muscle. Gas gangrene is a serious and potentially fatal disease. Antibiotics are used to treat the infection and surgical methods are used to remove the infected tissue. Amputation may be required to prevent spreading infection involving a limb. Hyperbaric oxygen therapy has been used, but clinical data supporting its efficacy have not been rigorously assessed.

Cellular Aging

Like adaptation and injury, aging is a process that involves the cells and tissues of the body. A number of theories have been proposed to explain the cause of aging. These theories are not mutually exclusive, and aging is most likely complex, with multiple causes. The main theories of aging can be categorized based on evolutionary, molecular, cellular, and systems-level explanations.[1]

The *evolutionary theories* focus on genetic variation and reproductive success. After the reproductive years have passed, it is not clear that continued longevity contributes to the fitness of the species. Thus, "antiaging" genes would not necessarily be selected, preserved, and prevalent in the gene pool.

The *molecular theories* of cellular aging focus more on mutations or changes in gene expression. Because the appearance, properties, and function of cells depend on gene expression, this aspect is likely to be involved in aging at some level. Recent attention is being given to the so-called aging genes identified in model systems.

There are a number of *cellular theories of senescence* that are currently under investigation, including those that focus on telomere shortening, free radical injury, and apoptosis. It has been known since the mid-1960s that many cells in culture exhibit a limit in replicative capacity, the so-called Hayflick limit of about 50 population doublings. This limit seems to be related to the length of the telomeres, which are DNA sequences at the ends of chromosomes. Each time a cell divides, the telomeres shorten until a critical minimal length is attained, senescence ensues, and further cell replication does not occur. Some cells have telomerase, an enzyme that "rebuilds" telomeres and lessens or prevents shortening. Cancer cells have high levels of telomerase, which prevents senescence and contributes to the cellular immortality that characterizes cancer. Telomere shortening appears to be related to other theories of cellular causes of aging. For example, free radicals and oxidative damage can kill cells and hasten telomere shortening. Caloric restriction, which appears to increase longevity, may be related to reduced mitochondrial free radical generation owing to reduced methionine or other dietary amino acid intake.[30]

Systems-level theories centre on a decline in the integrative functions of organ systems such as the immunologic and neuroendocrine systems, which are necessary for overall control of other body systems. The immune system may decline with age and be less effective in protecting the body from infection or cancer. In addition, mutations and manipulations of genes such as *daf*-2, which is similar to human insulin/IGF-1 receptor genes, in the aging worm model *Caenorhabditis elegans* cause significant changes in longevity.[31] Pathways related to *daf*-2 may be responsible for relationships between caloric restriction and prolonged life span in rodents and other animals. The mechanisms that regulate aging are likely to be complex and multifactorial, as will be any interventions to prolong aging.

IN SUMMARY

Cell injury can be caused by a number of mechanisms, including physical agents, chemicals, biologic agents, and nutritional factors. Among the physical agents that generate cell injury are mechanical forces that produce tissue trauma, extremes of temperature, electricity, radiation, and nutritional disorders. Chemical agents can cause cell injury through several mechanisms: they can block enzymatic pathways, cause coagulation of tissues, or disrupt the osmotic or ionic balance of the cell. Biologic agents differ from other injurious agents in that they are able to replicate and continue to produce injury. Among the nutritional factors that contribute to cell injury are excesses and deficiencies of nutrients, vitamins, and minerals.

Injurious agents exert their effects largely through generation of free radicals, production of cell hypoxia, or dysregulation of intracellular calcium levels. Partially reduced oxygen species called free radicals are important mediators of cell injury in many pathologic conditions. They are an important cause of cell injury in hypoxia and after exposure to radiation and certain chemical agents. Lack of oxygen underlies the pathogenesis of cell injury in hypoxia and ischemia. Hypoxia can result from inadequate oxygen in the air, cardiac or pulmonary disease, anemia, or the inability of the cells to use oxygen. Increased intracellular calcium activates a number of enzymes with potentially damaging effects.

Injurious agents may produce sublethal and reversible cellular damage or may lead to irreversible cell injury and death. Cell death can involve two mechanisms: apoptosis or necrosis. Apoptosis involves controlled cell destruction and is the means by which the body removes and replaces cells that have been produced in excess, developed improperly, have genetic damage, or are worn out. Necrosis refers to cell death that is characterized by cell swelling, rupture of the cell membrane, and inflammation.

Like adaptation and injury, aging is a process that involves the cells and tissues of the body. A number of theories have been proposed to explain the complex causes of aging, including those based on evolutionary mechanisms that explain aging as a consequence of natural selection, in which traits that maximize the reproductive capacity of an individual are selected over those that maximize longevity; molecular theories, such as those that explain aging as a result of changes in gene expression; cellular theories that explain cellular senescence in relation to telomere length or molecular events, free radical damage, accumulated wear-and-tear, or apoptosis; and systems theories that attribute cellular aging to a decline in the integrative functions of organ systems such as the neuroendocrine and immunologic systems.

REVIEW EXERCISES

1. A 30-year-old man sustained a fracture of his leg 2 months ago. The leg has been encased in a cast and he has just had it removed. He is amazed at the degree to which the muscles in his leg have shrunk.
   A. *Would you consider this to be a normal adaptive response? Explain.*

B. Will these changes have an immediate and/or long-term effect on the function of the leg?

C. What types of measures can be taken to restore full function to the leg?

2. A 45-year-old woman has been receiving radiation therapy for breast cancer.

A. Explain the effects of ionizing radiation in eradicating the tumour cells.

B. Why is the radiation treatment given in smaller divided, or fractionated, doses rather than as a single large dose?

C. Part way through the treatment schedule, the woman notices that her skin over the irradiated area has become reddened and irritated. What is the reason for this?

3. People who have had a myocardial infarction may experience additional damage once blood flow has been restored, a phenomenon referred to as reperfusion injury.

A. What is the proposed mechanism underlying reperfusion injury?

B. What factors might influence this mechanism?

4. Every day blood cells in our body become senescent and die without producing signs of inflammation, yet massive injury or destruction of tissue, such as occurs with trauma, produces significant signs of inflammation.

A. Explain.

References

1. Rubin E., Strayer D. S. (Eds.). (2012). *Rubin's pathology: Clinicopathologic foundations of medicine* (6th ed.). Philadelphia, PA: Lippincott Williams & Wilkins.
2. Kumar V., Abbas A. K., Fasutos N. (Eds.). (2010). *Robbins and Cotran pathologic basis of disease* (8th ed.). Philadelphia, PA: Elsevier Saunders.
3. Glass D. J. (2010). Signalling pathways perturbing muscle mass. *Current Opinion in Clinical Nutrition and Metabolic Care, 13*(3), 225–229.
4. Heszele M. F. C., Price S. R. (2004). Insulin-like growth factor 1: The yin and yang of muscle atrophy. *Endocrinology, 145*, 4803–4805.
5. Heineke J., Molkentin J. D. (2006). Regulation of cardiac hypertrophy by intracellular signalling pathways. *Nature Reviews: Molecular Cell Biology, 7*, 589–600.
6. Hunter J. J., Chien K. R. (1999). Signaling pathways in cardiac hypertrophy and failure. *New England Journal of Medicine, 341*, 1276–1283.
7. Barbera M., Fitzgerald R. C. (2009). Cellular mechanisms of Barrett's esophagus development. *Surgical Oncology Clinics of North America, 18*(3), 393–410.
8. Wright C. J., Kirpalania H. (2011). Targeting inflammation to prevent bronchopulmonary dysplasia: Can new insights be translated into therapies? *Pediatrics, 128*(1), 111–126.
9. Koumbourlis A. C. (2002). Electrical injuries. *Critical Care Medicine, 30*(11 Suppl), S424–S430.
10. Bickers D. R. (2012). Photosensitivity and other reactions to light. In Longo D., Fauci A., Kasper D. L., Hauser S. L. (Eds.), *Harrison's principles of internal medicine* (18th ed., pp. 350–355). New York: McGraw-Hill.
11. Chandran L., Cataldo R. (2010). Lead poisoning: Basics and new developments. *Pediatrics in Review, 31*(10), 399–406.
12. Abelsohn A. R., Sanborn M. (2010). Lead and children. *Canadian Family Physician, 56*, 531–535.
13. Health Canada. (2013). Risk management strategy for lead. Available online at: http://www.hc-sc.gc.ca/ewh-semt/pubs/contaminants/prms_lead-psgr_plomb/index-eng.php. Accessed December 30, 2013.
14. National Advisory Committee on Immunizations (NACI). (2003). Statement on thimerosal. *Canada Communicable Disease Report, 29*, 1–14.
15. Centers for Disease Control and Prevention. (2013). Lead. Available online at: http://www.cdc.gov/nceh/lead. Accessed December 30, 2013.
16. Clarkson T. W., Magos L., Myers G. J. (2003). The toxicity of mercury: Current exposures and clinical manifestations. *New England Journal of Medicine, 349*(18), 1731–1737.
17. Giustarini D., Dalle-Donne I., Tsikas D., Rossi R. (2009). Oxidative stress and human diseases: Origin, link, measurement, mechanisms, and biomarkers. *Critical Review in Clinical Laboratory Science, 46*(5-6), 241–281.
18. Martin I., Grotewiel M. S. (2006). Oxidative damage and age-related functional declines. *Mechanisms of Ageing and Development, 127*(5), 411–423.
19. Brenneistein P., Steinbrenner H., Seis H. (2005). Selenium, oxidative stress, and health aspects. *Molecular Aspects of Medicine, 26*, 256–267.
20. Comhair S. A., Erzurum S. C. (2005). The regulation and role of extracellular glutathione peroxidase. *Antioxidants and Redox Signaling, 7*, 72–79.
21. Vogt M. T., Farber E. (1968). On the molecular pathology of ischemic renal cell death: Reversible and irreversible cellular and mitochondrial metabolic alterations. *American Journal of Pathology, 53*, 1–26.
22. Shimoda L. A., Semenza G. L. (2011). HIF and the lung: Role of hypoxia-inducible factors in pulmonary development and disease. *American Journal of Respiratory and Critical Care Medicine, 183*(2), 152–156.
23. Vermeulen K., Van Bockstaele D. R., Berneman Z. N. (2005). Apoptosis: Mechanisms and relevance in cancer. *Annals of Hematology, 84*, 627–639.
24. Cruise M. W., Lukens J. R., Nguyen A. P., et al. (2006). Fas ligand is responsible for CXCR3 chemokine induction in CD4+ T cell-dependent liver damage. *Journal of Immunology, 176*, 6235–6244.
25. Malhi H., Gores G. J., Lemasters J. J. (2006). Apoptosis and necrosis in the liver: A tale of two deaths? *Hepatology, 43*(2 Suppl 1), S31–S44.
26. Ji X., Jiang C., Liu Y., et al. (2011). Fas ligand gene transfer effectively induces apoptosis in head and neck cancer cells. *Acta Oto-Laryngologica, 131*(8), 876–881.
27. Dorner T., Lipsky P. E. (2006). Signalling pathways in B cells: Implications for autoimmunity. *Current Topics in Microbiology and Immunology, 305*, 213–240.
28. Proskuryakov S. Y., Konoplyannikov A. G., Gabai V. L. (2003). Necrosis: A specific form of programmed cell death. *Experimental Cell Research, 283*, 1–16.
29. Bryant A. E., Stevens D. L. (2012). Gas gangrene and other clostridial infections. In Longo D., Fauci A., Kasper D. L., Hauser S. L. (Eds.), *Harrison's principles of internal medicine* (18th ed., pp. 903–908). New York: McGraw-Hill.
30. Sanz A., Caro P., Ayala V., et al. (2006). Methionine restriction decreases mitochondrial oxygen radical generation and leak as well as oxidative damage to mitochondrial DNA and proteins. *Federation of American Societies for Experimental Biology Journal, 20*, 1064–1073.
31. Halaschek-Wiener J., Khattra J. S., Pouzyrev A., et al. (2005). Analysis of long-lived C. elegans daf-2 mutants using serial analysis of gene expression. *Genome Research, 15*, 603–615.

Visit thePoint **http://thePoint.lww.com for animations, journal articles, and more!**

Genetic Control of Cell Function and Inheritance

6

Our genetic information is stored in the structure of *deoxyribonucleic acid* (DNA), an extremely stable macromolecule. Genetic information directs the function of our body cells, determines our appearance and how we respond to our environment, and serves as the unit of inheritance passed on from generation to generation. Genes also determine our disease susceptibility and how we react to drugs.

An understanding of the role that genetics plays in pathogenesis of disease has expanded greatly over the past century. It is now apparent that many diseases, including cancer, diabetes, and cardiovascular diseases, have a genetic component. In the case of cancer, recent genetic advances have led to new methods for early detection and more effective treatment. Advances in immunogenetics have made compatible blood transfusion and organ transplants a reality, and recombinant DNA technology has provided the methods for producing human insulin, growth hormone, and clotting factors. Perhaps the most extensive use of gene technology involved the Human Genome Project, begun in 1990 and completed in 2003, in which the entire human genetic complement (the genome) has been sequenced. Some of what was discovered was quite unexpected, including the revelation that humans have a mere 20,000 genes, rather than the predicted 140,000; and that on average any two individuals share 99.9% of their DNA sequence, indicating that the remarkable diversity among individuals is vested in about 0.1% of our DNA.[1]

This chapter includes discussions of genetic control of cell function, chromosomes, patterns of inheritance, and gene technology.

GENETIC CONTROL OF CELL FUNCTION

After completing this section of the chapter, you should be able to meet the following objectives:

* Relate the mechanisms of DNA repair to the development of a gene mutation.
* Describe the function of messenger RNA, ribosomal RNA, and transfer RNA as they relate to protein synthesis.

- Cite the effects of post-translational processing on protein structure and function.
- Explain the role of transcription factors in regulating gene activity.

The DNA that contains our genetic information is an extremely stable molecule. Because of its stable structure, the genetic information carried in DNA can survive the many stages of cell division and the day-to-day process of cell renewal and tissue growth. Its stable structure also allows information to survive the many processes of reduction division involved in gamete (*i.e.,* ovum and sperm) formation, the fertilization process, and the mitotic cell divisions involved in the formation of a new organism from the single-celled fertilized ovum called the *zygote.*

A second type of nucleic acid, *ribonucleic acid* (RNA), is involved in the actual synthesis of cellular proteins. The information contained in a given gene is first transcribed into an RNA molecule that, after being processed in the nucleus, carries the information to the cytoplasm, where it is translated and used in synthesizing proteins.

Although DNA and RNA have received a lot of attention, it is the proteins that the genes encode that make up the majority of cellular structures and perform most life functions. Proteins are responsible for the functional diversity of cells, they perform most biologic functions, and it is at their level that many regulatory processes take place, many disease processes occur, and most drug targets are found. The term *proteome* defines the complete set of proteins and their interactions encoded by a genome. *Proteomics,* the study of the proteome, uses highly sophisticated technological methods to examine the molecular and biochemical events in a cell.

FUNCTION OF DNA IN CONTROLLING CELL FUNCTION

- The information needed for the control of cell structure and function is embedded in the genetic information encoded in the stable DNA molecule.
- Although every cell in the body contains the same genetic information, each cell type uses only a portion of the information, depending on its structure and function.

DNA Structure and Function

The DNA molecule that stores the genetic information in the nucleus is a long, double-stranded, helical structure. DNA is composed of *nucleotides,* which consist of phosphoric acid, a five-carbon sugar called *deoxyribose,* and one of four nitrogenous bases (Fig. 6.1). These nitrogenous bases carry the genetic information and are divided into two groups: the *pyrimidine bases,* thymine (T) and cytosine (C), which have one nitrogen ring, and the *purine bases,* adenine (A) and guanine (G), which have two. The backbone of DNA consists of alternating groups of sugar and phosphoric acid, with the paired bases projecting inward from the sides of the sugar molecule.

Double Helix and Base-Pairing

The native structure of DNA, as elucidated by James Watson and Frances Crick in 1953, is that of a spiral staircase, with the

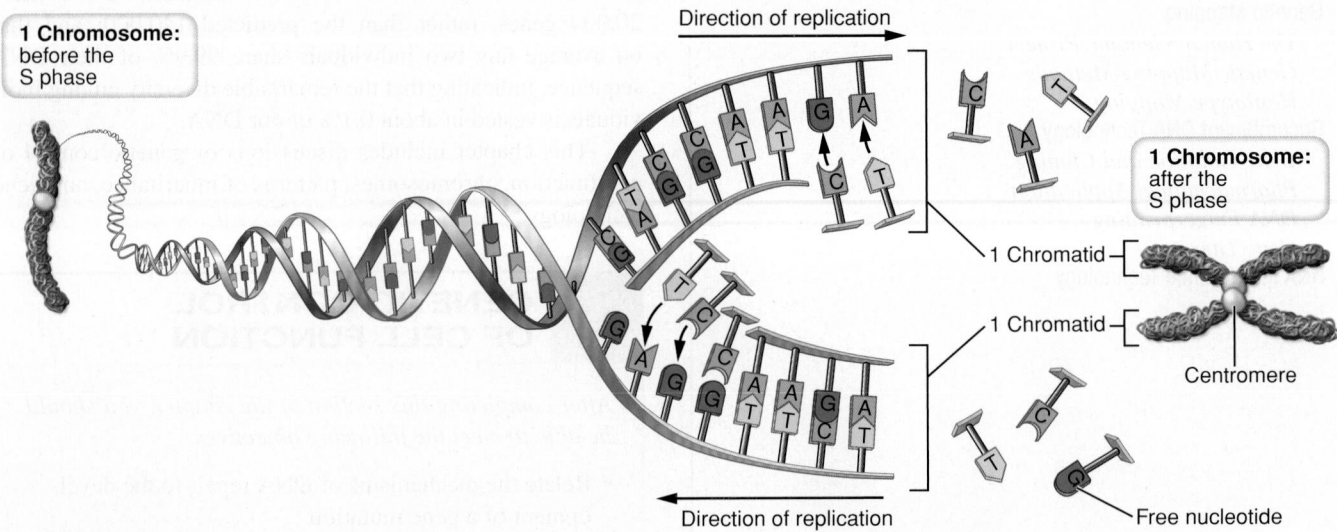

FIGURE 6.1 • A replicating DNA helix. The DNA helix is unwound, and base pairing rules (A with T and G with C) operate to assemble a new DNA strand on each original strand. After DNA replication is complete, each DNA molecule (chromatid) consists of an old strand a new synthesized strand. They are joined together at the centromere. (From McConnell T. H., Hull K. L. (2011). *Human form and human function: Essentials of anatomy and physiology* (p. 78). Philadelphia, PA: Lippincott Williams & Wilkins.)

paired bases representing the steps (Fig. 6.1). A precise complementary pairing of purine and pyrimidine bases occurs in the double-stranded DNA molecule in which A is paired with T and G is paired with C. Each nucleotide in a pair is on one strand of the DNA molecule, with the bases on opposite DNA strands bound together by hydrogen bonds that are extremely stable under normal conditions. The double-stranded structure of DNA molecules allows them to replicate precisely by separation of the two strands, followed by synthesis of two new complementary strands. Similarly, the base complementary pairing allows for efficient and correct repair of damaged DNA molecules.

Several hundred to almost one million base pairs can represent a gene, the size being proportional to the protein product it encodes. Of the two DNA strands, only one is used in transcribing the information for the cell's protein-building machinery. The genetic information of one strand is meaningful and is used as a template for transcription; the complementary code of the other strand does not make sense and is ignored. Both strands, however, are involved in DNA duplication. Before cell division, the two strands of the helix separate and a complementary molecule is duplicated next to each original strand. Two strands become four strands. During cell division, the newly duplicated double-stranded molecules are separated and placed in each daughter cell by the mechanics of mitosis. As a result, each of the daughter cells again contains the meaningful strand and the complementary strand joined together as a double helix. In 1958, Meselson and Stahl characterized this replication of DNA as *semiconservative,* as opposed to conservative replication in which the parental strands reassociate when the two strands are brought together (Fig. 6.2).[1,2]

Semiconservative Model   Conservative Model

▬▬▬ original strand of DNA
▬▬▬ newly synthesized strand of DNA

FIGURE 6.2 • Semiconservative versus conservative models of DNA replication as proposed by Meselson and Stahl in 1958. In semiconservative DNA replication, the two original strands of DNA unwind and a complementary strand is formed along each original strand.

Packaging of DNA

The genome or total genetic content is distributed in chromosomes. Each human somatic cell (cells other than the gametes [sperm and ovum]) has 23 pairs of different chromosomes, one pair derived from the individual's mother and the other from the father. One of the chromosome pairs consists of the sex chromosomes. Genes are arranged linearly along each chromosome. Each chromosome contains one continuous, linear DNA helix. The DNA in the longest chromosome is more than 7 cm in length. If the DNA of all 46 chromosomes were placed end-to-end, the total DNA would span a distance of about 2 m (more than 6 feet).

Because of their large size, DNA molecules are combined with several types of protein and small amounts of RNA into a coiled structure known as *chromatin.* The organization of DNA into chromatin is essential for controlling transcription and for packaging the molecule. Some DNA-associated proteins form binding sites for repressor molecules and hormones that regulate genetic transcription; others may block genetic transcription by preventing access of nucleotides to the surface of the DNA molecule.[1] A specific group of proteins called *histones* is thought to control the folding of the DNA strands.[3] Each double-stranded DNA molecule periodically coils around histones, forming regularly spaced spherical structures called *nucleosomes* that resemble beads on a string (Fig. 6.3). This string of beads further winds into filaments that make up the structure of chromatin.[1]

Although solving the structural problem of how to fit a huge amount of DNA into the nucleus, the chromatin fibre, when complexed with histones and folded into various levels of compaction, makes the DNA inaccessible during the processes of replication and gene expression. To accommodate these processes, chromatin must be induced to change its structure, a process called *chromatin remodelling.*[4] Several chemical interactions are now known to affect this process. One of these involves the acetylation of a histone amino acids group that is linked to the opening of the chromatin fibre and gene activation. Another important chemical modification involves the methylation of histone amino acids, which is correlated with gene inactivation.

Genetic Code

Four bases—guanine, adenine, cytosine, and thymine (uracil is substituted for thymine in RNA)—make up the alphabet of the genetic code. A sequence of three of these bases forms the fundamental triplet code used in transmitting the genetic information needed for protein synthesis. This triplet code is called a *codon* (Table 6.1). An example is the nucleotide sequence UGG (uracil, guanine, guanine), which is the triplet RNA code for the amino acid tryptophan. The genetic code is a universal language used by most living cells (*i.e.,* the code for the amino acid tryptophan is the same in a bacterium, a plant, and a human being). *Stop codes,* which signal the end of a protein molecule, are also present.[5] Mathematically, the 4 bases can be arranged in 64 different combinations. Sixty-one of the triplets correspond to particular amino acids, and

Dividing cell   Nondividing cell

Nucleoplasm   Chromatin

Chromosome   Chromatin

Histones

Chromosomal DNA

Double helix

FIGURE 6.3 • DNA strand organization. The DNA strands are shown in chromosomes for dividing cells and in chromatin for nondividing cells and are coiled around histones. (From McConnell T. H., Hull K. L. (2011). *Human form and human function: Essentials of anatomy and physiology* (p. 71, Figure 3.5). Philadelphia, PA: Lippincott Williams & Wilkins.)

three are stop signals. Only 20 amino acids are used in protein synthesis in humans. Several triplets code for the same amino acid; therefore, the genetic code is said to be *redundant* or *degenerate.* For example, AUG is a part of the initiation or start signal as well as the codon for the amino acid methionine. Codons that specify the same amino acid are called *synonyms.* Synonyms usually have the same first two bases but differ in the third base.

DNA Repair

Rarely, accidental errors in duplication of DNA occur. These errors are called *mutations.* Mutations result from the substitution of one base pair for another, the loss or addition of one or more base pairs, or rearrangements of base pairs. Many of these mutations occur spontaneously, whereas others occur because of environmental agents, chemicals, and radiation. Mutations may arise in somatic cells or in germ cells. Only those DNA changes that occur in germ cells can be inherited.

Considering the millions of base pairs that must be duplicated in each cell division, it is not surprising that random changes in replication occur. Most of these defects are corrected by DNA repair mechanisms. Several repair mechanisms exist, and each depends on specific enzymes called *endonucleases* that recognize local distortions of the DNA helix, cleave the abnormal chain, and remove the distorted region.[6] The gap is then filled when the correct deoxyribonucleotides, created by a DNA polymerase using the intact complementary strand as a template, are added to the cleaved DNA. The newly synthesized end of the segment is then joined to the remainder of the DNA strand by a DNA ligase. The normal regulation of these gene repair mechanisms is under the control of DNA repair genes. Loss of these gene functions renders the DNA susceptible to accumulation of mutations; when these affect proto-oncogenes or tumour suppressor genes, cancer may result (see Chapter 8).

Genetic Variability

As the Human Genome Project was progressing, it became evident that the human genome sequence is almost exactly (99.9%) the same in all people. It is the small variation (0.01%) in gene sequence (termed a *haplotype*) that is thought to account for the individual differences in physical traits, behaviours, and disease susceptibility. These variations are sometimes referred to as *polymorphisms* (from the existence of more than one morphologic or body form in a population). An international effort has been organized to develop a map (HapMap) of these variations with the intent of providing a link between genetic variations and common complex diseases such as cancer, heart disease, diabetes, and some forms of mental disease.[7]

Mitochondrial DNA

In addition to nuclear DNA, part of the DNA of a cell resides in the mitochondria. Mitochondrial DNA is inherited from the mother by her offspring (*i.e.,* matrilineal inheritance). It is a double-stranded closed circle, containing 37 genes, 24 of which are needed for mitochondrial DNA translation and 13 of which encode enzymes needed for oxidative metabolism.[8] Replication of mitochondrial DNA depends on enzymes encoded by nuclear DNA. Thus, the protein-synthesizing apparatus and molecular components for oxidative metabolism are jointly derived from nuclear and mitochondrial genes. Genetic disorders of mitochondrial DNA, although rare, commonly affect tissues such as those of the neuromuscular system that have a high requirement for oxidative metabolism (see Chapter 7).

From Genes to Proteins

Although DNA determines the type of biochemical product needed by the cell and directs its synthesis, it is RNA, through the processes of transcription and translation, that is responsible for the actual assembly of the products.

RNA Structure and Function

RNA, like DNA, is a large molecule made up of a long string of nucleotides. However, it differs from DNA in three aspects

TABLE 6.1 MESSENGER RNA TRIPLET CODES FOR AMINO ACIDS

AMINO ACID	RNA CODONS					
Alanine	GCU	GCC	GCA	GCG		
Arginine	CGU	CGC	CGA	CGG	AGA	AGG
Asparagine	AAU	AAC				
Aspartic acid	GAU	GAC				
Cysteine	UGU	UGC				
Glutamic acid	GAA	GAG				
Glutamine	CAA	CAG				
Glycine	GGU	GGC	GGA	GGG		
Histidine	CAU	CAC				
Isoleucine	AUU	AUC	AUA			
Leucine	CUU	CUC	CUA	CUG	UUA	UUG
Lysine	AAA	AAG				
Methionine	AUG					
Phenylalanine	UUU	UUC				
Proline	CCU	CCC	CCA	CCG		
Serine	UCU	UCC	UCA	UCG	AGC	AGU
Threonine	ACU	ACC	ACA	ACG		
Tryptophan	UGG					
Tyrosine	UAU	UAC				
Valine	GUU	GUC	GUA	GUG		
Start (CI)	AUG					
Stop (CT)	UAA	UAG	UGA			

of its structure. First, RNA is a single-stranded rather than a double-stranded molecule. Second, the sugar in each nucleotide of RNA is ribose instead of deoxyribose. Third, the pyrimidine base thymine in DNA is replaced by uracil in RNA.

Cells contain three types of RNA: messenger RNA (mRNA), ribosomal RNA (rRNA), and transfer RNA (tRNA).[9] All three types of RNA are synthesized in the nucleus by RNA polymerase enzymes and then moved into the cytoplasm, where protein synthesis takes place. *Messenger RNA* carries the instructions for protein synthesis, obtained from the DNA molecule, into the cytoplasm. *Transfer RNA* reads the instructions and delivers the appropriate amino acids to the ribosome, where *ribosomal RNA* translates the instructions and provides the machinery needed for protein synthesis.

Messenger RNA. mRNA is the template for protein synthesis. It is a long molecule containing several hundred to several thousand nucleotides. Each group of three nucleotides forms a codon that is exactly complementary to a nucleotide triplet of the DNA molecule. mRNA is formed by a process called *transcription*.[9] In this process, the weak hydrogen bonds of DNA are broken so that free RNA nucleotides can pair with their exposed DNA counterparts on the meaningful strand of the DNA molecule (Fig. 6.4). As with the base pairing of the DNA strands, complementary RNA bases pair with the DNA bases. In RNA, uracil (U) replaces thymine and pairs with adenine.

Ribosomal RNA. The ribosome is the physical structure in the cytoplasm where protein synthesis takes place. rRNA forms 60% of the ribosome, with the remainder of the ribosome composed of the structural proteins and enzymes needed for protein synthesis.[9] As with the other types of RNA, rRNA is synthesized in the nucleus. Unlike the two other types of RNA, rRNA is produced in a specialized nuclear structure called the *nucleolus.* The formed rRNA combines with ribosomal proteins in the nucleus to produce the ribosome, which is then transported into the cytoplasm. On reaching the cytoplasm, most ribosomes become attached to the endoplasmic reticulum and begin the task of protein synthesis.

Transfer RNA. tRNA is a clover-shaped molecule containing only 80 nucleotides, making it the smallest RNA molecule.[9] Its function is to deliver the activated form of an amino acid to the protein that is being synthesized in the ribosomes. At least 20 different types of tRNA are known, each of which recognizes and binds to only one type of amino acid. Each tRNA molecule has two recognition sites: the first is complementary for the mRNA anticodon, the second for the amino acid itself. Each type of tRNA carries its own specific amino acid to the ribosomes, where protein synthesis is taking place; there it recognizes the appropriate codon on the mRNA and delivers the amino acid to the newly forming protein molecule.

Understanding DNA-Directed Protein Synthesis

Deoxyribonucleic acid (DNA) directs the synthesis of the many thousands of proteins that are contained in the different cells of the body. Although some of the proteins are structural proteins, the majority are enzymes that catalyze the different chemical reactions in the cell. Because DNA is located in the cell's nucleus and protein synthesis takes place in the cytoplasm, a second type of nucleic acid—ribonucleic acid (RNA)—participates in the actual assembly of the proteins.

There are three types of RNA: messenger RNA (mRNA), ribosomal RNA (rRNA), and transfer RNA (tRNA) that participate in (1) the transcription of the DNA instructions for protein synthesis and (2) the translation of those instructions into the assembly of the polypeptides that make up the various proteins.

1 Transcription

Transcription involves copying the genetic code containing the instructions for protein synthesis from DNA to a complementary strand of mRNA. The genetic code is a triplet of four bases (adenine [A], thymine [T], guanine [G], and cytosine [C], with thymine in DNA being replaced with uracil [U] in RNA) that control the sequence of amino acids in a protein molecule that is being synthesized. (The triplet RNA code is called a *codon.*) Transcription is initiated by an enzyme called *RNA polymerase*, which binds to a promoter site on DNA. Many other proteins, including transcription factors, function to increase or decrease transcriptional activity of the genes. After mRNA has been transcribed, it detaches from DNA and is processed by cutting, removing, and splicing the internal RNA sequences to produce a variety of mRNA molecules from a single gene. Once mRNA has been processed, it diffuses through the nuclear pores into the cytoplasm, where it controls protein synthesis.

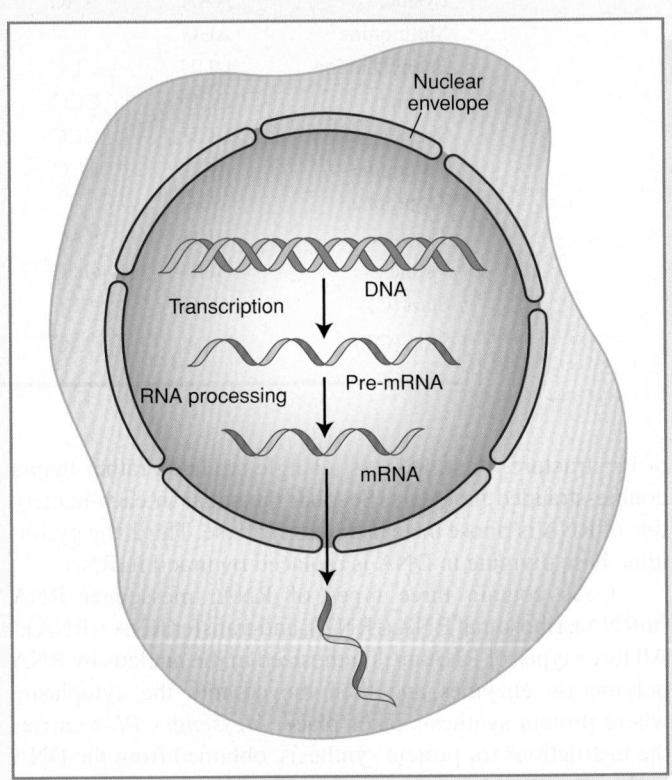

Transcription

Transcription occurs in the cell nucleus and involves the synthesis of RNA from a DNA template (Fig. 6.4).[9] Genes are transcribed by enzymes called *RNA polymerases* that generate a single-stranded RNA identical in sequence (with the exception of U in place of T) to one of the strands of DNA. It is initiated by the assembly of a transcription complex composed of RNA polymerase and other associated factors. This complex binds to the double-stranded DNA at a specific site called the *promoter region*. Within the promoter region the so-called TATA box is located. The TATA box contains the crucial thymine-adenine-thymine-adenine (TATA) nucleotide sequence

that RNA polymerase recognizes and binds to (Fig. 6.5). This binding also requires transcription factors, a transcription initiation site, and other proteins. Transcription continues to copy the meaningful strand into a single strand of RNA as it travels along the length of the gene, stopping only when it reaches a termination site with a stop codon (Fig. 6.5). On reaching the stop signal, the RNA polymerase enzyme leaves the gene and releases the RNA strand. The RNA strand then is processed.

Processing involves the addition of certain nucleic acids at the ends of the RNA strand and cutting and splicing of certain internal sequences. Splicing often involves the removal of stretches of RNA (Fig. 6.6). Because of the splicing process,

2 Translation

The process of translation involves taking the instructions transcribed from DNA to mRNA and transferring them to the rRNA of ribosomes located in the cytoplasm. When the mRNA carrying the instructions for a particular protein comes in contact with a ribosome, it binds to a small subunit of the rRNA. It then travels through the ribosome where the transcribed instructions are communicated to the tRNA, which delivers and transfers the correct amino acid to its proper position on the growing peptide chain. There are 20 types of tRNA, one for each of the 20 different types of amino acid. Each type of tRNA carries an anticodon complementary to the mRNA codon calling for the amino acid carried by the tRNA, and it is the recognition of the mRNA codon by the tRNA anticodon that ensures the proper sequence of amino acids in a synthesized protein.

In order to be functional, the newly synthesized protein must be folded into its functional form, modified further, and then routed to its final position in the cell.

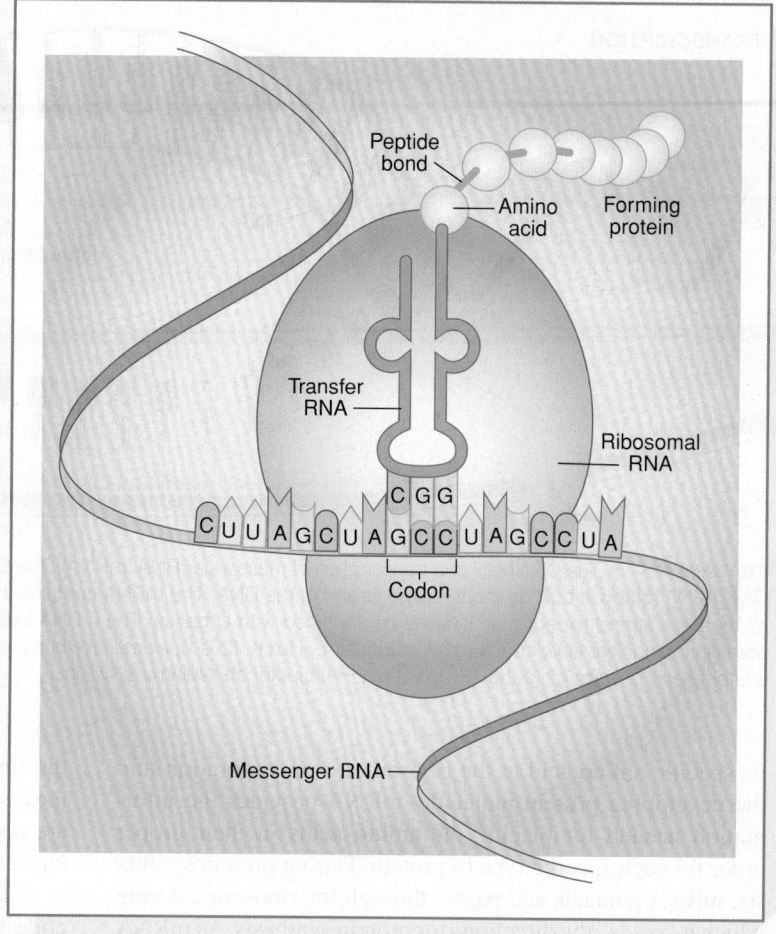

the final mRNA sequence is different from the original DNA template. The retained protein-coding regions of the mRNA sequences are called *exons* and the regions between exons are called *introns*.[10] The functions of the introns are unknown. They are thought to be involved in the activation or deactivation of genes during various stages of development.

Splicing permits a cell to produce a variety of mRNA molecules from a single gene. By varying the splicing segments of the initial mRNA, different mRNA molecules are formed. For example, in a muscle cell, the original tropomyosin mRNA is spliced in as many as 10 different ways, yielding distinctly different protein products. This permits different

proteins to be expressed from a single gene and reduces how much DNA must be contained in the genome.

Translation

Translation occurs in the cytoplasm of the cell and involves the synthesis of a protein using its mRNA template.[9] Proteins are made from a standard set of amino acids, which are joined end-to-end to form the long polypeptide chains of protein molecules. Each polypeptide chain may have as many as 100 to more than 300 amino acids in it. Besides rRNA, translation requires the coordinated actions of mRNA and tRNA (Fig. 6.7). Each of the 20 different tRNA molecules transports

TRANSCRIPTION

RNA polymerase creates RNA from the DNA template strand by matching with U/T and G with C.

DNA template strand

RNA

Free ribonucleotide

DNA sense strand

NUCLEUS

CYTOPLASM

FIGURE 6.4 • The DNA helix and transcription of messenger RNA (mRNA). The DNA helix unwinds and a new mRNA strand is built on the template strand of the DNA. The mRNA contains the same base sequence as the DNA strand except that T bases are replaced with U bases. The mRNA leaves the nucleus through pores in the nuclear envelope. (From McConnell T., Hull K. (2011). *Human form human function: Essentials of anatomy and physiology* (p. 83). Philadelphia, PA: Lippincott Williams & Wilkins.)

its specific amino acid to the ribosome for incorporation into the developing protein molecule. mRNA provides the information needed for placing the amino acids in their proper order for each specific type of protein. During protein synthesis, mRNA contacts and passes through the ribosome, during which it "reads" the directions for protein synthesis. As mRNA passes through the ribosome, tRNA delivers the appropriate amino acids for attachment to the growing polypeptide chain. The long mRNA molecule usually travels through and directs protein synthesis in more than one ribosome at a time. After

the first part of the mRNA is read by the first ribosome, it moves onto a second and a third. As a result, ribosomes that are actively involved in protein synthesis are often found in clusters called *polyribosomes.*

The process of translation is not over when the genetic code has been used to create the sequence of amino acids that constitute a protein. To be useful to a cell, this new polypeptide chain must fold up into its unique three-dimensional conformation. The folding of many proteins is made more efficient by special classes of proteins called *molecular*

FIGURE 6.5 • Transcription of messenger RNA from DNA involves attachment of RNA polymerase along with transcription factors and other proteins to a promoter region on DNA. This binding occurs at a specific nucleotide sequence, the "TATA" region (thymine-adenosine-thymine-adenosine). Other sites include a transcription initiation site and a termination site. (Courtesy of Edward W. Carroll.)

FIGURE 6.6 • RNA processing. In different cells, an RNA strand may eventually produce different proteins depending on the sequencing of exons during gene splicing. This variation allows a gene to code for more than one protein. (Courtesy of Edward W. Carroll.)

Forming protein

Peptide bond

Amino acid

Transfer RNA "head" bearing anticodon

Ribosome - large subunit

Direction of messenger RNA advance

Codon

Ribosome - small subunit

Messenger RNA

FIGURE 6.7 • Protein synthesis. A messenger RNA (mRNA) strand is shown moving along a small ribosomal subunit in the cytoplasm. As the mRNA codon passes along the ribosome, a new amino acid is added to the growing peptide chain by the transfer RNA (tRNA) bearing the anticodon for the mRNA-designated amino acid. As each amino acid is bound to the next by a peptide bond, its tRNA is released.

chaperones.[11] Typically the function of a chaperone is to assist a newly synthesized polypeptide chain to attain a functional conformation as a new protein and then to assist the protein's arrival at the site in the cell where the protein carries out its function. Molecular chaperones also assist in preventing the misfolding of existing proteins. Disruption of chaperoning mechanisms causes intracellular molecules to become denatured and insoluble. These denatured proteins tend to stick to one another, precipitate, and form inclusion bodies. The development of inclusion bodies is a common pathologic process in Parkinson, Alzheimer, and Huntington diseases.

A newly synthesized polypeptide chain may also need to combine with one or more polypeptide chains from the same or an adjacent chromosome, bind small cofactors for its activity, or undergo appropriate enzyme modification. During the post-translation process, two or more peptide chains may combine to form a single product. For example, two α-globin chains and two β-globin chains combine to form the $\alpha_2\beta_2$-hemoglobin molecule (see Chapter 14). The protein products may also be modified chemically by the addition of various types of functional groups. For example, fatty acids may be added, providing hydrophobic regions for attachment to cell membranes. Other modifications may involve cleavage of the protein, either to remove a specific amino acid sequence or to split the molecule into smaller chains. As an example, the two chains that make up the circulating active insulin molecule, one containing 21 and the other 30 amino acids, were originally part of an 82-amino-acid proinsulin molecule.

Regulation of Gene Expression

Only about 2% of the genome encodes instructions for synthesis of proteins; the remainder consists of noncoding regions that serve to determine where, when, and in what quantity proteins are made. The degree to which a gene or particular group of genes is active is called *gene expression.* A phenomenon termed *induction* is an important process by which gene expression is increased. *Gene repression* is a process by which a regulatory gene acts to reduce or prevent gene expression. Activator and repressor sites commonly monitor levels of the synthesized product and regulate gene transcription through a negative feedback mechanism. Whenever product levels decrease, gene transcription is increased, and when levels increase, it is repressed.

Although control of gene expression can occur in multiple steps, many regulatory events occur at the transcription level. The initiation and regulation of transcription require the collaboration of a battery of proteins, collectively termed *transcription factors.*[9] Transcription factors are a class of proteins that bind to their own specific DNA region and function to increase or decrease transcriptional activity of the genes. The role of transcription factors in gene expression explains why neurons and liver cells have completely different structures and functions although all the nucleated cells in a person contain the same DNA and thus the same genetic information. Some, referred to as *general transcription factors,* are required for transcription of all structural genes. Others, termed *specific transcription factors,* have more specialized roles, activating genes only at specific stages of development. For example, the PAX family of transcription factors is involved in the development of such embryonic tissues as the eye and portions of the nervous system.

Genetic Mediators of Embryonic Development

Regulation of gene expression also plays an essential role in the developing embryo. During embryonic development, many thousands of genes are expressed to control axial specification (*i.e.,* ventral/dorsal, anterior/posterior/medial/lateral, left/right), pattern formation (spatial arrangement of differentiated cells in body tissues and organs), and organogenesis (development of the different body organs). Many of these genes code transcription factors that produce signalling molecules, two examples being *sonic hedgehog* and *fibroblast growth factor.*[12] Signalling molecules bind to cells and are transported to the nucleus, where they initiate changes in gene expression. Depending on the embryonic tissue, these transcription factors and signalling molecules are produced temporally at various times during embryonic development.

Sonic hedgehog signalling is involved in many key developmental events at multiple times during embryogenesis.[12] It participates in such diverse developmental steps as establishment of the left-to-right axis responsible for the rostral–caudal orientation of the nervous system (see Chapter 48), the separation of the brain into two cerebral hemispheres, right and left eye orientation, and the separation and development of the correct number of fingers and toes. Fibroblast growth factors participate in a wide variety of developmental processes, including cell migration, growth, and differentiation. They are widely expressed in developing bone, and many autosomal dominant disorders of bone growth are mutations of fibroblast growth factor receptor genes. The most prevalent of these is a condition called *achondroplasia,* which is characterized by short stature with limbs that are disproportionately shorter than the trunk, and macrocephaly (large head).

IN SUMMARY

Genes are the fundamental unit of information storage in the cell. They determine the types of proteins and enzymes made by the cell and therefore control inheritance and day-to-day cell function. Genetic information is stored in a stable macromolecule called DNA. Genes transmit information contained in the DNA molecule as a triplet code. The genetic code is determined by the arrangement of the nitrogenous bases of the four nucleotides (*i.e.,* adenine, guanine, thymine [or uracil in RNA], and cytosine). Gene mutations represent accidental errors in duplication, rearrangement, or deletion of parts of the genetic code. Fortunately, most mutations are corrected by DNA repair mechanisms in the cell.

The transfer of stored information from DNA into production of cell products is accomplished through a second type of nucleotide called RNA. Messenger RNA transcribes the instructions for product synthesis from the DNA molecule and carries it into the cell's cytoplasm, where ribosomal RNA uses the information to direct protein synthesis. Transcription is initiated by RNA polymerase and other associated factors that bind to the double-stranded DNA at a specific site called the promoter region. Transfer RNA acts as a carrier system for delivering the appropriate amino acids to the ribosomes.

The degree to which a gene or particular group of genes is active is called gene expression. Gene expression involves a set of complex interrelationships among different levels of control, including RNA transcription and posttranslational processing. The initiation and regulation of RNA transcription are controlled by transcription factors that bind to specific DNA regions and function to regulate gene expression of the many different types of cells in the body. Post-translational processing involves the proper folding of the newly synthesized polypeptide chain into its unique three-dimensional conformation. Special classes of proteins called molecular chaperones make the folding of many proteins more efficient. Post-translational processing may also involve the combination of polypeptide chains from the same or an adjacent chromosome, the binding of small cofactors, or enzyme modification.

CHROMOSOMES

After completing this section of the chapter, you should be able to meet the following objectives:

- Define the terms autosomes, chromatin, meiosis, and mitosis.
- List the steps in constructing a karyotype using cytogenetic studies.
- Explain the significance of the Barr body.

Most genetic information of a cell is organized, stored, and retrieved in small intracellular structures called *chromosomes.* Although the chromosomes are visible only in dividing cells, they retain their integrity between cell divisions in the form of chromatin. The chromosomes are arranged in pairs; one member of the pair is inherited from the father, the other from the mother. Each species has a characteristic number of chromosomes. In the human, 46 single or 23 pairs of chromosomes are present. Of the 23 pairs of human chromosomes, 22 are called *autosomes* and are alike in both males and females. Each of the 22 pairs of autosomes has the same appearance in all individuals, and each has been given a numeric designation for classification purposes (Fig. 6.8).

In the diploid cell, each of the 22 autosomal chromosomes has a homolog. Homologous chromosomes contain a similar series of genes; that is, they have similar sequences. They are not identical, however, because one homolog comes from the haploid sperm of the father and one from the haploid

FIGURE 6.8 • Karyotype of human chromosomes. (From Rubin R., Strayer D. (Eds.). (2012). *Rubin's pathology: Clinicicopathologic foundations of medicine* (6th ed., p. 221). Philadelphia, PA: Lippincott Williams & Wilkins.)

ovum of the mother. The sex chromosomes, which make up the 23rd pair of chromosomes, determine the sex of a person. All males have an X and Y chromosome (*i.e.*, an X chromosome from the mother and a Y chromosome from the father); all females have two X chromosomes (*i.e.*, one from each parent). The much smaller Y chromosome contains the *male-specific region* (MSY) that determines sex. This region comprises more than 95% of the length of the Y chromosome.[13]

Only one X chromosome in the female is active in controlling the expression of genetic traits; however, both X chromosomes are activated during gametogenesis. In the female, the active X chromosome is invisible, but the inactive X chromosome can be visualized with appropriate nuclear staining. Inactivation is thought to involve the addition of a methyl group to the X chromosome. This inactive chromatin mass is seen as the *Barr body* in epithelial cells against the nuclear as the drumstick body in the chromatin of neutrophils.[14] The genetic sex of a child can

be determined by microscopic study of cell or tissue samples. The total number of X chromosomes is equal to the number of Barr bodies plus one (*i.e.*, an inactive plus an active X chromosome). For example, the cells of a normal female have one Barr body and therefore a total of two X chromosomes. A normal male has no Barr bodies. Males with Klinefelter syndrome, who have one Y and two X chromosomes (one active and one inactive), exhibit one Barr body (see Chapter 7). In the female, whether the active X chromosome is derived from the mother or father is determined within a few days after conception, the selection being random for each postmitotic cell line. Thus, the tissues of normal women have on average 50% maternally derived and 50% paternally derived active X chromosomes. This is known as the *Lyon principle*.[14]

Cell Division

Two types of cell division occur in humans and many other animals: mitosis and meiosis. Mitosis involves duplication of somatic cells in the body and is represented by the cell cycle (see Chapter 4). *Meiosis* is limited to replicating germ cells and takes place only once in a cell line. It results in the formation of gametes or reproductive cells (*i.e.*, ovum and sperm), each of which has only a single set of 23 chromosomes. Meiosis is typically divided into two distinct phases, meiosis I and meiosis II. Similar to mitosis, cells about to undergo the first meiotic division replicate their DNA during interphase (Fig. 6.9). During metaphase I, homologous autosomal chromosomes pair up, forming a synapsis or tetrad (two chromatids per chromosome). They are sometimes called *bivalents*. They do, however, pair up in several regions. The X and Y chromosomes are not homologs and do not form bivalents. While in metaphase I, an interchange of chromatid segments can occur. This process

FIGURE 6.10 • Crossing over of DNA at the time of meiosis.

FIGURE 6.9 • First and second meiotic divisions. (**Top**) Meiosis I, during which homologous chromosomes (A) approach each other and (B) pair; (C) intimately paired homologous chromosomes interchange chromatid fragments (crossing over); and (D) double-structured chromosomes pull apart. (E) Anaphase of first meiotic division. During meiosis II (F, G), the double-structured chromosomes pull apart at the centromere to form four single-stranded chromosomes (reduction division). (**Bottom**) Events occurring during meiosis I and II in female and male gametes. (A) The primitive female germ cell (oocyte) produces only one mature gamete, the mature oocyte. (B) The primitive male germ cell (primary spermatocyte) produces four spermatids, all of which develop into spermatozoa. (Adapted from Sadler R. W. (2014). *Langman's medical embryology* (13th ed., p. 16). Philadelphia, PA: Lippincott Williams & Wilkins.)

is called *crossing over* (Fig. 6.10). Crossing over allows for new combinations of genes, increasing genetic variability. After telophase I, each of the two daughter cells contains one member of each homologous pair of chromosomes and a sex

chromosome (23 double-stranded chromosomes). No DNA synthesis occurs before meiotic division II. During anaphase II, the 23 double-stranded chromosomes (two chromatids) of each of the two daughter cells from meiosis I divide at their centromeres. Each subsequent daughter cell receives 23 single-stranded chromosomes. Thus, a total of four daughter cells are formed by a meiotic division of one cell.

Meiosis, occurring only in the gamete-producing cells found in the testes or ovaries, has a different outcome in males and females. In males, meiosis (spermatogenesis) results in four viable daughter cells called *spermatids* that differentiate into sperm cells. In females, gamete formation or oogenesis is quite different. After the first meiotic division of a primary oocyte, a secondary oocyte and another structure called a *polar body* are formed. This small polar body contains little cytoplasm, but it may undergo a second meiotic division, resulting in two polar bodies. The secondary oocyte undergoes its second meiotic division, producing one mature oocyte and another polar body. Four viable sperm cells are produced during spermatogenesis, but only one ovum results from oogenesis.

Chromosome Structure

Cytogenetics is the study of the structure and numeric characteristics of the cell's chromosomes. Chromosome studies can be done on any tissue or cell that grows and divides in culture. Lymphocytes from venous blood are frequently used for this purpose. After the cells have been cultured, a drug called *colchicine* is used to arrest mitosis in metaphase. A chromosome spread is prepared by fixing and spreading the chromosomes on a slide. Subsequently, appropriate staining techniques show the chromosomal banding patterns so they can be identified. The chromosomes are photographed, and the photomicrographs of each of the chromosomes are cut out and arranged in pairs according to a standard classification system (see Fig. 6.8). The completed picture is called a *karyotype,* and the procedure for preparing the picture is called *karyotyping.* A uniform system of chromosome classification was originally formulated at the 1971 Paris Chromosome Conference and was later revised to describe the chromosomes as seen in more elongated prophase and prometaphase preparations.

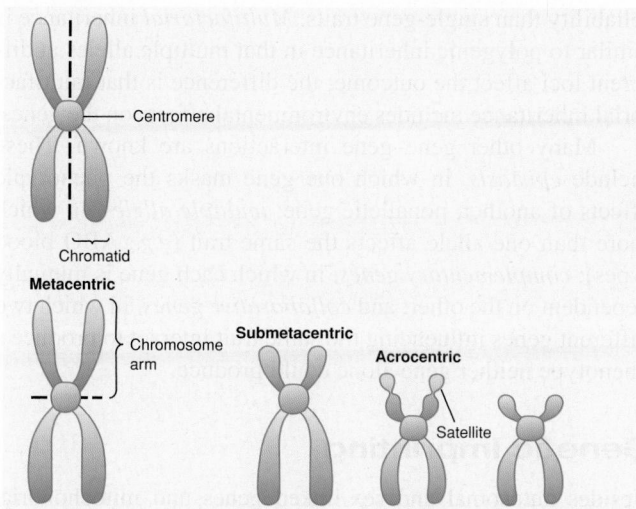

FIGURE 6.11 • Three basic shapes and the component parts of human metaphase chromosomes. The relative size of the satellite on the acrocentric chromosome is exaggerated for visibility. (Adapted from Cormack D. H. (1993). *Essential histology*. Philadelphia, PA: JB Lippincott.)

FIGURE 6.12 • The localization of inherited diseases as represented on the banded karyotype of the X chromosome. Notice the nomenclature of arms (p, q), regions (1, 2), and bands (*e.g.*, 22 = region 2, band 2). (Adapted from Rubin R., Strayer D. (Eds.). *Rubin's pathology: Clinicopathologic foundations of medicine* (6th ed., p. 251). Philadelphia, PA: Lippincott Williams & Wilkins.)

In the metaphase spread, each chromosome takes the form of chromatids to form an "X" or "wishbone" pattern. Human chromosomes are divided into three types according to the position of the centromere (Fig. 6.11). If the centromere is in the centre and the arms are of approximately the same length, the chromosome is said to be *metacentric;* if it is not centred and the arms are of clearly different lengths, it is *submetacentric;* and if it is near one end, it is *acrocentric.* The short arm of the chromosome is designated as "p" for "petite," and the long arm is designated as "q" for no other reason than it is the next letter of the alphabet.[14] The arms of the chromosome are indicated by the chromosome number followed by the p or q designation (*e.g.*, 15p). Chromosomes 13, 14, 15, 21, and 22 have small masses of chromatin called *satellites* attached to their short arms by narrow stalks. At the ends of each chromosome are special DNA sequences called *telomeres*. Telomeres allow the end of the DNA molecule to be replicated completely.

The banding patterns of a chromosome are used in describing the position of a gene on a chromosome. Each arm of a chromosome is divided into regions, which are numbered from the centromere outward (*e.g.*, 1, 2). The regions are further divided into bands, which are also numbered (Fig. 6.12). These numbers are used in designating the position of a gene on a chromosome. For example, Xp22 refers to band 2, region 2 of the short arm (p) of the X chromosome.

IN SUMMARY

The genetic information in a cell is organized, stored, and retrieved as small cellular structures called chromosomes. Forty-six chromosomes arranged in 23 pairs are present in the human being. Twenty-two of these pairs are autosomes. The 23rd pair is the sex chromosomes, which determine the person's sex. Two types of cell division occur, meiosis and mitosis. Meiosis is limited to replicating germ cells and results in the formation of gametes or reproductive cells (ovum and sperm), each of which has only a single set of 23 chromosomes. Mitotic division occurs in somatic cells and results in the formation of 23 pairs of chromosomes. A karyotype is a photograph of a person's chromosomes. It is prepared by special laboratory techniques in which body cells are cultured, fixed, and then stained to display identifiable banding patterns. A photomicrograph is then made. Often the photomicrographs of individual chromosomes are cut out and regrouped according to chromosome number.

PATTERNS OF INHERITANCE

After completing this section of the chapter, you should be able to meet the following objectives:

- Construct a hypothetical pedigree for a recessive and dominant trait according to Mendel's laws.
- Contrast genotype and phenotype.
- Define the terms allele, locus, expressivity, and penetrance.

The characteristics inherited from a person's parents are inscribed in gene pairs found along the length of the chromosomes. Alternate forms of the same gene are possible (*i.e.*, one inherited from the mother and the other from the father), and each may produce a different aspect of a trait.

Definitions

Genetics has its own set of definitions. The *genotype* of a person is the genetic information stored in the base sequence triplet code. The *phenotype* refers to the recognizable traits, physical or biochemical, associated with a specific genotype. Often, the genotype is not evident from available detection methods. More than one genotype may have the same phenotype. Some brown-eyed persons are carriers of the code for blue eyes, and other brown-eyed persons are not. Phenotypically, these two types of brown-eyed persons are the same, but genotypically they are different.

With regard to a genetic disorder, not all persons with a mutant gene are affected to the same extent. *Expressivity* refers to the manner in which the gene is expressed in the phenotype, which can range from mild to severe. *Penetrance* represents the ability of a gene to express its function. Seventy-five percent penetrance means 75% of persons of a particular genotype present with a recognizable phenotype. Syndactyly and blue sclera are genetic mutations that often do not exhibit 100% penetrance.

The position of a gene on a chromosome is called its *locus,* and alternate forms of a gene at the same locus are called *alleles.* When only one pair of genes is involved in the transmission of information, the term *single-gene trait* is used. Single-gene traits follow the mendelian laws of inheritance.

TRANSMISSION OF GENETIC INFORMATION

- The transmission of information from one generation to the next is vested in genetic material transferred from each parent at the time of conception.
- Alleles are the alternate forms of a gene (one from each parent), and the locus is the position that they occupy on the chromosome.
- The genotype of a person represents the sum total of the genetic information in the cells, and the phenotype the physical manifestations of that information.
- Penetrance is the percentage in a population with a particular genotype in which that genotype is phenotypically manifested, whereas expressivity is the manner in which the gene is expressed.
- Mendelian, or single-gene, patterns of inheritance include autosomal dominant and recessive traits that are transmitted from parents to their offspring in a predictable manner. Polygenic inheritance, which involves multiple genes, and multifactorial inheritance, which involves multiple genes as well as environmental factors, are less predictable.

Polygenic inheritance involves multiple genes at different loci, with each gene exerting a small additive effect in determining a trait. Most human traits are determined by multiple pairs of genes, many with alternate codes, accounting for some dissimilar forms that occur with certain genetic disorders. Polygenic traits are predictable, but with less reliability than single-gene traits. *Multifactorial* inheritance is similar to polygenic inheritance in that multiple alleles at different loci affect the outcome; the difference is that multifactorial inheritance includes environmental effects on the genes.

Many other gene–gene interactions are known. These include *epistasis,* in which one gene masks the phenotypic effects of another, nonallelic gene; *multiple alleles,* in which more than one allele affects the same trait (*e.g.,* ABO blood types); *complementary genes,* in which each gene is mutually dependent on the other; and *collaborative genes,* in which two different genes influencing the same trait interact to produce a phenotype neither gene alone could produce.

Genetic Imprinting

Besides autosomal and sex-linked genes and mitochondrial inheritance, it was found that certain genes exhibit a "parent of origin" type of transmission in which the parental genomes do not always contribute equally in the development of an individual (Fig. 6.13). The transmission of this phenomenon is called *genomic imprinting.* Although rare, it is estimated that approximately 100 genes exhibit genomic, or genetic, imprinting. Evidence suggests a genetic conflict occurs in the developing embryo: the male genome attempts to establish larger offspring, whereas the female prefers smaller offspring to conserve her energy for the current and subsequent pregnancies.

It was the pathologic analysis of ovarian teratomas (tumours made up of various cell types derived from an undifferentiated germ cell) and hydatidiform moles (gestational tumours made up of trophoblastic tissue) that yielded the first evidence of genetic imprinting. All ovarian teratomas were found to have a 46,XX karyotype. The results of detailed chromosomal polymorphism analysis confirmed that these tumours developed without the paternally derived genome. Conversely, analysis of hydatidiform moles suggested that they were tumours of paternal origin.

Well-known examples of genomic imprinting are the transmission of the mutations in Prader–Willi and Angelman syndromes.[15] Both syndromes exhibit mental retardation as a common feature. It was also found that both disorders had the same deletion in chromosome 15. When the deletion is inherited from the mother, the infant presents with Angelman ("happy puppet") syndrome; when the same deletion is inherited from the father, Prader–Willi syndrome results.

A related chromosomal disorder is *uniparental disomy.* This occurs when two chromosomes of the same number are inherited from one parent. Normally, this is not a problem except in cases where a chromosome has been imprinted by a parent. If imprinting inactivates an allele, the offspring will have only one working copy of the chromosome, resulting in possible problems.

Mendel's Laws

A main feature of inheritance is predictability: given certain conditions, the likelihood of the occurrence or recurrence of

FIGURE 6.13 • Pedigree of genetic imprinting. In generation I, male (**A**) has inherited a mutant allele from his affected mother (not shown); the gene is "turned off" during spermatogenesis, and therefore none of his offspring (generation II) will express the mutant allele, regardless of whether they are carriers. However, the gene will be "turned on" again during oogenesis in any of his daughters (**B**) who inherit the allele. All offspring (generation III) who inherit the mutant allele will be affected. All offspring of normal children (**C**) will produce normal offspring. Children of female (**D**) will all express the mutation if they inherit the allele.

Affected individuals

Have the mutant allele but are not affected

Do not have the mutant allele and are not affected

a specific trait is remarkably predictable. The units of inheritance are the genes, and the pattern of single-gene expression can often be predicted using Mendel's laws of genetic transmission. Techniques and discoveries since Gregor Mendel's original work was published in 1865 have led to some modification of the original laws.

Mendel discovered the basic pattern of inheritance by conducting carefully planned experiments with simple garden peas. Experimenting with several phenotypic traits in peas, Mendel proposed that inherited traits are transmitted from parents to offspring by means of independently inherited factors—now known as genes—and that these factors are transmitted as recessive and dominant traits. Mendel labelled dominant factors (his round peas) "A" and recessive factors (his wrinkled peas) "a." Geneticists continue to use capital letters to designate dominant traits and lowercase letters to identify recessive traits. The possible combinations that can occur with transmission of single-gene dominant and recessive traits can be described by constructing a figure called a *Punnett square* using capital and lowercase letters (Fig. 6.14).

The observable traits of single-gene inheritance are inherited by the offspring from the parents. During maturation, the primordial germ cells (*i.e.,* sperm and ovum) of both parents undergo meiosis, or reduction division, in which the number of chromosomes is divided in half (from 46 to 23). At this time, the two alleles from a gene locus separate so that each germ cell receives only one allele from each pair (*i.e.,* Mendel's first law). According to Mendel's second law, the alleles from the different gene loci segregate independently and recombine randomly in the zygote. Persons in whom the two alleles of a given pair are the same (AA or aa) are called *homozygotes.* *Heterozygotes* have different alleles (Aa) at a

gene locus. A *recessive trait* is one expressed only in a homozygous pairing; a *dominant trait* is one expressed in either a homozygous or a heterozygous pairing. All persons with a dominant allele (depending on the penetrance of the genes) manifest that trait. A *carrier* is a person who is heterozygous for a recessive trait and does not manifest the trait. For example, the genes for blond hair are recessive and those for brown

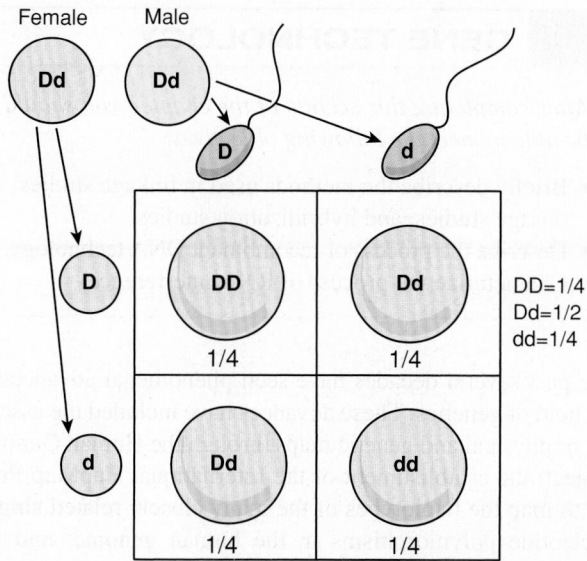

FIGURE 6.14 • The Punnett square showing all possible combinations for transmission of a single gene trait (dimpled cheeks). The example shown is when both parents are heterozygous (Dd) for the trait. The alleles carried by the mother are on the left and those carried by the father are on the top. The D allele is dominant and the d allele is recessive. The DD and Dd offspring have dimples and the dd offspring does not.

hair are dominant. Therefore, only persons with a genotype having two alleles for blond hair would be blond; persons with either one or two brown alleles would have dark hair.

Pedigree

A pedigree is a graphic method (Figs. 6.13 and 6.14) for portraying a family history of an inherited trait. It is constructed from a carefully obtained family history and is useful for tracing the pattern of inheritance for a particular trait (see Chapter 7).

IN SUMMARY

Inheritance represents the likelihood of the occurrence or recurrence of a specific genetic trait. The genotype refers to information stored in the genetic code of a person, whereas the phenotype represents the recognizable traits, physical and biochemical, associated with the genotype. Expressivity refers to the expression of a gene in the phenotype, and penetrance is the ability of a gene to express its function. The point on the DNA molecule that controls the inheritance of a particular trait is called a gene locus. Alternate forms of a gene at a gene locus are called alleles. The alleles at a gene locus may carry recessive or dominant traits. A recessive trait is one expressed only when two copies (homozygous) of the recessive allele are present. Dominant traits are expressed with either homozygous or heterozygous pairing of the alleles. A pedigree is a graphic method for portraying a family history of an inherited trait.

GENE TECHNOLOGY

After completing this section of the chapter, you should be able to meet the following objectives:

- Briefly describe the methods used in linkage studies, dosage studies, and hybridization studies.
- Describe the process of recombinant DNA technology.
- Characterize the process of RNA interference.

The past several decades have seen phenomenal advances in the field of genetics. These advances have included the assembly of physical and genetic maps through the Human Genome Project; the establishment of the International HapMap Project to map the haplotypes of the many closely related single-nucleotide polymorphisms in the human genome; and the development of methods for applying the technology of these projects to the diagnosis and treatment of disease.[1] Many health care professions also have established clinical competencies for their specific professions regarding genomics and genetics since the application of genetics is becoming more evident in all areas of disease screening and management.

There are multiple new genetic diagnostics advancing the ability to assess for various genetic alterations and to assist with planning individualized care including pharmacological disease management.

Genetic Mapping

Genetic mapping is the assignment of genes to specific chromosomes or parts of the chromosome. Another type of mapping strategy, the haplotype map, focuses on identifying the slight variations in the human genome that affect an individual's susceptibility to disease and responses to environmental factors such as microbes, toxins, and drugs.

There are two types of gene maps: genetic maps and physical maps. Genetic maps are like highway maps. They use linkage studies (*e.g.,* dosage, hybridization) to estimate the distances between chromosomal landmarks (*i.e.,* gene markers). Physical maps are similar to a surveyor's map. They make use of cytogenetic and molecular techniques to determine the actual, physical locations of genes on chromosomes. Genetic maps and physical maps have been refined over the decades. The earliest mapping efforts localized genes on the X chromosome (Fig. 6.12). The initial assignment of a gene to a particular chromosome was made in 1911 for the colour blindness gene inherited from the mother (*i.e.,* following the X-linked pattern of inheritance). In 1968, the specific location of the Duffy blood group on the long arm of chromosome 1 was determined.

The Human Genome Project

The Human Genome Project, initiated in 1990, sought to identify all the genes in the human genome. The international project was charged with developing genetic and physical maps that allowed the precise location of genes, and with exploring technologies that would enable the sequencing of large amounts of DNA with high accuracy and low cost. One of the surprising findings of the 2003 final report of the project was that humans have only 20,000 genes, much less than the previously estimated 80,000 to 140,000 genes.[1,16,17]

To date, the locations of more than 20,000 genes have been mapped to a specific chromosome, and most of them to a specific region on the chromosome. However, genetic mapping is continuing so rapidly that these numbers are constantly being updated. An excellent source of articles regarding specific chromosome sequencing in humans and a central database for mapped genes is the National Center for Biotechnology Information (NCBI) (www.ncbi.nlm.nih.gov/index.html).[16]

Genetic Mapping Methods

Many methods have been used for developing genetic maps. The most important ones are family linkage studies, gene dosage methods, and hybridization studies. Often, the specific assignment of a gene is made using information from several mapping techniques.

Linkage Studies. Linkage studies assume that genes occur in a linear array along the chromosomes. During meiosis, the paired chromosomes of the diploid germ cell exchange genetic material because of the crossing-over phenomenon (Fig. 6.10). This exchange usually involves more than one gene; large blocks of genes (representing large portions of the chromosome) are usually exchanged. Although the point at which one block separates from another occurs randomly, the closer together two genes are on the same chromosome, the greater the chance is that they will be passed on together to the offspring. When two inherited traits occur together at a rate greater than would occur by chance alone, they are said to be *linked*.

Several methods take advantage of the crossing over and recombination of genes to map a particular gene. In one method, any gene that is already assigned to a chromosome can be used as a marker to assign other linked genes. For example, it was found that an extra long chromosome 1 and the Duffy blood group were inherited as a dominant trait, placing the position of the blood group gene close to the extra material on chromosome 1. Colour blindness has been linked to classic hemophilia A (*i.e.,* lack of factor VIII) in some pedigrees; hemophilia A has been linked to glucose-6-phosphate dehydrogenase deficiency in others; and colour blindness has been linked to glucose-6-phosphate dehydrogenase deficiency in still others. Because the gene for colour blindness is found on the X chromosome, all three genes must be found in a small section of the X chromosome. Linkage analysis can be used clinically to identify affected persons in a family with a known genetic defect. Males, because they have one X and one Y chromosome, are said to be *hemizygous* for sex-linked traits. Females can be homozygous (normal or mutant) or heterozygous for sex-linked traits. Heterozygous females are known as *carriers* for X-linked defects.

One autosomal recessive disorder that has been successfully diagnosed prenatally by linkage studies using amniocentesis is congenital adrenal hyperplasia (due to 21-hydroxylase deficiency), which is linked to an immune response gene (human leukocyte antigen, HLA) type.[18] Postnatal linkage studies have been used in diagnosing hemochromatosis, which is closely linked to another HLA type.[19] Persons with this disorder are unable to metabolize iron, and it accumulates in the liver and other organs. It cannot be diagnosed by conventional means until irreversible damage has been done. Given a family history of the disorder, HLA typing can determine if the gene is present, and if it is present, dietary restriction of iron intake may be used to prevent organ damage.

Gene Dosage Studies. Dosage studies involve measuring enzyme activity. Autosomal genes are normally arranged in pairs, and normally both are expressed. If both alleles are present and both are expressed, the activity of the enzyme should be 100%. If one member of the gene pair is missing, only 50% of the enzyme activity is present, reflecting the activity of the remaining normal allele.

Hybridization Studies. A recent biologic discovery revealed that two somatic cells from different species, when grown together in the same culture, occasionally fuse to form a new

hybrid cell. Two types of hybridization methods are used in genomic studies: somatic cell hybridization and in situ hybridization.

Somatic cell hybridization involves the fusion of human somatic cells with those of a different species (typically, the mouse) to yield a cell containing the chromosomes of both species. Because these hybrid cells are unstable, they begin to lose chromosomes of both species during subsequent cell divisions. This makes it possible to obtain cells with different partial combinations of human chromosomes. The enzymes of these cells are then studied with the understanding that for an enzyme to be produced, a certain chromosome must be present and, therefore, the coding for the enzyme must be located on that chromosome.

In situ hybridization involves the use of specific sequences of DNA or RNA to locate genes that do not express themselves in cell culture. DNA and RNA can be chemically tagged with radioactive or fluorescent markers. These chemically tagged DNA or RNA sequences are used as probes to detect gene location. The probe is added to a chromosome spread after the DNA strands have been separated. If the probe matches the complementary DNA of a chromosome segment, it hybridizes and remains at the precise location (therefore the term *in situ*) on a chromosome. Radioactive or fluorescent markers are used to find the location of the probe.

Haplotype Mapping

As work on the Human Genome Project progressed, many researchers reasoned that identifying the common patterns of DNA sequence variations in the human genome would be possible. An international project, known as the *International HapMap Project*, was organized with the intent of developing a haplotype map of these variations.[1,7] One of the findings of the Human Genome Project was that the genome sequence was 99.9% identical for all people. It is anticipated that the 0.1% variation may greatly affect an individual's response to drugs, toxins, and predisposition to various diseases. Sites in the DNA sequence where individuals differ at a single DNA base are called *single nucleotide polymorphisms* (SNPs, pronounced "snips"). A haplotype consists of the many closely linked SNPs on a single chromosome that generally are passed as a block from one generation to another in a particular population (Fig. 6.15). One of the motivating factors behind the

FIGURE 6.15 • Two single nucleotide substitutions (SNPs) along DNA strand 2. At **A.,** the SNP replaces adenine (A) for guanine, whereas at **B.** guanine (G) is substituted for thymine. SNPs occur on average every 1,200 bases along the DNA molecule. It is estimated that a human genome contains about 10,000 SNPs. (Courtesy of Edward W. Carroll.)

HapMap Project was the realization that the identification of a few SNPs was enough to uniquely identify the haplotypes in a block. The specific SNPs that identify the haplotypes are called *tag SNPs.* A HapMap is a map of these haplotype blocks and their tag SNPs. This approach reduces the number of SNPs required to examine an entire genome and make genome scanning methods much more efficient in finding regions with genes that contribute to disease development.[1,17]

Much attention has focused on the use of SNPs to decide whether a genetic variant is associated with a higher risk of disease susceptibility in one population versus another. Pharmacogenetics addresses the variability of drug response due to inherited characteristics in individuals allowing identification of people who can be expected to respond favourably to a drug and those who can be expected to experience adverse reactions. This results in safer, more effective, and more cost-efficient use of medications.

Recombinant DNA Technology

The term *recombinant DNA* refers to a combination of DNA molecules that are not found together in nature. Recombinant DNA technology makes it possible to identify the DNA sequence in a gene and produce the protein product encoded by a gene. The specific nucleotide sequence of a DNA fragment can often be identified by analyzing the amino acid sequence and mRNA codon of its protein product. Short sequences of base pairs can be synthesized, radioactively labelled, and subsequently used to identify their complementary sequence. In this way, identifying normal and abnormal gene structures is possible.

Tests of DNA sequences are particularly useful in identifying polymorphisms, including the previously discussed SNPs, that are associated with various diseases. Because genetic variations are so distinctive, DNA fingerprinting (analysis of DNA sequence differences) can be used to determine family relationships or help identify persons involved in criminal acts. The methods of recombinant DNA technology can also be used in the treatment of disease. For example, recombinant DNA technology is used in the manufacture of human insulin that is used to treat diabetes mellitus.

Gene Isolation and Cloning

The gene isolation and cloning methods used in recombinant DNA technology rely on the fact that the genes of all organisms, from bacteria through mammals, are based on a similar molecular organization. Gene cloning requires cutting a DNA molecule apart, modifying and reassembling its fragments, and producing copies of the modified DNA, its mRNA, and its gene product. The DNA molecule is cut apart by using a bacterial enzyme, called a *restriction enzyme,* that binds to DNA wherever a particular short sequence of base pairs is found and cleaves the molecule at a specific nucleotide site. In this way, a long DNA molecule can be broken down into smaller, discrete fragments, one of which presumably contains the gene of interest. Many restriction enzymes are commercially available that cut DNA at different recognition sites.

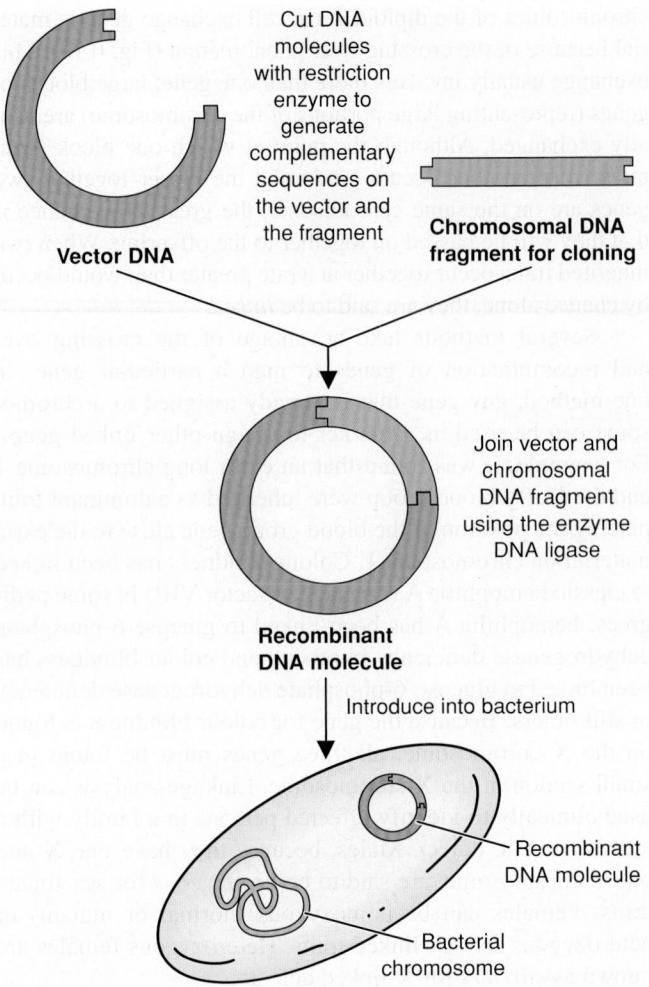

FIGURE 6.16 • Recombinant DNA technology. By fragmenting DNA of any origin and inserting it in the DNA of rapidly reproducing foreign cells, billions of copies of a single gene can be produced in a short time. DNA to clone is inserted into a plasmid (a small, self-replicating circular molecule of DNA) that is separate from chromosomal DNA. When the recombinant plasmid is introduced into bacteria, the newly inserted segment will be replicated along with the rest of the plasmid. (From the U.S. Department of Energy Genomic Image Gallery.)

The restrictive fragments of DNA can often be replicated through insertion into a unicellular organism, such as a bacterium (Fig. 6.16). To do this, a cloning vector such as a bacterial virus or a small DNA circle that is found in most bacteria, called a *plasmid,* is used. Viral and plasmid vectors replicate autonomously in the host bacterial cell. During gene cloning, a bacterial vector and the DNA fragment are mixed and joined by a special enzyme called a *DNA ligase.* The recombinant vectors formed are then introduced into a suitable culture of bacteria, and the bacteria are allowed to replicate and express the recombinant vector gene. Sometimes, mRNA taken from a tissue that expresses a high level of the gene is used to produce a complementary DNA molecule that can be used in the cloning process. Because the fragments of the entire DNA molecule are used in the cloning process, additional steps are taken to identify and separate the clone that contains the gene of interest.

Pharmaceutical Applications

Recombinant DNA technology has also made it possible to produce proteins that have therapeutic properties. One of the first products to be produced was human insulin. Recombinant DNA corresponding to the A chain of human insulin was isolated and inserted into plasmids that were in turn used to transform *Escherichia coli*. The bacteria then synthesized the insulin chain. A similar method was used to obtain the B chains. The A and B chains were then mixed and allowed to fold and form disulfide bonds, producing active insulin molecules. Human growth hormone has also been produced in *E. coli*. More complex proteins are produced in mammalian cell culture using recombinant DNA techniques. These include erythropoietin, which is used to stimulate red blood cell production; factor VIII, which is used to treat hemophilia; and tissue plasminogen activator (tPA), which may be administered for thrombotic strokes.

DNA Fingerprinting

The technique of DNA fingerprinting is based in part on those techniques used in recombinant DNA technology and on those originally used in medical genetics to detect slight variations in the genomes of different individuals.[20] Using restriction enzymes, DNA is cleaved at specific regions (Fig. 6.17). The DNA fragments are separated according to size by electrophoresis and denatured (by heating or treating chemically) so that all the DNA is single stranded. The single-stranded DNA is then transferred to nitrocellulose paper, baked to attach the DNA to the paper, and treated with series of radioactive probes. After the radioactive probes have been allowed to bond with the denatured DNA, radiography is used to reveal the labelled DNA fragments.

When used in forensic pathology, this procedure is applied to specimens from the suspect and the forensic specimen. Banding patterns are then analyzed to see if they match. With conventional methods of analysis of blood and serum enzymes, a 1 in 100 to 1,000 chance exists that the two specimens match because of chance. With DNA fingerprinting, these odds are 1 in 100,000 to 1 million.

When necessary, the polymerase chain reaction (PCR) can be used to amplify specific segments of DNA (see Chapter 16). It is particularly suited for amplifying regions of DNA for clinical and forensic testing procedures because only a small sample of DNA is required as the starting material. Regions of DNA can be amplified from a single hair or drop of blood or saliva.

Gene Therapy

Although quite different from inserting genetic material into a unicellular organism such as bacteria, techniques are available for inserting genes into the genome of intact multicellular plants and animals. Promising delivery vehicles for these genes are the adenoviruses. These viruses are ideal vehicles because their DNA does not become integrated into the host genome. However, repeated inoculations are often needed because the body's immune system usually targets cells expressing

FIGURE 6.17 • DNA fingerprinting. Restrictive enzymes are used to break chromosomal DNA into fragments, which are then separated by gel electrophoresis, denatured, and transferred to nitrocellulose paper; the DNA bands are labelled with a radioactive probe and observed using autoradiography. (Modified from Smith C., Marks A. D., Lieberman M. (2005). *Marks' basic medical biochemistry* (2nd ed., p. 309). Philadelphia, PA: Lippincott Williams & Wilkins.)

adenovirus proteins. Sterically stable liposomes also show promise as DNA delivery mechanisms.[21] This type of therapy is one of the more promising methods for the treatment of genetic disorders such as cystic fibrosis, certain cancers, and many infectious diseases.

Two main approaches are used in gene therapy: transferred genes can replace defective genes or they can selectively inhibit deleterious genes. Cloned DNA sequences are usually the compounds used in gene therapy. However, the introduction of the cloned gene into the multicellular organism can influence only the few cells that get the gene. An answer to this problem would be the insertion of the gene into a sperm or ovum; after fertilization, the gene would be replicated in all of the differentiating cell types. Even so, techniques for cell insertion are limited. Not only are moral and ethical issues involved, but these techniques cannot direct the inserted DNA to attach to a particular chromosome or supplant an existing gene by knocking it out of its place.

To date, gene therapy has been used successfully to treat children with severe combined immunodeficiency disease (see Chapter 20), and in a suicide gene transfer to facilitate treatment of graft-versus-host disease after donor lymphocyte infusion.

RNA Interference Technology

One approach of gene therapy focuses on the previously described replacement of missing or defective genes. However, several genetic disorders are not due to missing genes, but to faulty gene activity. With this in mind, some scientists are approaching the problem by using *RNA interference* (RNAi) to stop genes from making unwanted disease proteins.[22] RNAi is a naturally occurring process in which small pieces of double-stranded RNA (small interfering RNA [siRNA]) suppress gene expression. Scientists believe that RNAi may have originated as a defense against viral infections and potentially harmful genomic invaders. In viral infections, RNAi would serve to control the infection by preventing the synthesis of viral proteins.

With the continued refinement of techniques to silence genes, RNAi has already had a major impact on molecular biology. For example, it has given scientists the ability to practice reverse genomics, in which a gene's function can be inferred through silencing its expression. Increasingly, pharmaceutical companies are using RNAi to identify disease-related drug targets. There also is considerable interest in harnessing RNAi for therapeutic purposes, including the treatment of human immunodeficiency virus (HIV) infection and hepatitis C. Before this can occur, however, the therapeutic methods must be shown to be safe and effective, and obstacles to delivering the RNAi into targeted cells must be overcome. It is difficult for RNA to cross the cell membrane, and it is quickly broken down by enzymes in the blood.

IN SUMMARY

The genome is the gene complement of an organism. Genomic mapping is a method used to assign genes to particular chromosomes or parts of a chromosome. The most important ones used are family linkage studies, gene dosage methods, and hybridization studies. Often the specific assignment of a gene is determined by using information from several mapping techniques. Linkage studies assign a chromosome location to genes based on their close association with other genes of known location. Recombinant DNA studies involve the extraction of specific types of mRNA used in synthesis of complementary DNA strands. The complementary DNA strands, labelled with a radioisotope, bind with the genes for which they are complementary and are used as gene probes. A haplotype consists of the many closely linked SNPs on a single chromosome that generally are passed as a block from one generation to another in a particular population. The International HapMap Project has been developed to map the SNPs on the human genome with the anticipation that it may be useful in the prediction and management of disease.

Genetic engineering has provided the methods for manipulating nucleic acids and recombining genes (recombinant DNA) into hybrid molecules that can be inserted into unicellular organisms and reproduced many times over. As a result, proteins that formerly were available only in small amounts can now be made in large quantities once their respective genes have been isolated. DNA fingerprinting, which relies on recombinant DNA technologies and those of genetic mapping, is often used in forensic investigations. A newer strategy for management of genetic disorders focuses on gene silencing by using RNAi to stop genes from making unwanted disease proteins.

REVIEW EXERCISES

1. The human genome project has revealed that humans have only 20,000 to 25,000 genes. Only about 2% of the genome encodes instructions for protein synthesis, whereas 50% consists of repeat sequences that do not code proteins.
   A. *Use this information to explain how this small number of protein-encoding genes is able to produce the vast array of proteins needed for organ and structural development in the embryo, as well as those needed for normal function of the body in postnatal life.*
2. A child about to undergo surgery is typed for possible blood transfusions. His parents are told that

he is type O positive. Both his mother and father are type A positive.

A. *How would you explain this variation in blood type to the parents?*

3. The post-translational folding of proteins is essential to their proper functioning and degradation.

A. *Hypothesize how age-related changes in the folding of proteins in the central nervous system could contribute to the development of the neurofibrillary tangles that are characteristic of Alzheimer disease.*

4. It is estimated that more than 10,000 people die of adverse drug reactions each year; another 200,000 experience serious reactions, whereas others fail to respond at all to the therapeutic actions of drugs.

A. *Explain how the use of information about single nucleotide polymorphisms (SNPs) might be used to map individual variations in drug responses.*

5. Human insulin, prepared by recombinant DNA technology, is now available for the treatment of diabetes mellitus.

A. *Explain the techniques used for the production of a human hormone with this technology.*

References

1. National Human Genome Research Institute. (2011). Fact sheets on science, research, ethics and the institute. Available online at: http://www.genome.gov/10000202. Accessed December 30, 2013.
2. Holmes F. L. (2001). *Meselson, Stahl, and the replication of DNA: A history of "the most beautiful experiment in biology."* New Haven, CT: Yale University Press.
3. Gahan P. B. (2011). *Circulating nucleic acids in plasma and serum.* New York: Springer.
4. Wie C. (2004). *Methods in enzymology: Chromatin and chromatin remodeling enzymes, Part A.* St Louis, MO: Elsevier.
5. Sund J., Ander M. Aqvist J. (2010). Principles of stop-codon reading on the ribosome. *Nature, 465,* 947–950.
6. Jogland S. N. (2009). *Gene biotechnology.* New Delhi, India: Himalaya Publishing House.
7. Chung D. C., Haber D. A. (2010). *Principles of clinical cancer genetics: A handbook from the Massachusetts General Hospital.* New York: Springer.
8. Ahmad S. (2010). *Diseases of DNA repair.* New York: Springer.
9. Hall J. E. (2011). *Guyton and Hall textbook of medical physiology.* (12th ed.). Philadelphia, PA: Saunders Elsevier.
10. Primrose S. B., Twyman R. (2003). *Principles of genome analysis and genomics* (3rd ed.). Malden, MA: Wiley-Blackwell.
11. Wyttenbach A., O'Connor V. (Eds.). (2011). *Folding for the synapse.* New York: Springer.
12. Stanton B. Z., Peng L. F. (2010). Small molecule modulators of the Sonic Hedgehog signaling pathway. *Molecular Biosynthesis, 6*(1), 44–54.
13. Skaletsky H., Kuroda-Kawaguchi T., Minx P. J., et al. (2003). The male-specific region of the human Y chromosome is a mosaic of discrete sequence classes. *Nature, 423*(6942), 825–837.
14. Rubin R., Strayer D. (Eds.). (2012). *Rubin's pathology: Clinicopathologic foundations of medicine* (6th ed.). Philadelphia, PA: Lippincott.
15. Gurrieri F., Accadia M. (2009). Genetic imprinting: The paradigm of Prader-Willi and Angelman syndromes. *Endocrine Development, 14,* 20–28.
16. National Center for Biotechnology Information. (2009). *Human genome and maps.* Available online at: www.ncbi.nlm.nih.gov/index.html. Accessed December 31, 2013.
17. NSW Government. (2013). *Genetic fact sheets.* Available online at: http://www.genetics.edu.au/Publications-and-Resources/Genetics-Fact-Sheets. Accessed December 31, 2013.
18. Nimkarn S., Lin-Su K., New M. I. (2011). Steroid 21 hydroxylase deficiency congenital adrenal hyperplasia. *Pediatric Clinics of North America, 58*(5), 1281–1300.
19. McElroy V. (2009). Hemochromatosis: A literature review. *Journal of Diagnostic Medical Sonography, 25*(6), 325–330.
20. Laino C. (2008). Genetic Fingerprinting is changing clinical practice. *Oncology Times, 30*(15), 5–6.
21. Gregoriadis G. (2006). *Liposome technology Volume 1: Liposome preparation & related techniques.* London: Informa Healthcare.
22. Petrocca F., Lieberman J. (2011). Promise and challenge of RNA interference-based therapy for cancer. *Journal of Clinical Oncology, 29*(6), 747–754.

Visit thePoint **http://thePoint.lww.com for animations, journal articles, and more!**

Genetic and Congenital Disorders

7

Congenital defects, a term used synonymously with *birth defects,* are abnormalities of a body structure, function, or metabolism that are present at birth. In Canada approximately 380,000 children are born each year, and of these babies 3% to 5% will be born with a serious congenital anomaly. These major congenital anomalies remain the second leading cause of infant death after immaturity.[1] Birth defects may be caused by genetic factors (*i.e.,* single-gene or multifactorial inheritance or chromosomal aberrations) or environmental factors that are active during embryonic or fetal development (*e.g.,* maternal disease, infections, or drugs taken during pregnancy). Although congenital defects are present at birth, genetic disorders may make their appearance later in life. This chapter provides an overview of genetic and congenital disorders and is divided into three parts: (1) genetic and chromosomal disorders, (2) disorders due to environmental agents, and (3) diagnosis and counselling.

GENETIC AND CHROMOSOMAL DISORDERS

After completing this section of the chapter, you should be able to meet the following objectives:

- Define the terms congenital, allele, gene locus, gene mutation, genotype, phenotype, homozygous, heterozygous, polymorphism, gene penetrance, and gene expression.
- Describe three types of single-gene disorders and their patterns of inheritance.
- Contrast disorders due to multifactorial inheritance with those caused by single-gene inheritance.
- Describe three patterns of chromosomal breakage and rearrangement.

A genetic disorder can be described as a discrete event that affects gene expression in a group of cells related to each other by gene linkage. Most genetic disorders are caused by changes in the deoxyribonucleic acid (DNA) sequence that alters the synthesis of a single gene product. However, some genetic disorders are caused by chromosomal rearrangements that result in deletion or duplication of a group of closely linked genes, or by an abnormal number of chromosomes resulting from mistakes that occur during meiosis or mitosis.[2]

The genes on each chromosome are arranged in pairs and in strict order, with each gene occupying a specific location or *locus.* The two members of a gene pair, one inherited from the mother and the other from the father, are called *alleles.* If the members of a gene pair are identical (*i.e.,* code the exact same gene product), the person is *homozygous,* and if the two members are different, the person is *heterozygous.* The genetic composition of a person is called a *genotype,* whereas the *phenotype* is the observable expression of a genotype in terms of morphologic, biochemical, or molecular traits. If the trait is expressed in the heterozygote (one member of the gene pair codes for the trait), it is said to be *dominant;* if it is expressed only in the homozygote (both members of the gene pair code for the trait), it is *recessive.*

Although gene expression usually follows a dominant or recessive pattern, it is possible for both alleles (members) of a gene pair to be fully expressed in the heterozygote, a condition called *codominance.* Many genes have only one normal version, which geneticists call the *wild-type* allele. Other genes have more than one normal allele (alternate forms) at the same locus. This is called *polymorphism.* Blood group inheritance (*e.g.,* AO, BO, AB) is an example of codominance and polymorphism (see Chapter 14).

A gene *mutation* is a biochemical event, such as nucleotide change, deletion, or insertion, that produces a new allele. A single mutant gene may be expressed in many different parts of the body. Marfan syndrome, for example, is a defect in a connective tissue protein that has widespread effects involving skeletal, ocular, and cardiovascular structures. In other single-gene disorders, the same defect can be caused by mutations at several different loci. Childhood deafness can result from at least 16 different types of autosomal recessive mutations.

Genetic disorders can involve a single-gene trait, multifactorial inheritance, a chromosomal abnormality, or a

mitochondrial gene disorder. The disorder may be inherited as a family trait or arise as a sporadic case due to a new mutation.

Single-Gene Disorders

Single-gene disorders are caused by a defective or mutant allele at a single gene locus and follow mendelian patterns of inheritance described in Chapter 6. Single-gene disorders are primarily disorders of the pediatric age group. Less than 10% manifest after puberty, and only 1% after the reproductive years.[3]

Single-gene disorders are characterized by their patterns of transmission, which usually are obtained through a family genetic history. The patterns of inheritance depend on whether the phenotype is dominant or recessive and whether the gene is located on an autosomal or sex chromosome. In addition to disorders caused by mutations of genes located on the chromosomes located with the nucleus, another class of disorders with a maternal pattern of inheritance involves the mitochondrial genome.

Virtually all single-gene disorders lead to formation of an abnormal protein or decreased production of a gene product. The disorder can result in a defective enzyme or decreased amounts of an enzyme, defects in receptor proteins and their function, alterations in nonenzyme proteins, or mutations resulting in unusual reactions to drugs. Table 7.1 lists some of the common single-gene disorders and their manifestations.

Autosomal Dominant Disorders

In autosomal dominant disorders, a single mutant allele from an affected parent is transmitted to an offspring regardless of sex. The affected parent has a 50% chance of transmitting the disorder to each offspring (Fig. 7.1). The unaffected relatives of the parent or unaffected siblings of the offspring do not transmit the disorder. In many conditions, the age of onset is delayed, and the signs and symptoms of the disorder do not appear until later in life, as in Huntington chorea (see Chapter 53).

Autosomal dominant disorders also may manifest as a new mutation. Whether the mutation is passed on to the next generation depends on the affected person's reproductive

GENETIC AND CHROMOSOMAL DISORDERS

- Genetic disorders are inherited as autosomal dominant disorders, in which each child has a 50% chance of inheriting the disorder, or as autosomal recessive disorders, in which each child has a 25% chance of being affected, a 50% chance of being a carrier, and a 25% chance of being unaffected.
- Sex-linked disorders almost always are associated with the X chromosome and are predominantly recessive.
- Chromosomal disorders reflect events that occur at the time of meiosis and result from defective movement of an entire chromosome or from breakage of a chromosome with loss or translocation of genetic material.

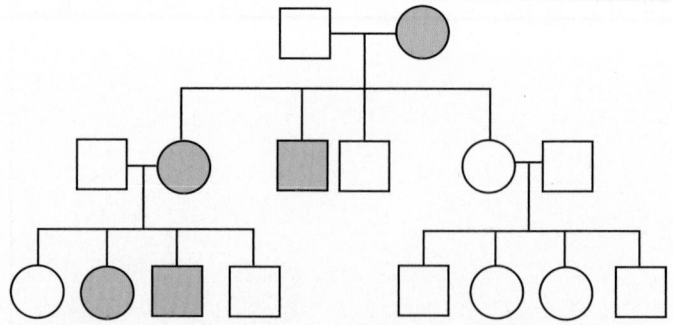

FIGURE 7.1 • Simple pedigree for inheritance of an autosomal dominant trait. The coloured circle or square represents an affected parent with a mutant gene. An affected parent with an autosomal dominant trait has a 50% chance of passing the mutant gene on to each child regardless of sex.

TABLE 7.1 SOME DISORDERS OF MENDELIAN OR SINGLE-GENE INHERITANCE AND THEIR SIGNIFICANCE

DISORDER	SIGNIFICANCE
Autosomal Dominant	
Achondroplasia	Short-limb dwarfism
Adult polycystic kidney disease	Chronic kidney disease
Huntington chorea	Neurodegenerative disorder
Familial hypercholesterolemia	Premature atherosclerosis
Marfan syndrome	Connective tissue disorder with abnormalities in the skeletal, ocular, and cardiovascular systems
Neurofibromatosis (NF)	Neurogenic tumours: fibromatous skin tumours, pigmented skin lesions, and ocular nodules in NF-1; bilateral acoustic neuromas in NF-2
Osteogenesis imperfecta	Brittle bone disease due to defects in collagen synthesis
Spherocytosis	Disorder of red blood cells
von Willebrand disease	Bleeding disorder
Autosomal Recessive	
Cystic fibrosis	Disorder of membrane transport of chloride ions in exocrine glands causing lung and pancreatic disease
Glycogen storage diseases	Excess accumulation of glycogen in the liver and hypoglycemia (von Gierke disease); glycogen accumulation in striated muscle in myopathic forms
Oculocutaneous albinism	Hypopigmentation of skin, hair, eyes as a result of inability to synthesize melanin
Phenylketonuria (PKU)	Lack of phenylalanine hydroxylase with hyperphenylalaninemia and impaired brain development
Sickle cell disease	Red blood cell defect
Tay–Sachs disease	Deficiency of hexosaminidase A; severe mental and physical deterioration beginning in infancy
X-Linked Recessive	
Bruton-type hypogammaglobulinemia	Immunodeficiency
Hemophilia A	Bleeding disorder
Duchenne dystrophy	Muscular dystrophy
Fragile X syndrome	Intellectual disability

capacity. Many new autosomal dominant mutations are accompanied by reduced reproductive capacity; therefore, the defect is not perpetuated in future generations. If an autosomal defect is accompanied by a total inability to reproduce, essentially all new cases of the disorder will be due to new mutations. If the defect does not affect reproductive capacity, it is more likely to be inherited.

Although there is a 50% chance of inheriting a dominant genetic disorder from an affected parent, there can be wide variation in gene penetration and expression. When a person inherits a dominant mutant gene but fails to express it, the trait is described as having *reduced penetrance*. Penetrance is expressed in mathematical terms: a 50% penetrance indicates that a person who inherits the defective gene has a 50% chance of expressing the disorder. The person who has a mutant gene but does not express it is an important exception to the rule that unaffected persons do not transmit an autosomal dominant trait. These persons can transmit the gene to their descendants and so produce a skipped generation. Autosomal dominant disorders also can display *variable expressivity*, meaning that they can be expressed differently among individuals. Polydactyly

or supernumerary digits, for example, may be expressed in either the fingers or the toes.

The gene products of autosomal dominant disorders usually are regulatory proteins involved in rate-limiting components of complex metabolic pathways or key components of structural proteins such as collagen.[4,5] Two disorders of autosomal inheritance, Marfan syndrome and neurofibromatosis (NF), are described in this chapter.

Marfan Syndrome. Marfan syndrome is an autosomal dominant disorder of the connective tissue, which gives shape and structure to other tissues in the body and holds them in place. The basic biochemical abnormality in Marfan syndrome affects *fibrillin I,* a major component of microfibrils found in the extracellular matrix.[5] These microfibrils form the scaffolding for the deposition of elastin and are considered integral components of elastic fibres. Fibrillin I is coded by the *FBN1* gene, which maps to chromosome 15q21.1. Over 100 mutations in the *FBN1* gene have been found, making genetic diagnosis unfeasible. The prevalence of Marfan syndrome is estimated to be 1 per 5,000. Approximately 70% to 85% of cases are familial and the remainder are sporadic, arising from new mutations in the germ cells of the parents.[5]

Marfan syndrome affects several organ systems, including the ocular system (eyes), the cardiovascular system (heart and blood vessels), and the skeletal system (bones, ligaments, and joints).[5–8] There is a wide range of variation in the expression of the disorder. Persons may have abnormalities of one or all three systems. The skeletal deformities, which are the most obvious features of the disorder, include a long, thin body with exceptionally long extremities and long, tapering fingers, sometimes called *arachnodactyly* or *spider fingers;* hyperextensible joints; and a variety of spinal deformities, including kyphosis and scoliosis (Fig. 7.2). Chest deformities, pectus excavatum (*i.e.,* deeply depressed sternum), or pigeon chest deformity, often are present and may require surgery. The most common eye disorder is bilateral dislocation of the lens due to weakness of the suspensory ligaments. Myopia and predisposition to retinal detachment also are common, the result of increased optic globe length due to altered connective tissue support of ocular structures. However, the most life-threatening aspects of the disorder are the cardiovascular defects, which include mitral valve prolapse, progressive dilation of the aortic valve ring, and weakness of the aorta and other arteries.[5] Dissection and rupture of the aorta may lead to premature death. In women, the risk of aortic dissection is increased in pregnancy.

The diagnosis of Marfan syndrome is based on major and minor diagnostic criteria that include skeletal, cardiovascular, and ocular deformities. There is no cure for Marfan syndrome; treatment plans include echocardiograms and electrocardiograms to assess the status of the cardiovascular system, periodic eye examinations, and evaluation of the skeletal system, especially in children and adolescents. The risks associated with participation in sports depend on which organ systems are involved.

Neurofibromatosis. Neurofibromatosis is a condition involving tumours that arise from Schwann cells and other elements of the peripheral nervous system.[4,5,9,10] There are at least two genetically and clinically distinct forms of the disorder: type 1 NF (NF-1), also known as *von Recklinghausen disease,* and type 2 bilateral acoustic NF (NF-2). Both of these disorders result from a genetic defect in a tumour suppressor gene that regulates cell differentiation and growth. The gene for NF-1 has been mapped to chromosome 17q11.2, and the gene for NF-2 to chromosome 22q12.

Type 1 NF is a relatively common disorder, with a frequency of 1 in 3,500.[4] In more than 90% of persons with NF-1, cutaneous and subcutaneous neurofibromas develop in late childhood or adolescence. The cutaneous neurofibromas, which vary in number from a few to many hundreds, manifest as soft, pedunculated lesions that project from the skin. They are the most common type of lesion, often are not apparent until puberty, and are present in greatest density over the trunk (Fig. 7.3). The subcutaneous lesions grow just below the skin; they are firm and round, and may be painful. Plexiform neurofibromas involve the larger peripheral nerves. They tend to form large tumours that cause severe disfigurement of the face, overgrowth of an extremity, or skeletal deformities such as scoliosis. Pigmented nodules of the iris (Lisch nodules), which are specific for NF-1, usually are present after 6 years of age. They do not present any clinical problem but are useful in establishing a diagnosis.[4,5]

A second major component of NF-1 is the presence of large (usually ≥15 mm in diameter), flat cutaneous pigmentations, known as *café au lait spots.* They are usually a uniform light brown in whites and darker brown in persons of colour, with sharply demarcated edges. Although small single lesions may be found in normal children, larger lesions or six or more spots larger than 1.5 cm in diameter suggest NF-1. The skin pigmentations become more evident with age as the melanosomes in the epidermal cells accumulate melanin.[4]

Children with NF-1 are also susceptible to neurologic complications. There is an increased incidence of learning disabilities, attention deficit disorders, and abnormalities of

EYE
Lens dislocation, myopia

SKELETAL DEFORMITY
Pectus carinatum (pigeon chest), pectus excavatum (funnel chest)

Vertebral deformity (kyphosis, scoliosis)

Long arms, arm span exceeds height

CARDIOVASCULAR
Aortic aneurysm, floppy valves

Dissecting aortic aneurysm with exsanguination

Joint hypermobility, especially fingers, wrists, and knees

FIGURE 7.2 • Clinical features of Marfan syndrome.

FIGURE 7.3 • Neurofibromatosis type 1. Multiple cutaneous neurofi-bromas are noted on the face and trunk. (From Rubin R., Strayer D. S. (Eds.). (2012). *Rubin's pathology: Clinicopathologic foundations of medicine* (6th ed., p. 238). Philadelphia, PA: Lippincott Williams & Wilkins.)

speech among affected children. Complex partial and general-ized tonic-clonic seizures are a frequent complication. Malig-nant neoplasms are also a significant problem in persons with NF-1. One of the major complications of NF-1, occurring in 3% to 5% of persons, is the appearance of a neurofibrosar-coma in a neurofibroma, usually a larger plexiform neurofi-broma.[4] NF-1 is also associated with increased incidence of other neurogenic tumours, including meningiomas, optic glio-mas, and pheochromocytomas.

Type 2 NF is characterized by tumours of the acoustic nerve. Most often, the disorder is asymptomatic through the first 15 years of life. This type of NF occurs less frequently at a rate of 1 in 50,000 people.[4] The most frequent symptoms are headaches, hearing loss, and tinnitus (*i.e.,* ringing in the ears). There may be associated intracranial and spinal menin-giomas. The condition is often made worse by pregnancy, and oral contraceptives may increase the growth and symptoms of tumours.[4] Persons with the disorder should be warned that severe disorientation may occur during diving or swimming underwater, and drowning may result. Surgery may be indi-cated for debulking or removal of the tumours.

Autosomal Recessive Disorders

Autosomal recessive disorders are manifested only when both members of the gene pair are affected. In this case, both parents may be unaffected but are carriers of the defective gene. Auto-somal recessive disorders affect both sexes. The occurrence

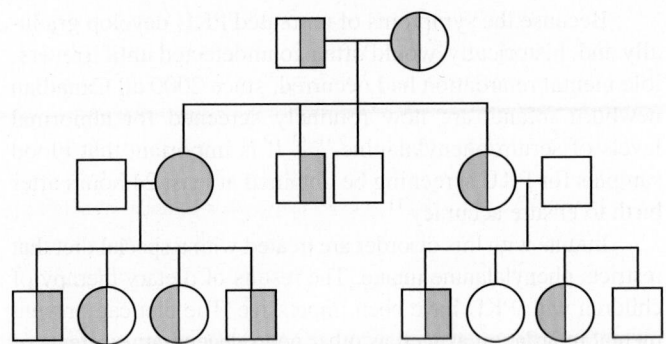

FIGURE 7.4 • Simple pedigree for inheritance of an autosomal recessive trait. The half-coloured circle and square represent carriers of a mutant gene. When both parents are carriers of a mutant gene, there is a 25% chance of having an affected child (full-coloured circle or square), a 50% chance of a carrier child, and a 25% chance of a nonaffected or noncarrier child, regardless of sex. All children (100%) of an affected parent are carriers.

risks in each pregnancy are one in four for an affected child, two in four for a carrier child, and one in four for a normal (noncarrier, unaffected), homozygous child (Fig. 7.4). *Con-sanguineous mating* (mating of two related individuals), or inbreeding, increases the chance that two people who mate will be carriers of an autosomal recessive disorder.[3]

With autosomal recessive disorders, the age of onset is frequently early in life; the symptomatology tends to be more uniform than with autosomal dominant disorders; and the dis-orders are characteristically caused by loss-of-function muta-tions, many of which impair or eliminate the function of an enzyme. In the case of a heterozygous carrier, the presence of a mutant gene usually does not produce symptoms because equal amounts of normal and defective enzymes are synthe-sized. This "margin of safety" ensures that cells with half their usual amount of enzyme function normally. By contrast, the inactivation of both alleles in a homozygote results in com-plete loss of enzyme activity. Autosomal recessive disorders include almost all inborn errors of metabolism. Enzyme dis-orders that impair catabolic pathways result in an accumula-tion of dietary substances (*e.g.,* phenylketonuria [PKU]) or cellular constituents (*e.g.,* lysosomal storage diseases). Other disorders result from a defect in the synthesis of an essential protein (*e.g.,* the cystic fibrosis transmembrane conductance regulator in cystic fibrosis; see Chapter 29). Two examples of autosomal recessive disorders that are not covered elsewhere in this book are PKU and Tay–Sachs disease.

Phenylketonuria. PKU is a rare autosomal recessive meta-bolic disorder that affects approximately 1 in every 12,000 to 15,000 infants in North America. The disorder is caused by a deficiency of the liver enzyme phenylalanine hydroxylase. As a result of this deficiency, toxic levels of the amino acid phenylalanine accumulate in the blood and other tissues.[11] If untreated, the disorder results in mental retardation, micro-cephaly, delayed speech, and other signs of impaired neuro-logic development.

Because the symptoms of untreated PKU develop gradually and, historically, would often go undetected until irreversible mental retardation had occurred, since 2000 all Canadian newborn infants are now routinely screened for abnormal levels of serum phenylalanine.[11-13] It is important that blood samples for PKU screening be obtained at least 24 hours after birth to ensure accuracy.[11]

Infants with this disorder are treated with a special diet that restricts phenylalanine intake. The results of dietary therapy of children with PKU have been impressive. The diet can prevent mental retardation as well as other neurodegenerative effects of untreated PKU. However, dietary treatment must be started early in neonatal life to prevent brain damage. Infants with elevated phenylalanine levels (>600 μmol/L) should begin treatment by 7 to 10 days of age, indicating the need for early diagnosis. Evidence suggests that high levels of phenylalanine even during the first 2 weeks of life can affect the structural development of the visual system, although visual deficits are usually mild.[12]

It is recommended that dietary control of phenylalanine levels be maintained throughout the lifetime of a person with PKU. Infants with PKU should have phenylalanine levels measured weekly during the first year of life; twice monthly from 1 to 12 years of age; and monthly after 12 years of age.[4] Women with PKU who wish to have children require careful attention to their diet, both before conception and during pregnancy, as a means of controlling both theirs and the unborn child's exposure to high phenylalanine levels.[4]

Tay–Sachs Disease. Tay–Sachs disease is a variant of a class of lysosomal storage diseases, known as the *gangliosidoses,* in which there is failure to break down the GM2 gangliosides of cell membranes. Tay–Sachs disease is inherited as an autosomal recessive trait and is predominantly a disorder of Eastern European (Ashkenazi) Jews, in which a carrier rate of 1 in 30 has been reported.[4,5]

The GM2 ganglioside accumulates in the lysosomes of all organs in Tay–Sachs disease, but is most prominent in the brain neurons and retina.[4,5] Microscopic examination reveals neurons ballooned with cytoplasmic vacuoles, each of which constitutes a markedly distended lysosome filled with gangliosides. In time, there is progressive destruction of neurons within the brain substance, including the cerebellum, basal ganglia, brain stem, spinal cord, and autonomic nervous system. Involvement of the retina is detected by ophthalmoscopy as a cherry-red spot on the macula.[4,5]

Infants with Tay–Sachs disease appear normal at birth but begin to manifest progressive weakness, muscle flaccidity, and decreased attentiveness at approximately 6 to 10 months of age. This is followed by rapid deterioration of motor and mental function, often with development of generalized seizures. Retinal involvement leads to visual impairment and eventual blindness. Death usually occurs before 4 to 5 years of age. Although there is no cure for the disease, analysis of the blood serum for the lysosomal enzyme, hexosaminidase A, which is deficient in Tay–Sachs disease, allows for accurate identification of genetic carriers for the disease.

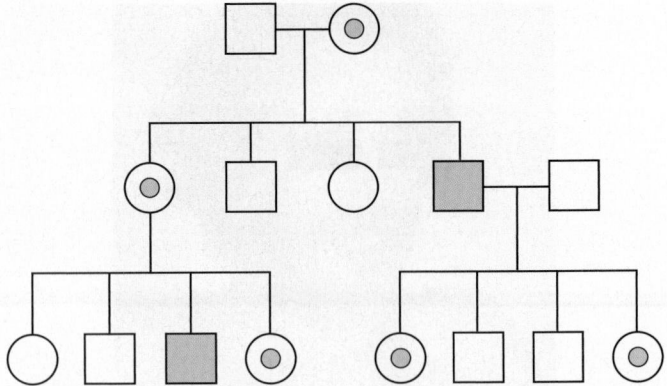

FIGURE 7.5 • Simple pedigree for inheritance of an X-linked recessive trait. X-linked recessive traits are expressed phenotypically in the male offspring. A small coloured circle represents the X chromosome with the defective gene in female carriers, and the larger coloured square the affected male. The affected male passes the mutant gene to all of his daughters, who become carriers of the trait and have a 50% chance of passing the gene; her daughters have a 50% chance of being carriers of the gene (sons cannot be carriers) and her sons have a 50% chance of being affected.

X-Linked Disorders

Sex-linked disorders are almost always associated with the X, or female, chromosome, and the inheritance pattern is predominantly recessive. Because of the presence of a normal X paired gene (XX) female heterozygotes rarely experience the effects of a defective gene, whereas all males who receive the gene (XY) typically affected. The common pattern of inheritance is one in which an unaffected mother carries one normal and one mutant allele on the X chromosome. This means that she has a 50% chance of transmitting the defective gene to her sons, and her daughters have a 50% chance of being carriers of the mutant gene (Fig. 7.5). When the affected son procreates, he transmits the defective gene to all of his daughters, who become carriers of the mutant gene. Because the genes of the Y chromosome are unaffected, the affected male does not transmit the defect to any of his sons, and they will not be carriers or transmit the disorder to their children. X-linked recessive disorders include glucose-6-phosphate dehydrogenase deficiency (see Chapter 14), hemophilia A (see Chapter 13), and X-linked agammaglobulinemia (see Chapter 19).

Fragile X Syndrome

Fragile X syndrome is a single-gene disorder in which the mutation is characterized by a long repeating sequence of three nucleotides within the fragile X gene. The disorder, which affects approximately 1 in 1,250 males and 1 in 2,500 females, is the most common form of inherited mental retardation. It is second only to Down syndrome as an identifiable cause of mental retardation.[4]

As with other X-linked disorders, fragile X syndrome affects boys more often than girls. Affected boys are intellectually disabled and share a common physical phenotype that includes a long face with large mandible and large, everted ears. Hyperextensible joints, a high-arched palate, and mitral valve prolapse, which are observed in some cases, mimic a connective tissue disorder. Some physical abnormalities may be subtle or absent. The most distinctive feature, which is present in 90% of prepubertal boys, is macroorchidism or large testes.[5] Because girls have two X chromosomes, they are more likely to have relatively normal cognitive development, or they may show a learning disability in a particular area, such as mathematics. Women with the disorder may also experience premature ovarian failure or begin menopause earlier than women who are not affected by fragile X syndrome.[5,14]

The fragile X gene has been mapped to a small area on the long arm of the X chromosome—Xq27, now designated the *FMR1* (fragile X mental retardation 1) site.[4,5] The gene product, the fragile X mental retardation protein (FMRP), is a widely expressed cytoplasmic protein. It is most abundant in the brain and testis, the organs most affected by the disorder. As discussed in Chapter 6, each gene contains an introduction or promoter region and an instruction region that carries the directions for protein synthesis. The promoter region of the *FMR1* gene contains repeats of a specific CGG (cytosine, guanine, guanine) triplet code that, when normal, controls gene activity. The mechanism by which the normal *FMR1* gene is converted to an altered, or mutant, gene capable of producing disease symptoms involves an increase in the number of CGG repeats in the promoter region of the gene. Once the repeat exceeds a threshold length, no FMRP is produced, resulting in the fragile X phenotype. People without fragile X syndrome have between 6 and 40 repeats. A gene with 55 to 200 repeats is generally considered a permutation, and one with more than 200 repeats, a full mutation.[5,14]

The inheritance of the *FMR1* gene follows the pattern of X-linked traits, with the father passing the gene on to all his daughters but not his sons. Approximately 20% of males who have been shown to carry the fragile X mutation are clinically and cytogenetically normal. Because these male carriers transmit the trait through all their daughters (who are phenotypically normal) to affected grandchildren, they are called *transmitting males.*

Diagnosis of fragile X syndrome is based on mental and physical characteristics. DNA molecular tests can be done to confirm the presence of an abnormal *FMR1* gene. Because the manifestations of fragile X syndrome may resemble those of other learning disorders, it is recommended that persons with mental retardation of unknown cause, developmental delay, learning disabilities, autism, or autism-like behaviours be evaluated for the disorder.[15]

Multifactorial Inheritance Disorders

Multifactorial inheritance disorders are caused by multiple genes and, in many cases, environmental factors.[4] The exact number of genes contributing to multifactorial traits is not known, and these traits do not follow the same clear-cut pattern of inheritance as do single-gene disorders. Disorders of multifactorial inheritance can be expressed during fetal life and be present at birth, or they may be expressed later in life.

Congenital disorders that are thought to arise through multifactorial inheritance include cleft lip or palate, clubfoot, congenital dislocation of the hip, congenital heart disease, pyloric stenosis, and urinary tract malformation. Environmental factors are thought to play a greater role in disorders of multifactorial inheritance that develop in adult life, such as coronary artery disease, diabetes mellitus, hypertension, and cancer.

Although multifactorial traits cannot be predicted with the same degree of accuracy as mendelian single-gene mutations, characteristic patterns exist. First, multifactorial congenital malformations tend to involve a single organ or tissue derived from the same embryonic developmental field. Second, the risk of recurrence in future pregnancies is for the same or a similar defect. This means that parents of a child with a cleft palate defect have an increased risk of having another child with a cleft palate, but not with spina bifida. Third, the increased risk (compared with the general population) among first-degree relatives of the affected person is 2% to 7%, and among second-degree relatives, it is approximately one half that amount.[4] The risk increases with increasing incidence of the defect among relatives. This means that the risk is greatly increased when a second child with the defect is born to a couple. The risk also increases with severity of the disorder and when the defect occurs in the sex not usually affected by the disorder.

Cleft Lip and Cleft Palate

Cleft lip with or without cleft palate is one of the most common birth defects, occurring in about 0.1% of all pregnancies.[4] It is also one of the more conspicuous birth defects, resulting in an abnormal facial appearance and defective speech. Cleft lip with or without cleft palate is more frequent among boys, whereas isolated cleft palate is twice as common among girls.

Developmentally, the defect has its origin at about the 35th day of gestation when the frontal prominences of the craniofacial structures fuse with the maxillary process to form the upper lip.[4] This process is under the control of many genes, and disturbances in gene expression (hereditary or environmental) at this time may result in cleft lip with or without cleft palate (Fig. 7.6). The defect may also be caused by teratogens (*e.g.,* rubella, anticonvulsant drugs) and is often encountered in children with chromosomal abnormalities.

Cleft lip and palate defects may vary from a small notch in the vermilion border of the upper lip to complete separation involving the palate and extending into the floor of the nose. The clefts may be unilateral or bilateral and may involve the alveolar ridge. The condition may be accompanied by deformed, supernumerary, or absent teeth. Isolated cleft palate occurs in the midline and may involve only the uvula or may extend into or through the soft and hard palates.

A child with cleft lip or palate may require years of special treatment by medical and dental specialists, including a plastic surgeon, pediatric dentist, orthodontist, speech therapist, and nurse specialist. The immediate problem in an infant with cleft palate is feeding. Nursing at the breast or nipple depends on suction developed by pressing the nipple against the hard palate with the tongue. Although infants with cleft lip

Unilateral   Bilateral

FIGURE 7.6 • Cleft lip and cleft palate.

usually have no problems with feeding, those with cleft palate usually require specially constructed, soft artificial nipples with large openings and a squeezable bottle.

Major advances in the care of children born with cleft lip and palate have occurred within the last quarter of the 20th century.[16] Surgical closure of the lip is usually performed by 3 months of age, with closure of the palate usually done before 1 year of age. Depending on the extent of the defect, additional surgery may be required as the child grows. Displacement of the maxillary arches and malposition of the teeth usually require orthodontic correction.[17]

Cleft lip and palate can also cause speech defects. The muscles of the soft palate and the lateral and posterior walls of the nasopharynx constitute a valve that separates the nasopharynx from the oropharynx during swallowing and in the production of certain sounds. If the valve does not function properly, it is difficult to build up sufficient pressure in the mouth to make explosive sounds such as *p, b, d, t, h,* and *y,* or the sibilants *s, sh,* and *ch.*[17] Although speech therapy is usually needed, early and more effective surgical procedures help to reduce the extent of the problem.

Chromosomal Disorders

Chromosomal disorders form a major category of genetic disease, accounting for a large proportion of reproductive wastage (early gestational abortions), congenital malformations, and mental retardation. Specific chromosomal abnormalities can be linked to more than 60 identifiable syndromes that are present in 0.7% of all live births, 2% of all pregnancies in women older than 35 years of age, and 50% of all first-term abortions.[4]

Prior to cell division (*i.e.,* mitosis) in nongerm cells, the chromosomes replicate so that each cell receives a full diploid number. In germ cells, a different form of division (*i.e.,*

meiosis) takes place (see Chapter 6). During meiosis, the double sets of 22 autosomes and the 2 sex chromosomes (normal diploid number) are reduced to single sets (haploid number) in each gamete. At the time of conception, the haploid number in the ovum and that in the sperm join and restore the diploid number of chromosomes.

Chromosomal abnormalities are commonly described according to the shorthand description of the karyotype. In this system, the total number of chromosomes is given first, followed by the sex chromosome complement, and then the description of any abnormality. For example, a male with trisomy 21 is designated 47,XY,+21.

The aberrations underlying chromosomal disorders may take the form of alterations in the structure of one or more chromosomes, or an abnormal number of chromosomes. Occasionally, mitotic errors in early development give rise to two or more cell lines characterized by distinctive karyotypes, a condition referred to as *mosaicism.* Mosaicism can result from mitotic errors during cleavage of the fertilized ovum or in somatic cells. Sometimes, mosaicism consists of an abnormal karyotype and a normal one, in which case the physical deformities caused by the abnormal cell line usually are less severe.

Structural Chromosomal Abnormalities

Structural changes in chromosomes usually result from breakage in one or more of the chromosomes followed by rearrangement or deletion of the chromosome parts. Among the factors believed to cause chromosome breakage are exposure to radiation sources, such as x-rays; influence of certain chemicals; extreme changes in the cellular environment; and viral infections.

Several patterns of chromosome breakage and rearrangement can occur (Fig. 7.7). There can be a *deletion* of the broken portion of the chromosome. When one chromosome is involved, the broken parts may be *inverted. Isochromosome formation* occurs when the centromere, or central portion, of the chromosome separates horizontally instead of vertically. *Ring formation* results when deletion is followed by uniting of the chromatids to form a ring. *Translocation* occurs when there are simultaneous breaks in two chromosomes from different pairs, with exchange of chromosome parts. With a balanced reciprocal translocation, no genetic information is lost; therefore, persons with translocations usually are normal. However, these persons are translocation carriers and may have normal or abnormal children.

A special form of translocation called a *centric fusion* or *robertsonian translocation* involves two acrocentric chromosomes in which the centromere is near the end, most commonly chromosomes 13 and 14 or 14 and 21. Typically, the break occurs near the centromere affecting the short arm in one chromosome and the long arm in the other. Transfer of the chromosome fragments leads to one long and one extremely short fragment. The short fragment is usually lost during subsequent divisions. In this case, the person has only 45 chromosomes, but the amount of genetic material that is lost is so small that it often goes unnoticed. Difficulty, however, arises

FIGURE 7.7 • Structural abnormalities in the human chromosome. (**A**) Deletion of part of a chromosome leads to loss of genetic material and shortening of the chromosome. (**B**) A reciprocal translocation involves two nonhomologous chromosomes, with exchange of the acentric segment. (**C**) Inversion requires two breaks in a single chromosome, with inversion to the opposite side of the centromere (pericentric) or with the fragment inverting but remaining on the same arm (paracentric). (**D**) In robertsonian translocation, two nonhomologous acrocentric chromosomes break near their centromeres, after which the long arms fuse to form one large metacentric chromosome. (**E**) Isochromosomes arise from faulty centromere division, which leads to duplication of the long arm and deletion of the short arm, or the reverse. (**F**) A ring chromosome forms with breaks in both telomeric portions of a chromosome, deletion of the acentric fragments, and fusion of the remaining centric portion. (From Rubin R., Strayer D. S. (Eds.). (2012). *Rubin's pathology: Clinicopathologic foundations of medicine* (6th ed., p. 223). Philadelphia, PA: Lippincott Williams & Wilkins.)

during meiosis; the result is gametes with an unbalanced number of chromosomes. The chief clinical importance of this type of translocation is that carriers of a robertsonian translocation involving chromosome 21 are at risk for producing a child with Down syndrome (to be discussed).

The manifestations of aberrations in chromosome structure depend to a great extent on the amount of genetic material that is lost or displaced. Many cells sustaining unrestored breaks are eliminated within the next few mitoses because of deficiencies that may in themselves be fatal. This is beneficial because it prevents the damaged cells from becoming a permanent part of the organism or, if it occurs in the gametes, from giving rise to grossly defective zygotes. Some altered chromosomes, such as those that occur with translocations, are passed on to the next generation.

Numeric Disorders Involving Autosomes

Having an abnormal number of chromosomes is referred to as *aneuploidy.* Among the causes of aneuploidy is a failure of the chromosomes to separate during oogenesis or spermatogenesis. This can occur in either the autosomes or the sex chromosomes and is called *nondisjunction* (Fig. 7.8). Nondisjunction gives rise to germ cells that have an even number of chromosomes (22 or 24). The products of conception formed from this even number of chromosomes have an uneven number of chromosomes, 45 or 47. *Monosomy* refers to the presence of only one member of a chromosome pair. The defects associated with monosomy of the autosomes are severe and usually cause abortion. Monosomy of the X chromosome (45,X), or Turner syndrome, causes less severe defects.

Polysomy, or the presence of more than two chromosomes to a set, occurs when a germ cell containing more than 23 chromosomes is involved in conception. A variety of trisomies involving autosomal chromosomes 8, 9, 12, 13, 18, and 22 have been described.[4,5] Trisomy 18 (Edwards syndrome) and trisomy 13 (Patau syndrome) share several karyotypic and clinical features with trisomy 21 (Down syndrome). In contrast to Down syndrome, however, the malformations are much more severe and wide-ranging. As a result, these infants rarely survive beyond the first years of life.[5]

Down Syndrome. First described in 1866 by John Langdon Down, trisomy 21, or Down syndrome, causes a combination of birth defects including some degree of intellectual disability, characteristic facial features, and other health problems.[4,5] It is the most common chromosomal disorder causing congenital anomalies worldwide and it occurs approximately one in every 800 births.[1]

Approximately 95% of cases of Down syndrome are caused by nondisjunction or an error in cell division during meiosis, resulting in a trisomy of chromosome 21. A rare form of Down syndrome can occur in the offspring of persons in whom there has been a robertsonian translocation (Fig. 7.7) involving the long arm of chromosome 21q and the long arm of one of the acrocentric chromosomes (most often 14 or 22). The translocation adds to the normal long arm of chromosome

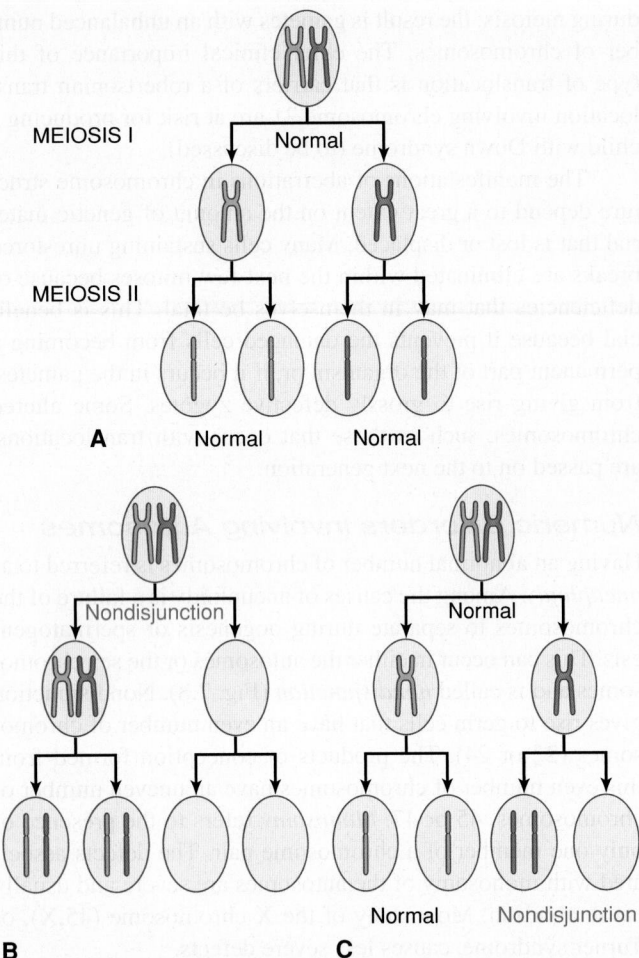

A Normal Normal

B Normal Nondisjunction

C Normal Nondisjunction

FIGURE 7.8 • Nondisjunction as a cause of disorders of chromosomal numbers. **A:** Normal distribution of chromosomes during meiosis I and II. **B:** If nondisjunction occurs at meiosis I, the gametes contain either a pair of chromosomes or a lack of chromosomes. **C:** If nondisjunction occurs at meiosis II, the affected gametes contain two of copies of one parenteral chromosome or a lack of chromosomes.

21; therefore, the person with this type of Down syndrome has 46 chromosomes, but essentially a trisomy of 21q.[4,5]

The risk of having a child with Down syndrome increases with maternal age—it is 1 in 1,250 at 25 years of age, 1 in 400 at 35 years, and 1 in 100 at 45 years of age.[18] The reason for the correlation between maternal age and nondisjunction is unknown, but is thought to reflect some aspect of aging of the oocyte. Although men continue to produce sperm throughout their reproductive lives, women are born with all the oocytes they ever will have. These oocytes may change as a result of the aging process. With increasing age, there is a greater chance of a woman having been exposed to damaging environmental agents such as drugs, chemicals, and radiation. Unlike trisomy 21, Down syndrome due to a chromosome (21;14) translocation shows no relation to maternal age but has a relatively high recurrence risk in families when a parent, particularly the mother, is a carrier.

The physical features of a child with Down syndrome are distinctive, and therefore the condition usually is apparent at birth.[4,5,19] These features include growth failure and a small and rather square head. There is a flat facial profile, with a small nose and somewhat depressed nasal bridge; small folds on the inner corners of the eyes (epicanthal folds) and upward slanting of the eyes; small, low-set, and malformed ears; a fat pad at the back of the neck; an open mouth; and a large, protruding tongue (Fig. 7.9). The child's hands usually are short and stubby, with fingers that curl inward, and there usually is only a single palmar (*i.e.,* simian) crease. There is excessive space between the large and second toes. Hypotonia and joint laxity also are present in infants and young children. There often are accompanying congenital heart defects and an increased risk of gastrointestinal malformations. Approximately 1% of persons with trisomy 21 Down syndrome have mosaicism (*i.e.,* cell populations with the normal chromosome number and trisomy 21); these persons may be less severely affected. There is a high correlation of the development of acute leukemia, both myeloid and lymphoblastic, among children with Down syndrome.[20] In addition, many of these children have a higher chance of acquiring cardiovascular disease plus there is an increased risk of Alzheimer disease among older people with Down syndrome.

There are several prenatal screening tests that can be done to determine the risk of having a child with Down

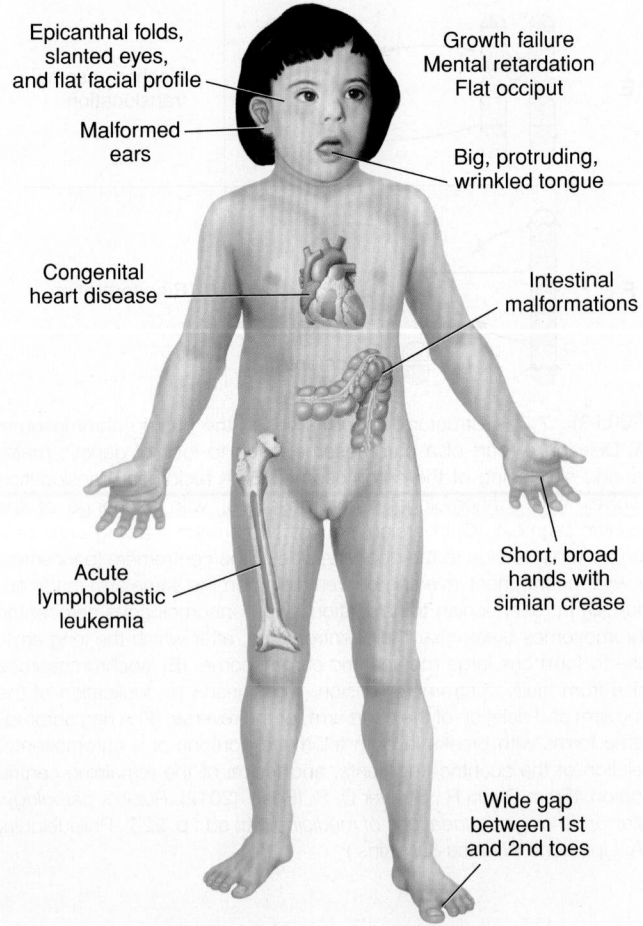

Epicanthal folds, slanted eyes, and flat facial profile

Growth failure
Mental retardation
Flat occiput

Malformed ears

Big, protruding, wrinkled tongue

Congenital heart disease

Intestinal malformations

Acute lymphoblastic leukemia

Short, broad hands with simian crease

Wide gap between 1st and 2nd toes

FIGURE 7.9 • Clinical features of a child with Down syndrome.

syndrome.[4,5,21] The most commonly used are blood tests that measure maternal serum levels of α-fetoprotein, human chorionic gonadotropin (hCG), unconjugated estriol, inhibin A, and pregnancy-associated plasma protein A (PAPP-A; see section on Diagnosis and Counselling). The results of three or four of these tests, together with the woman's age, often are used to determine the probability of a pregnant woman having a child with Down syndrome. Also correlated with the blood tests, fetal nuchal translucency (sonolucent space on the back of the fetal neck), is measured using ultrasonography and can be performed between 10 and 13 weeks' gestation. The fetus with Down syndrome tends to have a greater area of translucency compared with a chromosomally normal infant. The nuchal transparency test is usually used in combination with other screening tests. The only current way to accurately determine the presence of Down syndrome in the fetus is through chromosome analysis using invasive chorionic villus sampling, amniocentesis, or percutaneous umbilical blood sampling, but newer screening methods extracting cell-free fetal DNA (cffDNA) which is found circulating in maternal blood is showing promising results.[22]

Numeric Disorders Involving Sex Chromosomes

Chromosomal disorders associated with the sex chromosomes are much more common than those related to the autosomes, save for trisomy 21. Furthermore, imbalances (excess or deletions) are much better tolerated than those involving the autosomes. This is related in large part to two factors that are peculiar to the sex chromosomes: (1) the inactivation of all but one X chromosome, and (2) the modest amount of genetic material that is carried on the Y chromosome.

Although girls normally receive both a paternal and a maternal X chromosome, the clinical manifestations of X chromosome abnormalities can be quite variable because of the process of X inactivation (see discussion of the Lyon principle in Chapter 6). In somatic cells of females, only one X chromosome is transcriptionally active. The other chromosome is inactive. The process of X inactivation, which is random, occurs early in embryonic life and is usually complete at about the end of the first week of development. After one X chromosome has become inactivated in a cell, all cells descended from that cell have the same inactivated X chromosome. Although much of one X chromosome is inactivated in females, several regions contain genes that escape inactivation and continue to be expressed by both X chromosomes. These genes may explain some of the variations in clinical symptoms seen in cases of numeric abnormalities of the X chromosome, such as Turner syndrome.

It is well known that the Y chromosome determines the male sex. The gene that dictates testicular development (SRY: sex-determining region Y gene) has been located on its distal short arm.[5] Recent studies of the Y chromosome have yielded additional information about gene families in the so-called "male-specific Y" or MSY region. All of these are believed to be involved in spermatogenesis. A few additional genes with homologs on the X chromosome have been mapped to the Y chromosome, but to date, no disorders resulting from mutations in these genes have been described.

Turner Syndrome. Turner syndrome describes an absence of all (45,X/0) or part of the X chromosome.[23,24] Some women with Turner syndrome may have part of the X chromosome and some may display a mosaicism with one or more additional cells lines. This disorder affects approximately 1 of every 2,500 live births, and it has been estimated that almost all fetuses with the 45,X/0 karyotype are spontaneously aborted during the first trimester.[4]

Characteristically, the girl with Turner syndrome is short in stature, but her body proportions are normal (Fig. 7.10). Females with Turner syndrome lose the majority of their oocytes by the age of 2 years. Therefore, they do not menstruate and show no signs of secondary sex characteristics.[4] There are variations in the syndrome, with abnormalities ranging from essentially none to cardiac abnormalities such as a bicuspid aortic valve and coarctation of the aorta, problems with hearing and vision, a small size mandible, abnormal kidney development (i.e., abnormal location, abnormal vascular supply, or double collecting system), and a small webbed neck.[4] Although most women with Turner syndrome have normal

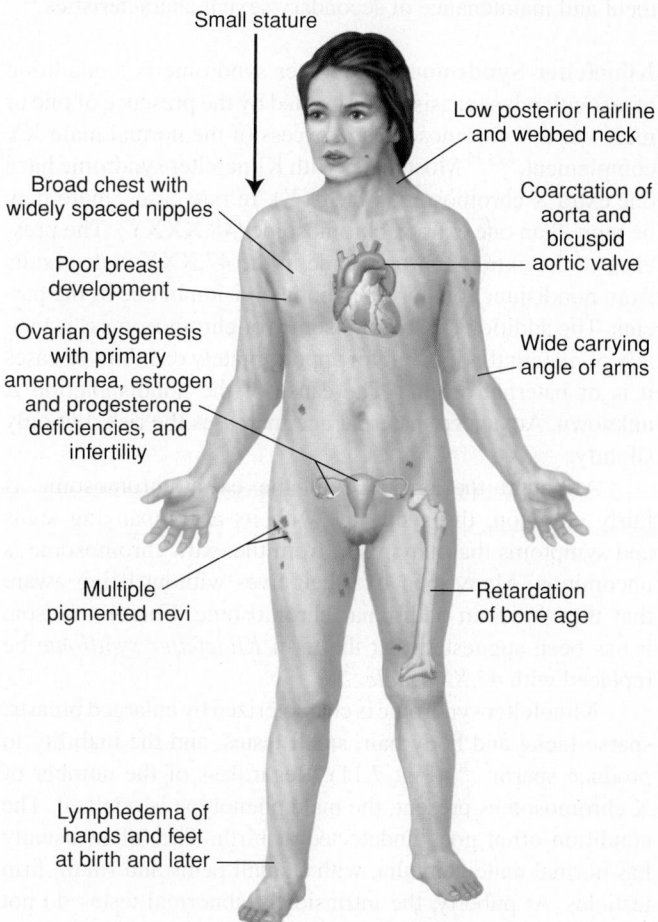

Small stature

Low posterior hairline and webbed neck

Broad chest with widely spaced nipples

Coarctation of aorta and bicuspid aortic valve

Poor breast development

Ovarian dysgenesis with primary amenorrhea, estrogen and progesterone deficiencies, and infertility

Wide carrying angle of arms

Multiple pigmented nevi

Retardation of bone age

Lymphedema of hands and feet at birth and later

FIGURE 7.10 • Clinical features of Turner syndrome.

intelligence, they may have problems with visuospatial organization (*e.g.,* difficulty in driving, nonverbal problem-solving tasks such as mathematics, and psychomotor skills) and attention deficit disorders.[23,24]

The diagnosis of Turner syndrome often is delayed until late childhood or early adolescence in girls who do not present with the classic features of the syndrome. Only about 20% to 33% of affected girls receive a diagnosis as a newborn because of puffy hands and feet or redundant nuchal skin; another 33% are diagnosed in mid-childhood because of short stature; and the rest are mainly diagnosed in adolescence when they fail to enter puberty.[23] Early diagnosis is an important aspect of treatment for Turner syndrome. It allows for counselling about the phenotypic characteristics of the disorder; screening for cardiac, renal, thyroid, and other abnormalities; and provision of emotional support for the girl and her family. Because of the potential for delay in diagnosis, it has been recommended that girls with unexplained short stature (height below the fifth percentile), webbed neck, peripheral lymphedema, coarctation of the aorta, or delayed puberty have chromosomal studies done.

The management of Turner syndrome begins during childhood and requires ongoing assessment and treatment. Growth hormone therapy generally can result in a gain of 6 to 10 cm in final height. Estrogen therapy, which is instituted around the normal age of puberty, is used to promote development and maintenance of secondary sexual characteristics.[23]

Klinefelter Syndrome. Klinefelter syndrome is a condition of testicular dysgenesis accompanied by the presence of one or more extra X chromosomes in excess of the normal male XY complement.[4,25,26] Most males with Klinefelter syndrome have one extra X chromosome (47,XXY). In rare cases, there may be more than one extra X chromosome (48,XXXY). The presence of the extra X chromosome in the 47,XXY male results from nondisjunction during meiotic division in one of the parents. The additional X chromosome (or chromosomes) is usually of maternal origin but for approximately one third of cases it is of paternal origin.[5] The cause of the nondisjunction is unknown. Advanced maternal age increases the risk, but only slightly.

Although the presence of the extra chromosome is fairly common, the syndrome with its accompanying signs and symptoms that may result from the extra chromosome is uncommon. Many men live their lives without being aware that they have an additional chromosome. For this reason, it has been suggested that the term *Klinefelter syndrome* be replaced with *47,XXY male.*[25]

Klinefelter syndrome is characterized by enlarged breasts, sparse facial and body hair, small testes, and the inability to produce sperm[25,26] (Fig. 7.11). Regardless of the number of X chromosomes present, the male phenotype is retained. The condition often goes undetected at birth. The infant usually has normal male genitalia, with a small penis and small, firm testicles. At puberty, the intrinsically abnormal testes do not respond to stimulation from the gonadotropins and undergo degeneration. This leads to a tall stature with abnormal body

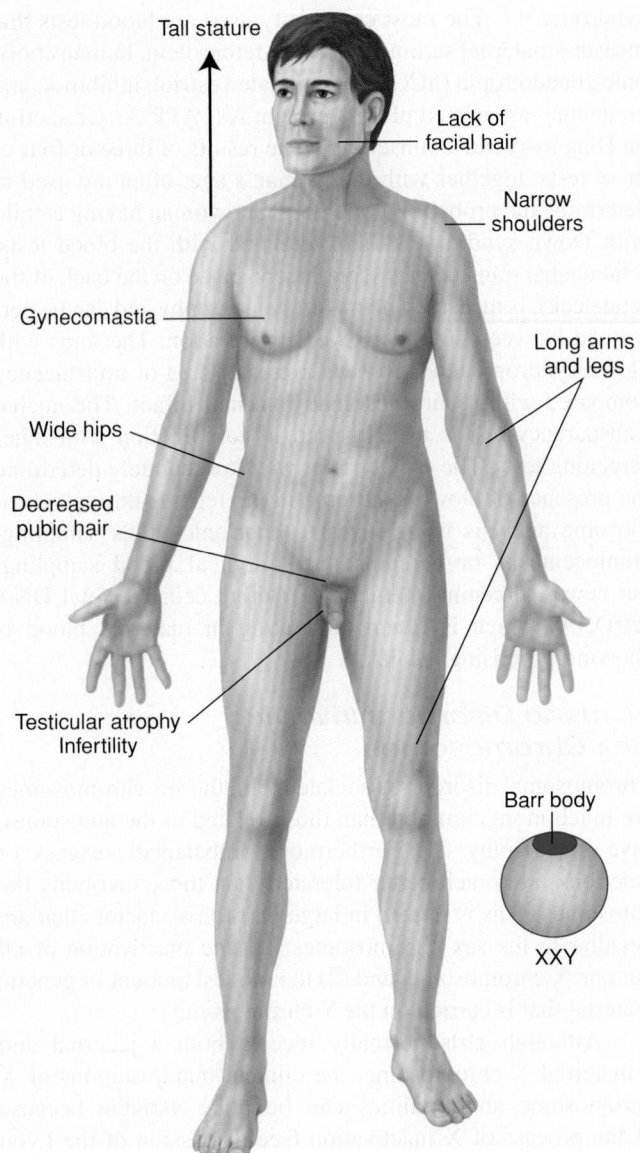

Tall stature

Lack of facial hair

Narrow shoulders

Gynecomastia

Long arms and legs

Wide hips

Decreased pubic hair

Testicular atrophy
Infertility

Barr body

XXY

FIGURE 7.11 • Clinical features of Klinefelter syndrome.

proportions in which the lower part of the body is longer than the upper part. Later in life, the body build may become heavy, with a female distribution of subcutaneous fat and variable degrees of breast enlargement. There may be deficient secondary male sex characteristics, such as a voice that remains feminine in pitch and sparse beard and pubic hair. Although the intellect usually is normal, most 47,XXY males have some degree of language impairment.

Adequate management of Klinefelter syndrome requires a comprehensive neurodevelopmental evaluation. In infancy and early childhood, this often includes a multidisciplinary approach to determine appropriate treatments such as physical therapy, infant stimulation programs, and speech therapy.[26] Men with Klinefelter syndrome have congenital hypogonadism, which results in an inability to produce normal amounts of testosterone accompanied by an increase in hypothalamic

TABLE 7.2 SOME DISORDERS OF ORGAN SYSTEMS ASSOCIATED WITH MITOCHONDRIAL DNA MUTATIONS

DISORDER	MANIFESTATIONS
Chronic progressive external ophthalmoplegia	Progressive weakness of the extraocular muscles
Deafness	Progressive sensorineural deafness, often associated with aminoglycoside antibiotics
Kearns-Sayre syndrome	Progressive weakness of the extraocular muscles of early onset with heart block, retinal pigmentation
Leber hereditary optic neuropathy	Painless, subacute, bilateral visual loss, with central blind spots (scotomas) and abnormal colour vision
Leigh disease	Proximal muscle weakness, sensory neuropathy, developmental delay, ataxia, seizures, dementia, and visual impairment due to retinal pigment degeneration
MELAS	*M*itochondrial *E*ncephalomyopathy (cerebral structural changes), *L*actic *A*cidosis, and *S*trokelike syndrome, seizures, and other clinical and laboratory abnormalities; may manifest only as diabetes mellitus
MERRF	*M*yoclonic *E*pilepsy, *R*agged *R*ed *F*ibres in muscle, ataxia, sensorineural deafness
Myoclonic epilepsy with ragged red fibres	Myoclonic seizures, cerebellar ataxia, mitochondrial myopathy (muscle weakness, fatigue)

gonadotrophic hormones (see Chapter 43). Androgen therapy is usually initiated around the age of 12 years when there is evidence of a testosterone deficit.[5] Because gynecomastia predisposes to breast cancer, breast self-examination should be encouraged for men with Klinefelter syndrome. Infertility is common in men with Klinefelter syndrome because of a decreased sperm count. If sperm are present, cryopreservation may be useful for future family planning. However, genetic counselling is advised because of the increased risk of autosomal and sex chromosomal abnormalities.

Mitochondrial Gene Disorders

The mitochondria contain their own DNA, which is distinct from the DNA contained in the cell nucleus. There are multiple disease-related rearrangements and point mutations have been identified.[3] Mitochondrial DNA, which is packaged in a double-stranded circular chromosome located inside the mitochondria, is often referred to as the "other human genome."[27] Mitochondrial DNA contains 37 genes: two ribosomal RNA (rRNA) genes; 22 transfer RNA (tRNA) genes; and 13 structural genes encoding subunits of the mitochondrial respiratory chain enzymes, which participate in oxidative phosphorylation and generation of adenosine triphosphate (see Chapter 4).[4]

In contrast to the mendelian pattern of inheritance of nuclear DNA, disorders of mtDNA are inherited on the maternal line. This can be explained by the fact that ova contain numerous mitochondria in their abundant cytoplasm, whereas spermatozoa contain few, if any, mitochondria. Thus, the mtDNA in the zygote is derived solely from the mother. The zygote and its daughter cells have many mitochondria, each of which contains multiple copies of the maternally derived mtDNA. During growth of the fetus or later, it is likely that some cells will contain only normal or mutant mtDNA (a situation called

homoplasmy), whereas others receive a mixture of normal and mutant DNA (*heteroplasmy*). In turn, the clinical expression of a disease produced by a given mutation of mtDNA depends on the total content of mitochondrial genes and the proportion that is mutant. The fraction of mutant mtDNA must exceed a critical value for a mitochondrial disease to become symptomatic. This threshold varies in different organs and is presumably related to the energy requirements of the cells.

Mitochondrial DNA mutations generally affect tissues that are dependent on oxidative phosphorylation to meet their high needs for metabolic energy. Thus, mtDNA mutations frequently affect the neuromuscular system and produce disorders such as encephalopathies, myopathies, retinal degeneration, loss of extraocular muscle function, and deafness.[27,28] The range of mitochondrial diseases is broad, however, and may include liver dysfunction, bone marrow failure, and pancreatic islet cell dysfunction and diabetes, among other disorders. Table 7.2 describes representative examples of disorders due to mutations in mtDNA.

IN SUMMARY

Genetic disorders can affect a single gene (mendelian inheritance) or several genes (polygenic inheritance). Single-gene disorders may be present on an autosome or on the X chromosome, and they may be expressed as a dominant or recessive trait. In autosomal dominant disorders, a single mutant allele from an affected parent is transmitted to an offspring regardless of sex. The affected parent has a 50% chance of transmitting the disorder to each offspring. Autosomal recessive disorders are manifested only when both members of the gene pair are affected. Usually, both parents are unaffected but are carriers of the defective gene. Their chances of having an affected child are one in four; of having a carrier child, two in four; and of having a noncarrier, unaffected child, one in four. Sex-linked disorders, which are associated with the X chromosome, are those in which an unaffected mother carries one normal and one mutant allele on the X chromosome. She has a 50% chance of transmitting the defective gene to her sons, who are affected, and her daughters have a 50% chance of being carriers of the mutant gene. Because of a normal paired gene, female heterozygotes rarely experience the effects of a defective gene. The fragile X syndrome is an inherited form of intellectual disability that results from a repeating sequence of three nucleotides on a single gene in the X chromosome. Multifactorial inheritance disorders are caused by multiple genes and, in many cases, environmental factors.

Chromosomal disorders result from a change in chromosome number or structure. A change in chromosome number is called aneuploidy. Monosomy involves the presence of only one member of a chromosome pair; it is seen in Turner syndrome, in which there is monosomy of the X chromosome. Polysomy refers to the presence of more than two chromosomes in a set. Klinefelter syndrome involves polysomy of the X chromosome. Trisomy 21 (*i.e.,* Down syndrome) is the most common form of chromosome disorder. Alterations in chromosome structure involve deletion or addition of genetic material, which may involve a translocation of genetic material from one chromosome pair to another.

The mitochondria contain their own DNA, which is distinct from nuclear DNA. This DNA, which is inherited maternally, is subject to mutations at a higher rate than nuclear DNA, and it has no repair mechanisms. Disorders of mitochondrial genes interfere with oxidative phosphorylation and the production of cellular energy. The range of mitochondrial gene disorders is diverse, with neuromuscular disorders predominating.

DISORDERS DUE TO ENVIRONMENTAL INFLUENCES

After completing this section of the chapter, you should be able to meet the following objectives:

- Cite the most susceptible period of intrauterine life for development of defects due to environmental agents.
- State the cautions that should be observed when considering use of drugs during pregnancy, including the possible effects of alcohol abuse, vitamin A derivatives, and folic acid deficiency on fetal development.

The developing embryo is subject to many nongenetic influences. After conception, development is influenced by the environmental factors that the embryo shares with the mother.

The physiologic status of the mother—her hormone balance, her general state of health, her nutritional status, and the drugs she takes—undoubtedly influences the development of the unborn child. For example, diabetes mellitus is associated with increased risk of congenital anomalies. Maternal smoking is associated with lower-than-normal neonatal weight. Maternal use of alcohol, in the context of chronic alcoholism, is known to cause fetal abnormalities. Some agents cause early abortion. Measles and other infectious agents cause congenital malformations. Other agents, such as radiation, can cause chromosomal and genetic defects and produce developmental disorders.

Period of Vulnerability

The embryo's development is most easily disturbed during the period when differentiation and development of the organs are taking place. This time interval, which is often referred to as the period of *organogenesis,* extends from day 15 to day 60 after conception. Environmental influences during the first 2 weeks after fertilization may interfere with implantation and result in abortion or early resorption of the products of conception. Each organ has a critical period during which it is highly susceptible to environmental derangements[4,29] (Fig. 7.12). Often, the effect is expressed at the biochemical level just before the organ begins to develop. The same agent may affect different organ systems that are developing at the same time.

Teratogenic Agents

A teratogenic agent is a chemical, physical or biologic agent that produces abnormalities during embryonic or fetal development. Maternal disease or altered metabolic state also can affect the development of the embryo or fetus. Theoretically, teratogenic agents can cause birth defects in three ways: by direct exposure of the pregnant woman and the embryo or fetus to the agent; through exposure of the soon-to-be-pregnant woman to an agent that has a slow clearance rate such that a teratogenic dose is retained during early pregnancy; or as a result of mutagenic effects of an environmental agent that occur before pregnancy, causing permanent damage to a woman's (or a man's) reproductive cells. For discussion purposes, teratogenic agents have been divided into three groups: radiation, drugs and chemical substances, and infectious agents. Chart 7.1 lists commonly identified agents in each of these groups.

Radiation

Heavy doses of ionizing radiation are teratogenic and mutagenic and have the capacity to effect inheritable changes in genetic materials. Specifically, excessive levels of radiation have been shown to cause microcephaly, skeletal malformations, and mental retardation. There is no evidence that diagnostic levels of radiation (*e.g.,* from a chest x-ray) cause congenital abnormalities. Additionally all efforts to shield the fetus are taken when possible. In situations where a study is necessary for the woman's health, the benefits to her of having proper diagnostic imaging outweigh potential theoretical risks

FIGURE 7.12 • Sensitivity of specific organs to teratogenic agents at critical periods in embryogenesis. Exposure to adverse influences in the preimplantation and early postimplantation stages of development (*far left*) leads to prenatal death. Periods of maximal sensitivity to teratogens (*horizontal bars*) vary for different organ systems, but overall are limited to the first 8 weeks of pregnancy. (From Rubin R., Strayer D. S. (Eds.). (2012). *Rubin's pathology: Clinicopathologic foundations of medicine* (6th ed., p. 2163). Philadelphia, PA: Lippincott Williams & Wilkins.)

to the fetus. Administration of therapeutic doses of radioactive iodine (^{131}I) during the 13th week of gestation, the time when the fetal thyroid is beginning to concentrate iodine, has been shown to interfere with thyroid development.

Chemicals and Drugs

Environmental chemicals and drugs can cross the placenta and cause damage to the developing embryo and fetus. It has been estimated that only 2% to 3% of developmental defects have a known drug or environmental origin. Some of the best-documented environmental teratogens are the organic mercurials, which cause neurologic deficits and blindness. Sources of exposure to mercury may include contaminated food (fish) and water. The precise mechanisms by which chemicals and drugs exert their teratogenic effects are largely unknown. They may produce cytotoxic (cell-killing), antimetabolic, or growth-inhibiting effects.

Drugs top the list of chemical teratogens, probably because they are regularly used at elevated doses. Many drugs can cross the placenta and expose the fetus to both the pharmacologic and teratogenic effects. Factors that affect placental drug transfer and drug effects on the fetus include the rate at which the drug crosses the placenta, the duration of exposure, and the stage of placental and fetal development at the time of exposure.[30] Lipid-soluble drugs tend to cross the placenta more readily and enter the fetal circulation. The molecular weight of a drug also influences the rate and amount of drug transferred across the placenta. Drugs with a molecular weight of less than 500 can cross the placenta easily, depending on lipid solubility and degree of ionization; those with a molecular weight of 500 to 1,000 cross the placenta with more difficulty; and those with molecular weights of more than 1,000 cross very poorly.[30]

A number of drugs are suspected of being teratogens, but only a few have been identified with certainty. Perhaps the best known of these drugs is thalidomide, which has been shown to give rise to a full range of malformations, including phocomelia (*i.e.,* short, flipper-like appendages) of all four extremities.

CHART 7.1 TERATOGENIC AGENTS[a]

Radiation
Drugs and Chemical Substances
Alcohol
Anticoagulants
   Warfarin
Anticonvulsants
Anticancer drugs
   Aminopterin
   Methotrexate
   6-Mercaptopurine
Antihypertensives
   ACE inhibitors
   Angiotensin II receptor blockers
Isotretinoin (Accutane)
Propylthiouracil
Tetracycline
Thalidomide

Infectious Agents
Viruses
   Cytomegalovirus
   Herpes simplex virus
   Measles (rubella)
   Mumps
   Varicella-zoster virus (chickenpox)
Nonviral factors
   Syphilis
   Toxoplasmosis

[a]Not inclusive.

Other drugs known to cause fetal abnormalities are the antimetabolites used in the treatment of cancer, the anticoagulant drug warfarin, several of the anticonvulsant drugs, ethyl alcohol, and cocaine. Some drugs affect a single developing structure; for example, propylthiouracil can impair thyroid development and tetracycline can interfere with the mineralization phase of tooth development. More recently, vitamin A and its derivatives (the retinoids) have been targeted for concern because of their teratogenic potential. Concern over the

TERATOGENIC AGENTS

- Teratogenic agents such as radiation, chemicals and drugs, and infectious organisms are agents that produce abnormalities in the developing embryo.
- The stage of development of the embryo determines the susceptibility to teratogens. The period during which the embryo is most susceptible to teratogenic agents is the time during which rapid differentiation and development of body organs and tissues are taking place, usually from days 15 to 60 postconception.

teratogenic effects of vitamin A derivatives arose with the introduction of the acne drug isotretinoin (Accutane).

In 1983, the U.S. Food and Drug Administration established a system, which Canada adopted, for classifying drugs according to probable risks to the fetus. According to this system, drugs are put into five categories: A, B, C, D, and X. Drugs in category A are the least dangerous, and categories B, C, and D are increasingly more dangerous. Those in category X are contraindicated during pregnancy because of proven teratogenicity.[30]

Because many drugs are suspected of causing fetal abnormalities, and even those that were once thought to be safe are now being viewed critically, it is recommended that women in their childbearing years avoid unnecessary use of drugs. This pertains to nonpregnant women as well as pregnant women because many developmental defects occur early in pregnancy. As happened with thalidomide, the damage to the embryo may occur before pregnancy is suspected or confirmed. A drug that is often abused and can have deleterious effects on the fetus is alcohol.

Fetal Alcohol Syndrome. The term *fetal alcohol syndrome* (FAS) refers to a constellation of physical, behavioural, and cognitive abnormalities resulting from maternal alcohol consumption.[31,32] Although there aren't any national statistics in Canada it is estimated that overall incidence for FAS is somewhere between 0.5 and 5.0 per 1,000 live births each year, with an increased prevalence for high-risk populations such as the First Nations and Inuit communities.[33] Alcohol, which is lipid soluble and has a molecular weight between 600 and 1,000, passes freely across the placental barrier; concentrations of alcohol in the fetus are at least as high as in the mother. Unlike other teratogens, the harmful effects of alcohol are not restricted to the sensitive period of early gestation but extend throughout pregnancy.

Alcohol has widely variable effects on fetal development, ranging from minor abnormalities to FAS. There may be prenatal or postnatal growth retardation; CNS involvement, including neurologic abnormalities, developmental delays, behavioural dysfunction, intellectual impairment, and skull and brain malformation; and a characteristic set of facial features that include small palpebral fissures (*i.e.,* eye openings), a thin vermilion border (upper lip), and an elongated, flattened midface and philtrum (*i.e.,* the groove in the middle of the upper lip)[33-36] (Fig. 7.13). The facial features of FAS may not be as apparent in the newborn but become more prominent as the infant develops. As the children grow into adulthood, the facial features become more subtle, making diagnosis of FAS in older individuals more difficult. Each of these defects can vary in severity, probably reflecting the timing of alcohol consumption in terms of the period of fetal development, amount of alcohol consumed, and hereditary and environmental influences.

In 2005, a subcommittee of the Public Health Agency of Canada's National Advisory Committee on Fetal Alcohol Spectrum Disorder published guidelines for the referral and diagnosis of FAS.[33] The criteria for FAS diagnosis require the documented presence of three of the following findings:

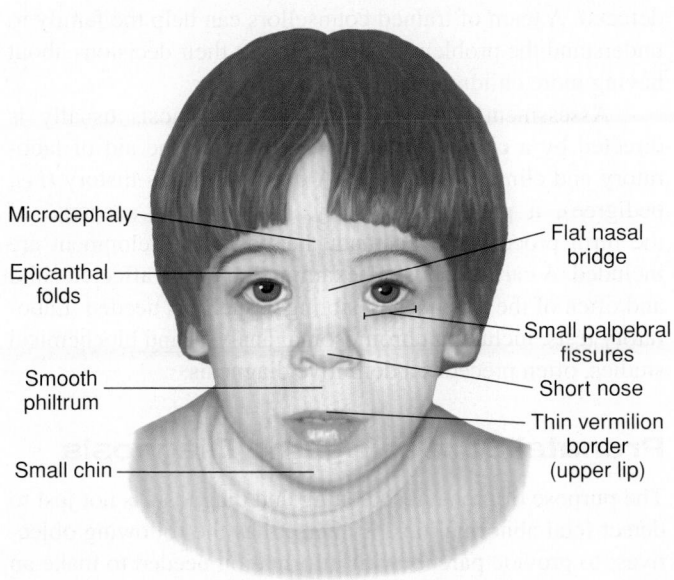

Microcephaly

Epicanthal folds

Smooth philtrum

Small chin

Flat nasal bridge

Small palpebral fissures

Short nose

Thin vermilion border (upper lip)

FIGURE 7.13 • Clinical features of fetal alcohol syndrome.

(1) three facial abnormalities (smooth philtrum, thin vermilion border on the upper lip, and small palpebral fissures); (2) growth deficits (prenatal or postnatal height or weight, at or below the 10th percentile); and (3) Neurobehavioural abnormalities (*e.g.*, head circumference below the 10th percentile, global cognitive or intellectual deficits, motor functioning delays, problems with attention or hyperactivity).

The amount of alcohol that can be safely consumed during pregnancy is unknown. Even small amounts of alcohol consumed during critical periods of fetal development may be teratogenic. For example, if alcohol is consumed during the period of organogenesis, a variety of skeletal and organ defects may result. If alcohol is consumed later in gestation, when the brain is undergoing rapid development, there may be behavioural and cognitive disorders in the absence of physical abnormalities. Chronic alcohol consumption throughout pregnancy may result in a variety of effects, ranging from physical abnormalities to growth retardation and compromised CNS functioning. Evidence suggests that short-lived high concentrations of alcohol, such as those that occur with binge drinking, may be particularly significant, with abnormalities being unique to the period of exposure. Because of the possible effect on the fetus, it is recommended that women abstain from alcohol during pregnancy.

Folic Acid Deficiency. Although most birth defects are related to exposure to a teratogenic agent, deficiencies of nutrients and vitamins also may be a factor. Folic acid deficiency has been implicated in the development of neural tube defects (*e.g.*, anencephaly, spina bifida, encephalocele). Studies have shown a reduction in neural tube defects when folic acid was taken before conception and continued during the first trimester of pregnancy.[37] Therefore, it is recommended that all women of childbearing age receive 0.4 mg of folic acid daily.[37] These recommendations are particularly important for

women who have previously had an affected pregnancy, for couples with a close relative with the disorder, and for women with diabetes mellitus or those taking anticonvulsant drugs as they are at increased risk for having infants with birth defects.

Since 1998, all enriched cereal grain products in Canada have been fortified with folic acid. To achieve an adequate intake of folic acid, pregnant women should couple a diet that contains folate-rich foods (*e.g.*, orange juice; dark, leafy green vegetables; and legumes) with sources of synthetic folic acid, such as fortified food products.[37]

Infectious Agents

Many microorganisms cross the placenta and enter the fetal circulation, often producing multiple malformations. The acronym TORCH stands for *t*oxoplasmosis, *o*ther, *r*ubella (*i.e.*, German measles), *c*ytomegalovirus, and *h*erpes, which are the agents most frequently implicated in fetal anomalies.[4] Other infections include varicella-zoster virus infection, listeriosis, leptospirosis, Epstein–Barr virus infection, tuberculosis, and syphilis.[4] Human immunodeficiency virus (HIV) and human parvovirus (B19) have been suggested as additions to the list. The TORCH screening test examines the infant's serum for the presence of antibodies to these agents. However, the titres for serum antibodies against the TORCH agents in the mother and newborn usually are not diagnostic, and the precise cause of the disorder often remains uncertain.

Infections with the TORCH agents are reported to occur in 1% to 5% of newborn infants and are among the major causes of neonatal morbidity and mortality.[4] Common clinical and pathologic manifestations include growth retardation and abnormalities of the brain (microcephaly, hydrocephalus), eye, ear, liver, hematopoietic system (anemia, thrombocytopenia), lungs (pneumonitis), and heart (myocarditis, congenital heart disorders).[4] These manifestations vary among symptomatic newborns, however, and only a few present with multisystem abnormalities.

Toxoplasmosis is a protozoal infection caused by *Toxoplasma gondii*. The infection can be contracted by eating raw or inadequately cooked meat or food that has come in contact with infected meat.[38] The domestic cat is known to carry this organism and excretes the protozoa in its feces. It has been suggested that pregnant women should avoid contact with excrement from the family cat. The introduction of the rubella vaccine has virtually eliminated the congenital rubella syndrome in most developed countries. Rubella remains endemic in many developing countries, however, where it is the major preventable cause of hearing impairment, blindness, and adverse neurodevelopmental outcome. The epidemiology of cytomegalovirus infection is largely unknown. Some infants are severely affected at birth, and others, although having evidence of the infection, have no symptoms. In some symptom-free infants, brain damage becomes evident over a span of several years. There also is evidence that some infants contract the infection during the first year of life, and in some of them the infection leads to retardation a year or two later. Herpes simplex virus type 2 infection is considered to be a genital infection and usually is transmitted through sexual contact. The infant acquires this infection in utero or in passage through the birth canal.

A teratogenic agent is one that produces abnormalities during embryonic or fetal life. It is during the early part of pregnancy (15 to 60 days after conception) that environmental agents are most apt to produce their deleterious effects on the developing embryo. A number of environmental agents can be damaging to the unborn child, including radiation, drugs and chemicals, and infectious agents. FAS is a risk for infants of women who regularly consume alcohol during pregnancy. Because many drugs have the potential for causing fetal abnormalities, often at an early stage of pregnancy, it is recommended that women of childbearing age avoid unnecessary use of drugs. It also has been shown that folic acid deficiency can contribute to neural tube defects. The acronym TORCH stands for *t*oxoplasmosis, *o*ther, *r*ubella, *c*ytomegalovirus, and *h*erpes, which are the infectious agents most frequently implicated in fetal anomalies.

DIAGNOSIS AND COUNSELLING

After completing this section of the chapter, you should be able to meet the following objectives:

- Describe the process of genetic assessment.
- Describe methods used in arriving at a prenatal diagnosis, including ultrasonography, amniocentesis, chorionic villus sampling, percutaneous umbilical fetal blood sampling, and laboratory methods to determine the biochemical and genetic makeup of the fetus.

The birth of a defective child is a traumatic event in any parent's life. Usually two issues must be resolved. The first deals with the immediate and future care of the affected child, and the second with the possibility of future children in the family having a similar defect. Genetic assessment and counselling can help to determine whether the defect was inherited and the risk of recurrence. Prenatal diagnosis provides a means of determining whether the unborn child has certain types of abnormalities.

Genetic Assessment

Effective genetic counselling involves accurate diagnosis and communication of the findings and of the risks of recurrence to the parents and other family members who need such information. Counselling may be provided after the birth of an affected child, or it may be offered to persons at risk for having defective children (*i.e.,* siblings of persons with birth

defects). A team of trained counsellors can help the family to understand the problem and can support their decisions about having more children.

Assessment of genetic risk and prognosis usually is directed by a clinical geneticist, often with the aid of laboratory and clinical specialists. A detailed family history (*i.e.,* pedigree), a pregnancy history, and detailed accounts of the birth process and postnatal health and development are included. A careful physical examination of the affected child and often of the parents and siblings usually is needed. Laboratory tests, including chromosomal analysis and biochemical studies, often precedes a definitive diagnosis.

Prenatal Screening and Diagnosis

The purpose of prenatal screening and diagnosis is not just to detect fetal abnormalities. Rather, it has the following objectives: to provide parents with information needed to make an informed choice about having a child with an abnormality; to provide reassurance and reduce anxiety among high-risk groups; and to allow parents at risk for having a child with a specific defect, who might otherwise forgo having a child, to begin a pregnancy with the assurance that knowledge about the presence or absence of the disorder in the fetus can be confirmed by testing.[3] Prenatal screening cannot be used to rule out all possible fetal abnormalities. It is limited to determining whether the fetus has (or probably has) designated conditions indicated by late maternal age, family history, or well-defined risk factors.

There are multiple methods that can assist in diagnosing a fetus regarding genetic disorders, including ultrasonography, maternal serum (blood) screening tests, amniocentesis, chorionic villus sampling, and percutaneous umbilical fetal blood sampling[3–5] (Fig. 7.14). Prenatal diagnosis can also provide the information needed for prescribing prenatal treatment for the fetus. For example, if congenital adrenal hyperplasia is diagnosed, the mother can be treated with adrenal cortical hormones to prevent masculinization of a female fetus.

Ultrasonography

Ultrasonography is a noninvasive diagnostic method that uses reflections of high-frequency sound waves to visualize soft tissue structures. Since its introduction in 1958, it has been used during pregnancy to determine number of fetuses, fetal size and position, amount of amniotic fluid, and placental location. It also is possible to assess fetal movement, breathing movements, and heart pattern. There is also good evidence that early ultrasonography (*i.e.,* before 14 weeks) accurately determines gestational age.

Improved resolution and real-time units have enhanced the ability of ultrasound scanners to detect congenital anomalies. With this more sophisticated equipment, it is possible to obtain information such as measurements of hourly urine output in a high-risk fetus. Ultrasonography makes possible the in utero diagnosis of hydrocephalus, spina bifida, facial defects, congenital heart defects, congenital diaphragmatic hernias,

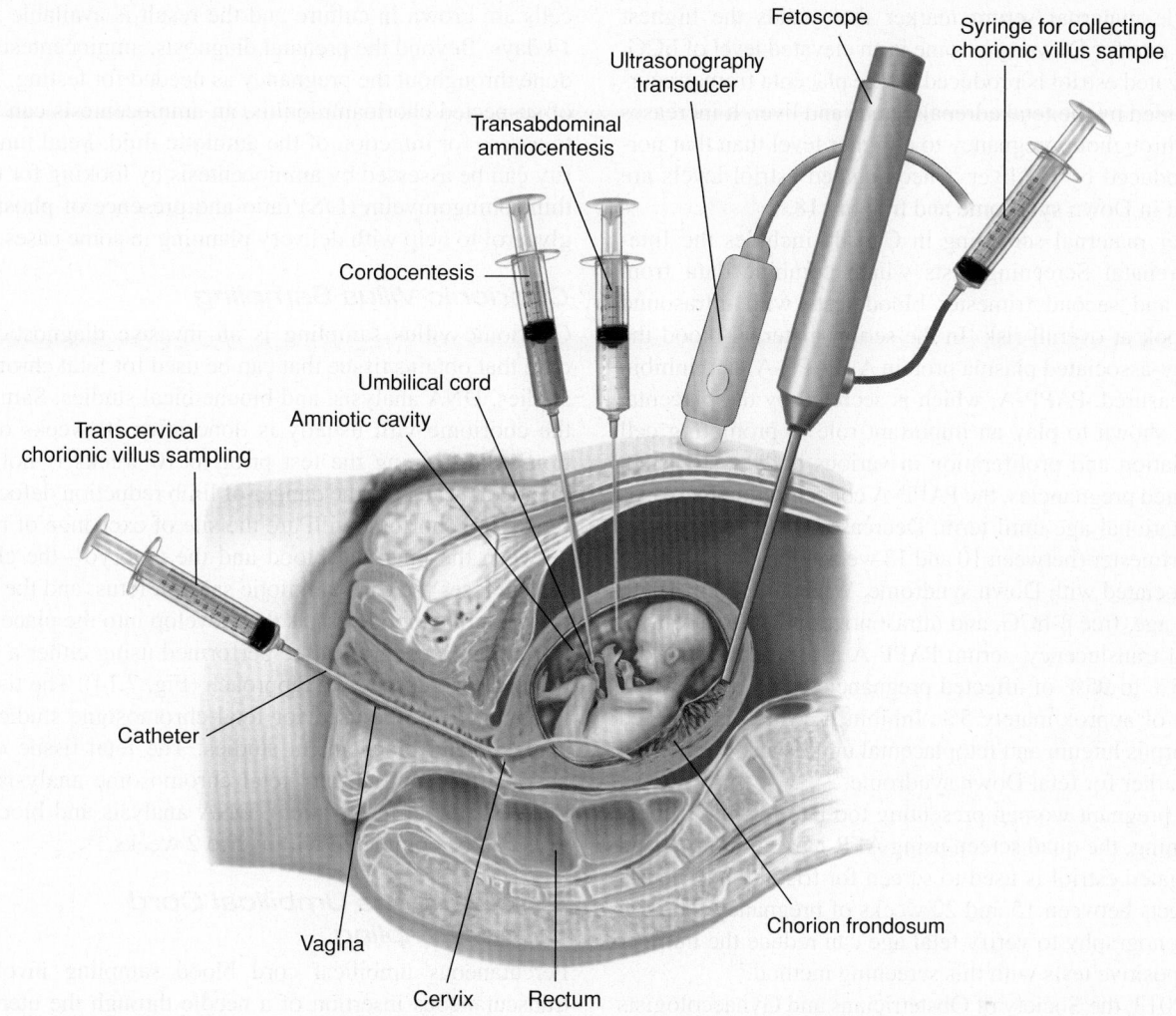

FIGURE 7.14 • Methods of prenatal screening.

Labels in figure: Fetoscope; Syringe for collecting chorionic villus sample; Ultrasonography transducer; Transabdominal amniocentesis; Cordocentesis; Umbilical cord; Amniotic cavity; Transcervical chorionic villus sampling; Catheter; Vagina; Cervix; Rectum; Chorion frondosum

disorders of the gastrointestinal tract, skeletal anomalies, and various other defects. Three-dimensional (3D) sonography has become useful in better assessing facial profiles and abdominal wall defects. A fetal echocardiogram can be done as follow-up for possible cardiac anomalies. Fetal MRI can be done to better assess skeletal, neurologic and other anomalies. Intrauterine diagnosis of congenital abnormalities permits better monitoring, further workup, and planning with appropriate specialities, preterm delivery for early correction, selection of cesarean section to reduce fetal injury, and, in some cases, intrauterine therapy.

Maternal Serum Markers

Maternal blood testing began in the early 1980s with the test for α-fetoprotein (AFP). Since that time, a number of serum factors have been studied as screening tests for fetal anomalies. Current maternal testing uses a variety of tests (*i.e.*, AFP, human chorionic gonadotropin [hCG], and unconjugated estriol) to screen for trisomy syndromes in high-risk women, while incorporating the detection of neural tube defects. The combined use of the three maternal serum markers between

15 and 22 weeks of pregnancy has been shown to detect as much as 60% of Down syndrome pregnancies.[3,39] The use of ultrasonography to verify fetal age can reduce the number of false-positive tests with this screening method.

AFP is a major fetal plasma protein and has a structure similar to the albumin found in postnatal life. AFP is made initially by the yolk sac, gastrointestinal tract, and liver. Fetal plasma levels peak at approximately 10 to 13 weeks' gestation and then decline progressively until term, whereas maternal levels peak in the third trimester. Maternal and amniotic fluid levels of AFP are elevated in pregnancies where the fetus has a neural tube defect (*i.e.*, anencephaly and open spina bifida) or certain other malformations such as an anterior abdominal wall defect in which the fetal integument is not intact. Although neural tube defects have been associated with elevated levels of AFP, decreased levels have been associated with Down syndrome.

A complex glycoprotein, hCG is produced exclusively by the outer layer of the trophoblast shortly after implantation in the uterine wall. It increases rapidly in the first 8 weeks of gestation, declines steadily until 20 weeks, and then plateaus.

The single maternal serum marker that yields the highest detection rate for Down syndrome is an elevated level of hCG. Unconjugated estriol is produced by the placenta from precursors provided by the fetal adrenal glands and liver. It increases steadily throughout pregnancy to a higher level than that normally produced by the liver. Unconjugated estriol levels are decreased in Down syndrome and trisomy 18.

Other maternal screening in Canada includes the Integrated Prenatal Screening tests which combine data from the first and second trimester blood tests with ultrasound data to look at overall risk. In the serum maternal blood the pregnancy-associated plasma protein A (PAPP-A) and inhibin A are measured. PAPP-A, which is secreted by the placenta, has been shown to play an important role in promoting cell differentiation and proliferation in various body systems. In complicated pregnancies, the PAPP-A concentration increases with gestational age until term. Decreased PAPP-A levels in the first trimester (between 10 and 13 weeks) have been shown to be associated with Down syndrome. When used along with maternal age, free β-hCG, and ultrasonographic measurement of nuchal translucency, serum PAPP-A levels can reportedly detect 85% to 95% of affected pregnancies with a false-positive rate of approximately 5%. Inhibin A, which is secreted by the corpus luteum and fetoplacental unit, is also a maternal serum marker for fetal Down syndrome.[39]

For pregnant women presenting too late for first trimester screening, the quad screen using AFP, hCG, inhibin A and unconjugated estriol is used to screen for trisomy and neural tube defects between 15 and 22 weeks of pregnancy. The use of ultrasonography to verify fetal age can reduce the number of false-positive tests with this screening method.[39]

In 2013, the Society of Obstetricians and Gynaecologists of Canada (SOGC) suggested that the newer non-invasive test looking at cell-free fetal DNA (cffDNA) in the maternal blood could be a potentially reliable alternative for pregnant women in their first trimester. This cffDNA testing accurately detects approximately 99% for the presence of Down syndrome, 98% for trisomy 18 and about 65% for trisomy 13 and may prove to be an alternative for women where more invasive tests are contraindicated.[22]

Amniocentesis

Amniocentesis is an invasive diagnostic procedure that involves the withdrawal of a sample of amniotic fluid from the pregnant uterus usually using a transabdominal approach (Fig. 7.14). The procedure is useful in women older than 35 years of age, who have an increased risk of giving birth to an infant with Down syndrome; in women with an elevated risk on maternal serum screening; in parents who have another child with chromosomal abnormalities; and in parents who are carriers or with a strong family history of an inherited disease. Ultrasonography is used to gain additional information and to guide the placement of the amniocentesis needle. The amniotic fluid and cells that have been shed by the fetus are studied. Amniocentesis is performed on an outpatient basis starting at 15 weeks gestational age. For chromosomal analysis, the fetal

cells are grown in culture and the result is available in 10 to 14 days. Beyond the prenatal diagnosis, amniocentesis can be done throughout the pregnancy as needed for testing. In cases of suspected chorioamnionitis, an amniocentesis can be done to assess for infection of the amniotic fluid. Fetal lung maturity can be assessed by amniocentesis by looking for the lecithin/sphingomyelin (L/S) ratio and presence of phosphatidyl glycerol to help with delivery planning in some cases.

Chorionic Villus Sampling

Chorionic villus sampling is an invasive diagnostic procedure that obtains tissue that can be used for fetal chromosome studies, DNA analysis, and biochemical studies. Sampling of the chorionic villi usually is done after 10 weeks of gestation.[40] Performing the test prior to 10 weeks is not recommended because of the danger of limb reduction defects in the fetus. The chorionic villi are the site of exchange of nutrients between the maternal blood and the embryo—the chorionic sac encloses the early amniotic sac and fetus, and the villi are the primitive blood vessels that develop into the placenta. The sampling procedure can be performed using either a transabdominal or transcervical approach (Fig. 7.14). The tissue that is obtained can be used for fetal chromosome studies, DNA analysis, and biochemical studies. The fetal tissue does not have to be cultured, and fetal chromosome analysis can be made available in 24 hours. DNA analysis and biochemical tests can be completed within 1 to 2 weeks.[40]

Percutaneous Umbilical Cord Blood Sampling

Percutaneous umbilical cord blood sampling involves the transcutaneous insertion of a needle through the uterine wall and into the umbilical artery. It is performed under ultrasonographic guidance and can be done any time after 16 weeks of gestation. It is used for prenatal diagnosis of hemoglobinopathies, coagulation disorders, metabolic and cytogenetic disorders, and immunodeficiencies. Fetal infections such as rubella and toxoplasmosis can be detected through measurement of immunoglobulin M antibodies or direct blood cultures. Results from cytogenetic studies usually are available within 48 to 72 hours. Because the procedure carries a greater risk of pregnancy loss than amniocentesis, it usually is reserved for situations in which rapid cytogenetic analysis is needed or in which diagnostic information cannot be obtained by other methods.

Fetal Biopsy

Fetal biopsy is done with a fetoscope under ultrasonographic guidance. It is used to detect certain genetic skin defects that cannot be diagnosed with DNA analysis. It also may be done to obtain muscle tissue for use in the diagnosis of Duchenne muscular dystrophy.

Cytogenetic and Biochemical Analyses

Amniocentesis and chorionic villus sampling yield cells that can be used for cytogenetic and DNA analyses. Biochemical analyses can be used to detect abnormal levels of AFP and abnormal biochemical products in the maternal blood and in specimens of amniotic fluid and fetal blood.

Cytogenetic studies are used for fetal karyotyping to determine the chromosomal makeup of the fetus. They are done to detect abnormalities of chromosome number and structure. Karyotyping also reveals the sex of the fetus. This may be useful when an inherited defect is known to affect only one sex.

Analysis of DNA is done on cells extracted from the amniotic fluid, chorionic villi, or fetal blood from percutaneous umbilical sampling to detect genetic defects such as inborn errors of metabolism. The defect may be established through direct demonstration of the molecular defect or through methods that break the DNA into fragments that can be studied to determine the presence of an abnormal gene. Direct demonstration of the molecular defect is done by growing the amniotic fluid cells in culture and measuring the enzymes that the cultured cells produce. Many of the enzymes are expressed in the chorionic villi; this permits earlier prenatal diagnosis because the cells do not need to be subjected to prior culture. DNA studies are used to detect genetic defects that cause inborn errors of metabolism, such as Tay–Sachs disease, glycogen storage diseases, and familial hypercholesterolemia. Prenatal diagnoses are possible for more than 70 inborn errors of metabolism.

IN SUMMARY

Genetic and prenatal diagnosis and counselling are done in an effort to determine the risk of having a child with a genetic or chromosomal disorder. They often involve a detailed family history (*i.e.,* pedigree), examination of any affected and other family members, and laboratory studies including chromosomal analysis and biochemical studies. They usually are done by a genetic counsellor and a specially prepared team of health care professionals. Prenatal screening and diagnosis are used to detect fetal abnormalities. Ultrasonography is used for fetal anatomic imaging. It is used for determination of fetal size and position and for the presence of structural anomalies. Maternal serum screening is used to identify pregnancies that are at increased risk of adverse outcomes such as Down syndrome and neural tube defects. Amniocentesis and chorionic villus sampling may be used to obtain specimens for cytogenetic and biochemical studies.

REVIEW EXERCISES

1. A 23-year-old woman with sickle cell disease and her husband want to have a child, but worry that the child will be born with the disease.
   A. *What is the mother's genotype in terms of the sickle cell gene? Is she heterozygous or homozygous?*

   B. *If the husband is found not to have the sickle cell gene, what is the probability of their child having the disease or being a carrier of the sickle cell trait?*
2. A couple has a child who was born with a congenital heart disease.
   A. *Would you consider the defect to be the result of a single gene or a polygenic trait?*
   B. *Would these parents be at greater risk of having another child with a heart defect or would they be at equal risk of having a child with a defect in another organ system, such as cleft palate?*
3. A couple has been informed that their newborn child has the features of Down syndrome and it is suggested that genetic studies be performed.
   A. *The child is found to have trisomy 21. Use Figure 7.7, which describes the events that occur during meiosis, to explain the origin of the third chromosome.*
   B. *If the child had been found to have the robertsonian chromosome, how would you explain the origin of the abnormal chromosome?*
4. An 8-year-old boy has been diagnosed with mitochondrial myopathy. His major complaints are those of muscle weakness and exercise intolerance. His mother gives a report of similar symptoms, but to a much lesser degree.
   A. *Explain the cause of this boy's symptoms.*
   B. *Mitochondrial disorders follow a nonmendelian pattern of inheritance. Explain. Define the terms homoplasmy and heteroplasmy in relation to the diversity of tissue involvement and symptoms in persons with mitochondrial disorders.*
5. A 26-year-old woman is planning to become pregnant.
   A. *What information would you give her regarding the effects of medications and drugs on the fetus? What stage of fetal development is associated with the greatest risk?*
   B. *What is the rationale for ensuring that she has an adequate intake of folic acid before conception?*
   C. *She and her husband have an indoor cat. What precautions should she use in caring for the cat?*

References

1. Public Health Agency of Canada. (2013). *Congenital anomalies in Canada in 2013: A perinatal health surveillance report.* Ottawa, Cat No. HP35–40/2013E-PDF.
2. Hall J. E. (2011). *Guyton and Hall textbook of medical physiology.* (12th ed.). Philadelphia, PA: Elsevier Saunders.
3. Nussbaum R. L., McInnes R. R., Willard H. F. (2007). *Thompson & Thompson genetics in medicine* (7th ed.). Philadelphia, PA: Elsevier Saunders.

4. Rubin R., Strayer D. (Eds.). (2012). *Pathology: Clinicopathologic foundations of medicine* (6th ed.). Philadelphia, PA: Lippincott Williams & Wilkins.

5. Kumar V., Abbas A. K., Fausto N., et al. (Eds.). (2010). Genetic disorders. *Robbins and Cotran pathologic basis of disease* (8th ed., pp. 135–182). Philadelphia, PA: Elsevier Saunders.

6. Judge N. P., Dietz H. C. (2005). Marfan's syndrome. *Lancet, 366*(9501), 1965–1976.

7. Gonzales E. A. (2009). Marfan syndrome. *Journal of the American Academy of Nurse Practitioners, 21*(12), 663–670.

8. Sponseller P. D., Erkula G., Skolasky R. L., et al. (2010). Improving clinical recognition of Marfan syndrome. *Journal of Bone & Joint Surgery, 92*(9), 1868–1875.

9. McClatchey A. I. (2007). Neurofibromatosis. *Annual Review of Pathology: Mechanism of Disease, 2,* 191–216.

10. Ferner R. E. (2007). Neurofibromatosis type 1 and 2. *Lancet Neurology. 6,* 340–351.

11. Targum S. D., Lang W. (2010). Neurobehavioral problem associated with PKU. *Psychiatry, 7*(12), 29–32.

12. Blau N., van Spronsen F. J., Levy H. L. (2010). Phenylketonuria. *Lancet, 376*(9750), 1417–1427.

13. Canadian PKU and Allied Disorders Inc. (CanPKU). (2013). Newborn screening in Canada status report. Available online at: http://raredisorders.ca/documents/CanadaNBSstatusupdatedJan.132012.pdf. Accessed February 1, 2014.

14. National Human Genome Research Institute. (2013). Learning about fragile X syndrome. Available online at: http://www.genome.gov/19518828. Accessed February 1, 2014.

15. U.S. National Library of Medicine. (2012). Fragile X syndrome. Available online at: http://ghr.nlm.nih.gov/condition/fragile-x-syndrome. Accessed February 2, 2014.

16. Agrawal K., Panda K. (2011). A modified surgical schedule for primary management of cleft lip and palate in developing countries. Available online at: http://www.cpcjournal.org/doi/pdf/10.1597/09-226. Accessed February 2, 2014.

17. Tinanoff N. (2011). Cleft lip and palate. In Kliegman R. M., Stanton B. F., St. Geme J. W. (Eds.), *Nelson textbook of pediatrics* (19th ed., pp. 1252–1254). Philadelphia, PA: Elsevier Saunders.

18. March of Dimes Foundation. (2009). Down syndrome. Available online at: www.marchofdimes.com/pnhec/4439_1214.asp. Accessed February 2, 2014.

19. Bacino C. A., Lee B. (2011). Cytogenetics. In Kliegman R. M., Stanton B. F., St. Geme J. W. (Eds.), *Nelson textbook of pediatrics* (19th ed., pp. 394–415). Philadelphia, PA: Elsevier Saunders.

20. Zwaan O. H., Reinhardt D., Hitzler J., Vyas P. (2010). Acute leukemias in children with Down syndrome. *Hematology/Oncology Clinics of North America, 24*(1), 19–34.

21. Koster M. P., Wortelboer E. J., Stoutenbeek P., et al. (2011). Modeling Down syndrome screening performance using first-trimester serum markers. *Ultrasound in Obstetrics & Gynecology, 38*(2), 134–139.

22. Langlois S., Brock J. (2013). Current status in non-invasive prenatal detection of Down syndrome, Trisomy 18, and Trisomy 13 using cell-free DNA in maternal plasma. *Journal of Obstetrics and Gynaecology Canada, 35*(2), 177–181.

23. Sybert V. P., McCauley E. (2004). Turner's syndrome. *New England Journal of Medicine, 351,* 1227–1238.

24. Gravholt C. H. (2004). Epidemiological, endocrine and metabolic features in Turner syndrome. *European Journal of Endocrinology, 151,* 657–687.

25. Lanfranco F., Kamischke A., Zitzmann M., Nieschlag E. (2004). Klinefelter syndrome. *Lancet, 364,* 273–283.

26. Wattendorf D. J., Muenke M. (2005). Klinefelter syndrome. *American Family Physician, 72,* 2259–2262.

27. Dimauro S., Davidzon G. (2005). Mitochondrial DNA and disease. *Annals of Medicine, 37,* 222–232.

28. Chaturvedi S., Bala K., Thakur G., Suri V. (2005). Mitochondrial encephalomyopathies: Advances in understanding. *Medical Science Monitor, 11,* RA238–RA246.

29. Brent R. L. (2004). Environmental causes of congenital malformations: The pediatrician's role in dealing with these complex clinical problems caused by a multiplicity of environmental and genetic factors. *Pediatrics, 113,* 957–968.

30. Young V. S. L. (2005). Teratogenicity and drugs in breast milk. In Koda-Kimble M. A., Young L. Y., Kradjan W. A. (Eds.), *Applied therapeutics: The clinical use of drugs* (8th ed., pp. 47-1–47-15). Philadelphia, PA: Lippincott Williams & Wilkins.

31. Bailey B. A., Sokol R. J. (2008). Pregnancy and alcohol use: Evidence and recommendations for prenatal care. *Clinical Obstetrics and Gynecology, 51*(2), 436–444.

32. Warren K. R., Hewitt B. G., Thomas J. D. (2011). Fetal alcohol spectrum disorders: Research challenges and opportunities. *Alcohol Research & Health, 34*(1), 4–14.

33. Chudley A. E., Conry J., Cook J. L., et al. (2005). Fetal alcohol spectrum disorder: Canadian guidelines for diagnosis. *Canadian Medical Association Journal, 172*(5 suppl) S1–S21.

34. Sokol R. J., Delaney-Black V., Nordstrom B. (2003). Fetal alcohol syndrome. *Journal of the American Medical Association, 290,* 2996–2999.

35. Wattendorf D. J., Muenke M. (2005). Fetal alcohol spectrum disorders. *American Family Physician, 72,* 279–285.

36. Riley E. P., McGee C. L. (2005). Fetal alcohol spectrum disorders: An overview with emphasis on changes in brain and behavior. *Experimental Biology and Medicine, 230,* 357–365.

37. Public Health Agency of Canada. (2008). Folic acid and prevention of neural tube defects. Available online at: http://www.phac-aspc.gc.ca/fa-af/fa-af08-eng.php. Accessed February 2, 2014.

38. Feldman D. M., Timms D., Borgida A. F. (2010). Toxoplasmosis, parvovirus, and cytomegalovirus in pregnancy. *Clinics in Laboratory Medicine, 30*(3), 709–720.

39. Summers A. M., Langlois S., Wyatt P., Wilson R. D.; Society of Obstetricians and Gynaecologists of Canada. (2007). Prenatal screening for fetal aneuploidy. *Journal of Obstetrics and Gynaecology Canada, 29*(2), 146–161.

40. Wilson R. D. (2000). Amniocentesis and chorionic villus sampling. *Current Opinion in Obstetrics and Gynecology, 12,* 81–86.

Visit the Point. **http://thePoint.lww.com for animations, journal articles, and more!**

Neoplasia

8

Cancer is the leading cause of death in Canada and, after heart disease, the second leading cause of death in the United States.[1,2] In Canada, for the year 2015, it was estimated that 196,900 people would be newly diagnosed with cancer and 78,000 people would die of the disease.[1] Trends in cancer survival demonstrate that relative 5-year survival rates have improved since the early 1960s. Although the mortality rate has decreased, the number of cancer deaths has increased due to the aging and expanding population. According to the Canadian Cancer Society, 43% of new cancer cases and 61% of deaths occur among people who are at least 70 years of age.[1]

Cancer is not a single disease. It can originate in almost any organ, with the skin being the most common site. Excluding skin cancers, the prostate is the most common site in men and the breast is the most common site in women (Fig. 8.1). The ability to cure cancer varies considerably and depends on the type of cancer and the extent of the disease at time of diagnosis. Cancers such as acute lymphoblastic leukemia, Hodgkin disease, testicular cancer, and osteosarcoma, which only a few decades ago had poor prognoses, are today cured in many cases. However, lung cancer, which is the leading cause of death in men and women in Canada and the United States,[1,2] is resistant to therapy, and although some progress has been made in its treatment, mortality rates remain high.

This chapter is divided into six sections: concepts of cell differentiation and growth, characteristics of benign and malignant neoplasms, etiology of cancer, clinical manifestations, screening, diagnosis and treatment, and childhood cancers. Hematologic malignancies (lymphomas and leukemias) are presented in Chapter 15.

CONCEPTS OF CELL DIFFERENTIATION AND GROWTH

After completing this section of the chapter, you should be able to meet the following objectives:

- Define neoplasm and explain how neoplastic growth differs from the normal adaptive changes seen in atrophy, hypertrophy, and hyperplasia.

- Distinguish between cell proliferation and differentiation.
- Describe the phases of the cell cycle.
- Explain the function of cyclins, cyclin-dependent kinases, and cyclin-dependent kinase inhibitors in terms of regulating the cell cycle.
- Describe the properties of stem cells.

Cancer is a disorder of altered cell differentiation and growth. The resulting process is called *neoplasia,* meaning "new growth," and the new growth is called a *neoplasm.* Unlike changes in tissue growth that occur with hypertrophy and hyperplasia, the growth of a neoplasm tends to be uncoordinated and relatively autonomous in that it lacks normal regulatory controls over cell growth and division. Neoplasms tend to increase in size and continue to grow after the stimulus that evoked the change has ceased or the needs of the organism have been met.

Normal tissue renewal and repair involves two components: cell proliferation and differentiation. *Proliferation,* or the process of cell division, is an inherent adaptive mechanism for cell replacement when old cells die or additional cells are needed. *Differentiation* is the process whereby cells become increasingly more specialized with each mitotic division. Apoptosis, which is discussed in Chapter 5, is a form of programmed cell death that eliminates senescent cells, cells with deoxyribonucleic acid (DNA) damage, or unwanted cells. In a given tissue, the size of a population of cells is determined by the rates of cell proliferation, differentiation, and death by apoptosis.[3,4]

CELL PROLIFERATION AND GROWTH

- Tissue growth and repair involve cell proliferation, differentiation, and apoptosis.
- Cell proliferation is the process whereby tissues acquire new or replacement cells through mitotic cell division.
- Cell differentiation is the orderly process in which proliferating cells are transformed into different, more specialized, mature cell types. It determines the microscopic characteristics of the cell, its functions, and its life span. Cells that are fully differentiated are no longer capable of cell division.
- Apoptosis is a form of programmed cell death that eliminates senescent, DNA-damaged, or unwanted cells.

The Cell Cycle

The cell cycle is an orderly sequence of events that occur as a cell duplicates its contents and divides. During the cell cycle, genetic information is duplicated and the duplicated chromosomes are appropriately aligned for distribution between two genetically identical daughter cells.

The cell cycle is divided into four distinct phases, referred to as G_1, S, G_2, and M. G_1 (*gap 1*) is the postmitotic phase during which DNA synthesis ceases while ribonucleic acid (RNA) and protein synthesis and cell growth take place.[5] During the *S phase,* DNA synthesis occurs, giving rise to two separate sets of chromosomes, one for each daughter cell. G_2 (*gap 2*) is the premitotic phase and is similar to G_1 in that DNA synthesis ceases while RNA and protein synthesis continue. Collectively G_1, S, and G_2 are referred to as *interphase.* The *M phase* is the phase of nuclear division or mitosis, and cytokinesis or cytoplasm division. Continually dividing cells, such as some cells in the stratified squamous epithelium of the skin, continue to cycle from one mitotic division to the next. When environmental conditions are adverse, such as nutrient or growth factor unavailability, or when cells are highly specialized, cells may exit the cell cycle, becoming mitotically quiescent, and reside in a special resting state known as G_0. Cells in G_0 may reenter the cell cycle in response to extracellular nutrients, growth factors, hormones, and other signals such as blood loss or tissue injury that trigger cell renewal.[5] Highly specialized and terminally differentiated cells, such as neurons, may permanently stay in G_0.

Within the cell cycle are checkpoints where pauses or arrests can be made if the specific events in the phases of

---

Estimated New Cases

Prostate (23.9%)	Breast (25.9%)
Colorectal (13.9%)	Lung (13.5%)
Lung (13.5%)	Colorectal (11.5%)
Bladder (6.1%)	Uterus (6.5%)
Non-Hodgkin lymphoma (4.5%)	Thyroid (5.0%)
Kidney (3.9%)	Non-Hodgkin lymphoma (3.8%)
Melanoma (3.6%)	Melanoma (3.2%)
Leukemia (3.5%)	Ovary (2.9%)
Oral (2.9%)	Leukemia (2.8%)
Pancreas (2.4%)	Pancreas (2.5%)
All other sites (21.7%)	All other sites (22.4%)

Estimated Deaths

Lung (26.6%)	Lung (27.0%)
Colorectal (12.4%)	Breast (13.6%)
Prostate (10.1%)	Colorectal (11.5%)
Pancreas (5.6%)	Pancreas (6.2%)
Bladder (4.0%)	Ovary (4.7%)
Esophagus (3.9%)	Non-Hodgkin lymphoma (3.3%)
Leukemia (3.8%)	Leukemia (3.1%)
Non-Hodgkin lymphoma (3.5%)	Uterus (2.8%)
Stomach (3.1%)	Brain/CNS (2.3%)
Brain/CNS (3.0%)	Stomach (2.1%)
All other sites (22.0%)	All other sites (23.4%)

Note: Percentages may not total 100 percent due to rounding.

FIGURE 8.1 • Canadian cancer incidence and mortality by site and sex.

Understanding ❯ The Cell Cycle

A cell reproduces by performing an orderly sequence of events called the *cell cycle*. The cell cycle is divided into four phases of unequal duration that include the (1) synthesis (S) and mitosis (M) phases that are separated by (2) two gaps (G_1 and G_2). There is also (3) a dormant phase (G_0) during which the cell may leave the cell cycle. Movement through each of these phases is mediated at (4) specific checkpoints that are controlled by specific enzymes and proteins called *cyclins*.

1. Synthesis and Mitosis

Synthesis (S) and mitosis (M) represent the two major phases of the cell cycle. The S phase, which takes about 10 to 12 hours, is the period of DNA synthesis and replication of the chromosomes. The M phase, which usually takes less than an hour, involves formation of the mitotic spindle and cell division with formation of two daughter cells.

2. Gaps 1 and 2

Because most cells require time to grow and double their mass of proteins and organelles, extra gaps (G) are inserted into the cell cycle. G_1 is the stage during which the cell is starting to prepare for DNA replication and mitosis through protein synthesis and an increase in organelle and cytoskeletal elements. G_2 is the premitotic phase. During this phase, enzymes and other proteins needed for cell division are synthesized and moved to their proper sites.

3. Gap 0

G_0 is the stage after mitosis during which a cell may leave the cell cycle and either remain in a state of inactivity or reenter the cell cycle at another time. Labile cells, such as blood cell precurors and those that line the gastrointestinal tract, do not enter G_0 but continue cycling. Stable cells, such as hepatocytes, enter G_0 after mitosis but can reenter the cell cycle when stimulated by the loss of other cells. Permanent cells, such as neurons that become terminally differentiated after mitosis, leave the cell cycle and are no longer capable of cell renewal.

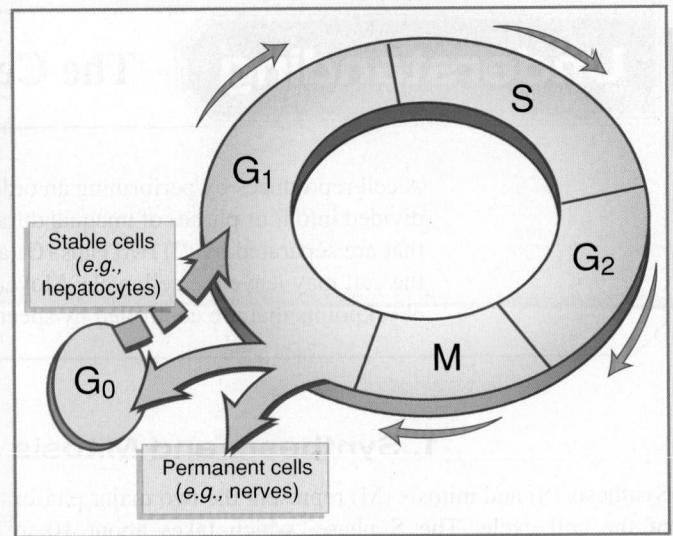

4. Checkpoints and Cylins

In most cells there are several checkpoints in the cell cycle, at which time the cycle can be arrested if previous events have not been completed. For example, the G_1/S checkpoint monitors whether the DNA in the chromosomes is damaged by radiation or chemicals, and the G_2/M checkpoint prevents entry into mitosis if DNA replication is not complete.

The cyclins are a family of proteins that control entry and progression of cells through the cell cycle. They function by activating proteins called *cyclin-dependent kinases* (CDKs). Different combinations of cyclins and CDKs are associated with each stage of the cell cycle. In addition to the synthesis and degradation of the cyclins, the cyclin-CDK complexes are regulated by the binding of CDK inhibitors. The CDK inhibitors are particularly important in regulating cell cycle checkpoints during which mistakes in DNA replication are repaired.

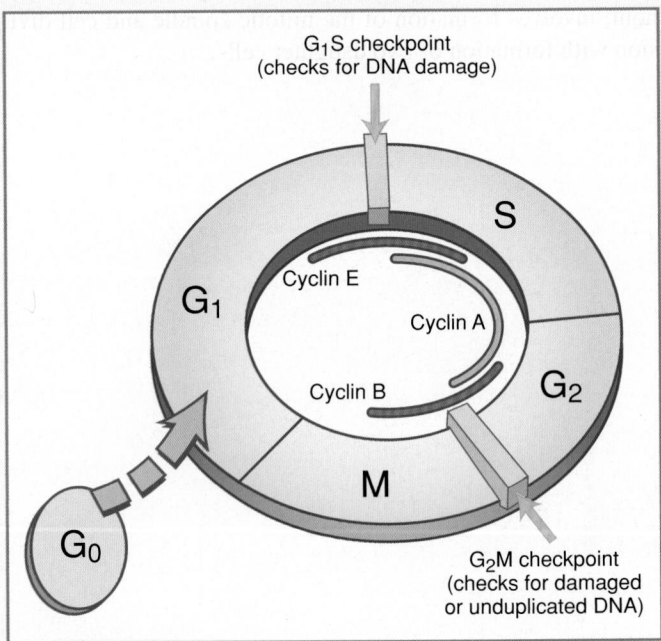

the cell cycle have not been completed. Mitosis is prevented until DNA is properly replicated. Chromosome separation in mitosis is delayed until all spindle fibres have properly attached to the chromosomes. There are also opportunities for ensuring the accuracy of DNA replication. These DNA damage checkpoints allow for any defects to be edited and repaired, thereby ensuring that each daughter cell receives a full complement of genetic information, identical to that of the parent cell.[5]

The cyclins are a family of proteins that control the entry and progression of cells through the cell cycle. Cyclins bind and activate proteins called *cyclin-dependent kinases* (CDKs).

Kinases are enzymes that phosphorylate proteins. The CDKs phosphorylate specific target proteins and are expressed continuously during the cell cycle but in an inactive form, whereas the cyclins are synthesized during specific phases of the cell cycle and then degraded by ubiquitination once their task is completed.[6] Different arrangements of cyclins and CDKs are associated with each stage of the cell cycle. For example, cyclin B and CDK1 control the transition from G_2 to M. As the cell moves into G_2, cyclin B is synthesized and binds to CDK1. The cyclin B–CDK1 complex then directs the events leading to mitosis, including DNA replication and assembly of the mitotic spindle. Although each phase of the cell cycle is monitored carefully, the transition from G_2 to M is believed to be one of the most important checkpoints in the cell cycle. In addition to the synthesis and degradation of the cyclins, the cyclin–CDK complexes are regulated by the binding of CDK inhibitors. The CDK inhibitors are particularly important in regulating cell cycle checkpoints during which mistakes in DNA replication are repaired. Manipulation of cyclins, CDKs, and CDK inhibitors serves as the basis for development of newer forms of drug therapy that can be used in cancer treatment.[7]

Cell Proliferation

Cell proliferation is the process of increasing cell numbers by mitotic cell division. In normal tissue, cell proliferation is regulated so that the number of cells actively dividing is equivalent to the number dying or being shed. In humans, there are two major categories of cells: gametes and somatic cells. The *gametes* (ovum and sperm) are *haploid,* having only one set of chromosomes from one parent, and are designed specifically for sexual fusion. After fusion, a *diploid* cell containing both sets of chromosomes is formed. This cell is the *somatic cell* that goes on to form the rest of the body.

In terms of cell proliferation, the 200 or more cell types of the body can be divided into three large groups: (1) the well-differentiated neurons and cells of skeletal and cardiac muscle that rarely divide and reproduce; (2) the progenitor or parent cells that continue to divide and reproduce, present among bone marrow, skin epidermal, and gastrointestinal epithelial cells; and (3) the undifferentiated stem cells that can be triggered to enter the cell cycle and produce large numbers of progenitor cells when the need arises. The rates of reproduction of cells vary greatly. White blood cells and cells that line the gastrointestinal tract live several days and must be replaced constantly. In most tissues, the rate of cell reproduction is greatly increased when tissue is injured or lost. Bleeding, for example, stimulates the renal production of erythropoietin which induces rapid reproduction of the blood-forming cells of the bone marrow. In some types of tissue, the genetic program for cell replication normally is suppressed, but can be reactivated under certain conditions. The liver, for example, has extensive regenerative capabilities under certain conditions, such as surgical partial hepatectomy.

Cell Differentiation

Cell differentiation is the process whereby proliferating cells become progressively more specialized cell types. This process results in a fully differentiated adult cell that has a specific set of structural, functional, and life expectancy characteristics. For example, the red blood cell is a terminally differentiated cell that has been programmed to develop into a concave disk that functions as a vehicle for oxygen transport and lives approximately 120 days.

During human embryogenesis, all of the different cell types of the body originate from a single cell—the fertilized ovum. As the embryonic cells increase in number, they engage in an orderly and coordinated process of differentiation that is necessary for the development of all the various organs of the body. The process of differentiation is regulated by a combination of internal processes involving the expression of specific genes and external stimuli provided by neighbouring cells, the extracellular matrix, exposure to substances in the maternal circulation, and a variety of growth factors, cytokines, oxygen, and nutrients.

What makes the cells of one organ different from those of another organ are the specific genes that are expressed and the particular pattern of gene expression. Although all cells have the same complement of genes, only a small number of these genes are expressed in postnatal life. When cells, such as those of the developing embryo, differentiate and give rise to committed cells of a particular tissue type, the appropriate genes are maintained in an active state, while the rest remain inactive. Normally, the rate of cell reproduction and the process of cell differentiation are precisely controlled in prenatal and postnatal life so that both of these mechanisms cease once the appropriate numbers and types of cells are formed.

The process of differentiation occurs in orderly steps. With each progressive step, increased specialization is exchanged for a loss of ability to develop different cell characteristics and different cell types. As a cell becomes more highly specialized, the stimuli that are able to induce mitosis become more limited. Neurons, which are highly specialized cells, lose their ability to divide and reproduce once development of the nervous system is complete. More importantly, there are very few remaining precursor cells to direct their replacement. However, appropriate numbers of these cell types are generated in the embryo such that loss of a certain percentage of cells does not affect the total cell population and specific functions.

In some tissues, such as the skin and mucosal lining of the gastrointestinal tract, a high degree of cell renewal continues throughout life. Even in these continuously renewing cell populations, the more specialized cells are unable to divide. These cell populations rely on *progenitor* or *parent cells* of the same lineage that have not yet differentiated to the extent that they have lost their ability to divide. These cells are sufficiently differentiated so that their daughter cells are limited to the same cell line, but they are insufficiently differentiated to preclude the potential for active proliferation. However, their cell renewal properties are restricted by growth factors required for cell division.

Another type of cell, called a *stem cell,* remains incompletely differentiated throughout life. Stem cells are reserve cells that remain quiescent until there is a need for cell replenishment, in which case they divide, producing other stem cells and cells that can carry out the functions of the differentiated cell. When a stem cell divides, one daughter cell retains the same genetic program and the stem cell characteristics, and the other daughter cell becomes a progenitor cell that proceeds through a process that leads to terminal differentiation (Fig. 8.2). The progeny of each progenitor cell follow

Stem cell

Stem cell

Progenitor cell

Daughter cells

Differentiated cells

FIGURE 8.2 • Mechanism of stem cell–mediated cell replacement. Division of a stem cell with an unlimited potential for proliferation results in one daughter cell, which retains the characteristics of a stem cell, and a second daughter cell that differentiates into a progenitor or parent cell, with a limited potential for differentiation and proliferation. As the daughter cells of the progenitor cell proliferate they become more differentiated, until they reach the stage where they are fully differentiated.

more restricted genetic programs, with the differentiating cells undergoing multiple mitotic divisions in the process of becoming a mature cell type and with each generation of cells becoming more specialized. In this way, a single stem cell can give rise to the many cells needed for normal tissue repair or blood cell production. When the dividing cells become fully differentiated, the rate of mitotic division is reduced. In the immune system, for example, appropriately stimulated B lymphocytes become progressively more differentiated as they undergo successive mitotic divisions, until they become mature plasma cells that no longer can divide but are capable of secreting large amounts of antibody.

Stem cells have two important properties, that of self-renewal and potency. *Self-renewal* means that the stem cells can undergo numerous mitotic divisions while maintaining an undifferentiated state.[8] The term *potency* is used to define the differentiation potential of stem cells. *Totipotent stem cells* are those produced by fertilization of the egg. The first few cells produced after fertilization are totipotent and can differentiate into embryonic and extraembryonic cells. Totipotent stem cells give rise to *pluripotent stem cells* that can differentiate into the three germ layers of the embryo. *Multipotent stem cells* are cells such as hematopoietic stem cells that give rise to a family of cells. Finally, *unipotent stem cells* produce only one cell type but retain the property of self-renewal.

It has become useful to categorize stem cells into two basic categories: embryonic stem cells and adult stem cells (sometimes called *somatic stem cells*).[9,10] *Embryonic stem cells* are pluripotent cells derived from the inner cell mass of the blastocyst stage of the embryo. These give rise to the three embryonic germ cell layers. As development progresses, the embryo forms germline stem cells for reproduction and somatic stem cells for organogenesis. Both the germline stem cells and the somatic stem cells retain the property of self-renewal. *Adult stem cells* reside in specialized microenvironments that differ depending on tissue type. These stem cells have important roles in homeostasis, as they contribute to tissue regeneration and replacement of cells lost to apoptosis.[10]

An important role of stem cells in the pathogenesis of cancer has been identified, and continues to be elucidated. Cancer stem cells (also called *tumour-initiating cells* [T-ICs]) have been identified in many common human cancers where they represent a small subpopulation of tumour cells. There is strong experimental support for the notion that, in certain cancers, cancer stem cells are the initial target for malignant transformation. If confirmed, these findings could have important implications for cancer treatment aimed at the elimination of proliferating cells.[9]

IN SUMMARY

The term neoplasm refers to an abnormal mass of tissue in which the growth exceeds and is uncoordinated with that of the normal tissues. Unlike normal cellular adaptive processes such as hypertrophy and hyperplasia, neoplasms do not obey the laws of normal cell growth. They serve no useful purpose, they do not occur in response to an appropriate stimulus, and they continue to grow at the expense of the host.

The process of cell growth and division is called the cell cycle. It is divided into four phases: G_1, the postmitotic phase, during which protein synthesis and cell growth take place; S, the phase during which DNA synthesis occurs, giving rise to two separate sets of chromosomes; G_2, the premitotic phase, during which RNA and protein synthesis continues; and M, the phase of cell mitosis or cell division. The G_0 phase is a resting or quiescent phase in which nondividing cells reside. The entry into and progression through the various stages of the cell cycle are controlled by cyclins, cyclin-dependent kinases, and cyclin-dependent kinase inhibitors.

Normal tissue renewal and repair involves cell proliferation, differentiation, and apoptosis. Proliferation, or the process of cell division, is an inherent adaptive mechanism for cell replacement when old cells die or additional cells are needed. Differentiation is the process of specialization whereby new cells acquire the structure and function of the cells they replace. Apoptosis is a form of programmed cell death that eliminates senescent cells, cells with damaged DNA, or unwanted cells. Body cells can be divided into two large groups: the well-differentiated neurons and cells of skeletal and cardiac muscle that rarely divide and reproduce, and the progenitor or parent cells that continue to divide and reproduce, such as blood cells, skin cells, and liver cells.

A third category of cells are the stem cells that remain quiescent until there is a need for cell replenishment, in which case they divide, producing other stem cells and cells that can carry out the functions of differentiated cells. Stem cells have two important properties, those of self-renewal and potency. Self-renewal means that the stem cells can undergo numerous mitotic divisions while maintaining an undifferentiated state. The term potency is used to define the differentiation potential of stem cells. There are two main categories of stem cells. Embryonic stem cells are pluripotent cells derived from the inner cell mass of the blastocyst stage of the embryo. Adult stem cells reside in specialized microenvironments and have important roles in homeostasis, as they contribute to tissue regeneration and replacement of cells lost to apoptosis. Cancer stem cells have been identified in breast, prostate, acute myeloid leukemia, and other cancers.

CONCEPTSin action**ANIMATION**

CHARACTERISTICS OF BENIGN AND MALIGNANT NEOPLASMS

After completing this section of the chapter, you should be able to meet the following objectives:

- Cite the method used for naming benign and malignant neoplasms.
- State at least five ways in which benign and malignant neoplasms differ.
- Relate the properties of cell differentiation to the development of a cancer cell clone and the behaviour of the tumour.
- Trace the pathway for hematologic spread of a metastatic cancer cell.
- Use the concepts of growth fraction and doubling time to explain the growth of cancerous tissue.

Body organs are composed of two types of tissue: parenchymal tissue and stromal or supporting tissue. The *parenchymal tissue cells* represent the functional components of an organ. The parenchymal cells of a tumour determine its behaviour and are the component for which a tumour is named. The *supporting tissue* includes the extracellular matrix and connective tissue that surround the parenchymal cells. It contains the lymphatic vessels and blood vessels that provide nourishment and support for the parenchymal cells.

Terminology

The term *tumour* is used to define a mass of cells that arises because of overgrowth. Although not synonymous, the terms *tumour* and *neoplasm* often are used interchangeably. Neoplasms usually are classified as benign or malignant. Neoplasms that contain well-differentiated cells that are clustered together in a single mass are considered to be *benign*. These tumours usually do not cause death unless their location or size

interferes with vital functions. In contrast, malignant neoplasms are less well differentiated and have the ability to break loose, enter the circulatory or lymphatic system, and form secondary malignant tumours at other sites. *Malignant neoplasms* frequently cause suffering and death if untreated or uncontrolled.

Tumours usually are named by adding the suffix *-oma* to the parenchymal tissue type from which the growth originated.[11] Thus, a benign tumour of glandular epithelial tissue is called an *adenoma,* and a benign tumour of bone tissue is called an *osteoma.* The term *carcinoma* is used to designate a malignant tumour of epithelial tissue origin. In the case of a malignant tumour of glandular epithelial tissue, the term *adenocarcinoma* is used. Malignant tumours of mesenchymal origin are called *sarcomas (e.g.,* osteosarcoma). *Blastoma* is a malignant cancer that is usually identified in infants and children. It originates from embryonic tissue consisting of immature or primitive precursor cells. *Papillomas* are benign, microscopic or macroscopic finger-like projections that grow on any surface. A *polyp* is a growth that projects from a mucosal surface, such as the intestine. Although the term usually implies a benign neoplasm, some malignant tumours also initially appear as polyps. Adenomatous polyps are considered precursors to adenocarcinomas of the colon. *Oncology* is the study of tumours and their treatment. Table 8.1 lists the names of selected benign and malignant tumours according to tissue types.

BENIGN AND MALIGNANT NEOPLASMS

- A neoplasm, benign or malignant, represents a new growth.
- Benign neoplasms are well-differentiated tumours that resemble the tissues of origin but have lost the ability to control cell proliferation. They grow by expansion, are enclosed in a fibrous capsule, and do not cause death unless their location is such that it interrupts vital body functions.
- Malignant neoplasms are less well-differentiated tumours that have lost the ability to control both cell proliferation and differentiation. They grow in a disorganized and uncontrolled manner to invade surrounding tissues, have cells that break loose and travel to distant sites to form metastases, and inevitably cause suffering and death unless their growth can be controlled through treatment.

Benign and malignant neoplasms usually are distinguished by their (1) cell characteristics, (2) rate of growth, (3) manner of growth, (4) capacity to invade and metastasize to other parts of the body, and (5) potential for causing death. The characteristics of benign and malignant neoplasms are summarized in Table 8.2.

Benign Neoplasms

Benign tumours are composed of well-differentiated cells that resemble the cells of the tissues of origin and are characterized

TABLE 8.1 NAMES OF SELECTED BENIGN AND MALIGNANT TUMOURS ACCORDING TO TISSUE TYPES

TISSUE TYPE	BENIGN TUMOURS	MALIGNANT TUMOURS
Epithelial		
Surface	Papilloma	Squamous cell carcinoma
Glandular	Adenoma	Adenocarcinoma
Connective		
Fibrous	Fibroma	Fibrosarcoma
Adipose	Lipoma	Liposarcoma
Cartilage	Chondroma	Chondrosarcoma
Bone	Osteoma	Osteosarcoma
Blood vessels	Hemangioma	Hemangiosarcoma
Lymph vessels	Lymphangioma	Lymphangiosarcoma
Lymph tissue	—	Lymphosarcoma
Muscle		
Smooth	Leiomyoma	Leiomyosarcoma
Striated	Rhabdomyoma	Rhabdomyosarcoma
Neural Tissue		
Nerve cell	Neuroma	Neuroblastoma
Glial tissue	Glioma	Glioblastoma, astrocytoma, medullo-blastoma, oligodendroglioma
Nerve sheaths	Neurilemmoma	Neurilemmal sarcoma
Meninges	Meningioma	Meningeal sarcoma
Hematologic		
Granulocytic	—	Myelocytic leukemia
Erythrocytic	—	Erythrocytic leukemia
Plasma cells	—	Multiple myeloma
Lymphocytic	—	Lymphocytic leukemia or lymphoma
Monocytic	—	Monocytic leukemia
Endothelial Tissue		
Blood vessels	Hemangioma	Hemangiosarcoma
Lymph vessels	Lymphangioma	Lymphangiosarcoma

TABLE 8.2 CHARACTERISTICS OF BENIGN AND MALIGNANT NEOPLASMS

CHARACTERISTICS	BENIGN	MALIGNANT
Cell characteristics	Well-differentiated cells that resemble cells in the tissue of origin	Cells are undifferentiated, with anaplasia and atypical structure that often bears little resemblance to cells in the tissue of origin
Rate of growth	Usually progressive and slow; may come to a standstill or regress	Variable and depends on level of differentiation; the more undifferentiated the cells, the more rapid the rate of growth
Mode of growth	Grows by expansion without invading the surrounding tissues; usually encapsulated	Grows by invasion, sending out processes that infiltrate the surrounding tissues
Metastasis	Does not spread by metastasis	Gains access to blood and lymph channels to metastasize to other areas of the body

by a slow, progressive rate of growth that may come to a standstill or regress. For unknown reasons, benign tumours have lost the ability to suppress the genetic program for cell proliferation but have retained the program for normal cell differentiation. They grow by expansion and remain localized to their site of origin, lacking the capacity to infiltrate, invade, or metastasize to distant sites. Because they expand slowly, they develop a surrounding rim of compressed connective tissue called a *fibrous capsule*.[11] The capsule is responsible for a sharp line of demarcation between the benign tumour and the adjacent tissues, a factor that facilitates surgical removal.

Benign tumours are usually much less of a threat to health and well-being than malignant tumours, and they usually do not cause death unless they interfere with vital functions because of their location. For instance, a benign tumour growing in the cranial cavity can eventually cause death by compressing brain structures. Benign tumours also can cause disturbances in the function of adjacent or distant structures by producing pressure on tissues, blood vessels, or nerves. Some benign tumours are also known for their ability to cause alterations in body function by abnormally producing hormones.

Malignant Neoplasms

Malignant neoplasms, which invade and destroy nearby tissue and spread to other parts of the body, tend to grow rapidly and spread widely, and have the potential to cause death. Because of their rapid rate of growth, malignant tumours may compress blood vessels and outgrow their blood supply, causing ischemia and tissue injury. Some malignancies secrete hormones, cytokines, enzymes, or toxins, some of which may induce an inflammatory response that injures normal tissue as well as the tumour itself. A number of malignancies secrete vascular endothelial cell growth factor, which increases the blood supply to the tumour and facilitates more rapid growth.

There are two categories of malignant neoplasms—solid tumours and hematologic cancers. Solid tumours initially are confined to a specific tissue or organ. As the growth of the primary solid tumour progresses, cells detach from the original tumour mass, invade the surrounding tissue, and enter the blood and lymph systems to spread to distant sites, a process termed *metastasis*. Hematologic cancers involve cells normally found in the blood and lymph, thereby making them disseminated diseases from the beginning.

Carcinoma in situ is a localized preinvasive lesion. As an example, in breast ductal carcinoma in situ, the cells have not crossed the basement membrane. Depending on its location, in situ lesions usually can be removed surgically or treated so that the chances of recurrence are small. For example, carcinoma in situ of the cervix is essentially 100% curable.

Cancer Cell Characteristics

Cancer cells are characterized by two main features: (1) abnormal and rapid proliferation; and (2) loss of differentiation so that they do not exhibit normal features and properties of differentiated cells, and hence are more similar to embryonic cells.

The term *anaplasia* describes the loss of cell differentiation in cancerous tissue.[11] Undifferentiated cancer cells are marked by a number of morphologic changes. Both the cells and nuclei display variations in size and shape, a condition referred to as *pleomorphism*. Their nuclei are variable in size and bizarre in shape, their chromatin is coarse and clumped, and their nucleoli are often considerably larger than normal (Fig. 8.3A). Frequently, the nuclei contain an abnormal number of chromosomes (*e.g.*, aneuploidy). The cells of undifferentiated tumours usually display greater numbers of cells in mitosis due to their high rate of proliferation. They also display atypical, bizarre mitotic figures, sometimes producing tripolar, tetrapolar, or multipolar spindles (Fig. 8.3B). Highly anaplastic cancer cells, whatever their tissue of origin, begin to resemble undifferentiated or embryonic cells more

FIGURE 8.3 • Anaplastic features of malignant tumours. **A:** The cells of this anaplastic carcinoma are highly pleomorphic (*i.e.,* they vary in size and shape). The nuclei are hyperchromatic and are large relative to the cytoplasm. Multinucleated tumour giant cells are present (*arrows*). **B:** A malignant cell in metaphase exhibits an abnormal mitotic figure. (From Rubin R., Strayer D. S. (Eds.). (2012). *Rubin's pathology: Clinicopathologic foundations of medicine* (6th ed., p. 162). Philadelphia, PA: Lippincott Williams & Wilkins.)

TABLE 8.3 COMPARISON OF NORMAL CELL CHARACTERISTICS WITH THOSE OF CANCER CELLS

CHARACTERISTIC	NORMAL CELLS	CANCER CELLS
Growth	Regulated	Unregulated
Differentiation	High	Low
Genetic stability	Stable	Unstable
Growth factor dependence	Dependent	Independent
Density-dependent inhibition	High	Low
Cell-to-cell adhesion	High	Low
Anchorage dependence	High	Low
Cell-to-cell communication	High	Low
Cell life span	Limited	Unlimited
Antigen expression	Absent	May be present
Substance production (*e.g.*, proteases, hormones)	Normal	Abnormal
Cytoskeletal composition and arrangement	Normal	Abnormal

than they do their tissue of origin. Some cancers display only slight anaplasia, whereas others display marked anaplasia. The cytologic/histologic grading of tumours is based on the degree of differentiation and the number of proliferating cells. The closer the tumour cells resemble comparable normal tissue cells, both morphologically and functionally, the lower the grade. Accordingly, on a scale ranging from grades I to IV, grade I neoplasms are well differentiated and grade IV are poorly differentiated and display marked anaplasia.[11]

The characteristics of altered proliferation and differentiation are associated with a number of other changes in cell characteristics and functions that distinguish cancer cells from their normally differentiated counterparts. These changes, which are listed in Table 8.3, include (1) genetic instability; (2) growth factor independence; (3) loss of cell density–dependent inhibition; (4) loss of cohesiveness and adhesion; (5) loss of anchorage dependence; (6) faulty cell-to-cell communication; (7) indefinite cell life span (immortality); (8) expression of altered tissue antigens; (9) abnormal secretion of degradative enzymes that enable invasion and metastatic spread, or ectopic production of hormones; and (10) abnormal cytoskeletal characteristics.

Genetic Instability. Most cancer cells exhibit a characteristic called *genetic instability* that is often considered to be a hallmark of cancer.[12] The concept arose after the realization that uncorrected mutations in normal cells are rare because of the numerous cellular mechanisms to prevent them. To account for the high frequency of mutations in cancer cells, it is thought that cancer cells have a "mutation phenotype" with genetic instability that contributes to the development and progression of cancer. Characteristics of genetic instability include aneuploidy, in which chromosomes are lost or gained; intrachromosomal instability, which includes insertions, deletions, and

amplifications; microsatellite instability, which involves short, repetitive sequences of DNA; and point mutations.

Growth Factor Independence. Another characteristic of cancer cells is the ability to proliferate even in the absence of growth factors. This characteristic is often observed when cancer cells are propagated in cell culture—the addition of serum, which is rich in growth factors, is unnecessary for the cancers to proliferate, whereas normal cells grown in culture often die without serum or growth factor addition. In some cases, this is because the cancer cells can rapidly divide without growth factor binding to its receptor. Breast cancer cells that do not express estrogen receptors are an example. These cancer cells grow even in the absence of estrogen, which is the normal growth stimulus for breast duct epithelial cells. Some cancer cells may produce their own growth factors and secrete them into the culture medium, whereas others have abnormal receptors or signalling proteins that may inappropriately activate growth signalling pathways in the cells.

Cell Density–Dependent Inhibition. Cancer cells often lose *cell density–dependent inhibition,* which is the cessation of growth after cells reach a particular density. This is sometimes referred to as *contact inhibition* because cells often stop growing when they come into contact with each other. In wound healing, contact inhibition causes tissue growth to cease at the point where the edges of the wound come together. Cancer cells, however, tend to grow rampantly without regard for adjacent tissue. Possible explanations for cancer cell loss of density-dependent contact inhibition include growth factor independence, oxidative mechanisms, and alterations in interactions between cell adhesion and cell growth signalling pathways (*e.g.,* surface integrin receptors, mitogen-activated protein [MAP] kinase, and focal adhesion kinase [FAK] phosphorylation).[12,13]

Cell Cohesiveness and Adhesion. The reduced tendency of cancer cells to stick together (*i.e.,* loss of cohesiveness and adhesiveness) permits shedding of the tumour's surface cells; these cells appear in the surrounding body fluids or secretions and often can be detected using cytologic methods. As discussed in Chapter 4, cadherins are adhesion molecules that link one cell with adjacent cells. Extracellularly, the cadherins of one cell bind to cadherins of adjacent cells, causing cell-to-cell attachment. Intracellularly, cadherins are connected to the actin cytoskeleton through protein intermediates, including the catenins. The cadherin–catenin–actin complex, acting with other proteins, has been proposed to be involved with cell migration, apoptosis, and cell cycle regulation. In some cancers, the cell adhesion molecule E-cadherin appears to play an important role in the lack of cohesiveness of cancer cells and the increased tendency for cancer cells to break free and migrate into the surrounding tissues. E-cadherin is reduced at the cell surface, whereas its partner protein β-catenin accumulates within the cancer cells and associates with the actin cytoskeletal-binding protein actinin-4. It has been postulated that the resulting β-catenin interaction with actinin-4 in the absence of E-cadherin may be the "switch" that shuts off cancer cell-to-cell adhesion and activates cancer cell motility and other mechanisms that facilitate invasion and metastasis.[14]

Anchorage Dependence. Cancer cells also differ from their normal counterparts in attaining anchorage independence. Normal epithelial cells must be anchored to either neighbouring cells or the underlying extracellular matrix to live and grow. If normal cells become detached, they often undergo a type of apoptosis known as *anoikis,* a term from the Greek for "homeless." Normal epithelial cells must be attached to either other cells or extracellular matrix to stay alive. Cancer cells, however, frequently remain viable and multiply without normal attachments to other cells and the extracellular matrix. Cancer cells often survive in microenvironments different from those of normal cells. Although the process of anchorage independence is complex and incompletely understood, recent studies have made progress in understanding the genes and mechanistic pathways involved.[15]

Cell-to-Cell Communication. Another characteristic of cancer cells is faulty cell-to-cell communication, a feature that may in turn contribute to other characteristics of cancer cells. Impaired cell-to-cell communication may interfere with formation of intercellular connections and responsiveness to membrane-derived signals. For example, changes in gap junction proteins, which enable cytoplasmic continuity and communication between cells, have been described in some types of cancer.[16]

Life Span. Cancer cells differ from normal cells by being *immortal,* with an unlimited life span. If normal, noncancerous cells are harvested from the body and grown under culture conditions, most cells divide a limited number of times, usually about 50 population doublings, then become senescent and fail to divide further. In contrast to the limited life span of normal cells, cancer cells may divide an infinite number of times, hence achieving immortality. Telomeres are short, repetitive nucleotide sequences at outermost extremities of chromosome arms (see Chapter 3). Telomeres shorten with each cell division and when the length is diminished sufficiently, chromosomes can no longer replicate and cell division will not occur. Most cancer cells maintain high levels of telomerase, an enzyme that prevents telomere shortening; this keeps telomeres from aging and attaining the critically short length that is associated with cellular replicative senescence.

Antigen Expression. Cancer cells also express a number of cell surface molecules or antigens that are immunologically identified as foreign. These *tissue antigens* are coded by the genes of a cell. Many transformed cancer cells revert to embryonic patterns of gene expression and produce antigens that are immunologically distinct from the antigens that are expressed by cells of the well-differentiated tissue from which the cancer originated. Some cancers express fetal antigens that are not produced by comparable cells in the adult. Tumour

antigens may be clinically useful as markers to indicate the presence, recurrence, or progressive growth of a cancer (to be discussed in Tumour Markers section).

Production of Enzymes, Hormones, and Other Substances. Cancer cells may produce substances that normal cells of the tissue of origin either do not produce or secrete in lesser amounts. They may also secrete degradative enzymes that enable invasion and metastatic spread. Cancer cells may also assume hormone synthesis or production and secretion of procoagulant substances that affect clotting mechanisms.

Cytoskeletal Changes. Finally, cancer cells may show cytoskeletal changes and abnormalities. These may involve the appearance of abnormal intermediate filament types or changes in actin filaments and microtubules that facilitate invasion and metastasis. Actin, microtubules, and their regulatory proteins remain the focus of many cancer-related investigations.

Invasion and Metastasis

Unlike benign tumours, which grow by expansion and usually are surrounded by a capsule, cancer spreads by direct invasion and extension, seeding of cancer cells in body cavities, and metastatic spread through the blood or lymph pathways. The word *cancer* is derived from the Latin word meaning "crablike" because cancers grow and spread by sending crablike projections into the surrounding tissues. Most cancers synthesize and secrete enzymes that break down proteins and contribute to the infiltration, invasion, and penetration of the surrounding tissues. The lack of a sharp line of demarcation separating them from the surrounding tissue makes the complete surgical removal of malignant tumours more difficult than removal of benign tumours. Often it is necessary for the surgeon to excise portions of seemingly normal tissue bordering the tumour for the pathologist to establish that cancer-free margins are present around the excised tumour and to ensure that the remaining tissue is cancer free.

The *seeding* of cancer cells into body cavities occurs when a tumour sheds cells into these spaces. Most often, the peritoneal cavity is involved, but other spaces such as the pleural cavity, pericardial cavity, and joint spaces may be involved. Seeding into the peritoneal cavity is particularly common with ovarian cancers. Similar to tissue culture, tumours in these sites grow in masses and are often associated with fluid accumulation (*e.g.,* ascites, pleural effusion).[11] The seeding of cancers is often a concern during the surgical removal of cancers where it is possible inadvertently to introduce free cancer cells into a body cavity such as the peritoneal cavity.[17]

The term *metastasis* is used to describe the development of a secondary tumour in a location distant from the primary tumour.[11,18] Because metastatic tumours frequently retain many of the characteristics of the primary tumour from which they were derived, it usually is possible to determine the site of the primary tumour from the cellular characteristics of the metastatic tumour. Some tumours tend to metastasize early in their developmental course, whereas others do not metastasize until later. Occasionally, a metastatic tumour will be found far advanced before the primary tumour becomes clinically detectable. Malignant tumours of the kidney, for example, may go completely undetected and be asymptomatic until a metastatic lesion is found in the lung.

Metastasis occurs through the lymph channels (*i.e.,* lymphatic spread) and the blood vessels (*i.e.,* hematogenic spread).[11,18] In many types of cancer, the first evidence of disseminated disease is the presence of tumour cells in the lymph nodes that drain the tumour area. When metastasis occurs by the lymphatic route, the tumour cells lodge first in the initial lymph node that receives drainage from the tumour site. Once in this lymph node, the cells may die because of the lack of a proper environment, grow into a discernible mass, or remain dormant for unknown reasons. If they survive and grow, the cancer cells may spread from more distant lymph nodes to the thoracic duct, and then gain access to the vasculature. Cancer cells also may gain access to the vasculature from the initial node and more distant lymph nodes through tumour-associated blood vessels infiltrating the tumour mass.[19]

The term *sentinel node* is used to describe the initial lymph node to which the primary tumour drains.[20] Because the initial metastasis in breast cancer is almost always lymphatic, lymphatic spread and therefore extent of disease may be determined through lymphatic mapping and sentinel lymph node biopsy. This is done by injecting a radioactive tracer and blue dye into the tumour to determine the first lymph node in the route of lymph drainage from the cancer. Once the sentinel lymph node has been identified, it is examined to determine the presence or absence of cancer cells. The procedure is also used to map the spread of melanoma and other cancers that have their initial metastatic spread through the lymphatic system.

With hematologic spread, the blood-borne cancer cells may enter the venous flow that drains the site of the primary neoplasm. Cancer cells may also enter tumour-associated blood vessels that either infiltrate the tumour or are found at the periphery of the tumour. Before entering the general circulation, venous blood from the gastrointestinal tract, pancreas, and spleen is routed through the portal vein to the liver. The liver is therefore a common site for metastatic spread of cancers that originate in these organs. Although the site of hematologic spread usually is related to vascular drainage of the primary tumour, some tumours metastasize to distant and unrelated sites. One explanation is that cells of different tumours tend to metastasize to specific target organs that provide suitable microenvironments containing substances such as cytokines or growth factors that are needed for their survival.[11] For example, transferrin, a growth-promoting substance isolated from lung tissue, has been found to stimulate the growth of malignant cells that typically metastasize to the lungs. Other organs that are preferential sites for metastasis contain particular cytokines, growth factors, and other microenvironmental characteristics that facilitate metastatic tumour survival and growth.

The selective nature of hematologic spread indicates that metastasis is a finely orchestrated, multistep process, and only a small, select clone of cancer cells has the right combination

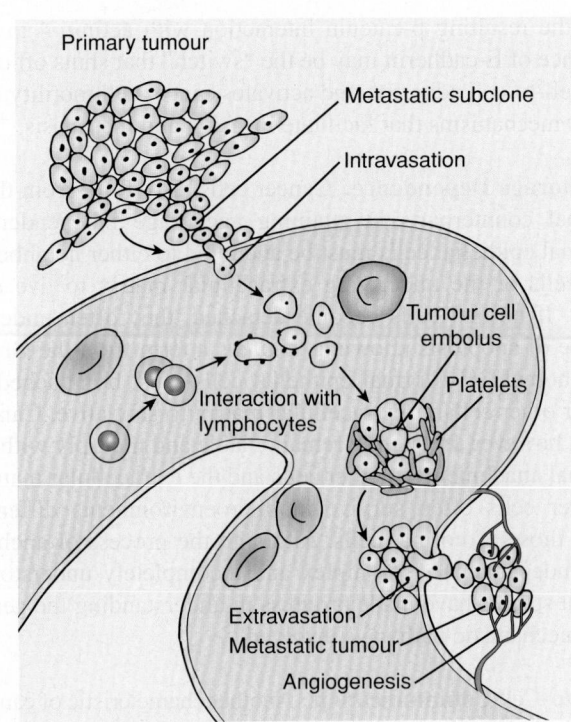

FIGURE 8.4 • The pathogenesis of metastasis. (Adapted from Kumar V., Abbas, A. K., Fausto, N., et al. (Eds.). (2010). *Robbins and Cotran pathologic basis of disease* (8th ed., p. 298). Philadelphia, PA: Elsevier Saunders.)

of gene products to perform all of the steps needed for establishment of a secondary tumour (Fig. 8.4). It has been estimated that fewer than 1 in 10,000 tumour cells that leave a primary tumour survives to start a secondary tumour.[21] To metastasize, a cancer cell must be able to break loose from the primary tumour, invade the surrounding extracellular matrix, gain access to a blood vessel, survive its passage in the bloodstream, emerge from the bloodstream at a favourable location, invade the surrounding tissue, begin to grow, and establish a blood supply. However, there is also growing evidence for the significant role of the tumour microenvironment—which includes but is not limited to the extracellular matrix, myoepithelial cells, endothelial cells, and macrophages—in enabling cancer cells to establish metastatic sites.[21]

Considerable evidence suggests that cancer cells capable of metastasis secrete enzymes that break down the surrounding extracellular matrix, allowing them to move through the degraded matrix and gain access to a blood vessel. Once in the circulation, the tumour cells are vulnerable to destruction by host immune cells. Some tumour cells gain protection from the antitumour host cells by aggregating and adhering to circulating blood components, particularly platelets, to form tumour emboli. Tumour cells that survive their travel in the circulation must be able to halt their passage by adhering to the vessel wall. Tumour cells express various cell surface attachment factors such as laminin receptors that facilitate their anchoring to laminin in the basement membrane. After attachment, the tumour cells secrete proteolytic enzymes such as type IV collagenase that degrade the basement membrane

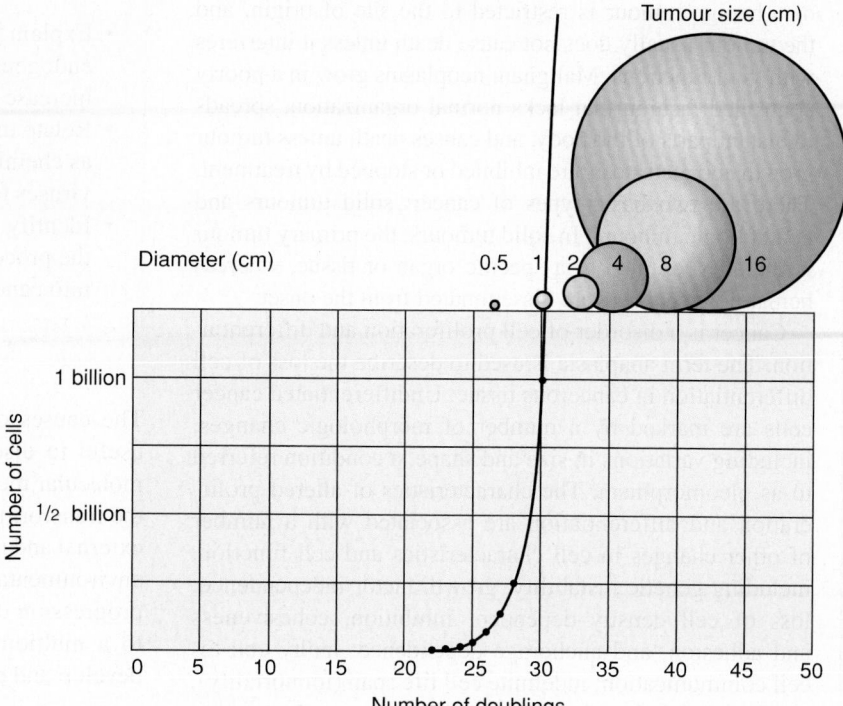

FIGURE 8.5 • Growth curve of a hypothetical tumour on arithmetic coordinates. Notice the number of doubling times before the tumour reaches an appreciable size. (Adapted from Collins V. P., Loeffler R. K., Tivey H. (1956). Observations on growth rates of human tumors. *American Journal of Roentgenology, Radium Therapy and Nuclear Medicine*, 76, 988.)

and facilitate the migration of the tumour cells through the capillary membrane into the interstitial area, where they subsequently establish growth of a secondary tumour.

Once in the distant tissue site, the process of metastatic tumour development depends on the establishment of blood vessels and specific growth factors that promote proliferation of the tumour cells. Tumour cells, as well as other cells in the microenvironment, secrete factors that enable the development of new blood vessels within the tumour, a process termed *angiogenesis*.[18] The presence of stimulatory or inhibitory growth factors correlates with the site-specific pattern of metastasis. For example, a potent growth-stimulating factor has been isolated from lung tissue, and stromal cells in bone have been shown to produce a factor that stimulates growth of prostatic cancer cells.[18]

Tumour Growth

Once cells have an adequate blood supply, the rate of tissue growth in normal and cancerous tissue depends on three factors: (1) the number of cells that are actively dividing or moving through the cell cycle, (2) the duration of the cell cycle, and (3) the number of cells that are being lost relative to the number of new cells being produced. One of the reasons cancerous tumours often seem to grow so rapidly relates to the size of the cell pool that is actively engaged in cycling. It has been shown that the cell cycle time of cancerous tissue cells is not necessarily shorter than that of normal cells. Rather, cancer cells do not die on schedule and growth factors prevent cells from exiting the cell cycle and entering the G_0 phase. Thus, a greater percentage of cells are actively engaged in cycling than occurs in normal tissue.

The ratio of dividing cells to resting cells in a tissue mass is called the *growth fraction*. The *doubling time* is the length of time it takes for the total mass of cells in a tumour to double. As the growth fraction increases, the doubling time decreases. When normal tissues reach their adult size, equilibrium between cell birth and cell death is reached. Cancer cells, however, continue to divide until limitations in blood supply and nutrients inhibit their growth. When this happens, the doubling time for cancer cells decreases. If tumour growth is plotted against time on a semilogarithmic scale, the initial growth rate is exponential and then tends to decrease or flatten out over time. This characterization of tumour growth is called the *Gompertzian model and is used for studying the effects of medications on cancer cells*.[22]

By conventional radiographic methods, a tumour usually is undetectable until it has doubled 30 times and contains more than 1 billion (10^9) cells. At this point, it is approximately 1 cm in size (Fig. 8.5). Methods to identify tumours at smaller sizes are under investigation; in some cases, the application of ultrasonography and magnetic resonance imaging (MRI) enable detection of tumours smaller than 1 cm. After 35 doublings, the mass contains more than 1 trillion (10^{12}) cells, which is a sufficient number to kill the host.

IN SUMMARY

Neoplasms may be either benign or malignant. Benign and malignant tumours differ in terms of cell characteristics, manner of growth, rate of growth, potential for metastasis, ability to produce generalized effects, tendency to cause tissue destruction, and capacity to cause death. The growth of a benign tumour is restricted to the site of origin, and the tumour usually does not cause death unless it interferes with vital functions. Malignant neoplasms grow in a poorly controlled fashion that lacks normal organization, spreads to distant parts of the body, and causes death unless tumour growth and metastasis are inhibited or stopped by treatment. There are two basic types of cancer: solid tumours and hematologic tumours. In solid tumours, the primary tumour is initially confined to a specific organ or tissue, whereas hematologic cancers are disseminated from the onset.

Cancer is a disorder of cell proliferation and differentiation. The term anaplasia is used to describe the loss of cell differentiation in cancerous tissue. Undifferentiated cancer cells are marked by a number of morphologic changes, including variations in size and shape, a condition referred to as pleomorphism. The characteristics of altered proliferation and differentiation are associated with a number of other changes in cell characteristics and cell function, including genetic instability; growth factor independence; loss of cell density–dependent inhibition, cohesiveness and adhesion, and anchorage dependence; faulty cell-to-cell communication; indefinite cell life span (immortality); expression of altered tissue antigens; abnormal secretion of degradative enzymes that enable invasion and metastatic spread, or ectopic production of hormones; and abnormal cytoskeletal characteristics.

The spread of cancer occurs through three pathways: direct invasion and extension, seeding of cancer cells in body cavities, and metastatic spread through vascular or lymphatic pathways. Only a proportionately small clone of cancer cells is capable of metastasis. To metastasize, a cancer cell must be able to break loose from the primary tumour, invade the surrounding extracellular matrix, gain access to a blood vessel, survive its passage in the bloodstream, emerge from the bloodstream at a favourable location, invade the surrounding tissue, and begin to grow. The rate of growth of cancerous tissue depends on the ratio of dividing to resting cells (growth fraction) and the time it takes for the total cells in the tumour to double (doubling time). A tumour is usually undetectable until it has doubled 30 times and contains more than 1 billion cells.

ETIOLOGY OF CANCER

After completing this section of the chapter, you should be able to meet the following objectives:

- Describe various types of cancer-associated genes and cancer-associated cellular and molecular pathways.
- Describe genetic events and epigenetic factors that are important in tumourigenesis.
- State the importance of cancer stem cells, angiogenesis, and the cell microenvironment in cancer growth and metastasis.

- Explain how host factors such as heredity, levels of endogenous hormones, and immune system function increase the risk for development of selected cancers.
- Relate the effects of environmental factors such as chemical carcinogens, radiation, and oncogenic viruses to the risk of cancer development.
- Identify concepts and hypotheses that may explain the processes by which normal cells are transformed into cancer cells by carcinogens.

The causes of cancers are very diverse and complex. It is useful to discuss causation in terms of (1) the genetic and molecular mechanisms that are involved and that characterize the transformation of normal cells to cancer cells; and (2) the external and more contextual factors such as age, heredity, and environmental agents that contribute to the development and progression of cancer. Together, both mechanisms contribute to a multidimensional web of causation by which cancers develop and progress over time.

Genetic and Molecular Basis of Cancer

The molecular pathogenesis of most cancers is thought to originate with genetic damage or mutation, with resultant changes in cell physiology that transform a normally functioning cell into a cancer cell. Epigenetic factors that involve silencing of a gene or genes may also be involved in the molecular pathogenesis of cancer. In recent years, an important role of cancer stem cells in the pathogenesis of cancer has been identified, and continues to be elucidated. Finally, the cellular microenvironment, which involves multiple cell types, the complex milieu of cytokines and growth factors, and the extracellular matrix, is now recognized as an important contributor to cancer development, growth, and progression.

Cancer-Associated Genes

Most cancer-associated genes can be classified into two broad categories based on whether gene overactivity or underactivity increases the risk for cancer. The category associated with gene overactivity involves *proto-oncogenes,* which are normal genes that become cancer-causing oncogenes if mutated. Proto-oncogenes encode for normal cell proteins such as growth factors, growth factor receptors, growth factor signalling molecules, and transcription factors that promote cell growth or increase growth factor–dependent signalling. The category associated with gene underactivity comprises the *tumour suppressor genes,* which, by being less active, create an environment in which cancer is promoted. Tumour suppressor genes include the retinoblastoma (*RB*) gene, which normally prevents cell division, and the *TP53* gene, which normally becomes activated in DNA-damaged cells to initiate apoptosis.[11] Loss of *RB* activity may accelerate the cell cycle and lead to increased cell proliferation, whereas inactivity of *TP53* may increase the survival of DNA-damaged cells. There are a number of genetic events that can lead to oncogene formation or loss of tumour suppressor gene function.

Genetic Events Leading to Oncogene Formation or Activation. One way genetic events can create or activate oncogenes is a point mutation, in which there is a single nucleotide base change due to an insertion, deletion, or substitution. An example of an oncogene caused by point mutations is the *ras* oncogene, which has been found in many cancers. Members of the *ras* proto-oncogene family are important signal-relaying proteins that transmit growth signals to the nucleus. Hence, activation of the *ras* oncogene can increase cell proliferation.

Chromosomal translocations have traditionally been associated with cancers such as Burkitt lymphoma and chronic myelogenous leukemia (CML). In Burkitt lymphoma, the *myc* proto-oncogene, which encodes a growth signal protein, is translocated from its normal position on chromosome 8 to chromosome 14, placing it at the site of an immunoglobulin gene.[11] The outcome of the translocation in CML is the appearance of the so-called *Philadelphia chromosome* involving chromosomes 9 and 22 and the formation of an abnormal fusion protein, a hybrid oncogenic protein (bcr–abl) that promotes cell proliferation (see Chapter 15, Fig. 15.8). Biotechnology and genomics are enabling the identification of gene translocations and an increased understanding of how these translocations, even within the same chromosome, contribute to tumourigenesis by the creation of abnormal fusion proteins that promote cell proliferation.

Another genetic event common in cancer is gene amplification. Multiple copies of certain genes may lead to overexpression, with higher-than-normal levels of proteins that increase cell proliferation. For example, the human epidermal growth factor receptor-2 (*HER-2/neu*) gene is amplified in up to 30% of breast cancers; its presence indicates an aggressive tumour with a poor prognosis. One of the agents used in treatment of *HER-2/neu*-overexpressing breast cancers is trastuzumab (Herceptin), a monoclonal antibody that selectively binds to HER-2, thereby inhibiting the proliferation of tumour cells that overexpress HER-2.[23]

Genetic Events Leading to Loss of Tumour Suppressor Gene Function. Tumour suppressor genes inhibit the proliferation of cells in a tumour. When this type of gene is inactivated, a genetic signal that normally inhibits cell proliferation is removed, thereby causing unregulated growth to begin. Numerous tumour suppressor genes have been identified and linked to inherited and sporadic forms of cancer.[11] Of particular interest in this group is the *TP53* gene. Located on the short arm of chromosome 17, it codes for the p53 protein, which functions as a suppressor of tumour growth. Mutations in the *TP53* gene have been implicated in the development of lung, breast, and colon cancer—the three leading causes of cancer death.[11] The *TP53* gene also appears to initiate apoptosis in radiation- and chemotherapy-damaged tumour cells.

Thus, tumours that retain normal *TP53* function are more likely to respond to such therapy than tumours that carry a defective *TP53* gene.[11]

Although a single mutation may play an important role in oncogene activation, the malfunction of tumour suppressor genes may require "two hits" to contribute to total loss of function, as suggested by the *two-hit hypothesis* of carcinogenesis[11,24] (Fig. 8.6). The first "hit" may be a point mutation in an allele of a particular chromosome; later, a second "hit" occurs that involves the companion allele of the gene. In hereditary cases, the first hit is inherited from an affected parent and is therefore present in all somatic cells of the body. In retinoblastoma, the second hit occurs in one of many retinal cells (all of which already carry the mutated gene). In sporadic (noninherited) cases, both mutations (hits) occur in a single somatic cell, whose progeny then form the cancer. In persons carrying an inherited mutation, such as a mutated *RB* allele, all somatic cells are perfectly normal, except for the increased risk of developing cancer. That person is said to be *heterozygous* at the gene locus. Cancer develops when a person becomes homozygous for the mutant allele, a condition referred to as *loss of heterozygosity* which confers a poor prognosis.[11] For example, loss of heterozygosity is known to occur in hereditary cancers, in which a mutated gene is inherited from a parent, and other conditions (*e.g.,* radiation exposure) are present that make individuals more susceptible to cancer.

Epigenetic Mechanisms

In addition to mechanisms that involve DNA and chromosomal structural changes, there are molecular and cellular mechanisms, termed *epigenetic mechanisms,* that involve changes in the patterns of gene expression without a change in the DNA. Epigenetic mechanisms may "silence" genes, such as tumour suppressor genes, so that even though the gene is present, it is not expressed and a cancer-suppressing protein is not made. One such mechanism of epigenetic silencing is by methylation of the promoter region of the gene, a change that prevents transcription and causes gene inactivity. Genes silenced by hypermethylation can be inherited, and epigenetic silencing of genes can be considered a first "hit" in the two-hit hypothesis described previously.[25] The epigenetic mechanisms that alter expression of genes associated with cancer are under intensive investigation, as are hypomethylating drugs to prevent or treat cancer.

Molecular and Cellular Pathways

There are numerous molecular and cellular mechanisms with a myriad of associated pathways and genes that are known or suspected to facilitate the development of cancer. Genes that increase susceptibility to cancer or facilitate cancer include defects in DNA repair mechanisms, defects in growth factor signalling pathways, evasion of apoptosis, avoidance of cellular senescence, development of sustained angiogenesis, and metastasis and invasion. In addition, associated genetic mutations are involved that enable invasion of and survival in neighbouring tissue, as well as evasion of immune detection and attack.

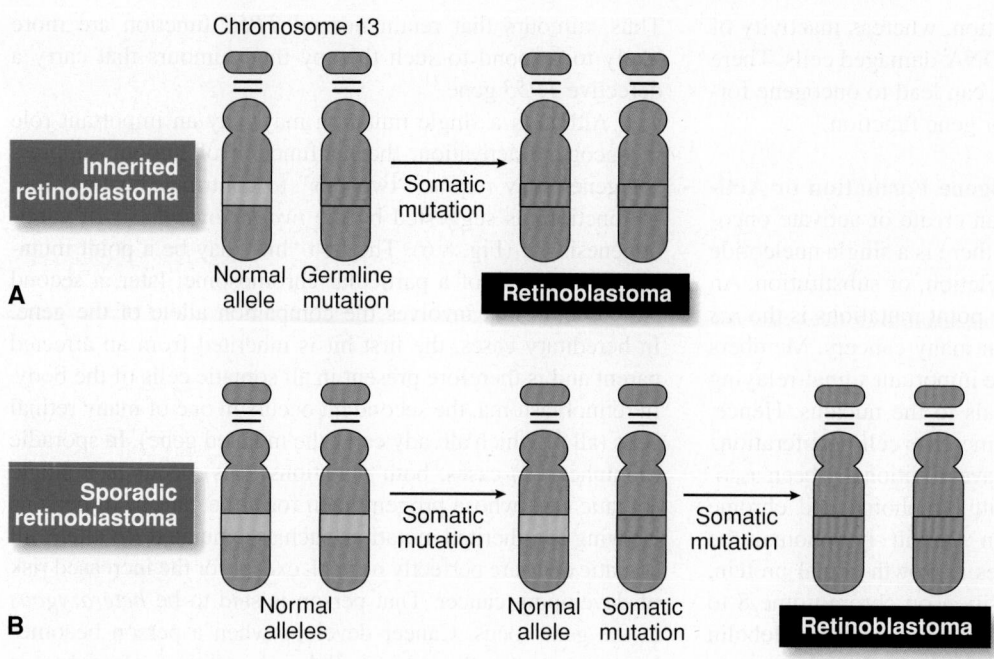

Chromosome 13

A Inherited retinoblastoma

Normal allele | Germline mutation → Somatic mutation → **Retinoblastoma**

B Sporadic retinoblastoma

Normal alleles → Somatic mutation → Normal allele | Somatic mutation → Somatic mutation → **Retinoblastoma**

FIGURE 8.6 • The "two-hit" origin of retinoblastoma. **A:** A child with an inherited form of retinoblastoma is born with a germline mutation in one allele of the retinoblastoma (*RB*) gene located on the long arm of chromosome 13. A second somatic mutation in the retina leads to inactivation of the normally functioning *RB* allele and subsequent development of retinoblastoma. **B:** In sporadic (non-inherited) cases of retinoblastoma, the child is born with two normal *RB* alleles. It requires two independent somatic mutations to inactivate *RB* gene function and allow for the appearance of a neoplastic clone. (From Rubin R., Strayer D. (2012). (Eds.). *Rubin's pathology: Clinicopathologic foundations of medicine* (6th ed., p. 178). Philadelphia, PA: Lippincott Williams & Wilkins.)

DNA Repair Defects. Genetic mechanisms that regulate repair of damaged DNA have been implicated in the process of oncogenesis (Fig. 8.7). The DNA repair genes affect cell proliferation and survival indirectly through their ability to

Carcinogenic agent → Normal cell

DNA repair (DNA repair genes)

DNA damage

Failure of DNA repair

• Activation of growth-promoting oncogenes
• Inactivation of tumour suppressor genes
• Alterations in genes that control apoptosis

Unregulated cell differentiation and growth

Malignant neoplasm

FIGURE 8.7 • Flow chart depicting the stages in the development of a malignant neoplasm resulting from exposure to an oncogenic agent that produces DNA damage. When DNA repair genes are present (*red arrow*), the DNA is repaired and gene mutation does not occur.

repair nonlethal damage in proto-oncogenes, tumour suppressor genes, and the genes that control apoptosis.[11] These genes have been implicated as the principal targets of genetic damage occurring during the development of a cancer cell.[26] Such genetic damage may be caused by the action of chemicals, radiation, or viruses, or it may be inherited in the germline. Significantly, it appears that the acquisition of a single-gene mutation is not sufficient to transform normal cells into cancer cells. Instead, cancerous transformation appears to require the activation of multiple independently mutated genes.

Defects in Growth Factor Signalling Pathways. A relatively common way in which cancer cells gain autonomous growth is through mutations in genes that control growth factor signalling pathways. These signalling pathways couple growth factor receptors to their nuclear targets.[11] Under normal conditions, cell proliferation involves the binding of a growth factor to its receptor on the cell membrane, activation of the growth factor receptor on the inner surface of the cell membrane, transfer of the signal across the cytosol to the nucleus by signal-transducing proteins that function as second messengers, induction and activation of regulatory factors that initiate DNA transcription, and entry of the cell into the cell cycle (Fig. 8.8). Many of the proteins involved in the signalling pathways that control the action of growth factors exert their effects through *kinases,* enzymes that phosphorylate proteins. In some types of cancer such as CML, mutation in a proto-oncogene controlling tyrosine kinase activity occurs, causing unregulated cell growth and proliferation.

Evasion of Apoptosis. Faulty apoptotic mechanisms have an important role in cancer. The failure of cancer cells to undergo apoptosis in a normal manner may be due to a number of problems. There may be altered cell survival signalling,

FIGURE 8.8 • Pathway for genes regulating cell growth and replication. Stimulation of a normal cell by a growth factor results in activation of the growth factor receptor and signalling proteins that transmit the growth-promoting signal to the nucleus, where it modulates gene transcription and progression through the cell cycle. Many of these signalling proteins exert their effects through enzymes called *kinases* that phosphorylate proteins. MAP, mitogen-activated protein.

overly active *ras* proteins, *TP53* mutations, down-regulation of death receptors (*e.g.,* TRAIL), stabilization of the mitochondria, inactivation of proapoptotic proteins (*e.g.,* methylation of caspase-8), overactivity of nuclear factor kappa B (NF-κB), heat-shock protein production, or failure of immune cells to induce cell death.[27] Alterations in apoptotic and antiapoptotic pathways, genes, and proteins have been found in many cancers. One example is the high levels of the antiapoptotic protein Bcl-2 that occur secondary to a chromosomal translocation in certain B-cell lymphomas. The mitochondrial membrane is a key regulator of the balance between cell death and survival. Proteins in the Bcl-2 family reside in the inner mitochondrial membrane and are either proapoptotic or antiapoptotic. Because apoptosis is considered a normal cellular response to DNA damage, loss of normal apoptotic pathways may contribute to cancer by enabling DNA-damaged cells to survive.

Evasion of Cellular Senescence. Another normal cell response to DNA damage is cellular senescence. As stated earlier, cancer cells are characterized by immortality due to high levels of telomerase that prevent cell aging and senescence (see Chapter 3). High levels of telomerase and prevention of telomere shortening may also contribute to cancer and its progression because senescence is considered to be a normal response to DNA damage in cells as well as a tumour suppressor mechanism, and in model systems, short telomeres limit cancer growth.[28,29]

Development of Sustained Angiogenesis. Even with all the aforementioned genetic abnormalities, tumours cannot grow unless angiogenesis occurs and supplies them with the blood vessels necessary for survival. Angiogenesis is required not only for continued tumour growth but for metastasis. The molecular basis for the angiogenic switch is unknown, but it appears to involve increased production of angiogenic factors or loss of angiogenic inhibitors. The normal *TP53* gene seems to inhibit angiogenesis by inducing the synthesis of an antiangiogenic molecule called *thrombospondin-1*.[11] With mutational inactivation of both *TP53* alleles (as occurs in many cancers), the levels of thrombospondin-1 drop precipitously, tilting the balance in favour of angiogenic factors. Angiogenesis is also influenced by hypoxia and release of proteases that are involved in regulating the balance between angiogenic and antiangiogenic factors. Because of the crucial role of angiogenic factors in tumour growth, much interest is focused on the development of antiangiogenesis therapy. Antiangiogenesis therapy is showing synergistic antitumour actions when combined with conventional forms of chemotherapy in the treatment of certain cancers.

Furthermore, antiangiogenesis therapy may have more broad-based actions. For example, it is now thought that cancer cells are a heterogeneous population of cells that include a cancer stem cell population characterized by mitotic quiescence and an increased ability to survive chemotherapy agents, which make cancer stem cells particularly difficult to treat. Cancer stem cells may reside close to blood vessels, where they receive signals for self-renewal. Use of antiangiogenesis therapy appears to destroy the niche where these stem cells reside.[30]

Invasion and Metastasis. Finally, multiple genes and molecular and cellular pathways are known to be involved in invasion and metastasis. There is evidence that cancer cells with invasive properties are actually members of the cancer stem cell population discussed previously. This evidence suggests that genetic programs that are normally operative in stem cells during embryonic development may become operative in cancer stem cells, enabling them to detach, cross tissue boundaries, escape death by anoikis, and colonize new tissues.[31] The *MET* proto-oncogene, which is expressed in both stem cells and cancer cells, is a key regulator of invasive growth. Findings suggest that adverse conditions such as tissue hypoxia, which are commonly present in cancerous tumours, trigger this invasive behaviour by activating the MET tyrosine kinase receptor.

Role of the Microenvironment

Traditionally, the molecular and cellular biology of cancer has focused on the cancer itself. More recently, the important role of the microenvironment in the development of cancer and metastasis has been described. The microenvironment of the cancer cell consists of multiple cell types, including macrophages, fibroblasts, endothelial cells, and a variety of immune and inflammatory cells; the extracellular matrix; and the primary signalling substances such as cytokines, chemokines, and hormones. For example, signalling of the cytokine transforming growth factor-beta (TGF-β) is known to be important in the cellular pathway leading to cancer cell formation or suppression.[32] The ability of TGF-β to cause the cancer to progress and metastasize, however, depends on the microenvironment of various cell types and cross-talk of signals among the cell types. In some cases, the phenotype of a cancer cell can actually normalize when it is removed from the tumour microenvironment and placed in a normal environment, and vice versa. Finally, essential steps needed for tumour growth and metastasis, such as angiogenesis and metastatic tumour survival, depend on the microenvironment.

Carcinogenesis

The process by which carcinogenic (cancer-producing) agents cause normal cells to become cancer cells is hypothesized to be a multistep mechanism that can be divided into three stages: initiation, promotion, and progression (Fig. 8.9). *Initiation* involves the exposure of cells to a carcinogenic agent that makes them susceptible to malignant transformation.[11] The carcinogenic agents can be chemical, physical, or biologic, and produce irreversible changes in the genome of a previously normal cell. Because the effects of initiating agents are irreversible, multiple divided doses may achieve the same effects as a single exposure to the same total dose or to small amounts of highly carcinogenic substances. The cells most susceptible to mutagenic alterations are those that are actively synthesizing DNA.

FIGURE 8.9 • The processes of initiation, promotion, and progression in the clonal evolution of malignant tumours. Initiation involves the exposure of cells to appropriate doses of a carcinogenic agent; promotion, the unregulated and accelerated growth of the mutated cells; and progression, the acquisition of malignant characteristics by the tumour cells.

Promotion involves the induction of unregulated accelerated growth in already initiated cells by various chemicals and growth factors.[11] Promotion is reversible if the promoter substance is removed. Cells that have been irreversibly initiated may be promoted even after long latency periods. The latency period varies with the type of agent, the dosage, and the characteristics of the target cells. Many chemical carcinogens are called *complete carcinogens* because they can initiate and promote neoplastic transformation. *Progression* is the process whereby tumour cells acquire malignant phenotypic changes that promote invasiveness, metastatic competence, autonomous growth tendencies, and increased karyotypic instability.

Host and Environmental Factors

Because cancer is not a single disease, it is reasonable to assume that it does not have a single cause. More likely, cancer occurs because of interactions among multiple risk factors or repeated exposure to a single carcinogenic agent. Among the traditional risk factors that have been linked to cancer are heredity, hormonal factors, immunologic mechanisms, and environmental agents such as chemicals, radiation, and cancer-causing viruses. More recently, there has been interest in obesity as a risk factor for cancer. A strong and consistent relationship has been reported between obesity and mortality from all cancers among men and women.[33] Obese persons tend to produce increased amounts of androgens, a portion of which is converted to the active form of estrogen in adipose tissue, causing a functional state of hyperestrogenism. Because of the association of estrogen with postmenopausal breast cancer and endometrial cancer (see Chapter 46), the relationship between obesity and cancer is stronger among women than among men.[33]

Heredity

A hereditary predisposition to approximately 50 types of cancer has been observed in families. Breast cancer, for example, occurs more frequently in women whose grandmothers, mothers, aunts, or sisters also have experienced a breast malignancy. A genetic predisposition to the development of cancer has been documented for a number of cancerous and precancerous lesions that follow mendelian inheritance patterns. Two tumour suppressor genes, called *BRCA1* (breast carcinoma 1) and *BRCA2* (breast carcinoma 2), have been implicated in genetic susceptibility to breast cancer.[11] Individuals carrying a *BRCA* mutation have a lifetime risk (if they live to the age of 85 years) of 80% for developing breast cancer. The lifetime risk for developing ovarian cancer is 10% to 20% for carriers of *BRCA2* mutations and 40% to 60% for *BRCA1* mutations.[11] These genes have also been associated with an increased risk of prostate, pancreatic, colon, and other cancers.

Several cancers exhibit an autosomal dominant inheritance pattern that greatly increases the risk of developing a tumour.[11] The inherited mutation is usually a point mutation occurring in a single allele of a tumour suppressor gene. Persons who inherit the mutant gene are born with one normal and one mutant copy of the gene. For cancer to develop, the normal gene must be inactivated, usually through a somatic mutation. Retinoblastoma, a rare childhood tumour of the retina, is an example of a cancer that follows an autosomal dominant inheritance pattern. Approximately 40% of retinoblastomas are inherited, and carriers of the mutant *RB* tumour suppressor gene have a 10,000-fold increased risk for developing retinoblastoma, usually with bilateral involvement.[5,11] Familial adenomatous polyposis of the colon also follows an autosomal dominant inheritance pattern. It is caused by mutation of another tumour suppressor gene, the *APC* gene.[5] In people who inherit this gene, hundreds of adenomatous polyps may develop, some of which inevitably become malignant.[11]

Hormones

Hormones have received considerable research attention with respect to cancer of the breast, ovary, and endometrium in women and of the prostate and testis in men. Although the link between hormones and the development of cancer is unclear, it has been suggested that it may reside with the ability of hormones to drive the cell division of a malignant phenotype. Neoplasms of tissues that are responsive to hormones are responsible for 30% to 35% of all newly diagnosed tumours in men and 40% to 43% of all newly diagnosed tumours in women in Canada and the United States.[1,2] Because of the evidence that endogenous hormones affect the risk of these cancers, concern exists regarding the effects on cancer risk if the same or closely related hormones are administered for therapeutic purposes.

Immunologic Mechanisms

There is substantial evidence for the immune system's participation in resistance against the progression and spread of cancer. The central concept, known as the *immune surveillance hypothesis,* first proposed by Paul Ehrlich in 1909, postulates that the immune system plays a central role in resistance against the development of tumours.[34] In addition to cancer–host interactions as a mechanism of cancer development, immunologic mechanisms provide a means for the detection, classification, and prognostic evaluation of cancers and a potential method of treatment. *Immunotherapy* (discussed later in this chapter) is a cancer treatment modality designed to heighten the patient's general immune responses in order to increase tumour destruction.

It has been suggested that the development of cancer might be associated with impairment or decline in the surveillance capacity of the immune system. For example, increases in cancer incidence have been observed in people with immunodeficiency diseases and in those with organ transplants who are receiving immunosuppressant drugs. The incidence of cancer also is increased in the elderly, in whom there is a known decrease in immune activity. The association of Kaposi sarcoma with acquired immunodeficiency syndrome (AIDS) further emphasizes the role of the immune system in preventing malignant cell proliferation.

It has been shown that most tumour cells have molecular configurations that can be specifically recognized by immune T cells or by antibodies and hence are termed *tumour antigens.* The most relevant tumour antigens fall into two categories: unique, tumour-specific antigens found only on tumour cells; and tumour-associated antigens found on tumour cells and normal cells. Quantitative and qualitative differences permit the use of tumour-associated antigens to distinguish cancer cells from normal cells.[11]

Virtually all of the components of the immune system have the potential for eradicating cancer cells, including T lymphocytes, B lymphocytes and antibodies, macrophages, and innate lymphoid natural killer (NK) cells (see Chapter 17). The T-cell response is undoubtedly one of the most important host responses for controlling the growth of antigenic tumour cells; it is responsible for direct killing of tumour cells and for activation of other components of the immune system. The T-cell immunity to cancer cells reflects the function of two subsets of T cells: the CD4+ helper T cells and the CD8+ cytotoxic T cells. The finding of tumour-reactive antibodies in the serum of people with cancer supports the role of the B cell as a member of the immune surveillance team. Antibodies can destroy cancer cells through complement-mediated mechanisms or through antibody-dependent cellular cytotoxicity, in which the antibody binds the cancer cell to another effector cell, such as the NK cell, that does the actual killing of the cancer cell. NK cells do not require antigen recognition and can lyse a wide variety of target cells. The cytotoxic activity of NK cells can be augmented by the cytokines interleukin (IL)-2 and interferon, and this activity can be amplified by immune T-cell responses. Macrophages are important in tumour immunity as antigen-presenting cells to initiate the immune response and as potential effector cells to participate in tumour cell lysis.

Chemical Carcinogens

A carcinogen is an agent capable of causing cancer. The role of environmental agents in causation of cancer was first noted in 1775 by Sir Percival Pott, who related the high incidence of scrotal cancer in chimney sweepers to their exposure to coal soot.[5,11] A few years later, based on this observation, the Danish Chimney Guild ruled that its members must bathe daily. Few public health measures since that time have so successfully controlled a form of cancer.[11] Over the next two centuries, many chemicals have been shown to transform cells in the laboratory and to be carcinogenic in animals (Chart 8.1). These agents include both natural (e.g., aflatoxin B_1) and artificial products (e.g., vinyl chloride).

Chemical carcinogens can be divided into two groups: (1) direct-reacting agents, which do not require activation in the body to become carcinogenic; and (2) indirect-reacting agents, called *procarcinogens or initiators,* which become active only after metabolic conversion. Direct- and indirect-acting initiators form highly reactive species (*i.e.,* electrophiles and free radicals) that bind with the nucleophilic residues on DNA, RNA, or cellular proteins. The action of these reactive species tends to cause cell mutation or alteration in synthesis of cell enzymes and structural proteins in a manner that alters cell replication and interferes with cell regulatory controls. The carcinogenicity of some chemicals is augmented by agents called *promoters* that, by themselves, have little or no cancer-causing ability. It is believed that promoters exert their effect by changing the expression of genetic material in a cell, increasing DNA synthesis, enhancing gene amplification (*i.e.,* number of gene copies that are made), and altering intercellular communication.

Exposure to many chemical carcinogens is associated with lifestyle risk factors, such as smoking, dietary factors, and alcohol consumption. Cigarette smoke contains both procarcinogens and promoters. It is directly associated with lung and laryngeal cancer and has been linked with cancers of the mouth, nasal cavities, pharynx, esophagus, pancreas, liver, kidney, uterus, cervix, and bladder, and with myeloid leukemias.[35] Chewing tobacco or tobacco products increases the risk of cancers of the oral cavity and esophagus. It has been estimated that 39% of all cancer deaths and 85% of lung cancer deaths in Canada are related to tobacco.[36,37] Not only is the smoker at risk, but others passively exposed to cigarette smoke are at increased risk. Environmental tobacco smoke has been classified as a "Group 1" human carcinogen based on the International Agency for Research on Cancer's system of carcinogen classification.[38] Each year in Canada, over 500 nonsmoking adults are diagnosed with lung cancer as a result of environmental tobacco smoke.[39]

There is strong evidence that certain elements in the diet contain chemicals that contribute to cancer risk. Most known dietary carcinogens occur either naturally in plants (*e.g.,* aflatoxins) or are produced during food preparation.[40] For example, benzo[a]pyrene and other polycyclic hydrocarbons are converted to carcinogens when foods are fried in fat that has been reused multiple times. Among the most potent of the procarcinogens are the polycyclic aromatic hydrocarbons. The polycyclic aromatic hydrocarbons are of particular interest because they are produced from animal fat in the process of charcoal-broiling meats and are present in smoked meats and fish. They also are produced in the combustion of tobacco and are present in cigarette smoke. Nitrosamines, which are powerful carcinogens, are formed in foods that are smoked, salted, cured, or pickled using nitrites or nitrates as preservatives.[40] Formation of nitrosamines may be inhibited by the presence of antioxidants such as vitamin C, found in fruits and vegetables. Cancer of the colon has been associated with high dietary intake of fat and red meat and a low intake of dietary fibre. A high-fat diet was thought to be carcinogenic because it increases the flow of primary bile acids that are converted to secondary bile acids in the presence of anaerobic bacteria in the colon, producing carcinogens or promoters. Recent studies have identified obesity and lowered physical activity with an increased risk of colon cancer.[5]

CHART 8.1 **CHEMICAL AND ENVIRONMENTAL AGENTS KNOWN TO BE CARCINOGENIC IN HUMANS**

Polycyclic Hydrocarbons
Soots, tars, and oils
Cigarette smoke

Industrial Agents
Aniline and azo dyes
Arsenic compounds
Asbestos
β-Naphthylamine
Benzene
Benzo[a]pyrene
Carbon tetrachloride
Insecticides, fungicides
Nickel and chromium compounds
Polychlorinated biphenyls
Vinyl chloride

Food and Drugs
Smoked foods
Nitrosamines
Aflatoxin B1
Diethylstilbestrol
Anticancer drugs (e.g., alkylating agents, cyclophosphamide, chlorambucil, nitrosourea)

Alcohol is associated with a variety of cancers; the causative mechanisms are very complex. The first and most toxic metabolite of ethanol is acetaldehyde, which is a known carcinogen that interferes with DNA synthesis and repair and causes point mutations in some cells.[41] In addition, ethanol can alter DNA methylation and interfere with retinoid metabolism, which is important in antioxidant mechanisms. The carcinogenic effect of cigarette smoke can be enhanced by concomitant consumption of alcohol; persons who smoke and drink considerable amounts of alcohol are at increased risk for development of cancer of the oral cavity, larynx, and esophagus.

The effects of carcinogenic agents usually are dose dependent—the larger the dose or the longer the duration of exposure, the greater the risk that cancer will develop. Some chemical carcinogens may act in concert with other carcinogenic influences, such as viruses or radiation, to induce neoplasia. There usually is a time delay ranging from 5 to 30 years from the time of chemical carcinogen exposure to the development of overt cancer. This is unfortunate because many people may have been exposed to the agent and its carcinogenic effects before the association was recognized. This occurred, for example, with the use of diethylstilbestrol, which was widely used in France and the United States from the mid-1940s to the mid-1970s to prevent miscarriages. But it was not until the late 1960s that many cases of vaginal adenosis and adenocarcinoma in young women were found to be the result of their exposure in utero to diethylstilbestrol.[42]

Radiation

The effects of *ionizing radiation* in carcinogenesis have been well documented in atomic bomb survivors, in patients diagnostically exposed, and in industrial workers, scientists, and physicians who were exposed during employment. Skin carcinomas and leukemia were significantly elevated in these populations. Between 1950 and 1970, the death rate from leukemia alone in the most heavily exposed population groups of atomic bomb survivors in Hiroshima and Nagasaki was 147 per 100,000 persons, 30 times the expected rate.[43]

The type of cancer that developed depended on the dose of radiation, the sex of the person, and the age at which exposure occurred. For instance, approximately 25 to 30 years after total-body or trunk irradiation, there were increased incidences of leukemia and cancers of the breast, lung, stomach, thyroid, salivary gland, gastrointestinal system, and lymphoid tissues. The length of time between exposure and the onset of cancer is related to the age of the individual. For example, children exposed to ionizing radiation in utero have an increased risk for developing leukemias and childhood tumours, particularly 2 to 3 years after birth. This latency period for leukemia extends to 5 to 10 years if the child was exposed after birth and to 20 years for certain solid tumours.[44] As another example, the latency period for the development of thyroid cancer in infants and small children who received radiation to the head and neck to decrease the size of the tonsils or thymus was as long as 35 years after exposure.

The association between sunlight and the development of skin cancer (see Chapter 61) has been reported for more than 100 years. *Ultraviolet radiation* consists of relatively low-energy rays that do not deeply penetrate the skin. The evidence supporting the role of ultraviolet radiation in the cause of skin cancer includes skin cancer that develops primarily on the areas of skin more frequently exposed to sunlight (*e.g.,* the head and neck, arms, hands, and legs), a higher incidence in light-complexioned individuals who lack the ultraviolet-filtering skin pigment melanin, and the fact that the intensity of ultraviolet exposure is directly related to the incidence of skin cancer, as evidenced by higher rates occurring in Australia and the American Southwest.[5,11] There also are studies that suggest intense, episodic exposure to sunlight, particularly during childhood, is more important in the development of melanoma than prolonged, low-intensity exposure. As with other carcinogens, the effects of ultraviolet radiation usually are additive, and there usually is a long delay between the time of exposure and detection of the cancer.

Oncogenic Viruses

An oncogenic virus is one that can induce cancer. It has been suspected for some time that viruses play an important role in the development of certain forms of cancer, particularly leukemia and lymphoma. Ellermann in 1908 and Rous in 1911 were the first to describe the transmissibility of avian leukemia and sarcoma, respectively.[45] Interest in the field of viral oncology, particularly in human populations, has burgeoned with the discovery of reverse transcriptase and the development of recombinant DNA technology, and more recently with the discovery of oncogenes and tumour suppressor genes.

Viruses, which are small particles containing genetic material (DNA or RNA), enter a host cell and become incorporated into its chromosomal DNA, taking control of the cell's machinery for the purpose of producing viral proteins. A large number of DNA and RNA viruses (*i.e.,* retroviruses) have been shown to be oncogenic in animals. However, only a few viruses have been linked to cancer in humans.

Four DNA viruses have been implicated in human cancers: the human papillomavirus (HPV), Epstein–Barr virus (EBV), hepatitis B virus (HBV), and human herpesvirus-8 (HHV-8).[11] HHV-8, which causes Kaposi sarcoma in persons with AIDS, is discussed in Chapter 20. There are over 60 genetically different types of HPV. Some types (*i.e.,* types 1, 2, 4, 7) have been shown to cause benign squamous papillomas (*i.e.,* warts). HPVs also have been implicated in squamous cell carcinoma of the cervix and anogenital region. HPV types 16 and 18 and, less commonly, HPV types 31, 33, 35, and 51 are found in approximately 85% of squamous cell carcinomas of the cervix and presumed precursors (*i.e.,* severe cervical dysplasia and carcinoma in situ).[11] A bivalent (for HPV types 16 and 18) and quadrivalent vaccine (for HPV types 6, 11, 16, and 18) are available to protect against HPV transmission, and vaccination of 9- to 26-year-old girls/women is being encouraged as a means of preventing cervical cancer (see Chapter 47). Only the quadrivalent vaccine has been approved for use in males ages 9 to 26 years, and for women up to the age of 45 years.[46]

EBV is a member of the herpesvirus family. It has been implicated in the pathogenesis of four human cancers: Burkitt lymphoma, nasopharyngeal cancer, B-cell lymphomas in immunosuppressed individuals such as those with AIDS, and in some cases of Hodgkin lymphoma. Burkitt lymphoma, a tumour of B lymphocytes, is endemic in parts of East Africa and occurs sporadically in other areas worldwide. In persons with normal immune function, the EBV-driven B-cell proliferation is readily controlled and the person becomes asymptomatic or experiences a self-limited episode of infectious mononucleosis (see Chapter 15). In regions of the world where Burkitt lymphoma is endemic, concurrent malaria or other infections cause impaired immune function, allowing sustained B-lymphocyte proliferation. The incidence of nasopharyngeal cancer is high in some areas of China, particularly southern China, and in the Cantonese population in Singapore. An increased risk of B-cell lymphomas is seen in individuals with drug-suppressed immune systems, such as individuals with transplanted organs.

HBV is the etiologic agent in the development of hepatitis B, cirrhosis, and hepatocellular carcinoma. There is a significant correlation between elevated rates of hepatocellular carcinoma worldwide and the prevalence of HBV carriers.[5,11] Other etiologic factors also may contribute to the development of liver cancer. Ingestion of aflatoxin and infection with HCV, the hepatitis C virus, have been implicated.[5,11] The precise mechanism by which HBV induces hepatocellular cancer has not been determined, although it has been suggested that it may be the result of prolonged HBV-induced liver damage and regeneration.

Although there are a number of retroviruses (RNA viruses) that cause cancer in animals, human T-cell leukemia virus-1 (HTLV-1) is the only known retrovirus to cause cancer in humans. HTLV-1 is associated with a form of T-cell leukemia that is endemic in parts of Japan and some areas of the Caribbean and Africa, and is found sporadically elsewhere, including the United States and Europe.[11] Similar to the human immunodeficiency virus (HIV) responsible for AIDS, HTLV-1 is attracted to CD4[+] T cells, and this subset of T cells is therefore the major target for cancerous transformation. The virus requires transmission of infected T cells through sexual intercourse, infected blood, or breast milk.

IN SUMMARY

The causes of cancer are highly complex and can be viewed from two perspectives: (1) the molecular and cellular origins and mechanisms; and (2) the external and contextual causative factors, including age, heredity, and environmental agents, that influence its inception and growth. In most cases, the molecular pathogenesis of cancer is thought to have its origin in genetic damage or mutation that changes cell physiology and transforms a normally functioning cell into a cancer cell. However, the complexity of the causation and pathogenesis of cancer is becoming increasingly apparent as more is learned about the roles of epigenetic mechanisms, cancer stem cells, and the microenvironment in tumourigenesis.

The types of genes involved in cancer are numerous, with the two main categories being the proto-oncogenes, which control cell growth and replication, and tumour suppressor genes, which are growth-inhibiting regulatory genes. Genetic and molecular mechanisms that increase susceptibility to cancer or facilitate cancer include defects in DNA repair mechanisms, defects in growth factor signalling pathways, evasion of apoptosis, avoidance of antiaging and senescence mechanisms, development of sustained angiogenesis, and invasion and metastasis. Because cancer is not a single disease, it is likely that multiple factors interact at the molecular and cellular levels to transform normal cells into cancer cells. Genetic and epigenetic damage may be the result of interactions between multiple risk factors or repeated exposure to a single carcinogenic (cancer-producing) agent. Among the risk factors that have been linked to cancer are heredity, hormonal factors, immunologic mechanisms, and environmental agents such as chemicals, radiation, and cancer-causing viruses.

CLINICAL MANIFESTATIONS

After completing this section of the chapter, you should be able to meet the following objectives:

- Describe the many possible ways by which cancer acts to disrupt organ function.
- Characterize the mechanisms involved in the anorexia and cachexia, fatigue and sleep disorders, anemia, and venous thrombosis experienced by patients with cancer.
- Define the term paraneoplastic syndrome and explain its pathogenesis and manifestations.

There probably is not a single body function left unaffected by the presence of cancer. Because tumour cells replace normally functioning parenchymal tissue, the initial manifestations of cancer usually reflect the primary site of involvement. For example, cancer of the lung initially produces impairment of respiratory function; as the tumour grows and metastasizes, other body structures become affected. Cancer also produces generalized manifestations such as fatigue, anorexia and cachexia, anemia, decreased resistance to infections, and symptoms unrelated to the tumour site (paraneoplastic syndromes). Many of these manifestations are compounded by the side effects of methods used to treat the disease. In its late stages, cancer often causes pain (see Chapter 49). Pain is one of the most dreaded aspects of cancer, and pain management is one of the major treatment concerns for persons with incurable cancers.

Tissue Integrity

Cancer disrupts tissue integrity. As cancers grow, they compress and erode blood vessels, causing ulceration and necrosis along with frank bleeding and sometimes hemorrhage. One of the early warning signals of colorectal cancer is blood in the stool. Cancer cells also may produce enzymes and metabolic toxins that are destructive to the surrounding tissues. Usually, tissue damaged by cancerous growth does not heal normally. Instead, the damaged area persists and often continues to grow; a wound that does not heal is another warning signal of cancer. Cancer has no regard for normal anatomic boundaries; as it grows, it invades and compresses adjacent structures. Abdominal cancer, for example, may compress the viscera and cause bowel obstruction.

The development of effusions (*i.e.*, fluid) in the pleural, pericardial, or peritoneal spaces may be the presenting sign of some tumours.[47] Direct involvement of the serous surface seems to be the most significant inciting factor, although many other mechanisms, such as obstruction of lymphatic flow, may play a role. It has been reported that almost 50% of undiagnosed effusions in persons not known to have cancer turn out to be due to malignancy. Lung cancers, breast cancers, and lymphomas account for about 75% of malignant pleural effusions.[47] Most persons with pleural effusions are symptomatic at presentation, with chest pain, shortness of breath, and cough. More than any other malignant neoplasms, ovarian cancers are associated with the accumulation of fluid in the peritoneal cavity. Abdominal discomfort, swelling and a feeling of heaviness, and increase in abdominal girth, which reflect the presence of peritoneal effusions or ascites, are the most common presenting symptoms in ovarian cancer, occurring in up to 65% of women with the disease.[48]

Systemic Manifestations

Many of the manifestations of cancer, including anorexia and cachexia, fatigue and sleep disorders, and anemia, are not directly related to the presence of a tumour mass but to altered metabolic pathways and the presence of circulating cytokines and other mediators. Although research has produced amazing insights into the causes and cures for cancer, efforts are also focused on the associated side effects of the disease.[49]

Anorexia and Cachexia

Many cancers are associated with weight loss and wasting of body fat and muscle tissue, accompanied by profound weakness, anorexia, and anemia. This wasting syndrome is often referred to as the *cancer anorexia–cachexia syndrome*.[49–53] It is a common manifestation of most solid tumours, with the exception of breast cancer. It has been estimated that it is a significant cause of morbidity and mortality in 80% of persons with advanced cancer, and responsible for death in up to one third of cases.[11] The condition is more common in children and elderly persons and becomes more pronounced as the disease progresses. Persons with cancer cachexia also respond less well to chemotherapy and are more prone to toxic side effects.

Although anorexia, reduced food intake, and abnormalities of taste are common in people with cancer and often are accentuated by treatment methods, the extent of weight loss and protein wasting cannot be explained in terms of diminished food intake alone. In contrast to starvation due to lack of food intake, where weight is preferentially lost from the fat compartment, in cachexia, it is lost from both the fat and skeletal muscle compartments.[52] Furthermore, the protein loss that occurs with starvation is divided equally between skeletal muscle and visceral proteins, whereas in cachexia, visceral proteins are relatively well preserved. Thus, there is a loss of liver mass in starvation, but an increase in cachectic persons because of hepatic recycling of nutrients and the acute-phase response. Finally, and more important, weight loss that occurs with starvation is usually reversed by refeeding, whereas oral or parenteral nutritional supplementation does not reverse cachexia. It has been suggested that the altered metabolism and weight loss seen in cancer cachexia more closely resembles that seen in persons suffering from severe sepsis or trauma rather than starvation.[52]

The mechanisms of cancer cachexia appear to reside in a hypermetabolic state and altered nutrient metabolism that are specific to the tumour-bearing state. Tumours tend to consume large amounts of glucose, with a resultant increase in lactate formation because the tumour oxygen levels are too low to support the citric acid cycle and mitochondrial oxidative phosphorylation (see Chapter 4). The lactate that is produced then circulates to the liver, where it is converted back to glucose. The production of glucose (gluconeogenesis) from lactate uses adenosine triphosphate (ATP) and is very energy inefficient, contributing to the hypermetabolic state of cachectic patients. Another mechanism for the increasing energy expenditure in cachectic persons is the increased expression of mitochondrial uncoupling proteins that uncouple the oxidative phosphorylation process, so that energy is lost as heat. Abnormalities in fat and protein metabolism have also been reported. During starvation in persons without cancer, ketones derived from fat replace the glucose normally used by the brain, leading to decreased gluconeogenesis from amino acids with conservation of muscle mass, whereas in persons with cancer cachexia, amino acids are not spared and there is depletion of lean body mass, a condition thought to contribute to decreased survival time.

Although the mechanisms of the cancer anorexia–cachexia syndrome remain incompletely understood, they are probably multifactorial, resulting from a persistent inflammatory response in conjunction with production of specific cytokines and catabolic factors by the tumour. The syndrome shows similarities to that of the acute-phase response seen with tissue injury, infection, or inflammation, in which liver protein synthesis changes from synthesis of albumin to acute-phase proteins such as C-reactive protein, fibrinogen, and α_1-antitrypsin (see Chapter 18). The acute-phase response is known to be activated by cytokines such as tumour necrosis factor-α (TNF-α) and IL-1 and IL-6, suggesting that they may also play a role in cancer cachexia.[49–53] High serum levels of these cytokines have been observed in persons with cancer, and their levels appear to correlate with progression of the tumour. TNF-α, secreted primarily by macrophages in response to tumour cell growth or gram-negative bacterial infections, was the first cytokine associated with cachexia and wasting to be identified. It causes anorexia by suppressing satiety centres in the hypothalamus and increasing the synthesis of lipoprotein lipase, an enzyme that facilitates the release of fatty acids from lipoproteins so that they can be used by tissues. IL-1 and IL-6 share many of the features of TNF-α in terms of the ability to initiate cachexia.

Fatigue and Sleep Disorders

Fatigue and sleep disturbances are two of the most frequent side effects experienced by persons with cancer.[54–57] Cancer-related fatigue is characterized by feelings of tiredness, weakness, and lack of energy, and is distinct from the normal tiredness experienced by healthy individuals in that it is not relieved by rest or sleep. It occurs both as a consequence of the cancer itself and as a side effect of cancer treatment. Cancer-related fatigue may be an early symptom of malignant disease and has been reported by as many as 40% of patients at the time of diagnosis.[56] Furthermore, the symptom often remains for months or even years after treatment.

The cause of cancer-related fatigue is largely unknown, but is probably multifactorial and involves the dysregulation of several interrelated physiologic, biochemical, and psychological systems. The basic mechanisms of fatigue have been broadly categorized into two components: peripheral and central.[55] Peripheral fatigue, which occurs in the neuromuscular junctions and muscles, results from the inability of the peripheral neuromuscular apparatus to perform a task in response to central stimulation. Mechanisms implicated in peripheral fatigue include a lack of ATP and the buildup of metabolic byproducts such as lactic acid. Central fatigue arises in the central nervous system (CNS) and is often described as difficulty in initiating or maintaining voluntary activities. One hypothesis proposed to explain cancer-related fatigue is that cancer and cancer treatments result in dysregulation of brain serotonin (5-hydroxytryptamine, 5-HT) levels or function. There is evidence that proinflammatory cytokines, such as TNF-α, can influence 5-HT metabolism.[55]

Although cancer-related fatigue and sleep disorders are distinct conditions, they are closely linked in terms of prevalence and symptoms.[57] Persons with cancer report poor sleep quality, disturbed initiation and maintenance of sleep, insufficient sleep, nighttime awakening, and restless sleep (see Chapter 52 for a discussion of sleep disorders). As with fatigue, precipitating factors include the diagnosis of cancer, type and stage of cancer, pain, and side effects of treatment (*e.g.,* nausea, vomiting). Once it begins, insomnia is often self-perpetuating because of the natural tendency to compensate for sleep loss by napping, going to bed earlier, and getting out of bed later. It may also be that the fatigue that occurs with cancer or anticancer therapy may, in fact, prompt persons to extend their sleep opportunity and thus becomes a contributing factor to ongoing insomnia. Correlations have also been noted between fatigue and daytime symptoms of sleep problems, such as daytime sleepiness and napping.

Anemia

Anemia is common in persons with various types of cancers. It may be related to blood loss, hemolysis, impaired red blood cell production, or treatment effects.[58,59] For example, drugs used in treatment of cancer are cytotoxic and can decrease red blood cell production. Also, there are many mechanisms through which erythrocyte production can be impaired in persons with malignancies, including nutritional deficiencies, bone marrow failure, and a blunted erythropoietin response to hypoxia. Inflammatory cytokines generated in response to tumours decrease erythropoietin production, resulting in a decrease in erythrocyte production.

Cancer-related anemia is associated with reduced treatment effectiveness, increased mortality, increased transfusion requirements, and reduced performance and quality of life. Hypoxia, a characteristic feature of advanced solid tumours, has been recognized as a critical factor in promoting tumour resistance to radiation therapy and some chemotherapeutic agents. Severe anemia may delay surgical interventions when preoperative transfusions are required. Similarly, low hemoglobin levels before or during chemotherapy may require dose reductions or delays in administration, resulting in a decrease in overall treatment effectiveness. Cancer-related anemia is often treated with recombinant human erythropoietin (EPO, epoetin alfa) (see Chapter 14).

Paraneoplastic Syndromes

In addition to signs and symptoms at the sites of primary and metastatic disease, cancer can produce manifestations in sites that are not directly affected by the disease. Such manifestations are collectively referred to as *paraneoplastic syndromes.*[60,61] Some of these manifestations are caused by the elaboration of hormones by cancer cells, and others from the production of circulating factors that produce hematopoietic, neurologic, and dermatologic syndromes (Table 8.4). These syndromes are most commonly associated with lung, breast, and hematologic malignancies.[11]

A variety of peptide hormones are produced by both benign and malignant tumours. Although not normally expressed, the biochemical pathways for the synthesis and release of peptide hormones (*e.g.,* antidiuretic [ADH], adrenocorticotropic [ACTH], and parathyroid [PTH] hormones) are present in most cells.[62] Thus, the three most common endocrine syndromes associated with cancer are the syndrome of inappropriate ADH secretion (see Chapter 31), Cushing syndrome due to ectopic ACTH production (see Chapter 41), and hypercalcemia (see Chapter 31).[61,62] Hypercalcemia of malignancy does not appear to be related to PTH but to a PTH-related protein that shares several biologic actions with PTH. Hypercalcemia also can be caused by osteolytic processes induced by cancers such as multiple myeloma or bony metastases from other cancers.

Some paraneoplastic syndromes are associated with the production of circulating mediators that produce hematologic complications.[61] For example, a variety of cancers may produce procoagulation factors that contribute to an increased risk for

TABLE 8.4 COMMON PARANEOPLASTIC SYNDROMES

TYPE OF SYNDROME	ASSOCIATED TUMOUR TYPE	PROPOSED MECHANISM
Endocrinologic		
Syndrome of inappropriate ADH	Small cell lung cancer, others	Production and release of ADH by tumour
Cushing syndrome	Small cell lung cancer, bronchial carcinoid cancers	Production and release of ACTH by tumour
Hypercalcemia	Squamous cell cancers of the lung, head, neck, ovary	Production and release of polypeptide factor with close relationship to PTH
Hematologic		
Venous thrombosis	Pancreatic, lung, other cancers	Production of procoagulation factors
Nonbacterial thrombolytic endocarditis	Advanced cancers	
Neurologic		
Lambert–Eaton syndrome	Small cell lung cancer	Autoimmune production of antibodies to motor end-plate structures
Myasthenia gravis	Thymoma	
Dermatologic		
Acanthosis nigricans	Gastric carcinoma	Possibly caused by production of growth factors (epidermal) by tumour cells

ADH, antidiuretic hormone; ACTH, adrenocorticotropic hormone; PTH, parathyroid hormone.

venous thrombosis and nonbacterial thrombotic endocarditis. Sometimes, unexplained thrombotic events are the first indication of an undiagnosed malignancy. The precise relationship between coagulation disorders and cancer is still unknown. Several malignancies, such as mucin-producing adenocarcinomas, release thromboplastin and other substances that activate the clotting system.

The symptomatic paraneoplastic neurologic disorders are relatively rare, with the exception of the Lambert–Eaton myasthenic syndrome, which affects about 3% of persons with small cell lung cancer; and myasthenia gravis, which affects about 15% of people with thymoma.[63] The *Lambert–Eaton syndrome,* or reverse myasthenia gravis, is seen almost exclusively in small cell lung cancer. It produces muscle weakness in the limbs rather than the initial bulbar and ocular muscle weakness seen in myasthenia gravis. The origin of paraneoplastic neurologic disorders is thought to be immune mediated.[63,64] The altered immune response is initiated by the production of onconeural antigens (*e.g.,* antigens normally expressed in the nervous system) by the cancer cells. The immune system, in turn, recognizes the onconeural antigens as foreign and mounts an immune response. In many cases, the immune attack controls the growth of the cancer. The antibodies and cytotoxic T cells are not sufficient to cause neurologic disease unless they cross the blood-brain barrier and react with neurons expressing the onconeural antigen.[63]

A wide variety of cutaneous syndromes is associated with malignancies and may precede, be concurrent with, or follow the discovery of cancer. Among the paraneoplastic dermatologic disorders is *acanthosis nigricans,* characterized by pigmented hyperkeratoses consisting of symmetric, verrucous, and papillary lesions that occur in skin flexures, particularly the axillary and perineal areas.[61] The lesions are usually symmetric and may be accompanied by pruritus. The condition is usually associated with adenocarcinomas of the gastrointestinal tract, particularly gastric carcinoma, but may be associated with a variety of adenocarcinomas, including lung, breast, ovarian, and even hematologic cancers. The pathogenesis of these lesions is uncertain.

The paraneoplastic syndromes may be the earliest indication that a person has cancer, and should be regarded as such.[60] They may also represent significant clinical problems, may be potentially lethal in persons with cancer, and may mimic metastatic disease and confound treatment. Diagnostic methods focus on both identifying the cause of the disorder and on locating the malignancy responsible. Techniques for precise identification of minute amounts of polypeptides may allow for early diagnosis of curable malignancies in asymptomatic individuals.[61] The treatment of paraneoplastic syndromes involves concurrent treatment of the underlying cancer and suppression of the mediator causing the syndrome.

IN SUMMARY

There probably is no single body function left unaffected by the presence of cancer. Because tumour cells replace normally functioning parenchymal tissue, the initial manifestations of cancer usually reflect the primary site of involvement. Cancer compresses blood vessels, obstructs lymph flow, disrupts tissue integrity, invades serous cavities, and compresses visceral organs. It may result in development of an effusion (*i.e.,* fluid) in the pleural, pericardial, or peritoneal spaces, and generalized manifestations such as anorexia and cachexia, fatigue and sleep disorders, and anemia. It may also produce paraneoplastic syndromes that arise from the ability of neoplasms to elaborate hormones and other chemical mediators to produce endocrine, hematopoietic, neurologic, and dermatologic syndromes. Many of these manifestations are compounded by the side effects of methods used to treat the disease.

SCREENING, DIAGNOSIS, AND TREATMENT

After completing this section of the chapter, you should be able to meet the following objectives:

- Cite three characteristics of an ideal screening test for cancer.
- Describe the four methods that are used in the diagnosis of cancer.
- Differentiate between the methods used for grading and staging of cancers.
- Explain the mechanism by which radiation exerts its beneficial effects in the treatment of cancer.
- Describe the adverse effects of radiation therapy.
- Differentiate between the action of direct DNA-interacting and indirect DNA-interacting chemotherapeutic agents and cell cycle–specific and cell cycle–independent drugs.
- Describe the three mechanisms whereby biotherapy exerts its effects.
- Describe three examples of targeted therapy used in the treatment of cancer.

Screening

Screening represents a secondary prevention measure for the early recognition of cancer in an otherwise asymptomatic population.[65] Screening can be achieved through observation (*e.g.,* skin, mouth, external genitalia), palpation (*e.g.,* breast, thyroid, rectum and anus, prostate, lymph nodes), and laboratory tests and procedures (*e.g.,* Papanicolaou [Pap] smear, colonoscopy, mammography). It requires a test that will specifically detect early cancers or premalignancies, is cost effective, and results in improved therapeutic outcomes.[65] For most cancers, stage at presentation is related to curability, with the highest rates reported when the tumour is small and there is no evidence of metastasis. For some tumours, however, metastasis tends to occur early, even from a small primary tumour. For other cancers, such as cancer of the pancreas, no screening methods are currently available. More sensitive screening methods such as tumour markers are being developed for these forms of cancer.

Cancers for which current screening or early detection has led to improvement in outcomes include cancers of the breast (mammography, discussed in Chapter 46), cervix (Pap smear, Chapter 46), colon and rectum (rectal examination, fecal occult blood test, and colonoscopy, Chapter 37), prostate (prostate-specific antigen [PSA] testing and transrectal ultrasonography, Chapter 44), and malignant melanoma (self-examination, Chapter 61). Although not as clearly defined, it is recommended that screening for other types of cancers such as cancers of the thyroid, testicles, ovaries, lymph nodes, and oral cavity be done at the time of periodic health examinations.

Diagnostic Methods

The methods used in the diagnosis and staging of cancer are determined largely by the location and type of cancer suspected. A number of procedures are used in the diagnosis of cancer, including blood tests for tumour markers, cytologic studies and tissue biopsy, endoscopic examinations, ultrasonography, x-ray studies, MRI, computed tomography (CT), and positron emission tomography (PET).

Tumour Markers

Tumour markers are antigens expressed on the surface of tumour cells or substances released from normal cells in response to the presence of tumours.[11,66] Some substances, such as hormones and enzymes that are produced normally by the involved tissue, become overexpressed as a result of cancer. Other tumour markers, such as oncofetal proteins, are produced during fetal development and are induced to reappear later in life as a result of benign and malignant neoplasms. Tumour markers are used for screening, establishing prognosis, monitoring treatment, and detecting recurrent disease. Table 8.5 identifies some of the more commonly used tumour markers and summarizes their source and the cancers associated with them.

The serum markers that have proved most useful in clinical practice are human chorionic gonadotropin (hCG), CA-125, PSA, α-fetoprotein (AFP), carcinoembryonic antigen (CEA), and CD blood cell antigens.[11] A hormone normally produced by the placenta, hCG, is used as a marker for diagnosing, prescribing treatment, and following the disease course in persons with high-risk gestational trophoblastic tumours. PSA is used as a marker in prostate cancer, and CA-125 is used as a marker in ovarian cancer. Markers for leukemia and lymphomas are grouped by the so-called *cluster of differentiation* (CD) antigens (see Chapter 15). The CD antigens help to distinguish among T and B lymphocytes, monocytes, granulocytes, and NK cells, and immature variants of these cells.[5,11]

Some cancers express fetal antigens that are normally present only during embryonal development.[11] The two that have proved most useful as tumour markers are AFP and CEA. AFP is synthesized by the fetal liver, yolk sac, and gastrointestinal tract and is the major serum protein in the fetus. Elevated levels are encountered in people with primary liver cancers

TABLE 8.5 TUMOUR MARKERS

MARKER	SOURCE	ASSOCIATED CANCERS
Oncofetal Antigens		
α-Fetoprotein (AFP)	Fetal yolk sac and gastrointestinal structures early in fetal life	Primary liver cancers, germ cell cancer of the testis
Carcinoembryonic antigen (CEA)	Embryonic tissues in gut, pancreas, and liver	Colorectal cancer and cancers of the pancreas, lung, and stomach
Hormones		
Human chorionic gonadotropin (hCG)	Hormone normally produced by placenta	Gestational trophoblastic tumours, germ cell cancer of testis
Calcitonin	Hormone produced by thyroid parafollicular cells	Thyroid cancer
Catecholamines (epinephrine, norepinephrine) and metabolites	Hormones produced by chromaffin cells of the adrenal gland	Pheochromocytoma and related tumours
Specific Proteins		
Monoclonal immunoglobulin	Abnormal immunoglobulin produced by neoplastic cells	Multiple myeloma
Prostate-specific antigen (PSA)	Produced by the epithelial cells lining the acini and ducts of the prostate	Prostate cancer
Mucins and Other Glycoproteins		
CA-125	Produced by müllerian cells of the ovary	Ovarian cancer
CA-19-9	Produced by alimentary tract epithelium	Cancer of the pancreas, colon
Cluster of Differentiation		
CD antigens	Present on leukocytes	Used to determine the type and level of differentiation of leukocytes involved in different types of leukemia and lymphoma

and have also been observed in some testicular, ovarian, pancreatic, and stomach cancers. CEA normally is produced by embryonic tissue in the gut, pancreas, and liver and is elaborated by a number of different cancers. Depending on the serum level adopted for significant elevation, CEA is elevated in colorectal, pancreatic, gastric and breast cancers.[11] As with most other tumour markers, elevated levels of CEA and AFP are found in other, noncancerous conditions, and elevated levels of both depend on tumour size, so that neither is useful as an early screening test for cancer.

As diagnostic tools, tumour markers have limitations. Nearly all markers can be elevated in benign conditions, and most are not elevated in the early stages of malignancy. Hence, tumour markers have limited value as screening tests. Furthermore, they are not in themselves specific enough to permit a diagnosis of a malignancy, but once a malignancy has been diagnosed and shown to be associated with elevated levels of a tumour marker, the marker can be used to assess response to therapy. Extremely elevated levels of a tumour marker can indicate a poor prognosis or the need for more aggressive treatment. Perhaps the greatest value of tumour markers is in monitoring therapy in people with widespread cancer. The level of most cancer markers tends to decrease with successful treatment and increase with recurrence or spread of the tumour.

Cytologic and Histologic Methods

Histologic and cytologic studies are laboratory methods used to examine tissues and cells. Several sampling approaches are available, including cytologic smears, tissue biopsies, and needle aspiration.[11]

Papanicolaou Test. The Pap test is a cytologic method used for detecting cancer cells. It consists of a microscopic examination of a properly prepared slide by a cytotechnologist or pathologist for the purpose of detecting the presence of abnormal cells. The usefulness of the Pap test relies on the fact that the cancer cells lack the cohesive properties and intercellular junctions that are characteristic of normal tissue; without these characteristics, cancer cells tend to exfoliate and become mixed with secretions surrounding the tumour growth. Although the Pap test is widely used as a screening test for cervical cancer, it can be performed on other body secretions, including nipple drainage, pleural or peritoneal fluid, and gastric washings.

Tissue Biopsy. Tissue biopsy, which is of critical importance in diagnosing the correct cancer and histology and for designing the treatment plan should cancer cells be found, involves the removal of a tissue specimen for microscopic study. Biopsies are obtained in a number of ways, including needle biopsy; endoscopic methods, such as bronchoscopy or cystoscopy, which involve the passage of an endoscope through an orifice and into the involved structure; or laparoscopic methods. In some instances, a surgical incision is made from which biopsy specimens are obtained. Excisional biopsies are those in which the entire tumour is removed. The tumours usually are small, solid, palpable masses. If the tumour is too large to be completely removed, a wedge of tissue from the mass can be excised for examination. Appropriate preservation of the specimen includes prompt immersion in a fixative solution such as formalin, with preservation of a portion of the specimen in a special fixative for electron microscopy, or prompt refrigeration to permit optimal hormone, receptor, and other types of molecular analysis. A quick frozen section may be done to determine the nature of a mass lesion or evaluate the margins of an excised tumour to ascertain that the entire neoplasm has been removed.[11]

Fine-needle aspiration is another approach that is widely used. The procedure involves aspirating cells and attendant fluid with a small-bore needle. The method is most commonly used for assessment of readily palpable lesions in sites such as the thyroid, breast, and lymph nodes. Modern imaging techniques have also enabled the method to be extended to deeper structures such as the pelvic lymph nodes and pancreas.

Immunohistochemistry. Immunohistochemistry involves the use of antibodies to facilitate the identification of cell products or surface markers.[11] For example, certain anaplastic carcinomas, malignant lymphomas, melanomas, and sarcomas look very similar under the microscope, but must be accurately identified because their treatment and prognosis are quite different. Antibodies against intermediate filaments have proved useful in such cases because tumour cells often contain intermediate filaments characteristic of their tissue of origin.[11] Immunohistochemistry can also be used to determine the site of origin of metastatic tumours. Many patients with cancer present with metastasis. In cases in which the origin of the metastasis is obscure, immunohistochemical detection of tissue-specific or organ-specific antigens can often help to identify the tumour source. Immunohistochemistry can also be used to detect molecules that have prognostic or therapeutic significance. For example, detection of estrogen receptors on breast cancer cells is of prognostic and therapeutic significance because these tumours respond to antiestrogen therapy.

Microarray Technology. Microarray technology uses "gene chips" that can simultaneously perform miniature assays to detect and quantify the expression of large numbers of genes.[11] The advantage of microarray technology is the ability to analyze a large number of changes in cancer cells to determine overall patterns of behaviour that could not be assessed by conventional means. DNA arrays are now commercially available to assist in making clinical decisions regarding cancer treatment. In addition to identifying tumour types, microarrays have been used for predicting prognosis and response

to therapy, examining tumour changes after therapy, and classifying hereditary tumours.[11]

Staging and Grading of Tumours

The two basic methods for classifying cancers are *grading* according to the histologic or cellular characteristics of the tumour and *staging* according to the clinical spread of the disease. Both methods are used to determine the course of the disease and aid in selecting an appropriate treatment or management plan. Grading of tumours involves the microscopic examination of cancer cells to determine their level of differentiation and the number of mitoses. Cancers are classified as grades I, II, III, and IV with increasing anaplasia or lack of differentiation. Staging of cancers uses methods to determine the extent and spread of the disease. Surgery may be used to determine tumour size and lymph node involvement.

The clinical staging of cancer is intended to group patients according to the extent of their disease at diagnosis. It is useful in determining the choice of treatment for individual patients, estimating prognosis, and comparing the results of different treatment regimens. The TNM system is the global classification system developed by the International Union Against Cancer (UICC) and is used by most cancer facilities.[67] This system, which is briefly described in Chart 8.2, classifies the disease into stages using three tumour components: *T* stands for the size and local spread of the primary tumour, *N* refers to the involvement of the regional lymph nodes, and *M* describes the extent of the metastatic involvement. The time of staging is indicated as clinical–diagnostic staging (cTNM), postsurgical resection–pathologic staging (pTNM), surgical–evaluative staging (sTNM), retreatment staging (rTNM), and autopsy staging (aTNM).[67]

CHART 8.2 TNM CLASSIFICATION SYSTEM

T (tumour)	
Tx	Tumour cannot be adequately assessed
T0	No evidence of primary tumour
Tis	Carcinoma in situ
T1–4	Progressive increase in tumour size or involvement
N (nodes)	
Nx	Regional lymph nodes cannot be assessed
N0	No evidence of regional node metastasis
N1–3	Increasing involvement of regional lymph nodes
M (metastasis)	
Mx	Not assessed
M0	No distant metastasis
M1	Distant metastasis present, specify sites

Cancer Treatment

The goals of cancer treatment methods fall into three categories: curative, control, and palliative. The most common modalities are surgery, radiation therapy, chemotherapy, hormonal therapy, and biotherapy. The treatment of cancer involves the use of a carefully planned program that combines the benefits of multiple treatment modalities and the expertise of an interdisciplinary team of specialists, including medical, surgical, and radiation oncologists; clinical nurse specialists; nurse practitioners; pharmacists; and a variety of ancillary personnel.

Surgery

Surgery is the oldest treatment for cancer and, until recently, the only treatment that could cure persons with cancer. Surgery is now used for diagnosis, staging of cancer, tumour removal, and palliation (*i.e.,* relief of symptoms) when a cure cannot be achieved. The type of surgery to be used is determined by the extent of the disease, the location and structures involved, the tumour growth rate and invasiveness, the surgical risk to the patient, and the quality of life the patient will experience after the surgery. Surgery is often thought of as the first line of treatment for solid tumours. If the tumour is small and has well-defined margins, the entire tumour often can be removed. If, however, the tumour is large or involves vital tissues, surgical removal may be difficult, if not impossible.

Surgery provides several approaches for cancer treatment. For example, it can be the primary, curative treatment for cancers that are locally or regionally contained, have not metastasized, or have not invaded major organs. It also is used as a component of adjuvant therapy in combination with chemotherapy or radiation therapy in other types of cancers. Surgical techniques also may be used to control oncologic emergencies such as gastrointestinal hemorrhages. Another approach includes using surgical techniques for cancer prophylaxis in families that have a high genetically confirmed risk for developing cancer. For instance, a total colectomy may be suggested for an individual with familial adenomatous polyposis coli because of the increased risk for developing cancer by 40 years of age.

Surgical techniques have expanded to include cryosurgery, chemosurgery, laser surgery, and laparoscopic surgery. *Cryosurgery* involves the instillation of liquid nitrogen into the tumour through a probe. It is used in treating cancers of the liver and prostate. *Chemosurgery* is used in skin cancers. It involves the use of a corrosive paste in combination with multiple frozen sections to ensure complete removal of the tumour. *Laser surgery* uses a laser beam to resect a tumour. It has been used effectively in retinal and vocal cord surgery. *Laparoscopic surgery* involves the performance of abdominal surgery through two or more small incisions—one for viewing within the cavity and the other(s) for insertion of the instruments to perform the surgery.

Cooperative efforts among cancer centres throughout the world have helped to standardize and improve surgical procedures, determine which cancers benefit from surgical intervention, and establish in what order surgical and other treatment modalities should be used. Increased emphasis also has been placed on the development of surgical techniques that preserve body image and form without compromising essential function. Nerve-sparing prostatectomy and limb-salvage surgery for soft tissue tumours preserve functional abilities while permitting complete removal of the tumour.[68,69]

Radiation Therapy

Radiation therapy is one of the most commonly used methods of cancer treatment.[70,71] It can be used alone as a primary method of therapy or as an adjuvant treatment with surgery, chemotherapy, or both. It can also be used as a palliative treatment to reduce symptoms such as bone pain resulting from metastasis in persons with advanced cancers. Radiation is used to treat oncologic emergencies such as superior vena cava syndrome, spinal cord compression, or bronchial obstruction.

Radiation therapy uses high-energy particles or waves to damage or destroy cancer cells. The absorption of energy from radiation in tissue leads to the ionization of molecules or creation of free radicals. Radiation can also produce effects indirectly by interacting with water (which makes up approximately 80% of a cell's volume) to produce free radicals, which damage cell structures (see Chapter 5). Radiation can immediately kill cells, delay or halt cell cycle progression, or, at dose levels commonly used in radiation therapy, produce damage to the cell's DNA, resulting in cell death after replication.[71] Radiation must produce double-stranded breaks in DNA to kill a cell, owing to the high capacity of cells for repairing single-stranded breaks.

The therapeutic effects of radiation therapy derive from the fact that the rapidly proliferating and poorly differentiated cells of a cancerous tumour are more likely to be injured than are the more slowly proliferating cells of normal tissue. To some extent, however, radiation is injurious to all rapidly proliferating cells, including those of the bone marrow and the mucosal lining of the gastrointestinal tract. Normal tissue usually is able to recover from radiation damage more readily than cancerous tissue. In addition to its lethal effects, radiation also produces sublethal injury. Recovery from sublethal doses of radiation occurs in the interval between the first dose of radiation and subsequent doses.[71,72] This is why large total doses of radiation can be tolerated when they are divided into multiple, smaller fractionated doses.[70–72]

The radiation dose that is chosen for treatment of a particular cancer is determined by factors such as the radiosensitivity of the tumour type, the size of the tumour, and, more important, the tolerance of the surrounding tissues.[71,72] The term *radiosensitivity* describes the inherent properties of a tumour that determine its responsiveness to radiation. It varies widely among the different types of cancers and is thought to vary as a function of their position in the cell cycle. Fast-growing cancers have cells that typically are more radiosensitive than slow-growing cancers. The combination of selected cytotoxic drugs with radiation has demonstrated a radiosensitizing effect on tumour cells by altering the cell cycle distribution, increasing DNA damage, and decreasing DNA repair. Radiosensitizers include 5-fluorouracil, capecitabine, paclitaxel, gemcitabine, and cisplatin.[73]

Radiation responsiveness describes the manner in which a radiosensitive tumour responds to irradiation. One of the major determinants of radiation responsiveness is tumour oxygenation, because oxygen is a rich source of free radicals that form and destroy essential cell components during irradiation.[72] Many rapidly growing tumours outgrow their blood supply and become deprived of oxygen. The hypoxic cells of these tumours are more resistant to radiation than normal or well-oxygenated tumour cells. Methods of ensuring adequate oxygen delivery, such as adequate hemoglobin levels, are important.

Dose–response curves, which express the extent of lethal tissue injury in relation to the dose of radiation, are determined by the number of cells that survive graded, fractional doses of radiation. The use of more frequent fractionated doses increases the likelihood that the cancer cells will be dividing and in the vulnerable period of the cell cycle during radiation administration. This type of dose also allows time for normal tissues to repair the radiation damage. An important focus of research has been the search for drugs to reduce the biologic effects of radiation on normal tissue. These drugs, known as *radioprotectants,* would preferentially protect normal cells from the cytotoxic effects of radiation. One drug, amifostine, is approved by Health Canada to reduce the incidence of dryness of the mouth (*i.e.,* xerostomia) due to the effects of radiation on salivary gland function in patients undergoing radiation therapy for head and neck cancers.[73]

Administration. Therapeutic radiation can be delivered in three ways: external beam or teletherapy, with beams generated at a distance and aimed at the tumour in a patient; brachytherapy, in which a sealed radioactive source is placed close to or directly in the tumour site; and systemic therapy, in which radioisotopes with a short half-life are given by mouth or injected into the tumour site.[71] Radiation from any source decreases in intensity as a function of the square of the distance from the source. Teletherapy, which is the most commonly used form of radiation therapy, maintains intensity over a large volume of tissue by increasing the source-to-surface distance. In brachytherapy, the source-to-surface distance is small; therefore, the effective treatment volume is small.

External-beam radiation is commonly delivered by a linear accelerator or a cobalt-60 machine.[71] The linear accelerator is the preferred machine because of its versatility and precision of dose distribution, as well as the speed with which treatment can be given. Linear accelerators produce ionizing radiation through a process in which electrons are accelerated at a very high rate, strike a target, and produce high-energy x-rays (photons). The linear accelerator can vary the level of radiation energy that is delivered so that different depths can be treated. Various beam-modifying approaches are used to define and shape the beam, thereby increasing the radiation

damage to the tumour site while sparing the normal surrounding tissues. Three-dimensional conformal radiation therapy (3D CRT) uses CT scans or MRI to construct an image of the tumour.[74,75] The patient is fitted with a plastic mold or cast to keep the body still, while radiation beams are delivered to the body from several directions. Intensity-modulated radiation therapy (IMRT) is another advanced form of external radiation therapy. As with 3D CRT, computer imaging techniques are used to calculate the most efficient dosages and combinations of radiation treatment. This precise mapping of the tumour allows for the delivery of radiation beams that conform to the contours of the tumour, reducing the dose and therefore the toxicity to adjacent normal tissue. Because of its precision, it is even more important that the patient remain in the right position and perfectly still during the treatment. This usually requires fabricating a special cast or mold before treatment to keep the body in place.

Brachytherapy involves the insertion of sealed radioactive sources into a body cavity (intracavitary) or directly into body tissues (interstitial). The term *brachytherapy* means "short therapy," implying that the radiation effect is limited to areas close to the radiation source.[76] Brachytherapy can be subdivided into high-dose radiation (HDR) and low-dose radiation (LDR) according to the rate at which the radiation is delivered. HDR uses a single highly radioactive source that is attached to a cable and housed in a robotic machine referred to as an HDR remote afterloader. When the treatment is delivered, the radiation source is pushed from the remote afterloader through a tube to a location near the tumour site. Remote afterloading machines make it possible to insert a radioactive material (*e.g.,* cesium-137, iridium-192) into a tumour area for a specific time and remove it while oncology personnel are outside the treatment room. This minimizes staff radiation exposure and decreases treatment times by allowing use of intermediate- and high-dose radioactive sources.[76] In contrast, the radiation source for LDR brachytherapy may be packed into catheter devices or sealed radiation sources (*e.g.,* beads, seeds) and placed directly in or near the area being treated. LDR therapy can be temporary or permanent. Temporary LDR brachytherapy can be accomplished as an inpatient procedure, with radiation applicators and sources remaining in the patient for a few days. Radioactive materials with a relatively short half-life, such as iodine-125 or palladium-103, are commonly encapsulated and used in permanent implants (*e.g.,* seed implants used to treat prostate cancer).

Unsealed internal radiation sources are injected intravenously or administered by mouth. Iodine-131, which is given by mouth, is used in the treatment of thyroid cancer. Strontium-89, administered intravenously, is given to control bone pain due to multiple skeletal metastases in patients with advanced breast, lung, or prostate cancer.[71] Stereotactic radiosurgery is a method of destroying brain tumours and brain metastases by delivering a single large dose of radiation through stereotactically directed narrow beams. Gamma knife radiosurgery allows the application of focused radiation for limited brain metastasis and is associated with fewer long-term complications, such as cognitive dysfunction, than whole-brain radiation.

Adverse Effects. Radiation cannot distinguish between malignant cells and rapidly proliferating cells of normal tissue.[71] During radiation treatment, injury to normal cells can produce adverse effects. Tissues within the treatment fields that are most frequently affected are the skin, the mucosal lining of the gastrointestinal tract, and the bone marrow. Anorexia, nausea, emesis, and diarrhea are common with abdominal and pelvic irradiation. These symptoms are usually controlled by medication and dietary measures. The primary systemic effect is fatigue. Most of these side effects are temporary and reversible.

Radiation can also cause bone marrow suppression, particularly when it is delivered to the bone marrow in skeletal sites. Subsequently, the complete blood count is affected, resulting in an initial decrease in the number of the leukocytes, followed by a decrease in thrombocytes (platelets) and, finally, red blood cells. This predisposes the individual to infection, bleeding, and anemia, respectively. Frequent blood counts are used during radiation therapy to monitor bone marrow function.

External-beam radiation must first penetrate the skin and, depending on the total dose and type of radiation used, skin reactions may develop. With moderate doses of radiation, the hair falls out spontaneously or when being combed after the 10th to the 14th day. With larger doses, erythema develops (much like sunburn) and may turn brown; and, at higher doses, patches of dry or moist desquamation may develop. Fortunately, reepithelialization takes place after the treatments have been stopped. Mucositis or desquamation of the oral and pharyngeal mucous membranes, which sometimes may be severe, may occur as a predictable side effect in people receiving head and neck irradiation. Pain and difficulty with eating and drinking can negatively affect the individual's nutritional status. Pelvic radiation can cause impotence or erectile dysfunction in men and vaginal irritation, dryness, and discharge, dyspareunia, and, as a late effect, vaginal stenosis in women.

Chemotherapy

Cancer chemotherapy has evolved to become one of the major systemic treatment modalities for cancer. Unlike surgery and radiation, chemotherapy is a systemic treatment that enables drugs to reach the site of the tumour as well as other distant sites. Chemotherapeutic drugs may be the primary form of treatment, or they may be used as part of a multimodal treatment plan. It is the primary treatment for most hematologic and some solid tumours, including choriocarcinoma, testicular cancer, acute and chronic leukemia, non-Hodgkin and Hodgkin lymphomas, and multiple myeloma. In persons with widespread disseminated disease, chemotherapy provides only palliative rather than curative therapy at present.

Cancer chemotherapeutic drugs exert their effects through several mechanisms. At the cellular level, they exert their lethal action by targeting processes that prevent cell growth and replication. These mechanisms include disrupting the production of essential enzymes; inhibiting DNA, RNA, and protein synthesis; and preventing cell mitosis.[71,77,78] Under ideal conditions, anticancer drugs would eradicate cancer cells without damaging normal tissues. Unfortunately, no cancer agents currently available are completely without toxic effects, and their clinical use involves weighing their beneficial effects against their toxicity.

For most chemotherapy drugs, the relationship between tumour cell survival and drug dose is exponential, with the number of cells surviving being proportional to the drug dose, and the number of cells at risk for exposure being proportional to the destructive action of the drug. Chemotherapeutic drugs are most effective in treating tumours that have a high growth fraction because of their ability to kill rapidly dividing cells. Exponential killing implies that a proportion or percentage of tumour cells is killed, rather than an absolute number.[5] This proportion is a constant percentage of the total number of cells. For this reason, multiple courses of treatment are needed if the tumour is to be eradicated.

A major problem in cancer chemotherapy is the development of cellular resistance. Acquired resistance develops in a number of drug-sensitive tumour types.[7,8] Experimentally, drug resistance can be highly specific to a single agent and is usually based on genetic changes in a given tumour cell. In other instances, a multidrug-resistant phenomenon encompassing anticancer drugs with differing structures occurs. This type of resistance often involves the increased expression of transmembrane transporter genes involved in drug efflux.

Chemotherapy drugs are commonly classified according to their site and mechanism of action. Chemotherapy drugs that have similar structures and effects on cell function usually are grouped together, and these drugs usually have similar side effect profiles. The major classifications of chemotherapy drugs are the direct DNA-interacting and indirect DNA-interacting agents.[78] Other systemic agents include hormonal and molecularly targeted agents. Cancer chemotherapy drugs may also be classified as either cell cycle-specific or cell cycle-nonspecific. Drugs are cell cycle-specific if they exert their action during a specific phase of the cell cycle. For example, methotrexate, an antimetabolite, acts by interfering with DNA synthesis and thereby interrupts the S phase of the cell cycle. Drugs that are cell cycle-nonspecific exert their effects throughout all phases of the cell cycle. The alkylating agents are cell cycle-nonspecific and act by disrupting DNA when the cells are in the resting state as well as when they are dividing. Because chemotherapy drugs differ in their mechanisms of action, cell cycle-specific and cell cycle-nonspecific agents are often combined to treat cancer.

Direct DNA-Interacting Agents. The direct DNA-interacting agents include the alkylating agents, antitumour antibiotics, and topoisomerase inhibitors. As a class, the alkylating agents exert their cytotoxic effects by transfer of their alkyl group to various cellular constituents.[71,78] Alkylation of DNA within the cell nucleus is probably the major interaction that causes cell death. Alkylating agents have direct vesicant effects and can damage tissues at the site of injection as well as produce systemic toxicity. Toxicities are generally dose related and occur particularly in rapidly proliferating tissues such as bone marrow, the gastrointestinal tract, and reproductive tissues.

The *antitumour antibiotics* are substances produced by bacteria that in nature appear to provide protection against hostile microorganisms. As a class they bind directly to DNA and frequently undergo electron transfer reactions to generate free radicals in close proximity to DNA, resulting in DNA damage in the form of single breaks or cross-links. All of the anticancer antibiotics now in clinical use are produced by the soil microbe *Streptomyces*. These include the anthracyclines, dactinomycin, bleomycin, and mitomycin. The anthracycline antibiotics (*e.g.,* doxorubicin and daunorubicin) are among the most widely used cytotoxic cancer drugs.[78] The main dose-limiting toxicity of all anthracyclines is cardiotoxicity and myelosuppression, with neutropenia more commonly observed than thrombocytopenia. Two forms of cardiotoxicity can occur—acute and chronic. The acute form occurs within the first 2 to 3 days of therapy and presents with arrhythmias, conduction disorders, other electrocardiographic changes, pericarditis, and myocarditis.[78] This form is usually transient and in most cases asymptomatic. The chronic form of cardiotoxicity results in a dose-dependent dilated cardiomyopathy (see Chapter 24). Efforts to minimize the toxicity profile of the antitumour antibiotics have resulted in the development of analog compounds (*e.g.,* idarubicin, epirubicin). Liposome technology has been used with two antitumour antibiotics (*i.e.,* doxorubicin and daunorubicin) to develop chemotherapy drugs that are encapsulated by coated liposomes. These drugs (*i.e.,* Myocet, Caelyx [doxorubicin], and DaunoXome [daunorubicin]) have been found to distribute more chemotherapy to the desired site with fewer side effects.[79]

The DNA *topoisomerase inhibitors* block cell division by interfering with the action of the topoisomerase enzymes that break and rejoin phosphodiester bonds in the DNA strands to prevent them from tangling during separation and unwinding of the double helix.[71,78] Topoisomerase I produces single-strand breaks (nicks) and topoisomerase II, double-strand breaks. The epipodophyllotoxins (etoposide and teniposide) are topoisomerase II inhibitors that block cell division in the late S-G2 phase of the cell cycle. The camptothecins (topotecan, irinotecan) inhibit the action of topoisomerase I, the enzyme responsible for cutting and rejoining single DNA strands. Inhibition of this enzyme interferes with resealing of the breaks and DNA damage.

Indirect DNA-Interacting Agents. The indirect DNA-interacting agents include the antimetabolites and mitotic spindle inhibitors. The antimetabolites (folic acid antagonists and purine and pyrimidine antagonists) interrupt the biochemical pathways relating to nucleotide and nucleic acid synthesis (see Chapter 6). Antimetabolites can cause DNA damage indirectly through misincorporation into DNA, abnormal timing or progression of DNA synthesis, or altered function of purine and pyrimidine biosynthetic enzymes.[77,78] They tend to convey their greatest effect during the S phase of the cell cycle. Because of their S-phase specificity, the antimetabolites have been shown to be more effective when given as a prolonged infusion. Common side effects include stomatitis, diarrhea, and myelosuppression.

The plant alkaloids, including the vinca alkaloids and taxanes, are drugs affecting the microtubule structures required for formation of the cytoskeleton and mitotic spindle[71,78] (see Chapter 4). Although each group of drugs affects the microtubule, their mechanism of action differs. The vinca alkaloids (*e.g.,* vinblastine, vincristine) inhibit tubulin polymerization, which disrupts assembly of microtubules. This inhibitory effect results in mitotic arrest in metaphase, bringing cell division to a stop, which then leads to cell death. Vinblastine is a potent vesicant and care must be taken in its administration. Toxicities include nausea and vomiting, bone marrow suppression, and alopecia. Despite similarities in their mechanisms of action, vincristine has a different spectrum of actions and toxicities than vinblastine. The main dose-limiting toxicity is neurotoxicity, usually expressed as a peripheral sensory neuropathy, although autonomic nervous system dysfunction (*e.g.,* orthostatic hypotension, sphincter problems, paralytic ileus), cranial nerve palsies, ataxia, seizures, and coma have been observed. The taxanes (*e.g.,* docetaxel, paclitaxel) differ from the vinca alkaloids in that they stabilize the microtubules against depolymerization. The stabilized microtubules are unable to undergo the normal changes necessary for cell cycle completion. These drugs are administered intravenously and require the use of a vehicle that can cause hypersensitivity reactions. In addition to hypersensitivity reactions, their side effect profile includes myelosuppression and peripheral neurotoxicity in the form of glove-and-stocking numbness, and paresthesia.

Combination Chemotherapy. Combination chemotherapy has been found to be more effective than treatment with a single drug. Combination chemotherapy creates a more hostile environment for tumour cell growth through higher drug concentrations and prevents the development of resistant clones of cancer cells. With this method, several drugs with different mechanisms of action, metabolic pathways, times of onset of action and recovery, side effects, and times of onset of side effects are used. Drugs used in combination must be individually effective against the tumour and may be synergistic with each other. Routes of administration and dosage schedules are carefully designed to ensure optimal delivery of the active forms of the drugs to a tumour during the sensitive phase of the cell cycle.

Administration. Many of the cancer chemotherapy drugs are administered intravenously. Venous access devices (VADs) often are used for people with poor venous access and those who require frequent or continuous intravenous therapy. The VAD can be used for home administration of chemotherapy drugs, blood sampling, and administration of blood components. These systems access the venous circulation either through an externalized catheter or an implanted catheter with access ports. In some cases, the drugs are administered by continuous infusion using an ambulatory infusion pump that allows the person to remain at home and maintain his or her activities. Newer drugs (*e.g.,* capecitabine, a pyrimidine antagonist) have been formulated for the oral route. Although adherence to a dosing schedule and reimbursement for oral drugs are a challenge, these drugs provide a more convenient administration form for the patient.

Adverse Effects. Chemotherapy is administered on a dose–response basis (*i.e.,* the more drug administered, the greater the number of cancer cells killed). Chemotherapeutic drugs affect neoplastic cells and the rapidly proliferating cells of normal tissue. The nadir (*i.e.,* lowest point) is the point of maximal toxicity for a given adverse effect of a drug and is stated in the time it takes to reach that point. Because many toxic effects of chemotherapeutic drugs persist for some time after the drug is discontinued, the nadir times and recovery rates are useful guides in evaluating the effects of cancer therapy. Some side effects appear immediately or after a few days (acute), some within a few weeks (intermediate), and others months to years after chemotherapy administration (long-term).

Most chemotherapeutic drugs cause pancytopenia due to bone marrow suppression, resulting in anemia, neutropenia, and thrombocytopenia.[71] With neutropenia, there is risk for developing serious infections, whereas thrombocytopenia increases the risk for bleeding. The availability of hematopoietic growth factors (*e.g.,* granulocyte colony-stimulating factor [G-CSF]; and IL-11, which stimulates platelet production) has shortened the period of myelosuppression, thereby reducing the need for hospitalizations due to infection and decreasing the need for blood products. However, when looking at the use of erythropoietin to stimulate red blood cell production, new clinical data suggests that replacing this factor might improve the quality of a person's life but conversely may also promote tumour progression and shorten survival. Analysis of the benefits and potential risks of treating chemotherapy induced anemia with erythropoietin should occur.[80]

Anorexia, nausea, and vomiting are common problems associated with cancer chemotherapy.[71,81] The severity of the vomiting is related to the emetic potential of the particular drug. These symptoms can occur within minutes or hours of drug administration and are thought to be due to stimulation of the chemoreceptor trigger zone in the medulla that initiates vomiting (see Chapter 36). The chemoreceptor trigger zone responds to levels of chemicals circulating in the blood. The acute symptoms usually subside within 24 to 48 hours and often can be relieved by antiemetics. The pharmacologic approaches to prevent chemotherapy-induced nausea and vomiting have greatly improved over the past several decades. The development of serotonin receptor (5-HT$_3$) antagonists (*e.g.,* ondansetron, granisetron, dolasetron,) has facilitated the use of highly emetic chemotherapy drugs by more effectively reducing the nausea and vomiting induced by these drugs. These antiemetics are effective when given by both the oral and intravenous routes. Aprepitant, a selective high-affinity antagonist of substance P/neuokinin-1 receptors, has been approved by Health Canada for use in treatment of nausea and vomiting associated with cancer chemotherapy. The drug, which is given orally, has been shown to inhibit both the acute and chronic phases of chemotherapy-induced nausea and vomiting.

Alopecia or hair loss results from impaired proliferation of the hair follicles and is a side effect of a number of cancer drugs; it usually is temporary, and the hair tends to regrow when treatment is stopped. The rapidly proliferating structures of the reproductive system are particularly sensitive to the action of cancer drugs. Women may experience changes in menstrual flow or have amenorrhea. Men may have a decreased sperm count (*i.e.,* oligospermia) or absence of sperm (*i.e.,* azoospermia). Many chemotherapeutic agents also may have teratogenic or mutagenic effects leading to fetal abnormalities.[82]

Chemotherapy drugs are toxic to all cells. The mutagenic, carcinogenic, and teratogenic potential of these drugs has been strongly supported by both animal and human studies. Because of these potential risks, special care is required when handling or administering the drugs. Drugs, drug containers, and administration equipment require special disposal as hazardous waste. Several organizations, including the Occupational Safety and Health Administration (OSHA), the Oncology Nursing Society (ONS), the Canadian Society of Hospital Pharmacists (CSHP), and the Canadian Cancer Society have developed special guidelines for the safe handling and disposal of antineoplastic drugs as well as for accidental spills and exposure.[81–84]

Epidemiologic studies have shown an increased risk for second malignancies such as acute leukemia after long-term use of alkylating agents, particularly procarbazine, for treatment of various forms of cancer.[78] These second malignancies are thought to result from direct cellular changes produced by the drug or from suppression of the immune response.

Hormonal Therapy

Hormonal therapy consists of administration of drugs designed to disrupt the hormonal environment of cancer cells. It is used for cancers that are responsive to or dependent on hormones for growth.[71,78] The actions of hormones and antihormones depend on the presence of specific receptors in the tumour. Among the tumours that are known to be responsive to hormonal manipulation are those of the breast, prostate, and endometrium. Other cancers, such as Kaposi sarcoma and renal, liver, ovarian, and pancreatic cancer, are also responsive to hormonal manipulation, but to a lesser degree.[85] The theory behind the majority of hormone-based cancer treatments is to deprive the cancer cells of the hormonal signals that otherwise would stimulate them to divide.

The therapeutic options for altering the hormonal environment in the woman with breast cancer or the man with prostate cancer include surgical and pharmacologic measures. Surgery involves the removal of the organ responsible for the hormone production that is stimulating the target tissue (*e.g.,* oophorectomy in women or orchiectomy in men). Pharmacologic methods focus largely on reducing circulating hormone levels or changing the hormone receptors so that they no longer respond to the hormone.

Pharmacologic suppression of circulating hormone levels can be effected through pituitary desensitization, as with the administration of androgens, or through the administration of *gonadotropin-releasing hormone* (GnRH) analogs that act at the level of the hypothalamus to inhibit gonadotropin production and release. Another class of drugs, the *aromatase inhibitors,* is used to treat breast cancer; these drugs act by interrupting the biochemical processes that convert the adrenal androgen androstenedione to estrone.[86] Aromatization of an androgenic precursor into an estrogen occurs in body fat. Because estrogen promotes the growth of breast cancer, estrogen synthesis in adipose tissue can be an important factor in breast cancer growth in postmenopausal women.

Hormone receptor function can be altered by the administration of pharmacologic doses of exogenous hormones that act by producing a decrease in hormone receptors, or by antihormone drugs (*i.e.,* antiestrogens [tamoxifen, fulvestrant] and antiandrogens [flutamide, bicalutamide, nilutamide]) that bind to hormone receptors, making them inaccessible to hormone stimulation. Initially, patients often respond favourably to hormonal treatments, but eventually the cancer becomes resistant to hormonal manipulation, and other approaches must be sought to control the disease.

Biotherapy

Biotherapy involves the use of immunotherapy and biologic response modifiers as a means of changing the person's own immune response to cancer.[78,87] The major mechanisms by which biotherapy exerts its effects are modifications of host responses or tumour cell biology.

Immunotherapy. Immunotherapy techniques include active and passive, or adoptive immunotherapy. *Active immunotherapy* involves nonspecific treatments such as bacille Calmette-Guérin (BCG). BCG is an attenuated strain of the bacterium that causes bovine tuberculosis. It acts as a nonspecific stimulant of the immune system and is instilled into the bladder as a means of treating superficial bladder cancer. *Passive or adoptive immunotherapy* involves the transfer of cultured immune cells into a tumour-bearing host. Early research efforts with adoptive immunotherapy involved the transfer of sensitized NK cells or T lymphocytes, combined with cytokines, to the tumour-bearing host in an attempt to augment the host's immune response. However, randomized clinical trials demonstrated no benefit from the addition of the cellular component beyond the benefit from the cytokines alone. Further research has focused on using antigen-presenting dendritic cells as delivery vehicles for tumour antigens. Dendritic cells are efficient at activating not only CD4+ helper T cells and CD8+ killer T cells but B cells and innate effectors such as NK cells.[5]

Biologic Response Modifiers. Biologic response modifiers can be grouped into three types: cytokines, which include the interferons and interleukins; monoclonal antibodies (mAB); and hematopoietic growth factors. Some agents, such as interferons, have more than one biologic function, including antiviral, immunomodulatory, and antiproliferative actions. The *interferons* are endogenous polypeptides that are synthesized by a number of cells in response to a variety of cellular or viral stimuli. The three major types of interferons are alpha (α), beta (β), and gamma (γ), each group differing in terms of their cell surface receptors.[88] The interferons appear to inhibit viral replication and also may be involved in inhibiting tumour protein synthesis and in prolonging the cell cycle, increasing the percentage of cells in the G_0 phase. Interferons stimulate NK cells and T-lymphocyte killer cells. Interferon-γ has been approved for the treatment of hairy cell leukemia, AIDS-related Kaposi sarcoma, and CML, and as adjuvant therapy for patients at high risk for recurrent melanoma.[88] Interferon-α has been used to treat some solid tumours (*e.g.,* renal cell carcinoma, colorectal cancer, carcinoid tumours, ovarian cancer) and hematologic neoplasms (e.g., B-cell and T-cell lymphomas, cutaneous T-cell lymphoma, and multiple myeloma).[88] Research now is focusing on combining interferons with other forms of cancer therapy and establishing optimal doses and treatment protocols.

The *interleukins* (IL) are cytokines that effect communication between cells by binding to receptor sites on the cell surface membranes of the target cells. Of the 18 known ILs (see Chapter 17), IL-2 has been the most widely studied.[89] A recombinant human IL-2 (rIL-2, aldesleukin) has been approved by Health Canada and is currently being used for the treatment of metastatic renal cell carcinoma and metastatic melanoma.

Monoclonal antibodies (mAbs) are highly specific antibodies (*e.g.,* IgG, which is the most commonly used immunoglobulin) derived from cloned cells or hybridomas.[90,91] Scientists have developed methods for producing large quantities of mAbs that are specific for tumour cells. For a mAB to be therapeutic as a cancer treatment modality, a specific target antigen should be present on cancer cells only. There are four types of therapeutic mAbs that are grouped according to their origin: murine (mouse), chimeric (mixed mouse and human), humanized, and human.[90] Chimeric antibodies essentially splice light- and heavy-chain regions of the murine antibody to human IgG, making a molecule that is 75% human and 25% murine IgG, whereas in a humanized antibody, the short segment of murine antibody that determines its specificity is grafted onto human IgG, making a molecule that is 5% murine.[90] A fully human IgG can be isolated from transgenic mice bred to produce human IgG. There has been recent interest in the development of technology for generating recombinant polyclonal antibodies capable of the multitargeting of tumour cells.[92]

Therapeutic monoclonal antibodies can be unconjugated (*i.e.,* "naked"), conjugated, or combined with a toxin, chemotherapy drug, or radioisotope.[90,93] A number of unconjugated mAbs are available, including alemtuzumab, a humanized mAB that targets the CD52 antigen of human B cells, T cells, NK cells, and monocyte-macrophages; rituximab, an anti-CD20 chimeric mAB; and trastuzumab, a humanized mAB that binds to the HER-2 receptor (a member of a family of receptor tyrosine kinases).[90,93] Other conjugated mAbs include gemtuzumab ozogamicin, a humanized antibody combined with an antitumour antibiotic; ibritumomab tiuxetan, a murine mAB combined with a radioisotope; and tositumomab, a murine anti-CD20 mAB bonded to radioactive iodine-131.[90,94]

Targeted Therapy

Targeted cancer therapy uses drugs that selectively attack malignant cells while leaving normal cells unharmed.[90] It focuses on altered molecules and signalling pathways that allow cancer cells to grow and spread in an uncontrolled manner. The first targeted therapies were the mAbs.

Other targeted therapies include small molecules that block specific enzymes and growth factors involved in cancer cell growth. The protein tyrosine kinases are intrinsic components of the signalling pathways for growth factors involved in the proliferation of lymphocytes and other cell types. Imatinib mesylate (Gleevec) is a protein tyrosine kinase inhibitor indicated in the treatment of CML (see Chapter 15). The epidermal growth factor receptor signalling pathway is an important mediator of cancer cell oncogenesis, proliferation, maintenance, and survival.[91] For this reason, it has long been proposed as a target for an anticancer drug. In the past several years, two agents, gefitinib and erlotinib, have made a significant impact on the understanding of non-small cell lung cancer and treatment options for persons with the neoplasm.[91] Angiogenesis is also being explored as a target for targeted cancer therapy.[90] One of the newly developed antiangiogenic agents, bevacizumab, targets and blocks vascular endothelial growth factor, which is released by many cancers to stimulate proliferation of new blood vessels. The combination of bevacizumab and chemotherapy was found to increase objective responses, median time to progression, and survival time of persons with metastatic colorectal cancer, compared with chemotherapy alone.[90]

Another class of drugs, the apoptosis-inducing drugs, causes cancer cells to undergo apoptosis by interfering with proteins involved in the process. Bortezomib is approved by Health Canada and the FDA to treat multiple myeloma that has not responded to other treatments.[91] It causes cancer cells to die by blocking enzymes known as proteosomes, which help regulate cell function and growth.

IN SUMMARY

The methods used in the diagnosis of cancer vary with the type of cancer and its location. Because many cancers are curable if diagnosed early, health care practices designed to promote early detection are important. Histologic studies are done in the laboratory using cells or tissue specimens. There are two basic methods of classifying tumours: grading according to the histologic or tissue characteristics and clinical staging according to spread of the disease.

The TNM system for clinical staging of cancer takes into account tumour size, lymph node involvement, and presence of metastasis.

Treatment plans that use more than one type of therapy, often in combination, are providing cures for a number of cancers that a few decades ago had a poor prognosis, and are increasing the life expectancy in other types of cancer. Surgical procedures are more precise and less invasive, preserving organ function and resulting in better quality-of-life outcomes. Newer radiation equipment and novel radiation techniques permit greater and more controlled destruction of cancer cells while sparing normal tissues. Cancer chemotherapy has evolved as one of the major systemic treatment modalities for cancer. Unlike surgery and radiation, chemotherapy is a systemic treatment that enables drugs to reach the site of the tumour as well as other distant sites. The major classifications of chemotherapy drugs are the direct DNA-interacting (alkylating agents, antitumour antibiotics, and topoisomerase inhibitors) and indirect DNA-interacting agents (antimetabolites and mitotic spindle inhibitors). Cancer chemotherapeutic drugs may also be classified as either cell cycle-specific or cell cycle-nonspecific depending on whether they exert their action during a specific phase of the cell cycle. Other systemic agents include hormonal and molecularly targeted agents that block specific enzymes and growth factors involved in cancer cell growth.

CHILDHOOD CANCERS

After completing this section of the chapter, you should be able to meet the following objectives:

- Cite the most common types of cancer affecting infants, children, and adolescents.
- Describe how cancers that affect children differ from those that affect adults.
- Discuss possible long-term effects of radiation therapy and chemotherapy on adult survivors of childhood cancer.

Cancer in children is relatively rare, accounting for about 1% of all malignancies in Canada and the United States.[1,2] Despite progressively improved 5-year survival rates, from 56% in 1974 to 75% in 2000, cancer is the leading cause of disease-related death among children 1 to 14 years of age in Canada and, after accidents, the second leading cause of death among children in the United States.[1,2] Leukemia (discussed in Chapter 15) accounts for 26% of the cases of childhood cancer and 28% of the expected deaths due to cancer in Canadian children.[2] Other forms of cancer that occur in children include non-Hodgkin and Hodgkin lymphomas (discussed in Chapter 15), and bone cancers (osteosarcoma and Ewing sarcoma, discussed in Chapter 57).

Incidence and Types

The spectrum of cancers that affect children differs markedly from those that affect adults. Although most adult cancers are of epithelial cell origin (*e.g.,* lung cancer, breast cancer, colorectal cancers), childhood cancers usually involve the hematopoietic system, nervous system, soft tissues, bone, and kidneys.[95,96] The incidence of childhood cancers is greatest during the first years of life, decreases during middle childhood, and then increases during puberty and adolescence.[95–97] During the first year of life, embryonal tumours such as Wilms tumour, retinoblastoma, and neuroblastoma are among the most common types of tumours. Embryonal tumours along with acute leukemia, non-Hodgkin lymphoma, and gliomas have a peak incidence in children 2 to 5 years of age. As children age, especially after they pass puberty, bone malignancies, Hodgkin lymphoma, gonadal germ cell tumours (testicular and ovarian carcinomas), and various carcinomas such as thyroid cancer and malignant melanoma increase in incidence.

Embryonal Tumours

A number of the tumours of infancy and early childhood are embryonal in origin, meaning that they exhibit features of organogenesis similar to that of embryonic development. Because of this characteristic, these tumours are frequently designated with the suffix "blastoma" (*e.g.,* nephroblastoma [Wilms tumour], retinoblastoma, neuroblastoma).[11] Wilms tumour (discussed in Chapter 33) and neuroblastoma are particularly illustrative of this type of childhood tumour.

Neuroblastoma. Neuroblastomas arise from the primordial neural crest tissue (see Chapter 48) of the sympathetic ganglia and adrenal medulla.[11,95] It is the second most common solid malignancy in childhood after brain tumours, accounting for 7% to 10% of pediatric malignancies and as much as 50% of neoplasms in infancy.[11] About 40% of neuroblastomas arise in the adrenal gland, with the remainder occurring anywhere along the sympathetic chain, most commonly in the paravertebral region of the abdomen and posterior mediastinum. Tumours may arise in numerous other sites, including the pelvis, neck, and within the brain. Clinical manifestations vary with the primary site and neuroendocrine function of the tumour. In children younger than 2 years of age, neuroblastoma generally presents with large abdominal masses, fever, and possibly weight loss. Bone pain suggests metastatic disease. In neonates, disseminated neuroblastoma may present as multiple cutaneous metastases with deep blue discolouration (sometimes designated as the "blueberry muffin baby").[11,95] About 90% of the tumours, regardless of location, secrete catecholamines, which is an important diagnostic feature (*i.e.,* elevated blood levels of catecholamines and elevated urine levels of catecholamine metabolites).[11]

As a group, these tumours demonstrate certain characteristics such as spontaneous or therapy-induced regression or differentiation to benign tumours.[11,95] Unfortunately, neuroblastoma, which is commonly diagnosed before the age of 5 years, is also an extremely malignant neoplasm, particularly in children with advanced disease. Although the 5-year survival rate has improved from 25% in the early 1960s to 55% in the mid-1990s, neuroblastoma continues to account for at least 15% of all childhood cancer deaths.[95] Infants tend to have a better prognosis than older children.

Biology of Childhood Cancers

As with adult cancers, there probably is no single cause of childhood cancer. Although a number of genetic conditions are associated with childhood cancer, such conditions are relatively rare, suggesting an interaction between genetic susceptibility and environmental exposures. The most notable heritable conditions that impart susceptibility to childhood cancer include Down syndrome (20- to 30-fold increased risk of acute lymphoblastic leukemia [ALL]),[1] neurofibromatosis (NF) type 1 (neurofibromas, optic gliomas, brain tumours), NF type 2 (acoustic neuroma, meningiomas), xeroderma pigmentosum (skin cancer), ataxia-telangiectasia (lymphoma, leukemia), and the Beckman–Wiedemann syndrome (Wilms tumour).[11,95]

Although constituting only a small percentage of childhood cancers, the biology of a number of these tumours illustrates several important biologic aspects of neoplasms, such as the two-hit theory of recessive tumour suppressor genes (*e.g., RB* gene mutation in retinoblastoma); defects in DNA repair; and the histologic similarities between organogenesis and oncogenesis. Syndromes associated with defects in DNA repair include xeroderma pigmentosa, in which there is increased risk of skin cancers owing to defects in repair of DNA damaged by ultraviolet light. The development of childhood cancers has also been linked to genomic imprinting, which is characterized by selective inactivation of one of the two alleles of a certain gene.[95] The inactivation is determined by whether the gene is inherited from the mother or father (see Chapter 6). For example, the maternal allele for the insulin-like growth factor-2 (IGF-2) gene normally is inactivated (imprinted). In some Wilms tumours, loss of imprinting (re-expression of the maternal allele) can be demonstrated by overexpression of the IGF-2 protein, which is an embryonal growth factor.[95] The Beckwith–Wiedemann syndrome is an overgrowth syndrome characterized by organomegaly, macroglossia (enlargement of the tongue), hemihypertrophy (muscular or osseous hypertrophy of one side of the body or face), renal abnormalities, and enlarged adrenal cells.[3,95] The syndrome, which reflects changes in the imprinting of IGF-2 genes located on chromosome 11, is also associated with increased risk of Wilms tumour, hepatoblastoma, rhabdomyosarcoma, and adrenal cortical carcinoma.

Diagnosis and Treatment

Because most childhood cancers are curable, early detection is imperative. In addition, there are several types of cancer for which less therapy is indicated than for more advanced disease. In fact, early detection often minimizes the amount and duration of treatment required for cure and may therefore not only increase the potential for cure but spare the child intensive or prolonged treatment.

Unfortunately, there are no early warning signs or screening tests for cancer in children. Prolonged fever, persistent lymphadenopathy, unexplained weight loss, growing masses (especially in association with weight loss), and abnormalities of CNS function should be viewed as warning signs of cancer in children. Because these signs and symptoms of cancer are often similar to those of common childhood diseases, they are frequently attributed to other causes.[95]

Diagnosis of childhood cancers involves many of the same methods used in adults. Histologic examination is usually an essential part of the diagnostic procedure. Accurate disease staging is especially beneficial in childhood cancers, in which the potential benefits of treatment must be carefully weighed against potential long-term effects.

The treatment of childhood cancers is complex, intensive, prolonged, and continuously evolving. It usually involves appropriate multidisciplinary and multimodal therapies, as well as the evaluation for recurrent disease and late effects of the disease and therapies used in its treatment. The treatment program should include specialized teams of health care providers with expertise in pediatric cancer care, such as pediatric oncologists, pathologists, radiologists, surgeons, nurses, and support staff, including nutritionists, social workers, psychologists, pharmacists, and other specialists.[95]

Two modalities are frequently used in the treatment of childhood cancer, with chemotherapy being the most widely used, followed, in order of use, by surgery, radiation therapy, and biologic agent therapy. Chemotherapy is more widely used in treatment of children with cancer than in adults because children better tolerate the acute adverse effects and, in general, pediatric tumours are more responsive to chemotherapy than adult cancers.[95] Radiation therapy tends to be used sparingly in children because they are more vulnerable to the late adverse effects.[95] As with care of adults, adequate pain management is critical.

Adult Survivors of Childhood and Adolescent Cancer

With improvement in treatment methods, the number of children who survive childhood cancer continues to increase. As a result of cancer treatment, almost 80% of children and adolescents with a diagnosis of cancer become long-term survivors.[1] Unfortunately, therapy may produce late sequelae, such as impaired growth, neurologic dysfunction, hormonal dysfunction, cardiomyopathy, pulmonary fibrosis, and risk for second malignancies. Thus, one of the growing challenges is providing appropriate health care to survivors of childhood and adolescent cancers.

In a large, retrospective cohort study that tracked the health status of 10,397 adult survivors of childhood cancer who were treated in the 1970s and 1980s and compared the results with 3,034 of their siblings, it was found that 62% had

at least one chronic health problem and 28% had a severe or life-threatening condition.[97] Three groups were at highest risk: survivors of bone tumours (severe musculoskeletal problems, congestive heart failure, and hearing loss), CNS tumours (cognitive impairment, seizure disorders, and various endocrinopathies), and Hodgkin lymphoma (cardiovascular disease, second cancers, lung disease, and thyroid disease). Many of the health problems of adult survivors of childhood cancer can be attributed to the late effects of radiation therapy and chemotherapy.

Radiation Therapy

The late effects of radiation therapy are influenced by the organs and tissues included in the treatment field, type of radiation administered, daily fractional and cumulative radiation dose, and age at treatment. Regardless of the region irradiated, the skin and musculoskeletal system are often involved.[98] There is increased risk for melanoma, squamous cell carcinoma, and basal cell carcinoma. Musculoskeletal changes are also common after radiation. In earlier days of radiation therapy, this often resulted in asymmetric growth of the spine and other structures. Even with current methods, survivors may have changes leading to pain and altered musculoskeletal function.

Cranial radiation therapy (CRT) has been used to treat brain tumours, ALL, head and neck soft tissue tumours, and retinoblastoma. The most common late effect of moderate- to high-dose whole-brain radiation is diminished intellectual function.[98] Brain tumour survivors treated at a younger age are particularly susceptible. Cranial radiation is also associated with neuroendocrine disorders, particularly growth hormone deficiency. Thus, children reaching adulthood after CRT may have reduced physical stature. The younger the age and the higher the radiation dose, the greater the deviation from normal growth. Growth hormone deficiency in adults is associated with increased prevalence of dyslipidemia, insulin resistance, and cardiovascular mortality. Moderate doses of CRT are also associated with obesity, particularly in female patients.[98] For many years, whole-brain radiation or CRT was the primary method of preventing CNS relapse in children with ALL. Recognition of cognitive dysfunction associated with CRT has led to the use of other methods of CNS prophylaxis.[98]

Radiation to the chest or mantle field (lymph nodes of neck, subclavicular, axillary, and mediastinal areas) is often used in treatment of Hodgkin and non-Hodgkin lymphomas and metastases to the lung. This field exposes the developing breast tissue, heart, and lungs to ionizing radiation. Female survivors who were treated with this type of radiation face significant risk for development of breast cancer.[98] Much of the heart is exposed in chest and mantle radiation fields, resulting in subsequent premature coronary artery, valvular, and pericardial disease. Exposure of the lungs to radiation therapy can result in a reduction in pulmonary function. Thyroid disease, particularly hypothyroidism, is common after mantle or neck radiation.

Childhood cancer survivors treated with abdominal or pelvic radiation are also at risk for a variety of late health problems involving the gastrointestinal tract, liver, spleen, kidneys, and genitourinary tract structures, including the gonads.[98] Gastrointestinal tract complications include chronic mucosal inflammation that interferes with absorption and digestion of nutrients. Chronic radiation injury to the kidneys may interfere with glomerular or tubular function, and fibrosis from pelvic radiation may adversely affect bladder capacity and function. The adverse effects of radiation on gonadal function vary by age, sex, and cumulative dose. Delayed sexual maturation in boys and girls can result from irradiation of the gonads. In boys, sperm production is reduced in a dose-dependent manner. In girls, radiation to the abdomen, pelvis, and spine is associated with increased risk of ovarian failure, especially if the ovaries are in the treatment field.

Chemotherapy

Chemotherapy also poses the risk of long-term effects for survivors of childhood cancer. Potential late effects of alkylating agents include dose-related gonadal injury (hypogonadism, infertility, and early menopause).[98] Alkylating agent therapy has also been linked to dose-related secondary acute myelogenous leukemia, pulmonary fibrosis, kidney disease, and bladder disorders. Anthracyclines, including doxorubicin and daunomycin, which are widely used in treatment of childhood cancers, can result in cardiomyopathy and eventual congestive heart failure.[98] The late effects of cisplatin and carboplatin, the most frequently used nonclassic alkylators, are nephrotoxicity, ototoxicity, and neurotoxicity. Although combination chemotherapy increases the effectiveness of treatment, it may also be associated with increased risk of side effects if the agents have a similar spectrum of toxicity. Intrathecal combination chemotherapy to prevent relapse of ALL in the CNS, which is a sanctuary for ALL cells, is known to cause significant and persistent cognitive impairment in many children.

IN SUMMARY

Although most adult cancers are of epithelial cell origin, most childhood cancers usually involve the hematopoietic system, nervous system, or connective tissue. Heritable forms of cancer tend to have an earlier age of onset, a higher frequency of multifocal lesions in a single organ, and bilateral involvement of paired organs or multiple primary tumours. The early diagnosis of childhood cancers often is missed because the signs and symptoms mimic those of other childhood diseases. With improvement in treatment methods, the number of children who survive childhood cancer is continuing to increase. As these children approach adulthood, there is continued concern that the life-saving therapy they received during childhood may produce late effects, such as impaired growth, cognitive dysfunction, hormonal dysfunction, cardiomyopathy, pulmonary fibrosis, and risk for second malignancies.

REVIEW EXERCISES

1. A 30-year-old woman has experienced heavy menstrual bleeding and is told she has a uterine tumour called a leiomyoma. She is worried she has cancer.
   A. *What is the difference between a leiomyoma and leiomyosarcoma?*
   B. *How would you explain the difference to her?*

2. Among the characteristics of cancer cells are lack of cell differentiation, impaired cell-to-cell adhesion, and loss of anchorage dependence.
   A. *Explain how each of these characteristics contributes to the usefulness of the Pap smear as a screening test for cervical cancer.*

3. A 12-year-old boy is seen at the pediatric cancer clinic with osteosarcoma. His medical history reveals that his father had been successfully treated for retinoblastoma as an infant.
   A. *Relate the genetics of the RB gene and the "two-hit" hypothesis to the development of osteosarcoma in this boy.*

4. A 48-year-old man presents at his health care clinic with complaints of leg weakness. He is a heavy smoker and has had a productive cough for years. Subsequent diagnostic tests reveal he has a small cell lung cancer with brain metastasis. His proposed plan of treatment includes chemotherapy and radiation therapy.
   A. *What is the probable cause of the leg weakness, and is it related to the lung cancer?*
   B. *Relate this man's smoking history to the development of lung cancer.*
   C. *Explain the mechanism of cancer metastasis.*
   D. *Explain the mechanisms whereby chemotherapy and irradiation are able to destroy cancer cells while having a lesser or no effect on normal cells.*

5. A 17-year-old-girl is seen by a guidance counsellor at her high school because of problems in keeping up with assignments in her math and science courses. She tells the counsellor that she had leukemia when she was 2 years old and was given radiation treatment to the brain. She confides that she has always had more trouble with learning than her classmates and thinks it might be due to the radiation. She also relates that she is shorter than her classmates, and this has been bothering her.
   A. *Explain the relationship between cranial radiation therapy and decreased cognitive function and short stature.*
   B. *What other neuroendocrine problems might this girl have as a result of the radiation treatment?*

References

1. Canadian Cancer Society's Advisory Committee (2015). *Canadian Cancer Statistics, 2015*. Toronto: Canadian Cancer Society.

2. American Cancer Society (2013). *Cancer Facts and Figures 2013*. Atlanta, GA: American Cancer Society.

3. Green D. R., Evan G. I. (2002). A matter of life and death. *Cancer Cell, 1*(1), 19–30.

4. Hipfner D. R., Cohen S. M. (2004). Connecting proliferation and apoptosis in development and disease. *Nature Reviews Molecular Cell Biology, 5*, 805–815.

5. Weinberg R. A. (2014). *The biology of cancer* (2nd ed.). New York: Garland Science Taylor & Francis Group.

6. Fung T. K., Poon R. Y. (2005). A roller coaster ride with the mitotic cyclins. *Seminars in Cell and Developmental Biology, 16*(3), 335–342.

7. Fischer P. M., Gianella-Borradori A. (2005). Recent progress in the discovery and development of cyclin-dependent kinase inhibitors. *Expert Opinion on Investigational Drugs, 14*(4), 457–477.

8. Vermeulen L., de Sousa e Melo F., Richel D. J., et al. (2012). The developing cancer stem-cell model: Clinical challenges and opportunities. *Lancet Oncology, 13*, e83–e89.

9. Ward R. J., Dirks P. B. (2007). Cancer stem cells: At the headwaters of tumor development. *Annual Review of Pathology, 2*, 175–189.

10. Li L., Xie T. (2005). Stem cell niche: Structure and function. *Annual Review of Cell and Developmental Biology, 21*, 605–631.

11. Stricker T. P., Kumar V. (2010). Neoplasia. In Kumar V., Abbas A. K., Fausto N., Aster J. (Eds.), *Robbins and Cotran Pathologic Basis of Disease* (8th ed., pp. 259–330), Philadelphia, PA: Elsevier Mosby Saunders.

12. Hanahan D., Weinberg R. A. (2011). Hallmarks of cancer: The next generation. *Cell, 144*(5), 646–674.

13. McClatchey A. I., Yap A. S. (2012). Contact inhibition (of proliferation) redux. *Current Opinion in Cell Biology, 24*(5), 685–694.

14. Hayashida Y., Honda K., Idogawa M., et al. (2005). E-cadherin regulates the association between β-catenin and actinin-4. *Cancer Research, 65*(19), 8836–8845.

15. Shen Y., Jia Z., Nagele R. G., et al. (2006). Src uses Cas to suppress Fhl1 in order to promote nonanchored growth and migration of tumor cells. *Cancer Research, 66*(3), 1543–1552.

16. Brooke M. A., Nitoiu D., Kelsell D. P. (2012). Cell-cell connectivity: Desmosomes and disease. *Journal of Pathology, 226*(2), 158–171.

17. Zanghi A., Cavallaro A., Piccolo G., et al. (2013). Dissemination metastasis after laparoscopic colorectal surgery versus conventional open surgery for colorectal cancer: A metanalysis. *European Review for Medical and Pharmacological Sciences, 17*(9), 1174–1184.

18. Minn A. J., Massague J. (2011). Molecular biology of cancer: Invasion and metastasis. In DeVita V. T., Hellman S., Rosenberg S. A. (Eds.), *Cancer: Principles and practice of oncology* (9th ed.). Philadelphia, PA: Lippincott Williams & Wilkins.

19. Tobler N. E., Detmar M. (2006). Tumor and lymph node lymphangiogenesis: Impact on cancer metastasis. *Journal of Leukocyte Biology, 80*(4), 691–696.

20. Chen S. L., Iddings D. M., Scheri R. P., Bilchik A. J. (2006). Lymphatic mapping and sentinel node analysis: Current concepts and applications. *CA: Cancer Journal for Clinicians, 56*(5), 292–307.

21. Langley R. R., Fidler I. J. (2011). The seed and soil hypothesis revisited–the role of tumor-stroma interactions in metastasis to different organs. *International Journal of Cancer, 128*(11), 2527–2535.

22. Haustein V., Schumacher U. (2012). A dynamic model for tumour growth and metastasis formation. *Journal of Clinical Bioinformatics, 2*, 11. doi:10.1186/2043-9113-2-11.

23. Gajria D., Chandarlapaty S. (2011). HER2-amplified breast cancer: Mechanisms of trastuzumab resistance and novel targeted therapies. *Expert Reviews of Anticancer Therapy, 11*(2), 263–275.

24. Berger A. H., Knudson A. G., Pandolfi P. P. (2011). A continuum model for tumour suppression. *Nature, 476*(7359), 163–169.

25. Baylin S. B. (2005). DNA methylation and gene silencing in cancer. *Nature Clinical Practice Oncology, 2*, S4–S11.

26. Curtin N. J. (2012). DNA repair dysregulation from cancer driver to therapeutic target. *Nature Reviews Cancer, 12*(12),801-817.

27. Schulze-Bergkamen H., Krammer P. H. (2004). Apoptosis in cancer: Implications for therapy. *Seminars in Oncology, 31*(1), 90–119.

28. Feldser D. M., Grieder C. W. (2007). Short telomeres limit tumor progression in vivo by inducing senescence. *Cancer Cell, 11*(5), 461–469.

29. Sedivy J. M. (2007). Telomeres limit cancer growth by inducing senescence: Long-sought in vivo evidence obtained. *Cancer Cell, 11*(5), 389–391.

30. Yang Z., Wechsler-Reya R. J. (2007). Hit 'em where they live: Targeting the cancer stem cell. *Cancer Cell, 11*(1), 3–5.

31. Boccaccio C., Comoglio P. M. (2006). Invasive growth: A MET-driven genetic programme for cancer and stem cells. *Nature Reviews Cancer, 6*, 637–645.

32. Bierie B., Moses H. L. (2006). TGFβ: The molecular Jekyll and Hyde. *Nature Reviews Cancer, 6*(7), 506–520.

33. Henderson K. D., Lu Y., Bernstein L. (2011). Obesity and physical activity. In DeVita V. T., Hellman S., Rosenberg S. A. (Eds.), *Cancer: Principles and practice of oncology* (9th ed.). Philadelphia, PA: Lippincott Williams & Wilkins.

34. Swann J. B., Smyth M. J. (2007). Immune surveillance of tumors. *Journal of Clinical Investigation, 117*(5), 1137–1146.

35. Cogliano V. J., Baan R., Straif K., et al. (2011). Preventable exposures associated with human cancers. *Journal of the National Cancer Institute, 103*(24), 1827–1839.

36. Kachuri L., De P., Ellison L. F., et al. (2013). Cancer incidence, mortality and survival trends in Canada, 1970–2007. *Chronic Diseases and Injuries in Canada, 33*(2), 69–80.

37. Illing E. M., Kaiserman M. J. (2004). Mortality attributable to tobacco use in Canada and its regions, 1998. *Canadian Journal of Public Health, 95*(1), 38–44.

38. World Health Organization, International Agency for Research on Cancer. (2004). *IARC monographs on the evaluation of carcinogenic risks to humans*. Volume 83: Tobacco smoke and involuntary smoking. Lyon, France

39. Baliunas D., Patra J., Rehm J., et al. (2007). Smoking-attributable morbidity: Acute care hospital diagnoses and days of treatment in Canada, 2002. *BioMed Central Public Health, 7*, 247. doi:10.1186/1471-2458-7-247.

40. Ferguson L. R. (2009). Role of dietary mutagens in cancer and atherosclerosis. *Current Opinion in Clinical Nutrition and Metabolic Care, 12*(4), 343–349.

41. Seitz H. K., Stickel F. (2007). Molecular mechanisms of alcohol-mediated carcinogenesis. *Nature Reviews Cancer, 7*(8), 599–612.

42. Laronda M. M., Unno K., Butler L. M., Kurita T. (2012). The development of cervical and vaginal adenosis as a result of diethylstilbestrol exposure in utero. *Differentiation, 84*(3), 252–260.

43. Little M. P. (2009). Cancer and non-cancer effects in Japanese atomic bomb survivors. *Journal of Radiological Protection, 29*(2A), A43–A59.

44. Wakeford R. (2013). The risk of childhood leukaemia following exposure to ionizing radiation–a review. *Journal of Radiological Protection, 33*(1). doi:10.1088/0952-4746/33/1/1.

45. Howley P. M., Ganem D., Kieff E. (2011). Etiology of cancer: Viruses. In DeVita V. T., Hellman S., Rosenberg S. A. (Eds.), *Cancer: Principles and practice of oncology* (9th ed.). Philadelphia, PA: Lippincott Williams & Wilkins.

46. Public Health Agency of Canada. (2011). Human papillomavirus (HPV) prevention and HPV vaccines: Questions and answers. Available online at: http://www.phac-aspc.gc.ca/std-mts/hpv-vph/hpv-vph-vaccine-eng.php. Accessed March 13, 2014.

47. Cornett P. A., Dea T. O. (2014). Cancer. In Papadakis M. A., McPhee S. J., Rabow M. V. (Eds.), *Current medical diagnosis and treatment 2014*. New York: McGraw-Hill.

48. Roett M. A., Evans P. (2009). Ovarian cancer: An overview. *American Family Physician, 80*(6), 609–616.

49. Sanchez O. H. (2004). Insights into novel biological mediators of clinical manifestations in cancer. *AACN Clinical Issues, 15*(1), 112–118.

50. Lagman R. L., Davis M. P., LeGrand S. B., Walsh D. (2005). Common symptoms of advanced cancer. *Surgical Clinics of North America, 85*(2), 237–255.

51. Argiles J. M., Busquets S., Garcia-Martinez C., López-Soriano FJ. (2005). Mediators involved in the cancer anorexia-cachexia syndrome: Past, present, and future. *Nutrition, 21*(9), 977–985.

52. Gordon J. N., Green S. R., Goggin P. M. (2005). Cancer cachexia. *Quarterly Journal of Medicine, 98*(11), 779–788.

53. Tisdale M. J. (2005). Molecular pathways leading to cancer cachexia. *Physiology, 20*, 340–348.

54. Patrick D. L., Ferketich S. L., Frame P. S., et al. (2003). National Institutes of Health State-of-the Science Conference Statement: Symptom management in cancer: pain, depression, and fatigue, July 15–17, 2002. *Journal of the National Cancer Institute, 95*(15), 1110–1117.

55. Ryan J. L., Carroll J. K., Ryan E. P., et al. (2007). Mechanisms of cancer-related fatigue. *Oncologist, 12*(Suppl 1), 22–34.

56. Hofman M., Ryan J. L., Fiqueroa-Moseley C. D., et al. (2007). Cancer-related fatigue: The scale of the problem. *Oncologist, 12*(Suppl 1), 4–10.

57. Roscoe J. A., Kaufman M. E., Matteson-Rusby S. E., et al. (2007). Cancer-related fatigue and sleep disorders. *Oncologist, 12*(Suppl 1), 35–42.

58. Knight K., Wade S., Balducci L. (2004). Prevalence and outcomes of anemia in cancer: A systematic review of the literature. *American Journal of Medicine, 116*(Suppl 7A), 11S–26S.

59. Hurter B., Bush N. J. (2007). Cancer-related anemia: Clinical review and management update. *Clinical Journal of Oncology Nursing, 11*(3), 349–359.

60. Boyiadzis M., Lieberman F. S., Geskin L. J., et al. (2011). Paraneoplastic syndromes. In DeVita V. T., Hellman S., Rosenberg S. A. (Eds.), *Cancer: Principles and practice of oncology* (9th ed.). Philadelphia, PA: Lippincott Williams & Wilkins.

61. Pelosof L. C., Gerber D. E. (2010). Paraneoplastic syndromes: An approach to diagnosis and treatment. *Mayo Clinic Proceedings, 85*(9), 838–854.

62. Shoback D., Funk J. (2011). Humoral manifestations of malignancy. In Gardner D. G., Shobeck D. (Eds.), *Greenspan's Basic and clinical endocrinology* (9th ed.). New York: McGraw-Hill.

63. Graus F., Dalmau J. (2012). Paraneoplastic neurological syndromes. *Current Opinion in Neurology, 25*, 795–801.

64. de Beukelarr J. W., Sllilevis Smitt P. A. (2006). Managing paraneoplastic neurologic disorders. *Oncologist, 11*(3), 292–305.

65. Smith R. A., Baptiste D., Brooks D., et al. (2014). Cancer screening in the United States, 2014: A review of current American Cancer Society guidelines and current issues in cancer screening. *CA: Cancer Journal for Clinicians, 64*(1), 30–51.

66. Duffy M. J. (2013). Tumor markers in clinical practice: A review focusing on common solid cancers. *Medical Principles and Practice, 22*(1), 4–11.

67. Sobin L. H., Gospodarowicz M. K., Wittekind C. (Eds.). (2010). *TNM Classification of Malignant Tumours* (7th ed). Hoboken, NJ: Wiley-Blackwell.

68. Rosenberg S. A. (2011). Cancer management: Principles of surgical oncology. In DeVita V. T., Hellman S., Rosenberg S. A. (Eds.), *Cancer: Principles and practice of oncology* (9th ed.). Philadelphia, PA: Lippincott Williams & Wilkins.

69. Fallowfield L. (2002). Quality of life: a new perspective for cancer patients. *Nature Reviews Cancer, 2*, 873–879.

70. Jeremic B. (2004). Radiation therapy. *Hematology/Oncology Clinics of North America, 18*(2), 297–307.

71. Sausville E. A., Longo D. L. (2012). Principles of cancer treatment. In Longo D. L., Fauci A. S., Kasper D. L., et al. (Eds.), *Harrison's principles of internal medicine* (18th ed.). New York: McGraw-Hill.

72. Willers H., Held K. D. (2006). Introduction to clinical radiation biology. *Hematology/Oncology Clinics of North America, 20*(1), 1–24.

73. Thomas C. T., Ammar A., Farrell J. J., Elsaleh H. (2006). Radiation modifiers: Treatment overview and future investigations. *Hematology/Oncology Clinics of North America, 20*(1), 119–139.

74. Smith R. P., Heron D. E., Huq M. S., Yue N. J. (2006). Modern radiation therapy: Treatment planning and delivery—From Röntgen to real time. *Hematology/Oncology Clinics of North America, 20*(1), 45–62.

75. Bucci M. K., Bevan A., Roach M. (2005). Advances in radiation therapy: Conventional to 3D, to IMRT, to 4D, and beyond. *CA: Cancer Journal for Clinicians, 55*(2), 117–134.

76. Patel R. R., Arthur D. W. (2006). The emergence of advanced brachytherapy techniques for common malignancies. *Hematology/Oncology Clinics of North America, 20*(1), 97–118.

77. Cheung-Ong K., Giaever G., Nislow C. (2013). DNA-damaging agents in cancer chemotherapy: Serendipity and chemical biology. *Chemistry and Biology, 20*(5), 648–659.

78. Chu E., Sartorelli A. C. (2012). Cancer chemotherapy. In Katzung B. G., Masters S. B., Trevor A. J. (Eds.), *Basic and clinical pharmacology* (12th ed.). New York: McGraw-Hill.

79. Torchilin V. P. (2007). Targeted pharmaceutical nanocarriers for cancer therapy and imaging. *AAPS Journal, 9*(2), E128–E146.

80. Milano M., Schneider M. (2007). EPO in cancer anemia: Benefits and potential risks. *Critical Reviews in Oncology/Hematology, 62*(2), 119–125.

81. Navari R. M. (2013). Management of chemotherapy-induced nausea and vomiting. *Drugs, 73*(3), 249–262.

82. Lindley C. (2012). Neoplastic disorders and their treatment. In Alldredge B. K., Corelli R. L., Ernst M. E., et al. (Eds.), *Koda-Kimble and Young's applied therapeutics: The clinical use of drugs* (10th ed.). Philadelphia, PA: Lippincott Williams & Wilkins.

83. U.S. Department of Labor, Office of Occupational Medicine, Occupational Safety and Health Administration (OSHA). (1986). *Work practice guidelines for personnel dealing with cytotoxic (antineoplastic) drugs.* Publication No. 8-1.1. Washington, DC: Author.

84. Polovich M. (2011). *Safe handling of hazardous drugs.* Pittsburgh, PA: Oncology Nursing Society.

85. Goetz M. P., Erlichman C., Kohli M., et al. (2011). Endocrine manipulation. In DeVita V. T., Hellman S., Rosenberg S. A. (Eds.), *Cancer: Principles and practice of oncology* (9th ed.). Philadelphia, PA: Lippincott Williams & Wilkins.

86. Altundag K., Ibrahim N. K. (2006). Aromatase inhibitors in breast cancer: An overview. *Oncologist, 11*(6), 553–562.

87. Kuroki M., Miyamoto S., Morisaki T., et al. (2012). Biological response modifiers used in cancer biotherapy. *Anticancer Research, 32*(6), 2229–2233.

88. Sondak V. K., Becker J. C., Hauschild A. (2011). Interferons. In DeVita V. T., Hellman S., Rosenberg S. A. (Eds.), *Cancer: Principles and practice of oncology* (9th ed.). Philadelphia, PA: Lippincott Williams & Wilkins.

89. Lotze M. T., Bates S. E. (2011). Interleukin Therapy. In DeVita V. T., Hellman S., Rosenberg S. A. (Eds.), *Cancer: Principles and practice of oncology* (9th ed.). Philadelphia, PA: Lippincott Williams & Wilkins.

90. Sharkey R. M., Goldenberg D. M. (2006). Targeted therapy of cancer: New prospects for antibodies and immunoconjugates. *CA: Cancer Journal for Clinicians, 56*(4), 226–243.

91. Marshall J. (2006). Clinical implications of the mechanism of epidermal growth factor receptor inhibitors. *Cancer, 107*(6), 1207–1218.

92. Sharon J., Liebman M. A., Williams B. R., (2005). Recombinant polyclonal antibodies for cancer treatment. *Journal of Cell Biochemistry, 96*(2), 305–313.

93. Sapra P., Shor B. (2013). Monoclonal antibody-based therapies in cancer: Advances and challenges. *Pharmacology and Therapeutics, 138*(3), 452–469.

94. Schmidt K. V., Wood B. A. (2003). Trends in cancer therapy: Role of monoclonal antibodies. *Seminars in Oncology Nursing, 19*, 169–179.

95. Kliegman R. M., Stanton B. F., St. Geme J. W., et al.. (Eds.). (2011). *Nelson textbook of pediatrics* (19th ed.). Philadelphia, PA: Elsevier Saunders.

96. Ries L. A., Smith M. A., Gurney J. G., et al.. (Eds.). (1999). Cancer incidence and survival among children and adolescents: United States SEER program 1975–1995. Available online at: http://seer.cancer.gov/archive/publications/childhood/childhood-monograph.pdf. Accessed March 13, 2014.

97. Oeffinger K. C., Mertens A. C., Sklar C. A., et al. (2006). Chronic health conditions in adult survivors of childhood cancer. *New England Journal of Medicine, 355*(15), 1572–1582.

98. Oeffinger K. C., Hudson M. M. (2004). Long-term complications following childhood and adolescent cancer: Foundations for providing risk-based health care for survivors. *CA: Cancer Journal for Clinicians, 54*(4), 208–236.

Visit thePoint **http://thePoint.lww.com for animations, journal articles, and more!**

Unit III

Disorders of Integrative Function

French physiologist Claude Bernard (1813–1878) was the first to theorize that, in a closely orchestrated process, the body strives to achieve and maintain a steady state. In the middle of the 19th century, Bernard proposed his concept of the *milieu intérieur,* or the stable internal environment, regulated by a multitude of interacting control mechanisms geared to maintain the body's chemical and physical status. He proposed that internal secretions functioned as a part of the body's regulatory mechanism, maintaining a balance in response to a range of changing conditions imposed by the external environment.

Through his experiments, Bernard discovered a number of mechanisms that were dedicated to maintaining homeostasis. One of his discoveries was the process by which internal temperature is kept constant. He was able to show that the nervous system responds to internal cold by sending chemical messages to the blood vessels to constrict in order to conserve body heat. The product of his considerable work is the classic *Introduction to the Study of Experimental Medicine* (1865).

Stress and Adaptation

9

Stress has become an increasingly discussed topic in today's world. The concept is discussed extensively in the health care fields, and it is found as well in economics, political science, business, and education. In the popular press, the physiologic response to stress is often implicated as a contributor to a variety of individual physical and mental challenges and societal problems.

Whether stress is more prevalent today than it was in centuries past is uncertain. Certainly, the pressures that existed in the past were equally challenging, although of a different type. Social psychologists Richard Lazarus and Susan Folkman related that as early as the 14th century the term was used to indicate hardship, straits, adversity, or affliction.[1] In the 17th century, *stress* and related terms appeared in the context of physical sciences: *load* was defined as an external force, *stress* as the ratio of internal force created by the load to the area over which the force acted, and *strain* was the deformation or distortion of the object.[1] These concepts are still used in engineering today.

The concepts of stress and strain survived, and throughout the 19th and early 20th centuries, stress and strain were thought to be the cause of "ill health" and "mental disease."[2] By the 20th century, stress had drawn considerable attention both as a health concern and as a research focus. In 1910, when Sir William Osler delivered his Lumleian Lectures on "Angina Pectoris," he described the relationship of stress and strain to angina pectoris.[3] Approximately 15 years later, Walter Cannon, well known for his work in physiology, began to use the word *stress* in relation to his laboratory experiments on the "fight-or-flight" response. It seems possible that the term emerged from his work on the homeostatic features of living organisms and their tendency to "bound back" and "resist disruption" when acted on by an "external force."[4] At about the same time, Hans Selye, who became known for his research (much of which was done in Canada) and publications on stress, began using the term *stress* in a very special way to mean an orchestrated set of bodily responses to any form of noxious stimulus.[5]

The content in this chapter has been organized into three sections: homeostasis, the stress response and adaptation to stress, and disorders of the stress response.

HOMEOSTASIS

After completing this section of the chapter, you should be able to meet the following objectives:

- Cite Cannon's four features of homeostasis.
- Describe the components of a control system, including the function of a negative feedback system.

The concepts of stress and adaptation have their origin in the complexity of the human body and the interactions between the body cells and its many organ systems. These interactions require that a level of homeostasis or constancy be maintained during the many changes that occur in the internal and external environments. In effecting a state of constancy, homeostasis requires feedback control systems that regulate cellular function and integrate the function of the different body systems.

Constancy of the Internal Environment

The environment in which body cells live is not the external environment that surrounds the organism, but rather the local fluid environment that surrounds each cell. Claude Bernard, a 19th century physiologist, was the first to describe clearly the central importance of a stable internal environment, which he termed the *milieu intérieur*. Bernard recognized that body fluids surrounding the cells (extracellular fluids) and the various organ systems provide the means for exchange between the external and the internal environments. It is from this internal environment that body cells receive their nourishment, and it is into this fluid that they secrete their wastes. Even the contents of the gastrointestinal tract and lungs do not become part of the internal environment until they have been absorbed into the extracellular fluid. A multicellular organism is able to survive only as long as the composition of the internal environment is compatible with the survival needs of the individual cells. For example, even a small change in the pH of the body fluids can disrupt the metabolic processes of the individual cells.

The concept of a stable internal environment was supported by Walter B. Cannon, who proposed that this kind of

HOMEOSTASIS

- Homeostasis is the purposeful maintenance of a stable internal environment by coordinated physiologic processes that oppose change.
- The physiologic control systems that oppose change operate by negative feedback mechanisms consisting of a sensor that detects a change, an integrator/comparator that sums and compares incoming data with a set point, and an effector system that returns the sensed function to within the range of the set point.

stability, which he called *homeostasis,* was achieved through a system of carefully coordinated physiologic processes that oppose change.[6] Cannon pointed out that these processes were largely automatic and emphasized that homeostasis involves resistance to both internal and external disturbances.

In his book *Wisdom of the Body,* published in 1939, Cannon presented four tentative propositions (*i.e.,* constancy, steady-state conditions, regulating systems, the unlikely probability that homeostasis occurs by chance, and together these are interconnected) to describe the general features of homeostasis.[6] With this set of propositions, Cannon emphasized that when a factor is known to shift homeostasis in one direction, it is reasonable to expect the existence of mechanisms that have the opposite effect. In the homeostatic regulation of blood sugar, for example, mechanisms that both raise and lower blood sugar would be expected to play a part. As long as the responding mechanism to the initiating disturbance can recover homeostasis, the integrity of the body and the status of normality are retained.

Control Systems

The ability of the body to function and maintain homeostasis under conditions of change in the internal and external environment depends on the thousands of physiologic *control systems* that regulate body function. A homeostatic control system consists of a collection of interconnected components that function to keep a physical or chemical parameter of the body relatively constant. The body's control systems regulate cellular function, control life processes, and integrate functions of the different organ systems.

Of recent interest have been the neuroendocrine control systems that influence behaviour. Biochemical messengers that exist in our brain serve to control nerve activity, regulate information flow, and, ultimately, influence behaviour. These control systems mediate the physical, emotional, and behavioural reactions to stressors that, taken together, are called the *stress response.*

Feedback Systems

Most control systems in the body operate by *negative feedback mechanisms,* which function in a manner similar to the thermostat on a heating system. When the monitored function or value decreases below the set point of the system, the feedback mechanism causes the function or value to increase; and when the function or value is increased above the set point, the feedback mechanism causes it to decrease (Fig. 9.1). For example, in the negative feedback mechanism that controls blood glucose levels, an increase in blood glucose stimulates an increase in insulin, which enhances the removal of glucose from the blood. When glucose has been taken up by cells and blood glucose levels fall, insulin secretion is inhibited and glucagon and other counter-regulatory mechanisms stimulate the release of glucose from the liver, which causes the blood glucose to return to normal.

The reason most physiologic control systems function under negative rather than *positive feedback mechanisms* is

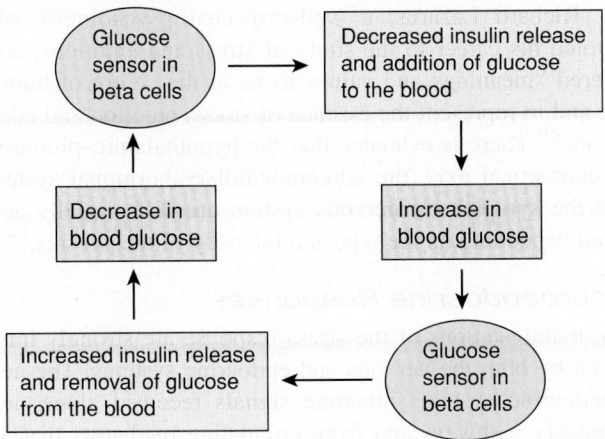

FIGURE 9.1 • Illustration of negative feedback control mechanisms using blood glucose as an example.

that a positive feedback mechanism interjects instability rather than stability into a system. It produces a cycle in which the initiating stimulus produces more of the same. For example, in a positive feedback system, exposure to an increase in environmental temperature would invoke compensatory mechanisms designed to increase rather than decrease body temperature.

IN SUMMARY

Physiologic and psychological adaptation involves the ability to maintain the constancy of the internal environment (homeostasis) and behaviour in the face of a wide range of changes in the internal and external environments. It involves negative feedback control systems that regulate cellular function, control life's processes, regulate behaviour, and integrate the function of the different body systems.

STRESS AND ADAPTATION

After completing this section of the chapter, you should be able to meet the following objectives:

- State Selye's definition of stress.
- Define *stressor.*
- Cite two factors that influence the nature of the stress response.
- Explain the interactions among components of the nervous system in mediating the stress response.
- Describe the stress responses of the autonomic nervous system, the endocrine system, the immune system, and the musculoskeletal system.
- Explain the purpose of adaptation.
- List at least six factors that influence a person's adaptive capacity.
- Propose a way by which social support may serve to buffer challenges to adaptation.

The increased focus on health promotion has heightened interest in the roles of stress and biobehavioural stress responses in the development of disease. Stress may contribute directly to the production or exacerbation of a disease, or it may contribute to the development of behaviours such as smoking, overeating, and drug abuse that increase the risk of disease.

The Stress Response

In the early 1930s, the world-renowned endocrinologist Hans Selye was the first to describe a group of specific anatomic changes that occurred in rats that were exposed to a variety of different experimental stimuli. He came to an understanding that these changes were manifestations of the body's attempt to adapt to stimuli. Selye described *stress* as "a state manifested by a specific syndrome of the body developed in response to any stimuli that made an intense systemic demand on it."[7] As a young medical student, Selye noticed that patients with diverse disease conditions had many signs and symptoms in common. He observed that "whether a man suffers from a loss of blood, an infectious disease, or advanced cancer, he loses his appetite, his muscular strength, and his ambition to accomplish anything; usually the patient also loses weight and even his facial expression betrays that he is ill."[8] Selye referred to this as the "syndrome of just being sick."

In his early career as an experimental scientist, Selye noted that a triad of adrenal enlargement, thymic atrophy, and gastric ulcers appeared in rats he was using for his studies. These same three changes developed in response to many different or nonspecific experimental challenges. He assumed that the hypothalamic–pituitary–adrenal (HPA) axis played a pivotal role in the development of this response. To Selye, the response to stressors was a process that enabled the rats to resist the experimental challenge by using the function of the system best able to respond to it. He labelled the response the *general adaptation syndrome* (GAS): *general* because the effect was a general systemic reaction, *adaptive* because the response was in reaction to a stressor, and *syndrome* because the physical manifestations were coordinated and dependent on each other.[7]

According to Selye, the GAS involves three stages: the alarm stage, the resistance stage, and the exhaustion stage. The *alarm stage* is characterized by a generalized stimulation of the sympathetic nervous system and the HPA axis, resulting in the release of catecholamines and cortisol. During the *resistance stage,* the body selects the most effective and economic channels of defence; thus, the increased cortisol levels that were present initially during the first stage drop because they are no longer needed. If the stressor is prolonged or overwhelms the ability of the body to defend itself, the *exhaustion stage* ensues, during which resources are depleted and signs of "wear and tear" or systemic damage appear.[9] Selye contended that many ailments, such as various emotional disturbances, mildly annoying headaches, insomnia, upset stomach, gastric and duodenal ulcers, certain types of rheumatic disorders, and cardiovascular and kidney diseases appear to be initiated or encouraged by the "body itself because of its faulty adaptive reactions to potentially injurious agents."[8]

The events or environmental agents responsible for initiating the stress response were called *stressors.* According to Selye, stressors could be endogenous, arising from within the body, or exogenous, arising from outside the body.[8] In explaining the stress response, Selye proposed that two factors determine the nature of the stress response: the properties of the stressor and the conditioning of the person being stressed. Selye indicated that not all stress was detrimental; hence, he coined the terms *eustress* and *distress.*[9] He suggested that mild, brief, and controllable periods of stress could be perceived as positive stimuli to emotional and intellectual growth and development. It is the severe, protracted, and uncontrolled situations of psychological and physical distress that are disruptive of health.[8] For example, the joy of becoming a new parent and the sorrow of losing a parent are completely different experiences, yet their stressor effect—the nonspecific demand for adjustment to a new situation—can be similar.

It is becoming increasingly clear that the physiologic stress response is far more complicated than can be explained fully by a classic stimulus–response mechanism. Stressors tend to produce different responses in different persons or in the same person at different times, indicating the influence of the adaptive capacity of the person, or what Selye called *conditioning factors.* These conditioning factors may be internal (*e.g.,* genetic predisposition, age, sex) or external (*e.g.,* exposure to environmental agents, life experiences, dietary factors, level of social support).[11] The relative risk for development of a stress-related pathologic process seems, at least in part, to depend on these factors.

Richard Lazarus, a well-respected psychologist who devoted his career to the study of stress and emotions, considered "meanings and values to be at the centre of human life and to represent the essence of stress, emotion and adaptation."[10] There is evidence that the hypothalamic–pituitary–adrenocortical axis, the adrenomedullary hormonal system, and the sympathetic nervous system are differentially activated depending on the type and intensity of the stressor.[11]

Neuroendocrine Responses

The manifestations of the stress response are strongly influenced by both the nervous and endocrine systems. The neuroendocrine systems integrate signals received along neurosensory pathways and from circulating mediators that are carried in the bloodstream. In addition, the immune system both affects and is affected by the stress response.[12] Table 9.1 summarizes the action of hormones involved in the neuroendocrine responses to stress. The results of the coordinated release of these neurohormones include the mobilization of energy, a sharpened focus and awareness, increased cerebral blood flow and glucose utilization, enhanced cardiovascular and respiratory functioning, redistribution of blood flow to the brain and muscles, modulation of the immune response, inhibition of reproductive function, and a decrease in appetite.[11]

The stress response is a normal, coordinated physiologic system meant to increase the probability of survival, but, importantly, also designed to be an acute response—turned on when necessary to bring the body back to a stable state and turned off when the challenge to homeostasis abates. Therefore, under normal circumstances, the neural responses and the hormones that are released during the response do not

TABLE 9.1 HORMONES INVOLVED IN THE NEUROENDOCRINE RESPONSES TO STRESS

HORMONES ASSOCIATED WITH THE STRESS RESPONSE	SOURCE OF THE HORMONE	PHYSIOLOGIC EFFECTS
Catecholamines (norepinephrine, epinephrine)	Locus ceruleus, adrenal medulla	Produces a decrease in insulin release and an increase in glucagon release resulting in increased glycogenolysis, gluconeogenesis, lipolysis, proteolysis, and decreased glucose uptake by the peripheral tissues; an increase in heart rate, cardiac contractility, and vascular smooth muscle contraction; and relaxation of bronchial smooth muscle
Corticotropin-releasing factor (CRF)	Hypothalamus	Stimulates ACTH release from the anterior pituitary and increased activity of neurons in locus ceruleus
Adrenocorticotropic hormone (ACTH)	Anterior pituitary	Stimulates the synthesis and release of cortisol
Glucocorticoid hormones (*e.g.,* cortisol)	Adrenal cortex	Potentiates the actions of epinephrine and glucagon; inhibits the release and/or actions of the reproductive hormones and thyroid-stimulating hormone; and produces a decrease in immune cells and inflammatory mediators
Mineralocorticoid hormones (*e.g.,* aldosterone)	Adrenal cortex	Increases sodium absorption by the kidney
Antidiuretic hormone (ADH, vasopressin)	Hypothalamus, posterior pituitary	Increases water absorption by the kidney; produces vasoconstriction of blood vessels; and stimulates the release of ACTH

persist long enough to cause damage to vital tissues. Since the early 1980s, the term *allostasis* has been used by some investigators to describe the physiologic changes in the neuroendocrine, autonomic, and immune systems that occur in response to either real or perceived challenges to homeostasis. The persistence or accumulation of these allostatic changes (*e.g.,* immunosuppression, activation of the sympathetic nervous and renin–angiotensin–aldosterone systems [RAASs]) has been called an *allostatic load,* and this concept has been used to measure the cumulative effects of stress on humans.[12]

The integration of the components of the stress response, which occurs at the level of the central nervous system (CNS), is complex as much of the focus is looking at the psychoneuroimmunologic components (or the integration of the consciousness with the endocrine and immune defences) and is not completely understood. It relies on communication along neuronal pathways of the cerebral cortex, the limbic system, the thalamus, the hippocampus, the amygdala, the hypothalamus, the pituitary gland, and the reticular activating system (RAS;

Fig. 9.2). The cerebral cortex is involved with vigilance, cognition, and focused attention, and the limbic system with the emotional components (*e.g.,* fear, excitement, rage, anger) of the stress response. The thalamus functions as the relay centre and is important in receiving, sorting out, and distributing sensory input. The amygdala, involved in the generation of fear or anger, with overstimulation can impair hippocampal function, which is involved in short and immediate term memory. Thus attention is focused on emotions, limiting the ability to absorb new information.[13] The hypothalamus coordinates the responses of the endocrine and autonomic nervous systems (ANS). The RAS modulates mental alertness, ANS activity, and skeletal muscle tone, using input from other neural structures. The musculoskeletal tension that occurs during the stress response reflects increased activity of the RAS and its influence on the reflex circuits that control muscle tone. Adding to the complexity of this system is the fact that the individual brain circuits that participate in the mediation of the stress response interact and regulate the activity of each other. For

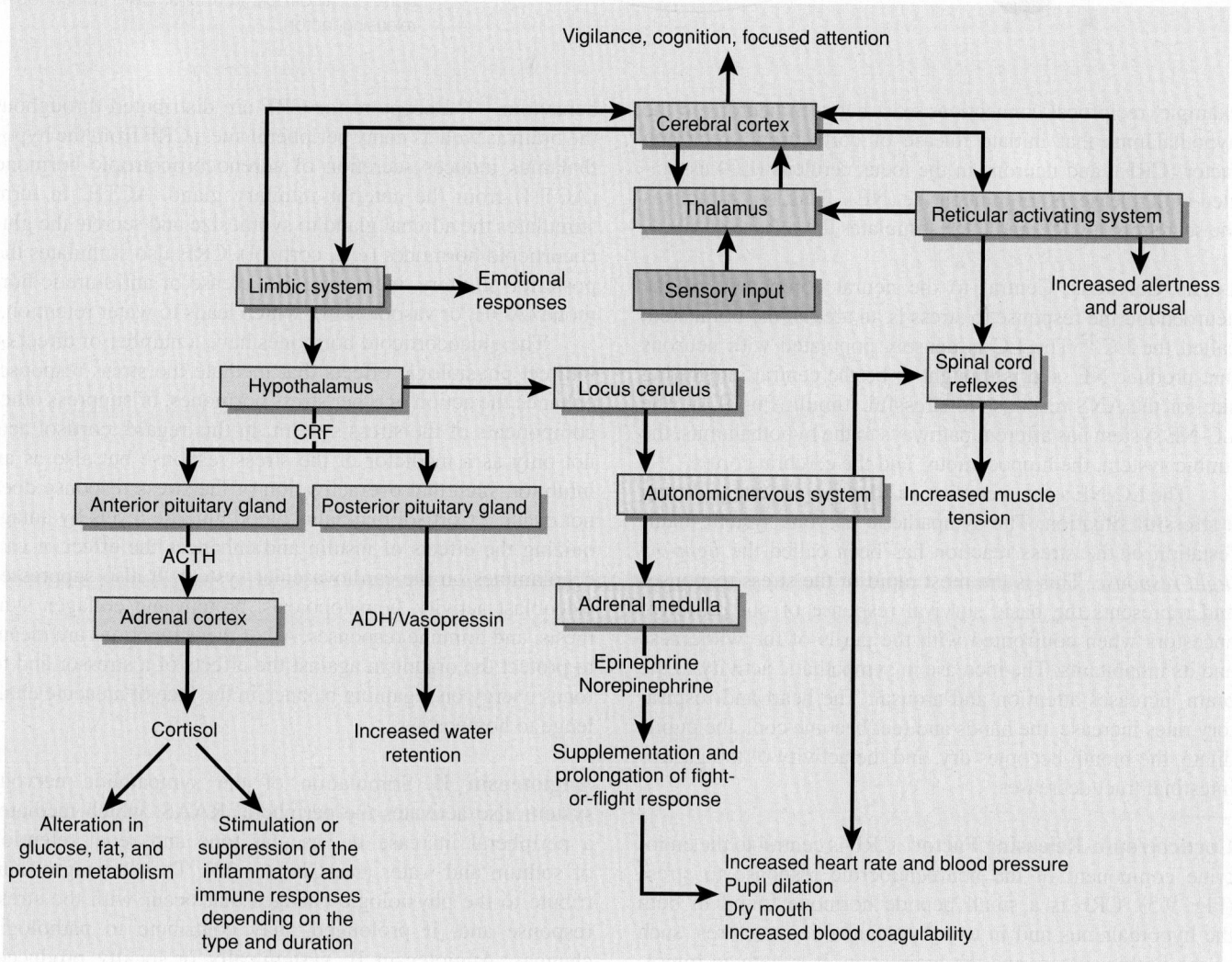

FIGURE 9.2 • Neuroendocrine pathways and physiologic responses to stress. (ACTH, adrenocorticotropic hormone; CRF, corticotropin-releasing factor).

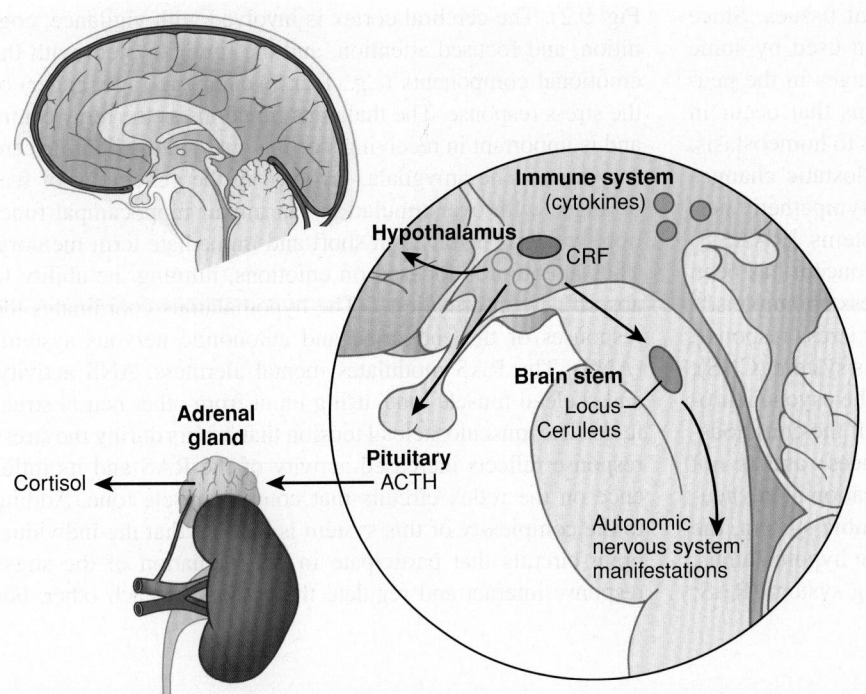

FIGURE 9.3 • Neuroendocrine–immune system regulation of the stress response. (ACTH, adrenocorticotropic hormone; CRF, corticotropin-releasing factor).

example, reciprocal connections exist between neurons in the hypothalamus that initiate release of corticotropin-releasing factor (CRF), and neurons in the locus ceruleus (LC) associated with release of norepinephrine (NE). Thus, NE stimulates the secretion of CRF, and CRF stimulates the release of NE.[14]

Locus Ceruleus. Central to the neural component of the neuroendocrine response to stress is an area of the brain stem called the LC.[12] The LC is densely populated with neurons that produce NE, and is thought to be the central integrating site for the ANS response to stressful stimuli (Fig. 9.3). The LC-NE system has afferent pathways to the hypothalamus, the limbic system, the hippocampus, and the cerebral cortex.

The LC-NE system confers an adaptive advantage during a stressful situation. The sympathetic nervous system manifestation of the stress reaction has been called the *fight-or-flight response*. This is the most rapid of the stress responses and represents the basic survival response of our primitive ancestors when confronted with the perils of the wilderness and its inhabitants. The increase in sympathetic activity in the brain increases attention and arousal. The heart and respiratory rates increase, the hands and feet become cool, the pupils dilate, the mouth becomes dry, and the activity of the gastrointestinal tract decreases.

Corticotropin-Releasing Factor. CRF is central to the endocrine component of the neuroendocrine response to stress (Fig. 9.3). CRF is a small peptide hormone found in both the hypothalamus and in extrahypothalamic structures, such as the limbic system and the brain stem. It is both an important endocrine regulator of pituitary and adrenal activity and a neurotransmitter involved in ANS activity, metabolism, and

behaviour.[12,14] Receptors for CRF are distributed throughout the brain as well as many peripheral sites. CRF from the hypothalamus induces secretion of adrenocorticotropic hormone (ACTH) from the anterior pituitary gland. ACTH, in turn, stimulates the adrenal gland to synthesize and secrete the glucocorticoid hormones (*e.g.,* cortisol). CRF also stimulates the posterior pituitary, increasing the release of antidiuretic hormone (ADH, or vasopressin), which leads to water retention.

The glucocorticoid hormones have a number of direct or indirect physiologic effects that mediate the stress response, enhance the action of other stress hormones, or suppress other components of the stress system. In this regard, cortisol acts not only as a mediator of the stress response but also as an inhibitor, such that overactivation of the stress response does not occur.[15] Cortisol maintains blood glucose levels by antagonizing the effects of insulin and enhances the effect of catecholamines on the cardiovascular system. It also suppresses osteoblast activity, hematopoiesis, protein and collagen synthesis, and immune responses. All of these functions are meant to protect the organism against the effects of a stressor and to focus energy on regaining balance in the face of an acute challenge to homeostasis.

Angiotensin II. Stimulation of the sympathetic nervous system also activates the peripheral RAAS, which mediates a peripheral increase in vascular tone and renal retention of sodium and water (see Chapter 23). These changes contribute to the physiologic changes that occur with the stress response and, if prolonged, may contribute to pathologic changes. Angiotensin II, systemically or locally produced, also has CNS effects; angiotensin II type 1 (AT$_1$) receptors are widely distributed in the hypothalamus and LC. Through these receptors, angiotensin II enhances CRF formation and release, contributes to the release of ACTH from the pituitary, enhances stress-induced release of ADH from the posterior pituitary, and stimulates the release of NE from the LC.[16]

Other Hormones. A wide variety of other hormones, including growth hormone, thyroid hormone, and the reproductive hormones, are responsive to stressful situations. Systems responsible for reproduction, growth, and immunity are directly linked to the stress system, and the hormonal effects of the stress response profoundly influence these systems.

Although growth hormone (or somatotropin) is initially elevated at the onset of stress, the prolonged presence of cortisol leads to suppression of growth hormone, insulin-like growth factor 1 (IGF-1), and other growth factors, exerting a chronically inhibitory effect on growth. In addition, CRF directly increases somatostatin, which in turn inhibits growth hormone secretion. Although the connection is speculative, the effects of stress on growth hormone may provide one of the vital links to understanding failure to thrive in children.

Stress-induced cortisol secretion also is associated with decreased levels of thyroid-stimulating hormone and inhibition of conversion of thyroxine (T_4) to the more biologically active triiodothyronine (T_3) in peripheral tissues (see Chapter 41). Both changes may serve as a means to conserve energy at times of stress.

The neurotransmitter *serotonin* or 5-hydroxytryptamine (5-HT) is hypothesized to play a role in the stress response through neurons that innervate the hypothalamus, amygdala, and other limbic structures. Administration of 5-HT receptor agonists to laboratory animals was shown to increase the secretion of several stress hormones. In addition, it has been demonstrated that CRF inhibits the firing of serotonergic neurons. Newer research is focusing on the genetic variants for serotonin transporters and receptor types and linking this to coping behaviours for stressful situations.[17]

Other hormones that have a possible role in the stress response include vasoactive intestinal peptide (VIP), neuropeptide Y, cholecystokinin (CCK), and substance P. These hormones have well-characterized physiologic roles in the periphery, but they are also found in the CNS and several studies suggest that they are involved in the stress response.[18]

The reproductive hormones (*e.g.,* estradiol, progesterone, testosterone) are inhibited by CRF at the hypophyseal level and by cortisol at the pituitary, gonadal, and target tissue levels.[8] Sepsis and severe trauma can induce anovulation and amenorrhea in women and decreased spermatogenesis and decreased levels of testosterone in men.

Immune Responses

The hallmark of the stress response, as first described by Selye, are the endocrine–immune interactions (*i.e.,* increased corticosteroid production and atrophy of the thymus) that are known to suppress the immune response. In concert, these two components of the stress system, through endocrine and neurotransmitter pathways, produce the physical and behavioural changes designed to adapt to acute stress. Much of the literature regarding stress and the immune response focuses on the causal role of stress in immune-related diseases. It has also been suggested that the reverse may occur; emotional and psychological manifestations of the stress response may be a reflection of alterations in the CNS resulting from the immune response (Fig. 9.3). Immune cells such as monocytes and lymphocytes can penetrate the blood–brain barrier and take up residence in the brain, where they secrete chemical messengers called *cytokines* that influence the stress response.[19,20]

The exact mechanism by which stress produces its effect on the immune response is unknown and probably varies from person to person, depending on genetic endowment and environmental factors. The most significant arguments for interaction between the neuroendocrine and immune systems derive from evidence that the immune and neuroendocrine systems share common signal pathways (*i.e.,* messenger molecules and receptors), that hormones and neuropeptides can alter the function of immune cells, and that the immune system and its mediators can modulate neuroendocrine function. Receptors for a number of CNS-controlled hormones and neuromediators reportedly have been found on lymphocytes. Among these are receptors for glucocorticoids, insulin, testosterone, prolactin, catecholamines, estrogens, acetylcholine, and growth hormone, suggesting that these hormones and neuromediators influence lymphocyte function. For example, cortisol is known to suppress immune function, and pharmacologic doses of cortisol are used clinically to suppress the immune response. There is evidence that the immune system, in turn, influences neuroendocrine function.[20] It has been observed that the HPA axis is activated by cytokines such as interleukin-1, interleukin-6, and tumour necrosis factor that are released from immune cells (see Chapter 17).

STRESS AND ADAPTATION

- Stress is a state manifested by symptoms that arise from the coordinated activation of the neuroendocrine and immune systems, which Selye called the general adaptation syndrome.
- The hormones and neurotransmitters (catecholamines and cortisol) that are released during the stress response function to alert the individual to a threat or challenge to homeostasis, to enhance cardiovascular and metabolic activity in order to manage the stressor, and to focus the energy of the body by suppressing the activity of other systems that are not immediately needed.
- Adaptation is the ability to respond to challenges of physical or psychological homeostasis and to return to a balanced state.
- The ability to adapt is influenced by previous learning, physiologic reserve, time, genetic endowment, age, health status and nutrition, sleep–wake cycles, and psychosocial factors.

A second possible route for neuroendocrine regulation of immune function is through the sympathetic nervous system and the release of catecholamines. The lymph nodes, thymus, and spleen are supplied with ANS nerve fibres. Centrally acting CRF activates the ANS through multisynaptic descending pathways, and circulating epinephrine acts synergistically with CRF and cortisol to inhibit the function of the immune system.

Not only is the quantity of immune expression changed because of stress, but also the quality of the response is changed. Stress hormones differentially stimulate the proliferation of subtypes of T-lymphocyte helper cells. Because these T-helper cell subtypes secrete different cytokines, they stimulate different aspects of the immune response. One subtype (T_H1) tends to stimulate T lymphocytes and the cellular-mediated immune response, whereas a second type (T_H2) tends to activate B lymphocytes and humoral-mediated immune responses.

Coping and Adaptation to Stress

The ability to adapt to a wide range of environments and stressors is not peculiar to humans. According to René Dubos (a microbiologist noted for his study of human responses to the total environment), "adaptability is found throughout life and is perhaps the one attribute that distinguishes most clearly the world of life from the world of inanimate matter."[21] Living organisms, no matter how primitive, do not submit passively to the impact of environmental forces. They attempt to respond adaptively, each in its own unique and most suitable manner. The higher functioning the organism is, the larger its repertoire of adaptive mechanisms and its ability to select and limit aspects of the environment to which it responds. The most advanced mechanisms are the social responses through which individuals or groups modify their environments, their habits, or both to achieve a way of life that is best suited to their needs.

Adaptation

Human beings, because of their highly developed nervous system and intellect, usually have alternative mechanisms for adapting and have the ability to control many aspects of their environment. Air conditioning and central heating limit the need to adapt to extreme changes in environmental temperature. The availability of antiseptic agents, immunizations, and antibiotics eliminates the need to respond to common infectious agents. At the same time, modern technology creates new challenges for adaptation and provides new sources of stress, such as increased noise, air pollution, exposure to harmful chemicals, and changes in biologic rhythms imposed by shift work and global travel.

Of particular interest are the differences in the body's response to events that threaten the integrity of the body's physiologic environment and those that threaten the integrity of the person's psychosocial environment. Many of the body's responses to physiologic disturbances are controlled on a moment-by-moment basis by feedback mechanisms that limit their application and duration of action. For example, the baroreflex-mediated rise in heart rate that occurs when a person moves from the recumbent to the standing position is almost instantaneous and subsides within seconds. Furthermore, the response to physiologic disturbances that threaten the integrity of the internal environment is specific to the threat; the body usually does not raise the body temperature when an increase in heart rate is needed. In contrast, the response to psychological disturbances is not regulated with the same degree of specificity and feedback control; instead, the effect may be inappropriate and sustained.

Factors Affecting the Ability to Adapt

Adaptation implies that an individual has successfully created a new balance between the stressor and the ability to deal with it. The means used to attain this balance are called *coping strategies* or *coping mechanisms*. Coping mechanisms are the emotional and behavioural responses used to manage threats to our physiologic and psychological homeostasis. According to Lazarus, how we cope with stressful events depends on how we perceive and interpret the event, including appraisal of the stressor and resources.[22] For example, is the event perceived as a threat of harm or loss? Is the event perceived as a challenge rather than a threat? Are there sufficient resources to meet the stressor? Physiologic reserve, time, genetic endowment and age, health status, nutrition, sleep–wake cycles, resilience, and psychosocial factors influence a person's appraisal of a stressor and the coping mechanisms used to adapt to the new situation (Fig. 9.4).

Physiologic and Anatomic Reserve. The safety margin for adaptation of most body systems is considerably greater than that needed for normal activities. The trained athlete is able to increase cardiac output six- to eightfold during exercise. The red blood cells carry more oxygen than the tissues can use, the liver and fat cells store excess nutrients, and bone tissue stores calcium in excess of that needed for normal neuromuscular

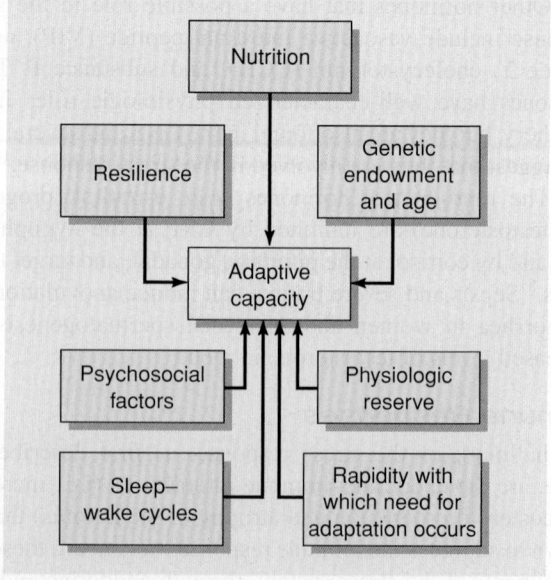

FIGURE 9.4 • Factors affecting adaptation.

function. The ability of body systems to increase their function given the need to adapt is known as the *physiologic reserve.* Many of the body organs, such as the lungs, kidneys, and adrenals, are paired to provide anatomic reserve as well. Both organs are not needed to ensure the continued existence and maintenance of the internal environment. Many persons function normally with only one lung or one kidney. In kidney disease, for example, signs of renal failure do not occur until approximately 75% of the functioning nephrons have been destroyed.

Time. Adaptation is most efficient when changes occur gradually rather than suddenly. It is possible, for instance, to lose a litre or more of blood through chronic gastrointestinal bleeding over a week without manifesting signs of shock. However, a sudden hemorrhage that causes rapid loss of an equal amount of blood is likely to cause hypotension and shock.

Genetics. Adaptation is further affected by the availability of adaptive responses and flexibility in selecting the most appropriate and economical response. The greater the number of available responses, the more effective is the capacity to adapt.

Genetic endowment can ensure that the systems that are essential to adaptation function adequately. Even a gene that has deleterious effects may prove adaptive in some environments. In Africa, the gene for sickle cell disease persists in some populations because it provides some resistance against the parasitic infection that causes malaria.

Age. The capacity to adapt is decreased at the extremes of age. The ability to adapt is impaired by the immaturity of an infant, much as it is by the decline in functional reserve that occurs with age. For example, the infant has difficulty concentrating urine because of immature renal structures and therefore is less able than an adult to cope with decreased water intake or exaggerated water losses. A similar situation exists in the elderly owing to age-related changes in renal function.

Gender. Within the last decade, primarily because females have been included in basic science and clinical investigations, differences between the sexes in cardiovascular, respiratory, endocrine, renal, and neurophysiologic function have been found, and it has been hypothesized that sex hormones are the basis of these biologic differences. Technological advances in cellular and molecular biology have made it clear, however, that there are fundamental differences in the locale and regulation of individual genes in the male and female genome. These differences have general implications for the prevention, diagnosis, and treatment of disease and specific implications for our understanding of the sex-based differences in response to life's stressors.

Given the nature of sex-based differences, it is not surprising that there are differences in the physiologic stress response in both the HPA axis and in the ANS.[23] For example, the male hypothalamus may produce more CRF and more ACTH than the female hypothalamus in response to a psychological stressor. However, the sensitivity to arginine vasopressin (AVP),

a hormone that has cardiovascular and renal effects and potentiates the release of ACTH, is greater in the female. Premenopausal women also tend to have a lower activation of the sympathetic nervous system than men in response to stressors. The phase of menstruation (luteal vs. follicular) as well as menopausal status can alter these responses and need to be taken into account when studying these responses.[23] These sex-based differences in activation of the stress response may partially explain differences in susceptibility to diseases in which the stress response may play a causal role. The neurobiological underpinnings of these differences are not definitive but are intriguing and continue to be explored.[23]

Health Status. Physical and mental health status determines physiologic and psychological reserves and is a strong determinant of the ability to adapt. For example, persons with heart disease are less able to adjust to stresses that require the recruitment of cardiovascular responses. Severe emotional stress often produces disruption of physiologic function and limits the ability to make appropriate choices related to long-term adaptive needs. Those who have worked with acutely ill persons know that the will to live often has a profound influence on survival during life-threatening illnesses.

Nutrition. There are 50 to 60 essential nutrients, including minerals, lipids, certain fatty acids, vitamins, and specific amino acids. Deficiencies or excesses of any of these nutrients can alter a person's health status and impair the ability to adapt. The importance of nutrition to enzyme function, immune response, and wound healing is well known. On a worldwide basis, malnutrition may be one of the most common causes of immunodeficiency.

Among the problems associated with dietary excess are obesity and alcohol abuse. Obesity is a common problem in Canada that predisposes an individual to a number of health problems, including atherosclerosis, hypertension, and joint injury. Alcohol is commonly used in excess. It acutely alters brain function and cognition and with long-term use can seriously impair the function of the liver, brain, and other vital structures, and diminish the immune response.

Sleep–Wake Cycles. Sleep is considered to be a restorative function in which energy is restored and tissues are regenerated.[24] Sleep occurs in a cyclic manner, alternating with periods of wakefulness and increased energy use (see Chapter 52). Biologic rhythms play an important role in adaptation to stress, development of illness, and response to medical treatment. Many rhythms such as rest and activity, work and leisure, and eating and drinking oscillate with a frequency similar to that of the 24-hour light–dark solar day. The term *circadian,* from the Latin *circa* ("about") and *dies* ("day"), is used to describe these 24-hour diurnal rhythms.

Sleep disorders and alterations in the sleep–wake cycle have been shown to alter immune function, the normal circadian pattern of hormone secretion, and physical and psychological functioning.[24,25] The two most common manifestations of an alteration in the sleep–wake cycle are insomnia and sleep deprivation or increased somnolence. In some persons, stress may produce sleep disorders, and in others, sleep disorders may lead to stress. Acute stress and environmental disturbances, loss of a loved one, recovery from surgery, and pain are common causes of transient and short-term insomnia. Air travel and jet lag constitute additional causes of altered sleep–wake cycles, as does shift work.

Psychological Resilience. Studies by social psychologists have focused on individuals' emotional reactions to stressful situations and their coping mechanisms to determine those characteristics that help some people remain healthy despite being challenged by high levels of stressors. For example, the concept of *resilience* describes a process of positively adapting in the face of adversity. Ordinary persons commonly have resilient abilities that involve behaviours, thoughts, and actions to recover from problems and challenges; those who lack these abilities are often capable of learning skills to help them. Many studies by nurses and social psychologists suggest that this kind of hardiness, or ability to conceptualize stressors as a challenge rather than a threat, is correlated with positive health outcomes.[26]

Psychosocial Factors. Several studies have related social connectedness and life events to illness. Scientific interest in the social environment as a cause of stress has gradually broadened to include the social environment as a resource that modulates the relation between stress and health. Presumably, persons who can mobilize strong supportive resources from within their social relationships are better able to withstand the negative effects of stress on their health. Studies suggest that social support has direct and indirect positive effects on health status and serves as a buffer or modifier of the physical and psychosocial effects of stress.[27]

Social networks contribute in a number of ways to a person's psychosocial and physical integrity. It seems that close relationships with others can involve positive effects as well as the potential for conflict and may, in some situations, leaving the person less able to cope with life stressors. Neurobiology is examining the interaction between the posterior pituitary hormones of oxytocic and vasopressin, and their link to behavioural and endocrine responses to social stress. Oxytocin has received increasing attention looking at its release and the potential ability to promote a stress-protective effect by encouraging people to seek contact or befriend others.[27,28] There is also evidence that persons who have social supports or social assets may live longer and have a lower incidence of somatic illness.

IN SUMMARY

The stress response involves the activation of several physiologic systems (sympathetic nervous system, the HPA axis, and the immune system) that work in a coordinated fashion to protect the body against damage from the intense demands made on it. Selye called this response the general adaptation

syndrome. The stress response is divided into three stages: the alarm stage, with activation of the sympathetic nervous system and the HPA axis; the resistance stage, during which the body selects the most effective defences; and the exhaustion stage, during which physiologic resources are depleted and signs of systemic damage appear.

The activation and control of the stress response are mediated by the combined efforts of the nervous and endocrine systems. The neuroendocrine systems integrate signals received along neurosensory pathways and from circulating mediators that are carried in the bloodstream. In addition, the immune system both affects and is affected by the stress response.

Adaptation is affected by a number of factors, including experience and previous learning, the rapidity with which the need to adapt occurs, genetic endowment and age, health status, nutrition, sleep–wake cycles, resilience, and psychosocial factors.

DISORDERS OF THE STRESS RESPONSE

After completing this section of the chapter, you should be able to meet the following objectives:

- Describe the physiologic and psychological effects of a chronic stress response.
- Describe the characteristic of post-traumatic stress disorder.
- List five nonpharmacologic methods of managing stress.

For the most part, the stress response is meant to be acute and time limited. The time-limited nature of the process renders the accompanying catabolic and immunosuppressive effects advantageous. It is the chronicity of the response that is thought to be disruptive to physical and mental health.

Stressors can assume a number of patterns in relation to time. They may be classified as acute time-limited, chronic intermittent, or chronic sustained. An acute time-limited stressor is one that occurs over a short time and does not recur; a chronic intermittent stressor is one to which a person is chronically exposed. The frequency or chronicity of circumstances to which the body is asked to respond often determines the availability and efficiency of the stress responses. The response of the immune system, for example, is more rapid and efficient on second exposure to a pathogen than it is on first exposure, but chronic exposure to a stressor can fatigue the system and impair its effectiveness, leading to immunopathology.[20]

Effects of Acute Stress

The reactions to acute stress are those associated with the ANS, the fight-or-flight response. The manifestations of the stress response—a pounding headache, cold, moist skin, a stiff neck—are all part of the acute stress response.[12] Centrally, there is facilitation of neural pathways mediating arousal, alertness, vigilance, cognition, and focused attention, as well as appropriate aggression. Increased alertness and cognitive functioning enable rapid processing of information and arrival at the most appropriate solution to the threatening situation. The acute stress response can result from either psychologically or physiologically threatening events. In situations of life-threatening trauma, these acute responses may be lifesaving in that they divert blood from less essential to more essential body functions.

However, for persons with limited coping abilities, either because of physical or mental health, the acute stress response may be detrimental. This is true of persons with pre-existing heart disease in whom an increase in the stress response and catecholamines can result in arrhythmias. For people with other chronic health problems, such as headache disorder, acute stress may precipitate a recurrence. In healthy individuals, the acute stress response can redirect attention from behaviours that promote health, such as attention to proper meals and getting adequate sleep. For those with health problems, it can interrupt adherence to medication regimens and exercise programs. In some situations, the acute arousal state actually can be life-threatening, physically immobilizing the person when movement would avert catastrophe (*e.g.,* not moving out of the way of a speeding car).

Effects of Chronic Stress

The stress response is designed to be an acute self-limited response in which activation of the ANS and the HPA axis is controlled in a negative feedback manner. As with all negative feedback systems, pathophysiologic changes can occur in the stress response system. Function can be altered in several ways, including when a component of the system fails; when the neural and hormonal connections among the components of the system are dysfunctional; and when the original stimulus for the activation of the system is prolonged or of such magnitude that it overwhelms the ability of the system to respond appropriately. In these cases, the system may become overactive or underactive.

Chronicity and excessive activation of the stress response can result from chronic illnesses as well as contribute to the development of long-term health problems. Chronic activation of the stress response is an important public health issue from both a health and a cost perspective.

The stress response is linked to a myriad of health disorders, such as diseases of the cardiovascular, gastrointestinal, immune, and neurologic systems, as well as depression, chronic alcoholism and drug abuse, eating disorders, injuries, and suicide.

Occurrence of the oral disease acute necrotizing gingivitis, in which the normal bacterial flora of the mouth become invasive, is known by dentists to be associated with acute stress, such as final examinations.[29] Similarly, herpes simplex virus type 1 infection (*i.e.,* cold sores) often develops during periods of inadequate rest, fever, ultraviolet radiation, and emotional distress. The resident herpes virus is kept in check by body defences, probably T lymphocytes, until a stressful event occurs that causes suppression of the immune system. Psychological stress is associated in a dose–response manner with an increased risk for development of the common cold, and this risk is attributable to increased rates of infection rather than frequency of symptoms after infection.[12]

In a study in which participants were infected with the influenza virus, those persons who reported the greatest amount of premorbid stress also reported the most intense influenza symptoms and had a statistically greater production of interleukin-6, a cytokine that acts as a chemotactic agent for immune cells.[30] Elderly caregivers of a spouse with dementia had a significantly higher score for emotional distress and higher salivary cortisol than matched control subjects. The higher stress was correlated with a decreased immune response to the influenza vaccine.[31] The experience of stress also has been associated with delays in wound healing.[32]

Post-Traumatic Stress Disorder

Post-traumatic stress disorder (PTSD) is characterized by a severe stress response as a result of experiencing a significant physical, emotional, or psychological traumatic event.[33] It was formerly called *battle fatigue* or *shell shock* because it was first characterized in soldiers returning from combat. Although war is still a significant cause of PTSD, other major catastrophic events, such as weather-related disasters (hurricanes and floods), airplane crashes, terrorist bombings, and rape or child abuse, also may result in development of the disorder. People who are exposed to such events are also at risk for development of major depression, panic disorder, generalized anxiety disorder, and substance abuse. They may also have bodily symptoms and physical illnesses, particularly hypertension, asthma, and chronic pain syndromes. PTSD became an official psychiatric diagnosis in 1980 in the third edition of the American Psychiatric Association's *Diagnostic and Statistical Manual of Mental Disorders (DSM-III)*.[33]

PTSD is characterized by multiple criteria: the presence of a stressor; symptoms of intrusion, avoidance, mood changes, and hyperarousal lasting longer than 1 month; a significant degree of impairment; and the lack of association between these alterations and other medical conditions (Box 9.1).[34] *Intrusion* refers to the occurrence of "flashbacks" during waking hours or nightmares in which the past traumatic event is relived, often in vivid and frightening detail. *Avoidance* refers to the emotional numbing that accompanies this disorder and disrupts important personal relationships. Because a person with PTSD has not been able to resolve the painful feelings associated with the trauma, depression is commonly a part of the clinical picture. Survivor guilt also may be a product of traumatic situations in which the person survived the disaster but loved ones did not. *Alterations in cognitions and mood,* newly added in the DSM 5, refers to the decline and profound changes in how the person sees themselves. These ruminative

---

BOX 9.1 POST-TRAUMATIC STRESS DISORDER

The eight criteria required for PTSD diagnosis in adult, adolescents, or children over the age of 6 years:

A. Must include actual or threatened exposure to a traumatic event(s) or stressor(s) (*e.g.*, death). The exposure can be in one or more of the following ways:
   - Direct
   - Witnessed
   - Indirect learning about close friend or relative's accidental or violent death
   - Repeated

B. Intrusion or re-experiencing (one required) of events such as:
   - Intrusive thoughts or memories
   - Nightmares or dreams
   - Flashbacks or images
   - Intense psychological distress or physical reactivity to reminders of events (*e.g.*, birthday)

C. Avoidance (one or both required). Persistent efforts to either:
   - Avoid thoughts, feelings, or conversations connected with traumatic event
   - Avoid people, places, or situations that may trigger reminders of the traumatic event

D. Negative alteration in mood or cognition (two or more required). A decline in mood or thought patterns, including:
   - Memory problems about specific traumatic event
   - Persistent and exaggerated negative beliefs about oneself or others
   - Distorted sense of blame about the cause of the event
   - Persistent negative emotional state
   - Significant diminished interest or participation in pre-trauma activities
   - Feeling of detachment or isolation from others
   - Persistent inability to experience positive emotions

E. Hyperarousal (two or more required). Symptoms worsening after traumatic event such as:
   - Irritability and increased temper or anger
   - Self-destructive behaviour
   - Hypervigilance
   - Exaggerated startle response
   - Concentration problems
   - Sleep disturbances

F. Duration of symptoms (B, C, D, and E) must be more than one month.

G. This disturbance must cause clinically significant distress or impairment in functioning.

H. This disturbance is not due to any other medical conditions or substance use.

Adapted from American Psychiatric Association. Posttraumatic stress disorder. (2013). In *Diagnostic and statistical manual of mental disorders: DSM-5*. Washington, DC: Author.

---

type symptoms can include blame for the event, anger, shame, and other negative emotions. *Hyperarousal* refers to the presence of increased irritability, difficulty concentrating, an exaggerated startle reflex, and increased vigilance. In addition, memory problems, sleep disturbances, and excessive anxiety are commonly experienced by persons with PTSD.

Although the pathophysiology of PTSD is not completely understood, the revelation of physiologic changes related to the disorder has shed light on why some people recover from the disorder, whereas others do not. It has been hypothesized that the intrusive symptoms of PTSD may arise from exaggerated sympathetic nervous system activation in response to the traumatic event. Persons with chronic PTSD have been shown to have increased levels of NE and increased activity of α_2-adrenergic receptors.

Recent neuroanatomic studies have identified alterations in two brain structures (the amygdala and hippocampus). Positron emission tomography and functional magnetic resonance imaging have shown increased reactivity of the amygdala and hippocampus and decreased reactivity of the anterior cingulate and orbitofrontal areas. These areas of the brain are involved in fear responses. The hippocampus also functions in memory processes. Differences in hippocampal function and memory processes suggest a neuroanatomic basis for the intrusive recollections and other cognitive problems that characterize PTSD.[33]

Persons with PTSD demonstrate decreased cortisol levels, increased sensitivity of cortisol receptors, and an enhanced negative feedback inhibition of cortisol release with the dexamethasone suppression test.[33] Dexamethasone is a synthetic glucocorticoid that mimics the effects of cortisol and directly inhibits the action of CRF and ACTH. This is in contrast to patients with major depression, who have a decreased sensitivity of glucocorticoid receptors, a high plasma level of cortisol, and decreased dexamethasone suppression. The hypersuppression of cortisol observed with the dexamethasone test suggests that persons with PTSD do not exhibit a classic stress response as described by Selye. Because this hypersuppression has not been described in other psychiatric disorders, it may serve as a relatively specific marker for PTSD.

Little is known about the risk factors that predispose people to the development of PTSD. Statistics indicate there is a need for studies to determine risk factors for PTSD as a means of targeting individuals who may need intensive therapeutic measures after a life-threatening event. Research also is needed to determine the mechanisms by which the disorder develops so that it can be prevented or, if that is not possible, so that treatment methods can be developed to decrease the devastating effects of this disorder on affected individuals and their families.[33]

Health care professionals need to be aware that clients who present with symptoms of depression, anxiety, and alcohol or drug abuse may in fact be suffering from PTSD. The client history should include questions concerning the occurrence of violence, major loss, or traumatic events in the person's life. In Canada it is estimated that up to 10% of soldiers stationed in combat missions will experience PTSD.[35] Also it has been noted that there is a sex-based difference in the type of trauma experienced. Women tend to report childhood physical and sexual abuse whereas men report combat or physical attacks, and women are twice as likely to develop PTSD after exposure to a traumatic event than men.[35] The cause for this sex-based difference is unclear, but it is surmised that the element of powerlessness in the event plays a role.

Debriefing, or talking about the traumatic event at the time it happens, often is an effective therapeutic tool. Crisis teams are often among the first people to attend to the emotional needs of those caught in catastrophic events. Some people may need continued individual or group therapy. Often concurrent pharmacotherapy with antidepressant and antianxiety agents is useful and helps the individual participate more fully in therapy.

Most important, the person with PTSD should not be made to feel responsible for the disorder or that it is evidence of a so-called character flaw. It is not uncommon for persons with this disorder to be told to "get over it" or "just get on with it, because others have." There is ample evidence to suggest that there is a physiologic basis for the individual differences in responses to traumatic events, and these differences need to be taken into account.

Treatment and Research of Stress Disorders

Treatment

The treatment of stress should be directed toward helping people avoid coping behaviours that impose a risk to their health and providing them with alternative stress-reducing strategies. Evidence suggests that early interventions can assist persons in adapting new and effective coping mechanisms to better manage stress in the future.[36] Purposeful priority setting and problem solving can be used by persons who are overwhelmed by the number of life stressors to which they have been exposed. Other nonpharmacologic methods used for stress reduction are relaxation techniques, guided imagery, music therapy, massage, and biofeedback.

Relaxation. Practices for evoking the relaxation response are numerous. They are found in virtually every culture and are credited with producing a generalized decrease in sympathetic system activity and musculoskeletal tension. According to Herbert Benson, a physician who worked in developing the technique, four elements are integral to the various relaxation techniques: a repetitive mental device, a passive attitude, decreased mental tonus, and a quiet environment.[37] Benson developed a noncultural method that is commonly used for achieving relaxation (Box 9.2).

Progressive muscle relaxation is another method of relieving tension. Tension can be defined physiologically as the inappropriate contraction of muscle fibres. The procedure, which has been modified by a number of therapists since its introduction, consists of systematic contraction and relaxation of major muscle groups. As the person learns to relax, the various muscle groups are combined. Eventually, the person learns to relax individual muscle groups without first contracting them.

BOX 9.2 **THE RELAXATION RESPONSE**

- Sit quietly in a comfortable position.
- Deeply relax all your muscles, beginning at your feet and progressing up to your face.
- Breathe through your nose. Become aware of your breathing. As you breathe out, say the word "one" silently to yourself. Continue for 20 minutes. When you have finished, sit quietly for several minutes, first with your eyes closed and then with them open.
- Do not worry about whether you are successful in achieving a deep level of relaxation. Maintain a positive attitude and permit the relaxation to occur at its own rate. Expect distracting thoughts, ignore them, and continue repeating "one" as you breathe out.

Modified from Benson H. L., Boro E. S. (1977). Systemic hypertension and the relaxation response. *New England Journal of Medicine.* 296(20), 1152–1156.

Imagery. Guided imagery is another technique that can be used to achieve relaxation. One method is scene visualization, in which the person is asked to sit back, close the eyes, and concentrate on a scene narrated by the therapist. Whenever possible, all five senses are involved: the person attempts to see, feel, hear, smell, and taste aspects of the visual experience. Other types of imagery involve imagining the appearance of each of the major muscle groups and how they feel during tension and relaxation.

Music Therapy. Music therapy is used for both its physiologic and psychological effects. It involves listening to selected pieces of music as a means of ameliorating anxiety or stress, reducing pain, decreasing feelings of loneliness and isolation, buffering noise, and facilitating expression of emotion. Music is defined as having three components: rhythm, melody, and harmony. Rhythm is the order in the movement of the music. Rhythm is the most dynamic aspect of music, and particular pieces of music often are selected because they harmonize with body rhythms such as heart rhythm, respiratory rhythm, or gait. The melody is created by the musical pitch and the distance (or interval) between the musical tones. The melody contributes to the listener's emotional response to the music. The harmony results from the way pitches are blended together, with the combination of sounds described as consonant or dissonant by the listener. Music usually is selected based on a person's musical preference and past experiences with music. Depending on the setting, headphones may be used to screen out other distracting noises. Radio and television music are inappropriate for music therapy because of the inability to control the selection of pieces that are played, the interruptions that occur (*e.g.*, commercials and announcements), and the quality of the reception.

Massage Therapies. Massage is the manipulation of the soft tissues of the body to promote relaxation and relief of muscle tension. The technique that is used may involve a gentle stroking along the length of a muscle (effleurage), application of pressure across the width of a muscle (petrissage), deep massage movements applied by a circular motion of the thumbs or fingertips (friction), squeezing across the width of a muscle (kneading), or use of light slaps or chopping actions (hacking). Massage may be administered by practitioners who have received special training in its use or by less-prepared persons such as parents of small children or caregivers of confused elders. It is often used as a means of physiologic relaxation and stress relief in critically ill patients.

Biofeedback. Biofeedback is a technique in which an individual learns to control physiologic functioning. It involves electronic monitoring of one or more physiologic responses to stress with immediate feedback of the specific response to the person undergoing treatment. Several types of responses are used: electromyographic (EMG), heart rate variability (HRV), electrothermal, and electrodermal.[38,39] The EMG response involves the measurement of electrical potentials from muscles, usually the forearm extensor or frontalis. This is used to gain control over the contraction of skeletal muscles that occurs with anxiety and tension. The HRV response works to balance the sympathetic and parasympathetic influences to control involuntary heart rate via breathing techniques. The electrothermal sensors monitor skin temperature in the fingers or toes. The sympathetic nervous system exerts significant control over blood flow in the distal parts of the body such as the digits of the hands and feet. Consequently, anxiety often is manifested by a decrease in skin temperature in the fingers and toes. Electrodermal sensors measure conductivity of skin (usually the hands) in response to anxiety. Fearful and anxious people often have cold and clammy hands, which lead to a decrease in conductivity.

Research

Research in stress has focused on personal reports of the stress situation and the physiologic responses to stress. Physiologic response can be difficult to quantify, as experiences of stress vary widely among individuals. As any stress responses are based on previous life experiences and availability of adaptive resources, it is difficult to find a stimulus that produces equivalent stress in all subjects in a study. A number of interview guides and written instruments are available for measuring the personal responses to stress and coping in adults and children. There are fewer methods available for measuring the physiologic responses to stress in humans because much of the research in the field of stress has been accomplished using animal models.

Some of the current methods for studying the physiologic manifestations of the stress response include electrocardiographic recording of heart rate, blood pressure measurement, electrodermal measurement of skin resistance associated with sweating, and biochemical analyses of hormone levels. Measurements of urinary and plasma catecholamines can be used as an index of ANS activation. Cortisol levels can be obtained from salivary samples. The effect of the stress response on the immune system can be studied through the use of blood tests to obtain immune cell (lymphocyte) counts and antibody levels.

Research that attempts to establish a link between the stress response and disease needs to be interpreted with caution owing to the influence that individual differences have in the way people respond to stress. Not everyone who experiences stressful life events develops a disease. The evidence for a link between the stress response system and the development of disease in susceptible persons is compelling but not conclusive. No study has established a direct cause-and-effect relationship between the stress response and disease occurrence. For example, depressive illness often is associated with an increase in both plasma cortisol and cerebrospinal fluid concentrations of CRF. The question that arises is whether this increased plasma cortisol is a cause or an effect of the depressive state. Although health care professionals continue to question the role of stressors and coping skills in the pathogenesis of disease states, we must resist the temptation to suggest that any disease is due to excessive stress or poor coping skills.

IN SUMMARY

Stress in itself is neither negative nor deleterious to health. The stress response is designed to be time limited and protective, but in situations of prolonged activation of the response because of overwhelming or chronic stressors, it could be damaging to health. PTSD is an example of chronic activation of the stress response as a result of experiencing a severe trauma. In this disorder, memory of the traumatic event seems to be enhanced. Flashbacks of the event are accompanied by intense activation of the neuroendocrine system.

Stress management should be aimed at helping people avoid behaviours that can adversely affect their health and providing them with other ways to reduce stress. Nonpharmacologic methods used in the alleviation of the stress response include relaxation techniques, guided imagery, music therapy, massage techniques, and biofeedback.

Research in stress has focused on personal reports of the stress situation and the physiologic responses to stress. A number of interview guides and written instruments are available for measuring the personal responses to acute and chronic stressors. Methods used for studying the physiologic manifestations of the stress response include electrocardiographic recording of heart rate, blood pressure measurement, electrodermal measurement of skin resistance associated with sweating, and biochemical analyses of hormone levels.

REVIEW EXERCISES

1. A 21-year-old college student notices that she frequently develops "cold sores" during the stressful final examination week.

A. What is the association between stress and the immune system?

B. One of her classmates suggests that she listen to music or try relaxation exercises as a means of relieving stress. Explain how these interventions might work in relieving stress.

2. A 75-year-old woman with congestive heart failure complains that her condition gets worse when she worries and is under a lot of stress.

A. Relate the effects stress has on the neuroendocrine control of cardiovascular function and its possible relationship to a worsening of the woman's congestive heart failure.

B. She tells you that she dealt with much worse stressors when she was younger and never had any problems. How would you explain this?

3. A 30-year-old woman who was rescued from a collapsed building has been having nightmares recalling the event, excessive anxiety, and loss of appetite, and is afraid to leave her home for fear something will happen.

A. Given her history and symptoms, what is the likely diagnosis?

B. How might she be treated?

References

1. Lazarus R. S., Folkman S. (1984). *Stress, appraisal, and coping.* New York, NY: Springer.
2. Hinkle L. E. (1977). The concept of "stress" in the biological and social sciences. In Lipowskin Z. J., Lipsitt D. R., Whybrow P. C. (Eds.), *Psychosomatic medicine* (pp. 27–49). New York, NY: Oxford University Press.
3. Osler W. (1910). The Lumleian lectures on angina pectoris. *Lancet, 175,* 696–700, 839–844, 974–977.
4. Cannon W. B. (1935). Stresses and strains of homeostasis. *American Journal of Medical Science, 189,* 13–14.
5. Selye H. (1946). The general adaptation syndrome and diseases of adaptation. *Journal of Clinical Endocrinology, 6,* 117–230.
6. Cannon W. B. (1939). *The wisdom of the body* (pp. 299–300). New York, NY: WW Norton.
7. Selye H. (1976). *The stress of life* (rev. ed.). New York, NY: McGraw-Hill.
8. Selye H. (1973). The evolution of the stress concept. *American Scientist, 61,* 692–699.
9. Selye H. (1974). *Stress without distress* (p. 6). New York, NY: New American Library.
10. Lazarus R. (1999). *Stress and emotion: A new synthesis* (p. 6). New York, NY: Springer.
11. McEwen B. S., Gianaros P. J. (2011). Stress- and allostasis-induced brain plasticity. *Annual Review of Medicine, 62,* 431–445.
12. Chrousos G. P. (2009). Stress and disorders of the stress system. *Nature Reviews Endocrinology, 5*(7), 374–381.
13. Goleman D. (2006). *Social intelligence: The new science of human relationships.* New York, NY: Bantam Books.
14. Hall J. E. (2011). *Textbook of medical physiology* (12th ed.). Philadelphia, PA: W. B. Saunders.
15. Bruce J., Gunnar M. R., Pears K. C., Fisher P. A. (2013). Early adverse care, stress neurobiology, and prevention science: Lessons learned. *Prevention Science, 14*(3), 247–256.
16. Herman J. P., McKlveen J. M., Solomon M. B., et al. (2012). Neural regulation of the stress response: Glucocorticoid feedback mechanisms. *Brazilian Journal of Medical and Biological Research, 45*(4), 292–298.
17. Puglisi-Allegra S., Andolina D. (2015). Sertonin and stress coping. *Behavioural Brain Research, 277,* 58–67.
18. Carrasco G. A., Van de Kar L. D. (2003). Neuroendocrine pharmacology of stress. *European Journal of Pharmacology, 463*(1–3), 235–272.
19. Bellavance M., Rivest S. (2012). The neuroendocrine control of the innate immune system in health and brain diseases. *Immunological Reviews, 248*(1), 36–55.
20. Dhabhar F. S. (2014). Effects of stress on immune function: The good, the bad, and the beautiful. *Immunology Research, 58*(2–3), 193–210.
21. Dubos R. (1965). *Man Adapting* (pp. 256, 258, 261, 264). New Haven, CT: Yale University Press.
22. Lazarus R. (2000). Evolution of a model of stress, coping, and discrete emotions. In: Rice V. H. (Ed.) *Handbook of stress, coping, and health* (pp. 195–222). Thousand Oaks, CA: Sage.
23. Verma R., Balhara Y. P. S., Gupta C. S. (2011). Gender differences in stress response: Role of developmental and biological determinants. *Industrial Psychiatry Journal, 20*(1), 4–10.
24. Elder G. J., Wetherell M. A., Barclay N. L., Ellis J. G. (2014). The cortisol awakening response: Application and implications for sleep medicine. *Sleep Medicine Reviews, 18*(3), 215–224.
25. Ganz F. D. (2012). Sleep and immune function. *Critical Care Nurse, 32*(2), e19–e25.
26. Crum A. J., Salovey P., Achor S. (2013). Rethinking stress: The role of mindsets in determining the stress response. *Journal of Personality and Social Psychology, 104*(4), 716–733.
27. Meyer-Lindenberg A., Domes G., Kirsch P., Henrichs M. (2011). Oxytocin and vasopressin in the human brain: Social neuropeptides for translational medicine. *Nature Reviews Neuroscience, 12*(9), 524–538.
28. Olff M., Frijling J. L., Kubzansky L. D., et al. (2013). The role of oxytocin in social bonding, stress regulation and mental health: An update on the moderating effects of context and interindividual differences. *Psychoneuroendocrinology, 38*(9), 1883–1894.
29. Dworkin S. F. (1969). Psychosomatic concepts and dentistry: Some perspectives. *Journal of Periodontology, 40*(11), 647–654.
30. Cohen S., Doyle W. J., Skoner D. P. (1999). Psychological stress, cytokine production, and severity of upper respiratory illness. *Psychosomatic Medicine, 61*(2), 175–180.
31. Vedhara K., Cox N. K., Wilcock G. K., et al. (1999). Chronic stress in elderly carers of dementia patients and antibody response to influenza vaccination. *Lancet, 353*(9153), 627–631.
32. Rozlog L. A., Kiecolt-Glaser J. K., Marucha P. T., et al. (1999). Stress and immunity: Implication for viral disease and wound healing. *Journal of Periodontology, 70*(7), 786–792.
33. Pitman R. K., Rasmusson A. M., Koenen K. C., et al. (2012). Biological studies of post-traumatic stress disorder. *Nature Reviews Neuroscience, 13*(11), 769–787.
34. O'Donnell M. L., Alkemade N., Nickerson A., et al. (2014). Impact of the diagnostic changes to post-traumatic stress disorder for DSM-5 and the proposed changes to ICD-11. *Brtish Journal of Psychiatry, 205*(3), 230–235.
35. Canadian Mental Health Association – British Columba Division. (2013). Post-traumatic stress disorder. Available: http://www.cmha.bc.ca/get-informed/mental-health-information/ptsd. Accessed on February 12, 2015.
36. Wilson K. R., Hansen D. J., Li M. (2011). The traumatic stress response in child maltreatment and resultant neuropsychological effects. *Aggression and Violent Behavior, 16*(2), 87–97.
37. Benson H. (1977). Systemic hypertension and the relaxation response. *The New England Journal of Medicine, 296*(20), 1152–1156.
38. Schoenberg P. L. A., David A. S. (2014). Biofeedback for psychiatric disorders: A systematic review. *Applied Psychophysiology and Biofeedback, 39*(2), 109–135.
39. Ratanasiripong P., Ratanasiripong N., Kathalae D. (2012). Biofeedback intervention for stress and anxiety among nursing students. *ISRN Nursing, 2012,* Article ID: 827972.

Visit thePoint **http://thePoint.lww.com for animations, journal articles, and more!**

Alterations in Temperature Regulation

10

BODY TEMPERATURE REGULATION

Body temperature, at any given point in time, represents a balance between heat gain and heat loss. Body heat is generated in the tissues of the body as a byproduct of metabolism, transferred to the skin surface by the blood, and then released into the environment surrounding the body. Body temperature rises in infection because of increased metabolic rate and cytokine-mediated changes in the set-point of the temperature-regulating centre in the hypothalamus. Hyperthermia may occur due to excessive heat production, inadequate heat dissipation, or a failure of thermoregulatory mechanisms. Body temperature falls during hypothermia caused by exposure to a cold environment. This chapter is organized into three sections: body temperature regulation, increased body temperature (fever and hyperthermia), and decreased body temperature (hypothermia).

BODY TEMPERATURE REGULATION

After completing this section of the chapter, you should be able to meet the following objectives:

- Differentiate between body core temperature and skin temperature and relate the differences to methods used for measuring body temperature.
- Describe the physiologic mechanisms that control the gain and loss of heat from the body.
- Define the terms *conduction, radiation, convection,* and *evaporation,* and relate them to the mechanisms for gain and loss of heat from the body.

Virtually all biochemical processes in the body are affected by changes in temperature. Metabolic processes speed up or slow down depending on whether body temperature is rising or falling. *Core body temperature (i.e.,* intracranial, intrathoracic, and intra-abdominal) normally is maintained within a range of 36.0° to 37.5°C.[1–5] Within this range, there are individual differences. For example, core temperature of most females increases approximately 0.5° to 1.0°C during the postovulation time of their menstrual cycle.[4] There are also diurnal variations as internal core temperatures reach their

FIGURE 10.1 • Normal diurnal variations in body temperature.

highest point in late afternoon and evening and their lowest point in the early morning hours (Fig. 10.1).

Body temperature reflects the difference between heat production and loss. It normally varies with exercise and extremes of environmental temperature. Properly protected, the body can function in environmental conditions that range from –50°C (–58°F) to +50°C (+122°F). Individual body cells, however, cannot tolerate such a wide range of temperatures: at –1°C ice crystals form, and at +45°C, cell proteins coagulate and/or aggregate.

Most of the body's heat is produced by the deeper core tissues (*i.e.*, muscles and viscera), which are insulated from the environment and protected against heat loss by an outer shell of subcutaneous tissues and skin (Fig. 10.2). Because the shell lies between the core and the environment, all heat leaving the body core, with the exception of that lost through

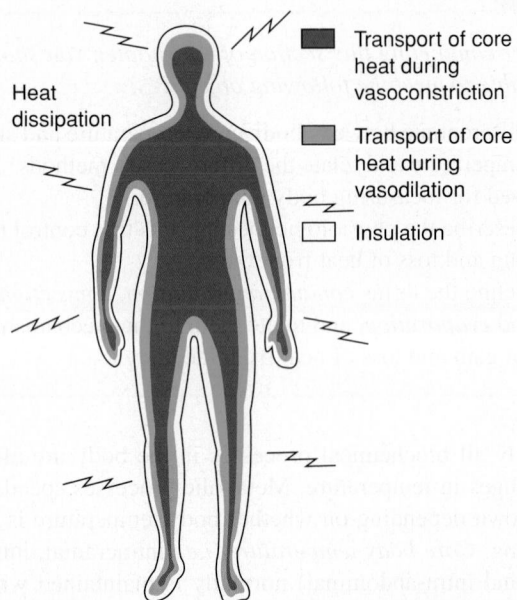

FIGURE 10.2 • Control of heat loss. Body heat is produced in the deeper core tissues of the body, which is insulated by the subcutaneous tissues and skin to protect against heat loss. During vasodilation, circulating blood transports heat to the skin surface, where it dissipates into the surrounding environment. Vasoconstriction decreases the transport of core heat to the skin surface, and vasodilation increases transport.

the respiratory tract, must pass through the outer shell.[2] The thickness of the shell depends on blood flow. In a warm environment, blood flow is increased to the periphery and the thickness of the outer shell is decreased, allowing for greater dissipation of heat. In a cold environment, the vessels supplying blood flow to the skin and underlying tissues, including those of the limbs and more superficial muscles of the neck and trunk, constrict. This increases the thickness of the shell and helps to minimize the loss of core heat for the body. The subcutaneous fat layer contributes to the insulation value of the outer shell because of its thickness and because it conducts heat only about one third as effectively as other tissues.

THERMOREGULATION

- Core body temperature is a reflection of the balance between heat gain and heat loss by the body. Metabolic processes produce heat, which must be dissipated.
- The hypothalamus is the thermal control centre for the body, receives information from peripheral and central thermoreceptors, and compares that information with its temperature set-point.
- Heat loss occurs through transfer of body core heat to the surface through the circulation. Heat is lost from the skin through radiation, conduction, convection, and evaporation.
- An increase in core temperature is effected by vasoconstriction and shivering, a decrease in temperature by vasodilation and sweating.

Thus, temperatures differ in various parts of the body, with core temperatures being higher than those at the skin surface. In general, the rectal or tympanic temperatures are used as a measure of core temperature. Core temperatures may also be obtained from the esophagus using a flexible thermometer, from a pulmonary artery catheter that is used for thermodilution measurement of cardiac output, or from a urinary catheter with a thermosensor that measures the temperature of urine in the bladder. Because of location, pulmonary artery and esophageal temperatures closely reflect the temperatures of the heart and thoracic organs.[3]

The oral temperature, taken sublingually, is usually 0.2° to 0.5°C lower than the rectal temperature; however, it usually follows changes in core temperature closely. The axillary temperature also can be used as an estimate of core temperature. However, the parts of the axillary fossa must be pressed closely together for an extended period (5 to 10 minutes for a glass thermometer) because this method requires considerable heat to accumulate before the final temperature is reached.

Ear-based thermometry uses an infrared sensor to measure the flow of heat from the tympanic membrane and ear canal.[5] It is popular because of its ease and speed of measurement, acceptability to parents and children, and cost savings in the personnel time that is required to take the temperature.

However, the debate continues regarding the accuracy of this method.[5] Pacifier thermometers and skin temperature strips have also raised concerns about accuracy, and are best used to monitor trends as opposed to absolute measurements.[5]

Core body and skin temperatures are sensed and integrated by thermoregulatory regions in the hypothalamus (particularly, the preoptic-anterior hypothalamic area) and other brain structures (*i.e.*, thalamus and cerebral cortex). Temperature-sensitive ion channels, identified as a subset of the transient receptor potential family (thermoTRPs), present in peripheral and central sensory neurons are activated by innocuous (warm and cool) and noxious (hot and cold) stimuli. Peripheral signals regarding temperature are initiated by changes in local membrane potentials that are transmitted to the brain through dorsal root ganglia.[6] The *set-point* of the hypothalamic thermoregulatory centre is set so that the temperature of the body core is regulated within the normal range of 36.0° to 37.5°C. When body temperature begins to rise above the set-point, the hypothalamus signals the central and peripheral nervous systems to initiate heat-dissipating behaviours. Likewise, when the temperature falls below the set-point, signals from the hypothalamus elicit physiologic behaviours that increase heat conservation and production. Core temperatures above 41°C or below 34°C usually mean that the body's ability to thermoregulate has been impaired (Fig. 10.3). For example, neurologic injuries may impair thermoregulation, resulting in fever. Body responses that produce, conserve, and dissipate heat are described in Table 10.1. Spinal cord injuries that transect the cord at T6 or above can seriously impair temperature regulation because the thermoregulatory centres in the hypothalamus can no longer control skin blood flow and sweating.

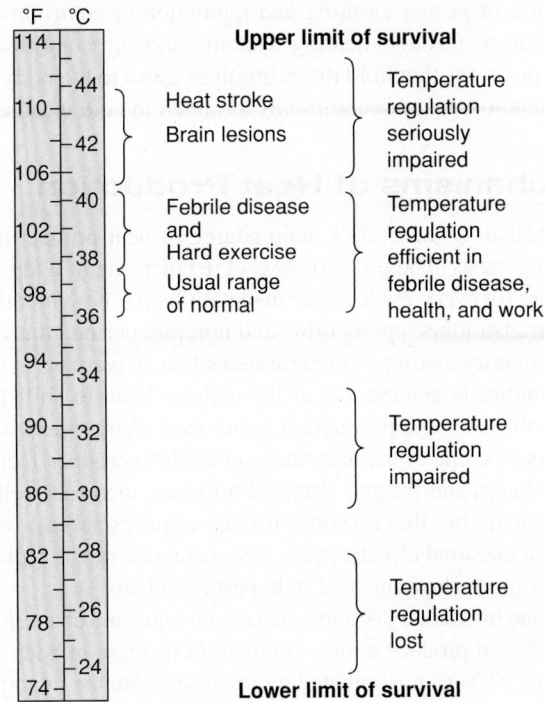

FIGURE 10.3 • Body temperatures under different conditions. (Adapted from Dubois E. F. [1948]. *Fever and the regulation of body temperature.* Springfield, IL: Charles C Thomas.)

In addition to reflexive and automatic thermoregulatory mechanisms, humans engage in voluntary behaviours to help regulate body temperature based on their conscious sensation of being too hot or too cold. These behaviours include the

TABLE 10.1 HEAT GAIN AND HEAT LOSS RESPONSES USED IN REGULATION OF BODY TEMPERATURE

HEAT GAIN		HEAT LOSS	
BODY RESPONSE	**MECHANISM OF ACTION**	**BODY RESPONSE**	**MECHANISM OF ACTION**
Vasoconstriction of the superficial blood vessels	Confines blood flow to the inner core of the body, with the skin and subcutaneous tissues acting as insulation to prevent loss of core heat	Dilation of the superficial blood vessels	Delivers blood containing core heat to the periphery where it is dissipated through radiation, conduction, and convection
Contraction of the pilomotor muscles that surround the hairs on the skin	Reduces the heat loss surface of the skin	Sweating	Increases heat loss through evaporation
Assumption of the huddle position with the extremities held close to the body	Reduces the area for heat loss		
Shivering	Increases heat production by the muscles		
Increased production of epinephrine	Increases the heat production associated with metabolism		
Increased production of thyroid hormone	Is a long-term mechanism that increases metabolism and heat production		

selection of proper clothing and regulation of environmental temperature through heating systems and air conditioning. Body positions that hold the extremities close to the body prevent heat loss and are commonly assumed in cold weather.

Mechanisms of Heat Production

Metabolism is the body's main source of heat production or thermogenesis. There is a 0.56°C (1°F) increase in body temperature for every 7% increase in metabolism. The sympathetic neurotransmitters, epinephrine and norepinephrine, plus other inflammatory mediators are released when an increase in body temperature is needed, act at the cellular level to shift body metabolism to heat production rather than energy generation. This may be one of the reasons fever tends to produce feelings of weakness and fatigue. Thyroid hormone increases cellular metabolism, but this response usually requires several weeks to reach maximal effectiveness. The metabolic rate is typically 45% or more above normal in hyperthyroidism.[2]

Fine involuntary actions such as shivering and chattering of the teeth can produce a three- to fivefold increase in body temperature. *Shivering* is initiated by impulses from the hypothalamus. The first muscle change that occurs with shivering is a general increase in muscle tone, followed by an oscillating rhythmic tremor involving the spinal-level reflex that controls muscle tone. The energy liberated by the metabolic processes from shivering is in the form of heat.[7] Physical exertion increases body temperature. Muscles convert most of the energy in the fuels they consume into heat rather than mechanical work. With strenuous exercise, more than three fourths of the increased metabolism resulting from muscle activity appears as heat within the body, and the remainder appears as mechanical work.

Mechanisms of Heat Loss

Most of the body's heat losses occur at the skin surface as heat from the blood moves to the skin and from there into the surrounding environment. There are numerous arteriovenous (AV) shunts or anastomoses under the skin surface that allow blood to move directly from the arterial to the venous system (Fig. 10.4).[1] These AV shunts are much like the radiators in a heating system. When the shunts are open, body heat is freely dissipated to the skin and surrounding environment; when the shunts are closed, heat is retained in the body. The blood flow in the AV shunts is controlled almost exclusively by the sympathetic nervous system in response to changes in core temperature and environmental temperature. Contraction of the *pilomotor muscles* of the skin, which raises skin hairs and produces goose bumps, also aids in heat conservation by reducing the surface area available for heat loss.

Heat is lost from the body through radiation, conduction, and convection from the skin surface; through the evaporation of sweat and insensible perspiration; through the exhalation of air that has been warmed and humidified; and through heat lost in urine and feces. Of these mechanisms, only heat losses that occur at the skin surface are directly under hypothalamic control.

FIGURE 10.4 • Skin circulation with arteriovenous shunts and venous plexuses that participate in transfer of core heat to the skin. (Adapted from Hall J. E. [2011]. *Textbook of medical physiology* [12th ed., p. 868]. Philadelphia, PA: W. B. Saunders.)

Radiation

Radiation is the transfer of heat through air or a vacuum. Heat from the sun is carried by radiation. Heat loss by radiation varies with the temperature of the environment. Environmental temperature must be less than that of the body for heat loss to occur. In a nude person sitting inside a normal-temperature room, approximately 60% of body heat typically is dissipated by radiation.[1]

Conduction

Conduction is the direct transfer of heat from one molecule to another. Blood carries, or conducts, heat from the inner core of the body to the skin surface. Normally only a small amount of body heat is lost through conduction to a cooler surface. Cooling blankets or mattresses that are used for reducing fever rely on conduction of heat from the skin to the cool surface of the mattress. Heat also can be conducted in the opposite direction—from the external environment to the body surface. For instance, body temperature may rise slightly after a hot bath.

Water has a specific heat several times greater than air, so water absorbs far greater amounts of heat than air does. The loss of body heat can be excessive and life-threatening in situations of cold water immersion or cold exposure in damp or wet clothing.

The conduction of heat to the body's surface is influenced by blood volume. In hot weather, the body compensates by increasing blood volume as a means of dissipating heat. A mild swelling of the ankles during hot weather (called *heat edema*) provides evidence of blood volume expansion. Exposure to cold produces a cold diuresis and a reduction in blood volume as a means of controlling the transfer of heat to the body's surface.

Convection

Convection refers to heat transfer through the circulation of air currents. Normally, a layer of warm air tends to remain near the body's surface; convection causes continual removal of the warm layer and replacement with air from the surrounding environment. The wind-chill factor that often is included in the weather report combines the effect of convection due to wind with the still-air temperature.

Evaporation

Evaporation involves the use of body heat to convert water on the skin to water vapour. Water that diffuses through the skin independent of sweating is called *insensible perspiration.* Insensible perspiration losses are greatest in a dry environment. Sweating occurs through the sweat glands and is controlled by the sympathetic nervous system. Unlike other sympathetically mediated functions, in which the catecholamines serve as neuromediators, sweating is mediated by acetylcholine. This means that anticholinergic drugs, such as atropine, can interfere with heat loss by interrupting sweating.

Evaporative heat losses involve insensible perspiration and sweating, with 0.58 calorie being lost for each gram of water that is evaporated.[1] As long as body temperature is greater than the atmospheric temperature, heat is lost through radiation. However, when the temperature of the surrounding environment becomes greater than skin temperature, evaporation is the only way the body can rid itself of heat. Any condition that prevents evaporative heat losses causes the body temperature to rise.

> **IN SUMMARY**
>
> Core body temperature is normally maintained within a range of 36.0° to 37.5°C. Core body and skin temperature are sensed and integrated by thermoregulatory regions in the hypothalamus and other brain structures that function to modify heat production and heat loss as a means of regulating body temperature. Most of the body's heat is produced by metabolic processes that occur within deeper core structures (*i.e.,* muscles and viscera) of the body. The sympathetic neurotransmitters (epinephrine and norepinephrine) and thyroid hormone act at the cellular level to shift body metabolism to heat production, whereas shivering and chattering of the teeth use the heat liberated from involuntary muscle movements to increase body temperature. Most of the body's heat losses occur at the skin surface as heat from the blood moves through the skin and from there into the surrounding environment. Heat is lost from the skin through radiation, conduction, convection, and evaporation of perspiration and sweat. Contraction of the pilomotor muscles of the skin aids in heat conservation by reducing the surface area available for heat loss.

INCREASED BODY TEMPERATURE

After completing this section of the chapter, you should be able to meet the following objectives:

- Characterize the physiology, patterns, and stages of fever.
- Differentiate between the physiologic mechanisms involved in fever and hyperthermia.

- State the definition of fever of unknown source in children 0 to 36 months of age.
- State the definition for fever in the elderly and cite possible mechanisms for altered febrile response in the elderly.
- Compare the characteristics of fevers caused by infectious agents and drug-related fevers.
- Compare the mechanisms of malignant hyperthermia and neuroleptic malignant syndrome.

Both fever and hyperthermia describe conditions in which body temperature is higher than the normal range. Fever is due to an upward displacement of the thermostatic set-point of the thermoregulatory centre in the hypothalamus, such as that which occurs with infection. This is in contrast to hyperthermia, in which the set-point is unchanged, but the mechanisms that control body temperature are ineffective in maintaining body temperature within a normal range during situations when heat production outpaces the ability of the body to dissipate that heat.

Fever

Fever, also referred to as *pyrexia,* describes an elevation in body temperature that is caused by an upward displacement of the thermostatic set-point of the hypothalamic thermoregulatory centre. Temperature is one of the most frequent physiologic responses to be monitored during illness.

Mechanisms

Many proteins, breakdown products of proteins, and certain other substances released from bacterial cell membranes can cause a change in the set-point to rise. Fever is resolved or "broken" when the condition that caused the increase in the set-point is removed. Fevers that are regulated by the

> **FEVER**
>
> - Fever represents an increase in body temperature that results from a cytokine-induced increase in the set-point of the thermostatic centre in the hypothalamus.
> - Fever is a nonspecific response that is mediated by endogenous pyrogens released from host cells in response to infectious or noninfectious disorders.
> - The development of fever involves a prodrome, a chill during which the temperature rises until it reaches the new hypothalamic set-point, a flush during which the skin vessels dilate and the temperature begins to fall, and a period of defervescence that is marked by sweating.
> - Fever is resolved when the condition causing the increase in the set-point of the thermostatic centre in the hypothalamus is resolved.

hypothalamus usually do not rise above 41°C, suggesting a built-in thermostatic safety mechanism. Temperatures above that level are usually the result of superimposed activity, such as convulsions, hyperthermic states, or direct impairment of the temperature control centre.

Pyrogens are exogenous or endogenous substances that produce fever. *Exogenous pyrogens* are derived from outside the body and include such substances as bacterial products, bacterial toxins, or whole microorganisms. Exogenous pyrogens induce host cells to produce fever-producing mediators called *endogenous pyrogens*. When bacteria or breakdown products of bacteria are present in blood or tissues, they are engulfed by phagocytic cells of the immune system (see Chapter 17). These phagocytic cells digest the bacterial products and then release pyrogenic cytokines, principally interleukin-1β (IL-1β), interleukin-6 (IL-6), interferon-γ (IFN-γ), and tumour necrosis factor-α (TNF-α), into the bloodstream for transport to the hypothalamus, where they exert their action.[8] Prostaglandin E_2 (PGE_2), which is a metabolite of arachidonic acid (an intramembrane fatty acid), is considered to be the final fever mediator in the hypothalamus, induced by these cytokines. PGE_2 binds to receptors in the hypothalamus to induce changes in its set-point through the second messenger cyclic adenosine monophosphate (cAMP).[1,8] In response to the increase in its thermostatic set-point, the hypothalamus initiates shivering and vasoconstriction that raise the body's core temperature to the new set-point, and fever is established.

Although the central role of PGE_2 in raising the set-point of the hypothalamic thermoregulatory centre and producing fever is not questioned, research suggests that the febrile response to invading gram-negative bacteria and their products (mainly endotoxic lipopolysaccharides) is mediated by peripherally rather than centrally produced PGE_2.

In addition to their fever-producing actions, the endogenous pyrogens mediate a number of other responses. For example, IL-1 and TNF-α are inflammatory mediators that produce other signs of inflammation such as leukocytosis, anorexia, and malaise (see Chapter 18). Many noninfectious disorders, such as myocardial infarction, pulmonary emboli, and neoplasms, produce fever. In these conditions, the injured or abnormal cells incite the production of endogenous pyrogens. For example, trauma and surgery can be associated with up to 3 days of fever. Some malignant cells, such as those of leukemia and Hodgkin disease, secrete chemical mediators that function as endogenous pyrogens.

A fever that has its origin in the central nervous system is sometimes referred to as a *neurogenic fever*. It usually is caused by damage to the hypothalamus due to central nervous system trauma, intracerebral bleeding, or an increase in intracranial pressure. Neurogenic fevers are characterized by a high temperature that is resistant to antipyretic therapy and is not associated with sweating.

Purpose

The purpose of fever is not completely understood. However, from a purely practical standpoint, fever is a valuable index to health status. For many, fever signals the presence of an infection and may legitimize the need for medical treatment. There is little research to support the belief that fever is harmful unless the temperature rises above 40°C. The main exception is the occurrence of fever in neurological injuries as the increase in temperature increases oxygen demand and cerebral blood flow. There is evidence that fever enhances the immune system. Animal studies have demonstrated a clear survival advantage in infected members with fever compared with animals that were unable to produce a fever. It has been shown that small elevations in temperature such as those that occur with fever enhance immune function. There is increased motility and activity of the white blood cells, stimulation of interferon production, production of cellular protective heat shock proteins, and activation of T cells.[8–11] Many of the microbial agents that cause infection grow best at normal body temperatures, and their growth is inhibited by temperatures in the fever range. For example, the rhinoviruses responsible for the common cold are cultured best at 33°C, which is close to the temperature in the nasopharynx; temperature-sensitive mutants of the virus that cannot grow at temperatures above 37.5°C produce fewer signs and symptoms.[10]

Patterns

The patterns of temperature change in persons with fever vary and may provide information about the nature of the causative agent.[11] These patterns can be described as intermittent, remittent, sustained, or relapsing (Fig. 10.5). An *intermittent fever* is one in which temperature returns to normal at least once every 24 hours. In a *remittent fever,* the temperature does not return to normal and varies a few degrees in either direction. In a *sustained* or *continuous fever,* the temperature remains above normal with minimal variations (usually less than 1°C). A *recurrent* or *relapsing fever* is one in which one or more episodes of fever occur, each as long as several days, with one or more days of normal temperature between episodes.[11]

Critical to the analysis of a fever pattern is the relation of heart rate to the level of temperature elevation. Normally, a 1°C rise in temperature produces a 10 beats/minute increase in heart rate.[12] Most persons respond to an increase in temperature with an appropriate increase in heart rate. The observation that a rise in temperature is not accompanied by the anticipated change in heart rate can provide useful information about the cause of the fever. For example, a heart rate that is slower than would be anticipated can occur with Legionnaire disease and drug fever, and a heart rate that is more rapid than anticipated can be symptomatic of hyperthyroidism and pulmonary emboli.

Manifestations

The physiologic behaviours that occur during the development of fever can be divided into four successive stages: a prodrome; a chill, during which the temperature rises; a flush; and defervescence (Fig. 10.6). During the *first* or *prodromal* period, there are nonspecific complaints such as mild headache and fatigue, general malaise, and fleeting aches and pains.

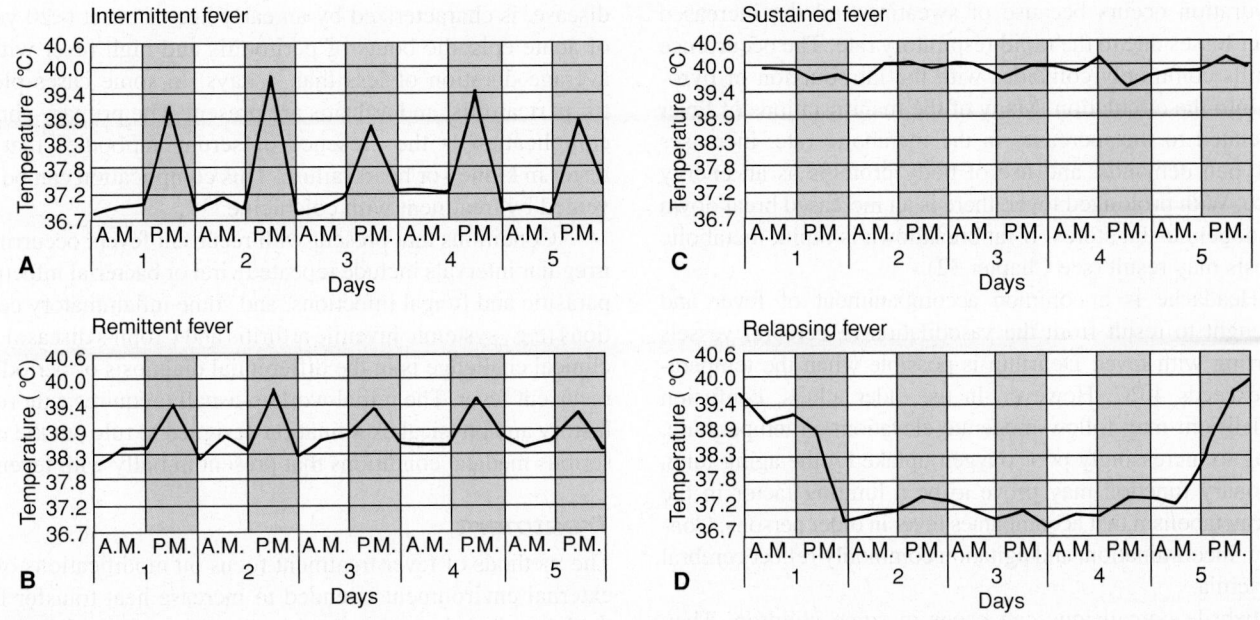

FIGURE 10.5 • Schematic representation of fever patterns: (**A**) intermittent, (**B**) remittent, (**C**) sustained, and (**D**) recurrent or relapsing.

During the *second stage* or *chill,* there is the uncomfortable sensation of being chilled and the onset of generalized shaking (rigours), although the temperature is rising. Vasoconstriction and piloerection usually precede the onset of shivering. At this point, the skin is pale and covered with goose flesh. There is a feeling of being cold and an urge to put on more clothing or covering and to curl up in a position that conserves body heat. When the shivering has caused the body temperature to reach the new set-point of the temperature control centre, the shivering ceases, and a sensation of warmth develops. At this point, the *third stage* or *flush* begins, during which cutaneous

vasodilation occurs and the skin becomes warm and flushed. The *fourth,* or *defervescence,* stage of the febrile response is marked by the initiation of sweating. Not all persons proceed through the four stages of fever development. Sweating may be absent, and fever may develop gradually with no indication of a chill or shivering.

Common manifestations that occur with fever are anorexia, myalgia, arthralgia, and fatigue, as they are initiated by similar inflammatory mediators. These manifestations are worse when the temperature rises rapidly or exceeds 39.5°C. Respiration is increased, and the heart rate usually is elevated.

FIGURE 10.6 • Mechanisms of fever. (1) Release of prostaglandin E₂ (PGE₂) or fever-producing cytokines from inflammatory cells; (2) resetting of the thermostatic set-point in the hypothalamus to a higher level (prodrome); (3) generation of hypothalamus-mediated responses that raise body temperature (chill); (4) development of fever with elevation of body to new thermostatic set-point; and (5) production of temperature-lowering responses (flush and defervescence) and return of body temperature to a lower level.

Hypothalamus:
Thermostatic
set point

4. Core body temperature
reaches new set point

2. Resetting
thermostatic
set point

1. Release of PGE₂
or fever-producing
cytokines from
inflammatory cells

3. Temperature-raising
responses:
Vasoconstriction
Shivering
Piloerection
Increased metabolism

5. Temperature-reducing
responses:
Vasodilation
Sweating
Increased ventilation

Fever

Dehydration occurs because of sweating and the increased vapour losses due to the rapid respiratory rate. The occurrence of chills commonly coincides with the introduction of pyrogens into the circulation. Many of the manifestations of fever are related to the increases in the metabolic rate, increases in oxygen demands, and use of body proteins as an energy source. With prolonged fever, there is an increased breakdown of endogenous fat stores. If fat breakdown is rapid, metabolic acidosis may result (see Chapter 32).

Headache is a common accompaniment of fever and is thought to result from the vasodilation of cerebral vessels occurring with fever. Delirium is possible when the temperature exceeds 40°C. However, in the older adults, confusion and delirium may follow moderate elevations in temperature. Owing to increasingly poor oxygen uptake by the aging lung, pulmonary function may prove to be a limiting factor in the hypermetabolism that accompanies fever in older persons. Confusion, incoordination, and agitation commonly reflect cerebral hypoxemia.

Febrile convulsions can occur in some children. They usually occur with rapidly rising temperatures or at a threshold temperature that differs with each child.[11,13]

The herpetic lesions, or fever blisters, that develop in some persons during fever are caused by a separate infection by the type 1 herpes simplex virus that has established latency in the regional ganglia and is reactivated by a rise in body temperature.

Differential Diagnosis

Most febrile illnesses are due to common infections and are relatively easy to diagnose. In certain instances, however, it is difficult to establish the cause of a fever. A prolonged fever for which the cause is difficult to ascertain is often referred to as *fever of unknown origin* (FUO). FUO is defined as a temperature elevation of 38.3°C or higher that is present for 3 weeks or longer and includes 1 week of comprehensive diagnostic testing that does not identify a diagnosis.[14] Among the causes of FUO are malignancies (*i.e.,* lymphomas, metastases to the liver and central nervous system); infections such as human immunodeficiency virus or tuberculosis, or abscessed infections; cirrhosis of the liver; and medications. Malignancies, particularly non-Hodgkin lymphoma, are important causes of FUO in the elderly.

Recurrent or periodic fevers may occur in predictable intervals or without any discernible time pattern. They may be associated with no discernible cause or they can be the presenting symptom of several serious illnesses, often preceding the other symptoms of those diseases by weeks or months. The PFAPA syndrome, which is characterized by *periodic fever, aphthous* (small ulcerative) stomatitis, *pharyngitis,* and cervical *adenopathy* reoccurring in 4- to 8-week periods, is the most common cause of recurrent fevers in children younger than 5 years of age.[15] Other conditions in which recurrent fevers occur but do not follow a strictly periodic pattern include genetic disorders such as familial Mediterranean fever.[15] Familial Mediterranean fever, an autosomal recessive

disease, is characterized by an early age of onset (<20 years) of acute episodic bouts of peritonitis and high fever with an average duration of less than 4 days. In some cases pleuritis, pericarditis, and arthritis are present. The primary chronic complication is the presence of serum antibodies that can result in kidney or heart failure. This complication can be prevented by treatment with colchicine.[15]

Conditions that present with recurrent fevers occurring at irregular intervals include repeated viral or bacterial infections, parasitic and fungal infections, and some inflammatory conditions (*e.g.,* systemic juvenile arthritis and Crohn's disease). The clinical challenge is in the differential diagnosis of periodic or recurrent fever. The initial workup usually requires a thorough history and physical examination designed to rule out the more serious medical conditions that present initially with fever.

Treatment

The methods of fever treatment focus on modifications of the external environment intended to increase heat transfer from the internal to the external environment, support of the hypermetabolic state that accompanies fever, protection of vulnerable body organs and systems, and treatment of the infection or condition causing the fever. Because fever is a disease symptom, its manifestation suggests the need for diagnosis and treatment of the primary cause.

Modification of the environment ensures that the environmental temperature facilitates heat transfer away from the body. Sponge baths with cool water can be used to increase evaporative heat losses. More profound cooling can be accomplished through the use of a cooling mattress, which facilitates the conduction of heat from the body into the coolant solution that circulates through the mattress. Care must be taken so that the cooling method does not produce vasoconstriction and shivering that decrease heat loss, increase heat production, and increase energy expenditure.

Adequate fluids and sufficient amounts of simple carbohydrates are needed to support the hypermetabolic state and prevent the tissue breakdown that is characteristic of fever. Additional fluids are needed for sweating and to balance the insensible water losses from the lungs that accompany an increase in respiratory rate. Fluids also are needed to maintain an adequate vascular volume for heat transport to the skin surface.

Antipyretic drugs, such as aspirin, ibuprofen, and acetaminophen, often are used to alleviate the discomforts of fever and protect vulnerable organs, such as the brain, from extreme elevations in body temperature. These drugs act by resetting the set-point of the temperature-regulating centre in the hypothalamus to a lower level, presumably by blocking the activity of cyclooxygenase, an enzyme that is required for the conversion of arachidonic acid to PGE_2.[16] Because of the risk of Reye syndrome, the Disease Prevention and Control of the Public Health Agency of Canada, Canada's Food and Drug Act, and the Canadian Paediatrics Society advise against the use of aspirin and other salicylates in children with viral illnesses such as influenza or chickenpox.

Fever in Children

Fever occurs frequently in infants and young children (*i.e.,* 1 day to 3 years of age) and is a common reason for visits to the clinic or emergency department.[16] Infants and young children have decreased immunologic function and are more commonly infected with virulent organisms. Also, the mechanisms for controlling temperature are not as well developed in infants as they are in older children and adults. Even though infants with fever may not appear ill, this does not imply an absence of bacterial disease. In infants younger than 3 months, a mild elevation in temperature (*i.e.,* rectal temperature of 38°C) can indicate serious infection that requires immediate medical attention.[17]

Although the differential diagnosis of fever is quite broad and includes both infectious and noninfectious causes, the majority of febrile children have an underlying infection. The most common causes are minor or more serious infections of the respiratory system, gastrointestinal tract, urinary tract, or central nervous system. The epidemiology of serious bacterial disease has changed dramatically with the introduction of the *Haemophilus influenzae* and *Streptococcus pneumoniae* vaccines in developed countries.[17] *H. influenzae* type b has substantially decreased, and the incidence of pneumococcal disease caused by vaccine and cross-reactive vaccine serotypes has declined substantially.

Although most children have identifiable causes for their fevers, many have fever without an apparent source. The American College of Emergency Physicians has developed clinical guidelines for use in the treatment of previously healthy infants and children 1 day to 3 years of age with fever without a source.[18] Based on this, the Canadian Association of Emergency Physicians have adopted a mandatory triage scale.[19] The guidelines define fever in this age group as an elevation in rectal temperature of at least 38°C. The reliability of other methods of temperature measurements is lower and must be considered when making decisions about the seriousness of the fever. In addition, bundling of infants may raise the skin temperature but not the rectal temperature.

Fever in infants and children can be classified as low risk or high risk, depending on the probability of the infection progressing to bacteremia or meningitis and signs of toxicity. Infants between the ages of 1 and 28 days with a fever should be considered to have a bacterial infection that can cause bacteremia or meningitis. Signs of toxicity include lethargy, poor feeding, hypoventilation, poor tissue oxygenation, and cyanosis. The response to antipyretic medications does not change the likelihood of the child having a serious bacterial infection and should not be used as an indicator of infection severity.[18] A white blood cell count and blood cultures usually are done in high-risk infants and children to determine the cause of fever. A lumbar puncture is usually performed on febrile neonates to rule out meningitis.[17]

A chest radiograph should be obtained in febrile infants younger than 3 months of age with at least one sign of a respiratory illness (*e.g.,* tachypnea, crackles, decreased breath sounds, wheezing, coughing).[17,18] Febrile children who are younger than 1 year of age and girls between 1 and 2 years of age should be considered at risk for a urinary tract infection (see Chapter 33).

Because of the significant sequelae associated with undiagnosed and untreated urinary tract infections, urine cultures are recommended for children aged younger than 2 years.[17,18]

The approach to treatment of the young child who has a fever without a known source varies depending on the age of the child. Antipyretics are used due to the risk of increased temperatures over 40°C. Because of the high rates of serious bacterial infections, febrile infants usually receive antibiotics.[17] High-risk infants and infants who are younger than 28 days are often hospitalized for evaluation of their fever and treatment.[17] Of children aged 3 to 36 months with fever without source, 1.5% to 2% will have occult bacteremia and only a small percentage will go on to develop serious sequelae. Antibiotic therapy should be considered if the fever of 39.0°C or greater is accompanied by a white blood cell count of 15.0×10^9/L or higher.[18]

Fever in Older Adults

In older adults, even slight elevations in temperature may indicate serious infection or disease. This is because the elderly often have a lower baseline temperature, and although their temperature increases during an infection, it may fail to reach a level that is equated with significant fever due to a lower immune response.[20] In addition, normal body temperature and the circadian pattern of temperature variation often are altered in the older adults. It has been suggested that 20% to 30% of elders with serious infections present with an absent or blunted febrile response.[21] It has been recommended that an older adult should be considered febrile when presenting with an elevated temperature of 1°C above their baseline values.[21]

When fever is present in the elderly, it usually indicates the presence of serious infection, most often caused by bacteria. The absence of fever may delay diagnosis and initiation of antimicrobial treatment. Unexplained changes in functional capacity, worsening of mental status, weakness and fatigue, and weight loss are additional indicators of infection in the elderly. They should be viewed as possible signs of infection and sepsis when fever is absent. A thorough history and physical examination are critically important. The probable mechanisms for the blunted fever response include a disturbance in sensing of temperature by the thermoregulatory centre in the hypothalamus, alterations in release of endogenous pyrogens, and the failure to elicit compensatory responses (*e.g.,* vasoconstriction of skin vessels, increased heat production, shivering to increase body temperature).

Another factor that may delay recognition of fever in the elderly is the method of temperature measurement. It has been suggested that rectal and tympanic membrane methods are more effective in detecting fever in older adults. This is because conditions such as mouth breathing, tongue tremors, and agitation often make it difficult to obtain accurate oral temperatures in older adults.

Hyperthermia

Hyperthermia describes an increase in body temperature that occurs without a change in the set-point of the hypothalamic thermoregulatory centre. It occurs when the thermoregulatory mechanisms are overwhelmed by heat production, excessive environmental heat, or impaired dissipation of heat.[20] It includes (in order of increasing severity) heat cramps, heat exhaustion, and heat stroke. Malignant hyperthermia describes a rare genetic disorder of anesthetic-related hyperthermia. Hyperthermia also may occur as the result of a drug reaction.

A number of factors predispose to hyperthermia. If muscle exertion is continued for long periods in warm weather, as often happens with athletes, military recruits, and labourers, excessive heat loads are generated. Because adequate circulatory function is essential for heat dissipation, elderly persons and those with cardiovascular disease are at increased risk for hyperthermia. Drugs that increase muscle tone and metabolism or reduce heat loss (*e.g.*, diuretics, neuroleptics, drugs with anticholinergic action) can impair thermoregulation. Infants and small children who are left in a closed car for even short periods in hot weather are potential victims of hyperthermia.

HYPERTHERMIA

- Hyperthermia is a pathologic increase in core body temperature without a change in the hypothalamic set-point. The thermoregulatory centre is overwhelmed by either excess heat production, impaired heat loss, or excessive environmental heat.
- Malignant hyperthermia is an autosomal dominant disorder in which an abnormal release of intracellular stores of calcium causes uncontrolled skeletal muscle contractions, resulting in a rapid increase in core body temperature. This usually is in response to an anesthetic.

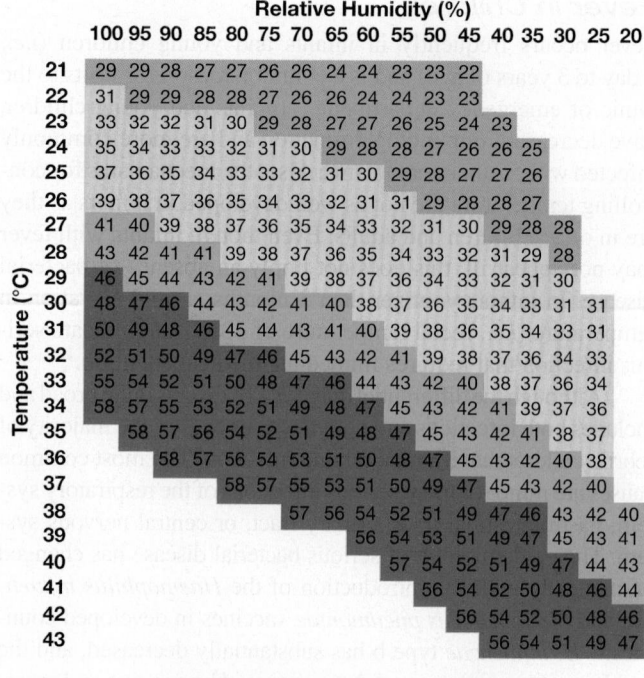

Humidex	Degree of Comfort
20–29	No discomfort
30–39	Some discomfort
40–45	Great discomfort; avoid exertion
46 and over	Dangerous; probable heat stroke

FIGURE 10.7 • Humidex: a combination of the measured temperature and relative humidity. (Source: Humidex table. Available: https://ec.gc.ca/meteo-weather/default.asp?lang=En&n=6C5D4990-1. © Environment Canada, 2015. Reproduced with permission.)

The best approach to heat-related disorders is prevention, primarily by avoiding activity in hot environments, increasing fluid intake, and wearing climate- and activity-appropriate clothing. The ability to tolerate a hot environment depends on both temperature and humidity. A high relative humidity retards heat loss through sweating and evaporation and decreases the body's cooling ability. The *humidex* is a measurement that combines the temperature and humidity to reflect the body's perceived temperature. Environment Canada identifies that with a humidex reading of less than 29 there is no discomfort but a reading greater than 46 is considered dangerous and if greater than 54 then heat stroke is imminent (Fig. 10.7).

Heat Cramps

Heat cramps are slow, painful, skeletal muscle cramps, and spasms, usually occurring in the muscles that are most heavily used and lasting for 1 to 3 minutes. Cramping results from salt depletion that occurs when fluid losses from heavy sweating are replaced by water alone.[22] The muscles are tender, and the skin usually is moist. Body temperature may be normal or slightly elevated. There almost always is a history of vigorous activity preceding the onset of symptoms.

Treatment consists of drinking an oral saline solution (commercially prepared electrolyte solutions or 1 tsp of salt in 500 ml of water), stretching the affected muscles, and resting in a cool environment.[23] Because absorption is slow and unpredictable, salt tablets are not recommended. Salt tablets also can cause gastric irritation, vomiting, and cerebral edema. Strenuous physical activity should be avoided for several days, while dietary sodium replacement is continued.

Heat Exhaustion

Heat exhaustion is related to a gradual loss of salt and water, usually after prolonged and heavy exertion in a hot environment. The symptoms include thirst, fatigue, nausea, oliguria, giddiness, and confusion. Gastrointestinal flulike symptoms are common. Hyperventilation in association with heat exhaustion may contribute to heat cramps and tetany by causing respiratory alkalosis (see Chapter 32). The skin is moist, the rectal temperature usually is higher than 37.8°C but below 40°C, and the heart rate is elevated, usually by more than half again the normal resting rate. Signs of heat cramps may accompany heat exhaustion.

Like heat cramps, heat exhaustion is treated by rest in a cool environment, the provision of adequate hydration, and salt replacement. Intravenous fluids are administered when adequate oral intake cannot be achieved. If the individual has water-depleted heat exhaustion and is hypernatremic, rehydration needs to occur at a regulated rate to reduce the development of iatrogenic cerebral edema (see Chapter 31).[23]

Heat Stroke

Heat stroke is a severe, life-threatening failure of thermoregulatory mechanisms resulting in an excessive rise in body temperature—a core temperature greater than 40°C, a hot, dry skin, absence of sweating, and characterized by central nervous system abnormalities such as delirium, convulsions, and loss of consciousness.[22–24] The risk of developing heat stroke in response to heat stress is increased in conditions (*i.e.*, alcoholism, obesity, diabetes mellitus, and chronic cardiac, renal, or mental disease) and with drugs (*i.e.*, alcohol, anticholinergics, beta blockers, or tricyclic antidepressants) that impair vasodilation and sweating.[22,23]

The pathophysiology of heat stroke is thought to result from the direct effect of heat on body cells and the release of cytokines (*e.g.*, interleukins, TNF-α, and interferon) from heat-stressed endothelial cells, leukocytes, and epithelial cells that protect against tissue injury. The net result is a combination of local and systemic inflammatory responses that may result in acute respiratory distress syndrome, acute renal failure, disseminated intravascular coagulation, multiorgan dysfunction, and rhabdomyolysis.[24]

Heat stroke may be designated as *classic* or *nonexertional* when it arises as a consequence of exposure to high environmental temperatures or as *exertional* when it arises as a consequence of strenuous exercise.[22–24] The classic or nonexertional form of heat stroke is seen most commonly at the extremes of age.[24] Infants and small children (younger than 5 years of age) lack sufficient body surface area to dissipate excess heat, have a lower rate of sweating, and a slower rate of acclimatization. In the elderly, the problem often is one of impaired heat loss and failure of homeostatic mechanisms, such that body temperature rises with any increase in environmental temperature. Older adults with a decreased ability to perceive changes in environmental temperature or decreased mobility are at particular risk because they also may be unable to take appropriate measures such as removing clothing, moving to a cooler environment, and increasing fluid intake. This is particularly true of older adults who live alone in small and poorly ventilated housing units and who may be too confused or weak to complain or seek help at the onset of symptoms.

Exertional heat stroke occurs most often in summer and mainly affects athletes and labourers who are exposed to high-temperature environments. Persons with exertional heat stroke often continue to perspire, a factor that often results in a delay in diagnosis. In addition, rhabdomyolysis and its complications (hyperkalemia, hyperphosphatemia, hypocalcemia, and myoglobinuria) contribute to the morbidity and mortality associated with the disorder.[23,24]

The symptoms of heat stroke include tachycardia, hyperventilation, dizziness, weakness, headache, emotional lability, nausea and vomiting, confusion, delirium, blurred vision, convulsions, collapse, and coma. The skin is hot and usually dry, and the pulse is typically strong initially. The blood pressure may be elevated at first, but hypotension develops as the condition progresses. As vascular collapse occurs, the skin becomes cool. Associated abnormalities include electrocardiographic changes consistent with cardiac injury, blood coagulation disorders, potassium and sodium depletion, and signs of liver damage.[24]

Treatment consists of measures to support the function of vital organs while instituting cooling procedures aimed at producing a rapid reduction in core temperature. Care must be taken that the cooling methods used do not produce vasoconstriction or shivering and thereby decrease the cooling rate or induce heat production. Cooling methods (*e.g.*, cold water, fans, ice packs) are important to reduce the temperature of vital structures such as the brain, heart and liver, because tissue damage ensues when core temperatures rise above 43°C.[24]

Drug Fever

Drug fever has been defined as fever coinciding with the administration of a drug and disappearing after the drug has been discontinued.[25] Drugs can induce fever by several mechanisms. They can interfere with heat dissipation; they can alter temperature regulation by the hypothalamic centres; they can act as direct pyrogens; they can injure tissues directly; or they can induce an immune response.

Exogenous thyroid hormone increases the metabolic rate and can increase heat production and body temperature. Peripheral heat dissipation can be impaired by atropine and anticholinergic drugs, antihistamines, phenothiazine antipsychotic drugs, and tricyclic antidepressants, which decrease sweating; or by amphetamines (especially ecstasy), cocaine, and sympathomimetic drugs, which produce peripheral vasoconstriction.[25] Bleomycin (an anticancer drug), amphotericin B (an antifungal drug), and vaccines that contain bacterial and viral products all can act to induce the release of pyrogens. Intravenously administered drugs can lead to infusion-related phlebitis with production of cellular pyrogens that produce fever. Treatment with anticancer drugs can cause the release of endogenous pyrogen from the cancer cells that are destroyed. Overdoses of serotonin reuptake inhibitors or use in persons taking monoamine oxidase (MOA) inhibitors can cause agitation, hyperactivity, and hyperthermia (serotonin syndrome).[25]

The most common cause of drug fever is a *hypersensitivity reaction*. Hypersensitivity drug fevers develop after several weeks of exposure to the drug, cannot be explained in terms of the drug's pharmacologic action, are not related to drug dose, disappear when the drug is stopped, and reappear when the drug is readministered.[25] The fever pattern is typically spiking in nature and exhibits a normal diurnal rhythm. Persons with drug fevers often experience other signs of hypersensitivity reactions, such as arthralgias, urticaria, myalgias, gastrointestinal discomfort, and rashes.

Temperatures of 38.9° to 40.0°C are common in drug fever. The person may be unaware of the fever and appear to be well for the degree of fever that is present. The absence of an appropriate increase in heart rate for the degree of temperature elevation is an important clue to the diagnosis of drug fever.[25] A fever often precedes other, more serious effects of a drug reaction; for this reason, the early recognition of drug fever is important. Drug fever should be suspected whenever the temperature elevation is unexpected and occurs despite improvement in the condition for which the drug was prescribed.

Malignant Hyperthermia

Malignant hyperthermia is a rare, autosomal dominant metabolic disorder in which heat generated by uncontrolled skeletal muscle contraction can produce severe and potentially fatal hyperthermia.[26] Generally, the mutation involves the *RYR1* gene on chromosome 19q13.1. The muscle contraction is caused by an abnormal release of intracellular calcium from the sarcoplasmic reticulum through calcium release channels or ryanodine receptors (see Chapter 4). The release of calcium at an abnormally high rate also leads to a sustained hypermetabolic rate and a subsequent loss of cellular integrity. The sustained hypermetabolism results in excess lactate production, high adenosine triphosphate (ATP) consumption, increased oxygen consumption and carbon dioxide production, and elevated heat production.[26]

In affected persons, an episode of malignant hyperthermia is triggered by exposure to certain stresses or general anesthetic agents. The syndrome most frequently is associated with the halogenated anesthetic agents and the depolarizing muscle relaxant succinylcholine. There also are various nonoperative precipitating factors, including trauma, exercise, environmental heat stress, and infection. The condition is particularly dangerous in a young person who has a large muscle mass to generate heat.[26]

During malignant hyperthermia, the body temperature can rise to as high as 43°C at a rate of 1°C every 15 minutes. In addition to a steady rise in end-tidal carbon dioxide levels, an initial sign of the disorder, when the condition occurs during anesthesia, is skeletal muscle rigidity. Cardiac arrhythmias and a hypermetabolic state follow in rapid sequence unless the triggering event is immediately discontinued. In addition to discontinuing the triggering agents, treatment includes measures to cool the body, cardiopulmonary support, and the administration of dantrolene, a muscle relaxant drug that acts by blocking the release of calcium from the sarcoplasmic reticulum.

At present, there is no accurate screening test for the condition. A family history of malignant hyperthermia should be considered when general anesthesia is needed because there are anesthetic agents available that do not trigger the hyperthermic response. A halothane–caffeine contracture test performed on muscle tissue obtained during biopsy can confirm the diagnosis; however, this test is performed only at selected centres. Molecular genetic testing for malignant hyperthermia remains difficult.

Neuroleptic Malignant Syndrome

The neuroleptic malignant syndrome is associated with neuroleptic (psychotropic) medications and may occur in as much as 0.01% to 3.2% of persons taking such drugs.[27] Research shows that virtually all neuroleptics, even the newer atypical antipsychotics, plus other medications affecting central dopaminergic neurotransmission are associated with this syndrome. These drugs block dopamine receptors in the basal ganglia and hypothalamus. Hyperthermia is thought to result from alterations in the function of the hypothalamic thermoregulatory centre caused by decreased dopamine levels or from uncontrolled muscle contraction like that occurring with anesthetic-induced malignant hyperthermia. Because many of the neuroleptic drugs produce an increase in muscle contraction similar to that of malignant hyperthermia, it has been suggested that the disorder may be caused by a spectrum of inherited defects in genes that are responsible for a variety of calcium regulatory mechanisms in sympathetic neurons (*e.g.,* dopaminergic neurons).

The syndrome usually has an explosive onset and is characterized by hyperthermia, muscle rigidity, alterations in consciousness, and autonomic nervous system dysfunction. The hyperthermia is accompanied by tachycardia, cardiac arrhythmias, labile blood pressure, postural instability, dyspnea, and tachypnea.[27]

Treatment for neuroleptic malignant syndrome includes the immediate discontinuance of the neuroleptic drug, measures to decrease body temperature, aggressive hydration, and treatment of dysrhythmias and other complications of the disorder. Bromocriptine (a dopamine agonist) and dantrolene (a muscle relaxant) may be used as part of the treatment regimen.[27]

IN SUMMARY

Fever and hyperthermia refer to an increase in body temperature outside the normal range. True fever is a disorder of thermoregulation in which there is an upward displacement of the set-point for temperature control. In hyperthermia, the set-point is unchanged, but the challenge to temperature regulation exceeds the thermoregulatory centre's ability to control body temperature. Fever can be caused by a number of factors, including microorganisms, trauma, and drugs or chemicals, all of which incite the release of endogenous pyrogens. The reactions that occur during fever consist of four stages: a prodrome, a chill, a flush, and defervescence. A fever can follow an intermittent, remittent, sustained, or recurrent pattern. The manifestations of fever are largely related to dehydration and an increased metabolic rate. Even a low-grade fever in high-risk infants or in the elderly can indicate serious infection.

The treatment of fever focuses on modifying the external environment as a means of increasing heat transfer to the external environment; supporting the hypermetabolic state that accompanies fever; protecting vulnerable body tissues; and treating the infection or condition causing the fever.

Hyperthermia, which varies in severity based on the degree of core temperature elevation and the severity of cardiovascular and nervous system involvement, includes heat cramps, heat exhaustion, and heat stroke. Among the factors that contribute to the development of hyperthermia are prolonged muscular exertion in a hot environment, disorders that compromise heat dissipation, and hypersensitivity drug reactions. Malignant hyperthermia is an autosomal dominant disorder that can produce a severe and potentially fatal increase in body temperature. The condition commonly is triggered by general anesthetic agents and muscle relaxants used during surgery. The neuroleptic malignant syndrome is associated with neuroleptic drug therapy and is thought to result from alterations in the function of the thermoregulatory centre or from uncontrolled muscle contraction.

DECREASED BODY TEMPERATURE

After completing this section of the chapter, you should be able to meet the following objectives:

- Define hypothermia.
- Compare the manifestations of mild, moderate, and severe hypothermia and relate them to changes in physiologic functioning that occur with decreased body temperature.
- Describe the causes of heat loss and hypothermia in the newborn infant and patient undergoing surgery.

HYPOTHERMIA

- Hypothermia is a pathologic decrease in core body temperature without a change in the hypothalamic set-point.
- The compensatory physiologic responses meant to produce heat (shivering) and retain heat (vasoconstriction) are overwhelmed by unprotected exposure to cold environments.

Hypothermia

Hypothermia is defined as a core temperature (*i.e.*, rectal, esophageal, or tympanic) less than 35°C. Core body temperatures in the range of 32° to 35°C are considered mildly hypothermic; 28° to 32°C, moderately hypothermic; and less than 28°C, severely hypothermic.[2,28]

Hypothermia may either be controlled or accidental. Controlled hypothermia may be used to decrease brain metabolism after brain injury, during certain types of surgery, and

post cardiac arrest. Accidental hypothermia may be defined as a spontaneous decrease in core temperature, usually in a cold environment and associated with an acute problem but without a primary disorder of the temperature-regulating centre. Systemic accidental hypothermia may result from exposure to prolonged cold (atmospheric or submersion). The term *submersion hypothermia* is used when cooling follows acute asphyxia, as occurs in drowning. In children, the rapid cooling process, in addition to the diving reflex that triggers apnea and circulatory shunting to establish a heart–brain circulation, may account for the surprisingly high survival rate after submersion. The longest time of submersion recorded was 66 minutes for a 2.5-year-old child who survived without neurological impairment.[28] The diving reflex is greatly diminished in adults.

The condition may develop in otherwise healthy persons in the course of accidental exposure to cold. Because water conducts heat more readily than air, body temperature drops rapidly when the body is submerged in cold water or when clothing becomes wet. In persons with altered homeostasis due to debility or disease, hypothermia may follow exposure to relatively small decreases in atmospheric temperature.

Many underlying conditions can contribute to the development of hypothermia. Malnutrition decreases the fuel available for heat generation and loss of body fat decreases tissue insulation. Alcohol and sedative drugs dull mental awareness to cold and impair judgment to seek shelter or put on additional clothing. Alcohol also inhibits shivering. Persons with cardiovascular disease, cerebrovascular disease, spinal cord injury, and hypothyroidism also are predisposed to hypothermia.

Neonatal Hypothermia

Infants are particularly at risk for hypothermia because of their high ratio of surface area to body mass. Relative to body weight, the body surface area of an infant is three times that of an adult, and in infants with low birth weight the insulating layer of subcutaneous fat is thinner. The newborn infant is particularly at risk. Under the usual delivery room conditions (20° to 25°C), an infant's skin temperature falls approximately 0.3°C/minute and deep body temperature by approximately 0.1°C/minute.[29] The heat loss occurs by convection to the cooler surrounding air; by conduction to cooler materials on which the infant is resting; by radiation to nearby cooler solid objects; and by evaporation from the moist skin. The unstable body temperature of a preterm infant can drop precipitously after delivery, and this hypothermia is associated with an increase in morbidity and mortality.

Perioperative Hypothermia

Persons who undergo surgical procedures are also at risk for hypothermia. Most open heart surgeries (adult and pediatric) involve intentionally induced hypothermia, whereas many other surgical patients undergoing general and regional anesthesia experience unintentional hypothermia. Perioperative hypothermia is the result of a cold environment and impaired thermoregulatory mechanisms brought about by anesthetics and other drugs. Among the environmental factors that contribute to the loss of body heat are the cool temperature of the operating room and its equipment, air turnover rates that increase convective losses, use of cold antiseptic solutions that are allowed to evaporate from the skin, instillation of cold fluids into body cavities, administration of cool intravenous infusions, and exposure of the inner cavity to the cool atmosphere.[30] Both general and regional anesthetic agents disrupt many of the body's thermoregulatory mechanisms. General anesthetic agents lower the metabolic rate and decrease vasoconstriction and shivering thresholds, whereas epidural and spinal anesthesia decrease the vasoconstriction and shivering thresholds. Postanesthetic shivering is a common complication of modern anesthesia, affecting up to 65% of patients. Apart from discomfort, postanesthesia shivering is associated with a number of potentially dangerous sequelae, including increased oxygen consumption and carbon dioxide production, increased cardiorespiratory effort, and effects of increased catecholamine (epinephrine and norepinephrine) release. These effects can pose a problem to recovery in vulnerable populations such as older adults and persons with marginal cardiopulmonary reserves, impaired oxygen-carrying capacity (anemia), and other health problems.

A number of methods are used to prevent heat loss during surgery. Core temperature monitoring, accompanied by passive and active methods to maintain normal body temperature, should be part of routine inoperative monitoring. In many cases, some form of active rewarming is required. At present, forced-air warming is the most effective method available.[31] When necessary, centrally active drugs (meperidine, chlorpromazine, clonidine) may be used to reduce postanesthesia shivering.

Manifestations

The signs and symptoms of hypothermia include poor coordination, stumbling, slurred speech, irrationality and poor judgment, amnesia, hallucinations, cyanosis and edema of the skin, dilation of the pupils, decreased respiratory rate, weak and irregular pulse, and altered level of consciousness. With mild hypothermia, intense shivering generates heat and sympathetic nervous system activity is raised to resist lowering of temperature. Vasoconstriction can be profound, heart rate is accelerated, and stroke volume is increased. Blood pressure increases slightly, and hyperventilation is common. Exposure to cold augments urinary flow (*i.e.,* cold diuresis) before there is any fall in temperature. Dehydration and increased hematocrit may develop within a few hours of even mild hypothermia, augmented by an extracellular-to-intracellular water shift.

With moderate hypothermia, shivering gradually decreases, and the muscles become rigid. Shivering usually ceases below 28°C.[2] Heart rate and stroke volume are reduced, and blood pressure falls.[5] There is a reduction in metabolic rate and an associated decrease in oxygen consumption and carbon dioxide production. There is roughly a 7% decrease in oxygen consumption for every 1°C decrease in temperature.[32] A decrease in carbon dioxide production leads to a decrease in respiratory rate. Respirations decrease as temperatures drop below 32°C.

Decreases in mentation, the cough reflex, and respiratory tract secretions may lead to difficulty in clearing secretions and aspiration. Consciousness usually is lost at 30°C.

In terms of cardiovascular function, a gradual decline in heart rate and cardiac output occurs as hypothermia progresses. Blood pressure initially rises and then gradually falls. There is increased risk of dysrhythmia developing, probably from myocardial hypoxia and autonomic nervous system imbalance. Ventricular fibrillation is a major cause of death in hypothermia.

Carbohydrate metabolism and insulin activity are decreased, resulting in a hyperglycemia that is proportional to the level of cooling. A cold-induced loss of cell membrane integrity allows intravascular fluids to move into the skin, giving the skin a puffy appearance. Acid-base disorders occur with increased frequency at temperatures below 25°C unless adequate ventilation is maintained. Extracellular sodium and potassium concentrations decrease, and chloride levels increase. There is a temporary loss of plasma from the circulation along with sludging of red blood cells and increased blood viscosity as the result of trapping in the small vessels and skin.[28]

Diagnosis and Treatment

Oral temperatures are markedly inaccurate during hypothermia because of severe vasoconstriction and sluggish blood flow. Electronic thermometers with flexible probes are available for measuring rectal, bladder, and esophageal temperatures. However, rectal and bladder temperatures often lag behind fluctuations in core temperature, and esophageal temperatures may be elevated during inhalation of heated air. Most clinical thermometers measure temperature only in the range of 35° to 42°C; a special thermometer that registers as low as 25°C or an electrical thermistor probe is needed for monitoring temperatures in persons with hypothermia.[28]

The treatment of hypothermia consists of rewarming, support of vital functions, and the prevention and treatment of complications.[28] There are three methods of rewarming: passive external rewarming, active external rewarming, and active core rewarming. *Passive external rewarming* is done by removing the person from the cold environment, covering with a blanket, supplying warm fluids (oral or intravenous), and allowing rewarming to occur at the person's own pace. Persons with mild hypothermia usually respond well to passive rewarming in a warm bed, but persons with moderate or severe hypothermia do not have the thermoregulatory shivering mechanism and require active rewarming. *Active external rewarming* involves immersing the person in warm water, using forced-air warming systems, or placing heating pads or hot water bottles on the surface of the body, including the extremities. *Active core rewarming* can be done by instilling warmed fluids into the gastrointestinal tract; through peritoneal dialysis; by extracorporeal blood warming, in which blood is removed from the body and passed through a heat exchanger and then returned to the body; or by inhalation of an oxygen mixture warmed to 42° to 46°C. It places a greater emphasis on rewarming the trunk, leaving the extremities, containing the major metabolic mass, cold until the inner core, including the heart, rewarms.

Therapeutic Hypothermia

Controlled hypothermia may be used after brain injury and during certain types of surgery to decrease inflammation and brain metabolism. Ideally, therapeutic hypothermia with a temperature of 32° to 34°C for 12 to 24 hours should be initiated as soon as possible after any potential neurologic injury.[32] This controlled therapeutic hypothermia has been found helpful for people who have had cardiac arrest due to ventricular fibrillation in terms of increasing the person's neurological outcomes. In cardiothoracic surgery, intraoperative patients are purposely kept hypothermic to decrease metabolic demands and prevent myocardial ischemia. While there are protective effects for this type of hypothermia (*e.g.*, decrease cellular and tissue oxygen consumption and glucose utilization, lower mortality), there are negative effects that include the need for intensive monitoring and equipment, overall electrolyte and glucose disturbances, infections, and coagulation complications.[32] Work continues in this area to develop guidelines identifying ideal clinical conditions for therapeutic hypothermia.

IN SUMMARY

Hypothermia is a potentially life-threatening disorder in which the body's core temperature drops below 35°C. Accidental hypothermia can develop in otherwise healthy persons in the course of accidental exposure and in older adults or disabled persons with impaired perception of or response to cold. Alcoholism, cardiovascular disease, malnutrition, and hypothyroidism contribute to the risk of hypothermia. Hypothermia is also a common occurrence in the operative patient and in newborn infants, particularly those born prematurely and can be used therapeutically for a variety of conditions. The greatest effect of hypothermia is a decrease in the metabolic rate, leading to a decrease in carbon dioxide production and respiratory rate. The signs and symptoms of hypothermia include poor coordination, stumbling, slurred speech, irrationality, poor judgment, amnesia, hallucinations, blueness and puffiness of the skin, dilation of the pupils, decreased respiratory rate, weak and irregular pulse, stupor, and coma. The treatment of hypothermia includes passive or active rewarming, support of vital functions, and the prevention and treatment of complications.

REVIEW EXERCISES

1. A 3-year-old child is seen in a pediatric clinic with a temperature of 39°C. Her skin is warm and flushed, her pulse is 120 beats/minute, and her respirations are shallow and rapid at 32 breaths/minute. Her mother states that her daughter has complained of a sore throat and has refused to drink or take medications to bring her temperature down.

   A. *Explain the physiologic mechanisms of fever generation.*

   B. *Are the warm and flushed skin, rapid heart rate, and respirations consistent with this level of fever?*

   C. *After receiving an appropriate dose of acetaminophen, the child begins to sweat, and the temperature drops to 37.2°C. Explain the physiologic mechanisms responsible for the drop in temperature.*

2. A 25-year-old man was brought to the emergency department after having been found unconscious in a snow bank. The outdoor temperature at the time he was discovered was –25°C. His car, which was stalled a short distance away, contained liquor bottles, suggesting that he had been drinking. His temperature on admission was 29.8°C. His heart rate was 40 beats/minute and his respirations 18 breaths/minute and shallow. His skin was cool, his muscles rigid, and his digits blue.

   A. *What factors might have contributed to this man's state of hypothermia?*

   B. *Is this man able to engage in physiologic behaviours to control loss of body heat (refer to Fig. 10.3)?*

   C. *Given two methods that are available for taking this man's temperature (oral or rectal), which would be more accurate? Explain.*

   D. *What precautions should be considered when deciding on a method for rewarming this man?*

References

1. Hall J. E. (2011). *Textbook of Medical Physiology* (12th ed.). Philadelphia, PA: W. B. Saunders.
2. Wizmann F. A. (2013). Chapter 28: Regulation of body temperature. In Rhoades R. A., Bell D. R. (Eds.). *Medical Physiology* (4th ed.). Philadelphia, PA: Lippincott Williams & Wilkins.
3. Gisolfi C. V., Mora F. (2000). *The hot brain: survival, temperature, and the human body.* Cambridge, MA: MIT Press.
4. Boron W. F., Boulpaep E. L. (2009). *Medical physiology* (2nd ed.). Philadelphia, PA: Saunders.
5. Davie A., Amoore J. (2010). Best practice in the measurement of body temperature. *Nursing Standard, 24*(42), 42–49.
6. Ferrandiz-Huertas C., Mathivanan S., Wolf C. J., et al. (2014). Trafficking of thermoTRP channels. *Membranes, 4*(3), 525–564.
7. Presciutti M., Bader M. K., Hepburn M. (2012). Shivering management during therapeutic temperature modulation: Nurses' perspective. *Critical Care Nurse, 32*(1), 33–42.
8. Rowsey P. J. (2013). Thermoregulation: cytokines involved in fever and exercise. *Annual Review of Nursing Research, 31*(1), 19–46.
9. Launey Y., Nesseler N., Mallédant Y., Seguin P. (2011). Clinical review: Fever in septic ICU patients, friend or foe? *Critical Care, 15*, 222.

10. Gern J. E., Palmenberg A. C. (2013). Chapter 18: Rhinoviruses. In Knipe D. M., Howley P. (Eds.). *Fields virology* (6th ed.). Philadelphia, PA: Lippincott Williams and Wilkins.

11. Ogoina D. (2011). Fever, fever patterns and diseases called 'fever'—a review. *Journal of Infection and Public Health, 4*(3), 108–124.

12. Davies P., Maconochie I. (2009). The relationship between body temperature, heart rate and respiratory rate in children. *Emergency Medicine Journal, 26*(9), 641–643.

13. Mittal R. (2014). Recent advances in febrile seizures. *Indian Journal of Pediatrics, 81*(9), 909–916.

14. Horowitz H. W. (2014). Fever of unknown origin or fever of too many origins? *The New England Journal of Medicine, 368*(3), 197–199.

15. Koyfman A., Lovallo E., Hazen M. M., Chiang V. W. (2013). A taste of periodic fever syndromes. *Pediatric Emergency Care, 29*(7), 842–851.

16. Sullivan J. E., Farrar H. C. (2011). Fever and antipyretic use in children. *Pediatrics, 127*(3), 580–587.

17. Hamilton J. L., John S. P. (2013). Evaluation of fever in infants and young children. *American Family Physician, 87*(4), 254–260.

18. American College of Emergency Physicians Clinical Policy Committee, American College of Emergency Physicians Clinical Policies Subcommittee on Pediatric Fever. (2003). Clinical policy for children younger than three years presenting to the emergency department with fever. *Annals of Emergency Medicine, 42*(4), 530–545.

19. Warren D. W., Jarvis A., LeBlanc L., et al. (2008). Revisions to the Canadian triage and acuity scale paediatric guidelines (PaedCTAS). *Canadian Journal of Emergency Medicine, 10*(3), 224–243.

20. Outzen M. (2009). Management of fever in older adults. *Journal of Gerontological Nursing, 35*(5), 17–23.

21. Auwaerter P. G. (2007). Chapter 31: Approach to the patient with fever. In Fiebach N. H., Kern D. E., Thomas P. A., et al. (Eds.). *Principles of ambulatory medicine* (6th ed.). Philadelphia, PA: Lippincott Williams & Wilkins.

22. Atha W. F. (2013). Heat-related illness. *Emergency Medicine Clinics of North America, 31*(4), 1097–1108.

23. Bergeron M. F. (2013). Reducing sports heat illness risk. *Pediatrics in Review, 34*(6), 270–279.

24. Horseman M. A., Rather-Conally J., Saavedra C., Surani S. (2013). A case of severe heat stroke and review of pathophysiology, clinical presentation, and treatment. *Journal of Intensive Care Medicine, 28*(6), 334–340.

25. Patel R. A., Gallagher J. C. (2010). Drug fever. *Pharmacotherapy, 30*(1), 57–69.

26. Schneiderbanger D., Johannsen S., Roewer N., Schuster F. (2014). Management of malignant hyperthermia: Diagnosis and treatment. *Therapeutics and Clinical Risk Management, 10*, 355–362.

27. Berman B. D. (2011). Neuroleptic malignant syndrome: A review for neurohospitalists. *Neurohospitalist, 1*(1), 41–47.

28. Brown D. J., Brugger H., Boyd J., Paal P. (2012). Accidental hypothermia. *The New England Journal of Medicine, 367*(20), 1930–1938.

29. Carlo W. A. (2011). Chapter 88: The newborn infant. In Kliegman R. M., Stanton B. F., St. Geme J. W., et al. (Eds.). *Nelson textbook of pediatrics* (19th ed.). Philadelphia, PA: Saunders Elsevier.

30. Sessler D. I. (2014). Temperature monitoring: The consequences and prevention of mild perioperative hypothermia. *Southern African Journal of Anaesthesia and Analgesia, 20*(1), 25–31.

31. John M., Ford J., Harper M. (2014). Peri-operative warming devices: Performance and clinical application. *Anaesthesia, 69*(6), 623–638.

32. Varon J., Marik P. E., Einav S. (2012). Therapeutic hypothermia: A state-of-the-art emergency medicine perspective. *American Journal of Emergency Medicine, 30*(5), 800–810.

Visit the Point. **http://thePoint.lww.com for animations, journal articles, and more!**

Activity Tolerance and Fatigue

Physical activity, including exercise, is a physiologic state, so common in its many forms that true physiologic rest is seldom achieved. Defined ultimately in terms of skeletal muscle contraction, exercise involves the coordinated responses of every body system to provide the energy needed for increased muscle activity. Fatigue represents the perceived lack of sufficient energy to engage fully in physical activities. Fatigue may be acute, as in that resulting from increased physical activity or it may be chronic, as in the chronic fatigue syndrome. Conditions that restrict physical activity, such as bed rest and immobility, can impair a person's exercise reserve and ability to perform work and other activities, and contribute to fatigue.

This chapter focuses on activity tolerance and exercise, activity intolerance and fatigue; and the physiologic and psychosocial responses to immobility and bed rest.

EXERCISE AND ACTIVITY TOLERANCE

After completing this section of the chapter, you should be able to meet the following objectives:

- Differentiate between aerobic, isometric, and flexibility exercises.
- Describe the physiologic and psychological responses to exercise.
- Define the term *maximal oxygen consumption* and state how it is measured.
- Describe methods that can be used to assess a person's activity tolerance and ability to engage in an exercise program.
- Describe the physiologic effects of exercise in the older adult population.

Physical activity is defined as any movement or force produced by skeletal muscles that requires energy expenditure. *Exercise* is a subset of physical activity consisting of planned, structured, and repetitive body movements.[1,2] Humans interact with their environment in a cyclic pattern involving periods of activity and rest, both of which have physical and psychological elements. Physical activity and exercise denote the process of skeletal muscle movement and energy expenditure, whereas rest is characterized by inactivity and minimal energy expenditure.

There is increasing interest in both the preventative and therapeutic effects of physical activity and exercise. A regular program of exercise is recommended as a means of maintaining weight control and cardiovascular fitness.[1-3] Exercise partnered with diet control also is becoming recognized as an integral part of the treatment regimen for many diseases. It is recommended as a means of slowing, or even halting, the progression of atherosclerotic coronary heart disease (CHD); of lowering low-density lipoproteins (LDL) and increasing high-density lipoproteins (HDL) in persons with hyperlipidemia; of providing better regulation of blood glucose in persons with diabetes; and of improving activity tolerance in persons with cardiovascular and respiratory diseases. Regular exercise can also have psychological benefits: it can improve self-esteem, remedy depressive moods, and enhance quality of life.[2]

ACTIVITY TOLERANCE

- Activity is the process of purposeful energy expenditure. Exercise, a form of activity that results in overall conditioning of the body, can be aerobic or resistance.
- Exercise depends on the availability of energy substrates, cardiovascular fitness, muscle strength and flexibility, and motivation.
- The cardiovascular response to exercise includes increased heart rate, stroke volume, and mean arterial pressure. An increased percentage of cardiac output is distributed to working muscle.
- Pulmonary perfusion and pulmonary ventilation increase in response to exercise.
- Psychological effects of exercise include an increase in energy and in the ability to adapt to stress.

Although there is a growing consensus regarding the importance of physical activity and exercise, there are questions regarding the type, intensity, frequency, and duration. A single episode of acute exercise may provoke responses quite different from the adaptations seen when exercise is chronic.

Types of Exercise

There are two main types of skeletal muscle exercise: aerobic and resistance. Another type—flexibility or stretching exercise—promotes flexibility and improved range of joint motion. Most exercise programs use a combination of all three types of exercise.

Aerobic Exercise

Aerobic, or *endurance, exercise* involves the body's ability to improve its use of oxygen for energy during prolonged strenuous exercise. It involves rhythmic changes in muscle length (contraction and elongation) during activities such as walking, running, bicycling, or swimming. During aerobic exercise that uses large muscle groups (*e.g.,* running), each person has a maximal oxygen uptake that cannot be exceeded, although it can be increased with appropriate training.[3,4] Although aerobic exercise training results in muscles that use oxygen more efficiently such that the body can do more work with less cardiac and respiratory effort, it does not promote significant increase in muscle mass, even though the exercise may go on for hours.

Whatever type of exercise a person chooses, the Canadian Society for Exercise Physiology (CSEP) recommends that adults strive for at least 150 minutes of moderate-intensity (*e.g.,* brisk walking, biking, dancing) to vigorous-intensity (*e.g.,* jogging, cross-country skiing) physical activity every week, in bouts of 10 minutes or more. CSEP also recommends adding muscle and bone strengthening activities at least 2 days per week.[5]

Resistance Exercise

In *resistance,* or *strength, exercise,* sustained muscle contraction is generated against a weight or load with no change in length of the involved muscle group or joint movement. It involves activities, such as weight lifting and repeated movement against low to moderate resistance, that improve overall muscle strength and tone and build muscle mass.

Although resistance training has long been accepted as a means of developing strength and muscle mass, its beneficial relationship to health factors and chronic diseases has only been recognized recently.[6] Despite the fact that the mechanisms may differ, both aerobic exercise and resistance training have similar effects on bone density, glucose tolerance, and insulin sensitivity. For weight control, aerobic exercise is considered a calorie burner; whereas resistance training assists the body in expending calories through an increase in lean body mass and basal metabolism.[6] Many leisure and occupational tasks require sustained muscle efforts, often involving the arms rather than the legs. Because the blood pressure response to resistance exercise is proportionate to the maximal voluntary contraction as well as muscle mass involved, increased muscle strength results in an attenuated heart rate and blood pressure response to a given load.

Flexibility Exercise

In contrast to aerobic and resistance exercises, stretching as an isolated activity increases neither strength nor endurance, but should be included in an overall fitness regimen.[5] Considerable evidence suggests that stretching exercises increase tendon flexibility, improve joint range of motion, and enhance muscular performance.[2,4] When properly performed, these exercises promote an overall improved general function. Thus, it is recommended that aerobic and resistance training be accompanied by a stretching program that exercises the major muscle or tendon groups at least 2 days per week.[4]

Physiologic and Psychological Responses

The physiologic and psychological benefits of exercise involve four major components: cardiopulmonary fitness; increased

FIGURE 11.1 • Beneficial effects of physical activity and exercise.

Improved self-esteem and increased quality of life

Improved cardiovascular and pulmonary fitness

More efficient use of energy substrates such as glucose and free fatty acids

Increased muscle strength, flexibility, and endurance

Improved health

muscle strength, flexibility, and endurance; availability of energy substrates to meet the increased energy demands imposed by increased physical activity; and motivation and mental endurance (Fig. 11.1). These benefits incorporate cardiopulmonary, neuromuscular, metabolic and thermal, and gastrointestinal responses; changes in hemostasis and immune function; and psychological behaviours that accompany physical activity and exercise.

Cardiopulmonary Responses

The cardiopulmonary responses to exercise involve the circulatory functions of the heart and blood vessels and the gas exchange functions of the respiratory system. Collectively, they function to supply oxygen and energy substrates to the working muscles and exchange oxygen and carbon dioxide with the atmosphere. Cardiopulmonary or aerobic exercise involves repetitive and rhythmic movements, uses large muscle groups, and results in the ability to perform vigorous exercise for an extended period.

The principal factor that determines how long and effectively a person will be able to exercise is the capacity of the heart, lungs, and circulation to deliver oxygen to the working muscles. The term *maximal oxygen consumption* ($\dot{V}O_2$ max) represents this principle. The $\dot{V}O_2$ max is determined by the rate at which oxygen is delivered to the working muscles, the oxygen-carrying capacity of blood, and the amount of oxygen extracted from the blood by the working muscles. It is measured as the volume of oxygen consumed, usually in litres or millilitres, per unit of

time (*i.e.,* litres/minute). The $\dot{V}O_2$ max is an important determinant of a person's capacity to perform work; in a very fit person participating in strenuous exercise, it can be 20 times the resting oxygen uptake.[2,4] An exercise training program can accelerate the rate of increased $\dot{V}O_2$ max so that the trained athlete has a more rapid increase in cardiac output and skeletal muscle blood flow during the first minute of exercise.

The cardiovascular responses to exercise are regulated by output from centres in the central nervous system (CNS) and autonomic nervous system to the heart and blood vessels in tandem with local mechanisms that further regulate cardiac output and muscle blood flow.[7,8] Recent research using brain mapping demonstrates specific areas of the brain, including the insular cortex and anterior cingulate cortex, that communicate with hypothalamic centres responsible for coordinating a pattern of increased sympathetic and decreased parasympathetic (vagal) outflow to the medullary cardiovascular centres (Fig. 11.2).[9] This leads to an increase in cardiac output and baroreceptor-mediated control of arterial blood pressure. Local control is derived from the release of metabolic end products (*e.g.,* lactic acid) and local vasoactive factors that dilate blood vessels. Local factors in the coronary blood vessels mediate vasodilation, whereas increased sympathetic activity produces vasoconstriction of renal and gastrointestinal vessels, reducing blood flow to these organs.[8,9]

Cardiac Output. Exercise produces an increase in heart rate and stroke volume (amount of blood pumped with each heart beat), which in turn increases cardiac output. During exercise,

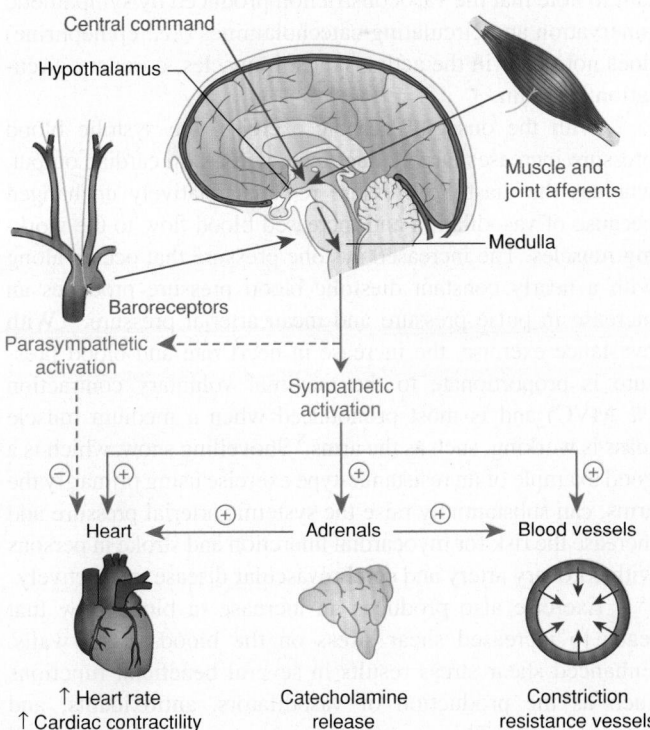

Central command

Hypothalamus

Muscle and joint afferents

Medulla

Baroreceptors

Parasympathetic activation

Sympathetic activation

Heart ← → Adrenals → Blood vessels

↑ Heart rate
↑ Cardiac contractility

Catecholamine release

Constriction resistance vessels

FIGURE 11.2 • Mechanisms of neural cardiovascular control during exercise.

the cardiac output may increase from a resting level of 4 to 8 L/minute to as high as 15 L/minute for the average woman and 22 L/minute for the average man; in highly trained endurance athletes, output can reach 40 L/min.[8] The increase in heart rate is mediated through neural, hormonal, and intrinsic cardiovascular mechanisms. With anticipation of exercise, cardiovascular centres in the brain stem are stimulated to initiate an increase in sympathetic activity concomitant with an inhibition of parasympathetic mechanisms. Stimulation of the sympathetic nervous system produces an increase in heart rate and cardiac contractility. At the start of exercise, the heart rate increases immediately and continues to increase until a plateau is reached. This plateau, or steady-state heart rate, is maintained until exercise is terminated. Release of epinephrine and norepinephrine from the adrenal glands helps to sustain the increased heart rate.[7]

Also contributing to the increased heart rate are mechanisms intrinsic to the heart. An increase in venous return stimulates right atrial stretch receptors that initiate an increase in heart rate, and an increase in ventricular filling stretches the myocardial fibres, resulting in a more forceful contraction and a more complete emptying of the ventricles with each beat through the *Frank–Starling mechanism* (see Chapter 21).[7,8]

Blood Pressure and Blood Flow. Blood pressure and blood flow also change with exercise. Increased sympathetic activity constricts the resistance vessels, leading to an increase in blood pressure; and it constricts the capacitance vessels in the visceral circulation, leading to an increase in venous return to the heart and maintenance of the cardiac output. It is important to note that the vasoconstriction produced by sympathetic innervation and circulating catecholamines (*i.e.,* epinephrine) does not occur in the active skeletal muscles, coronary circulation, or brain.

With the onset of aerobic exercise, the systolic blood pressure increases largely due to an increase in cardiac output, whereas the diastolic pressure remains relatively unchanged because of vasodilation and increased blood flow to the working muscles. The increased systolic pressure that occurs along with a nearly constant diastolic blood pressure produces an increase in pulse pressure and mean arterial pressure.[10] With resistance exercise, the increase in heart rate and blood pressure is proportionate to the maximal voluntary contraction (% MVC) and is most pronounced when a medium muscle mass is working, such as the arms.[8] Shovelling snow, which is a good example of an resistance-type exercise using primarily the arms, can substantially raise the systemic arterial pressure and increase the risk for myocardial infarction and stroke in persons with coronary artery and cerebrovascular disease, respectively.

Exercise also produces an increase in blood flow that leads to increased shear stress on the blood vessel walls. Enhanced shear stress results in several beneficial functions such as the production of vasodilators, antioxidants, and anticoagulants. This contributes to improved endothelial cell function, which results in vasodilation, inhibition of platelet activation, and increased fibrinolysis, thus leading to improved patency of the vasculature and maintenance of blood flow and vessel patency.[7,11] Adaptation to exercise also induces angiogenesis with an increased growth of vessels to support blood flow to the exercising muscle.[11] Because of the effects of exercise training on vascular function and angiogenesis, it has been proposed as a mechanism for improving blood flow and decreasing exercise-related leg pain (claudication) in persons with peripheral vascular disease.[10,12]

Respiratory Responses. The role of the respiratory system during exercise is to increase the rate of oxygen and carbon dioxide exchange. This takes place through a series of physiologic responses. With exercise, the respiratory rate increases four- to fivefold, tidal volume increases five- to sevenfold, and minute ventilation (respiratory rate × tidal volume) increases up to 20 to 30 times its resting value.[13] Also, the anticipation of physical activity contributes to the increase in respiratory rate (along with changes in sympathetics and joint proprioceptors) well before the pH or oxygen demands change. With the increase in cardiac output, a greater volume of blood under slightly increased pressure is delivered to the pulmonary vessels in the lungs. This results in the opening of more pulmonary capillary beds, producing better alveolar perfusion and more efficient exchange of oxygen and carbon dioxide. In addition to pulmonary perfusion being enhanced during exercise, pulmonary ventilation is increased, resulting in a more optimal ventilation–perfusion ratio. This response is controlled by chemoreceptors—located in the brain stem, aorta, and carotid arteries—that monitor pH, carbon dioxide, and oxygen. During exercise, decreases in pH and increases in carbon dioxide stimulate these receptors, producing an increase in both rate and depth of respiration, which results in an increase in minute ventilation.[8,13]

Neuromuscular Responses

The integration of the neurologic and musculoskeletal systems is essential for body movement and participation in activity. To initiate and sustain increased activity, muscle strength, flexibility, and endurance are needed. *Muscle strength* is defined as the ability of muscle groups to produce force against resistance. *Flexibility* involves the range of movement of joints, and *muscle endurance* refers to the ability of the body or muscle groups to perform increased activity for an extended time.

Types of Muscle. Skeletal muscle consists of two distinct types of muscle fibres based on differences in their size, speed, contractile properties, endurance, and metabolic characteristics: red (dark) slow-twitch (type I) and white (light) fast-twitch (type II) muscle fibres.[8,14] Both heredity and activity influence the distribution of fast-twitch and slow-twitch fibres. Heredity appears to contribute to differences in muscle fibre composition, such that some people have considerably more fast-twitch than slow-twitch fibres, and others have more slow-twitch than fast-twitch fibres. This could determine, to some extent, the area of athletics for which a person is best suited.[14]

The slow-twitch fibres, which are smaller than the fast-twitch fibres, tend to produce less overall force but are more energy efficient than fast-twitch fibres. They are better-suited biochemically to perform lower-intensity work for prolonged periods. These fibres have a high oxidative capacity as a result of high concentrations of mitochondria and myoglobin. Slow-twitch fibres are highly fatigue resistant and ideally suited for prolonged aerobic exercise or activity. Slow-twitch fibres predominate in the large muscle groups such as the leg muscles; therefore, they play a major role in sustaining activity during prolonged exercise or endurance activities. Periods of sustained inactivity, such as prolonged immobility or bed rest, primarily affect slow-twitch fibres, which quickly decondition.[8,14]

In contrast to slow-twitch fibres, fast-twitch fibres are larger and better suited for high-intensity work, but they fatigue more easily. These fibres have high myosin adenosine triphosphatase (ATPase) activity, few mitochondria, low myoglobin concentration, and high glycolytic capacity, resulting in dependence on anaerobic metabolism to supply adenosine triphosphate (ATP) for energy. Fast-twitch fibres predominate during activities in which short bursts of intense energy are required, such as sprinting or weight lifting. Anabolic steroids enhance fast-twitch fibre activity.[8,14]

Persons with heart failure typically experience symptoms of breathlessness, exertional fatigue, and exercise intolerance resulting in atrophy of skeletal muscles. When these individuals engage in exercise, there is a shift toward using fast-twitch muscle fibres. This causes an early dependence on anaerobic metabolism and excessive intramuscular acidification that leads to increased fatigability.[15] The increased reliance on anaerobic metabolism and subsequent vasoconstrictor response can also lead to an increase in afterload work (see Chapter 21) for an already compromised left ventricle. Thus, it is imperative that individuals with heart failure have their exercise regimens monitored closely.

Muscle Blood Flow. During aerobic activity, working muscles use 10 to 20 times more oxygen than nonworking muscles. This increased oxygen demand is met by an increase in cardiac output and muscle blood flow. Skeletal muscles receive 85% to 95% of the cardiac output during aerobic activities, and only 15% to 20% of the cardiac output at rest. The increased blood flow is achieved through two mechanisms: dilation of blood vessels in the working muscles and constriction of those in organs of low priority.[8,14]

Increased blood flow to working muscles is achieved by relaxation of the arterioles and the precapillary sphincters. Chemical changes such as decreased oxygen and pH and increased levels of potassium, adenosine, carbon dioxide, and phosphate contribute to the vasodilation during prolonged exercise and recovery from exercise.[14] Increased venous blood flow and central venous pressure are enhanced by the alternate contraction and relaxation of working muscles.

Another mechanism that increases blood flow to the working muscles is the diversion of blood from organs such as the kidneys and gastrointestinal structures that are less active than the working muscles.[7–9] The amount of blood flow diverted from the visceral organs is proportional to the level of exercise, and as exercise is increased, more blood is diverted to working muscles.

Metabolic and Thermal Responses

Skeletal muscles hypertrophy and undergo other anatomic changes in response to exercise training. "Trained muscles" have an increased number of capillaries surrounding each muscle fibre that facilitates the delivery of oxygen to the working muscle cells during exercise. They are able to use oxygen more efficiently, probably because of enhanced enzymatic activity that increases oxidative capacity. The mitochondria appear to adapt by increasing the transport of oxygen and other substrates to the inner regions of the muscle fibre.[8]

Unlike other tissues in the body, skeletal muscles switch between virtual inactivity when they are relaxed and using only minimal amounts of ATP, to extremes of physical activity during which they use ATP at a rapid rate. However, they have only enough ATP to power contraction for a few seconds. If strenuous exercise is to continue beyond this time, additional sources of ATP must be generated. The ATP that is used to power muscle contraction is obtained from three sources: creatine phosphate, glycogen, and fatty acids. Much like ATP, *creatine phosphate* (also known as *phosphocreatine*) contains high-energy phosphate bonds. It is unique to muscle fibres and is 8 to 10 times as abundant as ATP. Creatine is a small, amino acid-like molecule that is both synthesized in the body and derived from foods (Fig. 11.3). The enzyme creatine kinase (CK) catalyzes the transfer of the high-energy phosphate groups from ATP to creatine, forming creatine phosphate and adenosine diphosphate (ADP). When muscle contraction begins and ADP levels start to rise, CK catalyzes the transfer of a high-energy phosphate group back to ADP, thus forming new ATP molecules that can be used by the muscle for energy.

During exercise, particularly aerobic exercise, the body uses its energy sources in a characteristic pattern. The first sources for energy are stored ATP, creatine phosphate, and muscle glycogen. Short, intense periods of activity lasting 1 to 2 minutes exploit these energy sources through anaerobic

FIGURE 11.3 • The creatinine phosphokinase (CK) reaction. During increased muscle activity, the enzyme CK catalyzes the transfer of the high-energy phosphate group from creatine phosphate to adenosine diphosphate (ADP) to form adenosine triphosphate (ATP). During periods of inactivity, ATP transfers its high-energy phosphate group to creatine to form creatine phosphate. (The high-energy bond is indicated by a blue squiggle.) (From Lieberman M., Marks A. D., Peet A. (2013). *Marks' basic medical biochemistry* (4th ed., p. 892). Philadelphia, PA: Lippincott Williams & Wilkins.)

metabolism. If the activity is to be performed for longer periods, muscle glycogen and creatine phosphate are used to meet the energy requirements through both anaerobic and aerobic metabolism. For intense, prolonged periods of activity, aerobic metabolism and the use of glucose, fatty acids, and amino acids become essential.[8]

Nutritional and Hydration Status. To supply the energy needed for increased activity, a person must consume a balanced diet and have adequate hydration. Although proteins are not used for energy sources during increased activity, they have an essential role in the building and rebuilding of tissues and organs. During increased activity and exercise, it is essential that an individual maintain adequate hydration. Increased activity can result in loss of fluids from the vascular compartment. If this is allowed to progress, the person may experience severe dehydration that may lead to vascular collapse. Before and during vigorous activity, a person should replenish body fluids with water and electrolyte solutions.[8]

Temperature Regulation. Almost all the energy released from metabolic processes involved in muscle contraction is converted to heat. Under normal resting conditions, the body is able to maintain its temperature within a set range. It does this by two mechanisms. The first mechanism used by the body to regulate temperature is to change blood flow to the skin. When the blood vessels of the skin dilate, warm blood is shunted from the core tissues and organs to the skin surface, where heat is lost more easily to the surrounding environment (see Chapter 10). The second mechanism is through sweating, in which the evaporation of sweat from the skin surface contributes to the loss of body heat. Depending on training level and environmental conditions, the body may have difficulty regulating its temperature during vigorous exercise.[8,16] With sufficient training, the body adapts by increasing the rate of sweat production. As temperature regulation improves with training, the trained person begins to sweat sooner, often within 1 to 2 minutes of the start of exercise. Sweat production begins even before the core temperature rises, and a cooling effect is initiated soon after the start of exercise; the sweat produced is more dilute than that produced by a nontrained person. Sweat normally contains large amounts of sodium chloride; production of a dilute sweat allows evaporative cooling to take place while sodium chloride is conserved.[8]

During exercise, plasma proteins are shifted from the interstitial to the vascular compartment so that there is an increase in the amount of proteins in the blood. These proteins exert an osmotic force that draws fluid from the interstitial space into the vascular compartment. This contributes to an increase in vascular volume, which in turn is delivered to the working muscles and which also provides more efficient heat dissipation.[8]

Gastrointestinal Responses

The gastrointestinal system is affected by intense physical activity. During intense physical activity, blood flow is shunted away from the gastrointestinal tract toward the active skeletal muscles. As a result, gastrointestinal motility, secretory activity, and absorptive capacity are decreased. This can result in heartburn (reflux), vomiting, bloating, stomach pain, and gastrointestinal bleeding. It may also cause cramping, urge to defecate, and diarrhea. Although athletes may experience these symptoms, they are usually transient and do not have an effect on long-term health. Light and moderate exercise can benefit individuals with inflammatory bowel disease and liver disease. Evidence suggests that physical activity improves gastric emptying and lowers the risk of colon cancer and reduces the risks gastrointestinal hemorrhage and inflammatory bowel disease.[8,17]

Hemostasis and Immune Function

Increased physical activity affects both hemostasis and the immune system. Epinephrine levels increase during exercise and stimulate fibrinolysis, or the breakdown of fibrin strands in a blood clot. Thus, regular strenuous exercise prevents excessive coagulation of the blood.[8,14]

The response of the immune system to exercise is varied and depends on frequency, intensity, and duration of the exercise. The immune system is stimulated by regular, moderate exercise and impaired with regular, repetitive, intense exercise. A period of moderate-intensity exercise has been found to boost the immune system for several hours by producing an increase in circulating white blood cells, including neutrophils and lymphocytes. Of special note is the increased activity of natural killer cells. Chronic, intense, and exhausting exercise produces different effects on the immune system. Elevation in body temperature, cytokine release, and increased levels of various stress-related hormones (*e.g.*, epinephrine, growth hormone, cortisol) may result in a temporary depression of the body's innate immune defences. Strenuous exercise alters mucosal immunity of the upper respiratory tract. This may explain why elite athletes are susceptible to illness, especially upper respiratory tract infections.[8,18,19]

Psychological Responses

There is a mental component to the performance of increased activity and exercise. The mental aspect entails the motivation to initiate an activity, or exercise program, and the dedication to incorporate the regimen into one's lifestyle. Positive effects of regularly performed exercise include increased energy and motivation, positive self-image and self-esteem, decreased anxiety, and better management of stress.

Assessment of Activity and Exercise Tolerance

A person's ability to tolerate exercise and perform work can be assessed in several ways. One way is by having the person report his or her perceived response to different types of physical activity or exercise. This method is particularly useful in assessing persons for activity intolerance and fatigue (to be discussed). Another method, exercise stress testing, is used to measure aerobic fitness.

Activity Tolerance and Fatigue

One of the older methods of assessing activity tolerance involves the administration of paper-and-pencil tests in which participants describe their normal activities, their perceived level of activity tolerance, or their level of fatigue. Examples of paper-and-pencil tests include the following: the Human Activity Profile (HAP), which looks at the ability to perform common activities; the Fatigue Severity Scale, which describes nine statements ranking symptoms of fatigue; and the International Physical Activity Questionnaire (IPAQ), which reviews activity from the previous 7 days.

With advancements in technology, activity can be measured objectively using one-dimensional pedometers or the newer three-dimensional accelerometers, which can track motion, measure intensity, and provide digital feedback. Studies now show that accelerometers can capture activity that is often poorly reported in physical activity questionnaires.[20,21]

Aerobic Fitness

A number of tests are available to measure aerobic fitness, including the Rockport One Mile Test, the step test, and treadmill or bicycle ergometry. Often heart rate is used to estimate $\dot{V}O_2$ max without measuring oxygen consumption.[14,22]

Ergometry is a procedure for determining physical performance capacity. The ergometer is a specific tool that imposes a constant level of work. A specified workload, expressed in terms of watts or joules per second, is imposed while the person performs the task. Two examples of ergometers include the bicycle ergometer and the treadmill ergometer. A bicycle ergometer is a stationary bicycle that has a friction belt attached. The front wheel of the bicycle is rotated, and the braking force of the belt can be adjusted to alter the workload. A treadmill ergometer is used more frequently to assess workload performance, especially cardiac function. During treadmill testing, the person walks or runs on a moving belt. Changing the speed and incline of the treadmill alters the workload. This change usually is done in predetermined stages. During treadmill testing, the heart rate and electrocardiogram are monitored continuously, and the blood pressure is checked intermittently. Usually, the person being tested continues to exercise, completing successive stages of the test, until exhaustion intervenes or a predetermined or maximal heart rate is reached.

Maximal heart rate is estimated by age. Tables of maximal heart rate by age are available, but as a general rule, the predicted maximal heart rate can be estimated by subtracting age from 220 (*e.g.,* the target heart rate for a 40-year-old person would be 180 beats/minute). The person may continue to exercise until the predicted maximum heart rate is achieved, or until 85% to 90% of the predicted maximal rate is reached.

Metabolic Equivalents. Metabolic equivalents (METs), which are multiples of the basal metabolic rate, are commonly used to express workload at various stages of work. The energy expended in a resting position is equivalent to 1 MET and it changes as the type of activity performed (*e.g.,* walking, running) changes. For example, walking at 4 miles per hour (mph), cycling at 11 mph, playing tennis (singles), or doing carpentry requires 5 to 6 METs. Running at 6 mph requires 10 METs, and running at 10 mph requires 17 METs. Healthy sedentary persons seldom are able to exercise beyond 10 or 11 METs, whereas highly trained persons are able to achieve workloads of 16 METs or greater. In persons with coronary heart disease, workloads of 8 METs often produce angina.

During exercise stress testing, persons are asked to rate their subjective responses to the exercise experience. A commonly used tool to measure the person's perception of the amount of work being performed is the Borg Rating of Perceived Exertion (RPE) Scale, which is based on research that correlates heart rate to feelings of perceived exertion.[23] The original scale values range from 6 through 20 (*e.g.,* 7 represents very, very light; 9, very light; 13, somewhat hard; 15, hard; and 19 very, very hard). A newer category of scale has been developed with numbers ranging from 0 to 10, where 0 represents nothing; 0.5, very, very weak; and 10, very, very strong. With either scale, as the person is performing the exercise stress test, he or she is asked to select a number or expression that best corresponds to his or her feelings of exertion for the work being performed.[24]

Exercise and Activity Tolerance in Older Adults

As the population of older adults in Western societies increases, so does the concern over exercise and activity tolerance. Regular exercise benefits older adults through a variety of physical and psychosocial components.[5] These physical benefits include improved overall health and physical fitness, enhanced maximal aerobic capacity, prevention of a decline in the basal metabolic rate, gains in cerebral function, and improved balance and coordination. Psychologically, the older adult may experience a greater sense of well-being, increased opportunities for social interactions, lower rates of mortality, and fewer years of disability.

The capacity of older adults to undertake aerobic activities such as walking and running is adversely affected by advancing age. Current evidence supports a 5% to 15% decline per decade in $\dot{V}O_2$ max in men and women beginning at 25 years of age. Maximal heart rate decreases 6 to 10 beats/minute per decade, and it is this decrease in heart rate that is believed to contribute to a decreased cardiac output.[23,25] The decline in $\dot{V}O_2$ max seems to be due to both central and peripheral adaptations. Reductions in maximal heart rate, stroke volume, and lean body mass all contribute to a reduced $\dot{V}O_2$ max. Also contributing to a reduced $\dot{V}O_2$ max is a decrease in plasma volume, red blood cell count, and total blood volume.[23,26]

In terms of skeletal muscle function, there is a decrease in muscle mass (sarcopenia) and strength, flexibility and range of joint movement, and muscle endurance. There is a decrease in size of the individual muscles that occurs with aging, particularly beyond 60 years of age. Muscle strength and mass reportedly decline 30% to 50% between 30 and 80 years of age, with loss of muscle mass accounting for most of the decrease observed in muscle strength.[9,25] The most important factor in muscle atrophy in elderly persons is the reduction in type II fibres and the size of the muscle fibre areas. Muscle mass loss is subordinate to an age-related denervation of type II fibres, which removes the trophic effect on the fibres, leading to atrophy. Type I fibre collaterals expand to some of the denervated type II fibre areas in an attempt to lessen muscle fibre loss. This leads to an increase in type I motor neuron units at the expense of type II fibres, resulting in a reduction in muscle mass and muscle strength. There is also a slowing of muscle contraction and rate of force development, and reduced ability to accelerate limb movement. Changes in the elastic and collagen fibres of tendons and ligaments lead to decreased flexibility and loss of mobility and stability of the joints.[25]

As with exercise programs for younger persons, exercise programs for older persons should include an emphasis on aerobic activities, resistance training, flexibility or stretching exercises, and lifestyle changes.[5,23,25,26] Resistance exercise, which improves muscle strength, is particularly important for older adults. Most of the variance of walking speed in older adults is related to leg strength, and increased strength has been shown to increase walking endurance and stair climbing. Flexibility training is also important because limited range of motion in the hip, knee, and ankle joints increases the risk of falls and contributes to age-related changes in gait. Lifestyle modification involves finding opportunities within a person's existing routines to increase physical activity (*e.g.,* taking stairs rather than an elevator, parking farther from entrances).

IN SUMMARY

Physical activity and exercise denote the process of skeletal muscle movement and energy expenditure. There are two main types of exercise: aerobic and isometric. Aerobic, or endurance, exercise involves rhythmic changes in muscle length and increases the ability of muscles to use oxygen more efficiently so that the body can do more work with less cardiac and respiratory effort. Resistance, or strength, exercise involves the generation of force against low to moderate resistance, improves overall muscle strength and tone, and builds muscle mass. Flexibility, or stretching, exercise promotes flexibility and improves range of motion of the joints.

The body reacts to exercise by a series of physiologic responses that increase its level of performance. Heart rate, cardiac output, and stroke volume increase to deliver more blood to working muscles; minute ventilation and diffusion of oxygen and carbon dioxide increase to provide oxygen more efficiently to meet the rising metabolic demands; and local changes in the arterioles and capillaries contribute to enhanced perfusion of the working muscles. The maximal oxygen consumption ($\dot{V}O_2$ max), which is the volume of oxygen consumed (*i.e.,* litres/minute), is an important determinant of the person's capacity to perform work. Activity and exercise tolerance can be assessed in several ways, including through the use of paper-and-pencil tests

that measure subjective responses or through tests such as bicycle or treadmill ergometry that measure heart rate, $\dot{V}O_2$ max, and other responses during exercise.

The capacity of older adults to undertake aerobic activities such as walking and running is adversely affected by reductions in maximal heart rate, stroke volume, and $\dot{V}O_2$ max, along with a decrease in muscle mass and strength, flexibility and range of joint movement, and muscle endurance. Exercise programs for older persons should include an emphasis on aerobic activities, resistance training, flexibility or stretching exercises, and lifestyle changes.

ACTIVITY INTOLERANCE AND FATIGUE

After completing this section of the chapter, you should be able to meet the following objectives:

- Define fatigue and describe its manifestations.
- Differentiate acute from chronic fatigue.
- List at least four health problems that are associated with chronic fatigue.
- Define chronic fatigue syndrome and describe assessment findings, presenting symptoms, and laboratory values associated with the disorder.
- Discuss treatment modalities for chronic fatigue syndrome.

Activity intolerance can be viewed as not having sufficient physical or psychological energy reserve to endure or complete required or desired daily activities. Fatigue is the sensation that comes with having exhausted those energy reserves. It is a state that is experienced by everyone at some time in his or her life. Fatigue can be a normal physical response, such as that following extreme exercise in healthy people, or it can be a symptom that is experienced by people with limited exercise reserve, such as people with cardiac or respiratory disease, anemia, or malnutrition, or those on certain types of drug therapy. Fatigue also may be related to lack of sleep or mental stress.

Like nausea and pain, fatigue is a subjective symptom. It often is described as a feeling of tiredness or lack of energy and motivation that can vary in terms of intensity and duration and often is influenced by the time of day and a person's biorhythms. Fatigue is different from the normal tiredness that people experience at the end of the day. Tiredness is relieved by a good night's sleep, whereas fatigue persists despite sufficient or adequate sleep. Although fatigue is one of the most common symptoms reported to health care professionals, it is one of the least understood of all health problems. Ongoing research has expanded the understanding of both physiological and perceptual aspects; for example, fatigue has recently been differentiated along a continuum from tiredness to fatigue to exhaustion.[27]

Fatigue may be described in terms of its underlying physiologic basis, by its origin or cause, or by its patterns over time.[28] The physiologic basis of fatigue includes factors such as diaphragmatic, motor, and neurologic mechanisms. Diaphragmatic fatigue occurs in both acute and chronic respiratory conditions where the force and duration of muscle work exceeds muscle energy stores. Neuromuscular fatigue involves the loss of maximal capacity to generate force during exercise.

Mechanisms of Fatigue

The origin or cause of fatigue can be physiologic, psychological, pathologic, or unknown (*e.g.,* chronic fatigue syndrome). It can be caused by environmental factors (*e.g.,* excessive noise, temperature extremes, changes in weather); drug-related incidents (*e.g.,* use of tranquilizers, alcohol, toxic chemical exposure); treatment-related causes (*e.g.,* chemotherapy, radiation therapy, surgery, anesthesia, diagnostic testing); physical exertion (*e.g.,* exercise); and psychological factors (*e.g.,* stress, monotony).

ACTIVITY INTOLERANCE AND FATIGUE

- Activity intolerance is the inability of a person to complete activities because of insufficient psychological or physiologic energy.
- Fatigue is the sensation of having exhausted one's energy reserves.
- Acute fatigue is muscle fatigue with a rapid onset and duration limited to the duration of the exercise. The time it takes to develop acute fatigue at any level of exercise depends on conditioning.
- Chronic fatigue has an insidious onset, a long duration unrelated to duration of activity, and intensity not related to the intensity of activity.
- Chronic fatigue syndrome (CFS) is characterized by disabling fatigue and many nonspecific symptoms, including cognitive impairments, sleep disturbances, and musculoskeletal pain. The etiology of CFS is unknown, but it is associated with several chronic diseases such as fibromyalgia, depression, and irritable bowel syndrome.

Clinically, fatigue can be defined or described by its temporal patterns over time, such as acute (*e.g.,* less than 4 weeks) or chronic (*e.g.,* present for 50% of the day, or lasting 1 to 6 months or longer). It is thought that both acute and chronic fatigue can exist in the same person, similar to acute and chronic pain.

Acute Physical Fatigue

Acute fatigue has a rapid onset and is often defined as muscle fatigue associated with increased activity, or exercise, that is carried out to the point of exhaustion. It is relieved shortly after the activity ceases, and serves as a protective mechanism. It can also be associated with viral and bacterial infections and may present with other systemic symptoms such as fever

or malaise. Physical conditioning can influence the onset of acute fatigue. People who engage in regular exercise compared with sedentary persons are able to perform an activity for longer periods before acute fatigue develops. They probably are able to do so because their muscles use oxygen and nutrients more efficiently and their circulatory and respiratory systems are better able to deliver oxygen and nutrients to the exercising muscles.

Acute physical fatigue occurs more rapidly in deconditioned muscle. For example, acute fatigue often is seen in people who have been on bed rest because of a surgical procedure or in people who have had their activity curtailed because of chronic illness, such as heart or respiratory disease. In such cases, the acute fatigue often is out of proportion to the activity that is being performed (*e.g.,* dangling at the bedside, sitting in a chair for the first time). When resuming activity for the first time after a prolonged period of bed rest or inactivity, the person may experience tachycardia and hypotension. Unless these parameters are changed by medications such as β-adrenergic blocking drugs, heart rate and blood pressure become particularly sensitive indicators of activity tolerance or intolerance.

Another example of acute fatigue is that which occurs in people who require the use of assistive devices such as wheelchairs, walkers, or crutches. The upper arm muscles are less well adapted to prolonged exercise than the leg muscles. This is because arm muscles are primarily composed of type II muscle fibres. Type II muscle fibres, which are used when the body requires short bursts of energy, fatigue quickly. As a result, people who use wheelchairs or a pair of crutches may quickly experience fatigue until their arms become conditioned to the increased activity.

Chronic Fatigue

Chronic fatigue differs from acute fatigue in terms of onset, intensity, perception, duration, and relief. In contrast to acute fatigue, chronic fatigue has an insidious onset, is typically perceived as being unusually intense relative to the amount of activity performed, lasts longer than 1 month, has a cumulative effect, and is not relieved by cessation of activity.[29] It is one of the more common problems experienced by people with chronic health problems (Table 11.1). In the primary care setting, many patients present with chronic fatigue as their chief complaint. Some will have a primary cause for their fatigue, such as heart failure and emphysema, while others may have a primary psychiatric disorder. The remainder will either meet the criteria for diagnosis of chronic fatigue syndrome (to be discussed) or will remain undiagnosed.

Although acute fatigue often serves a protective function, chronic fatigue does not. It limits the amount of activity that a person can perform and may interfere with employment, the performance of activities of daily living, and the quality of life in general. Although fatigue often is viewed as a symptom of anxiety and depression, it is important to recognize that these psychological manifestations may be symptoms of the fatigue. For example, people with persistent fatigue due to a chronic

TABLE 11.1 CHRONIC ILLNESSES AND CAUSES OF CHRONIC FATIGUE

CHRONIC ILLNESS	CAUSE OF FATIGUE
Acquired immunodeficiency syndrome	Impaired immune function, anorexia, muscle weakness, and psychosocial factors associated with the disease
Anemia	Decreased oxygen-carrying capacity of blood
Arthritis	Pain and joint dysfunction lead to impaired mobility, loss of sleep, and emotional factors
Cancer	Presence of chemical products and catabolic processes associated with tumour growth; anorexia and difficulty eating; effects of chemotherapy and radiation therapy; and psychosocial factors such as depression, grieving, hopelessness, and fear
Cardiac disease	
Myocardial infarction	Death of myocardial tissue results in decreased cardiac output, poor tissue perfusion, and impaired delivery of oxygen and nutrients to vital organs
Heart failure	Impaired pumping ability of the heart results in poor perfusion of muscle tissue and vital organs
Neurologic disorders	
Multiple sclerosis	Demyelinating disease of CNS characterized by slowing of nerve conduction, resulting in lower extremity weakness and fatigue
Myasthenia gravis	Disorder of postsynaptic acetylcholine receptors of the myoneural junction, resulting in muscle weakness and fatigue
Chronic lung disease	Increased work of breathing and impaired gas exchange
Chronic renal failure	Accumulation of metabolic wastes; fluid, electrolyte, and acid–base disorders; decreased red blood cell count and oxygen-carrying capacity due to impaired erythropoietin production
Metabolic disorders	
Hypothyroidism	Decrease in basal metabolic rate manifested by fatigue
Diabetes mellitus	Impaired cellular use of glucose by muscle cells
Obesity	Imbalance in nutritional intake and energy expenditure; increased workload due to excess weight
Steroid myopathy	Glucocorticosteroids interfere with protein and glycogen synthesis, which leads to muscle wasting

illness may have to curtail their work schedules, decrease social activities, and limit their usual family responsibilities. These lifestyle changes may be the reasons for the depression rather than the depression being a cause of the fatigue.

Chronic fatigue occurs across a broad spectrum of disease states. It is a common complaint of persons with cancer, cardiac disease, end-stage renal disease, chronic lung disease, hepatitis C, arthritis, human immunodeficiency virus (HIV) infection and acquired immunodeficiency syndrome (AIDS), and neurologic disorders such as multiple sclerosis, postpolio syndrome, and Parkinson disease.

Chronic fatigue is almost a universal phenomenon in persons with cancer, with prevalence rates ranging from 40% to 100%, depending on the form of treatment and stage of disease.[30] Cancer-related fatigue may be caused by the disease itself, or it may be caused by treatment. In fact, the majority of persons undergoing cancer chemotherapy or radiation therapy have reported significant fatigue during the course of treatment.[30] Cancer-related fatigue involves a number of physiologic, sensory, affective, and cognitive dimensions. There is often a sensation of feeling unusually tired with generalized weakness and a greater need for rest. There may also be a disturbing lack of motivation, anxiety, and sadness as well as an inability to concentrate or difficulty in thinking.

There are several types of cancer-related factors that may cause fatigue, the most prominent of which are factors related to energy imbalance. They include anemia, cachexia,

stress, pain, infection, medications, and metabolic disorders.[30] The cytokine theory of cancer-related fatigue is based on the observation that patients receiving agents such as interferon-α as part of their treatment plan experienced devastating fatigue that appears to be dose limited. Interferon-α and other agents used to treat cancer also influence the release of other cytokines that are related to fatigue. Cancer cells and the immune system appear to produce or express a number of cytokines with the potential for manufacturing many of the factors that contribute to fatigue, particularly interleukin-1 (IL-1), tumour necrosis factor-α (TNF-α), and potentially interleukin-6 (IL-6).[31] TNF-α is thought to interfere with appetite, produce weight loss, and cause depletion of skeletal muscle protein stores. As a result, muscle wasting occurs, and people have to expend more energy to perform simple activities such as sitting and standing.

Management. Many pathologic factors associated with fatigue, including insomnia, anemia, psychological stress, and wasting or weakness, respond to appropriate treatment measures.[30] Anemia, which is common among persons with HIV/AIDS, patients with end-stage renal disease, and cancer patients receiving chemotherapy, causes fatigue by interfering with the oxygen-carrying capacity of the blood. It can often be treated with recombinant forms of erythropoietin (epoetin-alfa), an endogenous hormone normally produced by the kidney (see Chapter 14). Insomnia, which occurs for a number of reasons, including anxiety and depression, hot flashes, nocturia, and pain, is often amenable to nonpharmacologic and pharmacologic methods of treatment. Psychological disturbances, such as anxiety and depression, which are frequently associated with fatigue, can be treated with selected pharmacologic agents. Another cause of fatigue is loss of muscle mass, muscle strength, and endurance. This type of fatigue is common among persons with forced immobility, musculoskeletal disorders such as arthritis, neuromuscular disorders such as multiple sclerosis, and wasting syndromes such as HIV/AIDS. Aerobic exercise has been shown to decrease this type of fatigue.[2]

Chronic Fatigue Syndrome

Chronic fatigue syndrome (CFS)—also known as myalgic encephalomyelitis (ME) or the newly proposed term, Systemic Exertion Intolerance Disease (SEID)—is a condition of profound disabling fatigue that is typically accompanied by an array of self-reported, nonspecific symptoms such as cognitive impairments, sleep disturbances, and musculoskeletal pain. In the late 20th century and now into the 21st century, the disorder continues to be a relatively common problem in both adolescents and adults.[29,32–34]

Definition. Because the etiology of CFS is unknown, there are no biologic markers for the diagnosis of CFS, and there are no definitive treatments. Furthermore, the overlap of symptoms of CFS with other functional disorders such as fibromyalgia, multiple chemical sensitivities, depression, and irritable bowel syndrome, which also are characterized by fatigue, complicates the ability to define the syndrome with any degree of certainty. In fact, CFS may describe a group of similar symptoms that develop with different pathophysiologic disturbances.

Because of the need for diagnostic criteria, the case definition for CFS was established in 1988 by the US Center for Disease Control (CDC). The revised Canadian Clinical Case definition was established in 2010, and the latest criteria were released from the American Institute of Medicine in 2015.[34] To be classified as CFS, the fatigue must be clinically evaluated, cause severe mental and physical exhaustion, and result in a significant reduction in the individual's premorbid activity level. In addition, there must be evidence of cognitive impairment and/or orthostatic intolerance. The fatigue and concurrent symptoms must be of 6 months' duration or longer. Chart 11.1 outlines the newest criteria for diagnosis of this serious, complex, and multisystem disease, which is no longer a diagnosis of exclusion but can be applied to patients with other conditions (*e.g.*, fibromyalgia, depression).[34]

Pathophysiology. Theories of the pathogenesis of CFS include infections, psychological disorders, a dysfunction in the hypothalamic–pituitary–adrenal axis, or an alteration in the autonomic nervous system.[29,32,33] Despite much research and the development of several theories, the underlying pathophysiology of CFS remains elusive. Many people with CFS attribute the onset of their disease to an influenza-like infection. Thus, the link between infectious agents such as Epstein–Barr virus, human herpesvirus 6, enterovirus, and others has been

---

CHART 11.1 CRITERIA FOR DIAGNOSIS OF CHRONIC FATIGUE SYNDROME

The patient (child or adult) must have the following three symptoms:

- New onset of profound fatigue causing a significant decrease or impairment in the ability to engage in pre-illness levels of occupational, educational, social, or personal activities that persists for ≥6 months and is not due to ongoing excessive exertion or is not substantially alleviated by rest
- Post-exertional malaise (worsening of symptoms after physical, cognitive, or emotional activity)
- Unrefreshing sleep

The patient must also exhibit at least one of the following two symptoms:

- Cognitive impairment
- Orthostatic intolerance

Overall these symptoms should be present at least half the time with moderate, substantial, or severe intensity.

Developed from Committee on the diagnostic criteria for myalgic encephalomyelitis/chronic fatigue syndrome—Institute of Medicine. (2015). *Beyond myalgic encephalomyelitis/chronic fatigue syndrome redefining an illness.* Washington, DC: The National Academies Press.

---

extensively studied. To date, however, none of these agents has been conclusively linked in a cause-and-effect relationship with the development of CFS.[29,33] Several studies have also suggested that CFS may be due to a primary alteration in immune function. A number of immunologic abnormalities have been described in persons with CFS. It is hypothesized that the immune system may overreact to an environmental agent (most likely an infectious agent) or internal stimuli and be unable to self-regulate after the infectious insult is over. It has also been suggested that cytokines such as interleukin (IL)-6 might have an important role in CFS because they are also involved in the stress response and are crucial inducers of some of the manifestations of the disorder, such as sleepiness, anorexia, mild fever, and increased sensitivity to pain.[29]

Psychological disorders often are associated with CFS, especially anxiety and depression, but this is difficult to evaluate. Persons with CFS are more likely than the general population to have experienced a psychological disorder such as major depression or panic disorder before the development of CFS; however, it also is true that a significant proportion of those persons with CFS have not had such episodes, either before or after the development of CFS.[34]

Abnormalities of the hypothalamic–pituitary–adrenal axis, such as attenuated activity of corticotropin-releasing hormone and changes in the circadian rhythm of cortisol secretion, have been documented. However, these findings remain unexplained. Also, while it is noted that this disorder is more common in women, and a familial predisposition has been demonstrated, no definitive genetic abnormalities, including mitochondrial energy metabolism, have been identified.[29,32,33]

Manifestations. One of the most important findings in persons with CFS is the complaint of fatigue. Often, the symptom of fatigue is preceded by a cold or flulike illness. Frequently, the person describes the illness as recurring, with periods of exacerbations and remissions. With each subsequent episode of the illness, the fatigue increases.

Physical findings can include low-grade fever. The fever is intermittent and occurs only when the illness recurs. Other findings include nonexudative pharyngitis, palpable and tender cervical lymph nodes, a mildly enlarged thyroid gland, wheezing, splenomegaly, myalgia, arthralgia, and heme-positive stool with subsequent negative sigmoidoscopy.

Psychological problems include impaired cognition, which the person describes as an inability to concentrate and perform previously mundane tasks. There are reports of mood and sleep disturbances, balance problems, visual disturbances, and various degrees of anxiety and depression.

Diagnosis and Treatment. The diagnosis of CFS is based on integration of the entire clinical picture of the client's symptoms, physical assessment findings, and the results of diagnostic tests. Laboratory investigations are used to detect other disorders.[32]

Because there is no known cause of CFS, current treatment tends to remain symptomatic, with a focus on management rather than cure. It centres on education, emotional support, treatment of symptoms, and overall management of general health. Symptom management includes development of an exercise program that helps the person regain strength. Along with a structured activity program, persons should be encouraged to be as active as possible as they resume their activities of daily living.[29,32]

A holistic approach to the treatment of CFS is essential. With proper treatment and support, most persons with CFS demonstrate improvement. However, relapses can occur. Persons diagnosed with CFS must continue to receive follow-up care and treatment on a regular basis. Local and national support groups are available for persons who experience CFS.

IN SUMMARY

Fatigue is a nonspecific, self-recognized state of physical and psychological exhaustion. It results in the person's not being able to perform routine activities and is not relieved with sleep or rest. Acute fatigue results from excessive use of the body or specific muscle groups and often is related to depletion of energy sources. Chronic fatigue often is associated with a specific disease or chronic illness and may be relieved when the effects of the disease are corrected. CFS is a complex illness that has physiologic and psychological manifestations. It is characterized by debilitating fatigue. Diagnosis often is made by a process of elimination, and treatment requires a holistic approach.

BED REST AND IMMOBILITY

After completing this section of the chapter, you should be able to meet the following objectives:

- Describe the effects of immobility and prolonged bed rest on cardiovascular, pulmonary, renal, metabolic, musculoskeletal, gastrointestinal, and sensory functions.
- Describe the time course of the physiologic changes associated with immobility and prolonged bed rest.
- Identify physical assessment findings that are related to the effects of immobility and prolonged bed rest.
- Describe treatment interventions that counteract the negative effects of immobility and prolonged bed rest.

Bed rest is one of the oldest and most commonly used methods of treatment for various medical conditions. Historically, it was felt that bed rest was imperative for people convalescing from almost any illness. For example, before the 1940s, bed rest was prescribed for 2 weeks after childbirth, 3 weeks after herniorrhaphy, and 4 to 6 weeks after myocardial infarction. It was believed that the complex biochemical and physical demands of physical activity diverted energy from the restorative and reparative processes of healing. However when the cardiovascular, musculoskeletal, integumentary, and pulmonary manifestation of bed rest were identified, it was discovered that early mobilization lessened complications and improved patient outcomes.

Today it is known that bed rest and immobility are the antithesis of exercise and mobility. They defy the active use of skeletal muscles, movement against gravity, conservation of body fluids, normal distribution of blood flow, and maintenance of cardiopulmonary reserves. Immobility may be dictated by an injury that requires stabilization to facilitate the healing process, or it may result from conditions that limit physical reserve. The effects of immobility can be seen in a single extremity that has been stabilized by a cast; involve both legs, as in a person confined to a wheelchair; or involve the entire body, as in a person confined to bed rest. Bed rest and immobility are associated with various complications that include generalized weakness, orthostatic intolerance, atelectasis, pneumonia, thromboemboli, urinary retention, constipation, muscle atrophy, osteoporosis, and impaired sensory perception (Table 11.2).[35-39] This section of the chapter focuses on the physiologic changes that occur with bed rest and immobility and the interventions to counteract their effects.

Physiologic Effects of Bed Rest

The supine position that often accompanies immobility and bed rest interferes with the effects of gravity and exercise stimuli (Fig. 11.4). While in the upright position, the body compensates for the effects of gravity in a variety of ways. The skeletal muscles contract and exert pressure against veins and lymph vessels, counteracting the hydrostatic effects of

TABLE 11.2 COMPLICATIONS OF BED REST AND IMMOBILITY

SYSTEM	COMPLICATION
Cardiovascular	Increased heart rate; decreased cardiac output and stroke volume contributing to decreased aerobic capacity; decreased size of the heart; decreased left ventricular end-diastolic volume; unchanged systolic-diastolic blood pressure; decreased fluid volume; orthostatic intolerance; venous thrombophlebitis
Pulmonary	Mechanical resistance to breathing; reduced cardiopulmonary functional capacity; relative hypoxemia; pneumonia
Musculoskeletal	Muscle atrophy and loss of strength and endurance; decreased strength of tendons and ligaments and their insertions on bone; decreased muscle oxidative capacity contributing to decreased aerobic capacity; osteoporosis (bone loss); contractures; immobilization hypercalcemia; osteoarthritis
Gastrointestinal	Loss of appetite; constipation; dyspepsia
Genitourinary	Incontinence; renal calculi; urinary stasis and infection; electrolyte imbalance
Hematologic	Decreased total fluid volume; increased blood viscosity; thromboembolism
Metabolic and endocrine	Glucose intolerance; hyperglycemia; hyperinsulinemia; increased parathyroid hormone production
Skin	Pressure ulcers
Functional	Impaired ambulation and activity tolerance; impaired balance and coordination
Psychological	Sensory deprivation; altered sensory perception; confusion and disorientation; anxiety; depression; decreased intellectual capacity

Developed from information in Harper C. M., Lyles Y. M. (1988). Physiology and complications of bed rest. *Journal of the American Geriatrics Society,* 36:1047–1054.

FIGURE 11.4 • The effects of gravity and decreased use of the skeletal muscles during bed rest and assumption of the supine position on cardiovascular, respiratory, and renal function, and their impact on exercise tolerance and the risk of complications such as thromboembolism and postural hypotension.

BED REST AND IMMOBILITY

- The cardiovascular responses to bed rest include a redistribution of blood volume from the lower body to the central circulation, a deconditioning of the heart, and a reduction in total body water. Orthostatic intolerance may develop.
- Venous stasis due to bed rest encourages the development of deep vein thrombosis.
- Pulmonary changes due to bed rest include decreased tidal volume and functional residual capacity. Alveoli tend to collapse, resulting in areas of decreased pulmonary ventilation.
- Bed rest increases the risk for development of renal calculi and urinary tract infections.
- Muscle mass is reduced owing to disuse atrophy and bone mass is reduced because of an imbalance of activity between osteoclasts (bone resorption) and osteoblasts (bone generation).
- Pressure ulcers due to tissue ischemia may develop in areas in constant contact with the bed surface.
- Psychological effects of bed rest include anxiety and depression and decreased ability to concentrate and learn.

gravity that cause blood and fluid to pool in the lower extremities. Movement against the forces of gravity maintains muscle tone and bones remain stronger because longitudinal weight bearing keeps essential minerals, such as calcium, inside the structure of the bone.

Cardiovascular Responses

After a period of bed rest and assumption of the supine position, the cardiovascular system exhibits changes that reflect the loss of gravitational and exercise stimuli. These changes include (1) a redistribution and change in blood volume, (2) increased cardiac workload, (3) orthostatic hypotension, and (4) venous stasis with the potential for development of deep vein thrombosis.

One of the most striking responses to assumption of the supine position during bed rest is the redistribution of and change in blood volume. When a patient is maintained in the supine position longer than 24 hours, approximately 1 L of fluid is redistributed from the lower extremities to the central circulation. Most of this blood is diverted to the thoracic cavity; a smaller portion is diverted to the arms and head.[37–39] A major cardiovascular manifestation of bed rest is an increased workload on the heart. The increase in thoracic blood volume that occurs on assumption of the supine position results in an increase in central venous pressure and left ventricular end-diastolic volume, and an increase in stroke volume and cardiac output through the Frank–Starling mechanism (see Chapter 21). In the supine position, the normal cardiac output is 7 to 8 L/minute, compared with a cardiac output of 5 to 6 L/minute for a person in the standing position. Initially, the

increase in cardiac output is accompanied by a slight decrease in heart rate and systemic vascular resistance and maintenance of arterial blood pressure.

With extended periods of bed rest, there is an increase in venous distension; this leads to a decrease in venous return to the heart, along with a stabilization of the stroke volume and cardiac output. The heart rate, however, continues to increase. During periods of tachycardia, the diastolic filling time is decreased; as a result, the heart has to expend more energy and use more oxygen to perfuse vital organs and meet the metabolic demands of the body. This response is exaggerated when a person has to assume the upright position and begin activity after a prolonged period of bed rest. When a person begins submaximal exercise after prolonged bed rest, heart rate increases while stroke volume and cardiac output decrease. Between 5 and 10 weeks of reconditioning exercise is required for return of heart rate, stroke volume, and cardiac output parameters to their levels before bed rest.[37]

Bed rest also affects fluid balance. The increase in central blood volume results in an inhibition of antidiuretic hormone and aldosterone, with a resultant water and sodium diuresis. In the supine position, diuresis begins on the first day with the shift of blood from the lower extremities to the thoracic cavity. The loss of water and sodium results in an increase in hematocrit, hemoglobin, and red blood cell mass owing to the loss of plasma volume.[39] After approximately 4 days of bed rest, fluid losses reach an equilibrium. A possible explanation for this is that fluid is lost from the vascular compartment with a subsequent shift of fluid from the interstitial to the vascular fluid compartment. With a decrease in the interstitial fluid volume and the reestablishment of intravascular volume, the stimuli for salt and water diuresis are lost.

Orthostatic Hypotension. During bed rest, the forces of gravity and hydrostatic pressure are removed from the cardiovascular system. After 3 to 4 days of bed rest, resumption of the upright position results in orthostatic or postural intolerance. Standing after prolonged bed rest results in a decrease in central blood volume as blood is displaced to the lower extremities and dependent parts of the body. Decreases in stroke volume and cardiac output occur along with increases in heart rate and systemic vascular resistance. The signs and symptoms of postural intolerance include tachycardia, nausea, diaphoresis, and sometimes syncope or fainting (discussed in Chapter 23).[39]

The mechanism of orthostatic intolerance after bed rest involves multiple factors, including a decrease in vascular volume, a decline in skeletal muscle pump function, reduced sympathetic innervation of the resistance vessels, and resetting of the baroreceptors that control blood pressure. Because changes in plasma volume do not fully explain the orthostatic intolerance that occurs with bed rest, it is thought that the baroreceptors and sympathetic nervous system influence this response. It has also been suggested that the decrease in stroke volume that occurs with assumption of the upright position after bed rest may be due to a reduction in left ventricular size and distensibility that occurs in response to a decrease in loading conditions of the heart.[40]

Venous Stasis. Venous stasis in the legs results from a lack of the skeletal muscle pump function that promotes venous return to the heart. The skeletal muscle pump function decreases after assumption of the supine position, and there is mechanical compression of veins from the position of the lower extremities against the bed. This increased pressure can cause damage to the vessel intima, predisposing to platelet adherence and clot formation (see Chapter 13).[39]

The development of deep vein thrombosis (DVT) is a major complication of bed rest. It is believed that three factors (often referred to as the *Virchow triad*) combine to predispose a person to DVT (see Chapter 22). These factors are (1) stasis of venous flow due to inactivity of the skeletal muscle pumps, (2) a hypercoagulability state resulting from a decrease in vascular volume and an increase in blood viscosity and concentration of blood coagulation factors, and (3) vessel injury resulting from external pressure from the mattress against the veins. The development of DVT also predisposes to the development of pulmonary emboli. With resumption of activity, there is risk that large thrombi may dislodge, work their way through the circulatory system, and lodge in the pulmonary vessel.[39]

Pulmonary Responses

Assumption of the supine position produces changes in lung volumes and the mechanics of breathing that can contribute to respiratory complications such as atelectasis, accumulation of secretions, hypoxemia, and pneumonia.[39] In the supine position, breathing largely depends on the abdominal muscles rather than on movement of the chest cage; the diaphragm moves upward rather than downward, decreasing the size of the thoracic compartment, and chest and lung expansion are limited because of the resistance of the bed. As a result, the tidal volume and functional residual capacity are decreased, and the efficiency and effectiveness of ventilation are hindered. Thus, persons on bed rest need to work harder to breathe, and consequently they take fewer deep breaths.

A reduction in functional residual capacity predisposes to airway collapse, ventilation–perfusion inequalities, and impaired oxygen transport. Alveoli tend to collapse, resulting in areas of atelectasis and a decrease in the surface area for gas exchange (see Chapter 29). This may result in arteriovenous shunting along with a decrease in arterial oxygenation. Also, poor fluid intake and dehydration may cause secretions to become thick and tenacious. Stasis of secretions provides an ideal medium for bacterial growth and increases the risk for development of pneumonia. Reduced activity and the recumbent position inhibit coughing, foster the retention of secretions, and adversely affect secretion distribution in the airways. Coughing and deep breathing are necessary to prevent accumulation of secretions and airway collapse.

Urinary Tract Responses

The kidneys are designed to function optimally with the body in the erect position (Fig. 11.5). The anatomy of the kidney is such that urine flows from the kidney pelvis by gravity,

FIGURE 11.5 • Effect of body position on urine flow in the kidney.

whereas the action of peristalsis moves urine through the ureters to the bladder. Prolonged bed rest affects the renal system by altering the composition of body fluids and predisposing to the development of kidney stones. In the supine position, urine is not readily drained from the renal pelvis. Bed rest also may predispose to urinary tract infections and urinary incontinence because of positional changes and difficulty in emptying the bladder.[41]

A major complication of prolonged bed rest is the increased risk for development of kidney stones. Prolonged bed rest causes muscle atrophy, protein breakdown, and decalcification of bone with the development of hypercalcemia and hyperphosphatemia. Saturation of the urine with calcium salts (*i.e.,* calcium oxalate and calcium phosphate) coupled with urinary stasis increases the risk for the development of calcium-containing kidney stones (see Chapter 33). Dehydration further increases urine concentration of stone-forming elements and risk of kidney stone formation.[41]

Urinary tract infections and incontinence also may occur. The cause of incontinence is inadequate emptying of the bladder while the person is in the supine position. This position contributes to stagnation of urine in the bladder and may predispose the person to bladder and urinary tract infections.

Musculoskeletal Responses

Musculoskeletal responses to bed rest and immobility reflect changes associated with the loss of both gravitational and exercise stress. In addition to a loss of strength, muscles atrophy, change shape and appearance, and shorten when immobilized. Disuse atrophy can lead to loss of approximately one eighth of the muscle's strength with each week of disuse.[42] These changes affect individual muscle fibres and total muscle mass.

Immobilization also causes a reduction in force-generating capacity along with increased fatigability, primarily owing to a decrease in muscle mass and the cross-sectional area of muscle fibre. There also is a decrease in the oxidative capacity of the muscle mitochondria. Because of the decreased oxidative capacity of the mitochondria, muscles fatigue more easily.[38,42] The larger and better trained the muscle, the faster the loss of muscle strength and the quicker the deconditioning occurs.

Leg muscles tend to lose strength more rapidly than arm muscles, but it is not clear whether this is because legs are relatively better trained than arms, have a larger muscle mass, or because bed rest results in a greater decrease in activity for legs than arms.

Along with muscle, the supporting connective tissues undergo changes when subjected to immobility or bed rest. Periarticular connective tissue, ligaments, tendons, and articular cartilage require motion to maintain health. Changes in structure and function of connective tissue become apparent 4 to 6 days after immobilization and remain even after normal activity has been resumed. It is believed that changes in the structure of collagen fibres contribute to the connective tissue changes associated with immobility.[8,23,42]

Muscle atrophy and disuse not only contribute to wasting and weakening of muscle tissue, they play a role in the development of joint *contractures*. A contracture is the abnormal shortening of muscle tissue and connective tissue, rendering the muscle highly resistant to stretch. Contractures occur when muscles do not have the necessary strength to maintain their integrity (*i.e.*, their proper function and full range of motion). Contractures mainly develop over joints when there is an imbalance in the muscle strength of the antagonistic muscle groups. If allowed to progress, the contracture eventually involves the muscle groups, tendons, ligaments, and joint capsule. The joint becomes limited in its full use and range of motion.

Another consequence of prolonged immobility and bed rest for the musculoskeletal system is the loss of bone mineralization. Bone is a dynamic tissue that undergoes continual deposition and replacement of minerals in response to the dual stimuli of weight bearing and muscle pull. According to the Wolff law, the density of bone is directly proportional to the stress placed on it.

The maintenance of normal bone function depends on two types of cells: osteoblasts and osteoclasts. Osteoblasts function in building the osseous matrix of the bone, and osteoclasts function in the breakdown of the bone matrix (see Chapter 56). Osteoblasts depend on the stress of mobility and weight bearing to perform their function. During immobility and bed rest, the building of new bone stops, but the osteoclasts continue to perform their function. When bone experiences a lack of stress, as occurs with bed rest or immobility, there is a greater amount of bone resorption than bone formation, resulting in loss of bone mineralization.[42] The degree to which bone demineralization can be reversed is not known; however, permanent loss of bone mass and osteoporosis can result from long-term immobilization.

Osteoporosis represents an increase in skeletal porosity resulting from reduced bone mass. The bones may easily compress and become deformed. Because of the lack of structural firmness, the bones may easily fracture. The best measure to prevent the occurrence of osteoporosis is to begin weight-bearing exercises as soon as possible. The type of exercise that is performed is particularly important because load magnitude influences bone density more than the number of load cycles.

Metabolic, Endocrine, and Immune Responses

Metabolic Responses. Metabolic and endocrine changes reflect the absence of both gravitational and exercise stimulation during bed rest and immobility. The basal metabolic rate drops in response to decreased energy requirements of the body.[41] Anabolic processes are slowed, and catabolic processes become accelerated. Protein breakdown occurs and leads to a protein deficiency and a negative nitrogen balance. Persons in a negative nitrogen balance experience nausea and anorexia, which contribute to the catabolic state.

Endocrine Responses. In general, bed rest results in an uncoupling of hormonal stimulation and target organ unresponsiveness. Thyroid hormone concentrations tend to fluctuate; insulin levels are reduced, and cortisol levels tend to increase. A major hormonal change that occurs with prolonged periods of bed rest and immobility is an increase in the serum parathyroid hormone (PTH).[41] The increased level of PTH is related to the hypercalcemia that occurs secondary to immobility.

Persons who experience prolonged periods of bed rest often have changes in the circadian release of various hormones. Normally, insulin and growth hormone peak twice a day. In people who experienced 30 days of bed rest, a single daily peak of these hormones occurred. Other hormonal changes include an afternoon peak of epinephrine rather than the normal early morning peak, and an early morning peak of aldosterone rather than the usual noonday peak that is seen in normally active persons.

The person on bed rest also experiences an impaired responsiveness to the actions of insulin. The reason for this intolerance is not due to lack of insulin, but rather to an increased resistance to the action of insulin that then results in a hyperglycemic and hyperinsulinemic state. Possible reasons for the unresponsiveness of glucose to hyperinsulinemia include defects in suppression of hepatic glucose production, defects in insulin stimulation of glucose uptake by peripheral tissues, or both. Insulin also plays a role in regulating protein metabolism by inhibiting protein breakdown. This induced insulin resistance may explain the negative nitrogen balance seen in patients who experience prolonged bed rest.[41]

Immune Responses. The immune system also is subject to physiologic changes associated with bed rest or immobility. Research demonstrates that there is an increase in IL-1, IL-6, and TNF-α production (see Chapter 18). An increase in these mediators has been associated with hyperinflammatory reactions and tissue injury or wasting.[42,43] Increased IL-1 production contributes to the bone and mineral loss that occurs during bed rest. Also seen is decreased IL-2 secretion, which may play a part in the infectious diseases that often occur during periods of bed rest.[42]

Gastrointestinal Responses

Gastrointestinal responses to bed rest vary. Loss of appetite, slowed rate of absorption, and distaste for food combine to contribute to nutritional hypoproteinemia. Passage of food through the gastrointestinal tract is slowed when the person is placed in the supine position. In a supine position the transit time of food through the stomach decreases by 66%, and gastric secretions can collect and rest against the lower esophageal sphincter, leading to irritation and symptoms of dyspepsia. Also, the loss of plasma volume and dehydration can combine to exacerbate gastrointestinal problems. Thus, constipation and fecal impaction are frequent complications that occur when persons experience prolonged periods of immobility and bed rest. With inactivity, there is slowed movement of feces through the colon. The act of defecation requires the integration of the abdominal muscles, the diaphragm, and the levator ani. Muscle atrophy and loss of tone occur in the immobilized person and interfere with the normal act of defecation. Lack of privacy and the supine position may also compound problems with defecation.[41]

Sensory Responses

Bed rest and immobility reduce the quality and quantity of sensory information available from kinesthetic, visual, auditory, and tactile sensation. It also reduces the person's ability to interact with the environment and contributes to impaired sensory responses. Common occurrences include impaired sense of motion and limb movement, visual and auditory hallucinations, vivid dreams, inefficient thought processes, loss of contact with reality, and alteration in tactile stimulation.

In addition to sensory deprivation related to prolonged bed rest and immobility, persons may experience a sensory monotony from the hospital environment. Repetitious and meaningless sounds from cardiac monitors, respirators, and hospital personnel, along with an environment that may be void of a normal day–night cycle, also contribute to impaired sensory perception.

Skin Responses

Except for the soles of the feet, the skin is not designed for weight bearing. However, during bed rest, the large surface area of the skin bears weight and is in constant contact with the surface of the bed. Constant pressure is transmitted to the skin, subcutaneous tissue, and muscle, especially to those tissues over bony prominences. This constant contact causes increased pressure and impairs normal capillary blood flow, which interferes with the exchange of nutrients and waste products. Tissue ischemia and necrosis may result and lead to the development of pressure ulcers. Also contributing to the development of pressure ulcers is moisture from skin that is in constant contact with bed linens, along with the forces of friction and shear that occur when the person is repositioned in bed (see Chapter 61).[42]

Psychosocial Responses

Immobility often sets the stage for changes in the person's response to illness. Persons adapt to prolonged bed rest and immobility through a series of physiologic responses and through changes in affect, perception, and cognition. Affective changes include increased anxiety, fear, depression, hostility, rapid mood changes, and alterations in normal sleep patterns. These changes in mood occur with hospitalized patients who are subjected to periods of prolonged bed rest and immobility, and in persons in confinement, such as astronauts and prisoners. Research on immobilized or isolated persons has demonstrated that the motivation to learn decreases with periods of prolonged immobility, as does the ability to learn and retain new material and transfer newly learned material to a different situation.

Prolonged bed rest and immobility also contribute to the social isolation of the hospitalized person. Confined to a hospital bed, the person is unable to assume certain societal roles. The roles of spouse, parent, sibling, worker, and friend are altered either temporarily or permanently while the person is hospitalized. People may respond to this isolation by exhibiting various effective and ineffective coping behaviours, including increased anxiety, depression, restlessness, fear, and rapid mood changes.[42]

Time Course of Physiologic Responses

The deconditioning responses to the inactivity of immobility and bed rest affect all body systems. One of the important factors to keep in mind is the rapidity with which the changes occur and the length of time required to overcome these effects. The body responds in a characteristic pattern to the effects of the supine position and bed rest. During the first 3 days of bed rest, one of the first changes to occur is a massive diuresis. Accompanying the diuresis are increases in serum osmolality, hematocrit, venous compliance, and urinary sodium and chloride excretion. Fluid losses stabilize by approximately the fourth day. By days 4 to 7, there are changes in the hemolytic system. Fibrinogen and fibrinolytic activity increase, and clotting time is prolonged. The cardiovascular system responds with a decrease in cardiac output and stroke volume. The basal metabolic rate decreases and glucose intolerance and a negative nitrogen balance begin to develop.[39–42]

Additional effects on the hemolytic system are observed on days 8 to 14. Red blood cell number is decreased and the phagocytic ability of leukocytes is reduced. There is a decrease in lean body mass and, after 15 days of bed rest, osteoporosis and hypercalciuria occur. Aerobic power decreases, the cyclic excretion of some hormones is changed, and the person's thought patterns and sensory perception are altered.[39–42]

Interventions

A holistic approach should be taken when caring for persons who are immobile or require prolonged periods of bed rest. Interventions and treatment should include actions that address the person's physical and psychosocial needs. The goals of care for the immobilized person include structuring a safe environment in which the person is not at risk for complications; providing diversional activities to offset problems with sensory deprivation; and preventing complications of bed rest by implementing an interdisciplinary plan of care that includes repositioning schedules, prophylactic interventions to prevent DVT, and consultation with various disciplines to provide a comprehensive approach to care and treatment.

IN SUMMARY

During the last 75 years, the use of bed rest has undergone a complete reversal as a standard of treatment for a variety of medical conditions. Over time, research findings have described the deleterious consequences of inactivity. All body systems are affected by complications of immobility and prolonged bed rest.

The responses to bed rest and immobility affect all body systems. One of the important factors is the rapidity with which the changes occur and the long time required to overcome the effects of prolonged bed rest and immobility. Adverse effects of prolonged immobility and bed rest include a decreased cardiac output, orthostatic intolerance, dehydration, and sensory deprivation, as well as the potential for development of thrombophlebitis, pneumonia, kidney stones, and pressure ulcers.

REVIEW EXERCISES

1. A 60-year-old man sustains an acute myocardial infarction (heart attack). He has been discharged from the hospital and is about to enter a phase II cardiac rehabilitation program. On his first day of the program he is being examined for his tolerance to the exercise program.
    A. *One of the tests that he is scheduled to undergo is the treadmill stress test. How will this test contribute to the evaluation of his ability to engage in exercise?*
    B. *What other subjective tests might be used to determine his exercise tolerance?*

2. A 40-year-old woman who is being treated with chemotherapy for breast cancer complains of excessive fatigue and activity intolerance. She claims she has so little energy she can hardly get up in the morning and has difficulty concentrating and doing such simple activities as shopping.
    A. *What are some of the possible explanations for this woman's excessive fatigue?*
    B. *What types of medical tests might be done to identify possible causes of fatigue?*
    C. *What types of treatment might be used to alleviate some of her symptoms?*

3. A 23-year-old man, who has sustained multiple fractures and contusions in a motorcycle accident, is confined to bed rest in the supine position. He has been on bed rest for 2 days and has lost about 500 ml of extracellular fluid volume because of diuresis.
    A. *Explain the physiologic rationale for the excessive diuresis.*
    B. *Identify two complications of bed rest that might occur as the result of this loss of extracellular fluid volume.*
    C. *Upon getting out of bed on the fourth day he suddenly turns pale, has an increase in heart rate, and complains of dizziness. What has happened to this man?*

References

1. Thompson D., Karpe F., Lafontan M., Frayn K. (2012). Physical activity and exercise in the regulation of human adipose tissue physiology. *Physiological Reviews, 92*(1), 157–191.
2. Pescatello L. S., Arean R., Riebe D., et al. (2014). *ACSM's guidelines for exercise testing and prescription* (9th ed.). Philadelphia, PA: Lippincott Williams & Wilkins.
3. Witzmann F. A. (2013). Chapter 29: Exercise physiology. In Rhoades R. A., Bell D. R. (Eds.), *Medical physiology* (4th ed.). Philadelphia, PA: Lippincott Williams & Wilkins.
4. Garber C. E., Blissmer B., Deschenes M. R., et al. (2011). American college of sports medicine position stand. Quantity and quality of exercise for developing and maintaining cardiorespiratory, musculoskeletal, and neuromotor fitness in apparently healthy adults: Guidance for prescribing exercise. *Medicine and Science in Sports and Exercise, 43*(7), 1334–1359.
5. Canadian Society for Exercise Physiology (CSEP). (2015). *Canadian physical activity guidelines.* [Online] Available: http://www.csep.ca/english/view.asp?x=804. Accessed on February 14, 2015.
6. Westcott W. L. (2012). Resistance training is medicine: Effects of strength training on health. *Current Sports Medicine Reports, 11*(4), 209–216.
7. Smith D. L., Fernhall B. (2011). *Advanced cardiovascular exercise physiology.* Champaign, IL: Human Kinetics.
8. McArdle W. D., Katch F. I., Katch V. L. (2015). *Exercise physiology: Nutrition, energy and human performance* (8th ed.). Philadelphia, PA: Lippincott, Williams & Wilkins.
9. Klabunde R. E. (2012). *Cardiovascular physiology concepts* (2nd ed.). Philadelphia, PA: Lippincott Williams & Wilkins.
10. Delaney C. L., Miller M. D., Allan R. B., et al. (2014). The impact of different supervised exercise regimens on endothelial function in patients with intermittent claudication. *Vascular,* 1–9. doi: 10.1177/1708538114558329 [Epub ahead of print].
11. Padilla J., Simmons G. H., Bender S. B., et al. (2011). Vascular effects of exercise: Endothelial adaptations beyond active muscle beds. *Physiology(Bethesda), 26*(3), 132–145.
12. Hamburg N. M., Balady G. J. (2011). Exercise rehabilitation in peripheral artery disease. *Circulation, 123*(1), 87–97.
13. Booher M. A., Smith B. M. (2003). Physiological effects of exercise on the cardiopulmonary system. *Clinics in Sports Medicine, 22*(1), 1–21.
14. Wasserman K., Hansen J. E., Sue D. Y., et al. (2012). *Exercise testing and interpretation* (5th ed.). Philadelphia, PA: Lippincott Williams & Wilkins.
15. Downing J, Balady G. J. (2011). The role of exercise training in heart failure. *Journal of the American College of Cardiology, 58*(6), 561–569.
16. Gonzalez-Alonso J. (2012). Human thermoregulation and the cardiovascular system. *Experimental Physiology, 97*(3), 340–346.
17. Martin D. (2011). Physical activity benefits and risks on the gastrointestinal system. *Southern Medical Journal, 104*(12), 831–837.

18. Gleeson M., Bishop N. C., Stensel D. J., et al. (2011). The anti-inflammatory effects of exercise: Mechanisms and implications for the prevention and treatment of disease. *Nature Reviews Immunology, 11*(9), 607–615.

19. Walsh N. P., Gleeson M., Shephard R. J., et al. (2011). Position statement. Part one: Immune function and exercise. *Exercise Immunology Review, 17*, 6–63.

20. Plasqui G., Bonomi A. G., Westerterp K. R. (2013). Daily physical activity assessment with accelerometers: New insights and validation studies. *Obesity Reviews, 14*(6), 451–462.

21. Butte N. F., Ekelund U., Westerterp K. R. (2012). Assessing physical activity using wearable monitors: Measures of physical activity. *Medicine and Science in Sports and Exercise, 44*(Suppl 1), S5–S12.

22. Warburton D. E., Nicol C. W., Bredin S. S. (2006). Prescribing exercise as preventive therapy. *CMAJ: Canadian Medical Association Journal, 174*(7), 961–974.

23. Chodzko-Zajko W. J., Proctor D. N., Singh M. A. F., et al. (2009). American college of sports medicine position stand. Exercise and physical activity for older adults. *Medicine and Science in Sports and Exercise, 41*(7), 1510–1530.

24. Borg G. A. V. (1998). *Borg's rating of perceived exertion and pain scales.* Champaign, IL: Human Kinetics.

25. Mazzeo R. S. (2015). ACSM fact sheet: Exercise and the older adult. [Online] Available: https://www.acsm.org/docs/current-comments/exerciseandtheolderadult.pdf. Accessed on February 15, 2015.

26. Aronow W. S., Fleg J. L., Rich M. W. (2014). *Tresch and aronow's cardiovascular disease in the elderly* (5th ed.). Boca Raton, FL: Taylor & Francis Group.

27. Olsen K. (2007). A new way of thinking about fatigue: A reconceptualization. *Oncology Nursing Forum, 34*(1), 93–99.

28. Kluger B. M., Krupp L. B., Enoka R. M. (2013). Fatigue and fatigability in neurological illnesses: Proposal for a unified taxonomy. *Neurology, 80*(4), 409–416.

29. Prins J. B., van der Meer J. W., Bleijenberg G. (2006). Chronic fatigue syndrome. *Lancet, 367*(9507), 346–355.

30. Koornstra R. H. T., Peters M., Donofrio S., et al. (2014). Management of fatigue in patients with cancer: A practical overview. *Cancer Treatment Reviews, 40*(6), 791–799.

31. Bower J. E., Lamkin D. M. (2013). Inflammation and cancer-related fatigue: Mechanisms, contributing factors, and treatment implications. *Brain, Behavior, and Immunity, 30*(Suppl):S48–S57.

32. Yancey J. R., Thomas S. M. (2012). Chronic fatigue syndrome: Diagnosis and treatment. *American Family Physician, 86*(8), 741–746.

33. Fernandez A. A., Martin A. P., Martinez M. I., et al. Chronic fatigue syndrome: Aetiology, diagnosis and treatment. *BMC Psychiatry, 9*(Suppl 1), S1.

34. Committee on the diagnostic criteria for myalgic chronic fatigue syndrome – Institute of Medicine. (2015). *Beyond myalgic encephalomyelitis/chronic fatigue syndrome redefining an illness.* Washington, DC: The National Academies Press.

35. Winkelman C. (2009). Bed rest in health and critical illness: A body systems approach. *AACN Advanced Critical Care, 20*(3), 254–266.

36. Brower R. G. (2009). Consequences of bed rest. *Critical Care Medicine, 37*(10 Suppl):S422–S428.

37. Allen C., Glasziou P., Del Mar C. (1999). Bed rest: A potentially harmful treatment needing more careful evaluation. *Lancet, 354*(9186), 1229–1233.

38. Harper C. M., Lyules Y. M. (1988). Physiology and complications of bed rest. *Journal of the American Geriatrics Society, 36*(11), 1047–1054.

39. Knight J., Nigam Y., Jones A. (2009). Effects of bedrest 1: Cardiovascular, respiratory and haematological systems. *Nursing Times, 105*(21), 16–20.

40. Convertino V. A. (1997). Cardiovascular consequences of bed rest: Effect on maximal oxygen uptake. *Medicine and Science in Sports and Exercise, 29*(2), 191–196.

41. Knight J., Nigam Y., Jones A. (2009). Effects of bedrest 2: Gastrointestinal, endocrine, renal , reproductive and nervous system. *Nursing Times, 105*(22), 24–27.

42. Nigam Y., Knight J., Jones A. (2009). Effects of bedrest 3: Musculoskeletal and immune systems, skin and self-perception. *Nursing Times, 105*(23), 18–22.

43. Winkelman C. (2004). Inactivity and inflammation: selected cytokines as biologic mediators in muscle dysfunction during critical illness. *AACN Clinical Issues, 15*(1), 74–82.

Visit the Point **http://thePoint.lww.com for animations, journal articles, and more!**

Unit IV

Disorders of the Hematopoietic System

From ancient times, the importance of blood as a determinant of health was recognized. Its life-affecting powers are well described in the written treatises of Greek physician Galen (AD 130–200). Galen, who reigned as the foremost medical authority for nearly 1,500 years, believed that an individual stayed healthy as long as four body fluids—blood, phlegm, yellow bile, and black bile—remained in the right proportion. He also believed that the four humours determined one's basic temperament. Whether an individual was sanguine, sluggish and dull, quick to anger, or melancholy was determined by the degree to which one or another of the humours predominated. The most desirable personality type was achieved when blood was thought to predominate, yielding a warm and cheerful person.

The workings of blood were traced by Galen from its creation, which he believed took place in the liver, throughout the body. He came to believe that disease manifested itself if any one of the fluids was in excess or deficient and was carried in the blood. The theory led to bloodletting—the drawing of blood from the vein of a sick person so the disease could flow out with the blood. For many centuries, bloodletting was the standard treatment for a myriad of ills.

Unit IV

Disorders of the
Hematopoietic System

Blood Cells and the Hematopoietic System

12

Blood is unique in that it is the only liquid tissue in the body. Blood is a specialized connective tissue that consists of blood cells (red blood cells, white blood cells, and platelets) suspended in an extracellular fluid, known as *plasma*. Blood accounts for about 7% to 8% of total body weight. The total volume of blood in the average adult is about 5 to 6 L, and it circulates throughout the body within the confines of the circulatory system. Because blood circulates throughout the body, it is an ideal vehicle for transport of materials to and from the many cells of the body.

COMPOSITION OF BLOOD AND FORMATION OF BLOOD CELLS

After completing this section of the chapter, you should be able to meet the following objectives:

- Describe the composition and functions of plasma.
- Name the formed elements of blood and cite their function and life span.
- Trace the process of hematopoiesis from stem cell to mature blood cell.

When blood is artificially removed from the body for testing or when blood exits the body due to vascular injury, it clots within 30 to 60 minutes. The clot contains the blood's cellular components enmeshed in an insoluble fibrin network formed by the polymerization of the soluble plasma protein fibrinogen. The remaining fluid portion of clotted blood is the yellow liquid called *serum*. This serum no longer contains fibrinogen as the fibrinogen is consumed in the formation of the blood clot. Addition of an anticoagulant (*e.g.,* heparin, citrate) to blood removed from the circulation via phlebotomy creates a whole blood specimen. When a whole blood specimen is centrifuged, it will separate into three distinct layers (Fig. 12.1).

The bottom layer (approximately 42% to 47% of the whole-blood volume) contains the erythrocytes, or red blood cells (RBC), and is referred to as the *hematocrit*. The intermediate layer (approximately 1%), containing the leukocytes,

Plasma
(55% of
whole blood)

Buffy coat leukocytes
and platelets
(<1% of
whole blood)

Erythrocytes
(45% of
whole blood)

Formed
elements

FIGURE 12.1 • Layering of blood components in an anticoagulated and centrifuged blood sample.

or white blood cells (WBC), is white or grey and is called the *buffy layer*. Above the leukocytes is a thin layer of thrombocytes or platelets that is not discernible to the naked eye. The translucent, yellowish fluid that forms on the top of the cells is the *plasma,* which comprises approximately 55% of the total volume.

Plasma

Plasma, being a liquid, is 90% to 91% water by weight, 6.5% to 8% proteins by weight, and 2% other small molecular substances (Table 12.1). Unlike plasma, serum does not contain fibrinogen or clotting factors. Plasma water serves as a transport vehicle for materials carried in the blood. As a transport medium, plasma carries nutrients from the gastrointestinal tract and oxygen from the lungs to body cells while picking up waste products from the cells for delivery

TABLE 12.1 PLASMA COMPONENTS

PLASMA	PERCENTAGE OF PLASMA VOLUME	DESCRIPTION
Water	90–91	
Proteins	6.5–8	
Albumin		54% Plasma proteins
Globulins		38% Plasma proteins
Fibrinogen		7% Plasma proteins
Other substances	1–2	Hormones, enzymes, carbohydrates, fats, amino acids, gases, electrolytes, excretory products

COMPOSITION OF THE BLOOD

- The most abundant of the blood cells, the erythrocytes or RBCs, function in oxygen and carbon dioxide transport.
- The leukocytes, or WBCs, serve various roles in immunity and inflammation.
- Platelets are small cell fragments that are involved in blood clotting.

to excretory organs; it transports hormones and facilitates the exchange of chemical mediators; it participates in electrolyte and acid-base balance; and it contains the plasma proteins that contribute to the osmotic regulation of body fluids. In addition, because water has a high capacity to hold heat, plasma can absorb and distribute much of the heat that is generated in the body.

Plasma Proteins

The plasma proteins are the most abundant solutes in plasma. Except for the blood-borne hormones and gamma globulins, most plasma proteins are produced by the liver. The major types of plasma proteins are albumin, globulins, and fibrinogen. Albumin is the most abundant and makes up approximately 54% of the plasma proteins. It does not pass through the pores in the capillary wall to enter the interstitial fluid and therefore contributes to the plasma osmotic pressure and maintenance of blood volume (see Chapter 31). Albumin also serves as a carrier for certain substances and acts as a blood buffer. The globulins comprise approximately 38% of plasma proteins. There are three types of globulins: the *alpha globulins* that transport bilirubin and steroids, the *beta globulins* that transport iron and copper, and the *gamma globulins* that constitute the antibodies of the immune system. Fibrinogen makes up approximately 7% of the plasma proteins and is a key factor in blood clotting. The remaining 1% of the circulating proteins are hormones, enzymes, complement, and carriers for lipids.

Blood Cells

The blood cells include the erythrocytes, leukocytes, and platelets (Fig. 12.2). The blood cells, or formed elements, are not all true cells. Erythrocytes have no nuclei or organelles and platelets are just cell fragments. Most blood cells do not divide, so they must continually be renewed by division of cells in the bone marrow, where they originate. Table 12.2 lists the normal values for the blood cells.

Erythrocytes

The erythrocytes, or RBCs, are the most numerous of the formed elements. They are small, biconcave disks having an average diameter of 7.8 μm and a thickness of approximately 2.5 μm. The volume of an average RBC is approximately

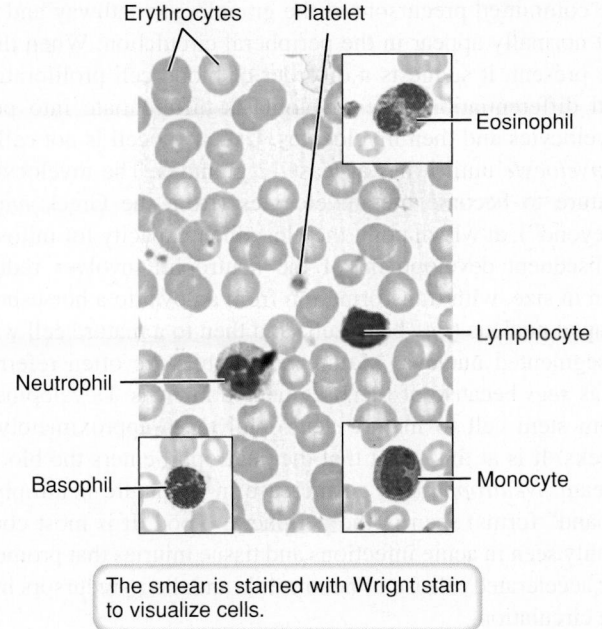

Erythrocytes Platelet

Eosinophil

Lymphocyte

Neutrophil

Basophil

Monocyte

The smear is stained with Wright stain to visualize cells.

FIGURE 12.2 • Photomicrograph of blood smear stained with Wright stain to allow the visualization of the components of blood. (From McConnell T. H., Hull K. L. (2011). *Human form human function: Essentials of anatomy & physiology* (pp. 380, Figure 10.2). Philadelphia, PA: Lippincott William & Wilkins.)

$90 \ \mu m^3$. RBCs have a large surface area and can easily deform (*i.e.,* change shape) to move through the small capillaries of the circulatory system. They contain large amounts of the oxygen-carrying protein, *hemoglobin,* that functions in the transport of oxygen.

Ninety percent of the erythrocytes, which have their origin in the bone marrow, live approximately 120 days in the circulation (see Chapter 14) and then are phagocytosed in the bone marrow, spleen, and liver. The other 10% of RBCs break down and excrete little amounts of hemoglobin into the circulatory system. Erythrocyte precursors in the bone marrow possess nuclei, but expel not only their nuclei but also all organelles before entering the circulation. Although erythrocytes have no organelles, they have soluble enzymes, including carbonic anhydrase, within their cytosol. This enzyme facilitates the formation of carbonic acid from carbon dioxide and water, which in turn dissociates into bicarbonate and hydrogen ions. Thus, erythrocytes also contribute to carbon dioxide transport and regulation of acid-base balance.

Leukocytes

The leukocytes, or WBCs, are 10 to 12 μm in diameter and thus much larger than RBCs. However, they constitute only 1% of the total blood volume. They originate in the bone marrow and circulate throughout the lymphoid tissues of the body. Leukocytes are crucial to our defence against disease. They are responsible for the immune response that protects against disease-causing microorganisms; they identify and destroy cancer cells; and they participate in the inflammatory response and wound healing. Leukocytes are commonly classified into two groups based on presence or absence of specific prominent granules in their cytoplasm (Fig. 12.3). Those containing specific granules (neutrophils, eosinophils, basophils) are classified as *granulocytes* and those that lack granules (lymphocytes and monocytes) as *agranulocytes.*

TABLE 12.2 BLOOD CELL COUNTS		
BLOOD CELLS	**NUMBER OF CELLS**	**PERCENTAGE OF WHITE BLOOD CELLS**
Red blood cell count	$4.2–5.4 \times 10^{12}$/L Male $3.6–5.0 \times 10^{12}$/L Female	
White blood cell count	$4.0–11.0 \times 10^{12}$/L	
Differential count		
Granulocytes		
Neutrophils		
Segs		47–63
Bands		0–4
Eosinophils		0–3
Basophils		0–2
Lymphocytes		24–40
Monocytes		4–9
Platelets	$150–400 \times 10^9$/L	

Granulocyte

Granules (lysosomes)

Lymphocyte

Lysosome

Monocyte/ Macrophage

Phagocytic vacuole

Lysosome

FIGURE 12.3 • White blood cells.

Granulocytes. Granulocytes are spherical and have distinctive multilobar nuclei. They are all phagocytic cells that are identifiable because of their cytoplasmic granules. They have two types of granules: the *specific granules* that bind neutral, basic, or acidic dye components, and *azurophilic granules.* The azurophilic granules stain purple and are lysosomes. The granulocytes are divided into three types—neutrophils, eosinophils, and basophils—according to the staining properties of their specific granules.

Neutrophils. The neutrophils, which normally constitute 55% to 65% of the total white blood cells, have granules that are neutral and hence do not stain with an acidic or a basic dye. Because these white cells have nuclei that are divided into three to five lobes, they are often called *polymorphonuclear leukocytes* or *PMNs*. Neutrophils are very mobile and are the first cells to go to an area of tissue damage. Their migration is a result of the release of adhesion molecules on the neutrophil surface, which connects with ligands on the endothelial cells.

The neutrophils are primarily responsible for maintaining normal host defences against invading bacteria and fungi, cell debris, and a variety of foreign substances. The cytoplasm of mature neutrophils has three types of granules: small specific granules that contain complement activators and bacteriostatic and bactericidal agents; larger azurophilic granules that contain peroxidases and other hydrolytic enzymes; and the newly discovered tertiary granules, which contain proteins thought to facilitate movement and migration of the neutrophil.

The neutrophils have their origin in the myeloblasts that are found in the bone marrow (Fig. 12.4). The myeloblasts are the committed precursors of the granulocyte pathway and do not normally appear in the peripheral circulation. When they are present, it suggests a disorder of blood cell proliferation and differentiation. The myeloblasts differentiate into promyelocytes and then myelocytes. Usually, a cell is not called a *myelocyte* until it has at least 12 granules. The myelocytes mature to become metamyelocytes (from the Greek *meta,* "beyond"), at which point they lose their capacity for mitosis. Subsequent development of the neutrophil involves reduction in size, with transformation from an oval to a horseshoe-shaped nucleus (*i.e.,* band cell) and then to a mature cell with a segmented nucleus. Mature neutrophils are often referred to as *segs* because of their segmented nucleus. Development from stem cell to mature neutrophil takes approximately 2 weeks. It is at this point that the neutrophil enters the bloodstream. *Neutrophilia* is an increase in immature neutrophils ("band" forms) seen in the peripheral blood. It is most commonly seen in acute infections and tissue injuries that promote the accelerated release of neutrophils and their precursors into the circulation.

After release from the marrow, the neutrophils spend only approximately 4 to 8 hours in the circulation before moving into the tissues. They survive in the tissues for approximately 4 to 5 days. They die in the tissues by discharging their phagocytic function or from senescence. The pool of circulating neutrophils (*i.e.,* those that appear in the blood count) is in a closely maintained equilibrium with a similar-sized pool of cells marginating along the walls of small blood vessels. These are the neutrophils that respond to chemotactic factors and migrate into the tissues toward the offending agent. Epinephrine, exercise, stress, and corticosteroid drug therapy can cause rapid increases in the circulating neutrophil count by shifting cells from the marginating to the circulating pool. Endotoxins or microbes have the opposite effect, producing a transient decrease in neutrophils by attracting neutrophils into the tissues.

Eosinophils. The specific cytoplasmic granules of the eosinophils stain red with the acidic dye eosin. These leukocytes constitute 1% to 3% of the total white blood cells and increase in number during allergic reactions and parasitic infections. It is thought that they release enzymes or chemical mediators that detoxify the agents associated with allergic reactions. In parasitic infections, the eosinophils use surface markers to attach themselves to the parasite and then release hydrolytic enzymes that kill it.

Basophils. The basophils are the least numerous of the white blood cells, accounting for only 0.3% to 0.5% of the total leukocytes. The specific granules of the basophils stain blue with a basic dye. These granules contain heparin, an anticoagulant; histamine, a vasodilator; and other mediators of inflammation. The basophil, which is a blood cell, is related, but not identical, to the connective tissue mast cell that contains similar granules. Both the basophils and mast cells are thought to be involved in allergic and hypersensitivity reactions.

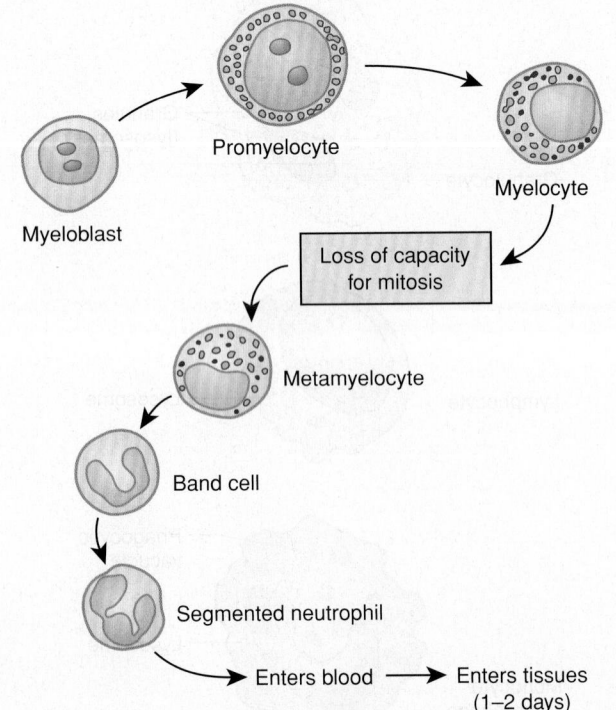

FIGURE 12.4 • Developmental stages of the neutrophil, which begins its development in the bone marrow as a myeloblast.

Lymphocytes. Lymphocytes are the most common agranulocytes and account for 20% to 30% of the total blood leukocytes. They originate in the bone marrow from lymphoid stem cells and are the main functional cells of the immune system. They move between blood and lymph tissue, where they may be stored for hours or years. Their function in the lymph nodes or spleen is to defend against microorganisms through the immune response (see Chapter 17).

There are three types of lymphocytes: B lymphocytes, T lymphocytes, and innate lymphoid cells such as natural killer cells. The *B lymphocytes (B cells)* account for 80% of the lymphocytes and are so named because they were first recognized as a separate population in the bursa of Fabricius in birds and bursa-equivalent organs (*e.g.,* bone marrow) in mammals. They differentiate to form antibody-producing plasma cells and are involved in humoral-mediated immunity. The *T lymphocytes (T cells)* account for 10% of lymphocytes and differentiate in the thymus. They activate other cells of the immune system (helper T cells) and are involved in cell-mediated immunity (cytotoxic T cells). The remaining 10% of lymphocytes are the *Natural killer (NK) cells,* which participate in innate or natural immunity and whose function is to destroy foreign cells. The lymphocytes of the three different subsets have unique surface markers that can be identified in order to define their function and diagnose disease (discussed in Chapters 17 and 18).

Monocytes and Macrophages. Monocytes are the largest of the white blood cells and constitute approximately 3% to 8% of the total leukocyte count. They are distinguished by a large amount of cytoplasm and a dark-stained nucleus in the shape of a kidney. The life span of the circulating monocyte is approximately 1 to 3 days, three to four times longer than that of the granulocytes. These cells migrate to tissues and survive for months to years after their maturation in the tissues. Monocytes, which are precursors of the mononuclear phagocyte system, are often referred to as *macrophages* when they enter the tissues. When the monocyte leaves the vascular system and enters the tissues, it functions as a macrophage with specific activity. It is estimated that 10% to 15% of most organs cells are comprised of macrophages. Types of macrophages are *histiocytes* in loose connective tissue, *microglial cells* in the brain, and *Kupffer cells* in the liver. Other macrophages function in the alveoli, lymph nodes, and other tissues.

The monocytes engulf more and larger foreign material than the neutrophils. These leukocytes play an important role in chronic inflammation and are also involved in the immune response by activating lymphocytes and by presenting antigen to T cells. Granulomatous inflammation is a distinctive pattern of chronic inflammation in which the macrophages form a capsule around insoluble materials that cannot be digested. Foreign body granulomas are incited by relatively inert foreign bodies, such as talc or surgical sutures. Immune granulomas are caused by insoluble particles that are capable of inciting a cell-mediated immune response. The tubercle that forms in primary tuberculosis infections is an example of an immune granuloma (see Chapter 28).

Thrombocytes

Thrombocytes, or platelets, are circulating cell fragments of the large megakaryocytes that are derived from the myeloid stem cell. They function to form the platelet plug to help control bleeding after injury to a vessel wall (see Chapter 13). Their cytoplasmic granules release mediators required for the blood coagulation process. Thrombocytes have a membrane but no nucleus, cannot replicate, and, if not used, last approximately 10 days in the circulation before they are removed by the phagocytic cells of the spleen.

Formation of Blood Cells (Hematopoiesis)

The generation of blood cells takes place in the *hematopoietic* (from the Greek *haima,* "blood," and *poiesis,* "making") system. The hematopoietic system encompasses all of the blood cells and their precursors, the bone marrow where blood cells have their origin, and the lymphoid tissues where some blood cells circulate as they develop and mature.

Hematopoiesis begins in the endothelial cells of the developing blood vessels during the fifth week of gestation and then continues in the liver and spleen. After birth, this function is gradually taken over by the bone marrow. Some hematopoiesis may also occur in the spleen and the liver. The marrow is a network of connective tissue containing immature blood cells. At sites where the marrow is hematopoietically active, it produces so many erythrocytes that it is red, hence the name *red bone marrow.* Fat cells are also present in bone marrow, but they are inactive in terms of blood cell generation. The fat cell can be visualized in the bone marrow in Figure 12.5. Marrow that is made up predominantly of fat cells is called *yellow bone marrow.* During active skeletal growth, red marrow is gradually replaced by yellow marrow in most of the long bones. In adults, red marrow is largely restricted to the flat bones of the pelvis, ribs, and sternum. When the demand for red cell replacement increases, as in hemolytic anemia, there can be resubstitution of red marrow for yellow marrow.

HEMATOPOIESIS

- White blood cells (granulocytes, monocytes, and lymphocytes) are formed from hematopoietic stem cells that differentiate into committed progenitor cells, which in turn develop into the myelogenous and lymphocytic lineages needed for the formation of the different types of white blood cell.
- The growth and reproduction of the different stem cells is controlled by CSFs and other cytokines and chemical mediators.
- The life span of white blood cells is relatively short so that constant renewal is necessary to maintain normal blood levels. Any conditions that decrease the availability of stem cells or hematopoietic growth factors produce a decrease in white blood cells.

FIGURE 12.5 • Structure of normal bone marrow. (From Rubin R., Strayer D. (Eds.). (2012). *Rubin's pathology: Clinicopathologic foundations of medicine*. (6th ed., pp. 948). Philadelphia, PA: Lippincott Williams & Wilkins.)

Labels: Adventitial cells; Endothelial cells; Megakaryocyte; Sinus; Fat cell; Arteriole; Endothelial cells; Erythroblastic islet

Blood Cell Precursors

The blood-forming population of bone marrow is made up of three types of cells: self-renewing stem cells, differentiated progenitor (parent) cells, and functional mature blood cells. All of the blood cell precursors of the erythrocyte (*i.e.,* red blood cell), myelocyte (*i.e.,* granulocyte or monocyte), lymphocyte (*i.e.,* T lymphocyte and B lymphocyte), and megakaryocyte (*i.e.,* platelet) series are derived from a small population of primitive cells called the *pluripotent stem cells* (Fig. 12.6). Their life-long potential for proliferation and self-renewal makes them an indispensable and lifesaving source of reserve cells for the entire hematopoietic system. Several levels of differentiation lead to the development of committed unipotential cells, which are the progenitors for each of the blood cell types. These cells are referred to as *colony-forming units* (CFUs). These progenitor cells have only limited capacity for self-renewal but retain the potential to differentiate into lineage-specific precursor cells. Precursor cells have morphologic characteristics that permit them to be recognized as the first cell of a particular cell line. They have lost their ability to self-renew but undergo cell division and differentiation, eventually giving rise to mature lymphocytes, myelocytes, megakaryocytes, or erythrocytes.

Disorders of hematopoietic stem cells include aplastic anemia and the leukemias. Today, potential cures for these and many other disorders use hematopoietic stem cell transplantation. Stem cell transplants correct bone marrow failure, immune deficiencies, hematologic defects and malignancies, and inherited errors of metabolism. Sources of the stem cells include bone marrow, peripheral blood, and umbilical cord blood, all of which replenish the recipient with a normal population of pluripotent stem cells. Bone marrow and peripheral blood transplants may be derived from the patient (autologous) or from a histocompatible donor (allogeneic). Autologous transplants are often used to replenish stem cells after high-dose chemotherapy or irradiation. Peripheral blood stem cells are harvested from the blood after the administration of a cytokine growth factor that increases the quantity and migration of the cells from the bone marrow. Umbilical cord blood from human leukocyte antigen (HLA)-matched donors is a transplant option for children and carries less risk of graft-versus-host disease. Methods of collecting, propagating, and preserving stem cells continue to be investigated.

Regulation of Hematopoiesis

Under normal conditions, the numbers and total mass for each type of circulating blood cell remain relatively constant. The blood cells are produced in different numbers according to needs and regulatory factors. This regulation of blood cells is thought to be at least partially controlled by hormone-like growth factors called *cytokines*. The cytokines are a family of short-lived mediators that stimulate the proliferation, differentiation, and functional activation of the various blood cells.

Many cytokines derived from lymphocytes or bone marrow stromal cells stimulate the growth and production of new

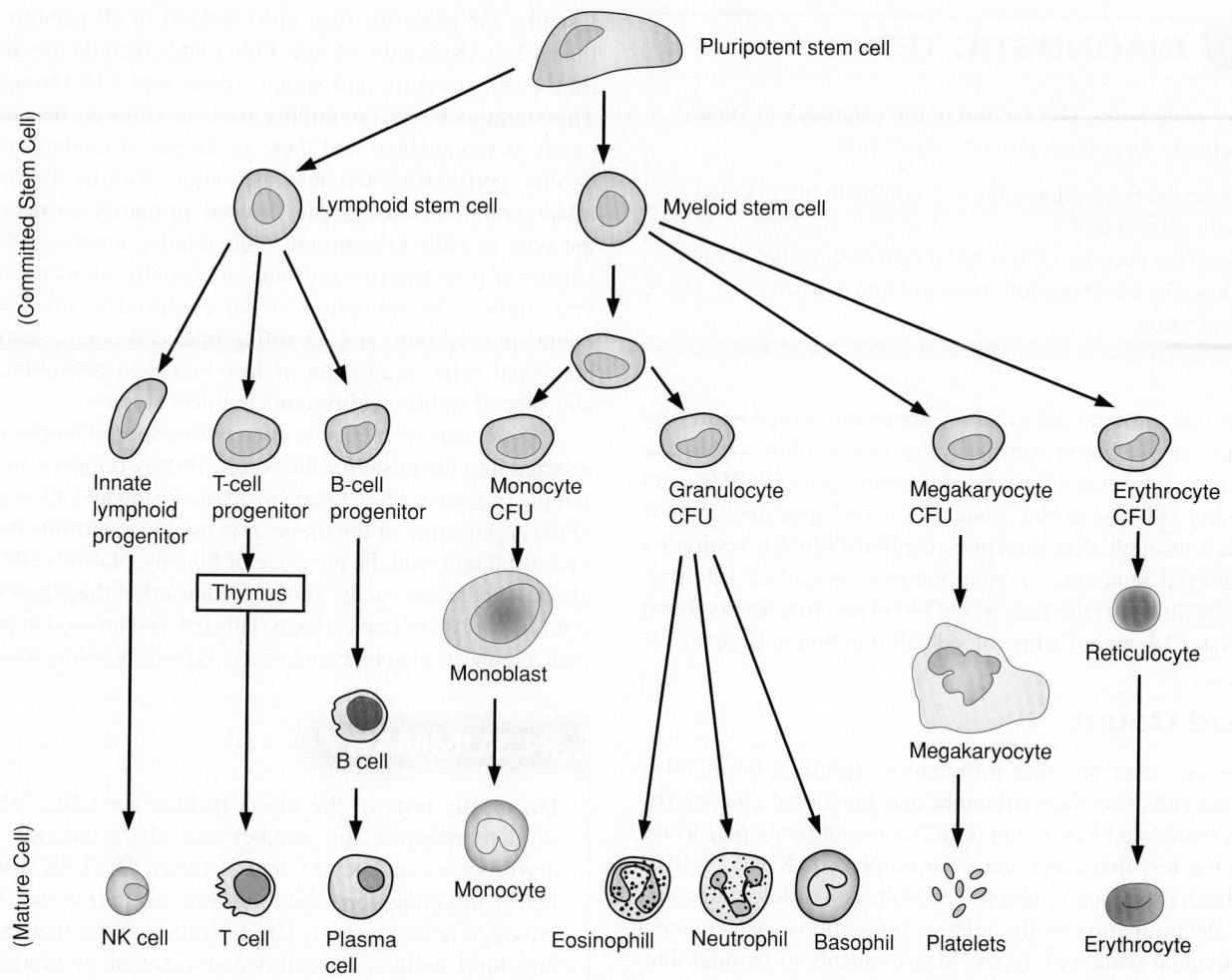

FIGURE 12.6 • Major maturational stages of blood cells. CFU, colony-forming unit; NK, natural killer cell.

blood cells. Several members of this family are called *colony-stimulating factors* (CSFs) because of their ability to promote the growth of hematopoietic cell colonies in the laboratory. The CSFs that act on committed progenitor cells include *erythropoietin* (EPO) which stimulates red blood cell production; *granulocyte–monocyte colony-stimulating factor* (GM-CSF) which stimulates progenitors for granulocytes, monocytes, erythrocytes, and megakaryocytes; *granulocyte colony-stimulating factor* (G-CSF) which promotes the proliferation of neutrophils; *macrophage colony-stimulating factor* (M-CSF), which induces macrophage colonies; and *thrombopoietin* (TPO) which stimulates the differentiation of platelets. Erythropoietin is primarily produced in the kidneys, thus normal red blood cell production is dependent upon normal renal function. Other cytokines, such as the interleukins, interferons, and tumour necrosis factor, support the proliferation of stem cells and the development of lymphocytes and act synergistically to aid the multiple functions of the CSFs (see Chapter 18).

The genes for most hematopoietic growth factors have been cloned and their recombinant proteins have been generated for use in a wide range of clinical problems. The clinically useful factors include EPO, TPO, G-CSF, and GM-CSF. They are used to treat bone marrow failure caused by chemotherapy or aplastic anemia, the anemia of kidney failure and cancer, hematopoietic neoplasms, infectious diseases such as acquired immunodeficiency syndrome (AIDS), and congenital and myeloproliferative disorders. Growth factors are used to increase peripheral stem cells for transplantation and to accelerate cell proliferation after bone marrow engraftment. Many of these uses are still investigational.

IN SUMMARY

Blood is composed of plasma, plasma proteins, fixed elements or blood cells, and substances such as hormones, enzymes, electrolytes, and byproducts of cellular waste. The blood cells consist of erythrocytes or RBCs, leukocytes or WBCs, and thrombocytes or platelets. Mature blood cells have a relatively short life span and must be continuously replaced. All of the different types of blood cells arise from pluripotent stem cells located in the bone marrow. The pluripotent stem cells, in turn, differentiate into unipotential CFUs, which are the progenitors for each of the blood cell types. Blood cell production is largely regulated by chemical messengers called cytokines (interleukins, interferons, and others) and growth factors (CSFs).

DIAGNOSTIC TESTS

After completing this section of the chapter, you should be able to meet the following objectives:

- Describe the components of a complete blood count with differential.
- State the purpose of the erythrocyte sedimentation rate.
- Describe the procedure used in bone marrow aspiration.

Blood tests provide information about the oxygen-carrying capacity of the blood (primarily by hemoglobin within the RBCs), the presence of infection or tissue injury (WBCs), and the ability of blood to clot (platelets). Blood specimens can be obtained through skin puncture (capillary blood), venipuncture, arterial puncture, or bone marrow aspiration. Information regarding specific tests of red blood cell function is found in Chapter 14, and of white blood cell function in Chapter 15.

Blood Count

The blood count provides information regarding the number of blood cells and their structural and functional characteristics. A complete blood count (CBC) is a commonly performed screening test that determines the number of RBCs, WBCs, and platelets per unit of blood. The white cell differential count is the determination of the relative proportions (percentages) of individual white cell types. Measurements of hemoglobin, hematocrit, mean corpuscular volume (MCV), mean corpuscular hemoglobin concentration (MCHC), and mean cell hemoglobin (MCH) are usually included in the CBC. These last three tests, MCV, MCHC, and MCH, are called the RBC indices. Inspection of the blood smear identifies morphologic abnormalities such as a change in size, shape, or colour of cells.

Erythrocyte Sedimentation Rate

The erythrocyte sedimentation rate (ESR) is a screening test for monitoring the fluctuations in the clinical course of a disease. In anticoagulated blood, red blood cells aggregate and sediment to the bottom of a tube. The rate of fall of the aggregates is accelerated in the presence of fibrinogen and other plasma proteins that are often increased in inflammatory diseases. The ESR is the distance in millimetres that a red cell column travels in 1 hour. Normal values are 0 to 15 mm/hr for men and 1 to 20 mm/hr for women.

Bone Marrow Aspiration and Biopsy

Tests of bone marrow function are done on samples obtained using bone marrow aspiration and/or bone marrow biopsy. Bone marrow aspiration is performed first with a special needle inserted into the bone marrow cavity, through which a sample of marrow (*i.e.,* fluid and cells only) is withdrawn.

Usually, the posterior iliac crest is used in all persons older than 12 to 18 months of age. Other sites include the anterior iliac crest, sternum, and spinous processes T10 through L4. The sternum is not commonly used in children because the cavity is too shallow and there is danger of mediastinal and cardiac perforation. Because aspiration disturbs the marrow architecture, this technique is used primarily to determine the type of cells present and their relative numbers. Stained smears of bone marrow aspirates are usually subjected to several studies: determination of the erythroid to myeloid cell count (normal ratio is 1:3), differential cell count, search for abnormal cells, evaluation of iron stores in reticulum cells, and special stains and immunochemical studies.

Bone marrow biopsy is done with a special biopsy needle inserted into the posterior iliac crest. Biopsy removes an actual sample of bone with the marrow tissue inside and allows study of the architecture of the tissue. It is used to determine the marrow-to-fat ratio and the presence of fibrosis, plasma cells, granulomas, and cancer cells. The major hazard of these procedures is the slight risk of hemorrhage. This risk is increased in persons with a reduced platelet count or any type of bleeding dyscrasia.

IN SUMMARY

Diagnostic tests of the blood include the CBC, which is used to describe the number and characteristics of the erythrocytes, leukocytes, and platelets. The ESR is used to detect inflammation. Bone marrow aspiration and biopsy are often done together. The aspiration of the marrow cells and fluid focuses on cellular assessment of morphology and determination of differential cell count whereas the biopsy removes a sample of solid bone marrow permitting study of the marrow's overall cellularity and extent of pathologic processes.

REVIEW EXERCISES

1. A 14-year-old boy is admitted to the emergency department with severe abdominal pain and a tentative diagnosis of appendicitis. His white blood cell count shows an elevated number of white blood cells with an increased percentage of "band cells."
   A. *Explain the significance of this finding.*
2. Many of the primary immunodeficiency disorders, in which there is a defect in the development of immune cells of T- or B-lymphocyte origin, can be cured with allogeneic stem cell transplantation from an unaffected donor.
   A. *Explain why stem cells are used rather than mature lymphocytes. You might want to refer to Figure 12.5.*
   B. *Describe how the stem cells would go about the process of repopulating the bone marrow.*

Bibliography

Ballen K. K., Gluckman E., Broxmeyer H. E. (2013). Umbilical cord blood transplantation: The first 25 years and beyond. *Blood, 122*(4), 491–498.

Fischbach F., Dunning M. (2009). *A manual of laboratory diagnostic tests* (8th ed.). Philadelphia, PA: Lippincott Williams & Wilkins.

Hall J. E. (2011). *Guyton and Hall Textbook of medical physiology* (12th ed.). Philadelphia, PA: Elsevier Saunders.

Kaushansky K. (2006). Lineage-specific hematopoietic growth factors. *New England Journal of Medicine, 354*, 2034–2045.

Koury M. J., Rhodes M. (2012). Howe to approach chronic anemia. *Hematology, 2012*(1), 183–190.

McConnell T. H., Hull K. L. (2011). *Human form human function: Essentials of anatomy and physiology.* Philadelphia, PA: Lippincott Williams & Wilkins.

Metcalf D. (2008). Hematopoietic cytokines. *Blood, 111*(2), 485–491.

Ross M. H., Pawlina W. (2011). *Histology: A text and atlas* (6th ed.). Philadelphia, PA: Lippincott Williams & Wilkins.

Tavian M., Péault B. (2005). Embryonic development of the human hematopoietic system. *International Journal of Developmental Biology, 49*, 243–250.

Tefferi A., Hanson C. A., Inwards D. J. (2005). How to interpret and pursue an abnormal complete blood count in adults. *Mayo Clinic Proceeding, 80*(7), 923–936.

Warren J. S., Bennett D. P., Pmerantz R. J. (2012). Hematopathology. In Rubin R., Strayer D. (Eds.), *Rubin's pathology: Clinicopathologic foundations of medicine* (6th ed.). Philadelphia, PA: Lippincott Williams & Wilkins.

Visit thePoint **http://thePoint.lww.com for animations, journal articles, and more!**

Disorders of Hemostasis

The term *hemostasis* refers to the stoppage of blood flow. The normal process of hemostasis is regulated by a complex array of activators and inhibitors that maintain blood fluidity and prevent blood from leaving the vascular compartment. Hemostasis is normal when it seals a blood vessel to prevent blood loss and hemorrhage. It is abnormal when it causes inappropriate blood clotting or when clotting is insufficient to stop the flow of blood from the vascular compartment. Disorders of hemostasis fall into two main categories: the inappropriate formation of clots within the vascular system (thrombosis) and the failure of blood to clot in response to an appropriate stimulus (bleeding or hemorrhage).

MECHANISMS OF HEMOSTASIS

After completing this section of the chapter, you should be able to meet the following objectives:

- Describe the five stages of hemostasis.
- Explain the formation of the platelet plug.
- State the purpose of blood coagulation.
- State the function of clot retraction.
- Trace the process of fibrinolysis.

Hemostasis is divided into five stages: (1) vessel spasm, (2) formation of the platelet plug, (3) blood coagulation or development of an insoluble fibrin clot, (4) clot retraction, and (5) clot dissolution.[1] During the process of hemostasis, hairlike fibrin strands glue the aggregated platelets together and intertwine to form the structural basis of the blood clot. In the presence of fibrin, plasma becomes gel-like and traps red blood cells and other formed elements in the blood (Fig. 13.1). Hemostasis is complete when fibrous tissue grows into the clot and seals the hole in the vessel. Breakdown or lysis of the clot is the final part of hemostasis.

Vessel Spasm

Vessel spasm constricts the vessel and reduces blood flow. It is a transient event that usually lasts less than 1 minute. Vessel spasm is initiated by endothelial injury and caused by local

FIGURE 13.1 • A scanning electron micrograph depicting a number of red cells enmeshed in a fibrinous matrix on the luminal surface of an indwelling catheter (magnification ×5698). (From the Centers for Disease Control and Prevention Public Images Library, Courtesy Janice Carr.)

and humoral mechanisms. Neural reflexes and thromboxane A₂ (TXA₂), a prostaglandin released from platelets, endothelin 1 released from vascular endothelial cells, and other mediators contribute to vasoconstriction. Prostacyclin, another prostaglandin released from the vessel endothelium, produces vasodilation and inhibits platelet aggregation in the surrounding uninjured endothelium.[1,2]

Formation of the Platelet Plug

The platelet plug, the second line of defence, is initiated as platelets come in contact with the vessel wall. Small breaks in the vessel wall are often sealed with the platelet plug rather than a blood clot.

Platelets, also called *thrombocytes,* are large fragments from the cytoplasm of bone marrow cells called *megakaryocytes.*[1] Each megakaryocyte releases 1,000 to 4,000 platelets into the circulation. The normal serum concentration is about 150 to 400 platelets ×10⁹/L of blood.[2] The platelets are released from the bone marrow, where their life span is only 8 to 10 days and then are broken down and eliminated by macrophages. Platelet production is controlled by a protein called

---

HEMOSTASIS

- Hemostasis is the orderly, stepwise process for stopping bleeding that involves vasospasm, formation of a platelet plug, and the development of a fibrin clot.
- The blood clotting process requires the presence of platelets produced in the bone marrow, von Willebrand factor generated by the vessel endothelium, and clotting factors synthesized in the liver, using vitamin K.
- The final step of the process involves fibrinolysis or clot dissolution, which prevents excess clot formation.

---

thrombopoietin that causes proliferation and maturation of megakaryocytes. The sources of thrombopoietin include the liver, kidney, smooth muscle, and bone marrow.[1–3]

Platelets have a cell membrane but no nucleus, and cannot reproduce. Although they lack a nucleus, they have many of the characteristics of a whole cell. The outer cell membrane is covered with a glycocalyx or coat of glycoproteins, glycosaminoglycans, and coagulation proteins (Fig. 13.2). One of the important glycoproteins is GPIIb/IIIa, which binds fibrinogen and bridges platelets to one another.[2] The platelet shape is maintained by microtubules and actin and myosin filaments that support the cell membrane. Platelets have mitochondria and enzyme systems capable of producing adenosine triphosphate (ATP) and adenosine diphosphate (ADP), and they have the enzymes needed for synthesis of the prostaglandin, TXA₂, required for their function in hemostasis.

Platelets contain two specific types of granules (α- and δ-granules) that release mediators for hemostasis.[2,4] The α-granules express the P-selectin, an adhesive protein, on their surface (see Chapter 4) and contain fibrinogen, von Willebrand factor (vWF), fibronectin, factors V and VIII, platelet factor 4 (a heparin-binding chemokine), platelet-derived growth factor (PDGF), transforming growth factor-α (TGF-α), and thrombospondin. The release of growth factors results in the proliferation and growth of vascular endothelial cells, smooth muscle cells, and fibroblasts and is important in vessel repair. The δ-granules, or dense granules, contain ADP and ATP, ionized calcium, histamine, serotonin, and epinephrine, which contribute to vasoconstriction.[2]

GPIIb/IIIa glycoprotein

Glycocalyx coat

Plasma membrane

Glycogen

Actin

Myosin II

α-Granules

δ-Granules

Mitochondria

Microtubules

FIGURE 13.2 • Platelet structure.

Platelet plug formation involves adhesion and aggregation of platelets. Platelets are attracted to a damaged vessel wall, become activated, and change from smooth disks to spiny spheres, exposing glycoprotein receptors on their surfaces. Platelet adhesion requires a protein molecule called *von Willebrand factor* (vWF).[1] This factor is produced by the endothelial cells of blood vessels and circulates in the blood as a carrier protein for coagulation factor VIII. Adhesion to the vessel subendothelial layer occurs when the platelet receptor binds to vWF at the injury site, linking the platelet to exposed collagen fibres.[2]

Platelet aggregation occurs soon after adhesion. It is mediated by the secretion of the contents of the platelet granules. The release of the dense body contents is particularly important because calcium is required for the coagulation component of hemostasis, and ADP is a mediator of platelet aggregation. ADP release also facilitates the release of ADP from other platelets, leading to amplification of the aggregation process. Besides ADP, platelets secrete the prostaglandin TXA_2, which is an important stimulus for platelet aggregation. The combined actions of ADP and TXA_2 lead to the expansion of the enlarging platelet aggregate, which becomes the primary hemostatic plug. Stabilization of the platelet plug occurs as the coagulation pathway is activated on the platelet surface and fibrinogen is converted to fibrin, thereby creating a fibrin meshwork that cements the platelets and other blood components together (Fig. 13.1). P-selectin also participates in platelet aggregation by binding leukocytes, which, with platelet substances such as PDGF, participate in the healing of the vessel wall.[2]

The platelet membrane plays an important role in platelet adhesion and the coagulation process. The coat of glycoproteins on its surface controls interactions with the vessel endothelium. Platelets normally avoid adherence to the endothelium but interact with injured areas of the vessel wall and the deeper exposed collagen.[1] When platelets are activated, Glycoprotein (GPIIb/IIIa) receptors on the platelet membrane bind with fibrinogen and link platelets together. Phospholipids, which are also present in the platelet membrane, provide critical binding sites for calcium and coagulation factors in the intrinsic coagulation pathway.

In addition to sealing vascular breaks, platelets play an almost continuous role in maintaining normal vascular integrity. They may supply growth factors for endothelial and arterial smooth muscle cells.[1] Defective platelet plug formation causes bleeding in people who are deficient in platelets or vWF. People with platelet deficiency have increased capillary permeability and sustain small skin hemorrhages from the slightest trauma or change in blood pressure.[2]

Platelet aggregation inhibitors, including aspirin, clopidogrel, and ticlopidine, can be used to prevent platelet aggregation and clot formation in people who are at risk for myocardial infarction, stroke, or peripheral artery disease. Low-dose aspirin therapy inhibits prostaglandin synthesis, including TXA_2. Clopidogrel and ticlopidine achieve their antiplatelet effects by inhibiting the ADP pathway in platelets. Unlike aspirin, these drugs have an effect on prostaglandin synthesis.

Both clopidogrel and ticlopidine inhibit clot formation and prolong the bleeding time. The most serious side effects of ticlopidine have been neutropenia and thrombotic thrombocytopenic purpura. Studies from randomized trials have shown that clopidogrel in combination with aspirin is associated with a reduction in major cardiac events, similar to ticlopidine plus aspirin, and appeared safer. In 2012 the Canadian Cardiovascular Society (CCS) updated the use of antiplatelet therapy guidelines specifically looking at drugs, indications, and potential drug interactions such as the use of proton pump inhibitors along with antiplatelet agents.[5]

The antiplatelet class of drugs that act as GPIIb/IIIa receptor inhibitors (tirofiban, eptifibatide, abciximab) have been developed for use in the treatment of acute myocardial infarction (see Chapter 24). However, acute and delayed thrombocytopenia has been reported after use of these agents, suggesting that further investigation is needed to understand the mechanisms leading to the thrombocytopenia and improve methods for detection for this complication.[5]

Blood Coagulation

The coagulation cascade is the third component of the hemostatic process. It is a stepwise process resulting in the conversion of the soluble plasma protein, fibrinogen, into fibrin. The insoluble fibrin strands create a meshwork that cements platelets and other blood components together to form the clot (*i.e.,* thrombus).

The coagulation process is controlled by many substances that promote clotting (procoagulation factors) or inhibit it (anticoagulation factors). Each of the procoagulation or coagulation factors, identified by Roman numerals, performs a specific step in the coagulation process. The activation of one procoagulation factor or proenzyme is designed to activate the next factor in the sequence (cascade effect). Because most of the inactive procoagulation factors are present in the blood at all times, the multistep process ensures that a massive episode of intravascular clotting does not occur by chance. It also means that abnormalities of the clotting process occur when one or more of the factors are deficient or when conditions lead to inappropriate activation of any of the steps.

Most of the coagulation factors are proteins synthesized in the liver. Vitamin K is necessary for the synthesis of factors II, VII, IX, and X, prothrombin, and protein C. If there is a deficiency of vitamin K or liver failure so that not enough prothrombin is created, a bleeding tendency will develop. Calcium (factor IV) is required in all but the first two steps of the clotting process.[1] The body usually has sufficient amounts of calcium for these reactions. Inactivation of the calcium ion prevents blood from clotting when it is removed from the body. The addition of citrate to blood stored for transfusion purposes prevents clotting by chelating ionic calcium. EDTA, another chelator, is often added to blood samples used for analysis in the clinical laboratory.

The coagulation process results from the activation of what have traditionally been designated the *intrinsic* and the

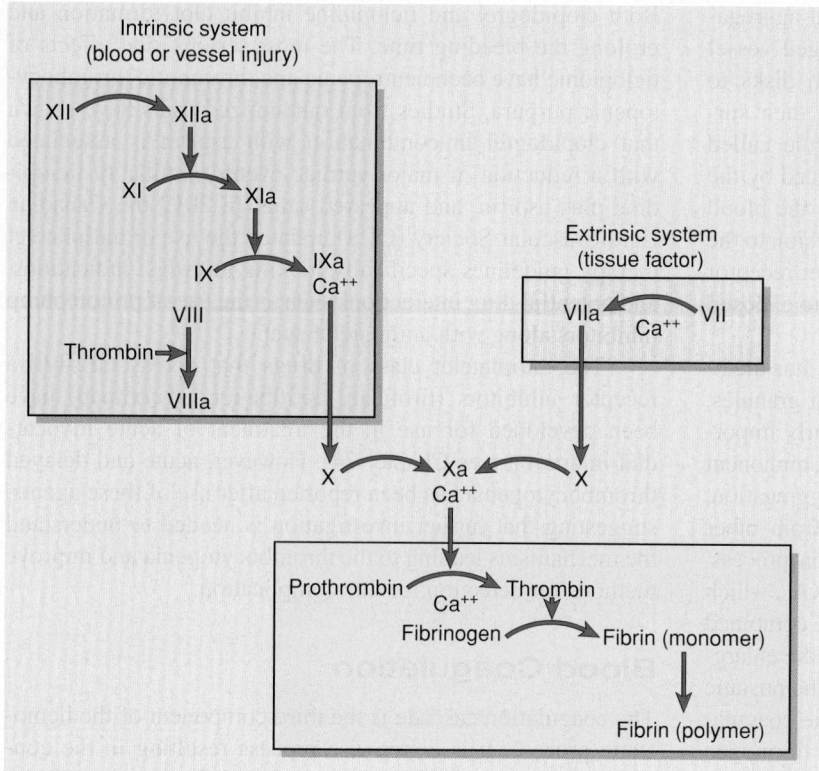

FIGURE 13.3 • The intrinsic and extrinsic coagulation pathways. The terminal steps in both pathways are the same. Calcium, factors X and V, and platelet phospholipids combine to form prothrombin activator, which then converts prothrombin to thrombin. This interaction causes conversion of fibrinogen into the fibrin strands that create the insoluble blood clot.

extrinsic pathways[1] (Fig. 13.3). The intrinsic pathway, which is a relatively slow process (can cause clotting in 1 to 6 minutes), begins in the circulation with the activation of factor XII. The extrinsic pathway, which is a much faster process (can cause clotting in 15 seconds), begins with injury to the blood vessel or surrounding tissues and the release of tissue factor, an adhesive lipoprotein, from the subendothelial cells.[1] The terminal steps in both pathways are the same: the activation of factor X and the conversion of prothrombin to thrombin. Thrombin then acts as an enzyme to convert fibrinogen to fibrin, the material that stabilizes the clot. Both pathways are needed for normal hemostasis, and many interrelations exist between them. Each system is activated when blood passes out of the vascular system. The intrinsic system is activated as blood comes in contact with collagen in the injured vessel wall; the extrinsic system is activated when blood is exposed to tissue extracts. However, bleeding that occurs because of defects in the extrinsic system usually is not as severe as that resulting from defects in the intrinsic pathway.[1]

Blood coagulation is regulated by several natural anticoagulants. Antithrombin III inactivates coagulation factors and neutralizes thrombin, the last enzyme in the pathway for the conversion of fibrinogen to fibrin. When antithrombin III is complexed with naturally occurring heparin, its action is accelerated to inactivate thrombin, factor Xa, and other coagulation factors. This complex activation provides protection against uncontrolled thrombus formation on the endothelial surface. Protein C, a plasma protein produced in the liver, acts as an anticoagulant by inactivating factors V and VIII. Protein deficiency

is 35% to 58% congenital, but it can also be acquired if one has severe liver failure, vitamin K deficiency, or malignancy. This inactive circulating protein C becomes activated (APC) when attached to thrombin and then with the normal cascade it inactivates coagulation factor V to slow down the clotting process. For people with factor V Leiden thrombophilia, factor V cannot be inactivated normally by APC and the clotting process continues longer with an increased chance for abnormal clots development.[6]

Protein S, another plasma protein, accelerates the action of protein C thus with a deficiency in either protein C or S the risk for thrombosis increases. A protein S test can be done to determine if the deficiency is inherited or acquired noting people with autoimmune disorders are at a higher risk for this deficiency.

Plasmin breaks down fibrin into fibrin degradation products that act as anticoagulants. It has been suggested that some of these natural anticoagulants may play a role in the bleeding that occurs with disseminated intravascular coagulation (DIC; discussed later).

The anticoagulant drugs warfarin (Coumadin) and heparin are used to prevent thromboembolic disorders, such as deep vein thrombosis and pulmonary embolism.[7] Warfarin acts by decreasing prothrombin and other procoagulation factors. It alters vitamin K in a manner that reduces its ability to participate in synthesis of the vitamin K–dependent coagulation factors in the liver. Warfarin is readily absorbed after oral administration. Its maximum effect takes 36 to 72 hours because of the varying half-lives of preformed clotting factors that remain in the circulation. Due to potential complications frequent laboratory testing of their anticoagulant time using the International Normalized Ratio (INR) test is required. Heparin is naturally formed and released in small amounts by mast cells in connective tissue surrounding capillaries. Pharmacologic preparations of heparin are extracted from animal tissues. Heparin binds to antithrombin III, causing a conformational change that increases the ability of antithrombin III to inactivate thrombin, factor Xa, and other clotting factors. By promoting the inactivation of clotting factors, heparin ultimately suppresses the formation of fibrin. Heparin is unable to cross the membranes of the gastrointestinal tract and must be given by injection, usually by subcutaneous or intravenous infusion. Low–molecular-weight heparins (LMWHs) have been developed that inhibit activation of factor X, but have little effect on thrombin and other coagulation factors. The LMWHs are given by subcutaneous injection and require less frequent administration and monitoring compared with the standard (unfractionated) heparin.[7]

Newer oral anticoagulant medications are available in Canada. The direct factor Xa inhibitors (rivaroxaban, apixaban) bind to the active side of factors Xa inhibiting thrombin formation and reducing fibrin formation. The direct thrombin inhibitors (dabigatran) binds to the active sites of factor IIa and inactivating both fibrin-bound and free thrombin thus inhibiting the clot formation.[7,8]

Clot Retraction

Clot retraction normally occurs within 20 to 60 minutes after a clot has formed, contributing to hemostasis by squeezing serum from the clot and joining the edges of the broken vessel. Platelets, through the action of their actin and myosin filaments, also contribute to clot retraction. Clot retraction therefore requires large numbers of platelets, and failure of clot retraction is indicative of a low platelet count.[1]

Clot Dissolution

The dissolution, or lysis, of a blood clot normally begins shortly after its formation. This allows blood flow to be reestablished and permanent tissue repair to take place. The process by which a blood clot dissolves is called *fibrinolysis*. As with clot formation, clot dissolution requires a sequence of steps controlled by activators and inhibitors. Plasminogen, the proenzyme for the fibrinolytic process, normally is present in the blood in its inactive form. It is converted to its active form, plasmin, by plasminogen activators formed in the vascular endothelium, liver, and kidneys. The plasmin formed from plasminogen digests the fibrin strands of the clot and certain clotting factors, such as fibrinogen, factor V, factor VIII, prothrombin, and factor XII. Circulating plasmin is rapidly inactivated by α_2-plasmin inhibitor, which limits the fibrinolytic process to the local clot and prevents it from occurring in the entire circulation.

Two naturally occurring plasminogen activators are tissue-type plasminogen activator and urokinase-type plasminogen activator. The liver, plasma, and vascular endothelium are the major sources of physiologic activators. These activators are released in response to a number of stimuli, including vasoactive drugs, venous occlusion, elevated body temperature, and exercise. The activators are unstable and rapidly inactivated by inhibitors synthesized by the endothelium and the liver. For this reason, chronic liver disease may cause altered fibrinolytic activity. A major inhibitor, plasminogen activator inhibitor-1, in high concentrations has been associated with deep vein thrombosis, coronary artery disease, and myocardial infarction.[7] Several tissue plasminogen activators (alteplase, reteplase, tenecteplase), produced by recombinant DNA technology, are available for use in treatment of acute myocardial infarction (see Chapter 24), acute ischemic stroke (see Chapter 51), and pulmonary embolism (see Chapter 29).

> ### IN SUMMARY
>
> Hemostasis is designed to maintain the integrity of the vascular compartment. The process is divided into five phases: vessel spasm, which constricts the size of the vessel and reduces blood flow; platelet adherence and formation of the platelet plug; formation of the fibrin clot, which cements the platelet plug together; clot retraction, which pulls the edges of the injured vessel together; and clot dissolution, which involves the action of plasmin to dissolve the clot and allow blood flow to be reestablished and tissue healing to take place. Blood coagulation requires the stepwise activation of coagulation factors, carefully controlled by activators and inhibitors.

CONCEPTS in action **ANIMATION**

HYPERCOAGULABILITY STATES

- Arterial thrombi are associated with conditions that produce turbulent blood flow and platelet adherence.
- Venous thrombi are associated with conditions that cause stasis of blood flow with increased concentrations of coagulation factors.

HYPERCOAGULABILITY STATES

After completing this section of the chapter, you should be able to meet the following objectives:

- Compare normal and abnormal clotting.
- Describe the causes and effects of increased platelet function.
- State two conditions that contribute to increased clotting activity.

Hypercoagulability represents an exaggerated form of hemostasis that predisposes to thrombosis and blood vessel occlusion. There are two general forms of hypercoagulability states: conditions that create increased platelet function and conditions that cause accelerated activity of the coagulation system. Chart 13.1 summarizes conditions commonly associated with hypercoagulability states. Arterial thrombi are usually due to turbulence and composed largely of platelet aggregates, whereas venous thrombi are usually due to stasis of flow and composed largely of platelet aggregates and fibrin complexes that result from activation of the coagulation cascade.

Hypercoagulability Associated With Increased Platelet Function

Hypercoagulability due to increased platelet function results in platelet adhesion, formation of platelet clots, and disruption of blood flow. The causes of increased platelet function are disturbances in flow, endothelial damage, and increased sensitivity of platelets to factors that cause adhesiveness and aggregation. Atherosclerotic plaques promote turbulent blood flow, causing endothelial damage and promoting platelet adherence. Platelets that adhere to the vessel wall release growth factors that cause proliferation of smooth muscle and thereby contribute to the development of atherosclerosis (discussed in Chapter 22). Smoking, elevated levels of blood lipids and cholesterol, hemodynamic stress, and diabetes mellitus predispose to vessel damage, platelet adherence, and eventual thrombosis.

Thrombocytosis

The term *thrombocytosis* is used to describe elevations in the platelet count above $1,000 \times 10^9$/L. Thrombocytosis can occur as a reactive process (secondary thrombocytosis) or as an essential process (primary thrombocytosis).[9]

Thrombopoietin is the key hormone in the regulation of megakaryocyte differentiation and platelet formation, although various cytokines (*e.g.*, interleukin-6 and interleukin-11) may play a role.[9] Megakaryocytes and their platelet progeny have receptors for thrombopoietin. Thrombopoietin is carried in the plasma attached to receptors on the surface of circulating platelets and in the unbound form is free to promote megakaryocyte proliferation. When the platelet count falls, more unbound thrombopoietin is available to stimulate megakaryocyte proliferation, and when the platelet count rises, less thrombopoietin is available to stimulate proliferation. Thus, megakaryocyte proliferation and platelet production are normally controlled in a negative feedback manner by the platelet count.[9]

The most common cause of secondary thrombocytosis is a disease state that stimulates thrombopoietin production. The result is increased megakaryocyte proliferation and platelet production. However, the platelet count seldom exceeds $1,000 \times 10^9$/L. The common underlying causes of secondary thrombocytosis include tissue damage due to surgery, infection, cancer, and chronic inflammatory conditions such as rheumatoid arthritis and Crohn's disease. Usually the only clinically apparent signs are those of the underlying disease. Thrombocytosis may also occur in other myeloproliferative disorders such as polycythemia vera (discussed in Chapter 14) and myelogenous leukemia (discussed in Chapter 15).

Primary or essential thrombocytosis represents a myeloproliferative (bone marrow) disorder of the hematopoietic stem cells.[9] Although thrombopoietin levels are often normal in essential thrombocytosis, abnormalities in the thrombopoietin receptor and platelet binding cause higher-than-expected levels of free thrombopoietin. This leads to increased megakaryocyte proliferation and platelet production. Dysfunction of the platelets produced contributes to the major clinical features of bleeding and thrombosis.

The common clinical manifestations of essential thrombocytosis are thrombosis and hemorrhage. Some people experience erythromelalgia, a painful throbbing and burning of the fingers caused by occlusion of the arterioles by platelet aggregates. Thrombotic events include deep vein thrombosis and pulmonary embolism, portal and hepatic vein thrombosis, and myocardial infarction. Typically, the disorder is characterized by long asymptomatic periods punctuated by occasional thrombotic episodes and hemorrhagic crises, both of which occur in people with very high platelet counts. Treatment includes the use of platelet-lowering drugs (*e.g.*, hydroxyurea) in high-risk cases.[9] Aspirin may be a highly effective adjunctive therapy in people with recurrent thrombotic complications.

Hypercoagulability Associated With Increased Clotting Activity

Thrombus formation due to activation of the coagulation system can result from primary (genetic) or secondary (acquired) disorders affecting the coagulation components of the blood clotting process (*i.e.*, an increase in procoagulation factors or a decrease in anticoagulation factors).

Understanding ▸ Hemostasis

Hemostasis, which refers to the stoppage of blood flow, is divided into five stages: (1) vessel spasm, (2) formation of the platelet plug, (3) development of a blood clot as a result of the coagulation process, (4) clot retraction, and (5) clot dissolution. The process involves the interaction of substrates, enzymes, protein cofactors, and calcium ions that circulate in the blood or are released from platelets and cells in the vessel wall.

1. Vessel Spasm

Injury to a blood vessel causes vascular smooth muscle in the vessel wall to contract. This instantaneously reduces the flow of blood from the vessel rupture. Both local nervous reflexes and local humoral factors such as thromboxane A_2 (TXA_2), which is released from platelets, contribute to the vasoconstriction.

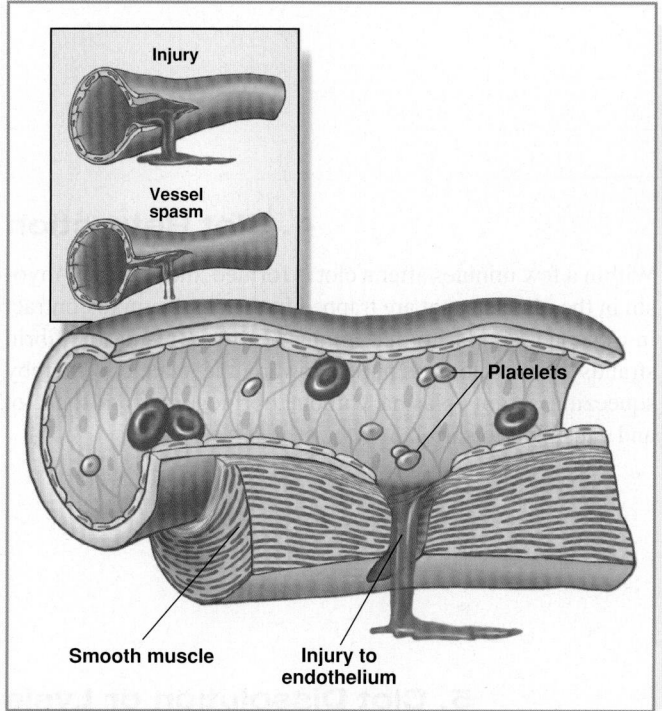

2. Formation of the Platelet Plug

Seconds after vessel injury, von Willebrand factor, released from the endothelium, binds to platelet receptors, causing adhesion of the platelets to the exposed collagen fibres *(inset)*. As the platelets adhere to the collagen fibres on the damaged vessel wall, they become activated and release adenosine diphosphate (ADP) and TXA_2. The ADP and TXA_2 attract additional platelets, leading to platelet aggregation.

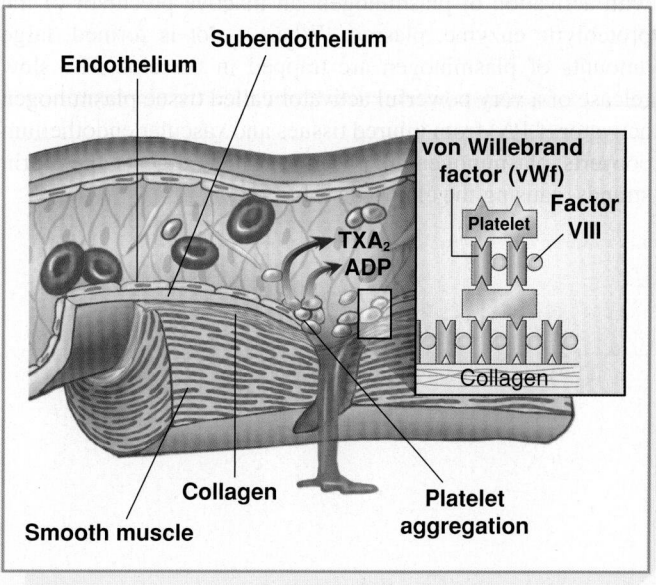

3. Blood Coagulation

Blood coagulation is a complex process involving the sequential activation of various factors in the blood. There are two coagulation pathways: (1) the intrinsic pathway begins in the circulation and is initiated by activation of circulating factor XII; and (2) the extrinsic pathway, which is activated by a cellular lipoprotein called *tissue factor* that becomes exposed when tissues are injured. Both pathways lead to the activation of factor X, the conversion of prothrombin to thrombin, and conversion of fibrinogen to the insoluble fibrin threads that hold the clot together.

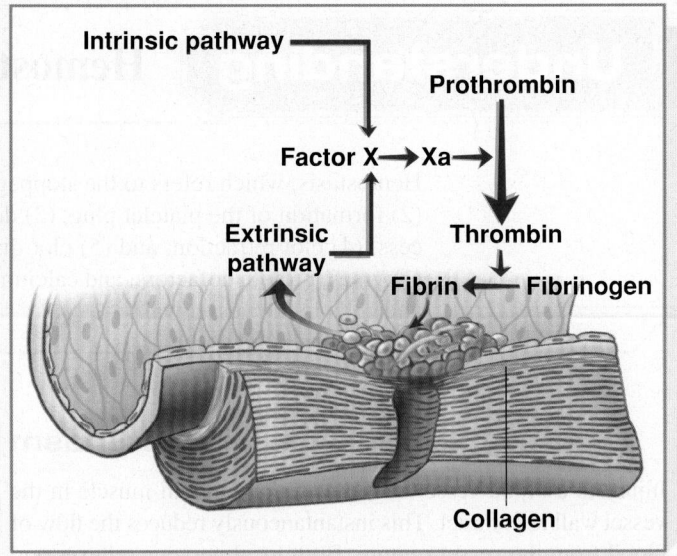

4. Clot Retraction

Within a few minutes after a clot is formed, the actin and myosin in the platelets that are trapped in the clot begin to contract in a manner similar to that in muscles. As a result, the fibrin strands of the clot are pulled toward the platelets, thereby squeezing serum (plasma without fibrinogen) from the clot and causing it to shrink.

5. Clot Dissolution or Lysis

Clot dissolution begins shortly after a clot is formed. It begins with activation of plasminogen, an inactive precursor of the proteolytic enzyme, plasmin. When a clot is formed, large amounts of plasminogen are trapped in the clot. The slow release of a very powerful activator called tissue plasminogen activator (t-PA) from injured tissues and vascular endothelium converts plasminogen to plasmin, which digests the fibrin strands, causing the clot to dissolve.

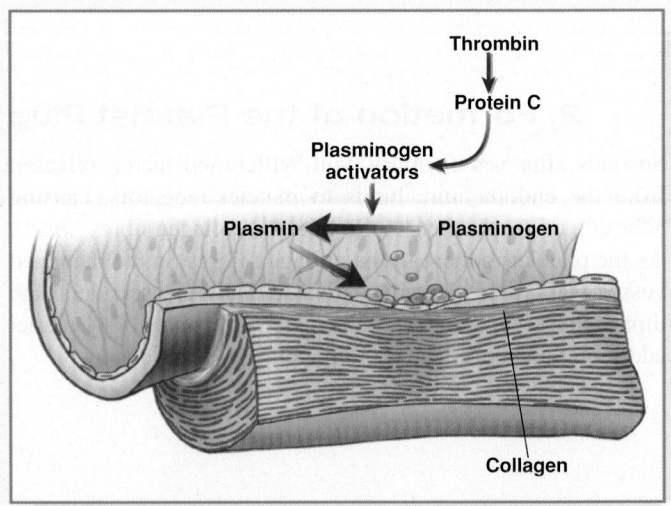

Inherited Disorders

Of the inherited causes of hypercoagulability, mutations in the factor V gene and prothrombin gene are the most common.[2] Approximately 2% to 15% of white people carry a specific factor V mutation (referred to as the *Leiden mutation,* because of the Dutch city where it was first discovered).[2] In persons with inherited defects in factor V, the mutant factor Va cannot be inactivated by protein C; as a result, an important antithrombotic counter-regulatory mechanism is lost. The defect predisposes to venous thrombosis, and among persons with recurrent deep vein thrombosis, the frequency of the mutation may be as high as 60%.[2] Women with factor V Leiden combined with the prothrombotic influence of pregnancy are at high risk for adverse pregnancy outcome such as venous thromboembolism disorders, preeclampsia, fetal loss, and placental abruption.[2]

A single nucleotide change in the prothrombin gene, which affects 1% to 2% of the population, is associated with elevated prothrombin levels and an almost threefold increase in venous thromboses. Less common primary hypercoagulable states include inherited deficiencies of anticoagulants such as antithrombin III, protein C, and protein S.[10] Another hereditary defect results in high circulating levels of homocysteine, which predisposes to venous and arterial thrombi by activating platelets and altering antithrombotic mechanisms.[2,10]

Acquired Disorders

Among the acquired or secondary factors that lead to increased coagulation and thrombosis are venous stasis due to prolonged bed rest and immobility, myocardial infarction, cancer, hyperestrogenic states, and oral contraceptives. Smoking and obesity promote hypercoagulability for unknown reasons.

Stasis of blood flow causes accumulation of activated clotting factors and platelets and prevents their interactions with inhibitors. Slow and disturbed flow is a common cause of venous thrombosis in the immobilized or postsurgical patient. Heart failure also contributes to venous congestion and thrombosis. Hyperviscosity syndromes (polycythemia) and deformed red blood cells in sickle cell disease increase the resistance to flow and cause small vessel stasis.

Elevated levels of estrogen increase hepatic synthesis of many coagulation factors and decrease the synthesis of antithrombin III.[11] The incidence of stroke, thromboemboli, and myocardial infarction is greater in women who use oral contraceptives, particularly those older than 35 years of age and those who are heavy smokers. Clotting factors are also increased during normal pregnancy. These changes, along with limited activity during the puerperium (immediate postpartum period), predispose to venous thrombosis.

Hypercoagulability is also common in cancer and sepsis. Many tumour cells are thought to release tissue factor molecules, which, along with the increased immobility and sepsis seen in patients with malignant disease, contribute to thrombosis in these patients.

Antiphospholipid Syndrome. Another cause of increased venous and arterial thrombi is the *antiphospholipid syndrome,* a condition associated with autoantibodies (primarily immunoglobulin G, IgG) directed against protein-binding phospholipids that results in increased coagulation activity.[12] The common features of antiphospholipid syndrome are venous and arterial thrombi, recurrent fetal loss, and thrombocytopenia. The disorder can be manifest as a primary condition occurring in isolation with signs of hypercoagulability, or as a secondary condition most often associated with connective tissue disorders, particularly systemic lupus erythematosus.[2]

People with the disorder present with a variety of clinical manifestations, typically those characterized by recurrent venous and arterial thrombi. Cardiac valvular vegetations associated with adherence of thrombi and thrombocytopenia due to excessive platelet consumption may also occur. Venous thrombosis, especially in the deep leg veins, occurs in up to 50% of persons with the syndrome, half of whom develop pulmonary emboli. Arterial thrombosis involves the brain in up to 50% of cases, causing transient ischemic attacks or strokes.[12] Other sites for arterial thrombosis are the coronary arteries of the heart and the retinal, renal, and peripheral arteries. Women with the disorder commonly have a history of recurrent pregnancy losses because of ischemia and thrombosis of the placental vessels. These women also have increased risk of giving birth to a premature infant owing to pregnancy-associated hypertension and uteroplacental insufficiency.

Although the mechanisms for this syndrome are unknown, several potential pathways have been identified. The antibodies may interfere with the coagulation cascade, leading to a hypercoagulability state; directly bind to the endothelial cell surface, causing secretion of cytokines that result in activation and aggregation of platelets; or target a serum phospholipid binding protein that functions as an anticoagulant. In addition to the action of the antibodies, it seems likely that other factors play a role in determining whether a person develops clinical manifestations of the disorder. Although speculative, these factors may include vascular trauma or the presence of infection that leads to cytokine production and endothelial cell activation.

In most people with antiphospholipid syndrome, the thrombotic events occur as a single episode at one anatomic site. In some people recurrences may occur months or years later and mimic the initial event. Occasionally, someone may present with multiple vascular occlusions involving many organ systems. This rapid onset condition is termed *catastrophic antiphospholipid syndrome* and is associated with a high mortality rate.[13]

Treatment of the syndrome focuses on removal or reduction in factors that predispose to thrombosis, including advice to stop smoking and counselling against use of estrogen-containing oral contraceptives by women. The acute thrombotic event is treated with anticoagulants (heparin and warfarin) and immune suppression in refractory cases. Aspirin and anticoagulant drugs may be used to prevent future thrombosis.[12] Bleeding disorders or impairment of blood coagulation can result from defects in any of the factors that contribute to hemostasis. Bleeding can occur as a result of disorders associated with platelet number or function, coagulation factors, and blood vessel integrity.

BLEEDING DISORDERS

After completing this section of the chapter, you should be able to meet the following objectives:

- Differentiate the mechanisms of drug-induced thrombocytopenia and idiopathic thrombocytopenia.
- Describe the manifestations of thrombocytopenia.
- State three common defects of coagulation factors and the causes of each.
- Differentiate between the mechanisms of bleeding in hemophilia A and von Willebrand disease.
- Describe the effect of vascular disorders on hemostasis.
- Explain the physiologic basis of acute disseminated intravascular coagulation.

Bleeding Associated With Platelet Disorders

Bleeding due to platelet disorders reflects a decrease in platelet number due to decreased production, increased destruction or impaired function of platelets. Spontaneous bleeding from platelet disorders most often involves small vessels of the mucous membranes and skin. Common sites of bleeding are the mucous membranes of the nose, mouth, gastrointestinal tract, and uterine cavity. Cutaneous bleeding is seen as pinpoint hemorrhages (petechiae) and purple areas of bruising (purpura) in dependent areas where the capillary pressure is higher (Fig. 13.4). Petechiae are seen almost exclusively

BLEEDING DISORDERS

- Bleeding disorders are caused by defects associated with platelets, coagulation factors, and vessel integrity.
- Disorders of platelet plug formation include a decrease in platelet numbers due to inadequate platelet production (bone marrow dysfunction), excess platelet destruction (thrombocytopenia), abnormal platelet function (thrombocytopathia), or defects in vWF.
- Impairment of the coagulation stage of hemostasis is caused by a deficiency in one or more of the clotting factors.
- Disorders of blood vessel integrity result from structurally weak vessels or vessel damage due to inflammation and immune mechanisms.

in conditions of platelet deficiency, not platelet dysfunction. Bleeding of the intracranial vessels is a rare but dangerous complication of severe platelet depletion.

Thrombocytopenia

A reduction in platelet number, also referred to as *thrombocytopenia,* is an important cause of generalized bleeding. Thrombocytopenia usually refers to a decrease in the number of circulating platelets to a level less than 150×10^9/L.[2] The greater the decrease in the platelet count, the greater the risk of bleeding. Thrombocytopenia can result from a decrease in platelet production, increased sequestration of platelets in the spleen, or decreased platelet survival.

Decreased platelet production due to loss of bone marrow function occurs in aplastic anemia (see Chapter 14); replacement of bone marrow by malignant cells, such as occurs

FIGURE 13.4 • Foot with acute purpura and petechiae. (From Hall B. J., Hall J. C. (Eds.). (2000). *Sauer's manual of skin diseases.* (10th ed., p. 139). Philadelphia, PA: Lippincott Williams & Wilkins.)

in leukemia, also results in decreased production of platelets. Radiation therapy and drugs such as those used in the treatment of cancer may depress bone marrow function and reduce platelet production. Infection with human immunodeficiency virus (HIV) or cytomegalovirus may suppress the production of megakaryocytes, the platelet precursors.

Production of platelets may be normal, but excessive pooling of platelets in the spleen may occur. Although the spleen normally sequesters 30% to 40% of the platelets before release into the circulation, the proportion can be as great as 90% when the spleen is enlarged in splenomegaly.[1] When necessary, hypersplenic thrombocytopenia may be treated with splenectomy.

Reduced platelet survival is caused by a variety of immune and nonimmune mechanisms. Platelet destruction may be caused by antiplatelet antibodies. The antibodies may be directed against platelet self-antigens or against antigens on the platelets from blood transfusions or pregnancy. The antibodies target the platelet membrane glycoproteins GPIIb/IIIa and GPIb/IX. Nonimmune destruction of platelets results from mechanical injury due to prosthetic heart valves or malignant hypertension, which results in small vessel narrowing. In acute disseminated intravascular coagulation (DIC) or thrombotic thrombocytopenic purpura (TTP), excessive platelet consumption leads to a deficiency. Massive blood or plasma transfusions may cause a dilutional thrombocytopenia because with prolonged blood storage the number of viable platelet is decreased.[2]

Drug-Induced Thrombocytopenia. Some drugs, such as quinine, quinidine, and certain sulfa-containing antibiotics, may induce thrombocytopenia. inducing an antigen–antibody response and formation of immune complexes that cause platelet destruction by complement-mediated lysis (see Chapter 17).[2] In people with drug-associated thrombocytopenia, there is a rapid fall in the platelet count within 2 to 3 days of resuming a drug, or 7 or more days (*i.e.,* the time needed to mount an immune response) after starting a drug for the first time. The platelet count rises rapidly after the drug is discontinued.

Heparin-Induced Thrombocytopenia. Heparin-induced thrombocytopenia (HIT) is associated with the anticoagulant drug heparin. Ten percent of patients treated with heparin develop a mild, transient thrombocytopenia within 2 to 5 days of starting the drug.[2] However, approximately 1% to 5% of heparin-treated patients experience life-threatening thromboembolic events 1 to 2 weeks after the start of therapy. HIT is caused by an immune reaction directed against a complex of heparin and platelet factor 4, a normal component of platelet granules that binds tightly to heparin. The binding of antibody to platelet factor 4 produces immune complexes that activate the remaining platelets, leading to thrombosis. In addition, prothrombotic platelet particles and induction of tissue factor continue to promote coagulation.[2]

The treatment of HIT requires the immediate discontinuation of heparin therapy and the use of alternative anticoagulants

to prevent thrombosis recurrence. The newer LMWH has been shown to be effective in reducing the incidence of heparin-induced complications compared with the older, high–molecular-weight form of the drug.

Immune Thrombocytopenic Purpura. Immune thrombocytopenic purpura (ITP), an autoimmune disorder, results in platelet antibody formation and excess destruction of platelets. The disorder can occur in the absence of any known risk factors (primary or idiopathic ITP) or as a secondary disorder due to an underlying disorder, and as an acute (duration of 6 months or less) or chronic disorder. Secondary forms of ITP may be associated with acquired immunodeficiency syndrome (AIDS), systemic lupus erythematosus, antiphospholipid syndrome, chronic lymphocytic leukemia, lymphoma, hepatitis C, and drugs such as heparin and quinidine.

About half of the cases of ITP occur as an acute primary disorder in children, affecting both boys and girls. The disorder occurs in young children (5 years of age) and usually follows a viral infection. It is characterized by sudden onset of petechiae and purpura and is usually a self-limited disorder requiring no treatment. Most children recover in a few weeks. In contrast, primary ITP is often a chronic disorder in adults with an insidious onset that seldom follows an infection. It is a disease of young people, with a peak incidence between the ages of 18 and 40 years, and is seen three times as often in women as in men.[2,10]

The thrombocytopenia that occurs in ITP is thought to result from multiple mechanisms, including antiplatelet antibodies against glycoproteins (IIb/IIIa and Ib/IX) in the platelet membrane. The platelets, which are made more susceptible to phagocytosis because of the antibody, are destroyed in the spleen. In addition, plasma levels of thrombopoietin, the major factor that stimulates growth and development of megakaryocytes, is not elevated in people with ITP, as opposed to people with thrombocytopenia from other causes such as chemotherapy or bone marrow failure.[2,14]

Manifestations of ITP include a history of bruising, bleeding from gums, epistaxis (*i.e.,* nosebleed), melena, and abnormal menstrual bleeding in those with moderately reduced platelet counts. Because the spleen is the site of platelet destruction, splenic enlargement may occur. The condition may be discovered incidentally or as a result of signs of bleeding, often into the skin (*i.e.,* purpura and petechiae) or oral mucosa. About half of adults with primary ITP present with a platelet count of less than 10×10^9/L and are at risk for internal hemorrhage.[15]

Diagnosis of ITP usually is based on severe thrombocytopenia (platelet counts less than 20 to 30×10^9/L), and exclusion of other causes. Tests for the platelet-bound antibodies are available but lack specificity (*e.g.,* they react with platelet antibodies from other sources). The secondary form of ITP sometimes mimics the idiopathic form of the disorder; therefore, the diagnosis is made only after excluding other known causes of thrombocytopenia.

The decision to treat ITP is based on the platelet count and the degree of bleeding. Many people with ITP do well without treatment. Corticosteroids are usually used as initial therapy. Other effective initial treatments include intravenous immune globulin. However, this treatment is expensive and the beneficial effect lasts only 1 to 2 weeks. Because the spleen is the major site of antibody formation and platelet destruction, splenectomy may be required for people who relapse or do not respond to drugs. Immunosuppressive therapy may be used for peoples who are refractory to other forms of treatment.

Thrombotic Thrombocytopenic Purpura. Thrombotic thrombocytopenic purpura (TTP) is a combination of thrombocytopenia, hemolytic anemia, renal failure, fever, and neurologic abnormalities. It is a rare disorder, occurring more commonly in adult women. The pathogenesis is elusive but likely results from introduction of platelet-aggregating substances into the circulation. The underlying cause of many cases is the deficiency of an enzyme (designated ADAMTS 13) that degrades large–molecular-weight multimers of vWF, allowing them to accumulate and cause platelet aggregation and adhesion to the endothelium.[2] The enzyme deficiency may be inherited or acquired as a result of antibody directed against the enzyme. TTP usually occurs in previously healthy peoples but may be associated with autoimmune collagen diseases, drugs, infections such as HIV, and pregnancy.[2] The disorder is similar to DIC but does not involve the clotting system. Toxins produced by some strains of *Escherichia coli* (e.g., *E. coli* O157:H7) cause endothelial injury and are responsible for a similar condition, *hemolytic uremic syndrome* (HUS).

The onset of TTP is abrupt and the outcome may be fatal. Widespread vascular occlusions result from thrombi in the arterioles and capillaries of many organs, including the heart, brain, and kidneys. Erythrocytes become fragmented as they circulate through the partly occluded vessels, causing hemolytic anemia and jaundice. The clinical manifestations include purpura, petechiae, vaginal bleeding, and neurologic symptoms ranging from headache to seizures and altered consciousness. Anemia is universal and may be marked.[2]

Emergency treatment for TTP includes *plasmapheresis*, a procedure that involves removal of plasma from withdrawn blood and replacement with fresh-frozen plasma. Plasma infusion provides the deficient enzyme. With plasmapheresis and plasma infusion treatment, there is a complete recovery in 80% of cases.[2]

Impaired Platelet Function

Impaired platelet function (also called *thrombocytopathia*) may result from inherited disorders of adhesion (e.g., von Willebrand disease) or acquired defects caused by drugs, disease, or surgery involving extracorporeal circulation (i.e., cardiopulmonary bypass). Defective platelet function is also common in uremia, presumably because of unexcreted waste products.

The use of aspirin and other nonsteroidal anti-inflammatory drugs (NSAIDs) is the most common cause of impaired platelet function. Aspirin produces irreversible acetylation of platelet cyclooxygenase activity and consequently impairs the synthesis of TXA_2, which is required for platelet

---

CHART 13.2 **DRUGS THAT MAY PREDISPOSE TO BLEEDING***

Interference With Platelet Production or Function
Acetazolamide
Antimetabolite and anticancer drugs
Antibiotics such as penicillin and the cephalosporins
Aspirin and salicylates
Carbamazepine
Clofibrate
Colchicine
Dipyridamole
Thiazide diuretics
Gold salts
Heparin
Nonsteroidal anti-inflammatory drugs (NSAIDs)
Quinine derivatives (quinidine and hydroxychloroquine)
Sulfonamides

Interference With Coagulation Factors
Amiodarone
Anabolic steroids
Warfarin
Heparin

Decrease in Vitamin K Levels
Antibiotics
Clofibrate

*This list is not intended to be inclusive.

---

aggregation. The effect of aspirin on platelet aggregation lasts for the life of the platelet—usually approximately 8 to 10 days. In contrast to the effects of aspirin, the inhibition of cyclooxygenase by other NSAIDs is reversible and lasts only for the duration of drug action. Low-dose aspirin (81 mg daily) is used to prevent formation of arterial thrombi and reduce the risk for myocardial infarction and stroke. Chart 13.2 lists other drugs that impair platelet function.

Bleeding Associated With Coagulation Factor Deficiencies

Blood coagulation defects can result from deficiencies or impaired function of one or more of the clotting factors, including vWF. Deficiencies can arise because of inherited disease, or defective synthesis or increased consumption of the clotting factors. Bleeding resulting from clotting factor deficiencies typically occurs after injury or trauma. Large bruises, hematomas, and prolonged bleeding into the gastrointestinal or urinary tracts or joints are common.

Inherited Disorders

Von Willebrand disease and hemophilia (A and B) are two of the most common inherited disorders of bleeding. Von

Willebrand disease is considered the most frequent inherited coagulopathy and affects up to 1% to 2% of the world's population. Hemophilia A (factor VIII deficiency) affects 1 in 5,000 male live births or approximately 2,500 Canadians. Hemophilia B, a deficiency of factor IX, occurs in approximately 1 in 20,000 persons, only accounting for 15% of people with hemophilia. It is genetically and clinically similar to hemophilia A.[2,10,16]

Hemophilia A and von Willebrand disease are caused by defects involving the factor VIII–vWF complex. Von Willebrand factor, which is synthesized by the endothelium and megakaryocytes, is required for platelet adhesion to the subendothelial matrix of the blood vessel. It also serves as the carrier for factor VIII, and is important for the stability of factor VIII in the circulation by preventing its proteolysis. Factor VIII coagulant protein, the functional portion, is produced by the liver and endothelial cells. Thus, factor VIII and vWF, synthesized separately, come together and circulate in the plasma as a unit that serves to promote clotting and adhesion of platelets to the vessel wall.[15–17]

Von Willebrand Disease. Von Willebrand disease is a relatively common hereditary bleeding disorder characterized by a deficiency or defect in vWF. As many as 20 variants of von Willebrand disease have been described. These variants can be grouped into two categories: types 1 and 3, which are associated with reduced levels of vWF; and type 2, which is characterized by defects in vWF.[2]

Type 1, an *autosomal dominant disorder,* accounts for approximately 70% of cases and is relatively mild. Type 2, also an autosomal dominant disorder, accounts for about 25% of cases and is associated with mild to moderate bleeding. Type 3, which is a relatively rare *autosomal recessive disorder,* is associated with extremely low levels of functional vWF and correspondingly severe clinical manifestations.

People with von Willebrand disease have a compound defect involving platelet function and the coagulation pathway. Clinical manifestations include spontaneous bleeding from the nose, mouth, and gastrointestinal tract, excessive menstrual flow, and a prolonged bleeding time in the presence of a normal platelet count. Most cases (*i.e.,* types 1 and 2) are mild and require no treatment, and many people with the disorder are diagnosed when surgery or dental extraction results in prolonged bleeding. In severe cases (*i.e.,* type 3), life-threatening gastrointestinal bleeding and joint hemorrhage may be similar to that seen in hemophilia.

The bleeding associated with von Willebrand disease is usually mild, and no treatment is routinely administered other than avoidance of aspirin. Desmopressin acetate (DDAVP), a synthetic analog of the hormone vasopressin, is used in the treatment of type 1 and 2A von Willebrand disease. DDAVP stimulates the endothelial cells to release stored vWF and plasminogen activator. The drug is available as an oral tablet and an intranasal spray. Factor VIII/vWF concentrate may be required as an alternative treatment or for any serious bleeding or major surgery in all types of the disease.[16]

Hemophilia A. Hemophilia A is an X-linked recessive disorder that primarily affects males. Although it is a hereditary disorder, there is no family history of the disorder in approximately 30% of newly diagnosed cases, suggesting that it has arisen as a new mutation in the factor VIII gene.[10] Approximately 90% of peoples with hemophilia produce insufficient quantities of the factor, and 10% produce a defective form. The percentage of normal factor VIII activity in the circulation depends on the genetic defect and determines the severity of hemophilia (*i.e.,* 6% to 30% in mild hemophilia, 2% to 5% in moderate hemophilia, and 1% or less in severe forms of hemophilia). In mild or moderate forms of the disease, bleeding usually does not occur unless there is a local lesion or trauma such as surgery or a dental procedure. The mild disorder may not be detected in childhood. In severe hemophilia, bleeding usually occurs in childhood (*e.g.,* it may be noticed at the time of circumcision) and is spontaneous and severe, often occurring several times a month.

Characteristically, bleeding occurs in soft tissues, the gastrointestinal tract, and the hip, knee, elbow, and ankle joints. Spontaneous joint bleeding usually begins when a child begins to walk. Often, a target joint is prone to repeated bleeding. The bleeding causes inflammation of the synovium, with acute pain and swelling. Without proper treatment, chronic bleeding and inflammation cause joint fibrosis and contractures, resulting in major disability. Muscle hematomas may be present in 10% to 25% of episodes, and intracranial hemorrhage, although uncommon, is an important cause of death.[18]

The prevention of trauma is important in peoples with hemophilia. Aspirin and other NSAIDs that affect platelet function should be avoided. Factor VIII replacement therapy (either recombinant or heat-treated concentrates from human plasma) administered at home has reduced the typical musculoskeletal damage. It is initiated when bleeding occurs or as prophylaxis with repeated bleeding episodes. The recombinant products and continuous-infusion pumps may allow prevention rather than therapy for hemorrhage. The development of inhibitory antibodies to recombinant factor VIII is still a major complication of treatment, as 10% to 15% of treated peoples produce high titres of antibodies that bind to and inhibit factor VIII.[10]

Current factor VIII products (both plasma derived and recombinant) are considered very safe as a result of technologic advances of the last two decades. Until the mid-1980s, before routine screening of blood for HIV antibodies was instituted, thousands of patients with hemophilia received plasma-derived factor VIII that was contaminated with HIV, and many developed AIDS.[10] Effective donor screening and development of purification and viral inactivation procedures now provide a safer product. In 2006, Health Canada approved a new recombinant factor VIII products (*i.e.,* Advate) that are produced without using additives derived from human or animal blood in the manufacturing process.[16]

The cloning of the factor VIII gene and progress in gene delivery systems have led to the hope that hemophilia A may be cured by gene replacement therapy. Carrier detection and prenatal diagnosis can now be done by analysis of direct gene mutation or DNA linkage studies. Prenatal amniocentesis or chorionic villus sampling is used to predict complications and determine therapy. It may eventually be used to select patients for gene addition.

Acquired Disorders

Coagulation factors V, VII, IX, X, XI, and XII, prothrombin, and fibrinogen are synthesized in the liver. In liver disease, synthesis of these clotting factors is reduced, and bleeding may result. Of the coagulation factors synthesized in the liver, factors II, VII, IX, and X and prothrombin require the presence of vitamin K for normal activity. In vitamin K deficiency, the liver produces the clotting factor, but in an inactive form. Vitamin K is a fat-soluble vitamin that is continuously being synthesized by intestinal bacteria. This means that a deficiency in vitamin K is not likely to occur unless intestinal synthesis is interrupted or absorption of the vitamin is impaired. Vitamin K deficiency can occur in the newborn infant before the establishment of the intestinal flora; it can also occur as a result of treatment with broad-spectrum antibiotics that destroy intestinal flora. Because vitamin K is a fat-soluble vitamin, its absorption requires bile salts. Vitamin K deficiency may result from impaired fat absorption caused by liver or gallbladder disease, and may also occur in chronic alcoholism.

Bleeding Associated With Vascular Disorders

Bleeding resulting from vascular disorders, sometimes called *nonthrombocytopenic purpura,* is relatively common and results in mild bleeding disorders.[10] These disorders may occur because of structurally weak vessel walls or because of damage to vessels by inflammation or immune responses. Most often they are characterized by easy bruising and the spontaneous appearance of petechiae and purpura of the skin and mucous membranes. In people with bleeding disorders caused by vascular defects, the platelet count and results of other tests for coagulation factors are normal.

Among the vascular disorders that cause bleeding are hemorrhagic telangiectasia, an uncommon autosomal dominant disorder characterized by thin-walled, dilated capillaries and arterioles; vitamin C deficiency (*i.e.,* scurvy), resulting in poor collagen synthesis and failure of the endothelial cells to be cemented together properly, which causes a fragile vascular wall; Cushing disease, causing protein wasting and loss of vessel tissue support because of excess cortisol; and senile purpura (*i.e.,* bruising in older adults), caused by impaired collagen synthesis in the aging process. Vascular defects also occur in the course of DIC or as a result of microthrombi and corticosteroid therapy.

Disseminated Intravascular Coagulation

Disseminated intravascular coagulation is a paradox in the hemostatic sequence and is characterized by widespread coagulation and bleeding in the vascular compartment. It is not a primary disease but occurs as a complication of a wide variety of conditions. DIC begins with massive activation of the coagulation sequence as a result of unregulated generation of thrombin, resulting in systemic formation of fibrin. In addition, levels of all the major anticoagulants are reduced (Fig. 13.5). The microthrombi that result cause vessel occlusion and tissue ischemia. Multiple organ failure may ensue. Clot formation consumes all available coagulation proteins and platelets, and severe hemorrhage results.

The disorder can be initiated by activation of the intrinsic or extrinsic pathway, or both. Activation through the extrinsic pathway occurs with liberation of tissue factor, and is associated with obstetric complications, trauma, bacterial sepsis, and cancers. The intrinsic pathway may be activated through extensive endothelial damage, with activation of factor XII. Endothelial damage may be caused by viruses, infections, immune mechanisms, stasis of blood, or temperature extremes. Impaired anticoagulation pathways are also associated with reduced levels of antithrombin and the protein C anticoagulant system in DIC. There is evidence that the underlying cause of DIC is infection or inflammation, and other proinflammatory cytokines (tumour necrosis factor, interleukin-1, and others) liberated in the process are the pivotal mediators.[10] These cytokines not only mediate inflammation, but can also increase the expression of tissue factor on endothelial cells and simultaneously decrease the expression of thrombomodulin. Thrombomodulin, a glycoprotein that is present on the cell membrane of endothelial cells, binds thrombin and acts as an additional regulatory mechanism in coagulation.[10]

Common clinical conditions that may cause DIC include obstetric disorders, accounting for 50% of cases, massive trauma, shock, sepsis, and malignant disease.[10] Chart 13.3 summarizes the conditions associated with DIC.

The factors involved in the conditions that cause DIC are often interrelated. In obstetric complications, tissue factor released from necrotic placental or fetal tissue or amniotic fluid may enter the circulation, inciting DIC. The hypoxia, shock, and acidosis that may coexist also contribute by causing endothelial injury. Gram-negative bacterial infections result in the release of endotoxins, which activate both the extrinsic pathway by release of tissue factor and the intrinsic pathway through endothelial damage. Endotoxins also inhibit the activity of protein C. Antigen–antibody complexes associated with infection can activate platelets through complement fragments.[10]

Although coagulation and formation of microemboli characterize DIC, its acute manifestations usually are more directly related to the bleeding problems that occur. The bleeding may be present as petechiae, purpura, oozing from puncture sites, or severe hemorrhage. Uncontrolled postpartum bleeding may indicate DIC. Microemboli may obstruct blood vessels and cause tissue hypoxia and necrotic damage to organ structures, such as the kidneys, heart, lungs, and brain. As a result, common clinical signs may be due to renal, circulatory, or respiratory failure, acute bleeding ulcers, or convulsions

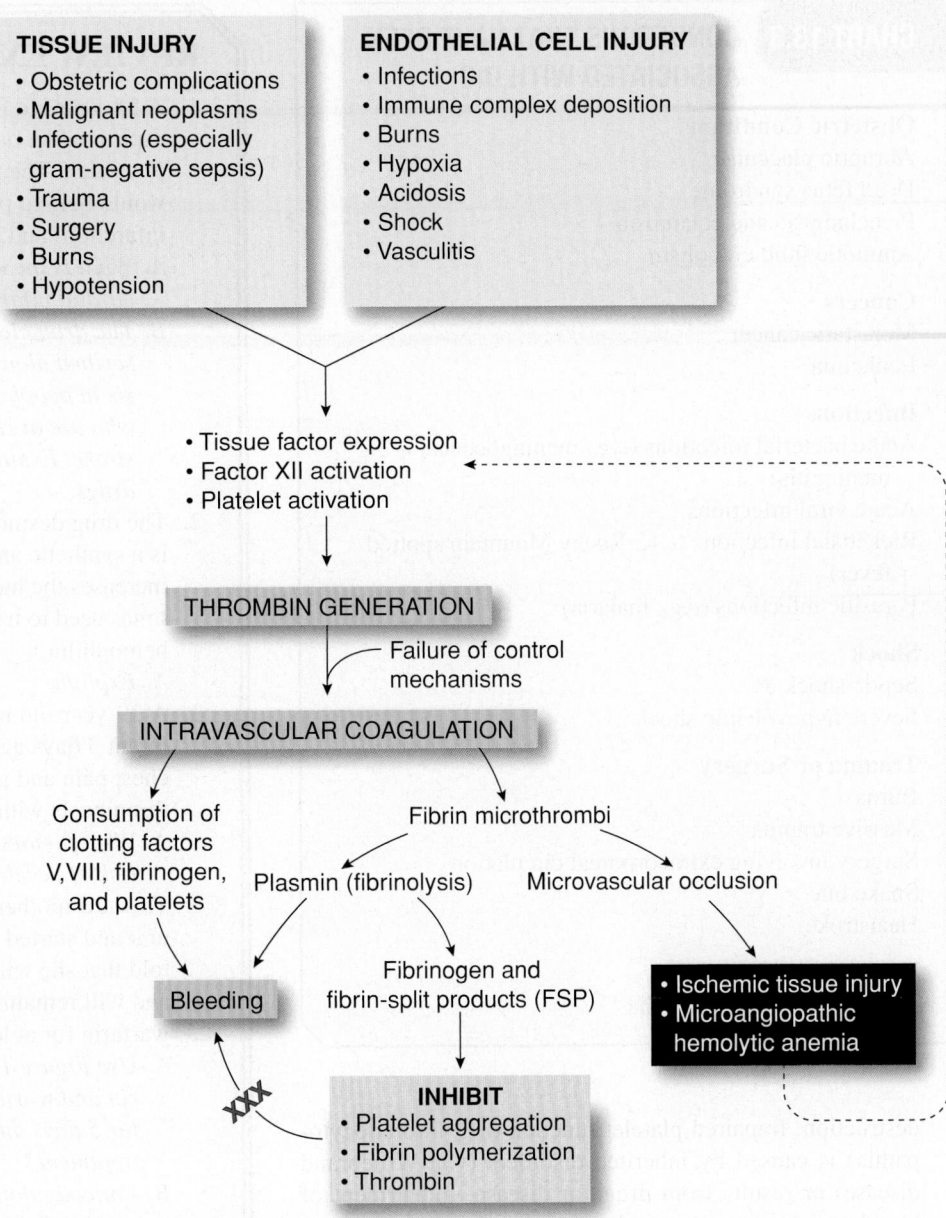

TISSUE INJURY
- Obstetric complications
- Malignant neoplasms
- Infections (especially gram-negative sepsis)
- Trauma
- Surgery
- Burns
- Hypotension

ENDOTHELIAL CELL INJURY
- Infections
- Immune complex deposition
- Burns
- Hypoxia
- Acidosis
- Shock
- Vasculitis

- Tissue factor expression
- Factor XII activation
- Platelet activation

THROMBIN GENERATION

Failure of control mechanisms

INTRAVASCULAR COAGULATION

Consumption of clotting factors V, VIII, fibrinogen, and platelets

Fibrin microthrombi

Plasmin (fibrinolysis)

Microvascular occlusion

Bleeding

Fibrinogen and fibrin-split products (FSP)

- Ischemic tissue injury
- Microangiopathic hemolytic anemia

INHIBIT
- Platelet aggregation
- Fibrin polymerization
- Thrombin

FIGURE 13.5 • Pathophysiology of disseminated intravascular coagulation. The DIC syndrome is triggered by tissue injury, endothelial cell injury, or a combination of the two. With the failure of normal mechanisms controlling hemostasis, intravascular coagulation occurs and is further potentiated by ongoing tissue ischemia (see dotted line). (Adapted from Rubin R., Strayer D. S. (Eds.). *Rubin's pathology: Clinicopathologic foundations of medicine.* (6th ed., p. 984). Philadelphia, PA: Lippincott Williams & Wilkins.)

and coma. A form of hemolytic anemia may develop as red cells are damaged passing through vessels partially blocked by thrombus.

The treatment of DIC is directed toward managing the primary disease, replacing clotting components, and preventing further activation of clotting mechanisms. Transfusions of fresh-frozen plasma, platelets, or fibrinogen-containing cryoprecipitate may correct the clotting factor deficiency. Heparin may be given to decrease blood coagulation, thereby interrupting the clotting process. Heparin therapy is controversial, however, and the risk of hemorrhage may limit its use to severe or chronic DIC cases. It typically is given as a continuous intravenous infusion that can be interrupted promptly if bleeding is accentuated. Administration of activated protein C (APC) was considered as an option but in 2011 drotrecogin

alfa was withdrawn from the market as it failed to show survival benefits. Tissue factor pathway inhibitors, antithrombin, recombinant thrombomodulin, and anti-inflammatory cytokines such as interleukin-10 are being evaluated in clinical trials as potential therapies.[19]

IN SUMMARY

Bleeding disorders or impairment of blood coagulation can result from defects in any of the factors that contribute to hemostasis: platelets, coagulation factors, or vascular integrity. The number of circulating platelets can be decreased (*i.e.*, thrombocytopenia) because of reduced bone marrow production, excess pooling in the spleen, or immune

CHART 13.3 CONDITIONS THAT HAVE BEEN ASSOCIATED WITH DIC

Obstetric Conditions
Abruptio placentae
Dead fetus syndrome
Preeclampsia and eclampsia
Amniotic fluid embolism

Cancers
Metastatic cancer
Leukemia

Infections
Acute bacterial infections (*e.g.,* meningococcal meningitis)
Acute viral infections
Rickettsial infections (*e.g.,* Rocky Mountain spotted fever)
Parasitic infections (*e.g.,* malaria)

Shock
Septic shock
Severe hypovolemic shock

Trauma or Surgery
Burns
Massive trauma
Surgery involving extracorporeal circulation
Snake bite
Heatstroke

Hematologic Conditions
Blood transfusion reactions

destruction. Impaired platelet function (*i.e.,* thrombocytopathia) is caused by inherited disorders (von Willebrand disease) or results from drugs or disease. Impairment of blood coagulation can result from deficiencies of one or more of the known clotting factors. Deficiencies can arise because of acquired disorders (*i.e.,* liver disease or vitamin K deficiency) or inherited diseases (*i.e.,* hemophilia A or von Willebrand disease). Bleeding may also occur from structurally weak vessels that result from impaired synthesis of vessel wall components (*i.e.,* vitamin C deficiency, excessive cortisol levels as in Cushing disease, or the aging process), or from damage by genetic mechanisms (*i.e.,* hemorrhagic telangiectasia), or the presence of microthrombi.

Disseminated intravascular coagulation (DIC) is characterized by the widespread imbalance between coagulation and bleeding in the vascular compartment. It begins with massive activation of the coagulation cascade and generation of microthrombi that cause vessel occlusion and tissue ischemia. Clot formation consumes all available coagulation proteins and platelets, and severe hemorrhage results.

REVIEW EXERCISES

1. A 55-year-old man has begun taking one 81-mg aspirin tablet daily on the recommendation of his physician. The physician had told him that this would help to prevent heart attack (myocardial infarction) and stroke.
   A. *What is the action of aspirin in terms of myocardial infarction and stroke prevention?*
   B. *The drug clopidogrel (Plavix) is often prescribed along with aspirin to prevent thrombosis in people with severe atherosclerotic disease who are at risk for myocardial infarction or stroke. Explain the rationale for using the two drugs.*
2. The drug desmopressin acetate (DDAVP), which is a synthetic analog of arginine vasopressin, increases the half-life of factor VIII and is sometimes used to treat bleeding in males with mild hemophilia.
   A. *Explain.*
3. A 29-year-old new mother, who delivered her infant 3 days ago, is admitted to the hospital with chest pain and is diagnosed as having venous thrombosis with pulmonary emboli.
   A. *What factors would contribute to this woman's risk of developing thromboemboli?*
4. The new mother is admitted to the intensive care unit and started on LMWH and warfarin. She is told that she will be discharged in a day or two and will remain on the heparin for 5 days and the warfarin for at least 3 months.
   A. *Use Figure 13.3 to explain the action of heparin and warfarin. Why is heparin administered for 5 days during the initiation of warfarin treatment?*
   B. *Anticoagulation with heparin and warfarin is not a definitive treatment for clot removal in pulmonary embolism, but a form of secondary prevention. Explain.*

References

1. Hall J. E. (2011). *Guyton and Hall textbook of medical physiology* (12th ed.). Philadelphia, PA: Elsevier Saunders.
2. Rubin R., Strayer D. S. (Eds.). (2012). *Rubin's pathology: Clinicopathologic foundations of medicine* (6th ed.). Philadelphia, PA: Lippincott Williams & Wilkins.
3. Rhoades R. A., Bell D. R. (2013). *Medical physiology: Principles for clinical medicine* (4th ed.). Philadelphia, PA: Lippincott Williams & Wilkins.
4. Ross M. H., Pawlina W. (2011). *Histology: A text and atlas with correlated cell and molecular biology* (6th ed., pp. 286–289.). Philadelphia, PA: Lippincott Williams & Wilkins.
5. Tanguay J., Bell A. D., Ackman M. L., et al.; Canadian Cardiovascular Society. (2012). Focused 2012 updated of the Canadian Cardiovascular Society guidelines for the use of antiplatelet therapy. *Canadian Journal of Cardiology, 29,* 1334–1345.

6. National Library of Medicine. (2013). Protein C deficiency. Available online at: http://ghr.nlm.nih.gov/condition/protein-c-deficiency. Accessed February 22, 2014.

7. Chrousos G. P. (2012). Chapter 40: The gonadal hormones and inhibitors. In Katzung B. G., Masters S. B., Trevor A. J. (Eds.), *Basic & clinical pharmacology* (12th ed.). Norwalk, CT: Appleton & Lange.

8. Thrombosis Canada. (2014). Clinical guides. Available online at: http://thrombosiscanada.ca/?page_id=18. Accessed February 22, 2014.

9. Schafer A. I. (2004). Thrombocytosis. *New England Journal of Medicine, 350*(12), 1211–1219.

10. Kumar V., Abbas A. K., Faustos N., et al. (Eds.). (2010). *Robbins and Cotran pathologic basis of disease* (8th ed.). Philadelphia, PA: Elsevier Saunders.

11. Zehnder J. L. (2012). Chapter 34: Drugs used in disorders of coagulation. In Katzung B. G., Masters S. B., Trevor A. J. (Eds.), *Basic & clinical pharmacology* (12th ed.). Norwalk, CT: Appleton & Lange.

12. Harper B. E., Willis R., Pierangeli S. S. (2011). Pathophysiological mechanisms in antiphospholipid syndrome. *International Journal of Clinical Rheumatology, 6*(2), 157–171.

13. Stojanovich L., Marisavljevic D., Rovensky J. et al. (2009). Clinical and laboratory features of the catastrophic antiphospholipid syndrome. *Clinical Reviews in Allergy & Immunology, 36*(2–3), 74–79.

14. Semple J. W., Provan D., Garvey M. B., Freedman J. (2010). Recent progress in understanding the pathogenesis of immune thrombocytopenia. *Current Opinion in Hematology, 17*(6), 590–595.

15. National Library of Medicine. (2012). Hemophilia. Available online at: http://ghr.nlm.nih.gov/condition/hemophilia. Accessed February 22, 2014.

16. Canadian Hemophilia Society. (2014). Bleeding disorders. Available online at: http://www.hemophilia.ca/en/bleeding-disorders/. Accessed February 22, 2014.

17. National Library of Medicine. (2012). Von Willebrand disease. Available online at: http://ghr.nlm.nih.gov/condition/von-willebrand-disease. Accessed February 22, 2014.

18. Sorensen B., Benson G. M., Bladen M., et al. (2012). Management of muscle haematomas in patients with severe haemophilia in an evidence-poor world. *Haemophilia, 18*, 598–606.

19. Wada H., Thachil J., Di Nisio M., et al.; The Scientific Standardization Committee on DIC of the International Society on Thrombosis Haemostasis. (2013). Guidance for diagnosis and treatment of disseminated intravascular coagulation from harmonization of the recommendations from three guidelines. *Journal of Thrombosis and Haemostasis, 11*, 761–767.

Visit thePoint **http://thePoint.lww.com for animations, journal articles, and more!**

Disorders of Red Blood Cells

14

Although the lungs provide the means for gas exchange between the external and internal environments, it is the hemoglobin in the red blood cells that transports oxygen to the tissues. The red blood cells also function as carriers of carbon dioxide and participate in acid-base balance. The function of the red blood cells, in terms of oxygen transport, is discussed in Chapter 27, and acid-base balance in Chapter 32. This chapter focuses on the red blood cell, anemia, blood types and transfusion therapy, polycythemia, and age-related changes in the red blood cells.

THE RED BLOOD CELL

After completing this section of the chapter, you should be able to meet the following objectives:

- Trace the development of a red blood cell from erythroblast to erythrocyte.
- Discuss the function of iron in the formation of hemoglobin.
- Describe the formation, transport, and elimination of bilirubin.
- Explain the function of the enzyme glucose-6-phosphate dehydrogenase in the red blood cell.
- State the meaning of the red blood cell count, percentage of reticulocytes, hemoglobin, hematocrit, mean corpuscular volume, and mean corpuscular hemoglobin concentration as they relate to the diagnosis of anemia.

The erythrocytes, 500 to 1,000 times more numerous than other blood cells, are the most common type of blood cell.[1] The mature red blood cell, the erythrocyte, is a nonnucleated, biconcave disk (Fig. 14.1). This unique shape contributes in two ways to the oxygen transport function of the erythrocyte. The biconcave shape provides a larger surface area for oxygen diffusion than would a spherical cell of the same volume, and the thinness of the cell membrane enables oxygen to diffuse rapidly between the exterior and the innermost regions of the cell (Fig. 14.2A).

Another structural feature that facilitates the transport function of the red blood cell is the flexibility of its

FIGURE 14.1 • A highly magnified (×11,397) scanning electron micrograph of a number of red blood cells found enmeshed in a fibrinous matrix on the luminal surface of an indwelling vascular catheter. Note the biconcave shape of each erythrocyte, which increases the surface area of these hemoglobin-filled cells, thus promoting more effective gas exchange. (Centers for Disease Control and Prevention Public Images Library, Courtesy Janice Carr.)

RED BLOOD CELLS

- The function of red blood cells, facilitated by the iron-containing hemoglobin molecule, is to transport oxygen from the lungs to the tissues.
- The production of red blood cells, which is regulated by erythropoietin, occurs in the bone marrow and requires iron, vitamin B_{12}, and folate.
- The red blood cell, which has a life span of approximately 120 days, is broken down in the spleen; the degradation products such as iron and amino acids are recycled.
- The heme molecule, which is released from the red blood cell during the degradation process, is converted to bilirubin and transported to the liver, where it is removed and rendered water soluble for elimination in the bile.

membrane. The biconcave shape and flexibility of the red cell membrane are maintained by a complex network of fibrous proteins, especially one called *spectrin* (Fig. 14.3). Spectrin forms an attachment with another protein, called *ankyrin,* that resides on the inner surface of the membrane and is anchored to an integral protein that spans the membrane. This unique arrangement of proteins imparts elasticity and stability to the membrane and allows it to deform (change shape) easily, which is required for the red blood cell to move through small capillaries to reach all peripheral body tissue.[2]

The function of the red blood cell, facilitated by the hemoglobin molecule, is to transport oxygen to the tissues. Because oxygen is poorly soluble in plasma, about 95% to 98% of the oxygen in arterial blood is carried bound to hemoglobin. The hemoglobin molecule is composed of two pairs of structurally different alpha (α) and beta (β) polypeptide chains (Fig. 14.2B). Each of the four polypeptide chains consists of

a globin (protein) portion and a heme unit, which surrounds an atom of iron that binds oxygen.[1] Thus, each molecule of hemoglobin can carry four molecules of oxygen. Hemoglobin is a natural pigment; because of its iron content, it appears reddish when oxygen is attached and has a bluish cast when deoxygenated. The production of each type of globin chain is controlled by individual structural genes with five different gene loci. Mutations, which can occur anywhere in these five loci, have resulted in over 550 types of abnormal hemoglobin molecules.[3]

The three types of normal hemoglobin are adult hemoglobin (both HbA and HbA_2) and fetal hemoglobin (HbF). The most common form of hemoglobin is HbA (consisting of a pair of α [alpha] and a pair of β [beta] chains) which represents approximately 97% of the total hemoglobin, HbA2 (with 2 α and 2 δ [delta] chains) which represents close to 2.5%, and HbF (with 2 α and 2 γ [gamma] chains) which represents approximately <1%. HbF is the predominant hemoglobin in the fetus from the third through the ninth months of gestation.

Plasma membrane
Hemoglobin

A Red blood cell
B Hemoglobin

FIGURE 14.2 • **A:** Biconcave structure of the red blood cell as shown in cross-section and in lateral surface view. **B:** Hemoglobin molecule, showing the four iron-containing heme subunits and their structure.

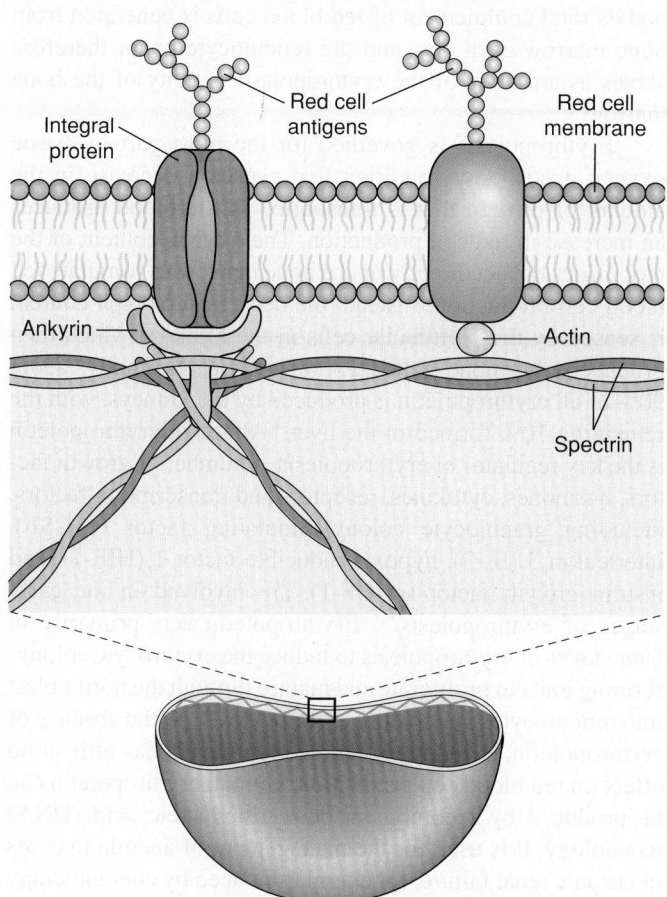

FIGURE 14.3 • Cross-sectional side view of the biconcave structure of the red blood cell and diagram showing the cytoskeleton and flexible network of spectrin proteins that attach to the ankyrin protein, a protein that resides on the inner surface of the membrane and is anchored to an integral protein that spans the membrane. Another transmembraneous protein is the Rh protein that would confirm if the red blood cell was Rh positive (not included in this diagram).

Because the γ is substituted for the α chain, HbF has a higher affinity for oxygen than either of the adult hemoglobins. This affinity facilitates the transfer of oxygen across the placenta from the HbA in the mother's blood to the HbF in the fetus's blood. HbF is replaced within 6 months of birth with HbA.[4]

Hemoglobin Synthesis

The rate at which hemoglobin is synthesized depends on the availability of iron for heme synthesis. A lack of iron results in relatively small amounts of hemoglobin in the red blood cells. The amount of iron in the body is approximately 2 g in women and up to 6 g in men.[5] Body iron is found in several compartments. Most iron (approximately 80%) is complexed to heme in hemoglobin, with small amounts found in the myoglobin of muscle, the cytochromes, and iron-containing enzymes. The other 20% is stored in the bone marrow, liver, spleen, and other organs. Iron in the hemoglobin compartment is recycled. When red blood cells age and are destroyed

in the spleen, the iron from their hemoglobin is released into the circulation and returned to the bone marrow for incorporation into new red blood cells or to the liver and other tissues for storage.[5]

Dietary iron also helps to maintain body stores. Iron, principally derived from meat, is absorbed in the small intestine, especially the duodenum (Fig. 14.4). When body stores of iron are diminished or erythropoiesis is stimulated, absorption is increased. In iron overload, excretion of iron is accelerated. Normally, some iron is sequestered in the intestinal epithelial cells and is lost in the feces as these cells slough off. The iron that is absorbed enters the circulation, where it immediately combines with an β-globulin, *apotransferrin*, to form *transferrin*, which is then transported in the plasma. From the plasma, iron can be deposited in tissues such as the liver, where it is stored as *ferritin*, a protein–iron complex, which can easily return to the circulation. Serum ferritin levels, which can be measured in the laboratory, provide an index of body iron stores.[2] Clinically, decreased ferritin levels usually indicate the need for prescription of iron supplements. Transferrin can also deliver iron to the developing red cell in bone marrow by binding to membrane receptors. This iron is

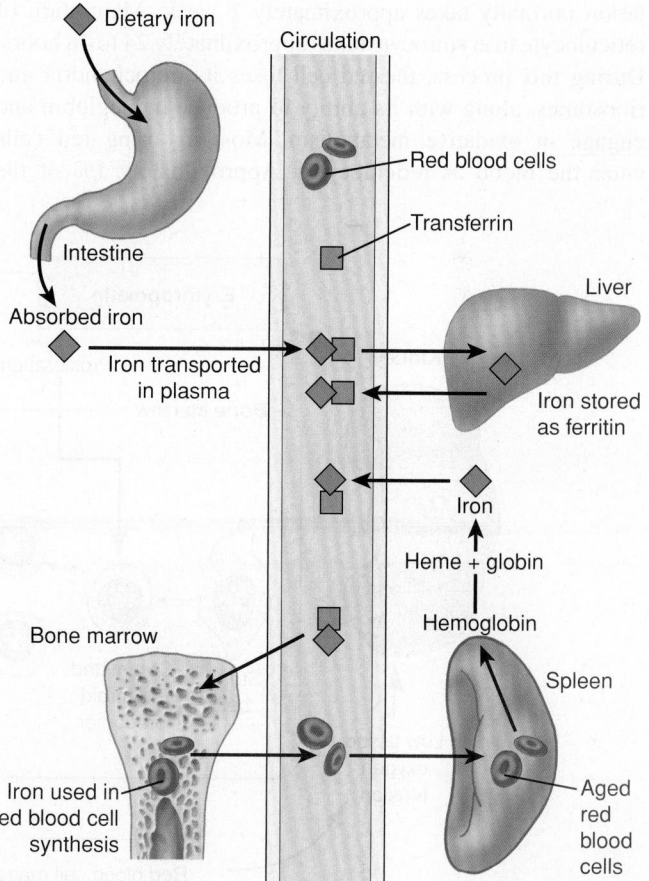

FIGURE 14.4 • Diagrammatic representation of the iron cycle, including its absorption from the gastrointestinal tract, transport in the circulation, storage in the liver, recycling from aged red cells destroyed in the spleen, and use in the bone marrow synthesis of red blood cells.

taken up by the developing red cell, where it is used in heme synthesis.

Red Cell Production

Erythropoiesis refers to the production of red blood cells. After birth, red cells are produced in the red bone marrow. Until 5 years of age, almost all bones produce red cells to meet the growth needs of a child, after which bone marrow activity gradually declines. After 20 years of age, red cell production takes place mainly in the membranous bones of the vertebrae, sternum, ribs, and pelvis. With this reduction in activity, the red bone marrow is replaced with fatty yellow bone marrow.

The red blood cells are derived from precursor cells called *erythroblasts,* which are formed continuously from the pluripotent stem cells in the bone marrow (Fig. 14.5). The red cell precursors move through a series of divisions, each producing a smaller cell as they continue to develop into mature red blood cells. Hemoglobin synthesis begins at the early erythroblast stage and continues until the cell becomes a mature erythrocyte. During its transformation from normoblast to reticulocyte, the red blood cell accumulates hemoglobin as the nucleus condenses and is finally lost. The period from stem cell to emergence of the reticulocyte in the circulation normally takes approximately 1 week. Maturation of reticulocyte to erythrocyte takes approximately 24 to 48 hours. During this process, the red cell loses its mitochondria and ribosomes, along with its ability to produce hemoglobin and engage in oxidative metabolism. Most maturing red cells enter the blood as reticulocytes. Approximately 1% of the body's total complement of red blood cells is generated from bone marrow each day, and the reticulocyte count therefore serves as an index of the erythropoietic activity of the bone marrow.

Erythropoiesis is governed for the most part by tissue oxygen needs. Any condition that causes a decrease in the amount of oxygen that is transported in the blood produces an increase in red cell production. The oxygen content of the blood does not act directly on the bone marrow to stimulate red blood cell production. Instead, the decreased oxygen content is sensed by the peritubular cells in the kidneys, which then produce a hormone called *erythropoietin.* Normally, about 90% of all erythropoietin is produced by the kidneys, with the remaining 10% formed in the liver.[2] Although erythropoietin is the key regulator of erythropoiesis, a number of growth factors, hormones, cytokines, receptors and transcription factors, including granulocyte colony-stimulating factor (G-CSF), interleukin 3 (IL-3), hypoxia inducible factor 1 (HIF-1), and insulin growth factor-1 (IGF-1), are involved in the early stages of erythropoiesis.[6,7] Erythropoietin acts primarily in later stages of erythropoiesis to induce the erythrocyte colony-forming units to proliferate and mature through the normoblast into reticulocytes and mature erythrocytes.[6,7] In the absence of erythropoietin, as in kidney failure, hypoxemia has little or no effect on red blood cell production. Human erythropoietin can be produced by recombinant deoxyribonucleic acid (DNA) technology. It is used for the management of anemia in cases of chronic renal failure, for anemias induced by chemotherapy in persons with malignancies, and in the treatment of anemia in human immunodeficiency virus (HIV)-infected persons.[3]

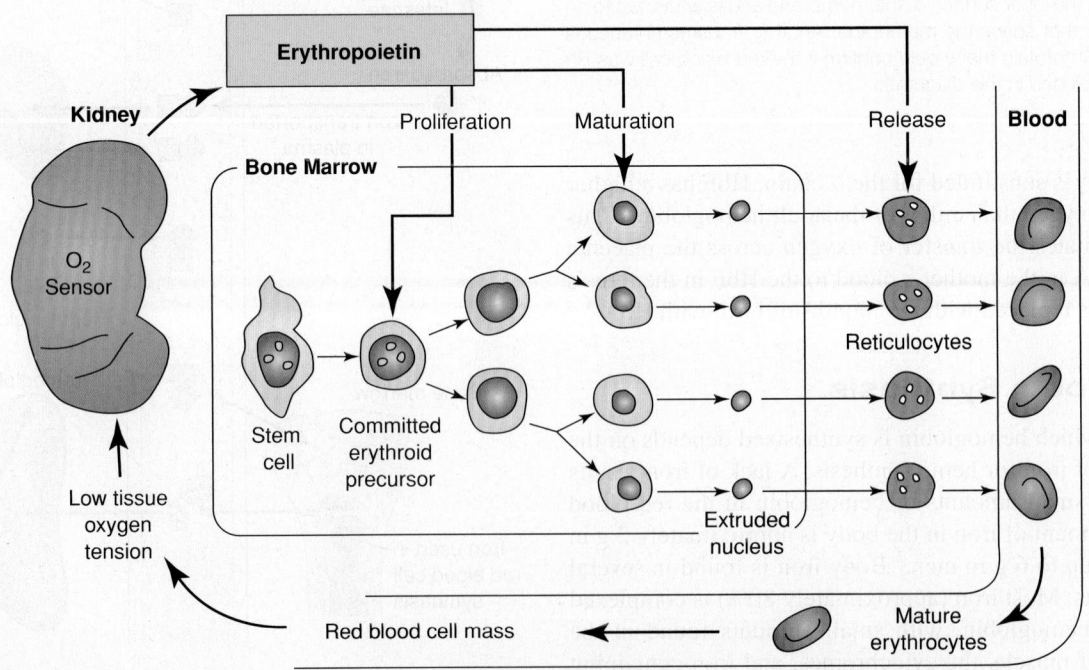

FIGURE 14.5 • Red blood cell development involves the proliferation and differentiation of committed bone marrow cells through the erythroblast and normoblast stages to reticulocytes, which are released into the bloodstream and finally become erythrocytes.

Because red blood cells are released into the blood as reticulocytes, the percentage of these cells is higher when there is a marked increase in red blood cell production. In some severe forms of anemia, the reticulocytes (normally about 1%) may account for as much as 30% of the total red cell count. In some situations, red cell production is so accelerated that numerous erythroblasts appear in the blood.[2]

Red Cell Destruction

Mature red blood cells have a life span of approximately 4 months or 120 days. As the red blood cell ages, a number of changes occur: metabolic activity in the cell decreases, enzyme activity declines, and adenosine triphosphate (ATP) decreases. Membrane lipids become reduced and the cell membrane becomes more fragile, causing the red cell to self-destruct as it passes through narrow places in the circulation and in the small trabecular spaces in the spleen.[2] The rate of red cell destruction (1% per day) normally is equal to the rate of red cell production, but in conditions such as hemolytic anemia, the cell's life span may be shorter.

The destruction of red blood cells is facilitated by a group of large phagocytic cells found in the spleen, liver, bone marrow, and lymph nodes. These phagocytic cells recognize old and defective red cells and then ingest and destroy them in a series of enzymatic reactions. During these reactions, the amino acids from the globulin chains and iron from the heme units are salvaged and reused (Fig. 14.6). The bulk of the heme unit is converted to bilirubin, the pigment of bile, which is insoluble in plasma and attaches to plasma proteins for transport. Bilirubin is removed from the blood by the liver and conjugated with glucuronide to render it water soluble so that it can be excreted in the bile. Excess elimination of bilirubin in the bile due to increased red cell destruction can lead to the development of bilirubin gallstones. The plasma-insoluble form of bilirubin is referred to as *unconjugated bilirubin* and the water-soluble form as *conjugated bilirubin*. Serum levels of conjugated and unconjugated bilirubin can be measured in the laboratory and are reported as direct and indirect, respectively. If red cell destruction and consequent bilirubin production are excessive, unconjugated bilirubin accumulates in the blood. This results in a yellow discolouration of the skin, called *jaundice*.[2]

When red blood cell destruction takes place in the circulation, as in hemolytic anemia, the hemoglobin remains in the plasma. The plasma contains a hemoglobin-binding protein called *haptoglobin*.[3] Other plasma proteins, such as albumin, can also bind hemoglobin. With extensive intravascular destruction of red blood cells, hemoglobin levels may exceed the hemoglobin-binding capacity of haptoglobin and other plasma proteins. When this happens, free hemoglobin appears in the blood (*i.e.,* hemoglobinemia) and is excreted in the urine (*i.e.,* hemoglobinuria). Because excessive red blood cell destruction can occur in hemolytic transfusion reactions, urine samples are tested for free hemoglobin after a transfusion reaction.

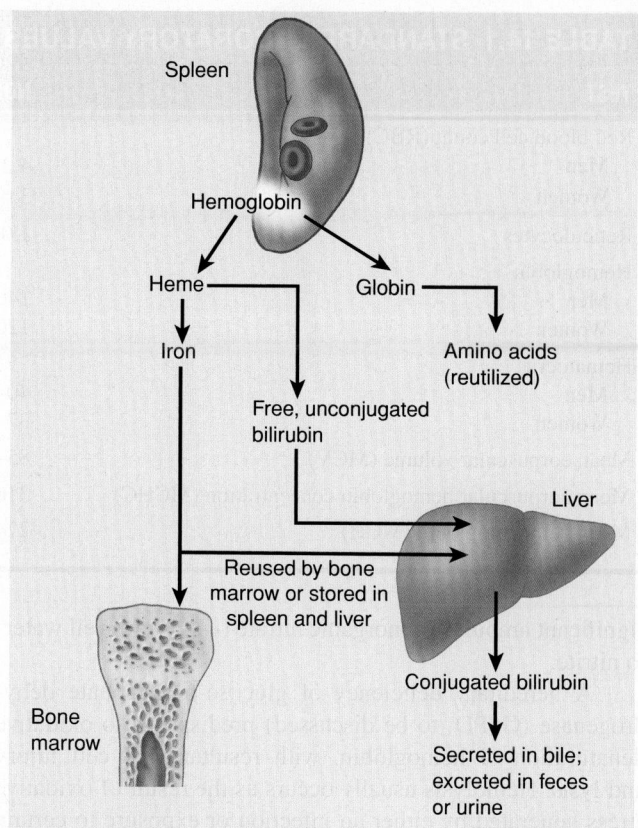

FIGURE 14.6 • Destruction of red blood cells and fate of hemoglobin.

Red Cell Metabolism and Hemoglobin Oxidation

The red blood cell, which lacks mitochondria, relies on glucose and the anaerobic glycolytic pathway for its metabolic needs (see Chapter 4). The enzyme-mediated anaerobic metabolism of glucose generates the ATP needed for normal membrane function and ion transport. The depletion of glucose or the functional deficiency of one of the glycolytic enzymes leads to the premature death of the red blood cell. An offshoot of the glycolytic pathway is the production of 2,3-diphosphoglycerate (2,3-DPG), which binds to the hemoglobin molecule and reduces the affinity of hemoglobin for oxygen. This facilitates the release of oxygen at the tissue level. An increase in the concentration of 2,3-DPG occurs in conditions of chronic hypoxemia such as occurs with chronic lung disease, anemia, and residence at high altitudes.[1]

The oxidation of hemoglobin—the combining of hemoglobin with oxygen—can be interrupted by certain chemicals (*e.g.,* nitrates and sulphates) and drugs that oxidize hemoglobin to an inactive form. The nitrite ion reacts with hemoglobin to produce *methemoglobin*, which has a low affinity for oxygen. Large doses of nitrites can result in high levels of methemoglobin, causing pseudocyanosis and tissue hypoxia. For example, sodium nitrate, which is used in curing meats, can produce methemoglobin when taken in large amounts. In nursing infants, the intestinal flora are capable of converting

TABLE 14.1 STANDARD LABORATORY VALUES FOR RED BLOOD CELLS

TEST	NORMAL VALUES	SIGNIFICANCE
Red blood cell count (RBC)		
Men	$4.2–5.4 \times 10^{12}/L$	Number of red cells in the blood
Women	$3.6–5.0 \times 10^{12}/L$	
Reticulocytes	1.0–1.5% of total RBC	Rate of red cell production
Hemoglobin		
Men	140–165 g/L	Hemoglobin content of the blood
Women	120–150 g/L	
Hematocrit		
Men	40–50%	Volume of cells in 100 ml of blood
Women	37–47%	
Mean corpuscular volume (MCV)	85–100 fL	Size of the red cell
Mean corpuscular hemoglobin concentration (MCHC)	310–350 g/L	Concentration of hemoglobin in the red cell
Mean cell hemoglobin (MCH)	27–34 pg	Red cell mass

significant amounts of inorganic nitrate (*e.g.*, from well water) to nitrite.

A hereditary deficiency of glucose-6-phosphate dehydrogenase (G6PD; to be discussed) predisposes to oxidative denaturation of hemoglobin, with resultant red cell injury and lysis. Hemolysis usually occurs as the result of oxidative stress generated by either an infection or exposure to certain drugs or foods.

Laboratory Tests

Red blood cells can be studied by means of a sample of blood (Table 14.1). In the laboratory, automated blood cell counters rapidly provide accurate measurements of red cell content and cell indices. The *red blood cell count* measures the total number of red blood cells in blood. The *percentage of reticulocytes* (normally approximately 1%) provides an index of the rate of red cell production. The *hemoglobin* (grams per litre [L] of blood) measures the hemoglobin content of the blood. The major components of blood are the red cell mass and plasma volume. The *hematocrit* measures the red cell mass in a 100-ml plasma volume. To determine the hematocrit, a sample of blood is placed in a glass tube, which is then centrifuged to separate the cells and the plasma. The hematocrit may be deceptive because it varies with the quantity of extracellular fluid, rising with dehydration and falling with overexpansion of extracellular fluid volume (Fig. 14.7).

Red cell indices are used to differentiate types of anemias by size or colour of red cells. The *mean corpuscular volume (MCV)* reflects the volume or size of the red cells. The MCV falls in microcytic (small cell) anemia and rises in macrocytic (large cell) anemia. Some anemias are normocytic (*i.e.*, cells are of normal size or MCV). The *mean corpuscular hemoglobin concentration (MCHC)* is the concentration of hemoglobin in each cell. Hemoglobin accounts for the colour of red blood cells. Anemias are described as *normochromic* (normal colour or MCHC) or *hypochromic* (decreased colour

or MCHC). *Mean cell hemoglobin* (MCH) refers to the mass of the red cell and is less useful in classifying anemias.[5]

A stained blood smear provides information about the size, colour, and shape of red cells and the presence of immature or abnormal cells. If blood smear results are abnormal, examination of the bone marrow may be indicated. Bone marrow commonly is aspirated with a special needle from the posterior iliac crest or the sternum. The aspirate is stained and observed for number and maturity of cells and abnormal types.

FIGURE 14.7 • Hematocrit. The hematocrit measures the percentage of cells in 100 ml of plasma: (**A**) normal, (**B**) decreased in anemia, and (**C**) increased in polycythemia.

The red blood cell provides the means for transporting oxygen from the lungs to the tissues. The biconcave shape of the red cell increases the surface area for diffusion of oxygen across the thin cell membrane. A complex cytoskeleton of proteins attached to the interior of the membrane maintains its shape and allows the cell to be deformed while passing through the small capillaries. The red cell contains extensive amounts of hemoglobin, a molecule composed of two polypeptide chains each consisting of a globin (protein) portion and a heme unit, which surrounds an iron atom that combines reversibly with oxygen. Red cells develop from stem cells in the bone marrow and are released as reticulocytes into the blood, where they become mature erythrocytes. Red blood cell production is regulated by the hormone erythropoietin, which is produced by the kidney in response to a decrease in oxygen levels.

The life span of a red blood cell is approximately 120 days. Red cell destruction normally occurs in the spleen, liver, bone marrow, and lymph nodes. In the process of destruction, the heme portion of the hemoglobin molecule is converted to bilirubin. Bilirubin, which is insoluble in plasma, attaches to plasma proteins for transport in the blood. It is removed from the blood by the liver and conjugated to a water-soluble form so that it can be excreted in the bile.

The red blood cell, which lacks mitochondria, relies on glucose and the glycolytic pathway for its metabolic needs. The end product of the glycolytic pathway, 2,3-DPG, increases the release of oxygen to the tissues during conditions of hypoxemia by reducing hemoglobin's affinity for oxygen.

In the laboratory, automated blood cell counters rapidly provide accurate measurements of red blood cell count and cell indices. A stained blood smear provides information about the size, colour, and shape of red cells, and the presence of immature or abnormal cells. If blood smear results are abnormal, examination of the bone marrow may be indicated.

ANEMIA

After completing this section of the chapter, you should be able to meet the following objectives:

- Describe the manifestations of anemia and their mechanisms.
- Explain the difference between intravascular and extravascular hemolysis.
- Compare the hemoglobinopathies associated with sickle cell disease and thalassemia.
- Explain the cause of sickling in sickle cell disease.
- Cite common causes of iron-deficiency anemia in infancy, adolescence, and adulthood.
- Describe the relation between vitamin B_{12} deficiency and megaloblastic anemia.
- List three causes of aplastic anemia.
- Compare characteristics of the red blood cells in acute blood loss, hereditary spherocytosis, sickle cell disease, iron-deficiency anemia, and aplastic anemia.

Anemia is defined as an abnormally low number of circulating red blood cells or level of hemoglobin, or both, resulting in diminished oxygen-carrying capacity. Anemia usually results from excessive loss (bleeding) or destruction (hemolysis) of red blood cells or from deficient red blood cell production because of a lack of nutritional elements or bone marrow failure.

Anemia is not a disease, but an indication of some disease process or alteration in body function. The effects of anemia can be grouped into three categories: (1) manifestations of impaired oxygen transport and the resulting compensatory mechanisms, (2) reduction in red cell indices and hemoglobin levels, and (3) signs and symptoms associated with the pathologic process that is causing the anemia. The manifestations of anemia depend on its severity, the rapidity of its development, and the person's age and health status.

In anemia, the overall oxygen-carrying capacity of hemoglobin is reduced, causing tissue hypoxia. Tissue hypoxia can give rise to fatigue, weakness, dyspnea, and sometimes angina. Hypoxia of brain tissue results in headache, faintness, and dim vision. The redistribution of the blood from cutaneous tissues or a lack of hemoglobin causes pallor of the skin, mucous membranes, conjunctiva, and nail beds. Tachycardia and palpitations may occur as the body tries to compensate for the low arterial oxygen content with an increase in cardiac output. A flow-type systolic heart murmur may result from changes

ANEMIA

- Anemia, which is a deficiency of red cells or hemoglobin, results from excessive loss (blood loss anemia), increased destruction (hemolytic anemia), or impaired production of red blood cells (iron-deficiency, megaloblastic, and aplastic anemias).
- Blood loss anemia is characterized by loss of iron-containing red blood cells from the body; hemolytic anemia involves destruction of red blood cells in the body with iron being retained in the body.
- Manifestations of anemia are caused by the decreased presence of hemoglobin in the blood (pallor), tissue hypoxia due to deficient oxygen transport (weakness and fatigue), and recruitment of compensatory mechanisms (tachycardia and palpitations) designed to increase oxygen delivery to the tissues.

in blood viscosity. Ventricular hypertrophy and high-output heart failure may develop in persons with severe anemia, particularly those with pre-existing heart disease. Erythropoiesis is accelerated and may be recognized by diffuse bone pain and sternal tenderness. In addition to the common anemic manifestations, hemolytic anemias are accompanied by jaundice caused by increased blood levels of bilirubin. In aplastic anemia, petechiae and purpura (*i.e.,* minute hemorrhagic spots and purplish areas on the skin caused by small vessel bleeding) are the result of reduced platelet function.[7]

Laboratory tests are useful in determining the severity and cause of the anemia. The red cell count and hemoglobin levels provide information about the severity of the anemia, whereas red cell characteristics such as size (normocytic, microcytic, macrocytic), colour (normochromic, hypochromic), and shape often provide information about the cause of anemia (Fig. 14.8).

Blood Loss Anemia

The clinical and red cell manifestations associated with blood loss anemia depend on the rate of hemorrhage and whether the bleeding loss is internal or external. With rapid blood loss, circulatory shock and circulatory collapse may occur. With more slowly developing anemia, the amount of red blood cells lost may reach 50% without the occurrence of signs and symptoms.[1,2]

The effects of acute blood loss are mainly due to loss of intravascular volume, which can lead to hypovolemic shock (see Chapter 26). A fall in the red blood cell count, hematocrit, and hemoglobin is caused by hemodilution resulting from movement of fluid into the vascular compartment. Initially, the red cells are normal in size and colour (normocytic, normochromic). The hypoxia that results from blood loss stimulates proliferation of committed erythroid stem cells in the bone marrow. It takes about 5 days for the progeny of stem cells to differentiate fully, an event that is marked by increased reticulocytes in the blood. If the bleeding is controlled and sufficient iron stores are available, the red cell concentration returns to normal within 3 to 4 weeks. External bleeding leads to iron loss and possible iron deficiency, which can hamper restoration of red cell counts.

Chronic blood loss does not affect blood volume but instead leads to iron-deficiency anemia when iron stores are depleted. It is commonly caused by gastrointestinal bleeding and menstrual disorders. Because of compensatory mechanisms, persons are commonly asymptomatic until the hemoglobin level is less than 80 g/L. The red cells that are produced have too little hemoglobin, giving rise to microcytic hypochromic anemia (Fig. 14.8).

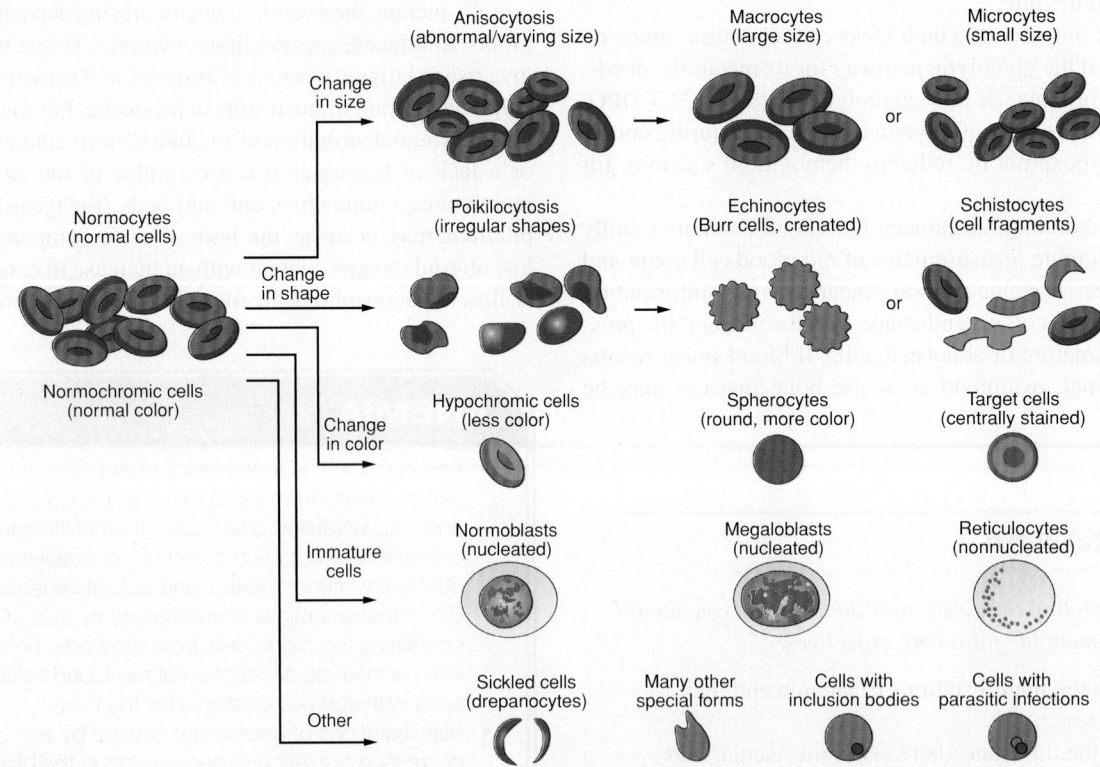

FIGURE 14.8 • Pathological changes in erythrocyte morphology. This synopsis of erythrocyte abnormalities presents a variety of possible deviations that are helpful for the diagnosis of anemias and other diseases. For example, a microcytic and hypochromic red cell is characteristic of iron deficiency anemia, or a macrocytic and misshaped red blood cell is characteristic of megaloblastic anemia. (From Rhoades, R. A., Bell, D. R. (2013). *Medical physiology: Principles for clinical medicine* (4th ed.). Philadelphia, PA: Lippincott Williams & Wilkins.)

Hemolytic Anemias

Hemolytic anemia is characterized by the premature destruction of red cells, the retention in the body of iron and the other products of hemoglobin destruction, and an increase in erythropoiesis. Almost all types of hemolytic anemia are distinguished by normocytic and normochromic red cells. Because of the red blood cell's shortened life span, the bone marrow usually is hyperactive, resulting in an increased number of reticulocytes in the circulating blood. As with other types of anemias, the person experiences signs and symptoms of impaired oxygen transport, such as fatigue, and compensatory mechanisms, which could include increases in both respiratory and heart rates.

In hemolytic anemia, red cell breakdown can occur within or outside the vascular compartment. Intravascular hemolysis is less common and occurs as a result of complement fixation in transfusion reactions, mechanical injury, or toxic factors. It is characterized by hemoglobinemia, hemoglobinuria, jaundice, and hemosiderinuria.[2] Extravascular hemolysis occurs when red cells become less deformable, making it difficult for them to traverse the splenic sinusoids. The abnormal red cells are sequestered and phagocytized by macrophages in the spleen. The manifestations of extravascular hemolysis include anemia and jaundice.

Another classification of hemolytic anemia is based on whether the cause is intrinsic or extrinsic. Intrinsic causes include defects of the red cell membrane, the various hemoglobinopathies, and inherited enzyme defects. Two main types of hemoglobinopathies can cause red cell hemolysis: the abnormal substitution of an amino acid in the hemoglobin molecule, as in sickle cell disease, and the defective synthesis of one of the polypeptide chains that form the globin portion of hemoglobin, as in the thalassemias.

Extrinsic or acquired forms of hemolytic anemia are caused by agents external to the red blood cell, such as drugs, bacterial and other toxins, antibodies, and physical trauma. Although all these factors can cause premature and accelerated destruction of red cells, they cannot all be treated in the same way. Some respond to splenectomy, others to treatment with corticosteroid hormones, and still others do not resolve until the primary disorder is corrected.

Inherited Hemolytic Anemias

There are also a group of inherited hemolytic anemias such as sickle cell anemia, thalassemia, and hereditary spherocytosis. People who inherit one of these anemias can have very different clinical manifestations, depending on the genotype they have. In fact, a person could be acutely ill or may have little to no clinical manifestations.

Inherited Disorders of the Red Cell Membrane. Hereditary spherocytosis, transmitted as an autosomal dominant trait in 75% of cases, is the most common inherited disorder of the red cell membrane.[4] The disorder is caused by abnormalities of defects in several membrane proteins including spectrin,

band 3, ankyrin, and protein 4.2 that lead to a gradual loss of the membrane surface.[7] The loss of membrane relative to cytoplasm causes the cell to become a tight sphere instead of a concave disk. Although the spherical cell retains its ability to transport oxygen, it is poorly deformable and susceptible to destruction as it passes through the venous sinuses of the splenic circulation. Clinical signs are variable but typically include mild hemolytic anemia, jaundice, splenomegaly, and bilirubin gallstones. A life-threatening aplastic crisis may occur when a sudden disruption of red cell production (often from a viral infection) causes a rapid drop in hematocrit and the hemoglobin level. The disorder usually is treated with splenectomy to reduce red cell destruction, and transfusions of concentrated or packed red cells may be required in a crisis.[1]

Sickle Cell Disease. Sickle cell disease is an inherited disorder in which an abnormal hemoglobin (hemoglobin S, HbS) leads to chronic hemolytic anemia, pain, and organ failure. The HbS gene is transmitted by recessive inheritance and can manifest as sickle cell trait (*i.e.*, heterozygote with one HbS gene) or sickle cell disease (*i.e.*, homozygote with two HbS genes). Sickle cell disease mostly affects people with African ancestry; however, other nationalities include Mediterranean, Middle Eastern, Indian, Caribbean, Hispanic, South and Central American and Asian. Although there are no Canadian statistics, it is estimated that 1 in 12 African Americans carry the trait.[8] In parts of Africa, where malaria is endemic, the gene frequency approaches 40%, attributed to the slight protective effect it confers against *Plasmodium falciparum* malaria.[1]

Pathogenesis. The abnormal structure of HbS results from a point mutation in the β chain of the hemoglobin molecule, with an abnormal substitution of a single amino acid, valine, for a hydrophobic glutamic acid (Fig. 14.9). In the heterozygote, only approximately 40% of the hemoglobin is HbS, but in the homozygote, 80% to 95% of the hemoglobin is HbS.[1,4] Variations in proportions exist, and the concentration of HbS correlates with the risk of sickling. In the homozygote with sickle cell disease, the HbS becomes sickled when deoxygenated or at a low oxygen tension. The deoxygenated hemoglobin aggregates and polymerizes in the cytoplasm, creating a semisolid gel that changes the shape and deformability of the cell. The sickled cell may return to normal shape with oxygenation in the lungs. However, after repeated episodes of deoxygenation, the cells remain permanently sickled. The person with sickle cell trait who has less HbS has little tendency to sickle, and is virtually asymptomatic. Fetal hemoglobin (HbF) inhibits the polymerization of HbS; therefore, most infants with sickle cell disease do not begin to experience the effects of the sickling until after 8 to 10 weeks of age, when the HbF has been replaced by HbS.[1]

There are two major consequences of red blood cell sickling: chronic hemolytic anemia and blood vessel occlusion. Premature destruction of the cells due to the rigid, nondeformable membrane occurs in the spleen, causing hemolysis and anemia from a decrease in red cell numbers. Vessel occlusion is a complex process involving an interaction among the sickled

FIGURE 14.9 • Mechanism of sickling and its consequences in sickle cell disease.

cells, endothelial cells, leukocytes, platelets, other plasma proteins.[7] The process is initiated by the abnormally adherent sickled cells to the vessel endothelium through adhesion molecules, causing endothelial activation with liberation of inflammatory mediators and substances that increase platelet activation and promote blood coagulation. The process also leads to the release of vasoconstrictor substances, whereas the liberation of nitric oxide, an important vasodilator, is impaired.[4,9]

Factors associated with sickling and vessel occlusion can include cold, stress, physical exertion, infection, and illnesses that lead to hypoxemia, dehydration, or acidosis. The rate of HbS polymerization is affected by the concentration of hemoglobin in the cell. Dehydration increases the hemoglobin concentration and contributes to the polymerization and resulting sickling. Acidosis reduces the affinity of hemoglobin for oxygen, resulting in more deoxygenated hemoglobin and increased sickling. Although sickling may be precipitated by these causes, in about half of the cases no precipitating factor is found.[7]

Clinical Course. Persons who are homozygous for the HbS gene experience severe hemolytic anemia, chronic hyperbilirubinemia, and vaso-occlusive crises. Hemolysis produces an

anemia with hematocrit values ranging from 18% to 30%.[5] The hyperbilirubinemia that results from the breakdown products of hemoglobin often leads to jaundice and the production of pigment stones in the gallbladder.

Blood vessel occlusion causes most of the severe complications. An acute pain episode results from vessel occlusion and hypoxia and can occur suddenly in almost any part of the body. Common sites obstructed by sickled cells include the abdomen, chest, bones, and joints. Many areas may be affected simultaneously. Infarctions caused by sluggish blood flow may cause chronic damage to the liver, spleen, heart, kidneys, retina, and other organs (Fig. 14.10). *Acute chest syndrome* is an atypical pneumonia resulting from pulmonary infarction. It is a leading cause of hospitalization in persons with sickle cell disease and is characterized by pulmonary infiltrates, shortness of breath, fever, chest pain, and cough.[10]

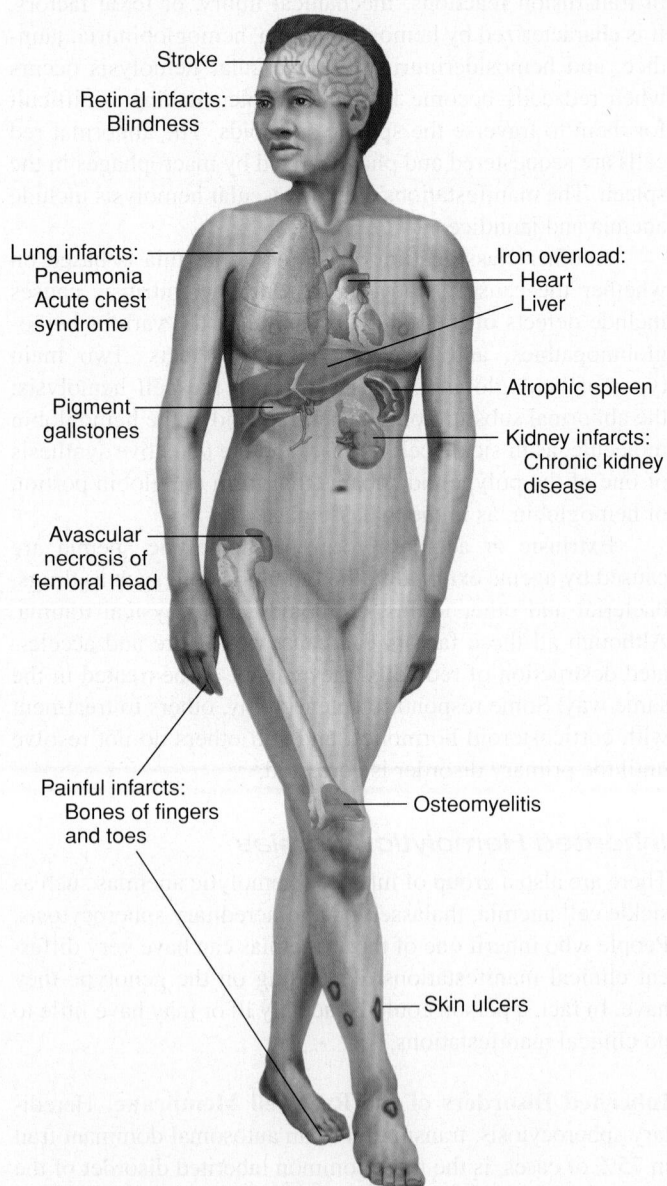

FIGURE 14.10 • Clinical manifestations of sickle cell disease.

The syndrome can cause chronic respiratory insufficiency and is a leading cause of death in sickle cell disease. Children may experience growth retardation and susceptibility to osteomyelitis. Painful bone crises may be caused by marrow infarcts of the bones of the hands and feet, resulting in swelling of those extremities. Approximately 11% of persons with sickle cell disease have overt stokes by the age of 20 years and transient ischemic attack or cerebral hemorrhage may precede the stroke.[11]

The spleen is especially susceptible to damage by HbS. Because of the spleen's sluggish blood flow and low oxygen tension, hemoglobin in red cells traversing the spleen becomes deoxygenated, causing ischemia. Splenic injury begins in early childhood, is characterized by intense congestion, and is usually asymptomatic. The congestion causes functional asplenia and predisposes the person to life-threatening infections by encapsulated organisms such as *Streptococcus pneumoniae, Haemophilus influenzae* type b, and *Klebsiella* species. Neonates and small children have not had time to create antibodies to these organisms and rely on the spleen for their removal. In the absence of specific antibody to the polysaccharide capsular antigens of these organisms, splenic activity is essential for removing these organisms when they enter the blood.

Diagnosis and Screening. Neonatal diagnosis of sickle cell disease is made on the basis of clinical findings and hemoglobin solubility results, which are confirmed by hemoglobin electrophoresis. Prenatal diagnosis can be done by the analysis of fetal DNA obtained by amniocentesis or in the future potentially using cell-free fetal DNA (cffDNA).

In Canada, some provinces universally offer screening programs to detect newborns with sickle cell disease and other hemoglobinopathies but these tests are not routinely done. Cord blood or heel-stick samples are subjected to electrophoresis to separate the HbF from the small amount of HbA and HbS. Other hemoglobins may be detected and quantified by further laboratory evaluation. In the United States, many states mandate screening of all newborns, regardless of ethnic origin.

Management. Currently there is no known cure for sickle cell disease; hence, treatment strategies focus on prevention of sickling episodes, symptom management, and treatment of complications. The person is advised to avoid situations that precipitate sickling episodes, such as infections, cold exposure, severe physical exertion, acidosis, and dehydration. Infections are aggressively treated, and blood transfusions may be warranted in a crisis or given chronically in severe disease.

Most children with sickle cell disease are at risk for fulminant septicemia from encapsulated organisms during the first 3 years of life. Prophylactic penicillin should be begun as early as 2 months of age and continued until at least 5 years of age. Maintaining full immunization, including *H. influenzae* vaccine and hepatitis B vaccine, is recommended. Canada's National Advisory Committee on Immunization also recommends administration of the 13-valent pneumococcal vaccine beginning at 2 to 6 months of age. This 13-valent vaccine should be followed by immunization with the 23-valent pneumococcal vaccine at 24 months of age or later.[12]

Hydroxyurea is a cytotoxic drug used to prevent complications of sickle cell disease. The drug allows synthesis of more HbF and less HbS, thereby decreasing sickling. Hydroxyurea reduces by 50% the pain episodes and pulmonary events in about 60% of the persons treated.[11] The others do not respond. Long-term effects regarding organ damage, growth and development, and risk of malignancies are unknown. Other therapies under investigation include drugs that affect globin gene expression; prevent polymerization, membrane damage, and cell dehydration; and inhibit sickle cell adhesion to endothelial cells and promote anticoagulation. Bone marrow or stem cell transplantation has the potential for cure in symptomatic children but carries multiple risks for complications. The bone marrow transplantation survival rate for human leukocyte antigen (HLA)–identical sibling donor transplants is about 93%.[9] Progress in gene therapy to treat sickle cell disease has been slow but promising, and may be a future option.

The Thalassemias

The thalassemias are a group of inherited disorders of hemoglobin synthesis. The majority of thalassemias involve the α- or β-globin chains of HbA; however, rare cases involving both chains (αβ) or all three (αδγ) do occur. β-Thalassemias are caused by deficient synthesis of the β chain and α-thalassemias by deficient synthesis of the α chain.[1,5] The defect is inherited as a mendelian trait, and a person may be heterozygous for the trait and have a mild form of the disease or be homozygous and have the severe form of the disease. Like sickle cell disease, the thalassemias occur with high degree of frequency in certain populations. The β-thalassemias, sometimes called *Cooley anemia* or *Mediterranean anemia,* are most common in the Mediterranean populations of southern Italy and Greece, and the α-thalassemias are most common among Asians. Both the α- and β-thalassemias are common in Africans and African Americans.

Two factors contribute to the anemia that occurs in thalassemia: low intracellular hemoglobin (hypochromia) due to the decreased synthesis of the affected chain, coupled with continued production and accumulation of the unaffected globin chain. The reduced hemoglobin synthesis results in a hypochromic, microcytic anemia, whereas the accumulation of the unaffected chain interferes with normal red cell maturation and contributes to membrane changes that lead to hemolysis and anemia.

The β-Thalassemias. The β-thalassemias result from 1 of nearly 200 point mutations in the β-globin gene causing a defect in β-chain synthesis.[14] In β-thalassemias, the excess α chains are denatured to form precipitates (*i.e.,* Heinz bodies) in the bone marrow red cell precursors. The Heinz bodies impair DNA synthesis and cause damage to the red cell membrane. Severely affected red cell precursors are destroyed in the bone marrow, and those that escape intramedullary death are at increased risk of destruction in the spleen. In addition to the anemia, persons with moderate to severe forms of the disease suffer from coagulation abnormalities.[1,5]

The clinical manifestations of the β-thalassemias are based on the severity of the anemia. The presence of one normal gene in heterozygous persons (thalassemia minor) usually results in sufficient normal hemoglobin synthesis to prevent severe anemia. Persons who are homozygous for the trait (thalassemia major) have severe, transfusion-dependent anemia that is evident at 6 to 9 months of age when the hemoglobin switches from HbF to HbA. If transfusion therapy is not started early in life, severe growth retardation occurs in children with the disorder.

In severe β-thalassemia, marked anemia produced by ineffective hematopoiesis and hemolysis lead to increased erythropoietin secretion and hyperplasia in the bone marrow and sites of extramedullary hematopoiesis. The expanding mass of erythropoietic marrow invades the bony cortex, impairs bone growth, and produces other bone abnormalities. There is thinning of the cortical bone, with new bone formation evident on the maxilla and frontal bones of the face (*i.e.,* chipmunk facies). The long bones, ribs, and vertebrae may become vulnerable to fracture because of osteoporosis or osteopenia, which contributes to increased morbidity in older adults. Enlargement of the spleen (splenomegaly) and liver (hepatomegaly) result from extramedullary hematopoiesis and increased red cell destruction.

Iron overload is a major complication of β-thalassemia. Excess iron stores, which accumulate from increased dietary absorption and repeated transfusions, are deposited in the myocardium, liver, and endocrine organs and induce organ damage. Cardiac, hepatic, and endocrine diseases are common causes of morbidity and mortality from *hemochromatosis* or iron overload. Disorders of the pituitary, thyroid, and adrenal glands and the pancreas result in significant morbidity and require hormone replacement therapy.[13]

Regular blood transfusions to maintain hemoglobin levels at 90 to 100 g/L improve growth and development and prevent most of the complications, and iron chelation therapy can reduce the iron overload and extend life expectancy. Bone marrow transplantation is a potential cure for low-risk patients, particularly in younger persons with no complications of the disease or its treatment, and has excellent results.[13] In the future, stem cell gene replacement may provide a cure for many with the disease.

The α-Thalassemias. The α-thalassemias are caused by a gene deletion that results in defective α-chain synthesis. Synthesis of the α-globin chains of hemoglobin is controlled by two pairs or four genes; hence, α-thalassemia shows great variation in severity related to the number of gene deletions. Silent carriers who have a deletion of a single α-globin gene are asymptomatic, and those with deletion of two genes have the α-thalassemia trait and exhibit mild hemolytic anemia. Deletion of three of the four α-chain genes leads to unstable aggregates of α chains called *hemoglobin H* (HbH). This

disorder is the most important clinical form and is common in Asians. The β chains are more soluble than the α chains, and their accumulation is less toxic to the red cells, so that senescent rather than precursor red cells are affected. Most persons with HbH have chronic moderate hemolytic anemia and may require transfusions in time of fever or illness or with certain medications.[14] The most severe form of α-thalassemia occurs in infants in whom all four α-globin genes are deleted and is called hydrops fetalis syndrome. Such a defect results in a hemoglobin molecule (Hb Bart) that is formed exclusively from the chains of HbF. Hb Bart, which has an extremely high oxygen affinity, cannot release oxygen in the tissues. Hydrops fetalis syndrome usually results in death *in utero* or shortly after birth.[14]

Inherited Enzyme Defects. The most common inherited enzyme defect that results in hemolytic anemia is a deficiency of glucose-6-phosphate dehydrogenase (G6PD). The gene that determines this enzyme is located on the X chromosome, and the defect is expressed only in males and homozygous females. There are more than 400 genetic variants of this disorder found in all populations, but particularly in African and Mediterranean groups. The African variant has been found in 10% to 15% of African Americans.[1] The disorder makes red cells more vulnerable to oxidants and causes direct oxidation of hemoglobin to methemoglobin, which cannot transport oxygen, and denaturing of the hemoglobin molecule to form Heinz bodies, which are precipitated in the red blood cell. Hemolysis usually occurs as the damaged red blood cells move through the narrow vessels of the spleen, causing hemoglobinemia, hemoglobinuria, and jaundice. The hemolysis is short-lived, occurring 2 to 3 days after the trigger event. In blacks, the defect is mildly expressed and is not associated with chronic hemolytic anemia unless triggered by oxidant drugs, acidosis, or infection.

The antimalarial drug primaquine, the sulfonamides, nitrofurantoin, aspirin, phenacetin, some chemotherapeutics, and other drugs cause hemolysis. For some people a potentially lethal hemolysis may occur after the ingestion of fava beans (favism). Free radicals generated by phagocytes during infections also are possible triggers. A more severe deficiency of G6PD is found in people of Mediterranean descent (*e.g.,* Sardinians, Sephardic Jews, Arabs). In some of these persons, chronic hemolysis occurs in the absence of exposure to oxidants. The disorder can be diagnosed through the use of a G6PD assay or screening test.

Acquired Hemolytic Anemias

Several acquired factors exogenous to the red blood cell produce hemolysis by direct membrane destruction or by antibody-mediated lysis.[1] Various drugs, chemicals, toxins, venoms, and infections such as malaria destroy red cell membranes. Hemolysis can also be caused by mechanical factors such as prosthetic heart valves, vasculitis, and severe burns. Obstructions in the microcirculation, as in disseminated intravascular coagulation (DIC), thrombotic thrombocytopenic purpura, and renal disease, may traumatize the red cells by producing turbulence and changing pressure gradients.

Many hemolytic anemias are immune mediated, caused by antibodies that destroy the red cell. Autoantibodies may be produced in response to drugs and disease. Alloantibodies come from an exogenous source and are responsible for transfusion reactions and hemolytic disease of the newborn.

The autoantibodies that cause red cell destruction are of two types: warm-reacting antibodies of the immunoglobulin G (IgG) type, which are maximally active at 37°C, and cold-reacting antibodies of the IgM type, which are optimally active at or near 4°C. The *warm-reacting antibodies* account for 80% of cases of hemolytic anemia.[1] They cause no morphologic or metabolic alteration in the red cell. Instead, they react with antigens on the red cell membrane, causing destructive changes that lead to spherocytosis, with subsequent phagocytic destruction in the spleen or reticuloendothelial system (RES). They lack specificity for the ABO antigens but may react with the Rh antigens. The hemolytic reactions associated with the warm-reacting antibodies affect women more frequently than men. The reactions have a rapid onset and may be severe and life-threatening. Fatigue is a common complaint and jaundice and moderate splenomegaly are present. Angina or congestive heart failure may also occur.

There are varied causes for this anemia; approximately 50% are idiopathic, and 50% are drug induced (*e.g.,* penicillin) or related to cancers of the lymphoproliferative system (*e.g.,* chronic lymphocytic leukemia, lymphoma), collagen diseases (*e.g.,* systemic lupus erythematosus), viral infections, and inflammatory disorders (*e.g.,* ulcerative colitis).[5] The drug-induced hemolysis is commonly benign.

The *cold-reacting antibodies* activate complement. Chronic hemolytic anemia caused by cold-reacting antibodies occurs with lymphoproliferative disorders and as an idiopathic disorder of unknown cause.[1] The hemolytic process occurs in distal body parts, where the temperature may fall below 30°C. Vascular obstruction by red cells results in pallor, cyanosis of the body parts exposed to cold temperatures, and Raynaud phenomenon (see Chapter 22). Hemolytic anemia caused by cold-reacting antibodies develops in only a few persons and is rarely severe.

The Coombs test, or antiglobulin test, is used to diagnose immune hemolytic anemias. It detects the presence of antibody or complement on the surface of the red cell. The direct antiglobulin test (DAT) detects the antibody on red blood cells. In this test, red cells that have been washed free of serum are mixed with anti-human globulin reagent. The red cells agglutinate if the reagent binds to and bridges the antibody or complement on adjacent red cells. The DAT result is positive in cases of autoimmune hemolytic anemia, erythroblastosis fetalis (Rh disease of the newborn), transfusion reactions, and drug-induced hemolysis. The indirect antiglobulin test detects antibody in the serum, and the result is positive for specific antibodies. It is used for antibody detection and crossmatching before transfusion.[15]

Anemias of Deficient Red Cell Production

Anemia may result from the decreased production of erythrocytes by the bone marrow. A deficiency of nutrients for hemoglobin synthesis (iron) or DNA synthesis (cobalamin or folic acid) may reduce red cell production by the bone marrow. A deficiency of red cells also results when the marrow itself fails or is replaced by nonfunctional tissue.

Iron-Deficiency Anemia

Iron deficiency is a common worldwide cause of anemia affecting persons of all ages. The anemia results from dietary deficiency, loss of iron through bleeding, or increased demands. Because iron is a component of heme, a deficiency leads to decreased hemoglobin synthesis and consequent impairment of oxygen delivery.

Body iron is used repeatedly. When red cells become senescent and are broken down, their iron is released and reused in the production of new red cells. Despite this efficiency, small amounts of iron are lost in the feces and need to be replaced by dietary uptake. Iron balance is maintained by the absorption of 1 to 2 mg daily to replace the iron lost in the feces. The average Western diet supplies about 20 mg.[1,4] The absorbed iron is more than sufficient to supply the needs of most individuals, but may be barely adequate in toddlers, adolescents, and women of child-bearing age. Dietary deficiency of iron is not common in developed countries except in certain populations. Most iron is derived from meat, and when meat is not available, as for deprived populations or individuals, or is not a dietary constituent, as for vegetarians, iron deficiency may occur.

The usual reason for iron deficiency in adults in the Western world is chronic blood loss because iron cannot be recycled to the pool. In men and postmenopausal women, blood loss may occur from gastrointestinal bleeding because of peptic ulcer, vascular lesions, intestinal polyps, hemorrhoids, or cancer. Excessive aspirin intake may cause undetected gastrointestinal bleeding. In women, menstruation may account for an average of 1.5 mg of iron lost per day, causing a deficiency.[4] Although cessation of menstruation removes a major source of iron loss in the pregnant woman, iron requirements increase at this time, and deficiency is common. The expansion of the mother's blood volume requires approximately 500 mg of additional iron, and the growing fetus requires approximately 280 mg during pregnancy. In the postnatal period, lactation requires approximately 1 mg of iron daily.[4]

A child's growth places extra demands on the body. Blood volume increases, with a greater need for iron. Iron requirements are proportionally higher in infancy (3 to 24 months) than at any other age, although they are also increased in childhood and adolescence. In infancy, the two main causes of iron-deficiency anemia are low iron levels at birth because of maternal deficiency and a diet consisting mainly of cow's milk, which is low in absorbable iron. Adolescents are also susceptible to iron deficiency because of high requirements due to growth spurts, dietary deficiencies, and menstrual loss.[16]

Iron-deficiency anemia is characterized by low hemoglobin and hematocrit, decreased iron stores, and low serum iron and ferritin. The red cells are decreased in number and are microcytic and hypochromic (Fig. 14.8). Poikilocytosis (irregular shape) and anisocytosis (irregular size) are also present. Laboratory values indicate reduced MCHC and MCV. Membrane changes may predispose to hemolysis, causing further loss of red cells.

The manifestations of iron-deficiency anemia are related to impaired oxygen transport and lack of hemoglobin. Depending on the severity of the anemia, fatigability, palpitations, dyspnea, angina, and tachycardia may occur. Epithelial atrophy is common and results in waxy pallor, brittle hair and nails, sometimes a spoon-shaped deformity of the fingernails called koilonychia, smooth tongue, sores in the corners of the mouth, and sometimes dysphagia and decreased acid secretion. A poorly understood symptom occasionally seen is pagophagia or pica, the bizarre, compulsive eating of ice, dirt, or other abnormal substances.

Prevention of iron deficiency is a primary concern in infants and children. Avoidance of cow's milk, iron supplementation at 4 to 6 months of age in breast-fed infants, and use of iron-fortified formulas and cereals are recommended for infants younger than 1 year of age. In the second year, a diet rich in iron-containing foods and use of iron-fortified vitamins will help prevent iron deficiency. The treatment of iron-deficiency anemia in children and adults is directed toward controlling chronic blood loss, increasing dietary intake of iron, and administering supplemental iron. Ferrous sulphate, which is the usual oral replacement therapy, replenishes iron stores in several months. Parenteral iron (iron dextran or sodium ferric gluconate) therapy may be used when oral forms are not tolerated or are ineffective. Because of the possibility of severe hypersensitivity reactions, an initial test dose should be done before administration of the first therapeutic dose of the drug. It is recommended that the test dose be administered in an environment equipped for treatment of severe allergic or anaphylactic reactions. Parenteral iron can be given intravenously or as a deep intramuscular injection by the Z-track method, in which the skin is pulled to one side before inserting the needle to prevent leakage into the tissues, with subsequent skin discolouration requiring rotation of the injected sites. In the future, gastric delivery systems may provide good therapy without side effects.

Megaloblastic Anemias

Megaloblastic anemias are caused by impaired DNA synthesis that results in enlarged red cells (MCV > 100 fL) due to impaired maturation and division. Vitamin B_{12} and folic acid deficiencies are the most common conditions associated with megaloblastic anemias. Because megaloblastic anemias develop slowly, there are often few symptoms until the anemia is far advanced.

Vitamin B_{12}-Deficiency Anemia. Vitamin B_{12}, also known as *cobalamin,* serves as a cofactor for two important reactions

in humans. It is essential for DNA synthesis and nuclear maturation, which in turn leads to normal red cell maturation and division.[17] Vitamin B_{12} is also involved in a reaction that prevents abnormal fatty acids from being incorporated into neuronal lipids. This abnormality may predispose to myelin breakdown and produce some of the neurologic complications of vitamin B_{12} deficiency.[5,17] Although this megaloblastic anemia can occur at any age, approximately 5% to 20% of older adults have B_{12} deficiency due to malabsorption, which can be impacted by several different factors such as medications (*i.e.,* proton pump inhibitors, metformin) or gastric bypass surgery.[4,17]

Vitamin B_{12} is found in all foods of animal origin. Dietary deficiency is rare and usually found only in strict vegetarians who avoid all dairy products as well as meat and fish. Normal body stores of 1,000 to 5,000 micrograms (μg) provide the daily requirement of 1 μg for a number of years.[1] Therefore, deficiency of vitamin B_{12} develops slowly. Vitamin B_{12} is absorbed by a unique process. After release from the animal protein, it is bound to intrinsic factor, a protein secreted by the gastric parietal cells (Fig. 14.11). The vitamin B_{12}–intrinsic factor complex protects vitamin B_{12} from digestion by intestinal enzymes. The complex travels to the ileum, where it binds to membrane receptors on the epithelial cells. Vitamin B_{12} is then separated from intrinsic factor and transported across the membrane into the circulation. There it is bound to its carrier protein, transcobalamin II, which transports vitamin B_{12} to its storage and tissue sites. Any defects in this pathway may cause a deficiency.

Pernicious anemia is a specific form of megaloblastic anemia caused by atrophic gastritis (see Chapter 37) and an attendant failure to produce intrinsic factor that leads to failure to absorb vitamin B_{12}. Pernicious anemia is believed to result from immunologically mediated, possibly autoimmune, destruction of the gastric mucosa. The resultant chronic atrophic gastritis

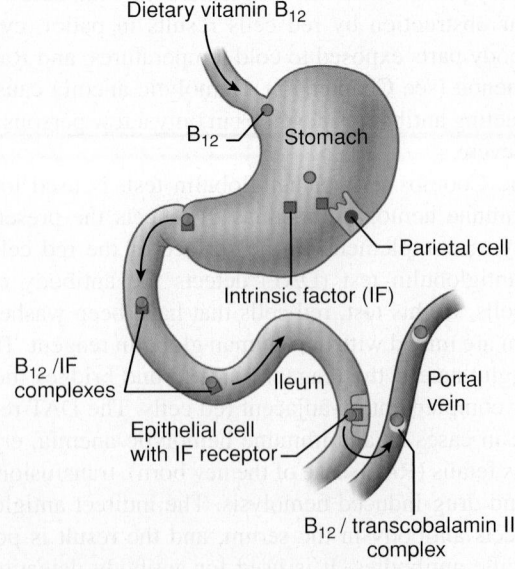

FIGURE 14.11 • Absorption of vitamin B_{12}.

is marked by loss of parietal cells and production of antibodies that interfere with binding of vitamin B_{12} to intrinsic factor. Other causes of vitamin B_{12}-deficiency anemia include gastrectomy, ileal resection, inflammation or neoplasms in the terminal ileum, and malabsorption syndromes in which vitamin B_{12} and other vitamin B compounds are poorly absorbed.

The hallmark of vitamin B_{12} deficiency is megaloblastic anemia. When vitamin B_{12} is deficient, the red cells that are produced are abnormally large because of excess cytoplasmic growth and structural proteins (Fig. 14.8). The cells have immature nuclei and show evidence of cellular destruction. They have flimsy membranes and are oval rather than biconcave. These oddly shaped cells have a short life span that can be measured in weeks rather than months. The loss of red cells results in a moderate to severe anemia and mild jaundice. The MCV is elevated, and the MCHC is normal.

Neurologic changes that accompany the disorder are caused by deranged methylation of myelin protein. Demyelination of the dorsal and lateral columns of the spinal cord causes symmetric paresthesias of the feet and fingers, loss of vibratory and position sense, and eventual spastic ataxia. In more advanced cases, cerebral function may be altered. In some cases, dementia and other neuropsychiatric changes may precede hematologic changes.

Diagnosis of vitamin B_{12} deficiency is made by finding an abnormally low vitamin B_{12} serum level. Previously the Schilling test, which measured the 24-hour urinary excretion of radiolabelled vitamin B_{12} administered orally, had been commonly used to document decreased absorption of vitamin B_{12}. Currently, the diagnosis of pernicious anemia is made by the detection of parietal cell and intrinsic factor antibodies. Lifelong treatment consisting of intramuscular injections or equally effective high oral doses of vitamin B_{12} reverses the anemia and improves the neurologic changes.[17]

Folic Acid–Deficiency Anemia. Folic acid is also required for DNA synthesis and red cell maturation, and its deficiency produces the same type of megaloblastic red cell changes that occur in vitamin B_{12}-deficiency anemia (*i.e.,* increased MCV and normal MCHC). Symptoms are also similar, but without the neurologic manifestations.

Folic acid is readily absorbed from the intestine. It is found in vegetables (particularly the green leafy types), fruits, cereals, and meats. Much of the vitamin, however, is lost in cooking. In Canada, most breakfast cereals and breads are fortified with folic acid. The most common causes of folic acid deficiency are malnutrition or dietary lack, especially in the elderly or in association with alcoholism. Total body stores of folic acid amount to 2,000 to 5,000 µg, and 50 µg is required in the daily diet.[1] A dietary deficiency may result in anemia in a few months. Malabsorption of folic acid may be due to syndromes such as celiac disease or other intestinal disorders. Some drugs used to treat seizure disorders (*e.g.,* primidone, phenytoin, phenobarbital) and triamterene, a diuretic, predispose to a deficiency by interfering with folic acid absorption. In neoplastic disease, tumour cells compete for folate, and

deficiency is common. Methotrexate, a folic acid analog used in the treatment of cancer, impairs the action of folic acid by blocking its conversion to the active form.[5]

Because pregnancy increases the need for folic acid 5- to 10-fold, a deficiency commonly occurs. Poor dietary habits, anorexia, and nausea are other reasons for folic acid deficiency during pregnancy. It is well known that there is an association between folate deficiency and neural tube defects in the growing fetus.[4] Health Canada recommends a daily folic acid intake of 400 µg for all women of childbearing age; this should be increased to 600 µg/day for pregnant women.[18] It is estimated that 50% of neural tube defects could thus be prevented. To facilitate adequate folate consumption, Health Canada mandated the addition of folate to cereal grain products in 1998.[19]

Aplastic Anemia

Aplastic anemia describes a disorder of pluripotential bone marrow stem cells that results in a reduction of all three hematopoietic cell lines—red blood cells, white blood cells, and platelets.[20] Pure red cell aplasia, in which only the red cells are affected, rarely occurs. Anemia results from the failure of the marrow to replace senescent red cells that are destroyed and leave the circulation, although the cells that remain are of normal size and colour. At the same time, because the leukocytes, particularly the neutrophils, and the thrombocytes have a short life span, a deficiency of these cells usually is apparent before the anemia becomes severe.[1]

The onset of aplastic anemia may be insidious, or it may strike with suddenness and great severity. It can occur at any age. The initial presenting symptoms include weakness, fatigability, and pallor caused by anemia. Petechiae (*i.e.,* small, punctate skin hemorrhages) and ecchymoses (*i.e.,* bruises) often occur on the skin, and bleeding from the nose, gums, vagina, or gastrointestinal tract may occur because of decreased platelet levels. The decrease in the number of neutrophils increases susceptibility to infection.

Among the causes of aplastic anemia are exposure to high doses of radiation, chemicals, and toxins that suppress hematopoiesis directly or through immune mechanisms. Chemotherapy and irradiation commonly result in bone marrow depression, which causes pancytopenia (anemia, thrombocytopenia, and neutropenia). Identified toxic agents include benzene, the antibiotic chloramphenicol, and the alkylating agents and antimetabolites used in the treatment of cancer (see Chapter 8). Aplastic anemia caused by exposure to chemical agents may be an idiosyncratic reaction because it affects only certain susceptible persons. It typically occurs weeks after a drug is initiated. Such reactions often are severe and sometimes irreversible and fatal. Aplastic anemia can develop in the course of many infections and has been reported most often as a complication of viral hepatitis, mononucleosis, and other viral illnesses, including acquired immunodeficiency syndrome (AIDS). In two thirds of cases, the cause is unknown, and these are called *idiopathic aplastic anemia.* The mechanisms underlying the pathogenesis of aplastic anemia are unknown. It is suggested that exposure to the chemicals, infectious agents, and other insults generates a cellular immune response resulting in production of cytokines by activated T cells. These cytokines (*e.g.,* interferon, tumour necrosis factor [TNF]) then suppress normal stem cell growth and development.[5,20]

Therapy for aplastic anemia in the young and severely affected includes stem cell replacement by bone marrow, peripheral blood transplantation, or immunosuppressive therapy. Histocompatible donors supply the stem cells to replace the patient's destroyed marrow cells. Graft-versus-host disease, rejection, and infection are major risks of the procedure, yet 75% or more survive. For those who are not transplantation candidates, immunosuppressive therapy with lymphocyte immune globulin (*i.e.,* antithymocyte globulin) prevents suppression of proliferating stem cells, producing remission but generally not as long lasting as bone marrow transplantation. Persons with aplastic anemia should avoid the offending agents and be treated with antibiotics for infection.[20,21]

Chronic Disease Anemias

Anemia often occurs as a complication of chronic infections, inflammation, and cancer. The most common causes of chronic disease anemias are acute and chronic infections, including AIDS and osteomyelitis; cancers; autoimmune disorders such as rheumatoid arthritis, systemic lupus erythematosus, and inflammatory bowel disease; and chronic kidney disease.[1] It is theorized that the short red cell life span, deficient red cell production, a blunted response to erythropoietin, and low serum iron are caused by actions of cytokines and cells of the reticuloendothelial system (RES). Microorganisms, tumour cells, and autoimmune dysregulation lead to T-cell activation and production of cytokines (*e.g.,* interleukin-1, interferon, and TNF) that suppress the erythropoietin response. In addition, macrophages take up iron and store it, thus reducing its availability for erythropoiesis. The mild anemia is normocytic and normochromic with low reticulocyte counts.

Chronic renal failure almost always results in anemia, primarily because of a deficiency of erythropoietin production. Unidentified uremic toxins and retained nitrogen also interfere with the actions of erythropoietin and with red cell production and survival.[1] Hemolysis and blood loss associated with hemodialysis and bleeding tendencies also contribute to the anemia of renal failure. Therapy for these anemias includes treatment for the underlying disease, short-term erythropoietin therapy, iron supplementation, and blood transfusions.

"Anemia of critical illness" is common in the intensive care unit, with more than 90% of patients having low hemoglobin levels secondary to their comorbidities. In critically ill persons, low erythropoietin concentrations and anemia also appear to be caused by inflammatory cytokines. Despite the prevalence of anemia in this population, it is suggested that red blood cell transfusions be restricted to reduce the risk of transmission of newer infectious agents and immune modulation (*e.g.,* immunosuppression).

IN SUMMARY

Anemia is a condition of an abnormally low number of circulating red blood cells or hemoglobin level, or both. It is not a disease, but a manifestation of a disease process or alteration in body function. The manifestations of anemia are those associated with impaired oxygen transport; alterations in red blood cell number, hemoglobin content, and cell structure, as well as the signs and symptoms of the underlying process causing the anemia.

Anemia can result from excessive blood loss, red cell destruction due to hemolysis, or deficient hemoglobin or red cell production. Blood loss anemia can be acute or chronic. With bleeding, iron and other components of the erythrocyte are lost from the body. Hemolytic anemia is characterized by the premature destruction of red cells, with retention in the body of iron and the other products of red cell destruction. Inherited hemolytic anemia can be caused by defects in the red cell membrane, hemoglobinopathies (sickle cell disease or thalassemia), or inherited enzyme defects (G6PD deficiency). Acquired forms of hemolytic anemia are caused by agents extrinsic to the red blood cell, such as drugs, bacterial and other toxins, antibodies, and physical trauma. Iron-deficiency anemia, which is characterized by decreased hemoglobin synthesis, can result from dietary deficiency, loss of iron through bleeding, or increased demands for red cell production. Vitamin B_{12} and folic acid deficiencies impair red cell production by interfering with DNA synthesis. Aplastic anemia is caused by bone marrow suppression and usually results in a reduction of white blood cells and platelets, as well as red blood cells. Chronic diseases such as inflammatory disorders (rheumatoid arthritis), cancers, and renal failure cause anemia through the production of inflammatory cytokines that interfere with erythropoietin production or response.

BLOOD TYPES AND TRANSFUSION THERAPY

After completing this section of the chapter, you should be able to meet the following objectives:

- Differentiate red cell antigens from antibodies in persons with type A, B, AB, or O blood.
- Explain the determination of the Rh factor.
- List the signs and symptoms of a blood transfusion reaction.

Anemias of various causes are treated with transfusions of whole blood or red blood cells only when oxygen delivery to the tissues is compromised, as evidenced by measures of oxygen transport and use, hemoglobin, and hematocrit. Current recommendations suggest transfusion for patients with hemoglobin levels less than 70 g/L, depending on age, illness, risk factors, and surgical procedures.[1,22] Persons with acute cardiac events require transfusion earlier to prevent reflex tachycardia and increased myocardial oxygen consumption. Acute massive blood loss usually is replaced with whole-blood transfusion. Most anemias, however, are treated with transfusions of red cell concentrates, which supply only the blood component that is deficient. Since the 1960s, devices that mechanically separate a unit of blood into its constituents have provided red cell components, platelets, fresh-frozen plasma, cryoprecipitate, and clotting factor concentrates. In this way, a unit of blood can be used efficiently for several recipients to correct specific deficiencies.

Several red cell components that are used for transfusion are prepared and stored under specific conditions and have unique uses, as described in Table 14.2. These red cell components are derived principally from voluntary blood donors. In the future, red cell substitutes, such as hemoglobin solutions, may be used, particularly in the trauma setting. The potential advantages are better storage, longer shelf life, and no risk of transfusion reaction.

The use of autologous donation and transfusion has been advocated since the early 1980s. Autologous transfusion refers to the procedure of receiving one's own blood—usually to replenish a surgical loss—thereby eliminating the risk of

TABLE 14.2 BLOOD AND BLOOD COMPONENTS USED IN TRANSFUSION THERAPY[a]

	COMPOSITION	INDICATIONS AND CONSIDERATIONS
Whole blood	Cells and plasma, hematocrit about 40%	Volume replacement and oxygen-carrying capacity; usually used only in significant bleeding (>25% blood volume lost)
Packed red blood cells (PRBCs)	RBCs with little plasma (hematocrit about 75%); some platelets and WBCs remain	↑ RBC mass Symptomatic anemia: platelets In the unit are not functional; WBCs in the unit may cause reaction and are not functional
Platelets—random	Platelets (5.5×10^{10} platelets/unit) Plasma; some RBCs, WBCs	Bleeding due to severe ↓ platelets Prevent bleeding when platelets <5,000–10,000/mm^3 Survival ↓ in presence of fever, chills, infection Repeated treatment → ↓ survival due to alloimmunization
Platelets—single donor	Platelets (3×10^{11} platelets/unit) 1 unit is equivalent to 6–8 units of random platelets	Used for repeated treatment: ↓ alloimmunization risk by limiting exposure to multiple donors
Plasma	Plasma; all coagulation factors Complement	Bleeding in patients with coagulation factor deficiencies; plasmapheresis
Granulocytes	Neutrophils (>1×10^{30}/unit); lymphocytes; some RBCs and platelets	Severe neutropenia in selected patients; controversial
Lymphocytes (WBCs)	Lymphocytes (number varies)	Stimulate graft-versus-host disease effect von Willebrand disease
Cryoprecipitate	Fibrinogen ≥150 mg/bag, AHF (VIII:C) 80–110 units/bag, von Willebrand factor; fibronectin	Hypofibrinogenemia Hemophilia A
Antihemophilic factor (AHF)	Factor VIII	Hemophilia A
Factor IX concentrate	Factor IX	Hemophilia B (Christmas disease)
Factor IX complex	Factors II, VII, IX, X	Hereditary factor VII, IX, X deficiency; hemophilia A with factor VII inhibitors
Albumin	Albumin 5%, 25%	Hypoproteinemia; burns; volume expansion by 5% to ↑ blood volume; 25% → ↓ hematocrit
Intravenous gamma globulin	IgG antibodies	Hypogammaglobulinemia (in CLL, recurrent infections); ITP; primary immunodeficiency states
Antithrombin III concentrate (AT III)	AT III (trace amounts of other plasma proteins)	AT III deficiency with or at risk for thrombosis

[a]The composition of each type of blood component is described as well as the most common indications for using a given blood component. RBCs, platelets, and fresh-frozen plasma are the blood products most commonly used. When transfusing these blood products, it is important to realize that the individual product is always "contaminated" with very small amounts of other blood products (*e.g.*, WBCs mixed in a unit of platelets). This contamination can cause some difficulties, particularly isosensitization, in certain patients.

AHF, antihemophilic factor; CLL, chronic lymphocytic leukemia; ITP, idiopathic thrombocytopenic purpura.

From Smeltzer S. C., Bare B. G., Hinkle J. L., et al. (2010). *Brunner & Suddarth's textbook of medical-surgical nursing* (12th ed.). Philadelphia, PA: Lippincott Williams & Wilkins; Table on p.964.

blood-borne disease or transfusion reaction. Autologous blood can be provided by several means: predeposit, hemodilution, and intraoperative salvage. A patient who is anticipating elective orthopedic, vascular, or open heart surgery may predeposit blood (*i.e.,* have the blood collected up to 6 weeks in advance and stored) for later transfusion during the surgery. Hemodilution involves phlebotomy before surgery with transfusion of the patient's blood at the completion of surgery. Intraoperative blood salvage is the collection of bloodshed from the operative site for reinfusion into the patient. Semiautomated devices are used to collect, anticoagulate, wash, and resuspend red cells for reinfusion during many procedures, including vascular, cardiac, and orthopedic surgery. Potential risks of autologous transfusion may include bacterial and other contamination, volume overload, and administrative errors.

Before a red cell or whole-blood transfusion from a volunteer donor source can occur, a series of procedures is required to ensure a successful transfusion. All Canadian donor samples are first tested for blood-borne diseases, such as hepatitis B and C viruses, HIV types 1 and 2, human T-cell lymphotropic viruses (HTLV-I and -II), syphilis, and West Nile Virus (WNV).[23] Donor and recipient samples are typed to determine ABO and Rh groups and screened for unexpected red cell antibodies. The cross-match is performed by incubating the donor cells with the recipient's serum and observing for agglutination. If none appears, the donor and recipient blood types are compatible.

ABO Blood Groups

ABO compatibility is essential for effective transfusion therapy and requires knowledge of ABO antigens and antibodies. There are four major ABO blood groups determined by the presence or absence of two red cell antigens (A and B). Persons who have neither A nor B antigens are classified as having type O blood; those with A antigens are classified as having type A blood; those with B antigens, as having type B blood; and those with A and B antigens, as having type AB blood (Table 14.3). The ABO blood groups are genetically determined. The type O gene is apparently functionless in production of a red cell antigen. Each of the other genes is expressed by the presence of a strong antigen on the surface of the red cell. Six genotypes, or gene combinations, result in four phenotypes, or blood type expressions. In Canada the

frequencies of ABO blood groups are approximately 46% for type O, 42% for type A, 9% for type B, and 3% for type AB.[24]

ABO antibodies predictably develop in the serum of persons whose red cells lack the corresponding antigen. Persons with type A antigens on their red cells develop type B antibodies; persons with type B antigens develop type A antibodies in their serum; persons with type O blood develop type A and type B antibodies; and persons with type AB blood develop neither A nor B antibodies. The ABO antibodies usually are not present at birth but begin to develop at 2 to 8 months of age and reach maximum levels between the ages of 5 and 10 years.[2]

Rh Types

Rh antigens are transmembranous proteins and an integral component of the red blood cells. While there are over 60 different RBC antigens that are capable of eliciting an immunogenic response, significant disease is associated with the D antigen of the Rh group. Rh antigens are routinely tested for transfusion compatibility. The Rh type antigens are coded by three gene pairs known as C, c; D, d; and E, e.[25] The D antigen is the most immunogenic and most predominant. Persons who express the D antigen are designated Rh positive, and those who do not express the D antigen are Rh negative. Unlike serum antibodies for the ABO blood types, which develop spontaneously after birth, Rh antibodies develop after exposure to one or more of the Rh antigens, usually through pregnancy or transfusions, and persist for many years.[2] More than 80% of Rh-negative persons develop the antibody to D antigen if they are exposed to Rh-positive blood.[26] Because it takes several weeks to produce antibodies, a reaction may be delayed and usually is mild. If subsequent transfusions of Rh-positive blood are given to a person who has become sensitized, the person may have a severe, immediate reaction.

Blood Transfusion Reactions

The seriousness of blood transfusion reactions prompts the need for extreme caution when blood is administered. Because most transfusion reactions result from administrative errors or misidentification, care should be taken to correctly identify the recipient and the transfusion source. The recipient's vital signs should be monitored before and during the transfusion, and careful observation for signs of transfusion reaction is imperative. The most feared and lethal transfusion reaction is the destruction of donor red cells by reaction with antibody in the recipient's serum.[22] This immediate hemolytic reaction usually is caused by ABO incompatibility. The signs and symptoms of such a reaction include sensation of heat along the vein where the blood is being infused, flushing of the face, urticaria, headache, pain in the lumbar area, chills, fever, constricting pain in the chest, cramping pain in the abdomen, nausea, vomiting, tachycardia, hypotension, and dyspnea.[22] If any of these adverse effects occur, the transfusion should be stopped immediately. Access to a vein should be maintained because it may be necessary to infuse intravenous solutions to ensure diuresis, administer medications, and take blood samples. The

TABLE 14.3 ABO SYSTEM FOR BLOOD TYPING			
GENOTYPE	RED CELL ANTIGENS	BLOOD TYPE	SERUM ANTIBODIES
OO	None	O	AB
AO	A	A	B
AA	A	A	B
BO	B	B	A
BB	B	B	A
AB	AB	AB	None

blood must be saved for studies to determine the cause of the reaction.

Hemoglobin that is released from the hemolyzed donor cells is filtered in the glomeruli of the kidneys. Two possible complications of a blood transfusion reaction are oliguria and renal shutdown because of the adverse effects of the filtered hemoglobin on renal tubular flow. The urine should be examined for the presence of hemoglobin, urobilinogen, and red blood cells. Delayed hemolytic reactions may occur more than 10 days after transfusion and are caused by undetected antibodies in the recipient's serum. The reaction is accompanied by a fall in hematocrit and jaundice, but most recipients are asymptomatic.

A febrile reaction, the most common transfusion reaction, occurs in approximately 1% of transfusions Recipient antibodies directed against the donor's white cells or platelets cause chills and fever. Antipyretics are used to treat this reaction. Future febrile reactions may be avoided by the use of leukocyte-reduced blood.[27]

Allergic reactions are caused by patient antibodies against donor proteins, particularly IgG. Urticaria and itching occur and can be relieved with antihistamines. Susceptible persons may be transfused with washed red cells to prevent reactions.

In rare cases, transfusion of packed cells results in acute lung injury, referred to as TRALI (see Chapter 29). The risk of TRALI increases with the number of packed cell infusions. The incidence of TRALI is low in Canada due to "washing" of packed cells. This process further filters and refines the plasma, which presumably reduces the amount of white blood cells and inflammatory mediators.

IN SUMMARY

Transfusion therapy provides the means for replacement of red blood cells and other blood components. Red blood cells contain surface antigens, and reciprocal antibodies are found in the serum. Four major ABO blood types are determined by the presence or absence of two red cell antigens: A and B. The D antigen determines the Rh-positive type; absence of the D antigen determines the Rh-negative type. At minimum, ABO and Rh types must be determined in recipient and donor blood before transfusion to ensure compatibility.

POLYCYTHEMIA

After completing this section of the chapter, you should be able to meet the following objectives:

- Define the term polycythemia.
- Compare causes of polycythemia vera and secondary polycythemia.
- Describe the manifestations of polycythemia.

Polycythemia is an abnormally high total red blood cell mass with a hematocrit greater than 54% in men and greater than 47% in women. A hematocrit greater than this can cause cardiac dysfunction and vascular obstruction, and levels greater than 60% can lead to hypoxia.[1] Polycythemia is categorized as *relative* or *absolute*. In *relative* polycythemia, the hematocrit rises because of a loss of plasma volume without a corresponding decrease in red cells. This may occur with water deprivation, excess use of diuretics, or gastrointestinal losses. Relative polycythemia is corrected by increasing the vascular fluid volume.[1]

Absolute polycythemia is a rise in hematocrit due to an increase in total red cell mass and is classified as primary or secondary. Primary polycythemia, or *polycythemia vera,* is a neoplastic disease of the pluripotent cells of the bone marrow characterized by an absolute increase in total red blood cell mass accompanied by elevated white cell and platelet counts. It most commonly is seen in men between 50 and 70 years of age, but may occur at any age.[28] In polycythemia vera, the manifestations are variable and are related to an increase in the red cell count, hemoglobin level, and hematocrit with increased blood volume and viscosity. Viscosity rises exponentially with the hematocrit and interferes with cardiac output and blood flow. Hypertension is common and there may be complaints of headache, dizziness, inability to concentrate, and some difficulty with hearing and vision because of decreased cerebral blood flow. Venous stasis gives rise to a plethoric appearance or dusky redness, even cyanosis, particularly of the lips, fingernails, and mucous membranes. Because of the increased concentration of blood cells, the person may experience itching and pain in the fingers or toes, and the hypermetabolism may induce night sweats and weight loss. Thromboembolism and hemorrhage, due to platelet abnormalities, are common complications that can be prevented by phlebotomy to reduce the hematocrit to less than 45.[28] The goal of treatment in primary polycythemia is to reduce blood viscosity. This can be done by withdrawing blood by periodic phlebotomy to reduce red cell volume. Low-dose aspirin may control the high platelet counts, and suppression of bone marrow function with chemotherapy (hydroxyurea) controls the elevated white cell count.[28]

Secondary polycythemia results from a physiologic increase in the level of erythropoietin, commonly as a compensatory response to hypoxemia. Conditions causing hypoxemia include living at high altitudes, chronic heart or lung disease, and smoking. The resultant release of erythropoietin by the kidney causes the increased formation of red blood cells in the bone marrow. Athletes injecting with exogenous erythropoietin (blood doping) or neoplasms that secrete erythropoietin may also experience a secondary polycythemia. Kidney disease such as hydronephrosis or renal cysts may obstruct blood flow, cause hypoxia, and lead to an increase in erythropoietin. Treatment of secondary polycythemia focuses on reducing the hematocrit or relieving hypoxemia. For example, continuous low-flow oxygen therapy can be used to correct the severe hypoxemia that occurs in some persons with chronic obstructive pulmonary disease. This form of treatment is thought to relieve the pulmonary hypertension and polycythemia and to delay the onset of cor pulmonale.

IN SUMMARY

Polycythemia describes a condition in which the red blood cell mass is increased. It can present as a relative, primary, or secondary disorder. Relative polycythemia results from a loss of vascular fluid and is corrected by replacing the fluid. Primary polycythemia, or polycythemia vera, is a proliferative disease of the bone marrow with an absolute increase in total red blood cell mass accompanied by elevated white cell and platelet counts. Secondary polycythemia results from increased erythropoietin levels caused by hypoxic conditions such as chronic heart and lung disease. Many of the manifestations of polycythemia are related to increased blood volume and viscosity that lead to hypertension and stagnation of blood flow.

AGE-RELATED CHANGES IN RED BLOOD CELLS

After completing this section of the chapter, you should be able to meet the following objectives:

- Cite the function of hemoglobin F in the neonate and describe the red blood cell changes that occur during the early neonatal period.
- Cite the factors that predispose to hyperbilirubinemia in the infant.
- Describe the pathogenesis of hemolytic disease of the newborn.
- Compare conjugated and unconjugated bilirubin in terms of production of encephalopathy in the neonate.
- Explain the action of phototherapy in the treatment of hyperbilirubinemia in the neonate.
- State the changes in the red blood cells that occur with aging.

Red Cell Changes in the Neonate

At birth, changes in the red blood cell indices reflect the transition to extrauterine life and the need to transport oxygen from the lungs. Hemoglobin concentrations at birth are high, reflecting the high synthetic activity in utero required to provide adequate oxygen delivery. Toward the end of the first postnatal week, hemoglobin concentration begins to decline, gradually falling to a minimum value at approximately 2 months of age. The red cell count, hematocrit, and MCV likewise fall. The factors responsible for the decline include reduced red cell production and plasma dilution caused by increased blood volume with growth. Neonatal red cells also have a shorter life span of 50 to 70 days, and are thought to be more fragile than those of older persons. During the early neonatal period, there is also a switch from HbF to HbA. The amount of HbF in term infants averages about 70% of the total hemoglobin and declines to trace amounts by 6 to 12 months of age.[29] The switch to HbA provides greater unloading of oxygen to the tissues because HbA has a lower affinity for oxygen compared with HbF. Infants who are small for gestational age or born to diabetic or smoking mothers or who experienced hypoxemia in utero have higher total hemoglobin levels, higher HbF levels, and a delayed switch to HbA.

A physiologic anemia of the newborn develops at approximately 2 months of age. It seldom produces symptoms and cannot be altered by nutritional supplements. Anemia of prematurity, an exaggerated physiologic response in infants with low birth weight, is thought to result from a poor erythropoietin response. A contributing factor is the frequent blood sampling often required in these infants. The hemoglobin level rapidly declines after birth to a low of 70 to 100 g/L at approximately 6 weeks of age. Signs and symptoms include apnea, poor weight gain, pallor, decreased activity, and tachycardia. In infants born before 33 weeks' gestation or those with hematocrits below 33%, the clinical features are more evident.

Anemia at birth, characterized by pallor, congestive heart failure, or shock, usually is caused by hemolytic disease of the newborn. Bleeding from the umbilical cord, internal hemorrhage, congenital hemolytic disease, or frequent blood sampling are other possible causes of anemia. The severity of symptoms and presence of coexisting disease may warrant red cell transfusion.

Hyperbilirubinemia in the Neonate

Hyperbilirubinemia, an increased level of serum bilirubin, is a common cause of jaundice in the neonate. A benign, self-limited condition, it most often is related to the developmental state of the neonate. Rarely, cases of hyperbilirubinemia are pathologic and may lead to kernicterus and serious brain damage.

In the first week of life, approximately 60% of term and 80% of preterm neonates are jaundiced.[30] This physiologic jaundice appears in term infants on the second or third day of life. Ordinarily, the indirect bilirubin in umbilical cord blood is less than 48 μmol/L and increases by no more than 85 μmol/L in 24 hours, giving rise to jaundice. The levels peak at 85 to 103 μmol/L between days 2 and 4 and decrease to less than 35 μmol/L by days 5 to 7.[30] The increase in bilirubin is related to the increased red cell breakdown and the inability of the immature liver to conjugate bilirubin. Premature infants exhibit a slower rise and longer duration of serum bilirubin levels, perhaps because of poor hepatic uptake and reduced albumin binding of bilirubin. Peak bilirubin levels of 140 to 205 μmol/L appear on days 5 to 7. Most neonatal jaundice resolves within 1 week and is untreated.

The cause of jaundice is made on the basis of history and clinical and laboratory findings. Generally, a search for the cause should be made when (1) the jaundice appears in the first 24 to 36 hours after birth and lasts more than 10 to 14 days, (2) serum bilirubin rises at a rate greater than 85 μmol/L per 24 hours, (3) serum bilirubin is greater than 205 μmol/L in a full-term infant or 170 to 240 μmol/L in a preterm infant, (4) or the direct-reacting bilirubin is greater than 85 μmol/L at any time.[30] Many factors cause elevated bilirubin levels in the neonate, including breast-feeding, hemolytic disease of the newborn, hypoxemia, infections, and acidosis. Bowel or biliary obstruction and liver disease are less common causes. Associated risk factors include prematurity, Asian ancestry, and maternal diabetes. Breast milk jaundice occurs in approximately 2% of breast-fed infants.[30] These neonates accumulate significant levels of unconjugated bilirubin 7 days after birth, with maximum levels of 170 to 515 µmol/L reached in the third week of life. It is thought that the breast milk contains fatty acids that inhibit bilirubin conjugation in the neonatal liver. A factor in breast milk is also thought to increase the absorption of bilirubin in the duodenum. This type of jaundice disappears if breast-feeding is discontinued. Nursing can be resumed in 3 to 4 days without any hyperbilirubinemia ensuing.

Hyperbilirubinemia places the neonate at risk for the development of a neurologic syndrome called *kernicterus*. This condition is caused by the accumulation of unconjugated bilirubin in brain cells. Unconjugated bilirubin is lipid soluble, crosses the permeable blood-brain barrier of the neonate, and is deposited in cells of the basal ganglia, causing brain damage. Asphyxia and hyperosmolality may also contribute by damaging the blood-brain barrier and allowing bilirubin to cross and enter the cells. The level of unconjugated bilirubin and the duration of exposure that will be toxic to the infant are unknown. The less mature infant, however, is at greater risk for kernicterus.[30]

Symptoms may appear 2 to 5 days after birth in term infants or by day 7 in premature infants. Lethargy, poor feeding, and short-term behavioural changes may be evident in mildly affected infants. Severe manifestations include rigidity, tremors, ataxia, and hearing loss. Extreme cases cause seizures and death. Most survivors are seriously damaged and by 3 years of age exhibit involuntary muscle spasm, seizures, mental retardation, and deafness.

Hyperbilirubinemia in the neonate is treated with phototherapy or exchange transfusion. Phototherapy is more commonly used to treat jaundiced infants and reduce the risk of kernicterus. Exposure to fluorescent light in the blue range of the visible spectrum (420- to 470-nm wavelength) reduces bilirubin levels. Bilirubin in the skin absorbs the light energy and is converted to a structural isomer that is more water soluble and can be excreted in the stool and urine. Effective treatment depends on the area of skin exposed and the infant's ability to metabolize and excrete bilirubin. Frequent monitoring of bilirubin levels, body temperature, and hydration are critical to the infant's care. Exchange transfusion is considered when signs of kernicterus are evident or hyperbilirubinemia is sustained or rising and unresponsive to phototherapy.

Hemolytic Disease of the Newborn

Erythroblastosis fetalis, or hemolytic disease of the newborn, occurs in Rh-positive infants of Rh-negative mothers who have been sensitized. The mother can produce anti-Rh antibodies from pregnancies in which the infants are Rh positive or by blood transfusions of Rh-positive blood. The Rh-negative mother usually becomes sensitized during the first few days after delivery (Fig. 14.12), when fetal Rh-positive red cells from the placental site are released into the maternal circulation. Because the antibodies take several weeks to develop, the first Rh-positive infant of an Rh-negative mother usually is not affected. Infants with Rh-negative blood have no antigens on their red cells to react with the maternal antibodies and are not affected.

After an Rh-negative mother has been sensitized, the Rh antibodies from her blood are transferred to subsequent infants through the placental circulation. These antibodies react with the red cell antigens of the Rh-positive infant, causing agglutination and hemolysis. This leads to severe anemia with compensatory hyperplasia and enlargement of the blood-forming organs, including the spleen and liver, in the fetus. Liver function may be impaired, with decreased production of albumin causing massive edema, called *hydrops fetalis*. If blood levels of unconjugated bilirubin are abnormally high because of red cell hemolysis, there is a danger of kernicterus developing in the infant, resulting in severe brain damage or death.

Several advances have significantly decreased the threat to infants born to Rh-negative mothers: prevention of sensitization, antenatal identification of the at-risk fetus, and intrauterine transfusion to the affected fetus. The injection of Rh immune globulin (*i.e.,* gamma-globulin containing Rh antibody) prevents sensitization in Rh-negative mothers who have given birth to Rh-positive infants if administered at 28 weeks' gestation and within 72 hours of delivery, abortion, genetic amniocentesis, or fetal-maternal bleeding. After sensitization has developed, the immune globulin is of no value. Since 1968, the year Rh immune globulin was introduced, the incidence of sensitization of Rh-negative women has dropped dramatically. Early prenatal care and screening of maternal blood continue to be important in reducing immunization. Efforts to improve therapy are aimed at production of monoclonal anti-D, the Rh antibody.

If hemolysis occurs the fetus can be treated by intrauterine transfusions of red cells through the umbilical cord. Postdelivery exchange transfusions are administered by removing and replacing the infant's blood volume with type O Rh-negative blood. The exchange transfusion removes most of the hemolyzed red cells and some of the total bilirubin, treating the anemia and hyperbilirubinemia.

Red Cell Changes With Aging

Anemia is an increasingly common health problem in the elderly. Its prevalence is known to increase with age, with the highest prevalence in men aged 85 years and older. Undiagnosed and untreated anemia can have severe complications and is associated with increased risk of mortality, cardiovascular disease, lower functional ability, self-care deficits, cognitive disorders, and reduced bone density that increases the risk for fractures with falls.[31]

Hemoglobin levels decline after middle age. In studies of men older than 60 years of age, mean hemoglobin levels ranged from 153 to 124 g/L, with the lowest levels found in the oldest persons. The decline is less in women, with mean levels ranging from 138 to 117 mg/L.[32] In most asymptomatic

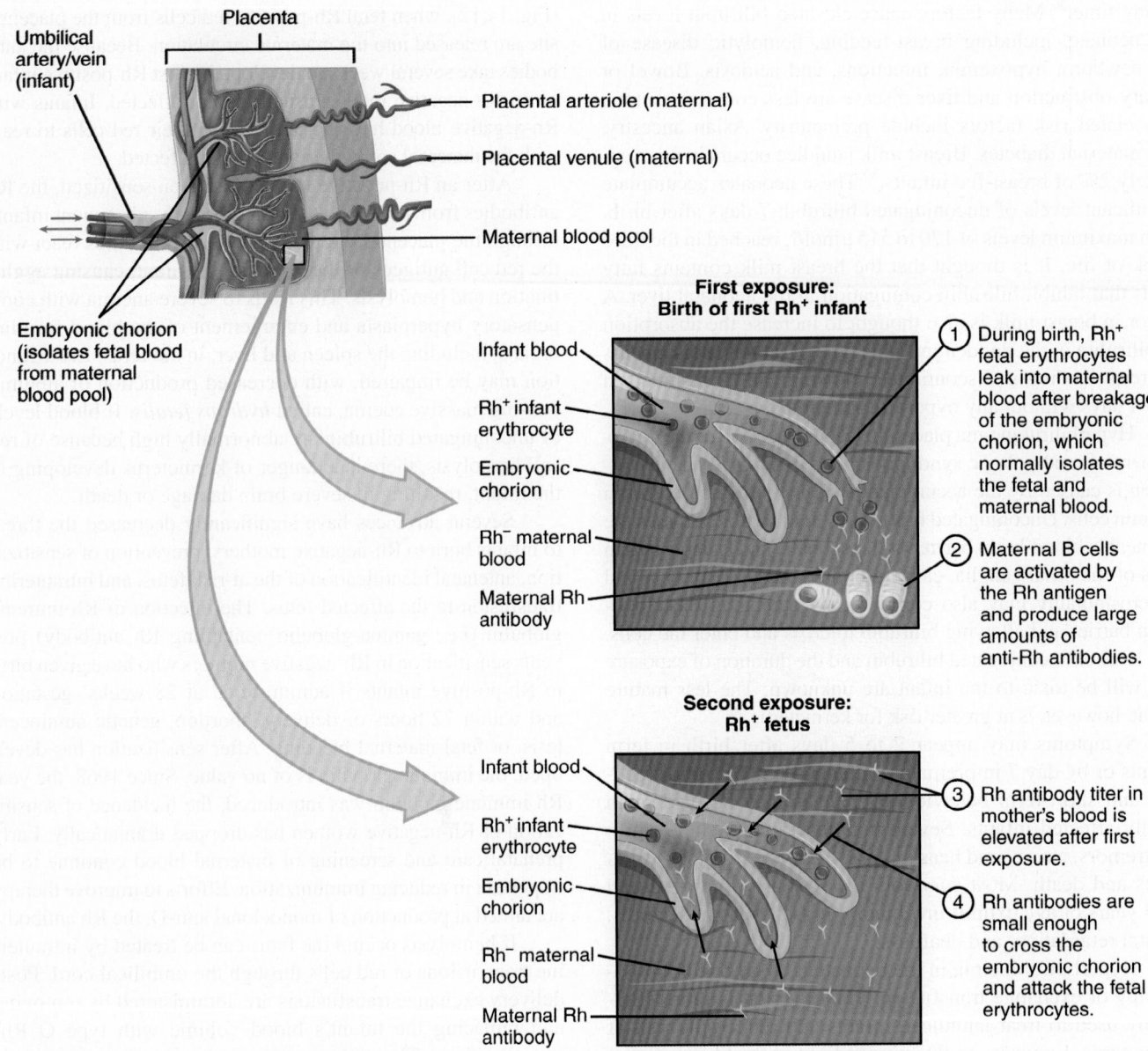

FIGURE 14.12 • The first exposure of an Rh⁻ mother to Rh⁺ erythrocytes during pregnancy induces sensitization. Anti-Rh antibodies begin to circulate in the mother's bloodstream. A second exposure occurs with a subsequent pregnancy with an Rh⁺ fetus in the uterus. Maternal anti-Rh antibodies may cross the placenta and enter the fetal bloodstream, causing agglutination and hemolysis of fetal erythrocytes leading to erythroblastosis fatalis. (From OpenStax College. (2015). Anatomy & Physiology–Connexions Website. [Online]. Available: http://cnx.org/content/m46708/latest/?collection=col11496/1.6. Accessed September 28, 2015.)

elderly persons, lower hemoglobin levels result from iron deficiency and anemia of chronic disease caused by inflammatory disease, malignancy or chronic kidney disease.[31]

As with other body systems, the capacity for red cell production changes with aging. The location of bone cells involved in red cell production shifts toward the axial skeleton, and the number of progenitor cells declines. Despite these changes, older adults are able to maintain hemoglobin and hematocrit levels within a range similar to that of younger adults. However, during a stress situation such as bleeding, the red blood cells of the elderly are not replaced as promptly as

those of their younger counterparts. This inability to replace red blood cells closely correlates with the increased prevalence of anemia in the elderly.

Although the age-associated decline in the hematopoietic reserve in the elderly is not completely understood, several factors seem to play a role, including a reduction in hematopoietic progenitors, reduced production of hematopoietic growth factors, and inhibition of erythropoietin or its interaction with its receptors. Inflammatory cytokines, which have been found to increase with age, may mediate this reduced sensitivity to erythropoietin.

The diagnosis of anemia in older adults requires a complete physical examination, a complete blood count, and studies to rule out comorbid conditions such as malignancy, gastrointestinal conditions that cause bleeding, and pernicious anemia. The CBC should include a peripheral blood smear and a reticulocyte count and index. The treatment of anemia in older adults should focus on the underlying cause and correction of the red cell deficit. Although erythropoietin remains the treatment of choice for anemias associated with cancer and renal disease, its potential use in treating anemias associated with aging remains to be established.

IN SUMMARY

Hemoglobin concentrations at birth are high, reflecting the in utero need for oxygen delivery; toward the end of the first postnatal week, these levels begin to decline, gradually falling to a minimum value at approximately 2 months of age. During the early neonatal period, there is a shift from fetal to adult hemoglobin. Many infants have physiologic jaundice because of hyperbilirubinemia during the first week of life, probably related to increased red cell breakdown and the inability of the infant's liver to conjugate bilirubin. The term kernicterus describes elevated levels of lipid-soluble, unconjugated bilirubin, which can be toxic to brain cells. Depending on severity, it is treated with phototherapy or exchange transfusions, or both. Hemolytic disease of the newborn occurs in Rh-positive infants of Rh-negative mothers who have been sensitized. It involves hemolysis of infant red cells in response to maternal Rh antibodies that have crossed the placenta. Administration of Rh immune globulin to the mother within 72 hours of delivery of an Rh-positive infant, abortion, or amniocentesis prevents sensitization.

Anemia is an increasingly common health problem in older adults. As with many other tissue cells, the capacity for red cell replacement decreases with aging. Although most elderly persons are able to maintain their hemoglobin and hematocrit levels within a normal range, they are unable to replace their red cells as promptly as their younger counterparts during a stress situation such as bleeding. This inability to replace red blood cells closely correlates with the increased prevalence of anemia in the elderly, which is usually the result of bleeding, infection, malignancy, or chronic disease.

REVIEW EXERCISES

1. A 29-year-old woman complains of generalized fatigue. Her physical examination reveals a heart rate of 115 beats/minute, blood pressure 115/75, respiratory rate 28 breaths/minute Her skin and nail beds are pale. Her laboratory results include red blood cell count 3.0×10^{12}/L, hematocrit 30%, hemoglobin 90 g/L, and a decrease in serum ferritin levels.
   A. *What disorder do you suspect this woman has?*
   B. *What additional data would be helpful in determining the etiology of her condition?*
   C. *Which of her signs reflect the body's attempt to compensate for the disorder?*
   D. *What is the significance of the low ferritin level, and how could it be used to make decisions related to her treatment?*

2. A 65-year-old woman is being seen in the clinic because of numbness in her lower legs and feet and difficulty walking. She has no other complaints. She takes a blood pressure pill, two calcium pills, and a multivitamin pill daily. Her laboratory results include red blood cell count 3.0×10^{12}/L, hematocrit 20%, hemoglobin 90 g/L, and a markedly elevated MCV.
   A. *What type of anemia does she have?*
   B. *What is the reason for her neurologic symptoms?*
   C. *What type of treatment would be appropriate?*

3. A 12-year-old boy with sickle cell disease presents in the emergency department with severe chest pain. His mother reports that he was doing well until he came down with a respiratory tract infection. She also states he insisted on playing basketball with the other boys in the neighbourhood even though he wasn't feeling well.
   A. *What is the most likely cause of pain in this boy?*
   B. *Infections and aerobic-type exercise that increase the levels of deoxygenated hemoglobin produce sickling in persons who are homozygous for the sickle cell gene and have sickle cell disease, but not in persons who are heterozygous and have sickle cell trait. Explain.*
   C. *People with sickle disease experience anemia but not iron deficiency. Explain.*

4. Forty students in a hematology class conducted a laboratory exercise that involved determining their blood type. In a subsequent laboratory discussion, they discovered that 16 students had type A blood, 20 had type O blood, 3 had type B blood, and only 1 had type AB blood.
   A. *What types of blood antigens and antibodies would students with type A, type O, and type AB blood have?*
   B. *What could be the possible blood types of the parents of students with type B blood, type O blood, and type AB blood?*
   C. *If these students required a blood transfusion, what type of blood could those with type A, type O, and type AB receive? (Assume the blood is of the same Rh type.)*

References

1. Valdez R., Zutter M., Florea A. D., Rubin R. (2012). Chapter 20: Hematopathology. In Rubin R., Stayer D. S. (Eds.), *Rubin's pathology: Clinicopathologic foundations of medicine* (6th ed.). Philadelphia, PA: Lippincott Williams & Wilkins.
2. Hall J. E. (2011). *Textbook of medical physiology* (12th ed.). Philadelphia, PA: W. B. Saunders.
3. Waite G. N. Blood components. In Rhoades R. A., Bell D. R. (Eds.), *Medical physiology* (4th ed.). Philadelphia, PA: Lippincott Williams & Wilkins.
4. Hoffman R., Benz E. J., Silberstein L. E., et al. (Eds.). (2013). *Hematology: Basic principles & practice* (6th ed.). Philadelphia, PA: Elsevier, Inc.
5. Kumar V., Abbas A. K., Fausto N., Aster J. C. (Eds.), (2010). *Robbins and Cotran pathophysiologic basis of disease* (8th ed.). Philadelphia, PA: Elsevier Saunders.
6. Hattangadi S. M., Wong P., Zhang L., et al. (2011). From stem to red cell: Regulation of erythropoiesis at multiple levels by multiple proteins, RNAs, and chromatic modifications. *Blood, 118*(24), 6258–6268.
7. Kaushansky K., Beulter E., Seligsohn U., et al. (Eds.). (2010). *Williams hematology* (8th ed.). New York: McGraw-Hill Companies, Inc.
8. WHO. (2014). Genes and human disease: Sickle cell anemia. Available online at: http://www.who.int/genomics/public/geneticdiseases/en/index2.html#SCA. Accessed February 26, 2014.
9. Rees D. C., Williams T. N., Gladwin M. T. (2010). Sickle-cell disease. *Lancet, 376*(9757), 2018–2031.
10. Pack-Mabien A., Haynes J. (2009). A primary care provider's guide to prevention and acute care management of adults and children with sickle cell disease. *Journal of the American Academy of Nurse Practitioners, 21*(5), 250–257.
11. Kassim A. A., DeBaun M. R. (2013). Sickle cell disease, vasculopathy, and therapeutics. *Annual Review of Medicine, 64*, 451–466.
12. National Advisory Committee on Immunization. (2012). Pneumococcal Vaccine. Available online at: http://www.phac-aspc.gc.ca/publicat/cig-gci/p04-pneu-eng.php#t2. Accessed March 2, 2014.
13. Galanello R., Origa R. (2010). Beta-thalassemia. *Orphanet Journal of Rare Diseases, 5*, 11.
14. Martin A., Thompson A. A. (2013). Thalassemias. *Pediatric Clinics of North America, 60*(6), 1383–1391.
15. Bass G. F., Tuscano E. T., Tuscano J. M. (2014). Diagnosis and classification of autoimmune hemolytic anemia. *Autoimmunity Reviews, 13*(4–5), 560–564.
16. Lerner M. B., Sills R. (2011). Iron deficiency anemia. In Kliegman R. M., Stanton B. F., St. Geme J. W., et al. (Eds.), *Nelson textbook of pediatrics* (19th ed., pp. 1655–1658). Philadelphia, PA: Elsevier Saunders.
17. Stabler S. P. (2013). Vitamin B$_{12}$ deficiency. *New England Journal of Medicine, 368*(2), 149–160.
18. Health Canada. (2010). Dietary reference intakes. Available online at: http://www.hc-sc.gc.ca/fn-an/nutrition/reference/table/ref_vitam_tbl_e.html. Accessed March 5, 2014.
19. Kinsman S. L., Johnston M. V. (2011). Congenital anomalies of the central nervous system. In Kliegman R. M., Stanton B. F., St. Geme J. W., et al. (Eds.), *Nelson textbook of pediatrics* (19th ed., pp. 1998–2013). Philadelphia, PA: Elsevier Saunders.
20. Kulasekararaj A. G., Mufti G. J., Marsh J. (2013). Bone marrow failure: Causes and complications. *Medicine, 41*(5), 257–260.
21. Scheinberg P., Young N. S. (2012). How I treat acquired aplastic anemia. *Blood, 120*(6), 1185–1196.
22. Collins T. A. (2011). Packed red blood cell transfusions in critically ill patients. *Critical Care Nurse, 31*(1), 25–34.
23. Goldman M., Scalia V., Devine D. (2015). Donor selection, transmissible disease testing and pathogen reduction. In Clarke G., Charge S. (Eds.), *Clinical guide to transfusion*. Canadian Blood Services. Available online at: http://www.transfusionmedicine.ca. Accessed August 3, 2015.
24. Canadian Blood Services. (2014). Percentage of blood types in Canada. Available online at: www.blood.ca. Accessed March 5, 2014.
25. International Society of Blood Transfusions. (2012). Blood group terminology. Available online at: http://www.isbtweb.org/working-parties/red-cell-immunogenetics-and-blood-group-terminology/blood-group-terminology. Accessed March 9, 2014.
26. Roback J. D., Grossman B. J., Harris T., et al. (Eds.). (2011). *Technical manual* (17th ed). Bethesda, MD: American Association of Blood Banks.
27. Public Health Agency of Canada. (2009). Noninfectious adverse events of transfusion. Available online at: http://www.phac-aspc.gc.ca/hcai-iamss/tti-it/noninfec-eng.php#fnhtr. Accessed March 5, 2014.
28. Tibes R., Mesa R. A. (2013). Emerging drugs for polycythemia vera. *Expert Opinion on Emerging Drugs, 18*(3), 393–404.
29. Maheshwari A., Carlo W. A. (2011). Blood disorders. In Kliegman R. M., Stanton B. F, St. Geme J. W, et al. (Eds.). *Nelson textbook of pediatrics* (19th ed., pp. 1655–1658). Philadelphia, PA: Elsevier Saunders.
30. Ambalavanan N., Carlo W. A. (2011). Jaundice and hyperbilirubinemia in the newborn. In Kliegman R. M., Stanton B. F., St. Geme J. W., et al. (Eds.), *Nelson textbook of pediatrics* (19th ed., pp. 1655–1658). Philadelphia, PA: Elsevier Saunders.
31. Andres E., Serraj K., Federici L. (2013). Anemia in elderly patients: New insight into an old disorder. *Geriatrics & Gerontology International, 13*(3), 519–527.
32. Balducci L. (2003). Epidemiology of anemia in the elderly: Information on diagnostic evaluation. *Journal of the American Geriatrics Society, 51*(Suppl 3), S2–S9.

Visit thePoint **http://thePoint.lww.com for animations, journal articles, and more!**

Disorders of White Blood Cells and Lymphoid Tissues

15

The white blood cells and the lymphoid tissues work to protect the body against invasion by foreign agents. Disorders of the white blood cells include leukopenia, in which there is a deficiency in leukocytes, and proliferative disorders, in which there is an expansion of leukocytes. The proliferative disorders may be reactive, as occurs with infection, or neoplastic, as occurs with malignant lymphomas and leukemia. This chapter focuses on leukopenia, infectious mononucleosis, malignant lymphomas, leukemias, and plasma cell dyscrasias (multiple myeloma).

HEMATOPOIETIC AND LYMPHOID TISSUES

After completing this section of the chapter, you should be able to meet the following objectives:

- Describe the different types of white blood cells and the structures of the lymphoid system where they circulate and mature.
- Trace the development of the different white blood cells from their origin in the pluripotent bone marrow stem cell to their circulation in the bloodstream.

The hematopoietic system encompasses all the blood cells and their precursors. It includes the myeloid or bone marrow tissue in which the blood cells are formed, and the lymphoid tissues of the lymph nodes, thymus, and spleen, in which the white blood cells circulate, mature and function. The development of the different blood cells involves interactions among precursor bone marrow cells and a variety of growth factors, cytokines (chemical messengers), and gene products such as transcription factors.

Leukocytes (White Blood Cells)

The white blood cells include the granulocytes (*i.e.*, neutrophils, eosinophils, and basophils), monocytes/macrophages, and lymphocytes. The granulocytes and the agranular monocytes/macrophages are derived from the myeloid stem cell in the bone marrow and circulate in the blood (Fig. 15.1). The T lymphocytes (T cells) and B lymphocytes (B cells) originate

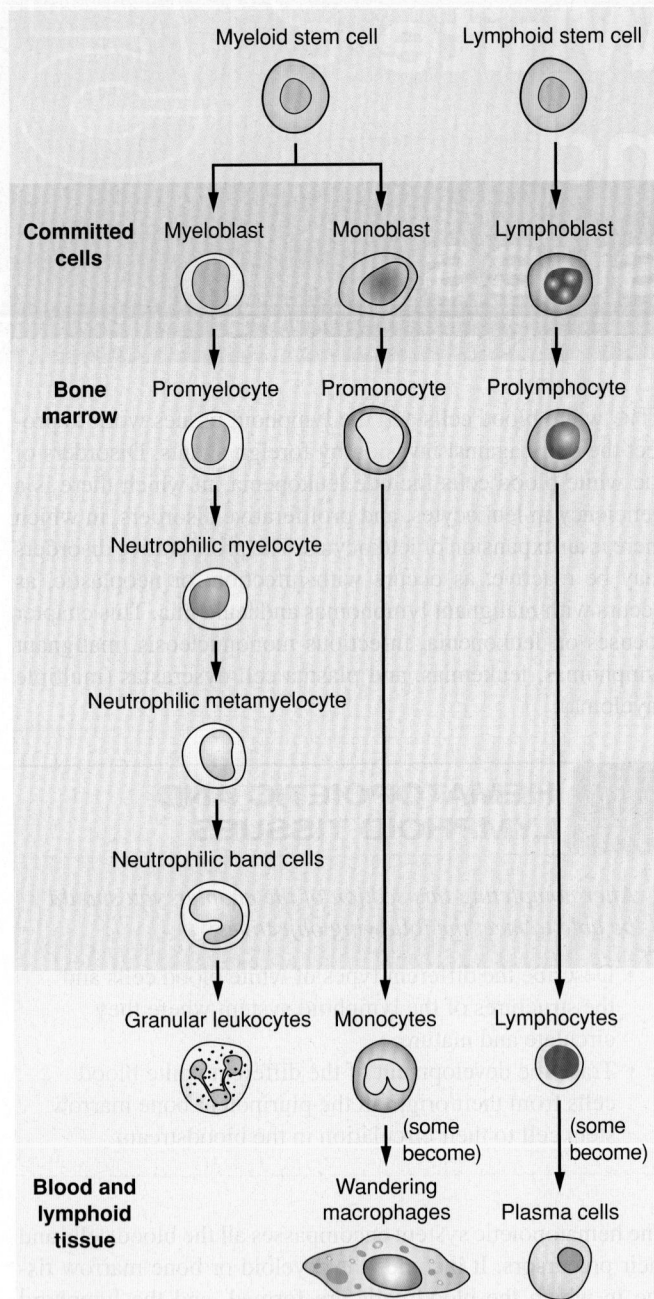

FIGURE 15.1 • Leukocytes originate from multipotential stem cells in the bone marrow. Granular leukocytes (neutrophils, eosinophils, basophils) have their origin in the myeloid stem cells and develop through a sequence involving myeloblasts. Monocytes, like granulocytes, are progeny of the myeloid stem cell line, but develop along a pathway involving monoblasts. Only lymphocytes originate from the lymphoid stem cell line. They develop through a sequence involving lymphoblasts and are released from the bone marrow as prolymphocytes, which undergo further differentiation in the lymphoid organs.

from lymphoid stem cells in the bone marrow and migrate between the blood and the lymphatic system (see Chapter 12). T lymphocytes mature in the thymus, and B lymphocytes in the bone marrow. The T lymphocytes differentiate to form CD4[+] helper T cells, which serve to orchestrate the immune

response, and CD8[+] cytotoxic T cells, which provide for cell-mediated immune responses (see Chapter 17). The B lymphocytes differentiate to form immunoglobulin-producing plasma cells. Another population of lymphocytes includes the innate lymphoid cell groups such as natural killer (NK) cells, which do not share the specificity or characteristics of the T or the B lymphocytes, but have the ability to destroy target cells.[1]

HEMATOPOIESIS

- The white blood cells are formed from hematopoietic stem cells that differentiate into committed progenitor cells that in turn develop into the myelocytic and lymphocytic lineages needed for the formation of the different types of white blood cells.
- The growth and reproduction of the different stem cells is controlled by colony-stimulating factors, other growth factors, and chemical mediators.
- The life span of white blood cells is relatively short so that constant renewal is necessary to maintain normal blood levels. Any conditions that decrease the availability of stem cells or hematopoietic growth factors produce a decrease in white blood cells.

Bone Marrow and Hematopoiesis

The entire hematopoietic system, with all its complexity, arises from a small number of stem cells that differentiate to form blood cells and replenish the bone marrow by a process of self-renewal. All the hematopoietic precursors, including the erythroid (red blood cell), myelocyte (granulocyte and monocyte), lymphocyte (T cell and B cell), and megakaryocyte (platelet) series, are derived from a small population of cells called *pluripotent stem cells.* These cells are capable of providing *progenitor cells (i.e.,* parent cells) for myelopoiesis and lymphopoiesis, processes by which myeloid and lymphoid blood cells are made. Several levels of differentiation lead to the development of committed *unipotent cells,* which are the progenitors for each of the different blood cell types.

Hematopoietic Growth Factors

Like erythropoiesis, which is described in Chapter 14, leukopoiesis, or production of white blood cells, is controlled by hematopoietic growth factors. The *hematopoietic growth factors* are a family of glycoproteins that support hematopoietic colony formation (see Chapter 12). These growth factors can be categorized into three functional groups: those that are involved in the development of a specific cell lineage, those that affect the early multipotential progenitor cells, and those that indirectly regulate hematopoiesis by inducing the expression of growth factor genes in other cells.[2] Cytokines or chemical messengers, such as interleukin (IL)-1, IL-3, IL-6, and interferon, act synergistically to support the functions of the growth factors.

There are several lineage-specific growth factors: erythropoietin, granulocyte-macrophage colony-stimulating factor (GM-CSF), and monocyte-macrophage colony-stimulating factor (M-CSF). Although the hematopoietic growth factors act at different points in the proliferation and differentiation pathway, their functions overlap. For example, GM-CSF stimulates the growth and function of granulocyte, macrophage, and eosinophil progenitor cells and induces IL-1 gene expression in neutrophils and peripheral mononuclear leukocytes. Cytokines, such as IL-3, act on the most immature bone marrow progenitor cells, thereby promoting the development of cells that can differentiate into a number of cell types. The identification and characterization of the various growth factors and cytokines has led to their use in treating a wide range of diseases, including bone marrow failure, hematopoietic neoplasms, infectious diseases, and congenital and myeloproliferative disorders.

Leukocyte Developmental Stages

Leukocyte development begins with the myeloid and lymphoid stem cells in the bone marrow. The granulocyte and monocyte cell lines derive from the myeloid stem cells and the lymphocytes from the lymphoid stem cells (Fig. 15.1). The immature precursor cells for each of the cell lines are called *blast cells. Myeloblasts,* which are the granulocytic precursor cells, have round to oval nuclei, with delicate chromatin and a blue to grey cytoplasm. During the next stage of development, the myeloblasts are transformed into *promyelocytes* with similar nuclei, but with a cytoplasm containing many primary granules. In the subsequent *metamyelocyte* stage, the nuclei distort and become arc-like, producing the band developmental stage. Maturation from metamyelocyte to mature neutrophil involves progressive condensation of nuclear chromatin, increasing nuclear lobulation, and the appearance of secondary (specific) granules. Eosinophils and basophils undergo similar developmental stages, but develop different secondary granules. Like granulocytes, monocytes develop from the granulocyte-monocyte progenitor cell and progress through a monoblast and promonocyte stage. By contrast, lymphocytes derive from lymphoid stem cells and progress through the lymphoblast and prolymphocyte stages. The prolymphocytes leave the bone marrow and travel to the lymphoid tissues, where further differentiation into T and B lymphocytes occurs. The names of the various leukocyte developmental stages are often used in describing blood cell changes that occur in hematopoietic disorders (*e.g.,* acute lymphoblastic leukemia, acute promyelocytic leukemia).

Lymphoid Tissues

The body's lymphatic system consists of the lymphatic vessels, lymphoid tissue and lymph nodes, thymus, and spleen (see Chapter 17). Although both precursor B and T lymphocytes begin their development in the bone marrow, they migrate to peripheral lymphoid structures to complete the differentiation process. B lymphocytes leave the bone marrow, differentiate into plasma cells, and then move to the lymph nodes, where they continue to proliferate and produce antibodies. T lymphocytes leave the bone marrow as precursor T lymphocytes and travel to the thymus, where they differentiate into CD4$^+$ helper T cells and CD8$^+$ cytotoxic T cells, after which many of them move to lymph nodes, where they undergo further proliferation.

Lymph nodes, the site at which many lymphomas originate, consist of organized collections of lymphoid tissue located along the lymphatic vessels.[3–5] Typically greyish-white and ovoid or bean-shaped, they range in size from 1 mm to about 1 to 2 cm in diameter. A fibrous capsule and radiating trabeculae provide a supporting structure, and a delicate reticular network contributes to internal support (Fig. 15.2). The parenchyma of the lymph node is divided into an outer or superficial cortex and an inner medulla. The superficial cortex contains well-defined B-cell and T-cell domains. The B-cell-dependent cortex consists of two types of follicles: immunologically inactive follicles, called *primary follicles,* and active follicles that contain germinal centres, called *secondary follicles.* Germinal centres contain large lymphocytes (centroblasts) and small lymphocytes with cleaved nuclei (centrocytes). The mantle zone is the small layer of B cells surrounding the germinal centres. The portion of the cortex between the medullary and superficial cortex is called the *paracortex.* This region contains most of the T cells in the lymph nodes.

Although some lymphocytes enter the lymph nodes through the afferent lymphatic channels, most enter through the wall of postcapillary venules located in the deep cortex. These vessels, which are lined with specialized endothelial cells that possess receptors for antigen-primed lymphocytes, signal lymphocytes to leave the circulation and migrate through the lymph nodes. Both B and T cells leave the bloodstream through these channels.[3] The T cells remain in the paracortex and the B cells migrate to the follicular area of the cortex. Most lymphocytes leave the lymph node by entering the lymphatic sinuses, from which they then enter the efferent lymphatic vessel.

The alimentary canal, respiratory passages, and genitourinary systems are guarded by accumulations of lymphoid tissue that are not enclosed in a capsule. This form of lymphoid tissue is called *diffuse lymphoid tissue* or *mucosa-associated lymphoid tissue* (MALT) because of its association with mucous membranes. Lymphocytes are found in the subepithelium of these tissues. Lymphomas can arise from MALT as well as from lymph node tissue.

IN SUMMARY

Leukocyte, or white blood cell, development begins with the myeloid and lymphoid stem cells in the bone marrow. The granulocyte and monocyte cell lines derive from the myeloid stem cells, and lymphocytes from the lymphoid stem cells. The immature precursor cells for each of the cell lines are called blast cells. The blast cells progress through subsequent maturational stages before becoming mature granulocytes, monocytes, or lymphocytes. The names of these developmental stages are often used in describing blood cell changes that occur in hematopoietic disorders.

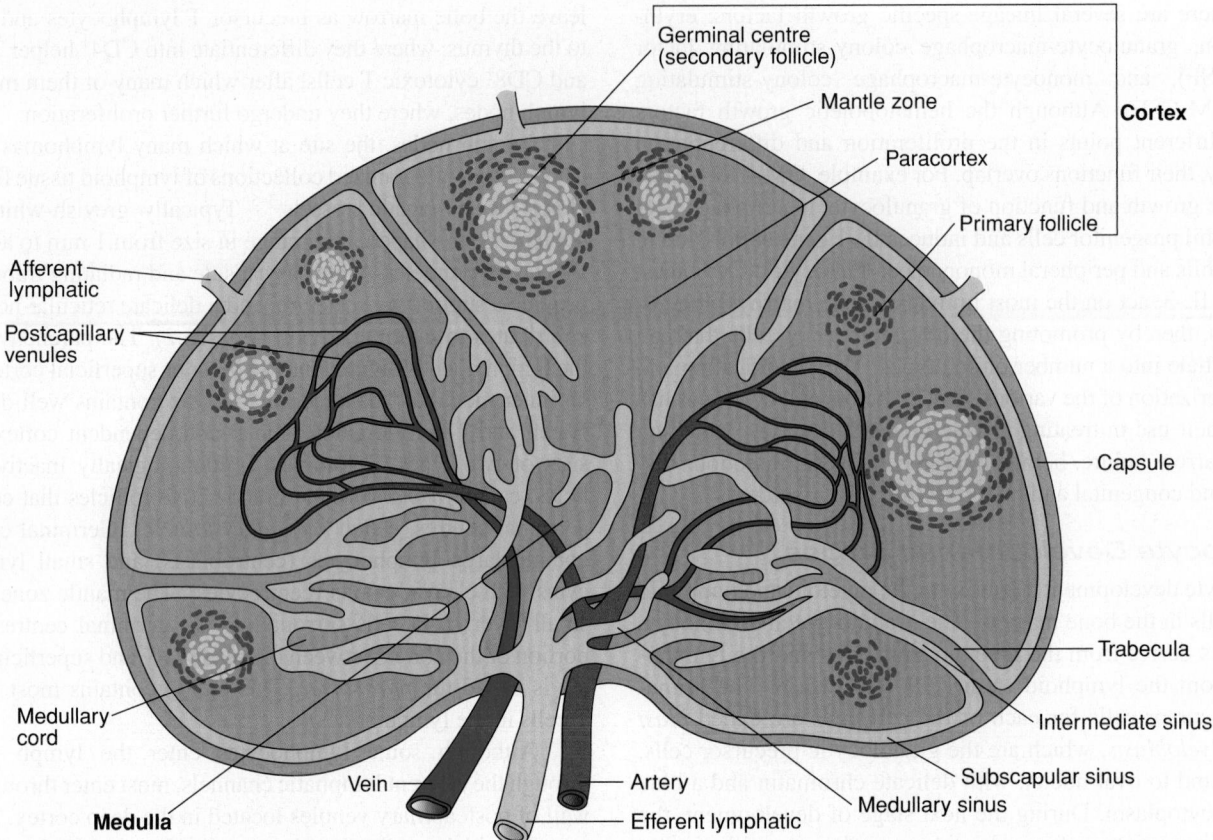

Germinal centre
(secondary follicle)

Mantle zone

Cortex

Paracortex

Primary follicle

Afferent
lymphatic

Postcapillary
venules

Capsule

Trabecula

Intermediate sinus

Medullary
cord

Subscapular sinus

Vein — Artery

Medulla Medullary sinus

Efferent lymphatic

FIGURE 15.2 • Structures of normal lymph node. (From Rubin R., Strayer D. S. (Eds.). (2012). *Rubin's pathology: Clinicopathologic foundations of medicine* (6th ed., p. 998). Philadelphia, PA: Lippincott Williams & Wilkins.)

The lymphatic system consists of a network of lymphatic vessels, nodes, and tissues where B and T lymphocytes complete their differentiation. Lymph nodes, the site at which many lymphomas originate, exhibit an outer or superficial cortex and an inner medulla. The cortex contains well-defined B-cell and T-cell domains. The B-cell-dependent cortex consists of two types of follicles: immunologically inactive follicles, called primary follicles, and active follicles that contain germinal centres, called secondary follicles. Most of the T cells are contained in the paracortex, the area between the medullary and superficial cortices.

NON-NEOPLASTIC DISORDERS OF WHITE BLOOD CELLS

After completing this section of the chapter, you should be able to meet the following objectives:

• Define the terms leukopenia, neutropenia, granulocytopenia, and aplastic anemia.

• Cite two general causes of neutropenia.

• Describe the mechanism of symptom production in neutropenia.

The number of leukocytes, or white blood cells, in the peripheral circulation normally ranges from 5 to 10×10^9 cells/L. The non-neoplastic disorders of white blood cells include a deficiency of leukocytes (leukopenia) and proliferative disorders in which there are increased numbers of leukocytes (leukocytosis).

Neutropenia (Agranulocytosis)

The term *leukopenia* describes a decrease in the absolute number of leukocytes in the blood. Although leukopenia may affect any of the specific types of white blood cells, it most often affects the neutrophil. Neutrophils constitute the majority of blood leukocytes and play a primary role in host defence mechanisms against infection. They migrate to sites of infection and engulf, digest, and destroy microorganisms. Thus a decrease in the number of neutrophils (neutropenia) places a person at risk for infection. The risk for and severity of neutropenia-associated infection are directly proportional to the absolute neutrophil count (ANC) and duration of the neutropenia.

Neutropenia refers specifically to an abnormally low number of neutrophils, and is commonly defined as a ANC of less than 1.5×10^9/L.[4–6] It can be further graded as mild (1.0×10^9/L), moderate (0.5 to 1.0×10^9/L), or severe (<0.5×10^9/L) based on absolute number of neutrophils circulating in the blood. *Agranulocytosis* denotes a virtual absence of neutrophils. In *aplastic anemia,* all of the myeloid stem cells are affected, resulting in individual decreases in red blood cells (anemia), platelets (thrombocytopenia), and neutrophils (agranulocytosis) or altogether can be denoted as pancytopenia.

Neutropenia can result from decreased neutrophil production, accelerated utilization or destruction, or a shift in neutrophils from the blood to the tissue compartments. It can be present at birth (congenital) or arise from a number of factors that occur later in life and does not have a hereditary component (acquired).

Congenital Neutropenia

Inherited disorders of proliferation and maturation of myeloid stem cell lines are relatively rare. Two of the more severe inherited types of congenital neutropenia are cyclic neutropenia and severe congenital neutropenia.[6-8] There are also several congenital immunodeficiency disorders that are accompanied by severe neutropenia, including the severe combined immunodeficiencies and common variable immunodeficiency (discussed in Chapter 19). In addition to the inherited forms of neutropenia that present in infancy, an alloimmune neonatal neutropenia can occur because of the transplacental transfer of maternal antibodies.

Alloimmune neonatal neutropenia is neutropenia that occurs after transplacental transfer of maternal alloantibodies directed at an infant's neutrophils, analogous to Rh hemolytic disease, discussed in Chapter 14. The disorder usually involves phagocytic destruction of antibody-coated neutrophils by splenic macrophages. Affected infants may present with delayed separation of the umbilical cord, mild skin infection, fever, and pneumonia within the first two weeks of life. These manifestations resolve with antimicrobial therapy.[7]

Periodic or *cyclic neutropenia* is a rare autosomal dominant disorder with variable expression that begins in infancy and persists for decades. The disorder arises from a regulatory abnormality involving early hematopoietic precursors and is associated with the neutrophil elastase (a protease that degrades virulent factors in bacteria) gene.[6,7] It is characterized by regular, periodic oscillations of peripheral neutrophils from normal to neutropenic values every 18 to 24 days.[7] During the neutropenic periods, most persons suffer from fever, stomatitis, and pharyngitis, occasionally associated with lymph node enlargement. Serious infections may occur occasionally. The cycles often become less noticeable in older persons, and the disorder then begins to resemble that of chronic neutropenia.

Severe congenital neutropenia, or *Kostmann syndrome,* is characterized by an arrest in myeloid maturation at the promyelocyte stage of development, resulting in an absolute neutrophil count of less than 0.2×10^9/L.[7] It can be inherited as either an autosomal dominant or autosomal recessive trait. The disease is usually associated with mutations in the neutrophil elastase gene, which in turn leads to apoptosis of bone marrow myeloid cells. The disorder is characterized by severe bacterial infections. Before the recombinant human G-CSFs or rhG-CSFs became available for clinical use, two thirds of children died of fatal infections before reaching adolescence.

CHART 15.1 PRINCIPAL CAUSES OF NEUTROPENIA

Congenital
- Alloimmune neonatal neutropenia (transfer of maternal antibodies)
- Cyclic neutropenia
- Kostmann syndrome (severe congenital neutropenia)

Acquired
Autoimmune
- Primary (rare, usually occurs in children and runs a benign course)
- Secondary
  - Systemic lupus erythematous
  - Felty syndrome in persons with rheumatoid arthritis
Infection-related
- Many types of infections agents, but most commonly viruses
- Mechanisms include increased consumption of neutrophils, production of autoantibodies, direct infiltration of hematopoietic cells, bone marrow suppression
Drug-related
- Cancer chemotherapeutic drugs (bone marrow depression)
- Immune-mediated reactions in which drugs act as haptens (e.g., penicillin, propylthiouracil)
- Accelerated apoptosis (clozapine [antipsychotic agent])
Radiation therapy to bone marrow
Hematologic malignancies

Approximately 20% of persons with the disorder will develop acute myelogenous leukemia (AML).[6-8]

Acquired Neutropenia

Acquired neutropenia encompasses a broad spectrum of causative processes and includes primary and secondary autoimmune neutropenia, infection-related neutropenia, and drug-induced neutropenia (Chart 15.1). It also may be caused by a number of bone marrow disorders, hematopoietic malignancies, and radiation therapy.

Autoimmune Neutropenia. Autoimmune neutropenia results from antibodies directed against neutrophil cell membrane antigens or bone marrow progenitors. The autoimmune forms of neutropenia may be classified as primary (*i.e.,* those not associated with other detectable pathologic processes) or secondary (*i.e.,* those associated with another disease condition).[6-8]

Primary autoimmune neutropenia is a rare disorder of early childhood, during which a moderate to severe neutropenia is observed. The condition is usually benign, with mild to moderate infections. Spontaneous remission usually occurs in children by 3 to 5 years of age.[8] The disorder is rare in adults.

Because primary autoimmune neutropenia is self-limiting, treatment is usually restricted to the use of antimicrobial agents for persons who experience recurrent infections.

Secondary immune-associated neutropenia is often associated with systemic autoimmune disorders, mainly rheumatoid arthritis (RA) and systemic lupus erythematosus (SLE).[6,8,9] Felty syndrome, a variant of RA, is a triad of splenomegaly, deforming RA, and neutropenia. The neutropenia is the result of antineutrophil antibodies and high levels of circulating immune complexes, which induce neutrophil apoptosis. Coupled with the end-organ manifestations of RA (discussed in Chapter 59), the majority of persons with Felty syndrome are susceptible to serious bacterial infection that sometimes leads to sepsis and poor clinical outcome.[9]

Several antibody-mediated mechanisms are believed to be responsible for the neutropenia seen in persons with SLE. These include the development of antineutrophil antibodies, along with increased neutrophil apoptosis, and decreased neutrophil production by the bone marrow. Similar to Felty syndrome, continued treatment of SLE to control symptoms is the preferred method of treatment.[9]

Infection-Related Neutropenia. Many different types of infectious diseases, including viral, bacterial, rickettsial, and parasitic, may cause neutropenia, the most common being viral. Infections may produce neutropenia by a variety of mechanisms, including production of autoantibodies that cause increased and premature destruction of neutrophils; direct infiltration of developing hematopoietic cell lines; loss of neutrophils by toxins; development of splenomegaly with increased neutrophil sequestration and destruction. Neutropenia is a common manifestation of acquired immunodeficiency syndrome (AIDS), in which a virus-induced suppression of marrow cell proliferation is often aggravated by infectious consumption of neutrophils and the action of antiviral drugs (*e.g.,* zidovudine).[4]

Drug-Related Neutropenia. The incidence of drug-induced neutropenia has increased significantly over the last several decades and is attributed primarily to a wider use of drugs in general and more specifically to the use of chemotherapeutic drugs in the treatment of cancer. Persons with almost any malignancy who receive chemotherapy with or without radiation therapy are at risk for development of chemotherapy-induced neutropenia.[5] The risk for development of chemotherapy-induced neutropenia is influenced by patient-, disease-, and treatment-related factors. One of the most important patient-related factors is age. Elderly patients are at greater risk than younger persons because of age-related cellular changes in neutrophils. Other patient-related factors include poor nutritional status and comorbid conditions such as kidney disease.[10] Disease-related factors include neoplastic bone involvement, type of cancer, and history of anemia or neutropenia with prior chemotherapy regimens. Treatment-related factors include radiation therapy to the bone marrow, extensive prior chemotherapy, and type of treatment regimen. Treatment regimens for hematologic malignancies are more likely to generate chemotherapy-induced neutropenia than some other treatment regimens.[5]

The term *idiosyncratic* is used to describe drug reactions that are different from the effect obtained in most persons and that cannot be explained in terms of allergy. A number of idiosyncratic cases of drug-induced neutropenia are thought to be caused by immunologic mechanisms, with the drug or its metabolites acting as antigens (*i.e.,* haptens) to incite the production of antibodies reactive against neutrophils.[10] In the case of hapten formation, discontinuation of the drug usually results in resolution of neutropenia within a week or two. Some drugs, such as the antipsychotic drug clozapine, have been shown to cause accelerated apoptosis of neutrophils. Clozapine has been shown to cause agranulocytosis in a small but significant number of persons. This serious, potentially fatal effect can develop rapidly, usually within the 6th to 18th weeks of therapy.[11] The reaction is reversible on discontinuation of the drug. Because of the risk of agranulocytosis, persons receiving clozapine must have weekly blood counts done for the first 6 months of therapy.

Other drugs, such as the β-lactam antibiotics (*e.g.,* cephalosporins), particularly when given in high doses, and some anticonvulsant drugs (*e.g.,* carbamazepine), may inhibit the colony-forming units of granulocytes and monocytes-macrophages in bone marrow. Suppression of myeloid precursors in the bone marrow also has been noted with administration of ticlopidine (an antiplatelet drug), sulfasalazine (an anti-inflammatory drug), and chlorpromazine (an antipsychotic drug).[10]

Clinical Course

The clinical features of neutropenia usually depend on the severity of neutropenia and the cause of the disorder.[8] Neutropenia from any cause increases the risk for infection by gram-positive and gram-negative bacteria and fungi.

Neutrophils provide the first line of defence against organisms that inhabit the skin and gastrointestinal tract. Thus early signs of infection due to neutropenia, particularly those associated with a mild to moderate decrease in neutrophils, include mild skin lesions, stomatitis, pharyngitis, and diarrhea. Signs and symptoms of more severe neutropenia include malaise, chills, and fever, followed in sequence by marked weakness and fatigability. Untreated infections can be rapidly fatal, particularly if the absolute neutrophil count drops below 0.25×10^9/L. With severe neutropenia, the usual signs of infection may not be present because of an insufficient number of neutrophils to produce an inflammatory response.

Antimicrobial agents are used to treat infections in situations in which neutrophil destruction cannot be controlled or the neutropoietic function of the bone marrow cannot be recovered. Hematopoietic growth factors such as rhG-CSF (*e.g.,* filgrastim, pegfilgrastim) may be used to stimulate the maturation and differentiation of the granulocyte cell lineage.[8] In patients receiving chemotherapy for solid tumours, lymphoma, and AML, these agents reduce the duration of severe neutropenia, decrease the incidence of febrile neutropenia, and facilitate on-time delivery of scheduled doses of chemotherapy.

Infectious Mononucleosis

Infectious mononucleosis is a self-limiting lymphoprolifera-tive disorder caused by the Epstein-Barr virus (EBV), a mem-ber of the herpesvirus family.[12–16] The term *EBV-associated infectious mononucleosis* (EBV IM) is often used to desig-nate infectious mononucleosis caused by EBV as opposed to non-EBV-associated clinical syndromes of infectious mono-nucleosis caused by other agents. Infectious mononucleosis may occur at any age, but occurs principally in adolescents and young adults in developed countries. In areas of the world where children often live in crowded conditions, asymptom-atic infection with EBV occurs in childhood and infectious mononucleosis is not encountered. Two thirds of persons newly infected with EBV after childhood develop clinically evident infectious mononucleosis.[12]

EBV spreads from person to person primarily through con-tact with infected oral secretions. Transmission requires close contact with infected persons. Thus, the virus spreads readily among young children in crowded conditions, where there is considerable sharing of oral secretions. Kissing is an effective mode of transmission, hence the term "kissing disease" among adolescents, although it is more readily spread when sharing items such as drinking glasses, water bottles, or cigarettes.[12]

Pathogenesis

Epstein-Barr virus initially penetrates the nasopharyngeal, oro-pharyngeal, and salivary epithelial cells. It then spreads to the underlying oropharyngeal lymphoid tissue and, more specifi-cally, to B lymphocytes, all of which have receptors for EBV. Infection of the B cells may take one of two forms—it may kill the infected B cell, or the virus may incorporate itself into the cell's genome. The B cells that harbour the EBV genome proliferate in the circulation and produce the well-known *het-erophil* antibodies that are used for the diagnosis of infectious mononucleosis.[12–15] A heterophil antibody is an immunoglobu-lin that reacts with antigens from another species—in this case, horse or sheep red blood cells. The Monospot screen is used to identify EBV and is based on identifying any clumping or agglutination of these heterophil antibodies.

The normal immune response is important in control-ling the proliferation of the EBV-infected B cells and cell free viruses. Most important in controlling the proliferation of EBV-infected B cells are the CD8[+] cytotoxic T cells and NK cells. These virus-specific T cells appear as large, atypical lymphocytes that are characteristic of the infection (Fig. 15.3). In otherwise healthy persons, the humoral and cellular immune responses serve to control viral shedding by limiting the num-ber of infected B cells rather than eliminating them.

Although infected B cells and free virions disappear from the blood after recovery from the disease, the virus remains in a few transformed B cells in the oropharyngeal region and is shed in the saliva. Once infected with the virus, persons remain asymptomatically infected for life, and a few such per-sons intermittently shed EBV.[12,14] Immunosuppressed persons shed the virus more frequently. Asymptomatic shedding of

FIGURE 15.3 • Infectious mononucleosis. Atypical lymphocytes are characteristic. (From Rubin R., Strayer D. S. (Eds.). (2012). *Rubin's pathology: Clinicopathologic foundations of medicine* (6th ed., p. 1002). Philadelphia, PA: Lippincott Williams & Wilkins.)

EBV by healthy persons is thought to account for most of the spread of infectious mononucleosis, despite the fact that it is not a highly contagious disease.

Clinical Course

The onset of infectious mononucleosis usually is insidious. The incubation period is estimated at 30 to 50 days.[14] A prodromal period, which lasts for several days, follows and is character-ized by malaise, anorexia, and chills. The prodromal period precedes the onset of fever, pharyngitis, and lymphadenopathy. Occasionally, the disorder comes on abruptly with a high fever. Most persons seek medical attention for severe pharyngitis, which usually is most severe on days 5 to 7 and persists for 7 to 14 days. The lymph nodes are typically enlarged through-out the body, particularly in the cervical, axillary, and groin areas. Hepatitis and splenomegaly are common manifestations of the disease and are thought to be immune mediated. Hepa-titis is characterized by hepatomegaly, nausea, anorexia, and jaundice. Although discomforting, it usually is a benign con-dition that resolves without causing permanent liver damage. The spleen may be enlarged two to three times its normal size, and rupture of the spleen is an infrequent complication. In less than 1% of cases, mostly in the adult age group, complications of the central nervous system (CNS) develop. These compli-cations include cranial nerve palsies, encephalitis, meningitis, transverse myelitis, and Guillain–Barré syndrome.

The peripheral blood usually shows an increase in the number of leukocytes, with a white blood cell count greater than 10×10^9/L, 60% of which are lymphocytes.[13] The rise in white blood cells begins during the first week, continues during the second week of the infection, and then returns to normal around the fourth week. Although leukocytosis is com-mon, leukopenia may be seen in some persons during the first 3 days of illness. Atypical lymphocytes are common, constitut-ing more than 20% of the total lymphocyte count. Heterophil antibodies usually appear during the second or third week and decline after the acute illness has subsided. They may, however, be detectable for up to 12 months after onset of the disease.

Most persons with infectious mononucleosis recover without incident. The acute phase of the illness usually lasts for 2 to 3 weeks, after which recovery occurs rapidly. Some degree of debility and lethargy may persist for 2 to 3 months. Treatment is primarily symptomatic and supportive, including rest and prevention of splenic injury. Analgesics such as acetaminophen or ibuprofen may be used to relieve fever, headache, and sore throat.[14–16]

In persons with immunodeficiency disorders that lead to defects in cellular immunity (*e.g.,* human immunodeficiency virus [HIV] infection, immunosuppressant-treated recipients of organ or bone marrow transplants), EBV infection may contribute to the development of lymphoproliferative disorders (*e.g.,* non-Hodgkin lymphoma).[12–16] These persons have impaired T-cell immunity and are unable to control the proliferation of EBV-infected B cells.

IN SUMMARY

Neutropenia, which represents a marked reduction in the absolute number of neutrophils, is one of the major disorders of the white blood cells. It can occur as a congenital or acquired disorder. Congenital neutropenia consists primarily of cyclic neutropenia, which is characterized by cyclic (18- to 24-day) oscillations of peripheral neutrophils, and severe congenital neutropenia or Kostmann syndrome, which is associated with severe bacterial infections. The acquired neutropenias encompass a wide spectrum of causative processes, including immunologically mediated bone marrow suppression or neutrophil injury and destruction; infection-mediated mechanisms, including increased peripheral utilization; and drug-mediated mechanisms, particularly those related to the use of cancer chemotherapeutic agents. Neutropenia may also be caused by a number of bone marrow conditions, hematopoietic malignancies, and radiation therapy. Because the neutrophil is essential to host defences against bacterial and fungal infections, severe and often life-threatening infections are common in persons with neutropenia.

Infectious mononucleosis is a self-limited lymphoproliferative disorder caused by the B-lymphotropic EBV, a member of the herpesvirus family. The highest incidence of infectious mononucleosis is found in adolescents and young adults, and it is seen more frequently in the upper socioeconomic classes of developed countries. The virus is usually transmitted in the saliva. The disease is characterized by fever, generalized lymphadenopathy, sore throat, and the appearance in the blood of atypical lymphocytes and several antibodies, including the well-known heterophil antibodies that are used in the diagnosis of infectious mononucleosis. Most persons with infectious mononucleosis recover without incident. Treatment is largely symptomatic and supportive.

NEOPLASTIC DISORDERS OF HEMATOPOIETIC AND LYMPHOID ORIGIN

After completing this section of the chapter, you should be able to meet the following objectives:

- Use the concepts regarding the central and peripheral lymphoid tissues to describe the site of origin of the malignant lymphomas, leukemias, and plasma cell dyscrasias.
- Explain how changes in chromosomal structure and gene function can contribute to the development of malignant lymphomas, leukemias, and plasma cell dyscrasias.
- Contrast and compare the signs, symptoms, and treatment of non-Hodgkin and Hodgkin lymphomas.
- Use the predominant white blood cell type and classification of acute or chronic to describe the four general types of leukemia.
- Explain the manifestations of leukemia in terms of altered cell differentiation.
- Describe the following complications of acute leukemia and its treatment: leukostasis, tumour lysis syndrome, hyperuricemia, and blast crisis.
- Relate the clonal expansion of immunoglobulin-producing plasma cells and accompanying destructive skeletal changes that occur with multiple myeloma in terms of manifestations and clinical course of the disorder.

The neoplastic disorders of hematopoietic and lymphoid origin represent the most important of the white blood cell disorders. They include the somewhat overlapping categories of the lymphomas (non-Hodgkin and Hodgkin lymphomas), acute and chronic leukemias, and plasma cell dyscrasias (multiple myeloma). The clinical features of these neoplasms are largely determined by their site of origin, the progenitor cell from which they originated, and the molecular events involved in their transformation into a malignant neoplasm (Fig. 15.4). The leukemias, which arise from hematopoietic precursors in the bone marrow, can involve the T and B lymphocytes, granulocytes, and other blood cells. The lymphomas originate in peripheral lymphoid structures such as the lymph nodes, where B and T lymphocytes undergo differentiation and proliferation as they interact with antigens. The plasma cell dyscrasias originate in the lymph node, where B cells differentiate into plasma cells. Because blood cells circulate throughout the body, these neoplasms are often disseminated from the onset.

Malignant Lymphomas

The lymphomas are a diverse group of solid tumours composed of neoplastic lymphoid cells that vary with respect to

FIGURE 15.4 • Origin of lymphoid neoplasms, showing the stages of B- and T-cell differentiation from which specific lymphoid tumours emerge. (Double-negative pre-T cells express neither CD4 nor CD8; double-positive T cells express both CD4 and CD8.) (Modified from Kumar V., Abbas A. K., Fausto N., et al. (Eds.). (2010). *Robbins and Cotran pathologic basis of disease* (8th ed., p. 599). Philadelphia, PA: Elsevier Saunders.)

molecular features, genetics, clinical presentation, and treatment. An estimated 9,200 new cases of lymphomas will be diagnosed in Canada in 2015, of which 8,200 will be non-Hodgkin lymphomas (NHLs) and 1,000 will be Hodgkin lymphoma (HL).[17] Since the early 1970s, the incidence rates for NHLs have nearly doubled. Although some of this increase was due to the AIDS related NHLs, for the most part the increase is unexplained. However, since 2000 the mortality rates have declined likely reflecting recent improvements in treatment (*i.e.*, immunotherapy, antiretroviral therapy).[17]

Non-Hodgkin Lymphomas

NHLs represent a clinically diverse group of either B-cell or T-cell neoplasms, the etiology of which is largely unknown. They represent the fifth most commonly diagnosed cancer in men (4.5%) and the sixth for women (3.8%) in Canada.[17–19]

As with most other malignancies, the cause of NHL is largely unknown. However, impairment of the immune system

MALIGNANT LYMPHOMAS

- The lymphomas represent malignancies that arise in the peripheral lymphoid tissues.
- Non-Hodgkin lymphomas (NHLs) represent a group of heterogeneous lymphocytic cancers that are multicentric in origin and spread to various tissues throughout the body, including the bone marrow.
- Hodgkin lymphoma (HL) is a group of cancers characterized by Reed–Sternberg cells that begins as a malignancy in a single lymph node and then spreads to contiguous lymph nodes.
- Both types of lymphomas are characterized by manifestations related to uncontrolled lymph node and lymphoid tissue growth, bone marrow involvement, and constitutional symptoms (fever, fatigue, weight loss) related to the rapid growth of abnormal lymphoid cells and tissues.

and infectious agents may play a role. There is evidence of the EBV infection in essentially all people with Burkitt lymphoma, which is endemic to some parts of Africa.[4,5,19] A second virus, the human T-cell lymphotropic virus (HTLV-1), notably more common in east Asia, has been associated with adult T-cell leukemia/lymphoma. The NHLs are also seen with increased frequency in persons infected with HIV, in those who have received chronic immunosuppressive therapy after organ transplantation, and in individuals with acquired or congenital immunodeficiencies. There is also a reported association between chronic *Helicobacter pylori* infection and low-grade MALT lymphoma of the stomach.[19]

Although the NHLs can originate in any of the lymphoid tissues, they most commonly originate in the lymph nodes. Like normal lymphocytes, transformed B and T cells tend to migrate to particular lymph node sites, leading to characteristic patterns of involvement. For example, B-cell lymphomas tend to proliferate in the B-cell areas of the lymph node, whereas T-cell lymphomas typically grow in the paracortical T-cell areas[4,5] (Fig. 15.4). All have the potential to spread to various lymphoid tissues throughout the body, especially the liver, spleen, and bone marrow.

NHLs can be classified according to the World Health Organization (WHO) system.[4,5,18,20] The current WHO classification scheme uses morphologic (cell type [B or T cell], level of maturation), immunophenotypic (presence of surface markers such as antigens, CD markers), genotypic (genetic makeup of cell) and clinical features including anatomic sites.[4] The NHLs are actually a complex group of almost 40 distinct entities.[4,5,19] Neoplasms of immature B cells include lymphoblastic leukemia/lymphoma (*i.e.*, acute lymphocytic leukemia, to be discussed). In addition, the specific types of lymphomas are sometimes grouped together into low-grade, aggressive, and very aggressive categories. The Ann Arbor Staging System is used in Canada to classify the spread of the disease. This system has four stages with subdivisions and identifies locations where the disease has spread, including extranodal lymph involvement.[17,19] Currently the International Prognostic Index (IPI) is preferred as it incorporates information from the WHO and Ann Arbor staging and is used as a means of predicting survival outcomes and guiding treatment decisions.[19]

Mature B-Cell Lymphomas. Mature (peripheral) B-cell lymphomas are the most common type of lymphoma in the Western world. The most common of the mature B-cell lymphomas are the follicular lymphomas (22%) and diffuse large B-cell lymphomas (31%). Small lymphocytic lymphoma, mantle cell lymphoma, peripheral T-cell lymphoma, and MALT lymphoma together account for 28% of NHLs.[4]

Follicular lymphomas are derived from germinal centre B cells and consist of a mixture of centroblasts and centrocytes. Follicular lymphomas are a particularly common neoplasm in North America, where they constitute about one third of all adult NHLs, with a peak incidence at 60 years of age. The lymphoma predominantly affects lymph nodes. Other sites of involvement include the spleen, bone marrow,

peripheral blood, head and neck region, gastrointestinal tract, and skin. Most persons have advanced disease at presentation and an indolent clinical course, with a median survival of 7 to 9 years.[5,18] Over time, 30 to 50% of follicular lymphomas transform into a fast-growing diffuse large B-cell lymphoma and the median survival after this transformation is less than 1 year.[4,5]

Diffuse large B-cell lymphomas are a heterogeneous group of aggressive germinal or postgerminal centre neoplasms. The disease occurs in all age groups but is most prevalent between 60 and 70 years of age. The cause of diffuse large B-cell lymphoma is unknown, but may involve EBV or HIV infections. It is a rapidly evolving, multifocal, nodal and extranodal tumour. Manifestations are typically seen at the time of presentation. As a group, diffuse large B-cell lymphomas are rapidly fatal if untreated. Approximately 30 to 40% of patients will relapse after initial chemotherapy and to potentially achieve remission high dose chemotherapy and stem cell transplantation regimens are used with limited success.[5,19]

Burkitt lymphoma, one of the most rapidly growing tumours of the NHLs, is also a disorder of germinal centre B cells. Endemic Burkitt lymphoma is the most common childhood cancer (peak age 3 to 7 years) in Central Africa, often beginning in the jaw[4] (Fig. 15.5). It occurs in regions of Africa where both EBV and malarial infection are common. Virtually 100% of patients with African Burkitt lymphoma have evidence of previous EBV infection and likely EBV has a direct causative role for the development of this lymphoma. Although the exact mechanism between EBV and B cells remains unknown, it is clear that the malaria induces the reactivation of the EBV with an over expression of oncogene (*MYC*) translocations.[20] A sporadic or nonendemic form of Burkitt lymphoma occurs less frequently in other parts of the world, and although these tumours are histologically

FIGURE 15.5 • African Burkitt lymphoma. A tumour of the jaw distorts the child's face. (From Rubin R., Strayer D. S. (Eds.). (2012). *Rubin's pathology: Clinicopathologic foundations of medicine* (6th ed., p. 1012). Philadelphia, PA: Lippincott Williams & Wilkins.)

similar to the endemic form, only about 20% carry the EBV genome. Both the endemic and sporadic forms have chromosomal translocation involving chromosome 8 that activates the *MYC* leading to uncontrolled tumour cell growth. Burkitt lymphoma is very aggressive but responds to short-term, high-dose chemotherapy, with a cure rate of up to 50%.[20]

Mantle cell lymphomas constitute less than 10% of NHLs and have their origin in the naive B cell. After the precursor stage, B cells undergo immunoglobulin (Ig) gene rearrangements and develop into surface IgM- and IgD-positive naive B cells (Fig. 15.4). These cells give rise to mantle cell lymphoma. Mantle cell lymphomas do not occur in children, but affect older persons (median age, 60 years). They have a rapid rate of progression, and half of persons affected do not survive 3 years.[19]

Marginal zone lymphomas involve late-stage memory B cells that reside in the marginal zone or outermost compartment of the lymph node follicle. Variants of marginal node lymphoma include splenic marginal zone lymphoma and MALT lymphomas of the stomach and other mucosal surfaces. *MALT lymphomas* constitute 5% to 10% of all B-cell NHLs. Most MALT lymphomas involve the stomach or other mucosal sites, including the respiratory system. MALT lymphomas tend to remain localized for prolonged periods and to follow an indolent course. Extranodal marginal B-cell lymphomas of the MALT type are curable by radiation or surgery when localized. MALT lymphomas that occur in the stomach secondary to *H. pylori* infection often respond to treatment with appropriate antimicrobial agents.

Clinical Manifestations. The manifestations of NHLs depend on lymphoma type (*i.e.*, indolent or aggressive) and the stage of the disease. Persons with indolent or slow-growing lymphomas usually present with painless lymphadenopathy, which may be isolated or widespread. Involved lymph nodes may be present in the retroperitoneum, mesentery, and pelvis. The indolent lymphomas are usually disseminated at the time of diagnosis, and bone marrow involvement is frequent. With or without treatment, the natural course of the disease may fluctuate over 5 to 10 or more years. Many low-grade lymphomas eventually transform into more aggressive forms of lymphoma/leukemia.

Persons with intermediate or more aggressive forms of lymphoma usually present with accompanying constitutional symptoms such as fever, drenching night sweats, or weight loss. Frequently, there is increased susceptibility to bacterial, viral, and fungal infections associated with hypogammaglobulinemia and a poor humoral antibody response, rather than the impaired cellular immunity seen with HL.

Diagnosis and Treatment. A lymph node biopsy is used to confirm the diagnosis of NHL and immunophenotyping to determine the lineage and clonality. Lymphomas can be grouped according to surface markers or phenotypic markers (*e.g.*, CD20).[21] Staging of the disease is important in selecting a treatment for persons with NHLs. Bone marrow biopsy,

blood studies, chest and abdominal computed tomography (CT) scans, magnetic resonance imaging (MRI), positron emission tomography (PET), gallium scans, and bone scans may be used to determine the stage of the disease.

Treatment of NHLs depends on the histologic type, stage of the disease, and clinical status of the person. For early-stage disease involving a single or limited node involvement, localized radiation may be used as a single treatment modality. However, because most people who present with indolent lymphoma have disseminated disease at the time of diagnosis, combination chemotherapy, combined adjuvant radiation therapy, or both are recommended. Persons with lymphomas that carry a risk of CNS involvement usually receive CNS prophylaxis with high doses of chemotherapeutic agents or cranial irradiation.

Monoclonal antibodies (mAbs) are used in the targeted treatment of NHLs. Rituximab (Rituxan), which was the first to be approved by the Canadian Food and Drug Act (FDA), recognizes and attaches to the CD20 antigen found on most B-cell lymphomas.[19,22,23] This mAb has been widely accepted because of its activity and favourable toxicity profile. Most adverse effects occur during infusion and consist mainly of chills, with occasional hypotension. For aggressive lymphomas, the combination of chemotherapy and rituximab has shown better response rates, indicating a synergistic effect.[19] Because lymphoma cells tend to be very sensitive to radiation, newer forms of mAbs have been developed that are similar to rituximab, but with a radioactive isotope such as radioactive iodine (Bexxar) or radioactive yttrium (Zevalin) attached. Another mAb (alemtuzumab) is directed at the CD52 antigen.[19] It is useful in some types of peripheral T-cell lymphomas. Bone marrow and peripheral stem cell transplantation are potentially curative treatments for people with highly resistant forms of the disease.

Hodgkin Lymphoma

Hodgkin lymphoma (HL), previously known as *Hodgkin disease,* is a specialized form of lymphoma that features the presence of an abnormal cell called a *Reed–Sternberg cell.*[4,5] Because of improved treatment methods, death rates have decreased by more than 60% since the early 1970s. Distribution of the disease is bimodal; it occurs more frequently in two separate groups, the first in early adulthood (15 to 40 years) and the second in older adulthood (55 years of age or older).[17] Only 10% to 15% if HL cases occur in children or adolescents.[22]

HL differs from NHLs in several respects. First, it usually arises in a single node or chain of nodes, whereas NHLs frequently originates at extranodal sites and spreads to anatomically contiguous nodes.[4,5] Second, HL is characterized by the presence of large, atypical, mononuclear tumour cells, called *Reed–Sternberg cells* (Fig. 15.6). These cells, which frequently constitute less than 1% of the total cell population, are a diagnostic hallmark of the disease.

Etiology and Pathogenesis. As with NHLs, the cause of HL is largely unknown. Although exposure to carcinogens and

FIGURE 15.6 • Classic Reed–Sternberg cell. Mirror-image nuclei contain large eosinophilic nucleoli. (From Rubin R., Strayer D. S. (Eds.). (2012). *Rubin's pathology: Clinicopathologic foundations of medicine* (6th ed., p. 1024). Philadelphia, PA: Lippincott Williams & Wilkins.)

viruses as well as genetic and immune mechanisms have been proposed as causes, none has been proved to be involved in the pathogenesis of the disease. It appears that people with a history of infectious mononucleosis are at increased risk for development of HL.[4,5]

The origin of the neoplastic Reed–Sternberg cell of HL has been difficult to study, in large part because these cells do not express many of the markers found on lymphocytes. It is only recently that methods have been developed that allow for the microanalysis of these cells and their variants. These studies have shown that the Reed–Sternberg cells of most individual cases harbour identical immunoglobulin genes that show evidence of mutation, establishing the cell of origin as a germinal centre or postgerminal centre B cell.

Classification. The WHO classification proposed classifying HL into two major categories: nodular lymphocyte-predominant HL and classic HL.[4,24] Nodular lymphocyte-predominant HL represents only a small portion of all cases of HL and is a unique form that generally exhibits a nodular growth pattern, with or without diffuse areas and with rare Reed–Sternberg cells called "popcorn" or "L&H" (lymphohistiocytic) cells. It is often localized rather than disseminated at the time of diagnosis, exhibits a slowly progressive course, and has an overall survival rate greater than 80%.[4]

Classic HL is characterized by clonal proliferation of typical mononuclear Hodgkin cells and multinucleated Reed–Sternberg cells with invariable expression of CD30. Four variants of classic HL have been described: nodular sclerosis, mixed cellularity, lymphocyte-rich, and lymphocyte-depleted. The nodular sclerotic type is the most common and is often found in adolescent and young adult women, 15 to 35 years of age. Lymphocyte-rich HL is rare, accounting for 5% of classic HL, and lymphocyte-depleted HL is very rarely diagnosed and accounts for less than 1% of classic HL cases.[4] At present, all subtypes of classic HL are treated in the similar manner.

Manifestations. Most persons with HL present with painless enlargement of a single node or group of nodes. The initial lymph node involvement typically is above the level of the diaphragm (*e.g.,* in the neck, supraclavicular area, or axilla). Mediastinal masses are frequent and are sometimes discovered on routine chest radiography. There may be complaints of chest discomfort with cough or dyspnea. Involvement of subdiaphragmatic lymph nodes at the time of presentation is unusual and more common in older men. Additional symptoms that suggest HL include fevers, chills, night sweats, and weight loss. Pruritus and intermittent fevers associated with night sweats are classic symptoms of HL.

Other symptoms such as fatigue and anemia are indicative of disease spread. In the advanced stages of HL, the liver, spleen, lungs, digestive tract, and, occasionally, the CNS may be involved (Fig. 15.7). As the disease progresses, the rapid proliferation of abnormal lymphocytes leads to an immunologic defect, particularly in cell-mediated responses, rendering the person more susceptible to viral, fungal, and protozoal infections. Anergy, or the failure to develop a positive response to skin tests such as the tuberculin test, is common early in the course of the disease.

Diagnosis and Treatment. A definitive diagnosis of HL requires that the Reed–Sternberg cell be present in a biopsy specimen of lymph node tissue. CT scans of the chest and abdomen commonly are used to assess for involvement of mediastinal, abdominal, and pelvic lymph nodes.[24] A bipedal lymphangiogram may detect structural changes in the lymph nodes too small to visualize on CT scan. If with initial screening the extent of lymph node involvement cannot be determined, PET imaging may be helpful.[24] A bilateral bone marrow biopsy is usually performed on patients who are suspected of having disseminated disease.

Using the Ann Arbor Staging System, persons with HF are staged according to the number of lymph nodes involved,

FIGURE 15.7 • Hodgkin lymphoma involving the spleen. Multinodular tumour masses replace the normal splenic tissue. (From Rubin R., Strayer D. S. (Eds.). (2012). *Rubin's pathology: Clinicopathologic foundations of medicine* (6th ed., p. 1027). Philadelphia, PA: Lippincott Williams & Wilkins.)

whether the lymph nodes are on one or both sides of the diaphragm, and whether there is disseminated disease involving the bone marrow, liver, lung, or skin. The staging of HL is of great clinical importance because the choice of treatment and the prognosis ultimately are related to the distribution of the disease.

Combined irradiation and chemotherapy are used in treating both localized and advanced disease.[24] As the accuracy of staging techniques, delivery of radiation, and curative efficacy of combination chemotherapy regimens have improved, the survival of people with HL also has improved. With modern treatment methods, a 5-year cure rate of 85% can be achieved.[17] As the cure rate for HL has risen and longer-term follow-up data have become available, the importance of the late effects of treatment, including secondary malignancies, has become more apparent.

Leukemias

The leukemias are malignant neoplasms of cells originally derived from hematopoietic precursor cells (Fig. 15.4). They are characterized by diffuse replacement of bone marrow with unregulated, proliferating, immature neoplastic cells. In most cases, the leukemic cells spill out into the blood, where they are seen in large numbers. The term *leukemia* (*i.e.,* "white blood") was first used by Virchow to describe a reversal of the usual ratio of red blood cells to white blood cells. The leukemic cells may also infiltrate the liver, spleen, lymph nodes, and other tissues throughout the body, causing enlargement of these organs.

Approximately 6,200 Canadians will be diagnosed with leukemia in 2015 and it is estimated for this year that approximately 2,700 Canadians will die of this disease.[17] Leukemia is the most common cause of cancer in children and adolescents. It accounts for about one third of cancers in children.[17,18] Although it commonly is thought of as a childhood disease, leukemia is diagnosed 10 times more frequently in adults than children.

LEUKEMIAS

- Leukemias are malignant neoplasms arising from the transformation of a single blood cell line derived from hematopoietic stem cells.
- The leukemias are classified as acute and chronic lymphocytic (lymphocytes) or myelocytic (granulocytes, monocytes) leukemias according to their cell lineage.
- Because leukemic cells are immature and poorly differentiated, they proliferate rapidly and have a long life span, they do not function normally, they interfere with the maturation of normal blood cells, and they circulate in the bloodstream, cross the blood–brain barrier, and infiltrate many body organs.

Classification

The leukemias commonly are classified according to their predominant cell type (*i.e.,* lymphocytic or myelocytic) and whether the condition is acute or chronic. Biphenotypic leukemias demonstrate characteristics of both lymphoid and myeloid lineages. A rudimentary classification system divides leukemia into four types: acute lymphocytic (lymphoblastic) leukemia (ALL), chronic lymphocytic leukemia (CLL), acute myelogenous (myeloblastic) leukemia (AML), and chronic myelogenous leukemia (CML).[17] The *lymphocytic leukemias* involve immature lymphocytes and their progenitors that originate in the bone marrow but infiltrate the spleen, lymph nodes, CNS, and other tissues. The *myelogenous leukemias,* which involve the pluripotent myeloid stem cells in bone marrow, interfere with the maturation of all blood cells, including the granulocytes, erythrocytes, and platelets.

Etiology and Molecular Biology

The causes of leukemia are largely unknown. The incidence of leukemia among persons who have been exposed to high levels of radiation is unusually high. An increased incidence of leukemia also is associated with exposure to benzene and the use of antitumour drugs (*e.g.,* mechlorethamine, procarbazine, cyclophosphamide, chloramphenicol, and the epipodophyllotoxins).[25] Leukemia may occur as a second cancer after aggressive chemotherapy for other cancers, such as HL. The existence of a genetic predisposition to development of acute leukemia is suggested by the increased leukemia incidence among a number of congenital disorders, including Down syndrome, neurofibromatosis, and Fanconi anemia. In individuals with Down syndrome, the incidence of acute leukemia is 10 to 20 times that of the general population.[21] There also are numerous reports of multiple cases of acute leukemia occurring within the same family.

The molecular biology of leukemia suggests that the event or events causing the disorders exert their effects through disruption or dysregulation of genes that normally regulate blood cell development, blood cell homeostasis, or both.[4] Cytogenetic studies have shown that recurrent chromosomal changes occur in over one half of all cases of leukemia. Most commonly, these are structural changes classified as translocations, written t(8;21), in which a part of one chromosome (*e.g.,* 8) becomes located on another chromosome (*e.g.,* 21) and vice versa; inversions, written inv(16), in which part of a chromosome (*e.g.,* 16) is upside down and now in reverse order, but still attached to the original chromosome; and deletions, written del(7) or −7, in which part of a chromosome (*e.g.,* 7) has been lost. It is the disruption or dysregulation of specific genes and gene products occurring at the site of these chromosome aberrations that contributes to the development of leukemia.[23] In many instances, these genes and their products have been shown to be directly or indirectly involved in the normal development or maintenance of the hematopoietic system. Thus, it would appear that leukemia results, at least in part, from disruption in the activity of genes that normally regulate blood cell development. Currently, several hundred recurring translocations have been described in hematologic malignancies. Advances in the understanding of the molecular biology of leukemia are beginning to provide a more complete

Normal chromosomes

Chromosome 22   Chromosome 9

BCR
locus

ABL
proto-
oncogene

Myelogenous leukemia

BCR
locus

BCR-ABL
hybrid gene

ABL
oncogene

ABL
protein

FIGURE 15.8 • The Philadelphia chromosome is formed by breaks at the ends of the long arms of chromosomes 9 and 22, allowing the *ABL* proto-oncogene on chromosome 9 to be translocated to the breakpoint cluster region (*BCR*) on chromosome 22. The result is a new fusion gene coding for the BCR-ABL protein, which is presumably involved in the pathogenesis of chronic myelogenous leukemia.

understanding of the molecular complexity of leukemia for the purposes of diagnosis, classification, treatment, and monitoring of clinical outcomes.

One of the more studied translocations is the *Philadelphia chromosome,* which was the first chromosomal abnormality identified in cancer. The *Philadelphia chromosome* translocation, t(9;22), represents a reciprocal translocation between the long arm of chromosome 22 and the long arm of chromosome 9.[4,5] During the translocation, a large portion of 22q is translocated to 9q, and a smaller piece of 9q is moved to 22q (Fig. 15.8). The portion of 9q that is translocated contains *ABL,* a proto-oncogene that is the cellular homolog of the Abelson murine leukemic virus. The *ABL* gene is received at a specific site on 22q called the *breakpoint cluster* (BCR). The resulting *BCR-ABL* fusion gene codes for a novel protein that differs from that of the normal *ABL* gene in that it possesses tyrosine kinase activity (a characteristic activity of transforming genes).[4,23,26] The presence of the tyrosine kinase generated by the fusion gene allows affected cells to bypass the regulated signals that control normal cell growth and differentiation, and instead undergo malignant transformation to become leukemic cells. The *Philadelphia chromosome* translocation is found in more than 90% of persons with CML and in some persons with acute leukemia. The development of tyrosine kinase inhibitors has contributed to the targeted approach for

treatment of leukemias that display the *Philadelphia chromosome* translocation.[26]

Acute Leukemias

The acute leukemias are cancers of the hematopoietic progenitor cells.[4,5] They usually have a sudden onset with signs and symptoms related to depressed bone marrow function (Table 15.1). There are two types of acute leukemia: ALL and AML. ALL occurs most frequently in children accounting for three of four cases of childhood cancer. However, about one third of cases of ALL occur in adults and most of the death from this disease occur in adults (about four out of five).[27] AML is mainly a disease of older adults, but is also seen in children and young adults. In 2010, 435 Canadians were diagnosed with ALL and 1,215 were diagnosed with AML.[17]

ALL encompasses a group of neoplasms composed of precursor B (pre-B) or T (pre-T) lymphocytes referred to as *lymphoblasts* (Fig. 15.4). Most cases (about 85% to 90%) of ALL are of pre-B-cell origin.[5] The majority of persons with ALL have numeric and structural changes in the chromosomes of their leukemic cells. They include hyperploidy (*i.e.,* more than 50 chromosomes), polyploidy (*i.e.,* 3 or more sets of chromosomes), and chromosomal translocations and deletions. Many of these chromosomal aberrations serve to dysregulate the expression and function of transcription factors required for normal hematopoietic cell development.

The AMLs are a diverse group of neoplasms affecting myeloid precursor cells in the bone marrow.[4,5,17,28] Most are associated with acquired genetic alterations that inhibit terminal myeloid differentiation. As a result, normal marrow elements are replaced by an accumulation of relatively undifferentiated blast cells with a resultant suppression of the remaining progenitor cells that leads to anemia, neutropenia, and thrombocytopenia. Specific chromosomal abnormalities, including translocations, are seen in a large number of AMLs. One subtype of AML, acute promyelocytic leukemia, which represents 10% of adult cases of AML, is associated with a t(15;17) chromosomal translocation.[29] This translocation produces a fusion gene that encodes a portion of the transcription factor, retinoic acid receptor-a (RARa), fused to a portion of another protein, PML. This change in the retinoic acid receptor produces a block in differentiation that can be overcome with pharmacologic doses of retinoic acid (to be discussed).

Clinical Manifestations. Although ALL and AML are distinct disorders, they typically present with similar clinical features. Both are characterized by an abrupt onset of symptoms, including fatigue resulting from anemia; low-grade fever, night sweats, and weight loss due to the rapid proliferation and hypermetabolism of the leukemic cells; bleeding due to a decreased platelet count; and bone pain and tenderness due to bone marrow expansion. Infection results from neutropenia, with the risk of infection rising steeply as the neutrophil count falls below 0.5×10^9/L. Generalized lymphadenopathy, splenomegaly, and hepatomegaly caused by infiltration of leukemic cells occur in all acute leukemias but are more common in ALL.[25]

TABLE 15.1 CLINICAL MANIFESTATIONS OF LEUKEMIA AND THEIR PATHOLOGIC BASIS[a]

CLINICAL MANIFESTATIONS	PATHOLOGIC BASIS
Bone marrow depression	
Malaise, easy fatigability	Anemia
Fever	Infection or increased metabolism by neoplastic cells
Bleeding	Decreased thrombocytes
Petechiae	
Ecchymosis	
Gingival bleeding	
Epistaxis	
Bone pain and tenderness upon palpation	Subperiosteal bone infiltration, bone marrow expansion, and bone resorption
Headache, nausea, vomiting, papilledema, cranial nerve palsies, seizures, coma	Leukemic infiltration of the central nervous system
Abdominal discomfort	Generalized lymphadenopathy, hepatomegaly, splenomegaly due to leukemic cell infiltration
Increased vulnerability to infections	Immaturity of the white cells and ineffective immune function
Hematologic abnormalities	Physical and metabolic encroachment of leukemia cells on red blood cells and thrombocyte precursors
Anemia	
Thrombocytopenia	
Hyperuricemia and other metabolic disorders	Abnormal proliferation and metabolism of leukemia cells

[a]Manifestations vary with the type of leukemia.

In addition to the common manifestations of acute leukemia (*i.e.,* fatigue, weight loss, fever, easy bruising), infiltration of malignant cells in the skin, gums, and other soft tissues is particularly common in the monocytic form of AML. The leukemic cells may also cross the blood–brain barrier and establish sanctuary in the CNS. CNS involvement is more common in ALL than AML, and is more common in children than adults. Signs and symptoms of CNS involvement include cranial nerve palsies, headache, nausea, vomiting, papilledema, and occasionally seizures and coma.

Leukostasis is a condition in which the circulating blast count is markedly elevated (usually 100×10^9/L). The high number of circulating leukemic blasts increases blood viscosity and predisposes to the development of leukoblastic emboli with obstruction of small blood vessels in the pulmonary and cerebral circulations. Occlusion of the pulmonary vessels leads to vessel rupture and infiltration of lung tissue, resulting in sudden shortness of breath and progressive dyspnea. Cerebral leukostasis leads to diffuse headache and lethargy, which can progress to confusion and coma. Once identified, leukostasis requires immediate and effective treatment to lower the blast count rapidly. Initial treatment uses apheresis to remove excess blast cells, followed by chemotherapy to stop leukemic cell production in the bone marrow.[30]

Hyperuricemia occurs as the result of increased proliferation or increased breakdown of purine nucleotides (*i.e.,* one of the components of nucleic acids) secondary to the leukemic cell death that results from chemotherapy. It may increase before and during treatment. Prophylactic therapy with rasburicase (Fasturtec), a recombinant version of a urate oxidase enzyme, is generally administered to prevent renal complications secondary to uric acid crystallization in the urine filtrate.[31,32]

Diagnosis. A definitive diagnosis of acute leukemia is based on blood and bone marrow studies; it requires the demonstration of leukemic cells in the peripheral blood, bone marrow, or extramedullary tissue. Laboratory findings reveal the presence of immature white blood cells (blasts) in the circulation and bone marrow, where they may constitute 60% to 100% of the cells. As these cells proliferate and begin to crowd the bone marrow, the development of other blood cell lines in the marrow is suppressed. Consequently, there is a loss of mature myeloid cells, such as erythrocytes, granulocytes, and platelets. Anemia is almost always present, and the platelet count is decreased. Immunophenotyping is performed to determine the lineage subtype of the leukemia.[23,28,33]

Bone marrow biopsy may be used to determine the molecular characteristics of the leukemia, the degree of bone marrow involvement, and the morphology and histology of the disease. Cytogenetic studies, which are used to determine chromosomal abnormalities, are one of the most powerful prognostic indicators in acute leukemia. Certain chromosomal abnormalities respond more favourably to certain types of treatment and have a better prognosis than other abnormalities.

In ALL, the staging includes a lumbar puncture to assess CNS involvement. Imaging studies that include CT scans of the chest, abdomen, and pelvis may also be obtained to identify additional sites of disease.[34]

Treatment. Treatment of ALL and AML consists of several phases and the likelihood of achieving a remission depends on a number of factors, including age, type of leukemia, and stage of the disease at time of presentation. Of these factors, age is probably the most significant prognostic variable.[28,35]

Treatment of ALL usually consists of four phases: induction therapy, CNS prophylaxis, consolidation or intensification therapy, and maintenance therapy. *Induction therapy* which is designed to elicit a remission incorporates a number of chemotherapeutic agents. The goal of induction therapy is the production of a severe bone marrow response with destruction of leukemic progenitor cells followed by normal bone marrow recovery. CNS prophylaxis may be accomplished through the administration of intrathecal chemotherapy by lumbar puncture or by cranial irradiation concurrent with systemic chemotherapy. Because of its side effects, CNS irradiation is being used less frequently than in the past. The use of high-dose chemotherapy that crosses the blood–brain barrier may make separate CNS treatment unnecessary in the future. Although CNS involvement is a major problem in children, the incidence in adults at the time of diagnosis is less than 10%. *Consolidation or intensification therapy* consists of high doses of chemotherapy given to patients who have achieved remission with their induction therapy. *Maintenance therapy* which serves to maintain the remission is usually accomplished with lower doses of chemotherapy given over a long period (*e.g.,* 2 years) to patients after consolidation therapy. Although almost 80% of children are cured of ALL, only about 30% to 40% of adults achieve long-term disease-free survival.[5,35]

Massive necrosis of malignant cells can occur during the initial phase of treatment. This phenomenon, known as *tumour lysis syndrome,* can lead to life-threatening metabolic disorders, including hyperkalemia, hyperphosphatemia, hyperuricemia, hypomagnesemia, hypocalcemia, and acidosis, with the potential for causing acute renal failure. Aggressive prophylactic hydration with alkaline solutions and administration of rasburicase to reduce uric acid levels are used to counteract these effects.[31,32]

As with ALL, treatment of AML consists of a number of phases. Treatment usually consists of induction therapy followed by intensive consolidation therapy. Induction therapy consists of intensive chemotherapy to effect aplasia of the bone marrow. During this period, supportive transfusion and treatment with antimicrobial agents often are needed. An mAbs conjugated with a chemotherapeutic agent (gemtuzumab ozogamicin) that targets the CD33 antigen found on 90% of AML blast cells is another treatment option for patients older than 60 years of age who are not candidates for intensive chemotherapy.[36] Acute promyelocytic leukemia is treated differently from other forms of AML. Induction therapy includes an anthracycline (*e.g.,* idarubicin) plus all-*trans*-retinoic acid (ATRA). This agent is an analog of vitamin A that leads to terminal differentiation of acute promyelocytic cells through an interaction with the abnormal retinoic acid receptor created by the specific chromosomal translocation that is a hallmark of this subtype of leukemia.[28]

Bone marrow or stem cell transplantation may be considered for persons with ALL and AML who have failed to

respond to other forms of therapy.[28,35] Because of the risk of complications, bone marrow transplantation is not usually recommended for patients older than 50 to 55 years of age.[23]

Chronic Leukemias

In contrast to acute leukemias, chronic leukemias are malignancies involving proliferation of more fully differentiated myeloid and lymphoid cells. As with acute leukemia, there are two major types of chronic leukemia: CLL and CML. CLL accounted for 2,195 new cases and 600 deaths in Canada in 2010.[17] It is mainly a disorder of older persons. The average age at time of diagnosis is approximately 72 years. It is rarely seen in people younger than 40 years of age, and is extremely rare in children.[37] CML accounted for approximately 590 new cases and 126 deaths in Canada in 2010.[17] As with CLL, it is predominantly a disorder of older adults, with an average age of approximately 64 years at time of diagnosis.[17,37]

Chronic Lymphocytic Leukemia. CLL, a clonal malignancy of B lymphocytes, is the most common form of leukemia in adults in the Western world. In the past, CLL was viewed as a homogeneous disease of immature, immune-incompetent, minimally self-renewing B cells, which accumulated because of faulty apoptotic mechanisms either due to chromosomal abnormalities or surface antigens. Some persons with CLL survive for many years without therapy and eventually succumb to unrelated diseases, whereas others have a rapidly fatal outcome despite aggressive therapy. One example of its heterogeneity is thought to reflect differences in immunoglobulin V-gene mutations, expression of cell surface CD markers (*e.g.,* CD38), and presence of the zeta-associated protein (ZAP-70). ZAP-70 is an intracellular protein that promulgates activation signals delivered to T cells and NK cells by their surface receptors for antigens. It is rarely present in normal B cells but is found in persons with CLL. Persons with leukemic cells having few or no V-gene mutations or with many CD38[+] or ZAP-70[+] B cells often have an aggressive course, whereas those with V-gene mutations but few CD38[+] or ZAP-70[+] B cells usually have a more indolent course.

The clinical signs and symptoms of CLL are largely related to the progressive infiltration of the bone marrow and lymphoid tissues by neoplastic lymphocytes and to secondary immunologic defects. Persons with the indolent form of CLL are often asymptomatic at the time of diagnosis, and lymphocytosis is noted on a complete blood count obtained for another, unrelated disorder. As the disease progresses, lymph nodes gradually increase in size and new nodes are involved, sometimes in unusual areas such as the scalp, orbit, pharynx, pleura, gastrointestinal tract, liver, prostate, and gonads. Persons with the aggressive form of CLL experience a more rapid sequence of clinical deterioration characterized by increasing lymphadenopathy, hepatosplenomegaly, fever, abdominal pain, weight loss, progressive anemia, and thrombocytopenia, with a rapid rise in lymphocyte count.

Hypogammaglobulinemia is common in CLL, especially in persons with advanced disease. An increased susceptibility to infection reflects an inability to produce specific antibodies and abnormal activation of complement. The most common infectious organisms are those that require opsonization for bacterial killing, such as *Streptococcus pneumoniae, Staphylococcus aureus,* and *Haemophilus influenzae.*

The diagnostic hallmark of CLL is isolated lymphocytosis. The white blood cell count is usually greater than $20 \times 10^9/L$ and may be elevated to several hundred thousand. Usually, 75% to 98% are lymphocytes. The hematocrit and platelet counts are usually normal at presentation. Tests to determine the presence of mutated forms of the immunoglobulin gene and expression of the C38 surface antigen and the ZAP-70 protein may be used to determine whether the leukemia is the indolent or aggressive type. Cytogenetic studies may also provide prognostic information. The finding of deletion of chromosome 17p or 11q is a poor prognostic indicator.[38]

Treatment of CLL usually depends on the presence of prognostic indicators.[17] Persons with the low-risk or indolent form of CLL usually do not require specific treatment for many years after diagnosis and eventually die of apparently unrelated causes. Reassurance that persons with the disorder can live a normal life for many years is important. Many persons with intermediate-risk disease may remain stable for many years as well, whereas others may develop complications and need treatment within a few months. Most persons with high-risk CLL require treatment at diagnosis.

The current treatment of choice is combination chemotherapy plus the mAb rituximab that targets CD20+ B lymphocytes. Alemtuzumab, a mAb directed against the CD52 antigen, may be used to treat persons who have not responded to chemotherapy. Complications such as autoimmune hemolytic anemia or thrombocytopenia may require treatment with corticosteroids or splenectomy.[39] Clinical trials are looking at medications to target different pathways such as the anti-apoptotic protein Bcl-2, or the B cell receptor (BCR) to manipulate the intracellular signalling and interactions.[39]

In younger patients with aggressive disease, an allogeneic ablative (destruction of bone marrow cells by irradiation or chemotherapy) or nonmyeloablative stem cell transplant is a treatment option. In a nonmyeloablative type of transplant, the goal is marrow suppression, destruction of leukemia cells by the donor's lymphocytes, known as "graft-versus-leukemia" effect, and marrow recovery with donor cells.

Chronic Myelogenous Leukemia. CML is a disorder of the pluripotent hematopoietic progenitor cell. It is characterized by excessive proliferation of marrow granulocytes, erythroid precursors, and megakaryocytes. The CML cells harbour a distinctive cytogenic abnormality, the previously described *Philadelphia chromosome.*[4,5] It is generally believed that CML develops when a single, pluripotent hematopoietic stem cell acquires a *Philadelphia chromosome.* Although CML originates in the pluripotent stem cells, granulocyte precursors remain the dominant leukemic cell type.

The clinical course of CML is commonly divided into three phases: (1) a chronic phase of variable length, (2) a short accelerated phase, and (3) a terminal blast crisis phase. The onset of the chronic phase is usually slow, with nonspecific symptoms such as weakness and weight loss. The most characteristic laboratory finding at the time of presentation is leukocytosis with immature granulocyte cell types in the peripheral blood. Anemia and, eventually, thrombocytopenia develop. Anemia causes weakness, easy fatigability, and exertional dyspnea. Splenomegaly is often present at the time of diagnosis; hepatomegaly is less common; and lymphadenopathy is relatively uncommon. Persons in the early chronic phase of CML generally are asymptomatic, but without effective treatment most will enter the accelerated phase within 4 years.[40]

The accelerated phase of CML is characterized by enlargement of the spleen and progressive symptoms. Splenomegaly often causes a feeling of abdominal fullness and discomfort. An increase in basophil count and more immature cells in the blood or bone marrow confirm transformation to the accelerated phase. During this phase, constitutional symptoms such as low-grade fever, night sweats, bone pain, and weight loss develop because of rapid proliferation and hypermetabolism of the leukemic cells. Bleeding and easy bruising may arise from dysfunctional platelets. Generally, the accelerated phase is short (6 to 12 months).

The terminal blast crisis phase of CML represents evolution to acute leukemia and is characterized by an increasing number of myeloid precursors, especially blast cells, in the blood (Fig. 15.9). Constitutional symptoms become more pronounced during this period, and splenomegaly may increase significantly. Isolated infiltrates of leukemic cells can involve the skin, lymph nodes, bones, and CNS. With very high blast counts ($>100 \times 10^9/L$), symptoms of leukostasis may occur. The prognosis for patients who are in the blast crisis phase and don't respond to chemotherapy is poor, with a median survival of 2 to 4 months.[41]

A diagnostic feature of CML is an elevated white blood count, with a median count of $150 \times 10^9/L$ at the time of diagnosis, although in some cases it is only modestly increased.

FIGURE 15.9 • Peripheral blood showing blast crisis in chronic myelogenous leukemia. (From Centers for Disease Control and Prevention. (2014). Public Health Image Library. Available online at: http://phil.cdc.gov/phil/home.asp.)

The hallmark of the disease is the presence of the BCR-ABL gene product, which can be detected in the peripheral blood. This is best done using the polymerase chain reaction (PCR), which has supplanted cytogenetics in identifying the *Philadelphia chromosome*. Bone marrow examination is not usually necessary for diagnosis, but is useful for prognosis and for detecting additional chromosomal abnormalities.

The goals of treatment for CML include a hematologic response characterized by normalized blood counts; a cytogenetic response demonstrated by the reduction or elimination of the Philadelphia chromosome from the bone marrow; and a molecular response confirmed by the elimination of the BCR-ABL fusion protein.[4,5,26] Since 2003, imatinib, a specifically designed inhibitor of the tyrosine kinase activity of the BCR-ABL oncogene product, remains the standard therapy for CML and newer agents (*e.g.,* dasatinib, nilotinib) can be used in cases of resistance or intolerance to imatinib. Their side effect profiles and ease of administration (oral route) have dramatically changed the treatment of CML.

The only available curative treatment for CML is allogeneic bone marrow or stem cell transplantation. In most transplantation centres, full myeloablative transplants are available to children and adults younger than 60 years of age who have an HLA-matched sibling donor or an unrelated molecular-matched donor. Nonmyeloablative or "mini-transplants" are available to patients younger than 70 years of age who have sibling HLA-matched or unrelated HLA-matched donors.

Plasma Cell Dyscrasias

Plasma cell dyscrasias are characterized by expansion of a single clone of immunoglobulin-producing plasma cells and a resultant increase in serum levels of a single monoclonal immunoglobulin or its fragments. The plasma cell dyscrasias include multiple myeloma; localized plasmacytoma (solitary myeloma); lymphoplasmacytic lymphoma; primary or immunocyte amyloidosis due to excessive production of light chains; and monoclonal gammopathy of undetermined significance. *Monoclonal gammopathy of undetermined significance* (MGUS) is characterized by the presence of monoclonal immunoglobulin in the serum without other findings of multiple myeloma. MGUS is considered a premalignant condition.[4,5,42] Approximately 1% per year of persons with MGUS will go on to develop a plasma cell dyscrasia (multiple myeloma, lymphoplasmacytic lymphoma, or amyloidosis). The strong link between MGUS and multiple myeloma suggests that a first oncogenic event produces MGUS and a second event results in multiple myeloma.[4]

Multiple Myeloma

Multiple myeloma is a B-cell malignancy of terminally differentiated plasma cells. It accounts for 1.3% of all cancers and 10% of all hematologic malignancies in whites and 20% in persons of African ancestry.[17,42] It occurs most frequently in persons older than 60 years of age, with the median age of patients with multiple myeloma being 65 years.[42]

The cause of multiple myeloma is unknown. Risk factors are thought to include chronic immune stimulation, autoimmune disorders, exposure to ionizing radiation, and occupational exposure to pesticides or herbicides (*e.g.,* dioxin). A number of viruses have been associated with the pathogenesis of myeloma. In the United States, myeloma has been associated with exposure to Agent Orange during the Vietnam War.

Pathogenesis. Multiple myeloma is characterized by proliferation of malignant plasma cells in the bone marrow and osteolytic bone lesions throughout the skeletal system. As with other hematopoietic malignancies, it is now recognized that multiple myeloma is associated with multiple chromosomal abnormalities, including deletions of 13q and translocations involving the IgG locus on chromosome 14. One fusion partner is a fibroblast growth factor receptor gene on chromosome 4, which is truncated to produce a constitutively active receptor. Changes also occur in the bone marrow microenvironment, including the induction of angiogenesis, the suppression of cell-mediated immunity, and the development of paracrine signalling loops involving cytokines such as IL-6 and vascular endothelial growth factor. Other growth factors that are implicated in multiple myeloma include granulocyte CSF, interferon-α, and IL-10. The development of bone lesions in multiple myeloma is thought to be related to an increase in expression by osteoblasts of the receptor activator of the nuclear factor-κB (NF-κB) ligand (RANKL) and the reduction of the level of its decoy receptor, osteoprotegerin[43] (see Chapter 58).

One of the characteristic features resulting from the proliferating osteoclasts in multiple myeloma is the unregulated production of a monoclonal antibody referred to as the *M protein* because it is detected as an M spike on protein electrophoresis. In most cases the M protein is either IgG (60%) or IgA (20% to 25%).[43] In the remaining 15% to 20% of cases, the plasma cells produce only abnormal proteins, termed *Bence Jones proteins,* that consist of light chains of the immunoglobulin molecule. Because of their low molecular weight, the Bence Jones proteins are readily excreted in the urine. Persons with this form of the disease (light-chain disease) have Bence Jones proteins in their serum, but lack the M component. However, up to 80% of myeloma cells produce both complete immunoglobulins as well as excess light chains; therefore, both M proteins and Bence Jones proteins are present. Many of the light-chain proteins are directly toxic to renal tubular structures, which may lead to tubular destruction and, eventually, to renal failure.

Manifestations. The main sites involved in multiple myeloma are the bones and bone marrow. In addition to the abnormal proliferation of marrow plasma cells, there is proliferation and activation of osteoclasts, which leads to bone resorption and destruction (Fig. 15.10). This increased bone resorption predisposes the individual to pathologic fractures and hypercalcemia. Paraproteins secreted by the plasma cells may cause a hyperviscosity of body fluids and may break down into

Failure of antibody production
• Recurrent infections

Osteolytic bone lesions
• Bone pain
• Hypercalcemia
• Pathologic fractures

Plasma cell secretion of paraproteins
• Hyperviscosity of body fluids
• Amyloid deposits in heart and kidney

Bone marrow infiltration
• Thrombocytopenia (purpura)

Renal failure

Proteinuria
• Bence Jones protein

Bone marrow infiltration
• Anemia (fatigue, pallor)
• Neutropenia (decreased resistance to infection)

M protein spike (serum)

Ab   a₁   a₂   b   g

FIGURE 15.10 • Clinical features of multiple myeloma.

amyloid, a proteinaceous substance deposited between cells, causing heart failure and nephropathy. Although multiple myeloma is characterized by excessive production of monoclonal immunoglobulin, levels of normal immunoglobulins are usually depressed. This contributes to a general susceptibility to recurrent bacterial infections.[36]

The malignant plasma cells also can form plasmacytomas (plasma cell tumours) in bone and soft tissue sites. The most common site of soft tissue plasmacytomas is the gastrointestinal tract. The development of plasmacytomas in bone tissue is associated with bone destruction and localized pain. Osteolytic lesions and compression fractures may be seen in the axial skeleton and proximal long bones. Occasionally, the lesions may affect the spinal column, causing vertebral collapse and spinal cord compression (Fig. 15.11).

Bone pain is one of the first symptoms to occur in approximately three fourths of all individuals diagnosed with multiple myeloma.[36] Bone destruction also impairs the production of erythrocytes and leukocytes and predisposes the patient to anemia and recurrent infections. Many patients experience weight loss and weakness. Renal insufficiency occurs in 50% of patients. Neurologic manifestations caused by neuropathy or spinal cord compression also may be present.

Diagnosis and Treatment. Diagnosis of multiple myeloma is based on clinical manifestations, blood tests, and bone marrow examination. The classic triad of bone marrow plasmacytosis (more than 10% plasma cells), lytic bone lesions, and either the serum M-protein spike or the presence of Bence Jones proteins in the urine is definitive for a diagnosis of multiple myeloma. Bone radiographs are important in establishing the presence of bone lesions. Anemia is almost universal. Other laboratory features include hypercalcemia, an elevated erythrocyte sedimentation rate, and signs of kidney failure. The strongest predictors of outcome are linked to the type of cytogenetic abnormalities of the myeloma cells, another predictor that is used to determine the staging of the disease is low serum beta-2 microglobulin (a small subunit of the major histocompatibility complex I molecule).

The treatment of multiple myeloma is changing rapidly. For several decades, melphalan (an alkylating agent) and prednisone were the cornerstone of treatment of multiple myeloma. Cumulative exposure to melphalan, however, is associated with increased risk of marrow toxicity, including myelodysplasia, acute leukemia, and impaired stem cell production. This is an important consideration in persons who are candidates for autologous stem cell transplants. Although the incorporation of new classes of medications in the treatment of multiple myeloma has seen a shift in the older treatment regimens, the conventional approaches have not been excluded.

Thalidomide combined with dexamethasone (a corticosteroid) has emerged as an active agent for use in the initial treatment of multiple myeloma.[36,42] The combination is given orally and has shown promising results in newly diagnosed patients. The exact mechanism of action of thalidomide is unknown. Proposed mechanisms include angiogenesis inhibition; immune modulation by increasing NK cell activity, IL-2, and interferon-γ; and increasing apoptosis. Thalidomide is

FIGURE 15.11 • Plasma cell myeloma. The vertebra illustrates several lytic bone lesions and these bones would be prone to pathologic fractures. (From Rubin R., Strayer D. S. (Eds.). (2012). *Rubin's pathology: Clinicopathologic foundations of medicine* (6th ed., p. 1019). Philadelphia, PA: Lippincott Williams & Wilkins.)

reasonably well tolerated; the toxicities include increased risk of venous thromboembolism (*i.e.,* deep vein thrombosis). Its efficacy as a front-line therapy has been supported by clinical trials. Because of its teratogenicity, the use of thalidomide in pregnant women is absolutely contraindicated. Lenalidomide, an oral agent, is an analog of thalidomide with both improved efficacy and reduced toxicity.

A reversible 26S proteosome inhibitor (bortezomib), is also used for treatment of multiple myeloma. Proteosomes are intracellular enzymes that degrade many proteins regulating the cell cycle, ribonucleic acid (RNA) transcription, apoptosis, cell adhesion, angiogenesis, and antigen presentation.[36] Proteolysis by the 26S proteosome is fundamental to multiple signalling pathways within the cell, and disruption of this homeostatic pathway by bortezomib can lead to cell death and a delay in tumour growth.

High-dose chemotherapy with autologous stem cell transplantation is now considered appropriate front-line therapy for patients younger than 70 years of age newly diagnosed with multiple myeloma. Allogeneic transplantation offers prolonged disease-free outcomes and potential cure, but at a high cost of treatment-related mortality. Because of this, "minitransplants" using nonmarrow-ablative chemotherapy may be used to provide sufficient immune suppression to allow donor engraftment and subsequent graft-versus-tumour effect.

IN SUMMARY

The lymphomas (NHL and HL) represent malignant neoplasms of cells native to lymphoid tissue that have their origin in the secondary lymphoid structures such as the lymph nodes and mucosa-associated lymphoid tissues. The NHLs are a group of neoplastic disorders that originate in the lymphoid tissues, usually the lymph nodes. The NHLs are multicentric in origin and spread early to various lymphoid tissues throughout the body, especially the liver, spleen, and bone marrow. HL is characterized by painless and progressive enlargement of a single node or group of nodes. It is believed to originate in one area of the lymphatic system and, if unchecked, spreads throughout the lymphatic network.

The leukemias are malignant neoplasms of the hematopoietic precursor cells that originate in the bone marrow. They are classified according to cell type (*i.e.,* lymphocytic or myelocytic) and whether the disease is acute or chronic. The lymphocytic leukemias involve immature lymphocytes and their progenitors that originate in the bone marrow but infiltrate the spleen, lymph nodes, CNS, and other tissues. The myelogenous leukemias involve the pluripotent myeloid stem cells in bone marrow and interfere with the maturation of all blood cells, including the granulocytes, erythrocytes, and thrombocytes.

The acute leukemias (*i.e.,* ALL, which primarily affects children, and AML, which primarily affects adults) have a sudden onset with symptoms of depressed bone marrow function (anemia, fatigue, bleeding, and infections); bone pain; and generalized lymphadenopathy, splenomegaly, and hepatomegaly. The chronic leukemias, which largely affect adults, have a more insidious onset. CLL often has the most favourable clinical course, with many persons living long enough to die of other, unrelated causes. The course of CML is slow and progressive, with transformation to a course resembling that of AML.

Multiple myeloma is a plasma cell dyscrasia characterized by expansion of a single clone of immunoglobulin-producing plasma cells and a resultant increase in serum levels of a single monoclonal immunoglobulin or its fragments. The main sites involved in multiple myeloma are the bones and bone marrow. In addition to the abnormal proliferation of marrow plasma cells, there is proliferation and activation of osteoclasts that leads to bone resorption and destruction, and predisposes to increased risk for pathologic fractures and development of hypercalcemia. Paraproteins secreted by the plasma cells may cause hyperviscosity of body fluids and may break down into amyloid, a proteinaceous substance deposited between cells that can cause heart failure and neuropathy. Bone marrow involvement leads to increased risk of infection due to suppressed humoral and cell-mediated immunity and anemia due to impaired red cell production.

REVIEW EXERCISES

1. Many of the primary immunodeficiency disorders, in which there is a defect in the development of the immune cells of T or B lymphocytes, can be cured by allogeneic stem cell transplantation from an unaffected donor.
   A. *Explain why stem cells are used rather than mature lymphocytes. You might want to refer to Figure 15.1.*
   B. *Explain how the stem cells would go about the process of repopulating the bone marrow.*
2. A mother brings her 4-year-old son into the pediatric clinic because of irritability, loss of appetite, low-grade fever, pallor, and complaints that his legs hurt. Blood tests reveal anemia, thrombocytopenia, and an elevated leukocyte count with atypical lymphocytes. A diagnosis of acute lymphocytic leukemia (ALL) is confirmed with bone marrow studies.
   A. *What is the origin of the anemia, thrombocytopenia, elevated leukocyte count, and atypical lymphocytes seen in this child?*
   B. *Explain the cause of the child's fever, pallor, increased bleeding, and bone pain.*
   C. *The parents are informed that the preferred treatment for ALL consists of aggressive chemotherapy with the purpose of achieving a remission. Explain the rationale for using chemotherapy to treat leukemia.*

D. The parents are told that the child will need intrathecal chemotherapy administered by a lumbar puncture. Why is this treatment necessary?

3. A 36-year-old man presents to his health care clinic with fever, night sweats, weight loss, and a feeling of fullness in his abdomen. Subsequent lymph node biopsy reveals a diagnosis of non-Hodgkin lymphoma (NHL).

A. Although lymphomas can originate in any of the lymphoid tissues of the body, most originate in the lymph nodes, and most (80% to 85%) are of B-cell origin. Hypothesize as to why B cells are more commonly affected than T cells.

B. Monoclonal antibodies are being used in the treatment of NHL. Explain how these agents exerts its effect and why they are specific for B-cell lymphomas.

References

1. Hall J. E. (2011). *Textbook of medical physiology* (12th ed.). Philadelphia, PA: W.B. Saunders.
2. Abbas A. K., Lichtman A. H., Pillai S. (2012). *Cellular and molecular immunology* (7th ed., pp. 1–35, 501). Philadelphia, PA: W.B. Saunders.
3. Ross M. H., Pawline W. (Eds.). (2011). Chapter 14: Lymphatic system. In *Histology: A text and atlas* (6th ed.). Philadelphia, PA: Lippincott Williams & Wilkins.
4. Valdez R., Zutter M., Florea A. D., Rubin R. (2012). Chapter 20: Hematopathology. In Rubin R., Strayer D. S. (Eds.), *Rubin's pathology: Clinicopathologic foundations of medicine* (6th ed.). Philadelphia, PA: Lippincott Williams & Wilkins.
5. Kumar V., Abbas A. K., Fausto N., et al. (Eds.). (2010). Chapter 13: Diseases of white blood cells, lymph nodes, spleen, and thymus. In *Robbins and Cotran pathologic basis of disease* (8th ed.). Philadelphia, PA: Elsevier Saunders.
6. Horwitz M. S., Corey S. J., Grimes H. L., Tidwell T. (2013). ELANE mutations in cyclic and severe congenital neutropenia. *Hematology/Oncology Clinics of North America, 27*(1), 19–41.
7. Boxer L. A. (2011). Chapter 125: Leukopenia. In Kliegman R. M., Stanton B. F., St. Geme J. W., et al. (Eds.), *Nelson textbook of pediatrics* (19th ed.). Philadelphia, PA: Saunders Elsevier.
8. Newburger P. E., Dale D. C. (2013). Evaluation and management of patients with isolated neutropenia. *Seminars in Hematology, 50*(3), 198–206.
9. Newman K. A., Akhtari M. (2011). Management of autoimmune neutropenia in Felty's syndrome and systemic lupus erythematosus. *Autoimmunity Reviews, 10*(7), 432–437.
10. Schwartzberg L. S. (2006). Neutropenia: Etiology and pathogenesis. *Clinical Cornerstone, 8*(Suppl 5), S5–S11.
11. Meltzer H. (2012). Chapter 29: Antipsychotic agents and lithium. In Katzung B. G., Masters S. B., Trevor A. J. (Eds.), *Basic and clinical pharmacology* (12th ed.). New York: McGraw-Hill Medical.
12. Schwartz D. A. (2012). Chapter 9: Infectious and parasitic diseases. In Rubin R., Strayer D. S. (Eds.), *Rubin's pathology: Clinicopathologic foundations of medicine* (6th ed.). Philadelphia, PA: Lippincott Williams & Wilkins.
13. McAdam A., Sharpe A. H. (2010). Chapter 8: Infectious diseases. In Kumar V., Abbas A. K., Fausto N., et al. (Eds.), *Robbins and Cotran pathologic basis of disease* (8th ed.). Philadelphia, PA: Elsevier Saunders.
14. Luzuriaga K., Sullivan J. L. (2010). Infectious mononucleosis. *New England Journal of Medicine, 362*(21), 1993–2000.
15. Vouloumanou E. K., Rafailidis P. I., Falagas M. E. (2012). Current diagnosis and management of infectious mononucleosis. *Current Opinion in Hematology, 19*(1), 14–20.
16. Roig I. L., Shandera W. X. (2014). Chapter 32: Viral and rickettsial infections. In Papadakis M. A., McPhee S. J., Rabow M. V. (Eds.), *Current medical diagnosis and treatment 2014.* New York: McGraw-Hill.
17. Canadian Cancer Society. (2014). Cancer statistics. Available online at: http://www.cancer.ca. Accessed July 12, 2015.
18. Canadian Cancer Society's Advisory Committee. (2013). *Canadian cancer statistics 2013.* Toronto: Canadian Cancer Society.
19. Shankland K. R., Armitage J. O., Hancock B. W. (2012). Non-Hodgkin lymphoma. *Lancet, 380*(9844), 848–857.
20. Molyneux E. M., Rochford R., Griffin B., et al. (2012). Burkitt's lymphoma. *Lancet, 379*(9822), 1234–1244.
21. National Cancer Institute. (2014). Children with Down syndrome. Available online at: http://www.cancer.gov/cancertopics/pdq/treatment/child AML/HealthProfessional/page8. Accessed May 4, 2014.
22. American Cancer Society. (2014). Hodgkin Disease. Available online at: http://www.cancer.org/cancer/hodgkindisease/index. Accessed May 4, 2014.
23. Raffel G. D., Cerny J. (2011). Chapter 130: Molecular biology of acute leukemias. In DeVita V. T., Hellman S., Rosenberg S. A. (Eds.), *Cancer: Principles and practice of oncology* (9th ed.). Philadelphia, PA: Lippincott Williams & Wilkins.
24. Townsend W., Linch D. (2012). Hodgkin's lymphoma in adults. *Lancet, 380*(9844), 836–847.
25. Ganzel C., Becker J., Mintz P. D., et al. (2012). Hyperleukocytosis, leukostasis and leukapheresis: Practice management. *Blood Reviews, 26,* 117–122.
26. O'Brien S., Abboud C. N., Akhtari M., et al.; National Comprehensive Cancer Network. (2012). Chronic myelogenous leukemia. *Journal of the National Comprehensive Cancer Network, 10,* 64–110.
27. American Cancer Society. (2014). Acute lymphocytic leukemia in adults. Available online at: http://www.cancer.org/cancer/leukemia-acutelymphocyticallinadults/index. Accessed May 4, 2014.
28. Rubnitz J. E., Gibson B., Smith F. O. (2010). Acute myeloid leukemia. *Hematology/Oncology Clinics of North America, 24*(1), 35–63.
29. U.S. National Library of Medicine. (2014). Acute promyelocytic leukemia. Available online at: http://ghr.nlm.nih.gov/condition/acute-promyelocytic-leukemia. Accessed May 4, 2014.
30. Grigoropoulos, N. F., Petter, R., Veer, M. B. V., et al. (2013). Leukaemia update part 2: Managing patients with leukaemia in the community. *Briish Medical Journal, 2013,* 346. doi: 10.1136/bmj.f1932.
31. Wilson F. P., Berns J. S. (2012). Onco-nephrology: Tumor lysis syndrome. *Clinical Journal of the American Society of Nephrology, 7*(10), 1730–1739.
32. Lopez-Olivo M. A., Pratt G., Palla S. L., Salahudeen A. (2013). Rasburicase in tumor lysis syndrome of the adult: A systematic review and meta-analysis. *American Journal of Kidney Disease, 62*(3), 481–492.
33. Grigoropoulos N. F., Petter R., Veer M. B. V., et al. (2013). Leukaemia update part 1: Diagnosis and management. *British Medical Journal, 346.* doi: 10.1136/bmj.f1660.
34. Canadian Cancer Society. (2014). Diagnosing leukemia. Available online at: http://www.cancer.ca. Accessed May 1, 2014.
35. Pieters R., Carroll W. L. (2010). Biology and treatment of acute lymphoblastic leukemia. *Hematology/Oncology Clinics of North America, 24*(1), 1–18.
36. Smith D., Yong K. (2013). Multiple myeloma. *British Medical Journal, 346.* doi: 10.1136/bmj.f3863.
37. American Cancer Society. (2014). Leukemia. Available online at: http://www.cancer.org/cancer/leukemia/index. Accessed May 12, 2014.
38. Rosenquist R., Cortese D., Bhoi S., et al. (2013). Prognostic markers and their clinical applicability in chronic lymphocytic leukemia: Where do we stand? *Leukemia & Lymphoma, 54*(11), 2351–2364.
39. Wierda W. G., O'brien S. (2011). Chapter 134: Chronic lymphocytic leukemias. In DeVita V. T., Hellman S., Rosenberg S. A. (Eds.), *Cancer: Principles and practice of oncology* (9th ed.). Philadelphia, PA: Lippincott Williams & Wilkins.

40. Breed C. D. (2003). Diagnosis, treatment, and nursing care of patients with chronic leukemia. *Seminars in Oncology Nursing, 19*(2), 109–117.

41. Karbasian E. M., Morris E. L., Dutcher J. P., Wiernik P. H. (2006). Blastic phase of chronic myelogenous leukemia. *Current Treatment Options in Oncology, 7*(3), 189–199.

42. Rajkumar S. V. (2011). Multiple myeloma: 2011 update on diagnosis, risk-stratification, and management. *American Journal of Hematology, 86*, 57–65.

43. Kyle R. A., Rajkumar S. V. (2004). Multiple myeloma. *New England Journal of Medicine, 351*, 1860–1873.

Visit the**Point** **http://thePoint.lww.com for animations, journal articles, and more!**

Unit V

Infection, Inflammation, and Immunity

The quest to understand the mechanism of disease and ways to prevent it permeates humankind's history. Many civilizations contributed to the storehouse of knowledge. Among the early accomplishments of the Chinese are a number of practices they developed to prevent disease, one of which took the form of inoculation.

The deadly smallpox had been one of the world's most dreaded diseases. During the Middle Ages, epidemics were frequent; they swept across Asia and other parts of the world, leaving widespread death in their wake. In the 1400s, the Chinese created a technique to protect themselves during an epidemic. They collected the crusts of smallpox sores and allowed them to dry. The dried material was ground into powder and inhaled. The procedure was found to be hazardous, but it remains one of the first attempts at vaccination.

Unit V

Infection, Inflammation, and Immunity

Mechanisms of Infectious Disease

16

All living creatures share two basic objectives in life: survival and reproduction. This doctrine applies equally to all members of the living world, including bacteria, viruses, fungi, and protozoa. To satisfy these goals, organisms must extract from the environment essential nutrients for growth and proliferation; for countless microscopic organisms, that environment includes the human body. Normally, the contact between humans and microorganisms is incidental and, in certain situations, may actually benefit both organisms. Under extraordinary circumstances, however, the invasion of the human body by microorganisms can produce harmful and potentially lethal consequences. These are collectively called *infectious diseases.*

INFECTIOUS DISEASES

After completing this section of the chapter, you should be able to meet the following objectives:

- Define the terms host, infectious disease, colonization, microflora, virulence, pathogen, and saprophyte.
- Describe the concept of host–microorganism interaction using the concepts of commensalism, mutualism, and parasitic relationships.
- Describe the structural characteristics and mechanisms of reproduction for prions, viruses, bacteria, fungi, and parasites.
- Use the concepts of incidence, portal of entry, source of infection, symptomatology, disease course, site of infection, agent, and host characteristics to explain the mechanisms of infectious diseases.

Terminology

All scientific disciplines evolve with a distinct vocabulary, and the study of infectious diseases is no exception. The most appropriate way to approach this subject is with a brief discussion of the terminology used to characterize interactions between humans and microbes.

Any organism capable of supporting the nutritional and physical growth requirements of another is called a *host.* Throughout this chapter, the term *host* most often refers to humans supporting the growth of microorganisms. Occasionally, *infection* and *colonization* may be used interchangeably; this is inappropriate, as the two terms differ in definition and manifestations. The term *infection* describes the presence and multiplication within a host of another living organism, with subsequent injury to the host, whereas *colonization* describes the act of establishing a presence, a step required in the multifaceted process of infection but which may not necessarily result in infection.

One common misconception should be dispelled from the start: Not all interactions between microorganisms and humans are detrimental. The internal and external exposed surfaces of the human body are normally and harmlessly inhabited by a multitude of bacteria, collectively referred to as the normal *microflora*. Although the colonizing bacteria acquire nutritional needs and shelter, the host is not adversely affected by the relationship. An interaction such as this is called *commensalism*, and the colonizing microorganisms are sometimes referred to as *commensal flora*. The term *mutualism* is applied to an interaction in which the microorganism and the host both derive benefits from the interaction. For example, certain inhabitants of the human intestinal tract extract nutrients from the host and secrete essential vitamin by-products of metabolism (*e.g.,* vitamin K) that are absorbed and used by the host. A *parasitic relationship* is one in which only the infecting organism benefits from the relationship and the host either gains nothing from the relationship or sustains injury from the interaction. If the host sustains injury or pathologic damage in response to a parasitic infection, the process is called an *infectious disease.*

The severity of an infectious disease can range from mild to life-threatening, depending on many variables, including the health of the host at the time of infection and the *virulence* (disease-producing potential) of the microorganism. A select group of microorganisms called *pathogens* are so virulent that they are rarely found in the absence of disease. Fortunately, there are few human pathogens in the microbial world. Most microorganisms are harmless *saprophytes,* free-living organisms obtaining their growth from dead or decaying organic material in the environment. All microorganisms, even saprophytes and members of the normal flora, can be *opportunistic pathogens,* capable of producing an infectious disease when the health and immunity of the host have been severely weakened by illness, malnutrition, or medical therapy. Table 16.1 illustrates common pathogens that invade humans.

TABLE 16.1 COMMON PATHOGENS

PATHOGEN	STRUCTURAL CHARACTERISTICS	FUNCTIONAL CHARACTERISTICS	TREATMENT	COMMON DISEASE
Viruses	DNA/RNA and protein coat	Cannot reproduce outside of cells	Antivirals, which slow viral replication	Influenza, the common cold, measles, HIV/AIDS
Bacteria	Microscopic cell without nucleus	Common on keyboards, water fountains, toilets	Antibiotics, which slow bacterial reproduction	Strep throat, some sinus and lung infections, some food poisoning
Fungi	Microscopic, unicellular (yeasts) or multicellular (molds)	Usually infect body surfaces and openings	Antifungals, which destroy the cell walls	Athlete's foot, yeast infections
Protozoa	Microscopic, unicellular	Common in water supplies of developing countries	Antiprotozoan drugs, which interfere with protozoan metabolism	Malaria, sleeping sickness
Worms	Multicellular	Prefer to live within body spaces and cells	Antihelminthics, which interfere with the worm's metabolism	Roundworms, tapeworms (helminths)

From McConnell T. H., Hull K. L. (2011). *Human form, human function: Essentials of anatomy & physiology* (p. 475). Philadelphia, PA: Lippincott Williams & Wilkins.

TABLE 16.2 COMPARISON OF CHARACTERISTICS OF HUMAN MICROBIAL PATHOGENS

ORGANISM	DEFINED NUCLEUS	GENOMIC MATERIAL	SIZE[a]	INTRACELLULAR OR EXTRACELLULAR	MOTILITY
Prions	No	Unknown	55 kDa	E	–
Viruses	No	DNA or RNA	0.02–0.3	I	–
Bacteria	No	DNA	0.5–15	I/E	±
Mycoplasmas	No	DNA	0.2–0.3	E	–
Spirochetes	No	DNA	6–15	E	+
Rickettsiaceae	No	DNA	0.2–2	I	–
Chlamydiaceae	No	DNA	0.3–1	I	–
Yeasts	Yes	DNA	2–60	I/E	–
Moulds	Yes	DNA	2–15 (hyphal width)	E	–
Protozoans	Yes	DNA	1–60	I/E	+
Helminths	Yes	DNA	2 mm to >1 m	E	+

[a]Micrometres unless indicated.

Agents of Infectious Disease

The agents of infectious disease include prions, viruses, bacteria, *Rickettsiaceae and Chlamydiaceae,* fungi, and parasites. A summary of the salient characteristics of these human microbial pathogens is presented in Table 16.2.

Prions

Previously microbiologists assumed that all infectious agents must possess a genetic master plan (a genome of either ribonucleic acid [RNA] or deoxyribonucleic acid [DNA]) that codes for the production of the essential proteins and enzymes necessary for survival and reproduction. However it is now known that prions, protein particles that lack any kind of a demonstrable genome, appear to be an exception to this rule. A number of prion-associated diseases have been identified, including Creutzfeldt–Jakob disease and kuru in humans, scrapie in sheep, chronic wasting disease in deer and elk, and bovine spongiform encephalopathy (BSE or mad cow disease) in cattle. The various prion-associated diseases produce very similar pathologic processes and symptoms in the hosts and are collectively called *transmissible neurodegenerative diseases.* All are characterized by a slowly progressive, noninflammatory neuronal degeneration, leading to loss of coordination (ataxia), dementia, and death over a period ranging from months to years. In fact, recent studies indicate that prion proteins (called PrP^{SC}) are actually altered or mutated forms of a normal host protein called PrP^{C}. Differences in the posttranslational structure cause the two proteins to behave differently. The PrP^{SC} is resistant to the action of proteases (enzymes that degrade excess or deformed proteins) and aggregates in the cytoplasm of affected neurons as amyloid fibrils. The normal PrP^{C} is protease sensitive and appears on the cell surface.

Prion diseases present significant challenges for management due to the pathogenic structure of PrP^{SC}. This protein molecule is very stable and resistant to conventional microbiology decontamination methods. Studies investigating transmission

AGENTS OF INFECTIOUS DISEASE

- The agents of infectious disease represent a diversity of microorganisms that are usually not visible to the human eye.
- Microorganisms can be separated into eukaryotes (fungi and parasites), organisms containing a membrane-bound nucleus, and prokaryotes (bacteria), organisms in which the nucleus is not separated.
- Eukaryotes and prokaryotes are organisms because they contain all the enzymes and biologic equipment necessary for replication and exploiting metabolic energy.
- Viruses, which are the smallest pathogens, have no organized cellular structure, but consist of a protein coat surrounding a nucleic acid core of DNA or RNA. Unlike eukaryotes and prokaryotes, viruses are incapable of replication outside of a living cell.
- Parasites (protozoa, helminths, and arthropods) are members of the animal kingdom that infect or colonize other animals, which then transmit them to humans or in some cases directly infect the human host.

of prion diseases in animals clearly demonstrate that prions replicate, leading researchers to investigate how proteins can reproduce in the absence of genetic material. Based on current models, it is believed that PrP^{SC} binds to the normal PrP^{C} on the cell surface, causing it to be processed into PrP^{SC}, which is released from the cell and then aggregates into amyloid-like plaques in the brain. The cell then replenishes the PrP^{C} and the cycle continues. As PrP^{SC} accumulates, it spreads within the axons of the nerve cells, causing progressively greater damage of host neurons and the eventual incapacitation of the host. In addition, because prions lack reproductive and metabolic functions, the currently available antimicrobial agents are useless against them.

A

Virion

Capsid

Nucleic acid genome
(DNA or RNA)

Envelope

B

FIGURE 16.1 • **A:** The basic structure of a virus includes a protein coat surrounding an inner core of nucleic acid (DNA or RNA). **B:** Some viruses may also be enclosed in a lipoprotein outer envelope.

Viruses

Viruses are the smallest obligate intracellular pathogens. They have no organized cellular structures but instead consist of a protein coat, or capsid, surrounding a nucleic acid core, or genome, of RNA or DNA—never both (Fig. 16.1). Some viruses are enclosed within a lipoprotein envelope derived from the cytoplasmic membrane of the parasitized host cell. Enveloped viruses include members of the herpesvirus group and paramyxoviruses, such as influenza and poxviruses. Certain enveloped viruses are continuously shed from the infected cell surface enveloped in buds pinched from the cell membrane.

The viruses of humans and animals have been categorized somewhat arbitrarily according to various characteristics. These include the type of viral genome (single-stranded or double-stranded DNA or RNA), physical characteristics (*e.g.*, size, presence or absence of a membrane envelope), the mechanism of replication (*e.g.*, retroviruses), the mode of transmission (*e.g.*, arthropod-borne viruses, enteroviruses), target tissue, and the type of disease produced (*e.g.*, hepatitis A, B, C, D, and E viruses), to name just a few.

Viruses are incapable of replication outside of a living cell. They must penetrate a susceptible living cell and use the biosynthetic machinery of the cell to produce viral progeny. The process of viral replication is shown in Figure 16.2. Not every viral agent causes lysis and death of the host cell during the course of replication. Some viruses enter the host cell and insert their genome into the host cell chromosome, where it remains in a latent, nonreplicating state for long periods without causing disease. Under the appropriate stimulation, the virus undergoes active replication and produces symptoms of disease months to years later. Members of the herpesvirus

group and adenovirus are the best examples of latent viruses. Herpesviruses include the viral agents of chickenpox and zoster (varicella-zoster), cold sores (herpes simplex virus [HSV] type 1), genital herpes (HSV type 2), cytomegalovirus infections, roseola (human herpesvirus 6), infectious mononucleosis (Epstein–Barr virus), and Kaposi sarcoma (herpesvirus 8). The resumption of the latent viral replication may produce symptoms of primary disease (*e.g.*, genital herpes) or cause an entirely different symptomatology (*e.g.*, shingles instead of chickenpox).

A family of viruses that has gained a great deal of attention in the media recently are the Orthomyxoviridae or flu viruses. Recent attention has focused on the H5N1 variant, commonly known as the *avian influenza virus,* and the H1N1 variant, commonly known as *swine flu.* These influenza viruses differ from the usual human influenza viruses by the hosts they normally infect. Avian influenza viruses typically infect wild birds; however, on occasion a new virus may result from genetic rearrangements that make it better fit to infect humans. When this occurs, the human population is more susceptible because the virus is unfamiliar to most of our immune systems.

Since the early 1980s, members of the retrovirus group have received considerable attention after identification of the human immunodeficiency viruses (HIV) as the causative agent of acquired immunodeficiency syndrome (AIDS). The retroviruses have a unique mechanism of replication. After entry into the host cell, the viral RNA genome is first translated into DNA by a viral enzyme called *reverse transcriptase* (see Chapter 20). The viral DNA copy is then integrated into the host chromosome where it exists in a latent state, similar to the herpesviruses. Reactivation and replication require a reversal of the entire process. Some retroviruses lyse the host cell during the process of replication. In the case of HIV, the infected cells regulate the immunologic defence system of the host and their lysis leads to a permanent suppression of the immune response.

In addition to causing infectious diseases, certain viruses also have the ability to transform normal host cells into

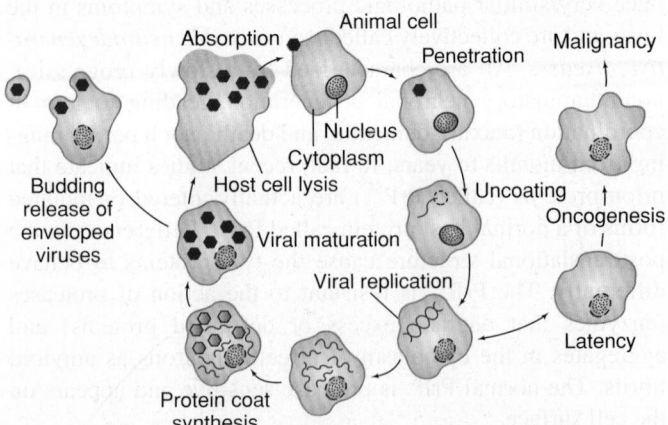

FIGURE 16.2 • Schematic representation of the many possible consequences of viral infection of host cells, including cell lysis (poliovirus), continuous release of budding viral particles, or latency (herpesviruses) and oncogenesis (papovaviruses).

malignant cells during the replication cycle. This group of viruses is referred to as *oncogenic* and includes certain retroviruses and DNA viruses, such as the herpesviruses, adenoviruses, and papovaviruses. Human papillomaviruses (HPVs), members of the papovavirus family, cause cutaneous and genital warts, and several genotypes are associated with cervical cancer (see Chapter 47). In June 2006, Health Canada approved the first vaccine (Gardasil) to prevent cervical cancer, precancerous genital lesions, and genital warts due to HPV types 6, 11, 16, and 18. All provinces and territories now offer this publically funded vaccine to girls in grades ranging from 4 to 9.

Bacteria

Bacteria are autonomously replicating unicellular organisms known as *prokaryotes* because they lack an organized nucleus. Compared with nucleated eukaryotic cells (see Chapter 4), the bacterial cell is small and structurally relatively primitive (Fig. 16.3). Similar to eukaryotic cells, but unlike viruses, bacteria contain both DNA and RNA. They contain no organized intracellular organelles, and the genome consists of only a single chromosome of DNA. Many bacteria transiently harbour smaller extrachromosomal pieces of circular DNA called *plasmids*. Occasionally, plasmids contain genetic information that increases the virulence or antibiotics resistance of the organism.

The prokaryotic cell is organized into an internal compartment called the *cytoplasm*, which contains the reproductive and metabolic machinery of the cell. The cytoplasm is surrounded by a flexible lipid membrane, called the *cytoplasmic membrane*. This in turn is enclosed within a rigid cell wall. The structure and synthesis of the cell wall determine the

FIGURE 16.3 • False-colour transmission electron micrograph of the rod-shaped, gram-negative bacterium *Escherichia coli*, showing the simple prokaryotic cell structure including the cytoplasm, the cytoplasmic membrane, and the rigid cell wall. (© Science Source/Photo Researchers.)

microscopic shape of the bacterium (*e.g.*, spherical [cocci], helical [spirilla], or elongate [bacilli]; Fig. 16.4). Most bacteria produce a cell wall composed of a distinctive polymer known as *peptidoglycan*. This polymer is produced only by prokaryotes and is therefore an attractive target for antibacterial therapy. Several bacteria synthesize an extracellular capsule composed of protein or carbohydrate. The capsule protects the organism from environmental hazards such as the immunologic defences of the host.

Certain bacteria are motile as the result of external whip-like appendages called *flagella*. The flagella rotate like a propeller, transporting the organism through a liquid environment. Bacteria can also produce hair-like structures projecting from the cell surface called *pili* or *fimbriae*, which enable the organism to adhere to surfaces such as mucous membranes or other bacteria.

Most prokaryotes reproduce asexually by simple cellular division. The manner in which an organism divides can influence the microscopic morphology. For instance, when the cocci divide in chains, they are called *streptococci;* in pairs, *diplococci*; and in clusters, *staphylococci*. The growth rate of bacteria varies significantly among different species and depends greatly on physical growth conditions and the availability of nutrients. In the laboratory, a single bacterium placed in a suitable growth environment, such as an agar plate, reproduces to the extent that it forms a visible colony composed of millions of bacteria within a few hours.

In nature, however, bacteria rarely exist as single cells floating in an aqueous environment. Rather, bacteria prefer to stick to and colonize environmental surfaces, producing structured communities called *biofilms*. The organization and structure of biofilms permit access to available nutrients and elimination of metabolic waste. Within the biofilm, individual organisms use chemical signalling as a form of primitive intercellular communication to represent the state of the environment. These signals inform members of the community when sufficient nutrients are available for proliferation or when environmental conditions warrant dormancy or evacuation. Examples of biofilms abound in nature and are estimated to cause 80% of chronic infections. Biofilms can be found on surfaces of aquatic environments and on humans. One has only to disassemble a clogged sink drain to see a perfect example of a bacterial biofilm.

The physical appearance of a colony of bacteria grown on an agar plate can be quite distinctive for different species. Some produce pigments that give colonies a unique colour. Some bacteria produce highly resistant spores when faced with an unfavourable environment. The spores can exist in a quiescent state almost indefinitely until suitable growth conditions are encountered, at which time the spores germinate and the organism resumes normal metabolism and replication.

Bacteria are extremely adaptable life forms. They are found not just in humans and other hosts, but in almost every environmental extreme on earth. However, each individual bacterial species has a well-defined set of growth parameters, including nutrition, temperature, light, humidity, and atmosphere. Bacteria with extremely strict growth requirements are called

FIGURE 16.4 • A sampling of microscopic morphology of bacteria demonstrating their variability in size and shape: (**A**) *Yersinia pestis;* (**B**) gram-positive diplococci typical of *Streptococcus pneumoniae;* (**C**) *Streptococcus species* (Gram stain); (**D**) *Escherichia coli* (Gram stain). (Public Images Library, Centers for Disease Control and Prevention. Available at http://phil.cdc.gov/phil/details.asp.)

fastidious. For example, *Neisseria gonorrhoeae*, the bacterium that causes gonorrhea, cannot live for extended periods outside the human body. Some bacteria require oxygen for growth and metabolism and are called *aerobes;* others cannot survive in an oxygen-containing environment and are called *anaerobes.* An organism capable of adapting its metabolism to aerobic or anaerobic conditions is called *facultatively anaerobic.*

In the laboratory, bacteria are generally classified according to the microscopic appearance and staining properties of the cell. The Gram stain, originally developed in 1884 by the Danish bacteriologist Christian Gram, is still the most widely used staining procedure. Bacteria are designated as *gram-positive* organisms if they are stained purple by a primary basic dye (usually crystal violet); those that are not stained by the crystal violet but are counterstained red by a second dye (safranin) are called *gram-negative* organisms. Staining characteristics and microscopic morphology are used in combination to describe bacteria. For example, *Streptococcus pyogenes,* the agent of scarlet fever and rheumatic fever, is a gram-positive streptococcal organism that is spherical, grows in chains, and stains purple by Gram stain. *Legionella*

pneumophila, the bacterium responsible for Legionnaires' disease, is a gram-negative rod.

Another means of classifying bacteria according to microscopic staining properties is the *acid-fast stain.* Because of their unique cell membrane fatty acid content and composition, certain bacteria are resistant to the decolourization of a primary stain (either carbol fuchsin or a combination of auramine and rhodamine) when treated with a solution of acid alcohol. These organisms are termed *acid-fast* and include a number of significant human pathogens, most notably *Mycobacterium tuberculosis* (the cause of tuberculosis) and other mycobacteria.

For purposes of taxonomy (*i.e.,* identification and classification), each member of the bacterial kingdom is categorized into a small group of biochemically and genetically related organisms called the *genus,* and further subdivided into distinct individuals within the genus called *species.* The genus and species assignment of the organism is reflected in its name (*e.g., Staphylococcus* [genus] *aureus* [species]).

Spirochetes. The spirochetes are an eccentric category of bacteria that are mentioned separately because of their unusual cellular morphology and distinctive mechanism of motility. Technically, the spirochetes are gram-negative rods but are unique in that the cell's shape is helical and the length of the organism is many times its width. A series of filaments are wound about the cell wall and extend the entire length of the cell. These filaments propel the organism through an aqueous environment in a corkscrew motion.

Spirochetes are anaerobic organisms and comprise three genera: *Leptospira, Borrelia,* and *Treponema.* Each genus has saprophytic and pathogenic strains. The pathogenic leptospires infect a wide variety of wild and domestic animals. Infected animals shed the organisms into the environment through the urinary tract. Transmission to humans occurs by contact with infected animals or urine-contaminated surroundings. Leptospires gain access to the host directly through mucous membranes or breaks in the skin and can produce a severe and potentially fatal illness called *Weil syndrome.* In contrast, the borreliae are transmitted from infected animals to humans through the bite of an arthropod vector such as lice or ticks. Included in the genus *Borrelia* are the agents of relapsing fever (*Borrelia recurrentis*) and Lyme disease (*Borrelia burgdorferi*). Pathogenic *Treponema* species require no intermediates and are spread from person to person by direct contact. The most important member of the genus is *Treponema pallidum,* the causative agent of syphilis.

Mycoplasmas. The mycoplasmas are unicellular prokaryotes capable of independent replication. These organisms are less than one third the size of bacteria and contain a small DNA genome approximately one half the size of the bacterial chromosome. The cell is composed of cytoplasm surrounded by a membrane but, unlike bacteria, the mycoplasmas do not produce a rigid peptidoglycan cell wall. As a consequence, the microscopic appearance of the cell is highly variable, ranging from coccoid forms to filaments, and the mycoplasmas are resistant to cell wall–inhibiting antibiotics such as penicillins and cephalosporins.

The mycoplasmas affecting humans are divided into three genera: *Mycoplasma, Ureaplasma,* and *Acholeplasma.* The first two require cholesterol from the environment to produce the cell membrane; the acholeplasmas do not. In the human host, mycoplasmas are commensals. However, a number of species are capable of producing serious diseases, including pneumonia (*Mycoplasma pneumoniae*), genital infections (*Mycoplasma hominis* and *Ureaplasma urealyticum*), and maternally transmitted respiratory infections in infants with low birth weight (*U. urealyticum*).

Rickettsiaceae, Chlamydiaceae, Anaplasmataceae, and Coxiella

This interesting group of organisms combines the characteristics of viral and bacterial agents to produce disease in humans. All are obligate intracellular pathogens, like the viruses, but produce a rigid peptidoglycan cell wall, reproduce asexually by cellular division, and contain RNA and DNA, similar to the bacteria.

The *Rickettsiaceae* depend on the host cell for essential vitamins and nutrients, but the *Chlamydiaceae* appear to scavenge intermediates of energy metabolism such as adenosine triphosphate (ATP). The *Rickettsiaceae* infect but do not produce disease in the cells of certain arthropods such as fleas, ticks, and lice. The organisms are accidentally transmitted to humans through the bite of the arthropod (*i.e.,* the vector) and produce a number of potentially lethal diseases, including Rocky Mountain spotted fever and epidemic typhus.

The *Chlamydiaceae* are slightly smaller than the *Rickettsiaceae* but are structurally similar and are transmitted directly between susceptible vertebrates without an intermediate arthropod host. Transmission and replication of *Chlamydiaceae* occur through a defined life cycle. The infectious form, called an *elementary body,* attaches to and enters the host cell, where it transforms into a larger *reticulate body.* This undergoes active replication into multiple elementary bodies, which are then shed into the extracellular environment to initiate another infectious cycle. Chlamydial diseases of humans include sexually transmitted genital infections (*Chlamydia trachomatis;* see Chapter 47); ocular infections and pneumonia of newborns (*C. trachomatis*); upper and lower respiratory tract infections in children, adolescents, and young adults (*Chlamydophila pneumoniae*); and respiratory disease acquired from infected birds (*Chlamydia psittaci*).

Organisms within the family *Anaplasmataceae* (including the reorganized genera *Ehrlichia, Anaplasma, Neorickettsia,* and *Wolbachia*) are also obligate intracellular organisms that resemble the *Rickettsiaceae* in structure and produce a variety of veterinary and human diseases, some of which have a tick vector. These organisms target host mononuclear and polymorphonuclear white blood cells for infection and, similar to the *Chlamydiaceae,* multiply in the cytoplasm of infected leukocytes within vacuoles called *morulae.* Unlike the *Chlamydiaceae,* however, the *Anaplasmataceae* do not have a defined life cycle and are independent of the host cell for energy production. *Ehrlichia sennetsu,* which is primarily restricted to Japan, produces a disease called *sennetsu fever* that resembles infectious mononucleosis. Disease produced by this species differs from other *Anaplasmataceae* because it is associated with eating raw fish infested with *E. sennetsu*–infected parasites. The most common infections caused by *Anaplasmataceae* are human monocytic and granulocytic ehrlichiosis. Human monocytic ehrlichiosis is a disease caused by *Ehrlichia chaffeensis* and *Ehrlichia canis* that is easily confused with Rocky Mountain spotted fever. Clinical disease severity ranges from mild to life-threatening. Manifestations include generalized malaise, anorexia and nausea, fever, and headache. Decreases in white blood cells (leukopenia) and platelets (thrombocytopenia) often occur. Severe sequelae include severe respiratory failure, encephalopathy, and acute renal failure. The disease is usually more severe in the older adults and persons with compromised immune function. Human granulocytic ehrlichiosis, which is caused by two species of *Ehrlichia* (*Anaplasma phagocytophilum* and *Ehrlichia ewingii*), is also transmitted by ticks. The symptoms are similar to those seen with human monocyto-tropic ehrlichiosis.

The genus *Coxiellai* contains only one species, *C. burnetii.* Like its rickettsial counterparts, it is a gram-negative intracel-lular organism that infects a variety of animals, including cattle, sheep, and goats. In humans, *Coxiellai* infection produces a disease called *Q fever,* characterized by a nonspecific febrile illness often accompanied by headache, chills, arthralgias, and mild pneumonia-like symptoms. The organism produces a highly resistant spore stage that is transmitted to humans when animal tissue is aerosolized (*e.g.,* during meat processing) or by ingestion of contaminated milk.

Fungi

The fungi are free-living, eukaryotic saprophytes found in every habitat on earth. Some are members of the normal human microflora. Fortunately, few fungi are capable of caus-ing diseases in humans, and most of these are incidental, self-limited infections of skin and subcutaneous tissue. Serious fungal infections are rare and usually initiated through punc-ture wounds or inhalation. Despite their normally harmless nature, fungi can cause life-threatening opportunistic diseases when host defence capabilities have been disabled.

The fungi can be separated into two groups, yeasts and moulds, based on rudimentary differences in their morphol-ogy (Fig. 16.5). The yeasts are single-celled organisms, approximately the size of red blood cells, that reproduce by a budding process. The buds separate from the parent cell and mature into identical daughter cells. Moulds produce long, hollow, branching filaments called *hyphae.* Some moulds produce cross walls, which segregate the hyphae into com-partments, and others do not. A limited number of fungi are capable of growing as yeasts at one temperature and as moulds at another. These organisms are called *dimorphic fungi* and include a number of human pathogens such as the agents of blastomycosis (*Blastomyces dermatitidis*), histoplasmosis (*Histoplasma capsulatum*), and coccidioidomycosis (*Coccidi-oides immitis*).

The appearance of a fungal colony tends to reflect its cellular composition. Colonies of yeast are generally smooth with a waxy or creamy texture. Moulds tend to produce cot-tony or powdery colonies composed of mats of hyphae col-lectively called a *mycelium.* The mycelium can penetrate the growth surface or project above the colony like the roots and branches of a tree. Yeasts and moulds produce a rigid cell wall layer that is chemically unrelated to the peptidoglycan of bacteria and is therefore not susceptible to the effects of penicillin-like antibiotics.

Most fungi are capable of sexual or asexual reproduction. The former process involves the fusion of zygotes with the production of a recombinant zygospore. Asexual reproduc-tion involves the formation of highly resistant spores called *conidia* or *sporangiospores,* which are borne by specialized structures that arise from the hyphae. Moulds are identified in the laboratory by the characteristic microscopic appearance of the asexual fruiting structures and spores.

Like the bacterial pathogens of humans, fungi can pro-duce disease in the human host only if they can grow at the temperature of the infected body site. For example, a number of fungal pathogens called *dermatophytes* are incapable of growing at core body temperature (37°C), and the infection is limited to the cooler cutaneous surfaces. Diseases caused by these organisms, including ringworm, athlete's foot, and jock itch, are collectively called *superficial mycoses.* Sys-temic mycoses are serious fungal infections of deep tissues and, by definition, are caused by organisms capable of growth at 37°C. Yeasts such as *Candida albicans* are commensal flora of the skin, mucous membranes, and gastrointestinal tract and are capable of growth at a wider range of temperatures. Intact immune mechanisms and competition for nutrients provided by the bacterial flora normally keep colonizing fungi in check. Alterations in either of these components by disease states or antibiotic therapy can upset the balance, permitting fungal overgrowth and setting the stage for opportunistic infections.

Parasites

In a strict sense, any organism that derives benefits from its biologic relationship with another organism is a parasite. In the study of clinical microbiology, however, the term *parasite* has evolved to designate members of the animal kingdom that infect and cause disease in other animals, and includes proto-zoa, helminths, and arthropods.

The protozoa are unicellular animals with a complete complement of eukaryotic cellular machinery, including a well-defined nucleus and organelles. Reproduction may be sexual or asexual, and life cycles may be simple or compli-cated, with several maturation stages requiring more than one host for completion. Most are saprophytes, but a few have adapted to the accommodations of the human environment and produce a variety of diseases, including malaria, amoebic dysentery, and giardiasis. Protozoan infections can be passed directly from host to host in a number of ways including sex-ual contact, indirectly through contaminated water or food, or by way of an arthropod vector. Direct or indirect transmission results from the ingestion of highly resistant cysts or spores that are shed in the feces of an infected host. When the cysts reach the intestine, they mature into vegetative forms called *trophozoites,* which are capable of asexual reproduction or cyst formation. Most trophozoites are motile by means of fla-gella, cilia, or amoeboid motion.

The helminths are a collection of worm-like parasites that include the nematodes or roundworms, cestodes or tape-worms, and trematodes or flukes. The helminths reproduce sexually within the definitive host, and some require an inter-mediate host for the development and maturation of offspring. Humans can serve as the definitive or intermediate host and, in certain diseases such as trichinosis, as both. Transmission of helminth diseases occurs primarily through the ingestion of fertilized eggs (ova) or the penetration of infectious lar-val stages through the skin—directly or with the aid of an arthropod vector. Helminth infections can involve many organ systems and sites, including the liver and lung, urinary and

FIGURE 16.5 • The microscopic morphology of fungal pathogens in humans. **A:** Histopathologic changes seen in histoplasmosis due to *Histoplasma capsulatum var. duboisii.* Note the presence of typical yeast cells, some of which are undergoing replication by budding. **B:** The moulds produce long-branched and unbranched filaments called *hyphae.* **C:** *Candida albicans* is a budding yeast that produces pseudohyphae both in culture and in tissues and exudate. (**A,** Public Images Library, Centers for Disease Control and Prevention. Available at http://phil.cdc.gov/phil/details.asp; **C,** © Science Source/Photo Researchers.)

intestinal tracts, circulatory and central nervous systems, and muscle. Although most helminth diseases have been eradicated from Canada and the United States, they are still a major health concern in developing nations.

The parasitic arthropods of humans and animals include the vectors of infectious diseases (*e.g.,* ticks, mosquitoes, biting flies) and the ectoparasites. The ectoparasites infest external body surfaces and cause localized tissue damage or inflammation secondary to the bite or burrowing action of the arthropod. The most prominent human ectoparasites are mites (scabies), chiggers, lice (head, body, and pubic), and fleas. Transmission of ectoparasites occurs directly by contact with immature or mature forms of the arthropod or its eggs found on the infested host or the host's clothing, bedding, or grooming articles such as combs and brushes. Many of the ectoparasites are vectors of other infectious diseases, including endemic typhus and bubonic plague (fleas) and epidemic typhus (lice).

IN SUMMARY

Throughout life, humans are continuously and harmlessly exposed to and colonized by a multitude of microscopic organisms. This relationship is kept in check by the intact defence mechanisms of the host (*e.g.,* mucosal and cutaneous barriers, normal immune function) and the innocuous nature of most environmental microorganisms. Those factors that weaken the host's resistance or increase the virulence of colonizing microorganisms can disturb the equilibrium of the relationship and cause disease. The degree to which the balance is shifted in favour of the microorganism determines the severity of illness.

There is an extreme diversity of prokaryotic and eukaryotic microorganisms capable of causing infectious diseases in humans. With the advent of immunosuppressive medical therapy and immunosuppressive diseases such as AIDS, the number and type of potential microbic pathogens, the so-called opportunistic pathogens, have increased dramatically. However, most infectious illnesses in humans continue to be caused by only a small fraction of the organisms that comprise the microscopic world.

MECHANISMS OF INFECTION

After completing this section of the chapter, you should be able to meet the following objectives:

- Differentiate between incidence and prevalence and among endemic, epidemic, and pandemic.
- Describe the stages of an infectious disease after the potential pathogen has entered the body.
- List the systemic manifestations of infectious disease.
- Explain how virulence factors enhance the microbe's ability to cause disease.

Epidemiology of Infectious Diseases

Epidemiology, in the context of this chapter, is the study of factors, events, and circumstances that influence the transmission of infectious diseases among humans. The ultimate goal of the epidemiologist is to devise strategies that interrupt or eliminate the spread of an infectious agent. To accomplish this, infectious diseases must be classified according to incidence, portal of entry, source, symptoms, disease course, site of infection, and virulence factors so that potential outbreaks may be predicted and averted or appropriately treated.

Epidemiology is a science of rates and statistics. The expected frequency of any infectious disease must be calculated

EPIDEMIOLOGY OF INFECTIOUS DISEASES

- Epidemiology is the study of factors, events, and circumstances that influence the transmission of infectious diseases in human populations.
- Epidemiology focuses on the incidence (number of new cases) and prevalence (number of active cases at any given time) of an infectious disease; the source of infection and its portal of entry, site of infection, and virulence factors of the infecting organism; and the signs and symptoms of the infection and its course.
- The ultimate goals of epidemiologic studies are the interruption of the spread of infectious diseases and their eradication.

so that gradual or abrupt changes in frequency can be observed. The term *incidence* is used to describe the number of new cases of an infectious disease that occur within a defined population (*e.g.,* per 100,000 persons) over an established period of time (*e.g.,* monthly, quarterly, yearly). Disease *prevalence* indicates the number of active cases at any given time. A disease is considered *endemic* in a particular geographic region if the incidence and prevalence are expected and relatively stable. An *epidemic* describes an abrupt and unexpected increase in the incidence of disease over endemic rates. A *pandemic* refers to the spread of disease beyond continental boundaries. The advent of rapid worldwide travel has increased the likelihood of pandemic transmission of pathogenic microorganisms.

As an illustration of these principles, an outbreak of a suspected respiratory viral illness—subsequently identified as severe acute respiratory syndrome (SARS)—was recognized in the Guangdong province in southern China beginning in November 2002. The illness was highly transmissible, as evidenced by the first recognized occurrence in Taiwan. Four days after returning to Taiwan from work in the Guangdong province, a businessman developed a febrile illness and was admitted to a local hospital. Within 1 month, a large nosocomial outbreak of SARS was documented to have affected approximately 3,000 people in Taipei City, Taiwan. Once the SARS outbreak had crossed these continental borders for the first time, its classification was changed from an epidemic to a pandemic.

Portal of Entry

The portal of entry refers to the process by which a pathogen enters the body, gains access to susceptible tissues, and causes disease. Among the potential modes of transmission are penetration, direct contact, ingestion, and inhalation. The portal of entry does not dictate the site of infection. Ingested pathogens may penetrate the intestinal mucosa, disseminate through the circulatory system, and cause diseases in other organs such as the lung or liver. Whatever the mechanisms of entry, the transmission of infectious agents is directly related to the number of infectious agents absorbed by the host.

Penetration

Any disruption in the integrity of the body's surface barrier—skin or mucous membranes—is a potential site for invasion of microorganisms. The break may be the result of an accidental injury causing abrasions, burns, or penetrating wounds; medical procedures such as surgery or catheterization; or a primary infectious process that produces surface lesions such as chickenpox or impetigo. Direct inoculation from intravenous drug use or an animal or arthropod bite also can occur.

Direct Contact

Some pathogens are transmitted directly from infected tissue or secretions to exposed, intact mucous membranes. This is especially true of certain sexually transmitted infections (STIs) such as gonorrhea, syphilis, chlamydia, and genital herpes, in which exposure of uninfected membranes to pathogens occurs during intimate contact (see Chapter 47).

The transmission of STIs is not limited to sexual contact. *Vertical transmission* of these agents, from mother to child, can occur across the placenta or during birth when the mucous membranes of the child come in contact with infected vaginal secretions of the mother. When an infectious disease is transmitted from mother to child during gestation or birth, it is classified as a *congenital infection*. The most frequently observed congenital infections include toxoplasmosis (caused by the parasite *Toxoplasma gondii*), syphilis, rubella, cytomegalovirus infection, and HSV infections (the so-called TORCH infections, discussed in Chapter 7); varicella-zoster (chickenpox); parvovirus B19; group B streptococci (*Streptococcus agalactiae*); and HIV. Of these, cytomegalovirus is by far the most common cause of congenital infection in Canada, affecting approximately 0.3% to 2.2% of all newborns.

The severity of congenital defects associated with these infections depends greatly on the gestational age of the fetus when transmission occurs, but most of these agents can cause profound mental retardation and neurosensory deficits, including blindness and hearing loss. HIV rarely produces overt signs and symptoms in the infected newborn, and it sometimes takes years for the effects of the illness to manifest.

Ingestion

The entry of pathogenic microorganisms or their toxic products through the oral cavity and gastrointestinal tract represents one of the more efficient means of disease transmission in humans. Many bacterial, viral, and parasitic infections, including cholera, typhoid fever, dysentery (amoebic and bacillary), food poisoning, traveller's diarrhea, cryptosporidiosis, and hepatitis A, are initiated through the ingestion of contaminated food and water. This mechanism of transmission necessitates that an infectious agent survive the low pH and enzyme activity of gastric secretions and the peristaltic action of the intestines in numbers sufficient to establish infection, deemed an *infectious dose*. Ingested pathogens also must compete successfully with the normal bacterial flora of the bowel for nutritional needs. Persons with reduced gastric acidity because of disease or medication are more susceptible to infection by this route

because the number of ingested microorganisms surviving the gastric environment is greater. Ingestion has also been postulated as a means of transmission of HIV infection from mother to child through breast-feeding.

Inhalation

The respiratory tract of healthy persons is equipped with a multitiered defence system to prevent potential pathogens from entering the lungs. The surface of the respiratory tree is lined with a layer of mucus that is continuously swept up and away from the lungs and toward the mouth by the beating motion of ciliated epithelial cells. Humidification of inspired air increases the size of aerosolized particles, which are effectively filtered by the mucous membranes of the upper respiratory tract. Coughing also aids in the removal of particulate matter from the lower respiratory tract. Respiratory secretions contain antibodies and enzymes capable of inactivating infectious agents. Particulate matter and microorganisms that ultimately reach the lung are cleared by phagocytic cells.

Despite this impressive array of protective mechanisms, a number of pathogens can invade the human body through the respiratory tract, including agents of bacterial pneumonia (*Streptococcus pneumoniae*, *L. pneumophila*), meningitis (*Neisseria meningitidis*, *Haemophilus influenzae*), and tuberculosis, as well as the viruses responsible for measles, mumps, chickenpox, influenza, and the common cold. Defective pulmonary function or mucociliary clearance caused by noninfectious processes such as cystic fibrosis, emphysema, or smoking can increase the risk of inhalation-acquired diseases.

Source

The source of an infectious disease refers to the location, host, object, or substance from which the infectious agent was acquired—essentially the "who, what, where, and when" of disease transmission. The source may be endogenous (acquired from the host's own microbial flora, as would be the case in an opportunistic infection) or exogenous (acquired from sources in the external environment, such as the water, food, soil, or air). The source of the infectious agent can also be another human being, as from mother to child during gestation (congenital infections); an inanimate object; an animal; or a biting arthropod. Inanimate objects that carry an infectious agent are known as *fomites*. For example, rhinoviruses and many other nonenveloped viruses can be spread by contact with contaminated fomites such as handkerchiefs and toys. Zoonoses are a category of infectious diseases passed from other animal species to humans. Examples of zoonoses include cat-scratch disease, rabies, and visceral or cutaneous larval migrans. The spread of infectious diseases such as Lyme disease through biting arthropod vectors is another route.

Source can denote a place. For instance, infections that develop in patients while they are hospitalized are called *nosocomial*, and those that are acquired outside of healthcare facilities are called *community acquired*. The source may also pertain to the body substance that is the most likely vehicle for transmission, such as feces, blood, body fluids, respiratory secretions, and urine. Infections can be transmitted from person to person through shared inanimate objects (fomites) contaminated with infected body fluids. An example of this mechanism of transmission would include the spread of the HIV and hepatitis B virus through the use of shared syringes by intravenous drug users. Infection can also be spread through a complex combination of source, portal of entry, and vector.

Symptomatology

The term *symptomatology* refers to the collection of signs and symptoms expressed by the host during the disease course. This is also known as the *clinical picture* or *disease presentation*, and can be characteristic of any given infectious agent. In terms of pathophysiology, symptoms are the outward expression of the struggle between invading organisms and the retaliatory inflammatory and immune responses of the host. The symptoms of an infectious disease may be specific and reflect the site of infection (*e.g.,* diarrhea, rash, convulsions, hemorrhage, and pneumonia). Conversely, symptoms such as fever, myalgia, headache, and lethargy are relatively nonspecific and can be shared by a number of diverse infectious diseases. The symptoms of a diseased host can be obvious, as in the cases of chickenpox or measles. Other covert symptoms, such as an increased white blood cell count, may require laboratory testing to detect. Accurate recognition and documentation of symptomatology can aid in the diagnosis of an infectious disease.

Disease Course

The course of any infectious disease can be divided into several distinguishable stages after the point when the potential pathogen enters the host. These stages are the incubation period, the prodromal stage, the acute stage, the convalescent stage, and the resolution stage (Fig. 16.6). The stages are based on the progression and intensity of the host's symptoms over time. The duration of each phase and the pattern of the overall illness can be specific for different pathogens, thereby aiding in the diagnosis of an infectious disease.

The *incubation period* is the phase during which the pathogen begins active replication without producing recognizable symptoms in the host. The incubation period may be short, as in the case of salmonellosis (6 to 24 hours), or prolonged, such as that of hepatitis B (50 to 180 days) or HIV (months to years). The duration of the incubation period can be influenced by additional factors, including the general health of the host, the portal of entry, and the infectious dose of the pathogen.

The hallmark of the *prodromal stage* is the initial appearance of symptoms in the host, although the clinical presentation during this time may be only a vague sense of malaise. The host may experience mild fever, myalgia, headache, and fatigue. These are constitutional changes shared by a great number of disease processes. The duration of the prodromal stage can vary considerably from host to host.

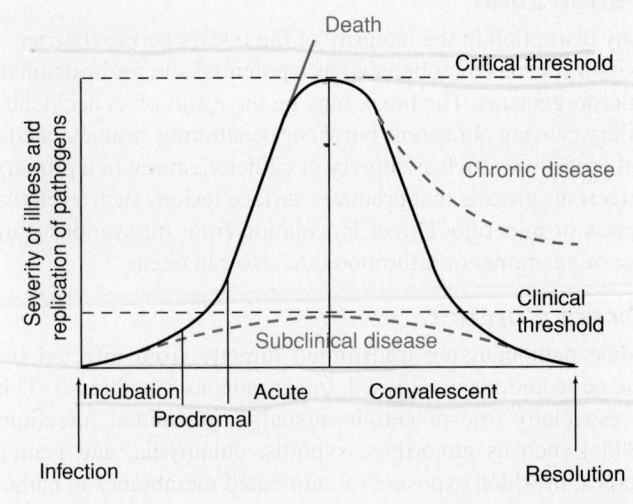

FIGURE 16.6 • Stages of a primary infectious disease as they appear in relation to the severity of symptoms and numbers of infectious agents. The clinical threshold corresponds with the initial expression of recognizable symptoms, whereas the critical threshold represents the peak of disease intensity.

The *acute stage* is the period during which the host experiences the maximum impact of the infectious process corresponding to rapid proliferation and dissemination of the pathogen. During this phase, toxic by-products of microbial metabolism, cell lysis, and the immune response mounted by the host combine to produce tissue damage and inflammation. The symptoms of the host are pronounced and more specific than in the prodromal stage, usually typifying the pathogen and sites of involvement.

The *convalescent period* is characterized by the containment of infection, progressive elimination of the pathogen, repair of damaged tissue, and resolution of associated symptoms. Similar to the incubation period, the time required for complete convalescence may be days, weeks, or months, depending on the type of pathogen and the voracity of the host's immune response. The *resolution* is the total elimination of a pathogen from the body without residual signs or symptoms of disease.

Several notable exceptions to the classic presentation of an infectious process have been recognized. Chronic infectious diseases have a markedly protracted and sometimes irregular course. The host may experience symptoms of the infectious process continuously or sporadically for months or years without a convalescent phase. In contrast, *subclinical or subacute illness* progresses from infection to resolution without clinically apparent symptoms. A disease is called *insidious* if the prodromal phase is protracted; a *fulminant illness* is characterized by abrupt onset of symptoms with little or no prodrome. Fatal infections are variants of the typical disease course.

Site of Infection

Inflammation of an anatomic location is usually designated by adding the suffix *-itis* to the name of the involved tissue (*e.g.,* bronchitis, infection of the bronchi and bronchioles; encephalitis, brain infection; carditis, infection of the heart). These are general terms, however, and they apply equally to inflammation from infectious and noninfectious causes. The suffix *-emia* is used to designate the presence of a substance in the blood (*e.g., bacteremia, viremia,* and *fungemia* describe the presence of these infectious agents in the bloodstream). The term *sepsis,* or *septicemia,* refers to the presence of microbial toxins in the blood.

The site of an infectious disease is determined ultimately by the type of pathogen, the portal of entry, and the competence of the host's immunologic defence system. Many pathogenic microorganisms are restricted in their capacity to invade the human body. *M. pneumoniae,* influenza viruses, and *L. pneumophila* rarely cause disease outside the respiratory tract; infections caused by *N. gonorrhoeae* are generally confined to the genitourinary tract; and shigellosis and giardiasis seldom extend beyond the gastrointestinal tract. These are considered localized infectious diseases. The bacterium *Helicobacter pylori* is an extreme example of a site-specific pathogen. *H. pylori* is a significant cause of gastric ulcers but has not been implicated in disease processes elsewhere in the human body. Bacteria such as *N. meningitidis,* a prominent pathogen of children and young adults; *Salmonella typhi,* the cause of typhoid fever; and *B. burgdorferi,* the agent of Lyme disease, tend to disseminate from the primary site of infection to involve other locations and organ systems. These are examples of systemic pathogens disseminated throughout the body by the circulatory system.

An *abscess* is a localized pocket of infection composed of devitalized tissue, microorganisms, and the host's phagocytic white blood cells: in essence, a stalemate in the infectious process. In this case, the dissemination of the pathogen has been contained by the host, but white cell function within the toxic environment of the abscess is hampered, and the elimination of microorganisms is retarded. Abscesses usually must be surgically drained to effect a complete cure. Similarly, infections of biomedical implants such as catheters, artificial heart valves, and prosthetic bone implants are seldom cured by the host's immune response and antimicrobial therapy. The infecting organism colonizes the surface of the implant, producing a dense matrix of cells, host proteins, and capsular material—a biofilm—necessitating the removal of the device.

Virulence Factors

Virulence factors are substances or products generated by infectious agents that enhance their ability to cause disease. Although a large number of microbial products fit this description, they can be grouped generally into four categories: toxins, adhesion factors, evasive factors, and invasive factors (Table 16.3).

Toxins

Toxins are substances that alter or destroy the normal function of the host or host's cells. Toxin production is a trait chiefly monopolized by bacterial pathogens, although certain fungal and protozoan pathogens also elaborate substances toxic to humans. Bacterial toxins have a diverse spectrum of activity and exert their effects on a wide variety of host target cells. For classification purposes, however, the bacterial toxins can be divided into two main types: *exotoxins* and *endotoxins*.

Exotoxins. Exotoxins are proteins released from the bacterial cell during growth. Bacterial exotoxins enzymatically inactivate or modify key cellular constituents, leading to cell death or dysfunction. Diphtheria toxin, for example, inhibits cellular protein synthesis; botulism toxin decreases the release of neurotransmitter from cholinergic neurons, causing flaccid paralysis; tetanus toxin decreases the release of neurotransmitter from inhibitory neurons, producing spastic paralysis; and cholera toxin induces fluid secretion into the lumen of

TABLE 16.3 EXAMPLES OF VIRULENCE FACTORS PRODUCED BY PATHOGENIC MICROORGANISMS

FACTOR	CATEGORY	ORGANISM	EFFECT ON HOST
Cholera toxin	Exotoxin	*Vibrio cholerae* (bacterium)	Secretory diarrhea
Diphtheria toxin	Exotoxin	*Corynebacterium diphtheriae* (bacterium)	Inhibits protein synthesis
Lipopolysaccharide	Endotoxin	Many gram-negative bacteria	Fever, hypotension, shock
Toxic shock toxin	Enterotoxin	*Staphylococcus aureus* (bacterium)	Rash, diarrhea, vomiting, hepatitis
Hemagglutinin	Adherence	Influenza virus	Establishment of infection
Pili	Adherence	*Neisseria gonorrhoeae* (bacterium)	Establishment of infection
Leukocidin	Evasive	*Staphylococcus aureus*	Kills phagocytes
IgA protease	Evasive	*Haemophilus influenzae* (bacterium)	Inactivates antibody
Capsule	Evasive	*Cryptococcus neoformans* (yeast)	Prevents phagocytosis
Collagenase	Invasive	*Pseudomonas aeruginosa* (bacterium)	Penetration of tissue
Protease	Invasive	*Aspergillus* (mould)	Penetration of tissue
Phospholipase	Invasive	*Clostridium perfringens* (bacterium)	Penetration of tissue
Botulinum toxin	Exotoxin	*Clostridium botulinum* (bacterium)	Neuroparalysis, inhibits acetylcholine release
Pneumolysin	Exotoxin	*Streptococcus pneumoniae* (bacterium)	Inhibition of respiratory ciliated and phagocytic cell function

the intestine, causing diarrhea. Other examples of exotoxin-induced diseases include pertussis (whooping cough), anthrax, traveller's diarrhea, toxic shock syndrome, and a host of food-borne illnesses (*i.e.,* food poisoning).

Bacterial exotoxins that produce vomiting and diarrhea are sometimes referred to as *enterotoxins.* There has been resurgent interest in streptococcal pyrogenic exotoxin A (SPEA), an exotoxin produced by certain strains of group A, beta-hemolytic streptococci (*S. pyogenes*) that causes a life-threatening toxic shock-like syndrome similar to the disease associated with tampon use produced by *S. aureus*. The strep-tococcal form of intoxication is sometimes called *Henson disease* because it was this infection that caused the death of the famous puppeteer Jim Henson. Other exotoxins that have gained notoriety include the Shiga toxins produced by *Escherichia coli* O157:H7 and other select strains. The inges-tion of undercooked hamburger meat or unpasteurized fruit juices contaminated with this organism produces hemorrhagic colitis and a sometimes fatal illness called *hemolytic uremic syndrome* (HUS), characterized by vascular endothelial dam-age, acute renal failure, and thrombocytopenia. HUS occurs primarily in infants and young children who have not devel-oped antibodies to the Shiga toxins. Over time, the incidence of disease caused by food-borne exotoxins has grown. One such event occurred in the late summer of 2006. Small clus-ters of infections appeared in sporadic locations throughout the United States. Epidemiologists identified fresh spinach from a Californian produce company as the suspected source of infection. This initiated a consumer advisory for all Ameri-cans and, soon afterward, Canadians. Another example was the Walkerton, Ontario, tragedy which occurred in 2000 when *E. coli* O157:H7 contaminated that city's water supply.

Endotoxins. In contrast to exotoxins, endotoxins do not con-tain protein, are not actively released from the bacterium dur-ing growth, and have no enzymatic activity. Rather, endotoxins are complex molecules composed of lipid and polysaccharides found in the cell wall of gram-negative bacteria. Studies of dif-ferent endotoxins have indicated that the lipid portion of the endotoxin confers the toxic properties to the molecule. Endo-toxins are potent activators of a number of regulatory systems in humans. A small amount of endotoxin in the circulatory system (endotoxemia) can induce clotting, bleeding, inflam-mation, hypotension, and fever. The sum of the physiologic reactions to endotoxins is sometimes called *endotoxic shock.*

Adhesion Factors

No interaction between microorganisms and humans can progress to infection or disease if the pathogen is unable to attach to and colonize the host. The process of microbial attachment may be site specific (*e.g.,* mucous membranes, skin surfaces), cell specific (*e.g.,* T lymphocytes, respira-tory epithelium, intestinal epithelium), or nonspecific (*e.g.,* moist areas, charged surfaces). In any of these cases, adhesion requires a positive interaction between the surfaces of host cells and the infectious agent.

The site to which microorganisms adhere is called a *receptor,* and the reciprocal molecule or substance that binds to the receptor is called a *ligand* or *adhesin*. Receptors may be proteins, carbohydrates, lipids, or complex molecules composed of all three. Similarly, ligands may be simple or complex mol-ecules and, in some cases, highly specific structures. Ligands that bind to specific carbohydrates are called *lectins*. After initial attachment, a number of bacterial agents become embedded in a gelatinous matrix of polysaccharides called a *slime* or *mucous layer.* The slime layer serves two purposes: it anchors the agent firmly to host tissue surfaces and it protects the agent from the immunologic defences of the host.

Many viral agents, including influenza, mumps, measles, and adenovirus, produce filamentous appendages or spikes called *hemagglutinins* that recognize carbohydrate receptors on the surfaces of specific cells in the upper respiratory tract of the host.

Evasive Factors

A number of factors produced by microorganisms enhance vir-ulence by evading various components of the host's immune system. Extracellular polysaccharides, including capsules, slime, and mucous layers, discourage engulfment and kill-ing of pathogens by the host's phagocytic white blood cells (*i.e.,* neutrophils and macrophages). Encapsulated organisms such as *S. agalactiae, S. pneumoniae, N. meningitidis,* and *H. influenzae* type b (before the vaccine) are a cause of signifi-cant morbidity and mortality in neonates and children who lack protective anticapsular antibodies. Certain bacterial, fun-gal, and parasitic pathogens avoid phagocytosis by excreting leukocidin C toxins, which cause specific and lethal damage to the cell membrane of host neutrophils and macrophages. Other pathogens, such as the bacterial agents of salmonellosis, listeriosis, and Legionnaire disease, are adapted to survive and reproduce within phagocytic white blood cells after ingestion, avoiding or neutralizing the usually lethal products contained within the lysosomes of the cell. *H. pylori,* the infectious cause of gastritis and gastric ulcers, produces a urease enzyme on its outer cell wall. The urease converts gastric urea into ammonia, thus neutralizing the acidic environment of the stomach and allowing the organism to survive in this hostile environment.

Other unique strategies used by pathogenic microbes to evade immunologic surveillance have evolved solely to avoid recognition by host antibodies. Strains of *S. aureus* produce a surface protein (protein A) that immobilizes immunoglobulin G (IgG), holding the antigen-binding region harmlessly away from the organisms. This pathogen also secretes a unique enzyme called *coagulase,* Coagulase converts soluble human coagulation factors into a solid clot, which envelops and pro-tects the organism from phagocytic host cells and antibod-ies. *H. influenzae* and *N. gonorrhoeae* secrete enzymes that cleave and inactivate secretory IgA, neutralizing the primary defence of the respiratory and genital tracts at the site of infec-tion. *Borrelia* species, including the agents of Lyme disease and relapsing fever, alter surface antigens during the disease course to avoid immunologic detection. It appears that the capability to devise strategic defence systems and stealth technologies is not limited to humans.

Some viruses, such as HIV, impair the function of immunoregulatory cells. Although this property increases the virulence of these agents, it is not considered a virulence factor in the true sense of the definition.

Invasive Factors

Invasive factors are products produced by infectious agents that facilitate the penetration of anatomic barriers and host tissue. Most invasive factors are enzymes capable of destroying cellular membranes (*e.g.,* phospholipases), connective tissue (*e.g.,* elastases, collagenases), intercellular matrices (*e.g.,* hyaluronidase), and structural protein complexes (*e.g.,* proteases). It is the combined effects of invasive factors, toxins, and antimicrobial and inflammatory substances released by host cells to counter infection that mediate the tissue damage and pathophysiology of infectious diseases.

IN SUMMARY

Epidemiology is the study of factors, events, and circumstances that influence the transmission of disease. Incidence refers to the number of new cases of an infectious disease that occur in a defined population, and prevalence to the number of active cases that are present at any given time. Infectious diseases are considered endemic in a geographic area if the incidence and prevalence are expected and relatively stable. An epidemic refers to an abrupt and unexpected increase in the incidence of a disease over endemic rates, and a pandemic to the spread of disease beyond continental boundaries.

The ultimate goal of epidemiology and epidemiologic studies is to devise strategies to interrupt or eliminate the spread of infectious disease. To accomplish this, infectious diseases are classified according to incidence, portal of entry, source, symptoms, disease course, site of infection, and virulence factors.

DIAGNOSIS AND TREATMENT OF INFECTIOUS DISEASES

After completing this section of the chapter, you should be able to meet the following objectives:

- State the two criteria used in the diagnosis of an infectious disease.
- Explain the differences among culture, serology, and antigen, metabolite, and molecular detection methods for diagnosis of infectious disease.
- Cite three general intervention methods that can be used in treatment of infectious illnesses.
- State four basic mechanisms by which antibiotics exert their action.
- Differentiate bactericidal from bacteriostatic.

Diagnosis

The diagnosis of an infectious disease requires two criteria: the recovery of a probable pathogen or evidence of its presence from the infected sites of a diseased host, and accurate documentation of clinical signs and symptoms (symptomatology) compatible with an infectious process. In the laboratory, the diagnosis of an infectious agent is accomplished using three basic techniques: culture, serology, or the detection of characteristic antigens, genomic sequences, or metabolites produced by the pathogen.

Culture

Culture refers to the propagation of a microorganism outside of the body, on or in artificial growth media such as agar plates or broth (Fig. 16.7). The specimen from the host is inoculated into broth or onto the surface of an agar plate, and the culture is placed in a controlled environment such as an incubator until the growth of microorganisms becomes detectable. In the case of a bacterial pathogen, identification is based on microscopic appearance and Gram stain reaction, shape, texture, and colour (*i.e.,* morphology) of the colonies, and by a panel of biochemical reactions that fingerprint salient biochemical characteristics of the organism. Certain bacteria such as *Mycobacterium leprae,* the agent of leprosy, and *T. pallidum,* the syphilis spirochete, do not grow on artificial media and require additional methods of identification. Fungi and mycoplasmas are cultured in much the same way as bacteria, but with more reliance on microscopic and colonial morphology for identification.

DIAGNOSIS AND TREATMENT OF INFECTIOUS DISEASES

- The definitive diagnosis of an infectious disease requires recovery and identification of the infecting organism by microscopic identification of the agent in stains of specimens or sections of tissue, culture isolation and identification of the agents, demonstration of antibody- or cell-mediated immune responses to an infectious agent, or DNA or RNA identification of infectious agents.
- Treatment of infectious disease is aimed at eliminating the infectious organism and promoting recovery of the infected person. Treatment is provided through the use of antimicrobial agents, immunotherapy, and, when necessary, surgical interventions.
- Prevention of infectious disease is accomplished through the use of immunization methods.

Chlamydiaceae, Rickettsiaceae, and all human viruses are obligate intracellular pathogens. As a result, the propagation of these agents in the laboratory requires the inoculation of eukaryotic cells grown in culture (cell cultures). A cell culture consists of a flask containing a single layer, or monolayer, of eukaryotic cells covering the bottom and overlaid with broth containing essential nutrients and growth factors. When

FIGURE 16.7 • Variability of the macroscopic appearance of bacteria cultured on solid, agar-containing medium and liquid broth medium. **A:** Photograph showing numerous *Legionella* species colonies that have been cultivated on an agar culture plate and illuminated using ultraviolet light. **B:** Bacteria cultured in broth form a variety of growth patterns, ranging from particulate to homogeneous, turbid suspensions. Anaerobic bacteria cultured in liquid medium tend to grow best at the bottom of the tube, where the concentration of molecular oxygen is lowest. (Public Images Library, Centers for Disease Control and Prevention. Available at http://phil.cdc.gov/phil/details.asp.)

a virus infects and replicates within cultured eukaryotic cells, it produces pathologic changes in the appearance of the cell called the *cytopathic effect* (CPE; Fig. 16.8). The CPE can be detected microscopically, and the pattern and extent of cellular destruction is often characteristic of a particular virus.

Although culture media can be used for the growth of certain human-infecting protozoa and helminths in the laboratory, the diagnosis of parasitic infectious diseases has traditionally relied on microscopic or, in the case of worms, visible identification of organisms, cysts, or ova directly from infected patient specimens.

Serology

Serology—literally, "the study of serum"—is an indirect means of identifying infectious agents by measuring serum antibodies in the diseased host. A tentative diagnosis can be made if the antibody level, also called *antibody titre*, against a specific pathogen rises during the acute phase of the disease and falls during convalescence. Serologic identification of an infectious agent is not as accurate as culture, but it may be a useful adjunct, especially for the diagnosis of diseases caused by pathogens such as the hepatitis B virus that cannot be cultured. The measurement of antibody titres has another advantage in that specific antibody types such as IgM and IgG are produced by the host during different phases of an infectious process. IgM-specific antibodies generally rise and fall during the acute phase of the disease, whereas the synthesis of the IgG class of antibodies increases during the acute phase and remains elevated until or beyond resolution. Measurements of class-specific antibodies are also useful in the diagnosis of congenital infections. IgM antibodies do not cross the placenta, but certain IgG antibodies are transferred passively from mother to child during the final trimester of gestation. Consequently, an elevated level of pathogen-specific IgM antibodies in the serum of a neonate must have originated from the child and therefore indicates congenital infection. A similarly increased IgG titre in the neonate does not differentiate congenital from maternal infection.

The technology of *antigen detection* has evolved rapidly over the past decade and in the process has revolutionized the diagnosis of certain infectious diseases. Antigen detection incorporates features of culture and serology but reduces to a fraction the time required for diagnosis. In principle, this method relies on purified antibodies to detect antigens of infectious agents in specimens obtained from the diseased host. The source of antibodies used for antigen detection can be animals immunized against a particular pathogen or *hybridomas*. Hybridomas are created by fusing normal antibody-producing spleen cells from an immunized animal with malignant myeloma cells; the resulting hybrid synthesizes large quantities of antibody. An antibody produced by a hybridoma is called a *monoclonal antibody,* and is highly specific for a single antigen and a single pathogen. Regardless of the source, the antibodies are labelled with a substance that allows microscopic or overt detection when bound

FIGURE 16.8 • The microscopic appearance of a monolayer of uninfected human fibroblasts grown in cell culture (**A**), and the same cells after infection with herpes simplex virus (**B**), demonstrating the cytopathic effect caused by viral replication and concomitant cell lysis.

to the pathogen or its products. In general, the three types of labels used for this purpose are fluorescent dyes, enzymes, and particles such as latex beads. Fluorescent antibodies allow visualization of an infectious agent with the aid of fluorescence microscopy. Depending on the type of fluorescent dye used, the organism may appear bright green or orange against a black background, making detection extremely easy. Enzyme-labelled antibodies function in a similar manner. The enzyme is capable of converting a colourless compound into a coloured substance, thereby permitting detection of antibody bound to an infectious agent without the use of a fluorescent microscope. Particles coated with antibodies clump together, or agglutinate, when the appropriate antigen is present in a specimen. Particle agglutination is especially useful when examining infected body fluids such as urine, serum, or spinal fluid.

DNA and RNA Sequencing

Methods for identifying infectious agents through the detection of DNA or RNA sequences unique to a single agent have recently seen rapid development and are widely used. Several techniques have been devised to accomplish this goal, each having different degrees of sensitivity regarding the number of organisms that need to be present in a specimen for detection. The first of these methods is called *DNA probe hybridization.* Small fragments of DNA are cut from the genome of a specific pathogen and labelled with compounds (photoemitting chemicals or antigens) that allow detection. The labelled DNA

probes are added to specimens from an infected host. If the pathogen is present, the probe attaches to the complementary strand of DNA on the genome of the infectious agent, permitting rapid diagnosis. The use of labelled probes has allowed visualization of particular agents within and around individual cells in histologic sections of tissue.

The preferred and most commonly used technique is a second and more sensitive method of DNA detection called the *polymerase chain reaction* (PCR; Fig. 16.9). This method incorporates two unique reagents: a specific pair of oligonucleotides (usually less than 25 nucleotides long) called *primers* and a heat-stable DNA polymerase. To perform the assay, the primers are added to the specimen containing the suspect pathogen, and the sample is heated to melt the DNA in the specimen and then allowed to cool. The primers locate and bind only to the complementary target DNA of the pathogen in question. The heat-stable polymerase begins to replicate the DNA from the point at which the primers attached, similar to two trains approaching one another on separate but converging tracks. After the initial cycle, DNA polymerization ceases at the point where the primers were located, producing a strand of DNA with a distinct size, depending on the distance separating the two primers. The specimen is heated again, and the process starts anew. After many cycles of heating, cooling, and polymerization, a large number of uniformly sized DNA fragments are produced only if the specific pathogen (or its DNA) is present in the specimen. The polymerized DNA fragments

Target DNA

5'
5'

↓ Heat

5'
5'

5'

↓ Primers

5'

5'

Extension of new DNA using Taq polymerase

↓ Repeat process multiple times

↓ Final amplified products

Detection probe

FIGURE 16.9 • Polymerase chain reaction. The target DNA is first melted using heat (generally around 94°C) to separate the strands of DNA. Primers that recognize specific sequences in the target DNA are allowed to bind as the reaction cools. Using a unique, thermostable DNA polymerase called Taq and an abundance of deoxynucleoside triphosphates, new DNA strands are amplified from the point of the primer attachment. The process is repeated many times (called *cycles*) until millions of copies of DNA are produced, all of which have the same length defined by the distance (in base pairs) between the primer binding sites. These copies are then detected by electrophoresis and staining or through the use of labelled DNA probes that, similar to the primers, recognize a specific sequence located in the amplified section of DNA.

are separated by electrophoresis and visualized with a dye or identified by hybridization with a specific probe.

A modification of PCR, known as real-time PCR, provides reliable, accurate, and fast detection of microbes. Real-time PCR uses the same principles as PCR, but includes a fluorescence-labelled probe that specifically binds a target DNA sequence between the oligonucleotide primers. As the DNA is replicated by the DNA polymerase, the level of fluorescence in the reaction is measured. If fluorescence increases beyond a minimum threshold, the PCR is considered positive and indicates the presence of the target DNA in a specimen.

Several variations of molecular gene detection techniques in addition to PCR have been developed and incorporated into diagnostic kits for use in the clinical laboratory, including ligase chain reaction (LCR), transcription-mediated amplification (TMA), strand displacement amplification, branched-chain

DNA signal amplification (bDNA), hybrid capture assays, and DNA sequencing.

Many of the newer gene detection technologies have been adapted for quantitation of the target DNA or RNA in serum specimens of patients infected with viruses such as HIV and hepatitis C. If the therapy is effective, viral replication is suppressed and the viral load (level of viral genome) in the peripheral blood is reduced. Conversely, if mutations in the viral genome lead to resistant strains or if the antiviral therapy is ineffective, viral replication continues and the patient's viral load rises, indicating a need to change the therapeutic approach.

Molecular biology has revolutionized medical diagnostics. Using techniques such as PCR, laboratories now can detect as little as one virus or bacterium in a single specimen, allowing for the diagnosis of infections caused by microorganisms that are difficult or impossible to grow in culture. These methods have increased sensitivity while decreasing the time required to identify the etiologic agent of infectious disease. For example, using standard viral culture, it can take days to weeks to grow a virus and correlate the CPE with the virus. Using molecular biologic techniques, laboratories are able to complete the same work in a few hours.

Treatment

The goal of treatment for an infectious disease is complete removal of the pathogen from the host and the restoration of normal physiologic function to damaged tissues. Most infectious diseases of humans are self-limiting in that they require little or no medical therapy for a complete cure. When an infectious process gains the upper hand and therapeutic intervention is essential, the choice of treatment may be medicinal through the use of antimicrobial agents; immunologic with antibody preparations, vaccines, or substances that stimulate and improve the host's immune function; or surgical by removing infected tissues. The decision about which therapeutic modality or combination of therapies to use is based on the extent, urgency, and location of the disease process, the pathogen, and the availability of effective antimicrobial agents.

Antimicrobial Agents

It was not until the advent of World War II, after the introduction of sulfonamides and penicillin that the development of antimicrobial compounds matured into a science of great consequence. Today, the comprehensive list of effective anti-infective agents is burgeoning. Most antimicrobial compounds can be categorized roughly according to mechanism of anti-infective activity, chemical structure, and target pathogen (*e.g.*, antibacterial, antiviral, antifungal, or antiparasitic agents).

Antibacterial Agents. Antibacterial agents are generally called *antibiotics*. Most antibiotics are actually produced by other microorganisms, primarily bacteria and fungi, as byproducts of metabolism, and usually are effective only against other prokaryotic organisms. An antibiotic is considered

TABLE 16.4 CLASSIFICATION AND ACTIVITY OF ANTIBACTERIAL AGENTS (ANTIBIOTICS)

FAMILY	EXAMPLE	TARGET SITE	SIDE EFFECTS
Penicillins	Ampicillin	Cell wall	Allergic reactions
Cephalosporins	Cephalexin	Cell wall	Allergic reactions
Monobactams	Aztreonam	Cell wall	Rash
Carbapenem	Imipenem	Cell wall	Nausea, diarrhea
Aminoglycosides	Gentamicin	Ribosomes (protein synthesis)	Hearing loss Nephrotoxicity
Tetracyclines	Doxycycline	Ribosomes (protein synthesis)	Gastrointestinal irritation Allergic reactions Teeth and bone dysplasia
Macrolides	Clarithromycin	Ribosomes (protein synthesis)	Colitis Allergic reactions
Glycopeptides	Vancomycin	Cell wall	Allergic reactions Hearing loss Nephrotoxicity
Quinolones	Ciprofloxacin	DNA synthesis	Gastrointestinal irritation Tendon rupture
Miscellaneous	Chloramphenicol	Ribosomes (protein synthesis)	Anemia
	Rifampin	Ribosomes (protein synthesis)	Hepatotoxicity
	Trimethoprim	Folic acid synthesis	Allergic reactions Same as sulfonamides
Sulfonamides	Sulfadiazine	Folic acid synthesis	Allergic reactions Anemia Gastrointestinal irritation
Oxazolidinone	Linezolid	Ribosomes (protein synthesis)	Diarrhea, thrombocytopenia
Streptogramin	Quinupristin/dalfopristin	Ribosomes (protein synthesis)	Muscle and joint aches
Glycylcycline	Tigecycline	Ribosomes	Nausea, vomiting, diarrhea
Polymyxins	Colistin	Membrane	Confusion, visual disturbances, vertigo, kidney damage
Lipopeptide	Daptomycin	Membrane depolarization	Nausea, vomiting, constipation, diarrhea, headache

bactericidal if it causes irreversible and lethal damage to the bacterial pathogen, and *bacteriostatic* if its inhibitory effects on bacterial growth are reversed when the agent is eliminated. Antibiotics can be classified into families of compounds with related chemical structure and activity (Table 16.4).

Not all antibiotics are effective against all pathogenic bacteria. Some agents are effective only against gram-negative bacteria, and others are specific for gram-positive organisms (*e.g.,* vancomycin). The so-called broad-spectrum antibiotics, such as the newest class of cephalosporins, are active against a wide variety of gram-positive and gram-negative bacteria. Members of the *Mycobacterium* genus, including *M. tuberculosis,* are extremely resistant to the effects of the major classes of antibiotics and require an entirely different spectrum of agents for therapy. The four basic mechanisms of the antibiotic action are interference with a specific step in bacterial cell wall synthesis (*e.g.,* penicillins, cephalosporins, glycopeptides, monobactams, carbapenems); inhibition of bacterial protein synthesis (*e.g.,* aminoglycosides, macrolides, ketolides, tetracyclines, chloramphenicol, oxazolidinones, streptogramins, and rifampin); interruption of nucleic acid synthesis (*e.g.,* fluoroquinolones, nalidixic acid); and interference with normal metabolism (*e.g.,* sulfonamides, trimethoprim).

Despite lack of antibiotic activity against eukaryotic cells, many agents cause unwanted or toxic side effects in humans, including allergic responses (penicillins, cephalosporins, sulfonamides, glycopeptides), hearing and kidney impairment (aminoglycosides), and liver or bone marrow toxicity (chloramphenicol, fluoroquinolones, vancomycin). Of greater concern is the increasing prevalence of bacteria resistant to the effects of antibiotics. The ways in which bacteria acquire resistance to antibiotics are becoming as numerous as the types of antibiotics. Bacterial-resistance mechanisms include the production of enzymes that inactivate antibiotics, such as β-lactamases; genetic mutations that alter antibiotic binding sites; alternative metabolic pathways that bypass antibiotic activity; and changes in the filtration qualities of the bacterial cell wall that prevent access of antibiotics to the target site in the organism.

Antiviral Agents. Until recently, few effective antiviral agents were available for treating human infections. The reason for this is host toxicity; viral replication requires the use of eukaryotic host cell enzymes, and the drugs that effectively interrupt viral replication are likely to interfere with host cell reproduction as well. However, in response to the AIDS epidemic, there has been massive, albeit delayed, development of antiretroviral agents. Almost all antiviral compounds are synthetic and, with few exceptions, the primary target of antiviral compounds is viral RNA or DNA synthesis. Agents such as acyclovir, ganciclovir, and ribavirin mimic the nucleoside building blocks of RNA and DNA. During active viral replication, the nucleoside analogs inhibit the viral DNA polymerase, preventing duplication of the viral genome and spread of infectious viral progeny to other susceptible host cells. Similar to the specificity of antibiotics, antiviral agents may be active against RNA viruses only, DNA viruses only, or occasionally both. Other nucleoside analogs such as zidovudine, lamivudine, didanosine, stavudine, and abacavir, and nonnucleoside inhibitors, including nevirapine, efavirenz, etravirine, rilpivirine, and delavirdine, were developed specifically for the treatment of AIDS by targeting the HIV-specific enzyme, reverse transcriptase, for inhibition. This key enzyme is essential for viral replication and has no counterpart in the infected eukaryotic host cells.

Another class of antiviral agents developed solely for the treatment of HIV infections is the *protease inhibitors* (e.g., indinavir, ritonavir, saquinavir, tipranavir, atazanavir, nelfinavir). These drugs inhibit an HIV-specific enzyme that is necessary for late maturation events in the virus life cycle.

Experimental approaches to antiviral therapy include compounds that inhibit viral attachment to susceptible host cells, drugs that prevent uncoating of the viral genome once inside the host cell, and agents that directly inhibit viral DNA polymerase. An example of drugs that prevent attachment is enfuvirtide, a peptide that binds to the docking glycopeptide (gp41) of HIV-1 and prevents its binding and fusion to the target $CD4^+$ lymphocyte (see Chapter 20). A class of antiviral agent that specifically inhibits influenza virus neuraminidase B, which is an essential enzyme for viral replication, includes zanamivir and oseltamivir, both approved for treatment of influenza A and B.

Although the treatment of viral infections with antimicrobial agents is a relatively recent endeavour, reports of viral mutations resulting in resistant strains are very common. This is especially troubling in the case of HIV, in which resistance to relatively new antiviral agents, including nucleoside analogs and protease inhibitors, has already been described, prompting the need for combination or alternating therapy with multiple antiretroviral agents.

Antifungal Agents. The target site of the two most important families of antifungal agents is the cytoplasmic membranes of yeasts or moulds. Fungal membranes differ from human cell membranes in that they contain the sterol ergosterol instead of cholesterol. The polyene family of antifungal compounds (e.g., amphotericin B, nystatin) preferentially binds to ergosterol and forms holes in the cytoplasmic membrane, causing leakage of the fungal cell contents and, eventually, lysis of the cell. The imidazole class of drugs (e.g., fluconazole, itraconazole, voriconazole, posaconazole) inhibits the synthesis of ergosterol, thereby damaging the integrity of the fungal cytoplasmic membrane. Both types of drugs bind to a certain extent to the cholesterol component of host cell membranes and elicit a variety of toxic side effects in treated patients. The nucleoside analog 5-fluorocytosine (5-FC) disrupts fungal RNA and DNA synthesis but without the toxicity associated with the polyene and imidazole drugs. Unfortunately, 5-FC demonstrates little or no antifungal activity against moulds or dimorphic fungi and is primarily reserved for infections caused by yeasts.

A novel class of antifungal compounds called *echinocandins* has received considerable attention because these drugs inhibit the synthesis of β-1,3-glucan, a major cell wall polysaccharide found in many fungi, including *C. albicans*, *Aspergillus* species, and *Pneumocystis carinii*. The drugs included in this class are caspofungin, micafungin, and anidulafungin. These inhibitors are available for treatment of patients with fungal infections, such as candidiasis or invasive aspergillosis, that are refractory to treatment with other antifungal agents.

Antiparasitic Agents. Because of the extreme diversity of human parasites and their growth cycles, a review of antiparasitic therapies and agents would be highly impractical and lengthy. Similar to other infectious diseases caused by eukaryotic microorganisms, treatment of parasitic illnesses is based on exploiting essential components of the parasite's metabolism or cellular anatomy that are not shared by the host. Any relatedness between the target site of the parasite and the cells of the host increases the likelihood of toxic reactions in the host.

Resistance among human parasites to standard, effective therapy is a major concern. In Africa, Asia, and South America, the incidence of chloroquine-resistant malaria (*Plasmodium falciparum*) is on the rise. Resistant strains require more complicated, expensive, and potentially toxic therapy with a combination of agents.

Immunotherapy

An exciting approach to the treatment of infectious diseases is immunotherapy. This strategy involves supplementing or stimulating the host's immune response so that the spread of a pathogen is limited or reversed. Several products are available for this purpose, including intravenous immune globulin (IVIG) and cytokines. IVIG is a pooled preparation of antibodies obtained from normal, healthy immune human donors that is infused as an intravenous solution. In theory, pathogen-specific antibodies present in the infusion facilitate neutralization, phagocytosis, and clearance of infectious agents above and beyond the capabilities of the diseased host. Hyperimmune immune globulin preparations, which are also commercially available, contain high titres of antibodies against specific pathogens, including hepatitis B virus, cytomegalovirus, rabies, and varicella-zoster virus.

Cytokines are substances produced by various cells that, in small quantities, stimulate white cell replication, phagocytosis, antibody production, and the induction of fever, inflammation, and tissue repair—all of which counteract infectious agents and hasten recovery (see Chapter 17). With the advent of genetic engineering and cloning, many cytokines, including interferons and interleukins, have been produced in the laboratory and are being evaluated experimentally as anti-infective agents. As we learn more about the action of cytokines, it becomes evident that some of the adverse reactions associated with infectious processes result from the body's own inflammatory response. Interventional therapies designed to inactivate certain cytokines such as tumour necrosis factor have proven to be helpful in animal models of infection. Potentially therapies based on the regulation of the inflammatory response will become widely used in human medicine over the next few years.

One of the most efficient but often overlooked means of preventing infectious diseases is immunization. Proper and timely adherence to recommended vaccination schedules in children and booster immunizations in adults effectively reduces the senseless spread of vaccine-preventable illnesses such as measles, mumps, pertussis, rubella, hepatitis B, and HPV, which still occur with alarming frequency. New strategies for the development of vaccines carried by harmless viral vectors are currently being developed that someday might lead to inexpensive and effective oral immunization against HIV, hepatitis C, malaria, and other potentially lethal infectious diseases.

Surgical Intervention

Before the discovery of antimicrobial agents, surgical removal of infected tissues, organs, or limbs was occasionally the only option available to prevent the demise of the infected host. Today, medicinal therapy with antibiotics and other anti-infective agents is an effective solution for most infectious diseases. However, surgical intervention is still an important option for cases in which the pathogen is resistant to available treatments. Surgical interventions may be used to hasten the recovery process by providing access to an infected site by antimicrobial agents (drainage of an abscess), cleaning the site (debridement), or removing infected organs or tissue (*e.g.,* appendectomy). In some situations, surgery may be the only means of effecting a complete cure, as in the case of endocarditis resulting in an infected heart valve, in which the diseased valve must be replaced with a mechanical or biologic valve to restore normal function. In other situations, surgical containment of a rapidly progressing infectious process such as gas gangrene may be the only means of saving a person's life.

IN SUMMARY

The ultimate outcome of any interaction between microorganisms and the human host is decided by a complex and ever-changing set of variables that take into account the overall health and physiologic function of the host and the virulence and infectious dose of the microbe. In many instances, disease is an inevitable consequence, but with continuing advances in science and technology, the majority of cases can now be eliminated or rapidly cured with appropriate therapy. It is the intent of those who study infectious diseases to understand thoroughly the pathogen, the disease course, the mechanisms of transmission, and the host response to infection. This knowledge will lead

to development of improved diagnostic techniques, revolutionary approaches to anti-infective therapy, and control or eradication of microscopic agents that cause frightening devastation and loss of life throughout the world.

BIOTERRORISM AND EMERGING GLOBAL INFECTIOUS DISEASES

After completing this section of the chapter, you should be able to meet the following objectives:

- List the infectious agents considered to pose the highest level of bioterrorism threat.
- Describe the effect of international travel on the spread of infection.
- State an important concept in containment of infections due to bioterrorism and global travel.

Bioterrorism

In October 2001, less than 1 month after the tragedy of September 11, the world became instantly acquainted with the term *bioterrorism.* By the end of November of that year, 22 cases of human anthrax (11 cutaneous and 11 inhalation) had been identified in the United States, resulting in five deaths, and all cases were associated with exposure to four intentionally contaminated envelopes delivered through the U.S. Postal Service. The reality of the 2001 outbreak brought a new sense of awareness concerning the use of microorganisms as weapons.

Anthrax is an ancient disease caused by the cutaneous inoculation, inhalation, or ingestion of the spores of *Bacillus anthracis,* a gram-positive bacillus. Anthrax is more commonly known as a disease of herbivores that can be transmitted to humans through contact with infected secretions, soil, or animal products. It is a rare disease, and so the sudden increase in American cases over a short time was a chilling indication that the spread of the organism had been intentional. Fortunately, the number of deaths was limited due to prompt recognition of cases and rapid initiation antimicrobial prophylaxis to exposed individuals.

To prepare for the possibility of Canadian bioterrorist attacks, Canada's Centre for Emergency Preparedness and Response works closely with Canada's National Microbiology Laboratory (NML). The NML consists of laboratories with ever-increasing expertise and responsibility, and houses the only Canadian Level 4 biocontainment facility that allows for the rapid and coordinated detection and identification of bioterrorism events under safe working conditions.

Potential agents of bioterrorism have been categorized into three levels (A, B, C) based on risk of use, transmissibility, invasiveness, and mortality rate. The agents placed in the highest bioterrorism threat level include *B. anthracis,* variola major virus (the cause of smallpox), *Yersinia pestis* (the cause of bubonic plague), *Francisella tularensis* (the cause of tularemia), and several hemorrhagic fever viruses (Ebola, Marburg, Lassa, and Junin). The toxin of the anaerobic gram-positive organism *Clostridium botulinum,* which causes the neuromuscular paralysis termed *botulism,* is also listed as a category A agent. Interestingly, purified *C. botulinum* toxins A and B are finding increasing use under the trade names Botox, Myobloc, and Neurobloc for various medicinal and cosmetic purposes. The category B agents include agents of food-borne and water-borne diseases (*Salmonella, Shigella, Vibrio cholerae, E. coli* O157:H7), agents of zoonotic infections (*Brucella* species, *C. burnetii, Burkholderia mallei*), viral encephalitides (Venezuelan, Western, and Eastern equine encephalitis viruses), as well as toxins from *S. aureus, Clostridium perfringens,* and *Ricinus communis* (the castor bean). Category C agents are defined as emerging pathogens and potential risks for the future, even though many of these organisms are causes of ancient diseases. Category C agents include *M. tuberculosis,* Nipah virus, hantavirus, tick-borne and yellow fever viruses, and the only protozoan of the group, *Cryptosporidium parvum.*

Global Infectious Diseases

Aided by a global market and the ease of international travel, the first years of the 21st century have witnessed the importation or emergence of a host of novel infectious diseases. During the late summer and early fall of 1999, West Nile virus (WNV an arthropod-borne flavivirus) was identified as the cause of an epidemic involving 56 American patients in the New York City area. This outbreak, which led to seven deaths (primarily in the elderly), marked the first time that WNV had been recognized in the Western Hemisphere since its discovery in Uganda nearly 60 years earlier. Because WNV is a mosquito-borne disease and is transmitted to a number of susceptible avian (*e.g.,* blue jays, crows, and hawks) and equine hosts, the potential for rapid and sustained spread of the disease across Canada was appreciated early. By 2002, the first Canadian case was detected. The disease ranges in intensity from a nonspecific febrile illness to fulminant meningoencephalitis. The Canadian national incidence varies dramatically from five cases in 2010 to the peak year of 2007 with 2,401 cases of WNV-associated illness identified, making this the largest arboviral meningoencephalitis outbreak ever described in the Western Hemisphere. Efforts to prevent further spread of the disease are currently centred on national surveillance of WNV-associated illness in birds, humans, and other mammals, as well as mosquito control, including use of mosquito repellent.

In the winter of 2002, SARS emerged as a global threat. The first inkling of the impending threat was when the Chinese Ministry of Health reported 305 cases of a mysterious and virulent respiratory tract illness that had appeared in Guangdong province in southern China in a 4-month period. The spread of the disease to household contacts of sick individuals and medical personnel caring for persons with the disease identified it as highly transmissible. In a very short time, patients with compatible symptoms were recognized in Hong Kong and Vietnam. The World Health Organization (WHO) promptly issued a global alert and started international surveillance for patients with typical symptomatology who had a history of travel to the endemic region. As of June 2003, more than 8,000 cases of SARS and 809 deaths from the disease in 29 countries were reported to the WHO, including 44 deaths in Toronto, Ontario. In a remarkable feat of molecular technology, the etiology of SARS was quickly determined to be a novel coronavirus, possibly of mammalian or avian origin, and its entire genome was sequenced by the end of May 2003.

In March 2014, the WHO first reported an outbreak of Ebola hemorrhagic fever in Guinea with suspected cases in Liberia and Sierra Leone. This highly contagious epidemic, largely contained to multiple West African countries and accounting for over 11,000 deaths, had the potential to spread to other global countries. This disease with a high mortality rate is caused by ebolavirus and is spread through direct skin or mucous membranes contact with infected bodily fluids or objects. Current antiviral medications are not effective against this disease and preliminarily results show that the Canadian newly developed Ebola vaccine is effective. As of 2015, the global alert and international surveillance for travellers with increased temperatures remains in effect.

These three scenarios highlight the rapidity with which novel or exotic diseases can be introduced into nonindigenous regions of the world and to a susceptible population. Although great strides in molecular microbiology have allowed for the rapid identification of new or rare microorganisms, the potential devastation in terms of human life and economic loss is great, underscoring the need to maintain resources for public health surveillance and intervention.

IN SUMMARY

The challenges associated with maintaining health throughout a global community are becoming increasingly apparent. Aided by a global market and the ease of international travel, the past decade has witnessed the importation and emergence of a host of novel infectious diseases. There is also the potential threat of the deliberate use of microorganisms as weapons of bioterrorism.

REVIEW EXERCISES

1. Newborn infants who have not yet developed an intestinal flora are routinely given an intramuscular injection of vitamin K to prevent bleeding due to a deficiency in vitamin K–dependent coagulation factors.
   A. *Use the concept of mutualism to explain why this is done.*
2. Persons with human granulocytic ehrlichiosis may be coinfected with Lyme disease.
   B. *Explain.*

3. Persons with chronic lung disease are often taught to contact their healthcare provider when they notice a change in the colour of their sputum (*i.e.,* from white or clear to yellow- or green-tinged) because it might be a sign of a bacterial infection. *C. Explain.*

4. Microorganisms are capable of causing infection only if they can grow at the temperature of the infected body site.
   D. Using this concept, explain the different sites of fungal infections due to the dermatophyte fungal species that cause tinea pedis (athlete's foot), and C. albicans, which causes infections of the mouth (thrush) and female genitalia (vulvovaginitis).

5. The threat of global infections, such as SARS and Ebola, continues to grow.
   E. What would you propose to be one of the most important functions of healthcare professionals in terms of controlling the spread of such infections?

Bibliography

Bennett J. E., Dolin R., Blaser M. J., et al. (Eds.). (2015). *Mandell, Douglas, and Bennett's principles and practice of infectious diseases* (8th ed.). Philadelphia, PA: Elsevier Saunders.

Boron W. F., Boulpaep E. L. (2009). *Medical Physiology* (2nd ed.). Philadelphia, PA: Saunders.

Centers for Disease Control and Prevention. (2014). Ebola (Ebola virus disease). Available online at: http://www.cdc.gov/vhf/ebola/index.html. Accessed November 20, 2014.

Dewar M., Harris T., McNeil S., et al. (2012). Update of human papillomavirus (HPV) vaccines. *Canada Communicable Disease Report, 38*, 1–62.

Hall J. E. (2011). *Textbook of medical physiology* (12th ed.). Philadelphia, PA: W. B. Saunders.

Henao-Restrepo A. M., Longini I. M., Egger M., et al. (2015). Efficacy and effectiveness of an rVSV-vectored vaccine expressing Ebola surface glycoprotein: Interim results from the Guinea ring vaccination cluster-randomised trial. *Lancet, 386*(9996), 857–866.

Hsueh P. R., Yang P. C. (2005). Severe acute respiratory syndrome epidemic in Taiwan, 2003. *Journal of Microbiology, Immunology and Infection, 38,* 82–88.

Kliegman R. M., Stanton B. F., St. Geme J. W., et al. (Eds.). (2011). *Nelson textbook of pediatrics* (19th ed.). Philadelphia, PA: Elsevier Saunders.

Knipe D. M., Howley P. (Eds.). (2013). *Fields virology* (6th ed.). Philadelphia, PA: Lippincott Williams and Wilkins.

Kumar V., Abbas A. K., Faustos N., et al. (Eds.). (2010). *Robbins and cotran pathologic basis of disease* (8th ed.). Philadelphia, PA: Elsevier Saunders.

Lampiris H. W., Maddix D. S. (2012). Chapter 51: Clinical use of antimicrobial agents. In Katzung B. G., Masters S. B., Trevor A. J. (Eds.), *Basic & clinical pharmacology* (12th ed.). Norwalk, CT: Appleton & Lange.

Montessory V., Harris M., Montaner J. S. G. (updated 2014). HIV infection. In Repchinsky C. (Ed.), *e-Therapeutics.* Ottawa: Canadian Pharmacists Association.

O'Brien K. K., Higdon M. L., Halverson J. J. (2003). Recognition and management of bioterrorism infections. *American Family Physician, 67*(9), 1927–1934.

Pritt B. S., Sloan L. M., Johnson D. K., et al. (2011). Emergence of a new pathogenic Ehrlichia species, Wisconsin and Minnesota, 2009. *The New England Journal of Medicine, 365*(5), 422–429.

Public Health Agency of Canada. (2010). HIV/AIDS Epi updates. Available online at: http://www.phac-aspc.gc.ca/aids-sida/publication/epi/2010/pdf/EN_Intro_Web.pdf. Accessed November 20, 2014.

Public Health Agency of Canada (PHAC). (2012). Bioterrorism and emergency preparedness. Available online at: http://www.phac-aspc.gc.ca/ep-mu/bioem-eng.php. Accessed November 20, 2014.

Rubin R., Strayer D. S. (Eds.). (2012). *Rubin's pathology: Clinicopathologic foundations of medicine* (6th ed.). Philadelphia, PA: Lippincott Williams & Wilkins.

Vaudry W., Lee B. E., Rosychuk R. J. (2014). Congenital cytomegalovirus infection in Canada: Active surveillance for cases diagnosed by paediatricians. *Paediatrics & Child Health, 19*(1), e1–e5.

Versalovic J., Carroll K. C., Funke G., Justice S. B. (Eds.). *Manual of clinical microbiology* (10th ed.). Washington, DC: American Society for Microbiology.

Weant K. A., Bailey A. M., Fleishaker E. L., Justice S. B. (2014a). Being prepared: Bioterrorism and mass prophylaxis part 1. *Advanced Emergency Nursing Journal, 36*(3), 226–238.

Weant K. A., Bailey A. M., Fleishaker E. L., Justice S. B. (2014b). Being prepared: Bioterrorism and mass prophylaxis part 2. *Advanced Emergency Nursing Journal, 36*(4), 307–317.

World Health Organization (WHO). (2014). Pandemic and epidemic diseases. Available online at: http://www.who.int/csr/disease/en./. Accessed November 20, 2014.

Zheng H., Drebot M. A., Coulthart M. B. (2014). West Nile virus in Canada: Ever-changing, but here to stay. *Canada Communicable Disease Report, 40*(10), 173–177.

Visit thePoint **http://thePoint.lww.com for animations, journal articles, and more!**

Innate and Adaptive Immunity

17

The human body is constantly exposed to potentially deleterious microorganisms and foreign substances. Therefore, it has evolved an interrelated system to defend against bacteria, viruses, and other foreign matter. Through recognition of molecular patterns, the body's immune system can distinguish itself from foreign substances and can discriminate potentially harmful from nonharmful agents. It also defends against abnormal cells and molecules that periodically develop. Although the immune response normally is protective, it also can produce undesirableeffects such as when the response is excessive, as in allergies, or when it recognizes self-tissue as foreign, as in autoimmune disease.

This chapter is divided into three parts: (1) immunity and the immune system, (2) innate immunity, and (3) adaptive immunity. The key cells, molecules, recognition systems, and effector responses integral to immunity are discussed.

IMMUNITY AND THE IMMUNE SYSTEM

After completing this section of the chapter, you should be able to meet the following objectives:

- Discuss the function of the immune system.
- Contrast and compare the general properties of innate and adaptive immunity.
- Describe the cells of the immune system.
- Characterize the chemical mediators that orchestrate the immune response.

The term *immunity* has come to mean the protection from disease and, more specifically, infectious disease. The collective, coordinated, multidimensional response initiated by the body's various defence systems is known as the *immune response*. Some of the responses become active almost immediately, while others develop slowly over time, but it is the coordinated interaction of these mechanisms that allows the body to maintain normal internal homeostasis. Although the relationship between microbes and infectious diseases dates far back in history, it has only been within the last 50 to 60 years that an understanding of the cellular and biochemical mechanisms

TABLE 17.1 FEATURES OF INNATE AND ADAPTIVE IMMUNITY

FEATURE	INNATE	ADAPTIVE
Time of response	Rapid (minutes/hours)	Slower (days/weeks)
Diversity	Limited to classes or groups of microbes	Very large; specific for each unique antigen
Microbe recognition	General patterns on microbes; nonspecific	Specific to microbes and antigens
Nonself recognition	Yes	Yes
Response to repeated infection	Similar with each exposure	Immunologic memory; more rapid and efficient with subsequent exposure
Defence	Barriers (skin, mucous membranes), phagocytes, inflammation, fever	Cell killing; tagging of antigen by antibody for removal
Cells	Phagocytes (macrophages, neutrophils), innate lymphoid cells (natural killer cells), dendritic cells	T and B lymphocytes, dendritic cells
Molecules	Cytokines, complement proteins, acute-phase proteins, soluble mediators	Antibodies, cytokines, complement proteins

involved has begun to emerge in both the innate and adaptive immune responses.

Innate and Adaptive Immunity

There are two host defences that cooperate to protect the body—the early, rapid responses of innate immunity and the very effective, but later responses of adaptive immunity (Table 17.1). As the first line of defence, *innate immunity* (also called *natural* or *native immunity*) consists of the physical, chemical, molecular, and cellular defences that are in place before infection and can function immediately as an effective barrier to microbes. *Adaptive* (also called *specific* or *acquired*) *immunity* is the second major immune defence, responding less rapidly than innate immunity but more effectively. Adaptive immunity uses focused recognition of each unique type of foreign agent followed in days by an amplified and effective response.

The major components of innate immunity are the skin and mucous membranes; phagocytic cells (mainly neutrophils and macrophages); specialized innate lymphoid cells (ILCs) that include *natural killer (NK) cells;* and several plasma proteins, including the proteins of the complement system. The innate immune system is able to distinguish self from nonself and is able to recognize and react against classes of microbial agents. The response of the innate immune system is rapid, usually within minutes to hours, and prevents the establishment of infection and deeper tissue penetration of microorganisms. The effector responses used by the innate immune system to eliminate the microbes are very similar for different classes of microorganisms. Although most innate responses are very effective in controlling and destroying the invader, pathogenic microbes have evolved several approaches to evade innate defences. The microorganisms not controlled by innate immunity are usually controlled by the more specific approaches of adaptive immunity.

The adaptive immune system consists of lymphocytes and their products, including antibodies. Whereas the cells of the innate immune system recognize structures shared by classes of microorganisms, the cells of the adaptive immune system (*i.e.,* lymphocytes) are capable of recognizing a vast array of substances produced by microorganisms as well as noninfectious substances and developing a specific immune response that differs with each substance. Substances that elicit adaptive immune responses are called *antigens.* A memory of the substance is also developed so that a repeat exposure to the same microbe or agent produces a quicker and more vigorous response. The practical aspect of immunization is based on this ability to generate an adaptive memory response. There are two types of adaptive immune responses: humoral and cell-mediated immunity. *Humoral immunity,* generated by *B lymphocytes,* is mediated by molecules called *antibodies* and is the principal defence against extracellular microbes and toxins. *Cell-mediated immunity,* or *cellular immunity,* is mediated by specific *T lymphocytes* (*e.g.,* T-helper and T-cytotoxic lymphocytes) and defends against intracellular microbes such as viruses.

An intact innate immune mechanism facilitates the initiation of the adaptive immune response, and cooperation between both systems is essential. Dendritic cells are integral to both innate and adaptive immunity and serve as a link between the two immune responses. As a result, innate immune cells are capable of communicating important information to lymphocytes involved in adaptive immunity the characteristics of the pathogen and information about its intracellular or extracellular location. The innate immune response also stimulates and influences the nature of adaptive immune responses. At the effector stage of immunity, the adaptive immune response amplifies and increases its efficiency by recruitment and activation of additional phagocytes and molecules of the innate immune system. Both innate and adaptive immunity destroy the invading agent by using the effector responses of phagocytosis and the complement system. Thus, immunity is truly an interactive, cooperative effort.

Cells of the Immune System

There are a large number of diverse cell types involved in the immune response, including phagocytic leukocytes, lymphocytes, and antigen-presenting cells (APCs). These cell

Understanding | Innate and Adaptive Immunity

The body's defence against microbes is mediated by two types of immunity: (1) innate immunity and (2) adaptive immunity. Both types of immunity are members of an integrated system in which numerous cells and molecules function cooperatively to protect the body against foreign invaders. The innate immune system stimulates adaptive immunity and influences the nature of the adaptive immune responses to make them more effective. Although they use different mechanisms of pathogen recognition, both types of immunity use many of the same effector mechanisms, including destruction of the pathogen by phagocytosis and the complement system.

1. Innate Immunity

Innate immunity (also called *natural immunity*) consists of the cellular and biochemical defences that are in place before an encounter with an infectious agent and provide rapid protection against infection. The major effector components of innate immunity include epithelial cells, which block the entry of infectious agents and secrete antimicrobial enzymes, proteins, and peptides; phagocytic neutrophils and macrophages, which engulf and digest microbes; innate lymphoid cells (ILCs) including natural killer (NK) cells, which kill intracellular microbes and foreign agents; and the complement system, which amplifies the inflammatory response and uses the membrane attack response to lyse microbes. The cells of the innate immune system also produce chemical messengers that stimulate and influence the adaptive immune response.

The innate immune system uses pattern recognition receptors (PRRs) that recognize microbial structures (*e.g.*, sugars, lipid molecules, proteins) that are shared by microbes and are often necessary for their survival, but are not present on human cells. Thus, the innate immune system is able to distinguish between self and nonself, but is unable to distinguish between agents.

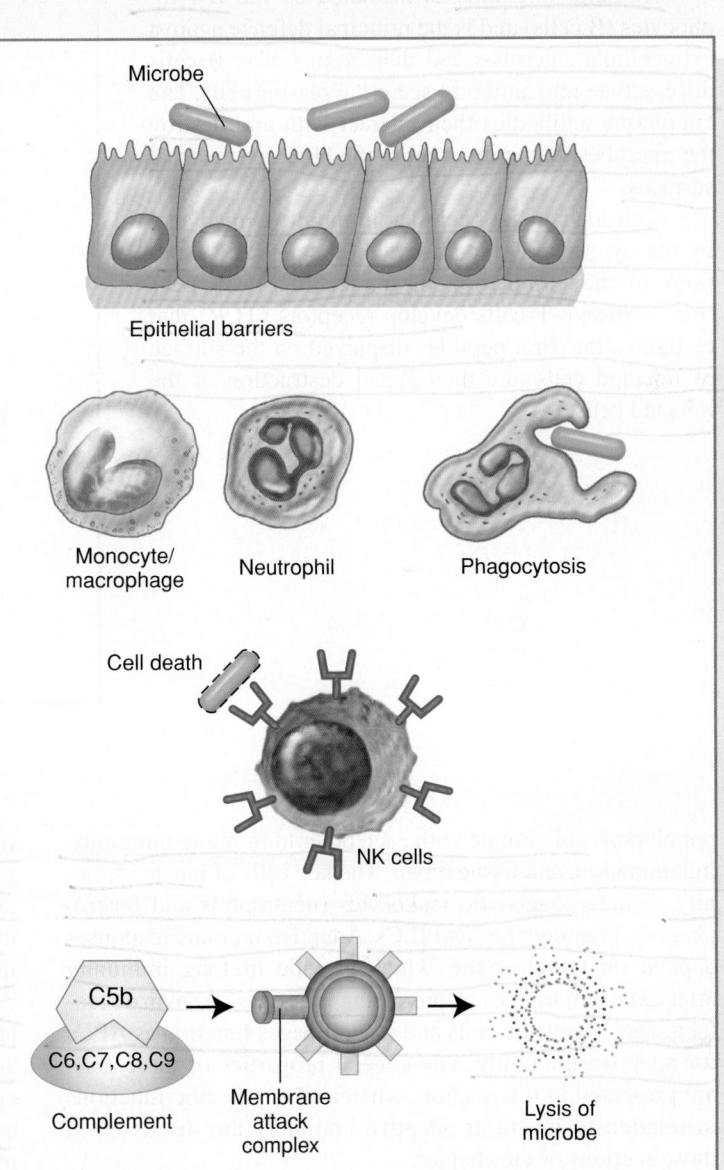

Microbe

Epithelial barriers

Monocyte/macrophage   Neutrophil   Phagocytosis

Cell death

NK cells

C5b

C6,C7,C8,C9

Complement

Membrane attack complex

Lysis of microbe

2. Adaptive Immunity

Adaptive immunity (also called *acquired immunity*) refers to immunity that is acquired through previous exposure to infectious and other foreign agents. A defining characteristic of adaptive immunity is the ability not only to distinguish self from nonself, but to recognize and destroy specific foreign agents based on their distinct antigenic properties. The components of the adaptive immune system are the T and B lymphocytes and their products. There are two types of adaptive immune responses, humoral and cell-mediated immunity, that function to eliminate different types of microbes.

Humoral immunity is mediated by the B lymphocytes (B cells) and is the principal defence against extracellular microbes and their toxins. The B cells differentiate into antibody-secreting plasma cells. The circulating antibodies then interact with and destroy the microbes that are present in the blood or mucosal surfaces.

Cell-mediated, or cellular, immunity is mediated by the cytotoxic T lymphocytes (T cells) and functions in the elimination of intracellular pathogens (*e.g.,* viruses). T cells develop receptors (TCR) that recognize the viral peptides displayed on the surface of infected cells and then signal destruction of the infected cells.

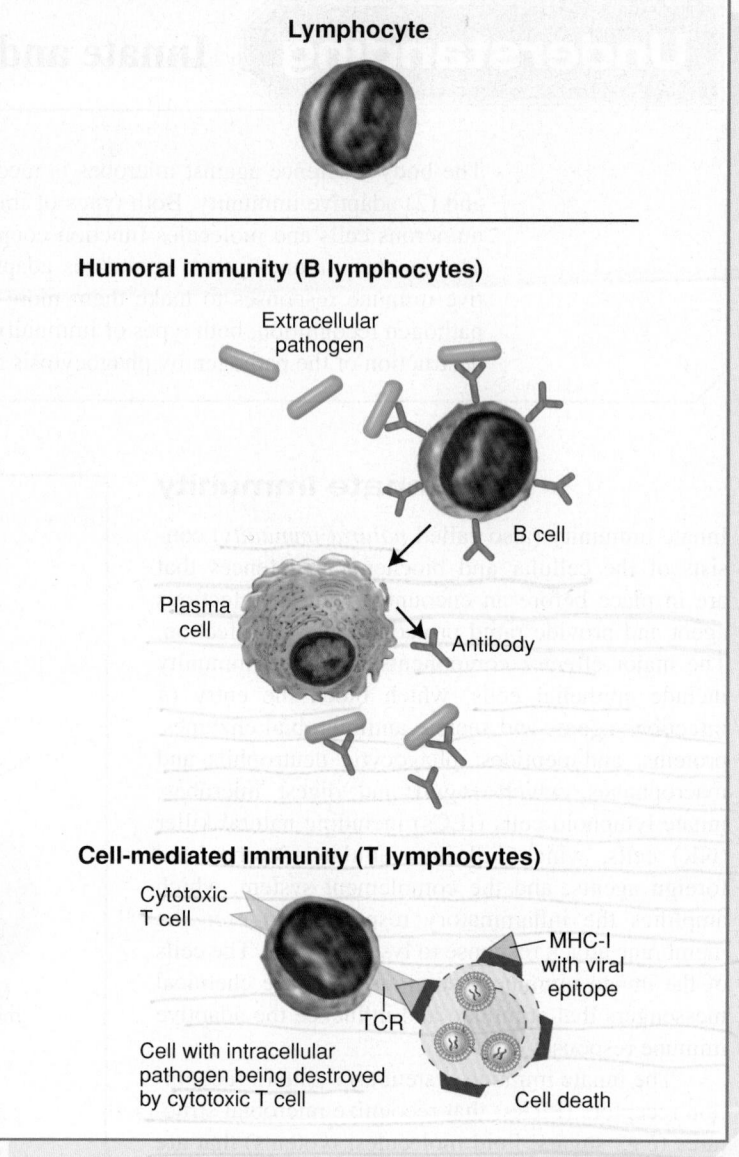

Lymphocyte

Humoral immunity (B lymphocytes)

Extracellular pathogen

B cell

Plasma cell

Antibody

Cell-mediated immunity (T lymphocytes)

Cytotoxic T cell

MHC-I with viral epitope

TCR

Cell with intracellular pathogen being destroyed by cytotoxic T cell

Cell death

populations collaborate with each other to promote immunity, inflammation, and tissue repair. The key cells of innate immunity include phagocytic leukocytes (neutrophils and macrophages), granulocytes, and ILCs. Adaptive immune responses depend on lymphocytes, which provide lifelong immunity after exposure to disease-producing microbes or environmental agents. Dendritic cells and macrophages function as APCs for adaptive immunity. The general properties of these cells are presented in this section, whereas their specific functions in relation to innate or adaptive immunity are discussed in those sections of the chapter.

Phagocytic Leukocytes

Leukocytes are subclassified into two general groups based on the presence or absence of specific staining granules in their cytoplasm. Cells containing granules are classified as granulocytes (neutrophils, eosinophils, and basophils) and cells that lack granules are classified as agranulocytes (lymphocytes, monocytes, and macrophages). Neutrophils, which are named for their neutral-staining granules, are the early-responding cells of innate immunity. Macrophages are part of the monocytic phagocyte system. During an inflammation response, the monocyte leaves the blood vessel, transforms into a tissue macrophage, and phagocytizes bacteria, damaged cells, and tissue debris (discussed in Chapter 18). Both neutrophils and macrophages are equipped with recognition receptors, phagocytic potential, antimicrobial molecules, and metabolic systems for producing toxic oxygen and nitrogen intermediates for killing infectious agents.

In addition to phagocytosis, macrophages function early in the immune response to amplify the inflammatory response and initiate adaptive immunity. Macrophages direct these processes through the secretion of cell communication molecules that initiate and coordinate the inflammatory response or activate lymphocytes. Macrophages also function at the end of an immune response as effector cells in both humoral and cell-mediated immune responses. Macrophages can remove antigen–antibody aggregates or, under the influence of T cells, they can destroy virus-infected cells or tumour cells.

Lymphocytes

There are three distinct subtypes of lymphocytes: B lymphocytes, T lymphocytes, and the most recently identified constituents, the ILCs, which include the NK cells. These subtypes are different in their functions and protein products but are morphologically similar.

T and B Lymphocytes. T and B lymphocytes represent 25% to 35% of blood leukocytes. They are the only cells in the body capable of specifically recognizing different antigenic determinants of microbial agents and other pathogens and therefore are responsible for two defining characteristics of adaptive immunity, specificity and memory.

Like other blood cells, T and B lymphocytes are generated from hematopoietic stem cells in the bone marrow. Undifferentiated immature lymphocytes congregate in the central lymphoid tissues, where they develop into distinct types of mature lymphocytes. One class of lymphocyte, the *B lymphocytes* (B cells), is essential for humoral immunity. The other class of lymphocyte, the *T lymphocytes*, is responsible for cell-mediated immunity, as well as aiding in antibody production. The various types of lymphocytes are distinguished by their function and response to antigen, cell membrane molecules and receptors, types of secreted proteins, and tissue location.

Lymphocyte Markers and the CD Nomenclature System. From the time that functionally distinct types of lymphocytes were first recognized, immunologists have worked to develop methods for distinguishing them. The development of laboratory reagents such as monoclonal antibodies allowed the recognition of distinct classes of lymphocytes based on their unique pattern of cell surface proteins. These identified proteins were then correlated with cell functions. The standard nomenclature for these proteins is the "CD" (clusters of differentiation) numeric designation (CD1, CD2), which is used to delineate surface proteins that define a particular cell type or stage of cell differentiation and are recognized by a cluster or group of antibodies. Although this nomenclature was originally developed for lymphocytes, it is now common practice to refer to homologous markers on cells other than lymphocytes by the same CD designation.

The classification of lymphocytes and other immune cells by CD antigen expression is now widely used in clinical medicine and experimental immunology. For example, the declining number of blood $CD4^+$ T cells is often used to follow the disease progression and response to treatment of persons with human immunodeficiency virus (HIV) infection. Further investigation of the CD molecules has shown that they are not merely phenotypic markers of cell type but

are themselves involved in a variety of lymphocyte functions, including promotion of cell-to-cell adhesion and transduction of signals that lead to lymphocyte activation.

Innate Lymphoid Cells. This most recently discovered class of cells is derived from a common lymphoid progenitor cell in the bone marrow, and while they have similar characteristic to the T cells, none of the three constituent groups (*i.e.,* innate lymphoid cells group 1 [ILC1s], ILC2s, ILC3s) has specific antigen receptors. Each of the groups produces different types of cytokines and plays a key role in innate immunity, inflammation, lymphoid tissue formation, and tissue remodelling and repair. The cytotoxic NK cells, the first and best described ILCs, are a subtype of ILC1s and do not bear T-cell receptors (TCRs) or cell surface immunoglobulins. Morphologically, they are somewhat larger than the smaller T and B lymphocytes and contain abundant cytoplasmic granules. NK cells are part of the innate immune system, and may be the first line of defence against viral infections. They also have the ability to recognize and kill tumour cells, abnormal body cells, and cells infected with *intracellular pathogens,* such as viruses and intracellular bacteria. Two cell surface molecules, CD16 and CD56, are widely used to identify NK cells. CD16 serves as a receptor for the immunoglobulin (Ig) G molecule, which provides NK cells with the ability to lyse IgG-coated target cells. ILC2s under the control of other cytokines produce a dynamic response to extracellular parasitic infections, and ILC3s seem to mediate the balance between intestinal microbiota and immunity. This robust area of research continues to generate new information and understanding of the complexities of immune responses.

Dendritic Cells

Dendritic cells are specialized, bone marrow–derived leukocytes found in lymphoid tissue that are another important intermediary between the innate and adaptive immune systems. Most dendritic cells are found as immature cells under epithelial tissue and in most organs, where they are poised to capture foreign agents and transport them to peripheral lymphoid organs. Once activated, they undergo a complex maturation process as they migrate to the first regional lymph node. These cells function as key APCs that are needed to initiate adaptive immunity, by processing and presenting molecules of the foreign antigen to the lymphocytes. Thus, the dendritic cell functions as an important intermediary between innate and adaptive immunity. Dendritic cells, like macrophages, also release several communication molecules that direct the nature of innate and adaptive immune responses.

Cytokines That Mediate and Regulate Immunity

Although cells of both the innate and adaptive immune systems communicate critical information by cell-to-cell contact, many interactions and effector responses depend on the secretion of short-acting, biologically active, soluble molecules

TABLE 17.2 CYTOKINES OF INNATE AND ADAPTIVE IMMUNITY

CYTOKINES	SOURCE	BIOLOGIC ACTIVITY
Interleukin-1 (IL-1)	Macrophages, endothelial cells, some epithelial cells	Wide variety of biologic effects; activates endothelium in inflammation; induces fever and acute-phase response; stimulates neutrophil production
Interleukin-2 (IL-2)	CD4$^+$, CD8$^+$ T cells	Growth factor for activated T cells; induces synthesis of other cytokines; activates cytotoxic T lymphocytes and NK cells
Interleukin-3 (IL-3)	CD4$^+$ T cells	Growth factor for progenitor hematopoietic cells
Interleukin-4 (IL-4)	CD4$^+$ T$_H$2 cells, mast cells	Promotes growth and survival of T, B, and mast cells; causes T$_H$2 cell differentiation; activates B cells and eosinophils and induces IgE-type responses
Interleukin-5 (IL-5)	CD4$^+$ T$_H$2 cells	Induces eosinophil growth and development
Interleukin-6 (IL-6)	Macrophages, endothelial cells, T lymphocytes	Stimulates the liver to produce mediators of acute-phase inflammatory response; also induces proliferation of antibody-producing cells by the adaptive immune system
Interleukin-7 (IL-7)	Bone marrow stromal cells	Primary function in adaptive immunity; stimulates pre-B cells and thymocyte development and proliferation
Interleukin-8 (IL-8)	Macrophages, endothelial cells	Primary function in adaptive immunity; chemoattracts neutrophils and T lymphocytes; regulates lymphocyte homing and neutrophil infiltration
Interleukin-10 (IL-10)	Macrophages, some T-helper cells	Inhibitor of activated macrophages and dendritic cells; decreases inflammation by inhibiting T$_H$1 cells and release of IL-12 from macrophages
Interleukin-12 (IL-12)	Macrophages, dendritic cells	Enhances NK cell cytotoxicity in innate immunity; induces T$_H$1 cell differentiation in adaptive immunity
Type I interferons (IFN-α, IFN-β)	Macrophages, fibroblasts	Inhibit viral replication, activate NK cells, and increase expression of MHC-I molecules on virus-infected cells
Interferon-γ (IFN-γ)	NK cells, CD4$^+$ and CD8$^+$ T lymphocytes	Activates macrophages in both innate immune responses and adaptive cell-mediated immune responses; increases expression of MHC-I and -II and antigen processing and presentation
Tumour necrosis factor-α (TNF-α)	Macrophages, T cells	Induces inflammation, fever, and acute-phase response; activates neutrophils and endothelial cells; kills cells through apoptosis
Chemokines	Macrophages, endothelial cells, T lymphocytes	Large family of structurally similar cytokines that stimulate leukocyte movement and regulate the migration of leukocytes from the blood to the tissues
Granulocyte-monocyte CSF (GM-CSF)	T cells, macrophages, endothelial cells, fibroblasts	Promotes neutrophil, eosinophil, and monocyte maturation and growth; activates mature granulocytes
Granulocyte CSF (G-CSF)	Macrophages, fibroblasts, endothelial cells	Promotes growth and maturation of neutrophils consumed in inflammatory reactions
Monocyte CSF (M-CSF)	Macrophages, activated T cells, endothelial cells	Promotes growth and maturation of mononuclear phagocytes

CD, cluster of differentiation; CSF, colony-stimulating factor; NK, natural killer; T$_H$1, T-helper type 1; T$_H$2, T-helper type 2; MHC, major histocompatibility complex.

called *cytokines*. Chemotactic cytokines or *chemokines* are a family of cytokines that direct leukocyte movement and migration, and colony-stimulating factors (CSFs) are cytokines that promote the proliferation and differentiation of bone marrow progenitor cells. The sources and properties of the main cytokines that participate in innate and adaptive immunity are summarized in Table 17.2.

General Properties of Cytokines

Cytokines are low–molecular-weight, regulatory, pro- or anti-inflammatory proteins that are produced by cells of the innate and adaptive immune systems and that mediate many of the actions of these cells. Cytokines were originally named for the general cell type that produced them (*e.g.,* monokines for

those produced by monocytes and lymphokines for those produced by lymphocytes). With the development of advanced technology, however, it became clear that the same protein can be produced by monocytes, lymphocytes, and a variety of tissue cells, including endothelial cells. Therefore, the generic term *cytokine* has become the preferred name for this class of mediators. Cytokines are also named for the biologic property that was first ascribed to them. For example, *interleukins* (ILs) are synthesized by leukocytes and act on other leukocytes, and *interferons* (IFNs) interfere with virus multiplication.

Although cytokines have many diverse actions, all share several important properties. All cytokines are secreted in a brief, self-limited manner. They are not usually stored as preformed molecules and their synthesis is limited to new gene transcription resulting from cellular activation. The actions of cytokines are often pleiotropic and redundant. Pleiotropism refers to the ability of a cytokine to act on different cell types. For example, IL-2, initially discovered as a T-cell growth factor, is also known to affect the growth of B cells and NK cells. Interferon-γ is the key macrophage-activating cytokine that functions in both innate and adaptive immune responses. Although pleiotropism allows cytokines to mediate diverse effects, it greatly limits their use for therapeutic purposes because of numerous unwanted side effects. Redundancy refers to the ability of different cytokines to stimulate the same or overlapping biologic functions. Because of this redundancy, antagonists against a single cytokine may not have functional consequences because other cytokines may compensate.

Not only are the actions of cytokines pleiotropic and redundant, but cytokines are produced by several different cell types. For example, IL-1 can be produced by virtually all leukocytes, endothelial cells, and fibroblasts. Cytokines often influence the synthesis and actions of other cytokines. The ability of one cytokine to stimulate the production of others often leads to cascades in which the second and third cytokines may mediate the biologic effects of the first. Cytokines may also serve as antagonists to inhibit the action of another cytokine or, in some cases, they may produce additive or greater-than-anticipated effects.

Cytokine actions may be local or systemic. Most cytokines act close to where they are produced, acting on the same cell that secreted the cytokine (autocrine mechanism), or they may influence the activity of nearby cells in a paracrine fashion. When produced in large amounts, cytokines may enter the bloodstream and exert their action on distant cells in an endocrine manner, the best examples being IL-1 and tumour necrosis factor-α (TNF-α), which produce the systemic acute-phase response during inflammation.

Cytokines generate their responses by binding to specific receptors on their target cells. Many cytokine receptors share a common structural shape and a cytoplasmic tail that interacts with a family of signalling proteins (Janus kinases [JAKs]). These signalling molecules then interact with cytoplasmic intermediary molecules (signal transducers and activators of transcription [STATs]) that are responsible for the induction of the genes for cell responses.

Chemokines

Chemokines are cytokines that stimulate the migration and activation of immune and inflammatory cells. Chemokines are synthesized as secretory proteins consisting of approximately 70 to 130 amino acids, and they are divided into subfamilies based on the molecular position of the first two cysteine residues and intermolecular disulfide bonds with or without amino acid placements. The major subclasses include C, CC, CX3C, and CXC chemokines. In the CC subclass, the first two cysteines are adjacent to each other; in CXC they are separated by an amino acid. The largest family, the CC chemokines attract mononuclear leukocytes to sites of chronic inflammation. The CXC chemokines attract neutrophils to sites of acute inflammation.

Chemokines are named according to structure, followed by "L" and the number of their gene (e.g., CCL1, CXCL1). Likewise, chemokine receptors are named according to the structure, followed by an "R" and a number (e.g., CCR1, CXCR1). Six receptors for CXC (CXCRs) and 10 for CC (CCRs) chemokines have been characterized in terms of their structure and function. Most receptors recognize more than one chemokine, and most chemokines recognize more than one receptor. Binding of a chemokine to a receptor can result in agonist or antagonist activity, with the same chemokine acting as an agonist at one type of receptor and as an antagonist at another.

Chemokines are implicated in a number of acute and chronic diseases, including atherosclerosis, rheumatoid arthritis, inflammatory bowel disease (Crohn's disease, ulcerative colitis), allergic asthma and chronic bronchitis, multiple sclerosis, systemic lupus erythematosus, and HIV infection. To enter target cells, HIV type 1 requires two distinct elements: the CD4 recognition molecule of the helper T cell and either the CXCR4 or CCR5 chemokine. The targeting of T cells and monocytes allows HIV-1 access to sanctuary sites throughout the body and also cripples the CD4+ T-helper cells that orchestrate antiviral immunity (discussed in Chapter 20). Genetic evidence of the central role of CCR5 in the pathogenesis of HIV-1 came from the identification of multiply exposed noninfected persons, who proved to be homozygous for a nonfunctional variant of CCR5. Drugs that target these chemokine receptors for HIV are currently in advanced clinical trials.

Colony-Stimulating Factors

Colony-stimulating factors (CSFs) are cytokines that stimulate bone marrow pluripotent stem and progenitor or precursor cells to produce large numbers of platelets, erythrocytes, lymphocytes, neutrophils, monocytes, eosinophils, basophils, and dendritic cells. The CSFs were named according to the type of target cell on which they act (see Table 17.2). GM-CSF acts on the granulocyte–monocyte progenitor cells to produce monocytes, neutrophils, and dendritic cells; G-CSF specifically induces neutrophil proliferation; and M-CSF directs the mononuclear phagocyte progenitor. Other cytokines, including IL-3, IL-7, and IL-11, also influence hematopoiesis (see Chapter 12). Recombinant CSF molecules are being used to increase the success rates of bone marrow transplantations. The availability of recombinant CSFs and cytokines offers the possibility of several clinical therapies where stimulation or inhibition of the immune response or cell production is desirable.

IN SUMMARY

Immunity is the resistance to a disease that is provided by the immune system. Immune mechanisms can be divided into two types: innate and adaptive immunity. Innate immunity is the first line of defence against microbial agents. It can distinguish between self and nonself through recognition of conserved broad patterns on microbes. Adaptive immunity involves humoral and cellular mechanisms that respond to a unique antigen, can amplify and sustain its responses, distinguish self from nonself, and remembers the antigen to quickly produce a heightened response on subsequent encounters with the same agent. There is a dynamic interplay between innate and adaptive immunity both in the early initiation stages and the final response to the foreign invader.

The cellular components of the innate and adaptive immunity include the T and B lymphocytes, ILCs (NK cells), dendritic cells, and phagocytic leukocytes (neutrophils and macrophages). The phagocytic leukocytes, ILCs, and dendritic cells participate in innate immunity. The T and B lymphocytes are the only cells in the body capable of specifically recognizing different antigenic determinants of microbial agents and other pathogens and therefore are responsible for two defining characteristics of adaptive immunity, specificity and memory.

Although cells of both the innate and adaptive immune systems communicate critical information about the invading microbe or pathogen by cell-to-cell contact, many interactions and effector responses depend on the secretion of chemical mediators (cytokines, chemokines, and CSFs). Cytokines are soluble proteins secreted by cells of both the innate and adaptive immune systems that mediate many of the functions of these cells. Chemokines are cytokines that stimulate the migration and activation of immune and inflammatory cells. CSFs stimulate the growth and differentiation of bone marrow progenitors of immune cells.

CONCEPTSin action**ANIMATION**

INNATE IMMUNITY

After completing this section of the chapter, you should be able to meet the following objectives:

- Characterize the function of the innate immune system.
- Describe components of the innate immune system, including epithelial barriers, soluble chemical agents, and cellular components.
- Describe the recognition systems for pathogens in innate immunity.
- State the types and functions of leukocytes that participate in innate immunity.
- Describe the functions of the various cytokines involved in innate immunity.
- Define the role of the complement system in immunity and inflammation.

The innate immune system consists of the epithelial barriers, phagocytic cells (mainly neutrophils and macrophages), ILCs, and several plasma proteins, including those of the complement system. These mechanisms are present in the body before an encounter with an infectious agent and are rapidly

INNATE IMMUNITY

- Innate immunity consists of physical, chemical, cellular, and molecular defences that are ready for activation and mediate rapid, initial protection against infection.
- Skin and mucous membranes are highly effective physical barriers against microorganisms. Antimicrobial molecules can effectively kill a wide variety of microbes.
- The cells of innate immunity express PRRs that bind with broad patterns shared by groups of microbes but not present on mammalian cells. Toll-like receptors, a major type of PRR, are expressed on phagocytes and are potent activators of innate immune system cells and molecules.
- The effector responses of innate immunity involve the inflammatory response, the complement system, ILCs, and phagocytosis by neutrophils and monocyte/macrophages.
- Cytokines released from activated leukocytes regulate the activity of other cells, amplify inflammation, stimulate the production of acute-phase proteins, and aid in the initiation of an adaptive immune response.

activated by microbes before the development of adaptive immunity. The innate immune system also interacts with and directs adaptive immune responses.

With the ever-expanding wealth of information on immune system function, it is becoming clear that the innate immune system not only protects against microbial agents, but may play a role in the pathogenesis of disease. Among the functions of the innate immune system is induction of a complex cascade of events known as the *inflammatory response* (discussed in Chapter 18). Recent evidence suggests that inflammation plays a key role in the pathogenesis of a number of disorders such as atherosclerosis and coronary artery disease, bronchial asthma, type 2 diabetes mellitus, rheumatoid arthritis, multiple sclerosis, and systemic lupus erythematosus.

Epithelial Barriers

Physical and chemical barriers against infection are found in all common portals of entry of microbes, namely, the skin and respiratory, gastrointestinal, and urogenital tracts. The intact skin is a formidable physical barrier because of its closely packed cells, multiple layering, continuous shedding of cells, and presence of the protective protein keratin. In addition to its barrier function, the skin has simple chemicals that create a nonspecific, salty, acidic environment and antibacterial proteins, such as the enzyme lysozyme, that inhibit the colonization of microorganisms and aid in their destruction.

The mucous membrane linings of the gastrointestinal, respiratory, and urogenital tracts are protected by sheets of tightly packed epithelial cells that block the entry of microbes and destroy them by secreting antimicrobial enzymes, proteins, and peptides. Specialized cells in these linings, such as the goblet cells in the gastrointestinal tract, secrete a viscous material consisting of high–molecular-weight glycoproteins known as mucins, which when hydrated form *mucus*. Mucus traps and washes away potential invaders, especially with the help of additional secretions such as saliva and excess mucus. Also in the lower respiratory tract, hairlike structures called *cilia* protrude through the epithelial cells. The synchronous action of the cilia moves many microbes trapped in the mucus toward the throat. The physiologic responses of coughing and sneezing further aid in their removal from the body.

Once microbes are trapped, various chemical defences come into play. These include lysozyme, a hydrolytic enzyme capable of cleaving the walls of bacterial cells; complement, which binds and aggregates bacteria to increase their susceptibility to phagocytosis or disrupt their lipid membrane; and members of the *collectin* family of surfactant proteins (*e.g.,* hydrophilic surfactants [SP]-A and SP-D) in the respiratory tract (see Chapter 27). Both SP-A and SP-D bind a variety of pathogens and are important defence molecules in the lung. The best-defined function of the collectins is their ability to opsonize pathogens, including bacteria and viruses, and to facilitate phagocytosis by innate immune cells such as macrophages. SP-A and SP-D also regulate production of inflammatory mediators. In the stomach and intestines, death of microbes results from the action of digestive enzymes, acidic conditions, and secretions of *defencins,* small cationic peptides that kill within minutes both gram-positive and gram-negative microorganisms by disrupting the microbial membrane.

Some pathogens can penetrate the anatomic layers of the host and cause physiologic changes that result in infectious disease. The subsequent innate immune response to the penetration of these invaders is initiated by various leukocytes through their recognition of common molecular motifs on microbes.

Cells of Innate Immunity

Several types of innate immune cells with receptors for recognition of general groups of microbes can provide an array of responses to the invader. The key cells of innate immunity include neutrophils, macrophages, dendritic cells, and ILCs.

Neutrophils and Macrophages

Several phagocytic cells recruited during an inflammatory response are innate immune cells that recognize and kill infectious invaders. The early-responding innate immune cell is the neutrophil, followed shortly by the more efficient, multifunctional macrophage. Phagocytes are activated to engulf and digest microbes that attach to their cell membrane. The initial attachment of the microbe to the phagocyte can be aided by pathogen-associated molecular pattern receptors (*i.e.,* Toll-like receptors), receptors for opsonins (*e.g.,* complement or antibodies), and receptors for lectins. Once the cell is activated and the microbe is ingested, the cell generates digestive enzymes

and toxic oxygen and nitrogen intermediates (*i.e.,* hydrogen peroxide or nitric oxide) through metabolic pathways. The phagocytic killing of microorganisms helps to contain infectious agents until adaptive immunity can be marshalled.

Innate Lymphoid Cells and Natural Killer Cells

Other cells involved in innate immunity include the family of lymphocytes that provide a quick response to nonspecific danger signals—namely the three groups of ILCs. ILCs have three key features: they do not express the specific, highly diverse receptors or antibodies associated with adaptive immunity; they lack dendritic cell markers; and they have characteristics of lymphoid morphology. Like other cells in the innate immune system, they can recognize only broad patterns associated with classes of microbes. Although many names have been used to denote cells within these groups (*i.e.,* NK cells, natural helper cells, intraepithelial lymphocytes, lymphoid tissue–inducer cells), the proposed classification for ILC populations is now based on their phenotypical and functional characteristics.

The ILC groups are analogous to the T-helper 1, T-helper 2, and T-helper 17 subsets of the CD4+ T lymphocytes that secrete some of the same cytokines. The ILCs generally are noncytotoxic and offer frontline protection, conversely the T-cell subsets are highly antigen specific, allowing them to target and destroy unwanted pathogens. When a pathogen is detected, the ILCs release high concentrations of their cytokines, which promotes the rapid mobilization of specific cells and mediators appropriate for the offending agents. Group 1 ILCs (ILC1s) are capable of producing interferon-γ (IFN-γ) and respond to intracellular bacteria, viruses, and tumour cells. ILC2s produce T-helper 2 lymphocyte cell–associated cytokines, which are adept at targeting helminths or parasitic infection. Finally, ILC3s produce T-helper 17 cell–associated cytokines that promote lymphoid tissue development, and work at an epithelial cell level with pro-inflammatory and tissue reparative functions.

Only NK cells, the most well-known and extensively studied subset of ILC1s, have cytotoxic capacity. They can control their responses by using both activating and inhibitory receptors. Their activating receptors (*i.e.,* killer cell receptors) recognize altered host molecules expressed on stressed tissue cells that may be infected with intracellular microbes. The inhibitory receptors on NK cells recognize molecules (major histocompatibility complex [MHC]-I, lectins) on normal host cells and function to stop the killing response of NK cells. This control ensures that normal body cells are not inappropriately destroyed. In contrast to the cytotoxic T lymphocyte, which needs to undergo amplification and maturation to become cytotoxic, the NK cell is programmed directly to kill foreign cells. Depending on the type or combination of NK cell receptors that are activated, the effect is cell death or no response. If an abnormal cell is correctly recognized, the NK cells will cause the death of the altered target cell by producing pore-forming proteins (*i.e.,* NK perforins), enzymes, and toxic cytokines.

Other ICLs, which express a receptor similar in general structure to the TCR, often recognize microbial lipids and other structures that are shared by microbes of the same type. Although they appear to function as early sentinels against infectious microbes at the epithelial layers, our knowledge of how they function continues to expand.

Pathogen Recognition

The ability of any of the leukocytes to participate in innate immunity depends on first recognizing the invader. The leukocyte receptors that bind these microbial molecules may be membrane-associated receptors or soluble pattern recognition molecules that first tag the microbes and subsequently bind to their complementary membrane receptors on the phagocytes. The impact of microbial binding to the leukocyte membrane receptors is cell activation, phagocytosis, and subsequent killing of the microorganisms. The key families of leukocyte PRRs involved in innate immunity include the Toll-like receptors and receptors for opsonins that promote phagocytosis.

Pattern Recognition

The cells of the innate immune system must recognize and react to invading microorganisms or damaged cells. The initial sensing of an organism's presence or cellular by-products is mediated by *PRRs*. They recognize molecular patterns present on pathogens (*pathogen-associated molecular patterns* or PAMPs) or products of cellular damage (*damage-associated molecular patterns* or DAMPs). The PAMPs are composed of combinations of sugars, lipid molecules, proteins, or patterns of modified nucleic acids. The recognized microbial structures are essential to the functioning, viability, and infectivity of the pathogen and are defined as "conserved." The microbes cannot, therefore, evade innate immune recognition through mutation or a lack of production of the microbial molecules because they would not survive. Humans inherit a limited number (approximately 1,000) of germline genes for PRRs that effectively recognize major groups of microbes. In contrast, the millions of somatically rearranged genes for the unique receptors involved in adaptive immunity allow recognition of fine details of molecular structure (Fig. 17.1).

The binding of pathogens to the PRRs on leukocytes initiates the signalling events that lead to innate immunity and the tissue changes associated with acute inflammation. After the inflammatory changes in the blood vessels near the site of infection, white blood cells, neutrophils, and monocytes are directed in their migration from the blood to the tissues, along with body fluids. The blood monocytes mature into macrophages as they traverse the tissues. Resident tissue macrophages and immature dendritic cells add to the responding cellular recruits. Triggering of PRRs on these new recruits amplifies the initial inflammatory response by inducing antimicrobial genes and secreting inflammatory cytokines. These cytokines amplify the production of soluble mediators of inflammation, including soluble PRRs and complement. The soluble pathogen sensors also tag pathogens to allow

Characteristics	Innate immunity	Adaptive immunity
Recognition	Molecular patterns common to microbes Different microbes Identical mannose receptor	Specific microbial molecules Different microbes Distinct antibodies
Receptors	Limited diversity expressed by germline genes Toll-like receptor Mannose receptor	Great diversity expressed through recombination of somatic genes B-cell receptor B cell → Plasma cell → Antibody
Cellular expression	Effector cell types express identical receptors (*e.g.*, neutrophils express Toll-like receptors).	Each clone of lymphocytes expresses unique receptors.
Self–nonself discrimination	Yes, by recognizing molecules unique to pathogen, NK cells recognize MHC-I self-recognizing molecules.	Yes, lymphocytes use MHC-I and -II and foreign peptides (*e.g.*, microbial peptides in recognition).

FIGURE 17.1 • Recognition systems of innate and adaptive immunity.

for activation of the complement system. In addition to these inflammatory and killing responses, activation of PRRs on macrophages and dendritic cells can lead to their maturation, secretion of cytokines, and expression of costimulatory molecules needed for activation of adaptive immunity.

Toll-Like Receptors

The main pathogen sensors important in innate immunity include the family of PRRs called *Toll-like receptors* (TLRs). Interestingly, the first protein to be identified in this family was the *Drosophila* Toll protein, which was found on the fruit fly *Drosophila,* where it functions in embryonic development as well as in protecting the fly from lethal fungal infections. Eleven different mammalian TLRs, TLR1 through TLR11, have so far been identified based on sequence homology to *Drosophila* Toll. All of these receptors are membrane-spanning proteins that contain an external horseshoe-shaped PAMP-binding structure and an internal signalling domain essential for activating the leukocyte. The TLRs are expressed on many different cell types that participate in innate immunity, including endothelial cells, neutrophils, macrophages, dendritic cells, and NK cells.

Human TLRs are involved in responses to widely divergent types of molecules that are commonly expressed by microbial but not mammalian cell types. For example, TLR4 is essential for phagocytic recognition and response to lipopolysaccharides (LPS or endotoxin) present in gram-negative bacteria; TLR2 binds to peptidoglycan, an essential component of the cell wall of gram-positive bacteria; and TLR5 can recognize the protein flagellin found in flagellated bacteria. Although most TLRs that recognize extracellular ligands on microbes are found on the surface of the leukocytes, a few are located on the membranes of intracellular compartments of the leukocyte, where they recognize viruses and intracellular pathogens such as *Mycobacterium.* Single-stranded ribonucleic acid (RNA), expressed during intracellular virus infections, is recognized by TLR7 and TLR8.

Ligand binding to the TLR at the cell surface leads to recruitment of cytoplasmic signalling molecules and eventual activation of transcription factors, notably nuclear factor κβ (NF-κβ). NF-κβ regulates the production of a number of proteins that are important components of innate immunity. These include inflammatory cytokines, endothelial adhesion molecules, and proteins involved in the antimicrobial activities of phagocytic leukocytes. Some TLRs function individually, whereas some dimerize to themselves (*e.g.,* TLR4–TLR4) or pair with other TLRs (*e.g.,* TLR2–TLR6) to expand their recognition of PAMPs. Recent research suggests that most TLRs need a coreceptor (*e.g.,* CD14 for TLR4) to serve as an accessory molecule, and some may recognize endogenous host molecules (*e.g.,* heat-shock proteins) for tissue regeneration and repair. Alterations in the structure of TLRs or mutations in the signalling system associated with TLRs have been suggested to play a pathologic role in disorders such as atherosclerosis, allergies, and certain autoimmune diseases.

Soluble Mediators of Innate Immunity

Although cells of the innate immune system can communicate critical information about the invader and self–nonself recognition through cell-to-cell contact, soluble mediators are essential for many other aspects of the innate immune response. Development of innate immunity and regulation of the behaviour of effector cells all depend on the secretion of soluble molecules such as opsonins, cytokines, and acute-phase proteins.

Opsonins

Various soluble molecules can tag microorganisms for more efficient recognition by phagocytes. The coating of particles, such as microbes, is called *opsonization,* and the coating materials are called *opsonins.* The opsonin bound to the microbe then activates the phagocyte after attachment to a complementary receptor on the phagocyte. Opsonins important in innate immunity and acute inflammation include acute-phase proteins, lectins, and complement. With the activation of adaptive humoral immunity, IgG and IgM antibodies can coat microbes and act as an opsonin by binding to Fc receptors on neutrophils and macrophages. The adaptive immune response can thus enhance the phagocytic function of innate cells.

Inflammatory Cytokines

A wide range of cytokines are involved in innate immunity, including TNF-α, the interleukins IL-1, IL-6, and IL-12, interferons (IFN-γ, IFN-α, IFN-β), and chemokines (see Table 17.2). These cytokines are part of an integrated signalling network with extension functions. They influence the events of inflammation and innate immunity by producing chemotaxis of leukocytes, stimulating acute-phase protein production, inhibiting virus replication, and affecting the development of cells of the innate and adaptive immune systems. A leukocyte exposed to an external stimulus (*i.e.,* bacteria) can be activated through appropriately triggered receptors (*e.g.,* TLRs) and respond by secreting small amounts of cytokines and other soluble mediators. If many cells are activated, the concentration of cytokines may be sufficient to influence the function of tissues distant from the site of infection, a true endocrine action. The biologic responses associated with cytokines are also regulated by the timing of cytokine receptor expression, which is affected by the stage of activation of a cell. The short half-life of cytokines ensures that an excessive immune response and systemic activation does not usually occur.

Other cytokines of innate immunity are the IFNs, so-named because of their ability to interfere with virus infections. Although ILC1s, macrophages, and NK cells are the major producers of these cytokines, they can also be secreted by tissue cells. IFN-α and IFN-β are classified as type I IFNs and are made by fibroblasts and macrophages. They function to inhibit the replication of viruses and improve the recognition of a virally infected cell by cells of the adaptive immune response. Type I IFNs interact with receptors on neighbouring

Understanding > The Complement System

The complement system provides one of the major effector mechanisms of both humoral and innate immunity. The system consists of a group of proteins (complement proteins C1 through C9) that are normally present in the plasma in an inactive form. Activation of the complement system is a highly regulated process, involving the sequential breakdown of the complement proteins to generate a cascade of cleavage products capable of proteolytic enzyme activity. This allows for tremendous amplification because each enzyme molecule activated by one step can generate multiple activated enzyme molecules at the next step. Complement activation is inhibited by proteins that are present on normal host cells; thus, its actions are limited to microbes and other antigens that lack these inhibitory proteins.

The reactions of the complement system can be divided into three phases: (1) the initial activation phase, (2) the early-step inflammatory responses, and (3) the late-step membrane attack responses.

1. Initial Activation Phase

There are three pathways for recognizing microbes and activating the complement system: (1) the alternative pathway, which is activated on microbial cell surfaces in the absence of antibody and is a component of innate immunity; (2) the classical pathway, which is activated by certain types of antibodies bound to antigen and is part of humoral immunity; and (3) the lectin pathway, which is activated by a plasma lectin that binds to mannose on microbes and activates the classical system pathway in the absence of antibody.

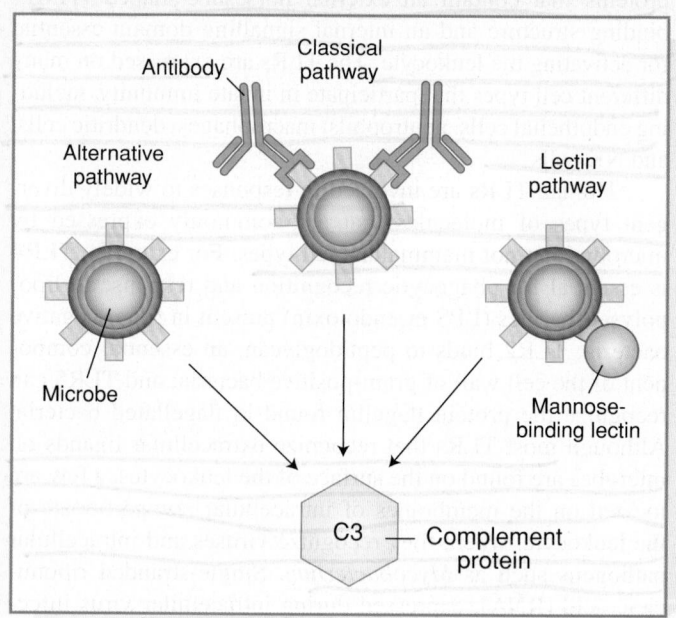

2. Early-Step Inflammatory Responses

The central component of complement for all three pathways is the activation of the complement protein C3 and its enzymatic cleavage into a larger C3b fragment and a smaller C3a fragment. The smaller 3a fragment stimulates inflammation by acting as a chemoattractant for neutrophils. The larger 3b fragment becomes attached to the microbe and acts as an opsonin for phagocytosis. It also acts as an enzyme to cleave C5 into two components: a C5a fragment, which produces vasodilation and increases vascular permeability; and a C5b fragment, which leads to the late-step membrane attack responses.

3. Late-Step Membrane Attack

In the late-step responses, C3b binds to other complement proteins to form an enzyme that cleaves C5, generating C5a and C5b fragments. C5a stimulates the influx of neutrophils and the vascular phase of acute inflammation. The C5b fragment, which remains attached to the microbe, initiates the formation of a complex of complement proteins C6, C7, C8, and C9 into a membrane attack complex protein, or pore, that allows fluids and ions to enter and cause cell lysis.

cells to stimulate the translation of an antiviral protein that affects viral synthesis and its spread to uninfected cells. The actions of type I IFNs are effective against different types of viruses and intracellular parasites and are thus part of innate immunity. IFN-γ can activate macrophages in innate immunity and regulates lymphocytes in adaptive immunity. IFN-γ is the most important cytokine produced by the ILC1s for the innate immune response and by the T-helper 1 subclass of T lymphocytes for the adaptive immune response. It is a potent activator of macrophages and enables them to destroy pathogens that proliferate in their vesicles. IFN-γ also stimulates the production of antibody isotypes that promote phagocytosis of microbes through the complement system.

Acute-Phase Proteins

The liver is the major source of acute-phase proteins. Two positive acute-phase proteins that increase plasma concentrations when defending against infections are the mannose-binding ligand (MBL) and C-reactive protein (CRP). MBL and CRP are produced by liver hepatocytes after cytokine activation and function as opsonins as well as activators of the alternative complement pathway. The binding of MBL to mannose residues and CRP to phospholipids and sugars on microbes and their subsequent binding to their complementary receptors on leukocytes lead to phagocytosis and immune cell activation.

The Complement System

The complement system is an important effector of both innate and humoral immunity that enables the body to localize and destroy infective agents. The complement system, like the blood coagulation system, consists of a group of proteins that are present in the circulation as functionally inactive precursors. These proteins, mainly proteolytic enzymes, make up 10% to 15% of the plasma proteins. For a complement reaction to occur, the complement components must be activated in the proper sequence. Uncontrolled activation of the complement system is prevented by inhibitor proteins and the instability of the activated complement proteins at each step of the process.

There are three parallel but independent pathways for recognizing microorganisms that result in activation of the complement system: the classical, the lectin, and the alternative pathways. The reactions of the complement systems can be divided into three phases: (1) initiation or activation, (2) amplification of inflammation, and (3) membrane attack response. The pathways differ slightly in the proteins used in the early stage of activation, but all converge in the process by acting on the key complement protein C3, essential for the amplification stage. Activated C3 then affects all subsequent complement molecules (C5 through C9). Inactive circulating complement proteins can be activated by microbial surface polysaccharides, MBL, and other soluble mediators in the lectin or alternative complement pathways that are integral to innate immunity, or by complement-fixing antibodies (IgG, IgM) of adaptive immunity that bind to microbial surfaces or other substances in the classical complement pathway. All activating pathways generate a series of enzymatic reactions that proteolytically cleave successive complement proteins in the pathway. New complement fragments (e.g., C3a, C3b) are regularly generated in this manner.

During the activation process, the enzymatic cleavage of C3 produces C3b, a key opsonin that coats microbes and allows them to be phagocytized after binding to the type 1 complement receptor on leukocytes. The small C3 complement fragment (C3a) can trigger an influx of neutrophils to enhance the inflammatory response. Production of C3a and C5a also leads to activation of basophils and mast cells and release of inflammatory mediators that produce smooth muscle contraction, increased vascular permeability, and changes in endothelial cells to enhance migration of phagocytes. The late phase of the complement cascade triggers the assembly of a membrane attack complex (MAC; C5 to C9) that leads to the lytic destruction of many kinds of cells, including bacteria and altered blood cells. The multiple functions of the complement system, including enhanced inflammatory responses, increased phagocytosis, and destruction and clearance of the pathogen from the body, make it an integral component of innate immunity and inflammation. Clinical changes associated with inherited deficiencies of complement range from increased susceptibility to infection to inflammatory tissue damage caused by complement-activated immune complexes not properly cleared by macrophages.

IN SUMMARY

The innate immune system consists of the epithelial cells of the skin and mucous membranes, phagocytic cells (neutrophils and macrophages), ILCs, and several plasma proteins, including those of the complement system. These defences are in place before an encounter with a microbial agent and are rapidly activated by microbes before the development of adaptive immunity. The epithelial cells of the skin and mucous membranes, which are the first line of defence, block the entry of infectious agents and secrete antimicrobial enzymes, proteins, and peptides.

The cells of the innate immunity include the phagocytic leukocytes (neutrophils and macrophages), which engulf and digest infectious agents, and ILCs, which kill microbes and foreign agents. These cells express PRRs on their membranes that bind broad patterns of molecules shared by microbes or damaged cells. TLRs, a major group of PRRs, are expressed on many cell types (neutrophils, macrophages,) and are potent activators of innate immune cells and molecules. TLRs are involved in responses to widely divergent types of molecules that are commonly expressed by microbial but not mammalian cell types.

Development of innate immunity and regulation of the behaviour of effector cells all depend on the secretion of soluble molecules, such as opsonins, cytokines, acute-phase proteins, and complement. Opsonins bind to and tag microorganisms for more efficient recognition by phagocytes. Activated leukocytes release cytokines that regulate innate immunity and inflammation by directing the migration of leukocytes, stimulating production of acute-phase proteins, and enhancing phagocytosis.

The complement system is a primary effector system for both the innate and adaptive immune systems and consists of a group of proteins that are activated by microbes and promote inflammation and destruction of the microbes. Recognition of microbes by complement occurs in three ways: by the classical pathway, which recognizes antibody bound to the surface of a microbe or other structure; by the alternative pathway, which recognizes certain microbial molecules; and by the lectin pathway, which uses a plasma protein called the mannose-binding protein to bind mannose residues on microbial glycoproteins or glycolipids.

 ## ADAPTIVE IMMUNITY

After completing this section of the chapter, you should be able to meet the following objectives:

- State the properties associated with adaptive immunity.
- Define and describe the characteristics of an antigen.
- Characterize the significance and function of major histocompatibility complex molecules.
- Describe the antigen-presenting functions of macrophages and dendritic cells.
- Contrast and compare the development and function of the T and B lymphocytes.
- State the function of the five classes of immunoglobulins.
- Differentiate between the central and peripheral lymphoid structures.
- Describe the function of cytokines involved in the adaptive immune response.
- Compare passive and active immunity.

The adaptive immune system is the final line of defence against foreign substances and is activated once the innate immune response initiates the inflammatory processes. In contrast to innate immunity, the adaptive immune response is able to recognize and react to a large number of microbes and nonmicrobial substances. Integral to the system is the ability to distinguish among different, even closely related, microbes and molecules and to "remember" the pathogen by quickly producing a heightened immune response on subsequent encounters with the same agent. The components of the adaptive immune system are lymphocytes and their products. Foreign substances that elicit specific responses are called *antigens*. There are two types of adaptive immune responses: humoral and cell-mediated immunity. *Humoral immunity* is mediated by secreted molecules and is the principal defence against extracellular microbes and toxins. *Cell-mediated immunity,* or *cellular immunity,* is mediated by specific T lymphocytes and defends against intracellular microbes such as viruses. By convention, the terms *immune response* and *immune system* usually refer to adaptive immunity.

Antigens

Before discussing the cells and responses inherent to adaptive immunity, it is important to understand the substances that elicit a response from the host. *Antigens, or immunogens,* are substances foreign to the body that can stimulate an immune response. These foreign molecules are recognized by receptors on immune cells and by secreted proteins, called *antibodies* or *immunoglobulins,* made in response to the antigen. Antigens include bacteria, fungi, viruses, protozoa, and parasites. Nonmicrobial agents such as plant pollens, poison ivy resin, insect venom, and transplanted organs can also act as antigens. Most antigens are macromolecules, such as proteins and polysaccharides, although lipids and nucleic acids occasionally can serve as antigens.

ADAPTIVE IMMUNITY

- The adaptive immune response involves a complex series of interactions between components of the immune system and the antigens of a foreign pathogen. It is able to distinguish between self and nonself, recognize and specifically react to large numbers of different microbes and pathogens, and remember the specific agents.
- Humoral immunity consists of protection provided by the B lymphocyte–derived plasma cells, which produce antibodies that travel in the blood and interact with circulating and cell surface antigens.
- Cell-mediated immunity consists of protection provided by cytotoxic T lymphocytes, which protect against virus-infected or cancer cells.
- Passive immunity represents a temporary type of immunity that is transferred from another source (*e.g.,* in utero transfer of antibodies from mother to infant), and active immunity is the response by the person's immune system that is acquired through immunization or actually having a disease.

Antigens, which in general are large and chemically complex, are biologically degraded into smaller chemical units or peptides. These discrete, immunologically active sites on antigens are called *antigenic determinants,* or *epitopes.* It is the unique molecular shape of an epitope that is recognized by a specific immunoglobulin receptor found on the surface of the lymphocyte or by an antigen-binding site of a secreted antibody (Fig. 17.2). A single antigen may contain multiple antigenic determinants, each stimulating a distinct clone of T and B lymphocytes. For example, different proteins that comprise the influenza virus may function as unique antigens (A, B, C, H, and N antigens), each of which contains several antigenic determinants. Hundreds of antigenic determinants are found on structures such as the bacterial cell wall.

Smaller substances (molecular masses <10,000 daltons) usually are unable to stimulate an adequate immune response by themselves. When these low–molecular-weight

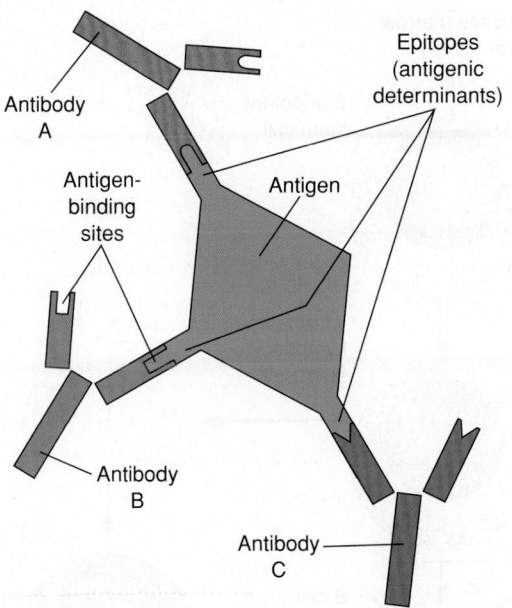

FIGURE 17.2 • Multiple epitopes on a complex antigen being recognized by their respective (A, B, C) antibodies.

compounds, known as *haptens,* combine with larger protein molecules, they function as antigens. The proteins act as carrier molecules for the haptens to form antigenic hapten–carrier complexes. An allergic response to the antibiotic penicillin is an example of a medically important reaction due to hapten–carrier complexes. Penicillin (molecular mass of approximately 350 daltons) is normally a nonantigenic molecule. However, in some individuals, it can chemically combine with body proteins to form larger complexes that can then generate a potentially harmful immune allergic response.

Cells of Adaptive Immunity

The principal cells of the adaptive immune system are the lymphocytes, APCs, and effector cells.

Lymphocytes

Lymphocytes are the cells that specifically recognize and respond to foreign antigens. Accessory cells, such as macrophages and dendritic cells, function as APCs by first processing a complex antigen into epitopes and then displaying the foreign and self-peptides on their membranes so that appropriate activation of lymphocytes occurs. Functionally, there are two types of immune cells: regulatory cells and effector cells. The *regulatory cells* assist in orchestrating and controlling the immune response. For example, helper T lymphocytes activate other lymphocytes and phagocytes, and regulatory T cells ensure that inappropriate and excessive immune responses do not occur. The final stages of the immune response are accomplished with the elimination of the antigen by *effector cells.* Cytotoxic T lymphocytes, macrophages, and other leukocytes function as effector cells in different immune responses.

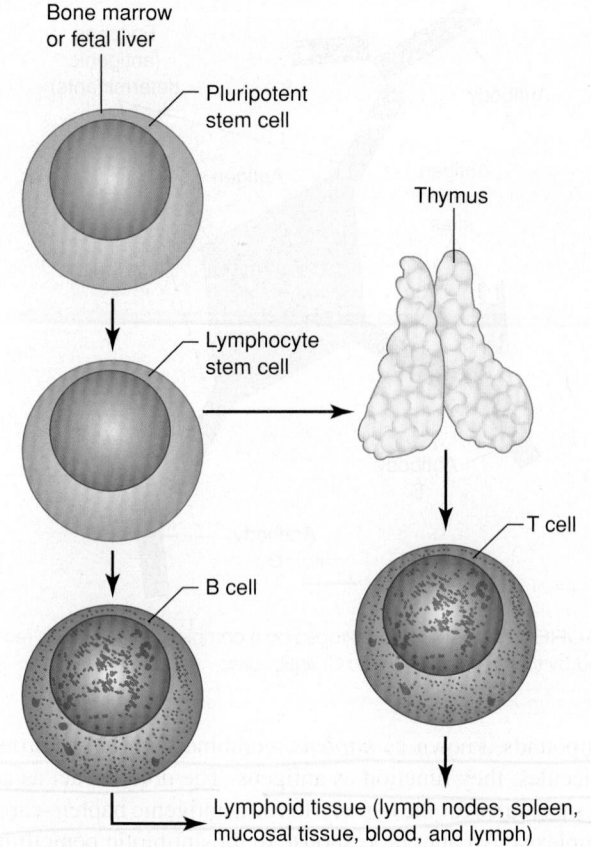

Bone marrow
or fetal liver

Pluripotent
stem cell

Thymus

Lymphocyte
stem cell

T cell

B cell

Lymphoid tissue (lymph nodes, spleen,
mucosal tissue, blood, and lymph)

FIGURE 17.3 • Pathway for T- and B-cell differentiation.

Like other blood cells, T and B lymphocytes are generated from stem cells in the bone marrow. Undifferentiated, immature lymphocytes congregate in the central lymphoid tissues, where they develop into distinct types of mature lymphocytes (Fig. 17.3). One class of lymphocyte, the *B lymphocytes* (B cells), matures in the bone marrow and is essential for *humoral*, or *antibody-mediated, immunity*. The other class of lymphocyte, the *T lymphocytes* (T cells), completes its maturation in the thymus and functions in the peripheral tissues to produce *cell-mediated immunity*, as well as aiding antibody production. The various types of lymphocytes are distinguished by their function and response to antigen, their cell membrane molecules and receptors, their types of secreted proteins, and their tissue location. High concentrations of mature T and B lymphocytes are found in the lymph nodes, spleen, skin, and mucosal tissues, where they can respond to antigens.

T and B lymphocytes possess all of the key properties associated with the adaptive immune response—specificity, diversity, memory, and self–nonself recognition. These cells can exactly recognize a particular microorganism or foreign molecule. Each lymphocyte targets a specific antigen and differentiates that invader from other substances that may be similar. The approximately 10^{12} lymphocytes in the body have tremendous diversity. They can respond to the millions of different kinds of antigens encountered daily. This diversity occurs because an enormous variety of lymphocyte populations

have been programmed and selected during development, each to respond to a different antigen. After lymphocytes have been stimulated by their antigen, they can acquire a memory response. The memory T and B lymphocytes that are generated remain in the body for a longer time and can respond more rapidly on repeat exposure than naive cells. Because of this heightened state of immune reactivity, the immune system usually can respond to commonly encountered microorganisms so efficiently that we are unaware of the response.

The key trigger for the activation of B and T cells is the recognition of the antigen by unique surface receptors. The B-cell antigen receptor consists of membrane-bound immunoglobulin molecules that can bind a specific epitope. The TCR recognizes a processed antigen peptide in association with a self-recognition protein, called a *major histocompatibility complex* (MHC) molecule (to be discussed). The appropriate recognition of MHC and self-peptides or MHC associated with foreign peptides is essential for lymphocytes to differentiate "self" from "foreign."

Activation of the lymphocytes depends on appropriate processing and presentation of antigen to T lymphocytes by APCs such as macrophages (Fig. 17.4). On recognition of antigen and after additional stimulation by cytokines, the B and T lymphocytes divide several times to form populations or clones of cells that continue to differentiate into several types of effector and memory cells. In an immune response, the effector cells destroy the antigens and the memory cells retain the potential needed for future encounters with the antigen.

Major Histocompatibility Complex Molecules

An essential feature of adaptive or specific immunity is the ability to discriminate between the body's own molecules and foreign antigens. Key recognition molecules essential for distinguishing self from nonself are the cell surface MHC molecules. These proteins, which in humans are coded by closely linked genes on chromosome 6, were first identified because of their role in organ and tissue transplantation. When cells are transplanted between individuals who are not identical for their MHC molecules, the immune system produces a vigorous response leading to rejection of the transferred cells or organs. MHC molecules did not evolve to reject transplanted tissues, a situation not encountered in nature. Rather, these molecules are essential for correct cell-to-cell interactions among immune and body cells.

The MHC molecules involved in self-recognition and cell-to-cell communication fall into two classes, class I and class II (Fig. 17.5). *Class I MHC* (MHC-I) molecules are cell surface glycoproteins that interact with the antigen receptor–foreign peptide complex and the CD8 molecule on T-cytotoxic lymphocytes. MHC-I molecules are found on nearly all nucleated cells in the body and hence are capable of alerting the immune system to any cellular changes due to viruses, intracellular bacteria, or cancer.

The MHC-I molecule contains a groove that accommodates a peptide fragment of antigen. T-cytotoxic cells can

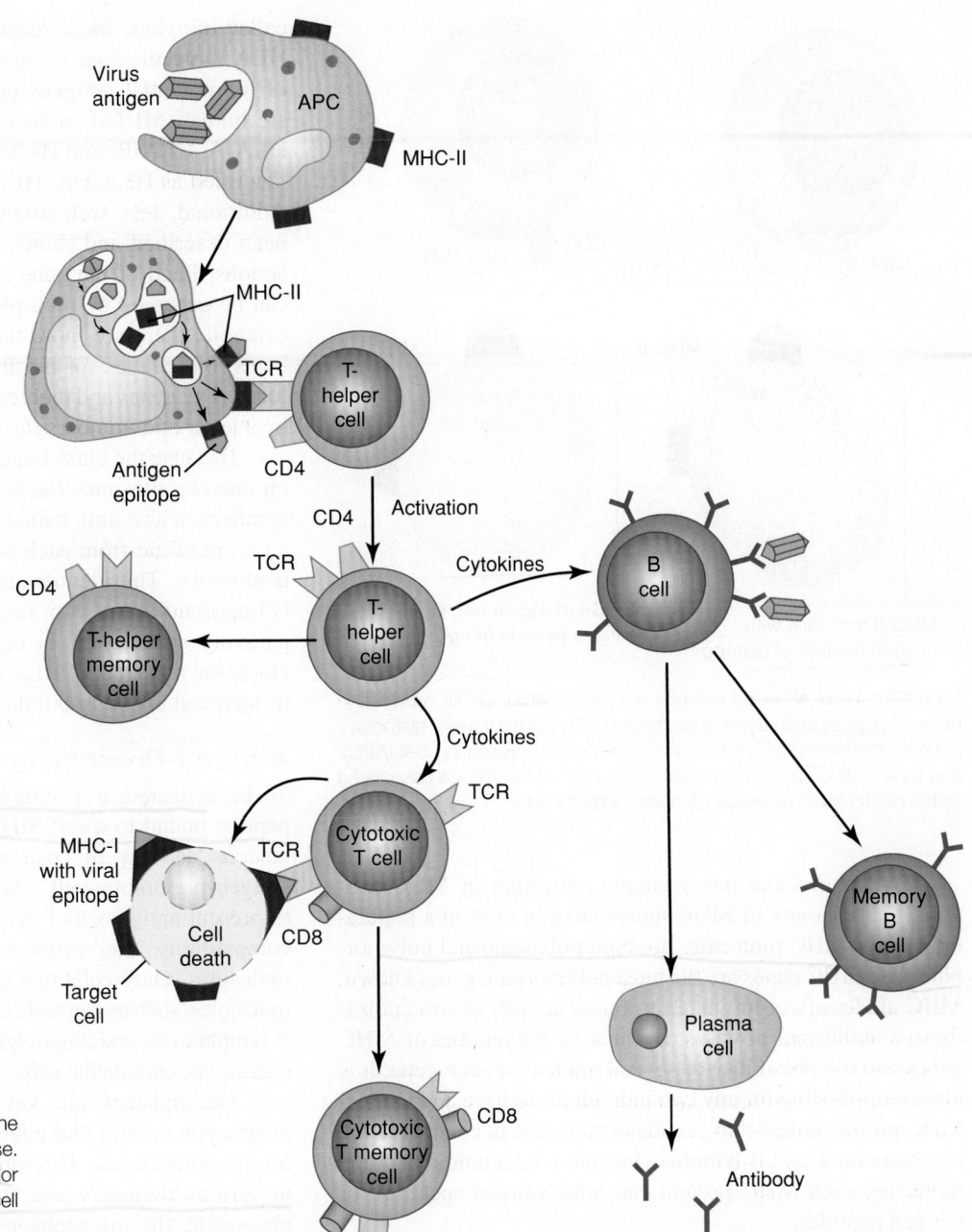

FIGURE 17.4 • Pathway for immune cell participation in an immune response. APC, antigen-presenting cell; MHC, major histocompatibility complex; TCR, T-cell receptor.

become activated only when they are presented with the foreign antigen peptide associated with the class I MHC molecule. During a typical viral infection of a cell, small peptides from degraded viral proteins associate with MHC-I molecules and are then transported to the infected cell membrane. This complex communicates to the T-cytotoxic cell that the cell must be destroyed for the overall survival of the host. *Class II MHC* (MHC-II) molecules, which are found primarily on APCs such as macrophages, dendritic cells, and B lymphocytes, communicate with the antigen receptor and CD4 molecule on T-helper lymphocytes.

Class II MHC molecules also have a groove or cleft that binds a fragment of antigen from pathogens that have been

engulfed and digested during the process of phagocytosis. The engulfed pathogen is degraded into peptide in cytoplasmic vesicles and then complexed with MHC-II molecules. T-helper cells recognize these complexes on the surface of APCs and become activated. These triggered T-helper cells multiply quickly and direct other immune cells to respond to the invading pathogen through the secretion of cytokines. A third group of genes located on the same chromosome near the class I and II MHC genes encode other proteins with diverse functions. Some complement and cytokines important for signalling an immune response are examples of class III MHC molecules. These secreted molecules are structurally and functionally unrelated to the class I and II MHC molecules.

FIGURE 17.5 • Recognition by a T-cell receptor (TCR) on a CD4⁺ helper T (T$_H$) cell of an epitope associated with a class II major histocompatibility complex (MHC) molecule on an antigen-presenting cell (APC); and by a TCR on a CD8⁺ cytotoxic T (T$_C$) cell of an epitope associated with a class I MHC molecule on a virus-infected cell.

Each individual has a unique collection of MHC proteins, and a variety of MHC molecules can exist in a population. Thus, MHC molecules are both polygenic and polymorphic. The MHC genes are the most polymorphic genes known. MHC alleles affect immune responses as well as susceptibility to a number of diseases. Because of the number of MHC genes and the possibility of several alleles for each gene, it is almost impossible for any two individuals to have an identical MHC profile, unless they are identical twins. In contrast to the receptors on T and B lymphocytes that bind a unique antigen molecule, each MHC protein can bind a broad spectrum of antigen peptides.

Human MHC proteins are called *human leukocyte antigens* (HLAs) because they were first detected on white blood cells. Because these molecules play a role in transplant rejection and are detected by immunologic tests, they are commonly called *antigens*. More recently, analysis of the genes for the HLA molecules has ensured a more complete identification of the potential antigens present in an individual. The classic human MHC-I molecules are divided into types called HLA-A, HLA-B, and HLA-C, and the MHC-II molecules are identified as HLA-DR, HLA-DP, and HLA-DQ (Table 17.3). Additional, less well-studied, nonclassic MHC genes have been described and shown to influence other immune interactions. Each of the gene loci that describe HLA molecules can be occupied by multiple alleles or alternative genes. For example, there are more than 350 possible alleles for the A locus, 650 alleles for the B locus, and 180 alleles for the C locus. The genes and their expressed molecules are designated by a letter and numbers (*i.e.,* HLA-B27).

Because the class I and II MHC genes are closely linked on one chromosome, the combination of HLA genes usually is inherited as a unit, called a *haplotype.* Each person inherits a chromosome from each parent and therefore has two HLA haplotypes. The identification or typing of HLA molecules is important in tissue or organ transplantation, forensics, and paternity evaluations. In organ or tissue transplantation, the closer the matching of HLA types, the greater is the probability of identical antigens and the lower the chance of rejection.

Antigen-Presenting Cells

To be activated, a T lymphocyte must recognize a foreign peptide bound to a self-MHC molecule. That requires simultaneous delivery of costimulatory signals by a specialized antigen-presenting cell (APC). APCs acquire the capacity to present antigens to T lymphocytes in the context of histocompatibility after cytokine-driven upregulation of MHC-II molecules. Only cells that can express both classes of MHC molecules, such as dendritic cells, monocytes, macrophages, and B lymphocytes residing in lymphoid follicles and, under certain conditions, endothelial cells, are able to function as APCs.

Macrophages are key members of the mononuclear phagocytic system that engulf and digest microbes and other foreign substances. The monocytes migrate from the blood to various tissues, where they mature into the major tissue phagocyte, the macrophages. As the general scavenger cells of the body, the macrophage can be fixed in a tissue or free to migrate from an organ to lymphoid tissues. The tissue macrophages are scattered in connective tissue or clustered in organs such as the lung (*i.e.,* alveolar macrophages), liver

TABLE 17.3 PROPERTIES OF CLASS I AND II MHC MOLECULES

PROPERTIES	HLA ANTIGENS	DISTRIBUTION	FUNCTIONS
Class I MHC	HLA-A, HLA-B, HLA-C	Virtually all nucleated cells	Present processed antigen to cytotoxic CD8⁺ T cells; restrict cytolysis to virus-infected cells, tumour cells, and transplanted cells
Class II MHC	HLA-DR, HLA-DP, HLA-DQ	Immune cells, antigen-presenting cells, B cells, and macrophages	Present processed antigenic fragments to CD4⁺ T cells; necessary for effective interaction among immune cells

HLA, human leukocyte antigen; MHC, major histocompatibility complex.

(*i.e.*, Kupffer cells), spleen, lymph nodes, peritoneum, central nervous system (*i.e.*, microglial cells), and other areas. When macrophages are activated, they engulf and break down complex antigens into peptide fragments for association with MHC-II molecules. Macrophages then present these complexes to the T-helper cell so that self–nonself recognition and activation of the immune response can occur.

Dendritic cells share with the macrophage the important task of presenting processed antigen to T lymphocytes. These distinctive, star-shaped cells with long extensions of their cytoplasmic membrane provide an extensive surface rich in MHC-II molecules and other membrane molecules important for initiation of adaptive immunity. Dendritic cells are found in most tissues where antigen enters the body and in the peripheral lymphoid tissues, where they function as potent APCs. In these different environments, dendritic cells can acquire specialized functions and appearances, as do macrophages. Langerhans cells are specialized dendritic cells in the skin, whereas follicular dendritic cells are found in the lymph nodes. Langerhans cells are constantly surveying the skin for antigen and can transport foreign material to a nearby lymph node. Skin dendritic cells and macrophages also are involved in cell-mediated immune reactions of the skin such as allergic contact dermatitis.

B Lymphocytes and Humoral Immunity

Humoral immunity is mediated by antibodies, which are produced by B lymphocytes and their progeny. It is the arm of the adaptive immune response that functions to eliminate extracellular microbes and microbial toxins. Humoral immunity is more important than cellular immunity in defending against microbes with capsules rich in polysaccharides and lipid toxins. The reason for this is that B cells respond to and produce antibodies specific for many types of molecules, whereas T cells, the mediators of cellular immunity, respond primarily to protein antigens.

B lymphocytes can be identified by the presence of membrane immunoglobulin that functions as the antigen receptor, class II MHC proteins, complement receptors, and specific CD molecules. During the maturation in the bone marrow, B-cell progenitors (pro-B and pre-B cells) develop into mature or naive B cells. Naive B cells express membrane-bound IgD and IgM that function as preceptors for antibody but do not secrete antibody. The mature B cell leaves the bone marrow, enters the circulation, and migrates to the various peripheral lymphoid tissues, where it is stimulated to respond to a specific antigen. Each of the stages of B-cell development is characterized by a specific pattern of Ig gene expression and the expression of other cell surface proteins that serve as phenotypic markers of these maturational stages.

The commitment of a B-cell line to a specific antigen is evidenced by the expression of the membrane-bound Ig receptors that recognize antigen. B cells that encounter antigen complementary to their surface immunoglobulin receptor and receive T-cell help undergo a series of changes that transform them into antibody-secreting plasma cells or into memory B cells (Fig. 17.6). The antibodies produced by the plasma cells are released into the lymph and blood, where they bind and remove their unique antigen with the help of other immune effector cells and molecules. The longer-lived memory B cells are distributed to the peripheral tissues in preparation for subsequent antigen exposure.

Immunoglobulins

Antibodies comprise a class of proteins called *immunoglobulins*. The immunoglobulins have been divided into five classes, IgG, IgA, IgM, IgD, and IgE, each with a different role in the immune defence strategy (Table 17.4). Immunoglobulins have a characteristic four-polypeptide structure consisting of at least two identical antigen-binding sites (Fig. 17.7). Each immunoglobulin is composed of two identical light (L) chains and two identical heavy (H) chains to form a "Y"-shaped molecule. The two forked ends of the immunoglobulin molecule bind antigen and are called *Fab* (*i.e.*, antigen-binding) fragments, and the tail of the molecule, which is called the *Fc*

FIGURE 17.6 • Pathway for B-cell differentiation.

TABLE 17.4 CLASSES AND CHARACTERISTICS OF IMMUNOGLOBULINS

FIGURE	CLASS	PERCENTAGE OF TOTAL	CHARACTERISTICS
	IgG	75.0	Displays antiviral, antitoxin, and antibacterial properties; only Ig that crosses the placenta; responsible for protection of newborn; activates complement and binds to macrophages
	IgA	15.0	Presents predominant Ig in body secretions, such as saliva, nasal and respiratory secretions, and breast milk; protects mucous membranes
	IgM	10.0	Forms the natural antibodies such as those for ABO blood antigens; prominent in early immune responses; activates complement
	IgD	0.2	Manifests in B lymphocytes; needed for maturation of B cells; protects upper respiratory mucosa
	IgE	0.004	Binds to mast cells and basophils; involved in parasitic infections, allergic and hypersensitivity reactions

fragment, determines the biologic properties that are characteristic of a particular class of immunoglobulins.

The amino acid sequence of the heavy and light chains shows constant (C) regions and variable (V) regions. The *constant regions* have sequences of amino acids that vary little among the antibodies of a particular class of immunoglobulin. The constant regions are the basis for the separation of immunoglobulins into classes (*e.g.,* IgM, IgG), and allow each class of antibody to interact with certain effector cells and molecules. For example, IgG can tag an antigen for recognition and destruction by phagocytes. The *variable regions* contain the antigen-binding sites of the molecule. The wide variation in the amino acid sequence of the variable regions seen from antibody to antibody allows this region to recognize its complementary epitope. A unique amino acid sequence in this region determines a distinctive three-dimensional pocket that is complementary to the antigen, allowing recognition and binding. Each B-cell clone produces an antibody with one

specific antigen-binding variable region or domain. During the course of the immune response, class switching (*e.g.,* from IgM to IgG) can occur, causing the B-cell clone to produce one of the different immunoglobulin types.

IgG (gamma globulin) is the most abundant of the circulating immunoglobulins. It is present in body fluids and readily enters the tissues. IgG is the only immunoglobulin that crosses the placenta and can transfer immunity from the mother to the fetus. This class of immunoglobulin protects against bacteria, toxins, and viruses in body fluids and activates the complement system. This antibody can also bind to target cells and Fc receptors on NK cells and macrophages, leading to lysis of the target cell. There are four subclasses of IgG (*i.e.,* IgG1, IgG2, IgG3, and IgG4), each of which has some restrictions in its response to certain types of antigens. For example, IgG2 appears to be responsive to bacteria that are encapsulated with a polysaccharide layer, such as *Streptococcus pneumoniae, Haemophilus influenzae,* and *Neisseria meningitidis.*

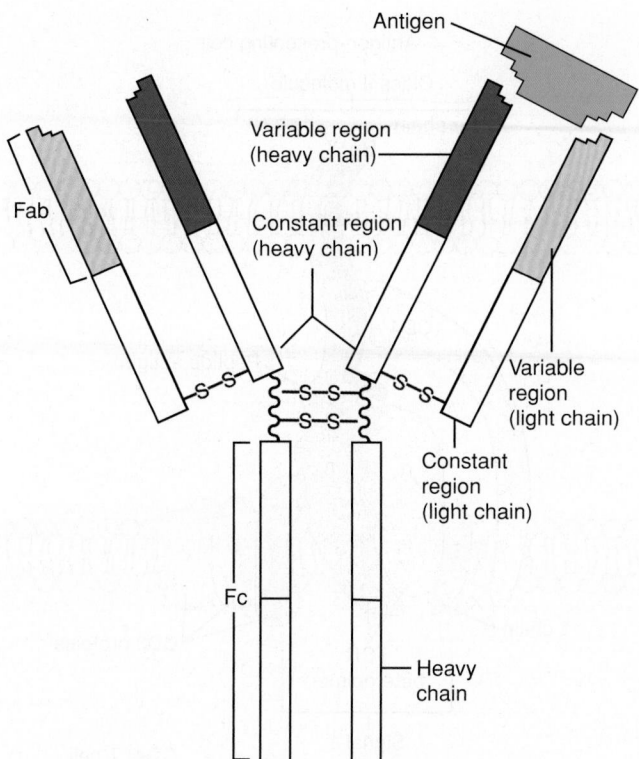

FIGURE 17.7 • Schematic model of an immunoglobulin G (IgG) molecule showing the constant and variable regions of the light and heavy chains.

IgA, a secretory immunoglobulin, is found in saliva, tears, colostrum (*i.e.,* first milk of a nursing mother), and bronchial, gastrointestinal, prostatic, and vaginal secretions. This dimeric secretory immunoglobulin is considered a primary defence against local infections in mucosal tissues. IgA prevents the attachment of viruses and bacteria to epithelial cells.

IgM is a macromolecule that forms a polymer of five basic immunoglobulin units. It cannot cross the placenta and does not transfer maternal immunity. It is the first circulating immunoglobulin to appear in response to an antigen and is the first antibody type made by a newborn. This is diagnostically useful because the presence of IgM suggests a current infection in the infant by a specific pathogen. The identification of newborn IgM rather than maternally transferred IgG to the specific pathogen is indicative of an in utero or newborn infection.

IgD is found primarily on the cell membranes of B lymphocytes. It also circulates in the blood serum where its function is essentially unknown. It serves as an antigen receptor for initiating the differentiation of B cells and apparently can bind to basophils and mast cells to activate and produce antimicrobial factors for mucosal respiratory immunity.

IgE is involved in inflammation, allergic responses, and combating parasitic infections. It binds to mast cells and basophils. The binding of antigen to mast cell–bound or basophil-bound IgE triggers these cells to release histamine and other mediators important in inflammation and allergies.

Humoral Immunity

Humoral immunity depends on maturation of B lymphocytes into plasma cells, which produce and secrete antibodies. The combination of antigen with antibody can result in several effector responses, such as precipitation of antigen–antibody complexes, agglutination or clumping of cells, neutralization of bacterial toxins and viruses, lysis and destruction of pathogens or cells, adherence of antigen to immune cells, facilitation of phagocytosis, and complement activation. For example, antibodies can neutralize a virus by blocking the sites on the virus that it uses to bind to the host cell, thereby negating its ability to infect the cell.

Two types of responses occur in the development of humoral immunity: a primary and a secondary response (Fig. 17.8). A *primary immune response* occurs when the antigen is first introduced into the body. During the primary response, there is a latent period or lag before the antibody can be detected in the serum. This latent period involves the processing of antigen by the APCs and its recognition by CD4$^+$ helper T cells. After the antigen receptors on CD4$^+$ helper T cells recognize the antigenic peptide–class II MHC complex, the T cells become activated and produce cytokines to further stimulate and direct the immune system. In humoral immunity, activated CD4$^+$ helper T cells trigger B cells to proliferate and differentiate into a clone of plasma cells that produce antibody. This activation process takes 1 to 2 weeks, but once generated, detectable antibody continues to rise for several weeks. Recovery from many infectious diseases occurs during the primary response when the antibody concentration is reaching its peak. The *secondary* or *memory response* occurs on second or subsequent exposures to the antigen. During the secondary response, the rise in antibody occurs sooner and reaches a higher level because of available memory cells.

During the primary response, B cells are activated to proliferate and differentiate into antibody-secreting plasma cells. A fraction of activated B cells does not differentiate into plasma cells but forms a pool of memory B cells. During the

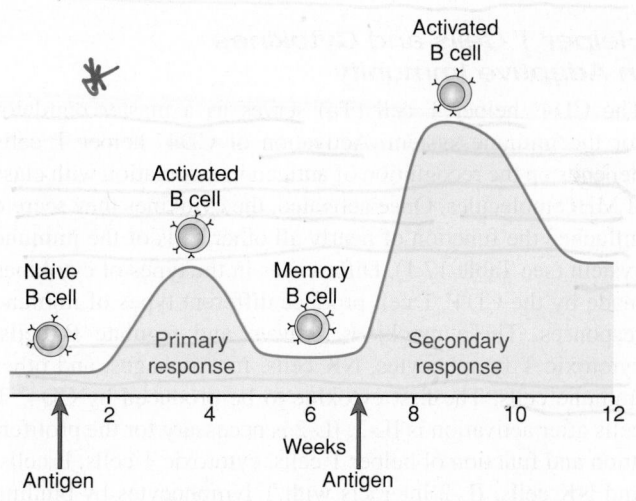

FIGURE 17.8 • Primary and secondary or memory phases of the humoral immune response to the same antigen.

secondary response, the memory cells recognize the antigen and respond more efficiently to produce the specific antibody. The booster immunization given for some diseases, such as tetanus, makes use of the memory response. For a person who has been previously immunized, administration of a booster shot causes an almost immediate rise in antibody to a level sufficient to prevent development of the disease. Activated T cells can also generate primary and secondary cell-mediated immune responses and the concurrent development of T memory cells.

T Lymphocytes and Cellular Immunity

T lymphocytes function in the activation of other T cells and B cells, in the control of intracellular viral infections, in the rejection of foreign tissue grafts, and in delayed hypersensitivity reactions (see Chapter 19). Collectively, these immune responses are referred to as *cell-mediated* or *cellular immunity*. The effector phase of cell-mediated immunity is carried out by T lymphocytes and macrophages.

T lymphocytes arise from bone marrow stem cells, but unlike B cells, pre-T cells migrate to the thymus for their maturation. There, the immature T lymphocytes undergo rearrangement of the genes needed for expression of a unique T-cell antigen receptor similar to but distinct from the B-cell receptor. The TCR is composed of two polypeptides that fold to form a groove that recognizes processed antigen peptide–MHC complexes (Fig. 17.9). The TCR–antigen–MHC complex is further stabilized during cell activation by the CD4 molecule on the helper T cell or the CD8 molecule on the cytotoxic T cell. The TCR is associated with other surface molecules known as the *CD3 complex* that aid cell signalling. Maturation of subpopulations of T cells (*i.e.,* CD4$^+$ and CD8$^+$) also occurs in the thymus. Mature T cells migrate to the peripheral lymphoid tissues and, on encountering antigen, multiply and differentiate into memory T cells and various mature T cells. The two main populations of mature T cells are CD4$^+$ (helper) and CD8$^+$ (cytotoxic or killer) T cells.

Helper T Cells and Cytokines in Adaptive Immunity

The CD4$^+$ helper T cell (T$_H$) serves as a master regulator for the immune system. Activation of CD4$^+$ helper T cells depends on the recognition of antigen in association with class II MHC molecules. Once activated, the cytokines they secrete influence the function of nearly all other cells of the immune system (see Table 17.1). Differences in the types of cytokines made by the CD4$^+$ T cell produce different types of immune responses. These cytokines activate and regulate B cells, cytotoxic T lymphocytes, NK cells, macrophages, and other immune cells. The first cytokine to be produced by CD4$^+$ T cells after activation is IL-2. IL-2 is necessary for the proliferation and function of helper T cells, cytotoxic T cells, B cells, and NK cells. IL-2 interacts with T lymphocytes by binding to specific membrane receptors that are present on activated T cells but not on resting T cells. The expression of high-affinity

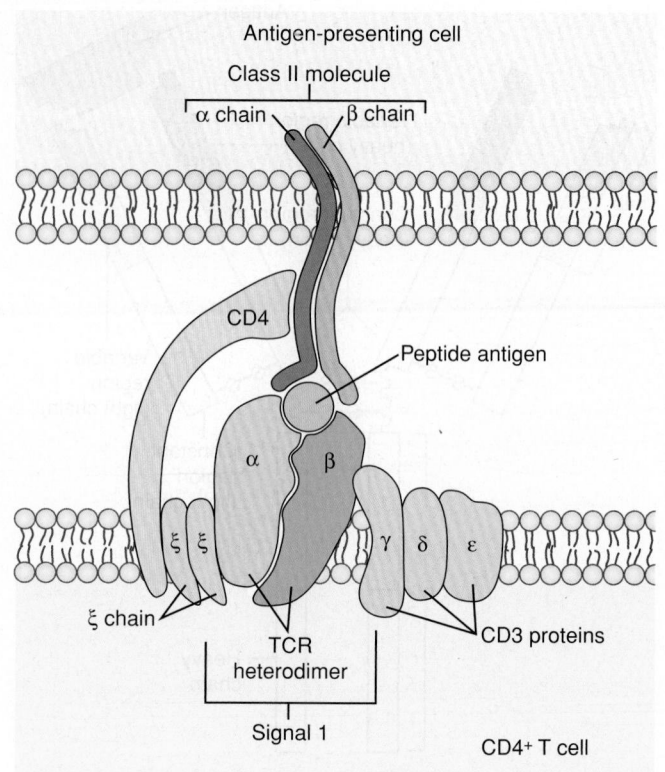

FIGURE 17.9 • The T-cell receptor (TCR) on a CD4$^+$ T cell and its interaction with the class II major histocompatibility complex (MHC) molecule on the antigen-presenting cell. Notice that the αβ TCR heterodimer recognizes a peptide fragment of antigen bound to the MHC class II molecule. The CD4 molecule binds to the nonpolymorphic portion of the class II MHC molecule, stabilizing the interaction. The CD3 proteins associated with the TCR aid in cell signalling. (Adapted from Kumar V., Abbas A. K., Faustos N., et al., (Eds). (2010). *Robbins and Cotran pathologic basis of disease* (8th ed., p. 186). Philadelphia, PA: Elsevier Saunders.)

IL-2 receptors can be triggered by specific antigen peptide–MHC-II interactions and other stimulatory signals. Sustained T-cell amplification relies on the presence of both IL-2 and IL-2 receptors; if either is missing, cell proliferation ceases. Severe combined immunodeficiency diseases have been associated with mutations in IL-2 and the IL-2 receptor, thereby documenting the importance of these molecules. Cyclosporine and tacrolimus are drugs used to prevent rejection of heart, kidney, and liver transplants, and function primarily by inhibiting the synthesis of IL-2.

The activated CD4$^+$ helper T cell can differentiate into distinct subpopulations of helper T cells (*i.e.,* T$_H$1, T$_H$2, T$_H$17) based on the cytokines secreted by the APC at the site of activation (Table 17.5). The cytokine IL-12 produced by macrophages and dendritic cells directs the maturation of CD4$^+$ helper T cells toward T$_H$1 cells. When a combination of IL-1 and IL-6 are secreted by the macrophages and dendritic cells, T$_H$17 cells are developed. IL-4 produced by mast cells and T cells induces differentiation toward T$_H$2 cells. The distinct pattern of cytokine secreted by mature T$_H$1, T$_H$2, and T$_H$17 cells defines these subpopulations of T$_H$ cells and determines

TABLE 17.5 COMPARISON OF PROPERTIES OF HELPER T-CELL SUBTYPES 1 (T_H1), 2 (T_H2), AND 17 (T_H17)

	T_H1	T_H2	T_H17
Stimulus for differentiation to T_H subtype	Intracellular pathogens	Allergens and parasitic worms	Extracellular bacteria and fungi
Cells and cytokines influencing T_H subtype maturation	IL-12 produced by macrophages and dendritic cells	IL-4 produced by mast cells and T cells	TGF-β and IL-6 by dendritic cells
Cytokines secreted by T_H subtype	IFN-γ, IL-2	IL-4, IL-5	IL-17
Effector functions	Phagocyte-mediated defence against infections, especially intracellular microbes; stimulates production of IgG	IgE- and eosinophil/mast cell–mediated immune reactions; stimulates production of IgE	Recruits neutrophils; mediates inflammation at mucosal surfaces; secretes cytotoxic proteins (defensins)

IL, interleukin, Ig, immunoglobulin, TGF-β, transforming growth factor-beta.

whether a humoral or cell-mediated response will occur. Activated T_H1 cells characteristically produce the IFN-γ cytokines, T_H2 cells produce IL-4 and IL-5, and T_H17 produces IL-17. Some of the cytokines (*e.g.,* IL-10) made by T_H2 cells inhibit macrophage activation and suppresses T_H1 responses.

IL-4 is the major regulatory molecule for the development of T_H2 cells, which direct B cells in the class switching needed to produce IgE antibodies. IL-4 can further expand T_H2 cell populations in an autocrine manner and at the same time inhibit T_H1-directed cell-mediated immunity. The detrimental impact of increased IL-4 on excessive IgE production is evident in allergic individuals. IL-5 is an activator of eosinophils that, along with IgE, functions in the control of helminth (intestinal parasite) infections. IL-17 plays an important protective role against certain pathogens at epithelial and mucosal barriers.

In most immune responses, a balanced response of T_H1 and T_H2 cells occurs, but immunization or exposure to antigen can skew the response to one or the other subset. For example, the extensive exposure to an allergen in atopic individuals has been shown to shift the naive T-helper cell toward a T_H2 response, with the production of the cytokines that influence IgE production and mast cell priming. An appreciation of these processes has led to clinical research that suggests redirection of an allergic T_H2 response to a nonallergic T_H1 response can occur in atopic individuals through modified immunization protocols.

Regulatory T Cells

Another type of T lymphocyte is the *regulatory T cell,* which has CD4 and CD25 expressed on its cell membrane. Regulatory T cells, in contrast to CD4+ helper T cells, suppress immune responses by inhibiting the proliferation of other potentially harmful self-reactive lymphocytes. The regulation by these cells is antigen specific and controlled through activation of a TCR by the antigen and subsequent secretion of the cytokines IL-10 and transforming growth factor-β (TGF-β). These cytokines inhibit the proliferation and activation of lymphocytes and macrophages, which adds restraint to the immune process and prevents an excessive response. There is also recent evidence of regulatory CD8+ T cells that can selectively downregulate T cells that are activated by either self or foreign antigens. These cells are thought to differentiate into effector cells during the primary immune response and function as suppressor cells during the secondary or memory phases of immunity, and are primarily involved in self–nonself discrimination. The potential clinical importance of regulatory T cells is suggested from animal studies showing inhibition of inflammatory bowel disease, experimental allergic encephalitis, and autoimmune diabetes by increased activity of regulatory T cells.

Cytotoxic T Cells

Activated CD8+ cytotoxic T cells become cytotoxic T lymphocytes after recognition of class I MHC–antigen complexes on target cell surfaces, such as body cells infected by viruses or transformed by cancer (Fig. 17.10). The recognition of class I MHC–antigen complexes on infected target cells ensures that neighbouring uninfected host cells, which express class I MHC molecules alone or with self-peptide, are not indiscriminately destroyed. The CD8+ cytotoxic T lymphocytes destroy target cells by releasing cytolytic enzymes, toxic cytokines, and pore-forming molecules (*i.e.,* perforins), or through programmed cell death of the target cell by triggering membrane molecules and intracellular apoptosis. *Apoptosis* or programmed cell death, is a normal cellular process enabling the controlled elimination of excessive, dangerous, or damaged cells. In addition, the perforin proteins can produce pores in the target cell membrane, allowing entry of toxic molecules and loss of cell constituents. The CD8+ T cells are especially important in controlling replicating viruses and intracellular bacteria because antibodies cannot readily penetrate the membrane of living cells.

Cell-Mediated Immunity

Cell-mediated immunity involves both CD4+ and CD8+ T lymphocytes. Activated CD4+ helper T cells release various

FIGURE 17.10 • Destruction of target cell by cytotoxic T cell. Cytokines released from the activated helper T cell enhance the potential of the cytotoxic T cell in destruction of the target cell.

cytokines (*i.e.,* IFN-γ) that recruit and activate other CD8⁺ cytotoxic T cells, macrophages, and inflammatory cells. Cytokines (*e.g.,* chemokines) can induce positive migration or chemotaxis of several types of inflammatory cells, including macrophages, neutrophils, and basophils. Activation of macrophages ensures enhanced phagocytic, metabolic, and enzymatic potential, resulting in more efficient destruction of infected cells. This type of defence is important against intracellular pathogens such as *Mycobacterium* species and *Listeria monocytogenes*. A similar sequence of T-cell and macrophage activation, but with sustained inflammation, is elicited in delayed hypersensitivity reactions. Contact dermatitis due to a poison ivy reaction or sensitivity to dyes is an example of delayed or cell-mediated hypersensitivity caused by hapten–carrier complexes.

In cell-mediated immunity, the actions of T lymphocytes and effector macrophages predominate. The most aggressive phagocyte, the macrophage, becomes activated after exposure to T-cell cytokines, especially IFN-γ. As in humoral immunity, the initial stages of cell-mediated immunity are directed by an APC displaying the antigen peptide–class II MHC complex to the CD4⁺ helper T cell. CD4⁺ helper T cells become activated after antigen recognition and by induction with IL-12. The activated helper T cell then synthesizes IL-2, IL-4, and other cytokines. These molecules drive the multiplication of clones of CD4⁺ helper T cells, which amplify the response. Further differentiation of the CD4⁺ helper T cells leads to production

of additional cytokines (*e.g.,* IFN-γ) that enhance the activity of cytotoxic T cells and effector macrophages.

Lymphoid Organs

The cells of the immune system are present in large numbers in the central and peripheral lymphoid organs. These organs and tissues are widely distributed in the body and provide different, but often overlapping, functions (Fig. 17.11). The central lymphoid organs, the bone marrow and the thymus, provide the environment for immune cell production and maturation. The structure and cells of the peripheral lymphoid organs function to concentrate antigen, aid processing of antigen, and promote cellular interactions necessary for development of adaptive immune responses. Lymph nodes, spleen, tonsils, appendix, Peyer patches in the intestine, and mucosa-associated lymphoid tissues in the respiratory, gastrointestinal, and reproductive systems comprise the peripheral lymphoid organs. The lymphoid organs are connected by networks of lymph channels, blood vessels, and capillaries. The immune cells continuously circulate through the various tissues and organs to seek out and destroy foreign material. The structure and organization of the cellular components of the peripheral

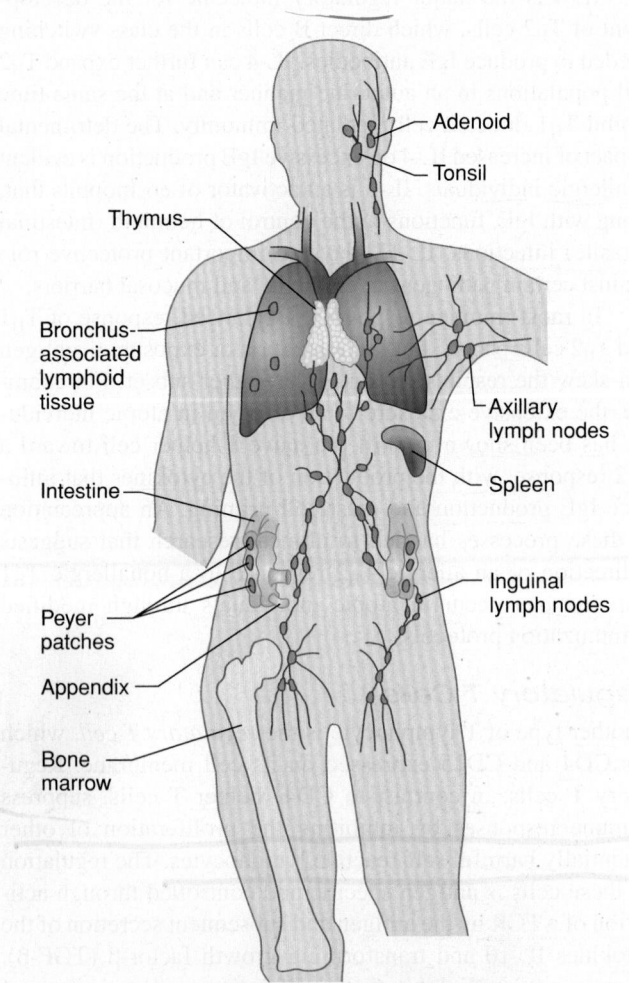

FIGURE 17.11 • Central and peripheral lymphoid organs and tissues.

lymphoid tissues ensure that the rare antigen-specific B and T cells will see each other and antigen peptide–MHC-coated APCs (*e.g.*, dendritic cells).

Thymus

The thymus is an elongated, bilobed structure located in the mediastinum above the heart. Each lobe is surrounded by a connective tissue capsule layer and is divided into lobules. Each lobule is composed of two compartments: an outer area or cortex, which is densely packed with thymocytes or immature T lymphocytes, and an inner, less dense area or medulla that contains fewer but more mature lymphocytes. The medulla also contains dendritic cells, macrophages, and the distinctive morphologic structure of the thymus, Hassall corpuscles (Fig. 17.12).

The function of the thymus is central to the development of the immune system because it generates mature, immunocompetent T lymphocytes expressing appropriate receptors. The thymus is a fully developed organ at birth, weighing approximately 15 to 20 g. At puberty, when the immune cells are well established in peripheral lymphoid tissues, the thymus begins slowly regressing and is replaced by adipose tissue. Nevertheless, some thymus tissue persists into old age. Precursor T (pre-T) cells enter the thymus as functionally and phenotypically immature T cells. They undergo cycles of proliferation and selection as they move from the cortical to

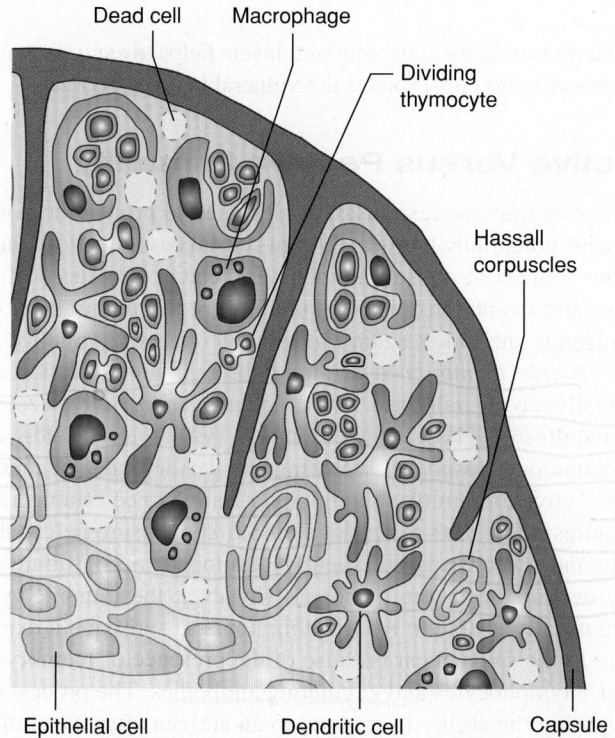

Dead cell Macrophage

Dividing thymocyte

Hassall corpuscles

Epithelial cell Dendritic cell Capsule

FIGURE 17.12 • Structural features of the thymus gland. The thymus gland is divided into lobules containing an outer cortex densely packed with dividing thymocytes or premature T cells and an inner medulla that contains mature T lymphocytes, macrophages, dendritic cells, and Hassall corpuscles.

medullary compartments of the thymus. Rapid cell multiplication, maturation, and selection occur in the cortex under the influence of the microenvironment, thymic hormones, and cytokines. As the T cells multiply and mature, they acquire TCRs, surface markers that distinguish among the different types of T cells, and antigens that distinguish them from nonself. More than 95% of the thymocytes die in the cortex and never leave the thymus because, in the random rearrangement of genes, cells are produced with inappropriate receptors. Only those T cells able to recognize foreign antigen displayed by self-MHC are allowed to mature. This process is called *thymic selection* or education. The thymus must be extremely thorough in eliminating self-reactive cells to ensure that autoimmune reactivity and disease do not result. Mature, immunocompetent T-helper and T-cytotoxic cells leave the thymus in 2 to 3 days and enter the peripheral lymphoid tissues through the bloodstream.

Lymph Nodes

Lymph nodes are small aggregates of lymphoid tissue located along lymphatic vessels throughout the body. Each lymph node processes lymph from a discrete, adjacent anatomic site. Many lymph nodes are in the axillae and groin, and along the great vessels of the neck, thorax, and abdomen. The lymph nodes are located along the lymph ducts, which lead from the tissues to the thoracic duct. Lymph nodes have two functions: removal of foreign material from lymph before it enters the bloodstream, and serving as centres for proliferation and response of immune cells.

A lymph node is a bean-shaped tissue surrounded by a connective tissue capsule. Lymph enters the node through multiple afferent lymph channels that penetrate the capsule, and leaves through the efferent lymph vessels located in the deep indentation of the hilus. Lymphocytes and macrophages flow slowly through the node, which allows trapping and interaction of antigen and immune cells. The reticular meshwork serves as a surface on which macrophages and dendritic cells can more easily present antigens.

A lymph node is divided into several specialized areas, an outer cortex, a paracortex, and an inner medulla (Fig. 17.13). The T lymphocytes are more abundant in the paracortex of the node, and the B lymphocytes are more abundant in the follicles and germinal centres located in the outer cortex. The T lymphocytes proliferate on antigenic stimulation and migrate to the follicles, where they interact with B lymphocytes. These activated follicles become germinal centres, containing macrophages, follicular dendritic cells, and maturing T and B cells. Activated B cells then migrate to the medulla, where they complete their maturation into plasma cells. These cells stay localized in the lymph node but release large quantities of antibodies into the circulation.

Spleen

The spleen is a large, ovoid secondary lymphoid organ located high in the left abdominal cavity. The spleen filters antigens from the blood and is important in the response to systemic

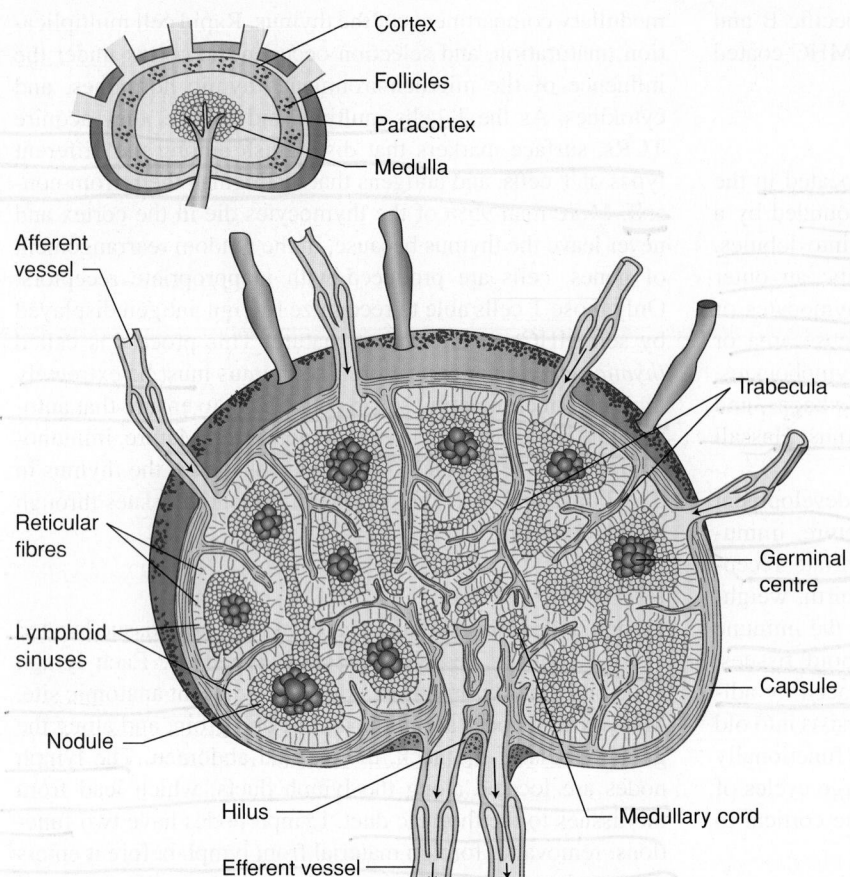

FIGURE 17.13 • Structural features of a lymph node. Bacteria that gain entry to the body are filtered out of the lymph as it flows through the node.

infections. The spleen is composed of red and white pulp. The red pulp is well supplied with arteries and is the area where senescent and injured red blood cells are removed. The white pulp contains concentrated areas of B and T lymphocytes permeated by macrophages and dendritic cells. The lymphocytes (primarily T cells) that surround the central arterioles form the area called the *periarterial lymphoid sheath*. The diffuse marginal zone contains follicles and germinal centres rich in B cells and separates the white pulp from the red pulp. A sequence of activation events similar to that seen in the lymph nodes occurs in the spleen.

Other Secondary Lymphoid Tissues

Other secondary lymphoid tissues include the *mucosa-associated lymphoid tissues*. These nonencapsulated clusters of lymphoid tissues are located around membranes lining the respiratory, digestive, and urogenital tracts. These gateways into the body must harbour the immune cells needed to respond to a large and diverse population of microorganisms. In some tissues, the lymphocytes are organized in loose clusters, but in other tissues such as the tonsils, Peyer patches in the intestine, and the appendix, organized structures are evident (Fig. 17.11). These tissues contain all the necessary cell components (*i.e.,* T cells, B cells, macrophages, and dendritic cells) for an immune response. Because of the continuous stimulation of the lymphocytes in these tissues by microorganisms constantly entering the body, large numbers of plasma cells are

evident. Immunity at the mucosal layers helps to exclude many pathogens and thus protects the vulnerable internal organs.

Active Versus Passive Immunity

Adaptive immune responses are designed to protect the body against potentially harmful foreign substances, infections, and other sources of nonself-antigens. Protection is induced after exposure to antigens (active immunity) or through transfer of protective antibodies against an antigen (passive immunity).

Active immunity is acquired through immunization or actually having a disease. It is called *active immunity* because it requires the host's own immune system to develop an immunologic response, including the development of memory. Active immunity, although long-lasting once established, requires a few days to weeks after a first exposure before the immune response is sufficiently developed to contribute to the destruction of the pathogen. However, the immune system usually is able to react within hours to subsequent exposure to the same agent because of the presence of memory B and T lymphocytes and circulating antibodies. The process of acquiring the ability to respond to an antigen after its administration by vaccine is known as *immunization*. An acquired immune response can improve on repeated exposures to an injected antigen (booster vaccines) or a natural infection.

Passive immunity is immunity transferred from another source. An infant receives passive immunity naturally from the transfer of antibodies from its mother in utero and through breast milk. Maternal IgG crosses the placenta and protects the newborn during the first few months of life. Normally, an infant has few infectious diseases during the first 3 to 6 months owing to the protection provided by the mother's antibodies, and this gives their own immune system time to mature. Passive immunity also can be artificially provided by the transfer of antibodies produced by other people or animals. Some protection against infectious disease can be provided by the injection of hyperimmune serum, which contains high concentrations of antibodies for a specific disease, or immune serum or gamma globulin, which contains a pool of antibodies from many individuals providing protection against many infectious agents. Passive immunity produces only short-term protection that lasts weeks to months.

Regulation of the Immune Response

Self-regulation is an essential property of the immune system. An inadequate or weakened immune response may lead to immunodeficiency, but an inappropriate or excessive response may lead to conditions varying from allergic reactions to autoimmune diseases. This regulation is not well understood and involves all aspects of the immune response—antigen, antibody, cytokines, regulatory T cells, and the neuroendocrine system.

With each exposure to antigen, the immune system must determine the branch of the immune system to be activated and the extent and duration of the immune response. After exposure to an antigen, the immune response to that antigen develops after a brief lag, reaches a peak, and then recedes. Normal immune responses are self-limited because the response eliminates the antigen, and the products of the response, such as cytokines and antibodies, have a short or limited life span and are secreted only for brief periods after antigen recognition. Evidence suggests that cytokine feedback from the helper T or regulatory T cells controls several aspects of the immune response.

Another facet of immune self-regulation is inhibition of immune responses by tolerance. The term *tolerance* is used to define the ability of the immune system to be nonreactive to self-antigens while producing immunity to foreign agents. Tolerance to self-antigens protects an individual from harmful autoimmune reactions. Exposure of an individual to foreign antigens may lead to tolerance and the inability to respond to potential pathogens that cause infection. Tolerance exists not only to self-tissues but to maternal–fetal tissues. Special regulation of the immune system is evident in defined privileged sites such as the brain, testes, ovaries, and eyes. Immune damage in these areas could result in serious consequences to the individual and the species.

IN SUMMARY

Adaptive immunity involves humoral and cellular mechanisms that respond to a unique antigen, can amplify and sustain its responses, distinguish self from nonself,

and remember the antigen to produce quickly a heightened response on subsequent encounters with the same agent. Antigens are substances foreign to the host that can stimulate an immune response. They have antigenic determinant sites or epitopes, which the adaptive immune system recognizes with specific receptors that distinguish the antigens as nonself and as unique foreign molecules.

The principal cells of the adaptive immune system are the lymphocytes, APCs, and effector cells that eliminate the antigen. There are two types of lymphocytes: T lymphocytes and B lymphocytes. B lymphocytes differentiate into plasma cells that produce antibodies and provide for the elimination of microbes in the extracellular fluid (humoral immunity). T lymphocytes differentiate into regulatory (helper T and regulatory T cells) and effector (cytotoxic T cells) cells. APCs consist of macrophages and dendritic cells that process and present antigen peptides to CD4$^+$ helper T cells.

Central to the identity of the immune cells are CD molecules that distinguish among the different immune cells and their level of differentiation. The regulatory CD4$^+$ helper T cells serve as a trigger for the immune response and are essential for the differentiation of B cells into antibody-producing plasma cells and the differentiation of T lymphocytes into effector CD8$^+$ cytotoxic T cells that eliminate intracellular microbes, such as viruses. Cytokines function as communication molecules for the cells of the adaptive immune system, activate their proliferation and differentiation, and ensure the appropriate development of T and B lymphocytes into effector and memory cells. The cell surface MHC molecules are key recognition molecules that the immune system uses in distinguishing self from nonself. Class I MHC molecules, which are present on body cells other than those of the immune system, interact with cytotoxic CD8$^+$ T cells in the destruction of cells that have been affected by intracellular pathogens or cancer. Class II MHC molecules, found on immune cells, aid in cell-to-cell communication between different cells of the immune system.

The cells of the immune system are present in large numbers in the central and peripheral lymphoid organs. The central lymphoid organs (bone marrow and thymus) provide the environment for immune cell production and maturation, whereas the peripheral lymphoid structures (lymph nodes, spleen, mucosa-associated lymphoid tissues in the respiratory, gastrointestinal, and reproductive systems) function to concentrate antigen, aid in the processing of antigen, and promote cellular interactions necessary for development of adaptive immune responses.

Adaptive immunity can be acquired actively through immunization or by having a disease (active immunity), or by receiving antibodies or immune cells from another source (passive immunity). An acquired immune response can improve with repeated exposure to an injected antigen or a natural infection.

DEVELOPMENTAL ASPECTS OF THE IMMUNE SYSTEM

After completing this section of the chapter, you should be able to meet the following objectives:

* Explain the transfer of passive immunity from mother to fetus and from mother to infant during breast-feeding.
* Characterize the development of active immunity in the infant and small child.
* Describe changes in the immune response that occur with aging.

Embryologically, the immune system develops in several stages, beginning at 5 to 6 weeks as the fetal liver becomes active in hematopoiesis. Development of the primary lymphoid organs (*i.e.,* thymus and bone marrow) begins during the middle of the first trimester and proceeds rapidly. Secondary lymphoid organs (*i.e.,* spleen, lymph nodes, and mucosa-associated lymphoid tissues) develop soon after. These secondary lymphoid organs are rather small but well developed at birth and mature rapidly after exposure to microbes during the postnatal period. The thymus at birth is the largest lymphoid tissue relative to body size and normally is approximately two thirds its mature weight, which it achieves during the first year of life.

Transfer of Immunity From Mother to Infant

Protection of a newborn against antigens occurs through transfer of maternal antibodies. Maternal IgG antibodies cross the placenta during fetal development and remain functional in the newborn for the first months of life (Fig. 17.14). IgG is the only class of immunoglobulins to cross the placenta. Levels of maternal IgG decrease significantly during the first 3 to 6 months of life, while infant synthesis of immunoglobulins increases. Maternally transmitted IgG is effective against most microorganisms and viruses. The largest amount of IgG crosses the placenta during the last weeks of pregnancy and is stored in fetal tissues, and infants born prematurely may be deficient. Because of transfer of IgG antibodies to the fetus, an infant born to a mother infected with HIV has a positive HIV antibody test result, although the child may not be infected with the virus.

Cord blood does not normally contain IgM or IgA. If present, these antibodies are of fetal origin and represent exposure to intrauterine infection. The infant begins producing IgM antibodies shortly after birth, in response to the immense antigenic stimulation of his or her new environment. Premature infants appear to be able to produce IgM as well as term infants. At approximately 6 days of age the IgM rises sharply, and this rise continues until approximately 1 year of age, when the adult level is achieved.

Serum IgA normally is first detected at approximately 13 days after birth. The level increases during early childhood until adult levels are reached between the sixth and seventh year. Maternal IgA also is transferred to the infant in colostrum or breast milk. These antibodies provide local immunity for the intestinal system and have been shown to decrease diarrheal infections in underdeveloped countries. These adaptations of the immune system have increased the survival of our species and optimized the development of other important organs in the early months of life.

Immune Response in Older Adults

Aging is characterized by a declining ability to adapt to environmental stresses. One of the factors thought to contribute to this problem is a decline in immune responsiveness referred to as *immunosenscence.* This includes changes in cell-mediated and humoral immune responses. Older adults tend to be more susceptible to infections, have more evidence of autoimmune and immune complex disorders than younger persons, and have a higher incidence of cancer. Experimental evidence suggests that vaccination is less successful in inducing immunization in older persons than in younger adults. However, the effect of altered immune function on the health of older adults is clouded by the fact that age-related changes or disease may affect the immune response.

The alterations in immune function that occur with advanced age are not fully understood. There is a decrease in the size of the thymus gland, which is thought to affect T-cell function. The size of the gland begins to decline shortly after sexual maturity, and by 50 years of age, it usually has diminished to 15% or less of its maximum size. There are conflicting reports regarding age-related changes in the peripheral lymphocytes. A suggested biologic clock in T cells that determines the number of times it divides may regulate cell number with age. Some researchers have reported a decrease in the absolute number of lymphocytes, and others have found

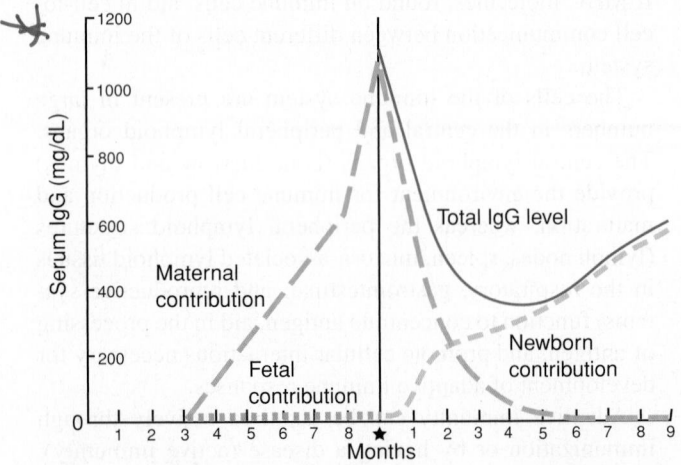

FIGURE 17.14 • Maternal/neonatal serum immunoglobulin G levels. (From Allansmith M., McClellan B. H., Butterworth M., et al. (1968). The development of immunoglobulin levels in man. *Journal of Pediatrics, 72,* 289.)

little, if any change. The most common finding is a slight decrease in the proportion of T cells to other lymphocytes and a decrease in $CD4^+$ and $CD8^+$ cells.

More evident are altered responses of the immune cells to antigen stimulation; increasing proportions of lymphocytes become unresponsive, whereas the remainder continue to function relatively normally. T and B cells show deficiencies in activation. In the T-cell types, the $CD4^+$ subset is most severely affected. Evidence indicates that aged T cells have a decreased rate of synthesis of the cytokines that drive the proliferation of lymphocytes and a diminished expression of the receptors that interact with those cytokines. For example, it has been shown that IL-2, IL-4, and IL-12 levels decrease with aging. Although B-cell function is compromised with age, the range of antigens that can be recognized is not diminished. If anything, the repertoire, including outgrowths of auto-reactive B-cell clones, is increased to the extent that B cells begin to recognize some self-antigens as foreign antigens. This may be the basis for the increased incidence of autoimmune disease in older adults.

IN SUMMARY

A newborn is protected against antigens in early life by passive transfer of maternal antibodies through the placenta (IgG) and in colostrum (IgA) through breast-feeding. Some changes are seen with aging, including an increase in autoimmune diseases. The impact of alterations in immune function that occur with aging is not fully understood.

REVIEW EXERCISES

1. The systemic manifestations (*e.g.,* generalized muscle aches, chills and fever, loss of appetite) that accompany a severe sore throat or acute respiratory infection are stimulated by reactions to cytokines of the innate immune system rather than by the antibodies or cell-mediated responses of the adaptive immune response.
   A. *Explain.*
2. A nursing student is working in a community clinic as a volunteer. Each time she enters the clinic, she suffers bouts of sneezing and runny nose. She has a history of mould allergy and her younger brother has asthma. Analysis at the allergy clinic indicates a strong reaction to latex. She is advised to avoid exposure to all forms of latex.
   A. *What class of immunoglobulin and what type of mediator cells are responsible for the symptoms expressed in this individual?*
   B. *What type of T-helper cell and cytokines direct the expression of this humoral immune response?*
   C. *Is this an example of active or passive immunity? Is this likely to be a primary or secondary immune response?*
3. A child of 5 months of age presents with thrush, a yeast infection of the mouth. In the last 2 months, he has had recurrent bouts of otitis media. His tonsils are very small. Laboratory analysis indicates a low lymphocyte count and no T lymphocytes. Further analysis indicates a genetic mutation in the T-cell receptor molecule complex (TCR–CD3) that affects maturation of all T cells. The final diagnosis is severe combined immunodeficiency disease. A bone marrow transplant is being pursued with cells from his HLA-matched sibling.
   A. *Why were infections not present in the first few months of this child's life?*
   B. *What would be the impact of an absence of T cells on both humoral and cell-mediated immunity?*
   C. *Why would it not be advisable to administer a live virus vaccine in this child?*

Bibliography

Abbas A. K., Lichtman A. H., Pillai S. (2015). *Cellular and molecular immunology* (8th ed.). Philadelphia, PA: Elsevier Saunders.

Akashi-Takamura S., Miyake K. (2006). Toll-like receptors (TLRs) and immune disorders. *Journal of Infection Chemotherapy, 12,* 233–240.

Annunziato F., Romagnani C., Romagnani S. (2015). The 3 major types of innate and adaptive cell-mediated effort immunity. *Journal of Allergy and Clinical Immunology, 135*(3), 626–635.

Artis D., Spits H. (2015). The biology of innate lymphoid cells. *Nature, 517*(7534), 293–301.

Chen K., Cerutti A. (2011). The function and regulation of immunoglobulin D. *Current Opinion in Immunology, 23*(3), 345–352.

Coulie P. G., Van den Eynde B. J., van der Bruggen P., et al. (2014). Tumour antigens recognized by T lymphocytes: At the core of cancer immunotherapy. *Nature Reviews Cancer, 14*(2), 135–146.

Hall J. E. (2011). *Textbook of medical physiology* (12th ed.). Philadelphia, PA: W. B. Saunders.

Jiang H., Chess L. (2006). Regulation of immune responses by T cells. *New England Journal of Medicine, 354,* 1166–1176.

Jin W., Dong C. (2013). IL-17 cytokines in immunity and inflammation. *Emerging Microbes and Infections, 2,* e60.

Josefowicz S. Z., Lu L., Rudensky A. Y. (2012). Regulatory T cells: Mechanisms of differentiation and function. *Annual Review of Immunology, 30,* 531–564.

Kliegman R. M., Stanton B. F., St. Geme J. W., et al. (Eds.). (2011). *Nelson textbook of pediatrics.* (19th ed.). Philadelphia, PA: Elsevier Saunders.

Kumar V., Abbas A. K., Faustos N., et al. (Eds.). (2010). *Robbins and Cotran pathologic basis of disease* (8th ed.). Philadelphia, PA: Elsevier Saunders.

Martinez-Sosa P., Mendoza L. (2013). The regulatory network that controls the differentiation of T lymphocytes. *BioSystems, 113*(2), 96–103.

Rhoades R. A., Bell D. R. (2013). *Medical physiology: Principles for clinical medicine* (4th ed.). Philadelphia, PA: Lippincott Williams & Wilkins.

Rubin R., Strayer D. S., (Eds.). (2012). *Rubin's pathology: Clinicopathologic foundations of medicine* (6th ed.). Philadelphia, PA: Lippincott Williams & Wilkins.

Solana R., Tarazona R., Gayoso I., et al. (2012). Innate immunosenescence: Effect of aging on cells and receptors of the innate immune system in humans. *Seminars in Immunology, 24*(5), 331–341.

Spits H., Artis D., Colonna M., et al. (2013). Innate lymphoid cells: A proposal for uniform nomenclature. *Nature Reviews Immunology, 13*(2), 145–149.

Spits H., Cupedo T. (2012). Innate lymphoid cells: Emerging insights in development, lineage relationships, and function. *Annual Review of Immunology, 30*, 647–675.

Takeuchi O., Akira S. (2010). Pattern recognition receptors and inflammation. *Cell, 140*(6), 805–820.

Tan Q., Zhu Y., Li J., et al. (2013). Structure of the CCR5 chemokine receptor – HIV entry inhibitor maraviroc complex. *Science, 341*(6152), 1387–1390.

Walker J. A., Barlow J. L., McKenzie A. N. J. (2013). Innate lymphoid cells: How did we miss them? *Nature Reviews Immunology, 13*(2), 75–87.

Walport M. J. (2001). Complement: Parts 1 and 2. *New England Journal of Medicine, 344*, 1058–1066, 1141–1144.

Ygberg S., Nilsson A. (2012). The developing immune system: From foetus to toddler. *Acta Paediatrica, 101*(2), 120–127.

Visit thePoint **http://thePoint.lww.com for animations, journal articles, and more!**

Inflammation, Tissue Repair, and Wound Healing

18

Inflammation is a protective response intended to eliminate the initial cause of cell injury, remove the damaged tissue, and generate new tissue. It accomplishes this by diluting, destroying, or otherwise neutralizing the harmful agents. It then sets the stage for the events that will eventually heal and reconstitute the damaged tissue. Thus, inflammation is intimately interwoven with the repair processes that replace damaged tissue or fill in the residual defects with fibrous scar tissue.

Although first described over 2,000 years ago, the inflammatory response has evoked renewed interest during the past several decades. As a result, a number of diseases are now known to be linked to the inflammatory response. For example, the role of the inflammatory response in bronchial asthma, rheumatoid arthritis, and atherosclerosis has been well established. There is also increasing evidence that the inflammatory response may play a role in the pathogenesis of a number of other diseases, such as diabetes mellitus, and Alzheimer disease.

This chapter focuses on the morphologic and functional manifestations of acute and chronic inflammation, tissue repair, and wound healing. The innate and adaptive immune response, which is closely intertwined with the inflammatory response, is discussed in Chapter 17.

THE INFLAMMATORY RESPONSE

After completing this section of the chapter, you should be able to meet the following objectives:

- List the cells involved in the inflammatory response and state their function.
- State the five cardinal signs of acute inflammation and describe the physiologic mechanisms involved in production of these signs.
- Describe the vascular changes in an acute inflammatory response.
- Characterize the interaction of adhesion molecules, chemokines, and cytokines in leukocyte adhesion, migration, and phagocytosis, which are part of the cellular phase of inflammation.

- List four types of inflammatory mediators and state their function.
- Contrast acute and chronic inflammation.
- Define the systemic manifestations of inflammation, including the characteristics of an acute-phase response.

General Features of Inflammation

Inflammation is the response of vascularized tissues to cell injury or death. It is characterized by the elaboration of inflammatory mediators and the movement of fluid and leukocytes from the blood into the extravascular tissues.[1-3] Although commonly perceived as a harmful reaction, it is actually a protective response that helps to rid the body of the initial cause of cell injury and the consequences of such injury.[2] This response localizes and eliminates microbes, foreign particles, and abnormal cells and paves the way for repair of the injured tissue. Inflammatory conditions are commonly named by adding the suffix *-itis* to the affected organ or system. For example, *appendicitis* refers to inflammation of the appendix, *pericarditis* to inflammation of the pericardium, and *neuritis* to inflammation of a nerve. More descriptive expressions of the inflammatory process might indicate whether the process was acute or chronic and what type of exudate was formed (*e.g.,* acute fibrinous pericarditis).

Inflammation can be divided into two types: acute and chronic.[1,2] *Acute inflammation* is triggered by noxious stimuli, such as infection or tissue injury, is rapid in onset (typically minutes), and is of relatively short duration, lasting from a few minutes to several days. It is characterized by the exudation of fluid and plasma components and emigration of leukocytes, predominantly neutrophils. *Chronic inflammation* is of a longer duration, lasting for days to years, and is associated with the proliferation of blood vessels, tissue necrosis, and fibrosis (scarring). Acute and chronic inflammation may coexist, with episodes of acute inflammation being superimposed on chronic inflammation.

Cells of Inflammation

Many cells and tissue components are involved in the inflammatory response, including the endothelial cells that line blood vessels, circulating platelets and leukocytes, connective tissue cells (mast cells, fibroblasts, tissue macrophages, and lymphocytes), and components of the extracellular matrix (ECM) (Fig. 18.1).[1,2,4] The principal leukocytes in acute inflammation are neutrophils, whereas macrophages, lymphocytes, eosinophils, and mast cells predominate in chronic infection. At the biochemical level, the inflammatory mediators, acting together or in sequence, amplify the initial response and influence its evolution by regulating the subsequent vascular and cellular responses.

Endothelial Cells. Endothelial cells, the single layer of cells that line the blood vessels, help to separate the intracellular and extracellular spaces.[4,5] They produce antiplatelet and antithrombotic agents that maintain vessel patency as well as vasodilators and vasoconstrictors that regulate blood flow. Endothelial cells are also key players in the inflammatory response. As such, they provide a selective permeability barrier to exogenous (microbial) and endogenous inflammatory stimuli; regulate leukocyte extravasation by expression of cell

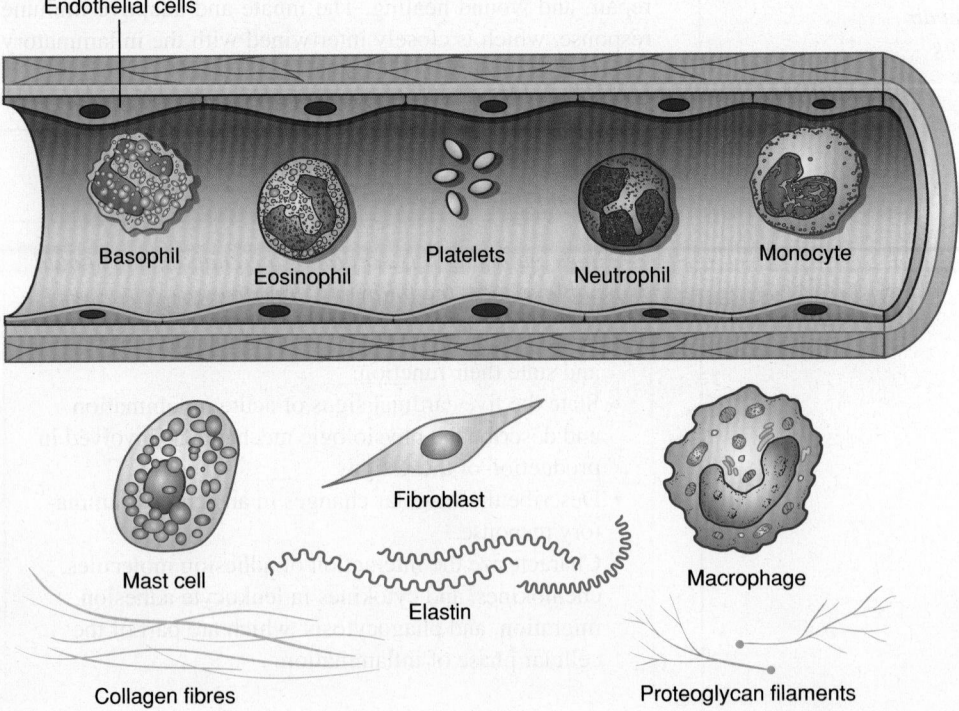

Endothelial cells

Basophil

Eosinophil

Platelets

Neutrophil

Monocyte

Mast cell

Fibroblast

Elastin

Macrophage

Collagen fibres

Proteoglycan filaments

FIGURE 18.1 • Cells involved in the inflammatory process.

adhesion molecules and receptors; contribute to the regulation and modulation of immune responses through synthesis and release of inflammatory mediators; and regulate immune cell proliferation through secretion of hematopoietic colony-stimulating factors (CSFs). Endothelial cells also participate in the repair process that accompanies inflammation through the production of growth factors that stimulate angiogenesis (formation of new blood vessels) and extracellular matrix synthesis.

Platelets. Platelets or thrombocytes are the cell fragments circulating in the blood that are involved in the cellular mechanisms of primary hemostasis (see Chapter 13). Activated platelets also release a number of potent inflammatory mediators, thereby increasing vascular permeability and altering the chemotactic, adhesive, and proteolytic properties of the endothelial cells.[6–8] When a platelet undergoes activation, over 300 proteins are released. Although only a relatively small proportion of these have been identified, it appears that a significant number are inflammatory mediators.[6] The association between the platelet and inflammatory diseases is highlighted by the number of inflammatory disease processes (*e.g.,* atherosclerosis, migraine headache, systemic lupus erythematosus) shown to be associated with platelet activation.[6]

Neutrophils and Monocytes/Macrophages. The neutrophils and macrophages are phagocytic leukocytes that are present in large numbers and are evident within hours at the site of inflammation.[9,10] Both types of leukocytes express a number of surface receptors and molecules that are involved in their activation. They include mannose receptors that bind glycoproteins of bacteria; Toll-like receptors that respond to different types and components of microbes; cell communication receptors that recognize specific cytokines and chemokines produced in response to infections and tissue injury; cell adhesion molecules that affect leukocyte adhesion; and complement receptors that recognize degraded fragments of complement deposited on the microbial surface (Fig. 18.2).

The *neutrophil* is the primary phagocyte that arrives early at the site of inflammation, usually within 90 minutes of injury. These leukocytes have nuclei that are divided into three to five lobes; therefore, they often are referred to as *polymorphonuclear neutrophils* (PMNs) or *segmented neutrophils (segs).* The neutrophil is classified as a granulocyte, a type of white blood cell identified by distinctive cytoplasmic granules. These cytoplasmic granules, which resist staining and remain a neutral colour in the neutrophil, contain enzymes and other antibacterial substances that are used in destroying and degrading engulfed microbes and dead tissue.[4,11] Neutrophils also have oxygen-dependent metabolic pathways that generate toxic oxygen (*e.g.,* hydrogen peroxide) and nitrogen (*e.g.,* nitric oxide) products that aid in the destruction of engulfed pathogens.

The neutrophil count in the blood often increases greatly during an inflammatory process, especially with bacterial infections. After being released from the bone marrow, circulating neutrophils have a life span of only approximately 4 to 10 hours and therefore must be constantly replaced if their numbers are to remain adequate.[2,9] This requires an increase in circulating white blood cells, a condition called *leukocytosis.* With excessive demand for phagocytes, immature forms of neutrophils are released from the bone marrow. These immature cells often are called *bands* because of the horseshoe shape of their nuclei.

Circulating monocytes have a single kidney-shaped nucleus, are the largest size of the circulating leukocytes, and constitute 5% to 6% of the white blood cell count.[9] They

FIGURE 18.2 • Leukocyte activation. Different classes of leukocyte cell surface receptors recognize different stimuli. The receptors initiate responses that mediate the functions of the leukocytes.

Understanding   Acute Inflammation

Acute inflammation is the immediate and early response to an injurious agent. The response, which serves to control and eliminate altered cells, microorganisms, and antigens, occurs in two stages: (1) the vascular stage, which leads to an increase in blood flow and changes in the small blood vessels of the microcirculation; and (2) the cellular stage, which leads to the migration of leukocytes from the circulation and their activation to eliminate the injurious agent. The primary function of inflammatory response is to limit the injurious effect of the pathologic agent and remove the injured tissue components, thereby allowing tissue repair to take place.

1. Vascular Stage

The vascular stage of acute inflammation is characterized by changes in the small blood vessels at the site of injury. It begins with momentary vasoconstriction followed rapidly by vasodilation. Vasodilation involves the arterioles and venules with a resultant increase in capillary blood flow, causing heat and redness, which are two of the cardinal signs of inflammation. This is accompanied by an increase in vascular permeability with outpouring of protein-rich fluid (exudate) into the extravascular spaces. The loss of proteins reduces the capillary osmotic pressure and increases the interstitial osmotic pressure. This, coupled with an increase in capillary pressure, causes a marked outflow of fluid and its accumulation in the tissue spaces, producing the swelling, pain, and impaired function that represent the other cardinal signs of acute inflammation. As fluid moves out of the vessels, stagnation of flow and clotting of blood occur. This aids in localizing the spread of infectious microorganisms.

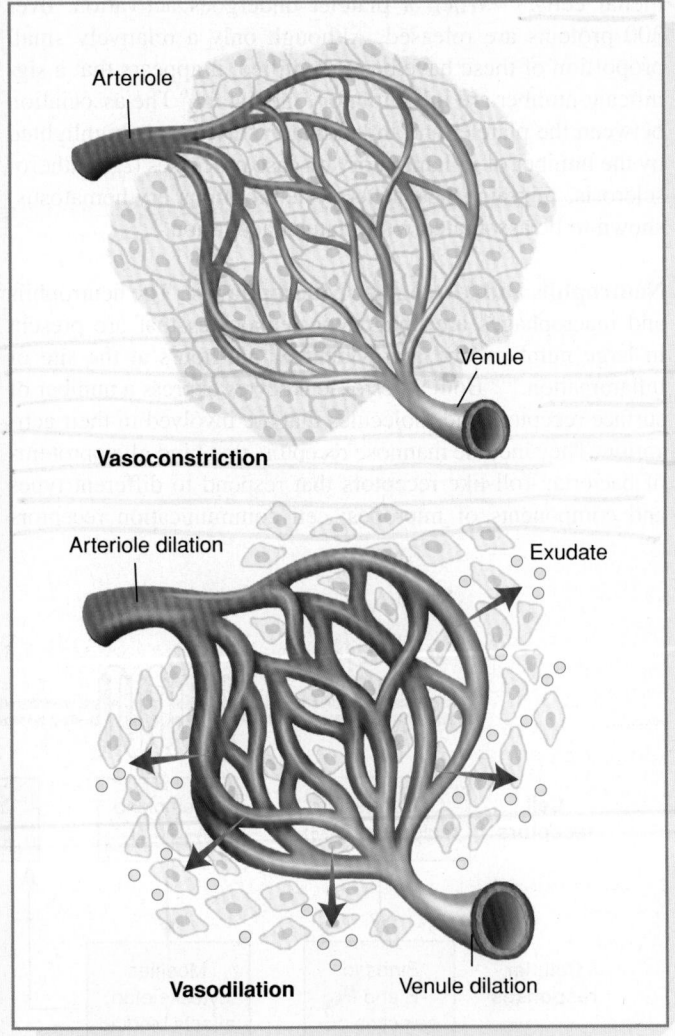

Arteriole

Venule

Vasoconstriction

Arteriole dilation

Exudate

Vasodilation   Venule dilation

are derived from the bone marrow and can exit the circulation in response to inflammatory stimuli and become tissue macrophages.[9,12] Within 24 hours, mononuclear cells arrive at the inflammatory site, where they are transformed into macrophages that phagocytose tissue debris, fibrin, bacteria, and dead neutrophils.

Monocytes and macrophages produce potent vasoactive mediators, including prostaglandins and leukotrienes,

2. Cellular Stage: Leukocyte Margination, Adhesion, and Transmigration

The cellular stage of acute inflammation involves the delivery of leukocytes, mainly neutrophils, to the site of injury so they can perform their normal functions of host defence. The delivery and activation of leukocytes can be divided into the following steps: adhesion and margination, transmigration, and chemotaxis. The recruitment of leukocytes to the precapillary venules, where they exit the circulation, is facilitated by the slowing of blood flow and margination along the vessel surface. Leukocyte adhesion and transmigration from the vascular space into the extravascular tissue is facilitated by complementary adhesion molecules (*e.g.,* selectins, integrins) on the leukocyte and endothelial surfaces. After extravasation, leukocytes migrate in the tissues toward the site of injury by chemotaxis, or locomotion oriented along a chemical gradient.

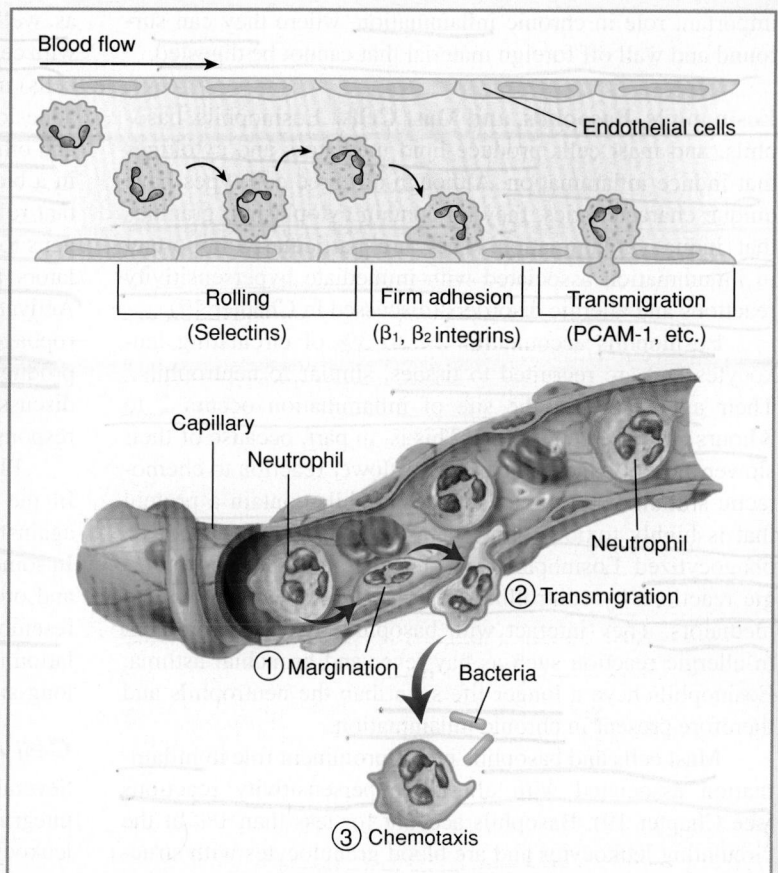

3. Leukocyte Activation and Phagocytosis

Once at the site of injury, the products generated by tissue injury trigger a number of leukocyte responses, including phagocytosis and cell killing. Opsonization of microbes (1) by complement factor C3b and antibody facilitates recognition by neutrophil C3b and the antibody Fc receptor. Receptor activation (2) triggers intracellular signalling and actin assembly in the neutrophil, leading to formation of pseudopods that enclose the microbe within a phagosome. The phagosome (3) then fuses with an intracellular lysosome to form a phagolysosome into which lysosomal enzymes and oxygen radicals (4) are released to kill and degrade the microbe.

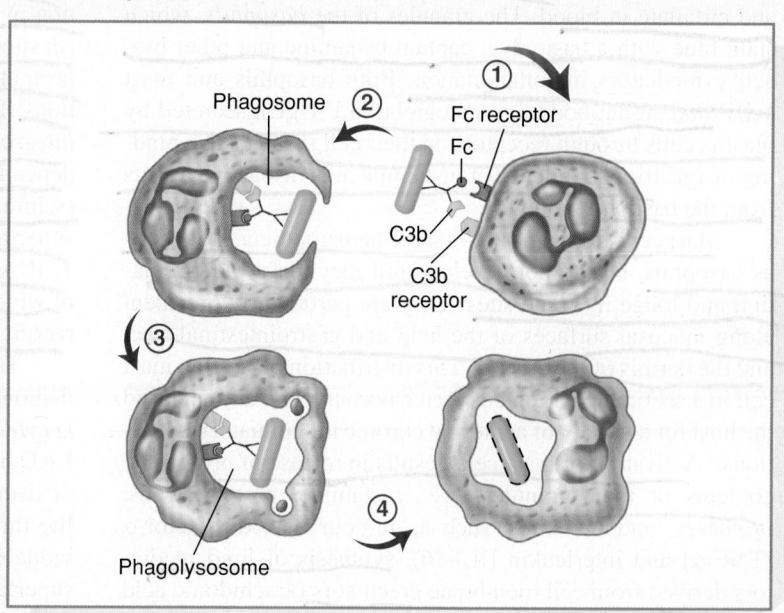

platelet-activating factor (PAF), inflammatory cytokines, and growth factors that promote regeneration of tissues. The macrophages engulf larger and greater quantities of foreign material than the neutrophils, and their circulating life span is three to four times longer. These longer-lived phagocytes help to destroy the causative agent, aid in the signalling processes of immunity, serve to resolve the inflammatory process, and contribute to initiation of the healing processes. They also play an important role in chronic inflammation, where they can surround and wall off foreign material that cannot be digested.

Eosinophils, Basophils, and Mast Cells. Eosinophils, basophils, and mast cells produce lipid mediators and cytokines that induce inflammation. Although all three cell types have unique characteristics, they all contain cytoplasmic granules that induce inflammation. They are particularly important in inflammation associated with immediate hypersensitivity reactions and allergic disorders (discussed in Chapter 19).

Eosinophils account for 2% to 3% of circulating leukocytes and are recruited to tissues, similar to neutrophils.[9] Their appearance at the site of inflammation occurs 2 to 3 hours after the neutrophils. This is, in part, because of their slower mobility and comparatively slower reaction to chemotactic stimuli. The granules of eosinophils contain a protein that is highly toxic to large parasitic worms that cannot be phagocytized. Eosinophils also play an important role in allergic reactions by controlling the release of specific chemical mediators. They interact with basophils and are prominent in allergic reaction such as hay fever and bronchial asthma. Eosinophils have a longer life span than the neutrophils and therefore present in chronic inflammation.

Mast cells and basophils play a prominent role in inflammation associated with allergic hypersensitivity reactions (see Chapter 19). Basophils account for less than 1% of the circulating leukocytes and are blood granulocytes with structural and functional similarities to mast cells of the connective tissue. They are derived from bone marrow progenitors and circulate in blood. The granules of the *basophils*, which stain blue with a basic dye, contain histamine and other bioactive mediators of inflammation. Both basophils and mast cells bind an antibody, immunoglobulin E (IgE), secreted by plasma cells through receptors on their cell surface. The binding of IgE triggers release of histamine and vasoactive agents from the basophil granules.

Mast cells derive from the same hematopoietic stem cells as basophils, but do not develop until they leave the circulation and lodge in tissue sites. They are particularly prevalent along mucosal surfaces of the lung and gastrointestinal tract and the dermis of the skin.[2,13] This distribution places the mast cell in a sentinel position between environmental antigens and the host for a variety of acute and chronic inflammatory conditions.[2] Activation of mast cells results in release of preformed contents of their granules (*e.g.*, histamine, proteoglycans, proteases, and cytokines such as tumour necrosis factor-α [TNF-α] and interleukin [IL]-16), synthesis of lipid mediators derived from cell membrane precursors (arachidonic acid metabolites, such as prostaglandins, and platelet-activating factor), and stimulation of cytokine and chemokine synthesis by other cells such as monocytes and macrophages.

Lymphoctyes and Plasma Cells. Lymphocytes are the smallest of the leukocytes and have a thin rim of cytoplasm surrounded by a deeply staining nucleus. They participate in immune-mediated inflammation caused by infectious agents

as well as non–immune-mediated inflammation associated with cell injury and death. Both T and B lymphocytes (T and B cells) migrate into inflammatory sites using some of the same adhesion molecules and chemokines that recruit neutrophils and other leukocytes. Lymphocytes and macrophages interact in a bidirectional way, and these interactions play an important role in chronic inflammation. Macrophages display antigens to T cells, express membrane molecules called costimulators, and produce cytokines that stimulate T-cell responses.[2] Activated T cells, in turn, produce cytokines that activate macrophages, increasing antigen presentation and further cytokine production. (Cytokines and other inflammatory mediators are discussed later in this chapter.) The result is a cycle of cellular responses that fuel and sustain chronic inflammation.

Plasma cells develop from activated B lymphocytes. In the inflammatory site, they produce antibodies directed against persistent antigens and altered tissue components.[1,2] In some intense, chronic inflammatory reactions, plasma cells and other lymphocytes may accumulate to form a mass that resembles a lymph node. This pattern of lymphocyte accumulation is often seen in the inflamed synovium of persons with long-standing rheumatoid arthritis.

Cell Adhesion Molecules

Several families of cell adhesion molecules, including selectins, integrins, and the immunoglobulin superfamily, are involved in leukocyte recruitment and trafficking.[2,14–16] The *selectins* are a family of three closely related proteins (E-selectin, L-selectin, P-selectin) that differ in their cellular distribution, but all function in adhesion of leukocytes to endothelial cells. The *integrin* superfamily consists of 30 structurally similar proteins that promote cell-to-cell and cell–to–extracellular matrix interactions. The name *integrin* derives from the hypothesis that they *integrate* the signals of extracellular ligands with cytoskeleton-dependent motility, shape change, and phagocytic responses of immune cells. *Adhesion* molecules of the immunoglobulin superfamily include intercellular adhesion molecules (ICAM)-1, ICAM-2, and vascular adhesion molecule (VCAM)-1, all of which interact with integrins on leukocytes to mediate their recruitment.

The importance of the leukocyte adhesion molecules is demonstrated in persons with a rare autosomal recessive *leukocyte adhesion deficiency (LAD)*.[16] Three different forms of LAD have been described to date. In *LAD type 1*, a deficiency of a member of the integrin superfamily leads to recurrent life-threatening infections. A similar deficiency is seen in individuals with impaired expression of a member of the selectin superfamily and has been labelled *LAD type 2*. There is also evidence that excessive expression of cell adhesion molecules or their receptors contributes to the pathogenesis of some chronic inflammatory diseases such as rheumatoid arthritis.

Acute Inflammation

Acute inflammation is the early or almost immediate reaction of local tissues and their blood vessels to injury. It typically occurs before adaptive immunity becomes established and is aimed primarily at removing the injurious agent and limiting the extent of tissue damage. Acute inflammation can be triggered by a variety of stimuli, including infections, immune reactions, blunt and penetrating trauma, physical or chemical agents (*e.g.,* burns, frostbite, irradiation, caustic chemicals), and tissue necrosis from any cause.

The classic description of inflammation has been handed down through the ages. In the first century ad, the Roman physician Celsus described the local reaction of injury in terms that are now known as the *cardinal signs* of inflammation.[1] These signs are *rubor* (redness), *tumour* (swelling), *calor* (heat), and *dolor* (pain). In the second century ad, the Greek physician Galen added a fifth cardinal sign, *functio laesa* (loss of function). In addition to the cardinal signs that appear at the site of injury, systemic manifestations (*e.g.,* fever) may occur as chemical mediators (*e.g.,* cytokines) produced at the site of inflammation gain entrance to the circulatory system. The constellation of systemic manifestations that may occur during acute inflammation is known as the *acute-phase response* (to be discussed).

THE INFLAMMATORY RESPONSE

- Inflammation represents the response of body tissue to immune reactions, injury, or ischemic damage.
- The classic response to inflammation includes redness, swelling, heat, pain or discomfort, and loss of function.
- The manifestations of an acute inflammatory response can be attributed to the immediate vascular changes that occur (vasodilation and increased capillary permeability), the influx of inflammatory cells such as neutrophils, and, in some cases, the widespread effects of inflammatory mediators, which produce fever and other systemic signs and symptoms.
- The manifestations of chronic inflammation are due to infiltration with macrophages, lymphocytes, and fibroblasts, leading to persistent inflammation, fibroblast proliferation, and scar formation.

Stages of Acute Inflammation

Acute inflammation has two stages: the vascular stage and the cellular stage. The vascular stage is characterized by increased blood flow (vasodilation) and structural changes (increased vascular permeability) that allow plasma proteins to leave the circulation. The cellular stage involves the emigration of leukocytes (mainly neutrophils) from the microcirculation and their accumulation at the site of injury or infection.

Vascular Stage. The vascular changes that occur with inflammation involve the arterioles, capillaries, and venules of the microcirculation. These changes begin almost immediately after injury and are characterized by vasodilation and changes in blood flow followed by increased vascular permeability and leakage of protein-rich fluid into the extravascular tissues.[1,2]

Vasodilation, which is one of the earliest manifestations of inflammation, follows a transient constriction of the arterioles, lasting a few seconds. Dilation begins in the arterioles and opens capillary beds in the area. As a result, the area becomes congested, causing the redness (erythema) and warmth associated with acute inflammation. Vasodilation is induced by the action of several mediators, most notably histamine and nitric oxide.

Vasodilation is quickly followed by increased permeability of the microvasculature, with the outpouring of a protein-rich fluid (exudate) into the extravascular spaces. The loss of fluid results in an increased concentration of blood constituents (red cells, leukocytes, platelets, and clotting factors), stagnation of flow, and clotting of blood at the site of injury. This aids in limiting the spread of infectious microorganisms. The loss of plasma proteins reduces the intracapillary osmotic pressure and increases the osmotic pressure of the interstitial fluid, causing fluid to move into the tissues and produce the swelling (*i.e.,* edema), pain, and impaired function that are the cardinal signs of acute inflammation. The exudation of fluid into the tissue spaces also serves to dilute the offending agent.

The increased permeability characteristic of acute inflammation results from formation of endothelial gaps in the venules of the microcirculation. Binding of the chemical mediators to endothelial receptors causes contraction of endothelial cells and separation of intercellular junctions. This is the most common mechanism of vascular leakage and is elicited by histamine, bradykinin, leukotrienes, and many other classes of chemical mediators.

Depending on the severity of injury, the vascular changes that occur with inflammation follow one of three patterns of responses.[2] The first pattern is an *immediate transient response*, which occurs with minor injury. It develops rapidly after injury and is usually reversible and of short duration (15 to 30 minutes). Typically, this type of leakage affects venules 20 to 60 μm in diameter, leaving capillaries and arterioles unaffected.[2] Although the precise mechanism for restriction of this effect to the venules is unknown, it may reflect the greater density of receptors in the endothelium of the venules. It has also been suggested that the later leukocyte events of inflammation (*i.e.,* adhesion and emigration) also occur predominantly in the venules of most organs.

The second pattern is *an immediate sustained response*, which occurs with more serious types of injury and continues for several days. It affects all levels of the microcirculation (arterioles, capillaries, and venules) and is usually due to direct damage of the endothelium by injurious stimuli, such as burns or the products of bacterial infections.[2] Neutrophils that adhere to the endothelium may also injure endothelial cells.

The third pattern is a *delayed hemodynamic response*, in which the increased permeability begins after a delay of 2 to 12 hours, lasts for several hours or even days, and involves venules as well as capillaries.[2] A delayed response often accompanies injuries due to radiation, such as sunburn. The mechanism of the leakage is unknown, but it may result from the direct effect of the injurious agent, leading to delayed endothelial cell damage.

Cellular Stage. The cellular stage of acute inflammation is marked by changes in the endothelial cells lining the vasculature and movement of phagocytic leukocytes into the area of injury or infection. Although attention has been focused on the recruitment of leukocytes from the blood, a rapid response also requires the release of chemical mediators from tissue cells (mast cells and macrophages) that are prepositioned in the tissues. The sequence of events in the cellular response to inflammation includes leukocyte (1) margination and adhesion to the endothelium, (2) transmigration across the endothelium, (3) chemotaxis, and (4) activation and phagocytosis.[1,2]

During the early stages of the inflammatory response, signalling between the blood leukocytes and the vascular endothelium defines the inflammatory event and ensures secure adhesion and arrest of the leukocytes along the endothelium. As a consequence, the leukocytes slow their migration, adhere tightly to the endothelium, and begin to move along the periphery of the blood vessels. This process of leukocyte accumulation is called *margination.* The subsequent release of cell communication molecules called *cytokines* causes the endothelial cells lining the vessels to express cell adhesion molecules, such as *selectins,* that bind to carbohydrates on the leukocytes. This interaction, which is called *tethering,* slows their flow and causes the leukocytes to move along the endothelial cell surface with a rolling movement, finally coming to rest and adhering strongly to ICAMs on the endothelium.[1] The adhesion causes the endothelial cells to separate, allowing the leukocytes to extend pseudopodia and *transmigrate* through the vessel wall and then, under the influence of chemotactic factors, migrate into the tissue spaces.

Chemotaxis is a dynamic and energy-directed process of directed cell migration.[1] Once leukocytes exit the capillary, they wander through the tissue guided by a gradient of secreted chemoattractants, such as chemokines, bacterial and cellular debris, and protein fragments generated from activation of the complement system (*e.g.,* C3a, C5a). Chemokines, an important subgroup of chemotactic cytokines, are small proteins that direct the trafficking of leukocytes during the early stages of inflammation or injury.[17,18] Several immune (*e.g.,* macrophages) and nonimmune cells secrete these chemoattractants to ensure the directed movement of leukocytes to the site of infection.

During the next and final stage of the cellular response, neutrophils, monocytes, and tissue macrophages are activated to engulf and degrade the bacteria and cellular debris in a process called *phagocytosis.*[1,2,19] Phagocytosis involves three distinct steps: (1) recognition and adherence, (2) engulfment, and (3) intracellular killing. Phagocytosis is initiated by the recognition and binding of particles by specific receptors on the surface of phagocytic cells. This binding is essential for trapping the agent, which triggers engulfment and activates the killing potential of the cell. Microbes can be bound directly to the membrane of phagocytic cells by several types of pattern

recognition receptors (*e.g.,* Toll-like and mannose receptors) or indirectly by receptors that recognize microbes coated with carbohydrate-binding lectins, antibody, or complement (see section on Innate Immunity, Chapter 17). The coating of an antigen with antibody or complement to enhance binding is called *opsonization.* Receptor-mediated endocytosis is triggered by opsonization and binding of the agent to phagocyte cell surface receptors. Endocytosis is accomplished through cytoplasmic extensions (pseudopods) that surround and enclose the particle in a membrane-bounded phagocytic vesicle or *phagosome.* Once inside the cell cytoplasm, the phagosome merges with a cytoplasmic lysosome containing antibacterial molecules and enzymes that can kill and digest the microbe.

Intracellular killing of pathogens is accomplished through several mechanisms, including toxic oxygen and nitrogen products, lysozymes, proteases, and defencins. The metabolic burst pathways that generate toxic oxygen and nitrogen products (*i.e.,* nitric oxide, hydrogen peroxide, and hypochlorous acid) require oxygen and metabolic enzymes such as myeloperoxidase, nicotinamide adenine dinucleotide phosphate (NADPH) oxidase, and nitric oxide (NO) synthetase. Oxygen-independent pathways generate several types of digestive enzymes and antimicrobial molecules (*e.g.,* defencins). Individuals born with genetic defects in some of these enzymes have immunodeficiency conditions that make them susceptible to repeated bacterial infection (discussed in Chapter 19).

Inflammatory Mediators

Although inflammation is precipitated by infection and injury, its signs and symptoms are produced by chemical mediators. Mediators can originate either from the plasma or from cells (Fig. 18.3). The *plasma-derived mediators,* which are synthesized in the liver, include the acute-phase proteins, coagulation factors (discussed in Chapter 13), and the complement proteins (discussed in Chapter 17). These mediators are present in the plasma in a precursor form that must be activated by a series of proteolytic processes to acquire their biologic properties. *Cell-derived mediators* are normally sequestered in intracellular granules that need to be secreted (*e.g.,* histamine from mast cells), or are newly synthesized (*e.g.,* cytokines) in response to a stimulus. Although the major sources of these mediators are platelets, neutrophils, monocytes/macrophages, and mast cells, most endothelial cells, smooth muscle, and fibroblasts can be induced to produce some of the mediators.

The production of active mediators is triggered by microbes or host proteins, such as those of the complement, kinin, or coagulation systems, that are themselves activated by microbes or damaged tissues. Mediators can act on one or a few target cells, have diverse targets, or have differing effects on different types of cells. Once activated and released from the cell, most mediators are short lived. They may be transformed into inactive metabolites, inactivated by enzymes, or scavenged or degraded.

Inflammatory mediators can be classified by function: (1) those with vasoactive and smooth muscle-constricting

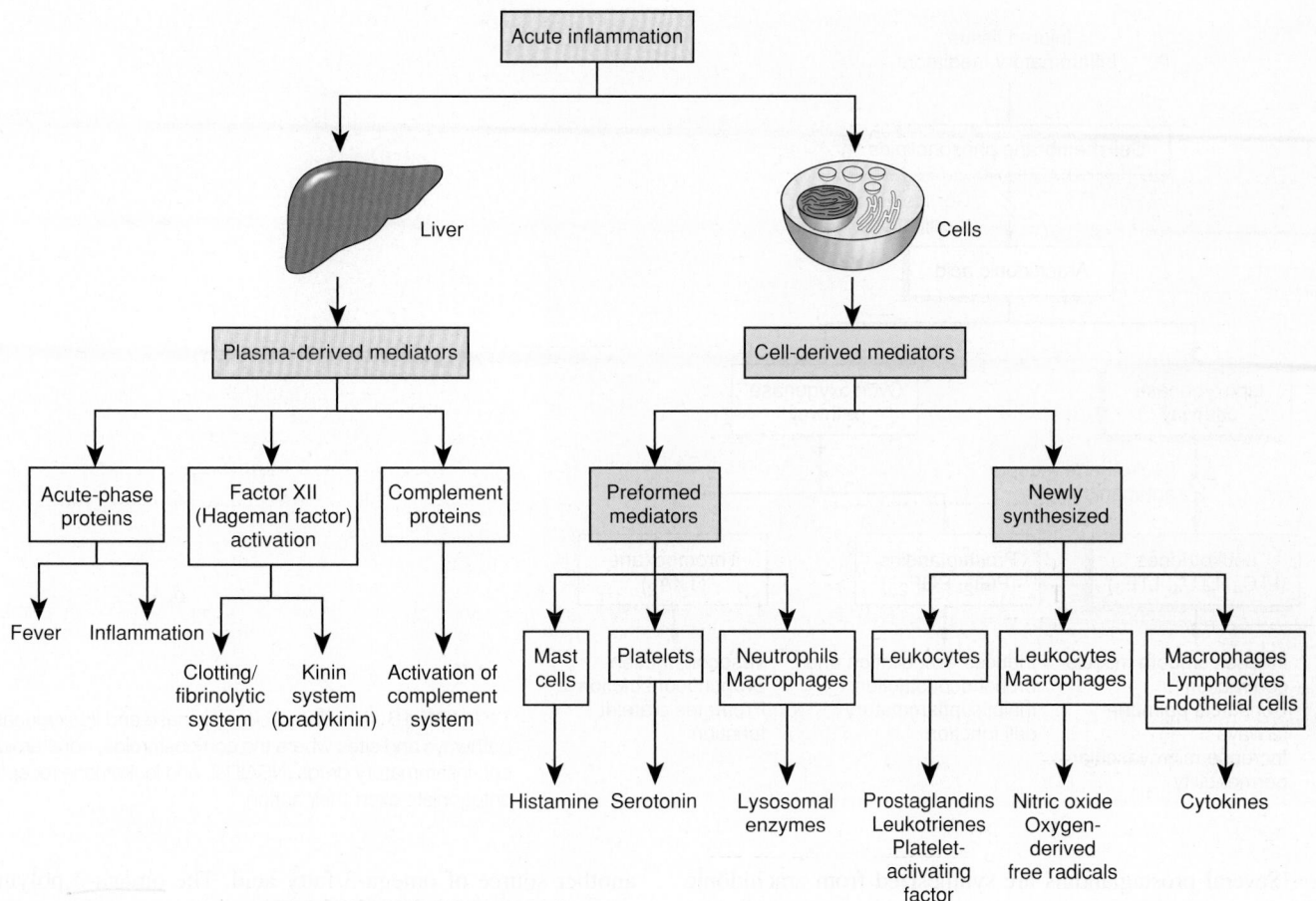

FIGURE 18.3 • Plasma- and cell-derived mediators of acute inflammation.

properties such as histamine, arachidonic acid metabolites (prostaglandins and leukotrienes), and platelet-activating factor; (2) plasma proteases that activate members of the complement system, coagulation factors of the clotting cascade, and vasoactive peptides of the kinin system; (3) chemotactic factors such as complement fragments and chemokines; and (4) reactive molecules and cytokines liberated from leukocytes, which when released into the extracellular environment can affect the surrounding tissue and cells.[1,2]

Histamine and Serotonin.   Histamine and serotonin are classified as *vasoactive amines,* meaning they are derived from amino acids (histamine from histidine, serotonin from tryptophan) and act by producing changes in blood vessel tone. Both histamine and serotonin are stored as preformed molecules in mast cells and other cells and are among the first mediators to be released during an acute inflammatory reaction.

Preformed histamine is widely distributed in tissues, the highest concentrations being found in the connective tissues adjacent to blood vessels.[1,2] It is also found in circulating platelets and basophils and is released in response to a variety of stimuli, including trauma and immune reactions involving binding of IgE to basophils and mast cells. Histamine produces dilation of arterioles and increases the permeability of venules. It acts at the

level of the microcirculation by binding to histamine type 1 (H₁) receptors on endothelial cells, and is considered the principal mediator of the immediate transient phase of increased vascular permeability in the acute inflammatory response. Antihistamine drugs (H₁ receptor antagonists), which bind to the H₁ receptors, act competitively to antagonize many of the effects of the immediate inflammatory response. Serotonin (5-hydroxytryptamin) is also a preformed vasoactive mediator, with effects similar to histamine. It is found primarily within platelet granules and is released during platelet aggregation.

Arachidonic Acid Metabolites.   Arachidonic acid is a 20-carbon unsaturated fatty acid found in phospholipids of cell membranes. Release of arachidonic acid by phospholipases initiates a series of complex reactions that lead to the production of the *eicosanoid* family inflammatory mediators (prostaglandins, leukotrienes and related metabolites).[1,2,20,21] Eicosanoid synthesis follows one of two pathways: the cyclooxygenase pathway, which culminates in the synthesis of prostaglandins, and the lipoxygenase pathway, which culminates in the synthesis of the leukotrienes (Fig. 18.4). The corticosteroid drugs block the inflammatory effects of both pathways by inhibiting phosphodiesterase activity and thus preventing the release of arachidonic acid.[22]

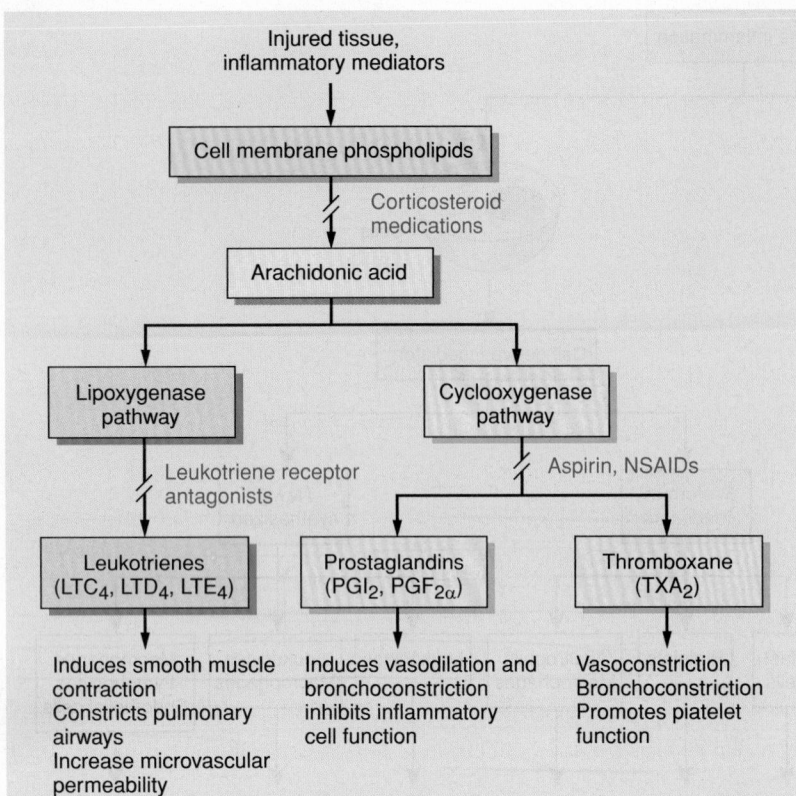

Injured tissue,
inflammatory mediators

Cell membrane phospholipids

Corticosteroid
medications

Arachidonic acid

Lipoxygenase
pathway

Cyclooxygenase
pathway

Leukotriene receptor
antagonists

Aspirin, NSAIDs

Leukotrienes
(LTC$_4$, LTD$_4$, LTE$_4$)

Prostaglandins
(PGI$_2$, PGF$_{2\alpha}$)

Thromboxane
(TXA$_2$)

Induces smooth muscle
contraction
Constricts pulmonary
airways
Increase microvascular
permeability

Induces vasodilation and
bronchoconstriction
inhibits inflammatory
cell function

Vasoconstriction
Bronchoconstriction
Promotes piatelet
function

FIGURE 18.4 • The cyclooxygenase and lipoxygenase pathways and sites where the corticosteroids, nonsteroidal anti-inflammatory drugs (NSAIDs), and leukotriene receptor antagonists exert their action.

Several prostaglandins are synthesized from arachidonic acid through the cyclooxygenase metabolic pathway.[21] The prostaglandins (*e.g.*, PGD$_2$, PGE$_2$, PGF$_{2\alpha}$, and PGI$_2$) induce inflammation and potentiate the effects of histamine and other inflammatory mediators. The prostaglandin thromboxane A$_2$ promotes platelet aggregation and vasoconstriction. Aspirin and the nonsteroidal anti-inflammatory drugs (NSAIDs) reduce inflammation by inactivating the first enzyme in the cyclooxygenase pathway for prostaglandin synthesis.

Like the prostaglandins, the leukotrienes are formed from arachidonic acid, but through the lipoxygenase pathway. Histamine and leukotrienes have similar functions; however, histamine is produced rapidly and transiently while the more potent leukotrienes are being synthesized. The leukotrienes also have been reported to affect the permeability of the postcapillary venules, the adhesion properties of endothelial cells, and the extravasation and chemotaxis of neutrophils, eosinophils, and monocytes. Leukotrienes C$_4$, LTD$_4$, and LTE$_4$, collectively known as the *slow-reacting substance of anaphylaxis* (SRS-A), cause slow and sustained constriction of the bronchioles and are important inflammatory mediators in bronchial asthma and anaphylaxis. Drugs such as LT receptor antagonists (*e.g.*, montelukast) target this pathway to limit inflammation and bronchoconstriction.

There has been interest in dietary modification of the inflammatory response through the use of omega-3 polyunsaturated fatty acids, specifically eicosapentaenoic acid and docosahexaenoic acid, which are present in oily fish and fish oil.[23,24] Alpha-linolenic acid, which is present in flax seed, canola oil, green leafy vegetables, walnuts, and soybeans, is

another source of omega-3 fatty acid. The omega-3 polyunsaturated fatty acids, which are considered antithrombotic and anti-inflammatory, are structurally different from the prothrombotic and proinflammatory omega-6 polyunsaturated fatty acids, which are present in most seeds, vegetable oils, and meats. Typically, the cell membranes of inflammatory cells contain high proportions of omega-6 arachidonic acid, which is the source of prostaglandin and LT inflammatory mediators. Eating oily fish and other foods that are high in omega-3 fatty acids results in partial replacement of arachidonic acid in inflammatory cell membranes by eicosapentaenoic acid, a change that leads to decreased production of arachidonic acid-derived inflammatory mediators. This response alone is a potentially beneficial effect of omega-3 fatty acids. However, omega-3 fatty acids have a number of other effects that might occur downstream of altered eicosanoid production or might be independent of this function. For example, animal and human research has shown that dietary fish oil results in suppressed production of proinflammatory cytokines and decreased expression of adhesion molecules that participate in the inflammatory response.

Platelet-Activating Factor. Originally named for its ability to cause platelet aggregation and granulation, PAF is another phospholipid-derived mediator with a broad spectrum of inflammatory effects.[1,2] PAF is generated from the membrane phospholipids of virtually all activated inflammatory cells and affects a variety of cell types. In addition to activating platelets, PAF stimulates neutrophils, monocytes/

macrophages, endothelial cells, and vascular smooth muscle. PAF-induced platelet aggregation and degranulation at the site of injury enhances serotonin release, thereby causing changes in vascular permeability. It also enhances leukocyte adhesion, chemotaxis, and leukocyte degranulation, and it stimulates the synthesis of other inflammatory mediators, especially the prostaglandins.

Plasma Proteins. A number of phenomena in the inflammatory response are mediated by plasma proteins that belong to three interrelated systems, the clotting, complement, and kinin systems.

The clotting system contributes to the vascular phase of inflammation, mainly through fibrinopeptides that are formed during the final steps of the clotting process (discussed in Chapter 13). The protease thrombin, which binds to receptors called *protease-activated receptors* (PARs), provides the final link between the coagulation system and inflammation. Engagement of the so-called type-1 receptor (PAR-1) by proteases, particularly thrombin, triggers several responses that induce inflammation, including production of chemokines, expression of endothelial adhesion molecules, induction of prostaglandin synthesis, and production of PAF.

The complement system consists of 20 component proteins (and their cleavage products) that are found in greatest concentration in the plasma (see Chapter 17). The complement proteins are present in inactive forms in the plasma. Many of them are activated to become proteolytic enzymes that degrade other complement proteins, thus forming a cascade that plays an important role in both immunity and inflammation. Complement fragments contribute to the inflammatory response by causing vasodilation, increasing vascular permeability, and enhancing the activity of phagocytes.[2]

The kinin system generates vasoactive peptides from plasma proteins called *kininogens,* by the action of proteases called *kallikreins.*[2] Activation of the kinin system results in release of bradykinin, which increases vascular permeability and causes contraction of smooth muscle, dilation of blood vessels, and stimulation of peripheral pain receptors (nociceptors). These effects are similar to those of histamine. The action of bradykinin is short lived because it is quickly inactivated by an enzyme called *kininase.* Any bradykinin that escapes inactivation by the kininase enzyme is degraded by the angiotensin-converting enzyme in the lung.

Cytokines and Chemokines. Cytokines are hormone-like, low–molecular-weight proteins that modulate the function of other cells. They are produced by many cell types (principally activated macrophages and lymphocytes, but also endothelium, epithelium, and connective tissue types).[1,2,18,19] Although well known for their role in immune responses, these proteins also play important roles in both acute and chronic inflammation.

TNF-α and IL-1 are two of the major cytokines that mediate inflammation. The major cellular source of TNF-α and IL-1 is activated macrophages (Fig. 18.5). IL-1 is also produced by many cell types other than macrophages, including

FIGURE 18.5 • Central role of interleukin (IL)-1 and tumour necrosis factor (TNF)-α in the acute inflammatory response. Lipopolysaccharide (LPS) and interferon (IFN)-γ activate macrophages to release inflammatory cytokines, principally IL-1 and TNF-α, responsible for directing both local and systemic inflammatory responses. (ACTH, adrenocorticotropic hormone) (From Rubin R., Strayer D. S. (Eds.). (2012). *Rubin's pathology: Clinicopathologic foundations of medicine* (6th ed., p. 60). Philadelphia, PA: Lippincott Williams & Wilkins.)

neutrophils, endothelial cells, and epithelial cells (*e.g.,* keratinocytes). The secretion of TNF-α and IL-1 can be stimulated by endotoxins and other microbial products, immune cells, injury, and a variety of inflammatory stimuli. TNF-α and IL-1 induce endothelial cells to express adhesion molecules and release cytokines, chemokines, and reactive oxygen species (ROSs). TNF-α induces priming and aggregation of neutrophils, leading to augmented responses of these cells to other mediators. IL-1 and TNF-α are also mediators of the acute-phase responses associated with infection or injury. Features of these systemic responses include fever, hypotension and increased heart rate, anorexia, release of neutrophils into the circulation, and increased levels of corticosteroid hormones.

Chemotactic cytokines, or *chemokines,* are a family of small proteins that act primarily as chemoattractants to recruit and direct the migration of immune and inflammatory cells[25] (see Chapter 17). Chemokines generate a chemotactic gradient by binding to proteoglycans on the surface of endothelial cells or in the ECM.[26] As a result, high concentrations of chemokines persist at sites of tissue injury or infection. Two classes of chemokines have been identified: inflammatory chemokines and homing chemokines. Inflammatory chemokines are produced in response to bacterial toxins and inflammatory cytokines (*i.e.,* IL-1, TNF-α). These chemokines recruit leukocytes during an inflammatory response. Homing chemokines are constitutively expressed and are up-regulated during inflammatory reactions and immune responses.

Nitric Oxide. Nitric oxide (NO), which is produced by a variety of cells, plays multiple roles in inflammation, including smooth muscle relaxation and antagonism of platelet adhesion, aggregation, and degranulation. It also serves as an endogenous regulator of leukocyte recruitment.[2] Blocking of NO production under normal conditions promotes leukocyte rolling and adhesion to postcapillary venules, and delivery of exogenous NO reduces leukocyte recruitment. Thus, production of NO appears to be a compensatory mechanism that reduces the cellular phase of inflammation. Impaired production of NO by vascular endothelial cells is implicated in the inflammatory changes that occur with atherosclerosis (see Chapter 22). NO and its derivatives also have antimicrobial actions and thus NO is also a host mediator against infection.

Oxygen-Derived Free Radicals. Oxygen free radicals may be released extracellularly from leukocytes after exposure to microbes, cytokines, and immune complexes, or during the phagocytic process that occurs during the cellular phase of the inflammatory process. The superoxide radical, hydrogen peroxide, and the hydroxyl radical (discussed in Chapter 5) are the major species produced in the cell. These species can combine with NO to form other reactive nitrogen intermediates. Extracellular release of low levels of these potent mediators can increase the expression of cytokines and endothelial adhesion molecules, amplifying the cascade that elicits the inflammatory process.[2] However, at higher levels, these potent mediators can produce endothelial cell damage, with a resultant increase in vascular permeability; inactivate antiproteases, such as α$_1$-antitrypsin, which protects against lung damage in smokers; and produce injury to other cell types, including red blood cells.[2] Thus, the influence of oxygen-derived free radicals in any inflammatory process depends on a balance between the generation and inactivation of these metabolites.

Local Manifestations

The local manifestations of acute inflammation, which are determined by severity of the reaction, its specific cause, and the site of involvement, can range from mild swelling and redness to abscess formation or ulceration. As part of the normal defence reaction, inflammation can also injure adjacent tissues.[2] In some infections such as tuberculosis and certain viral infections, the host response can cause more damage than the microbe itself. As a normal attempt to clear damaged and dead tissues (*e.g.,* after a myocardial infarction), the inflammatory response may prolong and exacerbate the injurious consequences of the infarction.

Characteristically, the acute inflammatory response involves the production of exudates. These exudates vary in terms of fluid type, plasma protein content, and the presence or absence of cells. They can be serous, hemorrhagic, fibrinous, membranous, or purulent. Often the exudate is composed of a combination of these types. *Serous exudates* are watery fluids low in protein content that result from plasma entering the inflammatory site. *Hemorrhagic exudates* occur when there is severe tissue injury that damages blood vessels or when there is significant leakage of red cells from the capillaries. *Fibrinous exudates* contain large amounts of fibrinogen and form a thick and sticky meshwork, much like the fibres of a blood clot. *Membranous* or *pseudomembranous exudates* develop on mucous membrane surfaces and are composed of necrotic cells enmeshed in a fibropurulent exudate.

A *purulent* or *suppurative exudate* contains pus, which is composed of degraded white blood cells, proteins, and tissue debris. The term *pyogenic* refers to "pus forming." Certain microorganisms, such as *Staphylococcus,* are more likely to induce localized suppurative inflammation than others. An *abscess* is a localized area of inflammation containing a purulent exudate (Fig. 18.6). Abscesses typically have a central necrotic core containing purulent exudates surrounded by a layer of neutrophils.[2] Fibroblasts may eventually enter the area and wall off the abscess. Because antimicrobial agents cannot penetrate the abscess wall, surgical incision and drainage may be required to effect a cure.

An *ulceration* refers to a site of inflammation where an epithelial surface (*e.g.,* skin or gastrointestinal epithelium) has become necrotic and eroded, often with associated subepithelial inflammation. Ulceration may occur as the result of traumatic injury to the epithelial surface (*e.g.,* peptic ulcer) or because of vascular compromise (*e.g.,* foot ulcers associated with diabetes). In chronic lesions where there is repeated insult, the area surrounding the ulcer develops fibroblastic proliferation, scarring, and accumulation of chronic inflammatory cells.[2]

Resolution

Although the manifestations of acute inflammation are largely determined by the nature and intensity of injury, the tissue affected, and the person's ability to mount a response, the outcome generally results in one of three processes: resolution, progression to chronic inflammation, or substantial scarring and fibrosis.[2] Resolution involves the replacement of any irreversibly injured cells and return of tissues to their normal structure and function.[27,28] It is seen with short-lived and minimal injuries and involves neutralization or degradation of inflammatory mediators, normalization of vascular permeability, and cessation of leukocyte infiltration. Progression to chronic inflammation may follow acute inflammation if the offending agent is not removed. Depending on the extent of injury, as well as the ability of the affected tissues to regenerate, chronic inflammation may be followed by restoration of normal structure and function. Scarring and fibrosis occurs when there is substantial tissue injury or when inflammation occurs in tissues that do not regenerate.

Although the mechanisms involved in the resolution of acute inflammation have remained somewhat elusive, emerging

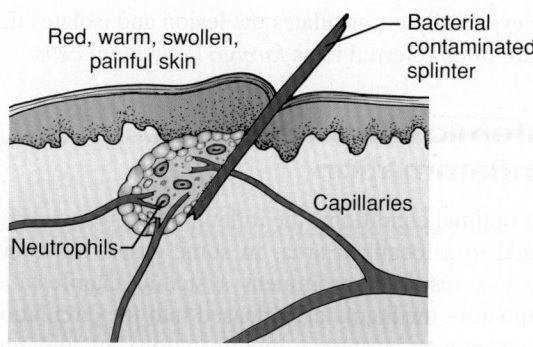

Red, warm, swollen, painful skin

Bacterial contaminated splinter

Capillaries

Neutrophils

A Inflammation
Capillary dilation, fluid exudation, neutrophil migration

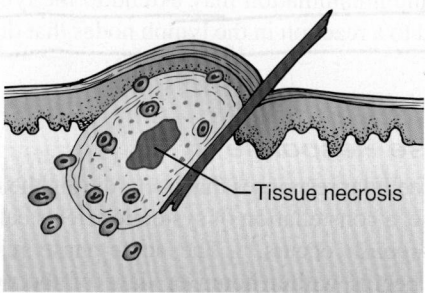

Tissue necrosis

B Suppuration
Development of suppurative or purulent exudate containing degraded neutrophils and tissue debris

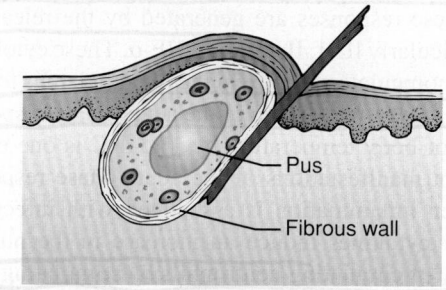

Pus

Fibrous wall

C Abscess formation
Walling off of the area of purulent (pus) exudate to form an abscess

FIGURE 18.6 • Abscess formation. (**A**) Bacterial invasion and development of inflammation. (**B**) Continued bacterial growth, neutrophil migration, liquefaction tissue necrosis, and development of a purulent exudate. (**C**) Walling off of the inflamed area and its purulent exudate to form an abscess.

evidence suggests that an active, coordinated program of resolution begins in the first hours after an inflammatory response begins.[2,28] Studies suggest that after entering the site of acute inflammation, neutrophils promote a switch from the previously described proinflammatory eicosanoids (*e.g.*, prostaglandins and leukotrienes) to other anti-inflammatory classes of eicosanoids, also generated from arachidonic acid. These eicosanoids initiate the termination sequence during which neutrophil recruitment ceases and programmed cell death by apoptosis commences. The apoptotic neutrophils then undergo phagocytosis by macrophages, leading to their clearance and

release of anti-inflammatory and reparative cytokines. Although much new information regarding the resolution of inflammation has been obtained over the past few years, many issues require further characterization. New therapeutic targets are currently being investigated and potential proresolution properties of existing drugs studied. These discoveries may bring profound advances in therapies aimed at reducing the adverse effects of persistent inflammation.

Chronic Inflammation

In contrast to acute inflammation, which is usually self-limited and of short duration, chronic inflammation is self-perpetuating and may last for weeks, months, or even years. It may develop as the result of a recurrent or progressive acute inflammatory process or from low-grade, smouldering responses that fail to evoke an acute response.[1,2] Instead of the vascular changes, edema, and predominantly neutrophilic infiltration as seen in acute inflammation, chronic inflammation is characterized by infiltration with mononuclear cells (macrophages, lymphocytes, and plasma cells) and attempted connective tissue repair involving new vessel formation (angiogenesis) and fibrosis. Chronic inflammation also involves the proliferation of fibroblasts instead of exudates. As a result, the risk of scarring and deformity usually is greater than in acute inflammation. This type of process is the cause of tissue damage in some of the most common disabling diseases such as atherosclerosis, chronic lung disease, rheumatoid arthritis, and inflammatory bowel disease.

There is also evidence that recurrent and persistent inflammation may induce, promote, or influence susceptibility to cancer by causing deoxyribonucleic acid (DNA) damage, inciting tissue reparative proliferation, and/or creating an environment that is enriched with cytokines and growth factors that favour tumour development and growth (see Chapter 7).[29] Among the cancers associated with chronic infection and inflammation are cervical cancer (human papillomavirus [HPV]), cancer of the stomach (*Helicobacter pylori*), and cancer of the gallbladder (chronic cholecystitis and cholelithiasis).

Causes of Chronic Inflammation

Agents that evoke chronic inflammation typically are low-grade, persistent infections or irritants that are unable to penetrate deeply or spread rapidly.[1,2] Among the causes of chronic inflammation are foreign bodies such as talc, silica, asbestos, and surgical suture materials. Many viruses provoke chronic inflammatory responses, as do certain bacteria, fungi, and larger parasites of moderate to low virulence. Examples are the tubercle bacillus, the treponeme of syphilis, and the *Actinomyces* species. The presence of injured tissue such as that surrounding a healing fracture also may incite chronic inflammation. Diseases that cause excessive and inappropriate activation of the immune system are increasingly being recognized as causes of chronic inflammation. Under certain conditions, immune reactions may develop against the person's own tissues, leading to autoimmune disease.

Obesity is a newly suspected cause of chronic inflammation.[30–32] During the last decade, white adipose tissue was recognized to be an active endocrine organ and a source of a number of proinflammatory mediators. Many of the mediators appear to play an important role in the pathogenesis of obesity-related diseases, including accelerated atherosclerosis and diabetes mellitus. The link between obesity and inflammation dates back to the discovery that adipose tissue was a source of the proinflammatory cytokine TNF-α and that adipose tissue TNF-α concentrations are correlated with insulin resistance both in persons with and without type 2 diabetes mellitus. It was later found that obesity is related not only to increased number and size of adipocytes, but also to infiltration of adipose tissue by macrophages that possess the ability to produce TNF-α, nitric oxide, and other inflammatory mediators. The mechanisms mediating the proinflammatory state associated with obesity are still unclear, but recent studies suggest that circulating free fatty acids may play a role.

Granulomatous Inflammation

A granulomatous lesion is a distinctive form of chronic inflammation.[1,2] A *granuloma* typically is a small, 1- to 2-mm lesion in which there is a massing of macrophages surrounded by lymphocytes. These modified macrophages resemble epithelial cells and sometimes are called *epithelioid cells*. Like other macrophages, these epithelioid cells are derived originally from blood monocytes. Granulomatous inflammation is associated with foreign bodies such as splinters, sutures, silica, and asbestos and with microorganisms that cause tuberculosis, syphilis, sarcoidosis, deep fungal infections, and brucellosis. These types of agents have one thing in common: they are poorly digested and usually are not easily controlled by other inflammatory mechanisms. The epithelioid cells in granulomatous inflammation may clump in a mass or coalesce, forming a multinucleated giant cell that attempts to surround the foreign agent (Fig. 18.7). A dense membrane of connective

FIGURE 18.7 • Foreign body giant cell. The numerous nuclei are randomly arranged in the cytoplasm. (From Rubin R., Strayer D. S. (Eds.). (2012). *Rubin's pathology: Clinicopathologic foundations of medicine* (6th ed., p. 9). Philadelphia, PA: Lippincott Williams & Wilkins.)

tissue eventually encapsulates the lesion and isolates it. These cells are often referred to as *foreign body giant cells.*

Systemic Manifestations of Inflammation

Under optimal conditions, the inflammatory response remains confined to a localized area. In some cases, however, local injury can result in prominent systemic manifestations as inflammatory mediators are released into the circulation. The most prominent systemic manifestations of inflammation include the acute-phase response, alterations in white blood cell count (leukocytosis or leukopenia), and fever. Localized acute and chronic inflammation may extend to the lymphatic system and lead to a reaction in the lymph nodes that drain the affected area.

Acute-Phase Response

Along with the cellular responses that occur during the inflammatory response, a constellation of systemic effects called the *acute-phase response* occurs.[1,2] The acute-phase response, which usually begins within hours or days of the onset of inflammation or infection, includes changes in the concentrations of plasma proteins (*i.e.*, acute-phase proteins), skeletal muscle catabolism, negative nitrogen balance, elevated erythrocyte sedimentation rate (ESR), and increased numbers of leukocytes. These responses are generated by the release of cytokines, particularly IL-1, IL-6, and TNF-α. These cytokines affect the thermoregulatory centre in the hypothalamus to produce fever, the most obvious sign of the acute-phase response. The elevation of body temperature by 1 to 4°C is one of the most prominent manifestations of the acute-phase response, especially when inflammation is associated with infection.[2] IL-1 and other cytokines induce an increase in the number and immaturity of circulating neutrophils by stimulating their production in the bone marrow. Other manifestations of the acute-phase response include anorexia, somnolence, and malaise, probably because of the actions of IL-1 and TNF-α on the central nervous system. The metabolic changes, including skeletal muscle catabolism, provide amino acids that can be used in the immune response and for tissue repair. In general, the acute-phase response serves to coordinate the various changes in body function to enable an optimal host response.

Acute-Phase Proteins. During the acute-phase response, the liver dramatically increases the synthesis of acute-phase proteins such as fibrinogen, C-reactive protein (CRP), and serum amyloid A protein (SAA), which serve several different defence functions.[1,2] The synthesis of these proteins is up-regulated by cytokines, especially TNF-α, IL-1 (for SAA), and IL-6 (for fibrinogen and CRP).

CRP was named because it precipitated with the C fraction (C-polypeptide) of pneumococci. The function of CRP is thought to be protective, in that it binds to the surface of invading microorganisms and targets them for destruction by complement and phagocytosis. Although everyone maintains a low level of CRP, this level rises when there is an acute inflammatory response.[33] Interest continues to focus on the use of high-sensitivity CRP (hsCRP) as a marker for increased risk of myocardial infarction in persons with coronary heart disease.[33,34] It is believed that inflammation involving atherosclerotic plaques in coronary arteries may predispose to thrombosis and myocardial infarction (see Chapter 22).

During the acute-phase response, SAA proteins largely produced by hepatocytes and adipocytes replace apolipoprotein A, a component of high-density lipoprotein (HDL) particles; this presumably increases the transfer of HDL from liver cells to macrophages, which can then use these particles for energy. The rise in fibrinogen causes red cells to form stacks (rouleaux) that sediment more rapidly than do individual erythrocytes. This is the basis for the accelerated ESR that occurs in disease conditions characterized by a systemic inflammatory response.

White Blood Cell Response

Leukocytosis, or the increase in white blood cells, is a frequent sign of an inflammatory response, especially those caused by bacterial infection. The white blood cell count commonly increases from a normal value of 4.0 to 10.0 × 10^9 cells/L to 15.0 to 20.0 × 10^9 cells/L in acute inflammatory conditions.[2] After being released from the bone marrow, circulating neutrophils have a life span of only about 10 hours and therefore must be constantly replaced if their numbers are to be adequate. With excessive demand for phagocytes, immature forms of neutrophils (bands) are released from the bone marrow. This phase, which is referred to as a *shift to the left* (or a left shift) in a white blood cell differential count, refers to the increase in immature neutrophils seen in severe infections.

Bacterial infections produce a relatively selective increase in neutrophils (neutrophilia), whereas parasitic and allergic responses induce eosinophilia. Viral infections tend to produce a decrease in neutrophils (neutropenia) and an increase in lymphocytes (lymphocytosis).[3] A decrease in white blood cells (leukopenia) may occur with overwhelming infections or an impaired ability to produce white blood cells.

Lymphadenitis

Localized acute and chronic inflammation may lead to a reaction in the lymph nodes that drain the affected area. This response represents a nonspecific response to mediators released from the injured tissue or an immunologic response to a specific antigen. Painful palpable nodes are more commonly associated with inflammatory processes, whereas nonpainful lymph nodes are more characteristic of neoplasms.

Systemic Inflammatory Response

In severe bacterial infections (sepsis), the large quantities of microorganisms in the blood result in an uncontrolled and overwhelming inflammatory response with the production and release of enormous quantities of inflammatory cytokines (most notably IL-1 and TNF-α) and development of what is referred to as the *systemic inflammatory response syndrome* or *SIRS*[35] (see Chapter 26). These cytokines cause generalized vasodilation, increased vascular permeability, intravascular fluid loss, myocardial depression, and circulatory shock.

IN SUMMARY

Inflammation describes a local response to tissue injury and can present as an acute or chronic condition. The classic signs of an acute inflammatory response are redness, swelling, local heat, pain, and loss of function. Acute inflammation is orchestrated by the endothelial cells that line blood vessels, phagocytic leukocytes (mainly neutrophils and monocytes) that circulate in the blood, and tissue cells (macrophages, mast cells) that direct the tissue responses. Acute inflammation involves a vascular stage, during which blood flow and capillary permeability are increased, and a cellular stage during which phagocytic white blood cells move into the area to engulf and degrade the inciting agent. The vascular stage of the inflammatory response is orchestrated by chemical mediators derived from three major protein cascades: the Kallikrien–Kininogen system, the coagulation system, and the complement system. Cell-derived mediators, including histamine, bradykinin, prostaglandins, PAF, reactive molecules, and many others, are released from cells at the site of inflammation. Acute inflammation may involve the production of exudates containing serous fluid (serous exudate), red blood cells (hemorrhagic exudate), fibrinogen (fibrinous exudate), or tissue debris and white blood cell breakdown products (purulent exudate).

In contrast to acute inflammation, which is self-limiting, chronic inflammation is prolonged and usually is caused by persistent irritants, most of which are insoluble and resistant to phagocytosis and other inflammatory mechanisms. Chronic inflammation involves the presence of mononuclear cells (lymphocytes and macrophages) rather than granulocytes. A granulomatous lesion is a distinctive form of chronic inflammation characterized by aggregates of epithelioid macrophages that wall off the causative agent. It is associated with foreign bodies such as splinters, sutures, silica, and asbestos, and with microorganisms such as those that cause tuberculosis and deep fungal infections.

The systemic manifestations of inflammation include the systemic effects of the acute-phase response, such as fever and lethargy; increased ESR and levels of CRP and other acute-phase proteins; leukocytosis or, in some cases, leukopenia; and enlargement of the lymph nodes that drain the affected area. In extreme cases, widespread inflammation can lead to an overwhelming systemic response.

CONCEPTS in action **ANIMATION**

TISSUE REPAIR AND WOUND HEALING

After completing this section of the chapter, you should be able to meet the following objectives:

- Compare labile, stable, and permanent cell types in terms of their capacity for regeneration.
- Describe healing by primary and secondary intention.
- Explain the effects of soluble mediators and the ECM on tissue repair and wound healing.
- Trace the wound healing process through the hemostasis, inflammatory, proliferative, and remodelling phases.
- Explain the effects of malnutrition; ischemia and oxygen deprivation; impaired immune and inflammatory responses; and infection, wound separation, presence of foreign bodies, and aging on wound healing.

Tissue Repair

Tissue repair, which overlaps the inflammatory process, is a response to tissue injury and represents an attempt to maintain normal body structure and function. It can take the form of regeneration in which the injured cells are replaced with cells of the same type, sometimes leaving no residual trace of previous injury, or it can take the form of replacement by connective tissue, which leaves a permanent scar. Both regeneration and repair by connective tissue replacement are determined by similar mechanisms involving cell migration, proliferation, and differentiation, as well as interaction with the extracellular matrix.

Tissue Regeneration

Body organs and tissues are composed of two types of structures: parenchymal and stromal. The parenchymal (from the Greek for "anything poured in") tissues contain the functioning cells of an organ or body part (*e.g.,* hepatocytes, renal tubular cells). The stromal tissues (from the Greek for "something laid out to lie on") consist of the supporting connective tissues, blood vessels, extracellular matrix, and nerve fibres.

Tissue regeneration involves replacement of the injured tissue with cells of the same type, leaving little or no evidence of the previous injury. The capacity for regeneration varies with the tissue and cell type. Body cells are divided into three types according to their ability to undergo regeneration: labile, stable, or permanent cells.[2,36]

Continuously dividing or *labile cells* are those continue to divide and replicate throughout life, replacing cells that are continually being destroyed. They include the hematopoietic cells of the bone marrow, surface epithelial cells of the skin, oral cavity, vagina, and cervix; the columnar epithelium of the gastrointestinal tract, uterus, and fallopian tubes; and the transitional epithelium of the urinary tract.

Stable cells are those that normally stop dividing when growth ceases and have minimal proliferative activity in their normal state. However, these cells are capable of undergoing regeneration when confronted with an appropriate stimulus and are thus capable of reconstituting the tissue of origin. This category includes the parenchymal cells of the liver and kidney, smooth muscle cells, and vascular endothelial cells. The liver, in particular, has a remarkable capacity to regenerate as demonstrated by its growth after a partial hepatectomy.

The cells of *permanent* or *fixed tissues* cannot undergo mitotic division. They are terminally differentiated and nonproliferative in postnatal life. The fixed cells include nerve cells, skeletal muscle cells, and cardiac muscle cells. These cells do not normally regenerate; once destroyed, they are replaced with fibrous scar tissue that lacks the functional characteristics of the destroyed tissue.

Restoration of normal tissue structure can occur only if the residual tissue is structurally and functionally intact. By contrast, if the entire tissue is damaged by infection or inflammation, regeneration is incomplete and accompanied by scarring.

Fibrous Tissue Repair

Severe or persistent injury with damage to both the parenchymal cells and ECM leads to a situation in which the repair cannot be accomplished with regeneration alone. When regeneration cannot occur, healing by replacement with a connective (fibrous) tissue occurs, a process that terminates in *scar formation*. The term *fibrosis* is often used to describe the extensive deposition of collagen that occurs in organs such as the lungs, liver, or kidney as a result of chronic inflammation or injury.[2] If fibrosis occurs in any tissue space occupied by an inflammatory exudate, it is called *organization*.[36] It occurs in serous cavities such as the pericardium and peritoneal cavities. In the pericardium, fibroblasts secrete and organize collagen within fibrous strands, thereby binding the visceral and parietal pericardia together. Fibrous strands sometimes become organized within the peritoneal cavity following abdominal surgery or peritonitis. These strands of collagen, called *adhesions,* can trap loops of bowel and cause obstruction.

Fibrogenesis involves the influx of activated fibroblasts. Activated fibroblasts secrete ECM components, including fibronectin, hyaluronic acid, proteoglycans, and collagen (to be discussed). Fibronectin and hyaluronic acid are the first to be deposited in the healing wound, and proteoglycans appear later. Because the proteoglycans are hydrophilic, their accumulation contributes to the edematous appearance of the wound. The initiation of collagen synthesis contributes to the subsequent formation of scar tissue.

Regulation of the Healing Process

Tissue healing is regulated by the actions of chemical mediators and growth factors that mediate the healing process as well as orchestrate the interactions between the extracellular and cell matrix.

Chemical Mediators and Growth Factors. Considerable research has contributed to the understanding of chemical mediators and growth factors that orchestrate the healing process.[2,36,37] These chemical mediators and growth factors are released in an orderly manner from many of the cells that participate in tissue regeneration and the healing process. The chemical mediators include the interleukins, interferons, TNF-α, and arachidonic acid derivatives (prostaglandins and leukotrienes) that participate in the inflammatory response.

The term *growth factor* is generally applied to small hormone-like proteins that increase cell size and cell division.[2] Growth factors are named for their tissue of origin (*e.g.,* platelet-derived growth factor [PDGF], fibroblast growth factor [FGF]), their biologic activity (*e.g.,* transforming growth factor [TGF]), or the cells on which they act (*e.g.,* epithelial growth factor [EGF]).

The growth factors are molecules that interact with specific cell surface receptors to control processes involved in tissue repair and wound healing. The growth factors control the proliferation, differentiation, and metabolism of cells during wound healing. They assist in regulating the inflammatory process; serve as chemoattractants for neutrophils, monocytes (macrophages), fibroblasts, and epithelial cells; stimulate angiogenesis; and contribute to the generation of the ECM. Many growth factors are produced by leukocytes recruited to the site of injury or activated at the site by the inflammatory process. They may act on adjacent cells or on the cell producing the growth factor. The sources and functions of selected growth factors are described in Table 18.1.

Extracellular Matrix. The understanding of tissue regeneration and repair has expanded over the past several decades to encompass the complex environment of the ECM.[2,36,38,39] The ECM is secreted locally and assembles into a network of spaces surrounding tissue cells. There are three basic components of the ECM: fibrous structural proteins (*e.g.,* collagen and elastin fibres), water-hydrated gels (*e.g.,* proteoglycans and hyaluronic acid) that permit resilience and lubrication, and adhesive glycoproteins (*e.g.,* fibronectin and laminin) that connect the matrix elements to each other and to cells (see Chapter 4). The ECM occurs in two basic forms: (1) the *basement membrane* that surrounds epithelial, endothelial, and smooth muscle cells; and (2) the *interstitial matrix,* which is present in the spaces between cells in connective tissue and between the epithelium and supporting cells of blood vessels.

The ECM provides turgor to soft tissue and rigidity to bone; it supplies the substratum for cell adhesion; it is involved in the regulation of growth, movement, and differentiation of the cells surrounding it; and it provides for the storage and presentation of regulatory molecules that control the repair process. The ECM also provides the scaffolding for tissue renewal. Although the cells in many tissues are capable of regeneration, injury does not always result in restoration of normal structure unless the ECM is intact. The integrity of the underlying basement membrane, in particular, is critical to the regeneration of tissue. When the basement membrane is disrupted, cells proliferate in a haphazard way, resulting in disorganized and nonfunctional tissues.

Critical to the process of wound healing is the transition from granulation tissue to scar tissue, which involves shifts in the composition of the ECM. In the transitional process, the ECM components are degraded by proteases (enzymes) that are secreted locally by a variety of cells (fibroblasts, macrophages, neutrophils, synovial cells, and epithelial cells). Some of the proteases, such as the collagenases, are highly specific, cleaving particular proteins at a small number of sites.[39] This allows for the structural integrity of the ECM to be retained

TABLE 18.1 GROWTH FACTORS INVOLVED IN TISSUE REGENERATION AND WOUND HEALING

GROWTH FACTOR	SOURCE	FUNCTION
Epidermal growth factor (EGF)	Activated macrophages, keratinocytes, and many other cells	Mitogenic for keratinocytes and fibroblasts; simulates keratinocyte migration and granulation tissue formation
Transforming growth factor-α (TGF-α)	Activated macrophages, T lymphocytes, keratinocytes, and many other cells	Similar to EGF; stimulates replication of hepatocytes and many epithelial cells
Transforming growth factor-β (TGF-β)	Platelets, macrophages, T lymphocytes, keratinocytes, smooth muscle cells, fibroblasts	Chemotactic for neutrophils, macrophages, fibroblasts, and smooth muscle cells; stimulates angiogenesis and production of fibrous tissue; inhibits proteinase production and keratinocyte proliferation
Vascular endothelial cell growth factor (VEGF)	Mesenchymal cells	Increases vascular permeability; mitogenic for endothelial cells of blood vessels
Platelet-derived growth factor (PDGF)	Platelets, macrophages, endothelial cells, keratinocytes, smooth muscle cells	Chemotactic for neutrophils, macrophages, fibroblasts, and smooth muscle cells; stimulates production of proteinases, fibronectin, and hyaluronic acid; stimulates angiogenesis and wound remodelling
Fibroblast growth factor (FGF)	Macrophages, mast cells, T lymphocytes, endothelial cells, fibroblasts, and many other tissues	Chemotactic for fibroblasts; mitogenic for fibroblasts and keratinocytes; stimulates angiogenesis, wound contraction, and matrix deposition
Keratinocyte growth factor (KGF)	Fibroblasts	Stimulates keratinocyte migration, proliferation, and differentiation

while cell migration occurs. Because of their potential to produce havoc in tissues, the actions of the proteases are tightly controlled. They are typically released in an inactive form that must be activated by chemical mediators that are present at the site of injury, and they are rapidly inactivated by tissue inhibitors. Recent research has focused on the unregulated action of the proteases in disorders such as cartilage matrix breakdown in arthritis and neuroinflammation in multiple sclerosis.[38]

TISSUE REPAIR AND WOUND HEALING

- Injured tissues can be repaired by regeneration of the injured tissue cells with cells of the same tissue or parenchymal type, or by connective repair processes in which scar tissue is used to effect healing.
- Regeneration is limited to tissues with cells that are able to undergo mitosis.
- Connective tissue repair occurs by primary or secondary intention and involves hemostatic, inflammatory, proliferative, and remodelling phases of the wound healing process.
- Wound healing is impaired by conditions that diminish blood flow and oxygen delivery, restrict nutrients and other materials needed for healing, and depress the inflammatory and immune responses; and by infection, wound separation, and the presence of foreign bodies.

Wound Healing

Injured tissues are repaired by regeneration of parenchymal cells or by connective tissue repair in which scar tissue is substituted for the parenchymal cells of the injured tissue. The primary objective of the healing process is to fill the gap created by tissue destruction and to restore the structural continuity of the injured part. When regeneration cannot occur, healing by replacement with a connective tissue scar provides the means for maintaining this continuity. Although scar tissue fills the gap created by tissue death, it does not repair the structure with functioning parenchymal cells. Because the regenerative capabilities of most tissues are limited, wound healing usually involves some connective tissue repair. The following discussion particularly addresses skin wounds.

Sequential Processes for Wound Repair

Repair by connective tissue deposition that follows tissue injury and the inflammatory process consists of sequential processes involving angiogenesis and ingrowth of granulation tissue, emigration of fibroblasts and deposition of connective tissue, and maturation and reorganization of the fibrous tissue (remodelling). It usually begins within 24 hours of injury and is evidenced by the migration of fibroblasts and the induction of fibroblast and endothelial cell proliferation.[2] By 3 to 5 days, a special type of tissue called *granulation tissue* is apparent.[2] The granulation tissue then progressively accumulates connective tissue, eventually resulting in the formation of a scar, which is then remodelled.

Angiogenesis and Ingrowth of Granulation Tissue. Granulation tissue is a glistening red, moist connective tissue that fills the injured area while necrotic debris is removed (Fig. 18.8).[2,36] It is composed of newly formed capillaries, proliferating fibroblasts, and residual inflammatory cells. The development of granulation tissue involves the growth of new capillaries (angiogenesis). Angiogenesis is a tightly regulated process that includes vasodilation in response to NO and increased permeability of pre-existing vessels, migration of endothelial cells to the site of tissue injury, and proliferation of endothelial cells, followed by fusion and remodelling of the endothelial cells into capillary tubes. Several growth factors induce angiogenesis, but the most important are vascular endothelial growth factor (VEGF) and basic FGF-2. In angiogenesis, VEGF stimulates both proliferation and motility of endothelial cells, thus initiating the process of capillary sprouting. FGF-2 participates in angiogenesis mainly by stimulating the proliferation of endothelial cells. New blood vessels during angiogenesis are leaky because of incompletely formed interendothelial cell junctions and because VEGF increases vascular permeability. This leakiness explains the edematous appearance of granulation tissue and accounts in part for the swelling that may persist in healing wounds long after the acute inflammation has subsided.

Emigration of Fibroblasts and Deposition of Connective Tissue. Scar formation builds on the granulation tissue framework of new vessels and loose ECM. The process occurs in two phases: emigration and proliferation of fibroblasts into the site of injury, and deposition of ECM by these cells.[40] Fibroblast are connective tissue cells that synthesize and secrete collagen and other intercellular elements needed for wound healing, as well as a family of growth factors that induce angiogenesis and endothelial cell proliferation and migration.[4] The recruitment

FIGURE 18.8 • Granulation tissue. A venous stasis leg ulcer illustrates exposed granulation tissue. (From Rubin R., Strayer D. S. (Eds.). (2012). *Rubin's pathology: Clinicopathologic foundations of medicine* (6th ed., p. 98). Philadelphia, PA: Lippincott Williams & Wilkins.)

and proliferation of fibroblasts is mediated by a number of growth factors including FGF-2 and transforming growth factor beta (TGF-β). These growth factors are released from endothelial cells and from inflammatory cells that are present at the site of injury.

As healing progresses, the number of proliferating fibroblasts and formation of new vessels decrease and there is increased synthesis and deposition of collagen. Collagen synthesis is important to the development of strength in the healing wound site. Ultimately, the granulation tissue scaffolding evolves into a scar composed of largely inactive spindle-shaped fibroblasts, dense collagen fibres, fragments of elastic tissue, and other ECM components.

Wound Contraction and Remodelling. As they heal, open wounds contract and deform, a process that is facilitated by a specialized cell, called the *myofibroblast*.[36,40] Myofibroblasts, which are modified fibroblasts usually begin to appear about the third day of wound healing, and gradually diminish over the next few weeks. Unlike fibroblasts, however, myofibroblasts express smooth muscle actin and other contractile elements that cause them to respond to agents that cause smooth muscle to contract and relax. A major function of the myofibroblast is to produce ECM proteins, most notably collagen types I, VI, and XVIII, glycoproteins, and proteoglycans needed for wound repair. In addition to producing matrix components, myofibroblasts also generate contractile forces that bring the edges of open wounds together and thereby facilitate wound closure. However, excessive myofibroblast activity, including excessive contraction and overproduction of ECM can lead to increased fibrosis and hypertrophic scaring, particularly in burn scars.

Phases of Cutaneous Wound Healing

The healing of skin wounds is different from the process of deep tissue and bone repair. Depending on the nature and size of the wound or the extent of tissue loss, wound closure and healing occurs by *primary* or *secondary intention* (Fig. 18.9).[2,36,41–46,47] A sutured surgical incision is an example of healing by primary intention. Larger wounds (*e.g.*, burns and large surface wounds) that have a greater loss of tissue and contamination heal by secondary intention. Healing by secondary intention is slower than healing by primary intention and results in the formation of larger amounts of scar tissue. A wound that might otherwise have healed by primary intention may become infected and heal by secondary intention.

Healing of cutaneous wounds is commonly divided into four phases: (1) hemostasis, (2) the inflammatory phase, (3) the proliferative phase, and (4) the maturational or remodelling phase.[2,36,41,42] The duration of the phases is fairly predictable in wounds healing by primary intention. In wounds healing by secondary intention, the process depends on the extent of injury and the healing environment.

Hemostasis. The first phase of wound healing starts immediately after an injury occurs. There is constriction of injured

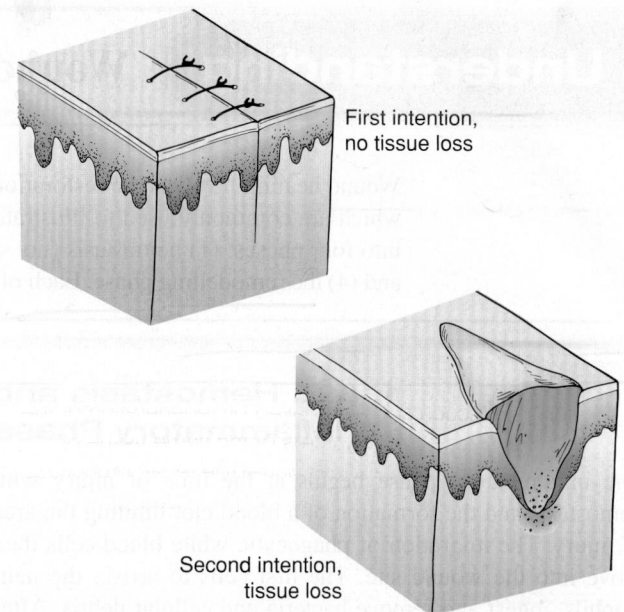

FIGURE 18.9 • Healing of a skin wound by first and second intention.

First intention, no tissue loss

Second intention, tissue loss

blood vessels and initiation of blood clotting through platelet activation and aggregation (see Chapter 13). After a brief period of constriction, the same vessels dilate and capillaries increase their permeability, allowing plasma and blood components to leak into the injured area. In small surface wounds, the clot loses fluid and becomes a hard, desiccated scab that protects the area.

Inflammatory Phase. The inflammatory phase of wound healing usually develops during the first 24 hours from time of injury and is a critical period because it prepares the wound environment for healing. It includes the vascular and cellular stages of inflammation. The cellular stage of inflammation is evidenced by the migration of phagocytic white blood cells that digest and remove invading organisms, fibrin, extracellular debris, and other foreign matter. The neutrophils are the first cells to arrive and are usually gone by day 3.[2] They ingest bacteria and cellular debris. After approximately 24 hours, macrophages, which are larger phagocytic cells, enter the wound area and remain for an extended period.[12,48] These cells, arising from blood monocytes, are essential to the healing process. Their functions include phagocytosis and release of growth factors that stimulate epithelial cell growth and angiogenesis, and attract fibroblasts. When a large defect occurs in deeper tissues, neutrophils and macrophages are required to remove the debris and facilitate wound closure. Although a wound may heal in the absence of neutrophils, it cannot heal in the absence of macrophages.

Proliferative Phase. The proliferative phase of healing usually begins within 2 to 3 days of injury and may last as long as 3 weeks in wounds healing by primary intention. The primary processes during this time focus on the building of new tissue to fill the wound space. The key cell during this phase

Understanding Wound Healing

Wound healing involves the restoration of the integrity of injured tissue. The healing of skin wounds, which are commonly used to illustrate the general principles of wound healing, is generally divided into four phases: (1) hemostasis (not shown), (2) the inflammatory phase, (3) the proliferative phase, and (4) the remodelling phase. Each of these phases is mediated through cytokines and growth factors.

1. & 2. Hemostasis and Inflammatory Phase

The inflammatory phase begins at the time of injury with hemostasis and the formation of a blood clot limiting the area of injury. The migration of phagocytic white blood cells then move into the wound site. The first cells to arrive, the neutrophils, ingest and remove bacteria and cellular debris. After 24 hours, the neutrophils are joined by macrophages, which continue to ingest cellular debris and play an essential role in the production of growth factors for the proliferative phase.

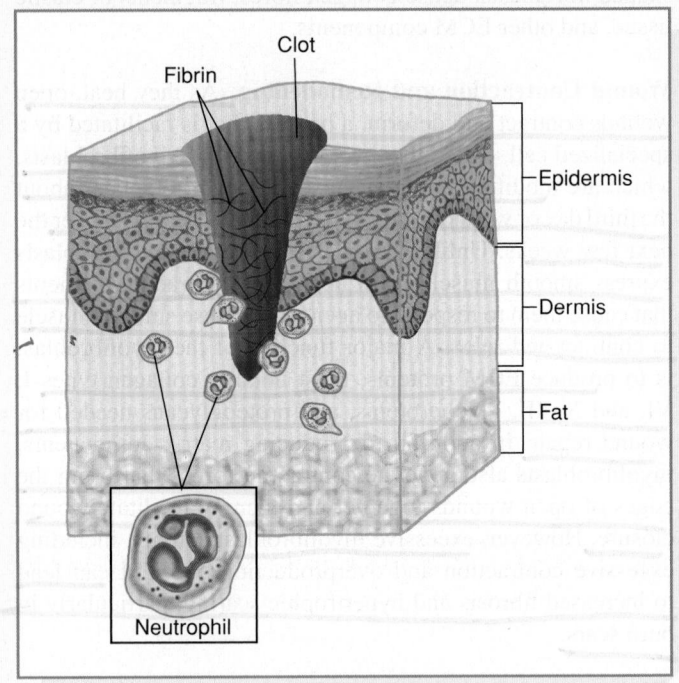

3. Proliferative Phase

The primary processes during this phase focus on the building of new tissue to fill the wound space. The key cell during this phase is the *fibroblast,* a connective tissue cell that synthesizes and secretes the collagen, proteoglycans, and glycoproteins needed for wound healing. Fibroblasts also produce a family of growth factors that induce angiogenesis (growth of new blood vessels) and endothelial cell proliferation and migration. The final component of the proliferative phase is epithelialization, during which epithelial cells at the wound edges proliferate to form a new surface layer that is similar to that which was destroyed by the injury.

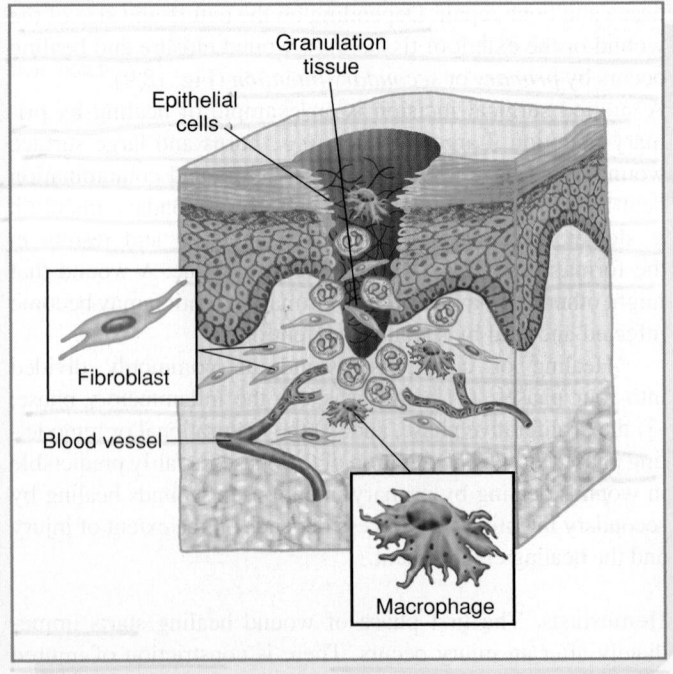

4. Remodelling Phase

This phase begins approximately 3 weeks after injury with the development of the fibrous scar, and can continue for 6 months or longer, depending on the extent of the wound. During this time, there is a decrease in vascularity and continued remodelling of scar tissue by simultaneous synthesis of collagen by fibroblasts and lysis by collagenase enzymes. As a result of these two processes, the architecture of the scar becomes reoriented to increase its tensile strength, and the scar shrinks so it is less visible.

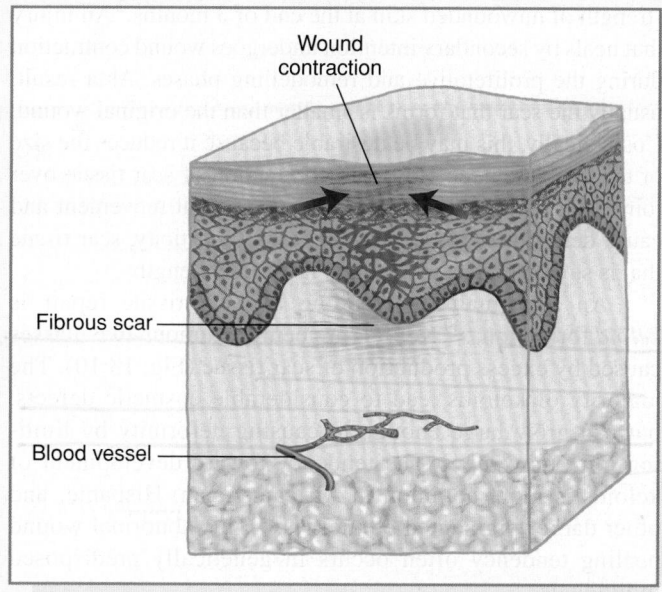

is the *fibroblast*. The fibroblast is a connective tissue cell that synthesizes and secretes collagen and other intercellular elements needed for wound healing. Fibroblasts also produce a family of growth factors that induce angiogenesis and endothelial cell proliferation and migration.

As early as 24 to 48 hours after injury, fibroblasts and vascular endothelial cells begin proliferating to form the granulation tissue that serves as the foundation for scar tissue development. This tissue is fragile and bleeds easily because of the numerous, newly developed capillary buds. Wounds that heal by secondary intention have more necrotic debris and exudate that must be removed, and they involve larger amounts of granulation tissue. The newly formed blood vessels are semipermeable and allow plasma proteins and white blood cells to leak into the tissues.

The final component of the proliferative phase is epithelialization, which is the migration, proliferation, and differentiation of the epithelial cells at the wound edges to form a new surface layer that is similar to the one destroyed by the injury. In wounds that heal by primary intention, these epidermal cells proliferate and seal the wound within 24 to 48 hours.[2] Because epithelial cell migration requires a moist vascular wound surface and is impeded by a dry or necrotic wound surface, epithelialization is delayed in open wounds until a bed of granulation tissue has formed. When a scab has formed on the wound, the epithelial cells migrate between it and the underlying viable tissue; when a significant portion of the wound has been covered with epithelial tissue, the scab lifts off.

At times, excessive granulation tissue, sometimes referred to as *proud flesh,* may form and extend above the edges of the wound, preventing reepithelialization from taking place. Surgical removal or chemical cauterization of the defect allows healing to proceed.

As the proliferative stage progresses, there is continued accumulation of collagen and proliferation of fibroblasts. Collagen synthesis reaches a peak within 5 to 7 days and continues for several weeks, depending on wound size. By the second week, the white blood cells have largely left the area, the edema has diminished, and the wound begins to blanch as the small blood vessels become thrombosed and degenerate.

Remodelling Phase. The third phase of wound healing, the remodelling process, begins approximately 3 weeks after injury and can continue for 6 months or longer, depending on the extent of the wound. The initial type III collagen which is more abundant in granulation tissue is replaced by the tougher type I collagen. Ultimately, the granulation tissue scaffolding evolves into a scar composed of largely inactive spindle-shaped fibroblasts, dense collagen fibres, fragments of elastic tissue, and other ECM components. As the scar matures, vascular degeneration eventually transforms the highly vascular granulation tissue into a pale, largely avascular scar. As the term implies, there is continued remodelling of scar tissue by simultaneous synthesis of collagen by fibroblasts and lysis by collagenase enzymes. As a result of these two processes, the architecture of the scar becomes reoriented to increase the tensile strength of the wound.

Most wounds do not regain the full tensile strength of unwounded skin after healing is completed. For primary intention healing, carefully sutured wounds done immediately after surgery have approximately 70% of the strength of unwounded skin, largely because of the placement of the sutures.[2] This allows persons to move about freely after surgery without fear of wound separation. When the sutures are removed, usually at the end of the first week, wound strength is approximately 10%. It increases rapidly over the next 4 weeks and then slows, reaching a plateau of approximately 70% to 80% of the tensile strength of unwounded skin at the end of 3 months.[2] An injury that heals by secondary intention undergoes wound contraction during the proliferative and remodelling phases. As a result, usually the scar that forms is smaller than the original wound. Cosmetically, this may be desirable because it reduces the size of the visible defect. However, contraction of scar tissue over joints and other body structures tends to limit movement and cause deformities. As a result of loss of elasticity, scar tissue that is stretched fails to return to its original length.

An abnormality in healing by scar tissue repair is *keloid* formation.[2,49] Keloids are benign, tumour-like masses caused by excess production of scar tissue (Fig. 18.10). The majority of keloids lead to considerable cosmetic defects, but can grow large enough to causing deformity by limiting joint movement. The tendency toward development of keloids is more common in African, Asian, Hispanic, and other darker pigmented ethnicities.[49] This abnormal wound healing tendency often occurs in genetically predisposed individuals.

Factors That Affect Wound Healing

Although many local and systemic factors impair wound healing, science has found only a few ways to promote wound repair. Among the causes of impaired wound healing are malnutrition; impaired blood flow and oxygen delivery; impaired inflammatory and immune responses; infection, wound separation, and foreign bodies.[2,50,51]

Nutritional Status. Successful wound healing depends in part on adequate supply of proteins, carbohydrates, fats, vitamins, and minerals. It is well recognized that malnutrition slows the healing process, causing wounds to heal inadequately or incompletely.[51–53] Protein deficiencies prolong the inflammatory phase of healing and impair fibroblast proliferation, collagen and protein matrix synthesis, angiogenesis, and wound remodelling. Carbohydrates are needed as an energy source for

FIGURE 18.10 • Keloid. A light-skinned black woman with keloid that developed after ear piercing. (From Rubin R., Strayer D. S. (Eds.). (2012). *Rubin's pathology: Clinicopathologic foundations of medicine* (6th ed., p. 113). Philadelphia, PA: Lippincott Williams & Wilkins.)

white blood cells. Carbohydrates also have a protein-sparing effect and help to prevent the use of amino acids for fuel when they are needed for the healing process. Fats are essential constituents of cell membranes and are needed for the synthesis of new cells.

Although most vitamins are essential cofactors for the daily functions of the body, vitamins play an essential role in the healing process. Vitamin C is needed for collagen synthesis. In vitamin C deficiency, improper sequencing of amino acids occurs, proper linking of amino acids does not take place, the byproducts of collagen synthesis are not removed from the cell, new wounds do not heal properly, and old wounds may fall apart. Administration of vitamin C rapidly restores the healing process to normal. Vitamin A functions in stimulating and supporting epithelialization, capillary formation, and collagen synthesis. Vitamin A also has been shown to counteract the anti-inflammatory effects of corticosteroid drugs and can be used to reverse these effects in persons who are on chronic steroid therapy. The B vitamins are important cofactors in enzymatic reactions that contribute to the wound healing process. All are water soluble and, with the exception of vitamin B_{12}, which is stored in the liver, all must be replaced daily. Vitamin K plays an indirect role in wound healing by preventing bleeding disorders that contribute to hematoma formation and subsequent infection.

The role of minerals in wound healing is less clearly defined. The macrominerals, including sodium, potassium, calcium, and phosphorus, as well as the microminerals such as copper and zinc, must be present for normal cell function. Zinc is a cofactor in a variety of enzyme systems responsible for cell proliferation. In animal studies, zinc has been found to aid in reepithelialization.

Blood Flow and Oxygen Delivery. For healing to occur, wounds must have adequate blood flow to supply the necessary nutrients and to remove the resulting waste, local toxins, bacteria, and other debris. Impaired wound healing due to poor blood flow may occur as a result of wound conditions (*e.g.*, swelling) or pre-existing health problems.[2,51,54,55] Arterial disease and venous pathology are well-documented causes of impaired wound healing. In situations of major trauma a decrease in blood volume may cause a reduction in blood flow to injured tissues.

Molecular oxygen is required for collagen synthesis and killing of bacteria by phagocytic white blood cells. It has been shown that even a temporary lack of oxygen can result in the formation of less stable collagen.[55] Wounds in ischemic tissue become infected more frequently than wounds in well-vascularized tissue. Neutrophils and macrophages require oxygen for destruction of microorganisms that have invaded the area. Although these cells can accomplish phagocytosis in a relatively anoxic environment, they cannot digest bacteria. Oxygen also contributes to signalling systems that support wound healing. Recent research suggests that almost all cells in the wound environment are equipped with specialized enzymes to convert oxygen to ROS.[55] These ROS function as cellular messengers that support wound healing, stimulating cytokine action, angiogenesis, cell motility, and ECM formation.

The availability of oxygen to wound tissues depends on vascular supply, vasomotor tone, the partial pressure of oxygen (PO_2) in arterial blood, and the diffusion distance for oxygen (see Chapter 21). The central area of a wound has the lower oxygen level, with dermal wounds ranging from 0 to 10 mm Hg centrally to 60 mm Hg in the periphery; the PO_2 of arterial blood is approximately 100 mm Hg.[55] Transcutaneous oxygen sensors are available for use in measuring wound oxygenation. From a therapeutic standpoint, oxygen can be given systemically or administered locally using a topical device. Although topical oxygen therapy is not likely to diffuse into the deeper tissues, it does have the advantage of oxygenating superficial areas of the wound not supported by intact vasculature. Hyperbaric oxygen therapy delivers 100% oxygen at two to three times the normal atmospheric pressure at sea level.[56] The goal of hyperbaric oxygen therapy is to increase oxygen delivery to tissues by increasing the PO_2 dissolved in the plasma. An increase in tissue oxygen tension by hyperbaric oxygen enhances wound healing by a number of mechanisms, including the increased killing of bacteria by neutrophils, impaired growth of anaerobic bacteria, and the promotion of angiogenesis and fibroblast activity. Hyperbaric oxygen is currently reserved for the treatment of problem wounds in which hypoxia and infection interfere with healing.

Impaired Inflammatory and Immune Responses. Inflammatory and immune mechanisms function in wound healing. Inflammation is essential to the first phase of wound healing, and immune mechanisms prevent infections that impair wound healing. Among the conditions that impair inflammation and immune function are disorders of phagocytic function, diabetes mellitus, and therapeutic administration of corticosteroid drugs.

Phagocytic disorders may be divided into extrinsic and intrinsic defects. Extrinsic disorders are those that reduce the total number of phagocytic cells, impair the attraction of phagocytic cells to the wound site, interfere with the engulfment of bacteria and foreign agents by the phagocytic cells (*i.e.,* opsonization), or suppress the total number of phagocytic cells (*e.g.,* immunosuppressive agents). Intrinsic phagocytic disorders are the result of enzymatic deficiencies in the metabolic pathway for destroying the ingested bacteria by the phagocytic cell. The intrinsic phagocytic disorders include chronic granulomatous disease (see Chapter 19), an X-linked inherited disease in which there is a deficiency of the myeloperoxidase, or NADPH oxidase enzymes. Deficiencies of these compounds prevent generation of superoxide and hydrogen peroxide needed for killing bacteria.

Wound healing is a problem in persons with diabetes mellitus, particularly those who have poorly controlled blood glucose levels.[2,50,57] Studies have shown delayed wound healing, poor collagen formation, and poor tensile strength in diabetic animals. Of particular importance is the effect of hyperglycemia on phagocytic function. Neutrophils, for example, have diminished chemotactic and phagocytic function, including engulfment and intracellular killing of bacteria, when exposed to altered glucose levels. Small blood vessel disease is also common among persons with diabetes, impairing the delivery of inflammatory cells, oxygen, and nutrients to the wound site.

The therapeutic administration of corticosteroid drugs decreases the inflammatory process and may delay the healing process.[50] These hormones decrease capillary permeability during the early stages of inflammation, impair the phagocytic property of the leukocytes, and inhibit fibroblast proliferation and function.

Infection, Wound Separation, and Foreign Bodies. Wound contamination, wound separation, and foreign bodies delay wound healing. Infection impairs all dimensions of wound healing.[50] It prolongs the inflammatory phase, impairs the formation of granulation tissue, and inhibits proliferation of fibroblasts and deposition of collagen fibres. All wounds are contaminated at the time of injury. Although body defences can normally handle the invasion of microorganisms at the time of injury, contaminated wounds can overwhelm host defences. Trauma and existing impairment of host defences also can contribute to the development of wound infections.

Approximation of the wound edges (*i.e.,* suturing of an incision type of wound) greatly enhances healing and prevents infection. Epithelialization of a wound with closely approximated edges occurs within 1 to 2 days. Large, gaping wounds tend to heal more slowly because it is often impossible to effect wound closure with this type of wound. Mechanical factors such as increased local pressure or torsion can cause wounds to pull apart, or *dehisce.*

Foreign bodies tend to invite bacterial contamination and delay healing. Fragments of wood, steel, glass, and other compounds may have entered the wound at the site of injury and can be difficult to locate when the wound is treated. Sutures are also foreign bodies, and although needed for the closure of surgical wounds, they are an impediment to healing. This is why sutures are removed as soon as possible after surgery. Wound infections are of special concern in persons with implantation of foreign bodies such as orthopedic devices (*e.g.,* pins, stabilization devices), cardiac pacemakers, and shunt catheters. These infections are difficult to treat and may require removal of the device.

Bite Wounds. Animal and human bites are particularly troublesome in terms of infection. The animal inflicting the bite, the location of the bite, and the type of injury are all important determinants of whether the wound becomes infected. Up to 80% of all cat bites become infected whereas dog bites become infected approximately 3% to 18% of the time. Cat bites have an increased rate of puncture wounds contaminating deep tissue, while dog bites are more frequently lacerations at the surface. In addition, cats have an increased amount and type of oral bacteria than dogs. Bites inflicted by children are usually superficial and seldom become infected, whereas bites inflicted by adults have a much higher rate of infection. Puncture wounds are more likely to become infected than lacerations, probably because lacerations are easier to irrigate and debride.

Treatment of bite wounds involves vigorous irrigation and cleansing as well as debridement or removal of necrotic tissue. Whether bite wounds are closed with sutures to promote healing by primary intention depends on the location of the bite and whether the wound is already infected. Wounds that are not infected and require closure for mechanical or cosmetic reasons may be sutured. Wounds of the hand are not usually sutured because closed-space infection of the hand can produce loss of function. Antibiotics are usually administered prophylactically to persons with high-risk bites (*e.g.,* cat bites in any location and human or animal bites to the hand). All persons with bites should be evaluated to determine if tetanus or rabies prophylaxis is needed.

Wound Healing in Older Adults

A number of structural and functional changes have been reported to occur in aging skin, including a decrease in dermal thickness, a decline in collagen content, and a loss of elasticity.[58,59] The observed changes in skin that occur with aging are complicated by the effects of sun exposure. Since the effects of sun exposure are cumulative, older persons show more changes in skin structure.

Wound healing is thought to be progressively impaired with aging. Older adults have alterations in wound healing, including hemostasis, inflammation, cell proliferation, and resolution. Keratinocytes, fibroblasts, and vascular endothelial cells display a reduced rate of proliferation. There is also a reported decrease in angiogenesis and collagen synthesis, impaired wound contraction, and slower reepithelialization of open wounds. Although wound healing may be delayed, most wounds heal, even in the debilitated older adult undergoing major surgical procedures.

Older adults are more vulnerable to chronic wounds than younger persons, and these wounds heal more slowly. However, these wounds are more likely due to other disorders such as immobility, diabetes mellitus, or vascular disease, rather than aging.

IN SUMMARY

The ability of tissues to repair damage due to injury depends on the body's ability to replace the parenchymal cells and to organize them as they were originally. Regeneration describes the process by which tissue is replaced with cells of a similar type and function. Healing by regeneration is limited to tissue with cells that are able to divide and replace the injured cells. Body cells are divided into types according to their ability to regenerate: continuously dividing or labile cells, such as the epithelial cells of the skin and gastrointestinal tract, which continue to regenerate throughout life; stable cells, such as those in the liver, which normally do not divide but are capable of regeneration when confronted with an appropriate stimulus; and permanent or fixed cells, such as nerve cells, which are unable to regenerate. Scar tissue repair involves the substitution of fibrous connective tissue for injured tissue that cannot be repaired by regeneration.

Cutaneous wound healing occurs by primary and secondary intention and is commonly divided into four phases: hemostasis, the inflammatory phase, the proliferative phase, and the maturational or remodelling phase. In wounds healing by primary intention, the duration of the phases is fairly predictable. In wounds healing by secondary intention, the process depends on the extent of injury and the healing environment. Wound healing can be impaired or complicated by factors such as malnutrition; restricted blood flow and oxygen delivery; diminished inflammatory and immune responses; infection, wound separation, and the presence of foreign bodies; and aging.

CONCEPTS in action **ANIMATION**

REVIEW EXERCISES

1. A 15-year-old boy presents with abdominal pain, a temperature of 38°C, and an elevated white blood cell count of 13.0×10^9 cells/L, with an increase in neutrophils. A tentative diagnosis of appendicitis is made.
   A. *Explain the significance of pain as it relates to the inflammatory response.*
   B. *What is the cause of the fever and elevated white blood cell count?*
   C. *What would be the preferred treatment for this boy?*

2. Aspirin and other NSAIDs are used to control the manifestations of chronic inflammatory disorders such as arthritis.
   A. *Explain their mechanism of action in terms of controlling the inflammatory response.*

3. After a heart attack, the area of heart muscle that has undergone necrosis because of a lack of blood supply undergoes healing by replacement with scar tissue.
   A. *Compare the functioning of the heart muscle that has been replaced by scar tissue with that of the normal surrounding heart muscle.*

4. A 35-year-old man presents with a large abscess on his leg. He tells you he injured his leg while doing repair work on his house and he thinks there might be a wood sliver in the infected area.
   A. *Explain the events that participate in formation of an abscess.*

B. He is told that incision and drainage of the lesion will be needed so healing can take place. Explain.

C. He is reluctant to have the procedure done and asks whether an antibiotic would work as well. Explain why antibiotics alone are usually not effective in eliminating the microorganisms contained in an abscess.

References

1. Murphy H. S. (2012). Chapter 2: Inflammation. In Rubin R., Strayer D. S. (Eds.), *Rubin's pathology: clinicopathologic foundations of medicine* (6th ed.). Philadelphia, PA: Lippincott Williams & Wilkins.
2. Kumar V., Abbas A. K., Fausto N., Aster J. (Eds.). (2010). *Robbins and Cotran pathologic basis of disease* (8th ed.). Philadelphia, PA: Elsevier Saunders.
3. Schmid-Schonbein G. W. (2006). Analysis of inflammation. *Annual Review of Biomedical Engineering, 8*, 93–131.
4. Ross M. H., Pawlina W. (2011). *Histology: A text and atlas* (6th ed.). Philadelphia, PA: Lippincott Williams & Wilkins.
5. Szekanecz Z., Koch A. E. (2004). Vascular endothelium and immune responses: Implications for inflammation and angiogenesis. *Rheumatic Diseases Clinics of North America, 30*(1), 97–114.
6. Steinhubl S. R. (2007). Platelets as mediators of inflammation. *Hematology/Oncology Clinics of North America, 21*(1), 115–121.
7. Morrell C. N., Aggrev A. A., Chapman L. M. (2014). Emerging roles for platelets as immune and inflammatory cells. *Blood, 123*(18), 2759–2767.
8. Stokes K. Y., Granger D. N. (2012). Platelets: A critical link between inflammation and microvascular dysfunction. *Journal of Physiology, 590*(5), 1023–1034.
9. Hall J. E. (2011). *Textbook of medical physiology* (12th ed.). Philadelphia, PA: W. B. Saunders.
10. Wright H. L., Moots R. J., Buchnall R. C., Edwards S. W. (2010). Neutrophil function in inflammation and inflammatory disease. *Rheumatology, 49*, 1618–1631.
11. Hongtao L., Pope R. M. (2004). Phagocytes: Mechanisms of inflammation and tissue destruction. *Rheumatic Diseases Clinics of North America, 30*, 19–30.
12. Koh T. J., DePietro L. A. (2013). Inflammation and wound healing: The role of the macrophage. *Expert Reviews in Molecular Medicine, 13*:e23, 1–12.
13. Bachelet I., Francesca L. S., Mekon Y. A. (2006). Mast cells: Not only in allergy. *Immunololgy and Allergy Clinics of North America, 26*(3), 407–425.
14. Frenette P. S, Wagner D. D. (1996). Adhesion molecules—Parts I and II. *New England Journal of Medicine, 334*(23), *335*(1), 1526–1529, 43–45.
15. Bochner B. S. (2004). Adhesion molecules as therapeutic targets. *Immunology and Allergy Clinics of North America, 24*(4), 615–630.
16. Langereis J. D. (2013). Neutrophil integrin affinity regulation in adhesion, migration, and bacterial clearance. *Cell Adhesion & Migration, 7*(6), 476–481.
17. Stein D. M., Nombela-Arrieta C. (2005). Chemokine control of lymphocyte trafficking: A general review. *Immunology, 116*, 1–12.
18. Roy I., Evans D., Dwinell M. B. (2014). Chemokines and chemokine receptors: Update on utility and challenges for the clinician. *Surgery, 155*(6), 961–973.
19. Underhill D. M., Ozinsky A. (2002). Phagocytosis of microbes. *Annual Review of Immunology, 20*, 825–852.
20. Simmons D. L., Botting R. M., Hla T. (2004). Cyclooxygenase isoenzymes: The biology of prostaglandin synthesis and inhibition. *Pharmacology Reviews, 56*(3), 387–437.
21. Ricclotti E., Fitzgerald G. A. (2011). Prostaglandins and inflammation. *Arteriosclerosis, Thrombosis, and Vascular Biology, 31*(5), 986–1000.
22. Barnes P. J. (2006). How corticosteroids control inflammation: Quintiles Prize Lecture 2005. *British Journal of Pharmacology, 148*(3), 245–254.
23. Covington M. B. (2004). Omega-3 fatty acids. *American Family Physician, 70*(1), 133–140.
24. Harper C. R., Jacobson T. A. (2005). Usefulness of omega-3 fatty acids and prevention of coronary heart disease. *American Journal of Cardiology, 96*, 1521–1529.
25. Gossain A., Gamelli R. L. (2005). A primer on cytokines. *Journal of Burn Care and Rehabilitation, 26*(1), 7–12.
26. Charo I., Ransohoff R. M. (2006). The many roles of chemokines and chemokine receptors in inflammation. *New England Journal of Medicine, 354*(6), 610–621.
27. Ortega-Gómez A., Perretti M., Soehnlein O. (2013). Resolution of inflammation: An integrated view. *EMBO Molecular Medicine, 5*(5), 661–674.
28. Serham C. N., Brain S. D., Buckley C. D., et al. (2007). Resolution of inflammation: State of the art, definitions and terms. *FASB Journal, 21*(2), 325–332.
29. Schottenfeld D., Beebe-Dimmer J. (2006). Chronic inflammation: A common and important factor in the pathogenesis of neoplasia. *CA: A Cancer Journal for Clinicians, 56*(2), 69–83.
30. Nathan C. (2008). Epidemic inflammation: Pondering obesity. *Molecular Medicine, 14*(7–8), 485–492.
31. Tateya S., Kim F., Tamoni Y. (2013). Recent advances in obesity-related inflammation and insulin resistance. *Frontiers in Endocrinology, 4*, 93.
32. Greenberg A. S., Obin M. S. (2006). Obesity and the role of adipose tissue in inflammation and metabolism. *American Journal of Clinical Nutrition, 83*(2), 461S–465S.
33. Ridker P. M. (2005). C-reactive protein, inflammation, and cardiovascular disease. *Current Issues in Cardiology, 32*(3), 384–386.
34. Bisoendial R., Boekholdt S. M., Vergeer M., et al. (2010). C-reactive protein as a mediator or cardiovascular disease. *European Heart Journal, 31*(17), 2087–2095.
35. Hotchiss R. S., Karl I. E. (2003). The pathophysiology and treatment of sepsis. *New England Journal of Medicine, 348*(2), 138–150.
36. Sephel G. C., Davidson J. M. (2012). Chapter 3: Repair, regeneration, and fibrosis. In Rubin R., Strayer D. S. (Eds.), *Rubin's pathology: Clinicopathologic foundations of medicine* (6th ed.). Philadelphia, PA: Lippincott Williams & Wilkins.
37. Werner S., Grose R. (2003). Regulation of wound healing by growth factors and cytokines. *Physiology Reviews, 83*, 835–870.
38. Daley W. P., Peters S. B., Larsen M. (2008). Extracellular matrix dynamics in development and regenerative medicine. *Journal of Cell Science, 121*(3), 255–264.
39. Olczyk P., Mencner L., Kosmosinka-Vassev K. (2014). The role of the extracellular matrix components in cutaneous wound healing. *BioMed Research International, 2014*, 747584.
40. Li B., Wang J. H. (2011). Fibroblasts and myofibroblasts in wound healing: Force generation and measurement. *Journal of Tissue Viability, 20*(4), 108–120.
41. Goldberg S. R., Dieglmann R. R. (2011). Wound healing primer. *Surgical Clinics of North America, 90*(6), 1113–1140.
42. Teller P., White T. K. (2009). The physiology of wound healing: Injury through maturation. *Surgical Clinics of North America, 89*, 598–610.
43. Whitney J. D. (2005). Overview: Acute and chronic wounds. *Nursing Clinics of North America, 40*, 191–205.
44. Bielefeld K. A., Amini-Nik S., Alman B. A. (2013). Cutaneous wound healing: Recruiting developmental pathways for regeneration. *Cellular and Molecular Life Sciences, 70*(12), 2059–2061.
45. Monaco J. L., Lawrence W. T. (2003). Acute wound healing: An overview. *Clinics in Plastic Surgery, 30*(1), 1–12.
46. Strecker-McGraw M. K., Jones T. R., Baer D. G. (2007). Soft tissue wounds and principles of healing. *Emergency Medicine Clinics of North America, 25*(1), 1–22.
47. Singer A. J., Clark R. A. (1999). Cutaneous wound healing. *The New England Journal of Medicine, 341*(10), 738–746.

48. Adamson R. (2009). Role of macrophages in normal wound healing: An overview. *Journal of Wound Care, 18*(8), 349–351.

49. Butler P. D., Longaker M. T., Yang G. P. (2008). Current progress in keloid research and treatment. *Journal of the American College of Surgeons, 208*(4), 731–741.

50. Guo D., DiPietro L. A. (2010). Factors affecting wound healing. *Journal of Dental Research, 89*(3), 2119–2229.

51. Burns J. L., Mancoll J. S., Phillips L. G. (2003). Impairments to wound healing. *Clinics in Plastic Surgery, 30*, 47–56.

52. Wild T., Raharnia A., Kellner M., et al. (2010). Basics in nutrition and wound healing. *Nutrition, 28*(5), 562–566.

53. Mechanick J. I. (2004). Practical aspects of nutrition support for wound-healing patients. *American Journal of Surgery, 188*(1A Suppl), 52–56.

54. Gordillo G. M., Sen C. K. (2003). Revisiting the essential role of oxygen in wound healing. *American Journal of Surgery, 186*, 259–263.

55. Tandara A. A., Mustoe T. A. (2004). Oxygen and wound healing—more than a nutrient. *World Journal of Surgery, 28*, 294–300.

56. Zamboni W. A., Browder L. K., Martinez J. (2003). Hyperbaric oxygen and wound healing. *Clinics in Plastic Surgery, 30*, 67–75.

57. Greenhalgh D. G. (2003). Wound healing and diabetes mellitus. *Clinics in Plastic Surgery, 30*, 37–45.

58. Sgonc R., Gruber J. (2013). Age-related aspects of cutaneous wound healing: A mini-review. *Gerontology, 59*, 159–164.

59. Gosain A., Dipietro L. A. (2004). Aging and wound healing. *World Journal of Surgery, 28*, 321–326.

Visit the**Point.** **http://thePoint.lww.com for animations, journal articles, and more!**

Disorders of the Immune Response

The immune system is a multifaceted defence network that is designed to protect against invading microorganisms or foreign substances, prevent the proliferation of cancer cells, and mediate the healing of damaged tissue. Under normal conditions, the immune response deters or prevents disease. Occasionally, however, the inadequate, inappropriate, or misdirected activation of the immune system can lead to debilitating or life-threatening illnesses, typified by immunodeficiency states, allergic or hypersensitivity reactions, transplantation rejection, and autoimmune disorders.

IMMUNODEFICIENCY DISORDERS

After completing this section of the chapter, you should be able to meet the following objectives:

- State the difference in causes of primary and secondary immunodeficiency disorders.
- Compare and contrast pathology and manifestations of humoral (B cell), cellular (T cell), and combined T- and B-cell immunodeficiency disorders.
- State the function of the complement system and relate it to the manifestations of complement deficiencies and hereditary angioneurotic edema.
- State the proposed mechanisms of dysfunction and manifestations of phagocytosis disorders.

Immunodeficiency can be defined as an abnormality in the immune system that renders a person susceptible to diseases normally prevented by an intact immune system. Immunodeficiency states can be classified as primary (*i.e.,* congenital or inherited) or secondary (acquired later in life).[1] Secondary immunodeficiency can be the result of malnutrition; disseminated cancers; infection of the cells of the immune system, most notably with human immunodeficiency virus (HIV), the etiologic agent of acquired immunodeficiency syndrome (AIDS); and treatment with immunosuppressive drugs (*e.g.,* corticosteroids or transplant rejection medications). The severity and symptoms of the various immunodeficiencies depend on the disorder and extent of immune system involvement. The various categories of immunodeficiency disorders

| CHART 19.1 | IMMUNODEFICIENCY STATES |

Humoral (B-Cell) Immunodeficiency
Primary
  X-linked hypogammaglobulinemia
  Common variable immunodeficiency
  Selective deficiency of IgG, IgA, IgM
Secondary
  Increased loss of immunoglobulin (nephrotic
    syndrome)

Cellular (T-Cell) Immunodeficiency
Primary
  Congenital thymic aplasia (DiGeorge syndrome)
  Hyper-IgM syndrome
Secondary
  Malignant disease (Hodgkin disease and others)
  Transient suppression of T-cell production and
    function due to acute viral infection
  HIV-AIDS

Combined B-Cell and T-Cell Immunodeficiency
Primary
  Severe combined immunodeficiency syndrome (SCID)
    X-linked
    Autosomal recessive (ADA deficiency, Jak3
      deficiency)
  Wiskott–Aldrich syndrome
  Ataxia-telangiectasia
  Combined immunodeficiency syndrome (CID)
Secondary
  Irradiation
  Immune suppression and cytotoxic drugs

Complement System Disorders
Primary
  Hereditary deficiency of complement proteins
  Hereditary deficiency of C1 inhibitor (angioneurotic
    edema)
Secondary
  Acquired disorders that consume complement factors

Disorders of Phagocytosis
Primary
  Chronic granulomatous disease
  Chédiak–Higashi syndrome
Secondary
  Drug-induced (corticosteroid and immuno-
    suppressive therapy)
  Diabetes mellitus
  End-stage renal disease

(see Chapter 17). The innate immune system uses the defences of the phagocytic leukocytes (*i.e.*, neutrophils, macrophages), innate lymphoid cells (natural killer [NK] cells), chemical mediators (cytokines, chemokines), and complement proteins. This arm responds rapidly to infections in a relatively nonspecific manner. The adaptive immune system differs from the innate immune system in its ability to exhibit memory for invading organisms and toxic substances. The adaptive immune response is composed mainly of T and B cells and responds to infections more slowly, but more specifically, than the innate immune system. The specificity of the adaptive immune response has enabled the ability of T and B cells to rearrange their receptors (T cells) and immunoglobulins (B cells) into billions of different combinations. This diversification, in turn, allows the adaptive immune system to recognize billions of different epitopes on infectious organisms.

The adaptive immune system is further divided into the humoral and cellular immune systems. The humoral immune system classically has been limited to B cells and their production of immunoglobulins or antibodies, whereas the cellular immune system has been restricted to T cells and their ability to produce various cytokines and, in the case of cytotoxic T cells, to kill cells infected with intracellular organisms. What has become clear in recent years is that the humoral and cellular immune systems are functionally dependent on each other for mounting an immune response.[2] B cells, for example, depend on certain cytokines produced by helper T cells to produce different classes of immunoglobulin (*i.e.*, IgG versus IgA). Likewise, cytotoxic T cells depend on specific immunoglobulins produced by B cells to clear viral infections effectively by destroying cell-free virus particles and preventing their spread to other cellular targets.

Although primary immunodeficiencies are thought to be rare, it has been estimated in Canada that this affects approximately 29,000 people.[3] Until recently, little was known about the causes of primary immunodeficiency diseases. However, this has changed with recent advances in genetic technology.[1–6] To date, there are more than 250 genetic defects and disorders of the immune system that are recognized as primary immunodeficiencies.[3] Most are transmitted as recessive traits, several of which are caused by mutations in genes on the X chromosome and others by mutations on autosomal chromosomes. Many of these disorders have been traced to mutations affecting signalling pathways (*e.g.*, cytokines and cytokine signalling, receptor subunits, and metabolic pathways) that dictate immune cell development and function. Furthermore, it has been shown that the immune system is a carefully balanced system that is designed to distinguish between self and nonself; therefore, symptoms of autoimmunity often are observed with primary immunodeficiency disease.[2]

Early detection is possible for most primary immunodeficiency diseases, is critical for the success of some treatments, and can be lifesaving. For infants with severe combined T- and B-cell immunodeficiency, early diagnosis is essential not only in terms of preventing life-threatening

are summarized in Chart 19.1. HIV/AIDS is discussed in Chapter 20.

The immune system is made up of two distinct but interrelated components: the innate and adaptive immune systems

- Four or more new ear infections within 1 year
- Two or more serious sinus infections within 1 year
- Two or more months on antibiotics with little effect
- Two or more pneumonias within 1 year
- Failure of an infant to gain weight or grow normally
- Recurrent, deep skin, or organ abscesses
- Persistent thrush in mouth or elsewhere on skin, after 1 year of age
- Need for intravenous antibiotics to clear infections
- Two or more deep-seated infections, including septicemia
- A family history of primary immunodeficiency

From the Jeffrey Modell Foundation. (2013). Available online at: www.info4pi.org

infections, but in preventing administration of live attenuated virus vaccines (*e.g.,* measles, mumps, rubella, varicella, bacillus Calmette–Guérin), which could prove fatal.[2] The first clinical clue for diagnosis of primary immunodeficiency disease is usually a history of infections that are persistent, difficult to treat, or caused by unusual microbes. The worldwide Jeffrey Modell Foundation/Immune Deficiency Foundation has developed a set of warning signs, one for children and another for adults, that serve as excellent tools for determining what should be considered abnormal (Chart 19.2).[7] Because these disorders are frequently inherited, a positive family history is also a key diagnostic tool. The type of infection can provide information regarding the type of defect that is present. Infections with bacterial organisms are frequently observed in cases of antibody deficiency, whereas severe viral, fungal, and opportunistic infections characterize T-cell deficiencies. Recurrent *Streptococcus pneumoniae* or *Neisseria* infections characterize persons with complement deficiencies, and recurrent infections with staphylococcal and other catalase-positive organisms indicate disorders of phagocytosis. Table 19.1 summarizes types of infections that occur with the different types of primary immunodeficiency disorders.

Humoral (B-Cell) Immunodeficiencies

Humoral immunodeficiencies involve B-cell function and immunoglobulin (*i.e.,* antibody) production. Defects in humoral immunity increase the risk of recurrent pyogenic infections, including those caused by *S. pneumoniae, Haemophilus influenzae, Staphylococcus aureus,* and gram-negative organisms such as *Pseudomonas* species. Humoral immunity usually is not as important in defending against intracellular bacteria (mycobacteria), fungi, and protozoa. Viruses usually are handled normally, except for the enteroviruses that cause gastrointestinal infections.

TABLE 19.1 INFECTIOUS ORGANISMS FREQUENTLY ASSOCIATED WITH MAJOR CATEGORIES OF IMMUNODEFICIENCY DISORDERS

IMMUNODEFICIENCY DISORDER	VIRUSES	BACTERIA	FUNGI	PROTOZOA
B-cell (humoral) immunodeficiency	Enteroviruses	*Streptococcus pneumoniae, Staphylococcus aureus, Haemophilus influenzae,* Encapsulated bacteria	No	*Giardia lamblia*
T-cell (cell-mediated) immunodeficiency	Herpesvirus	*Salmonella typhi,* all mycobacteria, intracellular bacteria	*Candida albicans, Coccidioides immitis, Histoplasma capsulatum, Aspergillus fumigatus*	*Strongyloides* spp, *Toxoplasma* spp
Combined T-cell and B-cell immunodeficiency	All	*S. pneumoniae, S. aureus, H. influenzae, Pseudomonas aeruginosa, Neisseria meningitidis, Mycoplasma hominis,* enteric flora	*C. albicans, Pneumocystis jiroveci* (formerly *carinii*)	*Toxoplasma gondii*
Complement system disorders		*S. aureus, S. pneumoniae, H. influenzae, N. meningitidis*		
Phagocytosis (neutrophils and monocytes) disorders		*S. aureus,* enteric flora, *P. aeruginosa,* all mycobacteria	*A. fumigatus, C. albicans, Nocardia asteroides*	

Information from Fishman J. A. (2015). Approach to the immunocompromised patient with fever and pulmonary infiltrates, Table: Organisms associated with infection in individuals with various immune deficits. *UpToDate*; Kumar V., Abbas A. K., Faustos, N., et al. (Eds.), (2010). *Robbins and Cotran pathologic basis of disease* (8th ed., p. 231). Philadelphia, PA: Elsevier Saunders; Verbsky J. W., Grossman W. J. (2006). Cellular and genetic basis of primary immune deficiencies. *Pediatric Clinics of North America, 53,* 649–684.

Transient Hypogammaglobulinemia of Infancy

During the first few months of life, infants are protected from infection by IgG antibodies that have been transferred from the maternal circulation during fetal life. IgA, IgM, IgD, and IgE do not normally cross the placenta. The presence of elevated levels of IgA or IgM in the infant cord blood suggests premature antibody production in response to an intrauterine infection. An infant's level of maternal IgG gradually declines over a period of approximately 6 months (see Chapter 17, Fig. 17.14). Concomitant with the loss of maternal antibody, the infant's immature humoral immune system begins to function, and between the ages of 1 and 2 years, the child's antibody production reaches adult levels.

Any abnormality that interferes with the production of immunoglobulin-producing plasma cells can produce a state of immunodeficiency. For example, certain infants may experience a delay in IgG production (IgM and IgA levels are normal) beyond 6 months of age. The total number and antigenic response of circulating B cells are normal, but the chemical communication between B and T cells that leads to clonal proliferation of antibody-producing plasma cells seems to be reduced.[6] This condition is referred to as *transient hypogammaglobulinemia of infancy*. The result of this condition usually is limited to repeated bouts of upper respiratory and middle ear infections. This condition usually resolves by the time the child is 2 to 4 years of age.

Primary Humoral Immunodeficiency Disorders

Of all the primary immunodeficiency diseases, those affecting antibody production are the most common.[6] Antibody production depends on the differentiation of hematopoietic stem cells into mature B lymphocytes and the antigen-dependent generation of immunoglobulin-producing plasma cells (Fig. 19.1). This maturation cycle initially involves the production of surface IgM, migration from the bone marrow to the peripheral lymphoid tissue, and switching to the production of specialized IgM-, IgA-, IgD-, IgE-, or IgG-secreting plasma cells after antigenic stimulation. Primary humoral immunodeficiency disorders can interrupt the production of one or all of the immunoglobulins.

X-Linked Agammaglobulinemia. X-linked (Bruton) agammaglobulinemia is a recessive trait that affects only boys.[2–6,8–11] As the name implies, persons with this disorder have essentially undetectable levels of all serum immunoglobulins. Therefore, they are susceptible to meningitis and recurrent otitis media and to sinus and pulmonary infections with encapsulated organisms such as *S. pneumoniae, H. influenzae* type b, *S. aureus,* and *Neisseria meningitidis.*[4]

The abnormal gene in X-linked agammaglobulinemia maps to the long arm of the X chromosome and encodes the B-cell protein tyrosine kinase (Bruton tyrosine kinase [*Btk*]). *Btk* appears to be necessary for pre-B-cell expansion and maturation into surface immunoglobulin-expressing B cells, but probably has a role in all stages of B-cell development. Mutation in the *Btk* gene results in an absence of mature circulating B cells and plasma cells.[8–11] T lymphocytes, however, are normal in number and function.

Most boys with the disorder remain asymptomatic until 6 to 9 months of life because of the presence of maternal antibodies. A clue to the presence of the disorder is the failure of an infection to respond completely and promptly to antibiotic therapy. Diagnosis is based on demonstration of low or absent serum immunoglobulins. Therapy consists of prophylaxis with intravenous or subcutaneous immunoglobulin and prompt antimicrobial therapy for suspected infections. The prognosis of this condition depends on the prompt recognition and treatment of infections. Chronic pulmonary disease is an ever-present danger.

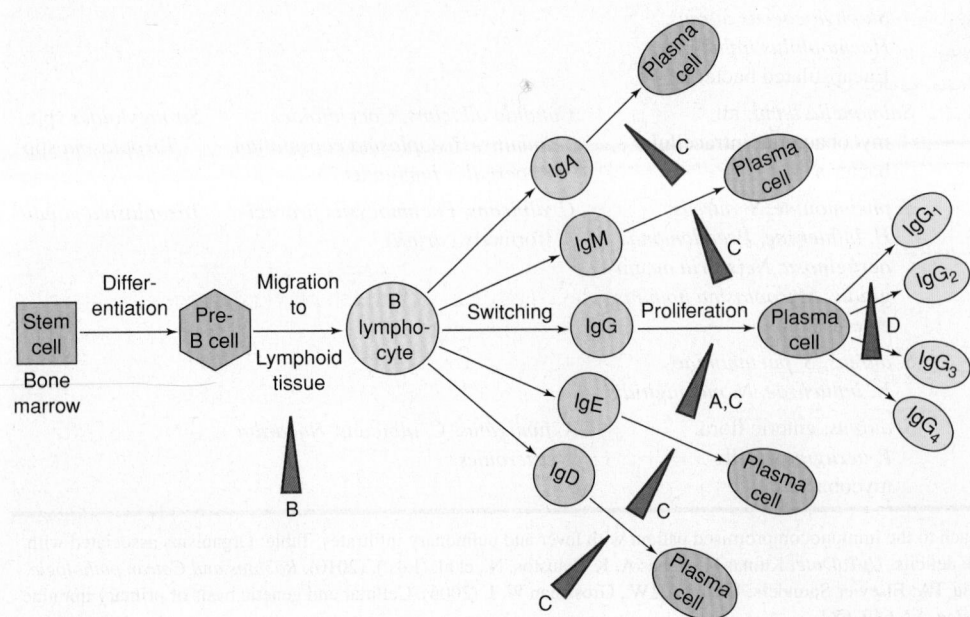

FIGURE 19.1 • Stem cells to mature immunoglobulin-secreting plasma cells. *Arrows* indicate the stage of the maturation process that is interrupted in **(A)** transient hypogammaglobulinemia, **(B)** X-linked agammaglobulinemia, **(C)** common variable immunodeficiency, and **(D)** IgG subclass deficiency.

Common Variable Immunodeficiency. Another disorder of B-cell maturation, which is similar to X-linked agammaglobulinemia, is a condition called *common variable immunodeficiency (CVID)*. In this syndrome, the terminal differentiation of mature B cells to plasma cells is blocked.[8] More than 80% of persons with this disorder have a normal number of B lymphocytes, but when the lymphocytes are presented with antigen, they fail to differentiate into antibody-secreting cells.[10] Some persons may also have increased apoptosis of helper T cells, and decreased T-cell function and signalling.

The symptomatology of CVID is similar to that of X-linked agammaglobulinemia (*i.e.,* recurrent otitis media and sinus and pulmonary infections with encapsulated organisms), but the onset of infections occurs much later, usually in the second to third decade of life. In contrast to X-linked agammaglobulinemia, the sex distribution in CVID is almost equal. Most persons with CVID have no identified molecular diagnosis. Because the disorder occurs in first-degree relatives of persons with IgA deficiency, and some persons with IgA deficiency develop agammaglobulinemia, these disorders may have a common genetic basis.

PRIMARY IMMUNODEFICIENCY DISORDERS

- Primary immunodeficiency disorders are congenital or inherited abnormalities of immune function that render a person susceptible to diseases normally prevented by an intact immune system.
- Disorders of B-cell function impair the ability to produce antibodies and defend against microorganisms and toxins that circulate in body fluids (IgM and IgG) or enter the body through the mucosal surface of the respiratory or gastrointestinal tract (IgA). Persons with primary B-cell immunodeficiency are particularly prone to pyogenic infections due to encapsulated organisms.
- Disorders of T-cell function impair the ability to orchestrate the immune response (CD4+ helper T cells) and to protect against fungal, protozoan, viral, and intracellular bacterial infections (CD8+ cytotoxic T cells). T cells also play an important role in surveillance against oncogenic viruses and tumours; hence, persons with impaired T-cell function are at increased risk for certain types of cancers.
- Combined T-cell and B-cell immunodeficiency states affect all aspects of immune function. Severe combined immunodeficiency (SCID) represents a life-threatening absence of immune function that requires bone marrow or stem cell transplantation for survival.

Persons with CVID often have autoantibody formation (about 30%), and up to 50% develop benign lymphoproliferation (*i.e.,* enlarged tonsils and lymph nodes), often presenting as splenomegaly.[10] They have an increased tendency toward development of interstitial lung disease, autoimmune disorders, hepatitis, and chronic diarrhea with associated intestinal malabsorption. There is also an increased risk of developing malignancies such as gastric cancer and non-Hodgkin B-cell lymphoma.

Treatment methods for CVID are similar to those used for X-linked agammaglobulinemia, with Ig therapy, either intravenous or subcutaneous, being the cornerstone of therapy. Anaphylaxis to IgA in the Ig infusions can occur in persons with CVID who are IgA deficient. The use of IgA-depleted Ig therapy has greatly reduced this risk.

Selective Immunoglobulin A Deficiency. Selective IgA deficiency is the most common type of immunoglobulin deficiency, affecting 1 in 300 to 1 in 600 persons.[3] The syndrome is characterized by moderate to marked reduction in levels of serum and secretory IgA. It is likely that the cause of this deficiency is a block in the pathway that promotes terminal differentiation of mature B cells to IgA-secreting plasma cells. The occurrence of IgA deficiency in both men and women and in members of successive generations within families suggests autosomal inheritance with variable expressivity. The disorder has also been noted in persons treated with certain drugs (*e.g.,* phenytoin, sulfasalazine), suggesting that environmental factors may trigger the disorder.[6]

Approximately two thirds of persons with selective IgA deficiency have no overt symptoms, presumably because IgG and IgM levels are normal and compensate for the defect. At least 50% of affected children overcome the deficiency by the age of 14 years. Persons with markedly reduced levels of IgA often experience repeated upper respiratory and gastrointestinal infections and have an increased incidence of allergic manifestations, such as asthma, and autoimmune disorders. Persons with IgA deficiency also can develop antibodies against IgA, which can lead to severe anaphylactic reactions when blood components containing IgA are given.[6] Therefore, only specially washed erythrocytes from normal donors or erythrocytes from IgA-deficient donors should be used.

There is no treatment available for selective IgA deficiency unless there is a concomitant reduction in IgG levels. Administration of IgA immune globulin is of little benefit because IgA has a short half-life and is not secreted across the mucosa. There also is the risk of anaphylactic reactions associated with IgA antibodies in the immune globulin.

Immunoglobulin G Subclass Deficiency. An IgG subclass deficiency can affect one or more of the IgG subtypes, despite normal levels or elevated serum concentrations of IgG. As discussed in Chapter 17, IgG immunoglobulins can be divided into four subclasses (IgG1 through IgG4) based on structure and function. Most circulating IgG belongs to the IgG1 (70%) and IgG2 (20%) subclasses. In general, antibodies directed against protein antigens belong to the IgG1 and IgG3 subclasses, and antibodies directed against carbohydrate and polysaccharide antigens are primarily IgG2 subclass. As a result, persons who are deficient in IgG2 subclass antibodies can be at greater risk for development of sinusitis, otitis media, and pneumonia caused by polysaccharide-encapsulated micro-organisms such as *S. pneumoniae*, *H. influenzae* type b, and *N. meningitidis*.

Children with mild forms of the deficiency can be treated with prophylactic antibiotics to prevent repeated infections. Immunoglobulins (IGIV or SCIG) can be given to children with severe manifestations of this deficiency. The use of conjugated vaccines in which the polysaccharide capsular protein is linked to a protein carrier can provide protection against some of these infections.

Secondary Humoral Immunodeficiency Disorders

Secondary deficiencies in humoral immunity can develop as a consequence of conditions that increase immunoglobulin loss, diseases that decrease immunoglobulin production, or drug-induced states that cause a decrease in immunoglobulin levels.

Abnormal immunoglobulin loss can occur with chronic kidney disease and protein-losing enteropathies. Such is the case in persons with nephrotic syndrome who, because of abnormal glomerular filtration, lose serum IgA and IgG in their urine. Because of its larger molecular size, IgM is not filtered into the urine, and serum levels remain normal. Protein-losing enteropathies that commonly present with decreased immuno-globulin levels include autoimmune enteropathy and intestinal lymphangiectasis (blocked interstitial lymphatics with loss of lymph fluid and immunoglobulins in the gastrointestinal tract).

Secondary humoral immunodeficiencies can also result from a number of malignancies, including chronic lymphocytic leukemia, lymphoma, and multiple myeloma, that interfere with normal immunoglobulin production. Medications that cause reversible secondary hypogammaglobulinemia include the disease-modifying antirheumatic drugs, corticosteroid agents, and the antiepileptic drugs phenytoin and carbamazepine.

Cell-Mediated (T-Cell) Immunodeficiencies

Unlike B cells, in which a well-defined series of differentiation steps ultimately leads to the production of immunoglobu-lins, mature T lymphocytes consist of distinct subpopulations whose immunologic assignments are diverse. T cells can be functionally divided into two main subtypes (CD4+ helper and CD8+ cytotoxic T cells). Collectively, T lymphocytes protect against fungal, protozoan, viral, and intracellular bacterial infections; control malignant cell proliferation; and are responsible for coordinating the overall immune response.

Primary Cell-Mediated Immunodeficiency Disorders

In general, persons with cell-mediated immunodeficiency disorders have infections or other clinical problems that are more severe than those seen with antibody disorders. Children with defects in this branch of the immune response rarely survive beyond infancy or childhood unless immunologic reconstitution is achieved through bone marrow transplantation.[6]

However, exceptions are being recognized as newer T-cell defects, such as the X-linked hyper-IgM syndrome, are identified. Other recently identified primary T-cell immunodeficiency disorders result from defective expression of the T-cell receptor (TCR) complex, defective cytokine production, and defects in T-cell activation.

For children with fatal forms of T-cell defects, transplantation of thymic tissue or major histocompatibility complex (MHC)–compatible bone marrow is currently the treatment of choice. Stem cell transplantation (to be discussed), an alternative to bone marrow transplantation, has also proved useful in treating some disorders. The major risk to recipients of bone marrow transplantation is that of graft-versus-host disease (GVHD). Gene replacement therapy remains a distant goal for most immunodeficiencies at present. The main obstacles to this type of therapy are purifying self-renewing stem cells, which are the ideal target for introduction of the replacement gene, and lack of methods for introducing the genes into the stem cell.

DiGeorge Syndrome. DiGeorge syndrome stems from an embryonic developmental defect. The defect is thought to occur before the 12th week of gestation, when the thymus gland, parathyroid gland, and parts of the head, neck, and heart are developing. The disorder affects both sexes. Because familial occurrence is rare, it seems unlikely that the disorder is inherited. Formerly thought to be caused by a variety of factors, including extrinsic teratogens, this defect has been traced to microdeletion of specific deoxyribonucleic acid (DNA) sequences from chromosome 22 (22q11).[6,8,12]

The clinical phenotype of DiGeorge syndrome varies considerably.[12] Infants born with this defect have partial or complete failure of development of the thymus and parathyroid glands and have congenital defects of the head, neck, and heart. The extent of immune and parathyroid abnormalities is highly variable, as are the other defects. Occasionally, a child has no heart defect. In some children, the thymus is not absent but is in an abnormal location and is extremely small. These infants can have partial DiGeorge syndrome, in which hypertrophy of the thymus occurs with development of normal immune function. The facial disorders can include hypertelorism (*i.e.*, increased distance between the eyes); micrognathia (*i.e.*, abnormally small jaw); low-set, posteriorly angulated ears; split uvula; and high-arched palate (Fig. 19.2). Urinary tract abnormalities also are common. The most frequent presenting sign is hypocalcemia and tetany that develop in the first 24 hours of life. It is caused by the absence of the parathyroid gland and is resistant to standard therapy.[13]

Children who survive the immediate neonatal period may have recurrent or chronic infections because of impaired T-cell immunity. Children also may have an absence of immunoglobulin production, caused by a lack of helper T-cell function. For children who do require treatment, thymus transplantation can be performed to reconstitute T-cell immunity. Bone marrow transplantation also has been successfully used to restore normal T-cell populations. If blood transfusions are

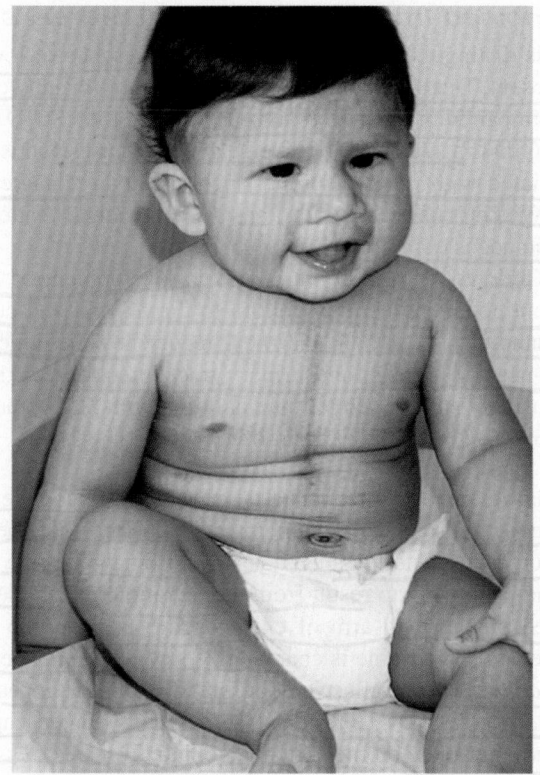

FIGURE 19.2 • An infant with DiGeorge syndrome. The surgical scar on the chest indicates repair of heart disease caused by truncus arteriosus or interrupted aortic arch, which is common in this syndrome. The infant also has the facial features of a child with DiGeorge syndrome, as illustrated by hypertelorism, low-set ears, hypoplastic mandible, and bowing upward of the upper lip. (From Roberts R. *Atlas of infectious diseases.* Edited by Gerald Mandell (series editor), Catherine M. Wilfert. © 1998 Current Medicine, Inc.)

needed, as during corrective heart surgery, special processing is required to prevent GVHD.

X-Linked Immunodeficiency With Hyper-IgM. The X-linked immunodeficiency of hyper-IgM, also known as the *hyper-IgM syndrome,* is characterized by low IgG and IgA levels with normal or, more frequently, high IgM concentrations. Being X-linked, the disorder is confined to boys. Formerly classified as a B-cell defect, it now has been traced to a T-cell defect.[14] The disorder results from the inability of T cells to signal B cells to undergo isotype switching to IgG and IgA; thus, they produce only IgM.[14] Although the disorder was identified on the basis of an antibody defect, its primary cause is a defect in cell-mediated immunity.

Like boys with X-linked agammaglobulinemia, affected boys become symptomatic during the first 2 years of life. They have recurrent pyogenic infections, including otitis media, sinusitis, tonsillitis, and pneumonia. They are also susceptible to opportunistic infections, especially *Pneumocystis jiroveci* (formerly *Pneumocystis carinii*), because of the defect in cell-mediated immunity. Persons with the syndrome are also at increased risk for development of autoimmune diseases of the

formed elements of the blood, including hemolytic anemia, thrombocytopenia, and recurrent severe neutropenia.[14]

Secondary Cell-Mediated Immunodeficiency Disorders

Secondary deficiencies of T-cell function are more common than primary deficiencies and have been described in conjunction with acute viral infections (*e.g.,* measles virus, cytomegalovirus) and with certain malignancies such as Hodgkin disease and other lymphomas. In the case of viruses, direct infection of specific T-lymphocyte subpopulations (*e.g.,* helper cells) by lymphotropic viruses such as HIV and human herpesvirus type 6 can lead to loss of cellular function and selective subtype depletion with a concomitant loss of immunologic function associated with that subtype. Persons with neoplastic disorders can have impaired T-cell function based on unregulated multiplication or dysfunction of one particular subclone of T cells. The outward expression of this may be an increased susceptibility to infections caused by normally harmless pathogens (*i.e.,* opportunistic infections) or failure to generate delayed-type hypersensitivity (DTH) reactions (*i.e.,* anergy). Persons with anergy have a diminished or absent reaction to a battery of skin test antigens, including *Candida* and the tuberculin test, even when infected with *Mycobacterium tuberculosis* (see Chapter 28).

Combined T-Cell and B-Cell Immunodeficiencies

Disorders that affect both B and T lymphocytes, with resultant defects in both humoral and cell-mediated immunity, fall under the broad classification of combined immunodeficiency syndrome (CIDS). A single mutation in any one of the many genes that influence lymphocyte development or response, including lymphocyte receptors, cytokines, or MHC antigens, could lead to combined immunodeficiency (CID). Regardless of the affected gene, the net result is a disruption in the normal communication system between B and T lymphocytes and deregulation of the immune response. The spectrum of disease resulting from CID disorders ranges from mild to severe to ultimately fatal forms.

Severe Combined Immunodeficiency Disorders

Combined B-cell and T-cell immunodeficiency disorders account for approximately 20% of primary immunodeficiency disorders. In the most pronounced forms of the disorder, often referred to as *SCID,* genetic mutations lead to absence of all T- and B-cell function and, in some cases, a lack of NK cells.[6,8,11,12] Affected infants have a disease course that resembles AIDS, with failure to thrive, chronic diarrhea, and opportunistic infections. Survival beyond the first year of life is rare without prompt immune reconstitution through bone marrow or hematopoietic stem cell transplantation. Early diagnosis is critical because the chances of successful treatment are highest in infants who have not experienced severe opportunistic infections. There is also hope that gene therapy will someday be available for some, if not all, forms of SCID.[9,12]

The first discovered cause of SCID, adenosine deaminase (ADA) deficiency, was reported in 1972. It was not until 21 years later, however, that a second cause, the molecular basis of X-linked SCID, was found. Since then, remarkable progress has been made in elucidating several other causes of SCID. It is now known that SCID can be caused by 14 different mutations. These mutations impact components of cytokine receptors that control T-cell differentiation (*i.e.,* γ chain, Janus kinase 3 [Jak3]); control aspects essential for rearrangement of antigen receptor genes (*i.e.,* kinases); and limit enzymes that prevent the accumulation of toxic metabolites causing T-cell destruction (*i.e.,* ADA).[8]

The most common form of SCID, accounting for half of all cases, is X-linked, and hence SCID is more common in boys than girls. It is caused by a genetic defect in the common gamma-chain subunit (γc) of cytokine receptors. This transmembrane receptor is a component of multiple interleukin (IL) receptors, including the IL-7 receptor, which is responsible for proliferation of T-lymphocyte precursors.[15] As a result of defective IL-7 signalling, there is a profound defect in the earliest stages of lymphocyte development with a greatly reduced number of T cells. Although the B cells are normal in number, antibody production is impaired because of a lack of T cell help. IL-15 is important for the maturation and proliferation of NK cells, and because the common γ chain is a component of the receptor for IL-15, this defect can lead to a deficiency of NK cells as well.[8]

The remaining cases of SCID show an autosomal recessive pattern of inheritance. The most common cause of autosomal recessive SCID is an ADA deficiency.[15] Absence of this enzyme leads to the accumulation of toxic metabolites that kill dividing and resting T cells. Infants with ADA-deficiency SCID usually have a much more profound lymphopenia than do infants with other forms of SCID, often manifesting as absolute lymphocyte counts of less than 500/mm³. The absolute numbers of both T and B cells are very low. Although the number of NK cells is low, their function is normal. Other distinguishing features of ADA deficiency include the presence of rib cage deformity and numerous skeletal deformities. Bone marrow transplantation has been successful in treating children with ADA-deficiency SCID.[6,8,12] Enzyme replacement therapy also may be used in the management of persons with this form of SCID. However, it should not be used if bone marrow transplantation is anticipated because it can predispose to graft rejection.[6,12]

Several other, less common causes of SCID are recombinase-activating gene (RAG) deficiencies, Jak3 deficiency, and mutations that impair the expression of class II MHC molecules.[6,8,12] Defects in RAG activity prevent the somatic gene rearrangements necessary for the assembly of the TCR and block the development of T and B cells. Jak3 is essential for signal transduction through the common γc, which is mutated in X-linked SCID. Therefore, mutations in Jak3 have the same effect as X-linked SCID. Mutations that impair expression of MHC II prevent the development of CD4+ helper T cells.

Combined Immunodeficiency Disorders

CID is distinguished from SCID by the presence of low, but not absent, T-cell function. Although antibody-forming capacity is impaired in most cases, it is not absent. Like SCID, however, CID is a syndrome of diverse genetic causes and is often associated with other disorders such as ataxia-telangiectasia and Wiskott–Aldrich syndrome. An autosomal pattern of inheritance is common.

Children with CID are prone to development of recurrent pulmonary infections, failure to thrive, oral and cutaneous candidiasis, chronic diarrhea, recurrent skin infections, gram-negative sepsis, and urinary tract infections. Although they usually survive longer than children with SCID, they fail to thrive and often die early in life.

Ataxia-Telangiectasia. Ataxia-telangiectasia is a complex syndrome of neurologic, immunologic, endocrinologic, hepatic, and cutaneous abnormalities. It is an autosomal recessive disorder that is thought to result from the mutation of a single gene located on the long arm of chromosome 11.[16] As the name implies, this syndrome is characterized by worsening cerebellar *ataxia* (*i.e.,* poor muscle coordination) and the appearance of *telangiectases* (*i.e.,* lesions consisting of dilated capillaries and arterioles) on the skin and conjunctival surfaces of the eye. The ataxia usually goes unnoticed until the child begins to walk and the telangiectases begin to develop, usually after the age of 3, especially on skin surfaces exposed to the sun. The ataxia progresses slowly and relentlessly to severe disability. Intellectual development is normal at first but seems to stop at the 10-year level in many of these children.

Children with ataxia-telangiectasia have deficiencies in both cellular and humoral immunity, including absolute lymphopenia and a decrease in the ratio of CD4+ helper T cells to CD8+ suppressor T cells. Approximately 60% have an IgA deficiency, and approximately 65% also have an IgG subclass deficiency. There is increased susceptibility to recurrent upper and lower respiratory tract infections (particularly those caused by encapsulated bacteria) and an increased risk for the development of malignancies. Death from malignant lymphoma is common.[16]

Wiskott–Aldrich Syndrome. The Wiskott–Aldrich syndrome is an X-linked recessive disorder that becomes symptomatic during the first year of life.[12,17] Infants with this syndrome are plagued by eczema, low platelet counts, and susceptibility to bacterial infections. Bleeding episodes or symptoms due to infection usually begin within the first 6 months of life. Abnormalities of humoral immunity include decreased serum levels of IgM and markedly elevated serum IgA and IgE concentrations. T-cell dysfunction initially is mild but progressively deteriorates, and persons with the disorder become increasingly susceptible to development of malignancies of the mononuclear phagocytic system, including Hodgkin lymphoma and leukemia. Children with Wiskott–Aldrich syndrome typically are unable to produce antibody to polysaccharide antigens and therefore are susceptible to infections caused by encapsulated microorganisms. They also are prone to septicemia and meningitis caused by these organisms. Varicella infection can be lethal to children with this condition.

Management of persons with Wiskott–Aldrich syndrome focuses on treatment of eczema, control of infections, and management of bleeding episodes. If an infection is suspected, careful evaluation for bacterial, viral, and fungal causes followed by administration of appropriate antimicrobial therapy is required. Bone marrow transplantation has been successful in children with Wiskott–Aldrich syndrome. Splenectomy, sometimes recommended for persons with thrombocytopenia, effectively stops the bleeding episodes, but increases the risk of septicemia.[17]

Disorders of the Complement System

The complement system is an integral part of the innate or non-specific immune response (see Chapter 17). The activation of the complement network through the classic, lectin-mediated, or alternative pathways promotes chemotaxis, opsonization, and phagocytosis of invasive pathogens, bacteriolysis, and anaphylactic reactions. Thus, alterations in normal levels of complement or the absence of a particular complement component can lead to enhanced susceptibility to infectious diseases and also to autoimmune diseases, particularly systemic lupus erythematosus (SLE).[2]

Primary Disorders of the Complement System

Primary disorders of the complement system can be transmitted as autosomal recessive, autosomal dominant, or autosomal codominant traits that can involve one or more complement components (the complement components are designated by "C" and enzyme subcomponents by "q," "r," and "s") and their regulators. Deficiencies that are transmitted as autosomal codominant occur when each parent transmits a gene that codes for half the serum level of the component. Because 50% activity is sufficient to prevent disease, persons who are heterozygous and have one normally functioning gene seldom have problems.[8] Primary disorders of the complement system can involve one or more proteins, receptors, and/or control molecules at any point along the complement cascade, and the clinical presentation is dependent upon the component(s) affects.

In general, persons with deficiencies in factors C1 (C1q, r, and s) and C4 are not necessarily at increased risk for recurrent infections because the lectin-mediated and alternative pathways can be activated normally through C3 (see Chapter 17). However, many of them acquire autoimmune diseases, particularly lupus-like syndromes.[2,18] Persons with primary deficiency of C1q have a high incidence of SLE, an SLE-like syndrome without typical SLE serology, a chronic rash with underlying vasculitis on biopsy, or membranoproliferative glomerulonephritis.[18] Like persons with C1q deficiency, persons with C1r, C1r/C1s, C4, C2, and C3 deficiencies have a high incidence of vasculitis syndromes, especially SLE or SLE-like syndrome.

A C2 deficiency causes a susceptibility to multiple and potentially life-threatening infections caused by encapsulated bacteria, especially *S. pneumoniae*. Similarly, persons with C3 deficiency are predisposed to infections that trigger the lectin-mediated or alternative pathway (*e.g.*, those caused by encapsulated bacteria and *S. aureus*) because of their inability to opsonize and lyse bacteria. Although persons with deficiencies in the terminal components of complement (C5 through C9) are susceptible to repeated episodes of meningitis and sepsis caused by *N. meningitidis* or systemic gonococcal disease, they are less likely to have autoimmune disorders than persons with other complement deficiencies.

Only supportive measures are available for treatment of primary disorders of the complement system. Measures to prevent bacterial infections are important. The affected person and close contacts should be immunized with vaccines for *S. pneumoniae, H. influenzae,* and *N. meningitidis*.

Hereditary Angioneurotic Edema. Hereditary angioneurotic edema is a particularly interesting form of complement deficiency. Persons with this disorder do not produce a functional C1 inhibitor or have a mutation in factor XII.[19–21] With a C1 inhibitor deficiency, activation of the classic complement pathway becomes uncontrolled, leading to increased breakdown of C4 and C2 with concomitant generation of bradykinin, a vasodilator. C1 inhibitor also functions as an inhibitor of coagulation, fibrinolytic, and kinin-generating pathways through the inactivation of plasma kallikrein and factor XIIa. With a mutation at the level of factor XII, this also can lead to the uncontrolled release of various vasoactive substances, particularity bradykinin that promotes vascular permeability. The net result is the development of episodic attacks of localized edema involving the face, neck, joints, abdomen, and sites of trauma. Swelling of the subcutaneous tissues, especially of the face, can be disfiguring, and swelling of the gastric mucosa causes nausea, vomiting, diarrhea, and even temporary bowel obstructions. If the trachea or larynx is involved, the episode can prove fatal. The attacks associated with this inherited disease can begin before the age of 2 years but usually are not severe until late childhood or adolescence. Symptoms can last from 1 to 5 days, and most persons with the disorder have more than one attack a month.

Management of the disorder involves emergency management in cases of severe airway obstruction, including emergency intubation or tracheotomy, recombinant C1 inhibitor concentrate, bradykinin receptor B2 antagonists, or kallikrein inhibitor. Preventative treatment usually involves the avoidance of precipitating influences, the administration of mild androgens and antifibrinolytics, or C1 inhibitor concentration.[18–21]

Secondary Disorders of the Complement System

Secondary complement deficiencies also can occur in persons with functionally normal complement systems because of rapid activation and turnover of complement components (as is seen in immune complex disease) or reduced synthesis of components, as would be the case in chronic cirrhosis of the liver or malnutrition.

Disorders of Phagocytosis

The phagocytic system is composed primarily of granulocytes (*i.e.,* neutrophils and eosinophils) and mononuclear phagocytes (*i.e.,* circulating monocytes and tissue and fixed [spleen] macrophages). The primary purpose of phagocytic cells is to migrate to the site of infection (*i.e.,* chemotaxis), aggregate around the affected tissue (*i.e.,* adherence), envelope invading microorganisms or foreign substances (*i.e.,* phagocytosis), and generate microbicidal substances (*e.g.,* enzymes or by-products of metabolism) to kill the ingested pathogens. A defect in any of these functions or a reduction in the absolute number of available cells can disrupt the phagocytic system. Patients with phagocytic disorders are particularly prone to infections by bacteria and often by *Candida* species and filamentous fungi, although the types of pathogens vary with different disorders.[22] As with other alterations in immune function, defects in phagocytosis can be primary or secondary disorders.

Primary Disorders of Phagocytosis

Primary disorders of phagocytosis include leukocyte adhesion deficiency disorders, defects in microbicidal activity (*e.g.,* chronic granulomatous disease [CGD]), and degranulation abnormalities (*e.g.,* Chédiak–Higashi syndrome).

Perhaps the best known of the primary disorders of phagocytosis is *CGD.* CGD represents a group of inherited disorders that greatly reduce or inactivate the ability of phagocytic cells to produce the so-called *respiratory burst* that results in the generation of toxic derivatives of oxygen (superoxide anion and hydrogen peroxide).[23] These oxygen species participate in creating an intracellular environment that kills ingested microorganisms. Recurrent infections, along with granulomatous lesions, in persons with CGD are thought to be due to persistence of viable microorganisms in impaired phagocytic cells. Other aspects of phagocyte function, such as engulfment of microorganisms, are normal. Although four mutations have been found to causes CGD, about 65% of persons with CGD are males who inherit their disorder as a result of mutations in the X chromosome.[23]

Children with CGD are subject to chronic and acute infections of the skin, liver, lung, bladder, and other soft tissues despite aggressive prophylactic and therapeutic antibiotic therapy. Severe facial acne and painful inflammation of the nares is common. Organisms responsible for the infections include *S. aureus, Serratia marcescens, Burkholderia cepacia, Nocardia* spp, *Escherichia coli, Candida albicans,* and *Aspergillus* species.[23] These infections usually begin during the first 2 years of life. The disorder is diagnosed by direct measurement of superoxide production or by examining the ability of a person's phagocytes to reduce a yellow dye (*i.e.,* nitroblue tetrazolium) to a blue compound during active respiration. Bone marrow transplantation is the only known cure

for CGD. Supportive care includes the use of recombinant interferon-gamma and prophylactic antimicrobial therapy.

Chédiak–Higashi syndrome is a rare autosomal recessive disorder characterized by increased susceptibility to infection owing to defective degranulation of neutrophils, a mild bleeding disorder, partial oculocutaneous albinism, progressive neurologic dysfunction, and a tendency to develop a life-threatening lymphoma-like syndrome.[24] The neutrophils (and other leukocytes) of persons with the disorder have giant granules, which can be seen on peripheral blood smears and which are thought to result from aberrant organelle fusion. In this syndrome, there is: reduced transfer of lysosomal enzymes to phagocytic vacuoles in phagocytes (causing susceptibility to infections); abnormalities in melanocytes (leading to albinism); changes in intracytoplasmic components of nerve cells such as astrocyte, satellite, Schwann, and ganglion cells (associated with nerve disorders); and dysfunctional platelets (generating bleeding disorders).[24]

Chédiak–Higashi syndrome manifests during infancy and early childhood, with at least half of the cases accompanied by a neural defect. Most cases have recurrent respiratory and skin infections, and 50% to 85% of people enter into a dangerous complication of the disease called the acceleration phase, characterized by fatal lymphocytic infiltration of all major organs. Bone marrow transplantation reconstitutes normal hematopoietic and immunologic function, but does not correct or prevent any of the associated complications.

Secondary Disorders of Phagocytosis

Secondary deficiencies of the phagocytic system can be caused by a number of conditions such as leukemia, malnutrition, viral infections, or diabetes mellitus. Persons with diabetes mellitus may demonstrate poor phagocytic function, primarily because of altered chemotaxis. The reason for this dysfunction is not understood, but it is unrelated to the person's age or the severity of the metabolic disorder. Apparently, this is a separate genetic disorder that is coinherited at a higher frequency among persons with diabetes and among family members. Other metabolic conditions (*e.g.,* end-stage renal disease with uremia) or drugs (*e.g.,* corticosteroids or cyclosporine) can impair or prevent inflammation and T-cell function and alter phagocytic response through modulation of cytokines.

HIV infection and AIDS represent another form of acquired or secondary deficiency of phagocytic function. However, in this case, the deficiency is due to direct infection and destruction of helper T cells and monocytes–macrophages by the virus (see Chapter 20).

Stem Cell Transplantation

Many of the primary immunodeficiency disorders in which the defect has been traced to the stem cell can be cured with allogeneic stem cell transplantation from an unaffected donor.[25,26] These include disorders such as SCID, Wiskott–Aldrich syndrome, and CGD.

It has been shown that stem cells can repopulate the bone marrow and reestablish hematopoiesis. For the procedure to be effective, the bone marrow cells of the host are destroyed by myeloablative doses of chemotherapy. The exception is children with SCID. Because of the profound cellular immune defect that is present in children with SCID, pretransplantation myeloablation may not be necessary.[25] After transplantation, a lineage-specific chimeric state usually develops in these children, in which the T-cell component is of donor origin and the B-cell component, although variable, remains largely of host origin.[25] Chronic immunoglobulin therapy may be necessary for transplant recipients who primarily retain B cells of host origin.

Stem cells can be collected from the bone marrow or peripheral blood. Donors with identical human leukocyte antigen (HLA) types (*i.e.*, matched for at least three of the six HLA loci) are associated with the least risk of GVHD or graft rejection. HLA-matched siblings usually produce the best results. Stem cell aspiration from the bone marrow is the most common form of allograft collection. Only a few (less than 1 in 100,000) nucleated bone marrow cells are true hematopoietic stem cells. These stem cells are separated from other bone marrow cells before transplantation. Peripheral blood offers a less invasive method for obtaining stem cells. Hematopoietic growth factors, such as granulocyte colony-stimulating factor, often are used to induce stem cells to move out of the bone marrow into the blood. Many of these stem cells can be collected from the blood using leukapheresis, a process that separates the stem cells from other blood cells. A third potential source of stem cells is umbilical cord blood. Umbilical cord blood is a rich source of primitive hematopoietic blood. Up to 250 ml of umbilical cord blood can be collected at the time of delivery without producing detrimental effects to the mother or newborn. Although reliable engraftment of bone marrow can be achieved in children, it is uncertain whether cord blood contains enough stem cells to engraft adult recipients.[25]

The newer role for gene therapy continues to be investigated with the hope of allowing a person's own cells, after being genetically altered and then reintroduced, to correct any cellular dysfunction or mutations. This treatment may be a potential option for patients with some of the primary or secondary immunodeficiencies who are unable to find a HLA match, are at high risk for GVHD, or who have other autoimmune disorders.[26]

IN SUMMARY

An immunodeficiency is defined as an absolute or partial loss of the normal immune response, which places a person in a state of compromise and increases the risk for development of infections or malignant complications. Immunodeficiency states can affect components of the innate or adaptive immune systems. The variety of defects known to involve the immune response can be classified as primary (*i.e.*, congenital or inherited) or secondary (*i.e.*, due another disease or condition). The extent to which any or all of these components are compromised dictates the severity of the immunodeficiency.

Immunodeficiency can affect the humoral or cellular components of the adaptive immune system. B-cell or humoral immunodeficiency disorders can selectively involve a single immunoglobulin (*e.g.*, IgA immunodeficiency) or all of the immunoglobulins (agammaglobulinemia). Defects in humoral immunity increase the risk of recurrent pyogenic infections but have less effect on the defence against intracellular bacteria (mycobacteria), fungi, protozoa, and viruses (except for the enteroviruses that cause gastrointestinal infections). T lymphocytes protect against fungal, protozoan, viral, and intracellular bacterial infections; control malignant cell proliferation; and are responsible for coordinating the overall immune response. T-cell or cellular immune disorders can present as selective T-cell immunodeficiency states or as combined T- and B-cell immunodeficiency disorders. Infants with SCID have a disease course that resembles AIDS, with failure to thrive, chronic diarrhea, and opportunistic infections. Survival beyond the first year of life is rare without prompt immune reconstitution through bone marrow or hematopoietic stem cell transplantation.

The complement system and phagocytosis are integral components of innate immunity. Activation of the complement system promotes chemotaxis, opsonization, and phagocytosis and destruction of invasive pathogens. Thus, deficiencies in normal levels of complement or the absence of a particular complement component can lead to enhanced susceptibility to infectious diseases and also to autoimmune diseases, particularly SLE. Persons with phagocytic disorders are particularly prone to infections by bacteria and often by *Candida* species and filamentous fungi, although the types of pathogens vary with different disorders. Primary disorders of phagocytosis include leukocyte adhesion deficiency disorders, degranulation abnormalities, and defects in microbicidal activity.

HYPERSENSITIVITY DISORDERS

After completing this section of the chapter, you should be able to meet the following objectives:

- Differentiate between adaptive immune responses that protect against microbial agents and hypersensitivity responses.
- Describe the immune mechanisms involved in a type I, type II, type III, and type IV hypersensitivity reaction.
- Describe the pathogenesis of common hypersensitivity reactions including allergic rhinitis, food allergy, serum sickness, Arthus reaction, contact dermatitis, and hypersensitivity pneumonitis.
- Characterize the differences in latex allergy caused by a type I, IgE-mediated hypersensitivity response and that caused by a type IV, cell-mediated response.

TABLE 19.2 CLASSIFICATION OF HYPERSENSITIVITY RESPONSES

TYPE OF HYPERSENSITIVITY	IMMUNE MECHANISM	MECHANISM OF INJURY
Type I, immediate hypersensitivity	IgE antibody	Immediate release of mast cell mediators; later recruitment of inflammatory cells
Type II, antibody mediated	IgM, IgG antibodies against cell surface or extracellular matrix	Phagocytosis and opsonization of cells; complement- and receptor-mediated recruitment and activation of inflammatory cells (neutrophils, macrophages); abnormalities in cellular functioning (e.g., receptor signalling)
Type III, immune complex mediated	Formation and deposition of immune complexes involving circulating antigens and IgM or IgG antibodies	Complement-mediated recruitment and activation of inflammatory cells
Type IV, T-cell mediated	CD4+ T cells (delayed-type hypersensitivity, or CD8+ cytotoxic T-cell–mediated cytolysis)	Macrophage activation of cytokine-mediated inflammation; direct target cell killing, cytokine-mediated inflammation

Hypersensitivity disorders refer to excessive or inappropriate activation of the immune system. Although activation of the immune system normally leads to production of antibodies and T-cell responses that protect the body against attack by microorganisms, it is also capable of causing tissue injury and disease. Disorders caused by immune responses are collectively referred to as *hypersensitivity reactions*.

Historically, hypersensitivity disorders have been subdivided into four types: type I, IgE-mediated disorders; type II, antibody-mediated disorders; type III, complement-mediated immune disorders; and type IV, T-cell–mediated disorders (Table 19.2).[1,8,11] These categories differ in terms of the type of immune response causing the injury and the nature and location of the antigen that is the target of the response. Latex allergy can result from an IgE-mediated or T-cell–mediated hypersensitivity

response. It is discussed separately at the end of this section. Transplant rejections and autoimmune disorders (discussed separately) may also be regarded as hypersensitivity responses.

Type I, Immediate Hypersensitivity Disorders

Type I hypersensitivity reactions are IgE-mediated reactions that begin rapidly, often within minutes of an antigen challenge. These types of reactions to antigens are often referred to as *allergic reactions*. In the context of an allergic response, the antigens usually are referred to as *allergens*. Typical allergens include the proteins in pollen, house dust mites, animal dander, foods, and chemicals like the antibiotic penicillin. Exposure to the allergen can be through inhalation, ingestion, injection, or skin contact. Depending on the portal of entry, type I reactions may occur as a local or atopic reaction that is merely annoying (*e.g.*, seasonal rhinitis) or severely debilitating (asthma), or as a systemic and potentially life-threatening reaction (anaphylaxis).

Cells that are central to a type I hypersensitivity reaction include type 2 helper T (T$_H$2) cells, mast cells, or basophils and eosinophils.[1,8,27] There are two main subsets of helper T cells (T$_H$1 and T$_H$2) that develop from the same precursor CD4+ T lymphocyte (see Chapter 17). T$_H$1 cells differentiate in response to microbes and stimulate the differentiation of B cells into IgM- and IgG-producing plasma cells. T$_H$2 cell differentiation occurs in response to allergens and helminths (intestinal parasites).[1] Cytokines (*i.e.*, IL-4, IL-5, IL-13) secreted by T$_H$2 cells stimulate differentiation of B cells into IgE-producing plasma cells, act as growth factors for mast cells, and recruit and activate eosinophils.

Mast cells, which are tissue cells, as well as basophils and eosinophils, which are blood cells, are derived from hematopoietic precursor cells. These cells have granules that contain mediators that are released to initiate the early events in type I hypersensitivity reactions. These mediators are preformed in the cell or activated through enzymatic processing. Mast cells normally are distributed throughout connective tissue,

---

ALLERGIC AND HYPERSENSITIVITY DISORDERS

- Hypersensitivity disorders result from immune responses to exogenous and endogenous antigens that produce inflammation and cause tissue damage.
- Type I hypersensitivity is an IgE-mediated immune response that leads to the release of inflammatory mediators for sensitized mast cells.
- Type II disorders involve humoral antibodies against cell surface or extracellular matrix antigens that result in complement-mediated phagocytosis or inflammation and cell injury, or, in some cases, abnormal physiologic responses without cell injury.
- Type III disorders result in generation of circulating immune complexes in which humoral antibodies bind antigen and activate complement. The fractions of complement attract inflammatory cells that release tissue-damaging products.
- Type IV disorders involve tissue damage in which cell-mediated immune responses with sensitized T lymphocytes cause cell and tissue injury.

especially in areas beneath the skin and mucous membranes of the respiratory, gastrointestinal, and genitourinary tracts, and adjacent to blood and lymph vessels.[27,28] This location places them near surfaces that are exposed to environmental antigens and parasites. Mast cells in different parts of the body and even in a single site can have significant differences in mediator content and sensitivity to agents that produce mast cell degranulation. Eosinophils contribute to the pathophysiology of asthma as they release leukotrienes, particularly at respiratory sites, and also produce mediators to help with T_H2 differentiation.

Type I hypersensitivity reactions begin with mast cell or basophil sensitization. During the sensitization or priming stage, allergen-specific IgE antibodies attach to receptors on the surface of mast cells and basophils. With subsequent exposure, the sensitizing allergen binds to the cell-associated IgE and triggers a series of events that ultimately lead to

degranulation of the sensitized mast cells or basophils, causing release of their preformed mediators (Fig. 19.3). Mast cells are also the source of lipid-derived membrane products (*e.g.*, prostaglandins and leukotrienes) and cytokines that participate in the continued response to the allergen.

Many type I hypersensitivity reactions such as bronchial asthma have two well-defined phases: (1) a primary or initial-phase response characterized by vasodilation, vascular leakage, and smooth muscle contraction; and (2) a secondary or late-phase response characterized by more intense infiltration of tissues with eosinophils and other acute and chronic inflammatory cells, as well as tissue destruction in the form of epithelial cell damage.[27]

The primary or initial-phase response usually occurs within 5 to 30 minutes of exposure to antigen and subsides within 60 minutes. It is mediated by mast cell degranulation and

FIGURE 19.3 • Type I, IgE-mediated hypersensitivity reaction. The stimulation of B-cell differentiation by an antigen-stimulated type 2 helper (T_H2) T cell leads to plasma cell production of IgE and mast cell sensitization. Subsequent binding of the antigen produces degranulation of the sensitized mast cell with release of preformed mediators that leads to a primary, or early-phase, response. T_H2 T-cell recruitment of eosinophils, along with the release of cytokines and membrane phospholipids from the mast cell, leads to a secondary, or late-phase, response.

the release of preformed mediators. These mediators include histamine, acetylcholine, adenosine, chemotactic mediators, and enzymes such as chymase and trypsin that lead to generation of kinins. Histamine is a potent vasodilator that increases the permeability of capillaries and venules and causes smooth muscle contraction and bronchial constriction. Acetylcholine produces bronchial smooth muscle contraction and dilation of small blood vessels. The kinins, which are a group of potent inflammatory peptides, require activation through enzymatic modification. Once activated, these peptide mediators produce vasodilation and smooth muscle contraction.

The secondary or late-phase response occurs about 2 to 8 hours later and lasts for several days. It results from the action of lipid mediators and cytokines involved in the inflammatory response. The lipid mediators are derived from mast cell membrane phospholipids, which are broken down to form arachidonic acid. Arachidonic acid, in turn, is the parent compound from which the leukotrienes and prostaglandins are synthesized (see Chapter 18). The leukotrienes and prostaglandins produce responses similar to histamine and acetylcholine, although their effects are delayed and prolonged by comparison. Mast cells also produce cytokines and chemotactic factors that prompt the influx of eosinophils and leukocytes to the site of allergen contact, contributing to the inflammatory response.

At this point, it is important to note that not all IgE-mediated responses produce discomfort and disease. Type I hypersensitivity, particularly the late-phase response, plays a protective role in the control of parasitic infections. IgE antibodies directly damage the larvae of these parasites by recruiting inflammatory cells and causing antibody-dependent cell-mediated cytotoxicity (ADCC). This type of type I hypersensitivity reaction is particularly important in developing countries where much of the population is infected with intestinal parasites.

Anaphylactic (Systemic) Reactions

Anaphylaxis is a systemic life-threatening hypersensitivity reaction characterized by widespread edema, vascular shock secondary to vasodilation, and dyspnea[8,27–30] (see section on Anaphylactic Shock, Chapter 26). It results from the presence of antigen introduced by injection, insect sting, or absorption across the epithelial surface of the skin or gastrointestinal mucosa. The level of severity depends on the level of sensitization. Even small amounts of antigen, such as the presence of residual amounts of peanut that remain on equipment used for preparing foods containing peanuts, can be sufficient to cause anaphylaxis in an extremely sensitive person. Within minutes after exposure, itching, hives, and skin erythema develop, followed shortly by bronchospasm and respiratory distress. Vomiting, abdominal cramps, diarrhea, and laryngeal edema and obstruction follow, and the person may go into shock and die within the hour.

The initial management of anaphylaxis focuses on establishment of a stable airway and intravenous access, and administration of epinephrine.[27,30] Persons with a history of anaphylaxis

should be provided with preloaded epinephrine syringes and instructed in their use. They should also be instructed to seek immediate professional help regardless of the initial response to self-treatment. Family members and caregivers of young children should be trained to inject epinephrine. Prevention of exposure to potential triggers that cause anaphylaxis is particularly important. Finally, all persons with potential for anaphylaxis should be advised to wear or carry a medical alert bracelet, necklace, or other identification to inform emergency personnel of the possibility of anaphylaxis.

Atopic (Local) Reactions

Local or atopic reactions usually occur when the antigen is confined to a particular site by virtue of exposure. The term *atopic* refers to a genetically determined hypersensitivity to common environmental allergens mediated by an IgE–mast cell reaction. Persons with atopic disorders commonly are allergic to more than one environmental allergen, and often to many. The most common atopic disorders are urticaria (hives), allergic rhinitis (hay fever), atopic dermatitis, food allergies, and some forms of asthma. The discussion in this section focuses on allergic rhinitis and food allergy. Allergic asthma is discussed in Chapter 29 and atopic dermatitis in Chapter 61.

The susceptibility to immediate hypersensitivity disorders tends to be genetically determined, and a positive family history of allergy is found in about 50% of atopic individuals.[8] The genetic basis of atopy is unclear; however, linkage studies suggest an association with cytokine genes on chromosome 5q that regulate the expression of circulating IgE and on 6p close to the HLA complex, suggesting certain HLA alleles facilitate reactivity.[8] Persons with atopic allergic conditions tend to have high serum levels of IgE and increased numbers of basophils and mast cells. Although the IgE-triggered response is likely a key factor in the pathophysiology of atopic allergic disorders, it is not the only factor and may not be responsible for conditions such as atopic dermatitis and certain forms of asthma.

Allergic Rhinitis. Allergic rhinitis is characterized by symptoms of sneezing, itching, and watery discharge from the nose and eyes (rhinoconjunctivitis) and affects between 20% and 40% of the western population.[31] Allergic rhinitis not only produces nasal symptoms but frequently is associated with other chronic airway disorders, such as sinusitis and bronchial asthma. Severe attacks may be accompanied by systemic malaise, fatigue, and muscle soreness from sneezing. Fever is absent. Sinus obstruction may cause headache. Typical allergens include pollens from ragweed, grasses, trees, and weeds; fungal spores; house dust mites; animal dander; and feathers. Allergic rhinitis can be divided into perennial and seasonal allergic rhinitis depending on the chronology of symptoms. Persons with the perennial type of allergic rhinitis experience symptoms throughout the year, but those with seasonal allergic rhinitis (*i.e.*, hay fever) are plagued with intense symptoms in conjunction with periods of high allergen (*e.g.*, pollens, fungal spores) exposure.[32] Symptoms that become worse at night suggest a household allergen, and symptoms that disappear on weekends suggest occupational exposure.

Diagnosis depends on a careful history and physical examination, microscopic identification of an increased number of eosinophils on a nasal smear, and skin testing to identify the offending allergens.[32] When possible, avoidance of the offending allergen is recommended. Treatment is symptomatic in most cases and includes the use of oral antihistamines and oral or topical decongestants.[33] Tolerance and rebound congestion may occur when topical decongestants are used for longer than 1 week. Intranasal corticosteroids often are effective when used appropriately. Intranasal cromolyn, a drug that stabilizes mast cells and prevents their degranulation, may be useful, especially when administered before expected contact with an offending allergen. A program of specific immunotherapy ("allergy shots") may be used when symptoms are particularly bothersome.[32,33] Desensitization involves frequent (usually weekly) injections of the offending antigens. The antigens, which are given in increasing doses, stimulate production of high levels of IgG, which acts as a blocking antibody by combining with the antigen before it can combine with the cell-bound IgE antibodies. Newer sublingual immunotherapy options, instead of the weekly injections, are available to Canadians for seasonal grass (*i.e.*, Oralair, Grastek) or ragweed pollen (*i.e.*, Ragwitek) allergic rhinitis, while others are currently in development.[34]

Food Allergies. Virtually any food can produce atopic or nonatopic allergies. The primary target of food allergy may be the skin, the gastrointestinal tract, or the respiratory system. The foods most commonly causing these reactions in children are milk, eggs, peanuts, soy, tree nuts, fish, and shellfish (*i.e.*, crustaceans and mollusks).[35,36] In adults, they are peanuts,[37] shellfish, and fish.[35] The allergenicity of a food may be changed by heating or cooking. Both acute reactions (hives and anaphylaxis) and chronic reactions (asthma, atopic dermatitis, and gastrointestinal disorders) can occur. Anaphylaxis occurs as a multiorgan response associated with IgE-mediated hypersensitivity. The foods most responsible for anaphylaxis are peanuts, tree nuts (*e.g.*, walnuts, almonds, pecans, cashews, hazelnuts), shellfish, milk, and egg.[35,36] One form of food-associated anaphylaxis occurs with exercise.[35,38,39] Food-associated, exercise-induced anaphylaxis may occur when exercise follows ingestion of a particular food to which IgE sensitivity has been demonstrated, or it may occur after ingestion of any food. Exercise without ingestion of the incriminated food does not produce symptoms.[36]

Food allergies can occur at any age but, similar to atopic dermatitis and rhinitis, they tend to manifest during childhood. The allergic response is thought to occur after contact between specific food allergens and sensitizing IgE in the intestinal mucosa causes local and systemic release of histamine and other mediators of the allergic response. In this disorder, allergens usually are food proteins and partially digested food products. Carbohydrates, lipids, or food additives, such as preservatives, colourings, or flavourings, also are potential allergens. Closely related food groups can contain common cross-reacting allergens. For example, some persons are allergic to all legumes (*i.e.*, beans, peas, and peanuts).

Diagnosis of food allergies usually is based on careful food history and provocative diet testing. Provocative testing involves careful elimination of a suspected allergen from the diet for a time to see if the symptoms disappear and reintroducing the food to see if the symptoms reappear. Only one food should be tested at a time. Treatment focuses on avoidance of the food or foods responsible for the allergy. However, avoidance may be difficult for persons who are exquisitely sensitive to a particular food protein because foods may be contaminated with the protein during processing or handling of the food. For example, contamination may occur when chocolate candies without peanuts are processed with the same equipment used for making candies with peanuts. Even using the same spatula to serve cookies with and without peanuts can cause enough contamination to produce a severe reaction.

Type II, Antibody-Mediated Disorders

Type II (antibody-mediated) hypersensitivity reactions are mediated by IgG or IgM antibodies directed against target antigens on cell surfaces or in connective tissues.[8,11] The antigens may be endogenous antigens that are present on the membranes of body cells or exogenous antigens that are adsorbed on the membrane surface. There are three different types of antibody-mediated mechanisms involved in type II reactions: opsonization and complement-mediated and antibody receptor–mediated phagocytosis, complement-mediated and antibody receptor–mediated inflammation, and antibody-mediated cellular dysfunction (Fig. 19.4).[8]

Complement- and Antibody-Mediated Cell Destruction

The deletion of cells targeted by antibody can occur by way of either the complement system or by antibody-dependent cell-mediated cytotoxicity (ADCC), which does not require complement. Complement-mediated cell destruction can occur because the cells are coated (opsonized) with molecules that make them attractive to phagocytes or because of the formation of membrane attack proteins that disrupt the integrity of the cell membrane and cause cell lysis (see Chapter 17, Understanding The Complement System). With ADCC destruction, cells that are coated with low levels of IgG antibody are killed by a variety of effector cells that bind to their target by their receptors for IgG, and cell lysis occurs without phagocytosis.

Examples of antibody-mediated cell destruction include mismatched blood transfusion reactions, hemolytic disease of the newborn due to ABO or Rh incompatibility (see Chapter 14), and certain drug reactions. In the latter, the binding of certain drugs or drug metabolites to the surface of red or white blood cells elicits an antibody response that lyses the drug-coated cell. Lytic drug reactions can produce transient anemia, leukopenia, or thrombocytopenia, which are corrected by the removal of the offending drug.

A Opsonization, MAC, phagocytosis

B Inflammation and tissue injury

C ↑ Thyroid hormone production and release

D Antibody inhibits binding of neurotransmitter to receptor

FIGURE 19.4 • Type II, hypersensitivity reactions result from binding of antibodies to normal or altered surface antigens. **A:** Opsonization and complement-mediated or antibody receptor–mediated phagocytosis or cell lysis through membrane attack complex (MAC). **B:** Complement-mediated and antibody receptor–mediated inflammation resulting from recruitment and activation of inflammation-producing leukocytes (neutrophils and monocytes). **C:** Antibody-mediated cellular dysfunction, in which antibody against the thyroid-stimulating hormone (TSH) receptor increases thyroid hormone production, and (**D**) antibody to acetylcholine receptor inhibits receptor binding of the neurotransmitter in myasthenia gravis. (ECM, extracellular matrix.)

Complement- and Antibody-Mediated Inflammation

When antibodies are deposited in the extracellular tissues, such as basement membranes and matrix, the injury is the result of inflammation rather than phagocytosis or cell lysis.[8,11] In this case, the deposited antibodies activate complement, generating chemotactic by-products (mainly C5a) that recruit and activate neutrophils and monocytes. The activated leukocytes release injurious substances, such as enzymes and reactive oxygen intermediates, that result in inflammation and tissue damage. Antibody-mediated inflammation is responsible for the tissue injury seen in some forms of glomerulonephritis, vascular rejection in organ grafts, and other diseases. In Goodpasture syndrome, for example, antibody binds to a major structural component of pulmonary and glomerular basement membranes, causing pulmonary hemorrhage and glomerulonephritis[11] (see Chapter 33).

Antibody-Mediated Cellular Dysfunction

In some type II reactions, antibody binding to specific target cell receptors does not lead to cell death, but to a change in cell function. In Graves disease, for example, autoantibody directed against thyroid-stimulating hormone (TSH) receptors

on thyroid cells stimulates thyroxine production, leading to hyperthyroidism[8,11] (discussed in Chapter 41). In contrast, in myasthenia gravis, autoantibodies to acetylcholine receptors on the neuromuscular endplates either block the action of acetylcholine or mediate internalization or destruction of receptors, leading to decreased neuromuscular function.

Type III, Immune Complex–Mediated Disorders

Immune complex allergic disorders are mediated by the formation of insoluble antigen–antibody complexes, complement fixation, and localized inflammation (Fig. 19.5).[8,11] Immune complexes formed in the circulation produce damage when they come in contact with the vessel lining or are deposited in tissues, including the renal glomerulus, skin venules, lung, and joint synovium. Once deposited, the immune complexes elicit an inflammatory response by activating complement, thereby leading to chemotactic recruitment of neutrophils and other inflammatory cells. The activation of these inflammatory cells by immune complexes and complement, accompanied by the release of potent inflammatory mediators, is directly responsible for the injury.

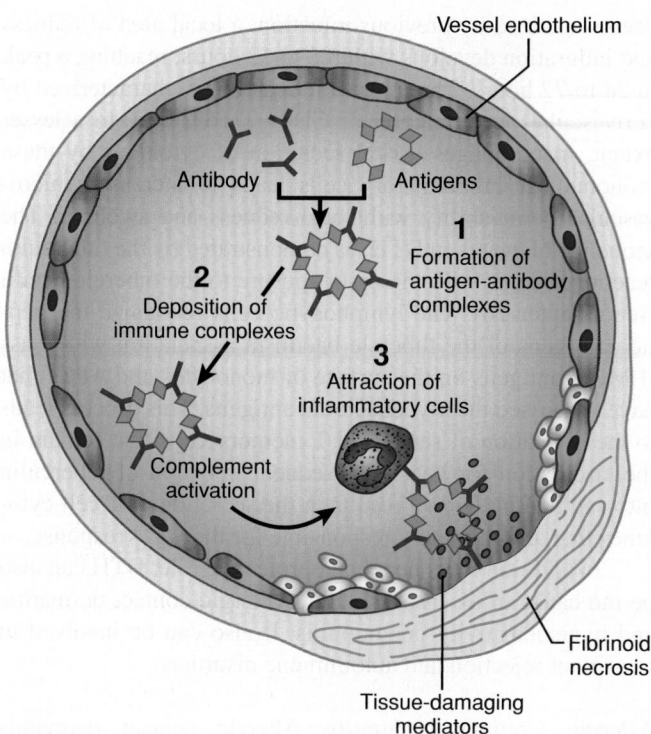

Vessel endothelium

Antibody

Antigens

1
Formation of antigen-antibody complexes

2
Deposition of immune complexes

3
Attraction of inflammatory cells

Complement activation

Fibrinoid necrosis

Tissue-damaging mediators

FIGURE 19.5 • Type III, immune complex reactions involving complement-activating IgG or IgM immunoglobulins with (**1**) formation of blood-borne immune complexes that are (**2**) deposited in tissues. Complement activation at the site of immune complex deposition (**3**) leads to attraction of leukocytes that are responsible for vessel and tissue injury.

Type III reactions are responsible for the vasculitis seen in certain autoimmune diseases such as SLE or the kidney damage seen with acute glomerulonephritis. Type III immune complex disorders can be systemic if the immune complexes are formed in the circulation and deposited in many organs, or localized to a particular organ or site, such as the kidney, joints, or small blood vessels of the skin.

Systemic Immune Complex Disorders

Serum sickness is a systemic immune complex disorder that is triggered by the deposition of insoluble antigen–antibody (IgM, IgG, and occasionally IgA) complexes in blood vessels, joints, and heart and kidney tissue.[8,11,37] The deposited complexes activate complement, increase vascular permeability, and recruit phagocytic cells, all of which can promote focal tissue damage and edema. Clinical manifestations include urticaria, patchy or generalized rash, extensive edema (usually of the face, neck, and joints), fever, generalized lymphadenopathy, and arthralgias, which usually begin approximately 1 to 2 weeks after the initial antigen exposure and subside upon withdrawal of the offending agent.[38] The term *serum sickness* was originally described in persons receiving foreign serum, such as horse serum, for treatment of diphtheria and scarlet fever. Although this therapy is not used today, the name remains. Today, large volume injections of foreign proteins are rarely indicated, but a variety of antigens are capable of causing

this reaction, including beta-lactam antibiotics, sulfonamides, NSAIDS, diuretics various foods, and insect venoms.

In most cases, the damage is temporary, and symptoms resolve within a few days. However, a prolonged and continuous exposure to the sensitizing antigen can lead to irreversible damage. In previously sensitized persons, severe and even fatal forms of serum sickness may occur immediately or within several days after the sensitizing drug or serum is administered.[37]

Treatment of serum sickness usually is directed toward removal of the sensitizing antigen and providing symptom relief. This may include aspirin for joint pain and antihistamines for pruritus. Epinephrine or systemic corticosteroids may be used for severe reactions.

Localized Immune Complex Reactions

The *Arthus reaction* is a term used by pathologists and immunologists to describe localized tissue necrosis (usually in the skin) caused by immune complexes.[39] An Arthus reaction can be caused by repeated local exposure to an antigen where high levels of preformed circulating antibodies exist. Within an hour symptoms usually begin and between 4 and 12 hours, a red, raised lesion appears on the skin at the site of the injection.[8] An ulcer often forms in the centre of the lesion. It is thought that the injected antigen diffuses into local blood vessels, where it comes in contact with specific antibody (IgG) to incite a localized vasculitis (*i.e.,* inflammation of a blood vessel). This experimental model of localized vasculitis is the prototype of many forms of vasculitis seen in humans, such as the cutaneous vasculitides that characterize certain drug reactions.

Type IV, Cell-Mediated Hypersensitivity Disorders

Type IV hypersensitivity reactions involve cell-mediated rather than antibody-mediated immune responses.[8,11] Cell-mediated immunity is the principal mechanism of response to a variety of microorganisms, including intracellular pathogens such as *M. tuberculosis* and viruses, as well as extracellular agents such as fungi, protozoa, and parasites. It can also lead to cell death and tissue injury in response to chemical antigens (contact dermatitis) or self-antigens (autoimmunity).

Type IV hypersensitivity reactions, which are mediated by specifically sensitized T lymphocytes, can be divided into two basic types: direct cell-mediated cytotoxicity and delayed-type hypersensitivity (Fig. 19.6).

Direct Cell-Mediated Cytotoxicity

In direct cell-mediated cytotoxicity, CD8+ cytotoxic T lymphocytes (CTLs) directly kill target cells that express peptides derived from cytosolic antigens that are presented in association with class I MHC molecules (see Chapter 17). In viral infections, CTL responses can lead to tissue injury by killing infected target cells even if the virus itself has no cytotoxic effects.[8] Some viruses directly injure infected cells and are said to be cytopathic, whereas other, noncytopathic viruses

FIGURE 19.6 • Type IV, cell-mediated hypersensitivity reactions, which include (**A**) direct cell-mediated cytotoxicity in which CD8+ T cells kill the antigen-bearing target cells, and (**B**) delayed-type hypersensitivity reactions in which presensitized CD4+ cells release cell-damaging cytokines.

do not. Because CTLs cannot distinguish between cytopathic and noncytopathic viruses, they kill virtually all infected cells regardless of whether the infection is harmful. In certain forms of hepatitis, for example, the destruction of liver cells is due to the host CTL response and not the virus.

Delayed-Type Hypersensitivity Disorders

Delayed-type hypersensitivity (DTH) reactions occur in response to soluble protein antigens and primarily involve antigen-presenting cells (APCs) such as macrophages and CD4+ helper T cells of the T_H1 and T_H17 subtypes. During the reaction T_H1 and T_H17 cells are activated and individually secrete their own array of cytokines that recruit and activate monocytes, lymphocytes, fibroblasts, and other inflammatory cells.[8] These T-cell–mediated responses require the synthesis of effector molecules and take 24 to 72 hours to develop, which is why they are called "delayed-type" hypersensitivity disorders.

The best-known DTH response is the reaction to the tuberculin test, in which inactivated tuberculin or purified protein derivative is injected under the skin. In a person who has

been sensitized by previous infection, a local area of redness and induration develops within 8 to 12 hours, reaching a peak in 24 to 72 hours. The tuberculin reaction is characterized by perivascular accumulation of CD4+ T cells and, to a lesser extent, macrophages. Local secretion of cytokines by these mononuclear inflammatory cells leads to increased microvascular permeability with local redness and swelling. The sequence of events in DTH, as demonstrated by the tuberculin reaction, begins with the first exposure to the tubercle bacilli (see Chapter 28). The lymphocytic cells recognize the peptide antigens of the tubercle bacilli in association with class II MHC antigens on the surface of monocytes and APCs that have processed the mycobacterial antigens. This process leads to the formation of sensitized T memory cells that remain in the circulation for years. Subsequent injection of tuberculin into such an individual results in the secretion of T-cell cytokines that are ultimately responsible for the DTH response.

In addition to its beneficial protective role, DTH can also be the cause of disease, including allergic contact dermatitis and hypersensitivity pneumonitis. It also can be involved in transplant rejection and autoimmune disorders.

Allergic Contact Dermatitis. Allergic contact dermatitis denotes an inflammatory response confined to the skin that is initiated by reexposure to an allergen to which a person had previously become sensitized (*e.g.*, cosmetics, hair dyes, metals, topical drugs).[40] The most common form of this condition is the dermatitis that follows an intimate encounter with poison ivy or poison oak antigens, although many other substances can trigger a reaction.

Contact dermatitis is characterized by erythematous, papular, and vesicular lesions associated with intense pruritus and weeping.[41] The affected area often becomes swollen and warm, with exudation, crusting, and development of a secondary infection. The location of the lesions often provides a clue about the antigen causing the disorder. The severity of the reaction associated with contact dermatitis ranges from mild to intense, depending on the person and the allergen. Because this condition follows the mechanism of a DTH response, the reaction does not become apparent for at least 12 hours and usually more than 24 hours after exposure. Depending on the antigen and the duration of exposure, the reaction may last from days to weeks.

Diagnosis of contact dermatitis is made by observing the distribution of lesions on the skin surface and associating a particular pattern with exposure to possible allergens. If a particular allergen is suspected, a patch test can be used to confirm the suspicion. Treatment usually is limited to removal of the irritant and application of topical preparations (*e.g.*, ointments, corticosteroid creams) to relieve symptomatic skin lesions and prevent secondary bacterial infections. Severe reactions may require systemic corticosteroid therapy.[40,41]

Hypersensitivity Pneumonitis. Hypersensitivity pneumonitis, which is associated with exposure to inhaled organic dusts or related occupational antigens, is another example of a DTH reaction.[42] The disorder is thought to involve a susceptible host and activation of pulmonary T cells, followed by the release of cytokine mediators of inflammation. The inflammatory response that ensues (usually several hours after exposure) produces laboured breathing, dry cough, chills and fever, headache, and malaise. The symptoms usually subside within hours after the sensitizing antigens are removed. A primary example of hypersensitivity pneumonitis is "farmer's lung," a condition resulting from inhaling dust and mouldy hay. Other sensitizing antigens include tree bark, sawdust, animal dander, and *Actinomycetes* bacteria that are occasionally found in humidifiers, hot tubs, and swimming pools. Exposure to small amounts of antigen for a long period may lead to chronic lung disease with minimal reversibility. This can happen to persons exposed to avian or animal antigens or a contaminated home air humidifier.

The most important element in the diagnosis of hypersensitivity pneumonitis is to obtain a good history (occupational and otherwise) of exposure to possible antigens. Treatment consists of identifying and avoiding the offending antigens. Severe forms of the disorder may be treated with systemic corticosteroid therapy.[42]

Latex Allergy

With the advent of HIV and other blood-borne diseases, the use of natural latex gloves has spiralled. Between 1988 and 1992, an estimated 11.8 billion examining gloves and 1.8 billion surgical gloves were used in the United States alone.[43] Along with the expanded use of latex gloves have come increased reports of latex allergy among healthcare workers. It has been estimated that 1% to 2% of the general population has some sensitivity or allergy to latex, and 8% to 12% of healthcare workers regularly exposed to latex develop sensitivity.[44,45] Other persons at high risk of sensitization are those with prolonged exposure to latex, including persons who have undergone repeated surgeries.

Exposure to latex may occur by cutaneous, mucous membrane, inhalation, internal tissue, or intravascular routes. Most severe reactions have resulted from latex proteins coming in contact with the mucous membranes of the mouth, vagina, urethra, or rectum. Although their allergen content is not very high, condoms can cause severe reactions because they come in contact with the mucous membranes.[44] Children with meningomyelocele (spina bifida) who undergo frequent examinations and treatments involving the mucosal surface of the bladder or rectum are at particular risk for development of latex allergy.[44] A large number of latex products are used in dentistry, and oral mucosal contact is common during dental procedures. Anaphylactic reactions have been caused by exposure of the internal organs to the surgeon's gloves during surgery.

Natural rubber latex, derived from the milky sap of the *Hevea brasiliensis* plant or rubber tree, is a milky mixture of proteins, phospholipids, and polyisoprene. Various accelerants, curing agents, antioxidants, and stabilizers are added to the liquid latex during the manufacturing process. Allergic reactions to latex products can be triggered by the latex proteins or by the additives used in the manufacturing process. Cornstarch powder is applied to the gloves during the manufacturing process to prevent stickiness and give the gloves a smooth feel. The cornstarch glove powder has an important role in the allergic response. Latex proteins are readily absorbed by glove powder and become airborne during removal of the gloves.[45] High-exposure areas such as operating rooms where powdered gloves are used contain sufficiently high levels of aerosolized latex to produce symptoms in sensitized persons.

The allergy to latex products can involve a type I, IgE-mediated hypersensitivity reaction or a type IV, T-cell–mediated response. Irritant dermatitis, which can result from glove use, is an entirely nonimmunologic response and should not be regarded as an allergy.[44,45] The distinction between type I and type IV reactions to latex products is not always clear. Affected individuals may experience both types of reactions. The most common type of reaction to latex gloves is contact dermatitis caused by a type IV, DTH response to the chemical additives used to process most gloves. It presents as a contact dermatitis that usually develops 48 to 96 hours after direct contact with latex additives. It often affects the dorsum of the hands and is characterized by a vesicular rash. When glove contact is continued, the area becomes crusted and thickened.

The type I, IgE-mediated hypersensitivity reactions occur in response to the latex proteins.[44] They may manifest as urticaria, rhinoconjunctivitis, asthma, or anaphylaxis. They are less common but far more serious than type IV responses. Persons with latex allergy commonly show cross-sensitivity to bananas, avocado, kiwi, and chestnuts, probably because latex proteins are similar to proteins in these products.[44] These foods have been responsible for anaphylactic reactions in latex-sensitive persons.

Diagnosis of latex allergy often is based on careful history and evidence of skin reactions due to latex exposure. Symptoms after use of a rubber condom or diaphragm should raise suspicion of latex allergy. Because many of the reported reactions to latex gloves have been the result of a nonimmunologic dermatitis, it is important to differentiate between nonallergic and allergic types of dermatitis. Latex skin-prick testing can be done, but it should be done in an allergy centre familiar with the test and with equipment available to treat possible anaphylactic reactions. Serum tests for latex-specific IgE antibodies also can be done. However, these tests may give false-positive or false-negative results. Thus, at this time, diagnosis usually is based on latex-specific symptoms of IgE-mediated reactions to latex exposure.[44]

Treatment of latex allergy consists of avoiding latex exposure. Use of powder-free gloves can reduce the amount of airborne latex particles. Healthcare workers with severe and life-threatening allergy may be forced to change employment. Patients at high risk for latex allergy (*e.g.*, children with spina bifida, healthcare workers with atopy) should be offered clinical testing for latex allergy before undergoing procedures that expose them to natural rubber latex. All surgical or other procedures on persons with latex allergy should be done in a latex-free environment in which no latex gloves are used in the room or surgical suite and no latex accessories (*e.g.*, catheters, adhesives, tourniquets, and anesthesia equipment) come in contact with the patient.[44] In healthcare settings, general use of latex gloves with negligible allergen content, powder-free latex gloves, and nonlatex gloves and medical articles should be considered to minimize latex exposure.[44]

IN SUMMARY

Hypersensitivity and allergic disorders are responses to environmental, food, or drug antigens that would not affect most of the population. There are four basic categories of hypersensitivity responses: (1) type I responses, which are mediated by the IgE-class immunoglobulins and include anaphylactic shock, hay fever, and bronchial asthma; (2) type II responses, which involve an antibody-mediated cell destruction (*e.g.*, transfusion reactions and hemolytic anemia), complement- and antibody-mediated inflammation (*e.g.*, some forms of glomerulonephritis), and antibody-mediated cell dysfunction (*e.g.*, Graves disease and myasthenia gravis); (3) type III hypersensitivity reactions, which involve the formation and deposition of insoluble antigen–antibody complexes, and are responsible for the vasculitis (seen in SLE or acute glomerulonephritis), systemic immune complex disease (serum sickness), and local immune complex disease (Arthus reaction); and (4) type IV cell-mediated hypersensitivity reactions, which include direct cell cytotoxicity, in which sensitized CD8+ T cells kill antigen-bearing target cells; and delayed-type hypersensitivity reactions, in which presensitized CD4+ T cells release cytokines that damage and kill antigen-containing cells.

Latex allergy can involve a type I, IgE-mediated reaction or a type IV, cell-mediated response. The most common type of allergic reaction to latex gloves is a contact dermatitis caused by a type IV, DTH reaction to rubber additives. The type I, IgE-mediated response to the latex protein is less common but can cause far more serious anaphylactic reactions.

TRANSPLANTATION IMMUNOPATHOLOGY

After completing this section of the chapter, you should be able to meet the following objectives:

- Discuss the rationale for matching of HLA or MHC types in organ transplantation.
- Compare the immune mechanisms involved in allogeneic transplant rejection.
- Describe the mechanisms and manifestations of GVHD.

Transplantation is the process of taking cells, tissues, or organs, called a *graft,* from one individual, and placing them into another individual (*i.e.*, allografts). Sometimes grafts are transplanted from another site in the same person (*i.e.*, autografts). The individual who provided the tissue is called the *donor,* and the individual who receives the graft is called either the *recipient* or the *host.* Transplantation rejection is discussed here because it involves several of the previously discussed immunologic reactions. A major barrier to transplantation is the process of rejection, in which the recipient's immune system recognizes the graft as foreign and attacks it.

The cell surface antigens that determine whether the tissue of transplanted organs is recognized as foreign are the MHC or *HLAs* (see Chapter 17). Transplanted tissue can be categorized as an *autologous* graft if donor and recipient are the same person, *syngeneic* graft if the donor and recipient are identical twins, and *allogeneic* (or allograft) if the donor and recipient are related or unrelated but share similar HLA types. The molecules that are recognized as foreign on allografts are called *alloantigens.* Donors of solid organ transplants can be living or dead (cadaver) and related or nonrelated (heterologous). The likelihood of rejection varies indirectly with the degree of MCH or HLA relatedness between donor and recipient.

Mechanisms Involved in Transplant Rejection

Rejection is a complex process that involves cell-mediated immunity and circulating antibodies. While T cells were thought to be of primary, perhaps exclusive, importance for transplant rejection and tolerance, it is now clear that many other cells, such as macrophages, natural killer cells, dendritic cells, and antibodies from B cells, impact the quality and quantity of the rejection process.[46–48] The critical role of T cells has been documented in both humans and experimental animals. T-cell–mediated graft rejection is called *cellular rejection* and is induced by two mechanisms: destruction of graft cells by CD8+ cytotoxic T cells and delayed hypersensitivity reactions triggered by CD4+ helper T cells.[8] The recipient's T cells recognize allogeneic antigens in the graft by two pathways: the direct and indirect pathways. It has been suggested that the direct pathway is the major pathway in acute rejection and the indirect pathway is more important in chronic rejection.[8]

In the *direct pathway,* T cells of the recipient recognize allogeneic MHC molecules on the surface of antigen-presenting cells on the graft. Both the CD4+ and CD8+ cells of the transplant recipient are involved in the reaction. CD8+ cells recognize class I MHC molecules and differentiate into mature CTLs. Once mature CTLs are generated, they kill the grafted tissue as they would any foreign substance. The CD4+ helper T-cell subset is triggered into proliferation and differentiation into T_H1, T_H2, and T_H17 effector cells by recognition of allogeneic class II MHC molecules. Multiple factors influence the T-cell differentiation, including the immune status of the recipient, the degree of ischemia-reperfusion injury, degree of donor/recipient mismatch, overall antigen load, and immunosuppression medications used to try to prevent any rejection.[46] As in delayed hypersensitivity reactions, cytokines secreted by activated CD4+ cells cause increased vascular permeability, local accumulation and activation of macrophages, and other immune responses, resulting in graft injury.

In the *indirect pathway,* recipient T lymphocytes recognize antigens of the graft donor after they have been presented by the recipient's own antigen-presenting cells. This process involves the uptake and processing of MHC molecules from the grafted organ by the host antigen-presenting cells. Thus, the indirect pathway is similar to the physiologic processing and presentation of other foreign (*i.e.,* microbial) antigens. It results in T cells that react with graft cells through cytokine production and delayed hypersensitivity responses.

Although there is little doubt that T cells are essential to the rejection process, antibodies evoked against alloantigens can also mediate rejection.[8] The process, which is called *humoral rejection,* can take one of two forms. *Hyperacute rejection* occurs when preformed antidonor antibodies are present in the circulation of the recipient. Such antibodies may be present if the recipient has already rejected a kidney transplant or received blood products with nonidentical HLA antigens. When preformed antidonor antibodies are present, rejection occurs immediately, within minutes to hours, after transplantation. The second form of antigen–antibody rejection occurs in recipients who were not previously sensitized, but who develop antibodies to graft alloantigens. The antibodies formed by the recipient may cause injury by several mechanisms, including complement-dependent cytotoxicity, inflammation, and antibody-dependent cell-mediated cytotoxicity. The initial target of these antibodies in rejection appears to be the graft vasculature.

Patterns of Rejection

The basic patterns of transplant rejection have historically been classified as hyperacute, acute, and chronic, based on the clinical tempo of the response and the pathologic mechanisms involved.[1,8,11] In actual practice, however, there is often an overlap in features. The diagnosis is further complicated by the effects of immunosuppressant drugs or recurrence of the original disease. The following section characterizes the rejection patterns in the context of renal transplantation. Similar responses occur with other types of organ transplants.

A *hyperacute reaction* occurs almost immediately after transplantation. In kidney transplants, it can often be seen at the time of surgery. As soon as blood flow from the recipient to the donor kidney begins, it takes on a cyanotic, mottled appearance. At other times, the reaction may take hours or days to develop. The hyperacute response is produced by existing recipient antibodies to graft antigens that initiate a type III, Arthus-type hypersensitivity reaction in the blood vessels of the graft. This can quickly lead to massive thrombosis in capillaries, preventing essential vascularization of transplanted tissue. These antibodies usually have developed in response to previous blood transfusions, pregnancies in which the mother makes antibodies to fetal antigens, or infections with bacteria or viruses possessing antigens that mimic MHC antigens.[48]

Acute rejection usually occurs within the first few months after transplantation and is evidenced by signs of organ failure. It also may occur suddenly months or even years later, after immunosuppression has been used and terminated. T lymphocytes play a central role in acute rejection, responding to antigens in the graft tissue. Also, donor dendritic cells (sometime called passenger leukocytes) can enter the circulation and present antigens to the host's immune system, further recruiting inflammation cytokines and leukocytes. Any activated T cells cause direct lysis of graft cells and recruit and activate inflammatory cells that injure the graft. In vascularized grafts such as kidney grafts, the endothelial cells of blood vessels are the earliest targets of acute rejection.

Chronic rejection occurs over a prolonged period due to both cell- and antibody-mediated reactions. It manifests with dense intimal fibrosis that can lead to scarring of blood vessels of the transplanted organ. In renal transplantation, it is characterized by a gradual rise in serum creatinine over a period of 4 to 6 months. The actual mechanism of this type of response is unclear but may include release of cytokines that stimulate fibrosis.

Graft-Versus-Host Disease

Graft-versus-host disease (GVHD) occurs when immunologically competent cells or precursors are transplanted into recipients who are immunologically compromised. Although GVHD occurs most often in persons who have undergone allogeneic bone marrow transplantation, it may also follow transplantation of organs rich in lymphoid tissue (*e.g.,* the liver) or follow sions with nonirradiated blood.[8,49]

Three basic requirements are necessary for GVHD to develop: (1) the transplant must have a functional cellular immune component; (2) the recipient tissue must bear antigens foreign to the donor tissue; and (3) recipient immunity must be compromised to the point that it cannot destroy the transplanted cells.[1,49] The primary agents of GVHD are the donor immunocompetent T cells derived from the donor marrow and the recipient tissue that they recognize as foreign and react against.[8] GVHD results in activation of both CD4+ and CD8+ T cells with ultimate generation of type IV DTH and CTL responses. The greater the difference in tissue antigens between the donor and recipient, the greater is the likelihood of GVHD.

GVHD can occur as an acute or chronic reaction. Acute GVHD, which develops within 100 days after transplantation, involves the epithelial cells of the skin, liver, and gastrointestinal tract.[8] The organ most commonly affected in acute GVHD is the skin. There is development of a pruritic, maculopapular rash, which begins on the palms and soles and frequently extends over the entire body, with subsequent desquamation. Involvement of the gastrointestinal tract usually parallels the development of skin and liver involvement.[50] Gastrointestinal symptoms include nausea, bloody diarrhea, and abdominal pain. GVHD of the liver is heralded by painless jaundice, hyperbilirubinemia, and abnormal liver function test results. Liver involvement can progress to development of veno-occlusive disease, drug toxicity, viral infection, iron overload, extrahepatic biliary obstruction, sepsis, and coma. *Veno-occlusive disease* is characterized by obliteration of the small hepatic veins and venules.[50] In acute veno-occlusive disease there is striking centrilobular congestion and hepatocellular necrosis. As the disease progresses, connective tissue is deposited in the lumen of venules and the centrilobular congestion becomes less evident.

GVHD is considered chronic if symptoms persist or begin 100 days or more after transplantation.[8,49] Chronic GVHD may follow acute GVHD or it may develop insidiously. Since persons in whom chronic GVHD develops are profoundly immunocompromised, they develop skin lesions resembling systemic sclerosis (discussed in Chapter 59) and manifestations mimicking other autoimmune diseases.

A second type of GVHD can follow the transplantation of genetically identical tissue (*i.e.,* syngeneic or autologous). This type of GVHD stems from the use of pretreatment conditioning regimens (*e.g.,* total-body irradiation or treatment with cytotoxic drugs). The conditioning therapy disrupts the normal immune surveillance system and allows "rogue" autoreactive T cells to proliferate and attack native tissue. This type of GVHD usually is self-limited and not severe.

GVHD can be prevented by blocking any of the three steps of pathogenesis. For example, donor T cells can be selectively removed from the transplanted tissue or destroyed using various treatments such as monoclonal antibodies with attached toxins, equivalent to heat-seeking missiles. Alternatively, immunosuppressive or anti-inflammatory drugs such as cyclosporine and tacrolimus or glucocorticoids can be used to block T-cell, B-cell, or NK cell proliferation and the action of cytokines (*e.g.,* TNF-α inhibitors, sirolimus).

IN SUMMARY

Transplantation is the process of taking cells, tissues, or organs, called a graft, from one individual (a donor), and placing them into another individual (recipient). A major barrier to transplantation is the process of rejection in which the recipient's immune system recognizes the graft as foreign and attacks it. Destruction of the cells or tissues of the graft can result from direct action of the recipient's cytotoxic T cells; from T-cell–generated cytokines and a delayed hypersensitivity reaction; or from antibodies generated against antigens in the graft. Hyperacute rejection occurs almost immediately after transplantation and is caused by existing recipient antibodies to graft antigens that initiate a type III, Arthus-type hypersensitivity reaction in the blood vessels of the graft. Acute rejection occurs within the first few months after transplantation and occurs when cytotoxic T cells cause direct lysis of graft cells and recruit and activate inflammatory cells that injure the graft. Chronic rejection occurs over a prolonged period and is caused by T-cell–generated cytokines that stimulate fibrosis of graft tissue.

GVHD occurs when immunologically competent cells or precursors are transplanted into recipients who are immunologically compromised. Three basic requirements are necessary for GVHD to develop: (1) the transplant must have a functional cellular immune component; (2) the recipient tissue must bear antigens foreign to the donor tissue; and (3) recipient immunity must be compromised to the point that it cannot destroy the transplanted cells.

AUTOIMMUNE DISEASE

After completing this section of the chapter, you should be able to meet the following objectives:

* Relate the mechanisms of self-tolerance to the possible explanations for development of autoimmune disease.
* Name four or more diseases attributed to autoimmunity.
* Describe three or more postulated mechanisms underlying autoimmune disease.
* State the criteria for establishing an autoimmune basis for a disease.

Autoimmune diseases represent a group of disorders that are caused by a breakdown in the ability of the immune system to differentiate between self- and nonself-antigens. Autoimmune diseases can affect almost any cell or tissue in the body. Some autoimmune disorders, such as Hashimoto thyroiditis, are tissue specific; others, such as SLE, affect multiple organs and systems. Chart 19.3 lists some of the probable autoimmune diseases. Many of these disorders are discussed elsewhere in this book.

Immunologic Tolerance

To function properly, the immune system must be able to differentiate foreign antigens from self-antigens. The ability of the immune system to differentiate self from nonself is called *self-tolerance*. It is the HLA antigens encoded by MHC genes that serve as recognition markers of self and nonself for the immune system (see Chapter 17). To elicit an immune response, an antigen must first be processed by an APC, such as a macrophage, which then presents the antigenic determinants along with an MHC II molecule to a CD4+ helper T cell. The dual recognition of the MHC–antigen complex by the TCR of the CD4+ helper T cell acts like a security check. Similar recognition checks occur between CD8+ cytotoxic T cells and the MHC I–antigen complex of tissue cells that have been targeted for elimination. A number of chemical messengers (*e.g.,* ILs) and costimulatory signals are essential to the activation of immune responses and the preservation of self-tolerance.

Several mechanisms have been postulated to explain the tolerant state, including central tolerance and peripheral tolerance.[8,51–53] *Central tolerance* refers to the elimination of

DISEASE[a]

Systemic
Mixed connective tissue disease
Polymyositis-dermatomyositis
Rheumatoid arthritis
Scleroderma
Sjögren syndrome
Systemic lupus erythematosus

Blood
Autoimmune hemolytic anemia
Autoimmune neutropenia and lymphopenia
Idiopathic thrombocytopenic purpura

Other Organs
Acute idiopathic polyneuritis
Atrophic gastritis and pernicious anemia
Autoimmune adrenalitis
Goodpasture syndrome
Hashimoto thyroiditis
Type 1 diabetes mellitus
Myasthenia gravis
Premature gonadal (ovarian) failure
Primary biliary cirrhosis
Sympathetic ophthalmia
Temporal arteritis
Thyrotoxicosis (Graves disease)
Crohn disease, ulcerative colitis

[a]Examples are not inclusive.

IMMUNOLOGIC TOLERANCE

- Immunologic tolerance is the ability of the immune system to differentiate self from nonself. It results from central and peripheral mechanisms that delete self-reactive immune cells that cause autoimmunity or render their response ineffective in destroying self-cells and self-tissue.
- Central tolerance involves the elimination of self-reactive T and B cells in the central lymphoid organs. Self-reactive T cells are deleted in the thymus and self-reactive B cells in the bone marrow.
- Peripheral tolerance derives from the deletion or inactivation of self-reactive T and B cells that escaped deletion in the central lymphoid organs. It involves mechanisms such as receptor editing, absence of necessary costimulatory signals, production of immunologic ignorance by separating self-reactive immune cells from target tissues, and the presence of suppressor immune cells.

self-reactive T cells and B cells in the central lymphoid organs (*i.e.,* the thymus for T cells and the bone marrow for B cells). *Peripheral tolerance* derives from the deletion or inactivation of autoreactive T cells or B cells that escaped elimination in the central lymphoid organs. *Anergy* represents the state of hyporesponsiveness or unresponsiveness to specific antigens. It may take the form of diminished immediate hypersensitivity or DTH, or both.

B-Cell Tolerance

Loss of self-tolerance with development of autoantibodies is characteristic of a number of autoimmune disorders. For example, hyperthyroidism in Graves disease is due to autoantibodies to the TSH receptor (see Fig. 19.4 and Chapter 41). Several mechanisms are available to filter autoreactive B cells out of the B-cell population: clonal deletion of immature B cells in the bone marrow; deletion of autoreactive B cells in the spleen or lymph nodes; functional inactivation or anergy; and receptor editing, a process that changes the specificity of a B-cell receptor when autoantigen is encountered. There is evidence that the B-cell peripheral tolerance requires help from T cells.[52]

T-Cell Tolerance

The central mechanisms of T-cell tolerance involve the deletion of self-reactive T cells in the thymus (Fig. 19.7). T cells develop from bone marrow–derived progenitor cells that migrate to the thymus, where they encounter self-peptides bound to MHC molecules. T cells that display the host's MHC antigens and TCRs for a nonself-antigen are allowed to mature in the thymus (*i.e.,* positive selection). T cells that have a high affinity for host cells are sorted out and undergo apoptosis or cell death (*i.e.,* negative selection). The deletion of self-reactive T cells in the thymus requires the presence of autoantigens. Because many autoantigens are not present in the thymus, self-reactive T cells may escape the thymus, so peripheral mechanisms that participate in T-cell tolerance are required.

Several peripheral mechanisms are available to control the responsiveness of self-reactive T cells in the periphery. Sometimes the host antigens are not available in the appropriate immunologic form or are separated from the T cells (*e.g.,* by the blood–brain barrier) so that corresponding T cells remain immunologically ignorant of their presence.[8] In other cases, the autoreactive T cell encounters its corresponding antigen in the absence of the costimulatory signals that are necessary for its activation. The peripheral activation of T cells requires two signals: recognition of the peptide antigen in association with the MHC molecules on the APCs and a set of secondary costimulatory signals. Because costimulatory signals are not strongly expressed on most normal tissues, the encounter of the autoreactive T cells and their specific target antigens frequently results in anergy.[8]

Another mechanism involves the apoptotic death of autoreactive T cells.[51–53] This type of apoptosis is mediated by an apoptotic cell surface receptor (called FAS) that is present on the T cell and a soluble membrane messenger molecule (FAS ligand) that binds to the apoptotic receptor and activates the death

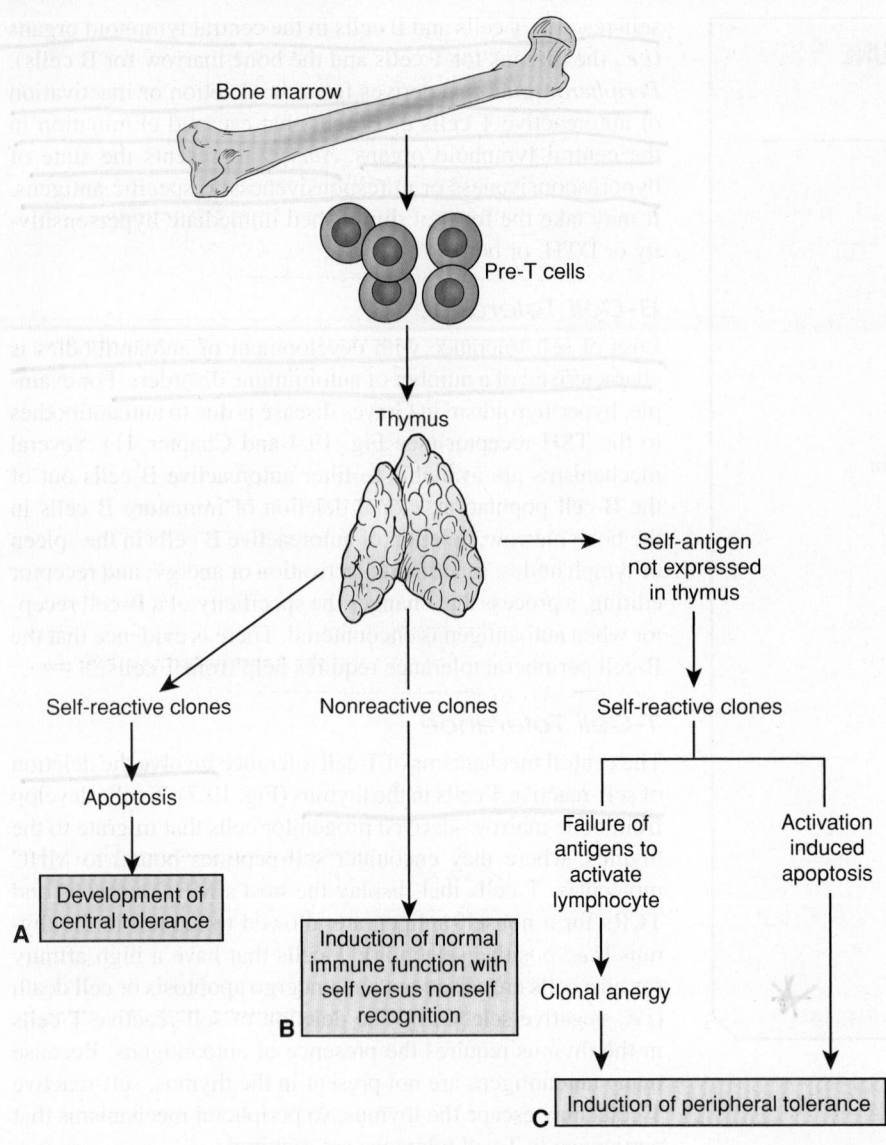

Bone marrow

Pre-T cells

Thymus

Self-antigen
not expressed
in thymus

Self-reactive clones   Nonreactive clones   Self-reactive clones

Apoptosis

A Development of
central tolerance

Induction of normal
immune function
with self versus nonself
recognition
B

Failure of
antigens to
activate
lymphocyte

Activation
induced
apoptosis

Clonal anergy

C Induction of peripheral tolerance

FIGURE 19.7 • Development of immunologic tolerance. **A:** Development of central tolerance with deletion of self-reactive T lymphocytes in the thymus. **B:** Nonreactive lymphocytes with development of normal immune function. **C:** Induction of peripheral tolerance in self-reactive cells that are not eliminated in the thymus.

program (see Chapter 5). The expression of the apoptotic FAS receptor is markedly increased in activated T cells; thus, coexpression of the FAS messenger molecule by the same cohort of activated autoreactive T cells may serve to induce their death.

Regulatory T cells (T_{reg}, previously called suppressor T cells) with the ability to down-regulate the function of autoreactive T cells are also thought to play an essential role in peripheral T-cell tolerance. These cells are believed to be a distinct subset of CD4$^+$ and CD8$^+$ T cells. The mechanism by which these T cells exert their suppressor function is unclear. They may secrete cytokines that suppress the activity of self-reactive immune cells, or they may delete the self-reactive T-cell clones.

Mechanisms of Autoimmune Disease

It is obvious that autoimmunity results from loss of self-tolerance. Just how this happens is largely unknown, but both inheritance of susceptibility genes that contribute to the

maintenance of self-tolerance and environmental factors, such as infections that promote the activation of self-reactive lymphocytes, are clearly important. Gender may also play a role in the development of autoimmune disorders. A number of autoimmune disorders such as SLE occur more commonly in women than men, suggesting that estrogens may play a role in the development of autoimmune disease. Estrogen has been shown to have strong immunomodulatory effects, including the stimulation of autoreactive B cells antibody production, increased leukocyte adhesion to endothelial cells, and increased cytokine production.[54] For example, estrogen stimulates a DNA sequence that promotes the production of interferon-γ, which is thought to assist in the induction of an autoimmune response. Because of the complexity of the immune system, it seems unlikely that autoimmune disorders arise from a single defect.

Heredity

Genetic factors can increase the incidence and severity of autoimmune diseases, as shown by the familial clustering of several autoimmune diseases and the observation that certain inherited HLA types occur more frequently in persons with a variety of immunologic and lymphoproliferative disorders.[8,52] For example, 90% of persons with ankylosing spondylitis carry the HLA-B27 antigen, compared with 10% of persons without the disease.[8] Other HLA-associated diseases are Reiter syndrome and HLA-B27, rheumatoid arthritis and HLA-DR4, and SLE and HLA-DR3 (see Chapter 59). The molecular basis for these associations is unknown. Persons with autoimmune disorders exhibit susceptibility genes that act in conjunction with environmental factors to increase a person's risk of developing the disease process.[52] Because autoimmunity does not develop in all persons with genetic predisposition, it appears that other factors such as a "trigger event" interact to precipitate the altered immune state. The event or events that trigger the development of an autoimmune response are unknown. It has been suggested that the "trigger" may be a virus or other microorganism, a chemical substance, or a self-antigen from a body tissue that has been hidden from the immune system during development.

Environmental Factors

Although environmental factors, such as infectious agents, appear to be involved in the pathogenesis of autoimmune disorders, their precise role in initiating or perpetuating the autoreactive response is largely unknown. Among the proposed mechanisms involved in loss of self-tolerance are breakdown of T-cell anergy, release of sequestered antigens, molecular mimicry, and superantigens.[52]

Breakdown in T-Cell Anergy. *Anergy* is a state of unresponsiveness to antigen. It involves the prolonged or irreversible inactivation of lymphocytes, such as that induced by an encounter with self-antigens. Activation of antigen-specific CD4[+] T cells requires two signals: (1) recognition of the antigen in association with class II MHC molecules on the surface of an antigen-presenting cells, and (2) a set of costimulatory signals provided by the antigen-presenting cells. If the second costimulatory signal is not delivered, the T cell becomes anergic. Most normal tissues do not express the costimulatory molecules and thus are protected from autoreactive T cells. However, this protection can be broken if the normal cells that do not normally express the costimulatory molecules are induced to do so. Some inductions can occur after an infection or in situations where there is tissue necrosis and local inflammation.

Release of Sequestered Antigens. Normally the body does not produce antibodies against self-antigens. Thus, any self-antigen that was completely sequestered during development and then reintroduced to the immune system is likely to be regarded as foreign. Among the sequestered tissues that could be regarded as foreign are spermatozoa and ocular antigens such as those found in uveal tissue. Posttraumatic uveitis and orchiditis after vasectomy may fall into this category.

Changes in antigen structure or release of hidden antigens may also account for the persistence of autoimmune

disorders. Once an autoimmune disorder has been induced, it tends to be progressive, sometimes with sporadic relapses and remissions. A possible mechanism for the persistence and evolution of autoimmunity is the phenomenon of epitope reading.[2] Infections, and even the initial autoimmune episode, may release and damage self-antigens and expose epitopes of the antigen that have been hidden from the immune system. The result is continued activation of new lymphocytes that recognize the previously hidden epitopes.

Molecular Mimicry. Many autoimmune diseases are associated with infections, and clinical flare-ups are often preceded by infectious processes. One proposed link between infections and autoimmunity is *molecular mimicry,* in which a microbe shares an immunologic epitope with the host. In rheumatic fever and acute glomerulonephritis, for example, a protein in the cell wall of group A, beta-hemolytic streptococci have considerable similarity with antigens in heart and kidney tissue, respectively. After infection, antibodies directed against the microorganism cause a classic case of mistaken identity, which leads to inflammation of the heart or kidney. Not everyone exposed to group A, beta-hemolytic streptococci has an autoimmune reaction. The reason that only certain persons are targeted for autoimmune reactions to a particular self-mimicry molecule may be determined by differences in HLA types. The HLA type determines exactly which fragments of a pathogen are displayed on the cell surface for presentation to T cells. One individual's HLA may bind self-mimicry molecules for presentation to T cells, and another's HLA type may not. In the spondyloarthropathies, particularly Reiter syndrome and reactive arthritis, there is a clear relationship between arthritis and a prior bacterial infection, combined with the inherited HLA-B27 antigens.[55,56]

Superantigens. Superantigens are a family of related substances, including staphylococcal and streptococcal exotoxins, that can short-circuit the normal sequence of events in an immune response, leading to inappropriate activation of CD4[+] helper T cells.[56] Superantigens do not require processing and presentation of antigen by antigen-presenting cells to induce a T-cell response. Instead, they are able to interact with a TCR outside the normal antigen-binding site. This distinctive mode of activation, together with the ability of superantigens to bind to a wide variety of MHC class II molecules, leads to activation of large numbers of T cells regardless of their MHC/peptide specificity. Superantigens are involved in several diseases, including food poisoning and toxic shock syndrome.[56]

Diagnosis and Treatment of Autoimmune Disease

The diagnosis of autoimmune disorders is not always easy. There are over 80 identified autoimmune disorders and many have overlapping clinical presentations. In addition, many of the manifestations are nonspecific and are frequently seen in other disease processes. Suggested criteria for determining that a disorder is an autoimmune disorder are evidence of an autoimmune reaction, determination that the immunologic findings are not secondary to another condition, and the lack of other identified causes for the disorder. Currently, the diagnosis of autoimmune disease is based primarily on history, clinical findings, and serologic testing. In the future, it is unlikely that autoimmune disorders will be diagnosed by directly identifying the genes responsible for the condition because of the multifactorial etiology.

The basis for most serologic assays is the demonstration of antibodies directed against tissue antigens or cellular components. For example, a child with chronic or acute history of fever, arthritis, and a macular rash along with high levels of antinuclear antibody has a probable diagnosis of SLE. The detection of autoantibodies in the laboratory usually is accomplished by one of three methods: indirect fluorescent antibody assays (IFA), enzyme-linked immunosorbent assay (ELISA), or particle agglutination of some kind. The rationale behind each of these methods is similar: the patient's serum is diluted and allowed to react with an antigen-coated surface (*i.e.,* whole, fixed cells for the detection of antinuclear antibodies). In the case of IFA and ELISA, a second "labelled" antibody is added, which binds to the patient's antibody and forms a visible reaction. Particle agglutination assays are much simpler—the binding of the patient's antibody to antigen-coated particles causes a visible agglutination reaction. For most serologic assays, the patient's serum is serially diluted until it no longer produces a visible reaction (*e.g.,* 1:100 dilution). This is called a *positive titre*. Healthy persons sometimes have low titres of antibody against cellular and tissue antigens, but their titres usually are far lower than in patients with autoimmune disease.

Treatment of autoimmune disease is based on the tissue or organ that is involved, the effector mechanism involved, and the magnitude and chronicity of the effector processes. Ideally, treatment should focus on the mechanism underlying the autoimmune disorder. Corticosteroids and immunosuppressive drugs may be used to arrest or reverse the downhill course of some autoimmune disorders. Purging autoreactive cells from the immune repertoire, through the use of plasmapheresis, is also an option in some severe cases of autoimmunity.

Recent research has focused on the cytokines involved in the inflammatory response that accompanies many of the autoimmune disorders. Notably, interferon beta for multiple sclerosis and tumour necrosis factor-α antibodies (*e.g.,* infliximab) for rheumatoid arthritis and Crohn disease are the first new treatments for autoimmunity in the past 20 years.[57] Other targeted monoclonal antibody therapies include rituximab (targets CD20 to deplete autoreactive B cells), tocilizumab (blocks T-cell differentiation or activation), belimumab (blocks B-cell growth factors), plus many others.[57,58] Finally, research into the development of vaccines that target critical pathways in the emergence of autoimmune responses is ongoing.

IN SUMMARY

Autoimmune diseases represent a disruption in self-tolerance that results in damage to body tissues by the immune system. Autoimmune diseases can affect almost any cell or tissue of the body. The ability of the immune system to differentiate self from nonself is called self-tolerance. Normally, self-tolerance is maintained through central and peripheral mechanisms that delete autoreactive B or T cells or otherwise suppress or inactivate immune responses that would be destructive to host tissues. Defects in any of these mechanisms could impair self-tolerance and predispose to development of autoimmune disease.

The ability of the immune system to differentiate foreign from self-antigens is the responsibility of HLA encoded by MHC genes. Antigen is presented to receptors of T cells in combination with MHC molecules. Among the possible mechanisms responsible for development of autoimmune disease are failure of T-cell–mediated immune suppression; aberrations in MHC–antigen–TCR interactions; molecular mimicry; and superantigens. The suggested criteria for determining that a disorder results from an autoimmune disorder are evidence of an autoimmune reaction, determination that the immunologic findings are not secondary to another condition, and the lack of other identifiable causes for the disorder.

REVIEW EXERCISES

1. A 20-year-old woman has been diagnosed with IgA deficiency. She has been plagued with frequent bouts of bronchitis and sinus infections.
   A. *Why are these types of infections particularly prominent in persons with an IgA deficiency?*
   B. *She has been told that she needs to be aware that she could have a severe reaction when given unwashed blood transfusions. Explain.*
2. Persons with impaired cellular immunity may not respond to the tuberculin test, even when infected with *M. tuberculosis*.
   A. *Explain.*
3. A 32-year-old man presents in the allergy clinic with complaints of allergic rhinitis or hay fever. His major complaints are those of nasal pruritus (itching), nasal congestion with profuse watery drainage, sneezing, and eye irritation. The physical examination reveals edematous and inflamed nasal mucosa and redness of the ocular conjunctiva. He relates that this happens every fall during "ragweed season."
   A. *Explain the immunologic mechanisms that are responsible for this man's symptoms.*
   B. *What type of diagnostic test might be used?*

> *C. What type of treatment(s) might be used to relieve his symptoms?*
> 4. Persons with intestinal parasites and those with allergies may both have elevated levels of eosinophils in their blood.
>   *A. Explain.*

References

1. Abbas A. K., Lichtman A. H., Pillai S. (2015). *Cellular and molecular immunology* (8th ed.). Philadelphia, PA: Elsevier Saunders.
2. Verbsky J. W., Grossman W. J. (2006). Cellular and genetic basis of primary immune deficiencies. *Pediatric Clinics of North America, 53,* 649–684.
3. Immunodeficiency Canada. (2015). Primary immunodeficiency. Available online at: http://immunodeficiency.ca/primary-immunodeficiency/primary-immunodeficiency-pi/. Accessed June 11, 2015.
4. Subbarayan A., Colarusso G., Hughes S. M., et al. (2011). Clinical features that identify children with primary immunodeficiency diseases. *Pediatrics, 127*(5), 810–816.
5. Younger E. M., Epland K., Zampelli A., Hintermeyer M. K. (2015). Primary immunodeficiency diseases: A primer of PCPs. *Nurse Practitioner, 40*(2), 1–7.
6. Buckley R. H., Newburger P. E., Boxer L. A., et al. (2011). Part 14: Immunology (Chapters 116–133). In Kliegman R. M., Stanton B. F., St. Geme J. W., et al. (Eds.), *Nelson textbook of pediatrics* (19th ed.). Philadelphia, PA: Saunders Elsevier.
7. The Jeffrey Modell Foundation Medical Advisory Board. (2013). Ten warning signs. Available online at: http://www.info4pi.org/library/educational-materials/10-warning-signs. Accessed June 15, 2015.
8. Kumar V., Abbas A. K., Fausto N. (2010). Chapter 6: Diseases of the immune system. In Kumar V., Abbas A. K., Fausto N., et al. (Eds.), *Robbins and Cotran pathologic basis of disease* (8th ed.). Philadelphia, PA: Elsevier Saunders.
9. Durandy A., Kracher S., Fischer A. (2013). Primary antibody deficiencies. *Nature Reviews Immunology, 13*(7), 519–533.
10. Salzer U., Warnatz K., Peter H. H. (2012). Common variable immunodeficiency: An update. *Arthritis Research & Therapy, 14*(5), 223.
11. Warren J. S., Bennett D. P. (2012). Chapter 4: Immunopathology. In Rubin R., Strayer D. S. (Eds.), *Rubin's pathology: Clinicopathologic foundations of medicine* (6th ed.). Philadelphia, PA: Lippincott Williams & Wilkins.
12. Kaushansky K., Beulter E., Seligsohn U., et al. (Eds.). (2010). *Williams hematology* (8th ed.). New York: McGraw-Hill Companies, Inc.
13. Fomin A. B., Pastorino A. C., Kim C. A., et al. (2010). DiGeorge syndrome: A not so rare disease. *Clinics (Sao Paulo), 65*(9), 865–869.
14. Qamer N., Fuleihan R. L. (2014). The hyper IgM syndromes. *Clinical Reviews in Allergy and Immunology, 46*(2), 120–130.
15. Roifman C. M., Somech R., Kavadas F., et al. (2012). Defining combined immunodeficiency. *Journal of Allergy and Clinical Immunology, 130*(1), 177–183.
16. Perreault S., Bernard G., Lortie A., et al. (2012). Ataxia-telangiectasia presenting with a novel immunodeficiency. *Pediatric Neurology, 46*(5), 322–324.
17. Ochs H. D., Thrasher A. J. (2006). The Wiskott-Aldrich syndrome. *Journal of Allergy and Clinical Immunology, 117,* 725–738.
18. Botto M., Kirschfink M., Macor P., et al. (2009). Complement in human diseases: Lessons from complement deficiencies. *Molecular Immunology, 46*(14), 2774–2783.
19. Frank M. M. (2010). Complement disorders and hereditary angioedema. *Journal of Allergy and Clinical Immunology, 125*(Suppl 2), S262–S271.
20. Caccia S., Suffritti C., Cicardi M. (2014). Pathophysiology of hereditary angioedema. *Pediatric Allergy, Immunology, and Pulmonology, 27*(4), 159–163.
21. Cicardi M., Aberer W., Banerji A., et al; HAWK under the patronage of EAACI (European Academy of Allergy and Clinical Immunology). (2014). Classification, diagnosis, and approach to treatment for angioedema: Consensus report from the hereditary angioedema international working group. *Allergy, 69*(5), 602–616.
22. Rosenzweig S. D., Holland S. M. (2004). Phagocyte immunodeficiencies and their infections. *Journal of Allergy and Clinical Immunology, 113,* 620–626.
23. Holland S. M. (2013). Chronic granulomatous disease. *Hematology/Oncology Clinics of North America, 27*(1), 89–99.
24. Ghaffari J., Rezaee S. A., Gharagozlou M. (2013). Chediak-Higashi syndrome. *Journal of Pediatrics Review, 1*(2), 80–87.
25. Horwitz M. E. (2000). Stem-cell transplantation for inherited immunodeficiency disorders. *Pediatric Clinics of North America, 47,* 1371–1384.
26. Immune Deficiency Foundation. (2013). Stem cell and gene therapy. Available online at: http://primaryimmune.org/treatment-information/stem-cell-and-gene-therapy/. Accessed June 15, 2015.
27. Barnes P. J. (2011). Pathophysiology of allergic inflammation. *Immunological Reviews, 242*(1), 31–50.
28. Lieberman P. (2006). Anaphylaxis. *Medical Clinics of North America, 90,* 77–95.
29. Simons F. E., Ardusso L. R., Dimov V., et al; World Allergy Organization. (2013). World allergy organization anaphylaxis guidelines: 2013 update of the evidence base. *International Archives of Allergy and Immunology, 162*(3), 193–204.
30. Simons F. E. (2011). Anaphylaxis pathogenesis and treatment. *Allergy, 66*(Suppl 95), 31–34.
31. Rondon C., Canto G., Blanca M. (2010). Local allergic rhinitis: A new entity, characterization and further studies. *Current Opinion in Allergy and Clinical Immunology, 10*(1), 1–7.
32. Greiner A. N., Hellings P. W., Rotiroti G., Scadding G. K. (2011). Allergic rhinitis. *Lancet, 378*(9809), 2112–2122.
33. Quillen D. M., Feller D. B. (2006). Diagnosis of rhinitis: Allergic vs. nonallergic. *American Family Physician, 73,* 1583–1590.
34. Kim H., Waserman S., Hebert J., et al. (2014). Efficacy and safety of ragweed sublingual immunotherapy in Canadian patients with allergic rhinoconjunctivitis. *Allergy, Asthma & Clinical Immunology, 10,* 55.
35. Sampson H. A. (2004). Update on food allergy. *Journal of Allergy and Clinical Immunology, 113,* 805–819.
36. Ho M., Wong W., Chang C. (2014). Clinical spectrum of food allergies: A comprehensive review. *Clinical Reviews in Allergy & Immunology, 46*(3), 225–240.
37. Pichler W. J., Adam J., Daubner B., et al. (2010). Drug hypersensitivity reactions: Pathomechanism and clinical symptoms. *Medical Clinics of North America, 94*(4), 645–664.
38. Kanji S., Chant C. (2010). Allergic and hypersensitivity reactions in the intensive care unit. *Critical Care Medicine, 38*(Suppl 6), S162–S168.
39. Male D., Brostoff J., Roth D. B., et al. (2013). *Immunology* (8th ed.). Philadelphia, PA: Elsevier Saunders.
40. Mark B. J., Slavin R. G. (2006). Allergic contact dermatitis. *Medical Clinics of North America, 90,* 169–185.
41. Becker D. (2013). Allergic contact dermatitis. *Journal of the German Society of Dermatology, 11*(7), 607–621.
42. Selman M., Pardo A., King T. E. (2012). Hypersensitivity pneumonitis: Insights in diagnosis and pathobiology. *American Journal of Respiratory and Critical Care Medicine, 186*(4), 314–324.
43. Sussman G. L. (1995). Allergy to latex rubber. *Annals of Internal Medicine, 122,* 43–46.
44. Pollart S. M., Warniment C., Mori T. (2009). Latex allergy. *American Family Physician, 80*(12), 1413–1418.
45. Canadian Centre for Occupational Health and Safety. (2015). Latex allergy. Available online at: http://www.ccohs.ca/oshanswers/diseases/latex.html. Accessed June 15, 2015.
46. Wood K. J., Goto R. (2012). Mechanisms of rejection: Current perspectives. *Transplantation, 93*(1), 1–10.
47. Murphy S. P., Porrett P. M., Turka L. A. (2011). Innate immunity in transplant tolerance and rejection. *Immunological Reviews, 241,* 39–48.

48. Montgomery R. A., Cozzi E., West L. J., Warren D. S. (2011). Humoral immunity and antibody-mediated rejection in sold organ transplantation. *Seminar in Immunology, 23,* 224–234.

49. Blazar B. R., Murphy W. J., Abedi M. (2012). Advances in graft-versus-host disease biology and therapy. *Nature Reviews Immunology, 12*(6), 443–458.

50. Gignan F., Clark A., Amrolia P., et al; Haemato-oncology Task Force of British Committee for Standards in Haematology; British Society for Blood and Marrow Transplantation. (2012). Diagnosis and management of acute graft-versus-host disease. *British Journal of Haematology, 158*(1), 30–45.

51. Sakaguchi S., Powrie F., Ransohoff R. M. (2012). Re-establishing immunological self-tolerance in autoimmune disease. *Nature Medicine, 18*(1), 54–58.

52. Wahren-Herlenius M., Dorner T. (2013). Immunopathogenic mechanisms of systemic autoimmune disease. *Lancet, 382*(9894), 819–831.

53. Medzhitov R., Schneider D. S., Soares M. P. (2012). Disease tolerance as a defense strategy. *Science, 335*(6071), 936–941.

54. Ryan M. J. (2009). The pathophysiology of hypertension in systemic lupus erythematosus. *American Journal of Physiology. Regulatory, Integrative and Comparative Physiology, 296*(4), R1258–R1267.

55. Cusick M. F., Libbey J. E., Fujinami R. S. (2012). Molecular mimicry as a mechanism of autoimmune disease. *Clinical Reviews in Allergy & Immunology, 42*(1), 102–111.

56. Sfriso P., Ghirardello A., Botsios C., et al. (2010). Infections and autoimmunity: The multifaceted relationship. *Journal of Leukocyte Biology, 87*(3), 385–395.

57. Repchinsky C. (Ed.). (2011). *e-Therapeutics.* [Online] Ottawa, ON: Canadian Pharmacists Association.

58. Bruno V., Battaglia G., Nicoletti F. (2011). The advent of monoclonal antibodies in the treatment of chronic autoimmune diseases. *Neurological Sciences, 31*(Suppl 3), S283–S288.

Visit thePoint **http://thePoint.lww.com for animations, journal articles, and more!**

Acquired Immunodeficiency Syndrome

The acquired immunodeficiency syndrome (AIDS) is a disease caused by infection with the human immunodeficiency virus (HIV) and is characterized by profound immunosuppression with associated opportunistic infections, malignancies, wasting, and central nervous system (CNS) degeneration. Because the disease affects an exceptionally high proportion of the population throughout the world, it is often referred to as a *pandemic*.[1]

20

THE AIDS EPIDEMIC AND TRANSMISSION OF HIV INFECTION

After completing this section of the chapter, you should be able to meet the following objectives:

- Briefly trace the history of the AIDS epidemic.
- State the virus responsible for AIDS and explain how it differs from most other viruses.
- Describe the mechanisms of HIV transmission and relate them to the need for public awareness and concern regarding the spread of AIDS.

As a national and global epidemic, the degree of morbidity and mortality caused by HIV, as well as its impact on healthcare resources and the economy, is tremendous and unrelenting. At the end of 2013, it was estimated that there were roughly 35.2 million people worldwide living with HIV/AIDS and that over 39 million had died of the infection (Table 20.1).[2] During the same year, 2.3 million people were newly infected with HIV, with women and young people (*i.e.,* those 15 to 24 years of age) accounting for nearly 50% of the infections. Because the reporting of cases is not uniform throughout the world, many countries may not be accurately represented in this number.

Most of the new infections worldwide are in people younger than 25 years of age who live in developing countries. Sub-Saharan Africa has been hardest hit by HIV. There are 25 million people living with HIV in Africa, with a reported 1.6 million new infections in 2013. Over 71% of all persons with HIV are living in sub-Saharan Africa. There are countries in Africa where more than 30% of the adults are infected with HIV. Because of the large number of infected people in Africa,

TABLE 20.1 ESTIMATED NUMBER OF ADULTS AND CHILDREN LIVING WITH HIV INFECTION/AIDS, NEW INFECTIONS, AND DEATHS AT THE END OF 2013

	LIVING WITH	NEW INFECTIONS	DEATHS
North America	1,300,000	48,000	20,000
Sub-Saharan Africa	25,000,000	1,600,000	1,200,000
Eastern Europe and Central Asia	1,300,000	130,000	91,000
East Asia and the Pacific	931,000	83,100	42,200
South and Southeast Asia	3,900,000	270,000	220,000
Western and Central Europe	860,000	29,000	7,600
Caribbean	250,000	12,000	11,000
Latin America	1,500,000	86,000	52,000
Middle East and North Africa	260,000	32,000	17,000
Total	35.2 million	2.3 million	1.6 million

Data from UNAIDS. (2013). 2013 Report on the Global AIDS epidemic. Available online at: http://www.unaids.org/en/resources/campaigns/globalreport2013/factsheet. Accessed May 25, 2015.

the average life expectancy is expected to drop from 59 to 45 years by 2005.[2] The death toll in sub-Saharan Africa represents 75% of global AIDS deaths.

Eastern Europe and central Asia have the world's fastest-growing HIV populations. Almost one third of all newly diagnosed HIV infections in Eastern Europe and central Asia are in people aged 15 to 24 years, with the Russian Federation and Ukraine accounting for 90% of all people living with HIV in this region.[2]

In Canada, 71,230 people were living with HIV by the end of 2011 with approximately 26% not aware of their condition. The number of deaths approximated 24,300 since 1987 with racial and ethnic minorities being disproportionately affected.[3] Although aboriginal people represent approximately 4.3% of the population in Canada, they account for 8.9% of people living with HIV and 12% of newly diagnosed HIV infections.[3]

Emergence of the AIDS Epidemic

Compared with other human pathogens, HIV evolved very recently. In 1981, clinicians in New York, San Francisco, and Los Angeles recognized a new immunodeficiency syndrome in homosexual men. Initially, the syndrome was called GRIDS, for "gay-related immunodeficiency syndrome." By the end of 1981, there had been several hundred cases reported, and the name was changed to *acquired immunodeficiency syndrome, or AIDS*.[4] It soon became apparent that this disease was not confined to one segment of the population, but was also occurring in intravenous drug users, people with hemophilia, blood transfusion recipients, infants born to infected mothers, and high-risk heterosexuals. Studies of these diverse groups led to the conclusion that AIDS was an infectious disease spread by blood, sexual contact, and perinatally from mother to child.

An understanding of the virology of AIDS progressed with amazing efficiency; within 3 years of the first cases being recognized, the virus that causes AIDS had been identified. The virus was initially known by various names, including human T-cell lymphotropic virus type 3 (HTLV-III), lymph-adenopathy-associated virus (LAV), and AIDS-associated retrovirus (ARV).[5] In 1986, the name *human immunodeficiency virus* became internationally accepted.[6]

Transmission of HIV Infection

HIV is a retrovirus that selectively attacks the CD4+ T lymphocytes, the immune cells responsible for orchestrating and coordinating the immune response to infection. As a consequence, persons with HIV infection have a deteriorating immune system, and thus are more susceptible to severe infections with ordinarily harmless organisms. The virus responsible for most HIV infection worldwide is called *HIV type 1* (HIV-1). A second type, *HIV type 2* (HIV-2), is endemic in many countries in West Africa but is rarely seen in other parts of the world.[7]

HIV is transmitted from one person to another through sexual contact, blood-to-blood contact, or perinatally. It is not transmitted through casual contact. Several studies involving more than 1,000 uninfected, nonsexual household contacts with persons with HIV infection (including siblings, parents, and children) have shown no evidence of casual transmission.[8] HIV is not spread by mosquitoes or other insect vectors.[6] Transmission can occur when infected blood, semen, or vaginal secretions from one person are deposited onto a mucous membrane or into the bloodstream of another person.

Sexual contact is the most frequent mode of HIV transmission. Worldwide, 75% to 85% of HIV infections are transmitted through unprotected sex.[9] HIV is present in semen and vaginal fluids. There is a risk of transmitting HIV when these fluids come in contact with a part of the body that lets them enter the bloodstream. This can include the vaginal mucosa, anal mucosa, and wounds or sores on the skin.[9] Contact with semen occurs during vaginal and anal sexual intercourse, oral sex (*i.e.,* fellatio), and donor insemination. Exposure to vaginal or cervical secretions occurs during vaginal intercourse and oral sex (*i.e.,* cunnilingus). Condoms are highly effective in preventing the transmission of HIV. In most cities in Canada, sexual transmission of HIV is primarily related to

PATHOPHYSIOLOGY OF HIV/AIDS

- The HIV is a retrovirus that destroys the body's immune system by taking over and destroying $CD4^+$ T cells.
- In the process of taking over the $CD4^+$ T cell, the virus attaches to receptors on the $CD4^+$ cell, fuses to and enters the cell, incorporates its RNA into the cell's DNA, and then uses the $CD4^+$ cell's DNA to reproduce large amounts of HIV, which are released into the blood.
- The three phases of HIV are primary HIV acute infection; latency, during which there are no signs or symptoms of disease; and overt AIDS, during which the $CD4^+$ cell count falls to low levels and signs of opportunistic infections and other disease manifestations develop.
- As the $CD4^+$ T-cell count decreases, the body becomes susceptible to opportunistic infections.

vaginal or anal intercourse. In Canada, about 47% of HIV infections are among men who have sex with men, and 17% are from heterosexual contact.[3] In the developing world, heterosexual transmission is the major route of HIV infection.[5]

Because HIV is found in blood, the use of needles, syringes, and other drug injection paraphernalia is a direct route of transmission. Of the reported cases of AIDS in Canada, almost 17% occurred among persons who injected drugs.[3] HIV-infected injecting drug users can pass the virus to their needle-sharing and sex partners and, in the case of pregnant women, to their infants.[6] Although alcohol, cocaine, and other noninjected drugs do not directly transmit infection, their use alters perception of risk and reduces inhibitions about engaging in behaviours that pose a high risk of transmitting HIV infection.

Increased potential transmission of HIV occurred in transfusions of whole blood, plasma, platelets, or blood cells before 1985, and since then, all blood donations in Canada have been screened for HIV greatly minimizing the transmission risk. The clotting factor used by persons with hemophilia is derived from the pooled plasma of hundreds of donors. Before HIV testing of plasma donors was implemented in 1985, the virus was transmitted to persons with hemophilia through infusions of these clotting factors.[6] Seventy percent to 80% of people with hemophilia who were treated with factor before 1985 became infected. Other blood products, such as gamma globulin or hepatitis B immune globulin, have not been implicated in the transmission of HIV.

Transmission from mother to infant is the most common way that children become infected with HIV. HIV may be transmitted from infected women to their offspring in utero, during labour and delivery, or through breast-feeding.[10,11] Ninety percent of infected children acquired the virus from their mother. As a result of scaled-up HIV prevention services worldwide, the number of newly infected children was estimated to be 260,000 in 2012, representing a 52% decrease since 2001.[2]

Occupational HIV infection among healthcare workers is uncommon. As of 2010, the Centers for Disease Control and Prevention (CDC) had received only 57 documented occupational HIV infections in the United States.[13] In Canada, only one documented and reported case of occupational HIV transmission has been directly linked to a needle stick injury whereas two other cases have been identified as possible occupational transmission.[14] Universal Blood and Body Fluid Precautions should be used in encounters with all patients in the healthcare setting because HIV status is not always known. Occupational risk of infection for healthcare workers most often is associated with percutaneous inoculation (*i.e.*, needle stick) of blood from a patient with HIV infection. Transmission is associated with the size of the needle, amount of blood present, depth of the injury, type of fluid contamination, stage of illness of the patient, and viral load of the patient. The average risk for HIV infection from percutaneous exposure to HIV-infected blood is about 0.3%, and about 0.9% after a mucous membrane exposure.[13–16]

People with other sexually transmitted infections (STIs) are at increased risk for HIV infection. The risk of HIV transmission is increased in the presence of genital ulcerative STIs (*i.e.*, syphilis, herpes simplex virus infection, and chancroid) and nonulcerative STIs (*i.e.*, gonorrhea, chlamydial infection, bacterial vaginosis, and trichomoniasis). HIV increases the duration and recurrence of STI lesions, treatment failures, and atypical presentation of genital ulcerative diseases because of the suppression of the immune system.[17–19]

The HIV-infected person is infectious even when symptoms are absent. The point at which an infected person converts from being negative for the presence of HIV antibodies in the blood to being positive is called *seroconversion*. Seroconversion typically occurs within 1 to 3 months after exposure to HIV, but can take up to 6 months. Recent data suggest that 50% of transmissions occur during primary HIV infection (PHI) and early HIV infection.[20] The time after infection and before seroconversion is known as the *window period*. During the window period, a person's HIV antibody test result will be negative. Rarely, infection can occur from transfused blood that was screened for HIV antibody and found negative because the donor was recently infected and still in the window period. Consequently, the Canadian Blood Services requires blood collection centres to screen potential donors through interviews designed to identify behaviours known to present a risk for HIV infection. In addition, in Canada, since 2001, the nucleic acid amplification testing (NAAT) of all blood donors has reduced the risk of transfusion transmission of HIV and hepatitis C virus to approximately 1 in 2.3 million blood units.[21]

IN SUMMARY

AIDS is an infectious disease of the immune system caused by HIV, a retrovirus that causes profound immunosuppression. First described in June 1981, the disease is one of the leading causes of morbidity and mortality worldwide. The severity of the clinical disease and the absence of a cure or preventive vaccine have increased public awareness and concern. Most recently, the greatest increase in incidence of the disease has been in women and young people 15 to 24 years of age.

HIV is transmitted from one person to another through sexual contact, blood-to-blood contact, or perinatally. Transmission occurs when the infected blood, semen, or vaginal secretions from one person are deposited onto a mucous membrane or into the bloodstream of another person. The primary routes of transmission are through sexual intercourse, intravenous drug use, and from mother to infant. Blood transfusions and other blood products continue to be routes of transmission in some underdeveloped countries. Occupational exposure in healthcare settings accounts for only a tiny percentage of HIV transmission. HIV infection is not transmitted through casual contact or by insect vectors. There is growing evidence of an association between HIV infection and other STIs. Infected individuals can transmit the virus to others before their own infections can be detected by antibody tests.

PATHOPHYSIOLOGY AND CLINICAL COURSE

After completing this section of the chapter, you should be able to meet the following objectives:

- Describe the structure of HIV and trace its entry and steps in replication within the CD4⁺ T lymphocyte.
- Describe the alterations in immune function that occur in persons with AIDS.
- Describe the HIV/AIDS classification system.
- Relate the altered immune function in persons with HIV infection and AIDS to the development of opportunistic infections, malignant tumours, nervous system manifestations, the wasting syndrome, and metabolic disorders.

Molecular and Biologic Features of HIV

HIV is a member of the lentivirus family of animal retroviruses.[22,23] Lentiviruses, including feline immunodeficiency virus, simian immunodeficiency virus, and the visna virus of sheep, are capable of long-term latency and short-term cytopathic effects. They can all produce slowly progressive fatal diseases that include wasting syndromes and CNS degeneration. Two genetically different but antigenically related forms of HIV, HIV-1, and HIV-2, have been isolated in people with AIDS. HIV-1 is the type most associated with AIDS in Canada, United States, Europe, and Central Africa, whereas HIV-2 causes a similar disease principally in West Africa. HIV-2 appears to be transmitted in the same manner as HIV-1; it can also cause immunodeficiency as evidenced by a reduction in the number of CD4⁺ T cells and the development of AIDS.

Although the spectrum of disease for HIV-2 is similar to that of HIV-1, it spreads more slowly and causes disease more slowly than HIV-1. Specific tests are now available for HIV-2, and blood collected for transfusion is routinely screened for HIV-2. The ensuing discussion focuses on HIV-1.

HIV infects a limited number of cell types in the body, including a subset of lymphocytes called CD4⁺ T lymphocytes (also known as *T-helper cells* or *CD4⁺ T cells*), macrophages, and dendritic cells[6] (see Chapter 17). The CD4⁺ T cells are necessary for normal immune function. Among other functions, the CD4⁺ T cell recognizes foreign antigens and helps activate antibody-producing B lymphocytes.[6] The CD4⁺ T cells also orchestrate cell-mediated immunity, in which cytotoxic CD8⁺ T cells and natural killer (NK) cells directly destroy virus-infected cells, tubercle bacilli, and foreign antigens. The phagocytic function of monocytes and macrophages is also influenced by CD4⁺ T cells.

Like other retroviruses, HIV carries its genetic information in ribonucleic acid (RNA) rather than deoxyribonucleic acid (DNA). The HIV virion is spherical and contains an electron-dense core surrounded by a lipid envelope (Fig. 20.1). The virus core contains the major capsid protein p24, two copies of the genomic RNA, and three viral enzymes (protease, reverse transcriptase, and integrase). Because p24 is the most readily detected antigen, it is the target for the antibodies used in screening for HIV infection. The viral core is surrounded by a matrix protein called p17, which lies beneath the viral envelope. The viral envelope is studded with two viral glycoproteins, gp120 and gp41, which are critical for the infection of cells.

Replication of HIV occurs in eight steps (Fig. 20.1).[22,23] Each of these steps provides insights into the development of methods used for preventing or treating the infection. The *first step* involves the binding of the virus to the CD4⁺ T cell. Once HIV has entered the bloodstream, it attaches to the surface of a CD4⁺ T cell by binding to a CD4 receptor that has a high affinity for HIV. However, binding to the CD4 receptor is not sufficient for infection; the virus must also bind with other surface molecules (chemokine coreceptors, such as CCR5 and CXCR4) that bind the gp120 and gp41 envelope glycoproteins. This process is known as *attachment*. The *second step* allows for the internalization of the virus. After attachment, the viral envelope peptides fuse to the CD4⁺ T-cell membrane. Fusion results in an *uncoating* of the virus, allowing the contents of the viral core (the two single strands of viral RNA and the reverse transcriptase, integrase, and protease enzymes) to enter the host cell. The chemokine coreceptors are critical components of the HIV infection process. It has been reported

THE AIDS EPIDEMIC AND TRANSMISSION OF HIV

- AIDS is caused by the HIV.
- HIV is transmitted through blood, semen, vaginal fluids, and breast milk.
- Persons with HIV infection are infectious even when asymptomatic.

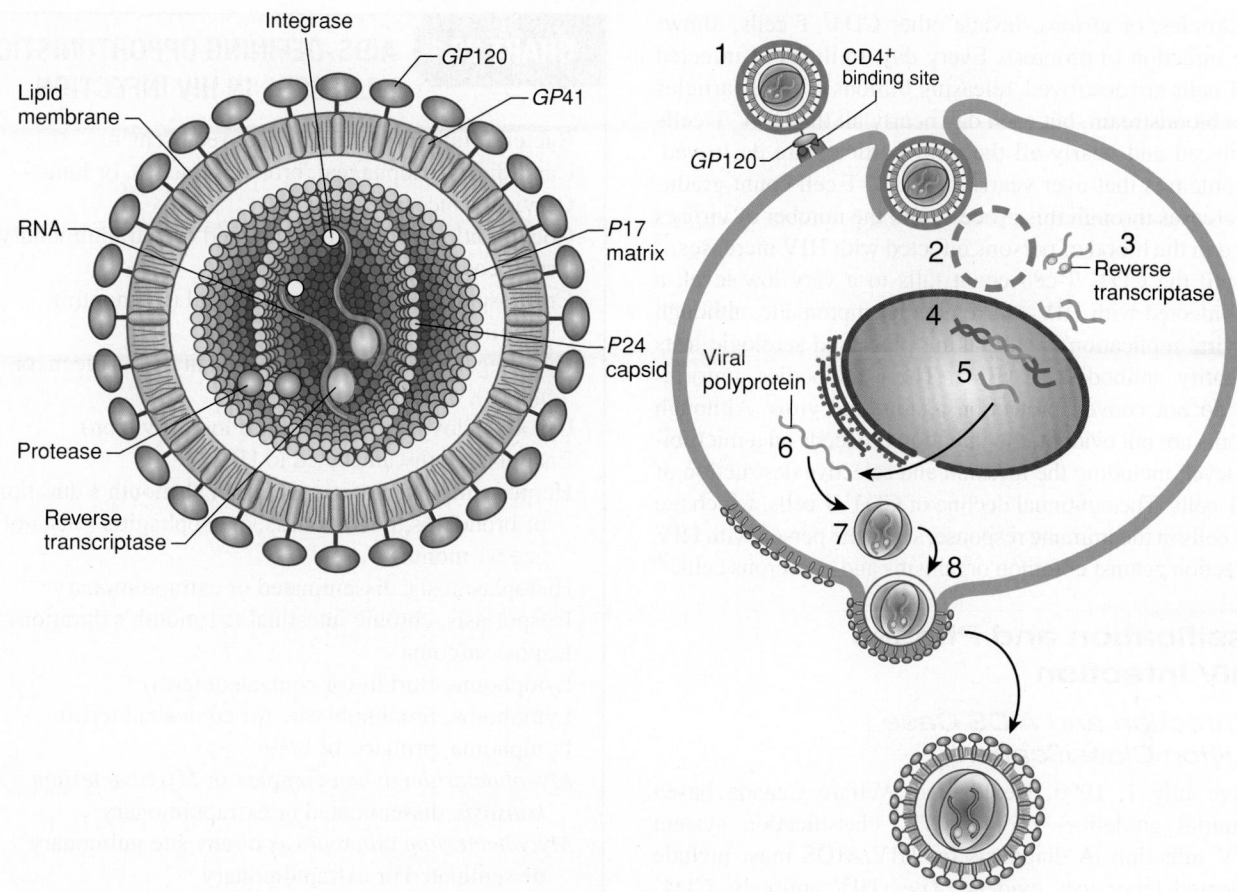

FIGURE 20.1 • Life cycle of the type 1 human immunodeficiency virus (HIV-1). (**1**) Attachment of the HIV to CD4$^+$ T-cell receptor; (**2**) internalization and uncoating of the virus with viral RNA and reverse transcriptase; (**3**) reverse transcription, which produces a mirror image of the viral RNA and double-stranded DNA molecule; (**4**) integration of viral DNA into host DNA using the integrase enzyme; (**5**) transcription of the inserted viral DNA to produce viral messenger RNA; (**6**) translation of viral messenger RNA to create viral polyprotein; (**7**) cleavage of viral polyprotein into individual viral proteins that make up the new virus; and (**8**) assembly and release of the new virus from the host cell.

that people with defective coreceptors are more resistant to development of HIV infection, despite repeated exposure.[24]

The *third step* consists of DNA synthesis. In order for HIV to reproduce, it must change its RNA into DNA. It does this by using the *reverse transcriptase* enzyme. Reverse transcriptase makes a copy of the viral RNA, and then in reverse makes another mirror-image copy. The result is double-stranded DNA that carries instructions for viral replication. The *fourth step* is called *integration*. During integration, the new DNA enters the nucleus of the CD4$^+$ T cell and, with the help of the enzyme integrase, is inserted into the cell's original DNA. The *fifth step* involves *transcription* of the double-stranded viral DNA to form a single-stranded messenger RNA (mRNA) with the instructions for building new viruses. Transcription involves activation of the T cell and induction of host cell transcription factors. The *sixth step* includes translation of mRNA. During *translation*, ribosomal RNA (rRNA) uses the instructions in the mRNA to create a chain of proteins and enzymes called a *polyprotein*. These polyproteins contain the components needed for the next stages in the construction of new viruses. The *seventh*

step is called *cleavage*. During cleavage, the protease enzyme cuts the polyprotein chain into the individual proteins that will make up the new viruses. Finally, during the *eighth step*, the proteins and viral RNA are assembled into new HIV viruses and released from the CD4$^+$ T cell.

Treatment of HIV/AIDS relies on the use of agents that interrupt steps of the HIV replication process. Currently, there are five classes of antiviral agents (discussed in the section on Treatment): nucleoside/nucleotide analog reverse transcriptase inhibitors (NRTIs/NtRTIs), nonnucleoside reverse transcriptase inhibitors (NNRTIs), protease inhibitors that interrupt the cleavage process, entry inhibitors that prevent HIV from entering or fusing with the CD4$^+$ cell, and integrase inhibitors that prevent the HIV genome from being integrated into the host's genome. The administration of highly active antiretroviral therapy (HAART), typically comprising a combination of at least three active antiretroviral agents, has become the current standard of care.

HIV replication involves the killing of the CD4$^+$ T cell and the release of HIV copies into the bloodstream. These viral particles, or *virions,* invade other CD4$^+$ T cells, allowing the infection to progress. Every day, millions of infected CD4$^+$ T cells are destroyed, releasing billions of viral particles into the bloodstream, but each day nearly all the CD4$^+$ T cells are replaced and nearly all the viral particles are destroyed. The problem is that over years, the CD4$^+$ T-cell count gradually decreases through this process, and the number of viruses detected in the blood of persons infected with HIV increases.[23]

Until the CD4$^+$ T-cell count falls to a very low level, a person infected with HIV can remain asymptomatic, although active viral replication is still taking place and serologic tests can identify antibodies to HIV.[25] These antibodies, unfortunately, do not convey protection against the virus. Although symptoms are not evident, the infection proceeds on a microbiologic level, including the invasion and selective destruction of CD4$^+$ T cells. The continual decline of CD4 T cells, which are pivotal cells in the immune response, strips the person with HIV of protection against common organisms and cancerous cells.[26]

Classification and Phases of HIV Infection

HIV Infection and AIDS Case Definition Classification

Effective July 1, 1993, Health and Welfare Canada based their initial guidelines on the CDC classification system for HIV infection. A diagnosis for HIV/AIDS must include documented laboratory evidence (*i.e.,* HIV antibody, CD4$^+$ counts) plus any one of the AIDS-defining illnesses.[27] The classification system defines three categories that correspond to CD4$^+$ cell counts of blood: *category 1,* >0.50×10^9/l (or >500 cells/µl); *category 2,* $0.20 - 0.49 \times 10^9$/l (or 200 to 499 cells/µl); and *category 3,* <0.20×10^9/l (or <200 cells/µl).

There also are three clinical categories. *Clinical category A* includes persons who are asymptomatic or have persistent generalized lymphadenopathy or symptoms of PHI (*i.e.,* acute seroconversion illness). *Clinical category B* includes persons with symptoms of immune deficiency not serious enough to be AIDS defining. *Clinical category C* includes AIDS-defining illnesses that are listed in the AIDS-defining conditions shown in Chart 20.1.[27] Each HIV-infected person has a CD4$^+$ T-cell count category and a clinical category. The combination of these two categorizations, CD4$^+$ cell count categories 1, 2, and 3 and clinical categories A, B, and C, was initially created to guide clinical and therapeutic decisions in the management of HIV infection. This classification scheme is rarely used in clinical practice today, but remains a tool for epidemiologic reporting.

Phases of HIV Infection

The typical course of HIV infection is defined by three phases, which usually occur over a period of 8 to 12 years. The three phases are the primary infection phase, chronic asymptomatic or latency phase, and overt AIDS phase (Fig. 20.2).[28]

Many persons, when they are initially infected with HIV, have an acute mononucleosis-like syndrome known as *primary infection.* This acute phase may include fever, fatigue, myalgias,

---

> **CHART 20.1** **AIDS-DEFINING OPPORTUNISTIC ILLNESSES IN HIV INFECTION**
>
> Bacterial infections, multiple or recurrent[a]
> Candidiasis. esophageal, bronchi, trachea, or lungs
> Cervical cancer, invasive[b]
> Coccidioidomycosis, disseminated or extrapulmonary
> Cryptococcosis, extrapulmonary
> Cryptosporidiosis, chronic intestinal (>1 month's duration)
> Cytomegalovirus disease (other than liver, spleen, or nodes), onset at age >1 month
> Cytomegalovirus retinitis (with loss of vision)
> Encephalopathy attributed to HIV[c]
> Herpes simplex: chronic ulcer(s) (>1 month's duration) or bronchitis, pneumonitis, or esophagitis (onset of age >1 month)
> Histoplasmosis, disseminated or extrapulmonary
> Isosporiasis, chronic intestinal (>1 month's duration)
> Kaposi sarcoma
> Lymphoma, Burkitt (or equivalent term)
> Lymphoma, immunoblastic (or equivalent term)
> Lymphoma, primary, of brain
> *Mycobacterium avium* complex or *Mycobacterium kansasii,* disseminated or extrapulmonary
> *Mycobacterium tuberculosis* of any site pulmonary[b] disseminated or extrapulmonary
> *Mycobacterium,* other species or unidentified species, disseminated or extrapulmonary
> *Pneumocystis jiroveci* (previously known as "*Pneumocystis carinii*") pneumonia
> Pneumonia, recurrent[b]
> Progressive multifocal leukoencephalopathy
> *Salmonella* septicemia, recurrent
> Toxoplasmosis of the brain, onset at age >1 month
> Wasting syndrome due to HIV[c]
>
> [a]Only among children aged <6 years.
> [b]Only among adults, adolescents, and children aged ≥6 years.
> [c]Suggested diagnostic criteria for these illnesses, which might be particularly important for HIV encephalopathy and HIV wasting syndrome.
> Developed from Centers for Disease Control and Prevention (CDC). (2014). Revised Surveillance Case Definition for HIV Infection—United States, 2014. *MMWR Recommendations and Reports, 63* (RR-03), 1–10.
> Also based on initial documentation from Health and Welfare Canada in 1987 and 1993. See Public Health Agency of Canada. (2013). Human immunodeficiency virus infections. Available online at: http://www.phac-aspc.gc.ca/std-mts/sti_its/cgsti-ldcits/section-5–8-eng.php/. Accessed May 25, 2015.

---

sore throat, night sweats, gastrointestinal problems, lymphadenopathy, maculopapular rash, and headache (Chart 20.2). Fever and malaise are the symptoms most commonly associated with primary infection.[29] During primary infection, there is an increase in viral replication, which leads to very high viral loads, sometimes greater than 1,000,000 copies/ml, and

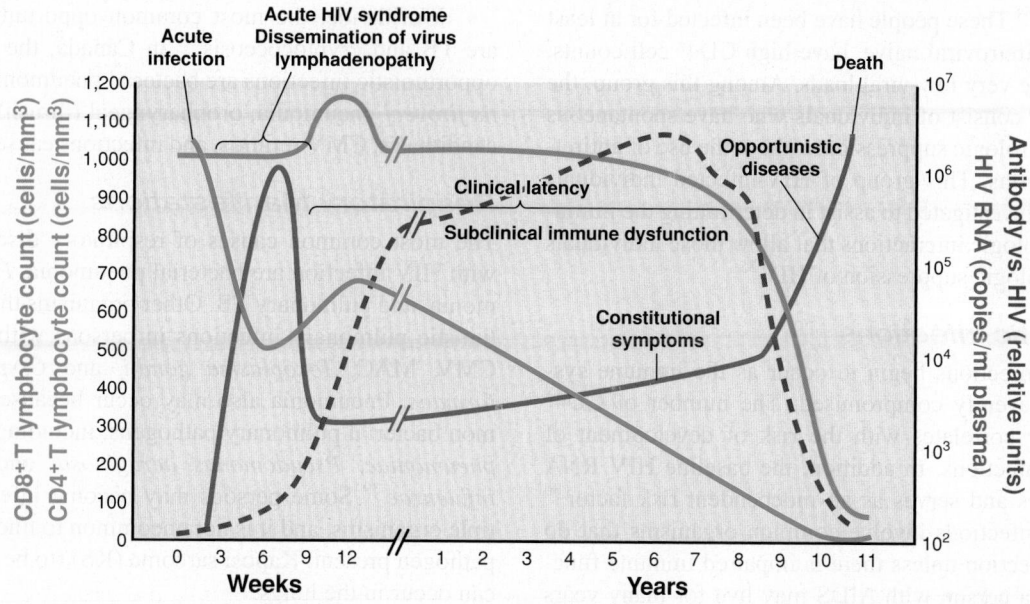

FIGURE 20.2 • Generalized viral load and CD4⁺ cell count during the phases of HIV infection. The time frame of important events in the development of an HIV infection are shown, including the clinical syndrome, virus loads, and CD4⁺ and CD8⁺ levels over time. (From Rubin R., Strayer D. S. (Eds.). (2012). *Rubin's pathology: Clinicopathologic foundations of medicine* (6th ed., p. 153). Philadelphia, PA: Lippincott Williams & Wilkins.)

a decrease in the CD4⁺ T-cell count. The signs and symptoms of PHI usually appear 1 to 4 weeks after exposure to HIV, and have an average duration of 7 to 10 days.[29] After several weeks, the immune system acts to control viral replication and reduces the viral load to a lower level, referred to as the "set point," where it often remains for several years.

People who are diagnosed with HIV infection while they are in the primary infection phase may have a unique opportunity for treatment. If started early, treatment may reduce the number of long-living HIV-infected reservoir cells (*e.g.,* CD4⁺ memory cells), reduce the risk of transmission to others, and preserve the immune system; however, these benefits are counterbalanced by the need for indefinite treatment, the cumulative risk of side effects, and the potential risk of resistance in those with incomplete adherence.[30,31] Early therapy may also protect the functioning of HIV-infected CD4⁺ T cells and cytotoxic T cells. Finally, early treatment could potentially help maintain a homogeneous viral population that will be better controlled by antiretroviral therapy and the immune system.

The primary phase is followed by a latent period during which the person has no signs or symptoms of illness. The median time of the latent period is about 10 years. During this time, the CD4⁺ T-cell count falls gradually from the normal range of 0.80 to $1.00 \times 10^9/l$ (800 to 1,000 cells/µl) to $0.20 \times 10^9/l$ (200 cells/µl) or lower. More recent data suggest that the CD4⁺ T-cell decline may not fall in an even slope based on level of HIV RNA levels, and the factors related to variability in the decline in CD4⁺ cells are under investigation.[32] Lymphadenopathy develops in some persons with HIV infection during this phase.[33] Persistent generalized lymphadenopathy usually is defined as lymph nodes that are chronically swollen for more than 3 months in at least two locations, not including the groin. The lymph nodes may be sore or visible externally.

The third phase, overt AIDS, occurs when a person has a CD4⁺ cell count of less than $0.20 \times 10^9/l$ (200 cells/µl) and an AIDS-defining illness.[28] Without antiretroviral therapy, this phase can lead to death within 2 to 3 years. The risk of opportunistic infections and death increases significantly when the CD4⁺ cell count falls below $0.20 \times 10^9/l$ (200 cells/µl).

Clinical Course

The clinical course of HIV varies from person to person. Most—60% to 70%—of those infected with HIV develop AIDS 10 to 11 years after infection. These people are the *typical progressors.*[28] Another 10% to 20% of those infected progress rapidly, with development of AIDS in less than 5 years, and are called *rapid progressors.* The final 5% to 15% are *slow progressors,* who do not progress to AIDS for more than 15 years. There is a subset of slow progressors, called *long-term nonprogressors,* who account for 2% to 5% of all

CHART 20.2	SIGNS AND SYMPTOMS OF ACUTE HIV INFECTION

- Fever
- Fatigue
- Rash
- Headache
- Lymphadenopathy
- Pharyngitis

- Arthralgia
- Myalgia
- Night sweats
- Gastrointestinal problems
- Aseptic meningitis
- Oral or genital ulcers

HIV infections.[34] These people have been infected for at least 8 years, are antiretroviral naive, have high CD4⁺ cell counts, and usually have very low viral loads. Among this group, the *elite controllers* consist of individuals who have spontaneous and sustained virologic suppression without the use of antiretroviral medications. This group of HIV-infected individuals continues to be investigated to assist in determining the immunologic and virologic interactions that allow those individuals to maintain virologic suppression of HIV.[35]

Opportunistic Infections

Opportunistic infections begin to occur as the immune system becomes severely compromised. The number of CD4⁺ T cells directly correlates with the risk of development of opportunistic infections. In addition, the baseline HIV RNA level contributes and serves as an independent risk factor.[36] Opportunistic infections involve common organisms that do not produce infection unless there is impaired immune function. Although a person with AIDS may live for many years after the first serious illness, as the immune system fails, these opportunistic illnesses become progressively more severe and difficult to treat.

Opportunistic infections are most often categorized by the type of organism (*e.g.,* fungal, protozoal, bacterial or mycobacterial, viral). Bacterial and mycobacterial opportunistic infections include bacterial pneumonia, salmonellosis, bartonellosis, *Mycobacterium tuberculosis* (TB), and *Mycobacterium avium* complex (MAC). Fungal opportunistic infections include candidiasis, coccidioidomycosis, cryptococcosis, histoplasmosis, penicilliosis, and pneumocystosis. Protozoal opportunistic infections include cryptosporidiosis, microsporidiosis, isosporiasis, and toxoplasmosis. Viral infections include those caused by cytomegalovirus (CMV), herpes simplex and zoster viruses, human papillomavirus (HPV), and JC virus, the causative agent of progressive multifocal leukoencephalopathy (PML).

Worldwide, the most common opportunistic infections are TB and cryptococcosis.[37] In Canada, the most common opportunistic infections are bacterial pneumonia, *Pneumocystis jiroveci* pneumonia, oropharyngeal (thrush) or esophageal candidiasis, CMV retinitis, and infections caused by MAC.[27,38]

Respiratory Manifestations

The most common causes of respiratory disease in persons with HIV infection are bacterial pneumonia, *P. jiroveci* pneumonia, and pulmonary TB. Other organisms that cause opportunistic pulmonary infections in persons with AIDS include CMV, MAC, *Toxoplasma gondii,* and *Cryptococcus neoformans*. Pneumonia also may occur because of more common bacterial pulmonary pathogens, including *Streptococcus pneumoniae, Pseudomonas aeruginosa,* and *Haemophilus influenzae*.[39] Some persons may become infected with multiple organisms, and it is not uncommon to find more than one pathogen present. Kaposi sarcoma (KS) (to be discussed) also can occur in the lungs.

Pneumocystis jiroveci **Pneumonia.** *P. jiroveci* (formerly known as *Pneumocystis carinii*) pneumonia (PCP) was the most common presenting manifestation of AIDS during the first decade of the epidemic. PCP is caused by *P. jiroveci,* an organism that is common in soil, houses, and many other places in the environment. In persons with healthy immune systems, *P. jiroveci* does not cause infection or disease. In persons with HIV infection, *P. jiroveci* can multiply quickly in the lungs and cause pneumonia. As the disease progresses, the alveoli become filled with a foamy, protein-rich fluid that impairs gas exchange (Fig. 20.3). Since HAART and prophylaxis for PCP were instituted, the incidence has decreased.[38] PCP still is common in people unaware of their HIV-positive status; those who choose not to treat their HIV infection or take prophylaxis; and in those with poor access to health care. The best predictor of PCP is a CD4⁺ cell count below $0.20 \times 10^9/l$ (200 cell/µl),[38]

FIGURE 20.3 • *Pneumocystis jiroveci* pneumonia. (**A**) The alveoli are filled with a foamy exudate, and the interstitium is thickened and contains a chronic inflammatory infiltrate. (**B**) A centrifuged bronchoalveolar lavage specimen impregnated with silver shows a cluster of *P. jiroveci* cysts. (From Rubin E., Farber J. L. (Eds.). (1994). *Pathology* (2nd ed.). Philadelphia, PA: Lippincott Williams & Wilkins.)

and it is at this point that prophylaxis with trimethoprim-sulfamethoxazole (or an alternative agent in the case of adverse reactions to sulpha compounds) is strongly recommended. Prophylaxis is also recommended if oral candidiasis (thrush) is present, regardless of the CD4[+] cell count.[40]

The symptoms of PCP may be acute or gradually progressive. Patients may present with complaints of a mild cough, fever, shortness of breath, and weight loss. Physical examination may demonstrate only fever and tachypnea, and breath sounds may be normal. The chest x-ray film may show interstitial infiltrates, but may be reported negative in up to 30% of cases.[41] Diagnosis of PCP is made by identifying the organism in pulmonary secretions. This can be done through examination of induced sputum, bronchoalveolar lavage, transbronchial biopsy, and, rarely, open lung biopsy.

Mycobacterium Tuberculosis. TB is the leading cause of death for people with HIV infection worldwide, and is often the first manifestation of HIV infection. At least one third of the 35 million people estimated to be living with HIV are likely to be infected with TB. TB cases in Canada have decreased since the 1950s and remain at a stable level of approximately 4.7 per 100,000. The incidence rate was the lowest in Prince Edward Island and the highest in Nunavut with 143.3 per 100,000 (see Chapter 28).[42] In the United States the number of TB cases have begun to increase and a number of factors have contributed to this increase, including changes in immigration patterns and increased numbers of people living in group settings like prisons, shelters, and nursing homes, but the most profound factor has been HIV infection.

The lungs are the most common site of *M. tuberculosis* infection, but extrapulmonary infection of the kidney, bone marrow, and other organs also occurs in people with HIV infection. Whether a person has pulmonary or extrapulmonary TB, most persons present with fever, night sweats, cough, and weight loss. Persons infected with *M. tuberculosis* (*i.e.,* those with positive tuberculin skin test results) are more likely to develop reactivated TB if they become infected with HIV. Coinfected individuals (*i.e.,* those with both HIV and TB infection) are also more likely to have a rapidly progressive form of TB. Equally important, HIV-infected persons with TB coinfection usually have an increase in viral load, which decreases the success of TB therapy. They also have an increased number of other opportunistic infections and an increased mortality rate.

Since the late 1960s, most persons with TB have responded well to therapy. However, in 1991, there were outbreaks of multidrug-resistant (MDR) TB. To be classified as MDR TB, the tubercle bacilli must be resistant to at least isoniazid and rifampin. The tubercle bacilli have recently developed more extensive resistance to include fluoroquinolones and other second-line agents, including capreomycin and kanamycin. These tuberculous strains are called extensively drug-resistant (XDR) TB.[43] Since the original outbreak of MDR TB in the early 1990s, new cases of MDR TB have declined, largely because of improved infection control practices and the expansion of directly observed therapy programs.

Gastrointestinal Manifestations

Diseases of the gastrointestinal tract are some of the most frequent complications of HIV infection and AIDS. Esophageal candidiasis, CMV infection, and herpes simplex virus infection are common opportunistic infections that cause esophagitis in people with HIV infection.[44] Aphthous ulcers presumed secondary to HIV are also common. Persons experiencing these infections usually complain of painful swallowing or retrosternal pain. The clinical presentation can range from asymptomatic to a complete inability to swallow resulting in dehydration. Endoscopy or barium esophagography is required for definitive diagnosis.

Diarrhea or gastroenteritis is a common complaint in persons with HIV infection. Patients should be evaluated for the same common causes of diarrhea as in the general population. The most common protozoal opportunistic infection that causes diarrhea is due to *Cryptosporidium parvum.* The clinical features of cryptosporidiosis can range from mild diarrhea to severe, watery diarrhea with a loss of up to several litres of water per day. The most severe form usually occurs in persons with a CD4[+] cell count of less than 0.05×10^9/l (50 cells/μl) and also can include malabsorption, electrolyte disturbances, dehydration, and weight loss.[25] Other organisms that cause gastroenteritis and diarrhea include *Salmonella,* CMV, *Clostridium difficile, Escherichia coli, Shigella, Giardia,* and microsporidia.[41] These organisms are often identified by examination of stool samples, cultures, or endoscopy.

Nervous System Manifestations

HIV infection, particularly in its late stages of severe immunocompromise, leaves the nervous system vulnerable to an array of neurologic disorders, including HIV-associated neurocognitive disorders (HAND), toxoplasmosis, and PML. These disorders can affect the peripheral nervous system or CNS and contribute to the morbidity and mortality of persons with HIV infection.

HIV-Associated Neurocognitive Disorders. In 2007, the American National Institute of Mental Health and the National Institute of Neurologic Disorders and Stroke developed a new classification with standardized diagnostic criteria which is used in Canada. The three conditions comprising HAND are HIV-associated asymptomatic neurocognitive impairment (ANI); HIV-associated mild neurocognitive disorder (MND); and HIV-associated dementia (HAD, formerly AIDS dementia complex).[45] HAND is a syndrome of cognitive impairment with motor dysfunction or behavioural/psychosocial symptoms associated with HIV infection itself.[45] HAD is usually a late complication of HIV infection. The clinical features of HAD are impairment of attention and concentration, slowing of mental speed and agility, slowing of motor speed, and apathetic behaviour. The diagnosis of HAD is one of exclusion, as all other potential etiologies need to be excluded. Treatment of HAD consists of HAART to decrease symptoms and may result in significant improvement of both motor and cognitive skills.

Toxoplasmosis. Toxoplasmosis is a common opportunistic infection in persons with AIDS. The organism responsible, *T. gondii*, is a parasite that most often affects the CNS.[46] Toxoplasmosis usually is a reactivation of a latent *T. gondii* infection that has been dormant in the CNS. The typical presentation includes fever, headaches, and neurologic dysfunction, including confusion and lethargy, visual disturbances, and seizures. Computed tomography scans or, preferably, magnetic resonance imaging (MRI) should be performed immediately to detect the presence of neurologic lesions. Prophylactic treatment with trimethoprim-sulfamethoxazole, dapsone-pyrimethamine, or atovaquone is effective against *T. gondii* when the CD4$^+$ cell count falls below 0.10×10^9/l (100 cells/µl). Given that these medications are also used for prevention of PCP, almost all persons in care with a CD4$^+$ count lower than 0.20×10^9/l (200 cells/µl) will be receiving effective toxoplasmosis prophylaxis. Since the use of trimethoprim-sulfamethoxazole and HAART began, the incidence of toxoplasmosis has decreased.[46]

Progressive Multifocal Leukoencephalopathy. PML is a demyelinating disease of the white matter of the brain caused by the John Cummingham or JC virus, a DNA polyomavirus that attacks the oligodendrocytes.[47] PML advances slowly, and it can be weeks to months before the patient seeks medical care. PML is characterized by progressive limb weakness, sensory loss, difficulty controlling the digits, visual disturbances, subtle alterations in mental status, hemiparesis, ataxia, diplopia, and seizures.[47] The mortality rate is high, and the average survival time is 2 to 4 months after diagnosis. The diagnosis is based on clinical findings and radiographic imaging (such as an MRI), and confirmed by the presence of the JC virus in the CNS.[47] There is no proven cure for PML, but improvement can occur after starting effective HAART. In patients who develop PML while on HAART, however, the outcome may be worse secondary to immune reconstitution syndrome (IRIS).[48]

Cancers and Malignancies

Persons with AIDS have a high incidence of certain malignancies, especially Kaposi sarcoma (KS), non-Hodgkin lymphoma, and noninvasive cervical carcinoma. The increased incidence of malignancies probably is a function of impaired cell-mediated immunity. As persons with HIV infection are living longer, there have been reports of the increasing incidence of age- and gender-specific malignancies.[49] Persons with HIV infection appear to have an increased risk of lung cancer even after adjusting for tobacco history. Non–AIDS-defining malignancies account for more morbidity and mortality than AIDS-defining malignancies in the antiretroviral therapy era. Traditional risk factors play a significant role in the increased risk of non–AIDS-defining malignancies for HIV-infected individuals, but do not entirely explain the excess cancer risk.[49] Increased incidences of lip cancer, penile cancer, and breast cancer have also been demonstrated in the post-HAART era.[50]

Kaposi Sarcoma. KS is a malignancy of the endothelial cells that line small blood vessels.[51] An opportunistic cancer, KS occurs in immunosuppressed persons (*e.g.,* transplant recipients or persons with AIDS). KS was one of the first opportunistic cancers associated with AIDS, and still is the most frequent malignancy related to HIV infection. It is 2,000 times more common in people infected with HIV than in the rest of the population.[51] Before 1981, most cases of KS were found in North America among elderly men of Mediterranean or Eastern European Jewish descent and in Africa among young black adults and children.[51]

There is evidence linking KS to a herpesvirus (herpesvirus 8, also called KS-associated herpes virus [KSHV]).[51] Over 95% of KS lesions, regardless of the source or clinical subtype, have reportedly been found to be infected with KSHV. The virus is readily transmitted through homosexual and heterosexual activities; however, there is a disproportionately higher incidence of KS in men who have sex with men compared with women and other men. Maternal–infant transmission also can occur. The virus has been detected in saliva from infected persons, and other modes of transmission are suspected.

The lesions of KS can be found on the skin and in the oral cavity, gastrointestinal tract, and the lungs. More than 50% of people with skin lesions also have gastrointestinal lesions. The disease usually begins as one or more macules, papules, or violet skin lesions that enlarge and become darker (Fig. 20.4). They may enlarge to form raised plaques or tumours. These irregularly shaped tumours can range from 2 to 4 cm in size. Tumour nodules frequently are located on the trunk, neck, and head, especially the tip of the nose. They usually are painless in the early stages, but discomfort may develop as the tumour develops. Invasion of internal organs, including the lungs, gastrointestinal tract, and lymphatic system, commonly occurs. Gastrointestinal tract KS is often asymptomatic, but can cause pain, bleeding, or obstruction.[51] Pulmonary KS usually is a late development of the disease and causes dyspnea, cough, and hemoptysis.[51] The tumours may obstruct organ function or rupture and cause internal bleeding. The progression of KS may be slow or rapid.

A presumptive diagnosis of KS usually is made based on visual identification of red or violet skin or oral lesions.[51] Biopsy of at least one lesion should be done to establish the diagnosis and to distinguish KS from other skin lesions that may resemble it. Diagnosis of solitary gastrointestinal or pulmonary KS is more difficult because endoscopy and bronchoscopy are needed for diagnosis and biopsy of such lesions is contraindicated because of the risk of severe bleeding. Effective HAART is the treatment of choice for localized KS. Local therapy with liquid nitrogen or vinblastine, chemotherapy, radiation, and interferon injections are the most common therapies for those with extensive or systemic disease.[40,51]

Non-Hodgkin Lymphoma. Non-Hodgkin lymphoma (see Chapter 15) develops in 3% to 4% of people with HIV infection. The clinical features are fever, night sweats, and weight loss. Because the manifestations of non-Hodgkin lymphoma

FIGURE 20.4 • Kaposi sarcoma. (**A**) Intraoral Kaposi sarcoma of the hard palate secondary to HIV infection. (**B**) Cutaneous brown Kaposi sarcoma lesions located over the maximal left ankle and foot. (From Centers for Disease Control and Prevention Public Image Library. Available online at: http://phil.cdc.gov/phil/details.asp.)

are similar to those of other opportunistic infections, diagnosis often is difficult. Diagnosis can be made by biopsy of the affected tissue. Treatment consists of aggressive combination chemotherapy that may include intrathecal chemotherapy. In the post-HAART era, outcomes of patients with non-Hodgkin lymphoma have significantly improved, with a 57% complete remission rate and median survival rates of 50% to 64% at 3 years, depending on the lymphoma subtype and tumour burden.[52,53]

Noninvasive Cervical and Anal Carcinoma. The HPV has been linked to the development of cervical carcinoma in both HIV-negative and -positive women, plus anal carcinoma for both HIV-positive men and women.[54] However women with HIV infection experience a higher incidence of cervical dysplasia than non–HIV-infected women.[55] HIV-infected women often experience persistent and recurrent HPV-associated

anogenital disease but may not be at a higher risk for development of invasive cervical cancer.[55] Occurrence of cervical dysplasia is detected by Papanicolaou smear and cervical colposcopy. Routine screening for anal intraepithelial neoplasia should be encouraged in all HIV-positive patients regardless of history of receptive anal intercourse.[56] In 2007, a quadrivalent vaccine to prevent HPV infection was approved by Health Canada.[57] The safety and immunogenicity of this vaccine among HIV-infected men and women continue to be studied; however, HPV vaccination may be administered to HIV-infected individuals according to routine vaccination schedules.[58]

Wasting Syndrome

Wasting syndrome is an AIDS-defining illness. Wasting is characterized by involuntary weight loss of at least 10% of baseline body weight in the presence of either diarrhea (more than two stools per day), or weakness plus a fever (intermittent or constant) for 30 days.[59] This diagnosis is made when no other opportunistic infections or neoplasms can be identified as causing these symptoms. Factors that contribute to wasting are anorexia, metabolic abnormalities, endocrine dysfunction, malabsorption, and cytokine dysregulation. Treatment for wasting includes nutritional interventions like oral supplements or enteral or parenteral nutrition. There also are numerous pharmacologic agents used to treat wasting, including appetite stimulants (such as megestrol acetate), cannabinoids, and recombinant human growth hormone.[60]

Metabolic and Morphologic Disorders

A wide range of metabolic and morphologic disorders is associated with HIV infection, including lipoatrophy and mitochondrial disorders, lipohypertrophy, hypercholesterolemia, hypertriglyceridemia, insulin resistance, and impaired glucose tolerance. The term *lipodystrophy* is frequently used to describe the body composition changes with or without the other metabolic derangements. Metabolic complications among people with HIV infection on HAART have been increasing since the introduction of potent HAART.[61] Insulin resistance and diabetes appear to be higher among those with HIV infection compared with the general population, although traditional risk factors contribute significantly.[62,63] Insulin resistance and diabetes also appear to be more associated with the use of specific nucleosides in combination with protease inhibitors rather than just the protease inhibitors, as initially thought. The one protease inhibitor exception is indinavir, which does alter the GLUT-4 transport system.[64,65] It is still not known why insulin resistance occurs in people with HIV infection, and most experts believe it is secondary to dysregulation of metabolic pathways or to indirect effects through mitochondrial toxicity linked to adipocyte toxicity. Treatment of insulin resistance is the same as for people without HIV infection—a healthy, balanced diet; exercise; and weight loss, if needed (see Chapter 42).

HIV and its therapies have been associated with dyslipidemia independent of HAART.[66] The severity of the dyslipidemia and the typical pattern of the lipid profile differ among and within the classes of antiretroviral agents.[67] The class of protease inhibitors is generally associated with elevated total cholesterol and triglyceride levels. The antiretroviral class of NNRTIs has been associated with elevated high-density lipoprotein (HDL) cholesterol and total cholesterol levels. NRTIs are a heterogeneous class in regard to lipids. Stavudine is more commonly associated with dyslipidemia with elevated total cholesterol, low-density lipoprotein (LDL) cholesterol, and triglyceride levels.

Before beginning antiretroviral therapy, a fasting lipid panel should be drawn, repeated in 3 to 6 months, and then repeated yearly. Currently, treatment of these lipid abnormalities is based on a modified version of the American National Cholesterol Education Program (NCEP) endorsed by the HIV Medicine Association.[68] One strategy in attempting to correct or reverse these abnormalities is to switch the HAART regimen to an equally suppressive one that contains medications less likely to cause dyslipidemia. It is important to carefully weigh the risks of potential loss of virologic suppression when alterations in HAART are made. One study compared the benefits of switching from a protease inhibitor to an NNRTI (efavirenz or nevirapine) with those of adding a lipid-lowering drug (pravastatin or bezafibrate), and found that lipid-lowering therapy was more effective than switching.[69] The statins (*e.g.*, atorvastatin, fluvastatin, pravastatin, simvastatin; discussed in Chapter 22) are the recommended medications to manage elevated LDL cholesterol. However, caution must be used because there can be serious drug-metabolizing interactions between the protease inhibitors, NNRTIs, and statins. Because increased triglycerides can lead to pancreatitis and may be an independent risk factor for coronary heart disease, the fibric acid derivatives (*e.g.*, fenofibrate), niacin, or fish oil may be prescribed as a means of decreasing triglyceride levels.[68]

Lipodystrophy. Lipodystrophy related to HIV infection includes symptoms that fall into two categories: changes in body composition and metabolic changes.[70] The alterations in body appearance are an increase in abdominal girth, buffalo hump development (abnormal enlargement of the dorsocervical fat pad), wasting of fat from the face and extremities, and breast enlargement in men and women. Most individuals experience either lipohypertrophy or lipoatrophy. Mixed patterns of fat changes are less common.[71] The metabolic changes include elevated serum cholesterol, low HDL cholesterol, elevated triglyceride levels, and insulin resistance. Originally attributed to the use of protease inhibitors, the pathogenesis of these metabolic derangements is complex and there may be multiple confounding factors.[72]

Diagnosis of lipodystrophy is difficult because it may depend on subjective measures of reports of alteration in body shape and also because the term has not been standardized. The Lipodystrophy Case Definition Study Group developed a definition that incorporated 10 clinical, metabolic, and body composition variables that can diagnose lipodystrophy with 80% accuracy.[73] The Study of Fat Redistribution and Metabolic Change in HIV Infection (FRAM) also developed a model to define lipodystrophy.[74] However, neither study's definitions have gained wide acceptance, and most clinicians prefer to describe the spectrum of signs and symptoms their patients experience. Therefore, it is critical when interpreting the vast number of clinical trials that one note the definition used for that particular study. There is no consensus on the best treatment for lipohypertrophy or lipoatrophy.[75] Some preliminary data are available on the use of recombinant human growth hormone to decrease visceral adipose tissue and subcutaneous adipose tissue. Metformin and thiazolidinedione, oral antidiabetic drugs, have also been studied; results have been inconsistent. Some experts recommend switching to a nonprotease inhibitor-based HAART regimen for treatment of lipohypertrophy, although this has not resulted in consistent results either. There is some evidence that switching from a thymidine analog to a nonthymidine analog may improve lipoatrophy. Surgical intervention (*e.g.*, liposuction, implantation or injection of synthetic substances) has been used with some success.

Mitochondrial Disorders. The mitochondria control many of the oxidative chemical reactions that release energy from glucose and other organic molecules. The mitochondria transform this newly released energy into adenosine triphosphate (ATP), which cells use as an energy source. In the absence of normal mitochondrial function, cells revert to anaerobic metabolism with generation of lactic acid. The mitochondrial disorders seen in persons with HIV infection are attributed to NRTIs, particularly the thymidine analogs.[76] The most common presentations are lipoatrophy and peripheral neuropathy, although patients may not experience both. Patients may also present with nonspecific gastrointestinal symptoms, including nausea, vomiting, and abdominal pain. They may develop altered liver function and lactic acidosis. Since the recognition of the ascending polyneuropathy syndrome and reports of hepatic failure due to combination therapy with stavudine and didanosine, reports of life-threatening events due to mitochondrial toxicities have dramatically decreased.

IN SUMMARY

HIV is a retrovirus that infects the body's CD4+ T cells and macrophages. HIV genetic material becomes integrated into the host cell DNA, so new HIV can be made.

Manifestations of infection, such as acute mononucleosis-like symptoms, may occur shortly after infection, and this is followed by a latent phase that may last for many years. The end of the latent period is marked by the onset of opportunistic infections and cancers as the person is diagnosed with AIDS. The complications of these infections can manifest throughout the respiratory, gastrointestinal, and nervous systems, and can include pneumonia, esophagitis, diarrhea, gastroenteritis, tumours, wasting syndrome, altered mental status, seizures, motor deficits, and metabolic disorders.

PREVENTION, DIAGNOSIS, AND TREATMENT

After completing this section of the chapter, you should be able to meet the following objectives:

- Discuss the transmission of HIV.
- Describe preventive strategies to decrease the transmission of HIV.
- Explain the possible significance of a positive antibody test for HIV infection.
- Differentiate between the enzyme immunoassay (EIA) (enzyme-linked immunosorbent assay [ELISA]) and Western blot antibody detection tests for HIV infection.
- Describe the methods used in the early management of HIV infection.
- Compare the actions of the reverse transcriptase inhibitors (*e.g.*, NRTIs/NtRTIs, NNRTIs), protease inhibitors, and fusion inhibitors in terms of controlling HIV replication.
- Enumerate some of the psychosocial issues associated with HIV infection/AIDS.

Since the first description of AIDS, considerable strides have been made in understanding the pathophysiology of the disease. The virus and its mechanism of action, HIV antibody screening tests, and some treatment methods were discovered within a few years after the recognition of the first cases. Further progress in understanding the pathophysiology of AIDS continues to be made, and more powerful treatments continue to be developed.

Prevention

Because there is no cure for HIV infection or AIDS, adopting risk-free or low-risk behaviour is the best protection against the disease. Abstinence or long-term, mutually monogamous sexual relationships between two uninfected partners are the best ways to avoid HIV infection and other STIs. Correct and consistent use of latex condoms can increase protection from HIV by not allowing contact with semen or vaginal secretions during intercourse.[10,27] Natural or lambskin condoms do not provide the same protection from HIV as latex because of the larger pores in the material. Only water-based lubricants should be used with condoms; petroleum (oil-based) products weaken the structure of the latex.

Injection of drugs provides another opportunity for HIV transmission. Avoiding recreational drug use and particularly avoiding the practice of using syringes that may have been used by another person are important to HIV prevention. Medical and public health authorities recommend that persons who inject drugs use a new sterile syringe for each injection, or if this is not possible, clean their syringes thoroughly with a household bleach mixture. Other substances that alter inhibitions can lead to risky sexual behaviour and increase the

risk of exposure to HIV. For example, smoking cocaine (*i.e.,* "crack") heightens the perception of sexual arousal, and this can influence the user to practice unsafe sexual behaviour.[77] The addictive nature of many recreational drugs can lead to an increase in the frequency of unsafe sexual behaviour and the number of partners as the user engages in sex in exchange for money or drugs. Persons concerned about their risk should be encouraged to get information and counselling and be tested to find out their infection status.

Public health programs in Canada have been profoundly affected by the HIV epidemic. Although standard methods for disease intervention and statistical analysis are applied to HIV infection, public health programs have become more responsive to community concerns, confidentiality, and long-term follow-up of clients as a direct result of the HIV epidemic. Canada now recommends that all individuals 13 to 64 years of age should be routinely screened and counselled, and mandatory consent be obtained before any HIV testing. Anyone who is at continued risk for HIV infection should be offered testing at least annually; those who are at high risk—injection drug users and their partners, persons who exchange sex for money or drugs, anyone who has had more than one sex partner since the last HIV test—should be tested more frequently. Whenever HIV testing is performed, pretest and posttest counselling should be offered. HIV prevention counselling should be culturally competent, sensitive to issues of sexual identity, developmentally appropriate, and linguistically relevant.[27]

The essential elements of any HIV prevention/counselling interaction include a personalized risk assessment and prevention plan.[27] Education and behavioural interventions continue to be the mainstays of HIV prevention programs. Individual risk assessment and education regarding HIV transmission and possible prevention techniques or skills are delivered to persons in clinical settings and to those at high risk of infection in community settings. Community-wide education is provided in schools, the workplace, and the media. Training for professionals can have an impact on the spread of HIV and is an important element of prevention. The constant addition of new information on HIV makes prevention an ever-changing and challenging endeavour.

Diagnostic Methods

The diagnostic methods used for HIV infection include laboratory methods to determine infection and clinical methods to evaluate the progression of the disease. The most accurate and inexpensive method for identifying HIV infection is the HIV antibody test. The first commercial assays for HIV were introduced in 1985 to screen donated blood. Since then, use of antibody detection tests has been expanded to include evaluating persons at increased risk for HIV infection. The HIV antibody test procedure consists of screening with an *EIA,* also known as *ELISA,* followed by a confirmatory test, the *Western blot* assay, which is performed if the EIA is positive.[68] In light of the psychosocial issues related to HIV infection and AIDS, sensitivity and confidentiality must be maintained whenever testing is implemented. Counselling before and after testing to allay fears, provide accurate information, ensure appropriate follow-up testing, and provide referral to needed medical and psychosocial services is essential.

The EIA detects antibodies produced in response to HIV infection.[26] In an EIA, when blood is added, antibodies to HIV bind to HIV antigens. The antigen–antibody complex is then detected using an anti-human immunoglobulin G (IgG) antibody conjugated to an enzyme such as alkaline phosphatase. A substrate is then added from which the enzyme produces a colour reaction. Colour development, indicating the amount of HIV antibodies found, is measured. The test is considered reactive, or positive, if colour is produced, and negative, or nonreactive, if there is no colour. EIA tests have high false-positive rates, so samples that are repeatedly reactive are tested by a confirmatory test such as the Western blot.

The Western blot test is more specific than the EIA, and in the case of a false-positive EIA result, the Western blot test can identify the person as uninfected. The Western blot is a more sensitive assay that looks for the presence of antibodies to specific viral antigens.[26] For the test, HIV antigens are separated by electrophoresis based on their weight, and then transferred to nitrocellulose paper and arranged in strips, with larger proteins at the top and smaller proteins at the bottom. The serum sample is then added. If HIV antibodies are present, they bind with the specific viral antigen on the paper. An enzyme and substrate then are added to produce a colour reaction as in the EIA. If there are no coloured bands present, the test is negative. A test is positive when certain combinations of bands are present. A test can be indeterminate if there are bands present but they do not meet the criteria for a positive test result. An indeterminate or false-positive test result can occur during the window period before seroconversion. When a serum antibody test result is reactive or borderline by EIA and positive by Western blot, the person is considered to be infected with HIV. When an EIA is reactive and the Western blot is negative, the person is not infected with HIV. Both tests are important because, in some situations, misinformation can be generated by EIA testing alone because there are many situations that can produce a false-positive (Chart 20.3) or a false-negative EIA result. The Western blot test therefore is essential to determine which persons with positive EIA results are truly infected.

Thousands of HIV antibody tests are performed in Canada each year. New technology has led to a new form of testing, namely the new rapid blood or saliva test. In October 2005, Health Canada regulated for rapid serum or saliva HIV testing to be done by healthcare professionals, giving preliminary results in minutes. There are three options for HIV testing and reporting in Canada: nominal (test is ordered using the patient's name), nonnominal (test is ordered using a code or initials that only the person ordering and the patient can identify), and anonymous (although not available in all provinces, the test is ordered so that only the person tested knows a unique code and the results cannot be linked to healthcare records).[27] In the United States home HIV testing kits can be bought over the counter. These kits, approved by the United States

---

> ## CHART 20.3 CAUSES OF FALSE-POSITIVE OR FALSE-NEGATIVE HIV ELISA TEST RESULTS
>
> **False-Positive Results**
> - Hematologic malignant disorders (*e.g.,* malignant melanoma)
> - DNA viral infections (*e.g.,* infectious mononucleosis [Epstein–Barr virus])
> - Autoimmune disorders
> - Primary biliary cirrhosis
> - Immunizations (*e.g.,* influenza, hepatitis)
> - Passive transfer of HIV antibodies (mother to infant)
> - Antibodies to class II leukocytes
> - Chronic renal failure/renal transplant
> - Stevens–Johnson syndrome
> - Positive rapid plasma reagin test
>
> **False-Negative Results**
> - "Window" period after infection
> - Immunosuppression therapy
> - Replacement transfusion
> - B-cell dysfunction
> - Bone marrow transplant
> - Contamination of specimen with starch powder from gloves
> - Use of kits that detect primary antibody to the p24 viral core protein

---

government, allow persons to collect their own blood sample through a finger-stick process, mail the specimen to a laboratory for EIA and confirmatory Western blot tests, and receive results by telephone in 3 to 7 days. There is also a quick version that uses a whole-blood specimen from a finger stick and can provide results in about 20 minutes.[78] Reactive, or positive, test results require confirmation using Western blot testing and persons with a reactive result are told that the preliminary test was positive, but that they need a confirmatory test. Since 2010, a fourth-generation screening test has been available in Canada and the United States. By combining the use of an ELISA with a p24 antigen detection assay, the window period for detection of HIV infection can be shortened to 2 to 3 weeks.[79]

Polymerase chain reaction (PCR) is a technique for detecting HIV DNA (see Chapter 16). PCR detects the presence of the virus rather than the antibody to the virus, which the EIA and Western blot tests detect. PCR is useful in diagnosing HIV infection in infants born to infected mothers because these infants have their mothers' HIV antibody regardless of whether the infants themselves are infected. Because the amount of viral DNA in the HIV-infected cell is small compared with the amount of human DNA, direct detection of viral genetic material is difficult. PCR is a method for amplifying the viral DNA up to 1 million times or more to increase the probability of detection.

Early Management

The management of HIV infection has changed dramatically since the mid-1990s. This change is due to a better understanding of the pathogenesis of HIV, the emergence of viral load testing, and the increased number of medications available to fight the virus. After HIV infection is confirmed, a baseline evaluation should be done.[68] This evaluation should include a complete history and physical examination and baseline laboratory tests. Routine follow-up care of a stable, asymptomatic HIV-infected patient should include a history and physical examination along with CD4[+] cell count and viral load testing every 3 to 4 months. Persons who are symptomatic may need to be seen more frequently.

Therapeutic interventions are determined by the level of disease activity based on the viral load, the degree of immunodeficiency based on the CD4[+] cell count, and the appearance of specific opportunistic infections. In January 2008, the Public Health Agency of Canada (PHAC) released recommendations for the initiation of antiretroviral therapy based on symptomatic disease and CD4[+] cell counts.[27] According to these guidelines, all symptomatic patients should be treated with antiretroviral therapy. If the individual is asymptomatic, therapy is recommended when the person's CD4[+] cell counts are $0.20 \times 10^9/l$ (200/μl) or less. For those who have a CD4[+] cell count greater than $0.35 \times 10^9/l$ (350/μl), antiretroviral therapy is generally not recommended. For those whose CD4[+] cell count is 0.20 to $0.35 \times 10^9/l$ (200–350/μl), antiretroviral therapy should be considered and a decision individualized to the patient should be made.[27] Because recent studies suggest that non–HIV-related conditions such as renal, liver, and heart disease may occur more frequently among those not on HAART, some experts are reverting back to previous recommendations to start therapy when the CD4[+] count is higher.[80,81] In the United States, current guidelines recommend treating all HIV-infected persons, regardless of symptoms and/or CD4+ cell count.[82] In addition, patients are more likely to experience toxicities due to HAART at lower CD4[+] counts compared with those who begin HAART at higher CD4[+] counts.[83] As HIV infection progresses, prophylaxis and treatment of opportunistic infections are critical.[40] Prophylaxis may differ based on geographic and environmental exposures and tolerability of medications, as well as the person's CD4[+] cell count. Early recognition of HIV infection is becoming more common, and medical intervention in the early stages may delay life-threatening symptoms and slow the progression of the disease.

Because of frequent advances in the management of HIV infection, primary care providers must be prepared to update their knowledge of diagnosis, testing, evaluation, and medical intervention. PHAC, Health Canada, and the Infectious Diseases Society of America/HIV Medicine Association regularly issue guidelines to assist clinicians in caring for persons with HIV infection.

Treatment

There is no cure for HIV infection. The medications that are currently available to treat HIV infection decrease the amount of virus in the body, but they do not eradicate HIV. The treatment of HIV infection is one of the most rapidly evolving fields in medicine. Because different drugs act on different stages of the replication cycle, optimal treatment includes a combination of at least three active drugs, often referred to as HAART.[82] The goal of HAART is sustained suppression of HIV replication, resulting in an undetectable viral load and an increasing CD4[+] cell count. In general, antiretroviral therapies are prescribed to slow the progression to AIDS and improve the overall survival time of persons with HIV infection.

The first drug that was approved by Health Canada for the treatment of HIV was zidovudine in 1987. Since then, an increasing number of therapeutics have been approved by Health Canada for treatment of HIV infection. There currently are five classes of HIV antiretroviral medications: nucleoside and NtRTIs; NNRTIs; protease inhibitors; entry inhibitors; and the newest class, integrase inhibitors (Table 20.2). Each type of agent attempts to interrupt viral replication at a different point.

Reverse transcriptase inhibitors inhibit HIV replication by acting on the enzyme reverse transcriptase. There are three types of HIV medications that work on this enzyme: NRTIs, NtRTIs, and NNRTIs. *NRTIs* and *NtRTIs* act by blocking the elongation of the DNA chain thereby stopping more nucleosides from being added. *NNRTIs* work by binding to the reverse transcriptase enzyme so it cannot copy the virus's RNA into DNA (Fig. 20.1).

Protease inhibitors bind to the protease enzyme and inhibit its action. This inhibition prevents the cleavage of the polyprotein chain into individual proteins, which would be used to construct the new virus. Because the information inside the nucleus is not put together properly, the new viruses that are released into the body are immature and noninfectious (Fig. 20.1).

The two newest classes of antiretroviral therapy are the *entry inhibitors* and *integrase inhibitors*. The entry inhibitors prevent HIV from entering or fusing with the CD4[+] cell, thus blocking the virus from inserting its genetic information into the CD4[+] T cell (Fig. 20.1).[84] There are two types of entry inhibitors: *fusion inhibitors* and *CCR5 antagonists*. Health Canada approved the first fusion inhibitor, enfuvirtide, in 2003. In September 2007, Health Canada approved the first CCR5 antagonist, maraviroc. *Integrase inhibitors* block the integration step of the viral cycle, thus preventing the HIV genome from integrating into the host's genome.[85] This is the newest class of inhibitors. Health Canada approved the first drug in this class, raltegravir, in November, 2007; approved elvitegravir (as a coformulation with cobicistat, tenofovir, and emtricitabine) in November 2012; and most recently approved dolutegravir in October 2013.

Preventive and therapeutic vaccines for HIV are also being investigated.[86] The preventive vaccine would be given to someone who is HIV negative, with the goal of preventing infection if exposed to HIV. These vaccines have focused mainly on inducing neutralizing antibodies to prevent infections. The second type of vaccine would be used in people

TABLE 20.2 ANTIVIRAL MEDICATIONS USED IN TREATMENT OF HIV INFECTION

MEDICATION (GENERIC NAME AND INITIALS) BY CLASSIFICATION	MEDICATION TRADE NAME	DOSING SCHEDULE
Nucleoside Reverse Transcriptase Inhibitors (NRTIs)		
Abacavir (ABC)	Ziagen	Once or twice daily
Didanosine (ddI)	Videx	Twice daily
Didanosine (ddI) enteric coated	Videx EC	Once daily
Emtricitabine (FTC)	Emtriva	Once daily
Lamivudine (3TC)	3TC	Once or twice daily
Stavudine (d4T)	Zerit	Twice daily
Zidovudine (AZT)	Retrovir	Twice daily
Nucleotide Reverse Transcriptase Inhibitor (NtRTI)		
Tenofovir (TDF)	Viread	Once daily
Nonnucleoside Reverse Transcriptase Inhibitors (NNRTIs)		
Delavirdine (DLV)	Rescriptor	Three times daily
Efavirenz (EFV)	Sustiva	Once daily
Etravirine (ETR)	Intelence	Twice daily
Nevirapine (NVP)	Viramune	Once or twice daily
Rilpivirine (RPV)	Edurant	Once daily
Protease Inhibitors (PIs)		
Atazanavir (ATV)[a]	Reyataz	Every 24 hours
Darunavir (DRV)[a]	Prezista	Every 12 hours
Fosamprenavir (FPV)[a]	Telzir	Every 12 or 24 hours
Indinavir (IDV)[a]	Crixivan	Every 8 or 12 hours
Lopinavir/Ritonavir (LPV/RTV)	Kaletra	Every 12 or 24 hours
Nelfinavir (NFV)	Viracept	Every 12 hours
Ritonavir (RTV)	Norvir	Varies
Saquinavir (SQV)[a]	Invirase	Every 12 or 24 hours
Tipranavir (TPV)[a]	Aptivus	Every 12 hours
Entry Inhibitors		
Enfuvirtide (T20, ENF)	Fuzeon	Every 12 hours
Maraviroc (MVC)	Celsentri	Every 12 hours
Integrase Inhibitor		
Dolutegravir (DTG)	Tivicay	Once or twice daily
Elvitegravir (EVG)	Stribild[b]	Once daily
Raltegravir (RAL)	Isentress	Every 12 hours
Combination Medications		
ABC + 3TC	Kivexa	Once daily
AZT + 3TC	Combivir	Twice daily
AZT + 3TC + ABC	Trizivir	Twice daily
TDF + FTC	Truvada	Once daily
TDF + FTC + EFV	Atripla	Once daily
TDF + FTC + RPV	Complera	Once daily
TDF + FTC + EVG + cobicistat	Stribild	Once daily

[a]Recommended to be boosted with ritonavir.
[b]Only available as part of coformulated compound (as of May 25, 2015).

who are already infected with HIV as a therapeutic strategy to control HIV replication. The goal of these vaccines would be to better control the HIV viremia by lowering the viral load set point, changing the viral load trajectories, and preserving immune function for longer periods of time. These vaccines have focused on bringing about cellular immune responses and preparing the immune system for the lysis of infected cells. To date, these strategies have proved disappointing.

Opportunistic infections occur as a consequence of immunodeficiency, which is caused by the progressive loss of CD4[+] T cells. Drugs and vaccines commonly are used for the prevention and treatment of opportunistic infections and conditions, including PCP, toxoplasmosis, MAC infection, candidiasis, CMV infection, influenza, hepatitis B, and *S. pneumoniae* infection.[40] Prophylactic medications are used once an individual's CD4[+] cell count has dropped below a certain level that indicates his or her immune system is no longer able to fight off opportunistic infections.[40]

Persons with HIV infection should be advised to avoid infections as much as possible and seek evaluation promptly when they occur. Immunization is important because persons infected with HIV are at risk for contracting other infectious diseases. Some of these diseases can be avoided by vaccination while the immune system's responsiveness is relatively intact. Persons with asymptomatic HIV infection and CD4[+] cell counts greater than $0.20 \times 10^9/l$ (200 cells/µl) should be vaccinated against measles, mumps, and rubella. Pneumococcal vaccine should be given once, as soon as possible after HIV infection is diagnosed, and then every 10 years, and influenza vaccine should be given yearly.[27,68] Hepatitis A and B vaccines appear to be more immunogenic when the HIV viral load is suppressed.[86–88] Customarily live-virus vaccines should not be given to persons with HIV infection; however, there is much interest in the possibility of vaccinating those HIV-infected persons with the live varicella-zoster virus (VZV) vaccine to decrease the risk of VZV reactivation disease, or shingles. A study conducted among children with HIV infection demonstrated virus-specific lymphocyte proliferative responses in all subjects by 4 weeks and in 90% by 1 year after VZV vaccination.[89] All subjects tolerated the vaccination without adverse reactions or rises in HIV viral load.

Psychosocial Issues

HIV infection and AIDS affect all spheres of life.[90] The psychological effects of HIV infection or AIDS may be just as significant as the physical effects. The dramatic impact of this illness is compounded by complex reactions on the part of the person with HIV or AIDS; his or her partner, friends, and family; members of the healthcare team; and the community. These reactions may be influenced by inadequate information, fear of contagion, shame, prejudices, and condemnation of risk behaviours.[91] Acknowledging a diagnosis of HIV infection or AIDS may be the first indication to family and colleagues of an otherwise hidden lifestyle (*e.g.*, unknown sexual partners, drug use). This increases the strain on relationships with important

support persons. Shock is a common reaction people have when they are diagnosed with HIV infection, often followed by anger at themselves or others and denial or guilt. In addition to the fear and grief associated with death, the person with HIV infection or AIDS also may experience uncertainty and may feel helpless, hopeless, stigmatized, and out of control.[90]

Many people with HIV infection have pre-existing mental health conditions such as depression or anxiety disorders as well as alcohol and other drug abuse (AODA). Appropriate diagnosis and treatment should be made available when mental health problems or AODA are evident. Diagnosis and treatment of cognitive and affective disorders are essential parts of ongoing care for the HIV-infected person.[90] The emotional stress, feelings of isolation, and sadness experienced by the person with HIV infection or AIDS can be overwhelming. Most persons, however, learn to cope and live with their HIV infection. Persons with the disease must have as much information and control as possible. They should be encouraged to direct their energies in a positive manner and continue with their social and group activities as long as such activities are helpful. Appropriate social support systems (*e.g.*, AIDS service organizations, community groups, religious organizations) should be called on to assist whenever possible. When they learn they can live with HIV infection, many persons acquire a positive outlook based on living their lives to the fullest.

To deal with these complex issues, the healthcare team must recognize and accept their own fears, prejudices, and emotions concerning those with HIV infection or AIDS. Personal feelings must not prevent caregivers from acknowledging the intrinsic human worth of all persons and their right to be treated with dignity and respect. Members of the healthcare team should have adequate support for their own emotional needs generated from working with persons with HIV infection. Grief, anxiety, and concern over stigmatization are normal feelings and should be acknowledged and dealt with through peer support or professional counselling to reduce burnout and emotional strain among members of the healthcare provider team.[91]

IN SUMMARY

Because there is no cure for HIV infection, risk-free or low-risk behaviour is the best protection against it. Abstinence or long-term, mutually monogamous sexual relationships between two uninfected partners, use of condoms, avoiding drug use, and the use of sterile syringes if drug use cannot be avoided are essential to halting the transmission of HIV.

HIV infection is diagnosed using the EIA or rapid test together with the Western blot assay, both of which are antibody detection tests. The emotional stress, feelings of isolation, and sadness experienced by the person with HIV infection or AIDS can be overwhelming, but most persons adjust to living with HIV infection. Diagnosis and treatment of cognitive and affective disorders are an essential part of ongoing care for the HIV-infected person. Appropriate treatment should be made available when alcohol or other drug dependence is noted.

The management of HIV infection/AIDS incorporates the use of HAART, early recognition and treatment of opportunistic infections and other clinical disorders, and acknowledgment and support of the psychosocial issues that are an ongoing concern for those who are infected with the virus.

HIV INFECTION IN PREGNANCY AND IN INFANTS AND CHILDREN

After completing this section of the chapter, you should be able to meet the following objectives:

- Discuss the vertical transmission of HIV from mother to child and recommended prevention measures.
- Cite problems with the diagnosis of HIV infection in the infant.
- Compare the progress of HIV infection in infants and children with HIV infection in adults.

Early in the epidemic, children who acquired HIV could have become infected through blood products or perinatally. Now, almost all of the children who become infected with HIV at a young age in Canada get the infection perinatally. Fortunately, the incidence of perinatally infected children in Canada has markedly decreased, with only two confirmed transmissions in 2013.[92] Infected women may transmit the virus to their offspring in utero, during labour and delivery, or through breast milk.[93] The risk of transmission is increased if the mother has advanced HIV disease as evidenced by low CD4$^+$ cell counts or high levels of HIV in the blood (high viral load); if there was prolonged time from rupture of membranes to delivery; if the mother breast-feeds the child; or if there is increased exposure of the fetus to maternal blood.[93,94]

Diagnosis of HIV infection in children born to HIV-infected mothers is complicated by the presence of maternal anti-HIV IgG antibody, which crosses the placenta to the fetus.[12] Consequently, infants born to HIV-infected women can be HIV antibody positive by ELISA for up to 18 months of age even though they are not infected with HIV. PCR testing for HIV DNA is used most often to diagnose HIV infection in infants younger than 18 months of age. Two positive PCR tests for HIV DNA are needed to diagnose a child with HIV infection. Children born to mothers with HIV infection are considered uninfected if they become HIV antibody negative after 6 months of age, have no other laboratory evidence of HIV infection, and have not met the surveillance case definition criteria for AIDS in children.

The landmark Pediatric AIDS Clinical Trials Group (PACTG) reported perinatal transmission could be lowered by two thirds, from 26% to 8%, by administering zidovudine to the mother during pregnancy, labour and delivery, and

HIV INFECTION IN PREGNANCY AND IN INFANTS AND CHILDREN

- HIV can be passed from mother to infant during labour and delivery or through breast-feeding.
- The course of HIV infection is different for children than adults.

to the newborn infant.[11] PHAC therefore recommends that HIV counselling and testing should be offered to all pregnant women.[27] The recommendations also stress that women who test positive for HIV antibodies should be informed of the perinatal prevention benefits of zidovudine therapy and offered HAART, which often includes zidovudine. This is done because it has now been found that women receiving antiretroviral therapy who also have a viral load of less than 1,000 copies/ml have very low rates of perinatal transmission. One caveat to antiretroviral therapy in pregnancy is that efavirenz should not be used during the first trimester because there may be an increased risk of neural tube defects. Benefits of voluntary testing for mothers and newborns include reduced morbidity because of intensive treatment and supportive health care, the opportunity for early antiretroviral therapy for mother and child, and the opportunity to provide information regarding the risk of transmission from breast milk.

Because pregnant women in less developed countries do not always have access to zidovudine, studies are being conducted in Africa to determine if other, simpler and less expensive antiretroviral regimens can be used to decrease transmission from mother to infant. One such study, HIVNET 012, evaluated single-dose nevirapine compared with zidovudine and found that nevirapine lowered the risk of HIV transmission by almost 50%.[95] However, this strategy could lead to nevirapine resistance, and other studies evaluating drug combinations and strategies are being conducted.

Children may have a different clinical presentation of HIV infection than adults. Failure to thrive, CNS abnormalities, and developmental delays are the most prominent primary manifestations of HIV infection in children.[12] Children born with HIV infection usually weigh less and are shorter than noninfected infants. A major cause of early mortality for HIV-infected children is PCP, which may also be transmitted vertically. As opposed to adults, in whom PCP occurs in the late stages, PCP occurs early in children, with the peak age of onset at 3 to 6 months. For this reason, prophylaxis with trimethoprim-sulfamethoxazole is started by 6 weeks for all infants born to HIV-infected mothers, regardless of their CD4$^+$ cell count or infection status.

IN SUMMARY

Infected women may transmit the virus to their offspring in utero, during labour and delivery, or through breast milk.

It is recommended that all pregnant women be tested for HIV at the time of diagnosis of pregnancy. Diagnosis of HIV infection in children born to HIV-infected mothers is complicated by the presence of maternal HIV antibody, which crosses the placenta to the fetus. This antibody usually disappears within 18 months in uninfected children. Administration of antiretroviral therapy to the mother during pregnancy, labour and delivery, and to the newborn infant decreases perinatal transmission.

REVIEW EXERCISES

1. A 29-year-old woman presents to the clinic for her initial obstetrics visit, about 10 weeks into her pregnancy.
   A. *This woman is in a monogamous relationship. Should an HIV test be a part of her initial blood work? Why?*
   B. *The woman's HIV test comes back positive. What should be done to decrease the risk of her passing on HIV to her infant?*
   C. *The infant is born, and its initial antibody test is positive. Does this mean the infant is infected? How is the diagnosis of HIV infection in an infant younger than 18 months made, and how is this different than the diagnosis for adults?*

2. A 40-year-old man presents to the clinic very short of breath, and based on radiography and examination, he is diagnosed with *P. jiroveci* pneumonia (PCP). His provider does an HIV test, which is positive. On further testing, the man's CD4$^+$ count is found to be 0.10×10^9/l (100 cells/µl) and his viral load is 250,000 copies/ml.
   A. *Why did the provider do an HIV test after the man was diagnosed with PCP?*
   B. *Is there a way to prevent PCP?*
   C. *What classification does this man fall into based on his CD4$^+$ count and symptomatology? Why?*

References

1. Quinn T. C. (2003). World AIDS Day: Reflections on the pandemic. *The Hopkins HIV Report, 15*(1), 12–14.
2. UNAIDS. (2013). Global report: UNAIDS report on the global AIDS epidemic 2013. Available online at: http://www.unaids.org/sites/default/files/en/media/unaids/contentassets/documents/epidemiology/2013/gr2013/UNAIDS_Global_Report_2013_en.pdf. Accessed May 25, 2015.
3. Public Health Agency of Canada. (2014). *HIV/AIDS Epi updates.* Available online at: http://www.phac-aspc.gc.ca/aids-sida/publication/epi/2010/1-eng.php. Accessed May 25, 2015.
4. Quinn T. C. (2001). The global HIV pandemic: Lessons from the past and glimpses into the future. *The Hopkins HIV Report, 13*(1), 4–5, 16.
5. Montagnier L., Alizon M. (1986). The human immune deficiency virus (HIV): An update. In Gluckman J. C., Vilmer E. (Eds.), *Proceedings of the Second International Conference on AIDS* (p. 13). Paris: Elsevier.
6. Friedland G. H., Klein R. S. (1987). Transmission of the human immunodeficiency virus. *New England Journal of Medicine, 317*, 1125–1135.
7. Gottlieb G. S. (2013). Changing HIV epidemics: What HIV-2 can teach us about ending HIV-1. *Acquired Immunodeficiency Syndrome, 27*(1), 135–137.
8. Gershon R. R., Vlahov D., Nelson K. E. (1990). The risk of transmission of HIV-1 through non-percutaneous, non-sexual modes: A review. *Acquired immune deficiency syndrome, 4*, 645–650.
9. Colpin H. (1999). Prevention of HIV transmission through behavioral changes and sexual means. In Armstrong D., Cohen J. (Eds.), *Infectious diseases* (Section 5, Chapter 2, pp. 1–4). London: Harcourt.
10. Connor E. M., Sperling R. S., Gelber R., et al. (1994). Reduction of maternal-infant transmission of human immunodeficiency virus type 1 with zidovudine treatment. Pediatric AIDS Clinical Trials Group Protocol 076 Study Group. *New England Journal of Medicine, 331*, 1173–1180.
11. McIntrye J. (2008). Chapter 35: Managing pregnant patients. In Dolin R., Masur H., Saag M., (Eds.) *AIDS therapy* (3rd ed.). London: Churchill Livingston.
12. Havens P. L. (1999). Pediatric AIDS. In Armstrong D., Cohen J. (Eds.), *Infectious diseases* (Section 5, Chapter 20). London: Harcourt.
13. Centers for Disease Control and Prevention. (2013). Occupational HIV transmission and prevention among health care workers. Available online at: www.cdc.gov/hiv/resources/factsheets/hcwprev.htm. Accessed May 25, 2015.
14. Canadian Centre for Occupational Health and Safety. (2005). Needlestick injuries. Available online at: http://www.ccohs.ca/oshanswers/diseases/needlestick_injuries.html. Accessed May 25, 2015.
15. Bell D. M. (1997). Occupational risk of HIV in health care workers: An overview. *American Journal of Medicine, 102*(5B), 9–15.
16. Ippolito G., Puro V., De Carli G. (1993). The risk of occupational human immunodeficiency virus infection in health care workers. Italian Multicenter Study. The Italian Study Group on Occupational Risk of HIV Infection. *Archives of Internal Medicine, 153*(12), 1451–1458.
17. Rottingen J. A., Cameron D. W., Garnett G. P. (2001). A systematic review of the epidemiologic interactions between classic sexually transmitted diseases and HIV: How much really is known? *Sexually Transmitted Diseases, 28*, 579–597.
18. Glynn J. R., Biraro S., Weiss H. A. (2009). Herpes simplex virus type 2: A key role in HIV incidence. *Acquired Immunodeficiency Syndrome, 23*, 1595–1598.
19. Atashili J., Poole C., Ndumbe P. M., et al. (2008). Bacterial vaginosis and HIV acquisition: A meta-analysis of published studies. *Acquired Immunodeficiency Syndrome, 22*, 1493–1501.
20. Brenner B. G., Roger M., Routy J. P., et al. (2007). High rates of forward transmission events after acute/early HIV-1 infection. *Journal of Infectious Disease, 195*, 951–959.
21. O'Brien S. F., Yi Q. L., Fan W., et al. (2007). Current incidence and estimated residual risk of transfusion-transmitted infections in donations made to Canadian Blood Services. *Transfusion, 47*(2), 316–325.
22. Abbas A. K. (2010). Chapter 6: Diseases of the immune systems. In Kumar V., Abbas A. K., Fausto N., et al. (Eds.), *Robbins and Cotran pathologic basis of disease* (8th ed.). Philadelphia, PA: Elsevier Saunders.
23. Warren J. S., Strayer D. S. (2012). Chapter 4: Immunopathology. In Rubin, R., Strayer, D. E. (Eds.), *Rubin's pathology: Clinicopathologic foundations of medicine* (6th ed.). Philadelphia, PA: Lippincott Williams & Wilkins.
24. Trecarichi E. M., Tumbarello M., de Gaetano Donati, K., et al. (2006). Partial protective effect of CCR5-delta 32 heterozygosity in a cohort of heterosexual Italian HIV-1 exposed uninfected individuals. *AIDS Research and Therapy, 3*, 22.
25. Fauci A. S. (1988). The human immunodeficiency virus: Infectivity and mechanisms of pathogenesis. *Science, 239*, 617–622.
26. Branson B. M., McDougal S. (2008). Chapter 1: Establishing the diagnosis of HIV infection. In Dolin R., Masur H., Saag M. S. (Eds.), *AIDS therapy* (3rd ed.). Philadelphia, PA: Churchill Livingstone.

27. Public Health Agency of Canada. (2013). Human immunodeficiency virus infections. Available online at: http://www.phac-aspc.gc.ca/std-mts/sti-its/cgsti-ldcits/section-5–8-eng.php. Accessed May 25, 2015.

28. Rizzardi G. P., Pantaleo, G. (1999). The immunopathogenesis of HIV-1 infection. In Armstrong D., Cohen J. (Eds.), *Infectious diseases* (Section 5, Chapter 6, pp. 1–12). London: Harcourt.

29. Hecht F. M., Busch M. P., Rawa,l B., et al. (2002). Use of laboratory tests and clinical symptoms for identification of primary HIV infections. *Acquired Immunodeficiency Syndrome, 16*, 1119–1129.

30. Hecht F. M., Wang L., Collier A, et al; AIEDRP Network. (2006). A multicenter observational study of potential benefits of initiating combination antiretroviral therapy during acute infection. *Journal of Infectious Disease, 194*, 725–733.

31. Ambrosioni J., Nicolas D., Sued O., et al. (2014). Update on antiretroviral treatment during primary HIV infection. *Expert Review of Anti-infective Therapy, 12*(7), 793–807.

32. Rodriguez B., Sethi,A. K., Cheruvu V. K. (2006). Predictive value of plasma HIV RNA level on rate of CD4 T-cell decline in untreated HIV infection. *Journal of the American Medical Association, 296*, 1498–1506.

33. Pantaleo G., Graziosi C., Fauci A. S. (1993). The immunopathogenesis of human immunodeficiency virus infection. *New England Journal of Medicine, 328*, 327–335.

34. Okulicz J. F., Marconi V. C., Landrum M. L., et al; Infectious Disease Clinical Research Program (IDCRP) HIV Working Group. (2009). Clinical outcomes of elite controllers, viremic controllers, and long-term nonprogressors in the US Department of Defense HIV Natural History Study. *Journal of Infectious Diseases, 200*, 1714–1723.

35. Walker B. (2007). Elite control of HIV infection: Implications for vaccine and treatment. *Top HIV MED, 15*(4), 134–136.

36. Kaplan J. E., Hanson D. L., Jones J. L., Dworkin M. S; Adult and Adolescent Spectrum of HIV Disease Project Investigators. (2001). Viral load as an independent risk factor for opportunistic infections in HIV-infected adults and adolescents. *Acquired Immunodeficiency Syndrome, 15*, 1831–1836.

37. Zanoni B. C., Gandhi R. T. (2014). Update on opportunistic infections in the era of effective antiretroviral therapy. *Infectious Disease Clinics of North America, 28*, 501–518.

38. Kaplan J. E., Hanson D., Dworkin M. S., et al. (2000). Epidemiology of HIV associated opportunistic infections in the United States in the era of highly active antiretroviral therapy. *Clinical Infectious Diseases, 30*(Suppl. 1), S5–S14.

39. Afessa B., Green B. (2000). Bacterial pneumonia in hospitalized patients with HIV. *Chest, 117*, 1017–1022.

40. Panel on Opportunistic Infections in HIV-Infected Adults and Adolescents. (2013). Guidelines for the prevention and treatment of opportunistic infections in HIV-infected adults and adolescents: Recommendations from the Centers for Disease Control and Prevention, the National Institutes of Health, and the HIV Medicine Association of the Infectious Diseases Society of America. Available online at: http://aidsinfo.nih.gov/contentfiles/lvguidelines/adult_oi.pdf. Accessed May 25, 2015.

41. Huang L., Stansell J., Osmond D. (1999). Performance of an algorithm to detect Pneumocystis carinii pneumonia in symptomatic HIV-infected persons. Pulmonary Complications of HIV Infection Study Group. *Chest, 115*, 1025–1032.

42. Public Health Agency of Canada. (2015). Tuberculosis in Canada 2013-Pre-release. Available online at: http://www.phac-aspc.gc.ca/tboc-latb/pubs/tbcan13pre/assets/pdf/tbcan13pre-eng.pdf. Accessed May 25, 2015.

43. Shah N. S., Wright A., Bai G. H., et al. (2007). Worldwide emergence of extensively drug-resistant tuberculosis. *Emerging Infectious Diseases, 13*(3), 380–387.

44. Wilcox C. M. (2004). Gastrointestinal manifestations of AIDS. *Nutrition in Clinical Practice, 19*, 356–364.

45. Antinori A., Arendt G., Becker J. T., et al. (2007). Updated research nosology for HIV-associated neurocognitive disorders. *Neurology, 69*, 1789–1799.

46. Dedicoat M., Livesley N. (2006). Management of toxoplasmic encephalitis in HIV-infected adults (with an emphasis on resource-poor settings). *Cochrane Database of Systematic Reviews, 3*, CD005420.

47. Berger J. R., Houff S. (2006). Progressive multifocal leukoencephalopathy: Lessons from AIDS and natalizumab. *Neurological Research, 28*, 299–305.

48. Roberts M. T. (2005). AIDS-associated progressive multifocal leukoencephalopathy: Current management strategies. *CNS Drugs, 19*, 671–682.

49. Silverberg M. J., Abrams D. I. (2007). AIDS-defining and non-AIDS-defining malignancies: Cancer occurrence in the antiretroviral therapy era. *Current Opinion in Oncology, 19*, 446–451.

50. Frisch M., Biggar R. J., Engels E. A. (2001). Association of cancer with AIDS-related immunosuppression in adults. *Journal of the American Medical Association, 285*, 1736–1745.

51. Antman K., Chang Y. (2000). Kaposi's sarcoma. *New England Journal of Medicine, 342*, 1027–1038.

52. Lim S. T., Karim R., Nathwani B. N., et al. (2005). AIDS-related Burkitt's lymphoma versus diffuse large-cell lymphoma in the pre-highly active antiretroviral therapy (HAART) and HAART eras: Significant differences in survival with standard chemotherapy. *Journal of Clinical Oncology, 23*, 4430–4438.

53. Mounier N., Spina M., Gisselbrecht C. (2007). Modern management of non-Hodgkin lymphoma in HIV-infected patients. *British Journal of Haematology, 136*, 685–698.

54. Einstein M. H., Kadish, A. S. (2004). Anogenital neoplasia in AIDS. *Current Opinion in Oncology, 16*, 455–462.

55. Massad L. S., Fazzari M. J., Anastos K., et al. (2007). Outcomes after treatment of cervical intraepithelial neoplasia among women with HIV. *Journal of Lower Genital Tract Disease, 11*, 90–97.

56. Abramowitz L., Benabderrahmane D., Ravaud P., et al. (2007). Anal squamous intraepithelial lesions and condyloma in HIV-infected heterosexual men, homosexual men and women: Prevalence and associated factors. *Acquired Immunodeficiency Syndrome, 21*, 1457–1465.

57. De Vuyst H., Franceschi S. (2007). Human papillomavirus vaccines in HIV-positive men and women. *Current Opinion in Oncology, 19*, 470–475.

58. Public Health Agency of Canada. (2013). Canadian Immunization Guide. Available online at http://www.phac-aspc.gc.ca/publicat/cig-gci/p03–07-eng.php. Accessed May 25, 2015.

59. Polsky B., Kotler D., Steinhart C. (2004). Treatment guidelines for HIV-associated wasting. *HIV Clinical Trials, 5*, 50–61.

60. Badowski M., Pandit N. S. (2014). Pharmacologic management of human immunodeficiency virus wasting syndrome. *Pharmacotherapy, 34*(8), 868–881.

61. Umeh O. C., Currier J. S. (2005). Lipids, metabolic syndrome, and risk factors for future cardiovascular disease among HIV-infected patients. *Current HIV/AIDS Reports, 2*, 132–139.

62. Brown T. T., Cole S. R., Li X., et al. (2005). Antiretroviral therapy and the prevalence and incidence of diabetes mellitus in the multicenter AIDS cohort study. *Archives of Internal Medicine, 165*, 1179–1184.

63. Howard A. A., Floris-Moore M., Arnsten J. H., et al. (2005). Disorders of glucose metabolism among HIV-infected women. *Clinical Infectious Diseases, 40*, 1492–1499.

64. Hertel J., Struthers H., Horj C. B., et al. (2004). A structural basis for the acute effects of HIV protease inhibitors on GLUT4 intrinsic activity. *Journal of Biological Chemistry, 279*, 55147–55152.

65. Koster J. C., Remedi M. S., Qiu H., et al. (2003). HIV protease inhibitors acutely impair glucose-stimulated insulin release. *Diabetes, 52*, 1695–1700.

66. Riddler S. A., Smit E., Cole S. R., et al. (2003). Impact of HIV infection and HAART on serum lipids in men. *Journal of the American Medical Association, 289*, 2978–2982.

67. Tungsiripat M., Aberg J. A. (2005). Dyslipidemia in HIV-infected individuals [invited review]. *Cleveland Clinic Journal of Medicine, 72*, 1113–1120.

68. Aberg J. A., Gallant J. E., Ghanem K. G., et al; Infectious Diseases Society of America. (2014). Primary care guidelines for the management of persons infected with HIV: 2013 update by the HIV Medicine Association of the Infectious Diseases Society of America. *Clinical Infectious Diseases, 58*(1), e1–e34.

69. Calza L., Manfredi R., Colangeli V., et al. (2005). Substitution of nevirapine or efavirenz for protease inhibitor versus lipid-lowering therapy for the management of dyslipidemia. *Acquired Immunodeficiency Syndrome, 19*, 1051–1058.

70. Tershakovec A. M., Frank I., Rader D. (2004). HIV-related lipodystrophy and related factors. *Atherosclerosis, 174*, 1–10.

71. Mulligan K., Parker R. A., Komarow L., et al. (2006). Mixed patterns of changes in central and peripheral fat following initiation of antiretroviral therapy in a randomized trial. *Journal of Acquired Immune Deficiency Syndromes, 41*, 590–597.

72. Grinspoon S., Carr A. (2005). Cardiovascular risk and body-fat abnormalities in HIV-infected adults. *New England Journal of Medicine, 352*, 48–62.

73. Carr A., Law M. (2003). HIV lipodystrophy case definition study group: An objective lipodystrophy severity grading scale derived from the lipodystrophy case definition score. *Journal of Acquired Immune Deficiency Syndromes, 33*, 571–576.

74. Tien P. C., Benson C., Zolopa A. R., et al. (2006). The study of fat redistribution and metabolic change in HIV Infection (FRAM): Methods, design, and sample characteristics. *American Journal of Epidemiology, 163*, 860–869.

75. Wohl D. A. (2004). Diagnosis and management of body morphology changes and lipid abnormalities associated with HIV Infection and its therapies. *Topics in HIV Medicine, 12*(3), 89–93.

76. McComsey G., Lonergan J. T. (2004). Mitochondrial dysfunction: Patient monitoring and toxicity management. *Journal of Acquired Immune Deficiency Syndromes, 37*(Suppl. 1), S30–S35.

77. Edlin B. R., Irwin K. L., Faruque, S., et al. (1994). Intersecting epidemics: Crack cocaine use and HIV infection among inner-city young adults. Multicenter Crack Cocaine and HIV Infection Study Team. *New England Journal of Medicine, 331*, 1422–1427.

78. Centers for Disease Control and Prevention. (2002). Notice to readers: Approval of a new rapid test for HIV antibody. *Morbidity and Mortality Weekly Report, 51*(46), 1051–1052.

79. Centers for Disease Control and Prevention. (2014). Laboratory testing for the diagnosis of HIV infection: Updated recommendations. Available online at http://stacks.cdc.gov/view/cdc/23447. Accessed May 25, 2015.

80. Strategies for management of antiretroviral therapy (SMART) study group, El-Sadr W. M., Lundgren J. D., et al. (2006). CD4+ count-guided interruption of antiretroviral treatment. *New England Journal of Medicine, 355*, 2283–2296.

81. Palella F. J., Deloria-Knoll M., Chmiel J. S., et al; HIV Outpatient Study Investigators. (2003). Survival benefit of initiating antiretroviral therapy in HIV-infected persons in different CD4+ cell strata. *Annals of Internal Medicine, 138*, 620–626.

82. Panel on Antiretroviral Guidelines for Adult and Adolescents. (2015). Guidelines for the use of antiretroviral agents in HIV-1-infected adults and adolescents. U.S. Department of Health and Human Services. Available online at: www.aidsinfo.nih.gov/ContentFiles/AdultandAdolescent GL.pdf. Accessed May 25, 2015.

83. Lichtenstein K., Armon C., Buchacz K., et al; HIV Outpatient Study (HOPS) Investigators. (2008). Initiation of antiretroviral therapy at higher CD4+ T cell counts ≥ 350 cells/mm^3 does not increase incidence or risk of peripheral neuropathy, anemia, or renal insufficiency. *Journal of Acquired Immune Deficiency Syndromes, 47*(1), 27–35.

84. Rusconi S., Scozzafava A., Mastrolorenzo A., Supuran C T. (2007). An update in the development of HIV entry inhibitors. *Current Topics in Medical Chemistry, 7*, 1273–1289.

85. Gardelli C., Nizi E., Muraglia E., et al. (2007). Discovery and synthesis of HIV integrase inhibitors: Development of potent and orally bioavailable N-methyl pyrimidones. *Journal of Medical Chemistry, 50*, 4953–4975.

86. Maplanka C. (2007). AIDS: Is there an answer to the global pandemic? The immune system in HIV infection and control. *Viral Immunology, 20*, 331–342.

87. Overton E. T., Sungkanuparph S., Powderly W. G., et al. (2005). Undetectable plasma HIV RNA load predicts success after hepatitis B vaccination in HIV-infected persons. *Clinical Infectious Diseases, 41*, 1045–1048.

88. Overton E. T., Nurutdinova D., Sungkanuparph S., et al. (2007). Predictors of immunity after hepatitis A vaccination in HIV-infected persons. *Journal of Viral Hepatitis, 14*, 189–193.

89. Armenian S. H., Han J. Y., Dunaway T. M., Church J A. (2006). Safety and immunogenicity of live varicella virus vaccine in children with human immunodeficiency virus type 1. *Pediatric Infectious Diseases Journal, 25*, 368–370.

90. O'Brien A. M., Oerlemans-Bunn M., Blachfield J. C. (1987). Nursing the AIDS patient at home. *AIDS Patient Care, 1*, 21.

91. Lippman S. W., James W. A., Frierson R. L. (1993). AIDS and the family: Implications for counseling. *AIDS Care, 5*, 71–78.

92. Public Health Agency of Canada. (2014). HIV and AIDS in Canada: Surveillance report to December 31, 2013. Available online at: http://www.phac-aspc.gc.ca/publication/survreport/2013/dec/index-eng.php. Accessed May 25, 2015.

93. Boyer P., Dillon M., Navaie M., et al. (1994). Factors predictive of maternal-fetal transmission of HIV-1. *Journal of American Medical Association, 271*, 1925–1930.

94. Panel on Treatment of HIV-Infected Pregnant Women and Prevention of Perinatal Transmission. (2014). Recommendations for use of antiretroviral drugs in pregnant HIV-1-infected women for maternal health and interventions to reduce perinatal HIV transmission in the United States. Available online at http://aidsinfo.nih.gov/contentfiles/lvguidelines/PerinatalGL.pdf. Accessed May 25, 2015.

95. Guay L., Muskoe P., Fleming T., et al. (1999). Intrapartum and neonatal single-dose nevirapine compared with zidovudine for prevention of mother-to-child transmission of HIV-1 in Kampala, Uganda: HIVNET 012 randomised trial. *Lancet, 354*, 795–802.

Visit thePoint **http://thePoint.lww.com for animations, journal articles, and more!**

Unit VI

Disorders of Cardiovascular Function

Of all body systems, the heart and circulation presented the most difficult puzzle to solve. From the fifth century BC, theories about blood and its movement were linked to the concept of the four elements (fire, earth, air, and water) and the *pneuma*, or life force. According to the Greek physician Galen (AD 130–200), the starting point of the circulatory system was the gut, where food was made into "chyle" and then carried to the liver where it was converted into blood. From the liver, which was believed to be the centre of the circulation, a small amount of blood was sent to the heart and lungs where heat from the heart and pneuma from the air were added, producing an ultimate concoction of "vital spirits" that was carried in the arteries to all parts of the body.

It was not until the work of the English physician William Harvey (1578–1657) that answers to the mysteries of the circulation began to emerge. It was he who first proposed that blood travelled in a circuitous route through the body, being pumped by the active phase of the heart's contraction, not relaxation as had previously been believed. In his studies, Harvey showed that a cut artery in an animal spurts during the heart's contraction. He also demonstrated that the atria of the heart had the same relationship to the ventricles as the ventricles do to the arteries and that blood from the heart was circulated through the lungs, where it was oxygenated. As strange as it may seem today, these concepts were so revolutionary to Harvey's contemporaries that the world's basic understanding of how the body functions was thrown into turmoil.

Structure and Function of the Cardiovascular System

21

The main function of the circulatory system, which consists of the heart and blood vessels, is that of transport. The circulatory system delivers oxygen and nutrients needed for metabolic processes to the tissues; carries waste products from the tissues to the kidneys and other excretory organs for elimination; and circulates electrolytes and hormones needed to regulate body function. It also plays an important role in body temperature regulation, which relies on the circulatory system for transport of core heat to the periphery, where it can be dissipated into the external environment.

ORGANIZATION OF THE CIRCULATORY SYSTEM

After completing this section of the chapter, you should be able to meet the following objectives:

- Compare the function and distribution of blood flow and blood pressure in the systemic and pulmonary circulations.
- State the relation between blood volume and blood pressure in arteries, veins, and capillaries of the circulatory system.

Pulmonary and Systemic Circulations

The circulatory system can be divided into two parts: the *pulmonary circulation,* which moves blood through the lungs and creates a link with the gas-exchange function of the respiratory system, and the *systemic circulation,* which supplies all the other tissues of the body (Fig. 21.1). The blood that is in the heart and pulmonary circulation is sometimes referred to as the *central circulation* and that outside the central circulation as the *peripheral circulation.*

Systemic circuit

Pulmonary circuit

Systemic circuit

Head and upper limbs

Lungs

Heart

Digestive tract

Kidneys

Trunk and lower limbs

FIGURE 21.1 • Systemic and pulmonary circulations. The right side of the heart pumps blood to the lungs, and the left side of the heart pumps blood to the systemic circulation.

The pulmonary circulation consists of the right side of the heart, the pulmonary trunk, the pulmonary arteries, the pulmonary capillaries, and the pulmonary veins. The large pulmonary vessels are unique in that the pulmonary artery is an artery that carries unoxygenated blood and the pulmonary veins are veins that carry oxygenated blood. The pulmonary circulation is considered low pressure and low resistance since it is a short system only involving blood to and from the lungs. The large surface area and low pressure of the pulmonary circulation allow blood to move through the lungs more slowly, which is important for gas exchange. The systemic circulation consists of the left side of the heart, the aorta and its branches, the capillaries that supply the brain and peripheral tissues, and the systemic venous system and the vena cava. The veins from the lower portion of the body merge to form the inferior vena cava and those from the head and upper extremities merge to form the superior vena cava, both of which empty into the right atrium. This systemic circulation is a high-pressure system, as it must transport blood to distant parts of the body, often against the effects of gravity and with much greater arterial vascular tone and resistance.

The heart, which propels blood through the circulatory system, consists of two pumps in series—the right side, which propels blood through the gas-exchange vessels in the lungs, and the left side, which propels blood through the vessels that supply all the other tissues in the body. Both sides of the heart are further divided into two chambers, an *atrium* and a *ventricle*. The atria function as collection chambers for blood returning to the heart and as auxiliary pumps that assist in filling the ventricles. The ventricles are the main pumping chambers of the heart. The right ventricle pumps blood through the pulmonary artery to the lungs and the left ventricle pumps blood through the aorta into the systemic circulation. The ventricular chambers of the right and left heart have inlet valves and outlet valves that act reciprocally (*i.e.*, one set of valves is open while the other is closed) to control the direction of blood flow through the cardiac chambers and into the arteries.

Because it is a closed system, the effective function of the circulatory system requires that the outputs of both sides of the heart must pump the same amount of blood over time. If the output of the left ventricle were to fall below that of the right ventricle, blood would accumulate in the pulmonary circulation. Likewise, if the right ventricle were to pump less effectively than the left ventricle, blood would accumulate in the systemic circulation. However, the left and right ventricles seldom eject exactly the same amount of blood with each beat. This is because blood returning to the heart is affected by activities of daily living such as taking a deep breath or moving from the seated to standing position. These beat-by-beat variations in cardiac output are accommodated by the large storage capabilities of the venous system that allow for temporary changes in blood volume. The accumulation of blood occurs only when the storage capacity of the venous system has been exceeded.

Volume and Pressure Distribution

Blood flow in the circulatory system depends on a blood volume that is sufficient to fill the blood vessels and a pressure difference across the system that provides the force to move blood forward. The total blood volume is a function of age and body weight, ranging from 85 to 90 ml/kg in the

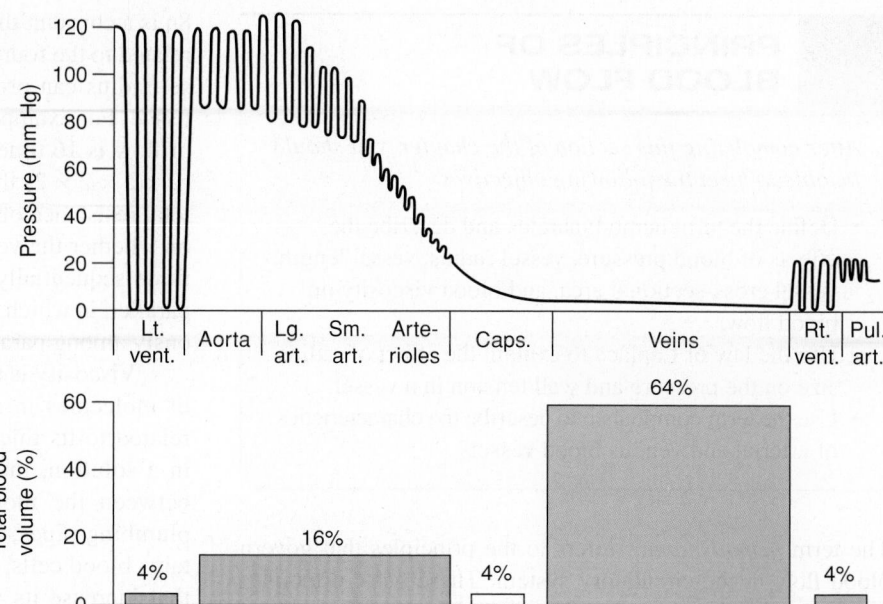

FIGURE 21.2 • Pressure and volume distribution in the systemic circulation. The graphs show the inverse relation between internal pressure and volume in different portions of the circulatory system. (From Smith J. J., Kampine J. P. (1990). *Circulatory physiology: The essentials* (3rd ed.). Baltimore, MD: Williams & Wilkins.)

neonate and from 70 to 75 ml/kg in the adult. As shown in Figure 21.2, approximately 4% of the blood at any given time is in the left heart, 16% is in the arteries and arterioles, 4% is in the capillaries, 64% is in the venules and veins, and 4% is in the right heart. The arteries and arterioles, which have thick, elastic walls and function as a distribution system, have the highest pressure. The capillaries are small, thin-walled vessels that link the arterial and venous sides of the circulation. Because of their small size and large surface area, the capillaries contain a small amount of blood. The venules and veins, which contain the largest amount of blood, are thin-walled, distensible vessels that function as a reservoir to collect blood from the capillaries and return it to the right atrium.

Blood moves from the arterial to the venous side of the circulation along a pressure gradient, moving from an area of higher pressure to an area of lower pressure. The pressure distribution in the different parts of the circulation is almost an inverse of the volume distribution (Fig. 21.2). Thus, the pressure in the arterial side of the systemic circulation, which contains only approximately one sixth of the blood volume, is much greater than the pressure on the venous side of the circulation, which contains approximately two thirds of the blood. This pressure and volume distribution is due in large part to the structure and relative elasticity of the arteries and veins. It is the pressure difference between the arterial and venous sides of the circulation (approximately 84 mm Hg) that provides the driving force for flow of blood in the systemic circulation. The pulmonary circulation has a similar arterial–venous pressure difference, albeit of a lesser magnitude, that facilitates blood flow.

Because the pulmonary and systemic circulations are connected and function as a closed system, blood can be shifted from one circulation to the other. In the pulmonary circulation, the blood volume, which approximates 450 ml in the average-size adult, can vary from as low as 50% of normal to as high as 200% of normal. An increase in intrathoracic pressure, which impedes venous return to the right atrium, can produce a transient shift from the pulmonary to the systemic circulation of as much as 250 ml of blood. Body position also affects the distribution of blood volume. In the recumbent position, approximately 25% to 30% of the total blood volume is in the central circulation. On standing, this blood is rapidly displaced to the lower part of the body due to the forces of gravity. Because the volume of the systemic circulation is approximately seven times that of the pulmonary circulation, a shift of blood from one system to the other has a much greater effect in the pulmonary than in the systemic circulation.

IN SUMMARY

The circulatory system functions as a transport system that circulates nutrients and other materials to the tissues and removes waste products. The circulatory system can be divided into two parts: the pulmonary circulation and the systemic circulation. The heart pumps blood throughout the system, and the blood vessels serve as tubes through which blood flows. The arterial system carries blood from the heart to the tissues and the veins carry it back to the heart. The cardiovascular system is a closed system with a right and left heart connected in series. The systemic circulation, which is served by the left ventricle, provides blood flow for all the tissues except the lungs, which are served by the right heart and the pulmonary circulation. Blood moves throughout the circulation along a pressure gradient, moving from the high-pressure arterial system to the low-pressure venous system. In the circulatory system, pressure is inversely related to volume. The pressure on the arterial side of the circulation, which contains only approximately one sixth of the blood volume, is much greater than the pressure on the venous side of the circulation, which contains approximately two thirds of the blood.

PRINCIPLES OF BLOOD FLOW

After completing this section of the chapter, you should be able to meet the following objectives:

- Define the term hemodynamics and describe the effects of blood pressure, vessel radius, vessel length, vessel cross-sectional area, and blood viscosity on blood flow.
- Use the law of Laplace to explain the effect of radius size on the pressure and wall tension in a vessel.
- Use the term compliance to describe the characteristics of arterial and venous blood vessels.

The term *hemodynamics* refers to the principles that govern blood flow in the circulatory system. These basic principles of physics are the same as those applied to the movement of fluid in general. The concepts of flow, pressure, resistance, and capacitance as applied to blood flow in the cardiovascular system will be used in subsequent chapters to describe the hemodynamic changes that occur with disorders of the cardiovascular system.

Relationships Between Blood Flow, Pressure, and Resistance

The most important factors governing the flow of blood in the cardiovascular system are *pressure, resistance,* and *flow.* Blood flow (Q) through a vessel or series of blood vessels is determined by the pressure difference (ΔP) between the two ends of a vessel (the inlet and the outlet) and the resistance (R) that blood must overcome as it moves through the vessel ($Q = \Delta P/R$). In the cardiovascular system, blood flow is represented by the cardiac output (CO). Resistance is the opposition to flow caused by friction between the moving blood and the stationary vessel wall. In the peripheral circulation, the collective resistance of all the vessels in that part of the circulation is referred to as the *peripheral vascular resistance* (PVR) or, more commonly, as the *systemic vascular resistance* (SVR). The flow, pressure, and resistance relationships also can be applied on a smaller scale to determine the blood flow and resistance to flow of a single organ.

Resistance to Flow

The blood vessels and the blood itself constitute resistance to flow. A helpful equation for understanding the relationship between resistance, blood vessel diameter (radius), and blood viscosity factors that affect blood flow was derived by the French physician Poiseuille more than a century ago. The equation $Q = \Delta P \times \pi \times r^4/8n \times L \times \eta$ expands on the previous equation, $Q = \Delta P/R$, by relating flow to several determinants of resistance—vessel length (L), radius (r), and blood viscosity (η). The length (L) of vessels does not usually change and

8n is a constant that does not change. Because flow is directly related to the fourth power of the radius, small changes in vessel radius can produce large changes in flow to an organ or tissue. For example, if the pressure remains constant, the rate of flow is 16 times greater in a vessel with a radius of 2 mm ($2 \times 2 \times 2 \times 2$) than in a vessel with a radius of 1 mm. The total resistance offered by a set of blood vessels also depends on whether the vessels are arranged in series, in which blood flows sequentially from one vessel to another, or arranged in parallel, in which the total blood flow is distributed simultaneously among parallel vessels.

Viscosity is the resistance to flow caused by the friction of molecules in a fluid. The viscosity of a fluid is largely related to its thickness. The more particles that are present in a solution, the greater the frictional forces that develop between the molecules. Unlike water that flows through plumbing pipes, blood is a nonhomogeneous liquid. It contains blood cells, platelets, fat globules, and plasma proteins that increase its viscosity. The red blood cells, which constitute 40% to 45% of the formed elements of the blood, largely determine the viscosity of the blood. A hematocrit measurement is performed in order to measure the proportion of red blood cells in a blood sample. For example, if a person has a hematocrit of 0.41, then 41% of the blood volume comprises red blood cells. If the hematocrit increases, the viscosity increases and vice versa. Also, under special conditions, temperature may affect viscosity. There is a 2% rise in viscosity for each 1°C decrease in body temperature, a fact that helps explain the sluggish blood flow seen in persons with hypothermia.

Velocity and Cross-Sectional Area

Velocity is a distance measurement. It refers to the rate of displacement of a particle of fluid with respect to time (*e.g.,* centimetres per second). *Flow* is a volume measurement. It refers to the displacement of a volume of fluid with respect to time (*e.g.,* millilitres per second). The flow is determined by the cross-sectional area of a vessel and the velocity of flow. When the flow through a given segment of the circulatory system is constant—as it must be for continuous flow—the velocity is inversely proportional to the cross-sectional area of the vessel (*i.e.,* the smaller the cross-sectional area, the greater the velocity of flow). This phenomenon can be compared with cars moving from a two-lane to a single-lane section of a highway. To keep traffic moving at its original pace, cars would have to double their speed in the single-lane section of the highway. So it is with blood flow in the circulatory system.

The linear velocity of blood flow in the circulatory system varies widely from 30 to 35 cm/second in the aorta to 0.2 to 0.3 mm/second in the capillaries. This is because even though each individual capillary is very small, the total cross-sectional area of all the systemic capillaries greatly exceeds the cross-sectional area of other parts of the circulation. As a result of this large surface area, the slower movement of blood allows ample time for exchange of nutrients, gases, and metabolites between the tissues and the blood.

Understanding   The Hemodynamics of Blood Flow

The term *hemodynamics* is used to describe factors such as (1) pressure and resistance, (2) vessel radius, (3) cross-sectional area and velocity of flow, and (4) laminar versus turbulent flow that affect blood flow through the blood vessels in the body.

1. Pressure, Resistance, and Flow

The flow (Q) of fluid through a tube, such as blood through a blood vessel, is directly related to a pressure difference ($P_1 - P_2$) between the two ends of the tube and inversely proportional to the resistance (R) that the fluid encounters as it moves through the tube.

The resistance to flow, in peripheral resistance units (PRU), is determined by the blood viscosity, vessel radius, and whether the vessels are aligned in series or in parallel. In vessels aligned in series, blood travels sequentially from one vessel to another such that the resistance becomes additive (*e.g.*, $2 + 2 + 2 = 6$ PRU). In vessels aligned in parallel, such as capillaries, the blood is not confined to a single channel but can travel through each of several parallel channels such that the resistance becomes the reciprocal of the total resistance (*i.e.*, $1/R$). As a result, there is no loss of pressure, and the total resistance (*e.g.*, $1/2 + 1/2 + 1/2 = 3/2$ PRU) is less than the resistance of any of the channels (*i.e.*, 2) taken separately.

P_i pressure in; P_o pressure out

2. Vessel Radius

In addition to pressure and resistance, the rate of blood flow through a vessel is affected by the fourth power of its radius (the radius multiplied by itself four times). Thus, blood flow in vessel B with a radius of 2 mm will be 16 times greater than in vessel A with a radius of 1 mm.

3. Cross-Sectional Area and Velocity of Flow

The velocity or rate of forward movement of the blood is affected by the cross-sectional area of a blood vessel. As the cross-sectional area of a vessel increases (sections 1 and 3), blood must flow laterally as well as forward to fill the increased area. As a result, the mean forward velocity decreases. In contrast, when the cross-sectional area is decreased (section 2), the lateral flow decreases and the mean forward velocity is increased.

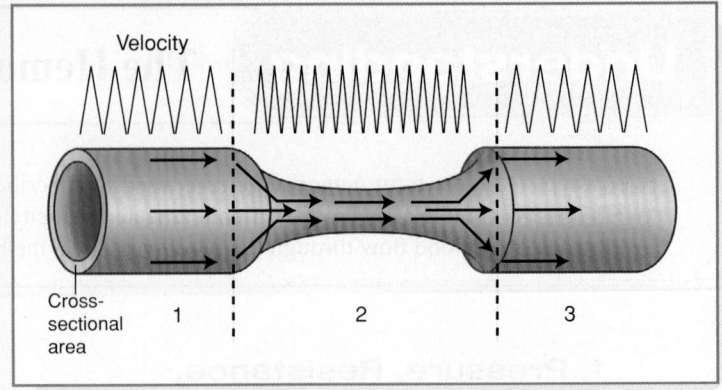

4. Laminar and Turbulent Flow

Blood flow is normally laminar, with platelets and blood cells remaining in the centre or axis of the bloodstream. Laminar blood flow can be described as layered flow in which a thin layer of plasma adheres to the vessel wall, while the inner layers of blood cells and platelets shear against this motionless layer. This allows each layer to move at a slightly faster velocity, with the greatest velocity occurring in the central part of the bloodstream.

Turbulent blood flow is flow in which the blood elements do not remain confined to a definite lamina or layer, but develop vortices (*i.e.*, a whirlpool effect) that push blood cells and platelets against the wall of the vessel. More pressure is required to force a given flow of blood through the same vessel (or heart valve) when the flow is turbulent rather than laminar. Turbulence can result from an increase in velocity of flow, a decrease in vessel diameter, or low blood viscosity. Turbulence is usually accompanied by vibrations of the fluid and surrounding structures. Some of these vibrations in the cardiovascular system are in the audible frequency range and may be detected as murmurs or bruits.

Laminar Versus Turbulent Flow

Ideally, blood flow is *laminar* or *streamlined,* with the blood components arranged in layers so that the plasma is adjacent to the smooth, slippery endothelial surface of the blood vessel, and the blood elements, including the platelets, are in the centre or *axis* of the bloodstream. This arrangement, also called the parabolic velocity profile, reduces friction by allowing the blood layers to slide smoothly over one another, with the axial layer having the most rapid rate of flow.

Under certain conditions, blood flow switches from laminar to turbulent (or disorderly) flow. In turbulent flow, the laminar stream is disrupted and the fluid particles become mixed radially (crosswise) and axially (lengthwise). Because energy is used in propelling blood both radially and axially, more energy (pressure) is required to drive turbulent flow than laminar flow. Turbulent flow can be caused by a number of factors, including high velocity of flow, change in vessel diameter, and low or high blood viscosity. The tendency for turbulence to occur is increased in direct proportion to the velocity of flow. Low blood viscosity allows the blood to move faster and accounts for the transient occurrence of heart murmurs in some persons who are severely anemic. Turbulence is often accompanied by vibrations of the blood and surrounding structures. Some of these vibrations are in the audible range and can be heard using a stethoscope. For example, a heart murmur results from turbulent flow through an impaired heart valve. Turbulent flow may also predispose to clot formation as platelets and other coagulation factors come in contact with the endothelial lining of the vessel.

Wall Tension, Radius, and Pressure

In a blood vessel, *wall tension* is the force in the vessel wall that opposes the distending pressure inside the vessel. The French astronomer and mathematician Pierre de Laplace described the relationship between wall tension, pressure, and the radius of a vessel or sphere more than 200 years ago. This relationship, which has come to be known as the *law of Laplace,* can be expressed by the equation, $P = T/r$, in which T is wall tension, P is the intraluminal pressure, and r is vessel radius. Accordingly, the internal pressure expands the vessel until it is exactly balanced by the tension in the vessel wall. The smaller the radius, the greater the pressure needed to balance the wall tension. The law of Laplace can also be used to express the effect of the radius on wall tension ($T = P \times r$). This correlation can be compared with a partially inflated balloon. Because the pressure in the balloon is equal throughout, the tension in the section with the smaller radius is less than the tension in the section with the larger radius. The same principle holds true for an arterial aneurysm, in which the tension and risk of rupture increase as the aneurysm expands (see Chapter 22).

The law of Laplace was later expanded to include wall thickness ($T = P \times r/\text{wall thickness}$). Wall tension is inversely related to wall thickness, such that the thicker the vessel wall, the lower the tension, and vice versa. In hypertension, arterial vessel walls hypertrophy and become thicker, thereby reducing the tension and minimizing wall stress. The law of Laplace can also be applied to the pressure required to maintain the patency of small blood vessels. Providing that the thickness of a vessel wall remains constant, it takes more pressure to overcome wall tension and keep a vessel open as its radius decreases in size. The *critical closing pressure* refers to the point at which blood vessels collapse so that blood can no longer flow through them. For example, in circulatory shock there is a decrease in blood volume and vessel radii, along with a drop in blood pressure. As a result, many of the small blood vessels collapse as blood pressure drops to the point where it can no longer overcome the wall tension. The collapse of peripheral veins often makes it difficult to insert venous lines that are needed for fluid and blood replacement.

Distension and Compliance

In the vascular system, *compliance* refers to the total quantity of blood that can be stored in a given portion of the circulation for each millimetre of mercury (mm Hg) rise in pressure. Compliance reflects the *distensibility* of the blood vessel. The distensibility of the aorta and large arteries allows them to accommodate the pulsatile output of the heart. The most distensible of all vessels are the veins, which can increase their volume with only slight changes in pressure, allowing them to function as a reservoir for storing large quantities of blood that can be returned to the circulation when it is needed. The compliance of a vein is approximately 24 times that of its corresponding artery because it is 8 times as distensible and has a volume 3 times as great.

IN SUMMARY

Blood flow is influenced by the pressure difference vessel length, radius and cross-sectional area, the viscosity of the blood, and tension of the vessel wall. The rate of flow is directly related to the pressure difference between the two ends of the vessel and the vessel radius and inversely related to vessel length and blood viscosity. The cross-sectional area of a vessel influences the velocity of flow; as the cross-sectional area decreases, the velocity is increased, and vice versa. Laminar blood flow is flow in which there is layering of blood components in the centre of the bloodstream. This reduces frictional forces and prevents clotting factors from coming in contact with the vessel wall. In contrast to laminar flow, turbulent flow is disordered flow, in which the blood moves crosswise and lengthwise in blood vessels. The relation between wall tension, transmural pressure, and radius is described by the law of Laplace, which states that the pressure needed to overcome wall tension becomes greater as the radius decreases. Wall tension is also affected by wall thickness; it increases as the wall becomes thinner and decreases as the wall becomes thicker. Vascular compliance refers to the distensibility of the vessels which affects changes in pressure in relation to changes in volume.

THE HEART AS A PUMP

After completing this section of the chapter, you should be able to meet the following objectives:

- Describe the structural components and function of the pericardium, myocardium, endocardium, and the heart valves and fibrous skeleton.
- Compare the cardiac cycle changes that occur during atrial and ventricular systole and diastole.
- Define the terms preload and afterload.
- State the formula for calculating the cardiac output and explain the effects that preload, afterload, contractility, and heart rate have on cardiac output.
- Describe the cardiac reserve and relate it to the Frank–Starling mechanism.

The heart is a four-chambered muscular pump approximately the size of a person's fist that beats an average of 70 times each minute, 24 hours each day, 365 days each year for a lifetime. In 1 day, this heart pumps more than 6,800 L of blood throughout the body.

Functional Anatomy of the Heart

The heart is located between the lungs in the mediastinal space of the intrathoracic cavity in a loose-fitting sac called the *pericardium.* It is suspended by the great vessels, with its

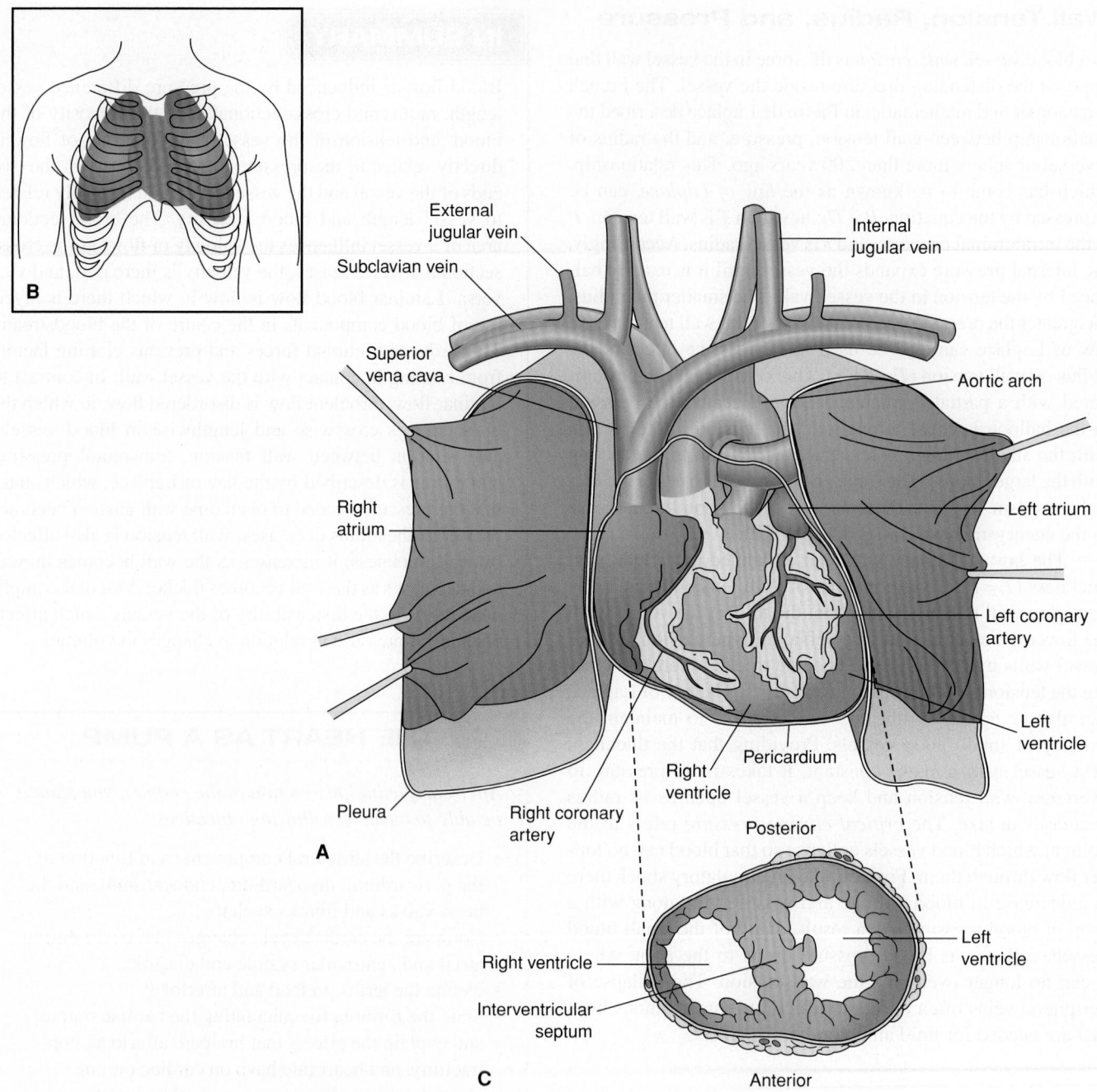

FIGURE 21.3 • **A:** Anterior view of the heart, lungs, and great vessels (note that the lungs, which normally fold over part of the heart's anterior, have been pulled back). **B:** The heart in relation to the sternum, ribs, and lungs. **C:** Cross section of the heart showing the increased thickness of the left ventricle compared with the right.

broader side (*i.e.,* base) facing upward and its tip (*i.e.,* apex) pointing downward, forward, and to the left. The heart is positioned obliquely, so that the right side of the heart is almost fully in front of the left side of the heart, with only a small portion of the lateral left ventricle on the frontal plane of the heart (Fig. 21.3). When the hand is placed on the thorax, the main impact of the heart's contraction is felt against the chest wall at a point between the fifth and sixth ribs, a little below the nipple and approximately 7 cm to the left of the midsternal line. This is called the *point of maximum impulse (PMI).*

The wall of the heart is composed of an outer epicardium, which lines the pericardial cavity; the myocardium or muscle layer; and the smooth endocardium, which lines the chambers of the heart (Fig. 21.4). A fibrous skeleton supports the valvular structures of the heart. The interatrial and interventricular septa divide the heart into a right and a left pump, each composed of two muscular chambers: A thin-walled atrium, which serves as a reservoir for blood coming into the heart, and a thick-walled ventricle, which pumps blood out of the heart. The increased thickness of the left ventricular wall compared

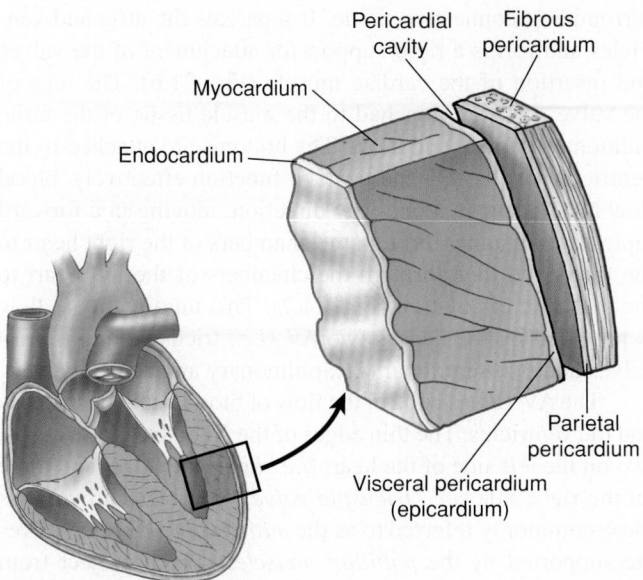

FIGURE 21.4 • Layers of the heart, showing the visceral pericardium, pericardial cavity, parietal pericardium, fibrous pericardium, myocardium, and endocardium.

to the right ventricle results from the additional work this ventricle is required to perform.

Pericardium

The pericardium forms a fibrous covering around the heart, holding it in a fixed position in the thorax and providing physical protection and a barrier to infection. The pericardium consists of a tough, outer fibrous layer and a thin, inner serous layer. The outer fibrous layer is attached to the great vessels that enter and leave the heart, the sternum, and the diaphragm. The fibrous pericardium is highly resistant to distension; it prevents acute dilation of the heart chambers and exerts a restraining effect on the left ventricle. The inner serous layer consists of a visceral layer and a parietal layer. The visceral layer, also known as the *epicardium,* covers the entire heart and great vessels and then folds over to form the parietal layer that lines the fibrous pericardium (Fig. 21.4). Between the visceral and parietal layers is the *pericardial cavity,* a potential space that contains 30 to 50 ml of serous fluid. This fluid acts as a lubricant to minimize friction as the heart contracts and relaxes.

Myocardium

The myocardium, or muscular portion of the heart, forms the wall of the atria and ventricles. Cardiac muscle cells, like skeletal muscle, are striated and composed of *sarcomeres* that contain actin and myosin filaments (see Chapter 4). They are smaller and more compact than skeletal muscle cells and contain numerous large mitochondria, reflecting their continuous energy needs.

The contractile properties of cardiac muscle are similar to those of skeletal muscle, except the contractions are involuntary and the duration of contraction is much longer. Unlike the orderly longitudinal arrangement of skeletal muscle fibres,

THE HEART

- The heart is a four-chambered pump consisting of two atria (the right atrium, which receives blood returning to the heart from the systemic circulation, and the left atrium, which receives oxygenated blood from the lungs) and two ventricles (a right ventricle, which pumps blood to the lungs, and a left ventricle, which pumps blood into the systemic circulation).
- Heart valves control the direction of blood flow from the atria to the ventricles (the atrioventricular [AV] valves), from the right side of the heart to the lungs (pulmonic valve), and from the left side of the heart to the systemic circulation (aortic valve).
- The myocardium, or muscle layer of the atria and ventricles, produces the pumping action of the heart. Intercalated disks between cardiac muscle cells contain gap junctions that allow for immediate communication of electrical signals from one cell to another so the cardiac muscle acts as a single unit, or syncytium.
- The cardiac cycle is divided into two major periods: Systole, when the ventricles are contracting, and diastole, when the ventricles are relaxed and filling.
- The cardiac output or amount of blood that the heart pumps each minute is determined by the amount of blood pumped with each beat (stroke volume [SV]) and the number of times the heart beats each minute (heart rate). Cardiac reserve refers to the maximum percentage of increase in cardiac output that can be achieved above the normal resting level.
- The work of the heart is determined by the volume of blood it pumps out (preload), the pressure that it must generate to pump the blood out of the heart (afterload), the strength of contraction, and the heart rate.

cardiac muscle cells are arranged as an interconnecting latticework, with their fibres dividing, recombining, and then dividing again (Fig. 21.5A). The fibres are separated from neighbouring cardiac muscle cells by dense structures called *intercalated disks.* The intercalated disks, which are unique to cardiac muscle, contain gap junctions that serve as low-resistance pathways for passage of ions and electrical impulses from one cardiac cell to another (Fig. 21.5B). Thus, the myocardium behaves as a single unit, or *syncytium,* rather than as a group of isolated units, as does skeletal muscle. When one myocardial cell becomes excited, the impulse travels rapidly so the heart can beat as a unit. The heart muscle has an atrial syncytium, which constitutes the walls of the atria, and a ventricular syncytium, which constitutes the walls of the ventricles. This allows the atria to contract prior to the ventricles for optimum heart filling and pumping.

As in skeletal muscle, cardiac muscle contraction involves actin and myosin filaments, which interact and slide along one another during muscle contraction. A number of important proteins regulate actin–myosin binding. These include tropomyosin and the troponin complex (see Chapter 4, Fig. 4.22). The

FIGURE 21.5 • A: Cardiac muscle fibres, showing their branching structure. **B:** Area indicated where cell junctions lie in the intercalated disks.

troponin complex consists of three subunits (troponin T, troponin I, and troponin C) that regulate calcium-mediated contraction in striated muscle. In clinical practice, the measurement of serum levels of the specific cardiac forms of either troponin T or troponin I are used in the diagnosis of myocardial infarction (see Chapter 24).

Although cardiac muscle cells require calcium for contraction, they have a less well-defined sarcoplasmic reticulum for storing calcium than skeletal muscle cells. Thus, cardiac muscle relies more heavily than skeletal muscle on an influx of extracellular calcium ions for contraction. The cardiac glycosides (*e.g.,* digoxin) are inotropic drugs that increase cardiac contractility by increasing the free calcium concentration in the vicinity of the actin and myosin filaments.

Endocardium

The endocardium is a thin, three-layered membrane that lines the heart. The innermost layer consists of smooth endothelial cells supported by a thin layer of connective tissue. The endothelial lining of the endocardium is continuous with the lining of the blood vessels that enter and leave the heart. The middle layer consists of dense connective tissue with elastic fibres. The outer layer, composed of irregularly arranged connective tissue cells, contains blood vessels and branches of the conduction system and is continuous with the myocardium.

Heart Valves and Fibrous Skeleton

An important structural feature of the heart is its fibrous skeleton, which consists of four interconnecting valve rings and

surrounding connective tissue. It separates the atria and ventricles and forms a rigid support for attachment of the valves and insertion of the cardiac muscle (Fig. 21.6). The tops of the valve rings are attached to the muscle tissue of the atria, pulmonary trunks, and aorta. The bottoms are attached to the ventricular walls. For the heart to function effectively, blood flow must occur in a one-way direction, moving in a forward (antegrade) manner through the chambers of the right heart to the lungs and then through the chambers of the left heart to the systemic circulation (Fig. 21.7). This unidirectional flow is provided by the heart's two AV (*i.e.,* tricuspid and mitral) valves and two semilunar (*i.e.,* pulmonary and aortic) valves.

The AV valves control the flow of blood between the atria and the ventricles. The thin edges of the AV valves form cusps, two on the left side of the heart (*i.e., bicuspid valve*) and three on the right side (*i.e., tricuspid valve*). The bicuspid valve is more commonly referred to as the *mitral valve*. The AV valves are supported by the *papillary muscles,* which project from the wall of the ventricles, and the *chordae tendineae,* which attach to the valve (Fig. 21.8). Contraction of the papillary muscles at the onset of systole ensures closure by producing

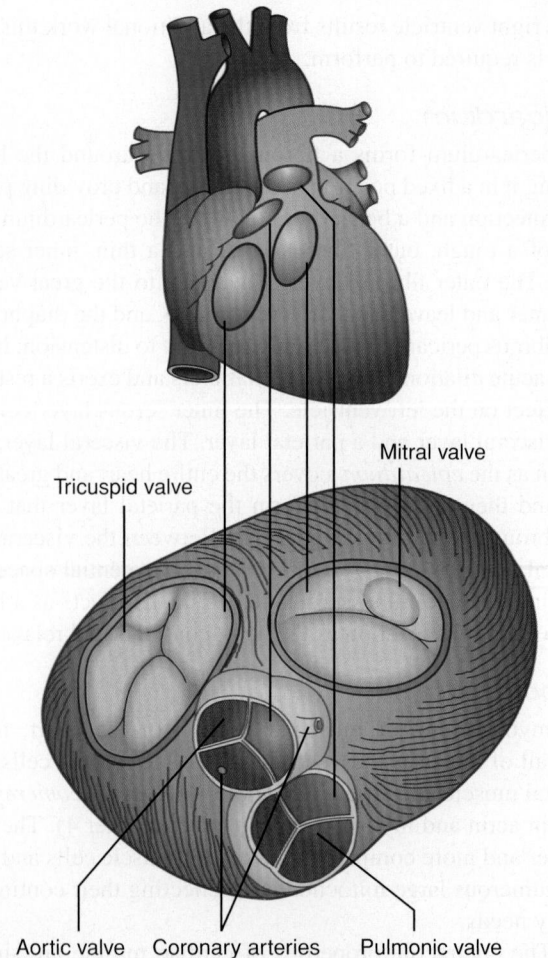

FIGURE 21.6 • Fibrous skeleton of the heart, which forms the four interconnecting valve rings and support for attachment of the valves and insertion of cardiac muscle.

FIGURE 21.7 • Valvular structures of the heart. *Arrows* show the course of blood flow through the heart chambers. The atrioventricular valves are in an open position, and the semilunar valves are closed. There are no valves to control the flow of blood at the inflow channels (*i.e.,* vena cava and pulmonary veins) to the heart. (Modified from Day R. A., Paul P., Williams B., et al. (2010). *Brunner and Suddarth's textbook of Canadian medical-surgical nursing* (2nd ed., p. 734). Philadelphia, PA: Lippincott Williams & Wilkins.)

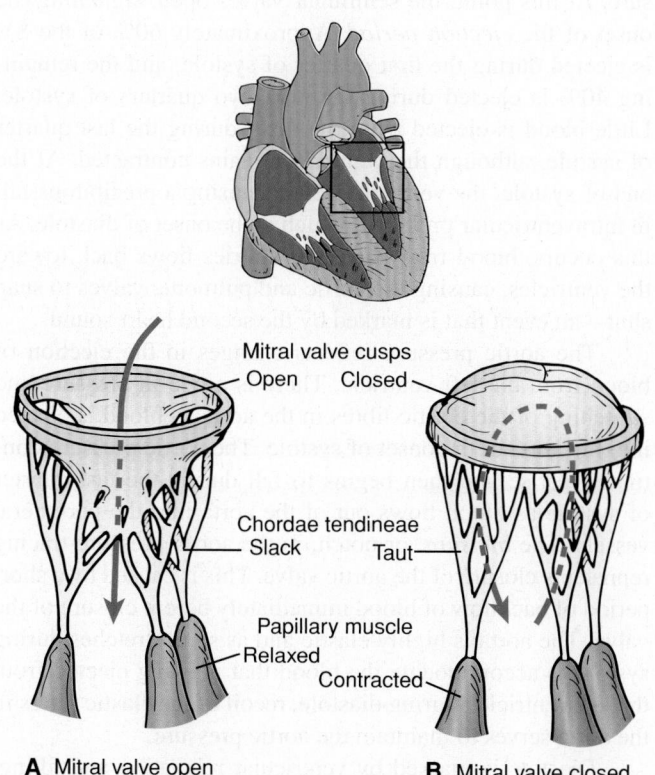

FIGURE 21.8 • The mitral (atrioventricular) valve showing the papillary muscles and chordae tendineae. **A:** The open mitral valve with relaxed papillary muscles and slack chordae tendineae. **B:** The closed mitral valve with contracted papillary muscles and taut chordae tendineae that prevent the valve cusps from everting into the atria.

tension on the leaflets of the AV valves before the full force of ventricular contraction pushes against them. The chordae tendineae are cord-like structures that support the AV valves and prevent them from everting into the atria during systole.

The *aortic* and *pulmonic valves* control the movement of blood out of the ventricles. The pulmonic valve, which is located between the right ventricle and the pulmonary artery, controls the flow of blood into the pulmonary circulation, and the aortic valve, located between the left ventricle and the aorta, controls the flow of blood into the systemic circulation. Because their flaps are shaped like half-moons, they are often referred to as the *semilunar valves*. These semilunar valves have three cup-like cusps that are attached to the valve rings (Fig. 21.9A). These cup-like structures collect the *retrograde,* or backward, flow of blood that occurs toward the end of systole, enhancing closure. For the development of a perfect seal along the free edges of the semilunar valves, each valve cusp must have a triangular shape, which is facilitated by a nodular thickening at the apex of each leaflet (Fig. 21.9B). Behind the semilunar valves are the *sinuses of Valsalva*. In these sinuses, eddy currents develop that tend to keep the valve cusps away from the vessel walls. The openings for the coronary arteries are located behind the right and left cusps, respectively, of the aortic valve. Were it not for the presence of the sinuses of Valsalva and the eddy currents, the coronary artery openings would be blocked by the valve cusps.

There are no valves at the atrial sites (*i.e.,* venae cavae and pulmonary veins) where blood enters the heart. In health, when the atria contract, the opening to the veins is essentially closed

Wall of aorta

Orifices of coronary arteries

Nodule at apex

Line of thickening

Valve leaflet

B

Left ventricle

A

FIGURE 21.9 • Diagram of the aortic valve. **A:** The appearance of the three leaflets of the aortic valve when the aorta is cut open and spread out flat. **B:** The position of the aortic valve at the base of the ascending aorta is indicated. (From Cormack D. H. (1987). *Ham's histology* (9th ed.). Philadelphia, PA: J.B. Lippincott.)

and minimal backflow occurs. However, excess blood is pushed back into the veins when the atria become distended. For example, the jugular veins typically become prominent in severe right-sided heart failure when they normally should be flat or collapsed. Likewise, the pulmonary venous system becomes congested when outflow from the left atrium is impeded.

Cardiac Cycle

The term *cardiac cycle* is used to describe the rhythmic pumping action of the heart. The cardiac cycle is divided into two parts: *Systole,* the period during which the ventricles are contracting, and *diastole,* the period during which the ventricles are relaxed and filling with blood. Simultaneous changes occur in left atrial pressure, left ventricular pressure, aortic pressure, ventricular volume, the electrocardiogram (ECG), and heart sounds during the cardiac cycle (Fig. 21.10).

The electrical activity, recorded on the ECG, precedes the mechanical events of the cardiac cycle. The small, rounded P wave of the ECG represents depolarization of the atrial muscle mass. The QRS complex represents depolarization of the ventricular conduction system and the ventricular muscle mass. The T wave on the ECG occurs during the last half of systole and represents repolarization of the ventricles. The cardiac conduction system and the ECG are discussed in detail in Chapter 25.

Ventricular Systole and Diastole

Ventricular systole is divided into two periods: the isovolumetric contraction period and the ejection period. The *isovolumetric contraction period,* which begins with closure of the AV valves and occurrence of the first heart sound, heralds the onset of systole. Immediately after closure of the AV valves, there is an additional 0.02 to 0.03 second during which the semilunar (pulmonary and aortic) valves remain closed. During this period (Fig. 21.10), the ventricular pressures rise

abruptly because the ventricles start to change shape and build tension. The volume does not change because both the AV and semilunar valves are closed and no blood is leaving the ventricles. The ventricles continue to contract until left ventricular pressure is slightly higher than aortic pressure and right ventricular pressure is higher than pulmonary artery pressure. At this point, the semilunar valves open, signalling the onset of the *ejection period.* Approximately 60% of the SV is ejected during the first quarter of systole, and the remaining 40% is ejected during the next two quarters of systole. Little blood is ejected from the heart during the last quarter of systole, although the ventricle remains contracted. At the end of systole, the ventricles relax, causing a precipitous fall in intraventricular pressures which is the onset of diastole. As this occurs, blood from the large arteries flows back toward the ventricles, causing the aortic and pulmonic valves to snap shut—an event that is marked by the second heart sound.

The aortic pressure reflects changes in the ejection of blood from the left ventricle. There is a rise in pressure and stretching of the elastic fibres in the aorta as blood is ejected into the aorta at the onset of systole. The aortic pressure continues to rise and then begins to fall during the last quarter of systole as blood flows out of the aorta into the peripheral vessels. The *incisura,* or notch, in the aortic pressure tracing represents closure of the aortic valve. This is caused by a short period of backflow of blood immediately before closure of the valve. The aorta is highly elastic and as such stretches during systole to accommodate the blood that is being ejected from the left ventricle. During diastole, recoil of the elastic fibres in the aorta serves to maintain the aortic pressure.

Diastole is marked by ventricular relaxation and filling. After closure of the semilunar valves, the ventricles continue to relax for another 0.03 to 0.06 second. During this time, which is referred to as the *isovolumetric relaxation period,* both the semilunar and AV valves remain closed and the ventricular volume remains the same, as the ventricular pressure drops until

FIGURE 21.10 • **(Top)** Events in the left side of the heart, showing changes in aortic pressure, left ventricular pressure, atrial pressure, left ventricular volume, the electrocardiogram (ECG), and heart sounds during the cardiac cycle. **(Bottom)** Position of the atrioventricular and semilunar valves during **(A)** isovolumetric contraction and ventricular ejection, **(B)** isovolumetric relaxation and ventricular filling, and **(C)** atrial contraction.

it becomes less than the atrial pressure (Fig. 21.10). As this occurs, the AV valves open and blood that has been accumulating in the atria during systole rapidly moves into the ventricles. Most of ventricular filling occurs during the first third of diastole, which is called the *rapid filling period.* During the middle third of diastole, inflow into the ventricles is almost at a standstill. The last third of diastole is marked by atrial contraction, also referred to as the *atrial kick,* which gives additional volume to ventricular filling. When audible, the third heart

sound is heard during the rapid filling period of diastole as blood flows into a distended ventricle. The fourth heart sound is always abnormal. It occurs during the last third of diastole when the atria contract into a noncompliant ventricle.

During diastole, the ventricles increase their volume to approximately 120 ml (*i.e.,* the *end-diastolic volume*), and at the end of systole, approximately 50 ml of blood (*i.e.,* the *end-systolic volume*) remains in the ventricles (Fig. 21.10). The difference between the end-diastolic and end-systolic volumes (approximately 70 ml) is called the *stroke volume*. The *ejection fraction*, which is the SV divided by the end-diastolic volume, represents the fraction or percentage of the end-diastolic volume that is ejected from the heart during systole. The left ventricular ejection fraction (normally about 55% to 75% when determined by echocardiography or angiocardiography) is frequently used to evaluate the cardiac function of persons with a variety of heart diseases.

Atrial Filling and Contraction

There are three main atrial pressure waves that occur during the cardiac cycle—the a, c, and v waves. The *a wave* occurs during the last part of ventricular diastole and is caused by atrial contraction. The *c wave* occurs as the ventricles begin to contract and their increased pressure causes the AV valves to bulge into the atria. The *v wave* occurs toward the end of systole when the AV valves are still closed and results from a slow buildup of blood in the atria. The right atrial pressure waves are transmitted to the internal jugular veins as pulsations. These pulsations can be observed visually or electronically, and may be used to assess cardiac function. For example, exaggerated a waves occur when the volume of the right atrium is increased because of impaired emptying into the right ventricle.

Because there are no valves between the junctions of the central veins (*i.e.*, venae cavae and pulmonary veins) and the atria, atrial filling occurs during both ventricular systole and diastole. During normal quiet breathing, right atrial pressure usually varies between –2 and +2 mm Hg. It is this low atrial pressure that maintains the movement of blood from the systemic circulation into the right atrium and from the pulmonary veins into the left atrium.

Right atrial pressure is regulated by a balance between the ability of the heart to move blood out of the right ventricle and through the left ventricle into the systemic circulation and the tendency of blood to flow from the peripheral circulation into the right atrium. When the heart pumps strongly, right atrial pressure is decreased and atrial filling is enhanced. Right atrial pressure is also affected by changes in intrathoracic pressure. It is decreased during inspiration when intrathoracic pressure becomes more negative, and it is increased during coughing or forced expiration when intrathoracic pressure becomes more positive. For example, venous return is a reflection of the amount of blood in the systemic circulation that is available for return to the right heart and the force that moves blood back to the right side of the heart. Venous return is increased when the blood volume is expanded or when right atrial pressure falls, and it is decreased in hypovolemic shock or when right atrial pressure rises.

Although the main function of the atria is to store blood as it enters the heart, these chambers also act as pumps that aid in ventricular filling. This function becomes more important during periods of increased activity when the diastolic filling time is decreased because of an increase in heart rate or when heart disease impairs ventricular filling. In these two situations, the cardiac output would fall drastically were it not for the action of the atria. It has been estimated that this atrial contraction can contribute as much as 30% to cardiac reserve during periods of increased need, while having little or no effect on cardiac output during rest.

Regulation of Cardiac Performance

The effectiveness of the heart as a pump is often measured in terms of *cardiac output* or the amount of blood the heart pumps each minute. The cardiac output (CO) is the product of the *stroke volume* (SV) and the *heart rate* (HR) and can be expressed by the equation: CO = SV × HR. The cardiac output varies with body size and the metabolic needs of the tissues. It increases with physical activity and decreases during rest and sleep. The average cardiac output in normal adults ranges from 3.5 to 8.0 L/minute. In the highly trained athlete, this value can increase to levels as high as 40 L/minute during maximum exercise.

The *cardiac reserve* refers to the maximum percentage of increase in cardiac output that can be achieved above the normal resting level. The normal young adult has a cardiac reserve of approximately 300% to 400%. Cardiac performance is influenced by the work demands of the heart and the ability of the coronary circulation to meet its metabolic needs.

The heart's ability to increase its output according to body needs mainly depends on four factors: the *preload*, or ventricular filling; the *afterload*, or resistance to ejection of blood from the heart; *cardiac contractility*; and the *heart rate*. Heart rate and cardiac contractility are strictly cardiac factors, meaning they originate in the heart, although they are controlled by various neural and humoral mechanisms. Preload and afterload, on the other hand, are mutually dependent on the behaviours of the heart and the vasculature. Not only do preload and afterload contribute to cardiac output, they are themselves determined by the cardiac output and certain vascular characteristics.

Preload

Preload is the work or load imposed on the ventricle immediately before the contraction begins. It is the volume of blood stretching the ventricle muscle at the end of diastole and is determined by the volume at the end of systole (*end-systolic volume*) and the venous return to the heart. During any given cardiac cycle, the maximum volume of blood filling the ventricle is present at the end of diastole. Known as the *end-diastolic volume*, this volume causes an increase in the length of the myocardial muscle fibres. Factors that influence preload include total blood volume, ventricular compliance, vascular tone, heart rate and rhythm, afterload, contractility, and valve competency.

The *Frank–Starling mechanism* or Starling law of the heart (Fig. 21.11) refers to the relationship between venous return and the force of contraction. Within limits, as preload increases, the stroke volume increases in accord with the Frank–Starling mechanism. Venous return affects ventricular end-diastolic volume (VEDV), muscle length, and therefore stroke volume. The anatomic arrangement of the actin and

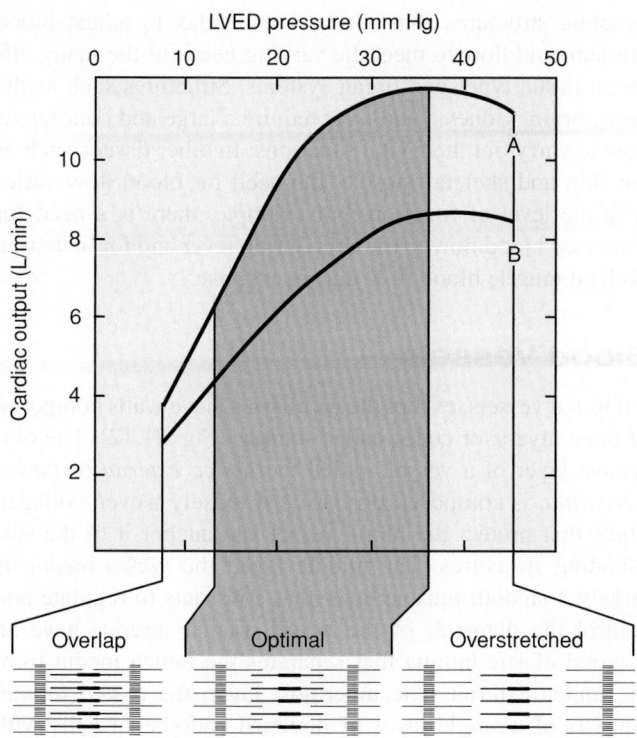

FIGURE 21.11 • The Frank–Starling ventricular function curve in a normal heart. (**Top**) An increase in left ventricular end-diastolic (LVED) pressure produces an increase in cardiac output (*curve B*) by means of the Frank–Starling mechanism. The maximum force of contraction and increased stroke volume are achieved when diastolic filling causes the muscle fibres to be stretched about two and one half times their resting length. In *curve A*, an increase in cardiac contractility produces an increase in cardiac output without a change in LVED volume and pressure. (**Bottom**) Stretching of the actin and myosin filaments at the different LVED filling pressures.

myosin filaments in the myocardial muscle fibres is such that the tension or force of contraction depends on the degree to which the muscle fibres are stretched just before the ventricles begin to contract. The maximum force of contraction and cardiac output is achieved when venous return produces an increase in ventricular end-diastolic filling (*i.e.,* preload) such that the muscle fibres are stretched to about two and one half times their normal resting length. When the muscle fibres are stretched to this degree, there is optimal overlap of the actin and myosin filaments needed for maximal contraction.

The Frank–Starling mechanism allows the heart to adjust its pumping ability to accommodate various levels of venous return. Thus, when a greater amount of blood flows into the ventricles, the heart accommodates with the cardiomyocytes being stretched to greater lengths. Conversely, cardiac output will be less when decreased filling causes excessive overlap of the actin and myosin filaments or when excessive filling causes the filaments to be pulled too far apart.

Afterload

Afterload is the pressure or tension work of the heart. It is the pressure that the ventricle must generate to move blood into the aorta. It is called the afterload because it is the work presented to the ventricle after the contraction has commenced. The systemic arterial blood pressure is the main source of afterload work on the left ventricle and the pulmonary arterial pressure is the main source of afterload work on the right ventricle. The afterload work of the left ventricle is also increased with narrowing (*i.e.,* stenosis) of the aortic valve. For example, in the late stages of aortic stenosis, the left ventricle may need to generate systolic pressures up to 300 mm Hg to move blood through the diseased valve.

Cardiac Contractility

Cardiac contractility refers to the ability of the heart to change its force of contraction without changing its resting (*i.e.,* diastolic) length. The contractile state of the myocardial muscle is determined by biochemical and biophysical properties that govern the actin and myosin interactions in the myocardial cells. It is strongly influenced by the number of calcium ions that are available to participate in the contractile process.

An *inotropic* effect is one that modifies the contractile state of the myocardium independent of the Frank–Starling mechanism (Fig. 21.11, top curve). For example, sympathetic stimulation produces a positive inotropic effect by increasing the calcium that is available for interaction between the actin and myosin filaments. Hypoxia exerts a negative inotropic effect by interfering with the generation of adenosine triphosphate (ATP), which is needed for muscle contraction.

Heart Rate

The heart rate determines the frequency with which blood is ejected from the heart. Therefore, as the heart rate increases, cardiac output tends to increase. As the heart rate increases, the time spent in diastole is reduced, and there is less time for the ventricles to fill. At a heart rate of 75 beats per minute, one cardiac cycle lasts 0.8 second, of which approximately 0.3 second is spent in systole and approximately 0.5 second in diastole. As the heart rate increases, the time spent in systole remains approximately the same, whereas that spent in diastole decreases. This leads to a decrease in stroke volume and, at excessively high heart rates (tachycardia), a decrease in cardiac output. One of the dangers of tachycardia is a reduction in cardiac output because the heart does not have time to fill adequately.

IN SUMMARY

The heart is a four-chambered muscular pump that lies in the pericardial sac within the mediastinal space of the intrathoracic cavity. The wall of the heart is composed of an outer epicardium, which lines the pericardial cavity; a fibrous skeleton; the myocardium, or muscle layer; and the smooth endocardium, which lines the chambers of the heart. The four heart valves control the direction of blood flow.

The cardiac cycle describes the pumping action of the heart. It is divided into two parts: Systole, during which the ventricles contract and blood is ejected, and diastole, during which the ventricles are relaxed and filling with blood. The stroke volume (approximately 70 ml) represents the difference between the end-diastolic volume (approximately 120 ml) and the end-systolic volume (approximately 50 ml). The electrical activity of the heart, as represented on the ECG, precedes the mechanical events of the cardiac cycle. The heart sounds signal the closing of the heart valves during the cardiac cycle. Atrial contraction occurs during the last third of diastole. Although the main function of the atria is to store blood as it enters the heart, atrial contraction acts to increase cardiac output during periods of increased activity when the filling time is reduced or in disease conditions in which ventricular filling is impaired.

The heart's ability to increase its output according to body needs depends on the preload, or filling of the ventricles (*i.e.,* end-diastolic volume); the afterload, or resistance to ejection of blood from the heart; cardiac contractility, which determines the force of contraction; and the heart rate, which determines the frequency with which blood is ejected from the heart. The maximum force of cardiac contraction occurs when an increase in preload stretches muscle fibres of the heart to approximately two and one half times their resting length (*i.e.,* Frank–Starling mechanism).

 CONCEPTSin action**ANIMATI☼N**

THE SYSTEMIC CIRCULATION AND CONTROL OF BLOOD FLOW

After completing this section of the chapter, you should be able to meet the following objectives:

- Compare the structure and function of arteries and veins.
- Describe the structure and function of vascular smooth muscle.
- Use the equation blood pressure = cardiac output × systemic vascular resistance to explain the regulation of arterial blood pressure.
- Define autoregulation and characterize mechanisms responsible for short-term and long-term regulation of blood flow.
- Describe mechanisms involved in the humoral control of blood flow.

The vascular system functions in the delivery of oxygen and nutrients and removal of waste products from the tissues. It consists of the arteries and arterioles, the capillaries, and the venules and veins. Although blood vessels of the vascular system are often compared with a system of rigid pipes and tubes, this analogy serves only as a starting point. Blood vessels are

dynamic structures that constrict and relax to adjust blood pressure and flow to meet the varying needs of the many different tissue types and organ systems. Structures such as the heart, brain, kidneys, and liver require a large and continuous flow to carry out their vital functions. In other tissues such as the skin and skeletal muscle, the need for blood flow varies with the level of function. For example, there is a need for increased blood flow to the skin during fever and for increased skeletal muscle blood flow during exercise.

Blood Vessels

All blood vessels, except the capillaries, have walls composed of three layers, or coats, called *tunicae* (Fig. 21.12). The outermost layer of a vessel, called the *tunica externa* or *tunica adventitia,* is composed primarily of loosely woven collagen fibres that protect the blood vessel and anchor it to the surrounding structures. The middle layer, the *tunica media,* is largely a smooth muscle layer that constricts to regulate and control the diameter of the vessel. Larger arteries have an external elastic lamina that separates the tunica media from the tunica externa. The innermost layer, the *tunica intima,* consists of a single layer of flattened endothelial cells with minimal underlying subendothelial connective tissue. The endothelial layer provides a smooth and slippery inner surface for the vessel. This smooth inner lining, as long as it remains intact, prevents platelet adherence and blood clotting.

The layers of the different types of blood vessels vary with vessel function. The walls of the arterioles, which control blood pressure, have large amounts of smooth muscle. Veins are thin-walled, distensible, and collapsible vessels.

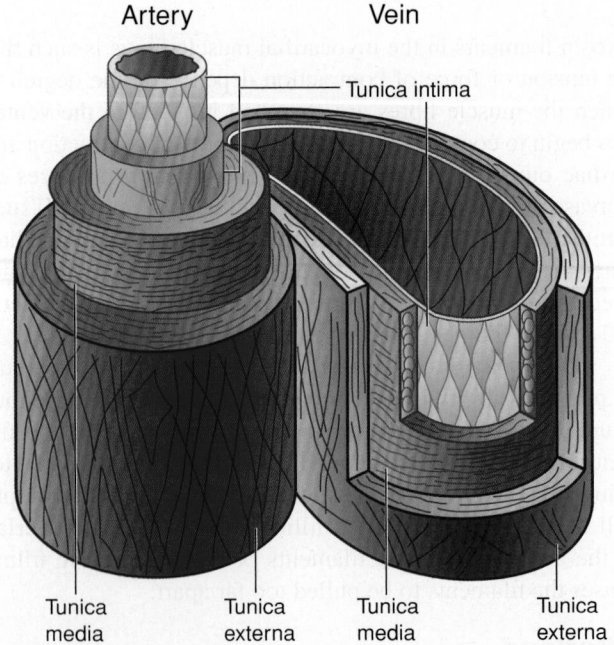

FIGURE 21.12 • Medium-sized artery and vein, showing the relative thicknesses of the three layers.

Capillaries are single-cell vessels designed for the exchange of gases, nutrients, and waste materials.

Vascular Smooth Muscle

Vascular smooth muscle cells, which form the predominant cellular layer in the tunica media, produce vasoconstriction or dilation of blood vessels. Smooth muscle contracts slowly and generates high forces for long periods with low-energy requirements; it uses only 1/10 to 1/300 the energy of skeletal muscle. These characteristics are important in structures, such as blood vessels, that must maintain their tone day in and day out.

Compared with skeletal and cardiac muscles, smooth muscle has less well-developed sarcoplasmic reticulum for storing intracellular calcium, and it has very few fast sodium channels. Depolarization of smooth muscle instead relies largely on extracellular calcium, which enters through calcium channels in the muscle membrane. Sympathetic nervous system control of vascular smooth muscle tone occurs through receptor-activated opening and closing of the calcium channels. In general, α-adrenergic receptors are excitatory in that they cause the channels to open and produce vasoconstriction, and β-adrenergic receptors are inhibitory in that they cause the channels to close and produce vasodilation. Calcium channel–blocking drugs cause vasodilation by blocking calcium entry through the calcium channels.

Smooth muscle contraction and relaxation also occur in response to local tissue factors such as lack of oxygen, increased hydrogen ion concentrations, and excess carbon dioxide. Nitric oxide (formerly known as the *endothelial relaxing factor*) acts locally to produce smooth muscle relaxation and regulate blood flow. These factors are discussed more fully in the section on Local and Humoral Control of Blood Flow.

Arterial System

The arterial system consists of the large and medium-sized arteries and the arterioles. Arteries are thick-walled vessels with large amounts of elastic fibres. The elasticity of these vessels allows them to stretch during systole, when the heart contracts and blood enters the circulation, and to recoil during diastole, when the heart relaxes. The arterioles, which are predominantly smooth muscle, serve as resistance vessels for the circulatory system. They act as control valves through which blood is released as it moves into the capillaries. Changes in the activity of sympathetic fibres that innervate these vessels cause them to constrict or to relax as needed to maintain blood pressure, flow, and perfusion.

Arterial Pressure Pulsations

The delivery of blood to the tissues of the body depends on pressure pulsations or waves of pressure that are generated by the intermittent ejection of blood from the left ventricle into the distensible aorta and large arteries of the arterial system. The arterial pressure pulse represents the energy that is transmitted from molecule to molecule along the length of the vessel (Fig. 21.13). In the aorta, this pressure pulse is transmitted at a velocity of 4 to 6 m/second, which is approximately 20 times faster than the flow of blood. Therefore, the pressure pulse has no direct relation to blood flow and could occur if there was no flow at all. When taking a pulse, it is the pressure

FIGURE 21.13 • Amplification of the arterial pressure wave as it moves forward in the peripheral arteries. This amplification occurs as a forward-moving pressure wave merges with a backward-moving reflected pressure wave. (*Inset*) The amplitude of the pressure pulse increases in the thoracic aorta, abdominal aorta, and dorsalis pedis.

THE VASCULAR SYSTEM AND CONTROL OF BLOOD FLOW

- The vascular system, which consists of the arterial system (a high-pressure system that delivers blood to the tissues), the venous system (a low-pressure system that collects blood from the capillaries), and the capillaries, functions in the delivery of oxygen and nutrients and in the removal of wastes from the tissues.

- Local control of blood flow is regulated by mechanisms that match blood flow to the metabolic needs of the tissue. Over the short term, the tissues autoregulate flow through the synthesis of vasodilators and vasoconstrictors derived from the tissue, smooth muscle, or endothelial cells; over the long term, blood flow is regulated by creation of a collateral circulation.

- Neural control of circulatory function occurs through the sympathetic and parasympathetic divisions of the autonomic nervous system (ANS). Sympathetic stimulation increases heart rate, cardiac contractility, and vessel tone (vascular resistance), whereas parasympathetic stimulation decreases heart rate.

pulses that are felt, and it is the pressure pulses that produce the Korotkoff sounds heard during blood pressure measurement. The tip or maximum deflection of the pressure pulsation coincides with the systolic blood pressure, and the minimum point of deflection coincides with the diastolic pressure. The pulse pressure is the difference between systolic and diastolic pressure. If all other factors are equal, the magnitude of the pulse pressure reflects the volume of blood ejected from the left ventricle in a single beat.

Both the pressure values and the conformation of the pressure wave change as it moves though the peripheral arteries, such that pulsations in the large arteries are even greater than those in the aorta (Fig. 21.13). In other words, systolic pressure and pulse pressure are higher in large arteries than in the aorta. The increase in pulse pressure in the "downstream" arteries is due to the fact that immediately after ejection from the left ventricle, the pressure wave travels at a higher velocity than the blood itself, augmenting the downhill pressure. Furthermore, at branch points of arteries, pressure points are reflected backward, which also tends to augment pressure at those sites. With peripheral arterial disease, there is a delay in the transmission of the reflected wave so that the pulse decreases rather than increases in amplitude.

After its initial amplification, the pressure pulse becomes smaller and smaller as it moves through the smaller arteries and arterioles, until it disappears almost entirely in the capillaries. This damping of the pressure pulse is caused by the resistance and distensibility characteristics of these vessels. The increased resistance of these small vessels impedes the transmission of the pressure waves, whereas their distensibility is great enough that any small change in flow does not cause a pressure change. Although the pressure pulses usually are not transmitted to the capillaries, there are situations in which this does occur. For example, injury to a finger or other area of the body often results in a throbbing sensation. In this case, extreme dilation of the small vessels in the injured area produces a reduction in the dampening of the pressure pulse. Capillary pulsations also occur in conditions that cause exaggeration of aortic pressure pulses, such as aortic regurgitation or patent ductus arteriosus (see Chapter 24).

Venous System

The venous system is a low-pressure system that returns blood to the heart. The venules collect blood from the capillaries, and the veins transport blood back to the right atrium. Blood from the systemic veins flows into the right atrium of the heart; therefore, the pressure in the right atrium is called the *central venous pressure*. Right atrial pressure is regulated by the ability of the right ventricle to pump blood into the lungs and the tendency of blood to flow from the peripheral veins into the right atrium. The normal right atrial pressure is about 0 mm Hg, which is equal to atmospheric pressure. It can increase to 20 mm Hg or higher in conditions such as right heart failure and when blood is rapidly transfused at a rate that greatly increases total blood volume. Both accumulate excessive quantities of blood within

FIGURE 21.14 • Portion of a femoral vein opened to show the valves. The direction of flow is upward. Backward flow closes the valve.

the systemic veins causing increasing pressure as the blood attempts to flow into the heart.

The veins and venules are thin-walled, distensible, and collapsible vessels. The veins are capable of enlarging and storing large quantities of blood, which can be made available to the circulation as needed. Even though the veins are thin walled, they are muscular. This allows them to contract or expand to accommodate varying amounts of blood. Veins are innervated by the sympathetic nervous system. When blood is lost from the circulation, the veins constrict as a means of maintaining intravascular volume.

Valves in the veins of extremities prevent retrograde flow (Fig. 21.14), and, with the help of skeletal muscles that surround and intermittently compress the leg veins in a milking manner, blood is moved forward to the heart. This pumping action is known as the *venous* or *muscle pump*. This facilitates blood flow return at low pressure back to the heart against gravity. There are no valves in the abdominal or thoracic veins, and blood flow in these veins is heavily influenced by the pressure in the abdominal and thoracic cavities, respectively.

Because the venous system is a low-pressure system, blood flow in the venous system must oppose the effects of gravity when a person is standing. In the standing position, the weight of the blood in the vascular column causes an increase of 1 mm Hg in pressure for every 13.6 mm of distance below the level of the heart. Were it not for the valves in the veins and the action of the skeletal muscles, the venous pressure in the feet would be about +90 mm Hg in the standing adult. Gravity has no effect on the venous pressure in a person in the recumbent position because the blood in the veins is then at the level of the heart.

Local and Humoral Control of Blood Flow

Tissue blood flow is regulated on a minute-to-minute basis in relation to tissue needs and on a longer-term basis through the development of collateral circulation. Neural mechanisms regulate the cardiac output and blood pressure needed to support these local mechanisms.

Short-Term Autoregulation

Local control of blood flow is governed largely by the nutritional needs of the tissue. For example, blood flow to organs such as the heart, brain, and kidneys remains relatively constant, even if the mean arterial blood pressure varies over a range of 60 to 180 mm Hg (Fig. 21.15). The ability of the tissues to regulate their own blood flow over a wide range of pressures is called *autoregulation*. Autoregulation of blood flow is mediated by changes in blood vessel tone due to changes in flow through the vessel or by local tissue factors, such as lack of oxygen or accumulation of tissue metabolites (*i.e.*, potassium, lactic acid, or adenosine, which is a breakdown product of ATP). Local control is particularly important in tissues such as skeletal muscle, which has blood flow requirements that vary according to the level of activity.

Reactive Hyperemia. An increase in local blood flow following a brief period of ischemia is called *reactive hyperemia*. The ability of tissues to increase blood flow in situations of increased activity, such as exercise, is called *functional*

FIGURE 21.15 • Effect of increasing arterial pressure on blood flow through a muscle. The *solid curve* shows the effect if pressure is raised over a few minutes. The *dashed curve* shows the effect if the arterial pressure is raised slowly over many weeks. (From Hall J.E. (2011). *Textbook of medical physiology* (12th ed., p. 194). Philadelphia, PA: W. B. Saunders.)

FIGURE 21.16 • Function of nitric oxide in smooth muscle relaxation.

hyperemia. When the blood supply to an area has been occluded and then restored, local blood flow through the tissues increases within seconds to restore the metabolic equilibrium of the tissues. The transient redness seen on an arm after leaning on a hard surface is an example of reactive hyperemia. Local control mechanisms rely on a continuous flow from the main arteries; therefore, hyperemia cannot occur when the arteries that supply the capillary beds are narrowed. For example, if a major coronary artery becomes occluded, the opening of channels supplied by that vessel cannot restore blood flow.

Endothelial Control of Vascular Function. One of the important functions of the endothelial cells lining the arterioles and small arteries is the synthesis and release of factors that control vessel dilation. Intact endothelium is able to produce a factor that causes relaxation of vascular smooth muscle. Originally this factor was called *endothelium-derived relaxing factor* and is now known as *nitric oxide*. The normal endothelium maintains a continuous release of nitric oxide, which is formed from L-arginine through the action of an enzyme called *nitric oxide synthase* (Fig. 21.16). The production of nitric oxide can be stimulated by a variety of endothelial *agonists*, including acetylcholine, bradykinin, histamine, and thrombin. *Shear stress* on the endothelium resulting from an increase in blood flow or blood pressure also stimulates nitric oxide production and vessel relaxation. Nitric oxide also inhibits platelet aggregation and secretion of platelet contents, many of which cause vasoconstriction. The fact that nitric oxide is released into the vessel lumen (to inactivate platelets) and away from the lumen (to relax smooth muscle) suggests that it protects against both thrombosis and vasoconstriction. Nitroglycerin, a medication which is used in the treatment of angina, produces its effects by being converted into nitric oxide in vascular smooth muscle of the target vessels.

The endothelium also produces a number of vasoconstrictor substances, including *angiotensin II,* vasoconstrictor prostaglandins, and a family of peptides called *endothelins.* There are at least three endothelins. Endothelin-1, made by all endothelial cells, is the most potent endogenous vasoconstrictor known. For example, after a blood vessel is damaged, local endothelin is released to constrict the vessel and prevent extensive bleeding.

Long-Term Regulation of Blood Flow

Collateral circulation is a mechanism for the long-term regulation of local blood flow. In the heart and other vital structures, anastomotic channels exist between some of the smaller arteries. These channels permit perfusion of an area by more than one artery. When one artery becomes occluded, these anastomotic channels increase in size, allowing blood from a patent artery to perfuse the area supplied by the occluded vessel. For example, persons with extensive obstruction of a coronary blood vessel may rely on collateral circulation to meet the oxygen needs of the myocardial tissue normally supplied by that vessel. As with other long-term compensatory mechanisms, the recruitment of collateral circulation is most efficient when obstruction of flow is gradual rather than sudden.

Humoral Control of Vascular Function

Humoral control of blood flow involves the effect of vasodilator and vasoconstrictor substances in the blood. Some of these substances are formed by special glands and transported in the blood throughout the entire circulation. Others are formed in local tissues and aid in the local control of blood flow. Among the most important of the humoral factors are norepinephrine and epinephrine, angiotensin II, histamine, serotonin, bradykinin, and the prostaglandins.

Norepinephrine and Epinephrine. Norepinephrine is an especially powerful vasoconstrictor; epinephrine is less so and in some tissues (*e.g.,* skeletal muscle) even causes mild vasodilation. Stimulation of the sympathetic nervous system during stress or exercise causes local constriction of veins and arterioles because of the release of norepinephrine from sympathetic nerve endings. In addition, sympathetic stimulation causes the adrenal medullae to secrete both norepinephrine and epinephrine into the blood. These catecholamines then circulate in the blood, causing direct sympathetic stimulation of blood vessels in all parts of the body.

Angiotensin II. Angiotensin II is another powerful vasoconstrictor substance. Angiotensin II is produced as a part of the renin–angiotensin–aldosterone system and normally acts on many arterioles simultaneously to increase the PVR, thereby increasing the arterial blood pressure (discussed in Chapter 23).

Histamine. Histamine has a powerful vasodilator effect on arterioles and has the ability to increase capillary permeability, allowing leakage of both fluid and plasma proteins into the tissues. Histamine is largely derived from mast cells in injured tissues and basophils in the blood. In certain tissues, such as skeletal muscle, the activity of the mast cells is mediated by the sympathetic nervous system; when sympathetic control is withdrawn, the mast cells release histamine.

Serotonin. Serotonin is liberated from aggregating platelets during the clotting process; it causes vasoconstriction and plays a major role in control of bleeding. Serotonin is found in brain and lung tissues, and there is some speculation that it may be involved in the vascular spasm associated with some allergic pulmonary reactions and migraine headaches.

Bradykinin. The kinins (*i.e.,* kallidins and bradykinin) are liberated from the globulin kininogen, which is present in body fluids. Bradykinin causes intense dilation of arterioles, increased capillary permeability, and constriction of venules. It is thought that the kinins play special roles in regulating blood flow and capillary leakage in inflamed tissues. It is also believed that bradykinin helps to regulate blood flow in the skin as well in the salivary and gastrointestinal glands.

Prostaglandins. Prostaglandins are synthesized from constituents of the cell membrane (*i.e.,* the long-chain fatty acid *arachidonic acid*). Tissue injury incites the release of arachidonic acid from the cell membrane, which initiates prostaglandin synthesis. There are several prostaglandins (*e.g.,* E_2, F_2, D_2), which are subgrouped according to their solubility; some produce vasoconstriction and some produce vasodilation. As a rule of thumb, those in the E group are vasodilators, and those in the F group are vasoconstrictors. The corticosteroid hormones produce an anti-inflammatory response by blocking the release of arachidonic acid, preventing prostaglandin synthesis.

IN SUMMARY

The walls of all blood vessels, except the capillaries, are composed of three layers: the tunica externa, tunica media, and tunica intima. The layers of the vessel vary with its function. Arteries are thick-walled vessels with large amounts of elastic fibres. The walls of the arterioles, which control blood pressure, have large amounts of smooth muscle. Veins are thin-walled, distensible, and collapsible vessels. Venous flow is designed to return blood to the right atrium. It is a low-pressure system and relies on venous valves and the action of muscle pumps to offset the effects of gravity.

The delivery of blood to the tissues of the body depends on pressure pulses that are generated by the intermittent ejection of blood from the left ventricle into the distensible aorta and large arteries of the arterial system. The combination of distensibility of the arteries and their resistance to flow reduces the pressure pulsations so that constant blood flow occurs by the time blood reaches the capillaries.

The mechanisms that control local blood flow are designed to ensure adequate delivery of blood to the capillaries in the microcirculation, where the exchange of cellular nutrients and wastes occurs. Local control is governed largely by the needs of the tissues and is regulated by local tissue factors such as lack of oxygen and the accumulation of metabolites. Hyperemia is a local increase in blood flow that occurs after a temporary occlusion of blood flow. It is a compensatory mechanism that decreases the oxygen debt of the deprived tissues. Collateral circulation is a mechanism for long-term regulation of local blood flow that involves the development of collateral vessels. The endothelial relaxing factor (mainly nitric oxide) and humoral factors, such as norepinephrine and epinephrine, angiotensin II, histamine, serotonin, bradykinin, and the prostaglandins, contribute to the regulation of blood flow.

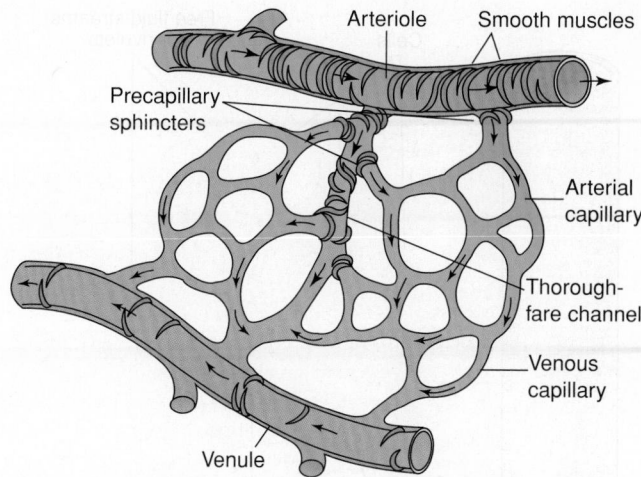

FIGURE 21.17 • Capillary bed. Precapillary sphincters control the flow of blood through the capillary network. Thoroughfare channels (*i.e.,* arteriovenous shunts) allow blood to move directly from the arteriole into the venule without moving through nutrient channels of the capillary.

THE MICROCIRCULATION AND LYMPHATIC SYSTEM

After completing this section of the chapter, you should be able to meet the following objectives:

- Define the term *microcirculation*.
- Describe the structure and function of the capillaries.
- Explain the forces that control the fluid exchange between the capillaries and the interstitial spaces.
- Describe the structures of the lymphatic system and relate them to the role of the lymphatics in controlling interstitial fluid volume.

The term *microcirculation* refers to the functions of the smallest blood vessels, the capillaries, and the neighbouring lymphatic vessels. The microcirculation is the site of exchange of gases, nutrients, and waste products in the tissues, as well as the site of vascular and interstitial fluid exchange.

Structure and Function of the Microcirculation

The structures of the microcirculation include the arterioles, capillaries, and venules. Blood enters the microcirculation through an arteriole, passes through the capillaries, and leaves through a small venule. The metarterioles serve as thoroughfare channels that link arterioles and capillaries (Fig. 21.17). Small cuffs of smooth muscle, the precapillary sphincters, are positioned at the arterial end of the capillary. The smooth muscle tone of the arterioles, venules, and precapillary sphincters serves to control blood flow through the capillary bed. Depending on venous pressure, blood flows through the capillary channels when the precapillary sphincters are open.

Capillary Structure and Function

Capillaries are microscopic vessels that connect the arterial and venous segments of the circulation. In each person, there are approximately 10 billion capillaries, with a total surface area of 500 to 700 m². The capillary wall is composed of a single layer of endothelial cells and their basement membrane (Fig. 21.18). The endothelial cells form a tube just large enough to allow the passage of red blood cells, one at a time.

Water-filled junctions, called the *capillary pores,* join the capillary endothelial cells and provide a pathway for passage of substances through the capillary wall. The size of the capillary pores varies with capillary function. In the brain,

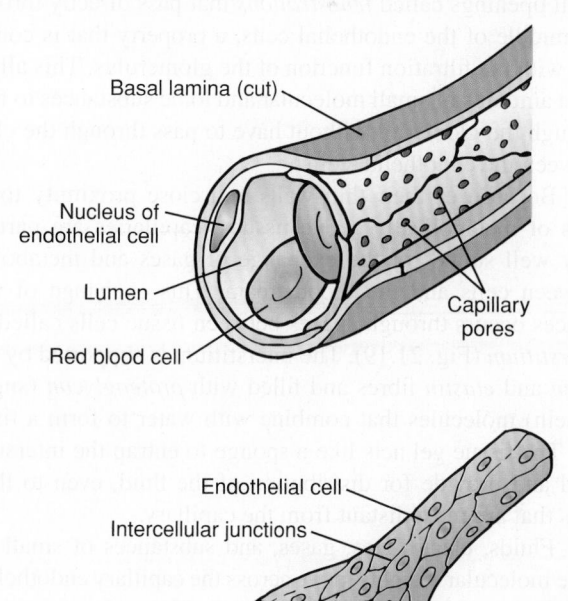

FIGURE 21.18 • Endothelial cells and intercellular junctions in a section of capillary.

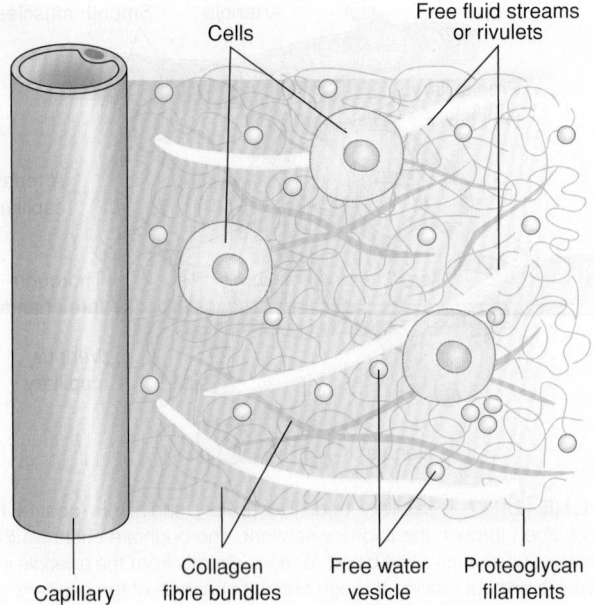

FIGURE 21.19 • Structure of the interstitium. Proteoglycan filaments are everywhere in the spaces between the collagen fibre bundles. Free water vesicles and small amounts of free fluid in the form of rivulets occasionally may occur. (From Hall J. E. (2011). *Textbook of medical physiology* (12th ed., p. 180). Philadelphia, PA: W. B. Saunders.)

the endothelial cells are joined by tight junctions that form the blood–brain barrier. This prevents substances that would alter neural excitability from leaving the capillary. In organs that process blood contents, such as the liver, capillaries have large pores so that substances can pass easily through the capillary wall. The glomerular capillaries in the kidney have small openings called *fenestrations* that pass directly through the middle of the endothelial cells, a property that is consistent with the filtration function of the glomerulus. This allows large amounts of small molecular and ionic substances to filter through the glomeruli without have to pass through the clefts between the endothelial cells.

Because of their thin walls and close proximity to the cells of metabolically active tissues, capillaries are particularly well suited for the exchange of gases and metabolites between cells and the bloodstream. This exchange of substances occurs through spaces between tissue cells called the *interstitium* (Fig. 21.19). The interstitium is supported by *collagen* and *elastin* fibres and filled with *proteoglycan* (sugar–protein) molecules that combine with water to form a tissue gel. The tissue gel acts like a sponge to entrap the interstitial fluid and provide for distribution of the fluid, even to those cells that are most distant from the capillary.

Fluids, electrolytes, gases, and substances of small and large molecular weights move across the capillary endothelium by diffusion, filtration, and pinocytosis. The exchange of gases and fluids across the capillary wall occurs by simple diffusion. Lipid-soluble substances such as oxygen and carbon dioxide readily exchange across the endothelial cells by diffusion. Water flows through the capillary endothelial cell membranes through water-selective channels called *aquaporins*. Water and

water-soluble substances such as electrolytes, glucose, and amino acids also diffuse between the endothelial cells in the capillary pores. Pinocytosis (discussed in Chapter 4) is responsible for the movement of white blood cells and large protein molecules.

Control of Blood Flow in the Microcirculation

Blood flow through capillary channels, designed for exchange of nutrients and metabolites, is called *nutrient flow*. In some parts of the microcirculation, blood flow bypasses the capillary bed, moving instead through a connection called an *arteriovenous shunt*, which directly connects an arteriole and a venule. This type of blood flow is called *nonnutrient flow* because it does not allow for nutrient exchange. Non-nutrient channels are common in the skin and are important in terms of heat exchange and temperature regulation (discussed in Chapter 10).

Capillary–Interstitial Fluid Exchange

The direction and magnitude of fluid movement across capillary walls are largely controlled by the hydrostatic and osmotic pressures of the capillary and interstitial fluids, as well as the permeability of the capillary wall. The direction of fluid movement can either be into or out of the capillary. When net fluid movement is out of the capillary into the interstitial spaces, it is called *filtration,* and when net movement is from the interstitium into the capillary, it is called *absorption* (Fig. 21.20).

The capillary hydrostatic pressure represents the fluid pressure that tends to push water and its dissolved substances

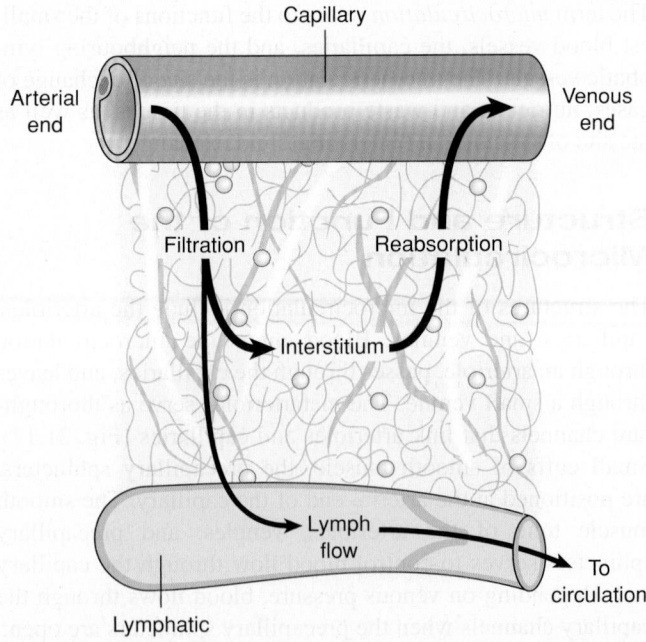

FIGURE 21.20 • Capillary filtration and lymph flow. Fluid is filtered out of the capillary and into the interstitium at the arterial end of the capillary. Most of the fluid is reabsorbed at the venous end of the capillary, with the rest of the fluid entering the terminal lymphatics for return to the circulation.

through the capillary pores into the interstitium. The osmotic pressure caused by the plasma proteins in the blood tends to pull fluid from the interstitial spaces back into the capillary. This pressure is termed *colloidal osmotic pressure* to differentiate the osmotic effects of the plasma proteins, which are suspended colloids, from the osmotic effects of substances such as sodium and glucose, which are dissolved crystalloids. Capillary permeability controls the movement of water and substances, such as the plasma proteins that influence osmotic pressure, into the interstitial spaces. Also important to this exchange mechanism is the lymphatic system, which removes excess fluid and osmotically active proteins and large particles from the interstitial spaces and returns them to the circulation.

Hydrostatic Forces

The capillary hydrostatic pressure is the principal force in capillary filtration. The hydrostatic pressure (blood pressure) within the capillaries is determined by both the arterial and venous pressures (the capillaries being interspersed between the arteries and veins). An increase in small artery and arterial pressure elevates capillary hydrostatic pressure, whereas a reduction in each of these pressures has the opposite effect. A change in venous pressure has a greater effect on the capillary hydrostatic pressure than does the same change in arterial pressure. About 80% of increased venous pressure, such as that caused by venous thrombosis or congestive heart failure, is transmitted back to the capillary. The previously discussed effects of gravity on venous pressure also affect capillary hydrostatic pressure, and when a person stands, the hydrostatic pressure is greater in the legs and lower in the head.

The interstitial hydrostatic pressure is the pressure exerted by the interstitial fluids outside the capillary. It can be positive or negative. A positive interstitial fluid pressure opposes capillary filtration and a negative interstitial fluid pressure increases the movement of fluid out of the capillary into the interstitium. In the normal nonedematous state, the interstitial hydrostatic pressure is close to zero or slightly negative (−1 to −4 mm Hg) and has very little effect on capillary filtration or outward movement of fluid.

Osmotic Forces

The key factor that restrains fluid loss from the capillaries is the colloidal osmotic pressure (approximately 28 mm Hg) generated by the plasma proteins. The plasma proteins are large molecules that disperse in the blood and occasionally escape into the tissue spaces. Because the capillary membrane is almost impermeable to the plasma proteins, these particles exert an osmotic force that pulls fluid into the capillary and offsets the pushing force of the capillary filtration pressure. The plasma contains a mixture of plasma proteins, including albumin, globulins, and fibrinogen. Albumin, which is the most abundant of the plasma proteins, accounts for approximately 70% of the total osmotic pressure. It is the number, not the size, of the particles in solution that controls the osmotic pressure. One gram of albumin (molecular weight of 69,000) contains almost six times as many molecules as 1 g of fibrinogen (molecular

weight of 400,000). (Normal values for albumin are 40 to 60 g/L; globulins, 23 to 35 g/L; and fibrinogen 2 to 4 g/L.)

Although the size of the capillary pores prevents most plasma proteins from leaving the capillary, small amounts escape into the interstitial spaces and exert an osmotic force that tends to pull fluid from the capillary into the interstitium. This amount is increased in conditions such as inflammation in which an increase in capillary permeability allows plasma proteins to escape into the interstitium. The lymphatic system is responsible for removing proteins from the interstitium. In the absence of a functioning lymphatic system, interstitial colloidal osmotic pressure increases, causing fluid to accumulate. Normally, a few white blood cells, plasma proteins, and other large molecules enter the interstitial spaces; these cells and molecules, which are too large to reenter the capillary, rely on the loosely structured wall of the lymphatic vessels for return to the vascular compartment.

Balance of Hydrostatic and Osmotic Forces

Normally, the movement of fluid between the capillary bed and the interstitial spaces is continuous. As Starling pointed out more than a century ago, a state of equilibrium exists as long as equal amounts of fluid enter and leave the interstitial spaces. The forces that contribute to the Starling equilibrium are illustrated in Figure 21.21. In the diagram, the hydrostatic pressure at the arterial end of the capillary is higher than at the venous end. The pushing force of the capillary hydrostatic pressure on the arterial end of the capillary, along with the pulling effects of the interstitial colloidal osmotic pressure, contributes to the net outward movement of fluid. The capillary colloidal osmotic pressure and opposing interstitial osmotic pressure determine the reabsorption of fluid at the venous end of the capillary. A slight imbalance in forces

FIGURE 21.21 • Capillary–interstitial fluid exchange equilibrium. Normally, the forces (capillary hydrostatic pressure, interstitial colloidal osmotic pressure, and the opposing interstitial fluid pressure) that control the outward movement of fluid from the capillary (filtration) are almost balanced by the forces (capillary colloidal osmotic pressure and interstitial colloidal osmotic pressure) that pull fluid back into the capillary (reabsorption).

causes slightly more filtration of fluid into interstitial spaces than absorption back into the capillary; it is this fluid that is returned to the circulation by the lymphatic system. Disorders of capillary fluid exchange are discussed in Chapter 31.

The Lymphatic System

The lymphatic system represents an accessory route through which fluid can flow back to the blood from interstitial spaces. This system, commonly called the *lymphatics,* serves almost all body tissues, except cartilage, bone, epithelial tissue, and tissues of the central nervous system (CNS). Most of these tissues, however, have prelymphatic channels that eventually flow into areas supplied by the lymphatics. Lymph is derived from interstitial fluids that flow through the lymph channels. It contains plasma proteins and other osmotically active particles that rely on the lymphatics for movement back into the circulatory system. The lymphatic system is also the main route for absorption of nutrients, particularly fats, from the gastrointestinal tract. The lymphatic system also filters the fluid at the lymph nodes and removes foreign particles such as bacteria. When lymph flow is obstructed, a condition called *lymphedema* occurs. Involvement of lymphatic structures by malignant tumours and removal of lymph nodes at the time of cancer surgery are common causes of lymphedema.

The lymphatic system is made up of vessels similar to those of the circulatory system. These vessels commonly travel along with an arteriole or venule or with its companion artery and vein. The terminal lymphatic vessels are made up of a single layer of connective tissue with an endothelial lining and resemble blood capillaries. The lymphatic vessels lack tight junctions and are loosely anchored to the surrounding tissues by fine filaments (Fig. 21.22). The loose junctions permit the entry of large particles, and the filaments hold the vessels open under conditions of edema, when the pressure of the surrounding tissues would otherwise cause them to collapse. The lymph capillaries drain into larger lymph vessels that ultimately empty into the right and left thoracic ducts (Fig. 21.23). The thoracic ducts empty into the circulation at the junctions of the subclavian and internal jugular veins. The total amount of lymph redirected back into the general circulation is 2 to 3 L/day in a healthy person.

Although the divisions are not as distinct as in the circulatory system, the larger lymph vessels show evidence of having intimal, medial, and adventitial layers similar to blood vessels. The intima of these channels contains elastic tissue and an endothelial layer, and the larger collecting lymph channels contain smooth muscle in their medial layer. Contraction of this smooth muscle assists in propelling lymph toward the thorax. External compression of the lymph channels by pulsating blood vessels in the vicinity and active and passive movements of body parts also aid in forward propulsion of lymph. The rate of flow through the lymphatic system through all of the various lymph channels, approximately 120 ml/hour, is determined by the interstitial fluid pressure and the activity of lymph pumps.

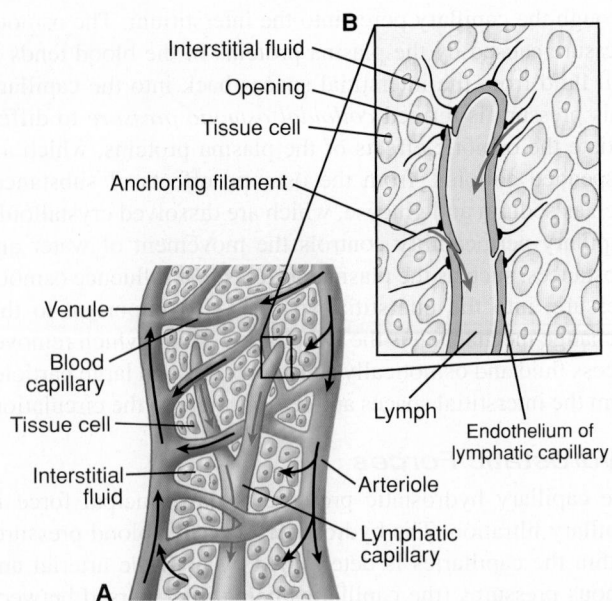

FIGURE 21.22 • A: Location of the lymphatic capillary. Fluid from the arterial side of the capillary bed moves into the interstitial spaces and is reabsorbed in the venous side of the capillary bed. **B:** Details of the lymphatic capillary with its anchoring filaments and overlapping edges that serve as valves and can be pushed open, allowing the inflow of interstitial fluid and its suspended particles.

IN SUMMARY

Exchange of fluids between the vascular compartment and the interstitial spaces occurs at the capillary level. The capillary hydrostatic pressure pushes fluids out of the capillaries, and the colloidal osmotic pressure exerted by the plasma proteins pulls fluids back into the capillaries. Albumin, which is the smallest and most abundant of the plasma proteins, provides the major osmotic force for return of fluid to the vascular compartment. Normally, slightly more fluid leaves the capillary bed than can be reabsorbed. This excess fluid is returned to the vascular circulation by way of the lymphatic channels.

NEURAL CONTROL OF CIRCULATORY FUNCTION

After completing this section of the chapter, you should be able to meet the following objectives:

- Describe the roles of the medullary vasomotor and cardioinhibitory centres in controlling the function of the heart and blood vessels.
- Relate the performance of baroreceptors and chemoreceptors in the control of cardiovascular function.
- Describe the distribution of the sympathetic and parasympathetic nervous systems in the innervation

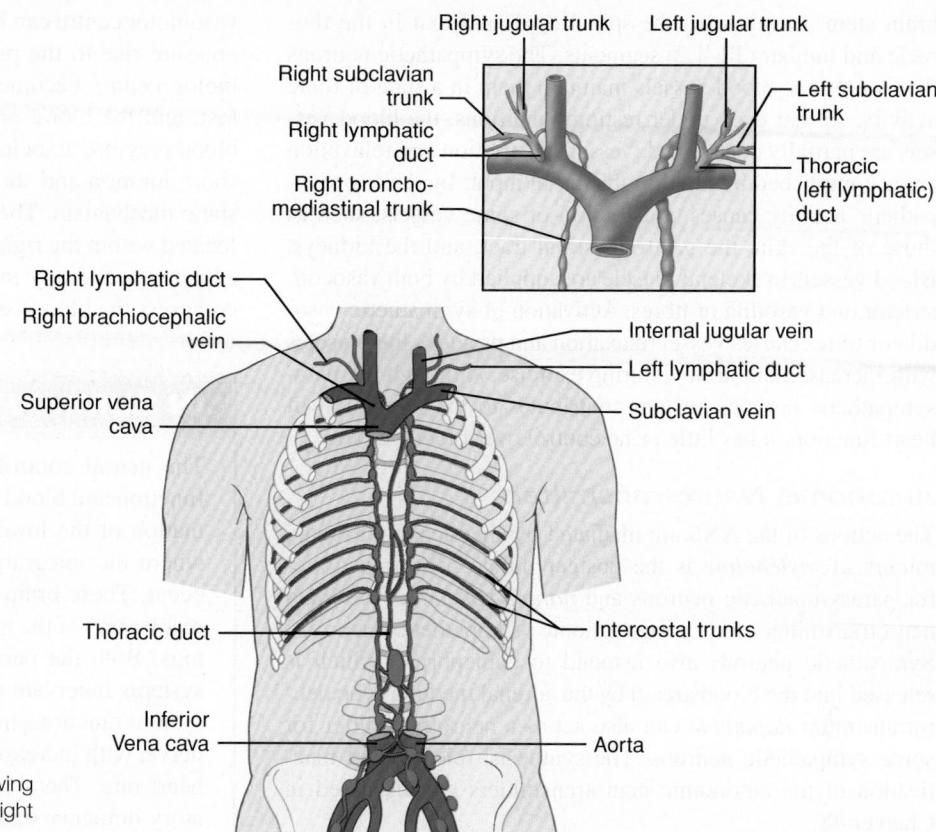

FIGURE 21.23 • Lymphatic system, showing the thoracic duct and position of the left and right lymphatic ducts (*inset*).

- of the circulatory system and their effects on heart rate and cardiac contractility.
- Relate the role of the CNS in terms of regulating circulatory function.

The neural control centres for the integration and modulation of cardiac function and blood pressure are located bilaterally in the medulla oblongata. The medullary cardiovascular neurons are grouped into three distinct pools that lead to sympathetic innervation of the heart and blood vessels and parasympathetic innervation of the heart. The first two, which control sympathetic-mediated acceleration of heart rate and blood vessel tone, are called the *vasomotor centre*. The third, which controls parasympathetic-mediated slowing of heart rate, is called the *cardioinhibitory centre*. These brain stem centres receive information from many areas of the nervous system, including the hypothalamus. The arterial baroreceptors and chemoreceptors provide the medullary cardiovascular centre with continuous information regarding changes in blood pressure (see Chapter 23).

Autonomic Nervous System Regulation

The neural control of the circulatory system occurs primarily through the *sympathetic* and *parasympathetic* divisions of the ANS. The ANS contributes to the control of cardiovascular function through modulation of cardiac (*i.e.,* heart rate and cardiac contractility) and vascular (*i.e.,* SVR) functions.

Autonomic Regulation of Cardiac Function

The heart is innervated by the parasympathetic and sympathetic nervous systems. Parasympathetic innervation of the heart is achieved by means of the *vagus nerve*. The parasympathetic outflow to the heart originates from the vagal nucleus in the medulla. The axons of these neurons pass to the heart in the cardiac branches of the vagus nerve. The effect of vagal stimulation on heart function is largely limited to heart rate, with increased vagal activity producing a slowing of the pulse. Sympathetic outflow to the heart and blood vessels arises from neurons located in the reticular formation of the brain stem. The axons of these neurons exit the thoracic segments of the spinal cord to synapse with the postganglionic neurons that innervate the heart. Cardiac sympathetic fibres are widely distributed to the sinoatrial and AV nodes and the myocardium. Increased sympathetic activity produces an increase in the heart rate, conduction through the AV node, and the velocity and force of cardiac contraction.

Autonomic Regulation of Vascular Function

The sympathetic nervous system serves as the final common pathway for controlling the smooth muscle tone of the blood vessels. Most of the sympathetic preganglionic fibres that control vessel function originate in the vasomotor centre of the brain stem, travel down the spinal cord, and exit in the thoracic and lumbar (T1–L2) segments. The sympathetic neurons that supply the blood vessels maintain them in a state of tonic activity, so that even under resting conditions, the blood vessels are partially constricted. Vessel constriction and relaxation are accomplished by altering this basal input. Increasing sympathetic activity causes constriction of some vessels, such as those of the skin, the gastrointestinal tract, and the kidneys. Blood vessels in skeletal muscle are supplied by both vasoconstrictor and vasodilator fibres. Activation of sympathetic vasodilator fibres causes vessel relaxation and provides the muscles with increased blood flow during exercise. Although the parasympathetic nervous system contributes to the regulation of heart function, it has little or no control over blood vessels.

Autonomic Neurotransmitters

The actions of the ANS are mediated by chemical neurotransmitters. *Acetylcholine* is the postganglionic neurotransmitter for parasympathetic neurons and *norepinephrine* is the main neurotransmitter for postganglionic sympathetic neurons. Sympathetic neurons also respond to epinephrine, which is released into the bloodstream by the adrenal medulla. The neurotransmitter *dopamine* can also act as a neurotransmitter for some sympathetic neurons. The synthesis, release, and inactivation of the autonomic neurotransmitters are discussed in Chapter 48.

Central Nervous System Responses

It is not surprising that the CNS, which plays an essential role in regulating vasomotor tone and blood pressure, would have a mechanism for controlling the blood flow to the cardiovascular centres that control circulatory function. When the blood flow to the brain has been sufficiently interrupted to cause ischemia of the vasomotor centre, these vasomotor neurons become strongly excited, causing massive vasoconstriction as a means of raising the blood pressure to levels as high as the heart can pump against. This response is called the *CNS ischemic response,* and it can raise the blood pressure to levels as high as 270 mm Hg for as long as 10 minutes. It is thought that the buildup of lactic acid and other acidic substances in the vasomotor centre also contributes to the CNS ischemic response as a last-ditch stand to preserve the blood flow to vital brain centres. It does not become activated until blood pressure has fallen to at least 60 mm Hg, and it is most effective in the range of 15 to 20 mm Hg. If the cerebral circulation is not reestablished within 3 to 10 minutes, the neurons of the vasomotor centre cease to function, so that the tonic impulses to the blood vessels stop and the blood pressure falls precipitously.

The *Cushing reflex* is a special type of CNS reflex resulting from an increase in intracranial pressure. When the intracranial pressure rises to levels that equal intra-arterial pressure, blood vessels to the vasomotor centre become compressed, initiating the CNS ischemic response. The purpose of this reflex is to produce a rise in arterial pressure to levels above intracranial pressure so that the blood flow to the vasomotor centre can be reestablished. Should the intracranial pressure rise to the point that the blood supply to the vasomotor centre becomes inadequate, vasoconstrictor tone is lost, and the blood pressure begins to fall. The elevation in blood pressure associated with the Cushing reflex is usually of short duration and should be considered a protective homeostatic mechanism. The brain and other cerebral structures are located within the rigid confines of the skull, with no room for expansion, and any increase in intracranial pressure tends to compress the blood vessels that supply the brain.

IN SUMMARY

The neural control centres for the regulation of cardiac function and blood pressure are located in the reticular formation of the lower pons and medulla of the brain stem, where the integration and modulation of ANS responses occur. These brain stem centres receive information from many areas of the nervous system, including the hypothalamus. Both the parasympathetic and sympathetic nervous systems innervate the heart. The parasympathetic nervous system functions in regulating heart rate through the vagus nerve, with increased vagal activity producing a slowing of heart rate. The sympathetic nervous system has an excitatory influence on heart rate and contractility, and it serves as the final common pathway for controlling the smooth muscle tone of the blood vessels.

REVIEW EXERCISES

1. In persons with atherosclerosis of the coronary arteries, symptoms of myocardial ischemia do not usually occur until the vessel has been 75% occluded.
   A. *Use the Poiseuille law to explain.*
2. Once an arterial aneurysm has begun to form, it continues to enlarge as a result of the increased tension in its wall.
   A. *Explain the continued increase in size using the law of Laplace.*
   B. *Using information related to cross-sectional area and velocity of flow, explain why there is stasis of blood flow with the tendency to form clots in aneurysms with a large cross-sectional area.*
3. Use events in the cardiac cycle depicted in Figure 21.10 to explain:
   A. *The effect of hypertension on the isovolumetric contraction period.*
   B. *The effect of an increase in heart rate on the time spent in diastole.*
   C. *The effect of an increase in the isovolumetric relaxation period on the diastolic filling of the ventricle.*

4. Use the Frank–Starling ventricular function curve depicted in Figure 21.11 to explain the changes in cardiac output that occur with changes in respiratory effort.

A. *What happens to cardiac output during increased inspiratory effort in which a marked decrease in intrathoracic pressure produces an increase in venous return to the right atrium?*

B. *What happens to cardiac output during increased expiratory effort in which a marked increase in intrathoracic pressure produces a decrease in venous return to the right atrium?*

C. *Given these changes in cardiac output that occur during increased respiratory effort, what would you propose as one of the functions of the Frank–Starling curve?*

Bibliography

Barrett K. E., Boitano S., Barman S. M., et al. (2012). *Ganong's review of medical physiology* (24th ed.). New York, NY: McGraw-Hill Medical.

Boron W. F., Boulpaep E. L. (2009). *Medical physiology* (2nd ed.). Philadelphia, PA: Saunders.

Forstermann U., Sessa W. C. (2012). Nitric oxide synthases: Regulation and function. *Eur Heart J, 33*(7), 829–837.

Hall J. E. (2011). *Textbook of medical physiology* (12th ed.). Philadelphia, PA: W. B. Saunders.

Klabunde R. E. (2011). *Cardiovascular physiology concepts* (2nd ed.). Philadelphia, PA: Lippincott Williams & Wilkins.

McConnell T. H., Hull K. L. (2011). *Human form human function: Essentials of anatomy & physiology.* Philadelphia, PA: Lippincott William & Wilkins.

Mohrman D. E., Heller L. J. (2014). *Cardiovascular physiology* (8th ed.). New York, NY: McGraw-Hill Education.

Pittman R. N. (2013). Oxygen transport in the microcirculation and its regulation. *Microcirculation, 20*(2), 117–137.

Pluim B. M., Zwinderman A. H., van der Laarse A., et al. (2000). The athlete's heart: A meta-analysis of cardiac structure and function. *Circulation, 101*(3), 336–344.

Rhoades R. A., Bell D. R. (2013). *Medical physiology: Principles for clinical medicine* (4th ed.). Philadelphia, PA: Lippincott Williams & Wilkins.

Wilcken D. E. L. (2014). Physiology of the normal heart. *Medicine, 42*(8), 409–412.

Visit thePoint **http://thePoint.lww.com for animations, journal articles, and more!**

Disorders of Blood Flow in the Systemic Circulation

22

Blood flow in the arterial and venous systems depends on a system of functional blood vessels and sufficient perfusion pressure. Unlike disorders of the respiratory system or central circulation that cause hypoxemia and impair oxygenation of tissues throughout the body, the effects of blood vessel disease usually are limited to local tissues supplied by a particular vessel or group of vessels. With arterial disorders, there is decreased blood flow to the tissues along with impaired delivery of oxygen and nutrients, and with venous disorders there is interference with the outflow of blood and removal of waste products.

Disturbances in blood flow can result from pathologic changes in the vessel wall (*e.g.,* atherosclerosis, vasculitis), acute vessel obstruction due to thrombus or embolus, vasospasm (*e.g.,* Raynaud phenomenon), or abnormal vessel dilation (*e.g.,* arterial aneurysms, varicose veins).

BLOOD VESSEL STRUCTURE AND FUNCTION

After completing this section of the chapter, you should be able to meet the following objectives:

- Describe the functions of the endothelial cells.
- Define the term *endothelial dysfunction.*
- Describe the function of vascular smooth muscle and its role in vascular repair.

Although the heart is at the centre of the cardiovascular system, it is the blood vessels that transport blood throughout the body. The walls of the arteries and veins, except for the very smallest, are composed of three distinct layers: an outer layer of loosely woven collagen tissue, the *tunica externa* (previously known as *tunica adventitia*) which is composed of loose connective tissue; a middle layer, the *tunica media,* which consists primarily of circumferentially arranged layers of smooth muscle cells; and an inner layer, the *tunica intima,* which consists of a single layer of endothelial cells that line the lumen of the vessel, and the underlying subendothelial connective tissue (Fig. 22.1).[1–3] As the main cellular components of the blood vessel wall, the endothelial and smooth muscle cells play an important role in the pathogenesis of many disorders of the arterial circulation.

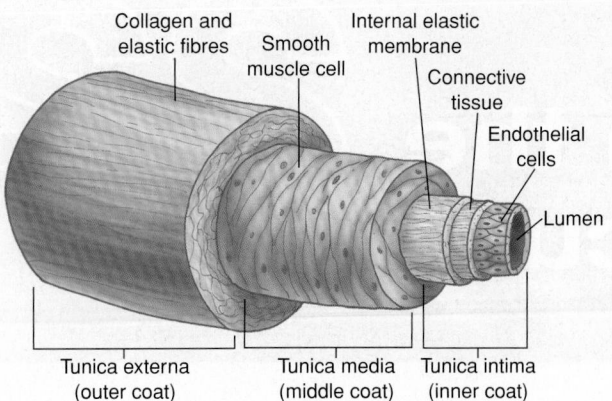

Collagen and elastic fibres
Smooth muscle cell
Internal elastic membrane
Connective tissue
Endothelial cells
Lumen
Tunica externa (outer coat)
Tunica media (middle coat)
Tunica intima (inner coat)

FIGURE 22.1 • Diagram of a typical artery showing the tunica intima, tunica media, and tunica externa (tunica adventitia).

Endothelial Cells

Endothelial cells form a continuous lining for the entire vascular system called the *endothelium*. This lining is made up of approximately 60,000 miles of squamous epithelium that lines the various-sized vessels.[2] The endothelium is a versatile, multifunctional tissue that plays an active role in controlling vascular function (Table 22.1).[1,2] As a semipermeable membrane, the endothelium controls the transfer of substances across the vascular wall. The endothelium plays a role in the control of platelet adhesion and blood clotting; modulation of blood flow and vascular resistance; metabolism of hormones; regulation of immune and inflammatory reactions; and elaboration of factors that influence the growth of other cell types, particularly vascular smooth muscle cells (see Chapter 21).

Endothelial Dysfunction

Structurally intact endothelial cells respond to various stimuli, regulating vascular reactivity and blood flow through levels of nitric oxide and other vasoactive dilating and constricting mediators.[1] The term *endothelial dysfunction* describes several types of potentially reversible changes in endothelial function that occur in response to environmental stimuli. Endothelial

dysfunction can reduce the availability of nitric oxide, causing a reduction in endothelial-dependent vasodilation or can cause an increase release of endothelins, which then increases vasoconstriction. Other stimuli include cytokines; inflammatory mediators; hemodynamic stressors such as hypertension; lipid products that are critical to the pathogenesis of atherosclerosis; and hypoxia. Dysfunctional endothelial cells, in turn, produce other cytokines, growth factors, procoagulant or anticoagulant substances, and a variety of other biologically active products.

Vascular Smooth Muscle Cells

Vascular smooth muscle cells, which form the predominant cellular layer in the tunica media, produce constriction or dilation of blood vessels. A network of vasomotor nerves of the sympathetic nervous system provides a mechanism for the smooth muscle surrounding the blood vessels to maintain vascular tone. Because vasomotor nerves do not enter the tunica media of the blood vessel, the nerves do not synapse directly on the smooth muscle cells. Instead, they release the neurotransmitter norepinephrine, which diffuses into the media and acts on the nearby smooth muscle cells. The resulting impulses are propagated along the smooth muscle cells through their gap junctions, causing contraction of the entire muscle cell layer and thus reducing the radius of the vessel lumen (vasoconstriction).

Vascular smooth muscle cells also synthesize collagen, elastin, and other components of the extracellular matrix (ECM) (material outside the cell), elaborate growth factors and cytokines; and migrate into the intima, causing cellular proliferation.[1] These processes contribute to normal cellular repair following vascular injury; however, they also contribute to excessive cellular proliferations in atherosclerosis. The migratory and proliferative activities of vascular smooth muscle cells are stimulated by growth promoters such as platelet-derived growth factor, fibroblast growth factor, and angiotensin II. A reduction in nitric oxide, which occurs with endothelial dysfunction, potentiates the proliferative action of the smooth muscle cells. Thus, smooth muscle cells play a key role in the

TABLE 22.1 ENDOTHELIAL CELL PROPERTIES AND FUNCTIONS	
MAJOR PROPERTIES	**ASSOCIATED FUNCTIONS/FACTORS**
Maintenance of a selective permeability barrier	Controls the transfer of small and large molecules across the vessel wall
Regulation of thrombosis	Elaboration of prothrombogenic molecules (von Willebrand factor, plasminogen activator) and antithrombotic molecules (prostacyclin, heparin-like molecules, plasminogen activator)
Modulation of blood flow and vascular reactivity	Elaboration of vasodilators (nitric oxide, prostacyclin) and vasoconstrictors (endothelins, angiotensin-converting enzyme)
Regulation of cell growth, particularly smooth muscle cells	Production of growth-stimulating factors (platelet-derived growth factor, hematopoietic colony–stimulating factor) and growth-inhibiting factors (heparin, transforming growth factor-β)
Regulation of inflammatory/immune responses	Expression of adhesion molecules that regulate leukocyte migration and release of inflammatory and immune system mediators (*e.g.*, interleukins, interferons)
Maintenance of the extracellular matrix	Synthesis of collagen, laminin, proteoglycans
Involvement in lipoprotein metabolism	Oxidation of very low–density lipoprotein, low-density lipoprotein, cholesterol

pathologic processes that occur with atherosclerosis, causing vascular remodelling, progressive vascular narrowing, and reductions in blood flow.

IN SUMMARY

The walls of the arteries and veins are composed of three layers: an outer layer of loosely woven collagen tissue, a middle layer of vascular smooth muscle, and an inner layer of endothelial cells. Endothelial dysfunction describes several types of potentially reversible changes in the endothelial function that occur in response to environmental stimuli that can lead to an imbalance between vasodilation and vasoconstriction primarily due to reduced availability of nitric oxide. Other alterations that are affected by and effect endothelial function are related to anti-inflammatory and antithrombogenic factors. Vascular smooth muscle cells not only control dilation and constriction of blood vessels, but elaborate growth factors and synthesize collagen, elastin, and other components of the ECM that are important in both normal vascular repair as well as in pathologic processes such as atherosclerosis.

DISORDERS OF THE ARTERIAL CIRCULATION

After completing this section of the chapter, you should be able to meet the following objectives:

- List the five types of lipoproteins and state their function in terms of lipid transport and development of atherosclerosis.
- Describe the role of lipoprotein receptors in removal of cholesterol from the blood.
- Cite the criteria for diagnosis of hypercholesterolemia.
- Describe possible mechanisms involved in the development of atherosclerosis, the risk factors associated with this, and vessel most commonly affected by atherosclerosis.
- State the signs and symptoms of acute arterial occlusion.
- Describe the pathology associated with the vasculitides and relate it to four associated disease conditions.
- Compare the mechanisms and manifestations of ischemia associated with atherosclerotic peripheral vascular disease, Raynaud phenomenon, and thromboangiitis obliterans (*e.g.,* Buerger disease).
- Distinguish between the pathology and manifestations of aortic aneurysms and dissection of the aorta.

The arterial system distributes blood to all the tissues in the body. There are three types of arteries: large elastic arteries, including the aorta and its distal branches; medium-sized arteries,

such as the coronary and renal arteries; and small arteries and arterioles that pass through the tissues. The large arteries function mainly in systemic transport of blood. The medium-sized arteries are composed predominantly of circular and spirally arranged smooth muscle cells. Their function is distribution of blood flow to the various organs and tissues of the body, which is controlled by contraction and relaxation of the smooth muscle of these vessels. The small arteries and arterioles regulate capillary blood flow. Each of these different types of arteries tends to be affected by different disease processes.

Disease of the arterial system affects body function by impairing blood flow. The effect of impaired blood flow on the body depends on the structures involved and the extent of altered flow. The term *ischemia* (*i.e.,* "holding back of blood") denotes a reduction in arterial flow to a level that is insufficient to meet the oxygen demands of the tissues. *Infarction* refers to an area of ischemic cell death or necrosis in an organ produced by significant deprivation of oxygen to tissues, most commonly the result of occlusion to its arterial blood supply (see Chapter 5). The discussion in this section focuses on blood lipids and hypercholesterolemia, atherosclerosis, vasculitis, arterial and venous disease of the extremities, and arterial aneurysms.

DISORDERS OF THE ARTERIAL CIRCULATION

- The arterial system delivers oxygen and nutrients to the tissues, and disorders of the arterial circulation produce ischemia owing to narrowing of blood vessels, thrombus formation associated with platelet adhesion, and weakening of the vessel wall.
- Atherosclerosis is a progressive disease characterized by the formation of fibrofatty plaques in the intima of large and medium-sized vessels, including the aorta, coronary arteries, and cerebral vessels. The major risk factors for atherosclerosis are hypercholesterolemia and inflammation.
- Vasculitis is an inflammation of the blood vessel wall resulting in vascular tissue injury and necrosis. Arteries, capillaries, and veins may be affected. The inflammatory process may be initiated by direct injury, infectious agents, or immune processes.
- Aneurysms represent an abnormal localized dilation of an artery due to a weakness in the vessel wall. As the aneurysm increases in size, the tension in the wall of the vessel increases and it may rupture. The increased size of the vessel also may exert pressure on adjacent structures.

Hyperlipidemia

Hyperlipidemia is an excess of lipids in the blood. Triglycerides, phospholipids, and cholesterol (the most common steroid), which are classified as lipids, are a diverse group of compounds that have many key biologic functions. Triglycerides, which are used in energy metabolism, are combinations of three fatty acids condensed with a single glycerol molecule. Phospholipids, which are a combination of two fatty acids and a phosphorous-containing group, are a chief component of cell membranes, contribute to blood clotting components, and are present in the myelin sheath. Although cholesterol is not composed of fatty acids, its steroid nucleus is synthesized from fatty acids and thus its chemical activity is similar to that of other lipid substances.[3] Unlike triglycerides, cholesterol is not used as an energy source but has important structural bases for bile salts, plasma membrane, and hormones (*e.g.*, sex and adrenal hormones).

Elevated levels of blood cholesterol (*hypercholesterolemia*) are implicated in the development of atherosclerosis, with its attendant risk of myocardial infarction, stroke and other cardiovascular events associated with atherosclerosis. This is a major public health issue; 38% of Canadians have elevated serum cholesterol levels, and an estimated 13 million Canadians have cholesterol levels above the recommended targets.[4]

Lipoproteins

Because lipids are insoluble in plasma, they are encapsulated by a stabilizing coat of water-soluble phospholipids and proteins (called *apoproteins*). These particles, which are called *lipoproteins,* transport cholesterol and triglycerides to various tissues for energy utilization, lipid deposition, steroid hormone production, and bile acid formation. Lipoproteins vary in their composition but all contain triglycerides, phospholipids, and cholesterol. Lipoproteins are classified according to their lipid densities; the higher the percentage of lipid the lower the density. The main lipoproteins are high-density lipoproteins (HDLs), intermediate-density lipoproteins (IDLs), low-density lipoproteins (LDLs), and very low–density lipoproteins (VLDLs). HDLs differ significantly from the other lipoproteins in that they are actually 50% protein (Fig. 22.2). *Chylomicrons* are a separate class of lipoproteins that are primarily made up of triglycerides (80% to 95%) and have the lowest density of all lipoproteins. Chylomicrons' function is to transport fat absorbed in the intestines.

Each type of lipoprotein consists of a large molecular complex of lipids combined with apoproteins.[5,6] The major lipid constituents are cholesterol esters, triglycerides, nonesterified (or free) cholesterol, and phospholipids. The insoluble cholesterol esters and triglycerides are located in the hydrophobic core of the lipoprotein macromolecule, surrounded by the soluble phospholipids, nonesterified cholesterol, and apoproteins (Fig. 22.3). Nonesterified cholesterol and phospholipids provide a negative charge that allows the lipoprotein to be soluble in plasma.

There are various types of apoproteins: A (*e.g.*, apoA-I, apoA-II, and apoA-IV), B (*e.g.*, apoB-48, apoB-100), C (*e.g.*, apoC-I, apoC-II, and apoC-III), plus others.[6] The apoproteins control the assembly and secretion, structural integrity, interactions, and ultimate metabolic fate of the lipoproteins. Some of the apoproteins activate or inhibit lipolytic enzymes that facilitate the removal of lipids from the lipoproteins; others serve as a reactive site that cellular receptors can recognize

FIGURE 22.2 • Lipoproteins are named based on their protein content, which is measured in density. Because fats are less dense than proteins, as the proportion of triglycerides decreases, the density increases.

and use in the endocytosis and metabolism of the lipoproteins.[6] The major apoprotein in LDL is apoB-100, whereas in HDL it is apoA-I. Research findings suggest that genetic defects in the apoproteins may be involved in hyperlipidemia and accelerated atherosclerosis.[5,6]

There are two sites of lipoprotein synthesis: the small intestine and the liver. The chylomicrons, which are the largest of the lipoprotein molecules, are synthesized in the wall of the

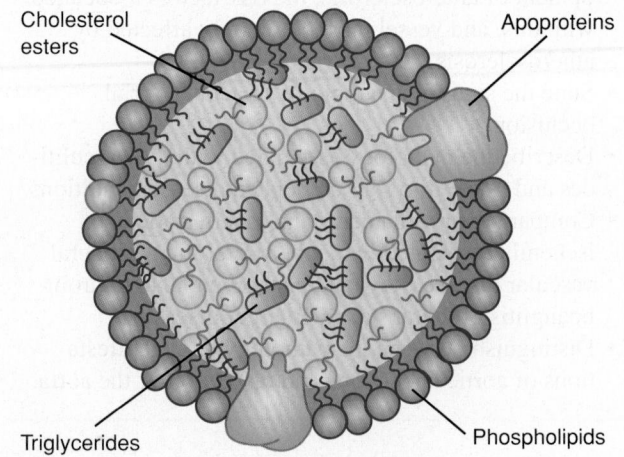

FIGURE 22.3 • General structure of a lipoprotein. The cholesterol esters and triglycerides are located in the hydrophobic core of the macromolecule, surrounded by phospholipids and apoproteins.

small intestine. They are involved in the transport of dietary (exogenous pathway), triglycerides, and cholesterol that have been absorbed from the gastrointestinal tract. Chylomicrons transfer their triglycerides to the cells of adipose and skeletal muscle tissue. The remnant chylomicron particles, which contain cholesterol, are then taken up by the liver and the cholesterol used in the synthesis of VLDL or excreted in the bile.

The liver synthesizes and releases VLDL and LDL. The VLDLs contain large amounts of triglycerides and lesser amounts of cholesterol esters.[1] They provide the primary pathway for transport of the endogenous triglycerides produced in the liver, as opposed to those obtained from the diet. They are also the body's main source of energy during prolonged fasting. Like chylomicrons, VLDLs carry their triglycerides to fat and muscle cells, where the triglycerides are removed. The resulting IDL fragments are reduced in triglyceride content and enriched in cholesterol. They are taken to the liver and recycled to form VLDL, or converted to LDL in the vascular compartment. The exogenous and endogenous pathways for triglyceride and cholesterol transport are shown in Figure 22.4.

LDL, sometimes referred to as the *bad cholesterol,* is the main carrier of cholesterol. LDL is removed from the circulation by either LDL receptors or by scavenger cells such as monocytes or macrophages. The majority of LDL is removed through the LDL receptor-dependent pathway, and the rest is removed by the scavenger pathway. Although LDL receptors are widely distributed, approximately 75% are located on hepatocytes; thus, the liver plays an extremely important role in LDL metabolism. LDL receptor-mediated removal involves binding of LDL to cell surface receptors, followed by *endocytosis,* a phagocytic process in which LDL is engulfed and moved into the cell in the form of a membrane-covered endocytic vesicle. Within the cell, the endocytic vesicles fuse with lysosomes, and the LDL molecule is enzymatically degraded, causing free cholesterol to be released into the cytoplasm.

Other, nonhepatic tissues (*e.g.,* adrenal glands, smooth muscle cells, endothelial cells, and lymphoid cells) also use the LDL receptor-dependent pathway to obtain cholesterol needed for membrane and hormone synthesis. These tissues can control their cholesterol intake by adding or removing

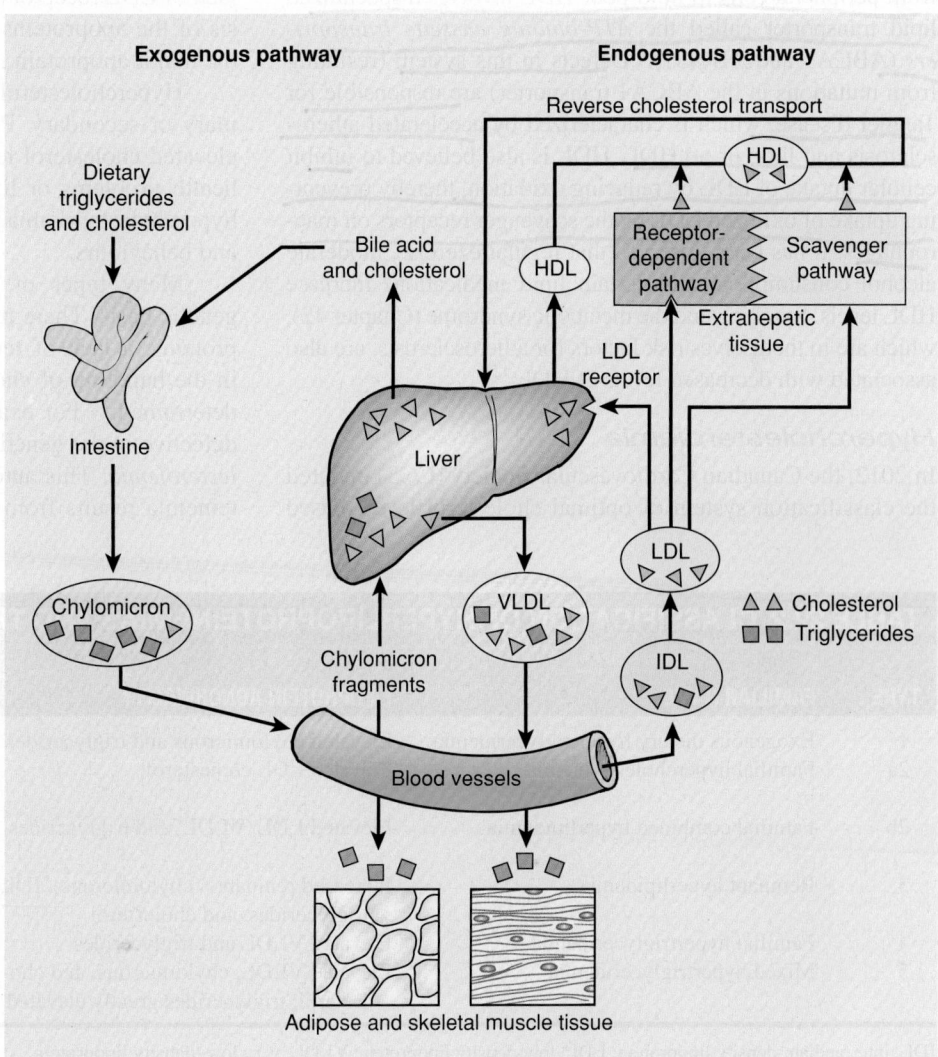

Exogenous pathway   **Endogenous pathway**

Reverse cholesterol transport

Dietary triglycerides and cholesterol

Bile acid and cholesterol

HDL

Receptor-dependent pathway

Scavenger pathway

Extrahepatic tissue

Intestine

Liver

LDL receptor

HDL

Chylomicron

VLDL

LDL

△ △ Cholesterol
▢ ▢ Triglycerides

Chylomicron fragments

IDL

Blood vessels

Adipose and skeletal muscle tissue

FIGURE 22.4 • Schematic representation of the exogenous and endogenous pathways for triglyceride and cholesterol transport.

LDL receptors. The scavenger pathway involves ingestion by phagocytic monocytes and macrophages. These scavenger cells have receptors that bind LDL that has been oxidized or chemically modified. The amount of LDL that is removed by the scavenger pathway is directly related to the plasma cholesterol level. When there is a decrease in LDL receptors or when LDL levels exceed receptor availability, the amount of LDL that is removed by scavenger cells is greatly increased. The uptake of LDL by macrophages in the arterial wall can result in the accumulation of insoluble cholesterol esters, the formation of *foam* cells, and the development of atherosclerosis.

HDL is synthesized in the liver and often is referred to as the *good cholesterol*. HDL participates in the reverse transport of cholesterol by carrying it from the peripheral tissues back to the liver. Epidemiologic studies show an inverse relation between HDL levels and the development of atherosclerosis.[7] It is thought that HDL, which is low in cholesterol and rich in surface phospholipids, facilitates the clearance of cholesterol from the periphery (including atheromatous plaques) and transports it to the liver, where it may be excreted rather than reused in the formation of VLDL (reverse cholesterol transport). The mechanism whereby HDL promotes the movement of cholesterol from peripheral cells to lipid-poor HDL involves a specialized lipid transporter called the *ATP-binding cassette transporters* (ABCA1 and ABCG1).[7] Defects in this system (resulting from mutations in the ABCA1 transporter) are responsible for Tangier disease, which is characterized by accelerated atherosclerosis and little or no HDL. HDL is also believed to inhibit cellular uptake of LDL by reducing oxidation, thereby preventing uptake of oxidized LDL by the scavenger receptors on macrophages. It has been observed that regular exercise, moderate alcohol consumption, and certain lipid medications increase HDL levels. Smoking and the metabolic syndrome (Chapter 42), which are in themselves risk factors for atherosclerosis, are also associated with decreased levels of HDL.[1,5,6]

Hypercholesterolemia

In 2012, the Canadian Cardiovascular Society (CCS) updated the classification system of optimal cholesterol levels based on an individual's overall risk of developing coronary artery disease.[8] The CCS recommends that all men over the age of 40 and women who are menopausal and/or 50 years and older should have a full fasting lipid profile (total cholesterol, LDL cholesterol, HDL cholesterol, and triglycerides) screening once every 1 to 5 years according to their Framingham risk score. Adults with risk factors for coronary artery disease (*e.g.,* diabetes, smoking, hypertension, abdominal obesity, family history, exertional chest discomfort) as well as individuals with chronic kidney disease, evidence of atherosclerosis, or manifestations of hyperlipidemia should be screened at any age. Children should be screened at any age if there is a family history of a monogenic lipid disorder.

Serum cholesterol levels may be elevated as a result of an increase in any of the lipoproteins—the chylomicrons, VLDL, IDL, LDL, or HDL. The commonly used classification system for hyperlipidemia is based on the type of lipoprotein involved (Table 22.2). Several factors, including nutrition, genetics, medications, comorbid conditions, and metabolic diseases, can raise blood lipid levels. Most cases of elevated levels of cholesterol are probably multifactorial. Some persons may have increased sensitivity to dietary cholesterol, others have a lack of LDL receptors, and still others have an altered synthesis of the apoproteins, including oversynthesis of apoB-100, the major apoprotein in LDL.

Hypercholesterolemia can be classified as either primary or secondary. Primary hypercholesterolemia describes elevated cholesterol levels that develop independent of other health problems or lifestyle behaviours, whereas secondary hypercholesterolemia is associated with other health problems and behaviours.

Many types of primary hypercholesterolemia have a genetic basis. There may be a defective synthesis of the apoproteins, a lack of receptors, defective receptors, or defects in the handling of cholesterol in the cell that are genetically determined.[5,6] For example, the LDL receptor is deficient or defective in the genetic disorder known as *familial hypercholesterolemia*. This autosomal dominant type of hyperlipoproteinemia results from a mutation in the gene specifying the

TABLE 22.2 CLASSIFICATION OF HYPERLIPOPROTEINEMIAS AND THEIR GENETIC BASIS

TYPE	FAMILIAR NAME	LIPOPROTEIN ABNORMALITY	KNOWN UNDERLYING GENETIC DEFECTS
1	Exogenous dietary hypertriglyceridemia	Elevated chylomicrons and triglycerides	Mutation in lipoprotein lipase gene
2a	Familial hypercholesterolemia	Elevated LDL cholesterol	Mutation in LDL receptor gene or in apoprotein B gene
2b	Familial combined hyperlipidemia	Elevated LDL, VLDL, and triglycerides	Mutation in LDL receptor gene or apoprotein B gene
3	Remnant hyperlipidemia	Increased remnants (chylomicrons), IDL triglycerides, and cholesterol	Mutation in apolipoprotein E2 gene
4	Familial hypertriglyceridemia	Elevated VLDL and triglycerides	Mutation in lipoprotein lipase gene
5	Mixed hypertriglyceridemia	Elevated VLDL, chylomicrons, and cholesterol; triglycerides greatly elevated	Mutation in apolipoprotein C-II gene

IDL, intermediate-density lipoprotein; LDL, low-density lipoprotein; VLDL, very low–density lipoprotein.

FIGURE 22.5 • Xanthomas in the skin and tendons (**A, C, D**). Arcus lipoides represents the deposition of lipids in the peripheral cornea (**B**). (From Rubin R., Strayer D. S. (Eds.). (2012). *Rubin's pathology: Clinicopathologic foundations of medicine* (6th ed., p. 459). Philadelphia, PA: Lippincott Williams & Wilkins.)

receptor for LDL. More than 1,000 different mutations in the LDL receptor gene have been described.[6] Because most of the circulating cholesterol is removed by receptor-dependent mechanisms, blood cholesterol levels are markedly elevated in persons with this disorder. The disorder is probably one of the most common of all mendelian disorders; the frequency of heterozygotes is 1 in 500 persons in the general population.[6] Plasma LDL levels in heterozygotes range between 6.5 and 13.0 mmol/L, whereas in homozygotes LDL cholesterol levels may rise to 26.0 mmol/L. Although heterozygotes commonly have an elevated cholesterol level from birth, they do not develop symptoms until adult life, when they often develop *xanthomas* (*i.e.,* cholesterol deposits) along the tendons and atherosclerosis appears (Fig. 22.5). Myocardial infarction before 40 years of age is common. Homozygotes are much more severely affected; they have cutaneous xanthomas in childhood and may experience myocardial infarction by as early as 2 to 4 years of age.[6,9]

Causes of secondary hyperlipoproteinemia include obesity with high calorie intake and diabetes mellitus. High-calorie diets increase the production of VLDL, with triglyceride elevation and high conversion of VLDL to LDL. Excess ingestion of cholesterol may reduce the formation of LDL receptors and thereby decrease LDL removal. Diets that are high in triglycerides and saturated fats increase cholesterol synthesis and suppress LDL receptor activity. In diabetes mellitus and the metabolic syndrome, typical dyslipidemia is seen with elevation of triglycerides, low HDL and minimal or modest elevation of LDL.[8] Other systemic disorders that can elevate lipids include hypothyroidism, nephrotic syndrome, and obstructive liver disease. Medications such as β blockers, estrogens, and protease inhibitors (used in the treatment of human immunodeficiency virus [HIV] infection), can also increase lipid levels.

Management of Hyperlipidemia. The CCS continues to identify reduction in LDL cholesterol as the primary target for cholesterol-lowering therapy, particularly in people at risk for CHD.[8] The major risk factors for CHD, that also modify LDL cholesterol goals include cigarette smoking, hypertension, family history of premature CHD in a first-degree relative, age (men ≥45 years; women ≥55 years), and a total cholesterol/HDL ratio greater than 6.0 mmol/L (Chart 22.1). The updated 2012 CCS

CHART 22.1 **RISK FACTORS FOR CORONARY HEART DISEASE IN ADULTS**

Nonmodifiable Risk Factors
- Men over age 45
- Women over the age 55 or postmenopausal
- Family history of cardiovascular disease
  - Males under age 55
  - Females under age 65
- First Nations people; African or South Asian ethnicity

Modifiable Risk Factors
- Hypertension
- Smoking
- Dyslipidemia
  - Low HDLs
  - Elevated LDLs
- Diabetes mellitus
- Obesity
- Excessive alcohol consumption
- Physical inactivity

Target Organ Damage
- Heart disease: left ventricular hypertrophy, coronary artery disease, heart failure
- Stroke or TIA (transient ischemic attack)
- Nephropathy
- Peripheral arterial disease

guidelines recommend that persons with no major risk factors should have an LDL cholesterol goal of 5.0 mmol/L or less; those with two or more of the major risk factors should have an LDL cholesterol goal of less than 3.5 mmol/L; persons with *high-risk* factors (*e.g.,* those with CHD, other forms of atherosclerotic disease, or diabetes) should have an LDL cholesterol goal of less than 2.0 mmol/L. These recommended target lipid levels are based on individual risk factors, determined by a risk assessment tool developed from the Framingham Heart Study data.

The management of hypercholesterolemia focuses on dietary and therapeutic lifestyle changes; when these are unsuccessful, pharmacologic treatment may be necessary. Therapeutic lifestyle changes include an increased emphasis on smoking cessation; maintenance of healthy body weight or weight reduction for people who are overweight; regular physical activity; and reduced intake of saturated fats and simple sugars.

Several dietary elements affect cholesterol and its lipoprotein fractions: (1) excess calorie intake, (2) saturated and trans fats, and (3) cholesterol. Excess calories consistently lower HDL and less consistently elevate LDL. There seems to be a linear relationship with saturated fats in the diet and plasma cholesterol concentrations, but subsequent research is focusing on the genetic polymorphisms of cholesterol transporters and individual responsiveness.[10] Trans fats, which are manufactured from vegetable oils and are used to enhance the taste and extend the shelf life of fast foods, are more atherogenic than saturated fats. Dietary cholesterol tends to increase LDL cholesterol.

The CCS guidelines focus on an overall plan of healthy food choices, maintenance of health body weight, and increased physical activity to decrease the risk for development of cardiovascular disease.[8] Exercise recommendations include 150 minutes of moderate to vigorous aerobic activity per week in bouts of 10 minutes or more. Also, resistance strengthening exercises should be added for at least 2 days per week. The aim of dietary therapy is to reduce total and LDL cholesterol levels and increase HDL cholesterol by a reduction in total calories, and to reduce the percentage of total calories from saturated fat and cholesterol. In general, the dietary guidelines emphasize an increased intake of fruits, vegetables, whole grain cereals, polyunsaturated and monounsaturated oils including omega 3 fatty acids, and decreased intake of saturated and trans fatty acids, simple sugars and refined carbohydrates. However, even with strict adherence to the diet, medication therapy is frequently necessary.

Lipid-lowering medications work in several ways, including decreasing cholesterol production, decreasing cholesterol absorption from the intestine, and removing cholesterol from the bloodstream. Drugs that act directly to decrease cholesterol levels also have the beneficial effect of further lowering cholesterol levels by stimulating the production of additional LDL receptors. Lifestyle management is the first step in managing individuals with low and moderate elevation of lipid levels; however, for individuals who fall into the high-risk category, medication treatment is started immediately along with therapeutic lifestyle changes.[8,11]

There currently are five major types of medications available for treating hypercholesterolemia: HMG-CoA reductase inhibitors (often referred to as "statins"), bile acid–binding resins, cholesterol absorption inhibitor agents, niacin or nicotinic acid, and the fibrates.[11]

Inhibitors of HMG-CoA reductase (*e.g.,* atorvastatin, rosuvastatin, simvastatin), a key enzyme in the cholesterol biosynthetic pathway, can reduce or block the hepatic synthesis of cholesterol and are considered first-line treatment for LDL-reducing therapy. HMG-CoA reductase inhibitors also reduce triglyceride levels.

The bile acid–binding resins (*e.g.,* cholestyramine, colesevelam, colestipol) bind and sequester cholesterol-containing bile acids in the intestine. This leads to increased production of LDL receptors by the liver, with resulting increased removal of cholesterol from the blood for synthesis of new bile acids. The cholesterol absorption inhibitor (ezetimibe) interferes with the absorption of cholesterol.[8,11] Both of these agents are typically used as adjuncts to HMG-CoA reductase inhibitor therapy for patients requiring further reductions in LDL.

Nicotinic acid, a niacin congener, blocks the synthesis and release of VLDL by the liver, thereby lowering not only VLDL levels but IDL and LDL levels. Nicotinic acid also increases HDL concentrations by up to 35%. The fibrates (*e.g.,* bezafibrate, fenofibrate, gemfibrozil) also decrease the synthesis of VLDL by the liver, and enhance the clearance of triglycerides from the circulation. The resulting decrease in triglycerides and increase in HDL with these agents are especially important in the treatment of metabolic syndrome.[11]

Atherosclerosis

Atherosclerosis is a type of arteriosclerosis or "hardening" of the arteries. The term *atherosclerosis,* which comes from the Greek words *atheros* ("gruel" or "paste") and *sclerosis* ("hardness"), denotes the formation of fibrofatty lesions in the intimal lining of the large and medium-sized arteries such as the aorta and its branches, coronary arteries, and large cerebral arteries (Fig. 22.6). Atherosclerosis begins as an insidious process, and clinical manifestations of the disease typically do not become evident for 20 to 40 years or more.

Although there has been a gradual decline in deaths from atherosclerosis over the past several decades, CHD remains the second leading cause of death among men and women in Canada.[12] The reported decline in death rate probably reflects new and improved methods of medical treatment and improved healthcare practices resulting from an increased public awareness of the factors that predispose to the development of this disorder. The major complications of atherosclerosis, including ischemic heart disease, stroke, and peripheral vascular disease, account for approximately 29% of all deaths in Canada (more than 69,5000 deaths per year).[13]

Risk Factors

In terms of healthcare behaviours, some of these risk factors can be affected by a change in behaviour (modifiable), and

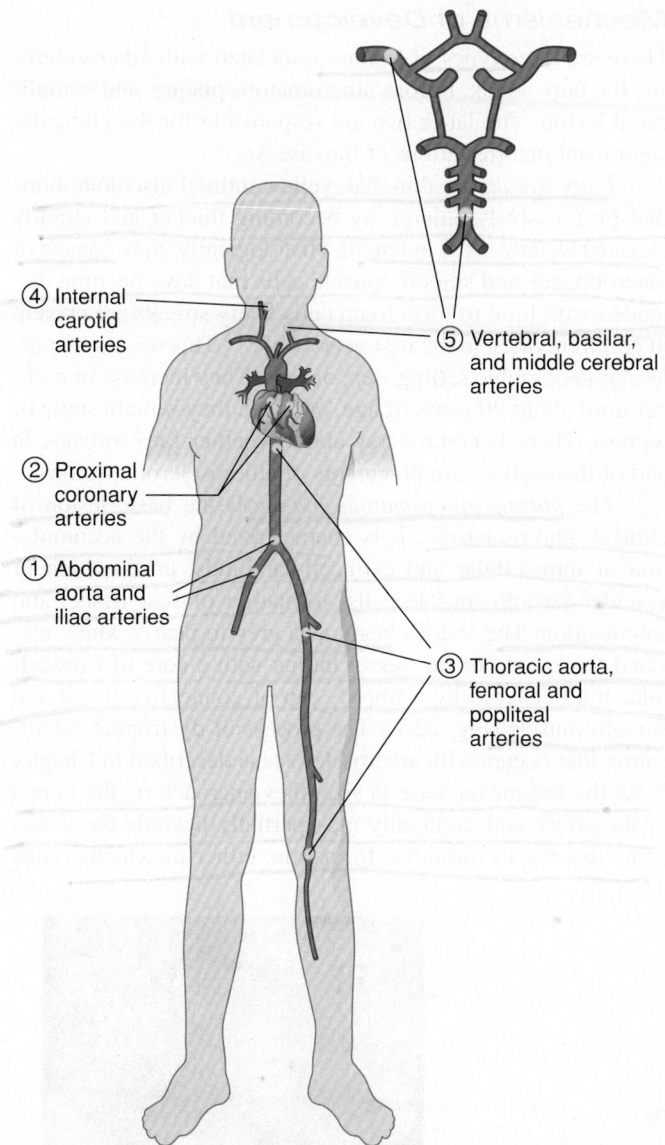

④ Internal carotid arteries

⑤ Vertebral, basilar, and middle cerebral arteries

② Proximal coronary arteries

① Abdominal aorta and iliac arteries

③ Thoracic aorta, femoral and popliteal arteries

FIGURE 22.6 • Sites of severe atherosclerosis in order of frequency. (From Rubin R., Strayer D. S. (Eds.). (2012). *Rubin's pathology: Clinicopathologic foundations of medicine* (6th ed., p. 452). Philadelphia, PA: Lippincott Williams & Wilkins.)

others cannot (nonmodifiable). A major risk factor for atherosclerosis is hypercholesterolemia. Nonlipid risk factors such as increasing age, family history of premature coronary heart disease, and male sex cannot be changed. The tendency toward the development of atherosclerosis appears to run in families. Persons who come from families with a strong history of heart disease or stroke due to atherosclerosis are at greater risk for developing atherosclerosis than those with a negative family history. Several genetically determined alterations in lipoprotein and cholesterol metabolism have been identified, and it seems likely that others will be identified in the future.[5] The incidence of atherosclerosis increases with age. Other factors being equal, men are at greater risk for development of CHD than are premenopausal women, probably because of

the protective effects of natural estrogens. After menopause, the incidence of atherosclerosis-related diseases in women increases, and at older ages actually exceeds that of men.[1]

When looking at risk factors it is estimated that 9 out of 10 Canadians have at least one modifiable risk factor.[13] These major risk factors that can be affected by a change in healthcare behaviours include cigarette smoking, central obesity, hypertension, high blood cholesterol levels, and diabetes mellitus (traditional cardiovascular risk factors). Cigarette smoking plays a strong role in CHD initiation, progression, and fatal cardiovascular outcomes. Components of cigarette smoke induce oxidative insult, leading to damage to the endothelial lining of blood vessels, production of oxidative pro-atherogenic lipids, and a shift toward a procoagulation state in the circulation.[14] Smoking cessation remains an effective measure to prevent smoking-caused cardiovascular events by significantly reducing the risk of endothelial damage.

Obesity, type 2 diabetes, nondiabetic individuals with glucose intolerance, metabolic syndrome (see Chapter 42), high blood pressure, and high blood cholesterol levels all contribute to risk factors and often can be controlled with a change in healthcare behaviours and medications. Women with high blood pressure have 3.5 times greater risk of developing heart disease compared with normotensive women; those who also have diabetes have a greater than eightfold risk of heart disease.[13] When looking at the evidence, an elevated serum cholesterol not only contributes to development of atherosclerotic lesions that block arteries, but interferes with vessel relaxation.

Not all atherothrombotic vascular disease can be explained by the established genetic and environmental risk factors. Other, so-called nontraditional, cardiovascular risk factors can be associated with an increased risk for development of atherosclerosis, including C-reactive protein (CRP), serum homocysteine, serum lipoprotein(a), and infectious agents.[5,15]

Considerable interest in the role of inflammation in the etiology of atherosclerosis has emerged over the last few years.[5,6,13,15] Of particular interest was CRP, a serum marker for systemic inflammation (see Chapter 18). More recent studies have demonstrated that CRP or high-sensitivity CRP (hs-CRP) levels do not show a direct causal relationship to CHD risk.[8] Despite the current limitations of CRP, in the JUPITER study, some patients with a normal LDL and an increase in hs-CRP did benefit from HMG-CoA reductase inhibitor therapy to decrease cardiovascular complications by 50%.[8] This was thought to be due to the anti-inflammatory effects of these agents and the premise that inflammation (as assessed by hs-CRP) could be reduced with certain lifestyle changes and by using medications (including HMG-CoA reductase inhibitors, fibrates, and thiazolidinediones). As atherosclerosis is primarily a disorder of inflammation, it is expected that more definitive information linking systemic inflammation to endothelial dysfunction will become available. Homocysteine is derived from the metabolism of dietary methionine, an amino acid that is abundant in animal protein. The normal metabolism of homocysteine requires adequate levels of folate, vitamin B$_6$, vitamin B$_{12}$, and riboflavin. Homocysteine inhibits elements of the anticoagulant cascade and is associated with endothelial damage, which is thought to be an important first step in the development of atherosclerosis.[5,16] However, supplementation with folic acid, vitamin B$_6$, and vitamin B$_{12}$ to decrease plasma homocysteine levels is not generally recommended for either primary or secondary prevention of cardiovascular disease based on recent clinical evidence.[17]

Lipoprotein(a) is similar to LDL in composition and is an independent risk factor for the development of premature coronary heart disease. Lipoprotein(a) can cause atherosclerosis by binding to macrophages through a high-affinity receptor that promotes foam cell formation and the deposition of cholesterol in atherosclerotic plaques. Routine measurement of lipoprotein(a) levels is not recommended but may be useful in persons who have premature coronary artery disease or a positive family history.[8]

Infectious agents—such as *Chlamydia pneumoniae*, periodontal organisms, *Helicobacter pylori*, cytomegalovirus, herpesvirus, and intestinal microflora—have been discussed as potential causes of atherosclerosis. The presence of these organisms in atheromatous lesions has been demonstrated by immunocytochemistry, but no conclusive causal relationship has been established. One possibility is the organisms play a role in lesion development by initiating and enhancing the inflammatory response, which leads to chronic unresolved inflammation in atherosclerotic plaques.[15]

Mechanisms of Development

There are three types of lesions associated with atherosclerosis: the fatty streak, fibrous atheromatous plaque, and complicated lesion. The latter two are responsible for the clinically significant manifestations of the disease.

Fatty streaks are thin, flat, yellow intimal discolourations that progressively enlarge by becoming thicker and slightly elevated as they grow in length. Histologically, they consist of macrophages and smooth muscle cells that have become distended with lipid to form foam cells. Fatty streaks are present in children, often in the first year of life.[1,5] This occurs regardless of geographic setting, sex, or race. They increase in number until about 20 years of age, and then they remain static or regress. There is controversy about whether fatty streaks, in and of themselves, are precursors of atherosclerotic lesions.

The *fibrous atheromatous plaque* is the basic lesion of clinical atherosclerosis. It is characterized by the accumulation of intracellular and extracellular lipids, proliferation of vascular smooth muscle cells, formation of scar tissue, and calcification. The lesions begin as a grey to pearly white, elevated thickening of the vessel intima with a core of extracellular lipid covered by a fibrous cap of connective tissue and smooth muscle (Fig. 22.7). The process of dystrophic calcification that occurs with atherosclerosis is described in Chapter 5. As the lesions increase in size, they encroach on the lumen of the artery and eventually may partially occlude the vessel or predispose to thrombus formation, either of which results

FIGURE 22.7 • Fibrofatty plaque of atherosclerosis. **A:** In this fully developed fibrous plaque, the core contains lipid-filled macrophages and necrotic smooth muscle cell debris. The "fibrous" cap is composed largely of smooth muscle cells, which produce collagen, small amounts of elastin, and glycosaminoglycans. Also shown are infiltrating macrophages and lymphocytes. Note that the endothelium over the surface of the fibrous cap frequently appears intact. **B:** The aorta shows discrete, raised, tan plaques. Focal plaque ulcerations are also evident. (From Rubin R., Strayer D. S. (Eds.). (2012). *Rubin's pathology: Clinicopathologic foundations of medicine* (6th ed., pp. 447, 448). Philadelphia, PA: Lippincott Williams & Wilkins.)

in a reduction of blood flow. Because blood flow is primarily related to vessel radius (see Chapter 21), the reduction in blood flow becomes increasingly greater as the disease progresses.

The more complicated lesions have thin, fragile caps and may contain a larger lipid core.[18] Therefore, they are more likely than stable lesions to develop ulceration, hemorrhage, and thrombosis. Thrombosis at the site of ulceration and hemorrhage are the most common complications of atherosclerosis. Ulceration may be caused by turbulence of blood flow as well as other factors such as endothelial injury, mediator release, and inflammation. Slowing of blood flow in the ulcerated area and accumulation of platelets, fibrin, and red blood cells enhance thrombus formation. The thrombus may cause occlusion of small vessels that can be life-threatening when it occurs in the heart and brain. Aneurysms may develop in arteries weakened by extensive plaque formation.

Although the risk factors associated with atherosclerosis have been identified through epidemiologic studies, many unanswered questions remain regarding the mechanisms by which these risk factors contribute to the development of atherosclerosis. The vascular endothelial layer, which consists of a single layer of cells with cell-to-cell attachments, normally serves as a selective barrier that protects the subendothelial layers by interacting with blood cells and other blood components. One hypothesis of plaque formation suggests that injury to the endothelial vessel layer is the initiating factor in the development of atherosclerosis.[1,5] A number of factors are regarded as possible injurious agents, including products associated with smoking, immune mechanisms, and mechanical stress such as that associated with hypertension. The fact that atherosclerotic lesions tend to form where vessels branch or where there is turbulent flow suggests that hemodynamic factors also play a role in endothelial injury.[19]

Hyperlipidemia, particularly LDL with its high cholesterol content, is believed to play an active role in the pathogenesis of the atherosclerotic lesion. Interactions between the endothelial layer of the vessel wall and white blood cells, particularly the monocytes (blood macrophages), normally occur throughout life; these interactions increase when blood cholesterol levels are elevated. One of the earliest responses to elevated cholesterol levels is the attachment of monocytes to the endothelium.[20] Monocytes have been observed to migrate through the cell-to-cell attachments of the endothelial layer into the subendothelial spaces, where they are transformed into macrophages. Modified or oxidized LDLs are thought to attract monocyte movement into the subendothelial spaces as well as promote the differentiation of monocytes to activated macrophages. There are a number of factors that contribute to the modification of LDLs in the subendothelial layer, oxidization being a significant contributor.

Activated macrophages release free radicals that oxidize LDL. Oxidized LDL is toxic to the endothelium, causing endothelial loss and exposure of the subendothelial tissue to blood components. This leads to platelet adhesion and aggregation and fibrin deposition. Platelets and activated macrophages release various factors that are thought to promote

growth factors that modulate the proliferation of smooth muscle cells and deposition of ECM in the lesions.[1,5] Activated macrophages also ingest oxidized LDL (by uptake through the scavenger receptor) to become foam cells, which are present in all stages of atherosclerotic plaque formation. Lipids released from necrotic foam cells accumulate to form the lipid core of unstable plaques. Unstable plaques typically are characterized histologically by a large central lipid core, inflammatory infiltrate, and a thin fibrous cap. These "vulnerable plaques" are at risk of rupture (plaque rupture), often at the shoulder of the plaque (Fig. 22.7A) where the fibrous cap is thinnest (because of the presence of local inflammatory cells and mediators that degrade the cap) and the mechanical stresses highest.[20] Thus, "active" atherosclerosis is associated with evidence of inflammation both systemically and at the level of the arterial wall.

Clinical Manifestations

The clinical manifestations of atherosclerosis usually occur late in the pathologic process, depend on the vessels involved and the extent of vessel obstruction. Atherosclerotic lesions produce their effects through narrowing of the vessel and production of ischemia; sudden vessel obstruction due to plaque rupture and hemorrhage; thrombosis and formation of emboli resulting from damage to the vessel endothelium; and aneurysm formation due to weakening of the vessel wall.[1] In larger vessels, such as the aorta, the important complications are those of thrombus formation and weakening of the vessel wall. In medium-sized arteries, such as the coronary and cerebral arteries, ischemia and infarction due to vessel occlusion are more common. Although atherosclerosis can affect any organ or tissue, the arteries supplying the heart, brain, kidneys, lower extremities, and small intestine are most frequently involved (Table 22.3).

TABLE 22.3 MAJOR MANIFESTATIONS OF ATHEROSCLEROSIS

Cardiovascular	Stable and unstable angina
	Myocardial infarction (with or without associated manifestations such as chest pain/discomfort)
	Heart failure
	Hypertension
	Sudden cardiac death
Neurologic	Stroke
	Weak carotid pulses
	Carotid bruits
	Transient ischemic attack (TIA)
	Aortic aneurysm
Peripheral vascular	Pallor and cyanosis
	Intermittent claudication
	Weak pulses
	Peripheral arterial bruits
	Ulcers
	Potential limb loss
Renovascular	Renal stenosis

Understanding The Development of Atherosclerosis

Atherosclerosis is characterized by the development of atheromatous lesions within the intimal lining of the large and medium-sized arteries that protrude into and can eventually obstruct blood flow. The development of atherosclerotic lesions is a progressive process involving (1) endothelial cell injury, (2) migration of inflammatory cells, (3) smooth muscle cell proliferation and lipid deposition, and (4) gradual development of the atheromatous plaque with a lipid core.

1. Endothelial Cell Injury

The vascular endothelium consists of a single layer of cells with cell-to-cell attachments, which normally protects the subendothelial layers from interacting with blood cells and other blood components. Factors, such as smoking, elevated LDL levels, immune mechanisms, and mechanical stress associated with hypertension, share the potential for causing endothelial injury with adhesion of monocytes and platelets.

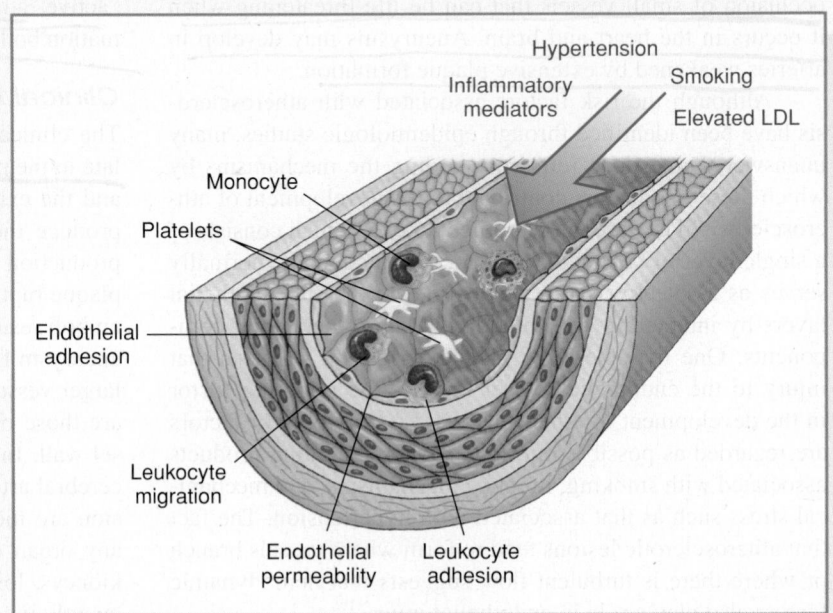

2. Migration of Inflammatory Cells

Early in the development of atherosclerotic lesions, endothelial cells begin to express selective adhesion molecules that bind monocytes and other inflammatory cells that initiate the atherosclerotic lesions. After monocytes adhere to the endothelium, they migrate between the endothelial cells to localize in the intima, transform into macrophages, and engulf lipoproteins, largely LDL.

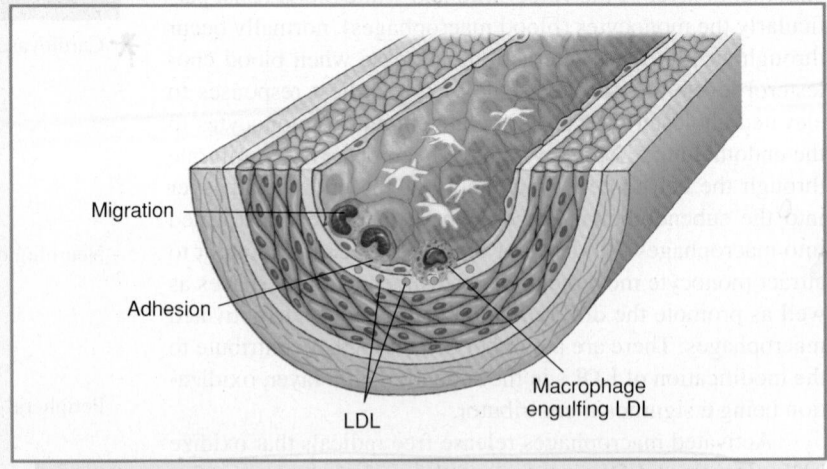

3. Lipid Accumulation and Smooth Muscle Cell Proliferation

Although the recruitment of monocytes, their differentiation into macrophages and subsequent ingestion of lipids, and their ultimate transformation into foam cells is protective in that it removes excess lipids from the circulation, progressive accumulation eventually leads to lesion progression. Activated macrophages release toxic oxygen species that oxidize LDL; they then ingest the oxidized LDL to become foam cells. They also produce growth factors that contribute to the migration and proliferation of smooth muscle cells and the elaboration of ECM.

4. Plaque Structure

Atherosclerotic plaques consist of an aggregation of smooth muscle cells, macrophages, and other leukocytes; ECM, including collagen and elastic fibres; and intracellular and extracellular lipids. Typically, the superficial fibrous cap is composed of smooth muscle cells and dense ECM. Immediately beneath and to the side of the fibrous cap is a cellular area (the shoulder) consisting of macrophages, smooth muscle cells, and lymphocytes. Below the fibrous cap is a central core of lipid-laden foam cells and fatty debris. Rupture, ulceration, or erosion of an unstable or vulnerable fibrous cap may lead to hemorrhage into the plaque or thrombotic occlusion of the vessel lumen.

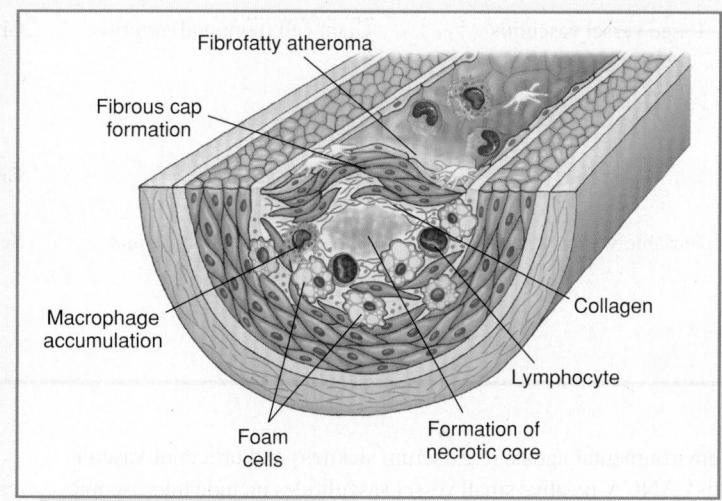

Vasculitis

The *vasculitides* are a group of vascular disorders that cause inflammatory injury and necrosis of the blood vessel wall. The vasculitides involve the endothelial cells and smooth muscle cells of the vascular wall.[21,22] Vessels of any type (arteries, veins, and capillaries) in virtually any organ can be affected. Because they may affect veins and capillaries, the terms *vasculitis, angiitis,* and *arteritis* often are used interchangeably. Clinical manifestations often include fever, myalgia, arthralgia, and malaise. Vasculitis may result from direct injury to the vessel, infectious agents, or immune processes, or they may be secondary to other disease states such as systemic lupus erythematosus. Secondary vascular injury may also occur from physical agents such as cold (*e.g.,* frostbite), irradiation (*e.g.,* sunburn), mechanical injury, and toxins, often leading to necrosis of the vessels. Small vessel vasculitides are sometimes associated with *antineutrophil cytoplasmic antibodies* (ANCA). ANCA are antibodies directed

against certain proteins in the cytoplasm of neutrophils. These autoantibodies may cause endothelial damage.[5] Serum ANCA titres, which can correlate with disease activity, may serve as a useful quantitative diagnostic marker for these disorders.[21]

The vasculitides are commonly classified based on etiology, pathologic findings, and prognosis. The newer classification system divides the conditions into multiple groups, including small vessel, medium-sized vessel, large vessel, variable vessel plus other vasculitides (Table 22.4).[22] Small vessel refers to small arteries (ANCA-associated disease only), arterioles, venules, and capillaries; medium vessels refer to medium- and small-sized arteries and arterioles; and large vessel refers to the aorta and its major tributaries. The small vessel vasculitides are involved in a number of different diseases, most of which are mediated by type III immune complex hypersensitivity reaction (see Chapter 19). They commonly involve the skin and are often a complication of an underlying disease (*e.g.,* vasculitis associated with neoplasms or connective tissue disease) and exposure to

TABLE 22.4 CLASSIFICATION OF THE VASCULITIDES

GROUP	EXAMPLES	CHARACTERISTICS
Small vessel vasculitis	Microscopic polyangiitis	Necrotizing vasculitis with few or no immune deposits affecting medium and small blood vessels, including capillaries, venules, arterioles; associated with antineutrophil cytoplasmic antibodies (ANCAs); necrotizing glomerulonephritis and involvement of the pulmonary capillaries is common
	Granulomatosis with polyangiitis (Wegener's)	Granulomatous inflammation involving the respiratory tract and necrotizing vasculitis affecting capillaries, venules, arterioles, and arteries; associated with ANCAs; necrotizing glomerulonephritis is common
Medium-sized vessel vasculitis	Polyarteritis nodosa	Necrotizing inflammation of medium-sized or small arteries without vasculitis in arteries, capillaries, or venules; not associated with ANCAs; usually associated with underlying disease or environmental agents
	Kawasaki disease	Involves medium-sized and small arteries (frequently the coronaries) and is associated with mucocutaneous lymph node syndrome; usually occurs in small children
Large vessel vasculitis	Giant cell (temporal) arteritis	Granulomatous inflammation of the aorta and its major branches with predilection for branches of carotid and vertebral arteries, often involves temporal artery; infiltration of vessel wall with giant cells and mononuclear cells; usually occurs in people older than 50 years of age and is often associated with polymyalgia rheumatica
	Takayasu arteritis	Granulomatous inflammation of the aorta and its branches; usually occurs in people younger than 50 years of age
Variable vessel vasculitis	Thromboangiitis obliterans (Buerger's)	Segmental, thrombosing, acute and chronic inflammation of the medium-sized and small arteries, principally the tibial and radial arteries but sometimes extending to the veins and nerves of the extremities; occurs almost exclusively in men who are heavy smokers

environmental agents (*e.g.*, serum sickness and urticarial vasculitis). ANCA-positive small vessel vasculitides include microscopic polyangiitis, granulomatosis with polyangiitis (Wegener's), and eosinophilic granulomatosis with polyangiitis (Churg–Strauss syndrome).[21,22] These ANCA-positive vasculitides are treated by similar regimens.

Medium-sized vessel vasculitides produce necrotizing damage to medium-sized muscular arteries of major organ systems. This group includes polyarteritis nodosa and Kawasaki disease (discussed in Chapter 24). Large vessel vasculitides involve large, elastic arteries. They include giant cell (temporal) arteritis and Takayasu arteritis. Variable vessel vasculitis, such as thromboangiitis obliterans (discussed in the section on Arterial Disease of the Extremities), can affect vessels of any size and type. The following discussion focuses on two of the vasculitides: polyarteritis nodosa and giant cell (temporal) arteritis.

Polyarteritis Nodosa

Polyarteritis nodosa, so named because of the numerous nodules found along the course of muscular arteries, is a primary multisystem inflammatory disease of smaller and medium-sized blood vessels, especially those of the kidney, liver, intestine, peripheral nerve, skin, and muscle. The disease is seen more commonly in men than women.

The cause of polyarteritis nodosa remains unknown. It can occur in drug abusers and may be associated with use of certain medications such as allopurinol and the sulfonamides. There is an association between polyarteritis nodosa and hepatitis B and C infection, with 10% to 30% of persons with the disease having antibodies to hepatitis B or C in their serum. This disease is becoming rare, in part because of the decrease in hepatitis B infections as a result of worldwide vaccination campaigns.[23] Other associations include parvovirus B19, HIV, and hairy cell leukemia. Persons with connective tissue diseases such as systemic lupus erythematosus, rheumatoid arthritis, and primary Sjögren syndrome may have manifestations similar to those of primary polyarteritis nodosa.

The onset of polyarteritis nodosa usually is abrupt, with complaints of anorexia, weight loss, fever, and fatigue often accompanied by signs of organ involvement. Clinical signs and symptoms may vary due to the widely varied vascular involvement. The kidney is the most frequently affected organ, and hypertension is a common manifestation of the disorder. Gastrointestinal involvement may manifest as abdominal pain, nausea, vomiting, or rectal bleeding. Myalgia, arthralgia, and arthritis are common, as are peripheral neuropathies such as paresthesias, pain, burning, and weakness. Central nervous system complications include thrombotic and hemorrhagic stroke. Cardiac manifestations result from involvement of the coronary arteries. Skin lesions also may occur and are highly variable. They include reddish-blue, mottled areas of discolouration of the skin of the extremities called *livedo reticularis,* purpura (*i.e.,* black and blue discolouration from bleeding into the skin), urticaria (*i.e.,* hives), and ulcers.[23]

Laboratory findings, although variable, include an elevated erythrocyte sedimentation rate, leukocytosis, anemia, and signs of organ involvement such as proteinuria and hematuria with kidney involvement and abnormal liver function test results. The diagnosis is confirmed through biopsy specimens demonstrating necrotizing vasculitis of the small and large arteries. Treatment involves use of high-dose corticosteroid therapy and often cytotoxic immunosuppressant agents (*e.g.,* azathioprine, cyclophosphamide). Before the availability of corticosteroids and immunosuppressive agents, the disease commonly was fatal. With the use of these agents, the 5-year survival rate is greater than 80%.[23] After the disease is under control, treatment usually is continued for 18 to 24 months and then gradually tapered. For persons with polyarteritis nodosa associated with hepatitis B or C, aggressive simultaneous treatment of the hepatitis is indicated.

Giant Cell Temporal Arteritis

Temporal arteritis (*e.g.,* giant cell arteritis), the most common of the vasculitides, is a focal inflammatory condition of medium-sized and large arteries. It is usually a self-limited condition lasting from months to 3 years. It predominantly affects branches of arteries originating from the aortic arch, including the superficial temporal, vertebral, ophthalmic, and posterior ciliary arteries. The disorder progresses to involve the entire artery wall with focal necrosis and granulomatous inflammation involving multinucleated giant cells (Fig. 22.8).

FIGURE 22.8 • Temporal arteritis. A cross-sectional photograph of a temporal artery shows inflammation throughout the wall, giant cells (*arrow*), and a lumen severely narrowed by intimal thickening. (From Rubin R., Strayer D. S. (Eds.). (2012). *Rubin's pathology: Clinicopathologic foundations of medicine* (6th ed., p. 466). Philadelphia, PA: Lippincott Williams & Wilkins.)

It is more common in elderly persons, with a 3:1 female-to-male ratio.[24] The cause is unknown, although an autoimmune origin has been suggested.

The disorder often is insidious in onset and may be heralded by the sudden onset of mild or severe localized headache; low-grade fever; tender, swollen, nodular, and erythematous superficial temporal artery with absent or decreased pulse; blurred vision or diplopia; and facial pain. Almost one half of affected persons have systemic involvement in the form of polymyalgia rheumatica (see Chapter 59).[25] Up to 10% of patients with giant cell arteritis go on to develop a major late complication of aortic aneurysm (especially thoracic).

Diagnosis is based on the clinical manifestations, a characteristically elevated erythrocyte sedimentation rate and CRP, and temporal artery biopsy. Treatment includes use of high-dose corticosteroids without delay because of the significant risk of visual loss. Before persons with the disorder were treated with corticosteroids, blindness developed in almost 80% of cases due to involvement of the posterior ciliary artery.

Arterial Disease of the Extremities

Disorders of the circulation in the extremities often are referred to as *peripheral vascular disorders.* In many respects, the disorders that affect arteries in the extremities are the same as those affecting the coronary and cerebral arteries in that they produce ischemia, pain, impaired function, and in some cases infarction and tissue necrosis. Not only are the effects similar, but the pathologic conditions that impair circulation in the extremities are identical. This section focuses on acute arterial occlusion of the extremities, atherosclerotic occlusive disease, thromboangiitis obliterans, and Raynaud disease and phenomenon.

Acute Arterial Occlusion

Acute arterial occlusion is a sudden event that interrupts arterial flow to the affected tissues or organ. Acute occlusion of peripheral arteries results in hypoperfusion to the limb tissue distal to the occlusion. Because of the sudden nature of acute arterial occlusion, collateral circulation is limited, thus increasing the risk of limb-threatening ischemia. Most acute arterial occlusions are the result of an embolus or a thrombus. Rarely, the tips of catheters that have been inserted into a vessel can break off and become emboli. Although much less common than emboli and thrombus, trauma or arterial spasm caused by arterial cannulation can be another cause of acute arterial occlusion.

An embolus is a freely moving particle such as a blood clot that breaks loose and travels in the larger vessels of the circulation until lodging in a smaller vessel and occluding blood flow. Most emboli arise in the heart and are caused by conditions that cause blood clots to develop on the wall of a heart chamber or valve surface. Emboli usually are a complication of heart disease: ischemic heart disease with or without infarction; atrial fibrillation, or endocarditis; valvular heart disease; and prostatic values. Arterial emboli can also originate from atherosclerostic plaque and from aneurysms. Other types of emboli are fat emboli that originate from bone marrow of fractured bones, air emboli from the lung, and amniotic fluid emboli that develop during childbirth.

A thrombus is a blood clot that forms on the wall of a vessel and continues to grow until reaching a size that obstructs blood flow. Thrombi often arise as the result of erosion or rupture of the fibrous cap of an arteriosclerotic plaque. A thrombus that breaks off and travels is called a thromboembolus. Thrombi may originate from vascular grafts, atherosclerosis or aneurysms, and are more likely to occur with hypercoagulable and low-flow states.

Manifestations. The signs and symptoms of acute arterial occlusion depend on the artery involved and the adequacy of the collateral circulation. Emboli tend to lodge in bifurcations of the major arteries, including the aorta and iliac, femoral, and popliteal arteries. The presentation of acute arterial embolism is often described as that of the seven "P's": (1) pistol shot (acute onset); (2) pallor; (3) polar (cold); (4) pulselessness; (5) pain; (6) paresthesia; and (7) paralysis. Occlusion in an extremity causes sudden onset of acute pain with numbness, tingling, weakness, pallor, and coldness. There often is a sharp line of demarcation between the oxygenated tissue above the line of obstruction and the ischemic tissue below the line of obstruction. Pulses are absent below the level of the occlusion. These changes are followed rapidly by cyanosis, mottling, and loss of sensory, reflex, and motor function. Tissue death occurs unless blood flow is restored.

Diagnosis and Treatment. Diagnosis of acute arterial occlusion is based on signs of impaired blood flow, namely visual assessment, palpation of pulses, and methods to assess blood flow. Treatment of acute arterial occlusion is aimed at restoring blood flow. The choice of treatment depends on the location of occlusion as well as acuity of the event, and risk factors. For example, an embolectomy—surgical removal of the embolus—is the best choice of intervention when the emboli are localized in a proximal large artery. Intra-arterial fibrinolytic therapy (*e.g.,* streptokinase or tissue plasminogen activator) may be used in an attempt to dissolve the clot. Anticoagulant therapy (*e.g.,* heparin) usually is given to prevent extension of the embolus and to prevent progression of the original thrombus. Application of cold should be avoided, and the extremity should be protected from injury resulting from hard surfaces and overlying bedclothes. If blood flow is not promptly restored, irreversible ischemia occurs and limb amputation may be inevitable.

Atherosclerotic Occlusive Disease

Atherosclerosis is an important cause of peripheral artery disease (PAD) and is seen most commonly in the vessels of the lower extremities. The condition is sometimes referred to as *arteriosclerosis obliterans*. The superficial femoral and popliteal arteries are the most commonly affected vessels. When lesions develop in the lower leg and foot, the tibial, common peroneal, or pedal vessels are the arteries most commonly

affected. The disease is seen most commonly in men and women over the age of 50.[26] Determining the precise number of people with PAD is difficult, but it is estimated that this affects 12% of the adult population and increases to 20% in persons over 70 years of age.[26]

The risk factors for this disorder are similar to those for atherosclerosis, namely diabetes, smoking, hypertension, and dyslipidemia. Cigarette smoking contributes to the progress of the atherosclerosis of the lower extremities and to the development of symptoms of ischemia. Persons with diabetes mellitus develop more extensive and rapidly progressive vascular disease than do nondiabetic individuals. Limb amputation occurs most often in individuals with renal disease and diabetes.[27]

Manifestations. As with atherosclerosis in other locations, the signs and symptoms of vessel occlusion are gradual. Usually, there is at least a 50% narrowing of the vessel before symptoms of ischemia arise. The gradual process of occlusion with atherosclerosis allows the development of collateral circulation. The primary symptom of chronic obstructive arterial disease is *intermittent claudication* or pain with walking.[26] Typically, persons with the disorder complain of calf pain because the gastrocnemius muscle has the highest oxygen consumption of any muscle group in the leg during walking. Some persons may complain of a vague aching feeling or numbness, rather than pain. Other activities such as swimming, bicycling, and climbing stairs use other muscle groups and may not incite the same degree of discomfort as walking. Other signs of ischemia include atrophic changes and thinning of the skin and subcutaneous tissues of the lower leg, and diminution in the size of the leg muscles. The foot often is cool, and the popliteal and pedal pulses are weak or absent. Limb colour blanches with elevation of the leg because of the effects of gravity on perfusion pressure, and becomes deep red when the leg is in the dependent position because of an autoregulatory increase in blood flow and a gravitational increase in perfusion pressure.

When blood flow is reduced to the extent that it no longer meets the minimal needs of resting muscle and nerves, ischemic pain at rest, ulceration, and gangrene develop. As tissue necrosis develops there typically is severe pain in the region of skin breakdown, which is worse at night with limb elevation and is improved with standing.[26]

Diagnosis and Treatment. Diagnostic methods include inspection of the limbs for signs of chronic low-grade ischemia such as subcutaneous atrophy, brittle toenails, hair loss, pallor, coolness, dependent rubor, and auscultation for bruits. Palpation of the femoral, popliteal, posterior tibial, and dorsalis pedis pulses allows for an estimation of the level and degree of obstruction. The ratio of ankle to arm (*e.g.,* tibial and brachial arteries) systolic blood pressure is used to detect significant obstruction, with a ratio of less than 0.9 indicating occlusion. Normally, systolic pressure in the ankle exceeds that in the brachial artery because systolic pressure and pulse pressure tend to increase as the pressure wave moves away from the heart (see Chapter 21). Blood pressures may be taken at various levels on the leg to determine the level of obstruction. A Doppler ultrasound stethoscope may be used for detecting pulses and measuring blood pressure. Ultrasound imaging, magnetic resonance imaging (MRI) arteriography, spiral computed tomographic (CT) arteriography, and invasive contrast angiography may also be used as diagnostic methods.[26]

The two goals of treatment in persons with PAD are (1) to decrease their considerable cardiovascular risk, and (2) to reduce symptoms. Patients should be evaluated for coexisting coronary and cerebrovascular atherosclerosis. The risk of death, mainly from coronary and cerebrovascular events, is high.[26] The other cardiovascular risk factors that should be addressed include smoking cessation, hypertension, lipid lowering, and diabetes. Medications that are useful include cholesterol-lowering agents (*e.g.,* HMG-CoA reductase inhibitors) and antiplatelet agents (*e.g.,* aspirin, dipyridamole, clopidogrel, cilostazol). Antiplatelet medications are used because of the key role platelets have in the pathogenesis of atherosclerosis.[26] The tissues of extremities affected by atherosclerosis are easily injured and slow to heal. Treatment includes measures directed at protection of the affected tissues and preservation of functional capacity. Walking (slowly) to the point of claudication usually is encouraged because it increases collateral circulation.

Percutaneous or surgical intervention is typically reserved for the patient with disabling claudication or limb-threatening ischemia. Surgery (*e.g.,* femoropopliteal bypass grafting using a section of saphenous vein) may be indicated in severe cases. In persons with diabetes, the peroneal arteries between the knees and ankles commonly are involved, making revascularization difficult. Thromboendarterectomy with removal of the occluding core of atherosclerotic tissue may be done if the section of diseased vessel is short. Percutaneous transluminal angioplasty and stent placement, in which a balloon catheter is inserted into the area of stenosis and the balloon inflated to increase vessel diameter, is another form of treatment.[26]

Thromboangiitis Obliterans

Thromboangiitis obliterans, or Buerger disease, is an inflammatory arterial disorder that causes thrombus formation. The disorder affects the small- and medium-sized arteries, usually the plantar and digital vessels in the foot and lower leg. Arteries in the arm and hand also may be affected. Although primarily an arterial disorder, the inflammatory process often extends to involve adjacent veins and nerves. Usually it is a disease of men between the ages of 25 and 40 years who are heavy cigarette smokers, but it is now also being reported with increasing frequency in young female smokers. The pathogenesis of Buerger disease remains speculative, although cigarette smoking and in some instances tobacco chewing seems to be involved. It has been suggested that the use of tobacco may trigger an immune response in susceptible persons or it may unmask a clotting defect, either of which could incite an inflammatory reaction of the vessel wall.[28]

Manifestations. Pain is the predominant symptom of the disorder. It usually is related to distal arterial ischemia. During the early stages of the disease, there is intermittent claudication in the feet, legs, hands, or arms.[28] In severe cases, pain is present even when the person is at rest. The impaired circulation increases sensitivity to cold. The peripheral pulses are diminished or absent, and there are changes in the colour of the extremity. In moderately advanced cases, the extremity becomes cyanotic when the person assumes a dependent position, and the digits may turn reddish-blue even when in a nondependent position. With lack of blood flow, the skin assumes a thin, shiny look and hair growth and skin nutrition suffer. Chronic ischemia causes thick, malformed nails. If the disease continues to progress, tissues eventually ulcerate and gangrenous changes arise that may necessitate amputation.

Diagnosis and Treatment. Diagnostic methods are similar to those for atherosclerotic disease of the lower extremities. As part of the treatment program for thromboangiitis obliterans, it is essential that the person stop smoking cigarettes or using tobacco. Even passive smoking and nicotine replacement therapy should be eliminated. Other treatment measures, are of secondary importance, focus on methods for producing vasodilation and preventing tissue injury. Sympathectomy may be done to alleviate the vasospastic manifestations of the disease.[28]

Raynaud Phenomenon

Raynaud phenomenon is a functional disorder caused by intense vasospasm of the arteries and arterioles in the fingers and, less often, the toes. This is a common disorder affecting 4 in every 10,000 Canadians, women more often than men. This disorder is divided into two types: the primary Raynaud phenomenon, previously called *Raynaud disease,* occurs without demonstrable cause, whereas the secondary Raynaud phenomenon is associated with other disease states or known causes of vasospasm.[29]

Vasospasm implies an excessive vasoconstrictor response to stimuli that normally produce only moderate vasoconstriction. In contrast to other regional circulations that are supplied by vasodilator and vasoconstrictor fibres, the cutaneous vessels of the fingers and toes are innervated only by sympathetic vasoconstrictor fibres. In these vessels, vasodilation occurs by withdrawal of sympathetic stimulation. Cooling of specific body parts such as the head, neck, and trunk produces a sympathetic-mediated reduction in digital blood flow, as does emotional stress.

Primary Raynaud's is seen in otherwise healthy young women, and it often is precipitated by exposure to cold or by strong emotions and usually is limited to the fingers. It also follows a more benign course than the rarer secondary Raynaud phenomenon, seldom causing tissue necrosis. The cause of vasospasm in primary Raynaud's is unknown.[29] Secondary Raynaud's is associated with previous vessel injury, such as frostbite, occupational trauma associated with the use of heavy vibrating tools, collagen diseases, neurologic disorders, and chronic arterial occlusive disorders. Another occupation-related cause is the exposure to alternating hot and

FIGURE 22.9 • Raynaud phenomenon. The tips of the fingers show marked pallor. (From Rubin R., Strayer D. S. (Eds.). (2012). *Rubin's pathology: Clinicopathologic foundations of medicine* (6th ed., p. 463). Philadelphia, PA: Lippincott Williams & Wilkins.)

cold temperatures such as that experienced by butchers and food preparers. This secondary type often is the first symptom of collagen diseases such as scleroderma and systemic lupus erythematosus.[5]

Manifestations. In primary and secondary Raynaud phenomenon, ischemia due to vasospasm causes changes in skin colour that progress from pallor to cyanosis, a sensation of cold, and changes in sensory perception, such as numbness and tingling. The colour changes usually are first noticed in the tips of the fingers, later moving into one or more of the distal phalanges (Fig. 22.9). After the ischemic episode, there is a period of hyperemia with intense redness, throbbing, and paresthesias. The period of hyperemia is followed by a return to normal colour. Although all of the fingers usually are affected symmetrically, in some cases only one or two digits are involved, or only a portion of the digit is affected.

In severe, progressive cases usually associated with secondary Raynaud's, trophic changes may develop. The nails may become brittle, and the skin over the tips of the affected fingers may thicken. Nutritional impairment of these structures may give rise to arthritis. Ulceration and superficial gangrene of the fingers, although infrequent, may occur.

Diagnosis and Treatment. The initial diagnosis is based on history of vasospastic attacks supported by other evidence of the disorder. Immersion of the hand in cold water may be used to initiate an attack as an aid to diagnosis. Laser Doppler flow velocimetry may be used to quantify digital blood flow during changes in temperature.

Treatment measures are directed toward eliminating factors that cause vasospasm and protecting the digits from trauma during an ischemic episode. Abstinence from smoking and protection from cold are priorities. The entire body must be protected from cold, not just the extremities. Avoidance of emotional stress is another important factor in controlling the

disorder because anxiety and stress may precipitate a vascular spasm in predisposed persons. Vasoconstrictor medications, such as the decongestants contained in allergy and cold preparations, should be avoided. Treatment with vasodilator drugs may be indicated, particularly if episodes are frequent, because frequency encourages the potential for development of thrombosis and gangrene. The calcium channel–blocking drugs (*e.g.,* nifedipine, diltiazem) do not change the progress of the condition but decrease the severity and frequency of attacks. Prazosin, an alpha-adrenergic receptor-blocking drug, also may be used. New research is suggesting that phosphodiesterase-5 inhibitors (*e.g.,* sildenafil, tadalafil, vardenafil) may also show a modest benefit for secondary Raynaud's by potentiating the effect of nitric oxide to promote vasodilation.[30] Surgical interruption of sympathetic nerve pathways (sympathectomy) may be used for persons with severe symptoms.[29]

Aneurysms and Dissection

An *aneurysm* is an abnormal localized dilation of a blood vessel. Aneurysms can occur in arteries and veins, but they are most common in the aorta. There are two types of aneurysms: true aneurysms and false aneurysms. A *true aneurysm* is one in which the aneurysm is bounded by a complete vessel wall with an increase in diameter of at least 50%.[31] The blood in a true aneurysm remains within the vascular compartment. A *false aneurysm* represents a localized rupture of the vascular wall of the artery with formation of an extravascular hematoma. Unlike true aneurysms, false aneurysms are bounded only by the supporting tissues such as the surrounding fascia and muscles.

Aneurysms can assume several forms and may be classified according to their cause, location, and anatomic features (Fig. 22.10). A *berry aneurysm* consists of a small, spherical dilation of the vessel at a bifurcation communicating with the main vessel by a small opening.[1,5] This type of aneurysm usually is found in the circle of Willis in the cerebral circulation. A *saccular aneurysm* has a weakness on one side of the vessel and is attached to the main vessel via a small stem appearing like a sac. A *fusiform aneurysm* involves the entire circumference of the vessel and is characterized by a gradual and progressive dilation of the vessel. These aneurysms, which vary in diameter (up to 20 cm) and length, may involve the entire ascending and transverse portions of the thoracic aorta or may extend over large segments of the abdominal aorta. A *dissecting aneurysm* is a false aneurysm resulting from a tear in the intimal layer of the vessel that allows blood to enter the vessel wall, dissecting its layers to create a blood-filled cavity.

The weakness that leads to aneurysm formation may be caused by several factors, including congenital defects, trauma, infections, and atherosclerosis. Once initiated, the aneurysm grows larger as the tension in the vessel increases. This is because the tension in the wall of a vessel is equal to the pressure multiplied by the radius (*e.g.,* tension = pressure × radius; see Chapter 21). In this case, the pressure in the segment of the vessel affected by the aneurysm does not change but remains the same as that of adjacent portions of the vessel.

Berry aneurysm

Aneurysm of abdominal aorta

Aortic dissection (longitudinal section)

A

B

C

FIGURE 22.10 • Three forms of aneurysms: (**A**) berry aneurysm in the circle of Willis, (**B**) aortic dissection, and (**C**) fusiform-type aneurysm of the abdominal aorta.

As an aneurysm increases in diameter, the tension in the wall of the vessel increases in direct proportion to its increased size. If untreated, the aneurysm may rupture because of the increased tension. Even an unruptured aneurysm can cause damage by exerting pressure on adjacent structures and interrupting blood flow.

Aortic Aneurysms

Aortic aneurysms may involve any part of the aorta: the ascending aorta, aortic arch, descending aorta, thoracoabdominal aorta, or abdominal aorta. Multiple aneurysms may be present. The two most common causes of aortic aneurysms are atherosclerosis and degeneration of the vessel media. Half of the people with aortic aneurysms have hypertension.[5] Aortic aneurysms usually develop in older males who smoke cigarettes and current recommendations support the routine screening for males smokers between the ages of 65 and 74.[31]

Manifestations. The signs and symptoms of aortic aneurysms depend on the size and location. An aneurysm also may be asymptomatic, with the first evidence of its presence being associated with vessel rupture. Aneurysms of the thoracic aorta are less common than abdominal aortic aneurysms. They account for less than 10% of aortic aneurysms and may present with substernal, back, and neck pain. There also may be dyspnea, stridor, or a brassy cough caused by pressure on the trachea. Hoarseness may result from pressure on the recurrent laryngeal nerve, and there may be difficulty swallowing because of pressure on the esophagus.[32] The aneurysm also may compress the superior vena cava, causing distension of neck veins and edema of the face and neck.

Abdominal aortic aneurysms are located most commonly below the level of the renal artery (>90%) and involve the bifurcation of the aorta and proximal end of the common iliac arteries.[1,5] The infrarenal aorta is normally 2 cm in diameter; an aneurysm is defined as an aortic diameter greater than 3 cm. They can involve any part of the vessel circumference (saccular) or extend to involve the entire circumference (fusiform). Most abdominal aneurysms are asymptomatic. Because an aneurysm is of arterial origin, a pulsating mass may provide the first evidence of the disorder. Typically, aneurysms larger than 4 cm are palpable. The mass may be discovered during a routine physical examination or the affected person may complain of its presence. Calcification, which frequently exists on the wall of the aneurysm, may be detected during abdominal radiologic examination. Pain may be present and varies from mild midabdominal or lumbar discomfort to severe abdominal and back pain. As the aneurysm expands, it may compress the lumbar nerve roots, causing lower back pain that radiates to the posterior aspects of the legs. The aneurysm may extend to and impinge on the renal, iliac, or mesenteric arteries, or to the vertebral arteries that supply the spinal cord. An abdominal aneurysm also may cause erosion of vertebrae. Stasis of blood favours thrombus formation along the wall of the vessel (Fig. 22.11), and peripheral emboli may develop, causing symptomatic arterial insufficiency.

With thoracic and abdominal aneurysms, the most dreaded complication is rupture. The likelihood of rupture correlates with increasing aneurysm size. The risk of rupture rises from less than 2% for small abdominal aneurysms (<4 cm in diameter) to 11% per year for aneurysms larger than 5 cm in diameter and 25% per year if greater than 6 cm in diameter.[1]

Diagnosis and Treatment. Diagnostic methods include use of ultrasonography, echocardiography, CT scans, and MRI. Currently repair is done either by open surgery with synthetic graft placement or by endovascular aneurysm repair (EVAR). EVAR is a device made of fabric and stent that is introduced under fluoroscopic control into the artery via a sheath. EVAR is minimally invasive and ideal for individuals who are not candidates for more invasive surgery.[33] The size of the aneurysm is the key determinant used to calculate the risk of rupture and the time when repair is recommended.[32,33]

Aortic Dissection

Aortic dissection (dissecting aneurysm) is an acute, life-threatening condition. It involves hemorrhage into the vessel wall

FIGURE 22.11 • Atherosclerotic aneurysm of the abdominal aorta. The aneurysm has been opened longitudinally to reveal a large thrombus in the lumen. The aorta and common iliac arteries display complicated lesions of atherosclerosis. (From Rubin R., Strayer D. S. (Eds.). (2012). *Rubin's pathology: Clinicopathologic foundations of medicine* (6th ed., p. 471). Philadelphia, PA: Lippincott Williams & Wilkins.)

with longitudinal tearing of the vessel wall to form a blood-filled channel (Fig. 22.10B). Unlike atherosclerotic aneurysms, aortic dissection often occurs without evidence of previous vessel dilation. The dissection can originate anywhere along the length of the aorta. The majority of dissections involve the ascending aorta.[5] The second most common site is the thoracic aorta just distal to the origin of the subclavian artery.

Aortic dissection is caused by conditions that weaken or cause degenerative changes in the elastic and smooth muscle of the layers of the aorta. It is most common in the 40- to 60-year-old age group and more prevalent in men than in women.[1] There are two risk factors that predispose to dissection: hypertension and degeneration of the medial layer of the vessel wall, noting that hypertension is present in approximately 75% of individuals with aortic dissection.[34] Aortic dissection also is associated with connective tissue diseases, such as Marfan syndrome. It may occur during pregnancy because of changes in the aorta that occur during this time. Other factors that predispose to dissection are congenital defects of the aortic valve (*e.g.*, bicuspid or unicuspid valve structures) and aortic coarctation. Aortic dissection is a potential complication of cardiac surgery or catheterization. Surgically related dissection may occur at the points where the aorta has been incised or cross-clamped; it also has been reported at the site where the saphenous vein was sutured to the aorta during coronary artery bypass surgery.

Aortic aneurysms are commonly classified into two types, type A and type B, as determined by the level of dissection. The more common (and potentially serious in terms of complications) proximal lesions, involving the ascending aorta only or both the ascending and descending aorta, are designated type A, whereas those not involving the ascending aorta and usually beginning distal to the subclavian artery are designated type B.[1] Dissections usually extend distally from the intimal tear. When the ascending aorta is involved, expansion of the wall of the aorta may impair closure of the aortic valve. There also is the risk of aortic rupture, with blood moving into the pericardium and compressing the heart. Although the length of dissection varies, it is possible for the abdominal aorta to be involved with progression into the renal, iliac, or femoral arteries. Partial or complete occlusion of the arteries that arise from the aortic arch or the intercostal or lumbar arteries may lead to stroke, ischemic peripheral neuropathy, or impaired blood flow to the spinal cord.

Manifestations. A major symptom of a dissecting aneurysm is the abrupt presence of excruciating pain, described as tearing or ripping. The location of the pain may point to the site of dissection.[1] Pain associated with dissection of the ascending aorta frequently is located in the anterior chest, and pain associated with dissection of the descending aorta often is located in the back. In the early stages, blood pressure typically is moderately or markedly elevated. Later, the blood pressure and the pulse rate become unobtainable in one or both arms as the dissection disrupts arterial flow to the arms. Syncope, hemiplegia, or paralysis of the lower extremities may occur because of occlusion of blood vessels that supply the brain or spinal cord. Heart failure may develop when the aortic valve is involved.

Diagnosis and Treatment. Diagnosis of aortic dissection is based on history and physical examination. Aortic angiography, transesophageal echocardiography, CT scans, and MRI studies aid in the diagnosis.[34]

The treatment of dissecting aortic aneurysm may be medical or surgical. Aortic dissection is a life-threatening emergency; persons with a probable diagnosis are stabilized medically even before the diagnosis is confirmed. Two important factors that participate in propagating the dissection are high blood pressure and the steepness of the pulse wave (related to force and velocity). Without intervention, these forces continue to cause extension of the dissection. Medical treatment therefore focuses on decreasing blood pressure and decreasing the force of systolic blood ejection from the heart. Two commonly used drugs, given in combination, are intravenous sodium nitroprusside and β-adrenergic blocking agents. Surgical treatment consists of resection of the involved segment of the aorta and replacement with a prosthetic graft. The mortality rate due to untreated dissecting aneurysm is high.[34]

IN SUMMARY

The arterial system distributes blood to all the tissues of the body, and lesions of the arterial system exert their effects through ischemia or impaired blood flow. There are two types of arterial disorders: diseases such as atherosclerosis, vasculitis, and peripheral arterial diseases that obstruct blood flow, and disorders such as aneurysms that weaken the vessel wall.

Cholesterol relies on lipoproteins (LDLs and HDLs) for transport in the blood. The LDLs, which are atherogenic, carry cholesterol to the peripheral tissues. The HDLs, which are protective, remove cholesterol from the tissues and carry it back to the liver for disposal (reverse cholesterol transport). LDL receptors play a major role in removing cholesterol from the blood; persons with reduced numbers of receptors are at particularly high risk for development of atherosclerosis.

Atherosclerosis, the second leading cause of death in Canada, affects large and medium-sized arteries, such as the coronary and cerebral arteries. It has an insidious onset, and its lesions usually are far advanced before symptoms appear. Although the mechanisms of atherosclerosis are uncertain, risk factors associated with its development have been identified. These include factors such as heredity, gender, and age, which cannot be controlled; and factors such as smoking, high blood pressure, high serum cholesterol levels, diabetes, obesity, and inflammation, which can be controlled or modified.

The vasculitides are a group of vascular disorders characterized by vasculitis or inflammation and necrosis of the blood vessels in various tissues and organs of the body. They can be caused by injury to the vessel, infectious agents, or immune processes, or can occur secondary to other disease states such as systemic lupus erythematosus.

Occlusive disorders interrupt arterial flow of blood and interfere with the delivery of oxygen and nutrients to the tissues. Occlusion of flow can result from a thrombus, emboli, vessel compression, vasospasm, or structural changes in the vessel. Peripheral arterial diseases affect blood vessels outside the heart and thorax. They include Raynaud phenomenon, caused by vessel spasm, and thromboangiitis obliterans (Buerger disease), characterized by an inflammatory process that involves small- and medium-sized arteries.

Aneurysms are localized areas of vessel dilation caused by weakness of the arterial wall. A berry aneurysm, most often found in the circle of Willis in the brain circulation, consists of a small, spherical vessel dilation. Fusiform and saccular aneurysms are most often found in the thoracic and abdominal aorta, and are characterized by gradual and progressive enlargement of the aorta. A dissecting aneurysm is an acute, life-threatening condition. It involves hemorrhage into the vessel wall with longitudinal tearing (dissection) of the vessel wall to form a blood-filled channel. The most serious consequence of aneurysms is rupture.

DISORDERS OF THE VENOUS CIRCULATION

After completing this section of the chapter, you should be able to meet the following objectives:

- Describe venous return of blood from the lower extremities, including the function of the muscle pumps and the effects of gravity, and relate to the development of varicose veins.
- Differentiate primary from secondary varicose veins.
- Characterize the pathology of venous insufficiency and relate to the development of stasis dermatitis and venous ulcers.
- List the four most common causes of lower leg ulcer.
- Cite risk factors associated with venous thrombosis and describe the manifestation of the disorder and its treatment.

Veins are low-pressure, thin-walled vessels that rely on the ancillary action of skeletal muscle pumps and changes in abdominal and intrathoracic pressure to return blood to the heart. Unlike the arterial system, the venous system is equipped with valves that prevent retrograde flow of blood. Although its structure enables the venous system to serve as a storage area for blood, it also renders the system susceptible to problems related to stasis and venous insufficiency. This section focuses on three common problems of the venous system: varicose veins, venous insufficiency, and venous thrombosis.

Venous Circulation of the Lower Extremities

The venous system in the legs consists of two components: the superficial veins (*e.g.,* saphenous vein and its tributaries) and the deep venous channels (Fig. 22.12A). Perforating or communicating veins connect these two systems. Blood from the skin and subcutaneous tissues in the leg collects in the superficial veins and is then transported across the communicating veins into the deeper venous channels for return to the heart. Venous valves prevent the retrograde flow of blood and play an important role in the function of the venous system. Although these valves are irregularly located along the length of the veins, they almost always are found at junctions where the communicating veins merge with the larger deep veins and where two veins meet. The number of venous valves differs somewhat from one person to another, as does their structural competence, factors that may help explain the familial predisposition to development of varicose veins.

The action of the leg muscles assists in moving venous blood from the lower extremities back to the heart. When a person walks, the action of the leg muscles serves to increase flow in the deep venous channels and return venous blood to the heart (Fig. 22.13). The function of the so-called *muscle pump,* located in the gastrocnemius and soleus muscles of the

FIGURE 22.12 • Superficial and deep venous channels of the leg. **A:** Normal venous structures and flow patterns. **B:** Varicosities in the superficial venous system are the result of incompetent valves in the communicating veins. The *arrows* in both views indicate the direction of blood flow. (Modified from Abramson D. I. (1974). *Vascular disorders of the extremities* (2nd ed.). New York: Harper & Row.)

lower extremities, can be compared with the pumping action of the heart.[5,35] During muscle contraction, which is similar to systole, valves in the communicating channels close to prevent backward flow of blood into the superficial system, as blood in the deep veins is moved forward by the action of the contracting muscles. During muscle relaxation, which is similar to diastole, the communicating valves open, allowing blood from the superficial veins to move into the deep veins.

DISORDERS OF THE VENOUS CIRCULATION

- Veins are thin-walled, distensible vessels that collect blood from the tissues and return it to the heart. The venous system is a low-pressure system that relies on the pumping action of the skeletal muscles to move blood forward and the presence of venous valves to prevent retrograde flow.
- Disorders of the venous system produce congestion of the affected tissues and predispose to clot formation because of stagnation of flow and activation of the clotting system.
- Varicose veins are dilated and tortuous veins that result from a sustained increase in pressure that causes the venous valves to become incompetent, allowing for reflux of blood and vein engorgement.
- Thrombophlebitis refers to thrombus formation in a vein and the accompanying inflammatory response in the vessel wall as a result of conditions that obstruct or slow blood flow, increase the activity of the coagulation system, or cause vessel injury. Deep vein thrombosis (DVT) may be a precursor to pulmonary embolism.

Disorders of the Venous Circulation of the Lower Extremities

Varicose Veins

Varicose, or dilated, tortuous veins of the lower extremities are common and often lead to secondary problems of venous insufficiency (Fig. 22.12B). Varicose veins are described as being primary or secondary. Primary varicose veins originate

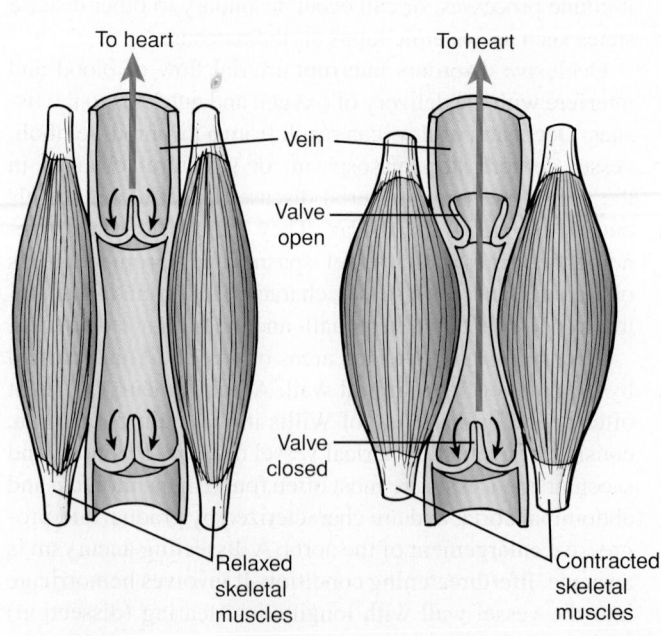

FIGURE 22.13 • The skeletal muscle pumps and their function in promoting blood flow in the deep and superficial calf vessels of the leg.

in the superficial saphenous veins, and secondary varicose veins result from impaired flow in the deep venous channels. Approximately 80% to 90% of venous blood from the lower extremities is transported through the deep channels. The development of secondary varicose veins becomes inevitable when flow in these deep channels is impaired or blocked. The most common cause of secondary varicose veins is DVT. Other causes include congenital or acquired arteriovenous fistulas, congenital venous malformations, and pressure on the abdominal veins caused by pregnancy or a tumour.

Varicose veins in Western nations occur in approximately one third of the adult population.[35] The prevalence increases with age and in obese persons, and it occurs more often in women, probably because of venous stasis caused by pregnancy.[5,35] More than 50% of persons with primary varicose veins have a family history of the disorder, suggesting that heredity may play a role.

Mechanisms of Development. Prolonged standing and increased intra-abdominal pressure are important contributing factors in the development of primary varicose veins. Prolonged standing increases venous pressure and causes dilation and stretching of the vessel wall. One of the most important factors in the elevation of venous pressure is the hydrostatic effect associated with the standing position. When a person is in the erect position, the full weight of the venous columns of blood is transmitted to the leg veins. The effects of gravity are compounded in persons who stand for long periods without using their leg muscles to assist in pumping blood back to the heart.

Because there are no valves in the inferior vena cava or common iliac veins, blood in the abdominal veins must be supported by the valves located in the external iliac or femoral veins. When intra-abdominal pressure increases, as it does during pregnancy, or when the valves in these two veins are absent or defective, the stress on the saphenofemoral junction is increased. The high incidence of varicose veins in women who have been pregnant also suggests a hormonal effect on venous smooth muscle contributing to venous dilation and valvular incompetence. Lifting also increases intra-abdominal pressure and decreases flow of blood through the abdominal veins. Occupations that require repeated heavy lifting also predispose to development of varicose veins.

Prolonged exposure to increased pressure causes the venous valves to become incompetent so they no longer close properly. When this happens, the reflux of blood causes further venous enlargement, pulling the valve leaflet apart and causing more valvular incompetence in sections of adjacent distal veins. Another consideration in the development of varicose veins is the fact that the superficial veins have only subcutaneous fat and superficial fascia for support, but the deep venous channels are supported by muscle, bone, and connective tissue. Obesity reduces the support provided by the superficial fascia and tissues, increasing the risk for development of varicose veins.

Manifestations. The signs and symptoms associated with primary varicose veins vary. Most women with superficial varicose veins complain of their unsightly appearance. In many cases, aching in the lower extremities and edema, especially after long periods of standing, may occur. The edema usually subsides at night when the legs are elevated. When the communicating veins are incompetent, symptoms are more common.

Diagnosis and Treatment. The diagnosis of varicose veins often can be made after physical inspection. Several procedures are used to assess the extent of venous involvement associated with varicose veins. In one of these, the Trendelenburg test, a tourniquet is applied to the affected leg while it is elevated and the veins are empty. The person then assumes the standing position, and the tourniquet is removed. If the superficial veins are involved, the veins distend quickly. To assess the deep channels, the tourniquet is applied while the person is standing and the veins are filled. The person then lies down and the affected leg is elevated. Emptying of the superficial veins indicates that the deep channels are patent. Other noninvasive testing includes the preferred venous duplex imaging, CT, or magnetic resonance venography. Invasive testing, if required, can include angiographic studies using a radiopaque contrast medium.[36]

After the venous channels have been repeatedly stretched and the valves rendered incompetent, little can be done to restore normal venous tone and function. Ideally, measures should be taken to prevent the development and progression of varicose veins. These measures centre on avoiding activities such as continued standing that produce prolonged elevation of venous pressure and promoting optimum body weight. Treatment measures for varicose veins focus on improving venous flow and preventing tissue injury. When correctly fitted, elastic support stockings or leggings compress the superficial veins and prevent distension. The most precise control is afforded by prescription stockings, measured to fit properly.[36] These stockings should be applied before the standing position is assumed, when the leg veins are empty.

Sclerotherapy, which often is used in the treatment of small residual varicosities, involves the injection of a sclerosing agent into the collapsed superficial veins to produce fibrosis of the vessel lumen. Surgical treatment consists of removing the varicosities and the incompetent perforating veins, but it is limited to persons with patent deep venous channels.[36]

Chronic Venous Insufficiency

The term *venous insufficiency* refers to the physiologic consequences of DVT, valvular incompetence, or a combination of both conditions. The most common cause is DVT, which causes deformity of the valve leaflets, rendering them incapable of closure. In the presence of valvular incompetence, effective unidirectional flow of blood and emptying of the deep veins cannot occur. The muscle pumps also are ineffective, often driving blood in retrograde directions. Secondary failure of the communicating and superficial veins subjects the subcutaneous tissues to high pressures.

With venous insufficiency, there are signs and symptoms associated with impaired blood flow. In contrast to the ischemia caused by arterial insufficiency, venous insufficiency

FIGURE 22.14 • Varicose veins of the legs. Severe varicosities of the superficial leg veins have led to stasis dermatitis and secondary ulcerations. (From Rubin R., Strayer D. S. (Eds.). (2012). *Rubin's pathology: Clinicopathologic foundations of medicine* (6th ed., p. 474). Philadelphia, PA: Lippincott Williams & Wilkins.)

leads to tissue congestion, edema, and eventual impairment of tissue nutrition.[36] The edema is exacerbated by long periods of standing. Necrosis of subcutaneous fat deposits occurs, followed by skin atrophy. Brown pigmentation of the skin caused by hemosiderin deposits resulting from the breakdown of red blood cells is common. Secondary lymphatic insufficiency occurs, with progressive sclerosis of the lymph channels in the face of increased demand for clearance of interstitial fluid.

In advanced venous insufficiency, impaired tissue nutrition causes stasis dermatitis and the development of stasis or venous ulcers (Fig. 22.14). Stasis dermatitis is characterized by the presence of thin, shiny, bluish-brown, irregularly pigmented desquamative skin that lacks the support of the underlying subcutaneous tissues. Minor injury leads to relatively painless ulcerations that are difficult to heal. The lower part of the leg is particularly prone to development of stasis dermatitis and venous ulcers. Most lesions are located medially over the ankle and lower leg, with the highest frequency just above the medial malleolus. Venous insufficiency is the most common cause of lower leg ulcers, accounting for nearly 80% of all cases.[37] The other common causes of lower extremity ulcers are arterial insufficiency, neuropathy (often due to diabetes), and pressure ulcers.

Treatment of venous ulcers includes compression therapy with dressings and inelastic or elastic bandages. Medications such as aspirin and pentoxifylline are sometimes used for symptom control, decreasing blood viscosity, and thereby improving blood flow. Occasionally skin grafting is required for large or slow-healing venous ulcers.[36] Growth factors (which are administered topically or by perilesional injection) may also be warranted.[37]

Venous Thrombosis

The term *venous thrombosis,* or *thrombophlebitis,* describes the presence of thrombus in a vein and the accompanying inflammatory response in the vessel wall. Thrombi can develop in the superficial or the deep veins. DVT most commonly occurs in the lower extremities. DVT of the lower extremity is a serious disorder, complicated by pulmonary embolism (see Chapter 29), recurrent episodes of DVT, and development of chronic venous insufficiency. Most postoperative thrombi arise in the soleal sinuses or the large veins draining the gastrocnemius muscles. Isolated calf thrombi often are asymptomatic. DVT is often associated with the risk of developing a pulmonary embolus.[5]

In 1846, Virchow described the triad that has come to be associated with venous thrombosis: stasis of blood, increased blood coagulability, and vessel wall injury.[1] Risk factors for venous thrombosis are summarized in Chart 22.2. Stasis of blood occurs with immobility of an extremity or the entire body. Bed rest and immobilization are associated with

---

CHART 22.2 **RISK FACTORS ASSOCIATED WITH VENOUS THROMBOSIS**[a]

Venous Stasis
Bed rest
Immobility
Spinal cord injury
Acute myocardial infarction
Congestive heart failure
Shock
Venous obstruction

Hyperreactivity of Blood Coagulation
Genetic factors
Stress and trauma
Pregnancy
Childbirth
Oral contraceptive and hormone replacement use
Dehydration
Cancer
Antiphospholipid syndrome
Hyperhomocysteinemia

Vascular Trauma
Indwelling venous catheters
Surgery
Massive trauma or infection
Fractured hip
Orthopedic surgery

[a]Many of these disorders involve more than one mechanism.

decreased blood flow, venous pooling in the lower extremities, and increased risk of DVT. Persons who are immobilized by a hip fracture, joint replacement, or spinal cord injury are particularly vulnerable to DVT. The risk of DVT is increased in situations of impaired cardiac function. This may account for the relatively high incidence in persons with acute myocardial infarction and congestive heart failure. Elderly persons are more susceptible than younger persons, probably because disorders that produce venous stasis occur more frequently in older persons. Long airplane travel poses a particular threat in persons predisposed to DVT because of prolonged sitting and increased blood viscosity due to dehydration.[1]

Hypercoagulability is a homeostatic mechanism designed to increase clot formation, and conditions that increase the concentration or activation of clotting factors predispose to DVT. Thrombosis also can be caused by inherited or acquired deficiencies in certain plasma proteins that normally inhibit thrombus formation, such as antithrombin III, protein C, and protein S. However, the most common inherited risk factors are the factor V Leiden and prothrombin gene mutations.[5,38] The postpartum state is associated with increased levels of fibrinogen, prothrombin, and other coagulation factors. The use of oral contraceptives and hormone replacement therapy appears to increase coagulability and predispose to venous thrombosis, a risk that is further increased in women who smoke. Certain cancers are associated with increased clotting tendencies, and although the reason for this is largely unknown, substances that promote blood coagulation may be produced by the tumour cells or released from the surrounding tissues in response to the cancerous growth. Immune interactions with cancer cells can result in the release of cytokines that can cause endothelial damage and predispose to thrombosis.[39] Aggressive antitumour therapy can also cause vascular damage. When body fluid is lost because of injury or disease, the resulting hemoconcentration causes clotting factors to become more concentrated. Other important risk factors include the antiphospholipid syndrome and hyperhomocysteinemia.[5]

Vessel injury can result from a trauma situation or from surgical intervention. It also may occur secondary to infection or inflammation of the vessel wall. Persons undergoing hip surgery and total hip replacement are at particular risk because of trauma to the femoral and iliac veins, and in the case of hip replacement, thermal damage from heat generated by the polymerization of the acrylic cement that is used in the procedure. Venous catheters are another source of vascular injury.

Manifestations. As many as 50% of persons with venous thrombosis are asymptomatic, and this is probably because the vein is not totally occluded or because of collateral circulation.[5] When present, the most common signs and symptoms of venous thrombosis are those related to the inflammatory process: pain, swelling, and deep muscle tenderness. Fever, general malaise, and an elevated white blood cell count and erythrocyte sedimentation rate are accompanying indications of inflammation. There may be tenderness and pain along the vein. Swelling may vary from minimal to maximal.

The site of thrombus formation determines the location of the physical findings. The most common site is in the venous sinuses in the soleus muscle and posterior tibial and peroneal veins. Swelling in these cases involves the foot and ankle, although it may be slight or absent. Calf pain and tenderness are common. Femoral vein thrombosis with calf thrombosis produces pain and tenderness in the distal thigh and popliteal area. Thrombi in iliofemoral veins produce the most profound manifestations, with swelling, pain, and tenderness of the entire extremity. With DVT in the calf veins, active dorsiflexion can produce calf pain (i.e., Homans sign).

Diagnosis and Treatment. The risk of pulmonary embolism emphasizes the need for early detection and treatment of DVT. Several tests are useful for this purpose: ascending venography, ultrasonography (e.g., real-time, B-mode, duplex), and plasma d-dimer assessment (see Chapter 29).

Whenever possible, venous thrombosis should be prevented in preference to being treated. Early ambulation after childbirth and surgery is one measure that decreases the risk of thrombus formation. Exercising the legs and wearing support stockings improve venous flow. A further precautionary measure is to avoid assuming body positions that favour venous pooling. Antiembolism stockings of the proper fit and length should be used routinely in persons at risk for DVT. Another strategy used for immobile persons at risk for development of DVT is a sequential pneumatic compression device. This consists of a plastic sleeve that encircles the legs and provides alternating periods of compression on the lower extremity. When properly used, these devices enhance venous emptying to augment flow and reduce stasis. Prophylactic anticoagulation often is used in persons who are at high risk for development of venous thrombi.

The objectives of treatment of venous thrombosis are to prevent the formation of additional thrombi, prevent extension and embolization of existing thrombi, and minimize venous valve damage. A 15- to 20-degree elevation of the legs prevents stasis. It is important that the entire lower extremity or extremities be carefully extended to avoid acute flexion of the knee or hip. Heat often is applied to the leg to relieve venospasm and to aid in the resolution of the inflammatory process. Bed rest usually is maintained until local tenderness and swelling have subsided. Gradual ambulation with elastic support is then permitted. Standing and sitting increase venous pressure and are to be avoided. Elastic support is needed for 3 to 6 months to permit recanalization and collateralization and to prevent venous insufficiency.

Anticoagulation therapy (e.g., heparin and warfarin) is used to treat and prevent venous thrombosis. Treatment typically is initiated with either continuous intravenous infusion of heparin followed by prophylactic therapy with oral anticoagulants to prevent further thrombus formation, or with subcutaneous injections of low–molecular-weight heparin (LMWH). LMWH may also be given on an outpatient basis. Fibrinolytic therapy (e.g., streptokinase, urokinase, or tissue plasminogen activator) may be used in an attempt to dissolve the clot.

Surgical removal of the thrombus may be undertaken in selected cases. Percutaneous (through the skin) insertion of intracaval filters may be done in persons at high risk for development of pulmonary emboli. This procedure prevents large clots from moving through the vessel. However, although filters prevent the development of pulmonary emboli, an increase in thrombosis occurs at the site of the filter itself in the absence of anticoagulation.

IN SUMMARY

The storage function of the venous system renders it susceptible to venous insufficiency, stasis, and thrombus formation. Varicose veins occur with prolonged distension and stretching of the superficial veins owing to venous insufficiency. Varicosities can arise because of defects in the superficial veins (*e.g.,* primary varicose veins) or because of impaired blood flow in the deep venous channels (*e.g.,* secondary varicose veins). Venous insufficiency reflects chronic venous stasis resulting from valvular incompetence. It is associated with stasis dermatitis and stasis or venous ulcers. Venous thrombosis describes the presence of thrombus in a vein and the accompanying inflammatory response in the vessel wall. It is associated with vessel injury, stasis of venous flow, and hypercoagulability states. Thrombi can develop in the superficial or deep veins (*e.g.,* DVT). Thrombus formation in deep veins is a precursor to venous insufficiency and embolus formation.

REVIEW EXERCISES

1. A 55-year-old male executive presents at the clinic for his regular checkup. He was diagnosed with hypertension 5 years ago and has been taking a diuretic and a β-adrenergic blocker to control his blood pressure. His blood pressure is currently being maintained at about 135/70 mm Hg. His total cholesterol level is 4.7 mmol/L and his HDL cholesterol is 0.7 mmol/L. He is otherwise well. He is a nonsmoker. He has recently read in the media about "inflammation" and the heart and expresses concern about his risk of coronary heart disease.
   A. *Discuss the risk factors that predispose this patient to developing myocardial infarction and coronary death. Find an online risk assessment tool based on the Framingham Heart Study and calculate this man's 10-year risk of developing coronary heart disease.*
2. A 62-year-old man presents at the emergency department of his local hospital with complaints of excruciating, "ripping" pain in his upper back. He has a history of poorly controlled hypertension. His radial pulse and blood pressure, which on admission were 92 and 140/80 mm Hg, respectively, become unobtainable in both arms. A transesophageal echocardiogram reveals a dissection of the descending aorta. Aggressive blood pressure control is initiated with the goal of reducing the systolic pressure and pulsatile blood flow (pulse pressure).
   A. *Explain how aortic dissection differs from a thoracic aorta aneurysm.*
   B. *Explain the role of poorly controlled hypertension as an etiologic factor in dissecting aneurysms.*
   C. *Why did his radial pulse and blood pressure become unobtainable?*
   D. *Explain the need for aggressive control of aortic pressure and pulsatile blood flow.*
3. A 34-year-old, otherwise healthy woman complains of episodes lasting several hours in which her fingers become pale and numb. This is followed by a period during which the fingers become red, throbbing, and painful.
   A. *What do you think is causing this woman's problem?*
   B. *She relates that the episodes often occur when her fingers become cold or when she becomes upset. Explain the possible underlying mechanisms.*
   C. *What types of measures could be used to treat this woman?*

References

1. Kumar V., Abbas A. K., Faustos N., et al. (Eds.). (2010). *Robbins and Cotran pathologic basis of disease* (8th ed.). Philadelphia, PA: Elsevier Saunders.
2. Ross M. H., Pawlina W. (2011). *Histology: A text and atlas* (6th ed.). Philadelphia, PA: Lippincott Williams & Wilkins.
3. Hall J. E. (2011). *Textbook of medical physiology* (12th ed.). Philadelphia, PA: W. B. Saunders.
4. Statistics Canada. (2013). Cholesterol levels of adults, 2012 to 2013. Available online at: http://www.statcan.gc.ca/pub/82–625-x/2014001/article/14122-eng.htm. Accessed February 28, 2015.
5. Rubin R., Strayer D. S. (Eds.). (2012). *Rubin's pathology: Clinicopathologic foundations of medicine* (6th ed.). Philadelphia, PA: Lippincott Williams & Wilkins.
6. Genest J., Libby P. (2014). Chapter 45: Lipoprotein disorders and cardiovascular disease. In Mann D. L., Zipes D. P., Libby P., et al. (Eds.), *Braunwald's heart disease: A textbook of cardiovascular medicine* (10th ed.). Philadelphia, PA: Elsevier/Saunders.
7. Westerterp M., Bochem A. E., Yvan-Charvet L., et al. (2014). ATP-binding cassette transporter, atherosclerosis, and inflammation. *Circulation Research, 114*(1), 157–170.
8. Anderson T., Gregoire J., Hegele R. A., et al. (2013). 2012 update of the Canadian Cardiovascular Society guidelines for the diagnosis and treatment of dyslipidemia for the prevention of cardiovascular disease in the adult. *Canadian Journal of Cardiology, 29*(2), 151–167.
9. Raal F. J., Santos R. D. (2012). Homozygous familial hypercholesterolemia: Current perspectives on diagnosis and treatment. *Atherosclerosis, 223*(2), 262–268.

10. Griffin J. D., Lichtenstein A. H. (2013). Dietary cholesterol and plasma lipoproteins profiles: Randomized-controlled trials. *Current Nutrition Reports, 2*(4), 274–282.

11. Roederer G. O. (updated 2014). Cardiovascular disorders: Dyslipidemias. In Repchinsky C. (Ed.). *e-Therapeutics*. Ottawa, ON: Canadian Pharmacists Association.

12. Statistics Canada. (2012). Mortality, summary list of causes. Available online at: http://www.statcan.gc.ca/pub/84f0209x/84f0209x2009000-eng.pdf. Accessed February 28, 2015.

13. Heart & Stoke Foundation. (2015). Statistics. Available online at: http://www.heartandstroke.com/site/c.ikIQLcMWJtE/b.3483991/k.34A8/Statistics.htm. Accessed February 28, 2015.

14. Messner B., Bernhard D. (2014). Smoking and cardiovascular disease. *Arteriosclerosis, Thrombosis, and Vascular Biology, 34*(3), 509–515.

15. Frostegard J. (2013). Immunity, atherosclerosis and cardiovascular disease. *BMC Medicine, 11*, 117.

16. Jensen M. K., Bertoia M. L., Cahill L. E., et al. (2014). Novel metabolic biomarkers of cardiovascular disease. *Nature Reviews Endocrinology, 10*(11), 659–672.

17. Debreceni B., Debreceni L. (2014). The role of homocysteine-lowering B-vitamins in the primary prevention of cardiovascular disease. *Cardiovascular Therapeutics, 32*(3), 130–138.

18. Yla-Herttuala S., Bentzon J. F., Daemen M., et al.; ESC Working Group of Atherosclerosis and Vascular Biology. (2013). Stabilization of atherosclerotic plaques: An update. *European Heart Journal, 34*(42), 3251–3258.

19. Ohayon J., Finet G., Le Floc'h S., et al. (2013). Biomechanics of atherosclerotic coronary plaque: Site, stability and in vivo elasticity modeling. *Annals of Biomedical Engineering, 42*(2), 269–279.

20. Libby P. (2012). Inflammation in atherosclerosis. *Arteriosclerosis, Thrombosis, and Vascular Biology, 32*(9), 2045–2051.

21. Jennette J. C. (2013). Overview of the 2012 revised international Chapel Hill consensus conference nomenclature of vasculitides. *Clinical and Experimental Nephrology, 17*(5), 603–606.

22. Jennette J. C., Falk R. J., Bacon P. A., et al. (2013). 2012 revised international Chapel Hill consensus conference nomenclature of vasculitides. *Arthritis & Rheumatism, 65*(1), 1–11.

23. Forbess L., Bannykh S. (2015). Polyarteritis nodosa. *Rheumatic Disease Clinics of North America, 41*(1), 33–46.

24. Smith J. H., Swanson J. W. (2014). Giant cell arteritis. *Headache, 54*(8), 1273–1289.

25. Chacko J. G., Chacho J. A., Salter M. W. (2015). Review of giant cell arteritis. *Saudi Journal of Ophthalmology, 29*(1), 48–52.

26. Olin J. W., Sealove B. A. (2010). Peripheral artery disease: Current insight into the disease and is diagnosis and management. *Mayo Clinic Proceedings, 85*(7), 678–692.

27. Lepantalo M., Fiengo L., Biancari F. (2012). Peripheral arterial disease in diabetic patient with renal insufficiency: A review. *Diabetes/Metabolism Research and Reviews, 28*(Suppl 1), 40–45.

28. Piazza G., Creager M. A. (2010). Thromboangiitis obliterans. *Circulation, 121*(16), 1858–1861.

29. Herrick A. L. (2012). The pathogenesis, diagnosis and treatment of Raynaud phenomenon. *Nature Reviews Rheumatology, 8*(8), 469–479.

30. Roustit M., Blaise S., Allanore Y., et al. (2013). Phosphodiesterase-5 inhibitors for the treatment of secondary Raynaud's phenomenon: Systematic review and meat-analysis of randomized trials. *Annals of the Rheumatic Disease, 72*(10), 1696–1699.

31. Nordon I. M., Hinchliffe R. J., Loftus I. M., Thompson M. M. (2011). Pathophysiology and epidemiology of abdominal aortic aneurysms. *Nature Reviews Cardiology, 8*(2), 92–102.

32. Isselbacher E. M. (2005) Thoracic and abdominal aortic aneurysms. *Circulation, 111*(6), 816–826.

33. Boodhwani M., Andelfinger G., Leipsic J., et al.; Canadian Cardiovascular Society. (2014). Canadian Cardiovascular Society position statement on the management of thoracic aortic disease. *Canadian Journal of Cardiology, 30*(6), 577–589.

34. Braverman A. C. (2010). Acute aortic dissection. *Circulation, 122*(2), 184–188.

35. Lim C. S., Davies A. H. (2009). Pathogenesis of primary varicose veins. *British Journal of Surgery, 96*(11), 1231–1242.

36. Eberhardt R. T., Raffetto J. D. (2014). Chronic venous insufficiency. *Circulation, 130*(4), 333–346.

37. Nelson E. A. (2011). Venous leg ulcers. *BMJ Clinical Evidence, 12*, Systematic review 1902.

38. Rosendaal F. R., Reitsma P. H. (2009). Genetics of venous thrombosis. *Journal of Thrombosis and Haemostasis, 7*(Suppl 1), 301–304.

39. Falanga A., Russo L., Verzeroli C. (2013). Mechanisms of thrombosis in cancer. *Thrombosis Research, 131*(Suppl 1), S59–S62.

Visit thePoint **http://thePoint.lww.com for animations, journal articles, and more!**

Disorders of Blood Pressure Regulation

23

Blood pressure is probably one of the most variable but best-regulated functions of the body. The control of blood pressure is required to provide sufficient blood flow to vital organs, such as the heart, brain, and kidneys, while increasing blood flow to organs and tissues, such as the skeletal muscle, when necessary. Without constant blood flow to the vital organs, death ensues within minutes or days. Although a decrease in flow produces an immediate threat to life, the continuous elevation of blood pressure that occurs with hypertension contributes to premature death and disability because of its effects on the heart, blood vessels, and kidneys.

The discussion in this chapter focuses on determinants of blood pressure and conditions of altered arterial pressure—hypertension and orthostatic hypotension.

THE ARTERIAL BLOOD PRESSURE

After completing this section of the chapter, you should be able to meet the following objectives:

- Define the terms systolic blood pressure, diastolic blood pressure, pulse pressure, and mean arterial blood pressure.
- Explain how cardiac output and peripheral vascular resistance interact in determining systolic and diastolic blood pressures.
- Describe the mechanisms for short-term and long-term regulation of blood pressure.
- Review the requirements for accurate and reliable blood pressure measurement.

The systemic arterial blood pressure reflects the rhythmic ejection of blood from the left ventricle into the aorta.[1,2] It rises during systole as the left ventricle contracts and falls as the heart relaxes during diastole. The contour of the arterial pressure tracing shown in Fig. 23.1 is typical of the pressure changes that occur in the large arteries of the systemic circulation. There is a rapid rise in the pulse contour during left ventricular contraction, followed by a slower rise to peak pressure. Approximately 70% of the blood that leaves the left ventricle is ejected during the first one third of systole, resulting in a rapid

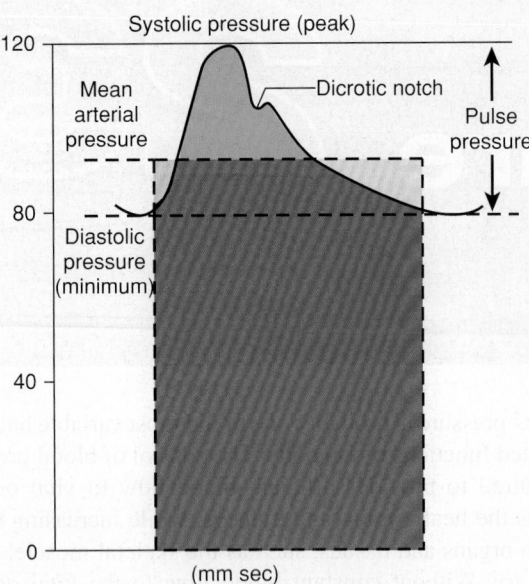

FIGURE 23.1 • Intra-arterial pressure tracing made from the brachial artery. Pulse pressure is the difference between systolic and diastolic pressures. The darker area represents the mean arterial pressure, which can be calculated by using the formula of mean arterial pressure = diastolic pressure + pulse pressure/3.

rise in the pressure contour. The end of systole is marked by a brief downward deflection and formation of the dicrotic notch, which occurs when ventricular pressure falls below that in the aorta. The sudden closure of the aortic valve is associated with a small rise in pressure caused by continued contraction of the aorta and other large vessels against the closed valve. As the ventricles relax and blood flows into the peripheral vessels during diastole, the arterial pressure falls rapidly at first and then declines slowly as the driving force decreases.

In adults, the pressure at the height of the pressure pulse, called the *systolic pressure*, is ideally less than 120 mm Hg, and the lowest pressure, called the *diastolic pressure*, is less than 80 mm Hg. The difference between the systolic and diastolic pressures (approximately 40 mm Hg) is called the *pulse pressure* (Fig. 23.1). The magnitude of the pulse pressure reflects the volume of blood ejected from the left ventricle during a single beat (stroke volume) and the total distensibility of the atrial tree. The *mean arterial pressure* (approximately 80 to 100 mm Hg), represents the average pressure in the arterial system during ventricular contraction and relaxation and is an overall indicator of tissue perfusion. The mean arterial pressure is not a simple mathematical average of systolic and diastolic pressures. This is because a great fraction of each cardiac cycle is spent in diastole rather than in systole. At normal heart rates this pressure can be estimated by adding one third of the pulse pressure to the diastolic pressure (*i.e.*, diastolic blood pressure + pulse pressure/3) or alternatively determining two times the diastolic pressure plus the systolic pressure all divided by 3 (*i.e.*, [2 × diastolic blood pressure + systolic blood pressure]/3).

The mean arterial blood pressure is determined mainly by the cardiac output (stroke volume × heart rate) and the systemic vascular resistance, and can also be expressed as the product of the two (mean arterial blood pressure = cardiac output × systemic vascular resistance). The systemic vascular resistance reflects changes in the radius of the arterioles as well as the viscosity or thickness of the blood (see Chapter 21 for a discussion of cardiac output and peripheral vascular resistance). The arterioles often are referred to as the resistance vessels because they can selectively constrict or relax to control the resistance to outflow of blood into the capillaries. The body maintains its blood pressure by adjusting the cardiac output to compensate for changes in systemic vascular resistance and changes the systemic vascular resistance to compensate for changes in cardiac output.

In hypertension and disease conditions that affect blood pressure, changes in blood pressure usually are described in terms of the systolic and diastolic pressures, pulse pressure, and mean arterial pressure. These pressures are influenced by the stroke volume, the rapidity with which blood is ejected from the heart, the elastic properties of the aorta and large arteries and their ability to accept various amounts of blood as it is ejected from the heart, and the properties of the resistance blood vessels that control the runoff of blood into the smaller vessels and capillaries that connect the arterial and venous circulations.

Mechanisms of Blood Pressure Regulation

Although some tissues in the body are able to regulate their own blood flow, it is necessary for the arterial pressure to remain relatively constant as blood shifts from one area of the body to another. The mechanisms used to regulate the arterial pressure depend on whether short-term or long-term adaptation is needed[2] (Fig. 23.2).

Short-Term Regulation

The mechanisms for short-term or rapid regulation of blood pressure, those acting over seconds or hours, are intended to correct temporary imbalances in blood pressure, such as occur during physical exercise and changes in body position. These mechanisms also are responsible for maintenance of blood pressure at survival levels during life-threatening situations such as during an acute hemorrhagic incident. The short-term regulation of blood pressure relies mainly on neural and humoral mechanisms, the most rapid of which are the neural mechanisms.

Neural Mechanisms. The neural control centres for the regulation of blood pressure are located in the reticular formation of the medulla and lower third of the pons, where integration and modulation of autonomic nervous system (ANS) responses occur.[2] This area of the brain contains the vasomotor and cardiac control centres and is often collectively referred to as the *cardiovascular centre*. The cardiovascular centre transmits parasympathetic impulses to the heart through the vagus nerve and sympathetic impulses to the heart and blood vessels through the spinal cord and peripheral

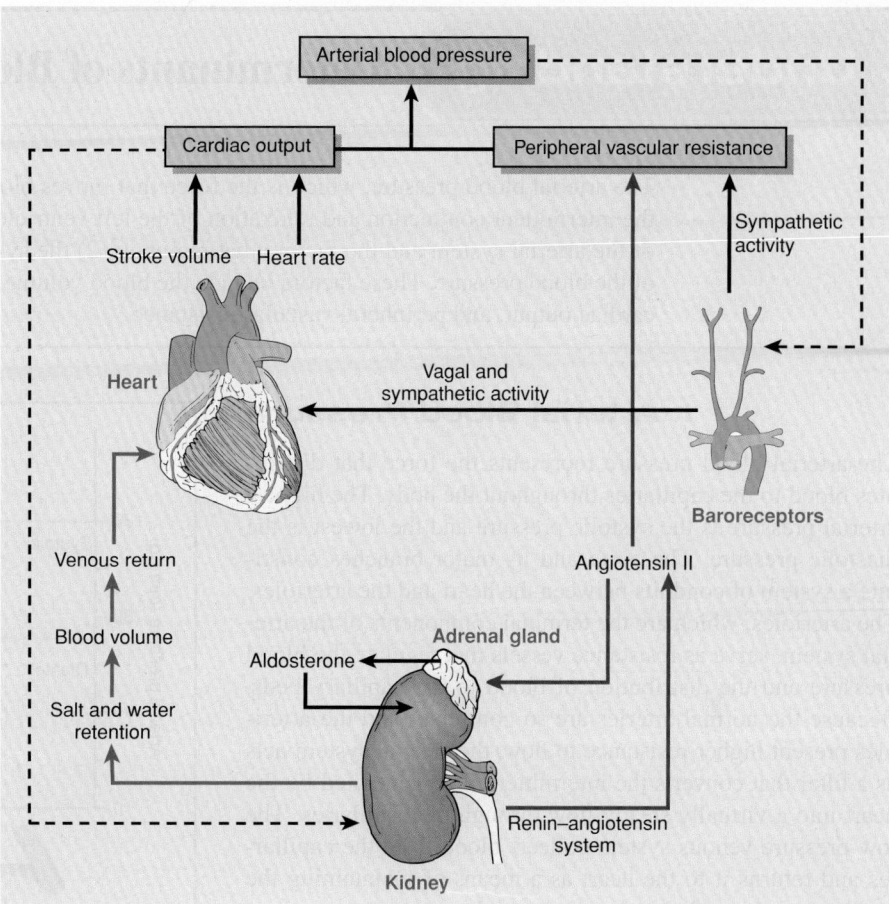

FIGURE 23.2 • Mechanisms of blood pressure regulation. The *solid lines* represent the mechanisms for renal and baroreceptor control of blood pressure through changes in cardiac output and peripheral vascular resistance. The *dashed lines* represent the stimulus for regulation of blood pressure by the baroreceptors and the kidneys.

sympathetic nerves. Vagal stimulation of the heart produces a slowing of heart rate, whereas sympathetic stimulation produces an increase in heart rate and cardiac contractility. Blood vessels are selectively innervated by the sympathetic nervous system. Increased sympathetic activity produces constriction of the small arteries and arterioles with a resultant increase in peripheral vascular resistance.

The ANS control of blood pressure is mediated through intrinsic circulatory reflexes, extrinsic reflexes, and higher neural control centres. The *intrinsic reflexes,* including the *baroreceptor* and *chemoreceptor reflexes,* are located in the circulatory system and are essential for rapid and short-term regulation of blood pressure. The sensors for *extrinsic reflexes* are found outside the circulation. They include blood pressure responses associated with factors such as pain and cold. The neural pathways for these reactions are more diffuse, and their responses are less consistent than those of the intrinsic reflexes. Many of these responses are regulated by the hypothalamus, which plays an essential role in the control of sympathetic nervous system responses. Among higher-centre responses are those caused by changes in mood and emotion.

The *baroreceptors* are pressure-sensitive receptors located in the walls of blood vessels and the heart. The carotid and aortic baroreceptors are located in strategic positions between the heart and the brain (Fig. 23.3). They respond to changes in the stretch of the vessel wall by sending impulses

to cardiovascular centres in the brain stem to effect appropriate changes in heart rate, force of contraction, and vascular smooth muscle tone. For example, the fall in blood pressure that occurs on moving from the lying to the standing position produces a decrease in the stretch of the baroreceptors with a resultant increase in heart rate, increasing contractility, and sympathetically induced vasoconstriction that together cause an increase in blood pressure.

The *arterial chemoreceptors* are chemosensitive cells that monitor the oxygen, carbon dioxide, and hydrogen ion content of the blood. They are located in the carotid bodies, which lie in the bifurcation of the two common carotids, and in the aortic bodies of the aorta (Fig. 23.3). Because of their location, these chemoreceptors are always in close contact with the arterial blood. Although the main function of the chemoreceptors is to regulate ventilation, they also communicate with cardiovascular centres in the brain stem and can induce widespread vasoconstriction. Whenever the arterial pressure drops below a critical level, the chemoreceptors are stimulated because of diminished oxygen supply or a buildup of carbon dioxide and hydrogen ions. In persons with chronic lung disease, systemic and pulmonary hypertension may develop because of hypoxemia (see Chapter 29). Persons with sleep apnea also may experience an increase in blood pressure because of the hypoxemia that occurs during the apneic periods.

Understanding ▸ Determinants of Blood Pressure

The arterial blood pressure, which is the force that moves blood through the arterial system, reflects the intermittent contraction and relaxation of the left ventricle. It is determined by (1) the properties of the arterial system and the factors that maintain (2) the systolic and (3) the diastolic components of the blood pressure. These factors include the blood volume, elastic properties of the blood vessels, cardiac output, and peripheral vascular resistance.

1. Arterial Blood Pressure

The arterial blood pressure represents the force that distributes blood to the capillaries throughout the body. The highest arterial pressure is the systolic pressure and the lowest is the diastolic pressure. The aorta and its major branches constitute a system of conduits between the heart and the arterioles. The arterioles, which are the terminal components of the arterial system, serve as resistance vessels that regulate the blood pressure and the distribution of blood to the capillary beds. Because the normal arteries are so compliant and the arterioles present higher resistance to flow, the arterial system acts as a filter that converts the intermittent flow generated by the heart into a virtually steady flow through the capillaries. The low-pressure venous system collects blood from the capillaries and returns it to the heart as a means of maintaining the cardiac output needed to sustain arterial pressure.

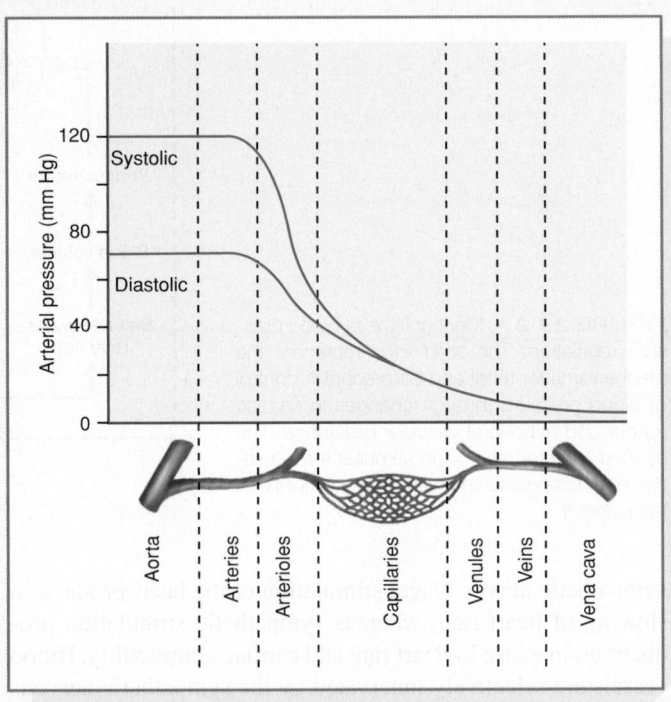

2. Systolic Pressure

The systolic blood pressure reflects the amount of blood (stroke volume) that is ejected from the heart with each beat, the rate and force with which it is ejected, and the elasticity or compliance of the aorta and large arteries. The blood that is ejected from the heart during systole does not move directly through the circulation. Instead, a substantial fraction of the stroke volume is stored in large arteries. Because the walls of these vessels are elastic, they can be stretched to accommodate a large volume of blood without an appreciable change in pressure. The systolic pressure often increases with aging as the aorta and large arteries lose their elasticity and become more rigid.

3. Diastolic Pressure

The diastolic blood pressure reflects the closure of the aortic valve, the underlying vascular tone, the total blood volume, the energy that has been stored in the elastic fibres of the large arteries during systole, and the resistance to flow through arterioles into the capillaries. Closure of the aortic valve at the onset of diastole and recoil of the elastic fibres in the aorta and large arteries continue to drive the blood forward, even though the heart is not pumping. These effects, largely restricted to the elastic vessels, convert the discontinuous systolic flow in the ascending aorta into a continuous flow in the peripheral arteries.

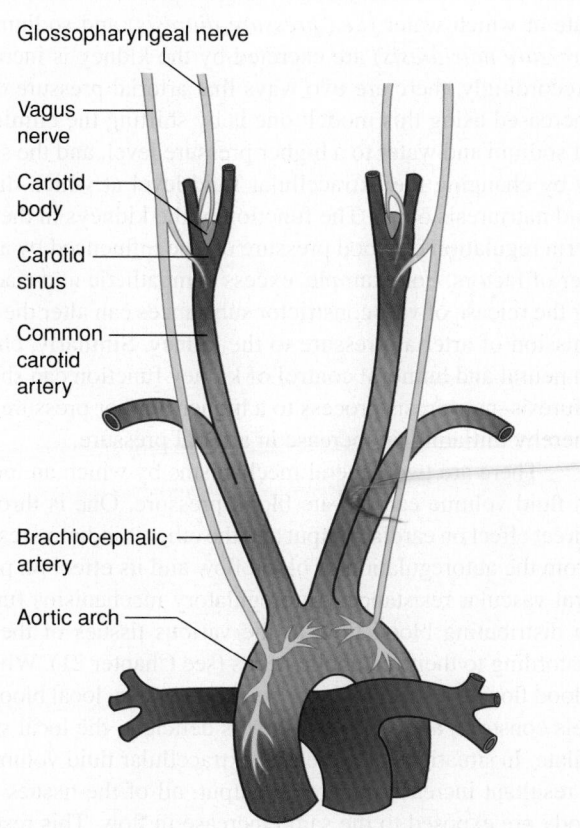

FIGURE 23.3 • Location and innervation of the aortic arch and carotid sinus baroreceptors and carotid body chemoreceptors.

Humoral Mechanisms. A number of humoral mechanisms contribute to blood pressure regulation, including the *renin–angiotensin–aldosterone system* and *vasopressin.*[1–3] Other humoral substances, such as epinephrine, a sympathetic neurotransmitter released from the adrenal gland, have the effect of directly stimulating an increase in heart rate, cardiac contractility, and vascular tone.

The *renin–angiotensin–aldosterone system* plays a central role in blood pressure regulation. Renin is an enzyme that is synthesized, stored, and released by the juxtaglomerular cells of the kidneys. Its release is increased in response to an increase in sympathetic nervous system activity or a decrease in blood pressure, extracellular fluid volume, or extracellular sodium concentration. Most of the renin that is released leaves the kidney and enters the bloodstream, where it acts enzymatically to convert an inactive circulating plasma protein made by the liver called *angiotensinogen* to angiotensin I (Fig. 23.4). Angiotensin I is then converted to angiotensin II. The conversion to angiotensin II occurs almost entirely in the lungs, while blood flows through the small vessels of the lung, catalyzed by an enzyme called the *angiotensin-converting enzyme* (ACE) that is present in the endothelium of the lung vessels. Although angiotensin II has a half-life of only several minutes, increases in renin persist in the circulation for 30 minutes to 1 hour and continue to cause production of angiotensin II during this time.

Angiotensin II functions in both the short- and long-term regulation of blood pressure. It is a strong vasoconstrictor,

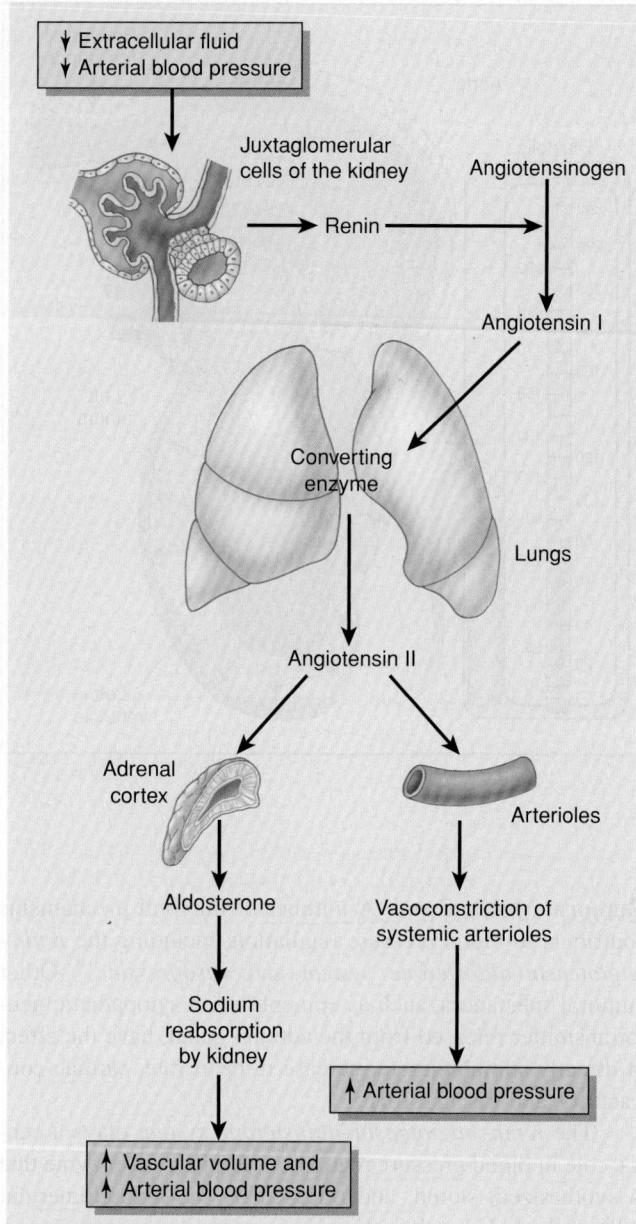

FIGURE 23.4 • Control of blood pressure by the renin–angiotensin–aldosterone system. Renin enzymatically converts the plasma protein angiotensinogen to angiotensin I; angiotensin-converting enzyme in the lung converts angiotensin I to angiotensin II; and angiotensin II produces vasoconstriction and increases salt and water retention through direct action on the kidney and through increased aldosterone secretion by the adrenal cortex.

particularly of arterioles and, to a lesser extent, of veins. Constriction of the arterioles increases the peripheral vascular resistance, thereby contributing to the short-term regulation of blood pressure. Angiotensin II also reduces sodium excretion by increasing sodium reabsorption by the proximal tubules of the kidney. A second major function of angiotensin II, stimulation of aldosterone secretion from the adrenal gland, contributes to the long-term regulation of blood pressure by increasing sodium and subsequent water retention by the kidney.

Vasopressin, also known as *antidiuretic hormone* (ADH), is released from the posterior pituitary gland in response to decreases in blood volume and blood pressure, an increase in the osmolality of body fluids, and other stimuli. The antidiuretic actions of vasopressin are discussed in Chapter 31. Vasopressin has a direct vasoconstrictor effect, particularly on the vessels of the splanchnic circulation that supplies the abdominal viscera. However, long-term increases in vasopressin cannot maintain an increase in blood pressure, and vasopressin does not enhance hypertension produced by sodium-retaining hormones or other vasoconstricting substances. It has been suggested that vasopressin plays a permissive role in hypertension through its water-retaining properties or as a neurotransmitter that serves to modify ANS function.

Long-Term Regulation

Long-term mechanisms control the daily, weekly, and monthly regulation of blood pressure. Although the neural and hormonal mechanisms involved in the short-term regulation of blood pressure act rapidly, they are unable to maintain their effectiveness over time. Instead, the long-term regulation of blood pressure is largely vested in the kidneys and their role in the regulation of the extracellular fluid volume.[2]

Extracellular fluid volume and arterial blood pressure are regulated around an equilibrium point, which represents the normal pressure for a given individual.[2] When the body contains excess extracellular fluids because of increased water and sodium intake, the arterial pressure rises, and the rate at which water (*i.e., pressure diuresis*) and sodium (*i.e., pressure natriuresis*) are excreted by the kidney is increased. Accordingly, there are two ways that arterial pressure can be increased using this model: one is by shifting the elimination of sodium and water to a higher pressure level, and the second is by changing the extracellular fluid level at which diuresis and natriuresis occur. The function of the kidneys in the long-term regulation of blood pressure can be influenced by a number of factors. For example, excess sympathetic nerve activity or the release of vasoconstrictor substances can alter the transmission of arterial pressure to the kidney. Similarly, changes in neural and humoral control of kidney function can shift the diuresis–natriuresis process to a higher fluid or pressure level, thereby initiating an increase in arterial pressure.

There are two general mechanisms by which an increase in fluid volume can elevate blood pressure. One is through a direct effect on cardiac output and the other is indirect, resulting from the autoregulation of blood flow and its effect on peripheral vascular resistance. Autoregulatory mechanisms function in distributing blood flow to the various tissues of the body according to their metabolic needs (see Chapter 21). When the blood flow to a specific tissue bed is excessive, local blood vessels constrict, and when the flow is deficient, the local vessels dilate. In situations of increased extracellular fluid volume and a resultant increase in cardiac output, all of the tissues of the body are exposed to the same increase in flow. This results in a generalized constriction of arterioles and an increase in both peripheral vascular resistance and blood pressure.

The role that the kidneys play in blood pressure regulation is emphasized by the fact that many antihypertensive medications produce their blood pressure–lowering effects by increasing sodium and water elimination.

Circadian Variations in Blood Pressure

These acute and chronic mechanisms attempt to regulate blood pressure around a particular set point. For most individuals, the blood pressure falls by an average of 10% to 20% in a characteristic circadian pattern, and this phenomenon is referred to as "dipping." Normally blood pressure tends to be higher shortly after awakening in the morning and then decreases gradually throughout the day and night, reaching the lowest point between approximately 2:00 AM and 5:00 AM. The term *dippers* is used to refer to people with a normal circadian blood pressure profile in which blood pressure falls during the night. The term *non-dippers* refers to individuals in whom the nocturnal decrease in blood pressures is blunted or does not decrease by ≤10% of daytime pressures. Nondippers often have higher mean nocturnal blood pressures. Finally, the *inverted dippers* are individuals whose nocturnal blood pressures actually increase.[4]

Blood Pressure Measurement

Arterial blood pressure measurements usually are obtained by the *indirect auscultatory method,* which uses a stethoscope and a well-calibrated sphygmomanometer. In the measurement of blood pressure, a cuff that contains an inflatable rubber bladder is placed around the upper arm. The bladder of the cuff is inflated to a point at which its pressure exceeds that of the artery, occluding the blood flow. The cuff is then slowly deflated at 2 mm Hg per second. At the point where the pressure in the vessel again exceeds the pressure in the cuff, a small amount of blood squirts through the partially obstructed artery. The sounds generated by the turbulent flow are called the *Korotkoff (K) sounds.* These low-pitched sounds are best heard with the bell of the stethoscope. Blood pressure is recorded in terms of systolic and diastolic pressures (*e.g.,* 120/70 mm Hg) unless sounds are heard to zero, in which case three readings are required (122/64/0 or K1/K4/K5). Systolic pressure is defined as the first of two or more Korotkoff sounds heard (K1). Diastolic pressure is recorded as the last sound heard (K5) unless sounds are heard to zero, in which case the muffling sound of K4 is used.[5,6]

It is important that the bladder of the cuff be appropriate for the arm size. The width of the bladder should be at least 40% of arm circumference and the length at least 80% of arm circumference.[5] Using a cuff with a bladder that is too small ("undercuffing") can cause blood pressure to be overestimated. This is because a cuff that is too small results in an uneven distribution of pressure across the arm, such that a greater cuff pressure is needed to occlude blood flow. Likewise, using a cuff with a bladder that is too large ("overcuffing") can cause an underestimation of blood pressure.

Automated or *semiautomated methods* of blood pressure measurement use a microphone, arterial pressure pulse sensor (oscillometric method), or Doppler equipment for detecting the equivalent of the Korotkoff sounds. Oscillometric measurement, the most commonly used method, depends on the detection of the pulsatile oscillations of the brachial artery in the blood pressure cuff. In contrast to the auscultatory method, this method determines the mean arterial pressure based on the amplitude of the arterial pulsations and then uses an algorithm to calculate the systolic and diastolic pressures.

Automated devices are useful for the self-monitoring of blood pressure and for 24-hour ambulatory monitoring of blood pressure.[5] Ambulatory blood monitors are fully automatic and can record blood pressure for 24 hours or longer while persons go about their normal activities. The monitors are typically programmed to take readings every 15 to 30 minutes throughout the day and night. The readings are stored and downloaded into a computer for analysis. Hypertension Canada has endorsed certain automated equipment for self-monitoring of blood pressure, and these devices can be found in most pharmacies and medical supply stores throughout the country. The equipment should use an appropriate-size cuff, and be checked at least once a year for accuracy.[7] The accuracy of an electronic device can be checked by comparing its readings with simultaneously obtained auscultatory measurements.

Intra-arterial methods provide for direct measurement of blood pressure. Intra-arterial measurement requires the insertion of a catheter into a peripheral artery. The arterial catheter is connected to a pressure transducer, which converts pressure into a digital signal that can be measured, displayed, and recorded. This type of blood pressure monitoring usually is restricted to critical care units.

IN SUMMARY

The alternating contraction and relaxation of the heart produces a pressure pulse that moves blood through the circulatory system. The elastic walls of the aorta stretch during systole and relax during diastole to maintain the diastolic pressure. The systolic blood pressure denotes the highest point of the pressure pulse and the diastolic pressure the lowest point. The pulse pressure, which reflects the pulsatile nature of arterial blood flow, is the difference between the systolic and diastolic pressures, and the mean arterial pressure, the average blood pressure in the systemic circulation. Systolic pressure is determined primarily by the characteristics of the stroke volume, whereas diastolic pressure is determined largely by the conditions of the arteries and arterioles and their abilities to accept the runoff of blood from the aorta.

The regulation of blood pressure involves both short- and long-term mechanisms. The short-term mechanisms are responsible for regulating blood pressure on a minute-by-minute or hour-by-hour basis during activities such as physical exercise and changes in body position. The short-term regulation of blood pressure relies mainly on neural and humoral mechanisms, the most rapid of which are the neural mechanisms. The long-term mechanisms, those maintaining blood pressure over days, weeks, and even years, are largely vested in the kidney and the regulation of extracellular fluid volume.

Arterial blood pressure measurements usually are obtained by the indirect auscultatory method, which uses a sphygmomanometer and a stethoscope. Automated or semiautomated methods of blood pressure measurement use a microphone, arterial pressure pulse sensor (oscillometric method), or Doppler equipment for detecting the equivalent of the Korotkoff sounds. Ambulatory and self-measurement of blood pressure may provide valuable information outside the clinician's office regarding a person's blood pressure and response to treatment. Accurate blood pressure measurement, whether by auscultatory or automated methods, requires the use of accurately calibrated equipment, a properly fitted cuff, and the proper level of cuff inflation and timing for cuff deflation.

HYPERTENSION

After completing this section of the chapter, you should be able to meet the following objectives:

- Cite the definition of hypertension put forth by the Canadian Hypertension Education Program.
- Differentiate essential, systolic, secondary, and malignant forms of hypertension.
- Describe the possible influence of genetics, age, race, obesity, diet and sodium intake, and alcohol consumption on the development of essential hypertension.
- Cite the risks of hypertension in terms of target-organ damage.
- Describe behaviour modification strategies used in the prevention and treatment of hypertension.
- List the different categories of drugs used to treat hypertension and state their mechanisms of action in the treatment of high blood pressure.
- Explain the changes in blood pressure that accompany normal pregnancy and describe the two classifications of hypertension that can occur during pregnancy.
- Cite the criteria for the diagnosis of high blood pressure in children.
- Define systolic hypertension and relate the circulatory changes that occur with aging that predispose to the development of systolic hypertension.

Hypertension is blood pressure above the normal range: systolic greater than 140 mm Hg or diastolic greater than 90 mm Hg. It is probably the most common of all health problems in adults and globally it is the leading risk factor for cardiovascular mortality.[8] Hypertension affects approximately 7.4 million Canadians[8] and 1 billion people worldwide. In Canada, approximately 20% of adults older than 20 years have hypertension. It is more common in younger men than in younger women, though the rates among postmenopausal women and men of the same age are similar. Hypertension is more common in people of African descent (compared to whites), in people from lower socioeconomic groups, and in older adults. Data suggest that persons who are normotensive at 55 years of age have a 90% lifetime risk for development of hypertension.[9] Thus, the problem of hypertension can be expected to become even greater with the aging of the "baby-boomer" population.

Hypertension is commonly divided into the categories of primary and secondary hypertension. Primary (essential or idiopathic) hypertension is the term applied to 95% of cases in which no cause for hypertension can be identified. In secondary hypertension, the elevation of blood pressure results from some other disorder, such as kidney disease.

Essential Hypertension

The recommendations for blood pressure management, diagnosis, and treatment by the Canadian Hypertension Education Program (CHEP) are completed yearly, and all updates and information are readily available on their website.[6] Included in the recommendations is an extensive discussion of modifiable and non-modifiable factors that contribute to hypertension, with consideration of both primary and secondary prevention.

Non-Modifiable Risk Factors

Although the causes of essential hypertension are largely unknown, both non-modifiable and modifiable lifestyle factors have been implicated, either singly or collectively, as contributing factors. The non-modifiable risk factors are those that

HYPERTENSION

- Hypertension represents an elevation in systolic and/or diastolic blood pressure.
- Essential hypertension is characterized by a chronic elevation in blood pressure that occurs without evidence of other disease, and secondary hypertension by an elevation of blood pressure that results from some other disorder, such as kidney disease.
- The pathogenesis of essential hypertension is thought to include modifiable and non-modifiable factors involving the kidney and its role in regulating extracellular fluid volume through sodium and water elimination, sympathetic nervous system hyperreactivity, renin–angiotensin system activity, or intracellular sodium and calcium levels. The medications that are used in the treatment of hypertension exert their effect through one or more of these mechanisms.
- Uncontrolled hypertension produces increased demands on the heart, resulting in left ventricular hypertrophy and heart failure, and on the vessels of the arterial system, leading to atherosclerosis, kidney disease, retinopathy, and stroke.

cannot be changed and include factors such as a family history of hypertension, gender, race, and age-related increases in blood pressure.[1]

Family History. The inclusion of heredity as a contributing factor in the development of hypertension is supported by the fact that hypertension is seen most frequently among persons with a family history of hypertension. The strength of the prediction depends on the definition of positive family history and the age of the person at risk. In studies of twins and family members in which the degree of familial aggregation is compared with the closeness of genetic sharing, the genetic contribution ranges from 30% to 70%.[15] Geneticists have failed to identify common genes with large effects on hypertension. Instead they have found over 1,500 genes at many loci, each with a small influence or contribution differing according to sex, race, age, and lifestyle, that have been related to blood pressure regulation, leaving much of the heritability of blood pressure unexplained currently.[10]

Age-Related Changes in Blood Pressure. Maturation and growth are known to cause predictable increases in blood pressure. For example, the arterial blood pressure in the newborn is approximately 50 mm Hg systolic and 40 mm Hg diastolic.[11] Sequentially, blood pressure increases with physical growth from a value of 78 mm Hg systolic at 10 days of age to 120 mm Hg at the end of adolescence.[11]

Findings reveal that systolic blood pressure increases significantly with age among both men and women but between the ages of 20 and 59 years it is lower among women than men. Diastolic blood pressure is greater for both men and women ages 49 to 59 years compared to those aged 20 to 39 years of age. Diastolic blood pressure is significantly lower among women than men between the ages of 40 and 79 years.[9]

In older persons, the arterial vasculature becomes increasingly stiffer and less compliant. Consequently, given an unchanged overall fluid volume and stroke volume, the systolic pressure will rise. Low diastolic pressure seen in many older adults may be caused by overall vascular stiffness and compromised cardiac function.[1]

Race. The Blood Pressure survey conducted in Ontario (ON-BP) in 2006 was the first Canadian adult population-based (between ages 20 and 79 years of age) study that measured blood pressures and determined hypertension rates among ethnic groups. This study showed that the ethnic groups consisting of South Asians (30%) and blacks (31%) in Canada are more likely to have hypertension in comparison to the primarily Caucasian population (21%) and East Asians are the least likely to have hypertension (19%).[12]

Reasons for the higher incidence of hypertension among the ethnic groups remain largely unknown. Studies have shown that many black persons with hypertension have lower renin levels than white persons with hypertension.[1,13] The suppression of renin has been considered a secondary

response to sodium retention and volume excess. Salt sensitivity, defined as an increase in blood pressure in response to a high-salt diet, is commonly described in both normotensive and hypertensive black persons. Recent research has focused on potential defects in renal sodium transport to explain this observation. Other factors, such as increased vasomotor function (*e.g.,* sympathetic nervous system overactivity) or abnormalities in endothelium-dependent vasodilation have also been suggested as possible contributing factors.[14,15]

Evidence suggests that blacks, when provided with equal access to diagnosis and treatment, can achieve overall reductions in blood pressure and experience fewer cardiovascular complications, similar to whites.[14,15] The ON-BP showed overall control rate of hypertension at 65.7%, with only minor variations seen by age, sex, ethnic groups and presence of diseases such as cardiovascular disease, diabetes, obesity, and high cholesterol.[12] The ON-BP study excluded the Canadian aboriginal group from their study with the intent to complete a separate study with this particular population.[12] Most of the research and prevalence of hypertension data available about the aboriginal population occurs within the context of diabetes. The incidence of diabetes in the aboriginal population in Canada is considerably higher in comparison to the rest of the Canadian population.[16] The incidence of hypertension in the aboriginal population with diabetes is at 42% compared to 10% in those without diabetes.[16] This is not a surprising percentage given that diabetes is a significant risk factor to the development of hypertension.

Barriers that limit access to health care include social isolation, which most often occurs as a result of oppression related to ethnicity/race, class, gender, disability, sexual orientation, immigrant status and religion; low income; and lack of access to culturally relevant health education about hypertension.[8] With salt sensitivity, obesity, and smoking being higher in some ethnic groups, health education and lifestyle modifications are important, as is the development of public policy and programs to ensure equal access to hypertension management.

Lifestyle Risk Factors (Modifiable Factors)

Lifestyle factors can contribute to the development of hypertension. Since atherosclerosis is associated with the development of hypertension, the factors that lead to atherosclerosis are considered significant for the development of hypertension. Modifiable risk factors include: sedentary lifestyle, poor dietary habits, abdominal obesity, impaired glucose tolerance or diabetes mellitus, smoking, dyslipidemia, and stress.[1,6] Other factors that may induce or aggravate hypertension include drugs (*e.g.,* NSAIDs, corticosteroids, erythropoietin, sympathomimetics, cocaine), salt, and excessive alcohol consumption. Although stress raises blood pressure acutely and affects behaviours such as alcohol consumption, physical activity, and poor nutrition, there is no strong evidence linking stress as an independent risk factor to hypertension.

High-Salt Intake. Increased salt intake has long been suspected as an etiologic factor in the development of hypertension.[17] Just how increased salt intake contributes to the development of hypertension is still unclear. It may be that salt causes an elevation in blood volume, increases the sensitivity of cardiovascular or renal mechanisms to sympathetic nervous system influences, or exerts its effects through some other mechanism such as the renin–angiotensin–aldosterone system. It has also been suggested that it may be the chloride rather than the sodium in salt that is responsible for the rise in blood pressure. This is difficult to study, however, because 95% of sodium in the diet is in the form of sodium chloride.[18]

Regardless of the mechanism, numerous studies have shown that a reduction in salt intake can lower blood pressure. The strongest data came from the INTERSALT study, which measured 24-hour urine sodium excretion (an indirect measure of salt intake) in men and women 20 to 59 years of age around the world.[17] Across all populations, there was a positive correlation between sodium excretion and both systolic and diastolic blood pressures. Furthermore, the association of sodium and blood pressure was greatest for older (40 to 59 years) subjects compared with younger (20 to 39 years) subjects in the study.

Health Canada estimates that Canadians consume approximately 150 mmol/day (3,400 mg/day), which is in excess of the recommended maximal intake of 87 mmol/day (2,000 mg/day) for adults.[6,16,19] Approximately 77% of salt intake comes from salt added in the processing and manufacturing of food; 11% from discretionary addition in cooking and at the table; and 12% from the natural sodium content of food.[16] The Dietary Approaches to Stop Hypertension (DASH) diet is a nutritional plan that emphasizes fruits, vegetables, low-fat dairy products, whole grains, poultry, fish, and nuts, and reduced red meat, fats, sweets, and sugar-containing beverages. Results from studies using the low-sodium DASH diet have shown significant reductions in both systolic and diastolic blood pressures.[20]

Dietary Habits. Vegetarians have a lower risk of developing hypertension in comparison to non-vegetarians. Possible reasons for this may be that vegetarian diets are higher in fibre as well as high in potassium, magnesium, and polyunsaturated fats and lower in saturated fats. Saturated fats contribute to the development of atherosclerosis and consequent hypertension. Increasing fibre in the diet for individuals with hypertension has been shown to decrease blood pressure.[21] Mechanisms that may help to explain the correlation between high fibre and reduction of blood pressure may include a weakened insulin response with an improved blood pressure regulation. High amounts of fibre may improve mineral absorption and indirectly affect blood pressure.

Low levels of dietary potassium have been linked to increased blood pressure. The strongest evidence comes from the INTERSALT study. In this study, a urinary excretion of 60 mmol/day or greater of potassium (an indirect measure of potassium intake) was associated with a reduction in systolic pressure of 3.4 mm Hg or more and a decrease in diastolic pressure of 1.9 mm Hg or more.[17] Various mechanisms have

been proposed to explain the influence of potassium on blood pressure, including a purported change in the ratio of sodium to potassium in the diet, a direct natriuretic effect, and suppression of the renin–angiotensin system.[22] In terms of food intake, a diet high in potassium usually is low in sodium. One of the major benefits of increased potassium intake is increased elimination of sodium through the renin–angiotensin–aldosterone mechanism.

The associations between high blood pressure and calcium and magnesium levels also have been investigated. Although there have been reports of high blood pressure in persons with low calcium intake or lowering of blood pressure with increased calcium intake, the link between low calcium and magnesium intake and hypertension is inconclusive.[23,24]

Recommended dietary changes to reduce hypertension or maintain a normal blood pressure consist of low saturated fat and cholesterol; plenty of fruits and vegetables; low-fat dairy products; dietary and soluble fibre; whole grains; and protein from plant sources.[6] Additional supplements of potassium, calcium, and magnesium are not recommended for the prevention or treatment of hypertension.[6]

Sedentary Lifestyle. There is increasing evidence that indicates that sedentary lifestyle (*i.e.,* low levels of physical activity) is an independent risk factor for hypertension.[25] Obesity appears to be a strongly interconnected risk factor with sedentary lifestyle, but obesity does not entirely account for blood pressure changes seen with inactivity. Examination of sedentary lifestyle and antecedents of cardiovascular disease in young adult men and women demonstrates that the arterial blood vessels of individuals who are sedentary and physically inactive are significantly less compliant in comparison to endurance-trained individuals.[26]

Abdominal Obesity. The prevalence of obesity in Canada is increasing at alarming rates, and excessive weight is commonly associated with hypertension. Weight reduction of as little as 2 kg can produce a decrease in blood pressure in a large proportion of overweight people with hypertension.[27] It has been suggested that fat distribution might be a more critical indicator of hypertension risk than actual overweight. The waist-to-hip ratio is commonly used to differentiate central or upper body obesity, that is, to differentiate fat cells located in the abdomen and viscera, from peripheral or lower body obesity, with fat cell deposits in the buttocks and legs (see Chapter 39). Studies have demonstrated an association between hypertension and increased waist-to-hip ratio (*i.e.,* central obesity), even when body mass index and skinfold thickness are taken into account.[28] Abdominal or visceral fat seems to be more insulin resistant than fat deposited over the buttocks and legs (see Chapter 42). There is also an evolving understanding of the neuroendocrine effects of excess adipose tissue on blood pressure. Recent evidence indicates that leptin, an adipocyte-derived hormone, may represent a link between adiposity and increased cardiovascular sympathetic activity. Besides its effect on appetite and metabolism, leptin acts on the hypothalamus to increase blood pressure through activation of the sympathetic nervous system.[29] High levels of circulating free fatty acids in obese people also appear to participate in activation of the sympathetic nervous system. There is also research supporting activation of the renin–angiotensin–aldosterone system by adipocyte-derived angiotensinogen and the ability of adipose tissue to increase aldosterone levels through the production of factors that induce aldosterone production. The recommended assessment of abdominal or visceral fat is by waist circumference. For the average Canadian, the CHEP guidelines recommend a waist circumference less than 102 cm for men and less than 88 cm for women, and attaining and maintaining a BMI between 18.5 and 24.9 kg/m[2].[6] Lower recommended waist measurements apply to some ethnic groups.

Insulin Resistance and Metabolic Abnormalities. Insulin resistance and an accompanying compensatory hyperinsulinemia have been suggested as possible etiologic links to the development of hypertension and associated metabolic disturbances such as impaired glucose tolerance, type 2 diabetes, hyperlipidemias, and obesity.[35–37] This clustering of cardiovascular risk factors has been named the *insulin resistance syndrome, cardiometabolic syndrome,* or *metabolic syndrome* (see Chapter 42).

Insulin resistance has been found to be more of an acquired trait than a genetic trait. For example, obesity plays an important role in the development of insulin resistance. Obesity affects the tissues' sensitivity towards insulin.[27,28] Nonpharmacologic interventions, such as caloric restriction, weight loss, and exercise, tend to decrease insulin resistance, sympathetic nervous system activity, and blood pressure.

Smoking. The evidence of smoking as a primary risk factor for hypertension is not clearly established. It is possible that smoking may enhance inflammation, affect vascular blood flow causing arterial stiffness, and contribute to the development of atherosclerosis. It does cause a temporary increase in blood pressure and heart rate.[30] An American comparison study between cigarette smoking and the incidence of hypertension in women demonstrated a significant correlation between smoking and development of hypertension, particularly for women who smoked 15 or more cigarettes per day. The overall impact of this risk was rated as modest and found mainly among women with a normal body mass index and lower initial blood pressures.[31]

Excess Alcohol Consumption. Regular heavy alcohol intake plays a role in the development of hypertension.[32] The effect is seen with different types of alcoholic drinks, in men and women, and in a variety of ethnic groups. Blood pressure may improve or return to normal when alcohol consumption is decreased or eliminated. Although the mechanism whereby alcohol exerts its effect on blood pressure is unclear, it is proposed that alcohol enhances the sympathetic system, increases heart rate, cardiac contraction and vasoconstriction, and may reduce the sensitivity of the baroreceptors that help to lower

blood pressure. It has also been suggested that lifestyle factors such as obesity and lack of exercise may be accompanying factors.

Cocaine. Use of cocaine causes acute hypertension.[33] The mechanism by which hypertension occurs may be multifactorial, explained by the stimulation of the sympathetic nervous system and endothelin-1, effects on the sodium channel, and reduced nitric oxide production.[33] Although cocaine has not been shown to cause chronic hypertension, the acute hypertension episodes are believed to contribute to a higher risk of cerebral infarction and intracranial hemorrhage. In addition, the frequent and severe episodes of hypertension associated with long-term use of cocaine can lead to target-organ damage such as end-stage renal failure and cardiomyopathy.

Target-Organ Damage

Primary (essential) hypertension is typically an asymptomatic disorder. When symptoms do occur, they are usually related to the long-term effects of hypertension on other organs and tissues, including the kidneys, heart, eyes, and blood vessels. CHEP uses the term *target-organ damage* to describe the heart, brain, peripheral vascular, kidney, and retinal complications associated with hypertension[6,8] (Chart 23.1). The excess morbidity and mortality related to hypertension is progressive

---

CHART 23.1 TARGET-ORGAN DAMAGE

Brain
- Cerebral vascular disease
- Stroke
- Dementia

Heart and Vasculature
- Coronary artery disease
- Angina pectoris
- Myocardial infarction
- Left ventricular dysfunction
- Heart failure
- Peripheral vascular disease
- Intermittent claudication

Eyes
- Hypertensive retinopathy

Kidneys
- Chronic renal disease
- Hypertensive nephropathy
- Albuminuria

Reproduction
- Erectile dysfunction

From the Canadian Hypertension Education Program (CHEP) recommendations for the management of hypertension.[6]

over the whole range of systolic and diastolic pressures, with target-organ damage varying markedly among persons with similar levels of hypertension.

Hypertension is a major risk factor for atherosclerosis since it promotes and accelerates plaque formation and possible rupture. It predisposes to all major atherosclerotic cardiovascular disorders, including coronary heart disease, heart failure, stroke, and peripheral artery disease. The risk for coronary artery disease and stroke depends to a great extent on other risk factors, such as obesity, smoking, and elevated cholesterol levels. In clinical trials, antihypertensive therapy has been associated with reductions in stroke incidence averaging 30% to 40%, myocardial infarction, 20% to 25%, and heart failure, more than 50%.

An elevation in blood pressure increases the workload of the left ventricle by increasing the pressure against which the heart must pump as it ejects blood into the systemic circulation.[1] As the workload of the heart increases, the left ventricular wall remodels and hypertrophies to compensate for the increased pressure work. Despite its adaptive advantage, left ventricular hypertrophy is a major risk factor for coronary heart disease, cardiac arrhythmias, sudden death, and congestive heart failure. Hypertensive left ventricular hypertrophy regresses with therapy. Regression is most closely related to systolic pressure reduction and does not appear to reflect the particular type of medication used.

Chronic hypertension leads to nephrosclerosis, a common cause of chronic kidney disease (see Chapter 33). Hypertensive kidney disease is more common in those of African descent. Hypertension also plays an important role in accelerating the course of other types of kidney disease, particularly diabetic nephropathy. Because of the risk for diabetic nephropathy, Canadian recommendations are that persons with diabetes maintain their blood pressure at levels less than 130/80 mm Hg.[6]

Dementia and cognitive impairment occur more commonly in persons with hypertension.[34] Hypertension, particularly systolic hypertension, is a major risk factor for ischemic stroke and intracerebral hemorrhage[1,35] (see Chapter 51). Narrowing and sclerosis of small penetrating arteries in the subcortical regions of the brain are common findings on autopsy in persons with chronic hypertension. These changes are thought to contribute to hypoperfusion, loss of autoregulation of blood flow, and impairment of the blood–brain barrier, ultimately leading to subcortical white matter demyelination.[34] Effective antihypertensive therapy strongly reduces the risk of development of significant white matter changes; however, existing white matter changes, once established, do not appear to be reversible.

Systemic hypertension is also associated with changes in the eye microvasculature and can lead to retinopathy and blindness. As hypertension initially increases vasomotor tone, this leads to generalized retinal arterial narrowing, vascular remodelling, and due to progressive arteriolar sclerosis the risk of arterial and venous occlusions, abnormal arteriovenous crossings, and/or microaneurysms increase. Another complication that is strongly linked to hypertension is the development of

ischemic optic neuropathy as the perfusion of the optic nerve can become compromised due to atherosclerotic lesions.[36]

Diagnosis

Unlike disorders of other body systems that are diagnosed by methods such as radiography and tissue examination, hypertension and other blood pressure disorders are determined by repeated blood pressure measurement and a thorough individual history and physical assessment. Laboratory tests, x-ray films, and other diagnostic tests are done to exclude secondary hypertension and determine the presence or extent of target-organ damage. The CHEP guidelines indicate that all Canadian adults should have ongoing assessment for hypertension, with an emphasis on management to decrease both hypertension and cardiovascular risk.

Blood pressure measurements should be taken when the person is relaxed, has rested for at least 5 minutes, and has not smoked or ingested caffeine within the preceding 30 minutes. The person should be seated in a chair (rather than on the examination table) with the feet on the floor and arm supported at heart level. Initially blood pressure should be taken in both arms. Subsequent blood pressures should be monitored using the same arm; if the blood pressure is higher in one arm then the arm with the higher measurement should be consistently used. If a blood pressure is 140/90 mm Hg or greater, at least two more readings should be done at the same visit, discarding the first reading and averaging the latter two. A repeat blood pressure measurement should be done within 1 month.[6,8] The number of repeated measurements that are recommended prior to diagnosis of hypertension depends on how significantly the blood pressure is elevated.[6,8] A diagnosis of hypertension is made when systolic blood pressure is greater than 160 mm Hg or diastolic blood pressure is greater than 100 mm Hg averaged across 3 visits. Hypertension is also diagnosed when a systolic blood pressure averages greater than 140 mm Hg or the diastolic blood pressure averages greater than 90 mm Hg across 4 to 5 visits.[6] Lower blood pressure values are used to diagnose hypertension if home or ambulatory blood pressures are available. For adults with diabetes mellitus, the optimal blood pressure goal has been lowered to less than 130/80 mm Hg. When a person has a very high blood pressure (*i.e.,* greater than 180/110) or displays organ damage from high blood pressure, the diagnosis can be made more quickly and appropriate treatment implemented. Examples of hypertensive urgencies that require immediate diagnosis and intervention include acute aortic dissection, acute left ventricular failure, and acute myocardial ischemia.[6]

The most significant changes made to the recent CHEP recommendations is first the emphasis on the risk of diabetes and hypertension, with the recommended blood pressure at less than 130/80 mm Hg, and second, the extensive description of how and when to incorporate ambulatory and home blood pressure monitoring as part of diagnosis and assessment of hypertension.[6] A systolic pressure of less than 120 mm Hg and a diastolic pressure of less than 80 mm Hg is considered an optimal blood pressure; blood pressures of 130–139/85–89 mm Hg are high normal in persons without diabetes, and high in those with diabetes. The new target for treatment of hypertension for the elderly (age ≥80 years) who do not have diabetes or target-organ damage is systolic blood pressure 160 mm Hg or higher.[6]

Home-Based and Ambulatory Blood Pressure Measurement. As previously discussed, ambulatory and self/home measurements of blood pressure may provide valuable information outside the clinician's office regarding the individual's blood pressure and response to treatment. Self/home measurements can help detect "white coat hypertension," a condition in which the blood pressure is consistently elevated in the healthcare provider's office but normal at other times. Home blood pressure measurements have a stronger association with cardiovascular risks and outcome than intermittent office-based readings. Home systolic pressure of 135 mm Hg or more, or diastolic pressure of 85 mm Hg or more, is associated with risks equal to office readings of systolic pressure of 140 mm Hg or diastolic pressure of 90 mm Hg or greater. In particular, home blood pressure monitoring should be implemented for individuals with diabetes type 2, chronic renal disease, suspected nonadherence to recommended therapy, demonstrated white coat syndrome, and masked hypertension (*i.e.,* normal B/P at the office but not at home). Duplicate blood pressure measures, morning and evening, for an initial 7-day period are recommended when assessing for intermittent hypertension or sustained hypertension. Also, 24-hour ambulatory blood pressure measurement (ABPM) can confirm the mean 24-hour blood pressure, incorporating information about alterations in circadian variations. Changes in the normal circadian blood pressure profile may occur in a number of conditions, including malignant hypertension, Cushing syndrome, preeclampsia, orthostatic hypotension, congestive heart failure, and sleep apnea.[4,37] There is increasing evidence that persons with a nondipping pattern of hypertension are at higher risk for development of target-organ damage than those with a dipping pattern; in addition, persons with an excessive morning surge in

blood pressure may also be at increased risk.[38] A mean 24-hour ABPM greater than 130/80 mm Hg or the mean awake ABPM of 135/85 mm Hg are considered hypertension.[6]

Treatment

The main objective for treatment of essential hypertension is to achieve and maintain arterial blood pressure below 140/90 mm Hg (home 135/85 mm Hg), with the goal of preventing morbidity and mortality. In persons with hypertension and diabetes or renal disease, the goal is below 130/80 mm Hg. The CHEP management approach for hypertension is individualized. Lifestyle modification and management strategies are first initiated, and include consideration of physical activity, weight, alcohol consumption, dietary approaches, salt intake, and stress management. Pharmacologic agents are used when necessary to achieve and maintain blood pressure within an optimal range; the target blood pressure and agent varies according to the individual.[6]

For persons with secondary hypertension, efforts are made to correct or control the disease condition causing the hypertension. Antihypertensive medications and other measures supplement the treatment of the underlying disease.

Lifestyle Modification. Lifestyle modification has been shown to reduce blood pressure, enhance the effects of antihypertensive drug therapy, and prevent cardiovascular risk. Major lifestyle modifications shown to lower blood pressure include weight reduction in persons who are overweight or obese, achieving ideal waist circumference, regular physical activity, adoption of a healthy eating plan, reduction of dietary sodium intake, limitation of alcohol intake, living in a smoke-free environment and stress management.[6] (See Table 23.1 for specific recommendations.)

Pharmacologic Treatment. The decision to initiate pharmacologic treatment is based on the severity of the hypertension,

TABLE 23.1 LIFESTYLE MODIFICATIONS TO PREVENT AND MANAGE HYPERTENSION

MODIFICATION	RECOMMENDATIONS
Dietary	High in fresh fruits and vegetables, low-fat dairy products, dietary and soluble fibre, whole grains and protein from plant sources Low in saturated fat, cholesterol, and salt (Canada's Guide to Healthy Eating. DASH diet[a])
Physical activity	Accumulation of 30–60 minutes of moderate intensity, dynamic exercise 4–7 times/week (*e.g.,* walking, jogging, cycling, swimming) in addition to daily activities
Alcohol consumption	≤2 drinks/day (<14/week for men and <9/week for women)
Body weight	Attaining and maintaining ideal body weight; BMI 18.5 to 24.9 kg/m^2 (diet education, increased activity, behaviour intervention)
Waist circumference	Caucasians, Europeans, Mediterraneans, Middle Eastern: Female <88 cm, Male <102 cm South Asians, Chinese, Japanese, South and Central Americans: Female <80 cm, Male <90 cm
Sodium consumption	Less than 2,000 mg/day (2,300 mg = 1 tsp)
Smoking	Smoke-free environment
Stress management	Cognitive and behavioural intervention if stress is a contributing factor to hypertension

Note: One standard drink is considered 13.6 g of alcohol, or approximately 41 ml of 80 proof (40%) of spirit, 150 ml of 12% wine or 340 ml of 5% beer.
[a]DASH, Dietary Approaches to Stop Hypertension.

the presence of target-organ disease, and the existence of other disease conditions and risk factors. The Canadian Hypertension Education Program (CHEP) has algorithms for pharmacologic treatment of hypertension available on their website: https://www.hypertension.ca/en/chep.

Among the drugs recommended for the treatment of hypertension are diuretics, β-adrenergic blocking agents, ACE inhibitors or angiotensin II receptor blockers, long-acting calcium channel blocking agents, α_1-adrenoreceptor antagonists, α_2-adrenergic agonists that act at the level of the central nervous system, and vasodilators. Preferably, initial therapy should be monotherapy followed by combination therapy if blood pressure remains uncontrolled.

Diuretics, such as the thiazides, loop diuretics, and the aldosterone antagonist (potassium-sparing) diuretics, lower blood pressure initially by decreasing vascular volume (by suppressing renal reabsorption of sodium and increasing salt and water excretion) and cardiac output. With continued therapy, a reduction in peripheral vascular resistance becomes a major mechanism of blood pressure reduction.

The β-*adrenergic blockers* are effective in treating hypertension because they decrease heart rate and cardiac output. These agents also decrease renin release, thereby decreasing the effect of the renin–angiotensin–aldosterone system on blood pressure. There are two types of β-adrenergic receptors: β_1 and β_2. The β_1-adrenergic blocking drugs are cardioselective, exerting their effects on the heart, whereas the β_2-adrenergic receptor blockers affect bronchodilation, relaxation of skeletal blood vessels, and other β-mediated functions. Both cardioselective (targeting β_1 receptors) and nonselective (targeting β_1 and β_2 receptors) β-adrenergic blockers are used in the treatment of hypertension. However, β-blockers are not recommended for management of isolated hypertension in individuals older than 60 years of age or persons with diabetic nephropathy.[6]

The *ACE inhibitors* act by inhibiting the conversion of angiotensin I to angiotensin II, thus decreasing angiotensin II levels and reducing its effect on vasoconstriction, aldosterone levels, intrarenal blood flow, and the glomerular filtration rate. They also inhibit the degradation of bradykinin and stimulate the synthesis of vasodilating prostaglandins. Because of their effect on the renin–angiotensin system, these drugs are contraindicated in persons with renal artery stenosis, in which the renin–angiotensin mechanism functions as a compensatory mechanism to maintain adequate renal perfusion. Because they inhibit aldosterone secretion, these agents also can increase serum potassium levels and cause hyperkalemia. *Angiotensin II receptor blocking* (ARB) agents block the receptors for angiotensin II in the arterial smooth muscle causing vasodilation and a decrease in blood pressure. Their effects on the arterial and renal system are similar to those of ACE inhibitors. Because ARBs do not inhibit bradykinin degradation in the lungs, they are less likely to produce a cough, which is a common and distressing side effect of ACE inhibitors, and angioedema, a rare but potentially life-threatening side effect.

The *calcium channel receptor blocking* (CCB) *drugs* inhibit the movement of calcium into cardiac and vascular

smooth muscle. They are thought to reduce blood pressure by several mechanisms, including a reduction of vascular smooth muscle tone in the venous and arterial systems. Each of the different agents in this group acts in a slightly different way. Some calcium channel blockers have a direct myocardial effect that reduces the cardiac output through a decrease in cardiac contractility and heart rate; others influence venous vasomotor tone and reduce the cardiac output through a decrease in venous return; still others influence arterial vascular smooth muscle tone by inhibiting either calcium transport across the cell membrane channels or the vascular response to norepinephrine or angiotensin.

The α_1-*adrenergic receptor antagonists* block postsynaptic α_1 receptors and reduce the effect of the sympathetic nervous system on the vascular smooth muscle tone of the blood vessels that regulate the peripheral vascular resistance. These drugs may produce a pronounced decrease in blood pressure after the first dose; therefore, treatment is initiated with a smaller dose given at bedtime. Postdosing palpitations, headache, and nervousness may continue with chronic treatment. These agents usually are more effective when used in combination with other agents. α-Blocking agents are not recommended as first-line therapy of isolated hypertension in individuals aged 60 years or older.[6]

The *centrally acting adrenergic agonists* block sympathetic outflow from the central nervous system. These agents are α_2-adrenergic agonists that act in a negative-feedback manner to decrease sympathetic outflow from presynaptic sympathetic neurons in the central nervous system. The α_2-adrenergic agonists are effective as a single therapy for some persons, but they often are used as second- or third-line agents because of the high incidence of side effects associated with them.

The *direct-acting smooth muscle vasodilators* (e.g., hydralazine) promote a decrease in peripheral vascular resistance by producing relaxation of vascular smooth muscle, particularly of the arterioles. These drugs often produce tachycardia because of an initial stimulation of the sympathetic nervous system, and salt and water retention owing to decreased filling of the vascular compartment. Vasodilators are most effective when used in combination with other antihypertensive drugs that oppose the compensatory cardiovascular responses (e.g., β-adrenergic blockers).

Long-acting nitrates (e.g., isosorbide) promote vascular smooth muscle relaxation similar to the endothelium-derived relaxing factor, nitric oxide. Nitrates cause relaxation of both the arterial and venous smooth muscles. Arterial relaxation reduces systemic vascular resistance and blood pressure. They are primarily used in conjunction with heart failure.

Factors to be considered when hypertensive drugs are prescribed include: the individual's lifestyle and the challenges of incorporating multiple doses into a busy schedule; demographics, with some drugs less effective in older adults or those of African descent; adherence to medications, with some drugs producing undesirable side effects; interactions with other disease conditions and therapies, including diabetic nephropathy or post myocardial infarction; safety in childbearing years and pregnancy; and financial resources. Adherence to pharmacological therapy must be continuously assessed and attempts made to tailor the regimen to fit the person's lifestyle. Educating clients and families about their hypertension and treatment regimens is necessary to facilitate involvement. Once-daily dosing helps to simplify the medication regimens and is generally preferable for individuals but, since these medications are more expensive, the simplicity must be balanced with the costs. Other strategies to simplify the medication regime include using fixed-dose combinations (*i.e.,* one pill containing two active agents), asking the pharmacy to package medications to be taken together (*i.e.,* blister packs) and the newest trials are looking at capsules containing multiple medications (*i.e.,* Polycap with a statin, ASA, ACE inhibitor, β-blocker, and diuretic together).

Systolic Hypertension

Systolic hypertension is defined as a systolic pressure of 140 mm Hg or greater and a diastolic pressure of less than 90 mm Hg. Historically, diastolic hypertension was thought to confer a greater risk for cardiovascular events than systolic hypertension.[39] However, there is evidence that elevated systolic blood pressure is at least as important as, if not more than, diastolic hypertension.[40]

There are two aspects of systolic hypertension that confer increased risk for cardiovascular events—one is the actual elevation in systolic pressure and the other is the disproportionate rise in pulse pressure. Elevated pressures during systole favour the development of left ventricular hypertrophy, increased myocardial oxygen demands, and eventual left ventricular failure. At the same time, the absolute or relative lowering of diastolic pressure is a limiting factor in coronary perfusion because coronary perfusion is greatest during diastole. Elevated pulse pressures produce greater stretch of arteries, causing damage to the elastic elements of the vessel, thus predisposing to aneurysms and intimal damage that leads to atherosclerosis and thrombosis.

Secondary Hypertension

Secondary hypertension, which describes an elevation in blood pressure due to another disease condition, accounts for 5% to 10% of hypertension cases.[1,41] Unlike primary hypertension, many of the conditions causing secondary hypertension can be corrected or cured by surgery or specific medical treatment. Secondary hypertension tends to be seen in persons younger than 30 and older than 50 years of age. Cocaine, amphetamines, and other illicit drugs can cause significant hypertension, as can sympathomimetic agents (decongestants, anorectics), erythropoietin, and licorice (including some chewing tobaccos with licorice as an ingredient). Obstructive sleep apnea (see Chapter 52) is an independent risk factor for secondary hypertension.

Among the most common causes of secondary hypertension are renal disease (*i.e.,* renovascular hypertension), adrenal cortical disorders, pheochromocytoma, and coarctation of the aorta. Oral contraceptive agents are also implicated as a cause of secondary hypertension. To avoid duplication in descriptions, the mechanisms associated with elevations of blood pressure in these disorders are discussed briefly, and a more detailed discussion of specific disease disorders is reserved for other sections of this book.

Renal Hypertension

With the dominant role that the kidney assumes in blood pressure regulation, it is not surprising that the largest single cause of secondary hypertension is renal disease. Most acute kidney disorders result in decreased urine formation, retention of salt and water, and hypertension. This includes acute glomerulonephritis, acute renal failure, and acute urinary tract obstruction. Hypertension also is common among persons with chronic pyelonephritis, polycystic kidney disease, diabetic nephropathy, and end-stage renal disease, regardless of cause. In older persons, the sudden onset of secondary hypertension often is associated with atherosclerotic disease of the renal blood vessels.

Renovascular hypertension refers to hypertension caused by reduced renal blood flow and activation of the renin–angiotensin–aldosterone system. It is the most common cause of secondary hypertension, accounting for 2% to 5% of all cases of hypertension.[1,41] The reduced renal blood flow that occurs with renovascular disease causes the affected kidney to release excessive amounts of renin, increasing circulating levels of angiotensin II. Angiotensin II, in turn, acts as a vasoconstrictor to increase peripheral vascular resistance and as a stimulus for increased aldosterone levels and sodium retention by the kidney. One or both of the kidneys may be affected. When the renal artery of only one kidney is involved, the unaffected kidney is subjected to the detrimental effects of the elevated blood pressure.

There are two major types of renovascular disease: atherosclerosis of the proximal renal artery and fibromuscular dysplasia, a noninflammatory vascular disease that affects the renal arteries and branch vessels.[1,41,42] Atherosclerotic stenosis of the renal artery accounts for up to 90% of cases and is seen most often in older adults, particularly those with diabetes, aortoiliac occlusive disease, coronary artery disease, or hypertension. Fibromuscular dysplasia is more common in women and tends to occur in younger age groups, often persons in their third decade. Genetic factors may be involved, and the incidence tends to increase with risk factors such as smoking and hyperlipidemia.

Renal artery stenosis should be suspected when hypertension develops in a previously normotensive person older than 50 (*i.e.,* atherosclerotic form) or younger than 30 (*i.e.,* fibromuscular dysplasia) years of age, or when accelerated hypertension occurs in a person with previously controlled hypertension. Hypokalemia (due to increased aldosterone levels), the presence of an abdominal bruit, the absence of a family history of hypertension, and a duration of hypertension of less than 1 year help to distinguish renovascular hypertension from primary hypertension.

Diagnostic tests for renovascular hypertension may include studies to assess overall renal function, physiologic studies to assess the renin–angiotensin system, perfusion studies to evaluate renal blood flow, and imaging studies to identify renal artery stenosis.[1,42] Renal arteriography remains the definitive test for identifying renal artery disease. Duplex ultrasonographic scanning, contrast-enhanced computed tomography (CT), and magnetic resonance angiography (MRA) are other tests that can be used to screen for renovascular hypertension.[1]

The goal of treatment of renal hypertension is to control the blood pressure and stabilize renal function. Angioplasty or revascularization has been shown to be an effective long-term treatment for the disorder. ACE inhibitors may be used in medical management of renal stenosis. However, these agents must be used with caution because of their potential to produce marked hypotension and renal dysfunction.[42]

Disorders of Adrenocortical Hormones

Increased levels of adrenocortical hormones also can give rise to hypertension. Primary hyperaldosteronism (excess production of aldosterone due to adrenocortical hyperplasia or adenoma) and excess levels of glucocorticoid (Cushing disease or syndrome) tend to raise the blood pressure[1,41] (see Chapter 41). These hormones facilitate sodium and water retention by the kidney; the hypertension that accompanies excessive levels of either hormone probably is related to this factor. For patients with primary hyperaldosteronism, a salt-restricted diet often produces a reduction in blood pressure. Because aldosterone acts on the distal renal tubule to increase sodium absorption in exchange for potassium elimination in the urine, persons with hyperaldosteronism usually have decreased potassium levels. Screening tests for primary hyperaldosteronism involve the determination of plasma aldosterone concentration and plasma renin activity. CT and MRI scans are used to localize the lesion. Persons with solitary adenomas are usually treated surgically.[1,6] Potassium-sparing diuretics, such as spironolactone, which is an aldosterone antagonist, often are used in the medical management of persons with bilateral hyperplasia.[1,43]

Licorice is an extract from the roots of the *Glycyrrhiza glabra* plant that has been used in medicine since ancient times. European licorice (not licorice flavouring) is associated with sodium retention, edema, hypertension, and hypokalemia. Licorice, which is an effective analog of the steroid 11β-dehydrogenase enzyme that modulates access to the aldosterone receptor in the kidney, produces a syndrome similar to primary hyperaldosteronism.[44]

Pheochromocytoma

A pheochromocytoma is a tumour of chromaffin tissue, which contains sympathetic nerve cells that stain with chromium salts. The tumour is most commonly located in the adrenal medulla but can arise in other sites, such as the sympathetic ganglia, where there is chromaffin tissue.[13,55] Although only 0.05% to 0.1% of persons with hypertension have an underlying pheochromocytoma, the disorder can cause serious hypertensive crises. The tumours are malignant 8% to 10% of the time.[41]

Like adrenal medullary cells, the tumour cells of a pheochromocytoma produce and secrete the catecholamines epinephrine and norepinephrine. The hypertension that develops is a result of the massive release of these catecholamines. Their release may be paroxysmal rather than continuous, causing periodic episodes of headache, excessive sweating, and palpitations. Headache is the most common symptom and can be quite severe. Nervousness, tremor, facial pallor, weakness, fatigue, and weight loss occur less frequently. Marked variability in blood pressure between episodes is typical. Approximately 50% of persons with pheochromocytoma have paroxysmal episodes of hypertension, sometimes to dangerously high levels. The other 50% have sustained hypertension, and some even may be normotensive.[1,41]

Several tests are available to differentiate hypertension due to pheochromocytoma from other forms of hypertension. The most commonly used diagnostic measure is the determination of urinary catecholamines and their metabolites. Although measurement of plasma catecholamines also may be used, other conditions can cause catecholamines to be elevated. After the presence of a pheochromocytoma has been established, the tumour needs to be located. MRI (preferable) and CT scans may be used for this purpose. Surgical removal of operable tumours is usually curative.[41] If surgical intervention is not possible, treatment with medications that block the action or synthesis of catecholamines can be used.

Coarctation of the Aorta

Coarctation represents a narrowing of the aorta. In the adult form of aortic coarctation, the narrowing most commonly occurs just distal to the origin of the subclavian arteries[1] (see Chapter 24). Because of the narrowing, blood flow to the lower parts of the body and kidneys is reduced. In the infantile form of coarctation, the narrowing occurs proximal to the ductus arteriosus, in which case heart failure and other problems may occur.

In the adult form of aortic coarctation, the ejection of an increased stroke volume into a narrowed aorta causes an increase in systolic blood pressure and blood flow to the upper part of the body. Blood pressure in the lower extremities may be normal, although it frequently is low. It has been suggested that the increase in stroke volume and maintenance of the pressure to the lower part of the body is achieved through the renin–angiotensin–aldosterone system in response to a decrease in renal blood flow. Pulse pressure in the legs almost always is narrowed, and the femoral pulses are weak. Because the aortic capacity is diminished, there usually is a marked increase in pressure (measured in the arms) during exercise, when the stroke volume and heart rate are increased. For this reason, blood pressures in both arms and one leg should be determined; a pressure that is 20 mm Hg more in the arms than in the legs suggests coarctation of the aorta. Involvement of the left subclavian artery or an anomalous origin of the right subclavian may produce decreased or absent left or right brachial pulses, respectively. Palpation of both brachial pulses and measurement of blood pressure in both arms are important.

Treatment consists of surgical repair or balloon angioplasty. Children require long-term follow-up to ensure vessel growth is matching demands and they may ultimately need a patch in the area due to strictures.

Oral Contraceptive Drugs

The use of oral contraceptive pills is probably the most common cause of secondary hypertension in young women.[44,45] Women taking oral contraceptive should have their blood pressure taken regularly. The cause of the increased blood pressure is largely unknown, although it has been suggested that the probable cause is volume expansion because both estrogens and synthetic progesterones used in oral contraceptive pills cause sodium retention. Various contraceptive drugs contain different amounts and combinations of estrogen and progestation agents, and these differences may contribute to the occurrence of hypertension in some women but not others. Fortunately, the hypertension associated with oral contraceptives usually disappears after the drug has been discontinued, although it may take as long as 3 months for this to happen.[45] However, in some women, the blood pressure may not return to normal, and they may be at risk for development of hypertension. The risk for hypertension-associated cardiovascular complications is found primarily in women older than 35 years of age and in those who smoke.

Malignant Hypertension

A small number of persons with hypertension develop an accelerated and potentially fatal form of the disease termed *malignant hypertension.*[1] This usually is a disease of younger persons, particularly young North American men of African descent, women with pre-existing or gestational hypertension with preeclampsia, and persons with renal and collagen diseases.

Malignant hypertension is characterized by sudden, marked elevations in blood pressure, with diastolic values above 120 mm Hg complicated by evidence of acute or rapidly progressive life-threatening organ dysfunction. There may be intense arterial spasm of the cerebral arteries with hypertensive encephalopathy. Cerebral vasoconstriction probably is an exaggerated homeostatic response designed to protect the brain from excesses of blood pressure and flow. The regulatory mechanisms often are insufficient to protect the capillaries, and cerebral edema frequently develops. As it advances, papilledema (*i.e.,* swelling of the optic nerve at its point of entrance into the eye) ensues, giving evidence of the effects of pressure on the optic nerve and retinal vessels. The patient may have headache, restlessness, confusion, stupor, motor and sensory deficits, and visual disturbances. In severe cases, convulsions and coma follow.[46]

Prolonged and severe exposure to exaggerated levels of blood pressure in malignant hypertension injures the walls of the arterioles, and intravascular coagulation and fragmentation of red blood cells may occur. The renal blood vessels are particularly vulnerable to hypertensive damage. Renal damage due to vascular changes probably is the most important prognostic determinant in malignant hypertension. Elevated levels of serum urea and creatinine, metabolic acidosis, hypocalcemia, and proteinuria provide evidence of renal impairment.

The complications associated with a hypertensive crisis demand immediate and rigorous medical treatment in an intensive care unit with continuous monitoring of arterial blood pressure. With proper therapy, the death rate from this cause can be markedly reduced, as can complications and additional episodes. Because chronic hypertension is associated with autoregulatory changes in coronary artery, cerebral artery, and kidney blood flow, care should be taken to avoid excessively rapid decreases in blood pressure, which can lead to hypoperfusion and ischemic injury. Therefore, the goal of initial treatment measures should be to obtain a partial reduction in blood pressure to a safer, less critical level, rather than to normotensive levels.[46]

Hypertension Disorders in Pregnancy

Hypertensive disorders of pregnancy complicate 5% to 10% of pregnancies and remain a major cause of maternal and neonatal mortality and morbidity worldwide.[47,48] Most adverse events are attributable directly to the preeclampsia syndrome, characterized by new-onset hypertension with proteinuria that develops in pregnancy. Women with chronic hypertension can also manifest adverse events.

Classification

The Society of Obstetricians and Gynaecologists of Canada (SOGC) classifies hypertensive disorders in pregnancies as pre-existing or gestational.[47] Pre-existing hypertension exists before pregnancy or appears before 20 weeks of pregnancy (see Table 23.2). Hypertension that is not pre-existing and occurs at or after 20 weeks of pregnancy is called gestational hypertension. Both pre-existing and gestational hypertension can be associated with comorbid conditions.

Defining the cause or causes of hypertension that occurs during pregnancy is difficult because of the normal circulatory changes that occur. Blood pressure normally decreases during the first trimester, reaches its lowest point during the second trimester, and gradually rises during the third trimester. The fact that there is a large increase in cardiac output during early pregnancy suggests the decrease in blood pressure that occurs during the first part of pregnancy results from a decrease in peripheral vascular resistance. Because the cardiac output remains high throughout pregnancy, the gradual rise in blood pressure that begins during the second trimester probably represents a return of the peripheral vascular resistance to normal. Pregnancy normally is accompanied by increased levels of renin, angiotensin I and II, estrogen, progesterone, prolactin, and aldosterone, all of which may alter vascular reactivity. Women who experience preeclampsia are thought to be particularly sensitive to the vasoconstrictor activity of the renin–angiotensin–aldosterone system. They also

TABLE 23.2 HYPERTENSION DISORDERS OF PREGNANCY CLASSIFICATION

CLASSIFICATION	DESCRIPTION
Pre-existing (chronic) hypertension • With or without comorbid conditions[a] • With preeclampsia after 20 weeks gestation	Hypertension diagnosed prior to 20 weeks gestation • Resistant hypertension *or* new or increased proteinuria *or* one or more adverse condition(s)[b]
Gestational hypertension • With comorbid conditions[a] • With preeclampsia after 20 weeks gestation	Hypertension diagnosed after 20 weeks gestation • New proteinuria *or* one or more adverse condition(s)

[a]Comorbid conditions include diabetes and renal disease.
[b]Adverse conditions include maternal signs or symptoms, or fetal signs or morbidity.
From the Society of Obstetricians and Gynecologists of Canada.[47]

are particularly responsive to other vasoconstrictors, including the catecholamines and vasopressin. It has been proposed that some of the sensitivity may be caused by a prostacyclin–thromboxane imbalance. Thromboxane is a prostaglandin with vasoconstrictor properties, and prostacyclin a prostaglandin with vasodilator properties. Emerging evidence suggests that insulin resistance, including that which occurs with diabetes, obesity, and the metabolic syndrome, may predispose to the hypertensive disorders of pregnancy.

Preeclampsia–Eclampsia. Preeclampsia–eclampsia is a pregnancy-specific syndrome with both maternal and fetal manifestations.[47,48] Women with either pre-existing or gestational hypertension may develop preeclampsia. The three criteria used to determine preeclampsia in Canada are hypertension (systolic blood pressure >140 mm Hg and diastolic blood pressure >90 mm Hg), proteinuria (>0.3 g/day in a 24-hour collection or urine creatinine of 30 mg/mmol in a spot [random] urine sample), and adverse conditions. Adverse conditions consist of symptoms such as persistent or new and unusual headache, visual disturbances, persistent abdominal or right, upper quadrant pain, severe nausea or vomiting, chest pain or dyspnea, signs of end organ dysfunction, abnormal laboratory test results (*e.g.,* elevated serum creatinine; elevated liver enzymes, alanine transaminase (ALT), aspartate transaminase (AST), lactate dehydrogenase (LDH), or bilirubin; low platelet count; low serum albumin; or feto-placental abnormalities.[47]

Preeclampsia occurs primarily during first pregnancies and during subsequent pregnancies in women with multiple fetuses, diabetes mellitus, collagen vascular disease, or underlying kidney disease.[47] It is also associated with a condition called a *hydatidiform mole* (*i.e.,* abnormal pregnancy caused by a pathologic ovum, resulting in a mass of cysts).[48] Women with chronic hypertension who become pregnant have an increased risk for preeclampsia and adverse neonatal outcomes, particularly when associated with proteinuria early in pregnancy.

The cause of gestational hypertension is largely unknown. The most popular theory is related to the mismatch between uteroplacental blood supply and fetal demands leading to maternal endothelial cell dysfunction.[47,48] Considerable evidence suggests that the placenta is the key component for all the manifestations because delivery is the only definitive cure

for this disease. Gestational hypertension is thought to involve a decrease in placental blood flow leading to the release of toxic mediators (*e.g.,* cytokines, prostaglandins, reactive oxygen radicals) that alter the function of endothelial cells in blood vessels throughout the body, including those of the kidney, brain, liver, and heart.[48] The endothelial changes result in signs and symptoms of preeclampsia and, in more severe cases, of intravascular clotting and hypoperfusion of vital organs. There is risk for development of disseminated intravascular coagulation (DIC; see Chapter 13), cerebral hemorrhage, generalized edema, hepatic failure, acute renal failure, cardiomyopathy, and acute respiratory distress syndrome.[47] Thrombocytopenia is the most common hematologic complication of preeclampsia. Platelet counts of less than 50×10^9/L signal serious disease. The cause of thrombocytopenia has been ascribed to platelet deposition at the site of endothelial injury. The renal changes that occur with preeclampsia include a decrease in glomerular filtration rate and renal blood flow. Sodium excretion may be impaired, although this is variable. Edema may or may not be present. Some of the severest forms of preeclampsia occur in the absence of edema. Even when there is extensive edema, the plasma volume usually is lower than that of a normal pregnancy. Liver damage, when it occurs, may range from mild hepatocellular necrosis with elevation of liver enzymes to the more ominous *H*emolysis, *E*levated *L*iver function test results, and *L*ow *P*latelet count (HELLP) syndrome that is associated with significant maternal mortality. Eclampsia, the convulsive stage of preeclampsia, is a significant cause of maternal mortality. The pathogenesis of eclampsia remains unclear but has been attributed to both increased blood coagulability and fibrin deposition in the cerebral vessels.

The decreased placental blood flow that occurs with preeclampsia also affects the fetus. It frequently results in intrauterine growth restriction and infants who are small for gestational age. Preeclampsia is one of the leading causes of prematurity because of frequent need for early delivery in affected women.

Chronic (Pre-existing) Hypertension. Chronic hypertension in pregnancy, referred to as pre-existing hypertension, is considered to be hypertension that is unrelated to the pregnancy. It is defined as a history of high blood pressure before pregnancy, identification of hypertension before 20 weeks of pregnancy, and hypertension that persists 6 weeks after pregnancy.[1,47] Hypertension that is diagnosed for the first time during pregnancy and does not resolve after pregnancy also is classified as pre-existing hypertension. In women with pre-existing hypertension, blood pressure often decreases in early pregnancy and increases during the last trimester (3 months) of pregnancy, resembling preeclampsia. Consequently, women with undiagnosed pre-existing hypertension who do not present for medical care until the later months of pregnancy may be incorrectly diagnosed as having preeclampsia.

Preeclampsia Superimposed on Pre-existing Hypertension. Women with pre-existing hypertension have an increased risk for the development of preeclampsia, in which case the prognosis for the mother and fetus tends to be worse than for either condition alone. Superimposed preeclampsia should be considered in women with hypertension before 20 weeks of gestation who develop new-onset proteinuria; women with hypertension and proteinuria before 20 weeks of gestation; women with previously well-controlled hypertension who experience a sudden increase in blood pressure; and women with pre-existing hypertension who develop thrombocytopenia or an increase in serum ALT or AST to abnormal levels.[48]

Diagnosis and Treatment

Early prenatal care is important in the detection of high blood pressure during pregnancy. It is recommended that all pregnant women, including those with hypertension, refrain from alcohol and tobacco use. Salt restriction usually is not recommended during pregnancy because pregnant women with hypertension tend to have lower plasma volumes than normotensive pregnant women and because the severity of hypertension may reflect the degree of volume contraction. The exception is women with pre-existing hypertension who have been following a salt-restricted diet.

In women with preeclampsia, delivery of the fetus is curative. The timing of delivery becomes a difficult decision in preterm pregnancies because the welfare of both the mother and the infant must be taken into account. Antihypertensive medications, when required, must be carefully chosen because of their potential effects on uteroplacental blood flow and on the fetus. For example, the ACE inhibitors can cause injury to and even death of the fetus when given during the second and third trimesters of pregnancy. Medications most commonly used for treatment of hypertensive disorders of pregnancy are labetalol and nifedipine.[47]

High Blood Pressure in Children and Adolescents

The estimated prevalence of hypertension among children is 1% to 5%, and this appears to be increasing.[49] This is due in part to increasing prevalence of obesity and other lifestyle factors, such as decreased physical activity and increased intake of high-calorie, high-salt foods.

Blood pressure is known to increase from infancy to late adolescence. The average systolic pressure at 1 day of age is approximately 70 mm Hg and increases to approximately 85 mm Hg at 1 month of age. Systolic blood pressure continues to increase with physical growth to about 120 mm Hg at the end of adolescence. During the preschool years, blood pressure begins to follow a pattern that tends to be maintained as the child grows older. This pattern continues into adolescence and adulthood, suggesting that the roots of essential hypertension have their origin early in life. A familial influence on blood pressure often can be identified early in life. Children of parents with high blood pressure tend to have higher blood pressures than do children with normotensive parents.

Blood pressure norms for children are based on age, height, and sex-specific percentiles. The American National High Blood Pressure Education Program (NHBPEP) first published its recommendations in 1977. Canadian recommendations are not available. The fourth NHBPEP Task Force report (published in 2004) recommended classification of blood pressure (systolic or diastolic) for age, height, and sex into four categories: normal (less than the 90th percentile), high normal (between the 90th and 95th percentiles), stage 1 hypertension (between the 95th and 99th percentiles plus 5 mm Hg), and stage 2 hypertension (greater than the 99th percentile plus 5 mm Hg).[50] The height percentile is determined by using the newly revised Centers for Disease Control and Prevention (CDC) growth charts.[51] High normal is now considered to be "prehypertensive" and is an indication for lifestyle modification. Children and adolescents with hypertension should be evaluated for target-organ damage.[50]

Secondary hypertension is the most common form of high blood pressure in infants and children. In later childhood and adolescence, essential hypertension is more common. Approximately 90% of secondary hypertension in children is caused by renovascular abnormalities.[52] Coarctation of the aorta is another cause of hypertension in children and adolescents. Endocrine causes of hypertension, such as pheochromocytoma and adrenal cortical disorders, are rare. Hypertension in infants is associated most commonly with high umbilical catheterization and renal artery obstruction caused by thrombosis. Most cases of essential hypertension are associated with obesity or a family history of hypertension.

A number of drugs of abuse, therapeutic agents, and toxins also may increase blood pressure. Alcohol should be considered as a risk factor in adolescents. Oral contraceptives may be a cause of hypertension in adolescent girls. The nephrotoxicity of the drug cyclosporine, an immunosuppressant used in transplant therapy, may cause hypertension in children (and adults) after bone marrow, heart, kidney, or liver transplantation. The coadministration of corticosteroids appears to increase the incidence of hypertension.[52]

Diagnosis and Treatment

The American Medical Association has recommended that children 3 years of age through adolescence should have their blood pressure taken once each year, but Canada has not adopted this screening recommendation. The auscultatory method using a cuff of an appropriate size for the child's upper arm is recommended.[50] Repeated measurements over time, rather than a single isolated determination, are required to establish consistent and significant observations. Children with high blood pressure should be referred for medical evaluation and treatment as indicated. Treatment includes nonpharmacologic methods and, if necessary, pharmacologic therapy.

High Blood Pressure in Older Adults

The prevalence of hypertension increases with advancing age to the extent that half of people aged 60 to 69 years and approximately three fourths of people 70 years and older are affected.[53] The age-related rise in systolic blood pressure is primarily responsible for the increase in hypertension that occurs with increasing age.

Among the aging processes that contribute to an increase in blood pressure are a stiffening of the large arteries, particularly the aorta; decreased baroreceptor sensitivity; increased peripheral vascular resistance; and decreased renal blood flow.[54] Systolic blood pressure rises almost linearly between 30 and 84 years of age, whereas diastolic pressure rises until 50 years of age and then levels off or decreases.[1] This rise in systolic pressure is thought to be related to increased stiffness of the large arteries. With aging, the elastin fibres in the walls of the arteries are gradually replaced by collagen fibres that render the vessels stiffer and less compliant.[54] Differences in the central and peripheral arteries relate to the fact that the larger vessels contain more elastin, whereas the peripheral resistance vessels have more smooth muscle and less elastin. Because of increased wall stiffness, the aorta and large arteries are less able to buffer the increase in systolic pressure that occurs as blood is ejected from the left heart, and they are less able to store the energy needed to maintain the diastolic pressure. As a result, the systolic pressure increases, the diastolic pressure remains unchanged or actually decreases, and the pulse pressure or difference between the systolic pressure and diastolic pressure widens.

Isolated systolic hypertension (systolic pressure ≥140 mm Hg and diastolic pressure <90 mm Hg) is recognized as an important risk factor for cardiovascular morbidity and mortality in older persons.[6] The treatment of hypertension in older adults has beneficial effects in terms of reducing the incidence of cardiovascular events such as stroke. Studies have shown a reduction in stroke, coronary heart disease, and congestive heart failure in persons who were treated for hypertension compared with those who were not.[54]

Diagnosis and Treatment

The recommendations for measurement of blood pressure in older adults are similar to those for the rest of the population.[6] Blood pressure variability is particularly prevalent among older persons, so it is especially important to obtain multiple measurements on different occasions to establish a diagnosis of hypertension. The effects of food, position, and other environmental factors also are exaggerated in older persons. Although sitting has been the standard position for blood pressure measurement, it is recommended that blood pressure also be taken in the supine and standing positions in older adults. In some older adults with hypertension, a silent interval, called the *auscultatory gap,* may occur between the end of the first and beginning of the third phases of the Korotkoff sounds, providing the potential for underestimating the systolic pressure, sometimes by as much as 50 mm Hg. Because the gap occurs only with auscultation, it is recommended that a preliminary determination of systolic blood pressure be made by palpation and the cuff be inflated 30 mm Hg above this value for auscultatory measurement of blood pressure. In some older persons, the indirect measurement using a blood pressure cuff and the Korotkoff sounds has been shown to give falsely elevated readings compared with the direct intra-arterial method. This is because excessive cuff pressure is needed to compress the rigid vessels of some older persons. Pseudohypertension should be suspected in older persons with hypertension in whom the radial or brachial artery remains palpable but pulseless at higher cuff pressures.

Recommendations for treating hypertension in the elderly are similar to those for the general population.[6] A conservative blood pressure target of less than 150/80 mm Hg in those over the age of 80 years is appropriate.[6] However, blood pressure should be reduced slowly and cautiously. When possible, appropriate lifestyle modification measures should be tried first. Antihypertensive medications should be prescribed carefully because the older person may have impaired baroreflex sensitivity and renal function. Usually, medications are initiated at smaller doses, and doses are increased more gradually. There is also the danger of adverse drug interactions in older persons, who may be taking multiple medications, including over-the-counter medications. β-Blockers and α-blockers are not recommended as first-line agents for persons aged 60 or older.[6]

IN SUMMARY

Hypertension (systolic pressure ≥140 mm Hg and/or diastolic pressure ≥90 mm Hg) is one of the most common cardiovascular disorders. It may occur as a primary disorder (*i.e.,* essential hypertension) or as a symptom of some other disease (*i.e.,* secondary hypertension). The incidence of primary hypertension increases with age; the condition is seen more frequently among persons of African descent, and it may be associated with a family history of high blood pressure, metabolic syndrome, obesity, and increased sodium intake. Causes of secondary hypertension include kidney disease and adrenal cortical disorders (hyperaldosteronism and Cushing disease), which increase sodium and water retention; pheochromocytomas, which increase catecholamine levels; and coarctation of the aorta, which produces an increase in blood flow and systolic blood pressure in the arms and a decrease in blood flow and systolic pressure in the legs.

Unlike disorders of other body systems that are diagnosed by methods such as radiography and tissue examination, hypertension and other blood pressure disorders are determined by repeated blood pressure measurements. Uncontrolled hypertension increases the risk of heart disease, renal complications, retinopathy, and stroke. Treatment of essential hypertension focuses on nonpharmacologic methods such as weight reduction, reduction of sodium intake, regular physical activity, and modification of alcohol intake. Among the drugs used in the treatment of hypertension are diuretics, β-adrenergic blocking agents, ACE inhibitors, calcium channel blocking agents, α_1-adrenergic blocking agents, centrally acting α_2 agonists, and vasodilator drugs.

The SOGC classify hypertensive disorders in pregnancies as pre-existing or gestational. Pre-existing hypertension exists before pregnancy or appears before 20 weeks of pregnancy. Gestational hypertension appears at or after 20 weeks of pregnancy. Both pre-existing and gestational hypertension can be associated with comorbid conditions. Three criteria that define preeclampsia are hypertension, proteinuria, and adverse conditions. Preeclampsia hypertension is thought to result from an imbalance of placental perfusion and fetal demands along with the release of toxic vasoactive substances that alter blood vessel tone and blood clotting mechanisms and poses a particular threat to the mother and the fetus. Pre-existing or chronic hypertension is considered to be hypertension that is unrelated to the pregnancy. It is defined as a history of high blood pressure before pregnancy, identification of hypertension before 20 weeks of pregnancy, and hypertension that persists 6 weeks after pregnancy.

The prevalence of hypertension in children and adolescents appear to be increasing, partly as a result of an increase in childhood obesity, and lifestyle factors such as physical inactivity and increased intake of high-calorie and high-salt foods. During childhood, blood pressure is influenced by growth and maturation; therefore, blood pressure norms have been established using percentiles specific to age, height, and sex to identify children for further follow-up and treatment. Although hypertension occurs infrequently in children, it is recommended that children 3 years of age through adolescence should have their blood pressure taken once each year.

The most common type of hypertension in older adults is isolated systolic hypertension (systolic pressure ≥140 mm Hg and diastolic pressure <90 mm Hg). Its pathogenesis is related to the loss of elastin fibres in the aorta and the inability of the aorta to stretch during systole. Untreated systolic hypertension is recognized as an important risk factor for stroke and other cardiovascular morbidity and mortality in older persons.

CONCEPTSin action **ANIMATION**

ORTHOSTATIC HYPOTENSION

After completing this section of the chapter, you should be able to meet the following objectives:

- Define the term orthostatic hypotension.
- Describe the cardiovascular, neurohumoral, and muscular responses that serve to maintain blood pressure when moving from the supine to standing position.
- Explain how fluid deficit, medications, aging, disorders of the ANS, and bed rest contribute to the development of orthostatic hypotension.

Orthostatic or postural hypotension, which is a physical finding and not a disease, is an abnormal drop in blood pressure on assumption of the standing position.[55,56] Orthostatic hypotension is defined as a drop in systolic pressure of 20 mm Hg or more or a drop in diastolic blood pressure of 10 mm Hg or more within 3 minutes of standing.[56]

ORTHOSTATIC HYPOTENSION

- Orthostatic or postural hypotension represents an abnormal drop in blood pressure on assumption of the upright position due to pooling of blood in the lower part of the body.
- Orthostatic hypotension may be accompanied by a decrease in cerebral perfusion that causes a feeling of lightheadedness, dizziness, and, in some cases, fainting. It poses a particular threat for falls in the elderly.
- The fall in blood pressure is caused by conditions that decrease vascular volume (dehydration), impair muscle pump function (bed rest and spinal cord injury), or interfere with the cardiovascular reflexes (medications that decrease heart rate or cause vasodilation, disorders of the ANS, effects of aging on baroreflex function).

Pathophysiology and Causative Factors

After the assumption of the upright posture from the supine position, approximately 700 ml of blood is momentarily shifted to the lower part of the body, with an accompanying decrease in central blood volume and arterial pressure.[56] Maintenance of blood pressure during position change is quite complex, involving the rapid initiation of cardiovascular, neurohumoral, and muscular responses. When the standing position is assumed in the absence of normal circulatory reflexes or blood volume, blood pools in the lower part of the body, cardiac output falls, blood pressure drops, and blood flow to the brain is inadequate. As a result, symptoms of decreased blood flow to the central nervous system may occur, including feelings of weakness, nausea, lightheadedness, dizziness, blurred vision, palpitations, and syncope (*i.e.*, fainting).

The decrease in blood pressure that occurs on standing is usually transient, lasting through several cardiac cycles. Normally, the baroreceptors located in the thorax and carotid sinus area sense the decreased pressure and initiate reflex constriction of the veins and arterioles and an increase in heart rate, which brings blood pressure back to normal (Fig. 23.5). The initial adjustment to orthostatic stress is mediated exclusively by the ANS.[56] Within a few minutes of standing, blood levels of ADH and sympathetic neuromediators increase as a secondary means of ensuring maintenance of normal blood pressure in the standing position. Under normal conditions,

the renin–angiotensin–aldosterone system is also activated when the standing position is assumed, and even more so in situations of hypotensive orthostatic stress.

Muscle movement in the lower extremities also aids venous return to the heart by pumping blood out of the legs. The unconscious slight body and leg movement during standing (postural sway) is recognized as an important factor in moving venous blood back to the heart. Crossing the legs, which involves contraction of the agonist and antagonist muscles, has been shown to be a simple and effective way of increasing cardiac output and, therefore, blood pressure.

Causes

A wide variety of conditions, acute and chronic, are associated with orthostatic hypotension. Although orthostatic hypotension can occur in all age groups, it is seen more frequently in the elderly, especially in persons who are sick and frail. Any disease condition that reduces blood volume, impairs mobility, results in prolonged inactivity, or impairs ANS function may also predispose to orthostatic hypotension. Adverse effects of medications are also commonly encountered causes of orthostatic hypotension.

Aging. Weakness and dizziness on standing are common complaints of elderly persons. Although orthostatic tolerance is well maintained in the healthy elderly, after 70 years of age there is an increasing tendency towards arterial pressure instability and postural hypotension. Although orthostatic hypotension may be either systolic or diastolic, that associated with aging seems more often to be systolic.[57] Several deficiencies in the circulatory response may predispose to this problem in the elderly, including diminished ability to produce an adequate increase in the heart rate, ventricular stroke volume, or peripheral vascular resistance; decreased function of the skeletal muscle pumps; and decreased blood volume. Because cerebral blood flow primarily depends on systolic pressure, patients with impaired cerebral circulation may experience symptoms of weakness, ataxia, dizziness, and syncope when their arterial pressure falls even slightly. This may happen in older persons who are immobilized for even brief periods or whose blood volume is decreased owing to inadequate fluid intake or overzealous use of diuretics.

Postprandial blood pressure often decreases in elderly persons.[58] The greatest postprandial changes occur after a meal high in simple carbohydrates. Although the mechanism responsible for these changes is not fully understood, it is thought to result from glucose-mediated impairment of baroreflex sensitivity and increased splanchnic blood flow mediated by insulin and vasoactive gastrointestinal hormones.[58]

Reduced Blood Volume. Orthostatic hypotension often is an early sign of reduced blood volume or fluid deficit. When blood volume is decreased, the vascular compartment is only partially filled; although cardiac output may be adequate when a person is in the recumbent position, it often decreases to the point of causing weakness and fainting when the person

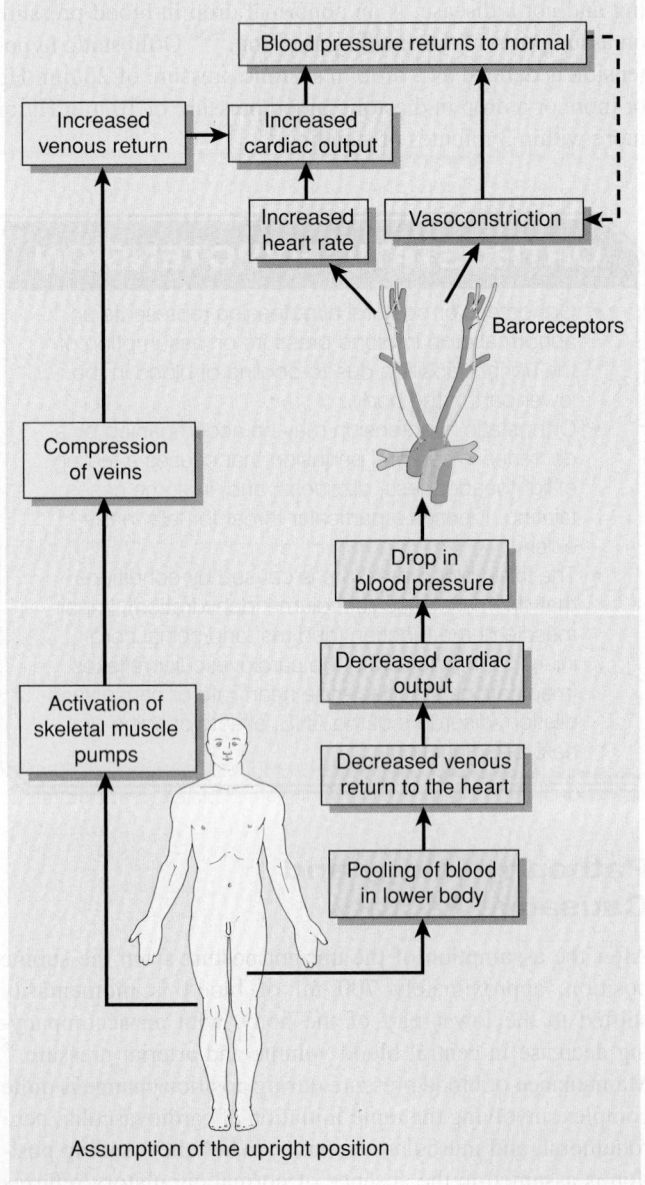

FIGURE 23.5 • Mechanisms of blood control on immediate assumption of the upright position.

assumes the standing position. Common causes of orthostatic hypotension related to hypovolemia are excessive use of diuretics, excessive diaphoresis, loss of gastrointestinal fluids through vomiting and diarrhea, and loss of fluid volume associated with prolonged bed rest.

Bed Rest and Impaired Mobility. Prolonged bed rest promotes a reduction in plasma volume, a decrease in venous tone, failure of peripheral vasoconstriction, and weakness of the skeletal muscles that support the veins and assist in returning blood to the heart (see Chapter 11). Physical deconditioning follows even short periods of bed rest. After 3 to 4 days, the blood volume is decreased. Loss of vascular and skeletal muscle tone is less predictable but probably becomes maximal after approximately 2 weeks of bed rest. Orthostatic intolerance is a recognized problem of space flight—a potential risk after reentry into the earth's gravitational field.

Drug-Induced Hypotension. Antihypertensives and psychotropics are the most common cause of chronic orthostatic hypotension. In most cases, the orthostatic hypotension is well tolerated. However, if the hypotension causes lightheadedness or syncope, the dosage of the drug is usually reduced or a different drug substituted.

Disorders of the Autonomic Nervous System. The sympathetic nervous system plays an essential role in adjustment to the upright position. Sympathetic stimulation increases heart rate and cardiac contractility and causes constriction of peripheral veins and arterioles. Orthostatic hypotension caused by altered autonomic function is common in peripheral neuropathies associated with diabetes mellitus, after injury or disease of the spinal cord, or as the result of a cerebral vascular accident in which sympathetic outflow from the brain stem is disrupted. The main forms of autonomic dysfunction (dysautonomia) include: pure autonomic failure, a peripheral degenerative disorder of the ANS leading to sporadic, idiopathic cause of persistent orthostatic hypotension and other manifestations of autonomic failure such as urinary retention, impotence, or decreased sweating; multiple-system atrophy (MSA), a progressive, neurodegenerative, adult-onset disorder with parkinsonism and ataxia features plus progressive autonomic failure; autoimmune autonomic neuropathy damaging autonomic ganglia receptors; and postural orthostatic tachycardia syndrome (POTS), a disturbance of the sympathetic system increasing heart rate.[8] MSA usually develops in middle to late life as orthostatic hypotension associated with uncoordinated movements, urinary incontinence, constipation, and other signs of neurologic deficits referable to the corticospinal, extrapyramidal, corticobulbar, and cerebellar systems.[59]

Diagnosis and Treatment

Orthostatic hypotension can be assessed with the auscultatory method of blood pressure measurement. Measurements should be made when the person is supine, after standing for

1 minute, and again after standing for 3 minutes.[57] Because it takes approximately 5 to 10 minutes for the blood pressure to stabilize after lying down, it is recommended that the patient be supine for this period before standing. It is strongly recommended that a second person be available when blood pressure is measured in the standing position to prevent injury should the person become faint. The seated position may be used in persons who are unable to stand; however, the postural blood pressure changes may be missed.

The detection of orthostatic hypotension may require numerous blood pressure measurements under different conditions.[57] The time of day is important because postural hypotension is often worse in the morning when the person rises from bed. Food and alcohol can also exacerbate orthostatic hypotension, as can activities that raise intrathoracic pressure (urination, defecation, coughing). An orthostatic hypotensive response may be immediate or delayed. Prolonged standing or a tilt table test may be needed to detect a delayed response. With a tilt table, the recumbent person can be moved to a head-up position without voluntary movement when the table is tilted. The tilt table also has the advantage of rapidly and safely returning persons with a profound postural drop in blood pressure to the horizontal position.

The heart rate response to postural change may provide valuable information about the cause of orthostatic hypotension.[57] A minimal increase in heart rate (<10 beats/minute) in the face of hypotension suggests impairment of baroreflex function, whereas tachycardia (>100 beats/minute) is suggestive of volume depletion or orthostatic intolerance. Because of the age-related decrease in baroreflex function, the absence of an increase in heart rate does not rule out volume depletion in the older person.[57]

Persons with a position-related drop in blood pressure sufficient to qualify as orthostatic hypotension should be evaluated to determine the cause and seriousness of the condition. A history should be taken to elicit information about symptoms, particularly dizziness and history of syncope and falls; medical conditions, particularly those such as diabetes mellitus that predispose to orthostatic hypotension; use of prescription and over-the-counter drugs; and symptoms of ANS dysfunction, such as erectile or bladder dysfunction. A physical examination should document blood pressure in both arms and the heart rate while in the supine, sitting, and standing positions and should note the occurrence of symptoms. Noninvasive, 24-hour ambulatory blood pressure monitoring may be used to determine blood pressure responses to other stimuli of daily life, such as food ingestion and exertion.

Treatment of orthostatic hypotension usually is directed towards alleviating the cause or, if this is not possible, towards helping people learn ways to cope with the disorder and prevent falls and injuries. Medications that predispose to postural hypotension should be avoided. Correcting the fluid deficit and trying a different antihypertensive medication are examples of measures designed to correct the cause. Measures designed to help persons prevent symptomatic orthostatic drops in blood pressure include gradual ambulation to allow the circulatory system to adjust (*e.g.,* sitting on the edge of the bed for several minutes and moving the legs to initiate skeletal muscle pump function before standing); avoidance of situations that encourage excessive vasodilation (*e.g.,* drinking alcohol, exercising vigorously in a warm environment); and avoidance of excess diuresis (*e.g.,* use of diuretics), diaphoresis, or loss of body fluids. Tight-fitting elastic support hose or an abdominal support garment may help prevent pooling of blood in the lower extremities and abdomen.[55,56,57]

Pharmacologic treatment may be used when nonpharmacologic methods are unsuccessful. A number of types of drugs can be used for this purpose.[55,56] Mineralocorticoids (*e.g.,* fludrocortisone) can be used to reduce salt and water loss and probably increase α-adrenergic sensitivity. Vasopressin-2 receptor agonists (desmopressin) may be used to reduce nocturnal polyuria. Sympathomimetic drugs that act directly on the resistance vessels (*e.g.,* phenylephrine, noradrenaline, clonidine, midodrine) or on the capacitance vessels (*e.g.,* dihydroergotamine) may be used. Many of these agents have undesirable side effects. Octreotide, a somatostatin analog that inhibits the release of vasodilatory gastrointestinal peptides, may prove useful in persons with postprandial hypotension.

IN SUMMARY

Orthostatic hypotension refers to an abnormal decrease in systolic and diastolic blood pressures that occurs on assumption of the upright position. An important consideration in orthostatic hypotension is the occurrence of dizziness and syncope. Among the factors that contribute to its occurrence are decreased fluid volume, medications, aging, defective function of the ANS, and the effects of immobility. Diagnosis of orthostatic hypotension relies on blood pressure measurements in the supine and upright positions, and a history of symptoms, medication use, and disease conditions that contribute to a postural drop in blood pressure. Treatment includes correcting the reversible causes and assisting the person to compensate for the disorder and prevent falls and injuries.

REVIEW EXERCISES

1. A 47-year-old African-American male, who is an executive in a law firm, has his blood pressure taken at a screening program and is told that his pressure is 142/90 mm Hg. His father and older brother have hypertension, and his paternal grandparents had a history of stroke and myocardial infarction. The patient enjoys salty foods and routinely uses a salt shaker to add salt to meals his wife prepares, drinks about four beers while watching television in the evening, and has gained 6 kg in the past year. Although his family has encouraged him to engage in physical activities with them, he states he is either too busy or too tired.
   A. *What are his risk factors for hypertension?*
   B. *Explain how an increased salt intake might contribute to his increase in blood pressure.*
   C. *What lifestyle changes would you suggest to the patient? Explain the rationale for your suggestions.*

2. A 36-year-old woman enters the clinic complaining of headache and not feeling well. Her blood pressure is 175/90 mm Hg. Her renal test results are abnormal, and follow-up tests confirm that she has a stricture of the left renal artery.
   A. *Would this woman's hypertension be classified as primary or secondary?*
   B. *Explain the physiologic mechanisms underlying her blood pressure elevation.*

3. A 75-year-old woman residing in an extended care facility has multiple health problems, including diabetes, hypertension, and heart failure. Lately, she has been feeling dizzy when she stands up, and she has almost fallen on several occasions. Her family is concerned and wants to know why this is happening and what they can do to prevent her from falling and injuring herself.
   A. *How would you go about assessing this woman for orthostatic hypotension?*
   B. *What are the causes of orthostatic hypotension in older adults?*
   C. *How might this woman's medical conditions and their treatment contribute to her orthostatic hypotension?*
   D. *The woman tells you that she feels particularly dizzy after she has eaten, yet staff members insist that she sit up and socialize with the other residents even though she would rather lie down and rest until the dizziness goes away. Explain the possible reason for her dizziness and what measures might be used to counteract the dizziness.*
   E. *The woman recently had an episode of vomiting and diarrhea on an extremely hot day. She told her family that she was so dizzy that she was sure she would fall. Explain why her dizziness was more severe under these conditions and what might be done to alleviate the situation.*

References

1. Mann D. L., Zipes D. P., Libby P., et al. (2014). *Braunwald's heart disease: A textbook of cardiovascular medicine* (10th ed.). Philadelphia, PA: Elsevier Saunders.
2. Hall J. E. (2011). *Textbook of medical physiology* (12th ed.). Philadelphia, PA: W. B. Saunders.

3. Chopra S., Baby C., Jacob J. J. (2011). Neuro-endocrine regulation of blood pressure. *Indian Journal of Endocrinology and Metabolism, 15*(Suppl 4), S281–S288.

4. Parati G., Ochoa J. E., Lombardi C., Bilo G. (2013). Assessment and management of blood-pressure variability. *Nature Reviews Cardiology, 10*(3), 143–155.

5. Hypertension Canada. (2014). Canadian Hypertension Education Program (CHEP) recommendations. Available online at: https://www.hypertension.ca/en/chep. Accessed March 2, 2015.

6. Dasgupta K., Quinn R. R., Zarnke K. B., et al.; Canadian Hypertension Education Program. (2014). The 2014 Canadian Hypertension Education Program recommendation for blood pressure measurement, diagnosis, assessment of risk, prevention, and treatment of hypertension. *Canadian Journal of Cardiology, 30*(5), 485–501.

7. Hypertension Canada. (2014). Devices endorsed by Hypertension Canada. Available online at: https://www.hypertension.ca/en/devices-endorsed-by-hypertension-canada. Accessed March 2, 2015.

8. Hypertension Canada. (2014). Hypertension Canada home page. Available online at: https://www.hypertension.ca/en. Accessed March 2, 2015.

9. Vassan R. S., Larson M. G., Leip E. P., et al. (2001). Assessment of frequency of progression to hypertension in non-hypertensive participants in the Framingham Heart Study: A cohort study. *Lancet, 358*(9294), 1682–1686.

10. Zhao Q., Kelly T. N., Li C., He J. (2013). Progress and future aspects in genetics of human hypertension. *Current Hypertension Reports, 15*(6), 676–686.

11. Burt V. L., Whelton P., Roccella E. J., et al. (1995). Prevalence of hypertension in the US adult population: Results from the third national health and nutrition examination survey, 1988–1991. *Hypertension, 25*(3), 305–313.

12. Leenen F. H., Dumais J., McInnis N. I., et al. (2008). Results of the Ontario survey on the prevalence and control of hypertension. *Canadian Medical Association Journal, 178*(11), 1441–1449.

13. Willimas S. F., Nicholas S. B., Vaziri N. D., Norris K. C. (2014). African Americans, hypertension and the renin angiotensin system. *World Journal of Cardiology, 6*(9), 878–889.

14. Rao S., Cherukuri M., Mayo H. G., Sehgal M. (2007). What is the best treatment of hypertension in African Americans? *Journal of Family Practice, 56*(2), 149–151.

15. Gadegbeku C. A., Lea J. P. Jamerson K. A. (2005). Update on disparities in the pathophysiology and management of hypertension: Focus on African Americans. *Medical Clinics of North America, 89*(5), 921–933.

16. Heart & Stroke Foundation. (2015). Statistics. Available online at: http://www.heartandstroke.com/site/c.ikIQLcMWJtE/b.3483991/k.34A8/Statistics.htm. Accessed March 2, 2016.

17. Adrogue H. J., Madias N. E. (2014). Impact of sodium and potassium on hypertension risk. *Seminars in Nephrology, 34*(3), 257–272.

18. Kotchen T. A. (2005). Contributions of sodium and chloride to NaCl-induced hypertension, *Hypertension, 45,* 849–850.

19. Garriguet D. (2010). Sodium consumption at all ages. *Health Reports, 18*(2), 47–52.

20. Sacks F. M., Svetkey L. P., Vollmer W. M., et al. (2001). Effects on blood pressure of reduced dietary sodium and the Dietary Approaches to Stop Hypertension (DASH) diet. *New England Journal of Medicine, 344*(1), 3–10.

21. Satija A., Hu F. B. (2012). Cardiovascular benefits of dietary fiber. *Current Atherosclerosis Reports, 14*(6), 505–514.

22. Adrogue H. J., Madias N. E. (2014). Sodium surfeit and potassium deficit: Keys to the pathogenesis of hypertension. *Journal of the American Society of Hypertension, 8*(3), 203–213.

23. Cunha A. R., Umbelino B., Correia M. L., et al. (2012). Magnesium and vascular changes in hypertension. *International Journal of Hypertension, 2012,* 754250. doi: 10.1155/2012/754250.

24. Hazari M. A., Arifuddin M. S., Muzzakar S., Reddy V. D. (2012). Serum calcium level in hypertension. *North American Journal of Medical Sciences, 4*(11), 569–572.

25. Kokkinos P. (2012). Physical activity, health benefits, and mortality risk. *International Scholarly Research Network Cardiology, 2012,* 718789, doi: 10.5402/2012/718789.

26. Izzard A. S. (2013). Aortic stiffening, cerebral resistance vessel function and structure, and cerebral perfusion. *Journal of Hypertension, 31*(12), 2337–2338.

27. Nguyen T., Lau D. C. (2012). The obesity epidemic and its impact on hypertension. *Canadian Journal of Cardiology, 28*(3), 326–333.

28. Kihara S., Matsuzawa Y. (2015). Fat distribution and cardiovascular disease risk. *Current Cardiovascular Risk Reports, 9,* 8, doi: 10.1007/s12170-015-0439-4.

29. Go O., Freeman R. H., Reams G. P., et al. (2014). Obesity hypertension: Pathophysiological role of leptin in neuroendocrine dysregulation. *American Journal of the Medical Sciences, 347*(6), 485–489.

30. Kubozono T., Miyata M., Ueyama K., et al. (2011). Acute and chronic effects of smoking on arterial stiffness. *Circulation Journal, 75*(3), 698–702.

31. Bowman T. S., Gaziano J. M., Buring J. E., Sesso H. D. (2007). A prospective study of cigarette smoking and risk of incident hypertension in women. *Journal of the American College of Cardiology, 50*(21), 2085–2092.

32. Briasoulis A., Agarwal V., Messerli F. H. (2012). Alcohol consumption and the risk of hypertension in men and women: A systematic review and meta-analysis. *Journal of Clinical Hypertension, 14*(11), 792–798.

33. Stankowski R. V., Kloner R. A., Rezkalla S. H. (2014). Cardiovascular consequences of cocaine use. *Trends in Cardiovascular Medicine, 25*(6), 517–526.

34. Duron E., Hanon O. (2010). Antihypertensive treatments, cognitive decline, and dementia. *Journal of Alzheimer's Disease, 20*(3), 903–914.

35. Endres M., Heuschmann P. U., Laufs U., Hakim A. M. (2011). Primary prevention of stroke: Blood pressure, lipids, and heart failure. *European Heart Journal, 32*(5), 545–555.

36. DellaCroce J. T., Vitale A. T. (2008). Hypertension and the eye. *Current Opinion in Ophthalmology, 19*(6), 493–498.

37. Staessen J. A., Wang J., Bianchi G., Birkenhäger W. H. (2003). Essential hypertension. *Lancet, 361*(9369), 1629–1641.

38. Mahabala C., Kamath P., Bhaskaran U., et al. (2013). Antihypertensive therapy: Nocturnal dippers and nondippers. Do we treat them differently? *Vascular Health and Risk Management, 9,* 125–133.

39. Arima H., Murakami Y., Lam T. H., et al.; Asia Pacific Cohort Studies Collaboration. (2012). Effects of prehypertension and hypertension subtype on cardiovascular disease in the Asia-Pacific region. *Hypertension, 59*(6), 1118–1123.

40. Griffith T. F., Klassen P. S., Franklin S. S. (2005). Systolic hypertension: An overview. *American Heart Journal, 149*(5), 769–775.

41. Sukor N. (2011). Secondary hypertension: A condition not to be missed. *Postgraduate Medical Journal, 87*(1032), 706–713.

42. Plouin P., Bax L. (2010). Diagnosis and treatment of renal artery stenosis. *Nature Reviews Nephrology, 6*(3), 151–159.

43. Chao C., Wu V., Kuo C., et al. (2013). Diagnosis and management of primary aldosteronism: An updated review. *Annals of Medicine, 45*(4), 375–383.

44. Grossman E., Messerli F. H. (2012). Drug-induced hypertension: An unappreciated cause of secondary hypertension. *American Journal of Medicine, 125*(1), 14–22.

45. August P. (2013). Hypertension in women. *Advances in Chronic Kidney Disease, 20*(5), 396–401.

46. Marik P. E., Rivera R. (2011). Hypertensive emergencies: An update. *Current Opinion in Critical Care, 17*(6), 569–580.

47. Magee L. A., Pels A., Helewa M., et al.; Canadian Hypertensive Disorders of Pregnancy Working Group. (2014). Diagnosis, evaluation, and management of the hypertensive disorders of pregnancy: Executive summary. *Journal of Obstetrics and Gynaecology Canada, 36*(5), 416–438.

48. Mustafa R., Ahmed S., Gupta A., et al. (2012). A comprehensive review of hypertension in pregnancy. *Journal of Pregnancy, 2012,* 105918. doi: 10.1155/2012/105918.

49. Assadi F. (2012). The growing epidemic of hypertension among children and adolescents: A challenging road ahead. *Pediatric Cardiology, 33*(7), 1013–1020.

50. National High Blood Pressure Education Program Working Group on Children and Adolescents. (2005). The fourth report on the diagnosis,

evaluation, and treatment of high blood pressure in children and adolescents. National Institutes of Health Publication No. 05–5267.

51. Centers for Disease Control and Prevention. (2010). Clinical growth charts. Available online at: http://www.cdc.gov/growthcharts/clinical_charts.htm. Accessed March 2, 2015.

52. Lande M. B. (2011). Chapter 439: Systemic hypertension. In Kliegman R. M., Stanton B. F., St. Geme J.W., et al. (Eds.), *Nelson textbook of pediatrics* (19th ed.). Philadelphia, PA: Saunders Elsevier.

53. Robitaille C., Dai S., Waters C., et al. (2012). Diagnosed hypertension in Canada: Incidence, prevalence and associated mortality. *Canadian Medical Association Journal, 184*(1), E49–E56.

54. Maddens M., Imam K., Ashkar A. (2005). Hypertension in the elderly. *Primary Care Clinics in Office Practice, 32*(3), 723–753.

55. Lanier J. B., Mote M. B., Clay E. C. (2011). Evaluation and management of orthostatic hypotension. *American Family Physician, 84*(5), 527–536.

56. Shibao C., Lipsitz L. A., Biaggioni I. (2013). ASH position paper: Evaluation and treatment of orthostatic hypotension. *Journal of Clinical Hypertension, 15*(3), 147–153.

57. Mukai S., Lipsitz L. A. (2002). Orthostatic hypotension. *Clinics in Geriatric Medicine, 18*(2), 253–268.

58. Trahair L. G., Horowitz M., Jones K. J. (2014). Postprandial hypotension: A systematic review. *Journal of American Medical Directors Association, 15*(6), 394–409.

59. Fanciulli A., Wenning G. K. (2015). Multiple-system atrophy. *New England Journal of Medicine, 372*(3), 249–263.

Visit the Point **http://thePoint.lww.com for animations, journal articles, and more!**

Disorders of Cardiac Function

Cardiovascular disease (CVD) is the second leading cause of death in men and women in Canada. It is estimated that the direct and indirect costs of CVD in Canada alone is approximately $20.9 billion per year.[1] To reduce this increase in morbidity, mortality, and cost, strategies such as population-based public health measures, preventative programs for high-risk subgroups, and the allocation of resources for treatments for CVD can be useful.[2]

In an attempt to focus on common heart problems that affect persons in all age groups, this chapter is organized into six sections: disorders of the pericardium, coronary artery disease, cardiomyopathies, infectious and immunologic disorders of the heart, valvular heart disease, and heart disease in infants and children.

DISORDERS OF THE PERICARDIUM

After completing this section of the chapter, you should be able to meet the following objectives:

- Characterize the function of the pericardium.
- Compare the clinical manifestations of acute pericarditis and chronic pericarditis.
- Describe the physiologic impact of pleural effusion on cardiac function and relate it to the life-threatening nature of cardiac tamponade.
- Relate the pathophysiology of constrictive pericarditis to its clinical manifestations.

DISORDERS OF THE PERICARDIUM

- The pericardium isolates the heart from other thoracic structures, maintains its position in the thorax, and prevents it from overfilling.
- The two layers of the pericardium are separated by a thin layer of serous fluid, which prevents frictional forces from developing between the visceral and parietal layers of the pericardium.
- Disorders that produce inflammation of the pericardium interfere with the friction-reducing properties of the pericardial fluid and produce pain.
- Disorders that increase the fluid volume of the pericardial sac interfere with cardiac filling and produce a subsequent reduction in cardiac output.

The pericardium, sometimes referred to as the *pericardial sac,* is a double-layered serous membrane that isolates the heart from other thoracic structures, maintains its position in the thorax, prevents it from overfilling, and serves as a barrier to infection. The pericardium consists of two layers: a thin inner layer, called the *visceral pericardium,* that adheres to the epicardium; and an outer fibrous layer, called the *parietal pericardium,* that is attached to the great vessels that enter and leave the heart, the sternum, and diaphragm (see Chapter 21, Figs. 21.3 & 21.4). These two layers of the pericardium are separated by a potential space, the *pericardial cavity,* that contains about 50 ml of serous fluid. This fluid acts as a lubricant that prevents frictional forces from developing as the heart contracts and relaxes. Although there is little blood supply to the pericardium, it is well innervated and inflammation can cause severe pain.[2]

The pericardium is subject to many of the same pathologic processes (*e.g.,* congenital disorders, infections, trauma, immune mechanisms, and neoplastic disease) that affect other structures of the body. Pericardial disorders frequently are associated with or result from another disease in the heart or the surrounding structures (Chart 24.1).

Acute Pericarditis

Pericarditis represents an inflammatory process of the pericardium. *Acute pericarditis,* defined as signs and symptoms resulting from a pericardial inflammation of less than 2 weeks, may occur as an isolated disease or as the result of systemic disease. Viral infections (especially infections with coxsackieviruses and echoviruses) are the most common cause of pericarditis and probably are responsible for many cases classified as idiopathic. Other causes of acute pericarditis include bacterial or mycobacterial infections, connective tissue diseases (*e.g.,* systemic lupus erythematosus, rheumatoid arthritis), uremia, postcardiac surgery, neoplastic invasion of the pericardium, radiation, trauma, drug toxicity, and contiguous inflammatory processes of the myocardium or lung.[2,3]

CHART 24.1 CLASSIFICATION OF DISORDERS OF THE PERICARDIUM

Inflammation
1. Acute inflammatory pericarditis
   a. Infectious
      - Viral (echovirus, coxsackievirus, and others)
      - Bacterial (*e.g.,* tuberculosis, *Staphylococcus, Streptococcus*)
      - Fungal
   b. Immune and collagen disorders
      Rheumatic fever
      Rheumatoid arthritis
      Systemic lupus erythematosus
   c. Metabolic disorders
      Uremia and dialysis
      Myxedema
   d. Ischemia and tissue injury
      Myocardial infarction
      Cardiac surgery
      Chest trauma
   e. Physical and chemical agents
      Radiation therapy
      Untoward reactions to drugs, such as hydralazine, procainamide, and anticoagulants
2. Chronic inflammatory pericarditis
   a. Can be associated with most of the agents causing an acute inflammatory response

Neoplastic Disease
1. Primary
2. Secondary (*e.g.,* carcinoma of the lung or breast, lymphoma)

Congenital Disorders
1. Complete or partial absence of the pericardium
2. Congenital pericardial cysts

Like other inflammatory conditions, acute pericarditis often is associated with increased capillary permeability. The capillaries that supply the serous pericardium become permeable, allowing plasma proteins, including fibrinogen, to leave the capillaries and enter the pericardial space. This results in an exudate that varies in type and amount according to the causative agent. Acute pericarditis frequently is associated with a fibrinous (fibrin-containing) exudate (Fig. 24.1), which heals by resolution or progresses to deposition of scar tissue and formation of adhesions between the layers of the serous pericardium. Inflammation also may involve the superficial myocardium and the adjacent pleura.

The manifestations of acute pericarditis include a triad of chest pain, pericardial friction rub, and electrocardiographic (ECG) changes. The clinical findings may vary according to the causative agent. Most persons with acute pericarditis have chest pain. The pain usually is abrupt in onset and

FIGURE 24.1 • Fibrinous pericarditis. The heart of a patient who died in uremia displays a shaggy, fibrinous exudate covering the visceral pericardium. (From Rubin R., Strayer D. S. (Eds.). (2012). *Rubin's pathology: Clinicopathologic foundations of medicine* (6th ed., p. 534). Philadelphia, PA: Lippincott Williams & Wilkins.)

sharp, occurring in the precordial area, and may radiate to the neck, back, abdomen, or side. Pain in the scapular ridge may be due to irritation of the phrenic nerve. The pain typically is worse with deep breathing, coughing, swallowing, and positional changes because of changes in venous return and cardiac filling. Many persons seek relief by sitting up and leaning forward. It is important that chest pain from pericarditis be differentiated from acute coronary syndrome (ACS) or pulmonary embolism.

Diagnosis of acute pericarditis is based on clinical manifestations, ECG, chest radiography, and echocardiography. A pericardial friction rub, often described as high-pitched or scratchy, results from the rubbing and friction between the inflamed pericardial surfaces. The friction rub is typically described as having three components, which correspond to atrial systole, ventricular systole, and rapid filling of the ventricle. Because it results from the rubbing together of the inflamed pericardial surfaces, large effusions are unlikely to produce a friction rub. Except in uremic pericarditis, the ECG changes in pericarditis typically evolve through four progressive stages: diffuse ST-segment elevations and PR-segment depression; normalization of the ST and PR segments; widespread T-wave inversions; and normalization of T waves. Laboratory markers of systemic inflammation may also be present, including an elevated white blood cell count, elevated erythrocyte sedimentation rate (ESR), and increased C-reactive protein (CRP). An elevated CRP is present in about

75% of cases and can be used to monitor disease activity and length of treatment needed.[3]

Acute idiopathic pericarditis is frequently self-limiting. Most cases are presumed to be viral, but testing for specific viruses is not routine. Symptoms are usually successfully treated with nonsteroidal anti-inflammatory drugs (NSAIDs).[2,3] Colchicine has also been shown to be of benefit, in combination with aspirin and prednisone, in management of acute pericarditis and for prevention of recurrences. Colchicine produces its anti-inflammatory effects by preventing the polymerization of microtubules, which leads to the inhibition of leukocyte migration and phagocytosis. When infection is present, antibiotics specific for the causative agent usually are prescribed. Corticosteroids may be used for treatment of persons with connective tissue disease or severely symptomatic pericarditis that is not responsive to NSAIDs and colchicine. Corticosteroids should be avoided if possible, as this medication can increase the risk of recurrence. However, if they cannot be avoided, only a short course should be initiated.[3]

Recurrent episodes of pericarditis can occur in up to 30% of persons with acute pericarditis.[2,3] A minority of these develop recurrent bouts of pericardial pain, which can sometimes be chronic and debilitating. The process commonly is associated with autoimmune disorders, such as systemic lupus erythematosus, rheumatoid arthritis, scleroderma, and myxedema but may also occur following viral pericarditis. Treatment includes the use of anti-inflammatory medications such as NSAIDs, corticosteroids, or colchicine. If the reoccurrence continues, prophylaxis over months may be warranted.

Pericardial Effusion and Cardiac Tamponade

Pericardial effusion refers to the accumulation of fluid in the pericardial cavity, usually as a result of an inflammatory or infectious process. It may also develop as the result of neoplasms, cardiac surgery, trauma, cardiac rupture due to myocardial infarction (MI), and dissecting aortic aneurysm. The pericardial cavity has little reserve volume. The pressure-volume relationship between the normal pericardial and cardiac volumes can be dramatically affected by only small amounts of fluid once critical levels of effusion are present. Because right ventricular filling pressures are lower than that of the left, increases in pressure are usually reflected in signs and symptoms of right-sided heart failure before equalization is achieved.

The amount of fluid, the rapidity with which it accumulates, and the elasticity of the pericardium determine the effect the effusion has on cardiac function. Small pericardial effusions may produce no symptoms or abnormal clinical findings. Even a large effusion that develops slowly may cause few or no symptoms, provided the pericardium is able to stretch and avoid compressing the heart. However, a sudden accumulation of even 200 ml may raise intracardiac pressure to levels that seriously limit the venous return to the heart. Symptoms of cardiac compression also may occur with relatively small accumulations of fluid if the pericardium has become thickened by scar tissue or neoplastic infiltrations.

Pericardial effusion can lead to a condition called *cardiac tamponade,* in which there is compression of the heart due to the accumulation of fluid, pus, or blood in the pericardial sac. This life-threatening condition can be caused by infections, neoplasms, and bleeding.[2,3] Cardiac tamponade results in increased intracardiac pressure, progressive limitation of ventricular diastolic filling, and reductions in stroke volume and cardiac output. The severity of the condition depends on the amount of fluid present and the rate at which it accumulates.

A significant accumulation of fluid in the pericardium results in increased adrenergic stimulation, which leads to tachycardia and increased cardiac contractility. There is elevation of central venous pressure, jugular vein distension, a fall in systolic blood pressure, narrowed pulse pressure, and signs of circulatory shock. The heart sounds may become muffled and difficult to hear because of the insulating effects of the pericardial fluid and reduced cardiac function. Persons with slowly developing cardiac tamponade usually appear acutely ill, but not to the extreme seen in those with rapidly developing tamponade.

A key diagnostic finding is *pulsus paradoxus,* or an exaggeration of the normal variation in the systemic arterial pulse volume with respiration.[2] Normally, the decrease in intrathoracic pressure that occurs during inspiration accelerates venous flow, increasing right atrial and right ventricular filling. This causes the interventricular septum to bulge to the left, producing a slight decrease in left ventricular filling, stroke volume output, and systolic blood pressure. In cardiac tamponade, the left ventricle is compressed from within by movement of the interventricular septum and from without by fluid in the pericardium (Fig. 24.2). This produces a marked decrease in left ventricular filling and left ventricular stroke volume output, often within a beat of the beginning of inspiration. Pulsus paradoxus can be determined by palpation, cuff sphygmomanometry, or arterial pressure monitoring. With pulsus paradoxus, the arterial pulse, as palpated at the carotid or femoral artery, becomes weakened or absent during inspiration and stronger during expiration. Palpation provides only a gross estimate of the degree of pulsus paradoxus. It is more sensitively estimated when the blood pressure cuff is used to compare the Korotkoff sounds during inspiration and expiration—a decline in systolic pressure greater than 10 mm Hg during inspiration is suggestive of tamponade. Arterial pressure monitoring allows visualization of the arterial pressure waveform and measurement of the decrease in blood pressure during inspiration.

The echocardiogram is a rapid, accurate, and widely used method of evaluating pericardial effusion. The ECG often reveals nonspecific T-wave changes and low QRS voltage. Usually only moderate to large effusions can be detected by chest radiography.

Treatment of pericardial effusions depends on the progression to cardiac tamponade. In small pericardial effusions or mild cardiac tamponade, NSAIDs, colchicine, or corticosteroids may minimize fluid accumulation. Pericardiocentesis,

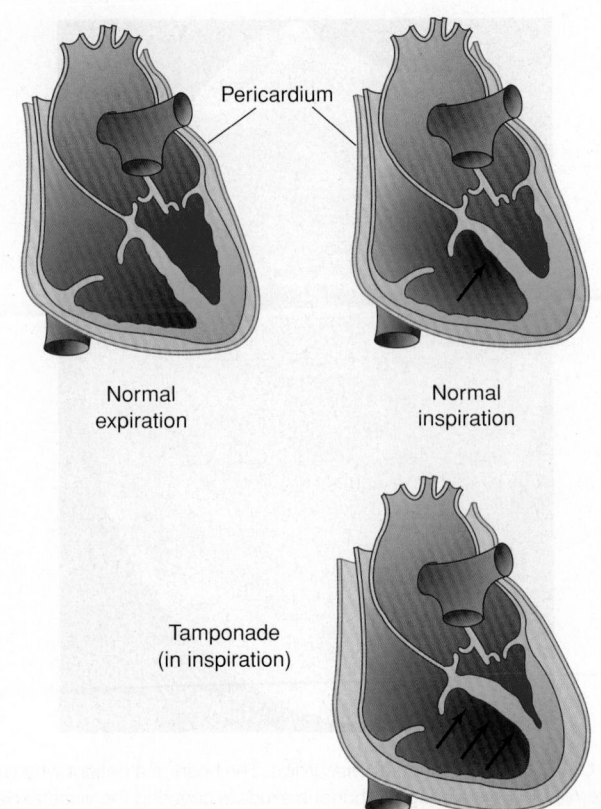

FIGURE 24.2 • Effects of respiration and cardiac tamponade on ventricular filling and cardiac output. During inspiration, venous flow into the right heart increases, causing the interventricular septum to bulge into the left ventricle. This produces a decrease in left ventricular volume, with a subsequent decrease in stroke volume output. In cardiac tamponade, the fluid in the pericardial sac produces further compression of the left ventricle, causing an exaggeration of the normal inspiratory decrease in stroke volume and systolic blood pressure.

or removal of fluid from the pericardial sac, often with the aid of echocardiography, is the initial treatment of choice. Closed pericardiocentesis, which is performed with a needle inserted through the chest wall, may be an emergency lifesaving measure in severe cardiac tamponade. Open pericardiocentesis may be used for recurrent or loculated effusions (*i.e.,* those confined to one or more pockets in the pleural space), during which biopsies can be obtained and pericardial windows created. Aspiration and laboratory evaluation of the pericardial fluid may be used to identify the causative agent.

Constrictive Pericarditis

In constrictive pericarditis, fibrous, calcified scar tissue develops between the visceral and parietal layers of the serous pericardium. In time, the scar tissue contracts and interferes with diastolic filling of the heart, at which point cardiac output and cardiac reserve become fixed. The equalization of end-diastolic pressures in all four cardiac chambers is the pathophysiologic hallmark of constrictive pericarditis.[2]

Long-standing inflammation from mediastinal radiation, cardiac surgery, or infection is usually the cause of constrictive pericarditis. Ascites is a prominent early finding and may be accompanied by pedal edema, dyspnea on exertion, and fatigue. The jugular veins also are distended. The Kussmaul sign is an inspiratory distension of the jugular veins caused by the inability of the right atrium, encased in its rigid pericardium, to accommodate the increase in venous return that occurs with inspiration. Exercise intolerance, muscle wasting, and weight loss develop in end-stage constrictive pericarditis.

Chest radiography and Doppler and transesophageal echocardiography are helpful in the diagnosis of constrictive pericarditis. The Doppler echocardiogram is especially useful in the differentiation of constrictive pericarditis from restrictive cardiomyopathy, as are computed tomography (CT) and magnetic resonance imaging (MRI). In chronic constrictive pericarditis, surgical removal or resection of the pericardium (*i.e.,* pericardiectomy) is often the treatment of choice.

Effusive–constrictive pericarditis, a combination of effusion-tamponade and constriction, is a syndrome that develops in a significant number of persons with pericardial disease. Because it occurs most often during a subacute or chronic course of pericardial disease, it is most likely due to a transition from acute pericarditis with pericardial effusion to constrictive pericarditis. It usually is detected when hemodynamic measurements fail to stabilize after pericardiocentesis. Persons with the disorder usually require pericardiectomy.[2]

IN SUMMARY

The pericardium is a two-layered membranous sac that isolates the heart from other thoracic structures, maintains its position in the thorax, and prevents it from overfilling; it also may help prevent infection. Disorders of the pericardium include acute and chronic pericarditis, pericardial effusion and cardiac tamponade, and constrictive and effusive–constrictive pericarditis. The major threat of pericardial disease is compression of the heart chambers.

Acute pericarditis may be infectious in origin or it may be due to systemic diseases. It is characterized by chest pain, ECG changes, and pericardial friction rub. Recurrent pericarditis is usually associated with autoimmune disorders, and symptoms may be minimal. Pericardial effusion, either acute or chronic, refers to the presence of an exudate in the pericardial cavity. It can increase intracardiac pressure, compress the heart, and interfere with venous return to the heart. The amount of exudate, the rapidity with which it accumulates, and the elasticity of the pericardium determine the effect the effusion has on cardiac function. Cardiac tamponade represents a life-threatening compression of the heart resulting from excess fluid in the pericardial sac. In constrictive pericarditis, scar tissue develops between the visceral and parietal layers of the serous pericardium. In time, the scar tissue contracts and interferes with cardiac filling.

CORONARY ARTERY DISEASE

After completing this section of the chapter, you should be able to meet the following objectives:

- Describe blood flow in the coronary circulation and relate it to the determinants of myocardial oxygen supply and demand.
- Define the term *acute coronary syndrome* and distinguish among chronic stable angina, unstable angina, non–ST-segment elevation myocardial infarction, and ST-segment elevation myocardial infarction in terms of pathology, symptomatology, ECG changes, and serum cardiac markers.
- Compare the treatment goals for stable angina and the acute coronary syndromes.

The term *coronary artery disease* (CAD) describes heart disease caused by impaired coronary blood flow. In most cases, CAD is caused by atherosclerosis, which affects not only the coronary arteries but arteries in other areas of the body. CAD is the second highest cause of mortality after cancer for both men and women in Canada as well as in other industrialized countries. In 2009, CVD accounted for approximately 21% of all deaths in Canada.[4] Approximately 70,000 MIs occur every year, 16,000 of which result in death.[5] It is estimated that over 35,800 deaths are related to ischemic heart disease per year.[4] Most of the deaths that occur with acute MI happen before hospital admission. In spite of these high numbers, mortality rates have been decreasing for the last decade, and this is attributed to the prevention efforts such as reduction in smoking and cholesterol as well as improvements in the acute care treatment. The Canadian Institute for Health Information (CIHI), reported in 2014 an improvement in the 30-day survival of individuals who had an acute MI compared to 31 other countries. The in-hospital death rate for Canada is 5.7 out of 100 patients admitted, compared to the average of 7.9 per 100 for the other countries.[5]

Major risk factors for CAD include diabetes, cigarette smoking, hypertension, elevated serum total and low-density lipoprotein (LDL) cholesterol, low serum high-density lipoprotein (HDL) cholesterol, advancing age, abdominal obesity, and decreased physical activity. Individuals with diabetes and metabolic syndrome (discussed in Chapter 42) are at particularly increased risk for development of CVD.[2] Risk factors for atherosclerosis and risk factor assessment are discussed in Chapter 22.

Coronary Circulation

The Coronary Arteries

The two main coronary arteries, the left and the right, arise from the coronary sinus just above the aortic valve[2,6,7] (Fig. 24.3). The left coronary artery extends for approximately

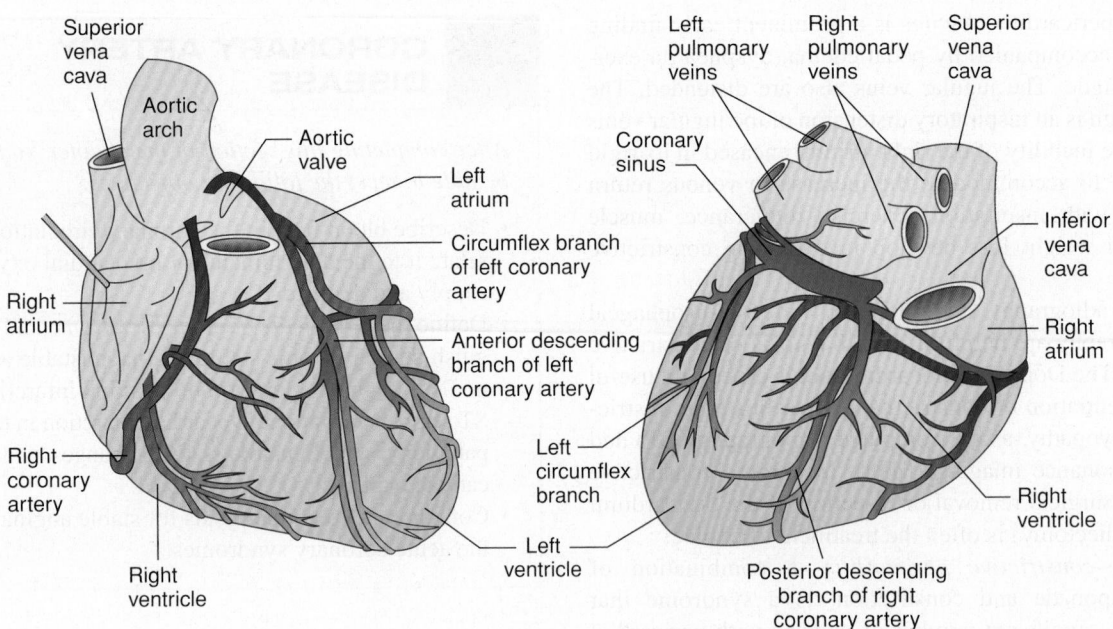

FIGURE 24.3 • Coronary arteries and some of the coronary sinus veins.

5 to 25 mm as the *left main coronary artery* and then divides into the left anterior descending and circumflex branches. The *left anterior descending artery* passes down through the groove between the two ventricles, giving off diagonal branches, which supply the anterior wall of the left ventricle, and perforating branches, which supply the anterior portion of the interventricular septum and the anterior papillary muscle of the left ventricle. The *circumflex branch* of the left coronary artery passes to the left and moves posteriorly in the groove that separates the left atrium and ventricle, giving off branches that supply the left lateral wall of the left ventricle.

The *right coronary artery* lies in the right atrioventricular (AV) groove, and its branches supply the right ventricle. The right coronary artery usually moves to the back of the heart, where it forms the *posterior descending artery,* which normally supplies the posterior portion of the heart, interventricular septum, sinoatrial (SA) and AV nodes, and posterior papillary muscle. By convention, the coronary artery that supplies the posterior third of the septum (either the right coronary artery or the left circumflex) is called *dominant.* In a right-dominant circulation, present in approximately four fifths of people, the left circumflex perfuses the lateral wall of the left ventricle, and the right coronary artery supplies the entire right ventricular free wall and the posterior third of the septum.[7] Thus, occlusion of the right as well as the left coronary artery can cause left ventricular damage.

The large epicardial coronary arteries lie on the surface of the heart, with smaller intramyocardial arteries branching and penetrating the myocardium before merging with a network or plexus of subendocardial vessels. Although there are no connections between the large coronary arteries, there are anastomotic channels that join the small arteries. With gradual occlusion of the larger vessels, the smaller collateral vessels increase in size and provide alternative channels for blood flow. One of the reasons CAD does not produce symptoms until it is far advanced is that the collateral channels develop at the same time the atherosclerotic changes are occurring.

Blood flow in the coronary arteries is controlled largely by physical, neural, and metabolic factors. The openings for the coronary arteries originate in the root of the aorta just outside the aortic valve. Thus, the main factor responsible for perfusion of the coronary arteries is the aortic blood pressure, which is generated by the heart itself. Myocardial blood flow, in turn, is largely regulated by the metabolic activity of the myocardium and autoregulatory mechanisms that control vessel dilation. In addition to generating the aortic pressure that moves blood through the coronary vessels, the contracting heart muscle influences its own blood supply by compressing the intramyocardial and subendocardial blood vessels during systole. The autonomic nervous system exerts its effects on coronary blood flow through changes in heart rate, cardiac contractility, and blood pressure.

Coronary blood flow is largely regulated by the need of the cardiac muscle for oxygen. Even under normal resting conditions, the heart extracts and uses 60% to 80% of oxygen in blood flowing through the coronary arteries, compared with the 25% to 30% extracted by skeletal muscle. Because there is little oxygen reserve in the blood, the coronary arteries must increase their flow to meet the metabolic needs of the myocardium during periods of increased activity. The normal resting blood flow through the coronary arteries averages approximately 225 ml/minute, or about 4% to 5% of the total cardiac output.[6] During strenuous exercise, coronary flow may increase three- to fourfold to meet the energy requirements of the heart.

One of the major determinants of coronary blood flow is the metabolic activity of the heart. Numerous agents, referred to as *metabolites,* are thought to act as mediators for the vasodilation that accompanies increased cardiac work. These substances, which include potassium ions, lactic acid, carbon dioxide, and adenosine, are released from working myocardial cells. Together these substances, promote the vasodilator effect, and adenosine is perhaps a key critical mediator of local blood flow.[6]

The endothelial cells line the blood vessels, including the coronary arteries. They form a selective barrier between the blood and the vascular wall, and regulate the flow of nutrient substances, molecules, and blood cells between the intravascular and the vascular tissue. They also synthesize several substances that, when released, can affect relaxation or constriction of the smooth muscle in the arterial wall. Potent vasodilators produced by the endothelium include nitric oxide, prostacyclin, and endothelium-derived hyperpolarizing factor (EDHF). The most important of these is nitric oxide (see Chapter 21). Most vasodilators and vasodilating stimuli exert their effects through nitric oxide. Products from aggregating platelets, thrombin, the products of mast cells, and increased shear force, which is responsible for the so-called flow-mediated vasodilation, stimulate the synthesis and release of nitric oxide.[2] The endothelium also is the source of vasoconstricting factors, the best known of which are the endothelins.

Myocardial Oxygen Supply and Demand

The coronary circulation supplies the heart muscle with the oxygen and nutrients it needs to pump blood out to the rest of the body. As the metabolic needs of the body change, cardiac function and coronary blood flow must adapt to meet these needs. If there is an imbalance in the myocardial oxygen supply and demand, myocardial ischemia, MI, or sudden death may occur. Angina is chest pain or discomfort associated with transient myocardial ischemia and MI is associated with prolonged ischemia and cell death.

Myocardial Oxygen Supply. Myocardial oxygen supply is determined by the coronary arteries and capillary inflow, and the ability of hemoglobin to transport and deliver oxygen to the heart muscle. Important factors in the transport and delivery of oxygen include the fraction of inspired oxygen in the blood and the number of red blood cells with normally functioning hemoglobin. Even with adequate coronary blood flow, myocardial hypoxia can occur in situations of hypoxemia, anemia, or carbon monoxide poisoning.[2]

Myocardial Oxygen Demand. There are three major determinants of myocardial oxygen demand (MVO_2): the heart rate, myocardial contractility, and myocardial wall stress or tension[2] (Fig. 24.4). The heart rate is the most important factor in myocardial oxygen demand, for two reasons: (1) as the heart rate increases, myocardial oxygen demand and consumption also increases; and (2) as noted previously, subendocardial coronary blood flow is reduced because of the decreased diastolic filling time with increased heart rates.[2,6]

Myocardial contractility is the intrinsic ability of the heart muscle to shorten and generate force. It reflects the interaction

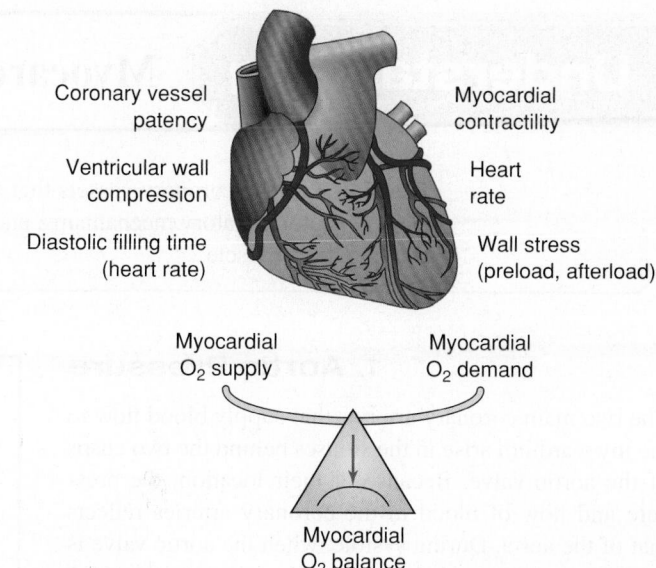

Coronary vessel patency

Ventricular wall compression

Diastolic filling time (heart rate)

Myocardial contractility

Heart rate

Wall stress (preload, afterload)

Myocardial O_2 supply

Myocardial O_2 demand

Myocardial O_2 balance

FIGURE 24.4 • Myocardial oxygen (O_2) balance is determined by factors that affect myocardial O_2 supply and myocardial O_2 demand.

between calcium ions and the contractile proteins (actin and myosin) of the muscle fibres[2] (see Chapter 4). It is normally determined by the rate of pressure development and muscle shortening. With increased myocardial contractility, the rate of change in wall stress is increased, which in turn increases myocardial oxygen uptake. Factors that increase contractility, such as exercise, sympathetic nervous system stimulation, and inotropic agents, all increase demand and MVO_2.[2]

Wall stress develops when tension is applied to a given area. Left ventricular wall stress can be thought of as the average tension that individual muscle fibres must generate to shorten against a developed intraventricular pressure. It is proportional to the product of the intraventricular pressure and ventricle radius, divided by the thickness of the ventricle wall. Thus, at a given pressure, wall stress is increased by an increase in radius (ventricular dilation) and it is increased by a decrease in wall thickness. The term *preload* is used to describe the distending force of the ventricular wall, which is highest at the end of diastole, just before contraction.[2,8] Changes in preload are assessed by using the left ventricular end-diastolic pressure. This can be measured indirectly by using the pulmonary artery occlusive (or wedge) pressure, obtained through a pulmonary artery catheter. *Afterload* is the "load" against which the heart must contract to eject blood. A major component of the left ventricular afterload is the aortic pressure, or pressure that the ventricle must generate to eject blood.[2,8] An increase in wall stress, whether caused by an increase in preload or afterload, increases MVO_2 because as cardiac muscle fibres develop more tension, they require a greater rate of adenosine triphosphate (ATP) use. Because wall stress is inversely related to wall thickness, ventricular hypertrophy serves as an adaptive mechanism by which the ventricle is able to offset the increase in wall stress that accompanies increased aortic pressure or aortic valve stenosis.

Understanding Myocardial Blood Flow

Blood flow in the coronary vessels that supply the myocardium is influenced by (1) the aortic pressure, (2) autoregulatory mechanisms, and (3) compression of the intramyocardial vessels by the contracting heart muscle.

1. Aortic Pressure

The two main coronary arteries that supply blood flow to the myocardium arise in the sinuses behind the two cusps of the aortic valve. Because of their location, the pressure and flow of blood in the coronary arteries reflects that of the aorta. During systole, when the aortic valve is open, the velocity of blood flow and position of the valve cusps cause the blood to move rapidly past the coronary artery inlets, and during diastole, when the aortic valve is closed, blood flow and the aortic pressure are transmitted directly into the coronary arteries.

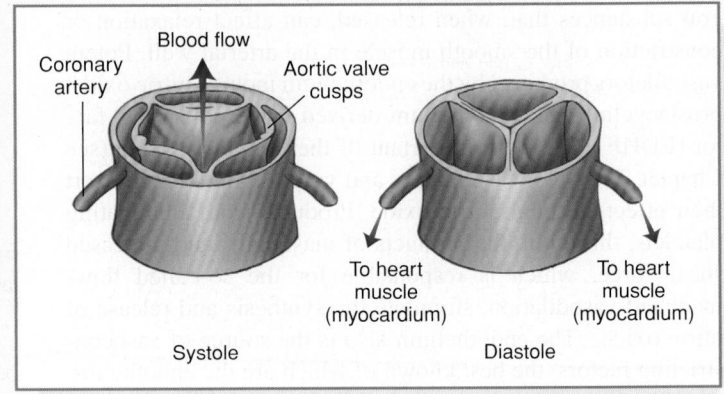

2. Autoregulatory Mechanisms

The heart normally extracts 60% to 80% of the oxygen in the blood delivered to it, leaving little in reserve. Accordingly, oxygen delivery during periods of increased metabolic demand depends on autoregulatory mechanisms that regulate blood flow through a change in vessel tone and diameter. During increased metabolic demand, vasodilation produces an increase in blood flow; during decreased demand, vasoconstriction or return of vessel tone to normal produces a reduction in flow. The mechanisms that link the metabolic activity of the heart to changes in vessel tone result from vasoactive mediators released from myocardial cells and the vascular endothelium.

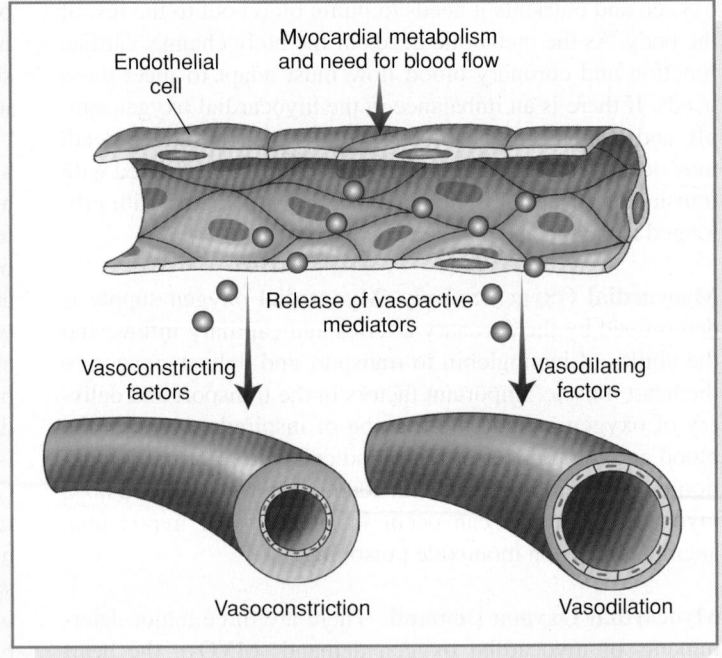

3. Vessel Compression

The large coronary arteries lie on the epicardial surface of the heart, with smaller intramyocardial vessels branching off and moving through the myocardium before merging with a plexus of vessels that supply the subendocardial muscle with blood. During systole, the contracting cardiac muscle has a squeezing effect on the intramyocardial vessels, while at the same time producing an increase in intraventricular pressure that pushes against and compresses the subendocardial vessels. As a result, blood flow to the subendocardial muscle is greatest during diastole. Because the time spent in diastole becomes shortened as the heart rate increases, myocardial blood flow can be greatly reduced during sustained periods of tachycardia.

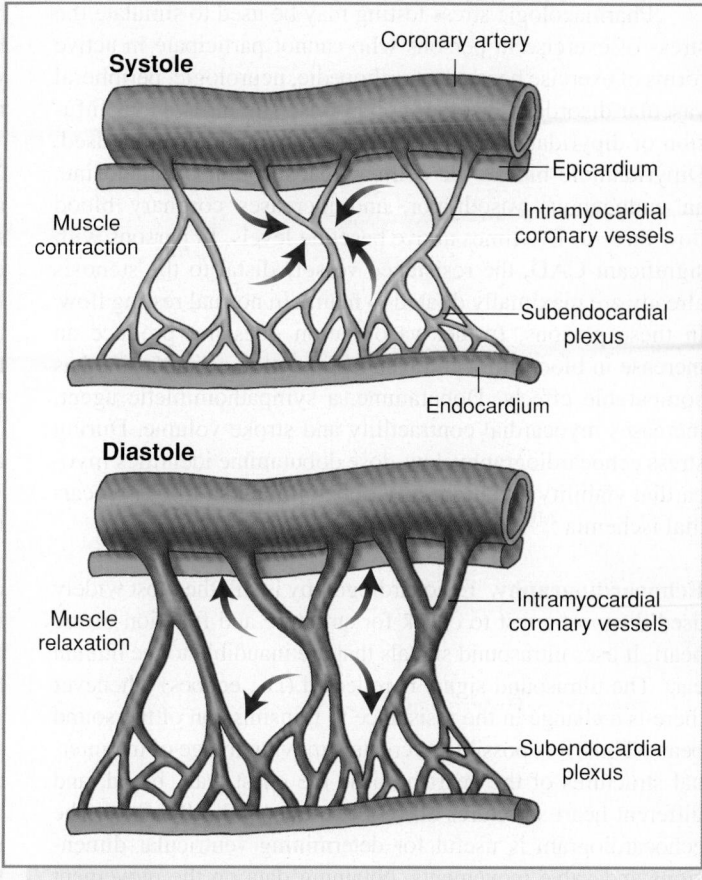

Assessment of Coronary Blood Flow and Myocardial Perfusion

Among the methods used in the evaluation of coronary blood flow and myocardial perfusion are ECG, exercise stress testing, echocardiography, and Doppler ultrasonographic imaging; cardiac MRI and CT; and cardiac catheterization and angiography. These assessment modalities vary widely and are undergoing constant technologic advances.

Electrocardiography. The 12-lead ECG is the most frequently used cardiovascular diagnostic procedure. It is indispensable not only for the diagnosis and treatment of CAD, but also for the identification of ventricular conduction defects, arrhythmias, electrolyte imbalances, drug effects, and genetically mediated electrical or structural abnormalities. The standard 12-lead ECG uses electrodes to record electrical potential differences, generated by ion currents (action potentials) during the cardiac cycle, between prescribed sites on the body (see Chapter 25). Electrode placement and patient position are important because they can change the recorded amplitudes and axes of the ECG.

Ambulatory ECG monitoring often is done to detect transient ST-segment and T-wave changes that occur and are not accompanied by symptoms (*i.e.,* silent ischemia). Continuous ambulatory ECG monitoring can be done using a Holter monitor

(see Chapter 25). Another method, called *signal-averaged* or *high-resolution ECG,* accentuates the QRS complex so that low-amplitude afterpotentials that correlate with high risk of ventricular arrhythmias and sudden death can be detected.

Exercise Stress Testing. Exercise stress testing is a means of observing cardiac function under stress and is typically performed in adults with symptoms of known or suspected ischemic heart disease. It is also used to check for physiologic response post MI or revascularization, functional capacity for an exercise program and/or employment capacity, efficacy of medication or surgical treatments, the severity of arrhythmias, preoperatively to assess functional status, and to evaluate intermitted claudication.[9,10]

Treadmill exercise, which is the most commonly used method of cardiovascular stress testing, requires higher levels of myocardial performance than other forms of exercise. The goal is to achieve a maximum level of exertion for the individual's age if possible. While trying to do this, blood pressure is monitored, and the ECG pattern is recorded for the purposes of determining heart rate and detecting myocardial ischemic changes. Chest pain, severe shortness of breath, arrhythmias, ST-segment changes on the ECG, or a decrease in blood pressure suggest CAD, and if one or more of these signs or symptoms is present, the test is usually terminated.

Pharmacologic stress testing may be used to simulate the stress of exercise in persons who cannot participate in active forms of exercise because of orthopedic, neurologic, peripheral vascular disorders, or other conditions. The intravenous infusion of dipyridamole, adenosine, or dobutamine can be used. Dipyridamole blocks the cellular reabsorption of adenosine, an endogenous vasodilator, and increases coronary blood flow three to five times above baseline levels. In persons with significant CAD, the resistance vessels distal to the stenosis already are maximally dilated to maintain normal resting flow. In these persons, further vasodilation does not produce an increase in blood flow. Intravenous injection of adenosine has comparable effects. Dobutamine, a sympathomimetic agent, increases myocardial contractility and stroke volume. During stress echocardiography, low-dose dobutamine identifies myocardial viability and high-dose dobutamine identifies myocardial ischemia.[2,10]

Echocardiography. Echocardiography is still the most widely used diagnostic test to check for structure and function of the heart. It uses ultrasound signals that are inaudible to the human ear.[2] The ultrasound signal is reflected (*i.e.,* echoes) whenever there is a change in the resistance to transmission of the sound beam. Thus, it is possible to create a moving image of the internal structures of the heart because the chest wall, blood, and different heart structures all reflect ultrasound differently. The echocardiogram is useful for determining ventricular dimensions and valve movements, obtaining data on the movement of the left ventricular wall and septum, estimating diastolic and systolic volumes, and viewing the motion of individual segments of the left ventricular wall during systole and diastole.

There are several different forms of echocardiography, including M-mode, two-dimensional (2D) imaging, Doppler, contrast echocardiography, and three-dimensional. M-mode echocardiography, which was the earliest form of cardiac ultrasonography, uses a stationary ultrasound beam to produce a one-dimensional or "ice-pick" view of the heart. *Two-dimensional echocardiography* uses a moving ultrasound beam to produce an integrated view of the heart comprising multiple pie-shaped images. *Doppler echocardiography* uses ultrasound to record blood flow within the heart. Using contrast has improved the delineation of structure on the left side of the heart. With the newer transducers, the *three-dimensional images* of the heart provide the ability to visualize valvular structures or congenital abnormalities, especially prior to surgical interventions.[2]

Transesophageal echocardiography uses a 2D echocardiography transducer placed at the end of a flexible endoscope to obtain echocardiographic images from the esophagus. Placement of the transducer in the esophagus allows echocardiographic images of cardiac structures to be obtained from different viewpoints, rather than only from the surface of the chest. Transesophageal echocardiography is particularly useful in assessing valve function. Stress echocardiography, with or without the use of pharmacologic agents, is used in conjunction with dynamic exercise. Rest and stress images are recorded, stored, and then analyzed for global and regional left ventricular size, shape, and function. Reduced systolic wall thickening seen on stress echocardiography identifies myocardial ischemia.

Nuclear Cardiac Imaging. Nuclear cardiac imaging techniques involve the use of radionuclides (*i.e.,* radioactive substances) and are essentially noninvasive. The main types of nuclear cardiology tests that are commonly used are the following: myocardial perfusion imaging, positron emission tomography (PET), and radionuclide angiocardiography. With these tests, a scintillation (gamma) camera is used to record the radiation emitted from the radionuclide. Single-photon emission computed tomography (SPECT), which uses a multiple-head camera to obtain a series of planar images over a 180- to 360-degree arc around the thorax, is the most widely used imaging technique at present.[2,11]

Myocardial perfusion imaging is used to visualize the regional distribution of blood flow. *Myocardial perfusion scintigraphy* uses thallium-201 or one of the newer technetium-based agents that are extracted from the blood and taken up by functioning myocardial cells. Thallium-201, an analog of potassium, is distributed to the myocardium in proportion to the magnitude of blood flow. After injection, an external detection device registers the distribution of the radioactive material. An ischemic area appears as a "cold spot" that lacks radioactive uptake. The most important application of this technique has been its use during stress testing for evaluation of ischemic heart disease.

Positron emission tomography (PET) uses positron-emitting agents to demonstrate either the perfusion or metabolic status of the myocardium. The radioisotopes used as positron emitters are the naturally occurring, small atomic weight atoms (*e.g.,* carbon, nitrogen, oxygen) that are the predominant constituents of organic compounds such as glucose. During ischemia, cardiac muscle shifts from fatty acid to glucose metabolism. Thus, a radioactive tracer such as fluorodeoxyglucose can be used to distinguish a transiently dysfunctional ("stunned") myocardium from scar tissue by showing persistent glucose metabolism in areas of reduced blood flow.

Radionuclide angiocardiography provides actual visualization of the ventricular structures during systole and diastole and a means for evaluating ventricular function during rest and exercise stress testing. A radioisotope such as technetium-labelled albumin, which does not leave the capillaries but remains in the blood and is not bound to the myocardium, is used for this type of imaging. This type of nuclear imaging can be used to determine right and left ventricular volumes, ejection fractions, regional wall motion, and cardiac contractility. This method also is useful in the diagnosis of intracardiac shunts.

Cardiac Magnetic Resonance Imaging and Computed Tomography. Cardiac MRI creates a spatially resolved map of radio signals and, compared with x-ray–based techniques, is much safer. Cardiac MRI uses gadolinium as a contrast agent and ECG gating to prevent artefacts and blurring from periodic cardiac cycles.[2] In nearly all scanners, this is achieved by gating (triggering) the acquisition of MRI data to the R wave of the ECG. Cardiac MRI is used for quantifying the volume, mass, and function of the ventricles. However, it cannot be used in persons with implanted metal pacemakers, defibrillators, or other devices.[2]

CT is an x-ray–based technique that obtains cross-sectional views of the body through rotation of the x-ray scanner around the patient. Several generations of CT technology have been developed, including conventional CT, contrast-enhanced CT, and electron-beam CT. CT cardiac imaging can be performed with or without injection of a contrast agent. Noncontrast CT studies are used primarily to assess coronary artery calcification. Contrast-enhanced studies can be used to assess cardiac chambers, great cardiac vessels, and sometimes the coronary artery lumen.[2] The electron-beam CT, developed specifically for cardiac imaging, is a useful technique for identifying persons with or at risk for CAD. Unlike conventional CT, in which the scanner moves around the patient, in electron-beam CT only the electron beam moves.

Cardiac Catheterization and Arteriography. Cardiac catheterization is one of the most widely used invasive procedures in the assessment of CAD.[2,10] Cardiac catheterization involves the passage of flexible catheters into the great vessels and chambers of the heart. In right heart catheterization, the catheter is inserted into a peripheral vein (usually the femoral) and then advanced into the right heart. The left heart catheter is inserted retrograde through a peripheral artery (usually the brachial or femoral) into the aorta and left heart. The cardiac catheterization laboratory, where the procedure is done, is equipped for viewing and recording fluoroscopic images of the heart and vessels in the chest and for measuring pressures in the heart and great vessels. It also has equipment for cardiac output studies and for obtaining samples of blood for blood gas analysis. Angiographic studies are done by injecting a radiographic contrast medium into the heart so that an outline of the moving structures can be visualized and filmed.

Coronary arteriography involves the injection of a radiographic contrast medium into the coronary arteries, permitting visualization of lesions in these vessels. It is used to identify and establish the extent of coronary artery narrowing, perform percutaneous coronary intervention and placement of coronary artery stents, and to determine appropriateness for coronary artery bypass graft surgery.[2] Intracoronary physiologic measurements (Doppler ultrasonography, fractional flow reserve) can also be obtained with new sensor guide wire technology.

Coronary Atherosclerosis and the Pathogenesis of Coronary Artery Disease

Atherosclerosis is by far the most common cause of CAD. It is slow and progressive, and can begin at a very young age (see Chapter 22). Atherosclerosis can affect one or all three of the major epicardial coronary arteries and their branches. Clinically significant lesions may be located anywhere in these vessels, but tend to predominate in the first several centimetres of the left anterior descending and left circumflex or the entire length of the right coronary artery.[2] Sometimes the major secondary branches also are involved.

Coronary artery disease is commonly divided into two types of disorders. The *acute coronary syndrome* (ACS) represents a spectrum of acute ischemic heart diseases ranging from unstable angina to MI (also known as a *heart attack*), and results from disruption of an atherosclerotic plaque that did not significantly compromise the coronary lumen before the event. Chronic ischemic heart disease is characterized by recurrent and transient episodes of myocardial ischemia and stable angina that result from narrowing of a coronary artery lumen due to atherosclerosis and/or vasospasm.

Stable Versus Unstable Plaque. There are two types of atherosclerotic lesions: the fixed or stable plaque, which reduces blood flow distal to the plaque, and the unstable or vulnerable plaque, which can rupture and cause platelet adhesion and thrombus formation. The fixed or stable plaque is commonly implicated in stable angina and the unstable plaque in ACS (*i.e.,* unstable angina and MI). In most cases the myocardial ischemia underlying ACS is precipitated by abrupt plaque disruptions (changes) by rupture followed by thrombosis. The major determinants of increased plaque vulnerability to rupture include a large lipid-rich core, a thin and unstable fibrous cap, the presence of inflammation, the lack of smooth muscle cells,[7] and the location at branch points or bends in the arteries (Fig. 24.5).

Any plaque rupture may occur spontaneously, but plaques with a thin fibrous cap overlaying a large lipid core are at high risk for rupture, and this is often triggered by hemodynamic factors such as blood flow characteristics and vessel tension. For example, a sudden surge of sympathetic activity with an increase in blood pressure, heart rate, force of cardiac contraction, and coronary blood flow is thought to increase the risk of plaque rupture. Indeed, many people with MI report a trigger event, most often emotional stress or physical activity.[7] Plaque rupture also has a diurnal variation, occurring most frequently during the first hour after arising, suggesting that physiologic factors such as surges in coronary artery tone and blood pressure may promote atherosclerotic plaque rupture and subsequent platelet deposition.[7] It has been suggested that the sympathetic nervous system is activated prior to and upon arising, resulting in changes in platelet aggregation and fibrinolytic activity that tend to favour thrombosis.

Thrombosis and Vessel Occlusion. Local thrombosis occurring after plaque rupture results from a complex interaction of the lipid core, smooth muscle cells, macrophages, and collagen. When the plaque ruptures, there is exposure to substances from the lipid core and these substances provide a stimulus for platelet aggregation and thrombus formation.[7,12] Both smooth muscle and foam cells in the lipid core contribute to the expression of tissue factor in unstable plaques. Once exposed to blood, tissue factor initiates the extrinsic coagulation pathway,

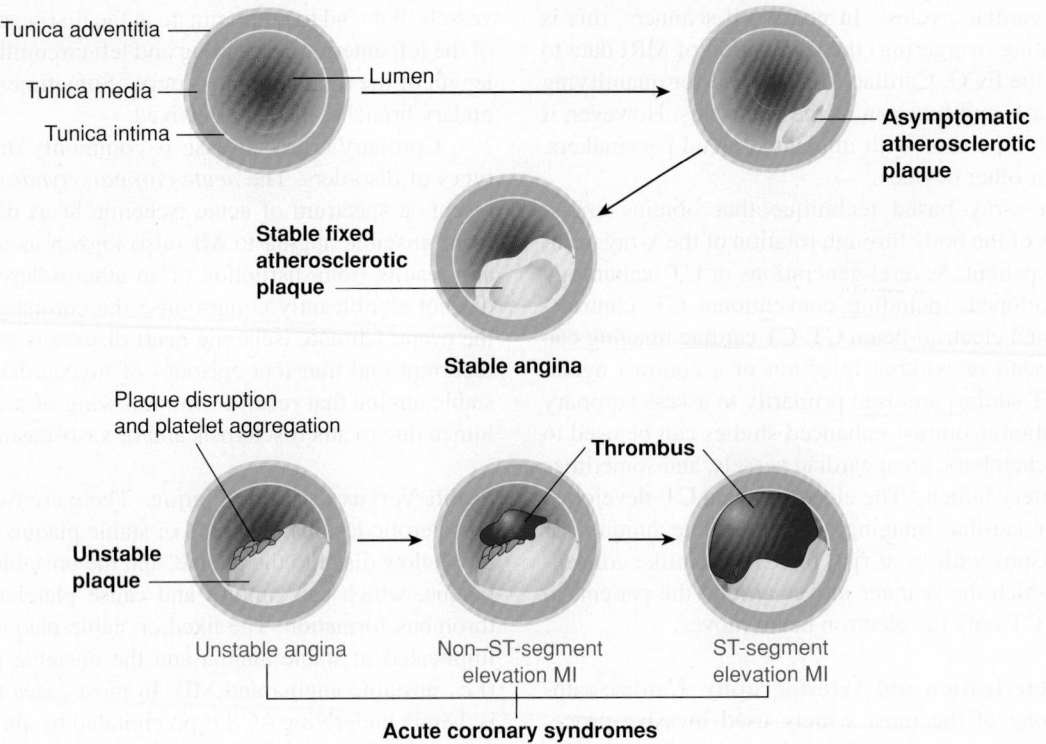

FIGURE 24.5 • Atherosclerotic plaque: stable fixed atherosclerotic plaque in stable angina and unstable plaque with plaque disruption and platelet aggregation in the acute coronary syndromes.

resulting in the local generation of thrombin and deposition of fibrin (see Chapter 13).

Platelets play an important role in linking plaque rupture to acute CAD. As a part of the response to plaque rupture, platelets adhere to the endothelium and release substances (*i.e.*, adenosine diphosphate [ADP], thromboxane A_2, and thrombin) that promote further aggregation of platelets and thrombus formation. The platelet membrane, which contains glycoprotein receptors that bind fibrinogen and link platelets together, contributes to thrombus formation. Platelet adhesion and aggregation occurs in several steps. First, release of ADP, thromboxane A_2, and thrombin initiates the aggregation process. Second, glycoprotein IIb/IIIa receptors on the platelet surface are activated. Third, fibrinogen binds to the activated glycoprotein receptors, forming bridges between adjacent platelets.

There are two types of thrombi formed as a result of plaque rupture—white platelet–containing thrombi and red fibrin–containing thrombi. The thrombi in unstable angina have been characterized as greyish-white and presumably platelet-rich.[13] Red thrombi, which develop with vessel occlusion in MI, are rich in fibrin and red blood cells superimposed on the platelet component and are extended by the stasis of blood flow.

Acute Coronary Syndrome

Acute coronary syndrome (ACS) includes unstable angina, non–ST-segment elevation myocardial infarction (NSTEMI/

non-STEMI), and ST-segment elevation myocardial infarction (STEMI). Persons with NSTEMI are those in whom the thrombotic coronary artery is partially occluded but remains patent, whereas those with STEMI are usually found to have complete coronary occlusion. Persons with an ACS are classified and managed according to the cardiac biomarkers (*i.e.*, acute infarction present or absent), the ECG (*i.e.*, changes in ST segment, T wave, or Q wave), and risk (*e.g.*, risk of heart failure).

Electrocardiographic Changes. The classic ECG changes that occur with ACS involve ST-segment elevation or depression, T-wave inversion, loss of R-wave progression, or development of an abnormal Q wave[2] (Fig. 24.6). The changes that occur may not be present with the onset of symptoms, and vary considerably depending on the duration of the ischemic event (acute versus changes that occur after the acute onset, referred to as an evolving MI), its extent (*i.e.*, subendocardial versus entire wall thickness, which is referred to as transmural, Fig. 24.6) and its location (*e.g.*, anterior versus inferior). Because these changes usually occur over time and are seen on the ECG leads that view the involved area of the myocardium, provision for continuous and serial 12-lead or 15-lead ECG monitoring is indicated (see Chapter 25 for a more complete discussion of the ECG).

The repolarization phase of the action potential (T wave and ST segment on the ECG) is usually the first to be altered during myocardial ischemia and injury. As the involved area become ischemic, myocardial repolarization is altered causing

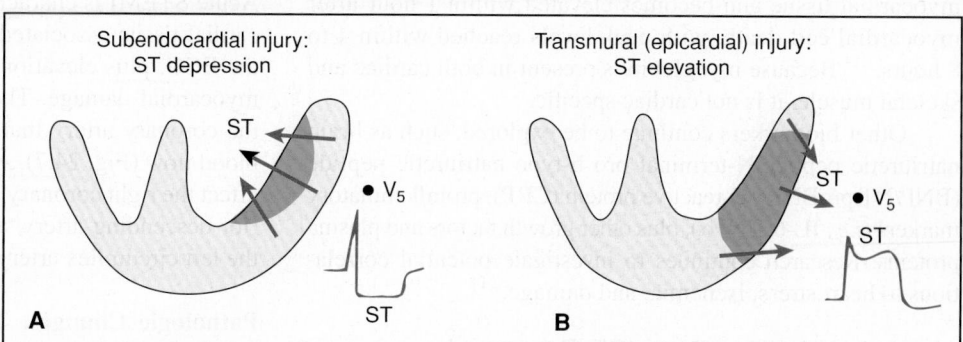

FIGURE 24.6 • **(Top) A:** ECG tracing showing normal P, Q, R, S, and T waves. **(B)** ST-segment elevation with acute ischemia. **C:** Q wave with acute myocardial infarction. **(Bottom)** Current-of-injury patterns with acute ischemia. **A:** With predominant subendocardial ischemia, the resultant ST segment is directed towards the inner layer of the affected ventricle and the ventricular cavity. Overlying leads therefore record ST-segment depression. **B:** With ischemia involving the outer ventricular layer (transmural or epicardial injury), the ST vector is directed outward. Overlying leads record ST-segment elevation. **(Bottom:** From Braunwald E., Zipes D. P., Libby P. (2002). *Heart disease: A textbook of cardiovascular medicine* (6th ed., p. 108). Philadelphia, PA: W.B. Saunders.)

changes in ST segment or the T wave (Fig. 24.6). This is usually represented by T-wave inversion, although a hyperacute T-wave elevation may occur as the earliest sign of ischemia. ST-segment changes occur with myocardial ischemia, injury, or infarct. Normally, the ST segment of the ECG is isoelectric (*i.e.,* flat along the baseline) because all healthy myocardial cells attain the same potential during early repolarization. Alterations in the resting membrane potentials and polarization may occur in acute ischemia, leading to altered current flow and a deviation from the isoelectric line of the ST segment on the ECG.[2,10,12] When the acute ischemia is transmural, the overall ST vector is shifted in the direction of the outer epicardium, resulting in ST-segment elevation[2] (Fig. 24.6). When the ischemia is confined primarily to the subendocardium, the overall ST segment is shifted towards the inner ventricular layer, resulting in an overall depression of the ST segment. It

is important to note that although ST changes represent acute ischemia, when biomarkers are elevated (*e.g.,* positive cardiac specific troponin), they indicate acute MI and are diagnosed and treated as either a non-STEMI or STEMI.

Additional ventricular depolarization (QRS) changes may occur in addition to the T-wave and ST-segment abnormalities. Abnormal Q waves (wide and deep) develop in the correlating leads because there is no depolarizing current conduction in the necrotic or dead tissue. In anterior MI, loss of R-wave progression occurs, again because of necrotic tissue and loss of conduction.

Serum Cardiac Biomarkers. Serum biomarkers for ACS include cardiac-specific troponin I (TnI) and troponin T (TnT), myoglobin, and creatine kinase MB (CK-MB).[14] As the myocardial cells become necrotic, their intracellular contents begin to diffuse into the surrounding interstitium and then into the blood. The rate at which the enzymes appear in the blood depends on their intracellular location, their molecular weight, and local blood flow. For example, they may appear at an earlier-than-predicted time in patients who have undergone successful reperfusion therapy.

The *troponin assays* have high specificity for myocardial tissue and have become the primary biomarker tests for the diagnosis of MI. The troponin complex, which is part of the actin filament, consists of three subunits (*i.e.,* TnC, TnT, and TnI) that regulate the calcium-mediated actin–myosin contractile process in striated muscle (see Chapter 4, Fig. 4.22). TnI and TnT, which are present in cardiac muscle, begin to rise within 3 hours after the onset of MI and may remain elevated for 7 to 10 days after the event. This is especially advantageous in the late diagnosis of MI.[2,14]

CORONARY ARTERY DISEASE

- The term *coronary artery disease* refers to disorders of myocardial blood flow due to stable or unstable coronary atherosclerotic plaques.
- Unstable atherosclerotic plaques tend to fissure or rupture, causing platelet aggregation and potential for thrombus formation with production of a spectrum of ACSs of increasing severity, ranging from unstable angina, to NSTEMI, to STEMI.
- Stable atherosclerotic plaques produce fixed obstruction of coronary blood flow with myocardial ischemia occurring during periods of increased metabolic need, such as in stable angina.

Creatine kinase is an intracellular enzyme found in muscle cells. There are three isoenzymes of CK, with the MB isoenzyme having higher specificity for myocardial tissue. CK-MB is used as a second-line biomarker when assessing for heart damage due to the decreased sensitivity and specificity compared to troponin. Serum levels of CK-MB exceed normal ranges within 4 to 8 hours of myocardial injury and decline to normal within 2 to 3 days.[2,14]

Myoglobin is an oxygen-carrying protein, similar to hemoglobin, that is normally present in cardiac and skeletal muscle. It is a small molecule that is released quickly from infarcted myocardial tissue and becomes elevated within 1 hour after myocardial cell death, with peak levels reached within 4 to 8 hours.[2,14] Because myoglobin is present in both cardiac and skeletal muscle, it is not cardiac specific.

Other biomarkers continue to be explored, such as brain natriuretic peptide/N-terminal pro b-type natriuretic peptide (BNP/NT-proBNP), C-reactive protein (CRP), proinflammatory markers (*i.e.*, IL-6, TNFα), plus other growth factors and plasma proteins. Research continues to investigate potential correlations to heart stress, ischemia, and damage.[2,14]

Unstable Angina/Non–ST-Segment Elevation Myocardial Infarction

Unstable angina (UA) and NSTEMI occur within the spectrum of ACS and have similar underlying pathophysiology and clinical manifestations. They differ in severity of ischemia and myocardial muscle damage. Ischemia that is severe enough to cause release of detectable cardiac markers is diagnostic of myocardial infarct and is indicative of NSTEMI; an absence of cardiac markers is indicative of UA.

The pathophysiologic process of UA/NSTEMI involves four processes: the rupture of unstable atheromatous plaque, coronary arterial vasoconstriction, imbalance between oxygen supply and demand for the myocardium, and gradual intraluminal narrowing of the coronary arteries because of progressive atherosclerosis. These processes may happen simultaneously, in any combination, and are not mutually exclusive.[15] Inflammation can play a prominent role in plaque instability, with inflammatory cells releasing cytokines that cause the fibrous cap to become thinner and more vulnerable to rupture or erosion (see Chapter 22). The acute ischemic event can be caused by an increase in myocardial oxygen demand precipitated by tachycardia or hypertension, or more commonly by a decrease in oxygen supply related to a reduction in coronary lumen diameter due to platelet-rich thrombi or vessel spasm.[15]

The pain associated with UA typically has a persistent and severe course and is characterized by at least one of three features: (1) it occurs at rest (or with minimal exertion), usually lasting more than 20 minutes (if not interrupted by nitroglycerin); (2) it is severe and described as frank pain and of new onset (*i.e.,* within 1 month); and (3) it is more severe, prolonged, or frequent than previously experienced.[15]

Risk stratification of persons presenting with UA/NSTEMI is important because the outcome can range from excellent to NSTEMI, or death. UA/NSTEMI is classified by severity based on clinical history, ECG pattern, and serum biomarkers. The ECG pattern in UA/NSTEMI may demonstrate normal or depressed ST-segment, transient ST-segment elevation, and T-wave changes. The degree of ST-segment deviation has been shown to be an important measure of ischemia and prognosis. Treatment will vary depending on risk, with more aggressive treatment indicated for persons with NSTEMI, and those with the highest risk for complications, reoccurring events, or potential death.

ST-Segment Elevation Myocardial Infarction

Acute STEMI is characterized by the ischemic death of myocardial tissue associated with elevation of the ST-segment of the ECG, plus elevation of serum cardiac markers indicating myocardial damage. The area of infarction is determined by the coronary artery that is affected and by its distribution of blood flow (Fig. 24.7). Approximately 30% to 40% of infarcts affect the right coronary artery, 40% to 50% affect the left anterior descending artery, and the remaining 15% to 20% affect the left circumflex artery.[7]

Pathologic Changes. The extent of an MI depends on the location and extent of occlusion, amount of heart tissue supplied by the vessel, duration of the occlusion, metabolic needs of the affected tissue, extent of collateral circulation, and other factors such as heart rate, blood pressure, and cardiac rhythm. An infarct may involve the endocardium, myocardium, epicardium, or a combination of these. Transmural infarcts involve the full thickness of the ventricular wall and most commonly occur when there is obstruction of a single artery (Fig. 24.8). Subendocardial infarcts involve the inner one third to one half of the ventricular wall and occur more frequently in the presence of severely narrowed but still patent arteries.

The principal biochemical consequence of MI is the conversion from aerobic to anaerobic metabolism with inadequate production of energy to sustain normal myocardial function. As a result, a striking loss of contractile function occurs within 60 seconds of onset.[7] Changes in cell structure (*i.e.,* glycogen depletion and mitochondrial swelling) develop within several minutes. These early changes are reversible if blood flow is restored and a minor infarcted area results. Although gross tissue changes are not apparent for hours after onset of MI, the ischemic area ceases to function within a matter of minutes, and irreversible damage to cells occurs in approximately 40 minutes. Irreversible myocardial cell death (necrosis) occurs after 20 to 40 minutes of severe ischemia. Microvascular injury occurs in approximately 1 hour and follows irreversible cell injury.[9] If the myocardial infarct is large enough, it depresses overall left ventricular function and pump failure ensues.

Multiple dynamic structural changes maintain cardiac function in persons with STEMI. Both the infarcted and noninfarcted areas of the ventricle undergo progressive changes in size, shape, and thickness, comprising early wall thinning, healing, hypertrophy, and dilation, collectively termed *ventricular remodelling.* As the nonfunctioning muscle in the infarcted area becomes thin and dilated, the muscle in the

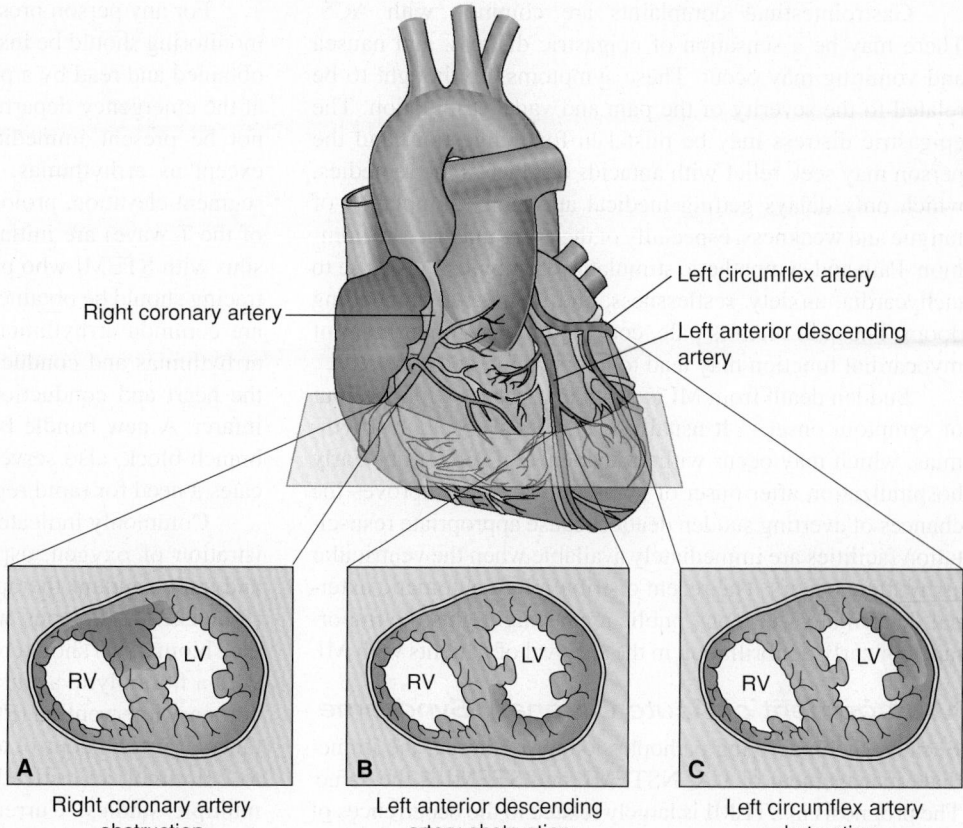

Right coronary artery

Left circumflex artery

Left anterior descending artery

FIGURE 24.7 • Areas of heart affected by occlusion of the (**A**) right coronary artery, (**B**) left anterior descending coronary artery, and (**C**) left circumflex coronary artery. RV, right ventricle; LV, left ventricle.

A Right coronary artery obstruction

B Left anterior descending artery obstruction

C Left circumflex artery obstruction

surrounding, noninfarcted area becomes thicker as it undergoes adaptive hypertrophy so it can take over the work of the muscle in the infarcted zone. However, the adaptive effect of remodelling may be overwhelmed by aneurysm formation or depression of myocardial function, causing further impairment of ventricular function.[2,7]

FIGURE 24.8 • Acute myocardial infarct. A cross section of the ventricles of a man who died a few days after the onset of severe chest pain shows a transmural infarct in the posterior and septal regions of the left ventricle. The necrotic myocardium is soft, yellowish, and sharply demarcated. (From Rubin R., Strayer D. S. (Eds.). (2012). *Rubin's pathology: Clinicopathologic foundations of medicine* (6th ed., p. 502). Philadelphia, PA: Lippincott Williams & Wilkins.)

Clinical Presentation of Acute Coronary Syndrome

The symptoms of ACS, encompassing UA, NSTEMI and STEMI, are very similar. The onset of ACS usually is abrupt, with pain as the significant symptom. Chest pain is the most common symptom for both men and women and may be severe and crushing, often described as being constricting, suffocating, pressure, or like "someone sitting on my chest." It usually is substernal, and may radiate to the left arm, neck, or jaw, although it may be experienced in other areas of the chest. Unlike that of stable angina, the pain associated with ACS is more prolonged, not relieved by rest or nitroglycerin, and opiates frequently are required. It is important to note that some persons may not experience the severe pain typically associated with an MI, describing it as "discomfort" rather than "pain." A large number of individuals who present with chest discomfort/pain may have additional "atypical" sensations such as shortness of breath, sweating, nausea, vomiting, syncope, and pain in other locations, including back, arm, shoulder, neck, or jaw.[16] Of greater concern are persons that experience no chest pain and present only with atypical sensations, which can be more difficult to detect and correctly diagnose. Persons most likely to experience atypical symptoms include the elderly, women, those with diabetes, and individuals with heart failure. A silent MI may occur when the person does not experience any symptoms at all or has only atypical symptoms.

Gastrointestinal complaints are common with ACS. There may be a sensation of epigastric distress, and nausea and vomiting may occur. These symptoms are thought to be related to the severity of the pain and vagal stimulation. The epigastric distress may be mistaken for indigestion, and the person may seek relief with antacids or other home remedies, which only delays getting medical attention. Complaints of fatigue and weakness, especially of the arms and legs, are common. Pain and sympathetic stimulation combine to give rise to tachycardia, anxiety, restlessness, and feelings of impending doom. The skin often is pale, cool, and moist. Impairment of myocardial function may lead to hypotension and shock.

Sudden death from MI is death that occurs within 1 hour of symptom onset.[2,7] It usually is attributed to fatal arrhythmias, which may occur without evidence of infarction. Early hospitalization after onset of symptoms greatly improves the chances of averting sudden death because appropriate resuscitation facilities are immediately available when the ventricular arrhythmia occurs. The recent distribution of automatic external defibrillators in many public arenas highlights the importance of early defibrillation in the survival of patients with MI.

Management of Acute Coronary Syndrome

Because the underlying pathophysiology is similar, the immediate management of UA, NSTEMI, and STEMI is the same. The prognosis in STEMI is largely related to the occurrences of two general complications—arrhythmias and mechanical complications (pump failure). The majority of deaths from STEMI are due to the sudden development of ventricular fibrillation. Therefore, the major elements in management of persons with STEMI are recognition of symptoms and prompt seeking of medical care; the prompt deployment of an emergency medical team capable of resuscitation procedures, including defibrillation; expeditious transport to a hospital equipped for managing arrhythmias and providing advanced cardiac life support; and expeditious implementation of reperfusion therapy.[2] Persons, particularly older adults, women, and persons of low socioeconomic status, who experience signs and symptoms of STEMI often delay seeking treatment, despite current public information regarding the benefits of early treatment. The development and revisions of algorithms for management of ACS is ongoing by organizations such as the Canadian Cardiovascular Society (CCS) in collaboration with the American Heart Association (AHA), the Canadian Heart Research Centre and other national and international organizations, with the goal of improving timely access and adherence to evidence-based therapies.[17]

The pre-emergency and emergency department goals for management of ACS include identification of persons who are candidates for reperfusion therapy. The history and physical examination should be conducted thoroughly but efficiently, so as not to delay reperfusion therapy. Prior episodes of cardiovascular disease, including ACS, coronary bypass surgery, or percutaneous coronary intervention, should be ascertained. Evaluation of the person's chief complaint, typically chest pain, along with other associated symptoms is essential in differentiating ACS from other diagnoses.

For any person presenting with symptoms of ACS, ECG monitoring should be instituted, and a 12-lead ECG should be obtained and read by a physician within 10 minutes of arrival at the emergency department. The typical ECG changes may not be present immediately after the onset of symptoms, except as arrhythmias. Diagnostic ECG tracings (*i.e.*, ST-segment elevation, prolongation of the Q wave, and inversion of the T wave) are initially absent in as many as half of persons with STEMI who present with chest pain, so serial ECG tracing should be obtained. Premature ventricular contractions are common arrhythmias after MI. The occurrence of other arrhythmias and conduction defects depends on the areas of the heart and conduction pathways that are included in the infarct. A new bundle branch block, particularly left bundle branch block, also serves as a criterion for STEMI and indicates a need for rapid reperfusion.

Commonly indicated treatment regimens include administration of oxygen, aspirin, nitrates, morphine, antiplatelet and anticoagulant therapy, and β-adrenergic blocking agents (β-blockers).[2] Persons with evidence of infarction (*i.e.*, cardiac biomarker) should receive immediate reperfusion therapy with a fibrinolytic agent (within 30 minutes) or percutaneous coronary intervention (PCI, within 90 minutes).[2,17] The importance of insulin control to maintain normal blood glucose (4.6 to 7.0 mmol) in critically ill patients has been supported by multiple studies. Current American College of Cardiology (ACC)/AHA guidelines recommend the maintenance of strict glucose control during STEMI.[18]

When present, chest pain gives rise to anxiety and recruitment of autonomic nervous system responses, both of which increase the work demands on the heart. Sudden increases in catecholamines may also play a role in plaque fissuring and thrombus propagation, as well as lowering the threshold for ventricular fibrillation.[7] Therefore, pain relief is a major objective in the treatment of ACS. Alleviation of pain is accomplished with a combination of nitrates, analgesics (*e.g.*, morphine), oxygen, and β-adrenergic blocking agents, and reperfusion measures for NSTEMI and STEMI.

Nitroglycerin is given because of its vasodilating effect, the ability to relieve coronary pain, and the ability to reduce the infarction size. The vasodilating effects are dose-dependent and include coronary artery dilation, decreased venous return (*i.e.*, reduced preload) and arterial blood pressure (*i.e.*, reduced afterload), thereby increasing oxygen delivery and reducing oxygen consumption. Nitroglycerin usually is administered sublingually initially, after which the need for intravenous infusion is assessed. The use of intravenous nitroglycerin may be indicated for treatment of ongoing ischemic pain, control of hypertension, or management of pulmonary congestion. Nitroglycerin should not be administered to patients with severe hypotension or to patients who have received a phosphodiesterase inhibitor for erectile dysfunction within the previous 24 hours due to the risk of a drop in blood pressure and a resultant decrease in coronary perfusion.[7]

Morphine is usually the agent of choice to treat pain associated with cardiac ischemia.[2,17,18] It usually is indicated if chest pain is unrelieved with oxygen and nitrates. The reduction in anxiety that accompanies the administration of morphine contributes to a decrease in restlessness and autonomic nervous system activity, with a subsequent decrease in the metabolic demands of the heart. It is given intravenously because of the rapid onset of action and because the intravenous route does not elevate enzyme levels. This route also bypasses the variable rate of absorption of subcutaneous or intramuscular sites, which often are underperfused because of the decrease in cardiac output that occurs after infarction.

The administration of oxygen augments the oxygen content of inspired air and increases the oxygen saturation of hemoglobin, which increases the oxygen content of the blood and delivery to the cardiac tissues. In patients with severe heart failure or cardiogenic shock, continuous positive-pressure ventilation or endotracheal intubation and support with mechanical ventilation may be necessary.

β-Adrenergic blocking drugs act as antagonists that block β-receptor–mediated functions of the sympathetic nervous system and thus decrease myocardial oxygen demand by reducing heart rate, cardiac contractility, and systemic arterial blood pressure. The lengthening of diastole caused by the slower heart rate may enhance myocardial perfusion, especially to the subendocardium. β-Blockers also alter resting myocardial membrane potentials and may decrease life-threatening ventricular arrhythmias. Because sympathetic nervous system activity increases the metabolic demands of the myocardium, oral or intravenous β-blockers are recommended for persons with ACS who do not have contraindications. They should not be given to persons with MI caused by cocaine use because they could accentuate coronary spasm. Other relative contraindications to β-blockers include symptomatic bradycardia, hypotension, moderate to severe left ventricular failure, shock, or second- or third-degree heart block.

Platelets play a major role in the thrombotic response to atherosclerotic plaque rupture; therefore, inhibition of platelet aggregation is an important aspect in the early treatment of ACS. Aspirin (*i.e.,* acetylsalicylic acid) is the preferred antiplatelet agent for preventing platelet aggregation in persons with ACS. Aspirin, which acts by inhibiting synthesis of the prostaglandin thromboxane A_2, is thought to promote reperfusion and reduce the likelihood of rethrombosis. The actions of aspirin are related to the presence of the acetyl group, which irreversibly acetylates the critical platelet enzyme, cyclooxygenase, which is required for thromboxane A_2 synthesis. Because the action is irreversible, the effect of aspirin on platelet function lasts for the lifetime of the platelet—approximately 8 to 10 days. For patients who are unable to take aspirin because of hypersensitivity or gastrointestinal intolerance, clopidogrel may be prescribed. Clopidogrel, prasugrel, and ticagrelor are thienopyridine derivatives that reduce platelet aggregation by inhibiting the $P2Y_{12}$ receptor. Unlike aspirin, it has no effect on prostaglandin synthesis. Results of several studies have resulted in recommendations for the use of clopidogrel along with aspirin for persons undergoing PCI.[17,19]

Another class of antiplatelet agents is the platelet receptor antagonists. In contrast to aspirin and clopidogrel, which target a single step in the aggregation process, the platelet glycoprotein IIb/IIIa (GP IIb/IIIa) receptor inhibitors (*e.g.,* tirofiban, eptifibatide, abciximab) block the GP IIb/IIIa receptor, which is involved in the final common pathway for platelet adhesion, activation, and aggregation. The GP IIb/IIIa receptor inhibitors are recommended in the treatment of patients with non-STEMI undergoing early invasive therapy (*e.g.,* PCI).

Antithrombin agents are also used in the treatment of patients with ACS. Anticoagulation therapy, which targets the coagulation pathway and formation of the fibrin clot, involves the use of either unfractionated or low–molecular-weight heparin (see Chapter 13). The rationale for the use of antithrombin therapy in patients with STEMI is the prevention of recoagulation of activated platelets, which can result in myocardial infarct extension.

Inhibition of the renin–angiotensin–aldosterone system should be considered for all patients with STEMI. ACE inhibitors, angiotensin receptor blockers (ARBs), or aldosterone are often used during the early and convalescent phases of STEMI, demonstrating a benefit in terms of decreased mortality rate and prevention of recurrent ischemic episodes. The greatest benefit is in those patients with previous infarctions, heart failure, and tachycardia. ACE inhibitors usually are started within the first 3 days, after fibrinolytic therapy has been completed. Therapy with ACE inhibitors is usually begun with low-dose oral administration and increased steadily to full dose.

Reperfusion Strategies. The term *reperfusion* refers to reestablishment of blood flow through use of pharmacologic agents (fibrinolytic therapy), PCI, or coronary artery bypass grafting. All patients presenting with ACS should be assessed for reperfusion therapy as soon as possible on entry into the healthcare system. Time since onset of symptoms, risk of STEMI, possible risks associated with fibrinolytic therapy, and time required for transport for PCI should all be considered.

Early reperfusion (within 30 minutes) after onset of MI due to coronary artery occlusion can prevent necrosis and improve myocardial perfusion in the infarct zone. Reperfusion after a longer interval can salvage some of the myocardial cells that would have died owing to longer periods of ischemia. It also may prevent the microvascular injury that occurs over a longer period. Even though much of the viable myocardium existing at the time of reflow, or reperfusion, ultimately recovers, critical abnormalities in biochemical function may persist, causing impaired ventricular function. The recovering area of the heart is often referred to as a *stunned myocardium*. Because myocardial function is lost before cell death occurs, a stunned myocardium may not be capable of sustaining life, and persons with large areas of dysfunctional myocardium may require life support until the stunned regions regain their function.[2,7,17]

Fibrinolytic Therapy. Fibrinolytic drugs break down blood and platelet clots and are used to reduce mortality, limit infarct size, encourage infarct healing and myocardial remodelling, and reduce the potential for life-threatening arrhythmias. These agents interact with plasminogen to generate plasmin, which lyses fibrin clots and digests clotting factors V and VIII, prothrombin, and fibrinogen (see Chapter 15). The fibrinolytic agents include streptokinase, alteplase (rtPA), reteplase, and tenecteplase (TNK). The best results occur if treatment is initiated within 30 minutes of symptom onset. The magnitude of the benefit declines after this period, but it is possible that some benefit can be achieved for up to 12 hours after the onset of pain. The person must be a low-risk candidate for complications caused by bleeding, with no intracranial hemorrhage or significant trauma within the last 3 months. The primary complication of fibrinolytic therapy is intracranial hemorrhage, which usually occurs within the first 24 hours of treatment.[2]

Percutaneous Coronary Intervention. Percutaneous coronary intervention (PCI) is indicated as an early invasive procedure for patients with ACS who have lesions amenable to PCI.[2,17] PCI includes percutaneous transluminal coronary angioplasty (PTCA), PTCA with stent implantation, atherectomy, and thrombectomy. The goal in PCI is to perform the procedure within 90 minutes of the patient's first medical contact (the "door-to-balloon interval").[2,17,18]

PTCA involves dilation of a stenotic atherosclerotic plaque with an inflatable balloon (Fig. 24.9). The procedure is similar to cardiac catheterization for coronary angiography, in that the double-lumen balloon dilation catheter is introduced percutaneously into the femoral, brachial, or radial artery and advanced under fluoroscopic view into the stenotic area of the affected coronary vessel. It differs in that the balloon is inflated to expand the coronary arterial lumen, thus stretching

FIGURE 24.9 • Balloon-expandable stent insertion. **A:** Insertion of a guide catheter with a collapsed balloon-expandable stent mounted over a guide wire into a coronary artery. **B:** Advancement of guide wire across the coronary lesion. **C:** Positioning of the balloon-expandable stent across the lesion. **D:** Balloon inflation with expansion of the stent. Once the stent is expanded, the balloon system is removed.

and breaking the atherosclerotic plaque and, to a lesser extent, by distributing the plaque along its longitudinal axis. This procedure is most often used in conjunction with the placement of stents, due to a high rate or reocclusion without stent implantation. Both acute and longer-term complications are rare. Acute complications include thrombosis and vessel dissection; longer-term complications involve restenosis of the dilated vessel.

The use of *coronary stenting* has been shown to improve short- and long-term outcomes compared with PTCA alone. Persons undergoing stent procedures are treated with antiplatelet and anticoagulant drugs to prevent thrombosis, which is a major risk of the procedure.[2] The self-expanding wire mesh stents that were used initially had high thrombosis rates and have largely been replaced by balloon-expandable stents. Drug-eluting stents (with sirolimus, paclitaxel, zotarolimus, and everolimus) are now being used to suppress local neointimal proliferation that causes restenosis of the coronary artery.[2] Bare metal stents are used in 10% to 30% of patients, most often because of an inability to take long-term antiplatelet therapy.[2]

Atherectomy (i.e., cutting of the atherosclerotic plaque with a high-speed circular blade from within the vessel) is a mechanical technique to remove atherosclerotic tissue during angioplasty. Laser angioplasty devices are also used. However, since the availability of stents, these procedures are rarely used. Thrombectomy (removal of the thrombus) involves the use of a special catheter device to fracture the thrombus into small pieces and then pull the fracture fragments into the catheter tip so they can be propelled proximally and removed. Recent research suggests this is not beneficial and that it carries an increased risk for an embolic stroke.[20]

Coronary Artery Bypass Grafting. Coronary artery bypass grafting (CABG) is one of the most common surgeries performed in the world, providing relief of angina, improvement in exercise tolerance, and prolongation of life. The procedure involves revascularization of the affected myocardium by placing a vein graft (e.g., saphenous vein) between the aorta and the affected coronary artery distal to the site of occlusion, or by using an artery (e.g., the internal mammary artery as a means of revascularizing the left anterior descending artery or its branches; Fig. 24.10). One to five distal anastomoses may be done.

Emergent or urgent CABG, as a reperfusion strategy, is indicated in situations such as failed PCI with persistent pain or hemodynamic instability, or for patients who are not candidates for PCI or fibrinolytic therapy.[2,21,22] In considering CABG as a treatment option, the risk for hospital mortality and other complications must be taken into account. Advanced age, poor left ventricular function, and the urgency with which surgery is performed increase the risk of early mortality. Serious complications, such as stroke, mediastinitis, and renal dysfunction, also increase the mortality and morbidity associated with CABG. The use of preoperative antibiotics and preoperative and postoperative administration of β-blockers help in reducing the incidence of postoperative infection and atrial fibrillation.

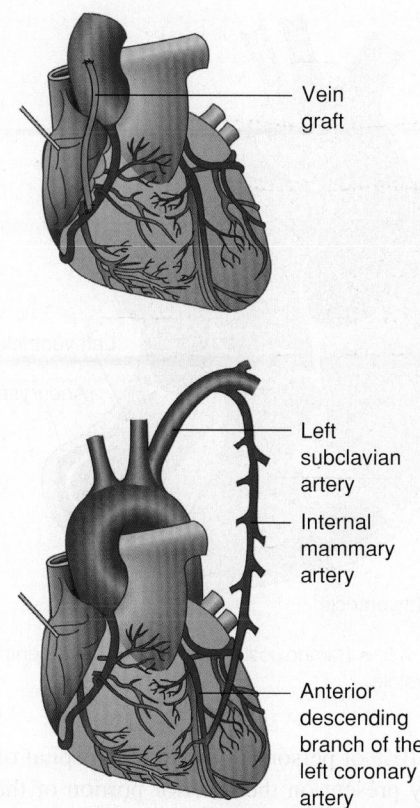

FIGURE 24.10 • Coronary artery revascularization. (**Top**) Saphenous vein bypass graft. The vein segment is sutured to the ascending aorta and the right coronary artery at a point distal to the occluding lesion. (**Bottom**) Mammary artery bypass graft. The mammary artery is anastomosed to the anterior descending left coronary artery, bypassing the obstructing lesion.

CABG does not alter the progress of the CAD, and although the incidence of return of angina is low for the first 5 years, about 50% of vein grafts are closed 10 years after CABG. The use of internal mammary artery grafts, however, has shown excellent late patency. Aspirin is the drug of choice for prophylaxis against early saphenous vein graft closure and is continued indefinitely.[17,19] New surgical techniques in the treatment of CAD continue to evolve in an effort to reduce adverse effects of the midline sternotomy incision, cardiopulmonary bypass, and global cardioplegic arrest. Some of these include "off-pump" CABG, the development of robotic coronary bypass, and transmyocardial laser revascularization.[2]

Postinfarction Recovery Period

After an MI, there usually are three zones of tissue damage: a zone of myocardial tissue that becomes necrotic because of an absolute lack of blood flow; a surrounding zone of injured cells, some of which will recover; and an outer zone in which cells are ischemic and can be salvaged if blood flow can be reestablished (Fig. 24.11). The boundaries of these zones may change with time after the infarction and with the success of treatment measures to reestablish blood flow. If blood flow can be restored within the 20- to 40-minute time frame, loss of cell viability does not occur or is minimal. The progression of ischemic

necrosis usually begins in the subendocardial area of the heart and extends through the myocardium to involve progressively more of the transmural thickness of the ischemic zone.

Myocardial cells that undergo necrosis are gradually replaced with scar tissue. An acute inflammatory response develops in the area of necrosis approximately 2 to 3 days after infarction. Thereafter, macrophages begin removing the necrotic tissue; the damaged area is gradually replaced with a growth of highly vascularized granulation tissue, which gradually becomes less vascular and more fibrous.[7] At approximately 4 to 7 days, the centre of the infarcted area is soft and yellow; if rupture of the ventricle, intraventricular septum, or valve structures occurs, it usually happens at this time. Replacement of the necrotic myocardial tissue usually is complete by the seventh week. Areas of the myocardium that have been replaced with scar tissue lack the ability to contract and initiate or conduct action potentials.

Complications. The stages of recovery from MI are closely related to the size of the infarct and the changes that have taken place in the infarcted area. Fibrous scar tissue lacks the contractile, elastic, and conductive properties of normal myocardial cells; the residual effects and the complications are determined essentially by the extent and location of the injury. Among the complications of MI are sudden death, pericarditis, stroke, thromboemboli, and mechanical defects (*e.g.,* mitral valve regurgitation, ventricular septal rupture, left ventricular wall rupture, and left ventricular aneurysm). Depending on its severity, MI has the potential for compromising the pumping action of the heart. Heart failure and cardiogenic shock are potential complications of MI (see Chapter 26).

Life-threatening arrhythmias can be the first symptom of an ACS, differing in mechanism from chronic stable angina. With ACS, mechanisms may be related to reentry, abnormal automaticity, and electrolyte imbalances, particularly potassium and magnesium (see Chapter 25). Symptomatic bradycardia and heart block are also complications of ACS and are treated according to the guidelines for implantation of cardiac pacemakers and antiarrhythmic devices.[23]

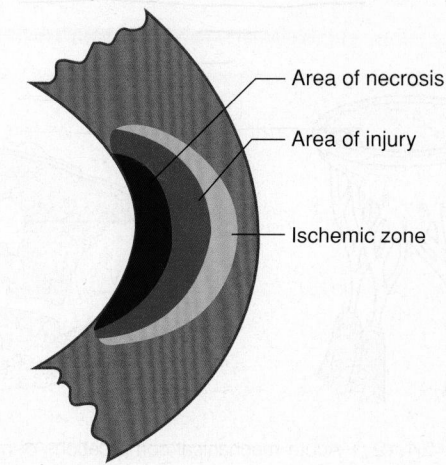

FIGURE 24.11 • Zones of tissue damage after myocardial infarction.

Pericarditis tends to occur in patients with large infarcts, a lower ejection fraction, and a higher occurrence of heart failure. It may appear as early as the second or third day postinfarction or up to several weeks later. This late complication, called *Dressler syndrome,* occurs weeks to months after MI, and is thought to be an autoimmune response. In contrast to the pain associated with MI, the pain with pericarditis is sharp and stabbing and aggravated by deep inspiration and positional changes. Because of reperfusion therapy, this complication has been greatly reduced.

Acute stroke is another complication of MI. Risk factors for stroke after an MI include hypertension, older age, history of previous stroke, decreased ejection fraction, and atrial fibrillation. Thromboemboli, presenting as deep vein thrombosis or pulmonary emboli, do not present as frequently as in the past because of the use of anticoagulant therapy.

Mechanical defects result from changes that occur in the necrotic and subsequently inflamed myocardium and include rupture of the ventricular septum, papillary muscle, or free ventricular wall[9] (Fig. 24.12). Partial or complete rupture of a papillary muscle is a rare but often fatal complication of transmural MI.[2] It is detected by the presence of a new systolic murmur and clinical deterioration, often with pulmonary edema. More frequently, postinfarction mitral valve regurgitation results from early ischemic dysfunction of the papillary muscle and underlying myocardium. Ventricular septal rupture occurs less frequently than in the past because of the use of reperfusion therapy.[2] Previously thought to require surgical intervention only in symptomatic patients, surgical repair is now recommended for all patients with ventricular septal rupture. Complete rupture of the free wall of the infarcted ventricle occurs in 1% to 6% of patients and usually results in immediate death.[7] It usually occurs 3 to 7 days postinfarction, usually involves the anterior wall, and is more frequent in older women. Incomplete or gradual rupture may be sealed off by the pericardium, creating a pseudoaneurysm. It requires early surgical intervention because delayed complete rupture is common.

A left ventricular aneurysm, a sharply delineated area of scar tissue that bulges paradoxically during systole (Fig. 24.13),

FIGURE 24.13 • Paradoxical movement of a left ventricular aneurysm during systole.

develops in 10% of persons dying in the hospital of STEMI.[2] They usually present on the anterior portion of the left ventricle after occlusion of the left anterior descending coronary artery and become evident 4 to 8 weeks after infarct. They rarely rupture but may be associated with arterial emboli, ventricular arrhythmias, and heart failure. Surgical resection may be performed for these indications when other treatment measures fail.[2]

Cardiac Rehabilitation

Cardiac rehabilitation programs are recommended for patients after ACS and incorporate strategies to improve adherence to medical therapies and lifestyle changes.[24] Components of cardiac rehabilitation include exercise, nutrition, smoking cessation, psychosocial management, and education. Education is an essential component of cardiac rehabilitation programs,

FIGURE 24.12 • Acute mechanical complications of myocardial infarction. **A:** Papillary muscle rupture. **B:** Interventricular septum rupture. **C:** Rupture of the free wall of the left ventricle with pseudoaneurysm formation. RA, right atrium; LA, left atrium; RV, right ventricle; LV, left ventricle.

and is often incorporated with other aspects of the program. This includes education related to exercise, nutrition, smoking cessation, and medications. Adherence to a cardiac rehabilitation program, or to any of its components, can be extremely difficult. Among the factors that influence participation and adherence are physician referral, reimbursement issues, distance and availability of transportation, and social support.[2,24]

An exercise program is an integral part of a cardiac rehabilitation program. It includes activities such as walking, swimming, and bicycling. These exercises involve changes in muscle length and rhythmic contractions of muscle groups. Most exercise programs are individually designed to meet each person's physical and psychological needs. The goal of the exercise program is to increase the maximal oxygen consumption by the muscle tissues, so that these persons are able to perform more work at a lower heart rate and blood pressure.[2,24]

In addition to exercise, cardiac risk factor modification incorporates strategies for smoking cessation, weight loss, stress reduction, and control of hypertension and diabetes (when present). Nutrition counselling has direct effects on weight, serum lipids, blood pressure, diabetes, and other factors. The choice of diet is based on beneficial effect, as well as the social and cultural needs of the patient. Dietary patterns are assessed and specific goals determined and communicated with the patient.[2] Cardiac rehabilitation programs should include an assessment of psychosocial problems, such as depression, anxiety, and social isolation. Behavioural therapy, such as stress management skills and individual or group counselling, can be provided, or referrals made to other experts.

Chronic Ischemic Heart Disease

Myocardial ischemia occurs when the ability of the coronary arteries to supply blood is inadequate to meet the metabolic demands of the heart. Limitations in coronary blood flow most commonly are the result of atherosclerosis, but vasospasm may serve as an initiating or contributing factor.[2] There are several types of chronic ischemic coronary artery disease: chronic stable angina, variant or vasospastic angina, and chest pain with normal coronary angiography. Silent myocardial ischemia can occur with either chronic stable angina or vasospastic angina.

Stable Angina

The classic chronic stable angina is associated with a fixed coronary obstruction that produces a disparity between coronary blood flow and metabolic demands of the myocardium. Stable angina is the initial manifestation of ischemic heart disease in approximately half of persons with CAD. Although most persons with stable angina have atherosclerotic heart disease, angina does not develop in a considerable number of persons with advanced coronary atherosclerosis. This probably is because of their sedentary lifestyle, the development of adequate collateral circulation, or the inability of these persons to perceive pain. In many instances, MI occurs without a history of angina.

FIGURE 24.14 • Areas of pain due to angina.

Angina pectoris usually is precipitated by situations that increase the work demands of the heart, such as physical exertion, exposure to cold, and emotional stress. The pain is typically described as a constricting, squeezing, or suffocating sensation. It usually is steady, increasing in intensity only at the onset and end of the attack. The pain of angina commonly is located in the precordial or substernal area of the chest; it is similar to MI in that it may radiate to the left shoulder, jaw, arm, or other areas of the chest (Fig. 24.14). In some persons, the arm or shoulder pain may be confused with arthritis; in others, epigastric pain is confused with indigestion. Angina commonly is categorized according to whether it occurs with exercise, occurs during rest, is of new onset, or is of increasing severity.

Typically, chronic stable angina is provoked by exertion or emotional stress and relieved within minutes by rest or the use of nitroglycerin. A delay of more than 5 to 10 minutes before relief is obtained suggests that the symptoms are not due to ischemia or that they are due to severe ischemia. Angina that occurs at rest, is of new onset, or is increasing in intensity or duration denotes an increased risk for MI and should be evaluated using the criteria for ACS.

Microvascular Angina

Exercise-induced angina pain with normal coronary angiography is called *microvascular angina* and is synonymous with *cardiac syndrome X*. This type of provoked chest pain is usually occurs in a stable pattern and linked to small coronary artery microvascular dysfunction. While the cause remains elusive, it is thought that functional abnormalities of the coronary flow reserve even with maximal adenosine stimulation leads to inadequacies with the microcirculation. Other factors potentially linked to this type of angina includes an increase in adrenergic activity, generalized systemic endothelial dysfunction, and the role of abnormal or enhanced cardiac pain perception.[25,26]

Variant (Vasospastic) Angina

Variant angina is also known as *vasospastic* or *Prinzmetal angina*. The causes of variant angina are not completely understood, but a combination of pathologic processes may be responsible. It has been suggested that it may result from endothelial dysfunction, hyperactive sympathetic nervous system responses, defects in the handling of calcium by vascular smooth muscle, or from an alteration in nitric oxide production.[25] In some persons it is associated with hypercontractility of vascular smooth muscle and is associated with migraine headaches or Raynaud phenomenon.

Unlike stable angina that occurs with exertion or stress, variant angina usually occurs during rest or with minimal exercise and frequently occurs nocturnally (between midnight and 8 AM). Arrhythmias often occur when the pain is severe, and most persons are aware of their presence during an attack. ECG changes are significant if recorded during an attack. These abnormalities include ST-segment elevation or depression, T-wave peaking, inversion of U waves, and rhythm disturbances. Persons with variant angina who have serious arrhythmias during spontaneous episodes of pain are at a higher risk of sudden death.

Silent Myocardial Ischemia

Silent myocardial ischemia occurs in the absence of anginal pain. The factors that cause silent myocardial ischemia appear to be the same as those responsible for angina: impaired blood flow from the effects of coronary atherosclerosis or vasospasm. Silent myocardial ischemia affects three populations: persons who are asymptomatic, without knowledge or diagnosis of CAD; persons who have had an MI and continue to have episodes of silent ischemia; and persons with angina who also have episodes of silent ischemia.[2,25,27] The reason for the painless episodes of ischemia is unclear. The episodes may be shorter and involve less myocardial tissue than those producing pain. Another explanation is that persons with silent angina have defects in decreased pain threshold or pain transmission, or autonomic neuropathy with sensory denervation. There is evidence of a 50% increased prevalence of silent myocardial ischemia in persons with diabetes mellitus, probably the result of autonomic neuropathy, which is a common complication of diabetes.[28]

Diagnosis and Treatment

The diagnosis of angina is based on a detailed pain history, the presence of risk factors, invasive and noninvasive studies, and laboratory studies. Noncoronary causes of chest pain, such as esophageal reflux or musculoskeletal disorders, are ruled out.

Noninvasive testing for chronic stable angina includes ECG, echocardiography, exercise stress testing, nuclear imaging studies, CT, and possibly cardiac MRI. Because the resting ECG is often normal, exercise testing is often used in evaluating persons with angina. Ischemia that is asymptomatic at rest is detected by precipitation of typical chest pain or ST-segment changes on the ECG. Although noninvasive testing is valuable in the diagnosis of chronic stable angina, cardiac catheterization and coronary arteriography are needed for definitive diagnosis.[25–28] Serum biochemical markers for MI are normal in patients with chronic stable angina. Metabolic abnormalities are frequently detected, such as hypercholesterolemia and other dyslipidemias, carbohydrate intolerance, and insulin resistance.

Comprehensive and individualized assessment, lifestyle changes, and treatments are needed for patients with chronic stable angina. The treatment goals for stable angina are directed towards symptom reduction and prevention of MI through nonpharmacologic strategies, pharmacologic therapy, and coronary interventions. PCI relieves symptoms for patients with chronic stable angina, but does not extend the life span. CABG may be indicated in patients with double- or triple-vessel disease.[25,27,28]

Nonpharmacologic methods are aimed at symptom control and lifestyle modifications to reduce risk factors for coronary disease. They include smoking cessation in persons who smoke, stress reduction, a regular exercise program, limiting dietary intake of cholesterol and saturated fats, weight reduction if obesity is present, and avoidance of cold or other stresses that produce vasoconstriction. Immediate cessation of activity often is sufficient to abort an angina attack. Sitting down or standing quietly may be preferable to lying down, because these positions decrease preload by producing pooling of blood in the lower extremities.

The goal of pharmacologic treatment of angina is to relieve ischemia and alleviate symptoms, prevent the development of ischemic cardiomyopathy, prevent MI and death, and improve the quality of life. With ongoing myocardial dysfunction and interruption in coronary arterial blood flow, the heart can develop ischemic cardiomyopathy, which may or may not be reversed. Pharmacologic agents used in chronic stable angina include aspirin or clopidogrel, β-blockers in persons without contraindications or calcium antagonists when β-blockers are contraindicated, and ACE inhibitors in patients who also have diabetes or left ventricular systolic dysfunction (see previous discussion in section on Acute Coronary Syndrome). In patients with established CAD, including chronic stable angina, the use of lipid-lowering agents or statins is recommended, even in the presence of mild to moderate elevations of LDL cholesterol (see Chapter 22).

Nitrates, both short acting and long acting, are vasodilators used in the treatment of chronic stable angina and in silent myocardial ischemia.[2] Nitrates exert their effect mainly through a decrease in venous return to the heart with a resultant decrease in intraventricular volume. Decreased intraventricular pressure and volume are associated with decreased wall tension and myocardial oxygen requirement.

Although they are not vasodilators, β-blocking drugs are extremely useful in management of angina associated with effort. The benefits of β-blocking agents are due primarily to their hemodynamic effects—decreased heart rate, blood pressure, and myocardial contractility—which decrease myocardial oxygen requirements at rest and during exercise. The calcium channel blocking drugs, also called *calcium antagonists,* block activated and inactivated L-type calcium channels in cardiac and smooth muscles. The therapeutic effects of the calcium channel blocking agents result from coronary and peripheral artery dilation and from decreased myocardial metabolism associated with the decrease in myocardial contractility. Persons with variant angina usually respond to treatment with calcium antagonists.

IN SUMMARY

CAD is a disorder of impaired coronary blood flow, usually caused by atherosclerosis. Myocardial ischemia occurs when there is a disparity between myocardial oxygen supply and demand and can present as chronic ischemic heart disease or ACS. Diagnostic methods for CAD include ECG, exercise stress testing, nuclear imaging studies, CT, MRI, and angiographic studies in the cardiac catheterization laboratory.

The ACS, which includes UA, non-STEMI, and STEMI, results from multiple pathophysiologic processes, including unstable atherosclerotic plaques, platelet aggregation, and thrombus formation. UA is an accelerated form of angina in which the pain occurs more frequently, is more severe, and lasts longer than in chronic stable angina. MI refers to the ischemic death of myocardial tissue associated with obstructed blood flow in the coronary arteries due to plaque rupture and occlusion of blood flow. Non-STEMI and STEMI differ in terms of extent of thrombus formation, but the management is similar. The complications of MI include potentially fatal arrhythmias, heart failure and cardiogenic shock, pericarditis, thromboemboli, rupture of cardiac structures, and ventricular aneurysms. Diagnostic methods include the use of ECG monitoring and serum biomarkers. Treatment goals focus on reestablishment of myocardial blood flow through rapid reperfusion of the occluded coronary artery, prevention of clot extension through use of aspirin and other antiplatelet and antithrombotic agents, alleviation of pain, administration of oxygen, and the use of vasodilators (nitroglycerin) and β-adrenergic blocking agents to reduce the work demands on the heart.

The chronic ischemic heart diseases include chronic stable angina, microvascular angina, variant (vasospastic) angina, and silent myocardial ischemia. Chronic stable angina is associated with a fixed atherosclerotic obstruction and pain that is precipitated by increased work demands on the heart and relieved by rest. Microvascular angina usually occurs during exercise; however angiography reveals normal coronary arteries. Variant angina can result from spasms of the coronary arteries or other dysfunctions. Silent myocardial ischemia occurs without symptoms.

CONCEPTSin action**ANIMATION**

CARDIOMYOPATHIES

After completing this section of the chapter, you should be able to meet the following objectives:

- Define the term *cardiomyopathy* as it relates to both the mechanical and electrical function of the myocardium.
- Describe the role of genetics in the etiology of the primary cardiomyopathies.
- Differentiate among the pathophysiologic changes that occur with hypertrophic cardiomyopathy, arrhythmogenic right ventricular cardiomyopathy, dilated cardiomyopathies, and myocarditis.
- List four causes of secondary cardiomyopathy.
- Describe the treatment strategies of both primary and secondary cardiomyopathy.

The definition and classification of the cardiomyopathies have evolved tremendously with the advance of molecular genetics. The definition and classification of cardiomyopathies were updated in an AHA scientific statement incorporating not only the advances of cardiac molecular genetics, but other newly diagnosed diseases, as well as ion channelopathies.[29] This scientific statement defines cardiomyopathies as

a heterogeneous group of diseases of the myocardium associated with mechanical and/or electrical dysfunction that usually (but not invariably) exhibit inappropriate ventricular hypertrophy or dilatation and are due to a variety of causes that frequently are genetic. Cardiomyopathies either are confined to the heart or are part of generalized systemic disorders, often leading to cardiovascular death or progressive heart failure-related disability. (p. 1809)[29]

Based on this definition, the classification of cardiomyopathies is divided into two major groups: *primary* and *secondary.* The primary cardiomyopathies represent heart disorders that are confined to the myocardium, whereas the secondary cardiomyopathies represent myocardial changes that occur with a variety of systemic (multiorgan) disorders. Cardiomyopathies are usually associated with disorders of myocardial performance, which may be mechanical (*e.g.,* heart failure) or electrical (*e.g.,* life-threatening arrhythmias).

Primary Cardiomyopathies

The primary cardiomyopathies are classified as genetic, mixed, or acquired, based on their etiology.[29] The genetic cardiomyopathies include hypertrophic cardiomyopathy, arrhythmogenic right ventricular cardiomyopathy, left ventricular noncompaction cardiomyopathy, inherited conduction system disorders, and ion channelopathies. The mixed cardiomyopathies, which include dilated cardiomyopathy, are of both genetic and nongenetic origin. Acquired cardiomyopathies include those that have their origin in the inflammatory process (*e.g.,* myocarditis), stress ("takotsubo" pericarditis), or pregnancy (peripartum cardiomyopathy). In many cases the cause is unknown, in which case it is referred to as an *idiopathic cardiomyopathy*.

Genetic Cardiomyopathies

Hypertrophic Cardiomyopathy. Hypertrophic cardiomyopathy (HCM) is characterized by unexplained left ventricular hypertrophy (sometimes involves the right ventricle) with disproportionate thickening of the ventricular septum, abnormal diastolic filling, cardiac arrhythmias, and, in some cases, intermittent left ventricular outflow obstruction[30,31] (Fig. 24.15). It is one of the most common types of cardiomyopathy, occurring in approximately 1 person in 500 of the general population.[30] HCM is the most common cause of sudden cardiac death (SCD) in young athletes. The propensity to sudden death seems to be genetic, and implantable cardioverter defibrillators (ICDs) have proved to be lifesaving. Other complications that occur include atrial fibrillation, stroke, and heart failure.

HCM is an autosomal dominant heart disease caused by mutations in the genes encoding proteins of the cardiac sarcomere (*i.e.,* muscle fibres). Histologically, HCM appears as myocyte hypertrophy with myofibril disarray and increased cardiac fibrosis. At least 11 different genes are associated with HCM, with the β-myosin heavy chain and the myosin-binding protein C genes being the most common. More than 1,400 individual mutations have been identified and are unique from family to family. Some phenotypic correlates can be made from specific mutations; however, there are many exceptions, indicating that genetic modifiers and environmental factors are also important.[30] Although HCM is inherited, it may present

anywhere from early childhood to late adulthood with a broad category of manifestations and variable clinical course.[31]

The basic physiologic abnormalities in HCM are reduced left ventricular chamber size; poor compliance with reduced stroke volume that results from impaired diastolic filling; and, in about 25% of cases, dynamic obstruction of left ventricular outflow.[7] The majority of people with HCM are asymptomatic. Clinical manifestations may include dyspnea, chest pain during exertion, or exercise intolerance, syncope, and palpitations.[30,31] Owing to massive hypertrophy, high left ventricular chamber pressure, and potentially abnormal intramural arteries, focal myocardial ischemia often develops even in the absence of CAD; thus, angina is common. HCM is frequently associated with the development of left ventricular outflow obstructions during rest or exertion, which is caused by systolic anterior motion of the mitral valve and contact of the mitral valve with the ventricular septum. SCD and atrial fibrillation are also complications of HCM. Clinical manifestations are highly variable and may progress to end-stage heart failure with left ventricular remodelling and systolic dysfunction.[30]

Diagnosis of HCM is frequently established with 2D echocardiography, demonstrating nondilated left ventricular hypertrophy, in the absence of other cardiac or systemic diseases. ECG, continuous ambulatory monitoring, and cardiac MRI can also be helpful. The value of electrophysiologic testing remains controversial. Genetic testing, through bidirectional deoxyribonucleic acid (DNA) sequence analysis, provides accurate diagnosis and precise identification of gene mutations, although with some limitations.[7,30]

Medical management of HCM is primarily focused on symptom management. The first-line approach to relief of symptoms is pharmacologic therapy designed to block the effects of catecholamines that exacerbate outflow obstruction and to slow the heart rate to enhance diastolic filling. β-Adrenergic blockers are generally the initial choice for persons with symptomatic HCM.[31] The calcium channel blocker verapamil can also be used, but it must be used cautiously as it can exacerbate left ventricular outflow obstruction and is not recommended for persons with severe outflow obstruction and pronounced symptoms.[30] Disopyramide may be used as an alternative strategy to control symptoms as it can reduce outflow gradients at rest for some persons.[30]

In obstructive HCM that is refractory to drug therapy, septal myectomy, alcohol ablation of the interventricular septum, and dual-chamber and biventricular pacing are alternative treatment options. Atrial fibrillation is treated with pharmacologic rate control, cardioversion, and anticoagulation. An implantable cardioverter–defibrillator (ICD) should be used for persons with HCM who have sustained ventricular tachycardia or ventricular fibrillation and are receiving optimal medical therapy.[30,31] About 5% of patients develop end-stage HCM and require standard therapy for advanced heart failure, including consideration for heart transplantation.

FIGURE 24.15 • Vertical section of the heart showing (**A**) normal heart and (**B**) a heart with hypertrophic cardiomyopathy in which disproportionate thickening of intraventricular septum causes intermittent left ventricular outflow obstruction.

Arrhythmogenic Right Ventricular Cardiomyopathy/Dysplasia. Arrhythmogenic right ventricular cardiomyopathy/dysplasia

(ARVC/D) is a heart muscle disease in which fibrofatty infiltration of the right ventricular myocardium occurs causing right-sided heart failure and various rhythm disturbances, particularly ventricular tachycardia.[32,33] It ranks second, after HCM, as the leading cause of SCD in young athletes. The incidence of ARVC/D varies from about 1 in 2,000 to 1 in 5,000.[32] It is inherited as an autosomal dominant trait in greater than 50% of cases, although often with incomplete penetrance and variable expression.[32,33] Defective desmosomal proteins impacting the cell-to-cell adhesion organelles have been implicated, but the exact pathogenesis of the disorder remains unclear.

The disorder is characterized by progressive loss of myocytes, with partial or complete replacement of the right ventricular muscle with fatty or fibrofatty tissue. The disorder is associated with reentrant ventricular tachyarrhythmias of right ventricular origin that are often precipitated by exercise-induced discharge of catecholamines. Clinical manifestations include palpitations, syncope, or cardiac arrest, usually in young or middle-aged adults. Other symptoms may include abdominal pain and mental confusion.

Diagnosis of ARVC/D is based on clinical, ECG (including standard 12 lead, Holter, and signal-average ECG [SAECG]), echocardiographic, cardiac MRI, and histologic findings. Characteristic findings on 12-lead ECG include ventricular tachycardia with left bundle branch block pattern, T-wave inversion in the right precordial leads, and epsilon waves (small deflections just beyond the QRS complex). Right ventricular bundle branch block may also be present. Other diagnostic studies that may be used in assessing ARVC/D include electrophysiologic studies, and right ventricular angiography. Clinical history noting personal and family history, including first- and second-degree relatives, is important.

Treatment for ARVC/D is aimed at prevention of SCD. Although ARVC/D cannot be cured, the goal of treatment is to control the arrhythmias with antiarrhythmic agents.[32,33] Combinations of various antiarrhythmic agents are often used. Radiofrequency ablation is used in drug-refractory cases, although it is completely successful in only 30% to 65% of cases, with multiple ablations sometimes needed. ICD placement is also indicated for drug-refractory cases and for those who have survived an SCD episode. ICD placement for others is debatable because no risk stratification system exists. Final options for treatment include ventriculotomy and heart transplantation.

Left Ventricular Noncompaction. Left ventricular noncompaction, also known as *spongy myocardium,* is a primary congenital cardiomyopathy that is thought to develop because of abnormal embryogenesis in which there is failure of trabecular compaction in the developing myocardium. The disorder may be isolated or associated with other congenital heart diseases.[34] Both familial and nonfamilial cases of left ventricular noncompaction have been identified, and mutations of several genes have been reported.[34]

Signs and symptoms are primarily related to arrhythmias, embolic events, and heart failure. Diagnosis is made primarily with 2D and colour echocardiography, but cardiac MRI or left ventricular angiography may also be helpful.[34] Treatment focuses on preventing symptoms of heart failure, arrhythmias, and systemic embolic events.

Ion Channelopathies. Ion channels are pore-forming proteins that provide pathways for movement of ions across cell membranes (see Chapter 4). Diseases caused by mutations in genes encoding ion channel subunits or proteins are called *ion channelopathies.*[29] In the heart, these ion channel disorders include the long QT syndrome (LQTS), short QT syndrome (SQTS), Brugada syndrome, and catecholaminergic polymorphic ventricular tachycardia (CPVT).

LQTS and SQTS are caused by sodium or potassium ion channel gene mutations. LQTS, which is probably the most common of the ion channelopathies, is identified on 12-lead ECG by a prolonged QT interval. It causes a polymorphic ventricular tachycardia known as *torsade de pointes* (discussed in Chapter 25). First described in 2000, the SQTS is characterized by short QT interval (<330 milliseconds) on the ECG, which can lead to ventricular tachycardia or fibrillation and SCD.[29]

Brugada syndrome was originally described in 1992 as a clinical entity related to a sodium channel gene mutation. It is associated with SCD in young people, particularly young Southeast Asian men who experience SCD during sleep. The disorder is characterized on ECG by right bundle branch block and ST-segment elevation in the anterior pericardial leads.[29] CPVT is caused by an abnormal receptor that regulates calcium release from the sarcoplasmic reticulum. It is triggered by vigorous physical activity or acute emotion, and leads to syncope, polymorphic ventricular tachycardia, and SCD. The resting ECG is usually normal.[29]

Mixed (Genetic and Nongenetic) Cardiomyopathies

Dilated Cardiomyopathy. Dilated cardiomyopathy (DCM), previously referred to as congestive cardiomyopathy, is a common cause of heart failure and the leading indication for heart transplantation. In 20% to 50% of cases, DCM is reported as familial and caused by inherited genetic abnormalities; that proportion may be even higher, as incomplete penetrance often makes it difficult to identify early or latent disease in family members.[7] Most familial cases appear to be transmitted as an autosomal dominant trait, but autosomal recessive, X-linked recessive, and mitochondrial inheritance patterns have been identified. Excessive alcohol consumption of longer than 10 years is a major risk factor for the development of DCM.[31] Other causes include infections (*i.e.,* viral, bacterial, fungal, mycobacterial, parasitic), toxins, long-term cocaine use, chemotherapeutic agents, metals, and multiple other disorders. Often no cause is found, in which case it is often referred to as *idiopathic DCM.*[7,35]

DCM is characterized by a flabby, hypocontracting heart with ventricular enlargement, a reduction in ventricular wall thickness, and impaired systolic function of one or both ventricles (Fig. 24.16). Histologically, DCM is characterized by

FIGURE 24.16 • Idiopathic dilated cardiomyopathy. A transverse section of the enlarged heart reveals conspicuous dilation of both ventricles. Although the ventricular wall appears thinned, the increased mass of the heart indicates considerable hypertrophy. (From Rubin R., Strayer D. S. (Eds.). (2012). *Rubin's pathology: Clinicopathologic foundations of medicine* (6th ed., p. 525). Philadelphia, PA: Lippincott Williams & Wilkins.)

atrophic and hypertrophic myocardial fibres and interstitial fibrosis. Cardiac myocytes, particularly those in the subendocardium, often show advanced degenerative changes. Interstitial fibrosis is present, also most prominently in the subendocardial zone. Scattered inflammatory cells may be present.

The most common clinical manifestations of DCM are those related to heart failure, such as dyspnea, orthopnea, and reduced exercise capacity. In the end stages, persons with DCM often have ejection fractions of less than 25% (normal is approximately 50% to 60%).[7] As the disease progresses, stasis of blood in the walls of the heart chambers can lead to thrombus formation and systemic emboli. Secondary mitral valve regurgitation and abnormal cardiac rhythms are common. Death is usually due to heart failure or arrhythmias, and can occur suddenly.

The treatment of DCM is directed towards relieving the symptoms of heart failure and reducing the work of the heart. Pharmacologic agents include diuretics to reduce preload, β-blockers to reduce heart rate and myocardial oxygen demand, afterload-reducing agents to improve contractility and decrease left ventricular filling pressures, and ACE inhibitors to prevent vasoconstriction. Anticoagulants to prevent thrombus formation and antiarrhythmics may also be used. Other treatments may include a biventricular pacemaker (cardiac resynchronisation therapy), an ICD, ventricular restoration surgery, and in cases that are refractory to treatment, cardiac transplantation.[35] Removing or avoiding causative agents (if identified); avoiding myocardial depressants, including alcohol; and pacing rest with asymptomatic levels of exercise or activity are also important.

Primary Restrictive Cardiomyopathy. Restrictive cardiomyopathy is a rare form of heart muscle disease in which ventricular filling is restricted because of excessive rigidity of the ventricular walls, although the contractile properties

of the heart remain relatively normal.[7] On examination, the ventricles appear normal or small with thickened walls and the atria are enlarged.[31] Restrictive cardiomyopathy can be idiopathic or associated with distinct diseases that affect the myocardium, principally radiation fibrosis, amyloidosis, sarcoidosis, or metastatic tumours. Genetics may also play a role because familial forms of restrictive cardiomyopathy have been reported.[29]

Symptoms of restrictive cardiomyopathy include dyspnea, paroxysmal nocturnal dyspnea, orthopnea, peripheral edema, ascites, fatigue, and weakness. The manifestations of restrictive cardiomyopathy resemble those of constrictive pericarditis. In the advanced form of the disease, all the signs of heart failure are present except cardiomegaly. The focus of treatment is on volume control to avoid overload of the ventricles, plus prevention of aggregating factors such as arrhythmias, hypertension, and ischemia.[31]

Acquired Cardiomyopathies

Myocarditis (Inflammatory Cardiomyopathy). Myocarditis can be defined simply as "an inflammation of the heart muscle," but the classification, diagnosis, and treatment are complex.[7,36] Clinical findings can vary greatly, from nonspecific symptoms, such as fever, myalgias, or exertional dyspnea, to hemodynamic collapse and sudden death. The incidence and prevalence of myocarditis have been difficult to ascertain because of the wide variation in clinical presentation.

Although there are a number of etiologies associated with myocarditis, in North America it is usually caused by a viral infection, commonly an enterovirus (coxsackievirus group B), adenovirus, and parvovirus B19.[7,35,36] Other etiologies include bacterial or fungal infections, hypersensitivity to certain drugs, and autoimmune diseases, such as systemic lupus erythematosus. Chagas cardiomyopathy is caused by the protozoan *Trypanosoma cruzi*. Although it is more commonly associated with endemic areas such as Mexico and Latin American countries, the incidence in other countries is changing. Myocarditis is a frequent pathologic cardiac finding in persons with acquired immunodeficiency syndrome (AIDS), although it is unclear whether it is due to the human immunodeficiency virus infection itself or to a secondary infection.

Acute viral myocarditis appears to progress through three phases: the acute viral infection, autoimmune activation, and ongoing myocardial injury, resulting in DCM.[37,38] The three phases present with varying clinical manifestations and varying indications for treatment. Phases 1 and 2 produce inflammatory responses to the initial viral infection. However, activation of the immune system in response to virus-specific antigens can also illicit inflammatory responses by the host, independent of the initial viral infection, which can lead to tissue damage in the host organism. As leukocytes, lymphocytes, and macrophages penetrate the myocardium, interstitial edema and focal myocyte necrosis lead to replacement fibrosis.[7] It has been suggested that autoreactive T cells and host-generated cytokines, including tumour necrosis factor-α (TNFα), interleukin-1, and interleukin-6, may play prominent roles in the myocardial changes that occur with myocarditis.[37] Some cases of myocarditis progress to phase 3, which is characterized by ongoing myocardial injury that ultimately results in acute or chronic DCM, severe left ventricular failure, or life-threatening arrhythmias.

The signs and symptoms of myocarditis vary from asymptomatic to cardiogenic shock. Some persons may present with fever, chills, nausea, vomiting, arthralgia, and myalgia, occurring up to 6 weeks before the diagnosis of myocarditis. Other persons may present with heart failure without antecedent symptoms. The onset of heart failure may be gradual or abrupt and fulminant. Emboli may occur because of the procoagulant effect of cytokines combined with decreased myocardial contractility. At times, the presentation may mimic ACS, with ST-segment and T-wave changes, positive cardiac markers, and regional wall motion abnormalities despite normal coronary arteries. Viral myocarditis in children or young adults is often nonspecific, with symptoms such as fever and poor eating.

Currently there are no established clinical practice guidelines to direct the diagnosis and treatment. Due to the wide variety of etiologies, histology, immunohistology and clinical presentations of myocarditis, specific criteria or guidelines used in the past are no longer adequate.[38]

Endomyocardial biopsy findings, obtained through cardiac catheterization, remain the gold standard for establishing the diagnosis of acute myocarditis, despite limited accuracy.[38] Other diagnostic methods include the use of serum cardiac biomarkers (*i.e.,* TnI, TnT, CK-MB), serum inflammation markers (*i.e.,* CRP, ESR), antimyosin antibodies, and immunohistochemical staining. Echocardiography is usually performed in the initial evaluation of suspected myocarditis, although the findings can be nonspecific. Cardiac MRI is a sensitive noninvasive test for confirmation of acute myocarditis.[38]

Many cases of myocarditis are mild and self-limiting, so first-line treatment remains largely supportive.[36–38] Initial treatments include supplemental oxygen, bed rest, and antibiotics, if needed. In persons with more severe myocarditis, hemodynamic support with vasopressors and positive inotropic agents may be needed. ACE inhibitors, β-blockers, and spironolactone (an aldosterone antagonist) may be used to prevent further clinical deterioration in persons with DCM due to myocarditis.[38] An ICD should be considered for those with documented life-threatening arrhythmias. Biventricular involvement usually indicates poorer prognosis. Immunosuppressive therapy continues to be investigated as a treatment for myocarditis.

Peripartum Cardiomyopathy. Peripartum cardiomyopathy is a rare heart muscle disorder that occurs during the last trimester of pregnancy or in the first 6 months of the postpartum period. This disorder is rare in Canada, but in other countries, such as South Africa and Haiti, it is more common. Although the etiology of peripartum cardiomyopathy is unknown, several causes have been proposed including infectious, immunologic, nutritional, drug-induced, and genetic factors. Some women exhibit inflammatory cells in heart biopsies taken during the symptomatic phase of the disorder, suggesting a disordered immune response.

Diagnosis of peripartum cardiomyopathy can be challenging because symptoms that can occur normally in late pregnancy are similar to the early signs of heart failure. The European Society of Cardiology in 2010 classified this as nonfamilial, nongenetic form of DCM heart failure due to left ventricular systolic dysfunction towards the end of pregnancy or in the months following delivery, where no identifiable cause of heart failure exists.[39,40]

Management of peripartum cardiomyopathy includes standard therapy for heart failure. However, potential teratogenic effects and excretion of drugs during breast-feeding need to be considered. Prognosis depends on resolution of the heart failure. About half of women with peripartum cardiomyopathy spontaneously recover normal cardiac function; the other half are left with persistent left ventricular dysfunction or progress to overt heart failure and early death.[39]

Stress or Takotsubo Cardiomyopathy. Stress cardiomyopathy was first described in Japan, where most cases have occurred, although cases have been described in the United States.[31,41] In Japan, it was called *tako-tsubo* after the fishing pot with a narrow neck and wide base used to trap octopus. The term *transient left ventricular apical ballooning* has also been used to describe this syndrome.

Stress or takotsubo cardiomyopathy has been identified in the clinical setting as a transient, reversible left ventricular dysfunction in response to profound psychological or emotional stress. The syndrome occurs primarily in middle-aged women who present with acute STEMI, but who, on cardiac catheterization, have no evidence of CAD. There is, however, impaired myocardial contractility characterized by apical ballooning of the left ventricle with hypercontractility of the basal left ventricle.

The mechanism for myocardial stunning in stress cardiomyopathy is unclear, although some theories suggest ischemia from coronary artery spasm, microvascular spasm, or direct myocyte injury. When catecholamine levels return to normal, the interventricular gradient resolves and left ventricular function recovers.[41] Treatment is the same as that for heart failure, and most patients demonstrate rapid improvement and an excellent prognosis.

Secondary Cardiomyopathies

Secondary cardiomyopathy is a heart muscle disease in the presence of a multisystem disorder. There are numerous conditions reported to involve the myocardium (Chart 24.2). Some of these disorders produce accumulation of abnormal substances between myocytes (extracellular), whereas others produce accumulation of abnormal substances within myocytes (intracellular).

Almost 100 distinct myocardial diseases can result in the clinical features of DCM. They include cardiomyopathies associated with drugs, diabetes mellitus, muscular dystrophy,

CHART 24.2   CONDITIONS ASSOCIATED WITH SECONDARY CARDIOMYOPATHIES[a]

Autoimmune Disorders
Systemic lupus erythematosus
Rheumatoid arthritis
Scleroderma
Polyarteritis nodosa

Endocrine Disorders
Acromegaly
Diabetes mellitus
Hypothyroidism and hyperthyroidism
Hyperparathyroidism
Obesity

Familial Storage Diseases
Glycogen storage disease
Mucopolysaccharidoses
Hemochromatosis

Infiltrative Disorders
Amyloidosis
Sarcoidosis
Radiation-induced fibrosis

Neuromuscular/Neurologic Disorders
Friedreich ataxia
Muscular dystrophy
Neurofibromatosis

Nutritional Deficiencies
Thiamine (beriberi)
Protein (kwashiorkor)

Toxins
Alcohol and its metabolites
Arsenic
Cancer chemotherapeutic agents (anthracyclines
    [doxorubicin, daunorubicin], cyclophosphamide)
Catecholamines
Hydrocarbons
Cocaine

[a]Not intended to be inclusive.

autoimmune disorders, and cancer treatment agents (radiation and cancer drugs).[31] Alcoholic cardiomyopathy is the single most common identifiable cause of DCM in North America and Europe. Doxorubicin (Adriamycin) and other anthracycline drugs, used in the treatment of cancer, are potent agents whose usefulness is limited by cumulative dose-dependent cardiac toxicity. Another cancer chemotherapeutic agent with cardiotoxic potential is cyclophosphamide (Cytoxan). Unlike the primary myocyte injury that occurs with doxorubicin, the principal insult with cyclophosphamide appears to be vascular, leading to myocardial hemorrhage.

IN SUMMARY

The cardiomyopathies involve both mechanical and electrical etiologies of myocardial dysfunction. They are currently identified as either primary or secondary cardiomyopathies, based on genetic or other organ system involvement. Symptoms related to most cardiomyopathies, whether primary or secondary, are those associated with heart failure and SCD. Treatments are related to symptom management and prevention of lethal arrhythmias.

The primary cardiomyopathies include genetic, mixed, or acquired types. The genetic cardiomyopathies include hypertrophic cardiomyopathy, arrhythmogenic right ventricular cardiomyopathy, left ventricular noncompaction cardiomyopathy, inherited conduction system disorders, and ion channelopathies. The mixed cardiomyopathies, which include DCM, are of both genetic and acquired origin. Acquired cardiomyopathies include those that have their origin in the inflammatory process (*e.g.,* myocarditis), stress (takotsubo pericarditis), or pregnancy (peripartum cardiomyopathy). In many cases the cause is unknown, in which case it is referred to as an idiopathic cardiomyopathy.

The secondary cardiomyopathies are heart diseases in which myocardial involvement occurs as part of a generalized systemic (multiorgan) disorder. They include cardiomyopathies associated with drugs, diabetes mellitus, muscular dystrophy, autoimmune disorders, and cancer treatment agents (radiation and chemotherapeutic drugs).

INFECTIOUS AND IMMUNOLOGIC DISORDERS

After completing this section of the chapter, you should be able to meet the following objectives:

- Distinguish between the roles of infectious organisms and the immune system in infective endocarditis and rheumatic fever.
- Describe the relation between the infective vegetations associated with infective endocarditis and the extracardiac manifestations of the disease.
- Describe the long-term effects of rheumatic fever and primary and secondary prevention strategies for rheumatic fever and rheumatic heart disease.

Infective Endocarditis

Infective endocarditis (IE) is a serious and potentially life-threatening infection of the inner surface of the heart. It is characterized by colonization or invasion of the heart valves and the mural endocardium by a microbial agent, leading to the formation of bulky, friable vegetations and destruction of underlying cardiac tissues.[7]

The incidence, demographics, and characteristics of IE have changed over the past decade. The classic picture of a person with pre-existing rheumatic heart disease and community-associated bacteremia no longer represents the majority of cases of IE. More common causes now are mitral valve prolapse, congenital heart disease, prosthetic heart valves, and contaminated implantable devices such as pacemakers and defibrillators. Neutropenia, immunodeficiency, malignancy, therapeutic immunosuppression, diabetes, hemodialysis, and alcohol or intravenous drug use are predisposing factors.[7] Infections of intracardiac, arterial, and venous devices are nosocomially acquired in medical centres throughout the developed world.[42]

Traditionally, IE has been classified on clinical grounds into acute or subacute–chronic forms, depending on the onset, etiology, and severity of the disease.[42] Usually, the onset of acute cases is rapid and involves patients with normal cardiac valves who are either healthy and perhaps have a history of intravenous drug use, or are debilitated. Subacute–chronic cases evolve over months; these patients usually have valve abnormalities. The development of drug-resistant strains of microorganisms due to the indiscriminate use of antibiotics and an increase in the number of immunocompromised persons have made classification of acute and subacute–chronic cases more difficult.[42]

Etiology and Pathogenesis

Staphylococcal infections have now emerged as the leading cause of IE, and together with streptococci accounts for 80% of cases of infective endocarditis.[42] Other causative agents include the so-called HACEK group (*Haemophilus* species, *Actinobacillus actinomycetemcomitans*, *Cardiobacterium hominis*, *Eikenella corrodens*, and *Kingella kingae*), gram-negative bacilli, and fungi.[7,42] The causative agents differ somewhat in the major high-risk groups. For example, *Staphylococcus aureus* is the major offender in intravenous drug abusers, whereas prosthetic heart valve IE tends to be caused by coagulase-negative staphylococci (*e.g., Staphylococcus epidermidis*).[7] Foremost among the factors leading to the development of IE is seeding of the blood with microbes. The portal of entry into the bloodstream may be an obvious infection, a dental or surgical procedure that causes transient bacteremia, injection of a contaminated substance directly into the blood by intravenous drug users, or an occult source in the oral cavity, gut, or a trivial injury.[7] Endothelial injury, bacteremia, and altered hemodynamics can all incite the formation of a fibrin–platelet thrombus along the endothelial lining. The thrombus is susceptible to bacterial seeding from transient bacteremia, causing continued monocyte activation and cytokine and tissue factor production. This results in progressive enlargement of infected valvular vegetations.

In both acute and subacute–chronic forms of IE, friable, bulky, and potentially destructive vegetative lesions form on the heart valves (Fig. 24.17). The aortic and mitral valves are the most common sites of infection, although the right heart valves may also be involved, particularly in intravenous drug abusers. These vegetative lesions consist of a collection

FIGURE 24.17 • Bacterial endocarditis. The mitral valve shows destructive vegetations, which have eroded through the free margin of the valve leaflet. (From Rubin R., Strayer D. S. (Eds.). (2012). *Rubin's pathology: Clinicopathologic foundations of medicine* (6th ed., p. 516). Philadelphia, PA: Lippincott Williams & Wilkins.)

of infectious organisms and cellular debris enmeshed in the fibrin strands of clotted blood. The lesions may be singular or multiple, may grow as large as several centimetres, and usually are found loosely attached to the free edges of the valve surface.[7] The infectious loci continuously release bacteria into the bloodstream and are a source of persistent bacteremia. As the lesions grow, they cause valve destruction, leading to valvular regurgitation, ring abscesses with heart block, pericarditis, aneurysm, and valve perforation.

The intracardiac vegetative lesions also have local and distant systemic effects.[7] The loose organization of these lesions permits the organisms and fragments of the lesions to form emboli and travel in the bloodstream, causing cerebral, systemic, or pulmonary emboli. The fragments may lodge in small blood vessels, causing small hemorrhages, abscesses, and infarction of tissue. The bacteremia also can initiate immune responses thought to be responsible for skin manifestations, polyarthritis, glomerulonephritis, and other immune disorders. Other complications from IE include heart failure, periannular extension of the infection, and mycotic aneurysms.

Clinical Features

Signs and symptoms of IE can include fever and signs of systemic infection (*e.g.,* positive blood cultures), anemia, change in the character of an existing heart murmur, and evidence of embolic distribution of the vegetative lesions.[42] In the acute form, the fever usually is spiking and accompanied by chills. In the subacute form, the fever usually is low grade, of gradual onset, and frequently accompanied by other systemic signs of inflammation, such as anorexia, malaise, and lethargy. Small petechial hemorrhages frequently result when emboli lodge in the small vessels of the skin, nail beds, and mucous membranes. Splinter hemorrhages (*i.e.,* dark red lines) under the nails of the fingers and toes are common. Cough, dyspnea, chest pain, blindness, paralysis, arthralgia or arthritis, diarrhea, and abdominal or flank pain may occur as the result of systemic emboli.[2,7,42]

Diagnosis. Infective endocarditis continues to pose major challenges in diagnosis and treatment, despite advances in its epidemiology and microbiology. The diagnosis of IE cannot be made through any single test, but rather includes the use of clinical assessment, laboratory (*e.g.*, WBC, C-Reactive protein, serum immunoglobulin, rheumatoid factor, blood cultures), and echocardiographic features.[2,7,42] The Duke criteria, which were modified by a committee of the AHA in 2005, provide healthcare professionals with a standardized assessment for persons with suspected IE that integrates blood culture evidence of infection, echocardiographic findings, clinical findings, and laboratory information.[42] The modified Duke criteria are classified into major criteria (positive blood culture for IE, evidence of endocardial involvement) and minor criteria (predisposition to IE, predisposing heart condition, or intravenous drug use; fever with a temperature greater than 38°C; vascular phenomena such as evidence of arterial emboli; immunologic phenomena such as glomerulonephritis; microbiologic evidence such as blood culture that does not meet major criteria). Cases are classified as "definite" if they fulfill two major criteria, one major criterion plus two minor criteria, or five minor criteria. Cases are defined as "possible" if they fulfill one major criterion and one minor criterion, or three minor criteria. Diagnosis of IE is rejected if an alternative diagnosis is made, the infection resolves with antibiotic treatment in 4 days or less, or there is no histologic evidence of infection.[42]

The blood culture remains the most definitive diagnostic procedure and is essential to guide treatment. Three separate sets of blood cultures from three separate venipuncture sites should be obtained within 24 hours. However, the indiscriminate use of antibiotics has made identifying the causative organism much more difficult. The modified Duke criteria recommend the inclusion of *S. aureus* as a major criterion, whether it is a nosocomial or a community-acquired infection. Serologic testing for *Coxiella burnetii*, *Chlamydia psittaci*, and *Bartonella* species should be considered if previous blood cultures are negative.[42] Negative blood cultures can occur delaying diagnosis and treatment and having a profound effect on outcome. This can occur because of prior antibiotic administration, or because the causative organisms are slow growing, require special culture media, or are not readily cultured.

Echocardiography is the primary technique for detection of vegetations and cardiac complications resulting from IE, and is an important tool in the diagnosis and management of disease. Echocardiographic evidence of endocardial involvement is now the major criterion in the modified Duke criteria. It is recommended that echocardiography be performed in all suspected cases of IE.

Treatment. Treatment of IE focuses on identifying and eliminating the causative microorganism, minimizing the residual cardiac effects, and treating the pathologic effect of emboli. The choice of antimicrobial therapy depends on the organism cultured and whether it occurs in a native or prosthetic valve. *S. aureus*, the most common cause of IE, is primarily the result of nosocomial infections from intravascular catheters, surgical wounds, and indwelling prosthetic devices. Guidelines for the prevention and management of nonvalvular cardiovascular device–related infections are presented in the literature.[42] The widespread emergence of multidrug-resistant organisms, including *S. aureus*, poses a serious challenge in the treatment of IE. In addition to antibiotic therapy, surgery may be needed for unresolved infection, severe heart failure, and significant emboli.

The majority of persons with IE are cured with medical or surgical treatment. Persons who have had infectious endocarditis should be educated about its signs and symptoms and informed of the possibility of relapse or recurrence. Immediate medical attention should be sought if signs or symptoms recur. Prevention of IE through the use of prophylactic antibiotics is controversial. The current recommendations conclude that only a very small number of persons with IE cases require antibiotic prophylaxis for dental procedures. Therefore, prophylaxis for dental procedures such as manipulation of gingival tissue or periapical region of teeth, and perforation of the oral mucosa is recommended only for persons with previous IE, congenital heart disease (*e.g.*, unrepaired cyanotic congenital heart disease including shunts and conduits), or prosthetic cardiac valves, as well as heart transplant recipients with valvulopathy. Treatment is not recommended based solely on an increased lifetime risk of acquiring IE.[43,44]

Prophylactic antibiotics may also be recommended to prevent wound infection in persons with high risk who have infections in the gastrointestinal or genitourinary tract. Persons who have enterococcal urinary tract infection and who are undergoing elective urinary tract manipulation (*e.g.*, cystoscopy) may also benefit from prophylactic antibiotics.[43]

Rheumatic Heart Disease

Rheumatic fever (RF) and rheumatic heart disease (RHD) are complications of the immune-mediated response to group A (β-hemolytic) streptococcal (GAS) throat infection.[7,45] The most serious aspect of RF is the development of chronic valvular disorders that produce permanent cardiac dysfunction and sometimes cause fatal heart failure years later. Although RF and RHD are rare in developed countries, they still exist in remote northern communities in Canada and continue to be major health problems in underdeveloped countries, where inadequate health care, poor nutrition, and crowded living conditions still prevail.[45,46]

Pathogenesis

β-Hemolytic streptococci are divided into several serologic groups based on their cell wall polysaccharide antigen. Group A is further subdivided into more than 130 distinct M types, which are responsible for the vast majority of infections. The M protein best defines the virulence of the bacterium, and has been studied most intensively with regard to cross-reactivity with heart tissue.[7] Although GAS causes both pharyngitis and skin (impetigo) infections, only the pharyngitis has been linked with RF and RHD.

The pathogenesis of RF is unclear. The time frame for development of symptoms in relation to the sore throat and the presence of antibodies to GAS strongly suggests an immunologic origin.[7,45] It is thought that antibodies directed against the M protein of certain strains of streptococci cross-react with glycoprotein antigens in the heart, joints, and other tissues to produce an autoimmune response through a phenomenon called *molecular mimicry* (see Chapter 19). The onset of symptoms 2 to 3 weeks after infection and the absence of streptococci in the lesion support this belief. Although only a small percentage of persons with untreated GAS pharyngitis develop RF, the incidence of recurrence with a subsequent untreated infection is substantially greater. These observations and more recent studies suggest a genetic predisposition to development of the disease.[7,45]

Clinical Features

Rheumatic fever can manifest as an acute, recurrent, or chronic disorder. The *acute stage* of RF includes a history of an initiating streptococcal infection and subsequent involvement of the connective tissue elements of the heart, blood vessels, joints, and subcutaneous tissues. Common to all is a lesion called the *Aschoff body*,[7] which is a localized area of tissue necrosis surrounded by immune cells. The *recurrent phase* usually involves extension of the cardiac effects of the disease. The *chronic phase* of RF is characterized by permanent deformity of the heart valves and is a common cause of mitral valve stenosis. Chronic RHD usually does not appear until at least 10 years after the initial attack, sometimes decades later.

Most persons with RF have a history of sore throat, headache, fever, abdominal pain, nausea, vomiting, swollen glands (usually at the angle of the jaw), and other signs and symptoms of streptococcal infection. Other clinical features associated with an acute episode of RF are related to the acute inflammatory process and the structures involved in the disease process. The course of the disease is characterized by a constellation of findings that includes migratory polyarthritis of the large joints, carditis, erythema marginatum, subcutaneous nodules, and Sydenham chorea.[7,45] Laboratory markers of acute inflammation include an elevated white blood cell count, ESR, and CRP. These elevated levels of acute-phase reactants are not specific for RF but provide evidence of an acute inflammatory response.

Polyarthritis. Polyarthritis is the most common, and frequently the first, manifestation of RF.[45] It may be the only major criterion in adolescents and adults. The arthritis, which may range from arthralgia to disabling arthritis, most often involves the larger joints, particularly the knees and ankles, and occurs less frequently in the wrists, elbows, shoulders, and hips. It is almost always migratory, affecting one joint and then moving to another. Untreated, the arthritis lasts approximately 4 weeks. A striking feature of rheumatic arthritis is the dramatic response (usually within 48 hours) to salicylates. Arthritis usually heals completely and leaves no functional residua.

Carditis. Acute rheumatic carditis, which complicates the acute phase of RF, can affect the endocardium, myocardium, or pericardium. Usually all three layers are involved. Both the pericarditis and myocarditis usually are self-limited manifestations of the acute stage of RF. The involvement of the endocardium and valvular structures produces the permanent and disabling effects of RF. Although any of the four valves can be involved, the mitral then the aortic valves are affected most often. During the acute inflammatory stage of the disease, the valvular structures become red and swollen, and small vegetative lesions develop on the valve leaflets. The acute inflammatory changes gradually proceed to development of fibrous scar tissue, which tends to contract and cause deformity of the valve leaflets and shortening of the chordae tendineae. In some cases, the edges or commissures of the valve leaflets fuse together as healing occurs.

Clinical features of endocarditis/valvulitis, without a history of RHD, include the presence of an apical holosystolic murmur of mitral regurgitation or a basal early diastolic murmur of aortic regurgitation. In someone with a history of RHD, a change in the character of these murmurs or a new murmur would indicate acute rheumatic carditis. In patients with recurrent carditis and a history of RHD, the condition is sometimes difficult to distinguish from acute endocarditis.

Subcutaneous Nodules, Erythema Marginatum, and Sydenham Chorea. *Subcutaneous nodules* are hard, painless, and freely movable and usually occur over the extensor muscles of the wrist, elbow, ankle, and knee joints, ranging in size from 0.5 to 2 cm. Subcutaneous nodules rarely occur alone in RF and occur most often in association with carditis.

Erythema marginatum lesions are maplike, macular areas most commonly seen on the trunk or inner aspects of the upper arm and thigh, but never on the face. They occur early in the course of a rheumatic attack and tend to occur with subcutaneous nodules as well as carditis. They are transitory and disappear during the course of the disease.

Sydenham chorea is the major central nervous system manifestation of RF. It is seen most frequently in young girls and rarely occurs after 20 years of age. There typically is an insidious onset of irritability and other behaviour problems. The child often is fidgety, cries easily, begins to walk clumsily, and drops things. The choreiform movements are spontaneous, rapid, purposeless, jerking movements that interfere with voluntary activities. Facial grimaces are common, and even speech may be affected. The chorea is self-limited, usually running its course within a matter of weeks or months, but recurrences are not uncommon. A previous streptococcal infection can be detected only in about two thirds of cases, making differential diagnosis more difficult.

Diagnosis. There are no specific laboratory tests that can establish a diagnosis of RF. Because of the variety of signs and symptoms, the Jones criteria for the diagnosis of RF, which were first proposed in 1944 and have undergone multiple reviews by the AHA and the World Health Organization (WHO), are designed to assist in standardizing the diagnosis of RF.[56,57] The Jones criteria divide the clinical features of RF into major and minor categories, based on prevalence and specificity. The presence of two major signs (*i.e.,* carditis, polyarthritis, chorea, erythema marginatum, or subcutaneous nodules) or one major and two minor signs (*i.e.,* arthralgia, fever, and elevated ESR, CRP, or leukocyte count), accompanied by evidence of a preceding GAS infection, indicates a high probability of RF. The latest review, in 2004 by the WHO, added the diagnostic categories of primary episode of RF, recurrent attacks of RF with or without RHD, rheumatic chorea, insidious onset of rheumatic carditis, and chronic RHD to inform the criteria.[48] The epidemiologic setting in which the diagnosis of RF is made is also considered important.

The use of echocardiography has enhanced the understanding of both acute and chronic RHD. It is useful in assessing the severity of valvular stenosis and regurgitation, chamber size and ventricular function, and the presence and size of pleural effusions. Doppler ultrasonography may be useful in identifying cardiac lesions in persons who do not show typical signs of cardiac involvement during an attack of RF, but these are not considered either a major or minor Jones criterion at this time.[47,49]

Treatment and Prevention. It is important that streptococcal infections be promptly diagnosed and treated to prevent RF. The gold standard for detecting a streptococcal infection is throat culture. However, it takes 24 to 48 hours to produce a result, delaying treatment. The development of rapid tests for direct detection of GAS antigens has provided at least a partial solution for this problem. Both the throat culture and the rapid antigen tests are highly specific for GAS infection but are limited in terms of their sensitivity (*e.g.,* the person may have a negative test result but have a streptococcal infection). A negative antigen test result should be confirmed with a throat culture when a streptococcal infection is suspected. The presence of GAS in the upper respiratory tract can indicate either a carrier or infectious state, the latter of which can be defined by a rising antibody response. Serologic examinations for streptococcal antibodies (antistreptolysin O and antideoxyribonuclease B) are measured for retrospective confirmation of recent streptococcal infections in persons thought to have acute RF. There is, however, no single specific laboratory test result that is pathognomonic for acute or recurrent RF.

Treatment of acute RF is designed to control the acute inflammatory response and prevent cardiac complications and recurrence of the disease. During the acute phase, antibiotics, anti-inflammatory drugs, and selective restriction of activities are prescribed. No clinical isolate of GAS is resistant to penicillin; therefore, penicillin, or another antibiotic in penicillin-sensitive patients, is the treatment of choice for GAS infection.[45] First-generation cephalosporins have also been given successfully. Salicylates and corticosteroids can be used to suppress the inflammatory response, but should not be given until the diagnosis of RF is confirmed. Surgery is indicated for chronic rheumatic valve disease, and is determined by the severity of the symptom or evidence that cardiac function is

significantly impaired. Procedures used include closed mitral commissurotomy, valve repair, and valve replacement.

The person who has had an attack of RF is at high risk for recurrence after subsequent GAS throat infections. Penicillin is the treatment of choice for secondary prophylaxis, but sulfadiazine or erythromycin may be used in penicillin-allergic individuals. The duration of prophylaxis depends on whether residual valvular disease is present or absent. It is recommended that persons with persistent valvular disease receive prophylaxis for at least 5 years after the last episode of acute RF or until the age of 21 years. Compliance with a plan for prophylactic administration of penicillin requires that the person and his or her family understand the rationale for such measures. They also need to be instructed to report possible streptococcal infections to their physicians and to inform their dentists about the disease so that they can be adequately protected during dental procedures that may traumatize the oral mucosa.

IN SUMMARY

Infective endocarditis involves the invasion of the endocardium by pathogens that produce vegetative lesions on the endocardial surface. The loose organization of these lesions permits the organisms and fragments of the lesions to be disseminated throughout the systemic circulation. Although several organisms can cause the condition, staphylococci have now become the leading cause of IE. Treatment of IE focuses on identifying and eliminating the causative microorganism, minimizing the residual cardiac effects, and treating the pathologic effect of emboli.

Rheumatic fever, which is associated with an antecedent GAS throat infection, is an important cause of heart disease. Its most serious and disabling effects result from involvement of the heart valves. Because there is no single laboratory test result, sign, or symptom that is pathognomonic for acute rheumatic fever, the Jones and WHO criteria are used to establish the diagnosis during the acute stage of the disease. Primary and secondary prevention strategies focus on appropriate antibiotic therapy.

VALVULAR HEART DISEASE

After completing this section of the chapter, you should be able to meet the following objectives:

- State the function of the heart valves and relate alterations in hemodynamic function of the heart that occur with valvular disease.
- Compare the effects of stenotic and regurgitant mitral and aortic valvular heart disease on cardiovascular function.
- Compare the methods of and diagnostic information obtained from cardiac auscultation and echocardiography as they relate to valvular heart disease.

The past several decades have brought remarkable advances in the treatment of and outlook for people with valvular heart disease. This is undoubtedly due to improved methods for noninvasive monitoring of ventricular function, improvement in prosthetic valves, advances in valve reconstruction procedures, and the development of useful guidelines to improve the timing of surgical interventions.[49] Nonetheless, valvular heart disease continues to produce considerable mortality and morbidity.

Hemodynamic Derangements

The function of the heart valves is to promote unidirectional flow of blood through the chambers of the heart. Dysfunction of the heart valves can result from a number of disorders, including congenital defects, trauma, ischemic damage, degenerative changes, and inflammation. Although any of the four heart valves can become diseased, the most commonly affected are the mitral and aortic valves. Disorders of the pulmonary and tricuspid valves are uncommon, probably because of the low pressure in the right side of the heart.

The heart valves consist of thin leaflets of tough, flexible, endothelium-covered fibrous tissue firmly attached at the base to the fibrous valve rings (see Chapter 21). Capillaries and smooth muscle are present at the base of the leaflet but do not extend up into the valve. The leaflets of the heart valves may be injured or become the site of an inflammatory process that can deform their line of closure. Healing of the valve leaflets often is associated with increased collagen content and scarring, causing the leaflets to shorten and become stiffer. The edges of the healing valve leaflets can fuse together so that the valve does not open or close properly.

Two types of mechanical disruptions occur with valvular heart disease: narrowing of the valve opening so it does not open properly, and distortion of the valve so it does not close properly (Fig. 24.18). *Stenosis* refers to a narrowing of the valve orifice and failure of the valve leaflets to open normally. Blood flow through a normal valve can increase by five to seven times the resting volume; consequently, valvular stenosis must be severe before it causes problems. Significant narrowing of the valve orifice increases the resistance to blood flow through the valve, converting the normally smooth laminar flow to a less efficient turbulent flow (see Chapter 21). This increases the volume and work of the chamber emptying through the narrowed valve—the left atrium in the case of mitral stenosis and the left ventricle in aortic stenosis. Symptoms usually are noticed first during situations of increased flow, such as exercise. An incompetent or regurgitant valve permits backward flow to occur when the valve should be closed—flowing back into the left ventricle during diastole when the aortic valve is affected and back into the left atrium during systole when the mitral valve is affected.

The effects of valvular heart disease on cardiac function are related to alterations in blood flow across the valve and to the resultant increase in work demands on the heart that the disorder generates. Many valvular heart defects are

A Thickened and stenotic valve leaflets   **B** Retracted fibrosed valve leaflets

FIGURE 24.18 • Disease of the aortic valve as viewed from the aorta. **A:** Stenosis of the valve opening. **B:** An incompetent or regurgitant valve that is unable to close completely.

characterized by heart murmurs resulting from turbulent blood flow through a diseased valve. Disorders in valve flow and heart chamber size for mitral and aortic valve disorders are illustrated in Figure 24.19.

Echocardiography, described earlier in the chapter, provides a means of visualizing valvular motion, patterns of flow, and closure patterns. Pulsed Doppler ultrasonography provides a semiquantitative or qualitative estimation of the severity of transvalvular gradients, right ventricular systolic pressure, and valvular regurgitation. Colour flow Doppler provides a visual pattern of flow velocities over the anatomic 2D echocardiographic image. This allows for demonstration of turbulence from stenotic and regurgitant valves.

Transesophageal echocardiography with Doppler ultrasonography is used to obtain more precise echocardiographic data when surface sound transmission is poor, particularly of the AV valves and prosthetic heart valves.

VALVULAR HEART DISEASE

- The heart valves determine the direction of blood flow through the heart chambers.
- Valvular heart defects exert their effects by obstructing flow of blood (stenotic valve disorders) or allowing backward flow of blood (regurgitant valve disorders).
- Stenotic valvular defects produce distension of the heart chamber that empties blood through the diseased valve and impaired filling of the chamber that receives blood that moves through the valve.
- Regurgitant valves allow blood to move back through the valve when it should be closed. This produces distension and places increased work demands on the chamber ejecting blood through the diseased valve.

Mitral Valve Disorders

The mitral valve controls the directional flow of blood between the left atrium and the left ventricle. The edges or cusps of the AV valves are thinner than those of the semilunar valves; they are anchored to the papillary muscles by the

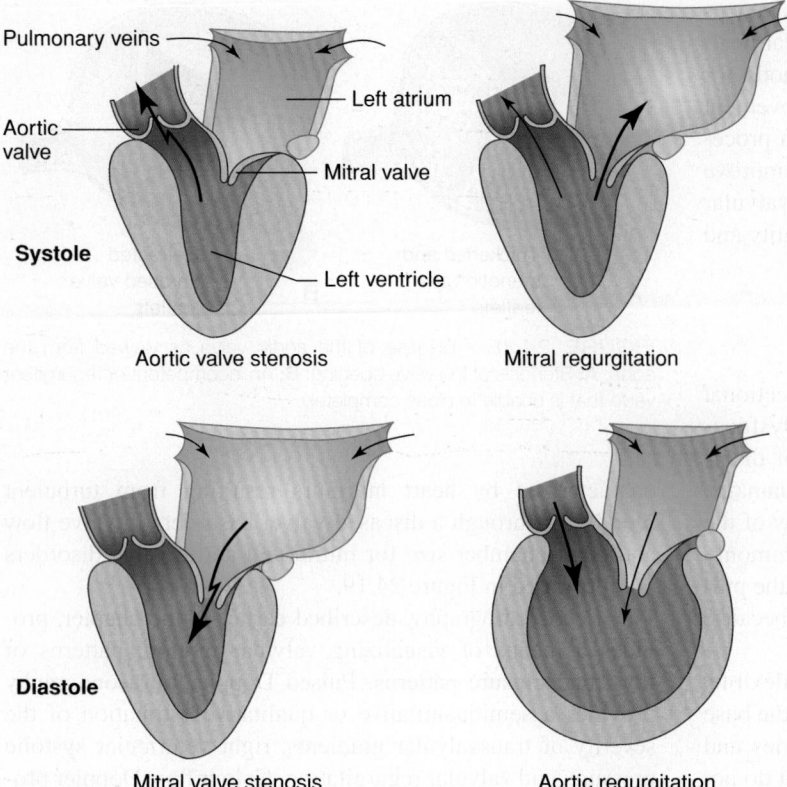

Systole

Pulmonary veins

Aortic valve

Left atrium

Mitral valve

Left ventricle

Aortic valve stenosis

Mitral regurgitation

Diastole

Mitral valve stenosis

Aortic regurgitation

FIGURE 24.19 • Alterations in hemodynamic function that accompany aortic valve stenosis, mitral valve regurgitation, mitral valve stenosis, and aortic valve regurgitation. The *thin arrows* indicate direction of normal flow, and *thick arrows* the direction of abnormal flow.

chordae tendineae. During much of systole, the mitral valve is subjected to the high pressure generated by the left ventricle as it pumps blood into the systemic circulation. During this period of increased pressure, the chordae tendineae prevent the eversion of the valve leaflets into the left atrium.

Mitral Valve Stenosis

Mitral valve stenosis represents the incomplete opening of the mitral valve during diastole, resulting in left atrial distension and impaired filling of the left ventricle. Mitral valve stenosis most commonly is the result of RF.[49,50] Less frequently, the defect is congenital and manifests during infancy or early childhood. Mitral valve stenosis is a continuous, progressive, lifelong disorder consisting of a slow, stable course in the early years and progressive acceleration in later years.

Mitral valve stenosis is characterized by fibrous replacement of valvular tissue, along with stiffness and fusion of the valve apparatus (Fig. 24.20). Typically, the mitral cusps fuse at the edges and involvement of the chordae tendineae causes shortening, which pulls the valvular structures more deeply into the ventricles. As the resistance to flow through the valve increases, the left atrium becomes dilated and left atrial pressure rises. The increased left atrial pressure eventually is transmitted to the pulmonary venous system, causing pulmonary congestion.

The rate of flow across the valve depends on the size of the valve orifice, the driving pressure (*i.e.,* atrial minus ventricular pressure), and the time available for flow during diastole. The normal mitral valve area is 4 to 6 cm². Narrowing

of the valve area to less than 2 cm² must occur before mild symptoms begin to develop.[50] As the condition progresses, symptoms of decreased cardiac output occur during extreme exertion or other situations that cause tachycardia and thereby reduce diastolic filling time. In the late stages of the disease, pulmonary vascular resistance increases with the development of pulmonary hypertension; this increases the pressure against

FIGURE 24.20 • Chronic rheumatic valvulitis. A view of the mitral valve from the left atrium shows rigid, thickened, and fused leaflets with a narrow orifice, creating the characteristic "fish mouth" appearance of rheumatic mitral stenosis. (From Rubin R., Strayer D. S. (Eds.). (2012). *Rubin's pathology: Clinicopathologic foundations of medicine* (6th ed., p. 513). Philadelphia, PA: Lippincott Williams & Wilkins.)

which the right heart must pump and eventually leads to right-sided heart failure.

The signs and symptoms of mitral valve stenosis depend on the severity of the obstruction and are related to the elevation in left atrial pressure and pulmonary congestion, decreased cardiac output owing to impaired left ventricular filling, and left atrial enlargement with development of atrial arrhythmias and mural thrombi. The symptoms are those of pulmonary congestion, including nocturnal paroxysmal dyspnea and orthopnea. Palpitations, chest pain, weakness, and fatigue are common complaints.

Premature atrial beats, paroxysmal atrial tachycardia, and atrial fibrillation may occur as a result of distension of the left atrium. Fibrosis of the internodal and interatrial tracts, along with damage to the SA node, may occur from the rheumatic process itself. Atrial fibrillation develops in 40% to 75% of persons with symptomatic mitral stenosis.[50] Together, the fibrillation and distension predispose to mural thrombus formation. The risk of arterial embolization, particularly stroke, is significantly increased in persons with atrial fibrillation.

The murmur of mitral valve stenosis is heard during diastole when blood is flowing through the constricted valve orifice; it is characteristically a low-pitched, rumbling murmur, best heard at the apex of the heart. The first heart sound often is accentuated and somewhat delayed because of the increased left atrial pressure; an opening snap may precede the diastolic murmur as a result of the elevation in left atrial pressure. The 2D and Doppler echocardiograms are most commonly used to diagnose mitral stenosis. These echocardiograms confirm the diagnosis of mitral stenosis, evaluate mitral valve morphology and hemodynamics, and measure pulmonary artery pressures. They also rule out other causes of mitral stenosis and assist in identifying the most appropriate treatment.

Medical treatment of mitral valve stenosis is aimed at relieving signs of decreased cardiac output and pulmonary congestion. In atrial fibrillation, the goals are to control ventricular rate and prevent systemic embolization with anticoagulation therapy. Antibiotic prophylaxis against recurrent RF is recommended. Surgical interventions, including commissurotomy, balloon valvotomy, and valve repair or replacement, may be used to treat degenerative and functional mitral valve disease and, in some cases, IE.[49,50]

Mitral valve commissurotomy can be performed percutaneously with a balloon catheter or surgically through a left thoracotomy. These procedures open the commissures that were fused by scar tissue, decreasing the gradient and increasing the valve area, and, as a result, improve clinical symptoms.[50] Mechanical or biologic prostheses can be used for mitral valve replacement. Because of the risk of thromboembolism, persons with mechanical prostheses usually require indefinite anticoagulation therapy.

Mitral Valve Regurgitation

Mitral valve regurgitation is characterized by incomplete closure of the mitral valve, with the left ventricular stroke volume being divided between the forward stroke volume that moves into the aorta and the regurgitant stroke volume that moves back into the left atrium during systole (Fig. 24.19). Mitral valve regurgitation can result from many processes. RHD is associated with a rigid and thickened valve that does not open or close completely. In addition to RHD, mitral regurgitation can result from rupture of the chordae tendineae or papillary muscles, papillary muscle dysfunction, or stretching of the valve structures due to dilation of the left ventricle or valve orifice. Mitral valve prolapse is a common cause of mitral valve regurgitation.

Acute mitral valve regurgitation may occur abruptly, such as with papillary muscle dysfunction after MI, valve perforation in IE, or ruptured chordae tendineae in mitral valve prolapse. In acute severe mitral regurgitation, acute volume overload increases left ventricular preload, allowing a modest increase in left ventricular stroke volume. However, the forward stroke volume (that moving through the aorta into the systemic circulation) is reduced and the regurgitant stroke volume leads to a rapid rise in left atrial pressure and pulmonary edema. Acute mitral valve regurgitation almost always is symptomatic; if severe, mitral valve replacement often is indicated.

The hemodynamic changes associated with chronic mitral valve regurgitation occur more slowly, allowing for recruitment of compensatory mechanisms. An increase in left ventricular end-diastolic volume permits an increase in total stroke volume, with restoration of forward flow into the aorta. Augmented preload and reduced or normal afterload (provided by unloading the left ventricle into the left atrium) facilitates left ventricular ejection. At the same time, a gradual increase in left atrial size allows for accommodation of the regurgitant volume at a lower filling pressure.

The increased volume work associated with mitral regurgitation is relatively well tolerated, and many persons with the disorder remain asymptomatic for many years, only developing symptoms between 6 and 10 years after diagnosis. The degree of left ventricular enlargement reflects the severity of regurgitation. As the disorder progresses, left ventricular function becomes impaired, the forward (aortic) stroke volume decreases, and the left atrial pressure increases, with the subsequent development of pulmonary congestion. Surgery should be performed before the onset of these symptoms.

A characteristic feature of mitral valve regurgitation is an enlarged left ventricle, a hyperdynamic left ventricular impulse, and a pansystolic (throughout systole) murmur. Mitral regurgitation, like mitral stenosis, predisposes to atrial fibrillation.

The 2D Doppler echocardiogram is useful in mitral regurgitation to evaluate left ventricular and atrial size, measure the ejection fraction, and assist in decision making regarding surgery through assessment of the severity of the regurgitation. In some patients with mitral regurgitation, preload reduction can be beneficial and may be treated with ACE inhibitors and biventricular pacing. Surgeries used in the treatment of mitral regurgitation include mitral valve repair and valve replacement with or without removal of the mitral apparatus. Mitral valve repair avoids the use of anticoagulation needed with artificial valves. Conservation of the mitral apparatus is always the goal in mitral valve replacement because it ensures competence of the mitral valve and preserves left ventricular function.

Mitral Valve Prolapse

Sometimes referred to as the *floppy mitral valve syndrome,* mitral valve prolapse occurs in 2% to 3% of the general population.[51] Familial mitral valve prolapse is transmitted as an autosomal trait, and several chromosomal loci have been identified. Although the exact cause of the disorder usually is unknown, it has been associated with Marfan syndrome, osteogenesis imperfecta, and other connective tissue disorders, and with cardiac, hematologic, neuroendocrine, metabolic, and psychological disorders.

Pathologic findings in persons with mitral valve prolapse include a myxedematous (mucinous) degeneration of mitral valve leaflets that causes them to become enlarged and floppy so that they prolapse or balloon back into the left atrium during systole[51] (Fig. 24.21). Secondary fibrotic changes reflect the stresses and injury that the ballooning movements impose on the valve. Certain forms of mitral valve prolapse may arise from disorders of the myocardium that place undue stress on the mitral valve because of abnormal movement of the ventricular wall or papillary muscle. Mitral valve prolapse may or may not cause mitral regurgitation.

Most persons with mitral valve prolapse are asymptomatic and the disorder is discovered during a routine physical examination, such as prenatal visits for young women. A minority of people have chest pain mimicking angina, dyspnea, fatigue, anxiety, palpitations, or lightheadedness. Unlike angina due to coronary artery disease, the chest pain often is prolonged, ill defined, and not associated with exercise or exertion. The pain has been attributed to ischemia resulting from traction of the prolapsing valve leaflets. The anxiety, palpitations, and arrhythmias may result from abnormal autonomic nervous system function that commonly accompanies the disorder. Rare cases of sudden death have been reported for persons with mitral valve prolapse, mainly those with a family history of similar occurrences.

The disorder is characterized by a spectrum of auscultatory findings, ranging from a silent form to one or more midsystolic clicks followed by a late systolic or holosystolic murmur. The clicks are caused by the sudden tensing of the mitral valve apparatus as the leaflets prolapse. Two-dimensional and Doppler echocardiography are valuable noninvasive studies used to diagnose mitral valve prolapse.

The treatment of mitral valve prolapse focuses on the relief of symptoms and the prevention of complications.[51] Persons with palpitations and mild tachyarrhythmias or increased adrenergic symptoms, and those with chest discomfort, anxiety, and fatigue often respond to therapy with the β-adrenergic blocking drugs. In many cases, the cessation of stimulants such as caffeine, alcohol, and cigarettes may be sufficient to control symptoms. IE is an uncommon complication in persons with a murmur; antibiotic prophylaxis are no longer recommended before dental or surgical procedures. Transient ischemic attacks occur more frequently in persons with mitral valve prolapse. Therefore, in persons with documented events who are in sinus rhythm with no atrial thrombi, daily aspirin therapy is recommended. Most persons with mitral valve prolapse are encouraged to participate in regular exercise and lead a normal life. Persons with severe valve dysfunction may require valve surgery.

Aortic Valve Disorders

The aortic valve is located between the left ventricle and the aorta. The aortic valve has three cusps and sometimes is referred to as the *aortic semilunar valve* because its leaflets are crescent or moon shaped (see Chapter 21, Fig. 21.9). The aortic valve has no chordae tendineae. Although their structures are similar, the cusps of the aortic valve are thicker than those of the mitral valve. The middle layer of the aortic valve is thickened near the middle, where the three leaflets meet, ensuring a tight seal. Between the thickened tissue and their free margins, the leaflets are more thin and flimsy.

An important aspect of the aortic valve is the location of the orifices for the two main coronary arteries, which are located behind the valve and at right angles to the direction of blood flow. It is the lateral pressure in the aorta that propels blood into the coronary arteries. During the ejection phase of the cardiac cycle, the lateral pressure is diminished by conversion of potential energy to kinetic energy as blood moves forward into the aorta. This process is grossly exaggerated in aortic valve stenosis because of the high flow velocities.

Aortic Valve Stenosis

Aortic valve stenosis, often referred to simply as *aortic stenosis,* is characterized by increased resistance to ejection of

FIGURE 24.21 • Mitral valve prolapse. A view of the mitral valve from the left atrium shows redundant and deformed leaflets that billow into the left atrial cavity. (From Rubin R., Strayer D. S. (Eds.). (2012). *Rubin's pathology: Clinicopathologic foundations of medicine* (6th ed., p. 518). Philadelphia, PA: Lippincott Williams & Wilkins.)

blood from the left ventricle into the aorta (Fig. 24.19). The most common causes of aortic valve stenosis are congenital valve malformations and acquired calcification of a normal tricuspid valve. Congenital malformations may result in unicuspid, bicuspid, or misshaped valve leaflets. Acquired aortic stenosis is usually the consequence of calcification associated with the normal "wear and tear" of either a previously normal aortic valve or congenitally bicuspid valves (with which approximately 1% of the population are born).[7] The incidence of acquired aortic valve stenosis is increasing with the rising average age of the population.[7]

The progression of calcific aortic stenosis is usually slow and varies widely among individuals. Valve changes range from mild thickening without obstruction to severe calcification with impaired leaflet motion and obstructed left ventricular outflow.[49] Processes in the development of calcific aortic valve disease have been shown to be similar to those in CAD. Both conditions are more common in men, older persons, and persons with hypercholesteremia; and both derive in part from an active inflammatory process.[49] Early lesions of aortic sclerosis show focal subendothelial plaquelike lesions, similar to the initial phases of an atherosclerotic lesion. Aortic sclerosis is distinguished from aortic stenosis by the degree of valve impairment. In aortic sclerosis the valve leaflets are abnormally thickened, but the obstruction to outflow is minimal, whereas in aortic stenosis the functional area of the valve has decreased enough to cause measurable obstruction to outflow. Calcification of the aortic valve progresses from the base of the cusps to the leaflets. This reduces leaflet motion and effective valve area, but without commissural fusion. As calcification progresses, the leaflets become more rigid, there is worsening obstruction to left ventricular outflow, and fusion of the commissures leads to aortic stenosis.

Because aortic stenosis develops gradually, the left ventricle has time to adapt. With increased systolic pressure from obstruction, the left ventricular wall becomes thicker, or hypertrophies, but a normal chamber volume is maintained. This increase in wall thickness can maintain a normal ejection fraction. Little hemodynamic disturbance occurs as the valve area is reduced by half its normal area (from a normal 3 to 4 cm^2 to 1.5 to 2 cm^2). However, an additional reduction in valve area from one half to one fourth of its normal size produces severe obstruction to flow and a progressive pressure overload on the left ventricle. At this point, the increased work of the heart begins to exceed the coronary blood flow reserve, causing both systolic and diastolic dysfunction and signs of heart failure.[49]

Aortic stenosis is usually first diagnosed with auscultation of a loud systolic ejection murmur or a single or paradoxically split second heart sound. Eventually, the classic symptoms of angina, syncope, and heart failure develop, although more subtle signs of a decrease in exercise tolerance or exertional dyspnea should be monitored closely. Angina occurs in approximately two thirds of persons with advanced aortic stenosis and is similar to that observed in CAD. Dyspnea, marked fatigability, peripheral cyanosis, and other signs of low-output heart failure usually are not prominent until late in the course

of the disease. Syncope (fainting) is most commonly due to the reduced cerebral circulation that occurs during exertion, when the arterial pressure declines consequent to vasodilation in the presence of a fixed cardiac output.

Echocardiography can be used to evaluate the severity and progression of calcified aortic lesions, left ventricular size and function, degree of ventricular hypertrophy, and presence of associated valve disorders, and plays a major part in decision making for aortic valve replacement.

There is no effective medical therapy for severe aortic stenosis, although statins and ACE inhibitors have been associated with delaying disease progression. In children with congenital aortic stenosis, the valve leaflets are merely fused and balloon valvulotomy may provide substantial benefit. However for all ages, valve replacement is the most effective treatment. Medical interventions are prescribed to relieve symptoms of heart failure for those patients who are ineligible for surgical intervention.

Aortic Valve Regurgitation

Aortic valve regurgitation (or *aortic regurgitation*) is the result of an incompetent aortic valve that allows blood to flow back to the left ventricle during diastole (Fig. 24.19). As a result, the left ventricle must increase its stroke volume to include blood entering from the lungs as well as that leaking back through the regurgitant valve. This defect may result from conditions that cause scarring of the valve leaflets or from enlargement of the valve orifice to the extent that the valve leaflets no longer meet. There are various causes of aortic regurgitation, including RF, idiopathic dilation of the aorta, congenital abnormalities, IE, and Marfan syndrome. Other causes include hypertension, trauma, and failure of a prosthetic valve.

Acute aortic regurgitation is characterized by the presentation of a sudden, large regurgitant volume to a left ventricle of normal size that has not had time to adapt to the volume overload. It is caused most commonly by disorders such as IE, trauma, or aortic dissection. Although the heart responds with use of the Frank–Starling mechanisms and an increase in heart rate, these compensatory mechanisms fail to maintain the cardiac output. As a result, there is severe elevation in left ventricular end-diastolic pressure, which is transmitted to the left atrium and pulmonary veins, culminating in pulmonary edema. A decrease in cardiac output leads to sympathetic stimulation and a resultant increase in heart rate and peripheral vascular resistance that cause the regurgitation to worsen. Death from pulmonary edema, ventricular arrhythmias, or circulatory collapse is common in severe acute aortic regurgitation.

Chronic aortic regurgitation, which usually has a gradual onset, represents a condition of combined left ventricular volume and pressure overload. As the valve deformity increases, regurgitant flow into the left ventricle increases, diastolic blood pressure falls, and the left ventricle progressively enlarges. Hemodynamically, the increase in left ventricular volume results in the ejection of a large stroke volume that usually is adequate to maintain the forward cardiac output until late in the course of the disease. Most persons remain asymptomatic during this compensated phase, which may last decades. The only sign for many years may be a soft systolic aortic murmur.

As the disease progresses, signs and symptoms of left ventricular failure begin to appear. These include exertional dyspnea, orthopnea, and paroxysmal nocturnal dyspnea. In aortic regurgitation, failure of aortic valve closure during diastole causes an abnormal drop in diastolic pressure. Because coronary blood flow is greatest during diastole, the drop in diastolic pressure produces a decrease in coronary perfusion. Although angina is rare, it may occur when the heart rate and diastolic pressure fall to low levels. Persons with severe aortic regurgitation often complain of an uncomfortable awareness of heartbeat, particularly when lying down, and chest discomfort due to pounding of the heart against the chest wall. Tachycardia, occurring with emotional stress or exertion, may produce palpitations, head pounding, and premature ventricular contractions.

The major physical findings relate to the widening of the arterial pulse pressure. Korotkoff sounds may persist to zero, even though intra-arterial pressure rarely falls below 30 mm Hg. The pulse has a rapid rise and fall (Corrigan pulse), with an elevated systolic pressure and low diastolic pressure owing to the large stroke volume and rapid diastolic runoff of blood back into the left ventricle.[58] The large stroke volume and wide pulse pressure may result in prominent carotid pulsations in the neck, head bobbing (de Musset sign), throbbing peripheral pulses, and a left ventricular impulse that causes the chest to move with each beat. The hyperkinetic pulse of more severe aortic regurgitation, called a *water-hammer pulse,* is characterized by distension and quick collapse of the artery. The turbulence of flow across the aortic valve during diastole produces a high-pitched or blowing sound.

The treatment for acute or severe chronic aortic regurgitation is aortic valve replacement. Surgery is recommended whenever patients are symptomatic, regardless of left ventricular function. In asymptomatic patients, valve replacement is controversial. However, in patients with left ventricular systolic dysfunction or with severe left ventricular dilation, valve replacement is also recommended, even if patients are asymptomatic.[49]

The goal of medical therapy is to improve forward stroke volume and reduce regurgitant volume, usually through the use of vasodilator therapy. This is indicated in symptomatic patients with severe aortic regurgitation when surgery is not recommended, or for short-term therapy to improve the hemodynamics of a patient preparing for valve replacement.[49]

IN SUMMARY

Dysfunction of the heart valves can result from a number of disorders, including congenital defects, trauma, ischemic heart disease, degenerative changes, and inflammation. Rheumatic endocarditis is a common cause. Valvular heart disease produces its effects through disturbances of blood flow. A stenotic valvular defect is one that causes a decrease in blood flow through a valve, resulting in impaired emptying and increased work demands on the heart chamber that empties blood across the diseased valve. A regurgitant valvular defect permits the blood flow to continue when the valve is closed. Valvular heart disorders produce blood flow turbulence and often are detected through cardiac auscultation.

HEART DISEASE IN INFANTS AND CHILDREN

After completing this section of the chapter, you should be able to meet the following objectives:

- Trace the flow of blood in the fetal circulation, state the function of the foramen ovale and ductus arteriosus, and describe the changes in circulatory function that occur at birth.
- Compare the effects of left-to-right and right-to-left shunts on the pulmonary circulation and production of cyanosis.
- Describe the anatomic defects and altered patterns of blood flow in children with atrial septal defects, ventricular septal defects, endocardial cushion defects, pulmonary stenosis, tetralogy of Fallot, patent ductus arteriosus, transposition of the great vessels, coarctation of the aorta, and single-ventricle anatomy.
- Describe the prevalence of the condition and issues of concern for adults with congenital heart disease.
- Describe the manifestations related to the acute, subacute, and convalescent phases of Kawasaki disease.

Congenital heart defects (CHDs) are present in about 1% of live births, making this the most common form of structural birth defect.[2,52] Compared to 60 years ago when fewer than 20% of infants with cardiac malformations reached adulthood, today with advances in diagnostic methods and surgical treatment more than 90% are expected to survive into adulthood. Surgical correction of most defects is now possible, often within the first weeks of life.

Although thousands of infants born each year will have a congenital heart disease, other children will develop an acquired heart disease, including Kawasaki disease. Two other acquired disorders that affect children, the cardiomyopathies and RF, were discussed earlier in the chapter.

Embryonic Development of the Heart

The heart is the first functioning organ in the embryo; its first pulsatile movements begin during the third week after conception. This early development of the heart is essential to the rapidly growing embryo as a means of circulating nutrients and removing waste products. Most of the development of the

22 ± 1 day   **23 ± 1 day**   **24 ± 1 day**

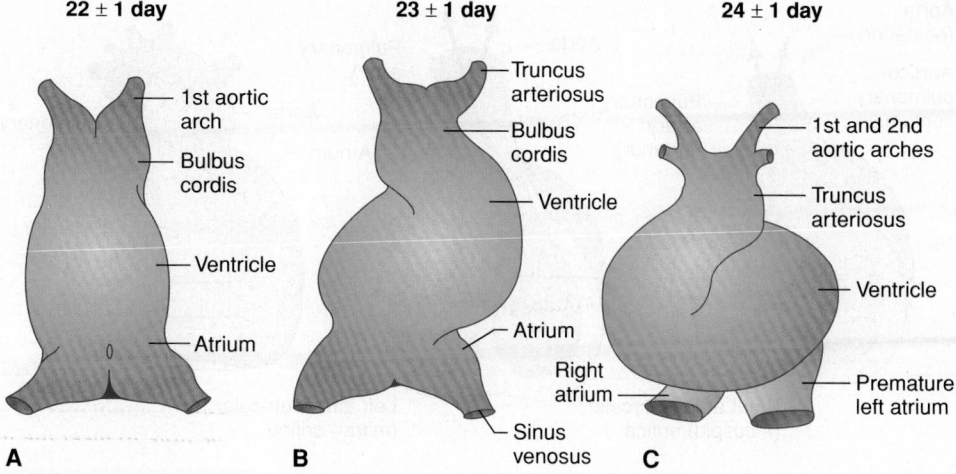

FIGURE 24.22 • Ventral view of the developing heart. **A:** Fusion of the heart tubes to form a single tube, it is at this stage that the heart begins to beat. **B:** Cardiac looping, in which the heart begins to bend ventrally and to the right, bringing the primitive ventricle leftward and in continuity with the sinus venosus (future left and right atria), with the future right ventricle being shifted rightward and in continuity with the bulbus cordis (future aorta and pulmonary artery), and **(C)** folding is complete. (Adapted from Moore K. L. (1977). *The developing human* (2nd ed.). Philadelphia, PA: W.B. Saunders.)

heart and blood vessels occurs between the third and eighth weeks of embryonic life.[53]

The developing heart begins as two endothelial tubes that fuse into a single tubular structure.[53] The early heart structures develop as the tubular heart elongates and forms alternating dilations and constrictions. A single atrium and ventricle along with the bulbus cordis develop first (Fig. 24.22). This is followed by formation of the truncus arteriosus and the sinus venosus, a large venous sinus that receives blood from the embryo and developing placenta. The early pulsatile movements of the heart begin in the sinus venosus and move blood out of the heart by way of the bulbus cordis, truncus arteriosus, and aortic arches.

A differential growth rate in the early cardiac structures, along with fixation of the heart at the venous and arterial ends, causes the tubular heart to bend over on itself. As the heart bends, the atrium and the sinus venosus come to lie behind the bulbus cordis, truncus arteriosus, and ventricle. This looping of the primitive heart results in the heart's alignment in the left side of the chest with the atrium located behind the ventricle. Malrotation during formation of the ventricular loop can cause various malpositions, such as dextroposition of the heart.

The embryonic heart undergoes further development as partitioning of the chambers occurs. Partitioning of the AV canal, atrium, and ventricle begins in the fourth week and essentially is completed by the fifth week. Septation of the heart begins as tissue bundles called the *endocardial cushions* form in the mid-portion of the dorsal and ventral walls of the heart in the region of the AV canal and begin to grow inward. Until septation begins, a single AV canal exists between the atria and the ventricles. As the endocardial cushions enlarge, they meet and fuse to form separate right and left AV canals (Fig. 24.23). The mitral and tricuspid valves develop in these canals. The endocardial cushions also contribute to formation of parts of the atrial and ventricular septa. Defects in endocardial cushion formation can result in atrial and ventricular septal defects, complete AV canal defects, and anomalies of the mitral and tricuspid valves.

Compartmentalization of the ventricles begins with the growth of the interventricular septum from the floor of the

ventricle moving upward towards the endocardial cushions. Fusion of the endocardial cushions with the interventricular septum usually is completed by the end of the seventh week.

Partitioning of the atrial septum is more complex and occurs in two stages, beginning with the formation of a thin, crescent-shaped membrane called the *septum primum* that emerges from the anterosuperior portion of the heart and grows towards the endocardial cushions, leaving an opening called the *foramen primum* between its lower edge and the endocardial cushions. A second membrane, called *septum secundum,* also begins to grow from the upper wall of the atrium on the right side of the septum primum. As this membrane grows towards the endocardial cushions, it gradually overlaps an opening in the upper part of the septum primum, forming an oval opening with a flap-type valve called the *foramen ovale* (Fig. 24.23). The upper part of the septum primum gradually disappears, with the remaining part becoming the

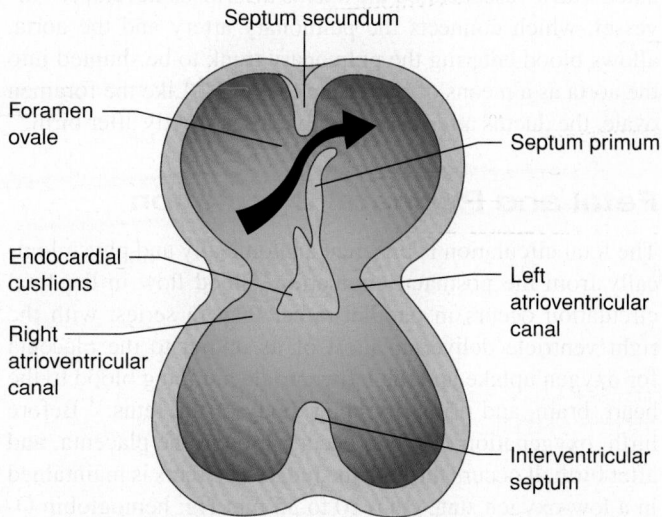

FIGURE 24.23 • Development of the endocardial cushions, right and left atrioventricular canals, interventricular septum, and septum primum and septum secundum of the foramen ovale. Note that blood from the right atrium flows through the foramen ovale to the left atrium.

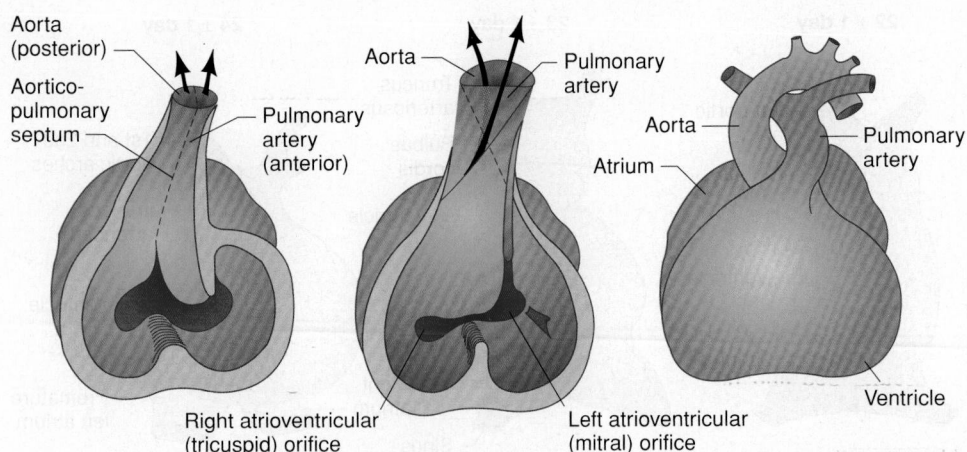

FIGURE 24.24 • Separation and twisting of the truncus arteriosus to form the pulmonary artery and aorta.

valve of the foramen ovale. The foramen ovale forms a communicating channel between the two upper chambers of the heart. This opening, which typically closes shortly after birth, allows blood from the umbilical vein to pass directly into the left heart, bypassing the lungs.

To complete the transformation into a four-chambered heart, provision must be made for separating the blood pumped from the right side of the heart, which is to be diverted into the pulmonary circulation, from the blood pumped from the left side of the heart, which is to be pumped to the systemic circulation. This separation of blood flow is accomplished by developmental changes in the outflow channels of the tubular heart, the *bulbus cordis* and the *truncus arteriosus*, which undergo spiral twisting and vertical partitioning (Fig. 24.24). As these vessels spiral and divide, the aorta takes up position posterior to and to the right of the pulmonary artery. Impaired spiralling during this stage of development can lead to defects such as *transposition of the great vessels.*

In the process of forming a separate pulmonary trunk and aorta, a vessel called the *ductus arteriosus* develops. This vessel, which connects the pulmonary artery and the aorta, allows blood entering the pulmonary trunk to be shunted into the aorta as a means of bypassing the lungs. Like the foramen ovale, the ductus arteriosus usually closes shortly after birth.[53]

Fetal and Perinatal Circulation

The fetal circulation is different anatomically and physiologically from the postnatal circulation. Blood flow in the fetal circulation occurs in parallel rather than in series, with the right ventricle delivering most of its output to the placenta for oxygen uptake and the left ventricle pumping blood to the heart, brain, and primarily upper body of the fetus.[54] Before birth, oxygenation of blood occurs through the placenta, and after birth, it occurs through the lungs. The fetus is maintained in a low-oxygen state (PO_2 30 to 35 mm Hg; hemoglobin O_2 saturation 60% to 70%). To compensate, fetal cardiac output is higher than at any other time in life (400 to 500 ml/kg/min) and fetal hemoglobin has a higher affinity for oxygen.[54] Also, the pulmonary vessels in the fetus are markedly constricted

because of the fluid-filled lungs and the heightened hypoxic stimulus for vasoconstriction that is present in the fetus. As a result, blood flow through the lungs is less than at any other time in life.

In the fetus, blood enters the circulation through the umbilical vein and returns to the placenta through the two umbilical arteries (Fig. 24.25). A vessel called the *ductus venosum* allows the majority of blood from the umbilical vein to bypass the hepatic circulation and pass directly into the inferior vena cava. From the inferior vena cava, blood flows into the right atrium, where approximately 40% of the blood volume moves through the foramen ovale into the left atrium. It then passes into the left ventricle and is ejected into the ascending aorta to perfuse the head and upper extremities. In this way, the best-oxygenated blood from the placenta is used to perfuse the brain. At the same time, venous blood from the

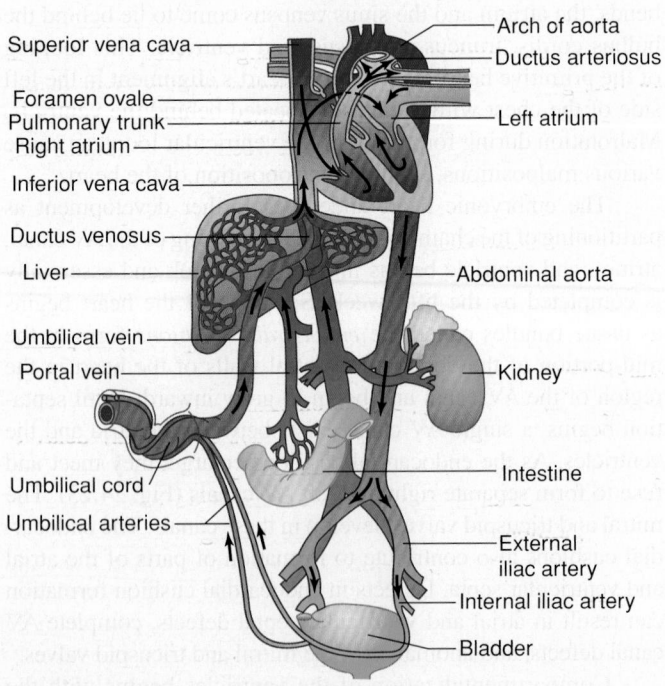

FIGURE 24.25 • Fetal circulation.

head and upper extremities returns to the right side of the heart through the superior vena cava, moves into the right ventricle, and is ejected into the pulmonary artery. Because of the very high pulmonary vascular resistance that is present, almost 90% of blood ejected into the pulmonary artery gets diverted through the ductus arteriosus into the descending aorta. This blood perfuses the lower extremities and is returned to the placenta by the umbilical arteries.

At birth, the infant takes its first breath and switches from placental to pulmonary oxygenation of the blood. The most dramatic alterations in the circulation after birth are the elimination of the low-resistance placental vascular bed and the marked pulmonary vasodilation that is produced by initiation of ventilation. Within minutes of birth, pulmonary blood flow increases from 35 ml/kg/minute to 160 to 200 ml/kg/min.[54] The pressure in the pulmonary circulation and the right side of the heart falls as fetal lung fluid is replaced by air and as lung expansion decreases the pressure transmitted to the pulmonary blood vessels. With lung inflation, the alveolar oxygen tension increases, causing reversal of the hypoxemia-induced pulmonary vasoconstriction of the fetal circulation. Cord clamping and removal of the low-resistance placental circulation produce an increase in systemic vascular resistance and a resultant increase in left ventricular pressure. The resultant decrease in right atrial pressure and increase in left atrial pressure produce closure of the foramen ovale flap valve. Reversal of the fetal hypoxemic state also produces constriction of ductal smooth muscle, contributing to closure of the ductus arteriosus. The foramen ovale and the ductus arteriosus normally close within the first day of life, effectively separating the pulmonary and systemic circulations.

After the initial precipitous fall in pulmonary vascular resistance, a more gradual decrease in pulmonary vascular resistance is related to regression of the medial smooth muscle layer in the pulmonary arteries. During the first 2 to 9 weeks of life, gradual thinning of the smooth muscle layer results in further decreases in pulmonary vascular resistance. By the time a healthy, term infant is several weeks old, the pulmonary vascular resistance has fallen to adult levels.

Several factors, including alveolar hypoxia, prematurity, lung disease, and congenital heart defects, may affect postnatal pulmonary vascular development. Alveolar hypoxia is one of the most potent stimuli of pulmonary vasoconstriction and pulmonary hypertension in the neonate. During this period, the pulmonary arteries remain highly reactive and can constrict in response to hypoxia, acidosis, hyperinflation of the alveoli, and hypothermia. Thus, hypoxia during the first days of life may delay or prevent the normal decrease in pulmonary vascular resistance.

Much of the development of the smooth muscle layer in the pulmonary arterioles occurs during late gestation; as a result, infants born prematurely have less medial smooth muscle. These infants follow the same pattern of smooth muscle regression, but because less muscle exists, the muscle layer may regress in a shorter time. The pulmonary vascular smooth muscle in premature infants also may be less responsive to hypoxia. For these reasons, a premature infant may demonstrate a larger decrease in pulmonary vascular resistance and a resultant shunting of blood from the aorta through the ductus arteriosus to the pulmonary artery within hours of birth.

Congenital Heart Defects

Congenital heart defects (CHD) affect 1% of Canadian newborns, making it the most common birth defect. There are an estimated total of 257,000 adults and children with CHD in Canada.[55]

The major development of the fetal heart occurs between the fourth and seventh weeks of gestation, and most CHDs arise during this time. Most CHDs are thought to be multifactorial in origin, resulting from an interaction between a genetic predisposition towards development of a heart defect and environmental influences.

Knowledge about the genetic basis of CHDs has grown dramatically in recent years. This area of research is particularly important as more individuals with congenital heart disease survive into adulthood and consider having children of their own. Recent knowledge suggests that the genetic contribution to congenital heart disease has been underestimated in the past.[56] Some heart defects, such as aortic stenosis, atrial septal defect of the secundum type, pulmonary valve stenosis, tetralogy of Fallot, and certain ventricular septal defects, have a stronger familial predisposition than others.

Chromosomal abnormalities are also associated with CHDs, as evidenced by the observation that as much as 20% of children with congenital heart disease have an associated chromosomal abnormality. Heart disease is found in over 90% of children with trisomy 18; 50% of those with trisomy 21; and 40% of those with Turner syndrome.[56] Other syndromes that commonly include cardiac malformations are DiGeorge syndrome (22q11 deletion), which is frequently associated with conotruncal defects such as interrupted aortic arch, truncus arteriosus, and tetralogy of Fallot; and Williams syndrome (7q11.23 microdeletion), which is associated with supravalvar aortic and pulmonary stenoses.[56]

As many as 30% of congenital cardiac defects may be attributable to identifiable and potentially modifiable risk factors, including teratogenic influences, and adverse maternal conditions such as febrile illnesses, systemic lupus erythematosus, diabetes mellitus, maternal alcohol ingestion, and treatment with anticonvulsant drugs, retinoids, lithium, and other prescription or nonprescription drugs. Periconceptive multivitamin intake with folic acid may reduce the risk of cardiac disease in the fetus.[57]

Pathophysiology

CHDs produce their effects mainly through abnormal shunting of blood, production of cyanosis, and disruption of pulmonary blood flow.

Abnormal Shunting of Blood. Shunting of blood refers to the diversion of blood flow from one system to the other—from the arterial to the venous system (*i.e.*, left-to-right shunt) or from the venous to the arterial system (*i.e.,* right-to-left shunt). The shunting of blood in CHDs is determined by the presence, position, and size of an abnormal opening between the right and left circulations and the degree of resistance to flow through the opening.

The vascular resistance of the systemic and pulmonary circulations influences the direction of shunting. Because of the high pulmonary vascular resistance in the neonate, atrial and ventricular septal defects usually do not produce significant shunt or symptoms during the first weeks of life.

As the pulmonary vascular smooth muscle regresses in the neonate, the resistance in the pulmonary circulation falls below that of the systemic circulation; in uncomplicated atrial or ventricular septal defects, blood shunts from the left side of the heart to the right. In more complicated ventricular septal defects, increased resistance to outflow may affect the pattern of shunting. For example, defects that increase resistance to aortic outflow (*e.g.,* aortic valve stenosis, coarctation of the aorta, hypoplastic left heart syndrome) increase left-to-right shunting, and defects that obstruct pulmonary outflow (*e.g.,* pulmonary valve stenosis, tetralogy of Fallot) increase right-to-left shunting. Crying, defecating, or even the stress of feeding may increase pulmonary vascular resistance and cause an increase in right-to-left shunting and cyanosis in infants with septal defects.

Cyanotic Versus Acyanotic Disorders. Congenital heart diseases are commonly divided into two categories: acyanotic and cyanotic. Defects that result in a left-to-right shunt are usually categorized as acyanotic disorders because they do not compromise oxygenation of blood in the pulmonary circulation.

Defects that produce shunting of blood from the right to the left side of the heart or result in obstruction of pulmonary blood flow are categorized as cyanotic disorders.[58,59] Cyanosis, a bluish colour of the skin, most notable in the nail beds and mucous membranes, develops when sufficient deoxygenated blood from the right side of the heart mixes with oxygenated blood in the left side of the heart. Abnormal colour becomes obvious when the oxygen saturation falls below 80% in the capillaries (equal to 50 g/L of deoxygenated hemoglobin).

A right-to-left shunt results in deoxygenated blood moving from the right side of the heart to the left side and then being ejected into the systemic circulation. With a left-to-right shunt, oxygenated blood intended for ejection into the systemic circulation is recirculated through the right side of the heart and back through the lungs. This increased volume distends the right side of the heart and pulmonary circulation and increases the workload placed on the right ventricle. A child with a defect that causes left-to-right shunting usually has an enlarged right side of the heart and pulmonary blood vessels. Of the congenital defects discussed in this chapter, patent ductus arteriosus, atrial and ventricular septal defects, endocardial cushion defects, pulmonary valve stenosis, and coarctation of the aorta are considered defects with little or no cyanosis; tetralogy of Fallot, transposition of the great vessels, and single-ventricle anatomy are considered defects with cyanosis.

Disruption of Pulmonary Blood Flow. Many of the complications of congenital heart disorders result from a decrease or an increase in pulmonary blood flow. Defects that reduce pulmonary blood flow (*e.g.,* pulmonary stenosis) typically cause symptoms of fatigue, dyspnea, and failure to thrive. In contrast to the arterioles in the systemic circulation, the arterioles in the pulmonary circulation are normally thin-walled vessels that can accommodate the various levels of stroke volume that are ejected from the right heart. The thinning of the pulmonary vessels occurs during the first weeks after birth, during which the vessel media thin and pulmonary vascular resistance decreases. In a term infant who has a CHD that produces markedly increased pulmonary blood flow (*e.g.,* ventricular septal defect), the increased flow stimulates pulmonary vasoconstriction and delays or reduces the normal involutional thinning of the small pulmonary arterioles. In most cases during early infancy, pulmonary vascular resistance is only slightly elevated, and the major contribution to pulmonary hypertension is the increased blood flow. However, in some infants with a large right-to-left shunt, the pulmonary vascular resistance never decreases.

CHDs that persistently increase pulmonary blood flow or pulmonary vascular resistance have the potential of causing pulmonary hypertension and producing irreversible pathologic changes in the pulmonary vasculature. When shunting of systemic blood flow into the pulmonary circulation threatens permanent injury to the pulmonary vessels, a surgical procedure should be done to reduce the flow temporarily or permanently. Pulmonary artery banding consists of placing a constrictive band around the main pulmonary artery, thereby increasing resistance to outflow from the right ventricle. The banding technique is a temporary measure to alleviate symptoms and protect the pulmonary vasculature in anticipation of later surgical repair of the defect.

Manifestations and Treatment

It is increasingly common for heart defects to be diagnosed prenatally. In this case, the infant can be evaluated shortly after birth to confirm the diagnosis and develop a treatment plan. Reliable diagnostic images of the fetal heart can be obtained as early as 16 weeks of gestation, and research using transvaginal ultrasonography is underway to view the heart even earlier. Among the disorders that can be diagnosed with certainty by fetal echocardiography are AV septal defects, hypoplastic left heart syndrome, aortic valve stenosis, hypertrophic cardiomyopathy, pulmonic valve stenosis, and transposition of the great arteries. Disorders that result in an abnormal four-chamber view, an image typically obtained during routine prenatal ultrasonography, are the most likely to be detected.

In the postnatal period, infants with CHDs may present with numerous signs and symptoms. Over 40 different types of CHDs have been described, and even individual lesions can vary along a spectrum of severity; therefore, there is no standard presentation for infants and children with congenital heart disease. Some defects, such as patent ductus arteriosus and small ventricular septal defects, close spontaneously. In other, less severe defects, there may be no obvious signs and symptoms and the disorder may be discovered during a routine health examination. Cyanosis, pulmonary congestion, cardiac failure, and decreased peripheral perfusion are the chief concerns in children with more severe defects. Such defects often cause problems immediately after birth or early in infancy. The infant may exhibit cyanosis, respiratory difficulty, and fatigability, and is likely to have difficulty with feeding and failure to thrive. A generalized cyanosis that persists longer than 3 hours after birth suggests congenital heart disease.

An oxygen challenge (administration of 100% oxygen for 5 to 10 minutes) can help to determine whether congenital heart disease is present in a cyanotic newborn. An arterial blood sample is taken during this time. If the partial pressure of oxygen (PO_2) is greater than 250 mm Hg, cyanotic heart disease can be ruled out; if the PO_2 is 160 to 250 mm Hg, heart disease is unlikely; failure of the PO_2 to rise to these levels is strongly suggestive of cyanotic heart disease.[60] Because infant cyanosis may appear as duskiness, it is important to assess the colour of the mucous membranes, fingernails, toenails, tongue, and lips. Pulmonary congestion in the infant causes an increase in respiratory rate, orthopnea, grunting, wheezing, coughing, and crackles. A chest radiograph can quickly differentiate infants who have reduced pulmonary vascular markings (densities) from those who have normal or increased markings. The infant whose peripheral perfusion is markedly decreased may be in a shocklike state.

Heart failure manifests itself as tachypnea or dyspnea at rest or on exertion. For the infant, this most commonly occurs during feeding. Recurrent respiratory infections and excessive sweating may also be reported. Growth failure results from unresolved heart failure.[59] The treatment plan usually includes supportive therapy (*e.g.,* digoxin, diuretics, and feeding supplementation) which is designed to help the infant compensate for the limitations in cardiac reserve and to prevent complications. Surgical intervention often is required for severe defects. It may be done in the early weeks of life or, conditions permitting, delayed until the child is older. A discussion of congestive heart failure in children is presented in Chapter 26.

Children with structural congenital heart disease and those who have had corrective surgery may have a higher-than-expected risk for development of IE. Prophylactic antibiotic therapy before dental procedures or other periods of increased risk for bacteremia is suggested for children with (1) unrepaired cyanotic heart disease, including those with palliative shunts and conduits; (2) completely repaired congenital heart disease with prosthetic material or device, whether placed by surgery or catheter intervention, during the first 6 months after the procedure; and (3) repaired congenital heart disease with residual defects at the site or adjacent to the site of a prosthetic patch or prosthetic device (which inhibit endothelialization).[43,44]

Types of Defects

CHDs can affect almost any of the cardiac structures or central blood vessels. Defects include communication between heart chambers, interrupted development of the heart chambers or

valve structures, malposition of heart chambers and great vessels, and altered closure of fetal communication channels. The particular defect reflects the embryo's stage of development at the time it occurred. It is common for multiple defects to be present in one child and for some congenital heart disorders, such as tetralogy of Fallot, to involve several defects.

The development of the heart is simultaneous and sequential; a heart defect may reflect the multiple developmental events that were occurring simultaneously or sequentially. Over 40 types of defects have been identified, the most common being patent ductus arteriosus (6% to 8%), atrial septal defects (6% to 8%), and ventricular septal defects (35% to 40%).[61]

Patent Ductus Arteriosus. The ductus arteriosus plays a vital role in diverting blood from the right side of the heart and away from the lungs to the systemic circulation during fetal life (Fig. 24.26G). With the onset of spontaneous respiration after birth, muscular constriction of the ductal tissue typically closes this vessel. The initiating step of ductal closure in the healthy infant is believed to be the sharp increase in arterial oxygen saturation and subsequent fall in pulmonary vascular resistance after birth. Additional factors that are thought to contribute to ductal closure are a fall in endogenous levels of prostaglandins and adenosine and the release of vasoactive substances. After constriction, the lumen of the ductus becomes permanently sealed with fibrous tissue within 2 to 3 weeks.

For 90% of full-term infants, the ductus is functionally closed by 48 hours of age.[62] Full-term infants with abnormalities of circulation or ventilation and premature infants are those most likely to exhibit persistent patency of the ductus arteriosus. Arterial oxygenation, circulating prostaglandins, genetic predetermination, and other, unknown factors interact to determine the mechanism of ductal closure. Circulating prostaglandin levels are directly related to gestational age, and the incidence of patent ductus arteriosus in infants with birth weights less than 1,000 g may be as high as 50%.[62]

Persistent patency of the ductus arteriosus is defined as a duct that remains open beyond 3 months in the full-term infant. The size of the persistent ductus and the difference between the systemic and pulmonary vascular resistance determine its clinical manifestations. Blood typically shunts across the ductus from the higher-pressure left side (systemic circulation) to the lower-pressure right side (pulmonary circulation). A murmur is typically detected within days or weeks of birth. The murmur is loudest at the second left intercostal space, is continuous through systole and diastole, and has a characteristic "machinery" sound.[59] A widened pulse pressure is common due to the continuous runoff of aortic blood into the pulmonary artery. Diagnostic methods include chest radiography and echocardiography. With a large shunt there are increased pulmonary markings on chest radiography and enlargement of the left heart from the increased pulmonary venous return, whereas for a small shunt the chest x-ray is normal.[59,63] Echocardiography is used to determine the presence, size, direction, (*i.e.,* left to right or right to left) and physical consequences of the shunt.

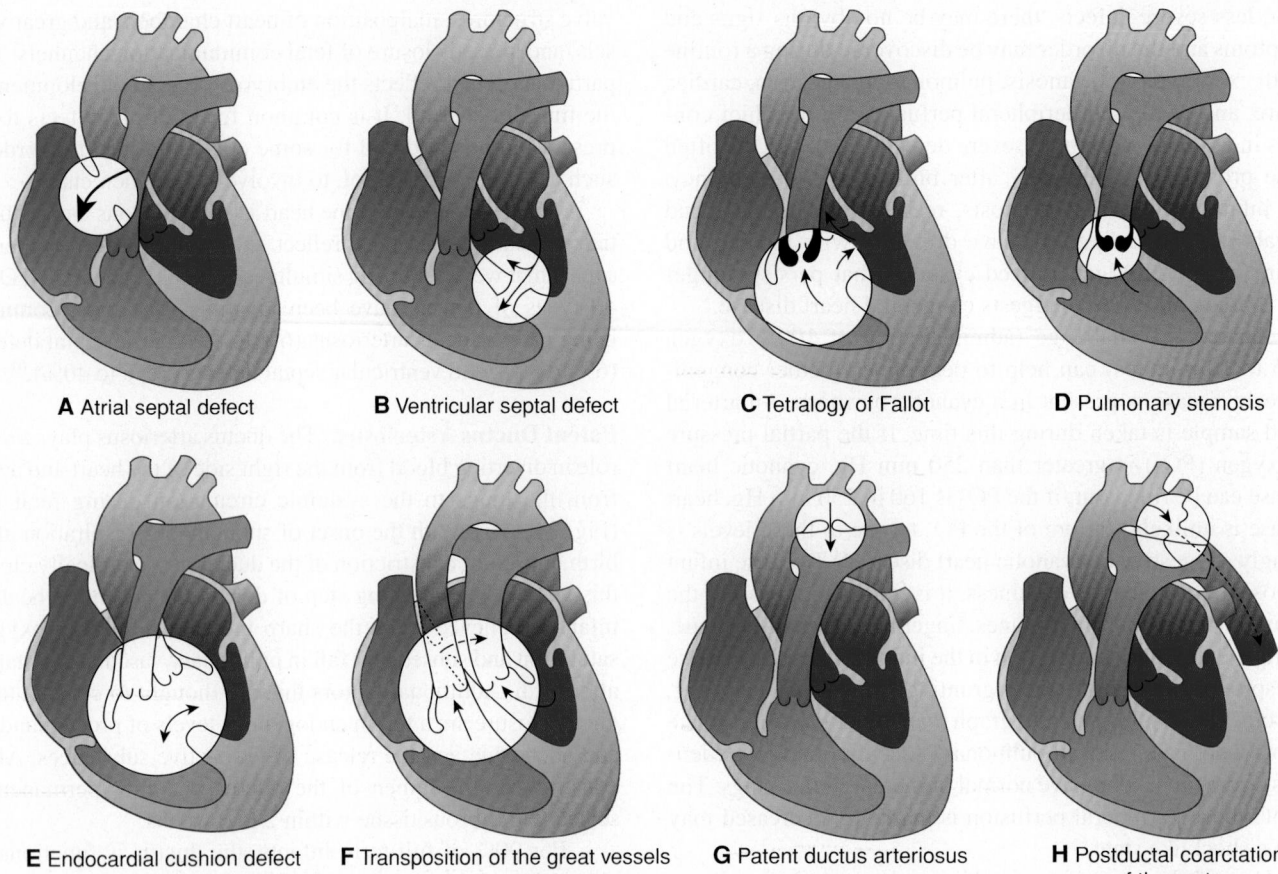

A Atrial septal defect **B** Ventricular septal defect **C** Tetralogy of Fallot **D** Pulmonary stenosis

E Endocardial cushion defect **F** Transposition of the great vessels **G** Patent ductus arteriosus **H** Postductal coarctation of the aorta

FIGURE 24.26 • Congenital heart defects. **A:** Atrial septal defect. Blood is shunted from left to right. **B:** Ventricular septal defect. Blood is usually shunted from left to right. **C:** Tetralogy of Fallot. This involves a ventricular septal defect, dextroposition of the aorta, right ventricular outflow obstruction, and right ventricular hypertrophy. Blood is shunted from right to left. **D:** Pulmonary stenosis, with decreased pulmonary blood flow and right ventricular hypertrophy. **E:** Endocardial cushion defects. Blood flows between the chambers of the heart. **F:** Transposition of the great vessels. The pulmonary artery is attached to the left side of the heart and the aorta to the right side. **G:** Patent ductus arteriosus. The high-pressure blood of the aorta is shunted back to the pulmonary artery. **H:** Postductal coarctation of the aorta.

An untreated patent ductus can result in important long-term complications that may include congestive heart failure, IE, pulmonary vascular disease, aneurysm formation, thromboembolism, and calcification.[59] The potential risk of complications and the extremely low procedural morbidity and mortality justify closure of a patent arterial ductus even when the shunt is small. In the full-term infant or older child, closure can be achieved with either surgical ligation or device occlusion. Surgery typically involves a small left thoracotomy or thoracoscopic approach that allows ligation of the vessel. Implantable devices, most commonly coils, have allowed successful ductus closure to be done in the catheterization laboratory on an outpatient basis. The anatomy of the ductus and the size of the patient are key determinants of the applicability of this technique. In the premature infant, a patent ductus can produce respiratory distress and impede weaning from mechanical ventilation. Indomethacin or ibuprofen, both inhibitors of prostaglandin synthesis, have proven effective in up to 79% of premature infants. Current research is evaluating

acetaminophen as another alternative to facilitate the ductus closure.[64] When this medical management fails, surgical intervention is recommended.

Although closure of a patent ductus is uniformly recommended when it is present as an isolated lesion, deliberate maintenance of ductal patency can be a lifesaving therapy for children with complex forms of congenital heart disease who have ductal-dependent pulmonary or systemic blood flow, or those with obligatory mixing of the arterial and venous circulations (i.e., transposition of the great arteries). Intravenous infusion of prostaglandin E_1 has proved extremely effective in maintaining ductal patency or reopening the ductus in newborns. Today, this therapy is routinely administered to newborns with suspected CHDs until they can be transported to a specialized centre where a diagnosis can be confirmed. The ductus has also been successfully stented to maintain patency in hypoplastic left heart syndrome, and implantation of a synthetic aortopulmonary shunt has been used to mimic the function of a patent ductus in other defects.

Atrial Septal Defects. Any persistent opening that allows shunting of blood across the atrial septum is considered an atrial septal defect. The defect may be single or multiple and vary from a small, asymptomatic opening to a large, symptomatic opening. The typology of the defect is determined by its position and may include a secundum atrial defect (the most common form), an ostium primum defect, a sinus venosus defect, or a patent foramen ovale (Fig. 24.26A). This type of defect occurs twice as frequently in girls than in boys.[59] As many as 50% of children with congenital heart disorders have an atrial septal defect as a part of their diagnosis.

Many atrial septal defects are asymptomatic and discovered inadvertently during a routine physical examination at a few years of age.[62] Intracardiac shunting is usually from left to right and may increase with age as the right ventricle becomes more compliant. In most cases there is a moderate shunt resulting in dilation of the right heart chambers and overperfusion of the pulmonary circulation. The increased volume of blood that must be ejected from the right heart prolongs closure of the pulmonary valve and produces a separation (fixed splitting) of the aortic and pulmonary components of the second heart sound. Children with undiagnosed atrial defects are at risk for pulmonary vascular disease, although this is a rare occurrence before 20 years of age. Rarely, infants with a large shunt may develop congestive heart failure and failure to thrive, prompting early closure of the defect.[59,62]

Atrial septal defects that measure 8 mm or more are unlikely to undergo spontaneous closure. Smaller defects may be observed for spontaneous closure in the young child. However, surgical or transcatheter closure is recommended in children with persistent defects to reduce the long-term risk of pulmonary vascular disease and atrial arrhythmias.[72] Both transcatheter device and surgical closure are effective and of low risk. Use of the transcatheter approach is determined by the position and size of the defect. Transcatheter device closure has been particularly effective for small to medium-sized secundum septal defects and patent foramen ovale. Sinus venosus defects, which are frequently associated with partial anomalous pulmonary venous return and ostium primum defects, require surgical closure. Surgery requires the use of cardiopulmonary bypass and mild hypothermia. Most defects are effectively closed using the patient's native septal tissue or a pericardial or synthetic patch. There is a very low incidence of residual sequelae or need for reintervention.

Ventricular Septal Defects. A ventricular septal defect is an opening in the ventricular septum that results from an incomplete separation of the ventricles during early fetal development (Fig. 24.26B). These defects may be single or multiple and may occur in any position along the ventricular septum. Ventricular septal defects are the most common form of CHD, accounting for up to 40% of congenital heart disorders.[65] Distribution between boys and girls is relatively even.[59] Ventricular septal defect may be the only cardiac defect, or it may occur in association with multiple cardiac anomalies.

The ventricular septum originates from two sources: the interventricular groove of the folded tubular heart that gives rise to the muscular part of the septum, and the endocardial cushions that extend to form the membranous portion of the septum. The upper membranous portion of the septum is the last area to close, typically by the seventh week of gestation, and it is here that most defects occur. Depending on the size of the opening and the pulmonary vascular resistance, the signs and symptoms of a ventricular septal defect may range from an asymptomatic murmur to congestive heart failure.[65]

The physical size of the ventricular septal defect is a major, but not the only, determinant of left-to-right shunt. The pulmonary vascular resistance in relation to systemic vascular resistance also determines the shunt's magnitude. In a small communicating defect (<0.5 cm^2), the higher pressure in the left ventricle drives the shunt to the left and the size of the defect limits the magnitude of the shunt. Most children with such defects are asymptomatic and have a low risk for development of pulmonary vascular disease.

In a larger, nonrestrictive shunt (usually >1 cm^2), right and left ventricular pressure is equalized and the degree of shunting is determined by the ratio of pulmonary to systemic vascular resistance. After birth in infants with large ventricular septal defects, pulmonary vascular resistance may remain higher than normal, and the size of the left-to-right shunt may initially be limited. As the pulmonary vascular resistance continues to fall in the first few weeks after birth because of normal involution of the media of the small pulmonary arterioles, the magnitude of the left-to-right shunt increases. Eventually, a large left-to-right shunt develops, and clinical symptoms (*e.g.,* tachypnea, diaphoresis, especially with feeding, and failure to thrive) become apparent. In most cases during infancy, pulmonary vascular pressure is only slightly elevated, and the major contributor to pulmonary hypertension is an increase in pulmonary blood flow. In some infants with a large septal defect, pulmonary arteriolar thickness never decreases. With continued exposure to high pulmonary blood flow, pulmonary vascular obstructive disease develops. In untreated patients, the pulmonary vascular resistance can eventually exceed the systemic resistance. In this case, a reversal of shunt flow occurs and the infant demonstrates progressive cyanosis as deoxygenated blood moves from the right to the left side of the heart. These symptoms, coupled with irreversible changes in the pulmonary vasculature, represent an end-stage form of congenital heart disease called *Eisenmenger syndrome.*

The treatment of a ventricular septal defect depends on the size of the defect, accompanying hemodynamic derangements, and symptomatology. Children with small or medium-sized defects may be followed without intervention if they remain free from signs of congestive heart failure or pulmonary hypertension. Ventricular defects do not increase in size, and some spontaneously close over time. Detailed 2D echocardiography is usually adequate to diagnose the size and position of a defect as well as to estimate pulmonary pressures. Cardiac catheterization is usually reserved for cases where it is necessary to confirm the degree and reversibility of pulmonary vascular resistance.[59,65]

Congestive heart failure is treated medically. Symptomatic infants may require feeding supplements or tube feeding to promote growth and development. In the symptomatic infant in whom complete repair cannot be achieved because of size or other complicating lesions, a palliative procedure may be performed to reduce symptoms. Placement of a synthetic band around the main pulmonary artery (pulmonary artery banding) can reduce pulmonary blood flow until complete repair can be accomplished. Surgical closure of the defect is completed by placement of a synthetic or autologous patch effectively to close the shunt across the ventricular septum. These procedures are typically done electively in the infant or young child, and are associated with low morbidity and mortality rates. Transcatheter device closure of ventricular septal defects remains an area of interest; however, difficulty with successful positioning of the devices and high rates of complete heart block have limited its applicability.

Atrioventricular Septal Defects or Endocardial Cushion Defects. The AV canal connects the atria to the ventricles during early cardiac development. The endocardial cushions surround this canal and contribute tissue to the lower part of the atrial septum, the upper part of the ventricular septum, the septal leaflet of the tricuspid valve, and the anterior leaflet of the mitral valve.[66] Any flaw in the development of these tissues results in an endocardial cushion defect or atrioventricular septal defects (AVSD). Approximately 4% of all CHDs are AVSD, with a nearly equal incidence in boys and girls. AVSD have a strong association with Down syndrome, and are seen in as many as 50% of children with Down syndrome.

Several variations of AVSD are possible. The defect may be described as *partial* or *complete.* The anatomy of the AV valve determines the classification. In partial AV canal defects, the two AV valve rings are complete and separate. The most common type of partial AV canal defect is an ostium primum defect, often associated with a cleft in the mitral valve. In a complete canal defect, there is a common AV valve orifice along with defects in both the atrial and ventricular septal tissue (Fig. 24.26E).[59] Other cardiac defects may be associated with AVSD and most commonly include cardiac malposition defects and tetralogy of Fallot.[59]

Physiologically, these defects result in abnormalities similar to those described for atrial or ventricular septal defects. The direction and magnitude of a shunt in a child with an AVSD are determined by the combination of defects and the child's pulmonary and systemic vascular resistance. The hemodynamic effects of an isolated ostium primum defect are those of the previously described atrial septal defect. These children are largely asymptomatic during childhood. With a complete AV canal defect, pulmonary blood flow is increased after pulmonary vascular resistance falls because of left-to-right shunting across both the ventricular and atrial septal defects. Children with complete defects often have effort intolerance, easy fatigability, failure to thrive, recurrent infections, and other signs of congestive heart failure, particularly when the shunt is large. Pulmonary hypertension and increased pulmonary vascular resistance result if the lesion is left untreated.

The timing of treatment for AVSD is determined by the severity of the defect and symptoms. With an ostium primum defect, surgical repair usually is planned on an elective basis before the child reaches school age. The defect in the atrial septum is closed with a patch and mitral valvuloplasty is performed if the valve is regurgitant. Corrective surgery is required for all complete AV canal defects. This is typically performed in infants at 3 to 6 months of age and requires patching of both the atrial and ventricular septal defects and separation of the AV valve apparatus to create competent mitral and tricuspid valves. Infants with severe symptoms may require a palliative procedure where the main pulmonary artery is banded to reduce pulmonary blood flow. This typically improves the infant's ability to grow and develop until a complete repair can be performed. Total surgical repair of complete AV canal defects can be accomplished with low operative risk. Reoperation may be required in approximately 10% to 12% of children. Late sequelae include AV valve regurgitation, subaortic stenosis, and arrhythmias.[59,67]

Pulmonary Stenosis. Obstruction of blood flow from the right ventricle to the pulmonary circulation is termed *pulmonary stenosis.* The obstruction can occur as an isolated valvular lesion, within the right ventricular chamber, in the pulmonary arteries, or as a combination of stenoses in multiple areas. It is a relatively common defect, estimated to account for approximately 10% of all congenital cardiac disease, and is often associated with other abnormalities.[59]

Pulmonary valvular defects, the most common type of obstruction, usually produce some impairment of pulmonary blood flow and increase the workload imposed on the right side of the heart (Fig. 24.26D). Most children with pulmonic valve stenosis have mild stenosis that does not increase in severity. These children are largely asymptomatic and are diagnosed by the presence of a systolic murmur. Moderate or greater stenosis has been shown to progress over time, particularly before 12 years of age, so these children require careful follow-up. Critical pulmonary stenosis in the neonate is evidenced by cyanosis due to right-to-left atrial-level shunting and right ventricular hypertension. These infants require prostaglandin E_1 to maintain circulation to the lungs through the ductus arteriosus.[59,68]

Pulmonary valvotomy is the treatment of choice for all valvular defects with pressure gradients from the right ventricle to the pulmonary circulation greater than 30 mm Hg. Transcatheter balloon valvuloplasty has been quite successful in this lesion. Stenosis in the peripheral pulmonary arteries can also be effectively treated with balloon angioplasty, with or without stent placement.[59,68]

Tetralogy of Fallot. Tetralogy of Fallot is the most common cyanotic CHD, accounting for approximately 5% to 7% of all CHDs. As the name implies, tetralogy of Fallot consists of four associated defects: (1) a ventricular septal defect involving the membranous septum and the anterior portion of the muscular septum; (2) dextroposition or shifting to the right of the aorta, so that it overrides the right ventricle and is in communication with the septal defect; (3) obstruction or narrowing of the pulmonary outflow channel, including pulmonic valve stenosis, a decrease in the size of the pulmonary trunk, or both; and (4) hypertrophy of the right ventricle because of the increased work required to pump blood through the obstructed pulmonary channels[59] (Fig. 24.26C). Variations of the defect can include complete atresia of the pulmonary valve or absence of pulmonary valve tissue altogether.

Cyanosis is caused by a right-to-left shunt across the ventricular septal defect. The degree of cyanosis is determined by the restriction of blood flow into the pulmonary bed. Right ventricular outflow obstruction causes deoxygenated blood from the right ventricle to shunt across the ventricular septal defect and be ejected into the systemic circulation. The degree of obstruction may be dynamic and can increase during periods of stress, causing hypercyanotic attacks ("tet spells"). These spells typically occur in the morning during crying, feeding, or defecating. These activities increase the infant's oxygen requirements. Crying and defecating may further increase pulmonary vascular resistance, thereby increasing right-to-left shunting and decreasing pulmonary blood flow. With the hypercyanotic spell, the infant becomes acutely cyanotic, hyperpneic, irritable, and diaphoretic. Later in the spell, the infant becomes limp and may lose consciousness. Placing the infant in the knee–chest position increases systemic vascular resistance, which increases pulmonary blood flow and decreases right-to-left shunting. During a hypercyanotic spell, toddlers and older children may spontaneously assume the squatting position, which functions like the knee–chest position to relieve the spell. Turbulent flow across the narrow right ventricular outflow track produces a characteristic harsh systolic ejection murmur. Auscultation during a hypercyanotic spell reveals a diminished or absent murmur due to the dramatic reduction in pulmonary blood flow.[59]

Total surgical correction is required for all children with tetralogy of Fallot. Early definitive repair in infancy is currently advocated in most centres experienced in intracardiac surgery in infants. When extreme cyanosis is present in a small infant or when there is associated marked hypoplasia of the pulmonary arteries, a palliative procedure to facilitate pulmonary blood flow may be necessary. This is accomplished by placing a prosthetic shunt between a systemic artery and the pulmonary artery (modified Blalock–Taussig shunt). Balloon dilation of the pulmonary valve may also afford palliation in some infants. Total correction is then carried out later in infancy or early childhood. Complete repair includes patch closure of the ventricular septal defect and relief of any right ventricular outflow tract obstruction. Repair is associated with a mortality rate of less than 3%; however, patients need long-term follow-up to monitor for residual lesions, right ventricular dilation or dysfunction, and arrhythmias.[59]

Transposition of the Great Arteries. In complete transposition of the great arteries, the aorta arises from the right ventricle, and the pulmonary artery arises from the left ventricle (Fig. 24.26F). Complete transposition occurs in 1 in 4,000 live births and is the most common reason for pediatric cardiology referral in the first 2 weeks of life. The defect is two to three times more common in boys.[59]

Cyanosis is the most common presenting symptom resulting from an anomaly that allows the systemic venous return to be circulated through the right heart and ejected into the aorta, and the pulmonary venous return to be recirculated to the lungs through the left ventricle and main pulmonary artery.[59] In infants born with this defect, survival depends on communication between the right and left sides of the heart in the form of a patent ductus arteriosus or septal defect. Ventricular septal defects are present in 50% of infants with transposition of the great arteries at birth and may allow effective mixing of blood. Prostaglandin E_1 should be administered to neonates when this lesion is suspected in an effort to maintain the patency of the ductus arteriosus. Balloon atrial septostomy may be done to increase the blood flow between the two sides of the heart. In this procedure, a balloon-tipped catheter is inserted into the heart through the vena cava and then passed through the foramen ovale into the left atrium. The balloon is then inflated and pulled back through the foramen ovale, enlarging the opening as it goes.

Corrective surgery is essential for long-term survival. An arterial switch procedure, the current operation of choice, has survival rates greater than 90%.[59] This procedure, which corrects the relation of the systemic and pulmonary blood flows, is preferably performed in the first 2 to 3 weeks of life, before the postnatal reduction in pulmonary vascular resistance occurs. The coronary arteries are moved to the left-sided great artery and any ventricular septal defects are closed during the same operation. Complications of the arterial switch procedure may include coronary insufficiency, supravalvar pulmonary stenosis, neoaortic regurgitation, and rhythm abnormalities.[69]

Coarctation of the Aorta. Coarctation of the aorta is a localized narrowing of the aorta, proximal to (preductal), distal to (postductal), or opposite the entry of the ductus arteriosus (juxtaductal; Fig. 24.26H). Approximately 98% of coarctations are juxtaductal. Constriction of aberrant ductal tissue extending into the aortic wall is believed to be the cause of obstruction.[62] The anomaly is frequently associated with other congenital cardiac lesions, most commonly bicuspid aortic valve, and approximately 45% of children with Turner syndrome have coarctation, suggesting a genetic linkage[59] (see Chapter 7).

The classic sign of coarctation of the aorta is a disparity in pulsations and blood pressures in the arms and legs. The femoral, popliteal, and dorsalis pedis pulsations are weak or delayed compared with the bounding pulses of the arms and carotid vessels. Normally, the systolic blood pressure in the legs obtained by the cuff method is 10 to 20 mm Hg higher than in the arms. In coarctation, the pressure in the legs is lower and may be difficult to obtain. Patients with coarctation are often identified during a diagnostic workup for hypertension. Most patients with moderate coarctation remain otherwise asymptomatic owing to collateral vessels that form around the area of narrowing. Left untreated, however, coarctation will result in left ventricular hypertension and hypertrophy and significant systemic hypertension (see Chapter 23). Infants with severe coarctation demonstrate early symptoms of heart failure and may present in critical condition upon ductal closure. Reopening of the duct with prostaglandin E₁, if possible, and emergent surgery are needed in this subgroup.[59]

Children with coarctation causing a blood pressure gradient between the arms and legs of 20 mm Hg or greater should ideally be treated by 2 years of age to reduce the likelihood of persistent hypertension. A surgical approach typically involves resection of the narrowed segment of the aorta and end-to-end anastomosis of healthy tissue. This can usually be accomplished without cardiopulmonary bypass, with a mortality rate near zero. Balloon angioplasty with or without stent placement has also been used, although the presence of residual gradients and the reliability of the surgical approach have limited this technique.[59,70] The most common complications after repair of coarctation are persistent hypertension and recoarctation.

Functional Single-Ventricle Anatomy. Several forms of complex congenital heart disease result in only one functional ventricle. There may be a single right or a single left ventricle, or a ventricle of indeterminate morphology. Functional single-ventricle anatomy is the most common form of congenital heart disease diagnosed during fetal life because of the inability to obtain a four-chamber cardiac view on routine prenatal ultrasonography. Hypoplastic left heart syndrome is the most common form of single right ventricular anatomy. Tricuspid valve atresia is the most common cause of a single left ventricle. Several other forms of double-inlet ventricle have been described; however, all forms of this disease result in similar pathologic effects and follow a common pathway of intervention.[59]

All forms of single-ventricle anatomy result in a common mixing chamber of pulmonary and systemic venous return and cause varying degrees of cyanosis. The single ventricle must supply both the pulmonary and systemic circulations.[71] The amount of blood flow to each circulation is determined by the resistance in each system. As pulmonary vascular resistance falls, flow to the pulmonary circulation will be preferential and systemic circulation will be compromised. In some defects, such as hypoplastic left heart syndrome, systemic flow depends on a patent ductus arteriosus. Neonates with this lesion typically present with extreme cyanosis and symptoms of heart failure as the duct begins to close.[71]

Although functional single-ventricle anatomy cannot be completely repaired, the surgical palliation of these defects has been one of the most innovative accomplishments in intervention for congenital heart disease. The goal of surgical palliation is to redirect systemic venous return directly to the pulmonary arteries and allow the single ventricle to deliver oxygenated blood to the systemic circulation. This is accomplished in a series of two- to three-staged surgical interventions during the child's first years of life. Currently a modified Fontan and Baudet approach is done surgically. The goal is to bypass the right side of the heart, so blood flow so systemic venous blood goes directly to the pulmonary arteries. This allows the single-ventricle chamber to pump into the systemic

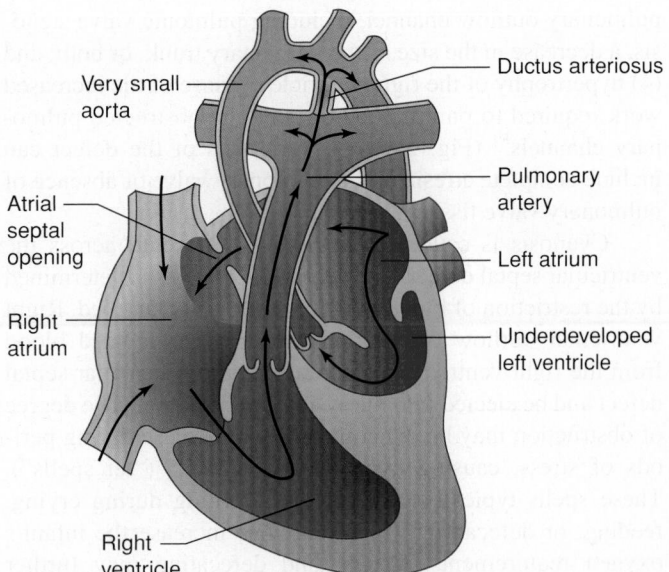

FIGURE 24.27 • Functional single-ventricle anatomy with an underdeveloped left ventricle and small ascending aorta. Because of the markedly decreased left ventricular compliance, most of the pulmonary venous blood returning to the left atrium shunts left to right at the atrial level. Pulmonary arterial blood flows into the pulmonary arteries as well as right to left across a patent ductus arteriosus into the aorta.

circulation (Fig. 24.27). Cardiac transplantation is also used as an intervention for the most complex forms of single-ventricle congenital heart disease.

Survival rates for children with complex forms of single-ventricle heart disease have improved markedly, but long-term outcomes remain uncertain. Ventricular dysfunction, arrhythmias, and thromboses plague this population of patients. Defining the optimal medical and surgical management strategies for these patients remains an active area of research in pediatric cardiology and cardiac surgery.[59,71]

Adults With Congenital Heart Disease

Successful treatment of congenital heart disease in the pediatric population has resulted in a growing number of adult survivors with a variety of repaired, unrepaired, and palliated congenital cardiac lesions. Approximately 90% of children born with CHD survive to adulthood. In Canada there are approximately 171,000 adults with CHD.[55]

Although the majority of adults with congenital heart disease will have undergone treatment and perhaps surgery as children, most CHDs must be considered chronic conditions requiring long-term surveillance and care. Only the simplest lesions, such as patent ductus arteriosus and uncomplicated secundum atrial septal defect, can be considered completely repaired.[72] Chronic physiologic concerns include arrhythmias, hemodynamic problems, complications of prolonged cyanosis, endocarditis, residual lesions, and the need for reoperation. The underlying heart defect can also have significant implications for other aspects of health, such as exercise tolerance, noncardiac surgery, and pregnancy. Several important psychosocial issues also require consideration, including neurocognitive achievement, employment, insurability, family planning, treatment adherence, and understanding of the underlying condition and risks. Life expectancy for some of the most complex lesions (*e.g.*, hypoplastic left heart syndrome) is unknown because the oldest survivors to date were born in the 1980s. A growing medical specialty has emerged, designed specifically to provide adults with congenital heart disease with the specialized services they need from practitioners, who understand both the complexities of their cardiac problems and other issues of adult health care.

Kawasaki Disease

Kawasaki disease, also known as *mucocutaneous lymph node syndrome,* is an acute febrile disease of young children. First described in Japan in 1967 by Dr. Tomisaku Kawasaki, the disease affects the skin, brain, eyes, joints, liver, lymph nodes, and heart. The disease is the most common cause of acquired heart disease in young children, with 15% to 25% of cases resulting in coronary artery aneurysms or ectasias that may lead to MI, sudden death, or chronic coronary insufficiency.[73,74] In Canada approximately 13 to 14 per 100,000 children under the age of five years are diagnosed with Kawasaki disease every year.[75] Approximately 85% of patients with Kawasaki disease are 5 years of age or younger.[74] Although most common in Japan, the disease affects children of many races, occurs worldwide, and is increasing in frequency.

The disease is characterized by a vasculitis (*i.e.*, inflammation of the blood vessels) that begins in the small vessels (*i.e.*, arterioles, venules, and capillaries) and progresses to involve some of the larger arteries, such as the coronaries. The exact etiology and pathogenesis of the disease remain unknown, but it is thought to be of infectious origin.[73] Infectious triggers are linked to immunologic abnormalities, including increased activation of helper T cells and increased levels of immune mediators and antibodies that destroy endothelial cells, have been detected during the acute phase of the disease. It has been hypothesized that an unknown infectious agent is an antigen that is responsible for triggering the immune response in a genetically predisposed child.

Manifestations and Clinical Course

The clinical course of the disease has been described in three phases: the acute, subacute, and convalescent phases.[73] The *acute phase* begins with an abrupt onset of fever, followed by conjunctivitis, rash, involvement of the oral mucosa, redness and swelling of the hands and feet, and enlarged cervical lymph nodes (Fig. 24.28). The fever typically is high, reaching 40°C or more, has an erratic spiking pattern, is unresponsive to antibiotics, and persists for 5 or more days. The conjunctivitis, which is bilateral, begins shortly after the onset of fever, persists throughout the febrile course of the disease, and may last as long as 3 to 5 weeks. There is no exudate, discharge, or conjunctival ulceration, differentiating it from many other types of conjunctivitis. The rash usually is deeply erythematous and may take several forms, the most common of which is

FIGURE 24.28 • Kawasaki disease. **A:** Rash of Kawasaki disease in a 7-month-old child on the 4th day of illness. **B:** Conjunctival injection, lip edema in a 2-year-old boy on the 6th day of illness. (From The Council on Cardiovascular Disease in Young, Committee on Rheumatic Fever, Endocarditis, and Kawasaki Disease. (2001). Diagnostic guidelines for Kawasaki disease. *Circulation, 103,* 335–336.)

a nonpruritic urticarial rash with large erythematous plaques, or a measles-type rash. Although the rash usually is generalized, it may be accentuated centrally or peripherally. Some children have a perianal rash with a diaper-like distribution. Oropharyngeal manifestations include fissuring of the lips, diffuse erythema of the oropharynx, and hypertrophic papillae of the tongue, creating a "strawberry" appearance. The hands and feet become swollen and painful, and have reddened palms and soles. The rash, oropharyngeal manifestations, and changes in hands and feet appear within 1 to 3 days of fever onset and usually disappear as the fever subsides. Lymph node involvement is the least constant feature of the disease. It is cervical and unilateral, with a single, firm, enlarged lymph node mass that usually is larger than 1.5 cm in diameter.

The *subacute phase* begins with defervescence and lasts until all signs of the disease have disappeared. During the subacute phase, desquamation (*i.e.*, peeling) of the skin of the fingers and toe tips begins and progresses to involve the entire surface of the palms and soles. Patchy peeling of skin areas other than the hands and feet may occur in some children. The convalescent stage persists from the complete resolution of symptoms until all signs of inflammation have disappeared. This usually takes approximately 8 weeks, although inflammatory changes in the coronary arteries may persist for as long as 4 years.

In addition to the major manifestations that occur during the acute stage of the illness, there are several associated, less specific characteristics of the disease, including arthritis, urethritis and pyuria, gastrointestinal manifestations (*e.g.,* diarrhea, abdominal pain), hepatitis, and hydrops of the gallbladder. Arthritis or arthralgia occurs in approximately 30% of children with the disease, characterized by symmetric joint swelling involving large and small joints. Central nervous system involvement occurs in almost all children and is characterized by pronounced irritability and lability of mood.

Cardiac involvement is the most important manifestation of Kawasaki disease. Coronary artery abnormalities develop in approximately 15% to 25% of children, manifested by coronary artery dilation and aneurysm formation as seen on 2D echocardiography. The manifestations of coronary artery involvement include signs and symptoms of myocardial ischemia or, rarely, overt MI or rupture of the aneurysm. Pericarditis, myocarditis, endocarditis, heart failure, and arrhythmias also may develop. Death from Kawasaki disease is estimated to occur in less than 1% of patients and is almost always cardiac in nature, most often occurring during the convalescent phase of the illness, usually from thromboses or coronary arterial aneurysms.[73]

Diagnosis and Treatment

No specific diagnostic test for Kawasaki disease is available; therefore, the diagnosis is made on clinical grounds following published guidelines.[73] The guidelines specify fever persisting at least 5 days or more without another source in association with at least four principal features, including oral changes that may include erythema or cracking of the lips, strawberry tongue, or erythema of the oral mucosa; bilateral, nonexudative conjunctivitis; polymorphous rash (which is generally truncal, nonvesicular); changes of extremities that may include erythema and edema of the hands or feet, desquamation of fingers and toes 1 to 3 weeks after onset of illness; and cervical lymphadenopathy, often unilateral, with at least one node that is 1.5 cm in size.[73] Chest radiographs, ECG tests, and 2D echocardiography are used to detect coronary artery involvement and follow its progress. Coronary angiography may be used to determine the extent of coronary artery involvement.

Intravenous gamma globulin and aspirin are considered the best therapies for prevention of coronary artery abnormalities in children with Kawasaki disease. During the acute phase of the illness, aspirin usually is given in larger doses (80 to 100 mg/kg/day divided in four doses) for its anti-inflammatory and antipyretic effects. After the fever is controlled, the aspirin dose is lowered (3 to 5 mg/kg/day, single dose), and the drug is given for its antiplatelet-aggregating effects for 6 to 8 weeks.[73]

Recommendations for cardiac follow-up evaluation (*i.e.,* stress testing and sometimes coronary angiography) are based on the level of coronary artery changes. Anticoagulant therapy may be recommended for children with multiple or large coronary aneurysms. Some restrictions in activities such as competitive sports may be advised for children with significant coronary artery abnormalities.[7]

IN SUMMARY

CHDs arise during fetal heart development, which occurs during weeks 3 through 8 after conception, and reflect the stage of development at the time the causative event occurred. Several factors contribute to the development of CHDs, including genetic and chromosomal influences, viruses, and environmental agents such as drugs and radiation. The exact cause of the defect often is unknown. These defects are relatively common and are the most common cause of death related to a birth defect.

CHDs may produce no effects, or they may markedly affect cardiac function. The defects may produce shunting of blood from the right to the left side of the heart or from the left to the right side of the heart. Left-to-right shunts typically increase the volume of the right side of the heart and pulmonary circulation, and right-to-left shunts transfer deoxygenated blood from the right side of the heart to the left side, diluting the oxygen content of blood that is being ejected into the systemic circulation and causing cyanosis. The direction and degree of shunt depend on the size and position of the defect that connects the two sides of the heart and the difference in resistance between the two sides of the circulation. CHDs often are classified as defects that produce cyanosis and those that produce little or no cyanosis. Depending on the severity of the defect, CHDs may be treated medically or surgically. Medical and surgical treatment often is indicated in children with severe defects.

Kawasaki disease is an acute febrile disease of young children that affects the skin, brain, eyes, joints, liver, lymph nodes, and heart. The disease can produce aneurysmal disease of the coronary arteries and is the most common cause of acquired heart disease in young children.

REVIEW EXERCISES

1. A 40-year-old man presents in the emergency department complaining of substernal chest pain that is also felt in his left shoulder. He is short of breath and nauseated. His blood pressure is 148/90 mm Hg and his heart rate is 110 beats/minute. His ECG shows an ST-segment elevation with T-wave inversion. He is given aspirin, morphine, nitroglycerin, and oxygen. Blood tests reveal elevated CK-MB and a positive troponin I.

    A. *What is the probable cause of the man's symptoms?*

    B. *Explain the origin of the left arm pain, nausea, and increased heart rate.*

C. What is the significance of the ST-segment changes and elevation in CK-MB and troponin I?

D. Relate the actions of aspirin, morphine, nitroglycerin, and oxygen to the treatment of this man's condition.

2. A 50-year-old woman presents with complaints of nocturnal paroxysmal dyspnea and orthopnea, palpitations, and fatigue. An echocardiogram demonstrates a thickened, immobile mitral valve with anterior and posterior leaflets moving together; slow early diastolic filling of the ventricle; and left atrial enlargement.

A. What is the probable cause of this woman's symptoms?

B. Explain the pathologic significance of the slow early diastolic filling, distended left atrium, and palpitations.

C. Given the echocardiographic data, what type of cardiac murmur would you expect to find in this woman?

D. Which circulation (systemic or pulmonary) would you expect to be affected as this woman's mitral valve disorder progresses?

3. A 4-month-old male infant is brought into the pediatric clinic by his mother. She reports that she noted over the past several weeks that her baby's lips, mouth, fingernails, and toenails have become a bluish-grey colour. She also states that he seems to tire easily and that even feeding seems to wear him out. Lately, he has had several spells where he has suddenly turned blue, has had difficulty breathing, and been very irritable. During one of these spells he turned limp and seemed to have passed out for a short time. An echocardiogram reveals a thickening of the right ventricular wall with overriding of the aorta, a large subaortic ventricular septal defect, and narrowing of the pulmonary outflow with stenosis of the pulmonary valve.

A. What is this infant's probable diagnosis?

B. Describe the shunting of blood that occurs with this disorder and its relationship to the development of cyanosis.

C. The mother is instructed to place the infant in the knee–chest position when he has one of the spells in which he becomes blue and irritable. How does this position help to relieve the cyanosis and impaired oxygenation of tissues?

D. The surgical creation of a shunt between the aorta and pulmonary artery may be performed as a palliative procedure for infants with marked hypoplasia of the pulmonary artery, with corrective surgery performed later in childhood. Explain how this procedure increases blood flow to the lungs.

References

1. Heart & Stroke Foundation. (2015). *Statistics*. Available online at: http://www.heartandstroke.com/site/c.ikIQLcMWJtE/b.3483991/k.34A8/Statistics.htm. Accessed March 24, 2015.

2. Mann D. L., Zipes D. P., Libby P., et al. (2015). *Braunwald's heart disease: A textbook of cardiovascular medicine* (10th ed.). Philadelphia, PA: Elsevier, Inc.

3. LeWinter M. M. (2014). Acute pericarditis. *New England Journal of Medicine, 371*(25), 2410–2416.

4. Statistics Canada. (2012). *Mortality, summary list of causes, 2009*. Ottawa: Minister of Industry. Catalogue No. 84F0209S.

5. Canadian Institute for Health Information (IHI). (2014). International comparisons: A focus on quality of care. Available online at: https://secure.cihi.ca/free_products/OECD_AFocusOnQualityOfCareAiB_EN.pdf. Accessed March 24, 2015.

6. Hall J. E. (2011). *Textbook of medical physiology* (12th ed.). Philadelphia, PA: W. B. Saunders.

7. Schoen F. J., Mitchell R. N. (2010). Chapter 12: The heart. In Kumar V., Abbas A. K., Fausto N., et al. (Eds.), *Robbins and Cotran pathologic basis of disease* (8th ed.). Philadelphia, PA: Elsevier Saunders.

8. Wilcken D. E. L. (2014). Physiology of the normal heart. *Medicine, 42*(8), 409–412.

9. Sprigings D., Graham A. (2014). Exercise electrocardiography in the management of obstructive coronary artery disease and other cardiac disorders. *Medicine, 42*(8), 436–441.

10. Woods S. L., Froelicher E. S. S., Motzer S. A., et al. (2010). *Cardiac nursing* (6th ed.). Philadelphia, PA: Lippincott Williams & Wilkins.

11. Loudon M., Sabharwal N. (2014). Nuclear imaging. *Medicine, 42*(8), 452–455.

12. Libby P. (2013). Mechanisms of acute coronary syndromes and their implications for therapy. *New England Journal of Medicine, 368*(21), 2004–2013.

13. Yunoki K., Naruko T., Sugioka K., et al. (2013). Thrombus aspiration therapy and coronary thrombus components in patients with acuter ST-elevation myocardial infarction. *Journal of Atherosclerosis and Thrombosis, 20*(6), 524–537.

14. Aldous S. J. (2013). Cardiac biomarkers in acute myocardial infarction. *International Journal of Cardiology, 164*(3), 282–294.

15. Giugliano R. P., Cannon C. P., Braunwald E. (2015). Chapter 53: Non-ST elevation acute coronary syndromes. In Mann D. L., Zipes D. P., Libby P., et al. (Eds.), *Braunwald's heart disease: A textbook of cardiovascular medicine* (10th ed.). Philadelphia, PA: Elsevier, Inc.

16. Kreatsoulas C., Shannon H. S., Giacomini M., et al. (2013). Reconstructing angina: Cardiac symptoms are the same in women and men. *JAMA Internal Medicine, 173*(9), 829–831.

17. Welsh R. C., Travers A., Huynh T., et al. (2009). Canadian Cardiovascular Society working group: providing a perspective on the 2007 focused update of the American College of Cardiology and American Heart Association 2004 guidelines for the management of ST elevation myocardial infarction. *Canadian Journal of Cardiology, 25*(1), 25–32.

18. Kushner F. G., Hand M., Smith S. C., et al. (2009). 2009 focused updates: ACC/AHA guidelines for the management of patients with ST-elevation myocardial infarction and the ACC/AHA/SCAI guidelines on percutaneous coronary intervention. *Journal of the American College of Cardiology, 54*(23), 2205–2241.

19. Tanguay J. F., Bell A. D., Ackman M. L., et al. (2013). Focused 2012 update of the Canadian Cardiovascular Society guidelines for the use of antiplatelet therapy. *Canadian Journal of Cardiology, 29*(11), 1334–1345.

20. Jolly S. S., Cairns J. A., Yusuf S., et al. (2015). Randomized trial of primary PCI with or without routine manual thrombectomy. *New England Journal of Medicine, 372*(15), 1389–1398.

21. Assmann A., Boeken U., Akhyari P., et al. (2012). Appropriate timing of coronary artery bypass grafting after acute myocardial infarction. *Thoracic and Cardiovascular Surgeon, 60*(7), 446–451.

22. Hillis L. D., Smith P. K., Anderson J. L., et al. (2011). 2011 ACCF/AHA guideline for coronary artery bypass graft surgery. *Circulation, 124*(23), e652–e735.

23. Tracy C. M., Epstein A. E., Darbar D., et al. (2012). 2012 ACCF/AHA/HRS focused update of the 2008 guidelines for device-based therapy of cardiac rhythm abnormalities. *Journal of the American College of Cardiology, 60*(14), 1297–1313.

24. Heran B. S., Chen J. M. H., Ebrahim S., et al. (2011). Exercise-based cardiac rehabilitation for coronary heart disease. *Cochrane Database System Reviews,* (7):CD001800.

25. Montalescot G., Sechtem U., Achenback S., et al. (2013). 2013 ESC guidelines on the management of stable coronary artery disease – web addenda. Available online at: http://www.escardio.org/guidelines-surveys/esc-guidelines/Pages/stable-angina-pectoris.aspx. Accessed March 23, 2015.

26. Mittal S. R. (2014). Etiopathogenesis of microvascular angina: Caveats in our knowledge. *Indian Heart Journal, 66*(6), 678–681.

27. Conti C. R., Bavry A. A., Petersen J. W. (2012). Silent ischemia: Clinical relevance. *Journal of the American College of Cardiology, 59*(5), 435–441.

28. Arenja N., Mueller C., Ehl N. F., et al. (2013). Prevalence, extent, and independent predictors of silent myocardial infarction. *The American Journal of Medicine, 126*(6), 515–522.

29. Maron B. J., Towbin J. A., Thiene G., et al. (2006). Contemporary definitions and classification of the cardiomyopathies. *Circulation, 113*(14), 1807–1816.

30. Maron B. J., Maron M. S. (2013). Hypertrophic cardiomyopathy. *Lancet, 381*(9862), 242–255.

31. Arnold J. M. O., Howlett J. G., Ducharme A., et al. (2008). Canadian Cardiovascular Society consensus conference guidelines on heart failure – 2008 updated: Best practices for the transition of care of heart failure patients, and the recognition, investigation and treatment of cardiomyopathies. *Canadian Journal of Cardiology, 24*(1), 21–40.

32. Basso C., Bauce B., Corrado D., et al. (2012). Pathophysiology of arrhythmogenic cardiomyopathy. *Nature Reviews Cardiology, 9*(4), 223–233.

33. Calkins H. (2013). Arrhythmogenic right ventricular dysplasia. *Current Problems in Cardiology, 38*(3), 103–123.

34. Udeoji D. U., Philip K. J., Morrissey R. P., et al. (2013). Left ventricular noncompaction cardiomyopathy: Updated review. *Therapeutic Advice's in Cardiovascular Disease, 7*(5), 260–273.

35. Jefferies J. L., Towbin J. A. (2010). Dilated cardiomyopathy. *Lancet, 375*(9716), 752–762.

36. Saffitz J. E. (2012). Chapter 11: The heart. In Rubin R., Strayer D. S. (Eds.). *Rubin's pathology: Clinicopathologic foundations of medicine* (6th ed.). Philadelphia, PA: Lippincott Williams & Wilkins.

37. Pinney S. P., Mancini D. M. (2011). Chapter 35: Myocarditis and specific cardiomyopathies. In Fuster V., Walsh R. A., Harrington, R. A., et al. *Hurst's the heart* (13th ed.). New York: McGraw Hill Companies.

38. Sager S., Liu P. P., Cooper L. T. (2012). Myocarditis. *Lancet, 379*(9817), 738–747.

39. Johnson-Coyle L., Jensen L., Sobey A. (2012). Peripartum cardiomyopathy: Review and practice guidelines. *American Journal of Critical Care, 21*(2), 89–98.

40. Sliwa K., Hilfiker-Kleiner D., Petrie M. C., et al. (2010). Current state of knowledge on aetiology, diagnosis, management, and therapy of peripartum cardiomyopathy: A European Society of Cardiology working group on peripartum cardiomyopathy. *European Journal of Heart Failure, 12*(8), 767–778.

41. Pelliccia F., Greco D., Vitale C., et al. (2014). Takotsubo syndrome (stress cardiomyopathy): An intriguing clinical condition in search of its identity. *The American Journal of Medicine, 127*(8), 699–704.

42. Hoen B., Duval X. (2013). Infective endocarditis. *New England Journal of Medicine, 368*(15), 1425–1433.

43. Allen U. D., Canadian Paediatric Society Infectious Disease and Immunization Committee. (2010). Infective endocarditis: Updated Guidelines – Reaffirmed 2014. *Paediatrics & Child Health, 15*(4), 205–208.

44. Canadian Dental Association. (2014). CDA position on prevention of infective endocarditis. Available online at: http://www.cda-adc.ca/_files/position_statements/infectiousEndocarditis.pdf. Accessed March 30, 2015.

45. Marijon E., Mirabel M., Celermajer D. S., et al. (2012). Rheumatic heart disease. *Lancet, 379*(9819), 953–964.

46. Madden S., Kelly L. (2009). Update on acute rheumatic fever. *Canadian Family Physician, 55*(5), 475–478.

47. Ferrieri P., Jones Criteria Working Group. (2002). Proceedings of the Jones criteria workshop. *Circulation, 106*(19), 2521–2527.

48. World Health Organization. (2004). Rheumatic fever and rheumatic heart disease: Report of a WHO expert consultation. Available online at: http://www.who.int/cardiovascular_diseases/resources/en/cvd_trs923.pdf. Accessed March 30, 2015.

49. Roberts, K., Colquhoun, S., Steer, A., et al. (2013). Screening for rheumatic heart disease: Current approaches and controversies. *Nature Reviews Cardiology, 10*, 49–58.

50. Chandrashekhar Y., Westaby S., Narula J. (2009). Mitral stenosis. *Lancet, 374*(9697), 1271–1283.

51. Guy T. S., Hill A. C. (2012). Mitral valve prolapse. *Annual Review of Medicine, 63*, 277–292.

52. Heart & Stroke Foundation. (2015). Congenital heart disease. Available online at: http://www.heartandstroke.com/site/c.ikIQLcMWJtE/b.3484063/k.E84C/Heart_disease__Congenital_heart_disease.htm. Accessed March 24, 2015.

53. Van Praagh R. (2006). Chapter 2: Embryology. In Keane J. F., Lock J. E., Fyler D. C. (Eds), *Nadas' pediatric cardiology* (2nd ed.). Philadelphia, PA: Elsevier Saunders.

54. Freed M. D. (2006). Chapter 6: Fetal and transitional circulation. In Keane J. F., Lock J. E., Fyler D. C. (Eds), *Nadas' pediatric cardiology* (2nd ed.). Philadelphia, PA: Elsevier Saunders.

55. Canadian Congenital Heart Alliance. (2014). Facts and issues. Available online at: http://www.cchaforlife.org/facts-issues. Accessed March 30, 2015.

56. Marian A. J., Brugada R., Roberts R. (2011). Chapter 82: Cardiovascular diseases caused by genetic abnormalities. In Fuster V., Walsh R. A., Harrington R. A., et al. *Hurst's the heart* (13th ed.). New York: McGraw Hill Companies.

57. Jenkins K. J., Correa A., Feinstein J. A., et al. (2007). Noninherited risk factors and congenital cardiovascular defects: Current knowledge. *Circulation, 115*(23), 2995–3014.

58. Fyler D. C. (2006). Chapter 8: Hypoxemia. In Keane J. F., Lock J. E., Fyler D. C. (Eds), *Nadas' pediatric cardiology* (2nd ed.). Philadelphia, PA: Elsevier Saunders.

59. Brown D. W., Fulton D. R. (2011). Chapter 83: Congenital heart disease in children and adolescents. In Fuster V., Walsh R. A., Harrington R. A., et al. *Hurst's the heart* (13th ed.). New York: McGraw Hill Companies.

60. Bernstein D. (2011). Chapter 423: Cyanotic congenital heart disease. In Kliegman R. M., Stanton B. F., St. Geme J. W., et al. (Eds.), *Nelson textbook of pediatrics* (19th ed.). Philadelphia, PA: Saunders Elsevier.

61. Bernstein D. (2011). Chapter 418: Epidemiology and genetic basis of congenital heart disease. In Kliegman R. M., Stanton B. F., St. Geme J. W., et al. (Eds.), *Nelson textbook of pediatrics* (19th ed.). Philadelphia, PA: Saunders Elsevier.

62. Keane J. F., Geva T., Fyler D. C. (2006). Chapter 34: Atrial septal defect. In Keane J. F., Lock J. E., Fyler D. C. (Eds.), *Nadas' pediatric cardiology* (2nd ed.). Philadelphia, PA: Elsevier Saunders.

63. Anikumar M. (2013). Patent ductus arteriosus. *Cardiology Clinics, 31*(3), 417–430.

64. Le J., Gales M. A., Gales B. J. (2015). Acetaminophen for patent ductus arteriosus. *The Annals of Pharmacotherapy, 49*(2), 241–246.

65. Penny D. J., Vick G. W. (2011). Ventricular septal defect. *Lancet, 377*(9771), 1103–1112.

66. Marx G. R., Fyler D. C. (2006). Chapter 38: Endocardial cushion defects. In Keane J. F., Lock J. E., Fyler D. C. (Eds.), *Nadas' pediatric cardiology* (2nd ed.). Philadelphia, PA: Elsevier Saunders.

67. Pontailler M., Kalfa D., Garcia E., et al. (2014). Preoperations for left atrioventricular valve dysfunction after repair of atrioventricular septal defect. *European Journal of Cardio-Thoracic Surgery, 45*(3), 557–563.

68. Rigby M. L. (2012). Severe aortic or pulmonary valve stenosis in premature infants. *Early Human Development, 88*(5), 291–294.

69. Fulton D. R., Fyler D. C. (2006). Chapter 37: D-transposition of the great arteries. In Keane J. F., Lock J. E., Fyler D. C. (Eds.), *Nadas' pediatric cardiology* (2nd ed.). Philadelphia, PA: Elsevier Saunders.

70. Tanous D., Benson L. N., Horlick E. M. (2009). Coarctation of the aorta: Evaluation and management. *Current Opinion in Cardiology, 24*(6), 509–515.

71. Jaquiss R. D. B., Imamura M. (2009). Single ventricle physiology: Surgical options, indications and outcomes. *Current Opinion in Cardiology, 24*(2), 113–118.

72. Aboulhosn J. A., Child J. S. (2011) Chapter 84: Congenital heart disease in adults. In Fuster V., Walsh R. A., Harrington R. A., et al. (Eds.), *Hurst's the heart* (13th ed.). New York: McGraw Hill Companies.

73. Son M. B., Newburger J. W. (2011). Chapter 160: Kawasaki disease. In Kliegman R. M., Stanton B. F., St. Geme J. W., et al. (Eds.), *Nelson textbook of pediatrics* (19th ed.). Philadelphia, PA: Saunders Elsevier.

74. Eleftheriou D., Levin M., Shingadia D., et al. (2014). Management of Kawasaki disease. *Archives of Disease in Childhood, 99*(1), 74–83.

75. Han R. K., Sinclair B., Newman A., et al. (2000). Recognition and management of Kawasaki disease. *Canadian Medical Association Journal, 162*(6), 807–812.

Visit thePoint **http://thePoint.lww.com for animations, journal articles, and more!**

Disorders of Cardiac Conduction and Rhythm

CARDIAC CONDUCTION SYSTEM
  Action Potentials
    Action Potential Phases
    Fast and Slow Responses
    Absolute and Relative Refractory Periods
  Electrocardiography
DISORDERS OF CARDIAC RHYTHM AND CONDUCTION
  Mechanisms of Arrhythmias and Conduction Disorders
  Types of Arrhythmias and Conduction Disorders
    Sinus Node Arrhythmias
    Arrhythmias of Atrial Origin
    Junctional Arrhythmias
    Disorders of Ventricular Conduction and Rhythm
    Long QT Syndrome and Torsades de Pointes
    Ventricular Arrhythmias
    Disorders of Atrioventricular Conduction
    Inherited Types of Arrhythmias
  Diagnostic Methods
    Signal-Averaged Electrocardiogram
    Holter Monitoring
    Implantable Loop ECG Recorder
    Exercise Stress Testing
    Electrophysiologic Studies
  Treatment
    Pharmacologic Treatment
    Electrical Interventions
    Ablation and Surgical Interventions

Heart muscle is unique in that it is capable of generating and rapidly conducting its own electrical impulses or action potentials. These action potentials result in excitation of muscle fibres throughout the myocardium. Impulse formation and conduction result in weak electrical currents that spread through the entire myocardium. It is these electrical impulses that are recorded on an electrocardiogram. Disorders of cardiac impulse generation and conduction range from benign arrhythmias to those causing serious disruption of heart function and sudden cardiac death.

CARDIAC CONDUCTION SYSTEM

After completing this section of the chapter, you should be able to meet the following objectives:

- Describe the cardiac conduction system and relate it to the mechanical functioning of the heart.
- Characterize the four phases of a cardiac action potential and differentiate between the fast and slow responses.
- Draw an electrocardiogram tracing and state the origin of the component parts of the tracing.
- Provide rationale for the importance of careful lead placement and monitoring of ischemic events.

In certain areas of the heart, the myocardial cells have been modified to form the specialized cells of the conduction system. Although most myocardial cells are capable of initiating and conducting impulses, it is the conduction system that maintains the sequential activation of myocardial tissue and the pumping efficiency of the heart. Specialized pacemaker cells generate impulses at a faster rate than other types of heart tissue, and the conduction tissue transmits these impulses more rapidly than other cardiac cell types. Because of these properties, the conduction system normally controls the rhythm of the heart. Blood reaches the conduction tissues by way of the coronary arteries. Coronary heart disease that interrupts blood flow through the arteries supplying tissues of the conduction system can induce serious and sometimes fatal disturbances in cardiac rhythm.

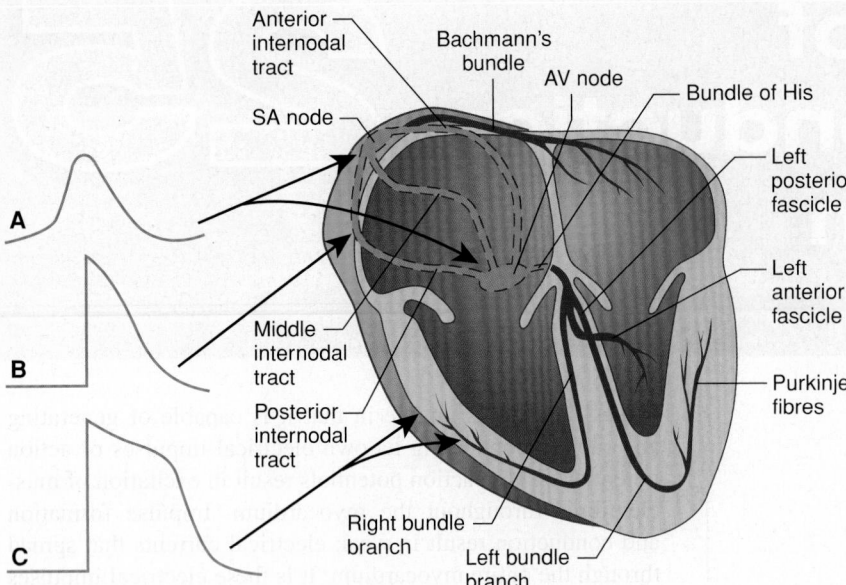

FIGURE 25.1 • Conduction system of the heart and action potentials. **A:** Action potential of sinoatrial (SA) and atrioventricular (AV) nodes. **B:** Atrial muscle action potential. **C:** Action potential of ventricular muscle and Purkinje fibres.

The specialized excitatory and conduction system of the heart consists of the sinoatrial (SA) node, in which the normal rhythmic impulse is generated; the internodal pathways between the atria and the ventricles; the atrioventricular (AV) node and bundle of His, which conduct the impulse from the atria to the ventricles; and the Purkinje fibres, which conduct the impulses to all parts of the ventricle (Fig. 25.1).

The heart essentially has two conduction systems: one that controls atrial activity and one that controls ventricular activity. The atrial conduction begins with the SA node, which has the fastest intrinsic rate of firing (60 to 100 beats/minute), normally serves as the pacemaker of the heart. It is a spindle-shaped strip of specialized muscle tissue, about 10 to 20 mm in length and 2 to 3 mm wide, located in the posterior wall of the right atrium just below the opening of the superior vena cava and less than 1 mm from the epicardial surface.[1] While the clusters of the SA cells work together to initiate electrical activity, this node is also richly supplied with nerves from both the sympathetic chains and the vagus nerve.

Impulses originating in the SA node travel through the atria to the AV node. Because of the anatomic location of the SA node, the progression of atrial depolarization occurs in an inferior, leftward, and somewhat posterior direction, and the right atrium is depolarized slightly before the left atrium.[2] There are three internodal pathways between the SA node and the AV node, including the anterior (Bachmann), middle (Wenckebach), and posterior (Thorel) internodal tracts. These three tracts anastomose with each other proximally to the AV node. Interatrial conduction appears to be accomplished through the Bachmann bundle. This large muscle bundle originates along the anterior border of the SA node and travels posteriorly around the aorta to the left atrium.[3]

The AV junction connects the two conduction systems and normally provides for a one-way conduction between the atria and ventricles. The AV node is a compact, ovoid structure measuring approximately $1 \times 3 \times 5$ mm and located slightly

beneath the right atrial endocardium, anterior to the opening of the coronary sinus, and immediately above the insertion of the septal leaflet of the tricuspid valve.[1,3] It is important to note that everywhere except for the AV node in a healthy heart, the atrial muscle is separated from the ventricular muscle in order to prevent cardiac impulses firing inappropriately.

The AV node is divided into three functional regions: the AN or transitional region, located between the atria and the rest of the node; the N or middle region (*i.e.,* the node proper); and the NH region, in which nodal fibres merge with the bundle of His, which is the upper portion of the specialized conduction system.[1,4] In the AN portion of the node, atrial fibres connect with very small junctional fibres of the node itself. The velocity of conduction through the AN and N fibres is very slow (approximately one half that of normal cardiac muscle), which greatly delays transmission of the impulse.[4,5] A further delay occurs as the impulse travels through the N region into the NH region, which connects with the *bundle of His* (also called the *AV bundle*). This delay provides a mechanical advantage whereby the atria complete their ejection of blood into the ventricles before ventricular contraction begins. Under normal circumstances, the AV node provides the only connection between the atrial and ventricular conduction systems as its main job is to coordinate atrial and ventricular conduction. The atria and ventricles beat independently of each other if the transmission of impulses through the AV node is blocked.

The *Purkinje system*, which initiates ventricular conduction, has large, specialized fibres that allow for rapid conduction and almost simultaneous excitation of the entire right and left ventricles (0.06 second).[5] This rapid rate of conduction throughout the Purkinje system is necessary for the swift and efficient ejection of blood from the heart. The Purkinje system originates in the AV node and proceeds to form the bundle of His, which extends through the fibrous tissue between the valves of the heart and into the ventricular system. Because of its proximity to the aortic valve and the mitral valve ring,

CARDIAC CONDUCTION SYSTEM

- The cardiac conduction system controls the rate and direction of electrical impulse conduction in the heart.
- Normally, impulses are generated in the SA node, which has the fastest rate of firing, and travel through the AV node to the Purkinje system in the ventricles.
- Cardiac action potentials are divided into five phases: phase 0, or the rapid upstroke of the action potential; phase 1, or early repolarization; phase 2, or the plateau; phase 3, or final repolarization period; and phase 4, or diastolic repolarization period.
- Cardiac muscle has two types of ion channels that function in producing the voltage changes that occur during the depolarization phase of the action potential: the fast sodium channels and the slow calcium channels.
- There are two types of cardiac action potentials: the fast response, which occurs in atrial and ventricular muscle cells and the Purkinje conduction system which uses the fast sodium channels; and the slow response of the SA and AV nodes, which uses the slow calcium channels.

the bundle of His is predisposed to inflammation and deposits of calcified debris that can interfere with impulse conduction.[5] There are fibres in the AV node or bundle of His, which together form the junctional area, most commonly referred to as the AV junction. The bundle of His almost immediately divides into *right* and *left bundle branches* that straddle the interventricular septum. Branches from the anterior and posterior descending coronary arteries provide the blood supply for the His bundle, making this conduction site less susceptible to ischemic damage, unless the damage is extensive.[1] The bundle branches move through the subendocardial tissues toward the papillary muscles and then subdivide into the Purkinje fibres, which branch out, forming a network of fibres into the outer walls of the ventricles. The main trunk of the left bundle branch extends for approximately 1 to 2 cm before fanning out as it enters the septal area and divides further into two segments: the *left posterior* and *anterior fascicles*.

The AV junctional fibres, when not stimulated by atrial depolarization, discharge at an intrinsic rate of 40 to 60 times a minute, and the Purkinje fibres discharge 15 to 40 times per minute. Although the AV junction and Purkinje system have the ability to control the rhythm of the heart, they do not normally do so because the discharge rate of the SA node is considerably faster. Each time the SA node discharges, its impulses are conducted into the AV node and Purkinje fibres, causing them to depolarize. The AV node can assume the pacemaker function of the heart, should the SA node fail to discharge, and the Purkinje system can assume the pacemaker function of the ventricles should the AV node fail to conduct impulses from the atria to the ventricles. Under these circumstances, the heart rate reflects the intrinsic firing rate of the prevailing structures.

Action Potentials

An action potential represents the sequential change in electrical potential that occurs across a cell membrane when excitation occurs (see Chapter 4, Understanding Membrane Potentials). These potential or voltage differences, often referred to as membrane potentials, represent the flow of current associated with the passage of ions through ion channels in the cell membrane. The sodium (Na^+), potassium (K^+), and calcium (Ca^{2+}) ions are the major charge carriers in cardiac muscle cells. Disorders of the ion channels, along with disruption in the flow of these current-carrying ions, are increasingly being linked to the generation of cardiac arrhythmias and conduction disorders.

Action potentials can be divided into three phases: the resting or unexcited state, depolarization, and repolarization. During the resting phase, cardiac cells exhibit a resting membrane potential that typically ranges from –60 to –90 millivolts (mV). The negative sign before the voltage indicates that the inside of the cell has a negative charge in relation to the outside (Fig. 25.2). Although different kinds of ions are found both inside and outside of the membrane, the membrane potential is determined largely by Na^+ and K^+ and the membrane is selectively permeable to K^+ and nearly impermeable to Na^+. As a result, K^+ diffuses out of the cell along its concentration gradient. In addition, Na^+/K^+ATPase pumps are unequal in their exchange of ions, with three sodium ions exiting the cell and two potassium ions entering the cell, resulting in a negative balance in charge. Sodium is strongly attracted to the interior of the cell by its concentration gradient, but because its ability to diffuse across the membrane is much less than that of K^+, the influx of Na^+ is inadequate to balance K^+ outflow. The result is an unequal distribution of Na^+ and K^+ across the membrane with a relative loss of positive ions from inside the membrane.

Depolarization represents the period of time (measured in either seconds or milliseconds) during which the polarity of the membrane potential is reversed and moves toward zero charge or even becomes positive. It occurs when the cell membrane suddenly becomes selectively permeable to a

FIGURE 25.2 • The flow of charge during impulse generation in excitable tissue. **A:** During the resting state, opposite charges are separated by the cell membrane. **B:** Depolarization represents the flow of charge across the membrane, and repolarization denotes the return of the membrane potential to its resting state (**C**).

current-carrying ion such as Na⁺, allowing it to move into the cell and change the membrane potential so the cell becomes positive on the inside and negative on the outside (Fig. 25.2B).

Repolarization involves reestablishment of the resting membrane potential. It is a complex and somewhat slower process in cardiac cells, involving the outward flow of electrical charges and the return of the membrane potential to its resting state.[6] During repolarization, membrane permeability for K⁺ again increases, allowing the positively charged K⁺ to move outward across the membrane. This outward movement removes positive charges from inside the cell; thus, the voltage across the membrane again becomes negative in the inside and positive on the outside (Fig. 25.2C). The adenosine triphosphatase (ATPase)-dependent sodium–potassium pump assists in repolarization by pumping positively charged Na⁺ out across the cell membrane and returning K⁺ to the inside of the membrane.[7]

Action Potential Phases

The action potentials in cardiac muscle cells are typically divided into five phases: *phase 0*—upstroke or rapid depolarization; *phase 1*—early repolarization period; *phase 2*—plateau; *phase 3*—final, rapid repolarization period; and *phase 4*—diastolic depolarization (Fig. 25.3B). Cardiac muscle cells have three types of membrane ion channels that contribute to the voltage changes that occur during the different phases of

the cardiac action potential. They are the fast Na⁺ channels, slow calcium (Ca²⁺) channels, and K⁺ channels. In contrast, the action potentials in the normal SA and AV nodes have a much slower upstroke and are mediated predominantly by slow Ca²⁺ channels.

During *phase 0,* in atrial and ventricular muscle and in the Purkinje system, the fast Na⁺ channels in the cell membrane are stimulated to open, resulting in the rapid influx of Na⁺. The point at which the Na⁺ channels open is called the *depolarization threshold.* When the cell has reached this threshold, a rapid influx of Na⁺ occurs. The exterior of the cell now is negatively charged in relation to the highly positive interior of the cell. This influx of Na⁺ produces a rapid, positively directed change in the membrane potential, resulting in the electrical spike and overshoot during phase 0 of the action potential.[6] The membrane potential shifts from a resting membrane potential of approximately –90 to +20 mV. The rapid depolarization that comprises phase 0 is responsible for the P wave and the QRS complex on the electrocardiogram (ECG), which represent atrial and ventricular muscle depolarization (Fig. 25.3A). Depolarization of a cardiac cell tends to cause adjacent cells to depolarize because the voltage spike of the cell's depolarization stimulates the Na⁺ channels in nearby cells to open. Therefore, when a cardiac cell is stimulated to depolarize, a wave of depolarization is propagated across the heart, cell by cell.

Phase 1 occurs at the peak of the action potential and signifies inactivation of the fast Na⁺ channels with an abrupt decrease in sodium permeability. The slight downward slope is thought to be caused by the influx of a small amount of negatively charged chloride ions and the efflux of potassium.[1] The decrease in intracellular charge reduces the membrane potential to a level near 0 mV, from which the plateau, or phase 2, arises.

Phase 2 represents the plateau of the action potential. If K⁺ permeability increased to its resting level at this time, as it does in nerve fibres or skeletal muscle, the cell would repolarize rapidly. Instead, K⁺ permeability is low, allowing the membrane to remain depolarized throughout the phase 2 plateau. A concomitant influx of Ca²⁺ into the cell through the slow Ca²⁺ channels contributes to the phase 2 plateau.[6] Calcium ions entering the muscle during this phase also play a key role in the contractile process.[1] These unique features of the phase 2 plateau cause the action potential of cardiac muscle (several hundred milliseconds [mSec]) to last 3 to 15 times longer than that of skeletal muscle and produce a corresponding increased period of contraction.[5] The phase 2 plateau of ventricular muscle cells coincides with the ST segment of the ECG.

Phase 3 reflects rapid repolarization and begins with the downslope of the action potential. During the phase 3 repolarization period, the slow Ca²⁺ channels close and the influx of Ca²⁺ and Na⁺ ceases. There is a sharp rise in K⁺ permeability, contributing to the rapid outward movement of K⁺ and reestablishment of the resting membrane potential (–90 mV). At the conclusion of phase 3, the distribution of K⁺ and Na⁺

FIGURE 25.3 • Relation between (**A**) the electrocardiogram and (**B**) phases of the ventricular action potential.

returns the membrane to the normal resting state. The T wave on the ECG corresponds with phase 3 of the action potential of ventricular muscle cells.

Phase 4 represents the resting membrane potential. During phase 4, the activity of the Na^+/K^+-ATPase pump contributes to maintaining the resting membrane polarity by transporting Na^+ out of the cell and moving K^+ back in. Phase 4 corresponds to ventricular diastole.[1]

Fast and Slow Responses

There are two main types of action potentials in the heart—the fast response and the slow response. The *fast response* occurs in the normal myocardial cells of the atria, the ventricles, and the Purkinje fibres (Fig. 25.4A). Depolarization is characterized by the opening of voltage-dependent Na^+ channels called the *fast sodium channels*. The fast-response cardiac cells do not normally initiate cardiac action potentials.

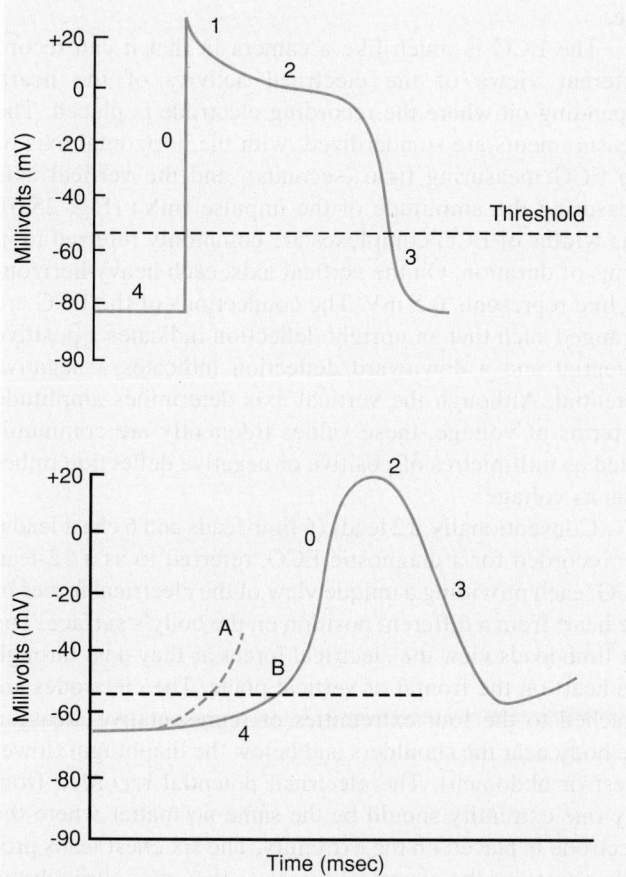

FIGURE 25.4 • Changes in action potential recorded from a fast response in cardiac muscle cell (**top**) and from a slow response recorded in the sinoatrial and atrioventricular nodes (**bottom**). The phases of the action potential are identified by numbers: phase 4, resting membrane potential; phase 0, depolarization; phase 1, brief period of repolarization; phase 2, plateau; phase 3, repolarization. The slow response is characterized by a slow, spontaneous rise in the phase 4 membrane potential to threshold levels; it has a lesser amplitude and shorter duration than the fast response. Increased automaticity (A) occurs when the rate of phase 4 depolarization is increased.

Instead, impulses originating in the specialized cells of the SA node are conducted to the fast-response myocardial cells, where they effect a change in the membrane potential to the threshold level. On reaching threshold, the voltage-dependent Na^+ channels open to initiate the rapid upstroke of the phase 1 action potential. The amplitude and the rate of rise of phase 1 are important to the conduction velocity of the fast response. Myocardial fibres with a fast response are capable of conducting electrical activity at relatively rapid rates (0.5 to 5.0 m/second), thereby providing a high safety factor for conduction.[8]

The *slow response* occurs in the SA node, which is the natural pacemaker of the heart, and the conduction fibres of the AV node (Fig. 25.4B). The hallmark of these pacemaker cells is a spontaneous phase 4 depolarization. The membrane permeability of these cells allows a slow inward leak of current to occur through the slow channels during phase 4. This leak continues until the threshold for firing is reached, at which point the cell spontaneously depolarizes. Under normal conditions, the slow response, sometimes referred to as the *calcium current,* does not contribute significantly to depolarization of the atria and ventricles. Its primary role in normal atrial and ventricular cells is to provide for the entrance of calcium for the excitation–contraction mechanism that couples the electrical activity with muscle contraction.

The rate of pacemaker cell discharge varies with the resting membrane potential and the slope of phase 4 depolarization (Fig. 25.4). Catecholamines (*i.e.,* epinephrine and norepinephrine) increase heart rate by increasing the slope or rate of phase 4 depolarization. Acetylcholine, which is released during vagal stimulation of the heart, slows the heart rate by decreasing the slope of phase 4.

The fast response of atrial and ventricular muscle can be converted to a slow pacemaker response under certain conditions. For example, such conversions may occur spontaneously in individuals with severe coronary artery disease, in areas of the heart where blood supply has been markedly compromised or curtailed. Impulses generated by these cells can lead to ectopic beats and serious arrhythmias.

Absolute and Relative Refractory Periods

The pumping action of the heart requires alternating contraction and relaxation periods, and there is a period in the action potential during which the membrane cannot be stimulated to generate another action potential (Fig. 25.5). This period, known as the *absolute refractory period,* includes phases 0, 1, and 2 and part of phase 3. During this time, the cell cannot depolarize again under any circumstances. This acts as a safety margin for the heart in order to prevent any stimulation or generation of any extra beats. When repolarization has returned the membrane potential to a level below the threshold potential, but not to the resting membrane potential, the cell is capable of responding to a greater-than-normal stimulus. This interval occurs at the end of phase 3 and is referred to as the *relative refractory*

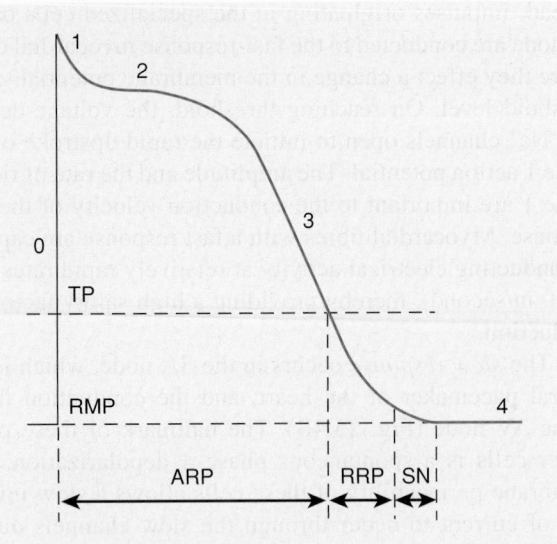

FIGURE 25.5 • Diagram of an action potential of a ventricular muscle cell, showing the threshold potential (TP), resting membrane potential (RMP), absolute refractory period (ARP), relative refractory period (RRP), and supernormal (SN) period.

period. The relative refractory period begins when the membrane potential in phase 3 reaches threshold level and ends just before the end of phase 3. After the relative refractory period is a short period called the *supernormal excitatory period*, during which a weak stimulus can evoke a response. The supernormal excitatory period extends from the terminal portion of phase 3 until the beginning of phase 4. It is during this period that cardiac arrhythmias may develop.[4,7,8]

In skeletal muscle, the refractory period is very short compared with the duration of contraction, such that a second contraction cannot be initiated before the first one is over, resulting in a summated tetanized contraction. In cardiac muscle, the absolute refractory period is almost as long as the contraction itself, ensuring that a second contraction cannot be stimulated until the first is complete. The longer length of the absolute refractory period of cardiac muscle is important in maintaining the alternating contraction and relaxation that are essential to the pumping action of the heart and for the prevention of fatal arrhythmias.

Electrocardiography

The electrocardiogram (ECG) is a graphic recording of the electrical activity of the heart. The electrical currents generated by the heart spread throughout the body and to the skin, where the current can be sensed by appropriately placed electrodes, amplified, and viewed on an oscilloscope or paper recorder.

The deflection points of an ECG are designated by the letters P, Q, R, S, and T. Figure 25.6 depicts the electrical activity of the conduction system on an ECG tracing. The P wave represents depolarization of the SA node and the atria;

the QRS complex (*i.e.,* beginning of the Q wave to the end of the S wave) depicts ventricular depolarization; and the T wave portrays ventricular repolarization. The isoelectric line between the P wave and the Q wave represents depolarization of the AV node, bundle branches, and Purkinje system. Atrial repolarization occurs during ventricular depolarization and is hidden in the QRS complex.

The ECG records the potential difference in charge between two electrodes as depolarization and repolarization waves move through the heart and are conducted to the skin surface. The shape of the recorder tracing is determined by the direction in which the impulse spreads through the heart muscle in relation to electrode placement. A depolarization wave that moves toward the recording electrode registers as a positive, or upward deflection. Conversely, if the impulse moves away from the recording electrode, the deflection is downward, or negative. When there is no flow of charge between electrodes, the potential is zero, and a straight line is recorded at the baseline of the chart, which is called the isoelectric line.

The ECG is much like a camera in that it can record different views of the electrical activity of the heart, depending on where the recording electrode is placed. The measurements are standardized, with the horizontal axis of the ECG measuring time (seconds), and the vertical axis measuring the amplitude of the impulse (mV) (Fig. 25.6). The widths of ECG complexes are commonly referred to in terms of duration. On the vertical axis, each heavy horizontal line represents 0.5 mV. The connections of the ECG are arranged such that an upright deflection indicates a positive potential and a downward deflection indicates a negative potential. Although the vertical axis determines amplitude in terms of voltage, these values frequently are communicated as millimetres of positive or negative deflection rather than as voltage.

Conventionally, 12 leads (6 limb leads and 6 chest leads) are recorded for a diagnostic ECG, referred to as a 12-lead ECG, each providing a unique view of the electrical forces of the heart from a different position on the body's surface. The six limb leads view the electrical forces as they pass through the heart on the frontal or vertical plane. The electrodes are attached to the four extremities or representative areas on the body near the shoulders and below the diaphragm (lower chest or abdomen). The electrical potential recorded from any one extremity should be the same no matter where the electrode is placed on the extremity. The six chest leads provide a view of the electrical forces as they pass through the heart on the horizontal plane. They are located on different positions on the chest, including the right and left sternal borders and the left anterior surface (Fig. 25.7). The right lower extremity lead is used as a ground electrode. When indicated, additional electrodes may be applied to the posterior and right anterior chest, to obtain either a 15-lead or 18-lead ECG.

Continuous cardiac monitoring reports one or two leads of the available 12 leads; conventionally, Leads V_1 and II are

FIGURE 25.6 • Diagram of the electrocardiogram (lead II) and representative depolarization and repolarization of the atria and ventricles. The P wave represents atrial depolarization, the QRS complex ventricular depolarization, and the T wave ventricular repolarization. Atrial repolarization occurs during ventricular depolarization and is hidden under the QRS complex.

FIGURE 25.7 • Electrode placement for limb leads and precordial leads. Limb electrodes can be placed anywhere on the arms and legs. Chest electrodes are purposely placed as follows: **V1,** fourth intercostal space, right sternal border; **V2,** fourth intercostal space, left sternal border; **V4,** fifth intercostal space, midclavicular line; **V3,** midway between V2 and V4; **V5,** fifth intercostal space, anterior axillary line; and **V6,** fifth intercostal space, midaxillary line. (From Woods S. L., Froelicher E. S., Motzer S. U., et al. (2010). *Cardiac nursing* (6th ed., p. 304). Philadelphia, PA: Lippincott, Williams & Wilkins.).

most commonly used. The goals of continuous bedside cardiac monitoring have shifted from simple heart rate and arrhythmia monitoring to identification of ST segment changes and advanced arrhythmia identification, diagnosis, and treatment. Many diagnostic criteria are lead specific. The monitoring leads selected must maximize the potential for accurately identifying anticipated arrhythmias and ischemic events on the basis of the person's underlying clinical situation.

Although accurate ECG placement and lead selection are important aspects of ECG monitoring, there have been many studies that identified two common errors: inaccurate electrode placement and inappropriate lead selection for individual clinical situations.[9] Improper lead placement can significantly change QRS morphology, resulting in misdiagnosis of cardiac arrhythmias or failure to detect existing conduction defects.

In persons with acute coronary syndromes (ACS), which include unstable angina and myocardial infarction, careful cardiac ECG monitoring is imperative[10] (see Chapter 24). Persons with ACS are at risk for development of extension of an infarcted area, ongoing myocardial ischemia, and life-threatening arrhythmias. Research has shown that ECG monitoring is more sensitive than a patient's report of symptoms for identifying transient ongoing myocardial ischemia. ECG monitoring also provides for more accurate and timely detection of ischemic events, essential for treatment options such as reperfusion strategies.[11] It is recommended that all 12 ECG leads be used for monitoring patients with ACS because ischemic changes that occur may be evident in different leads at different times.

IN SUMMARY

The rhythmic contraction and relaxation of the heart rely on the specialized cells of the heart's conduction system. Specialized cells in the SA node have the fastest inherent rate of impulse generation and act as the pacemaker of the heart. Impulses from the SA node travel through the atria to the AV node and then to the AV bundle and the ventricular Purkinje system. The AV node provides the only connection between the atrial and ventricular conduction systems. The atria and the ventricles function independently of each other when AV node conduction is blocked.

The action potential represents the sequential changes in electrical potentials that are associated with the movement of current-carrying ions through ion channels in the cell membrane. The action potentials of cardiac muscle are divided into five phases: phase 0 represents depolarization and is characterized by the rapid upstroke of the action potential; phase 1 is characterized by a brief period of repolarization; phase 2 consists of a plateau, which prolongs the duration of the action potential; phase 3 represents repolarization; and phase 4 is the resting membrane potential. After an action potential, there is a refractory period during which the membrane is resistant to a second stimulus. During the absolute refractory period, the membrane is insensitive to stimulation. This period is followed by the relative refractory period, during which a more intense stimulus is needed to initiate an action potential. The relative refractory period is followed by a supernormal excitatory period, during which a weak stimulus can evoke a response.

The ECG provides a means for monitoring the electrical activity of the heart. Conventionally, 12 leads (6 limb leads and 6 chest leads) are recorded for a diagnostic ECG, each providing a unique view of the electrical forces of the heart from a different position on the body's surface. This procedure allows for advanced arrhythmia detection, detection of wide-QRS-complex tachycardia, and early identification of ischemia- and infarction-related changes in persons with ASC.

DISORDERS OF CARDIAC RHYTHM AND CONDUCTION

After completing this section of the chapter, you should be able to meet the following objectives:

- Describe the possible mechanisms for arrhythmia generation.
- Compare sinus arrhythmias with atrial arrhythmias.
- Characterize the effects of atrial flutter and atrial fibrillation on heart rhythm.
- Describe the significance of long QT syndrome.
- Describe the characteristics of first-, second-, and third-degree heart block.
- Compare the effects of premature ventricular complexes, ventricular tachycardia, and ventricular fibrillation on cardiac function.
- Cite the types of cardiac conditions that can be diagnosed using the ECG.
- Describe the methods used in diagnosis of cardiac arrhythmias.
- Explain the mechanisms, criteria for use, and benefits of antiarrhythmic drugs, internal cardioverter-defibrillator therapy, ablation therapy, and surgical procedures in the treatment of persons with recurrent, symptomatic arrhythmias.

There are two types of disorders of the cardiac conduction system: disorders of impulse initiation and disorders of impulse conduction. The terms *dysrhythmia* and *arrhythmia* have sometimes been used interchangeably to describe disorders of cardiac rhythm. However, the term *dysrhythmia* has not been generally accepted and use of the term *arrhythmia* continues. Therefore, the term *arrhythmia* is used throughout this chapter.

There are many causes of cardiac arrhythmias and conduction disorders, including congenital defects or degenerative changes in the conduction system, myocardial ischemia and infarction, fluid and electrolyte imbalances, and the effects of pharmaceutical agents. Arrhythmias are not necessarily pathologic; they can occur in both healthy and diseased hearts. Disturbances in cardiac rhythms exert their harmful effects by interfering with the heart's pumping ability. Excessively rapid heart rates (tachyarrhythmias) reduce the diastolic filling time or impair ventricular contractility, causing a subsequent decrease in the stroke volume output and in coronary perfusion while increasing the myocardial oxygen needs. Abnormally slow heart rates (bradyarrhythmias) may impair blood flow to vital organs such as the brain.

Mechanisms of Arrhythmias and Conduction Disorders

The specialized cells in the heart manifest four inherent properties that contribute to the genesis of all cardiac rhythms, both normal and abnormal. They are automaticity, excitability, conductivity, and refractoriness. An alteration in any of these four properties may produce arrhythmias.

The ability of cells in the heart to spontaneously initiate an impulse or action potential is referred to as *automaticity*. The SA node has an inherent discharge rate of 60 to 100 times per minute. It normally acts as the primary or dominant pacemaker of the heart because it reaches the threshold for excitation before other parts of the conduction system have recovered sufficiently to be depolarized. If the SA node fires more slowly or SA node conduction is blocked, another site that is capable of automaticity takes over as pacemaker. Other regions that have intrinsic automaticity capabilities include the atrial fibres that have plateau-type action potentials, the AV junction, the bundle of His, and the bundle branch Purkinje fibres. These pacemakers have a slower rate of discharge than the SA node. The AV junction has an inherent firing rate of 40 to 60 times per minute, and the Purkinje system fires at a rate of 15 to 40 times per minute.[5] The SA node may be functioning properly, but because of additional precipitating factors, other cardiac cells can assume accelerated properties of automaticity and begin to initiate impulses. These additional factors might include injury, hypoxia, electrolyte disturbances, enlargement or hypertrophy of the atria or ventricles, and exposure to certain chemicals or drugs.

PHYSIOLOGIC BASIS OF ARRHYTHMIA GENERATION

- Cardiac arrhythmias represent disorders of cardiac rhythm related to alterations in automaticity, excitability, conductivity, or refractoriness of specialized cells in the conduction system of the heart.
- Automaticity refers to the ability of pacemaker cells in the heart to spontaneously generate an action potential. Normally, the SA node is the dominant pacemaker of the heart because of its intrinsic automaticity.
- Excitability is the ability of cardiac tissue to respond to an impulse and generate an action potential, whereas conductivity and refractoriness represent the ability of cardiac tissue to conduct action potentials.
- Whereas conductivity relates to the ability of cardiac tissue to conduct impulses, refractoriness represents temporary interruptions in conductivity related to the repolarization phase of the action potential.

An *ectopic pacemaker* is an excitable focus outside the normally functioning SA node. These pacemakers can reside in other parts of the conduction system or in muscle cells of the atria or ventricles. A premature complex occurs when an ectopic pacemaker initiates a beat. Premature complex do not follow the normal conduction pathways, they are not coupled with normal mechanical events, and they often render the heart refractory or incapable of responding to the next normal impulse arising in the SA node. They occur without incident in persons with healthy hearts in response to sympathetic nervous system stimulation or other stimulants, such as caffeine. In the diseased heart, premature complexes may lead to more serious arrhythmias.

Excitability describes the ability of a cell to respond to an impulse and generate an action potential. Myocardial cells that have been injured or replaced by scar tissue do not possess normal excitability. For example, during the acute phase of an ischemic event, involved cells become depolarized. These ischemic cells remain electrically coupled to the adjacent nonischemic area; current from the ischemic zone can induce reexcitation of cells in the nonischemic zone.

Conductivity is the ability to conduct impulses, and *refractoriness* refers to the extent to which the cell is able to respond to an incoming stimulus. The refractory period of cardiac muscle is the interval in the repolarization period during which an excitable cell has not recovered sufficiently to be reexcited. Disturbances in conductivity or refractoriness predispose the heart to arrhythmias.

Almost all tachyarrhythmias are the result of a phenomenon known as *reentry*.[4,5,7] Under normal conditions, an electrical impulse is conducted through the heart in an orderly, sequential manner. The electrical impulse then dies out and does not reenter adjacent tissue because that tissue has already been depolarized and is refractory to immediate stimulation. However, fibres that were not activated during the initial wave of depolarization can recover excitability before the initial impulse dies out, and they may serve as a link to reexcite areas of the heart that were just discharged and have recovered from the initial depolarization.[1] This activity disrupts the normal conduction sequence. For reentry to occur, there must be areas of slow conduction and a unidirectional conduction block (Fig. 25.8). For previously depolarized areas to repolarize adequately to conduct an impulse again, slow conduction is necessary. Unidirectional block is necessary to provide a one-way route for the original impulse to reenter, thereby blocking other impulses entering from the opposite direction from extinguishing the reentrant circuit.[4] Reentry requires a triggering stimulus such as an extrasystole. If sufficient time has elapsed for the refractory period in the reentered area to end, a self-perpetuating, circuitous movement can be initiated and an arrhythmia will occur.[1]

FIGURE 25.8 • The role of unidirectional block in reentry. **A:** An excitation wave traveling down a single bundle (S) of fibres continues down the left (L) and right (R) branches. The depolarization wave enters the connecting branch (**C**) from both ends and is extinguished at the zone of collision. **B:** The wave is blocked in the L and R branches. **C:** Bidirectional block exists in the R branch. **D:** The antegrade impulse is blocked, but the retrograde impulse is conducted through and reenters bundle S. (From Berne R. M., Levy M. N. (1988). *Physiology* (2nd ed., p. 417). St. Louis, MO: C.V. Mosby.).

Reentry may occur anywhere in the conduction system. The functional components of a reentry circuit can be large and include an entire specialized conduction system, or the circuit can be microscopic. It can include myocardial tissue, AV nodal cells, bundle of His, or the ventricles. Factors contributing to the development of a reentrant circuit include ischemia, infarction, and elevated serum potassium levels. Scar tissue interrupts the normally low-resistance paths between viable myocardial cells, slowing conduction, promoting asynchronous myocardial activation, and predisposing to unidirectional conduction block. Effects of drugs such as epinephrine can produce a shortened refractory period, thereby increasing the likelihood of reentrant arrhythmias.

There are several forms of reentry. The first is anatomic reentry. It involves an anatomic obstacle around which the circulating current must pass and results in an excitation wave that travels in a set pathway.[1] Arrhythmias that arise as a result of anatomic reentry are paroxysmal supraventricular tachycardias, as seen in Wolff–Parkinson–White syndrome, atrial fibrillation, atrial flutter, AV nodal reentry, and some ventricular tachycardias. Functional reentry does not rely on an anatomic structure to circle, but instead depends on the local differences in conduction velocity and refractoriness among neighbouring fibres that allow an impulse to circulate repeatedly around an area.[1,12,13] Spiral reentry is the most common form of this type of reentry. It is initiated by a wave of electrical current that does not propagate normally after meeting refractory tissue. The broken end of the wave curls, forms a vortex, and permanently rotates. This phenomenon suppresses normal pacemaker activity and in the atria can result in atrial fibrillation.[13,14] Arrhythmias observed with functional reentry are likely to be polymorphic because of changing circuits.[1] Reflection is sometimes considered another form of reentry that can occur in parallel pathways of myocardial tissue or the Purkinje network. With reflection, the cardiac impulse reaches an area of depressed conduction, triggers the surrounding tissue, and then returns in a retrograde direction through the severely depressed region. Reflection differs from true reentry in that the impulse travels along the same pathway in both directions and does not require a circuit.[1]

Types of Arrhythmias and Conduction Disorders

Sinus Node Arrhythmias

In a healthy heart driven by sinus node discharge, the rate ranges between 60 and 100 beats/minute. On the ECG, a P wave is observed to precede every QRS complex. Historically, normal sinus rhythm has been considered the "normal" rhythm of a healthy heart. In normal sinus rhythm, a P wave precedes each QRS complex and the RR intervals remain relatively constant over time (Fig. 25.9). Alterations in the function of the SA node lead to changes in rate or rhythm of the heartbeat.

Years ago, it was believed that sinus rhythm should be regular—that is, all RR intervals should be nearly equal. Today, it is accepted that a more optimal rhythm is respiratory

FIGURE 25.9 • Electrocardiographic tracings of rhythms originating in the sinus node. **A:** Normal sinus rhythm (60 to 100 beats/minute). **B:** Sinus bradycardia (less than 60 beats/minute). **C:** Sinus tachycardia (greater than 100 beats/minute). **D:** Respiratory sinus arrhythmia, characterized by gradual lengthening and shortening of RR intervals.

sinus arrhythmia. Respiratory sinus arrhythmia is a cardiac rhythm characterized by gradual lengthening and shortening of RR intervals (Fig. 25.9D). This variation in cardiac cycles is related to intrathoracic pressure changes that occur with respiration and resultant alterations in autonomic control of the SA node. Inspiration causes acceleration of the heart rate and expiration causes slowing. Respiratory sinus arrhythmia accounts for most heart rate variability in healthy individuals and does not require any treatment. Decreased heart rate variability has been associated with altered health states, including myocardial infarction, congestive heart failure, hypertension, diabetes mellitus, smoking, and prematurity in infants.[15]

Sinus Bradycardia. Sinus bradycardia describes a slow (less than 60 beats/minute) heart rate that has its origin in the SA node (Fig. 25.9B). In sinus bradycardia, a P wave precedes each QRS. A normal P wave and PR interval (0.12 to 0.20 second) indicates that the impulse originated in the SA node rather than in another area of the conduction system that has a slower inherent rate. Vagal stimulation decreases the firing rate of the SA node and conduction through the AV node to cause a decrease in heart rate. This rhythm may be normal in trained athletes, who maintain a large stroke volume, and during sleep. Sinus bradycardia may be an indicator of poor prognosis when it occurs in conjunction with acute myocardial infarction, particularly if associated with hypotension.

Sinus Tachycardia. Sinus tachycardia refers to a rapid heart rate (greater than100 beats/minute) that has its origin in the SA node (Fig. 25.9C). A normal P wave and PR interval should precede each QRS complex. The mechanism of sinus tachycardia is enhanced automaticity related to sympathetic stimulation or withdrawal of vagal tone. Sinus tachycardia is a normal response during fever and exercise, and in situations that incite sympathetic stimulation such as anxiety, blood loss, or pain. It may be associated with heart failure, myocardial infarction, and hyperthyroidism. Pharmacologic agents such as atropine, isoproterenol, epinephrine, and quinidine also can cause sinus tachycardia.

Sinus Arrest. Sinus arrest, or sinus pause, refers to failure of the SA node to discharge and may result in an irregular pulse. An escape rhythm develops as another pacemaker takes over. Sinus arrest may result in prolonged periods of asystole and often predisposes to other arrhythmias. Causes of sinus arrest include disease of the SA node, digitalis toxicity, myocardial infarction, acute myocarditis, excessive vagal tone, sleep apnea, quinidine, lidocaine, and hyperkalemia or hypokalemia.[16,17]

Sick Sinus Syndrome. Sick sinus syndrome is a term that describes a number of forms of cardiac impulse formation and intra-atrial and AV conduction abnormalities.[16,18,19] The syndrome most frequently is the result of total or subtotal destruction of the SA node, areas of nodal-atrial discontinuity, inflammatory or degenerative changes of the nerves and ganglia surrounding the node, or pathologic changes in the atrial wall.[19] In addition, occlusion of the sinus node artery may be a contributing factor. Sick sinus syndrome is most often idiopathic but can be seen in patients with coronary artery disease, fibrosis infective processes, or collagen vascular disease as well as in those taking certain drugs.[19] In children, the syndrome is most commonly associated with congenital heart defects, particularly after corrective cardiac surgery.[16]

The arrhythmias associated with the sick sinus syndrome include spontaneous persistent sinus bradycardia that is not drug induced or appropriate for the physiologic circumstances, prolonged sinus pauses, combinations of SA and AV node conduction disturbances, or alternating paroxysms of rapid regular or irregular atrial tachyarrhythmias and periods of slow atrial and ventricular rates (bradycardia-tachycardia syndrome).[19] Most commonly, the term sick sinus syndrome is used to refer to the *bradycardia-tachycardia syndrome*. The bradycardia is caused by disease of the sinus node (or other intra-atrial conduction pathways), and the tachycardia is caused by paroxysmal atrial or junctional arrhythmias. Individuals with this syndrome often are asymptomatic. Ironically, the development of atrial fibrillation may alleviate symptoms in persons who are symptomatic because heart rate can be controlled more consistently under these circumstances.

The most common manifestations of sick sinus syndrome are lightheadedness, dizziness, and syncope, and these symptoms are related to the bradyarrhythmias.[16,19] When persons with sick sinus syndrome experience palpitations, they are generally the result of tachyarrhythmias and are suggestive of the presence of bradycardia-tachycardia syndrome.

Treatment depends on the cause of the arrhythmia and frequently involves the implantation of a permanent pacemaker. Pacing for bradycardia, combined with drug therapy to treat tachycardia, often is required in the bradycardia-tachycardia syndrome.[16,19] Medications that affect SA node discharge must be used cautiously.

Arrhythmias of Atrial Origin

Impulses from the SA node pass through the conductive pathways in the atria to the AV node. Arrhythmias of atrial origin include premature atrial complexes, paroxysmal supraventricular tachycardia, atrial flutter, and atrial fibrillation (Fig. 25.10).

Premature Atrial Complexes. Premature atrial complexes (PACs) are complexes that originate in the atrial conduction pathways or atrial muscle cells and occur before the next expected SA node impulse. This impulse to contract usually is transmitted to the ventricle and back to the SA node. The location of the ectopic focus determines the configuration of the P wave. In general, the closer the ectopic focus is to the SA node, the more the ectopic complex resembles a normal sinus complex. The retrograde transmission to the SA node often interrupts the timing of the next sinus beat, such that a pause occurs between the two normally conducted beats. In healthy individuals, PACs may be the result of stress, tobacco, or caffeine. They also have been associated with myocardial infarction, digitalis toxicity, low serum potassium or magnesium levels, and hypoxia.

Paroxysmal Supraventricular Tachycardia. Paroxysmal supraventricular tachycardia refers to tachyarrhythmias that originate above the bifurcation of the bundle of His and have

FIGURE 25.10 • Electrocardiographic tracings of atrial arrhythmias. Atrial flutter (*first tracing*) is characterized by the atrial flutter (F) waves occurring at a rate of 240 to 450 beats/minute. The ventricular rate remains regular because of the conduction of every sixth atrial contraction. Atrial fibrillation (*second tracing*) has grossly disorganized atrial electrical activity that is irregular with respect to rate and rhythm. The ventricular response is irregular, and no distinct P waves are visible. The *third tracing* illustrates paroxysmal atrial tachycardia (PAT), preceded by a normal sinus rhythm. The *fourth tracing* illustrates a premature atrial complex (PAC).

a sudden onset and termination. The heart rate may be 140 to 240 beats/minute and be perfectly regular despite exercise or change in position. Most persons remain asymptomatic except for an awareness of the rapid heartbeat, but some may feel light-headed or short of breath, especially if the episodes are prolonged. The most common mechanism for paroxysmal supraventricular tachycardia is reentry. It may be the result of AV nodal reentry, Wolff–Parkinson–White syndrome (caused by an accessory conduction pathway between the atria and ventricles), or intra-atrial or sinus node reentry.

Atrial Flutter. Atrial flutter is a rapid atrial ectopic tachycardia, with a rate that ranges from 240 to 390 beats/minute. There are two types of atrial flutter.[16,20,21] Typical atrial flutter (sometimes called type I) is the result of a reentry rhythm in the right atrium that can be entrained and interrupted with atrial pacing techniques. The atrial rate in typical type I flutter usually is in the vicinity of 300 beats/minute, but it can range from 240 to 340 beats/minute. Other forms of atrial flutter (*i.e.*, the so-called atypical or type II flutters) are now recognized as distinct types and include atrial macro-reentry caused

by surgical scars, idiopathic fibrosis in areas of the atrium, or other anatomic or functional barriers in the atria. Because the barriers that constrain these flutters are variable, the ECG pattern of the atypical flutters can vary. Often, the flutter wave changes morphologically during the same episode of flutter, indicating multiple circuits or nonfixed conduction barriers.[16]

In typical atrial flutter, the ECG reveals a defined sawtooth pattern in leads aVF, V_1, and V_5.[21] The ventricular response rate and regularity are variable and depend on the AV conduction sequence. When regular, the ventricular response rate usually is a defined fraction of the atrial rate (*i.e.*, when conduction from the atria to the ventricles is 2:1, an atrial flutter rate of 300 would result in a ventricular response rate of 150 beats/minute). The QRS complex may be normal or abnormal, depending on the presence or absence of preexisting intraventricular conduction defects or aberrant ventricular conduction.

Atrial flutter rarely is seen in normal, healthy individuals. It may be seen in persons of any age in the presence of underlying atrial abnormalities. Subgroups that are at particularly high risk for development of atrial flutter include children, adolescents, and young adults who have undergone corrective surgery for complex congenital heart diseases.[16,21]

Atrial Fibrillation. Atrial fibrillation is characterized by chaotic impulses propagating in different directions and causing disorganized atrial depolarizations without effective atrial contraction.[21,22] In most cases multiple, small reentrant circuits are constantly arising in the atria, colliding, being extinguished, and arising again. Fibrillation occurs when the atrial cells cannot repolarize in time for the next incoming stimulus. Atrial fibrillation is characterized on the ECG by a grossly disorganized pattern of atrial electrical activity that is irregular with respect to rate and rhythm and the absence of discernible P waves. Atrial activity is depicted by fibrillatory (f) waves of varying amplitude, duration, and morphology. These f waves appear as random oscillation of the baseline. Because of the random conduction through the AV node, QRS complexes appear in an irregular pattern.

Atrial fibrillation is classified into three categories: paroxysmal, persistent, and permanent. Paroxysmal atrial fibrillation self-terminates and lasts no longer than 7 days, while persistent lasts greater than 7 days and usually requires intervention such as cardioversion. Permanent is considered when attempts to terminate have failed and the person remains in atrial fibrillation.[21] During atrial fibrillation the atrial rate typically ranges from 300 to 600 beats/minute, with many impulses blocked at the AV node.[22] The ventricular response is completely irregular, ranging from 80 to 180 beats/minute in the untreated state. Because of changes in stroke volumes resulting from varying periods of diastolic filling, not all ventricular beats produce a palpable pulse. The difference between the apical rate and the palpable peripheral pulses is called the *pulse deficit*. The pulse deficit increases when the ventricular rate is high.

Atrial fibrillation can be seen in persons without any apparent disease, or it may occur in individuals with coronary artery disease, mitral valve disease, ischemic heart disease, hypertension, myocardial infarction, pericarditis, heart failure, digitalis toxicity, and hyperthyroidism. Spontaneous conversion to sinus rhythm within 24 hours of atrial fibrillation is common, occurring in up to two thirds of persons with the disorder.[21] If the duration of atrial fibrillation exceeds 24 hours, the likelihood of conversion decreases, and after 1 week of persistent arrhythmia, spontaneous conversion is rare.[22]

Atrial fibrillation is the most common chronic arrhythmia, affecting 1% to 2% of the population, with an incidence and prevalence that increase with age. After the age of 55, the risk of developing atrial fibrillation doubles with each decade of life.[23]

The symptoms of chronic atrial fibrillation vary. Some people have minimal symptoms, and others have severe symptoms, particularly at the onset of the arrhythmia. The symptoms may range from palpitations to acute pulmonary edema. Fatigue and other nonspecific symptoms are common in older adults. The condition predisposes individuals to thrombus formation in the atria, with subsequent risk of embolic stroke.

The treatment of atrial fibrillation depends on its cause, recency of onset, and persistence. Anticoagulant medications may be used to prevent embolic stroke, and medications (*e.g.,* beta blockers, calcium channel blockers, digitalis, antiarrhythmics) may be used to control the ventricular rate in persons with persistent atrial fibrillation.[24] Cardioversion may be considered in some persons, particularly when pulmonary edema or unstable cardiac status is present. Because conversion to sinus rhythm is associated with increased risk of thromboembolism, anticoagulation therapy is usually administered for at least 3 weeks before cardioversion is attempted in persons in whom the duration of atrial fibrillation is unknown or exceeds 2 to 3 days.[24] Transesophageal echocardiography can be used to detect atrial thrombus, and transesophageal echo-guided cardioversion provides a means of ensuring that atrial thrombi are not present when cardioversion is attempted. Anticoagulant medication usually is continued after cardioversion.

Junctional Arrhythmias

The AV node can act as a pacemaker in the event the SA node fails to initiate an impulse. Junctional rhythms can be transient or permanent, and they usually have a rate of 40 to 60 beats/minute. Fibres in the AV node or bundle of His, which together form the junctional area, also can serve as ectopic pacemakers, producing premature junctional complexes. Another rhythm originating in the junctional tissues is nonparoxysmal junctional tachycardia. This rhythm usually is of gradual onset and termination. However, it may occur abruptly if the dominant pacemaker slows sufficiently. The rate associated with junctional tachycardia ranges from 70 to 130 beats/minute, but it may be faster.[1] The P waves may precede, be buried in, or follow the QRS complexes, depending on the site of the originating impulses. The clinical significance of nonparoxysmal junctional tachycardia is the same as for atrial tachycardias. Catheter ablation therapy has been used successfully to treat some individuals with recurrent or intractable junctional tachycardia. Nonparoxysmal junctional tachycardia is observed most frequently in individuals with underlying heart disease, such as inferior wall myocardial infarction or myocarditis, or after open heart surgery. It also may be present in persons with digitalis toxicity.

Disorders of Ventricular Conduction and Rhythm

The junctional fibres in the AV node join with the bundle of His, which divides to form the right and left bundle branches. The bundle branches continue to divide and form the Purkinje fibres, which supply the walls of the ventricles (Fig. 25.1). As the cardiac impulse leaves the junctional fibres, it travels through the AV bundle. Next, the impulse moves down the right and left bundle branches that lie beneath the endocardium on either side of the septum. It then spreads out through the walls of the ventricles. Interruption of impulse conduction through a bundle branch is called *bundle branch block*. These blocks usually do not cause alterations in the underlying rhythm of the heart. Instead, a bundle branch block interrupts the normal progression of ventricular depolarization, causing the ventricles to depolarize one after the other because the impulses must travel through muscle tissue rather than through the specialized conduction tissue. This prolonged conduction causes the QRS complex to be wider than the normal 0.08 to 0.12 second. The left bundle branch bifurcates into the left anterior and posterior fascicles. An interruption of one of these fascicles is referred to as a *hemiblock*.

Long QT Syndrome and Torsades de Pointes

The *long QT syndrome* (LQTS) is characterized by a prolongation of the QT interval that may result in a characteristic type of polymorphic ventricular tachycardia called *torsades de pointes* and possible sudden cardiac death (SCD).[16,25] *Torsades de pointes* (*i.e.,* "twisting or rotating around a point") is a specific type of ventricular tachycardia (Fig. 25.11). The term refers to the polarity of the QRS complex, which swings from positive to negative and vice versa. The QRS abnormality is characterized by large, bizarre, polymorphic QRS complexes that vary, often from beat to beat, in amplitude and direction, as well as in rotation of the complexes around the isoelectric line. The rate of tachycardia is 100 to 180, but it can be as fast as 200 to 300 per minute. The rhythm is highly unstable and may terminate in ventricular fibrillation or revert to sinus rhythm.

LQTS can be caused by various agents and conditions that reduce the magnitude of outward repolarizing potassium

FIGURE 25.11 • Torsades de pointes. (From Morton P. G., Fontaine D. K. (2009). *Critical care nursing: A holistic approach* (9th ed., p. 286). Philadelphia, PA: Lippincott, Williams & Wilkins.)

currents, enhance the magnitude of the inward depolarizing sodium and calcium currents, or both. Thus, there is delayed repolarization of the ventricles with development of early depolarizing afterpotentials that initiate the arrhythmia. Typically, the QT interval is measured in a lead in which the T wave is prominent and its end is easily distinguished, such as V_2 or V_3. Because the QT interval shortens with tachycardia and lengthens with bradycardia, it is typically corrected for heart rate and is noted as QT_c. Nonetheless, a QT_c greater than 440 mSec in men and greater than 460 mSec in women has been linked with episodes of sudden arrhythmia death syndromes. In addition, T-wave morphology frequently is abnormal in persons with LQTS.[1]

LQTSs have been classified into inherited and acquired forms, both of which are associated with the development of torsades de pointes and sudden cardiac death. The hereditary forms of LQTS are caused by disorders of membrane ion channel proteins, with either potassium channel defects or sodium channel defects.[1]

Acquired LQTS has been linked to a variety of conditions, including cocaine use, exposure to organophosphorus compounds, electrolyte imbalances, marked bradycardia, myocardial infarction, subarachnoid hemorrhage, autonomic neuropathy, human immunodeficiency virus infection, and protein-sparing fasting.[16] Medications linked to LQTS include digitalis, antiarrhythmic agents (*e.g.*, amiodarone, procainamide, and quinidine), verapamil (calcium channel blocker), haloperidol (antipsychotic agent), and erythromycin (antibiotic).[26] The acquired forms of LQTS often are classified as pause-dependent because the torsades de pointes associated with them generally occurs at slow heart rates or in response to short–long–short RR interval sequences. Treatment of acquired forms of LQTS is directed primarily at identifying and withdrawing the offending agent, although emergency measures that modulate the function of transmembrane ion currents can be lifesaving.

Ventricular Arrhythmias

Arrhythmias that arise in the ventricles generally are considered more serious than those that arise in the atria because they afford the potential for interfering with the pumping action of the ventricles.

Premature Ventricular Complexes. A premature ventricular complex (PVC) is caused by a ventricular ectopic pacemaker. After a PVC occurs, the ventricle usually is unable to repolarize sufficiently to respond to the next impulse that arises in the SA node. This delay, commonly referred to as a *compensatory pause,* occurs while the ventricle waits to reestablish its previous rhythm (Fig. 25.12). When a PVC occurs, the diastolic volume usually is insufficient for effective ejection of blood into the arterial system. As a result, PVCs usually do not produce a palpable pulse, or the pulse amplitude is significantly diminished. In the absence of heart disease, PVCs typically are not clinically significant. The incidence of PVCs is greatest with ischemia, acute myocardial infarction,

FIGURE 25.12 • Electrocardiographic (ECG) tracings of ventricular arrhythmias. Premature ventricular complexes (PVCs) (*top tracing*) originate from an ectopic focus in the ventricles, causing a distortion of the QRS complex. Because the ventricle usually cannot repolarize sufficiently to respond to the next impulse that arises in the sinoatrial node, a PVC frequently is followed by a compensatory pause. Ventricular tachycardia (*middle tracing*) is characterized by a rapid ventricular rate of 70 to 250 beats/minute and the absence of P waves. In ventricular fibrillation (*bottom tracing*), there are no regular or effective ventricular contractions, and the ECG tracing is totally disorganized.

history of myocardial infarction, ventricular hypertrophy, infection, increased sympathetic nervous system activity, or increased heart rate.[27] PVCs also can be the result of electrolyte disturbances or medications.

A special pattern of PVC called *ventricular bigeminy* is a condition in which each normal beat is followed by or paired with a PVC. This pattern often is an indication of digitalis toxicity or heart disease. The occurrence of frequent PVCs in the diseased heart predisposes to the development of other, more serious arrhythmias, including ventricular tachycardia and ventricular fibrillation.

Ventricular Tachycardia. Ventricular tachycardia describes a cardiac rhythm originating distal to the bifurcation of the bundle of His, in the specialized conduction system in ventricular muscle, or both.[1] It is characterized by a ventricular rate of 70 to 250 beats/minute, and the onset can be sudden or insidious. Usually, ventricular tachycardia is exhibited electrocardiographically by wide, tall, bizarre-looking QRS complexes that are longer than 0.12 second (Fig. 25.12). QRS complexes can be uniform in appearance (*e.g.*, monomorphic), or they can vary randomly, in a repetitive manner (*e.g.*, torsades de pointes), in an alternating pattern (*e.g.*, bidirectional), or in a stable but changing fashion (*e.g.*, polymorphic). Ventricular tachycardia can be sustained, lasting more than 30 seconds and requiring intervention, or it can be nonsustained and stop spontaneously. This rhythm is dangerous because it eliminates atrial kick and can cause a reduction in diastolic filling time to the point at which cardiac output is severely diminished or nonexistent, and there is no pulse.

Ventricular Fibrillation. This arrhythmia represents severe derangements of cardiac rhythm that terminate fatally within minutes unless corrective measures are taken promptly. In ventricular fibrillation, the ventricle quivers but does not contract. The classic ECG pattern of ventricular fibrillation is that of gross disorganization without identifiable waveforms or intervals (Fig. 25.12). When the ventricles do not contract, there is no cardiac output, and there are no palpable or audible pulses. Immediate defibrillation using a nonsynchronized, direct-current electrical shock is mandatory for ventricular fibrillation and for ventricular flutter that has caused loss of consciousness.[16]

Disorders of Atrioventricular Conduction

Under normal conditions, the AV junction, which consists of the AV node with its connections to the entering atrial internodal pathways, the AV bundle, and the nonbranching portion of the bundle of His, provides the only connection for transmission of impulses between the atrial and ventricular conduction systems. Junctional fibres in the AV node have high-resistance characteristics that cause a delay in the transmission of impulses from the atria to the ventricles. This delay provides optimal timing for the atrial contribution to ventricular filling and protects the ventricles from abnormally rapid rates that arise in the atria. Temporary conduction defects of the AV node are most commonly associated with ischemia; others are due to fibrosis or scar tissue in fibres of the conduction system. Conduction defects also may result from medications, including digoxin, β-adrenergic blocking agents, calcium channel blocking agents, and class 1A antiarrhythmic agents.[16] Additional contributing factors include electrolyte imbalances, inflammatory disease, or cardiac surgery. Some other less common causes include autoimmune, oncologic, and iatrogenic disorders.

Heart block refers to abnormalities of impulse conduction. It may be normal, physiologic (*e.g.,* in excessive vagal tone), or pathologic. It may occur in the AV nodal fibres or in the AV bundle (*i.e.,* bundle of His), which is continuous with the Purkinje conduction system that supplies the ventricles. The PR interval on the ECG corresponds with the time it takes for the cardiac impulse to travel from the SA node to the ventricular pathways. Normally, the PR interval ranges from 0.12 to 0.20 second.

First-Degree AV Block. First-degree AV block is characterized by a prolonged PR interval (greater than 0.20 second; Fig. 25.13). The prolonged PR interval indicates delayed AV conduction, but all atrial impulses are conducted to the ventricles. This condition usually produces a regular atrial and ventricular rhythm. Clinically significant PR interval prolongation can result from conduction delays in the AV node itself, in the His–Purkinje system, or both.[1] When the QRS complex is normal in contour and duration, the AV delay almost always occurs in the AV node and rarely in the bundle of His. In contrast,

FIGURE 25.13 • Electrocardiographic changes that occur with alterations in atrioventricular (AV) node conduction. The *top tracing* shows the prolongation of the PR interval, which is characteristic of first-degree AV block. The *middle tracing* illustrates Mobitz-type II second-degree AV block, in which the conduction of one or more P waves is blocked. In third-degree AV block (*bottom tracing*), impulses conducted through the AV node are completely blocked, and the atria and ventricles develop their own rates of impulse generation.

when the QRS complex is prolonged, showing a bundle branch block pattern, conduction delays may be in the AV node or the His–Purkinje system. First-degree block may be the result of disease in the AV node, such as ischemia or infarction, or of infections such as rheumatic fever or myocarditis.[16] Isolated first-degree heart block usually is not symptomatic, and temporary or permanent cardiac pacing is not indicated.

Second-Degree AV Block. Second-degree AV block is characterized by intermittent failure of conduction of one or more impulses from the atria to the ventricles. The nonconducted P wave can appear intermittently or frequently. A distinguishing feature of second-degree AV block is that conducted P waves relate to QRS complexes with recurring PR intervals; that is, the association of P waves with QRS complexes is not random.[1] Second-degree AV block has been divided into two types: type I (*i.e.,* Mobitz type I or Wenckebach phenomenon) and type II (*i.e.,* Mobitz type II). A *Mobitz type I* AV block is characterized by progressive lengthening of the PR interval until an impulse is blocked and the sequence begins again. It frequently occurs in persons with inferior wall myocardial infarction, particularly with concomitant right ventricular infarction.[1] The condition usually is associated with an adequate ventricular rate and rarely is symptomatic. It usually is transient and does not require temporary pacing.[16] In the *Mobitz type II* AV block, an intermittent block of atrial impulses occurs, with a constant PR interval (Fig. 25.13). It frequently accompanies anterior wall myocardial infarction and can require temporary or permanent pacing. This condition is associated with a high mortality rate. In addition, Mobitz type II AV block is associated with other types of organic heart disease and often progresses to complete heart block.

Third-Degree AV Block. Third-degree, or complete AV block, occurs when the conduction link between the atria and ventricles is lost, resulting in atrial and ventricular depolarization controlled by separate pacemakers (Fig. 25.13). The atrial pacemaker can be sinus or ectopic in origin. The ventricular pacemaker usually is located just below the region of the block. The atria usually continue to beat at a normal rate and the ventricles develop their own rate, which normally is slow (30 to 40 beats/minute). The atrial and ventricular rates are regular but dissociated. Third-degree AV block can result from an interruption at the level of the AV node, in the bundle of His, or in the Purkinje system. Third-degree blocks at the level of the AV node usually are congenital, whereas blocks in the Purkinje system usually are acquired. Normal QRS complexes, with rates ranging from 40 to 60 complexes per minute, usually are displayed on the ECG when the block occurs proximal to the bundle of His.

Complete heart block normally results in bradycardia and causes a decrease in cardiac output with possible periods of syncope (fainting), known as a *Stokes–Adams attack*.[1] Other symptoms include dizziness, fatigue, exercise intolerance, or acute heart failure.[17] Most persons with complete heart block require a temporary or permanent cardiac pacemaker.

Inherited Types of Arrhythmias

Cardiac arrhythmias most commonly occur in the presence of cardiac disease, electrolyte disorders, or other demonstrable abnormalities. Ischemic heart disease is the primary cause for the development of ventricular fibrillation, and structural heart defects such as hypertrophic and dilated cardiomyopathies account for most of the remaining cases. However, in what for many years was referred to as *idiopathic ventricular fibrillation,* 30% are unexplained after an autopsy.[28] Over the past several decades, considerable evidence has been collected indicating that these cases are genetically determined abnormalities of proteins in the ion channels that control the electrical activity of the heart. Multiple genes have now been associated with inherited arrhythmogenic cardiomyopathies (see Chapter 24), and it is expected that more will be identified and linked to sudden death in persons with apparently healthy hearts.[28] Among the inherited arrhythmogenic disorders are congenital LQTS, short QT syndrome, Brugada syndrome, and catecholamine polymorphic ventricular tachycardia.

Congenital Long QT Syndrome. Congenital LQTS is an inherited arrhythmogenic disease characterized by life-threatening ventricular arrhythmias. Three major forms of LQTS have been identified, accounting for approximately 90% of all genotype positive cases. Many other minor genes continue to be identified.[28]

The ECG marker for LQTS consists of a prolonged QT interval, abnormal morphology of the T wave, and a characteristic polymorphic ventricular tachycardia (torsades de pointes). Onset of symptoms is typically in the first two decades of life, including the neonatal period, where it can be misdiagnosed as sudden infant death.[28] The severity of the clinical manifestations in LQTS varies, ranging from full-blown disease with marked prolongation of the QT interval and recurrent syncope, to subclinical forms with borderline QT interval prolongation and no arrhythmias or syncopal episodes.

The hereditary forms of LQTS are typically considered adrenergic dependent because they are generally triggered by increased activity of the sympathetic nervous system.[25,28] Depending on which gene is affected, long-term treatment with β-adrenergic receptor blockers, permanent pacing, or left cardiac sympathetic denervation is frequently effective.[25,28] Placement of an implantable cardioverter-defibrillator (ICD) is recommended for persons in whom recurrent syncope, sustained ventricular arrhythmias, or sudden cardiac arrest occurs despite drug treatment.

Short QT Syndrome. Short QT syndrome (SQTS) is an inherited channelopathy that was first described in 2000 and is characterized by an abbreviated QT interval of less than 320 mSec.[29] This autosomal dominant pattern of inheritance is associated six susceptible genes responsible for potassium channels. Mutations in these genes increases the activity of the potassium ion channels and enhances the movement of potassium across the cardiac muscle cell membrane, leading to changes in electrical activity, arrhythmias, and sudden cardiac death. Up to 25% of persons first present with sudden death or cardiac arrest. Medications to elongate the QT interval and an implantable cardioverter defibrillator to prevent sudden death are current treatments as the research continues in this area.[29]

Brugada Syndrome. First described in 1992, Brugada syndrome is an autosomal dominant disorder characterized by ST segment elevation in precordial leads V_1 to V_3, right bundle branch block, and susceptibility to ventricular tachycardia.[28,29,30] It has so far been associated with genes encoding for the cardiac sodium channel. The disorder typically manifests in adulthood with very incomplete penetrance, and a high percentage of mutation carriers are asymptomatic.[31] Cardiac events typically occur during sleep or rest. Even though the disorder is inherited as an autosomal trait, a male-to-female ratio of 8:1 is observed in clinical manifestations.[28]

Catecholaminergic Polymorphic Ventricular Tachycardia. Catecholaminergic polymorphic ventricular tachycardia (CPVT) was first described in 1978.[29] It was reported that the disorder was characterized by ventricular tachycardia, syncope, and sudden death occurring in familial or sporadic cases in the absence of cardiac disease or ECG abnormalities.

The ECG of persons with CPVT is usually remarkably normal with the exception of sinus bradycardia reported in some persons. Physical activity and acute emotions are the specific triggers for arrhythmias in persons with CPVT. The complexity of the arrhythmias progressively increases with an increase in workload, from isolated premature beats to bigeminy to runs of ventricular tachycardia. Although clinical diagnosis of CPVT is rather elusive because of the absence of abnormal ECG findings, genetic analysis can identify the ryanodine receptors (RyR2) mutations in approximately 60% of persons with the disorder.[28,29] The ryanodine receptors play a key role in calcium regulation within the sarcoplasmic reticulum of cardiac cells. This is particularly important because if left untreated, the disorder is highly malignant, but the prognosis improves considerably once the disorder is correctly identified and treatment is implemented.

Antiadrenergic treatment with beta blockers is the cornerstone of therapy for CPVT. The use of an ICD may be necessary when exercise stress testing and Holter monitoring indicate that beta blockers do not provide complete arrhythmia protection.[28,29]

Diagnostic Methods

The diagnosis of disorders of cardiac rhythm and conduction usually is made on the basis of the surface ECG. Further clarification of conduction defects and cardiac arrhythmias can be obtained using exercise stress testing and electrophysiologic studies.

A resting surface ECG records the impulses originating in the heart as they are recorded at the body surface. These impulses are recorded for a limited time and during periods of inactivity. Although there are no complications related to the procedure, errors related to misdiagnosis may result in iatrogenic heart disease.[2] The resting ECG is the first approach to the clinical diagnosis of disorders of cardiac rhythm and conduction, but it is limited to events that occur during the period the ECG is being monitored.

Signal-Averaged Electrocardiogram

Signal-averaged ECG is a special type of ECG that is used to detect late ventricular potentials that are thought to originate from slow-conducting areas of the myocardium.[32] Late ventricular potentials are low-amplitude, high-frequency waveforms in the terminal QRS complex, and they persist for tens of milliseconds into the ST segment. The presence of late potentials indicates high risk for development of ventricular tachycardia and SCD. These late potentials are detectable from leads of the surface ECG when signal averaging is performed.

The intent of signal averaging is reduction of noise that makes surface ECG analysis more difficult to interpret. This technique averages multiple samples of QRS waveforms and creates a tracing that is an average of all the repetitive signals. Signal averaging can be carried out by using either temporal or spatial averaging. As a result, when several inputs that represent the same event are combined, the coherent signal will be reinforced and the noise will cancel itself.

Signal averaging is a computer-based process. Each electrode input is amplified, its voltage is sampled or measured at intervals of 1 mSec or less, and each sample is converted into a digital number with at least 12-bit precision.[32] The ECG

waveform is converted from an analog waveform to digital numbers that become a computer-readable ECG.

Holter Monitoring

Holter monitoring is one form of long-term monitoring during which a person wears a device that digitally records two or three ECG leads for up to 48 hours. During this time, the person keeps a diary of his or her activities or symptoms, which later are correlated with the ECG recording. Most recording devices also have an event marker button that can be pressed when the individual experiences symptoms, which assists the technician or physician in correlating the diary, symptoms, and ECG changes during analysis. Newer Holter recorders are capable of providing a derived 12-lead ECG. Holter monitoring is useful for documenting arrhythmias, conduction abnormalities, and ST segment changes. The interpretative accuracy of long-term Holter recordings varies with the system used and clinician expertise. Most computer software packages used to scan Holter recordings are sufficiently accurate to meet clinical demand. The majority of patients who have ischemic heart disease exhibit PVCs, particularly those who have recently experienced myocardial infarction.[32] The frequency of PVCs increases progressively over the first several weeks, and decreases approximately 6 months postinfarction. Holter recordings also are used to determine antiarrhythmic drug efficacy, episodes of myocardial ischemia, QT prolongation, and heart rate variability.

Intermittent ECG recorders also are used in the diagnosis of arrhythmias and conduction defects. There are two basic types of recorders that perform this type of monitoring.[32] The first continuously monitors rhythm and is programmed to recognize abnormalities. In the second variety, the unit does not continuously monitor the ECG and therefore cannot automatically recognize abnormalities. The latter form relies on the person to activate the unit when he or she is symptomatic. The data are stored in memory or transmitted telephonically to an ECG receiver, where they are recorded. These types of ECG recordings are useful in persons who have transient symptoms and are used for up to 30 days.

Implantable Loop ECG Recorder

If Holter and event monitors do no produce any diagnostic information, a loop recorder can be implanted. This device is implanted under the skin in the left upper chest area. It continuously monitors the person's ECG and can be programmed to store patient-activated events when they are symptomatic. The loop reorder can be in place for as long as 1 year. It is useful for documenting arrhythmias, antiarrhythmic drug efficacy, episodes of myocardial ischemia, QT prolongation, heart rate turbulence, and heart rate variability.

Exercise Stress Testing

The exercise stress test elicits the body's response to measured increases in acute exercise (see Chapter 24). This technique provides information about changes in heart rate, blood pressure, respiration, and perceived level of exercise. It is useful in determining exercise-induced alterations in hemodynamic response and ECG ischemic-type ST segment changes, and can detect and classify disturbances in cardiac rhythm and conduction associated with exercise. These changes are indicative of a poorer prognosis in persons with known coronary disease and recent myocardial infarction.

Electrophysiologic Studies

Electrophysiologic testing is used for the diagnosis and management of complex arrhythmias. It involves the passage of two or more electrode catheters into the right side of the heart. These catheters are inserted into the femoral, subclavian, internal jugular, or antecubital veins and positioned with fluoroscopy into the high right atrium near the sinus node, the area of the His bundle, the coronary sinus that lies in the posterior atrioventricular (AV) groove, and into the right ventricle.[6] The electrode catheters are used to stimulate the heart and record intracardiac ECGs. During the study, overdrive pacing, cardioversion, or defibrillation may be necessary to terminate tachycardia induced during the stimulation procedures.

The primary indications for electrophysiologic testing are to determine a person's potential for arrhythmia formation; evaluate recurrent syncope of cardiac origin when ambulatory ECG has not provided the diagnosis; differentiate supraventricular from ventricular arrhythmias; and locate arrhythmogenic foci for therapeutic interventions such as catheter ablation procedures or antitachycardia devices.[33] Testing can also define reproducible arrhythmia induction characteristics and hence can be used to evaluate the therapeutic efficacy of a particular treatment modality.

Electrophysiologic methods can also be used as interventions. These interventions may include pacing a person out of tachycardia or ablation therapy. Ablation therapy involves the destruction of myocardial tissue by delivering electrical energy over electrodes on a catheter placed next to an area related to the onset or maintenance of arrhythmias.

Risks associated with electrophysiologic testing are small. Most electrophysiologic studies do not involve left-sided heart access, and therefore the risk of myocardial infarction, stroke, or systemic embolism is less than observed with coronary arteriography. The addition of therapeutic manoeuvres, such as ablation therapy, to the procedure increases the risk of complications such as venous thrombosis and pulmonary emboli.

Treatment

The treatment of cardiac rhythm or conduction disorders is directed toward controlling the arrhythmia, correcting the cause, and preventing more serious or fatal arrhythmias. Correction may involve simply adjusting an electrolyte disturbance or withholding a medication such as digitalis. Preventing more serious arrhythmias often involves drug therapy, electrical stimulation, or surgical intervention.

Pharmacologic Treatment

Antiarrhythmic drugs act by modifying the disordered formation and conduction of impulses that induce cardiac muscle contraction. These drugs are classified into four major groups (Class I to Class IV) according to the drug's effect on the action potential of the cardiac cells.[7,33–36] Although drugs in one category have similar effects on conduction, they may vary significantly in their hemodynamic effects.

Class I drugs act by blocking the fast sodium channels. These drugs affect impulse conduction, excitability, and automaticity to various degrees and therefore have been divided further into three groups: IA, IB, and IC. Class IA drugs (*e.g.,* quinidine, procainamide, disopyramide) decrease automaticity by depressing phase 4 of the action potential, decrease conductivity by moderately prolonging phase 0, and prolong repolarization by extending phase 3 of the action potential.[7] Because these drugs are effective in suppressing ectopic foci and treating reentrant arrhythmias, they are used for supraventricular and ventricular arrhythmias. Class IB drugs (*e.g.,* lidocaine, mexiletine) decrease automaticity by depressing phase 4 of the action potential, have little effect on conductivity, decrease refractoriness by decreasing phase 2, and shorten repolarization by decreasing phase 3. These drugs have little or no effect on sodium channels in resting cells. However, they shorten the action potential and are powerful inhibitors of sodium-dependent conduction in depolarized cells, making them effective in depressing conduction in ischemic areas of the heart.[7] Drugs in this group are used for treating ventricular arrhythmias only and have little or no effect on myocardial contractility. Class IC drugs (*e.g.,* propafenone, flecainide) decrease conductivity by markedly depressing phase 0 of the action potential, but have little effect on refractoriness or repolarization. Their primary action is inhibition of sodium channel opening.[7] Drugs in this class are used for life-threatening ventricular arrhythmias and supraventricular tachycardias.

Class II agents (*e.g.,* atenolol, timolol, sotalol) are β-adrenergic blocking drugs that act by blunting the effect of sympathetic nervous system stimulation on the heart, thereby inhibiting calcium channel opening. These drugs decrease automaticity by depressing phase 4 of the action potential; they also decrease heart rate and cardiac contractility. These medications are effective for treatment of supraventricular arrhythmias and tachyarrhythmias secondary to excessive sympathetic activity, but they are not effective in treating ventricular arrhythmias such as recurrent ventricular tachycardia.[36]

Class III drugs (*e.g.,* amiodarone, sotalol, dronedarone) act by inhibiting the potassium current and repolarization, thereby extending the action potential and refractoriness. Intravenous amiodarone has Class I, II, and IV (see below) effects, and is used for several types of tachyarrhythmias. Sotalol has both β-adrenergic receptor blocking (class II) and action potential prolonging (class III) actions. These agents are used in the treatment of serious ventricular arrhythmias.

Class IV drugs (*e.g.,* verapamil, diltiazem, mibefradil) act by blocking the slow calcium channels, thereby depressing phase 4 and lengthening phases 1 and 2 of the action potential. By blocking the release of intracellular calcium ions, these agents reduce the force of myocardial contractility, thereby decreasing myocardial oxygen demand. These drugs are used to slow the SA node pacemaker and inhibit conduction in the AV node, slowing the ventricular response in atrial tachycardias, and to terminate reentrant paroxysmal supraventricular tachycardias when the AV node functions as a reentrant pathway.[33]

Two other types of antiarrhythmic drugs, the cardiac glycosides and adenosine, are not included in this classification schema. The cardiac glycosides (*i.e.,* digitalis drugs) slow the heart rate and are used in the management of arrhythmias such as atrial tachycardia, atrial flutter, and atrial fibrillation.[35] Adenosine, an endogenous nucleoside that is present in every cell, may be used to treat paroxysmal supraventricular tachycardia involving the AV node. It has a very short half-life and temporarily interrupts SA firing and AV node conduction.[36]

Electrical Interventions

The correction of conduction defects, bradycardias, and tachycardias can involve the use of an electronic pacemaker, cardioversion, or defibrillation. Electrical interventions can be used in emergency and elective situations.

Efforts directed at cardiac electrostimulation date back more than a century. Since then, tremendous strides have been made in the effectiveness of cardiac pacing. A *cardiac pacemaker* is an electronic device that delivers an electrical stimulus to the heart. It is used to initiate heartbeats in situations when the normal pacemaker of the heart is defective, with certain types of AV heart block, with symptomatic bradycardia in which the rate of cardiac contraction and consequent cardiac output are inadequate to perfuse vital tissues, and in other cardiac arrhythmias. A pacemaker may be used as a temporary or a permanent measure. Pacemakers can pace the atria, the ventricles, or the atria and ventricles sequentially, or overdrive pacing can be used. Overdrive pacing is used to treat recurrent ventricular tachycardia and reentrant atrial or ventricular tachyarrhythmias, and to terminate atrial flutter.

Temporary pacemakers are useful for treatment of symptomatic bradycardias and to perform overdrive pacing. They can be placed transcutaneously, transvenously, or epicardially. External temporary pacing, also known as *transcutaneous pacing,* involves the placement of large patch electrodes on the anterior and posterior chest wall, which then are connected by a cable to an external pulse generator. Many defibrillators today have transcutaneous pacing capabilities. Internal temporary pacing, also known as *transvenous pacing,* involves the passage of a venous catheter with electrodes on its tip into the right atrium or ventricle, where it is wedged against the endocardium. The electrode then is attached to an external pulse generator. This procedure is performed under fluoroscopic or electrocardiographic direction. During open thoracotomy procedures, *epicardial pacing wires* usually are anchored to epicardium of the right ventricle. These wires are brought out directly through the chest wall and also can be attached to an external pulse generator, if necessary. When the wires are no longer needed, they are removed by gentle traction.[37]

Permanent cardiac pacemakers may become necessary for a variety of reasons. Permanent pacemakers require a pulse generator and implantation of pacing wires into the epicardium. The pulse generator typically weighs approximately 25 to 30 g. Ongoing evaluation of the pacemaker's sensing, firing capabilities, and battery life is necessary.

Defibrillation and synchronized cardioversion are two reliable methods for treating ventricular tachycardia, and defibrillation is the definitive treatment for ventricular fibrillation. The discharge of electrical energy that is synchronized with the R wave of the ECG is referred to as *synchronized cardioversion,* and unsynchronized discharge is known as *defibrillation.* The goal of both of these techniques is to provide an electrical pulse to the heart in such a way as to depolarize the heart completely during passage of the current. This electrical current interrupts the disorganized impulses, allowing the SA node to regain control of the heart. Defibrillation and synchronized cardioversion can be delivered externally through large patch electrodes on the chest or internally through small paddle electrodes placed directly on the myocardium, patch electrodes sewn into the epicardium, or transvenous wires placed in the right ventricle. Electrical devices that combine antitachycardia pacing, cardioversion, defibrillation, and bradycardial pacing are under investigation.

Automatic implantable cardioverter-defibrillators (ICDs or AICDs) are being used successfully to treat individuals with life-threatening ventricular tachyarrhythmias by the use of intrathoracic electrical countershock.[38] Reliable sensing and detection of ventricular tachyarrhythmias are essential for proper functioning of the ICD. Sensing and detection are accomplished through endocardial leads. The ICD responds to ventricular tachyarrhythmia by delivering an electrical shock between intrathoracic electrodes within 10 to 20 seconds of its onset. This time frame provides nearly a 100% likelihood of reversal of the arrhythmia, supporting the utility of this device as a reliable and effective means of preventing SCD in survivors of out-of-hospital cardiac arrest.

Ablation and Surgical Interventions

Ablation therapy is used for treating recurrent, life-threatening supraventricular and ventricular tachyarrhythmias. Ablative therapy may be performed by catheter or surgical techniques. It involves localized destruction, isolation, or excision of cardiac tissue that is considered to be arrhythmogenic.[6,20,21,24]

The first catheter ablation procedures were performed using direct-current shocks, but this energy source has largely been replaced by radiofrequency (RF) energy, which is delivered by an external generator and destroys tissue by heat production.[14,20,21] Radiofrequency ablation uses radiofrequency waves to destroy defective or aberrant electrical conduction pathways. Cryoablation involves the direct application of an extremely cold probe to arrhythmogenic cardiac tissue. Catheter-delivered cryoablation causes damage by freezing cellular structures of defective or aberrant electrical conduction pathways.[39]

Additional surgical interventions such as coronary artery bypass surgery, ventriculotomy, and endocardial resection may be used to improve myocardial oxygenation, remove arrhythmogenic foci, or alter electrical conduction pathways. Coronary artery bypass surgery improves myocardial oxygenation by increasing blood supply to the myocardium. Ventriculotomy involves the removal of aneurysm tissue and the resuturing of the myocardial walls to eliminate the paradoxical ventricular movement and the foci of arrhythmias. In endocardial resection, endocardial tissue that has been identified as arrhythmogenic through the use of electrophysiologic testing or intraoperative mapping is surgically removed. Ventriculotomy and endocardial resection have been performed with cryoablation or laser ablation as an adjunctive therapy.

IN SUMMARY

Disorders of cardiac rhythm arise as the result of disturbances in impulse generation or conduction in the heart. Normal sinus rhythm and respiratory sinus arrhythmia (*i.e.*, heart rate speeds up and slows down in concert with respiratory cycle) are considered normal cardiac rhythms. Cardiac arrhythmias are not necessarily pathologic; they occur in healthy and diseased hearts. Sinus arrhythmias originate in the SA node. They include sinus bradycardia (heart rate less than 60 beats/minute); sinus tachycardia (heart rate greater than 100 beats/minute); sinus arrest, in which there are prolonged periods of asystole; and sick sinus syndrome, a condition characterized by periods of bradycardia alternating with tachycardia.

Atrial arrhythmias arise from alterations in impulse generation that occur in the conduction pathways or muscle of the atria. They include premature atrial complexes (PACs), atrial flutter (*i.e.*, atrial depolarization rate of 240 to 450 beats/minute), and atrial fibrillation (*i.e.*, grossly disorganized atrial depolarization that is irregular with regard to rate and rhythm). Atrial arrhythmias often go unnoticed unless they are transmitted to the ventricles.

Junctional rhythms are initiated in the AV junction and may occur normally as a back up pacemaker if the SA node fails to fire. The back up rate is between 40 and 60 beats/minute. Junctional tachycardias occur when the junction initiates the rhythm at a rate greater than 60 per minute.

Arrhythmias that arise in the ventricles are commonly considered more serious than those that arise in the atria because they afford the potential for interfering with the pumping action of the heart. The LQTS represents a prolongation of the QT interval that may result in torsades de pointes and sudden cardiac death. A premature ventricular complex (PVC) is caused by a ventricular ectopic pacemaker. Ventricular tachycardia is characterized by a ventricular rate of 70 to 250 beats/minute. Ventricular fibrillation (*e.g.*, ventricular rate greater than 350 beats/minute) is a fatal arrhythmia unless it is successfully treated with defibrillation. Arrhythmogenic cardiomyopathies are inherited disorders of the ion channels that control the electrical activity of the heart. Among the inherited arrhythmogenic disorders are congenital LQTS, SQTS, Brugada syndrome, and CPVT.

Alterations in the conduction of impulses through the AV node lead to disturbances in the transmission of impulses from the atria to the ventricles. There can be a delay in transmission (*i.e.*, first-degree heart block), failure to conduct one or more impulses (*i.e.*, second-degree heart block), or complete failure to conduct impulses between the atria and the ventricles (*i.e.*, third-degree heart block). Conduction disorders of the bundle branches, called bundle branch blocks, cause a widening of and changes in the configuration of the QRS complex of the ECG.

The diagnosis of disorders of cardiac rhythm and conduction typically is accomplished using surface electrodes or electrophysiologic studies. Surface electrodes can be used to obtain an intermittent or continuous 12-lead ECG, to continuously monitor the patient's rhythms at the bedside or by Holter monitoring, or for signal-averaged studies. Electrophysiologic studies use electrode catheters inserted into the right heart through a peripheral vein as a means of directly stimulating the heart while obtaining an intracardiac ECG recording.

Both electrical devices and medications are used in the treatment of arrhythmias and conduction disorders. Temporary and permanent cardiac pacemakers are used to treat symptomatic bradycardias or to provide overdrive pacing procedures. Defibrillation is used to treat atrial and ventricular fibrillation. Synchronized cardioversion procedures are carried out to treat ventricular tachycardia. These devices can be external or internally implanted. They deliver an electrical charge to the myocardium to depolarize the heart completely, supplying the SA node with an opportunity to take over as the dominant pacemaker of the heart. Radiofrequency ablation and cryoablation therapy are used to destroy specific irritable foci in the heart. Surgical procedures can be performed to excise irritable or dysfunctional tissue, replace cardiac valves, or provide better blood supply to the myocardial muscle wall.

REVIEW EXERCISES

1. A 63-year-old woman with a history of heart failure comes to the clinic complaining of feeling tired. Her heart rate is 97 beats/minute and the rhythm is irregular.
   A. *What type of arrhythmia do you think she might be having? If you were to obtain an ECG, what would it look like?*
   B. *What causes this irregularity?*
   C. *Why do you think she is feeling tired?*
   D. *What are some of the concerns with this type of arrhythmia?*

2. A 42-year-old man appears at the urgent care centre with complaints of chest discomfort, shortness of breath, and generally not feeling well. You assess his vital signs and find that his temperature is 38.5°C, blood pressure 166/90 mm Hg, pulse 87 and slightly irregular, and respiratory rate 26.

You do an ECG, and the readings from the anterior leads indicate that he is experiencing an ischemic episode.

A. *You attach him to a cardiac monitor and see that his underlying rhythm is normal sinus rhythm, but he is having frequent premature contractions that are more than 0.12 seconds in duration. What type of premature contractions do you suspect?*

B. *What would you expect his pulse to feel like?*

C. *What leads would you want to monitor?*

D. *What do you think the etiology of this arrhythmia might be? How might it be treated?*

References

1. Rubart M., Zipes D. P. (2015). Chapter 33: Genesis of cardiac arrhythmias. In Mann D. L., Zipes D. P., Libby P., et al. (Eds.), *Braunwald's heart disease: A textbook of cardiovascular medicine* (10th ed.). Philadelphia, PA: Elsevier, Inc.

2. Ho S. Y., Becker A. E. (2011). Chapter 37: Anatomy of electrophysiology. In Fuster V., Walsh R. A., Harrington R. A. et al. (Eds.), *Hurst's the heart* (13th ed.). New York: McGraw Hill Companies.

3. Malouf J. F., Edwards W. D., Tajik A. J., et al. (2011). Chapter 4: Functional anatomy of the heart. In Fuster V., Walsh R. A., Harrington R. A., et al. (Eds.), *Hurst's the heart* (13th ed.). New York: McGraw Hill Companies.

4. Pappano A. J., Wier W. G. (2013). *Cardiovascular physiology* (10th ed.). Philadelphia, PA: Elsevier/Mosby.

5. Hall J. E. (2011). *Textbook of medical physiology* (12th ed.). Philadelphia, PA: W. B. Saunders.

6. Fogoros R. N. (2012). *Electrophysiologic testing* (5th ed.). Hoboken, NJ: Wiley-Blackwell.

7. Katz A. M. (2011). *Physiology of the heart* (5th ed.). Philadelphia, PA: Lippincott Williams & Wilkins.

8. Klabunde R. E. (2012). *Cardiovascular physiology concepts* (2nd ed.). Philadelphia, PA: Lippincott Williams & Wilkins.

9. Rajaganeshan R., Ludlam C. L., Francis D. P., et al. (2008). Accuracy in ECG lead placement among technicians, nurses, general physicians and cardiologists. *International Journal of Clinical Practice, 62*(1), 65–70.

10. Mirvis D. M., Goldberger A. L. (2015). Chapter 12: Electrocardiography. In Mann D. L., Zipes D. P., Libby P., et al. (Eds.), *Braunwald's heart disease: A textbook of cardiovascular medicine* (10th ed.). Philadelphia, PA: Elsevier, Inc.

11. Ioannidis J. P., Salem D., Chew P. W., et al. (2001). Accuracy and clinical effect of out-of-hospital electrocardiography in the diagnosis of acute cardiac ischemia: A meta-analysis. *Annals of Emergency Medicine, 37*(5), 461–470.

12. Chun A. A., McGee S. R. (2004). Bedside diagnosis of coronary artery disease: A systematic review. *American Journal of Medicine, 117*(5), 334–343.

13. Yang M., Tran D. X., Weiss J. N., et al. (2007). The pinwheel experiment revisited: Effects of cellular electrophysiological properties on vulnerability to cardiac reentry. *American Journal of Physiology: Heart and Circulatory Physiology, 293*(3), H1781–H1790.

14. Lee G., Sanders P., Kalman J. M. (2012). Catheter ablation of atrial arrhythmias: State of the art. *Lancet, 380*(9852), 1509–1519.

15. Billman G. E. (2011). Heart rate variability: A historical perspective. *Frontiers in Physiology, 2*:86.

16. Olgin J. E., Zipes D. P. (2015). Chapter 37: Specific arrhythmias. In Mann D. L., Zipes D. P., Libby P., et al. (Eds.), *Braunwald's heart disease: A textbook of cardiovascular medicine* (10th ed.). Philadelphia, PA: Elsevier, Inc.

17. Bonvini R. F., Hendiri T., Anwar A. (2006). Sinus arrest and moderate hyperkalemia. *Annales de Cardiologie et d'Angeiologie (Paris), 55*(3), 161–163.

18. Ewy G. A. (2014). Sick sinus syndrome synopsis. *Journal of the America College of Cardiology, 64*(6), 539–540.

19. Semelka M., Gera J. (2013). Sick sinus syndrome: A review. *American Family Physician, 87*(10), 691–696.

20. Sawhney N. S., Anousheh R., Chen W., et al. (2009). Diagnosis and management of typical atrial flutter. *Cardiology Clinics, 27*(1), 55–67.

21. Prystowsky, E. N., Padanilam B. J., Waldo A. L. (2011). Chapter 40: Atrial fibrillation, atrial flutter, and atrial tachycardia. In Fuster V., Walsh R. A., Harrington R. A. et al. *Hurst's the heart* (13th ed.). New York: McGraw Hill Companies.

22. Morady F., Zipes D. P. (2015). Chapter 38: Atrial fibrillation: Clinical features, mechanisms, and managmeent. In Mann D. L., Zipes D. P., Libby P., et al. (Eds.), *Braunwald's heart disease: A textbook of cardiovascular medicine* (10th ed.). Philadelphia, PA: Elsevier, Inc.

23. Heart & Stroke Foundation. (2015). Statistics. Available online at: http://www.heartandstroke.com/site/c.ikIQLcMWJtE/b.3483991/k.34A8/Statistics.htm. Accessed May 4, 2015.

24. Verma A., Cairns J. A., Mitchell L. B., et al. (2014). 2014 focused update of the Canadian Cardiovascular Society guidelines for the management of atrial fibrillation. *Canadian Journal of Cardiology, 30*(10), 1114–1130.

25. Schwartz P. J., Crotti L., Insolia R. (2012). Long-QT syndrome: From genetics to management. *Circulation: Arrhythmia and Electrophysiology, 5*(4), 868–877.

26. Azcert Inc. (2013). QT drugs lists. Available online at: https://www.crediblemeds.org/healthcare-providers/. Accessed May 4, 2015.

27. Cantillon D. J. (2013). Evaluation and management of premature ventricular complexes. *Cleveland Clinic Journal of Medicine, 80*(6), 377–387.

28. Tester D. J., Ackerman M. J. (2015). Chapter 32: Genetics of cardiac arrhythmias. In Mann D. L., Zipes D. P., Libby P., et al. (Eds.), *Braunwald's heart disease: A textbook of cardiovascular medicine* (10th ed.). Philadelphia, PA: Elsevier, Inc.

29. Napolitano C., Bloise R., Monteforte N., et al. (2012). Sudden cardiac death and genetic ion channelopathies: Long QT, Brugada, short QT, CPVT, and idiopathic VF. *Circulation, 125*(16). 2027–2034.

30. Mizusawa Y., Wilde A. A. M. (2012). Brugada syndrome. *Circulation: Arrhythmia and Electrophysiology, 5*(3), 606–616.

31. Priori S. G., Napolitano C. (2006). Role of genetic analyses in cardiology: Part I: Mendelian diseases: cardiac channelopathies. *Circulation, 113*(8), 1130–1135.

32. Miller J. M., Zipes D. P. (2015). Chapter 34: Diagnosis of cardiac arrhythmias. In Mann D. L., Zipes D. P., Libby P., et al. (Eds.), *Braunwald's heart disease: A textbook of cardiovascular medicine* (10th ed.). Philadelphia, PA: Elsevier, Inc.

33. Bashore T. M., Granger C. B., Jackson K., et al. (2015). Chapter 10: Heart disease. In Papadakis M. A., McPhee S. J., Rabow M. V. (Eds.), *Current medical diagnosis and treatment 2015.* New York: McGraw-Hill.

34. Dorian P. (updated 2015). Cardiovascular disorders: Ventricular tachyarrhythmias. In Repchinsky C. (Ed.). *e-Therapeutics* [Online]. Ottawa: Canadian Pharmacists Association.

35. Frankel G., Kamrul R., Kosar L., et al. (2013). Rate versus rhythm control in atrial fibrillation. *Canadian Family Physician, 59*(2), 161–168.

36. Kowey P. R., Yan G. (2011). Chapter 45: Antiarrhythmic drugs. In Fuster V., Walsh R. A., Harrington R. A., et al. *Hurst's the heart* (13th ed.). New York: McGraw Hill Companies.

37. Reade M. C. (2007). Temporary epicardial pacing after cardiac surgery: A practical review. *Anaesthesia, 62*(3), 264–271.

38. Aronow W. S. (2010). Implantable cardioverter defibrillators. *American Journal of Therapeutics, 17*(6), e208–e220.

39. Miller J. M., Zipes D. P. (2015). Chapter 35: Therapy for cardiac arrhythmias. In Mann D. L., Zipes D. P., Libby P., et al. (Eds.), *Braunwald's heart disease: A textbook of cardiovascular medicine* (10th ed.). Philadelphia, PA: Elsevier, Inc.

Visit thePoint. **http://thePoint.lww.com** for **animations, journal articles, and more!**

Heart Failure and Circulatory Shock

26

Adequate perfusion of body tissues depends on four components: the pumping ability of the heart; a vascular system that transports blood to the cells and back to the heart; sufficient blood to fill the circulatory system; and tissues that are able to extract and use oxygen and nutrients from the blood. Heart failure and circulatory shock are separate conditions that reflect failure of the circulatory system in one or more of these components. Both conditions exhibit common compensatory mechanisms, even though they differ in terms of pathogenesis and causes.

 HEART FAILURE

After completing this section of the chapter, you should be able to meet the following objectives:

- Define heart failure.
- Describe the contractile properties of the myocardium.
- Explain how the Frank–Starling mechanism, sympathetic nervous system, renin–angiotensin–aldosterone system, natriuretic peptides, endothelins, and myocardial hypertrophy and remodelling function both as adaptive and maladaptive mechanisms in heart failure.
- Differentiate high-output versus low-output heart failure, systolic versus diastolic heart failure, and right-sided versus left-sided heart failure in terms of causes, impact on cardiac function, and major manifestations.
- Differentiate chronic heart failure from acute heart failure syndromes.
- Describe the manifestations of heart failure and relate to the function of the heart.
- Describe the methods used in diagnosis and assessment of cardiac function in persons with heart failure.
- Relate the pharmacologic actions of angiotensin-converting enzyme inhibitors and receptor blockers, β-adrenergic blockers, diuretics, digoxin, and vasodilatory agents to the treatment of heart failure.
- Relate the use of cardiac resynchronization, implantable cardioverter–defibrillators, left ventricular assist devices, heart transplantation, and other surgical alternatives to the treatment of selected types of heart failure.

Heart failure is defined as a complex syndrome resulting from any functional or structural disorder of the heart, in which the ventricle has an impaired ability to fill or eject blood.[1] There is a risk of developing manifestations of low cardiac output and/or pulmonary or systemic congestion, and it may be acute or chronic.[1,2] Not all affected individuals have congestion, so the term *heart failure* is preferred over the older term *congestive heart failure*. Heart failure affects more than an estimated 500,000 Canadians, with 50,000 new diagnoses per year and an annual mortality between 5% and 50%.[3] It remains one of the most prevalent acute care diagnoses and reasons for admission to hospital, with high risks of both morbidity and mortality. Heart failure can occur in any age group but primarily affects persons over 65 years of age. Although morbidity and mortality rates from other cardiovascular diseases have decreased over the past several decades, the incidence of heart failure is increasing. This change reflects improved treatment methods and increased survival from other forms of heart disease, plus an aging population.

HEART FAILURE

- The function of the heart is to move deoxygenated blood from the venous system through the right heart into the pulmonary circulation, and oxygenated blood from the pulmonary circulation through the left heart and into the arterial circulation.
- Systolic dysfunction represents a decrease in cardiac myocardial contractility and an impaired ability to eject blood from the left ventricle, whereas diastolic dysfunction represents an abnormality in ventricular relaxation and filling.
- Right-sided heart failure represents failure of the right ventricle to move unoxygenated blood from the venous system into the pulmonary circulation, with an eventual backup in the systemic venous circulation, whereas left-sided heart failure represents failure of the left ventricle to move oxygenated blood from the pulmonary circulation into the arterial circulation with eventual backup of blood in the lungs. Both types result in decreased forward flow, resulting in poor circulation of oxygenated blood in the body.

The syndrome of heart failure can be produced by any condition that reduces the pumping ability of the heart. Among the most common causes of heart failure are coronary artery disease, hypertension, dilated cardiomyopathy, and valvular heart disease.[1] Because many of the processes leading to heart failure are of long standing and progress gradually, heart failure can often be prevented by early detection and intervention. In 2007, the importance of prevention and management of heart failure including the identification of associated risk factors was emphasized by the Canadian Cardiovascular Society (CSS; see Chart 26.1).[2,4] Risk factors may vary with ethnocultural backgrounds. For example, the greatest risks for

---

CHART 26.1 | **RISK FACTORS FOR THE DEVELOPMENT OF HEART FAILURE**

- Hypertension[a]
- Ischemic heart disease[a]
- Diabetes Type 2 & the metabolic syndrome
- Hyperlipidemia[a]
- Smoking[a]
- Obesity
- Older age
- Sex
- Ethnicity
- Physical inactivity
- Heavy alcohol use
- Excessive salt intake
- Cardiotoxic agents
- Family history/genetic markers
- Low ejection fraction[a]
- Impaired diastolic function
- Left ventricular hypertrophy
- Elevated neurohormonal biomarkers
- Abnormal electrocardiogram
- Increased cardiothoracic ratio
- Microalbuminuria
- Elevated resting heart rate

[a]Most important targets for prevention.
Adapted from CCS Consensus Conference recommendations on heart failure update, 2007.[2]

Caucasians are acute coronary syndrome, diabetes, and aging, whereas hypertension and diabetes are significant factors in aboriginal, South Asian, Black, and Chinese populations. Diagnosis of clinical heart failure is made based on symptoms and signs of decreased cardiac output and increased body fluid volume measured by systolic or diastolic dysfunction. Once the presence of heart failure is established, the New York Heart Association Functional Classification of Patients with Heart Failure is frequently used to determine the severity of heart failure (Table 26.1).[1,2]

Pathophysiology of Heart Failure

Cardiac output is the amount of blood that the ventricles eject each minute. The heart has the amazing capacity to adjust its cardiac output to meet the varying needs of the body. During sleep, cardiac output declines, and during exercise or exertion it increases markedly. The ability to increase cardiac output during increased activity is called the *cardiac reserve*. For example, competitive swimmers and long-distance runners have large cardiac reserves. During exercise, the cardiac output of these athletes rapidly increases to as much as five to six times their resting level.[5] In sharp contrast with healthy

TABLE 26.1 NEW YORK HEART ASSOCIATION FUNCTIONAL CLASSIFICATION OF PATIENTS WITH HEART DISEASE

CLASSIFICATION	CHARACTERISTICS
Class I	Patients with cardiac disease but without the resulting limitations in physical activity. Ordinary activity does not cause undue fatigue, palpitation, dyspnea, or anginal pain.
Class II	Patients with heart disease resulting in slight limitations of physical activity. They are comfortable at rest. Ordinary physical activity results in fatigue, palpitation, dyspnea, or anginal pain.
Class III	Patients with cardiac disease resulting in marked limitation of physical activity. They are comfortable at rest. Less than ordinary physical activity causes fatigue, palpitation, dyspnea, or anginal pain.
Class IV	Patients with cardiac disease resulting in inability to carry on any physical activity without discomfort. The symptoms of cardiac insufficiency or of the anginal syndrome may be present even at rest. If any physical activity is undertaken, discomfort increases.

From Criteria Committee of the New York Heart Association. (1964). *Diseases of the heart and blood vessels: Nomenclature and criteria for diagnosis* (6th ed., pp. 112–113). Boston, MA: Little, Brown.

athletes, persons with heart failure often use their cardiac reserve at rest. For them, just climbing a flight of stairs may cause shortness of breath because they have exceeded their cardiac reserve.

Control of Cardiac Performance and Output

Cardiac output, which is the major determinant of cardiac performance, is determined by how often the heart beats each minute (heart rate) and how much blood it pumps with each beat (stroke volume). It can be expressed as the product of the heart rate and stroke volume (*i.e.,* cardiac output = heart rate × stroke volume). The heart rate is regulated by a balance between the activity of the sympathetic nervous system, which produces an increase in heart rate, and the parasympathetic nervous system, which slows it down, whereas the stroke volume is a function of preload, afterload, and myocardial contractility[5-7] (see Chapter 21). In heart failure, cardiac performance results in a decrease in stroke volume and consequently a decrease in cardiac output, even though heart rate may increase in an attempt to compensate. Stroke volume may be reduced due to systolic ventricular dysfunction, diastolic ventricular dysfunction, or a combination of systolic and diastolic dysfunction.

Preload and Afterload. The work that the heart performs consists mainly of ejecting blood that has returned to the ventricles during diastole into the pulmonary or systemic circulation. It is determined largely by the loading conditions, or what are called the *preload* and *afterload.*

Preload reflects the volume or loading conditions of the ventricle at the end of diastole, just before the onset of systole. It is the volume of blood stretching the heart muscle at the end of diastole and is determined mainly by the venous return to the heart. During any given cardiac cycle, the maximum volume of blood filling the ventricle is present at the end of diastole. Known as the *end-diastolic volume,* this volume causes an increase in the length of the myocardial muscle fibres. Within limits, as end-diastolic volume or preload increases, the stroke volume increases in accord with the Frank–Starling mechanism.

Afterload represents the force that the contracting heart muscle must generate to eject blood from the filled heart. The main components of afterload are the systemic (peripheral) or pulmonary vascular resistance and ventricular wall tension. For example, when the systemic vascular resistance is elevated, as with arterial hypertension, an increased intraventricular pressure must be generated to first open the aortic valve and then move blood out of the heart and into the systemic circulation. This increased pressure equates to an increase in ventricular wall stress or tension. As a result, excessive afterload may impair ventricular ejection and increase wall tension.

Myocardial Contractility. Myocardial contractility, also known as *inotropy,* refers to the contractile performance of the heart. It represents the ability of the contractile elements (actin and myosin filaments) of the heart muscle to interact and shorten against a load[5-7] (see Chapter 4, Fig. 4.22). Contractility increases cardiac output independent of preload and afterload.

The interaction between the actin and myosin filaments during cardiac muscle contraction (*i.e.,* cross-bridge attachment and detachment) requires the use of energy supplied by the breakdown of adenosine triphosphate (ATP) and the presence of calcium ions (Ca^{2+}). ATP provides the energy needed for cross-bridge formation during cardiac muscle contraction and for cross-bridge detachment during muscle relaxation.

As with skeletal muscle, when an action potential passes over the cardiac muscle fibre, the impulse spreads to the interior of the muscle fibre along the membranes of the transverse (T) tubules. The T tubule action potentials in turn act to cause release of Ca^{2+} from the sarcoplasmic reticulum (Fig. 26.1). These Ca^{2+} ions diffuse into the myofibrils and catalyze the chemical reactions that promote sliding of the actin and myosin filaments along one another to produce muscle shortening. In addition to the Ca^{2+} ions released from the sarcoplasmic reticulum, a large quantity of extracellular Ca^{2+} also diffuses into the sarcoplasm through voltage-dependent L-type Ca^{2+} channels in T tubules at the time of the action potential. Without the extra Ca^{2+} that enters through the L-type Ca^{2+} channels, the strength of the cardiac contraction would be considerably weaker. The Ca^{2+} channel protein is called the *dihydropyridine receptor* because it has a high affinity for this

FIGURE 26.1 • Schematic representation of the role of calcium ions (Ca^{2+}) in cardiac excitation–contraction coupling. The influx (site 1) of extracellular Ca^{2+} through the L-type Ca^{2+} channels in the T tubules during excitation triggers (site 2) release of Ca^{2+} by the sarcoplasmic reticulum. This Ca^{2+} binds to troponin C (site 3). The Ca^{2+}–troponin complex interacts with tropomyosin to unblock active sites on the actin and myosin filaments, allowing cross-bridge attachment and contraction of the myofibrils (systole). Relaxation (diastole) occurs as a result of calcium reuptake by the sarcoplasmic reticulum (site 4) and extrusion of intracellular Ca^{2+} by the sodium Na$^+$/Ca^{2+} exchange transporter or, to a lesser extent, by the Ca^{2+} ATPase pump (site 5). Mechanisms that raise systolic Ca^{2+} increase the level of developed force (inotropy). Binding of catecholamines to β-adrenergic receptors increases Ca^{2+} entry by phosphorylation of the Ca^{2+} channels through a cyclic adenosine monophosphate (cAMP)-dependent second messenger mechanism. The cardiac glycosides increase intracellular Ca^{2+} by inhibiting the Na$^+$/K$^+$-ATPase pump. The elevated intracellular Na$^+$ reverses the Na$^+$/Ca^{2+} exchange transporter (site 5), so less Ca^{2+} is removed from the cell. (Modified from Klabunde R. E. (2005). *Cardiovascular physiology concepts* (p. 46). Philadelphia, PA: Lippincott Williams & Wilkins.)

type of calcium blocking drug (*e.g.*, nifedipine). Opening of the L-type Ca^{2+} channels is facilitated by the second messenger cyclic adenosine monophosphate (cAMP), the formation of which is coupled to β-adrenergic receptors. The catecholamines (norepinephrine and epinephrine) exert their inotropic effects by binding to these receptors.

A number of factors interact in determining cardiac contractility, most of which act by altering systolic Ca^{2+} levels. For example, catecholamines (norepinephrine and epinephrine) increase Ca^{2+} entry into the cell by phosphorylation of the Ca^{2+} channels through a cAMP-dependent protein kinase. Another mechanism that can modulate inotropy is the sodium ion (Na$^+$)/Ca^{2+} exchange pump and the ATPase-dependent Ca^{2+} pump on the myocardial cell membrane (Fig. 26.1). These pumps transport Ca^{2+} out of the cell, thereby preventing the cell from becoming overloaded with Ca^{2+}. If Ca^{2+} extrusion is inhibited, the rise in intracellular Ca^{2+} can increase inotropy.

Systolic Versus Diastolic Dysfunction

Until recently, heart failure was viewed mainly in terms of backward and forward failure. *Backward failure* represented

failure of one of the ventricles effectively to empty the heart during systole, such that blood backs up in the venous system, causing congestion. *Forward failure* was characterized by impaired forward movement of blood into the arterial system emerging from the heart, resulting in reduced cardiac output.

A more recent classification separates the pathophysiology of heart failure into systolic and diastolic failure or dysfunction based on the ventricular ejection fraction.[2,8] *Ejection fraction* is the percentage of blood pumped out of the ventricles with each contraction. In systolic ventricular dysfunction, myocardial contractility is impaired, leading to a decrease in the ejection fraction and cardiac output. Diastolic ventricular dysfunction is characterized by a normal ejection fraction but impaired diastolic ventricular relaxation, leading to a decrease in ventricular filling that ultimately causes a decrease in preload, stroke volume, and cardiac output. Many persons with heart failure have combined elements of both systolic and diastolic ventricular dysfunction, and the division between systolic and diastolic dysfunction may be somewhat artificial, particularly as it relates to manifestations and treatment.[2,9] It is important to note that ventricular dysfunction is not synonymous with heart failure. It can, however, lead to heart failure.

With both systolic and diastolic ventricular dysfunction, compensatory mechanisms are usually able to maintain adequate resting cardiac function until the later stages of heart failure. Therefore, cardiac function measured at rest is a poor clinical indicator of the extent of cardiac impairment because cardiac output may be relatively normal at rest.[6]

Systolic Dysfunction. Systolic dysfunction is primarily defined as a decrease in myocardial contractility, most often characterized by an ejection fraction of less than 40%.[10] A normal heart ejects approximately 65% of the blood that is present in the ventricle at the end of diastole. In systolic heart failure, the ejection fraction declines progressively with increasing degrees of myocardial dysfunction. In very severe forms of heart failure, the ejection fraction may drop to a single-digit percentage. With a decrease in ejection fraction, there is a resultant increase in end-diastolic volume (preload), ventricular dilation, and ventricular wall tension and a rise in ventricular end-diastolic pressure.[8,10] This increased volume, added to the normal venous return, leads to an increase in ventricular preload. The rise in preload is thought to be a compensatory mechanism to help maintain stroke volume through the Frank–Starling mechanism despite a drop in ejection fraction (discussed later in the section on Compensatory Mechanisms). Although it serves as a compensatory mechanism, increased preload can also lead to one of the most deleterious consequences of systolic ventricular dysfunction—accumulation of blood in the atria and the venous system (which empties into the atria), causing either pulmonary or peripheral edema.

Systolic dysfunction commonly results from conditions that impair the contractile performance of the heart (*e.g.,* ischemic heart disease and cardiomyopathy), product of volume overload (*e.g.,* valvular insufficiency and anemia), or pressure overload (*e.g.,* hypertension and valvular stenosis) on the heart. The extent of systolic ventricular dysfunction can be estimated by measuring the cardiac output and ejection fraction and by assessment for manifestations of heart failure, particularly pulmonary congestion in left heart failure.

Diastolic Dysfunction. Although heart failure is commonly associated with impaired systolic function, in approximately 35% to 55% of cases systolic function has been preserved and heart failure occurs exclusively on the basis of left ventricular diastolic dysfunction.[11,12] Although such hearts contract normally, relaxation is abnormal. Cardiac output, especially during exercise, is compromised by the abnormal decrease in filling of the ventricle (*i.e.,* reduced preload). For any given ventricular volume, ventricular pressures are elevated, leading to signs of pulmonary and systemic venous congestion identical to those seen in persons with a dilated, poorly contracting heart. The prevalence of diastolic failure increases with age and is higher in women than men, and in persons with obesity, hypertension, or diabetes.[11,12]

Among the conditions that cause diastolic dysfunction are those that impede expansion of the ventricle (*e.g.,* pericardial

effusion, constrictive pericarditis), those that increase wall thickness and reduce chamber size (*e.g.,* myocardial hypertrophy, hypertrophic cardiomyopathy), and those that delay diastolic relaxation (*e.g.,* aging, ischemic heart disease).[12] Aging is often accompanied by a delay in relaxation of the heart during diastole; diastolic filling begins while the ventricle is still stiff and resistant to stretching to accept an increase in volume. A similar delay occurs in myocardial ischemia, resulting from a lack of energy to break the rigour bonds that form between the actin and myosin filaments and to move Ca^{2+} out of the cytosol and back into the sarcoplasmic reticulum.[12]

Diastolic function is further influenced by the heart rate, which determines how much time is available for ventricular filling. An increase in heart rate shortens the diastolic filling time.[12] Thus, diastolic dysfunction can be aggravated by tachycardia and improved by a reduction in heart rate, which allows the heart to fill over a longer period.

With diastolic dysfunction, blood is unable to move freely into the left ventricle, causing an increase in intraventricular pressure at any given volume. The elevated pressures are transferred *backward* from the left ventricle into the left atrium and pulmonary venous system, causing a decrease in lung compliance, which increases the work of breathing and evokes symptoms of dyspnea. Cardiac output is decreased, not because of a reduced ventricular ejection fraction as seen with systolic dysfunction, but because of a decrease in the volume (preload) available for adequate cardiac output. Inadequate cardiac output during exercise may lead to fatigue of the legs and the accessory muscles of respiration.

Right Versus Left Ventricular Dysfunction

Heart failure can be classified according to the side of the heart (right ventricular or left ventricular) that is primarily affected[10] (Fig. 26.2). Although the initial event that leads to heart failure may be primarily right- or left-ventricular in origin, long-term heart failure of one side usually leads to the failure of the other side. The pathophysiologic changes that occur in the myocardium itself, including the compensatory responses in conditions like myocardial infarction, are not significantly different between right and left ventricular dysfunction and are not addressed in detail in this section.

Right Ventricular Dysfunction. Right-sided heart failure impairs the ability to move deoxygenated blood from the systemic circulation into the pulmonary circulation. Consequently, when the right ventricle fails, there is a reduction in the amount of blood moved forward into the pulmonary circulation and then into the left side of the heart, ultimately causing a reduction of left ventricular cardiac output. Also, when the blood is not moved forward by the right ventricle, there is accumulation or congestion of blood into the systemic venous system. This causes an increase in right atrial, right ventricular end-diastolic, and systemic venous pressures. A major effect of right-sided heart failure is the development of peripheral edema (Fig. 26.2). Because of the effects of gravity, the edema is most pronounced in the dependent parts of the body—for

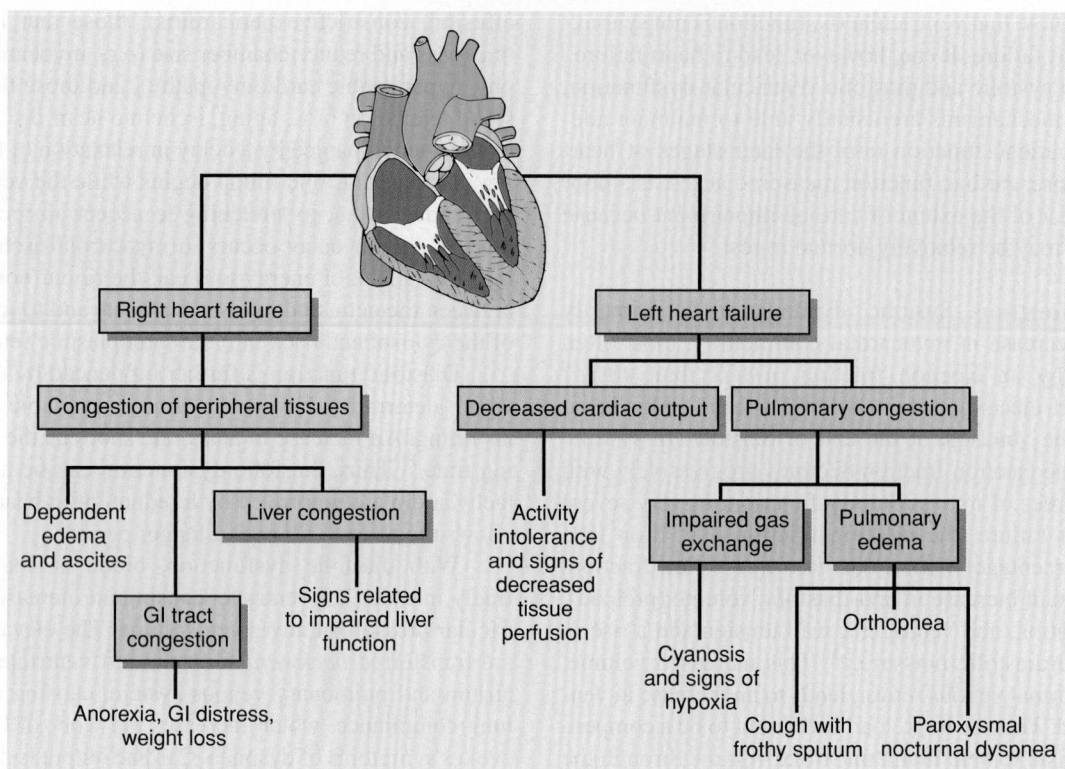

FIGURE 26.2 • Manifestations of left- and right-sided heart failure. GI, gastrointestinal.

example, in the lower extremities when the person is in the upright position and in the area over the sacrum when the person is supine. The accumulation of edema fluid is evidenced by a gain in weight, with each litre of water causing nearly 1 kg (2.2 lb) of weight gain. For example, 500 ml of accumulated fluid results in a 0.5 kg weight gain. Daily measurement of weight can be used as a means of assessing fluid accumulation in a patient with chronic heart failure. As a rule, a weight gain of more than 1.0 kg in 24 hours or 2.5 kg in 1 week is considered a sign of worsening failure.

Right-sided heart failure also produces congestion of the viscera. As venous distension progresses, blood backs up in the hepatic veins that drain into the inferior vena cava, and the liver becomes engorged. This may cause hepatomegaly and right upper quadrant pain. In severe and prolonged right-sided failure, liver function is impaired and hepatic cells may die. Congestion of the portal circulation also may lead to engorgement of the spleen and the development of ascites. Congestion of the gastrointestinal tract may interfere with digestion and absorption of nutrients, causing anorexia and abdominal discomfort. The jugular veins, which are above the level of the heart, are normally not visible in the standing position or when sitting with the head at higher than a 30-degree angle. In severe right-sided failure, the external jugular veins become distended and can be visualized when the person is sitting up or standing.

The causes of right ventricular dysfunction include conditions that impede blood flow into the lungs or compromise the pumping effectiveness of the right ventricle. Left ventricular

failure is the most common cause of right ventricular failure.[10] Sustained pulmonary hypertension also causes right ventricular dysfunction and failure. Pulmonary hypertension occurs in persons with chronic pulmonary disease, severe pneumonia, pulmonary embolus, or aortic or mitral stenosis. When the right heart failure occurs in response to acute or chronic pulmonary disease (*e.g.,* acute respiratory distress syndrome, pulmonary hypertension, chronic pulmonary disease), it is referred to as *cor pulmonale*[13] (see Chapter 29). Additional causes include stenosis or regurgitation of the tricuspid or pulmonic valves, right ventricular infarction, and cardiomyopathy. Right ventricular dysfunction with heart failure is also caused by congenital heart defects such as tetralogy of Fallot and ventricular septal defect (see Chapter 24).

Left Ventricular Dysfunction. Left-sided heart failure impairs the movement of blood from the low-pressure pulmonary circulation into the high-pressure arterial side of the systemic circulation. With impairment of left heart function, there is a decrease in cardiac output to the systemic circulation; blood accumulates in the left ventricle, left atrium, and pulmonary circulation, which causes elevated pulmonary venous pressure (Fig. 26.2). When the pressure in the pulmonary capillaries (normally approximately 10 mm Hg) exceeds the capillary osmotic pressure (normally approximately 25 mm Hg), there is a shift of intravascular fluid into the interstitium of the lung and development of pulmonary edema (Fig. 26.3). An episode of pulmonary edema often occurs at night, after the person has

Normal

Capillary
filtration
pressure
10 mm Hg

Arterial

Venous

Capillary
colloidal
osmotic
pressure
25 mm Hg

Pulmonary edema

Capillary
filtration
pressure
>25 mm Hg

Arterial

Venous

Capillary
colloidal
osmotic
pressure
25 mm Hg

FIGURE 26.3 • Mechanism of respiratory symptoms in left-sided heart failure. In the normal exchange of fluid in the pulmonary capillaries (**top**), the capillary filtration (hydrostatic) pressure that moves fluid out of the capillary into the lung is less than the capillary colloidal osmotic pressure that pulls fluid back into the capillary. Development of pulmonary edema (**bottom**) occurs when the capillary filtration (hydrostatic) pressure exceeds the capillary colloidal osmotic pressure that pulls fluid back into the capillary.

been reclining for some time and the gravitational forces have been removed from the circulatory system. It is then that the edema fluid that had been sequestered in the lower extremities during the day is returned to the vascular compartment and redistributed to the pulmonary circulation.

The most common causes of left ventricular dysfunction are hypertension, acute myocardial infarction, and cardiomyopathy. Left ventricular heart failure and pulmonary congestion can develop very rapidly in persons with acute myocardial infarction. Even when the infarcted area is small, there may be a surrounding area of ischemic tissue. This may result in large areas of ventricular wall hypokinesis or akinesis and rapid onset of pulmonary congestion and edema. Stenosis or regurgitation of the aortic or mitral valves also creates left-sided backflow that may result in pulmonary congestion. As pulmonary pressure rises as a result of pulmonary congestion, it may progress to produce right-sided heart failure. Pulmonary edema also may develop during rapid infusion of

intravenous fluids or blood transfusions in an elderly person or in a person with limited cardiac reserve.

High-Output Versus Low-Output Failure

High- and low-output heart failure are described in terms of cardiac output. *High-output failure* is an uncommon type of heart failure that is caused by an excessive need for cardiac output that is not attained. With high-output failure, the function of the heart may be greater than normal yet is inadequate due to excessive metabolic needs. Causes of high-output failure include severe anemia, sepsis, thyrotoxicosis, conditions that cause arteriovenous shunting, and Paget disease.

Low-output failure is caused by disorders that impair the pumping ability of the heart, such as ischemic heart disease and cardiomyopathy. Low-output failure is characterized by clinical evidence of systemic vasoconstriction with cold, pale, and sometimes cyanotic extremities.[2,10] In advanced forms of low-output failure, marked reductions in stroke volume are evidenced by a narrowing of the pulse pressure. In contrast, in high-output failure, the extremities are usually warm and flushed and the pulse pressure is widened or normal.

Compensatory Mechanisms

In heart failure, the cardiac reserve is largely maintained through compensatory or adaptive responses such as the Frank–Starling mechanism; activation of neurohumoral influences such as the sympathetic nervous system, the renin–angiotensin–aldosterone system, natriuretic peptides, and locally produced vasoactive substances; and myocardial hypertrophy and remodelling[5–7,14] (Fig. 26.4). The first two of these adaptations occur rapidly over minutes to hours of myocardial dysfunction and may be adequate to maintain the overall pumping performance of the heart at relatively normal levels. Myocardial hypertrophy and remodelling occur slowly over weeks to months and play an important role in the long-term adaptation to hemodynamic overload. In the failing heart, early decreases in cardiac function may go unnoticed because these compensatory mechanisms maintain the cardiac output. However, these mechanisms contribute not only to the adaptation of the failing heart but to the pathophysiology of the eventual heart failure.[14]

Length Tension/Frank–Starling Mechanism. The Frank–Starling mechanism operates through an increase in preload (Fig. 26.5). With increased diastolic filling, there is increased stretching of the myocardial fibres and more optimal approximation of the heads on the thick myosin filaments to the troponin binding sites on the thin actin filaments, with a resultant increase in the force of the next contraction (see Chapter 21). In the normally functioning heart, the Frank–Starling mechanism serves to match the outputs of the two ventricles. As illustrated in Figure 26.5, there is no one single Frank–Starling curve.[6] An increase in contractility, or inotropy, will increase cardiac output at any end-diastolic volume, causing the curve to move up and to the left, whereas a decrease in inotropy will cause the curve to move down and to the right. In heart failure, inotropy is decreased compared with normal; thus, cardiac

FIGURE 26.4 • Compensatory mechanisms in heart failure. The Frank–Starling mechanism, sympathetic reflexes, renin–angiotensin–aldosterone system, and myocardial hypertrophy function in maintaining cardiac output for the failing heart.

FIGURE 26.5 • Left ventricular function curves (Frank–Starling curves). *Curve A:* Normal function curve, with a normal cardiac output at optimal left ventricular end-diastolic filling pressures (capillary wedge pressure). *Curve B:* Compensated heart failure with normal cardiac output at higher filling pressures. *Curve C:* Decompensated heart failure with a decrease in cardiac output and elevated filling pressure. *Curve D:* Cardiogenic shock, with extremely depressed cardiac output and marked increase in filling pressures.

output will not be as high as with normal inotropy, regardless of the increase in preload.

In heart failure, a decrease in cardiac output and renal blood flow leads to increased sodium and water retention, a resultant increase in vascular volume and venous return to the heart, and an increase in ventricular end-diastolic volume. Within limits, as preload and ventricular end-diastolic volume increase, there is a resultant increase in cardiac output. Although this may preserve the resting cardiac output, the resulting chronic elevation of left ventricular end-diastolic pressure may be transmitted to the atria and the pulmonary circulation, causing pulmonary congestion.

An increase in muscle stretch, as occurs with the Frank–Starling mechanism, causes an increase in ventricular wall tension with a resultant increase in myocardial oxygen consumption. Because increased wall tension increases myocardial oxygen requirements, it can produce ischemia and contribute to further impairment of inotropy, moving the Frank–Starling curve further down and to the right (Fig. 26.5). In this situation, the increase in preload is no longer contributing to compensation but rather causing heart failure to worsen. The use of diuretics in persons with heart failure helps to reduce vascular volume and ventricular filling, thereby unloading the heart and reducing ventricular wall tension.

Sympathetic Nervous System Activity. Stimulation of the sympathetic nervous system plays an important role in the compensatory response to decreased cardiac output and in the pathogenesis of acute heart failure.[8,11,14,15] Both cardiac sympathetic tone and catecholamine (epinephrine and norepinephrine) levels are elevated in most forms of heart failure. By direct stimulation of heart rate and cardiac contractility, regulation of vascular tone, and enhancement of renal sodium and water retention, the sympathetic nervous system initially helps to maintain perfusion of the various body organs. In persons who progress to more severe heart failure, blood is diverted to the more critical cerebral and coronary circulations.

Although the sympathetic nervous system response is meant to augment blood pressure and cardiac output, it quickly becomes maladaptive and contributes to the deterioration of heart function. An increase in sympathetic activity can lead to tachycardia, vasoconstriction, and cardiac arrhythmias. Acutely, tachycardia significantly increases the workload of the heart, thus increasing myocardial oxygen demand and leading to cardiac ischemia, myocyte damage, and decreased contractility (inotropy).[15] Cardiac ischemia and cardiomyopathy both contribute to worsening of heart failure. By promoting arrhythmias, the catecholamines released with sympathetic nervous system stimulation also may contribute to the high rate of sudden death seen with heart failure.

There is evidence that prolonged sympathetic stimulation may also lead to desensitization of β-adrenergic receptors without affecting α-adrenergic receptors. As circulating norepinephrine levels are increased in persons with heart failure, the lack of functioning β-adrenergic receptors in relation to α-adrenergic receptors may lead to vasoconstriction and an increase in systemic vascular resistance. An increase in systemic vascular resistance causes an increase in cardiac afterload and ventricular wall stress, thus increasing myocardial oxygen consumption. Increased norepinephrine levels contribute to remodelling, fibrosis, ischemia, and apoptosis.[15] Other effects include decreased renal perfusion and additional augmentation of the renin–angiotensin–aldosterone system, as well as decreased blood flow to skin, muscle, and abdominal organs.[16]

Renin–Angiotensin–Aldosterone System. One of the most important effects of lowered cardiac output in heart failure is a reduction in renal blood flow and glomerular filtration rate, which leads to sodium and water retention. With decreased renal blood flow, there is an increase in renin secretion by the kidneys, with subsequent increases in circulating levels of angiotensin II. Angiotensin II contributes directly to a generalized and excessive vasoconstriction, as well as facilitating norepinephrine release and inhibiting reuptake of norepinephrine by the sympathetic nervous system.[6]

Angiotensin II also provides a powerful stimulus for aldosterone production by the adrenal cortex (see Chapter 23). Aldosterone increases tubular reabsorption of sodium, with an accompanying increase in water retention. Because aldosterone is metabolized in the liver, its levels are further increased when heart failure causes liver congestion. Angiotensin II also increases the level of antidiuretic hormone (ADH), which serves as a vasoconstrictor and inhibitor of water excretion

(see Chapter 31). In heart failure, the progressive accumulation of fluid leads to ventricular dilation and increased wall tension. As described earlier, the increased oxygen demand that accompanies increased wall tension eventually outweighs the compensatory Frank–Starling mechanism, reducing inotropy and exacerbating heart failure.

In addition to their individual effects on sodium and water balance, angiotensin II and aldosterone are also involved in regulating the inflammatory and reparative processes that follow tissue injury.[17] In this capacity, they stimulate inflammatory cytokine production (*e.g.,* tumour necrosis factor alpha [TNFα] and interleukin-6), attract immune cells (*e.g.,* neutrophils and macrophages), activate macrophages at sites of injury and repair, and stimulate the growth of fibroblasts and synthesis of collagen fibres. Fibroblast and collagen deposition results in ventricular hypertrophy and myocardial wall fibrosis, which decreases compliance (*i.e.,* increases stiffness), ultimately causing inappropriate remodelling of the heart and progression of both systolic and diastolic ventricular dysfunction.[18]

Aldosterone-synthesizing enzymes have been demonstrated in endothelial and vascular smooth muscle cells as well as in the adrenal gland, suggesting that these cells are capable of producing aldosterone as well as responding to it.[17] Thus, the progression of heart failure may be augmented by aldosterone-mediated vascular remodelling in the heart and other organs. In the International Randomized Aldactone Evaluation Study (RALES) trial involving more than 1,600 patients with moderately severe to severe heart failure, there was a 30% decrease in mortality from any cause among persons treated with standard therapy plus spironolactone (an aldosterone antagonist), compared with those who received a placebo plus standard therapy.[19] Spironolactone, the aldosterone antagonist available in Canada, is effective in severe heart failure post acute MI or acute episodes of chronic failure.[2]

Natriuretic Peptides. The heart muscle produces and secretes a family of related peptide hormones, the NPs, that have potent diuretic, natriuretic, and vascular smooth muscle effects. They interact with other neurohumoral mechanisms that affect cardiovascular function. Two of the four known NPs most commonly associated with heart failure are atrial natriuretic peptide (ANP) and brain natriuretic peptide (BNP).[20,21]

ANP is released from atrial cells in response to atrial stretch, pressure, or fluid overload. BNP, so named because it was originally found in extracts of porcine brain, is primarily secreted by cells in the right and left ventricles as a response to increased ventricular pressure or fluid overload in the heart. Although the NPs are not secreted from the same chambers in the heart, they have very similar functions. In response to increased chamber stretch and pressure, they promote rapid and transient natriuresis and diuresis through an increase in glomerular filtration rate resulting from dilation of afferent arterioles and constriction of efferent arterioles.

The NPs also facilitate complex interactions with the neurohormonal system, inhibiting the sympathetic nervous system, the renin–angiotensin–aldosterone system, endothelin inflammatory cytokines, and vasopressin.[22] Suppression of the sympathetic nervous system causes both venous and arterial dilation with consequent reduction in venous return to the heart (decreased preload) and cardiac filling pressures, and a decrease in afterload (arterial vasodilation). Inhibition of angiotensin II and vasopressin by the NPs decreases renal reabsorption of sodium and water. In addition, the NPs directly affect the central nervous system and the brain, inhibiting the secretion of vasopressin and the function of the salt appetite and thirst centre.[22]

Circulating levels of both ANP and BNP are elevated in persons with heart failure. The concentrations are well correlated with the extent of ventricular dysfunction, increasing up to 30-fold in persons with advanced heart disease.[20] Assays of BNP are used clinically in the diagnosis of heart failure and to predict the severity of the condition.

Endothelins. The endothelins, released from the endothelial cells throughout the circulation, are potent vasoconstrictors. Like angiotensin II, endothelin can also be synthesized and released by a variety of cell types, such as cardiac myocytes. Four endothelin peptides (endothelin-1 [ET-1], ET-2, ET-3, and ET-4) have been identified.[23] In addition to vasoconstrictor actions, the endothelins induce vascular smooth muscle cell proliferation and cardiac myocyte hypertrophy; increase the release of ANP, aldosterone, and catecholamines; and exert antinatriuretic effects on the kidneys. They have been shown to have a negative inotropic action in patients with heart failure.[24] Production of ET-1 is regulated by many factors that are significant for cardiovascular function and have implications for heart failure; for example, it is enhanced by angiotensin-II, vasopressin, and norepinephrine and by factors such as shear stress and endothelial stretching.[24] Plasma ET-1 levels also correlate directly with pulmonary vascular resistance, and it is thought that the peptide may play a role in mediating pulmonary hypertension in persons with heart failure. There are at least two types of endothelin receptors—type A and type B.[23] An endothelin receptor antagonist (e.g., bosentan) is available in Canada for pulmonary arterial hypertension. However, its effectiveness for chronic heart failure is not supported by evidence.[2,4]

Inflammatory Mediators. There is ongoing research examining the relationship between inflammatory markers, especially C-reactive protein (CRP), and heart failure. Elevated CRP levels have been associated with adverse consequences in persons with heart failure, and have been shown to be predictive of the development of heart failure in high-risk groups. Of particular interest are the interactions between CRP and the classic neurohormonal system including angiotensin II and norepinephrine. As previously mentioned, these associations relate to left ventricular dysfunction, ventricular hypertrophy and remodelling, progressive loss of myocardial cells through apoptosis (programmed cell death), and endothelial dysfunction. It has been suggested that many of the conventional treatments for heart failure (e.g., angiotensin-converting enzyme inhibitors and β-blockers) may work, at least in part, through modulation of the proinflammatory cytokines.[2,25]

Myocardial Hypertrophy and Remodelling. The development of myocardial hypertrophy constitutes one of the principal mechanisms by which the heart compensates for an increase in workload.[14,15] Ventricular hypertrophy improves the work performance of the heart, however, it is also an important risk factor for subsequent cardiac morbidity and mortality. Inappropriate hypertrophy and remodelling can result in changes in structure (e.g., muscle mass, chamber dilation) and function (i.e., impaired systolic or diastolic function) that often lead to further pump dysfunction and hemodynamic overload.

Myocardial hypertrophy and remodelling involve a series of complex events at both the molecular and cellular level. The myocardium is composed of myocytes, or muscle cells, and nonmyocytes. The myocytes are the functional units of cardiac muscle. Their growth is limited by an increment in cell size, as opposed to an increase in cell number. The nonmyocytes include cardiac macrophages, fibroblasts, vascular smooth muscle, and endothelial cells. These cells are present in the interstitial space, remain capable of an increase in cell number, and provide support for the myocytes. The nonmyocytes also determine many of the inappropriate changes that occur during myocardial hypertrophy. For example, uncontrolled cardiac fibroblast growth is associated with increased synthesis of collagen fibres, myocardial fibrosis, and ventricular wall stiffness. Not only does ventricular wall stiffness increase the workload of the heart, but the fibrosis and remodelling that occur lead to electrical conduction abnormalities in which the heart contracts in an uncoordinated manner, known as *cardiac dyssynchrony*, causing reduced systolic heart function.[26]

Recent research has focused on the type of hypertrophy that develops in persons with heart failure. At the cellular level, cardiac muscle cells respond to stimuli from stress placed on the ventricular wall by pressure and volume overload by initiating several different processes that lead to hypertrophy. These include stimuli that produce a *symmetric hypertrophy* with a proportionate increase in muscle length and width, as occurs in athletes; *concentric hypertrophy* with an increase in wall thickness, as occurs in hypertension; and *eccentric hypertrophy* with a disproportionate increase in muscle length, as occurs in dilated cardiomyopathy[27] (Fig. 26.6). When the primary stimulus for hypertrophy is *pressure overload*, the increase in wall stress leads to parallel replication of myofibrils, thickening of the individual myocytes, and concentric hypertrophy. Concentric hypertrophy may preserve systolic function for a time, but eventually the work performed by the ventricle exceeds the vascular reserve, predisposing to ischemia. When the primary stimulus is *ventricular volume overload*, the increase in wall stress leads to replication of myofibrils in series, elongation of the cardiac muscle cells, and eccentric hypertrophy. Eccentric hypertrophy leads to a decrease in ventricular wall thickness with an increase in diastolic volume and wall tension.

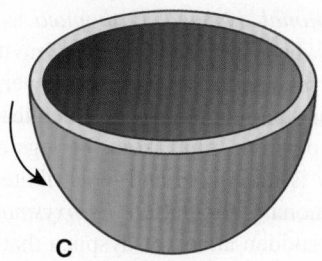

FIGURE 26.6 • Different types of myocardial hypertrophy. **A:** Normal symmetric hypertrophy with proportionate increases in myocardial wall thickness and length. **B:** Concentric hypertrophy with a disproportionate increase in wall thickness. **C:** Eccentric hypertrophy with a disproportionate decrease in wall thickness and ventricular dilation.

The stimuli for hypertrophy and remodelling are thought to reflect not only the mechanical stress placed on the myocytes, but growth signals provided by the release of substances such as norepinephrine, angiotensin II, ANP, and ET-1. It is hoped that further research into the signals that cause specific features of inappropriate myocardial hypertrophy and remodelling will lead to the identification of targets whose actions can be interrupted or modified.

Acute Heart Failure Syndromes

The acute heart failure syndromes (AHFSs) are "defined as gradual or rapid change in heart failure signs and symptoms resulting in a need for urgent therapy."[28] These symptoms are primarily the result of severe pulmonary edema due to elevated left ventricular filling pressures, with or without a low cardiac output.[28] The syndromes are among the most common disorders seen in emergency departments, and most patients have signs and symptoms of volume overload. Chronic heart failure, often complicated by episodes of acute failure (referred to as acute decompensated heart failure), is the most common cause of the syndrome. Until recently, the underlying cause of heart failure hospitalization was believed to be merely a problem with volume overload or low cardiac output precipitated by dietary indiscretions or medication nonadherence. Hospitalization therefore was considered to be an expected part of the chronic heart failure trajectory.

AHFS are thought to encompass three different types of conditions: (1) worsening of chronic systolic or diastolic dysfunction that appears to respond to treatment; (2) new-onset acute heart failure that occurs secondary to a precipitating event such as a large myocardial infarction or a sudden increase in blood pressure superimposed on a noncompliant left ventricle; and (3) worsening of end-stage/advanced heart failure that is refractory to treatment, with predominantly left ventricular systolic dysfunction associated with a low-output state.[28–30] The difference between new-onset AHFS and AHFS caused by chronic heart failure (*i.e.,* acute decompensated heart failure) is in the degree of physiologic response, which is more pronounced in the new-onset AHFS and more subtle in chronic heart failure because of the compensatory pathophysiology. For example, with new-onset AHFS, the person will have a stronger sympathetic response with enhanced pulmonary vascular permeability causing rapid and dramatic symptoms of pulmonary edema. Because many compensatory mechanisms operate in persons with chronic heart failure, they tolerate higher pulmonary vascular pressures. Chronic changes in neurohormonal regulation lead to stronger activation of the renin–angiotensin–aldosterone system with a resultant volume overload, and venous congestion is more prominent in both the systemic and pulmonary circulations.

Manifestations of Heart Failure

The manifestations of heart failure depend on the extent and type of cardiac dysfunction that is present and the rapidity with which it develops. A person with previously stable compensated heart failure may develop signs of heart failure for the first time when the condition has advanced to a critical point, such as with a progressive increase in pulmonary hypertension in a person with mitral valve regurgitation. Overt heart failure also may be precipitated by conditions such as infection, emotional stress, uncontrolled hypertension, or fluid overload.[8] Many persons with serious underlying heart disease, regardless of whether they have previously experienced heart failure, may be relatively asymptomatic as long they carefully adhere to their treatment regimen. A dietary excess of sodium is a frequent cause of sudden cardiac decompensation.[31]

The manifestations of heart failure reflect the physiologic effects of the impaired pumping ability of the heart, decreased renal blood flow, and activation of the sympathetic compensatory mechanisms. The severity and progression of symptoms depend on the extent and type of dysfunction that is present (systolic vs. diastolic, right- vs. left-sided). The signs and symptoms include shortness of breath and other respiratory manifestations, fatigue and limited exercise tolerance, fluid retention and edema, cachexia and malnutrition, and cyanosis. Persons with severe heart failure may exhibit diaphoresis and tachycardia.

Respiratory Manifestations

Shortness of breath due to congestion of the pulmonary circulation is one of the major manifestations of left-sided heart failure. Perceived shortness of breath (*e.g.,* breathlessness) is called *dyspnea.* Dyspnea related to an increase in activity is called *exertional dyspnea. Orthopnea* is shortness of breath that occurs when a person is supine. Gravitational forces cause fluid to become sequestered in the lower legs and feet when the person is standing or sitting. When the person assumes the recumbent position, fluid from the legs and dependent parts of the body is mobilized and redistributed to an already distended pulmonary circulation. *Paroxysmal nocturnal dyspnea* (PND) is a sudden attack of dyspnea that usually occurs during sleep. It disrupts sleep, and the person may awaken with significant feelings of shortness of breath, even feeling a sense of suffocation, plus coughing or wheezing.

A subtle and often overlooked symptom of heart failure is a chronic dry, nonproductive cough that becomes worse when the person is lying down. Bronchospasm due to congestion of the bronchial mucosa may cause wheezing and difficulty in breathing. This condition is sometimes referred to as *cardiac asthma* and is closely related to PND.[8]

Cheyne–Stokes Respiration. Cheyne–Stokes respiration is a pattern of periodic breathing characterized by gradual increase in depth (and sometimes rate) of breathing to a maximum, followed by a decrease resulting in apnea (see Chapter 27). Although no longer associated solely with heart failure, it is recognized as an independent risk factor for worsening of heart failure. During sleep, Cheyne–Stokes breathing causes recurrent awakening and thereby reduces slow-wave and rapid eye movement (REM) sleep. The recurrent cycling of hypoventilation/apnea and hyperventilation may also increase sympathetic activity and predispose to arrhythmias.

Acute Pulmonary Edema. Acute pulmonary edema is the most dramatic symptom of AHFS. It is a life-threatening condition in which capillary fluid moves into the alveoli.[8] The accumulated fluid in the alveoli and airways causes lung stiffness, makes lung expansion more difficult, and impairs the gas exchange function of the lung. With the decreased ability of the lungs to oxygenate the blood, the hemoglobin leaves the pulmonary circulation without being fully oxygenated, resulting in shortness of breath, fatigue, low oxygen saturations, and cyanosis.

The person with severe pulmonary edema is usually seen sitting and gasping for air. The pulse is rapid, the skin is moist and cool, and the lips and nail beds are cyanotic. As the pulmonary edema worsens and oxygen supply to the brain drops, confusion and altered cognition occur. Dyspnea and air hunger are accompanied by a productive cough with frothy (resembling beaten egg whites) and often blood-tinged sputum—the effect of air mixing with the serum albumin and red blood cells that have moved into the alveoli. The movement of air through the alveolar fluid produces fine crepitant sounds called *crackles,* which can be heard with chest auscultation. As fluid moves into the larger airways, the crackles become louder and coarser.

Fatigue, Weakness, and Mental Confusion

Fatigue and weakness often accompany diminished output from the left ventricle. Cardiac fatigue is different from general fatigue in that it usually is not present in the morning but appears and progresses as activity increases during the day.

In acute or severe left-sided failure, cardiac output may fall to levels that are insufficient to provide the brain with adequate oxygen, and there are indications of mental confusion and disturbed behaviour. Confusion, impairment of memory, anxiety, restlessness, and insomnia may occur in elderly persons with advanced heart failure, particularly in those with cerebral atherosclerosis. These symptoms may confuse the diagnosis of heart failure in the elderly because of the myriad other possible causes or disorders associated with aging.

Fluid Retention, Edema, and Renal Manifestations

Many of the manifestations of heart failure result from the increased capillary pressures (increased hydrostatic pressures) that develop in the peripheral circulation in persons with right-sided heart failure and in the pulmonary circulation in persons with left-sided heart failure. The increased capillary pressure reflects an overfilling of the vascular system because of increased sodium and water retention and venous congestion, referred to earlier as *backward* failure, resulting from impaired cardiac output.[8]

Nocturia is a nightly increase in urine output that occurs relatively early in the course of heart failure. It occurs because of the increased cardiac output, renal blood flow, and glomerular filtration rate that follow the increased blood return to the heart when the person is in a supine position. *Oliguria,* which is a decrease in urine output, is a late sign related to a severely reduced cardiac output and resultant renal failure.

Transudation of fluid into the pleural cavity (hydrothorax) or the peritoneal cavity (ascites) may occur in persons with advanced heart failure. Because the pleural veins drain into both the systemic and pulmonary venous beds, pleural effusion is observed more commonly in persons with hypertension involving both venous systems.[8] Pleural effusion occurs as the excess fluid in the lung interstitial spaces crosses the visceral pleura, which in turn overwhelms the capacity of the pulmonary lymphatic system. Ascites occurs in persons with increased pressure in the hepatic veins and veins draining the peritoneum. It usually reflects right ventricular failure and long-standing elevation of systemic venous pressure.[8]

The term cardiorenal syndrome (CRS) relays the interaction between the heart and the kidneys, with a complex combination of neurohormonal feedback mechanisms.[32] Persons with chronic heart disease are at risk for injury to the kidney, in part due to alterations in sodium, water, hemoglobin, and perfusion. In CRS, the primary organ failing can be either the heart or the kidney, with dysfunction in one inducing injury and dysfunction in the other.

Cachexia and Malnutrition

Cardiac cachexia is a loss of body weight, muscle, and fat that occurs as a complication in advanced heart failure. A number of factors probably contribute to its development, including anorexia, fatigue, and depression that interfere with food intake, congestion of the liver and gastrointestinal structures that impairs digestion and absorption and produces feelings of fullness, and the circulating toxins and mediators released from poorly perfused tissues that impair appetite and contribute to tissue wasting.[8] It is associated with right heart failure and increased mortality.[33]

Cyanosis

Cyanosis is the bluish discolouration of the skin and mucous membranes caused by excess desaturated hemoglobin in the blood; it often is a late sign of heart failure. Cyanosis may be central, caused by arterial desaturation resulting from impaired pulmonary gas exchange, or peripheral, caused by venous desaturation resulting from extensive extraction of oxygen at the capillary level. Central cyanosis is caused by conditions that impair oxygenation of the arterial blood, such as pulmonary edema, left heart failure, or right-to-left cardiac shunting. Peripheral cyanosis is caused by conditions such as low-output failure that result in delivery of poorly oxygenated blood to the peripheral tissues, or by conditions such as peripheral vasoconstriction that cause excessive removal of oxygen from the blood. Central cyanosis is best monitored in the lips and mucous membranes because these areas are not subject to conditions, such as a cold environment, that cause peripheral cyanosis. Persons with right- or left-sided heart failure may develop cyanosis especially around the lips and in the peripheral parts of the extremities.

Arrhythmias and Sudden Cardiac Death

Both atrial and ventricular arrhythmias (see Chapter 25) frequently occur in persons with heart failure. Atrial fibrillation is the most common arrhythmia. Manifestations associated with atrial fibrillation are related to loss of atrial contraction, tachycardia, irregular heart rate, and symptoms related to a drop in blood pressure.[2,10] There is also strong evidence that persons with heart failure are at increased risk for sudden cardiac arrest or death that occurs within 1 hour of the symptom onset. In persons with ventricular dysfunction, sudden death is caused most commonly by ventricular tachycardia or ventricular fibrillation.[26]

Diagnosis and Treatment

Diagnostic Methods

Diagnostic methods in heart failure are directed toward establishing the cause of the disorder and determining the extent of the dysfunction. Medical guidelines for diagnosis and treatment are clearly described in the Canadian Cardiovascular Society (CCS) guidelines for heart failure management.[1,2] Because heart failure represents the failure of the heart as a pump and can occur in the course of a number of heart diseases or other systemic disorders, the diagnosis of heart failure often is based on signs and symptoms related to the failing heart itself, such as shortness of breath and fatigue. The functional classification of the New York Heart Association (NYHA) is one guide to classifying the extent of dysfunction (Table 26.1).

The methods used in the diagnosis of heart failure include risk factor assessment, history and physical examination, laboratory studies, electrocardiography, chest radiography, and echocardiography. The history should include information related to dyspnea, cough, nocturia, generalized fatigue, and other signs and symptoms of heart failure. A complete physical examination includes assessment of heart rate, heart sounds, blood pressure, jugular veins for venous congestion, lungs for signs of pulmonary congestion, and lower extremities for edema. Laboratory tests are used in the diagnosis of anemia and electrolyte imbalances, and to detect signs of chronic liver congestion. Measurements of BNP are recommended to confirm the diagnosis of heart failure; to evaluate the severity of left ventricular compromise, estimate the prognosis, and predict future cardiac events such as sudden death; and to evaluate the effectiveness of treatment.[2]

Echocardiography plays a key role in assessing right and left ventricular wall motion (normal, akinesis, or hypokinesis), wall thickness, ventricular chamber size, valve function, heart defects, ejection fraction, and pericardial disease.[2] Electrocardiographic findings may indicate atrial or ventricular hypertrophy, underlying disorders of cardiac rhythm, or conduction abnormalities such as right or left bundle branch block. Radionuclide ventriculography and cardiac angiography are recommended if there is reason to suspect coronary artery disease as the underlying cause for heart failure. Chest x-rays provide information about the size and shape of the heart and pulmonary vasculature. The cardiac silhouette can be used to detect cardiac hypertrophy and dilation. Chest x-rays can indicate the relative severity of the failure by revealing whether pulmonary edema is predominantly vascular or interstitial, or has advanced to the alveolar and bronchial stages. Cardiac magnetic resonance imaging (CMRI) and cardiac computed tomography (CCT) are used to document ejection fraction, ventricular preload, and regional wall motion.

Invasive hemodynamic monitoring may be used for assessment in acute, life-threatening episodes of heart failure. These monitoring methods include central venous pressure (CVP), pulmonary artery pressure monitoring, thermodilution measurements of cardiac output, and intra-arterial measurements of blood pressure. CVP reflects the amount of blood returning to the right side of the heart, not the preload of the left side. Measurements of CVP are best obtained by a catheter inserted into the right atrium through a peripheral vein, or by the right atrial port (opening) in a pulmonary artery catheter. This pressure is decreased in hypovolemia and increased in right heart failure. The changes that occur in CVP over time usually are more significant than the absolute numeric values obtained during a single reading.

Ventricular volume pressures are obtained indirectly, such as by a flow-directed, balloon-tipped pulmonary artery catheter. This catheter is introduced through a peripheral or central vein and then advanced into the right atrium. The balloon is then inflated with air, enabling the catheter to float through the right ventricle into the pulmonary artery until it becomes wedged in a small pulmonary vessel (Fig. 26.7).

Pulmonary artery catheter

FIGURE 26.7 • Balloon-tipped pulmonary artery catheter positioned in a small pulmonary vessel. The pulmonary capillary wedge pressure, which reflects the left ventricular diastolic pressure, is measured with the balloon inflated.

With the balloon inflated, the catheter monitors pulmonary capillary pressures (also called *pulmonary wedge pressure* [PWP]) in direct communication with pressures from the left ventricle. The pulmonary capillary pressures provide a means of assessing preload and pumping ability of the left ventricle.

One type of pulmonary artery catheter is equipped with a thermistor probe to obtain *thermodilution measurements* of cardiac output. A known amount of solution of a known temperature (iced or room temperature) is injected into the right atrium through an opening in the catheter, and the temperature of the blood is measured downstream in the pulmonary artery by the thermistor probe located at the end of that catheter. A microcomputer calculates stroke volume from changes in the temperature of the blood as it flows past the thermistor, and multiplies by the heart rate to estimate cardiac output. Catheters with oximeters built into their tips that permit continuous monitoring of venous oxygen saturation (SvO_2) also are available.

Intra-arterial blood pressure monitoring provides a means for continuous monitoring of blood pressure. It is used in persons with acute heart failure when aggressive intravenous medication therapy or a mechanical assist device is required. Measurements are obtained through a small catheter inserted into a peripheral artery, usually the radial artery. The catheter is connected to a pressure transducer, and beat-by-beat measurements of blood pressure are recorded. The monitoring system displays the contour of the pressure waveform; the systolic, diastolic, and mean arterial pressures; and the pulse. Monitoring systems are available that estimate the cardiac output via flow in the artery, and may be used for high-risk persons in whom continuous monitoring of cardiac output is beneficial.

Treatment

The goals of treatment are determined by the rapidity of onset and severity of the heart failure. Persons with AHFSs require urgent therapy directed at stabilizing and correcting the cause of the cardiac dysfunction. For persons with chronic heart failure, the goals of treatment are directed toward relieving the symptoms, improving the quality of life, and reducing or eliminating risk factors (*e.g.,* hypertension, diabetes, obesity) with a long-term goal of slowing, halting, or reversing the cardiac dysfunction.[1,2]

Treatment measures for both acute and chronic heart failure include nonpharmacologic and pharmacologic approaches. Mechanical support devices, including the intra-aortic balloon pump (for acute failure) and the ventricular assist device (VAD), sustain life in persons with severe heart failure. Heart transplantation remains the treatment of choice for some persons with end-stage heart failure. However, less than 200 heart transplants are done per year in Canada,[34] in part due to a shortage of donors.

Nonpharmacologic Methods. Exercise intolerance is typical in individuals with chronic heart failure, yet exercise is an important component of management.[35] Consequently, individualized exercise training is important to maximize muscle conditioning; persons who are not accustomed to exercise and those with more severe heart failure are started at a lower intensity and shorter sessions than those who are mostly asymptomatic. Sodium and fluid restriction and weight management are important for all individuals with heart failure; the degree of sodium and fluid restriction is individualized to the severity of heart failure. Counselling, health teaching, and ongoing evaluation programs help persons with heart failure to manage and cope with their treatment regimen. Hypertension, hyperlipidemia, diabetes, and arrhythmias should be monitored and managed, with lifestyle modifications (*e.g.,* weight reduction, smoking cessation, avoidance of cardiotoxins such as alcohol) when appropriate.[2,10]

Pharmacologic Treatment. When heart failure is moderate to severe, pharmacologic in conjunction with nonpharmacologic management is important to prevent and treat acute heart failure and manage chronic heart failure. Evidence-based agents recommended for treatment and management include ACE inhibitors or angiotensin II receptor blockers, β-adrenergic blockers, and diuretics.[1,2,10,33,36] Although digoxin remains in use for specific populations, evidence of its benefit is both sparse and conflicting. The choice of pharmacologic agents is based on individual symptoms, responses, and comorbidities.

The *ACE inhibitors,* which prevent the conversion of angiotensin I to angiotensin II, have been used effectively in the treatment of chronic heart failure. The renin–angiotensin–aldosterone system is activated early in the course of heart failure and plays an important role in its progression. It results in an increase in angiotensin II, which causes vasoconstriction, unregulated ventricular remodelling, and increased aldosterone production with a subsequent increase in sodium and water retention by the kidneys. ACE inhibitors have been shown to limit these harmful complications. The *angiotensin II receptor blockers* appear to have similar but more limited beneficial effects. They have the advantage of not causing a cough, which is a troublesome side effect of the ACE inhibitors for many persons. Aldosterone has a number of deleterious effects in individuals with heart failure. *Aldosterone receptor antagonists* may be used in combination with other agents for persons with moderately severe to severe heart failure.

β*-Adrenergic receptor blocking drugs* are used to decrease left ventricular dysfunction associated with activation of the sympathetic nervous system. Large clinical trials have shown that long-term therapy with β-adrenergic receptor blocking agents reduces morbidity and mortality in persons with chronic heart failure. The mechanism of this benefit remains unclear, but it is likely that chronic elevations of catecholamines and sympathetic nervous system activity cause progressive myocardial damage, leading to a worsening of left ventricular function and a poorer prognosis in persons with heart failure. Large, landmark clinical trials of persons with stable NYHA class II and III heart failure have demonstrated significant reductions in the overall mortality rate with treatment with various β-adrenergic receptor blocking agents.[36,37]

Diuretics are frequently prescribed medications for moderate to severe heart failure.[1,2] They promote the excretion of fluid and help to sustain cardiac output and tissue perfusion by reducing preload and allowing the heart to operate at a more optimal part of the Frank–Starling curve. Aldosterone antagonists (spironolactone) and loop diuretics are used. In emergencies, such as acute pulmonary edema, loop diuretics such as furosemide can be administered intravenously. When given intravenously, these medications act quickly to reduce venous return through vasodilation so that right ventricular output and pulmonary vascular pressures are decreased. This response to intravenous medication administration is extrarenal and precedes the onset of diuresis.

Digitalis has been a recognized treatment for heart failure for over 200 years. The various forms of digitalis are called *cardiac glycosides*. The role of digitalis in the treatment of heart failure has been studied in clinical trials over the past several decades and remains somewhat controversial. Digitalis and related cardiac glycosides are inotropic agents that exert their effects by inhibiting the Na^+/K^+-ATPase pump, which increases intracellular Na^+; this in turn leads to an increase in intracellular Ca^{2+} through the Na^+/Ca^{2+} exchange pump. Therefore they act to improve cardiac function and stroke volume by increasing intracellular calcium and ventricular contractility. They are not recommended for individuals with adequate left ventricular ejection fraction.[2,38] Cardiac glycosides also decrease sinoatrial node activity and decrease conduction through the atrioventricular node; thus, they slow the heart rate (negative chronotropy) and increase diastolic filling time. For this reason glycosides may be used to control tachycardia, including rapid atrial fibrillation. However, the beneficial effect is minimal with activity, and β-adrenergic blockers have demonstrated greater effectiveness.[2,38]

Vasodilator drugs are included as recommended agents by the CCS Heart Failure Guidelines in combination therapy for heart failure.[2] Agents such as isosorbide dinitrate or hydralazine may be added to improve cardiac function.[2] Vasodilators such as nitroglycerin and nitroprusside are used in AHFS to improve left heart performance by decreasing the preload (through vasodilation) or reducing the afterload (through arteriolar dilation), or both.[2]

Oxygen Therapy. Oxygen therapy increases the oxygen content of the blood and is most often used in patients with acute episodes of heart failure. Either bilevel positive airway pressure (BiPAP) or continuous positive airway pressure (CPAP) are recommended to reduce the need for endotracheal intubation in patients with AHFS.[39] Because CPAP increases intrathoracic pressure, it also has the potential for decreasing venous return and left ventricular preload, thereby improving the cardiac ejection fraction and stabilizing the hemodynamic status in persons with severe heart failure.[40] BiPAP is similar to CPAP but delivers higher pressures during inspiration. It has been demonstrated to be of greater benefit than CPAP in that it decreases both pulmonary edema and respiratory work, thereby decreasing respiratory rate and heart rate and improving oxygenation more quickly or more substantially than CPAP.[2,40]

Cardiac Resynchronization and Implantable Cardioverter–Defibrillators. Some patients with heart failure have abnormal intraventricular conduction that results in dyssynchronous and ineffective contractions.[26] Cardiac resynchronization therapy (also called biventricular pacing) involves the placement of pacing leads into the right atrium and/or right ventricle with a separate lead wire positioned on the surface of the left ventricle via the coronary sinus vein. The leads are then able to coordinate or synchronize the ventricular contractions maximizing stroke volume. Cardiac resynchronization has been shown to improve ventricular function and blood pressure, increase the quality of life, and reduce the risk of death.[41]

Individuals with heart failure are at significant risk of sudden cardiac death from ventricular fibrillation or ventricular tachycardia. Implantation of a cardioverter–defibrillator is indicated in selected patients with heart failure to prevent sudden cardiac death.[2,41] A cardioverter–defibrillator is a programmable implanted device that monitors the cardiac rhythm. It has the capacity to pace the heart and deliver electrical energy to terminate lethal arrhythmias.

Mechanical Support and Heart Transplantation. Refractory heart failure reflects deterioration in cardiac function that is unresponsive to medical or surgical interventions. With improved methods of treatment, more people are reaching a point where a cure is unachievable and death is imminent without mechanical support or heart transplantation.

Since the early 1960s, significant progress has been made in improving the efficacy of *ventricular assist devices* (VADs), which are mechanical pumps used to support ventricular function. VADs are used to decrease the workload of the myocardium while maintaining cardiac output and systemic arterial pressure. This decreases the workload on the ventricle and allows it to rest and recover. Most VADs require an invasive open chest procedure for implantation. They may be used in patients who fail or have difficulty being weaned from cardiopulmonary bypass after cardiac surgery; those who develop cardiogenic shock after myocardial infarction; those with end-stage cardiomyopathy; and those who are awaiting cardiac transplantation. Earlier and more aggressive use of VADs as a bridge to transplantation and destination therapy (permanent support) has been shown to increase survival.[42] VADs that allow the patient to be mobile and managed at home are sometimes used for long-term or permanent support for treatment of end-stage heart failure, rather than simply as a bridge to transplantation. VADs can be used to support the function of the left ventricle, right ventricle, or both.[42]

Heart transplantation is the preferred treatment for patients with end-stage cardiac failure and otherwise good life expectancy.[2,44] In 2013, there were 2,611 Canadians living with a heart transplant. Survival rates for persons with heart transplants has increased significantly over the years, with a current rate of almost 90% at 8 years post transplant.[34,43] However, the number of heart transplants has remained relatively unchanged since 1995.[34,43] Despite the overall success of heart transplantation, donor availability remains a key problem, and many heart transplantation candidates are denied transplantation each year.

Other novel surgical therapies that are being explored include left ventricular remodelling and isolated cell transplantation or gene therapy.[44,45] Left ventricular remodelling is a surgical procedure designed to restore the size and shape of the ventricle, and is thought to be a viable surgical alternative to cardiac transplantation for persons with severe left ventricular dysfunction.[46]

IN SUMMARY

Heart failure occurs when the heart fails to pump sufficient blood to meet the metabolic needs of body tissues. The physiology of heart failure reflects the interplay between a decrease in cardiac output that accompanies impaired function of the failing heart and the compensatory mechanisms that preserve the cardiac reserve. Compensatory mechanisms include the Frank–Starling mechanism, sympathetic nervous system activation, the renin–angiotensin–aldosterone mechanism, NPs, the endothelins, and myocardial hypertrophy and remodelling. In the failing heart, early decreases in cardiac function may go unnoticed because these compensatory mechanisms maintain the cardiac output. Unfortunately, the mechanisms were not intended for long-term use, and in severe and prolonged heart failure the compensatory mechanisms no longer are effective, and instead contribute to the progression of heart failure.

Heart failure may be described in terms of systolic versus diastolic dysfunction and right ventricular versus left

ventricular dysfunction. With systolic dysfunction, there is impaired ejection of blood from the heart during systole; with diastolic dysfunction, there is impaired filling of the heart during diastole. Right ventricular dysfunction is characterized by congestion in the peripheral circulation, and left ventricular dysfunction by congestion in the pulmonary circulation. Heart failure can present as a chronic condition characterized by decreased cardiac function or as an AHFS. The AHFSs represent a gradual or rapid change in heart failure signs and symptoms, indicating need for urgent therapy. These symptoms are primarily the result of pulmonary congestion due to elevated left ventricular filling pressures with or without a low cardiac output.

The manifestations of heart failure include edema, nocturia, fatigue and impaired exercise tolerance, cyanosis, signs of increased sympathetic nervous system activity, and impaired gastrointestinal function and malnutrition. In right-sided failure, there is dependent edema of the lower parts of the body, engorgement of the liver, and ascites. In left-sided failure, pulmonary congestion with shortness of breath and chronic, nonproductive cough are common.

The diagnostic methods in heart failure are directed toward establishing the cause and extent of the disorder. Treatment is directed toward correcting the cause whenever possible, improving cardiac function, maintaining the fluid volume within a compensatory range, and developing an activity pattern consistent with individual limitations in cardiac reserve. Among the medications used in the treatment of heart failure are ACE inhibitors and angiotensin receptor blocking agents, β-adrenergic receptor blockers, diuretics, digoxin, and vasodilators. Mechanical support devices, including the VAD, sustain life in persons with severe heart failure. Heart transplantation remains the treatment of choice for many persons with end-stage heart failure.

CONCEPTS in action **ANIMATION**

CIRCULATORY FAILURE (SHOCK)

After completing this section of the chapter, you should be able to meet the following objectives:

- State a clinical definition of shock.
- Compare the causes, pathophysiology, and chief characteristics of cardiogenic, hypovolemic, obstructive, and distributive shock.
- Describe the complications of shock as they relate to the lungs, kidneys, gastrointestinal tract, and blood clotting.
- State the rationale for treatment measures to correct and reverse shock.
- Define multiple organ dysfunction syndrome and cite its significance in shock.

> **CHART 26.2** **CLASSIFICATION OF CIRCULATORY SHOCK**
>
> **Cardiogenic**
> Myocardial damage (myocardial infarction, contusion)
> Sustained arrhythmias
> Acute valve damage, ventricular septal defect
> Cardiac surgery
>
> **Hypovolemic**
> Loss of whole blood
> Loss of plasma
> Loss of extracellular fluid
>
> **Obstructive**
> Inability of the heart to fill properly (cardiac tamponade)
> Obstruction to outflow from the heart (pulmonary embolus, cardiac myxoma, pneumothorax, or dissecting aneurysm)
>
> **Distributive**
> Loss of sympathetic vasomotor tone (neurogenic shock)
> Presence of vasodilating substances in the blood (anaphylactic shock)
> Presence of inflammatory mediators (septic shock)

The function of the cardiovascular system is to perfuse body tissues and supply them with oxygen and nutrients, and remove waste products. Adequate perfusion of body tissues depends on the pumping ability of the heart, a vascular system that transports blood to the cells and back to the heart, and sufficient blood to fill the vascular system. As well, cells and tissues must be able to use and extract oxygen and nutrients from the blood.

Circulatory shock can be described as an acute failure of the circulatory system to supply the tissues and organs of the body with an adequate blood supply, resulting in cellular hypoxia.[5,47] Most often hypotension and hypoperfusion are present, but shock may occur in the presence of normal vital signs. Shock is not a specific disease but a syndrome that can occur in the course of many life-threatening traumatic conditions or disease states. It is often categorized by the predominant cause, including a decrease in blood volume (hypovolemic shock), an alteration in cardiac function (cardiogenic shock), an alteration of blood flow and maldistribution of blood due to increased and inappropriate vasodilation (distributive shock), or obstruction of blood flow through the circulatory system (obstructive shock).[47] The main types of shock are summarized in Chart 26.2 and depicted in Figure 26.8.

Pathophysiology of Circulatory Shock

Circulatory failure results in hypoperfusion of organs and tissues, which in turn results in insufficient supply of oxygen and nutrients for cellular function. There are initial compensatory physiologic responses that eventually decompensate into various shock states if the condition is not properly treated in a timely manner. The most immediate of the compensatory mechanisms are the sympathetic and renin systems, which are designed to maintain cardiac output and blood pressure.

There are two types of adrenergic receptors for the sympathetic nervous system: α and β. The α and β receptors are both further subdivided into α_1, α_2, β_1, and β_2 receptors. Overall, stimulation of the α_1 receptors causes vasoconstriction; stimulation of β_1 receptors, an increase in heart rate and force of myocardial contraction; and stimulation of β_2 receptors, vasodilation of the peripheral arteries and skeletal muscle beds and relaxation of the bronchioles. In shock, there is an increase in sympathetic outflow that results in increased epinephrine and norepinephrine release, and activation of both α and β receptors. Thus, increases in heart rate and vasoconstriction occur in most types of shock, although these compensatory mechanisms are impaired in distributive shock states. There is an increase in renin release, leading to an increase in angiotensin II, which augments vasoconstriction and leads to an aldosterone-mediated increase in sodium and water retention by the kidneys. In addition, there is local release of vasoconstrictors, including norepinephrine, angiotensin II, vasopressin, and endothelin, which contribute to arterial vasoconstriction, primarily in the peripheral circulation.

> **CIRCULATORY SHOCK**
>
> - Circulatory shock represents the inability of the circulation to adequately perfuse the tissues of the body.
> - It can result from failure of the heart as a pump, a loss of fluid from the vascular compartment (hypovolemic shock), obstruction of flow through the vascular compartment (obstructive shock), or an increase in the size of the vascular compartment that interferes with the distribution of blood (distributive shock).
> - The manifestations of shock reflect both the impaired perfusion of body tissues and the body's attempt to maintain tissue perfusion through conservation of water by the kidney, translocation of fluid from extracellular to the intravascular compartment, and activation of sympathetic nervous system mechanisms that increase heart rate and divert blood from the periphery to more essential body tissues and organs.

The compensatory mechanisms that the body recruits are not effective over the long term and become detrimental when the shock state is prolonged. The intense vasoconstriction causes a decrease in tissue perfusion and insufficient supply of oxygen. Cellular metabolism is impaired, vasoactive inflammatory mediators are released, production of oxygen free radicals is increased, and excessive lactic acid and hydrogen result in intracellular acidity.[5] Each of these factors promotes cellular dysfunction or death. If circulatory function is

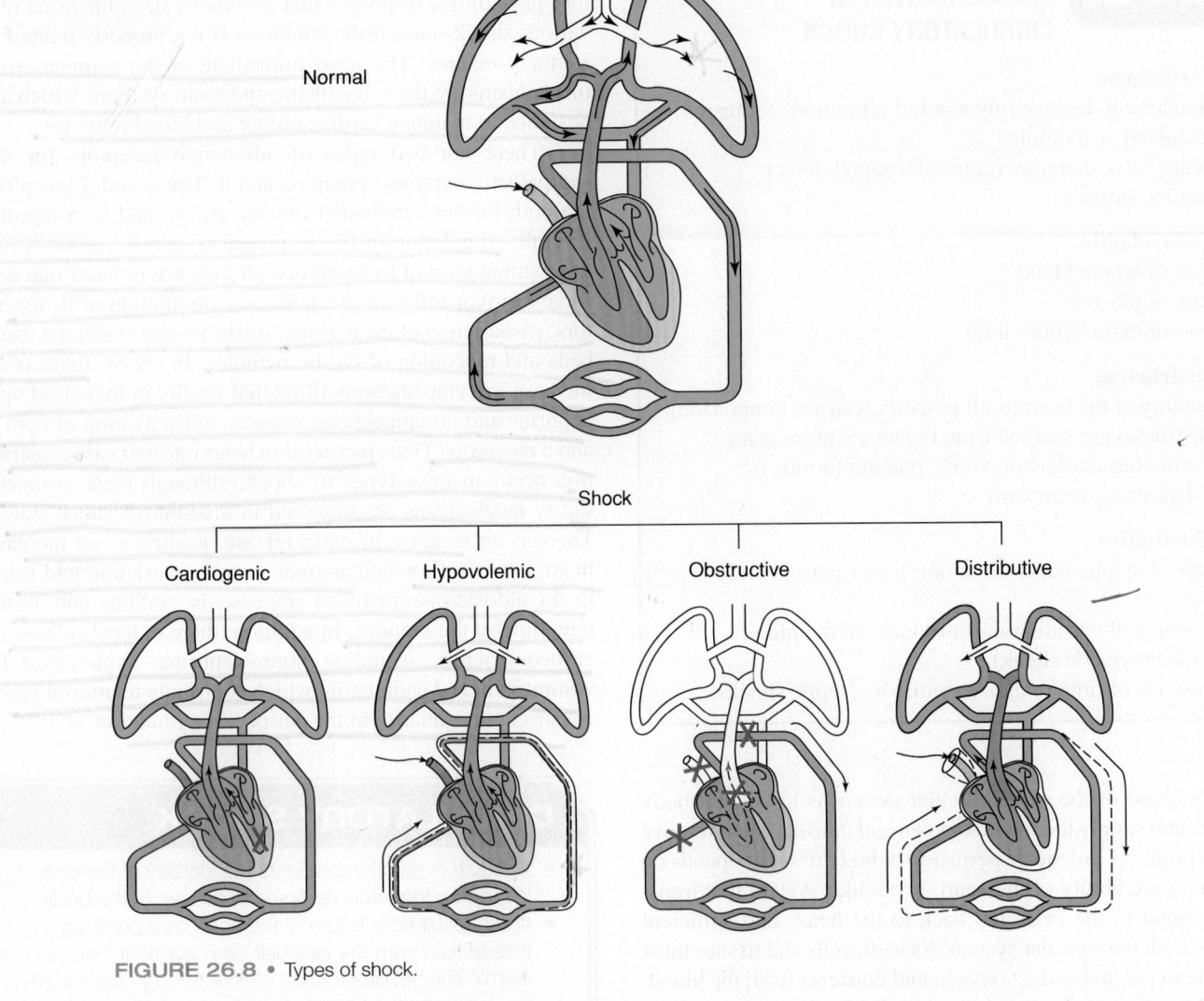

Normal

Shock

Cardiogenic   Hypovolemic   Obstructive   Distributive

FIGURE 26.8 • Types of shock.

reestablished, whether the shock is irreversible or the patient will survive is determined largely at the cellular level.

Shock ultimately exerts its effect at the cellular level, with failure of the circulation to supply cells, tissues, and organs with the oxygen and nutrients needed for production of ATP. The cell uses ATP for a number of purposes, including operation of the sodium–potassium membrane pump that moves sodium out of the cell and potassium back into the cell. The cell uses two pathways to convert nutrients to energy (see Chapter 4). The first is the anaerobic (nonoxygen-dependent) glycolytic pathway, which is located in the cytoplasm. Glycolysis converts glucose to ATP and pyruvate. The second pathway is the aerobic (oxygen-dependent) pathway, called the *citric acid cycle,* which is located in the mitochondria. When oxygen is available, pyruvate from the glycolytic pathway moves into the mitochondria and enters the citric acid cycle, where it is transformed into ATP and the metabolic byproducts carbon dioxide and water. When oxygen is lacking, pyruvate does not enter the citric acid cycle; instead, it is converted to lactic acid. The anaerobic pathway, although allowing energy

production to continue in the absence of oxygen, is relatively inefficient and produces significantly less ATP than the aerobic pathway.

In severe shock, cellular metabolic processes are essentially anaerobic owing to the decreased availability of oxygen. Excess amounts of lactic acid accumulate in the cellular and the extracellular compartments, and limited amounts of ATP are produced. Without sufficient energy production, normal cell function cannot be maintained. The sodium–potassium membrane pump is impaired, resulting in excess sodium inside the cells and potassium loss from cells. The increase in intracellular sodium results in cellular edema and increased cell membrane permeability. Mitochondrial activity becomes severely depressed and lysosomal membranes may rupture, resulting in the release of enzymes that cause further intracellular destruction. This is followed by cell death and the release of intracellular contents into the extracellular space. The destruction of the cell membrane activates the arachidonic acid cascade, release of inflammatory mediators, and production of oxygen free radicals that extend cellular damage.

The extent of the microvascular injury and organ dysfunction is primarily determined by the extent of the shock state and whether it is prolonged. Interventions are targeted at both prevention and early intervention, when possible.

Cardiogenic Shock

Cardiogenic shock occurs when the heart fails to pump blood sufficiently to meet the body demands (Fig. 26.8). It is defined as decreased cardiac output and cardiac index, hypotension with a systolic blood pressure of less than 90 mm Hg, and hypoperfusion to the tissues and organs, with indications of tissue hypoxia despite adequate intravascular volume.[48,49] Cardiogenic shock may occur suddenly from a number of causes, including myocardial infarction, myocardial contusion, sustained arrhythmias, and cardiac surgery. Cardiogenic shock also may ensue as an end-stage condition of coronary artery disease or cardiomyopathy.

Pathophysiology

The most common cause of cardiogenic shock is myocardial infarction, particularly ST segment elevation MI (STEMI). Most patients who die of cardiogenic shock have had extensive damage to the contracting muscle of the left ventricle because of a recent infarct or a combination of recent and old infarctions.[49] Cardiogenic shock can occur with other types of shock because of inadequate coronary blood flow, or it can develop because substances released from ischemic tissues impair cardiac function. One unidentified substance, called *myocardial depressant factor,* is thought to be released into the circulation during septic shock.[50] There are conflicting data on the identity of myocardial depressant factor; however, inflammatory mediators such as TNFα have been suggested as possible agents.[50] It has been hypothesized that the myocardial depressant factor produces severe but potentially reversible myocardial depression, ventricular dilation, and decreased left ventricular ejection fraction and diastolic pressure.[51]

Regardless of cause, persons with cardiogenic shock have a decrease in stroke volume and cardiac output, which results in insufficient perfusion to meet cellular demands for oxygen. The poor cardiac output is due to decreased myocardial contractility, increased afterload, and excessive preload. Mediators and neurotransmitters, including norepinephrine, produce an increase in systemic vascular resistance, which increases afterload and contributes to the deterioration of cardiac function. Preload, or the filling pressure of the heart, is increased as blood returning to the heart is added to blood that previously was not pumped forward, resulting in an excessive increase in left ventricular end-systolic volume. Activation of the renin–angiotensin–aldosterone system worsens both preload and afterload by producing an aldosterone-mediated increase in fluid retention and an angiotensin-II-mediated increase in vasoconstriction. The increased resistance (*i.e.,* afterload) to ejection of blood from the left ventricle, in combination with a decrease in myocardial contractility, results in an increase in end-systolic ventricular volume and preload, which further impairs the heart's ability to pump effectively.

There is an increase in intracardiac pressures due to volume overload and ventricular wall tension in both diastole and systole. Eventually, coronary artery perfusion is impaired because of the increased preload and afterload, and cardiac function decreases because of poor myocardial oxygen supply. Excessive pressures decrease coronary artery perfusion during diastole, and increased wall tension decreases coronary artery perfusion during systole. In addition to vasoconstriction resulting in organ dysfunction, alterations to the microcirculation occur that might not be as readily evident clinically. If treatment is unsuccessful, cardiogenic shock may result in a systemic inflammatory response syndrome (SIRS) (discussed in the section on Sepsis and Septic Shock), evidenced by increased white blood cell count, increased temperature, and release of inflammatory cytokines and neurohormonal mediators.[52]

Clinical Features

Manifestations. Signs and symptoms of cardiogenic shock include indications of hypoperfusion with hypotension, although a preshock state of hypoperfusion may occur with a normal blood pressure. The lips, nail beds, and skin may become cyanotic because of stagnation of blood flow and increased extraction of oxygen from the hemoglobin as it passes through the capillary bed. Mean arterial and systolic blood pressures decrease due to poor stroke volume, and there is a narrow pulse pressure and near-normal diastolic blood pressure because of arterial vasoconstriction.[49,51,52] Urine output decreases because of lower renal perfusion pressures and the increased release of aldosterone. Elevated preload is reflected in a rise in CVP and PWP. Neurologic changes, such as alterations in cognition or consciousness, may occur because of low cardiac output and poor cerebral perfusion.

Treatment. Treatment of cardiogenic shock requires striking a precarious balance between improving cardiac output, reducing the workload and oxygen needs of the myocardium, and increasing coronary perfusion. Fluid volume must be regulated within a level that optimizes filling pressure and stroke volume. Pulmonary edema and arrhythmias should be corrected or prevented to increase stroke volume and decrease the oxygen demands of the heart. Coronary artery perfusion is increased by promoting coronary artery vasodilation, increasing blood pressure, decreasing ventricular wall tension, and decreasing intracardiac pressures.

Pharmacologic treatment includes the use of vasodilators such as nitroprusside and nitroglycerin, unless hypotension is present. Both nitroprusside and nitroglycerin cause coronary artery dilation, which increases myocardial oxygen delivery. Nitroprusside causes arterial and venous dilation, producing a decrease in venous return to the heart and a reduction in arterial resistance against which the left heart must pump.[55] At lower doses, the main effects of nitroglycerin are on the venous vascular beds and coronary arteries; at high doses, it also dilates the arterial beds. Both medications may decrease diastolic arterial pressure, resulting in a lower systemic vascular resistance (afterload). The systolic arterial pressure is

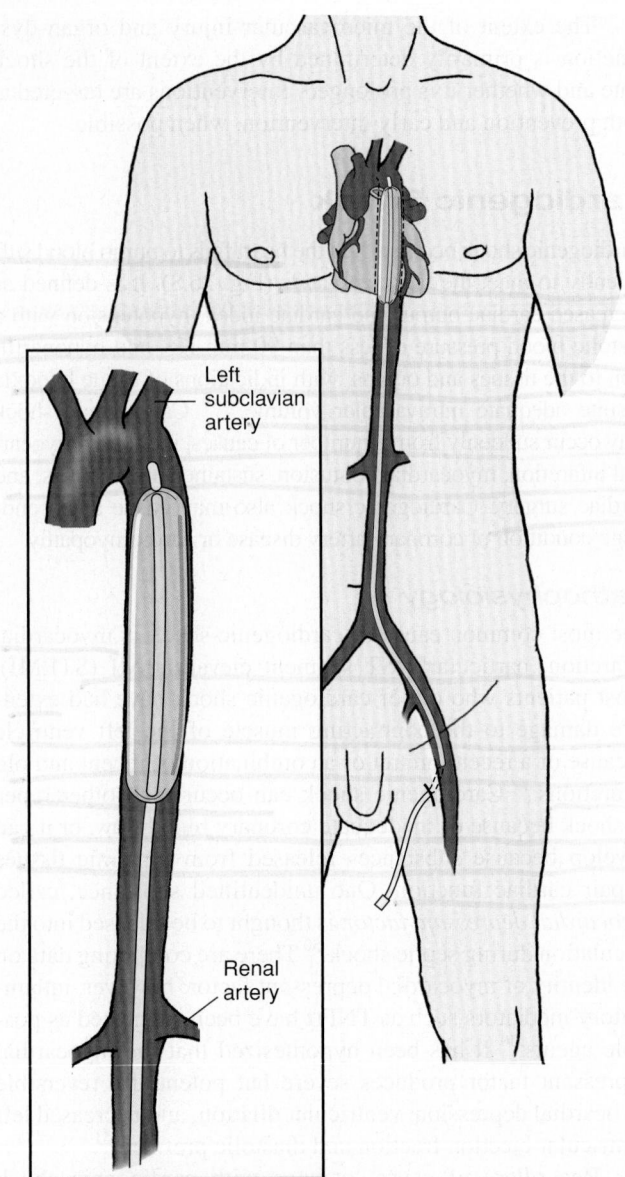

maintained by an increase in ventricular stroke volume, which is ejected against the lowered systemic vascular resistance. The improvement in heart function increases stroke volume and enables blood to be redistributed from the pulmonary vascular bed to the systemic circulation.

Positive inotropic agents are used cautiously to improve cardiac contractility. Both dobutamine and milrinone are effective medications in that they result in increased contractility and arterial vasodilation, which decreases afterload. Dobutamine is predominantly a β-adrenergic agonist which has greater inotropic than chronotropic effects. The combination tends to produce vasodilation and a positive inotropic action. Milrinone increases myocardial contractility by increasing the movement of Ca^{2+} into myocardial cells during an action potential (Fig. 26.1), and decreases Ca^{2+} in arterial vascular cells, resulting in increased contractility, decreased afterload, and increased stroke volume. The increase in stroke volume results in a decrease in end-systolic volume and a reduction in preload. With a decrease in preload pressures, coronary artery perfusion is improved during diastole. Thus, stroke volume and myocardial oxygen supply are improved with a minimal increase in myocardial oxygen demand. Catecholamines, such as epinephrine and dopamine, are also positive inotropes but must be used with extreme caution because they also result in arterial constriction and increased heart rates, which worsens the imbalance between myocardial oxygen supply and demand.

Mechanical circulatory support devices may assist in cardiac function and decrease workload.[50] The intra-aortic balloon pump, also referred to as *intra-aortic counterpulsation,* enhances coronary and systemic perfusion, yet decreases afterload and myocardial oxygen demands.[52,53] The device, which pumps in synchrony with the heart, consists of a balloon, approximately 26 cm long for an adult, that is inserted through a catheter into the descending aorta (Fig. 26.9). The balloon is timed to inflate during ventricular diastole and deflate just before ventricular systole. Diastolic inflation creates a pressure wave in the ascending aorta that increases coronary artery blood flow and a less intense wave in the lower aorta that enhances organ perfusion. The abrupt balloon deflation at the onset of systole results in a displacement of blood volume that lowers the resistance to ejection of blood from the left ventricle. Thus, the heart's pumping efficiency is increased, myocardial oxygen supply is increased, and myocardial oxygen consumption is decreased.

For end-stage renal failure a right or left VAD (R/LVAD) may be considered to reduce preload and support cardiac output.[50] The LVAD is most often inserted percutaneously in an acute event but can also be implanted. A pacemaker may be considered to maintain atrioventricular synchrony.[50]

When cardiogenic shock is caused by myocardial infarction, several aggressive interventions can be used successfully. Reperfusion of the coronary arteries improves myocardial function. Fibrinolytic therapy, percutaneous coronary intervention, or bypass surgery (see Chapter 24) may be used to prevent or treat cardiogenic shock.[54]

FIGURE 26.9 • Aortic balloon pump. Proper position of the intra-aortic balloon catheter illustrating percutaneous insertion. (From Morton P. G., Fontaine D. K. (2009). *Critical care nursing: A holistic approach* (9th ed., p. 369). Philadelphia, PA: J.B. Lippincott.)

Hypovolemic Shock

Hypovolemic shock is characterized by a significant decrease in blood or plasma volume such that there is inadequate filling of the vascular compartment and decreased cardiac output[5,55,56] (Fig. 26.8). Historically, hypovolemic shock has been well described, particularly in the context of trauma. It occurs when there is an acute loss of 20% or more of the circulating blood volume. The decrease may be caused by an external loss of whole blood (*e.g.,* hemorrhage), plasma (*e.g.,* severe burns), or extracellular fluid (*e.g.,* severe dehydration or loss of gastrointestinal fluids with vomiting or diarrhea). Hypovolemic shock also can result from an internal hemorrhage or from third-space losses, when extracellular fluid is

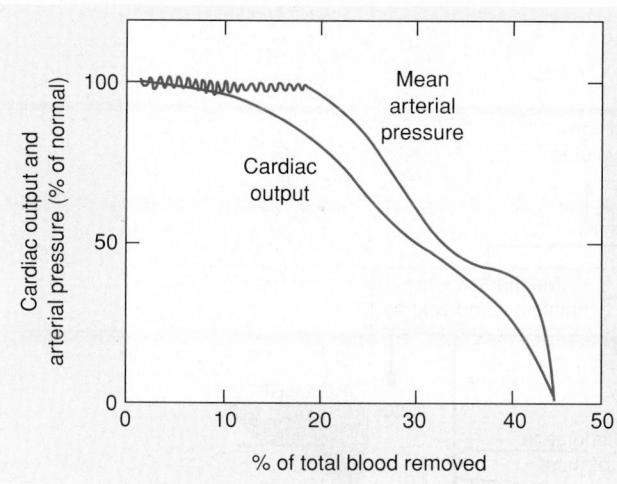

FIGURE 26.10 • Effect of hemorrhage on cardiac output and arterial pressure. (From Hall J. E. (2011). *Textbook of medical physiology* (12th ed., p. 274). Philadelphia, PA: W. B. Saunders.)

shifted from the vascular compartment to the interstitial space or compartment.

Pathophysiology

Hypovolemic shock, which has been the most widely studied type of shock, is often used as a prototype in discussions of the manifestations of shock. Figure 26.10 shows the effect of removing blood from the circulatory system over the course of approximately 30 minutes.[5] Approximately 10% of the total blood volume can be removed without changing cardiac output or arterial pressure. The average blood donor loses approximately 500 ml or 10% of their blood without experiencing adverse effects. As increasing amounts of blood (10% to 25%) are removed, the stroke volume falls but arterial pressure is maintained because of sympathetic-mediated increases in heart rate and vasoconstriction. Vasoconstriction results in an increased diastolic pressure and narrow pulse pressure. Blood pressure is the product of cardiac output and systemic vascular resistance (blood pressure = cardiac output × systemic vascular resistance). An increase in systemic vascular resistance maintains mean arterial pressure for a short time despite decreased cardiac output. Cardiac output and tissue perfusion decrease before signs of hypotension appear. Cardiac output and arterial pressure fall to zero when approximately 35% to 45% of the total blood volume has been removed.[5]

Compensatory Mechanisms. Without compensatory mechanisms to maintain cardiac output and blood pressure, the loss of vascular volume would result in a rapid progression from the initial to the progressive and irreversible stages of shock. The most immediate of the compensatory mechanisms are the sympathetic-mediated responses designed to maintain cardiac output and blood pressure (Fig. 26.11). Within seconds after the onset of hemorrhage or the loss of blood volume, tachycardia, increased cardiac contractility, vasoconstriction,

and other signs of sympathetic and adrenal medullary activity appear. The sympathetic vasoconstrictor response also mobilizes blood that has been stored in the venous side of the circulation as a means of increasing venous return to the heart. There is considerable capacity for blood storage in the large veins of the abdomen, and approximately 350 ml of blood that can be mobilized in shock is stored in the liver.[5] Sympathetic stimulation does not initially cause constriction of the cerebral and coronary vessels, and blood flow to the heart and brain is maintained at essentially normal levels as long as the mean arterial pressure remains above 70 mm Hg.[5]

Compensatory mechanisms designed to restore blood volume include absorption of fluid from the interstitial spaces, conservation of sodium and water by the kidneys, and thirst. Extracellular fluid is distributed between the interstitial spaces and the vascular compartment. When there is a loss of vascular volume, capillary pressures decrease and water is drawn into the vascular compartment from the interstitial spaces. The maintenance of vascular volume is further enhanced by renal mechanisms that conserve fluid. A decrease in renal blood flow and glomerular filtration rate results in activation of the renin–angiotensin–aldosterone system, which produces an increase in sodium reabsorption by the kidneys. The decrease in blood volume also stimulates centres in the hypothalamus that regulate ADH release and thirst. ADH, also known as *vasopressin,* greatly increases water retention by the kidneys and constricts the peripheral arteries and veins. Although the mechanism of ADH is more sensitive to changes in serum osmolality, a decrease of 10% to 15% in blood volume serves as a strong stimulus for thirst.[5] Due to the subtle signs and symptoms, combined with activation of the compensatory mechanisms, low volume accompanied by hypoperfusion may not be readily evident, leading to an increase in mortality.[55]

During the early stages of hypovolemic shock, vasoconstriction decreases the size of the vascular compartment and increases systemic vascular resistance. This response usually is all that is needed when the injury is slight and blood loss is minimal. As hypovolemic shock progresses, vasoconstriction of the blood vessels that supply the skin, skeletal muscles, kidneys, and abdominal organs becomes more severe, with a further decrease in blood flow and conversion to anaerobic metabolism, resulting in cellular injury.

Clinical Features

The signs and symptoms of hypovolemic shock depend on its severity and are closely related to low peripheral blood flow and excessive sympathetic stimulation. They include thirst, increased heart rate, cool and clammy skin, decreased arterial blood pressure, decreased urine output, and changes in mentation. Laboratory tests of hemoglobin and hematocrit provide information regarding the severity of blood loss or hemoconcentration due to dehydration. Serum lactate and arterial pH provide information about the severity of acidosis due to anaerobic metabolism. Metabolic acidosis revealed by arterial blood gas measurement is the gold standard diagnostic test.[56] Acute, fatal hemorrhagic shock is characterized by metabolic

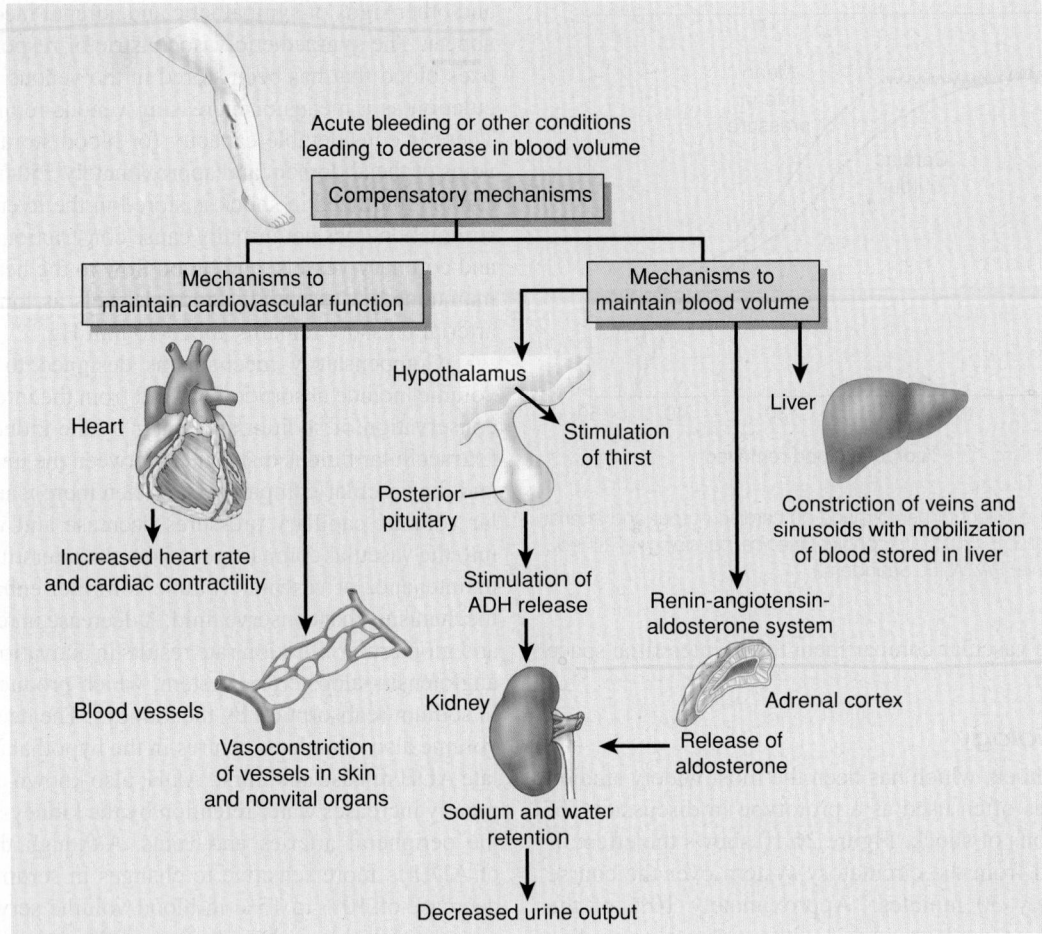

Acute bleeding or other conditions
leading to decrease in blood volume

Compensatory mechanisms

Mechanisms to
maintain cardiovascular function

Mechanisms to
maintain blood volume

Heart

Hypothalamus

Stimulation
of thirst

Liver

Posterior
pituitary

Constriction of veins and
sinusoids with mobilization
of blood stored in liver

Increased heart rate
and cardiac contractility

Stimulation of
ADH release

Renin-angiotensin-
aldosterone system

Blood vessels

Kidney

Adrenal cortex

Vasoconstriction
of vessels in skin
and nonvital organs

Release of
aldosterone

Sodium and water
retention

Decreased urine output

FIGURE 26.11 • Compensatory mechanisms used to maintain circulatory function and blood volume in hypovolemic shock. ADH, antidiuretic hormone.

acidosis, coagulopathy, and hypothermia, followed by circulatory failure.[56]

An increase in heart rate is an early sign of hypovolemic shock, as the body tries to maintain cardiac output despite the decrease in stroke volume. As shock progresses, the pulse becomes weak and thready, indicating vasoconstriction and reduced filling of the vascular compartment. Thirst is an early symptom in hypovolemic shock. Although the underlying cause is not fully understood, it probably is related to decreased blood volume and increased serum osmolality (see Chapter 31).

Arterial blood pressure is decreased in moderate to severe shock, with a near-normal diastolic and narrow pulse pressure due to vasoconstriction. However, controversy exists over the value of blood pressure measurements in the early diagnosis and management of shock. This is because compensatory mechanisms tend to preserve blood pressure until shock is relatively far advanced. Furthermore, a normal arterial pressure does not ensure adequate perfusion and oxygenation of vital organs at the cellular level. This does not imply that blood pressure should not be closely monitored in patients at risk for development of shock, but it does indicate the need for other assessment measures.

As shock progresses, the respirations become rapid and deep, to compensate for the increased production of acid and decreased availability of oxygen. Decreased intravascular volume results in decreased venous return to the heart and a decreased CVP. When shock becomes severe, the peripheral veins may collapse. Sympathetic stimulation leads to intense vasoconstriction of the skin vessels, which results in cool and mottled skin. In hemorrhagic shock, the loss of red blood cells results in pallor of the skin and mucous membranes.

Urine output decreases very quickly in hypovolemic shock due to decreased renal blood flow and increased renin release. Oliguria of 20 ml/hour or less with sufficient fluid replacement indicates inadequate renal perfusion. Continuous measurement of urine output is essential for assessing the circulatory and volume status of the person in shock.

Restlessness, agitation, and apprehension are common in early shock because of increased sympathetic outflow and increased levels of epinephrine. As the shock progresses and blood flow to the brain decreases, restlessness is replaced by altered arousal and mentation. Loss of consciousness may occur if the person does not receive or respond to treatment.

Treatment. The treatment of hypovolemic shock is directed toward correcting or controlling the underlying cause and restoring organ and tissue perfusion. Ongoing loss of blood, such as occurs in surgery or trauma, must be corrected. Oxygen is administered to increase oxygen delivery to the tissues. Medications usually are administered intravenously. Frequent measurements of heart rate and cardiac rhythm, blood pressure, and urine output are used to assess the severity of circulatory compromise and to monitor treatment.

In hypovolemic shock, the goal of treatment is to restore vascular volume.[55,56] This can be accomplished through intravenous administration of fluids and blood. The crystalloids (*e.g.,* isotonic saline and Ringer's lactate) are readily available and effective, at least temporarily. Plasma volume expanders (*e.g.,* hydroxyethyl starch and colloidal albumin) have a high molecular weight, do not necessitate blood typing, and remain in the vascular space for longer periods than crystalloids such as dextrose and saline. Blood or blood products (packed or frozen red cells) are administered based on hematocrit and hemodynamic findings. Fluids are best administered based on volume indicators such as CVP and urine output.

Vasoactive medications are agents capable of constricting or dilating blood vessels. Considerable controversy exists about the advantages or disadvantages related to the use of these drugs. As a general rule, vasoconstrictor agents are not used as a primary form of therapy in hypovolemic shock, and may be detrimental. These agents are given only when volume deficits have been corrected yet hypotension persists.

Distributive Shock

Distributive or vasodilatory shock is characterized by loss of blood vessel tone, enlargement of the vascular compartment, and displacement of the vascular volume away from the heart and central circulation.[57] In distributive shock, the capacity of the vascular compartment expands to the extent that a normal volume of blood does not fill the circulatory system (Fig. 26.8). Therefore, this type of shock is also referred to as *normovolemic shock.* Two main causes result in the loss of vascular tone: a decrease in the sympathetic control of vasomotor tone or the release of excessive vasodilator substances. It can also occur as a complication of vessel damage resulting from prolonged and severe hypotension due to hemorrhage, known as *irreversible* or *late-phase hemorrhagic shock.*[57] There are three shock states that share the basic circulatory pattern of distributive shock: neurogenic shock, anaphylactic shock, and septic shock.

Neurogenic Shock

Neurogenic shock is caused by decreased sympathetic control of blood vessel tone due to a defect in the vasomotor centre in the brain stem or the sympathetic outflow to the blood vessels.[5] The term *spinal shock* describes the neurogenic shock that occurs in persons with spinal cord injury (see Chapter 50). Output from the vasomotor centre can be interrupted by brain injury, the depressant action of drugs, general anesthesia, hypoxia, or lack of glucose (*e.g.,* insulin reaction). Fainting due to emotional causes is a transient form of impaired sy[...] outflow. Many general anesthetic agents can cause a neuro[...] shock-like reaction, especially during induction, because [...] interference with sympathetic nervous system function. Spinal anesthesia or spinal cord injury above the midthoracic region can interrupt the transmission of outflow from the vasomotor centre. In contrast to other shock states due to the loss of blood volume or impaired cardiac function, the heart rate in neurogenic shock is slower than normal, and the skin often dry and warm as the sympathetic response is impaired. This type of distributive shock is rare and usually transitory.

Anaphylactic Shock

Anaphylaxis is a clinical syndrome that represents the most severe systemic allergic reaction.[58–60] Most commonly it is mediated by IgE.[60] Anaphylactic shock results from an immunologically mediated reaction in which vasodilator substances such as histamine are released into the blood (see Chapter 19). These substances cause vasodilation of arterioles and venules along with a marked increase in capillary permeability. The vascular response in anaphylaxis is often accompanied by life-threatening laryngeal edema and bronchospasm, circulatory collapse, contraction of gastrointestinal and uterine smooth muscle, and urticaria (hives) or angioedema.

Among the most frequent causes of anaphylactic shock are reactions to medications, such as penicillin; foods, such as nuts and shellfish; and the venom of insects, such as bees. The most common cause is stings from insects of the order Hymenoptera (*i.e.,* bees, wasps, and fire ants). Latex allergy causes life-threatening anaphylaxis in a growing segment of the population (see Chapter 19). Healthcare workers and others who are exposed to latex may develop latex sensitivities that range from mild urticaria, contact dermatitis, and mild respiratory distress to anaphylactic shock.[61] Children with spina bifida also are at extreme risk for this serious and increasingly common allergy.

The onset and severity of anaphylaxis depend on the sensitivity of the person and the rate and quantity of antigen exposure. Signs and symptoms associated with impending anaphylactic shock include abdominal cramps and diarrhea; apprehension; warm or burning sensation of the skin, itching, and urticaria (*i.e.,* hives); and coughing, wheezing, chest tightness, or difficulty in breathing. After blood begins to pool peripherally or shifts to the gut, there is a precipitous drop in blood pressure and the pulse becomes so weak that it is difficult to detect. Life-threatening airway obstruction may ensue as a result of laryngeal angioedema or bronchial spasm. Anaphylactic shock often develops suddenly; death can occur within minutes unless appropriate medical intervention is promptly instituted.

Treatment includes immediate discontinuation of the inciting agent or institution of measures to decrease its absorption (*e.g.,* application of ice to the site of an insect bite); close monitoring of cardiovascular and respiratory function; and maintenance of respiratory gas exchange, cardiac output, and tissue perfusion. Epinephrine remains the medication of choice in an anaphylactic reaction because it constricts blood

...oth muscle in the bronchioles, thus ...ratory function.[55,59] Other treatment ...stration of fluids, oxygen, antihista-...teroids. The person should be placed ...romote venous return.[59]

... anaphylactic shock is preferable to ...son has been sensitized to an antigen, the risk of r... anaphylactic reactions with subsequent exposure is high. All healthcare providers should question patients regarding previous drug reactions and inform patients as to the name of the medication they are to receive before it is administered or prescribed. Persons with known hypersensitivities should wear Medic Alert jewellery and carry an identification card to alert medical personnel if they become unconscious or unable to relate this information. Persons who are at risk for anaphylaxis should be provided with emergency medications (*e.g.,* epinephrine autoinjector [Epipen or Allerject]) and instructed in procedures to follow in case they are inadvertently exposed to the offending antigen.[59]

Sepsis and Septic Shock

Septic shock, which is the most common type of vasodilatory shock, is most commonly associated with severe infection and the systemic response to infection.[62–69] The nomenclature related to sepsis and septic shock has been evolving.[62–64] *Systemic inflammatory response syndrome (SIRS)* is an overwhelming inflammatory response, which is not necessarily due to infection. The syndrome is associated with two or more alterations in temperature, heart rate, respiratory rate, or white blood cell count. *Sepsis* is currently defined as a suspected or proven infection, plus a systemic inflammatory response (*e.g.,* fever, tachycardia, tachypnea, and elevated white blood cell count, altered mental state, and hyperglycemia in the absence of diabetes).[68] *Severe sepsis* is defined as sepsis with organ dysfunction (*e.g.,* hypotension, hypoxemia, oliguria, metabolic acidosis, thrombocytopenia, or obtundation).[64] *Septic shock* is defined as severe sepsis with hypoperfusion, despite fluid resuscitation.[63–65]

The most common cause of sepsis is pneumonia, followed by intra-abdominal and urinary tract infections.[62] It is estimated that more than 750,000 cases of sepsis occur each year in the United States, leading to approximately 225,000 deaths.[64] Similar data is not available for Canada regarding incidence or mortality, as cause of death may be cited as pneumonia. In 2009, more than 30,500 patients in hospitals outside of Quebec were diagnosed with sepsis, resulting in 9,320 deaths: a 30% mortality.[65] Persons at risk for a higher mortality were elderly, had another comorbidity, or were female. With early intervention and advances in treatment methods, the mortality rate has decreased; however, the numbers of deaths has increased because of the increased prevalence.[65]

Mechanisms. The pathogenesis of sepsis involves a complex process of excessive inflammatory and immune responses followed by an impaired immune response.[66] Cellular activation results in the release of proinflammatory mediators

FIGURE 26.12 • Pathogenic mechanisms leading from infection to septic shock.

such as cytokines; activation of neutrophils, monocytes, and endothelial cells; involvement of neuroendocrine reflexes; and activation of complement, coagulation, and fibrinolytic systems (Fig. 26.12). Initiation of the response begins with activation of the innate immune system by pattern-recognition receptors (*e.g.,* Toll-like receptors [TLRs]) that interact with specific molecules present on microorganisms[63] (see Chapter 17). Binding of TLRs to epitopes on microorganisms stimulates transcription and release of a number of proinflammatory and anti-inflammatory mediators. Two of these mediators, TNF-α and interleukin-1β are involved in leukocyte adhesion, local inflammation, neutrophil activation, suppression of erythropoiesis, generation of fever, tachycardia, lactic acidosis, ventilation–perfusion abnormalities, and other signs of sepsis (see section on The Inflammatory Response, Chapter 18).

Although activated neutrophils kill microorganisms, they also injure the endothelium by releasing mediators that increase vascular permeability. In addition, activated endothelial cells release nitric oxide, a potent vasodilator that acts as a key mediator of septic shock.

Another important aspect of sepsis is an alteration of the procoagulation–anticoagulation balance with an increase in procoagulation factors and a decrease in anticoagulation factors. Lipopolysaccharide on the surface of microorganisms stimulates endothelial cells lining blood vessels to increase their production of tissue factor, thus activating coagulation[64] (see Chapter 13). Fibrinogen is then converted to fibrin, leading to the formation of microvascular thrombi that further amplify tissue injury. In addition, sepsis lowers levels of protein C, protein S, antithrombin III, and tissue factor pathway inhibitor, substances that modulate and inhibit coagulation. Lipopolysaccharide and TNF-α also decrease the synthesis of thrombomodulin and endothelial protein C receptor, impairing activation of protein C, and they increase the synthesis of plasminogen activator inhibitor-1, impairing fibrinolysis.[64]

Historically, the pathophysiology of sepsis focused on the presence, absence, or type of agent. Today, understanding has extended to encompass both the individual response and the characteristics of the pathogen, whether it be bacteria, virus, or fungi. The proinflammatory and anti-inflammatory immunosuppressive response to sepsis is influenced by pathogen factors, including load and virulence, and human factors such as the environment, genetics, stress response, age, comorbidities, and medications.[67]

Manifestations. Sepsis and septic shock typically manifest with hypotension and warm, flushed skin, in contrast to other forms of shock (*i.e.,* cardiogenic, hypovolemic, and obstructive), which are characterized by a compensatory increase in systemic vascular resistance. However, septic shock often presents with a decrease in systemic vascular resistance. The person has maldistribution of volume due to extensive arterial and venous dilation, and leakage of plasma into the interstitial spaces. Abrupt changes in cognition or behaviour are due to reduced cerebral blood flow, and may be early indications of septic shock. Regardless of the underlying cause, fever and increased leukocytes are present. An elevated serum lactate or metabolic acidosis indicates anaerobic metabolism due to tissue hypoxia or cellular dysfunction and altered cellular metabolism.[65] Tissue hypoxia produces continued production and activation of inflammatory mediators, resulting in further increases in vascular permeability, impaired vascular regulation, and altered hemostasis.

Treatment. The treatment of sepsis and septic shock focuses on control of the causative agent and support of the circulation. Early use of antibiotics is essential, followed by antibiotic therapy specific to the infectious agent.[68] However, antibiotics do not treat the inflammatory response to the infection; thus, the cardiovascular status of the patient must be supported to increase oxygen delivery to the cells and prevent further cellular injury.

Current recommendations to maintain perfusion and pressure are crystalloid fluid resuscitation targeted to outcomes, including hemodynamic data, urine output, and lactate levels. Hydroxyethyl starch solutions are not recommended. Vasoconstrictors are used when hypotension is unresponsive to fluids, with preference to norepinephrine and vasopressin. Phenylephrine and dopamine are not recommended.[67] A positive inotrope, such as dobutamine or milrinone, may be used to augment cardiac output and tissue perfusion. Ongoing assessment of CVP, central or mixed SvO_2, mean arterial pressure, urinary output, and laboratory measurements of serum lactate, base deficit, and pH are used to evaluate the progression of sepsis and adequacy of treatment.[63–65,68]

Earlier strategies for treatment of sepsis included use of intensive insulin therapy for hyperglycemia and the administration of recombinant human activated protein C. Hyperglycemia is potentially harmful because it acts as a procoagulant, induces apoptosis, impairs neutrophil function, increases the risk of infection, and impairs wound healing.[64] Although there is a consensus that hyperglycemia is detrimental, the optimal level and adverse effects of hypoglycaemia have created controversy regarding protocols for glycemic control.[69] Most protocols aim to achieve moderate blood glucose levels of less than 10 mmol/L, avoiding hypoglycemia, and low caloric feeding with enteral preference to parenteral administration. Recombinant activated Protein C is no longer recommended or available.[65]

The use of corticosteroids, once considered a mainstay in the treatment of sepsis, remains controversial. Use of high-dose corticosteroids, in particular, has not been shown to improve survival and may worsen outcomes by increasing the risk of secondary infections.

Obstructive Shock

The term *obstructive shock* describes circulatory shock that results from mechanical obstruction of the flow of blood through the central circulation (great veins, heart, or lungs; Fig. 26.8). Obstructive shock may be caused by a number of conditions, including dissecting aortic aneurysm, cardiac tamponade, pneumothorax, atrial myxoma, and evisceration of abdominal contents into the thoracic cavity because of a ruptured hemidiaphragm. The most frequent cause of obstructive shock is pulmonary embolism.

The primary physiologic result of obstructive shock is elevated right heart pressure due to impaired right ventricular function. Pressures are increased despite impaired venous return to the heart. Signs of right heart failure occur, including elevation of CVP and jugular venous distension. Treatment modalities focus on correcting the cause of the disorder, frequently with surgical interventions such as pulmonary embolectomy, pericardiocentesis (*i.e.,* removal of fluid from the pericardial sac) for cardiac tamponade, or the insertion of a chest tube for correction of a tension pneumothorax or hemothorax. In severe or massive pulmonary embolus, fibrinolytic drugs may be used to break down the clots causing the obstruction.

Complications of Shock

Carl Wiggers, a noted circulatory physiologist, stated, "Shock not only stops the machine, but it wrecks the machinery."[70] Many body systems are wrecked by severe shock. Five major complications of severe shock are pulmonary injury, acute renal failure, gastrointestinal ulceration, disseminated intravascular coagulation (DIC), and multiple organ dysfunction syndrome. These complications of shock are serious and often fatal.

Acute Respiratory Distress Syndrome

Acute respiratory distress syndrome (ARDS) is a potentially lethal form of pulmonary injury that may be either the cause or result of shock (see Chapter 29).

Acute Renal Failure

The renal tubules are particularly vulnerable to ischemia, and acute renal failure is an important factor in mortality due to severe shock. Most cases of acute renal failure are due to impaired renal perfusion or direct injury to the kidneys. The degree of renal damage is related to the severity and duration of shock. The normal kidney is able to tolerate severe ischemia for 15 to 20 minutes. The renal dysfunction most frequently seen after severe shock is acute tubular necrosis. Acute tubular necrosis usually is reversible, although return to normal renal function may require weeks or months (see Chapter 33). Continuous monitoring of urinary output during shock provides a means of assessing renal blood flow. Frequent monitoring of serum creatinine and urea (BUN) levels also provides valuable information regarding renal status.

Mediators implicated in septic shock are powerful vasoconstrictors capable of activating the sympathetic nervous system and causing intravascular clotting. They have been shown to trigger all the separate physiologic mechanisms that contribute to the onset of acute renal failure.

Gastrointestinal Complications

The gastrointestinal tract is particularly vulnerable to ischemia because of the changes in distribution of blood flow to its mucosal surface. In shock, there is widespread constriction of blood vessels that supply the gastrointestinal tract, causing a redistribution of blood flow and a severe decrease in mucosal perfusion. Patients may experience loss of appetite, nausea, or vomiting. Superficial mucosal lesions of the stomach and duodenum can develop within hours of severe trauma, sepsis, or burns leading to bacterial translocation from the lumen into the systemic circulation. Also bowel obstruction, necrosis, or bleeding may occur due to the decrease in perfusion in shock. Hemorrhage usually has its onset within 2 to 10 days after the original insult and often begins without warning.

Enteral feeding is recommended if tolerated. Proton pump inhibitors, histamine type 2 receptor antagonists, or sucralfate may be given prophylactically to prevent gastrointestinal ulcerations caused by shock.[71] Nasogastric tubes attached to intermittent or continuous suction also help to diminish the accumulation of hydrogen ions in the stomach.

Disseminated Intravascular Coagulation

Disseminated intravascular coagulation (DIC) is characterized by widespread activation of the coagulation system with resultant formation of fibrin clots and thrombotic occlusion of small and midsized vessels (see Chapter 13). The systemic formation of fibrin results from increased generation of thrombin, the simultaneous suppression of physiologic anticoagulation mechanisms, and the delayed removal of fibrin as a consequence of impaired fibrinolysis. As with other systemic inflammatory responses, the derangement of coagulation and fibrinolysis is thought to be mediated by inflammatory mediators and cytokines.

The contribution of DIC to morbidity and mortality in sepsis depends on the underlying clinical condition and the intensity of the coagulation disorder. Depletion of the platelets and coagulation factors increases the risk of bleeding. Deposition of fibrin in the vasculature of organs contributes to ischemic damage and organ failure. In a large number of clinical trials, the occurrence of DIC appeared to be associated with an unfavourable outcome and was an independent predictor of mortality. However, it remains uncertain whether DIC was a predictor of unfavourable outcome, or merely a marker of the seriousness of the underlying condition causing the DIC.[72]

The management of sepsis-induced DIC focuses on treatment of the underlying disorder and measures to interrupt the coagulation process. Anticoagulation therapy and administration of platelets and plasma may be used. Clinical trials have shown modest to marked reductions in mortality based on the dose of antithrombin III used. Other therapeutic options, aimed at interrupting the intrinsic coagulation pathway at the point where tissue factor complexes with factor VIIa, also are being investigated.[72]

Multiple Organ Dysfunction Syndrome

Multiple organ dysfunction syndrome (MODS) represents the presence of altered organ function in an acutely ill patient such that homeostasis cannot be maintained without intervention. As the name implies, MODS commonly affects multiple organ systems, including the kidneys, lungs, liver, brain, and heart. MODS is a particularly life-threatening complication of shock, especially septic shock. It has been reported as the most frequent cause of death in the noncoronary intensive care unit. Mortality rates vary from 30% to 100%, depending on the number of organs involved.[71] Mortality rates increase with an increased number of organs failing. A high mortality rate is associated with failure of the brain, liver, kidneys, and lungs. The pathogenesis of MODS is not clearly understood, and current management therefore is primarily supportive. Major risk factors for the development of MODS are severe trauma, sepsis, prolonged periods of hypotension, hepatic dysfunction, infarcted bowel, advanced age, and alcohol abuse.[71] Interventions for multiple organ failure are focused on support of the affected organs.

IN SUMMARY

Circulatory shock is an acute emergency in which body tissues are deprived of oxygen and cellular nutrients or are unable to use these materials in their metabolic processes. Circulatory shock may develop because the heart is unable to adequately pump blood through the circulatory system (*i.e.,* cardiogenic shock), there is insufficient blood in the circulatory system (*i.e.,* hypovolemic shock), there is a maldistribution of blood due to abnormalities in the vascular resistance (*i.e.,* distributive shock), or blood flow or venous return is obstructed (*i.e.,* obstructive shock). Three types of shock share the basic circulatory pattern of distributive shock: neurogenic shock, anaphylactic shock, and septic shock. Sepsis and septic shock, which is the most common of the three types, is associated with a severe, overwhelming inflammatory response and has a high mortality rate.

The manifestations of hypovolemic shock, which serves as a prototype for circulatory shock, are related to low peripheral blood flow and excessive sympathetic stimulation. The low peripheral blood flow produces thirst, changes in skin temperature, decreased blood pressure, increased heart rate, decreased venous pressure, decreased urine output, and changes in mentation. The intense vasoconstriction that serves to maintain blood flow to the heart and brain causes a decrease in tissue perfusion, impaired cellular metabolism, liberation of lactic acid, and, eventually, cell death. Whether the shock is irreversible or the patient will survive is determined largely by changes that occur at the cellular level.

The complications of shock result from the deprivation of blood flow to vital organs or systems, such as the lungs, kidneys, gastrointestinal tract, and blood coagulation system. Shock can cause or be accompanied by ARDS, which is characterized by changes in the permeability of the alveolar-capillary membrane with development of interstitial edema and severe hypoxemia that does not respond to oxygen therapy. The renal tubules are particularly vulnerable to ischemia, and acute renal failure is an important complication of shock. Gastrointestinal ischemia may lead to gastrointestinal bleeding and increased vascular permeability to intestinal bacteria, which can cause further sepsis and shock. DIC is characterized by formation of small clots in the circulation. It is thought to be caused by inappropriate activation of the coagulation cascade because of toxins or other products released as a result of the shock state. Multiple organ failure, perhaps the most ominous complication of shock, rapidly depletes the body's ability to compensate and recover from a shock state.

HEART FAILURE IN CHILDREN AND OLDER ADULTS

After completing this section of the chapter, you should be able to meet the following objectives:

- Describe the causes of heart failure in infants and children.
- Cite how the aging process affects cardiac function and predisposes to ventricular dysfunction.
- State how the signs and symptoms of heart failure may differ between younger and older adults.

Heart Failure in Infants and Children

As in adults, heart failure in infants and children results from the inability of the heart to maintain the cardiac output required to sustain metabolic demands.[73–75] The etiology of heart failure, however, is very different in children than in adults. Structural (congenital) heart defects are the most common cause of heart failure in children, who are most often diagnosed in infancy or even in gestation. The incidence drops sharply after the newborn state.[76] Surgical correction of congenital heart defects may cause heart failure as a result of intraoperative manipulation of the heart and resection of heart tissue, with subsequent alterations in pressure, flow, and resistance relations. Usually, the heart failure that results is acute and resolves after the effects of the surgical procedure have subsided. Another cause of heart failure in children is cardiomyopathy related to a genetic or inherited disorder, infectious disease, drugs, toxins, arrhythmias, or Kawasaki disease.[73–77] Chart 26.3 lists some of the more common causes of heart failure in children. Inflammatory heart disorders (*e.g.,* myocarditis, rheumatic fever, bacterial endocarditis, Kawasaki disease), cardiomyopathy, and congenital heart disorders are discussed in Chapter 24.

Clinical Features

Manifestations. Many of the signs and symptoms of heart failure in infants and children are similar to those in adults but may be missed without a careful history that considers the age of the child, normal development, and usual activities.[74] In children, overt symptoms of heart failure occur late in the disease process.[75,78] Breathlessness, tachypnea, and tachycardia felt as palpitations are the most common signs and symptoms.[75,78] Other symptoms include fatigue, effort intolerance, cough, anorexia, and abdominal pain. A subtle sign of cardiorespiratory distress in infants and children is a change in disposition or responsiveness, including irritability or lethargy. Children may decrease their activities to limit symptoms and unintentionally minimize the expression of their illness.[78] With worsening failure, sympathetic stimulation produces peripheral vasoconstriction and diaphoresis. Decreased renal blood flow often results in a decrease in urine output despite adequate fluid intake.

When right ventricular function is impaired, systemic venous congestion develops. Hepatomegaly due to liver

CHART 26.3 CAUSES OF HEART FAILURE IN CHILDREN

Newborn Period
Congenital heart defects
  Severe left ventricular outflow disorders
    Hypoplastic left heart
    Critical aortic stenosis or coarctation of the aorta
  Large arteriovenous shunts
    Ventricular septal defects
    Patent ductus arteriosus
  Transposition of the great vessels
Heart muscle dysfunction (secondary)
  Asphyxia
  Sepsis
  Hypoglycemia
Arrhythmias
Hematologic disorders (*e.g.,* anemia)

Infants 1 to 6 Months
Congenital heart disease
  Large arteriovenous shunts (ventricular septal
    defect)
Heart muscle dysfunction
  Myocarditis
  Cardiomyopathy
Pulmonary abnormalities
  Bronchopulmonary dysplasia
  Persistent pulmonary hypertension
Arrhythmias

Toddlers, Children, and Adolescents
Acquired heart disease
  Cardiomyopathy
  Viral myocarditis
  Rheumatic fever
  Endocarditis
  Systemic disease
    Sepsis
    Kawasaki disease
    Renal disease
    Sickle cell disease
Congenital heart defects
  Nonsurgically treated disorders
  Surgically treated disorders
Arrhythmias

---

failure. It results from rapid filling of a distended ventricle. However, it is difficult to distinguish at high heart rates.

Most commonly, children develop interstitial pulmonary edema rather than alveolar pulmonary edema. This reduces lung compliance and increases the work of breathing, causing tachypnea and increased respiratory effort. Older children display use of accessory muscles (*i.e.,* scapular and sternocleidomastoid). Head bobbing and nasal flaring may be observed in infants. Signs of respiratory distress often are the first and most noticeable indication of heart failure in infants and young children. Pulmonary congestion may be mistaken for bronchiolitis or lower respiratory tract infection. The infant or young child with respiratory distress often grunts with expiration. This grunting effort (essentially, exhaling against a closed glottis) is an instinctive effort to increase end-expiratory pressures and prevent collapse of small airways and the development of atelectasis. Respiratory crackles are uncommon in infants and usually suggest development of a respiratory tract infection. Wheezes may be heard, particularly if there is a large left-to-right shunt.

Infants with heart failure may show increased tachypnea, fatigue, and diaphoresis during feeding.[78] Weight gain is slow owing to high energy requirements and low calorie intake. Diaphoresis occurs because of increased sympathetic tone, particularly over the head and neck. They may have repeated lower respiratory tract infections. Peripheral perfusion usually is poor, with cool extremities; tachycardia is common (*e.g.,* resting heart rate >150 beats per minute); and the respiratory rate is increased (*e.g.,* resting rate >50 breaths per minute).[73]

Diagnosis and Treatment. Diagnosis of heart failure in infants and children is based on symptomatology, chest radiographic films, electrocardiographic findings, echocardiographic techniques to assess cardiac structures and ventricular function (*i.e.,* end-systolic and end-diastolic diameters), arterial blood gases to determine intracardiac shunting and ventilation–perfusion inequalities, and other laboratory studies to determine anemia and electrolyte imbalances.

Treatment of heart failure in infants and children includes measures aimed at improving cardiac function and eliminating excess intravascular fluid. Oxygen delivery must be supported and oxygen demands controlled or minimized. Whenever possible, the cause of the disorder is corrected (*e.g.,* medical treatment of sepsis and anemia, surgical correction of congenital heart defects). With congenital anomalies that are amenable to surgery, medical treatment often is needed for a time before surgery and usually is continued in the immediate postoperative period. For many children, only medical management can be provided.

Medical management of heart failure in infants and children is extrapolated from the adult, although it is tailored to the special developmental needs of the child.[74,75] ACE inhibitors and β-adrenergic blockers are frequently used to attenuate the renin–angiotensin–aldosterone response. Inotropic agents such as digitalis may be used to increase cardiac contractility. Diuretics may be given to reduce preload and vasodilating medications used to manipulate the afterload. Medication doses

congestion often is one of the first signs of systemic venous congestion in infants and children. However, dependent edema or ascites rarely is seen unless the CVP is extremely high. Because of their short necks, jugular venous distension is difficult to detect in infants; it is not a reliable sign until the child is of school age or older. A third heart sound, or gallop rhythm, is a common finding in infants and children with heart must be carefully tailored to control for the child's weight and conditions such as reduced renal function. Daily weighing and accurate measurement of intake and output are imperative during acute episodes of failure. Most children feel better in the semiupright position. An infant seat is useful for infants with chronic heart failure. Activity restrictions usually are designed to allow children to be as active as possible within the limitations of their heart disease. Infants with heart failure often have problems feeding. Small, frequent feedings usually are more successful than larger, less frequent feedings. Severely ill infants may lack sufficient strength to suck and may need to be tube fed.

The treatment of heart failure in children should be designed to allow optimal physical and psychosocial development. It requires the full involvement of the parents, who often are the primary care providers; therefore, parent education and support are essential.

Heart Failure in Older Adults

Heart failure is largely a disease of aging. It is one of the most common causes of disability in older adults and is the most frequent hospital discharge diagnosis for the elderly in Canada. An estimated 90% of people with heart failure are older than 60 years of age.[3] Among the factors that have contributed to the increased numbers of older people with heart failure are the improved therapies for ischemic and hypertensive heart disease.[79] Thus, persons who would have died from acute myocardial disease 20 years ago are now surviving, but with residual left ventricular dysfunction. Advances in treatment of other diseases, accompanied by the increased numbers of persons with hypertension, have also contributed indirectly to the rising prevalence of heart failure in the older population.

Coronary heart disease, hypertension, and valvular heart disease (particularly aortic stenosis and mitral regurgitation) are common causes of heart failure in older adults.[80,81] In contrast to the etiology in middle-aged persons with heart failure, factors other than systolic failure contribute to heart failure in the elderly. Preserved left ventricular function may be seen in 40% to 80% of older persons with heart failure.[81] Aging is associated with impaired left ventricular filling due to changes in myocardial relaxation and compliance. These alterations lead to a shift in the left ventricular pressure–volume relationship, such that small increases in left ventricular volume lead to greater increases in left ventricular diastolic pressure. This increase in diastolic pressure further compromises left ventricular filling and leads to increases in left atrial, pulmonary venous, and pulmonary capillary pressures, and thus predisposes to pulmonary congestion and heart failure.[80] Although diastolic heart failure accounts for less than 10% of heart failure cases in persons younger than 60 years of age, it accounts for greater than 50% of cases after 75 years of age.[80]

There are a number of changes associated with aging that contribute to the development of heart failure in older adults.[79–81] First, reduced responsiveness to β-adrenergic stimulation limits the heart's capacity to maximally increase heart rate and contractility. A second major effect of aging is increased vascular stiffness, which leads to a progressive increase in systolic blood pressure with advancing age, which in turn contributes to the development of left ventricular hypertrophy and altered diastolic filling. Third, in addition to increased vascular stiffness, the heart itself becomes stiffer and less compliant with age. The changes in diastolic stiffness result in important alterations in diastolic filling and atrial function. A reduction in ventricular filling not only affects cardiac output, but produces an elevation in diastolic pressure that is transmitted back to the left atrium, where it stretches the muscle wall and predisposes to atrial ectopic beats and atrial fibrillation. The fourth major effect of cardiovascular aging is altered myocardial metabolism at the level of the mitochondria. Although older mitochondria may be able to generate sufficient ATP to meet the normal energy needs of the heart, they may not be able to respond under stress.

Clinical Features

Manifestations. The manifestations of heart failure in older adults often are masked by other disease conditions.[2] Nocturia and nocturnal incontinence are early symptoms but may be caused by other conditions such as prostatic hypertrophy. Lower extremity edema may reflect venous insufficiency. Impaired perfusion of the gastrointestinal tract is a common cause of anorexia and profound loss of lean body mass. Loss of lean body mass may be masked by edema. Exertional dyspnea, orthopnea, and impaired exercise tolerance are cardinal symptoms of heart failure in both younger and older persons with heart failure. However, with increasing age, which is often accompanied by a more sedentary lifestyle, exertional dyspnea becomes less prominent. Instead of dyspnea, the prominent sign may be restlessness. Chart 26.4 summarizes the manifestations of heart failure in older adults.

Physical signs of heart failure, such as elevated jugular venous pressure, hepatic congestion, S_3 heart sound and pulmonary crackles, occur less commonly in the elderly, in part because of the increased incidence of diastolic failure, in which

---

CHART 26.4 MANIFESTATIONS OF HEART FAILURE IN OLDER ADULTS

Symptoms
Nocturia or nocturnal incontinence
Fatigue
Cognitive impairment (e.g., problem solving)
Depression
Restlessness/acute delirium
Sleep disturbance
History of falls
Loss of appetite

Signs
Pulmonary crackles
Dependent edema (ankles when sitting up and sacral edema when supine)

signs of right-sided heart failure are late manifestations and a third heart sound is typically absent.[81] Instead, behavioural changes and altered cognition such as short-term memory loss and impaired problem solving are more common.[2] With exacerbation of heart failure, older adults may present with acute delirium and dementia.[2] Depression is common in older adults with heart failure and shares the symptoms of weight gain, sleep disturbance, cognitive changes, and fatigue.[2]

Older adults also maintain a precarious balance between the managed symptom state and acute symptom exacerbation. During the managed symptom state, they are relatively symptom free while adhering to their treatment regimen. Acute symptom exacerbation, often requiring emergency medical treatment, can be precipitated by seemingly minor conditions such as infection, stress or poor adherence to sodium restriction. Failure to seek health care promptly is a common cause of progressive acceleration of symptoms.

Diagnosis and Treatment. The diagnosis of heart failure in older adults is based on the history, physical examination, chest radiograph, and ECG findings. However, the presenting symptoms of heart failure often are difficult to evaluate. Symptoms of dyspnea on exertion are often interpreted as a sign of "getting older" or attributed to deconditioning from other diseases. Ankle edema is not unusual in the elderly because of decreased skin turgor and the tendency of the elderly to be more sedentary with the legs in a dependent position.

Treatment of heart failure in older adults involves many of the same methods as in younger persons, with medication dose adaptations to reduce age-related adverse and toxic events.[2] ACE inhibitors may be particularly beneficial to preserve cognitive and functional capacities.[2] Activities are restricted to a level that is commensurate with the cardiac reserve. Seldom is bed rest recommended except in acute states. Bed rest causes rapid deconditioning of skeletal muscles and increases the risk of complications such as orthostatic hypotension and thromboemboli. Instead, carefully prescribed exercise programs can help to maintain activity tolerance. Even walking around a room usually is preferable to continuous bed rest. Sodium restriction usually is indicated.

IN SUMMARY

The mechanisms of heart failure in children and the elderly are similar to those in younger adults. However, the causes and manifestations may differ because of age. In children, heart failure is seen most commonly during infancy and immediately after heart surgery. It can be caused by congenital and acquired heart defects and is characterized by fatigue, effort intolerance, cough, anorexia, abdominal pain, and impaired growth. Treatment of heart failure in children includes correction of the underlying cause whenever possible. For congenital anomalies that are amenable to surgery, medical treatment often is needed for a time before surgery and usually is continued in the immediate postoperative period. For many children, only medical management can be provided.

In older adults, age-related changes in cardiovascular functioning contribute to heart failure but are not in themselves sufficient to cause heart failure. The manifestations of heart failure often are different and superimposed on other disease conditions; therefore, heart failure often is more difficult to diagnose in the elderly than in younger persons.

REVIEW EXERCISES

1. A 75-year-old woman with long-standing hypertension and angina due to coronary heart disease presents with ankle edema, nocturia, increased shortness of breath with activity, and a chronic nonproductive cough. Her blood pressure is 170/80 mm Hg and her heart rate 92. Electrocardiography and chest radiography indicate the presence of left ventricular hypertrophy.
   A. *Relate the presence of uncontrolled hypertension and coronary artery disease to the development of heart failure in this woman.*
   B. *Explain the significance of left ventricular hypertrophy in terms of both a compensatory mechanism and as a pathologic mechanism in the progression of heart failure.*
   C. *Use Figure 26.5 to explain this woman's symptoms, including shortness of breath and nonproductive cough.*

2. A 26-year-old man is admitted to the emergency department after an automobile injury with excessive blood loss. He is alert and anxious, his skin is cool and moist, his heart rate is 135, and his blood pressure is 100/85 mm Hg. He is receiving intravenous fluids, which were started at the scene of the accident by an emergency medical technician. He has been typed and cross-matched for blood transfusions and a urinary catheter has been inserted to monitor his urinary output. His urinary output has been less than 10 ml/hour since admission and his blood pressure has dropped to 85/70 mm Hg. Efforts to control his bleeding have been unsuccessful and he is being prepared for emergency surgery.
   A. *Use information regarding the compensatory mechanisms in circulatory shock to explain this man's presenting symptoms, including urinary output.*
   B. *Use Figure 26.11 to hypothesize about this man's blood loss and maintenance of blood pressure.*
   C. *The treatment of hypovolemic shock is usually directed at maintaining the circulatory volume through fluid resuscitation rather than maintaining the blood pressure through the use of vasoactive medications. Explain.*

References

1. Yancy C. W., Jessup M., Bozkurt, B., et al. (2013). 2013 ACCF/AHA guideline for the management of heart failure. *Journal of the American College of Cardiology, 62*(16), e147–e239.

2. McDonald M., McKelvie R., Harkness K., et al. (2014). CCS heart failure recommendations compendium, 2006–2013. Available online at: http://www.ccs.ca/index.php/en/resources/heart-failure-compendium. Accessed May 4, 2015.

3. Ross H., Howlett J., Arnold J. M., et al. (2006). Treating the right patient at the right time: Access to heart failure care. *Canadian Journal of Cardiology, 22*(9), 749–754.

4. Lepage S. (2008). Acute decompensated heart failure. *Canadian Journal of Cardiology, 24*(Suppl B), 6B–8B.

5. Hall J. E. (2011). *Textbook of medical physiology* (12th ed.). Philadelphia, PA: W. B. Saunders.

6. Klabunde R. E. (2005). *Cardiovascular physiology concepts.* Philadelphia, PA: Lippincott Williams & Wilkins.

7. Opie L. H., Bers D. M. (2015). Chapter 21: Mechanisms of cardiac contraction and relaxation. In Mann D. L., Zipes D. P., Libby P., et al. *Braunwald's heart disease: A textbook of cardiovascular medicine* (10th ed.). Philadelphia, PA: Elsevier, Inc.

8. Januzzi J. L., Mann D. L. (2015). Chapter 23: Clinical assessment of heart failure. In Mann D. L., Zipes D. P., Libby P., et al. *Braunwald's heart disease: A textbook of cardiovascular medicine* (10th ed.). Philadelphia, PA: Elsevier, Inc.

9. Wu E. B., Yu C. M. (2005). Management of diastolic heart failure: A practical review of pathophysiology and treatment trial data. *International Journal of Clinical Practice, 59*(10), 1239–1246.

10. Kemp C. D., Conte J. V. (2012). The pathophysiology of heart failure. *Cardiovascular Pathology, 21*(5), 365–371.

11. Aurigemma G. P., Gaasch W. H. (2004). Diastolic heart failure. *New England Journal of Medicine, 351*(11), 1095–1105.

12. Haney S., Sur D., Xu Z. (2005). Diastolic heart failure: A review and primary care perspective. *Journal of the American Board of Family Practice, 18*(3), 189–195.

13. Weitzenblum E., Chaouat A. (2009). Cor pulmonale. *Chronic Respiratory Disease, 6*(3), 177–185.

14. Hasenfuss G., Mann D. L. (2015). Chapter 22: Pathophysiology of heart failure. In Mann D. L., Zipes D. P., Libby P., et al. *Braunwald's heart disease: A textbook of cardiovascular medicine* (10th ed.). Philadelphia, PA: Elsevier, Inc.

15. Lymperopoulos A., Rengo G., Koch W. J. (2013). Adrenergic nervous system in heart failure: Pathophysiology and therapy. *Circulation Research, 113*(6), 739–753.

16. Adams K. F. (2004). Pathophysiologic role of the renin-angiotensin-aldosterone and sympathetic nervous system in HF. *American Journal of Health-System Pharmacy, 61*(Suppl. 2), S4–S13.

17. Weber K. T. (2001). Aldosterone in congestive heart failure. *New England Journal of Medicine, 345*(23), 1689–1697.

18. Struthers A. D. (2005). Pathophysiology of heart failure following myocardial infarction. *Heart, 91*(Suppl 2), 14–16.

19. Pitt B., Zannad F., Remme W. J., et al. (1999). The effect of spironolactone on morbidity and mortality in patients with severe heart failure. *New England Journal of Medicine, 341*(10), 709–717.

20. Levin E. R., Gardner D. G., Samson W. K. (1998). Natriuretic peptides. *New England Journal of Medicine, 339*(5), 321–328.

21. Baughman K. L. (2002). B-type natriuretic peptide: A window to the heart. *New England Journal of Medicine, 347*(3), 158–159.

22. Nathisuwan S., Talbert R. L. (2002). A review of vasopeptidase inhibitors: A new modality in the treatment of hypertension and chronic heart failure. *Pharmacotherapy, 22*(1), 27–42.

23. Spieker L. E., Lüscher T. F. (2003). Will endothelin receptor antagonists have a role in heart failure? *Medical Clinics of North America, 87*(2), 459–474.

24. Ergul A. (2002). Endothelin-1 and endothelin receptor antagonists as potential cardiovascular therapeutic agents. *Pharmacotherapy, 22*(1), 54–65.

25. Kardys I., Knetsch A. M., Bleumink G. S., et al. (2006). C-reactive protein and risk of heart failure: The Rotterdam Study. *American Heart Journal, 152*(3), 514–520.

26. Estes N. A. M. (2006). Implantable cardioverter defibrillator and cardiac resynchronization therapy in patients with left ventricular dysfunction: Evidence based medicine, economics, and guidelines: CME. Available online at: www.medscape.com/viewprogram/5242. Accessed May 4, 2015.

27. Hunter J. J., Chien K. R. (1999). Signaling pathways for cardiac hypertrophy and failure. *New England Journal of Medicine, 341*(17), 1276–1284.

28. Gheorghiade M., Zannad F., Sopko G., et al. (2005). Acute heart failure syndrome: Current state and framework for future research. *Circulation, 112*(25), 3958–3968.

29. Koniari K., Parissis J., Paraskevaidis I., et al. (2012). Treating volume overload in acutely decompensated heart failure: Established and novel therapeutic approaches. *European Heart Journal: Acute Cardiovascular Care, 1*(3), 256–268.

30. Filippatos G., Zannad F. (2007). An introduction to acute heart failure syndromes: Definition and classification. *Heart Failure Review, 12*(2), 87–90.

31. Arcand J., Ivanov J., Sasson A., et al. (2011). A high-sodium diet is associated with acute decompensated heart failure in ambulatory heart failure patients: A prospective follow-up study. *American Journal of Clinical Nutrition, 93*(2), 332–337.

32. Ronco C., Cicoira M., McCullough P. A. (2012). Cardiorenal syndrome type 1: Pathophysiological crosstalk leading to combined heart and kidney dysfunction in the setting of acutely decompensated heart failure. *Journal of the American College of Cardiology, 60*(12), 1031–1042.

33. Valentova M., von Haehling S., Krause C., et al. (2012). Cardiac cachexia is associated with right ventricular failure and liver dysfunction. *International Journal of Cardiology, 169*(3), 219–224.

34. Canadian Institute for Health Information. (2015). Canadian organ replacement register annual report: Treatment of end-stage organ failure in Canada, 2004 to 2013. Available online at: https://secure.cihi.ca/free_products/2015_CORR_AnnualReport_ENweb.pdf. Accessed May 4, 2015.

35. Piña I. L. (2003). Exercise and heart failure: A statement from the American Heart Association Committee on Exercise, Rehabilitation, and Prevention. *Circulation, 107*(4), 1210–1225.

36. Zile M. R., Little W. C. (2015). Chapter 27: Heart failure with a preserved ejection fraction. In Mann D. L., Zipes D. P., Libby P., et al. *Braunwald's heart disease: A textbook of cardiovascular medicine* (10th ed.). Philadelphia, PA: Elsevier, Inc.

37. MERIT-HF Study Group. (1999). Effect of metoprolol CR/XL in chronic heart failure: Metoprolol CR/XL Randomised Intervention Trial in Congestive Heart Failure (MERIT-HF). *Lancet, 353*(9169), 2001–2007.

38. van Veldhuisen D. J., Van Gelder I. C., Ahmed A., et al. (2013). Digoxin for patients with atrial fibrillation and heart failure: Paradise lost or not? *European Heart Journal, 34*(20), 1468–1470.

39. Stoltzfus S. (2006). The role of noninvasive ventilation: CPAP and BiPAP in the treatment of congestive heart failure. *Dimensions of Critical Care Nursing, 25*(2), 66–70.

40. Bendjelid K., Schutz N., Suter P. M., et al. (2005). Does continuous positive airway pressure by face mask improve patients with acute cardiogenic pulmonary edema due to left ventricular diastolic dysfunction? *Chest, 127*(3), 1053–1056.

41. Freeman J. V., Masoudi F. A. (2013). Effectiveness of implantable cardioverter defibrillators and cardiac resynchronization therapy in heart failure. *Heart Failure Clinic, 9*(1), 59–77.

42. Wheeldon D. R. (2003). Mechanical circulatory support: State of the art and future perspectives. *Perfusion, 18*(4), 233–243.

43. Heart & Stroke Foundation. (2011). Heart transplant surgery safe and effective: Canadian retrospective spanning three decades find survival rates now close to 90 per cent. Available online at: http://www.heartandstroke.com/site/apps/nlnet/content2.aspx?c=ikIQLcMWJtE&b=7799765&ct=11300869. Accessed May 4, 2015.

44. Menasche P. (2009). Stem cell therapy for heart failure. *Circulation, 119*(20), 2735–2740.

45. Giordano A., Galderisi U., Marino I. R. (2007). From the laboratory bench to the patient's bedside: An update on clinical trials with mesenchymal stem cells. *Journal of Cell Physiology, 211*(1), 27–35.

46. Patel N. D., Barreiro C. J., Williams J. A., et al. (2005). Surgical ventricular remodeling for patients with clinically advanced congestive heart failure and severe left ventricular dysfunction. *Journal of Heart and Lung Transplantation, 24*(12), 2202–2210.

47. Manji R. A., Wood K. E., Kumar A. (2009). The history and evolution of circulatory shock. *Critical Care Clinic, 25*(1), 1–29.

48. Aymong E. D., Ramanathan K., Buller C. E. (2007). Pathophysiology of cardiogenic shock complicating acute myocardial infarction. *Medical Clinics of North America, 91*(4), 701–712.

49. Mega J. L., Morrow D. A. (2015). Chapter 52: ST-Elevation myocardial infarction: Management. In Mann D. L., Zipes D. P., Libby P., et al. *Braunwald's heart disease: A textbook of cardiovascular medicine* (10th ed.). Philadelphia, PA: Elsevier, Inc.

50. Ng R., Yeghiazarians Y. (2011). Post myocardial infarction cardiogenic shock: A review of current therapies. *Journal of Intensive Care Medicine, 28*(3), 151–165.

51. Hollenberg S. M., Kavinsky C. J., Parrillo J. E. (1999). Cardiogenic shock. *Annals of Internal Medicine, 131*(1), 47–59.

52. Ashruf J. G., Bruining H. A., Ince C. (2013). New insights into the pathophysiology of cardiogenic shock: The role of the microcirculation. *Current Opinion in Critical Care, 19*(5), 381–386.

53. Aaronson K. D., Pagani F. D. (2015). Chapter 29: Mechanical circulatory support. In Mann D. L., Zipes D. P., Libby P., et al. *Braunwald's heart disease: A textbook of cardiovascular medicine* (10th ed.). Philadelphia, PA: Elsevier, Inc.

54. American College of Emergency Physicians; Society for Cardiovascular Angiography and Interventions, O'Gara P. T., Kushner F. G., et al. (2013). 2013 ACCF/AHA Guideline for the Management of ST-Elevation Myocardial Infarction. *Journal of the American College of Cardiology, 61*(4), e78–e140.

55. Wang J., Liang T., Louis L., et al. (2013). Hypovolemic shock complex in the trauma setting: A pictorial review. *Canadian Association of Radiologists Journal, 64*(2), 156–163.

56. Dutton R. P. (2007). Current concepts in hemorrhagic shock. *Anesthesiology Clinics, 25*(1), 23–34.

57. Landry D. W., Oliver J. A. (2001). The pathogenesis of vasodilatory shock. *New England Journal of Medicine, 345*(8), 588–595.

58. Lieberman P., Nicklas R. A., Oppenheimer J., et al. (2010). The diagnosis and management of anaphylaxis practice parameter: 2010 update. *Journal of Allergy and Clinical and Immunology, 126*(3), 477–480.

59. Brown S. G. (2007). The pathophysiology of shock in anaphylaxis. *Immunology and Allergy Clinics of North America, 27*(2), 165–175.

60. Simons F. E. (2010). Anaphylaxis. *Journal of Allergy and Clinical Immunology, 125*(Suppl 2), S161–S181.

61. Stankiewicz J., Ruta W., Gorski P. (1995). Latex allergy. *International Journal of Occupational Medicine and Environmental Health, 8*(2), 139–148.

62. Dellinger R. P., Levy M. M., Rhoades A., et al. (2008). Surviving sepsis campaign: International guidelines for management of severe sepsis and septic shock: 2012. *Critical Care Medicine, 41*(2), 580–637.

63. Nguyen H. B., Rivers E. P., Abrahamian F. M. (2006). Severe sepsis and septic shock: Review of the literature and emergency department management guidelines. *Annals of Emergency Medicine, 48*(1), 28–54.

64. Russell J. A. (2006). Management of sepsis. *New England Journal of Medicine, 355*(16), 1699–1713.

65. Canadian Institute for Health Information (CIHI). (2009). *In focus: A national look at sepsis.* Ottawa: CIHI.

66. Schulte W., Bernhagen J., Bucala R. (2013). Cytokines in sepsis: Potent immunoregulators and potential therapeutic targets–an updated view. *Mediators of Inflammation, 2013*, 165974.

67. Angus D. C., van der Poll T. (2013). Severe sepsis and septic shock. *New England Journal of Medicine, 369*(9), 840–851.

68. Rivers E. P., McIntyre L., Morro D. C., et al. (2005). Early and innovative interventions for severe sepsis and septic shock: Taking advantage of the window of opportunity. *CMAJ : Canadian Medical Association journal = journal de l'Association medicale canadienne, 173*(9), 1054–1065.

69. Weiss A. J., Mchanick J. I. (2011). Glycemic control: How tight in the intensive care unit? *Seminars of Thoracic Surgery, 23*(1), 1–4.

70. Smith J. J., Kampine J. P. (1980). *Circulatory physiology* (p. 298). Baltimore, MD: Williams & Wilkins.

71. Balk R. A. (2000). Pathogenesis and management of multiple organ dysfunction or failure in acute sepsis and septic shock. *Critical Care Clinics, 16*(2), 337–352.

72. Iba T. Saitoh D., Wada H., et al. (2014). Efficacy and bleeding risk of antithrombin supplementation in septic disseminated intravascular coagulation: A secondary survey. *Critical Care, 18*(5), 497.

73. Bernstein D. (2011). Chapter 436: Heart failure. In Kliegman R. M., Stanton B. F., St. Geme J. W., et al. (Eds.), *Nelson textbook of pediatrics* (19th ed.). Philadelphia, PA: Saunders Elsevier.

74. O'Connor M., Rosenthal D., Shaddy R. (2010). Outpatient management of pediatric heart failure. *Heart Failure Clinic, 6*(4), 515–529.

75. Simpson K., Canter C. (2012). Can adult heart failure regimens be applied to children: What works and what does not? *Current Opinion in Cardiology, 27*(2), 98–107.

76. Sundararaghavan S., Kumar R. K. (2013). Chapter 6: Heart failure in children. In Kumar R. K., Prabhu S. S., Ahamed M. Z. *IAP specialty series on pediatric cardiology* (2nd ed.). New Delhi: Jaypee Brothers Medical Publishers.

77. Berger S., Dubin A. (2010). Arrhythmogenic forms of heart failure in children. *Heart Failure Clinics, 6*(4), 471–481.

78. Rosenthal D., Chrisant M., Edens E., et al. (2004). International Society for Heart and Lung Transplantation: Practice guidelines for management of heart failure in children. *Journal of Heart and Lung Transplantation, 23*(12), 1313–1333.

79. Thomas S., Rich M. W. (2007). Epidemiology, pathophysiology, and prognosis of heart failure in the elderly. *Clinics in Geriatric Medicine, 23*(1), 1–10.

80. Schwartz J. B., Zipes D. P. (2015). Chapter 76: Cardiovascular disease in the elderly. In Mann D. L., Zipes D. P., Libby P., et al. *Braunwald's heart disease: A textbook of cardiovascular medicine* (10th ed.). Philadelphia, PA: Elsevier, Inc.

81. Rich M. W. (2006). Heart failure in older adults. *Medical Clinics of North America, 90*(5), 863–885.

Visit thePoint **http://thePoint.lww.com for animations, journal articles, and more!**

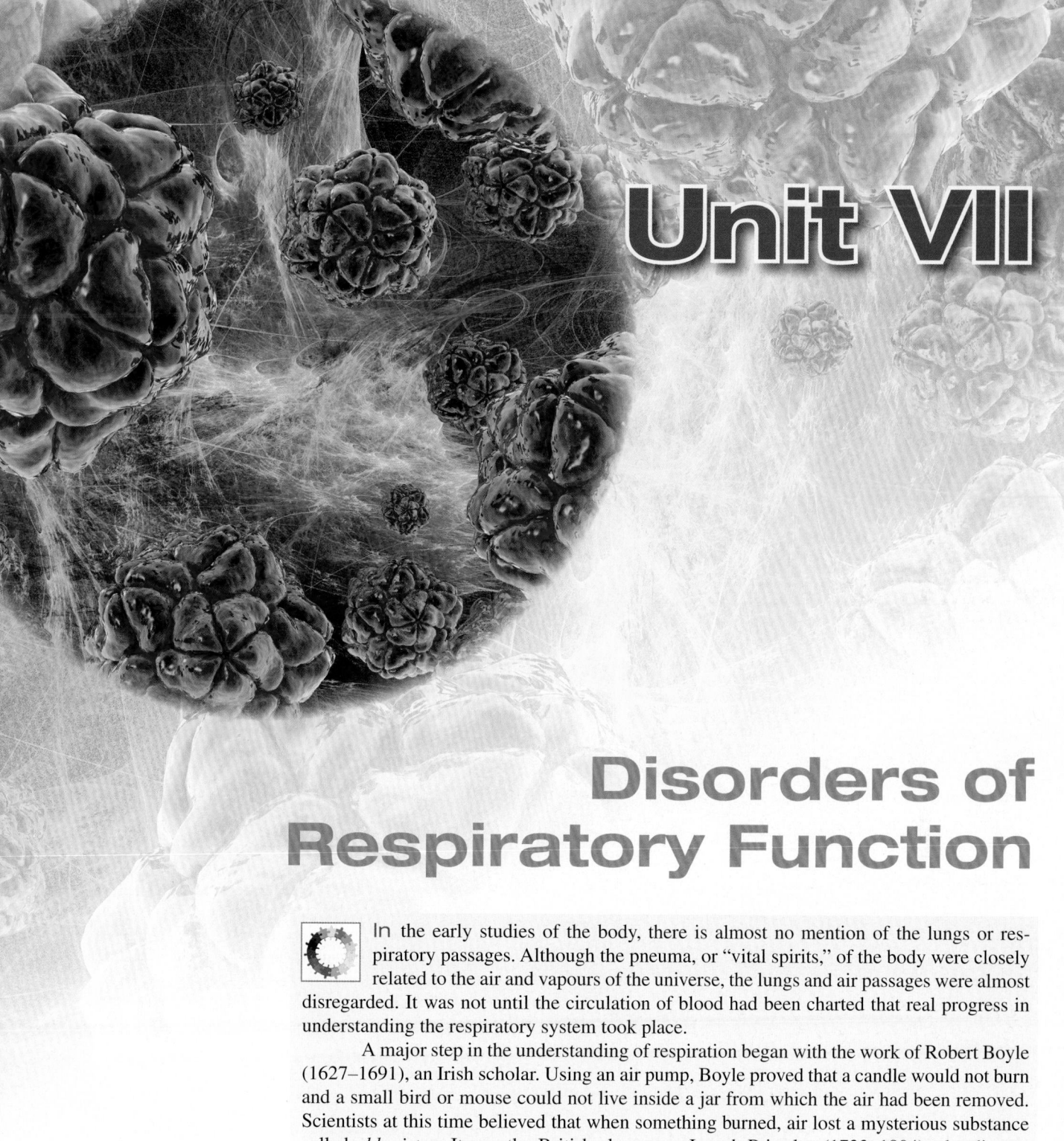

Unit VII

Disorders of Respiratory Function

In the early studies of the body, there is almost no mention of the lungs or respiratory passages. Although the pneuma, or "vital spirits," of the body were closely related to the air and vapours of the universe, the lungs and air passages were almost disregarded. It was not until the circulation of blood had been charted that real progress in understanding the respiratory system took place.

A major step in the understanding of respiration began with the work of Robert Boyle (1627–1691), an Irish scholar. Using an air pump, Boyle proved that a candle would not burn and a small bird or mouse could not live inside a jar from which the air had been removed. Scientists at this time believed that when something burned, air lost a mysterious substance called *phlogiston*. It was the British clergyman Joseph Priestley (1733–1804) who discovered that a gas made by heating oxide of mercury supported combustion. He called this gas, which later became known as oxygen, *dephlogisticated* air. Priestley showed that a mouse lived longer in a given volume of dephlogisticated air than it did in ordinary air. Antoine Lavoisier (1743–1794), a French chemist, confirmed that oxygen was present in inspired air and carbon dioxide in expired air and gave oxygen its name. In 1791, just 16 years after Priestley's discovery of oxygen, it was shown that blood contained both oxygen and carbon dioxide. From this point on, a detailed understanding of the respiratory system and its function proceeded rapidly.

Unit VII

Disorders of Respiratory Function

Structure and Function of the Respiratory System

27

Ventilation is the movement of air into and out of the lungs whereas respiration is the exchange and transport of oxygen and carbon dioxide. Exchange of these gases occurs at both the lung and tissue levels. Exchange of gases at the tissues is directly related to the consumption of oxygen and production of carbon dioxide by the mitochondria, referred to as cellular respiration or oxidative metabolism. The main focus of the respiratory system at the lung level is gas exchange at the alveoli and capillary level. Air is conducted to the respiratory zone of the lungs where oxygen diffuses into the capillary and carbon dioxide diffuses from the capillary into the alveoli. In addition to gas exchange, the lungs serve as a host defence by providing a barrier between the external environment and the inside of the body. The lung is also a metabolic organ that synthesizes and metabolizes different compounds.

This chapter focuses on the structural organization of the respiratory system; exchange of gases between the atmosphere and the lungs; exchange of gases in the lungs and its transport in the blood; and control of breathing. For discussion of the function of the red blood cell in the transport of oxygen see Chapter 14, and for discussion of the utilization of oxygen for cellular respiration see Chapter 4.

STRUCTURAL ORGANIZATION OF THE RESPIRATORY SYSTEM

After completing this section of the chapter, you should be able to meet the following objectives:

- Compare differences in function between the conducting and the respiratory airways.
- Describe the movement of air between the airways and alveoli, beginning in the nose and oropharynx.
- Describe the function of the mucociliary system.
- Compare the supporting structures of the large and small airways, including cartilage and smooth muscle.
- State the function of the two types of alveolar cells.
- Differentiate the function of the bronchial and pulmonary circulations that supply the lungs.

The respiratory system consists of the air passages, the two lungs, the blood vessels that supply them, and the structures that provide a ventilator mechanism that exchanges air between the respiratory zone and the atmosphere. The structures for ventilation include the rib cage and the respiratory muscles, of which the diaphragm is the principal respiratory muscle. Functionally, the airways can be divided into two types or zones: the *conducting zone,* which are the airways through which air moves as it passes between the atmosphere, and the *respiratory zone* in the final airways and the alveoli, where gas exchange occurs.

The lungs are soft, spongy, cone-shaped organs located side by side in the chest cavity (Fig. 27.1). They are separated from each other by the *mediastinum* (*i.e.,* the space between the lungs) and its contents—the heart, blood vessels, lymph nodes, nerve fibres, thymus gland, and esophagus. The upper part of the lung, which lies against the top of the thoracic cavity, is called the *apex,* and the lower part, which lies against the diaphragm, is called the *base.* The lungs are divided into lobes: three in the right lung and two in the left.

Conducting Airways

The conducting airways consist of the nasal passages, mouth and pharynx, larynx, trachea, bronchi, and bronchioles (Fig. 27.1).

CONDUCTING AND RESPIRATORY AIRWAYS

- Respiration requires ventilation, or movement of gases into and out of the lungs; perfusion, or movement of blood through the lungs; and diffusion of gases between the lungs and the blood.
- Ventilation depends on the conducting airways, including the nasopharynx and oropharynx, larynx, and tracheobronchial tree, which move air into and out of the lungs but do not participate in gas exchange.
- Gas exchange takes place in the respiratory airways zone of the lungs, where gases diffuse across the alveolar-capillary membrane as they are exchanged between the air in the lungs and the blood that flows through the pulmonary capillaries.

Besides functioning as a conduit for airflow, the conducting airways serve to "condition" the inspired air. The air we breathe is warmed, filtered, and moistened as it moves through these structures. Heat is transferred to the air from the blood flowing through the walls of the respiratory passages. The mucociliary

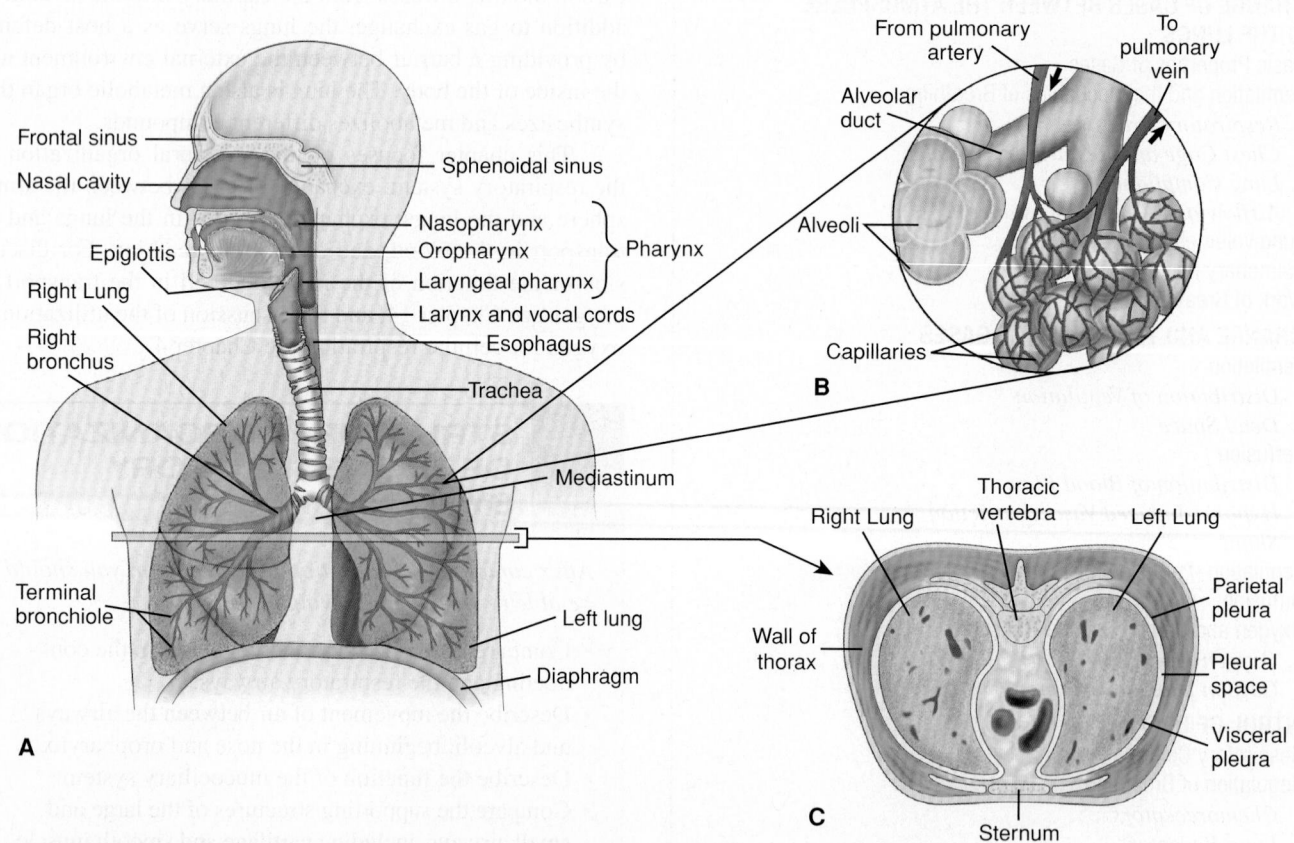

FIGURE 27.1 • The respiratory system. (**A**) Upper respiratory structures and the structures of the thorax, (**B**) alveoli, and (**C**) a horizontal cross-section of the lungs. (From Smeltzer C., Bare B. G., Hinkle J. L., et al. (2009). *Brunner & Siddarth's textbook of medical-surgical nursing* (12th ed., p. 488). Philadelphia, PA: Lippincott Williams & Wilkins.)

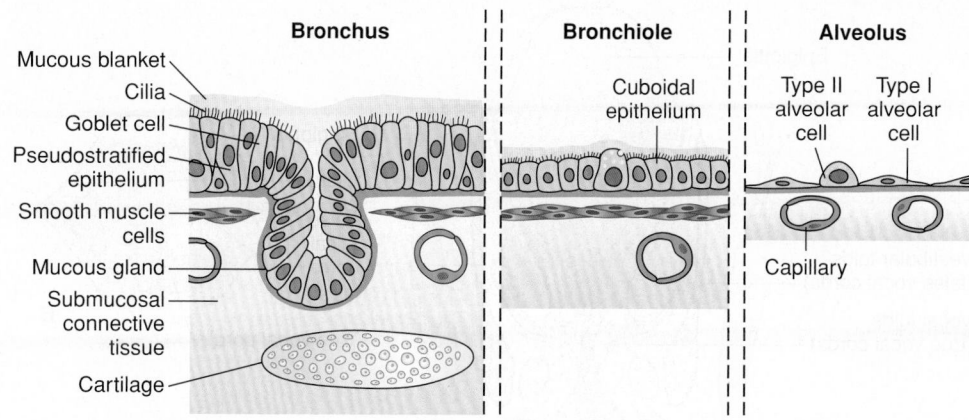

FIGURE 27.2 • Airway wall structure: bronchus, bronchiole, and alveolus. The bronchial wall contains pseudostratified epithelium, smooth muscle cells, mucous glands, connective tissue, and cartilage. In smaller bronchioles, a simple epithelium is found, cartilage is absent, and the wall is thinner. The alveolar wall is designed for gas exchange, rather than structural support. (From Porth, C. M. (2011). *Essential of pathophysiology* (3rd ed., p. 515). Philadelphia, PA: Lippincott Williams & Wilkins.)

blanket removes foreign materials, and water from the mucous membranes is used to moisten the air as it passes. Gas exchange does not occur in the conducting airways.

A combination of cartilage, elastic and collagen fibres, and smooth muscle provides the conducting airways with the combination of rigidity and flexibility needed to maintain airway patency and ensure an uninterrupted supply of air. Most of the conducting airways are lined with ciliated pseudostratified columnar epithelium, containing a mosaic of mucus-secreting glands, ciliated cells with hairlike projection, and serous glands that secrete a watery fluid containing antibacterial enzymes (Fig. 27.2). The epithelial layer gradually becomes thinner as it moves from the pseudostratified epithelium of the bronchi to the cuboidal epithelium of the bronchioles and then to the squamous epithelium of the alveoli.

The mucus produced by the epithelial cells in the conducting airways forms a layer called the *mucociliary system or blanket,* that protects the respiratory system by entrapping dust, bacteria, and other foreign particles that enter the airways. The cilia, which are in constant motion, move the mucus with its entrapped particles in an escalator-like fashion toward the oropharynx, where it is then expectorated or swallowed. The function of cilia in clearing the airways is optimal at normal oxygen levels and is impaired when oxygen levels are higher or lower than normal. It is also impaired by drying conditions, such as breathing heated but unhumidified indoor air during the winter months. Cigarette smoking slows down or paralyzes the motility of the cilia. This slowing allows the residue from tobacco smoke, dust, and other particles to accumulate in the lungs, decreasing the efficiency of this pulmonary defence system. As discussed in Chapter 29, these changes are thought to contribute to the development of chronic bronchitis and emphysema.

The conducting airways are kept moist by water contained in the mucous membranes of the upper airways and the tracheobronchial tree. The capacity of the air to contain moisture without condensation increases as the temperature rises. Thus, the air in the alveoli, which is maintained at body temperature, usually contains considerably more moisture than the atmosphere-temperature air that we breathe. The difference between the moisture contained in the air we breathe and that found in the alveoli is drawn from the moist surface of the mucous membranes that line the conducting airways and is a source of insensible water loss. Under normal conditions, approximately 500 ml of water per day is lost in humidifying the air breathed. When a person has a fever, water vapour in the lungs increases, causing more water to be lost from the respiratory mucosa. An increase in respiratory rate, tidal volume, or both will also increase the amount of air needing to be moisturized, which may be difficult to maintain. For example, fever, often accompanied by an increase in respiratory rate, may result in thicker respiratory secretions, which prevents free movement of the cilia and impairs the protective function of the mucociliary defence system. This is particularly true in persons whose water intake is inadequate or who are dehydrated.

Nasopharyngeal Airways

The nose is the preferred route for the entrance of air into the respiratory tract during normal breathing. As air passes through the nasal passages, it is filtered, warmed, and humidified. The outer nasal passages are lined with coarse hairs, which filter and trap dust and other large particles from the air. The upper portion of the nasal cavity is lined with a mucous membrane that contains a rich network of small blood vessels; this portion of the nasal cavity supplies warmth and moisture to the air from the air we breathe.

The mouth serves as an alternative airway when the nasal passages are plugged or when there is a need for the exchange of large amounts of air, as occurs during exercise. The oropharynx extends posteriorly from the soft palate to the epiglottis. The oropharynx is the only opening between the nose and mouth and the lungs. Both swallowed food on its way to the esophagus and air on its way to the larynx pass through it. Obstruction of the oropharynx leads to immediate cessation of ventilation. Neural control of the tongue and pharyngeal muscles may be impaired in coma and other neurologic disorders. In these conditions, the tongue falls back into the pharynx and obstructs the airway, particularly if the person is lying on his or her back. The presence of a foreign body or swelling of the pharyngeal structures caused by injury, infection, or severe allergic reaction also predispose a person to airway obstruction.

FIGURE 27.3 • **A:** Coronal section showing the position of the epiglottis, vestibular folds (true vocal cords), vocal folds (false vocal cords), and glottis. **(B)** Vocal cords viewed from above with glottis closed, and **(C)** with glottis open.

Larynx

The larynx connects the oropharynx with the trachea. The walls of the larynx are supported by firm cartilaginous structures that prevent collapse. The functions of the larynx can be divided into two categories: those associated with speech and those associated with protecting the lungs from substances other than air.

The cavity of the larynx is divided into two pairs of shelf-like folds stretching from front to back with an opening in the midline (Fig. 27.3). The upper pair of folds, called the *vestibular folds,* has a protective function. The lower pair of folds, called the *vocal folds,* produces the vibrations required for making vocal sounds. The vocal folds and the elongated opening between them are called the *glottis.* A complex set of muscles controls the opening and closing of the glottis. The *epiglottis,* which is located above the larynx, is a large, leaf-shaped piece of cartilage that is covered with epithelium. When only air is flowing through the larynx, the inlet of the larynx is open and the free edges of the epiglottis point upward. During swallowing, the larynx is pulled superiorly and the free edges of the epiglottis move downward to cover the larynx, thus routing liquids and foods into the esophagus.

In addition to opening and closing the glottis for speech, the vocal folds of the larynx can perform a sphincter function, closing off the airways. When confronted with substances other than air, the laryngeal muscles contract and close off the airway. At the same time, the cough reflex is initiated as a means of removing a foreign substance from the airway. If the swallowing mechanism is partially or totally paralyzed, food and fluids can enter the airways instead of the esophagus when a person attempts to swallow. These substances are not easily removed and when they are pulled into the lungs, they can result in a condition called *aspiration.*

Tracheobronchial Tree

The tracheobronchial tree, which consists of the trachea, bronchi, and bronchioles, can be viewed as a system of branching airways. It is similar to a tree whose branches become smaller and more numerous as they divide (Fig. 27.4A). There are approximately 23 levels or generations of branching, beginning with the conducting airways and ending with the respiratory airways and alveoli, where gas exchange takes place (Fig. 27.4B).

The trachea, commonly referred to as the "windpipe," connects the larynx and the major bronchi of the lungs. The walls of the trachea are supported by horseshoe- or C-shaped rings of hyaline cartilage, which prevent it from collapsing when the pressure in the thorax becomes negative (Fig. 27.5). The open part of the C ring, which is anterior to the esophagus, is connected by smooth muscle. Since this portion of the trachea is not rigid, the esophagus can expand anteriorly as swallowed food passes through it.

The trachea extends to the superior border of the fifth thoracic vertebra, where it divides to form the right and left main or primary bronchi. Between the main bronchi is a keel-like ridge, called the *carina* (Fig. 27.6A). The mucosa of the carina is highly sensitive and has numerous irritant receptors; extensive coughing is initiated when a foreign object (*e.g.,* suction catheter, food particles) makes contact with it. The structure of the primary bronchi is similar to that of the trachea in that these airways are lined with a mucosal surface and supported by cartilaginous rings. Each primary bronchus, accompanied by the pulmonary arteries, veins, and lymph vessels, enters the lung through a slit called the *hilum.*

Each primary bronchus divides into secondary or lobular bronchi that supply each of the lobes of the lung—three in the right lung and two in the left (Fig. 27.6B). The right middle lobe bronchus is of relatively small diameter and length and

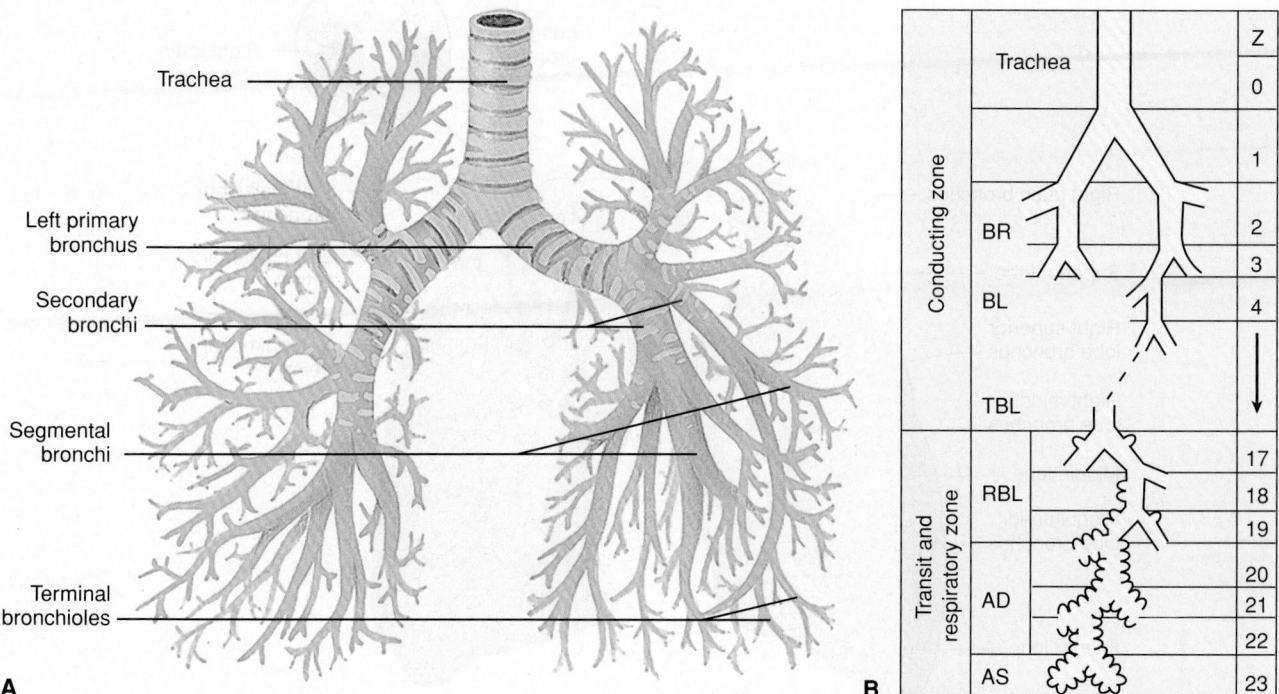

FIGURE 27.4 • A: Conducting and respiratory air pathways inferior to the larynx. (From The Anatomical Chart Company. (2001) *Atlas of Human Anatomy.* Springhouse, PA: Springhouse; 175.) **B:** Idealization of the human airways. The first 16 generations of branching (Z) make up the conducting airways, and the last 7 constitute the respiratory zone (or transitional and respiratory zone). BR, bronchus; BL, bronchiole; TBL, terminal bronchiole; RBL, respiratory bronchiole; AD, alveolar ducts; AS, alveolar sacs. (From Weibel E. R. (1962). *Morphometry of the human lung* (p. 111). Berlin, Germany: Springer-Verlag.)

FIGURE 27.5 • Cross-section of the trachea, illustrating its relationship to the esophagus, the position of the supporting hyaline cartilage rings in its wall, and the trachealis muscle connecting the free ends of the cartilage rings.

sometimes bends sharply near its bifurcation. It is surrounded by a collar of lymph nodes that drain the middle and the lower lobe, and is particularly subject to obstruction. The secondary bronchi, in turn, divide to form the segmental bronchi, which supply the bronchopulmonary segments of the lung. There are 10 segments on the right lung and 9 on the left (Fig. 27.7). These segments are identified according to their location in the lung (*e.g.*, the apical segment of the right upper lobe) and are the smallest named units in the lung. Lung disorders including atelectasis and pneumonia are often localized to a particular bronchopulmonary segment. The structure of the secondary and segmental bronchi is similar, for the most part, to that of the primary bronchi; however, the C-shaped cartilage rings are replaced by irregular plates of hyaline cartilage that completely surround the lumina of the bronchi, and there are two layers of smooth muscle spiralling in opposite directions (Fig. 27.8).

The segmental bronchi continue to branch, forming smaller bronchi, until they become the terminal bronchioles, the smallest of the conducting airways. As these bronchi branch and become smaller, their wall structure changes. The cartilage gradually decreases and there is an increase in smooth muscle and elastic tissue (with respect to the thickness of the wall). By the time the bronchioles are reached,

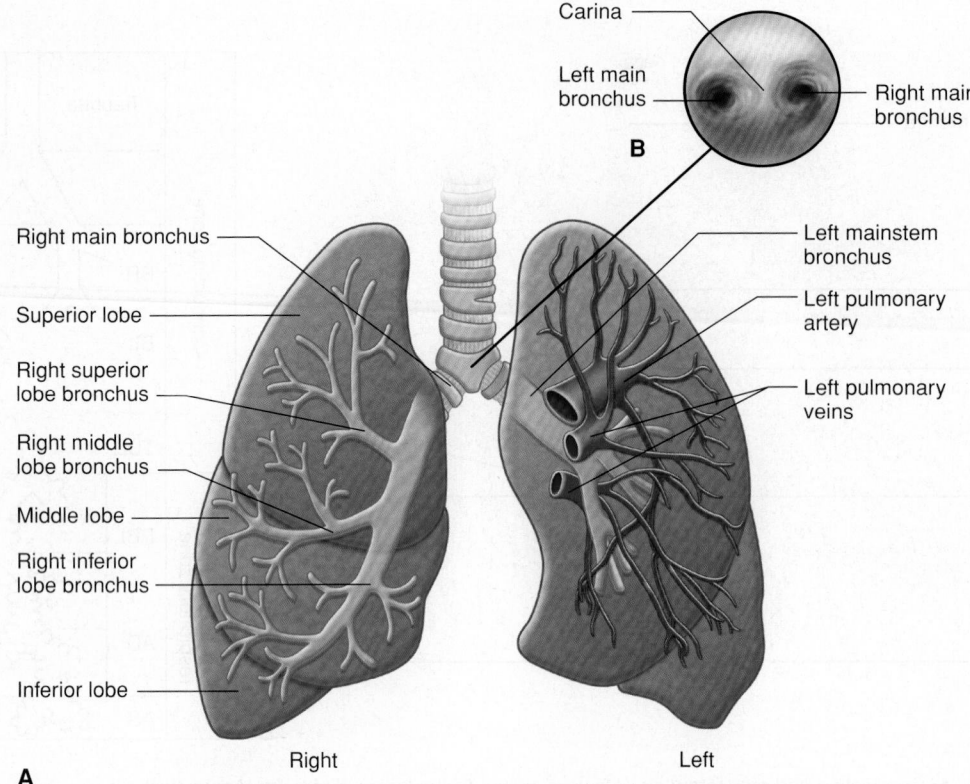

FIGURE 27.6 • **A:** Anterior view of respiratory structures, including the lobes of the lung, the larynx, the trachea, and the main bronchi on the left and the main pulmonary artery and vein on the right. **B:** The carina is located at the bifurcation of the right and left mainstem bronchi.

FIGURE 27.7 • Bronchopulmonary segments of the human lung. Left and right upper lobes: (**1**) apical, (**2**) posterior, (**3**) anterior, (**4**) superior lingular, and (**5**) inferior lingular segments. Right middle lobe: (**4**) lateral and (**5**) medial segments. Lower lobes: (**6**) superior (apical), (**7**) medial-basal, (**8**) anterior-basal, (**9**) lateral-basal, and (**10**) posterior-basal segments. The medial-basal segment (**7**) is absent in the left lung. (From Fishman A. P. (1980). *Assessment of pulmonary function* (p. 19). New York: McGraw-Hill.)

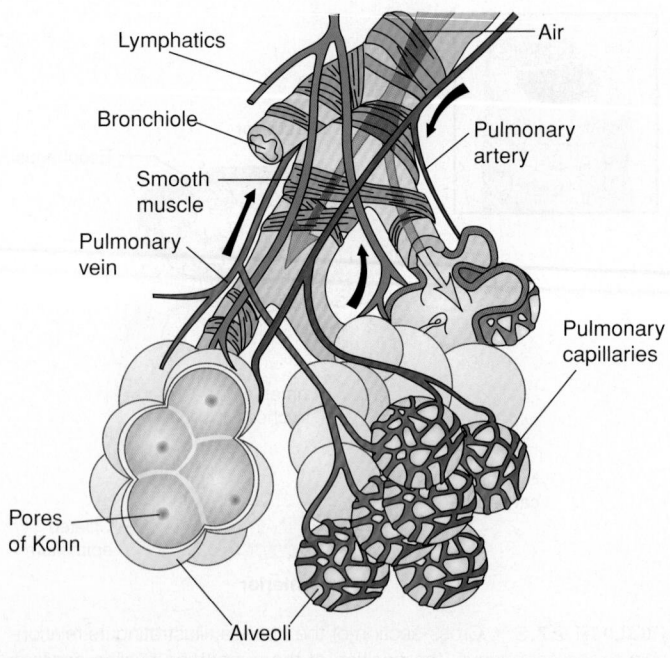

FIGURE 27.8 • Lobule of the lung, showing the bronchial smooth muscle fibres, pulmonary blood vessels, and lymphatics.

there is no cartilage present and their walls are composed mainly of smooth muscle and elastic fibres. Contraction of the smooth muscles causes narrowing of the bronchioles, referred to as bronchoconstriction, which impairs air flow. The elastic fibres, which radiate from the outer layer of the bronchial wall and connect with elastic fibres arising from other parts of the bronchial tree, exert tension on the bronchial walls. By pulling uniformly in all directions, the elastic fibres increase air flow on inspiration and help to maintain airway patency.

Lungs and Respiratory Airways

Gas exchange occurs in the lobules of the lungs. Each lobule, which is the smallest functional unit of the lung, is supplied by a branch of a terminal bronchiole, an arteriole, the pulmonary capillaries, and a venule (Fig. 27.8). Gas exchange takes place in the terminal respiratory bronchioles and the alveolar ducts and sacs, referred to as the respiratory zone. Blood enters the lobules through a pulmonary artery and exits through a pulmonary vein. Lymphatic structures surround the lobule and aid in the removal of plasma proteins and other particles from the interstitial spaces.

Unlike the larger bronchi, the respiratory bronchioles are lined with simple epithelium rather than ciliated pseudostratified epithelium (Fig. 27.2). The respiratory bronchioles also lack the cartilaginous support of the larger airways. Instead, they are attached to the elastic spongelike tissue that contains the alveolar air spaces.

In addition to their gas exchange function, the lungs have other functions. The pulmonary vascular system is the primary location where angiotensin I is converted to angiotensin II. Heparin-producing cells are particularly abundant in the capillaries of the lung. Vasoactive substances, such as bradykinin, are inactivated within the lungs and they serve also as a reservoir for blood storage.

Alveoli

The alveoli are the terminal air spaces of the respiratory tract and the primary site of gas exchange between the air and the blood. Each alveolus is a small outpouching of respiratory bronchioles, alveolar ducts, and alveolar sacs (Fig. 27.8). The alveolar sacs are cup-shaped, thin-walled structures that are separated from each other by thin alveolar septa. A single network of capillaries occupies most of the septa, so blood is exposed to alveolar air on both sides of the capillary. There are approximately 200 to 300 million alveoli in the adult lung, with a total surface area of approximately 50 to 100 m². Unlike the bronchioles, which are tubes with their own separate walls, the alveoli are interconnecting spaces that have no separate walls (Fig. 27.9). As a result of this arrangement, there is a continual mixing of air in the alveolar structures. Small holes in the alveolar walls, the pores of Kohn, also contribute to the mixing of air.

The alveolar epithelium is composed of two types of cells: type I and type II alveolar cells (Fig. 27.10). The alveoli also contain brush cells and macrophages. The brush cells, which

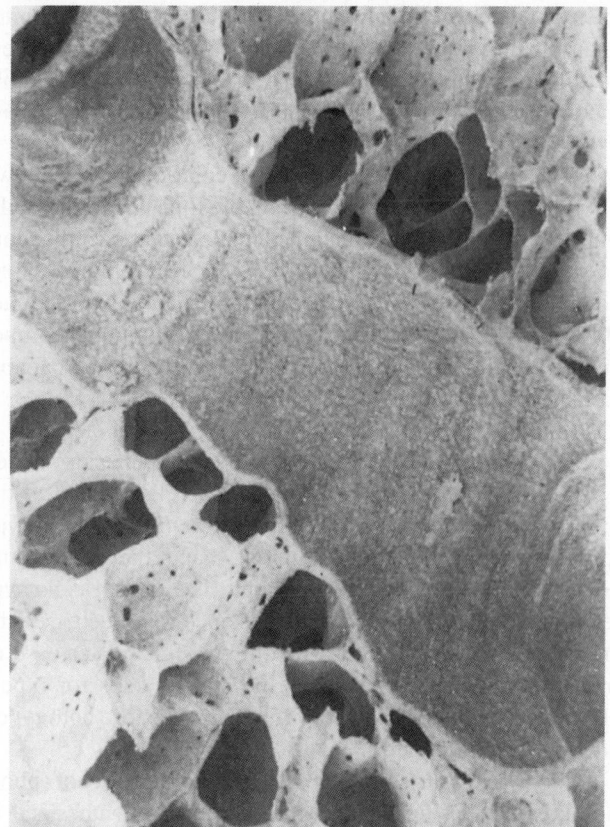

FIGURE 27.9 • Close-up of a cross-section of a small bronchus and surrounding alveoli. (Courtesy of Janice A. Nowell, University of California, Santa Cruz.)

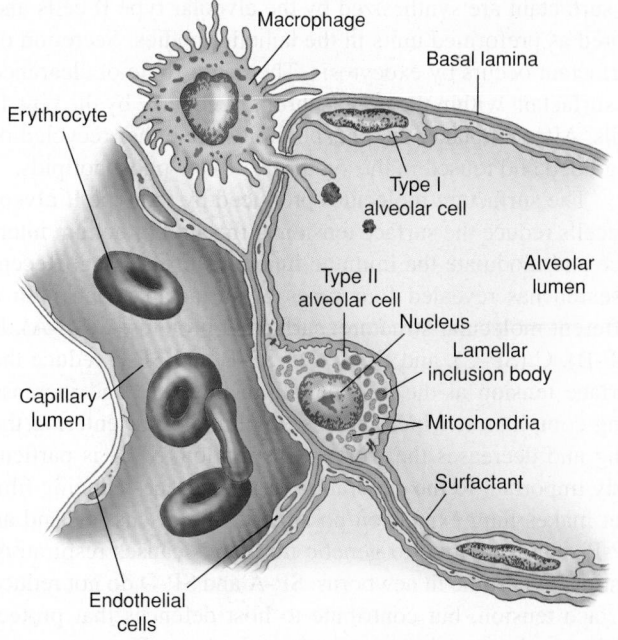

FIGURE 27.10 • Schematic illustration of type I and type II alveolar cells and their relationship to the alveoli and pulmonary capillaries. Type I alveolar cells comprise most of the alveolar surface. Type II alveolar cells, which produce surfactant, are located at the corners between adjacent alveoli. Also shown are the endothelial cells, which line the pulmonary capillaries, and an alveolar macrophage.

are few in number, are thought to act as receptors that monitor the air quality of the lungs. The macrophages, which are present in both the alveolar lumen and the septum of the alveoli, function to remove foreign substances from the alveoli.

Type I Alveolar Cells. The type I alveolar cells, also known as *type I pneumocytes,* are extremely thin squamous cells with a thin cytoplasm and flattened nucleus that occupy about 95% of the surface area of the alveoli. They are joined to one another and to other cells by occluding junctions. These junctions form an effective barrier between the air and the components of the alveolar wall. Type I alveolar cells are not capable of cell division.

Type II Alveolar Cells. The type II alveolar cells, also called *type II pneumocytes,* are small cuboidal cells located at the corners of the alveoli. Type II cells are as numerous as type I cells, but because of their different shape, they cover only about 5% of the alveolar surface area. The type II cells synthesize pulmonary surfactant, a substance that decreases the surface tension in the alveoli and allows for greater ease of lung inflation. They are also the progenitor cells for type I cells. After lung injury, they proliferate and restore both type I and type II alveolar cells.

Pulmonary surfactant is a complex mixture of phospholipids, neutral lipids, and proteins that is synthesized in the type II alveolar cells. Type II alveolar cells have numerous mitochondria and are metabolically active. Their apical cytoplasm contains stacks of parallel membrane sheets or lamellae, called the lamellar bodies. All of the components of surfactant are synthesized by the alveolar type II cells and stored as preformed units in the lamellar bodies. Secretion of surfactant occurs by exocytosis. The major route of clearance of surfactant within the lung is through reuptake by the type II cells. After reuptake, the phospholipids are either recycled or degraded and reused in the synthesis of new phospholipids.

The surfactant molecules produced by the type II alveolar cells reduce the surface tension at the air–epithelium interface and modulate the immune functions of the lung. Recent research has revealed four types of surfactant, each with a different molecular structure: surfactant proteins A (SP-A), B (SP-B), C (SP-C), and D (SP-D). SP-B and SP-C reduce the surface tension at the air–epithelium interface and increase lung compliance, which increases volume of air entering the lung and decreases the work of inspiration. SP-B is particularly important to the generation of the surface-reducing film that makes lung expansion possible (to be discussed) and an SP-B deficiency due to genetic mutations causes respiratory distress syndrome in newborns. SP-A and SP-D do not reduce surface tension, but contribute to host defences that protect against pathogens that have entered the lung. They are members of the collecting protein family that function as a part of the innate immune system (see Chapter 17). Collectively, they opsonize pathogens, including bacteria and viruses, to facilitate phagocytosis by macrophages. They also regulate the production of inflammatory mediators. Evidence also suggests that SP-A and SP-D are directly bactericidal, meaning they can kill bacteria in the absence of immune system effector cells.

Alveolar Macrophages. The macrophages, which are present in both the connective tissue of the septum and in the air spaces of the alveolus, are responsible for the removal of foreign substances from the alveoli. In the air spaces, they scavenge the surface to remove inhaled particulate matter, such as dust and pollen. Some macrophages move up the bronchial tree in the mucus and are disposed of by swallowing or coughing when they reach the pharynx. Others enter the septal connective tissue, where, filled with phagocytosed materials, they remain for life. Thus, at autopsy, smokers and urban dwellers usually show many alveolar macrophages filled with carbon and other polluting particles from the environment. The alveolar macrophages also phagocytose insoluble infectious agents such as *Mycobacterium tuberculosis.* The activated macrophages then aggregate to form a fibrin-encapsulated granuloma, called a *tubercle,* to contain the infection. The tubercle bacillus can remain dormant in this stage or be reactivated years later, when the person's immunologic tolerance wanes as the result of old age or immunosuppressive disease or therapy (see Chapter 28).

Pulmonary Vasculature and Lymphatic Supply

Pulmonary and Bronchial Circulations

The lungs are provided with a dual blood supply, the pulmonary and bronchial circulations. The pulmonary circulation arises from the pulmonary artery and provides for the gas exchange function of the lungs (Fig. 27.6). Blood that returns to the right atrium via the vena cava from the tissues has a lower oxygen content and is referred to as "deoxygenated." Deoxygenated blood leaves the right ventricle via the main pulmonary artery or pulmonary trunk, which quickly divides into a left pulmonary artery that enters the left lung and a right pulmonary artery that enters the right lung. As blood moves through the lungs, oxygen is picked up at the capillaries, and oxygenated blood is returned to the left side of the heart by the pulmonary veins, which empty into the left atrium. Oxygenated blood is subsequently pumped out into the systemic circulation by the left ventricle via the aorta. Other than in the fetus, where the umbilical artery carries deoxygenated blood and the umbilical vein oxygenated blood, the pulmonary circulation is the only portion of the circulation where arteries carry deoxygenated blood and veins carry oxygenated blood.

The bronchial circulation distributes blood to the conducting airways and the supporting structures of the lung. The bronchial circulation has a secondary function of warming and humidifying incoming air as it moves through the conducting airways. The bronchial arteries arise from the thoracic aorta and enter the lungs with the major bronchi, dividing and subdividing along with the bronchi as they move out into the lung, supplying them and other lung structures with oxygen.

The blood from the capillaries in the bronchial circulation drains into the bronchial veins, with the blood from the larger bronchial veins emptying into the vena cava. Blood from the smaller bronchial veins empties into the pulmonary veins. Because the bronchial circulation does not participate in gas exchange, this blood is deoxygenated. Although small in terms of volume, this deoxygenated blood slightly decreases the amount of oxygen in the blood returning to the left side of the heart through the pulmonary veins. This volume of blood that enters the left ventricle without being oxygenated is referred to as a normal or physiological shunt.

In the pulmonary circulation the bronchial blood vessels are the only ones that can undergo angiogenesis (formation of new vessels) and develop collateral circulation when vessels in the pulmonary circulation are obstructed, as in pulmonary embolism. If the pulmonary embolism is small or develops over time, the development of new blood vessels helps to keep lung tissue viable until the pulmonary circulation can be restored.

Lymphatic Circulation

The lungs are also supplied with lymphatic drainage that parallels that of their dual blood supply. One set of lymph vessels, the superficial vessels, drains the surface of the lung and travels in the connective tissue of the visceral pleura. A second set of lymph vessels, the deep lymphatic vessels, follows the pulmonary arteries, pulmonary veins, and bronchial tree down to the level of the respiratory bronchioles (Fig. 27.8). Both of these systems have numerous interconnections and form networks that drain into the hilar lymph nodes at the base of each lung. Particulate matter entering the lung is partly removed through these channels, as are the plasma proteins that have escaped from the pulmonary capillaries. The latter function is particularly important in keeping the lungs dry and in preventing the accumulation of fluid in the pleural cavity.

Innervation

There is no voluntary motor innervation of the lung, nor are there pain fibres. Pain fibres are found only in the pleura. The lung is innervated by the sympathetic and parasympathetic divisions of the autonomic nervous system. It is parasympathetic stimulation, through the vagus nerve, that is responsible for the slightly constricted smooth muscle tone in the normal resting lung. Parasympathetic innervation of the lung arises from the vagal nuclei in the medulla. Stimulation of the parasympathetic nervous system leads to airway constriction and increased glandular secretion. Preganglionic fibres from the vagal nuclei descend in the vagus nerve to ganglia adjacent to the airways and blood vessels of the lung. Postganglionic fibres from the ganglia then complete the network that innervates smooth muscle, blood vessels, and epithelial cells, including the goblet and submucosal glands. Both the preganglionic and postganglionic fibres contain excitatory (cholinergic) motor neurons that respond to acetylcholine. Parasympathetic innervation is greater in the large airways and diminishes toward the smaller airways.

Stimulation of the sympathetic nervous system causes smooth muscle relaxation, which results in airway dilation (*i.e.,* bronchodilation), pulmonary blood vessel dilation, and inhibition of glandular secretion. Sympathetic innervation arises from the cell bodies in paravertebral sympathetic ganglia. Neurotransmitters of the sympathetic nervous system include the catecholamine epinephrine, which activates β_2 receptors, resulting in vascular and bronchial dilation.

Pleura

A thin, transparent, double-layered serous membrane, called the *pleura,* lines the thoracic cavity and encases the lungs (Fig. 27.1). The outer parietal layer lines the pulmonary cavities and adheres to the thoracic wall, the mediastinum, and the diaphragm. The inner visceral pleura closely covers the lung and is adherent to all its surfaces. It is continuous with the parietal pleura at the hilum of the lung, where the major bronchus and pulmonary vessels enter and leave the lung. A thin film of serous fluid separates the two pleural layers, allowing the two layers to glide over each other and yet hold together, so there is no separation between the lungs and the chest wall. Normally lymphatic drainage exceeds that of fluid production and results in pressure within the pleural cavity that is lower than atmospheric pressure, which is referred to as a negative pressure. The pleural cavity is often called the pleural space, as there is a potential space in which serous fluid or inflammatory exudate can accumulate due to an imbalance in either fluid production or lymphatic drainage. The term *pleural effusion* is used to describe an abnormal collection of fluid or exudate in the pleural cavity.

IN SUMMARY

The respiratory system consists of the airways, blood vessels, and lung tissue. Functionally, the airways of the respiratory system can be divided into two parts: the conducting zone and the respiratory zone, where gas exchange actually takes place. The conducting airways include the nasal passages, mouth and nasopharynx, larynx, and tracheobronchial tree. The air we breathe is warmed, filtered, and humidified as it passes through these structures into the respiratory zone.

The lungs are the functional structures of the respiratory system. In addition to their gas exchange function, they inactivate vasoactive substances such as bradykinin; they convert angiotensin I to angiotensin II; and they serve as a reservoir for blood. The lobules, which are the functional units of the lung, consist of the respiratory bronchioles, alveoli, and pulmonary capillaries. It is here that gas exchange takes place. Oxygen from the alveoli diffuses across the alveolar capillary membrane into the capillary, and carbon dioxide diffuses from the capillary into the alveoli. There are two types of alveolar cells: type I and type II. Type I cells, which provide the gas exchange function of the lung, are extremely thin squamous cells lining most of the surface of the alveoli. Type II cells, which produce surfactant and serve as progenitor cells for type I cells, are small cuboidal cells. There are four types of surfactant protein (SP): SP-A, SP-B, SP-C, and SP-D. SP-B and SP-C provide the surface tension-lowering properties necessary for ease of lung inflation. SP-A and SP-D modulate the immune response to foreign pathogens and participate in local inflammatory responses.

The lungs are provided with a dual blood supply: the pulmonary circulation provides for the gas exchange function of the lungs and the bronchial circulation distributes blood to the conducting airways and supporting structures of the lung. The lungs are also supplied by a dual system of lymphatic vessels: a superficial system in the visceral pleura and a deep system that supplies deeper pulmonary structures, including the respiratory bronchioles.

The lung is innervated by the sympathetic and parasympathetic divisions of the autonomic nervous system. Parasympathetic innervation causes airway constriction and an increase in respiratory secretions, whereas sympathetic innervation causes bronchial dilation and a decrease in respiratory tract secretions. There is no voluntary motor innervation of the lung, nor are there pain fibres.

The lungs are encased in a thin, transparent, double-layered serous membrane called the pleura. A thin film of serous fluid separates the outer parietal and inner visceral pleural layers, allowing the two layers to glide over each other and yet hold together, so there is no separation between the lungs and the chest wall. The pleural cavity is a potential space in which fluid or air can accumulate.

 CONCEPTS in action **ANIMATION**

EXCHANGE OF GASES BETWEEN THE ATMOSPHERE AND THE LUNGS

After completing this section of the chapter, you should be able to meet the following objectives:

- Describe the basic properties of gases in relation to partial pressures and pressures in relation to volume and temperature.
- State the definitions of intrathoracic, intrapleural, and intra-alveolar pressures, and state how each of these pressures changes in relation to atmospheric pressure during inspiration and expiration.
- Use the law of Laplace to explain the need for surfactant in maintaining the inflation of small alveoli.
- Differentiate between the determinants of airway resistance and lung compliance and their effect on the work of breathing.
- Define tidal, minute, inspiratory reserve, expiratory reserve, vital capacity, residual, total lung, and forced expiratory lung volumes.

Basic Properties of Gases

The air we breathe is comprised of a mixture of gases, water, and small particles such as dust. These substances exert a combined pressure called the *atmospheric* or *barometric pressure*. The atmospheric pressure varies, primarily in relation to altitude. The atmospheric pressure is greatest at sea level, at 760 millimetres of mercury (mm Hg, or Torr), and decreases with increases in altitude. Nitrogen makes up the largest portion of the total gases, whereas the percentage of oxygen is approximately 21%.

The pressure exerted by a single gas in a mixture is called the *partial pressure* (P) of that particular gas. Dalton's law of partial pressures states that the total pressure of a mixture of gases is equal to the sum of the partial pressures of the different gases in the mixture. The capital letter "P" followed by the chemical symbol of the gas (*e.g.*, PO_2) is used to denote the partial pressure of oxygen. The percentage of oxygen does not vary within atmospheric air, but the partial pressure exerted by oxygen is dependent upon the total atmospheric pressure. Thus, to determine the partial pressure of oxygen, one multiplies the percentage of oxygen (expressed as a fraction) with the atmospheric pressure, conventionally measured in units of mm Hg or Torr. For example, the partial pressure of oxygen (PO_2) at 760 mm Hg is 159.6 mm Hg (760×0.21), and at 700 mm Hg is 147 mm Hg (700×0.21).

Water vapour is different from other types of gases; its partial pressure is affected by temperature but not by atmospheric pressure. The relative humidity refers to the percentage of moisture in the air compared with the amount that the air can hold without causing condensation (100% saturation). Warm air holds more moisture than cold air. This is the reason that precipitation in the form of rain or snow commonly occurs when the relative humidity is high and there is a sudden drop in atmospheric temperature. The air in the alveoli, which is 100% saturated at normal body temperature, has a water vapour pressure of 47 mm Hg. Water vapour pressure is a significant part of the sum of the total pressure of the gases in the alveoli. Therefore, the total pressure of the gases in the alveoli includes nitrogen, oxygen, carbon dioxide, and water. In other words, the total pressure of the gases in the alveoli is equal to the total pressure minus the pressure of water, for example, $760 - 47 = 713$ mm Hg.

Air moves between the atmosphere and the alveoli because of pressure differences on inspiration and expiration. According to Boyle's law of physics, the pressure of a gas varies inversely with the volume of its container, provided the temperature remains constant. If equal amounts of a gas were placed in two different-sized containers, the pressure of the gas in the smaller container would be greater than the pressure in the larger container. The movement of gases is always from the container with the greater pressure to the one with the lesser pressure. The chest cavity can be viewed as a volume container. During inspiration, the size of the chest cavity increases, which causes a decrease in pressure, and air moves into the lungs. During expiration, the size of the chest cavity decreases and pressure increases, and air moves out of the lungs.

Ventilation and the Mechanics of Breathing

Ventilation is concerned with the movement of air into and out of the lungs. It is a mechanical event that obeys the laws of physics as they relate to the behaviour of gases. It relies on a system of open airways and the respiratory pressures that are created when the respiratory muscles change the size of the chest cage. The degree to which the lungs inflate and deflate depends on the difference between atmospheric and alveolar pressures, plus airway resistance.

> ### VENTILATION AND GAS EXCHANGE
>
> - Ventilation refers to the movement of gases into and out of the lungs through a system of open airways and along a pressure gradient resulting from a change in chest volume.
> - During inspiration, air is drawn into the lungs as the respiratory muscles expand the chest cavity; during expiration, air moves out of the lungs as the chest muscles recoil and the chest cavity becomes smaller.
> - The ease with which air is moved into and out of the lung depends on the resistance of the airways, which is inversely related to the fourth power of the airway radius, and lung compliance, or the ease with which the lungs can be inflated.
> - The minute volume, which is normally determined by the metabolic needs of the body, is the amount of air that is exchanged each minute. It is the product of the tidal volume or amount of air exchanged with each breath multiplied by the respiratory rate.

Respiratory Pressures

The pressure inside the airways and alveoli of the lungs is called the *intrapulmonary pressure* or *alveolar pressure*. The gases in this area of the lungs are in communication with atmospheric pressure (Fig. 27.11). When the glottis is open and air is not moving into or out of the lungs, as occurs just before inspiration or expiration, the intrapulmonary pressure is zero, or equal to atmospheric pressure.

The pressure in the pleural cavity is called the *intrapleural pressure*. The intrapleural pressure of a normal inflated lung is always negative in relation to alveolar pressure, approximately –4 mm Hg between breaths when the glottis is open and the alveolar spaces are open to the atmosphere. The lungs and the chest wall have elastic properties, each pulling in the opposite direction. If removed from the chest, the lungs would contract to a smaller size, and the chest wall, if freed from the lungs, would expand. The opposing forces of the chest wall and lungs create a pull against the visceral and parietal layers of the pleura, causing the pressure in the pleural cavity to become negative. During inspiration, the elastic recoil of the lungs increases, causing intrapleural pressure to become more negative than during expiration. Without the negative

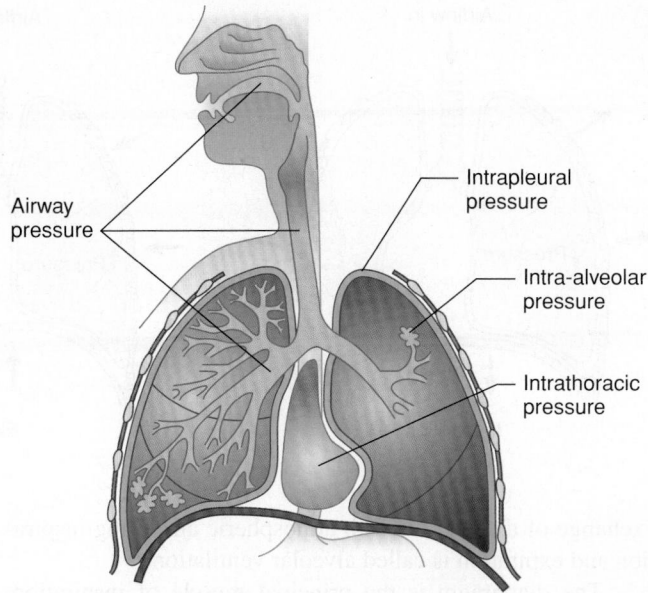

FIGURE 27.11 • Partitioning of respiratory pressures.

intrapleural pressure holding the lungs against the chest wall, their elastic recoil properties would cause them to collapse. Although intrapleural pressure is negative in relation to alveolar pressure, it may become positive in relation to atmospheric pressure (*e.g.,* during forced expiration and coughing). The *transpulmonary* (*trans* = "across") *pressure* is the difference between the alveolar and intrapleural pressures and is used in determining pulmonary compliance.

The *intrathoracic pressure* is the pressure in the thoracic cavity. It is essentially equal to the intrapleural pressure and is the pressure to which the lungs, heart, and great vessels are exposed. Forced expiration against a closed glottis, such as occurs during defecation, coughing, or the Valsalva maneuvre, produces marked increases in intrathoracic pressure and impedes venous return to the right atrium.

Chest Cage and Respiratory Muscles

The lungs and major airways share the chest cavity with the heart, great vessels, and esophagus. The chest cavity is a closed compartment with boundaries consisting of the neck muscles at the top of the cavity and the diaphragm at the bottom. The outer walls of the chest cavity are formed by 12 pairs of ribs, the sternum, the thoracic vertebrae, and the intercostal muscles that lie between the ribs. Mechanically, the act of breathing depends on the fact that the chest cavity is a closed compartment whose only opening to the external atmosphere is through the trachea.

Breathing consists of inspiration and expiration. During *inspiration,* the size of the chest cavity increases, the intrathoracic pressure becomes more negative, and air is drawn into the lungs. *Expiration* occurs as the elastic components of the chest wall and lung structures that were stretched during inspiration recoil, causing the size of the chest cavity to decrease and the pressure in the chest cavity to increase. The

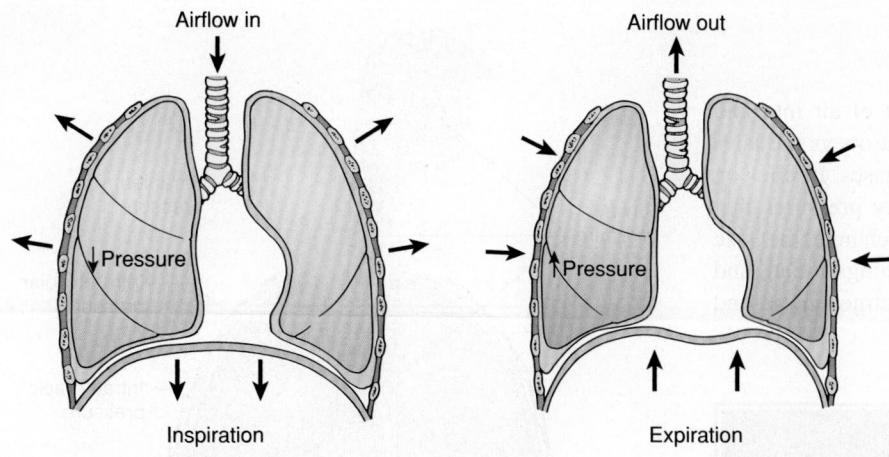

Airflow in

↓Pressure

Inspiration

Airflow out

↑Pressure

Expiration

FIGURE 27.12 • Movement of the diaphragm and changes in chest volume and pressure during inspiration and expiration. During inspiration, contraction of the diaphragm and expansion of the chest cavity produce a decrease in intrathoracic pressure, causing air to move into the lungs. During expiration, relaxation of the diaphragm and chest cavity produces an increase in intrathoracic pressure, causing air to move out of the lungs.

exchange of alveolar air with atmospheric air during inspiration and expiration is called alveolar ventilation.

The diaphragm is the principal muscle of inspiration. Inspiration is an active process requiring energy. When the diaphragm contracts, the abdominal contents are forced downward and the chest expands from top to bottom (Fig. 27.12). During normal levels of inspiration, the diaphragm moves approximately 1 cm, but this can be increased to 10 cm on forced inspiration. The diaphragm is innervated by the phrenic nerve roots, which arise from the cervical level of the spinal cord, mainly from C4 but also from C3 and C5. Persons who sustain spinal cord injury above C3 lose the function of the diaphragm and require mechanical ventilation (see Chapter 50). Paralysis of one side of the diaphragm causes the chest to move up on that side rather than down during inspiration because of the negative pressure in the chest. This is called *paradoxical movement.*

The external intercostal muscles, which also aid in inspiration, connect to the adjacent ribs and slope downward and forward (Fig. 27.13). When they contract, they raise the ribs and rotate them slightly so that the sternum is pushed forward; this enlarges the chest outward from side to side and front to back. The intercostal muscles receive their innervation from nerves that exit the central nervous system at the thoracic level of the spinal cord. Paralysis of these muscles usually does not

have a significant effect at rest because of the effectiveness of the diaphragm. However, coughing and deep inspiration may be impaired due to potentially lower tidal volumes.

The accessory muscles of inspiration include the scalene muscles and the sternocleidomastoid muscles. The scalene muscles elevate the first two ribs, and the sternocleidomastoid muscles raise the sternum to increase the size of the chest cavity. These muscles contribute little to quiet breathing but contract vigorously during exercise, during which the head commonly is bent backward so that the scalene and sternocleidomastoid muscles can elevate the ribs more effectively. Other muscles that play a minor role in inspiration are the *alae nasi,* which produce flaring of the nostrils during obstructed breathing.

Expiration is primarily passive. It occurs as the elastic components of the chest wall and lung structures that were stretched during inspiration recoil, causing air to leave the lungs as the intrathoracic pressure increases. When needed, the abdominal and the internal intercostal muscles can be used to increase expiratory effort (Fig. 27.13). The increase in intra-abdominal pressure that accompanies the forceful contraction of the abdominal muscles pushes the diaphragm upward and results in an increase in intrathoracic pressure. The internal intercostal muscles move inward, which pulls the chest downward, increasing expiratory effort.

Increased A-P diameter

Increased vertical diameter

External intercostals contracted

Diaphragmatic contraction

A Inspiration

Internal intercostals contracted

Diaphragm relaxed

Abdominals contracted

B Expiration

FIGURE 27.13 • Expansion and contraction of the chest cage during expiration and inspiration, demonstrating especially diaphragmatic contraction, elevation of the rib cage, and function of the **(A)** external and **(B)** internal intercostals.

Lung Compliance

Lung compliance refers to the ease with which the lungs can be inflated at a given pressure change. Compliance can be compared to the difficulty of blowing up a noncompliant new balloon that is stiff and resistant versus a compliant one that has been previously blown up and stretched. Specifically, lung compliance (C) describes the change in lung volume (ΔV) that can be accomplished with a given change in respiratory pressure (ΔP); thus, $C = \Delta V/\Delta P$. The change in pressure results in a change in volume. It takes more pressure to move the same amount of air into a noncompliant lung than it does into a compliant one.

Lung compliance is determined by the elastin and collagen fibres of the lung, its water content, and surface tension. It also depends on the compliance of the thoracic or chest cage. It is diminished by conditions that reduce the natural elasticity of the lung, block the bronchi or smaller airways, increase the surface tension in the alveoli, or impair the flexibility of the thoracic cage.

Lung tissue is made up of elastin and collagen fibres. The elastin fibres are easily stretched and increase the ease of lung inflation, whereas the collagen fibres resist stretching and make lung inflation more difficult. In lung diseases such as interstitial lung disease and pulmonary fibrosis, the lungs become stiff and noncompliant as the elastin fibres are replaced with scar tissue.

Elastic recoil describes the ability of the elastic components of the lung to recoil to their original position after having been stretched. Cellular damage in emphysema causes the elastic components of the lung to lose their recoil, making the lung easier to inflate but more difficult to deflate because of its inability to recoil.

Surface Tension. An important factor in lung compliance is the *surface tension* or attraction forces of the surface molecules in the alveoli. The alveoli are lined with a thin film of liquid, and it is at the interface between this liquid film and the alveolar air that surface tension develops. This is because the forces that hold the water molecules of the liquid film together are stronger than those that hold the air molecules in the alveoli together. In the alveoli, excess surface tension causes water molecules in the liquid film to pull inward, making lung inflation difficult, and decreasing compliance. For example, pulmonary congestion and edema produce a reversible decrease in pulmonary compliance.

The units of surface tension are those of force per unit length. The relationship between the pressure within a sphere such as an alveolus and the tension in the wall can be described using the law of Laplace (pressure = 2 × surface tension/radius). If the surface tension was equal throughout the lungs, the alveoli with the smallest radii would have the greatest pressure, and this would cause them to empty into the larger alveoli (Fig. 27.14). The reason this does not occur is because of special surface tension-lowering molecules, called *surfactant,* that line the inner surface of the alveoli.

Pulmonary surfactant is a complex mixture of phospholipids, neutral lipids, and proteins that is synthesized in the

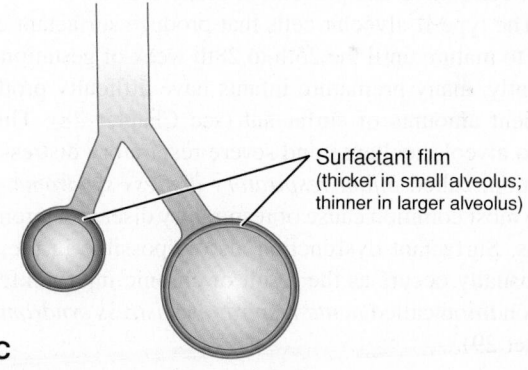

FIGURE 27.14 • **A:** The effect of the surface tension (forces generated at the fluid–air interface) and radius on the pressure and movement of gases in the alveolar structures. According to the law of Laplace (P = 2 T/r; P, pressure; T, tension; r, radius), the pressure generated within the sphere is inversely proportional to the radius. Air moves from the alveolus with a small radius and higher pressure to the alveolus with the larger radius and lower pressure. **B:** Surfactant molecules, showing their hydrophilic heads attached to the fluid lining of the alveolus and their hydrophobic tails oriented toward the air interface. **C:** The surfactant molecules form a monolayer (*shaded in blue*) that disrupts the intermolecular forces and lowers the surface tension more in the smaller alveolus with its higher concentration of surfactant than in the larger alveolus with the lower concentration.

type II alveolar cells. Substances that are termed surfactants consist of two parts with opposing properties that are irreversibly bound to each other. One part is polar and seeks aqueous fluid or hydrophilic (water-attracting) surfaces; the other is nonpolar and seeks oil, air, or hydrophobic (water-repelling) surfaces (Fig. 27.14B). Pulmonary surfactant forms a monolayer, with its hydrophilic surface binding to liquid film on the surface of the alveoli and its hydrophobic surface facing outward toward the gases in the alveolar air. It is this monolayer that interrupts the surface tension that develops at the air–liquid interface in the alveoli.

Pulmonary surfactant, particularly SP-B, exerts several important effects on lung inflation: it lowers the surface tension which increases lung compliance and ease of lung inflation. Without surfactant, lung inflation would be extremely difficult. In addition, surfactant helps to keep the alveoli dry and prevent pulmonary edema. This is because water is pulled out of the pulmonary capillaries into the alveoli when increased surface tension causes the alveoli to contract. Surfactant also provides for stability and more even inflation of the alveoli. Alveoli, except those at the pleural surface, are surrounded by other alveoli. Thus, the tendency of one alveolus to collapse is opposed by the traction exerted by the surrounding alveolus. The surfactant molecules are also more densely packed in small alveoli than in large alveoli (Fig. 27.14C). In immobilized persons, such as after surgery, shallow and quiet breathing impairs the spreading of surfactant. Encouraging these patients to cough and breathe deeply enhances the spreading of surfactant. This allows for a more even distribution of ventilation and prevention of atelectasis.

The type II alveolar cells that produce surfactant do not begin to mature until the 25th to 28th week of gestation; consequently, many premature infants have difficulty producing sufficient amounts of surfactant (see Chapter 28). This can lead to alveolar collapse and severe respiratory distress. This condition, called *infant respiratory distress syndrome,* is the single most common cause of respiratory disease in premature infants. Surfactant dysfunction also is possible in the adult. This usually occurs as the result of chronic injury, infection, or a condition called *acute respiratory distress syndrome* (see Chapter 29).

Airflow and Airway Resistance

The volume of air that moves into and out of the air exchange portion of the lungs is directly related to the pressure difference between the lungs and the atmosphere and inversely related to the resistance that the air encounters as it moves through the airways. Depending on the velocity and pattern of flow, airflow can be laminar or turbulent.

Laminar or *streamlined airflow* occurs at low flow rates in which the air stream is parallel to the sides of the airway. With laminar flow, the air at the periphery must overcome the resistance to flow, and as a result, the air in the centre of the airway moves faster. *Turbulent airflow* is disorganized flow in which the molecules of the gas move laterally, collide with one another, and change their velocities. Whether turbulence

develops depends on the radius of the airways, the interaction of the gas molecules, and the velocity of airflow. It is most likely to occur when the radius of the airways is large and the velocity of flow is high. Turbulent flow occurs regularly in the trachea. Turbulence of airflow accounts for the respiratory sounds that are heard during chest auscultation (*i.e.,* listening to chest sounds using a stethoscope).

In the bronchial tree with its many branches, laminar airflow probably occurs only in the very small airways, where the velocity of flow is low. Because the small airways contribute little resistance to airflow, they constitute a silent zone (to be discussed).

Airway Resistance. Airway resistance is the ratio of the pressure driving inspiration or expiration to airflow. The French physician Jean Léonard Marie Poiseuille first described the pressure-flow characteristics of laminar flow in a straight circular tube, a correlation that has become known as the *Poiseuille law.* According to the Poiseuille law, the resistance to flow is inversely related to the fourth power of the radius ($R = 1/r^4$). If the radius is reduced by one half, the resistance increases 16-fold ($2 \times 2 \times 2 \times 2 = 16$).

Airway resistance differs in large (*e.g.,* trachea and bronchi), medium-sized (*e.g.,* segmental), and small (*e.g.,* bronchioles) airways. Therefore, the total airway resistance is equal to the sum of the resistances in these three types of airways. The site of most of the resistance along the bronchial tree is the medium-sized bronchi, with the smallest airways contributing very little to the total airway resistance. This is because most of these airways are arranged in parallel and their resistances are added as reciprocals (*i.e.,* total combined resistance = 1/R + 1/R, etc.). Although the resistance of each individual bronchiole may be relatively high, their great number results in a large total cross-sectional area, causing their total resistance to be low. Many airway diseases, such as emphysema and chronic bronchitis, begin in the small airways. Early detection of these diseases is often difficult because a considerable amount of damage must be present before the usual measurements of airway resistance can detect them.

Airway resistance is greatly affected by lung volumes, being less during inspiration than expiration. This is due to the elastic fibres that connect the outside of the airways to the surrounding lung tissues. These airways are pulled open by the elastic fibres when the lungs expand during inspiration and increase in diameter. They subsequently become narrower as the lungs deflate during expiration (Fig. 27.15). This is one of the reasons why persons with conditions that increase airway resistance, such as bronchial asthma, initially have less difficulty during inspiration than during expiration.

Airway resistance is also affected by the bronchial smooth tone that controls airway diameter. The smooth muscles in the airway, from the trachea down to the terminal bronchioles, are under autonomic nervous system control. Stimulation of the parasympathetic nervous system causes bronchial constriction as well as increased mucus secretion, whereas sympathetic stimulation has the opposite effect.

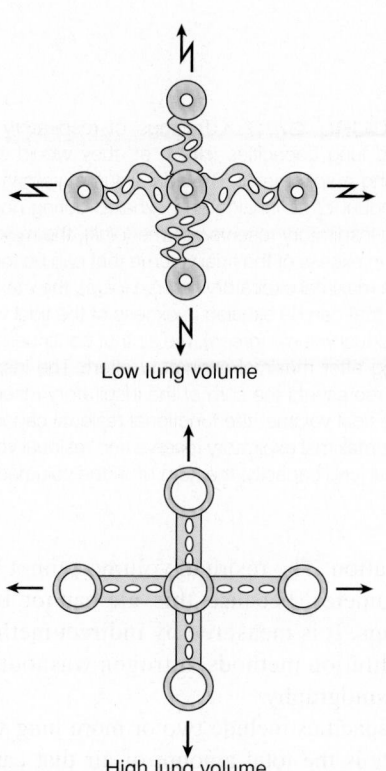

FIGURE 27.15 • Interaction of tissue forces on airways during low and high lung volumes. At low lung volumes, the tissue forces tend to fold and place less tension on the airways and they become smaller; during high lung volumes, the tissue forces are stretched and pull the airways open.

Airway Compression During Forced Expiration. Airway resistance does not change much during normal quiet breathing; however, it is significantly increased during forced expiration, such as in vigorous exercise. Airflow through the collapsible airways in the lungs depends on the distending airway (intrapulmonary) pressures that hold the airways open and the external (intrapleural or intrathoracic) pressures that surround and compress the airways. The difference between these two pressures (intrathoracic pressure minus airway pressure) is called the *transpulmonary pressure*. For airflow to occur, the distending pressure inside the airways must be greater than the compressing pressure outside the airways. During forced expiration, the transpulmonary pressure is decreased because of a disproportionate increase in the intrathoracic pressure compared with airway pressure. The resistance that air encounters as it moves out of the lungs causes a further drop in airway pressure. If this drop is sufficiently great, the surrounding intrathoracic pressure will compress the collapsible airways (*i.e.*, those that lack cartilaginous support), causing airflow to be interrupted and air to be trapped in the terminal airways (Fig. 27.16).

Although this type of airway compression usually is seen only during forced expiration in persons with normal respiratory function, it may occur during normal breathing in persons with lung diseases. For example, in conditions that increase airway resistance, such as chronic obstructive pulmonary disease (COPD), the pressure drop along the smaller airways is magnified, and an increase in intra-airway pressure is needed to maintain airway patency. Measures such as pursed-lip breathing increase airway pressure and improve expiratory flow rates in persons with COPD (discussed in Chapter 29). This is also the basis for using positive end-expiratory pressure in persons who are being mechanically ventilated. Infants who are having trouble breathing often grunt to increase their expiratory airway pressures and keep their airways open.

Lung Volumes

The amount of air that is or can be exchanged during ventilation can be subdivided into three components: (1) the

FIGURE 27.16 • Mechanism that limits maximal expiratory flow rate. **A:** Airway patency and airflow in the nonrigid airways of the lungs rely on a transpulmonary pressure gradient in which airway pressure is greater than intrapleural pressure. **B:** Airway resistance normally produces a drop in airway pressure as air moves out of the lungs. The increased intrapleural pressure that occurs with forced expiration produces airway collapse in the nonrigid airways at the point where intrapleural pressure exceeds airway pressure.

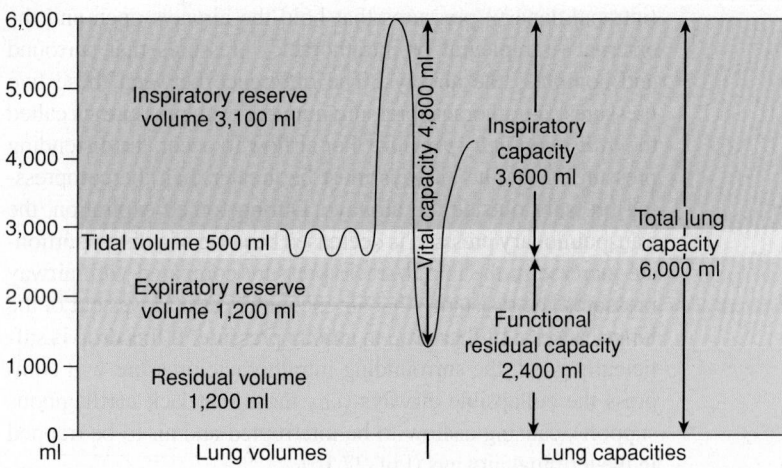

FIGURE 27.17 • Tracings of respiratory volumes (**left**) and lung capacities (**right**) as they would appear if made using a spirometer. The tidal volume (*yellow*) represents the amount of air inhaled and exhaled during normal breathing; the inspiratory reserve volume (*pink*), the maximal amount of air in excess of the tidal volume that can be forcefully inhaled; the maximal expiratory reserve (*blue*), the maximal amount of air that can be exhaled in excess of the tidal volume; and the residual volume (*green*), the air that continues to remain in the lung after maximal expiratory effort. The inspiratory capacity represents the sum of the inspiratory reserve volume and the tidal volume; the functional residual capacity, the sum of the maximal expiratory reserve and residual volumes; and the total lung capacity, the sum of all the volumes.

tidal volume, (2) the inspiratory reserve volume, and (3) the expiratory reserve volume (Fig. 27.17). These volumes can be measured using an instrument called a *spirometer.* The *tidal volume* (Vt) is the volume of air inspired (or exhaled) with each regular breath. It usually is about 500 ml in the average-sized adult and about 3 to 5 ml/kg in children. Tidal volume normally varies, particularly with exertion or metabolic activity, but also with age, gender, or body position. The maximum amount of air that can be inspired in addition to the tidal volume is called the *inspiratory reserve volume* (IRV), and the maximum amount that can be exhaled after expiration of the tidal volume is the *expiratory reserve volume* (ERV). A portion of the lung volume cannot be exhaled, thus approximately 1200 ml of air always remains in the lungs after forced expiration. This air is the *residual volume* (RV). The RV increases with age because there is more trapping of air in the lungs at the end of expiration. The residual volume cannot be measured with a spirometer, because this air cannot be expressed from the lungs. It is measured by indirect methods, such as the helium dilution methods, nitrogen washout methods, or body plethysmography.

Lung capacities include two or more lung volumes. The *vital capacity* is the total amount of air that can be exhaled after maximal inspiration. Therefore, it equals Vt, plus the IRV and the ERV. The *inspiratory capacity* is the amount of air a person can breathe in, beginning at the normal expiratory level and distending the lungs to the maximal amount. It equals the Vt plus the IRV. The *functional residual capacity* is the sum of the RV and ERV. It is the volume of air that remains in the lungs at the end of normal expiration, and is important for ongoing gas exchange. The *total lung capacity* is the sum of all the volumes in the lungs. Lung volumes and capacities are summarized in Table 27.1.

TABLE 27.1 LUNG VOLUMES AND CAPACITIES

VOLUME	SYMBOL	MEASUREMENT
Tidal volume (about 500 ml at rest)	Vt	Amount of air that moves into and out of the lungs with each breath
Inspiratory reserve volume (about 3,000 ml)	IRV	Maximum amount of air that can be inhaled from the point of maximal expiration
Expiratory reserve volume (about 1,100 ml)	ERV	Maximum volume of air that can be exhaled from the resting end-expiratory level
Residual volume (about 1,200 ml)	RV	Volume of air remaining in the lungs after maximal expiration. This volume cannot be measured with the spirometer; it is measured indirectly using methods such as the helium dilution method, the nitrogen washout technique, or body plethysmography.
Functional residual capacity (about 2,300 ml)	FRC	Volume of air remaining in the lungs at end-expiration (sum of RV and ERV)
Inspiratory capacity (about 3,500 ml)	IC	Sum of IRV and Vt
Vital capacity (about 4,600 ml)	VC	Maximal amount of air that can be forcibly exhaled from the point of maximal inspiration
Total lung capacity (about 5,800 ml)	TLC	Total amount of air that the lungs can hold; it is the sum of all the volume components after maximal inspiration. This value is about 20–25% less in females than in males.

TABLE 27.2 PULMONARY FUNCTION TESTS

TEST	SYMBOL	MEASUREMENT[a]
Maximal voluntary ventilation	MVV	Maximum amount of air that can be breathed in a given time
Forced vital capacity	FVC	Maximum amount of air that can be rapidly and forcefully exhaled from the lungs after full inspiration. The expired volume is plotted against time.
Forced expiratory volume achieved in 1 second	FEV_1	Volume of air expired in the first second of FVC
Proportion of forced vital capacity	FEV_1/FVC	Volume of air forcefully expired in the first second, over the total volume of air forcefully expired. Ratio often converted and expressed as a percentage.
Forced mid-expiratory flow rate	$FEF_{25-75\%}$	The forced mid-expiratory flow rate determined by locating the points on the volume-time curve recording obtained during FVC corresponding to 25% and 75% of FVC and drawing a straight line through these points. The slope of this line represents the average mid-expiratory flow rate.
Forced inspiratory flow rate	$FIF_{25-75\%}$	FIF is the volume inspired from RV at the point of measurement. $FIF_{25-75\%}$ is the slope of a line between the points on the volume pressure tracing corresponding to 25% and 75% of the inspired volume.

[a]By convention, all the lung volumes and rates of flow are expressed in terms of body temperature and pressure and saturated with water vapour (BTPS), which allows for a comparison of the pulmonary function data from laboratories with different ambient temperatures and altitudes.

Pulmonary Function Studies

The previously described lung volumes and capacities are anatomic or static measures determined by lung volumes and measured without relation to time. The spirometer is used to measure dynamic lung function (*i.e.,* ventilation with respect to time); these tests often are used in assessing pulmonary function. Pulmonary function measures include maximum voluntary ventilation, forced vital capacity, forced expiratory volumes and flow rates, and forced inspiratory flow rates (Table 27.2). Pulmonary function tests also include assessment of airway obstruction and oxygen diffusion. They are used for various clinical purposes, such as confirming respiratory disease diagnoses, evaluating abnormal radiologic or laboratory findings, monitoring ongoing chronic disease severity, optimizing pulmonary interventions, and assessing preoperative surgical and anesthetic risk.

The *maximum voluntary ventilation* measures the volume of air that a person can move into and out of the lungs during maximum effort lasting for 12 to 15 seconds. This measurement usually is converted to litres per minute. The *forced vital capacity* (FVC) is the amount of air forcefully expired, and involves full inspiration to total lung capacity followed by forceful maximal expiration. Abnormal obstruction of airways produces a lower FVC than that which occurs with slower expiration. The *forced expiratory volume* (FEV) is the expiratory volume achieved in a given time period. The FEV_1 is the volume of air that can be forcefully exhaled in 1 second. The FEV_1 will decrease with airway obstruction. The FEV_1 frequently is compared to the FVC and may be converted to a percentage (*e.g.,* an FEV_1 of 4 L and FVC of 5 L would be reported as 4 L/5 L = 80%). The FEV_1/FVC ratio is used in the diagnosis of obstructive lung disorders. Peak flow meters or chambers also provide information on airway obstruction,

with normal numbers varying with age, height and weight. Peak flow meters may be used for persons with asthma or obstructive lung disease to assess flow rate of air either in the emergency department or at home.

The *forced inspiratory vital flow* (FIF) measures the respiratory response during rapid maximal inspiration. Calculation of airflow during the middle half of inspiration ($FIF_{25\%-75\%}$) relative to the forced mid-expiratory flow rate ($FEF_{25\%-75\%}$) is used as a measure of respiratory muscle dysfunction because inspiratory flow depends more on effort than does expiration. The *negative inspired force* (NIF) is an indication of the person's ability to create a negative pressure upon inspiration. It reflects neuromuscular coupling for that time, not muscular endurance.

Work of Breathing

The *minute volume* is the amount of air that is exchanged in 1 minute, or the total alveolar ventilation in 1 minute. The minute volume is equal to the tidal volume (Vt) multiplied by the respiratory rate (RR), and conventionally converted to litres per minute (L/min). The minute volume in the average-sized adult at rest is normally about 6 L/min (500 ml Vt × RR rate of 12 breaths per minute = 6,000 ml/min). Normal minute volume fluctuates, with both rate and depth of breathing determined by neural centres and influenced by metabolic rate. The efficiency of breathing is determined by matching the Vt and respiratory rate to provide an optimal minute volume while minimizing the work of breathing.

The work of breathing is determined by the amount of effort required to move air through the conducting airways and by the ease of lung expansion, or compliance. There is resistance to airflow through the airways on both inspiration and expiration, referred to as either *resistance* or *friction* work of breathing. Expansion of the lungs is referred to the *elastic work* that is required on inspiration for the respiratory muscles to expand the chest and stretch the elastic fibres. There is no elastic work on expiration as the fibres recoil. Chest expansion is difficult for persons with stiff and noncompliant lungs, as in pulmonary fibrosis, or who are mechanically restricted, as with scoliosis. These persons usually find it easier to breathe if they keep their Vt low and breathe at a more rapid rate (*e.g.,* 300 × 20 = 6,000 ml = 6 L/min) to achieve their minute volume and meet their oxygen needs. In contrast, persons with obstructive airway disease usually find it less difficult to inflate their lungs but expend more energy in moving air through the airways. As a result, these persons take deeper breaths and breathe at a slower rate (*e.g.,* 600 × 10 = 6,000 ml = 6 L/min) to achieve their oxygen needs.

IN SUMMARY

The movement of air between the atmosphere and the lungs follows the laws of physics as they relate to gases. The air in the alveoli contains a mixture of gases, including nitrogen, oxygen, carbon dioxide, and water vapour. With the exception of water vapour, each gas exerts a pressure that varies. The partial pressure of oxygen and carbon dioxide are determined by the atmospheric pressure, the exchange of alveolar air with atmospheric air (ventilation), and the exchange of gases in the alveoli with capillary blood (diffusion). Water vapour pressure is affected by temperature but not atmospheric pressure. Air moves from the atmosphere into the airways and alveoli due to a pressure gradient. The pressure inside the airways and alveoli of the lungs is called intrapulmonary (or alveolar) pressure; the pressure in the pleural cavity is called pleural pressure; and the pressure in the thoracic cavity is called intrathoracic pressure.

Breathing allows the movement of gases between the atmosphere and the lungs. It requires a system of open airways and the pressure changes that result from the action of the respiratory muscles in changing the volume of the chest cage. The diaphragm is the principal muscle of inspiration, and is assisted by the external intercostal muscles. The scalene and sternocleidomastoid muscles elevate the ribs and act as accessory muscles for inspiration. The work of breathing primarily occurs during inspiration, and is due to muscle contraction and lung expansion. Expiration is largely passive, aided by the elastic recoil of the respiratory muscles that were stretched during inspiration. There is a small amount of resistance work of breathing on both inspiration and expiration due to air flow through the airways. When needed, the abdominal and internal intercostal muscles can be used to increase expiratory effort.

Lung compliance describes the ease with which the lungs can be inflated. It is determined by the elastic and collagen fibres of the lung, the water content, the surface tension of the alveoli, and the compliance of the chest cage.

Surface tension of the alveoli is normally decreased by surfactant molecules, produced by type II alveolar cells, which reduce the surface tension in the lungs. This decrease in surface tension increases lung compliance.

The volume of air that moves into and out of the airways and alveoli is directly related to the pressure difference between the alveoli and the atmosphere and inversely related to the resistance that the air encounters as it moves through the airways. Depending on the velocity and pattern of flow, airflow can be laminar or turbulent. Airway resistance refers to the impediment to flow that the air encounters as it moves through the airways. It differs with airway size, being greatest in the medium-sized bronchi and lowest in the smaller bronchioles.

Lung volumes and lung capacities reflect the amount of air that is exchanged during normal and forced breathing. The tidal volume (Vt) is the amount of air that moves into and out of the lungs with regular breaths; the inspiratory reserve volume (IRV) is the maximum amount of air that can be inspired in excess of the normal Vt; and the expiratory reserve volume (ERV) is the maximum amount that can be exhaled in excess of the normal Vt. The residual volume (RV) is the amount of air that remains in the lungs after forced expiration. Lung capacities include two or more lung volumes. The vital capacity equals the IRV plus the Vt plus the ERV and is the amount of air that can be exhaled from the point of maximal inspiration. The minute volume, which reflects alveolar ventilation, is the amount of air that is exchanged in 1 minute (*i.e.,* Vt × RR).

CONCEPTSin action **ANIMATION**

EXCHANGE AND TRANSPORT OF GASES

After completing this section of the chapter, you should be able to meet the following objectives:

* Trace the exchange of gases between the air in the alveoli and the blood in the pulmonary capillaries.
* Differentiate between pulmonary and alveolar ventilation.
* Explain why ventilation and perfusion must be matched.
* Cite the difference between dead air space and shunt.
* List four factors that affect the diffusion of gases in the alveoli.
* Explain the difference between PO_2 and hemoglobin-bound oxygen and O_2 saturation, and oxygen content.
* Explain the significance of a shift to the right and a shift to the left in the oxygen–hemoglobin dissociation curve.

The primary function of the lungs is gas exchange between the alveoli and pulmonary capillaries, namely the transfer of oxygen into the capillaries and removal of carbon dioxide. Pulmonary gas exchange is conventionally divided into three processes: ventilation, or the flow of gases into and out of the alveoli of the lungs; perfusion, or flow of blood through the adjacent pulmonary capillaries; and diffusion, or transfer of gases between the alveoli and the pulmonary capillaries. The efficiency of gas exchange requires that alveolar ventilation occur adjacent to perfused pulmonary capillaries.

Ventilation

Ventilation refers to the exchange of gases in the respiratory system. There are two types of ventilation: pulmonary and alveolar. *Pulmonary ventilation* refers to the total exchange of gases between the atmosphere and the lungs. *Alveolar ventilation* is the exchange of gases within the gas exchange portion of the lungs. Conventionally, the emphasis on alveolar ventilation is the removal of carbon dioxide and intake of oxygen into the alveoli. Ventilation requires a system of open airways and a pressure difference that moves air into and out of the lungs. It is affected by body position and lung volume as well as by disease conditions that affect the lungs, heart and neuromuscular function.

Distribution of Ventilation

The distribution of ventilation between the apex and base of the lung varies with body position and the effects of gravity on intrapleural pressure (Fig. 27.18). In the seated or standing position, gravity exerts a downward pull on the lung, causing

FIGURE 27.18 • Explanation of the regional differences in ventilation down the lung; the intrapleural pressure is less negative at the base than at the apex. As a consequence, the basal lung is relatively compressed in its resting state but expands more on inspiration than the apex. (From West J. B. (2012). *Respiratory physiology: The essentials* (9th ed., p. 106). Philadelphia, PA: Lippincott Williams & Wilkins.)

intrapleural pressure at the apex of the lung to become more negative than that at the base of the lung. As a result, the alveoli at the apex of the lung are more fully expanded than those at the base of the lung. The same holds true for dependent portions of the lung in the supine or lateral position. In the supine position, ventilation in the lowermost (posterior) parts of the lung exceeds that in the uppermost (anterior) parts. In the lateral position, the dependent lung is better ventilated (*i.e.,* when lying on the right side, the right lung is better ventilated).

The distribution of ventilation also is affected by lung volumes. As earlier stated, lung compliance reflects the change in volume that occurs with a change in pressure. Compliance is decreased in fully expanded alveoli, which have difficulty accommodating more air, and greater in alveoli that are less inflated. During full inspiration in the seated or standing position, the airways are pulled open and air moves into the more compliant portions of the lower lung. At the low lung volumes of functional residual capacity, the opposite occurs. In this case, the pleural pressure at the base of the lung exceeds airway pressure, compressing the airways so that ventilation is greatly reduced, while the airways in the upper part of the lung remain open so that the top of the lung is better ventilated than the bottom.

Even at low lung volumes, some air remains in the alveoli of the lower portion of the lungs, preventing their collapse. According to the law of Laplace (discussed previously), the pressure needed to overcome the tension in the wall of a sphere or an elastic tube is inversely related to its radius; therefore, the small airways close first, trapping some gas in the alveoli. There may be increased trapping of air in the alveoli of the lower part of the lungs in older persons and in those with lung disease (*e.g.,* emphysema). This condition is thought to result from a reduction in the elastic recoil properties of the lungs, so that the intrapleural pressure, created by the elastic recoil of the lung and chest wall, becomes less negative. In these persons, airway closure occurs at the end of normal instead of low lung volumes, trapping larger amounts of air with a resultant increase in the residual lung volume.

Dead Space

Dead space refers to the air that must be moved with each breath but does not participate in gas exchange. The movement of air which includes this dead space air contributes to the work of breathing but not to gas exchange. There are two types of dead space: that contained in the conducting airways, called the *anatomic dead space,* and that contained in the respiratory portion of the lung, called the *alveolar dead space.* The volume of anatomic airway dead space is normally fixed at approximately 150 to 200 ml, depending on body size. It constitutes air contained in the nose, pharynx, trachea, and bronchi. The creation of a tracheostomy (surgical opening in the trachea) decreases anatomic dead space ventilation because air does not have to move through the nasal and oral airways. Alveolar dead space, normally about 5 to 10 ml, constitutes alveolar air that does not participate in gas exchange. When alveoli are ventilated but poorly perfused, they are unable to contribute to gas exchange and thereby constitute alveolar dead space.

The *physiologic dead space* includes the anatomic dead space plus alveolar dead space. In persons with normal respiratory function, physiologic dead space is about the same as anatomic dead space. Only in lung disease does physiologic dead space increase. Alveolar ventilation is equal to the minute ventilation minus the physiologic dead space ventilation.

Perfusion

The primary function of the pulmonary circulation is to perfuse the alveoli, that is, to provide blood flow to the gas exchange portion of the lung and to facilitate gas exchange. The pulmonary circulation serves several important functions in addition to gas exchange. It filters all the blood that moves from the right to the left side of the circulation; it removes most of the thromboemboli that might form; and it serves as a reservoir of blood for the left side of the heart.

The gas exchange function of the lungs requires a continuous flow of blood through the respiratory portion of the lungs. Deoxygenated blood enters the lung through the pulmonary artery, which has its origin in the right ventricle and enters the lung at the hilus, along with the primary bronchus. The pulmonary arteries branch in a manner similar to that of the airways. The small pulmonary arteries accompany the bronchi as they move down the lobules and branch to supply the capillary network that surrounds the alveoli where it is oxygenated (Fig. 27.8). The oxygenated capillary blood is collected in the small pulmonary veins of the lobules, and then moves to the larger veins to be collected in the four large pulmonary veins that empty into the left atrium. Thus, deoxygenated blood leaves the right ventricle and oxygenated blood enters the left atrium.

The pulmonary blood vessels are thinner, more compliant, and offer less resistance to flow than those in the systemic circulation. Therefore, the pressures in the pulmonary system are much lower (*e.g.,* 25/10 mm Hg versus 120/70 mm Hg). The low pressure and low resistance of the pulmonary circulation accommodate the delivery of varying amounts of blood from the systemic circulation without increasing hydrostatic capillary pressure and movement of fluid from the capillary into the interstitial space. The volume in the pulmonary circulation is approximately 500 ml, with approximately 100 ml of this volume located in the pulmonary capillary bed. When the input of blood from the right heart and output of blood to the left heart are equal, pulmonary blood flow remains constant. Small differences between input and output can result in large changes in pulmonary volume if the differences continue for many heartbeats. The movement of blood through the pulmonary capillary bed requires that the mean pulmonary arterial pressure be greater than the mean pulmonary venous pressure. Pulmonary venous pressure increases in left-sided heart failure, resulting in increased pulmonary capillary pressures, which causes pulmonary edema (see Chapter 26).

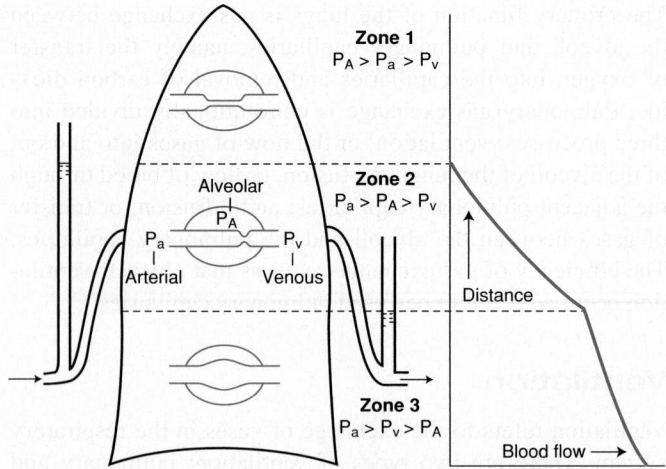

FIGURE 27.19 • The uneven distribution of blood flow in the lung results from different pressures affecting the capillaries, which are affected by body position and gravity. (From West J. B. (2012). *Respiratory Physiology: The Essentials* (9th ed., p. 45). Philadelphia, PA: Lippincott Williams & Wilkins.)

Distribution of Blood Flow

As with ventilation, the distribution of pulmonary blood flow is affected by body position and gravity. In the upright position, the distance of the upper apices of the lung above the level of the heart may exceed the perfusion capabilities of the mean pulmonary arterial pressure (approximately 15 mm Hg); therefore, blood flow in the upper part of the lungs is less than that in the base or bottom part of the lungs (Fig. 27.19). In the supine position, the lungs and the heart are at the same level, and blood flow to the apices and base of the lungs becomes more uniform. In this position, blood flow to the posterior or dependent portions (*e.g.,* bottom of the lung when lying on the side) exceeds flow in the anterior or nondependent portions of the lungs.

Hypoxia-Induced Vasoconstriction

The blood vessels in the pulmonary circulation are highly sensitive to alveolar oxygen levels and undergo marked vasoconstriction with alveolar hypoxia. The precise mechanism for this response is unclear. When alveolar oxygen levels drop below 60 mm Hg, marked vasoconstriction may occur, and at very low oxygen levels, the local flow may be almost abolished. In regional hypoxia, as occurs with atelectasis, vasoconstriction is localized to a specific region of the lung. In this case, vasoconstriction has the effect of directing blood flow away from the hypoxic regions of the lungs. When alveolar hypoxia no longer exists, blood flow is restored. This promotes the balance between alveolar ventilation and capillary perfusion.

Generalized alveolar hypoxia, such as occurs at high altitudes and in persons with chronic hypoxia due to lung disease, causes vasoconstriction throughout the lung. Prolonged hypoxia can lead to pulmonary hypertension and increased workload on the right heart (discussed in Chapter 29). A low blood pH produces a similar effect, particularly when alveolar hypoxia is present (*e.g.,* during circulatory shock).

Shunt

Shunt refers to blood that moves from the right to the left side of the circulation without being oxygenated. As with dead air space, there are two types of shunts: anatomic and physiologic. In *anatomic shunt,* blood moves from the venous to the arterial side of the circulation without moving through the lungs. Anatomic intracardiac shunting of blood due to congenital heart defects is discussed in Chapter 24. In a *physiologic shunt,* there is mismatching of ventilation and perfusion within the lung, resulting in insufficient ventilation to provide the oxygen needed to oxygenate the blood flowing through the alveolar capillaries. A small amount of physiologic shunt normally occurs in the bases of the lungs due to the differences in ventilation and perfusion.

Ventilation–Perfusion Mismatch

The gas exchange properties of the lung depend on matching ventilation and perfusion, ensuring that equal amounts of air and blood are entering the respiratory portion of the lungs. Both dead air space and shunt produce a mismatching of ventilation and perfusion, as depicted in Figure 27.20. With a shunt (depicted on the left), there is perfusion without ventilation, resulting in a low ventilation–perfusion ratio. It occurs in conditions in which there is decreased ventilation but ongoing perfusion, such as atelectasis or acute lung injury (see Chapter 29). With dead air space (depicted on the right), there is ventilation without perfusion, resulting in a high ventilation–perfusion ratio. It occurs in conditions such as pulmonary embolism, which impairs blood flow to a part of the lung. The arterial blood leaving the pulmonary circulation reflects mixing of blood from normally ventilated and perfused areas

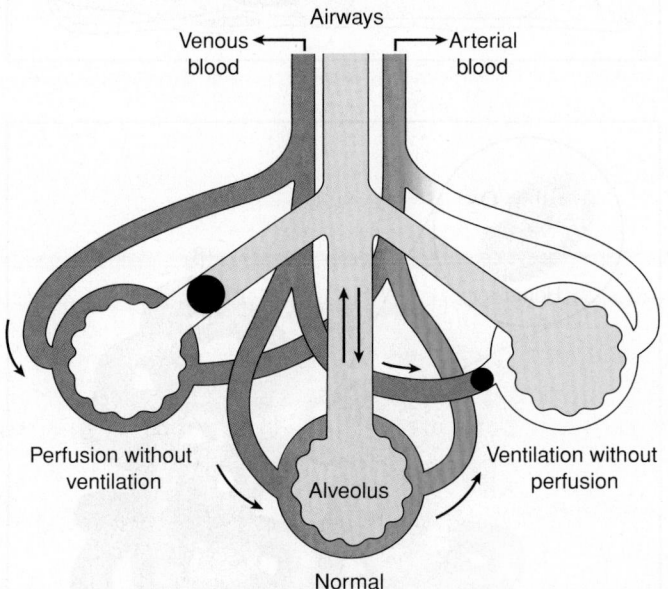

FIGURE 27.20 • Matching of ventilation and perfusion. (**Centre**) Normal matching of ventilation and perfusion; (**left**) perfusion without ventilation (*i.e.,* shunt); (**right**) ventilation without perfusion (*i.e.,* dead air space).

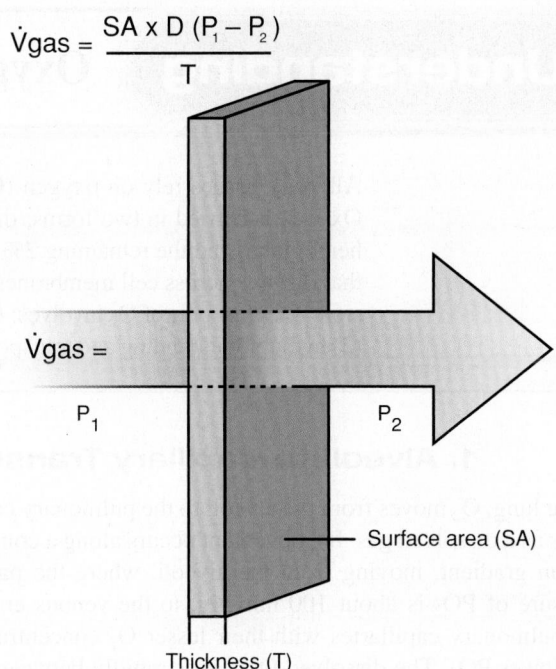

$$\dot{V}gas = \frac{SA \times D\,(P_1 - P_2)}{T}$$

FIGURE 27.21 • The Fick law of diffusion states that the diffusion of a gas ($\dot{V}gas$) across a sheet of tissue is related to the surface area (SA) of the tissue, the diffusion constant (D) for the gas, and the partial pressure difference ($P_1 - P_2$) on either side of the tissue, and is inversely proportional to the thickness (T) of the tissue.

of the lung as well as areas that are not ventilated (dead air space) or perfused (shunt). Many of the conditions that cause mismatching of ventilation and perfusion involve both dead air space and shunt. In chronic obstructive lung disease, for example, there may be impaired ventilation in one area of the lung and impaired perfusion in another area.

Diffusion

Diffusion occurs in the respiratory portions of the lung and refers to the movement of gases across the alveolar–capillary membrane. Gas diffusion in the lung can be determined by the *Fick law of diffusion.* The Fick law states that the volume of a gas ($\dot{V}gas$) diffusing across the membrane per unit time is directly proportional to the partial pressure difference of the gas ($P_1 - P_2$), the surface area (SA) of the membrane, and the diffusion coefficient (D), and is inversely proportional to the thickness (T) of the membrane (Fig. 27.21).

Several factors influence the diffusion of gases in the lung. The administration of supplemental oxygen increases the difference in partial pressure between the two sides of the membrane and increases oxygen diffusion. Diseases that destroy lung tissue (*i.e.,* decrease surface area for diffusion) or increase the thickness of the alveolar–capillary membrane adversely influence the diffusing capacity of the lungs. The removal of one lung, for example, reduces the diffusing capacity by one half. The thickness of the alveolar–capillary membrane and the distance for diffusion are increased in persons

Understanding Oxygen Transport

All body tissues rely on oxygen (O_2) that is transported in the blood to meet their metabolic needs. Oxygen is carried in two forms: dissolved and bound to hemoglobin. About 98% of O_2 is carried by hemoglobin and the remaining 2% is carried in the dissolved state. Dissolved oxygen is the only form that diffuses across cell membranes and produces a partial pressure (PO_2), which, in turn, drives diffusion. The transport of O_2 involves: (1) transfer from the alveoli to the pulmonary capillaries in the lung; (2) hemoglobin binding and transport; and (3) the dissociation from hemoglobin in the tissue capillaries.

1. Alveoli-to-capillary Transfer

In the lung, O_2 moves from the alveoli to the pulmonary capillaries as a dissolved gas. Its movement occurs along a concentration gradient, moving from the alveoli, where the partial pressure of PO_2 is about 100 mm Hg, to the venous end of the pulmonary capillaries with their lesser O_2 concentration and lower PO_2. The dissolved O_2 moves rapidly between the alveoli and the pulmonary capillaries, such that the PO_2 at the arterial end of the capillary is almost if not the same as that in the alveoli.

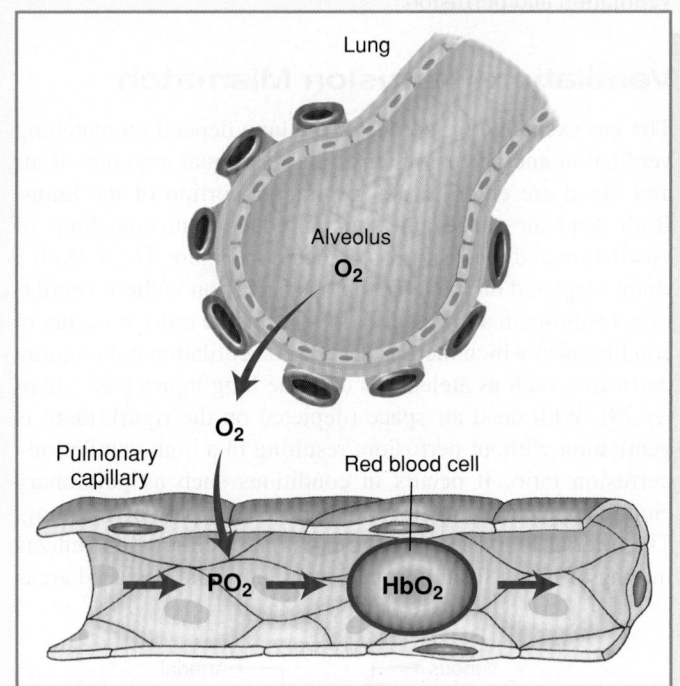

2. Hemoglobin Binding and Transport

Oxygen, which is relatively insoluble in plasma, relies on hemoglobin for transport in the blood. Once oxygen has diffused into the pulmonary capillary, it moves rapidly into the red blood cells and reversibly binds to hemoglobin to form HbO_2. The hemoglobin molecule contains four heme units, each capable of attaching an oxygen molecule. Hemoglobin is 100% saturated when all four units are occupied and is usually about 97% saturated in the systemic arterial blood. The capacity of the blood to carry O_2 is dependent both on hemoglobin levels and the ability of the lungs to oxygenate the hemoglobin.

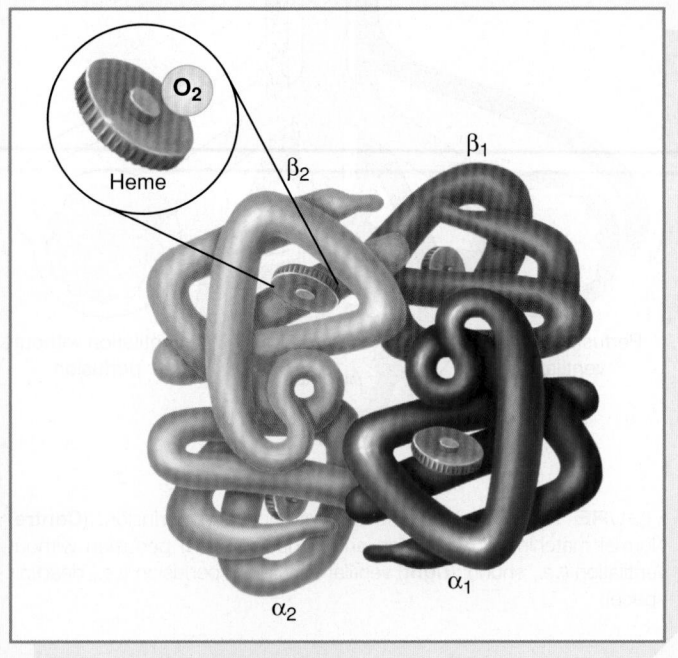

3. Oxygen Dissociation in the Tissues

The dissociation or release of O_2 from hemoglobin occurs in the tissue capillaries where the PO_2 is less than that of the arterial blood. As oxygen dissociates from hemoglobin, it dissolves in the plasma and then moves into the tissues where the PO_2 is less than that in the capillaries. The affinity of hemoglobin for O_2 is influenced by the carbon dioxide (PCO_2) content of the blood, the pH, temperature, and 2,3-diphosphoglycerate (2,3-DPG), a byproduct of glycolysis in red blood cells. Under conditions of high metabolic demand, in which the PCO_2 is increased and the pH is decreased, the binding affinity of hemoglobin is decreased, and O_2 is more easily released. During decreased metabolic demand, when the PCO_2 is decreased and the pH is increased, the affinity is increased.

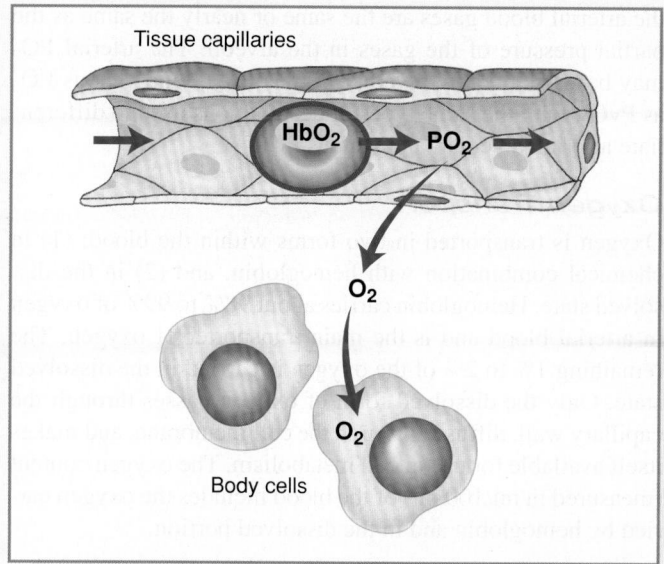

Tissue capillaries
HbO$_2$ PO$_2$
O$_2$
O$_2$
Body cells

MATCHING OF VENTILATION AND PERFUSION

- Exchange of gases between the air in the alveoli and the blood in pulmonary capillaries requires a matching of ventilation and perfusion.
- Dead air space refers to the volume of air that is moved with each breath but does not participate in gas exchange. Anatomic dead space is that contained in the conducting airways that normally do not participate in gas exchange. Alveolar dead space results from alveoli that are ventilated but not perfused.
- Shunt refers to blood that moves from the right to the left side of the circulation without being oxygenated. With an anatomic shunt, blood moves from the venous to the arterial side of the circulation without going through the lungs. Physiologic shunting results from blood moving through unventilated parts of the lung.
- The blood oxygen level reflects the mixing of blood from alveolar dead space and physiologic shunting areas as it moves into the pulmonary veins.

with pulmonary edema or pneumonia. The characteristics of the gas and its molecular weight and solubility constitute the diffusion coefficient and determine how rapidly the gas diffuses through the respiratory membranes. For example, carbon dioxide diffuses 20 times more rapidly than oxygen because of its greater solubility in the respiratory membranes. Therefore, any alterations in diffusion first result in decreased oxygen diffusion while carbon dioxide diffusion may remain normal.

The diffusing capacity provides a measure of the rate of gas transfer in the lungs per partial pressure gradient. Because the initial alveolar–capillary difference for oxygen cannot be

measured, carbon monoxide is used to determine the diffusing capacity. Carbon monoxide has several advantages: (1) its uptake is not limited by diffusion or blood flow; (2) there is essentially no carbon monoxide in venous blood; and (3) its affinity for hemoglobin is 210 times that of oxygen, ensuring that its partial pressure will remain essentially zero in the pulmonary capillary. The most common technique for making this measurement is the *single-breath test*. This test involves the inhalation of a single breath of dilute carbon monoxide (CO), followed by breath-hold of 10 seconds. The diffusing capacity can be calculated using the lung volume and the percentage of CO in the alveoli at the beginning and end of the 10-second breath-hold.

Oxygen and Carbon Dioxide Transport

Although the lungs are responsible for the exchange of gases with the external environment, it is the blood that transports these gases between the lungs and body tissues. The blood carries oxygen and carbon dioxide in the physically dissolved state and in combination with hemoglobin. Carbon dioxide also is converted to bicarbonate and transported in that form.

Dissolved oxygen and carbon dioxide exert a partial pressure that is designated in the same manner as the partial pressures in the gas state. In the clinical setting, blood gas measurements are used to determine the partial pressure of oxygen (PO_2) and carbon dioxide (PCO_2) in the blood. Arterial blood is used to assess diffusion of oxygen and carbon dioxide in the alveoli, whereas venous blood reflects the metabolic demands of the tissues rather than the gas exchange function of the lungs. The PO_2 of arterial blood normally varies slightly with altitude, and is above 80 mm Hg at sea level, and the PCO_2 is normally between 35 to 45 mm Hg. Normally, the arterial blood gases are the same or nearly the same as the partial pressure of the gases in the alveoli. The arterial PO_2 may be written PaO_2, alveolar PO_2 as PAO_2, and venous PO_2 as PvO_2, with the same types of designations used to differentiate arterial, alveolar, and venous PCO_2.

Oxygen Transport

Oxygen is transported in two forms within the blood: (1) in chemical combination with hemoglobin, and (2) in the dissolved state. Hemoglobin carries about 98% to 99% of oxygen in arterial blood and is the main transporter of oxygen. The remaining 1% to 2% of the oxygen is carried in the dissolved state. Only the dissolved form of oxygen passes through the capillary wall, diffuses through the cell membrane, and makes itself available for use in cell metabolism. The oxygen content (measured in ml/100 ml) of the blood includes the oxygen carried by hemoglobin and in the dissolved portion.

Hemoglobin Transport. Hemoglobin is a highly efficient carrier of oxygen. Hemoglobin bound with oxygen is called *oxyhemoglobin,* and when oxygen is removed, it is called *deoxygenated* or *reduced hemoglobin.* Each gram of hemoglobin carries approximately 1.34 ml of oxygen when it is fully saturated. This means that a person with a hemoglobin level of 140 g/L carries 188 ml of oxygen per litre or as commonly stated 18.8 ml of oxygen per 100 ml of blood.

In the lungs, oxygen diffuses across the alveolar–capillary membrane, through the plasma, and into the red blood cell, where it forms a loose and reversible bond with the hemoglobin molecule. In normal lungs, this process is rapid, so that even with a fast heart rate the hemoglobin is almost completely saturated with oxygen during the short time it spends in the pulmonary capillaries. Thus hemoglobin is approximately 95% to 100% saturated when the blood enters and leaves the left side of the heart. When oxygen moves out of the systemic capillaries in response to the needs of the tissues, the hemoglobin saturation drops to approximately 75%. The blood is now considered to be deoxygenated, and returns to the right side of the heart via the superior and inferior vena cavae.

Dissolved Oxygen. The partial pressure of oxygen represents the level of dissolved oxygen in plasma. The amount of dissolved oxygen depends on its partial pressure and its solubility in the plasma. In the normal lung at 760 mm Hg atmospheric pressure, the PO_2 of arterial blood is approximately 100 mm Hg. The solubility of oxygen in plasma is fixed and very small. For every 1 mm Hg of PO_2 present, 0.003 ml of oxygen becomes dissolved in 100 ml of plasma. This means that at a normal arterial PO_2 of 100 mm Hg, the blood carries only 0.3 ml of dissolved oxygen in each 100 ml of plasma. This amount (approximately 1% to 2%) is very small compared with the amount that can be carried in an equal amount of blood when oxygen is attached to hemoglobin.

Although the amount of oxygen carried in plasma under normal conditions is small, it determines the pressure gradient and attachment of oxygen to hemoglobin. Thus, we expect

more than 95% of the hemoglobin sites to be bound with oxygen at a PO_2 of greater than 80 mm Hg.

Binding Affinity of Hemoglobin for Oxygen. The efficiency of the hemoglobin transport system depends on the ability of the hemoglobin molecule to bind oxygen in the lungs and release it in the tissues. Oxygen that remains bound to hemoglobin cannot move out of the capillaries to participate in tissue metabolism. The term *affinity* refers to hemoglobin's ability to bind with oxygen. Hemoglobin binds with oxygen more readily when its affinity is increased and releases it more readily when its affinity is decreased.

As described in Chapter 14, the hemoglobin molecule is composed of four polypeptide chains with an iron-containing heme group. Because oxygen binds to the iron atom, each hemoglobin molecule can bind four molecules of oxygen when it is fully saturated. Oxygen binds cooperatively with the heme groups on the hemoglobin molecule. After the first molecule of oxygen binds to hemoglobin, the molecule undergoes a change in shape. As a result, the second and third molecules bind more readily, and binding of the fourth molecule is even easier. In a like manner, the unloading of the first molecule of oxygen enhances the unloading of the next molecule and so on. Thus, the affinity of hemoglobin for oxygen changes with hemoglobin saturation.

Hemoglobin's affinity for oxygen is influenced by pH, carbon dioxide concentration, temperature, and the enzyme 2,3-DPG. It binds with oxygen more readily under conditions of increased pH (alkalosis), decreased carbon dioxide concentration, or decreased temperature; however, less is available to be released at the tissues. Conversely, hemoglobin releases oxygen more readily under conditions of decreased pH (acidosis), increased carbon dioxide concentration, or increased temperature which decreases affinity. Increased tissue metabolism generates carbon dioxide and metabolic acids and thereby decreases the affinity of hemoglobin for oxygen. Heat also is a byproduct of tissue metabolism, explaining the effect of fever on increased oxygen availability to the tissues.

Red blood cells contain a metabolic intermediate called *2,3-diphosphoglycerate* (2,3-DPG) that also affects the affinity of hemoglobin for oxygen. An increase in 2,3-DPG enhances unloading of oxygen from hemoglobin at the tissue level. Conditions that increase 2,3-DPG include exercise, hypoxemia that occurs at high altitude, and hypoxemia due to chronic lung disease.

The Oxygen Dissociation Curve. The relationship between the PO_2 of the blood and the oxygen bound to hemoglobin is described by the *oxygen–hemoglobin dissociation curve,* which is shown in Figure 27.22. The x axis of the graph depicts the PO_2 or dissolved oxygen. This indicates the partial pressure of the oxygen in the blood. At sea level, the PO_2 is approximately 100 mm Hg when room air (*i.e.,* with 21% oxygen) is inspired. The left y axis (percentage) depicts hemoglobin saturation or the amount of oxygen that is carried by the hemoglobin. Note that hemoglobin can never be more than

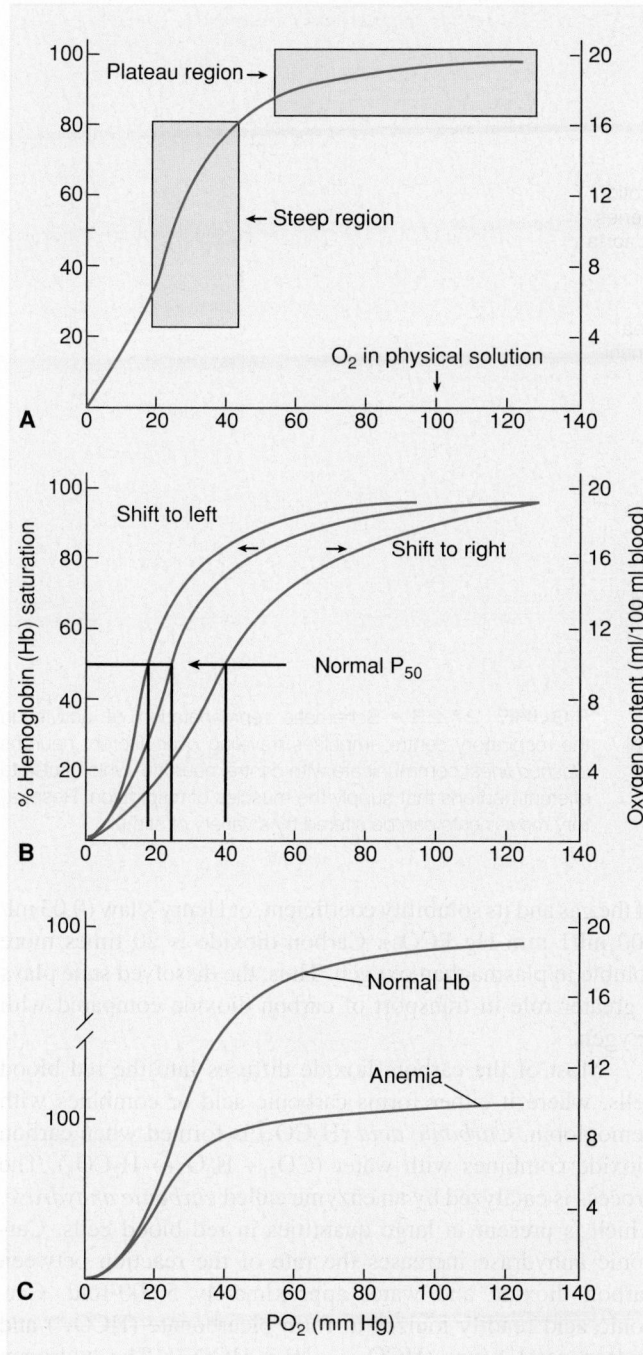

FIGURE 27.22 • Oxygen–hemoglobin dissociation curve. **A:** Left boxed area represents the steep portion of the curve where oxygen is released from hemoglobin (Hb) to the tissues, and the top boxed area the plateau of the curve where oxygen is loaded onto hemoglobin in the lung. **B:** The effect of body temperature, arterial PCO₂, and pH on hemoglobin affinity for oxygen as indicated by a shift in the curve and position of the P_{50}. A shift of the curve to the right due to an increase in temperature or PCO_2, or decreased pH, favours release of oxygen to the tissues. A decrease in temperature or PCO_2, or an increase in pH, shifts the curve to the left and has the opposite effect. The P_{50} is the partial pressure of oxygen required to saturate 50% of hemoglobin with oxygen. **C:** Effect of anemia on the oxygen-carrying capacity of blood. The hemoglobin can be completely saturated, but the oxygen content of the blood is reduced.

100% saturated; however, the PO_2 normally will increase to greater than 100 mm Hg with supplemental oxygen. The right y axis depicts oxygen content or total amount of the oxygen content being carried in the blood (ml O_2/100 ml blood).

The S-shaped oxygen dissociation curve has a plateau region representing binding of oxygen to hemoglobin in the pulmonary capillaries and a steep region representing release of oxygen into the tissue capillaries (Fig. 27.22A). The S shape of the curve reflects the effect that oxygen saturation has on the conformation of the hemoglobin molecule and its affinity for oxygen. At approximately 90 mm Hg PO_2, a plateau occurs, at which point the hemoglobin is nearly 100% saturated. Increasing the alveolar PO_2 above this level does not significantly increase the hemoglobin saturation. Even at high altitudes, when the partial pressure of oxygen is considerably decreased, the hemoglobin remains relatively well saturated. For example, at 60 mm Hg PO_2, the hemoglobin is still approximately 90% saturated.

The steep portion of the dissociation curve—between 60 and 40 mm Hg—represents the removal of oxygen from the hemoglobin as it moves through the tissue capillaries. This portion of the curve reflects the fact that there is considerable transfer of oxygen from hemoglobin to the tissues with only a small drop in PO_2, thereby ensuring a gradient for oxygen to move into body cells. The tissues normally remove approximately 5 ml of oxygen per 100 ml of blood, and the hemoglobin of venous blood is approximately 75% saturated when it returns to the right side of the heart. In this portion of the dissociation curve (saturation <75%), the rate at which oxygen is released from hemoglobin is determined largely by tissue uptake. During strenuous exercise, for example, the muscle cells may remove as much as 15 ml of oxygen per 100 ml of blood from hemoglobin due to factors that decrease affinity.

Hemoglobin can be regarded as a buffer system that regulates the delivery of oxygen to the tissues. In order to function as a buffer system, the affinity of hemoglobin for oxygen must change with the metabolic needs of the tissues. This change is represented by a shift to the right or left in the dissociation curve (Fig. 27.22B). A shift to the right indicates that the tissue PO_2 is greater for any given level of hemoglobin saturation and represents reduced affinity of the hemoglobin for oxygen at any given PO_2. It usually is caused by conditions that reflect increased tissue metabolism, such as increased temperature, acidosis, or increased PCO_2. High altitude and conditions such as pulmonary insufficiency, heart failure, and severe anemia also cause the oxygen dissociation curve to shift to the right. A shift to the left in the oxygen dissociation curve represents an increased affinity of hemoglobin for oxygen and occurs in situations associated with a decrease in tissue metabolism, such as alkalosis, decreased temperature, and decreased PCO_2 levels. The degree of shift can be determined by the P_{50}, or the partial pressure of oxygen that is needed to achieve a 50% saturation of hemoglobin. Returning to Figure 27.23B, the dissociation curve on the left has a P_{50} of approximately 20 mm Hg; the normal curve, a P_{50} of 26; and the curve on the right, a P_{50} of 40 mm Hg.

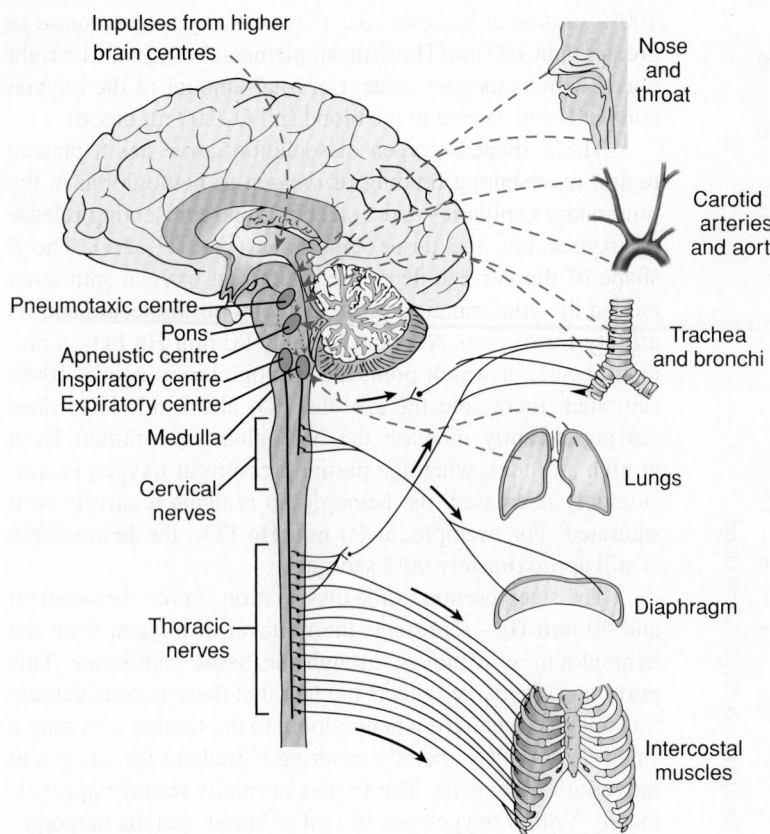

Impulses from higher
brain centres

Nose
and
throat

Carotid
arteries
and aorta

Pneumotaxic centre
Pons
Apneustic centre
Inspiratory centre
Expiratory centre
Medulla

Trachea
and bronchi

Cervical
nerves

Lungs

Diaphragm

Thoracic
nerves

Intercostal
muscles

FIGURE 27.23 • Schematic representation of activity in the respiratory centre. Impulses traveling over afferent neurons (*dashed lines*) communicate with central neurons, which activate efferent neurons that supply the muscles of respiration. Respiratory movements can be altered by a variety of stimuli.

The oxygen content (measured in ml/100 ml blood) represents the total amount of oxygen carried in the blood, including the dissolved oxygen and that carried by the hemoglobin (Fig. 27.22C). The amount of hemoglobin-bound oxygen is determined by the concentration of hemoglobin (in g/L), the oxygen-binding capacity of hemoglobin (1.34 ml O_2/g hemoglobin), and the percentage saturation of the hemoglobin. The dissolved oxygen content is the product of the oxygen solubility (0.003 ml O_2/100 ml) times the PO_2. Thus, an anemic person may have both a normal PO_2 and hemoglobin saturation level but actually have a decreased oxygen content because of the lower amount of hemoglobin available to bind with oxygen.

Carbon Dioxide Transport

Carbon dioxide is transported in the blood in three forms (see Understanding Carbon Dioxide Transport, Chapter 32): dissolved carbon dioxide, attached to hemoglobin, and as bicarbonate and hydrogen ions. Increased amounts of carbon dioxide are present in venous blood due to metabolism, with approximately 10% dissolved, 30% attached to hemoglobin, and 60% converted into bicarbonate and hydrogen. Acid-base balance is influenced by the amount of carbon dioxide in the blood.

As carbon dioxide is formed during the metabolic process, it diffuses out of cells into the tissue spaces and then into the capillaries. The amount of dissolved carbon dioxide that can be carried in plasma is determined by the partial pressure of the gas and its solubility coefficient, or Henry's law (0.03 ml/ 100 ml/1 mm Hg PCO_2). Carbon dioxide is 20 times more soluble in plasma than oxygen. Thus, the dissolved state plays a greater role in transport of carbon dioxide compared with oxygen.

Most of the carbon dioxide diffuses into the red blood cells, where it either forms carbonic acid or combines with hemoglobin. *Carbonic acid* (H_2CO_3) is formed when carbon dioxide combines with water ($CO_2 + H_2O \leftrightarrow H_2CO_3$). The process is catalyzed by an enzyme called *carbonic anhydrase,* which is present in large quantities in red blood cells. Carbonic anhydrase increases the rate of the reaction between carbon dioxide and water approximately 5,000-fold. Carbonic acid readily ionizes to form bicarbonate (HCO_3^-) and hydrogen (H^+) ions ($HCO_3 \leftrightarrow H^+ + HCO_3^-$). The hydrogen ion combines with the hemoglobin, which is a powerful acid-base buffer, and the bicarbonate ion diffuses into plasma in exchange for a chloride ion. This exchange is made possible by a special bicarbonate–chloride carrier protein in the red blood cell membrane. As a result of the bicarbonate–chloride shift, the chloride and water content of the red blood cell is greater in venous blood than in arterial blood.

In addition to the carbonic anhydrase-mediated reaction with water, carbon dioxide reacts directly with hemoglobin to form *carbaminohemoglobin*. The combination of carbon dioxide with hemoglobin is a reversible reaction that involves a loose bond, which allows transport of carbon dioxide from tissues to the lungs, where it is released into the alveoli for exchange with the external environment. The release of oxygen from hemoglobin in the tissues enhances the binding of carbon dioxide to hemoglobin; in the lungs, the combining of oxygen with hemoglobin displaces carbon dioxide. The binding of carbon dioxide to hemoglobin is determined by the acidic nature of hemoglobin. In the lungs, the highly acidic hemoglobin has a lesser tendency to form carbaminohemoglobin, and carbon dioxide is released from hemoglobin into the capillaries and diffuses into the alveoli. In the tissues, the release of oxygen from hemoglobin causes hemoglobin to become less acid, thereby increasing its ability to combine with carbon dioxide and form carbaminohemoglobin.

IN SUMMARY

The primary functions of the lungs are oxygenation of the blood and removal of carbon dioxide. Pulmonary gas exchange is conventionally divided into three processes: ventilation, or the flow of gases into the alveoli of the lungs; perfusion, or movement of blood through the adjacent pulmonary capillaries; and diffusion, or transfer of gases between the alveoli and the pulmonary capillaries.

Ventilation is the movement of air between the atmosphere and the lungs and perfusion is the flow of blood into and out of the gas exchange portions of the lung. Pulmonary ventilation refers to the total exchange of gases between the atmosphere and the lungs, and alveolar ventilation to ventilation in the gas exchange portion of the lungs. The distribution of alveolar ventilation and pulmonary capillary blood flow varies with lung volume and body position. In the upright position and at high lung volumes, ventilation is greatest in the upper parts of the lungs. The upright position also produces a decrease in blood flow to the upper parts of the lung, resulting from the distance above the level of the heart and the low mean arterial pressure in the pulmonary circulation. The efficiency of gas exchange requires matching of ventilation and perfusion, so that equal amounts of air and blood enter the respiratory portion of the lungs. Two conditions interfere with matching of ventilation and perfusion: dead air space, in which areas of the lungs are ventilated but not perfused, and shunt, in which areas of the lungs are perfused but not ventilated.

The diffusion of gases in the lungs is influenced by four factors: the surface area available for diffusion; the thickness of the alveolar–capillary membrane through which the gases diffuse; the differences in the partial pressure of the gas on either side of the membrane; and the diffusion characteristics of the gas.

The blood transports oxygen to the cells and returns carbon dioxide to the lungs through the systemic circulation. Oxygen is transported in two forms: in chemical combination with hemoglobin and physically dissolved in plasma (PO_2). Hemoglobin is an efficient carrier of oxygen, and approximately 98% to 99% of oxygen is transported in this manner. The relationship between the oxygen carried in

combination with hemoglobin and the PO_2 of the blood is described by the oxygen–hemoglobin dissociation curve. Carbon dioxide is carried in three forms: attached to hemoglobin (30%), dissolved carbon dioxide (10%), and bicarbonate (60%).

CONCEPTS in action **ANIMATION**

CONTROL OF BREATHING

After completing this section of the chapter, you should be able to meet the following objectives:

- Compare the neural control of the respiratory muscles, which control breathing, with that of cardiac muscle, which controls the pumping action of the heart.
- Describe the function of the chemoreceptors and lung receptors in the regulation of ventilation.
- Trace the integration of the cough reflex from stimulus to explosive expulsion of air that constitutes the cough.
- Describe the type of periodic breathing known as Cheyne-Stokes breathing.
- Define dyspnea and list three types of conditions in which dyspnea occurs.

Unlike the heart, which has inherent rhythmic properties and can beat independently of the nervous system, the muscles that control respiration require continuous input from the nervous system. Movement of the diaphragm, intercostal muscles, sternocleidomastoid, and other accessory muscles that control ventilation is integrated by neurons located in the pons and medulla. These neurons are collectively referred to as the *respiratory centre* (Fig. 27.23).

Respiratory Centre

The medullary respiratory centre consists of two dense, bilateral aggregates of respiratory neurons involved in initiating inspiration and expiration and incorporating afferent impulses into motor responses of the respiratory muscles. The first, or dorsal, group of neurons in the respiratory centre is concerned primarily with inspiration. These neurons control the activity of the phrenic nerves that innervate the diaphragm and drive the second, or ventral, group of respiratory neurons. They are thought to integrate sensory input from the lungs and airways into the ventilatory response. The second group of neurons, which contains inspiratory and expiratory neurons, controls the spinal motor neurons of the intercostal and abdominal muscles.

The control of rate, rhythms, and depth of breathing by the pontine respiratory centre results from the cycling of the two groups of respiratory neurons: the *pneumotaxic centre* in the upper pons and the *apneustic centre* in the lower pons (Fig. 27.23). These two groups of neurons contribute to the function of the respiratory centre in the medulla. The apneustic centre has an excitatory effect on inspiration, tending to prolong inspiration. The pneumotaxic centre switches inspiration off, assisting in the control of respiratory rate and inspiratory volume. Brain injuries that damage the connection between the pneumotaxic and apneustic centres result in an irregular breathing pattern that consists of prolonged inspiratory gasps interrupted by expiratory efforts.

Axons from the neurons in the respiratory centre cross in the midline and descend in the ventrolateral columns of the spinal cord. The tracts that control expiration and inspiration are spatially separated in the cord, as are the tracts that transmit specialized reflexes (*i.e.*, coughing and hiccupping) and voluntary control of ventilation. Only at the level of the spinal cord are the respiratory impulses integrated to produce a reflex response.

Regulation of Breathing

The control of breathing has involuntary and voluntary components. The involuntary or automatic regulation of breathing is controlled by input from two types of sensors or receptors: chemoreceptors and lung receptors. Chemoreceptors monitor blood levels of carbon dioxide, pH, and oxygen and adjust ventilation to meet the changing metabolic needs of the body. Lung receptors monitor breathing patterns and lung function.

Voluntary regulation integrates breathing with actions such as speaking, blowing, and singing. These actions, which are initiated by the motor and premotor cortex, cause a temporary suspension of automatic breathing. The involuntary and voluntary components of respiration are regulated by afferent impulses that are transmitted to the respiratory centre from a number of sources. Afferent input from higher brain centres is evidenced by the fact that a person can consciously and purposefully alter both depth and rate of respiration. Fever, pain, and emotion exert their influence through lower brain centres. Vagal afferents from sensory receptors in the lungs and airways are integrated in the dorsal area of the respiratory centre.

Chemoreceptors

Tissue needs for oxygen and the removal of carbon dioxide are regulated by chemoreceptors that monitor blood levels of these gases. Input from these sensors is transmitted to the respiratory centre, and breathing is adjusted to maintain the arterial blood gases within a normal range.

There are two types of chemoreceptors: central and peripheral. The most important chemoreceptors for sensing changes in the PCO_2 blood are the *central chemoreceptors,* which are located in chemosensitive regions near the respiratory centre in the medulla. The central chemoreceptors are surrounded by brain extracellular fluid and respond to changes in its hydrogen ion (H^+) concentration. The composition of

the extracellular fluid surrounding the chemoreceptors is governed by the cerebral spinal fluid (CSF), local blood flow, and tissue metabolism. Of these, the CSF is apparently the most important. The CSF is separated from the blood by the blood–brain barrier, which permits free diffusion of carbon dioxide but not bicarbonate (HCO_3^-) or H^+. When PCO_2 rises, carbon dioxide from the blood diffuses into the CSF, liberating H^+, which then stimulates the chemoreceptors. The central chemoreceptors are extremely sensitive to short-term changes in carbon dioxide. An increase in carbon dioxide levels produces an immediate increase in minute ventilation. The *peripheral chemoreceptors* are located in the carotid and aortic bodies, which are found at the bifurcation of the common carotid arteries and in the arch of the aorta, respectively (Fig. 27.23). These chemoreceptors monitor arterial blood oxygen levels. Although the peripheral chemoreceptors also monitor carbon dioxide, they play a much more important role in monitoring oxygen levels. These receptors exert little control over ventilation until the PO_2 has dropped below 60 mm Hg. In health, the primary mechanism to increase minute ventilation is the small increase in PCO_2 that is recognized by the central chemoreceptors. However, in persons with chronically elevated levels of carbon dioxide, the central chemoreceptors become less responsive to the higher than normal PCO_2, and hypoxemia becomes the main stimulus for increased ventilation.

Lung Receptors

Lung and chest wall receptors monitor the status of breathing in terms of airway resistance and lung expansion. There are three types of lung receptors: stretch, irritant, and juxtacapillary receptors.

Stretch receptors are located in the smooth muscle layers of the conducting airways. They respond to changes in pressure in the walls of the airways. When the lungs are inflated, these receptors inhibit inspiration and promote expiration. They are important in establishing breathing patterns and minimizing the work of breathing by adjusting respiratory rate and Vt to accommodate changes in lung compliance and airway resistance.

The *irritant receptors* are located between the airway epithelial cells. They are stimulated by noxious gases, cigarette smoke, inhaled dust, and cold air. Stimulation of the irritant receptors leads to airway constriction and a pattern of rapid, shallow breathing. This pattern of breathing protects respiratory tissues from the damaging effects of toxic inhalants. It also is thought that the mechanical stimulation of these receptors may ensure more uniform lung expansion by initiating periodic sighing and yawning. It is possible that these receptors are involved in the bronchoconstriction response that occurs in some persons with bronchial asthma when exposed to irritants such as tobacco smoke or perfume.

The *juxtacapillary* or *J receptors* are located in the alveolar wall, close to the pulmonary capillaries. It is thought that these receptors sense lung congestion. These receptors may be responsible for the rapid, shallow breathing that occurs with pulmonary edema, pulmonary embolism, and pneumonia.

Cough Reflex

Coughing is a neurally mediated reflex that protects the lungs from accumulation of secretions and from entry of irritating and destructive substances. It is one of the primary defence mechanisms of the respiratory tract. The cough reflex is initiated by receptors located in the tracheobronchial wall. These receptors are extremely sensitive to irritating substances and to the presence of excess secretions. Afferent impulses from these receptors are transmitted through the vagus to the medullary centre, which integrates the cough response.

Coughing itself requires the rapid inspiration of a large volume of air (usually about 2.5 L), followed by rapid closure of the glottis and forceful contraction of the abdominal and expiratory muscles, with higher than normal positive expiratory pressures. As these muscles contract, intrathoracic pressures are elevated to levels of 100 mm Hg or more. The rapid opening of the glottis at this point leads to an explosive expulsion of air.

Many conditions can interfere with the cough reflex and its protective function. The reflex is impaired in persons whose abdominal or respiratory muscles are weak. This problem can be caused by disease conditions that lead to muscle weakness or paralysis, and by prolonged inactivity, or can arise as an outcome of surgery involving these muscles. Bed rest interferes with expansion of the chest and limits the amount of air that can be taken into the lungs in preparation for coughing, making the cough weak and ineffective. Disease conditions that prevent effective closure of the glottis and laryngeal muscles interfere with production of the marked increase in intrathoracic pressure that is needed for effective coughing. The presence of a nasogastric tube, for example, may prevent closure of the upper airway structures and may fatigue the receptors for the cough reflex that are located in the area. The cough reflex also is impaired when there is depressed function of the medullary centres in the brain that integrate the cough reflex. Interruption of the central integration aspect of the cough reflex can arise as the result of disease of this part of the brain or the action of drugs that depress the cough centre.

Although the cough reflex is a protective mechanism, frequent and prolonged coughing can be exhausting and painful and can exert undesirable effects on the cardiovascular and respiratory systems and on the elastic tissues of the lungs. This is particularly true in young children and older adults.

Dyspnea

Dyspnea is a scientific term for the subjective sensation (*i.e.,* a person's perception) of difficulty in breathing that includes the perception of laboured breathing, or difficulty with breathing. The terms *dyspnea, breathlessness,* and *shortness of breath* (SOB) often are used interchangeably by health care professionals. Like other subjective symptoms, such as fatigue and pain, dyspnea is difficult to quantify because it describes the person's perception of the sensation. Dyspnea is frequently perceived in several acute or chronic states: lung disease such as pneumonia, asthma, and emphysema; heart disease that is characterized by pulmonary congestion; and neuromuscular disorders such as myasthenia gravis and muscular dystrophy that affect the respiratory muscles.

The physiological cause of perceiving difficulty or laboured breathing is unknown. Four types of mechanisms have been proposed to explain the sensation: stimulation of lung receptors; increased sensitivity to changes in ventilation perceived through central nervous system mechanisms; reduced ventilatory capacity or breathing reserve; and stimulation of neural receptors in the muscle fibres of the intercostals and diaphragm, and of receptors in the skeletal joints. The first of the suggested mechanisms is stimulation of lung receptors. These receptors are stimulated by the contraction of bronchial smooth muscle, the stretch of the bronchial wall, pulmonary congestion, and conditions that decrease lung compliance. The second category of proposed mechanisms focuses on central nervous system mechanisms that transmit information to the cortex regarding respiratory muscle weakness or a discrepancy between the increased effort of breathing and inadequate respiratory muscle contraction. The third type of mechanism focuses on a reduction in ventilatory capacity or breathing reserve. A reduction in breathing reserve (*i.e.,* maximum voluntary ventilation not being used during a given activity) to less than 65% to 75% may correlate with dyspnea on exertion. The fourth possible mechanism is stimulation of muscle and joint receptors in the respiratory musculature because of a discrepancy in the tension generated by these muscles and the Vt that results. When stimulated, these receptors transmit signals that bring about an awareness of the breathing discrepancy.

The most common method for measuring dyspnea is a retrospective determination of the level of daily activity at which a person experiences dyspnea. Several scales are available for use, such as visual analogs scales. The person being assessed selects a point on the scale that describes his or her perceived dyspnea with a given activity, such as walking a certain distance. This information can be used to assess dyspnea over time.

The treatment of dyspnea depends on the cause. For example, persons with impaired respiratory function may require oxygen therapy, and those with pulmonary edema may require measures to improve heart function or reduce fluid retention. Methods to decrease anxiety, breathing retraining, and energy conservation measures may be used to decrease the sensation of dyspnea.

IN SUMMARY

The respiratory system requires continuous input from the nervous system. Movement of the diaphragm, intercostal muscles, and other respiratory muscles is controlled by neurons of the respiratory centre located in the pons and medulla. The control of breathing has involuntary and voluntary components. The involuntary regulation of ventilation is controlled by two types of receptors: lung receptors, which protect respiratory structures, and chemoreceptors, which monitor the gas exchange function of the lungs by sensing changes in blood levels of carbon dioxide, oxygen, and pH. There are three types of lung receptors: stretch receptors, which monitor lung inflation; irritant receptors, which protect against the damaging effects of toxic inhalants; and J receptors, which are thought to sense lung congestion. There are two groups of chemoreceptors: central and peripheral. The central chemoreceptors are the most important in sensing changes in carbon dioxide levels, and the peripheral chemoreceptors function in sensing arterial blood oxygen levels.

Voluntary respiratory control is needed for integrating breathing and actions such as speaking, blowing, and singing. These acts, which are initiated by the motor and premotor cortex, cause temporary suspension of automatic breathing. The cough reflex protects the lungs from the accumulation of secretions and from the entry of irritating and destructive substances; it is one of the primary defence mechanisms of the respiratory tract. Dyspnea is a subjective sensation of difficulty in breathing that is seen in cardiac, pulmonary, and neuromuscular disorders that affect the respiratory muscles. It can also occur during strenuous work and exercise in healthy persons.

REVIEW EXERCISES

1. Calculate the *partial pressure* of oxygen (PO_2) in the alveoli at an atmospheric pressure near sea level in Montreal, Quebec (760 mm Hg); Whitehorse, Yukon at 702 m above sea level (700 mm Hg); and Banff, Alberta at 1580 m (580 mm Hg). Consider that the oxygen concentration is 21% and the water vapour pressure in the lungs is 47 mm Hg.

2. Use the solubility coefficient for oxygen and the oxygen dissociation curve depicted in Figure 27.22 to answer the following questions:

   A. *It is usually recommended that the hemoglobin saturation of persons with chronic lung disease be maintained at about 89% to 90% when they are receiving supplemental low-flow oxygen. What would their PO_2 be at this level of hemoglobin saturation and what is the rationale for keeping the PO_2 at this level?*

   B. *What is the oxygen content of a person with a hemoglobin level of 60 g/L who is breathing room air?*

   C. *What is the oxygen content of a person with carbon monoxide poisoning who is receiving 100% oxygen at 3 atmospheres' pressure in a hyperbaric chamber? Consider that most of the person's hemoglobin is saturated with carbon monoxide.*

Bibliography

Abdo W. F., Heunks L. M. (2012). Oxygen-induced hypercapnia in COPD: Myths and facts. *Critical Care, 16*(5), 323.

Barrett K. E., Boitano S., Barman S. M., et al. (2012). *Review of medical physiology* (24th ed.). New York: McGraw-Hill Company.

Boron W. F., Boulpaep E. L. (2009). *Medical physiology* (2nd ed.). Philadelphia, PA: Saunders.

Hall J. E. (2011). *Textbook of medical physiology* (12th ed.). Philadelphia, PA: Saunders.

Kliegman R. M., Stanton B. F., St. Geme J. W., et al. (Eds.). (2011). *Nelson textbook of pediatrics.* (19th ed.). Philadelphia, PA: Elsevier Saunders.

Moore K. L., Dalley A. F., Agur A. M. (2014). *Clinically oriented anatomy* (7th ed.). Philadelphia, PA: Lippincott Williams & Wilkins.

Prabhakar N. R., Peng Y. J. (2004). Peripheral chemoreceptors in health and disease. *Journal of Applied Physiology, 96*(1), 359–366.

Rhoades R. A., Bell D. R. (2013). *Medical physiology: Principles for clinical medicine* (4th ed.). Philadelphia, PA: Lippincott Williams & Wilkins.

Wert S. E., Whitsett J. A., Nogee L. M. (2009). Genetic disorder of surfactant dysfunction. *Pediatric and Developmental Pathology, 12*(4), 253–274.

West J. B. (2012). *Respiratory physiology: The essentials* (9th ed.). Philadelphia, PA: Lippincott Williams & Wilkins.

Wiebe B. M., Laursen H. (1995). Human lung volume, alveolar surface area, and capillary length. *Microscopy Research and Technique, 32*(3), 255–262.

Visit thePoint **http://thePoint.lww.com for animations, journal articles, and more!**

Respiratory Tract Infections, Neoplasms, and Childhood Disorders

28

Contagious respiratory illnesses represent one of the more common reasons for visits to physician, admission to hospital, and forced inactivity among all age groups. They include the common cold, influenza viruses, pneumonia, tuberculosis, and fungal infections. The common cold, although not usually serious, occurs often and results in many missed work and school days. Pneumonia is less common but is the eighth leading cause of death in Canada, particularly among the older adults and those with compromised immune function.[1] Tuberculosis (TB) remains one of the deadliest diseases in the world affecting one third of the world's population.[2] The rate of TB in Canada continues to decline slightly each year. In 2012, foreign-born individuals accounted for majority of reported cases (64%) but the incidence of cases in Canadian-born Aboriginal people (23%) remains disproportionate compared to Canadian-born non-Aboriginal cases (10%).[3] Lung cancer remains the leading cause of cancer death worldwide primarily affecting adults. Neonates, infants, and small children also have unique respiratory conditions and while some are common others can be life threatening or lead to chronic complications.

RESPIRATORY TRACT INFECTIONS

After completing this section of the chapter, you should be able to meet the following objectives:

- Describe the transmission of the common cold from one person to another.
- Describe the causes, manifestations, and treatment of acute and chronic sinusitis.
- Relate the characteristics of the influenza virus to its contagious properties and the need for a yearly immunization.
- Characterize community-acquired pneumonia, hospital-acquired pneumonia, and pneumonia in immunocompromised persons in terms of pathogens, manifestations, and prognosis.

- Describe the immunologic properties of the tubercle bacillus, and differentiate between primary tuberculosis and reactivated tuberculosis on the basis of their pathophysiology.
- State the mechanism for the transmission of fungal infections of the lung.

The respiratory tract is susceptible to infectious processes caused by many different types of microorganisms. Infections can involve the upper respiratory tract (*i.e.*, nose, oropharynx, and larynx), the lower respiratory tract (*i.e.*, lower airways and lungs), or the upper and lower airways. For the most part, the signs and symptoms of respiratory tract infections depend on the function of the structure involved, the severity of the infectious process, and the person's age and general health status. The discussion in this section of the chapter focuses on the common cold, rhinosinusitis, influenza, pneumonia, tuberculosis, and fungal infections of the lung. Acute respiratory infections in children are discussed in the last section of the chapter.

Viruses are the most frequent cause of respiratory tract infections. They can cause infections ranging from a self-limited cold to life-threatening pneumonia. Moreover, viral infections can damage bronchial epithelium, obstruct airways, and lead to secondary bacterial infections. Each viral species has its own pattern of respiratory tract involvement. Other microorganisms, such as bacteria (*e.g.*, pneumococci, staphylococci), mycobacteria (*e.g.*, *Mycobacterium tuberculosis*), fungi (*e.g.*, *Histoplasma capsulatum* [histoplasmosis], *Coccidioides immitis* [coccidioidomycosis], and *Blastomyces dermatitidis* [blastomycosis]), and opportunistic organisms (*e.g.*, *Pneumocystis jiroveci* [formerly *Pneumocystis carinii*]), also produce infections of the lung, many of which produce significant morbidity and mortality.

The Common Cold

The common cold is a viral infection of the upper respiratory tract. It occurs more frequently than any other respiratory tract infection. Most adults have 1 to 3 upper respiratory tract infections per year, whereas infants may experience up to 11 episodes per year, pre-school age up to 8 episodes, and at school age these infections usually decrease to approximately 4 episodes per year.[4,5] The condition usually begins with a feeling of dryness and stuffiness affecting mainly the nasopharynx, followed by excessive production of nasal secretions and tearing of the eyes (*i.e.*, rhinitis or coryza). Usually, the secretions remain clear and watery. The mucous membranes of the upper respiratory tract become reddened (erythematous), swollen (edematous), and bathed in secretions (leading to rhinorrhea). Involvement of the pharynx and larynx causes sore throat and hoarseness which can be further irritated by an accompanying post nasal drip (PND). The affected person may experience headache and generalized malaise. In severe cases, there may be chills, fever, and exhaustion. More than one third of

children can also present with an acute otitis media with the respiratory viral infections due to changes in middle ear pressure and eustachian tube function. The disease process is usually self-limited, lasting approximately 7 to 10 days.[4]

Initially thought to be caused by either a single "cold virus" or a group of them, the common cold is now recognized to be associated with a number of viruses. Up to 80% of cases are caused by rhinoviruses and other pathogens include parainfluenza viruses, respiratory syncytial virus (RSV), coronaviruses, and adenoviruses. The season of the year and the person's age and prior exposure are important factors in the type of virus causing the infection and the type of symptoms that occur. For example, outbreaks of colds due to rhinoviruses are most common in early fall and late spring; those due to RSV peak in the winter and spring months; and infections due to the adenoviruses and coronaviruses are more frequent during the winter and spring months. Infections resulting from RSV and parainfluenza viruses are most common and severe in children younger than 3 years of age. Infections occur less frequently and with milder symptoms with increasing age. Parainfluenza viruses often produce lower respiratory symptoms with first infections, but less severe upper respiratory symptoms with reinfections. The rhinoviruses are the most common cause of colds in persons between 5 and 40 years of age. Rhinoviruses have more than 100 different serotypes and a high-mutation rate during viral replication.[4] Although people acquire lifetime immunity to an individual serotype, it is unlikely to become immune to all serotypes.

The "cold viruses" rapidly spread from person to person. Children are the major reservoir of cold viruses, often acquiring a new virus from another child in school or day care. The fingers are the greatest source of spread, and the nasal mucosa and conjunctival surface of the eyes are the most common portals for entry of the virus. The most highly contagious period is during the first 3 days after the onset of symptoms, and the incubation period is approximately 5 days. Cold viruses have been found to survive for more than 5 hours on the skin and hard surfaces, such as plastic countertops.[6] Aerosol spread of colds through coughing and sneezing is much less important than the spread by fingers picking up the virus from contaminated surfaces and carrying it to the nasal membranes and eyes.[6] This suggests that careful attention to hand washing is one of the most important preventive measures for avoiding the common cold.

Treatment

Because the common cold is an acute and self-limited illness in persons who are otherwise healthy, symptomatic treatment with rest and antipyretic drugs is usually all that is needed. Antibiotics are ineffective against viral infections and are not recommended due to the increasing bacterial resistance. Many over-the-counter (OTC) remedies are available for treating symptoms of the common cold, without evidence of shortening the duration of the cold. Antihistamines are popular OTC drugs because of their action in drying nasal secretions. They alleviate some symptoms, but they may dry up bronchial secretions and worsen the cough, and may cause dizziness, drowsiness, and impaired judgment. Decongestant drugs (*i.e.,* sympathomimetic agents) are available in OTC nasal sprays, drops, and oral cold medications. These drugs constrict the blood vessels in the swollen nasal mucosa and reduce nasal swelling. Rebound nasal swelling can occur with indiscriminate use of nasal drops and sprays. Oral preparations containing decongestants may cause systemic vasoconstriction and elevation of blood pressure when given in doses large enough to relieve nasal congestion, and they should be avoided by persons with hypertension, heart disease, hyperthyroidism, diabetes mellitus, or other health problems.[4,6]

There is controversial interest regarding the use of vitamin C, zinc, ginseng, or Echinacea to reduce the incidence and severity of colds and influenza. Some studies have found vitamin C intake to be beneficial, and others have found it to be of questionable value. As with vitamin C, some studies have shown zinc lozenges to be beneficial, and others have not. Little research has been conducted on ginseng but it may be effective in enhancing the immune response and decreasing the incidence of acquiring the common cold as well as decreasing the severity of symptoms. Few studies have explored the prevention of the common cold with Echinacea; however, a Cochrane review concluded that intake after the onset of symptoms may be effective in shortening the duration or decreasing the severity of symptoms in adults.[4,6]

Rhinosinusitis

Rhinitis refers to inflammation of the nasal passages and sinusitis to inflammation of the paranasal sinuses. Although it has not been universally accepted, the suggestion has been made that the term *rhinosinusitis* is a more accurate term for what is commonly referred to as *sinusitis,* because the mucosa of the nasal cavities and paranasal sinuses are lined with a continuous mucous membrane layer and viral upper respiratory tract infections frequently precede or occur along with sinus infections.[7]

The paranasal sinuses are air sacs that develop during embryogenesis from a series of ridges and furrows within the cartilaginous capsule surrounding the developing nasal cavity. As development progresses, outpouchings from these furrows become lined with ciliated respiratory epithelium and invade the surrounding facial bones to become the major sinuses. Each sinus remains in constant communication with the nasal cavity through narrow openings or *ostia.* The sinuses are named for the bone in which in which they are located— frontal, ethmoid, maxillary, and sphenoidal (Fig. 28.1A). The *maxillary sinuses* are located inferior to the bony orbit and superior to the hard palate and their openings are located superiorly and medially in the sinus, a location that impedes drainage. The *frontal sinuses* open into the middle meatus of the nasal cavity. The *ethmoid sinuses* consist of 3 to 15 air cells on each side of the ethmoid, with each maintaining a separate path to the nasal chamber. The anterior ethmoid, frontal, and maxillary sinuses all drain into the nasal cavity through a

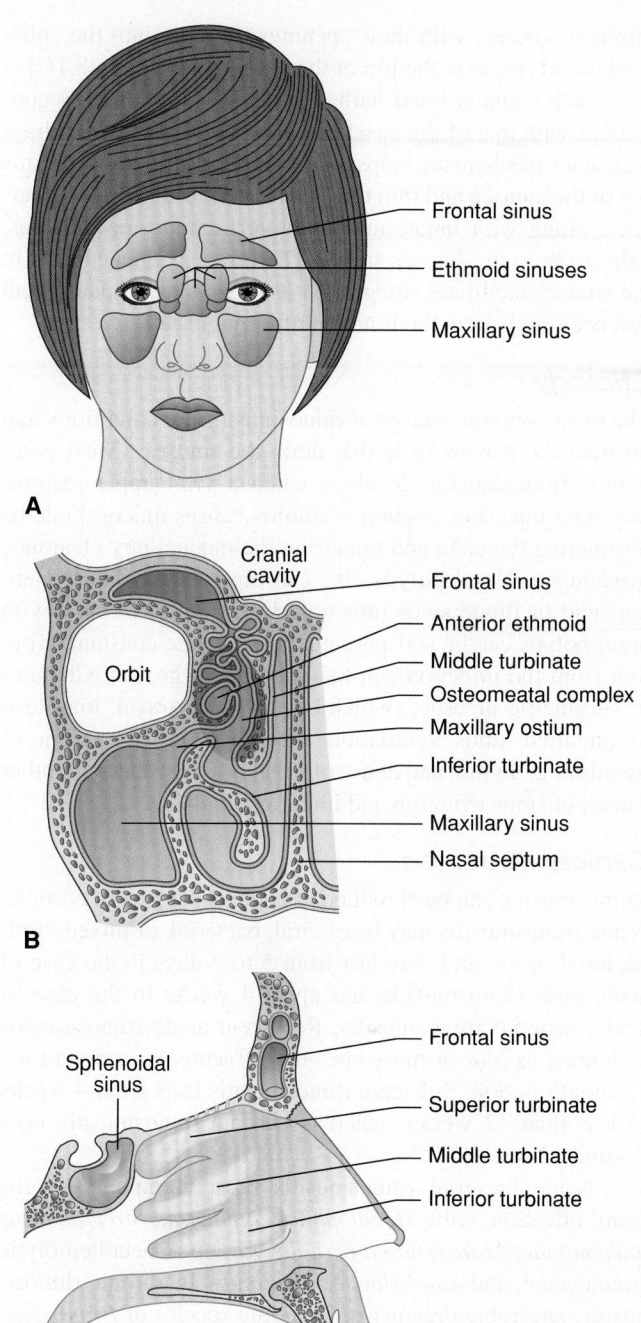

FIGURE 28.1 • Paranasal sinuses. **A:** Frontal view showing the frontal, ethmoid, and maxillary sinuses. **B:** Cross-section of nasal cavity (anterior view). The shaded area is the osteomeatal complex, which is the final common pathway for drainage of the anterior ethmoid, frontal, and maxillary sinuses. **C:** Lateral wall, left nasal cavity showing the frontal sphenoidal sinuses and the superior, middle, and inferior turbinates.

relatively convoluted and narrow passage called the *ostiomeatal complex* (Fig. 28.1B). Because of this anatomic configuration, any defects in the anterior ethmoid sinus can obstruct the ostiomeatal complex and cause secondary disease of the frontal or maxillary sinuses.[7,8] The *sphenoidal sinuses* are located just anterior to the pituitary fossa behind the posterior ethmoid sinuses, with their openings draining into the sphenoethmoid recess at the top of the nasal cavity (Fig. 28.1C).

Each sinus is lined with a mucosal surface that is continuous with that of the nasal passages. An active mucociliary clearance mechanism helps move fluid and microorganisms out of the sinuses and into the nasal cavity. Mucociliary clearance, along with innate and adaptive immune mechanisms, helps to keep the sinuses sterile. The lower oxygen content in the sinuses facilitates the growth of organisms, impairs local defences, and alters the function of immune cells.

Etiology

The most common causes of rhinosinusitis are conditions that obstruct the narrow ostia that drain the sinuses.[7] Most commonly, rhinosinusitis develops when a viral upper respiratory tract infection or allergic rhinitis causes mucosal edema obstructing the ostia and impairing the mucociliary clearance mechanism. Nasal polyps also can obstruct the sinus openings and facilitate sinus infection. Infections associated with nasal polyps can be self-perpetuating because constant irritation from the infection can facilitate polyp growth. Changes in barometric pressure, which occurs in air travel, may lead to impaired sinus ventilation and clearance of secretions. Swimming, diving, and abuse of nasal decongestants are other causes of sinus irritation and impaired drainage.

Clinical Features

Rhinosinusitis can be classified as acute, subacute, or chronic. Acute rhinosinusitis may be of viral, bacterial, or mixed viral-bacterial origin and may last from 5 to 7 days in the case of acute viral rhinosinusitis and up to 4 weeks in the case of acute bacterial rhinosinusitis. Recurrent acute rhinosinusitis is defined as four or more episodes of acute disease within a 12-month period. Subacute rhinosinusitis lasts from 4 weeks to less than 12 weeks, whereas chronic rhinosinusitis lasts beyond 12 weeks.[8]

Acute bacterial rhinosinusitis most commonly results from infection with *Haemophilus influenza, Streptococcus pneumoniae, Moraxella catarrhalis,* Group A beta-hemolytic streptococci, and *Staphylococcus aureus.*[9] In chronic rhinosinusitis, anaerobic organisms, including species of *Peptostreptococcus, Fusobacterium,* and *Prevotella,* tend to predominate, alone or in combination with aerobes such as the *Streptococcus* species or *Staphylococcus aureus.* In immunocompromised persons, such as those with human immunodeficiency virus (HIV) infection, the sinuses may become infected with gram-negative species (e.g., *Pseudomonas aeruginosa*) and opportunistic fungi. In this group, particularly in those with leukopenia, the disease may have a fulminant and even fatal course.

Manifestations. The symptoms of acute viral rhinosinusitis often are difficult to differentiate from those of the common cold and allergic rhinitis (discussed in Chapter 19). They include facial pain, headache, purulent nasal discharge, decreased sense of smell, and fever. A history of a preceding

common cold and the presence of purulent nasal drainage, pain on bending, unilateral maxillary pain, and pain in the teeth are common findings with involvement of the maxillary sinuses. The symptoms of acute viral rhinosinusitis usually resolve within 5 to 7 days without medical treatment. Acute bacterial rhinosinusitis is suggested by symptoms that worsen after 5 to 7 days or persist beyond 10 days, or symptoms that are out of proportion to those usually associated with a viral upper respiratory tract infection.[7–9] Persons who are immunocompromised, such as those with leukemia, aplastic anemia, a bone marrow transplant, or HIV infection, often present with fever of unknown origin, rhinorrhea, or facial edema. Often, other signs of inflammation such as purulent drainage are absent.

In persons with chronic rhinosinusitis, the only symptoms may be those such as nasal obstruction, a sense of fullness in the ears, postnasal drip, hoarseness, chronic cough, loss of taste and smell, or unpleasant breath.[7,8] Sinus pain often is absent; instead, the person may complain of a headache that is dull and constant. Persons with chronic rhinosinusitis may have superimposed bouts of acute rhinosinusitis. The epithelial changes that occur during acute and subacute forms of rhinosinusitis usually are reversible, but the mucosal changes that occur with chronic rhinosinusitis often are irreversible.

Diagnosis and Treatment. The diagnosis of rhinosinusitis usually is based on symptom history and a physical examination that includes inspection of the nose and throat.[7–9] Headache due to sinusitis needs to be differentiated from other types of headache. Sinusitis headache usually is exaggerated by bending forward, coughing, or sneezing. Physical examination findings in acute bacterial sinusitis include turbinate edema, nasal crusts, purulence of the nasal cavity, and failure of transillumination of the maxillary sinuses.[10] Transillumination is infrequently used because the findings do not always correlate with the condition and reproducibility between clinicians is poor.[9] Sinus radiographs and computed tomography (CT) scans are usually reserved for diagnosis of chronic rhinosinusitis or to exclude complications. Magnetic resonance imaging (MRI) is expensive and reserved for cases of suspected neoplasms or fungal sinusitis.

Treatment of rhinosinusitis depends on cause and includes appropriate use of antibiotics, topical corticosteroids, mucolytic agents, and symptom relief measures. About two thirds of persons with acute bacterial rhinosinusitis improve without antibiotic treatment, and most persons with viral upper respiratory infections improve within 7 days. Therefore, treatment with antibiotics is usually reserved for persons who have had symptoms for more than 7 days and who present with two or more manifestations of acute bacterial rhinosinusitis (*i.e.,* purulent nasal drainage; maxillary, tooth, or facial pain [especially if it is unilateral]; unilateral maxillary tenderness; or worsening of symptoms after initial improvement), or for those with severe symptoms. In addition to antibiotic therapy, the treatment of acute rhinosinusitis includes measures to promote adequate drainage by reducing nasal congestion. Oral and topical decongestants may be used for this purpose.

The use of intranasal decongestants should be limited to 3 to 5 days to prevent rebound vasodilation. Antihistamines tend to dry up secretions and are not recommended as adjunctive treatment in acute viral or bacterial rhinosinusitis. Mucolytic agents such as guaifenesin may be used to thin secretions. Topical corticosteroids are used to decrease inflammation in persons particularly with chronic or allergic rhinosinusitis. Nonpharmacologic measures include saline nasal sprays, nasal irrigation, and mist humidification.[8,9]

Surgical intervention directed at correcting obstruction of the ostiomeatal openings may be indicated in persons with chronic rhinosinusitis that is resistant to other forms of therapy. Indications for surgical intervention include obstructive nasal polyps and obstructive nasal deformities.

Complications. Because of the sinuses' proximity to the brain and orbital wall, sinusitis can lead to intracranial and orbital wall complications. Intracranial complications are seen most commonly with infection of the frontal and ethmoid sinuses because of their proximity to the dura and drainage of the veins from the frontal sinus into the dural sinus. Orbital complications can range from edema of the eyelids to orbital cellulitis and subperiosteal abscess formation. Facial swelling over the involved sinus, abnormal extraocular movements, protrusion

of the eyeball, periorbital edema, or changes in mental status may indicate intracranial complications and require immediate medical attention.[9]

Influenza

Influenza is one of the most important causes of acute upper respiratory tract infection in humans. In Canada, approximately 10% to 20% of the population becomes infected and 4,000 persons die each year of influenza-related illness.[10] Rates of infection are highest among children, but serious illness and death are highest among persons who are immunocompromised or who are 65 years of age or older, with deaths primarily due to secondary pneumonia.[10]

The viruses that cause influenza belong to the Orthomyxoviridae family, whose members are characterized by a segmented, single-stranded ribonucleic acid (RNA) genome[11] (Fig. 28.2). There are three types of influenza viruses that cause epidemics in humans: types A, B, and C. Influenza A differs in its ability to infect multiple species, including avian and mammalian species. The influenza A virus is further divided into subtypes based on two surface glycoproteins: hemagglutinin (HA) and neuraminidase (NA).[11] HA is an attachment protein that allows the virus to enter epithelial cells in the respiratory

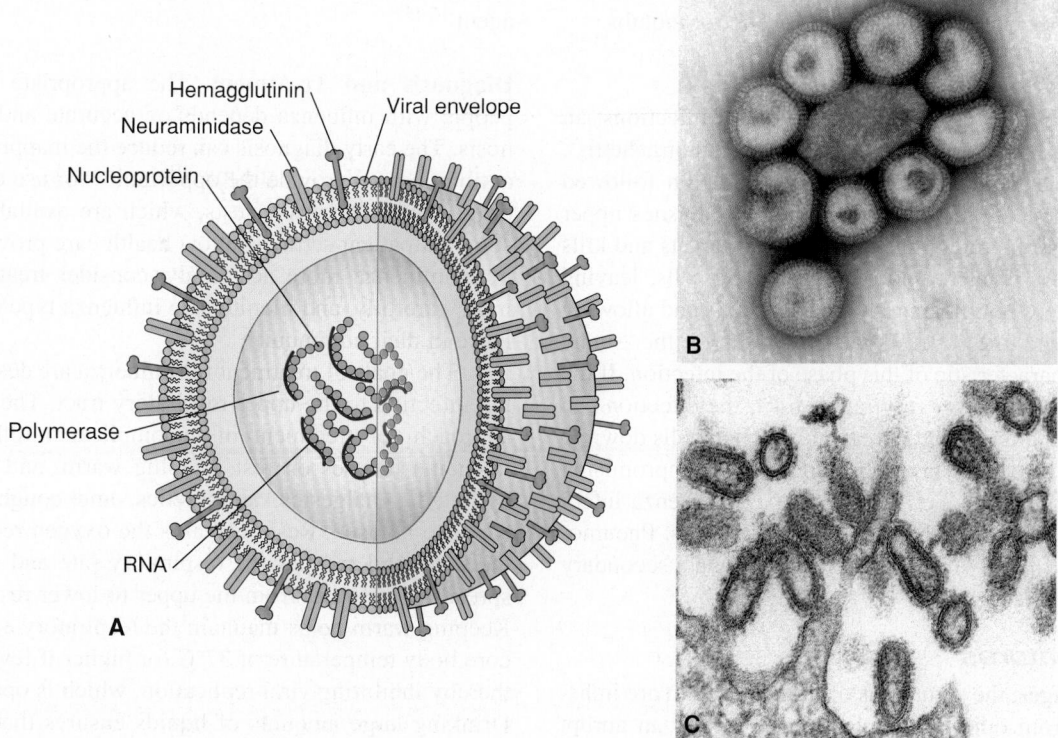

FIGURE 28.2 • Influenza type A virus. **A:** Model of the RNA influenza A virus, showing the hemagglutinin and neuraminidase envelope glycoproteins that provide access to host cells. **B:** Negative-stained transmission electron micrograph (TEM) depicting the ultrastructural details of a number of influenza viral particles, or "virions." **C:** TEM revealing ultrastructural features of the 1918 influenza pandemic virus virions. (**B** and **C** Courtesy Public Image Library, Centers for Disease Control and Prevention. Available online at: http://phil.cdc. gov/phil/home.asp.)

tract, and NA facilitates viral replication and release from the cell. Host antibodies to HA and NA prevent or ameliorate infection by the influenza virus. There are 17 known HA subtypes (*i.e.,* H1 to H17) and 9 known subtypes for NA (*i.e.,* N1 to N9). Contagion results from the ability of the influenza A virus to develop new HA and NA subtypes against which the population is not protected. An antigenic shift, which involves a major genetic rearrangement in either antigen, may lead to epidemic or pandemic infection. Lesser changes, called *antigenic drift,* find the population partially protected by cross-reacting antibodies. Influenza B and C undergo less frequent antigenic shifts than influenza A, probably because few related viruses exist in mammalian or avian species.[11]

As with many viral respiratory tract infections, influenza is more contagious than bacterial respiratory tract infections. In contrast to the rhinoviruses, transmission occurs by inhalation of droplet nuclei rather than by touching contaminated objects. Most infected people develop symptoms of the disease, increasing the likelihood of contagion through spread of infectious droplets. Young children are most likely to become infected and also to spread the infection. The incubation period for influenza is 1 to 4 days, with 2 days being the average. Persons become infectious starting 1 day before their symptoms begin and remain infectious through approximately 5 to 7 days after illness onset.[11] Children can be infectious for more than 10 days, and young children can shed the virus for up to 6 days before their illness onset. Severely immunocompromised persons can shed the virus for weeks or months.

Pathogenesis

The influenza viruses can cause three types of infections: an uncomplicated upper respiratory infection (rhinotracheitis), viral pneumonia, and a respiratory viral infection followed by a bacterial infection. Influenza initially establishes upper airway infection. In doing this, the virus first targets and kills mucus-secreting, ciliated, and other epithelial cells, leaving gaping holes between the underlying basal cells and allowing extracellular fluid to escape. This is the reason for the "runny nose" that is characteristic of this phase of the infection. If the virus spreads to the lower respiratory tract, the infection can cause severe shedding of bronchial and alveolar cells down to a single-cell-thick basal layer. In addition to compromising the natural defences of the respiratory tract, influenza infection promotes bacterial adhesion to epithelial cells. Pneumonia may result from a viral pathogenesis or from a secondary bacterial infection.[11]

Clinical Features

In the early stages, the symptoms of influenza often are indistinguishable from other viral infections. There is an abrupt onset of fever and chills, malaise, muscle aching, headache, profuse, watery nasal discharge, nonproductive cough, and sore throat.[11–14] One distinguishing feature of an influenza viral infection is the rapid onset, sometimes in as little as 1 to 2 minutes, of profound malaise. The symptoms of uncomplicated rhinotracheitis usually peak by days 3 to 5 and disappear by days 7 to 10. The aforementioned symptoms can be caused by any of the influenza A or B viruses. Influenza C virus infection causes symptoms similar to the common cold.

Viral pneumonia occurs as a complication of influenza, most frequently in the older adults or in persons with cardiopulmonary disease, but has been reported in pregnant women and in healthy, immunocompetent people. It typically develops within 1 day after onset of influenza and is characterized by rapid progression of fever, tachypnea, tachycardia, cyanosis, and hypotension.[12] The clinical course of influenza pneumonia progresses rapidly. It can cause hypoxemia and death within a few days of onset. Survivors often develop diffuse pulmonary fibrosis.

Secondary complications typically include sinusitis, otitis media, bronchitis, and bacterial pneumonia. Persons in whom secondary bacterial pneumonia develops usually report that they were beginning to feel better when they experienced a return of fever, shaking chills, pleuritic chest pain, and productive cough. The most common causes of secondary bacterial pneumonia are *S. pneumoniae, S. aureus,* and *H. influenzae.* This form of pneumonia commonly produces less cyanosis and tachypnea and is usually milder than primary influenza pneumonia. Influenza-related deaths can result from pneumonia as well as exacerbations of cardiopulmonary conditions and other disease. Reye syndrome (fatty liver with encephalitis) is a rare complication of influenza, particularly in young children who have been given aspirin as an antipyretic agent.[11–14]

Diagnosis and Treatment. The appropriate treatment of people with influenza depends on accurate and timely diagnosis. The early diagnosis can reduce the inappropriate use of antibiotics and provide the opportunity for use of an antiviral drug. Rapid diagnostic tests, which are available for use in some outpatient settings, allow health care providers to diagnose influenza more accurately, consider treatment options more carefully, and monitor the influenza type and its prevalence in their community.[14]

The goals of treatment for influenza are designed to limit the infection to the upper respiratory tract. The symptomatic approach for treatment of uncomplicated influenza rhinotracheitis focuses on rest, keeping warm, and keeping well hydrated. Analgesics, antipyretics, and cough medications can also be used. Rest decreases the oxygen requirements of the body and reduces the respiratory rate and the chance of spreading the virus from the upper to lower respiratory tract. Keeping warm helps maintain the respiratory epithelium at a core body temperature of 37°C (or higher if fever is present), thereby inhibiting viral replication, which is optimal at 35°C. Drinking large amounts of liquids ensures that the function of the epithelial lining of the respiratory tract is not further compromised by dehydration. Antiviral medications may be indicated in some persons. Antibacterial antibiotics should be reserved for bacterial complications. The use of aspirin to treat fever should be avoided in children because of the risk of Reye syndrome.

Three antiviral drugs are available for treatment of influenza: amantadine, zanamivir, and oseltamivir.[14] The first-generation antiviral drug amantadine (as well as rimantadine which is not available in Canada) is similarly effective against influenza A but not influenza B. These agents inhibit the uncoating of viral RNA in the host cells and prevent its replication. Both drugs are effective in prevention of influenza A in high-risk groups and in treatment of persons who acquire the disease. Unfortunately, resistance to the drugs develops rapidly and strains that are resistant to amantadine also are resistant to rimantadine.[11] Amantadine stimulates release of catecholamines, which can produce central nervous system side effects such as anxiety, depression, and insomnia.

The second-generation antiviral drugs zanamivir and oseltamivir are inhibitors of NA, a viral glycoprotein that is necessary for viral replication and release. These drugs, which have been approved for treatment of acute uncomplicated influenza infection, are effective against both influenza A and B viruses. Zanamivir and oseltamivir result in less resistance than amantadine and rimantadine.[11] Zanamivir is administered intranasally and oseltamivir is administered orally. Zanamivir can cause bronchospasm and is not recommended for persons with asthma or chronic obstructive lung disease.[14] To be effective, the antiviral drugs should be initiated as early as possible and up to 48 hours after onset of symptoms.

Influenza Immunization

Because influenza is so highly contagious, prevention relies primarily on hand washing and vaccination. In Canada, influenza vaccines are available and the formulation of these vaccines are changed yearly in response to antigenic changes in the influenza virus. The National Advisory Committee on Immunization (NACI) annually updates its recommendations for the composition of the vaccines. The influenza vaccines are contraindicated in persons with an anaphylactic response to a previous influenza vaccine or to other components of the vaccine (noting an egg allergy is no longer contraindicated), persons with a history of Guillain-Barré syndrome, and persons with acute febrile illness.[10]

Currently in Canada seven trivalent inactivated influenza vaccines (TIV) are administered by injection, and one live attenuated influenza vaccine (LAIV) is administered by intranasal spray.[10] These have become the mainstay for prevention of influenza. They have proved to be inexpensive and effective in reducing illness caused by influenza. Immunization is encouraged for all healthy children and adults and recommended for high-risk groups who, because of their age or underlying health problems, are unable to cope well with the infection and often require medical attention, including hospitalization. The effectiveness of the influenza vaccine in preventing and lessening the effects of influenza infection depends primarily on the age and immunocompetence of the recipient and the match between the virus strains included in the vaccine and those that circulate during the influenza season.[10] When there is a good match, the vaccine is effective in preventing the illness in approximately 80% of healthy persons younger than 65 years of age and with a vaccine mismatch potentially there is up to 50% efficacy.[10]

Swine Influenza (H1N1)

In June 2009, the World Health Organization declared a pandemic after identifying a novel virus spreading rapidly among humans and across different continents. This outbreak marked the first pandemic in more than 4 decades. A swine-origin influenza A H1N1 virus of the 2009 pandemic, abbreviated as A(H1N1)pdm09, was determined to be the cause. H1N1 presented with a range of symptoms from mild upper respiratory tract manifestations and uncharacteristic gastrointestinal symptoms to extremely high fevers with respiratory and multi-organ failure. It was especially serious for those aged 5 to 59 years, unlike other seasonal outbreaks. Other risk factors were pregnancy particularly the last trimester, other chronic diseases, and obesity.[12,13]

The first vaccine for influenza was developed by September 2009 and almost 15 million doses were distributed in Canada representing approximately 40% of the population. This mass vaccination program formed the basis for seasonal vaccine that now becomes available before the influenza season starts each year.[10]

Avian Influenza (Bird Flu)

Avian influenza, referred to as "bird flu," is an infection caused by the avian influenza virus. The normal hosts for avian influenza viruses are birds and occasionally pigs. The viruses occur naturally among birds, particularly those in the wild. Wild birds carry the viruses in their intestines, but usually are not affected by them. However, the virus is highly contagious among avian species and can infect and kill domestic poultry, such as chickens, ducks, and turkeys. Infected birds shed the virus in their saliva, nasal secretions, and feces. Susceptible birds become infected when they have contact with contaminated secretions or feces. Avian strains of the influenza virus do not usually cause outbreaks of disease in humans unless a reassortment of the virus genome has occurred within an intermediate mammalian host such as a pig. In this setting, a virus is produced that contains mammalian characteristics as well as avian characteristics, to which humans may not be immune. It is noteworthy that many of the pandemics of the past were thought to arise in Asia, where large human populations live in close proximity to ducks, chickens, and pigs, thus facilitating the phenomenon of viral reassortment.[11]

Recently, a highly pathogenic influenza A subtype, H5N1, was found in poultry in East and Southeast Asian countries.[10–13] Although the H5N1 strain is highly contagious from one bird to another, its transmission from human to human is relatively inefficient and not sustained. The result is only rare cases of person-to-person transmission. Most cases occur after exposure to infected poultry or surfaces contaminated with poultry droppings. Because infection in humans is associated with a high mortality rate, there is considerable concern that the H5N1 strain might mutate and initiate a new pandemic.

There currently is no commercially available vaccine to protect humans against the bird flu. Current commercial rapid diagnostic tests are not optimally sensitive or specific for detection of the virus. Most Asian H5N1 influenza strains are resistant to amantadine and rimantadine. The NA inhibitors, oseltamivir and zanamivir, would probably be effective if administered within 48 hours, but additional studies are needed to demonstrate their effectiveness.

Pneumonias

The term *pneumonia* describes inflammation of parenchymal structures of the lung, such as the alveoli and the bronchioles. Influenza and pneumonia are the eighth leading cause of death in Canada, and the most common cause of death from infectious disease, with an estimated 5,700 deaths in 2011.[1] Etiologic agents include infectious and noninfectious agents. Inhalation of irritating fumes or aspiration of gastric contents, although much less common than infectious causes, can result in subsequent bacterial infection and severe pneumonia.

Although antibiotics have significantly reduced the mortality rate from pneumonias, these diseases remain an important immediate cause of death of the older adults and persons with debilitating diseases. There have been subtle changes in the spectrum of microorganisms that cause infectious pneumonias, including a decrease in pneumonias caused by *S. pneumoniae* and an increase in pneumonias caused by other microorganisms such as *Pseudomonas, Candida* and other fungi, and nonspecific viruses. Many of these pneumonias occur in persons with impaired immune defences, including persons who are on immunosuppressant drugs to prevent rejection of a bone marrow or organ transplant.

Pneumonias can be commonly classified according to the type of agent (typical or atypical) causing the infection, distribution of the infection (lobar pneumonia or bronchopneumonia), and setting (community or hospital) in which it occurs. *Typical pneumonias* result from infection by bacteria that multiply extracellularly in the alveoli and cause inflammation and exudation of fluid into the air-filled spaces of the alveoli (Fig. 28.3). *Atypical pneumonias* are caused by viral and mycoplasma infections that involve the alveolar septum and the interstitium of the lung. They produce less striking symptoms and physical findings than bacterial pneumonia; there is a lack of alveolar infiltration and purulent sputum, leukocytosis, and lobar consolidation on the radiograph. Acute bacterial pneumonias can be classified as lobar pneumonia or bronchopneumonia, based on their anatomic pattern of distribution (Fig. 28.4). In general, *lobar pneumonia* refers to consolidation of a part or all of a lung lobe, and *bronchopneumonia* signifies a patchy consolidation involving more than one lobe (Fig. 28.4).

There is an overlap in symptomatology and changing spectrum of infectious organisms involved in pneumonias. To clarify risk factors and anticipate treatment, pneumonias are increasingly being classified as community-acquired and hospital-acquired (nosocomial) pneumonias.[15–18] Persons with

FIGURE 28.3 • Location of inflammatory processes in (**A**) typical and (**B**) atypical forms of pneumonia.

compromised immune function constitute a special concern in both categories.

Community-Acquired Pneumonia

The term *community-acquired pneumonia* is used to describe infections from organisms found in the community rather than in the hospital or nursing home. It is defined as an infection

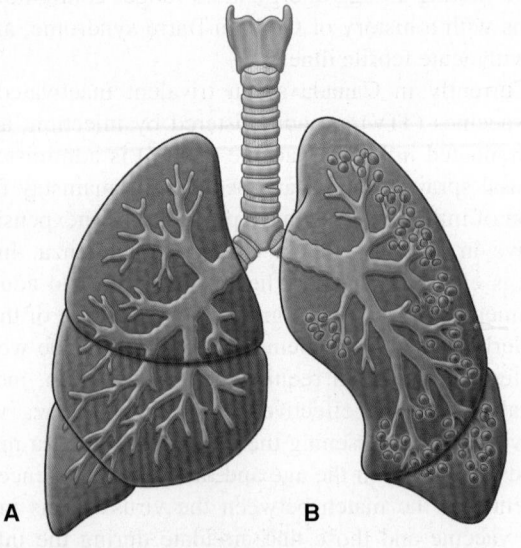

FIGURE 28.4 • Distribution of lung involvement in (**A**) lobar pneumonia and (**B**) bronchopneumonia.

> **PNEUMONIAS**
>
> - Pneumonias are respiratory disorders involving inflammation of the lung structures, such as the alveoli and bronchioles.
> - Pneumonia can be caused by infectious agents such as bacteria and viruses and noninfectious agents such as gastric secretions that are aspirated into the lungs.
> - The development of pneumonia is facilitated by an exceedingly virulent organism, large inoculum, and impaired host defences.
> - Pneumonias due to infectious agents commonly are classified according to the source of infection (community- vs hospital-acquired) and according to the immune status of the host (pneumonia in the immunocompromised person).

that begins outside the hospital or is diagnosed within 48 hours after admission to the hospital in a person who has not resided in a long-term care facility for 14 days or more before admission.[16] Community-acquired pneumonia may be further categorized according to risk of mortality and need for hospitalization based on age, presence of coexisting disease, and severity of illness, using physical examination, laboratory, and radiologic findings.[15]

Community-acquired pneumonia may be either bacterial or viral. The most common cause of infection in all categories is *S. pneumoniae*.[15–17] Other common pathogens include *H. influenzae*, *S. aureus*, *Klebsiella pneumoniae*, and *P. aeruginosa*. Less common agents are *Mycoplasma pneumoniae*, *Chlamydia* species, and viruses, sometimes called *atypical agents*. Common viral causes of community-acquired pneumonia include the influenza virus, RSV, adenovirus, and parainfluenza virus.

The methods used in the diagnosis of community-acquired pneumonia depend on age, coexisting health problems, and the severity of illness. In persons younger than 65 years of age and without coexisting disease, the diagnosis usually is based on history and physical examination, chest radiographs, and knowledge of the microorganisms currently causing infections in the community. Sputum specimens may be obtained for staining procedures and culture. Blood cultures may be done for persons requiring hospitalization.

Treatment involves the use of appropriate antibiotic therapy.[15–17] Empiric antibiotic therapy, based on knowledge regarding an antibiotic's spectrum of action and ability to penetrate bronchopulmonary secretions, often is used for persons with community-acquired pneumonia who do not require hospitalization. Hospitalization and more intensive care may be required depending on the person's age, preexisting health status, and severity of the infection.

Hospital-Acquired Pneumonia

Hospital-acquired, or nosocomial, pneumonia is defined as a lower respiratory tract infection that was not present or incubating on admission to the hospital. Usually, infections occurring 48 hours or more after admission are considered hospital acquired.[16,18] In Canada hospital-acquired pneumonia is the second most common cause of hospital-acquired infection and has a mortality rate up to 60%.[18] Persons with compromised immune function, chronic lung disease, and airway instrumentation, such as endotracheal intubation or tracheotomy, are particularly at risk. Persons requiring intubation and mechanical ventilation are also particularly at high risk for pneumonia, referred to as ventilator-associated pneumonia (VAP). Canadian guidelines to prevent VAP include effective infection control measures, oral versus nasal intubation, closed suction system and ongoing drainage of subglottic secretions, and head of bed positioning at 30 to 45 degrees.[18]

Most hospital-acquired infections are bacterial. The organisms are those present in the hospital environment and include *Pseudomonas aeruginosa*, *S. aureus*, *Enterobacter* species, *Klebsiella* species, *Escherichia coli*, and *Serratia* species. The organisms that are responsible for hospital-acquired pneumonias are different from those responsible for community-acquired pneumonias, and many of them have acquired antibiotic resistance and are more difficult to treat.

Pneumonia in Immunocompromised Persons

Pneumonia in immunocompromised persons remains a major source of morbidity and mortality. The term *immunocompromised host* usually is applied to persons with a variety of underlying defects in host defences.[19,20] It includes persons with primary and acquired immunodeficiency states, those who have undergone bone marrow or organ transplantation, persons with solid organ or hematologic cancers, and those on corticosteroid and other immunosuppressant drugs.

Although almost all types of microorganisms can cause pulmonary infection in immunocompromised persons, certain types of immunologic defects tend to favour certain types of infections.[19,20] Defects in humoral immunity predispose to bacterial infections against which antibodies play an important role, whereas defects in cellular immunity predispose to infections caused by viruses, fungi, mycobacteria, and protozoa. Neutropenia and impaired granulocyte function, as occur in persons with leukemia, chemotherapy, and bone marrow depression, predispose to infections caused by more opportunistic pathogens such as *S. aureus*, *Aspergillus*, *Pneumocystis jirovecii* (discussed in Chapter 20), gram-negative bacilli, and *Candida*. The time course of infection often provides a hint to the type of agent involved. A fulminant pneumonia usually is caused by bacterial infection, whereas an insidious onset usually is indicative of a viral, fungal, protozoal, or mycobacterial infection.

Acute Bacterial (Typical) Pneumonias

Bacterial pneumonias remain an important cause of mortality among older adults and people with debilitating illnesses. The lung below the main bronchi is normally sterile despite frequent entry of microorganisms into the air passages by

TABLE 28.1 RESPIRATORY DEFENCE MECHANISMS AND CONDITIONS THAT IMPAIR THEIR EFFECTIVENESS

DEFENCE MECHANISM	FUNCTION	FACTORS THAT IMPAIR EFFECTIVENESS
Glottic and cough reflexes	Protect against aspiration into tracheobronchial tree	Loss of cough reflex due to stroke or neural lesion, neuromuscular disease, abdominal or chest surgery, depression of the cough reflex due to sedation or anesthesia, presence of a nasogastric tube (tends to cause adaptation of afferent receptors)
Mucociliary blanket	Removes secretions, microorganisms, and particles from the respiratory tract	Smoking, viral diseases, chilling, inhalation of irritating gases
Phagocytic and bactericidal action of alveolar macrophages	Removes microorganisms and foreign particles from the lung	Tobacco smoke, chilling, alcohol, oxygen intoxication
Immune defences (IgA and IgG and cell-mediated immunity)	Destroy microorganisms	Congenital and acquired immunodeficiency states

inhalation during ventilation or by aspiration of nasopharyngeal secretions. Most people unknowingly aspirate small amounts of organisms that have colonized their upper airways, particularly during sleep. These organisms do not normally cause infection because of the small numbers that are aspirated and because of the respiratory tract's defence mechanisms, which prevent them from entering the distal air passages[19] (Table 28.1). Loss of the cough reflex, damage to the ciliated endothelium that lines the respiratory tract, or impaired immune defences predispose to colonization and infection of the lower respiratory system. Bacterial adherence also plays a role in colonization of the lower airways. The epithelial cells of critically and chronically ill persons are more receptive to binding microorganisms that cause pneumonia. Other clinical risk factors favouring colonization of the tracheobronchial tree include antibiotic therapy that alters the normal bacterial flora, diabetes, smoking, chronic bronchitis, and viral infection.

Bacterial pneumonias are commonly classified according to etiologic agent. This is because the clinical and morphologic features, and thus the therapeutic implications, often vary with the causative agent. The discussion in this section focuses on two types of bacterial pneumonia: pneumococcal pneumonia and Legionnaire disease.

Pneumococcal Pneumonia. *S. pneumoniae* (pneumococcus) remains the most common cause of bacterial pneumonia.[15–18,20–23] *S. pneumoniae* is a gram-positive diplococcus, possessing a capsule of polysaccharide. The virulence of the pneumococcus is a function of its capsule, which prevents or delays digestion by phagocytes. The polysaccharide is an antigen that primarily elicits a B-cell response with antibody production. In the absence of antibody, clearance of the pneumococci from the body relies on the reticuloendothelial system, with the macrophages in the spleen playing a major role in elimination of the organism. This, along with the spleen's role in antibody production, increases the risk for pneumococcal

bacteremia in persons who are anatomically or functionally asplenic, such as children with sickle cell disease. The initial step in the pathogenesis of pneumococcal infection is the attachment and colonization of the organism to the mucus and cells of the nasopharynx. Colonization does not equate with signs of infection. Perfectly healthy people can be colonized and carry the organism without evidence of infection. The spread of particular strains of pneumococci, particularly antibiotic-resistant strains, is largely by healthy colonized individuals.

The pathologic process of pneumococcal pneumonia can be divided into the four stages—edema, red hepatization, grey hepatization, and resolution[22] (Fig 28.5). During the first stage of pneumococcal pneumonia, the alveoli become filled with a protein-rich edema fluid containing numerous organisms (Fig. 28.6). Marked capillary congestion follows, leading to massive outpouring of polymorphonuclear leukocytes and red blood cells. Because the first consistency of the affected lung resembles that of the liver, this stage is referred to as the *red hepatization* stage. The next stage, occurring after 2 or more days depending on the success of treatment, involves the arrival of macrophages that phagocytose the fragmented polymorphonuclear cells, red blood cells, and other cellular debris. During this stage, which is termed the *grey hepatization* stage, the congestion has diminished but the lung is still firm. The alveolar exudate is then removed and the lung gradually returns to normal.[23]

The signs and symptoms of pneumococcal pneumonia vary widely, depending on the age and health status of the infected person. In previously healthy persons, the onset usually is sudden and is characterized by malaise, severe, shaking chills, and high fever. During the initial or congestive stage, coughing brings up watery sputum and breath sounds are limited, with fine crackles. As the disease progresses, the character of the sputum changes; it may be blood-tinged or rust-coloured, to purulent. Pleuritic pain, a sharp pain that is more severe with respiratory movements, is common. With

FIGURE 28.6 • Pneumococcal pneumonia. The alveoli are packed with an exudate composed of polymorphonuclear leukocytes and occasional macrophages. (From Rubin R., Strayer D. S. (Eds.). (2012). *Rubin's pathology: Clinicopathologic foundations of medicine* (6th ed., p. 547). Philadelphia, PA: Lippincott Williams & Wilkins.)

FIGURE 28.5 • Pathogenesis of pneumococcal lobar pneumonia. Pneumococci, characteristically in pairs (diplococci), multiply rapidly in the alveolar spaces and produce extensive edema. They incite an acute inflammatory response in which polymorphonuclear leukocytes and congestion are prominent (red hepatization). As the inflammatory process progresses, macrophages replace the polymorphonuclear leukocytes and ingest debris (grey hepatization). The process usually resolves, but complication may ensue. (PMN, polymorphonuclear neutrophil; RBC, red blood cell.) (From Rubin R., Strayer D. S. (Eds.). (2012). *Rubin's pathology: Clinicopathologic foundations of medicine* (6th ed., p. 547). Philadelphia, PA: Lippincott Williams & Wilkins.)

antibiotic therapy, fever usually subsides in approximately 48 to 72 hours, and recovery is uneventful.[23] Older adults are less likely to experience marked elevations in temperature; in these persons, the only sign of pneumonia may be a loss of appetite and deterioration in mental status.

Treatment includes the use of antibiotics that are effective against *S. pneumoniae*. In the past, *S. pneumoniae* was uniformly susceptible to penicillin. However, penicillin-resistant and multidrug-resistant strains have emerged in Canada, with a prevalence of approximately 20% penicillin-resistant strains.[24]

Pneumococcal pneumonia can be prevented through immunization. A 23-valent pneumococcal vaccine, composed of antigens from 23 types of *S. pneumoniae* capsular polysaccharides, is used. The capsular polysaccharides induce antibodies primarily by T-cell-independent mechanisms. The vaccine is recommended for persons 65 years of age or older and persons aged 2 to 65 years with chronic illnesses, particularly cardiovascular and pulmonary diseases, diabetes mellitus, and alcoholism, who sustain increased morbidity with respiratory infections. Immunization also is recommended for immunocompromised persons 2 years of age or older, including those with sickle cell disease, splenectomy, Hodgkin disease, multiple myeloma, renal failure, nephrotic syndrome, organ transplantation, and HIV infection. Immunization is also recommended for residents in special environments or social settings in which the risk for invasive pneumococcal disease is increased (*e.g.*, the aboriginal population, and residents of nursing homes and long-term care facilities).[21]

Because their immune system is immature, the antibody response to most pneumococcal capsular polysaccharides usually is poor or inconsistent in children younger than 2 years of age. In Canada a 13-valent pneumococcal polysaccharide-protein conjugate vaccine is used for infants and children.[21] *S. pneumoniae* is the leading cause of bacteremia, meningitis, bacterial pneumonia, and acute otitis media (AOM), and the National Advisory Committee on Immunizations (NACI) recommends this conjugate vaccine for all children aged 2 to 23 months and for children aged 24 months up to 17 years who are at increased risk for pneumococcal disease (*e.g.*, immunocompromised, chronic medical conditions).[21]

Legionnaire Disease. Legionnaire disease is a form of bronchopneumonia caused by a gram-negative rod, *Legionella pneumophila*.[19,25] Transmission from person to person has not been documented, and infection normally occurs by acquiring the organism from the environment. Infection typically occurs when water that contains the pathogen is aerosolized into appropriately sized droplets and is inhaled or aspirated by a susceptible host.[25] The disease was first recognized and received its name after an epidemic of severe and, for some, fatal pneumonia that developed among delegates to the 1976 American Legion convention held in a Philadelphia hotel. The spread of infection was traced to a water-cooled air-conditioning system. Although healthy persons can contract the infection, the risk is greatest among smokers, persons with chronic diseases, and those with impaired cell-mediated immunity.[19,25]

Symptoms of the disease typically begin approximately 2 to 10 days after infection. Onset is usually abrupt, with malaise, weakness, lethargy, fever, and dry cough. Other manifestations include disturbances of central nervous system function, gastrointestinal tract involvement, arthralgias, and elevation in body temperature.[23,26] The presence of pneumonia along with diarrhea, hyponatremia, hypophosphatemia, and confusion is characteristic of *Legionella* pneumonia. The disease causes consolidation of lung tissues and impairs gas exchange.[26]

Diagnosis is based on clinical manifestations, radiologic studies, and specialized laboratory tests to detect the presence of the organism. Of these, the *Legionella* urinary antigen test is a relatively inexpensive, rapid test that detects antigens of *L. pneumophila* in the urine.[25,26] The urine test usually is easier to obtain because people with legionellosis often have a nonproductive cough and the test results remain positive for weeks despite antibiotic therapy. The test is available as both a radioimmunoassay and an enzyme immunoassay.

Treatment consists of administration of antibiotics that are known to be effective against *L. pneumophila*. Delay in instituting antibiotic therapy significantly increases mortality rates; therefore, antibiotics known to be effective against *L. pneumophila* should be included in the treatment regimen for severe community-acquired pneumonia.[25,26]

Primary Atypical Pneumonia

The primary atypical pneumonias are caused by a variety of agents, the most common being *Mycoplasma pneumoniae*. Mycoplasma infections are particularly common among children and young adults. Other etiologic agents include viruses (*e.g.*, influenza virus, RSV, human metapneumovirus, adenoviruses, rhinoviruses, and the rubeola [measles] and varicella [chickenpox] viruses), *Coxiella burnetii*, and *Chlamydia pneumoniae*.[19,27] In some cases, the cause is unknown.

The atypical pneumonias are characterized by patchy involvement of the lung, largely confined to the alveolar septum and pulmonary interstitium. The term *atypical* denotes a lack of lung consolidation, production of moderate amounts of sputum, moderate elevation of white blood cell count, and lack of alveolar exudate.[19] The agents that cause atypical pneumonias damage the respiratory tract epithelium and impair respiratory tract defences, thereby predisposing to secondary bacterial infections. The sporadic form of atypical pneumonia is usually mild with a low mortality rate. It may, however, assume epidemic proportions with intensified severity and greater mortality, as in the influenza pandemics of 1915 and 1918.

The clinical course among persons with mycoplasmal and viral pneumonias varies widely from a mild infection (*e.g.*, influenza types A and B, adenovirus) that masquerades as a chest cold to a more serious and even fatal outcome (*e.g.*, chickenpox pneumonia). The symptoms may remain confined to fever, headache, and muscle aches and pains. Cough, when present, is characteristically dry, hacking, and nonproductive. The diagnosis is usually made based on history, physical findings, and chest radiographs.

Tuberculosis

Tuberculosis is the world's foremost cause of death from a single infectious agent. It is estimated that each year more than 8.6 million new cases of tuberculosis occur worldwide and approximately 1.4 million persons die of the disease.[2] In Canada, each year there are approximately 1,600 new cases and 130 deaths attributed to tuberculosis.[3,28] With the introduction of antibiotics in the 1950s, Western countries experienced a long decline in the number of infections until the mid-1980s. The rate of infection did not increase in Canada from the mid 1980s to early 1990s, although it did increase in the United States, particularly among HIV-infected people.[28] Tuberculosis is more common in Canada among foreign-born persons (64% of cases in 2012 occurred in foreign-born persons), with a higher incidence in Canadian-born persons (both aboriginal and non-aboriginal) in northern Canada.[3,28] Outbreaks of a drug-resistant form of tuberculosis have emerged, complicating the selection of drugs and affecting the duration of treatment.

Tuberculosis is an infectious disease caused by the mycobacterium, *M. tuberculosis*. The mycobacteria are slender, rod-shaped, aerobic bacteria that do not form spores (Fig. 28.6).

They are similar to other bacterial organisms except for an outer waxy capsule that makes them more resistant to destruction; the organism can persist in old necrotic and calcified lesions and remain capable of reinitiating growth. The waxy coat also causes the organism to retain red dye when treated with acid in acid-fast staining.[28,29] Thus, the mycobacteria are often referred to as *acid-fast bacilli.* Although *M. tuberculosis* can infect practically any organ of the body, the lungs are most frequently involved. The tubercle bacilli are strict aerobes that thrive in an oxygen-rich environment. This explains their tendency to cause disease in the upper lobe or upper parts of the lower lobe of the lung, where the ventilation and oxygen content are greatest.

M. tuberculosis hominis is the most frequent form of tuberculosis to threaten humans. Other mycobacteria, *M, avium* and *M. intracellulare* are similar species causing identical diseases and are grouped together as *Mycobacterium avium-intracellulare* complex. This complex is less virulent than *M. tuberculosis hominis* and rarely causes disease except in severely immunosuppressed persons, such as those with HIV infection.[29]

TUBERCULOSIS

- Tuberculosis is an infectious disease caused by *Mycobacterium tuberculosis,* a rod-shaped, aerobic bacterium that is resistant to destruction and can persist in necrotic and calcified lesions for prolonged periods and remain capable of reinstating growth.
- The organism is spread by inhaling the mycobacterium-containing droplet nuclei that circulate in the air. Overcrowded living conditions increase the risk of tuberculosis spread.
- The tubercle bacillus has no known antigens to stimulate an early immunoglobulin response; instead, the host mounts a delayed-type cell-mediated immune response.
- The cell-mediated response plays a dominant role in walling off the tubercle bacilli and preventing the development of active tuberculosis. People with impaired cell-mediated immunity are more likely to develop active tuberculosis when infected.
- A positive tuberculin skin test results from a cell-mediated immune response and implies that a person has been infected with *M. tuberculosis* and has mounted a cell-mediated immune response. It does not mean that the person has active tuberculosis.

M. tuberculosis hominis is an airborne infection spread by minute, invisible particles, called *droplet nuclei,* that are harboured in the respiratory secretions of persons with active tuberculosis. Coughing, sneezing, and talking all create respiratory droplets; these droplets evaporate, leaving the organisms (droplet nuclei), which remain suspended in the air and are circulated by air currents. Thus, living under crowded and confined conditions increases the risk for spread of the disease.

Pathogenesis

The pathogenesis of tuberculosis in a previously unexposed immunocompetent person is centred on the development of a cell-mediated immune response that confers resistance to the organism and development of tissue hypersensitivity to the tubercular antigens.[28–30] The destructive features of the disease, such as caseating necrosis and cavitation, result from the hypersensitivity immune response rather than the destructive capabilities of the tubercle bacillus.

Macrophages are the primary cell infected with *M. tuberculosis.* Inhaled droplet nuclei pass down the bronchial tree without settling on the epithelium and are deposited in the alveoli. Soon after entering the lung, the bacilli are phagocytosed by alveolar macrophages but resist killing, apparently because cell wall lipids of *M. tuberculosis* block fusion of phagosomes and lysosomes (see Chapter 18). Although the macrophages that first ingest *M. tuberculosis* cannot kill the organisms, they initiate a cell-mediated immune response that eventually contains the infection. As the tubercle bacilli multiply, the infected macrophages degrade the mycobacteria and present their antigens to T lymphocytes. The sensitized T lymphocytes, in turn, stimulate the macrophages to increase their concentration of lytic enzymes and ability to kill the mycobacteria. When released, these lytic enzymes also damage lung tissue. The development of a population of activated T lymphocytes and related development of activated macrophages capable of ingesting and destroying the bacilli constitutes the cell-mediated immune response, a process that takes about 3 to 6 weeks to become effective.

In persons with intact cell-mediated immunity, the cell-mediated immune response results in the development of a grey-white, circumscribed granulomatous lesion, called a *Ghon focus,* that contains the tubercle bacilli, modified macrophages, and other immune cells.[29,30] It is usually located in the subpleural area of the upper segments of the lower lobes or in the lower segments of the upper lobe. When the number of organisms is high, the hypersensitivity reaction produces significant tissue necrosis, causing the central portion of the Ghon focus to undergo soft, caseous (cheeselike) necrosis. During this same period, tubercle bacilli, free or inside macrophages, drain along the lymph channels to the tracheobronchial lymph nodes of the affected lung and there evoke the formation of caseous granulomas. The combination of the primary lung lesion and lymph node granulomas is called a *Ghon complex* (Fig. 28.7). The Ghon complex eventually heals, undergoing shrinkage, fibrous scarring, and calcification, the latter visible radiographically. However, small numbers of organisms may remain viable for years. Later, if immune mechanisms decline or fail, latent tuberculosis infection has the potential to develop into secondary tuberculosis.

Primary Tuberculosis

Primary tuberculosis is a form of the disease that develops in previously unexposed and therefore unsensitized people. It typically is initiated as a result of inhaling droplet nuclei that

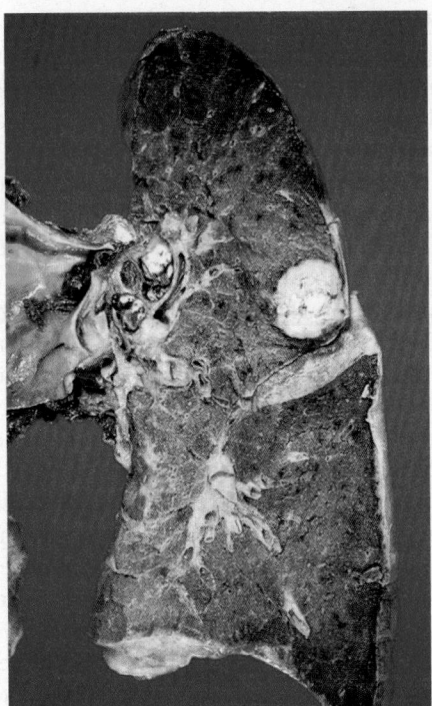

FIGURE 28.7 • Primary tuberculosis. A healed Ghon complex is represented by a subpleural nodule and involved hilar lymph nodes. (From Rubin R., Strayer D. S. (Eds.). (2012). *Rubin's pathology: Clinicopathologic foundations of medicine* (6th ed., p. 550). Philadelphia, PA: Lippincott Williams & Wilkins.)

contain the tubercle bacillus (Fig. 28.8). Most people with primary tuberculosis go on to develop *latent infection,* in which T lymphocytes and macrophages surround the organism in granulomas that limit their spread.[29,30] Individuals with latent tuberculosis do not have active disease and cannot transmit the organism to others.

In approximately 5% of newly infected people, the immune response is inadequate; these people go on to develop progressive primary tuberculosis with continued destruction of lung tissue and spread to multiple sites within the lung.[29] People with HIV infection and others with disorders of cell-mediated immunity are more likely to develop progressive tuberculosis if they become infected. In those who develop progressive disease, the symptoms are usually insidious and nonspecific, with fever, weight loss, fatigue, and night sweats.[28–30] Sometimes the onset of symptoms is abrupt, with high fever, pleuritis, and lymphadenitis. As the disease spreads, the organism gains access to the sputum, allowing the person to infect others.

In rare instances, tuberculosis may erode into a blood vessel, giving rise to hematogenic dissemination. *Miliary tuberculosis* describes minute lesions, resembling millet seeds, resulting from this type of dissemination that can involve almost any organ, particularly the brain, meninges, liver, kidney, and bone marrow.

Secondary Tuberculosis

Secondary tuberculosis represents either reinfection from inhaled droplet nuclei or reactivation of a previously healed

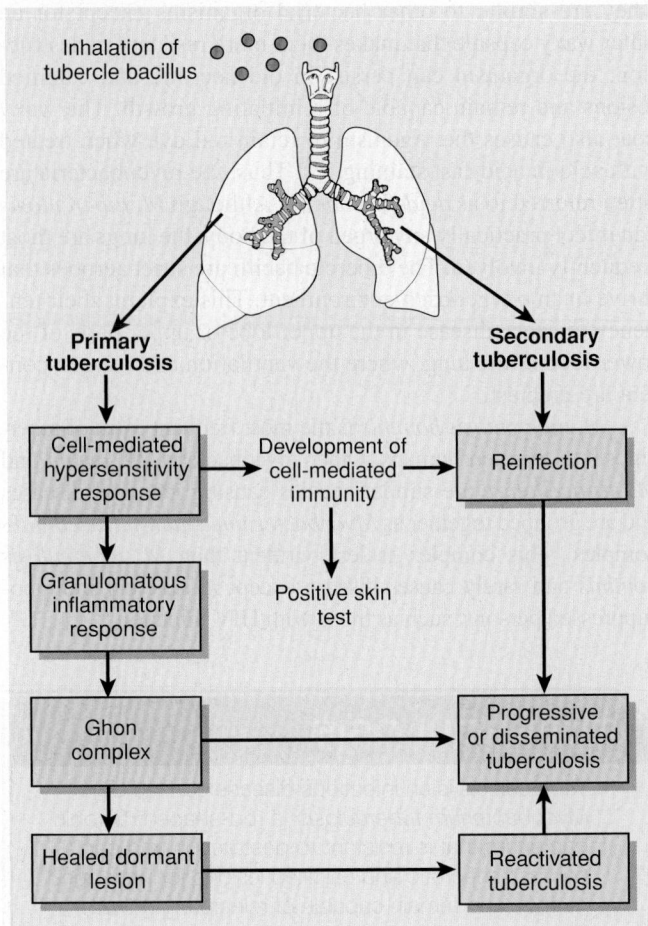

FIGURE 28.8 • Pathogenesis of tuberculosis infection.

primary lesion[29,30] (Fig. 28.8). It often occurs in situations of impaired body defence mechanisms. The partial immunity that follows primary tuberculosis affords protection against reinfection and to some extent aids in localizing the disease should reactivation occur. In secondary tuberculosis, the cell-mediated hypersensitivity reaction can be an aggravating factor, as evidenced by the frequency of cavitation and bronchial dissemination. The cavities may coalesce to a size of up to 10 to 15 cm in diameter[30] (Fig. 28.9). Pleural effusion and tuberculous empyema are common as the disease progresses.

Persons with secondary tuberculosis commonly present with low-grade fevers, night sweats, easy fatigability, anorexia, and weight loss.[30] A cough initially is dry but later becomes productive with purulent and sometimes blood-tinged sputum. Dyspnea and orthopnea develop as the disease advances.

Diagnosis

Diagnosing tuberculosis is challenging and can be easily missed if only non-specific symptoms are present. The most frequently used screening methods for pulmonary tuberculosis are the tuberculin skin tests and chest radiographic studies. The tuberculin skin test (TST) measures the delayed hypersensitivity (*i.e.,* cell-mediated, type IV) that follows exposure

FIGURE 28.9 • Cavitary tuberculosis in the apex of the left upper lobe of the lung. (From Rubin R., Strayer D. S. (Eds.). (2012). *Rubin's pathology: Clinicopathologic foundations of medicine* (6th ed., p. 550). Philadelphia, PA: Lippincott Williams & Wilkins.)

to the tubercle bacillus. Persons who become tuberculin positive usually remain so for the remainder of their lives. A positive reaction to the skin test does not mean that a person has active tuberculosis, only that there has been exposure to the bacillus and that cell-mediated immunity to the organism has developed. False-positive and false-negative skin test reactions can occur. False-positive reactions often result from cross-reactions with nontuberculosis mycobacteria, such as *M. avium-intracellulare* complex.[28] Because the hypersensitivity response to the tuberculin test depends on cell-mediated immunity, a false-negative test result can occur because of immunodeficiency states that result from HIV infection, immunosuppressive therapy, lymphoreticular malignancies, or aging. This is called *anergy*. In the immunocompromised person, a negative TST result can mean that the person has a true lack of exposure to tuberculosis or is unable to mount an immune response to the test. Because of the problem with anergy in persons with HIV infection and other immunocompromised states, immunologic interferon-γ release assays (IGRAs) can be used. While this blood test is not recommended for detection of active disease, it can detect the cell-mediated immune reactivity to *M. tuberculosis*. Although results can be obtained with 24 hours it is expensive and not available at all health care settings.[28]

A two-step testing procedure, which uses a "boosting" phenomenon, may be used to increase the reaction to a subsequent TST in persons who have been infected with tuberculosis.[28] If the first test result of the two-step procedure is negative, a second test is administered 1 week later. If the second test result is negative, the person is considered to be uninfected or anergic. If the second test result is positive, it is assumed to have occurred because of a boosted response. Use of the two-step test procedure for employee health or institutional screening only needs to be performed once and can reduce the likelihood that a boosted response in a subsequent test will not be interpreted as a recent infection.

Definitive diagnosis of active pulmonary tuberculosis requires identification of the organism from cultures or identification of the organism from deoxyribonucleic acid (DNA) or RNA amplification techniques.[28–30] Bacteriologic studies (*i.e.,* acid-fast stain and cultures) of early sputum specimens, gastric aspirations, or bronchial washings obtained during fibreoptic bronchoscopy may be used. Cultures of solid media to identify *M. tuberculosis* may take up to 8 weeks. Once mycobacteria have been grown in culture, nucleic acid probes or high-performance liquid chromatography can be used to identify the species within hours. Genotyping can be done to identify different strains of *M. tuberculosis*. It can be used to evaluate second episodes of tuberculosis to determine whether the second episode was due to relapse or reinfection. Genotyping also permits the evaluation of isolates with different patterns of drug susceptibility.[31] In addition, genotyping is useful in investigating outbreaks of infection and determining sites and patterns of *M. tuberculosis* transmission in communities.

Treatment

The goals of treatment are to eliminate all tubercle bacilli from an infected person while avoiding emergence of significant drug resistance. Treatment of active tuberculosis requires the use of multiple drugs.[28] Tuberculosis is an unusual disease in that chemotherapy is required for a relatively long period. The tubercle bacillus is an aerobic organism that multiplies slowly and remains relatively dormant in oxygen-poor caseous material. It undergoes a high rate of mutation and tends to acquire resistance to any one drug. For this reason, multidrug regimens are used for treating persons with active tuberculosis. Drug susceptibility tests are used to guide treatment in drug-resistant forms of the disease.

Two groups meet the criteria established for the use of antimycobacterial therapy for tuberculosis: persons with active tuberculosis and those who have had contact with cases of active tuberculosis and who are at risk for development of an active form of the disease. Prophylactic treatment is used for persons who are infected with *M. tuberculosis* but do not have active disease.[28] This group includes persons with a positive skin test result who have had close contact with active cases of tuberculosis; have converted from a negative to positive skin test result within 2 years; have a history of untreated or inadequately treated tuberculosis; have chest radiographs with evidence of tuberculosis but no bacteriologic evidence of the active disease; have special risk factors such as silicosis, diabetes mellitus, prolonged corticosteroid therapy, immunosuppression therapy, end-stage renal disease, chronic malnutrition from any cause, or hematologic or reticuloendothelial cancers; have a positive HIV test result or have AIDS; or are 35 years of age or younger with a positive reaction of unknown duration. These persons are considered to harbour a small number of microorganisms and usually are treated with isoniazid (INH).

The primary drugs used in the treatment of tuberculosis are INH, rifampin, pyrazinamide (PZA), ethambutol, floroquinolones, and streptomycin.[28] INH is remarkably potent against the tubercle bacillus and probably is the most widely used drug for tuberculosis. Although its exact mechanism of action is unknown, it apparently combines with an enzyme that is needed by the INH-susceptible strains of the tubercle bacillus. Resistance to the drug develops rapidly, and combination with other effective drugs delays the development of resistance. Rifampin inhibits RNA synthesis in the bacillus. Although ethambutol and PZA are known to inhibit the growth of the tubercle bacillus, their mechanisms of action are largely unknown. Floroquinolones (*e.g.*, moxifloxacin), currently considered second line drugs, target the mycobacterial DNA enzymes preventing replication but the concern about developing mutations and resistance continue to stimulate research.[32] Streptomycin, the first drug found to be effective against tuberculosis, must be given by injection, which limits its usefulness, particularly in long-term therapy. However, it remains an important drug in tuberculosis therapy and is used primarily in persons with severe, possibly life-threatening forms of tuberculosis.

Outbreaks of multidrug-resistant (MDR) and extensively drug resistant (XDR) tuberculosis continue to pose a problem for the prophylactic treatment of exposed persons, including health care workers.[28] Various treatment protocols are recommended, depending on the type of resistant strain that is identified. Success of chemotherapy for prophylaxis and treatment of tuberculosis depends on strict adherence to a lengthy drug regimen. This often is a problem, particularly for persons with asymptomatic tuberculosis infections and for poorly motivated groups such as intravenous drug users. Directly observed therapy, which requires that a health care worker observe while the person takes the antituberculosis drug, is recommended for some persons and for some types of treatment protocols.[28]

First administered to humans in 1921, the bacillus Calmette-Guérin (BCG) vaccine is used to prevent the development of tuberculosis in persons who are at high risk for infection. BCG is an attenuated strain of *M. tuberculosis bovis*.[21] It is administered only to persons who have a negative tuberculin skin test result. The vaccine, which is given intradermally, produces a local reaction that can last as long as 3 months and may result in scarring at the injection site. Persons who have been vaccinated with BCG usually have a positive tuberculin skin test result that wanes with time and is unlikely to persist beyond 10 years.

Today, more than 70 years after its development, BCG remains the only tuberculosis vaccine available. Currently, several candidate vaccines are being prepared or are already in the early stages of human testing. Worldwide, BCG is currently used as a major method of prevention for tuberculosis. Routine use of BCG vaccine is not recommended in any Canadian population because of the low prevalence of tuberculosis infection, the vaccine's interference with the ability to determine latent tuberculosis with skin tests, and variable effectiveness against pulmonary tuberculosis.[21,28] Vaccination may be considered for aboriginals in communities at high risk, health care workers in settings where patients are

infected with drug-resistant strains of tuberculosis, or travellers spending extensive time in areas of high TB incidence, particularly drug-resistant strains.[21]

Fungal Infections

Fungi are classified as yeasts and moulds. Yeasts are round and grow by budding. Moulds form tubular structures called *hyphae* and grow by branching and forming spores (see Chapter 16). Some fungi are *dimorphic*, meaning that they grow as yeasts at body temperatures and as moulds at room temperatures. A simple classification of mycoses or diseases caused by fungi divides them into superficial, cutaneous, subcutaneous, or deep (systemic) mycoses. The superficial, cutaneous, or subcutaneous mycoses cause disease of the skin, hair, and nails (discussed in Chapter 61). Deep fungal infections may produce pulmonary and systemic infections and are sometimes fatal. They are caused by virulent fungi that live free in nature or soil or in decaying organic matter and are frequently limited to certain geographic regions. The most common of these endemic infections are the dimorphic fungi, which include *Histoplasma capsulatum* (histoplasmosis), *Coccidioides immitis* (coccidioidomycosis), and *Blastomyces dermatitidis* (blastomycosis). These fungi form infectious spores, which enter the body through the respiratory system. Most people who become infected with these fungi develop only minor symptoms or none at all; only a small minority develop serious disease.

The host's cell-mediated immune response is paramount in controlling such infections. Pathologic fungi generally produce no toxins. In the host, they induce a delayed cell-mediated hypersensitivity response to their chemical constituents (see Chapter 19). Cellular immunity is mediated by antigen-specific T lymphocytes and cytokine-activated macrophages that assume fungicidal properties. The primary pulmonary lesions consist of aggregates of macrophages stuffed with organisms, with similar lesions developing in the lymph nodes that drain the area. These lesions develop into granulomas complete with giant cells and may develop central necrosis and calcification resembling that of primary tuberculosis.

Although most fungal infections are asymptomatic, they can be severe or even fatal in persons who have experienced a heavy exposure, have underlying immune deficiencies, or develop progressive disease that is not recognized or treated. Immunocompromised persons, particularly those with HIV infection, are particularly prone to development of disseminated infection.

Histoplasmosis

Histoplasmosis is caused by the dimorphic fungus *H. capsulatum*. In Canada, it is most prevalent along the St. Lawrence River, where 20 to 30 percent of persons may have acquired the fungus, but the incidence is unknown as most persons are asymptomatic.[33] The fungus grows in soil enriched with either bird or bat droppings; therefore, persons working with this soil are at the highest risk of acquiring the infection. The infection is acquired by inhaling the fungal spores that are released when the dirt or dust from the infected areas is disturbed. The spores convert to the parasitic yeast phase when exposed to body temperature in the alveoli. They are then carried to the regional lymphatics and from there are disseminated throughout the body in the bloodstream. Dissemination occurs during the first several weeks of infection before specific immunity has developed. After 2 to 3 weeks, cellular immunity develops, establishing the body's ability to control the infection.

Depending on the host's resistance and immunocompetence, the disease usually takes one of four forms: (1) latent asymptomatic disease, (2) self-limited primary disease, (3) chronic pulmonary disease, or (4) disseminated infection. The average incubation period for the infection is 5 to 18 days.[33] Most persons with *H. capsulatum* infection remain asymptomatic or have mild respiratory illness that is not diagnosed as histoplasmosis. Latent asymptomatic histoplasmosis is characterized by evidence of healed lesions in the lungs or hilar lymph nodes. Primary pulmonary histoplasmosis occurs in otherwise healthy persons as a mild, self-limited, febrile respiratory infection. During this stage of the disease, chest radiographs usually show single or multiple infiltrates.

Chronic histoplasmosis resembles reactivation tuberculosis. Infiltration of the upper lobes of one or both lungs occurs with cavitation. This form of the disease is more common in middle-aged men who smoke and in persons with chronic lung disease. In many persons, the disease is self-limited. In others, there is progressive destruction of lung tissue and dissemination of the disease.

Disseminated histoplasmosis can follow primary or chronic histoplasmosis but most often develops as an acute and fulminating infection in the very old or the very young or in persons who are immunocompromised, including persons who have undergone transplantations, those with hematologic malignancies, and persons with HIV/AIDS. Although the macrophages of the reticuloendothelial system can remove the fungi from the bloodstream, they are unable to destroy them. Characteristically, this form of the disease produces a high fever, generalized lymph node enlargement, hepatosplenomegaly, muscle wasting, anemia, leukopenia, and thrombocytopenia. There may be hoarseness, ulcerations of the mouth and tongue, nausea, vomiting, diarrhea, and abdominal pain. Often, meningitis becomes a dominant feature of the disease.

A number of laboratory tests, including cultures, fungal stain, antigen detection, and serologic tests for antibodies, are used in the diagnosis of histoplasmosis. The type of test that is used depends on the type of involvement that is present. Antigen tests can be performed on blood, urine, cerebrospinal fluid, or bronchoalveolar lavage fluid. A urine antigen assay is particularly useful in detecting disseminated histoplasmosis.

The antifungal drug, itraconazole, usually is the drug of choice for treatment of persons with disease severe enough to require treatment or those with compromised immune function who are at risk for the development of disseminated disease.[16] Amphotericin B, which is administered intravenously, usually is the drug of choice in severe disease. Persons with HIV-related histoplasmosis usually require lifelong suppression therapy with itraconazole.

Coccidioidomycosis

Coccidioidomycosis is a rare fungal infection caused by inhaling the spores of *C. immitis* or *C. posadasii*. The disease resembles tuberculosis, and its mechanisms of infection are similar to those of histoplasmosis. Cases in Canada and Europe are extremely rare and are associated with travel to the southwestern United States where it is more prevalent, principally in parts of California, Arizona, Nevada, New Mexico, and Texas. Because of its prevalence in the San Joaquin Valley, the disease is sometimes referred to as *San Joaquin fever* or *valley fever*. The *C. immitis* organism lives in the soil and any disruption (*e.g.,* construction, farming, dust storms) can establish new sites in the soil.[34]

The disease most commonly occurs as an acute, primary, self-limited pulmonary infection with or without systemic involvement, but in some cases it progresses to a disseminated disease. The incubation period is 1 to 3 weeks. About 60% of infected persons develop symptoms of primary coccidioidomycosis. The symptoms are usually those of a respiratory tract infection with fever, cough, and pleuritic pain. Erythema nodosum may occur 2 to 20 days after onset of symptoms. The skin lesions usually are accompanied by arthralgias or arthritis without effusion. The terms *desert bumps* and *desert arthritis* are used to describe these manifestations. The presence of skin and joint manifestations indicates strong host defences because persons who have had such manifestations seldom acquire disseminated disease.[34]

Radiologic studies, including chest radiographic studies and bone scans, are useful in determining disease but cannot distinguish coccidioidomycosis from other pulmonary diseases. A definitive diagnosis requires microscopic or serologic evidence that *Coccidioides* spp. is present in body tissues or fluids. Serologic tests can be done for immunoglobulin M (IgM) and IgG antibody detection.

Treatment depends on the severity of infection. Persons without associated risk factors such as HIV infection or without specific evidence of progressive disease usually can be managed without antifungal therapy. The oral antifungal drugs itraconazole and fluconazole are used for treatment of less severe forms of infection. Intravenous amphotericin B is used in the treatment of persons with progressive disease. Long-term treatment is often required.

Blastomycosis

Blastomycosis is a fungal infection caused by inhaling the spores of *B. dermatitidis*. The fungus is most commonly found in Manitoba, Ontario, and Quebec, including near the Great Lakes.[35] *B. dermatitidis* is most commonly found in soil containing decayed vegetation or decomposed wood. This rare disease occurs most often in men infected during occupational or recreational outdoor activities.

The infection is characterized by local suppurative (pus-forming) and granulomatous lesions of the lungs and skin.

The symptoms of acute infection, which are similar to those of acute histoplasmosis, include fever, cough, aching joints and muscles, and, uncommonly, pleuritic pain. In contrast to histoplasmosis, the cough in blastomycosis often is productive, and the sputum is purulent. Acute pulmonary infections may be self-limited or progressive. In persons with overwhelming pulmonary disease, diffuse intra-alveolar infiltrates and evidence of acute respiratory distress syndrome may develop (see Chapter 29). Extrapulmonary spread most commonly involves the skin, bones, or prostate. These lesions may provide the first evidence of the disease.

The definitive diagnostic test for *B. dermatitidis* infection is growth of the organism from sputum, tissue biopsy, or body fluid. It generally takes several weeks to grow in mould phase at room temperature. Once growth has occurred, laboratories that use the highly specific and sensitive DNA probe for *B. dermatitidis* can rapidly identify the organism.

Treatment of the progressive or disseminated form of the disease includes the use of itraconazole or amphotericin B.[35] Most persons with blastomycosis are identified and treated before the development of overwhelming or fatal disease.

IN SUMMARY

Respiratory infections are the most common cause of respiratory illness. They include the common cold, influenza, pneumonias, tuberculosis, and fungal infections. The common cold occurs more frequently than any other respiratory infection. The fingers are the usual source of transmission, and the most common portals of entry are the nasal mucosa and the conjunctiva of the eye. The influenza virus causes three syndromes: an uncomplicated rhinotracheitis, a respiratory viral infection followed by a bacterial infection, and viral pneumonia. The contagiousness of influenza results from the ability of the virus to mutate and form subtypes against which the population is unprotected.

Pneumonia describes an infection of the parenchymal tissues of the lung. Loss of the cough reflex, damage to the ciliated endothelium that lines the respiratory tract, or impaired immune defences predispose to pneumonia. Pneumonia can be classified according to the type of organism causing the infection (typical or atypical), location of the infection (lobar pneumonia or bronchopneumonia), and the setting in which it occurs (community- or hospital-acquired). Persons with compromised immune function constitute a special concern in both categories. Community-acquired pneumonia involves infections from organisms that are present more often in the community than in the hospital or nursing home. The most common cause of community-acquired pneumonia is *S. pneumoniae.* Hospital-acquired (nosocomial) pneumonia is defined as a lower respiratory tract infection occurring 48 hours or more after admission. Hospital-acquired pneumonia is the second most common cause of hospital-acquired infection. Acute typical pneumonias, including *S. pneumoniae* and

L. pneumophila pneumonia, are caused by organisms that multiply extracellularly in the alveoli and cause inflammation and transudation of fluid into the air-filled spaces of the alveoli. Atypical pneumonias are caused by a variety of agents, including *M. pneumoniae* and viruses that invade the alveolar septum and interstitium of the lung.

Tuberculosis is a chronic respiratory infection caused by *M. tuberculosis,* which is spread by minute, invisible particles called droplet nuclei. Tuberculosis is a particular threat among foreign-born persons from countries with a high incidence of tuberculosis and persons with HIV/AIDS. The tubercle bacillus incites a distinctive chronic inflammatory response referred to as granulomatous inflammation. The destructiveness of the disease results from the cell-mediated hypersensitivity response that the bacillus evokes rather than its inherent destructive capabilities. Cell-mediated immunity and hypersensitivity reactions contribute to the evolution of the disease. Although rare in Canada, the treatment of tuberculosis has been complicated by outbreaks of drug-resistant forms of the disease.

Endemic infections caused by the fungi *H. capsulatum* (histoplasmosis), *C. immitis* (coccidioidomycosis), and *B. dermatitidis* (blastomycosis) produce pulmonary manifestations that resemble tuberculosis. These infections are common but seldom serious unless they produce progressive destruction of lung tissue or the infection disseminates to organs and tissues outside the lungs.

CANCER OF THE LUNG

After completing this section of the chapter, you should be able to meet the following objectives:

- Cite risk factors associated with lung cancer.
- Compare small cell lung cancer and non-small cell lung cancer in terms of histopathology, prognosis, and treatment methods.
- Describe the manifestations of lung cancer and list two symptoms of lung cancer that are related to the invasion of the mediastinum.
- Define the term paraneoplastic and cite three paraneoplastic manifestations of lung cancer.
- Characterize the effect of age on treatment of lung cancer.

Lung cancer is the leading cause of cancer death among men and women in Canada.[36] The Canadian Cancer Society estimates that in 2014, there will be 26,100 new diagnoses of lung cancer and 20,500 Canadian deaths, which accounts for approximately 14% of cancer diagnoses and 27% of all cancer deaths.[36] Because smoking tobacco accounts for a majority of cases of lung cancer, it is also the most preventable type of cancer. The number of men who develop lung cancer is decreasing approximately 2% per year, and since 2006 the incidence for women has levelled off and with only minimal increases. These differences are attributed to past tobacco use over the late 30 years.[37] Because lung cancer usually is far advanced before it is discovered, the prognosis in general is poor, with an overall 5-year survival rate of about 17%.[36]

Smoking, which includes cigarettes, pipes, and exposure to second-hand smoke, is related to more than 85% of lung cancer cases in Canada.[36] The risk for lung cancer among cigarette smokers increases with duration of smoking and the number of cigarettes smoked per day. Cigarette smokers can benefit at any age from smoking cessation. However, even after periods of abstinence greater than 40 years, the risk for lung cancer among former smokers remains elevated compared with that of nonsmokers. Newer research looking at recreational and heavy marijuana smokers identifies an increased risk but not as strong as the risk between tobacco and smoking. Industrial hazards also contribute to the incidence of lung cancer. A commonly recognized hazard is exposure to asbestos, with the mean risk for lung cancer being significantly greater in asbestos workers than in the general population. There is also evidence to suggest a familial predisposition to lung cancer. This occurrence may be due to a genetic predisposition, with the trait being expressed only in the presence of its major predisposing factor—cigarette smoking.[36]

Histologic Subtypes and Pathogenesis

Most (about 95%) primary lung tumours are carcinomas that arise from the lung tissue.[19] The remaining 5% are a miscellaneous group that includes bronchial carcinoid tumours (neuroendocrine tumours), bronchial gland tumours, and other mesenchymal neoplasms. The lung is also a frequent site of metastasis from cancers in other parts of the body.

Lung cancers are aggressive, locally invasive, and widely metastatic tumours that arise from the epithelial lining of major bronchi. These tumours begin as small mucosal lesions that may follow one of several patterns of growth. They may form intraluminal masses that invade the bronchial mucosa and infiltrate the peribronchial connective tissue, or they may form large, bulky masses that extend into the adjacent lung tissue. Some large tumours undergo central necrosis and acquire local areas of hemorrhage, and some invade the pleural cavity and chest wall and spread to adjacent intrathoracic structures.[19] All types of lung cancer, especially small cell lung carcinoma, have the capacity to synthesize bioactive products and produce paraneoplastic syndromes.

Lung cancer is commonly subdivided into four major categories: squamous cell lung carcinoma (25% to 30%), adenocarcinoma (20% to 40%), small cell carcinoma (10% to 15%), and large cell carcinoma (10% to 15%).[14] For purposes of staging and treatment, lung cancers are commonly identified as small cell lung cancer (SCLC) or non-small cell lung cancer (NSCLC). The key reason for this classification is that the majority of SCLCs have metastasized by the time of diagnosis and hence are not amenable to cancer surgery. They are usually best treated with chemotherapy, with or without radiation.

Small Cell Lung Cancers

The SCLCs are characterized by a distinctive cell type—small round to oval cells that are approximately the size of a lymphocyte.[19,38] The cells grow in clusters that exhibit neither glandular nor squamous organization. Electron microscopic studies demonstrate the presence of neurosecretory granules in some of the tumour cells similar to those found in the bronchial epithelium of the fetus or neonate.[19,38] The presence of these granules, the ability of some of these tumours to secrete polypeptide hormones, and the presence of neuroendocrine markers such as neuron-specific enolase and parathormone-like and other hormonally active products suggest that these tumours may arise from the neuroendocrine cells of the bronchial epithelium. This cell type has the strongest association with cigarette smoking and is rarely observed in someone who has not smoked.[38]

The SCLCs are highly malignant, tend to infiltrate widely, disseminate early in their course, and rarely are resectable. About 70% have advanced disease with metastasis at the time of diagnosis.[19] Brain metastases are particularly common with SCLC and may provide the first evidence of the tumour.

This type of lung cancer is associated with several types of paraneoplastic syndrome, including the syndrome of inappropriate antidiuretic hormone secretion (SIADH; see Chapter 31), Cushing syndrome associated with ectopic production of adrenocorticotropic hormone (ACTH; see Chapter 41), and the Lambert-Eaton syndrome of neuromuscular disorder (see Chapter 8).[36,38]

Non-Small Cell Lung Cancers

The NSCLCs include squamous cell carcinomas, adenocarcinomas, and large cell carcinomas. Like the SCLCs, these cancers have the capacity to synthesize bioactive products and produce paraneoplastic syndromes.

Squamous Cell Carcinoma. Squamous cell carcinoma is found most commonly in men and is closely correlated with a smoking history. Squamous cell carcinoma tends to originate in the central bronchi as an intraluminal growth and is thus more amenable to early detection through cytologic examination of the sputum than other forms of lung cancer.[36] It tends to spread centrally into major bronchi and hilar lymph nodes and disseminates outside the thorax later than other types of bronchogenic cancers. Squamous cell carcinoma is associated with the paraneoplastic syndromes that produce hypercalcemia.

Adenocarcinoma. Currently, adenocarcinoma is the most common type of lung cancer in North America. Its association with cigarette smoking is weaker than that of squamous cell carcinoma. It is the most common type of lung cancer in women and nonsmokers. Adenocarcinomas can have their origin in either the bronchiolar or alveolar tissues of the lung.[36] These tumours tend to be located more peripherally than

FIGURE 28.10 • Adenocarcinoma of the lung. A peripheral tumour is located in the upper right lobe of the lung. (From Rubin R., Strayer D. S. (Eds.). (2012). *Rubin's pathology: Clinicopathologic foundations of medicine* (6th ed., p. 595). Philadelphia, PA: Lippincott Williams & Wilkins.)

squamous cell sarcomas and sometimes are associated with areas of scarring (Fig. 28.10). The scars may be due to old infarcts, metallic foreign bodies, wounds, and granulomatous infections such as tuberculosis. In general, adenocarcinomas have a poorer stage-for-stage prognosis than squamous cell carcinomas.[19]

Large Cell Carcinoma. Large cell carcinomas have large, polygonal cells. They constitute a group of neoplasms that are highly anaplastic and difficult to categorize as squamous cell carcinoma or adenocarcinoma. They tend to occur in the periphery of the lung, invading subsegmental bronchi and larger airways. They have a poor prognosis because of their tendency to spread to distant sites early in their course.[19]

Clinical Features

Manifestations

The manifestations of lung cancer can be divided into three categories: (1) those due to involvement of the lung and adjacent structures; (2) the effects of local spread and metastasis; and (3) nonmetastatic paraneoplastic manifestations involving endocrine, neurologic, and connective tissue function. As with other cancers, lung cancer also causes nonspecific symptoms such as anorexia and weight loss. Because its symptoms are similar to those associated with smoking and chronic bronchitis, they often are disregarded. Metastases already exist in many patients presenting with evidence of lung cancer. The most common sites of these metastases are the brain, bone, and liver.

Many of the manifestations of lung cancers result from local irritation and obstruction of the airways and from invasion of the mediastinum and pleural space. The earliest symptoms usually are chronic cough, shortness of breath, and wheezing because of airway irritation and obstruction. Hemoptysis (*i.e.,* blood in the sputum) occurs when the lesion erodes blood vessels. Pain receptors in the chest are limited to the parietal pleura, mediastinum, larger blood vessels, and peribronchial afferent vagal fibres. Dull, intermittent, poorly localized retrosternal pain is common in tumours that involve the mediastinum. Pain becomes persistent, localized, and more severe when the disease invades the pleura.

Tumours that invade the mediastinum may cause hoarseness because of the involvement of the recurrent laryngeal nerve and cause difficulty in swallowing because of compression of the esophagus. An uncommon complication called the *superior vena cava syndrome* occurs in some persons with mediastinal involvement. Interruption of blood flow in this vessel usually results from compression by the tumour or involved lymph nodes. The disorder can interfere with venous drainage from the head, neck, and chest wall. The outcome is determined by the speed with which the disorder develops and the adequacy of the collateral circulation. Tumours adjacent to the visceral pleura often insidiously produce pleural effusions. This effusions can compress the lung and cause atelectasis and dyspnea. It is less likely to cause fever, pleural friction rub, or pain than pleural effusion resulting from other causes.

Paraneoplastic disorders are those that are unrelated to metastasis (see Chapter 8) and occur in approximately 10% of persons with lung cancer.[39] These include hypercalcemia from secretion of parathyroid-like peptide, Cushing syndrome from ACTH secretion, SIADH, neuromuscular syndromes (*e.g.,* Lambert-Eaton syndrome), and hematologic disorders (*e.g.,* migratory thrombophlebitis, nonbacterial endocarditis, disseminated intravascular coagulation). Neurologic or muscular symptoms can develop 6 months to 4 years before the lung tumour is detected. One of the more common of these problems is weakness and wasting of the proximal muscles of the pelvic and shoulder girdles, with decreased deep tendon reflexes but without sensory changes. Hypercalcemia is seen most often in persons with squamous cell carcinoma, hematologic syndromes in persons with adenocarcinomas, and the remaining syndromes in persons with small-cell neoplasms. Manifestations of the paraneoplastic syndrome may precede the diagnosis of lung cancer leading to the discovery of an occult tumour, may appear late in the disease course, or may suggest recurrence.

Diagnosis and Treatment

The diagnosis of lung cancer is based on a careful history and physical examination and on other tests such as chest radiography, bronchoscopy, cytologic studies (Papanicolaou [Pap] test) of the sputum or bronchial washings, percutaneous needle biopsy of lung tissue, and scalene lymph node biopsy.[39] CT scans, MRI studies, and ultrasonography are used to locate lesions and evaluate the extent of the disease. Positron emission tomography (PET) is a noninvasive alternative for identifying metastatic lesions in the mediastinum or distant sites. Persons with SCLC should also have a CT scan or MRI of the brain for detection of metastasis.

Like other cancers, lung cancer is classified according to extent of disease. NSCLCs are usually classified according to cell type (*i.e.*, squamous cell carcinoma, adenocarcinoma, and large cell carcinoma) and staged according to the TNM international staging system[36] (see Chapter 8). SCLCs are not staged using the TNM system because micrometastases are assumed to be present at the time of diagnosis. Instead, they are usually classified as limited disease, when the tumour is limited to the unilateral hemithorax, or extensive disease, when it extends beyond these boundaries.[36]

Treatment methods for NSCLC include surgery, radiation therapy, and chemotherapy.[36–39] These treatments may be used singly or in combination. Surgery is used for the removal of small, localized NSCLC tumours. It can involve a lobectomy, pneumonectomy, or segmental resection of the lung. Radiation therapy can be used as a definitive or main treatment modality, as part of a combined treatment plan, or for palliation of symptoms. Because of the frequency of metastases, chemotherapy often is used in treating lung cancer. Combination chemotherapy, which uses a regimen of several drugs, usually is used. New targeted treatments are under development with the goal of increasing survival and ultimately providing a cure for this type of cancer.

Therapy for SCLC is based on chemotherapy and radiation therapy. Advances in the use of combination chemotherapy, along with thoracic irradiation, have improved the outlook for persons with SCLC. Because SCLC may metastasize to the brain, prophylactic cranial irradiation is often indicated. In most persons who achieve a complete remission from SCLC, the brain is the most frequent site of relapse. About half of such persons develop clinical metastasis within 2 years.[38] Newer combination chemotherapy regimens and targeted therapies are being developed in hopes of providing treatment alternatives that increase survival and produce fewer treatment liabilities.[40]

Management of Lung Cancer in Older Adults

At the time of diagnosis, 50% of people with lung cancer are older than 70 years of age.[41] Knowledge about the optimal treatment for older persons is limited because of underrepresentation in clinical trials and failure to evaluate younger versus older persons in randomized clinical trials. At present, it is recommended that the older adult should be treated based on their general physiologic rather than chronologic age. This includes an evaluation of functional status (ability to be independent in daily tasks at home and in the community), coexisting medical conditions, nutritional status, cognition, psychological functioning, social support, and medication review. Those with good performance status and normal renal and hematologic parameters may be treated surgically or receive standard chemoradiation for limited-stage disease and combination chemotherapy for extensive-stage disease.[41]

Surgery remains the mainstay for older persons with stages I to III NSCLC. Curative resection is feasible in older persons. The challenge for surgical treatment for older persons is age-related physiologic changes in cardiovascular and respiratory systems that may affect tolerance of surgery.

Radiation can be given with curative intent for older persons who are not surgical candidates. It may also be used for palliation of cancer-related symptoms. Evidence suggests that treatment tolerance and efficacy of thoracic radiation are similar in younger and older patients. Age is reported to have no effect on acute or late radiation toxicity, including nausea, dyspnea, esophagitis, or weakness. Older patients are more likely, however, to experience weight loss than younger patients.

Chemotherapy is the mainstay of treatment of SCLC. Older persons with good performance status may receive standard chemotherapy for limited disease and combination chemotherapy for extensive-stage disease. Some older persons may require dose reductions or be unable to complete the full chemotherapy course.

IN SUMMARY

Cancer of the lung is a leading cause of death among men and women in Canada. There is a higher incidence and mortality of lung cancer in persons older than 65 years of age. Because lung cancer develops insidiously, it often is far advanced before it is diagnosed, a fact that is used to explain the poor 5-year survival rate. The increased death rate from lung cancer has coincided with an increase in cigarette smoking. Industrial hazards, such as exposure to asbestos, increase the risk for development of lung cancer. Carcinoma, which accounts for 95% of all primary lung cancers, can be subdivided into four major categories: squamous cell carcinoma, adenocarcinoma, large cell carcinoma, and small cell carcinoma. For purposes of staging and treatment, lung cancer is divided into small cell lung cancer and non-small cell lung cancer. The main reason for this is that almost all small cell lung cancers have metastasized at the time of diagnosis and are not amenable to surgical resection.

The manifestations of lung cancer can be attributed to the involvement of the lung and adjacent structures, the effects of local spread and metastasis, and paraneoplastic syndromes involving endocrine, neurologic, and hematologic dysfunction. As with other cancers, lung cancer causes nonspecific symptoms such as anorexia and weight loss. Depending on the individual, treatment methods for lung cancer include surgery, irradiation, and chemotherapy to either cure, contain the growth, or provide symptom relief.

RESPIRATORY DISORDERS IN CHILDREN

After completing this section of the chapter, you should be able to meet the following objectives:

- Trace the development of the respiratory tract through the five stages of embryonic and fetal development.

- Cite the role of surfactant in lung function in the neonate.
- Cite the possible cause and manifestations of respiratory distress syndrome and bronchopulmonary dysplasia.
- Describe the physiologic basis for sternal and chest wall retractions and grunting, stridor, and wheezing as signs of respiratory distress in infants and small children.
- Compare croup, epiglottitis, and bronchiolitis in terms of incidence by age, site of infection, and signs and symptoms.
- List the signs of impending respiratory failure in small children.

Acute respiratory diseases are the most common cause of illness in infancy and childhood. This section focuses on (1) lung development, with an emphasis on the developmental basis for lung disorders in children; (2) respiratory disorders in the neonate; and (3) respiratory infections in children. A discussion of bronchial asthma in children and cystic fibrosis is included in Chapter 29.

Lung Development

Although other body systems are physiologically ready for extrauterine life as early as 25 weeks of gestation, the lungs require a much longer time. Immaturity of the respiratory system is a major cause of morbidity and mortality in infants born prematurely. Even at birth, the lungs are not fully mature, and additional growth and maturation continue well into childhood.

Lung development may be divided into five stages: embryonic period, pseudoglandular period, canalicular period, saccular period, and alveolar period[42] (Fig. 28.11). The development of the respiratory system begins with the *embryonic period* (weeks 4 to 6 of gestation), during which a rudimentary bronchial bud branches from the esophagus to begin formation of the airways and alveolar spaces. The bronchial bud divides into two lung buds that grow laterally; the right bud gives rise to two secondary bronchial buds and the left bud to one secondary bronchial bud. Consequently, at maturity, there are three main (primary) bronchi and three lung lobes on the right and only two main bronchi and two lung lobes on the left. Each secondary bronchial bud subsequently undergoes continuous branching. The tertiary (segmental) bronchi (10 in the right lung and 8 or 9 in the left lung) begin to form during the seventh week. The pulmonary vasculature is a mesenchymal derivative. Soon after their appearance, the bronchial buds are surrounded by a vascular plexus, which originates from the aorta and drains into the major somatic veins. This vascular plexus connects with the pulmonary artery and veins at the seventh week of gestation.

During the *pseudoglandular period* (weeks 5 to 16), the lungs resemble a gland. During this period, the conducting airways are formed. At 17 weeks, all of the major elements

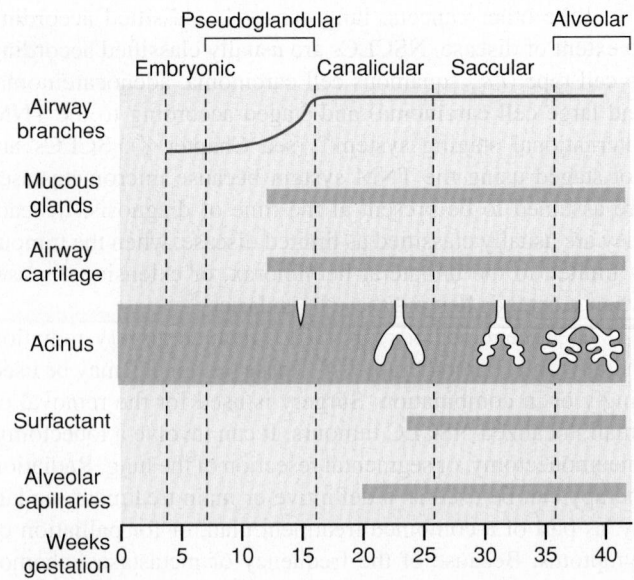

FIGURE 28.11 • Development of various respiratory structures during the five stages of lung development. (From Behrman R. E., Kliegman R. M., Jenson H. B. (Eds.). (2004). *Nelson textbook of pediatrics* (17th ed., p. 1358). Philadelphia, PA: Elsevier Saunders.)

of the lung have formed except the gas exchange structures. Respiration is not possible because the airways end in blind tubes. The *canalicular period* (weeks 17 to 26) marks the formation of the primitive alveoli. The lumina of the bronchi and bronchioles become much larger, and the lung tissue becomes more highly vascularized. By the 24th week, each bronchiole has given rise to two or more respiratory bronchioles. Respiration is possible at this time because some primitive alveoli have developed at the ends of the bronchioles.[42]

The *saccular period* (weeks 26 to 35) is devoted to the development of the terminal alveolar sacs, which facilitate gas exchange. During this period, the terminal sacs thin out, and capillaries begin to bulge into the terminal sacs. These thin cells are known as type I alveolar cells. By the 25th to 28th weeks, sufficient terminal sacs are present to permit survival. Before this time, the premature lungs are incapable of adequate gas exchange. It is not so much the presence of the thin alveolar epithelium as it is the adequate matching of pulmonary vasculature to it that is critical to survival.[42] Type II alveolar cells begin to develop at approximately 24 weeks. These cells produce surfactant, a substance capable of lowering the surface tension of the air–alveoli interface (see Chapter 27). By the 28th to 30th weeks, sufficient amounts of surfactant are available to prevent alveolar collapse when breathing begins.

The *alveolar period* (32 weeks to 8 years) marks the maturation and expansion of the alveoli. Starting as early as 30 weeks and usually by 36 weeks of gestation, the saccular structures become alveoli.[42,43] Alveolar development is characterized by thinning of the pulmonary interstitium and the appearance of a single-capillary network, in which one capillary bulges into each terminal alveolar sac. By the late fetal period, the lungs are capable of respiration because the alveolar–capillary membrane is sufficiently thin to allow for gas exchange.

Although transformation of the lungs from glandlike structures to highly vascular, alveoli-like organs occurs during the late fetal period, mature alveoli do not form for some time after birth. The growth of the lung during infancy and early childhood involves an increase in the number rather than the size of the alveoli. Only one eighth to one sixth of the adult number of alveoli are present at birth. There is a relative slowing of alveolar growth during the first 3 months after birth, and this is followed by a rapid increase in alveolar number during the rest of the first year of life, reaching approximately the adult number of 300 million alveoli by 8 years of age.[42]

Development of Breathing in the Fetus and Neonate

The fetal lung is a secretory organ, and fluids and electrolytes are secreted into the potential air spaces. This fluid appears to be important in stimulating alveolar development. For the fetus to complete the transition from intrauterine to extrauterine life, this fluid must be cleared from the lung soon after birth. Presumably with the onset of labour, the secretion of fluid ceases. During the birth process, pressure on the fetal thorax causes the fluid to be expelled from the mouth and nose. When the lungs expand after birth, the fluid moves into the tissues surrounding the alveoli and is then absorbed into the pulmonary capillaries or removed by the lymphatic system.

Fetal breathing movements occur in utero. These movements are irregular in rate and amplitude, ranging from 30 to 70 breaths per minute, and become more rapid as gestation advances. Because they are rapid and shallow, these movements do not result in movement of fluid into or out of the fetal lung. Instead, they are thought to condition the respiratory muscles and stimulate lung development. The breathing movements in the fetus become more rapid in response to an increase in carbon dioxide levels and become slower in response to hypoxia.

The major difference between respiration in the fetus and the neonate is that there is complete separation between gas exchange and breathing movements in the fetus. The gas supply and exchange depend entirely on maternal mechanisms controlling placental circulation. At birth, dependence on the placental circulation is terminated, and the infant must integrate the two previously separate functions of gas exchange and respiratory movements. Within seconds of the clamping of the umbilical cord, the infant takes its first breath, and rhythmic breathing begins and persists for life.

Effective ventilation requires coordinated interaction between the muscles of the upper airways, including those of the pharynx and larynx, the diaphragm, and the intercostal muscles of the chest wall. In infants, a specific sequence of upper airway nerve and muscle activity occurs before and early in inspiration: the tongue moves forward to prevent airway obstruction, and the vocal cord abducts, reducing laryngeal resistance. By moving downward, the action of the diaphragm increases chest volume in both the longitudinal and transverse directions. In the infant, the diaphragm inserts more horizontally than in the adult. As a result, contraction of the diaphragm tends to draw the lower ribs inward, especially if the infant is placed in the

FIGURE 28.12 • **A:** Normal inspiratory appearance of the chest during unobstructed breathing in the neonate. **B:** Sternal and intercostal retractions during obstructed breathing in the neonate.

horizontal position. The function of the intercostal muscles is to lift the ribs during inspiration. In the infant, however, the intercostal muscles are not fully developed, so they function largely to stabilize the chest rather than lift the chest wall.

The chest wall of the neonate is highly compliant; although this is advantageous during the birth process in that it allows for marked distortion to occur without damaging chest structures, it has implications for ventilation during the postnatal period. A striking characteristic of neonatal breathing is the paradoxical inward movement of the upper chest during inspiration, especially during active sleep. This occurs because of decreased activity of the intercostal muscles during active sleep, which allows the contracting diaphragm to pull the highly compliant chest wall inward. Under circumstances such as crying, the intercostal muscles of the neonate function together with the diaphragm to splint the chest wall and prevent its collapse.

Normally, the infant's lungs also are compliant; this is advantageous to the infant with a compliant chest cage because it takes only small changes in inspiratory pressure to inflate a compliant lung. When respiratory disease develops, lung compliance is reduced, and it takes more effort to inflate the lungs. The diaphragm must generate more negative pressure, causing the compliant chest wall structures to be sucked inward. *Retractions* are abnormal inward movements of the chest wall during inspiration; they may occur intercostally (between the ribs; Fig. 28.12), in the substernal or epigastric area, and in the supraclavicular spaces. Because the chest wall of the infant is compliant, substernal retractions become more obvious with small changes in lung function. Retractions can indicate airway obstruction or atelectasis.

Airway Resistance

Normal lung inflation requires uninterrupted movement of air through the extrathoracic airways (*i.e.,* nose, pharynx, larynx, and upper trachea) and intrathoracic airways (*i.e.,* bronchi and bronchioles). The neonate (0 to 4 weeks of age) breathes predominantly through the nose and does not adapt well to mouth breathing. Any obstruction of the nose or nasopharynx may increase upper airway resistance and increase the work of breathing.

The airways of the infant and small child are much smaller than those of the adult.[43] Because the resistance to airflow is inversely related to the fourth power of the radius (resistance = $1/r^4$), relatively small amounts of mucus secretion, edema, or airway constriction can produce marked increases in airway resistance and decreases in airflow. Nasal flaring is a method that infants use to take in more air. This method of breathing increases the size of the nares and decreases the resistance of the small airways.

Normally, the extrathoracic airways in the infant narrow during inspiration and widen during expiration, and the intrathoracic airways widen during inspiration and narrow during expiration.[43] This occurs because the pressure inside the extrathoracic airways reflects the intrapleural pressures that are generated during breathing, whereas the pressure outside the airways is similar to atmospheric pressure. Thus, during inspiration, the pressure inside becomes more negative, causing the airways to narrow, and during expiration it becomes more positive, causing them to widen. In contrast to the extrathoracic airways, the pressure outside the intrathoracic airways is equal to the intrapleural pressure. These airways widen during inspiration as the surrounding intrapleural pressure becomes more negative and pulls them open, and they narrow during expiration as the surrounding pressure becomes more positive.

Lung Volumes and Gas Exchange

The functional residual capacity, which is the air left in the lungs at the end of normal expiration, plays an important role in the infant's gas exchange. In the infant, the functional residual capacity occurs at a higher lung volume than in the older child or adult. This higher end-expiratory volume results from a more rapid respiratory rate, which leaves less time for expiration. However, the increased residual volume is important to the neonate for several reasons: (1) it holds the airways open throughout all phases of respiration, (2) it favours the reabsorption of intrapulmonary fluids, and (3) it maintains more uniform lung expansion and enhances gas exchange. During active sleep, the tone of the upper airway muscles is reduced, so that the time spent in expiration is shorter and the intercostal activity that stabilizes the chest wall is less. This results in a lower end-expiratory volume and less optimal gas exchange.

Control of Ventilation

Fetal arterial oxygen pressures (PO_2) normally range from 25 to 30 mm Hg, and carbon dioxide pressures (PCO_2) range from 45 to 50 mm Hg, independent of any respiratory movements. Any decrease in oxygen levels induces quiet sleep in the fetus with subsequent cessation of breathing movements, both of which lead to a decrease in oxygen consumption. Switching to oxygen derived from the aerated lung at birth causes an immediate increase in arterial PO_2 to approximately 50 mm Hg; within a few hours, it increases to approximately 70 mm Hg. These levels, which greatly exceed fetal levels, cause the chemoreceptors that sense arterial PO_2 levels to become silent for several days. Although the infant's arterial PO_2 may fluctuate during this critical time, the chemoreceptors

do not respond appropriately. It is not until several days after birth that the chemoreceptors "reset" their PO_2 threshold; only then do they become the major controller of breathing. However, the response seems to be biphasic, with an initial hyperventilation followed by a decreased respiratory rate and even apnea. In normal infants, especially those that are born prematurely, breathing patterns and respiratory reflexes depend on the arousal state.[43,44] Periodic breathing and apnea are characteristic of premature infants and reflect patterns of fetal breathing. The fact that they occur with sleep and disappear during wakefulness underscores the importance of arousal.

Alterations in Breathing

Most respiratory disorders in the infant or small child produce a decrease in lung compliance or an increase in airway resistance manifested by changes in breathing patterns, rib cage distortion (retractions), audible sounds, and use of accessory muscles.[43]

Children with restrictive lung disorders, such as pulmonary edema or respiratory distress syndrome, breathe at faster rates, and their respiratory excursions are shallow. *Grunting* is an audible noise emitted during expiration. An expiratory grunt is common as the child tries to raise the end-expiratory pressure and thus prolong the period of oxygen and carbon dioxide exchange across the alveolar–capillary membrane.

Increased airway resistance can occur in either the extrathoracic or intrathoracic airways. When the obstruction is in the extrathoracic airways, inspiration is more prolonged than expiration. *Nasal flaring* (enlargement of the nares) helps reduce the nasal resistance and maintain airway patency. It can be a sign of increased work of breathing and is a significant finding in an infant. *Inspiratory retractions,* or pulling in of the soft tissue surrounding the cartilaginous and bony thorax, is often observed with airway obstruction in infants and small children (Fig. 28.12). In conditions such as croup, the pressures distal to the point of obstruction must become more negative to overcome the resistance; this causes collapse of the distal airways, and the increased turbulence of air moving through the obstructed airways produces an audible crowing sound called a *stridor* during inspiration.

When the obstruction is in the intrathoracic airways, as occurs with bronchiolitis and bronchial asthma, expiration is prolonged and the child makes use of the accessory expiratory muscles (abdominals). Rib cage retractions may also be present. Intrapleural pressure becomes more positive during expiration because of air trapping; this causes collapse of intrathoracic airways and produces an audible wheezing or whistling sound during expiration.

Respiratory Disorders in the Neonate

The neonatal period is one of transition from placental dependency to air breathing. This transition requires functioning of the surfactant system, conditioning of the respiratory muscles, and establishment of parallel pulmonary and systemic circulations. Respiratory disorders develop in infants who are born prematurely or who have other problems that impair this transition. Among the respiratory disorders of the neonate are the respiratory distress syndrome, bronchopulmonary dysplasia, and persistent fetal circulation (*i.e.,* delayed closure of the ductus arteriosus and foramen ovale; see Chapter 24).

Respiratory Distress Syndrome

Respiratory distress syndrome (RDS), also known as *hyaline membrane disease,* is one of the most common causes of respiratory disease in premature infants.[45,46] In these infants, pulmonary immaturity, together with surfactant deficiency, leads to alveolar collapse (Fig. 28.13). The type II alveolar cells that produce surfactant do not begin to mature until approximately the 25th to 28th weeks of gestation; consequently, many premature infants are born with poorly functioning type II alveolar cells and have difficulty producing sufficient amounts of surfactant. The incidence of RDS is higher among preterm male infants, white infants, infants of diabetic mothers, and those subjected to asphyxia, cold stress, precipitous deliveries, and delivery by cesarean section (when performed before the 38th week of gestation).[46]

Surfactant synthesis is influenced by several hormones, including insulin and cortisol. Insulin tends to inhibit surfactant production; this explains why infants of insulin-dependent diabetic mothers are at increased risk for development of RDS. Cortisol can accelerate maturation of type II cells and formation of surfactant. The reason that premature infants born by cesarean section presumably are at greater risk for development of RDS is that they are not subjected to the stress of vaginal delivery, which is thought to increase the infants' cortisol levels. These observations have led to administration of corticosteroid drugs before delivery to mothers with infants at high risk for development of RDS.[45,46]

Surfactant reduces the surface tension in the alveoli, thereby equalizing the retractive forces in the large and small alveoli and reducing the amount of pressure needed to inflate and hold the alveoli open (see Chapter 27). Without surfactant, the large alveoli remain inflated, whereas the small alveoli become difficult to inflate. At birth, the first breath requires high inspiratory pressures to expand the lungs. With normal levels of surfactant, the lungs retain up to 40% of the residual volume after the first breath, and subsequent breaths require far lower inspiratory pressures. With a surfactant deficiency, the lungs collapse between breaths, making the infant work as hard with each successive breath as with the first breath. The airless portions of the lungs become stiff and noncompliant. A hyaline membrane forms inside the alveoli as protein- and fibrin-rich fluids are pulled into the alveolar spaces. The fibrin–hyaline membrane constitutes a barrier to gas exchange, leading to hypoxemia and carbon dioxide retention, a condition that further impairs surfactant production.

Infants with RDS present with multiple signs of respiratory distress, usually within the first 24 hours of birth. Central cyanosis is a prominent sign. Breathing becomes more difficult, and retractions occur as the infant's soft chest wall is pulled in as the diaphragm descends. Grunting sounds accompany expiration. As the tidal volume drops because of atelectasis, the respiration rate increases (usually to 60–120 breaths/minute) in an effort to maintain normal minute ventilation. Fatigue may develop rapidly because of the increased work of breathing. The stiff lungs of infants with RDS also increase the resistance to blood flow in the pulmonary circulation. As a result, a hemodynamically significant patent ductus arteriosus may develop in infants with RDS (see Chapter 24).

The basic principles of treatment for infants with suspected RDS focus on the provision of supportive care, including gentle handling and minimal disturbance.[46] An incubator or radiant warmer is used to prevent hypothermia and increased oxygen consumption. Continuous cardiorespiratory monitoring is needed. Monitoring of blood glucose and prevention of hypoglycemia are also recommended. Oxygen levels can be assessed through an arterial (umbilical) line or by a transcutaneous oxygen sensor. Treatment includes administration of supplemental oxygen, continuous positive airway pressure through nasal prongs, and often assisted mechanical ventilation.

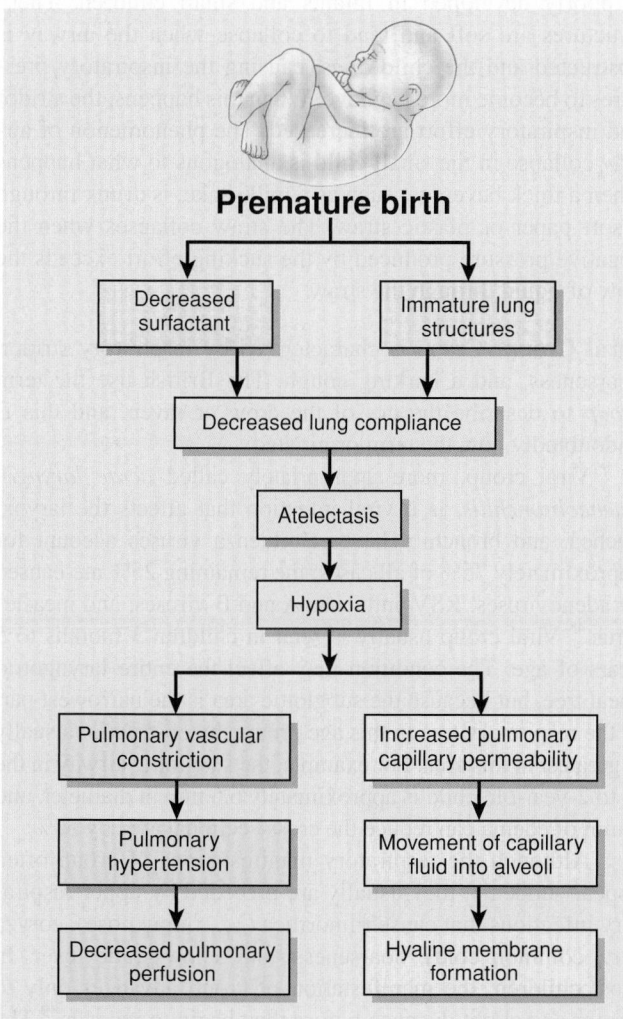

Premature birth

Decreased surfactant → Immature lung structures →

Decreased lung compliance →

Atelectasis →

Hypoxia →

Pulmonary vascular constriction → Increased pulmonary capillary permeability →

Pulmonary hypertension → Movement of capillary fluid into alveoli →

Decreased pulmonary perfusion → Hyaline membrane formation

FIGURE 28.13 • Pathogenesis of respiratory distress syndrome (RDS) in the infant.

Exogenous surfactant therapy is used to prevent and treat RDS. There are two types of surfactants used in Canada: natural surfactants prepared from animal sources and synthetic surfactants. The surfactants are suspended in saline and administered into the airways, usually through an endotracheal tube. The treatment often is initiated soon after birth in infants who are at high risk for RDS.

Bronchopulmonary Dysplasia

Bronchopulmonary dysplasia (BPD) is a chronic lung disease that develops in premature infants who were treated with mechanical ventilation, mainly for RDS.[31,47] The definition for BPD is if the neonate is oxygen dependent 28 days postnatally and the severity is graded based on supplemental oxygen requirements after 36 weeks gestation age. The disorder is thought to be a response of the premature lung to early injury. High inspired oxygen concentration and injury from positive-pressure ventilation (i.e., barotrauma) have been implicated.[31,47]

BPD is characterized by chronic respiratory distress, persistent hypoxemia when breathing room air, reduced lung compliance, increased airway resistance, and severe expiratory flow limitation. There is a mismatching of ventilation and perfusion with development of hypoxemia and hypercapnia. Pulmonary vascular resistance may be increased and pulmonary hypertension and cor pulmonale (i.e., right heart failure associated with lung disease) may develop. The infant with BPD often demonstrates a barrel chest, tachycardia, rapid and shallow breathing, chest retractions, cough, and poor weight gain.[31,47] Clubbing of the fingers occurs in children with severe disease. Hepatomegaly and periorbital edema may develop in infants with right heart failure.

The treatment of BPD includes mechanical ventilation and administration of supplemental oxygen. Weaning from ventilation is accomplished gradually, and some infants may require ventilation at home. Rapid lung growth occurs during the first year of life, and lung function usually improves. Adequate nutrition is essential for recovery of infants with BPD.[31]

Most adolescents and young adults who had severe BPD during infancy have some degree of pulmonary dysfunction, consisting of airway obstruction, airway hyperreactivity, or hyperinflation.

Respiratory Infections in Children

In children, respiratory tract infections are common, and although they are troublesome, they usually are not serious. Frequent infections occur because the immune systems of infants and small children have not been exposed to many common pathogens; consequently, they tend to contract infections with each new exposure. Although most of these infections are not serious, the small size of an infant's or child's airways tends to foster impaired airflow and obstruction. For example, an infection that causes only sore throat and hoarseness in an adult may result in serious airway obstruction in a small child.

Upper Airway Infections

Acute upper airway infections are important in infants and small children. They include viral croup (laryngotracheobronchitis), bacterial tracheitis, and epiglottitis.[48–53] Croup is the more common and usually is benign and self-limited, whereas bacterial tracheitis is an uncommon infection requiring antibiotics. Epiglottitis is a rapidly progressive and life-threatening condition. Characteristics of these infections are described in Table 28.2.

Obstruction of the upper airways because of infection tends to exert its greatest effect during the inspiratory phase of respiration. Movement of air through an obstructed upper airway, particularly the vocal cords in the larynx, causes stridor. Impairment of the expiratory phase of respiration also can occur, causing wheezing. With mild to moderate obstruction, inspiratory stridor is more prominent than expiratory wheezing because the airways tend to dilate with expiration. When the swelling and obstruction become severe, the airways no longer can dilate during expiration, and both stridor and wheezing occur.

Cartilaginous support of the trachea and the larynx is poorly developed in infants and small children. These structures are soft and tend to collapse when the airway is obstructed and the child cries, causing the inspiratory pressures to become more negative. When this happens, the stridor and inspiratory effort are increased. The phenomenon of airway collapse in the small child is analogous to what happens when a thick beverage, such as a milkshake, is drunk through a soft paper or plastic straw. The straw collapses when the negative pressure produced by the sucking effort exceeds the flow of liquid through the straw.

Viral Croup. Croup is characterized by inspiratory stridor, hoarseness, and a barking cough. The British use the term *croup* to describe the cry of the crow or raven, and this is undoubtedly how the term originated.

Viral croup, more appropriately called *acute laryngotracheobronchitis,* is a viral infection that affects the larynx, trachea, and bronchi. The parainfluenza viruses account for approximately 75% of all cases; the remaining 25% are caused by adenoviruses, RSV, influenza A and B viruses, and measles virus.[48] Viral croup usually is seen in children 3 months to 5 years of age. The condition may affect the entire laryngotracheal tree, but because the subglottic area is the narrowest part of the respiratory tree in this age group, the obstruction usually is greatest in this area. For example, the subglottic airway in the 1- to 2-year-old child is approximately 6.5 mm in diameter, and 1 mm of edema can reduce the cross-sectional area by 50%.

Although the respiratory manifestations of croup often appear suddenly, they usually are preceded by upper respiratory infections that cause rhinorrhea (i.e., runny nose), coryza (i.e., common cold), hoarseness, and a low-grade fever. In most children, the manifestation of croup advances only to stridor and slight dyspnea before they begin to recover.[49] The symptoms usually subside when the child is exposed to moist air. For example, letting the bathroom shower run and then

TABLE 28.2 CHARACTERISTICS OF CROUP, BACTERIAL TRACHEITIS, EPIGLOTTITIS, AND BRONCHIOLITIS IN SMALL CHILDREN

CHARACTERISTICS	CROUP	BACTERIAL TRACHEITIS	EPIGLOTTITIS	BRONCHIOLITIS
Common causative agent	Mainly parainfluenza virus	*Staphylococcus aureus* bacterium	*Haemophilus influenzae* type B bacterium	Respiratory syncytial virus (RSV)
Most commonly affected age group	3 months to 5 years	6 months to 8 years (peak 4–6 years)	2–7 years (peak 3–5 years)	Less than 2 years (most severe in infants younger than 6 months)
Onset and preceding history	Usually follows symptoms of a cold	Usually follows symptoms of a cold (similar to croup)	Sudden onset	Preceded by stuffy nose and other signs
Prominent features	Stridor and a wet, barking cough Usually occurs at night Relieved by exposure to cold or moist air	Fever, cough, stridor progressing to high fever, difficulty breathing Toxic appearance Does not respond to steroid treatment *Danger of airway obstruction and asphyxia*	Child appears very sick and toxic Sits with mouth open and chin thrust forward Low-pitched stridor, difficulty swallowing, fever, drooling, anxiety *Danger of airway obstruction and asphyxia*	Breathlessness, rapid, shallow breathing, wheezing, cough, and retractions of lower ribs and sternum during inspiration
Usual treatment	Mist tent or vaporizer Oxygen	Hospitalization Potential intubation Treatment with appropriate antibiotics	Hospitalization Intubation or tracheotomy Treatment with appropriate antibiotic	Supportive treatment, administration of oxygen and hydration

taking the child into the bathroom often brings prompt and dramatic relief of symptoms. Exposure to cold air also seems to relieve the airway spasm; often, the severe symptoms are relieved simply because the child is exposed to cold air on the way to the hospital emergency department. Viral croup does not respond to antibiotics; expectorants, bronchodilating agents, and antihistamines are not helpful. The child should be disturbed as little as possible and carefully monitored for signs of respiratory distress.

Airway obstruction may progress in some children. As obstruction increases, the stridor becomes continuous and is associated with nasal flaring with substernal and intercostal retractions. Agitation and crying aggravate the signs and symptoms, and the child prefers to sit up or be held upright. In the cyanotic, pale, or obstructed child, any manipulation of the pharynx, including use of a tongue depressor, can cause cardiorespiratory arrest and should be done only in a medical setting that has the facilities for emergency airway management. To decrease the laryngeal mucosal edema triggered by the viral infection, a single dose of dexamethasone (a long acting corticosteroid) can relieve the symptoms, reduce the severity, and decrease the risk of airway obstruction.[50] Establishment of an artificial airway may become necessary in severe airway obstruction.

Spasmodic Croup. Spasmodic croup manifests with symptoms similar to those of acute viral croup. Because the child is afebrile and lacks other manifestations of the viral prodrome, it is thought that it may have an allergic origin. Spasmodic croup characteristically occurs at night and tends to recur with respiratory tract infections. The episode usually lasts several hours and may recur several nights in a row.

Most children with spasmodic croup can be effectively managed at home. An environment of high humidification (*i.e.,* cold-water room humidifier or taking the child into a bathroom with a warm, running shower) lessens irritation and prevents drying of secretions.

Bacterial Tracheitis. This is an acute bacterial infection affecting children aged 6 months to 8 years (average age is 4–6 years) in the upper airway and is potentially life threatening. Bacterial tracheitis often follows a viral respiratory infection (especially laryngotracheitis), so it may be considered a bacterial complication of a viral disease, rather than a primary bacterial illness. Children can initially present with crouplike symptoms (barking cough, stridor) but they do not respond to standard therapy for croup. High fevers and a "toxic" appearance with increasing respiratory distress can precede acute respiratory decompensation. The usual pathogen is *S. aureus,* but others such as *Moraxella catarrhalis, H. influenzae,* and other anaerobic organisms have been implicated. Treatment with antibiotics and careful monitoring of airway patency is required as up to 50% of children will require intubation for airway management.[48,51,52]

Epiglottitis. Acute epiglottitis is a dramatic, potentially fatal condition characterized by inflammatory edema of the supraglottic area, including the epiglottis and pharyngeal structures, that comes on suddenly, bringing danger of airway obstruction and asphyxia.[48] In the past, the *H. influenzae* type B bacterium was the most commonly identified etiologic agent. It is seen less commonly since the widespread use of immunization against *H. influenzae* type B. Therefore, other agents such as *Streptococcus pyogenes, S. pneumoniae,* and *S. aureus* now represent the most common causes of pediatric epiglottitis.

The child appears pale, toxic, and lethargic and assumes a distinctive position—sitting up with the mouth open and the chin thrust forward. The child has difficulty in swallowing, a muffled voice, drooling, fever, and extreme anxiety. Moderate to severe respiratory distress is evident. There is inspiratory and sometimes expiratory stridor, flaring of the nares, and inspiratory retractions of the suprasternal notch and supraclavicular and intercostal spaces. Within a matter of hours, epiglottitis may progress to complete obstruction of the airway and death unless adequate treatment is instituted. Epiglottitis is a medical emergency and immediate establishment of an airway by endotracheal tube or tracheotomy usually is needed. If epiglottitis is suspected, the child should never be forced to lie down because this causes the epiglottis to fall backward and may lead to complete airway obstruction. Examination of the throat with a tongue blade or other instrument may cause cardiopulmonary arrest and should be done only by medical personnel experienced in intubation of small children. It also is unwise to attempt any procedure, such as drawing blood, that would heighten the child's anxiety because this also could precipitate airway spasm and cause death. Recovery from epiglottitis usually is rapid and uneventful after an adequate airway has been established and appropriate antibiotic therapy initiated.

Lower Airway Infections

Lower airway infections produce air trapping with prolonged expiration. Wheezing results from bronchospasm, mucosal inflammation, and edema. The child presents with increased expiratory effort, increased respiratory rate, and wheezing. If the infection is severe, there also are marked intercostal retractions and signs of impending respiratory failure.

Acute bronchiolitis is a viral infection of the lower airways, most commonly caused by the respiratory syncytial virus (RSV).[48,52] Other viruses, such as parainfluenza-3 virus and some adenoviruses, as well as mycoplasmas, also are causative. The infection produces inflammatory obstruction of the small airways and necrosis of the cells lining the lower airways. It occurs during the first 2 years of life, with a peak incidence between 3 and 6 months of age. The source of infection usually is a family member with a minor respiratory illness. Older children and adults tolerate bronchiolar edema much better than infants and do not manifest the clinical picture of bronchiolitis. Because the resistance to airflow in a tube is inversely related to the fourth power of the radius, even minor swelling of bronchioles in an infant can produce profound changes in airflow.

Most affected infants in whom bronchiolitis develops have a history of a mild upper respiratory tract infection. These symptoms usually last several days and may be accompanied by fever and diminished appetite. There is then a gradual development of respiratory distress, characterized by a wheezy cough, dyspnea, and irritability. The infant usually is able to take in sufficient air but has trouble exhaling it. Air becomes trapped in the lung distal to the site of obstruction and interferes with gas exchange. Hypoxemia and, in severe cases, hypercapnia may develop. Airway obstruction may produce air trapping and hyperinflation of the lungs or collapse of the alveoli. Infants with acute bronchiolitis have a typical appearance, marked by breathlessness with rapid respirations, a distressing cough, and retractions of the lower ribs and sternum. Crying and feeding exaggerate these signs. Wheezing and crackles may or may not be present, depending on the degree of airway obstruction. In infants with severe airway obstruction, wheezing decreases as the airflow diminishes. Usually, the most critical phase of the disease is the first 48 to 72 hours. Cyanosis, pallor, listlessness, and sudden diminution or absence of breath sounds indicate impending respiratory failure. The characteristics of bronchiolitis are described in Table 28.2.

Infants with respiratory distress usually are hospitalized. Treatment is supportive and includes administration of supplemental oxygen if the oxygen saturation consistently falls below 90%.[52] Elevation of the head facilitates respiratory movements and avoids airway compression. Handling is kept at a minimum to avoid tiring. Because the infection is viral, antibiotics are not effective and are given only for a secondary bacterial infection. Dehydration may occur as the result of increased insensible water losses because of the rapid respiratory rate and feeding difficulties, and measures to ensure adequate hydration are needed. If the child is in respiratory distress and adequate hydration cannot be achieved, the child should receive intravenous fluids.[48,52] Recovery usually begins after the first 48 to 72 hours and usually is rapid and complete. Adequate hand washing is essential to prevent the nosocomial spread of RSV.

Signs of Impending Respiratory Failure

Respiratory problems of infants and small children often originate suddenly, and recovery usually is rapid and complete. Children are at risk for the development of airway obstruction and respiratory failure resulting from obstructive disorders or lung infection. The child with epiglottitis is at risk for airway obstruction. The child with bronchiolitis is at risk for respiratory failure resulting from impaired gas exchange. Children with impending respiratory failure due to airway or lung disease have rapid breathing; exaggerated use of the accessory muscles; retractions, which are more pronounced in the child than in the adult because of more compliant chest; nasal flaring; and grunting during expiration. The signs and symptoms of impending respiratory failure are listed in Chart 28.1.

IN SUMMARY

Although other body systems are physiologically ready for extrauterine life as early as 25 weeks of gestation, the lungs take longer. Immaturity of the respiratory system is a major cause of morbidity and mortality in premature infants.

CHART 28.1 SIGNS OF RESPIRATORY DISTRESS AND IMPENDING RESPIRATORY FAILURE IN THE INFANT AND SMALL CHILD

- Severe increase in respiratory effort, including severe retractions or grunting, decreased chest movement
- Cyanosis that is not relieved by administration of oxygen (40%)
- Heart rate of 150 per minute or greater and increasing tachycardia
- Very rapid breathing (rate 60 per minute in the newborn to 6 months or above 30 per minute in children 6 months to 2 years)
- Very depressed breathing (rate 20 per minute or below)
- Retractions of the supraclavicular area, sternum, epigastrium, and intercostal spaces
- Extreme anxiety and agitation
- Fatigue
- Decreased level of consciousness

Lung development may be divided into five stages: embryonic period, pseudoglandular period, canalicular period, saccular period, and alveolar period. The first three phases are devoted to development of the conducting airways, and the last two phases are devoted to development of the gas exchange portion of the lung. By the 25th to 28th weeks of gestation, sufficient terminal air sacs are present to permit survival. It is also during this period that type II alveolar cells, which produce surfactant, begin to function. Lung development is incomplete at birth; an infant is born with only one-eighth to one-sixth the adult number of alveoli. Alveoli continue to be formed during early childhood, reaching the adult number of 300 million alveoli by 8 years of age.

Children with restrictive lung disease breathe at faster rates, and their respiratory excursions are shallow. An expiratory grunt is common as the child tries to raise the functional residual capacity by closing the glottis at the end of expiration. Obstruction of the extrathoracic airways often produces turbulence of airflow and an audible inspiratory crowing sound called stridor, and obstruction of the intrathoracic airways produces an audible expiratory wheezing or whistling sound. RDS is one of the most common causes of respiratory disease in premature infants. In these infants, pulmonary immaturity, together with surfactant deficiency, leads to alveolar collapse. BPD is a chronic pulmonary disease that develops in premature infants who were treated with mechanical ventilation.

Acute respiratory disease is the most common cause of illness in infancy and childhood, accounting for 50% of illnesses in children younger than 5 years of age and 30% of illnesses in children between 5 and 12 years of age. Because of the small size of the airway of infants and children, respiratory tract infections in these groups often are more serious. Infections that may cause only a sore throat and hoarseness in the adult may produce serious obstruction in the child. Among the respiratory tract infections that affect small children are croup, epiglottitis, and bronchiolitis. Epiglottitis is a life-threatening supraglottic infection that may cause airway obstruction and asphyxia.

REVIEW EXERCISES

1. It is flu season, and although you had a flu shot last year, you have not had one this year. Imagine yourself experiencing an abrupt onset of fever, chills, malaise, muscle aching, and nasal stuffiness.
   A. *Which of these symptoms would lead you to believe you are coming down with the flu?*
   B. *Because you hate to miss classes, you decide to go to the student health centre to get an antibiotic. After being seen by a health professional, you are told that antibiotics are ineffective against the flu virus, and you are instructed not to attend classes but instead to go home, take acetaminophen for your fever, go to bed and stay warm, and drink a lot of fluids. Explain the rationale for each of these recommendations.*
   C. *Explain why last year's flu shot did not protect you during this year's flu season.*
   D. *There is concern about the possibility of an influenza pandemic such as the one that occurred during the 1917–1918 season. What is the rationale for this concern?*
2. Bacterial (*e.g., S. pneumoniae*) pneumonia is commonly manifested by a cough productive of sputum, whereas with atypical (*e.g., Mycoplasma pneumoniae*) pneumonia, the cough is usually nonproductive or absent.
   A. *Explain.*
3. A 4-month-old infant is admitted to the pediatric intensive care unit with a diagnosis of bronchiolitis. The infant is tachypneic, with wheezing, nasal flaring, and retractions of the lower sternum and intercostal spaces during inspiration.
   A. *What is the usual pathogen in bronchiolitis? Would this infection be treated with an antibiotic?*
   B. *Explain the physiologic mechanism involved in the retraction of the lower sternum and intercostal spaces during inspiration.*
   C. *What would be the signs of impending respiratory failure in this infant?*

References

1. Statistics Canada. (2014). The 10 leading causes of death, 2011. Available online at: http://www.statcan.gc.ca/pub/82-625-x/2014001/article/11896-eng.htm. Accessed June 10, 2014.
2. World Health Organization. (2014). Tuberculosis. Available online at: http://www.who.int/mediacentre/factsheets/fs104/en. Accessed June 10, 2014.
3. Public Health Agency of Canada (PHAC). (2014). Tuberculosis in Canada 2012–Pre-release. 2014. Available online at: http://www.phac-aspc.gc.ca/tbpc-latb/pubs/tbcan12pre/index-eng.php. Accessed June 10, 2014.
4. Passioti M., Maggina P., Megremis S., Papadopoulos N. G. (2014). The common cold: Potential for future prevention or cure. *Current Allergy and Asthma Reports, 14*(2), 413.
5. Gruber C., Keil T., Kulig M., et al.; MAS-90 Study Group. (2008). History of respiratory infections in the first 12 yr among children from a birth cohort. *Pediatric Allergy and Immunology, 19*(6), 505–512.
6. Gern J. E., Palmenberg A. C. (2013). Chapter 18: Rhinoviruses. In Knipe D. M., Howley P. (Eds.), *Fields virology* (6th ed.). Philadelphia, PA: Lippincott Williams and Wilkins.
7. Dykewicz M. S., Hamilos D. L. (2010). Rhinitis and sinusitis. *Journal of Allergy and Clinical Immunology, 125*(Suppl 2), S103–S115.
8. Meltzer E. O., Hamilos D. L. (2011). Rhinosinusitis diagnosis and management for the clinician: A synopsis of recent consensus guidelines. *Mayo Clinic Proceedings, 86*(5), 427–443.
9. Brook I. (2013). Acute sinusitis in children. *Pediatric Clinics of North America, 60*(2), 409–424.
10. National Advisory Committee on Immunizations (NACI). (2013). Statement on seasonal influenza vaccine for 2013–2014. *CCDR, 39*(4), ISSN 1481–8531.
11. Wright P., Neumann G., Kawaoka Y. (2013). Chapter 41: Orthomyxoviruses. In: Knipe D. M., Howley P. (Eds.), *Fields virology* (6th ed.). Philadelphia, PA: Lippincott Williams and Wilkins.
12. Rothberg M. B., Haessler S. D. (2010). Complications of seasonal and pandemic influenza. *Critical Care Medicine, 38*(Suppl 4), e91–e97.
13. Ruuskanen O., Lahti E., Jennings L. C., Murdoch D. R. (2011). Viral pneumonia. *Lancet, 377*(9773), 1264–1275.
14. Aoki F. Y., Allen U. D., Stiver H. G., et al. (2013). The use of antiviral drugs for influenza: A foundation document for practitioners. *Canadian Journal of Infectious Diseases & Medical Microbiology, 24*(Suppl C), 1C–15C.
15. Remington L. T., Sligl W. I. (2014). Community-acquired pneumonia. *Current Opinion in Pulmonary Medicine, 20*(3), 215–224.
16. Weinberger S. E., Cockrill B. A., Mandel J. (2014). *Principles of pulmonary medicine* (6th ed.). Philadelphia, PA: Saunders Elsevier.
17. Wunderink R. G., Waterer G. W. (2014). Community-acquired pneumonia. *New England Journal of Medicine, 370*(6), 543–551.
18. Rotstein C. Evans G., Born A., et al. (2008). Clinical practice guidelines for hospital-acquired pneumonia and ventilator-associated pneumonia in adults. *Canadian Journal of Infectious Disease & Medical Microbiology, 19*(1), 19–53.
19. Husain AN. (2010). Chapter 15: The lung. In: Kumar V., Abbas A. K., Fausto N., Aster J. C. (Eds.), *Robbins and Cotran pathologic basis of disease* (8th ed). Philadelphia, PA: Elsevier Saunders.
20. Letourneau A., Issa N. C., Baden L. R. (2014). Pneumonia in the immunocompromised host. *Current Opinion in Pulmonary Medicine, 20*(3), 272–279.
21. PHAC. (2014). Canadian Immunization Guide. Available online at: http://www.phac-aspc.gc.ca/publicat/cig-gci/index-eng.php. Accessed June 11, 2014.
22. van der Poll T., Opal S. M. (2009). Pathogenesis, treatment, and prevention of pneumococcal pneumonia. *Lancet, 374*(9700), 1543–1556.
23. Beasley M. B., Travis W. D., Rubin E. (2012). Chapter 12: The respiratory system. In Rubin R., Strayer D. S. (Eds.), *Rubin's pathology: Clinicopathologic foundations of medicine* (6th ed.). Philadelphia, PA: Lippincott Williams & Wilkins.
24. Canadian Antimicrobial Resistance Alliance. (2014). Respiratory infections. Available online at: http://www.can-r.com/index.php. Accessed June 11, 2014.
25. Carratala J., Garcia-Vidal C. (2010). An update on Legionella. *Current Opinion in Infectious Diseases, 23*(2), 152–157.
26. Cunha B. A. (2008). Atypical pneumonias: Current clinical concepts focusing on Legionnaires' disease. *Current Opinion in Pulmonary Medicine, 14*(3), 183–194.
27. Basarab M., Macrae B., Curtis C. M. (2014). Atypical pneumonia. *Current Opinion in Pulmonary Medicine, 20*(3), 247–251.
28. PHAC. (2014). *Canadian tuberculosis standards* (7th ed.). Available online at: http://www.respiratoryguidelines.ca/tb-standards-2013. Accessed June 11, 2014.
29. McAdam A. J., Sharpe A. H. (2010). Chapter 8: Infectious diseases. In Kumar V., Abbas A. K., Fausto N., Aster J. C. (Eds.), *Robbins and Cotran pathologic basis of disease* (8th ed.). Philadelphia, PA: Elsevier Saunders.
30. Schwartz D. A. (2012). Chapter 9: Infectious and parasitic diseases. In Rubin R., Strayer D. S. (Eds.), *Rubin's pathology: Clinicopathologic foundations of medicine* (6th ed.). Philadelphia, PA: Lippincott Williams & Wilkins.
31. Lestrud S. (2011). Chapter 410: Bronchopulmonary dysplasia. In Kliegman R. M., Stanton B. F., St. Geme J. W., et al. (Eds.), *Nelson textbook of pediatrics.* (19th ed.). Philadelphia, PA: Saunders Elsevier; 2011.
32. Takiff H., Guerrero E. (2011). Current prospects for the fluoroquinolones as first-line tuberculosis therapy. *Antimicrobial Agents and Chemotherapy, 55*(12), 5421–5429.
33. Canadian Centre for Occupational Health and Safety. (2013). Histoplasmosis. Available online at: http://www.ccohs.ca/oshanswers/diseases/histopla.html. Accessed June 11, 2014.
34. PHAC. (2011). Coccidioides spp. Available online at: http://www.phac-aspc.gc.ca/lab-bio/res/psds-ftss/coccidioides-spp-eng.php. Accessed June 11, 2014.
35. Saccente M., Woods G. L. (2010). Clinical and laboratory update on blastomycosis. *Clinical Microbiology Reviews, 23*(2), 367–381.
36. Canadian Cancer Society. (2014). Lung cancer. Available online at: http://www.cancer.ca/en/cancer-information/cancer-type/lung/lung-cancer/?region=on. Accessed June 11, 2014.
37. Canadian Cancer Society's Advisory Committee. (2014). *Canadian cancer statistics.* Toronto, CA: Canadian Cancer Society.
38. van Meerbeeck J. P., Fennell D. A., De Ruysscher D. (2011). Small-cell lung cancer, *Lancet, 378*(9804), 1741–1755.
39. Collins L. G., Haines C., Perkel R., Enck R. E. (2007). Lung cancer: Diagnosis and management. *American Family Physician, 75*(1), 56–63.
40. Goldstraw P., Jett J. R., Chevalier T. L., et al. (2011). Non-small-cell lung cancer, *Lancet, 378*(9804), 1727–1740.
41. Blanco J. A. G., Toste I. S., Alvarez R. F., et al. (2008). Age, comorbidity, treatment decision and prognosis in lung cancer. *Age Ageing, 37*(6):715–718.
42. Moore K. L., Persaud T. V., Torchia M. G. (2013). *The developing human: Clinically oriented embryology* (9th ed.). Philadelphia, PA: Saunders Elsevier.
43. Sarnaik A. P., Heidemann S. M. (2011). Chapter 365: Respiratory pathophysiology and regulation. In Kliegman R. M., Stanton B. F., St. Geme J. W., et al. (Eds.), *Nelson textbook of pediatrics* (19th ed.). Philadelphia, PA: Saunders Elsevier.
44. Hillman N. H., Kallapur S. G., Jobe A. H. (2012). Physiology of transition from intrauterine to extrauterine life. *Clinics in Perinatology, 39*(4), 769–783.
45. Mattay M. A., Ware L. B., Zimmerman G. A. (2012). The acute respiratory distress syndrome. *Journal of Clinical Investigation, 122*(8), 2731–2740.
46. Carlo W. A. (2011). Chapter 95: Respiratory tract disorders. In Kliegman R. M., Stanton B. F., St. Geme J. W., et al. (Eds.), *Nelson textbook of pediatrics* (19th ed.). Philadelphia, PA: Saunders Elsevier.
47. Carraro S., Filippone M., Dalt L. D., et al. (2013). Bronchopulmonary dysplasia: The earliest and perhaps the longest lasting obstructive lung disease in humans. *Early Human Development, 89*(Suppl 3), S3–S5.
48. Roosevelt G. E. (2011). Chapter 377: Acute inflammatory upper airway obstruction. In Kliegman R. M., Stanton B. F., St. Geme J. W., et al. (Eds.), *Nelson textbook of pediatrics* (19th ed.). Philadelphia, PA: Saunders Elsevier.
49. Petrocheilou A., Tanou K., Kalampouka E., et al. (2014). Viral croup: Diagnosis and a treatment algorithm. *Pediatric Pulmonology, 49*(5), 421–429.
50. Russell K. F., Liang Y., O'Gorman K., et al. (2011). Glucocorticoids for croup. *Cochrane Database of Systematic Reviews, 1*, CD001955.
51. Sasidaran K., Bansal A., Singhi S. (2011). Acute upper airway obstruction. *Indian Journal of Pediatrics, 78*(10), 1256–1261.
52. Choi J., Lee G. L. (2012). Common pediatric respiratory emergencies. *Emergency Medicine Clinics of North America, 30*(2), 529–563.
53. Tibballs J., Watson T. (2011). Symptoms and signs differentiating croup and epiglottitis. *Journal of Paediatrics and Child Health, 47*(3), 77–82.

Visit the Point. **http://thePoint.lww.com for animations, journal articles, and more!**

Disorders of Ventilation and Gas Exchange

29

The major function of the lungs is to exchange oxygen and carbon dioxide to support the metabolic functions of the body's tissues. Gas exchange depends on a system of open airways, expansion of the lungs, an adequate surface area for diffusion, blood flow through the pulmonary capillary bed, and exchange of alveolar air with atmospheric air. Many types of disease are capable of disrupting the normal gas-exchanging function of the lungs. In some cases the disruption is temporary and in other cases it is permanent. This chapter focuses on disorders that disrupt ventilation and gas exchange. It is divided into six sections: the physiologic effects of altered ventilation and gas exchange, disorders of lung inflation, obstructive airway disorders, interstitial lung disorders, disorders of the pulmonary circulation, and acute respiratory disorders.

PHYSIOLOGIC EFFECTS OF VENTILATION AND DIFFUSION DISORDERS

After completing this section of the chapter, you should be able to meet the following objectives:

- Define the terms hypoxemia and hypercapnia.
- Characterize the mechanisms whereby disorders of ventilation and diffusion cause hypoxemia and hypercapnia.
- Compare the manifestations of hypoxemia and hypercapnia.

The primary function of the respiratory system is gas exchange between the alveoli and pulmonary capillaries. Oxygen (O_2) diffuses into the capillary from the alveoli, with carbon dioxide (CO_2) from the capillaries into the alveoli[1,2] (discussed in Chapter 27). Impaired respiratory function or gas exchange may cause O_2 levels to decrease, CO_2 levels to increase, or both. This section of the chapter provides a brief overview of the causes and manifestations of the hypoxemia and hypercapnia that develop as the result of the impaired ventilation and gas exchange that occurs with many of the disorders discussed in the chapter.

Alveolar ventilation involves the exchange of fresh atmospheric air (which is rich in O_2 and has virtually no CO_2) into the alveoli with stale alveolar air (which is lower in O_2 and higher in CO_2). Minute ventilation is the volume of air exchanged between the alveoli and atmosphere per minute, and is essentially equivalent to alveolar ventilation. It is determined by both the amount of air exchanged with each breath (tidal volume) and the respiratory rate (breaths per minute). *Gas exchange* within the lungs involves the exchange of O_2 and CO_2 at the alveolar level between the alveoli and the blood in the pulmonary capillaries. The process involves the diffusion or movement of O_2 from the alveolar air to the blood in the pulmonary capillaries and the transfer of CO_2 from the blood in the pulmonary capillaries. Adequate oxygenation of the blood and removal of CO_2 also depends on adequate circulation of blood through the pulmonary blood vessels (perfusion) and appropriate contact between ventilated alveoli and perfused capillaries of the pulmonary circulation (ventilation and perfusion matching) (Fig. 29.1).

As a general rule, diffusion of O_2 from the alveoli into the pulmonary capillaries depends primarily on the surface area and the distance (thickness), whereas diffusion of CO_2 primarily depends on minute ventilation and elimination of CO_2 from the alveoli. Thus, oxygenation refers to the diffusion of O_2 between the alveoli and pulmonary capillaries, whereas ventilation refers to the elimination of CO_2 by the alveoli.

Hypoxemia

Hypoxemia refers to a reduction in blood O_2 levels to below normal (designated as the partial pressure of oxygen, PO_2). Normal PO_2 is dependent upon several factors, primarily altitude, and therefore varies. Hypoxemia can result from an inadequate amount of O_2 in the air, disease of the respiratory system, dysfunction of the neurologic system, or alterations in circulatory function. The mechanisms whereby respiratory disorders lead to a significant reduction in PO_2 are impaired diffusion, inadequate circulation of blood through the pulmonary capillaries, and mismatching of ventilation and perfusion[2] (see Chapter 27). Hypoxemia may also occur if hypoventilation is severe; in this case O_2 diffusion is impaired due to the increase in alveolar PCO_2, which results in a decrease in alveolar PO_2. Often, more than one mechanism contributes to hypoxemia in a person with respiratory or cardiac disease.

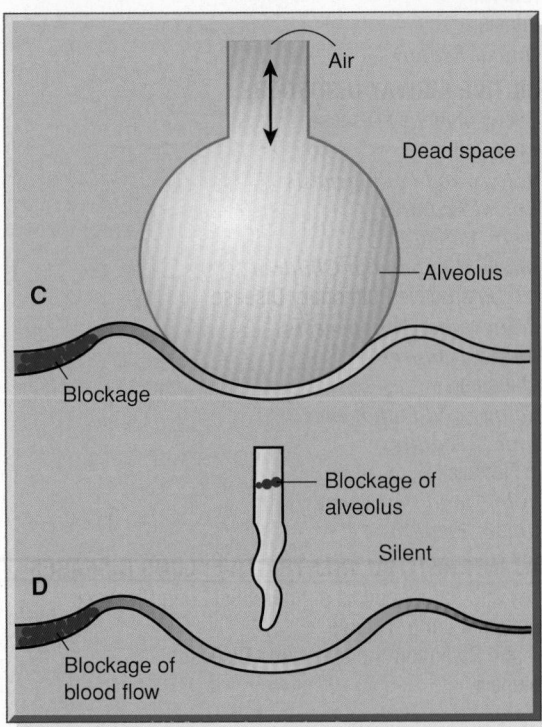

FIGURE 29.1 • Schema of various ventilation–perfusion situations. (From Day R. A., Paul P., Williams B., et al. (2010). *Brunner & Suddarth's Textbook of Canadian Medical-Surgical Nursing* (2nd ed., p. 527). Philadelphia, PA: Lippincott Williams & Wilkins.)

Clinical Manifestations and Treatment

Hypoxemia produces its effects through tissue hypoxia and the compensatory mechanisms that the body uses to adapt to the lowered oxygen level. Body tissues vary considerably in their vulnerability to hypoxia; those with the greatest need are the brain and heart. If the PO_2 of the tissues falls below a critical level, aerobic metabolism ceases and anaerobic metabolism takes over, with formation and release of lactic acid. This results in increased serum lactate levels and metabolic acidosis (see Chapter 32).

Mild hypoxemia produces few manifestations because hemoglobin saturation still is approximately 90% even when the PO_2 is only 60 mm Hg (see Chapter 27, Fig. 27.22). Sympathetic nervous system compensatory mechanisms result in an increase in heart rate, peripheral vasoconstriction, diaphoresis, and a mild increase in blood pressure. There may be slight impairment of mental performance and visual acuity and sometimes hyperventilation. More pronounced hypoxemia may produce restlessness, agitation, altered cognition, uncoordinated muscle movements, euphoria, impaired judgment, delirium, and, eventually, loss of consciousness and coma.

The manifestations of chronic hypoxemia may be insidious in onset and be attributed to other causes, particularly in persons with chronic lung disease. The body compensates for chronic hypoxemia by increased minute volume, pulmonary vasoconstriction, and a small increase in red blood cell production. Pulmonary vasoconstriction occurs as a local response to alveolar hypoxia increasing pulmonary arterial pressure with the goal of matching of ventilation and blood flow. Increased production of red blood cells results from the release of erythropoietin from the kidneys in response to hypoxemia (see Chapter 14). Polycythemia increases the red blood cell concentration and the oxygen-carrying capacity of the blood. Other adaptive mechanisms include a shift to the right in the oxygen dissociation curve (*e.g.*, acidosis) which increases O_2 release to the tissues (see Chapter 27).

Cyanosis refers to the bluish discolouration of the skin and mucous membranes that results from an excessive concentration of deoxygenated hemoglobin in the small blood vessels. It usually is most marked in the lips, nail beds, ears, and oral mucosa. The degree of cyanosis is modified by the amount of cutaneous pigment, skin thickness, and the state of the cutaneous capillaries. Cyanosis is more difficult to distinguish in persons with dark skin and in areas of the body with increased skin thickness. Although cyanosis may be evident in persons with respiratory failure, it often is a late sign.

The absolute quantity of reduced hemoglobin, rather than the relative quantity, is important in producing cyanosis. Persons with anemia and low hemoglobin levels are less likely to exhibit cyanosis (because they have less hemoglobin to deoxygenate), even though they may be relatively hypoxic because of their decreased ability to transport oxygen, than persons who have high hemoglobin concentrations. A person with a high hemoglobin level because of polycythemia may be cyanotic without being hypoxic.

Cyanosis can be divided into two types: central and peripheral. *Central cyanosis* is evident in the tongue and lips. It is caused by an increased amount of deoxygenated hemoglobin or an abnormal hemoglobin derivative in the arterial blood. Abnormal hemoglobin derivatives include *methemoglobin,* in

which the nitrite ion reacts with hemoglobin. Because methemoglobin has a low affinity for O_2, large doses of nitrites can result in cyanosis and tissue hypoxia. Although nitrites are used in treating angina, the therapeutic dose is too small to cause cyanosis. *Peripheral cyanosis* occurs in the extremities and on the tip of the nose or ears. It is caused by slower blood flow and increased extraction of oxygen from the blood. It may result from vasoconstriction and diminished peripheral blood flow, as occurs with cold exposure, shock, heart failure, or peripheral vascular disease.

Diagnosis. Diagnosis of hypoxemia is based on clinical observation and diagnostic measures of PO_2 levels. The analysis of arterial blood gases (PaO_2) provides a direct measure of the dissolved O_2 content of the blood and is the best indicator of the ability of the lungs to oxygenate the blood. Arterial oxygen saturation of hemoglobin (SaO_2) reflects the amount bound to the available hemoglobin, and is directly influenced by the PaO_2. Non-invasive measurements of arterial O_2 saturation of hemoglobin can be obtained using an instrument called the *pulse oximeter.* The conventional pulse oximeter uses light-emitting diodes and analysis of two wavelengths of light.[3] A red-wavelength light passes through oxygenated hemoglobin and is absorbed by deoxygenated hemoglobin, and an infrared-wavelength light is absorbed by oxygenated hemoglobin and passes through deoxygenated hemoglobin. The ratio is then calculated and provides a percentage of the hemoglobin that is oxygenated. Sensors require sufficient perfusion across the site, and can be placed on the ear, finger, toe, or forehead in adults, or also on the foot or palm of the hand in infants. Information is not conveyed as to the amount of carbon dioxide or acid-base balance, which requires an arterial blood gas. However, it does provide non-invasive and continuous monitoring of O_2 saturation, which is a useful indicator of oxygen status. The oxygen saturation must also be interpreted within the context of the amount of available hemoglobin to carry the oxygen.

The conventional pulse oximeter cannot distinguish between oxygen-carrying hemoglobin and other dyshemoglobins such as carbon monoxide-carrying hemoglobin or methemoglobin. However, new devices using up to eight wavelengths of light are able to accurately determine the percentage of carboxyhemoglobin (carbon monoxide bound to hemoglobin) and methemoglobin (iron in hemoglobin preventing release of bound oxygen to the tissues).[4] While a small portion of methemoglobin occurs in health, any increase by congenital defects or exposure to chemicals or medications can lead to cellular hypoxia. Carbon monoxide binds tightly to hemoglobin and is not easily released in the tissues.

The ratio between the arterial PO_2 and the fraction of inspired oxygen (FiO_2), termed the *PF ratio,* is an additional indicator of diffusion of O_2 at the lung level. The normal value of the PF ratio is greater than 300.[5] In determining this ratio, the PO_2 is divided by the FiO_2. For persons with a PO_2 of 80 when breathing room air, the PF ratio is 80 divided by 0.21 (21% of atmospheric air is O_2), which is 380 (a normal value). In contrast, if the person has a PO_2 of 80 and is receiving 40% O_2, the

P/F ratio is only 200 (80 divided by 0.40). This value indicates that although supplemental oxygen increases the PO_2 to normal, there is a diffusion problem. The PF ratio is useful for evaluating improvements or deteriorations in oxygen diffusion regardless of the amount of supplemental oxygen that is being administered. In addition, the PF ratio is a diagnostic indicator of acute respiratory distress syndrome (discussed later in the chapter).

Venous blood samples can be obtained either through a pulmonary artery catheter or a central line. The latter is less invasive but slightly less accurate because the blood has not yet been mixed in the right ventricle, and thus reflects a greater portion of the venous blood returning from the superior vena cava. Venous blood samples do not provide information regarding oxygenation, hypoxemia or lung function. Rather, comparison of venous oxygen saturation (SvO_2) with arterial oxygen saturation reflects the body's extraction and utilization of O_2 at the tissue level.

Treatment. Treatment of hypoxemia is directed toward correcting the cause of the disorder and increasing the gradient for diffusion through the administration of supplemental oxygen. Oxygen may be delivered by nasal cannula or mask, or administered directly into an endotracheal or tracheostomy tube. It may be provided by either high- or low-flow systems. A high-flow administration system is one in which the flow rate and reserve capacity are sufficient to meet the inspiratory effort.[6] A low-flow administration system delivers less than the total inspired air, and is variable depending upon the patient efforts.[6] The concentration of O_2 being administered (usually determined by the flow rate) is based on the actual and desired PO_2. High-flow oxygen can be provided by mask or high-flow nasal cannula systems which increase oxygen flow to meet that of the patient's inspirations.

Although oxygen is necessary and vital to life, there is the danger of oxygen toxicity with high concentrations of oxygen. Continuous breathing of oxygen at high concentrations can lead to diffuse parenchymal lung injury. Persons with healthy lungs begin to experience respiratory symptoms such as cough, sore throat, substernal distress, nasal congestion, and painful inspiration after breathing pure oxygen for 24 hours.[2] A high flow rate must be monitored in persons with chronic lung disease who chronically retain CO_2 because increases in PO_2 above 60 mm Hg may depress the ventilatory drive.

Hypercapnia

Hypercapnia, also called hypercarbia, refers to an increase in the carbon dioxide content of the arterial blood to a level greater than normal.[2] The carbon dioxide level in the arterial blood, or PCO_2, is inversely related to alveolar ventilation. The diagnosis of hypercapnia is based on physiologic manifestations, arterial pH, arterial blood gas levels, and end tidal capnography.

The diffusing capacity of carbon dioxide is 20 times that of oxygen; therefore, hypercapnia without hypoxemia is usually observed only in situations of hypoventilation.[2]

In severe hypoventilation, both hypercapnia and hypoxemia occur due to decreased alveolar oxygen levels. Hypercapnia that occurs with ventilation–perfusion mismatching is usually accompanied by a decrease in arterial PO_2 levels.

Conditions that increase carbon dioxide production, such as an increase in metabolic rate or a high-carbohydrate diet, can contribute to the degree of hypercapnia that occurs in persons with impaired respiratory function. Changes in the metabolic rate resulting from an increase in activity, fever, or disease can have profound effects on carbon dioxide production. Alveolar ventilation usually rises proportionally with these changes, and hypercapnia occurs only when minute volume is insufficient to exhale the CO_2.

The respiratory quotient (RQ), which is the ratio of carbon dioxide production to oxygen consumption (RQ = CO_2 production/O_2 consumption), varies with the type of food metabolized.[1] A characteristic of carbohydrate metabolism is an RQ of 1.0, with equal amounts of carbon dioxide being produced and oxygen being consumed. Because fats contain less oxygen than carbohydrates, their oxidation produces less carbon dioxide (RQ = 0.7). The metabolism of pure proteins (RQ = 0.81) results in the production of more carbon dioxide than the metabolism of fat, but less than the metabolism of carbohydrates. The type of food that is eaten or the types of nutrients that are delivered through enteral feedings (i.e., through a tube placed in the small intestine) or parenteral nutrition (i.e., through a venous catheter placed in the central vena cava) may influence PCO_2 levels in acute or critical illness.

Clinical Manifestations and Treatment

Hypercapnia affects a number of body functions, including kidney, nervous system, and cardiovascular function. An elevated level of PCO_2 alters acid-base balance due to the increased production of hydrogen ions, which decreases pH, and is called respiratory acidosis (see Chapter 32). Thus, a hallmark of hypoventilation is both an increase in CO_2 and a decrease in pH. Over time, the body normally compensates for an increase in PCO_2 by increasing renal bicarbonate (HCO_3^-) retention and increased H^+ excretion. This compensatory mechanism will result in an increase in serum HCO_3^- levels and a decrease in acidosis.

As long as the pH is within normal range, the main complications of hypercapnia are those resulting from the accompanying hypoxemia. Because the body adapts to chronic increases in blood levels of carbon dioxide, persons with chronic hypercapnia may not have symptoms until the PCO_2 becomes markedly elevated or O_2 falls significantly.

Treatment. The treatment of hypercapnia is directed at increasing the minute ventilation to eliminate the CO_2, namely increasing respiratory rate, tidal volume, or both. Increasing airway diameter through bronchodilators will increase air flow and tidal volumes. The use of intermittent therapy, such as nocturnal negative-pressure ventilation, in persons with chronic obstructive disease or chest wall disease may be effective in increasing the strength and endurance of the respiratory muscles, which increases the tidal volume and decreases the PCO$_2$. Respiratory muscle retraining aimed at improving respiratory muscle function, endurance, or both has been used to improve exercise tolerance and diminish the likelihood of respiratory fatigue. Although an increase in minute volume is required, this results in an increase in the work of breathing, risking diaphragmatic fatigue and worsened minute volume. Invasive or non-invasive positive pressure ventilation may become necessary in situations of acute hypercapnia (discussed in the section on Acute Respiratory Failure).

IN SUMMARY

The primary function of the respiratory system is to remove appropriate amounts of CO$_2$ from the pulmonary capillaries and transfer O$_2$ into the capillaries. This is accomplished through the process of ventilation, in which atmospheric air moves into and out of the lungs, and diffusion, in which the two gases move between the alveoli and the pulmonary capillaries. Although both diffusion and ventilation affect gas exchange, oxygenation of the blood largely depends on diffusion, and removal of carbon dioxide on ventilation.

Hypoxemia refers to a decrease in arterial blood oxygen levels below normal that results in a decrease in tissue oxygenation. Hypoxemia can occur as the result of diffusion impairment, marked hypoventilation, and ventilation–perfusion impairment (including shunt and dead space). Acute hypoxemia is manifested by increased respiratory effort, tachycardia, and impaired sensory and neurologic function. The body compensates for chronic hypoxemia through increased ventilation, pulmonary vasoconstriction, and increased production of red blood cells. If hypoxemia is not corrected, the person may experience chronic fatigue.

Hypercapnia refers to an increase in arterial blood carbon dioxide levels above normal. Hypercapnia results primarily from hypoventilation, such as occurs with abnormalities in function of the chest wall and respiratory muscles or changes in neural control of respiration. These alterations in respiratory function decrease minute volume, which is the most common cause of hypercapnia. The manifestations of hypercapnia consist of those associated with a decrease in pH (respiratory acidosis); vasodilation of blood vessels, including those in the brain; and depression of central nervous system function.

DISORDERS OF LUNG INFLATION

After completing this section of the chapter, you should be able to meet the following objectives:

- Characterize the pathogenesis and manifestations of transudative and exudative pleural effusion, chylothorax, and hemothorax.

- Differentiate among the causes and manifestations of spontaneous pneumothorax, secondary pneumothorax, and tension pneumothorax.
- Describe the causes of pleurisy and differentiate the characteristics of pleural pain from other types of chest pain.
- Describe the causes and manifestations of atelectasis.

Air entering through the airways inflates the lung, and the negative pressure in the pleural cavity keeps the lung from collapsing. Disorders of lung inflation are caused by conditions that obstruct the airways, cause lung compression, or produce lung collapse. There can be compression of the lung by an accumulation of fluid in the intrapleural space, complete collapse of an entire lung, as in pneumothorax, or collapse of a segment of the lung due to airway obstruction, as in atelectasis.

Disorders of the Pleura

The pleura is a thin, double-layered serous membrane that encases the lungs (Fig. 29.2). The outer *parietal layer* lines the thoracic wall and superior aspect of the diaphragm. It continues around the heart and between the lungs, forming the lateral walls of the mediastinum. The inner *visceral layer* covers the lung and is adherent to all its surfaces. The pleural cavity or space between the two layers contains a thin layer of serous fluid that lubricates the pleural surfaces and allows the parietal and visceral pleura to slide smoothly over each other during breathing movements. The pressure in the pleural cavity, which is negative in relation to atmospheric pressure, holds the lungs against the chest wall and keeps them from collapsing (see Chapter 27). Disorders of the pleura include pleural effusion, hemothorax, pneumothorax, and pleural inflammation.

Visceral pleura

Pleural space

Parietal pleura

FIGURE 29.2 • The relationship between the parietal and visceral pleurae and the pleural space, which is the site of fluid accumulation in pleural effusions.

Pleural Effusion

Pleural effusion refers to an abnormal collection of fluid in the pleural cavity.[7,8] As when fluid develops in other transcellular spaces in the body, pleural effusion occurs when the rate of fluid formation exceeds the rate of its removal (see Chapter 31). Normally, fluid enters the pleural space from capillaries in the parietal pleura and is removed by the lymphatics situated in the parietal pleura. Fluid can also enter from the interstitial spaces of the lung through the visceral pleura or from small holes in the diaphragm. The lymphatics have the capacity to reabsorb about 20 to 40 times the fluid that is formed.[7,8] Fluid may accumulate when there is excess fluid formation (from the interstitium of the lung, the parietal pleura, or peritoneal cavity) or when there is decreased removal by the lymphatics.

The fluid that accumulates in a pleural effusion may be transudate or exudate, purulent (containing pus), chyle, or sanguineous (bloody). An *exudate* is a pleural fluid that has a specific gravity greater than 1.020 and often contains inflammatory cells. The accumulation of a serous transudate (clear fluid) in the pleural cavity often is referred to as *hydrothorax*. The condition may be unilateral or bilateral. The most common cause of hydrothorax is congestive heart failure.[8] Other causes are renal failure, nephrosis, liver failure, and malignancy.

Transudative and exudative pleural effusions are distinguished by measuring the lactate dehydrogenase (LDH) and protein levels in the pleural fluid.[8] Exudative pleural effusion meets at least one of the following criteria: (1) a pleural fluid protein/serum protein ratio greater than 0.5; (2) a pleural fluid LDH/serum LDH ratio greater than 0.6; and (3) a pleural fluid LDH greater than two thirds of the upper limit of normal serum LDH.[7,8] LDH is an enzyme that is released by inflamed and injured pleural tissue. Because measurements of LDH are easily obtained from a sample of pleural fluid, it is a useful marker for diagnosis of exudative pleural disorders. Conditions that produce exudative pleural effusions are malignancies, bacterial pneumonia, viral infection, and pulmonary infarction.

Empyema refers to an infection in the pleural cavity that results in exudate containing glucose, proteins, leukocytes, and debris from dead cells and tissue.[8] It is caused by an adjacent bacterial pneumonia, rupture of a lung abscess into the pleural space, invasion from a subdiaphragmatic infection, or infection associated with trauma.

Chylothorax is the effusion of chyle in the thoracic cavity.[9] Chyle, a milky fluid containing chylomicrons, is found in the lymph fluid originating in the gastrointestinal tract. The thoracic duct transports chyle, which includes degraded dietary proteins and triglycerides, to the central circulation. Consequently, the exudate has a high triglyceride content (>1.2 mmol/L), with the exception in fasting or malnourishment.[9] Chylothorax results from trauma, inflammation, or malignant infiltration obstructing chyle transport from the thoracic duct into the central circulation. It is the most common cause of pleural effusion in the fetus and neonate, resulting from congenital malformation of the thoracic duct or lymph channels. Chylothorax also can occur as a complication of intrathoracic surgical procedures and use of the great veins for total parenteral nutrition and hemodynamic monitoring.

Manifestations. The manifestations of pleural effusion vary with the cause. Empyema may be accompanied by fever, increased white blood cell count, and other signs of inflammation. Fluid in the pleural cavity acts as a space-occupying mass; it causes a decrease in lung expansion on the affected side that is proportional to the amount of fluid collected. Characteristic signs of pleural effusion are dullness or flatness to percussion and diminished breath sounds. Hypoxemia may occur due to the decreased surface area and usually is corrected with supplemental oxygen. Dyspnea, the most common symptom, occurs when fluid compresses the lung, resulting in increased effort or rate of breathing and perception of being short of breath. Pleuritic pain usually occurs only when inflammation is present, although constant discomfort may be felt with large effusions.

Diagnosis and Treatment. Diagnosis of pleural effusion is based on chest radiographs, chest ultrasonography, and computed tomography (CT). Thoracentesis (aspiration of fluid from the pleural space) can be used to obtain a sample of pleural fluid for diagnosis. The treatment of pleural effusion is directed at the cause of the disorder. With large effusions, thoracentesis may be used to remove fluid from the intrapleural space and allow for reexpansion of the lung. Some malignant pleural effusions are managed through palliative measures.[10,11] One method is the injection of a sclerosing agent, (*e.g.*, talc, bleomycin), into the pleural cavity, which causes obliteration of the pleural space or *pleurodesis*, and prevents the reaccumulation of fluid. Another palliative method is insertion of a tunnelled pleural catheter with intermittent drainage to manage symptoms.[11]

Hemothorax

Hemothorax is a specific type of pleural effusion in which there is blood in the pleural cavity. Bleeding may be the result of chest injury, malignancies, rupture of a great vessel such as an aortic aneurysm, or a complication of chest surgery. Hemothorax may be classified as minimal, moderate, or massive.[12] For an adult, a minimal hemothorax involves the presence of 300 to 500 ml of blood in the pleural space. Small amounts of blood usually are absorbed from the pleural space, and the hemothorax usually clears in 10 to 14 days without complication. A moderate hemothorax (500 to 1,000 ml of blood) fills approximately one third of the pleural space and may produce signs of lung compression and loss of intravascular volume. It requires immediate drainage and replacement of intravascular fluids. A massive hemothorax fills one half or more of one side of the chest; it indicates the presence of 1500 ml or more of blood in the thorax and usually is caused by bleeding from a high-pressure vessel such as an intercostal or mammary artery. It requires immediate drainage and, if the bleeding continues, surgery to control the bleeding.

In addition to alterations in oxygenation, ventilation, respiration effort, and breath sounds, hemothorax may be accompanied by signs of blood loss, including increased heart rate and decreased blood pressure. Because hemothorax can be abrupt in onset, the manifestations are usually sudden and distressing. One of the complications of untreated moderate or large hemothorax is fibrothorax—the fusion of the pleural surfaces by fibrin, hyalin, and connective tissue—and in some cases, calcification of the fibrous tissue, which restricts lung expansion.

Diagnosis of hemothorax is based on chest radiographs, ultrasound, or computed tomography (CT). Drainage should be considered for any hemothorax,[12] and indicated if the person is symptomatic or oxygen exchange is compromised.

Pneumothorax

Pneumothorax refers to the presence of air in the pleural space. Pneumothorax causes partial or complete collapse of the affected lung. Pneumothorax can occur without an obvious cause or injury (*i.e.,* spontaneous pneumothorax) or as a result of direct injury to the chest or major airways (*i.e.,* traumatic pneumothorax). Tension pneumothorax describes a life-threatening condition in which pressure is increased within the pleural cavity and both respiratory and cardiac functions are impaired.

Spontaneous Pneumothorax. Spontaneous pneumothorax is hypothesized to occur due to the rupture of an air-filled bleb, bullae, or porous lesions on the surface of the lung.[13,14] Rupture of these blebs allows atmospheric air from the airways to enter the pleural cavity (Fig. 29.3). Because alveolar pressure normally is greater than pleural pressure, air flows from the alveoli into the pleural space, causing the involved portion of the lung to collapse as a result of its own recoil. Air continues to flow into the pleural space until a pressure gradient no longer exists

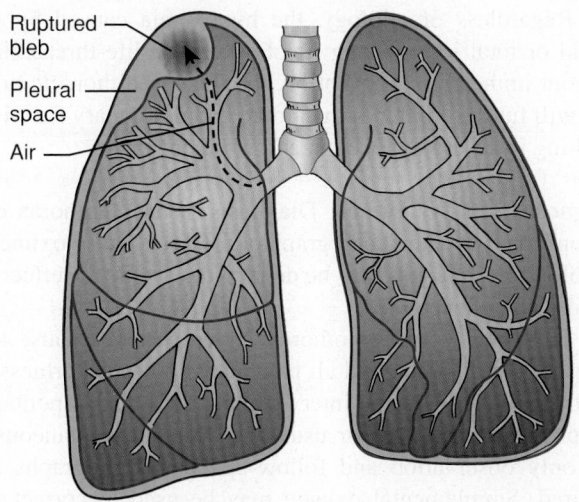

Ruptured bleb

Pleural space

Air

FIGURE 29.3 • Mechanism for development of spontaneous pneumothorax, in which an air-filled bleb on the surface of the lung ruptures, allowing atmospheric air from the airways to enter the pleural space.

or until the decline in lung size causes the leak to seal. Spontaneous pneumothoraces can be further divided into primary and secondary causes. Primary pneumothorax occurs in otherwise healthy persons, whereas secondary pneumothorax occurs in persons with underlying lung disease. Because of the risk for recurrence, persons with spontaneous pneumothorax should be advised against cigarette smoking, exposure to high altitudes, flying in nonpressurized aircraft, and scuba diving.

In primary spontaneous pneumothorax, the blebs usually are located at the top of the lungs.[13] The condition is seen most often in tall boys and young men between 10 and 30 years of age.[13,14] It has been suggested that the difference in pleural pressure from the top to the bottom of the lung is greater in tall persons and that this difference in pressure may contribute to the development of blebs. Smoking is another factor that has been associated with primary spontaneous pneumothorax. Inflammation of the small airways related to smoking probably contributes to the condition, and cessation of smoking may reduce the recurrence.[14,15]

Secondary spontaneous pneumothoraces occur in persons with lung disease. The most common cause of secondary spontaneous pneumothorax is chronic obstructive pulmonary disease. They are associated with many different types of lung conditions that cause trapping of gases and destruction of lung tissue, including asthma, tuberculosis, cystic fibrosis, sarcoidosis, bronchogenic carcinoma, and metastatic pleural diseases. Secondary spontaneous pneumothorax may be life-threatening because of the underlying lung injury and poor compensatory reserves.

Persons with *talc lung* are also highly susceptible to the occurrence of pneumothorax. Talc lung may result from inhalation of talc particles from household or industrial sources, but is more commonly associated with injected or inhaled talc powder, which is used as a filler with heroin, methamphetamine, or cocaine.[16]

Catamenial pneumothorax occurs in relation to the menstrual cycle and usually is recurrent. It typically occurs in women who are 30 to 40 years of age, usually affects the right lung and typically occurs between 24 to 72 hours of onset of menses. Risk factors include pelvic endometriosis, history of pelvic surgery, infertility, and familial history.[17] Although the cause of catamenial pneumothorax is unknown, it is hypothesized that air gains access to the peritoneal cavity during menstruation and then enter the pleural cavity through diaphragmatic perforations caused by endometrial implants.[17] Pleural and diaphragmatic endometriosis also have been implicated as causes of the condition.

Traumatic Pneumothorax. Traumatic pneumothorax may be caused by penetrating or blunt chest injuries. Fractured or dislocated ribs that penetrate the pleura are the most common cause of pneumothorax from chest injuries. Hemothorax may accompany these injuries. Pneumothorax also may accompany fracture of the trachea or major bronchus or rupture of the esophagus. Persons with pneumothorax due to penetrating chest trauma frequently have other complications and may require chest surgery. Medical procedures such as transthoracic needle aspirations, central line insertion, intubation, and positive-pressure ventilation or chest compressions occasionally cause pneumothoraces.

Tension Pneumothorax. Tension pneumothorax occurs when the intrapleural pressure exceeds atmospheric pressure. It is a life-threatening condition and occurs when injury to the chest or respiratory structures permits air to enter but not leave the pleural space (Fig. 29.4). This results in a rapid increase in pressure within the chest that causes compression atelectasis of the unaffected lung, a shift in the mediastinum to the opposite side of the chest, and compression of the vena cava, which results in a decrease in venous return to the heart and reduced stroke volume.[8] The intrathoracic pressure impedes cardiac contraction, further reducing stroke volume. Although tension pneumothorax can develop in persons with spontaneous pneumothoraces, it is seen most often in persons with traumatic pneumothoraces. It also may result from mechanical ventilation, particularly in patients with underlying lung disease.

Manifestations. The manifestations of pneumothorax depend on its size and the integrity of the underlying lung. In spontaneous pneumothorax, manifestations of the disorder include development of ipsilateral chest pain. There is an almost immediate increase in respiratory rate, often accompanied by dyspnea that occurs as a result of the activation of receptors that monitor lung volume. Asymmetry of the chest may occur because of the air trapped in the pleural cavity on the affected side. This asymmetry may be evidenced during inspiration as a lag in the movement of the affected side, with inspiration delayed until the unaffected lung reaches the same level of pressure as the lung with the air trapped in the pleural space. Percussion of the chest produces a more hyperresonant sound, and breath sounds are decreased or absent over the area of the pneumothorax.

With tension pneumothorax, the structures in the mediastinal space shift toward the opposite side of the chest (Fig. 29.3). When this occurs, the position of the trachea, normally located in the midline of the neck, deviates with the mediastinum. The position of the trachea can be used as a means of assessing for a mediastinal shift. Because of the increase in intrathoracic pressure, stroke volume is impaired to such an extent that cardiac output is decreased despite an increase in heart rate. There may be distension of the neck veins, subcutaneous emphysema (*i.e.,* presence of air in the subcutaneous tissues of the chest and neck), and clinical signs of shock due to impaired cardiac function, decreased venous return, and poor stroke volume.

Hypoxemia and oxygen desaturation usually develop immediately after a large pneumothorax. The hypoxemic vasoconstriction of the blood vessels in the affected lung causes the blood flow to shift to the unaffected lung. In persons with primary spontaneous pneumothorax that resolves, this mechanism may return oxygen saturation to near normal within 24 hours. Hypoxemia is usually more serious in persons with underlying lung disease in whom secondary spontaneous pneumothorax develops or in persons with underlying heart disease who are unable to compensate with an increase in heart rate and stroke volume.

Regardless of etiology, the hypoxemia caused by the partial or total loss of lung function can be life-threatening. Without immediate intervention, the increased thoracic pressure will further impair both cardiac and pulmonary function, resulting in severe hypoxemia and hypotension.

Diagnosis and Treatment. Diagnosis of pneumothorax can be confirmed by chest radiograph or CT scan. Pulse oximetry and blood gas analysis may be done to determine the effect on blood oxygen levels.

Treatment of pneumothorax varies with the cause and extent of the disorder, and all patients who have shortness of breath should have some intervention.[12] In a small spontaneous pneumothorax, the air usually reabsorbs spontaneously, and only observation and follow-up chest radiographs are required. Supplemental oxygen may be used to correct the hypoxemia until the air is reabsorbed. In a larger pneumothorax, the air is removed by a closed chest tube drainage system with or without suction. This type of drainage system uses a

Open Pneumothorax

Inspiration   Expiration

Tension Pneumothorax

Inspiration   Expiration

FIGURE 29.4 • Open or communicating pneumothorax **(top)** and tension pneumothorax **(bottom).** In an open pneumothorax, air enters the chest during inspiration and exits during expiration. There may be slight inflation of the affected lung because of a decrease in pressure as air moves out of the chest. In tension pneumothorax, air can enter but not leave the chest. As the pressure in the chest increases, the heart and great vessels are compressed and the mediastinal structures are shifted toward the opposite side of the chest. The trachea is pushed from its normal midline position toward the opposite side of the chest, and the unaffected lung is compressed.

one-way valve or a water-seal chamber to allow air to exit the pleural space and prevent it from re-entering the chest.

Emergency treatment of tension pneumothorax involves the prompt insertion of a large-bore needle into the affected side of the chest followed by continuous chest suction to aid in lung reexpansion. Sucking chest wounds, which allow air to pass in and out of the chest cavity, should be treated by promptly covering the area with an airtight covering (*e.g.,* Vaseline gauze, plastic) to prevent the formation of a tension pneumothorax. A Heimlich valve or chest tube should be inserted as soon as possible.

Pleuritis

Pleuritis (also called *pleurisy*) refers to inflammation of the pleura. Pleuritis is common in infectious processes such as respiratory infections that extend to involve the pleura. Pain is a frequent symptom, and most commonly, the pain is unilateral and abrupt in onset. When the central part of the diaphragm is irritated, the pain may be referred to the shoulder. The pain is usually made worse by chest movements such as deep breathing and coughing that exaggerate pressure changes in the pleural cavity and increase movement of the inflamed or injured pleural surfaces. Because breathing is painful, the person usually has small tidal volumes and a rapid respiratory rate to maintain minute volume. Reflex splinting of the chest muscles may occur, causing a lesser respiratory expansion on the affected side.

It is important to differentiate pleural pain from pain produced by other conditions, such as musculoskeletal strain of chest muscles, bronchial irritation, and myocardial disease. Musculoskeletal pain may occur as the result of frequent, forceful coughing. This type of pain usually is bilateral and located in the inferior portions of the rib cage, where the abdominal muscles insert into the anterior rib cage. It is made worse by movements associated with contraction of the abdominal muscles. The pain associated with irritation of the bronchi usually is substernal and dull in character rather than sharp. It is made worse with coughing but is not affected by deep breathing. Myocardial pain, which is discussed in Chapter 24, is usually located in the substernal area, although it may be referred to the arm, shoulder or neck, but is not usually affected by respiratory movements.

Treatment of pleuritis consists of treating the underlying disease and inflammation. Analgesics and nonsteroidal anti-inflammatory drugs (NSAIDs, *e.g.,* naproxen) may be used for pleural pain. Although these agents reduce pain and inflammation, they may not entirely relieve the discomfort associated with deep breathing and coughing.

Atelectasis

Atelectasis refers to an incomplete expansion of a lung or portion of a lung. It can be caused by airway obstruction, lung compression such as occurs in pneumothorax or pleural effusion, or increased recoil of the lung due to loss of pulmonary surfactant or increased secretions. The disorder may be

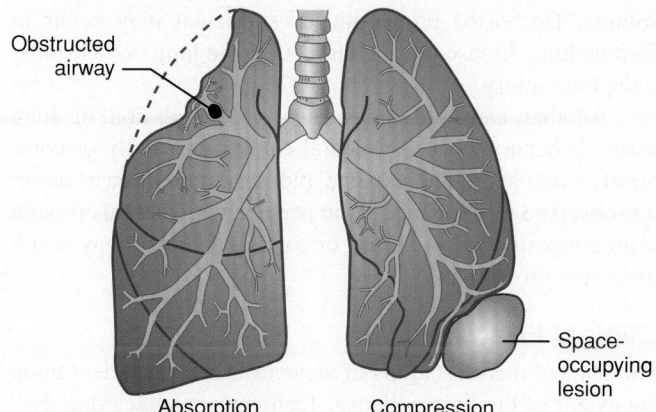

FIGURE 29.5 • Atelectasis caused by airway obstruction and absorption of air from the involved lung area **(left)** and by compression of lung tissue **(right)**.

present at birth (*i.e.,* primary atelectasis) or develop during the neonatal period or later in life (*i.e.,* acquired or secondary atelectasis).

Primary atelectasis of the newborn implies that the lung has never been inflated.[2] It is seen most frequently in premature and high-risk infants. A secondary form of atelectasis can occur in infants who established respiration and subsequently experienced impairment of lung expansion. Among the causes of secondary atelectasis in the newborn are the respiratory distress syndrome associated with lack of surfactant and airway obstruction due to aspiration of amniotic fluid or blood (see Chapter 28).

Acquired atelectasis occurs mainly in adults. It is caused most commonly by airway obstruction and lung compression (Fig. 29.5). Obstruction can be caused by a mucus plug in the airway or by external compression by fluid, tumour mass, exudate, or other matter in the area surrounding the airway. Portions of alveoli, a small segment of lung, or an entire lung lobe may be involved in obstructive atelectasis. Complete obstruction of an airway is followed by the absorption of air from the dependent alveoli and collapse of that portion of the lung. The danger of obstructive atelectasis increases after surgery. Anaesthesia, pain, administration of narcotics, and immobility tend to promote retention of viscid bronchial secretions and hence alveolar collapse and airway obstruction can occur. The encouragement of coughing and deep breathing, frequent change of position, adequate hydration, and early ambulation decrease the likelihood of atelectasis developing. Breathing high concentrations of oxygen increases the rate at which gases are absorbed from the alveoli and predisposes to alveolar collapse, referred to as absorption atelectasis. It rarely occurs in defined areas of the lung, but alveoli may not be ventilated. If the patient is receiving high oxygen concentration and mechanically ventilated, positive pressure ventilation at the end of expiration (PEEP) may decrease or prevent alveolar collapse and subsequent atelectasis.

Atelectasis may also occur with decreased production of surfactant or an increased amount of water that overwhelms the capability of the surfactant to maintain the alveolar volume. Decreased production of surfactant may occur in chronic lung disease (*e.g.*, asthma) or acute lung disease (*e.g.*, acute lung injury).

Another cause of atelectasis is compression of lung tissue. It occurs when the pleural cavity is partially or completely filled with fluid, exudate, blood, a tumour mass, or air. It is observed most commonly in persons with pleural effusion from congestive heart failure or cancer, and also may result from near drowning.

Clinical Features

The clinical manifestations of atelectasis are dependent upon the extent of the lung collapse. Tachypnea, tachycardia, dyspnea, cyanosis, signs of hypoxemia, diminished chest expansion, absence of breath sounds, and intercostal retractions may occur. Both chest expansion and breath sounds are decreased in the affected area. There may be intercostal retraction (pulling in of the intercostal spaces) over the involved area during inspiration. Signs of respiratory distress are proportional to the extent of lung collapse. If the collapsed area is large, the mediastinum and trachea shift to the affected side. In compression atelectasis, the mediastinum shifts away from the affected lung. The diagnosis of atelectasis is based on signs and symptoms. In addition, chest X-ray, bronchoscopy, or CT scans may be used to confirm the diagnosis and determine the location of the obstruction or area of collapse.

Treatment depends on the cause and extent of lung involvement. Strategies are directed at reducing the airway obstruction or lung compression and at reinflating the collapsed area of the lung. Ambulation, deep breathing and coughing, and body positions that promote increased lung expansion are used when appropriate. Administration of oxygen may be needed to correct the hypoxemia. Bronchoscopy may be used as both a diagnostic and a treatment method.

IN SUMMARY

Disorders of the pleura include pleural effusion, hemothorax, pneumothorax, and pleuritis. Pleural effusion refers to the abnormal accumulation of fluid in the pleural cavity. The fluid may be a transudate (*i.e.*, hydrothorax), exudate (*i.e.*, empyema), or chyle (*i.e.*, chylothorax). Hemothorax refers to the presence of blood in the pleural cavity. Pain is a common symptom of conditions that produce pleuritis or inflammation of the pleura. Characteristically, the pain is unilateral, abrupt in onset, and exaggerated by respiratory movements. Pneumothorax refers to an accumulation of air in the pleural cavity that causes partial or complete collapse of the lung. Pneumothorax can result from rupture of an air-filled bleb on the lung surface or from penetrating or nonpenetrating injuries. A tension pneumothorax is a life-threatening event in which air progressively accumulates in the thorax, collapsing the lung on the injured side and progressively shifting the mediastinum to the opposite side of the thorax, producing severe cardiac and respiratory impairment.

Atelectasis refers to an incomplete expansion of the lung. Primary atelectasis occurs most often in premature and high-risk infants. Acquired atelectasis occurs mainly in adults and is caused most commonly by a mucus plug in the airway or by external compression by fluid, tumour mass, exudate, or other matter in the area surrounding the airway.

OBSTRUCTIVE AIRWAY DISORDERS

After completing this section of the chapter, you should be able to meet the following objectives:

- Describe the physiology of bronchial smooth muscle as it relates to airway disease.
- Describe the interaction between heredity, alterations in the immune response, and environmental agents in the pathogenesis of bronchial asthma.
- Characterize the acute- or early-phase and late-phase responses in the pathogenesis of bronchial asthma and relate them to current methods for treatment of the disorder.
- Explain the changes in pulmonary function studies that occur with chronic airway disease.
- Explain the distinction between chronic bronchitis and emphysema in terms of pathology and clinical manifestations.
- State the chief manifestations of bronchiectasis.
- Describe the genetic abnormality responsible for cystic fibrosis and relate it to the manifestations of the disorder.

Obstructive airway disorders are caused by disorders that limit inspiratory or expiratory airflow, or both. Bronchial asthma represents an acute and reversible form of airway disease caused by narrowing of airways due to bronchospasm, inflammation, and increased airway secretions, that restricts air entry and may obstruct expiratory airflow. Chronic obstructive airway disorders include a variety of diseases, such as chronic obstructive pulmonary disease, bronchiectasis, and cystic fibrosis.

Physiology of Airway Disease

Air moves through the upper airways (*i.e.*, trachea and major bronchi) into the lower or pulmonary airways (*i.e.*, terminal bronchi and alveoli) of the lung. In the pulmonary airways, the cartilaginous layer that provides support for the trachea and major bronchi gradually disappears and is replaced with crisscrossing strips of smooth muscle (see Chapter 27). The contraction and relaxation of the smooth muscle layer, which is innervated by the autonomic nervous system, controls the diameter of the bronchial airways and consequent resistance to airflow. Parasympathetic stimulation, through the vagus nerve and cholinergic receptors, produces bronchial constriction, whereas sympathetic stimulation, through β_2-adrenergic receptors, increases bronchial dilation. At rest, a slight vagal-mediated bronchoconstrictor tone predominates. When there is need for increased airflow, as during exercise, the bronchodilator effects of the sympathetic nervous system are stimulated through β_2-adrenergic activation and the bronchoconstrictor effects of the parasympathetic nervous system are inhibited. Bronchial smooth muscle also responds to inflammatory mediators, such as histamine, that act directly on bronchial smooth muscle cells to produce constriction.

Bronchial Asthma

Asthma is a chronic inflammatory airway disorder, characterized by symptoms such as wheezing, shortness of breath, chest tightness, and cough.[18] Various triggers provoke inflammation and airway obstruction, including allergens (*e.g.,* animal dander), noxious stimuli or irritants (*e.g.,* perfume, cigarette smoke, cold air), infection, and exercise. In addition to the inflammatory response, the immune system is activated. Activated T-lymphocytes direct further release of inflammatory mediators from eosinophils, mast cells, and lymphocytes, and a subclass of helper T-lymphocytes that release cytokines, including pro-inflammatory interleukins (*e.g.,* IL-4, IL-5, IL-6, IL-13).[19]

AIRWAY DISORDERS

- Airway disorders affect airway patency and movement of atmospheric air into and out of the gas exchange portion of the lung.
- Changes in airway patency involve changes in airway diameter due to bronchial smooth muscle hyperreactivity or changes in bronchial wall structure, injury to the mucosal lining of the airways, or excess respiratory tract secretions.
- Bronchial asthma is a chronic disorder of the airways that causes episodes of airway obstruction due to bronchial smooth muscle hyperreactivity and airway inflammation. The episodes usually are reversible.
- Chronic obstructive pulmonary disease represents a group of disorders that cause chronic and recurrent obstruction of the pulmonary airways. These disorders can affect gas exchange due to altered ventilation, patency of the bronchial structures (chronic bronchitis), the gas-diffusing airspaces distal to the terminal bronchioles (emphysema), or a combination.

In 2012, approximately 8.1% of Canadians or 2.4 million Canadians over the age of 12 years reported that they had been diagnosed with asthma.[20,21] The highest rates are in the 12 to 19 and the 20 to 34 age groups, and the prevalence is generally greater in females.[21] Although the prevalence for asthma has stabilized over the past several decades, the reported incidence of asthma "attacks" have decreased during the past few years, suggesting a higher level of disease management.[22] The true incidence of asthma is unclear as respiratory symptoms in adults may be overdiagnosed and treated as asthma, when the disease is actually not present and there is likely a disproportionate number of obese people with dyspnea overdiagnosed.[23]

Symptomatic episodes of inflammation usually are initially reversible either spontaneously or with treatment. Additional exposure to triggers may result in an associated increase in bronchial responsiveness to a variety of stimuli. In susceptible persons, an acute episode of asthma, often referred to as an "attack," can be triggered by a variety of stimuli that do not normally cause immune and inflammatory responses. Decreasing the inflammatory response is important, either through avoidance of triggers or medication, or both, as the inflammatory and immune response can lead to long-term and even permanent damage and structural changes, referred to as remodelling.[24]

Asthma was differentiated as either extrinsic or intrinsic by Rackemann in 1947, based on whether a specific trigger could be identified.[25] Intrinsic asthma was further differentiated by a family history of allergies or a positive response to a serologic test to common allergens. Extrinsic asthma was identified as being a type I hypersensitivity [atopic] allergic response to an external antigen whereas intrinsic asthma was initiated by diverse nonimmune mechanisms, including respiratory tract infections, exercise, ingestion of aspirin, emotional upset, and exposure to bronchial irritants such as cigarette smoke. However, this distinction demonstrated to have more similarities than differences.

Etiology and Pathogenesis

The common denominator underlying all forms of asthma is an exaggerated hypersensitivity response to a variety of stimuli. Most current information suggests that airway inflammation manifested by the presence of inflammatory cells (including eosinophils, basal cells, lymphocytes, macrophages, and mast cells) and by damage to the bronchial epithelium contributes to the pathogenesis of the disease.[19] Epithelial cell activation and injury of the bronchi is a feature of asthma, and not predominant in other chronic inflammatory airway diseases.[20]

Research in the past 10 years has focused on the role of T lymphocytes in the pathogenesis of bronchial asthma. It is now known that there are subsets of T helper cells (*i.e.,* T_H1, T_H2) that develop from the same precursor CD4$^+$ T lymphocyte (see Chapter 17). T_H1 cells differentiate in response to microbes and stimulate the differentiation of B cells into immunoglobulin IgM- and IgG-producing plasma cells. T_H2 cells, on the other hand, respond to allergens and helminths (intestinal parasites) by stimulating the differentiation of B cells into IgE-producing plasma cells, acting as growth factors for mast cells, and recruiting and activating eosinophils (see Chapter 19, Fig. 19.3). In persons with allergic asthma, T-cell differentiation is skewed toward a proinflammatory T_H2 response. Although the molecular basis for this preferential differentiation is unclear, it seems likely that both genetic and environmental factors play a role.[26,27]

Cytokines have a significant role in the chronic inflammatory response and complications of asthma. Tumour necrosis factor (TNF)-α and interleukins (*e.g.*, IL-4, IL-5, IL-6, IL-13) mediate asthma symptoms and response through their effects on the bronchial epithelial and smooth muscle cells.[19,24] Studies suggest that TNF-α, an inflammatory cytokine that is stored in and released from mast cells, plays a critical role in the initiation and amplification of airway inflammation in persons with asthma. TNF-α is credited with increasing the migration and activation of inflammatory cells (*i.e.*, eosinophils and neutrophils) and contributing to all aspects of airway remodelling, including proliferation and activation of fibroblasts, increased production of extracellular matrix glycoproteins, and mucous cell hyperplasia.[24,28]

Extrinsic (Atopic) Asthma. Extrinsic or atopic asthma is typically initiated by a type I hypersensitivity reaction induced by exposure to an extrinsic antigen or allergen. It usually has its onset in childhood or adolescence and occurs in persons with a family history of atopic allergy (see Chapter 19). Candidate genes for predisposition to atopy and airway hyperresponsiveness are currently subjects for intensive research and include genes involved in antigen presentation, T-cell activation, regulation of cytokine production or function, and receptors for bronchodilating substances.[26] Also of interest is the early initiation and persistence of the inflammatory process, including risk factors such as respiratory viral infections.[24]

Persons with atopic asthma often have other allergic disorders, such as hay fever, urticaria, and eczema. Attacks are related to exposure to specific allergens. Among airborne allergens implicated in perennial (year-round) asthma are house dust, mite allergens, cockroach allergens, animal danders, and *Alternaria* (a fungus).

The mechanisms of response to antigens in atopic asthma can be described in terms of the early- or acute-phase response and the late-phase response[26] (Fig. 29.6). IgE-mediated hypersensitivity responses (discussed in Chapter 19) involve an initial antigen (allergen) sensitization, which leads to the production of presensitized IgE-coated mast cells. The symptoms of the *acute-phase response*, which usually develop within 10 to 20 minutes, are caused by the release of chemical mediators from the presensitized mast cells. In the case of airborne antigens, the reaction occurs when antigen binds to previously sensitized mast cells on the mucosal surface of the airways (Fig. 29.7). Mediator release results in the infiltration of inflammatory cells, opening of the mucosal intercellular junctions, and increased access of antigen to the more prevalent submucosal mast cells. In addition, there is bronchospasm caused by direct stimulation of parasympathetic receptors, mucosal edema caused by increased vascular permeability, and increased mucus secretions. Symptoms of an acute response usually can be inhibited or reversed by

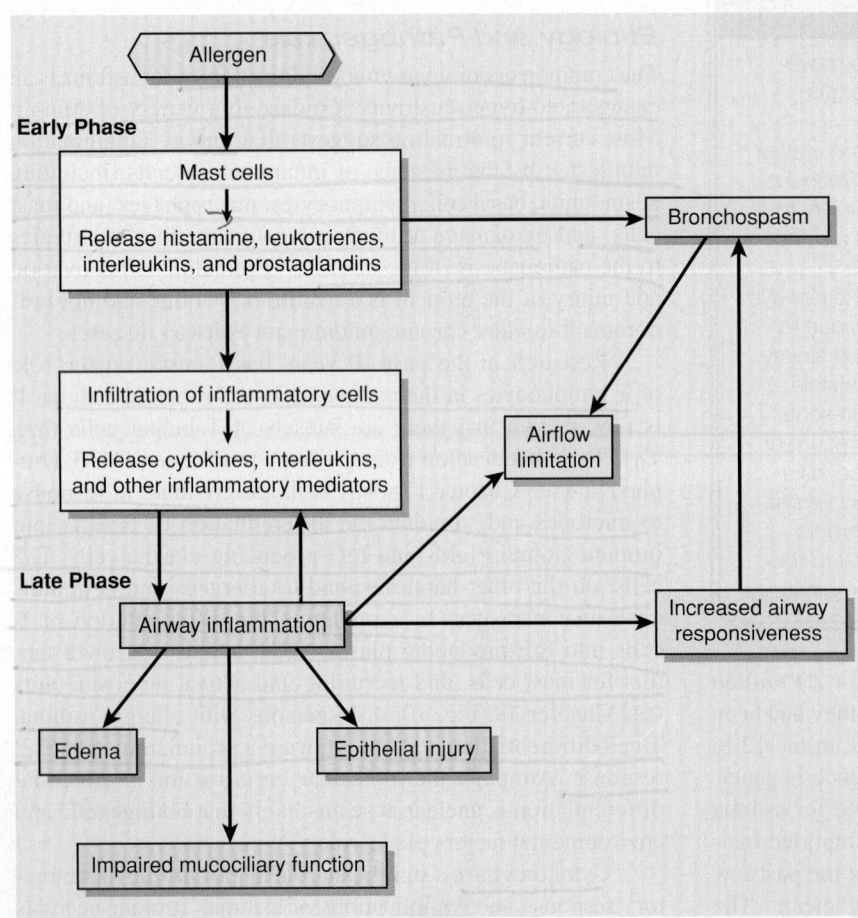

FIGURE 29.6 • Mechanisms of early- and late-phase IgE-mediated bronchospasm.

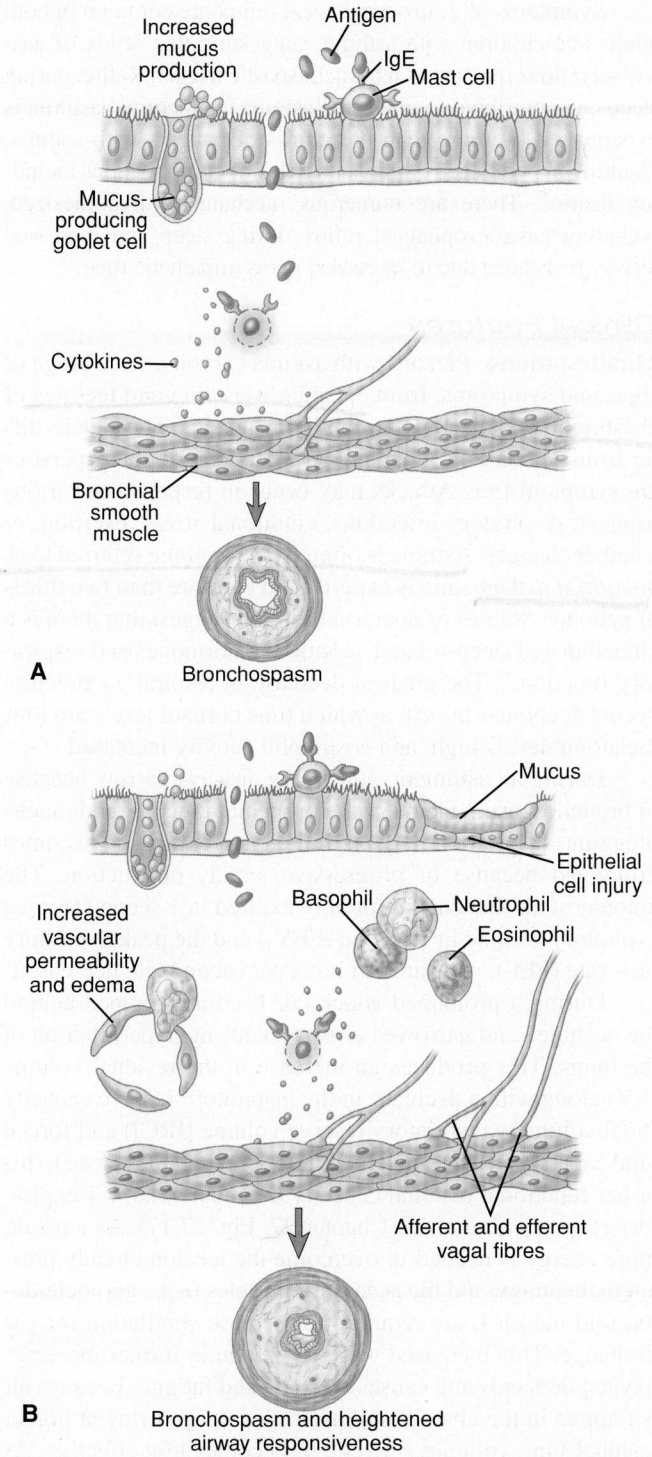

Increased mucus production

Antigen

IgE — Mast cell

Mucus-producing goblet cell

Cytokines

Bronchial smooth muscle

A Bronchospasm

Mucus

Epithelial cell injury

Basophil — Neutrophil

Eosinophil

Increased vascular permeability and edema

Afferent and efferent vagal fibres

B Bronchospasm and heightened airway responsiveness

FIGURE 29.7 • Pathogenesis of bronchial asthma. **A:** The immediate or early-phase response triggered by an IgE-mediated release of mediators from sensitized mast cells. The release of chemical mediators results in increased mucus production, opening of mucosal intercellular junctions with exposure of submucosal mast cells to antigen, and bronchospasm. **B:** The late-phase response involves epithelial cell injury with decreased mucociliary function and accumulation of mucus; release of inflammatory mediators with recruitment of neutrophils, eosinophils, and basophils; increased vascular permeability and edema; and increased airway responsiveness and bronchospasm.

bronchodilators, such as β_2-adrenergic agonists, but not by the anti-inflammatory actions of the corticosteroids.

The *late-phase response*, which develops 4 to 8 hours after exposure to an asthmatic trigger, involves inflammation and increased airway responsiveness that prolong the asthma attack and set into motion a vicious cycle of exacerbations, although the exact pathophysiology remains unclear. Typically, the response reaches a maximum within a few hours and may last for days or even weeks. An initial trigger in the late-phase response causes the release of inflammatory mediators from mast cells, macrophages, and epithelial cells. These substances induce the migration and activation of other inflammatory cells (*e.g.*, basophils, eosinophils, neutrophils), which then produce epithelial injury and edema, changes in mucociliary function and reduced clearance of respiratory tract secretions, and increased airway responsiveness (Fig. 29.7). Responsiveness to cholinergic mediators often is heightened, suggesting changes in parasympathetic control of airway function. Chronic inflammation can lead to airway remodelling, in which case airflow limitations may be only partially reversible.[24,28]

Intrinsic (Nonatopic) Asthma. Intrinsic or nonatopic asthma triggers include respiratory tract infections, exercise, hyperventilation, cold air, exercise, drugs and chemicals, hormonal changes and emotional upsets, airborne pollutants, and gastroesophageal reflux. Respiratory tract infections, especially those caused by viruses, may produce their effects by causing epithelial damage and stimulating the production of IgE antibodies directed toward the viral antigens. In addition to precipitating an asthmatic attack, viral respiratory infections increase airway responsiveness to other asthma triggers that may persist for weeks beyond the original infection. Exercise-induced bronchoconstriction (EIB) is the reversible narrowing of the lower airways that occurs during or after exercise. It is more prevalent in persons with bronchial asthma but can occur in the general population who do not have clinically recognized asthma.[29]

The cause of exercise-induced bronchoconstriction is unclear, but there are two main theories: osmotic and thermal but both are linked to the inspired air that is normally heated and humidified to a narrow range of temperature and water pressure before entering the lower airways. The osmotic theory proposes the loss of water from the upper and lower airways because of the need for humidifying large volumes of air creates a hyperosmotic environment that activate cellular inflammatory mechanisms.[29] The thermal theory proposed that vasoconstriction occurs when airways are cooled and subsequent vascular engorgement occurs when rewarmed stimulating release of mediators. However, EIB can occur in hot dry weather; therefore, the osmolar theory is the leading theory.[29] Warming up for up to 10 minutes and elevating the heart rate has a protective effect; wearing a mask or scarf over the nose and mouth in cold weather may minimize the attack or prevent it. Beta-2 agonists may prevent the attack but there is a risk of tolerance; small studies suggest that diet may decrease attacks, including fish oil, low salt, or ascorbic acid.[30]

It is important to consider avoidance of both irritants and allergens. Inhaled irritants, such as tobacco smoke and strong odours, are thought to induce bronchospasm by way of irritant receptors and a vagal reflex. Exposure to parental smoking has been reported to increase asthma severity in children.[31] High doses of irritant gases such as sulphur dioxide, nitrogen dioxide, and ozone may induce inflammatory exacerbations of airway responsiveness (*e.g.,* smog-related asthma), and correlate to emergency visits in Canadian cities.[31] Occupational asthma is stimulated by fumes and gases (*e.g.,* epoxy resins, plastics, toluene), organic and chemical dusts (*e.g.,* wood, cotton, platinum), and other chemicals (*e.g.,* formaldehyde) in the workplace. One group of chemicals that can provoke an asthmatic attack are sulphites, which are used in processing or preserving foods such as beer, wine, and fresh vegetables.

A small group of persons have the clinical triad of asthma, chronic rhinosinusitis with nasal polyps, and sensitivity to aspirin and other NSAIDs.[32] The mechanism of the hypersensitivity reaction is complex and related to an abnormality in arachidonic acid (AA) metabolism (see Chapter 18), not an immune mechanism. This non-allergic inflammatory response has numerous terms, including aspirin-induced asthma, aspirin-intolerant asthma, and aspirin-exacerbated respiratory disease, all of which name aspirin although the sensitivity may be to any NSAID.[32] Cyclooxygenase (COX), the rate-limiting enzyme in AA metabolism, exists in two main forms: COX-1 and COX-2. COX-1 is responsible for the synthesis of protective prostaglandins and COX-2 for the synthesis of mediators of inflammation and bronchoconstriction. The beneficial effects of aspirin and other NSAIDs are the inhibition of COX-1 and the subsequent decreased synthesis of COX-1 products. It has been hypothesized that in persons with aspirin-induced asthma, the inhibition of COX-1 shunts the metabolism of AA away from the production of protective prostaglandins and toward the generation of COX-2, lipoxygenase products, and other mediators of inflammation and bronchoconstriction. Aspirin-induced asthma is also associated with a late-onset activation of the eosinophils and release of IL-5.[32] Avoidance of aspirin and all NSAIDs is a necessary part of the prevention of a reaction.

Both emotional factors and changes in hormone levels are thought to contribute to an increase in asthma symptoms. Emotional factors produce bronchospasm by way of vagal pathways. They can act as a bronchospastic trigger, or they can increase airway responsiveness to other triggers through noninflammatory mechanisms. The role of sex hormones in asthma is unclear, although there is much circumstantial evidence to suggest that they may be important. Up to 40% of women with asthma report a premenstrual increase in asthma symptoms and severity.[33] Pregnancy is associated with a change in symptoms with about one third of pregnant women noticing an improvement in their asthma, one third worsening and one third staying the same.[34] Progesterone is hypothesized to increase cellular inflammation and reduce smooth muscle contractility; however, the underlying pathophysiology is not well understood.[34]

Symptoms of gastroesophageal reflux are common in both adults and children with asthma, suggesting that reflux of gastric secretions may act as a bronchospastic trigger. Reflux during sleep can contribute to nocturnal asthma.[35] Nocturnal asthma is experienced by more than two thirds of patients with asthma, resulting in poor sleep quality and a risk of complications including death.[35] There are numerous mechanisms hypothesized, including gastroesophageal reflux during sleep and increased airway resistance due to increased parasympathetic tone.[35]

Clinical Features

Manifestations. Persons with asthma exhibit a wide range of signs and symptoms, from episodic wheezing and feelings of chest tightness to acute, immobilizing attacks. The attacks differ from person to person, and between attacks, many persons are symptom free. Attacks may occur in response to various triggers, respiratory infections, emotional stress, exertion, or weather changes. Asthma is often worse at night, referred to as *nocturnal asthma,* and is experienced by more than two thirds of patients. Studies of nocturnal asthma suggest that there is a circadian and sleep-related variation in hormones and respiratory function.[35] The greatest decrease in respiratory function occurs at about 4:00 AM, at which time cortisol levels are low, melatonin levels high, and eosinophil activity increased.

During an asthmatic attack, the airways narrow because of bronchospasm, edema of the bronchial mucosa, and mucus plugging. Inspiration may be limited and expiration becomes prolonged because of progressive airway obstruction. The amount of air that can be forcibly expired in 1 second (forced expiratory volume in 1 second, FEV_1) and the peak expiratory flow rate (PEF), measured in litres per second, are decreased.

During a prolonged attack, air becomes trapped behind the occluded and narrowed airways, causing hyperinflation of the lungs. This produces an increase in the residual volume (RV) along with a decrease in the inspiratory reserve capacity (tidal volume + inspiratory reserve volume [IRC]) and forced vital capacity (FVC), such that the person breathes close to his or her functional residual capacity (residual volume + expiratory reserve volume; see Chapter 27, Fig. 27.17). As a result, more energy is needed to overcome the tension already present in the lungs, and the accessory muscles (*e.g.,* sternocleidomastoid muscles) are required to increase ventilation for gas exchange. This increased work of breathing further increases oxygen demands and causes dyspnea and fatigue. Because air is trapped in the alveoli and inspiration is occurring at higher residual lung volumes, the cough becomes less effective. As the condition progresses, the effectiveness of alveolar ventilation declines, and mismatching of ventilation and perfusion occurs, causing hypoxemia and hypercapnia. Pulmonary vascular resistance may increase as a result of the hypoxemia and hyperinflation, leading to a rise in pulmonary arterial pressure and increased work demands on the right heart.

The physical signs of bronchial asthma vary with the severity of the attack. A mild attack may produce a feeling of chest tightness, a slight increase in respiratory rate with prolonged expiration, and mild wheezing which may be inaudible without a stethoscope. A cough may accompany the wheezing. More severe attacks are accompanied by use of the accessory muscles, distant breath sounds due to air trapping, and loud wheezing. As the condition progresses, fatigue develops, the skin becomes moist, and anxiety and apprehension are obvious. Sensations of shortness of breath may be severe, and often the person is able to speak only one or two words before taking a breath. At the point at which airflow is markedly decreased, breath sounds become inaudible with diminished wheezing, and the cough becomes ineffective despite being repetitive and hacking. This point often marks the onset of respiratory failure.

Diagnosis. The diagnosis of asthma is based on a careful history and physical examination, laboratory findings, and pulmonary function studies (see Chapter 27). Spirometry provides a means for measuring FVC, FEV_1, PEF, tidal volume, expiratory reserve capacity, and inspiratory reserve capacity. The FEV_1/FVC ratio can then be calculated. Signs and symptoms of reversible airway narrowing are suggestive of asthma, which is supported by airway obstruction reversing with bronchodilators.[31] The level of airway responsiveness can be measured by inhalation challenge tests using methacholine (a cholinergic agonist) or histamine, or spirometry after exercise or exposure to a nonpharmacologic agent such as cold air. Methacholine is contraindicated if the FEV_1 is less than 60% of the predicted.[31]

Small, inexpensive, portable meters that measure PEF are available. Although not intended for use in diagnosis of asthma, they can be used in clinics and physicians' offices and in the home to provide frequent measures of flow rates. Day–night (circadian) variations in asthma symptoms and PEF variability can be used to indicate the severity of bronchial hyper responsiveness. The person's best performance is established from readings taken over several weeks. This often is referred to as the individual's *personal best* and is used as a reference to monitor changes in respiratory function, including triggers or medications.[18]

Treatment. The Canadian Thoracic Society (CTS) has classification systems intended for use in directing asthma treatment and identifying persons at high risk for development of life-threatening asthma attacks.[18,31] Criteria that demonstrate control of asthma include minimal symptoms per week, normal physical activity, fewer than 4 doses per week of a fast-acting β agonist inhaler and peak expiratory flow at 90% or greater of personal best. Based on these classifications systems, the panel recommends two categories for management and treatment of asthma: control of factors contributing to asthma severity and pharmacologic treatment.[18,31] See Table 29.1 to determine the level of control for asthma.

Measures to control factors contributing to asthma severity are aimed at prevention of exposure to irritants and factors that increase asthma symptoms and precipitate asthma exacerbations. They include education of the patient and family regarding measures to avoid exposure to irritants and allergens

TABLE 29.1 CONTROL OF ASTHMA

Inadequate control of asthma would be:
- Experiencing daytime symptoms more than 2 days per week
- Requiring the fast-acting inhaler (β₂ agonist) more than 2 times per week
- Awaking with nighttime symptoms (*e.g.,* cough) more than 2 nights per month
- Having more than 2 asthma exacerbations per year
- Refilling the fast-acting inhaler prescription more than 2 times per year

Adapted from Baylor Health Care System's Rule of Two ®.

that are known to induce or trigger an attack, including environmental tobacco smoke and air pollution.[31] A careful history often is needed to identify all the contributory factors. Factors such as nasal polyps, a history of aspirin sensitivity, and gastroesophageal reflux should be considered. Annual influenza vaccination is recommended for persons with persistent asthma.

Relaxation techniques and controlled breathing often help to allay the panic and anxiety that aggravate breathing difficulties. The hyperventilation that often accompanies anxiety and panic is known to act as an asthmatic trigger. In a child, measures to encourage independence as it relates to symptom control, along with those directed at helping to develop a positive self-concept, are essential.

A program of desensitization or immunotherapy may be undertaken in persons with persistent asthma who react to allergens, particularly those allergens that cannot be completely avoided, such as house dust mites. This involves the injection or newer oral medications of selected antigens (based on skin tests) to stimulate the production of IgG antibodies that block the IgE response. A course of allergen immunotherapy is long acting, and may minimize the need for medications and prevent acute events.[36] Newer research is looking at a potential antibody to block an epithelial protein called thymic stromal lymphopoeitin or TSLP, which is implicated with airway inflammation.[37]

Pharmacologic treatment is used to prevent or treat reversible airway obstruction and airway hyperresponsiveness caused by the inflammatory process. CTS recommends a stepwise approach to pharmacologic therapy based on frequency and severity of disease symptoms.[31] Medications used in the treatment of asthma include those with bronchodilator and anti-inflammatory actions. They are categorized into two general categories: fast acting medications and long-term control medications.

The *fast acting medications* include the short-acting β₂-adrenergic agonists, anticholinergic agents, and systemic corticosteroids. The short-acting β₂-adrenergic agonists (*e.g.,* salbutamol, fenoterol, terbutaline) relax bronchial smooth muscle and provide prompt relief of symptoms, usually within 30 minutes. They are administered by inhalation (*i.e.,* metered-dose inhaler [MDI] or nebulizer), and their recommended use is in alleviating acute attacks of asthma because regular use does not produce beneficial effects.[31] An increase in the use of short-acting β_2 agonists or use of more than one canister in a month indicates progression or inadequate control of the disease. The anticholinergic medications (e.g., ipratropium) block the postganglionic efferent vagal pathways that cause bronchoconstriction. These medications, which are administered by inhalation, produce bronchodilation by direct action on the large airways and do not change the composition or viscosity of the bronchial mucus. It is thought that they may provide some additive benefit for treatment of asthma exacerbations when administered with inhaled β_2-adrenergic agonists.[31] A short course of systemic corticosteroids, administered orally or parenterally, may be used for treating the inflammatory reaction associated with the late-phase response. Although their onset of action is slow (>4 hours), systemic corticosteroids may be used in the treatment of moderate to severe exacerbations because of their action in preventing the progression of the exacerbation, speeding recovery, and preventing early relapses.[31]

The *long-term medications* are taken on a daily basis to achieve and maintain control of persistent asthma symptoms. They include anti-inflammatory agents, long-acting beta agonists (LABAs), and leukotriene modifiers. The anti-inflammatory agents reduce inflammation in airway tissues and airway secretions (e.g., eosinophils, mast cells, activated lymphocytes, macrophages, cytokines or inflammatory mediators) and thus decrease the intensity of airway hyper responsiveness. The corticosteroids are considered the most effective anti-inflammatory agents for use in long-term treatment of asthma.[31] Inhaled corticosteroids (ICS) administered by MDI usually are preferred because of minimal systemic absorption and degree of disruption in hypothalamic-pituitary-adrenal function. In severe cases, intermittent oral or parenterally administered corticosteroids may be necessary. Health Canada has approved omalizumab, an anti-immunoglobulin IgE monoclonal antibody for treatment of moderate to severe persistent asthma.

The anti-inflammatory agents sodium cromolyn and nedocromil are also used to prevent asthmatic attacks, including exercise-induced bronchoconstriction. These agents act by stabilizing mast cells, thereby preventing release of the inflammatory mediators that cause an asthmatic attack. They are used prophylactically to prevent early and late responses but are of no benefit when taken during an attack.

The long-acting β_2-adrenergic agonists (LABAs), which are available for administration in inhaled (e.g., salmeterol, formoterol) or oral (e.g., albuterol sustained release) routes, act by relaxing bronchial smooth muscle. They are used as an adjunct to anti-inflammatory medications for providing long-term control of symptoms, especially nocturnal symptoms, and for preventing exercise-induced bronchospasm. The long-acting β_2 agonists have durations of action of at least 12 hours and should not be used to treat acute symptoms or exacerbations.[31]

Theophylline, a methylxanthine, is a bronchodilator that acts by relaxing bronchial smooth muscle. The sustained-release form of the drug is used as an adjuvant therapy and is particularly useful in relieving nighttime symptoms. It is rarely used but may be added to ICSs and LABAs when the asthma is not controlled by these drugs and by attempts to avoid triggers. Because elimination of this drug varies widely among persons, blood levels are required to ensure that the therapeutic, but not toxic, dose is achieved.[31]

Another group of medications available for use in the treatment of asthma are the *leukotriene modifiers or anti-leukotrienes*, as a second line when control is not attained by low doses of ICS.[31] Leukotrienes are potent biochemical mediators released from mast cells that cause bronchoconstriction, increased mucus secretion, and attraction and activation of inflammatory cells in the airways. There are two types of leukotriene modifiers: (1) those that act by inhibiting the binding of leukotrienes to their receptor in the target tissues (e.g., zafirlukast and montelukast), and (2) those that act by inhibiting 5-lipoxygenase (e.g., zileuton), an enzyme required for leukotriene synthesis. A particular advantage of the leukotriene modifiers is that they are taken orally to prevent the inflammatory response.

Severe Asthma

Previously, severe asthma was evidenced by high medication requirements to maintain good symptom control or persistent symptoms despite high medication use. More recently, severe asthma has been defined by the clinical control of symptoms and the risk of exacerbations and morbidity.[38] There are 3 groups of severe asthma: untreated; difficult to treat; and treatment resistant, in which control is not achieved despite the highest level of recommended treatment (refractory asthma) or control can only be maintained with the highest level of treatment. This approach is based on the underlying pathophysiology, including innate immunity, remodelling, epithelial dysfunction, eosinophilic activation, in addition to causative agents, comorbidity, and phenotyping.

Components of asthma severity including level of control, level of current treatment, responsiveness to treatment, and risk.[38] It has been proposed that because asthma is a disease involving multiple genes, mutations in genes regulating cytokines (e.g., IL-4), growth factors, or receptors for medications used in treatment of asthma (β_2-adrenergic agonist or glucocorticoid) could be involved. Environmental factors include both allergen and tobacco exposure, with the strongest response occurring in response to house dust, cockroach allergen, and *Alternaria* exposure. Infections may also play a role. Respiratory syncytial virus infections are implicated in children, and pathogens such as mycoplasma and chlamydiae may occur in adults. Gastroesophageal reflux and chronic sinusitis may also play a role.

Fatal and near-fatal asthma attacks have decreased over the past decade in Canada and are uncommon. Although the cause of death during an acute asthmatic attack is largely unknown, both cardiac arrhythmias and asphyxia due to severe airway obstruction, air trapping and barotrauma have been implicated. Deterioration often occurs rapidly during an acute attack, and underestimation of its severity may lead to a life-threatening delay in seeking medical attention. Frequent and repetitive use of β_2-adrenergic agonist inhalers in excess of the recommended doses may temporarily blunt symptoms and mask the severity of the condition.

Bronchial Asthma in Children

Asthma is a leading cause of chronic illness in children and is responsible for a significant number of lost school days. It is the most frequent admitting diagnosis in children's hospitals. The lifetime prevalence of asthma for Canadian children is approximately 11% to 16%.[39] Acute asthma attacks are associated with the severity of the disease, and poor control of asthma is associated with insufficient medication prescribed and taken.[38]

As with adults, asthma in children commonly is associated with an IgE-related reaction. It has been suggested that IgE directed against respiratory viruses in particular may be important in the pathogenesis of wheezing illnesses in infants (*i.e.*, bronchiolitis), which often precede the onset of asthma. The respiratory syncytial virus and parainfluenza viruses are the most commonly involved and are linked to the known spike of uncontrolled asthma cases that occurs around the third week of September (also referred to as Week 38).[40] Other contributing factors include exposure to environmental allergens such as pet dander, dust mite antigens, and cockroach allergens. Exposure to environmental tobacco smoke also contributes to asthma in children. Of particular concern is the effect of in utero exposure to maternal smoking on lung function and potential for asthma in infants and children.[34,39,40]

The signs and symptoms of asthma in infants and small children vary with the stage and severity of an attack. Because airway patency decreases at night, many children have acute signs of asthma at this time. Often, previously well infants and children develop what may seem to be a cold with rhinorrhea, rapidly followed by irritability, a tight and nonproductive cough, wheezing, tachypnea, dyspnea with prolonged expiration, and use of accessory muscles of respiration. Cyanosis, hyperinflation of the chest, and tachycardia indicate increasing severity of the attack. Wheezing may be absent in children with extreme respiratory distress. The symptoms may progress rapidly and require a trip to the emergency department or hospitalization.[39]

The Canadian Thoracic Society 2012 guidelines for management of asthma in children recommends ICSs as initial medications for mild asthma symptoms, combined with bronchodilators. Care of the child with asthma requires education of child and family, and regular assessment of control, triggers, adherence, and inhaler technique. Special delivery systems for administration of inhalation medications are available for infants and small children, including nebulizers with face masks and spacers and holding chambers for use with an MDI. For children younger than 2 years of age, nebulizer therapy is sometimes preferred. Children between 3 and 5 years of age should use an MDI with a spacer and holding chamber. The child's caregiver should be carefully instructed in the appropriate use of these devices. Active participation in physical activities, exercise, and sports should be encouraged.

Chronic Obstructive Pulmonary Disease

Chronic obstructive pulmonary disease (COPD) is a chronic pulmonary disease that is characterized by chronic, acute, and recurrent obstruction of airflow in the pulmonary airways, which may worsen over time.[41] Persistent inflammation of the pulmonary airways, parenchyma, and vasculature is present, which differs from that of asthma. Over time, lung inflation occurs due to airway obstruction on expiration.

COPD is a leading cause of morbidity and mortality worldwide, and although preventable it is anticipated to continue to increase over the next few decades. In 2011, chronic lower respiratory disease was the fourth leading cause of death in Canada.[42]

The risk factors for COPD include both host and environmental factors. The most common cause of COPD in Canada is smoking; other risk factors are occupational exposure such as coal or grain dust, second hand smoke or repeated childhood respiratory infections.[43] A less common contributing factor is a hereditary deficiency in α_1-antitrypsin, which may result in early onset and severe lung injury, with onset and severity worsened by smoking.[44] Other predisposing factors are asthma and airway hyperresponsiveness. Unfortunately, clinical findings are almost always absent during the early stages of COPD, and as many as 50% of smokers may have undiagnosed COPD.[41] Although 3.9% of Canadians over 35 years of age self-report having COPD, direct lung function measurement demonstrates that 13% have a airflow obstruction consistent with COPD.[45] By the time symptoms appear or are recognized, the disease is usually advanced. Early recognition, combined with smoking cessation, may prevent or delay the usually relentless progression of the disease.

Etiology and Pathogenesis

The mechanisms involved in the pathogenesis of COPD are multiple and include inflammation and fibrosis of the bronchial wall, hypertrophy of the submucosal glands, hypersecretion of mucus, and loss of elastic lung fibres and alveolar tissue[46] (Fig. 29.8). Inflammation and fibrosis of the bronchial wall, along with excess mucus secretion, obstruct airflow, decrease alveoli ventilation, and cause mismatching of ventilation and perfusion. Destruction of alveolar tissue decreases the surface area for gas exchange, and loss of elastic fibres impairs the expiratory flow rate, which increases air trapping and predisposes to airway collapse.

The term *chronic obstructive pulmonary disease* historically encompassed two types of obstructive airway disease: *emphysema*, with enlargement of airspaces and destruction of lung tissue; and *chronic obstructive bronchitis*, with increased mucus production, obstruction of small airways, and a chronic productive cough. While these terms can still be referred to in the literature, clinically persons with COPD often have overlapping features of both disorders.

Bronchial wall

Elastic fibres

Normal

A   B   C

FIGURE 29.8 • Mechanisms of airflow obstruction in chronic obstructive lung disease. **Top:** Normal bronchial airway with elastic fibres that provide traction and hold the airway open. **Bottom:** Obstruction of the airway caused by **(A)** hypertrophy of the bronchial wall, **(B)** inflammation and hypersecretion of mucus, and **(C)** loss of elastic fibres that hold the airway open.

Emphysema. Emphysema is characterized by a loss of lung elasticity and abnormal enlargement of the airspaces distal to the terminal bronchioles, with destruction of the alveolar walls and capillary beds (Fig. 29.9). Enlargement of the airspaces

leads to hyperinflation of the lungs and produces an increase in total lung capacity (TLC). Two of the recognized causes of emphysema are smoking, which incites lung injury, and an inherited deficiency of α_1-*antitrypsin,* an antiprotease enzyme that protects the lung from injury. Genetic factors other than an inherited α_1-antitrypsin deficiency also may play a role in smokers who develop COPD at an early age.[44,46]

Emphysema is thought to result from the breakdown of elastin and other alveolar wall components by enzymes, called *proteases,* that digest proteins. The proteases, particularly elastase, which is an enzyme that digests elastin, are released from polymorphonuclear leukocytes (*i.e.,* neutrophils), alveolar macrophages, and other inflammatory cells.[41] Normally, the lung is protected by antiprotease enzymes, including α_1-antitrypsin. Cigarette smoke and other irritants stimulate the movement of inflammatory cells into the lungs, resulting in increased release of elastase and other proteases. In smokers in whom COPD develops, antiprotease production and release may be inadequate to neutralize the excess protease production such that the process of elastic tissue destruction goes unchecked (Fig. 29.10).

A hereditary deficiency in α_1-antitrypsin accounts for approximately 1% to 5% of all cases of COPD and is more common in young persons with emphysema.[41] The type and amount of α_1-antitrypsin that a person has is determined by a pair of codominant genes referred to as *PI* (protein inhibitor) genes. An α_1-antitrypsin deficiency is inherited as an autosomal

FIGURE 29.9 • Panacinar emphysema. **A:** A whole mount of the left lung from a patient with severe emphysema reveals widespread destruction of pulmonary parenchyma that in some areas leaves behind a lacy network of supporting tissue. **B:** The lung from a patient with α_1-antitrypsin deficiency shows a panacinar pattern of emphysema. The loss of alveolar walls has resulted in markedly enlarged airspaces. (From Rubin R., Strayer D. S. (Eds.). (2012). *Rubin's Pathology: Clinicopathologic foundations of medicine.* (6th ed., p. 569). Philadelphia, PA: Lippincott Williams & Wilkins.)

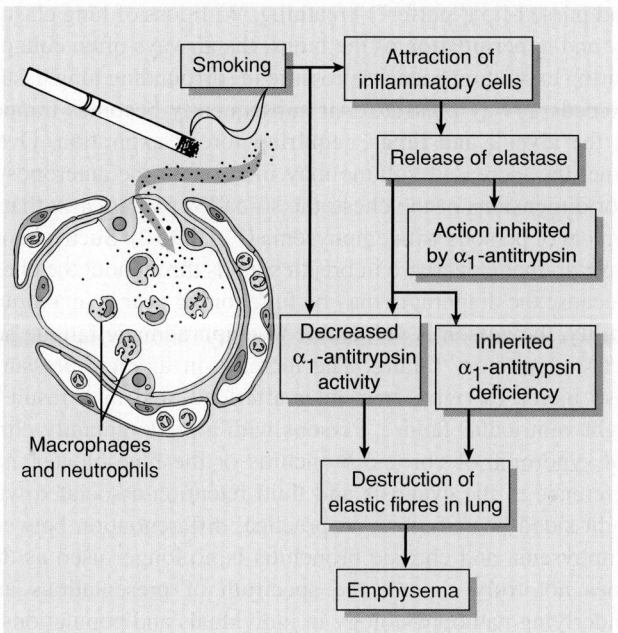

FIGURE 29.10 • Protease (elastase)–antiprotease (antitrypsin) mechanisms of emphysema. The effects of smoking and an inherited α_1-antitrypsin deficiency on the destruction of elastic fibres in the lung and development of emphysema are shown.

recessive disorder. There are more than 120 mutations of the gene located on the long arm of chromosome 14. Some of these mutations have minimal if any impact on α_1-antitrypsin production while others cause a significant deficiency of this protein. One of these, the *PIZ* variant, causes the most serious deficiency in α_1-antitrypsin. It is most common in persons of Scandinavian descent and is rare in Jews, blacks, and the Japanese.[44,46] Homozygotes who carry two defective *PIZ* genes have only about 15% to 20% of the normal plasma concentration of α_1-antitrypsin.[46] Most persons with clinically diagnosed emphysema before the age of 40 years have an α_1-antitrypsin deficiency. Smoking and repeated respiratory tract infections, which also decrease α_1-antitrypsin levels, contribute to the increased risk for emphysema in persons with α_1-antitrypsin deficiency. Laboratory methods are available for measuring α_1-antitrypsin levels. Human α_1-antitrypsin is available for replacement therapy in persons with a hereditary deficiency of the enzyme.

There are two commonly recognized types of emphysema: centriacinar or centrilobular, and panacinar (Fig. 29.11). The centriacinar type affects the bronchioles in the central part of the respiratory lobule, with initial preservation of the alveolar ducts and sacs.[46] It is the most common type of emphysema and is seen predominantly in male smokers. The panacinar

FIGURE 29.11 • Types of emphysema. The acinus is the unit gas-exchanging structure of the lung distal to the terminal bronchiole. It consists of (in order) respiratory bronchioles, alveolar ducts, alveolar sacs, and alveoli. In centrilobular (proximal acinar) emphysema, the destruction is confined to the terminal and respiratory bronchioles. In panacinar (panlobular) emphysema, the acinus is uniformly damaged. (From Rubin R., Strayer D. S. (Eds.). (2012). *Rubin's pathology: Clinicopathologic foundations of medicine* (6th ed., p. 568). Philadelphia, PA: Lippincott Williams & Wilkins.)

type produces initial involvement of the peripheral alveoli and later extends to involve the more central bronchioles. This type of emphysema is more common in persons with α_1-antitrypsin deficiency. It also is found in smokers in association with centriacinar emphysema. In such cases, the panacinar pattern tends to occur in the lower parts of the lung and centriacinar emphysema is seen in the upper parts of the lung.

Chronic Bronchitis. Chronic bronchitis represents airway inflammation and obstruction of the major and small airways.[46,47] The condition is seen most commonly in middle-aged men and is associated with chronic irritation from smoking and recurrent infections. A clinical diagnosis of chronic bronchitis requires the history of a chronic productive cough for at least 3 consecutive months over 2 consecutive years.[47] Typically, the cough has been present for many years, with a gradual increase in acute exacerbations that produce frankly purulent sputum.

The earliest feature of chronic bronchitis is hypersecretion of mucus in the large airways, associated with hypertrophy of the submucosal glands in the trachea and bronchi.[46,47] Although mucus hypersecretion in the large airways is the cause of sputum overproduction, it is now thought that accompanying changes in the small airways (small bronchi and bronchioles) are physiologically important in the airway obstruction that develops in chronic bronchitis. Histologically, these changes include a marked increase in goblet cells and excess mucus production with plugging of the airway lumen, inflammatory infiltration, and fibrosis of the bronchiolar wall. Submucosal hypertrophy in the larger airways and the increase in goblet cells in the smaller airways are activated in response to tobacco smoke and other pollutants, chronic and acute infections, and inflammatory epithelial receptors.[47] Unfortunately, the overproduction of mucus is compounded by the difficulty in effectively clearing secretions due to functional alterations in cilia, distal airways, and cough due to muscle weakness and low expiratory flow.[47]

Clinical Features

Clinical Manifestations. The clinical manifestations of COPD usually have an insidious onset. Patients characteristically seek medical attention in their fifth or sixth decade of life, with manifestations such as fatigue, exercise intolerance, cough, sputum production, or shortness of breath. The productive cough usually occurs in the morning. Frequent exacerbations of infection and respiratory insufficiency are common, causing absence from work and eventual disability. The late stages of COPD are characterized by limited activities of living, recurrent respiratory infections, and chronic respiratory failure. Death usually occurs during an exacerbation of illness associated with infection and respiratory failure.

The descriptors "pink puffer" and "blue bloater" have been used historically to differentiate the clinical manifestations of emphysema and chronic obstructive bronchitis. Persons with predominant emphysema, the *pink puffer*, is a reference to the lack of cyanosis, the use of accessory muscles,

and pursed-lip ("puffer") breathing. With loss of lung elasticity and hyperinflation of the lungs, the airways often collapse during expiration because pressure in surrounding lung tissues exceeds airway pressure. Air subsequently becomes trapped in the alveoli and lungs, requiring forced expiration. Overtime, the increased volume may increase in the anteroposterior dimensions of the chest, the so-called *barrel chest* that is typical of persons with emphysema (Fig. 29.12). Such persons have dramatic decrease in breath sounds throughout the chest. Because the diaphragm may be functioning near its maximum ability, the person is vulnerable to diaphragmatic fatigue and acute respiratory failure. The increase in thoracic pressures also increases right ventricular afterload, and may result in right ventricular failure. Persons with a predominantly clinical syndrome of chronic bronchitis or the blue bloater, is a reference to the cyanosis and fluid retention associated with right-sided heart failure. In practice, differentiation between emphysema and chronic bronchitis is no longer used as this does not truly capture the spectrum of presentations and underlying pathophysiology in individuals and populations.[48] This is because persons with COPD often have some degree of both types of disease processes.

The manifestations of COPD represent a progressive change in respiratory function. There is moderate to severe respiratory impairment due to obstruction of airflow, which is greater on expiration than inspiration, resulting in increased work of breathing but decreased effectiveness. The development of exertional dyspnea, often described as increased effort to breathe, heaviness, air hunger, or gasping, can be insidious. Activities involving significant arm work, particularly above the shoulders, are particularly difficult for persons with COPD. Activities that allow the person to brace the arms and use the accessory muscles are better tolerated. As the disease progresses, breathing becomes increasingly more laboured, even at rest. The expiratory phase of respiration is prolonged, and expiratory wheezes and crackles may be heard on auscultation. Persons with severe airflow obstruction may also exhibit use of the accessory muscles, sitting in the characteristic "tripod" position to facilitate use of the sternocleidomastoid, scalene, and intercostal muscles. Pursed-lip breathing enhances airflow because it increases the resistance to the outflow of air and helps to prevent airway collapse by increasing airway pressure. Eventually, persons with COPD are unable to maintain normal blood gases by increasing their breathing effort. Hypercapnia develops first due to impaired alveolar ventilation, followed by hypoxemia indicating impaired gas exchange.

Severe hypoxemia, in which arterial PO_2 levels fall below 55 mm Hg, causes reflex vasoconstriction of the pulmonary vessels and further impairment of gas exchange in the lung. Hypoxemia also stimulates red blood cell production, causing a mild polycythemia. The increase in pulmonary vasoconstriction and subsequent elevation in pulmonary artery pressure further increase the work of the right ventricle. As a result, persons with COPD may develop right-sided heart failure with peripheral edema (*i.e.,* cor pulmonale). However, signs of overt

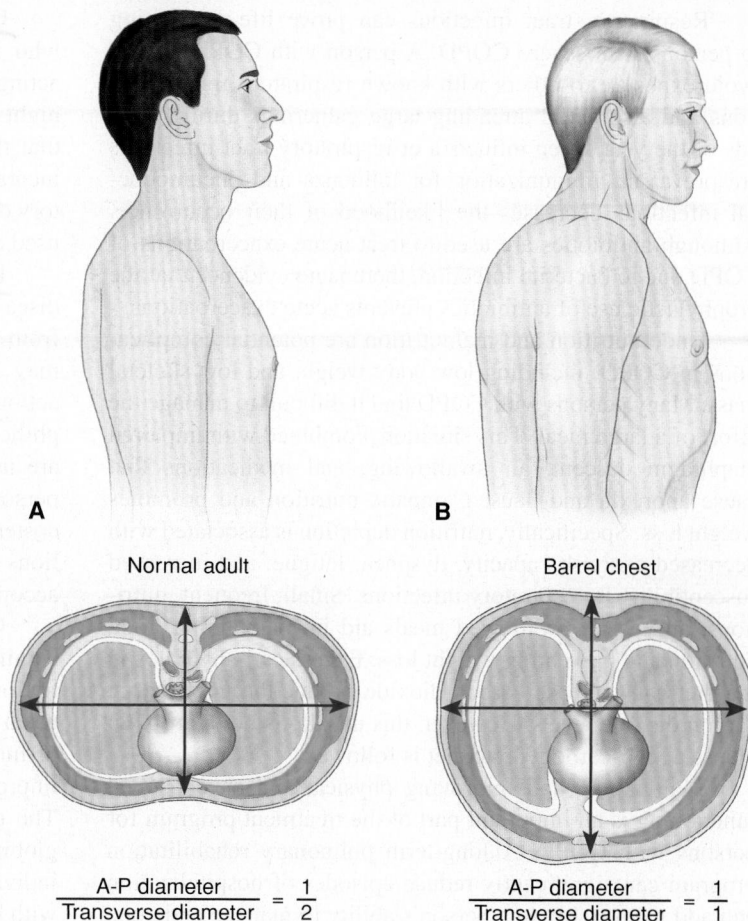

Normal adult   Barrel chest

A   B

$$\frac{\text{A-P diameter}}{\text{Transverse diameter}} = \frac{1}{2}$$ $$\frac{\text{A-P diameter}}{\text{Transverse diameter}} = \frac{1}{1}$$

FIGURE 29.12 • Characteristics of normal chest wall and chest wall in emphysema. The normal chest wall and its cross-section are illustrated on the left **(A)**. The barrel-shaped chest of emphysema and its cross-section are illustrated on the right **(B)**. (Adapted from Day R. A., Paul P., Williams B., et al. 2010. *Brunner & Suddarth's textbook of Canadian Medical-Surgical Nursing* (2nd ed., p. 640). Philadelphia, PA: Lippincott Williams & Wilkins.)

right-sided heart failure are seen less frequently if diagnosed and managed early with supplemental oxygen therapy.

Diagnosis

The diagnosis of COPD is based on a careful history and physical examination, pulmonary function studies, chest radiographs, and laboratory tests.[41,46] Airway obstruction prolongs the expiratory phase of respiration and affords the potential for impaired gas exchange because of hypoventilation and ventilation–perfusion mismatch. In an adult with normal respiratory function, the forced vital capacity (FVC), which is the amount of air that can be forcibly exhaled after maximal inspiration, should be achieved in 4 to 6 seconds. The ratio between the volume in one second (FEV_1) to the FVC (FEV_1/FVC) should be greater than 70%. In patients with chronic obstructive disease, the time required for FVC is increased, the FEV_1 is decreased, and the ratio of FEV_1 to FVC is decreased. In severe disease, the FVC is markedly reduced. Over time with progression of the disease, lung volume measurements reveal a marked increase in RV, an increase in TLC, and elevation of the RV-to-TLC ratio. These and other measurements of expiratory flow are determined by spirometry and are used in the diagnosis and follow-up of COPD (see Chapter 27, Fig. 27.17). Spirometry measurements can also be used in staging disease severity. For example, an FEV_1-to-FVC ratio of less than 70% with an FEV_1 of 80% or more, with or

without symptoms, indicates mild disease; and an FEV_1-to-FVC ratio of less than 70% with an FEV_1 of less than 50%, with or without symptoms, indicates severe disease.[41] Other diagnostic measures become important as the disease advances. Measures of exercise tolerance, nutritional status, hemoglobin saturation, and arterial blood gases can be used to assess the overall impact of COPD on health status and to direct treatment.

Treatment

The treatment of COPD depends on the stage of the disease and often requires an interdisciplinary approach. Smoking cessation is the only measure that slows the progression of the disease. Education of persons with COPD and their families is a key to successful management of the disease. Psychosocial rehabilitation must be individualized to meet the specific needs of persons with COPD and their families. These needs vary with age, occupation, financial resources, social and recreational interests, and interpersonal and family relationships. Persons in more advanced stages of the disease often require measures to maintain and improve physical and psychosocial functioning, pharmacologic interventions, and oxygen therapy. Avoidance of cigarette smoke and other environmental airway irritants is imperative. Wearing a cold-weather mask often decreases shortness of breath and bronchospasm due to cold air and wind exposure.

Respiratory tract infections can prove life-threatening to persons with severe COPD. A person with COPD should avoid exposure to others with known respiratory tract infections and also avoid attending large gatherings during periods of the year when influenza or respiratory tract infections are prevalent. Immunization for influenza and pneumococcal infections decreases the likelihood of their occurrence. Although antibiotics are used to treat acute exacerbations of COPD due to bacterial infection, there is no evidence that the prophylactic use of antibiotics prevents acute exacerbations.

Undernutrition and malnutrition are potential complications in COPD, including low body weight and low skeletal mass. Many persons with COPD find it difficult to manage the effort of a large meal. This situation, combined with impaired diaphragm descent, air swallowing, and medications that cause anorexia and nausea, impairs nutrition and promotes weight loss. Specifically, nutrition depletion is associated with decreased exercise capacity, dyspnea, fatigue, and increased susceptibility to respiratory infections. Small, frequent, nutritious, and easily swallowed meals aid in maintaining good nutrition and preventing weight loss. Excess carbohydrates in the diet can increase carbon dioxide production and arterial carbon dioxide levels. However, this usually is not a problem unless a high-carbohydrate diet is followed.

Maintaining and improving physical and psychosocial functioning is an important part of the treatment program for persons with COPD. A long-term pulmonary rehabilitation program can significantly reduce episodes of hospitalization and add measurably to a person's ability to manage and cope with his or her impairment in a positive way. This program includes breathing exercises that focus on restoring the function of the diaphragm, reducing the work of breathing, and improving gas exchange. Physical conditioning with appropriate exercise training increases maximal oxygen consumption and reduces ventilatory effort and heart rate for a given workload. Work simplification and energy conservation strategies may be needed when impairment is severe.

The pharmacologic treatment of COPD includes the use of bronchodilators, both short-acting and long-acting agents, ICSs, LABA, and anticholinergic agents as the disease worsens, and oxygen when it becomes severe.[41] It has been suggested that long-acting inhaled β_2-adrenergic agonists (LABAs) may be more effective than the short-acting forms of the drug. In addition to their action as bronchodilators, the long-acting β_2-adrenergic agonists are thought to reduce the adherence of bacteria such as *Haemophilus influenzae* to airway epithelial cells, thereby reducing the risk for infective exacerbations.[41] The anticholinergic drugs (*e.g.,* ipratropium, tiotropium), which are administered by inhalation, produce bronchodilation by blocking parasympathetic cholinergic receptors that produce contraction of bronchial smooth muscle. They also reduce the volume of sputum without altering its viscosity. Because these drugs have a slower onset and longer duration of action, they usually are used on a regular basis rather than on an as-needed basis. Inhalers that combine an anticholinergic drug with a β_2-adrenergic agonist are available.

Oral theophylline may be used in treatment of persons who fail to respond to inhaled bronchodilators. The long-acting theophylline preparations may be used to reduce overnight declines in respiratory function. There also is evidence that theophylline may improve respiratory muscle function, increase mucociliary clearance, and improve central respiratory drive.[41] When theophylline is prescribed, blood levels are used as a guide in arriving at an effective dose schedule.

Inhaled corticosteroids are not recommended until the disease is more severe, as the inflammation in COPD differs from that of asthma.[41] An explanation for this lack of effect may be related to the fact that corticosteroids prolong the action of neutrophils and hence do not suppress the neutrophilic inflammation seen in COPD. Because corticosteroids are useful in relieving asthma symptoms, they may benefit persons with asthma concomitant with COPD. Inhaled corticosteroids also may be beneficial in treating acute exacerbations of COPD, minimizing the undesirable effects that often accompany systemic use.

Oxygen therapy is prescribed for selected persons with significant hypoxemia (arterial PO_2 <55 mm Hg). Administration of continuous low-flow (1–3 L/minute) oxygen via nasal cannula to maintain arterial PO_2 levels between 55 and 65 mm Hg decreases dyspnea and pulmonary hypertension and improves neuropsychological function and activity tolerance. The overall goal of oxygen therapy is to maintain a hemoglobin oxygen saturation of 86% to 90% depending upon the individual.[41] Because the ventilatory drive may be associated with hypoxemic stimulation of the peripheral chemoreceptors does not occur until the arterial PO_2 has been reduced to about 60 mm Hg or less, increasing the arterial PO_2 above 65 mm Hg may depress the hypoxic stimulus for ventilation and lead to hypoventilation and carbon dioxide retention.[49] Portable oxygen administration units are usually used to allow mobility and the performance of activities of daily living. Transtracheal oxygen, delivered by a small-diameter percutaneous catheter placed in the trachea, can be used to supply increased amount of oxygen for persons with high oxygen requirements.[41] It also can be used to increase ambulation by eliminating the need to wear a nasal cannula.

Lung reduction surgery or bullectomy may prove useful for a limited number of persons. Lung volume reduction surgery involves the resection of the most distended areas of the lung as a means of improving respiratory function. Research studies are currently evaluating the minimally invasive technology of the lung volume reduction coil (LVRC) devices or endobronchial coils for the treatment of severe emphysema. Although not yet approved for use in Canada these coils are inserted endoscopically to gather and compress diseased lung tissue allowing for better expansion of surrounding healthier tissue.[50] Bullectomy is a surgical procedure that involves the removal of large emphysematous bullae that compress adjacent lung tissue and cause dyspnea. Lung transplantation is becoming an alternative treatment for persons with severe lung disease, limited life expectancy without transplantation, adequate functioning of other organ systems, and a good social support system.

Bronchiectasis

Bronchiectasis is an uncommon lung disorder characterized by a permanent dilation of the bronchi and bronchioles, which is caused by destruction of the muscle and elastic supporting tissue due to vicious cycles of infection and inflammation[51] (Fig. 29.13). It is not a primary disease but secondary to persisting infection, obstruction or genetic disorders such as cystic fibrosis. In the past, bronchiectasis often followed a necrotizing bacterial pneumonia that complicated measles, pertussis, or influenza.[51] Tuberculosis was also commonly associated with bronchiectasis. Thus, with the advent of antibiotics that more effectively treat respiratory infections such as tuberculosis, and with immunization against pertussis and measles, there has been a marked decrease in the prevalence of bronchiectasis.

Etiology and Pathogenesis

Two processes are critical to the pathogenesis of bronchiectasis: obstruction and chronic persistent infection.[51] Regardless of which may come first, both cause damage to the bronchial walls, leading to weakening and dilation. On gross examination, bronchial dilation is classified as saccular, cylindrical, or varicose. Saccular bronchiectasis involves the proximal third

FIGURE 29.13 • Bronchiectasis. The resected upper lobe shows widely dilated bronchi, with thickening of the bronchial walls and collapse and fibrosis of the pulmonary parenchyma. (From Rubin R., Strayer D. S. (Eds.). (2012). *Rubin's pathology: Clinicopathologic foundations of medicine* (6th ed., p. 545). Philadelphia, PA: Lippincott Williams & Wilkins.)

to fourth generation of bronchi[26,46] (see Chapter 27, Fig. 27.4). These bronchi become severely dilated and end blindly in dilated sacs, with collapse and fibrosis of more distal lung tissue. Cylindrical bronchiectasis involves uniform and moderate dilation of the sixth to eighth generations of airways. It is a milder form of disease than saccular bronchiectasis and leads to fewer symptoms. Varicose bronchiectasis involves the second through eighth branchings of bronchi and results in bronchi that resemble varicose veins. Bronchiolar obliteration is not as severe and symptoms are variable.

Bronchiectasis can present in either of two forms: a local obstructive process involving a lobe or segment of a lung or a diffuse process involving much of both lungs.[51] *Localized bronchiectasis* is most commonly caused by conditions such as tumours, foreign bodies, and mucus plugs that produce atelectasis and infection due to obstructed drainage of bronchial secretions. It can affect any area of the lung, the area being determined by the site of obstruction or infection. *Generalized bronchiectasis* usually is bilateral and most commonly affects the lower lobes. It is due largely to inherited impairments of host mechanisms or acquired disorders that permit introduction of infectious organisms into the airways. They include inherited conditions such as cystic fibrosis, in which airway obstruction is caused by impairment of normal mucociliary function; congenital and acquired immunodeficiency states, which predispose to respiratory tract infections; lung infection (*e.g.,* tuberculosis, fungal infections, lung abscess); and exposure to toxic gases that cause airway obstruction.

Clinical Features

Clinical Manifestations. Bronchiectasis is associated with a number of abnormalities that profoundly affect respiratory function, including atelectasis, obstruction of the smaller airways, and diffuse bronchitis. Affected persons have recurrent bronchopulmonary infection; coughing; production of copious amounts of foul-smelling, purulent sputum; and hemoptysis. Weight loss, fatigue, and anemia are common.

The manifestations of bronchiectasis are similar to those seen in chronic bronchitis and emphysema. As in the latter two conditions, chronic bronchial obstruction leads to marked dyspnea and cyanosis. Clubbing of the fingers is more common in moderate to advanced bronchiectasis than in other types of obstructive lung diseases.

Diagnosis and Treatment. Diagnosis is based on history and imaging studies. The condition is often evident on chest radiographs. High-resolution CT scanning of the chest allows for definitive diagnosis. Accuracy of diagnosis is important because interventional bronchoscopy or surgery may be palliative or curative in some types of obstructive disease.

Treatment consists of early recognition and treatment of infection along with regular postural drainage and chest physical therapy. Persons with this disorder benefit from many of the rehabilitation and treatment measures used for chronic bronchitis and emphysema.

Cystic Fibrosis

Cystic fibrosis (CF), which is the major cause of severe chronic respiratory disease in children, is an autosomal recessive disorder involving fluid secretion in the exocrine glands in the epithelial lining of the respiratory, gastrointestinal, and reproductive tracts.[52,53] In addition to chronic respiratory disease, CF is manifested by pancreatic exocrine deficiency and elevation of sodium chloride in the sweat. Nasal polyps, sinus infections, pancreatitis, and cholelithiasis also are common. Excessive loss of sodium in the sweat predisposes young children to salt depletion episodes. Most boys with CF have congenital bilateral absence of the vas deferens with azoospermia.

It is estimated that one in every 3,600 children born in Canada has cystic fibrosis, and currently approximately 4000 Canadians are registered with the CF foundation, ranging from children to adults.[54] Approximately one in 25 Canadians are asymptomatic carriers of the defective gene.[54] The gene is rare in blacks and Asians. Homozygotes (*i.e.,* persons with two defective genes) have all or substantially all of the clinical symptoms of the disease, compared with heterozygotes, who are carriers of the disease but have no recognizable symptoms. Previously, CF was a disease diagnosed in childhood with a poor prognosis to reach school age; with changes in treatment and life expectancy now almost half of the CF population is 18 years of age or older.[52,54]

Etiology and Pathogenesis

Cystic fibrosis is caused by mutations in a single gene on the long arm of chromosome 7 that encodes for the cystic fibrosis transmembrane regulator (CFTR), which functions as a chloride (Cl^-) channel in epithelial cell membranes.[52] Mutations in the *CFTR* gene render the epithelial membrane relatively impermeable to the chloride ion (Fig. 29.14). There are greater than 1,000 possible mutations in the *CFTR* gene that can occur. However, 70% of CF individuals have ΔF508, the most common mutation, which involves a three-base-pair deletion that codes for phenylalanine, and a more severe phenotype.[52] Others have a partial loss of CTFR function so their phenotype is less severe and often goes unnoticed until they have an acute injury or infection.

The impact on impaired Cl^- transport is relatively tissue specific. In the sweat glands, the concentration of sodium (Na^+) and Cl^- secreted into the lumen of the gland remains unaffected, whereas the reabsorption of Cl^- through the CFTR and accompanying reabsorption of Na^+ in the ducts of the gland fail to occur. This defect accounts for the high concentration of NaCl in the sweat of persons with CF.[52–54] In the normal airway epithelium, $Cl-$ is secreted into airway lumen through the CFTR. The impaired transport of Cl^- ultimately leads to a series of secondary events, including increased absorption of Na^+ and water from the airways into the blood. This lowers the water content of the mucociliary blanket coating the respiratory epithelium, causing it to become more viscid. The resulting dehydration of the mucous layer leads to defective mucociliary function and accumulation of viscid

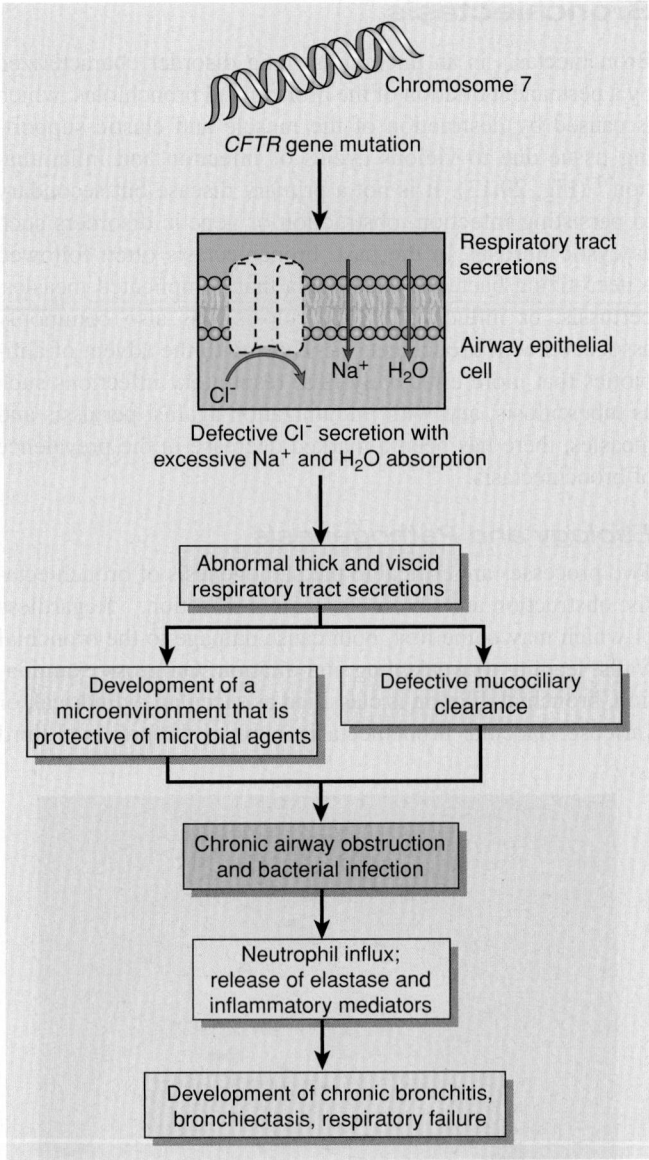

FIGURE 29.14 • Pathogenesis of cystic fibrosis.

secretions that obstruct the airways and predispose to recurrent pulmonary infections. Similar transport abnormalities and pathophysiologic events take place in the pancreatic and biliary ducts and in the vas deferens in boys.

Clinical Features

Respiratory manifestations of CF are caused by an accumulation of viscid mucus in the bronchi, impaired mucociliary clearance, and lung infections. Chronic bronchiolitis and bronchitis are the initial lung manifestations, but after months and years, structural changes in the bronchial wall lead to bronchiectasis. In addition to airway obstruction, the basic genetic defect that occurs with CF predisposes to chronic infection with a surprisingly limited number of organisms, the most common being *Pseudomonas aeruginosa, Burkholderia cepacia, Staphylococcus aureus,* and *Haemophilus influenzae.*[52–54] Soon after birth, initial infection with bacterial pathogens occurs and is associated with an excessive neutrophilic inflammatory response that appears to be independent of the infection itself. There is evidence that the CF airway epithelial cells or surface liquids provide a favourable environment for harbouring these organisms. *P. aeruginosa,* in particular, has a propensity to undergo mucoid transformation in this environment.[52] The complex polysaccharide produced by these organisms provides a hypoxic environment and generates a biofilm that protects *Pseudomonas* against antimicrobial agents. Pulmonary inflammation is another cause of decline in respiratory function in persons with CF and may precede the onset of chronic infection. Elevated levels of inflammatory mediators (*e.g.,* IL-1, IL-6, TNF-α), increase levels of T helper (T$_H$) 17 cell-associated cytokines, along with reduced levels of anti-inflammatory cytokines, have been found in the airways of persons with CF.[52]

Patients have a high risk for liver, hepatobiliary and pancreatic dysfunction.[52]

Steatorrhea, diarrhea, and abdominal pain or discomfort are common. In the newborn, meconium ileus may cause intestinal obstruction, a fatal condition if left untreated. The degree of pancreatic involvement is highly variable. In some children, the defect is relatively mild, and in others, the involvement is severe and impairs intestinal absorption. In addition to exocrine pancreatic insufficiency, hyperglycemia may occur, especially after 10 years of age and this is associated with higher mortality and morbidity rates.[52]

Diagnosis and Treatment. Early diagnosis and treatment are important in delaying the onset and severity of chronic illness in children with CF. Diagnosis is based on the presence of respiratory and gastrointestinal manifestations typical of CF, a history of CF in a sibling, or a positive newborn screening test result. Confirmatory laboratory tests include the sweat test, assessment of bioelectrical properties of respiratory epithelia by measurement of transepithelial potential differences in the nasal membrane, and genetic tests for *CFTR* gene mutations.[52,53] The *sweat test,* using pilocarpine iontophoresis to collect the sweat followed by chemical analysis of its chloride content, remains the standard approach to diagnosis. Newborns with CF have elevated blood levels of immunoreactive trypsinogen, presumably because of secretory obstruction in the pancreas. *Newborn screening* consists of a test for determination of immunoreactive trypsinogen. The test can be done on blood spots collected for routine newborn screening tests.

At present, there are no approved treatments for correcting the genetic defects in CF or reversing the ion transport abnormalities associated with the dysfunctional CFTR. Thus, treatment measures are directed toward slowing the progression of secondary organ dysfunction and sequelae such as chronic lung infection and pancreatic insufficiency.[52–54] They include the use of antibiotics to prevent and manage infections; the use of chest physical therapy (chest percussion and postural drainage) and mucolytic agents to prevent airway obstruction; and pancreatic enzyme replacement and nutritional therapy. Routine laboratory evaluations are key to assessing pulmonary

function and response to therapeutic interventions. These studies include radiologic examinations, pulmonary function testing, and microbiologic cultures of respiratory secretions.

Appropriate antibiotic therapy directed against bacterial pathogens isolated from the respiratory tract is an essential component in the management of CF lung disease. Antibiotics are initially used to prevent colonization with *P. aeruginosa;* they are used as maintenance therapy once the airways are colonized with *P. aeruginosa* and other organisms such as *S. aureus;* and they are administered as aggressive treatment during acute exacerbations of pulmonary symptoms caused by infections. To avoid adverse effects and to obtain high airway concentrations, the inhalation route is often used. Indications for oral antibiotics include the presence of respiratory tract symptoms and identification of pathogenic organisms in respiratory tract cultures. Intravenous antibiotics are used for progressive and unrelenting symptoms.

Up to 90% of patients with CF have complete loss of exocrine pancreas function and inadequate digestion of fats and proteins. They require diet adjustment, pancreatic enzyme replacement, and supplemental vitamins and minerals. Many individuals with CF have a higher-than-normal caloric need because of the increased work of breathing and perhaps because of the increased metabolic activity related to the basic defect. Pancreatic enzyme dosage and product type are individualized for each patient. Enteric-coated, pH-sensitive enzyme microspheres are available.[52] A low-fat, high-protein, high-calorie diet was generally recommended in the past. With the advent of improved pancreatic enzyme products, however, normal amounts of fat in the diet are usually tolerated and preferred.

Progress of the disease is variable. Improved medical management has led to longer survival. Today, many people with the disease can expect to live into their 30s, 40s, and beyond.[54] Lung transplantation is being used as a treatment for persons with end-stage lung disease. Current hopes reside in research that would make gene therapy a feasible alternative for persons with the disease.

> ## IN SUMMARY
>
> Obstructive ventilatory disorders are characterized by airway obstruction and limitation in expiratory airflow. Bronchial asthma is a chronic inflammatory disorder of the airways characterized by airway hyperreactivity and episodic attacks of airway narrowing. An asthmatic attack can be triggered by a variety of stimuli. Based on their mechanism of response, these triggers can be divided into two types: extrinsic (atopic) and intrinsic (nonatopic). Atopic asthma is typically initiated by a type I hypersensitivity reaction triggered by an extrinsic antigen or allergen and is linked to T$_H$2 proinflammatory response. Intrinsic asthma has triggers such as respiratory tract infections, exercise, drugs and chemicals, airborne pollutants, and gastroesophageal reflux. There are two types of responses in persons with asthma: the acute- or early-phase response

and the late-phase response. The acute-phase response results in immediate bronchoconstriction on exposure to an inhaled antigen and usually subsides within 90 minutes. The late-phase response usually develops 3 to 5 hours after exposure to an asthmatic trigger; it involves inflammation and increased airway responsiveness that prolong the attack and cause a vicious cycle of exacerbations.

Chronic obstructive pulmonary disease describes a group of conditions characterized by obstruction to airflow in the lungs. Among the conditions associated with COPD are emphysema, chronic bronchitis, and bronchiectasis. Emphysema is characterized by a loss of lung elasticity; abnormal, permanent enlargement of the airspaces distal to the terminal bronchioles; and hyperinflation of the lungs. Chronic bronchitis is caused by inflammation of major and small airways and is characterized by edema and hyperplasia of submucosal glands and excess mucus secretion into the bronchial tree. A history of a chronic productive cough that has persisted for at least 3 months and for at least 2 consecutive years in the absence of other disease is necessary for the diagnosis of chronic bronchitis. Emphysema and chronic bronchitis are manifested by eventual mismatching of ventilation and perfusion. As the condition advances, signs of respiratory distress and impaired gas exchange become evident, with development of hypercapnia and hypoxemia. Bronchiectasis is a less common form of COPD that is characterized by an abnormal dilation of the large bronchi associated with infection and destruction of the bronchial walls.

Cystic fibrosis is an autosomal recessive genetic disorder manifested by chronic lung disease, pancreatic exocrine deficiency, and elevation of sodium chloride in the sweat. The disorder is caused by a mutation of a single gene on the long arm of chromosome 7 that codes for the cystic fibrosis transmembrane regulator (CFTR), which functions in the transepithelial transport of the chloride ion. The defect causes exocrine gland secretions to become exceedingly viscid, and promotes colonization of the respiratory tract with *P. aeruginosa* and other organisms such as *S. aureus*. Accumulation of viscid mucus in the bronchi, impaired mucociliary function, and infection contribute to the development of chronic lung disease and a decreased life expectancy.

CONCEPTSin action **ANIMATION**

CHRONIC INTERSTITIAL (RESTRICTIVE) LUNG DISEASES

After completing this section of the chapter, you should be able to meet the following objectives:

- State the difference between chronic obstructive pulmonary diseases and chronic restrictive lung diseases in terms of their pathology and manifestations.

- Cite the characteristics of occupational dusts that determine their pathogenicity in terms of the production of pneumoconiosis.
- Describe the causes of hypersensitivity pneumonitis.
- Characterize the organ involvement in sarcoidosis.

The diffuse interstitial diseases are a diverse group of lung disorders that produce similar inflammatory and fibrotic changes in the interstitium or interalveolar septa of the lung. Because the interstitial lung diseases result in a stiff and noncompliant lung, they are commonly classified as restrictive lung disorders. In contrast to obstructive lung diseases, the lungs are stiff and difficult to expand, despite normally functioning airways.

Etiology and Pathogenesis of Interstitial Lung Diseases

The interstitial lung diseases may be acute or insidious in onset; they may be rapidly progressive, slowly progressive, or static in their course. They include occupational lung diseases such as the pneumoconioses, which are caused by the inhalation of inorganic dusts such as silica, coal dust, and asbestos; hypersensitivity pneumonitis[26,46] (see Chapter 19); lung diseases caused by exposure to toxic drugs (*e.g.,* the cancer drug, bleomycin; the antiarrhythmic drug, amiodarone) and radiation; and sarcoidosis. Some of the most common interstitial lung diseases are caused by exposure to inhaled dust and particles. In many cases, no specific cause can be found. Examples of interstitial lung diseases and their causes are listed in Chart 29.1.

INTERSTITIAL OR RESTRICTIVE LUNG DISEASES

- Interstitial lung diseases result from inflammatory conditions that affect the interalveolar structures of the lung and produce lung fibrosis and a stiff lung.
- A stiff and noncompliant lung is difficult to inflate, increasing the work of breathing and causing decreased exercise tolerance due to hypoxemia.
- Because of the increased effort needed for lung expansion, persons with interstitial lung disease tend to take small but more frequent breaths.

In contrast to the obstructive lung diseases, which primarily involve the airways of the lung, the interstitial lung disorders exert their effects on the collagen and elastic connective tissue found in the delicate interstitium of the alveolar walls. Many of these diseases also involve the airways, arteries, and veins. In general, these lung diseases share a pattern of lung dysfunction that includes diminished lung volumes, reduced diffusing capacity of the lung, and varying degrees of hypoxemia.

CHART 29.1 CAUSES OF INTERSTITIAL LUNG DISEASE[a]

Occupational and Environmental Inhalants

Pneumoconioses
 Coal miner's pneumoconiosis
 Silicosis
 Asbestosis
Hypersensitivity pneumonitis
 Farmer's lung
 Pigeon breeder's lung

Drugs and Therapeutic Agents

Cancer drugs
 Bleomycin
 Busulfan
 Cyclophosphamide
 Methotrexate
Amiodarone
Ionizing radiation (radiation therapy)

Immunologic Lung Disease

Sarcoidosis
Collagen vascular disease
 Systemic lupus erythematosus
 Rheumatoid arthritis
 Scleroderma

[a]This list is not intended to be inclusive.

Interstitial or diffuse parenchymal lung diseases can be challenging to diagnose and treat. Although some of these disorders are thought to be initiated by some type of injury to the alveolar epithelium, followed by an inflammatory process that involves the alveoli and interstitium of the lung, other mechanisms are novel or unknown.[55] Prolonged interstitial lung disease may progress to pulmonary fibrosis (to be discussed). In general, the interstitial lung diseases are characterized by clinical changes consistent with restrictive rather than obstructive changes in the lung. Persons with interstitial lung diseases have dyspnea, tachypnea, and eventual cyanosis, without evidence of wheezing or signs of airway obstruction. Usually, there is an insidious onset of breathlessness that initially occurs during exercise and may progress to the point at which the person is totally incapacitated. Typically, a person with a restrictive lung disease breathes with a tachypneic pattern of breathing, in which the respiratory rate is increased and the tidal volume is decreased. This pattern of breathing serves to maintain minute volume yet reduces the work of breathing because it takes less work to move air through the airways at an increased rate than it does to stretch a stiff lung to accommodate a larger tidal volume. A nonproductive cough may develop, particularly with continued exposure to the inhaled irritant. Clubbing of the fingers and toes may develop.

Lung volumes, including vital capacity and TLC, are reduced in interstitial lung disease. In contrast to COPD, in which expiratory flow rates are reduced, the FEV_1 usually is preserved, even though the ratio of FEV_1 to FVC may increase. Although resting arterial blood gases usually are normal early in the course of the disease, arterial PO_2 levels may fall during exercise. In persons with advanced disease, hypoxemia often is present, even at rest. In the late stages of the disease, hypercapnia and respiratory acidosis develop. Alterations in the alveolar–capillary membrane as well as an increase in shunt resulting from unventilated regions of the lung, are thought to cause the impaired diffusion of gases in people with interstitial lung disease. The diagnosis of interstitial lung disease requires a careful personal and family history, with particular emphasis on exposure to environmental, occupational, and other injurious agents. Chest radiographs may be used as an initial diagnostic method, and serial chest films often are used to follow the progress of the disease. A lung biopsy specimen for histologic study and culture may be obtained by surgical incision or bronchoscopy using a fibreoptic bronchoscope and is the preferred diagnostic examination.[55,56]

The treatment goals for persons with interstitial lung disease focus on identifying and removing the injurious agent, suppressing the inflammatory response, preventing progression of the disease, and providing supportive therapy for persons with advanced disease. In general, the treatment measures vary with the type of lung disease. Immunosuppressants and corticosteroid drugs frequently are used to suppress the inflammatory response. Many of the supportive treatment measures used in the late stages of the disease, such as oxygen therapy and measures to prevent infection, are similar to those discussed for persons with COPD. For some a lung transplant may be the only effective treatment.

Occupational Lung Disease

Two occupational lung diseases are the pneumoconioses and the hypersensitivity diseases. The *pneumoconioses* are caused by the inhalation of inorganic dusts and particulate matter, whereas the *hypersensitivity diseases* result from the inhalation of organic dusts and related occupational antigens.

Among the pneumoconioses are silicosis, found in hard-rock miners, foundry workers, sandblasters, pottery makers, and workers in the slate industry; coal miner's pneumoconiosis; asbestosis, found in asbestos miners, manufacturers of asbestos products, and installers and removers of asbestos insulation; talcosis, found in talc miners, millers, or drug abusers, and in infants or small children who accidentally inhale powder containing talc; and berylliosis, found in ore extraction workers and alloy production workers. The danger of exposure to asbestos dust is not confined to the workplace. The dust pervades the general environment because it was used in the construction of buildings and in other applications before its health hazards were realized. It has been mixed into paints and plaster, wrapped around water and heating pipes, used to insulate hair dryers, and woven into theatre curtains, hot pads, and ironing board covers.

Important etiologic determinants in the development of the pneumoconioses are the size of the dust particle, its chemical nature and ability to incite lung destruction, and the concentration of dust and the length of exposure to it. The most dangerous particles are those in the range of 1 to 5 μm.[26] These small particles are carried through the inspired air into the alveolar structures, whereas larger particles are trapped in the nose or mucous linings of the airways and removed by the mucociliary system. Exceptions are asbestos and talc particles, which range in size from 30 to 60 μm but find their way into the alveoli because of their density.

All particles in the alveoli must be cleared by the lung macrophages. Macrophages are thought to transport engulfed particles from the small bronchioles and the alveoli, which have neither cilia nor mucus-secreting cells, to the mucociliary system or to the lymphatic channels for removal from the lung. This clearing function is hampered when the function of the macrophage is impaired by factors such as cigarette smoking, consumption of alcohol, and hypersensitivity reactions. This helps to explain the increased incidence of lung disease among smokers exposed to asbestos. In silicosis, the ingestion of silica particles leads to the destruction of the lung macrophages and the release of substances resulting in inflammation and fibrosis.[26] Tuberculosis and other diseases caused by mycobacteria are common in persons with silicosis. Because the macrophages are responsible for protecting the lungs from tuberculosis, the destruction of macrophages accounts for an increased susceptibility to tuberculosis in persons with silicosis.

The concentration of some dusts in the environment strongly influences their effects on the lung. For example, acute silicosis is seen only in persons whose occupations entail intense exposure to silica dust over a short period. It is seen in sandblasters, who use a high-speed jet of sand to clean and polish bricks and the insides of corroded tanks; in tunnelers; and in rock drillers, particularly if they drill through sandstone. Acute silicosis is a rapidly progressive disease, usually leading to severe disability and death within 5 years of diagnosis. In contrast to acute silicosis, which is caused by exposure to extremely high concentrations of silica dust, the symptoms related to chronic, low-level exposure to silica dust usually do not begin to develop until after many years of exposure, and then the symptoms often are insidious in onset and slow to progress.

The hypersensitivity occupational lung disorders (*e.g.,* hypersensitivity pneumonitis or extrinsic allergic alveolitis) are caused by intense and often prolonged exposure to inhaled organic dusts and related occupational antigens. Affected persons have a heightened sensitivity to the antigen. The most common forms of hypersensitivity pneumonitis are farmer's lung, which results from exposure to mouldy hay or grain dust; pigeon breeder's lung, provoked by exposure to the serum, excreta, or feathers of birds; bagassosis, from contaminated sugar cane; and humidifier or air conditioner lung,

caused by mould in the water reservoirs of these appliances. Unlike bronchial asthma, this type of hypersensitivity reaction primarily involves the alveoli. These disorders cause progressive fibrotic lung disease, which can be prevented by the removal of the environmental agent.

Drug- and Radiation-Induced Lung Diseases

Drugs can cause a variety of both acute and chronic alterations in lung function. For example, some of the cytotoxic drugs (*e.g.,* bleomycin, busulfan, methotrexate, cyclophosphamide) used in treatment of cancer cause diffuse alveolar damage as a result of direct toxicity of the drug and by stimulating the influx of inflammatory cells into the alveoli.[26,46] Amiodarone, a drug used to treat cardiac arrhythmias, is preferentially sequestered in the lung and causes significant pneumonitis in 5% to 15% of persons receiving it.[26]

Radiation pneumonitis is a well-known complication of therapeutic radiation for pulmonary and other thoracic malignancies (esophageal, breast, mediastinal). It most often involves the lung in the radiation field but may extend to involve adjacent lung tissue or even the contralateral lung.[26] Two phases of the pulmonary response to radiation occur: an acute phase (radiation pneumonitis) and a chronic phase (radiation fibrosis).[46] Acute radiation pneumonitis occurs 1 to 6 months after completion of radiation and is characterized by insidious onset of dyspnea, dry cough, chest pain, weakness, and fever. Although the pathogenesis of acute radiation pneumonitis is unclear, there is speculation that hypersensitivity mechanisms are involved. Chronic radiation fibrosis develops insidiously usually following the acute diffuse alveolar damage and most persons are asymptomatic until progressive dyspnea may occur.[46]

Sarcoidosis

Sarcoidosis is a systemic disorder in which granulomas are found in affected tissues and organ systems, particularly the lung and lymphatic system.[57] An important qualification is that these granulomas occur in the absence of exogenous (infection or environmental) agents known to cause granulomatous inflammation. The disorder has a genetic susceptibility, and predominantly affects adults younger than 40 years of age, although it does occur in older persons.[57] The incidence is highest among North American blacks and northern European whites; among blacks, women are affected more frequently than men. The number of patients diagnosed with sarcoidosis is not reported in Canada, and due to higher prevalence in blacks and the lower number of blacks in Canada, it is not reliable to extrapolate the incidence of sarcoidosis in the United States to Canada.

Etiology and Pathogenesis

The characteristic lesion of sarcoidosis is the noncaseating granuloma. Unlike the granulomatous lesions that develop in tuberculosis and histoplasmosis, the collection of tissue macrophages composing the granulomas in sarcoidosis do not show evidence of necrosis or caseation. In addition to granulomas, in which multinuclear giant cells are frequently seen (see Chapter 5), there is often alveolitis or inflammation of the alveoli. The inflammation is composed largely of cytokine produced by T helper cells and tumour necrosis factor.[57]

The cause of sarcoidosis remains obscure. It is thought that the disorder may result from exposure of genetically predisposed persons to specific environmental agents.[57] Support for a genetic influence comes from epidemiologic studies that have demonstrated the higher incidence in blacks and Scandinavian populations. Additional evidence comes from familial clustering of the disease. Analysis of human leukocyte antigen (HLA) genes located in the major histocompatibility complex also suggests that unique HLA genes can be linked to disease susceptibility and prognosis. Despite advances, including the identification of sarcoidosis genetic factors, a specific etiologic agent has yet to be identified. Multiple lines of evidence suggest that the inciting agent triggers an immune response that depends on host susceptibility and is characterized by chronic inflammation, monocyte recruitment, and granuloma formation.

Clinical Features

Sarcoidosis has variable manifestations and an unpredictable course of progression in which any organ system can be affected. The systems that most commonly manifest symptoms are the lungs, skin, eyes and lymph nodes. Persons with sarcoidosis frequently seek health care either as a result of abnormalities detected on an incidental chest film or because of insidious onset of respiratory symptoms (shortness of breath, nonproductive cough, chest pain) or constitutional signs and symptoms (*e.g.,* fever, sweating, anorexia, weight loss, fatigue, myalgia).[26,57] Eye involvement (anterior uveitis) and skin involvement (skin papules and plaques) are particularly common extrathoracic manifestations, but there may be cardiac, neuromuscular, hematologic, hepatic, endocrine, and lymph node findings.[57]

Sarcoidosis follows an unpredictable course characterized by either progressive chronicity or periods of activity interspersed with remissions, sometimes permanent, that may be spontaneous or induced by corticosteroid therapy. Approximately 65% to 75% of persons recover with minimal clinical and radiographic abnormalities.[26] Other persons have persistent radiographic abnormalities and progression of their respiratory symptoms, with or without additional extrathoracic disease.[57]

The diagnosis of sarcoidosis is based on history and physical examination, tests to exclude other diseases, chest radiography, and biopsy to obtain confirmation of noncaseating granulomas.[57] The use of CT scans and magnetic resonance imaging (MRI) as routine methods for diagnosis of sarcoidosis remains controversial. A thorough ophthalmologic evaluation is recommended for most persons, even those without ocular symptoms.[58]

Treatment is directed at interrupting the granulomatous inflammatory process that is characteristic of the disease and managing the associated complications. When treatment is indicated, corticosteroid drugs are used. These agents produce clearing of the lung, as seen on the chest radiograph, and improve pulmonary function, but it is not known whether they affect the long-term outcome of the disease.

Pulmonary Fibrosis

Pulmonary fibrosis (IPF) is a chronic, progressive and irreversible interstitial restrictive lung disorder, that results in scarring of bilateral lung tissue, worsening lung function, and poor prognosis.[58,59] It primarily occurs in older adults, and is associated with a history of smoking and exposure to metal and wood dust. For a majority of cases the cause is unknown and is labelled idiopathic pulmonary fibrosis. It is estimated that 30,000 Canadians have pulmonary fibrosis, with 5,000 deaths per year.[56]

Inflammation has a pivotal role leading to fibrosis or scarring causing alveolar damage over time. Newer evidence indicates that abnormally activated alveolar epithelial cells are producing mediators and secreting excessive collagen which destroys the lung architecture. This "honeycomb" appearance can be seen on radiography and represents the fibrotic changes creating enlarged airspaces.[58]

The diagnosis requires exclusion of other known causes of interstitial lung disease, and is manifested by progressive dyspnea, chronic cough, fatigue, and weight loss symptoms and deteriorating pulmonary function. Although fatal, the trajectory is uncertain, the majority have a gradual decline over years whereas a minority decline rapidly. Unlike other fibrotic diseases, corticosteroids alone are not recommended but often combined with other immunosuppressants. Other novel medications are being reviewed as there are few treatment options. Lung transplant is the only treatment that can prolong life but risks and benefits must be examined.[58,59]

> **IN SUMMARY**
>
> The interstitial lung diseases are characterized by fibrosis and decreased compliance of the lung. They include the occupational lung diseases, lung diseases caused by toxic drugs and radiation, and lung diseases of unknown origin, such as sarcoidosis and idiopathic pulmonary fibrosis. These disorders are thought to result from an inflammatory process that begins in the alveoli and extends to involve the interstitial tissues of the lung. Unlike COPD, which affects the airways, interstitial lung diseases affect the supporting collagen and elastic tissues that lie between the airways and blood vessels. These lung diseases decrease lung volumes, reduce the diffusing capacity of the lung, and cause various degrees of hypoxemia. Because lung compliance is reduced, persons with this form of lung disease maintain their minute volume by a rapid, shallow breathing pattern.

DISORDERS OF THE PULMONARY CIRCULATION

After completing this section of the chapter, you should be able to meet the following objectives:

- State the most common cause of pulmonary embolism and the clinical manifestations of the disorder.
- Describe the pathophysiology of pulmonary arterial hypertension and state three causes of secondary pulmonary hypertension.
- Describe the alterations in cardiovascular function that are characteristic of cor pulmonale.

As blood moves through the pulmonary capillaries, oxygen content increases and carbon dioxide decreases. These processes depend on the matching of ventilation (*i.e.,* air flow) and perfusion (*i.e.,* blood flow). This section discusses two major problems of the pulmonary circulation: pulmonary embolism and pulmonary hypertension. Pulmonary edema, another major problem of the pulmonary circulation, is discussed in Chapter 26.

Pulmonary Embolism

Pulmonary embolism develops when a blood-borne substance lodges in a branch of the pulmonary artery and obstructs the flow. The embolism may consist of a thrombus (Fig. 29.15), air that has accidentally been injected during intravenous infusion, fat that has been mobilized from the bone marrow after a fracture or from a traumatized fat depot (see Chapter 58), or amniotic fluid that has entered the maternal circulation after rupture of the membranes at the time of delivery. The overall mortality rate of major pulmonary embolism is 30% or more, with the highest mortality occurring with massive pulmonary emboli or amniotic fluid emboli.[60–62]

Etiology and Pathogenesis

Almost all pulmonary emboli are thrombi that arise from deep vein thrombosis (DVT) in the lower extremities[60,61] (see Chapter 22). The presence of thrombosis in the deep veins of the legs or pelvis often is unsuspected until embolism occurs. The effects of emboli on the pulmonary circulation are related to mechanical obstruction of the pulmonary circulation and neurohumoral reflexes causing vasoconstriction. Obstruction of pulmonary blood flow causes reflex bronchoconstriction in the affected area of the lung, wasted ventilation and impaired gas exchange, and loss of alveolar surfactant. Pulmonary hypertension and right heart failure may develop when there is massive vasoconstriction because of a large embolus. Although small areas of infarction may occur, frank pulmonary infarction is uncommon.

Among the physiologic factors that contribute to venous thrombosis are venous stasis, venous endothelial injury, and

FIGURE 29.15 • Pulmonary embolism. The main pulmonary artery and its bifurcation have been opened to reveal a large saddle embolus. (From Rubin R., Strayer D. S. (Eds.). (2012). *Rubin's pathology: Clinicopathologic foundations of medicine* (6th ed., p. 275). Philadelphia, PA: Lippincott Williams & Wilkins.)

DISORDERS OF THE PULMONARY CIRCULATION

- The pulmonary circulation is a low-pressure system that links the systemic venous system and right heart with the left heart and the systemic arterial system and functions as a conduit for exchange between the dissolved gases in the blood and the ventilated air in the alveoli.
- Pulmonary thromboemboli are blood clots that originate in the systemic venous system and become lodged in a pulmonary blood vessel as they move from the right heart into and through the pulmonary circulation.
- Pulmonary hypertension is an elevated pulmonary arterial pressure. It may arise as a primary disorder of the pulmonary arteries in which an abnormal thickening of the vessel wall increases the resistance to blood flow, or as a secondary disorder due to chronic lung disorders or environmental conditions that produce hypoxemia and a resultant constriction of small pulmonary arteries, cardiac disorders that increase pulmonary venous pressure, or thromboembolic disorders that occlude pulmonary blood vessels.

hypercoagulability states (*i.e.*, Virchow triad). The thrombophilias (*e.g.*, antithrombin III deficiency, protein C and S deficiencies, factor V Leiden mutation) are a group of inherited disorders affecting coagulation that make an individual prone to development of venous thromboemboli.[60] Venous stasis and venous endothelial injury can result from prolonged bed rest, trauma, surgery, childbirth, fractures of the hip and femur, myocardial infarction and congestive heart failure, and spinal cord injury. Persons undergoing orthopedic surgery and gynecologic cancer surgery are at particular risk, as are immobilized persons. Venous stasis has also recently been noted to occur with prolonged sitting with extensive air travel, usually occurring in persons with other risks such as age, cancer, or history of vascular disease.[60] Hypercoagulability is related to various factors. Cancer cells can produce thrombin and synthesize procoagulation factors, increasing the risk for thromboembolism. Use of oral contraceptives, pregnancy, and hormone replacement therapy are thought to increase the resistance to endogenous anticoagulants. There is an increased risk for pulmonary embolism among users of oral contraceptives, and higher likelihood of complications in women who are older or are smokers.[60]

Clinical Features

Manifestations. The manifestations of pulmonary embolism depend on the size and location of the obstruction, and it may be overlooked or mistaken for other conditions.[60] Chest pain, dyspnea, and increased respiratory rate are the most frequent signs and symptoms of pulmonary embolism.[60,61] Pulmonary infarction often causes pleuritic pain that changes with respiration; it is more severe on inspiration and less severe on expiration. Moderate hypoxemia occurs as a result of impaired oxygen exchange. Diffusion and exhalation of carbon dioxide may be normal or even increased due to hyperventilation. Small emboli that become lodged in the peripheral branches of the pulmonary artery may go unrecognized unless the person is compromised, such as occurs in the elderly or acutely ill. Repeated small emboli gradually reduce the size of the pulmonary capillary bed, resulting in pulmonary hypertension. Persons with moderate-sized emboli often present with breathlessness accompanied by pleuritic pain, apprehension, slight fever, and cough productive of blood-streaked sputum. Tachycardia often occurs to compensate for decreased oxygenation, and the breathing pattern is rapid and shallow. Patients with massive emboli usually present with sudden collapse, crushing substernal chest pain, shock, and sometimes loss of consciousness. The pulse is rapid and weak, the blood pressure is low, the neck veins are distended, and the skin is cyanotic and diaphoretic. Massive pulmonary emboli often are fatal.

Diagnosis and Treatment. The diagnosis of pulmonary embolism is based on clinical signs and symptoms, blood gas determinations, venous thrombosis studies, D-dimer testing, lung scans, helical CT scans of the chest, and, in selected cases, pulmonary angiography.[60–62] Laboratory studies and radiologic films are useful in ruling out other conditions that might give rise to similar symptoms. Because emboli can cause an increase in pulmonary vascular resistance, the electrocardiogram (ECG) may be used to detect signs of right heart strain.

Because most thrombotic pulmonary emboli originate from DVT, venous studies such as *lower limb compression ultrasonography, impedance plethysmography,* and *contrast venography* are often used as initial diagnostic procedures. Of these, lower limb compression ultrasonography has become an important non-invasive means for detecting DVT. *D-dimer testing* involves the measurement of plasma D-dimer, a degradation product of coagulation factors that have been activated as the result of a thromboembolic event. Plasma D-dimers results are sensitive but non-specific, so a positive result is not definitive for a pulmonary embolus but a negative result (*i.e.*, normal value) will rule out any embolism.[60]

The *ventilation–perfusion scan* uses radiolabelled albumin, which is injected intravenously, and a radiolabelled gas, which is inhaled. A scintillation (gamma) camera is used to scan the various lung segments for blood flow and distribution of the radiolabelled gas. Ventilation–perfusion scans are useful only when their results are either normal or indicate a high probability of pulmonary embolism. *Helical (spiral) CT angiography* requires administration of an intravenous radiocontrast medium. It is sensitive for the detection of emboli in the proximal pulmonary arteries and provides another method of diagnosis. *Pulmonary angiography* involves the passage of a venous catheter through the right heart and into the pulmonary artery under fluoroscopy. Although it remains the most accurate method of diagnosis, it is an invasive procedure; therefore, its use is reserved for selected cases. An embolectomy sometimes is performed during this procedure.

The treatment goals for pulmonary emboli focus on preventing DVT and the development of thromboemboli, protecting the lungs from exposure to thromboemboli when they occur, and in the case of large and life-threatening pulmonary emboli, sustaining life and restoring pulmonary blood flow.[60,61] Fibrinolytic therapy using streptokinase, urokinase, or recombinant tissue plasminogen activator may be indicated in persons with multiple or large emboli. Fibrinolytic therapy is followed by administration of heparin to prevent clot reoccurrence.

Prevention. Prevention focuses on identification of persons at risk, avoidance of venous stasis and hypercoagulability states, and early detection of venous thrombosis.[60,61] Patients require mobilization as soon as possible after surgery or illness. For persons unable to be mobilized, either graded compression elastic stockings or intermittent pneumatic compression (IPC) boots should be used to prevent venous stasis. Both of these devices are safe and practical ways to prevent venous thrombosis. IPC boots provide intermittent inflation of air-filled sleeves that prevent venous stasis. Some devices produce sequential gradient compression that moves blood upward in the leg.

Pharmacologic prophylaxis involves the use of anticoagulant drugs (see Chapter 13). Anticoagulant therapy may be used to decrease the likelihood of deep vein thrombosis, thromboembolism, and fatal pulmonary embolism after major surgical procedures. Low-molecular-weight heparin, which can be administered subcutaneously, is often used either on an outpatient basis or in hospital for persons with increased risk. Oral anticoagulation drugs (*e.g.*, warfarin, rivaroxaban) may be used for persons with long-term risk for development of thromboemboli.[63]

Surgical placement of filters in the vena cava may be indicated when pulmonary embolism poses a life-threatening risk and there is a contraindication to anticoagulation medications.[61] The insertion of a filter or sieve, permits blood to flow while trapping the embolus but there is limited data demonstrating these prevent clinically important pulmonary embolisms.[63]

Pulmonary Hypertension

The pulmonary circulation is a low-pressure system designed to accommodate varying amounts of blood delivered from the right heart and to facilitate gas exchange. The main pulmonary artery and major branches are relatively thin-walled, compliant vessels. The distal pulmonary arterioles also are thin walled and have the capacity to dilate, collapse, or constrict depending on the presence of vasoactive substances released from the endothelial cells of the vessel, neurohumoral influences, flow velocity, oxygen pressure, and alveolar ventilation.

Pulmonary hypertension is a disorder characterized by an elevation of pressure within the pulmonary circulation, namely the pulmonary arterial system. The elevation in pressure may be acute or chronic, depending on the causative factors. A number of factors can contribute to the pathogenesis of pulmonary arterial hypertension, including a decrease in the cross-sectional area of the pulmonary arteries, a loss of blood vessels from either scarring or destructive processes affecting the alveolar walls, vasoconstriction in response to hypoxia, the need to accommodate excessive inflow of blood flow without any anatomic changes in the pulmonary arteries or arterioles, or the occlusion of outflow from the pulmonary circulation due to elevated pressures within the left atrium or ventricle. The disorder may be due to changes in the arterial wall, often referred to as *pulmonary arterial hypertension,* or it may occur as a secondary condition related to the occlusion of the pulmonary circulation by pulmonary emboli or to disruption of the pulmonary circulation due to heart or lung disease.

Pulmonary Arterial Hypertension

The term *pulmonary arterial hypertension* (PAH) is used to describe a type of pulmonary hypertension that has its origin in the pulmonary arteries. It includes primary (idiopathic or familial) pulmonary hypertension, as well as pulmonary hypertension associated with disease entities that clinically appear similar to primary pulmonary hypertension in presentation and response to treatment.[64,65] PAH is a rare and debilitating disorder characterized by abnormal proliferation and contraction of vascular smooth muscle, coagulation abnormalities, and marked intimal fibrosis leading to obliteration or obstruction of the pulmonary arteries and arterioles (Fig. 29.16). The resulting increase in pressure results in progressive right heart

FIGURE 29.16 • A: Normal pulmonary artery. **B:** Mild pulmonary hypertension with thickening of the media of the pulmonary artery. **C:** Pulmonary artery with extensive intimal fibrosis and thickening of vascular smooth muscle. **D:** Micrograph of a small pulmonary artery that is virtually occluded by concentrically thickened intimal fibrosis and thickening of the media due to pulmonary arterial hypertension. (From Rubin R., Strayer D. S. (Eds.). (2012). *Rubin's pathology: Clinicopathologic foundations of medicine* (6th ed., p. 592). Philadelphia, PA: Lippincott Williams & Wilkins.)

failure, low cardiac output, and death if left untreated. The number of Canadians who have pulmonary hypertension is anticipated to be as many as 10,000, much greater than the estimated 2,000 to 5,000 who have been diagnosed.[66] Despite advances in the treatment of PAH, with medical therapies targeting specific pathways believed to play pathogenetic roles in development of the disorder, PAH remains a serious, life-threatening condition.

The familial form of PAH appears to be inherited as an autosomal dominant trait with a variable but low penetrance, with some individuals inheriting the trait without exhibiting the disease. In 2000, the bone morphogenetic protein receptor type II gene (*BMPR2*), which codes for a member of the transforming growth factor-β (TGF-β) superfamily of receptors, was identified as causative of familial PAH.[64] Mutations in these receptors are thought to prevent TGF-β and related molecules from exerting an inhibitory effect on smooth muscle and endothelial cell proliferation.[64,65] Other conditions associated with PAH include collagen vascular disorders (*e.g.,* scleroderma), sarcoidosis, drugs and toxins, human immunodeficiency virus (HIV) infection, portal hypertension, and persistent pulmonary hypertension in the newborn.[64,65] A causal relationship has been established between several appetite suppressant drugs, including fenfluramine, and the development of PAH. Although the drug has been removed from the world market, there are still persons who were exposed to the drug and are at risk for PAH. The mechanism by which HIV infection produces PAH remains unknown, but treatment of HIV infection does not appear to affect the severity or natural history of the underlying pulmonary hypertension.

Although the specific mechanisms responsible for the vascular changes that occur in PAH remain unknown, a number of mechanisms have been proposed. These include enhanced expression of the serotonin transporter, diminished levels of nitric oxide and prostacyclin, and increased levels of several growth factors, including endothelin, vascular endothelial growth factor, and platelet-derived growth factor.[64,65]

The endothelium relaxing factor, nitric oxide, is a potent pulmonary vasodilator that is produced locally in the lung and has profound effects on smooth muscle relaxation and proliferation. Endothelin-1 is a peptide produced by the vascular endothelium that has potent vasoconstrictor and paracrine effects on vascular smooth muscle. The endothelium also produces prostacyclin (PGI2), an inhibitor of platelet aggregation and potent vasodilator. Results of studies relating these mechanisms to the structure and function of the pulmonary arterial circulation have already been translated into targeted therapies for PAH, with the probability that more will be investigated in the future.

PAH is defined by persistent elevation in pulmonary artery pressure with normal left-sided pressures, differentiating it from left-sided heart failure. Symptoms typically progress from shortness of breath and decreasing exercise tolerance to right heart failure, with marked peripheral edema and functional limitations. Other common symptoms include fatigue, angina, and syncope (fainting) or near-syncope. The diagnosis of primary pulmonary hypertension is based on an absence of disorders that cause secondary hypertension and mean pulmonary artery pressures greater than 25 mm Hg at rest or 30 mm Hg with exercise.

Treatment consists of measures to improve right heart function to reduce fatigue and peripheral edema. Supplemental oxygen may be used to increase exercise tolerance. The calcium channel blockers (nifedipine, diltiazem) may be effective early in the course of the disease but offer little in advanced stages. More advanced disease has been managed with epoprostenol, a prostacyclin that has potent pulmonary vasodilator effects.[67] Because of its short half-life (3–5 minutes), the drug must be administered by continuous infusion through an indwelling catheter with an automatic ambulatory pump. Properties of the drug other than its vasodilating effects include inhibition of platelet aggregation and beneficial vascular remodelling effects. This agent often improves symptoms, sometimes dramatically, in persons who have not responded to other vasodilators. Oral endothelin antagonists (*e.g.,* bosentan) have demonstrated to be effective in improving exercise capacity and hemodynamic markers over short periods of time.[68] Sildenafil (*e.g.,* Viagra), a highly selective phosphodiesterase-5 inhibitor, which acts in a manner similar to nitric oxide to produce vasodilation, is approved in Canada for treatment of pulmonary hypertension. Lung transplantation may be an alternative for persons who do not respond to other forms of treatment.

Secondary Pulmonary Hypertension

Although pulmonary hypertension can develop as a primary disorder, most cases develop secondary to conditions such as chronic hypoxemia due to COPD, interstitial lung disease, or sleep-disordered breathing; increased resistance to pulmonary venous drainage due to conditions such as diastolic dysfunction of the left heart or disorders of mitral or aortic valves; or chronic thromboembolic disorders.

Continued exposure of the pulmonary vessels to hypoxemia is a common cause of pulmonary hypertension. Unlike blood vessels in the systemic circulation, most of which dilate in response to hypoxemia and hypercapnia, the pulmonary vessels constrict. The stimulus for constriction seems to originate in the airspaces near the smaller branches of the pulmonary arteries. In regions of the lung that are poorly ventilated, the response is adaptive in that it diverts blood flow away from the poorly ventilated areas to those areas that are more adequately ventilated. This effect, however, becomes less beneficial as more and more areas of the lung become poorly ventilated. Pulmonary hypertension may develop with advanced COPD or interstitial lung disease. It also may develop at high altitudes in persons with normal lungs. Persons who experience marked hypoxemia during sleep (such as those with sleep apnea) often experience marked elevations in pulmonary arterial pressure.

Elevation of pulmonary venous pressure is common in conditions such as mitral valve disorders or left ventricular diastolic dysfunction. In each of these alterations, the elevated left atrial pressure is transmitted to the pulmonary circulation. Continued increases in left atrial pressure can lead to medial hypertrophy and intimal thickening of the small pulmonary arteries, causing sustained hypertension. Another cause of secondary pulmonary hypertension is obstruction of pulmonary blood flow due to pulmonary thromboemboli. Persons who are promptly treated for acute pulmonary thromboembolism with anticoagulants rarely develop pulmonary hypertension. However, in some persons chronic obstruction of the pulmonary vascular bed develops because of impaired resolution of the thromboemboli.

The signs and symptoms of secondary pulmonary hypertension reflect both the elevated pulmonary arterial pressure and the underlying heart or lung disease. As with primary pulmonary hypertension, diagnosis is based on radiographic findings, echocardiography, and Doppler ultrasonography. Treatment measures are directed toward the underlying disorder. Vasodilator therapy may be indicated for some persons.

Cor Pulmonale

The term *cor pulmonale* refers to right heart failure resulting from primary lung disease or pulmonary hypertension. The increased pressures and work result in hypertrophy and eventual failure of the right ventricle. The manifestations of cor pulmonale include the signs and symptoms of the primary lung disease and the signs of right-sided heart failure (see Chapter 26). Signs of right-sided heart failure include venous congestion, peripheral edema, shortness of breath, fatigue, and a productive cough that becomes worse during periods of heart failure. Plethora (*i.e.,* redness), cyanosis, and warm, moist skin may result from the compensatory polycythemia and desaturation of arterial blood that accompany chronic lung disease. Drowsiness and altered consciousness may occur as the result of carbon dioxide retention. Management of cor pulmonale focuses on the treatment of the lung disease and heart failure. Low-flow oxygen therapy may be used to reduce the pulmonary hypertension and polycythemia associated with severe hypoxemia caused by chronic lung disease.

IN SUMMARY

Pulmonary vascular disorders include pulmonary embolism and pulmonary hypertension. Pulmonary embolism develops when a blood-borne substance lodges in a branch of the pulmonary artery and obstructs blood flow. The embolus can consist of a thrombus, air, fat, or amniotic fluid. The most common form is thromboemboli arising from the deep veins of the lower extremities. Pulmonary hypertension is the elevation of pulmonary arterial pressure. It can be divided into two types: (1) pulmonary arterial hypertension, which has its origin in the pulmonary arteries and includes both primary (idiopathic or familial) pulmonary hypertension and pulmonary hypertension associated with disease entities that produce a similar pathologic process; and (2) pulmonary hypertension that develops secondary to lung disease and hypoxemia (*e.g.,* chronic lung diseases, sleep-disordered breathing, or chronic exposure to high altitude), conditions that elevate pulmonary venous pressures (left ventricular dysfunction, mitral valve disease), or chronic obstruction of the pulmonary vasculature due to thromboemboli. Cor pulmonale describes right heart failure caused by primary pulmonary disease or long-standing pulmonary hypertension.

ACUTE RESPIRATORY DISORDERS

After completing this section of the chapter, you should be able to meet the following objectives:

- Describe the pathologic lung changes that occur in acute respiratory distress syndrome and relate them to the clinical manifestations of a general definition of respiratory failure.
- Differentiate between the causes and manifestations of hypoxemic and hypercapnic/hypoxemic respiratory failure.
- Describe the treatment of respiratory failure.

The function of the respiratory system is to add oxygen to the blood and remove carbon dioxide. Disruptions in this function occur with acute respiratory distress syndrome and acute respiratory failure. Although the mechanisms that disrupt gas exchange may vary, both conditions represent a life-threatening situation with high risk of morbidity and mortality.

Acute Respiratory Distress Syndrome

Acute respiratory distress syndrome (ARDS) was first described in 1967 in adults, and initially called *adult respiratory distress syndrome*.[69] It later was renamed *acute respiratory distress syndrome* because it also affects children. In 2012 the term acute lung injury (ALI) was removed with the new Berlin classification of ARDS. Now ARDS is classified as mild (previously ALI), moderate, and severe according to the extent of impaired oxygen diffusion, as evaluated by the PF (PO_2 to FiO_2) ratio.[70] The incidence of ARDS is not consistently reported, although it is estimated to occur in approximately 150,000 to 200,000 persons each year in North America and has a mortality rate greater than breast cancer and HIV/AIDS combined. Despite the most sophisticated interventions in highly technologic environments, the mortality rate varies from 35% to 60% and morbidity is extensive, including physical, cognitive, and emotional sequelae.[71,72]

ARDS may result from a number of indirect and direct conditions, including aspiration of gastric contents, major trauma (with or without fat emboli), sepsis secondary to pulmonary or nonpulmonary infections, acute pancreatitis, hematologic disorders, metabolic events, and reactions to drugs and toxins (Chart 29.2). Chronic alcohol abuse increases both the risk for and severity of ARDS.[73] There is risk of transfusion-related acute lung injury (TRALI), which is rarer in Canada, Europe, Australia, and the United Kingdom owing to the standard practice of washing packed cells. It is hypothesized that levels of mediators and cytokines are higher in unwashed packed cells.[74] Other risk factors mitigated in Canada include limiting female plasma (due to alloimmunization during

CHART 29.2 CONDITIONS IN WHICH ARDS CAN DEVELOP[a]

Aspiration
Near drowning
Aspiration of gastric contents

Drugs, Toxins, Therapeutic Agents
Free-base cocaine smoking
Heroin
Inhaled gases (*e.g.,* smoke, ammonia)
Breathing high concentrations of oxygen
Radiation

Infections
Septicemia
Trauma and shock
Burns
Fat embolism
Chest trauma

Disseminated Intravascular Coagulation

Multiple Blood Transfusions

[a]This list is not intended to be inclusive.

pregnancies), whole blood or multiple transfusions to patients at risk for TRALI. Patient risk factors include higher interleukin-8, shock, liver surgery including transplantation, chronic alcohol abuse, positive fluid balance, peak airway pressures greater than 30 cm H2O if ventilated, and current smoking history.[75]

Etiology and Pathogenesis

Although numerous conditions may lead to ARDS, all result in pathologic diffuse epithelial cell injury with increased permeability of the alveolar–capillary membrane and an acute systemic inflammatory response (Fig. 29.17). The increased permeability permits fluid, plasma proteins, and blood cells to move out of the vascular compartment into the interstitium and alveoli of the lung.[76,77] Diffuse alveolar cell damage leads to accumulation of fluid, surfactant inactivation, and formation of a hyaline membrane that is impervious to gas exchange. As the disease progresses, the work of breathing becomes greatly increased as the lung stiffens and becomes more difficult to inflate. There is increased intrapulmonary shunting of blood, impaired gas exchange, and hypoxemia despite high supplemental oxygen therapy. Gas exchange is further compromised by alveolar collapse resulting from abnormalities in surfactant production. When injury to the alveolar epithelium is severe, disorganized epithelial repair may lead to fibrosis. Most persons who do not survive ARDS die during the phase of capillary thrombosis and fibroproliferation.[76]

The pathogenesis of ARDS is unclear, although both pulmonary and systemic inflammatory responses occur. Neutrophils accumulate and are activated early by cytokines, and subsequently synthesize and release a variety of products, including proteolytic enzymes, reactive oxygen species, and phospholipid products.[76,77] These products increase the inflammatory response and cause direct injury to the capillary endothelium and alveolar epithelium.

Clinical Features

Clinically, ARDS is marked by a rapid onset of respiratory distress, usually within 12 to 18 hours of the initiating event, with an increase in respiratory rate and signs of respiratory

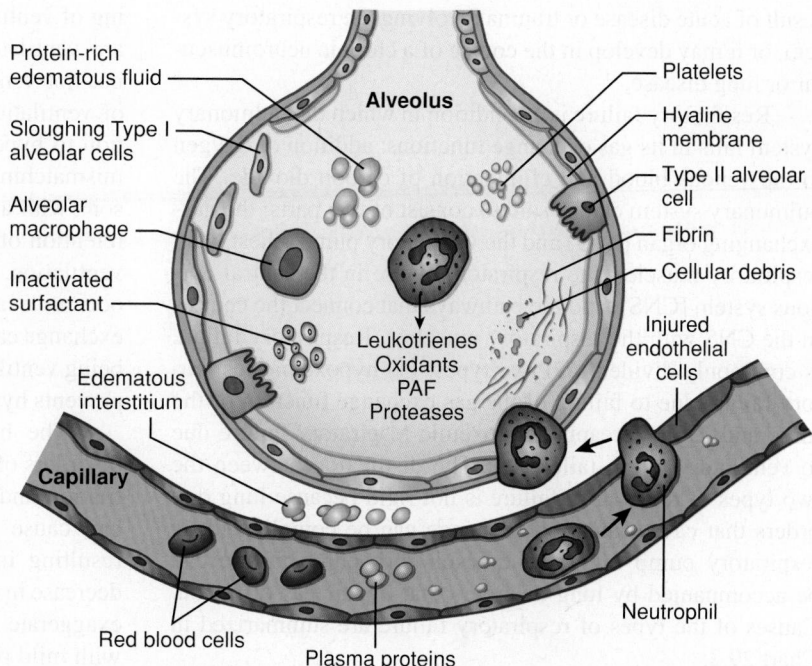

FIGURE 29.17 • The mechanism of lung changes in ARDS. Injury and increased permeability of the alveolar capillary membrane allow fluid, protein, cellular debris, platelets, and blood cells to move out of the vascular compartment and enter the interstitium and alveoli. Activated neutrophils release a variety of products that damage the alveolar cells and lead to edema, surfactant inactivation, and formation of a hyaline membrane. PAF, platelet-activating factor.

failure. Chest radiography shows diffuse bilateral infiltrates of the lung tissue in the absence of cardiac dysfunction. Diffusion of oxygen is impaired and results in a decrease in the PF ratio, and marked hypoxemia occurs that is refractory to treatment with supplemental oxygen therapy. Pulmonary hypertension may occur as a result of hypoxia or vasoconstrictive mediators, worsening diffusion.[77] As the inflammatory mediators are transported throughout the body, many persons with ARDS have a systemic response that results in multiple organ failure, particularly of the renal, gastrointestinal, cardiovascular, and central nervous systems.

Treatment. The treatment goals in ARDS are to supply oxygen to vital organs and provide supportive care until the condition causing the pathologic process has been reversed and the lungs have had a chance to heal. Assisted ventilation using high concentrations of oxygen may be required to address or correct the hypoxemia (to be discussed). Positive end-expiratory pressure (PEEP), which increases the pressure in the alveoli at the end of expiration, may be used to assist in maintaining alveolar volume by either preventing collapse or reinflating the collapsed areas of the lung to improve the matching of ventilation and perfusion. Extensive research has been done to determine optimal pressures and volumes to correct the hypoxemia while preventing further lung injury due to the mechanics of ventilation.[76]

Acute Respiratory Failure

Respiratory failure can be viewed as a failure in gas exchange due to lung failure. It is not a specific disease, but can occur in the course of a number of conditions that impair ventilation, compromise the matching of ventilation and perfusion, or impair gas diffusion. It has numerous potential causes and factors and may occur in previously healthy persons as the result of acute disease or trauma involving the respiratory system, or it may develop in the course of a chronic neuromuscular or lung disease.

Respiratory failure is a condition in which the pulmonary system fails in its gas exchange functions: addition of oxygen to the venous blood and elimination of carbon dioxide. The pulmonary system can be said to consist of two parts: the gas-exchanging organ (lung) and the ventilatory pump (chest wall, respiratory muscles, the respiratory centre in the central nervous system [CNS], and the pathways that connect the centres in the CNS with the respiratory muscles). Respiratory failure is commonly divided into two types: (1) hypoxemic respiratory failure due to failure of the gas exchange function of the lung, and (2) hypercapnic/hypoxemic respiratory failure due to ventilatory pump failure.[77,78] The distinction between the two types of respiratory failure is not rigid because lung disorders that cause impaired exchange can be complicated by respiratory pump failure, and respiratory pump failure can be accompanied by lung disorders that impair gas diffusion. Causes of the types of respiratory failure are summarized in Chart 29.3.

CHART 29.3 | CAUSES OF RESPIRATORY FAILURE[a]

Hypoxemic Respiratory Failure
Restrictive lung disease
Severe pneumonia
Atelectasis

Hypercapnic/Hypoxemic Respiratory Failure
Upper airway obstruction
Infection (*e.g.*, epiglottitis)
Laryngospasm
Tumours
Weakness or paralysis of respiratory muscles
Brain injury
Drug overdose
Guillain-Barré syndrome
Muscular dystrophy
Spinal cord injury
Chest wall injury
Chronic obstructive pulmonary disease
Asthma

Impaired Diffusion
Pulmonary edema
Acute respiratory distress syndrome

[a]This list is not intended to be inclusive.

Hypoxemic Respiratory Failure

In persons with hypoxemic respiratory failure, two major pathophysiologic factors contribute to the lowering of arterial PO_2—ventilation–perfusion mismatching or impaired diffusion.

Mismatching of Ventilation and Perfusion. The mismatching of ventilation and perfusion occurs when areas of the lung are ventilated but not perfused or when areas are perfused but not ventilated. Usually the hypoxemia seen in situations of ventilation–perfusion mismatching is more severe in relation to hypercapnia than that seen in hypoventilation. Severe mismatching of ventilation and perfusion often is seen in persons with advanced COPD. These disorders contribute to the retention of carbon dioxide by reducing the effective alveolar ventilation, even when total ventilation is maintained. This occurs because a region of the lung is not perfused and gas exchange cannot take place or because an area of the lung is not being ventilated. Maintaining a high ventilation rate effectively prevents hypercapnia but also increases the work of breathing.

The hypoxemia associated with ventilation–perfusion disorders often is exaggerated by conditions such as hypoventilation and decreased cardiac output. For example, sedation can cause hypoventilation in persons with severe COPD, resulting in further impairment of ventilation. Likewise, a decrease in cardiac output because of myocardial infarction can exaggerate the ventilation–perfusion impairment in a person with mild pulmonary edema or COPD.

The beneficial effect of oxygen administration on PO_2 levels in ventilation–perfusion disorders depends on the degree of mismatching that is present. Because oxygen administration increases the diffusion gradient in ventilated portions of the lung, it usually is effective in raising arterial PO_2 levels. However, there may be clinical consequences of oxygen toxicity if high concentrations of oxygen are delivered over prolonged periods of time and in persons with chronic lung disease, the risk of high-flow oxygen may decrease the respiratory drive.

Impaired Diffusion. Impaired diffusion describes a condition in which gas exchange between the alveolar air and pulmonary blood is impeded because of an increase in the distance for diffusion or a decrease in the permeability or surface area of the respiratory membranes to the movement of gases. It most commonly occurs in conditions such as interstitial lung disease, ARDS, pulmonary edema, and pneumonia.

Conditions that impair diffusion may produce severe hypoxemia but no hypercapnia because of the increase in ventilation and greater diffusion rate of carbon dioxide. Hypoxemia resulting from impaired diffusion can be partially or completely corrected by the administration of high concentrations of oxygen. In this case, the high concentration of oxygen serves to overcome the decrease in diffusion by establishing a larger alveolar-to-capillary diffusion gradient.

Hypercapnic/Hypoxemic Respiratory Failure

In the hypercapnic form of respiratory failure, patients are unable to maintain a level of alveolar ventilation sufficient to eliminate CO_2 and keep arterial O_2 levels within normal range. Because ventilation is determined by a sequence of events ranging from generation of impulses in the CNS to movement of air through the conducting airways, there are several stages at which problems can adversely affect the total minute ventilation.

Hypoventilation or ventilatory failure occurs when the volume of "fresh" air moving into and out of the lung is significantly reduced. It is commonly caused by conditions outside the lung such as depression of the respiratory centre (*e.g.,* drug overdose, brain injury), diseases of the nerves supplying the respiratory muscles (*e.g.,* Guillain-Barré syndrome, spinal cord injury), disorders of the respiratory muscles (*e.g.,* muscular dystrophy), exacerbation of chronic lung disease (*e.g.,* COPD, asthma), or thoracic cage disorders (*e.g.,* severe scoliosis or crushed chest).

Hypoventilation has two important effects on arterial blood gases. First, it causes an increase in PCO_2. The rise in PCO_2 is directly related to the level of ventilation: reducing the ventilation by one half causes a doubling of the PCO_2. Thus, the PCO_2 level is a good diagnostic measure for hypoventilation. Second, it may cause hypoxemia when severe, although the hypoxemia that is caused by hypoventilation can be readily corrected by the administration of supplemental oxygen.

Clinical Features

Acute respiratory failure is usually manifested by varying degrees of hypoxemia and hypercapnia. There is no absolute definition of the levels of PO_2 and PCO_2 that indicate respiratory failure. Respiratory failure is conventionally defined by an arterial PO_2 of less than 60 mm Hg on room air (at sea level), an arterial PCO_2 of more than 45 mm Hg, or both, when prior blood values have been normal.[78] It is important to emphasize that these cut-off values are not rigid, but serve as a guide in combination with history and physical assessment information. The signs and symptoms of acute respiratory failure are those of the underlying disease combined with signs of hypoxemia and hypercapnia/hypoxemia. Respiratory acidosis is usually present because the person is not yet compensating for the retention of CO_2 and increased production of acids.

Hypoxemia is accompanied by increased respiratory drive and increased sympathetic tone. Potential signs of hypoxemia include cyanosis, restlessness, confusion, anxiety, delirium, fatigue, tachypnea, hypertension, cardiac arrhythmias, and tremor. The initial cardiovascular effects are tachycardia with increased cardiac output and increased blood pressure. Serious arrhythmias may be triggered. The pulmonary vasculature constricts in response to low alveolar PO_2. Thus, hypoxemia may have signs similar to those of cor pulmonale (*i.e.,* jugular vein distension, dependent edema). Profound acute hypoxemia can cause convulsions, retinal hemorrhages, and permanent brain damage. Hypotension and bradycardia often are preterminal events in persons with hypoxemic respiratory failure, indicating the failure of compensatory mechanisms.

Many of the adverse consequences of hypercapnia are the result of respiratory acidosis. Direct effects of acidosis include depression of cardiac contractility, decreased respiratory muscle contractility, and arterial vasodilation (see Chapter 32). Raised levels of PCO_2 greatly increase cerebral blood flow, which may result in headache, increased cerebrospinal fluid pressure, and sometimes papilledema (see Chapter 54, Fig. 54.14). The headache is due to dilation of the cerebral vessels. Additional indicators of hypercapnia are warm and flushed skin and hyperemic conjunctivae. Hypercapnia has nervous system effects similar to those of an anesthetic—hence the term *carbon dioxide narcosis*. There is progressive somnolence, disorientation, and, if the condition is untreated, coma. Mild to moderate increases in blood pressure are common. Air hunger and rapid breathing occur when alveolar PCO_2 levels rise to approximately 60 to 75 mm Hg; as PCO_2 levels reach 80 to 100 mm Hg, the person becomes lethargic, disorientated, and sometimes semicomatose.

Treatment. The treatment of the person with acute respiratory failure consists of specific therapy directed toward the underlying disease, respiratory supportive care directed toward maintenance of adequate gas exchange, and general supportive care. A number of treatment modalities are available, including the establishment of an airway, use of bronchodilating drugs, and antibiotics for respiratory infections. The main therapeutic goal in acute hypoxemic respiratory failure is to ensure adequate oxygenation of vital organs. This is accomplished through administration of supplemental oxygen.

Mechanical Ventilation. When alveolar ventilation is inadequate to maintain PCO_2 or PO_2 levels because of impaired respiratory function or neurologic failure, mechanical ventilation may be necessary. There are non-invasive forms of mechanical ventilation that use a face mask to deliver positive-pressure ventilation. Bilevel positive airway pressure (BiPAP) ventilation mode senses inspiratory effort and delivers a higher pressure during inspiration, which decreases work and increases effectiveness of breathing.[78] This external mode of mechanical ventilation has been demonstrated to be effective in patients who are conscious, and have minimal airway secretions and a normal blood pressure. It is recommended within Canadian clinical practice guidelines for first consideration for the person with acute respiratory failure, and underlying COPD or cardiogenic edema.[79] There is insufficient evidence to support recommendation of use in asthma, severe community-acquired pneumonia or chest trauma.[79,80]

If mechanical ventilation is required, either an endotracheal or tracheal tube is required to establish the airway. There are two basic types of positive-pressure mechanical ventilators: pressure-cycled units and volume-cycled units. In each type, the tidal volume and respiratory rate are adjusted to maintain ventilation at a given minute volume, and the patient does minimal or no work of breathing when fully ventilated or supported. The pressure-cycled unit delivers a preset pressure, whereas the tidal volume is determined by the airway pressure with a controlled flow rate. The volume-cycled ventilator delivers a preset tidal volume, but the pressure may vary. Thus, either pressure or volume is controlled. Both of these modes of ventilation deliver the pressure or volume at a minimum set rate per minute, and the person may initiate additional breaths at that preset volume or pressure. Thus, ventilators deliver a breath triggered by the patient or independently if such an effort does not occur.

Mandatory volume ventilation may be intermittent and synchronized to the patient, which is called *synchronized intermittent mandatory ventilation* (SIMV). In this mode, the patient receives periodic positive-pressure ventilation from the ventilator at a preset volume and rate, and pressure-support ventilation, in which the ventilator delivers a set pressure rather than volume to augment each spontaneous respiratory effort. Ventilators also can be programmed to supply positive pressure for support during inspiration (PSV) or continuous positive airway pressure (CPAP) in spontaneously breathing patients. In each of these, the work of breathing is supported by the ventilator, but the patient also provides some effort.

IN SUMMARY

The hallmark of acute respiratory distress syndrome is a pronounced inflammatory response that affects the lung and may result in systemic organ failure. The acute inflammatory response results in damage and dysfunction of the alveolar–capillary membrane of the lung. Classically, there is interstitial edema of lung tissue, an increase in surface tension caused by inactivation of surfactant, collapse of the alveolar structures, a stiff and noncompliant lung that is difficult to inflate, and impaired diffusion of the respiratory gases with severe hypoxia that is resistant to oxygen therapy.

Acute respiratory failure is a condition in which the lungs fail to oxygenate the blood adequately (hypoxemic respiratory failure) or prevent undue retention of carbon dioxide (hypercapnic/hypoxemic respiratory failure). The causes of respiratory failure are many. It may arise acutely in persons with previously healthy lungs, or it may be superimposed on chronic lung disease. Treatment of acute respiratory failure is directed toward treatment of the underlying disease, maintenance of adequate gas exchange and tissue oxygenation, and general supportive care. When alveolar ventilation is inadequate to maintain PO_2 or PCO_2 levels because of impaired respiratory function or neurologic failure, mechanical ventilation may be necessary.

REVIEW EXERCISES

1. A 30-year-old man is brought to the emergency department with a knife wound to the chest. On visual inspection, asymmetry of chest movement during inspiration, displacement of the trachea, and absence of breath sounds on the side of the wound are noted. His neck veins are distended, his blood pressure is low, and his pulse is rapid and thready. A rapid diagnosis of tension pneumothorax is made.
   A. *Explain the observed respiratory and cardiovascular function in terms of the impaired lung expansion and the air that has entered the chest as a result of the injury.*
   B. *What type of emergent treatment is necessary to save this man's life?*

2. A 10-year-old boy who is having an acute asthmatic attack is brought to the emergency department by his parents. The boy is observed to be sitting up and struggling to breathe. His breathing is accompanied by use of the accessory muscles, a weak cough, and audible wheezing sounds. His pulse is rapid and weak and both heart and breath sounds are distant on auscultation. His parents relate that his asthma began to worsen after he developed a "cold," and now he doesn't even get relief from his salbutamol inhaler.
   A. *Explain the changes in physiologic function underlying this boy's signs and symptoms.*
   B. *What is the most probable reason for the progression of this boy's asthma in terms of the early- and late-phase responses?*
   C. *The boy is treated with a systemic corticosteroid and inhaled anticholinergic and β_2-adrenergic agonist and then transferred to the intensive care unit. Explain the action of each of these medications in terms of relieving this boy's symptoms.*

3. A 62-year-old man with an 8-year history of chronic bronchitis reports to his health care provider with complaints of increasing shortness of breath, ankle swelling, and a feeling of fullness in his upper abdomen. The expiratory phase of his respirations is prolonged and expiratory wheezes and crackles are heard on auscultation. His blood pressure is 160/90 mm Hg, his red blood cell count is 6.0×10^{12}/L (normal 4.2 to 5.4×10^{12}/L), his hematocrit is 65% (normal male value 40% to 50%), his arterial PO_2 is 55 mm Hg, and his O_2 saturation, which is 85% while he is resting, drops to 82% during walking exercise.

   A. *Explain the physiologic mechanisms responsible for his edema, hypertension, and elevated red blood cell count.*

   B. *His arterial PO_2 and O_2 saturation indicate that he is a candidate for continuous low-flow oxygen. Explain the benefits of this treatment in terms of his activity tolerance, blood pressure, and red blood cell count.*

   C. *Explain why the oxygen flow rate for persons with COPD is normally titrated to maintain the arterial PO_2 between 60 and 65 mm Hg.*

4. An 18-year-old woman is admitted to the emergency department with a suspected drug overdose. Her respiratory rate is slow (4–6 breaths/minute) and shallow. Arterial blood gases reveal a PCO_2 of 80 mm Hg and a PO_2 of 60 mm Hg.

   A. *What is the cause of this woman's high PCO_2 and low PO_2?*

   B. *Hypoventilation almost always causes an increase in PCO_2. Explain.*

   C. *Even though her PO_2 increases to 90 mm Hg with institution of oxygen therapy, her PCO_2 remains elevated. Explain.*

References

1. Hall J. E. (2011). *Textbook of medical physiology* (12th ed.). Philadelphia, PA: W. B. Saunders.
2. West J. B. (2013). *Pulmonary pathophysiology: The essentials* (8th ed.). Philadelphia, PA: Lippincott Williams & Wilkins.
3. Casey G. (2011). Pulse oximetry: What are we really measuring? *Nursing New Zealand, 17*(3), 24–29.
4. Zaouter C., Zavorsky G. S. (2012). The measurement of carboxyhemoglobin and methemoglobin using a non-invasive pulse CO-oximeter. *Respiratory Physiology and Neurobiology, 182*(2-3), 88–92.
5. ARDS Definition Task Force, Ranieri V. M., Rubenfeld G. D., Thompson B. T., et al. (2012). Acute respiratory distress syndrome: The Berlin definition. *Journal of the American Medical Association, 307*(23), 2526–2533.
6. Walter E. C. (2013). High-flow nasal cannula: What is it, how does it work, and do we know if it works? *Critical Care Alert, 21*(1), 1–4.
7. Ahmad Z., Krishnadas R., Froeschle P. (2009). Pleural effusion: Diagnosis and management. *Journal of Perioperative Practice, 19*(8), 242–247.
8. Light R. W. (2012). Chapter 263: Disorders of the pleura and mediastinum. In Longo D. L., Fauci A. S., Kasper D. L., Hauser S. (Eds.), *Harrison's principles of internal medicine* (18th ed.). New York: McGraw-Hill.
9. Skouras V., Kalomenidis I. (2010). Chylothorax: Diagnostic approach. *Current Opinion in Pulmonary Medicine, 16*(4), 387–393.
10. Roberts M. E., Neville E., Berrisford R. G., et al.; BTS Pleural Disease Guideline Group. (2010). Management of a malignant pleural effusion: British Thoracic Society pleural disease guideline 2010. *Thorax, 65*(Suppl 2), ii32–ii40.
11. Boshuizen R. C., Thomas R., Lee Y. C. G. (2013). Advantages of indwelling pleural catheters for management of malignant pleural effusions. *Current Respiratory Care Reports, 2*(2), 93–99.
12. Mowery N. T., Gunter O. L., Collier B. R., et al. (2011). Practice management guidelines for management of hemothorax and occult pneumothorax. *The Journal of Trauma, Injury, Infection, and Critical Care, 70*(2), 510–518.
13. Henry M., Arnold T., Harvey J.; Pleural Diseases Group, Standards of Care Committee, British Thoracic Society. (2003). BTS guidelines for the management of spontaneous pneumothorax. *Thorax, 58*(Suppl 2), ii39–ii52.
14. Noppen M. (2010). Spontaneous pneumothorax: Epidemiology, pathophysiology and cause. *European Respiratory Review, 19*(117), 217–219.
15. Baumann M. H., Noppen M. (2004). Invited review: Pneumothorax. *Respirology, 9*, 157–164.
16. Siddiqui M. F., Saleem S., Badireddi S. (2013). Pulmonary talcosis with intravenous drug abuse. *Respiratory Care, 58*(10), e126–e128.
17. Rousset-Jablonski C., Alifano M., Plu-Bureau G., et al. (2011). Catamenial pneumothorax and endometriosis-related pneumothorax: Clinical features and risk factors. *Human Reproduction, 26*(9), 2322–2329.
18. Lougheed M. D., Lemiere C., Ducharme F. M., et al.; Canadian Thoracic Society Asthma Clinical Assembly. (2012). Canadian Thoracic Society 2012 guideline update: Diagnosis and management of asthma in preschoolers, children and adults. *Canadian Respiratory Journal, 19*(2), 127–164.
19. Robinson D. S. (2010). The role of the T cell in asthma. *Journal of Allergy and Clinical Immunology, 126*(6), 1081–1091.
20. Statistics Canada. (2013). Asthma, by sex, provinces and territories. Available online at: http://www.statcan.gc.ca/tables-tableaux/sum-som/l01/cst01/health50a-eng.htm. Accessed June 25, 2014.
21. Statistics Canada. (2013). Asthma, 2012. Available online at: http://www.statcan.gc.ca/pub/82-625-x/2013001/article/11834-eng.htm. Accessed June 25, 2014.
22. Garner R., Kohen D. (2008). Changes in the prevalence of asthma among Canadian children. *Health Reports, 19*(2), No. 82-003-XIE, 45–50. 23.
23. Aaron S. D., Vandemheen K. L., Bouet L., et al.; Canadian Respiratory Clinical Research Consortium. (2008). Overdiagnosis of asthma in obese and nonobese adults. *CMAJ, 179*(11), 1121–1131.
24. Cardinale F., Giordano P., Chinellato I., Tesse R. (2013). Respiratory epithelial imbalances in asthma pathophysiology. *Allergy and Asthma Proceedings, 34*(2), 143–149.
25. Pillai P., Corrigan C. J., Ying S. (2011). Airway epithelium in atopic and nonatopic asthma: Similarities and differences. *International Scholarly Research Network Allergy, 2011*(195846), doi:10.5402/2011/195846.
26. Husain A. N. (2010). Chapter 15: The lung. In Kumar V., Abbas A. K., Fausto, N., et al. (Eds.), *Robbins and Cotran pathologic basis of disease* (8th ed.), Philadelphia, PA: Elsevier Saunders.
27. Holgate S. T. (2011). Pathophysiology of asthma: What has our current understanding taught us about new therapeutic approaches? *Journal of Allergy and Clinical Immunology, 128*(3), 495–505.
28. Berry M. A., Hargadon B., Shelley M., et al. (2006). Evidence of a role of tumor necrosis factor-alpha in refractory asthma. *New England Journal of Medicine, 354*(7), 697–708.
29. Pongdee T., Li J. T. (2013). Exercise-induced bronchoconstriction. *Annals of Allergy, Asthma & Immunology, 110*(5), 311–315.
30. Spector S., Tan R. (2012). Exercise-induced bronchoconstriction update: Therapeutic management. *Allergy and Asthma Proceedings, 33*(1), 7–12.
31. Lougheed M. D., Lemiere C., Dell S. D., et al. (2010). Canadian Thoracic Society asthma management continuum: 2010 consensus summary for children six years of age and over, and adults. *Canadian Respiratory Journal, 17*(1), 15–24.
32. Velazquez J. R., Teran L. M. (2013). Aspirin-intolerant asthma: A comprehensive review of biomarkers and pathophysiology. *Clinical Reviews in Allergy & Immunology, 45*(1), 75–86.

33. Dratva J., Schindler C., Curjuric I., et al. (2010). Perimenstrual increase in bronchial hyperactivity in premenopausal women: Results from the population-based SAPALDIA 2 cohort. *Journal of Allergy and Clinical Immunology, 125*(4), 823–829.

34. Virchow J. C. (2012). Pregnancy and asthma. *Seminars in Respiratory and Critical Care Medicine, 33*(6), 630–644.

35. Greenberg H., Cohen R. I. (2012). Nocturnal asthma. *Current Opinion in Pulmonary Medicine, 18*(1), 57–62.

36. Abramson M. J., Puy R. M., Weiner J. M. (2010). Injection allergen immunotherapy for asthma. *Cochrane Database of Systematic Reviews,* (8). No. CD001186.

37. Gauvreau G. M., O'Bryne P. M., Boulet L. P., et al. (2014). Effects of an anti-TSLP antibody on allergen-induced asthmatic responses. *New England Journal of Medicine, 370*(22), 2102–2110.

38. Bousquet J., Mantzouranis E., Cruz A. A., et al. (2010). Uniform definition of asthma severity, control and exacerbations: Document presented for the World Health Organization consultation on severe asthma. *Journal of Allergy and Clinical Immunology, 126*(5), 926–938.

39. Ortiz-Alvarez O., Mikrogianakis A. (2012). Managing the paediatric patient with an acute asthma exacerbation. *Paediatrics & Child Health, 17*(5), 251–255.

40. Lui A. H., Covar R. A., Spahn J. D., et al. (2011). Chapter 138: Childhood asthma. In Kliegman R. M., Stanton B. F., St. Geme J. W., et al. (Eds.), *Nelson textbook of pediatrics* (19th ed.). Philadelphia, PA: Saunders Elsevier.

41. O'Donnell D. E., Hernandez P., Kaplan A., et al. (2008). Canadian Thoracic Society recommendations for management of chronic obstructive pulmonary disease, 2008 update, highlights for primary care. *Canadian Respiratory Journal, 15*(Suppl A), 1A–8A.

42. Statistics Canada. (2015). The 10 leading causes of death, 2011. Available online at: http://www.statcan.gc.ca/pub/82-625-x/2014001/article/11896-eng.htm. Accessed August 5, 2015.

43. Public Health Agency of Canada. (2011). Fast facts about Chronic Obstructive Pulmonary Disease (COPD) 2011. Available online at: http://www.phac-aspc.gc.ca/cd-mc/publications/copd-mpoc/ff-rr-2011-eng.php. Accessed June 25, 2014.

44. Kelly E., Greene C. M., Carroll T. P., et al. (2010). Alpha-1 antitrypsin deficiency. *Respiratory Medicine, 104*(6), 763–772.

45. Statistics Canada. (2013). *Chronic obstructive pulmonary disease in Canadians, 2009 to 2011.* Available online at: http://www.statcan.gc.ca/pub/82-625-x/2012001/article/11709-eng.htm. Accessed June 25, 2014.

46. Beasley M. B., Travis W. D., Rubin E. (2012). Chapter 12: The respiratory system. In Rubin R., Strayer D. S. (Eds.), *Rubin's pathology: Clinicopathologic foundations of medicine* (6th ed.). Philadelphia, PA: Lippincott Williams & Wilkins.

47. Kim V., Criner G. J. (2013). Chronic bronchitis and chronic obstructive pulmonary disease. *American Journal of Respiratory and Critical Care Medicine, 187*(3), 228–237.

48. Rennard S. I. (2011). COPD heterogeneity: What this will mean in practice. *Respiratory Care, 56*(8), 1181–1187.

49. Abdo W. F., Heunks L. M. A. (2012). Oxygen-induced hypercapnia in COPD: Myths and facts. *Critical Care, 16*(5), 323. doi:10.1186/cc11475.

50. Shah P. L., Zoumot Z., Singh S., et al. (2013). Endobronchial coils for the treatment of severe emphysema with hyperinflation (RESET). *Lancet Respiratory Medicine, 1*(3), 233–240.

51. Rademacher J., Welte T. (2011). Bronchiectasis: Diagnosis and treatment. *Deutsches Ärzteblatt International, 108*(48), 809–815.

52. Lobo J., Rojas-Balcazar J. M., Noone P. G. (2012). Recent advances in cystic fibrosis. *Clinics in Chest Medicine, 33*(2), 307–328.

53. Jain M., Goss C. H. (2014). Update in cystic fibrosis 2013. *American Journal of Respiratory and Critical Care Medicine, 189*(10), 1181–1186.

54. Cystic Fibrosis Canada. (2013). What is cystic fibrosis? Available online at: http://www.cysticfibrosis.ca/about-cf/what-is-cystic-fibrosis/?lang=en. Accessed June 25, 2014.

55. Harari S., Caminati A. (2010). Update on diffuse parenchymal lung disease. *European Respiratory Review, 19*(116), 97–108.

56. Canadian Pulmonary Fibrosis Foundation. (2014). About pulmonary fibrosis. Available online at: http://www.canadianpulmonaryfibrosis.ca/about-pulmonary-fibrosis. Accessed June 25, 2014.

57. Chen E. S., Moller D. R. (2011). Sarcoidosis: Scientific progress and clinical challenges. *Nature Reviews Rheumatology, 7*(8), 457–467.

58. King T. E., Pardo A., Selman M. (2011). Idiopathic pulmonary fibrosis, *Lancet, 378*(9807), 1949–1961.

59. Rafii R., Juarez M. M., Albertson T. E., et al. (2013). A review of current and novel therapies for idiopathic pulmonary fibrosis. *Journal of Thoracic Disease, 5*(1), 48–73.

60. Kostadima E., Zakynthinos E. (2007). Pulmonary embolism: Pathophysiology, diagnosis, treatment. *Hellenic Journal of Cardiology, 48*(2), 94–107.

61. Agnelli G., Becattini C. (2010). Acute pulmonary embolism. *The New England Journal of Medicine, 363*(3), 266–274.

62. Montagnana M., Cervellin G., Franchini M., et al. (2011). Pathophysiology, clinics and diagnostics of non-thrombotic pulmonary embolism. *Journal of Thrombosis and Thrombolysis, 31*(4), 436–444.

63. Thrombosis Canada. (2014). Clinical guides. Available online at: http://thrombosiscanada.ca. Accessed July 1, 2014.

64. McLaughlin V. V., McGoon M. D. (2006). Pulmonary arterial hypertension. *Circulation, 114*(13), 1417–1431.

65. Kherbeck N., Tamby M.C., Bussone G., et al. (2013). The role of inflammation and autoimmunity in the pathophysiology of pulmonary arterial hypertension. *Clinical Reviews in Allergy & Immunology, 44*(1), 31–38.

66. Pulmonary Hypertension Association of Canada. (2014). About pulmonary hypertension. Available online at: http://www.phacanada.ca/en/about-ph. Accessed July 1, 2014.

67. Nagai T., Kohsaka S., Anzai T., et al. (2012). Low incidence of catheter-related complications in patients with advanced pulmonary arterial hypertension undergoing continuous epoprostenol infusion. *Chest, 141*(1), 272–273.

68. Liu C., Chen J., Gao Y., et al. (2013). Endothelin receptor antagonists for pulmonary arterial hypertension(update). *Cochrane Database of Systematic Reviews, 2*:No. CD004434.

69. Ashbaugh D. G., Bigelow D. B., Petty T. L., et al. (1967). Acute respiratory distress in adults. *Lancet, 2*(7511), 319–323.

70. The ARDS Definition Task Force. (2012). Acute respiratory distress syndrome: The Berlin definition. *The Journal of the American Medical Association, 307*(23), 2526–2533.

71. Rubenfeld G. D., Caldwell E., Peabody E., et al. (2005). Incidence and outcomes of acute lung injury. *The New England Journal of Medicine, 353*(16), 1685–1693.

72. Masclans J. R., Roca O., Muñoz X., et al. (2011). Quality of life, pulmonary function, and tomographic scan abnormalities after ARDS. *Chest, 139*(6), 1340–1346.

73. Moss M., Burnham E. L. (2003). Chronic alcohol abuse, acute respiratory distress syndrome, and multiple organ dysfunction. *Critical Care Medicine, 31*(Suppl 4), S207–S212.

74. Lin Y., Saw C. L., Hannach B., et al. (2012). Transfusion-related acute lung injury prevention measures and their impact at Canadian Blood Services. *Transfusion, 52*(3), 567–574.

75. Sayah D. M., Looney M. R., Toy P. (2012). Transfusion reactions: Newer concepts on the pathophysiology, incidence, treatment, and prevention of transfusion-related acute lung injury. *Critical Care Clinics, 28*(3), 363–372.

76. Villar J. (2011). What is the acute respiratory distress syndrome? *Respiratory Care, 56*(10), 1539–1545.

77. Pierrakos C., Karanikolas M., Scolletta S., et al. (2012). Acute respiratory distress syndrome: Pathophysiology and therapeutic options. *Journal of Clinical Medicine Research, 4*(1), 7–16.

78. Schneider J., Sweberg T. (2013). Acute respiratory failure. *Critical Care Clinics, 29*(2), 167–183.

79. Keenan S. P., Sinuff T., Burns K. E. A., et al. (2011). Clinical practice guidelines for the use of noninvasive positive-pressure ventilation and noninvasive continuous positive airway pressure in the acute care setting. *Canadian Medical Association Journal, 183*(3), E195–E214.

80. Berg K. M., Clardy P., Donnino M. W. (2012). Noninvasive ventilation for acute respiratory failure: A review of the literature and current guidelines. *Internal and Emergency Medicine, 7*(6), 539–545.

Visit thePoint **http://thePoint.lww.com for animations, journal articles, and more!**

Unit VIII

Disorders of Renal Function and Fluids and Electrolytes

Throughout the earlier part of the Middle Ages, one of the major concerns of the physician was examination of the urine. Many physicians of this time thought that most diseases could be diagnosed by careful examination of the urine. Numerous illustrations taken from this period show early physicians holding up flasks of urine to study its colour, cloudiness, and other properties. It was thought that if the cloudiness was at the top of the urine, the problem was in the head, and if it was at the bottom, the problem was in the legs.

From the 16th century on, anatomists began to acquire a fairly good understanding of the gross structure of the kidney, ureters, and bladder. The first great discovery of the minute structures of the kidney was made by Marcello Malpighi (1628–1694), one of the earliest microscopists, who described the ball-shaped structure of the glomerulus. The work of Malpighi was followed by that of Sir William Bowman (1816–1892), who described the urine collecting capsule of the nephron, Bowman's capsule. Bowman also described the relationship between the glomerulus and the tubules. German pathologist Friedrich Henle (1809–1885) described the long U-shaped loop, called the loop of Henle, that contributes to the concentrating abilities of the kidney. Once this structure of the kidney was established, other scientists began to focus on the chemical composition of urine and on the function of the kidney in the regulation of blood pressure.

Structure and Function of the Kidney

It is no exaggeration to say that the composition of the blood is determined not so much by what the mouth takes in as by what the kidneys keep.

—HOMER SMITH, *FROM FISH TO PHILOSOPHER*

The kidneys are remarkable organs. Each is smaller than a person's fist, but in a single day the two organs process approximately 1,700 L of blood and combine its waste products into approximately 1.5 L of urine. As part of their function, the kidneys filter physiologically essential substances, such as sodium (Na^+) and potassium (K^+) ions, from the blood and selectively reabsorb those substances that are needed to maintain the normal composition of internal body fluids. Substances that are not needed or are in excess of those needed for this purpose pass into the urine. In regulating the volume and composition of body fluids, the kidneys perform excretory and endocrine functions. The renin–angiotensin–aldosterone system participates in the regulation of blood pressure and the maintenance of circulating blood volume, and erythropoietin stimulates red blood cell production. The discussion in this chapter focuses on the structure and function of the kidneys, tests of renal function, and the physiologic action of diuretics.

KIDNEY STRUCTURE AND FUNCTION

After completing this section of the chapter, you should be able to meet the following objectives:

- Describe the location and gross structure of the kidney.
- Explain why the kidney receives such a large percentage of the cardiac output and describe the mechanisms for regulating renal blood flow.
- Describe the structure and function of the glomerulus and tubular components of the nephron in terms of regulating the composition of the extracellular fluid compartment.
- Explain the function of sodium in terms of tubular transport mechanisms.
- Describe how the kidney produces concentrated or dilute urine.

- Characterize the function of the juxtaglomerular complex.
- Relate the function of the kidney to drug elimination.
- Explain the endocrine functions of the kidney.
- Relate the sodium reabsorption function of the kidney to the action of diuretics.

Gross Structure and Location

The kidneys are paired, bean-shaped organs that lie outside the peritoneal cavity in the back of the upper abdomen, one on each side of the vertebral column at the level of the 12th thoracic to 3rd lumbar vertebrae (Fig. 30.1). The right kidney normally is situated lower than the left, presumably because of the position of the liver. In the adult, each kidney is approximately 10 to 12 cm long, 5 to 6 cm wide, and 2.5 cm deep, and weighs approximately 113 to 170 g. The medial border of the kidney is indented by a deep fissure called the *hilus*. It is here that blood vessels and nerves enter and leave the kidney. The ureters, which connect the kidneys with the bladder, also enter the kidney at the hilus.

The kidney is a multilobular structure, composed of up to 18 lobes. Each lobe is composed of nephrons, which are the functional units of the kidney. Each nephron has a glomerulus that filters the blood and a system of tubular structures that selectively reabsorb material from the filtrate back into the blood and secrete materials from the blood into the filtrate as urine is being formed.

On longitudinal section, a kidney can be divided into an outer cortex and an inner medulla (Fig. 30.2). The cortex, which is reddish-brown, contains the glomeruli and convoluted tubules of the nephron and blood vessels. The medulla consists of light-coloured, cone-shaped masses—the renal

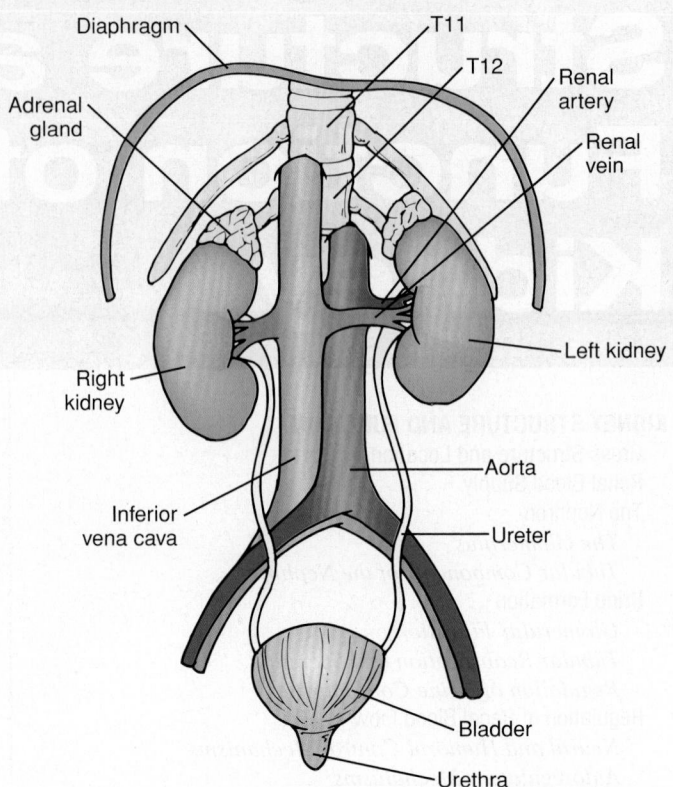

FIGURE 30.1 • Kidneys, ureters, and bladder. (The right kidney is usually lower than the left.)

pyramids—that are divided by the columns of the cortex (columns of Bertin) that extend into the medulla. Each pyramid, topped by a region of cortex, forms a lobe of the kidney. The apices of the pyramids form the papillae (8 to 18 per kidney, corresponding to the number of lobes), which are perforated by the openings of the collecting ducts. The renal pelvis is a

FIGURE 30.2 • Internal structure of the kidney.

wide, funnel-shaped structure at the upper end of the ureter. It is made up of the calyces or cuplike structures that drain the upper and lower halves of the kidney.

The kidney is sheathed in a fibrous external capsule and surrounded by a mass of fatty connective tissue, especially at its ends and borders. The adipose tissue protects the kidney from mechanical blows and assists, together with the attached blood vessels and fascia, in holding the kidney in place. Although the kidneys are relatively well protected, they may be bruised by blows to the loin or by compression between the lower ribs and the ileum. Because the kidneys are located outside the peritoneal cavity, injury and rupture do not produce the same threat of peritoneal involvement as that of other organs such as the liver or spleen.

Renal Blood Supply

Each kidney is supplied by a single renal artery that arises on either side of the aorta. As the renal artery approaches the kidney, it divides into five segmental arteries that enter the hilus of the kidney. In the kidney, each segmental artery branches into several lobular arteries that supply the upper, middle, and lower parts of the kidney. The lobular arteries further subdivide to form the interlobular arteries at the level of the corticomedullary junction (Fig. 30.3). These arteries give off branches, the arcuate arteries, that arch across the top of the pyramids. Small intralobular arteries radiate from the arcuate arteries to supply the cortex of the kidney. The afferent arterioles that supply the glomeruli arise from the intralobular arteries.

Although nearly all the blood flow to the kidneys passes through the cortex, less than 10% is directed to the medulla and only approximately 1% goes to the papillae. Under conditions of decreased perfusion or increased sympathetic nervous system stimulation, blood flow is redistributed away from the cortex toward the medulla. This redistribution of blood flow decreases glomerular filtration while maintaining

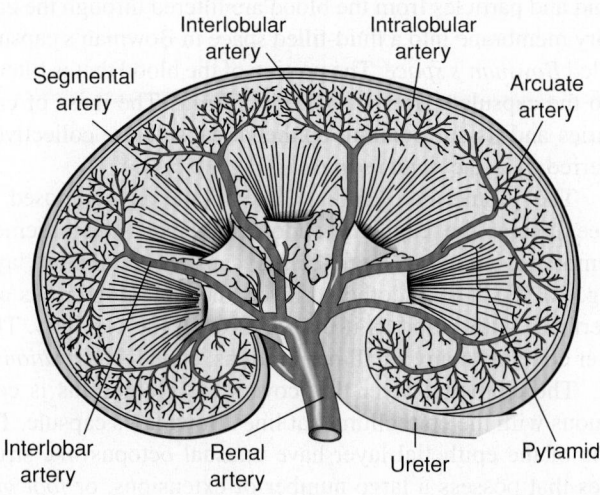

Interlobular artery Intralobular artery
Segmental artery
Arcuate artery
Interlobar artery Renal artery Ureter Pyramid

FIGURE 30.3 • Simplified illustration of the arterial supply of the kidney. (From Cormack D. H. (1987). *Ham's histology* (9th ed.). Philadelphia, PA: J.B. Lippincott.)

the urine-concentrating ability of the kidneys, a factor that is important during conditions such as shock.

The Nephron

Each kidney is composed of 80,000 to 1,000,000 tiny, closely packed functional units called *nephrons* (Fig. 30.4A). The kidney has no ability to regenerate nephrons. Therefore, with aging, there is a generalized decrease in functioning nephrons. In fact, adults tend to lose approximately 10% of their nephrons each decade beginning at 40 years of age.

Each nephron consists of a glomerulus, where blood is filtered, the proximal convoluted tubule, loop of Henle, distal convoluted tubule, and collecting duct. In the tubular network, substances needed to maintain the constancy of the internal environment (*e.g.,* water, nutrients, ions) are reabsorbed into the bloodstream while other, unneeded substances (*e.g.,* acids, creatinine) are secreted into the tubular filtrate for elimination.

Nephrons can be roughly grouped into two categories. Approximately 85% of the nephrons originate in the superficial part of the cortex and are called *cortical nephrons* (Fig. 30.4B). They have short, thick loops of Henle that penetrate only a short distance into the medulla. The remaining 15% are called *juxtamedullary nephrons*. They originate deeper in the cortex and have longer and thinner loops of Henle that penetrate the entire length of the medulla. The juxtamedullary nephrons are largely concerned with urine concentration.

The nephrons are supplied by two capillary systems, the glomerulus and the peritubular capillary network (Fig. 30.4A). The *glomerulus* is a unique, high-pressure capillary filtration system located between two arterioles, the afferent and the efferent arterioles. Because the arterioles are high-resistance vessels and the afferent arteriole has a larger diameter than the efferent arteriole, the blood pressure in the glomerulus is extraordinarily high for a capillary bed and easily forces fluid and solutes out of the blood into the glomerular capillary along its entire length. The *peritubular capillaries* originate from the efferent arteriole. They are low-pressure vessels that are adapted for reabsorption rather than filtration. These capillaries surround all portions of the tubules, an arrangement that permits rapid movement of solutes and water between the fluid in the tubular lumen and the blood in the capillaries. In the deepest part of the renal cortex, the efferent arterioles serving the juxtaglomerular also continue into long, thin-walled looping vessels called the *vasa recta*. The vasa recta accompany the long loops of Henle in the medullary portion of the kidney to assist in exchange of substances flowing in and out of that portion of the kidney. The peritubular capillaries rejoin to form the venous channels by which blood leaves the kidneys and empties into the inferior vena cava.

The Glomerulus

The glomerulus consists of a compact tuft of capillaries encased in a thin, double-walled capsule called *Bowman's capsule.* Blood flows into the glomerular capillaries from the afferent arteriole and flows out of the glomerular capillaries into the efferent arteriole, which leads into the peritubular capillaries.

FIGURE 30.4 • **A:** Nephron, showing the glomerular and tubular structures along with the blood supply.
B: Comparison of differences in location of tubular structures of the cortical and juxtamedullary nephrons.

THE NEPHRON

- The nephron, which is the functional unit of the kidney, is composed of a vascular component, which connects to the circulatory system, and a tubular component, which has connections to both the circulatory system and the elimination functions of the kidney.
- The vascular component of the nephron consists of two arterioles closely associated with two capillary beds: the glomerulus (where water-soluble nutrients, wastes, and other small particles are filtered from the blood) and the peritubular capillaries (which surround the tubular structures).
- The tubular portion of the nephron processes the glomerular filtrate (urine), facilitating the reabsorption of substances from the tubular fluid into the peritubular capillaries and the secretion of substances from the peritubular capillaries into the urine filtrate.

Fluid and particles from the blood are filtered through the capillary membrane into a fluid-filled space in Bowman's capsule, called *Bowman's space*. The portion of the blood that is filtered into the capsule space is called the *filtrate*. The mass of capillaries and its surrounding epithelial capsule are collectively referred to as the *renal corpuscle* (Fig. 30.5A).

The glomerular capillary membrane is composed of three layers: the capillary endothelial layer, the basement membrane, and the single-celled capsular epithelial layer (Fig. 30.5B). The endothelial layer lines the glomerulus and interfaces with blood as it moves through the capillary. This layer contains many small perforations, called *fenestrations*.

The epithelial layer that covers the glomerulus is continuous with the epithelium that lines Bowman's capsule. The cells of the epithelial layer have unusual octopus-like structures that possess a large number of extensions, or *foot processes (i.e., podocytes)*, which are embedded in the basement membrane (Fig. 30.5B). These foot processes form *slit pores* through which the glomerular filtrate passes.

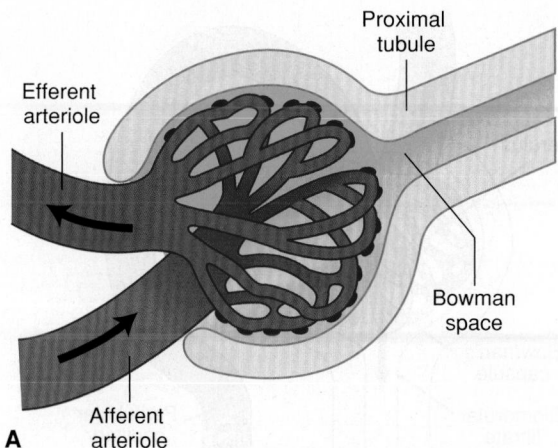

Efferent arteriole

Proximal tubule

Bowman space

Afferent arteriole

A

Mesangial matrix   Mesangial cell

Epithelial podocytes

Endothelial cell

Basement membrane

Glomerular capsule   Bowman space

B

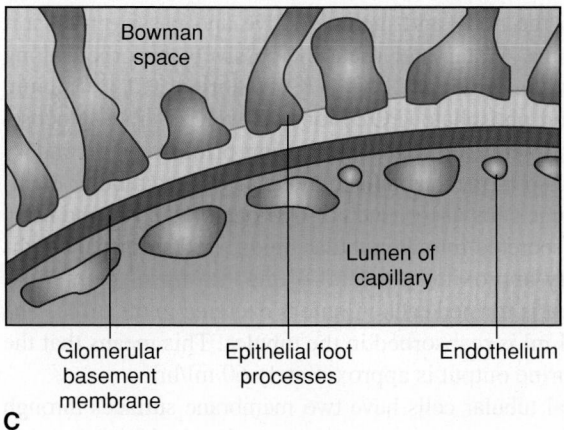

Bowman space

Lumen of capillary

Glomerular basement membrane   Epithelial foot processes   Endothelium

C

FIGURE 30.5 • Renal corpuscle. **A:** Structures of the glomerulus. **B:** Cross section of the glomerular membrane showing the position of the endothelium, basement membrane, and epithelial foot processes. **C:** Position of the mesangial cells in relation to the capillary loops and Bowman capsule.

The basement membrane consists of a homogeneous acellular meshwork of collagen fibres, glycoproteins, and mucopolysaccharides (Fig. 30.5C). Because the endothelial and epithelial layers of the glomerular capillary have porous structures, the basement membrane determines the permeability of the glomerular capillary membrane. The spaces between the fibres that make up the basement membrane represent the pores of a filter and determine the size-dependent permeability barrier of the glomerulus. The size of the pores in the basement membrane normally prevents red blood cells and plasma proteins from passing through the glomerular membrane into the filtrate. There is evidence that the epithelium plays a major role in producing the basement membrane components, and the epithelial cells probably are active in forming new basement membrane material throughout life. Alterations in the structure and function of the glomerular basement membrane are responsible for the leakage of proteins and blood cells into the filtrate that occurs in many forms of glomerular disease.

Another important component of the glomerulus is the *mesangium.* In some areas, the capillary endothelium and the basement membrane do not completely surround each capillary. Instead, the mesangial cells, which lie between the capillary tufts, provide support for the glomerulus in these areas (Fig. 30.5B). The mesangial cells produce an intercellular substance similar to that of the basement membrane. This substance covers the endothelial cells where they are not covered by basement membrane. The mesangial cells possess (or can develop) phagocytic properties and remove macromolecular materials that enter the intercapillary spaces. Mesangial cells also exhibit contractile properties in response to neurohumoural substances and are thought to contribute to the regulation of blood flow through the glomerulus. In normal glomeruli, the mesangial area is narrow and contains only a small number of cells. Mesangial hyperplasia and increased mesangial matrix occur in a number of glomerular diseases.

Tubular Components of the Nephron

The nephron tubule is divided into four segments: a highly coiled segment called the *proximal convoluted tubule,* which drains Bowman's capsule; a thin, looped structure called the *loop of Henle;* a distal coiled portion called the *distal convoluted tubule;* and the final segment, called the *collecting tubule,* which joins with several tubules to collect the filtrate. The filtrate passes through each of these segments before reaching the pelvis of the kidney.

The proximal tubule is a highly coiled structure that dips toward the renal pelvis to become the descending limb of the loop of Henle. The ascending loop of Henle returns to the region of the renal corpuscle, where it becomes the distal tubule. The distal convoluted tubule, which begins at the juxtaglomerular complex, is divided into two segments: the *diluting segment* and the *late distal tubule.* The late distal tubule fuses with the collecting tubule. Like the distal tubule, the collecting duct is divided into two segments: the *cortical collecting tubule* and the *inner medullary collecting tubule.*

Throughout its course, the tubule is composed of a single layer of epithelial cells resting on a basement membrane. The structure of the epithelial cells varies with tubular function. The cells of the proximal tubule have a fine, villous structure that increases the surface area for reabsorption; they also are rich in mitochondria, which support active transport processes. The epithelial layer of the thin segment of the loop of Henle has few mitochondria, indicating minimal metabolic activity and reabsorptive function.

Urine Formation

Urine formation involves the filtration of blood by the glomerulus to form an *ultrafiltrate of urine* and the tubular reabsorption of electrolytes and nutrients needed to maintain the constancy of the internal environment while eliminating waste materials.

Glomerular Filtration

Urine formation begins with the filtration of essentially protein-free plasma through the glomerular capillaries into Bowman's space. The movement of fluid through the glomerular capillaries is determined by the same factors (*i.e.,* capillary filtration pressure, colloidal osmotic pressure, and capillary permeability) that affect fluid movement through other capillaries in the body (see Chapter 21). The glomerular filtrate has a chemical composition similar to plasma, but it contains almost no proteins because large molecules do not readily cross the glomerular wall. Approximately 125 ml of filtrate is formed each minute. This is called the *glomerular filtration rate (GFR)*. This rate can vary from a few millilitres per minute to as much as 200 ml/min.

The location of the glomerulus between two arterioles allows for maintenance of a high-pressure filtration system. The capillary filtration pressure (approximately 60 mm Hg) in the glomerulus is approximately two to three times higher than that of other capillary beds in the body. The filtration pressure and the GFR are regulated by the constriction and relaxation of the afferent and efferent arterioles. Constriction of the efferent arteriole increases resistance to outflow from the glomeruli and increases the glomerular pressure and the GFR. Constriction of the afferent arteriole causes a reduction in the renal blood flow, glomerular filtration pressure, and GFR. The afferent and the efferent arterioles are innervated by the sympathetic nervous system and are sensitive to vasoactive hormones or substances, such as angiotensin II, or endothelin. During periods of intense sympathetic stimulation, such as shock, constriction of the afferent arteriole causes a marked decrease in renal blood flow and thus glomerular filtration pressure. Consequently, urine output can fall almost to zero.

Tubular Reabsorption and Secretion

From Bowman's capsule, the glomerular filtrate moves into the tubular segments of the nephron. In its movement through the lumen of the tubular segments, the glomerular filtrate is changed considerably by the tubular transport of water and solutes. Tubular transport can result in reabsorption of substances from the tubular fluid into the peritubular capillaries or secretion of substances into the tubular fluid from the blood in the peritubular capillaries (Fig. 30.6).

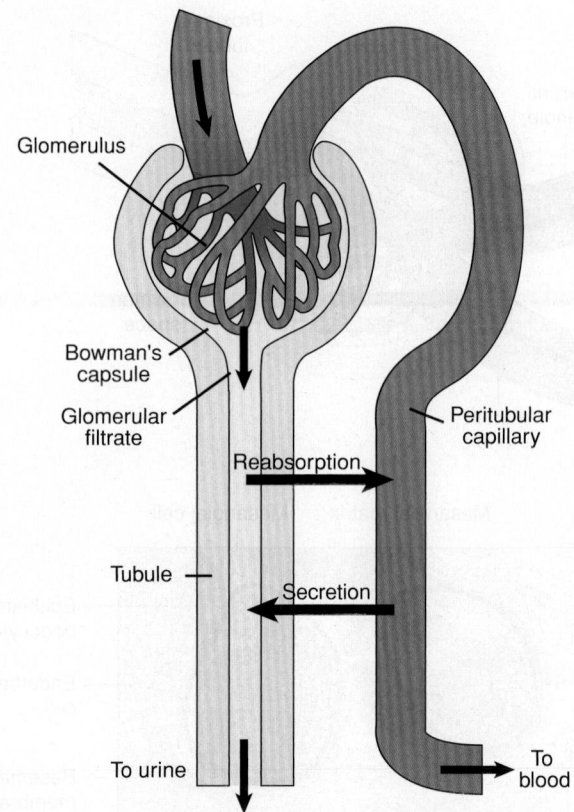

FIGURE 30.6 • Reabsorption and secretion of substances between the renal tubules and peritubular capillaries.

The basic mechanisms of transport across the tubular epithelial cell membrane are similar to those of other cell membranes in the body and include active and passive transport mechanisms. Water and urea are passively absorbed along concentration gradients. Na^+, K^+, chloride (Cl^-), calcium (Ca^{2+}), and phosphate (PO_4^-) ions, as well as urate, glucose, and amino acids are reabsorbed using primary or secondary active transport mechanisms to move across the tubular membrane. Some substances, such as hydrogen (H^+), K^+, and urate ions, are secreted into the tubular fluids. Under normal conditions, only approximately 1 ml of the 125 ml of glomerular filtrate that is formed each minute is excreted in the urine. The other 124 ml is reabsorbed in the tubules. This means that the average urine output is approximately 60 ml/hr.

Renal tubular cells have two membrane surfaces through which substances must pass as they are reabsorbed from the tubular fluid. The outside membrane that lies adjacent to the interstitial fluid is called the *basolateral membrane,* and the side that is in contact with the tubular lumen and tubular filtrate is called the *luminal membrane.* In most cases, substances move from the tubular filtrate into the tubular cell along a concentration gradient, but they require facilitated transport or carrier systems to move across the basolateral membrane into the interstitial fluid, where they are absorbed into the peritubular capillaries.

The bulk of energy used by the kidney is for active sodium transport mechanisms that facilitate sodium reabsorption and

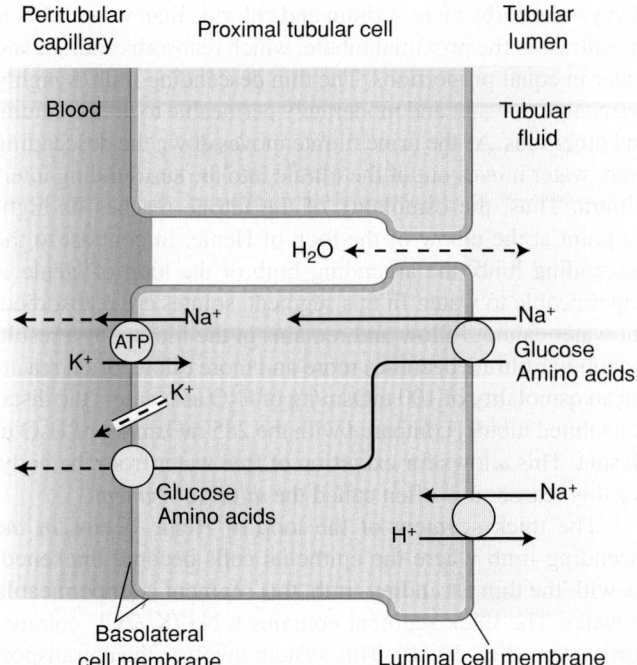

FIGURE 30.7 • Mechanism for secondary active transport or cotransport of glucose and amino acids in the proximal tubule. The energy-dependent sodium-potassium pump on the basal lateral surface of the cell maintains a low intracellular gradient that facilitates the downhill movement of sodium and glucose or amino acids (cotransport) from the tubular lumen into the tubular cell and then into the peritubular capillary.

cotransport of other electrolytes and substances such as glucose and amino acids. This is called *secondary active transport* or *cotransport* (Fig. 30.7). Secondary active transport depends on the energy-dependent Na^+/K^+-adenosine triphosphatase (ATPase) pump on the basolateral side of renal tubular cells. The pump maintains a low intracellular sodium concentration that facilitates the downhill (*i.e.*, from a higher to lower

concentration) movement of sodium from the filtrate across the luminal membrane. Cotransport uses a carrier system in which the downhill movement of one substance such as sodium is coupled to the uphill movement (*i.e.*, from a lower to higher concentration) of another substance such as glucose or an amino acid. A few substances, such as the H^+ ion, are secreted into the tubule using countertransport, in which the movement of one substance, such as sodium, enables the movement of a second substance in the opposite direction.

Proximal Tubule. Approximately 65% of all reabsorptive and secretory processes that occur in the tubular system take place in the proximal tubule. There is almost complete reabsorption of nutritionally important substances, such as glucose, amino acids, lactate, and water-soluble vitamins (Fig. 30.8). Electrolytes, such as Na^+, K^+, Cl^-, and bicarbonate (HCO_3^-), are 65% to 90% reabsorbed. As these solutes move into the tubular cells, their concentration in the tubular lumen decreases, providing a concentration gradient for the osmotic reabsorption of water and urea. The proximal tubule is highly permeable to water, and the osmotic movement of water occurs so rapidly that the concentration difference of solutes on either side of the membrane seldom is more than a few milliosmoles.

Many substances, such as glucose, are freely filtered in the glomerulus and reabsorbed by energy-dependent cotransport carrier mechanisms. The maximum amount of substance that these transport systems can reabsorb per unit time is called the *transport maximum*. The transport maximum is related to the number of carrier proteins (*i.e.*, sodium-glucose cotransporters [SGLT] 1, SGLT2) that are available for transport and usually is sufficient to ensure that all of a filtered substance such as glucose can be reabsorbed rather than being eliminated in the urine. The plasma level at which the substance appears in the urine is called the *renal threshold* (Fig. 30.9). Under some circumstances, the amount of substance filtered in the glomerulus exceeds the transport maximum. For example, when the

FIGURE 30.8 • Sites of tubular water (H_2O), glucose, amino acids, Na+ (sodium), Cl^- (chloride), HCO_3^- (bicarbonate), K^+ (potassium), Ca^{2+} (calcium), and Mg^{2+} (magnesium) reabsorption; and organic acids and bases, H^+ (hydrogen), and K^+ secretion.

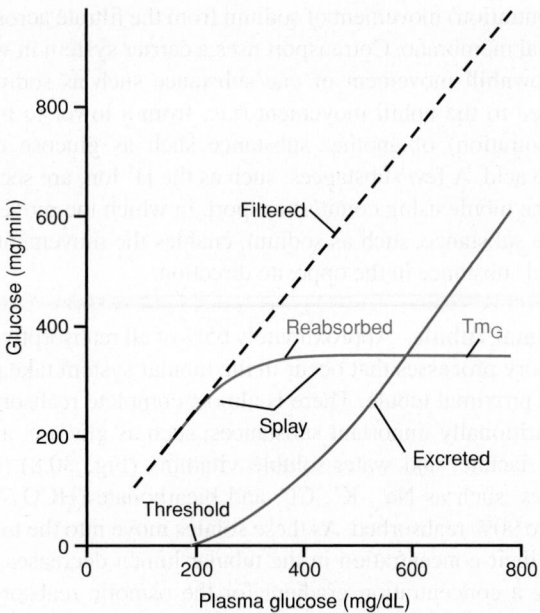

FIGURE 30.9 • Relations among the filtered load of glucose (*broken line*), the rate of glucose reabsorption by the renal tubules (*red line*), and the rate of glucose excretion in the urine (*new colour line*). The tubular transport maximum for glucose (Tm$_G$) is the maximum rate at which glucose can be reabsorbed from the tubules. The *threshold* for glucose refers to the filtered load of glucose at which glucose first begins to appear in the urine. The splay or rounding of the graph represents the fact that some nephrons reach their tubular maximum before others do. Note: Conversion to SI units—200 mg/dL = 11.1 mmol/L; 400 mg/dL = 22.2 mmol/L; 600 mg/dL = 33.3 mmol/L. (From Rhoades R. A., Bell D. R. (2013). *Medical physiology*. (4th ed., p. 406). Philadelphia, PA: Lippincott Williams & Wilkins.)

blood glucose level is elevated in uncontrolled diabetes mellitus, the amount that is filtered in the glomerulus may exceed the transport maximum at approximately 18 mmol/L, and glucose spills into the urine.

In addition to *reabsorbing* solutes and water, cells in the proximal tubule also *secrete* organic cations and anions into the urine filtrate (Figs. 30.6 and 30.8). Many of these organic anions and cations are end products of metabolism (*e.g.,* urate, oxalate) that circulate in the plasma. The proximal tubule also secretes exogenous organic compounds such as penicillin, aspirin, and morphine. Many of these compounds can be bound to plasma proteins and are not freely filtered in the glomerulus. Therefore, excretion by filtration alone eliminates only a small portion of these potentially toxic substances from the body.

The Loop of Henle. The loop of Henle plays an important role in controlling the concentration of the urine. It does this by establishing a high concentration of osmotically active particles in the interstitium surrounding the medullary collecting tubules where the antidiuretic hormone (ADH) exerts its effects (to be discussed).

The loop of Henle is divided into three segments: the thin descending segment, the thin ascending segment, and thick ascending segment. The loop of Henle, taken as a whole, always reabsorbs more sodium and chloride than water. This is in contrast to the proximal tubule, which reabsorbs sodium and water in equal proportions. The thin descending limb is highly permeable to water and moderately permeable to urea, sodium, and other ions. As the urine filtrate moves down the descending limb, water moves out of the filtrate into the surrounding interstitium. Thus, the osmolality of the filtrate reaches its highest point at the elbow of the loop of Henle. In contrast to the descending limb, the ascending limb of the loop of Henle is impermeable to water. In this segment, solutes are reabsorbed, but water cannot follow and remains in the filtrate; as a result, the tubular filtrate becomes more and more dilute, often reaching an osmolality of 100 mOsm/kg of H$_2$O as it enters the distal convoluted tubule, compared with the 285 mOsm/kg of H$_2$O in plasma. This allows for excretion of free water from the body. For this reason, it is often called the *diluting segment.*

The thick segment of the loop of Henle begins in the ascending limb where the epithelial cells become thickened. As with the thin ascending limb, this segment is impermeable to water. The thick segment contains a Na$^+$/K$^+$/2Cl$^-$ cotransport system (Fig. 30.10). This system involves the cotransport of a positively charged Na$^+$ and a positively charged K$^+$ ion accompanied by two negatively charged Cl$^-$ ions. The gradient for the operation of this cotransport system is provided by the basolateral Na$^+$/K$^+$-ATPase pump, which maintains a low intracellular sodium concentration. Approximately 20% to 25% of the filtered load of sodium, potassium, and chloride is reabsorbed in the thick loop of Henle. Movement of these ions out of the tubule leads to the development of a transmembrane potential that favours the passive reabsorption of small divalent cations such as calcium and magnesium. The thick

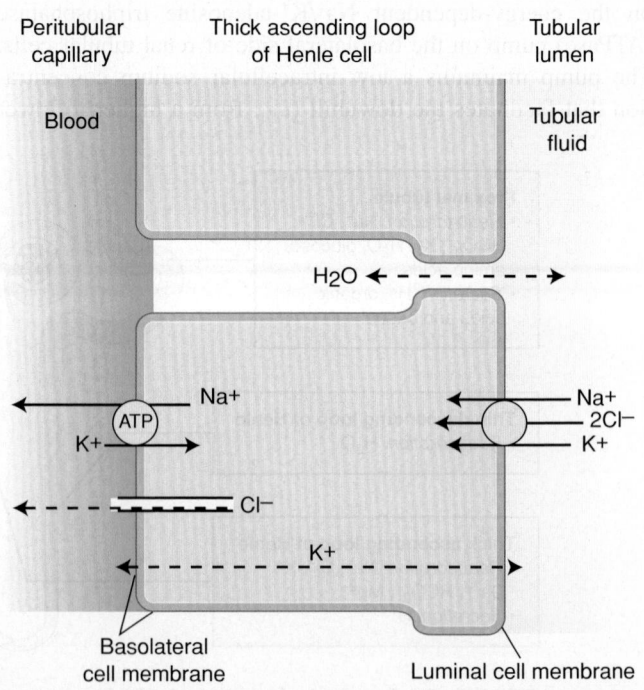

FIGURE 30.10 • Sodium, chloride, and potassium reabsorption in the thick segment of the loop of Henle.

ascending loop of Henle is the site of the powerful "loop" diuretics (*e.g.,* furosemide [Lasix]), which exert their action by inhibiting the $Na^+/K^+/2Cl^-$ cotransporters (to be discussed).

Distal and Collecting Tubules. Like the thick ascending loop of Henle, the distal convoluted tubule is relatively impermeable to water, and reabsorption of sodium chloride from this segment further dilutes the tubular fluid. Sodium reabsorption occurs through a Na^+/Cl^- cotransport mechanism. Approximately 5% of filtered sodium chloride is reabsorbed in this section of the tubule. Unlike the thick ascending loop of Henle, neither Ca^{2+} nor Mg^{2+} is passively absorbed in this segment of the tubule. Instead, Ca^{2+} ions are actively reabsorbed in a process that is largely regulated by parathyroid hormone and possibly by vitamin D. The thiazide diuretics (to be discussed) exert their action by inhibiting sodium chloride reabsorption in this segment of the renal tubules.

The late distal tubule and the cortical collecting tubule constitute the site where aldosterone exerts its action on sodium reabsorption and potassium secretion and elimination. Although responsible for only 2% to 5% of sodium chloride reabsorption, this site is largely responsible for determining the final sodium concentration of the urine. The late distal tubule with the cortical collecting tubule also is the major site for regulation of potassium excretion by the kidney. When the body is confronted with a potassium excess, as occurs with a diet high in potassium content, the amount of potassium secreted at this site may exceed the amount filtered in the glomerulus.

The mechanism for sodium reabsorption and potassium secretion in this section of the nephron is distinct from other tubular segments. This tubular segment is composed of two types of cells, the *intercalated cells,* where potassium is reabsorbed and hydrogen is secreted, and the *principal cells,* where aldosterone exerts its action. The secretion of H^+ ions into the tubular fluid by the intercalated cells is accompanied by the reabsorption of HCO_3^- ions. The intercalated cells can also reabsorb K^+ ions. The principal cells reabsorb Na^+ and facilitate the movement of K^+ into the urine filtrate (Fig. 30.11). Under the influence of aldosterone, sodium moves from the urine filtrate into principal cells; from there, it moves into the surrounding interstitial fluid and peritubular capillaries. Potassium moves from the peritubular capillaries into the principal cells and then into the urine filtrate.

Regulation of Urine Concentration

The kidney responds to changes in the osmolality of the extracellular fluids by producing either concentrated or dilute urine. The ability of the kidney to respond in this manner depends on the establishment of a high concentration of osmotically active particles (approximately 1,200 mOsm/kg of H_2O) in the interstitium of the kidney medulla and the action of the antidiuretic hormone (ADH) in regulating the water permeability of the surrounding medullary collecting tubules (see Understanding How the Kidney Concentrates Urine).

In approximately one fifth of the juxtamedullary nephrons, the loops of Henle and special hairpin-shaped capillaries

FIGURE 30.11 • Mechanism of sodium reabsorption and potassium secretion by principal cells of the late distal and collecting tubules. Aldosterone exerts its action by increasing the activity of the Na^+/K^+-ATPase pump that transports sodium outward through the basolateral membrane of the cell and into the blood at the same time it pumps potassium into the cell. Aldosterone also increases the permeability of the luminal membrane for potassium.

called the *vasa recta* descend into the medullary portion of the kidney, forming a countercurrent system that controls water and solute movement so that water is kept out of the area surrounding the tubule and solutes are retained. The term *countercurrent* refers to a flow of fluids in opposite directions in adjacent structures. In this case, there is an exchange of solutes between the adjacent descending and ascending loops of Henle and between the ascending and descending sections of the vasa recta. Because of these exchange processes, a high concentration of osmotically active particles (approximately 1,200 mOsm/kg of H_2O) collects in the interstitium of the kidney medulla. The presence of these osmotically active particles in the interstitium surrounding the medullary collecting tubules facilitates the ADH-mediated reabsorption of water.

ADH assists in maintenance of the extracellular fluid volume by controlling the permeability of the medullary collecting tubules. Osmoreceptors, located in the hypothalamus, sense an increase in osmolality of extracellular fluids and stimulate the release of ADH from the posterior pituitary gland. In exerting its effect, ADH, also known as *vasopressin,* binds to receptors on the basolateral side of the tubular cells. Binding of ADH to the vasopressin receptors causes water channels, known as *aquaporin-2 channels,* to move into the luminal side of the tubular cell membrane, producing a marked increase in water permeability. At the basolateral side of the membrane, water exits the tubular cell into the hyperosmotic interstitium of the medullary area, where it enters the

Understanding How the Kidney Concentrates Urine

The osmolarity of body fluids relies heavily on the ability of the kidney to produce dilute or concentrated urine. Urine concentration depends on three factors: (1) the osmolarity of interstitial fluids in the urine-concentrating part of the kidney, (2) the antidiuretic hormone (ADH), and (3) the action of ADH on the cells in the collecting tubules of the kidney.

1. Osmolarity

In approximately one fifth of the juxtamedullary nephrons, the loops of Henle and special hairpin-shaped capillaries called the vasa recta descend into the medullary portion of the kidney to form a countercurrent system—a set of parallel passages in which the contents flow in opposite directions. The countercurrent design serves to increase the osmolarity in this part of the kidney by promoting the exchange of solutes between the adjacent descending and ascending loops of Henle and between the descending and ascending sections of the vasa recta. Because of these exchange processes, a high concentration of osmotically active particles (approximately 1,200 mOsm/kg of H_2O) collects in the interstitium surrounding the collecting tubules where the ADH-mediated reabsorption of water takes place.

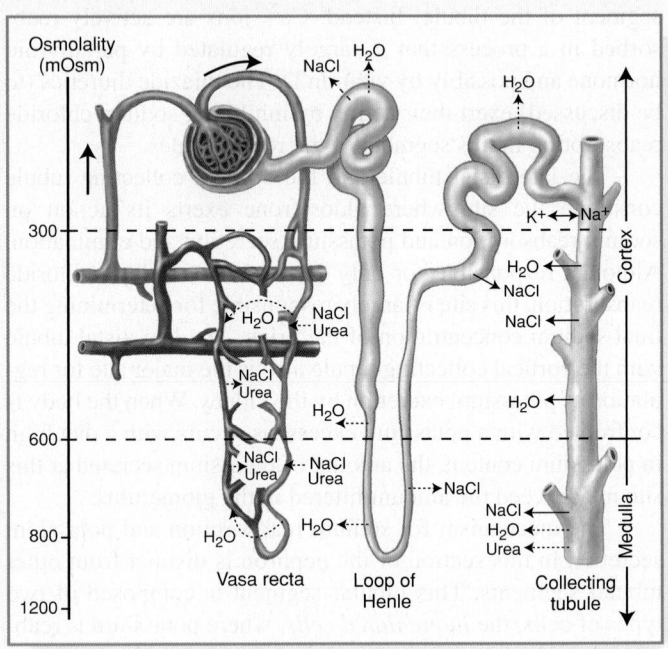

2. Antidiuretic Hormone

ADH, which regulates the ability of the kidneys to concentrate urine, is synthesized by neurons in the hypothalamus and transported down their axons to the posterior pituitary gland and then released into the circulation. One of the main stimuli for synthesis and release of ADH is an increase in serum osmolarity. ADH release is also controlled by cardiovascular reflexes that respond to changes in blood pressure or blood volume.

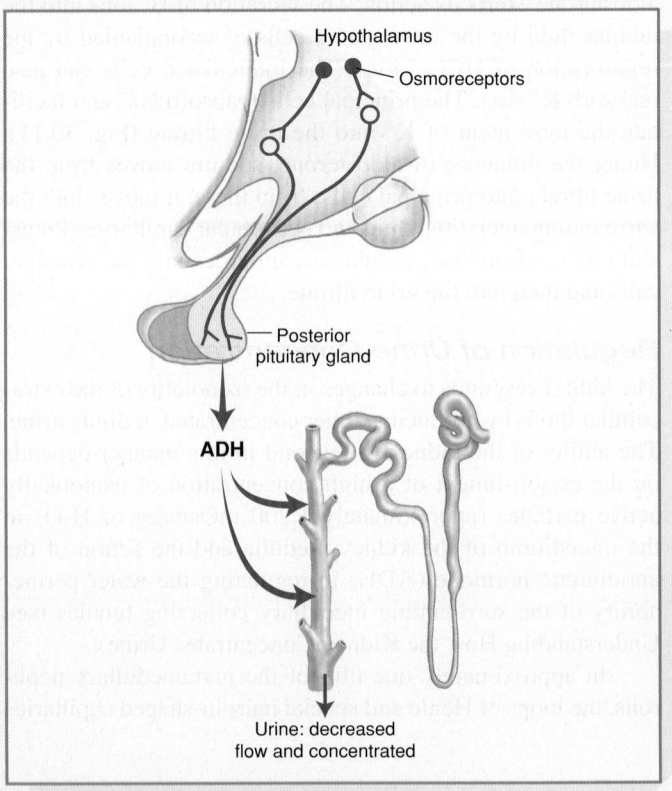

3. Action of ADH

ADH, also known as vasopressin, acts at the level of the collecting tubule to increase water absorption. It exerts its action by binding to vasopressin receptors on the basolateral membrane of the tubular cell. Binding of ADH to the vasopressin receptors causes water channels (aquaporin-2 channels) to move into the luminal side of the cell membrane, which is normally impermeable to water. Insertion of the channels allows water from the tubular fluids to move into the tubular cell and then out into the surrounding hyperosmotic interstitial fluid on the basolateral side of the cell, and from there it moves into the peritubular capillaries for return to the circulatory system. Thus, when ADH is present, the water that moved from the blood into the urine filtrate in the glomeruli is returned to the circulatory system, and when ADH is absent, the water is excreted in the urine.

peritubular capillaries for return to the vascular system. The aquaporin-2 channels are thought to have a critical role in inherited and acquired disorders of water reabsorption by the kidney (*e.g.,* diabetes insipidus).

Regulation of Renal Blood Flow

In the adult, the kidneys are perfused with 1,000 to 1,300 ml of blood per minute, or 20% to 25% of the cardiac output. This large blood flow is mainly needed to ensure a sufficient GFR for the removal of waste products from the blood, rather than for the metabolic needs of the kidney. Feedback mechanisms, both intrinsic (*e.g.,* autoregulation, local hormones) and extrinsic (*e.g.,* sympathetic nervous system, systemic hormones), normally keep blood flow and GFR constant despite changes in arterial blood pressure.

Neural and Humoral Control Mechanisms

The kidney is richly innervated by the sympathetic nervous system. Increased sympathetic activity causes constriction of the afferent and efferent arterioles and thus a decrease in renal blood flow. Intense sympathetic stimulation such as occurs in shock and trauma can produce marked decreases in renal blood flow and GFR, even to the extent of causing blood flow to cease altogether.

Several humoral substances, including angiotensin II, ADH, and the endothelins, produce vasoconstriction of renal vessels. The endothelins are a group of peptides released from damaged endothelial cells in the kidney and other tissues. Although not thought to be an important regulator of renal blood flow during everyday activities, endothelin I may play a role in reduction of blood flow in conditions such as post-ischemic acute renal failure (see Chapter 34). In this situation endothelin is a potent vasoconstrictor and can exacerbate the acute renal failure.

Other substances such as dopamine, nitric oxide, and prostaglandins (*i.e.,* E_2 and I_2) produce vasodilation. Nitric oxide, a vasodilator produced by the vascular endothelium, appears to be important in preventing excessive vasoconstriction of renal blood vessels and allowing normal excretion of sodium and water. Prostaglandins are a group of mediators of cell function that are produced locally and exert their effects locally. Although prostaglandins do not appear to be of major importance in regulating renal blood flow and GFR under normal conditions, they may protect the kidneys against the vasoconstricting effects of sympathetic stimulation and angiotensin II. Nonsteroidal anti-inflammatory drugs (NSAIDs) that inhibit prostaglandin synthesis may cause reduction in renal blood flow and GFR under certain conditions risking the development of renal impairment or failure.

Autoregulatory Mechanisms

The constancy of renal blood flow is maintained by a process called *autoregulation*. Normally, autoregulation of blood flow is designed to maintain blood flow at a level consistent with the metabolic needs of the tissues. In the kidney, autoregulation of blood flow also allows for precise regulation of solute and water excretion. For autoregulation to occur, the resistance to blood flow through the kidneys must be varied in direct proportion to the arterial pressure. The exact mechanisms responsible for the intrarenal regulation of blood flow are unclear. One of the proposed mechanisms is a direct effect on vascular smooth muscle that causes the blood vessels to relax when there is an increase in blood pressure, and to constrict when there is a decrease in pressure. A second proposed mechanism is the juxtaglomerular complex or apparatus.

The Juxtaglomerular Apparatus. The juxtaglomerular apparatus (JGA) is thought to represent a feedback control system that links changes in the GFR with renal blood flow. The JGA is located at the site where the distal tubule extends back to the glomerulus and passes between the afferent and efferent arterioles (Fig. 30.12A). The distal tubular site that is nearest the glomerulus is characterized by densely nucleated cells called the *macula densa*. In the adjacent afferent arteriole, the smooth muscle cells of the media are modified as special secretory cells called *juxtaglomerular cells*. These cells contain granules of inactive renin, an enzyme that functions in the conversion of angiotensinogen to angiotensin. Renin functions by means of angiotensin II to produce vasoconstriction of the efferent arteriole as a means of preventing large decreases in the GFR. Angiotensin II also increases sodium reabsorption indirectly by stimulating aldosterone secretion from the adrenal gland, and directly by increasing sodium reabsorption by the proximal tubule cells.

Because of its location between the afferent and efferent arterioles, the JGA plays an essential feedback role in linking the level of arterial blood pressure and renal blood flow to the GFR and fine-tuning the composition of the distal tubular fluid (Fig. 30.12B). It is thought to monitor the systemic arterial blood pressure by sensing the stretch of the afferent arteriole and the concentration of sodium chloride in the tubular filtrate as it passes through the macula densa. This information is then used in determining how much renin should be released to keep the arterial blood pressure in its normal range and maintain a relatively constant GFR. Studies suggest that a decrease in the GFR slows the flow rate of the urine filtrate in the ascending loop of Henle, thereby increasing sodium and chloride reabsorption. This, in turn, decreases the delivery of sodium chloride to the macula densa. The decrease in delivery of sodium chloride to the macula densa has two effects: it decreases resistance in the afferent arterioles, which raises glomerular filtration pressure, and it increases the release of renin from the juxtaglomerular cells. The renin from these cells functions as an enzyme to convert angiotensinogen to angiotensin I, which is converted to angiotensin II (see Chapter 23, Fig. 23.4). Finally, angiotensin II acts to constrict the efferent arteriole as a means of producing a further increase in the glomerular filtration pressure and thereby returning the GFR to a more normal range.

A

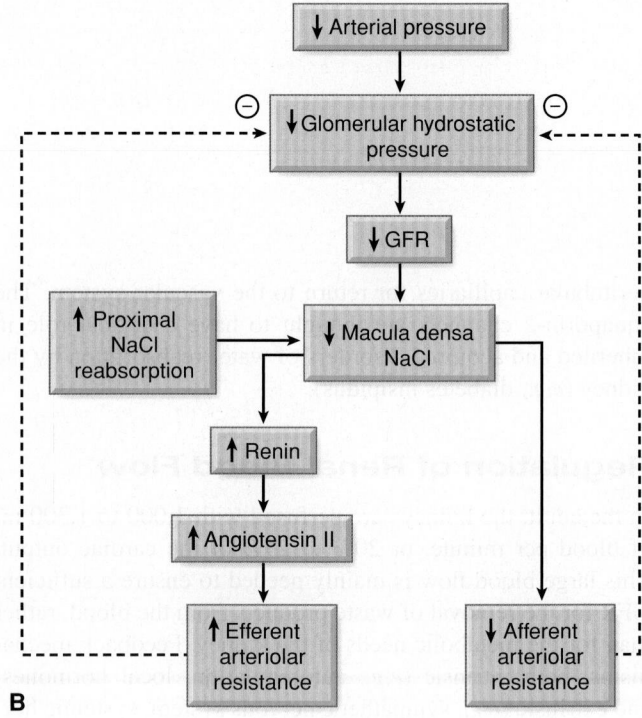

B

FIGURE 30.12 • **A:** Juxtaglomerular apparatus, showing the close contact of the distal tubule with the afferent arteriole, the macula densa, and the juxtaglomerular cells. **B:** Flow chart depicting the macula densa feedback mechanism for autoregulation of glomerular hydrostatic pressure and glomerular filtration rate (GFR) during changes in renal arterial pressure. (From Hall J. E. (2011). *Textbook of medical physiology* (12th ed., p. 320). Philadelphia, PA: Elsevier Saunders.)

Effect of Increased Protein and Glucose

Even though renal blood flow and glomerular filtration are relatively stable under most conditions, two conditions can increase renal blood flow and glomerular filtration. These are an increased amount of protein in the diet and an increase in blood glucose. With ingestion of a high-protein diet, renal blood flow increases 20% to 30% within 1 to 2 hours. Although the exact mechanism for this increase is uncertain, it is thought to be related to the fact that amino acids and sodium are absorbed together in the proximal tubule (secondary active transport). As a result, delivery of sodium to the macula densa is decreased, which elicits an increase in renal blood flow through the JGA feedback mechanism. The resultant increase in blood flow and GFR allows sodium excretion to be maintained at a near-normal level while increasing the excretion of the waste products of protein metabolism, such as urea. The same mechanism is thought to explain the large increases in renal blood flow and GFR that occur with high blood glucose levels in persons with uncontrolled diabetes mellitus.

Elimination Functions of the Kidney

The functions of the kidney focus on elimination of water, waste products, excess electrolytes, and unwanted substances from the blood. Blood tests can provide valuable information about the kidneys' ability to remove metabolic wastes and maintain the blood's normal electrolyte and pH composition. As renal function declines, there is an increase in serum levels of substances such as urea, creatinine, phosphate, and potassium. The effect of renal failure on the concentration of serum electrolytes and metabolic end products is discussed in Chapter 34.

Renal Clearance

Renal clearance is the volume of plasma that is completely cleared each minute of any substance that finds its way into the urine. It is determined by the ability of the substance to be filtered in the glomeruli and the capacity of the renal tubules to reabsorb or secrete the substance. Every substance has its own clearance rate, the units of which are always stated in terms of volume of plasma per unit time. It can be determined by measuring the amount of a substance that is excreted in the urine (*i.e.,* urine concentration × urine flow rate in millilitres per minute) and dividing by its plasma concentration. Inulin (not to be confused with insulin) is a large polysaccharide which is freely filtered in the glomeruli and neither reabsorbed nor secreted by the tubular cells. After intravenous injection, the amount that appears in the urine is equal to the amount that is filtered in the glomeruli (*i.e.,* the clearance rate is equal to the GFR). Because of these properties, inulin can be used as a laboratory measure of the GFR. Some substances, such as urea, are freely filtered in the glomeruli, but the volume that is cleared from the plasma is less than the GFR, indicating that at least some of the substance is being reabsorbed. At normal plasma levels, glucose has a clearance of zero because it is reabsorbed in the tubules and none should appear in the urine.

Regulation of Sodium and Potassium Elimination

Elimination of sodium and potassium is regulated by the GFR and by Humoral agents that control their reabsorption. Aldosterone functions in the regulation of sodium and potassium

elimination. Atrial natriuretic peptide (ANP) contributes to the regulation of sodium elimination. Sodium reabsorption in the distal tubule and collecting duct is highly variable and depends on the presence of aldosterone, a hormone secreted by the adrenal gland. In the presence of aldosterone, almost all the sodium in the distal tubular fluid is reabsorbed, and the urine essentially becomes sodium free. In the absence of aldosterone, virtually no sodium is reabsorbed from the distal tubule. The remarkable ability of the distal tubular and collecting duct cells to alter sodium reabsorption in relation to changes in aldosterone allows the kidneys to excrete urine with sodium levels that range from a few tenths of a gram to 40 g per day.

Like sodium, potassium is freely filtered in the glomerulus, but unlike sodium, potassium is reabsorbed from and secreted into the tubular fluid. The secretion of potassium into the tubular fluid occurs in the distal tubule and, like that of sodium, is regulated by aldosterone. Only approximately 70 mmol of potassium is delivered to the distal tubule each day, but the average person consumes this much potassium and more in the diet. Excess potassium that is not filtered in the glomerulus and delivered to the collecting tubule therefore must be secreted (*i.e.,* transported from the blood) into the tubular fluid for elimination from the body. In the absence of aldosterone (as in Addison disease; see Chapter 41), potassium secretion becomes minimal. In these circumstances, potassium reabsorption exceeds secretion, and blood levels of potassium increase.

The natriuretic peptides, of which atrial natriuretic peptide (ANP) was the first to be discovered in 1981, are hormones that have important roles in salt and water excretion by the kidney. ANP is synthesized in muscle cells of the atria of the heart and released when the atria are stretched. Brain natriuretic peptide (BNP) was first discovered in ventricles in the brain of animals, but is now known to be released by cardiac ventricles in humans in response to stretch and volume. The actions of the natriuretic peptides include vasodilation of the afferent and efferent arterioles, which results in an increase in renal blood flow and GFR; inhibition of sodium reabsorption from the collecting tubules through indirect action on aldosterone and direct action on the tubular cells; inhibition of ADH release from the posterior pituitary gland; and inhibition of the sympathetic system. Thus, increased atrial or ventricular volume increases release of ANP and BNP, which promote both natriuresis and diuresis.

Regulation of pH

The kidneys regulate body pH by conserving base bicarbonate (HCO_3^-) and eliminating acid hydrogen ions (H^+). Neither the blood buffer systems nor the respiratory control mechanisms for carbon dioxide elimination can eliminate hydrogen ions from the body. This is accomplished by the kidneys. The average North American diet results in the liberation of 40 to 80 mmol of hydrogen ions each day. Virtually all the hydrogen ions excreted in the urine are secreted into the tubular fluid by means of tubular secretory mechanisms. The lowest tubular fluid pH that can be achieved is 4.4 to 4.5. The ability of the

THE FUNCTIONS OF THE KIDNEY

- The kidney regulates the composition and pH of body fluids through the reabsorption and elimination or conservation of sodium, potassium, hydrogen, chloride, and bicarbonate ions.
- It functions in the elimination of metabolic wastes (urea, uric acid, creatinine) and drugs and their metabolites.
- It serves to regulate the osmolality of the extracellular fluid through the action of antidiuretic hormone (ADH).
- It plays a central role in blood pressure regulation through the renin–angiotensin–aldosterone mechanism and the regulation of salt and water elimination.
- It contributes to the metabolic functions of the skeletal system through activation of vitamin D and regulation of calcium and phosphate conservation and elimination.
- It controls the production of red blood cells in the bone marrow through the production of erythropoietin.

kidneys to excrete hydrogen ions depends on buffers in the urine that combine with the hydrogen ion. The three major urine buffers are bicarbonate (HCO_3^-), phosphate (HPO_4^{2-}), and ammonia (NH_3). Bicarbonate ions, which are present in the urine filtrate, combine with hydrogen ions that have been secreted into the tubular fluid; this results in the formation of carbon dioxide and water. The carbon dioxide is then absorbed into the tubular cells and bicarbonate is regenerated. The phosphate ion is a metabolic end product that is filtered into the tubular fluid; it combines with a secreted hydrogen ion and is not reabsorbed. Ammonia is synthesized in tubular cells by deamination of the amino acid glutamine; it diffuses into the tubular fluid and combines with the hydrogen ion. An important aspect of this buffer system is that the deamination process increases whenever the body's hydrogen ion concentration remains elevated for 1 to 2 days. These mechanisms for pH regulation are described more fully in Chapter 32.

pH-Dependent Elimination of Organic Ions

The proximal tubule actively secretes large amounts of different organic anions. Foreign anions (*e.g.,* salicylates, penicillin) and endogenously produced anions (*e.g.,* bile acids, uric acid) are actively secreted into the tubular fluid. Most of the anions that are secreted use the same transport system, allowing the kidneys to rid the body of many different drugs and environmental agents. Because the same transport system is shared by different anions, there is competition for transport such that elevated levels of one substance tend to inhibit the secretion of other anions. The proximal tubules also possess an active transport system for organic cations that is analogous to that for foreign cations.

Uric Acid Elimination

Uric acid is a product of purine metabolism (see Chapter 59). Excessively high blood levels (*i.e.,* hyperuricemia) can cause gout, and excessive urine levels can cause kidney stones. Uric acid is freely filtered in the glomerulus and is reabsorbed and secreted into the proximal tubules. Uric acid is one of the anions that use the previously described anion transport system in the proximal tubule. Tubular reabsorption normally exceeds secretion, and the net effect is removal of uric acid from the filtrate. Although the rate of reabsorption exceeds secretion, the secretory process is homeostatically controlled to maintain a constant plasma level. Many persons with elevated uric acid levels secrete less uric acid than do persons with normal uric acid levels.

Uric acid uses the same transport systems as anion medications, such as aspirin, sulfinpyrazone, and probenecid. Small doses of aspirin compete with uric acid for secretion into the tubular fluid and reduce uric acid secretion, and large doses compete with uric acid for reabsorption and increase uric acid excretion in the urine. Because of its effect on uric acid secretion, aspirin is not recommended for treatment of gouty arthritis. Thiazides (*e.g.,* indapamide, hydrochlorothiazide) and loop diuretics (*e.g.,* ethacrynic acid, furosemide) also can cause hyperuricemia and gouty arthritis, presumably through a decrease in extracellular fluid volume and enhanced uric acid reabsorption.

Urea Elimination

Urea is an end product of protein metabolism. The normal adult produces 25 to 30 g per day; the quantity rises when a high-protein diet is consumed, when there is excessive tissue breakdown, or in the presence of gastrointestinal bleeding. With gastrointestinal bleeding, the blood proteins are broken down to form ammonia in the intestine; the ammonia is then absorbed into the portal circulation and converted to urea by the liver before being released into the bloodstream. The kidneys, in their role as regulators of urea (also referred to as blood urea nitrogen or BUN) levels, filter urea in the glomeruli and then reabsorb it in the tubules. This enables maintenance of a normal urea level, which is in the range of 2.9 to 7.1 mmol/L. During periods of dehydration, the blood volume and GFR drop, and urea levels increase. The renal tubules are permeable to urea, which means that the longer the tubular fluid remains in the kidneys, the greater is the reabsorption of urea into the blood. Only small amounts of urea are reabsorbed into the blood when the GFR is high, but relatively large amounts of urea are returned to the blood when the GFR is reduced.

Drug Elimination

Many drugs are eliminated in the urine. These drugs are selectively filtered in the glomerulus and reabsorbed or secreted into the tubular fluid. Only drugs that are not bound to plasma proteins are filtered in the glomerulus and therefore able to be eliminated by the kidneys. Many drugs are weak acids or weak bases and are present in the renal tubular fluid partly as water-soluble ions and partly as nonionized lipid-soluble molecules. The nonionized lipid-soluble form of a drug diffuses more readily through the lipid membrane of the tubule and then back into the bloodstream, whereas the water-soluble ionized form remains in the urine filtrate. The ratio of ionized to nonionized drug depends on the pH of the urine. For example, aspirin is highly ionized in alkaline urine and in this form is rapidly excreted in the urine. Aspirin is largely nonionized in acidic urine and is reabsorbed rather than excreted. Alkaline or acid diuresis may be used to increase elimination of drugs in the urine, particularly in situations of drug overdose.

Endocrine Functions of the Kidney

In addition to their function in regulating body fluids and electrolytes, the kidneys function as an endocrine organ in their production of chemical mediators that travel through the blood to distant sites where they exert their actions. The kidneys participate in control of blood pressure through the renin–angiotensin–aldosterone system (RAAS), in regulating red blood cell production through the synthesis of erythropoietin, and in calcium metabolic by activating vitamin D.

The Renin–Angiotensin–Aldosterone System

The renin–angiotensin–aldosterone system (RAAS) plays an important role in both short-term and long-term regulation of blood pressure (see Chapter 23). Renin is an enzyme synthesized and stored in the juxtaglomerular cells of the kidney. This enzyme is thought to be released in response to a decrease in renal blood flow, a change in the composition of the distal tubular fluid, or an increase in sympathetic nervous system stimulation. Renin itself has no direct effect on blood pressure. Rather, it acts enzymatically to convert a circulating plasma protein called *angiotensinogen* to angiotensin I (see Chapter 23, Fig. 23.4). Angiotensin I, which has few vasoconstrictor properties, leaves the kidneys and enters the circulation; as it is circulated, *angiotensin-converting enzyme* (ACE) catalyzes the conversion of angiotensin I to angiotensin II. Although ACE has been found in a variety of locations (*i.e.,* vascular endothelium, renal tubular epithelial cells), it is expressed in high amounts in the lung capillaries. Angiotensin II is a potent vasoconstrictor, and acts directly on the kidneys to decrease Na^+ and water excretion. Both mechanisms have relatively short periods of action. Angiotensin II also stimulates aldosterone secretion from the adrenal cortex in the adrenal gland. Aldosterone acts on the distal tubule to increase Na^+ reabsorption and exerts a longer-term effect on the maintenance of blood pressure. Angiotensin II also produces constriction of the efferent arteriole to prevent a serious decrease in glomerular filtration pressure.

Erythropoietin

Erythropoietin is a polypeptide hormone that regulates the differentiation of red blood cells in the bone marrow (see Chapter 14). Between 89% and 95% of erythropoietin is formed in the kidneys. The synthesis of erythropoietin is stimulated by renal tissue hypoxia, which may result from impaired oxygenation due to anemia, hypoxemia, or ischemia. Persons with end-stage kidney disease often are anemic because of an inability of the kidneys to produce erythropoietin. This anemia usually is managed by the administration of a recombinant erythropoietin (epoetin alfa) produced through DNA technology, to stimulate erythropoiesis.

Vitamin D

Activation of vitamin D occurs in the kidneys. Vitamin D increases calcium absorption from the gastrointestinal tract and helps to regulate calcium deposition in bone. It also has a weak stimulatory effect on renal calcium absorption. Although vitamin D is not synthesized and released from an endocrine gland, it often is considered as a hormone because of its pathway of molecular activation and mechanism of action.

Vitamin D is a fat-soluble vitamin that exists in several forms but the two major forms are natural vitamin D (cholecalciferol or D_3), which results from ultraviolet irradiation of the skin, and synthetic vitamin D (ergocalciferol or D_2), which is derived from irradiation of ergosterol. The active form of vitamin D is 1,25-dihydroxycholecalciferol. Cholecalciferol and ergocalciferol must undergo chemical transformation to become active: first to 25-hydroxycholecalciferol in the liver and then to 1,25-dihydroxycholecalciferol in the kidneys. Persons with end-stage renal disease are unable to transform vitamin D to its active form and may require pharmacologic preparations of the active vitamin (calcitriol) for maintaining mineralization of their bones.

Action of Diuretics

Diuretics are drugs that increase urine volume. Many diuretic agents (loop diuretics, thiazide diuretic, and potassium-sparing diuretics) exert their effects by blocking Na^+ reabsorption in the renal tubules, resulting in loss of both sodium and water. Others exert osmotic effects that prevent water reabsorption in the water-permeable parts of the nephron.

Diuretics That Block Sodium Reabsorption

Most diuretics share the same mechanism of action—blockade of sodium and chloride reabsorption. By blocking the reabsorption of these solutes, diuretics create an osmotic pressure gradient within the nephron that prevents the passive reabsorption of water. Thus, diuretics cause water and sodium to be retained in the nephron, thereby promoting the excretion of both. The increase in urine flow that a diuretic produces is related to the amount of sodium and chloride reabsorption that it blocks. Because the amount of sodium becomes progressively less as the urine filtrate flows from the proximal tubule to the collecting ducts, drugs that act early in the nephron have the opportunity to block the greatest amount of sodium reabsorption. Approximately 65% of sodium that is filtered in the glomeruli of the kidney is reabsorbed in the proximal tubule, 20% is reabsorbed in the thick ascending loop of Henle, 10% in the early distal convoluted tubule, and 2% to 5% is reabsorbed in the late distal and cortical collecting tubules (Fig 30.13).

The so-called *loop diuretics* exert their effect in the thick ascending loop of Henle. Because of their site of action, these drugs are the most effective diuretic agents available. These

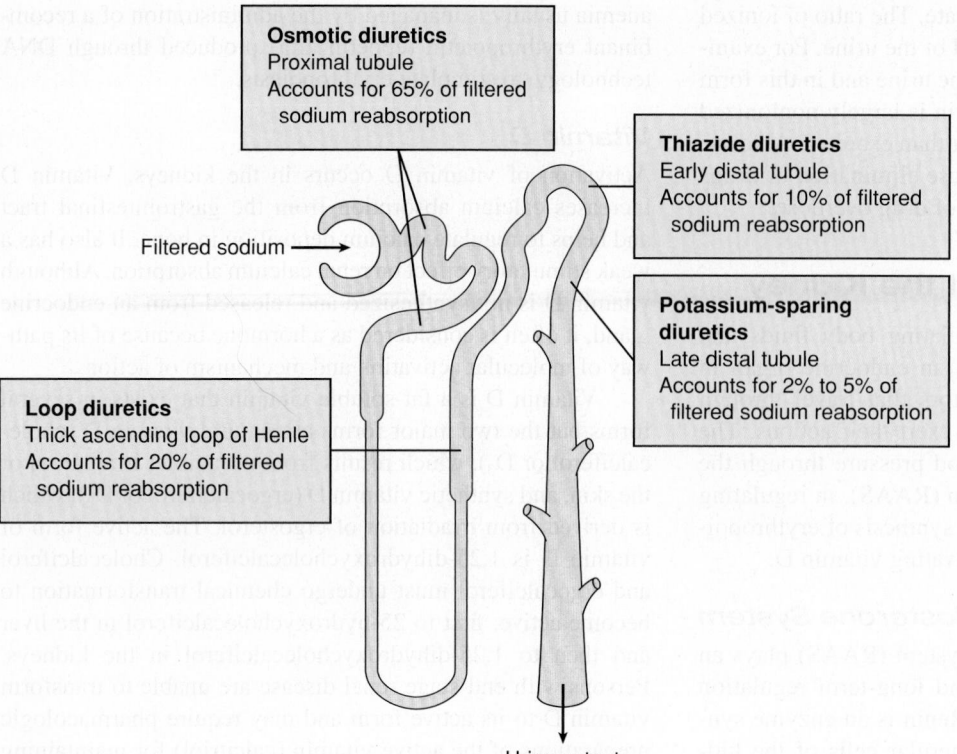

Osmotic diuretics
Proximal tubule
Accounts for 65% of filtered sodium reabsorption

Thiazide diuretics
Early distal tubule
Accounts for 10% of filtered sodium reabsorption

Filtered sodium →

Potassium-sparing diuretics
Late distal tubule
Accounts for 2% to 5% of filtered sodium reabsorption

Loop diuretics
Thick ascending loop of Henle
Accounts for 20% of filtered sodium reabsorption

Urine output

FIGURE 30.13 • Tubular sites of diuretic action and percentage of sodium reabsorption.

drugs inhibit the coupled $Na^+/K^+/2Cl^-$ transport system on the luminal side of the ascending loop of Henle (Fig. 30.10). By inhibiting this transport system, they reduce the reabsorption of sodium chloride, decrease potassium reabsorption, and increase calcium and magnesium elimination. Prolonged use can cause significant loss of magnesium in some persons. Because calcium is actively reabsorbed in the distal convoluted tubule, loop diuretics usually do not cause hypocalcemia. The loop diuretics may also increase uric acid retention and impair glucose tolerance.

The *thiazide diuretics* act by preventing the reabsorption of sodium chloride in the early distal convoluted tubule. Because of their site of action, the thiazide diuretics are less effective than loop diuretics in terms of effecting diuresis. The thiazide diuretics produce increased losses of potassium in the urine, uric acid retention, and some impairment in glucose tolerance. In contrast to the situation in the loop of Henle, where the loop diuretics inhibit calcium reabsorption, the thiazide diuretics actually enhance calcium reabsorption in the distal convoluted tubule.

The *aldosterone antagonists,* also called *potassium-sparing diuretics,* reduce sodium reabsorption and decrease potassium secretion in the late distal tubule and cortical collecting tubule site regulated by aldosterone (Fig. 30.11). Because potassium secretion is linked to sodium reabsorption in this segment of the tubule, these agents are also effective in reducing potassium excretion and may, in some cases, cause severe hyperkalemia. These agents also tend to interfere with secretion of hydrogen ions in the collecting duct, explaining

in part the metabolic acidosis sometimes seen with the use of these agents.

There are two types of potassium-sparing diuretics: those that act as direct aldosterone antagonists and those that act independently of aldosterone. The first type (*e.g.,* spironolactone) binds to the mineralocorticoid receptor in the tubule, preventing aldosterone from entering the cell and exerting its effects. The second type (*e.g.,* amiloride) does not bind to the receptor, but instead directly interferes with sodium entry through the sodium-selective ion channel. The potassium-sparing diuretics produce only mild diuresis because they inhibit such a small percentage of sodium reabsorption. However, as the name implies, their main use is in combination with other diuretics to inhibit K^+ secretion by the principal cells. These diuretics may also be used during states of mineralocorticoid (*i.e.,* aldosterone) excess.

Osmotic Diuretics

The osmotic diuretics act in the proximal tubule and ascending loop of Henle, both of which are highly permeable to water. In contrast to the loop, thiazide, and potassium-sparing diuretics that exert their effects by blocking specific tubular Na^+ transport mechanisms, the osmotic diuretics, which are filtered but not reabsorbed, cause water to be retained in the urine filtrate and promote water diuresis. One such agent, mannitol, is used mainly to reduce increased intracranial pressure, but is occasionally used to promote prompt removal of toxins. Because it is not absorbed, mannitol must be given parenterally to act as a diuretic. If given orally, it causes osmotic diarrhea.

IN SUMMARY

The kidneys perform excretory and endocrine functions. In the process of excreting wastes, the kidneys filter the blood and then selectively reabsorb those materials that are needed to maintain a stable internal environment. The kidneys rid the body of metabolic wastes, regulate fluid volume, regulate the concentration of electrolytes, assist in maintaining acid-base balance, aid in regulation of blood pressure through the RAAS and control of extracellular fluid volume, regulate red blood cell production through erythropoietin, and aid in calcium metabolism by activating vitamin D.

The nephron is the functional unit of the kidney. It is composed of a glomerulus, which filters the blood, and a tubular component, where electrolytes and other substances needed to maintain the constancy of the internal environment are reabsorbed back into the bloodstream while unneeded materials are secreted into the tubular filtrate for elimination. Urine concentration occurs in the collecting tubules under the influence of ADH. ADH maintains extracellular volume by returning water to the vascular compartment, producing concentrated urine by removing water from the tubular filtrate.

The GFR is the amount of filtrate that is formed each minute as blood moves through the glomeruli. It is regulated by the arterial blood pressure and renal blood flow in the normally functioning kidney. The juxtaglomerular apparatus is thought to represent a feedback control system that links changes in the GFR with renal blood flow. Renal clearance is the volume of plasma that is completely cleared each minute of any substance that finds its way into the urine. It is determined by the ability of the substance to be filtered in the glomeruli and the capacity of the renal tubules to reabsorb or secrete the substance.

Diuretics are drugs that increase urine volume. Many diuretic agents (loop diuretics, thiazide diuretics, and potassium-sparing diuretics) exert their effect by blocking the reabsorption of sodium at specific sites in the renal tubules. Others exert osmotic effects that prevent water reabsorption in the water-permeable parts of the nephron. The effectiveness of a diuretic is related to its site of action; accordingly, diuretics such as the loop diuretics that act in the thick ascending loop of Henle, where approximately 20% of sodium reabsorption takes place, produce the greatest diuresis.

CONCEPTS in action **ANIMATION**

TESTS OF RENAL FUNCTION

After completing this section of the chapter, you should be able to meet the following objectives:

- Describe the characteristics of normal urine.
- Explain the significance of casts in the urine.
- Explain the value of urine specific gravity in evaluating renal function.
- Explain the concept of the glomerular filtration rate.
- Explain the value of serum creatinine levels in evaluating renal function.
- Describe the methods used in cystoscopic examination of the urinary tract, ultrasonographic studies of the urinary tract, computed tomographic scans, magnetic resonance imaging studies, excretory urography, and renal angiography.

The function of the kidneys is to filter the blood, selectively reabsorb those substances that are needed to maintain the constancy of body fluid, and excrete metabolic wastes. The composition of urine and blood provides valuable information about the adequacy of renal function. Radiologic tests, endoscopy, and renal biopsy afford means for viewing the gross and microscopic structures of the kidneys and urinary system.

Urine Tests

Urine is a clear, amber-coloured fluid that is approximately 95% water and 5% dissolved solids. The kidneys normally produce approximately 1.5 L of urine each day. Normal urine contains metabolic wastes and few or no plasma proteins, blood cells, or glucose molecules. Urine tests can be performed on a single (or spot) urine specimen or on a 24-hour urine specimen. First-voided morning specimens are useful for qualitative protein and specific gravity testing. A freshly voided specimen is most reliable. Urine specimens that have been left standing may contain lysed red blood cells, disintegrating *casts*, and rapidly multiplying bacteria. Table 30.1 describes urinalysis values for normal urine.

Casts are particles from the nephron lumen. A gel-like substance called *Tamm–Horsfall mucoprotein,* which is formed in the tubular epithelium, is the major protein constituent of urinary casts. Casts composed of this gel but devoid of cells are called *hyaline casts.* These casts develop when the protein concentration of the urine is high (as in nephrotic syndrome), urine osmolality is high, and urine pH is low. The inclusion of granules or cells in the matrix of the protein gel leads to the formation of various other types of casts.

Proteinuria represents excessive protein excretion in the urine. Because of the glomerular capillary filtration barrier, less than 150 mg/L of protein is excreted in the urine over 24 hours in a healthy person. Urine tests for proteinuria are used to detect abnormal filtering of albumin in the glomeruli or defects in its reabsorption in the renal tubules. A protein reagent dipstick can be used as a rapid screening test for the presence of proteins in the urine. Once the presence of proteinuria has been detected, a 24-hour urine test is often used to quantify the amount of protein that is present.

Albumin, which is the smallest of the plasma proteins, is filtered more readily than globulins or other plasma proteins.

TABLE 30.1 NORMAL VALUES FOR ROUTINE URINALYSIS

GENERAL CHARACTERISTICS AND MEASUREMENTS	CHEMICAL DETERMINATIONS	MICROSCOPIC EXAMINATION OF SEDIMENT
Colour: yellow-amber Turbidity: clear to slightly hazy Specific gravity: 1.010–1.025 with a normal fluid intake pH: 4.5–8.0 Volume: 600–2,500 ml/24 hr	Glucose: negative Ketones: negative Blood: negative Protein: negative Bilirubin: negative Urobilinogen: 0.9–7.2 µmol/day Nitrate for bacteria: negative Leukocyte esterase: negative	Casts negative: occasional hyaline casts Red blood cells: negative or rare Crystals: negative (none) White blood cells: negative or rare Epithelial cells: few

Adapted from Fischbach F., Dunning M. B. (2009). *A manual of laboratory and diagnostic tests* (8th ed., p. 199). Philadelphia, PA: Lippincott Williams & Wilkins.

Thus, *microalbuminuria* tends to occur long before clinical proteinuria becomes evident. A dipstick test for microalbuminuria is available for screening purposes. The microalbuminuria dipstick method, however, only indicates an increase in urinary albumin that is below the detectable range of the standard proteinuria test. It does not specify the amount of albumin that is present in the urine. Therefore, a 24-hour urine collection is the standard method for detecting microalbuminuria (an albumin excretion >30 mg/day is abnormal).

The *specific gravity* of urine varies with its concentration of solutes. Urine specific gravity provides a valuable index of the hydration status and functional ability of the kidneys. Healthy kidneys can produce concentrated urine with a specific gravity of 1.030 to 1.040. During periods of marked hydration, the specific gravity can approach 1.000. With diminished renal function, there is a loss of renal-concentrating ability, and the urine specific gravity may fall to levels of 1.006 to 1.010 (usual range is 1.010 to 1.025 with normal fluid intake). These low levels are particularly significant if they occur during periods that follow a decrease in water intake (*e.g.,* during the first urine specimen on arising in the morning).

Urine osmolality, which depends on the number of particles of solute in a unit of solution, is a more exact measurement of urine concentration than specific gravity. More information concerning renal function can be obtained if the serum and urine osmolality tests are done at the same time. The normal ratio between urine and serum osmolality is 3:1. A high urine-to-serum ratio is seen in concentrated urine. With poor concentrating ability, the ratio is low.

Glomerular Filtration Rate

The GFR provides a gauge of renal function. It can be measured clinically by collecting timed samples of blood and urine. *Creatinine,* a product of creatine metabolism by the muscle, is filtered by the kidneys but not reabsorbed in the renal tubule. Creatinine levels in the blood and urine can be used to measure GFR. The clearance rate for creatinine is the amount that is completely cleared by the kidneys in 1 minute. The formula is expressed as C = UV/P, in which C is the clearance rate (ml/min), U is the urine concentration (µmol/L), V is the urine volume excreted (ml/min or 24 hours), and P is plasma concentration (µmol/L).

Normal creatinine clearance varies between men and women, and is approximately 80 to 110 ml/min for females and 90 to 140 for males, with low-normal values for elderly persons. The calculation must include correction for age and body surface area, which reflects the muscle mass where creatinine metabolism takes place. There is an expected age-related decline in creatinine clearance in older adults because muscle mass and the GFR decline with age (see Chapter 34). The test may be done on a 24-hour basis, with blood being drawn when the urine collection is completed. In another method, two 1-hour urine specimens are collected, and a blood sample is drawn in between.

Blood Tests

Blood tests can provide valuable information about the kidneys' ability to remove metabolic wastes from the blood and maintain normal electrolyte and pH composition of the blood. Normal blood values are listed in Table 30.2. Serum levels of potassium, phosphate, urea, and creatinine increase in renal failure. Serum pH, calcium, and bicarbonate levels decrease in renal failure. The effect of renal failure on the concentration of serum electrolytes and metabolic end products is discussed in Chapter 34.

Serum Creatinine

Serum creatinine levels reflect the GFR. Because these measurements are easily obtained and relatively inexpensive, they often are used as a screening measure of renal function. Creatinine is a product of creatine metabolism in muscles; its formation and release are relatively constant and proportional to the amount of muscle mass present. Creatinine is freely filtered in the glomeruli, is not reabsorbed from the tubules into the blood, and is only minimally secreted into the tubules from the blood; therefore, its blood values depend closely on the GFR.

TABLE 30.2 NORMAL BLOOD CHEMISTRY LEVELS

SUBSTANCE	NORMAL VALUE[a]
Urea	2.9–7.1 mmol/L
Creatinine	50–100 μmol/L
Sodium	135–145 mmol/L
Chloride	98–106 mmol/L
Potassium	3.5–5.0 mmol/L
Carbon dioxide (CO$_2$ content)	24–29 mmol/L
Calcium	2.1–2.6 mmol/L
Phosphate	0.8–1.45 mmol/L
Uric acid	
Male	140–440 μmol/L
Female	80–350 μmol/L
pH	7.35–7.45

[a]Values may vary among laboratories, depending on the method of analysis used.

The normal creatinine value varies depending upon the lab, and the person's age and muscle mass. Normal serum creatinine is approximately 25 to 65 micromol/L (μmol/L) for a child, 45 to 100 μmol/L for an adult woman, 55 to 110 μmol/L for an adult man, and 60 to 130 μmol/L for a muscular adult man. A normal serum creatinine level usually indicates normal renal function. In addition to its use in calculating the GFR, the serum creatinine level is used in estimating the functional capacity of the kidneys (Fig. 30.14). In an adult, a value of 120 to 150 μmol/L represents a loss of filtration function of more than 50%. However, serum creatinine is a poor indicator of renal filtration function in elderly persons, resulting in a delayed or lack of diagnosis and treatment (see Chapter 34).

Recently it has been proposed that another serum protein, *cystatin-C* (a cysteine protease inhibitor), could be useful as a marker of GFR because it has a stable production rate, is freely filtered at the glomerulus, and in several studies has shown a greater sensitivity in detecting a decreased GFR. Further clinical studies are needed to determine the clinical efficacy of cystatin-C as a marker, predictor for disease, and to determine whether there is an advantage to its use compared with creatinine.

Urea

Urea is formed in the liver as a byproduct of protein metabolism and is eliminated entirely by the kidneys. Urea therefore is related to the GFR but, unlike creatinine, also is influenced by protein intake, gastrointestinal bleeding, and hydration status. In gastrointestinal bleeding, the blood is broken down by the intestinal flora, and the nitrogenous waste is absorbed into the portal vein and transported to the liver, where it is converted to urea. During dehydration, elevated urea levels result from increased concentration. Approximately two thirds of renal function must be lost before a significant rise in the urea level occurs.

The urea is less specific for renal insufficiency than creatinine, but the *urea–creatinine ratio* may provide useful diagnostic information. The ratio normally is between 40:1 and 100:1 in adults. Ratios greater than 100:1 represent prerenal conditions that produce an increase in urea but not in creatinine, such as dehydration, congestive heart failure and upper gastrointestinal tract bleeding.

Cystoscopy

Cystoscopy provides a means for direct visualization of the urethra, bladder, and ureteral orifices. It relies on the use of a cystoscope, an instrument with a lighted lens. The cystoscope is inserted through the urethra into the bladder. Biopsy specimens, lesions, small stones, and foreign bodies can be removed from the bladder. Urethroscopy may be used to remove stones from the ureter and aid in the treatment of ureteral disorders such as ureteral strictures.

Ultrasonography

Ultrasonographic studies use the reflection of ultrasonic (high-frequency) waves to visualize the deep structures of the body. The procedure is painless and noninvasive and requires no patient preparation. Ultrasonography is used to visualize the structures of the kidneys and has proved useful in the diagnosis of many urinary tract disorders, including congenital anomalies, renal abscesses, hydronephrosis, and kidney stones. It can differentiate a renal cyst from a renal tumour. The use of ultrasonography also enables accurate placement of needles for renal biopsy and catheters for percutaneous nephrostomy.

Radiologic and Other Imaging Studies

Radiologic studies include a simple flat plate of the kidneys, ureters, and bladder that can be used to determine the size, shape, and position of the kidneys and observe any radiopaque stones that may be in the kidney pelvis or ureters. In excretory urography, or *intravenous pyelography,* a radiopaque dye is injected into a peripheral vein; the dye is then filtered by the

FIGURE 30.14 • Relation between the percentage of renal function and serum creatinine levels.

glomerulus and excreted into the urine, and x-ray films are taken as it moves through the kidneys and ureters.

Urography is used to detect space-occupying lesions of the kidneys, pyelonephritis, hydronephrosis, vesicoureteral reflux, and kidney stones. Some persons are allergic to the dye used for urography and may have an anaphylactic reaction after its administration. Every person undergoing urographic studies should be questioned about previous reactions to the dye or to similar dyes. If the test is considered essential in such persons, premedication with antihistamines and corticosteroids may be used. The dye also reduces renal blood flow; acute renal failure can occur, particularly in persons with vascular disease or pre-existing renal insufficiency.

Other diagnostic tests include computed tomographic (CT) scans, magnetic resonance imaging (MRI), radionuclide imaging, and renal angiography. CT scans may be used to outline the kidneys and detect renal masses and tumours. MRI is used in imaging the kidneys, retroperitoneum, and urinary bladder. It is particularly useful in evaluating vascular abnormalities in and around the kidneys. Radionuclide imaging involves the injection of a radioactive material that subsequently is detected externally by a scintillation camera, which detects the radioactive emissions. Radionuclide imaging is used to evaluate renal function and structures, as well as the ureters and bladder. It is particularly useful in evaluating the function of kidney transplants. Renal angiography provides x-ray pictures of the blood vessels that supply the kidneys. It involves the injection of a radiopaque dye directly into the renal artery. A catheter usually is introduced through the femoral artery and advanced under fluoroscopic view into the abdominal aorta. The catheter tip then is manoeuvred into the renal artery, and the dye is injected. This test is used to evaluate persons suspected of having renal artery stenosis, abnormalities of renal blood vessels, or vascular damage to the renal arteries after trauma.

IN SUMMARY

Urinalysis and blood tests that measure serum levels of pH, electrolytes, and byproducts of metabolism provide valuable information about renal function. Urine specific gravity is used to assess the kidneys' ability to concentrate urine. Dipstick and 24-hour urine tests for proteinuria and microalbuminuria are used to detect abnormal filtering of albumin in the glomeruli or defects in its reabsorption in the renal tubules. Creatinine is a product of creatine metabolism in muscles that is continually produced and then cleared by the kidneys. It is freely filtered in the glomeruli and secreted into the tubules, but not reabsorbed in the tubules. Serum creatinine levels are commonly used to estimate the GFR because it is freely filtered. Urea is formed in the liver as a byproduct of protein metabolism and is eliminated entirely by the kidneys. Urea is therefore related to the GFR but, unlike creatinine, also is influenced by protein intake, gastrointestinal bleeding, hydration status, and liver function.

Cystoscopic examinations can be used for direct visualization of the urethra, bladder, and ureters. Ultrasonography can be used to determine kidney size, and renal radionuclide imaging can be used to evaluate the kidney structures. Radiologic methods such as excretory urography provide a means by which kidney structures such as the renal calyces, pelvis, ureters, and bladder can be outlined. Other diagnostic tests include CT scans, MRI, radionuclide imaging, and renal angiography.

REVIEW EXERCISES

1. A 32-year-old woman with diabetes is found to have a positive result on a urine dipstick test for microalbuminuria. A subsequent 24-hour urine specimen reveals an albumin excretion of 50 mg (an albumin excretion >30 mg/day is abnormal).
   A. *Use the structures of the glomerulus in Figure 30.5 to provide a possible explanation for this finding. Why specifically test for the albumin rather than the globulins or other plasma proteins?*
   B. *Strict control of blood sugars and treatment of hypertension have been shown to decrease the progression of kidney disease in persons with diabetes. Explain the physiologic rationale for these two types of treatments.*

2. A 10-year-old boy with bed-wetting was placed on an ADH nasal spray at bedtime as a means of treating the disorder.
   A. *Explain the rationale for using ADH to treat bed-wetting.*

3. A 54-year-old man, seen by his physician for an elevated blood pressure, was found to have a serum creatinine of 176 μmol//L. He complains that he has been urinating more frequently than usual and his first morning urine specimen reveals a dilute urine with a specific gravity of 1.010.
   A. *Explain the elevation of serum creatinine in terms of renal function.*
   B. *Explain the inability of persons with early renal failure to produce a concentrated urine as evidenced by the frequency of urination and the low specific gravity of his first morning urine specimen.*

4. A 60-year-old woman with a diagnosis of hypertension is being treated with a thiazide diuretic.
   A. *What diuretic effect would you expect the woman to have based on the percentage of sodium reaching the site where the diuretic exerted its action?*
   B. *What type of effects might be expected in terms of renal losses of potassium and calcium?*

Bibliography

Bargnoux A. S., Cavalier E., Cristol J. P., et al. (2011). Cystatin C is a reliable marker for estimation of glomerular filtration rate in renal transplantation: Validation of a new turbidimetric assay using monospecific sheep antibodies. *Clinical Chemistry & Laboratory Medicine, 49*(2), 265–270.

Barrett K. E., Boitano S., Barman S. M., et al. (Eds.). (2012). *Ganong's review of medical physiology* (24th ed.). New York: McGraw Hill Companies.

Bernstein K. E., Ong F. S., Blackwell W. B., et al. (2013). A modern understanding of the traditional and nontraditional biological functions of the angiotensin-converting enzyme. *Pharmacological Reviews, 65*(1), 1–46.

Boron W. F., Boulpaep E. L. (2009). *Medical physiology.* (2nd ed.). Philadelphia, PA: Saunders Elsevier.

Cunningham J., Zehnder D. (2011). New vitamin D analogs and changing therapeutic paradigms. *Kidney International, 79*(7), 702–707.

Eaton D. C., Pooler J. P. (2013). *Vander's renal physiology* (8th ed.). New York: McGraw-Hill Education.

Fain J. A. (2009). Understanding diabetes mellitus and kidney disease. *Nephrology Nursing Journal, 36*(5), 465–470.

Fischbach F., Dunning M. (2009). *A manual of laboratory and diagnostic tests* (8th ed.). Philadelphia, PA: Lippincott Williams & Wilkins.

Hall J. E. (2011). *Textbook of medical physiology* (12th ed.). Philadelphia, PA: W.B. Saunders.

Koeppen B. M., Stanton B. A. (Eds.). (2013). *Renal physiology* (5th ed.). Philadelphia, PA: Elsevier Mosby.

Lehne R. A. (2010). *Pharmacology for nursing care* (7th ed.). St. Louis, MO: Elsevier.

Loonen A. J., Knoers N., van Os C. H., Deen P. M. (2008). Aquaporin 2 mutations in nephrogenic diabetes insipidus. *Seminars in Nephrology, 28*(3), 252–265.

Peralta C. A., Shlipak M. G., Judd S., et al. (2011). Detection of chronic kidney disease with creatinine, cystatin C, and urine albumin-to-creatinine ratio and association with progression to end-stage renal disease and mortality. *Journal of the American Medical Association, 304*(15), 1545–1552.

Pratt N., Roughead E. E., Ryan P., Gilbert A. L. (2010). Differential impact of NSAIDs on rate of adverse events that require hospitalization in high-risk and general veteran populations: A retrospective cohort study. *Drugs & Aging, 27*(1), 63–71.

Rennke H. G., Denker B. M. (2010). *Renal pathophysiology: The essentials* (3rd ed.). Philadelphia, PA: Lippincott Williams & Wilkins.

Ross M., Pawlina W. (2011). *Histology: A text and atlas with correlated cell and molecular biology.* (6th ed.) Philadelphia, PA: Lippincott Williams & Wilkins.

Rubin R., Strayer D. S. (Eds.). (2012). *Rubin's pathology: Clinicopathologic foundations of medicine* (6th ed.). Philadelphia, PA: Lippincott Williams & Wilkins.

Visit thePoint **http://thePoint.lww.com for animations, journal articles, and more!**

Disorders of Fluid and Electrolyte Balance

31

Fluids and electrolytes are present in body cells, in the tissue spaces between the cells, and in the blood that fills the vascular compartment. Body fluids transport gases, nutrients, and wastes; help generate the electrical activity needed to power body functions; take part in the transforming of food into energy; and otherwise maintain the overall function of the body. Although fluid volume and composition remain relatively constant in the presence of a wide range of changes in intake and output, conditions such as environmental stresses and disease can impair intake, increase losses, and otherwise interfere with mechanisms that regulate fluid volume, composition, and distribution.

This chapter is divided into four sections: (1) Composition and Compartmental Distribution of Body Fluids, (2) Sodium and Water Balance, (3) Potassium Balance, and (4) Calcium, Phosphorus, and Magnesium Balance. The mechanisms of edema formation are discussed in the section on composition and compartmental distribution of body fluids.

COMPOSITION AND COMPARTMENTAL DISTRIBUTION OF BODY FLUIDS

After completing this section of the chapter, you should be able to meet the following objectives:

- Define the terms electrolyte, ion, and nonelectrolytes.
- Differentiate the intracellular from the extracellular fluid compartments in terms of distribution and composition of water, electrolytes, and other osmotically active solutes.
- Cite the rationale for the use of concentration rather than absolute values in describing electrolyte content of body fluids.

- Relate the concept of a concentration gradient to the processes of diffusion and osmosis.
- Describe the control of cell volume and the effect of isotonic, hypotonic, and hypertonic solutions on cell size.
- Describe factors that control fluid exchange between the vascular and interstitial fluid compartments and relate them to the development of edema and third spacing of extracellular fluids.
- Describe the manifestations and treatment of edema.

Body fluids are distributed between the intracellular (ICF) and extracellular fluid (ECF) compartments. The *ICF compartment* consists of fluid contained within all of the billions of cells in the body. It is the larger of the two compartments, with approximately two thirds of the body water in healthy adults. The remaining one third of body water is in the *ECF compartment,* which contains all the fluids outside the cells, including those in the interstitial or tissue spaces and blood vessels (Fig. 31.1).

The ECF, including blood plasma and interstitial fluids, contains large amounts of sodium and chloride, moderate amounts of bicarbonate, but only small quantities of potassium, magnesium, calcium, and phosphorus. In contrast to the ECF, the ICF contains almost no calcium; small amounts of sodium, chloride, bicarbonate, and phosphorus; moderate amounts of magnesium; and large amounts of potassium (Table 31.1). It is the ECF levels of electrolytes in the blood or blood plasma that are measured clinically. Although blood levels usually are representative of the total body levels of an electrolyte, this is not always the case, particularly with potassium, which is approximately 28 times more concentrated inside the cell than outside.[1]

The cell membrane serves as the primary barrier to the movement of substances between the ECF and ICF compartments. Lipid-soluble substances (*e.g.,* oxygen [O_2] and carbon

FIGURE 31.1 • Distribution of body water. The extracellular space includes the vascular compartment and the interstitial spaces.

dioxide [CO_2]), which dissolve in the lipid bilayer of the cell membrane, pass directly through the membrane, whereas many ions (*e.g.,* sodium [Na^+] and potassium [K^+]) rely on transport mechanisms such as the Na^+/K^+ pump, located in the cell membrane, for movement across the membrane.[2] Because the Na^+/K^+ pump relies on adenosine triphosphate (ATP) and the enzyme ATPase for energy, it is often referred to as the Na^+/K^+-ATPase membrane pump. Water crosses the cell membrane by osmosis using special transmembrane protein channels called *aquaporins.*[3]

Introductory Concepts

Dissociation of Electrolytes

Body fluids contain water and electrolytes. Electrolytes are substances that dissociate in solution to form charged particles, or *ions.* For example, a sodium chloride (NaCl) molecule dissociates to form a positively charged Na^+ and a negatively charged Cl^- ion. Particles that do not dissociate into ions such as glucose and urea are called *nonelectrolytes.* Positively charged ions are called *cations* because they are attracted to the cathode of a wet electric cell, and negatively charged ions are called *anions* because they are attracted to the anode. The ions found in body fluids carry one charge (*i.e.,* monovalent ion) or two charges (*i.e.,* divalent ion). Because of their attraction forces, positively charged cations are always accompanied by negatively charged anions. Thus, all body fluids contain equal amounts of anions and cations. However, cations and anions may be exchanged one for another, providing they carry the same charge. For example, a positively charged H^+ ion may be exchanged for a positively charged K^+ ion, and a negatively charged HCO_3^- ion may be exchanged for a negatively charged Cl^- ion.

TABLE 31.1	CONCENTRATIONS OF EXTRACELLULAR AND INTRACELLULAR ELECTROLYTES IN ADULTS	
ELECTROLYTE	**EXTRACELLULAR CONCENTRATION**[a] **SI UNITS (mmol/L)**	**INTRACELLULAR CONCENTRATION**[a] **SI UNITS (mmol/L)**
Sodium	135–145	10–14
Potassium	3.5–5.0	140–150
Chloride	98–106	3–4
Bicarbonate	24–31	7–10
Calcium	2.1–2.6	<0.25
Phosphorus	0.8–1.45	Variable
Magnesium	0.70–1.25	20

[a]Values may vary among laboratories, depending on the method of analysis used.

[b]Values vary among various tissues and with nutritional status.

Diffusion, Osmosis, and Tonicity

Diffusion. *Diffusion* is the movement of charged or uncharged particles along a concentration gradient. All molecules and ions, including water and dissolved molecules, are in constant random motion. It is the motion of these particles, each colliding with one another, that supplies the energy for diffusion. Because there are more molecules in constant motion in a concentrated solution, particles move from an area of higher concentration to one of lower concentration.

Osmosis. *Osmosis* is the movement of water across a semipermeable membrane (*i.e.,* one that is permeable to water but impermeable to most solutes). As with particles, water diffuses down its concentration gradient, moving from the side of the membrane with the lesser number of particles and greater concentration of water to the side with the greater number of particles and lesser concentration of water (Fig. 31.2). As water moves across the semipermeable membrane, it generates a pressure called the *osmotic pressure*. The magnitude of the osmotic pressure represents the hydrostatic pressure (measured in millimetres of mercury [mm Hg]) needed to oppose the movement of water across the membrane.

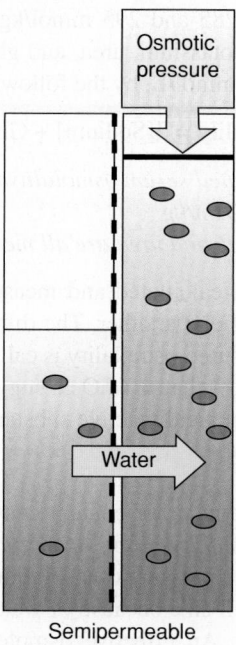

FIGURE 31.2 • Movement of water across a semipermeable membrane. Water moves from the side that has fewer nondiffusible particles to the side that has more. The osmotic pressure is equal to the hydrostatic pressure needed to oppose water movement across the membrane.

Measurement Units

The amount of electrolytes and solutes in body fluids is expressed as a concentration or amount of solute in a given volume of fluid, such as millimoles per litre (mmol/L; used in Canada), milliequivalents per litre (mEq/L) or milligrams per decilitre (mg/dL; used in United States). The *millimoles per litre* measurement unit expresses the weight of the solute (one thousandth of a mole) in a litre or 1,000 ml of solution. In Canada, the concentration of electrolytes (*e.g.,* potassium, calcium, phosphate) is expressed in mmol/L from the metric or International System of Units (*i.e.,* abbreviated SI from *Le Système International d'Unitées*).

The *milliequivalent* is used to express the charge equivalency for a given weight of an electrolyte. Electroneutrality requires that the total number of cations in the body equals the total number of anions. When cations and anions combine, they do so according to their ionic charge, not according to their atomic weight. Thus, 1 mEq of sodium has the same number of charges as 1 mEq of chloride, regardless of molecular weight (although sodium is positive and chloride is negative). The number of millimoles of an electrolyte in a litre of solution can be calculated using the following equation:

$$mmol/L = \frac{mEq/L}{valence}$$

For monovalent electrolytes such as sodium and potassium, the mmol and mEq values are identical. For example 140 mEq is equal to 140 mmol of sodium.

The osmotic activity that nondiffusible particles exert in pulling water from one side of the semipermeable membrane to the other is measured by a unit called an *osmole*. The osmole is derived from the gram molecular weight of a substance (*i.e.,* 1 g molecular weight of a nondiffusible and nonionizable substance is equal to 1 Osm). In the clinical setting, osmotic activity usually is expressed in milliosmoles (one thousandth of an osmole) per litre. Each nondiffusible particle, large or small, is equally effective in its ability to pull water through a semipermeable membrane. Thus, it is the number, rather than the size, of the nondiffusible particles that determines the osmotic activity of a solution.

The osmotic activity of a solution may be expressed in terms of either its osmolarity or osmolality. *Osmolarity* refers to the osmolar concentration in 1 L of solution (mOsm/L) and *osmolality* to the osmolar concentration in 1 kg of water (mOsm/kg of H_2O). Osmolarity is usually used when referring to fluids outside the body and osmolality for describing fluids inside the body. Because 1 L of water weighs 1 kg, the terms *osmolarity* and *osmolality* are often used interchangeably.

The predominant osmotically active particles in the extracellular fluid are Na^+ and its attendant anions (Cl^- and HCO_3^-), which together account for 90% to 95% of the osmotic pressure. Urea (blood urea nitrogen or BUN) and glucose, which also are osmotically active, account for less than 5% of the total osmotic pressure in the extracellular compartment.[2] This can change, however, as when blood glucose levels are elevated in persons with diabetes mellitus or when urea levels change rapidly in persons with chronic kidney disease. Serum osmolality, which normally ranges between 285 and 295 mOsm/kg (or also referred to as 285 and 295 mmol/kg) can be calculated using the sodium, potassium, urea, and glucose values which are all expressed in mmol/L, by the following equation:

$$\text{Serum Osmolality} = 2[\text{Sodium}] + \text{Glucose} + \text{Urea}$$

Note: Calculated serum osmolality can be expressed in mmol/kg or mOsm/kg
Sodium, glucose and urea are all measured in mmol/L

Ordinarily, the calculated and measured osmolality are within 10 mOsm of one another. The difference between the calculated and measured osmolality is called the *osmolar gap*. An osmolar gap larger than 10 mOsm suggests the presence of an unmeasured, osmotically active substance such as alcohol, acetone, or mannitol.

Tonicity. A change in water content causes cells to swell or shrink. The term *tonicity* refers to the tension or effect that the effective osmotic pressure of a solution with impermeable solutes exerts on cell size because of water movement across the cell membrane. An effective osmole is one that exerts an osmotic force and cannot permeate the cell membrane, whereas an ineffective osmole is one that exerts an osmotic force but crosses the cell membrane. Tonicity is determined solely by effective solutes such as glucose that cannot penetrate the cell membrane, thereby producing an osmotic force that pulls water out of the cell. In contrast, urea, which is osmotically active but lipid soluble, tends to distribute equally across the cell membrane. Therefore, when ECF levels of urea are elevated, ICF levels also are elevated. Urea is therefore considered to be an ineffective osmole. It is only when extracellular levels of urea change rapidly, as during hemodialysis treatment, that urea affects tonicity.

Solutions to which body cells are exposed can be classified as isotonic, hypotonic, or hypertonic depending on whether they cause cells to swell or shrink (Fig. 31.3). Cells

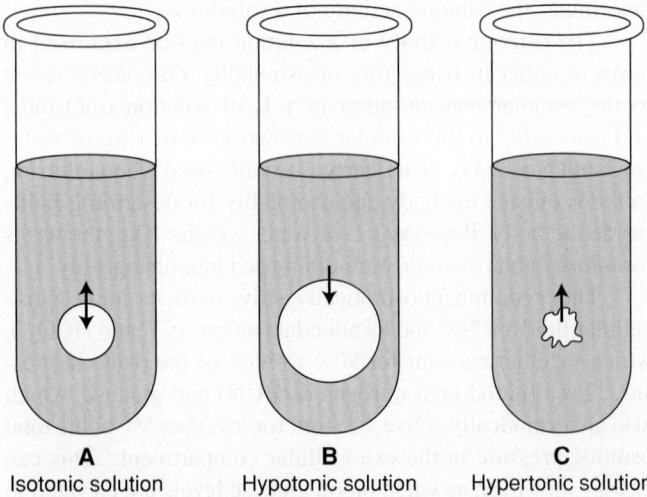

A
Isotonic solution

B
Hypotonic solution

C
Hypertonic solution

FIGURE 31.3 • Osmosis. (**A**) Red cells undergo no change in size in isotonic solutions. (**B**) They increase in size in hypotonic solutions and (**C**) decrease in size in hypertonic solutions.

placed in an isotonic solution, which has the same effective osmolality as the ICF (*i.e.*, 280 mOsm/kg), neither shrink nor swell. An example of an isotonic solution is 0.9% sodium chloride. When cells are placed in a hypotonic solution, which has a lower effective osmolality than the ICF, they swell as water moves into the cell, and when they are placed in a hypertonic solution, which has a greater effective osmolality than the ICF, they shrink as water is pulled out of the cell. However, an iso-osmotic solution is not necessarily isotonic. For example, the intravenous administration of a solution of 5% dextrose in water, which is iso-osmotic, is equivalent to the infusion of a hypotonic solution of distilled water because the glucose is rapidly metabolized to carbon dioxide and water.

Urine Osmolality
Urine osmolality reflects the kidneys' ability to produce concentrated or diluted urine based on serum osmolality and the need for water conservation or excretion. The ratio of urine osmolality to serum osmolality in a 24-hour urine sample normally exceeds 1:1, and after a period of overnight water deprivation, it should be greater than 3:1. A dehydrated person (one who has a loss of water) may have a urine–serum ratio approaching 4:1. In these persons, urine osmolality may exceed 1,000 mOsm/kg H_2O. In those who have difficulty concentrating their urine (*e.g.*, those with diabetes insipidus or chronic renal failure), the urine–serum ratio often is less than or equal to 1:1.

Urine specific gravity compares the weight of urine with that of water, providing an index for solute concentration. Water is considered to be 1.000. A change in specific gravity of 1.010 to 1.020 is an increase of 400 mOsm/kg H_2O. In the sodium-depleted state, the kidneys usually try to conserve sodium, urine specific gravity is normal, and urine sodium and chloride concentrations are low.

Compartmental Distribution of Body Fluids

Total body water (TBW) in an average adult male is about 60% of body weight and this water is distributed between the ICF and ECF compartments. Because adult females have more adipose tissue, approximately 50% of their body weight is made up of body water.[2] In the adult, the fluid in the ICF compartment constitutes approximately 40% of body weight, and the ECF 20%. The fluid in the ECF compartment is further divided into two major subdivisions: the plasma compartment, which constitutes approximately 5% of body weight, and the interstitial fluid compartment, which constitutes approximately 14% of body weight (Fig. 31.4).

A third, usually minor, subdivision of the ECF compartment is the transcellular compartment. It includes the cerebrospinal fluid and fluid contained in the various body spaces,

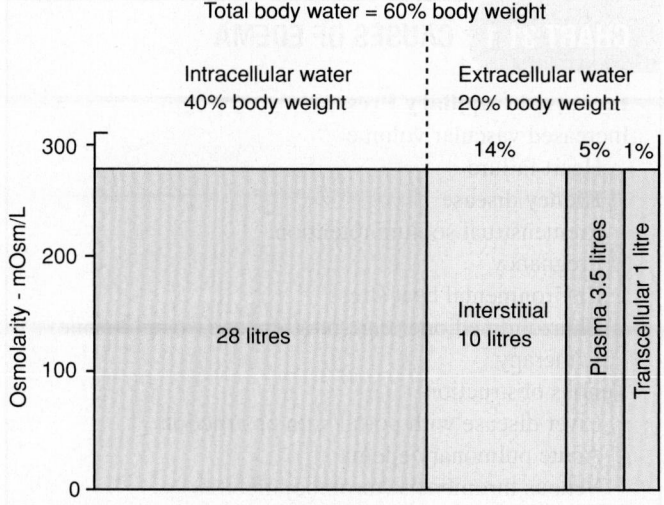

Total body water = 60% body weight

Intracellular water
40% body weight

Extracellular water
20% body weight

14%   5% 1%

FIGURE 31.4 • Approximate sizes of body compartments in a 70-kg adult.

such as the peritoneal, pleural, and pericardial cavities; the joint spaces; ocular fluid; and the gastrointestinal tract. Normally, only approximately 1% of ECF is in the transcellular space. This amount can increase considerably in conditions such as ascites, in which large amounts of fluid are sequestered in the peritoneal cavity. When the transcellular fluid compartment becomes considerably enlarged, it is referred to as a *third space,* because this fluid is not readily available for exchange with the rest of the ECF.

Intracellular Fluid Volume

The ICF volume is regulated by proteins and organic compounds within the body cells and by water and solutes that move between the ECF and ICF. The membrane in most cells is freely permeable to water; therefore, water moves between the ECF and ICF as a result of osmosis. In contrast, osmotically active proteins and other organic compounds cannot pass through the membrane. Water entry into the cell is regulated by these osmotically active substances as well as by solutes such as sodium and potassium that pass through the cell membrane. Many of the intracellular proteins are negatively charged and attract positively charged ions such as K^+, accounting for its higher concentration in the ICF. Na^+, which has a greater concentration in the ECF than the ICF, tends to enter the cell by diffusion. Na^+ is osmotically active and, if left unchecked, its entry would pull water into the cell until it ruptured. The reason this does not occur is because the Na^+/K^+-ATPase membrane pump continuously removes three Na^+ ions from the cell for every two K^+ ions that are moved back into the cell. Situations that impair the function of the Na^+/K^+-ATPase pump, such as hypoxia, cause cells to swell because of an accumulation of Na^+ ions.

The ICF volume is also affected by the concentration of osmotically active substances in the ECF that cannot cross the cell membrane. In diabetes mellitus, for example, glucose cannot enter the cell and its increased concentration in the ECF pulls water out of the cell. Some cells, such as those in

the central nervous system (CNS), defend against significant shifts in fluid volume through a change in osmotically active intracellular molecules. As an initial compensatory mechanism to preserve cell volume, there is a shift of sodium, potassium, chloride, and water out of brain cells in response to a decrease in ECF osmolality and into brain cells in response to an increase in ECF osmolality. After 48 to 72 hours, a slower adaptive process takes place, during which brain cells mobilize organic osmolytes, composed mainly of amino acids, in an effort to maintain a normal cellular volume.

Extracellular Fluid Volume

The ECF is divided between the vascular, interstitial, and transcellular fluid compartments. The vascular compartment contains blood, which is essential to the transport of substances such as electrolytes, gases, nutrients, and waste products throughout the body. The fluid in the interstitial spaces acts as a transport vehicle for gases, nutrients, wastes, and other materials that move between the vascular compartment and body cells. Interstitial fluid also provides a reservoir from which the vascular volume can be maintained during periods of hemorrhage or loss of vascular fluid. A tissue gel, which is a spongelike material composed of large quantities of proteoglycan filaments, fills the tissue spaces and aids in even distribution of interstitial fluid[2] (Fig. 31.1). Normally, most of the fluid in the interstitium is in gel form. The tissue gel is supported by collagen fibres that hold the gel in place. The tissue gel, which has a firmer consistency than water, opposes the outflow of water from the capillaries and helps to prevent the accumulation of free water in the interstitial spaces.

Capillary–Interstitial Fluid Exchange

The transfer of water between the vascular and interstitial compartments occurs at the capillary level. Four forces control the movement of water between the capillary and interstitial spaces:

1. the capillary filtration pressure, which pushes water out of the capillary into the interstitial spaces;
2. the capillary colloidal osmotic pressure, which pulls water back into the capillary;
3. the interstitial hydrostatic pressure, which opposes the movement of water out of the capillary; and
4. the tissue colloidal osmotic pressure, which pulls water out of the capillary into the interstitial spaces.[2]

Normally, the combination of these four forces is such that only a small excess of fluid remains in the interstitial compartment. This excess fluid is removed from the interstitium by the lymphatic system and returned to the systemic circulation. The capillary–interstitial fluid exchange and lymphatic system are further discussed in Chapter 21.

Capillary filtration refers to the movement of water through capillary pores because of a mechanical, rather than an osmotic, force. The capillary filtration pressure (approximately

30 to 40 mm Hg at the arterial end, 10 to 15 mm Hg at the venous end, and 25 mm Hg in the middle), sometimes called the *capillary hydrostatic pressure,* is the pressure pushing water out of the capillary into the interstitial spaces. It reflects the arterial and venous pressures, the precapillary (arterioles) and postcapillary (venules) resistances, and the force of gravity.[2] A rise in arterial or venous pressure increases capillary pressure. The force of gravity increases capillary pressure in the dependent parts of the body. In a person who is standing absolutely still, the weight of blood in the vascular column causes an increase of 1 mm Hg in pressure for every 13.6 mm of distance from the heart.[2] This pressure results from the weight of water and is therefore called *hydrostatic pressure.* In the adult who is standing absolutely still, the pressure in the veins of the feet can reach 90 mm Hg. This pressure is then transmitted to the capillaries.

The *capillary colloidal osmotic pressure* (approximately 28 mm Hg) is the osmotic pressure generated by the plasma proteins that are too large to pass through the pores of the capillary wall.[2] The term *colloidal osmotic pressure* differentiates this type of osmotic pressure from the osmotic pressure that develops at the cell membrane from the presence of electrolytes and nonelectrolytes. Because plasma proteins do not normally penetrate the capillary pores and because their concentration is greater in the plasma than in the interstitial fluids, it is the capillary colloidal osmotic pressure that pulls fluids back into the capillary.

The interstitial fluid pressure (approximately −3 mm Hg) and the tissue colloidal osmotic pressure (approximately 8 mm Hg) contribute to movement of water into and out of the interstitial spaces.[2] The interstitial fluid pressure, which is normally negative, contributes to the outward movement of water into the interstitial spaces. The tissue colloidal osmotic pressure, which reflects the small amount of plasma proteins that normally escape into the interstitial spaces from the capillary, also pulls water out of the capillary into the tissue spaces.

The lymphatic system represents an accessory route whereby fluid from the interstitial spaces can return to the circulation. More important, the lymphatic system provides a means for removing plasma proteins and osmotically active particulate matter from the tissue spaces, neither of which can be reabsorbed into the capillaries.

Edema

Edema can be defined as palpable swelling produced by expansion of the interstitial fluid volume. Clinically edema becomes evident when the interstitial volume has been increased by 2 to 3 L but the interstitial fluid spaces can actually contract to hold an additional 10 to 30 L of fluid.[2,4] The physiologic mechanisms that contribute to edema formation include factors that (1) increase the capillary filtration pressure, (2) decrease the capillary colloidal osmotic pressure, (3) increase capillary permeability, or (4) produce obstruction to lymph flow.[2,4] The causes of edema are summarized in Chart 31.1.

CHART 31.1 | **CAUSES OF EDEMA**

Increased Capillary Pressure
Increased vascular volume
   Heart failure
   Kidney disease
   Premenstrual sodium retention
   Pregnancy
   Environmental heat stress
   Thiazolidinedione (e.g., pioglitazone, rosiglitazone)
     therapy
Venous obstruction
   Liver disease with portal vein obstruction
   Acute pulmonary edema
   Venous thrombosis (thrombophlebitis)
Decreased arteriolar resistance
   Calcium channel–blocking drug responses

Decreased Colloidal Osmotic Pressure
Increased loss of plasma proteins
   Protein-losing kidney diseases
   Extensive burns
Decreased production of plasma proteins
   Liver disease
   Starvation, malnutrition

Increased Capillary Permeability
Inflammation
Allergic reactions (e.g., hives, angioneurotic edema)
Malignancy (e.g., ascites, pleural effusion)
Tissue injury and burns

Obstruction of Lymphatic Flow
Malignant obstruction of lymphatic structures
Surgical removal of lymph nodes

Increased Capillary Filtration Pressure. As the capillary filtration pressure rises, the movement of vascular fluid into the interstitial spaces increases. Among the factors that increase capillary pressure are (1) increased arterial pressure or decreased resistance to flow through the precapillary sphincters, (2) an increase in venous pressure or increased resistance to outflow at the postcapillary sphincter, and (3) capillary distension due to increased vascular volume.

Edema can be either localized or generalized. The localized edema that occurs with urticaria (*i.e.,* hives) or other allergic or inflammatory conditions results from the release of histamine and other inflammatory mediators that cause dilation of the precapillary sphincters and arterioles that supply the swollen lesions. Thrombophlebitis obstructs venous flow, producing an elevation of venous pressure and edema of the affected part, usually one of the lower extremities.

Generalized edema (termed *anasarca*) is generally the result of increased vascular volume. The swelling of hands and feet that occurs in healthy persons during hot weather is an example of edema that is caused by the vasodilation of superficial blood vessels along with sodium and water retention. Generalized edema is common in conditions such as congestive heart failure that produce fluid retention and venous congestion. In right-sided heart failure, blood dams up throughout the entire venous system, causing organ congestion and edema of the dependent extremities (discussed in Chapter 26).

Because of the effects of gravity, edema resulting from increased capillary pressure commonly causes fluid to accumulate in the dependent parts of the body, a condition referred to as *dependent edema*. For example, edema of the ankles and feet becomes more pronounced during prolonged periods of standing.

Decreased Capillary Colloidal Osmotic Pressure. Plasma proteins exert the osmotic force needed to pull fluid back into the capillary from the tissue spaces. The plasma proteins constitute a mixture of proteins, including albumin, globulins, and fibrinogen. Albumin, the smallest of the plasma proteins, has a molecular weight of 69,000; globulins have molecular weights of approximately 140,000; and fibrinogen has a molecular weight of 400,000.[2] Because of its lower molecular weight, 1 g of albumin has approximately twice as many osmotically active molecules as 1 g of globulin and almost six times as many osmotically active molecules as 1 g of fibrinogen. Also, the concentration of albumin (approximately 45 g/L) is greater than that of the globulins (25 g/L) and fibrinogen (3 g/L).

Edema due to decreased capillary colloidal osmotic pressure usually is the result of inadequate production or abnormal loss of plasma proteins, mainly albumin. The plasma proteins are synthesized in the liver. In persons with severe liver failure, the impaired synthesis of albumin results in a decrease in colloidal osmotic pressure. In starvation and malnutrition, edema develops because there is a lack of amino acids for plasma protein synthesis.

The most common site of plasma protein loss is the kidney. In kidney diseases such as glomerulonephritis, the glomerular capillaries become permeable to the plasma proteins, particularly albumin, which is the smallest of the proteins. When this happens, large amounts of albumin are filtered out of the blood and lost in the urine. An excessive loss of plasma proteins also occurs when large areas of skin are injured or destroyed. Edema is a common problem during the early stages of a burn, resulting from capillary injury and loss of plasma proteins.[1]

Because the plasma proteins are evenly distributed throughout the body and are not affected by the force of gravity, edema due to a decrease in capillary colloidal osmotic pressure tends to affect tissues in nondependent as well as dependent parts of the body. There is swelling of the face as well as the legs and feet.

Increased Capillary Permeability. When the capillary pores become enlarged or the integrity of the capillary wall is damaged, capillary permeability is increased. When this occurs, plasma proteins and other osmotically active particles leak into the interstitial spaces, increasing the tissue colloidal osmotic pressure and thereby contributing to the accumulation of interstitial fluid. Among the conditions that increase capillary permeability are burn injury, capillary congestion, inflammation, and immune responses.

Obstruction of Lymph Flow. Osmotically active plasma proteins and other large particles that cannot be reabsorbed through the pores in the capillary membrane rely on the lymphatic system for movement back into the circulatory system. Edema due to impaired lymph flow is commonly referred to as *lymphedema*.[5] Malignant involvement of lymph structures and removal of lymph nodes at the time of cancer surgery are common causes of lymphedema. Another cause of lymphedema is infection and trauma involving the lymphatic channels and lymph nodes.

Manifestations. The effects of edema are determined largely by its location. Edema of the brain, larynx, or lungs is an acute, life-threatening condition. Although not life-threatening, edema may interfere with movement, limiting joint motion. Swelling of the ankles and feet often is insidious in onset and may or may not be associated with disease. At the tissue level, edema increases the distance for diffusion of oxygen, nutrients, and wastes. Edematous tissues usually are more susceptible to injury and development of ischemic tissue damage, including pressure ulcers. Edema can also compress blood vessels. The skin of a severely swollen finger can act as a tourniquet, shutting off the blood flow to the finger. Edema can also be disfiguring, causing psychological effects and disturbances in self-concept. It can also create problems with obtaining proper-fitting clothing and shoes.

Pitting edema occurs when the accumulation of interstitial fluid exceeds the absorptive capacity of the tissue gel. In this form of edema, the tissue water becomes mobile and can be translocated with pressure exerted by a finger. *Nonpitting edema* usually reflects a condition in which plasma proteins have accumulated in the tissue spaces and coagulated. It is seen most commonly in areas of localized infection or trauma. The area often is firm and discoloured. *Brawny edema* is a type of nonpitting edema in which the skin thickens and hardens.

Assessment and Treatment. Methods for assessing edema include daily weight, visual assessment, measurement of the affected part, and application of finger pressure to assess for pitting edema. Daily weight performed at the same time each day with the same amount of clothing provides a useful index of water gain due to edema (1 L of water weighs 1 kg). Visual inspection and measurement of the circumference of an extremity can also be used to assess the degree of swelling. This is particularly useful when swelling is due to thrombophlebitis. Finger pressure can be used to assess the degree of pitting edema. If an indentation remains after the finger has been removed, pitting edema is identified. It is evaluated on a scale of +1 (minimal) to +4 (severe; Fig. 31.5).

Distinguishing lymphedema from other forms of edema can be challenging, especially early in its course. Papillomatosis, a characteristic honeycomb appearance of the skin due

Understanding Capillary Fluid Exchange

Movement of fluid between the vascular compartment and the interstitial fluid compartment surrounding the body cells occurs at the capillary level. The direction and amount of fluid that flows across the capillary wall are determined by (1) the hydrostatic pressure of the two compartments, (2) the colloidal osmotic pressures of the two compartments, and (3) the removal of excess fluid and osmotically active particles from the interstitial spaces by the lymphatic system.

1. Hydrostatic Pressure

The hydrostatic pressure is the pushing force exerted by a fluid. Inside the capillaries, the hydrostatic pressure is the same as the capillary filtration pressure, about 30 mm Hg at the arterial end and 10 mm Hg at the venous end. The interstitial fluid pressure is the force of fluid in the interstitial spaces pushing against the outside of the capillary wall. Evidence suggests that the interstitial pressure is slightly negative (–3 mm Hg), contributing to the outward movement of fluid from the capillary.

2. Colloidal Osmotic Pressure

The colloidal osmotic pressure is the pulling force created by the presence of evenly dispersed particles, such as the plasma proteins, that cannot pass through the pores of the capillary membrane. The capillary colloidal osmotic pressure is normally about 28 mm Hg throughout the length of the capillary bed. The interstitial colloidal osmotic pressure (approximately 8 mm Hg) represents the pulling pressure exerted by the small amounts of plasma proteins that leak through the pores of the capillary wall into the interstitial spaces. The capillary colloidal osmotic pressure, which is greater than both the hydrostatic pressure at the venous end of the capillary and the interstitial colloidal osmotic pressure, is largely responsible for the movement of fluid back into the capillary.

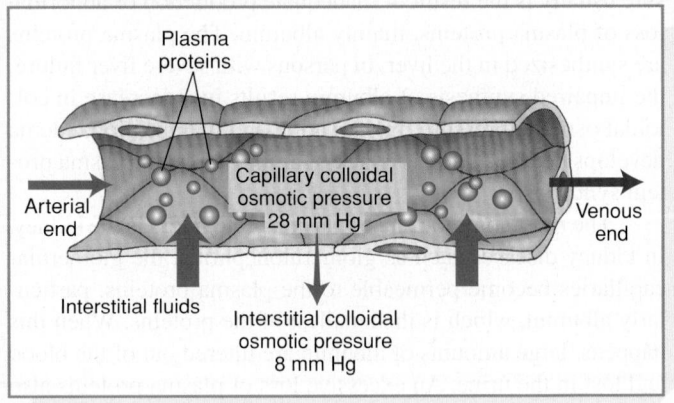

to dilated lymph vessels that are enveloped in fibrotic tissue, distinguishes lymphedema from other edemas. Computed tomography (CT) or magnetic resonance imaging (MRI) may be used to confirm the diagnosis.[5,6]

Treatment of edema usually is directed toward maintaining life when the swelling involves vital structures, correcting or controlling the cause, and preventing tissue injury. Edema of the lower extremities may respond to simple measures such as elevating the feet. Diuretic therapy commonly is used to treat edema associated with an increase in ECF volume. Serum albumin levels can be measured, and albumin may

be administered intravenously to raise the plasma colloidal osmotic pressure when edema is caused by hypoalbuminemia.

Elastic support stockings and sleeves increase interstitial fluid pressure and resistance to outward movement of fluid from the capillary into the tissue spaces. These support devices typically are prescribed for patients with conditions such as lymphatic or venous obstruction and are most efficient if applied before the tissue spaces have filled with fluid—in the morning, for example, before the effects of gravity have caused fluid to move into the ankles. Moderate to severe lymphedema is usually treated with light-pressure massage

3. Lymph Drainage

The lymphatic system represents an accessory system by which fluid can be returned to the circulatory system. Normally the forces moving fluid out of the capillary into the interstitium are greater than those returning fluid to the capillary. Any excess fluids and osmotically active plasma proteins that may have leaked into the interstitium are picked up by vessels of the lymphatic system and returned to the circulation. Without the function of the lymphatic system, excessive amounts of fluid would accumulate in the interstitial spaces.

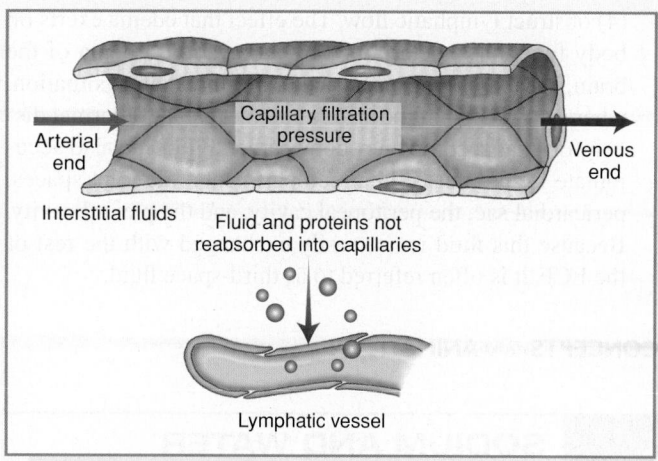

designed to increase lymph flow by encouraging opening and closing of lymph vessel valves; compression garments or pneumatic compression pumps; range-of-motion exercises; and scrupulous skin care to prevent infection.[5,6]

Third-Space Accumulation

Third spacing represents the loss into or trapping of ECF in the transcellular space. The serous cavities are part of the transcellular compartment (*i.e.,* third space) located in strategic body areas where there is continual movement of body structures—the pericardial sac, the peritoneal cavity, and the pleural cavity. The exchange of ECF between the capillaries, the interstitial spaces, and the transcellular space of the serous cavity uses the same mechanisms as capillaries elsewhere in the body. The serous cavities are closely linked with lymphatic drainage systems. The milking action of the moving structures, such as the lungs, continually forces fluid and plasma proteins back into the circulation, keeping these cavities empty. Any

obstruction to lymph flow causes fluid accumulation in the serous cavities. As with edema fluid, third-space fluids represent an accumulation or trapping of body fluids that contribute to body weight but not to fluid reserve or function.

The prefix *hydro-* may be used to indicate the presence of excessive fluid, as in *hydrothorax,* which means excessive fluid in the pleural cavity. The accumulation of fluid in the peritoneal cavity is called *ascites.* The transudation of fluid into the serous cavities is also referred to as *effusion.* Effusion can contain blood, plasma proteins, inflammatory cells (*i.e.,* pus), and ECF.

IN SUMMARY

Body fluids, which contain water and electrolytes, are distributed between the ICF and ECF compartments of the body. Two thirds of body fluid is contained in the body cells of the ICF compartment and one third is contained in the vascular compartment, interstitial spaces, and third-space areas of the ECF compartment. The ICF has high concentrations of potassium, calcium, phosphorus, and magnesium, and the ECF high concentrations of sodium, chloride, and bicarbonate.

Electrolytes and nonelectrolytes move by diffusion across cell membranes that separate the ICF and ECF compartments. Water crosses the cell membrane by osmosis, using special protein channels called aquaporins. It moves from the side of the membrane that has the lesser number of particles and greater concentration of water to the side that has the greater number of particles and lesser concentration of water. The osmotic tension or effect that a solution exerts on cell volume in terms of causing the cell to swell or shrink is called tonicity.

Edema represents an increase in interstitial fluid volume. The physiologic mechanisms that contribute to the development of edema include factors that (1) increase capillary filtration pressure, (2) decrease capillary colloidal osmotic pressure, (3) increase capillary permeability, and

FIGURE 31.5 • 3+ pitting edema of the left foot. (Used with permission for Bickley L. S. (2013). *Bates' guide to physical examination and history taking* (11th ed., p. 505). Philadelphia, PA: Lippincott Williams & Wilkins.)

(4) obstruct lymphatic flow. The effect that edema exerts on body function is determined by its location. Edema of the brain, larynx, or lungs is an acute, life-threatening situation, whereas swelling of the ankles and feet can be a normal discomfort that accompanies hot weather. Fluid can also accumulate in the transcellular compartment—the joint spaces, pericardial sac, the peritoneal cavity, and the pleural cavity. Because this fluid is not easily exchanged with the rest of the ECF, it is often referred to as third-space fluid.

 CONCEPTS in action ANIMATION

SODIUM AND WATER BALANCE

After completing this section of the chapter, you should be able to meet the following objectives:

- State the functions and physiologic mechanisms controlling body water levels and sodium concentration, including the effective circulating volume, sympathetic nervous system, renin—angiotensin–aldosterone system, and antidiuretic hormone.
- Describe measures that can be used in assessing body fluid levels and sodium concentration.
- Describe the causes, manifestations, and treatment of psychogenic polydipsia.
- Describe the relationship between antidiuretic hormone and aquaporin-2 channels in reabsorption of water by the kidney.
- Compare the pathology, manifestations, and treatment of diabetes insipidus and the syndrome of inappropriate antidiuretic hormone.
- Compare and contrast the causes, manifestations, and treatment of isotonic fluid volume deficit, isotonic fluid volume excess, hyponatremia with water excess, and hypernatremia with water deficit.

The movement of body fluids between the ICF and ECF compartments occurs at the cell membrane and depends on ECF levels of water and sodium. Water provides approximately 90% to 93% of the volume of body fluids and sodium salts approximately 90% to 95% of ECF solutes.[2] Normally, equivalent changes in sodium and water are such that the volume and osmolality of ECF are maintained within a normal range. Because it is the concentration of sodium that primarily controls ECF osmolality, changes in sodium are usually accompanied by proportionate changes in water volume.

Body Water Balance

Total body water varies with sex and weight. These differences can be explained by differences in body fat, which is essentially water free (*i.e.,* fat is approximately 10% water

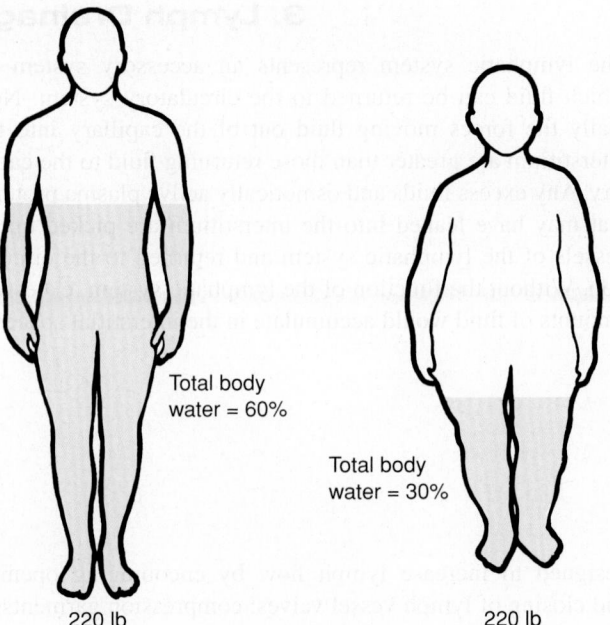

FIGURE 31.6 • Body composition of a lean and an obese individual. (Adapted with permission from Statland H. (1963). *Fluids and electrolytes in practice* (3rd ed.). Philadelphia, PA: J.B. Lippincott.)

by composition, compared with 75% for skeletal muscle). In men, TBW approximates 60% of body weight during young adulthood and decreases to approximately 50% in old age; in young women it is approximately 50% and in elderly women approximately 40%.[7] Obesity produces further decreases in TBW, sometimes reducing these levels to values as low as 30% to 40% of body weight in adults (Fig. 31.6).

Infants normally have more TBW than older children or adults. TBW constitutes approximately 75% to 80% of body weight in full-term infants and an even greater proportion in premature infants.[1] In addition to having proportionately more body water than adults, infants have relatively more water in their ECF compartment. Infants have more than half of their TBW in the ECF compartment, whereas adults have only approximately one third. The greater ECF water content of an infant can be explained in terms of its higher metabolic rate, larger surface area in relation to body mass, and its inability to concentrate urine because of immature kidney structures. Because ECFs are more readily lost from the body, infants are more vulnerable to fluid deficit than older children and adults. As an infant grows older, TBW decreases, and by the second year of life, the percentages and distribution of body water approach those of an adult.[7,8]

Gains and Losses

Regardless of age, all healthy persons require approximately 100 ml of water per 100 calories metabolized for dissolving and eliminating metabolic wastes. This means that a person who expends 1,800 calories for energy requires approximately 1,800 ml of water for metabolic purposes. The metabolic rate increases with fever; it rises approximately 12% for every

TABLE 31.2 SOURCES OF BODY WATER GAINS AND LOSSES IN THE ADULT

GAINS		LOSSES	
Oral intake		Urine	1,500 ml
As water	1,000 ml	Insensible losses	
In food	1,300 ml	Lungs	300 ml
Water of	200 ml	Skin	500 ml
oxidation		Feces	200 ml
Total	2,500 ml	Total	2,500 ml

1°C increase in body temperature.[2] Fever also increases the respiratory rate, resulting in additional loss of water vapour through the lungs.

The main source of water gain is through oral intake and metabolism of nutrients. Water, including that obtained from liquids and solid foods, is absorbed from the gastrointestinal tract. Tube feedings and parenterally administered fluids are also sources of water gain. Metabolic processes also generate a small amount of water. The amount of water gained from these processes varies from 150 to 300 ml/day, depending on the metabolic rate.

Normally, the largest loss of water occurs through the kidneys, with lesser amounts being lost through the skin, lungs, and gastrointestinal tract. Even when oral or parenteral fluids are withheld, the kidneys continue to produce urine as a means of ridding the body of metabolic wastes. The urine output that is required to eliminate these wastes is called the *obligatory urine output*. The obligatory urine loss is approximately 300 to 500 ml/day. Water losses that occur through the skin and lungs are referred to as *insensible water losses* because they occur without a person's awareness. The gains and losses of body water are summarized in Table 31.2.

Sodium Balance

Sodium is the most abundant cation in the body, averaging approximately 60 mmol/kg of body weight.[1] Most of the body's sodium is in the ECF compartment (135 to 145 mmol/L), with only a small amount (10 to 14 mmol/L) located in the ICF compartment. The resting cell membrane is relatively impermeable to sodium; sodium that enters the cell is transported out of the cell against an electrochemical gradient by the Na$^+$/K$^+$-ATPase membrane pump.

Sodium functions mainly in regulating the ECF volume. As the major cation in the ECF compartment, Na$^+$ and its attendant anions (Cl$^-$ and HCO$_3^-$) account for approximately 90% to 95% of the osmotic activity in the ECF. Because sodium is part of the sodium bicarbonate molecule, it is important in regulating acid–base balance. As a current-carrying ion, Na$^+$ contributes to the function of the nervous system and other excitable tissue.

Gains and Losses

Sodium normally enters the body through the gastrointestinal tract and is eliminated by the kidneys or lost from the gastrointestinal tract or skin. Sodium intake normally is derived from dietary sources. Body needs for sodium usually can be met by as little as 500 mg/day. The average salt intake in Canada is approximately 6 to 15 g/day, or 12 to 30 times the daily requirement. Dietary intake, which frequently exceeds the amount needed by the body, is often influenced by culture and food preferences rather than need. As package labels indicate, many commercially prepared foods and soft drinks contain considerable amounts of sodium. Other sources of sodium are intravenous saline infusions and medications that contain sodium.

Most sodium losses occur through the kidneys. The kidneys are extremely efficient in regulating sodium output, and when sodium intake is limited or conservation of sodium is needed, the kidneys are able to reabsorb almost all the sodium that has been filtered by the glomerulus. This results in essentially sodium-free urine. Conversely, urinary losses of sodium increase as intake increases.

Usually less than 10% of sodium intake is lost through the gastrointestinal tract and skin. Although the sodium concentration of fluids in the upper part of the gastrointestinal tract approaches that of the ECF, sodium is reabsorbed as the fluids move through the lower part of the bowel, so that the concentration of sodium in the stool is only approximately 40 mmol/L. Sodium losses increase with conditions such as vomiting, diarrhea, fistula drainage, and gastrointestinal suction that remove sodium from the gastrointestinal tract. Irrigation of gastrointestinal tubes with distilled water removes sodium from the gastrointestinal tract, as do repeated tap water enemas.

Sodium leaves the skin through the sweat glands. Sweat is a hypotonic solution containing both sodium and chloride. Although sodium losses due to sweating are usually negligible, they can increase greatly during exercise and periods of exposure to a hot environment. A person who sweats profusely can lose up to 15 to 30 g of salt each day for the first few days of exposure to a hot environment. This amount usually drops to less than 3 to 5 g a day after 4 to 6 weeks of acclimatization.[2]

Mechanisms of Regulation

The major regulator of sodium and water balance is the maintenance of the *effective circulating volume* (also termed the *effective arterial blood volume*), which can be described as that portion of the ECF that fills the vascular compartment and is "effectively" perfusing the tissues. A low effective circulating volume activates feedback mechanisms that produce an increase in renal sodium and water retention, and a high effective circulating volume triggers feedback mechanisms that decrease sodium and water retention.

The effective circulating volume is monitored by a number of sensors that are located in both the vascular system and the kidney. These sensors are commonly referred to as *baroreceptors* because they respond to pressure-induced stretch of the vessel walls in which they are located.[1] There are baroreceptors located in the low-pressure venous and atrial side of the circulation (in the walls of the cardiac atria and large pulmonary vessels) that respond primarily to changes in blood volume.

Baroreceptors are also present in the high-pressure arterial side of the circulation (aortic arch and carotid sinus) that respond primarily to changes in the arterial pressure or fullness of the circulation. The activity of both types of receptors regulates renal sodium and water elimination by modulating sympathetic nervous system outflow and antidiuretic hormone (ADH) secretion.[1] The sympathetic nervous system responds to changes in arterial blood pressure and blood volume by adjusting the glomerular filtration rate and thus the rate at which sodium is filtered from the blood. Sympathetic activity also regulates tubular reabsorption of sodium and renin release. An additional mechanism related to renal sodium excretion is the natriuretic peptides (ANP and BNP), which are released from atrial and ventricular cells in the heart in response to increased volume, stretch and filling. The natriuretic peptides provide a counter-regulation to the baroreceptors, ANS, ADH as they increase sodium and water excretion by the kidney[1] (see Chapter 30).

Pressure-sensitive receptors in the kidney, particularly in the afferent arterioles, respond directly to changes in arterial pressure through stimulation of the sympathetic nervous system and release of renin with activation of the renin–angiotensin–aldosterone system (RAAS).[1] The RAAS exerts its action through angiotensin II and aldosterone. Renin is a small protein enzyme that is released by the kidney in response to changes in arterial pressure, the glomerular filtration rate, and the amount of sodium in the tubular fluid. Most of the renin that is released leaves the kidney and enters the blood-stream, where it interacts enzymatically to convert a circu-lating plasma protein called *angiotensinogen* to angiotensin I (see Chapter 23, Fig. 23.4).

Angiotensin I is rapidly converted to angiotensin II by the angiotensin-converting enzyme (ACE), primarily in the small blood vessels of the lung, but also locally in vascular endothelial cells. Angiotensin II acts directly on the renal tubules to increase sodium reabsorption. It also acts to con-strict renal blood vessels, thereby decreasing the glomerular filtration rate and slowing renal blood flow so that less sodium is filtered and more is reabsorbed.

Angiotensin II is also a powerful regulator of *aldoste-rone*, a hormone secreted by the adrenal cortex. Aldosterone acts at the level of the cortical collecting tubules of the kidneys to increase sodium reabsorption while increasing potassium elimination. The sodium-retaining action of aldosterone can be inhibited by blocking the actions of aldosterone with potas-sium-sparing diuretics (*e.g.*, spironolactone, amiloride), by suppressing renin release (*e.g.*, β-adrenergic blocking drugs), by inhibiting the conversion of angiotensin I to angiotensin II (*i.e.*, ACE inhibitors), or by blocking the action of angioten-sin II on the angiotensin receptor (*i.e.*, angiotensin II receptor blockers, ARBs).[1]

Disorders of Thirst and Antidiuretic Hormone

Two other mechanisms that contribute directly to the regula-tion of body water and indirectly to the regulation of sodium

FIGURE 31.7 • Top: Sagittal section through the pituitary and ante-rior hypothalamus. Antidiuretic hormone (ADH) is formed primarily in the supraoptic nucleus and to a lesser extent in the paraventricular nucleus of the hypothalamus. It is then transported down the hypothalamohypo-physial tract and stored in secretory granules in the posterior pituitary, where it can be released into the blood. **Bottom:** Pathways for regula-tion of extracellular water volume by thirst and ADH.

are thirst and ADH. Thirst is primarily a regulator of water intake and ADH a regulator of water output. Both mechanisms respond to changes in extracellular osmolality and the effec-tive circulating volume[1] (Fig. 31.7).

Disorders of Thirst

Like appetite and eating, thirst and drinking behaviour are two separate entities. Thirst is the conscious sensation of the need to obtain and drink fluids high in water content. Drinking of water or other fluids often occurs as the result of habit or for reasons other than those related to thirst. Most people drink without being thirsty, and water is consumed before it is needed. As a result, thirst is basically an emergency response. It usually occurs only when the need for water has not been anticipated.

Thirst is controlled by the thirst centre in the hypothala-mus. There are two stimuli for true thirst based on water need:

(1) cellular dehydration caused by an increase in ECF osmolality and (2) a decrease in blood volume, which may or may not be associated with a decrease in serum osmolality. Sensory neurons, called *osmoreceptors,* which are located in or near the thirst centre in the hypothalamus, respond to changes in ECF osmolality by swelling or shrinking (Fig. 31.7). Thirst normally develops when there is as little as a 1% to 2% change in serum osmolality.[9] The previously described stretch receptors in the vascular system that monitor the effective circulating volume also aid in the regulation of thirst. Thirst is one of the earliest symptoms of hemorrhage and is often present before other signs of blood loss appear.

A third important stimulus for thirst is angiotensin II, levels of which increase in response to low blood volume and low blood pressure. The renin–angiotensin mechanism contributes to nonosmotic thirst. This system is considered a backup system for thirst should other systems fail. Because it is a backup system, it probably does not contribute to the regulation of normal thirst. However, elevated levels of angiotensin II may lead to thirst in conditions such as chronic kidney disease and congestive heart failure, in which renin levels may be elevated.

Dryness of the mouth, such as the thirst a lecturer experiences during speaking, produces a sensation of thirst that is not necessarily associated with the body's hydration status. Thirst sensation also occurs in those who breathe through their mouths, such as smokers and persons with chronic respiratory disease or hyperventilation syndrome.

Hypodipsia. Hypodipsia represents a decrease in the ability to sense thirst. It is commonly associated with lesions in the area of the hypothalamus (*e.g.,* head trauma, meningiomas, occult hydrocephalus, subarachnoid hemorrhage). There is also evidence that thirst is decreased, and therefore water intake reduced, in elderly persons, despite higher plasma sodium and osmolality levels.[10] The inability to perceive and respond to thirst is compounded in older adults who have had a stroke and may be further influenced by confusion, sensory deficits, and motor disturbances.

Polydipsia. Polydipsia, or excessive thirst, is normal when it accompanies conditions of water deficit. Increased thirst and drinking behaviour can be classified into three categories: (1) symptomatic or true thirst, (2) inappropriate or false thirst that occurs despite normal levels of body water and serum osmolality, and (3) compulsive water drinking. *Symptomatic thirst* develops when there is a loss of body water and resolves after the loss has been replaced. Among the most common causes of symptomatic thirst are water losses associated with diarrhea, vomiting, diabetes mellitus, and diabetes insipidus (DI). *Inappropriate or excessive thirst* may persist despite adequate hydration. It is a common complaint in persons with congestive heart failure and chronic kidney disease. Although the cause of thirst in these persons is unclear, it may result from increased angiotensin levels. Thirst is also a common complaint in persons with dry mouth caused by decreased salivary function or

treatment with drugs with an anticholinergic action (*e.g.,* antihistamines, atropine) that lead to decreased salivary flow.

Psychogenic polydipsia involves compulsive water drinking and is usually seen in persons with psychiatric disorders, most commonly schizophrenia.[11] Persons with the disorder drink large amounts of water and excrete large amounts of urine. The cause of excessive water drinking in these persons is uncertain. The condition may be compounded by antipsychotic medications that increase ADH levels and interfere with water excretion by the kidneys. Cigarette smoking, which is common among persons with psychiatric disorders, also stimulates ADH secretion. Excessive water ingestion coupled with impaired water excretion (or rapid ingestion at a rate that exceeds renal excretion) in persons with psychogenic polydipsia can lead to water intoxication (see section on hyponatremia). Treatment usually consists of water restriction and behavioural measures aimed at decreasing water consumption. Measurements of body weight can be used to provide an estimate of water consumption.

Disorders of Antidiuretic Hormone

The reabsorption of water by the kidneys is regulated by ADH, also known as *vasopressin.* ADH is synthesized by cells in the supraoptic and paraventricular nuclei of the hypothalamus and then transported along a neural pathway (*i.e.,* hypothalamo-hypophysial tract) to the posterior pituitary gland, where it is stored. When the supraoptic and paraventricular nuclei in the hypothalamus are stimulated by increased serum osmolality or other factors, nerve impulses travel down the hypothalamo-hypophysial tract to the posterior pituitary gland, causing the stored ADH to be released into the circulation[12] (Fig. 31.7).

ADH exerts its effects through two types of vasopressin (V) receptors—V_1 and V_2. V_1 receptors, which are located in vascular smooth muscle, cause vasoconstriction—hence the name *vasopressin.* Although ADH can increase blood pressure through V_1 receptors, this response occurs only when ADH levels are very high. The V_2 receptors, which are located on the tubular cells of the cortical collecting duct, control water reabsorption by the kidney. These renal mechanisms for water reabsorption are responsible for maintaining the osmolality of body fluids.[2]

Without ADH, the luminal membranes of the tubular epithelial cells of the collecting ducts are almost impermeable to water. In the presence of ADH, pores or water channels, called *aquaporins,* are inserted into the membrane of these tubular cells, making them permeable to water (see Understanding Urine Concentration, Chapter 30). The specific water channel that is controlled by ADH is aquaporin-2.[2,13]

As with thirst, ADH levels are controlled by ECF volume and osmolality. Osmoreceptors in the hypothalamus sense changes in ECF osmolality and stimulate the production and release of ADH. A small increase in serum osmolality of 1% is sufficient to cause ADH release.[2] Likewise, stretch receptors that are sensitive to changes in blood pressure and the effective circulating volume aid in the regulation of ADH release (*i.e.,* nonosmotic ADH secretion). A blood volume decrease of 5% to 10% produces a maximal increase in ADH levels. As with

TABLE 31.3 DRUGS THAT AFFECT ANTIDIURETIC HORMONE LEVELS[a]

DRUGS THAT DECREASE ADH LEVELS/ACTION	DRUGS THAT INCREASE ADH LEVELS/ACTION
Amphotericin B	Anticancer drugs (vincristine and
Demeclocycline	cyclophosphamide)
Ethanol	Carbamazepine
Foscarnet	Chlorpropamide
Lithium	Clofibrate
Morphine antagonists	General anesthetics (most)
	Narcotics (morphine and meperidine)
	Nicotine
	Nonsteroidal anti-inflammatory drugs
	Phenothiazine antipsychotic drugs
	Selective serotonin reuptake inhibitors
	Thiazide diuretics (chlorothiazide)
	Thiothixene (antipsychotic drug)
	Tricyclic antidepressants

ADH, antidiuretic hormone.
[a]List not inclusive.

many other homeostatic mechanisms, acute conditions produce greater changes in ADH levels than do chronic conditions.

The abnormal synthesis and release of ADH occurs in a number of stress situations. Severe pain, nausea, trauma, surgery, certain anesthetic agents, and some narcotics (*e.g.,* morphine and meperidine) increase ADH levels.[2] Among the drugs that affect ADH are nicotine, which stimulates its release, and alcohol, which inhibits it (Table 31.3). Two important conditions alter ADH levels: DI and inappropriate secretion of ADH.

Diabetes Insipidus. Diabetes insipidus is caused by a deficiency of or a decreased response to ADH.[14,15] Persons with DI are unable to concentrate their urine during periods of water restriction and they excrete large volumes of urine, usually 3 to 20 L/day, depending on the degree of ADH deficiency or renal insensitivity to ADH. This large urine output is accompanied by excessive thirst. As long as the thirst mechanism is normal and fluid is readily available, there is little or no alteration in the fluid levels of persons with DI. The danger arises when the condition develops in someone who is unable to communicate the need for water or is unable to secure the needed water. In such cases, inadequate fluid intake rapidly leads to hypertonic dehydration and increased serum osmolality.

There are two types of DI: neurogenic or central DI, which occurs because of a defect in the synthesis or release of ADH, and nephrogenic DI, which occurs because the kidneys do not respond to ADH.[14,16] In neurogenic DI, loss of 80% to 90% of ADH-secreting neurons is necessary before polyuria becomes evident. Most persons with neurogenic DI have an incomplete form of the disorder and retain some ability to concentrate their urine. Temporary neurogenic DI may follow head injury or surgery near the hypothalamohypophysial tract. Nephrogenic DI is characterized by impairment of urine-concentrating ability and free-water conservation. It may be due to a genetic trait

that affects the V_2 receptor that binds ADH, or the aquaporin-2 protein that forms the water channels in the collecting tubules.[16] Other, acquired causes of nephrogenic DI are drugs such as lithium and electrolyte disorders such as potassium depletion or chronic hypercalcemia. Lithium and the electrolyte disorders are thought to interfere with the postreceptor actions of ADH on the permeability of the collecting ducts.

Diagnosis of DI usually starts by attempting to document the total 24-hour urine output. Also, it must be documented that an osmotic diuresis is not caused by glucose or such disorders as kidney disease. Further evaluation is based on measurement of ADH levels along with plasma and urine osmolality before and after a period of fluid deprivation or hypertonic saline infusion. Persons with neurogenic DI do not increase their ADH levels in response to increased plasma osmolality. Another diagnostic approach is to conduct a carefully monitored trial of a pharmacologic form of ADH. Persons with nephrogenic DI do not respond to pharmacologic preparations of the hormone. When central DI is suspected, diagnostic methods such as MRI studies of the pituitary–hypothalamic area are used to determine the cause of the disorder. MRI studies localize the normal posterior pituitary as a high-intensity signal on T1-weighted images. Research reports indicate the "bright spot" is related to the content of stored ADH. This high-intensity signal is present in most (but not all) normal subjects and is absent in most (but not all) patients with DI.[14]

The management of central DI depends on the cause and severity of the disorder. Many persons with incomplete neurogenic DI maintain near-normal water balance when permitted to ingest water in response to thirst. Pharmacologic preparations of ADH are available for persons who cannot be managed by conservative measures. The preferred drug for treating chronic DI is desmopressin acetate (DDAVP). It is usually given orally, but is also available in parenteral and nasal forms. The oral antidiabetic agent chlorpropamide may be used to stimulate ADH release in partial neurogenic DI. It is usually reserved for special cases because of its ability to cause hypoglycemia. Both neurogenic and nephrogenic forms of DI respond partially to the thiazide diuretics (*e.g.,* hydrochlorothiazide). These diuretics are thought to act by increasing sodium excretion by the kidneys, leading to ECF volume contraction, a decrease in the glomerular filtration rate (along with filtered load of sodium), and an increase in sodium and water reabsorption. It also has been postulated that the thiazide diuretics increase water permeability in the collecting tubules.[16]

Syndrome of Inappropriate Antidiuretic Hormone. The syndrome of inappropriate ADH (SIADH) results from a failure of the negative feedback system that regulates the release and inhibition of ADH.[17] In persons with this syndrome, ADH secretion continues even when serum osmolality is decreased, causing marked water retention and dilutional hyponatremia.

SIADH may occur as a transient condition, as in a stress situation, or as a chronic condition, resulting from disorders such as lung or brain tumours. Stimuli such as surgery, pain, stress, and temperature changes are capable of triggering ADH release through action of the CNS. Drugs induce SIADH in different ways. Some drugs are thought to increase hypothalamic production and release of ADH, and others are believed to act directly on the renal tubules to enhance the action of ADH. More chronic forms of SIADH may result from lung tumours, chest lesions, and CNS disorders. Tumours, particularly bronchogenic carcinomas and cancers of the lymphoid tissue, prostate, and pancreas, are known to produce and release ADH independent of normal hypothalamic control mechanisms (examples of paraneoplastic conditions are described in Chapter 8). Other intrathoracic conditions, such as advanced tuberculosis, severe pneumonia, and positive-pressure ventilation, also cause SIADH. The suggested mechanism for SIADH in positive-pressure ventilation is activation of baroreceptors (*e.g.,* aortic baroreceptors, cardiopulmonary receptors) that respond to marked changes in intrathoracic pressure. Disease and injury to the CNS can cause direct pressure on or direct involvement of the hypothalamic-posterior-pituitary structures.[18] Examples include brain tumours, hydrocephalus, head injury, meningitis, and encephalitis. Human immunodeficiency virus (HIV) infection is an established cause of SIADH, related to associated infections, tumours, or drugs.

The manifestations of SIADH are those of dilutional hyponatremia (discussed next). Urine osmolality is high and serum osmolality is low. Urine output decreases despite adequate or increased fluid intake. Hematocrit and the plasma sodium and urea levels are all decreased because of the expansion of the ECF volume. The diagnosis of SIADH should be considered only if the five cardinal features are fulfilled: (1) hypotonic hyponatremia, (2) natriuresis (>20 mmol/L), (3) urine osmolality in excess of plasma osmolality, (4) absence of edema and volume depletion, and (5) normal renal, thyroid, and adrenal function.[17]

The treatment of SIADH depends on its severity. In mild cases, treatment consists of fluid restriction. If fluid restriction is not sufficient, diuretics such as mannitol and furosemide (Lasix) may be given to promote diuresis and free-water clearance. Lithium and the antibiotic demeclocycline inhibits the action of ADH on the renal collecting ducts and may be used in treating the disorder.[7] In cases of severe water intoxication, a hypertonic (*e.g.,* 3%) sodium chloride solution may be administered intravenously. The recently developed antagonists to the antidiuretic action of ADH (aquaretics) offer a new therapeutic approach to the treatment of euvolemic hyponatremia.[13] These agents (*e.g.,* conivaptan) are specific ADH V_2 receptor antagonists and result in aquaresis (*i.e.,* the electrolyte-sparing excretion of free water).

Disorders of Sodium and Water Balance

Disorders of sodium and water balance can be divided into two main categories: (1) isotonic contraction or expansion of ECF volume and (2) hypotonic dilution (hyponatremia) or hypertonic concentration (hypernatremia) of extracellular sodium brought about by changes in extracellular water (Fig. 31.8). Isotonic disorders usually are confined to the ECF compartment, producing a contraction (fluid volume deficit)

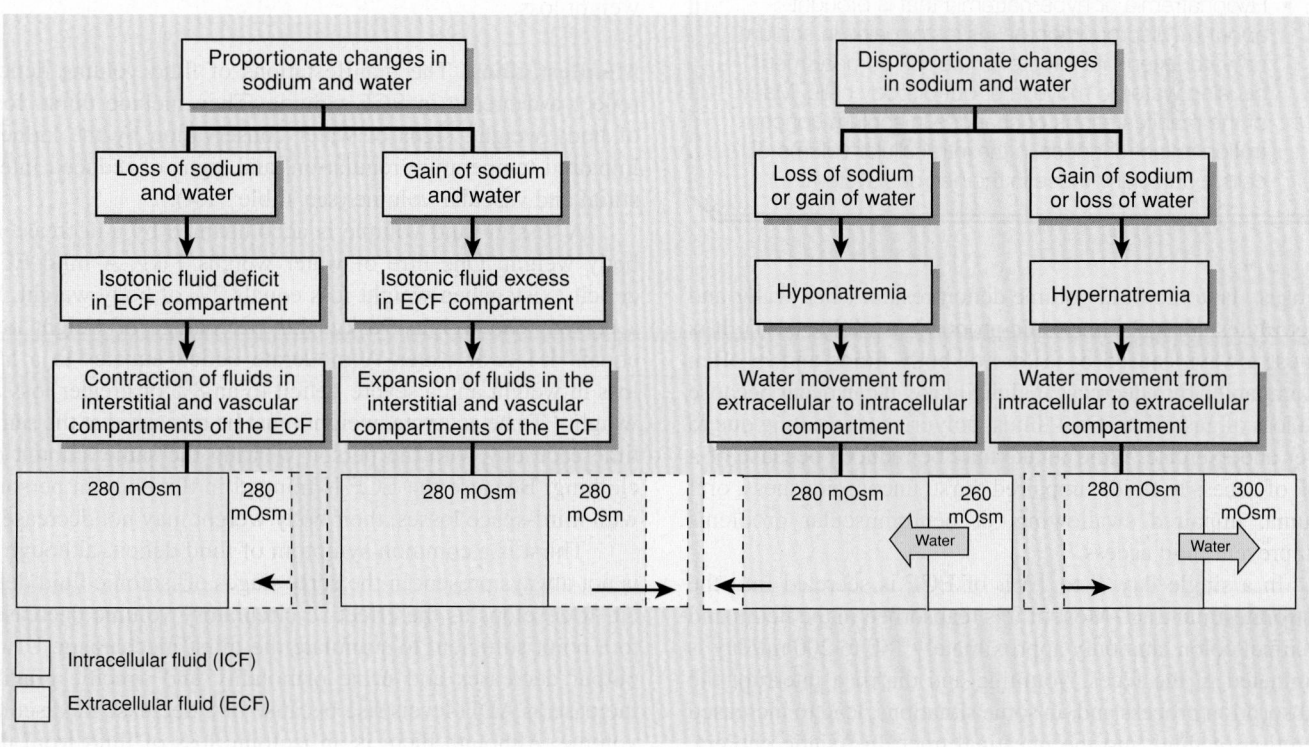

FIGURE 31.8 • Effect of isotonic fluid excess and deficit and of hyponatremia and hypernatremia on movement of water between the extracellular (ECF) and intracellular fluid (ICF) compartments.

or expansion (fluid volume excess) of the interstitial and vascular fluids. Disorders of sodium concentration produce a change in the osmolality of the ECF, with movement of water from the ECF compartment into the ICF compartment (hyponatremia) or from the ICF compartment into the ECF compartment (hypernatremia).

Isotonic Fluid Volume Deficit

Fluid volume deficit is characterized by a decrease in the ECF, including the circulating blood volume. The term *isotonic fluid volume deficit* is used to differentiate the type of fluid deficit in which there are proportionate losses in sodium and water from water deficit and the hyperosmolar state associated with hypernatremia. Unless other fluid and electrolyte imbalances are present, the concentration of plasma electrolytes remains essentially unchanged. When the effective circulating blood volume is compromised, the condition is often referred to as *hypovolemia*.

> ## SODIUM AND WATER BALANCE
>
> - It is the amount of water and its effect on sodium concentration in the ECF that serves to regulate the distribution of fluid between the ICF and the ECF compartments.
> - Isotonic changes in body fluids that result from proportionate gains or losses of sodium and water are largely confined to the ECF compartment. Many of the manifestations of isotonic fluid deficit or excess reflect changes in vascular and interstitial fluid volume.
> - Hyponatremia or hypernatremia that is brought about by disproportionate losses or gains in sodium or water exerts its effects on the ICF compartment, causing water to move in or out of body cells. Many of the manifestations of changes in sodium concentration reflect changes in the intracellular volume of cells, particularly those in the nervous system.

Causes. Isotonic fluid volume deficit results when water and electrolytes are lost in isotonic proportions (Table 31.4). It is almost always caused by a loss of body fluids and is often accompanied by a decrease in fluid intake. It can occur because of a loss of gastrointestinal fluids, polyuria, or sweating due to fever and exercise. Fluid intake may be reduced because of a lack of access to fluids, impaired thirst, unconsciousness, oral trauma, impaired swallowing, or neuromuscular problems that prevent fluid access.

In a single day, 8 to 10 L of ECF is secreted into the gastrointestinal tract. Most of it is reabsorbed in the ileum and proximal colon, and only approximately 150 to 200 ml/day is eliminated in the feces. Vomiting and diarrhea interrupt the reabsorption process and, in some situations, lead to increased secretion of fluid into the intestinal tract. In Asiatic cholera, death can occur within a matter of hours as the cholera organism causes excessive amounts of fluid to be secreted into the

bowel. These fluids are then lost as vomitus or excreted as diarrheal fluid. Gastrointestinal suction, fistulas, and drainage tubes can remove large amounts of fluid from the gastrointestinal tract.

Excess sodium and water losses can also occur through the kidney. Certain forms of kidney disease are characterized by salt wasting due to impaired sodium reabsorption. Fluid volume deficit can also result from osmotic diuresis or injudicious use of diuretic therapy. Glucose in the urine filtrate prevents reabsorption of water by the renal tubules, causing a loss of sodium and water. In Addison disease, a condition of chronic adrenocortical insufficiency, there is unregulated loss of sodium in the urine with a resultant loss of ECF (see Chapter 41). This is accompanied by increased potassium retention.

The skin acts as an exchange surface for heat and as a vapour barrier to prevent water from leaving the body. Body surface losses of sodium and water increase when there is excessive sweating or when large areas of skin have been damaged. Hot weather and fever increase sweating. In hot weather, water losses through sweating may be increased by as much as 1 to 3 L/hour, depending on acclimatization.[2] The respiratory rate and sweating usually are increased as body temperature rises. As much as 3 L of water may be lost in a single day as a result of fever. Burns are another cause of excess fluid loss. Evaporative losses can increase 10-fold with severe burns, up to 3 to 5 L/day.[2]

Third-space losses cause sequestering of ECF in the serous cavities, extracellular spaces in injured tissues, or lumen of the gut.[7] Because the fluid remains in the body, fluid volume deficit caused by third spacing does not usually cause weight loss.

Manifestations. The manifestations of fluid volume deficit reflect a decrease in ECF volume. They include thirst, loss of body weight, signs of water conservation by the kidney, impaired temperature regulation, and signs of reduced interstitial and vascular volume (see Table 31.4).

A loss in fluid volume is accompanied by a decrease in body weight. One litre of water weighs 1 kg. A mild ECF deficit exists when weight loss equals 2% of body weight. In a person who weighs 70 kg, this percentage of weight loss equals 1.4 L of water. A moderate deficit equates to a 5% loss in weight and a severe deficit to an 8% or greater loss in weight.[7] To be accurate, weight must be measured at the same time each day with the person wearing the same amount of clothing. Because the ECF is trapped in the body in persons with third-space losses, their body weight may not decrease.

Thirst is a common symptom of fluid deficit, although it is not always present in the early stages of isotonic fluid deficit. It develops as the effective circulatory volume decreases to a point sufficient to stimulate the thirst mechanism. Urine output decreases and urine osmolality and specific gravity increase as ADH levels rise because of a decrease in vascular volume. Although there is an isotonic loss of fluid from the vascular compartment, other blood components such as red blood cells and urea (or BUN) become more concentrated.

TABLE 31.4 CAUSES AND MANIFESTATIONS OF ISOTONIC FLUID VOLUME DEFICIT

CAUSES	MANIFESTATIONS
Inadequate Fluid Intake	**Acute Weight Loss (% body weight)**
Oral trauma or inability to swallow	Mild fluid volume deficit: 2%
Inability to obtain fluids	Moderate fluid volume deficit: 2–5%
(e.g., impaired mobility)	Severe fluid deficit: 8% or greater
Impaired thirst sensation	**Compensatory Increase in Antidiuretic**
Therapeutic withholding of fluids	**Hormone**
Unconsciousness or inability to	Decreased urine output
express thirst	Increased osmolality and specific gravity
Excessive Gastrointestinal Fluid Losses	**Increased Serum Osmolality**
Vomiting	Thirst
Diarrhea	Increased hematocrit and blood urea
Gastrointestinal suction	nitrogen
Draining gastrointestinal fistula	**Decreased Vascular Volume**
Excessive Renal Losses	Postural hypotension
Diuretic therapy	Tachycardia, weak and thready pulse
Osmotic diuresis (hyperglycemia)	Decreased vein filling and increased vein
Adrenal insufficiency (Addison disease)	refill time
Salt-wasting kidney disease	Hypotension and shock
Excessive Skin Losses	**Decreased Extracellular Fluid Volume**
Fever	Depressed fontanel in an infant
Exposure to hot environment	Sunken eyes and soft eyeballs
Burns and wounds that remove skin	**Impaired Temperature Regulation**
Third-Space Losses	Elevated body temperature
Intestinal obstruction	
Edema	
Ascites	
Burns (first several days)	

The fluid content of body tissues decreases as fluid is removed from the interstitial spaces. The eyes assume a sunken appearance and feel softer than normal as the fluid content in the anterior chamber of the eye is decreased. Fluids add resiliency to the skin and underlying tissues that is referred to as *skin* or *tissue turgor*. Tissue turgor is assessed by pinching a fold of skin between the thumb and forefinger. The skin should immediately return to its original configuration when the fingers are released.[7,19] If 3% to 5% of body water is lost in infants, there is fairly normal turgor, whereas with 6% to 9% loss of body water, there is poor turgor and a sunken anterior fontanelle.[8] Decreased tissue turgor is less predictive of fluid deficit in older persons (>65 years) because of the loss of tissue elasticity. In infants, fluid deficit may be evidenced by depression of the anterior fontanel due to a decrease in cerebrospinal fluid.[7]

Arterial and venous volumes decline during periods of fluid deficit, as does filling of the capillary circulation. As the volume in the arterial system declines, blood pressure decreases, heart rate increases, and the pulse becomes weak and thready. Postural hypotension (a drop in blood pressure on standing) is an early sign of fluid deficit. On the venous side of the circulation, the veins become less prominent. When

volume depletion becomes severe, signs of hypovolemic shock and vascular collapse appear (see Chapter 26).

Diagnosis and Treatment. Diagnosis of fluid volume deficit is based on a history of conditions that predispose to sodium and water losses, weight loss, and observations of altered physiologic function indicative of decreased fluid volume. Intake and output measurements afford a means for assessing fluid balance. However, these measurements may not represent actual losses and gains, largely because accurate measurements of intake and output often are difficult to obtain and insensible losses are difficult to estimate.

Measurement of heart rate and blood pressure provides useful information about vascular volume. A simple test to determine venous refill time consists of compressing the distal end of a vein on the dorsal aspect of the hand when it is not in the dependent position. The vein is then emptied by "milking" the blood toward the heart. The vein should refill almost immediately when the occluding finger is removed. In the case of decreased venous volume, as occurs in fluid deficit, venous refill time increases. Capillary refill time is also increased. Capillary refill can be assessed by applying pressure to a fingernail for 5 seconds and then releasing the pressure and observing the time (normally 1 to 2 seconds) it takes for the colour to return to normal.[20]

Treatment of fluid volume deficit consists of fluid replacement and measures to correct the underlying cause. Usually, isotonic electrolyte solutions are used for fluid replacement. Acute hypovolemia and hypovolemic shock can cause renal damage; therefore, prompt assessment of the degree of fluid deficit and adequate measures to resolve the deficit and treat the underlying cause are essential.

Isotonic Fluid Volume Excess

Fluid volume excess represents an isotonic expansion of the ECF compartment with increases in both interstitial and vascular volumes. Although increased fluid volume is usually the result of a disease condition, this is not always true. For example, a compensatory isotonic expansion of body fluids can occur in healthy persons during hot weather as a mechanism for increasing body heat loss.

Causes. Isotonic fluid volume excess almost always results from an increase in total body sodium that is accompanied by a proportionate increase in body water. Although it can occur as the result of excessive sodium intake, it is most commonly caused by a decrease in sodium and water elimination by the kidney.

Among the causes of decreased sodium and water elimination are disorders of renal function, heart failure, liver failure, and corticosteroid excess (Table 31.5). Heart failure (see Chapter 26) produces a decrease in the effective circulating volume and renal blood flow and a compensatory increase in sodium and water retention. Persons with severe congestive heart failure maintain a precarious balance between sodium and water intake and output. Even small increases in sodium intake can precipitate a state of fluid volume excess and a worsening of heart failure. A condition called *circulatory overload* results from an increase in blood volume; it can occur during infusion of intravenous fluids or transfusion of blood if the amount or rate of administration is excessive. Liver failure (*e.g.*, cirrhosis of the liver) impairs aldosterone metabolism and decreases effective circulating volume and renal perfusion, leading to increased salt and water retention. The corticosteroid hormones increase sodium reabsorption by the kidneys. Persons taking corticosteroid medications and those with Cushing disease (see Chapter 41) often have problems with sodium retention.

Manifestations. Isotonic fluid volume excess is manifested by an increase in interstitial and vascular fluids. It is characterized by weight gain over a short period of time. Mild fluid volume excess represents a 2% gain in weight; moderate fluid volume excess, a 5% gain in weight; and severe fluid volume excess, a gain of 8% or more in weight[7] (Table 31.5). The presence of edema is characteristic of isotonic fluid excess. When the excess fluid accumulates gradually, as often happens in debilitating diseases and starvation, edema fluid may mask the loss of tissue mass. There may be a decrease in urea and hematocrit as a result of dilution due to expansion of the plasma volume. An increase in vascular volume may be evidenced by distended neck veins, slow-emptying peripheral veins, a full and bounding pulse, and an increase in central venous pressure. When excess fluid accumulates in the lungs (*i.e.*, pulmonary edema), there are complaints of shortness of breath and difficult breathing, respiratory crackles, and

TABLE 31.5 CAUSES AND MANIFESTATIONS OF ISOTONIC FLUID VOLUME EXCESS	
CAUSES	**MANIFESTATIONS**
Inadequate Sodium and Water Elimination	**Acute Weight Gain (% Body Weight)**
Congestive heart failure	Mild fluid volume excess: 2%
Renal failure	Moderate fluid volume excess: 5%
Increased corticosteroid levels	Severe fluid volume excess: 8% or greater
Hyperaldosteronism	**Increased Interstitial Fluid Volume**
Cushing disease	Dependent and generalized edema
Liver failure (*e.g.*, cirrhosis)	
	Increased Vascular Volume
Excessive Sodium Intake in Relation to Output	Full and bounding pulse
Venous distension	Pulmonary edema
Excessive dietary intake	Shortness of breath
Excessive ingestion of sodium-containing	Dyspnea
medications or home remedies	
Crackles	
Excessive administration of sodium-	
containing parenteral fluids	
Cough	
Excessive Fluid Intake in Relation to Output	
Ingestion of fluid in excess of elimination	
Administration of parenteral fluids or	
blood at an excessive rate	

a productive cough. Ascites and pleural effusion may occur with severe fluid volume excess.

Diagnosis and Treatment. Diagnosis of fluid volume excess is usually based on a history of factors that predispose to sodium and water retention, weight gain, and manifestations such as edema and cardiovascular symptoms indicative of an expanded ECF volume.

The treatment of fluid volume excess focuses on providing a more favourable balance between sodium and water intake and output. A sodium-restricted diet is often prescribed as a means of decreasing extracellular sodium and water levels. Diuretic therapy is commonly used to increase sodium elimination. When there is a need for intravenous fluid administration or transfusion of blood components, the procedure requires careful monitoring to prevent fluid overload.

Hyponatremia

The normal plasma concentration of sodium ranges from 135 to 145 mmol/L. Plasma sodium values reflect the sodium concentration which is expressed in millimoles (or milliequivalents) per litre, rather than an absolute amount. Because sodium and its attendant anions account for 90% to 95% of the osmolality of ECF, changes in normal serum osmolality (normal range, 275 to 295 mOsm/kg) usually occur due to changes in plasma sodium concentration. However, serum osmolality also is significantly influenced by amounts of albumin and glucose.

Hyponatremia represents a plasma sodium concentration below 135 mmol/L. It is one of the most common electrolyte disorders seen in general hospital patients and is also common in the outpatient population, particularly in the elderly.[7] A number of age-related events make the elderly population more vulnerable to hyponatremia, including a decrease in renal function accompanied by limitations in sodium conservation. Although older people maintain body fluid homeostasis under most circumstances, the ability to withstand environmental, drug-related, and disease-associated stresses becomes progressively limited.

Types and Causes. Because of the effects of osmotically active particles such as glucose, hyponatremia can present as a hypotonic or hypertonic state.[21] *Hypertonic (translocational) hyponatremia* results from an osmotic shift of water from the ICF to the ECF compartment, such as occurs with hyperglycemia. In this case, the sodium in the ECF becomes diluted as water moves out of cells in response to the osmotic effects of the elevated blood glucose level. *Hypotonic (dilutional) hyponatremia,* by far the most common type of hyponatremia, is caused by water retention. It can be classified as hypovolemic, euvolemic, or hypervolemic based on accompanying ECF fluid volumes.[12,21] Because of its effect on both sodium and water elimination, diuretic therapy can cause either hypovolemic or euvolemic hyponatremia.

Hypovolemic hypotonic hyponatremia occurs when water is lost along with sodium, but to a lesser extent. Among the causes of hypovolemic hyponatremia are excessive sweating in hot weather, particularly during heavy exercise, which leads to loss of salt and water. Hyponatremia develops when water, rather than electrolyte-containing liquids, is used to replace fluids lost in sweating. Another potential cause of hypovolemic hyponatremia is the loss of sodium from the gastrointestinal tract caused by frequent gastrointestinal irrigations with distilled water. Iso-osmotic fluid loss, such as occurs in vomiting or diarrhea, does not usually lower plasma sodium levels unless these losses are replaced with disproportionate amounts of orally ingested or parenterally administered water. Gastrointestinal fluid loss and ingestion of excessively diluted formula are common causes of acute hyponatremia in infants and children. Hypovolemic hyponatremia is also a common complication of adrenal insufficiency and is attributable to a decrease in aldosterone levels. A lack of aldosterone increases renal losses of sodium and a cortisol deficiency leads to increased release of ADH with water retention.

Euvolemic or *normovolemic hypotonic hyponatremia* represents retention of water with dilution of sodium while maintaining the ECF volume within a normal range. It is usually the result of SIADH. The risk of normovolemic hyponatremia is increased during the postoperative period. During this time ADH levels are often high, producing an increase in water reabsorption by the kidney (see section on SIADH). Although these elevated levels usually resolve in about 72 hours, they can persist for as long as 5 days. The hyponatremia becomes exaggerated when electrolyte-free fluids (*e.g.,* 5% glucose in water) are used for fluid replacement.

Hypervolemic hypotonic hyponatremia is seen when hyponatremia is accompanied by edema-associated disorders such as decompensated heart failure, advanced liver disease, and renal disease. Although the total body sodium is increased in heart failure, the effective circulating volume is often sensed as inadequate by the baroreceptors (*i.e.,* relative arterial under-filling), resulting in increased ADH levels (nonosmotic ADH secretion).[22]

Abuse of methylenedioxymethamphetamine (MDMA), also known as "ecstasy," can lead to severe neurologic symptoms, including seizures, brain edema, and herniation due to severe hyponatremia. MDMA and its metabolites have been shown to cause enhanced release of ADH from the hypothalamus.[23]

Manifestations. The manifestations of hypotonic hyponatremia are largely related to sodium dilution (Table 31.6). Serum osmolality is decreased and cellular swelling occurs owing to the movement of water from the ECF to the ICF compartment. The manifestations of hyponatremia depend on the rapidity of onset and the severity of the sodium dilution. The signs and symptoms may be acute (*i.e.,* onset within 48 hours), as in severe water intoxication, or more insidious in onset and less severe, as in chronic hyponatremia. Because of water movement, hyponatremia produces an increase in intracellular water, which is responsible for many of the clinical manifestations of the disorder. Fingerprint edema is a sign of excess intracellular water. This phenomenon is demonstrated by pressing the finger firmly over the bony surface of the sternum

TABLE 31.6 CAUSES AND MANIFESTATIONS OF HYPONATREMIA

CAUSES	MANIFESTATIONS
Hypotonic Hyponatremia	**Laboratory Values**
Hypovolemic (Decreased Serum Sodium With Decreased ECF Volume)	Serum sodium levels below 135 mmol/L
Use of excessively diluted infant formula	Hypotonic hyponatremia
Administration of sodium-free parenteral solutions	Serum osmolality <280 mOsm/kg
Gastrointestinal losses	Dilution of blood components, including hematocrit, urea
Vomiting, diarrhea (sweating, with sodium-free fluid replacement)	Hypertonic hyponatremia
Repeated irrigation of body cavities with sodium-free solutions	Serum osmolality >280 mOsm/kg
Irrigation of gastrointestinal tubes with distilled water	**Signs Related to Hypo-osmolality of Extracellular Fluids and Movement of Water Into Brain Cells and Neuromuscular Tissue**
Tap water enemas	Muscle cramps
Use of nonelectrolyte irrigating solutions during prostate surgery	Weakness
Third-spacing (paralytic ileus, pancreatitis)	Headache
Diuretic use	Depression
Mineralocorticoid deficiency (Addison disease)	Apprehension, feeling of impending doom
Salt-wasting nephritis	Personality changes
Euvolemic (Decreased Serum Sodium With Normal ECF Volume)	Lethargy
Increased ADH levels	Stupor, coma
Trauma, stress, pain	**Gastrointestinal Manifestations**
Syndrome of inappropriate ADH	Anorexia, nausea, vomiting
Use of medications that increase ADH	Abdominal cramps, diarrhea
Diuretic use	**Increased Intracellular Fluid**
Glucocorticoid deficiency	Fingerprint edema
Hypothyroidism	Manifestations largely related to hyperosmolality of extracellular fluids
Psychogenic polydipsia	
Endurance exercise	
Methylenedioxymethamphetamine ("ecstasy") abuse	
Hypervolemic (Decreased Serum Sodium With Increased ECF Volume)	
Decompensated heart failure	
Advanced liver disease	
Kidney failure without nephrosis	
Hypertonic Hyponatremia (Osmotic Shift of Water From the ICF to the ECF Compartment)	
Hyperglycemia	

for 15 to 30 seconds. When excess intracellular water is present, a fingerprint similar to that observed when pressing on a piece of modelling clay is seen.[7]

Muscle cramps, weakness, and fatigue reflect the effects of hyponatremia on skeletal muscle function and are often early signs of hyponatremia. These effects commonly are observed in persons with hyponatremia that occurs during heavy exercise in hot weather. Gastrointestinal manifestations such as nausea and vomiting, abdominal cramps, and diarrhea may develop.

The cells of the brain and nervous system are most seriously affected by increases in intracellular water. Symptoms include apathy, lethargy, and headache, which can progress to disorientation, confusion, gross motor weakness, and depression of deep tendon reflexes. Seizures and coma occur when plasma sodium levels reach extremely low levels. These severe effects, which are caused by brain swelling, may be irreversible. If the condition develops slowly, signs and symptoms do not develop until plasma sodium levels approach 120 mmol/L (*i.e.,* severe hyponatremia).[21-24] The term *water intoxication* is often used to describe the neurologic effects of acute hypotonic hyponatremia.

Diagnosis and Treatment. Diagnosis of hyponatremia is based on laboratory reports of a decreased plasma sodium concentration, plasma and urine osmolality, and urine sodium concentration; assessment of the person's volume status; presence of conditions that predispose to sodium loss or water retention; and signs and symptoms indicative of the disorder.

The treatment of hyponatremia with water excess focuses on the underlying cause. When hyponatremia is caused by water intoxication, limiting water intake or discontinuing medications that contribute to SIADH may be sufficient. The administration of a saline solution orally or intravenously may be needed when hyponatremia is caused by sodium deficiency. Symptomatic hyponatremia (*i.e.,* neurologic manifestations) is often treated with hypertonic saline solution and a loop diuretic, such as furosemide, to increase water elimination. This combination allows for correction of plasma sodium levels while ridding the body of excess water. Specific ADH V_2 receptor antagonists to the antidiuretic action of ADH (aquaretics) offer a newer therapeutic approach to the treatment of euvolemic hyponatremia.[25]

There is concern about the rapidity with which plasma sodium levels are corrected, particularly in persons with chronic symptomatic hyponatremia. Cells, particularly those in the brain, tend to defend against changes in cell volume caused by changes in ECF osmolality by increasing or decreasing their concentration of organic osmolytes.[23–25] In the case of prolonged water intoxication, brain cells reduce their concentration of osmolytes as a means of preventing an increase in cell volume. It takes several days for brain cells to restore the osmolytes lost during hyponatremia. Thus, treatment measures that produce rapid changes in serum osmolality may cause a dramatic change in brain cell volume. One of the reported effects of rapid treatment of hyponatremia is an osmotic demyelinating condition called *central pontine myelinolysis,* which produces serious neurologic sequelae and sometimes causes death.[24] This complication occurs more commonly in premenopausal women and in hypoxic patients.

Hypernatremia

Hypernatremia represents a plasma sodium level above 145 mmol/L and a serum osmolality greater than 295 mOsm/kg. Because sodium is functionally an impermeable solute, it contributes to tonicity and induces movement of water across cell membranes. Hypernatremia is characterized by hypertonicity of ECF and almost always causes cellular dehydration. Although this condition is often seen in older adults, hospital-acquired hypernatremia occurs in all ages and is an independent risk factor for an increase in mortality.[7,26]

Causes. Hypernatremia represents a deficit of water in relation to the body's sodium stores. It can be caused by net loss of water or sodium gain. Net water loss can occur through the urine, gastrointestinal tract, lungs, or skin. A defect in thirst or inability to obtain or drink water can interfere with water replacement. Excessive intake of sodium is rare; examples include taking excess salt tablets or near-drowning in salt water, which produces a disproportionate gain in sodium compared to water (Table 31.7).

Hypernatremia almost always follows a loss of body fluids that have a lower-than-normal concentration of sodium so that water is lost in excess of sodium. This can result from increased losses from the respiratory tract during fever or strenuous exercise, from watery diarrhea, or when osmotically active tube feedings are given with inadequate amounts of water. With pure water loss, each body fluid compartment loses an equal percentage of its volume. Because approximately one third of the water is in the ECF compartment, compared with the two thirds in the ICF compartment, more actual water volume is lost from the ICF than the ECF compartment.[2]

Normally, water deficit stimulates thirst and increases water intake. Therefore, hypernatremia is more likely to occur in infants and in persons who cannot express their thirst or obtain water to drink. With hypodipsia, or impaired thirst, the need for fluid intake does not activate the thirst response. Hypodipsia is particularly prevalent among the elderly. In persons with DI, hypernatremia can develop when thirst is impaired or access to water is impeded.

The therapeutic administration of sodium-containing solutions may also cause hypernatremia. For example, the administration of sodium bicarbonate during cardiopulmonary resuscitation increases body sodium levels because each 50-ml ampule of 7.5% sodium bicarbonate contains 892 mmol of sodium. Hypertonic saline solution intended for intra-amniotic instillation for therapeutic abortion may inadvertently be injected intravenously, causing hypernatremia.[7]

Manifestations. The clinical manifestations of hypernatremia caused by water loss are largely those of ECF loss and cellular dehydration (Table 31.7). The severity of signs and symptoms is greatest when the increase in plasma sodium is large and occurs rapidly. Body weight is decreased in proportion to the amount of water that has been lost. Because blood plasma is roughly 90% to 93% water, the concentrations of blood cells and other blood components increase as ECF water decreases.

Thirst is an early symptom of water deficit, occurring when water losses are equal to 0.5% of body water. Urine output is decreased and urine osmolality increased because of renal water-conserving mechanisms. Body temperature frequently is elevated, and the skin becomes warm and flushed. The vascular volume decreases, the pulse becomes rapid and thready, and the blood pressure drops. Hypernatremia produces an increase in serum osmolality and results in water being pulled out of body cells. As a result, the skin and mucous membranes become dry, and salivation and lacrimation are decreased. The mouth becomes dry and sticky, and the tongue becomes rough and fissured. Swallowing is difficult. The subcutaneous tissues assume a firm, rubbery texture. Most significantly, water is pulled out of the cells in the CNS, causing decreased reflexes,

TABLE 31.7 CAUSES AND MANIFESTATIONS OF HYPERNATREMIA

CAUSES	MANIFESTATIONS
Excessive Water Losses Watery diarrhea Excessive sweating Increased respirations due to conditions such as tracheobronchitis Hypertonic tube feedings Diabetes insipidus	**Laboratory Values** Serum sodium level above 145 mmol/L Increased serum osmolality Increased hematocrit and urea
Decreased Water Intake Unavailability of water Oral trauma or inability to swallow Impaired thirst sensation Withholding water for therapeutic reasons Unconsciousness or inability to express thirst	**Thirst and Signs of Increased ADH Levels** Polydipsia Oliguria or anuria High urine specific gravity **Intracellular Dehydration** Dry skin and mucous membranes Decreased tissue turgor Tongue rough and fissured Decreased salivation and lacrimation

Excessive Sodium Intake
Rapid or excessive administration of
    sodium-containing parenteral solutions
Near-drowning in salt water
	**Signs Related to Hyperosmolality of
	    Extracellular Fluids and Movement
	    of Water Out of Brain Cells**
	Headache
	Agitation and restlessness
	Decreased reflexes
	Seizures and coma
	
	**Extracellular Dehydration and Decreased
	    Vascular Volume**
	Tachycardia
	Weak and thready pulse
	Decreased blood pressure
	Vascular collapse

agitation, headache, and restlessness. Coma and seizures may develop as hypernatremia progresses.

Diagnosis and Treatment. The diagnosis of hypernatremia is based on history, physical examination findings indicative of dehydration, and results of laboratory tests. The treatment of hypernatremia includes measures to treat the underlying cause of the disorder and fluid replacement therapy to treat the accompanying dehydration. Replacement fluids can be given orally or intravenously. The oral route is preferable. Oral glucose-electrolyte replacement solutions are available for the treatment of infants with diarrhea[27] (see Chapter 37). Until recently, these solutions were used only early in diarrheal illness or as a first step in reestablishing oral intake after parenteral replacement therapy. These solutions are now widely available in grocery stores and pharmacies for use in the treatment of diarrhea and other dehydrating disorders in infants and young children.

One of the serious aspects of fluid volume deficit is dehydration of brain and nerve cells. Serum osmolality should be corrected slowly in cases of chronic hypernatremia. As mentioned previously, brain cells mobilize organic osmolytes to protect against changes in cell volume.[23–25] If hypernatremia is corrected too rapidly before the osmolytes have had a chance to dissipate, the plasma may become relatively hypotonic

in relation to brain cell osmolality. When this occurs, water moves into the brain cells, causing cerebral edema and potentially severe neurologic impairment.

IN SUMMARY

Body fluids are distributed between the ICF and ECF compartments. Regulation of fluid volume, solute concentration, and distribution between the two compartments depends on water and sodium balance. Water provides approximately 90% to 93% of fluid volume, and sodium salts, approximately 90% to 95% of extracellular solutes. Both water and sodium are absorbed from the gastrointestinal tract and eliminated by the kidneys. The main regulator of sodium and water is the maintenance of the effective circulating blood volume, which is monitored by stretch receptors in the vascular system, which exert their effects through ADH and the sympathetic nervous system; and those in the kidney, which exert their effects through the sympathetic nervous system and the RAAS. Body water and serum osmolality are also regulated by thirst, which controls water intake, and ADH, which controls urine concentration and renal output.

Isotonic fluid disorders result from contraction or expansion of ECF volume brought about by proportionate losses of sodium and water. Isotonic fluid volume deficit is characterized by a decrease in ECF volume. It causes thirst, decreased vascular volume and circulatory function, decreased urine output, and increased urine specific gravity. Isotonic fluid volume excess is characterized by an increase in ECF volume. It is manifested by signs of increased vascular volume and edema.

Alterations in extracellular sodium concentration are brought about by a disproportionate gain (hyponatremia) or loss (hypernatremia) of water. As the major cation in the ECF compartment, sodium controls the ECF osmolality and its effect on cell volume. Hyponatremia can present as a hypertonic (translocational) hyponatremia in which water moves out of the cell in response to elevated blood glucose levels, or as a hypotonic (dilutional) hyponatremia that is caused by retention of water by the body in excess of sodium. Hypotonic hyponatremia, which can present as a hypovolemic, euvolemic, or hypervolemic state, is characterized by water being pulled into the cell from the ECF compartment, causing cells to swell. It is manifested by muscle cramps and weakness; nausea, vomiting, abdominal cramps, and diarrhea; and CNS signs such as headache, lethargy, depression of deep tendon reflexes, and in severe cases seizure and coma.

Hypernatremia represents a disproportionate loss of body water in relation to sodium. It is characterized by intracellular water being pulled into the ECF compartment, causing cells to shrink. It is manifested by thirst and decreased urine output; dry mouth and decreased tissue turgor; signs of decreased vascular volume (tachycardia, weak and thready pulse); and CNS signs, such as decreased reflexes, agitation, headache, and in severe cases seizures and coma.

POTASSIUM BALANCE

After completing this section of the chapter, you should be able to meet the following objectives:

- Characterize the distribution of potassium in the body and explain how extracellular potassium levels are regulated in relation to body gains and losses.
- State the causes of hypokalemia and hyperkalemia in terms of altered intake, output, and transcellular shifts.
- Relate the functions of potassium to the manifestations of hypokalemia and hyperkalemia.
- Describe methods used in diagnosis and treatment of hypokalemia and hyperkalemia.

Regulation of Potassium Balance

Potassium is the second most abundant cation in the body and the major cation in the ICF compartment. Approximately 98% of body potassium is contained within body cells, with an intracellular concentration of 140 to 150 mmol/L.[1] The potassium content of the ECF (3.5 to 5.0 mmol/L) is considerably lower. Because potassium is an intracellular ion, total body stores of potassium are related to body size and muscle mass. In adults, total body potassium is approximately 50 mmol/kg of body weight. Approximately 75% of potassium is in muscle cells. Thus, potassium content declines with age, mainly as a result of a decrease in muscle mass.[2,28]

Gains and Losses

Potassium intake is normally derived from dietary sources. In healthy persons, potassium balance usually can be maintained by a daily dietary intake of 50 to 100 mmol. Additional amounts of potassium are needed during periods of trauma and stress. The kidneys are the main source of potassium loss. Approximately 80% to 90% of potassium losses occur in the urine, with the remainder being lost in stools or sweat.

Mechanisms of Regulation

Normally, the ECF concentration of potassium is precisely regulated at about 4.2 mmol/L. The precise control is necessary because many cell functions are sensitive to even small changes in ECF potassium levels. Either an increase or decrease of 1.0 to 2.0 mmol/L outside the normal range can cause serious neurological complications, cardiac dysrhythmias and even death.[2]

Plasma potassium is largely regulated through two mechanisms: (1) renal mechanisms that conserve or eliminate potassium and (2) a transcellular shift between the ICF and ECF compartments.

POTASSIUM BALANCE

- Potassium is mainly an intracellular ion with only a small, but vital, amount being present in the extracellular fluids.
- The distribution of potassium between the intracellular and extracellular compartments regulates electrical membrane potentials controlling the excitability of nerve and muscle cells as well as contractility of skeletal, cardiac, and smooth muscle tissue.
- Because of its vital role in regulating neuromuscular excitability, potassium regulation must be extremely efficient.
- Two major mechanisms function in the control of serum potassium: (1) renal mechanisms that conserve or eliminate potassium and (2) transcellular buffer systems that remove potassium from and release it into the serum as needed. Conditions that disrupt the function of either mechanism can result in a serious alteration in serum potassium levels.

Renal Regulation. The major route for potassium elimination is the kidney. Unlike other electrolytes, the regulation of potassium elimination is controlled by secretion from the blood into the tubular filtrate rather than through reabsorption from the tubular filtrate into the blood. Potassium is filtered in the glomerulus, reabsorbed along with sodium and water in the proximal tubule and with sodium and chloride in the thick ascending loop of Henle, and then secreted into the late distal and cortical collecting tubules for elimination in the urine. The latter mechanism serves to "fine-tune" the concentration of potassium in the ECF.

Aldosterone plays an essential role in regulating potassium elimination by the kidney. The effects of aldosterone on potassium elimination are mediated through an Na^+/K^+ exchange mechanism located in the late distal and cortical collecting tubules of the kidney (see Chapter 30). In the presence of aldosterone, Na^+ is transported back into the blood and K^+ is secreted in the tubular filtrate for elimination in the urine. The rate of aldosterone secretion by the adrenal gland is strongly controlled by plasma potassium levels. For example, an increase of less than 1 mmol/L of potassium causes aldosterone levels to triple.[2] The effect of plasma potassium on aldosterone secretion is an example of the powerful feedback regulation of potassium elimination. In the absence of aldosterone, as occurs in persons with Addison disease, renal elimination of potassium is impaired, causing plasma potassium levels to rise to dangerously high levels. Aldosterone is often referred to as a *mineralocorticoid hormone* because of its effect on sodium and potassium. The term *mineralocorticoid activity* is used to describe the aldosterone-like actions of other adrenocortical hormones, such as cortisol.

There is also a K^+/H^+ exchange mechanism in the cortical collecting tubules of the kidney (see Chapter 30). When plasma potassium levels are increased, K^+ is secreted into the urine and H^+ is reabsorbed into the blood, producing a decrease in pH and metabolic acidosis. Conversely, when potassium levels are low, K^+ is reabsorbed and H^+ is secreted in the urine, leading to metabolic alkalosis.

Extracellular–Intracellular Shifts. To avoid an increase in extracellular potassium levels during this time, excess potassium is temporarily shifted into red blood cells and other cells such as those of muscle, liver, and bone. This movement is controlled by the function of the Na^+/K^+-ATPase membrane pump and the permeability of the ion channels in the cell membrane.

Among the factors that alter the intracellular–extracellular distribution of potassium are serum osmolality, acid–base disorders, insulin, and β-adrenergic stimulation. Acute increases in serum osmolality cause water to leave the cell. The loss of cell water produces an increase in intracellular potassium, causing it to move out of the cell into the ECF.

The H^+ and K^+ ions, which are positively charged, can be exchanged between the ICF and ECF in a cation shift (Fig. 31.9). In metabolic acidosis, for example, H^+ moves into body cells for buffering, causing K^+ to leave and move into the ECF.[7,8] Both insulin and the catecholamines (*e.g.,* epinephrine) increase cellular uptake of K^+ by increasing the activity of the Na^+/K^+-ATPase membrane pump.[29] Insulin produces an increase in cellular uptake of potassium after a meal. The catecholamines, particularly epinephrine, facilitate the movement of potassium into muscle tissue during periods of physiologic

FIGURE 31.9 • Mechanisms regulating transcellular shifts in potassium.

stress. β-Adrenergic agonist drugs, such as pseudoephedrine and salbutamol, have a similar effect on potassium distribution.

Exercise also produces compartmental shifts in potassium. Repeated muscle contraction releases potassium into the ECF. Although the increase usually is small with modest exercise, it can be considerable during exhaustive exercise. Even the repeated clenching and unclenching of the fist during a blood draw can cause potassium to move out of cells and artificially elevate plasma potassium levels.

Disorders of Potassium Balance

As the major intracellular cation, potassium is critical to many body functions. It is involved in a wide range of body functions, including the maintenance of the osmotic integrity of cells, acid–base balance, and the kidney's ability to concentrate urine. Potassium is necessary for growth and it contributes to the intricate chemical reactions that transform carbohydrates into energy, change glucose into glycogen, and convert amino acids to proteins. Potassium also plays a critical role in conducting nerve impulses and the excitability of skeletal, cardiac, and smooth muscle (see Chapter 4). It does this by regulating (1) the resting membrane potential, (2) the opening of the sodium channels that control the flow of current during the action potential, and (3) the rate of membrane repolarization. Changes in nerve and muscle excitability are particularly important in the heart, where alterations in plasma potassium can produce serious cardiac arrhythmias and conduction defects. Changes in plasma potassium also affect skeletal muscles and the smooth muscle in blood vessels and the gastrointestinal tract.

The *resting membrane potential* is determined by the ratio of ICF to ECF potassium concentration (Fig. 31.10). A decrease in plasma potassium causes the resting membrane potential to become more negative, moving it further away

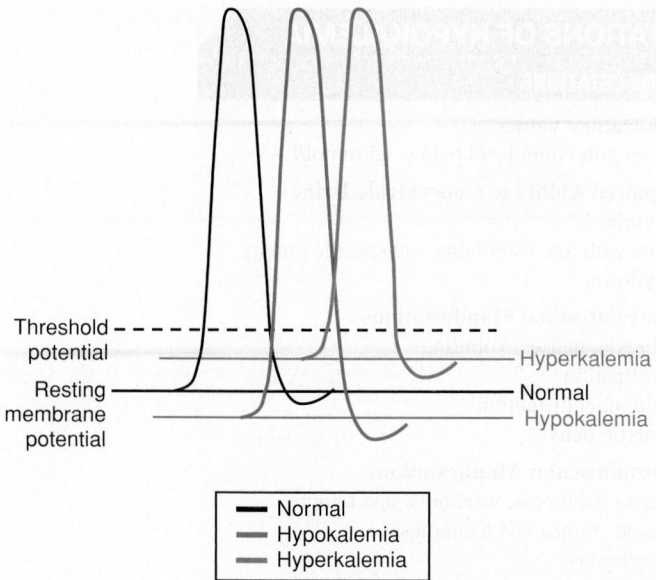

FIGURE 31.10 • Effect of changes in plasma hypokalemia (*red*) and hyperkalemia (*blue*) on the resting membrane potential, activation and opening of the sodium channels at threshold potential, and the rate of repolarization during a nerve action potential.

from the threshold for excitation (see Chapter 4). Thus, it takes a greater stimulus to reach threshold and open the sodium channels that are responsible for the action potential. An increase in plasma potassium has the opposite effect; it causes the resting membrane potential to become more positive, moving it closer to threshold. With severe hyperkalemia, the resting membrane approaches the threshold potential, causing sustained subthreshold depolarization with a resultant inactivation of the sodium channels and a net decrease in excitability. The *rate of repolarization* also varies with plasma potassium levels. It is more rapid in hyperkalemia and delayed in hypokalemia. Both the inactivation of the sodium channels and the rate of membrane repolarization are important clinically because they predispose to cardiac arrhythmias or conduction defects (see Chapter 25).

Hypokalemia

Hypokalemia refers to a decrease in plasma potassium levels below 3.5 mmol/L. Because of transcellular shifts, temporary changes in plasma potassium may occur as the result of movement between the ICF and ECF compartments.

Causes. The causes of potassium deficit can be grouped into three categories: (1) inadequate intake; (2) excessive gastrointestinal, renal, and skin losses; and (3) redistribution between the ICF and ECF compartments (Table 31.8).[30]

Inadequate Intake. Inadequate intake is a frequent cause of hypokalemia. A potassium intake of at least 40 to 50 mmol/day is needed to compensate for obligatory urine losses.[7] Insufficient dietary intake (typically <40 mmol/day) may result from the inability to obtain or ingest food or from a diet that is low

in potassium-containing foods. Potassium intake is often inadequate in persons on fad diets and those who have eating disorders. Older adults are particularly likely to have potassium deficits. They may have poor eating habits as a consequence of living alone; limited income, which makes buying foods high in potassium difficult; difficulty chewing many foods that have high potassium content because of dental problems; or problems with swallowing.

Excessive Losses. The kidneys are the main source of potassium loss. Approximately 80% to 90% of potassium losses occur in the urine, with the remaining losses occurring in the stool and sweat. The kidneys do not have the homeostatic mechanisms needed to conserve potassium during periods of insufficient intake. After trauma and in stress situations, urinary losses of potassium are greatly increased, sometimes approaching levels of 150 to 200 mmol/L.[30] This means that a potassium deficit can develop rather quickly if intake is inadequate. Renal losses also can be increased by medications, metabolic alkalosis, magnesium depletion, and increased levels of aldosterone. Some antibiotics, particularly amphotericin B and gentamicin, are impermeable anions that require the presence of positively charged cations for elimination in the urine; this causes potassium wasting.

Diuretic therapy, with the exception of potassium-sparing diuretics, is the most common cause of hypokalemia. Both thiazide and loop diuretics increase the loss of potassium in the urine. The degree of hypokalemia is directly related to diuretic dose and is greater when sodium intake is higher.[31] Magnesium depletion causes renal potassium wasting. Magnesium deficiency often coexists with potassium depletion due to diuretic therapy or disease processes such as diarrhea. Importantly, the ability to correct potassium deficiency is impaired when magnesium deficiency is present.

Renal losses of potassium are accentuated by aldosterone and cortisol. Increased potassium losses occur in situations such as trauma and surgery that produce a stress-related increase in these hormones. Primary aldosteronism, caused by either a tumour or hyperplasia of the cells of the adrenal cortex that secrete aldosterone, produces severe potassium losses and a decrease in plasma potassium levels. Cortisol binds to aldosterone receptors and exerts aldosterone-like effects on potassium elimination. Licorice-induced hypokalemia results from inhibition of the enzyme that inactivates cortisol.

Other rare, genetic disorders that can also result in hypokalemia are the Bartter, Gitelman, and Liddle syndromes. *Bartter syndrome,* which involves the $Na^+/K^+/2Cl^-$ cotransporter in the thick loop of Henle, is manifested by metabolic alkalosis, hypercalciuria or excessive loss of calcium in the urine, and *normal* blood pressure.[32] Because the loop diuretics act at the same site in the kidney, these features are identical to those seen with chronic loop diuretic ingestion. The manifestations of *Gitelman syndrome,* which involves the Na^+/Cl^- transporter in the distal tubule, are similar to those of Bartter syndrome, but with hypocalciuria and hypomagnesemia due to renal magnesium wasting.[33] Because this is the site where

TABLE 31.8 CAUSES AND MANIFESTATIONS OF HYPOKALEMIA

CAUSES	MANIFESTATIONS
Inadequate Intake Diet deficient in potassium Inability to eat Administration of potassium-free parenteral solutions	**Laboratory Values** Serum potassium level below 3.5 mmol/L
	Impaired Ability to Concentrate Urine Polyuria Urine with low osmolality and specific gravity Polydipsia
Excessive Renal Losses Diuretic therapy (except potassium-sparing diuretics) Diuretic phase of renal failure Increased mineralocorticoid levels Primary hyperaldosteronism Treatment with corticosteroid drugs	**Gastrointestinal Manifestations** Anorexia, nausea, vomiting Constipation Abdominal distention Paralytic ileus
Excessive Gastrointestinal Losses Vomiting Diarrhea Gastrointestinal suction Draining gastrointestinal fistula	**Neuromuscular Manifestations** Muscle flabbiness, weakness, and fatigue Muscle cramps and tenderness Paresthesias Paralysis
Transcompartmental Shift Administration of β-adrenergic agonist (*e.g.,* salbutamol) Administration of insulin for treatment of diabetic ketoacidosis Alkalosis, metabolic or respiratory	**Cardiovascular Manifestations** Postural hypotension Increased sensitivity to digitalis toxicity Changes in electrocardiogram Cardiac dysrhythmias
	Central Nervous System Manifestations Confusion Depression
	Acid–base disorders Metabolic Alkalosis

the thiazide diuretics exert their action, these manifestations are identical to those seen with chronic thiazide diuretic ingestion. *Liddle syndrome* has manifestations similar to Bartter syndrome, but with *high* blood pressure due to excessive sodium reabsorption.[34]

Although potassium losses from the skin and the gastrointestinal tract usually are minimal, these losses can become excessive under certain conditions. For example, burns increase surface losses of potassium. Losses due to sweating increase in persons who are acclimated to a hot climate, partly because increased secretion of aldosterone during heat acclimatization increases the loss of potassium in urine and sweat. Gastrointestinal losses also can become excessive; this occurs with vomiting and diarrhea and when gastrointestinal suction is being used. The potassium content of liquid stools, for example, is approximately 40 to 60 mmol/L.

Transcellular Shifts. Because of the high ratio of intracellular to extracellular potassium, conditions that produce a redistribution of potassium from the ECF to the ICF compartment can cause a marked decrease in plasma potassium levels (Fig. 31.9). Insulin increases the movement of glucose and potassium into cells; therefore, potassium deficit often develops during treatment of diabetic ketoacidosis. A wide variety of β₂-adrenergic agonist drugs (*e.g.,* decongestants and bronchodilators) shift

potassium into cells and cause transient hypokalemia. For example, standard doses of nebulized salbutamol (a bronchodilator) can reduce plasma potassium up to 1 mmol/L.[35]

Manifestations. The manifestations of hypokalemia include alterations in renal, gastrointestinal, cardiovascular, and neuromuscular function (Table 31.8). These manifestations reflect both the intracellular functions of potassium as well as the body's attempt to regulate ECF potassium levels within the very narrow range needed to maintain the normal electrical activity of excitable tissues such as nerve and muscle cells. The signs and symptoms of potassium deficit seldom develop until plasma potassium levels have fallen to levels below 3 mmol/L. They are typically gradual in onset, and therefore the disorder may go undetected for some time.

The renal processes that conserve potassium during hypokalemia interfere with the kidney's ability to concentrate urine. Urine output and plasma osmolality are increased, urine specific gravity is decreased, and complaints of polyuria, nocturia, and thirst are common (an example of nephrogenic DI). Metabolic alkalosis and renal chloride wasting are signs of severe hypokalemia.

There are numerous signs and symptoms associated with gastrointestinal function, including anorexia, nausea, and vomiting. Atony of the gastrointestinal smooth muscle can cause constipation, abdominal distension, and, in severe hypokalemia, paralytic ileus. When gastrointestinal symptoms occur gradually and are not severe, they often impair potassium intake and exaggerate the condition.

The most serious effects of hypokalemia are those affecting cardiovascular function. Postural hypotension is common. Most persons with plasma potassium levels below 3 mmol/L demonstrate electrocardiographic (ECG) changes typical of hypokalemia. These changes include prolongation of the PR interval, depression of the ST segment, flattening of the T-wave, and appearance of a prominent U-wave (Fig. 31.11). Normally, potassium leaves the cell during the repolarization phase of the action potential, returning the membrane potential to its normal resting value. Hypokalemia reduces the permeability of the cell membrane to potassium and thus produces a decrease in potassium efflux that prolongs the rate of repolarization and lengthens the relative refractory period. The U-wave normally may be present on the ECG but should

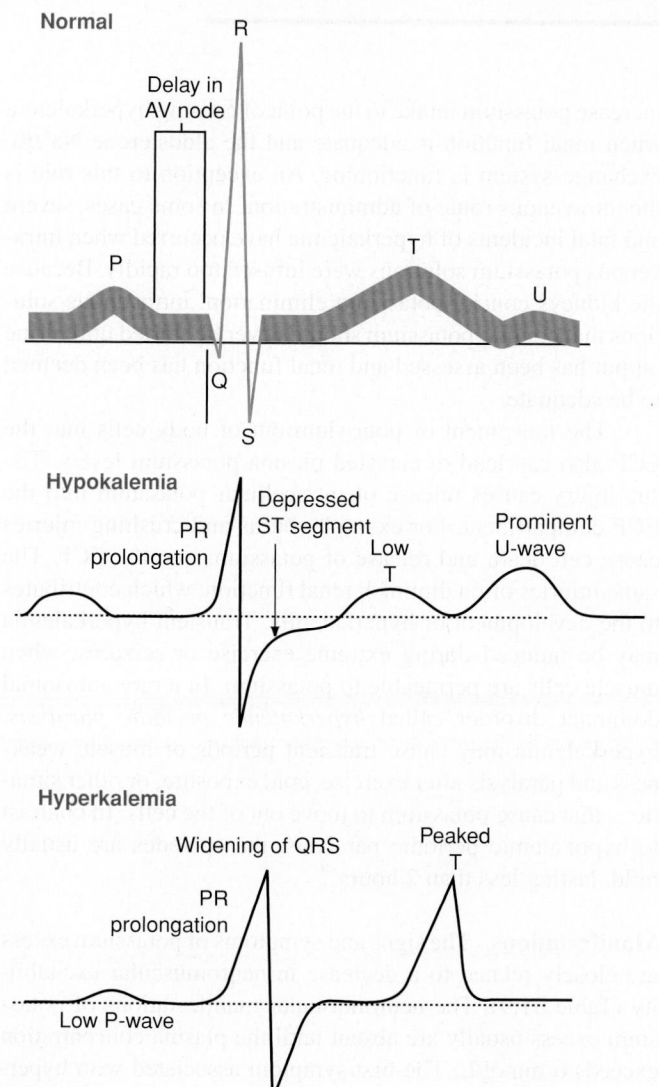

FIGURE 31.11 • Electrocardiographic changes with hypokalemia and hyperkalemia.

be of lower amplitude than the T-wave. With hypokalemia, the amplitude of the T-wave decreases as the U-wave amplitude increases. Although these changes in electrical cardiac activity usually are not serious, they may predispose to sinus bradycardia and ectopic ventricular arrhythmias (see Chapter 25 for additional information on the ECG and cardiac arrhythmias). Digitalis toxicity can be provoked in persons treated with this drug and there is an increased risk of ventricular arrhythmias, particularly in persons with underlying heart disease. The dangers associated with digitalis toxicity are compounded in persons who are receiving diuretics that increase urinary losses of potassium.

Complaints of weakness, fatigue, and muscle cramps, particularly during exercise, are common in moderate hypokalemia (plasma potassium 2.5 to 3 mmol/L). Muscle paralysis with life-threatening respiratory insufficiency can occur with severe hypokalemia (plasma potassium <2.5 mmol/L). Leg muscles, particularly the quadriceps, are most prominently affected. Some persons complain of muscle tenderness and paresthesias rather than weakness. In chronic potassium deficiency, muscle atrophy may contribute to muscle weakness.

In a rare genetic condition called *hypokalemic familial periodic paralysis*, episodes of hypokalemia cause attacks of flaccid paralysis that last 6 to 48 hours if untreated.[36] The paralysis may be precipitated by situations that cause severe hypokalemia by producing an intracellular shift in potassium, such as ingestion of a high-carbohydrate meal or administration of insulin, epinephrine, or glucocorticoid drugs. The paralysis often can be reversed by potassium replacement therapy. A similar condition can occur with poorly controlled hyperthyroidism (thyrotoxic hypokalemic periodic paralysis), especially in Asian persons. Treatment is with potassium replacement and appropriate therapy for the underlying thyroid disorder.[37]

Treatment. When possible, hypokalemia caused by potassium deficit is treated by increasing the intake of foods high in potassium content—meats, dried fruits, fruit juices (particularly orange juice), and bananas. Oral potassium supplements are prescribed for persons whose intake of potassium is insufficient in relation to losses. This is particularly true of persons who are receiving diuretic therapy and those who are taking digitalis.

Potassium may be given intravenously when the oral route is not tolerated or when rapid replacement is needed. Magnesium deficiency may impair potassium correction; in such cases, magnesium replacement is indicated.[38] The rapid infusion of a concentrated potassium solution can cause death from cardiac arrest. Health personnel who assume responsibility for administering intravenous solutions that contain potassium should be fully aware of all the precautions pertaining to their dilution and flow rate.

Hyperkalemia

Hyperkalemia refers to an increase in plasma levels of potassium in excess of 5.0 mmol/L. It seldom occurs in healthy persons because the body is extremely effective in preventing excess potassium accumulation in the ECF.

TABLE 31.9 CAUSES AND MANIFESTATIONS OF HYPERKALEMIA

CAUSES	MANIFESTATIONS
Excessive Intake	**Laboratory Values**
Excessive oral intake	Serum potassium level above 5.0 mmol/L
Treatment with oral potassium supplements	**Gastrointestinal Manifestations**
Excessive or rapid infusion of potassium-containing parenteral fluids	Nausea and vomiting
	Intestinal cramps
Release From Intracellular Compartment	Diarrhea
Tissue trauma	**Neuromuscular Manifestations**
Burns	Paresthesias
Crushing injuries	Weakness, dizziness
Extreme exercise or seizures	Muscle cramps
Inadequate Elimination by Kidneys	**Cardiovascular Manifestations**
Renal failure	Changes in electrocardiogram
Adrenal insufficiency (Addison disease)	Risk of cardiac arrest with severe excess
Treatment with potassium-sparing diuretics	
Treatment with angiotensin-converting enzyme inhibitors or angiotensin II receptor blockers	

Causes. The three major causes of potassium excess are (1) decreased renal elimination, (2) excessively rapid administration, and (3) movement of potassium from the ICF to ECF compartment[39] (Table 31.9). A pseudohyperkalemia can occur secondary to release of potassium from intracellular stores after a blood sample has been collected, hemolysis of red blood cells from excessive agitation of a blood sample, traumatic venipuncture, or prolonged application of a tourniquet during venipuncture.[39]

The most common cause of hyperkalemia is decreased renal function. Chronic hyperkalemia is almost always associated with renal failure. Usually, the glomerular filtration rate must decline to less than 10 ml/min before hyperkalemia develops. Some renal disorders, such as sickle cell nephropathy, lead nephropathy, and systemic lupus nephritis, can selectively impair tubular secretion of potassium without causing renal failure. Acidosis further diminishes potassium elimination by the kidney. Persons with acute renal failure accompanied by lactic acidosis or ketoacidosis are at increased risk for development of hyperkalemia. Correcting the acidosis usually helps to correct the hyperkalemia.

Aldosterone acts at the level of the distal tubular Na$^+$/K$^+$ exchange system to increase potassium excretion while facilitating sodium reabsorption. A decrease in aldosterone-mediated potassium elimination can result from adrenal insufficiency (*i.e.,* Addison disease), depression of aldosterone release due to a decrease in renin or angiotensin II, or impaired ability of the kidneys to respond to aldosterone. Potassium-sparing diuretics (*e.g.,* spironolactone, amiloride) can produce hyperkalemia by means of the latter mechanism. Because of their ability to decrease aldosterone levels, the ACE inhibitors and ARBs can also produce an increase in plasma potassium levels.

Potassium excess can result from excessive oral ingestion or intravenous administration of potassium. It is difficult to increase potassium intake to the point of causing hyperkalemia when renal function is adequate and the aldosterone Na$^+$/K$^+$ exchange system is functioning. An exception to this rule is the intravenous route of administration. In some cases, severe and fatal incidents of hyperkalemia have occurred when intravenous potassium solutions were infused too rapidly. Because the kidneys control potassium elimination, intravenous solutions that contain potassium should never be started until urine output has been assessed and renal function has been deemed to be adequate.

The movement of potassium out of body cells into the ECF also can lead to elevated plasma potassium levels. Tissue injury causes release of intracellular potassium into the ECF compartment. For example, burns and crushing injuries cause cell death and release of potassium into the ECF. The same injuries often diminish renal function, which contributes to the development of hyperkalemia. Transient hyperkalemia may be induced during extreme exercise or seizures, when muscle cells are permeable to potassium. In a rare autosomal dominant disorder called *hyperkalemic periodic paralysis,* hyperkalemia may cause transient periods of muscle weakness and paralysis after exercise, cold exposure, or other situations that cause potassium to move out of the cells. In contrast to hypokalemic periodic paralysis, the episodes are usually mild, lasting less than 2 hours.[40]

Manifestations. The signs and symptoms of potassium excess are closely related to a decrease in neuromuscular excitability (Table 31.9). The neuromuscular manifestations of potassium excess usually are absent until the plasma concentration exceeds 6 mmol/L. The first symptom associated with hyperkalemia typically is paresthesia. There may be complaints of generalized muscle weakness or shortness of breath secondary to respiratory muscle weakness.

The most serious effect of hyperkalemia is on the heart. As potassium levels increase, disturbances in cardiac conduction occur. The earliest changes are peaked, narrow T-waves and widening of the QRS complex. If plasma levels continue to rise, the PR interval becomes prolonged, followed by disappearance of P-waves (Fig. 31.11). The heart rate may be slow. Ventricular fibrillation and cardiac arrest are terminal events. Detrimental effects of hyperkalemia on the heart are most pronounced when the plasma potassium level rises rapidly.

Diagnosis and Treatment. Diagnosis of hyperkalemia is based on complete history, physical examination to detect muscle weakness and signs of volume depletion, plasma potassium levels, and ECG findings. The history should include questions about dietary intake, use of potassium-sparing diuretics, history of kidney disease, and recurrent episodes of muscle weakness.

The treatment of potassium excess varies with the degree of increase in plasma potassium and whether there are ECG and neuromuscular manifestations. Calcium antagonizes the potassium-induced decrease in membrane excitability, restoring excitability toward normal. The protective effect of calcium administration is usually short-lived (15 to 30 minutes), and it must be accompanied by other therapies to decrease the ECF potassium concentration. The administration of sodium bicarbonate, β-adrenergic agonists (*e.g.,* salbutamol), or insulin distributes potassium into the ICF compartment and rapidly decreases the ECF concentration. Intravenous infusions of insulin and glucose are often used for this purpose.

Less emergent measures focus on decreasing or curtailing intake or absorption, increasing renal excretion, and increasing cellular uptake. Decreased intake can be achieved by restricting dietary sources of potassium. The major ingredient in most salt substitutes is potassium chloride, and such substitutes should not be given to patients with renal problems. Increasing potassium output often is more difficult. Patients with renal failure may require hemodialysis or peritoneal dialysis to reduce plasma potassium levels. Sodium polystyrene sulfonate, a cation exchange resin, also may be used to remove K$^+$ ions from the colon. The Na$^+$ ions in the resin are exchanged for K$^+$ ions, and the potassium-containing resin is eliminated in the stool.

IN SUMMARY

Potassium is the major ICF cation. It contributes to the maintenance of intracellular osmolality; plays a critical role in conducting nerve impulses and in the excitability of skeletal, cardiac, and smooth muscle; and influences acid–base balance. Potassium is ingested in the diet and eliminated through the kidney. Because potassium is poorly conserved by the kidney, an adequate daily intake is needed. A transcellular shift can produce a redistribution of potassium between the ECF and ICF compartments, causing blood levels to increase or decrease.

Hypokalemia represents a decrease in plasma potassium to levels below 3.5 mmol/L. It can result from inadequate intake, excessive losses, or redistribution between the ICF and ECF compartments. The manifestations of potassium deficit include alterations in renal, skeletal muscle, gastrointestinal, and cardiovascular function, reflecting the crucial role of potassium in cell metabolism and neuromuscular function.

Hyperkalemia represents an increase in plasma potassium to levels plasma greater than 5.0 mmol/L. It seldom occurs in healthy persons because the body is extremely effective in preventing excess potassium accumulation in the ECF. The major causes of potassium excess are decreased elimination of potassium by the kidney, excessively rapid intravenous administration of potassium, and a transcellular shift of potassium out of the cell to the ECF compartment. The most serious effect of hyperkalemia is cardiac arrest.

CALCIUM, PHOSPHORUS, AND MAGNESIUM BALANCE

After completing this section of the chapter, you should be able to meet the following objectives:

- Describe the associations among intestinal absorption, renal elimination, bone stores, and the functions of vitamin D and parathyroid hormone in regulating calcium, phosphorus, and magnesium levels.
- State the difference between ionized and bound or chelated forms of calcium in terms of physiologic function.
- Describe the mechanisms of calcium gain and loss and relate them to the causes and manifestations of hypocalcemia and hypercalcemia.
- Describe the mechanisms of phosphorus gain and loss and relate them to causes and manifestations of hypophosphatemia and hyperphosphatemia.
- Describe the mechanisms of magnesium gain and loss and relate them to the causes and manifestations of hypomagnesemia and hypermagnesemia.

Mechanisms Regulating Calcium, Phosphorus, and Magnesium Balance

Calcium, phosphorus, and magnesium are the major divalent cations in the body. They are ingested in the diet, absorbed from the intestine, filtered in the glomerulus of the kidney, reabsorbed in the renal tubules, and eliminated in the urine. Approximately 99% of calcium, 85% of phosphorus, and 50% to 60% of magnesium are found in bone. Most of the remaining calcium (approximately 1%), phosphorus (approximately 14%), and magnesium (approximately 40% to 50%)

are located inside cells. Only a small amount of these three ions is present in ECF. This small, but vital, amount of ECF calcium, phosphorus, and magnesium is directly or indirectly regulated by vitamin D and parathyroid hormone. Calcitonin, a hormone produced by C-cells in the thyroid, is thought to act on the kidney and bone to remove calcium from the extracellular circulation. The roles of vitamin D, parathyroid hormone (PTH), and calcitonin in skeletal function are discussed further in Chapters 57 and 59.

Vitamin D

Although classified as a vitamin, vitamin D functions as a hormone. It acts to sustain normal plasma levels of calcium and phosphorus by increasing their absorption from the intestine, and it is also necessary for normal bone formation. Vitamin D_3 (cholecalciferol) is synthesized by ultraviolet irradiation of 7-dehydrocholesterol, which is present in the skin or obtained from foods in the diet, many of which are fortified with vitamin D_2 (ergocalciferol). The synthesized or ingested forms of vitamin D are essentially prohormones that lack biologic activity and must undergo metabolic transformation to achieve potency. Once vitamin D enters the circulation from the skin or intestine, it is concentrated in the liver. There it is hydroxylated to form 25-hydroxyvitamin D [25-(OH)D_3], also called *calcidiol*. It is then transported to the kidney, where it is transformed into active 1,25-(OH)$_2D_3$. The major action of the activated form of vitamin D, also called *calcitriol*, is to increase the absorption of calcium from the intestine. Calcitriol also sensitizes bone to the resorptive actions of PTH. There is evidence that vitamin D controls parathyroid gland growth and suppresses the synthesis and secretion of PTH.[41] The formation of 1,25-(OH)$_2D_3$ in the kidneys is regulated in feedback fashion by plasma calcium and phosphorus levels. Low calcium levels lead to an increase in PTH, which then increases vitamin D activation. A lowering of plasma phosphorus also augments vitamin D activation. Additional control of renal activation of vitamin D is exerted by a negative feedback loop that monitors 1,25-(OH)$_2D_3$ levels.[41] Vitamin D deficiency is further discussed in Chapter 59.

Parathyroid Hormone

Parathyroid hormone, a major regulator of plasma calcium and phosphorus, is secreted by the parathyroid glands. There are four parathyroid glands located on the dorsal surface of the thyroid gland. The dominant regulator of PTH is the plasma calcium concentration. A unique calcium receptor on the parathyroid cell membrane (extracellular calcium-sensing receptor) responds rapidly to changes in plasma calcium levels.[42] When the plasma calcium level is high, PTH is inhibited and the calcium is deposited in the bones. When the level is low, PTH secretion is increased and calcium is mobilized from the bones. The response to a decrease in plasma calcium is prompt, occurring within seconds. phosphorus does not exert a direct effect on PTH secretion. Instead, it acts indirectly by forming a complex with calcium, thereby decreasing the plasma calcium concentration.

The secretion, synthesis, and action of PTH are also influenced by magnesium. Magnesium serves as a cofactor in the generation of cellular energy and is important in the function of second messenger systems. Magnesium's effects on the synthesis and release of PTH are thought to be mediated through these mechanisms. Because of its function in regulating PTH release, severe and prolonged hypomagnesemia can markedly inhibit PTH levels.

The main function of PTH is to maintain the calcium concentration of the ECF. It performs this function by promoting the release of calcium from bone, increasing the activation of vitamin D as a means of enhancing intestinal absorption of calcium, and stimulating calcium conservation by the kidney while increasing phosphorus excretion (Fig. 31.12). PTH acts on bone to accelerate the mobilization and transfer of calcium to the ECF. The skeletal response to PTH is a two-step process. There is an immediate response in which calcium that is present in bone fluid is released into the ECF, and a second, more slowly developing response in which completely mineralized bone is resorbed, resulting in the release of both calcium and phosphorus. The actions of PTH in terms of bone resorption require normal levels of both vitamin D and magnesium. The

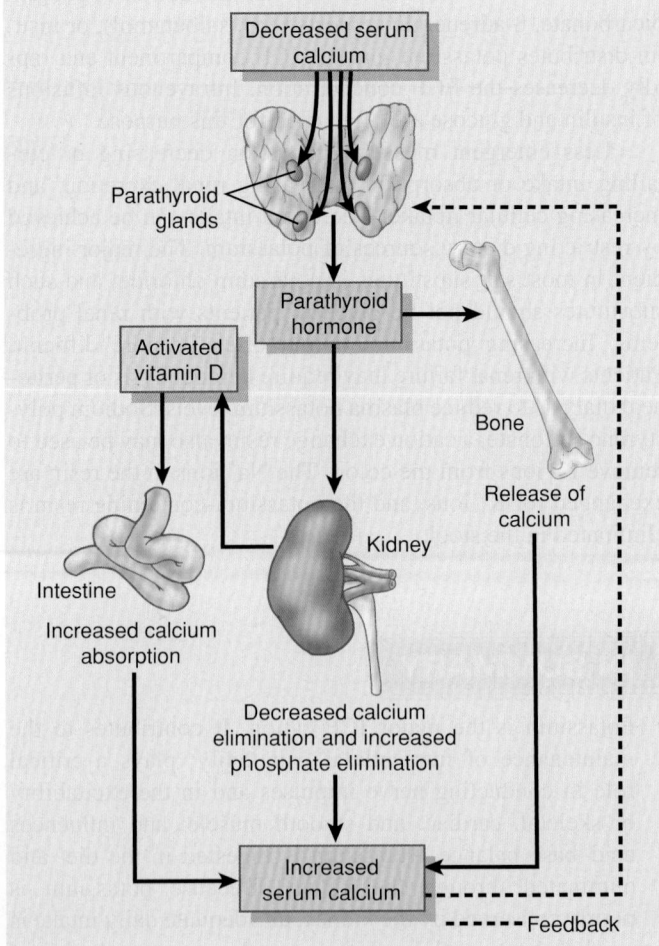

FIGURE 31.12 • Regulation of plasma calcium concentration by parathyroid hormone.

activation of vitamin D by the kidney is enhanced by the presence of PTH; it is through the activation of vitamin D that PTH increases intestinal absorption of calcium and phosphorus as well as acting on the kidney to increase tubular reabsorption of calcium and magnesium while increasing phosphorus elimination. The accompanying increase in phosphorus elimination ensures that the phosphorus released from bone does not produce hyperphosphatemia and increase the risk of soft tissue deposition of calcium phosphate crystals.

Hypoparathyroidism. Hypoparathyroidism reflects deficient PTH secretion, resulting in hypocalcemia. PTH deficiency may be caused by a congenital absence of all of the parathyroid glands, as in DiGeorge syndrome (see Chapter 19). An acquired deficiency of PTH may occur after neck surgery, particularly if the surgery involves removal of a parathyroid adenoma, thyroidectomy, or bilateral neck resection for cancer. A transient form of PTH deficiency, occurring within 1 to 2 days and lasting up to 5 days, may occur after thyroid surgery owing to parathyroid gland suppression.[7,43] Hypoparathyroidism also may have an autoimmune origin. Antiparathyroid antibodies have been detected in some persons with hypoparathyroidism, particularly those with multiple autoimmune disorders such as type 1 diabetes, Graves disease, and vitiligo (autoimmune destruction of melanocytes resulting in the development of totally white areas of skin). Other causes of hypoparathyroidism include heavy metal damage such as occurs with Wilson disease, metastatic tumours, and surgery. Functional impairment of parathyroid function occurs with magnesium deficiency. Correction of the hypomagnesemia results in rapid disappearance of the condition.

Manifestations of acute hypoparathyroidism, which result from a decrease in plasma calcium, include tetany with muscle cramps, carpopedal spasm, and convulsions (see section on Hypocalcemia). Paresthesias, such as tingling of the circumoral area and the hands and feet, are almost always present. Low calcium levels may cause prolongation of the QT interval, resistance to digitalis, hypotension, and refractory heart failure. Symptoms of chronic PTH deficiency include lethargy, anxiety state, and personality changes. There may be blurring of vision because of cataracts, which develop over a number of years. Extrapyramidal signs, such as those seen with Parkinson disease, may occur because of calcification of the basal ganglia. Successful treatment of the hypocalcemia may improve the disorder and is sometimes associated with a decrease in basal ganglia calcification on radiography. Teeth may be defective if the disorder occurs during childhood.

Diagnosis of hypoparathyroidism is based on low plasma calcium levels, high plasma phosphorus levels, and low plasma PTH levels. Plasma magnesium levels usually are measured to rule out hypomagnesemia as a cause of the disorder. Acute hypoparathyroid tetany is treated with intravenous calcium gluconate followed by oral administration of calcium salts and vitamin D. Magnesium supplementation is used when the disorder is caused by magnesium deficiency. Persons with chronic hypoparathyroidism are treated with oral calcium and

vitamin D. Plasma calcium levels are monitored at regular intervals (at least every 3 months) as a means of maintaining plasma calcium within a slightly low but asymptomatic range. Maintaining plasma calcium within this range helps to prevent hypercalciuria and kidney damage.

Pseudohypoparathyroidism is a rare familial disorder characterized by target tissue resistance to PTH. It is characterized by hypocalcemia, increased parathyroid function, and a variety of congenital defects in the growth and development of the skeleton, including short stature and short metacarpal and metatarsal bones. There are variants in the disorder, with some persons having pseudohypoparathyroidism with the congenital defects and others having the congenital defects with normal calcium and phosphorus levels. The manifestations of the disorder are due primarily to chronic hypocalcemia. Treatment is similar to that for hypoparathyroidism.

Hyperparathyroidism. Hyperparathyroidism is caused by hypersecretion of PTH. Hyperparathyroidism can manifest as a primary disorder caused by hyperplasia (15%), an adenoma (85%), and, rarely, carcinoma of the parathyroid glands, or as a secondary disorder seen in persons with chronic renal failure or chronic malabsorption of calcium. Parathyroid adenomas and hyperplasia can occur in several distinct familial diseases (including multiple endocrine neoplasia [MEN] types 1 and 2a).[44]

Primary hyperparathyroidism is seen more commonly after 50 years of age and is more common in women than men.[44,45] Primary hyperparathyroidism causes hypercalcemia and an increase in calcium in the urine filtrate, resulting in hypercalciuria and the potential for development of kidney stones. Chronic bone resorption may produce diffuse demineralization, pathologic fractures, and cystic bone lesions. A dual-energy x-ray absorptiometry (DEXA) bone scan may be used to assess bone mineral density (BMD). Signs and symptoms of the disorder are related to skeletal abnormalities, exposure of the kidney to high calcium levels, and elevated plasma calcium levels (see section on Hypercalcemia). At present, most patients with primary hyperparathyroidism manifest an asymptomatic disorder that is discovered in the course of routine biochemical testing.[45]

Diagnostic procedures, which include plasma calcium levels and intact PTH levels, are used to differentiate between the two most common causes of hypercalcemia: primary hyperparathyroidism and hypercalcemia of malignancy. Assays of intact PTH use two antibodies that bind to different sites on PTH and are specifically designed to measure the intact, biologically active hormones. In primary hyperparathyroidism the intact PTH levels are elevated in 75% to 90% of affected persons or are inappropriately "normal" in the face of hypercalcemia, when they should be suppressed. In hypercalcemia of malignancy, the intact PTH levels are suppressed. Imaging studies of the parathyroid area may be used to identify a parathyroid adenoma. Parathyroid surgery is usually the treatment of choice.[45]

Secondary hyperparathyroidism involves hyperplasia of the parathyroid glands and occurs primarily in persons with renal failure[46,47] (see Chapter 34). In early renal failure, an increase in PTH results from decreased plasma calcium and activated vitamin D levels. As the disease progresses, there is a decrease in vitamin D and calcium receptors, making the parathyroid glands more resistant to feedback regulation by plasma calcium and vitamin D level. At this point, elevated plasma phosphorus levels induce hyperplasia of the parathyroid glands independent of calcium and activated vitamin D. The bone disease seen in persons with secondary hyperparathyroidism due to renal failure is known as *chronic kidney disease–mineral and bone disorder (CKD-MBD)*. The traditional term, renal osteodystrophy, is a single measure looking at the alteration in bone morphology, whereas the systemic disorder of CKD-MBD encompasses abnormal mineral metabolism (*i.e.*, calcium, phosphate, vitamin D, or PTH), abnormalities in bone turnover, plus any extraskeletal calcification[48] (see Chapter 34).

Treatment of hyperparathyroidism includes resolving the hypercalcemia with increased fluid intake. Persons with mild disease are advised to keep active and drink adequate fluids. They are also advised to avoid calcium-containing antacids, vitamin D, and thiazide diuretics, which increase reabsorption of calcium by the kidney. Parathyroidectomy may be indicated in persons with symptomatic hyperparathyroidism, kidney stones, or bone disease. Avoiding hyperphosphatemia may lessen the problems of CKD-MBD caused by secondary hyperparathyroidism in renal failure. Calcium acetate or a calcium-free agent (sevelamer HCl [Renagel]) can be given with meals to bind phosphorus.[49] Calcitriol, the activated form of vitamin D, may be used to control parathyroid hyperplasia and suppress the synthesis and secretion of PTH. However, because of its potent effect on intestinal absorption and bone mobilization, calcitriol can cause hypercalcemia. Newer analogs of activated vitamin D are being developed that retain the ability to suppress parathyroid function while having minimal effects on calcium or phosphorus reabsorption. Calcimimetics (*e.g.*, cinacalcet), which increase the sensitivity of the parathyroid calcium-sensing receptor to extracellular calcium, have been introduced to control secondary hyperparathyroidism in patients with chronic kidney disease.[46]

Disorders of Calcium Balance

Calcium enters the body through the gastrointestinal tract, is absorbed from the intestine under the influence of vitamin D, stored in bone, and excreted by the kidney. Approximately 99% of body calcium is found in bone, where it provides strength and stability for the skeletal system and serves as an exchangeable source to maintain extracellular calcium levels. Most of the remaining calcium (approximately 1%) is located inside cells, and only approximately 0.1% to 0.2% (approximately 2.1 to 2.6 mmol/L) of the remaining calcium is present in the ECF.

The ECF calcium exists in three forms: (1) protein-bound, (2) complexed, and (3) ionized (Fig. 31.13). Approximately 40% of ECF calcium is bound to plasma proteins, mostly albumin, and cannot diffuse or pass through the capillary wall

FIGURE 31.13 • Distribution of body calcium between bone and the intracellular (ICF) and extracellular fluid (ECF) compartments. The percentages of free, complexed, and protein-bound calcium in extracellular fluids are indicated.

to leave the vascular compartment. Another 10% is complexed (*i.e.*, chelated) with substances such as citrate, phosphorus, and sulphate. This form is not ionized. The remaining 50% of ECF calcium is present in the ionized form. It is the ionized form of calcium that is free to leave the vascular compartment and participate in cellular functions. The total plasma calcium level fluctuates with changes in plasma albumin and pH.[50] The equation to correct total serum calcium levels is:

Calcium (corrected, mmol/L)
= Calcium (measured) + 0.02 [40 – Albumin (measured)]

*calcium—serum level in mmol/L
*albumin—serum level in g/L

Ionized calcium serves a number of functions. It participates in many enzyme reactions; exerts an important effect

CALCIUM BALANCE

- About 99% of body calcium is stored in bone; 1% is located inside cells; and 0.1% is found in the extracellular fluid.
- Extracellular fluid calcium levels are made up of free (ionized), complexed, and protein-bound fractions. Only the ionized Ca^{2+} plays an essential role in neuromuscular and cardiac excitability.
- Serum calcium levels are regulated by parathyroid hormone and by renal mechanisms in which serum levels of calcium and phosphate are reciprocally regulated to prevent the damaging deposition of calcium phosphate crystals in the soft tissues of the body.

on membrane potentials and neuronal excitability; is necessary for contraction in skeletal, cardiac, and smooth muscle; participates in the release of hormones, neurotransmitters, and other chemical messengers; influences cardiac contractility and automaticity through the slow calcium channels; and is essential for blood clotting.[50,51] The use of calcium channel blocking drugs in circulatory disorders demonstrates the importance of Ca^{2+} ions in the normal function of the heart and blood vessels. Calcium is required for all but the first two steps of the intrinsic pathway for blood coagulation. Because of its ability to bind calcium, citrate often is used to prevent clotting in blood that is to be used for transfusions.

Gains and Losses

The major Canadian dietary sources of calcium are milk and milk products. However, only 30% to 50% of dietary calcium is absorbed from the duodenum and upper jejunum; the remainder is eliminated in the stool. There is a calcium influx of approximately 150 mg/day into the intestine from the blood. Net absorption of calcium is equal to the amount that is absorbed from the intestine less the amount that moves into the intestine. Calcium balance can become negative when dietary intake (and calcium absorption) is less than intestinal secretion.

Calcium is stored in bone and excreted by the kidney. Approximately 60% to 65% of filtered calcium is passively reabsorbed in the proximal tubule, driven by the reabsorption of sodium chloride; 15% to 20% is reabsorbed in the thick ascending loop of Henle, driven by the $Na^+/K^+/2Cl^-$ cotransport system; and 5% to 10% is reabsorbed in the distal convoluted tubule (see Chapter 30). The distal convoluted tubule is an important regulatory site for controlling the amount of calcium that enters the urine. PTH and possibly vitamin D stimulate calcium reabsorption in this segment of the nephron. Thiazide diuretics, which exert their effects in the distal convoluted tubule, enhance calcium reabsorption. Other factors that may influence calcium reabsorption in the distal convoluted tubule are phosphorus, glucose, and insulin levels.

Hypocalcemia

Hypocalcemia represents a plasma calcium level of less than 2.1 mmol/L. Hypocalcemia occurs in many forms of critical illness and affects as many as 70% to 90% of patients in intensive care units.[52]

Causes. The causes of hypocalcemia can be divided into four categories: (1) impaired ability to mobilize calcium from bone stores, (2) abnormal losses of calcium from the kidney, (3) increased protein binding or chelation such that greater proportions of calcium are in the nonionized form, and (4) soft tissue sequestration (Table 31.10). A pseudohypocalcemia is caused by hypoalbuminemia. It results in a decrease in protein-bound, rather than ionized, calcium and usually is asymptomatic.

Plasma calcium exists in a dynamic equilibrium with calcium in bone. The ability to mobilize calcium from bone depends on adequate levels of PTH. Decreased levels of PTH may result from primary or secondary forms of hypoparathyroidism. Suppression of PTH release may also occur when

TABLE 31.10 CAUSES AND MANIFESTATIONS OF HYPOCALCEMIA	
CAUSES	**MANIFESTATIONS**
Impaired Ability to Mobilize Calcium From Bone	**Laboratory Values**
Hypoparathyroidism	Serum calcium level below 2.1 mmol/L
Resistance to the actions of parathyroid hormone	**Neuromuscular Manifestations (Increased Neuromuscular Excitability)**
Hypomagnesemia	Paresthesias, especially numbness and tingling
Decreased Intake or Absorption	Skeletal muscle cramps
Malabsorption	Abdominal spasms and cramps
Vitamin D deficiency	Hyperactive reflexes
Failure to activate	Carpopedal spasm
Liver disease	Tetany
Kidney disease	Laryngeal spasm
Medications that impair activation of vitamin D (*e.g.,* phenytoin)	Positive Chvostek and Trousseau signs
Abnormal Renal Losses	**Cardiovascular Manifestations**
Renal failure and hyperphosphatemia	Hypotension
	Signs of cardiac insufficiency
Increased Protein Binding or Chelation	Failure to respond to drugs that act by calcium-mediated mechanisms
Increased pH	Prolongation of QT interval predisposes to ventricular arrhythmias
Increased fatty acids	
Rapid transfusion of citrated blood	**Skeletal Manifestations (Chronic Deficiency)**
Increased Sequestration	Osteomalacia
Acute pancreatitis	Bone pain, deformities, fracture

vitamin D levels are elevated. The activated form of vitamin D (calcitriol) can be used to suppress the secondary hyperparathyroidism that occurs in persons with chronic renal disease. Magnesium deficiency inhibits PTH release and impairs the action of PTH on bone resorption. This form of hypocalcemia is difficult to treat with calcium supplementation alone and requires correction of the magnesium deficiency.

There is an inverse relation between calcium and phosphorus excretion by the kidneys. Phosphorus elimination is impaired in chronic kidney disease, causing plasma calcium levels to decrease. Hypocalcemia and hyperphosphatemia occur when the glomerular filtration rate falls below 59 ml/min (normal values, which are related to age, sex, and body size, are approximately 120 ml/min in young women and 130 ml/min in young men; see Chapter 34).

Only the ionized form of calcium is able to leave the capillary and participate in body functions. A change in pH alters the proportion of calcium that is in the bound and ionized forms. An acid pH decreases binding of calcium to protein, causing a proportionate increase in ionized calcium, whereas total plasma calcium remains unchanged. An alkaline pH has the opposite effect. For example, hyperventilation sufficient to cause respiratory alkalosis can produce tetany because of increased protein binding of calcium. Free fatty acids also increase binding of calcium to albumin, causing a reduction in ionized calcium. Elevations in free fatty acids sufficient to alter calcium binding may occur during stressful situations that cause elevations of epinephrine, glucagon, growth hormone, and adrenocorticotropic hormone levels. Heparin, β-adrenergic drugs (*i.e.*, epinephrine, isoproterenol, and norepinephrine), and alcohol can also produce elevations in free fatty acid levels sufficient to increase calcium binding.

Citrate, which complexes with calcium, is often used as an anticoagulant in blood transfusions. Theoretically, excess citrate in donor blood could combine with the calcium in a recipient's blood, producing a sharp drop in ionized calcium. This normally does not occur because the liver removes the citrate within a matter of minutes. When blood transfusions are administered at a slow rate, there is little danger of hypocalcemia caused by citrate binding.

Hypocalcemia is a common finding in patients with acute pancreatitis. Inflammation of the pancreas causes release of proteolytic and lipolytic enzymes. It is thought that the Ca^{2+} combines with free fatty acids released by lipolysis in the pancreas, forming soaps and removing calcium from the circulation.

Calcium deficit due to dietary deficiency exerts its effects on bone stores rather than extracellular calcium levels. A dietary deficiency of vitamin D is still seen today despite many foods being fortified with vitamin D. Vitamin D deficiency is more likely to occur in malabsorption states, such as biliary obstruction, pancreatic insufficiency, and celiac disease, in which the ability to absorb fat and fat-soluble vitamins is impaired. Failure to activate vitamin D is another cause of hypocalcemia. Anticonvulsant medications, particularly phenytoin, can impair initial activation of vitamin D in the liver. The final step in activation of vitamin D is impaired in persons

with chronic kidney disease (see Chapter 34). Fortunately, the activated form of vitamin D, calcitriol, has been synthesized and is available for use in the treatment of calcium deficit in persons with chronic kidney disease.[51]

Manifestations. Hypocalcemia can manifest as an acute or chronic condition. The manifestations of acute hypocalcemia reflect the increased neuromuscular excitability and cardiovascular effects of a decrease in ionized calcium (Table 31.10). Ionized calcium stabilizes neuromuscular excitability, thereby making nerve cells less sensitive to stimuli. Nerves exposed to low ionized calcium levels show decreased thresholds for excitation, repetitive responses to a single stimulus, and, in extreme cases, continuous activity. The severity of the manifestations depends on the underlying cause, rapidity of onset, accompanying electrolyte disorders, and extracellular pH. Increased neuromuscular excitability can manifest as paresthesias (*i.e.*, tingling around the mouth and in the hands and feet) and tetany (*i.e.*, spasms of the muscles of the face, hands, and feet).[53] Severe hypocalcemia can lead to laryngeal spasm, seizures, and even death.

Cardiovascular effects of acute hypocalcemia include hypotension, cardiac insufficiency, cardiac arrhythmias (particularly heart block and ventricular fibrillation), and failure to respond to drugs such as digitalis, norepinephrine, and dopamine that act through calcium-mediated mechanisms.

The Chvostek and Trousseau tests can be used to assess for an increase in neuromuscular excitability and tetany[7,53] (Fig. 31.14). The Chvostek sign is elicited by tapping the face just below the temple at the point where the facial nerve emerges. Tapping the face over the facial nerve causes spasm of the lip, nose, or face when the test result is positive. An

A   **B**

FIGURE 31.14 • A: The Chvostek sign: a contraction of the facial muscles elicited in response to a light tap over the facial nerve in front of the ear. **B:** The Trousseau sign: a carpopedal spasm induced by inflating a blood pressure cuff above systolic blood pressure. (Adapted from Bullock B. A., Henze R. J. (2000). *Focus on pathophysiology* (p. 173). Philadelphia, PA: Lippincott Williams & Wilkins.)

inflated blood pressure cuff is used to test for the Trousseau sign. The cuff is inflated 10 mm Hg above systolic blood pressure for 3 minutes. Contraction of the fingers and hands (*i.e.,* carpopedal spasm) indicates the presence of tetany.

Chronic hypocalcemia is often accompanied by skeletal manifestations and skin changes. There may be bone pain, fragility, deformities, and fractures. The skin may be dry and scaling, the nails brittle, and hair dry. Development of cataracts is common.

Treatment. Acute hypocalcemia is an emergency, requiring prompt treatment. An intravenous infusion containing calcium (*e.g.,* calcium gluconate, calcium chloride) is used when tetany or acute symptoms are present or anticipated because of a decrease in the plasma calcium level.[54]

Chronic hypocalcemia is treated with oral intake of calcium. One glass of milk contains approximately 300 mg of calcium. Oral calcium supplements of carbonate, gluconate, or lactate salts may be used. Long-term treatment may require the use of vitamin D preparations, especially in persons with hypoparathyroidism and chronic kidney disease. The active form of vitamin D is administered when the liver or kidney mechanisms needed for hormone activation are impaired.

Synthetic PTH (1-34) can be administered by subcutaneous injection as replacement therapy in hypoparathyroidism.

Hypercalcemia

Hypercalcemia represents a total plasma calcium concentration greater than 2.6 mmol/L. Falsely elevated levels of calcium can result from prolonged drawing of blood with an excessively tight tourniquet. Increased plasma proteins (*e.g.,* hyperalbuminemia, hyperglobulinemia) may elevate the total plasma calcium but not affect the ionized calcium concentration.

Causes. A plasma calcium excess (*i.e.,* hypercalcemia) results when calcium movement into the circulation overwhelms the calcium regulatory hormones or the ability of the kidney to remove excess calcium ions (Table 31.11). The two most common causes of hypercalcemia are increased bone resorption due to neoplasms and hyperparathyroidism.[55] These two etiologies account for over 90% of all persons with hypercalcemia. Hypercalcemia is a common complication of malignancy, occurring in approximately 10% to 30% of persons with advanced disease.[56] A number of malignant tumours, including carcinoma of the lungs, have been associated with hypercalcemia. Some tumours destroy the bone,

TABLE 31.11 CAUSES AND MANIFESTATIONS OF HYPERCALCEMIA

CAUSES	MANIFESTATIONS
Increased Intestinal Absorption	**Laboratory Values**
Excessive vitamin D	Serum calcium level above 2.6 mmol/L
Excessive calcium in the diet	**Impaired Ability to Concentrate Urine and Expo-**
Milk-alkali syndrome	**sure of Kidney to Increased Concentration of**
Increased Bone Resorption	**Calcium**
Increased levels of parathyroid	Polyuria
hormone	Polydipsia
Malignant neoplasms	Flank pain
Prolonged immobilization	Signs of acute and chronic renal insufficiency
Decreased Elimination	Signs of kidney stones
Thiazide diuretics	**Gastrointestinal Manifestations**
Lithium therapy	Anorexia
	Nausea, vomiting
	Constipation
	Neuromuscular Manifestations (Decreased
	Neuromuscular Excitability)
	Muscle weakness and atrophy
	Ataxia, loss of muscle tone
	Skeletal Manifestations
	Osteopenia
	Osteoporosis
	Central Nervous System Manifestations
	Lethargy
	Personality and behavioural changes
	Stupor and coma
	Cardiovascular Manifestations
	Hypertension
	Shortening of the QT interval
	Atrioventricular block on electrocardiogram

whereas others produce humoral agents that stimulate osteoclastic activity, increase bone resorption, or inhibit bone formation. Approximately 80% of patients with hypercalcemia of malignancy produce PTH-related protein (PTH-rP). PTH and PTH-rP have marked homology, or structural similarity, at their amino terminal ends, with 8 of the first 13 amino acids in the same positions. This homology results in both PTH and PTH-rP binding to the same receptor (PTH/PTH-rP receptor). PTH-rP is produced by several tumours, including cancers of the lung, breast, kidney, head and neck, and ovary.[56]

Less frequent causes of hypercalcemia are prolonged immobilization, increased intestinal absorption of calcium, excessive doses of vitamin D, or the effects of drugs such as lithium and thiazide diuretics. Prolonged immobilization and lack of weight bearing cause demineralization of bone and release of calcium into the bloodstream. Intestinal absorption of calcium can be increased by excessive doses of vitamin D or as a result of a condition called the *milk-alkali syndrome*. The milk-alkali syndrome is caused by excessive ingestion of calcium (often in the form of milk) and absorbable antacids. Because of the availability of nonabsorbable antacids, the condition is seen less frequently than in the past, but it may occur in women who are overzealous in taking calcium preparations for osteoporosis prevention. Discontinuance of the antacid repairs the alkalosis and increases calcium elimination.

A variety of drugs elevate calcium levels. The use of lithium to treat bipolar disorders has caused hypercalcemia and hyperparathyroidism. The thiazide diuretics increase calcium reabsorption in the distal convoluted tubule of the kidney. Although the thiazide diuretics seldom cause hypercalcemia, they can unmask hypercalcemia from other causes such as underlying bone disorders and conditions that increase bone resorption.

Manifestations. The signs and symptoms associated with calcium excess reflect (1) changes in neural excitability, (2) alterations in smooth and cardiac muscle function, and (3) exposure of the kidneys to high concentrations of calcium (Table 31.11). Neural excitability is decreased in patients with hypercalcemia. There may be a dulling of consciousness, stupor, weakness, and muscle flaccidity. Behavioural changes may range from subtle alterations in personality to acute psychoses. The heart responds to elevated levels of calcium with increased contractility and ventricular arrhythmias. Digitalis accentuates these responses. Gastrointestinal symptoms reflect a decrease in smooth muscle activity and include constipation, anorexia, nausea, and vomiting. High calcium concentrations in the urine impair the ability of the kidneys to concentrate urine by interfering with the action of ADH (an example of nephrogenic DI). This causes salt and water diuresis and an increased sensation of thirst. Hypercalciuria also predisposes to the development of renal calculi. Pancreatitis is another potential complication of hypercalcemia and is probably related to stones in the pancreatic ducts.

Hypercalcemic crisis describes an acute increase in the plasma calcium level.[57] Malignant disease and hyperparathyroidism are the major causes of hypercalcemic crisis. In hypercalcemic crisis, cardiac arrhythmias, polyuria, excessive thirst, volume depletion, fever, altered levels of consciousness, azotemia (*i.e.*, nitrogenous wastes in the blood), and a disturbed mental state accompany other signs of calcium excess.[57,58] Symptomatic hypercalcemia is associated with a high mortality rate; death often is caused by cardiac arrest.

Treatment. Treatment of calcium excess usually is directed toward rehydration and use of measures to increase urinary excretion of calcium and inhibit release of calcium from bone.[55–58] Fluid replacement is needed in situations of volume depletion. The excretion of sodium is accompanied by calcium excretion. Diuretics and sodium chloride can be administered to increase urinary elimination of calcium after the ECF volume has been restored. Loop diuretics commonly are used rather than thiazide diuretics, which increase calcium reabsorption. Initial lowering of calcium levels is followed by measures to inhibit bone reabsorption. Drugs that are used to inhibit calcium mobilization include bisphosphonates, calcitonin, corticosteroids, mithramycin, and gallium nitrate. The bisphosphonates (*e.g.*, pamidronate, zoledronate), which act mainly by inhibiting osteoclastic activity, provide a significant reduction in calcium levels with relatively few side effects. Calcitonin inhibits osteoclastic activity, thereby decreasing resorption. The corticosteroids and mithramycin inhibit bone resorption and are used to treat hypercalcemia associated with cancer. The long-term use of mithramycin, an antineoplastic drug, is limited because of its potential for nephrotoxicity and hepatotoxicity. Gallium nitrate is highly effective in the treatment of severe hypercalcemia associated with malignancy. It is a chemical compound that inhibits bone resorption, although the precise mechanism of action is unclear. Dialysis can be used in hypercalcemic patients with renal failure and in patients with heart failure in whom fluid overload is a concern.

Disorders of Phosphorus Balance

Phosphorus is mainly an intracellular anion. Approximately 85% of phosphorus is contained in bone, and most of the remainder (approximately 14%) is located in cells. Only about 1% is in the ECF compartment, and of that, only a minute proportion is in the plasma. In the adult, the normal plasma phosphorus level ranges from 0.8 to 1.45 mmol/L. These values are slightly higher in infants (1.2 to 2.7 mmol/L) and children (1.3 to 1.7 mmol/L), probably because of increased growth hormone and decreased gonadal hormones.

Phosphorus exists in two forms within the body: inorganic and organic. The inorganic form (phosphate [H_2PO^- or HPO_4^{2-}]) is the principal circulating form that is routinely measured and reported for laboratory purposes.[2] Most of the intracellular phosphorus is in the organic form (*e.g.*, nucleic acids, phospholipids, ATP). Entry of phosphorus into cells is enhanced after glucose uptake because phosphorus is incorporated into the phosphorylated intermediates of glucose metabolism. Cell injury or atrophy leads to a loss of cell components that contain organic phosphorus; regeneration of these cellular

PHOSPHORUS BALANCE

- Approximately 85% of the phosphorus is contained in bone. Most of the remaining phosphorus is incorporated into organic compounds such as nucleic acids, high-energy compounds (*e.g.,* ATP), and coenzymes that are critically important for cell function.
- Many of the manifestations of hypophosphatemia are related to a decrease in cell energy due to ATP depletion.
- Serum phosphorus levels are regulated by the kidneys, which eliminate or conserve phosphate as serum levels change. Serum levels of calcium and phosphate are reciprocally regulated to prevent the damaging deposition of calcium phosphate crystals in the soft tissues of the body. Many of the manifestations of hyperphosphatemia reflect a decrease in serum calcium levels.

components results in withdrawal of inorganic phosphorus from the ECF compartment.

Phosphorus is essential to many bodily functions. It plays a major role in bone formation; is essential to certain metabolic processes, including the formation of ATP and the enzymes needed for metabolism of glucose, fat, and protein; is a necessary component of several vital parts of the cell, being incorporated into the nucleic acids of DNA and RNA and the phospholipids of the cell membrane; and serves as an acid–base buffer in the ECF and in the renal excretion of hydrogen ions. Delivery of oxygen by the red blood cell depends on organic phosphates in ATP and 2,3-diphosphoglycerate. Phosphorus is also needed for normal function of other blood cells, including the white blood cells and platelets.

Gains and Losses

Phosphorus is ingested in the diet and eliminated in the urine. Phosphorus is derived from many dietary sources, including milk and meats. Approximately 80% of ingested phosphorus is absorbed in the intestine, primarily in the jejunum. Absorption is diminished by concurrent ingestion of substances that bind phosphorus, including calcium, magnesium, and aluminum.

Phosphorus is not bound to plasma proteins and essentially all of the phosphorus that is present in the plasma is filtered in the glomerulus.[59] Renal elimination of phosphorus is then regulated by an overflow mechanism in which the amount of phosphorus lost in the urine is directly related to phosphorus concentrations in the blood. Essentially all the filtered phosphorus is reabsorbed when phosphorus levels are low; when plasma phosphorus levels rise above a critical level, the excess phosphorus is eliminated in the urine. Phosphorus is reabsorbed from the filtrate into the proximal tubular epithelial cells through the action of a sodium-phosphorus cotransporter (NPT2). PTH can play a significant role in regulating phosphorus reabsorption by inhibiting the synthesis and expression of the NPT2 transporter. Thus, whenever PTH is increased, tubular reabsorption of phosphorus is decreased and more phosphorus is lost in the urine. NPT2 is also inhibited by the recently identified hormones called *phosphatonins*.[59] The best defined phosphatonin is fibroblast growth factor 23 (FGF23) and when this hormone is overproduced, as in tumour-induced osteomalacia, marked hypophosphatemia occurs. In addition, increased phosphatonins cause excessive calcitriol (active vitamin D) degradation, resulting in osteomalacia or rickets[59,60] (see Chapter 57).

Hypophosphatemia

Hypophosphatemia is commonly defined by a plasma phosphorus level of less than 0.8 mmol/L in adults; it is considered severe at concentrations of less than 0.32 mmol/L.[2] Hypophosphatemia may occur despite normal body phosphorus stores as a result of movement from the ECF into the ICF compartment. Serious depletion of phosphorus may exist with low, normal, or high plasma concentrations.

Causes. The most common causes of hypophosphatemia are depletion of phosphorus because of insufficient intestinal absorption, transcompartmental shifts, and increased renal losses (Table 31.12). Often, more than one of these mechanisms is active. Unless food intake is severely restricted, dietary intake and intestinal absorption of phosphorus are usually adequate. Intestinal absorption may be inhibited by administration of glucocorticoids, high dietary levels of magnesium, and hypothyroidism. Prolonged ingestion of antacids may also interfere with intestinal absorption. Antacids that contain aluminum hydroxide, aluminum carbonate, and calcium carbonate bind with phosphorus, causing increased phosphorus losses in the stool. Because of their ability to bind phosphorus, calcium-based antacids are sometimes used therapeutically to decrease plasma phosphorus levels in persons with chronic kidney disease.

Alcoholism is a common cause of hypophosphatemia. The mechanisms underlying hypophosphatemia in the person addicted to alcohol may be related to malnutrition, increased renal excretion rates, or hypomagnesemia. Malnutrition and diabetic ketoacidosis increase phosphorus excretion and phosphorus loss from the body. Refeeding of malnourished patients increases the incorporation of phosphorus into nucleic acids and phosphorylated compounds in the cell.[61] The same thing happens when diabetic ketoacidosis is reversed with insulin therapy. Urinary losses of phosphorus may be caused by drugs, such as theophylline, corticosteroids, and loop diuretics, which increase renal excretion.

Hypophosphatemia also can occur during prolonged courses of glucose administration or hyperalimentation. Glucose administration causes insulin release, with transport of glucose and phosphorus into the cell. The catabolic events that occur with diabetic ketoacidosis also deplete phosphorus stores. Usually the hypophosphatemia does not become apparent, however, until insulin and fluid replacement have reversed the dehydration and glucose has started to move back into the cell. Administration of hyperalimentation solutions

TABLE 31.12 CAUSES AND MANIFESTATIONS OF HYPOPHOSPHATEMIA

CAUSES	MANIFESTATIONS
Decreased Intestinal Absorption Antacids (aluminum and calcium) Severe diarrhea Lack of vitamin D	**Laboratory Values** Serum level below 0.8 mmol/L in adults and 1.3 mmol/L in children
Increased Renal Elimination Alkalosis Hyperparathyroidism Diabetic ketoacidosis Renal tubular absorption defects	**Neural Manifestations** Intention tremor Ataxia Paresthesias Confusion, stupor, coma Seizures
Malnutrition and Intracellular Shifts Alcoholism Total parenteral hyperalimentation Recovery from malnutrition Administration of insulin during recovery from diabetic ketoacidosis	**Musculoskeletal Manifestations** Muscle weakness Joint stiffness Bone pain Osteomalacia
	Blood Disorders Hemolytic anemia Platelet dysfunction with bleeding disorders Impaired white blood cell function

without adequate phosphorus can cause a rapid influx of phosphorus into the body's muscle mass, particularly if treatment is initiated after a period of tissue catabolism. Because only a small amount of total-body phosphorus is in the ECF compartment, even a small redistribution between the ECF and ICF compartments can cause hypophosphatemia, even though total phosphorus levels have not changed.

Respiratory alkalosis due to prolonged hyperventilation can produce hypophosphatemia through decreased levels of ionized calcium from increased protein binding, increased PTH release, and increased phosphorus excretion. Clinical conditions associated with hyperventilation include gram-negative septicemia, alcohol withdrawal, heat stroke, and primary hyperventilation.

Manifestations. The manifestations of phosphorus deficiency result from a decrease in cellular energy stores due to deficiency in ATP and impaired oxygen transport due to a decrease in red blood cell 2,3-diphosphoglycerate (2,3-DPG). Hypophosphatemia results in altered neural function, disturbed musculoskeletal function, and hematologic disorders (Table 31.12).

Red blood cell metabolism is impaired by phosphorus deficiency; the cells become rigid, undergo increased hemolysis, and have diminished ATP and 2,3-DPG levels (see Chapter 14). The chemotactic and phagocytic functions of white blood cells and the hemostatic functions of the platelets are also impaired. Acute severe hypophosphatemia (0.03 to 0.06 mmol/L) can lead to acute hemolytic anemia with increased erythrocyte fragility, increased susceptibility to infection, and platelet dysfunction with petechial hemorrhages. Anorexia and dysphagia can occur. Neural manifestations (intention tremors, paresthesias,

hyporeflexia, stupor, coma, and seizures) are uncommon but serious manifestations. Respiratory insufficiency resulting from impaired function of the respiratory muscles can develop in patients with severe hypophosphatemia.

Chronic phosphorus depletion interferes with mineralization of newly formed bone matrix. In growing children, this process causes abnormal endochondral growth and clinical manifestations of rickets. In adults, the condition leads to joint stiffness, bone pain, and skeletal deformities consistent with osteomalacia (see Chapter 59).

Treatment. The treatment of hypophosphatemia is usually directed toward prophylaxis. This may be accomplished with dietary sources high in phosphorus (one glass of milk contains approximately 250 mg of phosphorus) or with oral or intravenous replacement solutions. Phosphorus supplements usually are contraindicated in hyperparathyroidism, chronic kidney disease, and hypercalcemia because of the increased risk of extracellular calcifications.

Hyperphosphatemia

Hyperphosphatemia represents a plasma phosphorus concentration in excess of 1.45 mmol/L in adults. Children normally have plasma phosphorus levels higher than those of adults.

Causes. Hyperphosphatemia results from failure of the kidneys to excrete excess phosphorus, rapid redistribution of intracellular phosphorus to the ECF compartment, and excessive intake of phosphorus.[62] The most common cause of hyperphosphatemia is impaired renal function (Table 31.13).

Hyperphosphatemia is a common electrolyte disorder in persons with chronic kidney disease. The increase in

TABLE 31.13 CAUSES AND MANIFESTATIONS OF HYPERPHOSPHATEMIA

CAUSES	MANIFESTATIONS
Acute Phosphate Overload	**Laboratory Values**
Laxatives and enemas containing phosphorus	Serum level above 1.45 mmol/L in adults and 1.7 mmol/L in children
Intravenous phosphate supplementation	
Intracellular-to-Extracellular Shift	**Neuromuscular Manifestations (Reciprocal Decrease in Serum Calcium)**
Massive trauma	Paresthesias
Heat stroke	Tetany
Seizures	
Rhabdomyolysis	**Cardiovascular Manifestations**
Tumour lysis syndrome	Hypotension
Potassium deficiency	Cardiac arrhythmias
Impaired Elimination	
Kidney failure	
Hypoparathyroidism	

phosphorus levels in persons with chronic renal disease occurs despite compensatory increases in PTH. Evidence shows an increase in soft tissue calcification (vascular and cardiac calcification especially) and mortality among patients with chronic kidney disease with hyperphosphatemia.[62] Release of intracellular phosphorus can result from conditions such as massive tissue injury, rhabdomyolysis, heat stroke, potassium deficiency, and seizures. Chemotherapy can raise plasma phosphorus levels because of the rapid destruction of tumour cells (tumour lysis syndrome).

The administration of excess phosphorus-containing antacids, laxatives, or enemas can be another cause of hyperphosphatemia, especially when there is a decrease in vascular volume and a reduced glomerular filtration rate. phosphorus-containing laxatives and enemas predispose to hypovolemia and a decreased glomerular filtration rate by inducing diarrhea, thereby increasing the risk of hypophosphatemia. Serious and even fatal hyperphosphatemia has resulted from administration of a sodium phosphate solution enterally or as an enema (*i.e.*, Fleet).[63]

Manifestations. Hyperphosphatemia is accompanied by a decrease in plasma calcium. Many of the signs and symptoms of a phosphorus excess are related to a calcium deficit (Table 31.13). Inadequately treated hyperphosphatemia in chronic disease can lead to secondary hyperparathyroidism, renal osteodystrophies, and extraosseous calcifications in soft tissues.

Treatment. The treatment of hyperphosphatemia is directed at the cause of the disorder. Dietary restriction of foods that are high in phosphorus may be used. Calcium-based phosphorus binders are useful in chronic hyperphosphatemia. Sevelamer, a calcium- and aluminium-free phosphorus binder, is as effective as a calcium-based binder, but lacks its adverse manifestations such as elevation of the calcium × phosphorus product, hypercalcemia, and vascular and cardiac calcifications.[49] Hemodialysis is used to reduce phosphorus levels in persons with chronic renal disease.

Disorders of Magnesium Balance

Magnesium is the fourth most abundant cation in the body and the second most abundant intracellular cation after potassium. The average adult has approximately 24 g of magnesium distributed throughout the body. Of the total magnesium content, approximately 50% to 60% is stored in bone, 39% to 49% is contained in the body cells, and the remaining 1% is dispersed in the ECF.[2] Approximately 20% to 30% of ECF magnesium is protein bound, and only a small amount of ICF magnesium (15% to 30%) is exchangeable with the ECF. The normal plasma concentration of magnesium is 0.70 to 1.25 mmol/L.

Only recently has the importance of magnesium to the overall function of the body been recognized. Magnesium acts as a cofactor in many intracellular enzyme reactions, including the transfer of high-energy phosphorus groups in the generation of ATP from adenosine diphosphate (ADP). It is essential to all reactions that require ATP, for every step related to replication and transcription of DNA, and for the translation of messenger RNA. It is required for cellular energy metabolism, functioning of the Na^+/K^+-ATPase membrane pump, membrane stabilization, nerve conduction, ion transport, and potassium and calcium channel activity.[64] Potassium channels, including the acetylcholine-sensitive potassium channel, depend on adequate intracellular magnesium levels. Magnesium blocks the outward movement of potassium in cardiac cells; when magnesium levels are low, the channel permits outward flow of potassium, resulting in low levels of intracellular potassium. Many calcium channels are also magnesium dependent. Higher ICF magnesium concentrations inhibit calcium transport into the cell and its release from the sarcoplasmic reticulum. Therefore, magnesium tends to act as a smooth muscle relaxant by altering calcium levels that are responsible for muscle contraction.[64] In addition, it has been suggested that magnesium has an anticonvulsant effect. The suggested mechanism of action is cerebral vasodilation or prevention of ischemic neuronal damage by blockade of *N*-methyl-D-aspartate

(NMDA) receptors in the brain (see Chapter 51). Magnesium is the first-line drug in the treatment of eclampsia in pregnant women.[65] Newer evidence is looking at administering magnesium sulphate for imminent preterm births (less than 32 gestational weeks) for fetal neuroprotection to reduce the risk of cerebral palsy for surviving infants.[66]

MAGNESIUM BALANCE

- Most of the body's magnesium is located within cells, where it functions in regulation of enzyme activity, generation of ATP, and calcium transport. Magnesium is necessary for parathyroid hormone function and hypomagnesemia is a common cause of hypocalcemia.
- Elimination of magnesium occurs mainly through the kidney, which adjusts urinary excretion as a means of maintaining serum magnesium levels. Diuretics tend to disrupt renal regulatory mechanisms and increase urinary losses of magnesium.
- There is an interdependency between intracellular concentrations of magnesium and potassium such that a decrease in one is accompanied by a decrease in the other. Magnesium deficiency contributes to cardiac arrhythmias that occur with hypokalemia.

Gains and Losses

Magnesium is ingested in the diet, absorbed from the intestine, and excreted by the kidneys. Intestinal absorption is not closely regulated, and approximately 25% to 65% of dietary magnesium is absorbed. Magnesium is contained in all green vegetables, grains, nuts, meats, and seafood. Magnesium is also present in much of the groundwater in North America.

The kidney is the principal organ of magnesium regulation. The kidneys filter about 70% to 80% of the plasma magnesium and excrete about 6%, although this amount can be influenced by other conditions and medications.[2,64] Magnesium is a unique electrolyte in that only approximately 12% to 20% of the filtered amount is reabsorbed in the proximal tubule.[67] The greatest quantity, approximately 70%, is passively reabsorbed in the thick ascending loop of Henle. The major driving force for magnesium absorption in the thick ascending loop of Henle is the positive voltage gradient created in the tubular lumen by the $Na^+/K^+/2Cl^-$ cotransport system (see Chapter 30). Inhibition of this transport system by loop diuretics lowers magnesium reabsorption. Active reabsorption of magnesium takes place in the distal convoluted tubule and accounts for about 10% of the filtered load. Magnesium reabsorption is stimulated by PTH and is decreased in the presence of increased plasma levels of magnesium and calcium.

Hypomagnesemia

Magnesium deficiency refers to depletion of total body stores, whereas severe hypomagnesemia describes a plasma magnesium concentration below 0.70 mmol/L.[68] It is seen in conditions that limit intake or increase intestinal or renal losses, and it is a common finding in emergency departments and intensive care units.

Causes. Magnesium deficiency can result from insufficient intake, excessive losses, or movement between the ECF and ICF compartments (Table 31.14). It can result from conditions that directly limit intake, such as malnutrition, starvation, or prolonged maintenance of magnesium-free parenteral nutrition. Other conditions, such as diarrhea, malabsorption syndromes, prolonged nasogastric suction, or laxative abuse, decrease intestinal absorption. Another common cause of magnesium deficiency is chronic alcoholism. Many factors contribute to hypomagnesemia in alcoholism, including low intake and gastrointestinal losses from diarrhea. The effects of hypomagnesemia are exaggerated by other electrolyte disorders, such as hypokalemia, hypocalcemia, and metabolic acidosis.

TABLE 31.14 CAUSES AND MANIFESTATIONS OF HYPOMAGNESEMIA

CAUSES	MANIFESTATIONS
Impaired Intake or Absorption	**Laboratory Values**
Alcoholism	Serum magnesium level below 0.70 mmol/L
Malnutrition or starvation	**Neuromuscular Manifestations**
Malabsorption	Personality change
Small bowel bypass surgery	Athetoid or choreiform movements
Parenteral hyperalimentation with inadequate amounts of magnesium	Nystagmus
	Tetany
High dietary intake of calcium without concomitant amounts of magnesium	Positive Babinski, Chvostek, Trousseau signs
Increased Losses	**Cardiovascular Manifestations**
Diuretic therapy	Tachycardia
Hyperparathyroidism	Hypertension
Hyperaldosteronism	Cardiac arrhythmias
Diabetic ketoacidosis	
Magnesium-wasting kidney disease	

Although the kidneys are able to defend against hypermagnesemia, they are less able to conserve magnesium and prevent hypomagnesemia. Urine losses are increased in diabetic ketoacidosis, hyperparathyroidism, and hyperaldosteronism. Some drugs increase renal losses of magnesium, including both loop and thiazide diuretics and nephrotoxic drugs such as aminoglycoside antibiotics, cyclosporine, cisplatin, and amphotericin B. Several rare, genetic disorders can also result in hypomagnesemia (*i.e.*, Gitelman and Bartter syndromes; see discussion in section on hypokalemia).[64]

Relative hypomagnesemia may also develop in conditions that promote movement of magnesium between the ECF and ICF compartments, including rapid administration of glucose, insulin-containing parenteral solutions, and alkalosis. Although transient, these conditions can cause serious alterations in body function.

Manifestations. Magnesium deficiency usually occurs in conjunction with hypocalcemia and hypokalemia, producing a number of related neurologic and cardiovascular manifestations (Table 31.14). Hypocalcemia is typical of severe hypomagnesemia. Most persons with hypomagnesemia-related hypocalcemia have decreased PTH levels, probably as a result of impaired magnesium-dependent mechanisms that control PTH release and synthesis. There is also evidence that hypomagnesemia decreases both the PTH-dependent and PTH-independent release of calcium from bone. In hypomagnesemia, magnesium ions (Mg^{2+}) are released from bone in exchange for increased uptake of calcium from the ECF.

Hypomagnesemia leads to a reduction in intracellular potassium and impairs the ability of the kidney to conserve potassium. When hypomagnesemia is present, hypokalemia is unresponsive to potassium replacement therapy.

Magnesium is vital to carbohydrate metabolism and the generation of both aerobic and anaerobic metabolisms. Many of the manifestations of magnesium deficit are due to related electrolyte disorders such as hypokalemia and hypocalcemia. Hypocalcemia may be evidenced by personality changes and neuromuscular irritability along with tremors, athetoid or choreiform movements, and positive Chvostek or Trousseau signs (Fig. 31.14). Cardiovascular manifestations include tachycardia, hypertension, and ventricular arrhythmias. There may be ECG changes such as widening of the QRS complex, appearance of peaked T-waves, prolongation of the PR interval, T-wave inversion, and appearance of U-waves. Ventricular arrhythmias, particularly in the presence of digitalis, may be difficult to treat unless magnesium levels are normalized.

Persistent magnesium deficiency has been implicated as a risk factor for osteoporosis and osteomalacia, particularly in persons with chronic alcoholism, diabetes mellitus, and malabsorption syndrome.

Treatment. Hypomagnesemia is treated with magnesium replacement. The route of administration depends on the severity of the condition. Symptomatic, moderate to severe magnesium deficiency is treated by parenteral administration. Treatment must be continued for several days to replace stored and plasma levels. In conditions of chronic intestinal or renal loss, maintenance support with oral magnesium may be required. Magnesium often is used therapeutically to treat cardiac arrhythmia, myocardial infarct, angina, bronchial asthma, and pregnancy complicated by preeclampsia or eclampsia. Caution to prevent hypermagnesemia is essential; patients with any degree of renal failure must be carefully monitored to prevent magnesium excess.

Hypermagnesemia

Hypermagnesemia represents an increase in total body magnesium and a plasma magnesium concentration in excess of 1.25 mmol/L. Because of the ability of the normal kidney to excrete magnesium, hypermagnesemia is rare.[69]

Causes. When hypermagnesemia does occur, it is usually related to renal insufficiency and the injudicious use of magnesium-containing medications such as antacids, mineral supplements, or laxatives (Table 31.15). The elderly are particularly at risk because they have age-related reductions in renal function and tend to consume more magnesium-containing

TABLE 31.15 CAUSES AND MANIFESTATIONS OF HYPERMAGNESEMIA

CAUSES	MANIFESTATIONS
Excessive Intake	**Laboratory Values**
Intravenous administration of magnesium for treatment of preeclampsia	Serum magnesium level above 1.25 mmol/L
Excessive use of oral magnesium-containing medications	**Neuromuscular Manifestations**
	Lethargy
	Hyporeflexia
Decreased Excretion	Confusion
Kidney disease	Coma
Glomerulonephritis	**Cardiovascular Manifestations**
Tubulointerstitial kidney disease	Hypotension
Acute renal failure	Cardiac arrhythmias
	Cardiac arrest

medications, including antacids and laxatives. Magnesium sulphate is used to treat toxemia of pregnancy and premature labour; in these cases, careful monitoring for signs of hypermagnesemia is essential.

Manifestations. Hypermagnesemia affects neuromuscular and cardiovascular function (Table 31.15). Because magnesium tends to suppress PTH secretion, hypocalcemia may accompany hypermagnesemia. Signs and symptoms usually occur only when plasma magnesium levels exceed 2 mmol/L.

Hypermagnesemia diminishes neuromuscular function, causing hyporeflexia, muscle weakness, and confusion. Magnesium decreases acetylcholine release at the myoneural junction and may cause neuromuscular blockade and respiratory paralysis. Cardiovascular effects are related to the calcium channel blocking effects of magnesium. Blood pressure is decreased, and the ECG shows shortening of the QT interval, T-wave abnormalities, and prolongation of the QRS and PR intervals. Severe hypermagnesemia (>5.0 mmol/L) is associated with muscle and respiratory paralysis, complete heart block, and cardiac arrest.

Treatment. The treatment of hypermagnesemia includes cessation of magnesium administration. Calcium is a direct antagonist of magnesium, and intravenous administration of calcium may be used. Peritoneal dialysis or hemodialysis may be required.

Magnesium is the second most abundant ICF cation. It acts as a cofactor in many intracellular enzyme reactions and is required for cellular energy metabolism, functioning of the Na^+/K^+-ATPase membrane pump, nerve conduction, ion transport, and potassium and calcium channel activity. Magnesium blocks the outward movement of potassium in cardiac cells; when magnesium levels are low, the channel permits outward flow of potassium, resulting in low levels of intracellular potassium. It acts on calcium channels to inhibit the movement of calcium into cells. Magnesium deficiency can result from insufficient intake, excessive losses, or movement between the ECF and ICF compartments. Hypomagnesemia impairs PTH release and the actions of PTH; it leads to a reduction in ICF potassium and impairs the ability of the kidney to conserve potassium. Hypermagnesemia usually is related to renal insufficiency and the injudicious use of magnesium-containing medications such as antacids, mineral supplements, or laxatives. It can cause neuromuscular dysfunction with hyporeflexia, muscle weakness, and confusion. Magnesium decreases acetylcholine release at the myoneural junction and may cause neuromuscular blockade and respiratory paralysis.

CONCEPTS in action **ANIMATION**

IN SUMMARY

Calcium, phosphorus, and magnesium are major divalent ions in the body. Calcium is a major divalent cation. Approximately 99% of body calcium is found in bone; less than 1% is found in the ECF compartment. The calcium in bone is in dynamic equilibrium with ECF calcium. Of the three forms of ECF calcium (*i.e.,* protein-bound, complexed, and ionized), only the ionized form can cross the cell membrane and contribute to cellular function. Ionized calcium has a number of functions. It contributes to neuromuscular function, plays a vital role in the blood clotting process, and participates in a number of enzyme reactions. Alterations in ionized calcium levels produce neural effects; neural excitability is increased in hypocalcemia and decreased in hypercalcemia.

Phosphorus is largely an ICF anion. It is incorporated into the nucleic acids and ATP. The most common causes of altered levels of ECF phosphorus are alterations in intestinal absorption, transcompartmental shifts, and disorders of renal elimination. Phosphorus deficit causes signs and symptoms of neural dysfunction, disturbed musculoskeletal function, and hematologic disorders. Most of these manifestations result from a decrease in cellular energy stores due to a deficiency in ATP and oxygen transport by 2,3-diphosphoglycerate in the red blood cell. Phosphorus excess occurs with renal failure and PTH deficit; it is associated with decreased plasma calcium levels.

REVIEW EXERCISES

1. A 40-year-old man with advanced acquired immunodeficiency syndrome (AIDS) presents with an acute chest infection. Investigations confirm a diagnosis of *Pneumocystis jiroveci* (formerly *P. carinii*) pneumonia. Although he is being treated appropriately, his plasma sodium level is 118 mmol/L. Results of adrenal function tests are normal.
   A. *What is the likely cause of his electrolyte disturbance?*
   B. *What are the five cardinal features of this condition?*
2. A 70-year-old woman who is taking furosemide (a loop diuretic) for congestive heart failure complains of weakness, fatigue, and cramping of the muscles in her legs. Her plasma potassium is 2.0 mmol, and her plasma sodium is 140 mmol/L. She also complains that she notices a "strange heartbeat" at times.
   A. *What is the likely cause of this woman's symptoms?*
   B. *An ECG shows depressed ST segment and low T-wave changes. Explain the physiologic mechanism underlying these changes.*
   C. *What would be the treatment for this woman?*

3. A 50-year-old woman presents with symptomatic hypercalcemia. She has a recent history of breast cancer treatment.
   A. *How do you evaluate her with the increased plasma calcium levels in mind?*
   B. *What is the significance of the recent history of malignancy?*
   C. *What further tests may be indicated?*

References

1. Rhoades R. A., Bell D. R. (2013). *Medical physiology: Principles for clinical medicine.* (4th. ed.). Philadelphia, PA: Lippincott Williams & Wilkins.
2. Hall J. E. (2011). *Guyton and Hall Textbook of medical physiology* (12th ed.). Philadelphia, PA: Elsevier Saunders.
3. Nielsen S., Kwon T. H., Frokiaer J., Agre P. (2007). Regulation and dysregulation of aquaporins in water balance disorders. *Journal of Internal Medicine, 261*(1), 53–64.
4. Koeppen B. M., Stanton B. A. (2013). *Renal physiology* (5th ed.). Philadelphia, PA: Elsevier Mosby.
5. Poaage E., Singer M., Armer J., et al. (2008). Demystifying lymphedema: Development of the lymphedema putting evidence into practice card. *Clinical Journal of Oncology Nursing, 12*(6), 951–964.
6. Zuther J. E. (2005). *Lymphedema management: The comprehensive guide for practitioners.* New York: Thieme Medical Publishers.
7. Metheny N. M. (2012). *Fluid and electrolyte balance: Nursing considerations* (5th ed.). Sudbury, MA: Jones & Bartlett Learning.
8. Ball J., Bindler R., Cowen K. (2012). *Principles of pediatric nursing: Caring for children* (5th ed.). Boston, MA: Pearson.
9. McKinley M. J., Johnson A. K. (2004). The physiological regulation of thirst and fluid intake. *News in Physiological Sciences, 19*, 1–6.
10. Zizza C. A., Ellison K. J., Wernette C. M. (2009). Total water intakes of community living of middle-old and oldest-old adults. *Journal of Gerontological Series A: Biological Sciences & Medical Sciences, 64A*(4), 481–486.
11. Valente S., Fisher D. (2010). Recognizing and managing psychogenic polydipsia in mental health. *Journal for Nurse Practitioners, 6*(7), 546–550.
12. Lin M., Liu S. J., Lim I. T. (2005). Disorders of water imbalance. *Emergency Medicine Clinics of North America, 23*, 749–770.
13. Palm C., Pistrosch F., Herbrig K., Gross P. (2006). Vasopressin antagonists as aquaretic agents for the treatment of hyponatremia. *American Journal of Medicine, 119*(7 Suppl 1), S87–S92.
14. Makaryus A. N., McFarlane S. I. (2006). Diabetes insipidus: Diagnosis and treatment of a complex disease. *Cleveland Clinic Journal of Medicine, 73*, 65–71.
15. Eknoyan G. (2010). A history of diabetes insipidus: Paving the road to internal water balance. *American Journal of Kidney Diseases, 56*(6), 1175–1183.
16. Sands J. M., Bichet D. G. (2006). Nephrogenic diabetes insipidus. *Annals of Internal Medicine, 144*, 186–194.
17. Robertson G. L. (2006). Regulation of arginine vasopressin in the syndrome of inappropriate antidiuresis. *American Journal of Medicine, 119*(7 Suppl 1), S36–S42.
18. Decauyo G. (2009). The syndrome of inappropriate secretion of antidiuretic hormone. *Seminars in Nephrology, 29*(3), 239–256.
19. de Vries Feyens C., de Jager C. P. (2011). Images in clinical medicine: Decreased skin turgor. *New England Journal of Medicine, 364*(4), e6.
20. Jensen S. (2011). *Nursing health assessment: A best practice approach.* Philadelphia, PA: Lippincott Williams & Wilkins.
21. Gohl K. P. (2004). Management of hyponatremia. *American Family Physician, 69*, 2387–2394.
22. Schrier R. W. (2006). Water and sodium retention in edematous disorders: Role of vasopressin and aldosterone. *American Journal of Medicine, 119*(7 Suppl 1), S47–S53.
23. Keane M. (2014). Recognising and managing acute hyponatraemia. *Emergency Nurse, 29*(9), 32–36.
24. Haskal R. (2007). Current issues for nurse practitioners: Hyponatremia. *Journal of American Academy of Nurse Practitioners, 19*(11), 563–579.
25. Elhassan E. A., Schrier R. W. (2011). Hyponatremia: Diagnosis, complications, and Management including V_2 receptor antagonists. *Current Opinion in Nephrology & Hypertension, 20*(2), 161–168.
26. Adrogue H. J., Madias N. E. (2000). Hypernatremia. *New England Journal of Medicine, 342*, 1493–1499.
27. Rao M. C. (2004). Oral rehydration therapy. *Annual Review of Physiology, 66*, 183–417.
28. Schaefer T. J., Wolford R. W. (2005). Disorders of potassium. *Emergency Medicine Clinics of North America, 23*, 723–747.
29. Lehnhardt A., Kemper M. J. (2011). Pathogenesis, diagnosis, and management of hyperkalemia. *Pediatric Nephrology, 26*(3), 377–384.
30. Palmer B. F. (2010). A physiologic based approach to the evaluation of a patient with hypokalemia. *American Journal of Kidney Disease, 56*(6), 1184–1190.
31. Reungjul S., Pratipanwatr T., Johnson R. J., Nakagawa T. (2008). Do thiazides worsen metabolic syndrome and renal disease? The pivotal roles for hyperuricemia and hypokalemia. *Current Opinion in Nephrology & Hypertension, 17*(5), 470–476.
32. Yamazaki H., Nozu K., Narita I., et al. (2009). Atypical phenotype of type I Bartter syndrome accompanied by focal segmental glomerulosclerosis. *Pediatric Nephrology, 24*(2), 415–418.
33. Slovacek L. (2009). Gitelman's syndrome: A hereditary disorder characterized by hypokalemia and hypomagnesemia. *European Journal of General Medicine, 6*(2), 127–130.
34. Tapolyai M., Uysal A., Dossabhoy N. R., et al. (2010). High prevalence of Liddle syndrome phenotype among hypertensive US veterans in northwest Louisiana. *Journal of Clinical Hypertension, 12*(11), 856–860.
35. Sahan M., Yilmaz M., Gokel Y., et al. (2013). Nebulized salbutamol for asthma: Effects on serum potassium and phosphate levels at the 60 min. *Portuguese Journal of Pulmonology, 19*(5), 200–203.
36. Kim J. B., Lee G. M., Kim S. J., et al. (2011). Expression patterns of two potassium channel genes in skeletal muscle cells of patient with familial hypokalemic periodic paralysis. *Neurology India, 59*(4), 527–531.
37. Cope T. E., Samaraweera A. P., Burn D. J. (2013). Thyrotoxic periodic paralysis: Correct hypokalemia with caution. *The Journal of Emergency Medicine, 45*(3), 338–340.
38. Unwin R. J., Luft F. C., Shirley D. G. (2011). Pathophysiology and management of hypokalemia: A clinical perspective. *Nature Reviews Nephrology, 7*(2), 75–84.
39. Hollander-Rodriguez J. C., Calvert J. F. (2006). Hyperkalemia. *American Family Physician, 73*(2), 283–290.
40. Barker M. C. (2010). Combined spinal/general anesthesia with postop femoral nerve block for total potassium replication in a patient with familial hyperkalemic periodic paralysis: A case report. *American Association of Nurse Anesthetists, 78*(3), 191–194.
41. Bienaime F., Prie D., Friedlander G., Souberbielle J. C.. (2011). Vitamin D metabolism and activity in the parathyroid gland. *Molecular and Cellular Endocrinology, 347*(1-2), 30–41.
42. Quarles L. D. (2003). Extracellular calcium-sensing receptors in the parathyroid gland, kidney, and other tissues. *Current Opinion in Nephrology and Hypertension, 12*, 349–355.
43. Karamanakos S. N., Markou K. B., Panagopoulos K., et al. (2010). Complications and risk factors related to the extent of surgery in thyroidectomy. Results from 2,043 procedures. *Hormones, 9*(4), 318–325.
44. Taniegra E. D. (2004). Hyperparathyroidism. *American Family Physician, 69*(2), 333–340.
45. Marcocci C., Cetani F. (2011). Primary hyperparathyroidism. *New England Journal of Medicine, 365*(25), 2389–2397.
46. Cunningham J., Locatelli F., Rodriguez M. (2011). Secondary hyperparathyroidism: Pathogenesis, disease progression, and therapeutic options. *Clinical Journal of the American Society of Nephrology, 6*(4), 913–921.
47. Eddington H., Kalra P. A. (2010). The association of chronic kidney disease-mineral bone disorder and cardiovascular risk. *Journal of Renal Care, 36*(Suppl.1), 61–67.

48. Kidney Disease: Improving Global Outcomes (KDIGO) CKD-MBD Work Group. (2009). KDIGO clinical practice guideline for the diagnosis, evaluation, prevention, and treatment of chronic kidney disease-mineral and bone disorder (CKD-MBD). *Kidney International, 76*(Suppl 113), S1–S130.

49. Hervas J. G., Prados D., Cerezo S. (2003). Treatment of hyperphosphatemia with sevelamer hydrochloride in hemodialysis patients. *Kidney International, 85*, 69–72.

50. Egi M., Kim I., Nichol A., et al. (2011). Ionized calcium concentration and outcome in critical illness. *Critical Care Medicine, 39*(2), 314–321.

51. Peacock M. (2010). Calcium metabolism in health and disease. *Clinical Journal of the American Society of Nephrology, 5*(Suppl 1), S23–S30.

52. Buckley M. S., Leblanc J. M., Cawley M. J. (2010). Electrolyte disturbances associated with commonly prescribed medications in the intensive care unit. *Critical Care Medicine, 38*(Suppl), S253–S264.

53. Dunphy L. M., Winland-Brown J. E., Porter B. O., et al. (2011). *Primary care: The art and science of advanced practice nursing* (3rd ed.). Philadelphia, PA: F.A. Davis Company.

54. Lehne R. (2012). *Pharmacology for nursing care* (8th ed.). St. Louis, MO: Elsevier Saunders.

55. Assadi F. (2009). Hypercalcemia: An evidence-based approach to clinical cases. *Iranian Journal of Kidney Disease, 3*(2), 71–79.

56. Fojo A. T. (2011). Chapter 146: Metabolic emergencies. In DeVita V. T., Hellman S., Rosenberg S. A. (Eds.), *Cancer: Principles and practice of oncology* (9th ed.). Philadelphia, PA: Lippincott Williams & Wilkins.

57. Wang C. C., Chen Y. C., Shiang J. C., et al. (2009). Hypercalcemic crisis successfully treated with prompt calcium-free hemodialysis. *American Journal of Emergency Medicine, 27*(9), 1174 (e1-e3).

58. Starker L. F., Bjorklund P., Theoharis C., et al. (2011). Clinical histopathological characteristic of hyperparathyroidism-induced hypercalcemic crisis. *World Journal of Surgery, 35*(2), 331–335.

59. Penido M. G., Alon U. S. (2012). Phosphate homeostasis and is role in bone health. *Pediatric Nephrology, 27*(11), 2039–2048.

60. Berndt T. J., Schiavi S., Kumar R. (2005). "Phosphatonins" and the regulation of phosphorus homeostasis. *American Journal of Physiology: Renal Physiology, 289*(6), F1170–1182.

61. Marinella M. A. (2009). Refeeding syndrome: An important aspect of supportive oncology. *Journal of Supportive Oncology, 7*(1), 11–16.

62. Roman-Garcia P., Carullo-Lopez N., Cannata-Andia J. B. (2009). Pathogenesis of bone and mineral related disorders in chronic kidney disease: Key role of hyperphosphatemia. *Journal of Renal Care, 35*(Suppl 1), 34–38.

63. Jacobson R. M., Perry J., Thompson W. O., et al. (2010). Serum electrolytes shifts following administration of sodium phosphates enema. *Gastroenterology Nursing, 33*(3), 191–201.

64. Romani A. M. P. (2011). Cellular magnesium homeostasis. *Archives of Biochemistry and Biophysics, 512*(1), 1–23.

65. Hunter L. A., Gibbins K. L. (2011). Magnesium sulfate: Past, present, and future. *Journal of Midwifery & Women's Health, 56*(6), 566–574.

66. Magee L., Sawchuk D., Synnes A., von Dadelszen P. (2011). SOGC Clinical practice guideline. Magnesium sulphate for fetal neuroprotection. *Journal of Obstetrics and Gynaecology Canada, 33*(5), 516–529.

67. Konrad M., Schlingmann K. P., Gundermann T. (2003). Insights into the molecular nature of magnesium homeostasis. *American Journal of Physiology: Renal Physiology, 286*, F599–F605.

68. Assadi F. (2010). Hypomagnesemia: An evidence-based approach to clinical cases. *Iranian Journal of Kidney Diseases, 4*(1), 13–19.

69. Topf J. M., Murray P. T. (2003). Hypomagnesemia and hypermagnesemia. *Reviews in Endocrine and Metabolic Disorders, 4*, 195–206.

Visit thePoint. **http://thePoint.lww.com for animations, journal articles, and more!**

Disorders of Acid–Base Balance

32

The need for precise regulation of hydrogen ion (H^+) balance is similar in many ways to that of other ions in the body. Membrane excitability, enzyme systems, and chemical reactions all depend on the H^+ concentration being regulated within a narrow physiologic range to function in an optimal way. Many conditions, pathologic or otherwise, can alter H^+ concentration and acid–base balance. This chapter has been organized into two sections: Mechanisms of Acid–Base Balance and Disorders of Acid–Base Balance.

MECHANISMS OF ACID–BASE BALANCE

After completing this section of the chapter, you should be able to meet the following objectives:

- State the definition of an acid and a base.
- Cite the source of metabolic acids.
- Describe the three forms of carbon dioxide transport and their contribution to acid–base balance.
- Define pH and use the Henderson–Hasselbalch equation to calculate pH and to compare compensatory mechanisms for regulating pH.
- Describe the intracellular and extracellular mechanisms for buffering changes in body pH.
- Compare the role of the kidneys and respiratory system in regulation of acid–base balance.
- Explain how interactions between potassium and hydrogen cations and between bicarbonate and chloride anions contribute to the regulation of pH.

Normally, the concentration of body acids and bases is regulated so that the pH of extracellular body fluids is maintained within a very narrow range of 7.35 to 7.45. This balance is maintained through mechanisms that generate, buffer, and eliminate acids and bases. This section of the chapter focuses on acid–base chemistry, the production and regulation of metabolic acids and bicarbonate, calculation of pH, and laboratory tests of acid–base balance.

MECHANISMS OF ACID–BASE BALANCE

- The pH is determined by the ratio of the bicarbonate (HCO_3^-) base to the volatile carbonic acid ($H_2CO_3 \rightleftharpoons H^+ + HCO_3^-$). At a normal pH of 7.4, the ratio is 20:1.
- The pH is regulated by extracellular (carbonic acid [H_2CO_3]/bicarbonate [HCO_3^-]) and intracellular (proteins) systems that buffer changes in pH that would otherwise occur because of the metabolic production of volatile (CO_2) and nonvolatile (*i.e.,* sulphuric and phosphoric) acids.
- The respiratory system regulates the concentration of the volatile carbonic acid ($CO_2 + H_2O \rightleftharpoons H_2CO_3 \rightleftharpoons H^+ + HCO_3^-$) by changing the rate and depth of respiration.
- The kidneys regulate the plasma concentration of HCO_3^- by two processes: reabsorption of the filtered HCO_3^- and generation of new HCO_3^- or the elimination of H^+ ions that have been buffered by tubular systems (phosphate and ammonia) to maintain a luminal pH of at least 4.5.

Acid–Base Chemistry

An *acid* is a molecule that can release an H^+ and a *base* is an ion or molecule that can accept or combine with an H^+.[1–6] For example, hydrochloric acid (HCl) dissociates in water to form H^+ and chloride (Cl^-) ions. A base, such as the bicarbonate ion (HCO_3^-), is a base because it can combine with H^+ to form carbonic acid (H_2CO_3). Most of the body's acids and bases are weak acids and bases, the most important being H_2CO_3, which is a weak acid derived from carbon dioxide (CO_2), and *bicarbonate* (HCO_3^-), which is a weak base.

Acids and bases exist as buffer pairs or systems—a mixture of a weak acid and its conjugate base or a weak base and its conjugate acid. When an acid (HA) is added to water, it dissociates reversibly to form H^+ and its conjugate anion (A^-), for example, $HA \leftrightarrow H^+ + A^-$. The degree to which an acid dissociates and acts as an H^+ donor determines whether it is a strong or weak acid. *Strong acids,* such as sulphuric acid, dissociate completely; *weak acids,* such as acetic acid, dissociate only to a limited extent. The same is true of a base and its ability to dissociate and accept an H^+.

The concentration of H^+ in body fluids is low compared with other ions. For example, the sodium ion (Na^+) is present at a concentration approximately 3.5 million times that of H^+. Because it is cumbersome to work with such a small number, the H^+ concentration is commonly expressed in terms of the *pH.* Specifically, pH represents the negative logarithm (log_{10}) of the H^+ concentration expressed in millimoles per litre (mmol/L). Thus, a pH value of 7.0 implies an H^+ concentration of 10^{-7} (0.0000001 mmol/L). Because the pH is inversely related to the H^+ concentration, a low pH indicates a high concentration of H^+, and a high pH indicates a low concentration.

The *dissociation constant* (K_a) is used to describe the degree to which an acid or base in a buffer system dissociates. The symbol pK_a refers to the negative log_{10} of the dissociation constant for an acid and represents the pH at which an acid is 50% dissociated.[4] Use of a negative log_{10} for the dissociation constant allows pH to be expressed as a positive value. Each acid in an aqueous solution has a characteristic pK_a that varies slightly with temperature and pH. At normal body temperature, the pK_a for the HCO_3^- buffer system of the extracellular fluid compartment is 6.1.[1–4]

Metabolic Acid and Bicarbonate Production

Acids are continuously generated as byproducts of metabolic processes (Fig. 32.1). Physiologically, these acids fall into two groups: the *volatile acid* H_2CO_3 and all other *nonvolatile*

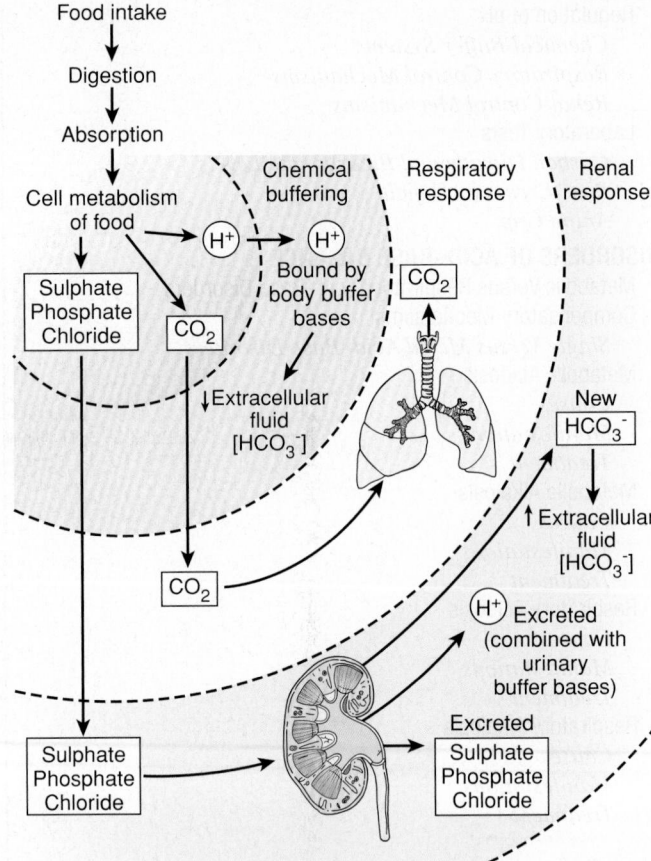

FIGURE 32.1 • The maintenance of normal blood pH by chemical buffers, the respiratory system, and the kidneys. On a mixed diet, pH is threatened by the production of strong acids (sulphuric, hydrochloric, and phosphoric) mainly as the result of protein metabolism. These strong acids are buffered in the body by chemical buffer bases, such as extracellular fluid (ECF) bicarbonate (HCO_3^-). The respiratory system disposes of carbon dioxide (CO_2). The kidneys eliminate hydrogen ions (H^+) combined with urinary buffers and anions in the urine. At the same time, they add new HCO_3^- to the ECF, to replace the HCO_3^- consumed in buffering strong acids. (From Rhoades R. A., Bell D. R. (2013). *Medical physiology: Principles for clinical medicine* (4th ed., p. 454). Philadelphia, PA: Lippincott Williams & Wilkins.).

or *fixed acids*. The difference between the two types of acids arises because H_2CO_3 is in equilibrium with CO_2 ($H_2CO_3 \leftrightarrow CO_2 + H_2O$), which is volatile and leaves the body by way of the lungs. Therefore, the H_2CO_3 concentration is determined by the lungs and their capacity to exhale CO_2. The fixed or *nonvolatile acids* (*e.g.,* sulphuric, hydrochloric, phosphoric) are not eliminated by the lungs. Instead, they are buffered by body proteins or extracellular buffers, such as HCO_3^-, and then eliminated by the kidney.

Carbon Dioxide and Bicarbonate Production

Body metabolism results in the production of approximately 13,000 to 20,000 mmol of CO_2 each day.[4] Carbon dioxide is transported in the circulation in three forms: (1) as a dissolved gas, (2) as bicarbonate, and (3) as carbaminohemoglobin (see Understanding Carbon Dioxide Transport). Collectively, dissolved CO_2 and HCO_3^- account for approximately 77% of the CO_2 that is transported in the extracellular fluid; the remaining CO_2 travels as carbaminohemoglobin (CO_2 bound to amino acids in hemoglobin).[2] Although CO_2 is a gas and not an acid, a small percentage of the gas combines with water to form H_2CO_3. The reaction that generates H_2CO_3 from CO_2 and water is catalyzed by an enzyme called *carbonic anhydrase,* which is present in large quantities in red blood cells, renal tubular cells, and other tissues in the body. The rate of the reaction between CO_2 and water is increased approximately 5,000 times by the presence of carbonic anhydrase. Were it not for this enzyme, the reaction would occur too slowly to be of any significance.

Because it is almost impossible to measure H_2CO_3, CO_2 measurements are commonly used when calculating pH. The H_2CO_3 content of the blood can be calculated by multiplying the partial pressure of CO_2 (PCO_2) by its solubility coefficient, which is 0.03. This means that the concentration of H_2CO_3 in the arterial blood, which normally has a PCO_2 of approximately 40 mm Hg, is 1.20 mmol/L ($40 \times 0.03 = 1.20$), and that for venous blood, which normally has a PCO_2 of approximately 45 mm Hg, is 1.35 mmol/L.

Production of Fixed or Nonvolatile Acids and Bases

The metabolism of dietary proteins and other substances results in the generation of fixed or nonvolatile acids and bases.[2–4] Oxidation of the sulphur-containing amino acids (*e.g.,* methionine, cysteine) results in the production of sulphuric acid. Oxidation of arginine and lysine produces hydrochloric acid, and oxidation of phosphorus-containing nucleic acids yields phosphoric acid. Incomplete oxidation of glucose results in the formation of lactic acid and incomplete oxidation of fats, the production of ketoacids. The major sources of base are the metabolism of amino acids such as aspartate and glutamate and the metabolism of certain organic anions (*e.g.,* citrate, lactate, acetate). Acid production normally exceeds base production, with the net effect being the addition of approximately 1 mmol/kg body weight of nonvolatile or fixed acid to the body each day. Consumption of a vegetarian diet,

which contains large amounts of organic anions, results in the net production of base.[3]

Calculation of pH

The plasma pH can be calculated using an equation called the *Henderson–Hasselbalch equation.*[1–3] This equation uses the pK_a of the bicarbonate buffer system, which is 6.1, and $\log_{10}$ of the HCO_3^- to dissolved CO_2 (H_2CO_3) ratio:

$$pH = 6.1 + \log_{10}(HCO_3^-/PCO_2 \times 0.03)$$

It should be noted that it is the ratio rather than the absolute values for bicarbonate and dissolved CO_2 that determines pH (*e.g.,* when the ratio is 20:1, the pH = 7.4). Plasma pH decreases when the ratio is less than 20:1, and it increases when the ratio is greater than 20:1 (Fig. 32.2). Because it is the ratio rather than the absolute values of HCO_3^- or CO_2 that determines pH, the pH can remain within a relatively normal range as long as changes in HCO_3^- are accompanied by similar changes in CO_2, or vice versa. For example, the pH will remain at 7.4 when plasma HCO_3^- has increased from 24 to 48 mmol/L as long as CO_2 levels are also doubled. Likewise, the pH will remain at 7.4 when plasma HCO_3^- has decreased from 24 to 12 mmol/L as long as CO_2 levels are also reduced by one half.

Regulation of pH

The pH of body fluids is regulated by three major mechanisms: (1) chemical buffer systems of the body fluids, which immediately combine with excess acids or bases to prevent large changes in pH; (2) the lungs, which control the elimination of CO_2 through minute ventilation; and (3) the kidneys, which excrete H^+ and both reabsorb and generate HCO_3^- (Fig. 32.1).

Chemical Buffer Systems

The moment-by-moment regulation of pH depends on chemical buffer systems of the intracellular (ICF) and extracellular fluids (ECF). As previously discussed, a *buffer system* consists of a weak base and its conjugate acid pair, or a weak acid and its conjugate base pair. In the process of preventing large changes in pH, the system trades a strong acid for a weak acid or a strong base for a weak base.

The three major buffer systems that protect the pH of body fluids are (1) the bicarbonate buffer system, (2) proteins, and (3) the transcellular H^+/K^+ exchange system.[1–5] These buffer systems are immediately available to combine with excess acids or bases and prevent large changes in pH from occurring during the time it takes for the respiratory and renal mechanisms to become effective.

Bone represents an additional source of acid–base buffering.[3] Excess H^+ ions can be exchanged for Na^+ and K^+ on the bone surface, and dissolution of bone minerals with release of compounds such as sodium bicarbonate ($NaHCO_3$) and calcium carbonate ($CaCO_3$) into the ECF can be used for buffering excess acids. It has been estimated that as much as 40% of buffering of an acute acid load takes place in bone. The

$$pH = 6.1 + \log_{10} (\text{ratio } HCO_3^- : H_2CO_3)$$

FIGURE 32.2 • Normal and compensated states of pH and acid–base balance represented as a balance scale. **A:** When the ratio of bicarbonate (HCO_3^-) to carbonic acid (H_2CO_3, arterial $CO_2 \times 0.03$) = 20:1, the pH = 7.4. **B:** Metabolic acidosis with a HCO_3^-:H_3CO_3 ratio of 10:1 and a pH of 7.1. **C:** Respiratory compensation lowers the H_3CO_3 to 0.6 mmol/L and returns the HCO_3^-:H_3CO_3 ratio to 20:1 and the pH to 7.4. **D:** Respiratory alkalosis with a HCO_3^-:H_3CO_3 ratio of 40:1 and a pH of 7.7. **E:** Renal compensation eliminates HCO_3^-, reducing serum levels to 12 mmol/L, returning the HCO_3^-:H_3CO_3 ratio to 20:1 and the pH to 7.4. Normally, these compensatory mechanisms are capable of buffering large changes in pH, but do not return the pH completely to normal as illustrated here.

role of bone buffers is even greater in the presence of chronic acidosis. The consequences of bone buffering include demineralization of bone and predisposition to development of kidney stones because of increased urinary excretion of calcium. Persons with chronic kidney disease are at particular risk for reduction in bone calcium due to acid retention.

Bicarbonate Buffer System. The HCO_3^- buffer system, which is the principal ECF buffer, uses H_2CO_3 as its weak acid and a bicarbonate salt such as sodium bicarbonate ($NaHCO_3$) as its weak base.[1–3] It substitutes the weak H_2CO_3 for a strong acid such as hydrochloric acid ($HCl + NaHCO_3 \leftrightarrow H_2CO_3 + NaCl$)

or the weak bicarbonate base for a strong base such as sodium hydroxide ($NaOH + H_2CO_3 \leftrightarrow NaHCO_3 + H_2O$). The bicarbonate buffer system is a particularly efficient system because its components can be readily added or removed from the body.[1–3] Metabolism provides an ample supply of CO_2, which can replace any H_2CO_3 that is lost when excess base is added, and CO_2 can be readily eliminated when excess acid is added. Likewise, the kidney can conserve or form new HCO_3^- when excess acid is added, and it can excrete HCO_3^- when excess base is added.

Protein Buffer Systems. Proteins are the largest buffer system in the body.[1–3] Proteins are *amphoteric*, meaning that they can function either as acids or bases. They contain many ionizable groups that can release or bind H^+. The protein buffers are largely located in cells, and H^+ ions and CO_2 diffuse across cell membranes for buffering by intracellular proteins. Albumin and plasma globulins are the major protein buffers in the vascular compartment.

Hydrogen–Potassium Exchange. The transcompartmental exchange of H^+ and potassium ions (K^+) provides another important system for regulation of acid–base balance. Both ions are positively charged, and both ions move freely between the ICF and ECF compartments (see Chapter 31). When excess H^+ is present in the ECF, it moves into the ICF in exchange for K^+, and when excess K^+ is present in the ECF, it moves into the ICF in exchange for H^+. Thus, alterations in potassium levels can affect acid–base balance, and changes in acid–base balance can influence potassium levels. Potassium shifts tend to be more pronounced in metabolic acidosis than in respiratory acidosis.[3] Also, metabolic acidosis caused by an accumulation of nonorganic acids (*e.g.*, hydrochloric acid that occurs in diarrhea or phosphoric acid that occurs in chronic kidney disease) produces a greater increase in extracellular K^+ levels than does acidosis caused by an accumulation of organic acids (*e.g.*, lactic acid, ketoacids).

Respiratory Control Mechanisms

The second line of defence against acid–base disturbances is the control of CO_2 by the lungs. Increased ventilation decreases PCO_2, whereas decreased ventilation increases PCO_2. The blood PCO_2 and pH are important regulators of ventilation. Chemoreceptors in the brain stem and the peripheral chemoreceptors in the carotid and aortic bodies sense changes in PCO_2 and pH and alter the ventilatory rate to maintain acid–base balance.

The respiratory control of pH is rapid, occurring within minutes, and is maximal within 12 to 24 hours.[1-3] Although the respiratory response is rapid, it does not completely return the pH to normal. It is only about 50% to 75% effective as a buffer system.[2] This means that if the pH falls from 7.4 to 7.0, the respiratory system can return the pH to a value of about 7.2 to 7.3.[2] In acting rapidly, however, it prevents large changes in pH from occurring while waiting for the much more slowly reacting kidneys to respond.

Although CO_2 readily crosses the blood–brain barrier, there is a lag for entry of HCO_3^-. Thus, blood levels of HCO_3^- levels change more rapidly than those of the cerebrospinal fluid (CSF). In metabolic acidosis, for example, there is often a primary decrease in pH of the cerebral fluids and a slower decrease in HCO_3^-. When metabolic acid–base disorders are corrected rapidly, the respiratory response may persist because of a delay in adjustment of HCO_3^- levels in CSF.

Renal Control Mechanisms

The kidneys play three fundamental roles in regulating acid–base balance.[1-6] The first is accomplished through the reabsorption of the HCO_3^- that is filtered in the glomerulus so

this important buffer is not lost in the urine. The second is through the excretion of H^+ from fixed acids that result from protein and lipid metabolism. The third is the generation of new HCO_3^- released into the blood.[2] The renal mechanisms for regulating acid–base balance cannot adjust the pH within minutes, as respiratory mechanisms can, but they continue to function for days until the pH has returned to normal or near-normal range.

Hydrogen Ion Elimination and Bicarbonate Conservation. The kidney regulates pH by excreting excess H^+ and reabsorbing or regenerating HCO_3^-. Bicarbonate is freely filtered in the glomerulus (approximately 4,300 mmol/day) and reabsorbed in the tubules.[2] Loss of even small amounts of HCO_3^- impairs the body's ability to buffer its daily load of metabolic acids. Because the amount of H^+ that can be filtered in the glomeruli is relatively small compared with HCO_3^-, its elimination relies on secretion of H^+ from the blood into the urine filtrate in the tubules.

Most (80% to 90%) of the H^+ secretion and reabsorption of HCO_3^- takes place in the proximal tubule.[1-3] The process begins with a coupled Na^+/H^+ transport system in which H^+ is secreted into the tubular fluid and Na^+ is reabsorbed into the tubular cell (Fig. 32.3). The secreted H^+ combines with filtered HCO_3^- to form H_2CO_3. The H_2CO_3 then decomposes into CO_2 and H_2O, catalyzed by a brush border carbonic anhydrase. The CO_2 and H_2O that are formed readily cross the luminal membrane and enter the tubular cell. Inside the tubular cell, the reactions occur in reverse. The CO_2 and H_2O combine to form H_2CO_3, in a carbonic anhydrase-mediated reaction. The H_2CO_3, in turn, is converted to HCO_3^- and H^+. The HCO_3^- is then reabsorbed into the blood along with Na^+,

FIGURE 32.3 • Hydrogen ion (H^+) secretion and bicarbonate ion (HCO_3^-) reabsorption in a renal tubular cell. Carbon dioxide (CO_2) diffuses from the blood or urine filtrate into the tubular cell, where it combines with water in a carbonic anhydrase (CA)—catalyzed reaction that yields carbonic acid (H_2CO_3). The H_2CO_3 dissociates to form H^+ and HCO_3^-. The H^+ is secreted into the tubular fluid in exchange for Na^+. The Na^+ and HCO_3^- enter the extracellular fluid (ATP, adenosine triphosphate).

Understanding Carbon Dioxide Transport

Body metabolism results in a continuous production of carbon dioxide (CO_2). As CO_2 is formed during the metabolic process, it diffuses out of body cells into the tissue spaces and then into the circulation. It is transported in the circulation in three forms: (1) dissolved in the plasma, (2) as bicarbonate, and (3) attached to hemoglobin.

1. Plasma

A small portion (about 10%) of the CO_2 that is produced by body cells is transported in the dissolved state to the lungs and then exhaled. The amount of dissolved CO_2 that can be carried in plasma is determined by the partial pressure of the gas (PCO_2) and its solubility coefficient (0.03 ml/100 ml plasma for each 1 mm Hg PCO_2). Thus, each 100 ml of arterial blood with a PCO_2 of 40 mm Hg would contain 1.2 ml of dissolved CO_2. It is the carbonic acid (H_2CO_3) formed from hydration of dissolved CO_2 that contributes to the pH of the blood.

Body cell

CO_2

CO_2 dissolved in plasma

10% transported as CO_2 dissolved in plasma

---

and the newly generated H^+ is secreted into the tubular fluid to begin another cycle. Normally, only a few of the secreted H^+ ions remain in the tubular fluid because the secretion of H^+ is roughly equivalent to the number of HCO_3^- ions filtered in the glomerulus.

Tubular Buffer Systems. Because an extremely acidic urine filtrate would be damaging to structures in the urinary tract, the minimum urine pH is about 4.5.[1-3] Once the urine pH reaches this level of acidity, H^+ secretion ceases. This limits the amount of unbuffered H^+ that can be excreted by the kidney. When the amount of free H^+ secreted into the tubular fluid threatens to cause the pH of the urine to become too acidic, it must be carried in another form. This is accomplished by combining H^+ ions with intratubular buffers before they are excreted in the urine. There are two important intratubular buffer systems: the phosphate and ammonia buffer systems.[2] The HCO_3^- that is generated by these two buffer systems is new bicarbonate, demonstrating one of the ways that the kidney is able to replenish the ECF stores of HCO_3^-.

The *phosphate buffer system* uses HPO_4^- and $H_2PO_4^-$ that are present in the tubular filtrate. Both forms of phosphate

become concentrated in the tubular fluid because of their relatively poor absorption and because of reabsorption of water from the tubular fluid. Another factor that makes phosphate so effective as a urinary buffer is the fact that urine pH is close to the pK of the phosphate buffer system. The process of H^+ secretion in the tubules is the same as that used for reabsorption of HCO_3^-. As long as there is excess HCO_3^- in the tubular fluid, most of the secreted H^+ combines with HCO_3^-. However, once all the HCO_3^- has been reabsorbed and is no longer available to combine with H^+, any excess H^+ combines with HPO_4^{2-} to form $H_2PO_4^-$ (Fig. 32.4). After H^+ combines with HPO_4^{2-}, it can be excreted as NaH_2PO_4, carrying the excess H^+ with it.

Another important but more complex buffer system is the *ammonia buffer system*. The excretion of H^+ and generation of HCO_3^- by the ammonia buffer system occurs in three major steps: (1) the synthesis of ammonium (NH_4^+) from the amino acid glutamine in the proximal tubule, (2) the reabsorption and recycling of NH_4^+ within the medullary portion of the kidney, and (3) the buffering of H^+ ions by NH_3 in the collecting tubules.[1-5] The metabolism of glutamate in the proximal tubule results in the formation of two NH_4^+

2. Bicarbonate

Carbon dioxide in excess of that which can be carried in the plasma moves into the red blood cells, where the enzyme carbonic anhydrase (CA) catalyzes its conversion to carbonic acid (H_2CO_3). The H_2CO_3, in turn, dissociates into hydrogen (H^+) and bicarbonate (HCO_3^-) ions. The H^+ combines with hemoglobin and the HCO_3^- diffuses into plasma, where it participates in acid–base regulation. The movement of HCO_3^- into the plasma is made possible by a special transport system on the red blood cell membrane in which HCO_3^- ions are exchanged for chloride ions (Cl^-).

3. Hemoglobin

The remaining CO_2 in the red blood cells combines with hemoglobin to form carbaminohemoglobin ($HbCO_2$). The combination of CO_2 with hemoglobin is a reversible reaction characterized by a loose bond, so that CO_2 can be easily released in the alveolar capillaries and exhaled from the lung.

FIGURE 32.4 • The renal phosphate buffer system. The monohydrogen phosphate ion (HPO_4^2) enters the renal tubular fluid in the glomerulus. An H^+ combines with the HPO_4^{2-} to form $H_2PO_4^-$ and is then excreted into the urine in combination with Na^+. The HCO_3^- moves into the extracellular fluid along with the Na^+ that was exchanged during secretion of the H^+ (ATP, adenosine triphosphate; CA, carbonic anhydrase).

and two HCO_3^- ions[2] (Fig. 32.5A). The two NH_4^+ ions are secreted into the tubular fluid by a countertransport mechanism in exchange for Na^+. The two HCO_3^- ions move out of the tubular cell along with the reabsorbed Na^+ to enter the peritubular capillary system. Thus, for each molecule of glutamine metabolized in the proximal tubule, two NH_4^+ ions are secreted into the tubular filtrate, and two HCO_3^- ions are reabsorbed into the blood. The HCO_3^- generated by this process constitutes new HCO_3^-.

A significant portion of the NH_4^+ secreted by the proximal tubular cells is reabsorbed in the thick ascending loop of Henle, where the NH_4^+ substitutes for K^+ on the $Na^+/K^+/2Cl^-$ cotransporter (discussed in Chapter 30). The NH_4^+ that is reabsorbed by the thick ascending loop of Henle accumulates in the medullary interstitium of the kidney, where it exists in equilibrium with NH_3 (Fig. 32.5B). Although both NH_4^+ and NH_3 are present in the medullary interstitial fluid, only NH_3 is lipid soluble and can diffuse across the collecting duct cells into the tubular fluid. Once in the tubular fluid, NH_3 combines with secreted H^+ to form NH_4^+ (Fig. 32.5C). NH_4^+ is not lipid soluble, and thus is trapped in the tubular fluid and excreted in urine. Note that the source of the H^+ secreted by the cells

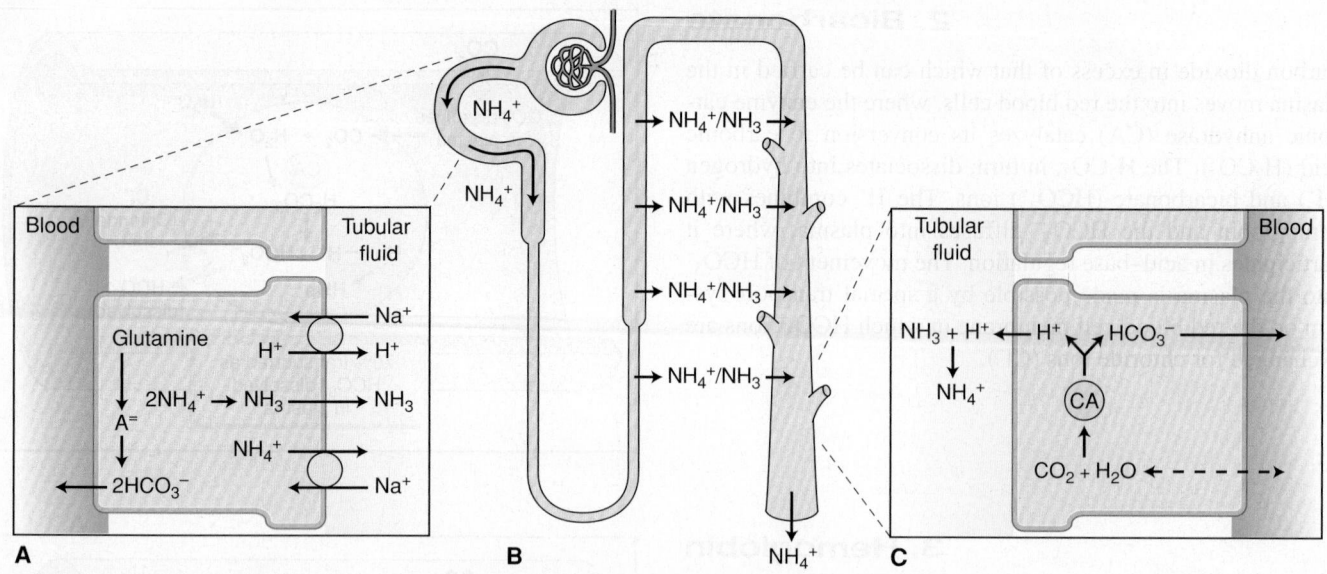

FIGURE 32.5 • Production, transport, and excretion of ammonium (NH_4^+) by the kidney. **A:** Glutamine is metabolized in the proximal tubule to produce two NH_4^+ and two bicarbonate ions (HCO_3^-). The two NH_4^+ are secreted into the tubular fluid and the two HCO_3^- ions, which represent new HCO_3^-, are returned to the circulation. **B:** A significant portion of the secreted NH_4^+ is reabsorbed in the medullary interstitium, where it exists as both NH_4^+ and NH_3. **C:** The NH_3 diffuses into the tubular fluid of the collecting tubule, where it interacts with secreted hydrogen ions (H^+) to form NH_4^+, which is eliminated in the urine. For each NH_4^+ excreted in the urine, another HCO_3^- is returned to the circulation (CA, carbonic anhydrase). (From Berne R. M., Levy M. N. (2000). *Principles of Physiology* (3rd ed., p. 474). St. Louis: Mosby.)

of the collecting tubules is CO_2 and H_2O. Thus, for each H^+ that is produced in the cells and secreted, an additional new HCO_3^- is generated and added to the blood.

One of the most important features of the ammonia buffer system is that it is subject to physiologic control. Under normal conditions, the amount of H^+ eliminated by the ammonia buffer system is about 50% of the acid excreted and new HCO_3^- regenerated.[2] However, with chronic acidosis, it can become the dominant mechanism for H^+ excretion and new HCO_3^- generation. The urine anion gap (discussed in the section on Laboratory Tests), which is an indirect method for assessing urine NH_4^+ levels, can be used to assess kidney function in terms of H^+ elimination.

Potassium–Hydrogen Exchange. Plasma K^+ levels influence renal elimination of H^+ and vice versa. Hypokalemia is a potent stimulus for H^+ secretion and HCO_3^- reabsorption. When plasma K^+ levels fall, there is movement of K^+ from the ICF into the ECF compartment and a reciprocal movement of H^+ from the ECF into the ICF compartment. A similar process occurs in the distal tubules of the kidney, where the H^+/K^+-adenosine triphosphatase (ATPase) exchange pump actively reabsorbs K^+ as well as secreting H^+. An elevation in plasma K^+ levels has the opposite effect. Plasma K^+ levels are similarly altered by acid–base balance. Thus, acidosis tends to increase H^+ elimination and decrease K^+ elimination, with a resultant increase in plasma potassium levels, whereas alkalosis tends to decrease H^+ elimination and increase K^+ elimination, with a resultant decrease in plasma potassium levels.[3]

Aldosterone also influences H^+ elimination by the kidney. It acts in the collecting duct to stimulate H^+ secretion indirectly, while increasing Na^+ reabsorption and K^+ secretion (see Chapter 30). Thus, hyperaldosteronism tends to lead to a decrease in plasma K^+ levels and an increase in pH because of increased H^+ secretion, whereas hypoaldosteronism has the opposite effect.

Chloride–Bicarbonate Exchange. Another mechanism that the kidney uses in regulating HCO_3^- is the chloride–bicarbonate anion exchange that occurs in association with Na^+ reabsorption. Normally, Cl^- is absorbed along with Na^+ throughout the tubules. In situations of volume depletion due to vomiting and chloride depletion, the kidney is forced to substitute HCO_3^- for the Cl^- anion, thereby increasing its absorption of HCO_3^-. *Hypochloremic alkalosis* refers to an increase in pH induced by excess HCO_3^- reabsorption due to a decrease in Cl^- levels, and *hyperchloremic acidosis* refers to a decrease in pH because of decreased HCO_3^- reabsorption due to an increase in Cl^- levels.[1]

Laboratory Tests

Laboratory tests that are used in assessing acid–base balance include arterial blood gases and pH, CO_2 content and HCO_3^- levels, base excess or deficit, and blood and urine anion gaps (Table 32.1). Although useful in determining whether acidosis or alkalosis is present, measurements of the blood pH provide little information about the cause of an acid–base disorder.

TABLE 32.1 BLOOD GAS VALUES		
SOURCE	**ARTERIAL**	**VENOUS**
pH	7.35–7.45	7.31–7.41
pO_2	80–100 mm Hg	30–40 mm Hg
pCO_2	35–45 mm Hg	41–57 mm Hg
HCO_3^-	22–26 mmol/L	17–23 mmol/L
BE	±2 mmol/L	±2 mmol/L
O_2 sats	>94%	>70%

Adapted from Fischbach F. T., Dunning M. B. (2015). *A Manual of Laboratory and Diagnostic Tests* (9th ed.) Philadelphia, PA: Lippincott Williams & Wilkins.

Carbon Dioxide and Bicarbonate Levels

The PCO_2 of the arterial blood gases provide a means of assessing the respiratory component of acid–base balance. Arterial blood gases are used because the CO_2 in arterial blood reflects the amount of CO_2 after it has diffused into the alveoli and been exhaled. In addition, venous blood gases are highly variable, depending on metabolic demands of the various tissues that empty into the vein from which the sample is being drawn. The H_2CO_3 levels can be determined from arterial blood gas measurements using the PCO_2 and the solubility coefficient for CO_2 (normal arterial PCO_2 is 35 to 45 mm Hg). Arterial blood gases also provide a measure of blood oxygen (PO_2) levels. This can be important in assessing lung function, such as diffusion.

The CO_2 content refers to the total CO_2 in the blood, including dissolved CO_2, that contained in HCO_3^-, and that attached to hemoglobin (carbaminohemoglobin [CO_2HHb]). The normal range of values for arterial $HCO3^-$ concentration is 22 to 26 mmol/L and venous is 24 to 31 mmol/L.

Base Excess or Deficit

The total base excess or deficit, also referred to as the *whole blood buffer base*, measures the level of all the buffer systems of the blood—hemoglobin, protein, phosphate, and HCO_3^-. The base excess or deficit describes the amount of a fixed acid or base that must be added to a blood sample to achieve a pH of 7.4 (normal ± 2 mmol/L).[7] For clinical purposes, base excess or deficit can be viewed as a measurement of bicarbonate excess or deficit. A base excess indicates metabolic alkalosis, and a base deficit indicates metabolic acidosis.

Anion Gap

The anion gap describes the difference between the plasma concentration of the major measured cation (Na^+) and the sum of the measured anions (Cl^- and HCO_3^-).[8] This difference represents the concentration of unmeasured anions, such as phosphates, sulphates, organic acids, and proteins (Fig. 32.6). Normally, the anion gap ranges between 12 +/– 4 mmol/L (a value of 16 +/– 4 mmol/L is normal if both sodium and potassium concentrations are used in the calculation).[7] Because albumin is an anion, it is often measured and used in determining the anion gap in persons with decreased albumin levels. For every 10 g/L decline in plasma albumin concentration, 2.5

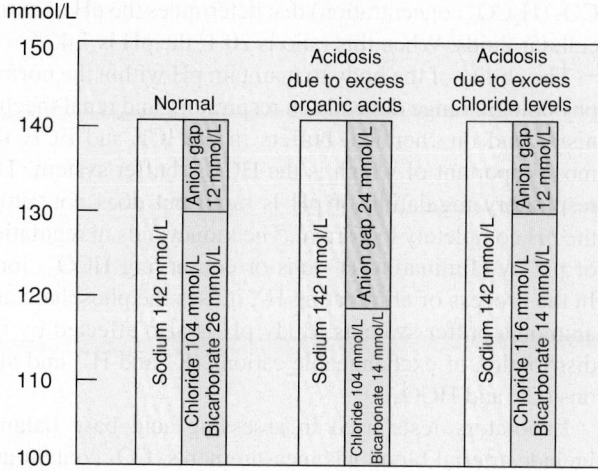

FIGURE 32.6 • The anion gap in acidosis due to excess metabolic acids and excess plasma chloride levels. Unmeasured anions such as phosphates, sulphates, and organic acids increase the anion gap because they replace bicarbonate. This assumes there is no change in sodium content.

should be added to the gap that is calculated from the formula $Na^+ - (Cl^- + HCO_3^-)$.[9] The anion gap is increased in conditions such as lactic acidosis and ketoacidosis that result from elevated levels of metabolic acids. A low anion gap is found in conditions that produce a fall in unmeasured anions (primarily albumin) or rise in unmeasured cations. The latter can occur in hyperkalemia, hypercalcemia, hypermagnesemia, lithium intoxication, or multiple myeloma, in which an abnormal immunoglobulin is produced.[1]

The anion gap of urine is a useful measure as a diagnostic tool.[1,8] Urine electrolyte determinations do not include bicarbonate. Instead, the urine anion gap uses the difference between the measurable cations (Na^+ and K^+) and anions (Cl^-) to provide an estimate of ammonium (NH_4^+) excretion. Because ammonium is a cation, the value of the anion gap becomes more negative as the ammonium level increases. In normal persons secreting 20 to 40 mmol of ammonium per litre, the urine anion gap is close to zero. In metabolic acidosis, the amount of unmeasured NH_4^+ should increase if renal excretion of H^+ is intact; as a result, the urine anion gap should become more negative.

IN SUMMARY

Normal body function depends on the precise regulation of acid–base balance. The pH of the extracellular fluid is normally maintained within the narrow physiologic range of 7.35 to 7.45. Metabolic processes produce volatile and fixed or nonvolatile metabolic acids that must be buffered and eliminated from the body. The volatile acid, H_2CO_3, is in equilibrium with dissolved CO_2, which is eliminated through the lungs. The nonvolatile metabolic acids, which are derived mainly from protein metabolism and incomplete carbohydrate and fat metabolism, are excreted by the kidneys. It is the ratio of the HCO_3^- concentration to dissolved

CO_2 (H_2CO_3 concentration) that determines the pH of extracellular fluids. When this ratio is 20:1, the pH is 7.4.

The ability of the body to maintain pH within the normal physiologic range depends on respiratory and renal mechanisms and on chemical buffers in the ICF and ECF, the most important of which is the HCO_3^- buffer system. The respiratory regulation of pH is rapid but does not return the pH completely to normal. The kidney aids in regulation of pH by eliminating H^+ ions or conserving HCO_3^- ions. In the process of eliminating H^+, it uses the phosphate and ammonia buffer systems. Body pH is also affected by the distribution of exchangeable cations (K^+ and H^+) and anions (Cl^- and HCO_3^-).

Laboratory tests used in assessing acid–base balance include arterial blood gas measurements, CO_2 content and HCO_3^- levels, base excess or deficit, and the anion gap. The base excess or deficit describes the amount of a fixed acid or base that must be added to a blood sample to achieve a pH of 7.4. The anion gap describes the difference between the plasma concentration of the major measured cation (Na^+) and the sum of the anions (Cl^- and HCO_3^-). This difference represents the concentration of unmeasured anions, such as phosphates, sulphates, and organic acids, that are present. The urine anion gap uses the difference between the measurable cations (Na^+ and K^+) and anions (Cl^-) to provide an estimate of ammonium (NH_4^+) excretion and the ability of the kidney to rid the body of excess H^+.

DISORDERS OF ACID–BALANCE BALANCE

After completing this section of the chapter, you should be able to meet the following objectives:

- Differentiate the terms acidemia, alkalemia, acidosis, and alkalosis.
- Describe a clinical situation involving an acid–base disorder in which both primary and compensatory mechanisms are present.
- Define metabolic acidosis, metabolic alkalosis, respiratory acidosis, and respiratory alkalosis.
- Explain the use of the plasma anion gap in differentiating types of metabolic acidosis.
- List common causes of metabolic and respiratory acidosis and metabolic and respiratory alkalosis.
- Contrast and compare the clinical manifestations and treatment of metabolic and respiratory acidosis and of metabolic and respiratory alkalosis.

The terms *acidosis* and *alkalosis* describe the clinical conditions that arise as a result of changes in dissolved CO_2 and HCO_3^- concentrations. An alkali represents a combination of one or more alkali metals, such as sodium or potassium, with a highly basic ion such as a hydroxyl ion (OH^-). Sodium bicarbonate is the main alkali in the extracellular fluid. Although the definitions differ somewhat, the terms *alkali* and *base* are often used interchangeably. Hence, the term *alkalosis* has come to mean the opposite of *acidosis.*

Metabolic Versus Respiratory Acid–Base Disorders

There are two types of acid–base disorders: metabolic and respiratory (Table 32.2). *Metabolic disorders* produce an alteration in the plasma HCO_3^- concentration and result from the addition to or loss from the ECF of nonvolatile acid or alkali. A reduction in pH due to a decrease in HCO_3^- is called *metabolic acidosis,* and an elevation in pH due to increased HCO_3^- levels is called *metabolic alkalosis. Respiratory disorders* involve an alteration in the PCO_2, reflecting an increase or decrease in alveolar ventilation, best indicated by minute volume (respiratory rate multiplied by tidal volume). *Respiratory acidosis* is characterized by a decrease in pH, reflecting a decrease in ventilation and an increase in PCO_2. *Respiratory alkalosis* involves an increase in pH, resulting from an increase in ventilation and a decrease in PCO_2.

Compensatory Mechanisms

Acidosis and alkalosis typically involve a *primary* or *initiating event* and a *compensatory* or *adaptive state* that results from homeostatic mechanisms that attempt to correct or prevent large changes in pH. For example, a person may have a primary metabolic acidosis as a result of overproduction of ketoacids and respiratory alkalosis because of a compensatory increase in ventilation (Table 32.2).

Compensatory mechanisms provide a means to control pH when correction is impossible or cannot immediately be achieved. Often, compensatory mechanisms are interim measures that permit survival while the body attempts to correct the primary disorder. Compensation requires the use of mechanisms that are different from those that caused the primary disorder. For example, the lungs cannot compensate for respiratory acidosis that is caused by lung disease, nor can the kidneys compensate for metabolic acidosis that occurs because of chronic kidney disease. The body can, however, use renal mechanisms to compensate for respiratory-induced changes in pH, and it can use respiratory mechanisms to compensate for metabolically induced changes in acid–base balance. Because compensatory mechanisms become more effective with time, there are often differences between the level of pH change that is present in acute and chronic acid–base disorders.[3]

Single Versus Mixed Acid–Base Disorders
Thus far we have discussed acid–base disorders as if they existed as a single primary disorder, such as metabolic acidosis, accompanied by a predicted compensatory response (*i.e.,* hyperventilation and respiratory alkalosis). It is not uncommon, however, for persons to present with more than

TABLE 32.2 SUMMARY OF SINGLE ACID–BASE DISTURBANCES AND THEIR COMPENSATORY RESPONSES

ACID–BASE IMBALANCE	PRIMARY DISTURBANCE	RESPIRATORY COMPENSATION AND PREDICTED RESPONSE[a]	RENAL COMPENSATION AND PREDICTED RESPONSE[a,b]
Metabolic acidosis	↓plasma pH and HCO_3^-	↑ventilation and ↓PCO_2 *1 mmol/L ↓HCO_3^- → 1 to 1.5 mm Hg ↓PCO_2*	↑H^+ excretion and ↑HCO_3^- reabsorption if no renal disease
Metabolic alkalosis	↑plasma pH and HCO_3^-	↓ventilation and ↑PCO_2 *1 mmol/L ↑HCO_3^- → 0.25 to 1.0 mm Hg ↑PCO_2*	↓H^+ excretion and ↓HCO_3^- reabsorption if no renal disease
Respiratory acidosis	↓plasma pH and ↑PCO_2	None	↑H^+ excretion and ↑HCO_3^- reabsorption *Acute: 1 mm Hg ↑PCO_2 → 0.1 mmol/L ↑HCO_3^- Chronic: 1 mm Hg ↑PCO_2 → 0.4 mmol/L ↑HCO_3^-*
Respiratory alkalosis	↑plasma pH and ↓PCO_2	None	↓H^+ excretion and ↓HCO_3^- reabsorption *Acute: 1 mm Hg ↓PCO_2 → 0.2 mmol/L ↓HCO_3^- Chronic: 1 mm Hg ↓PCO_2 → 0.4 mmol/L ↓HCO_3^-*

Note: Predicted compensatory responses are in *italics*.
[a]If blood values are the same as predicted compensatory values, a single acid–base disorder is present; if values are different, a mixed acid–base disorder is present.
[b]Acute renal compensation ≤48 hours, chronic renal compensation >48 hours.

one primary disorder or a mixed disorder.[3,10] For example, a person may present with a low plasma HCO_3^- concentration due to metabolic acidosis and a high PCO_2 due to chronic lung disease. Values for the predicted renal or respiratory compensatory responses can be used in the diagnosis of these mixed acid–base disorders[3,11] (Table 32.2). If the values for the compensatory response fall outside the predicted plasma values, it can then be concluded that more than one disorder (*i.e.,* a mixed disorder) is present. Because the respiratory response to changes in HCO_3^- occurs almost immediately, there is only one predicted compensatory response for primary metabolic acid–base disorders. This is in contrast to the primary respiratory

disorders, which have two ranges of predicted values, one for the acute and one for the chronic response. Renal compensation takes several days to become fully effective. The acute compensatory response represents the HCO_3^- levels before renal compensation has occurred, and the chronic response after it has occurred. Thus, the values for the plasma pH tend to be more normal in the chronic phase.

Metabolic Acidosis

Metabolic acidosis involves a decreased plasma HCO_3^- concentration along with a decrease in pH. In metabolic acidosis, the body compensates for the decrease in pH by increasing the respiratory rate in an effort to decrease PCO_2 and H_2CO_3 levels. The PCO_2 can be expected to fall by 1 to 1.5 mm Hg for each 1 mmol/L fall in HCO_3^-.[3,11]

Causes

Metabolic acidosis can be caused by one or more of the following four mechanisms: (1) increased production of fixed metabolic acids or ingestion of fixed acids such as salicylic acid, (2) inability of the kidneys to excrete the fixed acids produced from normal metabolism, (3) excessive loss of bicarbonate through the kidneys or gastrointestinal tract, or (4) increased plasma Cl^- concentration.[1–3] The anion gap is often useful in determining the underlying cause of the metabolic acidosis (Chart 32.1). The presence of excess metabolic acids produces an increase in the anion gap as sodium bicarbonate is replaced by the sodium salt of the offending acid (*e.g.,* sodium lactate). When the acidosis results from an increase in plasma Cl^- levels (*e.g.,* hyperchloremic acidosis), the anion gap remains within normal levels. The causes of metabolic acidosis are summarized in Table 32.3.

METABOLIC ACID–BASE IMBALANCE

- Metabolic acid–base disorders represent a primary change in the plasma HCO_3^- ion concentration.
- Metabolic acidosis can be defined as a decrease in plasma HCO_3^- and pH that is caused by an excess of production or accumulation of fixed acids or loss of HCO_3^- ion. Compensatory responses include an increase in ventilation and elimination of CO_2 and the reabsorption and generation of bicarbonate by the kidney.
- Metabolic alkalosis can be defined as an increase in plasma HCO_3^- and pH that is initiated by excess H^+ ion loss or HCO_3^- ion gain and maintained by conditions that impair the ability of the kidney to excrete the excess HCO_3^- ion. Compensatory responses include a decreased respiratory rate with retention of PCO_2 and increased elimination of HCO_3^- by the kidney.

CHART 32.1 THE ANION GAP IN DIFFERENTIAL DIAGNOSIS OF METABOLIC ACIDOSIS

Decreased Anion Gap (<8 mmol/L)

Hypoalbuminemia (decrease in unmeasured anions)

Multiple myeloma (increase in unmeasured cationic IgG paraproteins)

Increased unmeasured cations (hyperkalemia, hypercalcemia, hypermagnesemia, lithium intoxication)

Increased Anion Gap (>16 mmol/L)

Presence of unmeasured metabolic anion

    Diabetic ketoacidosis

    Alcoholic ketoacidosis

    Lactic acidosis

    Starvation

    Renal insufficiency

Presence of drug or chemical anion

    Salicylate poisoning

    Methanol poisoning

    Ethylene glycol poisoning

Normal Anion Gap (8–16 mmol/L)

Loss of bicarbonate

    Diarrhea

    Pancreatic fluid loss

    Ileostomy (unadapted)

Chloride retention

    Renal tubular acidosis

    Ileal loop bladder

    Parenteral nutrition (arginine and lysine)

TABLE 32.3 CAUSES AND MANIFESTATIONS OF METABOLIC ACIDOSIS

CAUSES	MANIFESTATIONS
Excess Metabolic Acids (Increased Anion Gap)	**Blood pH, HCO_3^-, CO_2**
Excessive production of metabolic acids	pH decreased
Lactic acidosis	HCO_3^- (primary) decreased
Diabetic ketoacidosis	PCO_2 (compensatory) decreased
Alcoholic ketoacidosis	**Gastrointestinal Function**
Fasting and starvation	Anorexia
Poisoning (*e.g.,* ethylene glycol, isoniazid, methanol, paraldehyde, salicylate)	Nausea and vomiting
	Abdominal pain
Impaired elimination of metabolic acids	**Neural Function**
	Weakness
Kidney failure or dysfunction (uremia)	Lethargy
	General malaise
Excessive Bicarbonate Loss (Normal Anion Gap)	Confusion
	Stupor
	Coma
Loss of intestinal secretions	Depression of vital functions
Diarrhea (severe)	**Cardiovascular Function**
Intestinal suction	Peripheral vasodilation
Intestinal or biliary fistula	Decreased heart rate
Increased renal losses	Cardiac arrhythmias
Renal tubular acidosis	**Skin**
Treatment with carbonic anhydrase inhibitors	Warm and flushed
	Skeletal system
Hypoaldosteronism	Bone disease (*e.g.,* chronic acidosis)
Increased Chloride Levels (Normal Anion Gap)	**Signs of Compensation**
	Increased rate and depth of respiration (*i.e.,* Kussmaul breathing)
Excessive reabsorption of chloride by the kidney	Hyperkalemia
Sodium chloride infusions	Acid urine
Treatment with ammonium chloride	Increased ammonia in urine
Parenteral hyperalimentation	

Lactic Acidosis. Acute lactic acidosis is the most common cause of metabolic acidosis in hospitalized patients and develops when there is excess production or diminished removal of lactic acid from the blood. Lactic acid is produced by the anaerobic metabolism of glucose (see Understanding Cell Metabolism, Chapter 4). Most cases of lactic acidosis are caused by inadequate oxygen delivery or impaired tissue perfusion, as in shock or cardiac arrest.[12] Such conditions not only increase lactic acid production, but they tend to impair lactic acid clearance because of poor liver and kidney perfusion. Mortality rates are high for persons with lactic acidosis due to shock and tissue hypoxia.[13] Lactic acidosis can also occur during periods of intense exercise in which the metabolic needs of the exercising muscles outpace their aerobic capacity for production of ATP, causing them to revert to anaerobic metabolism and the production of lactic acid.[12]

Lactic acidosis is also associated with disorders in which tissue hypoxia does not appear to be present. It has been reported in patients with leukemia, lymphomas, and other cancers; those with poorly controlled diabetes; and persons with severe liver failure.[12] Mechanisms causing lactic acidosis in these conditions are poorly understood. Some conditions such as neoplasms may produce local increases in tissue metabolism and lactate production or they may interfere with blood flow to noncancerous cells.

Lactic acidosis may also occur in genetic mitochondrial disorders that impair oxidative metabolism (see Chapter 7).[12,14] One of these disorders, referred to by the acronym MELAS, involves mitochondrial encephalopathy (ME), lactic acidosis (LA), and strokelike episodes (S). Children with the disorder develop normally for the first few years of life and then begin to display impaired motor and cognitive development. The mitochondrial defect also leads to short stature, seizure disorders, and multiple strokes. Lowering the plasma lactate level of children with severe lactic acidosis may result in marked clinical improvement. A variety of drugs can also produce life-threatening lactic acidosis by inhibiting mitochondrial function. These drugs include the biguanide antidiabetic drugs (*e.g.,* metformin)[14,15] and the antiretroviral nucleoside analogs (*e.g.,* zidovudine [AZT]) that are used to treat the acquired immunodeficiency syndrome (AIDS).[12]

A unique form of lactic acidosis, called D-lactic acidosis, can occur in persons with intestinal disorders that involve the generation and absorption of D-lactic acid (L-lactic acid is the usual cause of lactic acidosis). It can occur in persons with jejunoileal bypass, small bowel resection, or short bowel syndrome, in which there is impaired absorption of carbohydrate in the small intestine.[16] In these cases, the unabsorbed carbohydrate is delivered to the colon, where it is converted to D-lactic acid by an overgrowth of gram-positive anaerobes. Persons with D-lactic acidosis experience episodic periods of metabolic acidosis often brought on by eating a meal high in carbohydrates. Manifestations include confusion, cerebellar ataxia, slurred speech, and loss of memory. They may complain of feeling (or appear) intoxicated. Treatment includes use of antimicrobial agents to decrease the number of D-lactic acid-producing microorganisms in the bowel along with a low-carbohydrate diet.[16]

Ketoacidosis. Ketoacids (*i.e.,* acetoacetic and β-hydroxybutyric acid), produced in the liver from fatty acids, are the source of fuel for many body tissues. An overproduction of ketoacids occurs when carbohydrate stores are inadequate or when the body cannot use available carbohydrates as a fuel. Under these conditions, fatty acids are mobilized from adipose tissue and delivered to the liver, where they are converted to ketones. Ketoacidosis develops when ketone production by the liver exceeds tissue use.[17]

The most common cause of ketoacidosis is uncontrolled diabetes mellitus, in which an insulin deficiency leads to the release of fatty acids from adipose cells with subsequent production of excess ketoacids (see Chapter 42). Ketoacidosis may also develop as the result of fasting or food deprivation, during which the lack of carbohydrates produces a self-limited state of ketoacidosis.

Ketones are also formed during the oxidation of alcohol, a process that occurs in the liver. A condition called *alcoholic ketoacidosis* can develop in persons who engage in excess alcohol consumption.[18] It usually follows prolonged alcohol ingestion, particularly if accompanied by decreased food intake and vomiting—conditions that result in using fatty acids as an energy source. Ketone formation may be further enhanced by the hypoglycemia that results from alcohol-induced inhibition of glucose synthesis (*i.e.,* gluconeogenesis) by the liver and impaired ketone elimination by the kidneys because of dehydration. An ECF volume deficit caused by vomiting and decreased fluid intake often contributes to the acidosis. Numerous other factors, such as elevations in cortisol, growth hormone, glucagon, and catecholamines, mediate free fatty acid release and thereby contribute to the development of alcoholic ketoacidosis.

Salicylate Toxicity. Salicylates are another potential source of metabolic acids. Aspirin (acetylsalicylic acid) is rapidly converted to salicylic acid in the body.[19] Although aspirin is the most common cause of salicylate toxicity, other salicylate preparations such as methyl salicylate, sodium salicylate, and salicylic acid may produce similar effects. Salicylate overdose produces serious toxic effects, including death. A fatal overdose can occur if 300 to 500 mg/kg is ingested.

A variety of acid–base disturbances occur with salicylate toxicity. The salicylates cross the blood–brain barrier and directly stimulate the respiratory centre, causing hyperventilation and respiratory alkalosis. The kidneys compensate by secreting increased amounts of HCO_3^-, K^+, and Na^+, thereby contributing to the development of metabolic acidosis. Salicylates also interfere with carbohydrate metabolism, which results in increased production of metabolic acids.

One of the treatments for salicylate toxicity is *alkalinization* of the plasma. Salicylic acid, which is a weak acid, exists in equilibrium with the alkaline salicylate anion. It is the salicylic acid that is toxic because of its ability to cross cell membranes and enter brain cells. The salicylate anion crosses membranes poorly and is less toxic. With alkalinization of the extracellular fluids, the ratio of salicylic acid to salicylate is greatly reduced. This allows salicylic acid to move out of cells into the extracellular fluid along a concentration gradient. The renal elimination of salicylates follows a similar pattern when the urine is alkalinized.[19]

Methanol and Ethylene Glycol Toxicity. Ingestion of methanol and ethylene glycol results in the production of metabolic acids and causes metabolic acidosis. Both produce an osmolar gap because of their small size and osmotic properties. Methanol (wood alcohol) is a component found in shellac, varnish, de-icing solutions, Sterno (a canned heating fuel), and other commercial products. Methanol can be absorbed through the skin or gastrointestinal tract or inhaled through the lungs. A dose as small as 30 ml can be fatal. In addition to metabolic acidosis, methanol produces severe optic nerve and central nervous system toxicity.[1] Organ system damage occurs after a 24-hour period in which methanol is converted to formaldehyde and formic acid.

Ethylene glycol is a solvent found in products ranging from antifreeze and de-icing solutions to carpet and fabric cleaners. It tastes sweet and is intoxicating, factors that contribute to its abuse potential. It is rapidly absorbed from the intestine, making treatment with gastric lavage and syrup of ipecac ineffective. Acidosis occurs as ethylene glycol is converted to oxalic and lactic acid. Manifestations of ethylene glycol toxicity occur in three stages: neurologic symptoms ranging from drunkenness to coma, which appear during the first 12 hours; cardiorespiratory disorders such as tachycardia and pulmonary edema; and flank pain and acute renal failure caused by plugging of the tubules with oxalate crystals (from excess oxalic acid production).[20]

The enzyme *alcohol dehydrogenase* metabolizes methanol and ethylene glycol into their toxic metabolites. This is the same enzyme that is used in the metabolism of ethanol. Because alcohol dehydrogenase has an affinity for ethanol

10 times its affinity for methanol or ethylene glycol, intravenous or oral ethanol is used as an antidote for methanol and ethylene glycol poisoning. Extracellular volume expansion and hemodialysis are also used. Since 2001 Fomepizole was approved by Health Canada, as an antidote for methanol and ethylene glycol poisoning. In a manner similar to ethanol, it is thought to act as an inhibitor of alcohol dehydrogenase, thereby preventing the formation of the toxic ethylene glycol metabolites. [20]

Decreased Renal Function. Chronic kidney disease is the most common cause of chronic metabolic acidosis. The kidneys normally conserve HCO_3^- and secrete H^+ ions into the urine as a means of regulating acid–base balance. In chronic kidney disease, there is loss of both glomerular and tubular function, with retention of nitrogenous wastes and metabolic acids. In a condition called *renal tubular acidosis,* glomerular function is normal, but the tubular secretion of H^+ or reabsorption of HCO_3^- is abnormal[1] (discussed in Chapter 33).

Increased Bicarbonate Losses. Increased HCO_3^- losses occur with the loss of bicarbonate-rich body fluids or with impaired conservation of HCO_3^- by the kidney. Intestinal secretions have a high HCO_3^- concentration. Consequently, excessive loss of HCO_3^- occurs with severe diarrhea; small bowel, pancreatic, or biliary fistula drainage; ileostomy drainage; and intestinal suction. In diarrhea of microbial origin, HCO_3^- is also secreted into the bowel as a means of neutralizing the metabolic acids produced by the microorganisms causing the diarrhea. Creation of an ileal bladder, which is done for conditions such as neurogenic bladder or surgical removal of the bladder because of cancer, involves the implantation of the ureters into a short, isolated loop of ileum that serves as a conduit for urine collection. With this procedure, contact time between the urine and ileal bladder is normally too short for significant anion exchange, and HCO_3^- is lost in the urine.[21]

Hyperchloremic Acidosis. Hyperchloremic acidosis occurs when Cl^- levels are increased. Because Cl^- and HCO_3^- are exchangeable anions, the plasma HCO_3^- decreases when there is an increase in Cl^-. Hyperchloremic acidosis can occur as the result of abnormal absorption of Cl^- by the kidneys or as a result of treatment with chloride-containing medications (*i.e.,* sodium chloride, amino acid–chloride hyperalimentation solutions, and ammonium chloride). Ammonium chloride is broken down into NH_4^+ and Cl^-. The ammonium ion is converted to urea in the liver, leaving the Cl^- free to react with H^+ to form HCl. The administration of intravenous sodium chloride or parenteral hyperalimentation solutions that contain an amino acid–chloride combination can cause acidosis in a similar manner. With hyperchloremic acidosis, the anion gap remains within the normal range, whereas plasma Cl^- levels are increased and HCO_3^- levels are decreased.[1-3]

Manifestations

Metabolic acidosis is characterized by a decrease in plasma pH (<7.35) and HCO_3^- levels (<22 mmol/L) due to either a gain in H^+ or loss of HCO_3^-. Acidosis typically produces a compensatory increase in respiratory rate with a decrease in PCO_2.

The manifestations of metabolic acidosis fall into three categories: (1) signs and symptoms of the disorder causing the acidosis; (2) changes in body function related to recruitment of compensatory mechanisms; and (3) alterations in cardiovascular, neurologic, and musculoskeletal function resulting from the decreased pH (Table 32.3). The signs and symptoms of metabolic acidosis usually begin to appear when the plasma HCO_3^- concentration falls to 20 mmol/L or less. A fall in pH to less than 7.1 to 7.2 can reduce cardiac contractility and predispose to potentially fatal cardiac arrhythmias.[11]

Metabolic acidosis is seldom a primary disorder; it usually develops during the course of another disease. The manifestations of metabolic acidosis frequently are superimposed on the symptoms of the contributing health problem. With diabetic ketoacidosis, which is a common cause of metabolic acidosis, there is an increase in blood and urine glucose and a characteristic smell of ketones to the breath. In the metabolic acidosis that accompanies chronic kidney disease, urea (BUN) levels are elevated and other tests of renal function yield abnormal results.

Manifestations related to respiratory and renal compensatory mechanisms usually occur early in the course of metabolic acidosis. In situations of acute metabolic acidosis, the respiratory system compensates for a decrease in pH by increasing ventilation to reduce PCO_2; this is accomplished through deep and rapid respirations. In diabetic ketoacidosis, this breathing pattern is referred to as *Kussmaul breathing.* For descriptive purposes, it can be said that Kussmaul breathing resembles the hyperpnea of exercise—the person breathes as though he or she had been running. There may be complaints of difficult breathing or dyspnea with exertion; with severe acidosis, dyspnea may be present even at rest. Respiratory compensation for acute acidosis tends to be somewhat greater than for chronic acidosis. When kidney function is normal, H^+ excretion increases promptly in response to acidosis, and the urine becomes more acid.

Changes in pH have a direct effect on body function that can produce signs and symptoms common to most types of metabolic acidosis, regardless of cause. A person with metabolic acidosis often complains of weakness, fatigue, general malaise, and a dull headache. They also may have anorexia, nausea, vomiting, and abdominal pain. Tissue turgor is impaired, and the skin is dry when fluid deficit accompanies acidosis. In persons with undiagnosed diabetes mellitus, the nausea, vomiting, and abdominal symptoms may be misinterpreted as being caused by gastrointestinal flu or other abdominal disease, such as appendicitis. Acidosis depresses neuronal excitability and it decreases binding of calcium to plasma proteins so that more free calcium is available to decrease neural activity. As acidosis progresses, the level of consciousness declines, and stupor and coma develop. The skin is often warm and flushed because blood vessels in the skin become less responsive to sympathetic nervous system stimulation and lose their tone.

When the pH falls to 7.1 to 7.2, cardiac contractility and cardiac output decrease, the heart becomes less responsive to catecholamines (*i.e.,* epinephrine and norepinephrine), and arrhythmias, including fatal ventricular arrhythmias, can develop. A decrease in ventricular function may be particularly important in perpetuating shock-induced lactic acidosis, and partial correction of the acidemia may be necessary before tissue perfusion can be restored.[11]

Chronic acidemia, as in chronic kidney disease, can lead to a variety of musculoskeletal problems, some of which result from the release of calcium and phosphate during bone buffering of excess H^+ ions.[11] Of particular importance is impaired growth in children. In infants and children, acidemia may be associated with a variety of nonspecific symptoms such as anorexia, weight loss, muscle weakness, and listlessness.[2] Muscle weakness and listlessness may result from alterations in muscle metabolism.

Treatment

The treatment of metabolic acidosis focuses on correcting the condition that caused the disorder and restoring the fluids and electrolytes that have been lost from the body. The treatment of diabetic ketoacidosis is discussed in Chapter 42.

The use of supplemental sodium bicarbonate ($NaHCO_3$) may be indicated in the treatment of some forms of normal anion gap acidosis. However, its use in treatment of metabolic acidosis with an increased anion gap is controversial, particularly in cases of impaired tissue perfusion.[17] In most patients with circulatory shock, cardiac arrest, or sepsis, impaired oxygen delivery is the primary cause of lactic acidosis. In these situations, the administration of large amounts of $NaHCO_3$ does not improve oxygen delivery and may produce hypernatremia, hyperosmolality, and decreased oxygen release by hemoglobin because of a shift in the oxygen dissociation curve.[11]

Metabolic Alkalosis

Metabolic alkalosis is a systemic disorder caused by an increase in plasma pH due to a primary excess in HCO_3^-.[1-6] It is reported to be the second most common acid–base disorder in hospitalized adults, accounting for about 32% of all acid–base disorders.

Causes

Metabolic alkalosis can be caused by factors that generate a loss of fixed acids or a gain of bicarbonate and those that maintain the alkalosis by interfering with excretion of the excess bicarbonate (Table 32.4). They include (1) a gain of base through the oral or intravenous route; (2) loss of fixed acids from the stomach; and (3) maintenance of the increased bicarbonate levels by contraction of the ECF volume, hypokalemia, and hypochloremia.

TABLE 32.4 CAUSES AND MANIFESTATIONS OF METABOLIC ALKALOSIS

CAUSES	MANIFESTATIONS
Excessive Gain of Bicarbonate or Alkali	**Blood pH, HCO_3^-, CO_2**
Ingestion or administration of sodium bicarbonate	pH increased
Administration of hyperalimentation solutions containing acetate	HCO_3^- (primary) increased
Administration of parenteral solutions containing lactate	PCO_2 (compensatory) increased
Administration of citrate-containing blood transfusions	**Neural Function**
	Confusion
Excessive Loss of Hydrogen Ions	Hyperactive reflexes
Vomiting	Tetany
Gastric suction	Convulsions
Binge-purge syndrome	**Cardiovascular Function**
Potassium deficit	Hypotension
Diuretic therapy	Arrhythmias
Hyperaldosteronism	**Respiratory Function**
Milk/calcium-alkali syndrome	Respiratory acidosis due to decreased respiratory rate
Increased Bicarbonate Retention	**Signs of Compensation**
Loss of chloride with bicarbonate retention	Decreased rate and depth of respiration
	Increased urine pH
Volume Contraction	
Loss of body fluids	
Diuretic therapy	

Excess Base Loading. Because the normal kidney is extremely efficient at excreting bicarbonate, excess base intake is rarely a cause of significant chronic metabolic alkalosis. Transient acute alkalosis, on the other hand, is a rather common occurrence during or immediately after excess oral ingestion of bicarbonate-containing antacids (*e.g.,* Alka-Seltzer) or intravenous infusion of $NaHCO_3$ or base equivalent (*e.g.,* acetate in hyperalimentation solutions, lactate in Ringer's lactate, and citrate in blood transfusions). A classic condition called the *milk-alkali syndrome* was a condition in which the chronic ingestion of milk or calcium carbonate antacids leads to hypercalcemia, metabolic alkalosis, and hyperphosphatemia. As the antacids increased the plasma HCO_3^- concentration the hypercalcemia prevented the urinary excretion of HCO_3^-. After histamine-2 blockers and proton pump inhibitors medications were introduced to treat the dyspepsia, the incidence of this syndrome decreased. Now the modern version, called the calcium-alkali syndrome, has emerged with hypercalcemia and metabolic alkalosis. Over the last 20 years increasing calcium supplements (*e.g.,* calcium carbonate) used to prevent or treat osteoporosis and dyspepsia remain the main cause of this syndrome.[22]

Loss of Fixed Acid. The loss of fixed acids occurs mainly through the loss of acid from the stomach and the loss of chloride in the urine. Vomiting and removal of gastric secretions by nasogastric suction are common causes of metabolic alkalosis in acutely ill or hospitalized patients. Bulimia nervosa with self-induced vomiting also is associated with metabolic alkalosis. Gastric secretions contain high concentrations of HCl and lesser concentrations of potassium chloride (KCl). As Cl^- is taken from the blood and secreted into the stomach, it is replaced by HCO_3^-. Under normal conditions, each 1 mmol of H^+ that is secreted into the stomach generates 1 mmol of plasma HCO_3^-. Thus, the loss of gastric secretions through vomiting or gastric suction is a common cause of metabolic alkalosis. The accompanying ECF volume depletion, hypochloremia, and hypokalemia serve to maintain the metabolic alkalosis by increasing HCO_3^- reabsorption by the kidneys (Fig. 32.7).[1]

The loop (*e.g.,* furosemide) and thiazide (*e.g.,* hydrochlorothiazide) diuretics are commonly associated with metabolic alkalosis, the severity of which varies directly with the degree of diuresis. The volume contraction and loss of H^+ in the urine contribute to the problem. The latter is primarily due to the enhanced H^+ secretion in the distal tubule that results from an interplay between the diuretic-induced increase in Na^+ delivery to the distal tubule and collecting duct, where an accelerated excretion of H^+ and K^+ takes place, and an increase in aldosterone secretion resulting from the volume contraction. Although aldosterone blunts the loss of Na^+, it also accelerates the secretion of K^+ and H^+. The resulting loss of K^+ also accelerates HCO_3^- reabsorption.

Metabolic alkalosis can also occur with abrupt correction of respiratory acidosis in persons with chronic respiratory acidosis. Chronic respiratory acidosis is associated with a compensatory loss of H^+ and Cl^- in the urine along with HCO_3^- retention. When respiratory acidosis is corrected abruptly, as with mechanical ventilation, a "posthypercapnic" metabolic alkalosis may develop because although the PCO_2 drops rapidly, the plasma HCO_3^-, which must be eliminated through the kidney, remains elevated.

Maintenance of Metabolic Alkalosis. Maintenance of metabolic alkalosis resides within the kidney and its inability to rid the body of excess HCO_3^-. Many of the conditions that accompany the development of metabolic alkalosis, such as contraction of the ECF volume, hypochloremia, and hypokalemia, also increase reabsorption of HCO_3^- by the kidney, thereby contributing to its maintenance.

Depletion of the ECF causes a decline in the glomerular filtration rate with a subsequent increase in Na^+ and H_2O reabsorption. When there is Cl^- depletion from loss of HCl, the available anion for reabsorption with Na^+ is HCO_3^-. Hypokalemia, which generally accompanies metabolic alkalosis, also contributes to its maintenance. This is due partly to the direct effect of alkalosis on potassium excretion by the kidney and partly to a secondary hyperaldosteronism resulting from volume depletion. In hypokalemia, the distal tubular reabsorption of K^+ is accompanied by an increase in H^+ secretion.[23] The secondary hyperaldosteronism, in turn, promotes extensive reabsorption of Na^+ from the distal and collecting tubules and at the same time stimulates the secretion of H^+ from cells in the collecting tubules. Hypokalemia induced in this manner further worsens the metabolic alkalosis by increasing HCO_3^- reabsorption in the proximal tubule and H^+ secretion in the distal tubule.

Manifestations

Metabolic alkalosis is characterized by an increase in plasma pH (>7.45), plasma HCO_3^- (>26 mmol/L), and base excess (>2 mmol/L) (Table 32.4). Persons with metabolic alkalosis often are asymptomatic or have signs related to ECF volume depletion or hypokalemia. Neurologic signs and symptoms (*e.g.,* hyperexcitability) occur less frequently with metabolic alkalosis than with other acid–base disorders because HCO_3^- enters the CSF more slowly than CO_2. When neurologic manifestations do occur, as in acute and severe metabolic alkalosis, they include mental confusion, hyperactive reflexes, tetany, and carpopedal spasm. Metabolic alkalosis also leads to a compensatory hypoventilation with development of various degrees of hypoxemia and respiratory acidosis. Significant morbidity occurs with severe metabolic alkalosis (pH >7.55), including respiratory failure, cardiac arrhythmias, seizures, and coma.

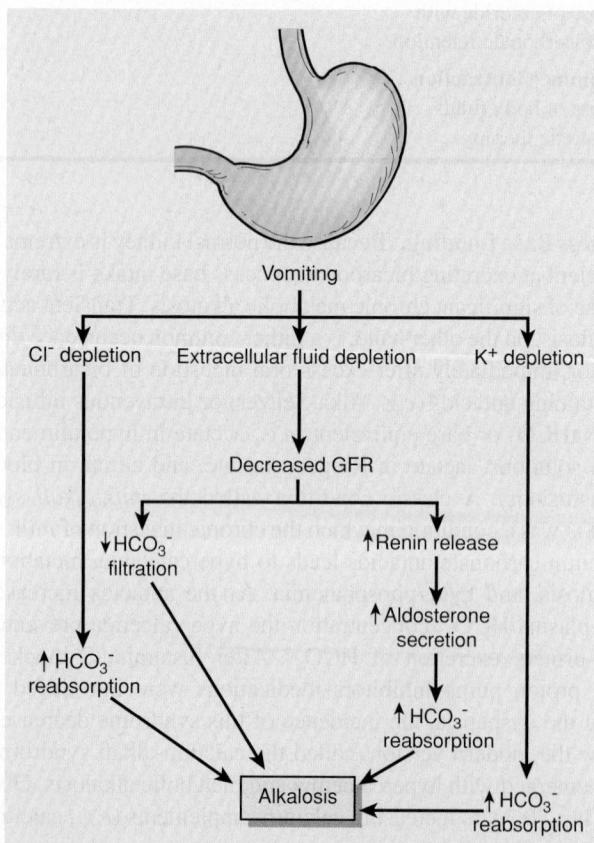

FIGURE 32.7 • Renal mechanisms for bicarbonate (HCO_3^-) reabsorption and maintenance of metabolic alkalosis after depletion of extracellular fluid volume, chloride (Cl^-), and potassium (K^+) due to vomiting (GFR, glomerular filtration rate).

Treatment

The treatment of metabolic alkalosis usually is directed toward correcting the cause of the condition. A chloride deficit requires correction. Potassium chloride usually is the treatment of choice when there is an accompanying K^+ deficit. When KCl is used as a therapy, the Cl^- anion replaces the HCO_3^- anion and the K^+ corrects the potassium deficit, allowing the kidneys to retain H^+ while eliminating K^+. Fluid replacement with normal saline or one-half normal saline often is used in treatment volume contraction alkalosis.

Respiratory Acidosis

Respiratory acidosis occurs in conditions that impair alveolar ventilation and cause an increase in plasma PCO_2, also known as *hypercapnia,* along with a decrease in pH. Respiratory acidosis can occur as an acute or chronic disorder, but occurs most often as a result of decreased ventilation. Acute respiratory failure is associated with a rapid rise in arterial PCO_2 with a minimal increase in plasma HCO_3^- and large decrease in pH. Chronic respiratory acidosis is characterized by a sustained increase in arterial PCO_2, resulting in renal adaptation with a more marked increase in plasma HCO_3^- and a lesser decrease in pH.[1-6]

RESPIRATORY ACID–BASE IMBALANCE

- Respiratory acid–base imbalances are due to a primary disturbance in PCO_2, reflecting an increase or decrease in alveolar ventilation.
- Respiratory acidosis, or hypercapnia, represents an increase in PCO_2 and a decrease in plasma pH, resulting from a decrease in effective alveolar ventilation. Compensatory mechanisms include increased conservation and generation of HCO_3^- and elimination of H^+ by the kidney.
- Respiratory alkalosis, or hypocapnia, represents a decrease in PCO_2 and an increase in plasma pH, resulting from increased alveolar ventilation. Compensatory mechanisms include increased elimination of HCO_3^- and conservation of H^+ by the kidney.

Causes

Respiratory acidosis occurs in acute or chronic conditions that impair effective alveolar ventilation and cause an accumulation of PCO_2 (Table 32.4). Impaired ventilation can occur as the result of decreased respiratory drive, lung disease, or disorders of chest wall and respiratory muscles. Less commonly, it results from excess CO_2 production.

Acute Disorders of Ventilation. Acute respiratory acidosis can be caused by impaired function of the respiratory centre in the medulla (as in narcotic overdose), lung disease, chest injury, weakness of the respiratory muscles, or airway obstruction. Almost all persons with acute respiratory acidosis are hypoxemic if they are breathing room air. In many cases, signs of hypoxemia develop before those of respiratory acidosis because CO_2 diffuses across the alveolar capillary membrane 20 times more rapidly than oxygen.[1,2]

Chronic Disorders of Ventilation. Chronic respiratory acidosis is a relatively common disturbance in patients with chronic obstructive lung disease. In these persons, the persistent elevation of PCO_2 stimulates renal H^+ secretion and HCO_3^- reabsorption. The effectiveness of these compensatory mechanisms can often return the pH to near-normal values as long as oxygen levels are maintained within a range that does not unduly suppress chemoreceptor control of respirations.

An acute episode of respiratory acidosis can develop in persons with chronic lung disease who receive oxygen therapy at a flow rate that is sufficient to raise their PO_2 to a level that produces a decrease in ventilation (discussed in Chapter 29). In these persons, the medullary respiratory centre has adapted to the elevated levels of CO_2 and no longer responds to increases in PCO_2. Instead, a decrease in the PO_2 becomes the major stimulus for respiration. If oxygen is administered at a flow rate that is sufficient to suppress this stimulus, the rate and depth of respiration decrease, and the PCO_2 increases. That being said, any person who is in need of additional oxygen must have it administered, albeit at a flow rate that does not depress the respiratory drive or at higher percentages under close supervision.

Increased Carbon Dioxide Production. Carbon dioxide is a product of the body's metabolic processes, generating a substantial amount of acid that must be excreted by the lungs or kidneys to prevent acidosis. An increase in CO_2 production can result from numerous processes, including exercise, fever, sepsis, and burns. Nutrition also affects the production of carbon dioxide. A carbohydrate-rich diet produces larger amounts of CO_2 than one containing reasonable amounts of protein and fat. Although excess CO_2 production can lead to an increase in PCO_2, it seldom does. In healthy persons, an increase in CO_2 is usually matched by an increase in CO_2 elimination by the lungs. In contrast, persons with respiratory diseases may be unable to eliminate the excess CO_2.

Manifestations

Respiratory acidosis is associated with a decrease in plasma pH (<7.35) and an increase in arterial PCO_2 (>45 mm Hg, Table 32.5). The signs and symptoms of respiratory acidosis depend on the rapidity of onset and whether the condition is acute or chronic. Because respiratory acidosis often is accompanied by hypoxemia, the manifestations of respiratory acidosis often are intermixed with those of oxygen deficit. Carbon dioxide readily crosses the blood–brain barrier, exerting its effects by changing the pH of brain fluids. Elevated levels of CO_2 produce vasodilation of cerebral blood vessels, causing headache, blurred vision, irritability, muscle twitching, and psychological disturbances. If the

TABLE 32.5 CAUSES AND MANIFESTATIONS OF RESPIRATORY ACIDOSIS

CAUSES	MANIFESTATIONS
Depression of Respiratory Centre	**Blood pH, CO_2, HCO_3^-**
Drug overdose	pH decreased
Head injury	PCO_2 (primary) increased
Lung Disease	HCO_3^- (compensatory) increased
Bronchial asthma	
Emphysema	**Neural Function**
Chronic bronchitis	Dilation of cerebral vessels and depression of neural function
Pneumonia	
Pulmonary edema	Headache
Respiratory distress syndrome	Weakness
Airway Obstruction, Disorders of Chest Wall and Respiratory Muscles	Behaviour changes
	Confusion
	Depression
Paralysis of respiratory muscles	Paranoia
	Hallucinations
Chest injuries	Tremors
Kyphoscoliosis	Paralysis
Extreme obesity	Stupor and coma
Treatment with paralytic drugs	**Skin**
	Skin warm and flushed
Breathing Air With High CO_2 Content	**Signs of Compensation**
	Acid urine

condition is severe and prolonged, it can cause an increase in CSF pressure and papilledema. Impaired consciousness, ranging from lethargy to coma, develops as the PCO_2 rises to extreme levels. Respiratory depression may occur, and even paralysis of the extremities. Less severe forms of acidosis often are accompanied by warm and flushed skin, weakness, and tachycardia.

Treatment

The treatment of acute and chronic respiratory acidosis is directed toward improving ventilation. In severe cases, mechanical ventilation may be necessary. The treatment of respiratory acidosis due to respiratory failure is discussed in Chapter 29.

Respiratory Alkalosis

Respiratory alkalosis is a systemic acid–base disorder characterized by a primary decrease in plasma PCO_2, also referred to as *hypocapnia*, which produces an elevation in pH and a subsequent decrease in HCO_3^-.[24] Because respiratory alkalosis can occur suddenly, a compensatory decrease in bicarbonate level may not occur before respiratory correction has taken place.

Causes

Respiratory alkalosis is caused by hyperventilation or a respiratory rate in excess of that needed to maintain normal plasma PCO_2 levels (Table 32.6). Although it rarely occurs as a result

of a physical pathologic condition it may occur as the result of central stimulation of the medullary respiratory centre or stimulation of peripheral (*e.g.,* carotid chemoreceptor) pathways to the medullary respiratory centre.[2]

Mechanical ventilation may produce respiratory alkalosis if the rate and tidal volume are set so that CO_2 elimination exceeds CO_2 production. Carbon dioxide crosses the alveolar capillary membrane 20 times more rapidly than oxygen. Therefore, increased minute ventilation may be necessary to maintain adequate oxygen levels while producing a concomitant decrease in CO_2 levels. In some cases, respiratory alkalosis may be induced through mechanical ventilation as a means of controlling disorders such as severe intracranial hypertension.[24]

Central stimulation of the medullary respiratory centre occurs with anxiety, pain, pregnancy, febrile states, sepsis, encephalitis, and salicylate toxicity. Respiratory alkalosis has long been recognized as a common acid–base disorder in critically ill patients, and is a consistent finding in septic shock, systemic inflammatory response syndrome, pulmonary embolism, and congestive heart failure[24] (see Chapter 26). Progesterone increases ventilation in women; during the progesterone or luteal phase of the menstrual cycle, normal women decrease their PCO_2 values by 3 to 8 mm Hg.[25] Women also develop substantial hypocapnia during pregnancy, most notably during the last trimester, with PCO_2 values of 28 to 30 mm Hg.[25]

One of the most common causes of respiratory alkalosis is hyperventilation syndrome, which is characterized by recurring episodes of increased minute volume, and is often associated with anxiety. Persons experiencing panic attacks frequently present in the emergency department with manifestations of acute respiratory alkalosis.

TABLE 32.6 CAUSES AND MANIFESTATIONS OF RESPIRATORY ALKALOSIS

CAUSES	MANIFESTATIONS
Excessive Ventilation	**Blood pH, CO_2, HCO_3^-**
Anxiety and psychogenic hyperventilation	pH increased
	PCO_2 (primary) decreased
Hypoxia and reflex stimulation of ventilation	HCO_3^- (compensatory) decreased
Lung disease that causes a reflex stimulation of ventilation	**Neural Function**
	Constriction of cerebral vessels and increased neuronal excitability
Stimulation of respiratory centre	Dizziness, panic, lightheadedness
Elevated blood ammonia level	Tetany
Salicylate toxicity	Numbness and tingling of fingers and toes
Encephalitis	Positive Chvostek and Trousseau signs
Fever	Seizures
Mechanical ventilation	
	Cardiovascular Function
	Cardiac arrhythmias

A physiologic type of respiratory alkalosis can occur when a person climbs in high altitudes. The lower oxygen content in the air stimulates the respiratory rate. As the rate increases more CO_2 is released resulting in a mild form of respiratory alkalosis. Typically the body will compensate for this through the kidneys to increase HCO_3^- excretion.[2]

Manifestations

Respiratory alkalosis manifests with an increase in plasma pH (>7.45), a decrease in PCO_2 (<35 mm Hg) and a compensatory deficit in HCO_3^- (<22 mmol/L, Table 32.6).

The signs and symptoms of respiratory alkalosis are associated with hyperexcitability of the nervous system and a decrease in cerebral blood flow. Alkalosis increases protein binding of extracellular calcium. This reduces ionized calcium levels, causing an increase in neuromuscular excitability. A decrease in the CO_2 content of the blood causes constriction of cerebral blood vessels. Because CO_2 crosses the blood–brain barrier rather quickly, the manifestations of acute respiratory alkalosis are usually of sudden onset. The person often experiences lightheadedness, dizziness, tingling, and numbness of the fingers and toes. These manifestations may be accompanied by sweating, palpitations, panic, air hunger, and dyspnea. Chvostek and Trousseau signs may be positive (see Chapter 31), and tetany and convulsions may occur. Because CO_2 provides the stimulus for short-term regulation of respiration, short periods of apnea may occur in persons with acute episodes of hyperventilation.

Treatment

Since respiratory alkalosis is typically a compensatory state the treatment focuses on measures to correct the underlying cause. Hypoxia may be corrected by administration of supplemental oxygen. Changing ventilator settings may be used to prevent or treat respiratory alkalosis in persons who are being mechanically ventilated. Persons with hyperventilation syndrome may benefit from reassurance, rebreathing from a paper bag during symptomatic attacks, and attention to the psychological stress.[25]

IN SUMMARY

Acidosis describes a decrease in pH and alkalosis an increase in pH. Acid–base disorders may be caused by alterations in the body's volatile acids (*i.e.,* respiratory acidosis or respiratory alkalosis) or nonvolatile or fixed acids (*i.e.,* metabolic acidosis or metabolic alkalosis). Acidosis and alkalosis typically involve a primary or initiating event and a compensatory or adaptive state that results from homeostatic mechanisms that attempt to prevent or correct large changes in pH. A mixed acid–base disorder is one in which there is both a primary and a compensatory change in acid–base balance.

Metabolic acidosis is defined as a decrease in pH due to a decrease in the HCO_3^- level, and metabolic alkalosis as an increase in pH due to an increase in the HCO_3^- level. It is caused by an increased production of nonvolatile metabolic acids such as lactic acid or ketoacids, decreased acid excretion by the kidney, excessive loss of HCO_3^- as in diarrhea, or an increase in Cl^-. Metabolic acidosis may present with an increased anion gap in which sodium bicarbonate is replaced by the sodium salt of the offending anion, or with a normal anion gap as when HCO_3^- is replaced by Cl^-. Metabolic alkalosis involves generation of the increased pH and HCO_3^- levels through a loss of H^+ or gain of HCO_3^-, and the maintenance of the alkalotic state because of the kidney's failure to eliminate the excess HCO_3^- owing to an accompanying ECF volume contraction, increased aldosterone levels, and decreased Cl^- and K^+ levels.

Respiratory acidosis reflects an increase in PCO_2 levels and is caused by conditions that impair alveolar ventilation. It can occur as an acute disorder in which there is a rapid rise in PCO_2, a minimal increase in plasma HCO_3^-, and a large decrease in pH. Respiratory alkalosis is caused by conditions that cause hyperventilation and a reduction in PCO_2 levels. Because respiratory alkalosis often occurs suddenly, a compensatory decrease in HCO_3^- levels may not occur before corrections have been accomplished.

The signs and symptoms of acidosis and alkalosis reflect alterations in body function associated with the disorder causing the acid–base disturbance, the effect of the change of pH on body function, and the body's attempt to correct and maintain the pH within a normal physiologic range. In general, neuromuscular excitability is decreased in acidosis and increased in alkalosis.

REVIEW EXERCISES

1. A 34-year-old woman with diabetes is admitted to the emergency department in a stuporous state. Her skin is flushed and warm, her breath has a sweet odour, her pulse is rapid and weak, and her respirations are rapid and deep. Her initial laboratory tests indicate a blood sugar of 18 mmol/L, serum HCO_3^- of 12 mmol/L (normal, 22 to 26 mmol/L), and a pH of 7.1 (normal, 7.35 to 7.45).
   A. *What is the most likely cause of her lowered pH and bicarbonate levels?*
   B. *How would you account for her rapid and deep respirations?*
   C. *Using the Henderson–Hasselbalch equation and the solubility coefficient for CO_2 given in this chapter, what would you expect her PCO_2 to be?*
   D. *How would you explain her warm, flushed skin, and stuporous mental state?*
2. Explain the use of the urine anion gap to determine the kidney's ability to compensate for acid–base disorders by secreting and eliminate H^+ ions.

3. A 16-year-old girl is seen by her primary care provider because of her parents' concern over her binge eating and their recent discovery that she engages in self-induced vomiting. A tentative diagnosis of bulimia nervosa is made. Initial laboratory tests reveal a plasma K^+ of 3 mmol/L (normal is 3.5 to 5.0 mmol/L) and a Cl^+ of 93 mmol/L (normal is 98 to 106 mmol/L).

   A. *Explain her low K^+ and Cl^-.*

   B. *What type of acid–base abnormality would you expect her to have?*

4. A 65-year-old man with chronic obstructive lung disease has been using low-flow oxygen therapy because of difficulty in maintaining adequate oxygenation of his blood. He has recently had a severe respiratory tract infection and has had difficulty breathing. He is admitted to the emergency department because he became increasingly lethargic and his wife has had trouble arousing him. His respirations are 12 breaths/minute. She relates that he had "turned his oxygen way up" because he was "trying to get his breath."

   A. *What is the most likely cause of this man's problem?*

   B. *How would you explain the lethargy and difficulty in arousal?*

   C. *Arterial blood gases, drawn on admission to the emergency department, indicated a PO_2 of 85 mm Hg (normal at this elevation, 90 to 98 mm Hg) and a PCO_2 of 90 mm Hg (normal, 35 to 45 mm Hg). His serum HCO_3^- was 34 mmol/L (normal, 22 to 26 mmol/L). What is his pH?*

   D. *What would be the main goal of treatment for this man in terms of acid–base balance?*

References

1. Taal M. W., Chertow G. M., Marden P. A., et al. (Eds.). (2012). *Brenner and Rector's the kidney* (9th ed.). Philadelphia, PA: Elsevier Saunders.
2. Hall J. E. (2011). *Textbook of medical physiology* (12th ed.). Philadelphia, PA: Saunders Elsevier.
3. Tanner G. A. (2013). Chapter 24: Acid-base homeostasis. In Rhoades R. A., Bell D. R. *Medical physiology: Principles for clinical medicine* (4th ed.). Philadelphia, PA: Lippincott Williams & Wilkins.
4. Costanzo L. S. (2014). *Physiology* (5th ed.). Philadelphia, PA: Saunders Elsevier.
5. Reddi A. S. (2014). *Fluid, electrolytes and acid-base disorders*. New Jersey: Springer.
6. Metheny N. M. (2012). *Fluid and electrolyte balance: Nursing considerations* (5th ed.). Sudbury, MA: Jones & Bartlett Learning.
7. Fischbach F. T., Dunning M. B. (2015). *A manual of laboratory and diagnostic test* (9th ed.). Philadelphia, PA: Lippincott Williams & Wilkins.
8. Reddy P., Mooradian A. D. (2009). Clinical utility of anion gap in deciphering acid-base disorders. *International Journal of Clinical Practice, 63*(10), 1516–1525.
9. Feldman M., Soni N., Dickson B. (2005). Influence of hypoalbuminemia or hyperalbuminemia on the serum anion gap. *The Journal of Laboratory and Clinical Medicine, 146*(6), 318–320.
10. Adrogue H. J., Gennari F. J., Galla J. H., Madias N. E. (2009). Assessing acid-base disorders. *Kidney International, 76*(12), 1239–1247.
11. Kraut J. A., Madias N. E. (2010). Metabolic acidosis: Pathophysiology, diagnosis and management. *Nature Reviews Nephrology, 6*(5), 274–285.
12. Vernon C., LeTourneau J. L. (2010). Lactic acidosis: Recognition, kinetics, and associated prognosis. *Critical Care Clinics, 26*(2), 255–283.
13. Gunnerson K. J., Saul M., He S., Kellum J. A. (2006). Lactate versus non-lactate metabolic acidosis: A retrospective outcome evaluation of critically ill patients. *Critical Care, 10*(1), R22–R32.
14. Seidowsky A., Nseir S., Houdret N., Fourrier F. (2009). Metformin-associated lactic acidosis: A prognostic and therapeutic study. *Critical Care Medicine, 37*(7), 2191–2196.
15. Fitzgerald E., Mathieu S., Ball A. (2009). Metformin associated lactic acidosis. *British medical journal (Clinical research ed.), 339*, b3660.
16. Petersen C. (2005). D-lactic acidosis. *Nutrition in Clinical Practice, 20*(6), 634–645.
17. Lu J., Zello G. A., Randell E., et al. (2011). Closing the anion gap: Contribution of D-lactate to diabetic ketoacidosis. *Clinica Chimica Acta, 412*(3-4), 286–291.
18. Allison M. G., McCurdy M. T. (2014). Alcoholic metabolic emergencies. *Emergency Medicine Clinics of North America, 32*(2), 293–301.
19. Vale A. (2012). Salicylates. *Medicine, 40*(3), 156–157.
20. McQuade D. J., Dargan P. I., Wood D. M. (2014). Challenges in the diagnosis of ethylene glycol poisoning. *Annals of Clinical Biochemistry, 51*(2), 167–178.
21. Van der Aa F., Joniau S., Braden M., et al. (2011). Metabolic changes after urinary diversion. *Advances in Urology, 2011*, 764325.
22. Soifer J. T., Kim H. T. (2014). Approach to metabolic alkalosis. *Emergency Medicine Clinics of North America, 32*(2), 453–463.
23. Harvey S., Jordan S. (2010). Diuretic therapy: Implications for nursing practice. *Nursing Standard, 24*(43), 40–50.
24. Palmer B. F. (2012). Evaluation and treatment of respiratory alkalosis. *American Journal of Kidney Disease, 60*(5), 834–838.
25. Krapf R., Hulter H. N. (2005). Chapter 21: Respiratory alkalosis. In Gennari F. J., Adrogue H. J., Galla J. H., et al. (Eds.), *Acid-base disorders and their treatment*. Boca Raton, FL: Taylor & Francis Group.

Visit thePoint **http://thePoint.lww.com for animations, journal articles, and more!**

Disorders of Renal Function

33

Kidney disease continues to be a major cause of work loss, physician visits, and hospitalization among both men and women. Urinary tract infections (UTIs) and kidney stones are the two most commonly occurring kidney disorders, with an estimated 60% of North American women having a UTI and one in ten Canadians having a kidney stone in their lifetime.[1,2] The kidneys filter blood from all parts of the body, and although many forms of kidney disease originate in the kidneys, others develop secondary to disorders such as hypertension, diabetes mellitus, and systemic lupus erythematosus (SLE). The content in this chapter focuses on congenital disorders of the kidneys, obstructive disorders, UTIs, disorders of glomerular function, tubulointerstitial disorders, and neoplasms of the kidneys. Acute renal failure and chronic kidney disease are discussed in Chapter 34, and disorders that predominantly affect the lower urinary tract and bladder in Chapter 35.

CONGENITAL AND INHERITED DISORDERS OF THE KIDNEYS

After completing this section of the chapter, you should be able to meet the following objectives:

- Define the terms agenesis, hypoplasia, and dysgenesis, and discuss them as they refer to the development of the kidney.
- Cite the effect of urinary obstruction in the fetus.
- Describe the inheritance, pathology, and manifestations of the different types of polycystic kidney disease.

Congenital anomalies of the kidney and urinary tract (CAKUT) occur in 1 in 500 newborns and play a causative role in 30%

to 50% for chronic renal disease in children.[3,4] Anomalies in shape and position are the most common. Less common are disorders involving a decrease in renal mass (*e.g.,* agenesis, hypogenesis) or a change in renal structure (*e.g.,* renal dysplasia). The kidneys can be visualized as early as 12 weeks' gestation by ultrasonography, allowing many fetal urinary abnormalities to be detected before birth.

Congenital Disorders of the Kidneys

The kidneys begin to develop early in the fifth week of gestation and start to function approximately 4 weeks later. Formation of urine is thought to begin in the 9th to 12th weeks of gestation; by the 32nd week, fetal production of urine reaches approximately 25 ml/hr. The urine that is produced is excreted into the amniotic cavity and is one of the constituent of amniotic fluid. Thus, the relative amount of amniotic fluid can provide information about the status of fetal renal function. In pregnancies that involve infants with nonfunctional kidneys or outflow obstruction of urine from the kidneys, the amount of amniotic fluid is small—a condition called *oligohydramnios.* The condition causes compression of the developing fetus and is often associated with impaired development of lungs and other fetal structures.[4–6]

Agenesis and Hypoplasia

The term *dysgenesis* refers to a failure of an organ to develop normally, and *agenesis* refers to failure of an organ to develop at all. Unilateral renal agenesis is relatively common, being present in about 1 of 1,000 to 5,000 newborn infants. Boys are affected more often than girls, and the left kidney is the one that is usually absent.[6] Usually unilateral agenesis does not cause symptoms and is not discovered during infancy because the other kidney often undergoes compensatory hypertrophy and performs the functions of the missing kidney.

Total agenesis of both kidneys is incompatible with extrauterine life. Infants are stillborn or die shortly after birth of pulmonary hypoplasia. Newborns with renal agenesis often have characteristic facial features, termed *Potter syndrome,* resulting from the effects of oligohydramnios.[6] The eyes are widely separated and have epicanthic folds, the ears are low set, the nose is broad and flat, the chin is receding, and limb defects are often present.[6]

In *renal hypoplasia,* the kidneys do not develop to normal size. Like agenesis, hypoplasia more commonly affects only one kidney. When both kidneys are affected, there is progressive development of renal failure. It has been suggested that true hypoplasia is extremely rare; most cases probably represent acquired scarring due to vascular, infectious, or other kidney diseases rather than an underlying developmental failure.[3–6]

Renal Dysplasia

Renal dysplasia is caused by an abnormality in the differentiation of kidney structures during embryonic development. It is characterized by undifferentiated tubular structures surrounded by primitive embryonic tissue.[4,6] The disorder may result in small, aplastic kidneys or cysts that form from the abnormal tubules. If cysts are present, the condition is referred to as *cystic dysplasia.* One or both kidneys may be involved, and the affected kidney may be abnormally large or very small. Many forms of dysplasia are accompanied by other urinary tract abnormalities, especially disorders that cause obstruction of urine flow (*e.g.,* ureteral agenesis or atresia; ureteropelvic junction obstruction).[4]

A multicystic kidney is one in which the kidney is replaced by cysts and does not function. The kidney does not have the usual kidney shape, but is rather a mass of cysts. Unilateral multicystic renal dysplasia is the most common cause of an abdominal mass in newborns. The function of the opposite kidney is usually normal and such children have an excellent prognosis after surgical removal of the affected kidney. Bilateral renal dysplasia causes oligohydramnios and the resultant Potter facies, pulmonary hypoplasia, and renal failure.

Alterations in Kidney Position and Form

The development of the kidneys during embryonic life can result in *ectopic kidneys* that lie outside their normal position. One or both kidneys may be in an abnormal position. Most ectopic kidneys are located just above the pelvic brim or within the pelvis, but some lie in the inferior part of the abdomen. Because of the abnormal position, kinking of the ureters and obstruction of urinary flow may occur.[4]

One of the most common alterations in kidney form is an abnormality called a *horseshoe kidney.* This abnormality occurs in approximately 1 of every 500 to 1,000 persons.[3] In this disorder, the upper or lower poles of the two kidneys are fused, producing a horseshoe-shaped structure that is continuous along the midline of the body anterior to the great vessels. Most horseshoe kidneys are fused at the lower pole[6] (Fig. 33.1). The condition usually does not cause problems unless there is an associated defect in the renal pelvis or other urinary structures that obstructs urinary flow.[3,4]

Cystic Kidney Diseases

Cystic kidney diseases are a group of kidney disorders characterized by fluid-filled sacs or segments that have their origin in the tubular structures of the kidney. The cysts may be single or multiple and can vary in size from microscopic to several centimetres in diameter. Although they may arise as a developmental abnormality or be acquired later in life, most forms are hereditary. The inherited polycystic kidney diseases, which are single-gene disorders and are inherited as mendelian traits, include autosomal dominant and recessive polycystic kidney disease and nephronophthisis–medullary cystic disease.[7] In the autosomal dominant form of polycystic kidney disease (ADPKD), thousands of large cysts are derived from every segment of the nephron (Fig. 33.2A). The tubule wall, which is lined by a single layer of tubular cells, expands and then rapidly closes the cyst off from the tubule of origin. In the autosomal recessive form of polycystic kidney disease

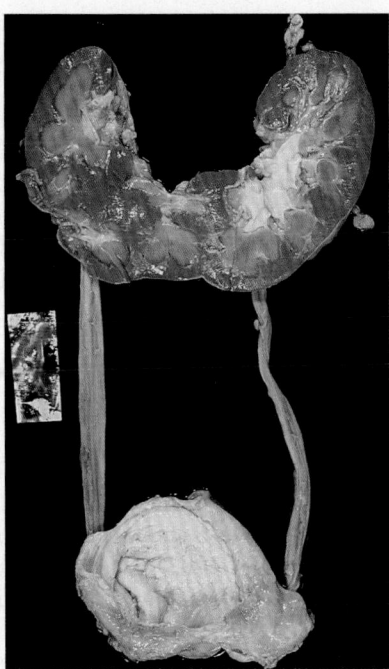

FIGURE 33.1 • Horseshoe kidney. The kidneys are fused at the lower poles. (From Rubin R., Strayer D. S. (Eds.). (2012). *Rubin's pathology: Clinicopathologic foundations of medicine* (6th ed., p. 757). Philadelphia, PA: Lippincott Williams & Wilkins.)

A Autosomal dominant polycystic disease

B Autosomal recessive polycystic disease

C Medullary cystic disease

D Simple cyst

FIGURE 33.2 • Cystic diseases of the kidney. **A:** Autosomal dominant polycystic kidney disease, cystic outpouchings arise in every tubule segment and rapidly close off the tubule from the nephron of origin. **B:** Autosomal recessive polycystic kidney disease, cysts are derived from collecting tubules, which remain connected to the nephron of origin. **C:** Nephronophthisis–medullary, cysts predominantly around corticomedullary junction. **D:** Simple fluid-filled cyst. (Adapted from Rubin R., Strayer D. S. (Eds.). (2012). *Rubin's pathology: Clinicopathologic foundations of medicine* (6th ed., p. 759). Philadelphia, PA: Lippincott Williams & Wilkins.)

(ARPKD), small, elongated cysts form in the collecting ducts and maintain contact with the nephron of origin (Fig. 33.2B). In nephronophthisis–medullary cystic kidney disease, the cysts are restricted to the corticomedullary border. Simple cysts are acquired cysts that develop in the kidney as a consequence of aging, dialysis, or other conditions that affect tubular function.[4,7]

Autosomal Dominant Polycystic Kidney Disease

Autosomal dominant polycystic kidney disease, also known as *adult polycystic disease*, is the most common form of renal cystic disease. The disorder, which is inherited as an autosomal trait, results in the formation of destructive fluid-filled cysts in the kidney and other organs. ADPKD affects one in 500 persons worldwide. The disease accounts for 5% of all cases of chronic kidney disease that require dialysis or transplantation.[4,7,8]

There are two types of ADPKD: type I, which is caused by mutations in the *PKD1* gene and accounts for 85% of cases; and type II, which is caused by mutations in the *PKD2* gene and accounts for most of the remaining 15% of cases.[7,8] Recent research has shown that the products of these genes, polycystin-1 and polycystin-2, are found in the primary cilia that line the apical surface of the tubular epithelium. These primary cilia are thought to act as sensors of urinary flow and as signal transducers for tubular cell proliferation, differentiation, and apoptosis.[4,7,8]

Although the precise pathogenesis of ADPKD remains unclear, it is thought that the cysts arise in segments of the renal tubules from a few epithelial cells that proliferate abnormally. The epithelial cells lining the cysts of ADPKD have a high proliferation rate and are relatively undifferentiated. Concomitantly, a defective basement membrane immediately underlying the abnormal epithelium allows for dilation and cyst formation. Cysts frequently detach from the tubule and grow by active fluid secretion from the epithelial lining cells. Historically, it was thought that chronic kidney disease resulted from pressure exerted by expanding cysts on the normal surrounding kidney tissue. However, it is now appreciated that cysts arise in less than 2% of nephrons, and that factors other than compression by the expanding cysts account for loss of functioning renal tissue. Apoptotic loss of renal tubular cells and accumulation of inflammatory mediators are now thought to contribute to the destruction of normal kidney tissue.[7–10]

Mutations in the *PKD1* and *PKD2* genes produce identical renal and extrarenal disease, but disease progression is typically more rapid in people with type I disease.[7] The kidneys are usually enlarged in persons with ADPKD and may achieve enormous sizes (Fig. 33.3). The external contours of the kidneys are distorted by numerous cysts, some as large as

FIGURE 33.3 • Gross pathology of polycystic kidneys. (From Centers for Disease Control and Prevention Public Images Library. Available online at: http://phil.cdc.gov/phil/details.asp.)

5 cm in diameter, which are filled with straw-coloured fluid.[6] Cysts may also be found in the liver and, less commonly, the pancreas and spleen. Mitral valve prolapse and other valvular heart diseases occur in 20% to 25% of persons with ADPKD, but most are asymptomatic.[10] Many persons with polycystic disease also develop colonic diverticula. One of the most devastating extrarenal manifestations is a weakness in the walls of the cerebral arteries that can lead to aneurysm formation.[9]

Clinical Features. The manifestations of ADPKD include pain from the enlarging cysts that may reach debilitating levels, episodes of gross hematuria from bleeding into a cyst, infected cysts from ascending UTIs, and hypertension resulting from compression of intrarenal blood vessels with activation of the renin–angiotensin mechanism. The progress of the disease is slow, and end-stage renal disease is uncommon before 40 years of age. Extrarenal manifestations are frequent, underscoring the systemic nature of the disease. Hepatic cysts occur in 40% of persons.[10] Cysts are generally asymptomatic, and liver function is normal. Approximately 15% of persons with polycystic kidney disease have an associated aneurysm, and subarachnoid hemorrhage is a frequent cause of death.[9]

Serum creatinine levels have not been found to be an effective predictive marker for worsening ADPKD; however more recently urine albumin excretion has been determined to be more reliable.[11] Ultrasonography usually is the preferred technique for diagnosis of ADPKD in symptomatic patients and for screening of asymptomatic family members. Computed tomography (CT) may be used for detection of small cysts. Genetic linkage studies are now available for diagnosis of ADPKD, but are usually reserved for cases in which radiographic imaging is negative and the need for a definitive diagnosis is essential, such as when screening family members for potential kidney donation.

Currently the treatment of ADPKD is largely supportive and aimed at delaying progression of the disease. Control of hypertension and prevention of ascending UTIs are important. Pain is a common complaint of persons with ADPKD, and a systematic approach is needed to differentiate the etiology of the pain and define an approach for management. In 2012 Tolvaptan, a selective vasopressin (V2) receptor antagonist, was approved for the treatment of ADPKD in Canada. This medication has been shown to decrease the overall kidney volume by inhibiting cyst formation thus slowing disease progression and preserving kidney function.[12] Dialysis and kidney transplantation are reserved for those who progress to kidney failure.

Autosomal Recessive Polycystic Kidney Disease

Autosomal recessive polycystic kidney disease is characterized by cystic dilation of the cortical and medullary collecting tubules[7,8] (Fig. 33.2B). It is rare compared with ADPKD, occurring in 1 to 20,000. ARPKD is caused by mutations in the *PKHD1* gene. The gene product, fibrocystin, is found in the kidney, liver, and pancreas and appears to be involved in the regulation of cell proliferation and adhesion.[4]

Clinical Features. The typical infant with ARPKD presents with bilateral flank masses, accompanied by severe renal failure, signs of impaired lung development, and variable degrees of liver fibrosis and portal hypertension.[4] Potter facies and other defects associated with oligohydramnios may be present. Hypertension is usually noted within the first few weeks of life and is often severe. Approximately 25% of infants die during the perinatal period, often of pulmonary hypoplasia.[4] Exceptional cases of ARPKD manifest in older children and adults.

The treatment of ARPKD is largely supportive. Aggressive ventilatory support is often necessary in the neonatal period because of pulmonary hypoplasia and hypoventilation. Modern neonatal respiratory techniques and renal replacement therapy have increased the 10-year survival rate of children surviving beyond the first year of life to approximately 80%.[7] Morbidity and mortality in the older child is related to complications from chronic renal failure and liver disease.

Nephronophthisis–Medullary Cystic Disease Complex

The nephronophthisis–medullary cystic disease complex is a group of renal disorders that have their onset in childhood.[4,7–10] Common characteristics are small and shrunken kidneys and the presence of a variable number of cysts, usually concentrated at the corticomedullary junction. The initial insult involves the distal tubules, with tubular basement membrane disruption followed by chronic and progressive tubular atrophy involving both the medulla and cortex. Although the presence of medullary cysts is important, the cortical and tubular damage is the eventual cause of chronic kidney disease and failure.

As a complex, the disorders account for 10% to 25% of renal failure in childhood. Affected children present first with polyuria, polydipsia, and enuresis (bed-wetting), which reflect impaired ability of the kidneys to concentrate urine. Other manifestations of the disorders include salt wasting, growth retardation, anemia, and progressive renal insufficiency. Some juvenile forms of nephronophthisis have extrarenal complications, including ocular motor abnormalities, retinitis pigmentosa, liver fibrosis, and cerebellar abnormalities. Progressive azotemia and renal failure follow, usually within 5 to 10 years.[10]

Simple and Acquired Renal Cysts

Simple cysts are a common disorder of the kidney. The cysts may be single or multiple, unilateral or bilateral, and they usually are less than 1 cm in diameter, although they may grow larger. Most simple cysts do not produce signs or symptoms or compromise renal function. When symptomatic, they may cause flank pain, hematuria, infection, and hypertension related to ischemia-produced stimulation of the renin–angiotensin system. They are most common in older persons. Although the cysts are benign, they may be confused clinically with renal cell carcinoma.

An acquired form of renal cystic disease occurs in persons with end-stage renal failure who have undergone prolonged dialysis treatment. The cysts, which measure 0.2 to 2 cm in diameter, probably develop as a result of tubular obstruction. Although the condition is largely asymptomatic, the cysts may bleed, causing hematuria. Tumours, usually adenomas but occasionally adenosarcomas, may develop in the walls of these cysts.[10]

IN SUMMARY

Approximately 3% to 4% of infants are born with potentially significant malformations of the urinary system. These abnormalities can range from bilateral renal agenesis, which is incompatible with life, to hypogenesis of one kidney, which usually causes no problems unless the function of the remaining kidney is impaired. Renal dysplasia is caused by an abnormality in the differentiation of kidney structures during embryonic development. A dysplastic multicystic kidney is one in which the kidney is replaced by cysts and does not function. The horseshoe kidney is a developmental disorder in which the upper or lower poles of the two kidneys are fused, producing a horseshoe-shaped structure.

Renal cystic disease is a condition in which there is dilation of tubular structures with cyst formation. Cysts may be single or multiple. Polycystic kidney disease is an inherited form of renal cystic disease; it can be inherited as an autosomal dominant or recessive trait. The autosomal dominant form of the disease (ADPKD) results in the formation of numerous fluid-filled cysts in the tubular structures of both kidneys with the threat of progression to chronic renal failure. Other manifestations of the disease include hypertension, cardiovascular abnormalities, cerebral aneurysms, and cysts in other organs such as the liver and pancreas. The ARPKD is characterized by cystic transformation of

the collecting ducts. It is rare compared with ADPKD, and usually presents as severe renal dysfunction during infancy. The nephronophthisis–medullary cystic disease complex is a group of hereditary disorders that usually have their onset during childhood and are characterized by the presence of cysts in the medullary portion of the kidney, renal atrophy, and eventual kidney failure. Single or multiple simple renal cysts most commonly occur in persons older than 50 years of age.

OBSTRUCTIVE DISORDERS

After completing this section of the chapter, you should be able to meet the following objectives:

- List four common causes of urinary tract obstruction.
- Define the term hydronephrosis and relate it to the destructive effects of urinary tract obstruction.
- Describe the role of urine supersaturation, nucleation, and inhibitors of stone formation in the development of kidney stones.
- Explain the mechanisms of pain and infection that occur with kidney stones.
- Describe methods used in the diagnosis and treatment of kidney stones.

Urinary obstruction can occur in persons of any age and can involve any level of the urinary tract, from the urethra to the renal pelvis (Fig. 33.4). Obstruction may be sudden or insidious, partial or complete, unilateral or bilateral, and may occur

FIGURE 33.4 • Locations and causes of urinary tract obstruction.

TABLE 33.1 CAUSES OF URINARY TRACT OBSTRUCTION

LEVEL OF OBSTRUCTION	CAUSE
Renal pelvis	Renal calculi
	Papillary necrosis
Ureter	Renal calculi
	Pregnancy
	Tumours that compress the ureter
	Ureteral stricture
	Congenital disorders of the uretero-vesical junction and ureteropelvic junction strictures
Bladder and urethra	Bladder cancer
	Neurogenic bladder
	Bladder stones
	Prostatic hyperplasia or cancer
	Urethral strictures
	Congenital urethral defects

at any level of the urinary tract. The conditions that cause urinary tract obstruction include congenital anomalies, urinary calculi (*i.e.,* stones), pregnancy, benign prostatic hyperplasia, scar tissue resulting from infection and inflammation, tumours, and neurologic disorders such as spinal cord injury. The causes of urinary tract obstructions are summarized in Table 33.1.

Obstructive uropathy is usually classified according to site, degree, and duration of obstruction. Lower urinary tract obstructions are located below the ureterovesical junction and are bilateral in nature. Upper urinary tract obstructions are located above the ureterovesical junction and are usually unilateral. The condition causing the obstruction can cause complete or partial occlusion of urine outflow. When the obstruction is of short duration (*i.e.,* less than a few days), it is said to be acute and is usually caused by conditions such as renal calculi. An obstruction that develops slowly and is longer lasting is said to be chronic and is usually caused by conditions such as congenital ureterovesical abnormalities. Bilateral acute urinary tract obstruction causes acute renal failure. Because many causes of acute obstruction are reversible, prompt recognition is important. When left untreated, an obstructed kidney undergoes atrophy, and in the case of bilateral obstruction, results in chronic renal failure.

Mechanisms of Renal Damage

The destructive effects of urinary obstruction on kidney structures are determined by the degree (*i.e.,* partial versus complete, unilateral versus bilateral) and the duration of the obstruction. The two most damaging effects of urinary obstruction are stasis of urine, which predisposes to infection and stone formation; and progressive dilation of the renal collecting ducts and renal tubular structures, which causes destruction and atrophy of renal tissue.

A common complication of urinary tract obstruction is infection. Stagnation of urine predisposes to infection, which may spread throughout the urinary tract. When present, urinary calculi serve as foreign bodies and contribute to the infection. Once established, the infection is difficult to treat. It often is caused by urea-splitting organisms (*e.g., Proteus,* staphylococci) that increase ammonia production and cause the urine to become alkaline.[10] Calcium salts precipitate more readily in stagnant alkaline urine; thus, urinary tract obstructions also predispose to stone formation.

In situations of severe partial or complete obstruction, the impediment to the outflow of urine causes dilation of the renal pelvis and calices associated with progressive atrophy of the kidney. Even with complete obstruction, glomerular filtration continues for some time. Because of the continued filtration, the calices and pelvis of the affected kidney become dilated, often markedly so. The high pressure in the renal pelvis is transmitted back through the collecting ducts of the kidney, compressing renal vasculature and causing renal atrophy. Initially, the functional alterations are largely tubular, manifested primarily by impaired urine-concentrating ability. Only later does the glomerular filtration rate (GFR) begin to diminish.

Hydronephrosis

Hydronephrosis refers to urine-filled dilation of the renal pelvis and calices associated with progressive atrophy of the kidney due to obstruction of urine outflow. The degree of hydronephrosis depends on the duration, degree, and level of obstruction. In far-advanced cases, the kidney may be transformed into a thin-walled cystic structure with parenchymal atrophy, total obliteration of the pyramids, and thinning of the cortex (Fig. 33.5). The condition is usually unilateral. Bilateral hydronephrosis occurs only when the obstruction is below the level of the ureterovesical junction. When the obstruction affects the outflow of urine from the distal ureter, the increased pressure dilates the ureter, a condition called *hydroureter* (Fig. 33.6). Bilateral hydroureter may develop as

FIGURE 33.5 • Hydronephrosis. Bilateral urinary tract obstruction has led to conspicuous dilation of the ureters, pelves, and calices. The kidney on the right shows severe cortical atrophy. (From Rubin R., Strayer D. S. (Eds.). (2012). *Rubin's pathology: Clinicopathologic foundations of medicine* (6th ed., p. 801). Philadelphia, PA: Lippincott Williams & Wilkins.)

FIGURE 33.6 • Hydroureter caused by ureteral obstruction in a woman with cancer of the uterus.

a complication of bladder outflow obstruction due to prostatic hyperplasia (see Chapter 44).

Clinical Features

The manifestations of urinary obstruction depend on the site of obstruction, the cause, and the rapidity with which the condition developed. Most of the early symptoms are produced by the underlying pathologic process. Urinary tract obstruction encourages the growth of microorganisms and should be suspected in persons with recurrent UTIs.

Complete or partial unilateral hydronephrosis may remain silent for long periods because the unaffected kidney can maintain adequate kidney function. Obstruction may provoke pain due to distension of the collecting system and renal capsule. Acute supravesical obstruction, such as that due to a kidney stone lodged in the ureter, is associated with excruciatingly severe pain. By contrast, more insidious causes of obstruction, such as narrowing of ureteropelvic junction, may produce little pain but cause total destruction of the kidney.

Complete bilateral obstruction results in oliguria, anuria, and renal failure. Acute bilateral obstruction may mimic prerenal failure. With partial bilateral obstruction, the earliest manifestation is an inability to concentrate urine, reflected by polyuria and nocturia. Hypertension is an occasional complication of urinary tract obstruction. It is more common in cases of unilateral obstruction in which renin secretion is enhanced, probably secondary to impaired renal blood flow. In these circumstances, removal of the obstruction often leads to a reduction in blood pressure. When hypertension accompanies bilateral obstruction, it is volume related. The relief of bilateral obstruction leads to a loss of volume and a decrease in blood pressure. In some cases, relieving the obstruction does not correct the hypertension.

Diagnosis and Treatment. Early diagnosis of urinary tract obstruction is important because the condition usually is treatable and a delay in therapy may result in permanent damage to the kidneys. Diagnostic methods vary with the symptoms. Ultrasonography has proved to be the single most useful noninvasive diagnostic modality for urinary obstruction. Radiologic methods, CT scans, and intravenous urography may also be used. Other diagnostic methods, such as urinalysis, are used to determine the extent of renal involvement and the presence of infection.

Treatment of urinary tract obstruction depends on the cause. Urinary stone removal may be necessary, or surgical treatment of structural defects may be indicated. Treatment of complicating UTIs due to urinary stasis is also important.

> ### KIDNEY STONES
>
> - Kidney stones are polycrystalline structures that form from components of the urine.
> - Stones require a nidus to form and a urinary environment that supports continued crystallization of stone components.
> - The development of kidney stones is influenced by the concentration of stone components in the urine, the ability of the stone components to complex and form stones, and the presence of substances that inhibit stone formation.

Renal Calculi

The most common cause of upper urinary tract obstruction is urinary calculi. Although stones can form in any part of the urinary tract, most develop in the kidneys. Renal calculi or kidney stones are a common disorder of the urinary tract affecting one in every ten Canadians. The highest in incidence is in Caucasian males between 40 and 60 years of age.[2]

Kidney stones are polycrystalline aggregates composed of materials that the kidneys normally excrete in the urine. The etiology of urinary stone formation is complex. It is thought to encompass a number of factors, including increases in blood and urinary levels of stone components and interactions among the components; anatomic changes in urinary tract structures; metabolic and endocrine influences; fluid intake; dietary and intestinal absorption factors; and UTIs. Adding to the mystery of stone formation is the fact that although both kidneys are exposed to the same urinary constituents, kidney stones tend to form in only one kidney. Several factors are used to explain stone formation, including a supersaturated urine, presence of a nucleus for crystal formation, and deficiency of inhibitors of stone formation.[4,13]

Kidney stone formation requires a supersaturated urine and an environment that allows the stone to grow. The risk for stone formation is increased when the urine is supersaturated with stone components (*e.g.,* calcium salts, uric acid, magnesium ammonium phosphate, cystine). Supersaturation depends on urinary pH, solute concentration, ionic strength, and complexation. The greater the concentration of two ions, the more likely they are to precipitate. Complexation influences the availability of specific ions. For example, oxalate complexes with sodium and decreases the availability of its free ionic form that participates in stone formation.

In addition to a supersaturated urine, kidney stone formation requires a nidus or nucleus that facilitates crystal aggregation. In supersaturated urine, stone formation begins with small clusters of crystals such as calcium oxalate. Most small clusters tend to disperse because the internal forces that hold them together are too weak to overcome the random tendency of ions to move apart. Larger ion clusters form nuclei and remain stable because the attraction forces balance surface losses. Once they are stable, nuclei can grow at levels of supersaturation below that needed for their creation. Organic materials, such as mucopolysaccharides derived from the epithelial cells that line the tubules, are also thought to act as nuclei for stone formation by lowering the level of supersaturation required for crystal aggregation.[4,13]

The fact that many people experience supersaturation of their urine without development of kidney stones is believed to be a result of the presence of natural stone inhibitors, including magnesium, citrate, pyrophosphate, and the Tamm–Horsfall mucoprotein. Urine citrate reduces supersaturation by binding calcium, and inhibits nucleation and growth of calcium crystals. Citrate is a normal byproduct of the citric acid cycle in renal cells. Metabolic stimuli that consume this product (as with metabolic acidosis due to fasting or hypokalemia) reduce the urinary concentration of citrate. Citrate supplementation (potassium citrate) may be used in the treatment of some forms of hypocitraturic kidney stones.

Types of Stones

There are four basic types of kidney stones: calcium stones (*i.e.,* oxalate or phosphate), magnesium ammonium phosphate stones, uric acid stones, and cystine stones.[13,14] The causes and treatment measures for each of these types of renal stones are described in Table 33.2. Most kidney stones (70% to 80%) are calcium stones—calcium oxalate, calcium phosphate, or a combination of the two materials. Calcium stones usually are associated with increased concentrations of calcium in the blood and urine. Excessive bone resorption caused by immobility, bone disease, hyperparathyroidism, and renal tubular acidosis all are contributing conditions. High oxalate concentrations in the blood and urine predispose to formation of calcium oxalate stones.[9,10,13,14]

Magnesium ammonium phosphate stones, also called *struvite stones,* form only in alkaline urine (pH >7.2) and in the presence of bacteria that possess an enzyme called *urease,* which splits the urea in the urine into ammonia and carbon dioxide. The ammonia that is formed takes up a hydrogen ion to become an ammonium ion, increasing the pH of the urine so that it becomes more alkaline. Because phosphate levels are increased in alkaline urine and because magnesium always is present in the urine, struvite stones form. These stones enlarge

TABLE 33.2 COMPOSITION, CONTRIBUTING FACTORS, AND TREATMENT OF KIDNEY STONES

TYPE OF STONE	CONTRIBUTING FACTORS	TREATMENT
Calcium (oxalate and phosphate)	Hypercalcemia and hypercalciuria Immobilization	Treatment of underlying conditions Increased fluid intake Thiazide diuretics
	Hyperparathyroidism Vitamin D intoxication Diffuse bone disease Milk–alkali syndrome Renal tubular acidosis	
	Hyperoxaluria Intestinal bypass surgery	Dietary restriction of foods high in oxalate
Magnesium ammonium phosphate (struvite)	Urea-splitting urinary tract infections	Treatment of urinary tract infection Acidification of the urine Increased fluid intake
Uric acid (urate)	Formed in acid urine with pH of approximately 5.5	Increased fluid intake
	Gout High-purine diet	Allopurinol for hyperuricosuria Alkalinization of urine
Cystine	Cystinuria (inherited disorder of amino acid metabolism)	Increased fluid intake Alkalinization of urine

FIGURE 33.7 • Staghorn stones. The kidney shows hydronephrosis and stones that are casts of the dilated calices. (From Rubin R., Strayer D. S. (Eds.). (2012). *Rubin's pathology: Clinicopathologic foundations of medicine* (6th ed., p. 800). Philadelphia, PA: Lippincott Williams & Wilkins.)

as the bacterial count grows, and they can increase in size until they fill an entire renal pelvis (Fig. 33.7). Because of their shape, they often are called *staghorn stones*. They almost always are associated with UTIs and persistently alkaline urine. Because these stones act as a foreign body, treatment of the infection often is difficult. Struvite stones usually are too large to be passed and require lithotripsy or surgical removal.[4,13]

Uric acid stones develop in conditions of gout and high concentrations of uric acid in the urine. Hyperuricosuria may also contribute to calcium stone formation by acting as a nucleus for calcium oxalate stone formation. Unlike radiopaque calcium stones, uric acid stones are not visible on x-ray films. Uric acid stones form most readily in urine with a pH less than 5.8. Thus, these stones can be treated by raising the urinary pH to 6 to 6.5 with potassium alkali salts.[15,16]

Cystine stones account for less than 1% of kidney stones overall but represent a significant proportion of childhood calculi. They are seen in cystinuria, which results from a genetic defect in renal transport of cystine. These stones resemble struvite stones except that infection is unlikely to be present.[4,13]

Clinical Features

One of the major manifestations of kidney stones is pain. Depending on location, there are two types of pain associated with kidney stones: renal colic and noncolicky renal pain.[4,9,10,13–15] *Renal colic* is the term used to describe the colicky pain that accompanies stretching of the collecting system

or ureter. The symptoms of renal colic are caused by stones 1 to 5 mm in diameter that can move into the ureter and obstruct flow. Classic ureteral colic is manifested by acute, intermittent, and excruciating pain in the flank and upper outer quadrant of the abdomen on the affected side. The pain may radiate to the lower abdominal quadrant, bladder area, perineum, or scrotum in the man. The skin may be cool and clammy, and nausea and vomiting are common. Noncolicky pain is caused by stones that produce distension of the renal calyces or renal pelvis. The pain usually is a dull, deep ache in the flank or back that can vary in intensity from mild to severe. The pain is often exaggerated by drinking large amounts of fluid.

Diagnosis and Treatment. Patients with kidney stones often present with acute renal colic, and the diagnosis is based on symptomatology and diagnostic tests, which include urinalysis, plain film radiography, intravenous pyelography (IVP), and abdominal ultrasonography.[14] Urinalysis provides information related to hematuria, infection, the presence of stone-forming crystals, and urine pH. Most stones are radiopaque and readily visible on a plain radiograph of the abdomen. The noncontrast spiral CT scan is the imaging modality of choice in persons with acute renal colic.[14] IVP uses an intravenously injected contrast medium that is filtered in the glomeruli to visualize the collecting system of the kidneys and ureters. Abdominal ultrasonography is highly sensitive to hydronephrosis, which may be a manifestation of ureteral obstruction. A new imaging technique called *nuclear scintigraphy* uses bisphosphonate markers as a means of imaging stones. The method has been credited with identifying stones that are too small to be detected by other methods.

Treatment of acute renal colic usually is supportive. Pain relief may be needed during acute phases of obstruction, and antibiotic therapy may be necessary to treat UTIs. Most stones that are less than 5 mm in diameter pass spontaneously. All urine should be strained during an attack in the hope of retrieving the stone for chemical analysis and determination of type. This information, along with a careful history and laboratory tests, provides the basis for long-term preventive measures.[17]

A major goal of treatment in persons who have passed kidney stones or have had them removed is to prevent their recurrence. Prevention requires investigation into the cause of stone formation using urine tests, blood chemistries, and stone analysis. Underlying disease conditions, such as hyperparathyroidism, are treated. Adequate fluid intake reduces the concentration of stone-forming crystals in the urine and needs to be encouraged. Depending on the type of stone that is formed, dietary changes, medications, or both may be used to alter the concentration of stone-forming elements in the urine. For example, persons who form calcium oxalate stones may need to decrease their intake of foods that are high in oxalate (*e.g.,* spinach, Swiss chard, cocoa, chocolate, pecans, peanuts). Calcium supplementation with calcium salts such as calcium carbonate and calcium phosphate may also be used to bind oxalate in the intestine and decrease its absorption. Thiazide diuretics lower urinary calcium by increasing tubular reabsorption so that less remains in the urine. Drugs that bind calcium in the gut (*e.g.,* cellulose phosphate) may be used to inhibit calcium absorption and urinary excretion.[16]

Measures to change the pH of the urine also can influence kidney stone formation. In persons who lose the ability to lower the pH of (or acidify) their urine, there is an increase in the divalent and trivalent forms of urine phosphate that combine with calcium to form calcium phosphate stones. The formation of uric acid stones is increased in acid urine; stone formation can be reduced by raising the pH of urine to 6.0 to 6.5 with potassium alkali (*e.g.,* potassium citrate) salts. Table 33.2 summarizes measures for preventing the recurrence of different types of kidney stones.

In some cases, stone removal may be necessary. Several methods are available for removing kidney stones: ureteroscopic removal, percutaneous removal, and extracorporeal lithotripsy.[14] All these procedures eliminate the need for an open surgical procedure, which is another form of treatment. Open stone surgery may be required to remove large calculi or those that are resistant to other forms of removal.

Ureteroscopic removal involves the passage of an instrument through the urethra into the bladder and then into the ureter. The development of high-quality optics has improved the ease with which this procedure is performed and its outcome. The procedure, which is performed under fluoroscopic guidance, involves the use of various instruments for dilating the ureter and for grasping, fragmenting, and removing the stone. Preprocedure radiologic studies using a contrast medium (*i.e.,* excretory urography) are done to determine the position of the stone and direct the placement of the ureteroscope.[17]

Percutaneous nephrolithotomy is the treatment of choice for removal of renal or proximal ureteral calculi.[14,17] It involves the insertion through the flank of a small-gauge needle into the collecting system of the kidney; the needle tract is then dilated, and an instrument called a *nephroscope* is inserted into the renal pelvis. The procedure is performed under fluoroscopic guidance. Preprocedure radiologic and ultrasonographic examinations of the kidney and ureter are used to determine the placement of the nephroscope. Stones up to 1 cm in diameter can be removed through this method. Larger stones must be broken up with an electrohydraulic or ultrasonic lithotriptor (*i.e.,* stone breaker).

A nonsurgical treatment, called *extracorporeal shock-wave lithotripsy,* uses acoustic shock waves to fragment calculi into sandlike particles that are passed in the urine over the next few days. Because of the large amount of stone particles that are generated during the procedure, a ureteral stent (*i.e.,* a tubelike device used to hold the ureter open) may be inserted to ensure adequate urine drainage.

IN SUMMARY

Obstruction of urine flow can occur at any level of the urinary tract. Among the causes of urinary tract obstruction are developmental defects, pregnancy, infection and inflammation,

kidney stones, neurologic defects, and prostatic hypertrophy. Obstructive disorders produce stasis of urine, increase the risk for infection and calculi formation, and produce progressive dilation of the renal collecting ducts and renal tubular structures, which causes renal atrophy.

Hydronephrosis refers to urine-filled dilation of the renal pelvis and calices associated with progressive atrophy of the kidney due to obstruction of urine outflow. Unilateral hydronephrosis may remain silent for long periods because the unaffected kidney can maintain adequate kidney function. With partial bilateral obstruction, the earliest manifestation is an inability to concentrate urine, reflected by polyuria and nocturia. Complete bilateral obstruction results in oliguria, anuria, and renal failure.

Kidney stones are a major cause of upper urinary tract obstruction. There are four types of kidney stones: calcium (*i.e.,* oxalate and phosphate) stones, which are associated with increased serum calcium levels; magnesium ammonium phosphate (*i.e.,* struvite) stones, which are associated with UTIs; uric acid stones, which are related to elevated uric acid levels; and cystine stones, which are seen in cystinuria. A major goal of treatment for persons who have passed kidney stones or have had them removed is to identify stone composition and prevent their recurrence. Treatment measures depend on stone type and include adequate fluid intake to prevent urine saturation, dietary modification to decrease intake of stone-forming constituents, treatment of UTI, measures to change urine pH, and the use of diuretics that decrease the calcium concentration of urine.

URINARY TRACT INFECTIONS

After completing this section of the chapter, you should be able to meet the following objectives:

- Cite the organisms most responsible for UTIs and state why urinary catheters, obstruction, and reflux predispose to infections.
- List three physiologic mechanisms that protect against UTIs.
- Describe the signs and symptoms of UTIs.
- Describe factors that predispose to UTIs in children, sexually active women, pregnant women, and older adults.
- Compare the manifestations of UTIs in different age groups, including infants, toddlers, adolescents, adults, and older adults.
- Cite measures used in the diagnosis and treatment of UTIs.

UTIs are the second most common type of bacterial infection seen by healthcare providers, with respiratory tract infections being the first. UTIs include several distinct entities, including asymptomatic bacteriuria, symptomatic infections, lower

UTIs such as cystitis, and upper UTIs such as pyelonephritis. Because of their ability to cause renal damage, upper UTIs are considered more serious than lower UTIs. Acute pyelonephritis (discussed in the section on Tubulointerstitial Disorders) represents an infection of the renal parenchyma and renal pelvis. Improperly treated, it can lead to sepsis, renal abscesses, and chronic pyelonephritis.

URINARY TRACT INFECTIONS

- UTIs involve host–agent interactions that pit the defences of the host against the virulence of the infectious agent.
- Infection is facilitated by host conditions that disrupt washout of the agent from the UT through urine flow, change the protective properties of the mucin lining of the UT, disrupt the protective function of the normal bacterial flora, or impair the function of the immune system.
- Virulence of the agent is derived from its ability to gain access to and thrive in the UT environment, adhere to the tissues of the lower or upper UT, evade the destructive effects of the host's immune system, and develop resistance to antimicrobial agents.

Etiologic Factors

Most uncomplicated lower UTIs are caused by *Escherichia coli*. Other uropathic pathogens include *Staphylococcus saprophyticus* in uncomplicated UTIs, and both non-*E. coli* gram-negative rods (*i.e.*, *Proteus mirabilis*, *Klebsiella* species, *Enterobacter* species, and *Pseudomonas aeruginosa*) and gram-positive cocci (*i.e.*, *Staphylococcus aureus*) in complicated UTIs.[4,18–21] Most UTIs are caused by bacteria that enter through the urethra. Bacteria can also enter through the bloodstream, usually only in immunocompromised persons and neonates. Although the distal portion of the urethra often contains pathogens, the urine formed in the kidneys and found in the bladder normally is sterile or free of bacteria. This is because of the *washout phenomenon,* in which urine from the bladder normally washes bacteria out of the urethra. When a UTI occurs, it is usually from bacteria that have colonized the urethra, vagina, or perianal area.

There is an increased risk for UTIs in persons with urinary obstruction and reflux, in people with neurogenic disorders that impair bladder emptying, in women who are sexually active, in postmenopausal women, in men with diseases of the prostate, and in older adults. Instrumentation and urinary catheterization are the most common predisposing factors for nosocomial UTIs. UTIs occur more commonly in women with diabetes than in women without the disease. People with diabetes are also at increased risk for complications associated with UTIs, including pyelonephritis, and they are more susceptible to fungal infections (particularly *Candida* species) and infections with gram-negative pathogens other than *E. coli*.

Host–Agent Interactions

Because certain people tend to be predisposed to development of UTIs, considerable interest has been focused on host–pathogen interactions and factors that increase the risk for UTI.[4,18–20] UTIs are more common in women than men, specifically at 16 to 35 years of age, at which time they are more than 35 times likely to develop a UTI than age-matched men.[18] In men, the longer length of the urethra and the antibacterial properties of the prostatic fluid provide some protection from ascending UTIs until approximately 50 years of age.[4] After this age, prostatic hypertrophy becomes more common, and with it may come obstruction and increased risk for UTI (see Chapter 44).

Host Defences. In the development of a UTI, host defences are matched against the virulence of the pathogen. The host defences of the bladder have several components, including the washout phenomenon, in which bacteria are removed from the bladder and urethra during voiding; the protective mucin layer of the uroepithelium that lines the bladder and protects against bacterial invasion; and local immune responses.[4] In the ureters, peristaltic movements facilitate the movement of urine from the renal pelvis through the ureters and into the bladder. Immune mechanisms, particularly secretory immunoglobulin (Ig) A, appear to provide an important antibacterial defence. Phagocytic blood cells further assist in the removal of bacteria from the urinary tract.

There continues to be appreciation of the protective function of the bladder's mucin layer.[4] It is thought that the epithelial cells that line the bladder synthesize protective substances that subsequently become incorporated into the mucin layer that adheres to the bladder wall. One theory proposes that the mucin layer acts by binding water, which then constitutes a protective barrier between the bacteria and the bladder epithelium. Elderly and postmenopausal women produce less mucin than younger women, suggesting that estrogen may play a role in mucin production in women.

Other important host factors include the normal flora of the periurethral area in women and prostate secretions in men.[4] In women, the normal flora of the periurethral area, which consists of organisms such as *Lactobacillus*, provides defence against the colonization of uropathic bacteria. Alterations in the periurethral environment, such as occurs with a decrease in estrogen levels during menopause or the use of antibiotics, can alter the protective periurethral flora, allowing uropathogens to colonize and enter the urinary tract. In men, the prostatic fluid has antimicrobial properties that protect the urethra from colonization.

Pathogen Virulence. Not all bacteria are capable of adhering to and infecting the urinary tract. Of the many strains of *E. coli*, only those with increased ability to adhere to the epithelial cells of the urinary tract are able to produce UTIs. These bacteria have fine protein filaments, called *pili* or *fimbriae,* that help them adhere to receptors on the lining of urinary tract structures.[4,18] The two main types of pili (types 1 and P) found on

E. coli that cause UTIs are morphologically similar but differ in their ability to mediate hemagglutination in the presence of mannose. Type P pili are mannose resistant and were named because of their high incidence in *E. coli* that cause pyelonephritis and because of their association with the P blood group system. P pili have been observed in over 90% of *E. coli* strains causing pyelonephritis but in less than 20% of strains causing lower UTIs.[21]

Obstruction and Reflux

Obstruction and reflux are other contributing factors in the development of UTIs. Any microorganisms that enter the bladder normally are washed out during voiding. When outflow is obstructed, urine remains in the bladder and acts as a medium for microbial growth; the microorganisms in the contaminated urine can then ascend along the ureters to infect the kidneys. The presence of residual urine correlates closely with bacteriuria and with its recurrence after treatment. Another aspect of bladder outflow obstruction and bladder distension is increased intravesical pressure, which compresses blood vessels in the bladder wall, leading to a decrease in the mucosal defences of the bladder.

In UTIs associated with stasis of urine flow, the obstruction may be anatomic or functional. Anatomic obstructions include urinary tract stones, prostatic hyperplasia, pregnancy, and malformations of the ureterovesical junction. Functional obstructions include neurogenic bladder, infrequent voiding, detrusor (bladder) muscle instability, and constipation.

Reflux occurs when urine from the urethra moves into the bladder (*i.e.*, urethrovesical reflux). In women, *urethrovesical reflux* can occur during activities such as coughing or squatting, in which an increase in intra-abdominal pressure causes the urine to be squeezed into the urethra and then to flow back into the bladder as the pressure decreases. This also can happen when voiding is abruptly interrupted. Because the urethral orifice frequently is contaminated with bacteria, the reflux mechanism may cause bacteria to be drawn back into the bladder.

A second type of reflux mechanism, *vesicoureteral reflux*, occurs at the level of the bladder and ureter.[9] Normally, the distal portion of the ureter courses between the muscle layer and the mucosal surface of the bladder wall, forming a flap (Fig. 33.8). The flap is compressed against the bladder wall during micturition, preventing urine from being forced into the ureter. In persons with vesicoureteral reflux, the ureter enters the bladder at an approximate right angle such that urine is forced into the ureter during micturition. It is seen most commonly in children with UTIs and is believed to result from congenital defects in length, diameter, muscle structure, or innervation of the submucosal segment of the ureter. Vesicoureteral reflux also is seen in adults with obstruction to bladder outflow, primarily due to increased bladder volume and pressure.

Catheter-Induced Infection

Urinary catheters are tubes made of latex or plastic. They are inserted through the urethra into the bladder for the purpose of

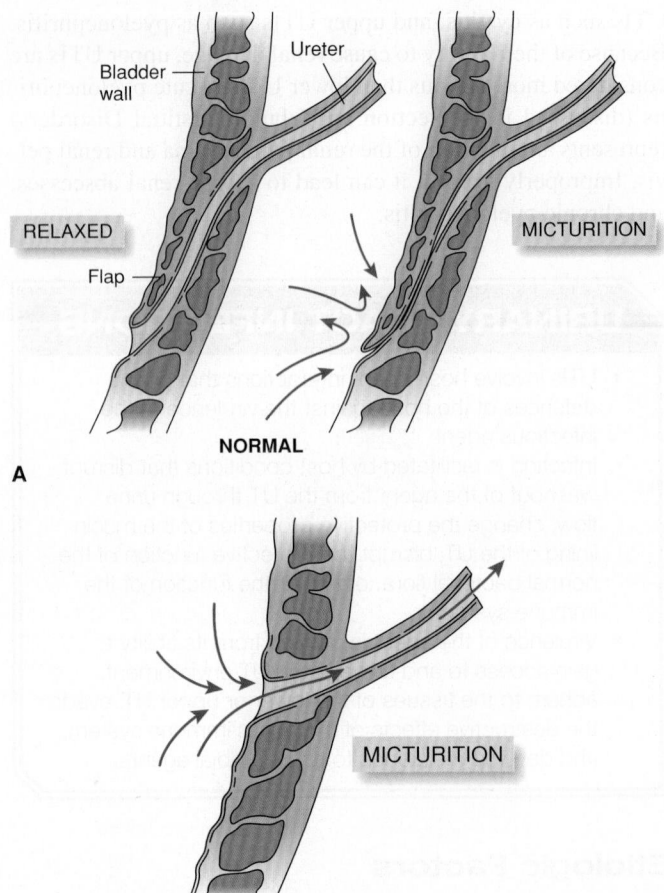

FIGURE 33.8 • Anatomic features of the ureter and bladder and their relationship to vesicoureteral reflux. **A:** In the normal bladder, the distal portion of the intravesical ureter courses between the mucosa and the muscularis of the bladder. A mucosal flap is thus formed. On micturition, the elevated intravesicular pressure compresses the flap against the bladder wall, thereby occluding the lumen. **B:** Persons with a congenitally short intravesical ureter have no mucosal flap because the entry of the ureter into the bladder approaches a right angle. Thus, micturition forces urine into the ureter. (From Rubin R., Strayer D. S. (Eds.). (2012). *Rubin's pathology: Clinicopathologic foundations of medicine* (6th ed., p. 795). Philadelphia, PA: Lippincott Williams & Wilkins; Courtesy of Dmitri Karetnikov, artist.)

draining urine. They are a source of urethral irritation and provide a means for entry of microorganisms into the urinary tract.

Catheter-associated bacteriuria remains the most frequent cause of gram-negative septicemia in hospitalized patients. Studies have shown that bacteria adhere to the surface of the catheter and initiate the growth of a biofilm that then covers the surface of the catheter.[22] The biofilm tends to protect the bacteria from the action of antibiotics and makes treatment difficult. A closed drainage system (*i.e.*, closed to air and other sources of contamination) and careful attention to perineal hygiene (*i.e.*, cleaning the area around the urethral meatus) help to prevent infections in persons who require an indwelling catheter. Careful handwashing and early detection and treatment of UTIs also are essential.

Clinical Features

The manifestations of UTI depend on whether the infection involves the lower (bladder) or upper (kidney) urinary tract and whether the infection is acute or chronic. The majority of UTIs are acute uncomplicated bladder infections that occur in women. Upper UTIs affect the parenchyma and pelvis of the kidney (pyelonephritis, to be discussed). They are less common and occur more frequently in children and adults with urinary tract obstructions or other predisposing conditions such as diabetes.

An acute episode of cystitis (bladder infection) is characterized by frequency of urination, lower abdominal or back discomfort, and burning and pain on urination (*i.e.*, dysuria).[18–22] Occasionally, the urine is cloudy and foul smelling. In adults, fever and other signs of infection usually are absent. If there are no complications, the symptoms disappear within 48 hours of treatment. The symptoms of cystitis may also represent urethritis caused by *Chlamydia trachomatis, Neisseria gonorrhoeae,* or herpes simplex virus, or vaginitis attributable to *Trichomonas vaginalis* or *Candida* species[18–20] (see Chapter 47).

Diagnosis and Treatment

The diagnosis of UTI usually is based on symptoms and on examination of the urine for the presence of microorganisms. Urine tests are used to establish the presence of bacteria in the urine and a diagnosis of UTI. A commonly accepted criterion for diagnosis of a UTI is the presence of 100,000 colony-forming units (CFU) or more bacteria per millilitre of urine.[4] Colonization usually is defined as the multiplication of microorganisms in or on a host without apparent evidence of invasiveness or tissue injury. Pyuria (the presence of less than five to eight leukocytes per high-power field) indicates a host response to infection rather than asymptomatic bacterial colonization. A Gram stain may be done to determine the type (gram-positive or gram-negative) of organism that is present. A urine culture may be done to confirm the presence of pathogenic bacteria in urine specimens, allow for their identification, and permit the determination of their sensitivity to specific antibiotics. When necessary, x-ray films, ultrasonography, and CT and renal scans are used to identify contributing factors, such as obstruction.[4]

Chemical screening (urine dipstick) for markers of infection may provide useful information but is less sensitive than microscopic analysis.[21,23] These tests are relatively inexpensive, easy to perform, and can be done in the clinic setting or even in the home. Bacteria reduce nitrates in the urine to nitrites, providing a means for chemical analysis. Similarly, activated leukocytes secrete leukocyte esterase, which can be detected chemically. Leukocyte esterase is specific (78% to 87%) and reliably sensitive (79% to 83%) for detecting uropathogens equivalent to 100,000 CFU/ml urine.[23] Nitrite tests may be negative if the causative organism is not nitrate producing (*e.g.*, enterococci, *S. saprophyticus*). Therefore, the sensitivity of nitrite tests ranges from 49% to 53%, but the specificity is 98%.[21,23] The nitrite test can also be negative if the urine specimen is too diluted.

The treatment of UTI is based on the pathogen causing the infection, and the presence of contributing host–agent factors. Other considerations include whether the infection is acute, recurrent, or chronic. Most acute lower UTIs, which occur mainly in women and are generally caused by *E. coli,* are treated successfully with a short course of antimicrobial therapy. Forcing fluids may relieve signs and symptoms, and this approach is used as an adjunct to antimicrobial treatment. The selection of empiric therapy is based on suspected or known local resistance patterns and the patient's own tolerance and medication history.

Recurrent lower UTIs are those that occur again after a course of treatment. They are due either to bacterial resistance, persistence or reinfection. Bacterial persistence usually is curable by removal of the infectious source (*e.g.*, urinary catheter or infected bladder stones). Reinfection is managed principally through education regarding pathogen transmission and prevention measures. Cranberry juice has been suggested as a preventive measure for persons with frequent UTIs with the assumption that this juice prevents bacterial adherence to the epithelial lining of the urinary tract but studies do not support this.[24]

Chronic UTIs are more difficult to treat. Because they often are associated with obstructive uropathy or reflux flow of urine, diagnostic tests usually are performed to detect such abnormalities. When possible, the condition causing the reflux flow or obstruction is corrected. Most persons with recurrent UTIs are treated with antimicrobial agents for 10 to 14 days in doses sufficient to maintain high urine levels of the drug, and they are examined for obstruction or other causes of infection. Men in particular should be investigated for obstructive disorders or a prostatic focus of infection.

Infections in Special Populations

UTIs affect persons of all ages. In infants, they occur more often in boys than in girls. After the first year of life UTIs occur more often in girls. This is because of the shorter length of the female urethra and because the vaginal vestibule can be contaminated easily with fecal flora. Approximately half of all adult women have at least one UTI during their lifetime.[1,4,18] The major risk factors for women 16 to 35 years of age are related to sexual intercourse and use of spermicidal agents. The anterior urethra usually is colonized with bacteria; urethral massage or sexual intercourse can force these bacteria back into the bladder.

Urinary Tract Infections in Pregnant Women

Pregnant women are at increased risk for UTIs. Normal changes in the functioning of the urinary tract that occur during pregnancy predispose to UTIs.[18] These changes involve the collecting system of the kidneys and include dilation of the renal calyces, pelves, and ureters that begins during the first trimester and becomes most pronounced during the third trimester. This dilation of the upper urinary system is accompanied by a reduction in the peristaltic activity of the ureters that is thought to result from the muscle-relaxing effects of progesterone-like hormones and mechanical obstruction from the enlarging uterus. In addition to the changes in the kidneys and ureters, the bladder becomes displaced from its pelvic position to a more abdominal position, producing further changes in ureteral position.

Asymptomatic UTIs are common, with a prevalence of 2% to 14% in pregnant women. The complications of asymptomatic UTIs during pregnancy include persistent bacteriuria, acute and chronic pyelonephritis, and preterm delivery of infants with low birth weight. Evidence suggests that few women become bacteriuric during pregnancy. Rather, it appears that symptomatic UTIs during pregnancy reflect pre-existing asymptomatic bacteriuria and that changes occurring during pregnancy simply permit the prior urinary colonization to progress to symptomatic infection and invasion of the kidneys. Incidence of pyelonephritis during pregnancy is approximately 1% to 2%. However, 20% to 40% of women with untreated bacteriuria will develop pyelonephritis during pregnancy.[21,25] Because bacteriuria may occur as an asymptomatic condition in pregnant women, it is recommended that a urine culture be obtained early in the pregnancy, between 12 and 16 weeks' gestation. A repeat culture should be obtained during the third trimester. Women with bacteriuria should be followed closely, and infections should be properly treated to prevent complications. The choice of antimicrobial agent should address the common infecting organisms and should be safe for the mother and fetus.

Urinary Tract Infections in Children

UTIs occur in 1% to 3% of female and 1% of male children.[26] In girls, the average age at first diagnosis is 5 years or younger, with peaks during infancy and toilet training. In boys, most UTIs occur during the first year of life; they are more common in uncircumcised than in circumcised boys. Children who are at increased risk for bacteriuria or symptomatic UTIs are premature infants discharged from neonatal intensive care units; children with systemic or immunologic disease or urinary tract abnormalities such as neurogenic bladder or vesicoureteral reflux; those with a family history of UTI or urinary tract anomalies with reflux; and girls younger than 5 years of age with a history of UTI.[26]

UTIs in children frequently involve the upper urinary tract (pyelonephritis). In children in whom renal development is not complete, pyelonephritis can lead to renal scarring and permanent kidney damage. Most UTIs that lead to scarring and diminished kidney growth occur in children younger than 4 years, especially infants younger than 1 year of age. The incidence of scarring is greatest in children with gross vesicoureteral reflux or obstruction, in children with recurrent UTIs, and in those with a delay in treatment.

Unlike adults, children frequently do not present with the typical signs of a UTI.[23,26] Many neonates with UTIs have bacteremia and may show signs and symptoms of septicemia, including fever, hypothermia, apneic spells, poor skin perfusion, abdominal distension, diarrhea, vomiting, lethargy, and irritability. Older infants may present with feeding problems, failure to thrive, diarrhea, vomiting, fever, and foul-smelling urine. Toddlers often present with abdominal pain, vomiting,

diarrhea, abnormal voiding patterns, foul-smelling urine, fever, and poor growth. In older children with lower UTIs, the classic features—enuresis, frequency, dysuria, and suprapubic discomfort—are more common. Fever is a common sign of UTI in children, and the possibility of UTI should be considered in any child with unexplained fever.

Diagnosis is based on a careful history of voiding patterns and symptomatology; physical examination to determine fever, hypertension, abdominal or suprapubic tenderness, and other manifestations of UTI; and urinalysis to determine bacteriuria, pyuria, proteinuria, and hematuria. A positive urine culture that is obtained correctly is essential for the diagnosis. Additional diagnostic methods may be needed to determine the cause of the disorder. Vesicoureteral reflux is the most commonly associated abnormality in UTIs, and reflux nephropathy is an important cause of end-stage renal disease in children and adolescents. Children with a relatively uncomplicated first UTI may turn out to have significant reflux. Therefore, even a single documented UTI in a child requires careful diagnosis. Urinary symptoms in the absence of bacteriuria suggest vaginitis, urethritis, sexual molestation, use of irritating bubble baths, pinworms, or viral cystitis. In adolescent girls, a history of dysuria and vaginal discharge makes vaginitis or vulvitis a consideration.[23,26]

The approach to treatment is based on the clinical severity of the infection, the site of infection (*i.e.,* lower versus upper urinary tract), the risk for sepsis, and the presence of structural abnormalities.[23,26] The immediate treatment of infants and young children is essential. Most infants with symptomatic UTIs and many children with clinical evidence of acute upper UTIs require hospitalization, rehydration, and intravenous antibiotic therapy. Follow-up is essential for children with febrile UTIs to ensure resolution of the infection. Follow-up urine cultures are done 1 to 2 weeks after the treatment has ended to make certain the offending organism has been eradicated. Imaging studies often are recommended for all children after their first UTI to detect renal scarring, vesicoureteral reflux, or other abnormalities.

Urinary Tract Infections in the Older Adults

UTIs are relatively common in elderly persons.[20] They are the second most common form of infection, after respiratory tract infections, among otherwise healthy community-dwelling older adults. They are particularly prevalent in older adults living in nursing homes or extended care facilities.[20]

Most of these infections follow invasion of the urinary tract by the ascending route. Several factors predispose older adults to UTIs, including immobility resulting in poor bladder emptying; bladder outflow obstruction caused by prostatic hyperplasia or kidney stones; bladder ischemia caused by urine retention; constipation; senile vaginitis; and diminished bactericidal activity of urine and prostatic secretions. Added to these risks are other health problems that necessitate instrumentation of the urinary tract. UTIs develop in 1% of ambulatory patients after a single catheterization and within 1 week in essentially all patients with indwelling catheters have bacteriuria.[27]

Elderly persons with bacteriuria have varying symptoms, ranging from the absence of symptoms to the presence of typical UTI symptoms. Even when symptoms of lower UTIs are present, they may be difficult to interpret because elderly persons without UTIs commonly experience urgency, frequency, and incontinence. Alternatively, elderly persons may have vague symptoms such as anorexia, fatigue, weakness, or change in mental status. Even with more serious upper UTIs (*e.g.*, pyelonephritis), the classic signs of infection such as fever, chills, flank pain, and tenderness may be altered or absent in elderly persons.[20] Sometimes, no symptoms occur until the infection is far advanced, as in the case of urosepsis.

IN SUMMARY

UTI is the second most common type of bacterial infection seen by healthcare professionals. Infections can range from asymptomatic bacteriuria to severe kidney infections that cause irreversible kidney damage. Predisposition to infection is determined by host defences and pathogen virulence. Host defences include the washout phenomenon associated with voiding, the protective mucin lining of the bladder, and the local immune defences. Pathogen virulence is enhanced by the presence of pili that facilitate adherence to structures in the urinary tract, lipopolysaccharides that bind to host cells and elicit an inflammatory reaction, and enzymes that break down red blood cells and make iron available for bacterial metabolism and multiplication.

Most UTIs ascend from the urethra and bladder. A number of factors interact in determining the predisposition to development of UTIs, including urinary tract obstruction, urine stasis and reflux, pregnancy-induced changes in urinary tract function, age-related changes in the urinary tract, changes in the protective mechanisms of the bladder and ureters, impaired immune function, and virulence of the pathogen. Urinary tract catheters and urinary instrumentation contribute to the incidence of UTIs. Early diagnosis and treatment of UTI are essential to preventing permanent kidney damage.

DISORDERS OF GLOMERULAR FUNCTION

After completing this section of the chapter, you should be able to meet the following objectives:

- Describe the two types of immune mechanisms involved in glomerular disorders.
- Use the terms proliferation, sclerosis, membranous, diffuse, focal, segmental, and mesangial to explain changes in glomerular structure that occur with glomerulonephritis.

- Relate the proteinuria, hematuria, pyuria, oliguria, edema, hypertension, and azotemia that occur with glomerulonephritis to changes in glomerular structure.
- Briefly describe the difference among the nephritic syndromes, rapidly progressive glomerulonephritis, nephrotic syndrome, asymptomatic glomerular disorders, and chronic glomerulonephritis.

The glomeruli are tufts of capillaries that lie between the afferent and efferent arterioles. The capillaries of the glomeruli are arranged in lobules and supported by a stalk consisting of mesangial cells and a basement membrane-like extracellular matrix (Fig. 33.9A). The glomerular capillary membrane is composed of three structural layers: an endothelial cell layer that lines the inner surface of the capillary, a basement membrane made up of a network of matrix proteins, and a layer of epithelial cells that surrounds the outer surface of the capillary and lines the inner surface of the Bowman capsule (see Chapter 30, Fig. 30.5). The epithelial cells are attached to the

FIGURE 33.9 • Schematic representations of a glomerulus. **A:** Normal. **B:** Localization of immune deposits (mesangial, subendothelial, subepithelial) and changes in glomerular architecture associated with injury. WBC, white blood cell. (From Whitley K., Keane W. F., Vernier R. L. (1984). Acute glomerulonephritis: A clinical overview. *Medical Clinics of North America, 68*, 263.)

FIGURE 33.10 • Algorithm demonstrating the integration of pathologic findings with clinical data to make a diagnosis of a specific form of primary or secondary glomerulonephritis. Note that an important initial categorization is as anti-glomerular basement membrane (GBM), immune complex or antineutrophil cytoplasmic autoantibody (ANCA) glomerulonephritis. Once this determination is made, more specific diagnoses depend on additional clinical or pathologic observations. (From Rubin R., Strayer D. S. (Eds.). (2012). *Rubin's pathology: Clinicopathologic foundations of medicine* (6th ed., p. 765). Philadelphia, PA: Lippincott Williams & Wilkins.)

basement membrane by long, footlike processes (*podocytes*) that encircle the outer surface of the capillaries. The glomerular capillary membrane is selectively permeable, allowing water and small particles (*e.g.*, electrolytes and dissolved particles, such as glucose and amino acids) to leave the blood and enter the Bowman space, and preventing larger particles (*e.g.*, plasma proteins and blood cells) from leaving the blood.[4]

Glomerulonephritis is an inflammatory process that involves glomerular structures and is the third leading cause of kidney failure in Canada after diabetes and hypertension.[28] There are many causes of glomerular disease. The disease may occur as a primary condition in which the glomerular abnormality is the only disease present, or it may occur as a secondary condition in which the glomerular abnormality results from another disease, such as diabetes mellitus or SLE (Fig. 33.10).

Etiology and Pathogenesis of Glomerular Injury

The causative agents or triggering events that produce glomerular injury include immunologic, nonimmunologic, and hereditary mechanisms. Most cases of primary and many cases of secondary glomerular disease probably have an immune origin.[4,9,10] Although many glomerular diseases are driven by immunologic events, a variety of nonimmunologic metabolic (*e.g.*, diabetes), hemodynamic (*e.g.*, hypertension), and toxic

(*e.g.*, drugs, chemicals) stresses can induce glomerular injury, either alone or in concert with immunologic mechanisms. Hereditary glomerular diseases such as Alport syndrome, although relatively rare, are an important category of glomerular disease because of their association with progressive loss of renal function and transmission to future generations.

Two types of immune mechanisms have been implicated in the development of glomerular disease: (1) injury resulting from antibodies reacting with fixed glomerular antigens or antigens planted within the glomerulus, and (2) injury resulting from circulating antigen–antibody complexes that become trapped in the glomerular membrane (Fig. 33.11). Antigens responsible for development of the immune response may be of endogenous origin, such as autoantibodies to deoxyribonucleic acid (DNA) in SLE, or they may be of exogenous origin, such as streptococcal membrane antigens in poststreptococcal glomerulonephritis. Frequently, the source of the antigen is unknown.

The cellular changes that occur with glomerular disease include increases in glomerular or inflammatory cell number (proliferative or hypercellular), basement membrane thickening (membranous), and changes in noncellular glomerular components (sclerosis and fibrosis). An increase in cell numbers is characterized by one or more of the following: proliferation of endothelial and mesangial cells, leukocyte infiltration (neutrophils, monocytes, and in some cases lymphocytes),

FIGURE 33.11 • Immune mechanisms of glomerular disease. **A:** Antiglomerular membrane antibodies leave the circulation and interact with antigens that are present in the basement membrane of the glomerulus. **B:** Antigen–antibody complexes circulating in the blood become trapped as they are filtered in the glomerulus.

Labels in figure: Epithelial cell; Foot process; Basement membrane; Subendothelial deposit; Circulating antigen–antibody complexes; Antigen; Antibody. **A** Antiglomerular membrane antibodies. **B** Circulating antigen–antibody complex deposition

and formation of crescents (half-moon-shaped collections of proliferating epithelial cells and infiltrating leukocytes) in the Bowman space.[4,9,10] *Basement membrane thickening* involves deposition of dense noncellular material on the endothelial and epithelial sides of the basement membrane or within the membrane itself. *Sclerosis* refers to an increase in the amount of extracellular material in the mesangial, subendothelial, or subepithelial tissue of the glomerulus, and *fibrosis* refers to the deposition of collagen fibres. Glomerular changes can be *diffuse,* involving all glomeruli and all parts of the glomeruli; *focal,* in which only some glomeruli are affected and others are essentially normal; *segmental,* involving only a certain segment of each glomerulus; or *mesangial,* affecting only mesangial cells.[10] Figure 33.9B illustrates the location of lesions associated with various types of glomerular disease.

Types of Glomerular Disease

The clinical manifestations of glomerular disorders generally fall into one of five categories: nephritic syndromes, rapidly progressive glomerulonephritis, the nephrotic syndrome, asymptomatic disorders of urinary sediment (*i.e.,* hematuria, proteinuria), and chronic glomerulonephritis[4,9,10] (Table 33.3). The nephritic syndromes produce a proliferative inflammatory response, whereas the nephrotic syndrome produces increased permeability of the glomerulus. Because most glomerular disorders can produce mixed nephritic and nephrotic syndromes, a definitive diagnosis often requires renal biopsy.

Acute Nephritic Syndrome

The acute nephritic syndrome is the clinical correlate of acute glomerular inflammation. In its most dramatic form, the acute nephritic syndrome is characterized by sudden onset of hematuria (either microscopic or grossly visible, with red cell casts), variable degrees of proteinuria, diminished GFR, oliguria, and signs of impaired renal function. It is caused by inflammatory processes that occlude the glomerular capillary lumen and damage the capillary wall, permitting red blood cells to escape into the urine and producing hemodynamic changes that decrease the GFR. Extracellular fluid accumulation,

TABLE 33.3 CLASSIFICATION AND MANIFESTATIONS OF GLOMERULAR SYNDROMES	
CLASSIFICATION	**MANIFESTATIONS**
Acute nephritic syndrome	Recent onset of hematuria and proteinuria, impairment of kidney function (azotemia), and salt and water retention causing edema and hypertension
Rapidly progressive glomerulonephritis	Progression of renal failure over days to weeks, in most cases in the context of nephritic presentation, typically associated with pathologic finding of extensive glomerular crescent formation on renal biopsy
Nephrotic syndrome	Nephrotic-range proteinuria (>3.5 g in 24 hours), hypoalbuminemia, hyperlipidemia, and lipiduria
Asymptomatic hematuria or proteinuria	Subnephrotic-range proteinuria, or hematuria, not accompanied by acute manifestations of impaired kidney function, edema, or hypertension
Chronic glomerulonephritis	Persistent proteinuria with or without hematuria and slowly progressive impairment of kidney function

FIGURE 33.12 • Acute postinfectious glomerulonephritis. An immunofluorescence micrograph demonstrates granular staining for complement C3 in capillary walls and the mesangium. (From Rubin R., Strayer D. S. (Eds.). (2012). *Rubin's pathology: Clinicopathologic foundations of medicine* (6th ed., p. 776). Philadelphia, PA: Lippincott Williams & Wilkins.)

hypertension, and edema develop because of the decreased GFR and enhanced tubular reabsorption of salt and water.

The acute nephritic syndrome may occur in such systemic diseases as SLE. Typically, however, it is associated with acute proliferative glomerulonephritis such as postinfectious glomerulonephritis.

Acute Postinfectious Glomerulonephritis. Acute postinfectious glomerulonephritis usually occurs after infection with certain strains of group A β-hemolytic streptococci and is caused by deposition of immune complexes.[4,9,10,29] It may also occur after infections by other organisms, including other positive bacteria (*e.g.,* staphylococci) gram negative bacteria (*e.g., Meningococcus, Hemophilus*), viral agents (*i.e.,* viruses responsible for hepatitis B, measles, chicken pox), fungal (*e.g., Candida albicans*) and parasitic pathogens (*e.g.,* malaria).[29] This type of glomerular disease is decreasing in frequency in North America but continues to be a common disorder worldwide. Although the disease is seen primarily in children, persons of any age can be affected.[29]

The acute phase of postinfectious glomerulonephritis is characterized by diffuse glomerular enlargement and hypercellularity. The hypercellularity is caused by infiltration of leukocytes, both neutrophils and monocytes; proliferation of endothelial and mesangial cells; and in severe cases, formation of crescents. There is also swelling of endothelial cells, and the combination of proliferation, swelling, and leukocyte infiltration obliterates the glomerular capillary lumens. There may be interstitial edema and inflammation, and the tubules often contain red blood cells. In the first weeks of disease, immunofluorescence microscopy typically reveals granular deposits of varying levels IgG and significant amounts of the complement component C3 in the mesangium and along the basement membrane (Fig. 33.12).[4,9]

The classic case of poststreptococcal glomerulonephritis follows a streptococcal infection by approximately 7 to 12 days—the time needed for the development of antibodies. The primary infection usually involves the pharynx (pharyngitis) but can also result from a skin infection (impetigo).

Oliguria, which develops as the GFR decreases, is one of the first symptoms. Proteinuria and hematuria follow because of increased glomerular capillary wall permeability. The red blood cells are degraded by materials in the urine, and cola-coloured urine may be the first sign of the disorder. Sodium and water retention gives rise to edema (particularly of the face and hands) and hypertension. Important laboratory findings include an elevated antistreptococcal antibody (ASO) titre, a decline in serum concentrations of C3 and other components of the complement cascade, and cryoglobulins (*i.e.,* large immune complexes) in the serum.

Treatment of acute poststreptococcal glomerulonephritis includes elimination of the streptococcal infection with antibiotics and providing supportive care. The disorder carries an excellent prognosis and rarely causes chronic kidney disease.[9] In children, spontaneous resolution of the glomerular lesion and nephritic syndrome is usually the norm and occurs within 6 to 8 weeks. Adults tend to recover more slowly; approximately 20% have some degree of persistent proteinuria or compromise of GFR 1 year after presentation.

Rapidly Progressive Glomerulonephritis

Rapidly progressive glomerulonephritis, also referred to as crescentic glomerulonephritis, is a clinical syndrome characterized by signs of severe glomerular injury that does not have a specific cause. As its name indicates, this type of glomerulonephritis is rapidly progressive, often within a matter of months. The disorder involves focal and segmental proliferation of glomerular cells and recruitment of monocytes and macrophages with formation of crescent-shaped structures that obliterate the Bowman space.[30] Three types of rapidly proliferative glomerulonephritis may be caused by a number of immunologic disorders, some systemic and others restricted to the kidney. The forms of this glomerulonephritis are Type 1—associated

FIGURE 33.13 • Antiglomerular basement membrane glomerulonephritis. Linear immunofluorescence for IgG is seen along the glomerular basement membrane. Contrast this with the granular pattern of immunofluorescence typical of most types of immune complex deposition within the capillary wall. (From Rubin R., Strayer D. S. (Eds.). (2012). *Rubin's pathology: Clinicopathologic foundations of medicine* (6th ed., p. 782). Philadelphia, PA: Lippincott Williams & Wilkins.)

FIGURE 33.14 • Pathophysiology of the nephrotic syndrome.

with anti-glomerular basement membrane (GBM) antibodies (*e.g.*, Goodpasture syndrome), Type 2—as a result of immune complex deposition (*e.g.*, SLE) and Type 3, also called pauci-immune type, is associated with ANCA and small vessel vasculitides (*e.g.*, microscopic polyangiitis).[4,10,30]

Goodpasture Syndrome. Goodpasture syndrome (Type 1) is an immune disorder with an uncommon and aggressive form of glomerulonephritis caused by antibodies to GMB. The anti-GBM antibodies cross-react with the pulmonary alveolar basement membrane to produce the syndrome of pulmonary hemorrhage associated with renal failure. The pathologic hallmark of anti-GBM glomerulonephritis is diffuse linear staining of GBMs for IgG (Fig. 33.13). The cause of the disorder is unknown, although influenza infection and exposure to hydrocarbon solvent (found in paints and dyes) have been implicated in some persons, as have various drugs and cancers. There is a high prevalence of certain human leukocyte antigen subtypes (*e.g.*, HLA-DRB1) in those affected, suggesting a genetic predisposition. Treatment includes plasmapheresis to remove circulating anti-GBM antibodies and immunosuppressive therapy (*i.e.*, corticosteroids and cyclophosphamide) to inhibit antibody production.[9,30]

Nephrotic Syndrome

The nephrotic syndrome is characterized by massive proteinuria (>3.5 g/day) and lipiduria (*e.g.*, free fat, oval bodies, fatty casts), along with an associated hypoalbuminemia (<30 g/L), generalized edema, and hyperlipidemia (cholesterol >6 mmol/L).[4,9,10] The nephrotic syndrome is not a specific glomerular disease, but a constellation of clinical findings that result from an increase in glomerular permeability and loss of plasma proteins in the urine (Fig. 33.14).

The glomerular membrane acts as a size and charge barrier through which the glomerular filtrate must pass. Any increase in permeability allows proteins to escape from the plasma into the glomerular filtrate. Massive proteinuria results leading to hypoalbuminemia. Generalized edema, which is a hallmark of the nephrotic syndrome, results from the loss of colloidal osmotic pressure of the blood with subsequent accumulation of fluid in the interstitial tissues.[9,10] There is also salt and water retention, which aggravates the edema. This appears to be due to several factors, including a compensatory increase in aldosterone, stimulation of the sympathetic nervous system, and a reduction in secretion of natriuretic factors. Initially, the edema presents in dependent parts of the body such as the lower extremities, but becomes more generalized as the disease progresses. Dyspnea due to pulmonary edema, pleural effusions, and diaphragmatic compromise due to ascites can develop in persons with nephrotic syndrome.

The hyperlipidemia that occurs in persons with nephrosis is characterized by elevated levels of triglycerides and low-density lipoproteins (LDLs). Levels of high-density lipoproteins (HDLs) usually are normal. It is thought that these abnormalities are related, at least in part, to increased synthesis of lipoproteins in the liver secondary to a compensatory increase in albumin production. Because of the elevated LDL levels, persons with nephrotic syndrome are at increased risk for development of atherosclerosis.

The largest proportion of protein lost in the urine is albumin, but globulins may be lost in some diseases. As a result, persons with nephrosis may be vulnerable to infections, particularly those caused by staphylococci and pneumococci.[10]

This decreased resistance to infection probably is related to loss of both immunoglobulins and low-molecular-weight complement components in the urine. Many binding proteins also are lost in the urine. Consequently, the plasma levels of many ions (iron, copper, zinc) and hormones (thyroid and sex hormones) may be low because of decreased binding proteins. Many drugs require protein binding for transport. Hypoalbuminemia reduces the number of available protein-binding sites, thereby producing a potential increase in the amount of free (active) drug that is available.

Thrombotic complications also have evolved as a risk in persons with nephrotic syndrome. These disorders reflect a disruption in the function of the coagulation system brought about by a loss of coagulation and anticoagulation factors. Renal vein thrombosis, once thought to be a cause of the disorder, is more likely a consequence of the hypercoagulable state.[10] Other thrombotic complications include deep vein thrombosis and pulmonary emboli.

Causes. The glomerular derangements that occur with nephrosis can develop as a primary disorder or secondary to changes caused by systemic diseases such as diabetes mellitus and SLE. Among the primary glomerular lesions leading to nephrotic syndrome are minimal-change disease (lipoid nephrosis), focal segmental glomerulosclerosis, and membranous glomerulonephritis. The relative frequency of these causes varies with age. In children younger than 17 years of age, nephrotic syndrome almost always is caused by primary idiopathic glomerular disease, whereas in adults, it often is a secondary disorder.[4,10]

Minimal-Change Disease (Lipoid Nephrosis). Minimal-change disease is characterized by diffuse loss (through fusion) of the foot processes of cells in the epithelial layer of the glomerular membrane. It is most commonly seen in children (peak incidence at 2 to 6 years of age),[10] but may occasionally occur in adults. The cause of minimal-change nephrosis is unknown. Although minimal-change disease does not progress to renal failure, it can cause significant complications, including predisposition to infection with gram-positive organisms, a tendency toward thromboembolic events, hyperlipidemia, and protein malnutrition. There usually is a dramatic response to corticosteroid therapy.[10]

Membranous Glomerulonephritis. Membranous glomerulonephritis is the most common cause of primary nephrosis in adults. The disorder is caused by diffuse thickening of the GBM due to deposition of immune complexes. The disorder may be idiopathic or associated with a number of disorders, including autoimmune diseases such as SLE and thyroiditis, infections such as chronic hepatitis B, and use of certain drugs such as gold compounds, penicillamine, and captopril. The presence of immunoglobulins and complement in the subendothelial deposits suggests that the disease represents a chronic immune complex-mediated disorder.[4,10]

The disorder usually begins with insidious onset of the nephrotic syndrome or, in a small percentage of patients, with

non-nephrotic proteinuria. Hematuria and mild hypertension may be present. The progress of the disease is variable. The nephrotic syndrome remits spontaneously in about one third of patients, and 40% progress to end stage renal failure after 10 years.[31] Spontaneous remissions and a relatively benign outcome occur more commonly in women and those with proteinuria in the non-nephrotic range. Treatment is controversial. Because of the variable course of the disease, the overall effectiveness of corticosteroids and other immunosuppressive therapy in controlling the progress of the disease has been difficult to evaluate.[4,10]

Focal Segmental Glomerulosclerosis. Focal segmental glomerulosclerosis is characterized by sclerosis (i.e., increased collagen deposition) of some but not all glomeruli, and in the affected glomeruli, only a portion of the glomerular tuft is involved. The disorder has increased in prevalence so that it now is accounting for as many as 40% of cases of nephrotic syndrome in adults.[32]

Although focal segmental sclerosis often is an idiopathic syndrome, viruses (e.g., HIV), drugs (e.g., interferon, heroin), serum permeability factors, and reduced oxygen in the blood (e.g., sickle cell disease and cyanotic congenital heart disease) are implicated as potential causes, or it may occur as a secondary event reflecting glomerular scarring due to other forms of glomerulonephritis or reflux nephropathy.[9,32]

The presence of hypertension and decreased renal function distinguishes focal sclerosis from minimal-change disease. The disorder usually is treated with corticosteroids. Most persons with the disorder progress to kidney failure within 5 to 20 years.[9]

Asymptomatic Hematuria or Proteinuria

Many cases of glomerulonephritis result in mild asymptomatic illness that is not recognized or brought to the attention of a healthcare professional, and therefore remains undiagnosed. Population-based screening studies have shown that kidney damage as evidenced by proteinuria, hematuria, low GFR, or a combination of these features is present in 16% of persons in Australia and a similar proportion in the United States.[33] Canadian data is not available, but is estimated to be similar, with an increased incidence in older adults, or those with diabetes, hypertension, or heart failure. Disorders such as Henoch–Schönlein purpura often resolve without permanent kidney damage, whereas others, such as IgA nephropathy and Alport syndrome, can progress to chronic kidney disease and renal failure.

Immunoglobulin A Nephropathy. Immunoglobulin A nephropathy (i.e., Berger disease) is a primary glomerulonephritis characterized by the presence of glomerular complement component 3 (C3) and IgA immune complex deposits. It can occur at any age, but most commonly has its onset in the second and third decades of life. The disease occurs more commonly in men than women and is the most common cause of glomerular nephritis in Asians.[4,9,34]

The disorder is characterized by the granular deposition of IgA-containing immune complexes in the mesangium of the glomerulus. Once deposited in the kidney, these complexes are associated with glomerular inflammation likely activating complement by the alternative pathway as evidence by the C3 microscopic findings. The cause of the disorder is unknown. Some persons with the disorder have elevated serum IgA levels. Recent studies have focused on potential abnormalities of the IgA molecule as a factor in the pathogenesis of the disorder.[4]

Early in the disease, many persons with the disorder have no obvious symptoms and are unaware of the problem. In these persons, IgA nephropathy is suspected during routine screening or examination for another condition. In other persons, the disorder presents with gross hematuria that is preceded by upper respiratory tract infection, gastrointestinal tract symptoms, or a flulike illness. The hematuria usually lasts 2 to 6 days. Approximately one half of the persons with gross hematuria have a single episode, whereas the remainder experience a gradual progression in the disease with recurrent episodes of hematuria and mild proteinuria. Progression usually is slow, extending over several decades.

Immunofluorescence microscopy is essential for diagnosis of IgA nephropathy.[4] The diagnostic finding is mesangial staining for IgA with C3 and occasionally IgG or IgM (Fig. 33.15). At present, there are no satisfactory treatment measures for IgA nephropathy. The role of immunosuppressive drugs such as steroids and cytotoxic drugs is not clear. There has been recent interest in the use of omega-3 fatty acids (*i.e.,* fish oil) in delaying the progression of the disease.[4]

Henoch–Schönlein Purpura Nephritis. Henoch–Schönlein purpura is a small vessel vasculitis (see Chapter 22) that causes a purpuric rash largely of the lower extremities, arthritis or arthralgia, abdominal pain, and renal involvement identical

FIGURE 33.15 • IgA nephropathy. An immunofluorescence micrograph shows deposits of IgA in the mesangial areas. (From Rubin R., Strayer D. S. (Eds.). (2012). *Rubin's pathology: Clinicopathologic foundations of medicine* (6th ed., p. 781). Philadelphia, PA: Lippincott Williams & Wilkins.)

to that of IgA nephropathy. The disease is seen most commonly in children (peak age 4 to 7 years) but can also occur in adults.[4,35,36] Renal involvement is not always present initially, but its incidence increases with time and is more common in older children who have associated abdominal pain and a persistent rash. Although hematuria and proteinuria are the most common presentation, some persons present with manifestations of acute nephritis and others may present with combined nephritis and nephrotic manifestations. Corticosteroids effectively decrease the duration and intensity of abdominal and joint pain with most persons recovering fully over a period of several weeks.

Alport Syndrome. Alport syndrome represents a hereditary defect of the GBM that results in hematuria and may progress to chronic renal failure due to the genetic mutations of type IV collagen chains.[37] Approximately 85% of cases are inherited as an X-linked autosomal dominant trait, whereas others have autosomal dominant and recessive patterns of inheritance. In X-linked pedigrees, boys are usually affected more seriously than girls. Affected boys usually progress to renal failure as adults, but progression may occur during adolescence. Although many girls never have more than mild hematuria with or without mild proteinuria, some have more significant disease and may even progress to kidney failure.[37]

Diagnosis of Alport syndrome is often made after urinalysis of a child from a family with multiple cases of hereditary nephritis. Children may initially present with heavy microscopic hematuria (large amount of blood on dipstick), followed by the development of proteinuria. Many, but not all, persons with Alport syndrome have sensorineural deafness and various eye disorders, including lens dislocation, posterior cataracts, and corneal dystrophy. The hearing loss is bilateral and often is first detected during adolescence.[37]

Chronic Glomerulonephritis

Chronic glomerulonephritis represents the chronic phase of a number of specific types of glomerulonephritis.[10] Some forms of acute glomerulonephritis (*e.g.,* poststreptococcal glomerulonephritis) undergo complete resolution, whereas others progress at variable rates to chronic glomerulonephritis. Some persons who present with chronic glomerulonephritis have no history of glomerular disease. These cases may represent the end result of relatively asymptomatic forms of glomerulonephritis. Histologically, the condition is characterized by small kidneys with sclerosed glomeruli. In most cases, chronic glomerulonephritis develops insidiously and slowly progresses to chronic kidney disease over a period of years (see Chapter 34).

Glomerular Lesions Associated With Systemic Disease

Many immunologic, metabolic, or hereditary systemic diseases are associated with glomerular injury. In some diseases, such as SLE, diabetes mellitus, and hypertension, the glomerular involvement may be a major clinical manifestation.

Systemic Lupus Erythematosus Glomerulonephritis

Renal involvement is clinically evident in 25% to 50% people with the onset of SLE and up to 60% will develop renal disease. It is seen more commonly in African or Hispanic women.[4,38] The pathogenesis of SLE (discussed in Chapter 59) is uncertain, but seems to be related to dysregulated B-cell immunity with production of autoantibodies to a variety of nuclear, cytoplasmic, extracellular matrix, and cell membrane components. Most glomerular injury is triggered by the formation of immune complexes within the glomerular capillary wall.

The clinical manifestations of lupus nephritis depend on the site of immune complex-mediated injury. Immune complexes confined to the mesangium cause less inflammation than subendothelial immune complexes, which have greater exposure to inflammatory cells and mediators in the blood, and which therefore are more likely to produce inflammation. The World Health Organization (WHO) classifies the renal glomerular lesions of SLE as class I, normal; class II, mesangial proliferation; class III, focal and segmental proliferation; class IV, diffuse proliferation; and class V, membranous proliferation.[4]

Because of the high risk for kidney disease, all persons with SLE should undergo routine urinalysis to monitor for the appearance of hematuria or proteinuria. If urinary abnormalities are noted, renal biopsy is often performed. Treatment depends on the extent of glomerular involvement. Individuals with class I or II glomerulonephritis usually require no treatment. Progression to higher classes is usually accompanied by an increase in lupus serology activity and evidence of deteriorating renal function (*i.e.,* rising serum creatinine, decrease in calculated GFR). Oral corticosteroids and angiotensin-converting enzyme (ACE) inhibitors are the mainstays of treatment. Persons with more advanced disease may require treatment with immunosuppressive agents (*e.g.,* intravenous cyclophosphamide or oral mycophenolate mofetil). Clinical trials using other immunosuppressant agents are ongoing.[4]

Diabetic Glomerulosclerosis

Diabetic nephropathy is a major cause of chronic kidney disease and the most common cause of kidney failure treated by renal replacement therapy in both Canada and the United States.[39] It occurs in both types 1 and 2 diabetes mellitus. In North America, it is more prevalent among aboriginal, black, and Asian persons. Among persons starting renal replacement therapy in Canada due to end-stage renal disease (ESRD), the incidence of diabetes and end-stage renal disease have continued to increase slowly since 1996.

The lesions of diabetic nephropathy most commonly involve the glomeruli. Widespread thickening of the glomerular capillary basement membrane occurs in almost all persons with diabetes and can occur without evidence of proteinuria. This is followed by a diffuse increase in mesangial matrix, with mild proliferation of mesangial cells. As the disease progresses, the mesangial cells impinge on the capillary lumen, reducing the surface area for glomerular filtration. In nodular glomerulosclerosis, also known as *Kimmelstiel–Wilson syndrome,* there is nodular deposition of hyaline in the mesangial portion of the glomerulus. As the sclerotic process progresses in the diffuse and nodular forms of glomerulosclerosis, there is complete obliteration of the glomerulus, with impairment of renal function.[9,10]

Although the mechanisms of glomerular change in diabetes are uncertain, they are thought to represent enhanced or defective synthesis of the GBM and mesangial matrix with an inappropriate incorporation of glucose into the noncellular components of these glomerular structures. Alternatively, hemodynamic changes that occur secondary to elevated blood glucose levels may contribute to the initiation and progression of diabetic glomerulosclerosis.[10] It has been hypothesized that elevations in blood glucose produce an increase in GFR and glomerular pressure that leads to enlargement of glomerular capillary pores by a mechanism that is, at least partly, mediated by angiotensin II. This enlargement results in an increase in the protein content of the glomerular filtrate, which in turn requires increased endocytosis of the filtered proteins by tubular endothelial cells, a process that ultimately leads to nephron destruction and progressive deterioration of renal function.

The clinical manifestations of diabetic glomerulosclerosis are closely linked to those of diabetes. The increased GFR that occurs in persons with early alterations in renal function is associated with *microalbuminuria,* defined as urinary albumin excretion of 30 to 300 mg in 24 hours.[4] Microalbuminuria is an important predictor of future diabetic nephropathies.[4,10] In many cases, these early changes in glomerular function can be reversed by careful control of blood glucose levels (see Chapter 42). Inhibition of angiotensin by ACE inhibitors or angiotensin receptor blockers (ARBs) has been shown to have a beneficial effect, possibly by reversing increased glomerular pressure. Hypertension and cigarette smoking have been implicated in the progression of diabetic nephropathy. Thus, control of blood pressure (to levels of 130/80 mm Hg or less) and smoking cessation are recommended as primary and secondary prevention strategies in persons with diabetes.[4]

Hypertensive Glomerular Disease

It is believed that mild to moderate hypertension causes sclerotic changes in renal arterioles and small arteries, referred to as *benign nephrosclerosis.* The condition has been identified in approximately 15% of persons with benign hypertension (hypertension is discussed in Chapter 23).[9,10] However it is unclear whether hypertensive nephropathy is directly associated with a number of changes in kidney structure and function or the increased pressure accelerates the rate of progression of preexisting renal disease. Usually the kidneys are smaller than normal and are usually affected bilaterally. On histologic examination, there is narrowing of the arterioles and small arteries, caused by thickening and hyalinization of the vessel walls. As the vascular structures thicken and perfusion diminishes, blood flow to the nephron decreases, causing patchy tubular atrophy, interstitial fibrosis, and a variety of changes in glomerular structure and function.[4,9,10]

Although uncomplicated hypertensive nephrosclerosis is not usually associated with significant abnormalities in renal function, a few persons may progress to end-stage renal disease. Three groups of people are at particular risk for development of renal failure: blacks, persons with more severe blood pressure elevations, and persons with a second underlying disease, such as diabetes.[10]

IN SUMMARY

Glomerulonephritis, an inflammatory process that involves glomerular structures, is the third leading cause of kidney failure after diabetes and hypertension as a cause of chronic kidney disease in Canada. The disease may occur as a primary condition in which the glomerular abnormality is the only disease present, or it may occur as a secondary condition in which the glomerular abnormality results from another disease, such as hypertension or SLE. Most cases of primary and many cases of secondary glomerular disease probably have an immune origin.

The clinical manifestations of glomerular disorders generally fall into one of five categories: the nephritic syndromes, rapidly progressive glomerulonephritis, nephrotic syndrome, asymptomatic disorders (*i.e.*, hematuria, proteinuria), and chronic glomerulonephritis. The nephritic syndrome evokes an inflammatory response in the glomeruli and is characterized by hematuria with red cell casts in the urine, a diminished GFR, azotemia, oliguria, and hypertension. The nephrotic syndrome affects the integrity of the glomerular capillary membrane and is characterized by massive proteinuria, hypoalbuminemia, generalized edema, lipiduria, and hyperlipidemia. Asymptomatic hematuria and proteinuria represent glomerular disorders that are not recognized or brought to the attention of a healthcare professional, and therefore remain undiagnosed. Chronic glomerulonephritis represents the chronic phase of a number of specific types of glomerulonephritis. Secondary causes of glomerular kidney disease include SLE, diabetes mellitus, and hypertension.

TUBULOINTERSTITIAL DISORDERS

After completing this section of the chapter, you should be able to meet the following objectives:

- Cite a definition of tubulointerstitial kidney disease.
- Differentiate between the defects in tubular function that occur in proximal and distal tubular acidosis.
- Explain the pathogenesis of kidney damage in acute and chronic pyelonephritis.
- Explain the vulnerability of the kidneys to injury caused by drugs and toxins.

Several disorders affect renal tubular structures, including the proximal and distal tubules. Most of these disorders also affect the interstitial tissue that surrounds the tubules. These disorders, sometimes are referred to as *tubulointerstitial disorders,* include acute tubular necrosis (see Chapter 34), renal tubular acidosis, acute and chronic pyelonephritis, and the effects of drugs and toxins.

Tubulointerstitial renal diseases may be divided into acute and chronic disorders. The acute disorders are characterized by their sudden onset and by signs and symptoms of interstitial edema; they include acute pyelonephritis and acute hypersensitivity reaction to drugs. The chronic disorders produce interstitial fibrosis, atrophy, and mononuclear infiltrates. Most persons are asymptomatic until late in the course of the disease. In the early stages, tubulointerstitial diseases commonly are manifested by fluid and electrolyte imbalances that reflect subtle changes in tubular function. These manifestations can include inability to concentrate urine, as evidenced by polyuria and nocturia; interference with acidification of urine, resulting in metabolic acidosis; and diminished tubular reabsorption of sodium and other substances.[10]

Renal Tubular Acidosis

Renal tubular acidosis (RTA) refers to a group of tubular defects in reabsorption of bicarbonate ions (HCO_3^-) or excretion of hydrogen ions (H^+) that result in metabolic acidosis and its subsequent complications, including metabolic bone disease, kidney stones, and growth failure in children. There are two main types of RTA: proximal tubular disorders that affect bicarbonate reabsorption, and distal tubular defects that affect the secretion of fixed metabolic acids. A third type of RTA results from aldosterone deficiency or resistance to its action that leads to impaired reabsorption of sodium ions (Na^+) with decreased elimination of H^+ and potassium ions (K^+).[39] Renal acidosis also occurs in kidney failure (see Chapter 34).

Proximal Renal Tubular Acidosis

Proximal RTA involves a defect in proximal tubular reabsorption, the nephron site where 85% of filtered HCO_3^- is reabsorbed (see Chapter 32). With the onset of impaired tubular HCO_3^- reabsorption, there is a loss of HCO_3^- in the urine that reduces plasma HCO_3^- levels. The concomitant loss of Na^+ in the urine leads to contraction of the extracellular fluid volume with increased aldosterone secretion and a resultant decrease in serum K^+ levels (see Chapter 31). With proximal tubular defects in acid-base regulation, the distal tubular sites for secretion of the fixed acids into the urine continue to function, and the reabsorption of HCO_3^- eventually resumes, albeit at a lower level of serum HCO_3^-. Whenever serum levels rise above this decreased level, HCO_3^- is lost in the urine. Persons with proximal RTA generally have plasma HCO_3^- levels greater than 15 mmol/L and seldom develop severe acidosis.[39]

Proximal RTA may occur as a hereditary or acquired disorder and may involve an isolated defect in HCO_3^- reabsorption or accompany other defects in proximal tubular function

(Fanconi syndrome). Isolated defects in HCO_3^- reabsorption are relatively rare. The term *Fanconi syndrome* is used to describe a generalized proximal tubular dysfunction in which the RTA is accompanied by excessive amounts of glucose, amino acids, phosphate, uric acid and protein in urine. Children with Fanconi syndrome are likely to have growth retardation, rickets, osteomalacia, and abnormal vitamin D metabolism in addition to mild acidosis associated with proximal RTA.[4,39]

Children and infants with proximal RTA require alkali therapy because of the high incidence of growth retardation due to acidemia. Potassium supplements are also needed because of increased loss of potassium that occurs with alkali therapy.[39] Adults may also require alkali therapy. Vitamin D and phosphate are appropriate treatments for rickets and hypophosphatemia.

Distal Renal Tubular Acidosis

Distal RTA has its origin in the distal convoluted tubule and the collecting duct, where about 15% of the filtered bicarbonate is reabsorbed. The clinical syndrome of distal RTA includes hypokalemia, hyperchloremic metabolic acidosis, inability to acidify the urine, nephrocalcinosis, and nephrolithiasis. Additional features include osteomalacia or rickets.

Distal RTA results from a distal tubular defect in H^+ secretion with failure to acidify the urine. Because the secretion of H^+ in the distal tubules is linked to sodium reabsorption, failure to secrete H^+ results in a net loss of sodium bicarbonate in the urine. This results in contraction of fluids in the extracellular fluid compartment, a compensatory increase in aldosterone levels, and development of hypokalemia. The persistent acidosis, which requires buffering by the skeletal system, causes calcium to be released from bone. Increased losses of calcium in the urine lead to increased levels of parathyroid hormone, osteomalacia, bone pain, impaired growth in children, and development of kidney stones and nephrocalcinosis.[39]

Long-term treatment of distal RTA requires alkali supplementation. Greater amounts are needed for children because of the need for base deposition in growing bone and because bicarbonate wastage is greater in children than in adults. Alkali therapy generally allows for correction of potassium wasting and hypokalemia. It also decreases the calcium concentration in the urine and increases citrate excretion, both of which serve to decrease the incidence of nephrocalcinosis and nephrolithiasis.

Pyelonephritis

Pyelonephritis refers to infection of the kidney parenchyma and renal pelvis. There are two forms of pyelonephritis: acute and chronic.

Acute Pyelonephritis

Acute pyelonephritis represents an infection of the upper urinary tract, specifically the renal parenchyma and renal pelvis. Risk factors for complicated acute pyelonephritis are those that increase the host's susceptibility or reduce the host response to infection. Persons with diabetes mellitus are at increased risk.

A less frequent and more serious type of acute pyelonephritis, called *necrotizing pyelonephritis,* is characterized by necrosis of the renal papillae. It is particularly common in persons with diabetes and may also be a complication of acute pyelonephritis when there is significant urinary tract obstruction.

Gram-negative bacteria, including *E. coli* and *Proteus, Klebsiella,* and *Enterobacter* species, are the most common causative agents. The infection usually ascends from the lower urinary tract, with the exception of *S. aureus,* which is usually spread through the bloodstream. Factors that contribute to the development of acute pyelonephritis are catheterization and urinary instrumentation, vesicoureteral reflux, pregnancy, and neurogenic bladder.[9,10]

Hematogenous acute pyelonephritis occurs most often in debilitated, chronically ill persons and those receiving immunosuppressive therapy. Immunosuppression favours the development of subclinical (silent) pyelonephritis and infections caused by nonenteric, aerobic, gram-negative rods, and *Candida.* Metastatic staphylococcal or fungal infections may spread to the kidney from distant foci in the skin or bone.

Clinical Features. Acute pyelonephritis tends to present with an abrupt onset of shaking chills, moderate to high fever, and a constant ache in the loin area of the back that is unilateral or bilateral. Lower urinary tract symptoms, including dysuria, frequency, and urgency, also are common. There may be significant malaise, and the person usually looks and feels ill. Nausea and vomiting may occur along with abdominal pain. Palpation or percussion over the costovertebral angle on the affected side usually causes pain. Pyuria occurs but is not diagnostic because it also occurs in lower UTIs. The development of necrotizing papillitis is associated with a much poorer prognosis. These persons have evidence of overwhelming sepsis with frequent development of renal failure.[1,4,10,18,19]

Acute pyelonephritis is treated with appropriate antimicrobial drugs. Unless obstruction or other complications occur, the symptoms usually disappear within several days. Treatment with an appropriate antimicrobial agent usually is continued for 7 to 14 days. Persons with complicated acute pyelonephritis and those who do not respond to outpatient treatment may require hospitalization.[4]

Chronic Pyelonephritis

Chronic pyelonephritis represents a progressive process. There is scarring and deformation of the renal calyces and pelvis[9,10] (Fig. 33.16). The disorder appears to involve a bacterial infection superimposed on obstructive abnormalities or vesicoureteral reflux. Chronic obstructive pyelonephritis is associated with recurrent bouts of inflammation and scarring, which eventually lead to chronic pyelonephritis. Reflux, which is the most common cause of chronic pyelonephritis, results from superimposition of infection on congenital vesicoureteral reflux or intrarenal reflux. Reflux may be unilateral with involvement of a single kidney or bilateral, leading to scarring and atrophy of both kidneys with the eventual development of chronic renal insufficiency.

FIGURE 33.16 • Chronic pyelonephritis. **A:** The cortical surface contains many irregular, depressed scars (reddish areas). **B:** There is marked dilation of calices caused by inflammatory destruction of papillae, with atrophy and scarring of the overlying cortex. (From Rubin R., Strayer D. S. (Eds.). (2012). *Rubin's pathology: Clinicopathologic foundations of medicine* (6th ed., p. 797). Philadelphia, PA: Lippincott Williams & Wilkins.)

Clinical Features. Chronic pyelonephritis may cause many of the same symptoms as acute pyelonephritis, or its onset may be insidious. Often there is a history of recurrent episodes of UTI or acute pyelonephritis. Loss of tubular function and the ability to concentrate urine give rise to polyuria and nocturia, and mild proteinuria is common. Severe hypertension often is a contributing factor in the progress of the disease. Chronic pyelonephritis is a significant cause of renal failure.

Drug-Related Nephropathies

Drug-related nephropathies involve functional or structural changes in the kidneys that occur after exposure to a drug. Because of their large blood flow and high filtration pressure, the kidneys are exposed to any substance that is in the blood. The kidneys also are active in the metabolic transformation of drugs and therefore are exposed to a number of toxic metabolites. The tolerance to drugs varies with age and depends on renal function, state of hydration, blood pressure, and the pH of the urine. Older adults are particularly susceptible to kidney damage caused by drugs and toxins. The dangers of nephrotoxicity are increased when two or more potentially nephrotoxic drugs or toxins are given at the same time.

Drugs and toxic substances can damage the kidneys by causing a decrease in renal blood flow, obstructing urine flow, directly damaging tubulointerstitial structures, or producing hypersensitivity reactions. Some drugs, such as diuretics, high-molecular-weight radiocontrast media, the immunosuppressive drugs cyclosporine and tacrolimus, and the nonsteroidal anti-inflammatory drugs (NSAIDs), can cause acute prerenal failure by decreasing renal blood flow[40] (see Chapter 34). Persons at particular risk are those who already have compromised renal blood flow. Other drugs such as sulfonamides and vitamin C (due to oxalate crystals) can form crystals that cause kidney damage by obstructing urinary flow in the tubules. Also aminoglycosides (*e.g.,* gentamicin, tobramycin, amikacin) and glycopeptides (*e.g.,* vancomycin) are known to cause nephrotoxicity and acute renal failure (Chapter 34).

Acute drug-related hypersensitivity reactions produce tubulointerstitial nephritis, with damage to the tubules and interstitium. This condition was observed initially in persons who were sensitive to the sulfonamide drugs; currently, it is observed most often with the use of methicillin and other synthetic antibiotics, and with the use of furosemide and the thiazide diuretics in persons sensitive to these drugs. The condition begins approximately 15 days (range, 2 to 40 days) after exposure to the drug.[10] At the onset, there is fever, eosinophilia, hematuria, mild proteinuria, and in approximately one fourth of cases, a rash. In approximately 50% of cases, signs and symptoms of acute renal failure develop. Withdrawal of the drug commonly is followed by complete recovery, but there may be permanent damage in some persons, usually in older persons. Drug nephritis may not be recognized in its early stage because it is relatively uncommon.

Chronic analgesic nephritis, which is associated with analgesic abuse, causes interstitial nephritis with renal papillary necrosis. When first observed, it was attributed to phenacetin, a then-common ingredient of over-the-counter medications containing aspirin, phenacetin, and caffeine. Although phenacetin is no longer contained in these preparations, it has been suggested that other ingredients, such as aspirin and acetaminophen, may also contribute to the disorder. How much analgesic it takes to produce papillary necrosis is unknown. NSAIDs also have the potential for damaging renal structures, including medullary interstitial cells. Prostaglandins (particularly PGI_2 and PGE_2) contribute to the regulation of tubular blood flow. The deleterious effects of NSAIDs on the kidney are thought to result from their ability to inhibit prostaglandin synthesis. Persons particularly at risk are the elderly because of age-related changes in renal function, individuals who are dehydrated or have a decrease in blood volume, and those with pre-existing kidney disease or renal insufficiency.

IN SUMMARY

Tubulointerstitial diseases affect the tubules and the surrounding interstitium of the kidneys. These disorders include renal tubular acidosis, acute and chronic pyelonephritis, and the effects of drugs and toxins. Renal tubular acidosis describes a form of systemic acidosis that results from tubular defects in bicarbonate reabsorption or hydrogen ion secretion. Pyelonephritis, or infection of the kidney and kidney pelvis, can occur as an acute or a chronic condition. Acute pyelonephritis typically is caused by ascending bladder infections or infections that come from the bloodstream; it usually is successfully treated with appropriate antimicrobial drugs. Chronic pyelonephritis is a progressive disease that produces scarring and deformation of the renal calyces and pelvis. Drug-induced impairment of tubulointerstitial structure and function usually is the result of direct toxic injury, decreased blood flow, or hypersensitivity reactions.

MALIGNANT TUMOURS OF THE KIDNEY

After completing this section of the chapter, you should be able to meet the following objectives:

- Characterize Wilms tumour in terms of age of onset, possible oncogenic origin, manifestations, and treatment.
- Cite the risk factors for renal cell carcinoma, describe its manifestations, and explain why the 5-year survival rate has been so low.

There are two major groups of malignant tumours of the kidney: embryonic kidney tumours (*i.e.,* Wilms tumour), which occur during childhood, and renal cell carcinoma, which occurs in adults.

Wilms Tumour

Wilms tumour (nephroblastoma) is one of the most common primary neoplasms of young children. It usually presents between 2 and 5 years of age and is the most common malignant abdominal tumour in children.[9,41] It may occur in one or both kidneys; the incidence of bilateral Wilms tumour is 7%.[41]

Histologically, the tumour is composed of elements that resemble normal fetal tissue: blastemic, stromal, and epithelial. An important feature of Wilms tumour is its association

FIGURE 33.17 • Wilms tumour. A cross-section of a pale tan neoplasm attached to a residual portion of the kidney. (From Rubin R., Strayer D. S. (Eds.). (2012). *Rubin's pathology: Clinicopathologic foundations of medicine* (6th ed., p. 805). Philadelphia, PA: Lippincott Williams & Wilkins.)

with other congenital anomalies, including aniridia (absence of the iris), hemihypertrophy (enlargement of one side of the face or body), and other congenital anomalies, usually of the genitourinary system. Several chromosomal abnormalities have been associated with Wilms tumour. One Wilms tumour gene, *WT1,* which is located on chromosome 11, encodes a transcription factor that is critical for normal kidney development. Roughly 10% to 20% of all Wilms tumours carry *WT1* mutations.[41]

Wilms tumour usually is a solitary mass that occurs in any part of the kidney. It usually is sharply demarcated and variably encapsulated (Fig. 33.17). The tumours grow to a large size, distorting kidney structure. The tumours usually are staged using the National Wilms' Tumour Study Group classification.[41] Stage I tumours are limited to the kidney and can be excised with the capsular surface intact. Stage II tumours extend into the renal capsule but can be excised. In stage III, extension of the tumour occurs but is confined to the abdomen, and in stage IV, hematogenous metastasis most commonly involves the lung.

The common presenting signs are a large asymptomatic abdominal mass and hypertension.[10,41] The tumour is often discovered inadvertently, and it is not uncommon for the mother to discover it while bathing the child. Some children may present with abdominal pain, vomiting, or both. Microscopic and gross hematuria is present in 15% to 25% of children. CT scans are used to confirm the diagnosis.[41]

Treatment involves surgery, chemotherapy, and sometimes radiation therapy. Long-term survival rates have increased to more than 70% for all stages and to 89% to 96% for stages I through III.[41]

Renal Cell Carcinoma

Cancer of the kidney in Canada is the 6th leading malignancy among men and the 11th among women, increasing each year about 2.6% for males and 1.9% for females.[42] Renal cell carcinoma is more common in males (2:1 ratio) and typically presents after the age of 50 with a median age of 60 years.[43] The increased use of imaging procedures such as ultrasonography, CT scanning, and magnetic resonance imaging (MRI) has contributed significantly to earlier diagnosis and more accurate staging of kidney cancers.[4,43]

Renal cell carcinoma accounts for approximately 80% to 90% of kidney tumours.[9] The tumour may arise from any portion of the kidney, but most commonly affects the poles, most commonly the upper pole (Fig. 33.18). The cause of renal cell carcinoma remains unclear. Epidemiologic evidence suggests correlation between the risk factors of heavy smoking, obesity or hypertension and the development of kidney cancer. The risk for renal cell carcinoma also is increased in persons with acquired cystic kidney disease associated with chronic renal insufficiency.[9,43]

There are pathologic variants of renal cell carcinoma that reflect differences in cellular pathology, genetic profile, and clinical features ranging from benign to highly malignant. Categories include clear cell carcinoma (70% to 80% of cases), papillary tumours (105% to 15%), chromophobic tumours (53% to 105%), oncocytomas (2% to 4%), and collecting duct tumours (<1%).[4,43] Clear cell tumours have a clear cytoplasm, usually show chromosome 3 deletion, and arise from proximal tubular epithelial cells. Papillary renal cell tumours tend to be bilateral and multifocal, show trisomy 7 or 17, and arise from proximal tubular cells. Chromophobic tumours are characterized by multiple chromosomal losses but do not exhibit 3 deletions or trisomy 7 or 17, have an indolent clinical course, and appear to arise from intercalated cells of the collecting tubules. Collecting duct tumours arise from the collecting ducts within the renal medulla, are very rare, affect younger individuals, and are very aggressive. Oncocytomas do not exhibit chromosomal changes and are considered benign.[4,9,43]

Kidney cancer is largely a silent disorder during its early stages, and symptoms usually denote advanced disease. The classic triad of hematuria, flank pain, and presence of a palpable flank mass occurs in fewer than 10% of cases. Gross or microscopic hematuria is usually observed only when the tumour has invaded the collecting system.[4] It is, however, intermittent and may be microscopic; as a result, the tumour may reach considerable size before it is detected. Because of the widespread use of ultrasonography and CT scanning for diverse indications, renal tumours are being detected incidentally in persons with no urologic symptoms.

Kidney cancer is suspected when there are findings of hematuria and a renal mass. Ultrasonography and CT scanning are used to confirm the diagnosis. MRI may be used when involvement of the inferior vena cava is suspected. Renal cancer is commonly staged using the global International Union Against Cancer (UICC) system described in Chapter 8.[44]

Surgery (radical nephrectomy with lymph node dissection) is the treatment of choice for all resectable tumours. Nephron-sparing surgery may be done when both kidneys are involved or when the contralateral kidney is threatened by an associated disease such as hypertension or diabetes mellitus. Single-agent and combination chemotherapies have been used with limited success. Immunotherapy involving interferon-alfa and interleukin-2 had been used with some success but the newer vascular endothelial growth factor (VEGF) inhibiting drugs (*e.g.,* sunitinib, sorafenib) are preferred. The 5-year survival rate is 90% if the tumour has not extended beyond the renal capsule, but drops to 20% if metastasis has occurred.[44]

FIGURE 33.18 • Gross pathology of bisected kidney showing large renal cell carcinoma. Much of the kidney has been replaced by grey and yellow tumour tissue. A little remaining renal cortex and pericapsular fat are visible at the bottom of this surgical specimen. (From Centers for Disease Control and Prevention Public Images Library. Available online at: http://phil.cdc.gov/phil/details.asp.)

IN SUMMARY

There are two major groups of renal neoplasms: embryonic kidney tumours (*i.e.,* Wilms tumour) that occur during childhood and adult renal cell carcinomas. Wilms tumour is one of the most common malignant tumours that occur in children. The most common presenting signs are a large abdominal mass and hypertension. Treatment is surgery, chemotherapy, and sometimes radiation therapy. The long-term survival rate for children with Wilms tumour is approximately 90%, with an aggressive plan of treatment.

Renal cancer typically presents after the age of 50 and accounts for about 2% to 3% of all cancers. Renal cell carcinoma accounts for 80% to 90% of kidney tumours. These tumours are characterized by a lack of early warning signs, diverse clinical manifestations, and resistance to chemotherapy and radiation therapy. Because of the widespread use of ultrasonography and CT scanning for diverse indications, renal tumours are being detected incidentally in persons with no urologic symptoms. Diagnostic methods include ultrasonography and CT scans. The treatment of choice is surgical resection. Prognosis depends on the stage of the cancer; the 5-year survival rate is 90% if the tumour has not extended beyond the renal capsule, but drops to considerably if metastasis has occurred.

REVIEW EXERCISES

1. A 36-year-old man is admitted to the emergency department with a sudden onset of severe, intermittent, cramping pain that makes him feel nauseated. He describes the pain as originating in the left groin and radiating toward the flank. Microscopic examination of his urine reveals the presence of red blood cells. His temperature is normal, and he does not exhibit signs of sepsis.
   A. *What is the probable cause of this man's pain?*
   B. *What diagnostic measure could be used to confirm the cause of his pain?*
   C. *A plain-film radiograph reveals a 4 to 5 mm kidney stone in the left ureter. What are the chances that this man will pass the stone spontaneously?*
   D. *What type of medications and other treatments should this man receive?*
   E. *Once the stone has been passed, what type of measures can he use to prevent stone recurrence?*

2. A 6-year-old boy is diagnosed with acute glomerulonephritis that developed after a streptococcal throat infection. At this time, the following manifestations are noted: a decrease in urine output, increasing lethargy, hyperventilation, and generalized edema. Trace amounts of protein are detected in his urine. Blood analysis reveals the following: pH = 7.35, HCO_3 = 18 mmol/L, hematocrit = 29%, Na = 132 mmol/L, K = 5.6 mmol/L, urea (BUN) = 21 mmol/L, creatinine = 86 µmol/L, and albumin = 20 g/L.
   A. *What is the probable cause of this boy's glomerular disease?*
   B. *Use the laboratory values in the Appendix to interpret his laboratory test results. Which values are significant and why?*
   C. *Is he progressing to uremia? How can you tell?*

3. A 26-year-old woman makes an appointment with her healthcare provider, complaining of urinary frequency, urgency, and burning. She reports that her urine is cloudy and smells abnormal. Her urine is cultured, and she is given a prescription for antibiotics.
   A. *What is the most likely cause of the woman's symptoms?*
   B. *What microorganism is most likely responsible for the infection?*
   C. *What factors may have predisposed her to this disorder?*
   D. *What could this woman do to prevent future infection?*

References

1. Nicolle L. E. (2008). Uncomplicated urinary tract infection in adults including uncomplicated pyelonephritis. *Urologic Clinics of North America, 35*(1), 1–12.
2. Kidney Foundation of Canada. (2013). Kidney stones. Available online at: http://www.kidney.ca/page.aspx?pid=328. Accessed May 24, 2014.
3. Schedl A. (2007). Renal abnormalities and their developmental origin. *Nature Reviews Genetics, 8*(10), 791–802.
4. Taal M. W., Chertow G. M., Marden P. A., et al. (Eds). (2012). *Brenner and Rector's the kidney* (9th ed.). Philadelphia, PA: Elsevier Saunders.
5. Underwood M. A., Gilbert W. M., Sherman M. P. (2005). Amniotic fluid: Not just fetal urine anymore. *Journal of Perinatology, 25*, 341–348.
6. Moore K. L., Persaud T. V., Torchia M. G. (2013). *The developing human: Clinical oriented embryology* (9th ed.). Philadelphia, PA: Saunders Elsevier.
7. Loftus H., Ong A. C. (2013). Cystic kidney diseases: Many ways to form a cyst. *Pediatric Nephrology, 28*(1), 33–49.
8. Harris P. S., Torres V. E. (2009). Polycystic kidney disease. *Annual Review of Medicine, 60*, 321–337.
9. Rubin R., Strayer D. S. (Eds.). (2012). *Rubin's pathology: Clinicopathologic foundations of medicine* (6th ed.). Philadelphia, PA: Lippincott Williams & Wilkins.
10. Alpers C. E. (2010). Chapter 20: The kidney. In Kumar V., Abbas A. K., Fausto N., et al. (Eds.), *Robbins and Cotran pathologic basis of disease* (8th ed.). Philadelphia, PA: Elsevier Saunders.
11. Meijer E., Boertien W. E., Nauta F. L., et al. (2010). Association of urinary biomarkers with disease severity in patients with ADPKD. *American Journal of Kidney Diseases, 56*(5), 883–895.
12. Torres V. E., Chapman A. B., Devuyst O., et al. (2010). Tolvaptan inpatients with autosomal dominant polycystic kidney disease. *New England Journal of Medicine, 367*, 2407–2418.
13. Sakhaee K., Maalouf N. M., Sinnott B. (2012). Kidney stones 2012: Pathogenesis, diagnosis, and management. *Journal of Clinical Endocrinology and Metabolism, 97*(6), 1847–1860.
14. Frassetto L., Kohlstadt I. (2011). Treatment and prevention of kidney stones: An update. *American Family Physician, 84*(11), 1234–1242.
15. Sakhaee K. (2014). Epidemiology and clinical pathophysiology of uric acid kidney stones. *Journal of Nephrology, 27*(3), 241–245.
16. Xu H., Zisman A. L., Coe F. L., et al. (2013). Kidney stones: An update on current pharmacological management and future directions. *Expert Opinion in Pharmacotherapy, 14*(4), 435–447.
17. Worcester E. M., Coe F. L. (2010). Calcium kidney stones. *New England Journal of Medicine, 363*(10), 954–963.
18. Dielubanza E. J., Schaeffer A. J. (2011). Urinary tract infections in women. *Medical Clinical of North America, 95*(1), 27–41.
19. Raynor M. C., Carson C. C. (2011). Urinary infections in men. *Medical Clinical of North America, 95*(1), 43–54.
20. Woodford H. J., George J. (2011). Diagnosis and management of urinary infections in older people. *Clinical Medicine, 11*(1), 80–83.

21. McAninch J. W., Lue T. F. (2013). *Smith & Tanagho's general urology* (18th ed.). New York: McGraw Hill.

22. Nicolle L. E. (2012). Urinary catheter-associated infections. *Infectious Disease Clinics of North America, 26*(1), 13–27.

23. White B. (2011). Diagnosis and treatment of urinary tract infections in children. *American Family Physician, 83*(4), 409–415.

24. Jepson R. G., Williams G., Craig J. C. (2013). Cranberries for preventing urinary tract infections. *Cochrane Library, 2012*(10), CD001321.

25. Mittal P., Wing D. A. (2005). Urinary tract infections in pregnancy. *Clinics in Perinatology, 32*(3), 749–764.

26. Elder J. S. (2011). Chapter 532: Urinary tract infections. In Kliegman R. M., Stanton B. F., St Geme J. W., et al. (Eds.), *Nelson textbook of pediatrics* (19th ed.). Philadelphia, PA: Elsevier Saunders.

27. Mohajer M. A., Darouiche R. O. (2013). Prevention and treatment of urinary catheter-associated infections. *Current Infectious Disease Report, 15*(2), 116–123.

28. Kidney Foundation of Canada. (2014). Common causes of chronic kidney disease. Available online at: http://www.kidney.ca/page.aspx?pid=321. Accessed May 27, 2014.

29. Kanjanabuch T., Kittikowit W., Eiam-Ong S. (2009). An update on acute postinfectious glomerulonephritis worldwide. *Nature Reviews Nephrology, 5*(5), 259–269.

30. Moroni G., Ponticelli C. (2014). Rapidly progressive crescentic glomerulonephritis: Early treatment is a must. *Autoimmunity Reviews, 13*(7), 723–729.

31. Ronco P., Debiec H. (2010). Membranous glomerulopathy: The evolving story. *Current Opinion in Nephrology & Hypertension, 19*(3), 254–253.

32. D'Agati V. D., Kaskel F. J., Falk R. J. (2011). Focal segmental glomerulosclerosis. *New England Journal of Medicine, 365*(25), 2398–2411.

33. Chadban S. J., Briganti E. M., Kerr P. G., et al. (2003). Prevalence of kidney damage in Australian adults: The AusDiab kidney study. *Journal of the American Society of Nephrology, 14*(Suppl 2), S131–S138.

34. Kiryluk K., Novak J., Gharavi A. G. (2013). Pathogenesis of Immunoglobulin A nephropathy. *Annual Review of Medicine, 64*, 339–356.

35. Reamy B. V., Williams P. M., Lindsay T. (2009). Henoch–Schonlein purpura. *American Family Physician, 80*(7), 697–704.

36. Punnoose A. R., Lynm C., Golub R. M. (2012). Henoch-Schonlein purpura patient page. *Journal of American Medical Association, 307*(7), 742.

37. Heidet L., Gubler M. (2009). The renal lesions of Alport syndrome. *Journal of the American Society of Nephrology, 20*(6), 1210–1215.

38. Canadian Institute for Health Information. (2014). Treatment of end-stage organ failure in Canada 2003-2012. Available online at: https://secure.cihi.ca/free_products/2014_CORR_Annual_Report_EN.pdf. Accessed May 28, 2014.

39. Basu G., Sudhakar G., Mohapatra A. (2013). Renal tubular acidosis. *Clinical queries: Nephrology, 2*(4), 166–178.

40. John R., Herzenberg A. M. (2009). Renal toxicity of therapeutic drugs. *Journal of Clinical Pathology, 62*(6), 505–515.

41. Anderson P. M., Dhamne C. A., Huff V. (2011). Chapter 493: Neoplasms of the kidney. In Kliegman R. M., Stanton B. F., St Geme J. W., et al. (Eds.), *Nelson textbook of pediatrics* (19th ed.). Philadelphia, PA: Elsevier Saunders.

42. Canadian Cancer Society's Advisory Committee on Cancer Statistics. (2013). *Canadian cancer statistics 2013.* Toronto, ON.

43. Rini B. I., Campbell S. C., Escudier B. (2009). Renal cell carcinoma. *Lancet, 373*(9669), 1119–1132.

44. Canadian Cancer Society. Kidney cancer. (2014). Available online at: http://www.cancer.ca/en/cancer-information/cancer-type/kidney/kidney-cancer/?region=on. Accessed May 28, 2014.

Visit thePoint **http://thePoint.lww.com for animations, journal articles, and more!**

Acute Renal Injury and Chronic Kidney Disease

34

Renal failure is a condition in which the kidneys fail to remove metabolic end products from the blood and regulate the fluid, electrolyte, and pH balance of the extracellular fluids. The underlying cause may be renal disease, systemic disease, or urologic defects of nonrenal origin. Renal failure can occur as an acute or a chronic disorder. Acute renal failure is abrupt in onset and often is reversible if recognized early and treated appropriately. In contrast, chronic kidney disease (CKD) is the end result of irreparable damage to the kidneys. It develops slowly, usually over the course of a number of years.

ACUTE RENAL INJURY

After completing this section of the chapter, you should be able to meet the following objectives:

- Describe the causes, treatment, and outcomes of acute and chronic renal failure.
- Differentiate the prerenal, intrinsic, and postrenal forms of acute renal injury in terms of the mechanisms of development and manifestations.
- Cite the two most common causes of acute tubular necrosis (ATN) and describe the course of the disease in terms of the initiation, maintenance, and recovery phases.

Acute renal injury (formally known as acute renal failure) is a syndrome characterized by a rapid decline in kidney function sufficient to increase blood levels of nitrogenous wastes and impair fluid and electrolyte balance whereas acute renal failure is now limited to situations in the acute setting requiring renal replacement therapy.[1–8] Unlike CKD and failure, acute renal injury is potentially reversible if the precipitating factors can be corrected or removed before permanent kidney damage has occurred.

Acute renal injury is a common threat to seriously ill persons in intensive care units, with a reported hospital mortality rate ranging from 40% to 90% in the United States and a worldwide mortality of approximately 2 million people.[1,2,7] Although treatment methods such as dialysis and renal replacement therapies are effective in correcting life-threatening fluid and electrolyte disorders, the mortality rate from acute renal injury remains virtually unchanged for the past 50 years.[5] This

ACUTE RENAL INJURY

- Acute renal injury is caused by conditions that produce an acute decrease in or cessation of renal function.
- It can result from decreased blood flow to the kidney (prerenal), disorders that disrupt the structures in the kidney (intrinsic or intrarenal), or disorders that interfere with the elimination of urine from the kidney (postrenal).
- Acute renal injury, although it causes an accumulation of products normally cleared by the kidney, is a potentially reversible process if the factors causing the condition can be corrected.

CHART 34.1   CAUSES OF ACUTE RENAL INJURY

Prerenal
Hypovolemia
   Hemorrhage
   Dehydration
   Excessive loss of gastrointestinal tract fluids
   Excessive loss of fluid due to burn injury
Decreased vascular filling
   Anaphylactic shock
   Septic shock
Heart failure or cardiogenic shock
Hepatorenal syndrome
Decreased renal perfusion due to sepsis, vasoactive
   mediators, drugs, diagnostic agents

Intrinsic or Intrarenal
Acute tubular necrosis
   Prolonged renal ischemia
   Exposure to nephrotoxic drugs, heavy metals, and
     organic solvents
   Intratubular obstruction and tubular injury resulting
     from hemoglobinuria, myoglobinuria, myeloma
     light chains, or uric acid casts
Acute interstitial nephritis
   Allergic reaction to a variety of drugs including
     antibiotics
Acute glomerulonephritis
Renovascular causes
   Large-vessel involvement such as renal artery throm-
     bosis or stenosis
   Small-vessel involvement such as thrombotic throm-
     bocytopenia purpura, hemolytic uremic syndrome,
     scleroderma renal crisis (rare), etc.

Postrenal
Bilateral ureteral obstruction
Bladder outlet obstruction
Prostatic hyperplasia

---

probably is because acute renal injury is seen more often than before in older persons, and because it frequently superimposed on other life-threatening conditions, such as trauma, shock, and sepsis and comorbidities such as cardiovascular disease, diabetes, and respiratory disease.

The most common indicator of acute renal injury is *azotemia,* an accumulation of nitrogenous wastes (urea nitrogen, uric acid, and creatinine) in the blood, and a decrease in the glomerular filtration rate (GFR). As a result, excretion of nitrogenous wastes is reduced and fluid and electrolyte balance cannot be maintained.

Types of Acute Renal Injury

Acute renal injury can be caused by several types of conditions, including a decrease in blood flow without ischemic injury; ischemic, toxic, or obstructive tubular injury; and obstruction of urinary tract outflow. The causes of acute renal injury commonly are categorized as prerenal, intrinsic, and postrenal[1–8] (Fig. 34.1). Collectively, prerenal and intrinsic

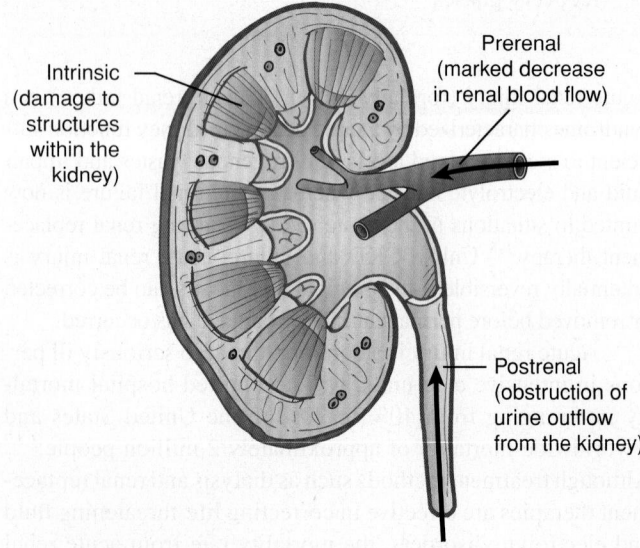

Intrinsic (damage to structures within the kidney)

Prerenal (marked decrease in renal blood flow)

Postrenal (obstruction of urine outflow from the kidney)

FIGURE 34.1 • Types of acute renal failure.

causes account for 80% to 95% of acute renal injury cases.[6] Causes of renal injury within these categories are summarized in Chart 34.1.

Prerenal Injury

Prerenal injury, the most common form of acute renal injury, is characterized by a marked decrease in renal blood flow. It is reversible if the cause of the decreased renal blood flow can be identified and corrected before kidney damage occurs. Causes of prerenal injury include profound depletion of vascular volume (*e.g.,* hemorrhage, loss of extracellular fluid volume), impaired perfusion due to heart failure and cardiogenic shock, and decreased vascular filling because of increased vascular capacity (*e.g.,* anaphylaxis or sepsis). Older adults are particularly at risk because of their predisposition to hypovolemia and their high prevalence of renal vascular disorders.

Some vasoactive mediators, drugs, and diagnostic agents stimulate intense intrarenal vasoconstriction and may induce glomerular hypoperfusion and prerenal injury. Examples include endotoxins, radiocontrast agents such as those used for cardiac catheterization, cyclosporine (an immunosuppressant drug that is used to prevent transplant rejection), amphotericin B (an antifungal agent), and oral administration of phosphate solution (bowel cathartic) prior to colonoscopy or bowel surgery.[6] Many of these drugs may also cause ATN (discussed later). In addition, several commonly used classes of drugs impair renal adaptive mechanisms and can convert compensated renal hypoperfusion into prerenal injury. Angiotensin-converting enzyme (ACE) inhibitors and angiotensin receptor blockers (ARBs) reduce the effects of renin on renal blood flow; when combined with diuretics, they may cause prerenal injury in persons with decreased blood flow due to large-vessel or small-vessel kidney disease. Prostaglandins have a vasodilatory effect on renal blood vessels. Nonsteroidal anti-inflammatory drugs (NSAIDs) may reduce renal blood flow through inhibition of prostaglandin synthesis and may precipitate prerenal injury in persons with diminished renal perfusion.[1,6,7]

Normally, the kidneys receive 20% to 25% of the cardiac output. This large blood supply is required to remove metabolic wastes and regulate body fluids and electrolytes. Fortunately, the normal kidney can tolerate relatively large reductions in blood flow before renal damage occurs. As renal blood flow is reduced, the GFR decreases, the amount of sodium and other substances that are filtered by the glomeruli is reduced, and the need for energy-dependent mechanisms to reabsorb these substance is also reduced (see Chapter 30). As the GFR and urine output approach zero, oxygen consumption by the kidney approximates that required to keep renal tubular cells alive. When blood flow falls below this level, which is about 25% of normal, ischemic changes occur.[9] Because of their high metabolic rate, the tubular epithelial cells are most vulnerable to ischemic injury. Improperly treated, prolonged renal hypoperfusion can lead to ischemic tubular necrosis with significant morbidity and mortality.

Prerenal injury is manifested by a sharp decrease in urine output and a disproportionate elevation of serum urea in relation to creatinine levels. The kidney normally responds to a decrease in the GFR with a decrease in urine output. Thus, an early sign of prerenal injury is a sharp decrease in urine output. When faced with decreased renal blood flow, the renal tubules respond appropriately by retaining sodium. Water follows sodium in the kidneys, so sodium retention leads to overall fluid volume expansion in an effort to improve renal blood flow. Sodium retention by the kidney can be measured by the "fractional excretion of sodium" ([urinary sodium × serum creatinine/serum sodium × urinary creatinine] × 100). A low fractional excretion of sodium (<1%) suggests that oliguria is due to decreased renal perfusion. A fractional excretion of sodium >1% in the setting of acute kidney injury is suggestive of acute tubular injury. The serum markers of renal filtration function

are handled differently by the renal tubules. Urea is reabsorbed along with sodium whereas creatinine is not reabsorbed and in fact is secreted by the tubules into the urine. Therefore, in the setting of prerenal acute kidney injury where the tubules are avidly reabsorbing sodium, there will be a disproportionate elevation in the ratio of serum urea to serum creatinine, from a normal value of 40:1 to a ratio greater than 100:1.

Intrinsic Renal Injury

Intrinsic or intrarenal renal injury results from conditions that cause damage to structures within the kidney—glomerular, tubular, interstitium, or blood vessels.[6,7] The major causes of intrarenal injury are ischemia associated with prerenal injury, toxic insult to the tubular structures of the nephron, and intratubular obstruction. Acute interstitial nephritis can occur as a result of an allergic inflammatory response to medication. Acute glomerulonephritis is a rare intrarenal cause of injury. Even more rare is acute renal failure caused by injury to the small blood vessels of the kidney by diseases such as hemolytic uremic syndrome. Injury to the tubular structures of the nephron (ATN) is the most common cause and often is ischemic or toxic in origin.

Acute Tubular Necrosis. ATN is characterized by the destruction of tubular epithelial cells with acute reduction of renal function (Fig. 34.2). ATN can be caused by a variety of conditions, including acute tubular damage due to ischemia,

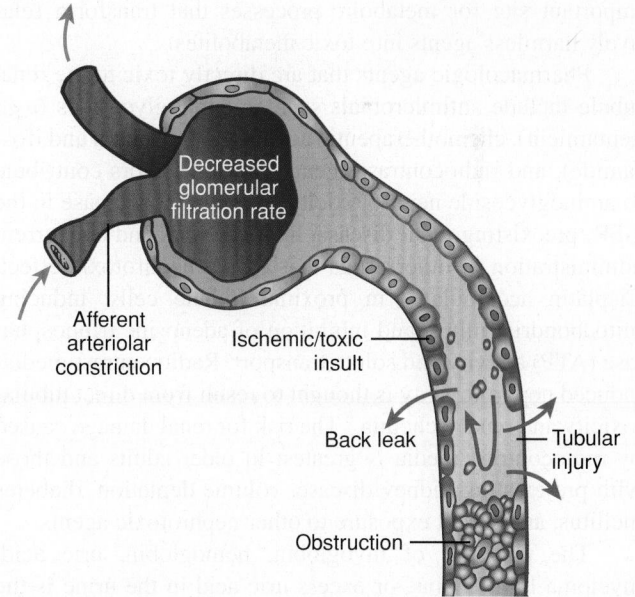

FIGURE 34.2 • Pathogenesis of AKI caused by acute tubular injury (ATN). Sloughing and necrosis of tubular epithelial cells lead to obstruction and increased intraluminal pressure, which reduce glomerular filtration. Afferent arteriolar vasoconstriction caused in part by tubuloglomerular feedback mechanisms results in decreased glomerular capillary filtration pressure. Tubular injury and increased intraluminal pressure cause fluid to move from the tubular lumen into the interstitium (back leak). (From Rubin R., Strayer D. S. (Eds.). (2012). *Rubin's Pathology: Clinicopathologic foundations of medicine* (6th ed., p. 792). Philadelphia, PA: Lippincott Williams & Wilkins.)

sepsis, nephrotoxic effects of drugs, tubular obstruction, rhabdomyolysis, and toxins from infection related sepsis.[1-8] Tubular epithelial cells are particularly sensitive to ischemia and also are vulnerable to toxins. The tubular injury that occurs in ATN frequently is reversible. The process depends on recovery of the injured cells, removal of the necrotic cells and intratubular casts, and regeneration of renal cells to restore the normal continuity of the tubular epithelium.[6,7]

Ischemic ATN occurs most frequently in persons who have had major surgery, severe hypovolemia, or overwhelming sepsis, trauma, or burns.[6] Sepsis produces ischemia by provoking a combination of systemic vasodilation and intrarenal hypoperfusion. In addition, sepsis results in the generation of toxins that sensitize renal tubular cells to the damaging effects of ischemia. ATN that complicates trauma and burns is frequently multifactorial in origin, resulting from the combined effects of hypovolemia, myoglobinuria, and from other toxins released from damaged tissue. In contrast to prerenal injury, the GFR does not improve with the restoration of renal blood flow in acute renal injury caused by ischemic ATN.

Nephrotoxic ATN complicates the administration of or exposure to many structurally diverse drugs and other nephrotoxic agents. These agents cause tubular injury by inducing varying combinations of renal vasoconstriction, direct tubular damage, or intratubular obstruction. The kidney is particularly vulnerable to nephrotoxic injury because of its rich blood supply and ability to concentrate toxins to high levels in the medullary portion of the kidney. In addition, the kidney is an important site for metabolic processes that transform relatively harmless agents into toxic metabolites.

Pharmacologic agents that are directly toxic to the renal tubule include antimicrobials such as aminoglycosides (*e.g.,* gentamicin), chemotherapeutic agents (*e.g.,* cisplatin and ifosfamide), and radiocontrast agents. Several factors contribute to aminoglycoside nephrotoxicity, including a decrease in the GFR, preexisting renal disease, hypovolemia, and concurrent administration of other drugs that have a nephrotoxic effect. Cisplatin accumulates in proximal tubule cells, inducing mitochondrial injury and inhibition of adenosine triphosphatase (ATP) activity and solute transport. Radiocontrast media-induced nephrotoxicity is thought to result from direct tubular toxicity and renal ischemia.[6] The risk for renal damage caused by radiocontrast media is greatest in older adults and those with pre-existing kidney disease, volume depletion, diabetes mellitus, and recent exposure to other nephrotoxic agents.

The presence of myoglobin, hemoglobin, uric acid, myeloma light chains, or excess uric acid in the urine is the most frequent cause of ATN due to intratubular obstruction. Both myeloma cast nephropathy and acute urate nephropathy usually are seen in the setting of widespread malignancy or massive tumour destruction by therapeutic agents.[6] Hemoglobinuria results from blood transfusion reactions and other hemolytic crises. Skeletal and cardiac muscles contain myoglobin, which corresponds to hemoglobin in function, serving as an oxygen reservoir in the muscle fibres. Myoglobin normally is not found in the serum or urine. If it is released

into the circulation, it is rapidly filtered in the glomerulus as it has a low molecular weight of 17,000 daltons. Myoglobinuria most commonly results from muscle trauma, but may result from extreme exertion, hyperthermia, sepsis, prolonged seizures, potassium or phosphate depletion, and alcoholism or drug abuse. A potentially life-threatening condition, known as *rhabdomyolysis,* occurs when increased myoglobinuria levels cause myoglobin to precipitate in the renal tubules, leading to obstruction and damage to surrounding tubular cells.[10] Both myoglobin and hemoglobin discolour the urine, which may range from the colour of tea, which is most commonly associated with myoglobin, to red, brown, or black.

The course of ATN can be divided into three phases: the onset or initiating phase, the maintenance phase, and the recovery or convalescent phase. The *onset* or *initiating phase,* which lasts hours or days, is the time from the onset of the precipitating event (*e.g.,* ischemic phase of prerenal injury or toxin exposure) until tubular injury occurs.

The *maintenance phase* of ATN is characterized by a marked decrease in the GFR, causing sudden retention of endogenous metabolites, such as urea, hydrogen ions, potassium, sulphate, and creatinine, that normally are cleared by the kidneys. The urine output usually is lowest at this point. Fluid retention gives rise to edema, water intoxication, and pulmonary congestion. If the period of oliguria is prolonged, hypertension frequently develops and with it signs of uremia. Renal replacement therapy should be initiated in this phase. When untreated, the neurologic manifestations of uremia progress from neuromuscular irritability to seizures, somnolence, coma, and death. Hyperkalemia usually is asymptomatic until the serum potassium level rises above 6.0 mmol/L, at which point characteristic electrocardiographic changes and symptoms of muscle weakness may be seen.

Formerly, most patients with ATN were considered to be oliguric (*i.e.,* urine output <400 ml/day). During the past several decades, a nonoliguric form (*i.e.,* urine output of >400 ml/day) of ATN has become increasingly prevalent. Persons with nonoliguric injury have higher levels of glomerular filtration and excrete more nitrogenous waste, water, and electrolytes in their urine than persons with acute oliguric renal injury. Abnormalities in blood chemistry levels usually are milder and cause fewer complications. The decrease in oliguric ATN probably reflects early recognition of renal injury and treatment of poor cardiac performance and circulatory failure that focus on vigorous plasma volume expansion.

The *recovery phase* is the period during which repair of renal tissue takes place. Its onset usually is heralded by a gradual increase in urine output and a fall in serum creatinine, indicating that the nephrons have recovered to the point at which urine excretion is possible. Diuresis often occurs before renal function has fully returned to normal. Consequently, serum urea and creatinine, potassium, and phosphate levels may remain elevated or continue to rise even though urine output is increased. In some cases, the diuresis may result from impaired nephron function and may cause excessive loss of water and electrolytes. Eventually, renal tubular function is restored with improvement in concentrating ability. At about the same time, the urea and creatinine begin to return to normal. In some persons, mild to severe kidney damage persists.

Postrenal Injury

Postrenal injury results from obstruction of urine outflow from the kidneys. The obstruction can occur in the ureter (*i.e.,* calculi and strictures), bladder (*i.e.,* tumours or neurogenic bladder), or urethra (*i.e.,* prostatic hyperplasia). Prostatic hyperplasia is the most common underlying problem. Because both ureters must be occluded to produce renal injury, obstruction of the bladder rarely causes acute renal injury unless one of the kidneys already is damaged or a person has only one kidney. The treatment of acute postrenal injury consists of treating the underlying cause of obstruction so that urine flow can be reestablished before permanent nephron damage occurs.[6]

Diagnosis and Treatment

Given the high morbidity and mortality rates associated with acute renal injury, attention should be focused on prevention and early diagnosis. This includes assessment measures to identify persons at risk for development of acute renal injury, including those with pre-existing renal insufficiency and diabetes. These persons are particularly at risk for development of acute renal failure due to nephrotoxic drugs (*e.g.,* aminoglycosides and radiocontrast agents), or drugs such as the NSAIDs that alter intrarenal hemodynamics.[6] Older adults are susceptible to all forms of acute renal injury because of the effects of aging on renal reserve.

Careful observation of urine output is essential for persons at risk for development of acute renal injury. Urine tests that measure urine osmolality, urinary sodium concentration, and fractional excretion of sodium help differentiate prerenal azotemia, in which the reabsorptive capacity of the tubular cells is maintained, from tubular necrosis, in which these functions are lost. One of the earliest manifestations of tubular damage is the inability to concentrate the urine.

The RIFLE criteria (*r*isk, *i*njury, *f*ailure, *l*oss and *e*nd state renal disease) is another diagnostic tool using the combination of serum creatinine, GFR and urine output to classify acute kidney injury (Box 34.1).[1–3] End-stage renal disease (ESRD) is acute or chronic kidney failure that persists for more than 3 months, and requires dialysis or renal replacement therapy.

Further diagnostic information that can be obtained from the urinalysis includes evidence of proteinuria, hemoglobinuria, myoglobinuria, and casts or crystals in the urine. Blood tests for urea and creatinine provide information regarding the ability to remove nitrogenous wastes from the blood. It also is important to exclude urinary obstruction by ensuring a Foley catheter is inserted and an ultrasound is carried out that will identify hydronephrosis, a hallmark of urinary tract obstruction.

Research is now focusing on new biomarkers for assessing acute kidney injury earlier than conventional parameters. Interleukin (IL)-18 is an inflammatory cytokine produced in the proximal tubule after an ischemic injury and an increase in

BOX 34.1	RIFLE CLASSIFICATION FOR ACUTE RENAL FAILURE	
Category	**GFR Criteria**	**Urine Output Criteria**
Risk	↑ Cr × 1.5 GFR <25%	<0.5 ml/kg/hour × 6 hours
Injury	↑ Cr × 2 GFR <50%	<0.5 ml/kg/hour × 12 hours
Failure	↑ Cr × 3 GRF <75%	<0.3 ml/kg/hour × 24 hours or no urine output for 12 hours
Loss	Complete loss of kidney function >4 weeks	No urine output >4 weeks
ESRD	Complete loss of kidney function >3 months	No urine output >3 months

CR, serum creatinine; ESRD, end stage renal disease.
Adapted from Bellomo R., Ronco C., Kellum J. A., et al. (2006). Acute renal failure—definition, outcome measures, animal models, fluid therapy and information technology need. (Figure 1). Available online at: http://ccforum.com/content/8/4/R204. Accessed June 7, 2014.

this urinary marker is predictive of acute kidney injury often 24 hours prior to any increase in creatinine levels. Neutrophil gelatinin–associated lipocalin (NGAL) is another well-studied biomarker that is found in several organs including the kidneys. Increased levels of urinary NGAL excretion are associated with kidney tubular stress or injury however extrarenal stressors can also lead to higher NGAL urinary levels and this lack of specificity is a disadvantage. Other arising biomarkers continue to be studied.[1–8]

A major concern in the treatment of acute renal injury is identifying and correcting the cause (*e.g.,* improving renal perfusion, discontinuing nephrotoxic drugs). Fluids are carefully regulated in an effort to maintain normal fluid volume and electrolyte concentrations. Adequate caloric intake is needed to prevent the breakdown of body proteins, which increases nitrogenous wastes.[1–3,6–8,10] Because secondary infections are a major cause of death in persons with acute renal injury, constant effort is needed to prevent and treat such infections.

Intermittent hemodialysis or continuous renal replacement therapy (CRRT) may be indicated when nitrogenous wastes and the water and electrolyte balance cannot be kept under control by other means.[6–8] CRRT may have an advantage in treating acute renal injury in patients who are hemodynamically unstable and unable to tolerate intermittent hemodialysis but clinical trials suggest both treatments are equivocal.[6,11]

IN SUMMARY

Acute renal injury is an acute, potentially reversible decrease in kidney function. Acute renal injury is characterized by a decrease in GFR, accumulation of nitrogenous wastes in the blood (*i.e.*, azotemia), and alterations in body fluids and electrolytes. Acute renal injury is classified as prerenal, intrinsic or intrarenal, or postrenal in origin. Prerenal injury is caused by decreased blood flow to the kidneys; postrenal injury by obstruction to urine output; and intrinsic renal injury by disorders in the kidney itself. ATN, due to ischemia, sepsis, or nephrotoxic agents, is the most common cause of acute intrinsic renal injury. ATN typically progresses through three phases: the initiation phase, during which tubular injury is induced; the maintenance phase, during which the GFR falls, nitrogenous wastes accumulate, and urine output decreases; and the recovery or reparative phase, during which the GFR, urine output, and blood levels of nitrogenous wastes return to normal.

Because of the high morbidity and mortality rates associated with acute renal injury, identification of persons at risk is important to clinical decision making. Acute renal injury often is reversible, making early identification and correction of the underlying cause (*e.g.*, improving renal perfusion, discontinuing nephrotoxic drugs) important. Treatment includes the judicious administration of fluids and potentially renal replacement therapy.

CHRONIC KIDNEY DISEASE

After completing this section of the chapter, you should be able to meet the following objectives:

- State the most common causes of CKD.
- Describe the five stages of CKD.
- Describe the methods used to arrive at an accurate estimation of the GFR and explain the rationale for its use in defining the stages of CKD.
- Explain the physiologic mechanisms underlying the common problems associated with CKD, including alterations in fluid and electrolyte balance and disorders of skeletal, hematologic, cardiovascular, immune system, neurologic, skin, and sexual function.
- State the basis for adverse drug reactions in patients with CKD.
- Describe the scientific principles underlying dialysis treatment, and compare hemodialysis with peritoneal dialysis.
- Cite the possible complications of kidney transplantation.
- State the goals for dietary management of persons with CKD.

CKD is a worldwide problem affecting people of all ages, races, and economic groups. The prevalence and incidence of the disease, which mirrors that of conditions such as diabetes, hypertension, and obesity, is rising. In Canada, the number of Canadians being treated for kidney failure has more than tripled in 20 years, with approximately 1 in 10 people or

2.9 million Canadians with CKD of whom approximately 23,400 require a form of dialysis.[12,13]

Definition and Classification

In 2002, the Kidney Disease Outcome Quality Initiative (K/DOQI) of the National Kidney Foundation (NKF) published clinical practice guidelines for CKD.[14] The goals of the Work Group that developed the guidelines were to define CKD and classify its stages, to evaluate laboratory measures used for assessment of kidney disease, and to associate the level of kidney function with the complications of CKD. The K/DOQI definition and classification were later accepted by participants in an International Controversies Conference on Kidney Disease: Improving Global Outcomes (KDIGO).[15] Canada has accepted these definitions and classifications, which use the GFR to classify CKD into six stages, beginning with kidney damage with normal or elevated GFR, progressing to CKD and, potentially, to kidney failure (Table 34.1).[15] It is anticipated that early detection of kidney damage along with implementation of aggressive measures to decrease its progression can delay or prevent the onset of kidney failure.

CHRONIC KIDNEY DISEASE

- CKD represents the progressive decline in kidney function due to the permanent loss of nephrons.
- CKD can result from a number of conditions, including diabetes, hypertension, glomerulonephritis, and other kidney diseases.
- The GFR is considered the best measure of kidney function.
- The Kidney Disease: Improving Global Outcomes (KDIGO) divide CKD into five stages based on GFR, beginning with minimal loss of renal function (stage 1) and progressing to kidney failure (stage 5).
- The Practice Guidelines are intended to encourage the early diagnosis of CKD so that measures to delay or prevent its progression are instituted.

GFR is used as it is much more sensitive than serum creatinine. Kidney damage that is present but undetected due to a normal GFR is classified as stage 1. Individuals with a mild decrease in GFR (60 to 89 ml/min/1.73 m² body surface area) are stratified as stage 2.[15] Decreased GFR without recognized markers of kidney damage can occur in infants and older adults, and is usually considered to be normal for age. Other causes of chronically decreased GFR without kidney damage in adults include removal of one kidney, extracellular fluid volume depletion, and systemic illnesses associated with reduced kidney perfusion, such as heart failure and cirrhosis.[15] With these factors, there is often a characteristic loss of renal reserve and poorer outcomes.

CKD is defined as kidney damage or a GFR less than 60 ml/min/1.73 m² for 3 months or longer.[14-17] CKD can

TABLE 34.1 STAGES OF CHRONIC KIDNEY DISEASE

STAGE	DESCRIPTION	GFR (ml/min/1.73 m²)
1	Kidney damage with normal or increased GFR	≥90
2	Kidney damage with mild decrease in GFR	60–89
3a	Mild to moderate decrease in GFR	45–59
3b	Moderate to severe decrease in GFR	30–44
4	Severe decrease in GFR	15–29
5	Kidney failure/ESRD	<15 (or dialysis)

Chronic kidney disease is defined as either kidney damage or GFR <60 ml/min/1.73 m² for ≥3 months. Kidney damage is defined as pathologic abnormalities or markers of damage, including abnormalities in blood or urine tests or imaging studies.

ESRD, end-stage renal disease denoting need for renal replacement therapy.

Adapted Kidney Disease Improving Global Outcomes (KDIGO). (2013). KDIGO 2012 Clinical practice guidelines for the evaluation and management of chronic kidney disease. *Kidney International Supplements, 3*(1), 1–150.

result from a number of conditions that cause permanent loss of nephrons, including diabetes, hypertension, glomerulonephritis, systemic lupus erythematosus, and polycystic kidney disease. Diabetes mellitus and hypertension are the two greatest risk factors for CKD in Canada.[12,13]

The KDIGO Clinical Practice Guidelines define kidney failure "as either (1) a GFR of less than 15 ml/min/1.73 m², usually accompanied by most of the signs and symptoms of uremia, or (2) a need to start renal replacement therapy (dialysis or transplantation)."[15] These guidelines point out that CKD is not synonymous with ESRD, which is a clinical description to denote the requirement of a form of renal replacement therapy (*e.g.,* dialysis, transplantation).

Regardless of cause, CKD represents a loss of functioning kidney nephrons with progressive deterioration of glomerular filtration, tubular reabsorptive capacity, and endocrine functions of the kidneys (Fig. 34.3). All forms of CKD are characterized by a reduction in the GFR, reflecting a corresponding reduction in the number of functional nephrons. The rate of nephron destruction differs across individuals, ranging from several months to many years. Typically, the signs and symptoms of CKD occur gradually and do not become evident until the disease is far advanced. This is because of the amazing compensatory ability of the kidneys. Diagnosis is often delayed until damage is far advanced due to the non-specific and slow onset of symptoms, reliance upon serum creatinine, and compensation by the kidneys.[6] As kidney structures are destroyed, the remaining nephrons undergo structural and functional hypertrophy, each increasing its function as a means of compensating for those that have been lost. In the process, each of the remaining nephrons must filter more solute particles from the blood. It is only when the few remaining nephrons are destroyed that the manifestations of kidney failure become more evident.

Assessment of Glomerular Filtration Rate and Other Indicators of Renal Function

The GFR is considered the best measure of overall function of the kidney. The normal GFR, which varies with age, sex, and body size, is approximately 120 to 130 ml/min/1.73 m² for normal young healthy adults.[15–18] Although GFR is usually estimated using serum creatinine concentration in clinical practice, it is recommended that creatinine clearance be estimated using the Cockcroft–Gault formula. This provide a more accurate indication of renal function because GFR varies with age, sex, ethnicity, muscle mass, and body size.[15]

FIGURE 34.3 • Relation of renal function and nephron mass. Each kidney contains about 1 million tiny nephrons. A proportional relation exists between the number of nephrons affected by a disease process and the resulting glomerular filtration rate.

BOX 34.2 **PREDICTION OF CREATININE CLEARANCE USING SERUM CLEARANCE**

Cockroft and Gault Equation

$$\text{Creatinine clearence (ml/min)} = \frac{(140 - \text{age}) \times (\text{body weight in kg})}{\text{serum creatinine in } \mu\text{mol/L}} \times 1.23$$

The equation result should be multiplied by a factor of 0.85 for women.

Modification of Diet in Renal Diseases (MDRD)[a]

$$\text{GFR} = 175 \times \frac{(\text{serum Cr})^{-1.154}}{88.4} \times (\text{age})^{-0.203} \times 0.742 \text{ if patient is female} \times 1.212 \text{ if patient is black}$$

Note: GFR, ml/min/1.73 m²; Cr, creatinine.

[a]Levey A. S., Coresh J., Greene T., et al. (2006). Chronic kidney disease epidemiology collaboration: Using standardized serum creatinine values in the modification of diet in renal disease study equation for estimating glomerular filtration rate. *Annals of Internal Medicine, 145*(4), 247–254.

The Cockroft–Gault formula or the alterative Modification of Diet in Renal Diseases (MDRD) equations take these factors into account and are used for estimating the GFR based on serum creatinine levels[15–18] (Box 34.2). However, neither serum creatinine nor creatinine clearance accurately reflect GFR because at low levels of GFR, creatinine secretion by the tubules can make up to 10% of the loss of creatinine by the kidneys but does not represent glomerular filtration. Thus, GFR may be overestimated at low levels of renal function.

Albuminuria serves as a key adjunctive tool for assessing nephron injury and repair. Urine normally contains small amounts of protein. However, a persistent increase in protein excretion usually is a sign of kidney damage. The type of protein (*e.g.,* low–molecular-weight proteins or albumin) depends on the type of kidney disease. Increased excretion of low–molecular-weight proteins is a marker of tubulointerstitial disease, and excretion of albumin is a marker of glomerular injury resulting from a range of disorders such as hypertension, diabetes mellitus, or chronic glomerulonephritis. In adults and postpubertal children with diabetes, urinary albumin excretion is a risk factor for progressive CKD.[15] In most cases, urine dipstick tests are acceptable for detecting albuminuria. If the urine dipstick test is positive (1+ or greater), albuminuria is usually confirmed by quantitative measurement of the albumin-to-creatinine ratio in a spot (untimed) urine specimen.[15,17] Populations at risk for CKD (*i.e.,* those with hypertension, or family history of kidney disease) should be screened for albuminuria, at least annually, as part of their health examination.[15] Microalbuminuria, which is an early sign of diabetic kidney disease, refers to albumin excretion that is above the normal range, but below the range normally detected by tests of total protein excretion in the urine (see Chapter 42). Patients with diabetes should be screened annually with a more sensitive urine protein assay to detect microalbuminuria.

Other markers of kidney damage include abnormalities in urine sediment (red and white blood cells) and abnormal

findings on imaging studies.[15,17] Ultrasonography is particularly useful for detecting a number of kidney disorders, including urinary tract obstructions, infections, stones, and polycystic kidney disease. Novel biomarkers continue to be studied such as urinary excretion of cystatin C and its use in detecting early CKD.[6,17]

Clinical Manifestations

The manifestations of CKD include an accumulation of nitrogenous wastes; alterations in water, electrolyte, and acid–base balance; mineral and skeletal disorders; anemia and coagulation disorders; hypertension and alterations in cardiovascular function; gastrointestinal disorders; neurologic complications; disorders of skin integrity; and disorders of immunologic function[6,16,17] (Fig. 34.4). The point at which these disorders make their appearance and the severity of the manifestations are determined largely by the extent of renal function that is present and the coexisting disease conditions. Many of them make their appearance before the GFR has reached the kidney failure stage.

Accumulation of Nitrogenous Wastes

The accumulation of nitrogenous wastes in the blood, or azotemia, is an early sign of kidney failure, usually occurring before other symptoms become evident. Urea is one of the first nitrogenous wastes to accumulate in the blood, and this level becomes increasingly elevated as CKD progresses. The normal concentration of urea in the plasma is approximately 2.9 to 7.1 mmol/L. In kidney failure, this level may rise as high as 100 mmol/L. Creatinine, a byproduct of muscle metabolism, is freely filtered in the glomerulus and is not reabsorbed in the renal tubules. It is produced at a relatively constant rate, and essentially all the creatinine that is filtered in the glomerulus is excreted in the urine rather than being reabsorbed into the blood. Thus, serum creatinine can be used as an indirect

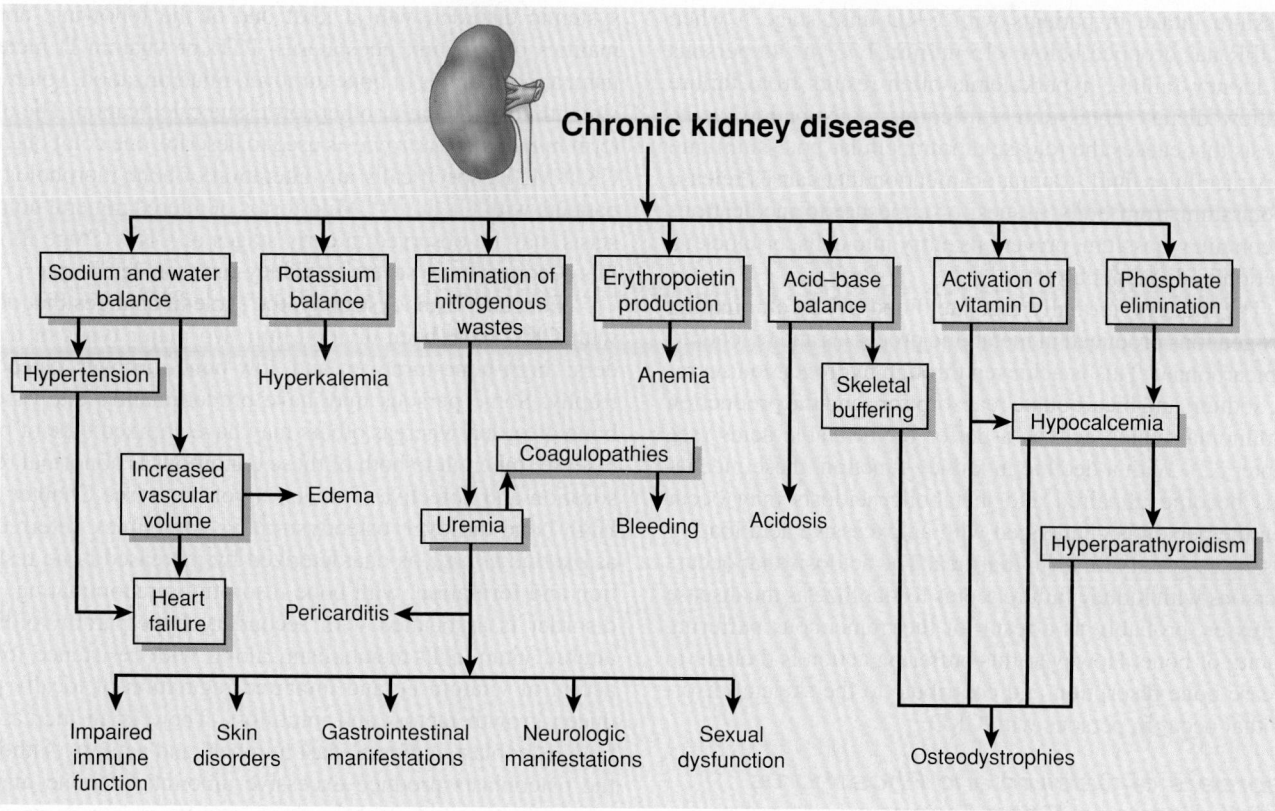

FIGURE 34.4 • Mechanisms and manifestations of chronic kidney disease.

method for assessing the GFR and the extent of kidney damage that has occurred in CKD but as previously mentioned because of secretion of creatinine by the tubules, the serum creatinine overestimates GFR at low levels of renal function.

Uremia, which literally means "urine in the blood," is the term used to describe the clinical manifestations of kidney failure. Few symptoms of uremia appear until at least two thirds of the kidney's nephrons have been destroyed. Uremia differs from azotemia, which merely indicates the accumulation of nitrogenous wastes in the blood and can occur without symptoms. Uremia refers to the symptoms associated with decreased renal clearance of nitrogenous wastes and includes uremic encephalopathy, peripheral neuropathy, pruritus, and serositis. At an advanced stage, virtually every organ and structure in the body is affected. The symptoms at the onset of uremia (*e.g.,* weakness, fatigue, nausea, apathy) often are subtle. More severe symptoms include extreme weakness, frequent vomiting, lethargy, and confusion. Without treatment, coma and death follow. The uremic symptoms occur concomitantly with other signs and symptoms of renal failure that include altered fluid, electrolyte, and acid–base balance; alterations in regulatory functions (*e.g.,* blood pressure control, production of red blood cells, and impaired vitamin D synthesis).

Fluid, Electrolyte, and Acid–Base Disorders

The kidneys function in the regulation of extracellular fluid volume. They do this by either eliminating or conserving sodium and water. CKD can produce dehydration or fluid overload, depending on the pathologic process of the kidney disease. In addition to volume regulation, the ability of the kidneys to concentrate the urine is diminished. One of the earliest symptoms of kidney damage is *isosthenuria,* or polyuria with urine that is almost isotonic with plasma (*i.e.,* specific gravity of 1.008 to 1.012) and varies little from voiding to voiding.

As renal function declines further, the ability to regulate sodium excretion is reduced. The kidneys normally tolerate large variations in sodium intake while maintaining normal serum sodium levels. In CKD, they lose the ability to regulate sodium excretion. There is impaired ability to adjust to a sudden reduction in sodium intake and poor tolerance of an acute sodium overload. Volume depletion with an accompanying decrease in the GFR can occur with a restricted sodium intake or excess sodium loss caused by diarrhea or vomiting. In advanced stages of CKD, the ability of the kidneys to excrete salt often falls below the level of dietary salt intake leading to fluid volume expansion, edema, and hypertension. Diuretics and salt restriction are often required to maintain sodium balance.

Approximately 90% of potassium excretion is through the kidneys.[6,9] In kidney failure, potassium excretion by each nephron increases as the kidneys adapt to a decrease in the GFR. In addition, excretion in the gastrointestinal tract is increased. As a result, hyperkalemia usually does not develop until kidney function is severely compromised. Because of this adaptive mechanism, it usually is not necessary to restrict potassium intake in patients with CKD until stage 5 when the GFR has dropped below <15 ml/min/1.73 m². In persons with kidney failure, hyperkalemia often results from failure to follow dietary potassium restrictions; constipation; acute acidosis that causes the release of intracellular potassium into the extracellular fluid; trauma or infection that causes release of potassium from body tissues; or exposure to medications that contain potassium, prevent its entry into cells, or block its secretion in distal nephrons.

The kidneys normally regulate blood pH by eliminating hydrogen ions produced in metabolic processes and regenerating bicarbonate. This is achieved through hydrogen ion secretion, sodium and bicarbonate reabsorption, and the production of ammonia, which acts as a buffer for titratable acids (see Chapter 32). With a decline in kidney function, these mechanisms become impaired and metabolic acidosis may occur when the person is challenged with an excessive acid load or loses excessive alkali, as in diarrhea. The acidosis that occurs in persons with kidney failure seems to stabilize as the disease progresses, probably as a result of the tremendous buffering capacity of bone. However, this buffering action is thought to increase bone resorption and contribute to the skeletal disorders that occur in persons with CKD.

Disorders of Calcium and Phosphorus Metabolism and Bone Disease

Abnormalities of calcium and phosphorus metabolism occur early in the course of CKD.[19–24] The regulation of serum phosphate levels requires a daily urinary excretion of an amount equal to that ingested in the diet. With deteriorating renal function, phosphate excretion is impaired, and as a result serum phosphate levels rise. At the same time, serum calcium levels, which are inversely regulated in relation to serum phosphate levels, fall (see Chapter 31). The drop in serum calcium, in turn, stimulates parathyroid hormone (PTH) release, with a resultant increase in calcium resorption from bone. Although serum calcium levels are maintained through increased PTH function, this adjustment is accomplished at the expense of the skeletal system and other body organs.

Vitamin D synthesis also is impaired in CKD. The kidneys regulate vitamin D activity by converting the inactive form of vitamin D (25[OH] vitamin D_3) to calcitriol (1,25[OH] vitamin D_3), the active form of vitamin D.[6,15] Calcitriol is known to have a direct suppressive effect on PTH production; therefore, reduced levels of calcitriol cause elevated levels of PTH. In addition, reduced calcitriol levels lead to impaired calcium absorption from the gastrointestinal tract. Vitamin D also regulates osteoblast differentiation, thereby affecting bone replacement.

Most persons with CKD develop a secondary hyperparathyroidism, the result of chronic stimulation of the parathyroid glands. It is recommended that serum level of calcium, phosphate, and PTH measurements are done for all CKD patients with Stage 3b or higher (Table 34.1)[15,23,24] (see Chapter 31).

Skeletal Disorders. The newer term Chronic Kidney Disease–Mineral (and) Bone Disorder (CKD-MBD) describes the systemic disorder with at least one of the following: abnormalities of calcium, phosphorus, PTH or vitamin D metabolism; abnormalities of bone turnover, mineralization, volume or strength; or vascular or other soft tissue calcification. The older term *renal osteodystrophy* is used to describe one component of CKD-MBD, specifically any alteration of bone morphology in patients with CKD.[6,15,21] Mild forms of altered mineral homeostasis may be observed in early stages of CKD (Stage 2), and this becomes more severe as kidney function deteriorates.

For renal osteodystrophy, the skeletal changes that occur with CKD have been divided into two major types of disorders: high-bone-turnover and low-bone-turnover osteodystrophy. Some persons may have predominantly one type of bone disorder, whereas others may have a mixed type of bone disease. Inherent to both of these conditions is abnormal reabsorption and defective remodelling of bone (see Chapter 58). High-bone-turnover osteodystrophy, sometimes referred to as *osteitis fibrosa,* is characterized by increased bone resorption and formation, with bone resorption predominating. The disorder is associated with secondary hyperparathyroidism; altered vitamin D metabolism, along with resistance to the action of vitamin D; and impaired regulation of locally produced growth factors and inhibitors. There is an increase in both osteoblast and osteoclast numbers and activity. Although the osteoblasts produce excessive amounts of bone matrix, mineralization fails to keep pace, and there is a decrease in bone density and formation of porous and coarse-fibred bone. Cortical bone is affected more severely than cancellous bone. Bone marrow fibrosis is another component of osteitis fibrosa; it occurs in areas of increased bone cell activity. In advanced stages of the disorder, cysts may develop in the bone, a condition called *osteitis fibrosa cystica.*[6]

Low-bone-turnover osteodystrophy is characterized by decreased numbers of osteoblasts and low or reduced numbers of osteoclasts, a low rate of bone turnover, and an accumulation of unmineralized bone matrix. There are two forms of low-turnover osteodystrophy: osteomalacia and adynamic osteodystrophy. *Osteomalacia* is characterized by a slow rate of bone formation and defects in bone mineralization, which may be caused by vitamin D deficiency, excess aluminum deposition, or metabolic acidosis. Metabolic acidosis is thought to have a direct effect on both osteoblastic and osteoclastic activity, as well as on the mineralization process, by decreasing the availability of trivalent phosphate. Until the 1980s, the osteomalacia seen in CKD resulted mainly from aluminum intoxication. Aluminum intoxication causes decreased and defective mineralization of bone by existing osteoblasts and more long-term inhibition of osteoblast differentiation. During the 1970s and 1980s, it was discovered that accumulation of aluminum from water used in dialysis and aluminum salts used as phosphate binders caused osteomalacia and adynamic bone disease. This discovery led to a change in the composition of dialysis solutions and the substitution of calcium carbonate for aluminum salts as phosphate binders. As a result, the prevalence of osteomalacia in persons with CKD has declined.[6,22]

The second type of low-bone-turnover osteodystrophy, *adynamic osteodystrophy,* is characterized by a few or no osteoblasts, with the osteoclast number being normal or reduced. Adynamic bone disease is characterized by reduced bone volume and mineralization that may result, in part, from excessive suppression of PTH production with calcitriol however the specific etiology remains unknown. Other contributory factors are diabetes, aging, and malnutrition.[6,22]

Regardless of the cause of skeletal abnormalities in CKD, bone disease can lead to bone tenderness and muscle weakness. Bone fractures complicate both high- and low-turnover types of bone disease. However, it is now recognized that persons with adynamic bone disease may be more predisposed to fractures than those with osteitis fibrosa cystica. In the latter disorder, however, PTH-associated proximal muscle weakness in the lower extremities often coexists, giving rise to gait abnormalities and making it difficult to get out of a chair or climb stairs.

Early treatment of hyperphosphatemia and hypocalcemia is important to prevent or slow the development of skeletal complications. Milk products and other foods high in phosphorus content are restricted in the diet. Phosphate-binding antacids (aluminum salts, calcium carbonate, or calcium acetate) may be prescribed to decrease absorption of phosphate from the gastrointestinal tract. Calcium-containing phosphate binders can lead to hypercalcemia, thus worsening soft tissue calcification, especially in persons receiving vitamin D therapy. Aluminum-containing antacids are no longer used as they contribute to the development of osteodystrophy. Sevelamer and the newer lanthanum carbonate are non–calcium-based phosphate binders approved by Health Canada to manage hyperphosphatemia. Sevelamer is a hydrogel that is resistant to digestive degradation and is not absorbed; however despite its high cost few benefits have been demonstrated for patients.[6,15,24]

Activated pharmacologic forms of vitamin D (*e.g.,* calcitriol) often are used to increase serum calcium levels and at least partially reverse the secondary hyperparathyroidism and osteitis fibrosis that occur with CKD. Although calcitriol is effective in controlling PTH overproduction, its stimulatory effects on intestinal absorption of calcium and phosphorus, along with its suppressive effects on bone turnover, predispose to hypercalcemia and hyperphosphatemia and to an increase in the calcium–phosphate (Ca × P) product (see Chapter 31). Hypercalcemia and an elevated Ca × P product increase the risk for metastatic calcification, a complication associated with cardiac dysfunction and death; the risk is greater in patients who are also taking calcium-based phosphate binders.[20–24] Two medications have been approved by Health Canada for treatment of secondary hyperparathyroidism. Paricalcitol is a vitamin D analogue and cinacalcet activates the calcium-sensing receptor on the parathyroid gland.

Hematologic Disorders

Anemia. Chronic anemia, defined as hemoglobin levels <135 g/L in adult men and <120 g/L in adult women, is the most profound hematologic alteration that accompanies CKD.[25] The prevalence of anemia increases as GFR declines and becomes almost universal in Stage 5. The KDIGO guidelines recommend that those persons with a GFR less than 60 ml/min/1.73 m^2 should be evaluated for anemia. The assessment for anemia and its causes includes measures of hemoglobin, hematocrit, and iron stores (direct measurement of iron in a bone marrow biopsy is the gold standard but rarely done, indirect measures include serum ferritin, or transferrin saturation levels, vitamin B$_{12}$, and folate; see Chapter 14).[26]

The anemia of CKD is due to several factors, including chronic blood loss, hemolysis, bone marrow suppression due to retained uremic factors, and decreased red cell production due to impaired production of erythropoietin and iron deficiency. The kidneys are the primary site for the production of the hormone *erythropoietin,* which controls red blood cell production.[6,26,27] In renal failure, erythropoietin production usually is insufficient to stimulate adequate red blood cell production by the bone marrow. Among the causes of iron deficiency in persons with CKD are anorexia and dietary restrictions that limit intake, and the blood loss that occurs during dialysis.[6]

When untreated, anemia causes or contributes to weakness, fatigue, depression, insomnia, and decreased cognitive function. There also is an increasing concern regarding the physiologic effects of anemia on cardiovascular function.[26,27] The anemia of renal failure produces a decrease in blood viscosity and a compensatory increase in heart rate. The decreased blood viscosity also exacerbates peripheral vasodilation and contributes to decreased vascular resistance. Cardiac output increases in a compensatory fashion to maintain tissue perfusion. Anemia also limits myocardial oxygen supply, particularly in persons with coronary heart disease, leading to angina pectoris and other ischemic events. It has also been suggested that anemia may contribute to the progression of CKD by subjecting the functioning nephrons that remain to increased hypoxic and oxidative stress.

Normalization of hemoglobin has not been demonstrated to have benefits regarding cardiovascular outcomes but increases the risk of other vascular events such as stroke. Partial correction may alleviate symptoms of fatigue. Guidelines from the Canadian Society of Nephrology recommend a target hemoglobin of 110 g/L with use of erythropoiesis-stimulating agents, with an acceptable range of 100 to 120 g/L.[28] Recombinant human erythropoietin (rhEPO) has been used to help maintain hemoglobin levels in persons with kidney failure.[26,27] More recently, a novel erythropoiesis-stimulating protein has been introduced for treatment of anemia in CKD. This protein, darbepoetin alpha, is a hyperglycosylated analog of rhEPO that possesses great biologic activity and a prolonged half-life.[27] Secondary benefits of treating anemia with rhEPO, previously attributed to the correction of uremia, include improvements in appetite, energy level, sexual function, skin colour, and hair and nail growth, and reduced cold intolerance. Because worsening of hypertension and seizures have occurred when the hematocrit was raised too suddenly, frequent measurements of hematocrit are necessary.

Because iron deficiency is common among persons with CKD, iron supplementation often is needed, and should be the first line of treatment for anemia.[15,26] Iron can be given orally or intravenously. Intravenous iron (iron dextran, iron sucrose, or ferric sodium gluconate) is used for treatment of persons who are not able to maintain adequate iron status with oral iron. Because intravenously administered iron may cause serious immediate and delayed hypersensitivity reactions, including life-threatening anaphylactic reactions, care is required when prescribing and administering these drugs.[6,26]

Coagulopathies. Bleeding disorders are manifested by epistaxis, menorrhagia, gastrointestinal bleeding, and bruising of the skin and subcutaneous tissues. Although platelet production often is normal in CKD, platelet function is impaired. Coagulative function improves with dialysis but does not completely normalize, suggesting that uremia contributes to the problem. Persons with CKD also have greater susceptibility to thrombotic disorders, particularly if their underlying disease was characterized by a nephrotic presentation.[6]

Cardiovascular Disorders

The overall mortality rate from cardiovascular disease in people with CKD is significantly increased compared to the general population. Even after stratification for age, the incidence of cardiovascular disease remains 10 to 20 times higher in persons with CKD especially when accompanied by albuminuria than in the general population.[6] Furthermore, the major risk for persons with CKD is death from cardiovascular complications, with the second greatest risk from complications due to diabetes. Thus, the Canadian Society of Nephrology's guidelines for the management of CKD are aligned with those of the Canadian Cardiovascular Society, the Canadian Hypertension Education Program, and the Canadian Diabetes Association.[28]

Hypertension. Hypertension commonly is an early manifestation of CKD. The mechanisms that produce hypertension in CKD are multifactorial. They include an increased vascular volume, elevation of peripheral vascular resistance, decreased levels of renal vasodilator prostaglandins, and increased activity of the renin–angiotensin–aldosterone system.

Early identification and aggressive treatment of hypertension has been shown to slow the progression of renal impairment in many types of kidney disease.[17,26] Treatment involves salt and water restriction and the use of antihypertensive medications to control blood pressure. Many persons with CKD need to take several antihypertensive medications to control blood pressure (see Chapter 23).

Heart Disease. The spectrum of cardiovascular disease due to CKD includes left ventricular hypertrophy and ischemic heart disease. People with CKD tend to have an increased prevalence of left ventricular dysfunction, with both depressed left ventricular ejection fraction, as in systolic dysfunction, and impaired ventricular filling, as in diastolic failure[6] (see Chapter 26). Multiple factors lead to development of left ventricular

dysfunction, including extracellular fluid overload, shunting of blood through an arteriovenous fistula for dialysis, and anemia. Anemia, in particular, has been correlated with the presence of left ventricular hypertrophy. PTH also may play a role in the pathogenesis of cardiomyopathy in renal failure. These abnormalities, coupled with the hypertension that often is present, cause increased myocardial work and oxygen demand, with eventual development of heart failure.

Heart failure and pulmonary edema tend to occur in the late stages of kidney failure. Coexisting conditions that have been identified as contributing to the burden of cardiovascular disease include hypertension, anemia, diabetes mellitus, dyslipidemia, and coagulopathies.

Pericarditis. Pericarditis occurs in approximately 20% of persons receiving chronic dialysis.[29] It can result from metabolic toxins associated with the uremic state or from dialysis. The manifestations of uremic pericarditis resemble those of viral pericarditis, with all its potential complications, including cardiac tamponade (see Chapter 24). The presenting signs include mild to severe chest pain with respiratory accentuation and a pericardial friction rub. Fever is variable in the absence of infection and is more common in dialysis than uremic pericarditis.

Gastrointestinal Disorders

Anorexia, nausea, and vomiting are common in patients with uremia, along with a metallic taste in the mouth that further depresses the appetite.[6] Early morning nausea and hiccups are common. Ulceration and bleeding of the gastrointestinal mucosa may develop. A possible cause of nausea and vomiting is the decomposition of urea by intestinal flora, resulting in a high concentration of ammonia. PTH increases gastric acid secretion and contributes to gastrointestinal problems. Nausea and vomiting often improve with restriction of dietary protein and after initiation of dialysis, and disappear after kidney transplantation.

Neuromuscular Disorders

Many persons with CKD have alterations in peripheral and central nervous system function.[6,25] Peripheral neuropathy, or involvement of the peripheral nerves, affects the lower limbs more frequently than the upper limbs. It is symmetric and affects both sensory and motor function. Neuropathy is caused by atrophy and demyelination of nerve fibres, possibly caused by uremic toxins. Restless legs syndrome is a manifestation of peripheral nerve involvement and can be seen in as many as two thirds of patients on dialysis. This syndrome is characterized by creeping, prickling, and itching sensations that typically are more intense at rest. Temporary relief is obtained by moving the legs. A burning sensation in the feet, which may be followed by muscle weakness and atrophy, is a manifestation of uremia.

The central nervous system disturbances in uremia are similar to those caused by other metabolic and toxic disorders. Sometimes referred to as *uremic encephalopathy,* the condition is poorly understood and may result, at least in part, from an excess of toxic organic acids that alter neural function. Electrolyte abnormalities, such as sodium shifts, also may contribute. The manifestations are more closely related to the progress of the uremic disorder than to the level of the metabolic end products. Reductions in alertness and awareness are the earliest and most significant indications of uremic encephalopathy. These often are followed by an inability to fix attention, loss of recent memory, and perceptual errors in identifying persons and objects. Delirium and coma occur late; seizures are the preterminal event.

Disorders of motor function commonly accompany the neurologic manifestations of uremic encephalopathy. During the early stages, there often is difficulty in performing fine movements of the extremities; the gait becomes unsteady and clumsy with tremulousness of movement. Asterixis (dorsiflexion movements of the hands and feet) typically occurs as the disease progresses. It can be elicited by having the person hyperextend his or her arms at the elbow and wrist with the fingers spread apart. If asterixis is present, this position causes side-to-side flapping movements of the fingers.[25]

Altered Immune Function

Infection is a common complication and cause of hospitalization and death for persons with kidney failure. Immunologic abnormalities decrease the efficiency of the immune response to infection.[6] All aspects of inflammation and immune function may be affected adversely by the high levels of urea and metabolic wastes, including a decreased granulocyte count, impaired humoral and cell-mediated immunity, and defective phagocyte function. The acute inflammatory response and delayed-type hypersensitivity response are impaired. Although persons with CKD have normal humoral responses to vaccines, a more aggressive immunization program may be needed. Skin and mucosal barriers to infection also may be defective. In persons who are maintained on dialysis, vascular access devices are common portals of entry for pathogens. Many persons with CKD fail to mount a fever with infection, making the diagnosis more difficult.

Disorders of Skin Integrity

Skin manifestations are common in persons with kidney failure.[6] The skin often is pale owing to anemia and may have a sallow, yellow-brown hue. The skin and mucous membranes often are dry, and subcutaneous bruising is common. Skin dryness or *xerosis* is caused by a reduction in perspiration owing to the decreased size of sweat glands and the diminished activity of oil glands. Up to 90% of persons on hemodialysis experience pruritus. The pathophysiology is poorly understood but risk factors include inadequate dialysis, secondary hyperparathyroidism and increased serum phosphate. Severe scratching and repeated needle sticks, especially with hemodialysis, break the skin integrity and increase the risk for infection. In the advanced stages of untreated kidney failure, urea crystals may precipitate on the skin as a result of the high urea concentration in body fluids (*i.e.,* calciphylaxis).

Sexual Dysfunction

The cause of sexual dysfunction in men and women with CKD is unclear. The cause probably is multifactorial and may result from high levels of uremic toxins, neuropathy, altered endocrine function, psychological factors, and medications (*e.g.,* antihypertensive drugs). Alterations in physiologic sexual responses, reproductive ability, and libido are common.[6]

Erectile dysfunction occurs in as much as 70% to 80% of male patients with CKD.[6] Derangements of the pituitary and gonadal hormones, such as decreases in testosterone levels and increases in prolactin and luteinizing hormone levels, are common and cause erectile difficulties and decreased spermatocyte counts. Loss of libido may result from chronic anemia and decreased testosterone levels. Sildenafil improves erectile dysfunction caused by both psychogenic and organic factors. Other drugs, such as exogenous testosterone and bromocriptine, have been used in an attempt to return hormone levels to normal.

Impaired sexual function in women is manifested by abnormal levels of progesterone, luteinizing hormone, and prolactin. Hypofertility, menstrual abnormalities, decreased vaginal lubrication, and various orgasmic problems have been described. Amenorrhea is common among women who are on dialysis therapy.[30]

Elimination of Drugs

The kidneys are responsible for the elimination of many drugs and their metabolites. CKD and its treatment can interfere with the absorption, distribution, and elimination of drugs.[6,15] The administration of large quantities of phosphate-binding antacids to control hyperphosphatemia and hypocalcemia in patients with advanced renal failure interferes with the absorption of some drugs. Many drugs are bound to plasma proteins, such as albumin, for transport in the body; the unbound portion of the drug is available to act at the various receptor sites and is free to be metabolized. The decrease in plasma proteins, particularly albumin, that occurs in many persons with CKD results in less protein-bound drug and greater amounts of free drug.

In the process of metabolism, some drugs form intermediate metabolites that are toxic if not eliminated. Some pathways of drug metabolism, such as hydrolysis, are slowed with uremia. In persons with diabetes, for example, insulin requirements may be reduced as renal function deteriorates. Decreased elimination by the kidneys allows drugs or their metabolites to accumulate in the body and requires that drug dosages be adjusted accordingly. This is particularly true of certain antibiotics where the dosing interval is increased. Some drugs are cleared rapidly by hemodialysis and a supplemental dose is given at the end of this treatment. Some drugs contain unwanted nitrogen, sodium, potassium, and magnesium and must be avoided in patients with renal failure. Penicillin, for example, contains potassium. Nitrofurantoin and ammonium chloride add to the body's nitrogen pool. Many antacids contain magnesium. Because of problems with drug dosing and elimination, persons with CKD should be cautioned against the use of over-the-counter remedies.

Treatment

CKD is treated by conservative management to prevent or slow the rate of nephron destruction, to manage symptoms and quality of life, and, when necessary, by hemodialysis or kidney transplantation.

Measures to Slow Progression of the Disorder

Conservative treatment can often delay the progression of CKD.[6,31] It includes measures to retard deterioration of renal function and assist the body in managing the effects of impaired function. Urinary tract infections should be treated promptly and medication with renal damaging potential should be avoided. It should be noted that these strategies are complementary to the treatment of the original cause of the renal disorder, which is of the utmost importance and needs to be continually addressed.

Blood pressure control is important, as is control of blood glucose in persons with diabetes mellitus. Glycemic control (hemoglobin A_{1C} <7.0%; fasting plasma glucose 4 to 6 mmol/L) in persons with diabetes helps to prevent the development of microalbuminuria and retards the progression of diabetic nephropathy[26,28] (see Chapter 42). In addition to reduction in cardiovascular risk, antihypertensive therapy in persons with CKD aims to slow the progression of nephron loss by lowering intraglomerular hypertension and hypertrophy.[6] Elevated blood pressure also increases proteinuria due to a corresponding elevated pressure in the glomeruli. This is the basis for the treatment guideline establishing less than 140/90 mm Hg as the target blood pressure for persons with nondiabetic CKD or 130/90 for CKD *and* diabetes[32] (see Chapter 23). The ACE inhibitors and ARBs, which have a unique effect on the glomerular microcirculation (*i.e.,* dilation of the efferent arteriole), should be first line medications used in the treatment of hypertension and proteinuria, particularly in persons with diabetes.[32]

It has become apparent that smoking has a negative impact on kidney function, and it is one of the most remedial risk factors for CKD.[6,17] The mechanisms of smoking-induced renal damage appear to include both acute hemodynamic effects (*i.e.,* increase in blood pressure, intraglomerular pressure, and urinary albumin excretion) and chronic effects (endothelial cell dysfunction).[33] Smoking is particularly nephrotoxic in elderly persons with hypertension and in those with diabetes. Importantly, the adverse effects of smoking appear to be independent of the underlying kidney disease thus smoking cessation should be encouraged to reduce the risk of CKD and also the risk of cardiovascular disease progression. Additional lifestyle modifications to decrease the cardiovascular risk in persons with CKD include a healthy body weight (BMI 25 or less) and waist circumference (<102 cm for men, <88 cm for women), low-risk alcohol consumption (not exceeding 15 drinks per week for men and 10 drinks for women), and moderate exercise.[34]

Dialysis and Transplantation

Dialysis or renal replacement therapy is indicated when advanced uremia or serious electrolyte imbalances are present.

In Canada, there are approximately 23,400 persons receiving dialysis, and over 4,500 persons waiting for kidney transplant.[13] In 2012 although 2,225 kidney transplants were done in Canada approximately 230 persons died while waiting for kidney transplant.[35]

The choice between dialysis and transplantation is dictated by age, related health problems, donor availability, and personal preference. Although transplantation often is the preferred treatment, dialysis plays a critical role as a treatment method for ESRD. It is life-sustaining for persons who are not candidates for transplantation or who are awaiting transplantation. There are two broad categories of dialysis: hemodialysis and peritoneal dialysis.

Hemodialysis. The basic principles of hemodialysis have remained unchanged over the years, although new technology has improved the efficiency and speed of dialysis.[6,36] A hemodialysis system, or artificial kidney, consists of three parts: a blood delivery system, a dialyzer, and a dialysis fluid delivery system. The dialyzer is usually a hollow cylinder composed of bundles of capillary tubes through which blood circulates, while the dialysate travels on the outside of the tubes. The walls of the capillary tubes in the dialysis chamber are made up of a semipermeable membrane material that allows all molecules except blood cells and plasma proteins to move freely in both directions—from the blood into the dialyzing solution and from the dialyzing solution into the blood. The direction of flow is determined by the concentration of the substances contained in the two solutions. The waste products and excess electrolytes in the blood normally diffuse into the dialyzing solution. If there is a need to replace or add substances, such as bicarbonate, to the blood, these can be added to the dialyzing solution (Fig. 34.5).[6,36]

During dialysis, blood moves from a dialysis access in the patient through the tubing and blood chamber in the dialysis machine and then back into the body. Access to the vascular system is accomplished through a central venous catheter or, preferably, through an arteriovenous fistula (*i.e.,* anastomosis of a vein to an artery, usually in the forearm). Heparin is used to prevent clotting during the dialysis treatment; it can be administered continuously or intermittently. Problems that may occur during dialysis, depending on the rates of blood flow and solute removal, include hypotension, nausea, vomiting, muscle cramps, headache, chest pain, and disequilibrium syndrome.

Most persons are dialyzed three times each week for 3 to 4 hours; treatment is determined by kinetic profiles of solute removal, referred to as Kt/V values, which is influenced by dialyzer size, dialysate, flow rate, time of dialysis, and body size. Hemodialysis can be done in hospitals, community dialysis centres, or at home depending on variety of individual factors (*e.g.,* acuity, comorbidities).[6]

Peritoneal Dialysis. Peritoneal dialysis was introduced in the mid-1970s. Improvements in technology and the ability to deliver adequate dialysis resulted in improved outcomes and the acceptance of peritoneal dialysis as a renal replacement therapy.

FIGURE 34.5 • Schematic diagram of a hemodialysis system. The blood compartment and dialysis solution compartment are separated by a semipermeable membrane. This membrane is porous enough to allow all the constituents, except the plasma proteins and blood cells, to diffuse between the two compartments.

The same principles of diffusion, osmosis, and ultrafiltration that apply to hemodialysis apply to peritoneal dialysis.[6,36] The thin serous membrane of the peritoneal cavity serves as the dialyzing membrane. A silastic catheter is surgically implanted in the peritoneal cavity below the umbilicus to provide access. The catheter is tunnelled through subcutaneous tissue and exits on the side of the abdomen (Fig. 34.6). The

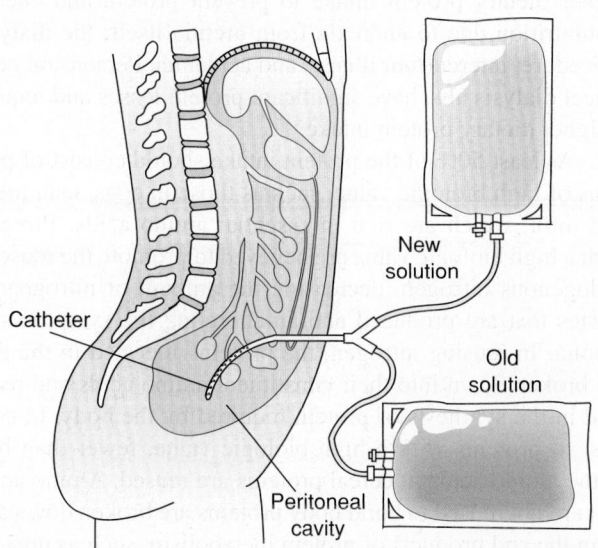

FIGURE 34.6 • Peritoneal dialysis. A semipermeable membrane, richly supplied with small blood vessels, lines the peritoneal cavity. With dialysate dwelling in the peritoneal cavity, waste products diffuse from the network of blood vessels into the dialysate.

dialysis process involves instilling a sterile dialyzing solution (usually 1 to 3 L) through the catheter over a period of approximately 10 minutes. The solution then is allowed to remain, or *dwell,* in the peritoneal cavity for a prescribed amount of time, during which the metabolic end products and extracellular fluid diffuse into the dialysis solution. At the end of the dwell time, the dialysis fluid is drained out of the peritoneal cavity by gravity into a sterile bag. Glucose in the dialysis solution accounts for water removal. Commercial dialysis solution is available in 1.5%, 2.5%, and 4.25% dextrose concentrations. Solutions with higher dextrose levels increase osmosis, causing more fluid to be removed. As with hemodialysis, Kt/V values are used to evaluate adequacy of peritoneal dialysis.

Peritoneal dialysis is usually performed at home and can be carried out by continuous ambulatory peritoneal dialysis (CAPD) or continuous cyclic peritoneal dialysis (CCPD). Individual preference, manual ability, lifestyle, knowledge of the procedure, and physiologic response to treatment are used to determine the type of dialysis that is used. The most common method is CCPD, where exchanges are performed in an automated manner, usually at night, with the person connected to an automatic cycler, which then performs four or five cycles while the person sleeps. In the morning, the person, with the last exchange remaining in the abdomen, is disconnected from the cycler and goes about his or her usual activities. CAPD involves instilling the dialysate into the peritoneal cavity and then disconnecting so that the patient is free. After the dwell time is completed (usually 4 to 6 hours during the day), the patient reconnects to a drain bag, allowing the waste-containing dialysis solution to drain from the peritoneal cavity into the bag. A fresh bag of dialysate is then instilled, starting the cycle over again. Each exchange, which involves draining the solution and infusing a new solution, requires approximately 30 to 45 minutes. Four exchanges usually are performed each day. Potential problems with peritoneal dialysis include infection, catheter malfunction, dehydration caused by excessive fluid removal, hyperglycemia, and hernia. The most serious complication is infection, which can occur at the catheter exit site, in the subcutaneous tunnel, or in the peritoneal cavity (*i.e.*, peritonitis).[6,36]

Transplantation. Greatly improved success rates have made kidney transplantation the treatment of choice for many patients with ESRD. The availability of donor organs continues to limit the number of transplantations performed each year.[35] Donor organs are obtained from cadavers and living related donors (*e.g.*, parent, sibling). Transplants from living unrelated donors (*e.g.*, spouse, friend) have been used in cases of suitable ABO blood type and tissue compatibility. Living donor kidney transplantation has more than doubled over the past 15 years, with regional and provincial variation.

The success of transplantation depends on multiple variables such as the general health of the recipient, the degree of histocompatibility with the donor, adequate organ preservation, and immunologic management. Maintenance immunosuppressive therapy typically consists of corticosteroids, immunosuppressants (*i.e.*, mycophenolate, azathioprine), calcineurin inhibitors (*i.e.*, tacrolimus, cyclosporine,) and/or sirolimus (inhibits the mTOR pathway). Interleukin(IL)-2, a cytokine, plays an essential role in T- and B-cell activation (see Chapter 17). Cyclosporine and tacrolimus inhibit IL-2 synthesis, and sirolimus inhibits the T-cell response to IL-2. Genetically engineered antibodies that selectively target interleukin receptors also are available. Antilymphocyte antibodies which target the T-cells directly may be used as induction therapy. Because of the increased number of effective immunosuppressive agents that have become available, lower corticosteroid doses are used, resulting in reduced cushingoid effects after transplantation.[37]

Rejection, which is categorized as either acute or chronic, can occur at any time (see Chapter 19). Acute rejection most commonly occurs during the first several months after transplantation and involves a cellular response with the proliferation of T lymphocytes. Chronic rejection can occur months to years after transplantation. Because chronic rejection is caused by both cellular and humoral immunity, it does not respond well to increased immunosuppressive therapy.

Maintenance immunosuppressive therapy and increased use of immunosuppression to treat rejection predispose the person to a spectrum of infectious complications. Prophylactic antimicrobials may be prescribed to decrease the incidence of common infections, such as candidiasis, herpesvirus infections, and *Pneumocystis jiroveci* (formerly *P. carinii*) pneumonia. Other infections, such as cytomegalovirus infection and aspergillosis, are seen with chronic immunosuppression.

Direct infection of the kidney with subsequent injury and loss of allograft function has been seen with BK virus, one of the polyoma viruses.[38]

Dietary Management

A major component in the treatment of CKD is dietary management.[6,17] The goal of dietary treatment is to provide optimum nutrition while maintaining tolerable levels of metabolic wastes. The specific diet prescription depends on the type and severity of renal disease and on the dialysis modality. Because of the severe restrictions placed on food and fluid intake, these diets may be complicated and unappetizing. After kidney transplantation, some dietary restrictions still may be necessary, even when renal function is normal, to control the adverse effects from immunosuppressive medication.

Protein. Restriction of dietary proteins may decrease the progress of renal impairment in persons with advanced renal disease. Proteins are broken down to form nitrogenous wastes, and reducing the amount of protein in the diet lowers the urea levels and reduces symptoms. Moreover, a high-protein diet is high in phosphates and inorganic acids. The Modification of Diet in Renal Disease (MDRD) Study, which was conducted in 15 university hospital outpatient nephrology clinics and included 255 patients between the ages of 18 and 70 years, demonstrated a slower decline in GFR among patients randomized to the very–low-protein diet compared with patients on a low-protein diet.[39]

Considerable controversy exists over the degree of restriction needed. If the diet is too low in protein, protein malnutrition can occur, with a loss of strength, muscle mass, and body weight. Canadian guidelines recommend a protein controlled diet of 0.80 to 1.0 g of protein per kilogram of body weight per day.[28] Persons on hemodialysis usually require a higher dietary protein intake to prevent protein and energy malnutrition due to anorexia from uremia itself, the dialysis procedure, intercurrent illness, and acidemia. Persons on peritoneal dialysis also have significant protein losses and require a higher dietary protein intake.

At least 50% of the protein intake should consist of proteins of high biologic value, such as those in eggs, lean meat, and milk, which are rich in essential amino acids. Proteins with a high biologic value are believed to promote the reuse of endogenous nitrogen, decreasing the amount of nitrogenous wastes that are produced and ameliorating the symptoms of uremia. In reusing nitrogen, the proteins ingested in the diet are broken down into their constituent amino acids and recycled in the synthesis of protein required by the body. In contrast to proteins with a high biologic value, fewer than half of the amino acids in cereal proteins are reused. Amino acids that are not reused to build body proteins are broken down and form the end products of protein metabolism, such as urea.

Carbohydrates, Fat, and Calories. With CKD, adequate calories in the form of carbohydrates and fat are required to meet energy needs. This is particularly important when the protein content of the diet is severely restricted. If sufficient calories are not available, the limited protein in the diet goes into energy production, or body tissue itself is used for energy purposes. Caloric intake for persons on peritoneal dialysis includes food intake and calories absorbed from the dialysis solution.

Fluid and Electrolytes. The sodium and fluid restrictions depend on the kidneys' ability to excrete sodium and water and must be individually determined. Renal disease of glomerular origin is more likely to contribute to sodium retention, whereas tubular dysfunction causes salt wasting. Fluid intake in excess of what the kidneys can excrete causes circulatory overload, edema, and water intoxication. Thirst is a common problem among patients on hemodialysis, often resulting in large weight gains between treatments. Inadequate intake, on the other hand, causes volume depletion and hypotension and can cause further decreases in the already compromised GFR. It is common practice to allow a daily fluid intake of 500 to 800 ml, which is equal to insensible water loss plus a quantity equal to the 24-hour urine output.

When the GFR falls to extremely low levels in kidney failure or during hemodialysis therapy, dietary restriction of potassium becomes mandatory. Using salt substitutes that contain potassium, or ingesting fruits, fruit juice, chocolate, potatoes, or other high-potassium foods can cause hyperkalemia. Most persons on peritoneal dialysis do not need to limit potassium intake and often may even need to increase intake.

Persons with CKD are usually encouraged to limit their dietary phosphorus as a means of preventing secondary hyperthyroidism, renal osteodystrophy, and metastatic calcification. Unfortunately, many processed and convenience foods contain considerable amounts of phosphorus additives. The most notable products using phosphorus additives are restructured meats (*e.g.,* chicken nuggets, hot dogs), processed and spreadable cheeses, instant products (*e.g.,* puddings, sauces), refrigerated bakery products, and beverages. These phosphorus additives are highly absorbable. In a typical diet of grains, meats, and dairy products, only about 60% of phosphorus is absorbed, whereas phosphorus additives (*e.g.,* polyphosphates, pyrophosphates) are almost 90% absorbed.[40] Identifying these newer phosphorus-containing foods is often challenging because manufacturers are no longer required to list the phosphorus content on food labels.

IN SUMMARY

CKD results from the destructive effects of many forms of renal disease. Regardless of the cause, the consequences of nephron destruction in CKD are alterations in the filtration, reabsorption, and endocrine functions of the kidneys. Chronic disease is defined as either diagnosed kidney damage or GFR of less than 60 ml/min/1.73 m^2 for 3 months or more, and kidney failure as a GFR of <15 ml/min/1.73 m^2, usually accompanied by most of the signs and symptoms of uremia, and a need for renal replacement therapy.

CKD affects almost every body system. It causes an accumulation of nitrogenous wastes (*i.e.,* azotemia), alters sodium and water excretion, and alters regulation of body levels of potassium, phosphate, calcium, and magnesium. It also causes skeletal disorders, anemia, cardiovascular disorders, neurologic disturbances, gastrointestinal dysfunction, immunosuppression, and discomforting skin changes.

The treatment measures for CKD can be divided into two types: conservative treatment measures and renal replacement therapy. Conservative treatment consists of measures to prevent or retard deterioration in remaining renal function and assist the body in compensating for the existing impairment. Interventions that have been shown to retard the progression of CKD include blood pressure normalization and control of blood glucose in persons with diabetes. Activated vitamin D can be used to increase calcium absorption and control secondary hyperparathyroidism. Recombinant human erythropoietin is used to treat the profound anemia that occurs in persons with CKD. Renal replacement therapy (dialysis or kidney transplantation) is indicated when advanced uremia and serious electrolyte problems are present.

CHRONIC KIDNEY DISEASE IN CHILDREN AND OLDER ADULTS

After completing this section of the chapter, you should be able to meet the following objectives:

* List the causes of CKD in children and describe the special problems of children with kidney failure.
* State why CKD is more common in the older adults and describe measures to prevent or delay the onset of kidney failure in this population.
* Describe the treatment of CKD in children and the older adults.

Although the spectrum of CKD among children and older adults is similar to that of adults, several unique issues affecting these groups warrant further discussion.

Chronic Kidney Disease in Children

The true incidence of CKD in infants and children is unknown. Data suggests that 1% to 2% of persons with CKD are in the pediatric age range with this trend increasing worldwide.[6] The causes of CKD in children include congenital malformations, inherited disorders, acquired diseases, and metabolic syndromes. The underlying cause correlates closely with the age of the child.[6,41] In children younger than 5 years of age, CKD is commonly the result of congenital malformations such as renal dysplasia or obstructive uropathy. After 5 years of age, acquired diseases (*e.g.,* glomerulonephritis) and inherited disorders (*e.g.,* familial juvenile nephronophthisis) predominate. CKD related to metabolic disorders such as hyperoxaluria and inherited disorders such as polycystic kidney disease may present throughout childhood.[6,42]

The stages for progression of CKD in children over 2 years of age are similar to those for adults: Stages 1 to 5 that identify the reduction of GFR, and kidney failure with a GFR of less than 15 ml/min/1.73 m[2], or a need for renal replacement therapy. Because the GFR is much lower in infancy and undergoes gradual changes in relation to body size during the first 2 years of life, these values apply only to children older than 2 years of age.[42,43]

The manifestations of CKD in children are quite varied and depend on the underlying disease condition. Features of CKD that are marked during childhood include severe growth impairment, developmental delay, delay in sexual maturation, bone abnormalities, and development of psychosocial problems. Critical growth periods occur during the first 2 years of life and during adolescence. Physical growth and cognitive development occur at a slower rate as consequences of renal disease, especially among children with congenital renal disease.[42] Puberty usually occurs at a later age in children with renal failure, partly because of endocrine abnormalities. Renal osteodystrophies are more common and extensive in children than in adults. The most common condition seen in children is high-bone-turnover bone disease caused by secondary hyperparathyroidism. Some hereditary renal diseases, such as medullary cystic disease, have patterns of skeletal involvement that further complicate the problems of renal osteodystrophy. Clinical manifestations of renal osteodystrophy include muscle weakness, bone pain, and fractures with minor trauma.[42] In growing children, rachitic changes, varus and valgus deformities of long bones, and slipped capital femoral epiphysis may be seen (see Chapter 58).

Factors related to impaired growth include deficient nutrition, anemia, renal osteodystrophy, chronic acidosis, and cases of nephrotic syndrome that require high-dose corticosteroid therapy. Success of treatment depends on the level of bone maturation at the initiation of therapy. Nutrition is believed to be the most important determinant during infancy. During childhood, growth hormone is important, and gonadotropic hormones become important during puberty. Parental heights provide a means of assessing growth potential (see Chapter 41). For many children, catch-up growth is important because a growth deficit frequently is established during the first months of life. Recombinant human growth hormone therapy has been used to improve growth in children with CKD.[42]

All forms of renal replacement therapy can be safely and reliably used for children. Age is a defining factor in dialysis modality selection; 88% of infants and children from birth to 5 years of age are treated with peritoneal dialysis, whereas 54% of children older than 12 years of age are treated with hemodialysis.[42] The majority of North American children are treated with CCPD, which leaves the child and family free of dialysis demands during waking hours, with the exchanges being performed automatically during sleep by the machine.

Renal transplantation is considered the best alternative for children.[42] Early transplantation in young children is regarded as the best way to promote physical growth, improve cognitive function, and foster psychosocial development. Immunosuppressive therapy in children is similar to that used in adults. All of these immunosuppressive agents have side effects, including increased risk for infection. Corticosteroids, which have been the mainstay of chronic immunosuppressive therapy for decades, carry the risk of hypertension, orthopedic complications (especially aseptic necrosis of the hip), cataracts, and growth retardation.

Chronic Kidney Disease in Older Adults

The incidence of CKD in older adults, including those requiring hemodialysis, is increasing and is now more common in males. There was a threefold increase from 1994 to 2002 in Canada particularly in the over 75 age group but since 2003 this has remained constant.[35] However, the true prevalence or outcomes of CKD in older adults have not been verified or systematically studied, in part due to lack of detection and referral. As well, the presentation and course of CKD in the older adult may be altered because of age-related changes in the kidneys and concurrent medical conditions, increasing the risk of delayed diagnosis.

Normal aging is associated with a minor decline in the GFR and subsequently with reduced homeostatic regulation under stressful conditions. This reduction in GFR makes older adults more susceptible to the detrimental effects of nephrotoxic drugs, such as radiographic contrast compounds. The reduction in GFR related to aging is not accompanied by a parallel rise in the serum creatinine level because the serum creatinine level, which results from muscle metabolism, is significantly reduced in older adults because of diminished muscle mass and other age-related changes. The NKF and Canadian Society of Nephrology guidelines suggest that the same criteria for establishing the presence of CKD in younger adults be used for the older adults as creatinine clearance measurements are adjusted for age.[28]

The prevalence of chronic disease affecting the cerebrovascular, cardiovascular, and skeletal systems is higher in this age group. Because of concurrent disease, the presenting symptoms of kidney disease in older adults may be less typical than those observed in younger adults. For example, congestive heart failure and hypertension may be the dominant clinical features with the onset of acute glomerulonephritis, whereas oliguria and discoloured urine more often are the first signs in younger adults. The course of kidney failure may be more complicated in older patients with numerous chronic diseases.

Clinical interventions for older adults with CKD should be based on diagnosis, severity of kidney function impairment, and stratification of risk for progression to renal failure and cardiovascular disease. Persons with low risk may require only modification of dosages of medications excreted by the kidney, monitoring of blood pressure, avoidance of drugs and procedures that increase the risk of acute renal injury, and lifestyle modification to reduce the risk of cardiovascular disease.

Older adults with more severe impairment of kidney function may require renal replacement therapy. Treatment options for renal failure in older adults include hemodialysis, peritoneal dialysis, transplantation and palliation. The mode of renal replacement therapy should be individualized, taking into account underlying medical and psychosocial factors. Age alone does not preclude either hemodialysis or renal transplantation.[43] With increasing experience, many transplantation centres have increased the age for acceptance on transplant waiting lists. Reluctance to provide transplantation as an alternative may have been due, at least in part, to the scarcity of available organs and the view that younger persons are more likely to benefit for a longer time. The general reduction in T-lymphocyte function that occurs with aging has been suggested as a beneficial effect that increases transplant graft survival.

Because initiation of dialysis in an older adult, especially where there is decreased functional capacity, can lead to a significant decline in quality of life, palliative and supportive care is increasingly recognized as a reasonable alternative to dialysis. In this course of treatment, the patient and/or caregivers are aware that the goal is not to prolong life at the expense of quality of life.[43]

IN SUMMARY

Available data suggest that 1% to 2% of patients with CKD are in the pediatric age range. The causes of renal failure include congenital malformations (*e.g.*, renal dysplasia and obstructive uropathy), inherited disorders (*e.g.*, polycystic kidney disease), acquired diseases (*e.g.*, glomerulonephritis), and metabolic syndromes (*e.g.*, hyperoxaluria). Problems associated with renal failure in children include growth impairment, delay in sexual maturation, and more extensive bone abnormalities than in adults. Although all forms of renal replacement therapy can be safely and reliably used in children, CAPD or transplantation optimizes growth and development.

Normal aging is associated with a decline in the GFR, which makes older adults more susceptible to the detrimental effects of nephrotoxic drugs and other conditions that compromise renal function. Current guidelines for diagnosis of CKD and stratification of risk for progression to kidney failure are the same as for younger adults. Renal replacement options for kidney failure in older adults are also similar to those for younger adults with the focus on quality of life.

REVIEW EXERCISES

1. A 55-year-old man with diabetes and coronary heart disease, who had undergone cardiac catheterization with the use of a radiocontrast agent 2 days ago, is admitted to the emergency department with a flulike syndrome including chills, nausea, vomiting, abdominal pain, fatigue, and pulmonary congestion. His serum creatinine is elevated, and he has protein in his urine. He is admitted to the intensive care unit with a tentative diagnosis of acute renal injury due to radiocontrast nephropathy.
   A. *Radiocontrast agents are thought to exert their effects through decreased renal perfusion and through direct toxic effects on renal tubular structures. Explain how each of these phenomena contributes to the development of acute renal failure.*
   B. *Explain the elevated serum creatinine, proteinuria, and presence of pulmonary congestion.*

2. A 35-year-old, 70-kg white man with diabetes mellitus is seen in the diabetic clinic for his 6-month checkup. His serum creatinine, which was slightly elevated at his last visit, is now 140 μmol/L. Use the following website to estimate his GFR: www.kidney.org/professionals/KDOQI/gfr_calculator.cfm.
   A. *Would he be classified as having CKD?*
   B. *If so, what stage? What might be done to delay or prevent further deterioration of his kidney function?*

3. *CKD* is accompanied by hyperphosphatemia, hypocalcemia, impaired activation of vitamin D, hyperparathyroidism, and skeletal complications.
   A. *Explain the impaired activation of vitamin D and its consequences on calcium and phosphate homeostasis, parathyroid function, and mineralization of bone in persons with renal failure.*
   B. *Explain the possible complications of the administration of activated forms of vitamin D on parathyroid function and calcium and phosphate homeostasis (e.g., calcium × phosphate product).*

References

1. Bellomo R., Kellum J. A., Ronco C. (2012). Acute kidney injury. *Lancet, 380*(9843), 756–766.
2. Murugan R., Kellum J. A. (2011). Acute kidney injury: What's the prognosis? *Nature Reviews Nephrology, 7*(4), 209–217.
3. Hilton R. (2011). Defining acute renal failure. *Canadian Medical Association Journal, 183*(10), 1167–1169.
4. Obermuller N., Gieger H., Weipert C., Urbschat A. (2014). Current development in early diagnosis of acute kidney injury. *International Urology and Nephrology, 46*(1), 1–7.
5. Vanmassenhove J., Vanholder R., Ngaler E., Van Biesen W. (2013). Urinary and serum biomarkers for the diagnosis of acute kidney injury: An in-depth review of the literature. *Nephrology Dialysis Transplantation, 28*(2), 254–273.
6. Taal M. W., Chertow G. M., Marden P. A., et al. (Eds.). (2012). *Brenner and Rector's the kidney* (9th ed.). Philadelphia, PA: Elsevier Saunders.

7. Bonventre J. V., Yang L. (2011). Cellular pathophysiology of ischemic acute kidney injury. *Journal of Clinical Investigation, 121*(11), 4210–4221.

8. Dirkes S. (2011). Acute kidney injury: Not just acute renal failure anymore? *Critical Care Nurse, 31*(1), 37–50.

9. Hall J. E. (2011). *Textbook of medical physiology* (12th ed.). Philadelphia, PA: W.B. Saunders.

10. Cervellin G., Comelli I., Lippi G. (2010). Rhabdomyolysis: Historical background, clinical, diagnostic and therapeutic features. *Clinical Chemistry and Laboratory Medicine, 48*(6), 749–756.

11. Lins R. L. (2012). RRT treatment for AKI: Is more always better? *Nephrology Dialysis Transplantation, 27*(12), 4252–4255.

12. Arora P., Vasa P., Brenner D., et al. (2013). Prevalence estimates of chronic kidney disease in Canada: Results of a nationally representative survey. *Canadian Medical Association Journal, 185*(9), E417–E423.

13. The Kidney Foundation of Canada. (2013). Facing the facts. Available online at: http://www.kidney.ca/document.doc?id=4083. Accessed June 5, 2014.

14. Hemmelgarn B. R., Manns B. J., Tonelli M. (2012). A decade after the KDOQI CKD guidelines: A perspective from Canada. *American Journal of Kidney Disease, 60*(5), 723–724.

15. Kidney Disease Improving Global Outcomes (KDIGO). (2013). KDIGO 2012 Clinical practice guidelines for the evaluation and management of chronic kidney disease. *Kidney International Supplements, 3*(1), 1–150.

16. Levey A. S., Coresh J. (2012). Chronic kidney disease. *Lancet, 379*(9811), 165–180.

17. James M. T., Hemmelgarn B. R., Tonelli M. (2010). Early recognition and prevention of chronic kidney disease. *Lancet, 375*(9722), 1296–1309.

18. Abboud H., Henrich W. L. (2010). Stage IV chronic kidney disease. *New England Journal of Medicine, 362*(1), 56–65.

19. Waheed A. A., Pedraza F., Lenz O., Isakova T. (2013). Phosphate control in end-stage renal disease: Barriers and opportunities. *Nephrology Dialysis Transplantation, 28*(12), 2961–2968.

20. Elder G. J. (2012). Pathophysiology of CKD-MBD. *Clinical Reviews in Bone and Mineral Metabolism, 10*(3), 128–141.

21. Kiattisunthorn K., Moe S. M. (2012). Chronic kidney disease-mineral bone disorder: Definitions and rationale for a systemic disorder. *Clinical Reviews in Bone and Mineral Metabolism, 10*(3), 119–127.

22. Morrow B., Qunibi W. (2012). Specific bone and mineral disorders in patients with chronic kidney disease. *Clinical Reviews in Bone and Mineral Metabolism, 10*(3), 184–208.

23. Heymann E. P., Jenkins M., Goldsmith D. (2012). Clinical features and manifestations of CKD-MBD. *Clinical Reviews in Bone and Mineral Metabolism, 10*(3), 142–148.

24. Covic A., Apetrii M., Heymann E. P., Goldsmith D. (2012). Medical and surgical management (including diet). *Clinical Reviews in Bone and Mineral Metabolism, 10*(3), 174–183.

25. Seifter J. L., Samuels M. A. (2011). Uremic encephalopathy and other brain disorders associated with renal failure. *Seminars in Neurology, 31*(2),139–143.

26. Kidney Disease Improving Global Outcomes (KDIGO). (2012). KDIGO Clinical practice guideline for anemia in chronic kidney disease. *Kidney International Supplements, 2*(4), 279–335.

27. Magwood J. S., Lebby A., Chen B., et al. (2013). Emerging drugs for treatment of anemia of chronic kidney disease. *Expert Opinion on Emerging Drugs, 18*(4), 421–429.

28. Levin A., Hemmelgarn B., Culleton B., et al.; Canadian Society of Nephrology. (2008). Guidelines for the management of chronic kidney disease. *CMAJ, 179*, 1154–1162.

29. Gunukula S., Spodick D. H. (2001). Pericardial disease in renal failure. *Seminars in Nephrology, 21*(1), 52–56.

30. Rathi M., Ramachandran R. (2012). Sexual and gonadal dysfunction in chronic kidney disease: Pathophysiology. *Indian Journal of Endocrinology and Metabolism, 16*(2), 214–219.

31. Turner J. M., Bauer C., Abramowitz M. K., et al. (2012). Treatment of chronic kidney disease. *Kidney International, 81*(4), 351–362.

32. Dasqupta K., Quinn R. R., Zarnke K. B., et al.; Canadian Hypertension Education Program. (2014). The 2014 Canadian hypertension education program recommendations for blood pressure measurement, diagnosis, assessment of risk, prevention, and treatment of hypertension. *Canadian Journal of Cardiology, 30*(5), 485–501.

33. Maeda I., Hayashi T., Sato K. K., et al. (2011). Cigarette smoking and the association with glomerular hyperfiltration and proteinuria in healthy middle-aged men. *CJASN, 6*(10), 2462–2469.

34. Beirness D., Gliksman L., Paradis C., Stockwell T. (2011). *Alcohol and health in Canada: A summary of evidence and guidelines for low risk drinking.* Ottawa: Canadian Centre of Substance Abuse.

35. Canadian Institute for Health Information. (2014). *Canadian organ replacement register annual report: Treatment of end-stage organ failure in Canada, 2003–2012.* Ottawa: CIHI/CORR.

36. Fleming G. M. (2011). Renal replacement therapy review. *Organogenesis, 7*(1), 2–12.

37. Menon M. C., Murphy B. (2013). Maintenance immunosuppression in renal transplantation. *Current Opinion in Pharmacology, 13*(4), 662–671.

38. Balba G. P., Javaid B., Timpone J. G. (2013). BK polyomavirus infection in the renal transplant recipient. *Infectious Disease Clinics of North America, 27*(2), 271–283.

39. Karalis M. (2005). Hidden phosphorus in popular beverages: Part 1; at breakfast: Part II, and enhanced meats: Part IV. *Journal of Renal Nutrition, 15*(2, 3, 4), e1–e6, e1–e6, e1–e4.

40. Kalnatar-Zadeh K., Gutekunst L., Mehrotra R., et al. (2010). Understanding sources of dietary phosphorus in the treatment of patients with chronic kidney disease. *CJASN, 5*(3), 519–530.

41. Staples A., Wong C. (2010). Risk factors for progression of chronic kidney disease. *Current Opinion in Pediatrics, 22*(2), 161–169.

42. Sreedharan R., Avner E. D. (2011). Chapter 529: Renal failure. In Kliegman R. M., Stanton B. F., St. Geme J. W., et al. (Eds.), *Nelson textbook of pediatrics* (19th ed.). Philadelphia, PA: Saunders Elsevier.

43. Whyte D. A., Fine R. N. (2008). Chronic kidney disease in children. *Pediatrics in Review, 29*(10), 335–341.

Visit thePoint **http://thePoint.lww.com for animations, journal articles, and more!**

Disorders of the Bladder and Lower Urinary Tract

35

Although the kidneys control the formation of urine and regulate the composition of body fluids, it is the bladder that stores urine and controls its elimination from the body. Alterations in the storage and expulsion functions of the bladder can result in incontinence, with its accompanying social and hygienic problems, or obstruction of urinary flow, which has deleterious effects on ureteral flow and, ultimately, renal function. The discussion in this chapter focuses on the normal control of urine elimination, urinary obstruction and stasis, neurogenic bladder, incontinence, and bladder cancer. Urinary tract infections are discussed in Chapter 33.

CONTROL OF URINE ELIMINATION

After completing this section of the chapter, you should be able to meet the following objectives:

- Trace the ascending sensory and descending motor impulses between the detrusor muscle and external urinary sphincter and the spinal cord, pontine micturition centre, and cerebral cortex.
- Explain the mechanism of low-pressure urine storage in the bladder.
- List at least three classes of autonomic drugs and explain their potential effect on bladder function.
- Describe at least three urodynamic studies that can be used to assess bladder function.

Bladder Structure

The bladder, also known as the *urinary vesicle,* is a freely movable organ located retroperitoneally on the pelvic floor, just posterior to the pubic symphysis. It consists of two main components: the body in which urine collects and the neck, which is a funnel-shaped extension of the body that connects with the urethra.[1-6] In the male, the urethra continues anteriorly through the penis, with the prostate gland surrounding the neck of the bladder where it empties into the urethra. In the female, the bladder is located anterior to the vagina and uterus.

BLADDER FUNCTION

- The functions of the bladder are storage and emptying of urine.
- The control of the storage and emptying functions of the bladder involves both involuntary (autonomic nervous system) and voluntary (somatic nervous system) control.
- The parasympathetic nervous system promotes bladder emptying. It produces contraction of the smooth muscle of the bladder wall and relaxation of the internal sphincter.
- The sympathetic nervous system promotes bladder filling. It produces relaxation of the smooth muscle of the bladder wall and contraction of the internal sphincter.
- The striated muscles in the external sphincter and pelvic floor, which are innervated by the somatic nervous system, provide for the voluntary control of urination and maintenance of continence.

Urine passes from the kidneys to the bladder through the ureters. The interior of the bladder has openings for both the ureters and the urethra. The smooth triangular area that is bounded by these three openings is called the *trigone* (Fig. 35.1). There are no valves at the ureteral openings, but as the pressure of the urine in the bladder rises, the ends of the ureters are compressed against the bladder wall to prevent the backflow of urine.

The bladder is composed of four layers. The first is an outer serosal layer, which covers the upper surface and is continuous with the peritoneum. The second is a network of smooth muscle fibres called the *detrusor muscle*. The third is

FIGURE 35.1 • Diagram of the bladder, showing the detrusor muscle, ureters, trigone area, and urethral orifice. Note the flattening of epithelial cells when the bladder is full and the wall is stretched.

a submucosal layer of loose connective tissue, and the fourth is an inner mucosal lining of transitional epithelium (urothelium). This stratified epithelium is essentially impermeable to salts and water. The tonicity and composition of the urine often is quite different from that of the blood, and the epithelial lining of the bladder acts as an effective barrier to prevent the passage of water and other urine elements between the bladder and the blood. The epithelial lining of the bladder is six or more layers thick in the empty bladder. However, when the bladder is distended, as few as two or three layers are seen. This change reflects the ability of these cells to flatten and unfold to accommodate the increased surface area of a distended bladder (Fig. 35.1).

The detrusor muscle is the muscle of micturition (passage of urine). When it contracts, urine is expelled from the bladder. Muscles in the bladder neck, sometimes referred to as the *internal urethral sphincter,* are a continuation of the detrusor muscle. They run down obliquely behind the proximal urethra, forming the posterior urethra in males and the entire urethra in females. When the bladder is relaxed, these circular muscle fibres are closed and act as a sphincter. When the detrusor muscle contracts, the sphincter is pulled open as the shape of the bladder changes. In the female, the urethra (approximately 4 cm) is shorter than in the male (approximately 22.3 cm), and usually affords less resistance to urine outflow.[5]

Another muscle important to bladder function is the *external sphincter,* a circular muscle composed of striated muscle fibres that surrounds the urethra distal to the base of the bladder. The external sphincter operates as a reserve mechanism to stop micturition when it is occurring and to maintain continence in the face of unusually high bladder pressure. The skeletal muscle of the pelvic floor also contributes to the support of the bladder and the maintenance of continence.

Neural Control of Bladder Function

Normal bladder function requires the coordinated interaction between the sensory and motor components of the involuntary autonomic and voluntary somatic nervous systems. The motor component of the neural reflex that causes bladder emptying is controlled by the parasympathetic nervous system, whereas the relaxation and storage function of the bladder is controlled by the sympathetic nervous system. The somatic nervous system provides for the voluntary control of the external sphincter and pelvic floor muscles. These functions are controlled by three neurologic centres: the spinal cord reflex centres, the micturition centre in the pons, and the cortical and subcortical centres.[2]

Spinal Cord Centres

The centres for reflex control of bladder function are located in the sacral (S1 through S4) and thoracolumbar (T11 through L2) segments of the spinal cord[1–6] (Fig. 35.2). The parasympathetic lower motor neurons (LMNs) for the detrusor muscle of the bladder are located in the sacral segments of the spinal cord; their axons travel to the bladder by way of the *pelvic nerve.* LMNs for the external sphincter are also located in the

Afferent fibres
Efferent motor
Efferent inhibitory

Sympathetic neurons

T11
T12
L1
L2

Hypogastric nerve

Parasympathetic pelvic nerves

S1
S2
S3

S2
S3
S4

Detrusor muscle
Internal sphincter
External sphincter

Somatic pudendal nerve

FIGURE 35.2 • Nerve supply to the bladder and the urethra.

sacral segments of the spinal cord. These LMNs receive their control from the motor cortex through the corticospinal tract and send impulses to the external sphincter through the *pudendal nerve*. The bladder neck and trigone area of the bladder, because of their different embryonic origins, receive sympathetic outflow from the thoracolumbar (T11 to L2) segments of the spinal cord. In the male, the seminal vesicles, ampulla, and vas deferens also receive sympathetic innervation from the thoracolumbar segments of the cord.

The afferent input from the bladder and urethra is carried to the central nervous system (CNS) by fibres that travel with the parasympathetic (pelvic), somatic (pudendal), and sympathetic (hypogastric) nerves. The pelvic nerve carries sensory fibres from the stretch receptors in the bladder wall; the pudendal nerve carries sensory fibres from the external sphincter and pelvic muscles; and the hypogastric nerve carries sensory fibres from the trigone area.[3]

Pontine Micturition Centre

The immediate coordination of the normal micturition reflex occurs in the micturition centre in the pons, facilitated by descending input from the forebrain and ascending input from the reflex centres in the spinal cord[1-3] (Fig. 35.3). This centre is thought to coordinate the activity of the detrusor muscle and the external sphincter. As bladder filling occurs, ascending spinal afferents relay this information to the micturition centre, which also receives important descending information from the forebrain concerning behavioural cues for bladder emptying and urine storage. Descending pathways from the pontine micturition centre produce coordinated inhibition or relaxation of the external sphincter. Disruption of pontine

control of micturition, as in spinal cord injury, results in uninhibited spinal reflex-controlled contraction of the bladder without relaxation of the external sphincter, a condition known as *detrusor–sphincter dyssynergia.*

Cortical and Subcortical Centres

Cortical brain centres enable inhibition of the micturition centre in the pons and conscious control of urination. Neural influences from the subcortical centres in the basal ganglia modulate the contractile response. They modify and delay the detrusor contractile response during filling and then modulate the expulsive activity of the bladder to facilitate complete emptying.

Micturition and Maintenance of Continence

To maintain continence, or retention of urine, the bladder must function as a low-pressure storage system, with the pressure in the bladder being lower than that in the urethra. To ensure that this condition is met, the increase in intravesical pressure that accompanies bladder filling is almost imperceptible. For example, an increase in bladder volume from 10 to 400 ml may be accompanied by only a 5 cm H_2O increase in pressure.[6] Abnormal sustained elevations in intravesical pressures (>40 to 50 cm H_2O) often are associated with vesicoureteral reflux (*i.e.,* backflow of urine from the bladder into the ureter) and the development of ureteral dilation (see Chapter 33). Although the pressure in the bladder is maintained at low levels, sphincter pressure remains high (45 to 65 cm H_2O) as a means of preventing loss of urine as the bladder fills.

Micturition, or the act of bladder emptying, involves both sensory and motor functions associated with bladder emptying. When the bladder is distended to 150 to 250 ml in the adult, the sensation of fullness is transmitted first to the spinal cord and then to the cerebral cortex. At approximately 400 to 500 ml the person will sense fullness of the bladder.[3] During the act of micturition, the detrusor muscle of the bladder fundus and bladder neck contract down on the urine; the ureteral orifices are forced shut; the bladder neck is widened and shortened as it is pulled up by the globular muscles in the bladder fundus; the resistance of the internal sphincter in the bladder neck is decreased; and the external sphincter relaxes as urine moves out of the bladder.

Neuromediator Control of Micturition

The autonomic nervous system (ANS) and its neuromediators play a central role in micturition. Parasympathetic innervation of the bladder is mediated by the neurotransmitter acetylcholine. Two types of cholinergic receptors, nicotinic and muscarinic, affect various aspects of micturition. *Nicotinic* (N) receptors are found in the synapses between the preganglionic and postganglionic neurons of the sympathetic and the parasympathetic system, as well as in the neuromuscular endplates of the striated muscle fibres of the external sphincter and pelvic muscles. *Muscarinic* (M) receptors are found in the postganglionic parasympathetic endings of the detrusor muscle. Several subtypes of M receptors have been identified.

FIGURE 35.3 • Pathways and central nervous system centres involved in the control of bladder emptying (**left**) and storage (**right**) functions. Efferent pathways for micturition (**left**) and urine storage (**right**) are also shown.

Both M_2 and M_3 receptors appear to mediate detrusor muscle activity, with the M_3 subtype mediating direct activation of detrusor muscle contraction. The M_2 subtype appears to act indirectly by inhibiting sympathetically mediated detrusor muscle relaxation.[2–4,7] The identification of muscarinic receptor subtypes has facilitated the development of medications that selectively target bladder structures while minimizing undesired side effects.

Although sympathetic innervation is not essential to the act of micturition, it allows the bladder to store a large volume without the involuntary escape of urine—a mechanism that is consistent with the fight-or-flight function subserved by the sympathetic nervous system. The bladder is supplied with α_1- and β_2-adrenergic receptors. The β_2-adrenergic receptors are found in the detrusor muscle; they produce relaxation of the detrusor muscle, increasing the bladder volume at which the micturition reflex is triggered. The α_1-adrenergic receptors are found in the trigone area, including the intramural ureteral musculature, bladder neck, and internal sphincter. The activation of α_1-adrenergic receptors produces contraction of these

muscles. Sympathetic activity ceases when the micturition reflex is activated. During male ejaculation, which is mediated by the sympathetic nervous system, the musculature of the trigone area and that of the bladder neck and prostatic urethra contract and prevent the backflow of seminal fluid into the bladder.

Because of their effects on bladder function, drugs that selectively activate or block ANS outflow or receptor activity can alter urine elimination. Table 35.1 indicates the action of drug groups that can impair bladder function or can be used in the treatment of micturition disorders. Many of the nonprescription cold preparations contain α-adrenergic agonists and antihistamine agents that have anticholinergic properties. These drugs can cause urinary retention. Many of the antidepressant and antipsychotic drugs also have anticholinergic actions that influence urination.

Continence in Children

In infants and young children, micturition is an involuntary act that is triggered by a spinal cord reflex; when the bladder fills to a given capacity, the detrusor muscle contracts, and

TABLE 35.1 ACTION OF DRUG GROUPS ON BLADDER FUNCTION

FUNCTION	DRUG GROUPS	MECHANISM OF ACTION
Detrusor Muscle		
Increased tone and contraction	Cholinergic drugs	Stimulate parasympathetic receptors that cause detrusor contraction
Inhibition of detrusor muscle relaxation during filling	β_2-Adrenergic blockers	Block β_2 receptors that produce detrusor muscle relaxation
Decreased tone	Anticholinergic drugs and drugs with an anticholinergic action	Block the muscarinic receptors that cause detrusor muscle contraction
	Calcium channel blockers	May interfere with influx of calcium to support contraction of detrusor smooth muscle
Internal Bladder Sphincter		
Increased tone	α_1-Adrenergic agonists	Activate α_1 receptors that produce contraction of the smooth muscle of the internal sphincter
Decreased tone	α_1-Adrenergic blockers	Block contraction of the smooth muscle of the internal sphincter
External Sphincter		
Decreased tone	Skeletal muscle relaxants	Decrease the tone of the external sphincter by acting at the level of the spinal cord or by interfering with release of calcium in the muscle fibres

the external sphincter relaxes.[8] As the child grows, the bladder gradually enlarges with approximately 30 ml capacity in the neonatal period and increases by approximately 30 ml/year for the first 8 years of life. However due to the many anatomical variables (e.g., height, weight) this can only be rough estimation.[9] As the bladder grows and increases in capacity, the tone of the external sphincter muscle increases. Toilet training begins at about 2 to 4 years of age when the child becomes conscious of the need to urinate. Conscious control of bladder function depends on (1) normal bladder growth, (2) myelination of the ascending afferents that signal awareness of bladder filling, (3) development of cortical control and descending communication with the sacral micturition centre, (4) ability consciously to tighten the external sphincter to prevent incontinence, and (5) motivation of the child to stay dry. Girls typically achieve continence before boys, and bowel control is typically achieved before bladder control. By 5 years of age, 90% to 95% of children are continent during the day and 80% to 85% are continent at night.[10]

Diagnostic Methods of Evaluating Bladder Function

Bladder structure and function can be assessed by a number of methods.[9,10] Reports or observations of frequency, hesitancy, straining to urinate or void, and a weak or interrupted stream are suggestive of outflow obstruction. Palpation and percussion provide information about bladder distension.

Physical Examination

Postvoidal residual (PVR) urine volume provides information about bladder emptying. It can be estimated by abdominal palpation and percussion. Catheterization and ultrasonography can be used to obtain specific measurements of PVR. A PVR value of less than 50 ml suggests adequate bladder emptying and more than 200 ml indicates inadequate bladder emptying.[11]

Pelvic examination is used in women to assess perineal skin condition, perivaginal muscle tone, genital atrophy, pelvic prolapse (e.g., cystocele, rectocele, uterine prolapse), pelvic mass, or other conditions that may impair bladder function. Bimanual examination (i.e., pelvic and abdominal palpation) can be used to assess PVR volume. Rectal examination is used to test for perineal sensation, sphincter tone, fecal impaction, and rectal mass. It is also used to assess the contour of the prostate in men.

Laboratory and Radiologic Studies

Urine tests provide information about kidney function and urinary tract infections (discussed in Chapter 33). The presence of bacteriuria or pyuria suggests urinary tract infection and the possibility of urinary tract obstruction. Blood tests (i.e., urea and creatinine) provide information about renal function.

Bladder structures can be visualized indirectly by taking x-ray films of the abdomen and by using excretory urography, which involves the use of a radiopaque dye, computed tomographic (CT) scanning, magnetic resonance imaging (MRI), or ultrasonography. Cystoscopy enables direct visualization of the urethra, bladder, and ureteral orifices.[11]

Ultrasonographic Bladder Scan. The ultrasonographic bladder scan provides a noninvasive method for estimating bladder volume.[11] The device uses ultrasonic reflections to differentiate the urinary bladder from the surrounding tissue. A computer system calculates and displays bladder volume. The device can be used to determine the need for catheterization, for evaluation and diagnosis of urinary retention, to measure PVR volumes, and for facilitating volume- or time-dependent catheterization or toileting programs.

Urodynamic Studies

Urodynamic studies are used to study bladder function and voiding problems. Three aspects of bladder function can be assessed by urodynamic studies: bladder, urethral, and intra-abdominal pressure changes; characteristics of urine flow; and the activity of the striated muscles of the external sphincter and pelvic floor.[1] Specific urodynamic tests include uroflowmetry, cystometry, urethral pressure profile, and sphincter electromyography (EMG). It often is advantageous to evaluate several components of bladder function simultaneously.

Uroflowmetry. Uroflowmetry measures the flow rate (millilitres per minute) during urination.[10] It commonly is done using a weight-recording device located at the bottom of a commode receptacle unit. As the person being tested voids, the weight of the commode receptacle unit increases. This weight change is electronically recorded and then analyzed as volume (weight converted to millilitres) versus time.[1]

Cystometry

Cystometry is used to measure bladder pressure during filling and voiding. It provides valuable information about total bladder capacity, intravesical pressures during bladder filling, the ability to perceive bladder fullness and the desire to urinate, the ability of the bladder to contract and sustain a contraction, uninhibited bladder contractions, and the ability to inhibit urination. Bladder pressure is measured using gas or water to transfer pressure to a transducer near a polygraph, or a pressure-tipped catheter to transfer the pressure recording directly to a polygraph. The test can be done by allowing physiologic filling of the bladder with urine and recording intravesical pressure throughout a voiding cycle, or by using a catheter to fill the bladder with water and measuring intravesical pressure against the volume of water instilled into the bladder.

In a normally functioning bladder, the sensation of bladder fullness is first perceived when the bladder contains 100 to 200 ml of urine while bladder pressure remains constant at approximately 8 to 15 cm H_2O. The desire to void occurs when the bladder is full (normal capacity is approximately 400 to 500 ml). At this point, a definite sensation of fullness occurs, the pressure rises sharply to 40 to 100 cm H_2O, and voiding occurs around the catheter. Urinary continence requires that urethral pressure exceed bladder pressure. If the urethral resistance is high because of obstruction, greater pressure is required, a condition that can be detected by cystometry.

Urethral Pressure Profile. The urethral pressure profile is used to evaluate the intraluminal pressure changes along the length of the urethra with the bladder at rest. It provides information about smooth muscle activity along the length of the

urethra. This test can be done using the infusion method (most commonly used), the membrane catheter method, or the microtip transducer. The infusion method involves the insertion of a small double-lumen urethral catheter, followed by the infusion of water into the bladder and measurement of the changes in urethral pressure as the catheter is slowly withdrawn.

Sphincter Electromyography. Sphincter EMG allows the activity of the striated (voluntary) muscles of the perineal area to be studied. Activity is recorded using an anal plug electrode, a catheter electrode, adhesive skin electrodes, or needle electrodes.[1] Electrode placement is based on the muscle groups that need to be tested. The test usually is done along with urodynamic tests such as cystometry and uroflowmetry.

IN SUMMARY

Although the kidneys function in the formation of urine and the regulation of body fluids, it is the bladder that stores and controls the elimination of urine. Micturition is a function of the peripheral ANS, subject to facilitation or inhibition from higher neurologic centres. The parasympathetic nervous system controls the function of the detrusor muscle and internal sphincter; its cell bodies are located in S1 through S3 of the spinal cord and communicate with the bladder through the pelvic nerve. Efferent sympathetic control originates at the thoracolumbar level (T11 through L2) of the spinal cord and produces relaxation of the detrusor muscle and contraction of the internal sphincter. Skeletal muscle found in the external sphincter and the pelvic muscles that support the bladder are supplied by the pudendal nerve, which exits the spinal cord at the sacral level (S2 through S4) of the spinal cord. The pontine micturition centre coordinates the action of the detrusor muscle and the external sphincter, whereas cortical centres permit conscious control of micturition.

Bladder structure and function can be evaluated using physical examination, laboratory and radiologic studies, urodynamic studies that measure bladder, urethral, and abdominal pressures; urine flow characteristics; and skeletal muscle activity of the external sphincter.

ALTERATIONS IN BLADDER FUNCTION

After completing this section of the chapter, you should be able to meet the following objectives:

- Describe the causes of and compensatory changes that occur with urinary tract obstruction.
- Differentiate lesions that produce storage dysfunction associated with spastic bladder from those that produce emptying dysfunction associated with

flaccid bladder in terms of the level of the lesions and their effects on bladder function.
- Describe methods used in treatment of neurogenic bladder.
- Define incontinence and differentiate between stress incontinence, overactive bladder/urge incontinence, and overflow incontinence.
- Describe behavioural, pharmacologic, and surgical methods used in treatment of the different types of incontinence.
- List the treatable causes of incontinence in older adults.

Alterations in bladder function include urinary obstruction with retention or stasis of urine and urinary incontinence with involuntary loss of urine. Although the two conditions have almost opposite effects on urination, they can have similar causes. Both can result from structural changes in the bladder, urethra, or surrounding organs or from impairment of neurologic control of bladder function.

Lower Urinary Tract Obstruction and Stasis

Urinary tract obstructions are classified according to cause (congenital or acquired), degree (partial or complete), duration (acute or chronic), and level (upper or lower urinary tract).[1] In lower urinary tract obstruction and stasis, urine is produced normally by the kidneys but is retained in the bladder. Because it has the potential to produce vesicoureteral reflux and cause kidney damage, lower urinary tract obstruction and stasis is a serious disorder.

The common sites of congenital obstructions are the external meatus (*i.e.,* meatal stenosis) in boys and just inside the external urinary meatus in girls. Another congenital cause of urinary stasis is the damage to sacral nerves that is seen in spina bifida and meningomyelocele.

The acquired causes of lower urinary tract obstruction and stasis are numerous. In males, the most important cause of urinary obstruction is external compression of the urethra caused by the enlargement of the prostate gland. In males and females gonorrhea and other sexually transmitted infections contribute to the incidence of infection-produced urethral strictures. Bladder tumours and secondary invasion of the bladder by tumours arising in structures that surround the bladder and urethra can compress the bladder neck or urethra and cause obstruction. Because of the proximity of the involved structures, constipation and fecal impaction can compress the urethra and produce urethral obstruction. This can be a particular problem in elderly persons.

Compensatory and Decompensatory Changes

The body compensates for the obstruction of urine outflow with mechanisms designed to prevent urine retention. These mechanisms can be divided into two stages: a compensatory stage and a decompensatory stage.[1] The degree to which these changes occur and their effect on bladder structure and urinary function depend on the extent of the obstruction, the rapidity with which it occurs, and the presence of other contributing factors, such as neurologic impairment and infection.

NEUROGENIC BLADDER DISORDERS

- Neurogenic disorders of the bladder commonly are manifested by a spastic bladder dysfunction, in which there is failure to store urine, or as flaccid bladder dysfunction, in which bladder emptying is impaired.
- Spastic bladder dysfunction results from neurologic lesions above the level of the sacral cord that allow neurons in the micturition centre to function reflexively without control from higher CNS centres.
- Flaccid bladder dysfunction results from neurologic disorders affecting the motor neurons in the sacral cord or peripheral nerves that control detrusor muscle contraction and bladder emptying.

During the early stage of obstruction, the bladder begins to hypertrophy and becomes hypersensitive to afferent stimuli arising from stretch receptors in the bladder wall. The ability to suppress urination is diminished, and bladder contraction can become so strong that it virtually produces bladder spasm. There is urgency, sometimes to the point of incontinence, and frequency during the day and at night.

With continuation and progression of the obstruction, compensatory changes begin to occur. There is further hypertrophy of the bladder muscle, the thickness of the bladder wall may double, and the pressure generated by detrusor contraction can increase dramatically to overcome the resistance from the obstruction. As the force needed to expel urine from the bladder increases, compensatory mechanisms may become ineffective, causing muscle fatigue before complete emptying can be accomplished. After a few minutes, voiding can again be initiated and completed, accounting for the frequency of urination.[1]

The inner bladder surface forms smooth folds. With continued outflow obstruction, this smooth surface is replaced with coarsely woven structures (*i.e.,* hypertrophied smooth muscle fibres) called *trabeculae*. Small pockets of mucosal tissue, called *cellules,* commonly develop between the trabecular ridges. These pockets form diverticula when they extend between the actual fibres of the bladder muscle (Fig. 35.4). Because the diverticula have no muscle, they are unable to contract and expel their urine into the bladder, and secondary infections caused by stasis are common.

Along with hypertrophy of the bladder wall, there is hypertrophy of the trigone area and the interureteric ridge, which is located between the two ureters. This causes backpressure on the ureters, the development of hydroureters (*i.e.,* dilated, urine-filled ureters), and, eventually, kidney damage

Diverticulum

Cellulae

Benign
prostatic
hyperplasia

FIGURE 35.4 • Destructive changes of the bladder wall with development of diverticulum caused by benign prostatic hypertrophy.

(see Chapter 33). Stasis of urine predisposes to urinary tract infections.

When compensatory mechanisms no longer are effective, signs of decompensation begin to appear. The period of detrusor muscle contraction becomes too short to expel the urine completely, and residual urine remains in the bladder. At this point, the symptoms of obstruction—frequency of urination, hesitancy, need to strain to initiate urination, a weak and small stream, and termination of the stream before the bladder is completely emptied—become pronounced. With progressive decompensation, the bladder may become severely overstretched, with a residual urine volume of 1,000 to 3,000 ml.[1] At this point, it loses its power of contraction and overflow incontinence occurs. The signs of outflow obstruction and urine retention are summarized in Chart 35.1.

CHART 35.1 **SIGNS OF OUTFLOW OBSTRUCTION AND URINE RETENTION**

Bladder distension
Hesitancy
Straining when initiating urination
Small and weak stream
Frequency
Feeling of incomplete bladder emptying
Overflow incontinence

Treatment

The immediate treatment of lower urinary tract obstruction and stasis is directed toward relief of bladder distension. This usually is accomplished through urinary catheterization (to be discussed). Constipation or fecal impaction should be corrected. Long-term treatment is directed toward correcting the problem causing the obstruction.

Neurogenic Bladder Disorders

The urinary bladder is unique in that it is probably the only autonomically innervated visceral organ that is under CNS control. The neural control of bladder function can be interrupted at any level. It can be interrupted at the level of the peripheral nerves that connect the bladder to the reflex micturition centre in the sacral cord, the ascending and descending tracts in the spinal cord, the pontine micturition centre, or the cortical centres that are involved in voluntary control of micturition[1–4,12,13] (Fig. 35.3).

Neurogenic disorders of bladder function commonly are manifested in one of two ways: failure to store urine (spastic bladder dysfunction) or failure to empty (flaccid bladder dysfunction). Spastic bladder dysfunction usually results from neurologic lesions located above the level of the sacral micturition reflexes, whereas flaccid bladder dysfunction results from lesions at the level of the sacral micturition reflexes or the peripheral nerves that innervate the bladder. In addition to disorders of detrusor muscle function, disruption of micturition occurs when the neurologic control of external sphincter function is disrupted. Some disorders, such as stroke and Parkinson disease, may affect both the storage and emptying functions of the bladder. Table 35.2 describes the characteristics of neurogenic bladder according to the level of the lesion.

Spastic Bladder: Failure to Store Urine

Failure to store urine results from conditions that cause reflex bladder spasm and a decrease in bladder volume. It commonly is caused by conditions that produce partial or extensive neural damage above the micturition reflex centre in the sacral cord (Fig. 35.3). As a result, bladder function is regulated by segmental reflexes, without control from higher brain centres. The degree of bladder spasticity and dysfunction depends on the level and extent of neurologic dysfunction. Usually, both the ANS neurons controlling bladder function and the somatic neurons controlling the function of the striated muscles in the external sphincter are affected. In some cases, there is a detrusor–sphincter dyssynergia with uncoordinated contraction and relaxation of the detrusor and external sphincter muscles. The most common causes of spastic bladder dysfunction are spinal cord lesions such as spinal cord injury, herniated intervertebral disk, vascular lesions, spinal cord tumours, and myelitis. Other neurologic conditions that affect voiding are stroke, multiple sclerosis, and brain tumours.

Bladder Dysfunction Caused by Spinal Cord Injury. One of the most common types of spinal cord lesions is spinal cord injury (see Chapter 50). The immediate and early effects of

TABLE 35.2 TYPES AND CHARACTERISTICS OF NEUROGENIC BLADDER

LEVEL OF LESION	CHANGE IN BLADDER FUNCTION	COMMON CAUSES
Sensory cortex, motor cortex, or corticospinal tract	Loss of ability to perceive bladder filling; low-volume, physiologically normal micturition that occurs suddenly and is difficult to inhibit	Stroke and advanced age
Basal ganglia or extrapyramidal tract	Detrusor contractions are elicited suddenly without warning and are difficult to control; bladder contraction is shorter than normal and does not produce full bladder emptying	Parkinson disease
Pontine micturition centre or communicating tracts in the spinal cord	Storage reflexes are provoked during filling, and external sphincter responses are heightened; uninhibited bladder contractions occur at a lower volume than normal and do not continue until the bladder is emptied; antagonistic activity occurs between the detrusor muscle and the external sphincter	Spinal cord injury
Sacral cord or nerve roots	Areflexic bladder fills but does not contract; loss of external sphincter tone occurs when the lesion affects the α-adrenergic motor neurons or pudendal nerve	Injury to sacral cord or spinal roots
Pelvic nerve	Increased filling and impaired sphincter control cause increased intravesicular pressure	Radical pelvic surgery
Autonomic peripheral sensory pathways	Bladder overfilling occurs owing to a loss of ability to perceive bladder filling	Diabetic neuropathies, multiple sclerosis

spinal cord injury on bladder function are quite different from those that follow recovery from the initial injury. During the period immediately after spinal cord injury, a state of spinal shock develops, during which all the reflexes, including the micturition reflex, are depressed. During this stage, the bladder becomes atonic and cannot contract. Catheterization is necessary to prevent injury to urinary structures associated with over-distension of the bladder. Aseptic intermittent catheterization is the preferred method of catheterization. Depression of reflexes lasts from a few weeks to 6 months (usually 2 to 3 months), after which the spinal reflexes return and become hyperactive.[13]

After the acute stage of spinal cord injury, the micturition response changes from a long-tract reflex to a segmental reflex. Because the sacral reflex arc remains intact, stimuli generated by bladder stretch receptors during filling produce frequent spontaneous contractions of the detrusor muscle. This creates a small, hyperactive bladder subject to high-pressure and short-duration uninhibited bladder contractions. Voiding is interrupted, involuntary, or incomplete. Dilation of the internal sphincter and spasticity of the external sphincter and perineal muscles innervated by upper motor neurons occur, producing resistance to bladder emptying. Hypertrophy of the trigone develops, often leading to vesicoureteral reflux and risk for renal damage.

Spastic bladder due to spinal cord injuries at the cervical level is often accompanied by a condition known as *autonomic hyperreflexia* (see Chapter 50). Because the injury interrupts CNS control of sympathetic reflexes in the spinal cord, severe hypertension, bradycardia, and sweating can be triggered by insertion of a catheter or mild overdistension of the bladder.

Uninhibited Neurogenic Bladder. A mild form of reflex neurogenic bladder, sometimes called *uninhibited bladder,* can develop after a stroke, during the early stages of multiple sclerosis, or as a result of lesions located in the inhibitory centres of

the cortex or the pyramidal tract. With this type of disorder, the sacral reflex arc and sensation are retained, the urine stream is normal, and there is no residual urine. Bladder capacity is diminished, however, because of increased detrusor muscle tone and spasticity.

Detrusor–Sphincter Dyssynergia. Depending on the level of the lesion, the coordinated activity of the detrusor muscle and the external sphincter may be affected. Lesions that affect the micturition centre in the pons or impair communication between the micturition centre and spinal cord centres interrupt the coordinated activity of the detrusor muscle and the external sphincter. This is called *detrusor–sphincter dyssynergia.* Instead of relaxing during micturition, the external sphincter becomes more constricted. This condition can lead to elevated intravesical pressures, vesicoureteral reflux, and kidney damage.[12]

Treatment. Among the methods used to treat spastic bladder and detrusor–sphincter dyssynergia are the administration of anticholinergic medications to decrease bladder hyperactivity (to be discussed) and urinary catheterization to produce bladder emptying. A sphincterotomy (surgical resection of the external sphincter) or implantable urethral stent may be used to decrease outflow resistance in a person who cannot be managed with medications and catheterization procedures. An alternative to surgical resection of the external sphincter is the injection of botulinum toxin type A (BTX-A) to produce paralysis of the striated muscles in the external sphincter. The effects of the injection last from 6 to 12 months, after which the injection must be repeated.[1,14,15]

Flaccid Bladder: Failure to Empty Urine

Failure to empty the bladder can be due to flaccid bladder dysfunction, peripheral neuropathies that interrupt afferent or efferent communication between the bladder and the spinal cord, or conditions that prevent relaxation of the external sphincter (Fig. 35.3).

Flaccid Bladder Dysfunction. Detrusor muscle areflexia, or flaccid neurogenic bladder, occurs when there is injury to the micturition centre of the sacral cord, the cauda equina, or the sacral nerves that supply the bladder.[1] Atony of the detrusor muscle and loss of the perception of bladder fullness permit the overstretching of the detrusor muscle that contributes to weak and ineffective bladder contractions. External sphincter tone and perineal muscle tone are diminished. Voluntary urination does not occur, but fairly efficient emptying usually can be achieved by increasing the intra-abdominal pressure or applying manual suprapubic pressure. Among the causes of flaccid neurogenic bladder are trauma, tumours, and congenital anomalies (*e.g.,* spina bifida, meningomyelocele).[1]

Bladder Dysfunction Caused by Peripheral Neuropathies. In addition to CNS lesions and conditions that disrupt bladder function, disorders of the peripheral (pelvic, pudendal, and hypogastric) nerves that supply the muscles of micturition can occur. These neuropathies can selectively interrupt sensory or motor pathways for the bladder or involve both pathways.

Bladder atony with dysfunction is a frequent complication of diabetes mellitus.[16,17] The disorder initially affects the sensory axons of the urinary bladder without involvement of the pudendal nerve. This leads to large residual volumes after micturition, sometimes complicated by infection. There frequently is a need for straining, accompanied by hesitation, weakness of the stream, dribbling, and a sensation of incomplete bladder emptying. The chief complications are vesicoureteral reflux and ascending urinary tract infection. Because persons with diabetes are already at risk for development of kidney disease, urinary stasis and reflux can have serious effects on renal function (see Chapter 33). After control blood glucose levels, treatment consists of client education, including the need for frequent voiding (*e.g.,* every 3 to 4 hours while awake), use of abdominal compression to effect more complete bladder emptying, and intermittent catheterization when necessary.[17]

Nonrelaxing External Sphincter

Another condition that affects micturition and bladder function is the nonrelaxing external sphincter. This condition usually is related to a delay in maturation, developmental regression, psychomotor disorders, or locally irritative lesions. Inadequate relaxation of the external sphincter can be the result of anxiety or depression. Any local irritation can produce spasms of the sphincter through afferent sensory input from the pudendal nerve, including vaginitis, perineal inflammation, and inflammation or irritation of the urethra. In men, chronic prostatitis contributes to impaired relaxation of the external sphincter.

Treatment

The goals of treatment for neurogenic bladder disorders focus on preventing bladder overdistension, urinary tract infections,

and potentially life-threatening renal damage; and reducing the undesirable social and psychological effects of the disorder. The methods used in treatment of neurogenic bladder disorders are individualized based on the type of neurologic lesion that is involved; information obtained through the health history, including fluid intake; report or observation of voiding patterns; presence of other health problems; urodynamic studies when indicated; and the ability of the person to participate in the treatment. Treatment methods include catheterization, bladder training, pharmacologic manipulation of bladder function, and surgery.

Catheterization. Catheterization involves the insertion of a small-diameter latex or silicone tube into the bladder through the urethra.[18] The catheter may be inserted on a one-time basis to relieve temporary bladder distension, left indwelling (*i.e.,* retention catheter), or inserted intermittently. Historically it was thought that with acute overdistension of the bladder, no more than 1,000 ml of urine should be removed from the bladder at one time but updated studies do not support this.[18,19]

Permanent indwelling catheters sometimes are used when there is urine retention or incontinence in persons who are ill or debilitated or when conservative or surgical methods for the correction of incontinence are not feasible. The use of permanent indwelling bladder catheters in patients with spinal cord injury has been shown to produce a number of complications, including urinary tract infections, pyelonephritis, and kidney stones. Because urethral catheters often produce urethral irritation and injury, a suprapubic catheter may be inserted in persons requiring long-term catheter drainage.[12,13]

Intermittent catheterization is used to treat urine retention or incomplete emptying secondary to various neurologic or obstructive disorders.[12] Properly used, it prevents bladder overdistension and urethral irritation, allows more freedom of activity, and provides periodic distension of the bladder to prevent muscle atony. It often is used with pharmacologic manipulation to achieve continence; when possible, it is learned and managed as a self-care procedure (*i.e.,* intermittent self-catheterization).[20] It may be carried out as an aseptic (sterile) or a clean procedure. Aseptic intermittent catheterization is used in persons with spinal shock, in those who need short-term catheterization, and any persons who are acutely ill or immunocompromised.

The clean procedure typically is used for self-catheterization. It is performed at 3- to 4-hour intervals to prevent overdistension of the bladder. The best results are obtained if only 300 to 400 ml is allowed to collect in the bladder between catheterizations. The use of the clean instead of the sterile procedure has been defended on the basis that most urinary tract infections are caused by some underlying abnormality of the urinary tract that leads to impaired mucosal resistance to bacterial infection, the most common cause of which is decreased blood flow to the bladder wall because of bladder overdistension.[20]

Bladder Retraining. Bladder retraining differs with the type of disorder.[21] Methods used to supplement bladder retraining include monitoring fluid intake to prevent urinary tract infections and control urine volume and osmolality, developing scheduled times for urination, and using body positions that facilitate micturition. Adequate fluid intake also is needed to prevent urinary tract infections, the irritating effects of which increase bladder irritability and the risk for urinary incontinence and renal damage. Fluid intake must be balanced to prevent bladder overdistension from occurring during the night. Developing scheduled times for urinating prevents overdistension of the bladder.

The methods used for bladder retraining depend on the type of lesion causing the disorder.[21] In spastic neurogenic bladder, methods designed to trigger the sacral micturition reflex are used; in flaccid neurogenic bladder, manual methods that increase intravesical pressure are used. Credé manoeuvres, which are used with the person in a sitting position, consists of applying pressure with four fingers of one hand or both hands to the suprapubic area as a means of increasing intravesical pressure. The Valsalva manoeuvre (*i.e.*, bearing down by exhaling against a closed glottis) increases intra-abdominal pressure and aids in bladder emptying. This manoeuvre is repeated until the bladder is empty. For the best results, the person must be able to cooperate fully with the procedures and, if possible, learn to perform them independently.

Biofeedback methods have been useful for teaching some aspects of bladder control. They involve the use of EMG or cystometry as a feedback signal for training a person to control the function of the external sphincter or raise intravesical pressure enough to overcome outflow resistance.

Pharmacologic Manipulation. Pharmacologic manipulation includes the use of drugs to alter the contractile properties of the bladder, decrease the outflow resistance of the internal sphincter, and relax the external sphincter. The usefulness of drug therapy often is evaluated during cystometric studies. Antimuscarinic drugs, such as oxybutynin, tolterodine, and propantheline, decrease detrusor muscle tone and increase bladder capacity in persons with spastic bladder dysfunction[1,7] (discussed in the section on Overactive Bladder/Urge Incontinence). Cholinergic drugs that stimulate parasympathetic receptors, such as bethanechol, provide increased bladder tonus and may prove helpful in the symptomatic treatment of milder forms of flaccid neurogenic bladder. Muscle relaxants, such as diazepam and baclofen, may be used to decrease the tone of the external sphincter.

Surgical Procedures. Among the surgical procedures used in the management of neurogenic bladder are sphincterectomy, reconstruction of the sphincter, nerve resection of the sacral reflex nerves that cause spasticity or the pudendal nerve that controls the external sphincter, and urinary diversion. Urinary diversion can be done by creating an ileal or a colon loop into which the ureters are anastomosed; the distal end of the loop is brought out and attached to the abdominal wall.[9] Research is being conducted on methods of restoring voluntary control of the storage and evacuation functions of the bladder through the use of implanted electrodes.

Urinary Incontinence

The International Continence Society and the Canadian Continence Foundation have defined urinary incontinence as the involuntary loss or leakage of urine.[22,23] Urinary incontinence is a common problem, particularly in older adults, affecting as many as 3.3 million Canadians.[24]

Incontinence can be caused by a number of conditions. It can occur without the person's knowledge; at other times, the person may be aware of the condition but be unable to prevent it. The Canadian Continence Foundation has identified four main types of incontinence: stress incontinence, urge incontinence, overflow incontinence, and mixed incontinence, which is a combination of stress and urge incontinence.[24] Recently, the term *urge incontinence* has been expanded to include *overactive bladder* (*i.e.*, overactive bladder/urge incontinence). Another type is functional incontinence caused by cognitive, environmental, or physical barriers making toileting difficult. Table 35.3 summarizes the characteristics of the different types of incontinence.[25]

Stress Incontinence

Stress incontinence is the involuntary loss of urine during coughing, laughing, sneezing, or lifting that increases intra-abdominal pressure.[23–25] With severe urinary stress incontinence, any strain or increase in bladder pressure leads to urinary leakage.

In women, the angle between the bladder and the posterior proximal urethra (*i.e.*, urethrovesical junction) is important to continence.[26] This angle normally is 90 to 100 degrees, with at least one third of the bladder base contributing to the angle when not voiding (Fig. 35.5). During the first stage of voiding, this angle is lost as the bladder descends. In women, diminution of muscle tone can cause weakness of the pelvic floor muscles and result in stress incontinence by obliterating the critical

TABLE 35.3 TYPES AND CHARACTERISTICS OF URINARY INCONTINENCE

TYPE	CHARACTERISTICS
Stress	Involuntary loss of urine associated with activities, such as coughing, that increase intra-abdominal pressure
Overactive bladder/ urge incontinence	Urgency and frequency associated with hyperactivity of the detrusor muscle; may or may not involve involuntary loss of urine
Overflow	Involuntary loss of urine when intra-vesical pressure exceeds maximal urethral pressure in the absence of detrusor activity
Functional	Loss of urine due to cognitive impairment preventing understanding when the bladder is full, environmental barriers preventing ability to access toilet, physical barriers preventing mobility to get to the toilet

INCONTINENCE

- Incontinence represents the involuntary loss of urine due to increased bladder pressures (overactive bladder with urge incontinence or overflow incontinence) or decreased ability of the vesicourethral sphincter to prevent the escape of urine (stress incontinence).
- Stress incontinence is caused by the decreased ability of the vesicourethral sphincter to prevent the escape of urine during activities, such as lifting and coughing, that raise bladder pressure above the sphincter closing pressure.
- Overactive bladder/urge incontinence is caused by neurogenic or myogenic disorders that result in hyperactive bladder contractions.
- Overflow incontinence results from overfilling of the bladder with escape of urine.

posterior urethrovesical angle. The loss of muscle tone is associated with normal aging, childbirth, or surgical procedures. In these women, loss of the posterior urethrovesical angle, descent and funnelling of the bladder neck, and backward and downward rotation of the bladder occur, so that the bladder and urethra are already in an anatomic position for the first stage of voiding. Any activity that causes downward pressure on the bladder is sufficient to allow the urine to escape involuntarily.

Another cause of stress incontinence is intrinsic urethral deficiency, which may result from congenital sphincter weakness, as occurs with meningomyelocele. It also may be acquired as a result of trauma, irradiation, or sacral cord lesions. Stress incontinence in men may result from a congenital defect or from trauma or surgery to the bladder outlet, as

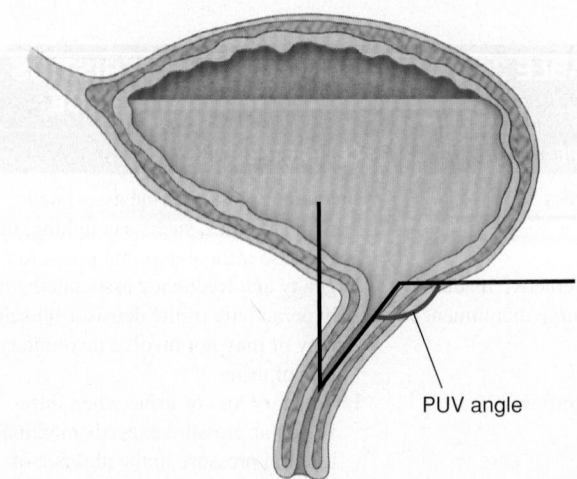

FIGURE 35.5 • Normal 90° to 100° posterior urethrovesical (PUV) angle. In the presence of a normal PUV angle, sudden changes in intra-abdominal pressure are transmitted optimally to all sides of the proximal urethra, ensuring that intraurethral pressure remains higher than intravesical pressure. Loss of the PUV angle results in displacement of the vesicle neck to the most dependent portion of the bladder, preventing the equal transmission of sudden increases in intra-abdominal pressure.

occurs with prostatectomy. Neurologic dysfunction, as occurs with impaired sympathetic innervation of the bladder neck, impaired pelvic nerve innervation to the intrinsic sphincter, or impaired pudendal nerve innervation to the external sphincter, may also be contributing factors.

Overactive Bladder/Urge Incontinence

The Canadian Continence Foundation has defined urge incontinence as the involuntary loss of urine associated with a strong desire to void (*i.e.,* urgency).[23–25] Urgency is a key symptom of overactive bladder.[27] Nocturia often occurs and is associated with sleep disruption. Although overactive bladder often is associated with urge incontinence, it can occur without incontinence. Nearly 1 in 5 Canadians over the age of 35 suffer from overactive bladder and despite recent media coverage of overactive bladder and advances in treatment, many people continue to suffer in silence, probably because they are embarrassed or think it is an inevitable consequence of aging.[24]

The symptoms of overactive bladder, which are caused by involuntary bladder contractions during filling, may occur alone or in any combination, and they constitute overactive bladder when they occur in the absence of other pathologic processes. Regardless of the primary cause of overactive bladder, two types of mechanisms are thought to contribute to its symptomatology: those involving CNS and neural control of bladder sensation and emptying (neurogenic), and those involving the smooth muscle of the bladder itself (myogenic).[7,28,29]

The neurogenic theory for overactive bladder postulates that the CNS functions as an on–off switching circuit for voluntary control of bladder function. Therefore, damage to the CNS inhibitory pathways may trigger bladder overactivity owing to uncontrolled voiding reflexes. Neurogenic causes of overactive bladder include stroke, Parkinson disease, and multiple sclerosis. Other neurogenic causes of overactive bladder include increased sensitization of the afferent nerves that sense bladder filling or increased sensitivity to efferent nerves that produce bladder emptying.[26,29]

The myogenic causes of overactive bladder are thought to result from changes in the properties of the smooth muscle of the bladder itself. One example is overactive bladder associated with bladder outlet obstruction. It is hypothesized that the sustained increase in intravesical pressure that occurs with the outlet obstruction causes a partial destruction of the nerve endings that control bladder excitability. This partial denervation results in increased excitability of the individual muscle cells. The result is urgency and frequency of urination due to spontaneous bladder contractions resulting from detrusor muscle hyperexcitability.[26] Disorders of detrusor muscle structure and excitability also can occur as the result of the aging process or disease conditions such as diabetes mellitus. Overactive bladder symptoms usually are exaggerated by incomplete bladder emptying, a common accompaniment of overactive bladder.

Overflow Incontinence

Overflow incontinence is an involuntary loss of urine that occurs when intravesical pressure exceeds the maximal urethral pressure because of bladder distension in the absence of detrusor activity. It can occur with retention of urine owing to nervous system lesions or obstruction of the bladder neck. With this type of incontinence, the bladder is distended, and small amounts of urine are passed, particularly at night. In men, one of the most common causes of obstructive incontinence is enlargement of the prostate gland. Another cause that commonly is overlooked is fecal impaction (*i.e.,* dry, hard feces in the rectum). When a large bolus of stool forms in the rectum, it can push against the urethra and block the flow of urine.

Other Causes of Incontinence

Other causes of incontinence include decreased bladder compliance or distensibility. This abnormal bladder condition may result from radiation therapy, radical pelvic surgery, or interstitial cystitis. Many persons with this disorder have severe urgency related to bladder hypersensitivity that results in loss of bladder elasticity, such that any small increase in bladder volume or detrusor function causes a sharp rise in bladder pressure and severe urgency.

Incontinence may occur as a transient and correctable phenomenon, or it may not be totally correctable and occur with various degrees of frequency. Among the transient causes of urinary incontinence are recurrent urinary tract infections; medications that alter bladder function or perception of bladder filling and the need to urinate; diuretics and conditions that increase bladder filling; stool impaction; restricted mobility; and confusional states.

Incontinence also may be caused by factors outside the lower urinary tract, such as the inability to locate, reach, or receive assistance in reaching an appropriate place to void. This may be a particular problem for elderly persons, who may have problems with mobility and manual dexterity or find themselves in unfamiliar surroundings. It occurs when a person cannot find or reach the bathroom or manipulate clothing quickly enough. Failing vision may contribute to the problem. Embarrassment in front of other persons at having to use the bathroom, particularly if the timing seems inappropriate, may cause a person to delay emptying the bladder and may lead to incontinence. Treatment with drugs such as diuretics may cause the bladder to fill more rapidly than usual, making it difficult to reach the bathroom in time if there are problems with mobility or if a bathroom is not readily available. Night sedation may cause a person to sleep through the signal that normally would waken a person so that he or she could get up and empty the bladder and avoid wetting the bed.

Diagnosis and Treatment

Urinary incontinence is not a single disease but a symptom with many possible causes. As a symptom, it requires full investigation to establish its cause.[1,9,24–29] This usually is accomplished through a careful history, physical examination, blood tests, and urinalysis. A voiding record (*i.e.,* diary) may be used to determine the frequency, timing, and amount of voiding, as well as other factors associated with the incontinence. Because many drugs affect bladder function, a full drug history is essential. Estimation of PVR volume is recommended for all persons with incontinence.[30] Provocative stress testing is done when stress incontinence is suspected. This test is done by having the person relax and then cough vigorously while the examiner observes for urine loss. The test usually is done in the lithotomy position; if no leakage is observed, it is repeated in the standing position. Urodynamic studies may be needed to provide information about urinary pressures and urine flow rates.

Treatment or management depends on the type of incontinence, accompanying health problems, and the person's age. It includes behavioural measures, exercises to strengthen the pelvic muscles, pharmacologic measures, and surgical correction of pelvic relaxation disorders associated with stress incontinence.[31] When urine flow cannot be controlled, noncatheter devices to obstruct urine flow or collect urine as it is passed may be required. Indwelling catheters (discussed earlier), although a solution to the problem of urinary incontinence, usually are considered only after all other treatment methods have failed. In some types of incontinence, such as that associated with spinal cord injury or meningomyelocele, self-catheterization may provide the best means for controlling urine elimination (see Chapter 51).

Behavioural Measures. Behavioural methods include fluid management, timed/prompted voiding, bladder retraining, and toileting assistance. Bladder retraining and biofeedback techniques seek to reestablish cortical control over bladder function by having the person ignore urgency and respond only to cortical signals during waking hours. Toileting assistance techniques are caregiver-dependent techniques used to treat persons with cognitive and motor dysfunction.

Pelvic Exercises. Muscle-tensing exercises of the pelvic muscles may prove effective in treatment of stress incontinence for men and more commonly used for women. These exercises were first advocated by Kegel, and they commonly are called *Kegel exercises.*[32] Two groups of muscles are strengthened: those of the back part of the pelvic floor (*i.e.,* muscles used to contract the anus and control the passing of stool) and the front muscles of the pelvic floor (*i.e.,* muscles used to stop the flow of urine during voiding). In learning the exercises, a woman concentrates on identifying the muscle groups and learning how to control contraction.[33] After this has been accomplished, she can start an exercise program that consists of slowly contracting the muscles, beginning at the front and working to the back while counting to four and then releasing. The exercises can be done while sitting or standing and usually are performed in repetitions of 10, three to five times each day. A vaginal cone, a tampon-like device, may be used to enhance the benefits of the exercise. The cone is placed in the vagina, and the woman is instructed to hold it in place by contracting the proper inner muscles.[24]

Pharmacologic Treatment. Pharmacologic treatment is aimed at using drugs to alter the physiologic mechanisms that contribute to the neurogenic or myogenic causes of incontinence.[30,31] They include the use of drugs that increase sphincter tone in stress incontinence, decrease hyperreactivity of the detrusor muscle in overactive bladder/urge incontinence, or relieve outflow obstruction in overflow incontinence.

The α-adrenergic agonist drugs, such as pseudoephedrine, increase sympathetic relaxation of the detrusor muscle and internal sphincter tone and may be used in treating stress incontinence. The tricyclic antidepressants (particularly imipramine hydrochloride) are useful in facilitating urine storage because they decrease bladder contractility and increase outlet resistance. Although these drugs have a weak anticholinergic effect on smooth muscle, it has recently been postulated that their beneficial effects may be caused by increased serotonin activity (due to reuptake blockade) in the CNS. This may involve a direct inhibition of normal excitatory pathways or a depression of afferent ascending neural activity. Duloxetine, a selective serotonin and norepinephrine reuptake inhibitor, is thought to increase external sphincter tone by stimulation of the pudendal motor α$_1$-adrenergic receptors and serotonin-2 receptors. Because serious side effects (*e.g.*, CNS effects, postural hypotension, cardiac arrhythmias) can occur with imipramine and other tricyclic antidepressants, these agents need to be used with caution.

Acetylcholine is the neurotransmitter that mediates detrusor contraction in overactive bladder. Therefore, anticholinergic medications are used to suppress these contractions. Some of the antimuscarinic drugs (*e.g.*, oxybutynin, tolterodine, trospium, darifenacin, solifenacin) have greater selectivity for the M$_3$ muscarinic receptors and produce fewer side effects than some of the older agents (*e.g.*, propantheline). All anticholinergic drugs can have bothersome side effects. Although dry mouth is the most common, constipation, gastroesophageal reflux, blurred vision, urinary retention, and cognitive effects can occur. The use of controlled-release (*e.g.*, oxybutynin, tolterodine) or transdermal drug delivery (*e.g.*, oxybutynin) can reduce but not completely eliminate side effects. Botulinum toxin (BTX-A) injection into the bladder was recently introduced as an alternative treatment for persons with overactive bladder who do not respond to anticholinergic agents or cannot tolerate their side effects.[15,30,31] The duration of the injection's effect seems to be at least 6 to 12 months.

The primary treatment of overflow incontinence that results from benign prostatic hypertrophy is relief of outflow obstruction. α-Adrenergic blocker therapy is based on the hypothesis that clinical manifestations of prostatic hyperplasia are caused partly by α$_1$-adrenergic–mediated contraction of prostatic smooth muscle, resulting in bladder outlet obstruction. Bladder outlet obstruction contributes to overfilling of the bladder and large-volume contraction, or frequency of urination resulting from incomplete bladder emptying. α-Adrenergic antagonists such as alfuzosin, doxazosin, tamsulosin, and terazosin are treatment options for men with symptomatic prostatic hyperplasia[34] (see Chapter 44). The primary adverse effects of α-adrenergic blocker therapy are orthostatic hypotension, dizziness, fatigue, ejaculatory problems, and nasal congestion.

Surgical Treatment of Stress Incontinence. Surgical intervention may be considered when other treatment methods have proven ineffective. Three types of surgical procedures are used: procedures that increase outlet resistance, decrease detrusor muscle instability, or remove outflow obstruction to reduce overflow incontinence and detrusor muscle instability. There are several surgeries (*e.g.*, colposuspension/Burch procedure, retropubic suspension, sacral colpopexy) that reposition the bladder, urethra, and/or vagina and are done under general anesthetic. Newer treatments of stress incontinence for women are the tension-free vaginal tape (TVT) procedure or other forms of midurethral slings. These procedures, which are minimally invasive and performed under local anesthesia, involve recreating suburethral support with a polypropylene mesh. Evidence suggests that the synthetic suburethral sling procedures are effective with limited long-term information. Long-term data about types of tape material used and incidences of complications (*e.g.*, erosion of mesh through the vaginal wall) is limited.[35–38] Another minimally invasive procedure for the treatment of stress incontinence is the periurethral injection of a bulking agent (glutaraldehyde cross-linked bovine collagen or carbon-coated beads). Both of these agents typically require multiple treatment sessions to achieve a cure.[24,30,39]

Noncatheter Devices. Two types of noncatheter devices commonly are used in the management of urinary incontinence: one obstructs flow, and the other collects urine as it is passed. Obstruction of urine flow is achieved by compressing the urethra or stimulating contraction of the pelvic floor muscles. Penile clamps are available that occlude the urethra without obstructing blood circulation to the penis. Clamps must be removed at 3-hour intervals to empty the bladder. Complications such as penile and urethral erosion can occur if clamps are used incorrectly. In women, compression of the urethra usually is accomplished by intravaginal devices.[40]

Surgically implanted artificial sphincters are available for use in men and women. These devices consist of an inflatable cuff that surrounds the proximal urethra. The cuff is connected by tubing to an implanted fluid reservoir and an inflation bulb. Pressing the bulb, which is placed in the scrotum in men, inflates the cuff. It is emptied in a similar manner.[30,39]

When urinary incontinence cannot be prevented, various types of urine collection devices or protective pads are used. Men can be fitted with collection devices (*i.e.*, condom or sheath urinals) that are worn over the penis and attached to a container at the bedside or fastened to the body. There are no effective external collection devices for women. Pants and pads usually are used. Dribbling bags (men) and pads (women) in which the urine changes to a nonpourable gel are available for occasional dribbling but are unsuitable for considerable wetting.[40]

Special Needs of Older Adults

Urinary incontinence is a common problem in older adults, both male and female with an estimated 30% to 60% of people over 65 years of age experiencing urinary incontinence and this increases exponentially with age.[30] Incontinence increases social isolation, frequently leads to institutionalization of older adults, and predisposes to infections and skin breakdown. In Canada, the total direct health care cost (*e.g.,* pads, linens, medications) for incontinence is estimated to be $1.9 billion per year with over 51% prevalence in the older adult population.[22,30]

Many factors contribute to incontinence in older adults, a number of which can be altered. The overall capacity of the bladder is reduced with aging, as is the urethral closing pressure. Detrusor muscle function also tends to decline with aging; thus, there is a trend toward a reduction in the strength of bladder contraction and impairment in emptying that leads to larger PVR volumes. It has been proposed that many of these changes are due to degenerative detrusor muscle changes rather than neurologic changes, as was once thought. The combination of involuntary detrusor contraction (detrusor hyperactivity) leading to urge incontinence, along with impaired contractile function, leads to incomplete bladder emptying. Urge incontinence is the most frequent type of incontinence in older men. In about 50% of these men, detrusor overactivity is found; the urge to urinate comes on suddenly, without warning, accompanied by an uncontrolled detrusor contraction causing incontinence.[1,41]

Furthermore, advancing age often results in restricted mobility, an increasing number of medications being taken, comorbid illness, infection, and stool impaction, all of which can precipitate urinary incontinence.[41–43] More than half of normal older adults experience nocturia and many have difficulty getting to the toilet in time. This can be caused by arthritis that makes walking or removing clothing difficult or by failing vision that makes trips to the bathroom precarious, especially in new and unfamiliar surroundings.

Medication prescribed for other health problems may prevent a healthy bladder from functioning normally.[41–43] Potent, fast-acting diuretics are known for their ability to cause urge incontinence. Impaired thirst or limited access to fluids predisposes to constipation with urethral obstruction and overflow incontinence and to concentrated and infected urine, which increases bladder excitability. Drugs such as hypnotics, tranquilizers, and sedatives can interfere with the conscious inhibition of voiding, leading to urge incontinence. Diuretics, particularly in older adults, increase the flow of urine and may contribute to incontinence, particularly in persons with diminished bladder capacity and in those who have difficulty reaching the toilet.

Diagnosis and Treatment. As with urinary incontinence in younger persons, incontinence in older adults requires a thorough history and physical examination to determine the cause of the problem. A voiding history is important. A voiding diary provides a means for the person to provide objective information about the number of bathroom visits, the number of protective pads used, and even the volume of urine voided. A medication history is also important because medications can affect bladder function.

There are many nonurologic conditions that predispose to urinary incontinence. The transient and often treatable causes of urinary incontinence in elderly persons may best be remembered with the acronym DIAPPERS, in which the *D* stands for dementia/dementias, *I* for infection (urinary or vaginal), *A* for atrophic vaginitis, *P* for pharmaceutical agents, *P* for psychological causes, *E* for endocrine conditions (diabetes), *R* for restricted mobility, and *S* for stool impaction.[25] These eight transient causes of incontinence should be identified and treated before other treatment options are considered.

Treatment may involve changes in the physical environment so that the older person can reach the bathroom more easily or remove clothing more quickly. Habit training with regularly scheduled toileting—usually every 2 to 4 hours—often is effective. Many older adults who void on a regular schedule can gradually increase the interval between toileting while improving their ability to suppress bladder instability. The treatment plan may require dietary changes to prevent constipation or a plan to promote adequate fluid intake to ensure adequate bladder filling and prevent urinary stasis and symptomatic urinary tract infections.[1,25,41–43]

IN SUMMARY

Alterations in bladder function include urinary obstruction with retention of urine, neurogenic bladder, and urinary incontinence with involuntary loss of urine. Urine retention occurs when the outflow of urine from the bladder is obstructed because of urethral obstruction or impaired bladder innervation. Urethral obstruction causes bladder irritability, detrusor muscle hypertrophy, formation of trabeculae and diverticula, development of hydroureters, and eventual renal failure.

Neurogenic bladder is caused by interruption in the innervation of the bladder. It can result in spastic bladder dysfunction caused by failure of the bladder to fill or flaccid bladder dysfunction caused by failure of the bladder to empty. Spastic bladder dysfunction usually results from neurologic lesions that are above the level of the sacral micturition reflex centre; flaccid bladder dysfunction results from lesions at the level of the sacral micturition reflexes or peripheral innervation of the bladder. A third type of neurogenic disorder involves a nonrelaxing external sphincter.

Urinary incontinence is the involuntary loss of urine in amounts sufficient to be a problem. It may manifest as stress incontinence, in which the loss of urine occurs as a result of coughing, sneezing, laughing, or lifting; overactive bladder/urge incontinence, characterized by urgency, frequency, and nocturia associated with hyperactive bladder contractions; or overflow incontinence, which results when intravesical pressure exceeds the maximal urethral pressure because of bladder distension. Other causes of incontinence include a small, contracted bladder or external environmental conditions that make it difficult to access proper toileting facilities. Diagnosis usually is accomplished through a careful history (including a voiding record and full drug history), physical examination, blood tests and urinalysis, and in some cases urodynamic studies. Treatment methods include correction of the underlying cause, such as obstruction due to prostatic hyperplasia; behavioural methods that focus on bladder and habit training; exercises to improve pelvic floor function; pharmacologic methods to improve bladder and external sphincter tone; surgical intervention; and the use of catheters and urine collection devices.

Urinary incontinence is a common problem in older adults. Many factors, including health problems, medications, and changes in bladder structure and function, contribute to incontinence in older adults. The acronym DIAPPERS— *D* (dementia), *I* (infection), *A* (atrophic vaginitis), *P* (pharmaceutical), *P* (psychological), *E* (endocrine), *R* (restricted mobility), and *S* (stool impaction)—emphasizes the transient and often treatable causes of incontinence in the elderly.

CANCER OF THE BLADDER

After completing this section of the chapter, you should be able to meet the following objectives:

- Discuss the difference between superficial and invasive bladder cancer in terms of bladder involvement, extension of the disease, and prognosis.
- State the most common sign of bladder cancer.

Bladder cancer is the most frequent form of urinary tract cancer. It is estimated in 2014 that 8,000 new cases will be diagnosed and 2,200 deaths will occur, with a greater occurrence in men than women.[44] This type of cancer predominantly affects Canadians over the age of 70 years and occurs more commonly in the Atlantic provinces. Approximately 90% of bladder cancers are derived from the transitional (urothelium) cells that line the bladder.[1,44,46] These tumours can range from low-grade noninvasive tumours to high-grade tumours that invade the bladder wall and metastasize frequently. The low-grade tumours, which may recur after resection, have an excellent prognosis, with only a small number (<5%) progressing to higher-grade tumours, whereas 15% to 40% of persons with high-grade tumours progress to invasive disease even with extensive follow up.[1] As the ureters are lined with urothelium, most cancers of the ureters (*i.e.,* ureteric cancer) have similar characteristics as transitional cell carcinoma. There are other rarer types of bladder cancers such as squamous cell carcinoma, adenocarcinoma, and small cell carcinoma which differ in the ability to invade surrounding tissues.

Etiology and Pathophysiology

Although the cause of bladder cancer is unknown, evidence suggests that its origin is related to local influences, such as carcinogens that are excreted in the urine and stored in the bladder. These include the breakdown products of aromatic amines used in the dye industry, and products used in the manufacture of rubber, textiles, paint, chemicals, and petroleum. Smoking also deserves attention. Thirty to 50% of all bladder cancers are associated with cigarette smoking. Chronic bladder irritation caused by urinary tract infections or bladder stones also increase the risk for bladder cancer.[1,44-46]

Manifestations

The most common sign of bladder cancer is painless hematuria.[44,46] Gross hematuria is a presenting sign in 75% of persons with the disease, and microscopic hematuria is present in most others. Frequency, urgency, and dysuria occasionally accompany the hematuria. Because hematuria often is intermittent, the diagnosis may be delayed. Periodic urine cytology is recommended for all persons who are at high risk for the development of bladder cancer because of exposure to urinary tract carcinogens. Ureteral invasion leading to bacterial and obstructive renal disease and dissemination of the cancer are potential complications and ultimate causes of death. The prognosis depends on the histologic grade of the cancer and the stage of the disease at the time of diagnosis.[46]

Diagnosis and Treatment

Diagnostic methods include cytologic studies, excretory urography, cystoscopy, and biopsy. Ultrasonography, CT scans, and MRI are used as aids for staging the tumour. Cytologic studies performed on biopsy tissues or cells obtained from bladder washings may be used to detect the presence of malignant cells.[1] A technique called *fluorescence cystoscopy* is helpful in screening persons at high risk for the disease and for monitoring the results of therapy. In fluorescence cystoscopy, porphyrins (a chemical that glows when exposed to blue light) are inserted into the bladder. This chemical is taken up by cancer cells allowing easier identification. Other cell markers (*e.g.,* bladder tumour antigen), proteins (*e.g.,* NMP22) and chromosomal abnormalities are also being used to help identify and monitor progress of the cancer.[1,44,46]

The treatment of bladder cancer depends on the extent of the lesion and the health of the patient. Endoscopic resection usually is done for diagnostic purposes and may be used as a treatment for superficial lesions. Diathermy (*i.e.,* electrocautery) may be used to remove the tumours. Segmental surgical resection may be used for removing a large single lesion. When the tumour is invasive, cystectomy with resection of the pelvic lymph nodes frequently is the treatment of choice. In men, the prostate and seminal vesicles often are removed as well. Until the 1980s, most men who underwent radical cystectomy became impotent. Newer surgical approaches designed to preserve erectile function now are being used. Cystectomy requires urinary diversion, an alternative reservoir, usually created from the ileum (*e.g.,* an ileal loop), that is designed to collect the urine. Traditionally, the ileostomy reservoir drains urine continuously into an external collecting device. External-beam radiation therapy is an alternative to radical cystectomy in some patients with deeply infiltrating bladder cancer.

Although a number of chemotherapeutic drugs have been used in the treatment of bladder cancer, no chemotherapeutic regimens for the disease have been established. Perhaps of more importance is the increasing use of intravesical chemotherapy, in which the cytotoxic drug is instilled directly into the bladder, thereby avoiding the side effects of systemic therapy. These drugs can be instilled prophylactically, after surgical resection of all the demonstrable tumour tissue, or therapeutically, in the presence of residual disease. Among the chemotherapeutic drugs that have been used for this purpose are thiotepa, mitomycin C, doxorubicin, and gemcitabine. The intravesical administration of bacillus Calmette–Guérin (BCG) vaccine, made from a strain of *Mycobacterium bovis* that formerly was used to protect against tuberculosis, causes a significant reduction in the rate of relapse and prolongs relapse-free interval in persons with cancer in situ. The vaccine is thought to act as a nonspecific stimulator of cell-mediated immunity. It is not known whether the effects of BCG are immunologic or include a component of direct toxicity. Several strains of this agent exist, and it is not known which strains are the most active and least toxic.

Newer target therapies are looking at the role of monoclonal antibodies that interfere with tumour angiogenesis and overall growth but further research is ongoing.

IN SUMMARY

Cancer of the bladder is the most common cause of urinary tract cancer in Canada. Bladder cancers fall into two major groups: low-grade noninvasive tumours and high-grade invasive tumours that are associated with metastasis and a worse prognosis. Although the cause of cancer of the bladder is unknown, evidence suggests that carcinogens excreted in the urine may play a role. Microscopic and gross, painless hematuria are the most frequent presenting signs of bladder cancer. The methods used in treatment of bladder cancer depend on the cytologic grade of the tumour and the lesion's degree of invasiveness. The methods include surgical removal of the tumour, radiation therapy, and chemotherapy. In many cases, chemotherapeutic or immunotherapeutic agents can be instilled directly into the bladder, thereby avoiding the side effects of systemic therapy.

REVIEW EXERCISES

1. A 23-year-old man is recovering after the acute phase of a cervical (C6) spinal cord injury with complete loss of motor and sensory function below the level of injury. He is now experiencing spastic bladder contractions with involuntary and incomplete urination. Urodynamic studies reveal spastic contraction of the external sphincter with urine retention and high bladder pressures.
   A. *Explain the reason for the involuntary urination and incomplete emptying of the bladder despite high bladder pressures.*
   B. *What are possible complications associated with overdistension and high pressure within the bladder?*
2. A 66-year-old woman complains of leakage of urine during coughing, sneezing, laughing, or squatting down.
   A. *Explain the source of this woman's problem.*
   B. *One of the recommended treatments for stress incontinence is the use of Kegel exercises, which focus on strengthening the muscles of the pelvic floor. Explain how these exercises contribute to the control of urine leakage in women with stress incontinence.*

References

1. McAninch J. W., Lue T. F. (2013). *Smith & Tanagho's general urology* (18th ed.). New York: McGraw Hill Company.
2. Benarroch E. E. (2010). Neural control of the bladder: Recent advance and neurologic implications. *Neurology, 75*, 1839–1846.
3. Hall J. E. (2011). *Textbook of medical physiology* (12th ed.). Philadelphia, PA: W.B. Saunders.
4. Fowler C. J., Griffiths D., de Groat W. C. (2008). The neural control of micturition. *Nature Reviews Neuroscience, 9*(6), 453–466.
5. Jung J., Ahn H. K., Huh Y. (2012). Clincial and functional anatomy of the urethral sphincter. *International Neurourology Journal, 16*(3), 102–106.
6. Rhoades R. A., Bell D. R. (2013). *Medical physiology: Principles for clinical medicine* (4th ed.). Philadelphia, PA: Lippincott Williams & Wilkins.
7. Cipullo L., Cosimato C., Filippelli A., et al. (2014). Pharmacological approach to overactive bladder and urge urinary incontinence in women: An overview. *European Journal of Obstetrics & Gynecology and Reproductive Biology, 174*(2), 27–34.
8. de Jong T. P., Klijn A. J. (2009). Urodynamic studies in pediatric urology. *Nature Reviews Urology, 6*(11), 585–594.
9. Gearhart J. P., Rink R. C., Mouriquand P. D. (2010). *Pediatric urology* (2nd ed.). Philadelphia, PA: Elsevier.
10. Kliegman R. M., Stanton B. F., St. Geme J. W., et al. (Eds.). (2011). *Nelson textbook of pediatrics* (19th ed.). Philadelphia, PA: Elsevier Saunders.
11. Goroll A. H., Mulley A. G. (2009). *Primary care medicine: Office evaluation and management of the adult patient* (2nd ed.). Philadelphia, PA: Lippincott Williams & Wilkins.
12. Klausner A. P., Steers W. D. (2011). The neurogenic bladder: An update with management strategies for primary care physicians. *Medical Clinics of North America, 95*(1), 111–120.
13. Jeong S. J., Cho S. Y., Oh S. (2010). Spinal cord/brain injury and the neurogenic bladder. *Urological Clinics of North America, 37*(4), 537–546.
14. Cameron A. P. (2010). Pharmacologic therapy for the neurogenic bladder. *Urological Clinics of North America, 37*(4), 495–506.
15. Orasanu B., Mahajan S. T. (2013). The use of botulinum toxin for the treatment of overactive bladder syndrome. *Indian Journal of Urology, 29*(1), 2–11.
16. Karampini J. E., Pucci M., Burbridge W., et al. (2011). Diabetic cystopathy: Do we recognise this in our patient? *Practical Diabetes International, 28*(3), 129–131.

17. Miyazato M., Yoshimura N., Chancellor M. B. (2013). The other bladder syndrome: Underactive bladder. *Reviews in Urology, 15*(1), 11–22.

18. Boettcher S., Brandt A. S., Roth S., et al. (2013). Urinary retention: Benefit of gradual bladder decompression – Myth or truth? A randomized controlled trial. *Urologic International, 91*, 140–144.

19. Nyman M. A., Schwenk N. M., Silverstein M. D. (1997). Management of urinary retention: Rapid versus gradual decompression and risk of complications. *Mayo Clinic Proceedings, 72*, 951–956.

20. Newman D. K., Willson M. M. (2011). Review of intermittent catheterization and current best practices. *Urologic Nursing, 31*(1), 12–29, 48.

21. Roe B., Ostaszkiewicz J., Milne J., Wallace S. (2007). Systematic review of bladder training and voiding programmes in adults: A synopsis of findings from data analysis and outcomes using metastudy techniques. *Journal of Advanced Nursing, 27*(1), 15–31.

22. The Canadian Continence Foundation. (2009). Impacts of incontinence in Canada. Available online at: http://www.canadiancontinence.ca/pdfs/impacts-of-incontinence-in-canada.pdf. Accessed May 29, 2014.

23. International Continence Society. (2013). ICS Fact Sheets. Available online at: file:///C:/Users/Ruth%20Hannon/Desktop/Documents/Downloads/ICS_Factsheets_2013_Edition.pdf. Accessed May 29, 2104.

24. The Canadian Continence Foundation. (2014). Bladder Health / Diagnosis & Treatment. Available online at: http://www.canadiancontinence.ca/EN/index.php. Accessed May 29, 2014.

25. Khandelwal C., Kistler C. (2013). Diagnosis of urinary incontinence. *American Family Physician, 87*(8), 543–550.

26. Ismail M., Hashim H., Abrams P. (2012). Update on the management of overactive bladder syndrome. *European Urological Review, 7*(1), 70–73.

27. Abrams P., Andersson K. E., Birder L., et al. (2009). 4th International Consultation on Incontinence: Evaluation and treatment of urinary incontinence, pelvic organ prolapse and faecal incontinence. Available online at: http://www.ics.org/Publications/ICI_4/files-book/recommendation.pdf. Accessed May 29, 2014.

28. Lutz A. T., Winters J. C. (2013). Guidelines and practice standardization for female stress urinary incontinence (SUI). *Current Bladder Dysfunction Reports, 8*(1), 38–44.

29. Shah M. B., Weiss J. P. (2013). Medical causes of overactive bladder. *Current Bladder Dysfunction Reports, 8*(1), 51–56.

30. Bettez M., Tu L. M., Carlson K., et al. (2012). 2012 Update: Guidelines for adult urinary incontinence. Available online at: http://www.cua.org/guidelines_e.asp. Accessed May 29, 2014.

31. Deng D. Y. (2011). Urinary incontinence in women. *Medical Clinics of North America, 95*(1), 101–109.

32. Kegal A. H. (1948). Progressive resistance exercises in the functional restoration of the perineal muscles. *American Journal of Obstetrics and Gynecology, 56*, 238–248.

33. Bo K., Hilde G. (2013). Does it work in the long term? A systematic review on pelvic floor muscle training for female stress urinary incontinence. *Neurourology and Urodynamics, 32*(3), 215–223.

34. Nickel J. C., Mendez-Probst C. E., Whelan T. F., et al. (2010). 2010 Update: Guidelines for the management of benign prostatic hyperplasia. Available online at: http://www.cua.org/guidelines_e.asp. Accessed May 29, 2014.

35. Schulz J. A., Chan M. C., Farrell S. A.; Sub-Committee on Urogynaecology. (2008). Midurethral minimally invasive sling procedure for stress urinary incontinence. *Journal of Obstetrics and Gynaecology Canada, 30*(8), 728–733.

36. Walter J. (2011). Transvaginal mesh procedures for pelvic organ prolapse. *Journal of Obstetrics and Gynaecology Canada, 33*(2), 168–174.

37. Ogah J., Cody J. D., Rogerson L. (2010). Minimally invasive synthetic suburethral sling operations for stress urinary incontinence in women (Review). *Cochrane Database of Systamatic Reviews, 7*(4), CD006375.

38. Pushkar D., Kasyan G. (2013). The bladder neck sling: What role remains? *Current Bladder Dysfunction Reports, 8*(1), 32–37.

39. Cornu J., Peyrat L., Haab F. (2013). Update in management of male urinary incontinence. *Current Opinion in Urology, 23*(6), 536–539.

40. Moore K. C., Lucas M. G. (2010). Management of male urinary incontinence. *Indian Journal of Urology, 26*(2), 236–244.

41. Kraus S. R., Bavendam T., Brake T., Griebling T. L. (2010). Vulnerable elderly patients and overactive bladder syndrome. *Drugs & Aging, 27*(9), 697–713.

42. Wagg A., Gibson W., Johnson T., et al. (2014). Urinary incontinence in frail elderly persons: Report form the 5th international consultation on incontinence. *Neurourology and Urodynamics, 34*(5), 398–406.

43. Guzzo T. J., Drach G. W. (2011). Major urologic problems in geriatrics: Assessment and management. *Medical Clinics of North America, 95*(1), 253–264.

44. Canadian Cancer Society. (2014). Bladder cancer. Available online at: http://www.cancer.ca/en/cancer-information/cancer-type/bladder/bladder-cancer/?region=on. Accessed June 1, 2014.

45. Canadian Cancer Society. (2014). Canadian Cancer Statistics 2014. Available online at: http://www.cancer.ca/~/media/cancer.ca/CW/cancer%20information/cancer%20101/Canadian%20cancer%20statistics/Canadian-Cancer-Statistics-2014-EN.pdf. Accessed June 1, 2014.

46. Kaufman D. S., Shipley W. U., Feldman A. S. (2009). Bladder cancer. *Lancet, 374*(9685), 239–249.

Visit thePoint. **http://thePoint.lww.com for animations, journal articles, and more!**

Disorders of Gastrointestinal Function

The study of the gastrointestinal system aroused none of the philosophical interest that surrounded the elements, humours, and pneuma of Galen's time. During ancient times, the gut was thought merely to provide the chyle that was turned into blood by the liver. Although the structures of the gut had been fairly well described, perhaps owing to observations made during the slaughtering of animals, it was not until the 18th and 19th centuries that the function of the gastrointestinal tract began to unfold.

One of the breakthroughs in gastrointestinal physiology came as the result of an accident. In 1822, William Beaumont (1785–1853), a self-trained surgeon in the United States Army, was called upon to render aid to Alexis St. Martin, a Canadian traveller who had suffered a large gunshot wound to the chest and abdomen. Although not expected to live, young St. Martin rallied and his wounds healed; however, he was left with a permanent fistula that opened to his stomach. Beaumont became intrigued with this patient's unique defect, using this living laboratory to study the process of digestion. He would have St. Martin swallow different types of food and then collect the stomach contents by means of a tube passed into the fistula. Beaumont described the movement of the stomach, and he confirmed the presence of hydrochloric acid and a ferment, later shown to be the result of the protein-breaking enzyme pepsin. Because of an unfortunate accident, both Beaumont and St. Martin gained a place in the history of gastrointestinal physiology.

Unit IX

Disorders of Gastrointestinal Function

Structure and Function of the Gastrointestinal System

36

In the digestive system, food is dismantled and its nutrients absorbed, wastes are collected and eliminated, vitamins are synthesized, and enzymes are produced. The gastrointestinal (GI) tract is also becoming increasingly recognized as an endocrine organ that produces and augments hormones that contribute to the regulation of appetite and nutrient intake and function in the use and storage of nutrients. The GI tract has multiple collections of specialized cells interspersed throughout GI tissue that secrete these types of hormones.

As a matter of semantics, the GI tract also is referred to as the *digestive tract,* the *alimentary canal,* and, at times, the *gut.* The intestinal portion also may be called the *bowel.* For the purposes of this text, the liver and pancreas (discussed in Chapter 38), which produce secretions that aid in digestion, are considered *accessory organs.*

STRUCTURE AND ORGANIZATION OF THE GASTROINTESTINAL TRACT

After completing this section of the chapter, you should be able to meet the following objectives:

- Describe the anatomic structures of the upper, middle, and lower gastrointestinal tract.
- List the four layers of the gastrointestinal tract wall and describe their function.
- Characterize the structure and function of the peritoneum and describe its attachment to the abdominal wall.

The major physiologic functions of the GI system are to digest food and absorb nutrients into the bloodstream. It carries out these functions by motility, secretion, digestion, and absorption. In the digestive tract, food and other materials move slowly along its length as they are systematically broken down into ions and molecules that can be absorbed into the body. In the large intestine, unabsorbed nutrients and wastes are collected for later elimination.

Structurally, the GI tract is a long, hollow tube, the lumen (*i.e.,* hollow centre) of which is an extension of the external environment (Fig. 36.1). Nutrients do not become part of the internal

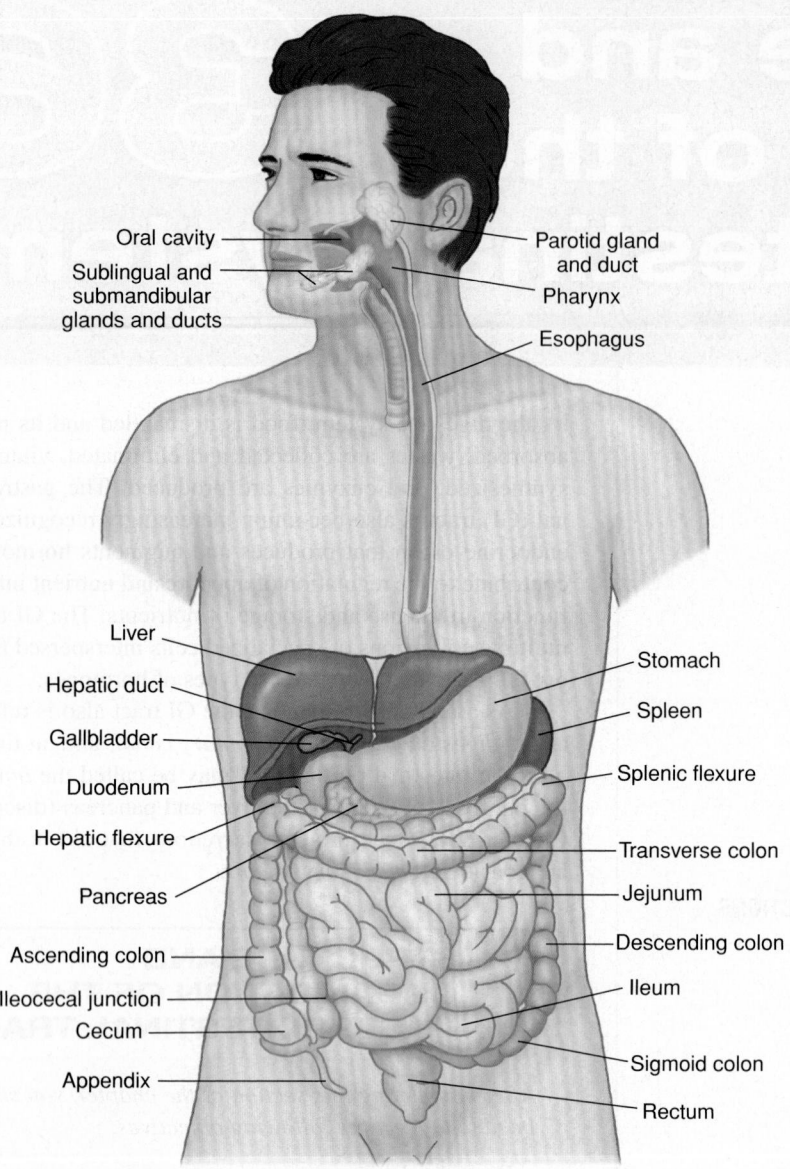

Oral cavity

Sublingual and submandibular glands and ducts

Parotid gland and duct

Pharynx

Esophagus

Liver

Hepatic duct

Gallbladder

Duodenum

Hepatic flexure

Pancreas

Ascending colon

Ileocecal junction

Cecum

Appendix

Stomach

Spleen

Splenic flexure

Transverse colon

Jejunum

Descending colon

Ileum

Sigmoid colon

Rectum

FIGURE 36.1 • The digestive system.

environment until they have passed through the intestinal wall and have entered the blood or lymph channels. For simplicity and understanding, the GI tract can be divided into three parts. The upper part—the mouth, esophagus, and stomach—acts as an intake source and receptacle through which food passes and in which initial digestive processes take place. The middle portion—the duodenum, jejunum, and ileum—is where most digestive and absorptive processes occur. The lower segment—the cecum, colon, and rectum—serves as a storage channel for the efficient elimination of waste. The accessory organs, which include the salivary glands, liver, and pancreas, produce secretions that aid in digestion.

Upper Gastrointestinal Tract

The mouth forms the entryway into the GI tract for food; it contains the teeth, used in the mastication or mechanical breakdown of food, and the tongue and other structures needed to direct food toward the pharyngeal structures and the esophagus. The mouth also serves as a receptacle for saliva produced by the salivary glands. Saliva moistens and lubricates food so it is easier to swallow, and contains enzymes involved in the initial digestion of lipids and starches.

Esophagus

The esophagus is a straight, collapsible tube, about 25 cm in length, which lies behind the trachea and connects the oropharynx with the stomach. The esophagus functions primarily as a conduit for the passage of food from the pharynx to the stomach. Its structure is uniquely designed for this purpose: the smooth muscle layers provide the peristaltic movements needed to move food along its length, and the mucosal and submucosal glands secrete mucus, which protects its surface and aids in lubricating food.

STRUCTURE AND FUNCTION OF THE GASTROINTESTINAL TRACT

- The gastrointestinal tract is a long, hollow tube that extends from the mouth to the anus; food and fluids that enter the gastrointestinal tract do not become part of the internal environment until they have been broken down and absorbed into the blood or lymph channels.
- The wall of the GI tract is essentially a four-layered tube: an inner mucosal layer; a supporting submucosal layer; a muscularis layer consisting of an inner circular layer and outer longitudinal layer of smooth muscle that functions propel to its contents in a proximal-to-distal direction, and an outer serosa layer that covers those parts of the GI tract that are suspended in the abdominopelvic cavity.
- The nutrients contained in ingested foods and fluids must be broken down into molecules that can be absorbed across the wall of the intestine. Gastric acids and pepsin from the stomach begin the digestive process: bile from the liver, digestive enzymes from the pancreas, and brush border enzymes break carbohydrates, fats, and proteins into molecules that can be absorbed from the intestine.

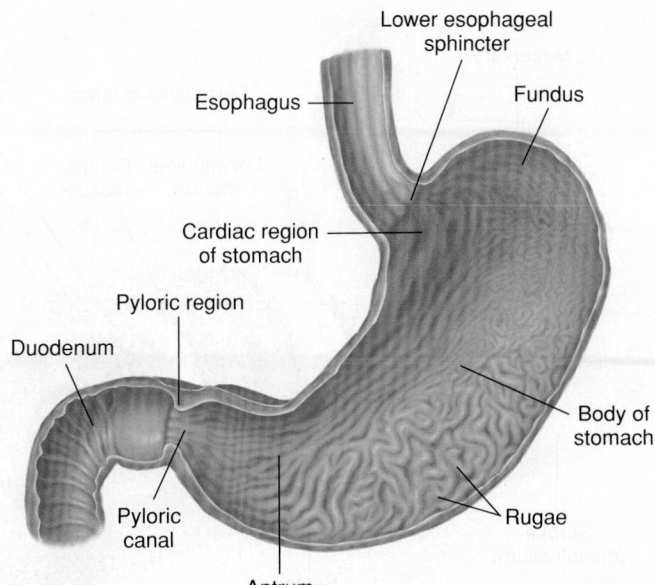

FIGURE 36.2 • Structures of the stomach.

The wider and more superior part of the pyloric region, the *antrum*, narrows to form the pyloric channel as it approaches the small intestine. At the end of the pyloric channel, the circular layer of smooth muscle thickens to form the *pyloric sphincter*. This muscle serves as a valve that controls the rate of stomach emptying and prevents the regurgitation of intestinal contents back into the stomach.

Middle Gastrointestinal Tract

The small intestine, which forms the middle portion of the digestive tract, consists of three subdivisions: the duodenum, jejunum, and ileum (Fig. 36.1). The duodenum, which is approximately 25 cm long, connects the stomach to the jejunum and contains the opening for the common bile duct and the main pancreatic duct. Bile and pancreatic juices enter the intestine through these ducts. The jejunum and ileum together are approximately 3 m long due to muscle tone but in a cadaver can be stretched out to 7 m. These must be folded onto themselves to fit into the abdominal cavity and this is where food is digested and absorbed.

Lower Gastrointestinal Tract

The large intestine, which forms the lower GI tract, is approximately 1.5 m long and 6 to 7 cm in diameter. It is divided into the cecum, colon, rectum, and anal canal (Fig. 36.1). The cecum is a blind pouch that projects down at the junction of the ileum and the colon. The ileocecal valve lies at the upper border of the cecum and prevents the return of feces from the cecum into the small intestine. The appendix arises from the cecum approximately 2.5 cm from the ileocecal valve. The colon is further divided into ascending, transverse, descending, and sigmoid portions. The ascending colon extends from the cecum to the undersurface of the liver, where it turns abruptly to form the right

There are sphincters at either end of the esophagus. The upper esophageal sphincter, the *pharyngoesophageal* sphincter, consists of a circular layer of striated muscle. It keeps air from entering the esophagus and stomach during breathing. The lower esophageal sphincter, the *gastroesophageal sphincter* or *cardiac sphincter*, lies just above the area where the esophagus joins the stomach. The circular muscle in this area normally remains tonically contracted, creating a zone of high pressure that serves to prevent reflux of gastric contents into the esophagus. During swallowing, there is "receptive relaxation" of the lower esophageal sphincter, which allows easy propulsion of the esophageal contents into the stomach. The lower esophageal sphincter passes through an opening, or *hiatus*, in the diaphragm as it joins with the stomach, which is located in the abdomen. The portion of the diaphragm that surrounds the lower esophageal sphincter helps to maintain the zone of high pressure needed to prevent reflux of stomach contents into the esophagus.

Stomach

The stomach is a pouch-like structure that lies in the left upper quadrant of the abdomen and serves as a food storage reservoir during the early stages of digestion. The esophagus opens into the stomach through an opening called the *cardiac orifice*, so named because of its proximity to the heart. The small part of the stomach that surrounds the cardiac orifice is called the *cardiac region*, the dome-shaped region that bulges above the cardiac region is called the *fundus*, the middle portion is called the *body*, and the funnel-shaped portion that connects with the small intestine is called the *pyloric region* (Fig. 36.2).

FIGURE 36.3 • Transverse section of the digestive system.

colic (hepatic) flexure. The transverse colon crosses the upper half of the abdominal cavity from right to left and then curves sharply downward beneath the lower end of the spleen, forming the left colic (splenic) flexure. The descending colon extends from the colic flexure to the rectum. The rectum extends from the sigmoid colon to the anus. The anal canal passes between the two medial borders of the levator ani muscles. Powerful sphincter muscles guard against fecal incontinence.

Gastrointestinal Wall Structure

The digestive tract, below the upper third of the esophagus, is essentially a four-layered tube (Fig. 36.3).

Mucosal Layer. The inner *mucosal layer* is made up of a lining of epithelium, an underlying connective tissue called the lamina propria, and the muscularis mucosae composed of smooth muscle cells that can contract and change the shape and surface area of the mucosal layer. This mucosal layer performs numerous functions in its role as an interface between the body and the environment, including production of the mucus that lubricates and protects the inner surface of the alimentary canal, secretion of the digestive enzymes, and substances that break down food, absorption of the breakdown products of digestion, and maintenance of a barrier to prevent the entry of noxious substances and pathogenic organisms; the lymphatics within the mucosa serve as the body's first line of immune defence. The epithelial cells in the mucosal layer have a rapid turnover rate and are replaced every 4 to 5 days. Because of the regenerative capabilities of the mucosal layer, injury to this layer heals rapidly without leaving scar tissue.

Submucosal Layer. The *submucosal (second) layer* consists of dense connective tissue and aggregates of adipose tissue.

It contains the blood vessels, nerves, and structures responsible for secreting digestive enzymes. The submucosal glands either deliver their secretions directly to the lumen of the mucosal glands or via ducts that pass through the mucosa to the luminal surface.

Muscularis Externa Layer. The third layer, the *muscularis externa,* consists of an inner layer of circularly arranged smooth muscle cells and outer layer of longitudinally arranged smooth muscle layers, which facilitates movement of contents of the GI tract.

Fourth Layer. In the abdominal cavity the fourth or *serosal layer* is a serous membrane consisting of a layer of simple squamous epithelium, called the *mesothelium,* and a small amount of underlying connective tissue. It is equivalent to the visceral peritoneum and is the most superficial layer of those parts of the digestive tract that are suspended in the peritoneal cavity. For the esophagus which lies in the thoracic cavity, the fourth layer is the adventitia layer consisting of fibrous connective tissue binding the esophagus to surrounding structures. Retroperitoneal organs have both serosa and adventitia layers, serosa if facing the peritoneal cavity and adventitia to adhere to the dorsal wall.

The peritoneum is the largest serous membrane in the body, having a surface area approximately equal to that of the skin. The peritoneum consists of two continuous layers: the *parietal peritoneum,* which lines the wall of the abdomino-pelvic cavity, and the *visceral peritoneum,* which covers most abdominal organs such as the stomach and intestines. Between the two layers is the *peritoneal cavity,* a potential space containing fluid secreted by the serous membranes. This serous fluid forms a moist and slippery surface that prevents friction between the continuously moving abdominal structures.

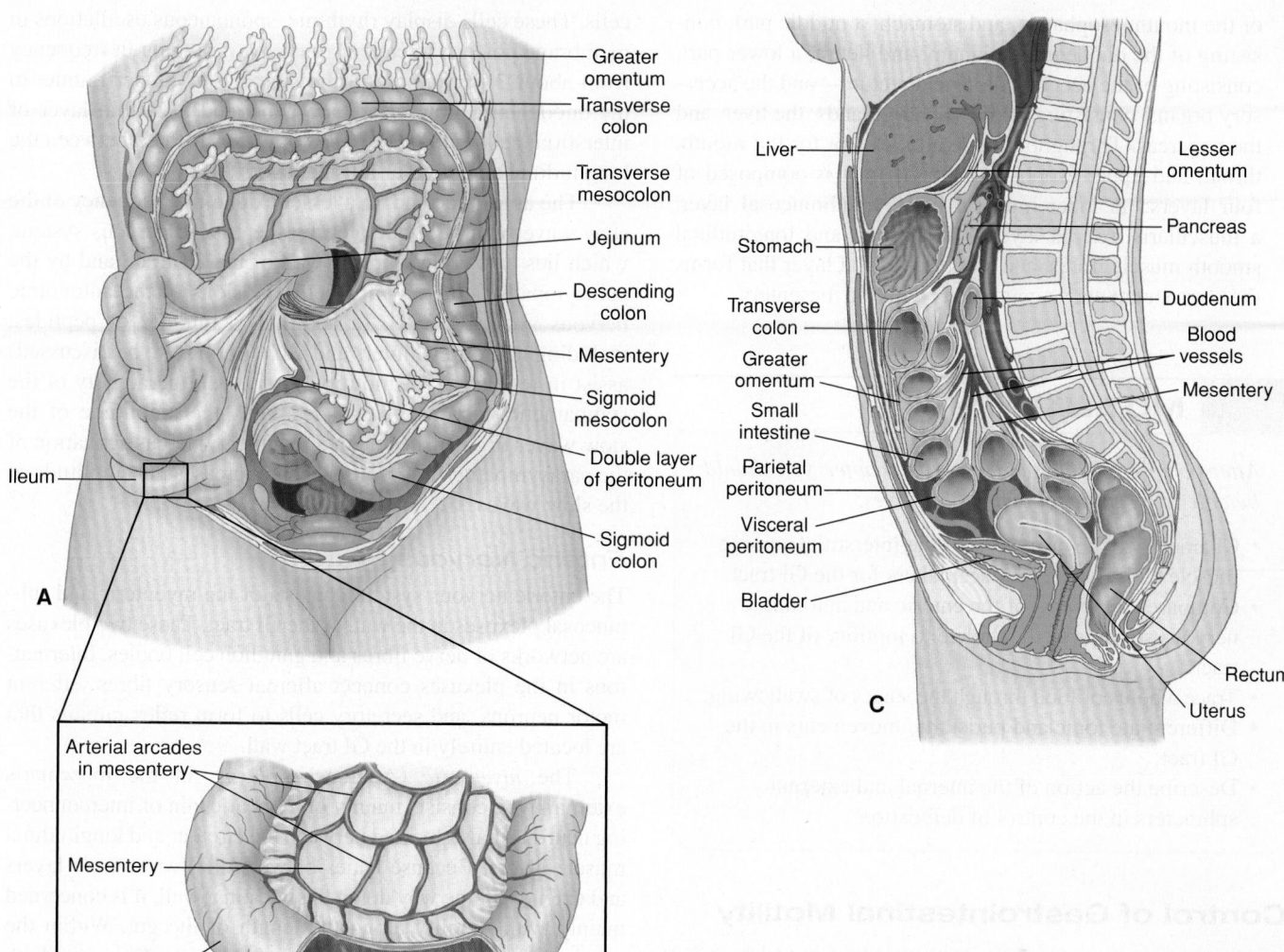

FIGURE 36.4 • Mesenteries of the abdominal cavity. **A:** The greater omentum has been reflected superiorly to reveal the mesentery attachments to the small and large intestines. **B:** The attachment of the mesentery to the small bowel. The mesentery contains the blood vessels, nerves, and lymphatic vessels that supply the intestinal wall. **C:** Sagittal section of the abdominopelvic cavity in a woman, showing the relationships of the peritoneal attachments and the greater and lesser omentums.

The *mesentery* is the double layer of peritoneum that encloses a portion or all of one of the abdominal viscera and attaches it to the abdominal wall (Fig. 36.4A). The mesentery contains the blood vessels, nerves, and lymphatic vessels that supply the intestinal wall (Fig. 36.4B). It also holds the organs in place and stores fat. There are dorsal as well as ventral mesenteries; however, in most places the mesentery is dorsal and attaches to the posterior abdominal wall. The mesentery that attaches to the jejunum and ileum is gathered in folds that attach to the dorsal abdominal wall along a short line of insertion, giving a fan-shaped appearance, with the intestines at the edge.

An *omentum* is a double-layered extension or fold of peritoneum that passes from the stomach or proximal part of the duodenum to adjacent organs in the abdominal cavity or abdominal wall. The *greater omentum* extends from the stomach to cover the transverse colon and the folds of the intestine, whereas the *lesser omentum* extends between the transverse fissure of the

liver and the lesser curvature of the stomach (Fig. 36.4C). The greater omentum always contains some fat, which in obese persons can be a considerable amount. It has considerable mobility and moves around in the peritoneal cavity with the peristaltic movements of the intestines. It often forms adhesions (*i.e.,* bands of fibrous scar tissue) adjacent to inflamed organs such as the appendix, walling off the infection and thereby preventing its spread. The greater omentum also cushions the abdominal organs against injury and provides insulation against the loss of body heat.

IN SUMMARY

The GI tract is a long, hollow tube, the lumen of which is an extension of the external environment. The digestive tract can be divided into three parts—an upper part, consisting of the mouth, esophagus, and stomach; a middle part, consisting of the duodenum, jejunum, and ileum; a lower part, consisting of the cecum, colon, and rectum—and the accessory organs, consisting of the salivary glands, the liver, and the pancreas. Throughout its length, except for the mouth, throat, and upper esophagus, the GI tract is composed of four layers: an inner mucosal layer, a submucosal layer, a muscularis externa layer with circular and longitudinal smooth muscle fibres, and an outer serosal layer that forms the peritoneum and is continuous with the mesentery.

MOTILITY

After completing this section of the chapter, you should be able to meet the following objectives:

- Characterize the properties of the interstitial smooth muscle cells that act as pacemakers for the GI tract.
- Compare the actions of the enteric and autonomic nervous systems as they relate to motility of the GI tract.
- Trace a bolus of food through the stages of swallowing.
- Differentiate tonic and peristaltic movements in the GI tract.
- Describe the action of the internal and external sphincters in the control of defecation.

Control of Gastrointestinal Motility

The motility of the GI tract propels food and fluids along its length, from mouth to anus, in a manner that facilitates digestion and absorption. The movements of the GI tract can be either rhythmic or tonic. The *rhythmic movements* consist of intermittent contractions that are responsible for mixing and moving food along the digestive tract. Rhythmic movements are found in the esophagus, antrum of the stomach, and small intestine. The *tonic movements* consist of a constant level of contraction or tone without regular periods of relaxation. They are found in the lower esophagus, the upper region of the stomach, the ileocecal valve, and the internal anal sphincter.

Pacemaker-Generated Slow-Wave Activity

All of the contractile tissue in the GI tract is smooth muscle, except for that in the pharynx, the upper third of the esophagus, and the external anal sphincter. Although the smooth muscle found in each region of the GI tract exhibits structural and functional differences, certain basic properties are common to all of the muscle cells. All of the smooth muscle of the GI tract is unitary smooth muscle, in which the cells are electrically coupled by gap junctions so that electrical signals initiating muscle contractions can move rapidly from one fibre to the next within each bundle.

Like the self-excitable cardiac muscle cells in the heart, some smooth muscle cells of the GI tract function as pacemaker cells. These cells display rhythmic, spontaneous oscillations in membrane potentials, called *slow waves,* ranging in frequency from about 3 per minute in the stomach to 12 per minute in the duodenum. Slow waves are generated by a thin layer of interstitial cells (*interstitial cells of Cajal*) located between the longitudinal and circular muscle layers.

The amplitude and, to a lesser extent, the frequency of the slow waves can be modulated by the enteric nervous system, which lies entirely within the wall of the GI tract, and by the parasympathetic and sympathetic divisions of the autonomic nervous system (ANS). In addition, a number of peptides, including neurotransmitters and GI hormones (to be discussed) assist in regulating GI motility. In general, the activity of the sympathetic nervous system decreases the amplitude of the slow waves or abolishes them altogether, whereas activation of the parasympathetic nervous system increases the amplitude of the slow waves.

Enteric Nervous System

The enteric nervous system consists of the myenteric and submucosal plexuses in the wall of the GI tract. These two plexuses are networks of nerve fibres and ganglion cell bodies. Interneurons in the plexuses connect afferent sensory fibres, efferent motor neurons, and secretory cells to form reflex circuits that are located entirely in the GI tract wall.

The *myenteric (Auerbach) plexus,* in the muscularis externa layer, consists mainly of a linear chain of interconnecting neurons that is located between the circular and longitudinal muscle layers. Because it lies between the two muscle layers and extends all the way down the intestinal wall, it is concerned mainly with motility along the length of the gut. Within the submuscosa layer is the *submucosal (Meissner) plexus* which is mainly concerned with controlling the function of each segment of the intestinal tract. It integrates signals received from the mucosal layer into local control of motility, intestinal secretions, and absorption of nutrients.

The activity of the neurons in the myenteric and submucosal plexuses is regulated by local influences, input from the ANS, and by interconnecting fibres that transmit information between the two plexuses. Mechanoreceptors monitor the stretch and distension of the GI tract wall, and chemoreceptors monitor the chemical composition (*i.e.,* osmolality, pH, and digestive products of protein and fat metabolism) of its contents. These receptors can communicate directly with ganglionic cells in the intramural plexuses or with visceral afferent fibres that influence ANS control of GI function.

Autonomic Nervous System Innervation. The autonomic innervation of the GI system is mediated by both the sympathetic and parasympathetic nervous systems (Fig. 36.5). Parasympathetic innervation to the stomach, small intestine, cecum, ascending colon, and transverse colon occurs through the vagus nerve. The remainder of the colon is innervated by parasympathetic fibres that exit the sacral segments of the spinal cord, by way of the pelvic nerves. Preganglionic parasympathetic fibres can synapse with intramural plexus neurons, or

Understanding Intestinal Motility

Motility of the small intestine is organized to optimize the digestion and absorption of nutrients and the propulsion of undigested material toward the colon. Peristaltic movements mix the ingested foodstuffs with digestive enzymes and secretions and circulate the intestinal contents to facilitate contact with the intestinal mucosa. The regulation of motility results from an interplay of input from the (1) enteric and (2) autonomic nervous (ANS) systems and the intrinsic pacemaker activity of the (3) intestinal smooth muscle cells.

1. Enteric Nervous System Innervation

The gastrointestinal system has its own nervous system, called the *enteric nervous system*. The enteric nervous system is composed mainly of two plexuses: (1) the outer *myenteric (Auerbach) plexus* that is located between the longitudinal and circular layers of smooth muscle cells, and (2) an inner *submucosal (Meissner) plexus* that lies between the mucosal and circular muscle layers. The myenteric plexus controls mainly intestinal movements along the length of the gut, whereas the submucosal plexus is concerned mainly with controlling the function within each segment of the intestine. Fibres in the submucosal plexus also use signals originating from the intestinal epithelium to control intestinal secretion and local blood flow.

2. ANS Innervation

The intestine is also innervated by the parasympathetic and sympathetic branches of the ANS (Fig. 36.5). *Parasympathetic innervation* is supplied mainly by the vagus nerve with postganglionic neurons located primarily in the myenteric and submucosal plexuses. Stimulation of these parasympathetic nerves causes a general increase in both intestinal motility and secretory activity. *Sympathetic innervation* is supplied by nerves that run between the spinal cord and the prevertebral ganglia and between these ganglia and the intestine. Stimulation of the sympathetic nervous system is largely inhibitory, producing a decrease in intestinal motility and secretory activity.

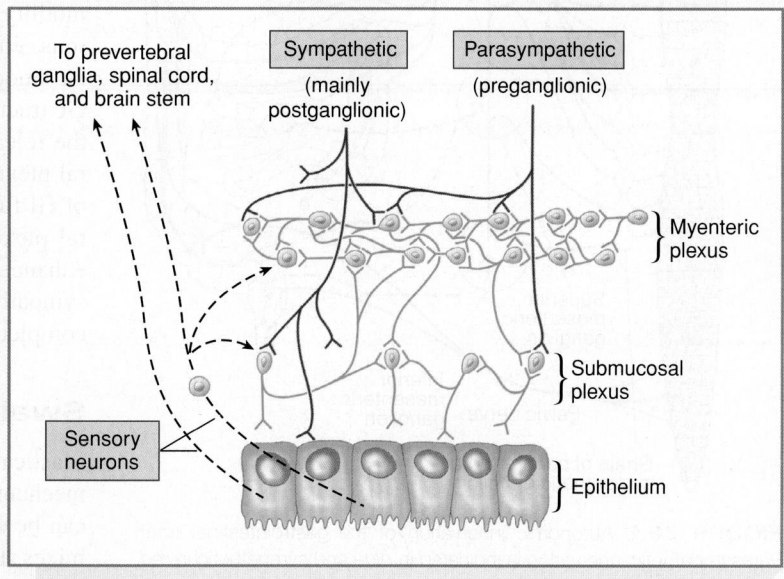

3. Intestinal Smooth Muscle

Intestinal smooth muscle has its own intrinsic slow-wave activity, which varies from about 12 per minute in the duodenum to 8 or 9 per minute in the ileum. This slow-wave activity is thought to reside in a network of specialized pacemaker cells, the *interstitial cells of Cajal,* that are interposed between the smooth muscle cells. Slow waves are not action potentials and they do not directly induce muscle contraction; instead, they are rhythmic, wavelike fluctuations in the membrane potential that cyclically bring the membrane closer to threshold. If the peak voltage of the slow wave exceeds the cell's threshold potential, one or more action potentials may be triggered. Because action potentials occur at the peak of a smooth wave, slow-wave frequency determines the rate of smooth muscle contractions. Stretching the intestinal smooth muscle and parasympathetic nervous system stimulation increase excitability of the smooth muscle cells, whereas sympathetic stimulation decreases excitability.

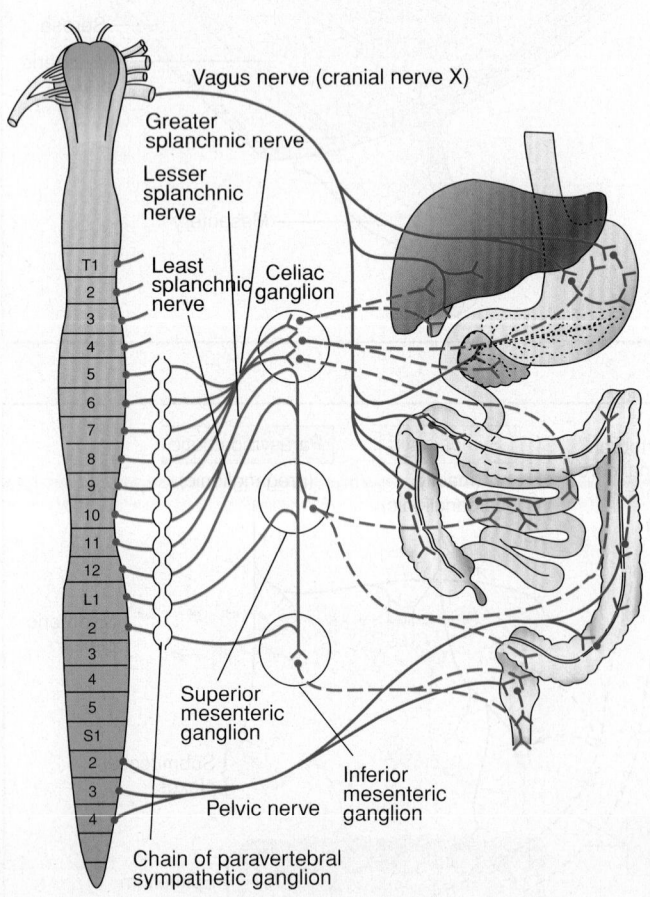

FIGURE 36.5 Autonomic innervation of the gastrointestinal tract. Parasympathetic innervation is indicated in *blue* and sympathetic in *red*.

they can act directly on intestinal smooth muscle. In addition, these same nerve bundles provide many afferent nerves whose receptors lie within the various tissues of the gut. Their nerves project to the spinal cord and brain to provide sensory input for integration. Most parasympathetic innervation is excitatory. Numerous vagovagal reflexes influence motility and secretions of the digestive tract.

Sympathetic innervation occurs through the thoracic chain of sympathetic ganglia and the celiac, superior mesenteric, and inferior mesenteric ganglia. The sympathetic nervous system exerts several effects on GI function. It controls the extent of mucus secretion by the mucosal glands, reduces motility by inhibiting the activity of intramural plexus neurons, enhances sphincter function, and increases the vascular smooth muscle tone of the blood vessels that supply the GI tract. The effect of sympathetic stimulation is to block the release of the excitatory neuromediators in the intramural plexuses, thus inhibiting GI motility. Sympathetic control of GI function is largely mediated by activity in the intramural plexuses. For example, when gastrointestinal motility is enhanced because of increased vagal activity, stimulation of sympathetic centres in the hypothalamus promptly, and often completely, inhibits motility.

Swallowing and Esophageal Motility

Mastication or chewing begins the digestive process; it mechanically breaks the food into particles of a size that can be swallowed, lubricates it by mixing it with saliva, and mixes starch-containing food with salivary amylase. Although chewing usually is considered a voluntary act, it can be carried out involuntarily by a person who has lost the function of the cerebral cortex.

The swallowing reflex is a rigidly ordered sequence of events that results in the propulsion of food from the mouth to the stomach through the esophagus. Although swallowing is initiated as a voluntary activity, it becomes involuntary as food or fluid reaches the pharynx. Sensory impulses for the reflex begin at tactile receptors in the pharynx and esophagus and are integrated with the motor components of the response in an area of the reticular formation of the medulla and lower pons called the *swallowing centre*. The motor impulses for the oral and pharyngeal phases of swallowing are carried in the trigeminal (V), glossopharyngeal (IX), vagus (X), and hypoglossal (XII) cranial nerves, and impulses for the esophageal phase are carried by the vagus nerve. Diseases that disrupt these brain centres or their cranial nerves disrupt the coordination of swallowing and predispose an individual to food and fluid lodging in the trachea and bronchi, leading to risk of asphyxiation or aspiration pneumonia.

Swallowing consists of three phases: an oral or voluntary phase, a pharyngeal phase, and an esophageal phase (Fig. 36.6). During the *oral phase,* the bolus is collected at the back of the

mouth so the tongue can lift the food upward until it touches the posterior wall of the pharynx (Fig. 36.6A). At this point, the *pharyngeal phase* of swallowing is initiated. The soft palate is pulled upward, the palatopharyngeal folds are pulled together so that food does not enter the nasopharynx, the vocal cords are pulled together, and the epiglottis is moved so that it covers the larynx (Fig. 36.6B). Respiration is inhibited, and the bolus is moved backward into the esophagus by constrictive movements of the pharynx. Although the striated muscles of the pharynx are involved in the second stage of swallowing, it is an involuntary stage.

The third phase of swallowing is the *esophageal stage* (Fig. 36.6C). As food enters the esophagus and stretches its walls, local and central nervous system (CNS) reflexes that initiate peristalsis are triggered. There are two types of peristalsis—primary and secondary. Primary peristalsis is controlled by the swallowing centre in the brain stem and begins when food enters the esophagus. Secondary peristalsis is partially mediated by smooth muscle fibres in the esophagus and occurs when primary peristalsis is inadequate to move food through the esophagus. Peristalsis begins at the site of distension and moves downward. Before the peristaltic wave reaches the stomach, the lower esophageal sphincter relaxes to allow the bolus of food to enter the stomach. The pressure

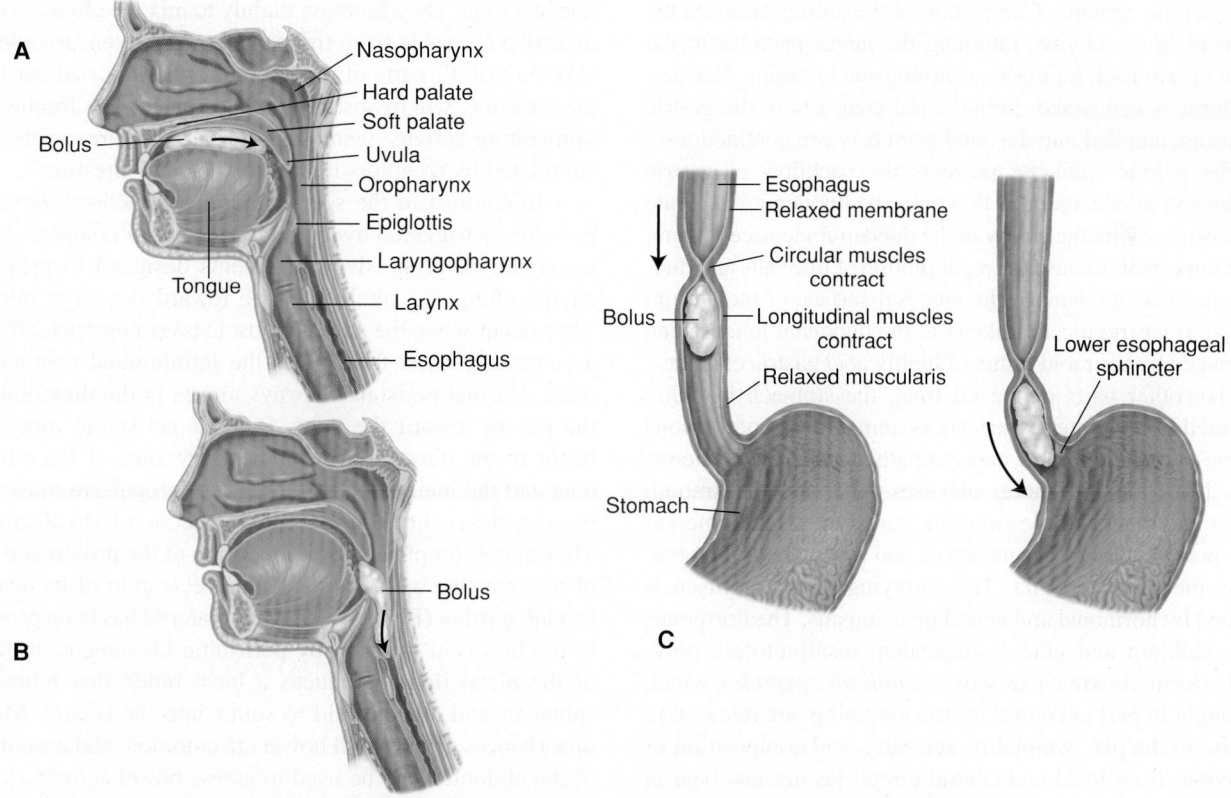

FIGURE 36.6 • Steps in the swallowing reflex. (**A**) The *oral* or *voluntary phase* during which the bolus is collected at the back of the mouth so the tongue can lift the food upward and into the pharynx; (**B**) the *pharyngeal phase* during which food movement into the respiratory passages is prevented as the tongue is elevated and pressed against the soft palate closing the epiglottis, the upper esophageal sphincter relaxes, and the superior constrictor muscle contracts forcing food into the esophagus; and (**C**) the *esophageal phase* during which peristalsis moves food through the esophagus and into the stomach.

in the lower esophageal sphincter normally is greater than that in the stomach, an important factor in preventing the reflux of gastric contents. The lower esophageal sphincter is innervated by the vagus nerve. Increased levels of parasympathetic stimulation increase the constriction of the sphincter. The hormone gastrin also increases constriction of the sphincter. Gastrin provides the major stimulus for gastric acid production, and its action on the lower esophageal sphincter protects the esophageal mucosa when gastric acid levels are elevated.

Gastric Motility

The stomach serves as a food storage reservoir where the chemical breakdown of proteins begins and food is converted to a creamy mixture called *chyme*. Although an empty stomach has a volume of about 50 ml, it can expand to as much as 1,000 ml before the intraluminal pressure begins to rise.

Motility of the stomach results in the churning and mixing of solid foods and regulates the emptying of the gastric contents, or chyme, into the duodenum. Peristaltic mixing and churning contractions begin in a pacemaker area in the middle of the stomach and move toward the antrum. They occur at a frequency of 3 to 5 contractions per minute, each lasting 2 to 20 seconds. As the peristaltic wave approaches the antrum, it speeds up, and the entire terminal 5 to 10 cm of the antrum contracts, occluding the pyloric opening. Contraction of the antrum reverses the movement of the chyme, returning the larger particles to the body of the stomach for further churning and kneading. Because the pylorus is contracted during antral contraction, the gastric contents are emptied into the duodenum between contractions.

The pyloric sphincter prevents the backflow of gastric contents and allows them to flow into the duodenum at a rate commensurate with the ability of the duodenum to accept them. This is important because the regurgitation of bile salts and duodenal contents can damage the mucosal surface of the antrum and lead to gastric ulcers. Likewise, the duodenal mucosa can be damaged by the rapid influx of highly acid gastric contents.

Like other parts of the GI tract, the stomach is richly innervated by the enteric nervous system and its connections with the sympathetic and parasympathetic nervous systems. Axons from the intramural plexuses innervate the smooth muscles and glands of the stomach. Parasympathetic innervation is provided by the vagus nerve and sympathetic innervation by the celiac ganglia. The emptying of the stomach is regulated by hormonal and neural mechanisms. The hormones cholecystokinin and glucose-dependent insulinotropic polypeptide (formerly known as *gastric inhibitory peptide*), which are thought in part to control gastric emptying, are released in response to the pH, osmolality, and fatty acid composition of the chyme. Both local and central circuitries are involved in the neural control of gastric emptying. Afferent receptor fibres synapse with the neurons in the intramural plexus or trigger intrinsic reflexes through vagal or sympathetic pathways that participate in extrinsic reflexes.

Disorders of gastric motility can occur when the rate is too slow or too fast (see Chapter 37). A rate that is too slow leads to gastric retention. It can be caused by obstruction or gastric atony. Obstruction can result from the formation of scar tissue in the pyloric area after a peptic ulcer. Another example of obstruction is *hypertrophic pyloric stenosis*, which can occur in infants with an abnormally thick muscularis externa layer in the terminal pylorus. Myotomy, or surgical incision of the muscular ring, may be done to relieve the obstruction. Gastric atony can occur as a complication of visceral neuropathies in diabetes mellitus. Surgical procedures that disrupt vagal activity also can result in gastric atony. Abnormally fast emptying occurs in the dumping syndrome, which is a consequence of certain types of gastric operations. This condition is characterized by the rapid dumping of highly acidic and hyperosmotic gastric secretions into the duodenum and jejunum.

Small Intestinal Motility

The small intestine is the major site for the digestion and absorption of food; its movements are mixing and propulsive. There are two patterns of contractions in the small intestine: segmentation and peristaltic contractions. With *segmentation waves,* slow contractions of the circular muscle layer occlude the lumen and drive the contents forward and backward (Fig. 36.7A). Most of the contractions that produce segmentation waves are local events involving only 1 to 4 cm of intestine at a time. They function mainly to mix the chyme with the digestive enzymes from the pancreas and to ensure adequate exposure of all parts of the chyme to the mucosal surface of the intestine, where absorption takes place. The frequency of segmenting activity increases after a meal. Presumably, it is stimulated by receptors in the stomach and intestine.

In contrast to the segmentation contractions, *peristaltic movements* triggered by the *migrating motor complex* (MMC) are rhythmic propulsive movements designed to propel the chyme along the small intestine toward the large intestine. They occur when the smooth muscle layer constricts, forming a contractile band that forces the intraluminal contents forward. Normal peristalsis always moves in the direction from the mouth toward the anus. Regular peristaltic movements begin in the duodenum near the entry sites of the common duct and the main hepatic duct. These propulsive movements occur with synchronized activity in a section 10 to 20 cm long. They are accomplished by contraction of the proximal portion of the intestine with the sequential relaxation of its distal, or caudal, portion (Fig. 36.7B). After material has been propelled to the ileocecal junction by peristaltic movement, stretching of the distal ileum produces a local reflex that relaxes the sphincter and allows fluid to squirt into the cecum. Motility disturbances of the small bowel are common, and auscultation of the abdomen can be used to assess bowel activity. Inflammatory changes often increase motility. In many instances, it is not certain whether changes in motility occur because of inflammation or are secondary to toxins or unabsorbed nutrients. Delayed passage of chyme in the small intestine also can be a problem. Transient interruption of intestinal motility often occurs after GI surgery, thus gastric suction often is

FIGURE 36.7 • Two types of small intestine movements. (**A**) Mixing *segmentation waves* in which slow contractions of the circular muscle layer occlude the lumen and drive the contents forward and backward and (**B**) propulsive *peristaltic movements* in which segmental contractions followed by sequential relaxation moves the contents forward.

required to remove the accumulating intestinal contents and gases until activity is resumed.

Colonic Motility and Defecation

The storage function of the colon dictates that movements in this section of the gut are different from those in the small intestine. Movements in the colon are of two types. First are the segmental mixing movements, called *haustral churning,* so named because they occur within sacculations called *haustra.* These movements produce a local digging-type action, moving contents from one haustra to the next which ensures that all portions of the fecal mass are exposed to the intestinal surface. Second are the more intense propulsive *mass movements,* in which a large segment of the colon (≥20 cm) contracts as a unit, moving the fecal contents forward as a unit. Mass movements last approximately 30 seconds, followed by a 2- to 3-minute period of relaxation, after which another contraction occurs. A series of mass movements lasts only for 10 to 30 minutes and may occur only several times a day. Defecation normally is initiated by the mass movements. The normal colonic transit time is 24 to 48 hours, and normal stool is comprised of 75% water and 25% solid matter.

Defecation is controlled by the action of two sphincters, the internal and external anal sphincters (Fig. 36.8). The internal sphincter is a several-centimetres-long, circular thickening of smooth muscle that lies inside the anus. The external sphincter, which is composed of striated voluntary muscle, surrounds the internal sphincter. The external sphincter is controlled by nerve fibres in the pudendal nerve, which is part of the somatic nervous system and therefore under voluntary control. Defecation is controlled by defecation reflexes. One of these reflexes is the intrinsic myenteric reflex mediated by the local enteric nervous system. It is initiated by distension of the rectal wall, with initiation of reflex peristaltic waves that spread through the descending colon, sigmoid colon, and rectum. A second defecation reflex, the parasympathetic reflex, is integrated at the level of the sacral cord. When the nerve endings in the rectum are stimulated, signals are transmitted first to the sacral cord and then reflexively back to the descending colon, sigmoid colon, rectum, and anus by the pelvic nerves. These impulses greatly increase peristaltic movements as well as relax the internal sphincter.

To prevent involuntary defecation from occurring, the external anal sphincter is under the conscious control of the cortex. As afferent impulses arrive at the sacral cord, signalling the presence of a distended rectum, messages are transmitted to the cortex. If defecation is inappropriate, the cortex initiates impulses that constrict the external sphincter and inhibit efferent parasympathetic activity. Normally, the afferent impulses in this reflex loop fatigue easily, and the urge to defecate soon ceases. At a more convenient time, contraction

FIGURE 36.8 • Interior of the rectum and anal canal.

of the abdominal muscles compresses the contents in the large bowel, reinitiating afferent impulses to the cord.

IN SUMMARY

Motility of the GI tract propels food products and fluids along its length from the mouth to anus. Although the activity of GI smooth muscle is self-propagating and can continue without input from the nervous system, its rate and strength of contractions are regulated by a network of intramural neurons that receive input from the ANS and local receptors that monitor wall stretch and the chemical composition of luminal contents. Parasympathetic innervation occurs through the vagus nerve and nerve fibres from sacral segments of the spinal cord; it increases GI motility. Sympathetic activity occurs through thoracolumbar output from the spinal cord, its paravertebral ganglia, and celiac, superior mesenteric, and inferior mesenteric ganglia. Sympathetic stimulation enhances sphincter function and reduces motility by inhibiting the activity of intramural plexus neurons.

HORMONAL, SECRETORY, AND DIGESTIVE FUNCTIONS

After completing this section of the chapter, you should be able to meet the following objectives:

- State the source and function of water and electrolytes that are secreted in digestive secretions.
- Explain the protective function of saliva.
- Describe the function of the gastric secretions in the process of digestion.
- List three major GI hormones and cite their function.
- Describe the site of gastric acid and pepsin production and secretion in the stomach.
- Describe the function of the gastric mucosal barrier.
- Describe the functions of the secretions of the small and the large intestines.
- Discuss the function of gut flora in terms of metabolic activities, trophic effects, and protection against invasion by pathogenic microorganisms.

Gastrointestinal Hormones

The GI tract is the largest endocrine organ in the body. It produces hormones that act locally, pass into the general circulation for distribution to more distant sites, and interact with the CNS through the enteric and autonomic nervous systems. Among the multiple hormones produced by the GI tract are gastrin, ghrelin, secretin, cholecystokinin, motilin, serotonin, somatostatin, and incretin hormones (glucagon-like peptide-1 [GLP-1] and glucose-dependent insulinotropic polypeptide [GIP]). These hormones influence appetite, GI motility, enzyme activity,

electrolyte levels, and the secretion and actions of hormones such as growth hormone, insulin, and glucagon. The actions of many of these hormones overlap: two or more GI hormones may affect the same process in the same direction, or they may inhibit each other. Some of the GI tract hormones and their functions are summarized in Table 36.1.

The stomach is the source of two important GI hormones: gastrin and ghrelin. Gastrin is produced by G cells, located predominantly in the antrum of the stomach. The primary function of *gastrin* is the stimulation of gastric acid secretion. Gastrin also has a trophic, or growth-producing, effect on the mucosa of the small intestine, colon, and acid-secreting area of the stomach. Removal of the tissue that produces gastrin results in atrophy of these structures. *Ghrelin* is another peptide hormone produced by endocrine cells in the mucosal layer of the fundus of the stomach. It displays potent growth hormone–releasing activity and has a stimulatory effect on food intake and digestive function, while reducing energy expenditure. The isolation of this hormone has led to new insights into the gut–brain regulation of growth hormone secretion and energy balance.

The intestine is the source of secretin, cholecystokinin, and incretin hormones. *Secretin,* which is secreted by S cells in the mucosa of the duodenum and jejunum, inhibits gastric acid secretion. The entry of an acid chyme into the intestine stimulates the release of secretin, which inhibits the release of gastrin. Secretin also stimulates the pancreas to secrete large quantities of fluid with a high bicarbonate concentration and low chloride concentration. The primary function of *cholecystokinin* (CCK), secreted by I cells in the intestinal mucosa, is the stimulation of pancreatic enzyme secretion. It potentiates the action of secretin, increasing the pancreatic bicarbonate response to low circulating levels of secretin, stimulates biliary secretion of fluid and bicarbonate, and regulates gallbladder contraction and gastric emptying. CCK has also been shown to inhibit food intake and to be an important mediator for the appetite and control of meal size.

Several gut-derived hormones have been identified as having what is termed an *incretin* effect, meaning that they increase insulin release after an oral glucose load. This suggests that gut-derived factors can stimulate insulin secretion after a predominantly carbohydrate meal. The two hormones that account for about 90% of the incretin effect are GLP-1, which is released from L cells in the distal small bowel, and GIP, which is released by K cells in the upper gut (mainly the jejunum). Because increased levels of GLP-1 and GIP can lower blood glucose levels by augmenting insulin release in a glucose-dependent manner (*i.e.,* at low blood glucose levels no further insulin is secreted, minimizing the risk of hypoglycemia), now GLP-1 is used to treat diabetes (see Chapter 42). Moreover, GLP-1 can exert other metabolically beneficial effects, including suppression of glucagon release, slowing of gastric emptying, augmenting of net glucose clearance, and decreasing appetite and body weight.

Other hormones have excitatory or inhibitory effects on motility. Motilin increases intestinal contraction by stimulating the MMC both with duodenum distension and between meals to prevent colonic bacteria re-entering the ileum.

TABLE 36.1 SELECTED GASTROINTESTINAL HORMONES AND THEIR ACTIONS

HORMONE	ENTEROENDOCRINE CELL SITE OF SECRETION	STIMULUS FOR SECRETION	ACTION
Cholecystokinin (CCK)	Cell: I cell Duodenum, jejunum	Products of protein digestion and long-chain fatty acids	Stimulates contraction of gallbladder and secretion of pancreatic enzymes; slows gastric emptying; inhibits food intake
Gastrin	Cell: G cell Antrum of stomach, duodenum	Vagal stimulation; epinephrine; neutral amino acids; calcium-containing foods such as milk; alcohol Secretion inhibited by acid content of stomach antrum (pH <2.5)	Stimulates secretion of gastric acid and pepsinogen; increases gastric blood flow; stimulates gastric smooth muscle contractions; stimulates growth of gastric and intestinal mucosal cells
Ghrelin	Cell: P/D1 cell Stomach	Nutritional (fasting) and hormonal (decreased levels of growth hormone)	Stimulates secretion of growth hormone; acts as an appetite-stimulating signal from stomach when an increase in metabolic efficiency is necessary
Glucagon-like peptide-1 (GLP-1)	Cell: Intestinal L cell Small and large intestine, mainly ileum	High-carbohydrate meal	Augments insulin release; suppresses glucagon release; slows gastric emptying; decreases appetite and body weight
Glucose-dependent insulin-otropic polypeptide or gastric inhibitory peptide (GIP)	Cell: K cell Small intestine, mainly jejunum	High-carbohydrate meal	Augments insulin release
Motilin	Cell: M cell Duodenum, jejunum	Duodenal alkaline pH Vagal stimulation	Increases migrating motor complexes
Secretin	Cell: S cell Duodenum	Acid pH or chyme entering duodenum (pH <3.0)	Stimulates secretion of bicarbonate-containing fluids by pancreas and liver
Serotonin	Cell: Intestinal enterochro-maffin cell Throughout intestines	Chyme in duodenum Intraluminal distension Vagal stimulation	Motility of intestinal tract
Somatostatin	Cell: D cell Mainly antrum stomach, small intestine	High carbohydrate and protein meal Sympathetic stimulation	Inhibits release of all GI hormones Inhibits hydrogen secretion

Approximately 90% of the body's serotonin is found in the GI tract and it used to help regulate intestinal contractions. Somatostatin is an inhibitory hormone essentially suppresses the release of all GI hormones including gastric, duodenal, pancreatic, and liver secretions plus decreasing motility which ultimately slows the digestive process.

Gastrointestinal Secretions

Throughout the GI tract, secretory glands serve two basic functions: (1) production of mucus to lubricate and protect the mucosal layer of the GI tract wall and (2) secretion of fluids and enzymes to aid in the digestion and absorption of nutrients. Each day, approximately 7,000 ml of fluid is secreted into the GI tract (Table 36.2). Approximately 100 to 200 ml of this fluid leaves the body in the stool; the remainder is reabsorbed in the small and large intestines. These secretions are mainly water and have sodium and potassium concentrations similar to those of extracellular fluid. Because water and electrolytes

for digestive tract secretions are derived from the extracellular fluid compartment, excessive secretion or impaired absorption can lead to extracellular fluid deficit.

The secretory and digestive functions of the gut are influenced by local, humoral, and neural influences. Neural control of GI secretory activity is mediated through the ANS. Secretory

TABLE 36.2 SECRETIONS OF THE GASTROINTESTINAL TRACT*

SECRETIONS	AMOUNT DAILY (ml)
Salivary	1,200
Gastric	2,000
Pancreatic	1,200
Biliary	700
Intestinal	2,000
Total	7,100

*approximate amounts.

activity, like motility, is increased with parasympathetic stimulation and inhibited with sympathetic activity. Many of the local influences, including the pH, osmolality, and chyme, consistently act as stimuli for neural and humoral mechanisms.

Salivary Secretions

Saliva is secreted by the salivary glands. The salivary glands consist of the parotid, submaxillary, sublingual, and buccal glands. Saliva has three functions. The first is protection and lubrication. Saliva is rich in mucus, which protects the oral mucosa and coats the food as it passes through the mouth, pharynx, and esophagus. The sublingual and buccal glands produce only mucus-type secretions. The second function of saliva is its protective antimicrobial action. The saliva cleans the mouth and contains the enzyme lysozyme, which has an antibacterial action. Third, saliva contains ptyalin and amylase, which initiate the digestion of dietary starches. Secretions from the salivary glands are primarily regulated by the ANS. Parasympathetic stimulation increases flow and sympathetic stimulation decreases flow. The dry mouth that accompanies anxiety attests to the effects of sympathetic activity on salivary secretions.

Mumps, or parotitis, is an infection of the parotid glands. Although most of us associate mumps with the contagious viral form of the disease, inflammation of the parotid glands can also occur in the seriously ill person who does not receive adequate oral hygiene and who is unable to take fluids orally.

Gastric Secretions

In addition to mucus-secreting cells that line the entire surface of the stomach, the stomach mucosa has several other types of cells, including the parietal (or oxyntic) cells, chief cells, and G cells. The parietal and chief cells are located in the proximal

80% (body and fundus) of the stomach. There are approximately 1 billion parietal cells in the stomach, which secrete hydrochloric acid (HCl) and intrinsic factor. The chief cells secrete pepsinogen, an enzyme that initiates proteolysis or breakdown of proteins. The antrum is located in the distal 20% of the stomach. This area contains the G cells, which secrete gastrin.

The luminal surface and gastric pits of the stomach are lined with mucus-producing epithelial cells, with the parietal and chief cells situated in the bases of the gastric pits (Fig. 36.9). There are approximately 1 billion parietal cells in the stomach; together they produce and secrete approximately 20 mmol of HCl in several hundred millilitres of gastric juice each hour. The pepsinogen that is secreted by the chief cells is rapidly converted to pepsin when exposed to the low pH of the gastric juices. Intrinsic factor, which is produced by the parietal cells, is necessary for the absorption of vitamin B_{12} (see Chapter 14).

One of the important characteristics of the gastric mucosa is resistance to the highly acid secretions that it produces. When the gastric mucosa is damaged by aspirin, nonsteroidal anti-inflammatory drugs (NSAIDs), ethyl alcohol, or bile salts, this barrier is disrupted, and hydrogen ions move into the tissue. As the hydrogen ions accumulate in the mucosal cells, intracellular pH decreases, enzymatic reactions become impaired, and cellular structures are disrupted. The result is local ischemia, vascular stasis, hypoxia, and tissue necrosis. The mucosal surface is further protected by prostaglandins. Aspirin and NSAIDs inhibit prostaglandin synthesis by inhibition of cyclooxygenase, which also impairs the integrity of the mucosal surface.

Gastric Acid Secretion. The cellular mechanism for HCl secretion by the parietal cells in the stomach involves the hydrogen (H^+)/potassium (K^+) adenosine triphosphatase (ATPase)

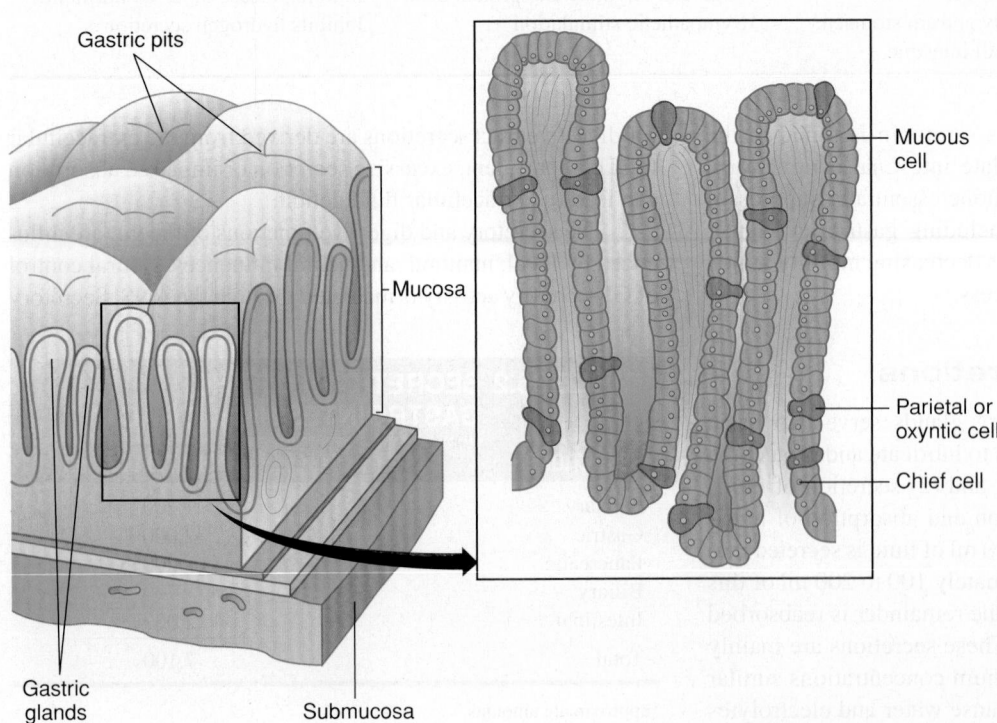

Gastric pits

Mucosa

Gastric glands

Submucosa

Mucous cell

Parietal or oxyntic cell

Chief cell

FIGURE 36.9 • Gastric pit from body of the stomach.

FIGURE 36.10 • Mechanism of gastric acid secretion by the parietal cells in the stomach.

transporter and chloride (Cl^-) channels located on their luminal membrane (Fig. 36.10). During the process of H^+ and Cl^- secretion, carbon dioxide (CO_2) produced by aerobic metabolism combines with water (H_2O), catalyzed by carbonic anhydrase, to form carbonic acid (H_2CO_3), which readily dissociates into H^+ and bicarbonate (HCO_3^-). The H^+ is secreted with Cl^+ into the stomach, and the HCO_3^- moves out of the cell and into blood from the basolateral membrane. The absorbed HCO_3^- is responsible for the alkaline tide (increased pH) that occurs after a meal. At the luminal side of the membrane, H^+ is secreted into the stomach by the H^+/K^+-ATPase transporter (also known as the *proton pump*). Chloride follows H^+ into the stomach by diffusing through Cl^- channels in the luminal membrane and combines making HCl in the stomach lumen. The proton pump inhibitors (*e.g.,* omeprazole), which are used in treatment of acid reflux and peptic ulcer, inhibit gastric acid secretion by binding irreversibly to the sulfhydryl groups of the H^+/K^+-ATPase transporter.

Three substances stimulate HCl secretion by the parietal cells: acetylcholine, gastrin, and histamine. Although each substance binds to different receptors on the parietal cell and has a different mechanism of action, they all serve to stimulate an increase in H^+ secretion through the H^+/K^+-ATPase transporter. Acetylcholine is released from vagal nerves innervating the stomach and binds to acetylcholine receptors on the parietal cells. Gastrin is secreted by G cells in the antrum of the stomach

and reaches the parietal cells through the circulation. It binds to cholecystokinin type 2 (CCK2) receptors on the parietal cells. Histamine is released from special endocrine cells in the gastric mucosa and diffuses to nearby parietal cells, where it binds to histamine-2 (H_2) receptors. H_2 receptor blockers (*e.g.,* ranitidine), used in treatment of peptic ulcer and gastroesophageal reflux, bind to H_2 receptors and block the action of histamine on parietal cells. In contrast to these acid-stimulatory factors, prostaglandin E_2 (after binding to its receptor) inhibits acid secretion and stimulates mucus production. Hence, it is an important factor in the maintenance and protection of the gastric mucosal barrier. Gastric acid secretion and its relation to gastroesophageal reflux and peptic ulcer are discussed further in Chapter 37.

Mucosal Barrier. One of the important characteristics of the gastric mucosa is its resistance to the highly corrosive acidic secretions it produces. This gel-like mucosal barrier consists of a thick coat of rich bicarbonate mucus. Tight junctions between epithelial cells aid to prevent gastric juice from gain access to deeper tissues and these epithelial cells shed every 3 to 6 days. In contrast to generating an acidic environment, prostaglandin E_2 (after binding to its receptor) has cytoprotective properties to inhibit acid secretion and stimulate mucus production.

When aspirin, NSAIDs, *Helicobacter pylori,* or alcohol damage the gastric mucosa, this protective barrier is disrupted and hydrogen ions can come in direct contact with the surface epithelial cells. If this occurs the initial inflammatory response of gastritis can occur but with ongoing damage can further develop into an erosion or ulcer.

Intestinal Secretions

The small intestine secretes digestive juices and receives secretions from the liver and pancreas (see Chapter 38). An extensive array of mucus-producing glands, called *Brunner glands,* is concentrated at the site where the contents from the stomach and secretions from the liver and pancreas enter the duodenum. These glands secrete large amounts of alkaline mucus that protect the duodenum from the acid content in the gastric chyme and from the action of the digestive enzymes. The activity of Brunner glands is strongly influenced by ANS activity. For example, sympathetic stimulation causes a marked decrease in mucus production, leaving this area more susceptible to irritation. Between 75% and 80% of peptic ulcers occur at this site.

In addition to mucus, the intestinal mucosa produces two other types of secretions. The first is a serous fluid (pH 6.5 to 7.5) secreted by specialized cells (*i.e.,* crypts of Lieberkühn) in the intestinal mucosal layer. This fluid, which is produced at the rate of 2,000 ml/day, acts as a vehicle for absorption. The second type of secretion consists of surface or brush border enzymes that aid absorption. These enzymes are the peptidases, or enzymes that separate amino acids, and the disaccharidases, or enzymes that split sugars.

The large intestine usually secretes only mucus. ANS activity strongly influences mucus production in the bowel, as in other parts of the digestive tract. During intense parasympathetic stimulation, mucus secretion may increase to the point that the stool contains large amounts of obvious mucus. Although the bowel normally does not secrete water or electrolytes, these substances are lost in large quantities when the bowel becomes irritated or inflamed.

Intestinal Flora

The gut is the natural habitat of a large and diverse bacterial community. The major functions of the gut microflora include metabolic activities that salvage energy and absorbable nutrients, trophic effects on intestinal epithelial cells, and protection of the colonized host against invasion by pathogenic organisms.

The stomach and small intestine contain only a few species of bacteria, probably because of the composition of luminal contents (*i.e.,* acids, bile, pancreatic secretions), which kills most ingested microorganisms, and the propulsive movements of this area, which impedes their colonization. The large intestine, on the other hand, contains a large and complex microbial ecosystem. It has been estimated that each individual has 300 to 500 different species of intestinal bacteria, with anaerobic bacteria outnumbering aerobic bacteria by a large percentage.

Colonization of the GI tract begins shortly after birth and is influenced by passage through the birth canal and the type of diet (breast milk versus formula) the infant receives. Other environmental factors such as neonatal care, stress, pH and immunologic status also have a role because differences exist between the intestinal flora of infants born in industrialized countries and those born in developing countries.

The major metabolic function of colonic microflora is the fermentation of undigestible dietary residue and endogenous mucus produced by the epithelial cells. The genetic diversity of the microorganisms in the gut provides various enzymes and biochemical pathways that are distinct from those of the host. Fermentation of nondigestible carbohydrates, including resistant starches, cellulose, pectins, and unabsorbed sugars, is a major source of energy in the colon. The metabolic end point is the generation of short-chain fatty acids, which play a major role in epithelial cell growth and differentiation. Colonic microorganisms also play a role in vitamin synthesis and in absorption of calcium, magnesium, and iron. Vitamin K, for example, is synthesized by the colonic flora; the newborn infant does not synthesize adequate amounts of vitamin K for the first week or so of life until the normal colonic bacterial flora becomes established. Last, the resident gut flora provide a crucial line of resistance to colonization by exogenous microbes, and therefore are highly protective against invasion of tissues by pathogens. Colonization resistance also applies to opportunistic bacteria that are present in the gut but whose growth is restricted. The administration of broad-spectrum antibiotics can disrupt the microbial balance and allow overgrowth of species with potential pathogenicity, such as *Clostridium difficile* (see Chapter 37).

The role of probiotics as a supplement to the normal diet and as a treatment for several disease states has become increasingly recognized. Probiotics are live microorganisms that, when ingested, can modify the composition of enteric microflora. Commonly used probiotics are lactobacilli, bifidobacteria, and nonpathogenic *Escherichia coli*. Probiotics have shown value in several diseases, such as maintaining remission in ulcerative colitis.

The increasing use of fecal transplants have successfully reintroduced a more balanced composition of microorganisms. This strategy has been implemented for protracted cases especially when a *C. difficile* infection does not respond to medications and has become overwhelming for the patient.

IN SUMMARY

The secretions of the GI tract include saliva, gastric juices, bile, and pancreatic and intestinal secretions. Each day, more than 7,000 ml of fluid is secreted into the digestive tract; all but 100 to 200 ml of this fluid is reabsorbed. Water, derived from the extracellular fluid compartment, is the major component of GI tract secretions. Neural, humoral, and local mechanisms contribute to the control of these secretions. The parasympathetic nervous system increases secretion, and sympathetic activity exerts an inhibitory effect. In addition to secreting fluids containing digestive enzymes, the GI tract produces and secretes hormones, such as gastrin, ghrelin, secretin, CCK, and the incretin hormones (GLP-1 and GIP) that influence appetite, GI motility, enzyme activity and the secretions. They also affect the actions of hormones such as growth hormone, insulin, and glucagon.

The gut is also the natural habitat of a large and diverse bacterial community. The major functions of the gut microflora include metabolic activities that salvage energy and absorbable nutrients, impart trophic effects on intestinal epithelial cells, and protect the colonized host against invasion by pathogenic organisms.

DIGESTION AND ABSORPTION

After completing this section of the chapter, you should be able to meet the following objectives:

- Differentiate digestion from absorption.
- Relate the characteristics of the small intestine to its absorptive function.
- Explain the function of intestinal brush border enzymes.
- Compare the digestion and absorption of carbohydrates, fats, and proteins.

Digestion is the process of dismantling foods into their constituent parts. Digestion requires hydrolysis, enzyme cleavage, and fat emulsification. Hydrolysis is the breakdown of a compound that involves a chemical reaction with water. The importance of hydrolysis to digestion is evidenced by the amount of water (7 to 8 L) that is secreted into the GI tract daily. The intestinal mucosa is impermeable to most large molecules: most proteins, fats, and carbohydrates must be broken down into smaller particles before they can be absorbed. Although some digestion of carbohydrates and proteins begins in the stomach, digestion takes place mainly in the small intestine. The breakdown of fats to free fatty acids and monoglycerides takes place entirely in the small intestine. The liver, with its production of bile, and the pancreas, which supplies a number of digestive enzymes, play important roles in digestion.

Absorption is the process of moving nutrients and other materials from the external environment in the lumen of the GI tract into the internal environment. Absorption is accomplished by active transport and diffusion. The absorptive function of the large intestine focuses mainly on water reabsorption. A number of substances require a specific carrier or transport system. For example, vitamin B_{12} is not absorbed in the absence of intrinsic factor, which is secreted by the parietal cells of the stomach. Transport of amino acids and glucose occurs mainly in the presence of sodium. Water is absorbed passively along an osmotic gradient.

The distinguishing characteristic of the small intestine is its large surface area, which in the adult is estimated to be approximately 250 m². Anatomic features that contribute to this enlarged surface area are the circular folds that extend into the lumen of the intestine and the villi, which are finger-like projections of mucous membrane, numbering as many as 25,000, that line the entire small intestine (Fig. 36.11). Each

FIGURE 36.11 • The mucous membrane of the small intestine. Note the numerous villi on a circular fold.

villus is equipped with an artery, vein, and lymph vessel (*i.e.,* lacteal), which bring blood to the surface of the intestine and transport the nutrients and other materials that have passed into the blood from the lumen of the intestine (Fig. 36.12). Fats rely largely on the lymphatics for absorption.

Each villus is covered with cells called *enterocytes* that contribute to the absorptive and digestive functions of the small bowel, and goblet cells that provide mucus. The crypts of Lieberkühn are glandular structures that open into the spaces between the villi. The enterocytes have a life span of approximately 3 to 5 days, and it is believed that replacement cells differentiate from progenitor cells located in the area of the crypts. The maturing enterocytes migrate up the villus and eventually are extruded from the tip.

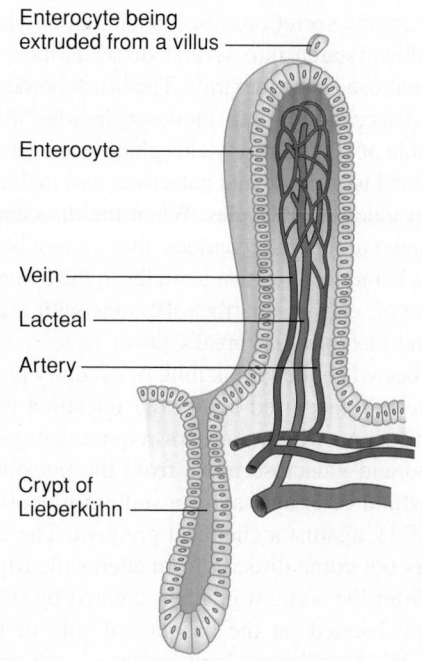

FIGURE 36.12 • A single villus from the small intestine.

TABLE 36.3 ENZYMES USED IN DIGESTION OF CARBOHYDRATES

DIETARY CARBOHYDRATES	ENZYME	MONOSACCHARIDES PRODUCED
Lactose	Lactase	Glucose and galactose
Sucrose	Sucrase	Fructose and glucose
Starch	Amylase	Maltose, maltotriase, and α-dextrins
Maltose and maltotriose	Maltase	Glucose and glucose
α-Dextrins	α-Dextrinase	Glucose and glucose

The enterocytes secrete enzymes that aid in the digestion of carbohydrates and proteins. These enzymes are called *brush border enzymes* because they adhere to the border of the villus structures. In this way, they have access to the carbohydrates and protein molecules as they come in contact with the absorptive surface of the intestine. This mechanism of secretion places the enzymes where they are needed and eliminates the need to produce enough enzymes to mix with the entire contents of the lumen of the small bowel. The digested molecules diffuse through the membrane or are actively transported across the mucosal surface to enter the blood or, in the case of fatty acids, the lacteal. These molecules are then transported through the portal vein or lymphatics into the systemic circulation.

Carbohydrate Absorption

Carbohydrates must be broken down into monosaccharides, or single sugars, before they can be absorbed from the small intestine. The average daily intake of carbohydrate in the Canadian diet is approximately 350 g to 400 g accounting for approximately 21% of their daily calories. However, a large percentage of these carbohydrates come from simple sugars (*i.e.,* sucrose or table sugar).

Digestion of starch begins in the mouth with the action of amylase. Pancreatic secretions also contain an amylase. Amylase breaks down starch into several disaccharides, including maltose, isomaltose, and α-dextrins. The brush border enzymes convert the disaccharides into monosaccharides that can be absorbed (Table 36.3). Sucrose yields glucose and fructose, lactose is converted to glucose and galactose, and maltose is converted to two glucose molecules. When the disaccharides are not broken down to monosaccharides, they cannot be absorbed but remain as osmotically active particles in the contents of the digestive system, causing diarrhea. Persons with a deficiency of lactase, the enzyme that breaks down lactose, experience cramps diarrhea when they drink milk or eat dairy products.

Fructose is transported across the intestinal mucosa by facilitated diffusion, which does not require energy expenditure. Glucose and galactose move from the intestinal lumen into the intestinal cells by way of a sodium-glucose cotransporter (SGLT-1), against a chemical gradient. The energy for this step does not come directly from adenosine triphosphate (ATP), but from the sodium gradient created by the Na^+/K^+-ATPase pump located on the basolateral side of the membrane (Fig. 36.13). Glucose and galactose are transported from the cell into the blood across the basolateral membrane

by facilitated diffusion using a glucose transporter-2 (GLUT-2) protein. Water absorption from the intestine is linked to absorption of osmotically active particles, such as glucose and sodium. It follows that an important consideration in facilitating the transport of water across the intestine (and decreasing diarrhea) after temporary disruption in bowel function is to include sodium and glucose in the fluids that are consumed.

Fat Absorption

The average adult eating a Western diet consumes approximately 100 to 140 g of fat daily, principally as triglycerides. The first step in digestion of lipids is to break the large globules of

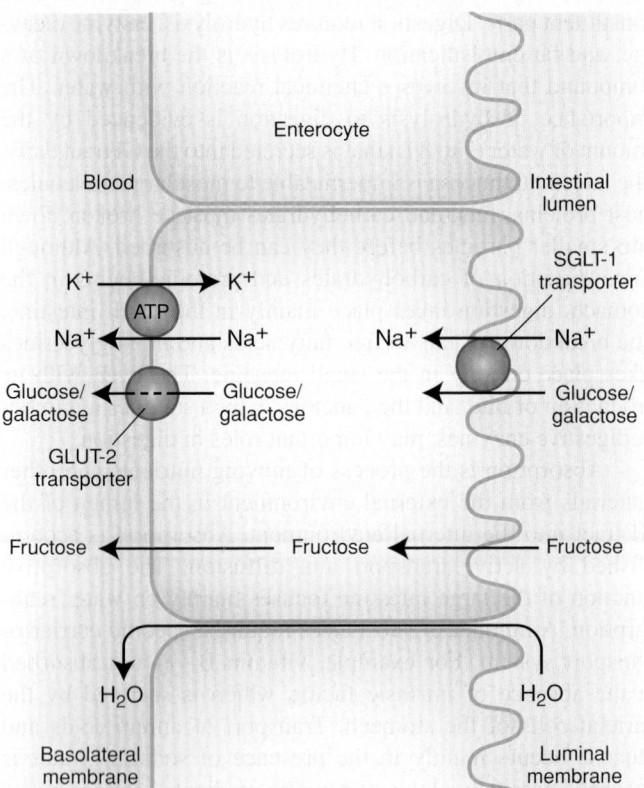

FIGURE 36.13 • Intestinal transport of glucose, galactose, and fructose. Glucose and galactose are transported across the apical membrane by the sodium-glucose cotransporter (SGLT-1). Glucose moves out of the intestinal cell and into the blood using a glucose transporter-2 (GLUT-2) protein. Sodium is transported out of the cell by the Na^+/K^+-ATPase sodium pump. This creates the gradient needed to operate the transport system. Fructose is passively transported across the apical and basolateral membranes of the intestinal cell.

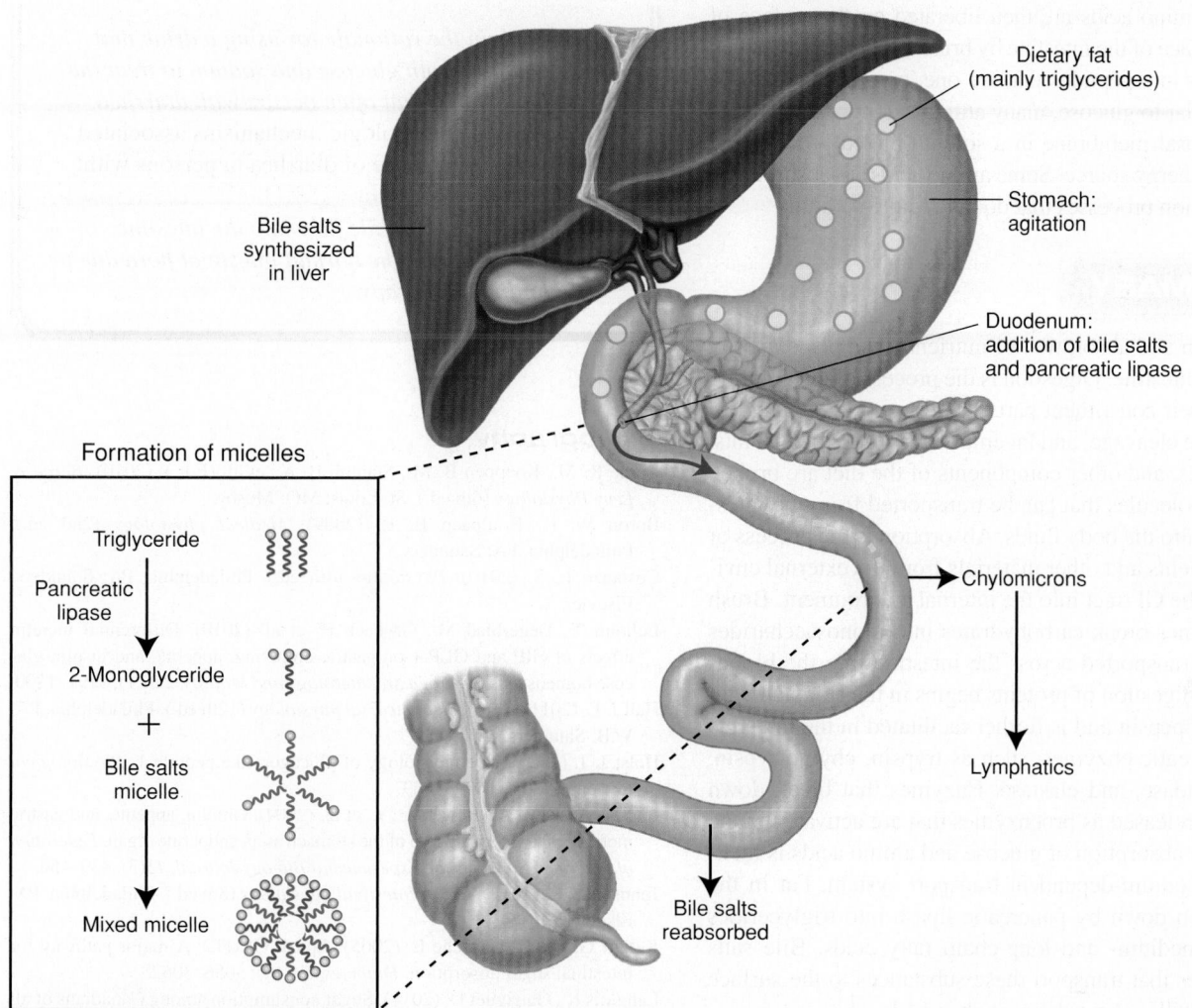

Dietary fat
(mainly triglycerides)

Stomach:
agitation

Duodenum:
addition of bile salts
and pancreatic lipase

Bile salts
synthesized
in liver

Formation of micelles

Triglyceride

Pancreatic
lipase

2-Monoglyceride

+

Bile salts
micelle

Mixed micelle

Chylomicrons

Lymphatics

Bile salts
reabsorbed

FIGURE 36.14 • Mechanisms for dietary fat absorption. During digestion, agitation in the stomach and bile from the liver break large globules of dietary fat into small particles that facilitate the action of pancreatic lipase in splitting triglycerides into free fatty acids and monoglycerides (glycerol with one fatty acid chain attached). Bile salts also facilitate the formation of micelles that transport the monoglycerides and fatty acids to the intestinal mucosa, where they are absorbed and converted to chylomicrons for transport in the lymphatic system.

dietary fat into smaller particles so that water-soluble digestive enzymes can act on the surface molecules. This process, which is called *emulsification,* begins in the stomach with agitation of the globules and continues in the duodenum under the influence of bile from the liver (Fig. 36.14). Emulsification greatly increases the number of triglyceride molecules exposed to pancreatic lipase, which splits triglycerides into free fatty acids and monoglycerides. Bile salts play an additional role by forming micelles that transport these substances to the surface for the intestinal villi, where they are taken into the epithelial cells and used to form new triglycerides. These new triglycerides are then released into the lymphatic system as chylomicrons. Small quantities of short- and medium-chain fatty acids are absorbed directly into the portal blood rather than being converted into triglycerides and absorbed by way of the lymphatics.

Fat that is not absorbed in the intestine is excreted in the stool. *Steatorrhea* is the term used to describe fatty stools. It usually indicates that there is more than 7 g of fecal fat per

24 hours. Normally, a chemical test is done on a 72-hour stool collection, during which time the diet is restricted to 50 to 150 g of fat per day.

Protein Absorption

Protein digestion begins in the stomach with the action of pepsin. Pepsinogen, the enzyme precursor of pepsin, is secreted by the chief cells in response to a meal and acid pH. Acid in the stomach is required for the conversion of pepsinogen to pepsin. Pepsin is inactivated when it enters the intestine by the alkaline pH.

Proteins are broken down further by pancreatic enzymes, such as trypsin, chymotrypsin, carboxypeptidase, and elastase. As with pepsin, the pancreatic enzymes are secreted as precursor molecules. Trypsinogen, which lacks enzymatic activity, is activated by an enzyme located on the brush border cells of the duodenal enterocytes. Activated trypsin activates additional trypsinogen molecules and other pancreatic precursor proteolytic enzymes. The amino acids are then liberated on the surface of the mucosal surface of the intestine by brush border enzymes that degrade proteins into peptides that are one, two, or three amino acids long. Similar to glucose, many amino acids are transported across the mucosal membrane in a sodium-linked process that uses ATP as an energy source. Some amino acids are absorbed by facilitated diffusion processes that do not require sodium.

IN SUMMARY

The digestion and absorption of nutrients take place mainly in the small intestine. Digestion is the process of dismantling foods into their constituent parts. Digestion requires hydrolysis, enzyme cleavage, and fat emulsification. Proteins, fats, carbohydrates, and other components of the diet are broken down into molecules that can be transported from the intestinal lumen into the body fluids. Absorption is the process of moving nutrients and other materials from the external environment of the GI tract into the internal environment. Brush border enzymes break carbohydrates into monosaccharides that can be transported across the intestine into the bloodstream. The digestion of proteins begins in the stomach with the action of pepsin and is further facilitated in the intestine by the pancreatic enzymes, such as trypsin, chymotrypsin, carboxypeptidase, and elastase. Enzymes that break down proteins are released as proenzymes that are activated in the GI tract. The absorption of glucose and amino acids is facilitated by a sodium-dependent transport system. Fat in the diet is broken down by pancreatic lipase into triglycerides containing medium- and long-chain fatty acids. Bile salts form micelles that transport these substances to the surface of intestinal villi, where they are absorbed.

REVIEW EXERCISES

1. Persons receiving chemotherapeutic agents, which interfere with mitosis of cancer cells as well as the cells of other rapidly proliferating tissues in the body, often experience disorders such as ulcerations in the mucosal tissues of the mouth and other parts of the GI tract. These disorders are resolved once the chemotherapy treatment has been completed.
   A. *Explain.*
2. People with gastroesophageal reflux (movement of gastric contents into the esophagus) often complain of heartburn that becomes worse as the pressure in the stomach increases.
   A. *Use information on hormonal control of gastric emptying to explain why eating a meal that is high in fat content often exaggerates the problem.*
3. Infections of the GI tract, such as the "GI flu," often cause profound diarrhea.
   A. *Describe the neural mechanisms involved in the increase in GI motility that produces the diarrhea.*
   B. *Explain the rationale for using a drink that contains both glucose and sodium to treat the fluid deficit that often occurs with diarrhea.*
4. Explain the physiologic mechanisms associated with the occurrence of diarrhea in persons with:
   A. *Lactase deficiency.*
   B. *Obstruction of bile flow into the intestine.*
   C. *Disruption of the normal intestinal flora due to antibiotic therapy.*

Bibliography

Berne R. M., Koeppen B. M., Stanton B. A., et al. (Eds.). (2010). *Berne & Levy Physiology* (6th ed.). St. Louis, MO: Mosby.

Boron W. F., Boulpaep E. L. (2009). *Medical physiology* (2nd ed.). Philadelphia, PA: Saunders.

Costanzo L. S. (2010). *Physiology* (4th ed.). Philadelphia, PA: Saunders/Elsevier.

Edholm T., Degerblad M., Gryback P., et al. (2010). Differential incretin effects of GIP and GLP-1 on gastric emptying, appetite, and insulin-glucose homeostasis. *Neurogastroenterology and Motility, 22*(11), 1191–1200.

Hall J. E. (2011). *Textbook of medical physiology* (12th ed.). Philadelphia, PA: W.B. Saunders.

Holst J. J. (1987). The physiology of glucagon-like peptide 1. *Physiological Reviews, 87*(4), 1409–1439.

Inul A., Asakawa A., Bowers C. Y., et al. (2004). Ghrelin, appetite, and gastric motility: The emerging role of the stomach as an endocrine organ. *Federation of American Societies for Experimental Biology Journal, 18*(3), 439–456.

Johnson L. R. (2013). *Gastrointestinal physiology* (8th ed.). Philadelphia, PA: Elsevier/Mosby.

Kellert G. L., Brot-Larche E. (2005). Apical GLUT2: A major pathway for intestinal sugar absorption. *Diabetes, 54*(10), 3056–3062.

Langlois K., Garriguet D. (2011). Sugar consumption among Canadians of all ages. *Health Reports, 22*(3). Statistics Canada Catalogue No. 82–003-X.

Manocha M., Khan W. I. (2012). Serotonin and GI disorders: An update on clinical and experimental studies. *Clinical and Translational Gastroenterology, 3*, (e13), doi: 10.1038/stg.2012.8.

Marieb E. N., Hoehn K. (2013). *Human anatomy & physiology* (9th ed.). Glenview, IL: Pearson Education.

Moore K. L., Dalley A. F., Agur A. M. (2014). *Clinically oriented anatomy* (7th ed.). Philadelphia, PA: Lippincott Williams & Wilkins.

Neary M. T., Batterham R. L. (2009) Gut hormones: Implications for the treatment of obesity. *Pharmacology & Therapeutics, 124*(1), 44–56.

Rhoades R. A., Bell D. R. (2013). *Medical physiology: Principles for clinical medicine* (4th ed.). Philadelphia, PA: Lippincott Williams & Wilkins.

Sanders K. M., Koh S. D., Ward M. (2006). Interstitial cells of Cajal in the gastrointestinal tract. *Annual Review of Physiology, 68*, 307–343.

Sang L. X., Chang B., Zhang W. L., et al. (2010). Remission induction and maintenance effect of probiotics on ulcerative colitis: A meta-analysis. *World Journal of Gastroenterology, 16*(15), 1908–1915.

Soybel D. I. (2005). Anatomy and physiology of the stomach. *Surgical Clinics of North America, 85*(5), 875–894.

Tortora G. J., Derrickson B. (2014). *Principles of anatomy & physiology* (14th ed.). Hoboken, NJ: John Wiley & Sons.

Turner J. R. (2010). The gastrointestinal tract. In Kumar V., Abbas A. K., Fausto N., et al., (Eds.), *Robbins and cotran pathologic basis of disease* (8th ed.). Philadelphia, PA: Elsevier Saunders.

Visit thePoint. **http://thePoint.lww.com for animations, journal articles, and more!**

Disorders of Gastrointestinal Function

37

Gastrointestinal (GI) disorders are not cited as a leading cause of death in Canada, nor do they receive the same publicity as heart disease and cancer. However, according to Health Canada, digestive diseases rank sixth in the total economic burden of illness, resulting in considerable human suffering, personal expenditures for treatment, and lost working hours, as well as a drain on the nation's economy.[1] In Canada the total economic burden of direct and indirect healthcare costs for digestive diseases is approximately $18 billion per year and these diseases contribute to 10% of all hospitalizations.[2] Even more important is the fact that proper nutrition or a change in health practices could prevent or minimize many of these disorders.

Disruption in structure and function can occur at any level of the GI tract, from the esophagus to the colon and rectum. This chapter is divided into four sections: (1) common manifestations of GI disorders, (2) disorders of the esophagus, (3) disorders of the stomach, and (4) disorders of the small and large intestines. Disorders of the hepatobiliary system and exocrine pancreas are discussed in Chapter 38.

ANOREXIA, NAUSEA, AND VOMITING

After completing this section of the chapter, you should be able to meet the following objectives:

• Characterize the relationship among anorexia, nausea, retching, and vomiting.
• Describe the neural structures involved in vomiting and their mediators.

Anorexia, nausea, and vomiting are physiologic responses common to many GI disorders. These responses are protective to the extent that they signal the presence of disease and, in the case of vomiting, remove noxious agents from the GI tract. They can also contribute to impaired intake or loss of fluids and nutrients.

Anorexia

Anorexia represents a loss of appetite. Several factors influence appetite. One is hunger, which is stimulated by contractions of the empty stomach. Appetite or the desire for food intake is regulated by the hypothalamus and other associated centres in the brain. Smell plays an important role, as evidenced by the fact that appetite can be stimulated or suppressed by the smell of food. Loss of appetite is associated with emotional factors, such as fear, depression, frustration, and anxiety. Many drugs and disease states cause anorexia. For example, in uremia the accumulation of nitrogenous wastes in the blood contributes to the development of anorexia. Anorexia often is a forerunner of nausea, and most conditions that cause nausea and vomiting also produce anorexia.

Nausea

Nausea is an ill-defined and unpleasant subjective sensation. It is the conscious sensation resulting from stimulation of the medullary vomiting centre that often precedes or accompanies vomiting. Nausea usually is preceded by anorexia, and stimuli such as foods and drugs that cause anorexia in small doses usually produce nausea when given in larger doses. A common cause of nausea is distension of the duodenum or upper small intestinal tract. Nausea is frequently accompanied by autonomic nervous system manifestations such as watery salivation and vasoconstriction with pallor, sweating, and tachycardia. Nausea may function as an early warning signal of a pathologic process.

Retching and Vomiting

Retching consists of the rhythmic spasmodic movements of the diaphragm, chest wall, and abdominal muscles. It usually precedes or alternates with periods of vomiting. Vomiting or emesis is the sudden and forceful oral expulsion of the contents of the stomach. It is usually preceded by nausea. The contents that are expelled are called *vomitus*. Vomiting, as a basic physiologic protective mechanism, limits the possibility of damage from ingested noxious agents by emptying the contents of the stomach and portions of the small intestine. Nausea and vomiting may represent a total-body response to drug therapy, including overdose, cumulative effects, toxicity, and side effects.

Vomiting involves two functionally distinct medullary centres: the *vomiting centre* and the *chemoreceptor trigger zone*. The act of vomiting is thought to be a reflex that is integrated in the vomiting centre, which is located in the dorsal portion of the reticular formation of the medulla near the sensory nuclei of the vagus[3] (Fig. 37.1). The chemoreceptor trigger zone is located in a small area on the floor of the fourth ventricle, where it is exposed to both blood and cerebrospinal fluid. It is thought to mediate the emetic effects of blood-borne drugs and toxins.

The act of vomiting consists of taking a deep breath, closing the airways, and producing a strong, forceful contraction

FIGURE 37.1 • Physiologic events involved in vomiting. CSF, cerebrospinal fluid.

of the diaphragm and abdominal muscles along with relaxation of the gastroesophageal sphincter. Respiration ceases during the act of vomiting. Vomiting may be accompanied by dizziness, lightheadedness, a decrease in blood pressure, and bradycardia.

The vomiting centre receives input from the GI tract and other organs; from the cerebral cortex and thalamus; from the vestibular apparatus, which is responsible for motion sickness; and from the chemoreceptor trigger zone, which is activated by many drugs and endogenous and exogenous toxins[4] (Fig. 37.1). Hypoxia exerts a direct effect on the vomiting centre, producing nausea and vomiting. This direct effect probably accounts for the vomiting that occurs during periods of decreased cardiac output, shock, environmental hypoxia, and brain ischemia caused by increased intracranial pressure. Inflammation of any of the intra-abdominal organs, including the liver, gallbladder, or urinary tract, can cause vomiting because of the stimulation of the visceral afferent pathways that communicate with the vomiting centre. Distension or irritation of the GI tract also causes vomiting through the stimulation of visceral afferent neurons.

Several neurotransmitters and receptor subtypes are implicated as neuromediators in nausea and vomiting.[4] Dopamine, serotonin, and opioid receptors are found in the GI tract and in the vomiting centre and chemoreceptor trigger zone. Dopamine antagonists, such as prochlorperazine, depress vomiting caused by stimulation of the chemoreceptor trigger zone. Serotonin is believed to be involved in the nausea and emesis associated with cancer chemotherapy and radiation therapy. Serotonin antagonists (*e.g.,* granisetron, ondansetron) are effective in treating the nausea and vomiting associated with these stimuli. Motion sickness appears to be a central nervous system (CNS) response to vestibular stimuli. Norepinephrine and acetylcholine receptors are located in the vestibular centre. The acetylcholine receptors are thought to mediate the impulses responsible for exciting the vomiting centre; norepinephrine receptors may have a stabilizing influence that resists motion sickness. Many of the motion sickness drugs (*e.g.,* dimenhydrinate) have a strong CNS anticholinergic effect and act on the receptors in the vomiting centre and areas related to the vestibular system.

IN SUMMARY

The signs and symptoms of many GI tract disorders are manifested by anorexia, nausea, and vomiting. Anorexia, or loss of appetite, may occur alone or may accompany nausea and vomiting. Nausea, which is an ill-defined, unpleasant sensation, signals the stimulation of the medullary vomiting centre. It often precedes vomiting and frequently is accompanied by autonomic responses, such as salivation and vasoconstriction with pallor, sweating, and tachycardia. The act of vomiting, which is integrated by the vomiting centre, involves the forceful oral expulsion of the gastric contents. It is a basic physiologic mechanism that rids the GI tract of noxious agents.

DISORDERS OF THE ESOPHAGUS

After completing this section of the chapter, you should be able to meet the following objectives:

- Define and cite the causes of dysphagia, odynophagia, and achalasia.
- Relate the pathophysiology of gastroesophageal reflux to measures used in the diagnosis and treatment of the disorder in adults and children.
- State the reason for the poor prognosis associated with esophageal cancer.

The esophagus is a tube that connects the oropharynx with the stomach. It lies posterior to the trachea and larynx and extends through the mediastinum, intersecting the diaphragm at the level of the 11th thoracic vertebra.

The esophagus functions primarily as a conduit for passage of food and liquid from the pharynx to the stomach. The walls of the esophagus consist of a mucosal, submucosal, muscularis externa, and adventitial layer, reflecting the general structural organization of the GI tract. The inner mucosal layer contains nonkeratinized stratified epithelium. At the esophageal–stomach junction, the abrasion-resistant epithelium changes abruptly to the simple columnar epithelium of the stomach. The submucosal layer contains mucus-secreting glands that provide the mucin-containing fluids that lubricate the esophageal wall and aid in the passage of food. The muscularis externa layer consists of skeletal muscle in the superior third of the esophagus, a mixture of skeletal and smooth muscle in its middle third, and entirely smooth muscle in its lower third. The outer fibrous adventitial layer of the esophagus is composed entirely of connective tissue, which adheres to surrounding structures along its route.

There are sphincters at either end of the esophagus: an upper esophageal sphincter and a lower esophageal sphincter. The upper esophageal, or pharyngoesophageal, sphincter consists of a circular layer of striated muscle, the cricopharyngeal muscle. The lower esophageal, or gastroesophageal, sphincter is an area approximately 3 cm above the junction with the stomach. The gastroesophageal sphincter is a physiologic rather than a true anatomic sphincter. That is, it acts as a valve, but the only structural evidence of a sphincter is a slight thickening of the circular smooth muscle. The smooth muscle in this portion of the esophagus normally remains tonically constricted, creating an intraluminal pressure of about 30 mm Hg, in contrast to the mid-portion of the esophagus, which normally remains relaxed.[3] The lower esophageal sphincter passes through an opening, or *hiatus,* in the diaphragm as it joins with the stomach, which is located in the abdomen. The portion of the diaphragm that surrounds the lower esophageal sphincter helps to maintain the zone of high pressure needed to prevent reflux of stomach contents.

Congenital Anomalies

Congenital anomalies of the esophagus require early detection and correction because they are incompatible with life. Esophageal atresia (EA) and tracheoesophageal fistula (TEF) are the two most common congenital anomalies of the esophagus.[5,6] EA, which is the most common congenital anomaly, affects about 1 in 4,000 neonates.[6] Of these, more than 90% have an associated TEF. In the most common form of EA, the upper esophagus ends in a blind pouch and the TEF is connected to the trachea (Fig. 37.2). This defect now has a survival rate greater than 90% owing largely to early recognition and improved neonatal intensive care units. Infants weighing less than 1,500 g have the greatest risk for mortality, as do neonates with other congenital anomalies.[6]

The newborn infant with EA/TEF typically has frothing and bubbling at the mouth and nose and episodes of coughing, cyanosis, and respiratory distress. Feeding exacerbates these manifestations, causes regurgitation, and precipitates aspiration. The inability to pass a catheter into the stomach provides further evidence of the disorder. The infant with isolated TEF may develop respiratory symptoms at a later age.

Treatment of EA and TEF is surgical. Surgical ligation of the TEF and end-to-end anastomosis of the esophagus is performed when possible. Temporary ligation of the TEF and insertion of a gastrostomy tube may be used to delay the need

FIGURE 37.2 • Congenital tracheoesophageal fistulas. **A:** The most common type (85% of cases) is a communication between the trachea and the lower portion of the esophagus. The upper segment of the esophagus ends in a blind sac. **B:** In a few cases, the proximal esophagus communicates with the trachea. **C:** H type is a fistula between a continuous esophagus and the trachea. **D:** Tracheal fistulas to both a proximal esophageal pouch and distal esophagus. (From Rubin R., Strayer D. S. (Eds.). (2012). *Rubin's pathology: Clinicopathologic foundations of medicine* (6th ed., p. 607). Philadelphia, PA: Lippincott Williams & Wilkins.)

for primary closure in preterm infants and those with more complicated lesions. The main goal of preoperative management is to maintain the airway and prevent lung damage from aspiration of gastric contents. Prone positioning minimizes movement of gastric secretions into a distal fistula and esophageal suctioning minimizes the risk of aspiration from a blind pouch.

Dysphagia

The act of swallowing depends on the coordinated action of the tongue and pharynx. These structures are innervated by cranial nerves V, IX, X, and XII. *Dysphagia* refers to difficulty in swallowing. If swallowing is painful, it is referred to as *odynophagia*. Dysphagia can result from disorders that produce narrowing of the esophagus, lack of salivary secretion, weakness of the muscular structures that propel the food bolus, or disruption of the neural networks coordinating the swallowing mechanism.[7] Lesions of the CNS, such as a stroke, often involve the cranial nerves that control swallowing. Cancer of the esophagus and strictures resulting from scarring can reduce the size of the esophageal lumen and make swallowing difficult. Scleroderma, an autoimmune disease that causes fibrous replacement of tissues in the muscularis layer of the GI tract, is another important cause of dysphagia.[8] Persons

with dysphagia usually complain of choking, coughing, or an abnormal sensation of food sticking in the back of the throat or upper chest when they swallow.

In a condition called *achalasia,* the lower esophageal sphincter fails to relax due to a disruption in the input from the enteric neural plexus and the vagus nerve. This results in difficulty passing food into the stomach, and the esophagus above the lower esophageal sphincter becomes enlarged. One or several meals may lodge in the esophagus and pass slowly into the stomach over time. There is danger of aspiration of esophageal contents into the lungs when the person lies down.

Endoscopy, barium esophagoscopy, and videoradiography may be used to determine the site and extent of a swallowing disorder. Esophageal manometry, a procedure in which a small pressure-sensing catheter is inserted into the esophagus, may be done to measure pressures in different parts of the esophagus. Treatment of swallowing disorders depends on the cause and type of altered function that is present. Treatment of dysphagia often involves a multidisciplinary team of health professionals, including a speech therapist. Mechanical dilation or surgical procedures may be done to enlarge the lower esophageal sphincter in persons with esophageal strictures.

Esophageal Diverticulum

A diverticulum of the esophagus is an outpouching of the esophageal wall caused by a weakness of the muscularis layer.[8,9] An esophageal diverticulum tends to retain food. Complaints that the food stops before it reaches the stomach are common, as are reports of gurgling, belching, coughing, and foul-smelling breath. The trapped food may cause esophagitis and ulceration. Because the condition usually is progressive, correction of the defect requires surgical intervention.

Tears (Mallory–Weiss Syndrome)

Longitudinal tears in the esophagus at the esophagogastric junction are termed *Mallory–Weiss tears.*[10] They are most often encountered in persons with chronic alcoholism after a bout of severe retching or vomiting, but may also occur during acute illness with severe vomiting. The presumed pathogenesis is inadequate relaxation of the esophageal sphincter during vomiting, with stretching and tearing of the esophageal junction at the moment of propulsive expulsion of gastric contents. Tears may involve only the mucosa or may penetrate the wall of the esophagus. Infection may lead to inflammatory ulcer or mediastinitis.

Most often bleeding is not severe and does require surgical intervention. Severe bleeding usually responds to vasoconstrictive medications, transfusions, and balloon compression. Healing is usually prompt, with minimal or no residual effects.

Hiatal Hernia

Hiatal hernia is characterized by a protrusion or herniation of the stomach through the esophageal hiatus of the diaphragm. There

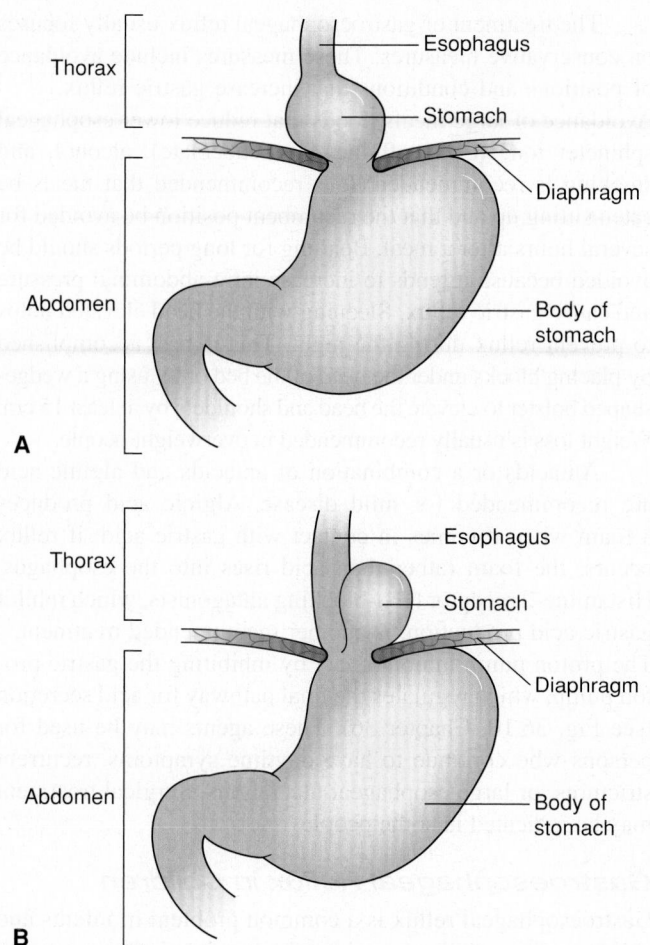

FIGURE 37.3 • Hiatal hernia. **A:** Sliding hiatal hernia. **B:** Paraesophageal hiatal hernia.

are two anatomic patterns of hiatal herniation: axial, or sliding, and nonaxial, or paraesophageal.[8,9] The sliding hiatal hernia is characterized by a bell-shaped protrusion of the stomach above the diaphragm (Fig. 37.3). Small sliding hiatal hernias are common and considered to be of no significance in asymptomatic people. However, in cases of severe erosive esophagitis where gastroesophageal reflux and a large hiatal hernia coexist, the hernia may retard esophageal acid clearance and contribute to the more severe esophagitis, especially Barrett esophagus (to be discussed). In paraesophageal hiatal hernias, a separate portion of the stomach, usually along the greater portion of the stomach, enters the thorax through a widened opening. The hernia progressively enlarges, and increases in size. In extreme cases, most of the stomach herniates into the thorax. Large paraesophageal hiatal hernias may require surgical treatment.

Gastroesophageal Reflux

The term *reflux* refers to backward or return movement. In the context of gastroesophageal reflux, it refers to the backward movement of gastric contents into the esophagus, a condition that causes heartburn or pyrosis.[11,12] It probably is the most common disorder originating in the GI tract and is estimated that approximately 5 million Canadian experience heartburn at least once week.[2] Such symptoms usually occur soon after eating, are short lived, and seldom cause more serious problems.

The lower esophageal sphincter regulates the flow of food from the esophagus into the stomach. Both internal and external mechanisms function in maintaining the antireflux function of the lower esophageal sphincter. The circular muscles of the distal esophagus constitute the internal mechanisms, and the portion of the diaphragm that surrounds the esophagus constitutes the external mechanism. The oblique muscles of the stomach, located below the lower esophageal sphincter, form a flap that contributes to the antireflux function of the internal sphincter.[8] Relaxation of the lower esophageal sphincter is a brain stem reflex that is mediated by the vagus nerve in response to a number of afferent stimuli. Transient relaxation with reflux is common after meals. Gastric distension and meals high in fat increase the frequency of relaxation. Normally, refluxed material is returned to the stomach by secondary peristaltic waves in the esophagus and swallowed saliva neutralizes and washes away the refluxed acid.

Gastroesophageal Reflux Disease

The persistent reflux of gastric contents into the esophagus is referred to as *gastroesophageal reflux disease* (GERD). It is thought to be associated with transient relaxations of weak or incompetent lower esophageal sphincter that allows reflux to occur, the irritant effects of the refluxate, and decreased clearance of the refluxed acid from the esophagus after it has occurred[11,12] (Fig. 37.4). In most cases, reflux occurs during transient relaxation of the esophagus. Delayed gastric emptying also may contribute to reflux by increasing gastric volume and pressure with greater chance for reflux. Esophageal mucosal injury is related to the destructive nature of the refluxate and the amount of time it is in contact with mucosa. Acidic gastric fluids (pH <4.0) are particularly damaging. The gastroesophageal reflux is normally cleared and neutralized

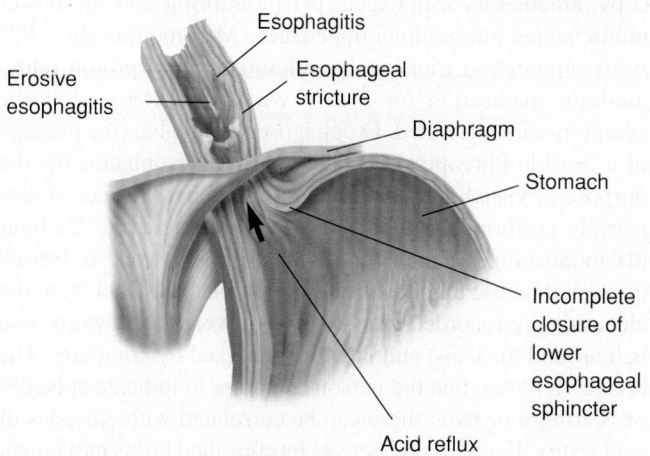

FIGURE 37.4 • Gastroesophageal junction and site of gastroesophageal reflux. (From Anatomical Chart Company. (2004). *Atlas of pathophysiology* (p. 171). Springhouse, PA: Springhouse.)

by esophageal peristalsis and salivary bicarbonate. Decreased salivation and salivary buffering capacity may contribute to impaired clearing of acid reflux from the esophagus.

Clinical Features. The most frequent symptom of GERD is heartburn. It is frequently severe, occurring 30 to 60 minutes after eating. It is often made worse by bending at the waist and recumbency and is usually relieved by sitting upright. The severity of heartburn is not indicative of the extent of mucosal injury; only a small percentage of people who complain of heartburn have mucosal injury. Often, the heartburn occurs during the night. Antacids give prompt, although transient, relief. Other symptoms include belching and chest pain. The pain usually is located in the epigastric or retrosternal area and often radiates to the throat, shoulder, or back. Because of its location, the pain may be confused with angina. The reflux of gastric contents also may produce respiratory symptoms such as asthma, chronic cough, and laryngitis.[12] The proposed mechanisms of reflux-associated asthma and chronic cough include microaspiration, macroaspiration, laryngeal injury, and vagal-mediated bronchospasm.

Reflux esophagitis involves mucosal injury to the esophagus, hyperemia, and inflammation. Complications such as strictures and a condition called *Barrett esophagus* can result from persistent reflux, which produces a cycle of mucosal damage that causes hyperemia, edema, and erosion of the luminal surface.[11–13] Strictures are caused by a combination of scar tissue, spasm, and edema. They produce narrowing of the esophagus and cause dysphagia when the lumen becomes sufficiently constricted. Barrett esophagus is characterized by a reparative process in which the squamous mucosa that normally lines the esophagus gradually is replaced by columnar epithelium resembling that in the stomach or intestines.[8,9,13] It is associated with increased risk for development of esophageal cancer.

Diagnosis of gastroesophageal reflux depends on a history of reflux symptomatology and use of diagnostic methods, including acid suppression trial with medication, radiographic studies using a contrast medium such as barium, esophagoscopy, ambulatory esophageal pH monitoring and the newer multichannel intraluminal impedance (MII) monitoring.[11,12,14] Acid suppression trial involve administering a proton pump inhibitor medication for 2 to 8 weeks to determine if the symptoms are alleviated. Esophagoscopy involves the passage of a flexible fibreoptic endoscope into the esophagus for the purpose of visualizing the lumen of the upper GI tract. It also permits performance of a biopsy, if indicated. For 24-hour pH monitoring, a small tube with a pH electrode is passed through the nose and down into the esophagus. Data from the electrode are recorded in a small, lightweight box worn on a belt around the waist and later are analyzed by computer. The box has a button that the person can press to indicate episodes of heartburn or pain; these can be correlated with episodes of acid reflux. For MII, this detects intraluminal bolus movement through the esophagus without radiation and when combined with pH monitoring provides useful information for persons with ongoing GERD symptoms despite medical treatment.[14]

The treatment of gastroesophageal reflux usually focuses on conservative measures. These measures include avoidance of positions and conditions that increase gastric reflux.[11,12,14] Avoidance of large meals, foods that reduce lower esophageal sphincter tone (*e.g.,* caffeine, fats, chocolate), alcohol, and smoking is recommended. It is recommended that meals be eaten sitting up and that the recumbent position be avoided for several hours after a meal. Bending for long periods should be avoided because it tends to increase intra-abdominal pressure and cause gastric reflux. Sleeping with the head elevated helps to prevent reflux during the night. This is best accomplished by placing blocks under the head of the bed or by using a wedge-shaped bolster to elevate the head and shoulders by at least 15 cm. Weight loss is usually recommended in overweight people.

Antacids or a combination of antacids and alginic acid are recommended for mild disease. Alginic acid produces a foam when it comes in contact with gastric acid; if reflux occurs, the foam rather than acid rises into the esophagus. Histamine-2 receptor (H_2)-blocking antagonists, which inhibit gastric acid production, is another recommended treatment.[12] The proton pump inhibitors act by inhibiting the gastric proton pump, which regulates the final pathway for acid secretion (see Fig. 36.10, Chapter 36). These agents may be used for persons who continue to have daytime symptoms, recurrent strictures, or large esophageal ulcerations. Surgical treatment may be indicated in some people.

Gastroesophageal Reflux in Children

Gastroesophageal reflux is a common problem in infants and children. The small reservoir capacity of an infant's esophagus coupled with frequent spontaneous reductions in sphincter pressure contributes to reflux. At least one episode of regurgitation a day occurs in as much as half of infants ages 0 to 4 months. By 6 months of age it becomes less frequent, and it abates by 2 years of age as the child assumes a more upright posture and eats solid foods.[3,6,14] Although many infants have minor degrees of reflux, complications can occur in children with more frequent or persistent episodes. The condition occurs more frequently in children with cerebral palsy, Down syndrome, and other neurologic disorders.

In most cases, infants with simple reflux are thriving and healthy, and symptoms resolve between 9 and 24 months of age. Pathologic reflux is classified into three categories: (1) regurgitation and malnutrition with failure to thrive, (2) esophagitis, and (3) respiratory problems.

Clinical Features. Symptoms of reflux esophagitis include evidence of pain when swallowing, hematemesis, anemia due to esophageal bleeding, heartburn, irritability, and sudden or inconsolable crying. Parents often report feeding problems in their infants.[6,14] These infants often are irritable and demonstrate early satiety. Sometimes the problems progress to actual resistance to feeding. Tilting of the head to one side and arching of the back may be noted in children with severe reflux. The head positioning is thought to represent an attempt to protect the airway or reduce the pain-associated reflux.

Sometimes regurgitation is associated with dental caries and recurrent otalgia. The ear pain is thought to occur through referral from the vagus nerve in the esophagus to the ear.

A variety of respiratory symptoms are caused by damage to the respiratory mucosa when gastric reflux enters the esophagus. Reflux may cause laryngospasm, apnea, and bradycardia. Asthma may co-occur with GERD in about 50% of asthmatic children. Asthmatic children who are particularly likely to have GERD as a provocative factor are those with symptoms of reflux, those with refractory or steroid-dependent asthma, and those with nocturnal worsening of symptoms[3] (see Chapter 29 for a discussion on childhood asthma).

Diagnosis of gastroesophageal reflux in infants and children often is based on parental and clinical observations. The diagnosis may be confirmed by esophageal pH or MII probe studies or barium fluoroscopic esophagography. In severe cases, esophagoscopy may be used to demonstrate reflux and obtain a biopsy.

Various treatment methods are available for infants and children with gastroesophageal reflux. Small, frequent feedings are recommended because of the association between gastric volume and transient relaxation of the esophagus. Thickening an infant's feedings has not been found to decrease the amount of regurgitation occurrences but potentially decreases the volume of reflux. However it does increase the calorie density of the formula.[3,14] In infants, keeping them upright for 2 hours after feeding seems to decrease reflux. Prone positioning may decrease the likelihood of symptoms but it has been associated with increase the risk for sudden infant death syndrome so should be reserved for infants who are observed and awake or greater than the age of 1. In older infants and children, raising the head of the bed and keeping the child upright may help. Medications usually are not added to the treatment regimen until pathologic reflux has been documented by diagnostic testing. Antacids are the most commonly used antireflux therapy and weight based dosing of H_2-receptor antagonists and proton pump inhibitors may be used in children with persistent reflux. Prokinetic agents (*e.g.,* metoclopramide, a dopamine-2 and 5-hydroxytryptamine [$5-HT_3$] receptor antagonist; bethanechol chloride, a cholinergic agonist) are associated with significant side effects and only used in selected cases.[14]

Cancer of the Esophagus

Carcinoma of the esophagus represents almost 1% of all new cancers.[15] It is more common in persons over the age of 60 years. This disease occurs three times more frequently in men than women and in 2015, and estimated 2,200 new cases will be diagnosed and approximately 2,100 Canadians will die from this disease.[1,5]

There are two types of esophageal cancers: squamous cell carcinoma and adenocarcinoma. Most squamous cell esophageal carcinomas are attributable to alcohol and tobacco use. Worldwide, squamous cell carcinomas are the most common esophageal cancers, but in Canada, the squamous cell carcinomas are decreasing.[16,17] However there has been an exponential increase in adenocarcinomas associated with Barrett esophagus.[16] Molecular studies have suggested that the pathogenesis of adenocarcinoma from Barrett esophagus is a multistep process, with the development of dysplasia being a critical step in the process.[8] Thus, endoscopic surveillance of persons with Barrett esophagus provides the means for detecting adenocarcinoma at an earlier stage, when it is most amenable to curative surgical resection.[13]

Progressive dysphagia is by far the most frequent complaint of persons with esophageal cancer. It is apparent first with ingestion of bulky food, later with soft food, and finally with liquids. Unfortunately, it is a late manifestation of the disease. Unintentional weight loss, anorexia, fatigue, and pain on swallowing also may occur.

Treatment of esophageal cancer depends on tumour staging. Surgical resection provides a means of cure when done in early disease and palliation when done in late disease. Radiation may be used as an alternative to surgery. Chemotherapy may be used before surgery to decrease the size of the tumour or it may be used along with irradiation and surgery in an effort to increase survival.

The long-term survival rate for persons with cancer of the esophagus, although poor, has improved.[17] Even with modern forms of therapy, however, the prognosis is limited because, in many cases, the disease has already metastasized by the time the diagnosis is made.

IN SUMMARY

The esophagus is a tube that connects the oropharynx with the stomach; it functions primarily as a conduit for passage of food from the pharynx to the stomach. Although relatively uncommon, congenital anomalies (*i.e.,* EA and TEFs) must be corrected early because they cause aspiration of gastric and oral secretions and are incompatible with life. Dysphagia refers to difficulty in swallowing; it can result from altered nerve function or from disorders that produce narrowing of the esophagus. A diverticulum of the esophagus is an outpouching of the esophageal wall caused by a weakness of the muscularis layer. Longitudinal tears (Mallory–Weiss tears) at the esophagogastric junction can occur with severe bouts of retching or vomiting. They are most often encountered in persons with chronic alcoholism, but may also occur during acute illness with severe vomiting. Hiatal hernia is characterized by a protrusion or herniation of the stomach through the esophageal hiatus of the diaphragm. There are two anatomic patterns of herniation: (1) the axial or sliding hiatal hernia, which is the most common type and is characterized by bell-shaped protrusion of the stomach above the diaphragm; and (2) the nonaxial or paraesophageal hernia, in which a portion of the stomach enters the thorax through a widened opening.

Gastroesophageal reflux refers to the backward movement of gastric contents into the esophagus, a condition that causes heartburn. Although most persons experience occasional gastroesophageal reflux and heartburn, persistent reflux can result in a cycle of mucosal damage that causes hyperemia, edema, erosion luminal surface, and Barrett esophagus. Reflux can cause respiratory symptoms, including chronic cough, and serve as a potential trigger for asthma. Gastroesophageal reflux is a common problem in infants and children. Reflux commonly corrects itself with age, and symptoms abate in most children by 2 years of age. Although many infants have minor degrees of reflux, some infants and small children have significant reflux that interferes with feeding, causes esophagitis, and results in respiratory symptoms and other complications.

Carcinoma of the esophagus is more common in older persons and occurs more frequently in men than women. There are two types of esophageal cancer: squamous cell carcinoma and adenocarcinoma. Most squamous cell carcinomas are attributable to alcohol and tobacco use, whereas adenocarcinomas are more closely linked to gastroesophageal reflux and Barrett esophagus.

DISORDERS OF THE STOMACH

After completing this section of the chapter, you should be able to meet the following objectives:

- Describe the anatomic and physiologic factors that contribute to the gastric mucosal barrier.
- Differentiate between the causes and manifestations of acute and chronic gastritis.
- Characterize the proposed role of *Helicobacter pylori* in the development of chronic gastritis and peptic ulcer and cite methods for diagnosis and treatment of the infection.
- Describe the predisposing factors in development of peptic ulcer and cite the three complications of peptic ulcer.
- Describe the goals for pharmacologic treatment of peptic ulcer disease.
- Cite the etiologic factors in ulcer formation related to Zollinger–Ellison syndrome and stress ulcer.
- List risk factors associated with gastric cancer.

The stomach is a reservoir for contents entering the digestive tract. It lies in the upper abdomen, anterior to the pancreas, splenic vessels, and left kidney. Anteriorly, the stomach is bounded by the anterior abdominal wall and the left inferior lobe of the liver. While in the stomach, food is churned and mixed with hydrochloric acid and pepsin before being released into the small intestine. Normally, the mucosal surface of the stomach provides a barrier that protects it from the hydrochloric acid and pepsin contained in gastric secretions. Disorders of the stomach include gastritis, peptic ulcer, and gastric carcinoma.

Gastric Mucosal Barrier

The stomach lining usually is impermeable to the acid it secretes, a property that allows the stomach to contain acid and pepsin without having its walls digested. Several factors contribute to the protection of the gastric mucosa, including an impermeable epithelial cell surface covering, mechanisms for the selective transport of hydrogen and bicarbonate ions, and the characteristics of gastric mucus.[18] These mechanisms are collectively referred to as the *gastric mucosal barrier*.

The cells of the gastric epithelia are connected by tight junctions that prevent acid penetration, and they are covered with an impermeable hydrophobic lipid layer that prevents diffusion of ionized water-soluble molecules. Aspirin, which is nonionized and lipid soluble in acid solutions, rapidly diffuses across this lipid layer, increasing mucosal permeability and damaging epithelial cells. Gastric irritation and occult bleeding due to gastric irritation occur in a significant number of persons who take aspirin on a regular basis. Alcohol, which also is lipid soluble, disrupts the mucosal barrier; when aspirin and alcohol are taken in combination, as they often are, there is increased risk of gastric irritation.[18] Bile acids also attack the lipid components of the mucosal barrier and afford the potential for gastric irritation when there is reflux of duodenal contents into the stomach.

DISRUPTION OF THE GASTRIC MUCOSA AND ULCER DEVELOPMENT

- The stomach is protected by a mucosal barrier that prevents gastric secretions and other destructive agents from injuring the epithelial and deeper layers of the stomach wall.
- The integrity of the mucosal layer is maintained by tight cellular junctions and the presence of a protective mucus layer.
- Two of the major causes of gastric irritation and ulcer formation are aspirin or nonsteroidal anti-inflammatory drugs (NSAIDs) and infection with *H. pylori*.
- Aspirin and NSAIDs exert their destructive effects by irritating the stomach and inhibiting prostaglandin synthesis.
- *H. pylori* is an infectious agent that thrives in the acid environment of the stomach and disrupts the mucosal barrier that protects the stomach from the harmful effects of its digestive enzymes.

Normally, the secretion of hydrochloric acid by the parietal cells of the stomach is accompanied by secretion of bicarbonate ions (HCO_3^-). For every hydrogen ion (H^+) that is secreted, an HCO_3^- is produced, and as long as HCO_3^- production is equal to H^+ secretion, mucosal injury does not occur. Changes in gastric blood flow, as in shock, tend to decrease HCO_3^- production. This is particularly true in situations in which decreased blood flow is accompanied by acidosis. Aspirin and the nonsteroidal anti-inflammatory drugs (NSAIDs), such as indomethacin and ibuprofen, also impair HCO_3^- secretion by limiting the cyclooxygenase (COX)-1 enzyme.[18]

The mucus that protects the gastric mucosa is of two types: water insoluble and water soluble.[19] Water-insoluble mucus forms a thin, stable gel that adheres to the gastric mucosal surface and provides protection from the proteolytic (protein-digesting) actions of pepsin. It also forms an unstirred layer that traps bicarbonate, forming an alkaline interface between the luminal contents of the stomach and its mucosal surface. The water-soluble mucus is washed from the mucosal surface and mixes with the luminal contents; its viscid nature makes it a lubricant that prevents mechanical damage to the mucosal surface. In addition to their effects on mucosal permeability and bicarbonate production, damaging agents such as aspirin and the NSAIDs inhibit and modify the characteristics of gastric mucus.

Prostaglandins, chemical messengers derived from cell membrane lipids, play an important role in protecting the gastric mucosa from injury.[8] The prostaglandins are thought to exert their effect through improved mucosal blood flow, decreased acid secretion, increased bicarbonate ion secretion, and enhanced mucus production. The fact that drugs such as aspirin and the NSAIDs inhibit prostaglandin synthesis may contribute to their ability to produce gastric irritation.

Gastritis

Gastritis refers to inflammation of the gastric mucosa. There are many causes of gastritis, most of which can be grouped as either acute or chronic gastritis.

Acute Gastritis

Acute gastritis is characterized by an acute mucosal inflammatory process, usually transient in nature. The inflammation may be accompanied by hemorrhage into the mucosa and, in severe cases, by sloughing of the superficial mucosa. This erosive form is an important cause of acute GI bleeding. The condition is most commonly associated with local irritants such aspirin or other NSAIDs, alcohol, or bacterial toxins.[8] Oral administration of corticosteroids may also be complicated by acute hemorrhagic gastritis. Any serious illness or trauma that is accompanied by profound physiologic stress that requires substantial medical or surgical treatment renders the gastric mucosa more vulnerable to acute hemorrhagic gastritis because of mucosal injury (discussed under stress ulcers).[9] Uremia, treatment with cancer chemotherapy drugs, and gastric radiation are other causes of acute gastritis.

The complaints of persons with acute gastritis vary. Persons with aspirin-related gastritis can be totally unaware of the condition or may complain only of heartburn or sour stomach. Gastritis associated with excessive alcohol consumption is often a different situation; it often causes transient gastric distress, which may lead to vomiting and, in more severe situations, to bleeding and hematemesis. Gastritis caused by the toxins of infectious organisms, such as the staphylococcal enterotoxins, usually has an abrupt and violent onset, with gastric distress and vomiting ensuing approximately 5 hours after the ingestion of a contaminated food source. Acute gastritis usually is a self-limiting disorder, with complete regeneration and healing occurring within several days of removal of the inciting agent.

Chronic Gastritis

Chronic gastritis is a separate entity from acute gastritis. It is characterized by the absence of grossly visible erosions and the presence of chronic inflammatory changes leading eventually to atrophy of the glandular epithelium of the stomach and/or associated mucosal injury. Chronic gastritis is usually develops because of infectious (*e.g.*, *H. pylori* gastritis) or autoimmune causes although it can result from other prolonged drug or hypersensitivity reactions. Reactive or chemical gastropathy suggests underlying chemical injury from sources such as bile reflux or NSAIDs, rather than an infectious process.[8,9]

Helicobacter pylori **Gastritis.** *H. pylori* infection is the most common cause of chronic gastritis It is estimated that 50% to 70% of the world's population has *H. pylori* infection.[8,9,20] In Canada, the overall prevalence is estimated at 30% but this is significantly increased for Inuit (51% to 56%) and First Nations communities (up to 95%).[21] It has been suggested that transmission in industrialized countries is largely person-to-person by vomitus, saliva, or feces, whereas additional transmission routes such as water may be important in developing countries. In industrialized countries, the rate of infection with *H. pylori* has decreased substantially over the past several decades owing to improved sanitation.

H. pylori gastritis is a chronic inflammatory disease of the antrum and body of the stomach. Chronic infection with *H. pylori* can lead to gastric atrophy and peptic ulcer, and is associated with increased risk of gastric adenocarcinoma and low-grade B-cell gastric lymphoma (MALToma [mucosa-associated lymphoid tissue] which can transform into lymphoma).[9]

H. pylori are small, curved, gram-negative rods (protobacteria) that can colonize the mucus-secreting epithelial cells of the stomach[8,9,20] (Fig. 37.5). *H. pylori* have multiple flagella, which allow them to move through the mucous layer of the stomach, and they secrete urease, which enables them to produce sufficient ammonia to buffer the acidity of their immediate environment. These properties help to explain why the organism is able to survive in the acidic environment of the stomach. *H. pylori* produce enzymes and toxins that have the capacity to interfere with the local protection of the gastric mucosa against acid, produce intense inflammation, and elicit an immune response. There is increased production of proinflammatory cytokines that serve to recruit and activate neutrophils. Several *H. pylori* proteins are immunogenic and they evoke an intense immune response in the mucosa. Both T- and B-cells can be seen in the chronic gastritis caused by *H. pylori*. Although the role of T- and B-cells in causing epithelial injury has not been established, T-cell-driven activation of B-cells may be involved in the pathogenesis of gastric lymphomas.[9]

FIGURE 37.5 • Infective gastritis. *H. pylori* appear on silver staining as small, curved rods on the surface of the gastric mucosa. (From Rubin R., Strayer D. S. (Eds.). (2012). *Rubin's pathology: Clinicopathologic foundations of medicine* (6th ed., p. 619). Philadelphia, PA: Lippincott Williams & Wilkins.)

Why some people with *H. pylori* infection develop clinical disease and others do not is unclear. Scientists are studying the different strains of the bacteria in an attempt to establish whether certain strains are more virulent than others and whether host and environmental factors contribute to the development of clinical disease.[9]

Methods for establishing the presence of *H. pylori* infection include the carbon (C) urea breath test using a radioactive carbon isotope (^{13}C or ^{14}C), the stool antigen test, and endoscopic biopsy for urease testing.[22,23] Blood tests to obtain serologic titres of *H. pylori* antibodies also can be done. The serologic test can establish that a person has been infected with *H. pylori*, but the results are limited as it cannot distinguish how recently the infection occurred.

Eradication of *H. pylori* has proved difficult.[24] Treatment requires combination therapy that includes the use of two antibiotics with a proton pump inhibitor or bismuth subsalicylate. Treatment is usually continued for 7 to 14 days. *H. pylori* mutate rapidly to develop antibiotic-resistant strains.[25] The combination of two or more antimicrobial agents increases the rates of cure and reduces the risk of resistant strains developing. The antibiotics that have shown the greatest efficacy against *H. pylori* are amoxicillin, clarithromycin, metronidazole, and tetracycline. The proton pump inhibitors have direct antimicrobial properties against *H. pylori*, and by raising the intragastric pH they suppress bacterial growth and optimize antibiotic efficacy. Bismuth subsalicylate has a direct antibacterial effect against *H. pylori*.[25]

Chronic Autoimmune and Multifocal Gastritis. *Autoimmune gastritis*, which accounts for less than 10% of cases of chronic gastritis, is a diffuse form of gastritis that is limited to the body and fundus of the stomach, with a lack or minimal involvement of the antrum. The disorder results from the presence of autoantibodies to components of gastric gland parietal cells and intrinsic factor. Gastric gland and mucosal atrophy lead to a loss of acid production. In the most severe cases, production of intrinsic factor is lost, leading to a vitamin B_{12} deficiency and pernicious anemia (see Chapter 14). This type of chronic gastritis frequently is associated with other autoimmune disorders such as Hashimoto thyroiditis, type I diabetes, and Addison disease.[8]

Multifocal atrophic gastritis is a disorder of uncertain etiology that affects the antrum and adjacent areas of the stomach. It is more common than autoimmune gastritis, and is seen more frequently in whites than in other races. It is particularly common in Asia, Scandinavia, and parts of Europe and Latin America.[9] As with autoimmune gastritis, it is associated with reduced gastric acid secretion, but achlorhydria and pernicious anemia are uncommon.

Chronic autoimmune gastritis and multifocal atrophic gastritis usually cause few symptoms related directly to gastric changes. When severe parietal cell loss occurs in the presence of autoimmune gastritis, hypochlorhydria or achlorhydria and hypergastrinemia are characteristically present. More important is the relationship of chronic gastritis to the development of peptic ulcer and an increased risk of gastric carcinoma.

Chemical Gastropathy. Chemical or reactive gastropathy is a chronic gastric injury resulting from prolonged NSAIDs use, reflux of alkaline duodenal contents, pancreatic secretions, and bile into the stomach. It is most commonly seen in persons who have had gastroduodenostomy or gastrojejunostomy surgery. A milder form may occur in persons with gastric ulcer, gallbladder disease, or various motility disorders of the distal stomach.

Peptic Ulcer Disease

Peptic ulcer is a term used to describe a group of ulcerative disorders that occur in areas of the upper GI tract that are exposed to acid–pepsin secretions.[8,9,19] The most common forms of peptic ulcer are duodenal and gastric ulcers. Peptic ulcer disease, with its remissions and exacerbations, is a chronic health problem. Approximately 10% of the population have or will develop peptic ulcer.[9] Duodenal ulcers occur four times more commonly than gastric ulcers. The peak age for peptic ulcer has progressively increased in the last 50 years, and is now between 30 and 60 years of age for duodenal ulcers, although the disorder can occur in persons of any age. Gastric ulcers are more prevalent among middle-aged and older adults. For duodenal ulcers there is a male predominance, whereas the incidence of gastric ulcers is more equally distributed between men and women.[9]

Peptic Ulcers

A peptic ulcer can affect one or all layers of the stomach or duodenum (Fig. 37.6). The ulcer may penetrate only the mucosal

FIGURE 37.6 • Gastric and duodenal ulcers. **A:** Gastric ulcer: the stomach has been opened to reveal a sharply demarcated, deep peptic ulcer on the lesser curvature. **B:** Duodenal ulcer. There are two sharply demarcated duodenal ulcers surrounded by inflamed duodenal mucosa. The gastroduodenal junction is in the midportion of the photograph. (From Rubin R., Strayer D. S. (Eds.). (2012). *Rubin's pathology: Clinicopathologic foundations of medicine* (6th ed., p. 625). Philadelphia, PA: Lippincott Williams & Wilkins.)

surface, or it may extend into the smooth muscle layers. Occasionally, an ulcer penetrates the outer wall of the stomach or duodenum. Spontaneous remissions and exacerbations are common. Healing of the muscularis externa layer involves replacement with scar tissue; although the mucosal layers that cover the scarred muscle layer regenerate, the regeneration often is less than perfect, which contributes to repeated episodes of ulceration.

A variety of risk factors have been shown to have an association with peptic ulcer disease. The two most important are infection with the bacteria *H. pylori* and use of aspirin and other NSAIDs.[19] Both *H. pylori* infection and exposure to NSAIDs have been shown to impair the mechanisms that protect the gastric mucosa from the destructive effects of the corrosive acid that is continually challenging the upper GI tract mucosa, and ulceration reflects a failure of these mechanisms.

The exact mechanism by which *H. pylori* promotes the development of peptic ulcer has not been fully elucidated. *H. pylori*'s ability to induce inflammation and stimulate the release of cytokines and other mediators of inflammation contributes to mucosal damage. Infection, predominantly in the antrum of the stomach, leads to hypergastrinemia and an increased acid production. Acid injury to the duodenum is thought to promote the development of gastric metaplasia, allowing the organism to colonize these areas and promote the development of duodenal ulcers.

The pathogenesis of NSAID-induced ulcers is thought to involve mucosal injury and inhibition of prostaglandin synthesis.[19] Aspirin appears to be the most ulcerogenic of the NSAIDs. Ulcer development in NSAID users is dose dependent, but some risk occurs even with aspirin doses as low as 81 mg/day.[19] In contrast to peptic ulcer from other causes, NSAID-induced gastric injury often is without symptoms, and life-threatening complications can occur without warning. There is reportedly less gastric irritation with the newer class of NSAIDs that selectively inhibit cylcooxygenase-2 (COX-2-selective NSAIDs), the principal enzyme involved in prostaglandin synthesis at the site of inflammation, than with the nonselective NSAIDs that also inhibit COX-1, the enzyme involved in prostaglandin production in the gastric mucosa.

Epidemiologic studies have identified independent factors that augment the effect of *H. pylori* infection and NSAID-produced peptic ulcer disease. These factors include advancing age, a prior history of peptic ulcer, multiple NSAID use, and concurrent use of warfarin (an anticoagulant) and corticosteroid drugs. Smoking and alcohol may augment the risk of peptic ulcer by impairing healing but on their own are not ulcerogenic agents. There is no convincing evidence that dietary factors play a role in development of peptic ulcer. There is increased incidence of peptic ulcer in families. This finding is likely due to familial clustering of *H. pylori* infection, and inherited genetic factors reflecting responses to the organism likely play a secondary role.[19]

Clinical Features. The clinical manifestations of uncomplicated peptic ulcer focus on discomfort and pain. The pain, which is described as burning, gnawing, or cramplike, is usually rhythmic and frequently occurs when the stomach is empty—between meals and at 1 or 2 o'clock in the morning. The pain is usually located over a small area near the midline in the epigastrium near the xiphoid, and may radiate below the costal margins, into the back, or, rarely, to the right shoulder. Superficial and deep epigastric tenderness and voluntary muscle guarding may occur with more extensive lesions. An additional characteristic of ulcer pain is periodicity. The pain tends to recur at intervals of weeks or months. During an exacerbation, it occurs daily for a period of several weeks and then remits until the next recurrence. Characteristically, the pain is relieved by food or antacids.

The most common complications of peptic ulcer are hemorrhage, perforation and penetration, and gastric outlet obstruction. Hemorrhage is caused by bleeding from granulation tissue or from erosion of an ulcer into an artery or vein. It occurs in up to 20% of persons with peptic ulcer.[8] Evidence of bleeding may consist of hematemesis or melena. Bleeding may be sudden, severe, and without warning, or it may be insidious, producing only occult blood in the stool. Up to 20% of persons with bleeding ulcers have no antecedent symptoms of pain; this is particularly true in persons using NSAIDs. Acute hemorrhage is evidenced by the sudden onset of weakness; dizziness; thirst; cold, moist skin; the desire to defecate; and the passage of loose, tarry, or even red stools and coffee-ground emesis. Signs of circulatory shock develop depending on the amount of blood lost.

Perforation occurs when an ulcer erodes through all the layers of the stomach or duodenum wall. Perforation develops in approximately 5% of persons with peptic ulcers, usually from ulcers on the anterior wall of the stomach or duodenum.[8] With perforation, GI contents enter the peritoneum and cause peritonitis. Radiation of the pain into the back, severe night distress, and inadequate pain relief from eating foods or taking antacids in persons with a long history of peptic ulcer may signify perforation.[7,19] Penetration is a process similar to perforation, but with penetration the ulcer crater erodes into adjacent organs, including the small bowel, pancreas, liver, or biliary tree. Typically it has a subtle presentation marked by a gradual increase in severity and frequency of pain.

Outlet obstruction is caused by edema, spasm, or contraction of scar tissue and interference with the free passage of gastric contents through the pylorus or adjacent areas. The presentation of an obstruction is typically insidious, with symptoms of early satiety, feeling of epigastric fullness and heaviness after meals, gastroesophageal reflux, weight loss, and abdominal pain. With severe obstruction, there is vomiting of undigested food.

Diagnosis and Treatment. Diagnostic procedures for peptic ulcer include history taking, laboratory tests, radiologic imaging, and endoscopic examination. The history should include careful attention to aspirin and NSAID use. Peptic ulcer should be differentiated from other causes of epigastric pain. Laboratory findings of hypochromic anemia and occult blood in the stools indicate bleeding. Endoscopy (*i.e.*, gastroscopy and duodenoscopy) can be used to visualize the ulcer area and obtain biopsy specimens to test for *H. pylori* and exclude malignant disease. X-ray studies with a contrast medium such as barium are used to detect the presence of an ulcer crater and to exclude gastric carcinoma.

The treatment of peptic ulcer has changed dramatically over the past several decades and now aims to eradicate the cause and promote a permanent cure for the disease. Pharmacologic treatment focuses on eradicating *H. pylori,* relieving ulcer symptoms, and healing the ulcer crater. Acid-neutralizing, acid-inhibiting drugs and mucosa-protective agents are used to relieve symptoms and promote healing of the ulcer crater. There is no evidence that special diets are beneficial in treating peptic ulcer. Aspirin and NSAID use should be avoided when possible.

There are two pharmacologic methods for reducing gastric acid content. The first involves the neutralization of gastric acid through the use of antacids, and the second a decrease in gastric acid production through the use of H_2-receptor antagonists or proton pump inhibitors. Essentially three types of antacids are used to relieve gastric acidity: calcium carbonate, aluminum hydroxide, and magnesium hydroxide. Many antacids contain a combination of ingredients, such as magnesium aluminum hydroxide. *Calcium preparations* are constipating and may cause hypercalcemia and the milk-alkali syndrome (see Chapter 31). *Magnesium hydroxide* is a potent antacid that also has laxative effects. Approximately 5% to 10% of the magnesium in this preparation is absorbed from the intestine; because magnesium is excreted through the kidneys, this formulation should not be used in persons with renal failure. *Aluminum hydroxide* reacts with hydrochloric acid to form aluminum chloride. It combines with phosphate in the intestine, and prolonged use may lead to phosphate depletion and osteoporosis. Because antacids can decrease the absorption, bioavailability, and renal elimination of a number of drugs, this should be considered when antacids are administered with other medications.

Histamine is the major physiologic mediator for hydrochloric acid secretion (see Chapter 36, Fig. 36.10). The H_2-receptor antagonists block gastric acid secretion stimulated by histamine, gastrin, and acetylcholine. The volume of gastric secretion and the concentration of pepsin also are reduced. The proton pump inhibitors block the final stage of hydrogen ion secretion by blocking the action of the gastric parietal cell proton pump.[19]

Among the agents that enhance mucosal defences are sucralfate and prostaglandin analogs. The drug sucralfate, which is a complex salt of sucrose containing aluminum and sulphate, selectively binds to necrotic ulcer tissue and serves as a barrier to acid, pepsin, and bile. Sucralfate also can directly absorb bile salts and initiate secretion of bicarbonate and mucus. The drug is not absorbed systemically. The drug requires an acid pH for activation and should not be administered with antacids or an H_2 antagonist. Misoprostol, a prostaglandin E derivative, promotes ulcer healing by stimulating mucus and bicarbonate secretion and by modestly inhibiting acid secretion. Health Canada has approved this drug for the prevention of NSAID-induced ulcers. Side effects may be dose-dependent diarrhea, and because of its stimulant effect on the uterus, it is contraindicated in women of childbearing age.[26]

The current surgical management of peptic ulcer disease is largely limited to treatment of complications. When surgery is needed, it usually is performed using minimally invasive methods. With bleeding ulcers, hemostasis often can be achieved by endoscopic methods, and endoscopic balloon dilation often is effective in relieving outflow obstruction.

Zollinger–Ellison Syndrome

The Zollinger–Ellison syndrome is a rare condition caused by a gastrin-secreting tumour (gastrinoma). In persons with this disorder, gastric acid secretion reaches such levels that ulceration becomes inevitable.[27] The tumours may be single or multiple; although most tumours are located in the pancreas, some develop in the submucosa of the stomach or most arise from duodenum. Over half of gastrin-producing tumours are malignant and have already metastasized at the time of diagnosis. The increased gastric secretions cause similar symptoms as peptic ulcer but most of these ulcers develop in the distal duodenum or proximal jejunum (unlike *H. pylori* or NSAID locations). Diarrhea may result from hypersecretion or from the inactivation of intestinal lipase and impaired fat digestion that occur with a decrease in intestinal pH.[27]

Hypergastrinemia may also occur in an autosomal dominant disorder called the *multiple endocrine neoplasia type 1 (MEN 1) syndrome,* which is characterized by multiple endocrine neoplasms. The syndrome is characterized by hyperparathyroidism and multiple endocrine tumours, including gastrinomas. Approximately 20% of gastrinomas are due to MEN 1.[27]

The diagnosis of the Zollinger–Ellison syndrome is based on elevated serum gastrin and basal gastric acid levels and elimination of the MEN 1 syndrome as a cause of the disorder. Computed tomography (CT), abdominal ultrasonography, and selective angiography are used to localize the tumour and determine if metastatic disease is present.

Treatment of Zollinger–Ellison syndrome involves control of gastric acid secretion by proton pump inhibitors. Over half of gastrin-producing tumours are locally invasive or have already metastasized at the time of diagnosis. Surgical removal is indicated when the tumour is malignant and has not metastasized.

Stress Ulcers

A stress ulcer, sometimes called a *Curling ulcer,* refers to GI ulcerations that develop in relation to major physiologic stress.[9] Persons at high risk for development of stress ulcers include those with large-surface-area burns, trauma, sepsis, acute respiratory distress syndrome, severe liver failure, and major surgical procedures. These lesions occur most often in the fundus of the stomach and proximal duodenum and are thought to result from ischemia, tissue acidosis, and bile salts entering the stomach in critically ill persons with decreased GI tract motility.[8,28] Another form of stress ulcer, called *Cushing ulcer,* consists of gastric, duodenal, and esophageal ulcers arising in persons with elevated intracranial pressure due to intracranial injury, operations, or tumours. They are thought to be caused by hypersecretion of gastric acid resulting from stimulation of vagal nuclei by increased intracranial pressure. These ulcers are associated with a high incidence of perforation.[28]

Persons admitted to hospital intensive care units are at particular risk for development of stress ulcers. H_2-receptor antagonists and proton pump inhibitors are used in the prevention and treatment of stress ulcers.[28]

Cancer of the Stomach

Gastric carcinoma is the second most common tumour in the world. However, its incidence varies widely, being particularly high in countries such as Japan, Korea, and China. It is more common in lower socioeconomic groups and exhibits a male-to-female ratio of about 2:1. Although it is responsible for only 3% of all cancer deaths in Canada, it is the second leading cause of cancer mortality worldwide.[2,8,15,22]

Factors thought to increase the risk of gastric cancer include genetic factors, carcinogenic factors in the diet (*e.g., N*-nitroso compounds and benzopyrene found in smoked and preserved foods), autoimmune gastritis, and gastric adenomas or polyps. The incidence of stomach cancer continue to decline in Canada, presumably because of improved storage of food with decreased consumption of salted, smoked, and preserved foods.[8,15] Chronic infection with *H. pylori* appears to serve as a cofactor in some types of gastric carcinomas. The bacterial infection causes gastritis, followed by atrophy, intestinal metaplasia, and carcinoma. This sequence of cellular events depends on both the presence of the bacterial proteins and the host immune response, with the latter being influenced by the host genetic background. In addition to genetics, the likelihood of developing gastric cancer from an *H. pylori* infection is related to the strain of the microbe, environmental factors, and the duration of the infection.[7] Autoimmune gastritis, like *H. pylori* infection, increases the risk of gastric cancer, presumably due to chronic inflammation and intestinal metaplasia.[8]

Between 50% and 60% of gastric cancers occur in the pyloric region or adjacent to the antrum. Compared with a benign ulcer, which has smooth margins and is concentrically shaped, gastric cancers tend to be larger, are irregularly shaped, and have irregular margins.

Clinical Features

Unfortunately, stomach cancers often are asymptomatic until late in their course. Symptoms, when they do occur, usually are vague and include indigestion, anorexia, weight loss, vague epigastric pain, vomiting, and an abdominal mass. Because these symptoms are essentially nonspecific, early detection is difficult.

Diagnosis of gastric cancer is accomplished by a variety of techniques, including barium x-ray studies, endoscopic studies with biopsy, and cytologic studies (*e.g.,* Papanicolaou smear) of gastric secretions.[23] Cytologic studies can prove particularly useful as routine screening tests for persons with atrophic gastritis or gastric polyps. CT and endoscopic ultrasonography often are used to delineate the spread of a diagnosed stomach cancer.

Depending on the location and extent of the lesion, surgery in the form of radical subtotal gastrectomy usually is the treatment of choice. Irradiation and chemotherapy have not proved particularly useful as primary treatment modalities in stomach cancer. These methods are usually used for palliative purposes or to control metastatic spread of the disease.

IN SUMMARY

Disorders of the stomach include gastritis, peptic ulcer, and cancer of the stomach. Gastritis refers to inflammation of the gastric mucosa. Acute gastritis refers to a transient inflammation of the gastric mucosa; it is associated most commonly with local irritants such as bacterial endotoxins, caffeine, alcohol, and aspirin. Chronic gastritis is characterized by the absence of grossly visible erosions and the presence of chronic inflammatory changes leading eventually to atrophy of the glandular epithelium of the stomach. There are three main types of chronic gastritis: *H. pylori* gastritis, autoimmune gastritis and multifocal atrophic gastritis, and chemical gastropathy. *H. pylori* is an "S"-shaped bacterium that colonizes the mucus-secreting epithelial cells of the stomach. Infection increases the risk of chronic gastritis, peptic ulcer, gastric carcinoma, and low-grade B-cell lymphoma. Treatment of *H. pylori* infection involves the use of multidrug therapy aimed at increasing the pH of gastric secretions and antimicrobial agents designed to eradicate the organism.

Peptic ulcer is a term used to describe a group of ulcerative disorders that occur in areas of the upper GI tract that are exposed to acid–pepsin secretions, most commonly the duodenum and stomach. There are two main causes of peptic ulcer: *H. pylori* infection and aspirin or NSAID use. The treatment of peptic ulcer focuses on eradication of *H. pylori,* avoidance of gastric irritation from NSAIDs, and conventional pharmacologic treatment directed at symptom relief and ulcer healing.

The Zollinger–Ellison syndrome is a rare condition caused by a gastrin-secreting tumour in which gastric acid secretion reaches such levels that ulceration becomes inevitable. Stress ulcers (Curling ulcers) occur in relation to major physiologic stresses such as burns and trauma and are thought to result from ischemia, tissue acidosis, and bile salts entering the stomach in critically ill persons with decreased GI tract motility. Another form of stress ulcer, Cushing ulcer, occurs in persons with intracranial trauma or surgery and is thought to be caused by hypersecretion of gastric acid resulting from stimulation of vagal nuclei by increased intracranial pressure.

Although the incidence of cancer of the stomach has declined over the past 50 years in Canada, it remains the second leading cause of death worldwide. Because there are few early symptoms with this form of cancer, the disease often is far advanced at the time of diagnosis.

DISORDERS OF THE SMALL AND LARGE INTESTINES

After completing this section of the chapter, you should be able to meet the following objectives:

- State the diagnostic criteria for irritable bowel syndrome.
- Compare the characteristics of Crohn's disease and ulcerative colitis.
- Relate the use of a high-fibre diet in the treatment of diverticular disease to the etiologic factors for the condition.
- Describe the pathogenesis of the symptoms associated with appendicitis.

- Compare the causes and manifestations of small-volume diarrhea and large-volume diarrhea.
- Explain why a failure to respond to the defecation urge may result in constipation.
- List five causes of fecal impaction.
- Differentiate between mechanical and paralytic intestinal obstruction in terms of cause and manifestations.
- Describe the characteristics of the peritoneum that increase its vulnerability to and protect it against the effects of peritonitis.
- List three causes of intestinal malabsorption and describe their manifestations.
- List the risk factors associated with colorectal cancer and cite the screening methods for detection.

There are many similarities in conditions that disrupt the integrity and function of the small and large intestines. The walls of the small and large intestines consist of four layers (see Chapter 36, Fig. 36.3): an inner mucosal layer, which lines the lumen of the intestine; a submucosal layer; a muscularis externa layer, which is subdivided into a layer of circular and a layer of longitudinal muscle fibres; and an outer serosal layer. Among the conditions that cause altered intestinal function are irritable bowel syndrome (IBS), inflammatory bowel disease (IBD), diverticulitis, appendicitis, disorders of bowel motility (*i.e.,* diarrhea, constipation, and bowel obstruction), malabsorption syndrome, and cancer of the colon and rectum.

Irritable Bowel Syndrome

The term *irritable bowel syndrome* is used to describe a functional GI disorder characterized by a variable combination of chronic and recurrent intestinal symptoms not explained by structural or biochemical abnormalities. Canada has one of the highest rates of IBS in the world with up to 5 million suffering from this disorder.[2]

Irritable bowel syndrome is characterized by persistent or recurrent symptoms of abdominal pain, altered bowel function, and varying complaints of flatulence, bloating, nausea and anorexia, constipation or diarrhea, and anxiety or depression. A hallmark of IBS is abdominal pain that is relieved by defecation and associated with a change in consistency or frequency of stools. Abdominal pain usually is intermittent, cramping, and in the lower abdomen. It does not usually occur at night or interfere with sleep. The condition is believed to result from dysregulation of intestinal motor and sensory functions modulated by the CNS. Persons with IBS tend to experience increased motility and abnormal intestinal contractions in response to psychological and physiologic stresses. The role that psychological factors play in the disease is uncertain. Although changes in intestinal activity are normal responses to stress, these responses appear to be exaggerated in persons with IBS. Women tend to be affected more often than men.[29] Menarche is often associated with onset of the disorder. Women frequently notice an exacerbation of symptoms during the premenstrual period, suggesting a hormonal component.

Because IBS lacks anatomic or physiologic markers, diagnosis is usually based on signs and symptoms of abdominal pain or discomfort, bloating, and constipation or diarrhea, or alternating bouts of constipation and diarrhea. A commonly used Rome III criteria requires continuous or recurrent symptoms of at least 3 days per month in the last 3 months of abdominal discomfort or pain, with two of three accompanying features: relief with defecation, onset associated with a change in bowel frequency, and associated with a change in form (appearance) of stool.[30] Other symptoms that support the diagnosis of IBS include abnormal stool frequency (more than three times per day or less than three times per week), abnormal stool form (lumpy/hard or loose/watery), abnormal stool passage (straining, urgency, or feeling of incomplete evacuation), passage of mucus, and bloating or feeling of abdominal distension.[29] A history of lactose intolerance should be considered because intolerance to lactose and other sugars may be a precipitating factor in some persons. The acute onset of symptoms raises the likelihood of organic disease, as does weight loss, anemia, fever, occult blood in the stool, nighttime symptoms, or signs and symptoms of malabsorption. These signs and symptoms require additional investigation.

The treatment of IBS focuses on methods of stress management, particularly those related to symptom production. Reassurance is important. Usually, no special diet is indicated, although adequate fibre intake usually is recommended. Avoidance of offending dietary substances such as fatty and gas-producing foods, alcohol, and caffeine-containing beverages may be beneficial. Various pharmacologic agents, including antispasmodic and anticholinergic and antidepressant drugs, have been used with varying success in treatment of the disorder.[29]

Inflammatory Bowel Disease

The term *inflammatory bowel disease* is used to designate two related inflammatory intestinal disorders: Crohn's disease and ulcerative colitis. It is estimated that approximately 200,000

Crohn disease   **Ulcerative colitis**

FIGURE 37.7 • Distribution patterns of disease with (**A**) skip lesions in Crohn's disease and (**B**) continuous involvement of the colon, beginning with the rectum, in ulcerative colitis.

Canadians have IBD and Canada has the highest rates of IBD in the world.[31] Although the two diseases differ sufficiently to be distinguishable, they have many features in common. Both diseases produce inflammation of the bowel, both lack confirming evidence of a proven causative agent, both have a pattern of familial occurrence, and both can be accompanied by systemic manifestations. Crohn's disease most commonly affects the distal small intestine and proximal colon, but can affect any area of the GI tract from the esophagus to the anus, whereas ulcerative colitis is confined to the colon and rectum (Fig. 37.7).[32] The distinguishing characteristics of Crohn's disease and ulcerative colitis are summarized in Table 37.1.

The clinical manifestations of both Crohn's disease and ulcerative colitis are ultimately the result of activation of inflammatory cells with elaboration of inflammatory mediators that cause nonspecific tissue damage. Both diseases are characterized by remissions and exacerbations of diarrhea, fecal urgency, and weight loss. Acute complications, such as intestinal obstruction, may develop during periods of fulminant disease.

A number of systemic manifestations have been identified in persons with Crohn's disease and ulcerative colitis. These include axial arthritis affecting the spine and sacroiliac

TABLE 37.1 DIFFERENTIATING CHARACTERISTICS OF CROHN'S DISEASE AND ULCERATIVE COLITIS		
CHARACTERISTIC	**CROHN'S DISEASE**	**ULCERATIVE COLITIS**
Types of inflammation	Granulomatous	Ulcerative and exudative
Level of involvement	Primarily submucosal	Primarily mucosal
Extent of involvement	Skip lesions	Continuous
Areas of involvement	Primarily ileum, secondarily colon	Primarily rectum and left colon
Diarrhea	Common	Common
Rectal bleeding	Rare	Common
Fistulas	Common	Rare
Strictures	Common	Rare
Perianal abscesses	Common	Rare
Development of cancer	Uncommon	Relatively common

joints and oligoarticular arthritis affecting the large joints of the arms and legs; inflammatory conditions of the eye, usually uveitis; skin lesions, especially erythema nodosum; stomatitis; and autoimmune anemia, hypercoagulability of blood, and sclerosing cholangitis.[8,9] Occasionally, these systemic manifestations may herald the recurrence of intestinal disease. In children, growth retardation may occur, particularly if the symptoms are prolonged and nutrient intake has been poor.

Etiology and Pathogenesis

A remarkable feature of the GI tract is that the mucosal immune system is always ready to respond against ingested pathogens but is unresponsive to the normal intestinal microflora. According to the currently accepted hypothesis, this normal state of homeostasis is disrupted in IBD, leading to unregulated and exaggerated immune responses against bacteria in the normal intestinal flora of genetically susceptible individuals.[33] Thus, as in many other autoimmune disorders, the pathogenesis of Crohn's disease and ulcerative colitis involves a failure of immune regulation, genetic predisposition, and an environmental trigger, especially microbial flora.[8]

Genetic Susceptibility. The genetic basis of IBD has long been suspected and approximately 30% of the genetic loci susceptibilities are similar between Crohn's and ulcerative colitis suggesting these diseases may share a common pathway despite distinct clinical features.[33] When looking at the concordance rate for monozygotic twins studies, for Crohn's disease this was up to 50% but with ulcerative colitis this genetic component was found to be weaker, with a rate of only 16%.[8] These associations clearly indicate that genetic susceptibility plays an important role in the development of IBD. However, classic mendelian inheritance patterns are not seen, and IBD therefore cannot be attributed to a single gene. Utilizing the genome-wide association studies many candidate genes are known to be associated with, and likely to contribute to, the development of IBD. Accumulating evidence also suggests that both Crohn's disease and ulcerative colitis are associated with profound disorders of mucosal immunity. The IBD1 locus on chromosome 16 has been shown to contribute to Crohn's disease.[8,9,32,33] The product of the implicated gene, NOD2 (so named because the coded protein has a nucleotide oligomerization domain) binds to intracellular bacterial peptidoglycan and then activates the nuclear kappa beta (NFκβ) transcription factor. On binding microbial products, it triggers the NFκβ pathway, which leads to the production of cytokines and other proteins involved in the innate immune defence against microorganisms. The NOD2 mutations that are associated with Crohn's disease likely reduce the activity of the protein, resulting in persistence of intracellular microbes and prolonged immune responses. Multiple gene mutations being studied include CARD9, an adaptor protein for integrating signals from pathogens and activating pro-inflammatory cytokines, ATG16L1 and IRGM, both proteins linked to autophagy and intracellular pathogens.[8,33] Other research is studying adaptive immune regulation and the potential imbalance of different T-cell populations and their links to cytokines, metabolites, and microbial signals.[32,33]

Role of Environmental Factors. Animal studies have definitively established the importance of the gut flora in IBD. The sites affected by IBD, the distal ileum and the colon, are awash with bacteria. Although it is unlikely that IBD is caused by microbes, it seems likely that microbes may provide the antigen trigger for an unregulated immune response.

Interestingly, smoking tobacco has the opposite effect on the two forms of IBD. Crohn's disease is more commonly associated with smokers while ulcerative colitis is associated with nonsmokers or those who have quit.[32] Smoking also increases the likelihood of disease exaggeration and need for surgery in people with Crohn's disease.

Crohn's Disease

Crohn's disease is a recurrent, granulomatous type of inflammatory response that can affect any area of the GI tract. In nearly 40% of persons with the disease, the lesions are restricted to the small intestine; in 30%, only the large bowel is affected; and in the remaining 30%, both the large and small bowel are affected.[8] It is a slowly progressive, relentless, and often disabling disease. The disease usually strikes people in their twenties or thirties, with women being affected slightly more often than men.

A characteristic feature of Crohn's disease is the sharply demarcated, granulomatous lesions that are surrounded by normal-appearing mucosal tissue. When the lesions are multiple, they often are referred to as *skip lesions* because they are interspersed between what appear to be normal segments of the bowel. All the layers of the bowel are involved, with the submucosal layer affected to the greatest extent. The surface of the inflamed bowel usually has a characteristic "cobblestone" appearance resulting from the fissures and crevices that develop, surrounded by areas of submucosal edema[8,9] (Fig. 37.8). There usually is a relative sparing of the smooth muscle layers of the bowel, with marked inflammatory and fibrotic changes of the submucosal layer. The bowel wall, after a time, often becomes thickened and inflexible; its appearance has been likened to a lead pipe or rubber hose. The adjacent mesentery may become inflamed, and the regional lymph nodes and channels may become enlarged.

Clinical Features. The clinical course of Crohn's disease is variable; often, there are periods of exacerbations and remissions, with symptoms being related to the location of the lesions. The principal symptoms include intermittent diarrhea, colicky pain (usually in the lower right quadrant), weight loss, fluid and electrolyte disorders, malaise, and low-grade fever.[8] Because Crohn's disease affects the submucosal layer to a greater extent than the mucosal layer, there is less bloody diarrhea than with ulcerative colitis. Ulceration of the perianal skin is common, largely because of the severity of the diarrhea. The absorptive surface of the intestine may be disrupted; nutritional deficiencies may occur, related to the specific segment of the

Serosa

Muscularis

Uninvolved (skipped) area

Hyperplastic lymph node

Linear ulceration

Narrow lumen

Thickened wall

Perforation

Abscess

Granuloma

Lymphoid follicle

Fistula into loop
of small bowel

Transmural chronic
inflammation

Granulomatous lymphadenitis

A

B

FIGURE 37.8 • Crohn's disease. (**A**) A schematic representation of the major features of Crohn disease in the small intestine. (**B**) The mucosal surface of the colon displays a "cobblestone" appearance owing to the presence of linear ulcerations and edema and inflammation of the intervening tissue. (From Rubin R., Strayer D. S. (Eds.) (2012). *Rubin's pathology: Clinicopathologic foundations of medicine.* (6th ed., p. 654, 655). Philadelphia, PA: Lippincott Williams & Wilkins.)

intestine involved. When Crohn's disease occurs in childhood, one of its major manifestations may be retardation of growth and physical development.

Complications of Crohn's disease include fistula formation, abdominal abscess formation, and intestinal obstruction. Fistulas are tubelike passages that form connections between different sites in the GI tract. They also may develop between other sites, including the bladder, vagina, urethra, and skin. Perineal fistulas that originate in the ileum are relatively common. Fistulas between segments of the GI tract may lead to malabsorption, syndromes of bacterial overgrowth, and diarrhea. They also can become infected and cause abscess formation.

The diagnosis of Crohn's disease requires a thorough history and physical examination. Colonoscopy is used for direct visualization of the affected areas and to obtain biopsies. Measures are taken to exclude infectious agents as the cause of the disorder. This usually is accomplished by the use of stool cultures and examination of fresh stool specimens for ova and parasites. In persons suspected of having Crohn's disease, radiographic contrast studies provide a means for determining the extent of involvement of the small bowel and establishing the presence and nature of fistulas. CT scans may be used to detect an inflammatory mass or abscess.

Treatment methods focus on terminating the inflammatory response and promoting healing, maintaining adequate nutrition, and preventing and treating complications. Several medications have been successful in suppressing the inflammatory reaction, including the corticosteroids, sulfasalazine, metronidazole, azathioprine, 6-mercaptopurine, methotrexate, and infliximab. Surgical resection of damaged bowel, drainage of abscesses, or repair of fistula tracts may be necessary.

Sulfasalazine is a topically active agent that has a variety of anti-inflammatory effects. The beneficial effects of sulfasalazine are attributable to one component of the drug, 5-aminosalicylic acid (5-ASA). Agents containing 5-ASA affect multiple sites in the arachidonic acid pathway critical to the pathogenesis of inflammation. Sulfasalazine contains 5-ASA with sulfapyridine linked to an azo bond. The drug is poorly absorbed from the intestine, and the azo linkage is broken down by the bacterial flora in the ileum and colon to release 5-ASA. Metronidazole is an antibiotic used to treat bacterial overgrowth in the small intestine. Azathioprine, 6-mercaptopurine, and methotrexate are immunomodulating drugs that are used in the approximately one third of persons who do not respond to other forms of therapy.

Infliximab is a monoclonal antibody that targets the destruction of tumour necrosis factor (TNFα), a mediator of the inflammatory response that is known to be important in granulomatous inflammatory processes such as Crohn's disease.[34] It is the first drug approved specifically for Crohn's disease and is used in the treatment of persons with active moderate to severe disease who have had an inadequate response to corticosteroids or other immune modulators. Although infliximab is currently the only anti-TNF agent approved for treatment of persons with IBD, controlled studies of other anti-TNF and immunomodulating agents are ongoing.

Nutritional deficiencies are common in Crohn's disease because of diarrhea, steatorrhea, and other malabsorption problems. A nutritious diet that is high in calories, vitamins, and proteins is recommended. Because fats often aggravate the diarrhea, it is recommended that they be avoided. Elemental diets, which are nutritionally balanced but residue free and bulk free, may be given during the acute phase of the illness. These diets are largely absorbed in the jejunum and allow the inflamed bowel to rest. Total parenteral nutrition (*i.e.,* parenteral hyperalimentation) consists of intravenous administration of hypertonic glucose solutions to which amino acids and fats may be added. This form of nutritional therapy may be needed when food cannot be absorbed from the intestine. Because of the hypertonicity of these solutions, they must be administered through a large-diameter central vein.

Ulcerative Colitis

Ulcerative colitis is a nonspecific inflammatory condition of the colon. The disease is more common in Canada, the United States, and Western countries. The disease may arise at any age, with a peak incidence between ages 20 and 25 years.[8] Unlike Crohn's disease, which can affect various sites in the GI tract, ulcerative colitis is confined to the rectum and colon. The disease usually begins in the rectum and spreads proximally, affecting primarily the mucosal layer, although it can extend into the submucosal layer. The length of proximal extension varies. It may involve the rectum alone (ulcerative proctitis), the rectum and sigmoid colon (proctosigmoiditis), or the entire colon (pancolitis). The inflammatory process tends to be confluent and continuous instead of skipping areas, as it does in Crohn's disease.

Characteristic of the disease are the lesions that form in the crypts of Lieberkühn in the base of the mucosal layer (see Chapter 36, Fig. 36.12). The inflammatory process leads to the formation of pinpoint mucosal hemorrhages, which in time suppurate and develop into *crypt abscesses.* These inflammatory lesions may become necrotic and ulcerate. Although the ulcerations usually are superficial, they often extend, causing large denuded areas (Fig. 37.9). As a result of the inflammatory process, the mucosal layer often develops tonguelike projections that resemble polyps and therefore are called *pseudopolyps.* The bowel wall thickens in response to repeated episodes of colitis.

Clinical Features. Ulcerative colitis typically presents as a relapsing disorder marked by attacks of diarrhea. The diarrhea may persist for days, weeks, or months and then subside, only to recur after an asymptomatic interval of several months to years or even decades. Because ulcerative colitis affects the mucosal layer of the bowel, the stools typically contain blood and mucus. Nocturnal diarrhea usually occurs when daytime symptoms are severe. There may be mild abdominal cramping and fecal incontinence. Anorexia, weakness, and fatigability are common.

Based on clinical and endoscopic findings, the disease is characterized by its severity and extent. Severity is defined

FIGURE 37.9 • Ulcerative colitis. Prominent erythema and ulceration of the colon begin in the ascending colon and are most severe in the rectosigmoid area. (From Rubin R., Strayer D. S. (Eds.). (2012). *Rubin's pathology: Clinicopathologic foundations of medicine* (6th ed., p. 656). Philadelphia, PA: Lippincott Williams & Wilkins.)

as mild, moderate, severe, or fulminant.[35] The most common form of the disease is the mild form, in which the person has less than four stools daily, with or without blood, no systemic signs of toxicity, and a normal erythrocyte sedimentation rate (ESR). Persons with moderate disease have more than four stools daily, but have minimal signs of toxicity. Severe disease is manifested by more than six bloody stools daily, and evidence of toxicity as demonstrated by fever, tachycardia, anemia, and elevated ESR. Persons with fulminant disease have features that include more than 10 bowel movements a day, continuous bleeding, fever and other signs of toxicity, abdominal tenderness and distension, need for blood transfusions, and colonic dilation on abdominal radiographs.[35] These persons are at risk for development of toxic megacolon, which is characterized by dilation of the colon and signs of systemic toxicity. It results from extension of the inflammatory response, with involvement of neural and vascular components of the bowel.

Diagnosis of ulcerative colitis is based on history and physical examination. The diagnosis usually is confirmed by colonoscopy, sigmoidoscopy, biopsy, and by negative stool examinations for infectious or other causes. Colonoscopy should not be performed on persons with severe disease because of the danger of perforation, but may be performed after demonstrated improvement to determine the extent of disease and need for subsequent cancer surveillance.

Treatment depends on the extent of the disease and severity of symptoms. It includes measures to control the acute manifestations of the disease and prevent recurrence. Some people with mild to moderate symptoms are able to control their symptoms simply by avoiding caffeine, lactose (milk), highly spiced foods, and gas-forming foods. Fibre supplements may be used to decrease diarrhea and rectal symptoms. Surgical treatment (*i.e.,* removal of the rectum and entire colon) with the creation of an ileostomy or ileoanal anastomosis may be required for persons who do not respond to medications and conservative methods of treatment.

The medications used in treatment of ulcerative colitis are similar to those used in the treatment of Crohn's disease. They include the nonabsorbable 5-ASA compounds (*e.g.,* mesalamine, olsalazine, etc.).[34] The corticosteroids are used selectively to lessen the acute inflammatory response. Many of these medications can be administered rectally by suppository or enema. Immunomodulating drugs and anti-TNF therapies may be used to treat persons with severe colitis.

Cancer of the colon is one of the feared complications of ulcerative colitis. Ulcerative colitis is characterized by deoxyribonucleic acid (DNA) damage with microsatellite instability in mucosa cells. More recently, genomic instability was detected in nondysplastic areas of persons with ulcerative colitis, suggesting that these persons have DNA repair deficiency and genomic instability throughout the intestinal tract. The risk for development of cancer is related to: the duration, with a sharp increase after 8 to 10 years after disease initiation; the anatomic extent of colitis, with an increase in pancolitis compared to only life-sided disease; and greater frequency and severity of microscopic inflammation over time may increase risk.[8] Because of this relatively high risk for development of cancer, regular annual or biannual surveillance colonoscopies with multiple biopsies are recommended for persons with extensive colitis, beginning 8 to 10 years after diagnosis.[35]

Infectious Enterocolitis

A number of microbial agents, including viruses, bacteria, and protozoa, can infect the GI tract, causing diarrhea and sometimes ulcerative and inflammatory changes in the small or large intestine. Infectious enterocolitis is a global problem, causing more than 12,000 deaths per day among children in developing countries.[8] Although far less common in industrialized countries, these disorders still have infection rates second only to the common cold. Most infections are spread by the oral-fecal route, often through contaminated water or food.

Viral Infection

Most viral infections affect the superficial epithelium of the small intestine, destroying these cells and disrupting their absorptive function. Repopulation of the small intestinal villi with immature enterocytes and preservation of crypt secretory cells leads to net secretion of water and electrolytes compounded by incomplete absorption of nutrients and osmotic diarrhea. Symptomatic disease is caused by several distinct viruses, including the rotavirus, which most commonly affects children 6 to 24 months of age; the Norwalk virus, which is responsible for the majority of nonbacterial food-borne epidemic gastroenteritis in all age groups: and enteric adenoviruses, which primarily affect children.[7]

Rotavirus. Worldwide, rotavirus is estimated to cause more than 140 million cases of diarrhea per year in children younger than 5 years of age. This infection is considered the most common cause of severe childhood diarrhea and diarrheal mortality worldwide. Epidemiological studies show that all children will have at least one episode of this gastroenteritis infection by the time they are 5 years of age. The disease tends to be most severe in children 3 to 24 months of age and many of these children will require hospitalization due to prolonged diarrhea and malnutrition.[36] Infants younger than 3 months of age are relatively protected by transplacental antibodies and possibly by breastfeeding. The virus is spread by a fecal–oral route and outbreaks are common in children in daycare centres. The virus is shed before and for days after clinical illness. Very few infectious virions are needed to cause disease in a susceptible host.[8]

Rotavirus infection typically begins after an incubation period of less than 24 hours, with mild to moderate fever and vomiting, followed by onset of frequent watery stools. The fever and vomiting usually disappear on about the second day, but the diarrhea continues for 5 to 7 days. Dehydration may develop rapidly, particularly in infants.

Treatment is largely supportive. Avoiding and treating dehydration are the main goals. Since 2008, two live oral vaccine for rotavirus (RotaTeq, Rotarix) have been approved by the Health Canada and are recommended by the National Advisory Committee on Immunizations (NACI).[37] As of 2014, most provinces and territories cover this vaccine at 2 and 4 months as part of the routine childhood vaccines.[38] Recent data suggests that the rotavirus vaccines are effective and can reduce the burden of illness, namely decreasing healthcare provider visits, hospitalizations, and complications.[37]

Bacterial Infection

Infectious enterocolitis can be caused by a number of bacteria. There are several pathogenic mechanisms for bacterial enterocolitis: ingestion of preformed toxins that are present in contaminated food; infection by toxigenic organisms that proliferate in the gut lumen and produce an enterotoxin; and infection by enteroinvasive organisms, which proliferate in the lumen and invade and destroy mucosal epithelial cells. The pathogenic effects of bacterial infections depend on the ability of the organism to adhere to the mucosal epithelial cells, elaborate enterotoxins, then invade the mucosal epithelial cells.

In general, bacterial infections produce more severe effects than viral infections. The complications of bacterial enterocolitis result from massive fluid loss or destruction of intestinal mucosa and include dehydration, sepsis, and perforation. Among the organisms that cause bacterial enterocolitis are *Staphylococcus aureus* (toxins associated with "food poisoning"), *Escherichia coli*, *Shigella* species, *Salmonella*, and *Campylobacter.* Two particularly serious forms of bacteria enterocolitis are caused by *Clostridium difficile* and *E. coli* O157:H7.

***Clostridium difficile* Colitis.** *C. difficile* colitis is associated with antibiotic therapy.[39] *C. difficile* is a gram-positive, spore-forming bacillus that is part of the normal flora in 1% to 3% of healthy adults.[39] The spores are resistant to the acid environment of the stomach and convert to vegetative forms in the colon. Treatment with broad-spectrum antibiotics predisposes

to disruption of the normal protective bacterial flora of the colon, leading to colonization by *C. difficile* along with the release of toxins that cause mucosal damage and inflammation. Almost any antibiotic may cause *C. difficile* colitis, but broad-spectrum antibiotics with activity against gram-negative enteric bacteria are the most frequent agents. After antibiotic therapy has made the bowel susceptible to infection, colonization by *C. difficile* occurs by the oral–fecal route. *C. difficile* infection usually is acquired in the hospital, where the organism is commonly encountered.

In general, *C. difficile* is noninvasive. Development of *C. difficile* colitis and diarrhea requires an alteration in the normal gut flora, acquisition and germination of the spores, overgrowth of *C. difficile,* and toxin production. The toxins bind to and damage the intestinal mucosa, causing hemorrhage, inflammation, and necrosis. The toxins also interfere with protein synthesis, attract inflammatory cells, increase capillary permeability, and stimulate intestinal peristalsis. The infection commonly manifests with diarrhea that is mild to moderate and sometimes is accompanied by lower abdominal cramping. Typically symptoms begin within 1 to 2 weeks after an antibiotic treatment has been started, although presentation varies from 1 day to 6 weeks.[39] In most cases, systemic manifestations are absent, and the symptoms subside after the antibiotic has been discontinued.

A more severe form of colitis, *pseudomembranous colitis,* is characterized by an adherent inflammatory membrane overlying the areas of mucosal injury. It is a life-threatening form of the disease. Persons with the disease are acutely ill, with lethargy, fever, tachycardia, abdominal pain and distension, and dehydration. The smooth muscle tone of the colon may be lost, resulting in toxic dilation of the colon. Prompt therapy is needed to prevent perforation of the bowel.

The diagnosis of *C. difficile*-associated diarrhea requires a careful history, with particular emphasis on antibiotic use. Diagnostic findings include a history of antibiotic use and laboratory tests that confirm the presence of *C. difficile* toxins in the stool. Treatment includes the immediate discontinuation of antibiotic therapy. Specific treatment aimed at eradicating *C. difficile* is used when symptoms are severe or persistent. Metronidazole is the drug of first choice, with vancomycin being reserved for persons who cannot tolerate metronidazole, do not respond to the drug, or more severe cases. Ideally both drugs are given orally.[39] Metronidazole is absorbed from the upper GI tract and may cause side effects. Vancomycin is poorly absorbed, and its actions are limited to the GI tract. For recurrent or refractory disease, bacteriotherapy (*i.e.*, fecal transplantation) is very effective at reestablishing the gut microbiota but underutilized for aesthetic and logistical reasons.[39,40]

***Escherichia coli* O157:H7 Infection.** *E. coli* O157:H7 has become recognized as an important cause of epidemic and sporadic colitis.[41] An unfortunate example of an *E. coli* O157:H7 outbreak occurred in Walkerton, Ontario, where almost 1,300 cases were identified and 7 people died in May 2000.[42] *E. coli* O157:H7 is a strain of *E. coli* found in the feces and contaminated milk of healthy dairy and beef cattle, but it also has been found in contaminated pork, poultry, and lamb. Infection usually is by food-borne transmission, often by the ingestion of undercooked hamburger. The organism also can be transferred to nonmeat products such as fruits and vegetables. Transmission has also been reported in persons swimming in a fecally contaminated lake as well as among visitors to farms and petting zoos, where children are in direct contact with animals. Person-to-person transmission may occur, particularly in nursing homes, daycare settings, and hospitals. The very young and the very old are particularly at risk for the infection and its complications.

The infection may cause no symptoms or cause a variety of manifestations, including acute, nonbloody diarrhea; hemorrhagic colitis; hemolytic uremic syndrome; and thrombotic thrombocytopenic purpura. The infection often presents with abdominal cramping and watery diarrhea and subsequently may progress to bloody diarrhea.[43] The diarrhea commonly lasts 3 to 7 days or longer. Fever occurs in up to one third of the cases.

Most strains of E. coli are harmless; however, enterohemorrhagic E. coli can release Shigella-like toxins that attach to and damage the mucosal lining of the intestine, causing bloody diarrhea.[43] Subsequently, the Shigella-like toxins gain access to the circulatory system and travel in the plasma and on the surface of platelets and monocytes. The Shigella-like toxins bind to high-affinity galactose-containing receptors called Gb3, in the membranes of glomerular, cerebral, or microvascular endothelial cells; renal mesangial and tubular cells; and monocytes and platelets.[43] Two complications of the infection, hemolytic uremic syndrome and thrombotic thrombocytopenic purpura, reflect the effects of the Shigella-like toxins. The hemolytic uremic syndrome is characterized by hemolytic anemia, thrombocytopenia, and renal failure. It occurs predominantly in infants and young children and is the most common cause of acute renal failure in children. It has a mortality rate of 3% to 5%. Thrombotic thrombocytopenic purpura is manifested by thrombocytopenia, renal failure, fever, and neurologic manifestations. It often is regarded as the severe end of the disease that leads to hemolytic uremic syndrome plus neurologic problems.

No specific therapy is available for E. coli O157:H7 infection. Treatment is largely symptomatic and directed toward treating the effects of complications. The use of antibiotics or antimotility/antidiarrheal agents are discouraged in the early stages of diarrhea as they have been shown to increase the risk of hemolytic uremic syndrome because the gut is exposed to a greater amount of toxins for a longer time.[43]

Because of the seriousness of the infection and its complications, education of the public about techniques for decreasing primary transmission of the infection from animal sources is important. Undercooked meats and unpasteurized milk are sources of transmission. The Canadian Food Inspection Agency recommends a minimal internal temperature of 71°C (160°F) for cooked hamburger.[44] Food handlers and consumers should be aware of the proper methods for handling uncooked meat to prevent cross-contamination of other foods. Particular attention

should be paid to hygiene in daycare centres and nursing homes, where the spread of infection to the very young and very old may result in severe complications.

Protozoan Infection

Amebiasis refers to an infection by *Entamoeba histolytica* involving the colon and occasionally the liver. Humans are the only known reservoir for E. histolytica, which reproduce in the colon and pass in the feces. Although E. histolytica infection occurs worldwide, it is more common and more severe in tropical and subtropical areas, where crowding and poor sanitation prevail.[8,45] Intestinal amebiasis ranges from completely asymptomatic infection to serious dysenteric disease.

E. histolytica has two distinct stages: the trophozoites (amoeboid form) and cysts. The trophozoites thrive in the colon and feed on bacteria and human cells. They may colonize any portion of the large bowel, but the area of maximum disease is usually the cecum. Persons with symptomatic disease pass both cysts and trophozoites in their feces, but the latter survive only briefly outside the body. Only the cysts are infectious because they survive gastric acidity, which destroys the trophozoites. Once established, the trophozoites invade the crypts of colonic glands and burrow down into the submucosa; the organism then fans out to create a flask-shaped ulcer with a narrow neck and broad base. E. histolytica that have invaded into the submucosal veins of the colon enter the portal vein and embolize to the liver to produce solitary and, less often, multiple discrete hepatic abscesses.[8]

Some people have an acute onset of diarrhea as early as 8 days (commonly 2 to 4 weeks) after infection.[46] Others may be asymptomatic or have only mild intestinal symptoms for months or several years before either intestinal symptoms or liver abscesses appear. Manifestations include abdominal discomfort, tenderness, cramps, and fever, often accompanied by nausea, vomiting, and passage of malodorous flatus. There may be frequent passage of liquid stools containing bloody mucus, but the duration of diarrhea is not usually so prolonged as to cause dehydration. The infection often persists for months or years, causing emaciation and anemia. In severe cases, massive destruction of the colonic mucosa may lead to hemorrhage, perforation, or peritonitis. Persons with amebic liver abscesses often present with severe right upper quadrant pain, low-grade fever, and weight loss.[45]

Diagnostic methods include microscopic examination of the stool for E. histolytica, serum antibody tests, and colonoscopy with specimen collection or biopsy. Treatment includes use of the metronidazole or tinidazole, which act against the trophozoites, followed by a course of luminal amebicides such as iodoquinol or paromomycin which are effective against the cysts.[45]

Diverticular Disease

Diverticulosis is a condition in which the mucosal layer of the colon herniates through the muscularis externa layer. There are often multiple diverticula, most of which occur in the sigmoid

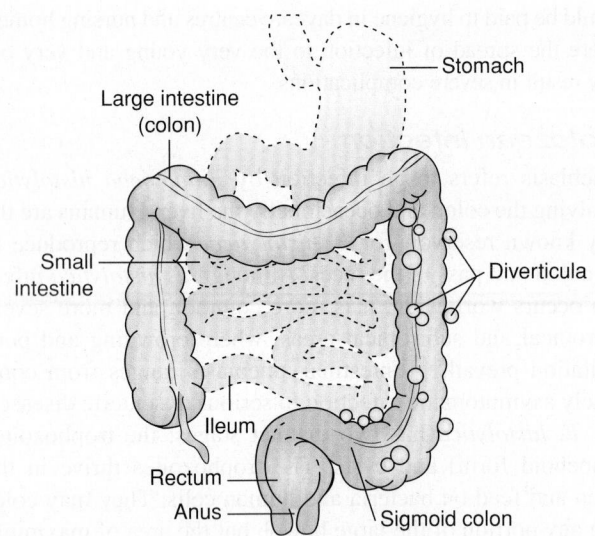

FIGURE 37.10 • Location of diverticula in the sigmoid colon.

colon (Fig. 37.10).[9] Diverticular disease refers to the complications of diverticulosis and is common in Western society, affecting approximately 5% of the population older than 40 years of age and almost 65% of those older than 85 years.[47] Although the disorder is prevalent in the developed countries of the world, it is almost nonexistent in many African nations and underdeveloped countries. This suggests that factors such as lack of fibre in the diet, a decrease in physical activity, and poor bowel habits (*e.g.*, neglecting the urge to defecate), along with the effects of aging, contribute to the development of the disease.

In the colon, the longitudinal muscle does not form a continuous layer, as it does in the small bowel. Instead, there are three separate longitudinal bands of muscle called the *teniae coli*. In a manner similar to the small intestine, bands of circular muscle constrict the large intestine. As the circular muscle contracts at each of these points (approximately every 2.5 cm), the lumen of the bowel becomes constricted, so that it is almost occluded. The combined contraction of the circular muscle and the lack of a continuous longitudinal muscle layer cause the intestine to bulge outward into pouches called *haustra*. Diverticula develop between the longitudinal muscle bands of the haustra, in the area where the blood vessels pierce the circular muscle layer to bring blood to the mucosal layer. An increase in intraluminal pressure in the haustra provides the force for creating these herniations. The increase in pressure is thought to be related to the volume of the colonic contents. The scantier the contents, the more vigorous are the contractions and the greater is the pressure in the haustra.

Most persons with diverticular disease remain asymptomatic.[47] The disease often is found when x-ray studies are done for other purposes. When symptoms do occur, they often are attributed to IBS or other causes. Ill-defined lower abdominal discomfort, a change in bowel habits (*e.g.*, diarrhea, constipation, etc.), bloating, and flatulence are common.

Diverticulitis is a complication of diverticulosis in which there is inflammation and gross or microscopic perforation of

the diverticulum.[48] One of the most common complaints of diverticulitis is pain in the lower left quadrant, accompanied by nausea and vomiting, tenderness in the lower left quadrant, a slight fever, and an elevated white blood cell count. These symptoms usually last for several days, unless complications occur, and usually are caused by localized inflammation of the diverticula with perforation and development of a small, localized abscess. Up to 25% of persons with acute diverticulitis will develop complications including perforation with peritonitis, hemorrhage, and bowel obstruction. Fistulas can form, usually involving the bladder (*i.e.*, vesicosigmoid fistula) but sometimes involving the skin, perianal area, or small bowel. Pneumaturia (*i.e.*, air in the urine) is a sign of vesicosigmoid fistula.

The diagnosis of diverticular disease is based on history and presenting clinical manifestations. The disease may be confirmed by CT scans or ultrasonographic studies. CT scans are the safest and most cost-effective method. Although barium enema was used in the past, it is no longer recommended because of the risk of extravasation of contrast material if perforation has occurred.[48] Flat abdominal radiographs may be used to detect complications associated with acute diverticulitis.

The usual treatment for diverticular disease is to prevent symptoms and complications. This includes increasing the bulk in the diet and bowel retraining so that the person has at least one bowel movement each day. The increased bulk promotes regular defecation and increases colonic contents and colon diameter, thereby decreasing intraluminal pressure. Acute diverticulitis is treated by withholding solid food and administering a broad-spectrum antibiotic. Other agents being investigated are 5-aminosalicylic acid (5-ASA) and/or probiotics and the potential effectiveness to manage diverticular disease. Hospitalization may be required for persons who show significant inflammation, are unable to tolerate oral fluids, are older adults, or have significant comorbid conditions. Surgical treatment is reserved for complications.[48]

Appendicitis

Acute appendicitis is extremely common. It is seen most frequently in the 15- to 30-year-old age group, but it can occur at any age. The appendix becomes inflamed, swollen, and gangrenous, and it eventually perforates if not treated. Although the cause of appendicitis is unknown, it is thought to be related to intraluminal obstruction with a fecalith (*i.e.*, hard piece of stool), gallstones, tumours, parasites, or to twisting.[8,49]

Appendicitis usually has an abrupt onset, with pain referred to the epigastric or periumbilical area. This pain is caused by stretching of the appendix during the early inflammatory process. At approximately the same time that the pain appears, there are one or two episodes of nausea. Initially, the pain is vague, but over a period of 2 to 12 hours, it gradually increases and may become colicky. When the inflammatory process has extended to involve the serosal layer of the appendix and the peritoneum, the pain becomes localized to the lower right quadrant. There usually is an elevation in temperature and a white blood cell count greater than $10.0 \times 10^9/L$, with 75% or more polymorphonuclear cells.[49] Palpation of the abdomen usually reveals a deep tenderness in the lower right quadrant, which is confined to a small area around McBurney's point. It usually is located at approximately the site of the inflamed appendix. The person with appendicitis often is able to place his or her finger directly over the tender area. Rebound tenderness, which is pain that occurs when pressure is applied to the area and then released, and spasm of the overlying abdominal muscles are common.[8,49]

Diagnosis is usually based on history and findings on physical examination. Ultrasonography or CT may be used to confirm the diagnosis.[49] Treatment usually consists of surgical removal of the appendix but newer evidence is supporting the use of antibiotics instead of surgery for uncomplicated acute appendicitis.[50] Complications include peritonitis, localized periappendiceal abscess formation, and septicemia.

DISORDERS OF GASTROINTESTINAL MOTILITY

- The luminal contents move down the GI tract as a result of peristaltic movements regulated by a complex interaction of electrical, neural, and hormonal control mechanisms.
- Local irritation and the composition and constituents of GI contents influence motility through the submucosal afferent neurons of the enteric nervous system. GI wall distension, chemical irritants, osmotic gradients, and bacterial toxins exert many of their effects on GI motility through these afferent pathways.
- Autonomic influences generated by factors such as medications, trauma, and emotional experiences interact with the enteric nervous system to alter GI motility.

Alterations in Intestinal Motility

The movement of contents through the GI tract is controlled by neurons located in the submucosal and myenteric plexuses of the gut (see Chapter 36). The axons from the cell bodies in the myenteric plexus innervate the circular and longitudinal smooth muscle layers of the gut. These neurons receive impulses from local receptors located in the mucosal and muscle layers of the gut and extrinsic input from the parasympathetic and sympathetic nervous systems. As a general rule, the parasympathetic nervous system tends to increase the motility of the bowel, whereas sympathetic stimulation tends to slow its activity.

The colon has sphincters at both ends: the ileocecal sphincter, which separates it from the small intestine, and the anal sphincter, which prevents the movement of feces to the outside of the body. The colon acts as a reservoir for fecal material. Normally, approximately 400 ml of water, 55 mmol of sodium, 30 mmol of chloride, and 15 mmol of bicarbonate are absorbed each day in the colon. At the same time, approximately 5 mmol of potassium is secreted into the lumen of the colon. The amount of water and electrolytes that remains in the stool reflects the absorption or secretion that occurs in the colon. The average adult ingesting a typical Canadian diet evacuates approximately 100 to 300 g of stool each day.

Diarrhea

The usual definition of *diarrhea* is excessively frequent passage of loose or unformed stools. The complaint of diarrhea is a general one and can be related to a number of pathologic and nonpathologic factors.[51] Diarrhea can be acute or chronic and can be caused by infectious organisms, food intolerance, drugs, or intestinal disease. Acute diarrheas that last less than 4 days are predominantly caused by infectious agents and follow a self-limited course.

Acute Diarrhea. Diarrhea that is acute in onset and persists for less than 2 weeks is commonly caused by infectious agents (see previous discussion of infectious enterocolitis).[51] Acute diarrhea is commonly divided into noninflammatory (large-volume) and inflammatory (small-volume) diarrhea, based on the characteristics of the diarrheal stool.[52] Enteric organisms cause diarrhea by several ways. Some are noninvasive and do not cause inflammation, but secrete toxins that stimulate fluid secretion. Others invade and destroy intestinal epithelial cells, thereby altering fluid transport so that secretory activity continues while absorption activity is halted.

Noninflammatory diarrhea is associated with large-volume watery and nonbloody stools, periumbilical cramps, bloating, and nausea or vomiting. It is commonly caused by toxin-producing bacteria (*e.g.*, enterotoxigenic *E. coli*, *S. aureus*, *Vibrio cholerae*, etc.) or other agents (*e.g.*, viruses, *Giardia*) that disrupt the normal absorption or secretory process in the small bowel. Prominent vomiting suggests viral enteritis or *S. aureus* food poisoning. Although typically mild, the diarrhea (which originates in the small intestine) can be voluminous and result in dehydration with hypokalemia and metabolic acidosis (*i.e.*, cholera). Because tissue invasion does not occur, leukocytes are not present in the feces.

Inflammatory diarrhea is usually characterized by the presence of fever and bloody diarrhea (dysentery). It is caused by invasion of intestinal cells (*e.g.*, *Shigella*, *Salmonella*, *Yersinia*, and *Campylobacter*) or the toxins associated with the previously described *C. difficile* or *E. coli* O157:H7 infection.[53] Because infections associated with these organisms predominantly affect the colon, the diarrhea is small in volume (<1 L/day) and is associated with left lower quadrant cramps, urgency, and tenesmus (or feeling of incomplete defecation). Infectious dysentery must be distinguished from acute ulcerative colitis, which may present with bloody diarrhea, fever, and abdominal pain. Diarrhea that persists for 14 days is not attributable to bacterial pathogens (except for *C. difficile*), and the person should be evaluated for chronic diarrhea.

Chronic Diarrhea. Diarrhea is considered to be chronic when the symptoms persist for 4 or more weeks. Chronic diarrhea is often associated with conditions such as IBD, IBS, malabsorption syndrome, endocrine disorders (hyperthyroidism, diabetic autonomic neuropathy), or radiation colitis. There

CHART 37.1	CHRONIC DIARRHEA

Hyperosmotic diarrhea
    Saline cathartics
    Lactase deficiency
Secretory diarrhea
    Acute infectious diarrhea
    Failure to absorb bile salts
    Fat malabsorption
    Chronic laxative abuse
    Carcinoid syndrome
    Zollinger–Ellison syndrome
    Fecal impaction
Inflammatory bowel disease
    Crohn's disease
    Ulcerative colitis
Infectious disease
    Shigellosis
    Salmonellosis
Irritable colon

are four major causes of chronic diarrhea: presence of hyperosmotic luminal contents, increased intestinal secretory processes, inflammatory conditions, and infectious processes[13] (Chart 37.1). Factitious diarrhea is caused by indiscriminate use of laxatives or excessive intake of laxative-type foods.

In *osmotic diarrhea,* water is pulled into the bowel by the hyperosmotic nature of its contents and the colon is unable to reabsorb the excess fluid. It occurs when osmotically active particles are not absorbed. In persons with lactase deficiency, the lactose in milk cannot be broken down and absorbed. Magnesium salts, which are contained in milk of magnesia and many antacids, are poorly absorbed and cause diarrhea when taken in sufficient quantities. Another cause of osmotic diarrhea is decreased transit time, which interferes with absorption. Osmotic diarrhea usually disappears with fasting.[51]

Secretory diarrhea occurs when the secretory processes of the bowel are increased. Secretory diarrhea also occurs when excess bile acids remain in the intestinal contents as they enter the colon. This often happens with disease processes of the ileum because bile salts are absorbed there. It also may occur with bacterial overgrowth in the small bowel, which interferes with bile absorption. Some tumours, such as those of the Zollinger–Ellison syndrome and carcinoid syndrome, produce hormones that cause increased secretory activity of the bowel.[51]

Inflammatory diarrhea commonly is associated with acute or chronic inflammation or intrinsic disease of the colon, such as ulcerative colitis or Crohn's disease. Inflammatory diarrhea usually is evidenced by frequency, urgency, and colicky abdominal pain. It commonly is accompanied by tenesmus, fecal soiling of clothing, and awakening during the night with the urge to defecate.[51]

Chronic parasitic infections may cause chronic diarrhea through a number of mechanisms. Pathogens most commonly associated with chronic diarrhea include the protozoans *Giardia, E. histolytica,* and *Cyclospora.* Immunocompromised persons are particularly susceptible to infectious organisms that can cause acute and chronic diarrhea (see Chapter 20), including *Cryptosporidium,* cytomegalovirus (CMV), and *Mycobacterium avium-intracellulare* complex.

Diagnosis and Treatment. The diagnosis of diarrhea is based on complaints of frequent stools and a history of accompanying factors such as concurrent illnesses, medication use, and exposure to potential intestinal pathogens. Disorders such as IBD and celiac disease should be considered. If the onset of diarrhea is related to travel outside Canada, the possibility of traveller's diarrhea must be considered.

Although most acute forms of diarrhea are self-limited and require no treatment, diarrhea can be particularly serious in infants and small children, persons with other illnesses, elderly persons, and even previously healthy persons if it continues for any length of time. Thus, the replacement of fluids and electrolytes is considered to be a primary therapeutic goal in the treatment of diarrhea.[53]

Drugs used in the treatment of diarrhea include diphenoxylate (Lomotil) and loperamide (Imodium), which are opiumlike drugs. These drugs decrease GI motility and stimulate water and electrolyte absorption. Adsorbents, such as kaolin and pectin, adsorb irritants and toxins from the bowel. These ingredients are included in many over-the-counter antidiarrheal preparations because they adsorb toxins responsible for certain types of diarrhea. Bismuth subsalicylate (Pepto-Bismol) can be used to reduce the frequency of unformed stools and increase stool consistency, particularly in cases of traveller's diarrhea. The drug is thought to inhibit intestinal secretion caused by enterotoxigenic *E. coli* and cholera toxins. Antidiarrheal medications should not be used in persons with bloody diarrhea, high fever, or signs of toxicity because of the risk of worsening the disease. Antibiotics should be reserved for use in persons with identified enteric pathogens.[51,53]

Acute Diarrheal Disease in Children. In developing countries, diarrhea is a common cause of mortality among children younger than 5 years of age, with an estimated 1.9 million deaths annually.[53] Although diarrheal diseases are less prevalent in Canada than in other countries, they place a burden on the healthcare system. More than 200,000 hospitalizations for dehydration related to acute gastroenteritis were recorded annually in the United States, with comparable rates in Canada.[36]

The causes of acute diarrhea in children vary with location, time of year, and population studied. There is increasing recognition of a widening array of enteric pathogens that cause acute diarrhea in children. Viruses are the most common pathogen causing diarrheal illness in Canada. Rotaviruses and noroviruses are the frequently observed pathogens.[8] Other viruses that have been observed in the stools of children include astroviruses and enteric adenoviruses. Many of these pathogens are transmitted easily through food and water or from one person to another. Prevention remains the most vital measure in managing diarrheal disease in children. Important measures to prevent spread of pathogens include proper sanitation methods for food processing and preparation, sanitary water supplies, proper hand hygiene, exclusion of infected people from handling food or providing healthcare, and exclusion of people with diarrhea from using public recreational water (*i.e.,* swimming pools, ponds, and lakes).

The main objectives in the approach to a child with acute diarrhea are to assess the degree of dehydration, prevent spread of the infection, determine the nature of the etiologic agent, and provide specific therapy as needed. The hydration status of children can be assessed on the basis of easily observed signs and symptoms. Questions about oral intake, frequency and volume of stool output, general appearance and activity of the child, and frequency of urination provide essential information about hydration. Thirst, dry mucous membranes, and decreased skin turgor are the common symptoms of dehydration.[51–53] Data should be obtained about daycare attendance, recent travel to a diarrhea-endemic area, use of antimicrobial drugs, and exposure to contaminated water, unwashed fruits or vegetables, or improperly cooked meats because they may indicate the cause of the disorder. Fever is suggestive of an inflammatory process, but also occurs with dehydration.

Management of dehydration remains the cornerstone of treatment of children with diarrhea.[53] Infants in particular are more susceptible to dehydration because of their greater surface area, higher metabolic rate, and inability effectively to concentrate their urine. Oral replacement therapy (ORT) is usually the method of choice for infants and children with uncomplicated diarrhea that can be treated at home.

First applied to the treatment of diarrhea in developing countries, ORT can be regarded as a case of reverse technology, in which the protocols originally implemented in these countries have changed healthcare in industrialized countries as well.[53] Complete ORT solutions contain carbohydrate, sodium, potassium, chloride, and base to replace that lost in the diarrheal stool. Commonly used beverages such as apple juice and cola drinks, which have increased osmolarity because of their high carbohydrate content and low electrolyte content, are not recommended. The effectiveness of ORT is based on the coupled transport of sodium and glucose or other actively transported small organic molecules (see Chapter 36). Bottled ORT solutions are available but can be costly, particularly in cases where large amounts of replacement fluids are needed. The cost can represent a sizable burden for socioeconomically disadvantaged families. Less expensive, premeasured packets and recipes for preparing replacement solutions are available. The use of ORT for treatment of diarrhea in infants and small children is often labour intensive, requiring frequent feeding, sometimes using a spoon.[51,53] More importantly, the diarrhea does not promptly cease after ORT has been instituted; this can be discouraging for parents and caregivers who desire early results from their efforts. Children who are severely dehydrated with changes in vital signs or mental status require emergency intravenous fluid resuscitation. After initial treatment with intravenous fluids, these children can be given ORT.

Evidence suggests that feeding should be continued during diarrheal illness, particularly in children.[53] It has been shown that unrestricted diets do not worsen the course or symptoms of mild diarrhea and can decrease stool output. Starch and simple proteins are thought to provide cotransport molecules with little osmotic activity, increasing fluid and electrolyte uptake by intestinal cells. The luminal contents associated with early refeeding are also a known growth factor for enterocytes and help facilitate repair after injury. It is recommended that children who require rehydration therapy because of diarrhea be fed an age-appropriate diet. Although there is little agreement on which foods are best, fatty foods and foods high in simple sugars are best avoided. No data suggest that a diet consisting of only bananas, rice, applesauce, and toast (the BRAT diet) speeds recovery from diarrheal illnesses.[54] Almost all infants with acute gastroenteritis can tolerate breast-feeding. For formula-fed infants, diluted formula does not provide an advantage over full-strength formula.

Constipation

Constipation can be defined as the infrequent, incomplete, or difficult passage of stools.[41,51] The difficulty with this definition arises from the many individual variations of function that are normal. What is considered normal for one person (*e.g.,* two or three bowel movements per week) may be considered evidence of constipation by another. Constipation can occur as a primary disorder of intestinal motility, as a side effect of drugs, as a problem associated with another disease condition, or as a symptom of obstructing lesions of the GI tract. Some common causes of constipation are failure to respond to the urge to defecate, inadequate fibre in the diet, inadequate fluid intake, weakness of the abdominal muscles, inactivity and bed rest, pregnancy, and hemorrhoids. The pathophysiology of constipation can be classified into three broad categories: normal-transit constipation, slow-transit constipation, and disorders of defecatory or rectal evacuation.[41] Normal-transit constipation (or functional constipation) is characterized by perceived difficulty in defecation and usually responds to increased fluid and fibre intake. Slow-transit constipation, which is characterized by infrequent bowel movements, is often caused by alterations in intestinal innervation impacting colonic motor function. Hirschsprung disease is an extreme form of slow-transit constipation in which the ganglion cells in the distal bowel are absent because of a defect that occurred during embryonic development; the bowel narrows at the area that lacks ganglionic cells. Although most persons with this disorder present in infancy or early childhood, some with a relatively short segment of involved colon do not have symptoms until later in life. Defecatory disorders are most commonly due to dysfunction of the pelvic floor or anal sphincter.

Diseases associated with chronic constipation include neurologic diseases such as spinal cord injury, Parkinson disease, and multiple sclerosis; endocrine disorders such as hypothyroidism; and obstructive lesions in the GI tract.[51] Drugs such as narcotics, anticholinergic agents, calcium channel blockers, diuretics, calcium (antacids and supplements), iron supplements, and aluminum antacids tend to cause constipation. Elderly people with long-standing constipation may develop dilation of the rectum, colon, or both. This condition allows large amounts of stool to accumulate with little or no sensation. Constipation, in the context of a change in bowel habits, may be a sign of colorectal cancer.

Diagnosis of constipation usually is based on a history of infrequent stools, straining with defecation, the passing of hard and lumpy stools, or the sense of incomplete evacuation with defecation. Rectal examination is used to determine whether fecal impaction, anal stricture, or rectal masses are present. Constipation as a sign of another disease condition should be ruled out. Tests that measure colon transit time and defecatory function are reserved for refractory cases.

The treatment of constipation usually is directed toward relieving the cause. A conscious effort should be made to respond to the defecation urge. A time should be set aside after a meal, when mass movements in the colon are most likely to occur, for a bowel movement. Adequate fluid intake and bulk in the diet should be encouraged. Moderate exercise is essential, and persons on bed rest benefit from passive and active exercises. Laxatives and enemas should be used judiciously. They should not be used on a regular basis to treat simple constipation because they interfere with the defecation reflex and actually may damage the rectal mucosa.[41]

Fecal Impaction

Fecal impaction is the retention of hardened or putty-like stool in the rectum and colon, which interferes with normal passage of feces. If not removed, it can cause partial or complete bowel obstruction. It may occur in any age group but is more common in incapacitated older adults.[55] Fecal impaction may result from painful anorectal disease, tumours, or neurogenic disease; use of constipating antacids or bulk laxatives; a low-residue diet; drug-induced colonic stasis; or prolonged bed rest and debility. In children, a habitual neglect of the urge to defecate because it interferes with play may promote impaction.

The manifestations may be those of severe constipation, but frequently there is a history of watery diarrhea, fecal soiling, and fecal incontinence.[55] This is caused by increased secretory activity of the bowel, representing the body's attempt to break up the mass so that it can be evacuated. The abdomen may be distended, and there may be blood and mucus in the stool. The fecal mass may compress the urethra, giving rise to urinary incontinence. Fecal impaction should be considered in an elderly or immobilized person who develops watery stools with fecal or urinary incontinence.[55]

Digital examination of the rectum is done to assess for the presence of a fecal mass. The mass may need to be broken up and dislodged manually or with the use of a sigmoidoscope. Oil enemas often are used to soften the mass before removal. The best treatment is prevention.

Intestinal Obstruction

Intestinal obstruction designates an impairment of movement of intestinal contents in a cephalocaudad direction. The causes

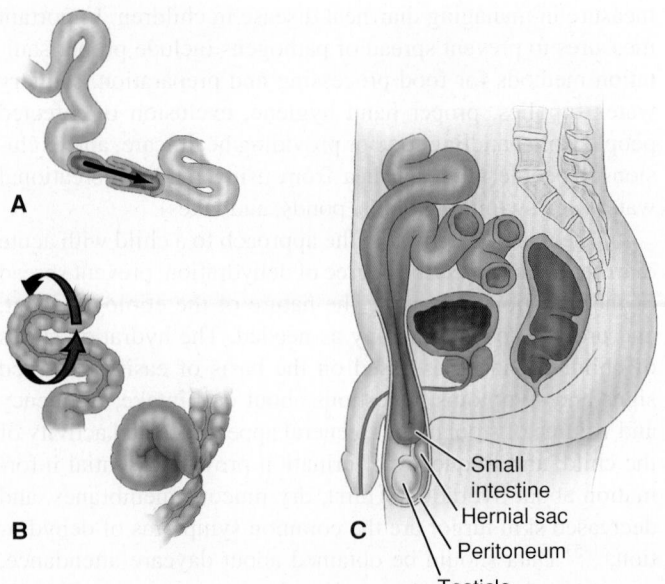

FIGURE 37.11 • Three causes of intestinal obstruction. **A:** Intussusception with invagination or shortening of the bowel caused by movement of one segment of the bowel into another. **B:** Volvulus of the sigmoid colon; the twist is counterclockwise in most cases. Note the edematous section of bowel. **C:** Hernia (inguinal). The sac of the hernia is a continuation of the peritoneum of the abdomen. The hernial contents are intestine, omentum, or other abdominal contents that pass through the hernial opening into the hernial sac. (From Day R. A., Paul P., Williams B., et al. (2010). *Brunner & Suddarth's textbook of Canadian medical-surgical nursing* (2nd ed., p. 1188). Philadelphia, PA: Lippincott Williams & Wilkins.)

can be categorized as mechanical or paralytic. Strangulation with necrosis of the bowel may occur and lead to perforation, peritonitis, and sepsis.[56,57]

Mechanical obstruction can result from a number of conditions, intrinsic or extrinsic, that encroach on the patency of the bowel lumen (Fig. 37.11). Major inciting causes include external postoperative adhesions, tumours, and, hernia (*i.e.,* inguinal, femoral, or umbilical).[56] Less common causes are strictures, IBD, foreign bodies, intussusception, and volvulus.

Intussusception involves the telescoping of bowel into the adjacent segment (Fig. 37.12). It is the most common cause of intestinal obstruction in children younger than 2 years of age.[46] The most common form is intussusception of the terminal ileum into the right colon, but other areas of the bowel may be involved. In most cases, the cause of the disorder is unknown. The condition can also occur in adults when an intraluminal mass or tumour acts as a traction force and pulls the segment along as it telescopes into the distal segment.[8] Volvulus refers to a complete twisting of the bowel on an axis formed by its mesentery (Fig. 37.11B). It can occur in any portion of the GI tract, but most commonly involves the sigmoid colon, followed by the cecum.[8] Mechanical bowel obstruction may be a simple obstruction, in which there is no alteration in blood flow, or a strangulated obstruction, in which there is impairment of blood flow and necrosis of bowel tissue.

FIGURE 37.12 • Intussusception. A cross-section through the area of the obstruction shows "telescoped" small intestine surround by dilated small intestine. (From Rubin R., Strayer D. S. (Eds.). (2012). *Rubin's pathology: Clinicopathologic foundations of medicine* (6th ed., p. 645). Philadelphia, PA: Lippincott Williams & Wilkins.)

Paralytic, or adynamic, obstruction results from neurogenic or muscular impairment of peristalsis.[57] Paralytic ileus is seen most commonly after abdominal surgery. It also accompanies inflammatory conditions of the abdomen, intestinal ischemia, pelvic fractures, and back injuries. It occurs early in the course of peritonitis and can result from chemical irritation caused by bile, bacterial toxins, electrolyte imbalances as in hypokalemia, and vascular insufficiency.[57]

The major effects of both types of intestinal obstruction are abdominal distension and loss of fluids and electrolytes (Fig. 37.13).[56–58] Gases and fluids accumulate in the area; if

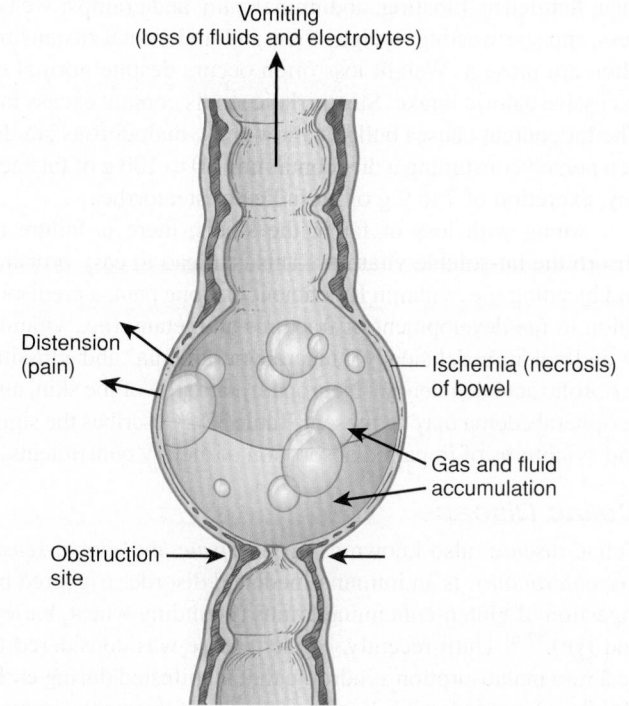

FIGURE 37.13 • Pathophysiology of intestinal obstruction.

untreated, the distension resulting from bowel obstruction tends to perpetuate itself by causing atony of the bowel and further distension.[58] Distension is further aggravated by the accumulation of gases. Approximately 70% of these gases are derived from swallowed air.[57] As the process continues, the distension moves proximally (*i.e.,* toward the mouth), involving additional segments of bowel. Either form of obstruction eventually may lead to strangulation (*i.e.,* interruption of blood flow), gangrenous changes, and, ultimately, perforation of the bowel. The increased pressure in the intestine tends to compromise mucosal blood flow, leading to necrosis and movement of blood into the luminal fluids. This promotes rapid growth of bacteria in the obstructed bowel. Anaerobes grow rapidly in this favourable environment and produce a lethal endotoxin.

The manifestations of intestinal obstruction depend on the degree of obstruction and its duration. With acute obstruction, the onset usually is sudden and dramatic. With chronic conditions, the onset often is more gradual. The cardinal symptoms of intestinal obstruction are pain, absolute constipation, abdominal distension, and vomiting. With mechanical obstruction, the pain is severe and colicky, in contrast with the continuous pain and silent abdomen of paralytic ileus. There also is borborygmus (*i.e.,* rumbling sounds made by propulsion of gas in the intestine); audible, high-pitched peristalsis; and peristaltic rushes.[58] Visible peristalsis may appear along the course of the distended intestine. Extreme restlessness and conscious awareness of intestinal movements are experienced along with weakness, perspiration, and anxiety. Should strangulation of the bowel occur, the symptoms change. The character of the pain shifts from the intermittent colicky pain caused by the hyperperistaltic movements of the intestine to a severe and steady type of pain. Vomiting and fluid and electrolyte disorders occur with both types of obstruction.[57–58]

Diagnosis of intestinal obstruction usually is based on history and physical findings. Plain film radiography of the abdomen may be used to detect the presence of a gas-filled bowel. CT scans and ultrasonography may also be used to detect the presence of mechanical obstruction.

Treatment depends on the cause and type of obstruction. Most cases of adynamic obstruction respond to decompression of the bowel through nasogastric suction and correction of fluid and electrolyte imbalances. Strangulation and complete bowel obstruction require surgical intervention.[56,57]

Peritonitis

Peritonitis is an inflammatory response of the serous membrane that lines the abdominal cavity and covers the visceral organs. It can be caused by bacterial invasion or chemical irritation.[8,9] Most commonly, enteric bacteria enter the peritoneum because of a defect in the wall of one of the abdominal organs. Causes of peritonitis include perforated peptic ulcer, ruptured appendix, perforated diverticulum, gangrenous bowel, pelvic inflammatory disease, and gangrenous gallbladder. Other causes are abdominal trauma, wounds, and ingesting foreign bodies. Generalized peritonitis, although no longer the overwhelming problem it once was, is still a leading cause of death after abdominal surgery.

The peritoneum has several characteristics that increase its vulnerability to or protect it from the effects of peritonitis. One weakness of the peritoneal cavity is that it is a large, unbroken space that favours the dissemination of contaminants. For the same reason, it has a large surface that permits rapid absorption of bacterial toxins into the blood. The peritoneum is particularly well adapted for producing an inflammatory response as a means of controlling infection. It tends, for example, to exude a thick, sticky, and fibrinous substance that adheres to other structures, such as the mesentery and omentum, and that seals off the perforated viscus and aids in localizing the process. Localization is enhanced by sympathetic stimulation that limits intestinal motility. Although the diminished or absent peristalsis that occurs tends to give rise to associated problems, it does inhibit the movement of contaminants throughout the peritoneal cavity.

One of the most important manifestations of peritonitis is the translocation of extracellular fluid into the peritoneal cavity (through weeping or serous fluid from the inflamed peritoneum) and into the bowel as a result of bowel obstruction. Nausea and vomiting cause further losses of fluid. The fluid loss may encourage development of hypovolemia and shock. The onset of peritonitis may be acute, as with a ruptured appendix, or it may have a more gradual onset, as occurs in pelvic inflammatory disease. Pain and tenderness are common symptoms. The pain usually is more intense over the inflamed area. The person with peritonitis usually lies still because any movement aggravates the pain. Breathing often is shallow to prevent movement of the abdominal muscles. The abdomen usually is rigid and sometimes described as boardlike because of reflex muscle guarding. Vomiting is common. Fever, an elevated white blood cell count, tachycardia, and hypotension are common. Hiccups may develop because of irritation of the phrenic nerve. Paralytic ileus occurs shortly after the onset of widespread peritonitis and is accompanied by abdominal distension. Peritonitis that progresses and is untreated leads to toxemia and shock.

Treatment. Treatment measures for peritonitis are directed toward preventing the extension of the inflammatory response, correcting the fluid and electrolyte imbalances that develop, and minimizing the effects of paralytic ileus and abdominal distension. All oral fluids are avoided as surgical intervention may be needed to remove an acutely inflamed appendix or close the opening in a perforated peptic ulcer.. Nasogastric suction, which entails the insertion of a tube placed through the nose into the stomach or intestine, is used to decompress the bowel and relieve the abdominal distension. Fluid and electrolyte replacement is essential and these fluids are prescribed on the basis of frequent blood chemistry determinations. Antibiotics are given to combat infection. Narcotics often are needed for pain relief.

Alterations in Intestinal Absorption

Malabsorption is the failure to transport dietary constituents, such as fats, carbohydrates, proteins, vitamins, and minerals, from the lumen of the intestine into the extracellular fluid compartment for transport to the various parts of the body. It can selectively affect a single component, such as vitamin B_{12} or lactose, or its effects can extend to all the substances absorbed in a specific segment of the intestine. When one segment of the intestine is affected, another may compensate. For example, the ileum may compensate for malabsorption in the proximal small intestine by absorbing substantial amounts of fats, carbohydrates, and amino acids. Similarly, the colon, which normally absorbs water, sodium, chloride, and bicarbonate, can compensate for small intestine malabsorption by absorbing additional end products of bacterial carbohydrate metabolism.

The conditions that impair one or more steps involved in digestion and absorption of nutrients can be divided into three broad categories: intraluminal maldigestion, disorders of transepithelial transport, and lymphatic obstruction. Intraluminal maldigestion involves a defect in processing of nutrients in the intestinal lumen. The most common causes are pancreatic insufficiency, hepatobiliary disease, and intraluminal bacterial growth. Disorders of transepithelial transport are caused by mucosal lesions that impair uptake and transport of available intraluminal nutrients across the mucosal surface of the intestine. They include disorders such as celiac disease and Crohn's disease. Lymphatic obstruction interferes with the transport of the products of fat digestion to the systemic circulation after they have been absorbed by the intestinal mucosa. The process can be interrupted by congenital defects, neoplasms, trauma, and selected infectious diseases.

Malabsorption Syndrome

Persons with intestinal malabsorption usually have symptoms directly referable to the GI tract that include diarrhea, steatorrhea, flatulence, bloating, abdominal pain, and cramps. Weakness, muscle wasting, weight loss, and abdominal distension often are present. Weight loss often occurs despite normal or excessive caloric intake. Steatorrheic stools contain excess fat. The fat content causes bulky, yellow-grey, malodorous stools. In a person consuming a diet containing 80 to 100 g of fat each day, excretion of 7 to 9 g of fat indicates steatorrhea.

Along with loss of fat in the stools, there is failure to absorb the fat-soluble vitamins. This can lead to easy bruising and bleeding (*i.e.*, vitamin K deficiency), bone pain, a predisposition to the development of fractures and tetany (*i.e.*, vitamin D and calcium deficiency), macrocytic anemia, and glossitis (*i.e.*, folic acid deficiency). Neuropathy, atrophy of the skin, and peripheral edema may be present. Table 37.2 describes the signs and symptoms of impaired absorption of dietary constituents.

Celiac Disease

Celiac disease, also known as *celiac sprue* and *gluten-sensitive enteropathy*, is an immune-mediated disorder triggered by ingestion of gluten-containing grains (including wheat, barley, and rye).[59–61] Until recently, celiac disease was considered to be a rare malabsorption syndrome that manifested during early childhood, but today it is known to be one of the most common genetic diseases, with a mean prevalence of 1% globally.[59,60]

TABLE 37.2 SITES OF AND REQUIREMENTS FOR ABSORPTION OF DIETARY CONSTITUENTS AND MANIFESTATIONS OF MALABSORPTION

DIETARY CONSTITUENT	SITE OF ABSORPTION	REQUIREMENTS	MANIFESTATIONS
Water and electrolytes	Mainly small bowel	Osmotic gradient	Diarrhea Dehydration Cramps
Fat	Upper jejunum	Pancreatic lipase Bile salts Functioning lymphatic channels	Weight loss Steatorrhea Fat-soluble vitamin deficiency
Carbohydrates			
Starch	Small intestine	Amylase Maltase Isomaltase α-dextrins	Diarrhea Flatulence Abdominal discomfort
Sucrose	Small intestine	Sucrase	
Lactose	Small intestine	Lactase	
Maltose	Small intestine	Maltase	
Fructose	Small intestine		
Protein	Small intestine	Pancreatic enzymes (*e.g.,* trypsin, chymotrypsin, elastin, etc.)	Loss of muscle mass Weakness Edema
Vitamins			
A	Upper jejunum	Bile salts	Night blindness Dry eyes Corneal irritation
Folic acid	Duodenum and jejunum	Absorptive; may be impaired by some drugs (*i.e.,* anticonvulsants)	Cheilosis Glossitis Megaloblastic anemia
B₁₂	Ileum	Intrinsic factor	Glossitis Neuropathy Megaloblastic anemia
D	Upper jejunum		Bone pain Fractures Tetany
E	Upper jejunum	Bile salts	Uncertain
K	Upper jejunum	Bile salts	Easy bruising and bleeding
Calcium	Duodenum	Bile salts	Bone pain Fractures Tetany
Iron	Duodenum and jejunum	Vitamin D and parathyroid hormone Normal pH (hydrochloric acid secretion)	Iron-deficiency anemia Glossitis

The disease results from an inappropriate T-cell–mediated immune response against ingested α-gliadin (a component of gluten protein) in genetically predisposed people. Almost all persons with the disorder share the major histocompatibility complex class II allele HLA-DQ2 or HLA-DQ8. Persons with the disease have increased levels of antibodies to a variety of antigens, including transglutaminase, endomysium, and gliadin. The resultant immune response produces an intense inflammatory reaction that results in loss of absorptive villi from the small intestine (Fig. 37.14).[59] When the resulting lesions are extensive, they may impair absorption of macronutrients (*i.e.,* proteins, carbohydrates, fats) and micronutrients (*i.e.,* vitamins and minerals). Small bowel involvement is most prominent in the proximal part of the small intestine, where the exposure to gluten is greatest.

There are a number of populations who are at higher risk for celiac disease. These include persons with type 1 diabetes mellitus, other autoimmune endocrinopathies, first- and second-degree relatives of persons with celiac disease, and individuals with Turner syndrome.[59–61] Various malignancies also appear to be a direct result of celiac disease, in that the increased incidence seen in persons with celiac disease returns to that of the general population after several years of a gluten-free diet. These malignancies include head and neck squamous cell carcinoma, small intestinal adenocarcinoma, and non-Hodgkin lymphoma.

FIGURE 37.14 • Celiac disease. **A:** Microscopic view of the normal proximal small intestine showing tall, slender villi with crypts present at the base. **B:** A mucosal biopsy from a patient with advanced celiac disease showing complete loss of the villi with infiltration of the lamina propria by lymphocytes and plasma cells. (From Rubin R., Strayer D. S. (Eds.). (2012). *Rubin's pathology: Clinicopathologic foundations of medicine* (6th ed., p. 643). Philadelphia, PA: Lippincott Williams & Wilkins.)

The classic form of celiac disease presents in infancy and manifests as failure to thrive, diarrhea, abdominal distension, and, occasionally severe malnutrition. Beyond infancy, the manifestations tend to be less dramatic. Older children may present with anemia, constitutional short stature, dental enamel defects, and constipation. In adults, GI symptoms may manifest as diarrhea, constipation, or other symptoms of malabsorption such as bloating, flatus, or belching.

The diagnosis of celiac disease is based on clinical manifestations and confirmed by serologic tests and intestinal biopsy. Based on very high sensitivities, the best available tests are the immunoglobulin (Ig) A antihuman tissue transglutaminase (TTG) and IgA endomysial antibody immunofluorescence (EMA) tests. Biopsies of the proximal small bowel are indicated in persons with a positive celiac disease antibody test. Usually, additional laboratory tests are done to determine if the disorder has resulted in nutritional disorders such as iron-deficiency anemia.[59–61]

The primary treatment of celiac disease consists of life-long removal of gluten and related proteins from the diet. Gluten is the primary protein in wheat, barley, and rye. Oat products, which are nontoxic, may be contaminated with wheat during processing. Many gluten-free types of bread, cereals, cookies, and other products are available. Meats, vegetables, fruits, and dairy products are free of gluten as long as they are not contaminated during processing. Complete exclusion of dietary gluten generally results in rapid and complete healing of the intestinal mucosa.

Neoplasms

Epithelial cell tumours of the intestines are a major cause of morbidity and mortality worldwide. The colon, including the rectum, is the site of more primary neoplasms than any other organ in the body.[8] Although the small intestine accounts for approximately 75% of the length of the GI tract, it is an uncommon site of benign or malignant tumours.

Adenomatous Polyps

By far the most common types of neoplasms of the intestine are adenomatous polyps. A GI polyp can be described as a mass of colonic epithelium that protrudes into the lumen of the gut.[8,9] Polyps can be subdivided according to their attachment to the bowel wall (sessile [raised mucosal nodules] or pedunculated [attached by a stalk]); their histopathologic appearance (hyperplastic or adenomatous); and their neoplastic potential (benign or malignant).[9]

Adenomatous polyps (adenomas) are benign neoplasms that arise from the mucosal epithelium of the intestine. They are composed of neoplastic cells that have proliferated in excess of those needed to replace the cells that normally are shed from the mucosal surface (Fig. 37.15). The pathogenesis of adenoma formation involves neoplastic alteration in the replication of the crypt epithelial cells. There may be diminished apoptosis (see Chapter 5), persistence of cell replication, and failure of cell maturation and differentiation of the cells that migrate to the surface of the crypts.[9] Normally, DNA synthesis ceases as the cells reach the upper two thirds of the crypts, after which they mature, migrate to the surface, and become senescent. They then become apoptotic and are shed from the surface.[9] Adenomas arise from a disruption in this sequence, such that the epithelial cells retain their proliferative ability throughout the entire length of the crypt. Alterations in cell differentiation can lead to dysplasia and progression to the development of invasive carcinoma.

More than half of all adenomatous polyps are located in the rectosigmoid colon and can be detected by rectal examination or sigmoidoscopy.[9] The remainder are evenly distributed throughout the rest of the colon. Adenomas can range in size

FIGURE 37.15 • The histogenesis of adenomatous polyps of the colon. The initial proliferative abnormality of the colonic mucosa, the extension of the mitotic zone in the crypts, leads to accumulation of mucosal cells. The formation of adenomas may reflect epithelial–mesenchymal interactions. (From Rubin R., Strayer D. S. (Eds.). (2012). *Rubin's pathology: Clinicopathologic foundations of medicine* (6th ed., p. 663). Philadelphia, PA: Lippincott Williams & Wilkins.)

from a barely visible nodule to a large, sessile mass. They can be classified as tubular, villous, or tubulovillous adenomas.

Tubular adenomas, which constitute approximately 65% of benign large bowel adenomas, typically are smooth-surfaced spheres, usually less than 2 cm in diameter, that are attached to the mucosal surface by a stalk.[9] Although most tubular adenomas display little epithelial dysplasia, approximately 20% show a range of dysplastic changes, from mild nuclear changes to frank invasive carcinoma. *Villous adenomas* constitute 10% of adenomas of the colon.[9] They are found predominantly in the rectosigmoid colon. They typically are broad-based, elevated lesions, with a shaggy, cauliflower-like surface. In contrast to tubular adenomas, villous adenomas are more likely to contain malignant cells. When invasive carcinoma develops, there is no stalk to isolate the tumour and invasion is directly into the wall of the colon. *Tubulovillous adenomas* manifest both tubular and villous architecture. They are intermediate between tubular and villous adenomas in terms of invasive carcinoma risk.

Most cases of colorectal cancer begin as benign adenomatous colonic polyps. The frequency of polyps increases with age, and the prevalence of adenomatous polyps significantly increases after 60 years of age.[24] Men and women are equally affected. The peak incidence of adenomatous polyps precedes by some years the peak for colorectal cancer. Programs that provide careful follow-up for persons with adenomatous polyps and removal of all suspect lesions have substantially reduced the incidence of colorectal cancer.

Colorectal Cancer

According to Canadian Cancer Society, colorectal cancer is the second leading cause of cancer mortality for males and the third leading cause for females in Canada. For 2015 it is estimated that approximately 25,100 Canadians will be diagnosed with colorectal cancer and there will be approximately 9,300 deaths.[62] The death rate for colorectal cancer has been steadily declining since the early 1980s.[15] This may due to a decreased number of cases, earlier diagnosis, and improved treatments.

The cause of cancer of the colon and rectum is largely unknown. Its incidence increases with age, as evidenced by the fact that approximately 90% of persons who develop this form of cancer are older than 50 years of age.[15] Its incidence is increased among persons with a family history of cancer, persons with Crohn's disease or ulcerative colitis, and those with familial adenomatous polyposis of the colon. Persons with a familial risk—those who have two or more first- or second-degree relatives (or both) with colorectal cancer—make up approximately 20% of all persons with colorectal cancer. Familial adenomatous polyposis is a rare autosomal dominant trait linked to a mutation of the *APC* gene on the long arm of chromosome 5.[9] Persons with the disorder develop multiple adenomatous polyps of the colon at an early age.[8,9,63] Carcinoma of the colon is inevitable, often by 40 years of age, unless a total colectomy is performed.

Diet also is thought to play a role.[62] Attention has focused on dietary fat intake, refined sugar intake, fibre intake, and the adequacy of such protective micronutrients as vitamins A, C, and E in the diet. It has been hypothesized that a high level of fat in the diet increases the synthesis of bile acids in the liver, which may be converted to potential carcinogens by the bacterial flora in the colon. Bacterial organisms in particular are suspected of converting bile acids to carcinogens; their proliferation is enhanced by a high dietary level of refined sugars. Dietary fibre is thought to increase stool bulk and thereby dilute and remove potential carcinogens. Refined diets often contain reduced amounts of vitamins A, C, and E, which may act as oxygen free radical scavengers.

Reports indicate that aspirin may protect against colorectal cancer.[64] Although the mechanism of aspirin's action is unknown, it may be related to its effect on the synthesis of prostaglandins, one or more of which may be involved in signal systems that influence cell proliferation or tumour growth. Aspirin inhibits cyclooxygenase, the enzyme which catalyzes the conversion of arachidonic acid in cell membranes to prostaglandins. One form of cyclooxygenase, COX-2, promotes inflammation and cell proliferation, and colorectal cancers often overexpress this enzyme. Regular use of aspirin appears to reduce the risk of colorectal cancers that overexpress COX-2 but not the risk of colorectal cancers with weak or absent expression of COX-2.[64] Supplemental folate and calcium, selected vitamins, and postmenopausal hormone replacement therapy (estrogen) also have been proposed as potential chemoprotective agents.[62] All of these agents will require more extensive study before they can be recommended for long-term chemoprevention of colorectal cancer.

Usually, cancer of the colon and rectum is present for a long time before it produces symptoms. Bleeding is a highly significant early symptom, and usually is the one that causes persons to seek medical care. Other symptoms include a change in bowel habits, diarrhea or constipation, and sometimes a sense of urgency or incomplete emptying of the bowel. Pain usually is a late symptom.

The prognosis for persons with colorectal cancer depends largely on the extent of bowel involvement and on the presence of metastasis at the time of diagnosis. Colorectal cancer commonly is classified into four tumour, node, and metastasis (TNM) stages. In this system, a stage I tumour is limited to invasion of the mucosal and submucosal layers of the colon and has a 5-year survival rate of 90% to 100%. A stage II (lymph node-negative) tumour infiltrates into, but not through, the muscularis externa, and has a 5-year survival rate of 70% to 85%. With a stage III (lymph node-positive) tumour, in which there is invasion of the serosal layer and regional lymph node involvement, the 5-year survival rate is 40% to 60%. Stage IV (metastatic) tumours penetrate the serosa or adjacent organs and have a much poorer prognosis.[62]

Screening, Diagnosis, and Treatment. The single most important prognostic indicator of colorectal cancer is the extent (stage) of the tumour at time of diagnosis.[62] Therefore, the challenge is to discover the tumours at their earliest stages. Among the methods used for the detection of colorectal cancers are the digital rectal examination and the fecal occult blood test, usually done during routine physical examinations; x-ray studies using barium (*e.g.,* barium enema); and flexible sigmoidoscopy and colonoscopy.[5,8,65] Digital rectal examinations are most helpful in detecting neoplasms of the rectum. Rectal examination should be considered a routine part of a good physical examination. The Canadian Cancer Society recommends that all asymptomatic men and women, beginning at 50 years of age, should have a fecal occult blood test at least every 2 years. With any positive test, individuals should follow up with a colonoscopy, double contrast barium enema, and/or a flexible sigmoidoscopy.[62] People with increased risk for colorectal cancer should be screened earlier and more often. Colonoscopy is recommended whenever a screening test is positive.[62]

Almost all cancers of the colon and rectum bleed intermittently, although the amount of blood is small and usually not apparent in the stools. It therefore is feasible to screen for colorectal cancers using commercially prepared tests for occult blood in the stool.[62] Two slides must be prepared from three consecutive bowel movements. To reduce the likelihood of false-positive test results, persons are instructed to avoid NSAIDs such as ibuprofen and aspirin for 7 days before testing; to avoid vitamin C in excess of 250 mg from either supplements or citrus fruits for 3 days before testing; and to avoid red meats for 3 days before testing. The most commonly used tests are guaiac-based fecal occult blood tests, which are uncomplicated and can be processed in local medical laboratories. There are also immunochemistry-based tests that may be processed in a laboratory or in the healthcare provider's office, but they are less commonly used. Persons with a positive fecal occult blood test should be referred to their healthcare provider for further study. Usually, a physical examination, rectal examination, and flexible sigmoidoscopy or colonoscopy are done.

Flexible sigmoidoscopy involves examination of the rectum and sigmoid colon with a hollow, lighted tube that is inserted through the rectum. The procedure is performed without sedation and is well tolerated. Approximately 40% of cancers and polyps are out of the reach of the sigmoidoscope, emphasizing the need for fecal occult blood tests. Polyps can be removed or tissue can be obtained for biopsy during the procedure.

Colonoscopy provides a means for examining the entire bowel, with the examination ending at the cecum.[66] The colonoscope is a tubelike instrument with sufficient flexibility to maneuver through the bends and folds of the colon. The instrument is far more complex than a sigmoidoscope because it must be capable of insufflation, irrigation, suction and passage of biopsy forceps or polypectomy snare. Like sigmoidoscopes, the tip of the instrument is equipped with a small video camera and a light to provide high-resolution visualization of the bowel wall. Colonoscopy is used for screening persons at high risk for development of cancer of the colon (*e.g.,* those with ulcerative colitis and for those with symptoms). It is also used for obtaining a biopsy and for removing polyps. Although this method is one of the most accurate for detecting early colorectal cancers, it is expensive and time consuming and must be done by a person who is highly trained in the use of the instrument.

The only recognized treatment for cancer of the colon and rectum is surgical removal. Preoperative radiation therapy may be used and has in some cases demonstrated increased 5-year survival rates. Postoperative adjuvant chemotherapy may be used. Radiation therapy and chemotherapy are used as palliative treatment methods.

Disorders of the small and large intestines include IBS, IBD, diverticular disease, disorders of motility (*i.e.,* diarrhea, constipation, fecal impaction, and intestinal obstruction), alterations in intestinal absorption, and colorectal cancer.

Irritable bowel syndrome is a functional disorder characterized by a variable combination of chronic and recurrent intestinal symptoms not explained by structural or biochemical abnormalities. The term inflammatory bowel disease is used to designate two inflammatory conditions: Crohn's disease, which affects the small and large bowel, and ulcerative colitis, which affects the colon and rectum. Both are chronic diseases characterized by remissions and exacerbations of diarrhea, weight loss, fluid and electrolyte disorders, and systemic signs of inflammation.

Infectious forms of enterocolitis include viral (*e.g.,* rotavirus), bacterial (*e.g., C. difficile* and *E. coli* O157:H7), and protozoal (*E. histolytica*) infections. Diverticular disease includes diverticulosis, which is a condition in which the mucosal layer of the colon herniates through the muscularis layer, and diverticulitis, in which there is inflammation and gross or microscopic perforation of the diverticulum.

Diarrhea and constipation represent disorders of intestinal motility. Diarrhea is characterized by excessively frequent passage of stools. It can be acute or chronic and can be caused by infectious organisms, food intolerance, drugs, or intestinal disease. Acute diarrheas that last less than 4 days are predominantly caused by infectious agents and follow a self-limited course. Chronic diarrhea persists beyond 4 weeks and is caused by the presence of hyperosmotic luminal contents, increased intestinal secretory processes, inflammatory conditions, and infectious processes. Constipation can be defined as the infrequent passage of stools; it is commonly caused by failure to respond to the urge to defecate, inadequate fibre or fluid intake, weakness of the abdominal muscles, inactivity and bed rest, pregnancy, hemorrhoids, and GI disease. Fecal impaction is the retention of hardened or putty-like stool in the rectum and colon, which interferes with normal passage of feces. Intestinal obstruction designates an impairment of movement of intestinal contents in a cephalocaudad direction as the result of mechanical or paralytic mechanisms. Peritonitis is an inflammatory response of the serous membrane that lines the abdominal cavity and covers the visceral organs. It can be caused by bacterial invasion or chemical irritation resulting from perforation of the viscera or abdominal organs.

Malabsorption results from the impaired absorption of nutrients and other dietary constituents from the intestine. It can involve a single dietary constituent, such as vitamin B_{12}, or extend to involve all the substances absorbed in a particular part of the small intestine. Malabsorption can result from disease of the small bowel and disorders that impair digestion and, in some cases, obstruct the lymph flow by which fats are transported to the general circulation. Celiac disease is an immune-mediated disorder triggered by ingestion of gluten-containing grains (including wheat, barley, and rye).

Colorectal cancer remains one of the leading causes of cancer deaths in Canada and is seen most commonly in persons older than 50 years of age. Most, if not all, cancers of the colon and rectum arise in pre-existing adenomatous polyps. Programs that provide careful follow-up for persons with adenomatous polyps and removal of all suspect lesions have substantially reduced the incidence of colorectal cancer.

REVIEW EXERCISES

1. Anticholinergic drugs are often effective in treating the nausea and vomiting that accompany motion sickness but are relatively ineffective in treating the nausea and vomiting associated with chemotherapy agents used in the treatment of cancer.

   A. *Explain.*

2. A 40-year-old man reports to his healthcare provider complaining of "heartburn" that occurs after eating and also wakes him up at night. He is overweight, admits to enjoying fatty foods, and usually lies down on the sofa and watches TV after dinner. He also complains that lately he has been having a cough and some wheezing. A diagnosis of GERD was made.

   A. *Explain the cause of heartburn and why it becomes worse after eating.*

   B. *Persons with GERD are advised to lose weight, avoid eating fatty foods, remain sitting after eating, and to sleep with their head slightly elevated. Explain the possible relationship between these situations and the occurrence of reflux.*

   C. *Explain the possible relationship between GERD and the respiratory symptoms this man is having.*

3. A 36-year-old woman who has been taking aspirin for back pain experiences a sudden episode of tachycardia and feeling faint, accompanied by the vomiting of a coffee-ground emesis and the passing of a tarry stool. She relates that she has not had any signs of a "stomach ulcer" such as pain or heartburn.

   A. *Relate the mucosal protective effects of prostaglandins to the development of peptic ulcer associated with aspirin or NSAID use.*

   B. *Explain the apparent suddenness of the bleeding and the fact that the woman did not experience pain as a warning signal.*

4. A 29-year-old woman has been diagnosed with Crohn's disease. Her medical history reveals that she began having symptoms of the disease at 24 years of age and that her mother died of complications of the disease at 54 years of age. She complains of diarrhea and chronic cramping abdominal pain.

A. *Define the term inflammatory bowel disease (IBD) and compare the pathophysiologic processes and manifestations of Crohn's disease and ulcerative colitis.*

B. *Describe the possible association between genetic and environmental factors in the pathogenesis of Crohn's disease.*

C. *Relate the use of the monoclonal antibody infliximab to the pathogenesis of the inflammatory lesions that occur in Crohn's disease.*

References

1. PHAC. (2009). Investing in prevention the economic perspective. Available online at: http://www.phac-aspc.gc.ca/ph-sp/preveco-index-eng.php. Accessed July 6, 2014.

2. Canadian Digestive Health Foundation. (2009). The Canadian digestive health foundation national digestive disorders prevalence & impact study report. Available online at: http://cdhf.ca/en/news. Accessed July 6, 2014.

3. Hall J. E. (2011). *Textbook of medical physiology* (12th ed.). Philadelphia, PA: W. B. Saunders.

4. Becker D. E. (2010). Nausea, vomiting, and hiccups: A review of mechanisms and treatment. *Anesthesia Progress, 57*(4), 150–157.

5. El-Gohary Y., Gittes G. K., Tovar J. A. (2010). Congenital anomalies of the esophagus. *Seminars in Pediatric Surgery, 19*(3), 186–193.

6. Khan S., Orenstein S. R. (2011). Section 3: The esophagus. In Kliegman R. M., Stanton B. F., St. Geme J. W., et al. (Eds.), *Nelson textbook of pediatrics.* (19th ed.). Philadelphia, PA: Saunders Elsevier.

7. DeVault K. R. (2010). Chapter 12: Symptoms of esophageal disease. In Feldman M., Friedman L. S., Brandt L. J, (Eds.), (*Sleisenger and fordtran's gastrointestinal and liver disease* (9th ed.). Philadelphia, PA: Saunders Elsevier.

8. Turner J. R. (2010). Chapter 17: The gastrointestinal tract. In Kumar V., Abbas A. K., Fausto N., et al. (Eds.), *Robbins and cotran pathologic basis of disease.* (8th ed.). Philadelphia, PA: Elsevier Saunders.

9. Rubin R. (2012). Chapter 13: The gastrointestinal tract. In Rubin, R., Strayer D. S. (Eds.), (*Rubin's pathology: Clinicopathologic foundations of medicine* (6th ed.). Philadelphia, PA: Lippincott Williams & Wilkins.

10. Feinman M., Haut E. R. (2014). Upper gastrointestinal bleeding. *Surgical Clinics of North America, 94*(1), 43–53.

11. Kandulski A., Malfertheiner P. (2012). Gastroesophageal reflux disease: From reflux episodes to mucosal inflammation. *Nature Reviews Gastroenterology & Hepatology, 9*(1), 15–22.

12. Katz P. O., Gerson L. B., Vela M. F. (2013). Guidelines for the diagnosis and management of gastroesophageal reflux disease. *American Journal of Gastroenterology, 108*(3), 308–328.

13. Badreddine R. J., Wang K. K. (2010). Barrett esophagus: An update. *Nature Reviews Gastroenterology & Hepatology, 7*(7), 369–378.

14. Lightdale J. R., Gremse D. A. (2013). Gastroesophageal reflux: Management guidance for the pediatrician. *Pediatrics, 131*(5), e1684–e1695.

15. Canadian Cancer Society's Advisory Committee. (2015). *Canadian Cancer Statistics, 2015.* Toronto, ON: Canadian Cancer Society.

16. Canadian Cancer Society. (2014). Esophageal cancer. Available online at: http://www.cancer.ca/en/cancer-information/cancer-type/esophageal/esophageal-cancer/?region=on. Accessed July 6, 2014.

17. Otterstatter M. C., Brierley J. D., De P., et al. (2012). Esophageal cancer in Canada: Trends according to morphology and anatomical location. *Canadian Journal of Gastroenterology, 26*(10), 723–728.

18. Wallace J. L. (2008). Prostaglandins, NSAIDs, and gastric mucosal protection: Why doesn't the stomach digest itself? *Physiological Reviews, 88*(4), 1547–1565.

19. Malfertheiner P., Chan F. K., McColl K. E. (2009). Peptic ulcer disease. *Lancet, 374*(9677), 1449–1461.

20. McColl K. E. (2010). Clinical practice. Helicobacter pylori infection. *New England Journal Medicine, 362*(17), 1597–1604.

21. Goodman K. J., Jacobson K., Zanten S. V. (2008). Helicobacter pylori infection in Canadian and related arctic aboriginal populations. *Canadian Journal of Gastroenterology, 22*(3), 289–295.

22. Krejs G. J. (2010). Gastric cancer: epidemiology and risk factors. *Digestive Diseases, 28*(4–5), 600–603.

23. Canadian Cancer Society. (2014). Stomach cancer. Available online at: http://www.cancer.ca/en/cancer-information/cancer-type/stomach/stomach-cancer/?region=on. Accessed July 6, 2014.

24. Seddik H., Ahid S., El Adioui T. E., et al. (2013). Sequential therapy versus standard triple-drug therapy for Helicobacter pylori eradication: A prospective randomized study. *European Journal of Clinical Pharmacology, 69*(9), 1709–1715.

25. Greenberg D. E, Muraca M. (Eds.). (2008). *Canadian clinical practice guidelines 2008 – H. pylori.* Toronto, ON: Elsevier.

26. Targownik L. (2014). Gastrointestinal disorders: Dyspepsia and peptic ulcer disease. Available online at: http://www.e-therapeutics.ca. Accessed July 7, 2014.

27. Epelboym I., Mazeh H. (2013). Zollinger–Ellison syndrome: Classical considerations and current controversies. *The Oncologist, 19*(1), 44–50.

28. Valle J. D. (2012). Chapter 293: Peptic ulcer disease and related disorders. In Longo D. L., Fauci A. S., Kasper D. L., et al., (Eds.), *Harrison's principles of internal medicine* (18th ed.). New York: McGraw-Hill Company.

29. Canadian Digestive Health Foundation. (2014). Irritable bowel syndrome. Available online at: http://www.cdhf.ca/en/disorders/details/id/12. Accessed July 7, 2014.

30. Rome Foundation, Inc. (2013). Rome III disorders and criteria. Available online at: http://www.theromefoundation.org/criteria/. Accessed July 7, 2014.

31. Canadian Digestive Health Foundation. (2014). Inflammatory bowel disease. Available online at: http://www.cdhf.ca/en/disorders/details/id/22. Accessed July 7, 2014.

32. Abraham C., Cho J. H. (2009). Inflammatory bowel disease. *New England Journal Medicine, 361*(21), 2066–2078.

33. Khor B., Gardet A., Xavier R. J. (2011). Genetics and pathogenesis of inflammatory bowel disease. *Nature, 474*(7351), 307–317.

34. Chami G. (updated 2014). Gastrointestinal disorders: Inflammatory bowel disease. In Repchinsky C., (Ed.). *e-Therapeutics.* [Online] Ottawa: Canadian Pharmacists Association.

35. Kornbluth A., Sachar D. B. (2009). Ulcerative colitis practice guidelines in adults: American College of Gastroenterology, practice parameters committee. *American Journal of Gastroenterology, 105*(3), 500–524.

36. Goldman R. D. (2012). Effectiveness of rotavirus vaccine in preventing severe acute gastroenteritis in children. *Canadian Family Physician, 58*(2), 270–271.

37. National Advisory Committee on Immunization. (2010). Updated statement on the use of rotavirus vaccines. *Canada Communicable Disease Report, 36*(4), 1–37.

38. Public Health Agency of Canada. (2014). Provincial and territorial web sites and immunizations schedules. Available online at: http://www.phac-aspc.gc.ca/im/is-pi-eng.php. Accessed July 9, 2014.

39. Higa J. T., Kelly C. P. (2014). New drugs and strategies for management of Clostridium difficile colitis. *Journal of Intensive Care Medicine, 29*(4), 190–199.

40. Van Nood E., Speelman P., Nieuwdorp M., et al. (2014). Fecal microbiota transplantation: Facts and controversies. *Current Opinion in Gastroenterology, 30*(1), 34–39.

41. Bharucha A. E., Dorn S. D., Lembo A., Pressman A.; American Gastroenterological Association. (2013). American Gastroenterological

Association medial position statement on constipation. *Gastroenterology, 144*(1), 211–217.

42. Liu Z., Calvin S., Middleton D. (2007). Descriptive epidemiology of verotoxin-producing E. coli reported in Ontario, 1996–2005. *Canada Communicable Disease Report, 33*(7), 69–76.

43. Croxen M. A., Law R. J., Scholz R., et al. (2013). Recent advances in understanding enteric pathogenic Escherichia coli. *Clinical Microbiology Reviews, 26*(4), 822–880.

44. Canadian Food Inspection Agency. (2013). Safe internal cooking temperatures. Available online at: http://www.inspection.gc.ca/food/information-for-consumers/fact-sheets/food-handling/eng/1331871496701/1331871695247. Accessed July 9, 2014.

45. Rosenthal P. J. (2014). Chapter 35: Protozoal & helminthic infections. In Papadakis M. A., McPhee S. J., Rabow M. V., (Eds.), (*Current medical diagnosis and treatment 2014.* New York: McGraw-Hill.

46. Chus A., Liacouras C. A. (2011). Chapter 325: Ileus, adhesions, intussusception, and closed-loop obstructions. In Kliegman R. M., Stanton B. F., St. Geme J. W., et al. (Eds.), *Nelson textbook of pediatrics* (19th ed.). Philadelphia, PA: Saunders Elsevier.

47. Weizman A. V., Nguyen G. C. (2011). Diverticular disease: Epidemiology and management. *Canadian Journal of Gastroenterology, 25*(7), 385–389.

48. Humes D. J., Spiller R. C. (2014). Review article: The pathogenesis and management of acute colonic diverticulitis. *Alimentary Pharmacology and Therapeutics, 39*(4), 359–370.

49. Petroianu A. (2012). Diagnosis of acute appendicitis. *International Journal of Surgery, 10*(3), 115–119.

50. Salminen P., Paajanen H., Rautio T., et al. (2015). Antibiotic therapy vs appendectomy for treatment of uncompleted acute appendicitis. *Journal of the American Medical Association, 313*(23), 2340–2348.

51. Camilleri M., Murray J. A. (2012). Chapter 40: Diarrhea and constipation. In Longo D., Fauci A., Kasper D. L., et al. (Eds.), *Harrison's principles of internal medicine* (18th ed.). New York: McGraw-Hill.

52. Schiller L. R., Sellin J. H. (2010). Chapter 15: Diarrhea. In Feldman M., Friedman L. S., Brandt L. J. *Sleisenger and fordtran's gastrointestinal and liver disease* (9th ed.). Philadelphia, PA: Saunders Elsevier.

53. Farthing M., Salam M. A., Lindberg G., et al. (2013). Acute diarrhea in adults and children: A global perspective. *Journal of Clinical Gastroenterology, 47*(1), 12–20.

54. Duro C., Duggan D. (2007). The BRAT diet for acute diarrhea in children: Should it be used? *Practical Gastroenterology, June 2007,* Series 51, 60–68.

55. Craft L., Prahlow J. A. (2011). From fecal impaction to colon perforation. *American Journal of Nursing, 111*(8), 38–43.

56. Jackson P. G., Raiji M. T. (2011). Evaluation and management of intestinal obstruction. *American Family Physician, 83*(2), 159–165.

57. Silen W. (2012). Chapter 299: Acute intestinal obstruction. In Longo D., Fauci A., Kasper D. L., et al. (Eds.), *Harrison's principles of internal medicine* (18th ed.). New York, NY: McGraw-Hill.

58. Turnage R. H., Heldmann M. (2010). Chapter 119: Intestinal obstruction. In Feldman M., Friedman L. S., Brandt L. J. *Sleisenger and fordtran's gastrointestinal and liver disease* (9th ed.). Philadelphia, PA: Saunders Elsevier.

59. Fasano A., Catassi C. (2012). Celiac disease. *New England Journal Medicine, 367*(25), 2419–2426.

60. Gujral N., Freeman H. J., Thomson A. B. (2012). Celiac disease: Prevalence, diagnosis, pathogenesis and treatment. *World Journal of Gastroenterology, 18*(42), 6036–6059.

61. Kupfer S. S., Jabri B. (2012). Celiac disease pathophysiology. *Gastrointestinal Endoscopy Clinics of North American, 22*(4), 639–660.

62. Canadian Cancer Society. (2015). Colorectal cancer. Available online at: http://www.cancer.ca/en/cancer-information/cancer-type/colorectal/colorectal-cancer/?region = bc. Accessed September 20, 2015.

63. Jasperson K. W., Tuohy T. M., Neklason D. W., et al. (2010). Hereditary and familial colon cancer. *Gastroenterology, 138*(6), 2044–2058.

64. Tougeron D., Sha D., Manthravadi S., et al. (2014). Aspirin and colorectal cancer: Back to the future. *Clinical Cancer Research, 20*(5), 1087–1094.

65. Korownyk C., Kolber M. R. (2012). Is quadruple therapy the new triple therapy for H pylori? *Canadian Family Physician, 58*(1), 58.

66. Zauber A. G., Winawer S. J., O'Brien M. J., et al. (2012). Colonoscopic polypectomy and long-term prevention of colorectal cancer deaths. *New England Jouranl of Medicine, 366*(8), 687–696.

Visit thePoint **http://thePoint.lww.com for animations, journal articles, and more!**

Disorders of Hepatobiliary and Exocrine Pancreas Function

38

The liver, the gallbladder, and the exocrine pancreas are classified as accessory organs of the gastrointestinal tract. In addition to producing digestive secretions, the liver and the pancreas have other important functions. The endocrine pancreas, for example, supplies the insulin and glucagon needed in cell metabolism, whereas the liver synthesizes glucose, plasma proteins, and blood clotting factors and is responsible for the degradation and elimination of drugs and hormones, among other functions. This chapter focuses on functions and disorders of the liver, the biliary tract and gallbladder, and the exocrine pancreas.

THE LIVER AND HEPATOBILIARY SYSTEM

After completing this section of the chapter, you should be able to meet the following objectives:

- Describe the lobular structures of the liver.
- Describe the function of the liver in terms of carbohydrate, protein, and fat metabolism.
- Characterize the function of the liver in terms of bilirubin elimination and describe the pathogenesis of unconjugated and conjugated hyperbilirubinemia.
- Relate the mechanism of bile formation and elimination to the development of cholestasis.
- List four laboratory tests used to assess liver function and relate them to impaired liver function.

The liver is the largest visceral organ in the body, weighing approximately 1.5 kg in the adult.[1] It is located below the diaphragm and occupies much of the right hypochondrium (Fig. 38.1). The liver is surrounded by a tough fibroelastic capsule called the *Glisson capsule*. The liver is anatomically divided into two large lobes (the right and left lobes) and two smaller lobes (the caudate and quadrate lobes). Except

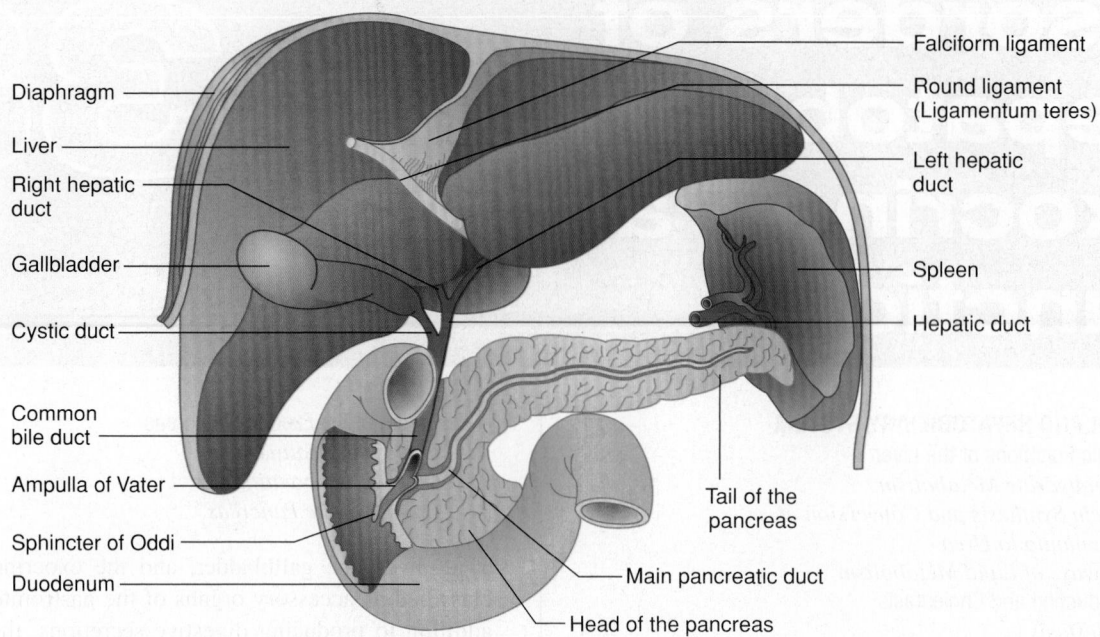

FIGURE 38.1 • The liver and biliary system, including the gallbladder and bile ducts.

Labels (clockwise from top left): Diaphragm, Liver, Right hepatic duct, Gallbladder, Cystic duct, Common bile duct, Ampulla of Vater, Sphincter of Oddi, Duodenum, Head of the pancreas, Main pancreatic duct, Tail of the pancreas, Hepatic duct, Spleen, Left hepatic duct, Round ligament (Ligamentum teres), Falciform ligament

for the portion that is in the epigastric area, the liver is contained within the rib cage, and cannot normally be palpated in healthy persons.

The liver is unique among the abdominal organs in having a dual blood supply consisting of a venous (portal) supply through the hepatic portal vein and an arterial supply through the hepatic artery. Approximately 300 ml of blood per minute enters the liver through the hepatic artery; another 1,050 ml/minute enters by way of the valveless portal vein and overall represents 25% of the resting cardiac output.[1] The venous blood delivered by the hepatic portal vein comes from the digestive tract and major abdominal organs, including the pancreas and spleen (Fig. 38.2). The portal blood supply carries nutrient and toxic materials absorbed in the intestine, blood cells, and their breakdown products from the spleen, and insulin and glucagon from the pancreas. Although the blood from the portal vein is incompletely saturated with oxygen, it supplies approximately 60% to 70% of the oxygen needs of the liver.

The venous outflow from the liver is carried by the valveless hepatic veins, which empty into the inferior vena cava just below the level of the diaphragm. The pressure difference between the hepatic vein and the portal vein normally is such that the liver stores approximately 450 ml of blood or almost 10% of the body's total blood volume.[1] This blood can be shifted back into the general circulation during periods of hypovolemia and shock. In right heart failure in which the pressure in the vena cava increases, blood backs up and accumulates in the liver.

The *lobules* are the functional units of the liver. Each lobule is a cylindrical structure that measures approximately 0.8 to 2 mm in diameter and several millimetres in length. There are approximately 50,000 to 100,000 lobules in the liver.[1] Each lobule is organized around a central vein that empties into the hepatic veins and from there into the vena cava. The portal

triad consists of the terminal bile ducts and small branches of the portal vein and hepatic artery; they are located at the periphery of the lobule. Plates of hepatic cells radiate centrifugally from the central vein like spokes on a wheel (Fig. 38.3). These hepatic plates are separated by wide, thin-walled sinusoidal capillaries, called *sinusoids,* that extend from the periphery of the lobule to its central vein. The sinusoids are supplied by blood from the portal vein and hepatic artery. The sinusoids are in intimate contact with the hepatocytes and provide for the exchange of substances between the blood and liver cells. The sinusoids are lined with two types of cells: the typical capillary endothelial cells and Kupffer cells. *Kupffer cells* are reticuloendothelial cells that are capable of removing and phagocytizing old and defective blood cells, bacteria, and other foreign material from the portal blood as it flows through the sinusoid.[1] This phagocytic action removes enteric bacilli and other harmful substances that filter into the blood from the intestine.

A major exocrine function of the liver is bile secretion. The lobules also are supplied by small tubular channels, called *bile canaliculi,* that lie between the cell membranes of adjacent hepatocytes. The bile produced by the hepatocytes flows into the canaliculi and then to the periphery of the lobules, draining into progressively larger ducts, until it reaches the right and left hepatic ducts. The intrahepatic and extrahepatic bile ducts often are collectively referred to as the *hepatobiliary tree.* These ducts unite to form the common duct (Fig. 38.1). The common duct, which is approximately 10 to 15 cm long, descends and passes behind the pancreas and enters the descending duodenum. The pancreatic duct joins the common duct at a short dilated tube called the *hepatopancreatic ampulla* (ampulla of Vater), which empties into the duodenum through the duodenal papilla. Muscle tissue at the junction of the papilla, sometimes called the *sphincter of*

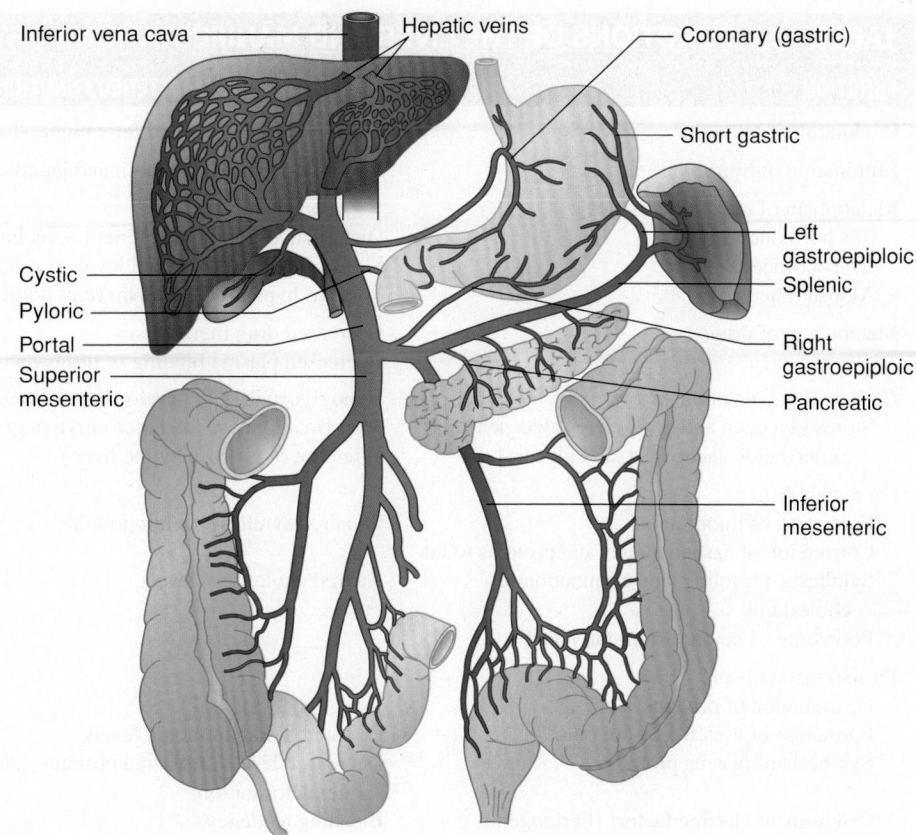

FIGURE 38.2 • The portal circulation. Blood from the gastrointestinal tract, spleen, and pancreas travels to the liver through the portal vein before moving into the vena cava for return to the heart.

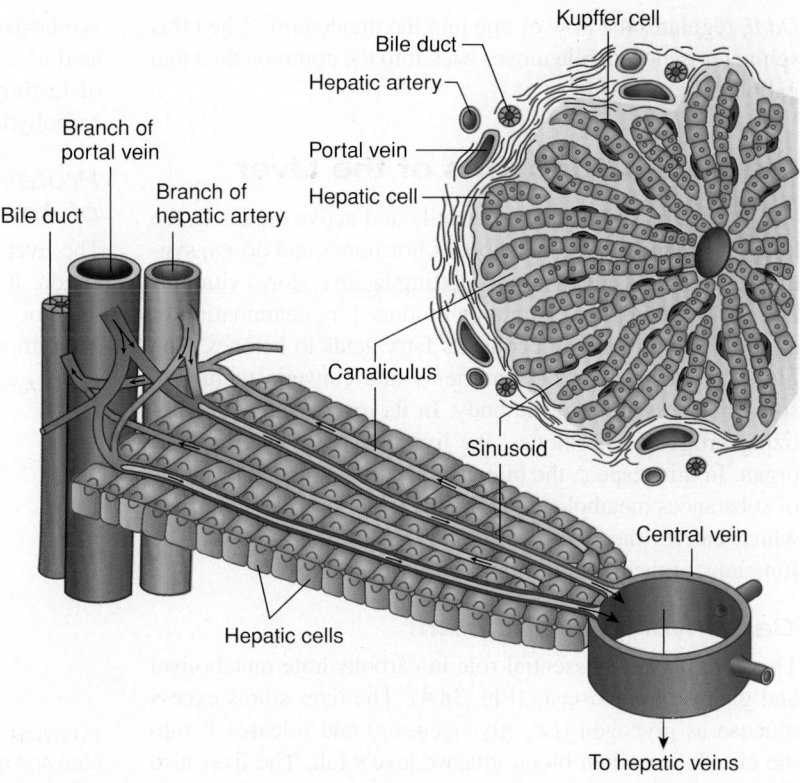

FIGURE 38.3 • A section of liver lobule showing the location of the hepatic veins, hepatic cells, liver sinusoids, and branches of the portal vein and hepatic artery.

TABLE 38.1 FUNCTIONS OF THE LIVER AND MANIFESTATIONS OF ALTERED FUNCTION

FUNCTION	MANIFESTATIONS OF ALTERED FUNCTION
Production of bile salts	Malabsorption of fat and fat-soluble vitamins
Elimination of bilirubin	Elevation in serum bilirubin and jaundice
Metabolism of steroid hormones	
Sex hormones	Disturbances in gonadal function, including gynecomastia in the male
Glucocorticoids	Signs of increased cortisol levels (*i.e.,* Cushing syndrome)
Aldosterone	Signs of hyperaldosteronism (*e.g.,* sodium retention and hypokalemia)
Metabolism of drugs	Decreased drug metabolism
	Decreased plasma binding of drugs owing to a decrease in albumin production
Carbohydrate metabolism	Hypoglycemia may develop when glycogenolysis and gluconeogenesis are impaired
Stores glycogen and synthesizes glucose from amino acids, lactic acid, and glycerol	Abnormal glucose tolerance curve may occur because of impaired uptake and release of glucose by the liver
Fat metabolism	
Formation of lipoproteins	Impaired synthesis of lipoproteins
Conversion of carbohydrates and proteins to fat	
Synthesis, recycling, and elimination of cholesterol	Altered cholesterol levels
Formation of ketones from fatty acid	
Protein metabolism	
Deamination of proteins	
Formation of urea from ammonia	Elevated blood ammonia levels
Synthesis of plasma proteins	Decreased levels of plasma proteins, particularly albumin, which contributes to edema formation
Synthesis of clotting factors (fibrinogen, prothrombin, factors V, VII, IX, X)	Bleeding tendency
Storage of minerals and vitamins	Signs of deficiency of fat-soluble and other vitamins that are stored in the liver
Filtration of blood and removal of bacteria and particulate matter by Kupffer cells	Increased exposure of the body to colonic bacteria and other foreign matter

Oddi, regulates the flow of bile into the duodenum. When this sphincter is closed, bile moves back into the common duct and gallbladder.

Metabolic Functions of the Liver

The liver is one of the most versatile and active organs in the body. It produces bile; metabolizes hormones and drugs; synthesizes proteins, glucose, and clotting factors; stores vitamins and minerals; changes ammonia produced by deamination of amino acids to urea; and converts fatty acids to ketones. The liver also degrades excess nutrients and converts them into substances essential to the body. In its capacity for metabolizing drugs and hormones, the liver serves as an excretory organ. In this respect, the bile, which carries the end products of substances metabolized by the liver, is much like the urine, which carries the body wastes filtered by the kidneys. The functions of the liver are summarized in Table 38.1.

Carbohydrate Metabolism

The liver plays an essential role in carbohydrate metabolism and glucose homeostasis (Fig. 38.4). The liver stores excess glucose as glycogen (*i.e.,* glycogenesis) and releases it into the circulation when blood glucose levels fall. The liver also

synthesizes glucose from amino acids, glycerol, and lactic acid as a means of maintaining blood glucose during periods of fasting or increased need. The liver also converts excess carbohydrates to triglycerides for storage in adipose tissue.

Protein Synthesis and Conversion of Ammonia to Urea

The liver is an important site for protein synthesis and degradation. It produces the proteins for its own cellular needs, and secretory proteins that are released into the circulation. The most important of these secretory proteins is albumin. Albumin

FIGURE 38.4 • Hepatic pathways for storage and synthesis of glucose and conversion of glucose to fatty acids.

FIGURE 38.5 • Hepatic pathways for conversion of amino acids to proteins, nucleic acids, ketoacids, and glucose. The urea cycle converts ammonia generated by the deamination of amino acids to urea. Acetyl CoA, acetyl-coenzyme A; ATP, adenosine triphosphate.

during deamination is rapidly removed from the blood by the liver and converted to urea. Essentially all urea formed in the body is synthesized by the urea cycle in the liver and then excreted by the kidneys.[2] Although urea is mostly excreted by the kidneys, some diffuses into the intestine, where it is converted to ammonia by enteric bacteria. The intestinal production of ammonia also results from bacterial deamination of unabsorbed amino acids and proteins derived from the diet, exfoliated cells, or blood in the gastrointestinal tract. Ammonia produced in the intestine is absorbed into the portal circulation and transported to the liver, where it is converted to urea before being released into the systemic circulation. Intestinal production of ammonia is increased after ingestion of high-protein foods and gastrointestinal bleeding. In advanced liver disease, urea synthesis often is impaired, leading to an accumulation of blood ammonia.

Pathways of Lipid Metabolism

Although most cells of the body metabolize fat, certain aspects of lipid metabolism occur mainly in the liver, including the oxidation of free fatty acids to ketoacids that supply energy for other body functions; synthesis of cholesterol, phospholipids, and lipoproteins; and formation of triglycerides from carbohydrates and proteins (Fig. 38.6). To derive energy from triglycerides, the molecule must first be split into glycerol and fatty acids, and then the fatty acids split into two-carbon acetyl-coenzyme A (acetyl-CoA) units by a process called *beta*

contributes significantly to the plasma colloidal osmotic pressure (see Chapter 31) and to the binding and transport of numerous substances, including some hormones, fatty acids, bilirubin, and other anions. The liver also produces other important proteins, such as fibrinogen and the blood clotting factors.

Through a variety of anabolic and catabolic processes, the liver is the major site of amino acid interconversion (Fig. 38.5). Hepatic catabolism and degradation involve two major reactions: transamination and deamination.[1] In *transamination*, an amino group (NH$_2$) is transferred to an acceptor substance. As a result of transamination, amino acids can participate in the intermediary metabolism of carbohydrates and lipids. During periods of fasting or starvation, amino acids are used for producing glucose (*i.e.*, gluconeogenesis). Most of the nonessential amino acids are synthesized in the liver by transamination. The process of transamination is catalyzed by *aminotransferases*, enzymes that are found in high amounts in the liver.

Oxidative *deamination* involves the removal of the amino groups from amino acids and conversion of amino acids to ketoacids and ammonia. This occurs mainly by transamination, in which the amino groups are removed and then transferred to another acceptor substance. The acceptor substance can then transfer the amino group to still another substance or release it as ammonia. Because ammonia is very toxic to body tissues, particularly neurons, the ammonia that is released

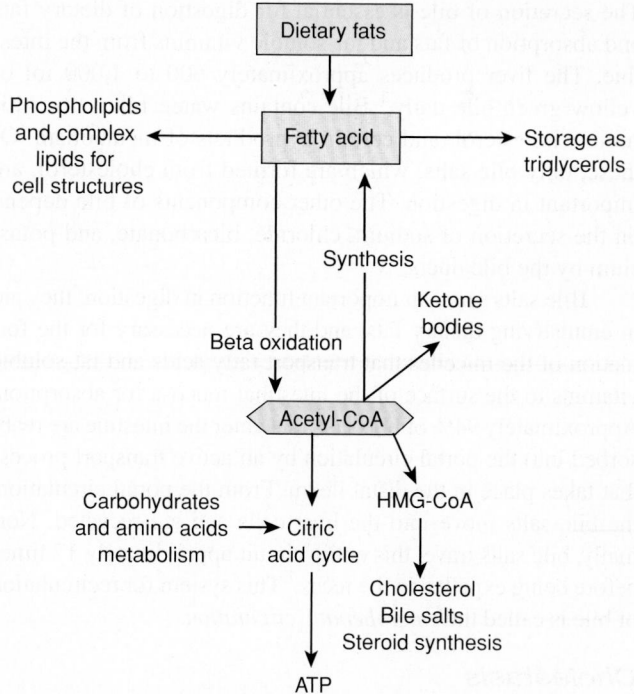

FIGURE 38.6 • Hepatic pathways for fat metabolism. Beta oxidation breaks fatty acids into two-carbon acetyl-coenzyme A (acetyl-CoA) units that are used in the citric acid cycle to generate adenosine triphosphate (ATP), or are used in the synthesis of cholesterol of ketoacids that are released into the blood for use by other tissues as an energy source.

oxidation. Acetyl-CoA is readily channelled into the citric acid cycle to produce adenosine triphosphate (ATP). Because the liver cannot use all the acetyl-CoA that is formed, it converts the excess into acetoacetic acid, a highly soluble ketoacid that is released into the bloodstream and transported to other tissues, where it is used for energy. During periods of starvation, ketones become a major source of energy as fatty acids released from adipose tissue are converted to ketones by the liver.

Acetyl-CoA units from fat metabolism also are used to synthesize cholesterol and bile acids in the liver. Cholesterol can be used in several ways by the liver. It can be esterified and stored; it can be exported bound to lipoproteins; or it can be converted to bile acids. The rate-limiting step in cholesterol synthesis is that which is catalyzed by 3-hydroxy-3-methyl-glutaryl-coenzyme A reductase (HMG-CoA reductase). The HMG-CoA reductase inhibitors, or statins (atorvastatin, fluvastatin, lovastatin, pravastatin, simvastatin, rosuvastatin), are used to treat high cholesterol levels by inhibiting this step in cholesterol synthesis (see Chapter 22).

Almost all the fat synthesis in the body from carbohydrates and proteins occurs in the liver. Whenever a greater quantity of carbohydrates enters the body than can be immediately used, the excess is converted to triglycerides in the liver. The triglycerides formed in the liver are transported mainly in low-density lipoproteins (LDLs) to the adipose tissue, where they are stored.

Bile Production and Cholestasis

The secretion of bile is essential for digestion of dietary fats and absorption of fats and fat-soluble vitamins from the intestine. The liver produces approximately 600 to 1,000 ml of yellow-green bile daily.[1] Bile contains water, bile salts, bilirubin, cholesterol, and certain byproducts of metabolism. Of these, only bile salts, which are formed from cholesterol, are important in digestion. The other components of bile depend on the secretion of sodium, chloride, bicarbonate, and potassium by the bile ducts.

Bile salts serve an important function in digestion; they aid in emulsifying dietary fats, and they are necessary for the formation of the micelles that transport fatty acids and fat-soluble vitamins to the surface of the intestinal mucosa for absorption. Approximately 94% of bile salts that enter the intestine are reabsorbed into the portal circulation by an active transport process that takes place in the distal ileum. From the portal circulation, the bile salts move into the liver cells and are recycled. Normally, bile salts travel this entire circuit approximately 17 times before being expelled in the feces.[1] This system for recirculation of bile is called the *enterohepatic circulation.*

Cholestasis

Cholestasis represents a decrease in bile flow through the intrahepatic canaliculi and a reduction in secretion of water, bilirubin, and bile acids by the hepatocytes. As a result, the materials normally transferred to the bile, including bilirubin, cholesterol, and bile acids, accumulate in the blood.[3,4] The condition may be caused by intrinsic liver disease, in which case it is referred to as *intrahepatic cholestasis,* or by obstruction of the large bile ducts, a condition known as *extrahepatic cholestasis.*

A number of mechanisms are implicated in the pathogenesis of cholestasis. Primary biliary cirrhosis and primary sclerosing cholangitis are caused by disorders of the small intrahepatic canaliculi and bile ducts. In the case of extrahepatic obstruction, which can be caused by conditions such as cholelithiasis, common duct strictures, or obstructing neoplasms, the effects begin with increased pressure in the large bile ducts. Genetic disorders involving the transport of bile into the canaliculi also can result in cholestasis (*e.g.,* Alagille syndrome, progressive familial intrahepatic cholestasis).

The morphologic features of cholestasis depend on the underlying cause. Common to all types of obstructive and hepatocellular cholestasis is the accumulation of bile pigment in the liver. Elongated green-brown plugs of bile are visible in the dilated bile canaliculi. Rupture of the canaliculi leads to extravasation of bile and subsequent degenerative changes in the surrounding hepatocytes. Prolonged obstructive cholestasis leads not only to fatty changes in the hepatocytes but to destruction of the supporting connective tissue, giving rise to bile lakes filled with cellular debris and pigment.[3] Unrelieved obstruction leads to biliary tract fibrosis and ultimately to end-stage biliary cirrhosis.

Pruritus is the most common presenting symptom in persons with cholestasis, probably related to an elevation in plasma bile acids. Skin xanthomas (focal accumulations of cholesterol) may occur, the result of hyperlipidemia and impaired excretion of cholesterol. A characteristic laboratory finding is an elevated serum alkaline phosphatase level, an enzyme present in the bile duct epithelium and canalicular membrane of hepatocytes. Other manifestations of reduced bile flow relate to intestinal absorption, including nutritional deficiencies of the fat-soluble vitamins A, D, and K.

Bilirubin Elimination and Jaundice

Bilirubin is the substance that gives bile its colour. It is formed from senescent red blood cells. In the process of degradation, the hemoglobin from the red blood cell is broken down to form biliverdin, which is rapidly converted to free bilirubin (Fig. 38.7). Free bilirubin, which is insoluble in plasma, is transported in the blood attached to plasma albumin. Even when it is bound to albumin, this bilirubin is still called *free bilirubin,* to distinguish it from conjugated bilirubin. As it passes through the liver, free bilirubin is absorbed through the hepatocytes' cell membrane and released from its albumin carrier molecule. Inside the hepatocytes, free bilirubin is converted to conjugated bilirubin, making it soluble in bile. Conjugated bilirubin is secreted as a constituent of bile, and in this form it passes through the bile ducts into the small intestine. In the intestine, approximately one half of the bilirubin is converted into a highly soluble substance called *urobilinogen* by the intestinal flora. Urobilinogen is either absorbed into the portal circulation or excreted in the feces. Most of the urobilinogen that is absorbed is returned to the liver to be reexcreted into the bile. A

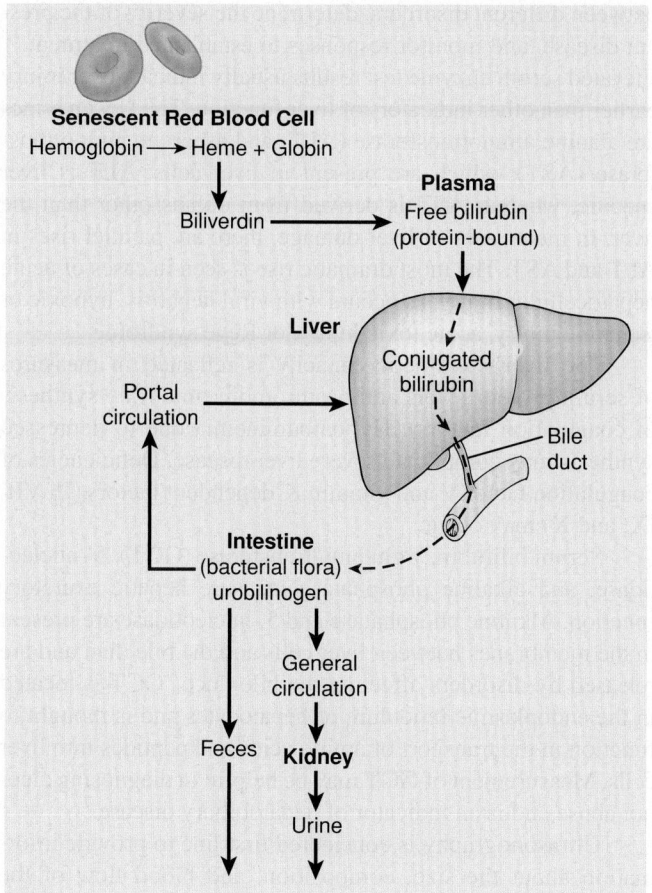

FIGURE 38.7 • The process of bilirubin formation, circulation, and elimination.

FIGURE 38.8 • Jaundice in a person with hepatitis A. (From Centers for Disease Control and Prevention. (2014). Public Health Image Library No. 2860. Available online at: http://phil.cdc.gov/phil/details.asp)

of bile flow in the canaliculi of the hepatic lobules or in the intrahepatic or extrahepatic bile ducts. From an anatomic standpoint, jaundice can be categorized as prehepatic, intrahepatic, and posthepatic. Chart 38.1 lists the common causes of prehepatic, hepatic, and posthepatic jaundice.

The major cause of prehepatic jaundice is excessive hemolysis of red blood cells. Hemolytic jaundice occurs when red blood cells are destroyed at a rate in excess of the liver's

small amount of urobilinogen, approximately 5%, is absorbed into the general circulation and then excreted by the kidneys.[1]

Usually, only a small amount of bilirubin is found in the blood; the normal level of total serum bilirubin is 2 to 20 µmol/L. Laboratory measurements of bilirubin usually measure the free and the conjugated bilirubin as well as the total bilirubin. These are reported as the direct (conjugated) bilirubin and the indirect (unconjugated or free) bilirubin.

Jaundice

Jaundice (*i.e.,* icterus) results from an abnormally high accumulation of bilirubin in the blood, as a result of which there is a yellowish discolouration to the skin and deep tissues. Jaundice becomes evident when the serum bilirubin levels rise above 34 to 50 µmol/L.[3–5] Because normal skin has a yellow cast, the early signs of jaundice often are difficult to detect, especially in persons with dark skin. Bilirubin has a special affinity for elastic tissue. The sclera of the eye, which contains a high proportion of elastic fibres, usually is one of the first structures in which jaundice can be detected (Fig. 38.8).

The four major causes of jaundice are excessive destruction of red blood cells, impaired uptake of bilirubin by the liver cells, decreased conjugation of bilirubin, and obstruction

---

CHART 38.1 **CAUSES OF JAUNDICE**

Prehepatic (Excessive Red Blood Cell Destruction)
Hemolytic blood transfusion reaction
Hereditary disorders of the red blood cell
   Sickle cell disease
   Thalassemia
   Spherocytosis
Acquired hemolytic disorders
Hemolytic disease of the newborn
Autoimmune hemolytic anemias

Intrahepatic
Decreased bilirubin uptake by the liver
Decreased conjugation of bilirubin
Hepatocellular liver damage
   Hepatitis
   Cirrhosis
   Cancer of the liver
Drug-induced cholestasis

Posthepatic (Obstruction of Bile Flow)
Structural disorders of the bile duct
Cholelithiasis
Congenital atresia of the extrahepatic bile ducts
Bile duct obstruction caused by tumours

ability to remove the bilirubin from the blood. It may follow a hemolytic blood transfusion reaction, due to the decreased lifespan of the donated red blood cells, or may occur in diseases such as hereditary spherocytosis, in which the red cell membranes are defective, or in hemolytic disease of the newborn (see Chapter 14). Neonatal hyperbilirubinemia results from increased production of bilirubin in newborn infants and their limited ability to excrete it.[6] Premature infants are at particular risk because their red cells have a shorter life span and higher turnover rate. In prehepatic jaundice, there is mild jaundice, the unconjugated bilirubin is elevated, the stools are of normal colour, and there is no bilirubin in the urine.

Intrahepatic or hepatocellular jaundice is caused by disorders that directly affect the ability of the liver to remove bilirubin from the blood or conjugate it so it can be eliminated in the bile. Gilbert disease is inherited as a dominant trait and results in a reduced removal of bilirubin from the blood; the disorder is benign and fairly common. Affected persons have no symptoms other than a slightly elevated unconjugated bilirubin and mild jaundice. Conjugation of bilirubin is impaired whenever liver cells are damaged, when transport of bilirubin into liver cells becomes deficient, or when the enzymes needed to conjugate the bile are lacking. Liver diseases such as hepatitis and cirrhosis are the most common causes of intrahepatic jaundice. Drugs such as the anesthetic agent halothane, oral contraceptives, estrogen, anabolic steroids, isoniazid, and chlorpromazine may also be implicated in this type of jaundice. Intrahepatic or hepatocellular jaundice usually interferes with all phases of bilirubin metabolism—uptake, conjugation, and excretion. Both conjugated and unconjugated bilirubin are elevated, the urine often is dark because of bilirubin in the urine, and the serum alkaline phosphatase is slightly elevated.

Posthepatic or obstructive jaundice, also called *cholestatic jaundice,* occurs when bile flow is obstructed between the liver and the intestine, with the obstruction located at any point between the junction of the right or left hepatic duct and the point where the bile duct opens into the intestine. Among the causes are strictures of the bile duct, gallstones, and tumours of the bile duct or the pancreas. Conjugated bilirubin levels usually are elevated; the stools are clay coloured because of the lack of bilirubin in the bile; the urine is dark; the levels of serum alkaline phosphatase are markedly elevated; and the aminotransferase levels are slightly increased. Blood levels of bile acids often are elevated in obstructive jaundice. As the bile acids accumulate in the blood, pruritus develops. A history of pruritus preceding jaundice is common in obstructive jaundice.

Tests of Hepatobiliary Function

The history and physical examination, in most instances, provide clues about liver function. Diagnostic tests help to evaluate liver function and the extent of liver damage. Laboratory tests commonly are used to assess liver function and confirm the diagnosis of liver disease.

Liver function tests, including serum levels of liver enzymes, are used to assess injury to liver cells, differentiate between different disorders, determine the severity of the present disease, and monitor responses to established treatment.[7,8] Elevated serum enzyme test results usually indicate liver injury earlier than other indicators of liver function. The key enzymes are alanine aminotransferase (ALT) and aspartate aminotransferase (AST), which are present in liver cells. ALT is liver specific, whereas AST is derived from organs other than the liver. In most cases of liver damage, there are parallel rises in ALT and AST. The most dramatic rise is seen in cases of acute hepatocellular injury, as occurs with viral hepatitis, hypoxic or ischemic injury, acute toxic injury, or Reye syndrome.

The liver's synthetic capacity is reflected in measures of serum protein levels and prothrombin time (*i.e.,* synthesis of coagulation factors). Hypoalbuminemia due to depressed synthesis may complicate severe liver disease. Deficiencies of coagulation factor V and vitamin K-dependent factors (II, VII, IX, and X) may occur.

Serum bilirubin, γ-glutamyltransferase (GGT), 5′-nucleotidase, and alkaline phosphatase measure hepatic excretory function. Alkaline phosphatase and 5′-nucleotidase are present in the membranes between liver cells and the bile duct and are released by disorders affecting the bile duct.[7] GGT is located in the endoplasmic reticulum of hepatocytes and is thought to function in the transport of amino acids and peptides into liver cells. Measurement of GGT may be helpful in diagnosing alcohol abuse and is an indicator of hepatobiliary disease.[7]

Ultrasonography is considered first line to provide information about the size, composition, and blood flow of the liver. It has largely replaced cholangiography in detecting stones in the gallbladder or biliary tree. Computed tomography (CT) scanning provides information similar to that obtained by ultrasonography. Magnetic resonance imaging (MRI) has proved to be useful in some disorders.[5] Selective angiography of the celiac, superior mesenteric, or hepatic artery may be used to visualize the hepatic or portal circulation. A liver biopsy affords a means of examining liver tissue without surgery. There are several methods for obtaining liver tissue: percutaneous liver biopsy, which uses a suction, cutting, or spring-loaded cutting needle; laparoscopic liver biopsy; and fine-needle biopsy, which is performed under ultrasonographic or CT guidance. The type of method used is based on the number of specimens needed and the amount of tissue required for evaluation. Laparoscopic liver biopsy provides the means for examining abdominal masses, evaluating ascites of unknown cause, and staging liver cancers.

IN SUMMARY

The hepatobiliary system consists of the liver, gallbladder, and bile ducts. The liver is the largest and, in terms of function, one of the most versatile organs in the body. It is located between the gastrointestinal tract and the systemic circulation; venous blood from the intestine flows through the liver before it is returned to the heart. In this way, nutrients can be removed for processing and storage, and bacteria and other foreign matter can be removed by Kupffer cells before the blood is returned to the systemic circulation.

The liver synthesizes fats, glucose, and plasma proteins. Other important functions of the liver include the deamination of amino acids, conversion of ammonia to urea, and the interconversion of amino acids and other compounds that are important to the metabolic processes of the body. The liver produces approximately 600 to 1,000 ml of yellow-green bile daily. Bile serves as an excretory vehicle for bilirubin, cholesterol, and certain products of organic metabolism and it contains bile salts that are essential for digestion of fats and absorption of fat-soluble vitamins. The liver also removes, conjugates, and secretes bilirubin into the bile. Jaundice occurs when bilirubin accumulates in the blood. It can occur because of excessive red blood cell destruction, failure of the liver to remove and conjugate the bilirubin, or obstructed biliary flow.

Liver function tests, including serum aminotransferase levels, are used to assess injury to liver cells. Serum bilirubin, GGT, 5'-nucleotidase, and alkaline phosphatase are used as measures of hepatic excretory function. Ultrasonography, CT scans, and MRI are used to evaluate liver structures. Angiography may be used to visualize the hepatic or portal circulation, and a liver biopsy obtains tissue specimens for microscopic examination.

DISORDERS OF HEPATIC AND BILIARY FUNCTION

After completing this section of the chapter, you should be able to meet the following objectives:

- State the three ways by which drugs and other substances are metabolized or inactivated in the liver and provide examples of liver disease related to the toxic effects of drugs and chemical agents.
- Compare hepatitis A, B, C, D, and E in terms of source of infection, incubation period, acute disease manifestations, development of chronic disease, and the carrier state.
- Define chronic hepatitis and compare the pathogenesis of chronic autoimmune and chronic viral hepatitis.
- Characterize the metabolism of alcohol by the liver and state metabolic mechanisms that can be used to explain liver injury.
- Summarize the three patterns of injury that occur with alcohol-induced liver disease.
- Describe the pathogenesis of intrahepatic biliary tract disease.
- Characterize the liver changes that occur with cirrhosis.
- Describe the physiologic basis for portal hypertension and relate it to the development of ascites, esophageal varices, and splenomegaly.

- Relate the functions of the liver to the manifestations of liver failure.
- Characterize etiologies of hepatocellular cancer and state the reason for the poor prognosis in persons with this type of cancer.

The structures of the hepatobiliary system are subject to many of the same pathologic conditions that affect other body systems: injury from drugs and toxins; infection, inflammation, and immune responses; metabolic disorders; and neoplasms. This section focuses on alterations in liver function due to drug-induced injury; viral and autoimmune hepatitis; intrahepatic biliary tract disorders; alcohol-induced liver disease; cirrhosis, portal hypertension, and liver failure; and cancer of the liver.

Hepatotoxic Disorders

By virtue of its many enzyme systems that are involved in biochemical transformations and modifications, the liver has an important role in the metabolism of many drugs and chemical substances. The liver is particularly important in terms of metabolizing lipid-soluble substances that cannot be directly excreted by the kidneys. Because the liver is central to the metabolic disposition of virtually all drugs and foreign substances, drug-induced liver toxicity is a potential complication of many medications.

Drug and Hormone Metabolism

Two major types of reactions are involved in the hepatic detoxification and metabolism of drugs and other chemicals: phase 1 reactions, which involve chemical modification or inactivation of a substance, and phase 2 reactions, which involve conversion of lipid-soluble substances to water-soluble derivatives.[9] Often, the two types of reactions are linked. Many phase 1 reactants are not water soluble and must therefore undergo a subsequent phase 2 reaction to be eliminated. These reactions, which are called *biotransformations,* are important considerations in drug therapy.

Phase 1 Reactions. *Phase 1 reactions* result in chemical modification of reactive drug groups by oxidation, reduction, hydroxylation, or other chemical reactions. Most drug-metabolizing enzymes are located in the lipophilic membranes of the smooth endoplasmic reticulum of liver cells (see Chapter 4). When these membranes are broken down and separated in the laboratory, they re-form into vesicles called *microsomes.* The enzymes in these membranes are often referred to as *microsomal enzymes.* The enzymes involved in most phase 1 oxidation–reduction processes are products of a gene superfamily that has nearly 300 members. These genes code for a group of microsomal isoenzymes that make up the cytochrome (CYP) P450 system. (The name *cytochrome P450* is derived from the spectral properties [absorbing light at 450 nm] of the hemoproteins that participate in oxidation–reduction processes.) The gene products of many of the *CYP* genes have been identified and traced to the metabolism of specific drugs and to potential interactions among drugs. Each family of genes is responsible for certain drug-metabolizing processes, and each member of the family undertakes specific drug-metabolizing functions. For example, the *CYP3* gene family contains an A subfamily and several genes numbered 1, 2, 3, and so forth. It is noteworthy that CYP 3A4 alone is responsible for the metabolism of over 50% of clinically prescribed drugs metabolized by the liver.[9]

Many gene members of the *CYP* system can have their activity induced or suppressed as they undergo the task of metabolizing drugs. For example, drugs such as alcohol and barbiturates can induce certain members to increase enzyme production, accelerating drug metabolism and decreasing the pharmacologic action of the drug and of coadministered drugs that use the same member of the CYP system. In the case of drugs metabolically transformed to reactive intermediates, enzyme induction may exacerbate drug-mediated tissue toxicity. Enzymes in the cytochrome system also can be inhibited by drugs. For example, imidazole-containing drugs such as cimetidine (a histamine type 2 receptor blocking drug that is used to reduce gastric acid secretion) and ketoconazole (an antifungal agent) effectively inhibit the metabolism of testosterone.[9] Environmental pollutants also are capable of inducing *CYP* gene activity. For example, exposure to benzo[*a*]pyrene, which is present in tobacco smoke, charcoal-broiled meat, and other organic pyrolysis products, is known to induce members of the *CYP* family and alter the rates of metabolism of some drugs.

Phase 2 Reactions. *Phase 2 reactions,* which involve the conversion of lipid-soluble derivatives to water-soluble substances, may follow phase 1 reactions or proceed independently. Conjugation, catalyzed by endoplasmic reticulum enzymes that couple the drug with an activated endogenous compound to render it more water soluble, is one of the most common phase 2 reactions. Although many water-soluble drugs and endogenous substances are excreted unchanged in the urine or bile, lipid-soluble substances tend to accumulate in the body unless they are converted to less active compounds or water-soluble metabolites. In general, the conjugates are more soluble than the parent compound and are pharmacologically inactive. Because the endogenous substrates used in the conjugation process are obtained from the diet, nutrition plays a critical role in phase 2 reactions.

An alternative cytochrome P450-dependent conjugation pathway is important in detoxifying reactive metabolic intermediates. This pathway uses a thiol, or sulphur-containing substance, called *glutathione,* which is used in conjugating drugs that form potentially harmful electrophilic groups. Glutathione is depleted in the detoxification process and must be constantly replenished by compounds from the diet or by cysteine-containing drugs such as *N*-acetylcysteine.[9] The glutathione pathway is central to the detoxification of a number of compounds, including the over-the-counter pain medication acetaminophen (*e.g.,* Tylenol). Acetaminophen metabolism involves a phase 2 reaction. Normally, the capacity of the phase 2 reactants is much greater than that required for metabolizing recommended doses of the drug. However, in situations of acetaminophen overdose, the capacity of the phase 2 system is exceeded and the drug is transformed into toxic metabolites that can cause necrosis of the liver if allowed to accumulate. In this situation, the glutathione pathway plays a critical role in the detoxification of these metabolites. Because the glutathione stores are rapidly depleted, the drug *N*-acetylcysteine, which serves as a glutathione substitute, is used as an antidote for acetaminophen overdose. Chronic alcohol ingestion decreases glutathione stores and increases the risk of acetaminophen toxicity.[10]

In addition to its role in metabolism of drugs and chemicals, the liver also is responsible for hormone inactivation or modification. Insulin and glucagon are inactivated by proteolysis or deamination. Thyroxine and triiodothyronine are metabolized by reactions involving deiodination. Steroid hormones such as the glucocorticoids are first inactivated by a phase 1 reaction and then conjugated by a phase 2 reaction.

***P*-Glycoproteins.** While the liver is considered the principle organ for drug metabolism, other tissues such as gastrointestinal tract, lungs, skin, kidneys, placenta, brain plus the liver have *P-glycoproteins* (Pgp) that are specialized for expelling foreign molecules. Pgp, also referred to as multidrug resistance type 1 (MDR1) transporter, is a plasma membrane protein powered by ATP and is capable of transporting drugs, natural products, and peptides out of the cell. Because the Pgp transporter protein is located on the luminal surface, it is able to limit the cellular update of substrates from the intestinal lumen into epithelial cells or from the blood circulation into the brain or across the placenta. This active exportation of drugs can limited the overall availability of the drug and the need for metabolism within the liver. However, there seems to be an overlap between CYP substrates and Pgp in the intestine, kidney, and liver suggesting interaction between the sites. For example a drug metabolized by the liver and excreted in the bile might be prevented for being reabsorbed in the intestine by the Pgp. Another area of interest is the increased expression of these transporter proteins due to genetic polymorphisms potentially contributing resistance to certain drugs such as anticancer and digoxin. As more research is done in this area, the list of medications known to be exported out of the human cells by the Pgp increases.[9,11]

Drug-Induced Liver Disease

As the major drug-metabolizing and detoxifying organ in the body, the liver is subject to potential damage from the enormous array of pharmaceutical and environmental chemicals. Many of the widely used therapeutic drugs, including over-the-counter "natural" products, can cause hepatic injury. Of the numerous remedies, medicinal agents, chemicals, and herbal remedies in existence, more than 600 are recognized as being capable of producing hepatic injury.[12]

Numerous host factors contribute to the susceptibility of drug-induced liver disease, including genetic predisposition, age differences, underlying chronic liver disease, diet and alcohol consumption, and the use of multiple interacting drugs.[13] For unknown reasons, women generally predominate among persons with drug-induced liver disease. Early identification of drug-induced liver disease is important because withdrawal of the drug is curative in most cases.

Drugs and chemicals can exert their effects by causing hepatocyte injury and death or by cholestatic liver damage due to injury of biliary drainage structures.[13] Drug reactions can be predictable based on the drug's chemical structure and metabolites or unpredictable (idiosyncratic) based on individual characteristics of the person receiving the drug.

Direct Hepatotoxic Injury. Some drugs are known to have toxic effects on the liver based on their chemical structure and the way they are metabolized in the liver. Direct hepatic damage often is age and dose dependent. Direct hepatotoxic reactions usually are a recognized characteristic of certain drugs. They usually result from drug metabolism and the generation of toxic metabolites. Because of the greater activity of the drug-metabolizing enzymes in the central zones of the liver, these agents typically cause centrilobular necrosis. Examples of drugs that cause direct hepatotoxicity are acetaminophen, isoniazid, and phenytoin, as well as a number of chemical agents, including carbon tetrachloride. Acetaminophen toxicity produces the most common form of acute liver failure in adults in the United States, accounting for 50% of cases.[13] The injury is characterized by marked elevations in ALT and AST values with minimally elevated alkaline phosphatase. Bilirubin levels invariably are increased, and the prognosis often is worse when hepatocellular necrosis is accompanied by jaundice.[10]

Idiosyncratic Reactions. In contrast to direct hepatotoxic drug reactions, idiosyncratic reactions are unpredictable, not related to dose, and sometimes accompanied by features suggesting an allergic reaction. In some cases, the reaction results directly from a metabolite that is produced only in certain persons based on a genetic predisposition.[13] For example, certain people are capable of rapid acetylation of isoniazid, an antituberculosis drug.

Cholestatic Reactions. Cholestatic drug reactions result in decreased secretion of bile or obstruction of the biliary tree.[13] Acute intrahepatic cholestasis is one of the most frequent types of idiosyncratic drug reactions. Among the drugs credited with causing cholestatic drug reactions are estradiol; chlorpromazine, an antipsychotic drug; and some of the antibiotics, including amoxicillin/clavulanic acid and erythromycin. Typically, cholestatic drug reactions are characterized by an early onset of jaundice and pruritus, with little alteration in the person's general feeling of well-being. Most instances of acute drug-induced cholestasis subside once the drug is withdrawn.

Chronic Hepatitis. Some drugs produce a more indolent form of liver damage that closely resembles autoimmune

---

DISEASES OF THE LIVER

- Diseases of the liver can affect the hepatocytes or the biliary drainage system.
- Diseases of hepatocytes impair the metabolic and synthetic functions of the liver, causing disorders in carbohydrate, protein, and fat metabolism; metabolism and removal of drugs, hormones, toxins, ammonia, and bilirubin from the blood; and the interconversion of amino acids and synthesis of proteins. Elevations in serum aminotransferase levels signal the presence of hepatocyte damage.
- Diseases of the biliary drainage system obstruct the flow of bile and interfere with the elimination of bile salts and bilirubin, producing cholestatic liver damage because of the backup of bile into the lobules of the liver. Elevations in bilirubin and alkaline phosphatase signal the presence of cholestatic liver damage.

---

hepatitis. Early identification of drug-related chronic hepatitis often is difficult. Cirrhosis may develop before the hepatitis is diagnosed. In addition, identifying the drug that caused the liver damage may be difficult retrospectively if the person has been consuming alcohol or taking several drugs.

Viral Hepatitis

Hepatitis refers to inflammation of the liver. It can be caused by hepatotropic viruses that primarily affect liver cells or hepatocytes, autoimmune mechanisms, or reactions to drugs and toxins, or be secondary to other systemic disorders. Viruses causing systemic disease that can involve the liver include Epstein–Barr virus (infectious mononucleosis), which may cause a mild hepatitis during the acute phase; cytomegalovirus (particularly in newborns and immunosuppressed persons); herpesviruses; and enteroviruses.

The known hepatotropic viruses include hepatitis A virus (HAV), hepatitis B virus (HBV), the hepatitis B-associated delta virus (HDV), hepatitis C virus (HCV), and hepatitis E virus (HEV). Although all of these viruses cause acute hepatitis, they differ in the mode of transmission and incubation period; mechanism, degree, and chronicity of liver damage; and ability to evolve to a carrier state. The presence of viral antigens and their antibodies can be determined through laboratory tests. Epidemiologic studies have indicated that some cases of infectious hepatitis are due to other agents. A viral agent similar to HCV has been cloned and was identified as hepatitis G virus (HGV), also referred to as GBV-C. Evidence of HGV has been found in 1% to 4% of blood donors in Canada. However, HGV is not linked to liver disease or exacerbations of liver disease.[3,14–17]

There are two mechanisms of liver injury in viral hepatitis: direct cellular injury and induction of immune responses against the viral antigens. The mechanisms of injury have been most closely studied in HBV. It is thought that the extent of inflammation and necrosis depends on the individual's immune response. Accordingly, a prompt immune response during the acute phase of the infection would be expected to cause cell injury but at the same time eliminate the virus. Thus, people who respond with fewer symptoms and a marginal immune response are less likely to eliminate the virus, and hepatocytes expressing the viral antigens persist, leading to the chronic or carrier state. Fulminant hepatitis would be explained in terms of an accelerated immune response with severe liver necrosis.

The clinical course of viral hepatitis involves a number of syndromes, including asymptomatic infection with only serologic evidence of disease; acute hepatitis; the carrier state without clinically apparent disease or with chronic hepatitis; chronic hepatitis with or without progression to cirrhosis; or fulminating disease (<1% to 4%) with rapid onset of liver failure.[16] Not all hepatotoxic viruses provoke each of the clinical syndromes.

The manifestations of acute viral hepatitis can be divided into three phases: the prodromal or preicterus period, the icterus period, and the convalescent period. The manifestations of the prodromal period vary from abrupt to insidious, with general malaise, myalgia, arthralgia, easy fatigability, and anorexia.[17] Gastrointestinal symptoms such as nausea, vomiting, and diarrhea or constipation may occur. Abdominal pain is usually mild and felt on the right side. Chills and fever may mark an abrupt onset. In persons who smoke, there may be a distaste for smoking that parallels the anorexia. Serum levels of AST and ALT show variable increases during the preicterus phase of acute hepatitis and precede a rise in bilirubin that accompanies the onset of the icterus or jaundice phase of infection. The icterus phase, if it occurs, usually follows the prodromal phase by 1 to 2 weeks. Jaundice is less likely to occur with HCV infection. The prodromal symptoms may become worse with the onset of jaundice, followed by progressive clinical improvement. Severe pruritus and liver tenderness are common during the icterus period. The convalescent phase is characterized by an increased sense of well-being, return of appetite, and disappearance of jaundice. The acute illness usually subsides gradually over a 2- to 12-week period, with complete clinical recovery in 1 to 4 months depending on the type of hepatitis.[17]

Infection with HBV and HCV can produce a *carrier state* in which the person does not have symptoms but harbours the virus and can therefore transmit the disease. Evidence also indicates a carrier state for HDV infection. There is no carrier state for HAV infection. There are two types of carriers: healthy carriers who have few or no ill effects, and those with chronic disease who may or may not have symptoms. Factors that increase the risk of becoming a carrier are age at time of infection and immune status. The carrier state for infections that occur early in life, as in infants of HBV-infected mothers, may be as high as 90%, compared with 1% to 10% of infected adults.[3,18] Other persons at high risk of becoming carriers are those with impaired immunity, those who have received multiple transfusions or blood products, those who are on hemodialysis, and drug addicts.

Hepatitis A

Hepatitis A is caused by the Hepatitis A virus (HAV), a small, unenveloped, single-stranded ribonucleic acid (RNA) virus. It usually is a benign, self-limited disease, although it can cause acute fulminant hepatitis and death from liver failure in rare cases.[3,17,19,20] The onset of symptoms usually is abrupt and includes fever, malaise, nausea, anorexia, abdominal discomfort, dark urine, and jaundice. The likelihood of having symptoms is related to age. Children younger than 6 years often are asymptomatic.[20] The illness in older children and adults usually is symptomatic and jaundice occurs in approximately 70% of cases.[19] Symptoms usually last approximately 2 months but can last longer. HAV does not cause chronic hepatitis or induce a carrier state.

Hepatitis A is contracted primarily by the fecal-oral route.[17,19,20] It has a brief incubation period (15 to 50 days), with an average of 28 days. The virus replicates in the liver, is excreted in the bile, and shed in the stool. The fecal shedding of HAV occurs up to 2 weeks before the development of symptoms and ends as the immunoglobulin M (IgM) levels rise.[3] The disease often occurs sporadically or in epidemics.[19,20] Drinking contaminated milk or water and eating shellfish from infected waters are fairly common routes of transmission. At special risk are persons travelling abroad who have not previously been exposed to the virus. Because young children are asymptomatic, they play an important role in the spread of the disease. Institutions housing large numbers of persons (usually children) sometimes are stricken with an epidemic of hepatitis A. Oral behaviour and lack of toilet training promote viral infection among children attending preschool daycare centres, who then carry the virus home to older siblings and parents. Hepatitis A usually is not transmitted by transfusion of blood or plasma derivatives, presumably because its short period of viremia usually coincides with clinical illness, so that the disease is apparent and blood donations are not accepted.

Serologic Markers. Antibodies to HAV (anti-HAV) appear early in the disease and tend to persist in the serum (Fig. 38.9). The IgM antibodies (see Chapter 17) usually appear during the first week of symptomatic disease and begin to decline in a few months.[3] Their presence coincides with a decline in fecal shedding of the virus. Peak levels of IgG antibodies occur after 1 month of illness and may persist for years; they provide long-term protective immunity against reinfection. The presence of IgM anti-HAV is indicative of acute hepatitis A, whereas IgG anti-HAV merely documents past infection.[3]

Immunization. A hepatitis A vaccine is available in Canada.[20] Immunization is intended to replace the use of immune globulin in persons at high risk for HAV exposure. These include international travellers to regions where sanitation is poor and endemic HAV infections are high, children living in communities with high rates of HAV infection, homosexually active men, and users of illicit drugs. Persons with pre-existing chronic liver disease also may benefit from immunization. A public health benefit also may be derived from vaccinating

FIGURE 38.9 • The sequence of fecal shedding of the hepatitis A virus (HAV), HAV viremia, and HAV antibody (IgM and IgG anti-HAV) changes in hepatitis A.

persons with increased potential for transmitting the disease (*e.g.,* food handlers). Because the vaccine is of little benefit in prevention of hepatitis in persons with known HAV exposure, immune globulin (IgG) is recommended for these persons.[20]

Hepatitis B

Hepatitis B is caused by the Hepatitis B virus (HBV), a double-stranded deoxyribonucleic acid (DNA) virus.[3,17,21] The complete virion, also called a *Dane particle,* consists of an outer envelope and an inner nucleocapsid that contains HBV DNA and DNA polymerase (Fig. 38.10). HBV infection can produce acute hepatitis, chronic hepatitis, progression of chronic hepatitis to cirrhosis, fulminant hepatitis with massive hepatic necrosis, and the carrier state. It also participates in the development of hepatitis D (delta hepatitis).

Hepatitis B affects more than 360 million people worldwide.[3,15,21] In Canada, the incidence of acute hepatitis B has declined steadily since the late 1980s and has virtually disappeared in the cohorts who benefited from the universal vaccination implemented in the early 1990s. In 2008, estimations of overall incidence was 1.7 cases per 100,000; incidence rate for men were twice as high as women, and peak incidence rates occurred between the ages of 20 and 39. This shows the benefits of the current school-based vaccination programs and reinforces the need for vaccination programs that target high-risk populations.[21]

Hepatitis B has a longer incubation period and represents a more serious health problem than hepatitis A. The virus usually is transmitted through inoculation with infected blood or serum. However, the viral antigen can be found in most body secretions and can be spread by oral or sexual contact. In Canada, most persons with hepatitis B acquire the infection as adults or adolescents. The disease is highly prevalent among injecting drug users, heterosexuals with multiple sex partners, and men who have sex with men.[17,21] Healthcare workers are at risk owing to blood exposure and accidental needle

injuries. Although the virus can be spread through transfusion or administration of blood products, routine screening methods have appreciably reduced transmission through this route. The risk of hepatitis B in infants born to HBV-infected mothers ranges from 10% to 85%, depending on the mother's HBV status. Infants who become infected have a 90% risk of becoming chronic carriers, and up to 25% will die of chronic liver disease as adults.[22]

Serologic Markers. Three well-defined antigens are associated with the virus: a core antigen, HBcAg, which is contained in the nucleocapsid; a longer polypeptide transcript with pre-core and core regions, designated HBeAg; and a surface antigen, HBsAg, which is found in the outer envelope of the virus. The precore region directs the HBeAg polypeptide toward the blood, whereas the HBcAg remains in the hepatocytes to direct the assembly of new virions.

The HBV antigens evoke specific antibodies: anti-HBs, anti-HBc, and anti-HBe. These antigens (HBcAg does not circulate freely in the blood) and their antibodies serve as serologic markers for following the course of the disease[3,23] (see Fig. 38.10). The *HBsAg* is the viral antigen measured most routinely in blood. It appears before onset of symptoms, peaks during overt disease, and then declines to undetectable levels in 3 to 6 months. Persistence beyond 6 months indicates

FIGURE 38.10 • **A:** The hepatitis B virus. **B:** The sequence of hepatitis B virus (HBV) viral antigens (HBsAg, HBeAg), HBV DNA, and HBV antibody (IgM, IgG, anti-HBc, and anti-HBs) changes in acute resolving hepatitis B.

continued viral replication, infectivity, and risk of chronic hepatitis. HBeAg appears in the serum soon after HBsAg and signifies active viral replication. IgM anti-HBc becomes detectable shortly before the onset of symptoms, concurrent with onset of an elevation in serum transaminases. Over the months, the IgM antibody is replaced by IgG anti-HBc. Anti-HBe is detectable shortly after the disappearance of HBeAg, and its appearance signals the onset of resolution of the acute illness. IgG anti-HBs, a specific antibody to HBsAg, occurs in most individuals after clearance of HBsAg. Development of anti-HBs signals recovery from HBV infection, noninfectivity, and protection from future HBV infection. Anti-HBs is the antibody present in persons who have been successfully immunized against HBV.

The presence of viral DNA (HBV DNA) in the serum is the most certain indicator of hepatitis B infection. It is transiently present during the presymptomatic period and for a brief time during the acute illness. The presence of DNA polymerase, the enzyme used in viral replication, usually is transient but may persist for years in persons who are chronic carriers, and is an indication of continued infectivity.

Immunization. Hepatitis B vaccine provides long-term protection against HBV infection.[21,24] HBsAg is the antigen used for hepatitis B vaccines. Vaccines available in Canada use recombinant DNA technology to express HBsAg in yeast, which is then purified by biochemical and biophysical methods. The vaccine is available as a single-antigen formulation and also in fixed combination with other vaccines. The effectiveness of immunization was evidenced by a significant decline in overall incidence of acute hepatitis B from 1990 to 2008, with the most drastic declines occurring in the cohort of children in whom recommendations for routine infant and adolescent vaccination were implemented. A hepatitis B immune globulin (HBIG) is available. Prepared from plasma donors with high concentrations of anti-HBs, it is used as an adjunct to hepatitis B vaccine for postexposure immunoprophylaxis to prevent HBV infection.

Health Canada recommends vaccination of all children 0 to 18 years of age as a means of preventing HBV transmission.[24] The vaccine also is recommended for all unvaccinated adults (1) who are at high risk for infection by sexual exposure, including sex partners of HBsAg-positive persons, sexually active persons who are not in a long-term mutually monogamous relationship, persons seeking evaluation for treatment of sexually transmitted diseases, and men who have sex with men; (2) who are at high risk for infection by percutaneous or mucosal exposure to blood, including current and recent injecting drug abusers, household contacts of HBsAg-positive persons, residents and staff of institutions for the developmentally disabled, healthcare and public safety workers with reasonably anticipated risk for exposure to blood or blood-contaminated body fluids, and persons with chronic kidney disease (predialysis, hemodialysis, peritoneal dialysis, and home dialysis patients); and (3) others, including international travellers to regions with high or intermediate

levels of endemic HBV infection, persons with chronic liver disease, persons with human immunodeficiency virus (HIV) infection, and all other persons seeking protection from HBV infection.[21] Public Health Agency of Canada (PHAC) and the Society of Obstetricians and Gynaecologists (SOGC) also recommend that all pregnant women be routinely tested for HBsAg during an early prenatal visit and that infants born to HBsAg-positive mothers receive appropriate doses of HBIG and hepatitis B vaccine.[24]

HBIG may be effective for unvaccinated persons who are exposed to the infection if given within 7 days of exposure. Hepatitis vaccination is recommended for pre-exposure and postexposure prophylaxis.

Hepatitis C

Hepatitis C is the most common cause of chronic hepatitis, cirrhosis, and hepatocellular cancer in the world. Approximately 250,000 Canadians, or 0.7% of the population, are infected with Hepatitis C and it is estimated that potentially 50,000 of these people are unaware that they are infected.[3,15,25] Before 1990, the main route of transmission of Hepatitis C virus (HCV) was through contaminated blood transfusions or blood products. With implementation of HCV testing in blood banks, the risk of HCV infection from blood transfusion is almost nonexistent in Canada and other developed countries.[26,27] However, unsafe medical procedures and unscreened blood transfusions may be the most important sources of HCV infections in less developed countries of the world. Currently, recreational injecting drug use is the most common mode of HCV transmission in Canada and the United States.[26] High-risk sexual behaviour, defined as having sex with multiple partners or sex with an HCV-infected partner, is currently the second most common risk factor in Canada. The rate of transmission to infants born to HCV RNA-positive mothers ranges from 4.6% to 10%.[27] HCV also can be spread through exposure in the healthcare setting, primarily through needle-stick injuries. There also is concern that transmission of small amounts of blood during tattooing, acupuncture, and body piercing may facilitate the transmission of HCV.

HCV is a single-stranded RNA virus with properties similar to those of the flaviviruses, a genus of the family of *Flaviviridae* that includes yellow fever and St. Louis encephalitis viruses.[17] The genome contains a single open reading frame that encodes a polyprotein of about 3,000 amino acids. The transcript is cleaved into single proteins, including three structural proteins (one core and two envelope proteins) and four nonstructural proteins. The virus is genetically unstable, which leads to multiple genotypes and subtypes. Six different genotypes and more than 70 subtypes of the virus have been recognized.[3,28] Genotype 1a and b account for 60% to 75% of all infections in Canada and the United States and is associated with the lower rate of response to therapy.[3,28] It is likely that the wide diversity of genotypes contributes to the pathogenicity of the virus, allowing it to escape the actions of host immune mechanisms and antiviral medications, and to difficulties in developing a preventive vaccine.[28] Development of a vaccine and treatment measures has also been hampered by the lack of a reliable, reproducible, and efficient culture system for propagating the virus.

The incubation period for HCV infection ranges from 2 to 26 weeks (average, 2 to 12 weeks).[3,29] Children and adults who acquire the infection usually are asymptomatic (80%), or have a nonspecific clinical disease characterized by fatigue, malaise, anorexia, and weight loss.[29] Jaundice is uncommon, and only 10% to 20% of symptomatic adults have jaundice.[4] These symptoms usually last for 2 to 12 weeks. Fulminant hepatic failure is rare and only a few cases have been reported. A minority of persons who are newly infected with HCV will clear the infection, but most (50% to 80%) go on to develop chronic hepatitis.[4] Factors associated with spontaneous clearing of HCV infection appear to include younger age, female sex, and certain histocompatibility genes. The most serious consequences of chronic HCV infection are progressive liver fibrosis leading to cirrhosis, end-stage liver disease, and hepatocellular cancer. Host factors that may exacerbate the progression of liver disease include older age at onset of infection, male sex, an immunosuppressed state, concurrent HBV infection, alcohol consumption, and hepatotoxic medications.

Serologic Markers. Both antibody and viral tests are available for detecting the presence of HCV infection (Fig. 38.11). False-negative results can occur in immunocompromised people and early in the course of the disease before antibodies develop. Direct measurement of HCV in the serum remains the most accurate test for infection. The viral tests are highly sensitive and specific, but more costly than antibody tests. With newer antibody testing methods, infection often can be detected as early as 6 to 8 weeks after exposure, and as early as 1 to 2 weeks with viral tests that use polymerase chain reaction methods (see Chapter 16). Unlike hepatitis A and B, antibodies to HCV are not protective, but they serve as markers for the disease.

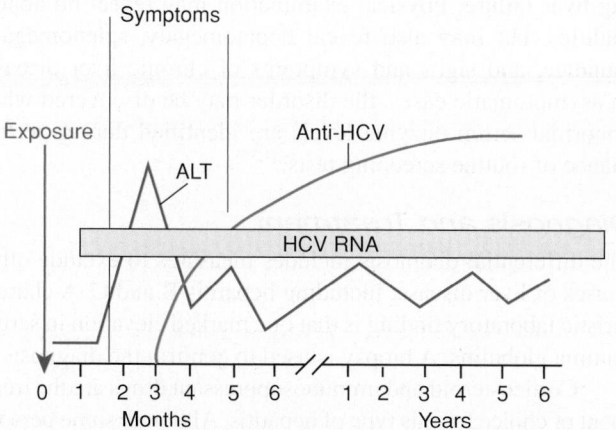

FIGURE 38.11 • The sequence of serologic changes in chronic hepatitis C, with persistence of hepatitis C virus (HCV) RNA and exacerbations and remissions of clinical symptoms indicated by changes in serum alanine aminotransferase (ALT) levels.

Hepatitis D and E

Hepatitis D Virus. Hepatitis D virus (HDV), or the delta hepatitis agent, is a defective RNA virus. It can cause acute or chronic hepatitis. Infection depends on concomitant infection with HBV, specifically the presence of HBsAg. Acute hepatitis D occurs in two forms: coinfection that occurs simultaneously with acute hepatitis B, and a superinfection in which hepatitis D is imposed on chronic hepatitis B or a hepatitis B carrier state.[3,4,15] The delta agent often increases the severity of HBV infection. It can convert mild HBV infection into severe, fulminating hepatitis, cause acute hepatitis in asymptomatic carriers, or increase the tendency for progression to chronic hepatitis and cirrhosis.

The routes of transmission of hepatitis D are similar to those for hepatitis B. In Canada, infection is restricted largely to persons at high risk for HBV infection, particularly injecting drug users. The greatest risk is in HBV carriers; these persons should be informed about the dangers of HDV superinfection. Worldwide of the persons infected with hepatitis B approximately 5% are also infected with hepatitis D.[15] Hepatitis D is diagnosed by detection of antibody to HDV (anti-HDV) in the serum or HDV RNA in the serum. There is no specific treatment for hepatitis D. Because the infection is linked to hepatitis B, prevention of hepatitis D should begin with prevention of hepatitis B through vaccination.

Hepatitis E Virus. Hepatitis E virus (HEV) is an unenveloped, single-stranded RNA virus. It is transmitted by the fecal-oral route and causes manifestations of acute hepatitis that are similar to hepatitis A.[30,31] Its distinguishing feature is the high mortality rate (approximately 20%) among pregnant women, owing to the development of fulminant hepatitis. The infection occurs primarily in developing areas such as India, other Southeast Asian countries, parts of Africa, and Mexico. China has produced a vaccine but this currently is not available globally.[3,30] Hepatitis E is rarely seen in Canada.

Chronic Viral Hepatitis

Chronic hepatitis is defined as a chronic inflammatory reaction of the liver of more than 3 to 6 months' duration. It is characterized by persistently elevated serum aminotransferase levels and characteristic histologic findings on liver biopsy.[32] The clinical features of chronic viral hepatitis are highly variable and not predictive of outcome. The most common symptoms are fatigue, malaise, loss of appetite, and occasional bouts of jaundice. Elevation of serum aminotransferase concentrations depends on the level of disease activity.

Chronic viral hepatitis is the principal cause of chronic liver disease, cirrhosis, and hepatocellular cancer in the world and now ranks as the chief reason for liver transplantation in adults.[33] Of the hepatotropic viruses, only three are known to cause chronic hepatitis—HBV, HCV, and HDV. Hepatitis B, which is less likely than hepatitis C to progress to chronic infection, accounts for 5% to 10% of chronic liver disease and cirrhosis.[18] It is characterized by the persistence of HBV DNA and usually by HBeAg in the serum, indicating active viral replication. Many persons are asymptomatic at the time of diagnosis, and elevated serum aminotransferase levels are the first sign of infection. Chronic hepatitis D infection depends on concurrent infection with HBV.

Chronic hepatitis C accounts for most cases of chronic viral hepatitis. HCV infection becomes chronic in 60% to 85% of cases.[27] Chronic HCV infection often smoulders over a period of years, silently destroying liver cells. Most persons with chronic hepatitis C are asymptomatic, and diagnosis usually follows a finding of elevated serum aminotransferase levels or complaints of fatigue or nonspecific weakness. Because the course of acute hepatitis C often is mild, many persons do not recall the events of the acute infection.[32]

Treatment. There are no simple and effective treatment methods for chronic viral hepatitis. Drugs used in the treatment of chronic HBV include interferons (recombinant interferon-2α and peginterferon) and the nucleotide and nucleotide analog antiretroviral agents (lamivudine, entecavir, tenofovir).[32] Persons with active viral replication may be treated with peginterferon (pegylated interferon alfa-2a). Peginterferons have a prolonged serum half-life and are given once a week. Up to 40% of treated patients respond with sustained normalization of liver enzyme levels, disappearance of HBeAg and HBV DNA from the serum, appearance of anti-HBe, and improved survival.[32] Nucleoside and nucleotide analogs may be used instead of interferon for treatment of chronic HBV infection, and are better tolerated. Lamivudine can be given orally and usually is well tolerated, but has a higher rate of viral resistance, a lower durable rate of response, and a greater need for prolonged therapy compared with interferon. Entecavir, another nucleoside analog, can be used in the treatment of persons who are resistant to lamivudine or have cirrhosis. Tenofovir, a drug used for treatment of HIV infection, also has considerable activity against HBV. Other antiviral agents and combination strategies continue to be studied. In persons with concurrent hepatitis D infection, interferon therapy may lead to normalization of aminotransferase levels, histologic improvement, and elimination of HDV RNA from the serum in approximately 50% of cases, but relapse is common after the therapy is stopped.[32] Lamivudine is not effective in chronic hepatitis D.

The current treatment for untreated persons with chronic hepatitis C is a combination of the new pegylated forms of interferon (alfa-2b or alfa-2a) plus ribavirin (a nucleoside analog).[32,33] Treatment with peginterferon and ribavirin is costly, and side effects, which include flulike symptoms, are almost universal. More serious side effects, which include neurotoxicities (*e.g.,* depression, confusion, seizures), thyroid dysfunction, and bone marrow depression, are less common.[9,32] Adding protease inhibitors such as telaprevir or boceprevir has been shown to increase the efficacy of preinterferon and ribavirin for some genotypes of hepatitis C.[33] Although most persons with HCV infection are candidates for treatment, many have other health problems that are contraindications to therapy.

Liver transplantation is a treatment option for end-stage liver disease due to viral hepatitis. Liver transplantation has been more successful in persons with hepatitis C than in those with hepatitis B. Although the graft often is reinfected, the disease seems to progress more slowly.[33]

Autoimmune Hepatitis

Autoimmune hepatitis is a severe type of chronic hepatitis of unknown etiology that is associated with high levels of serum transaminases (AST, ALT more than bilirubin, GGT and AP), immunoglobulins, including autoantibodies with histologic changes.[4,32,34] Although the disorder is usually seen in young women, it can occur in either sex at any age.

Clinical and laboratory observations have led to the hypothesis that autoimmune hepatitis is a multifactorial disorder, with genetic and environmental factors playing important roles. Most knowledge of the genetics of the disease comes from the human leukocyte antigen (HLA) genes that reside in the major histocompatibility complex (MHC), located on the short arm of chromosome 6 (see Chapter 17). The environmental agents assumed to induce autoimmune hepatitis have not been delineated, but include viruses and chemical agents.[34]

Two distinct types of autoimmune hepatitis have been identified. Type I autoimmune hepatitis, the most common form of the disease, is characterized by increased levels of anti-smooth muscle and antinuclear autoantibodies. Approximately 78% of cases occur in women and 38% have other autoimmune diseases. Susceptibility to type I autoimmune hepatitis resides mainly with the *HLA-DRB1* gene. Type II autoimmune hepatitis occurs mainly in children 2 to 14 years of age and is characterized by the presence of antibody to liver and kidney microsomes and liver cytosol. The disorder is often accompanied by other autoimmune disorders, especially ulcerative colitis and thyroiditis. The genetic component for this type of autoimmune hepatitis is less well defined.[34,35]

Clinical Manifestations

Clinical manifestations of the disorder cover a spectrum that extends from no apparent symptoms to the signs accompanying liver failure. Physical examination may reveal no abnormalities, but may also reveal hepatomegaly, splenomegaly, jaundice, and signs and symptoms of chronic liver disease. In asymptomatic cases, the disorder may be discovered when abnormal serum enzyme levels are identified during performance of routine screening tests.[34,35]

Diagnosis and Treatment

The differential diagnosis includes measures to exclude other causes of liver disease, including hepatitis B and C. A characteristic laboratory finding is that of a marked elevation in serum gamma globulins. A biopsy is used to confirm the diagnosis.

Corticosteroid and immunosuppressant drugs are the treatment of choice for this type of hepatitis. Although some persons remain in remission after drug treatment is withdrawn, most require long-term maintenance treatment. Liver transplantation may be required for persons who are refractory to or intolerant of immunosuppressive therapy and in whom end-stage liver disease develops. Unfortunately the autoimmune hepatitis recurs in approximately 30% of patients.[34]

Intrahepatic Biliary Disorders

Intrahepatic biliary diseases disrupt the flow of bile through the liver, causing cholestasis and biliary cirrhosis. Among the causes of intrahepatic biliary disease are primary biliary cirrhosis and secondary biliary cirrhosis.

Primary Biliary Cirrhosis

Primary biliary cirrhosis is a chronic disease of the liver characterized by the autoimmune destruction of the small intrahepatic bile ducts, cholestasis, and in some cases cirrhosis.[36] The disease is seen most commonly in women 30 to 65 years of age.[4] Familial occurrences of the disease are found between parents and children and among siblings. Like other autoimmune disorders there is likely a genetic component that contributes to the autoreactivity of T-cell populations and currently up to 25 genetic regions are being investigated for their association with this disease. Antimitochondrial antibodies are found in approximately 90% to 95% of persons with the disease, but their role in the pathogenesis of the disease is unclear. As with other autoimmune disorders, possible environmental triggers include infectious and chemical agents.[3,36]

Clinical Manifestations. The disorder is characterized by an insidious onset and progressive scarring and destruction of liver tissue. The liver becomes enlarged and takes on a green hue because of the accumulated bile. The earliest symptoms are unexplained pruritus or itching, weight loss, and fatigue, followed by dark urine and pale stools. Osteopenia (a precursor to osteoporosis) occurs in up to one third of persons with the disorder.[36] Jaundice is a late manifestation of the disorder, as are other signs of liver failure. Serum alkaline phosphatase levels are elevated in persons with primary biliary cirrhosis.

Treatment. Treatment is largely symptomatic. Cholestyramine, a bile acid-binding drug, or rifampin, an antibiotic, may prove beneficial for treatment of pruritus. There is no generally accepted treatment for the underlying disease. Ursodeoxycholic acid (ursodiol), a drug that increases bile flow and decreases the toxicity of bile contents, has been shown to decrease the rate of clinical deterioration. Colchicine, which acts to prevent leukocyte migration and phagocytosis, and methotrexate, a drug with immunosuppressive properties, have also resulted in reported benefits in terms of symptom relief. Due to the high rate of osteopenia and osteoporosis, supplementation of vitamin D may be required and monitoring of other fat-soluble vitamins is advised. However, liver transplantation remains the only treatment for advanced disease. Primary biliary cirrhosis rarely recurs after liver transplantation if appropriate immunosuppression is used.[36]

Secondary Biliary Cirrhosis

Secondary biliary cirrhosis results from prolonged obstruction of the extrabiliary tree. The most common cause is cholelithiasis. Other causes of secondary biliary cirrhosis are malignant neoplasms of the biliary tree or head of the pancreas and strictures of the common duct caused by previous surgical procedures. Extrahepatic biliary cirrhosis may benefit from surgical procedures designed to relieve the obstruction.

Alcohol-Induced Liver Disease

The spectrum of alcoholic liver disease includes fatty liver disease, alcoholic hepatitis, and cirrhosis. Most deaths from alcoholic cirrhosis are attributable to liver failure, bleeding esophageal varices, or kidney failure. It has been estimated that about 10% of Canadians are dependent on alcohol at some time in their lives.[37] Only approximately 15% of alcoholics develop cirrhosis, however, suggesting that other conditions such as genetic and environmental factors contribute to its occurrence.[4]

Metabolism of Alcohol

Alcohol is absorbed readily from the gastrointestinal tract; it is one of the few substances that can be absorbed from the stomach. As a substance, alcohol fits somewhere between a food and a drug. It supplies calories but cannot be broken down or stored as protein, fat, or carbohydrate. As a food, alcohol yields 7.1 kcal/g, compared with the 4 kcal/g produced by metabolism of an equal amount of carbohydrate. Between 80% and 90% of the alcohol a person drinks is metabolized by the liver. The rest is excreted through the lungs, kidneys, and skin.

Alcohol (ethyl alcohol or ethanol) metabolism proceeds simultaneously by two pathways: the alcohol dehydrogenase (ADH) system, located in the cytoplasm of the hepatocytes; and the microsomal ethanol-oxidizing system (MEOS), located in the hepatic endoplasmic reticulum.[38–40] The ADH and MEOS pathways produce specific metabolic and toxic disturbances. A third and minor pathway, the catalase pathway, located in the peroxisomes, can break down ethanol in unusual circumstances.[40]

The major pathway for ethanol metabolism involves ADH, an enzyme that catalyzes the conversion of alcohol to acetaldehyde. In the ADH-mediated oxidation of alcohol, both acetaldehyde and hydrogen are produced. The hydrogen (H^+) is transferred to the cofactor nicotinamide adenine dinucleotide (NAD), which is converted to its reduced form (NADH). The formed acetaldehyde again loses hydrogen and is metabolized to acetate, much of which is released in the bloodstream. As a result, ethanol metabolism generates an excess of NADH, which is thought to contribute to the liver damage that often accompanies excess alcohol consumption.

NAD is also necessary for many other metabolic processes, including the metabolism of pyruvates, urates, and fatty acids. Because alcohol competes for the use of NAD, it tends to disrupt other metabolic functions of the liver. The preferential use of NAD for alcohol metabolism can result in increased production and accumulation of lactic acid in the blood. By reducing the availability of NAD, alcohol also impairs the liver's ability to form glucose from amino acids and other glucose precursors (*i.e.,* can prevent gluconeogenesis). Alcohol-induced hypoglycemia can develop when excessive alcohol ingestion occurs during periods of depleted liver glycogen stores.

The MEOS pathway, which is located in the smooth endoplasmic reticulum, produces acetaldehyde and free radicals. Prolonged and excessive alcohol ingestion results in enzyme induction and increased activity of the MEOS. One of the most important enzymes of the MEOS, a member of the CYP P450 system, also oxidizes a number of other compounds, including various drugs (*e.g.,* acetaminophen, isoniazid), toxins (*e.g.,* carbon tetrachloride, halothane), vitamins A and D, and carcinogenic agents (*e.g.,* aflatoxin, nitrosamines). Increased activity of this system enhances the susceptibility of persons with heavy alcohol consumption to the hepatotoxic effects of industrial toxins, anesthetic agents, chemical carcinogens, vitamins, and the pain reliever acetaminophen.[40]

The metabolic end products of alcohol metabolism (*e.g.,* acetaldehyde, free radicals) are responsible for a variety of metabolic alterations that can cause liver injury. Acetaldehyde, for example, has multiple toxic effects on liver cells and liver function. Age and sex play a role in metabolism of alcohol and production of harmful metabolites. The ADH system is depressed by testosterone. Thus, women tend to produce greater amounts of acetaldehyde and are more predisposed to alcohol-induced liver damage than men.[40] Age also appears to affect the alcohol-metabolizing abilities of the liver and the resistance to hepatotoxic effects. Furthermore, genetic factors may influence the severity of alcohol-induced liver disease. ADH has multiple isoenzymes, the genetic polymorphism currently being studied in terms of possible clinical implications.[40]

Alcoholic Liver Disease

The metabolism of alcohol leads to chemical attack on certain membranes of the liver, but whether the damage is caused by acetaldehyde or other metabolites is unknown. Acetaldehyde is known to impede the mitochondrial electron transport system, which is responsible for oxidative metabolism and generation of ATP; as a result, the hydrogen ions that are generated in the mitochondria are shunted into lipid synthesis and ketogenesis.[40] Abnormal accumulations of these substances are found in hepatocytes (*i.e.,* fatty liver) and blood. Binding of acetaldehyde to other molecules impairs the detoxification of free radicals and synthesis of proteins. Acetaldehyde also promotes collagen synthesis and fibrogenesis. The lesions of hepatocellular injury tend to be most prevalent in the centrilobular area that surrounds the central vein, where the pathways for alcohol metabolism are concentrated. This is the part of the lobule that has the lowest oxygen tension; it is thought that the low oxygen concentration in this area of the liver may contribute to the damage.

The amount of alcohol required to produce chronic liver disease varies widely, depending on body size, age, sex, and ethnicity, but the high end of the range seems to be about 80 g/day (*e.g.,* 237 ml or 8 ounces of 86 proof [41% alcohol] whiskey, two 750 ml bottles of wine, or six 341 ml bottles of beer) for 10 to 12 years.[4,41] Even after alcohol intake has stopped and all alcohol has been metabolized, the processes that damage liver cells may continue for many weeks and months. Clinical and chemical effects often become worse before the disease resolves. The accumulation of fat usually disappears within a few weeks, and cholestasis and inflammation also subside with time. However, fibrosis and scarring remain. The liver lobules become distorted as new liver cells regenerate and form nodules.

Although the mechanism by which alcohol exerts its toxic effects on liver structures is somewhat uncertain, the changes that develop can be divided into three stages: fatty changes, alcoholic hepatitis, and cirrhosis.[3,4]

Fatty liver is characterized by the accumulation of fat in hepatocytes, a condition called *steatosis* (Fig. 38.12). The liver becomes yellow and enlarges owing to excessive fat accumulation. The pathogenesis of fatty liver is not completely understood and can depend on the amount of alcohol consumed, dietary fat content, body stores of fat, hormonal status, and other factors. There is evidence that ingestion of large amounts of alcohol can cause fatty liver changes even with an adequate diet. For example, young, nonalcoholic volunteers had fatty liver changes after 2 days of consuming an excess amount of alcohol, even though adequate carbohydrates, fats, and proteins were included in the diet.[42] The fatty changes that occur with ingestion of alcohol usually do not produce symptoms and are reversible after the alcohol intake has been discontinued.

FIGURE 38.12 • Alcoholic fatty liver. A photomicrograph shows the cytoplasm of almost all the hepatocytes to be distended by fat, which displaces the nucleus to the periphery (*arrows*). Note the absence of inflammation and fibrosis. (From Rubin R., Strayer D. (Eds.). (2012). *Rubin's pathology: Clinicopathologic foundations of medicine* (6th ed., p. 708). Philadelphia, PA: Lippincott-Raven)

Alcoholic hepatitis is the intermediate stage between fatty changes and cirrhosis. It often is seen after an abrupt increase in alcohol intake and is common in binge drinkers. Alcoholic hepatitis is characterized by inflammation and necrosis of liver cells. This stage usually is characterized by hepatic tenderness, pain, anorexia, nausea, fever, jaundice, ascites, and liver failure, but some individuals may be asymptomatic. The condition is always serious and sometimes fatal. The immediate prognosis correlates with severity of liver cell injury. In some cases, the disease progresses rapidly to liver failure and death. The mortality rate in the acute stage is about 10% to 20%.[4] In persons who survive and continue to drink, the acute phase often is followed by persistent alcoholic hepatitis with progression to cirrhosis in a matter of 1 to 2 years.

Alcoholic cirrhosis is the end result of repeated bouts of drinking-related liver injury and designates the onset of end-stage alcoholic liver disease. The gross appearance of the early cirrhotic liver is one of fine, uniform nodules on its surface. The condition has traditionally been called *micronodular* or *Laennec cirrhosis*. With more advanced cirrhosis, regenerative processes cause the nodules to become larger and more irregular in size and shape. As this occurs, the nodules cause the liver to become relobulized through the formation of new portal tracts and venous outflow channels. The nodules may compress the hepatic veins, curtailing blood flow out of the liver and producing portal hypertension, extrahepatic portosystemic shunts, and cholestasis.

Nonalcoholic Fatty Liver Disease

The term *nonalcoholic fatty liver disease* (NAFLD) is often used to describe fatty liver disease with the potential for progression to cirrhosis and end-stage liver disease arising from causes other than alcohol.[43–46] The condition can range from simple steatosis (fatty infiltration of the liver) to nonalcoholic steatohepatitis (steatosis with inflammation and hepatocyte necrosis). Although steatosis alone does not appear to be progressive, approximately 20% of persons with nonalcoholic steatohepatitis progress to cirrhosis.[3,47] Obesity, type 2 diabetes, the metabolic syndrome, and hyperlipidemia are coexisting conditions frequently associated with fatty liver disease (see Chapter 42). The condition is also associated with other nutritional abnormalities, surgical conditions, drugs, and occupational exposure to toxins. Both rapid weight loss and parenteral nutrition may lead to NAFLD. Jejunoileal bypass, a surgical procedure used for weight loss, has largely been abandoned for this reason.

Pathogenesis. The pathogenesis of NAFLD is thought to involve both lipid accumulation within hepatocytes and formation of free radicals, in a manner similar to that which occurs with alcohol metabolism. The primary metabolic abnormalities leading to lipid accumulation are poorly understood but are thought to include alterations in pathways for uptake, synthesis, degradation, or secretion of hepatic lipids resulting from insulin resistance. Obesity increases the synthesis and reduces the oxidation of free fatty acids. Type 2 diabetes or insulin resistance also increases adipose tissue lipolysis and the subsequent production of free fatty acids.[47] When the capacity of the liver to export triglyceride is exceeded, excess fatty acids contribute to the formation of fatty liver. Both ketones and free fatty acids are inducers of previously described CYP P450 enzymes of the MEOS pathway, which results in free radical formation, including hydrogen peroxide and superoxide (see Chapter 5). Abnormal lipid peroxidation ensues, followed by direct hepatocyte injury, release of toxic byproducts, inflammation, and fibrosis.

Clinical Manifestations. NAFLD is usually asymptomatic, although fatigue and discomfort in the right upper quadrant of the abdomen may be present. Mildly to moderately elevated serum levels of AST, ALT, or both are the most common and often the only abnormal laboratory findings. Other abnormalities, including hypoalbuminemia, a prolonged prothrombin time, and hyperbilirubinemia, may be present in persons with cirrhotic-stage liver disease. The diagnosis of NAFLD requires liver biopsy and exclusion of alcohol as a cause of the disorder.[47]

Treatment. The aim of treatment is to slow progression of NAFLD and to prevent liver-related illness. Both weight loss and exercise improve insulin resistance and are recommended in conjunction with treatment of associated metabolic disturbances. Alcohol use should be avoided. Disease progression is slow and the magnitude of disease-related morbidity and mortality is uncertain. Liver transplantation is an alternative for some persons with end-stage liver disease, but NAFLD may reoccur or develop after liver transplantation.[48]

Cirrhosis, Portal Hypertension, and Liver Failure

Cirrhosis

Cirrhosis represents the end stage of chronic liver disease in which much of the functional liver tissue has been replaced by fibrous tissue. Although cirrhosis usually is associated with alcoholism, it can develop in the course of other disorders, including viral hepatitis, toxic reactions to drugs and chemicals, biliary obstruction, and NAFLD. Cirrhosis also accompanies metabolic disorders that cause the deposition of minerals in the liver. Two of these disorders are hemochromatosis (*i.e.,* iron deposition) and Wilson disease (*i.e.,* copper deposition).

Cirrhosis is characterized by diffuse fibrosis and conversion of normal liver architecture into nodules containing proliferating hepatocytes encircled by fibrosis. The formation of nodules, which vary in size from very small (<3 mm, micronodules) to large (several centimetres, macronodules), represents a balance between regenerative activity and constrictive scarring.[3,4] The fibrous tissue that replaces normally functioning liver tissue forms constrictive bands that disrupt flow in the vascular channels and biliary duct systems of the liver. The disruption of vascular channels predisposes to portal hypertension and its complications; obstruction of biliary channels and exposure to the destructive effects of bile stasis; and loss of liver cells, leading to liver failure.

Clinical Manifestations. The manifestations of cirrhosis are variable, ranging from asymptomatic hepatomegaly to hepatic failure (Fig. 38.13). Often there are no symptoms until the disease is far advanced.[3,4] The most common signs and symptoms of cirrhosis are weight loss (sometimes masked by ascites), weakness, and anorexia. Diarrhea frequently is present, although some persons may complain of constipation. Hepatomegaly and jaundice also are common signs of cirrhosis. There may be abdominal pain because of liver enlargement or stretching of the Glisson capsule. This pain is located in the epigastric area or in the upper right quadrant and is described as dull, aching, and causing a sensation of fullness.

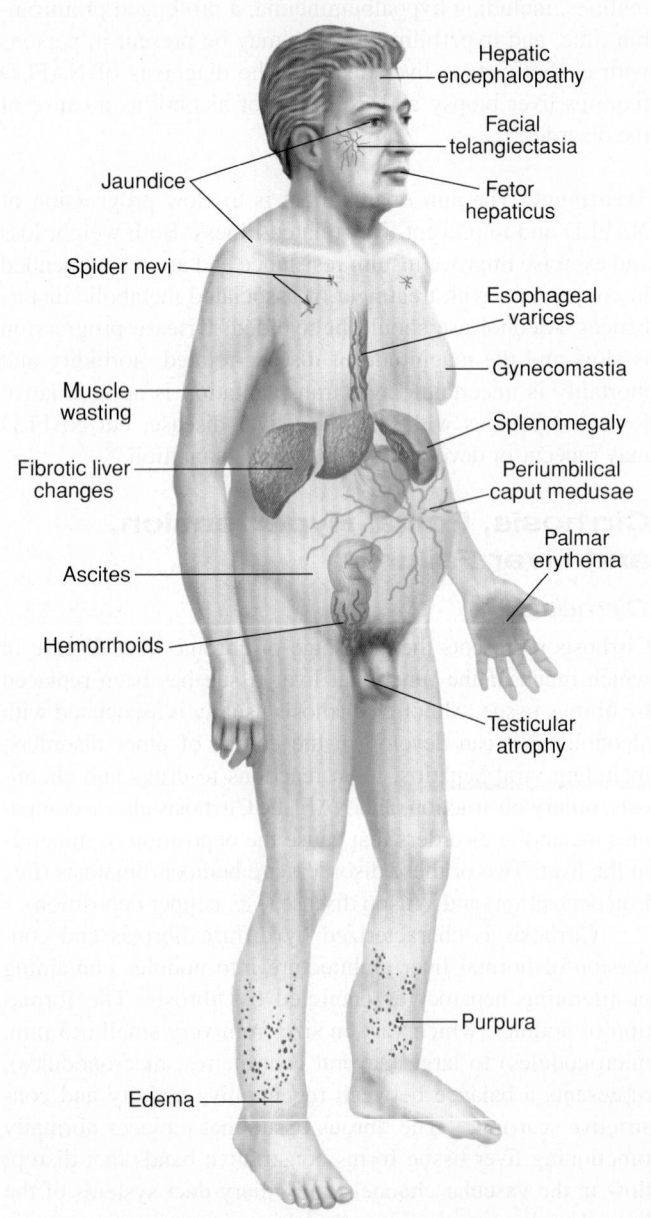

FIGURE 38.13 • Clinical manifestations of cirrhosis.

Labels: Hepatic encephalopathy; Facial telangiectasia; Fetor hepaticus; Jaundice; Spider nevi; Esophageal varices; Gynecomastia; Muscle wasting; Splenomegaly; Fibrotic liver changes; Periumbilical caput medusae; Palmar erythema; Ascites; Hemorrhoids; Testicular atrophy; Purpura; Edema

The late manifestations of cirrhosis are related to portal hypertension and liver cell failure. Splenomegaly, ascites, and portosystemic shunts (*i.e.,* esophageal varices, hemorrhoids, and caput medusae) result from portal hypertension. Other complications include bleeding due to decreased clotting factors, thrombocytopenia due to splenomegaly, gynecomastia and a feminizing pattern of pubic hair distribution in men because of testicular atrophy, spider angiomas, palmar erythema, and encephalopathy with asterixis and neurologic signs.

Portal Hypertension

Portal hypertension is characterized by increased resistance to flow in the portal venous system and sustained portal vein pressure above 12 mm Hg (normal, 5 to 10 mm Hg).[4,43] Normally, venous blood returning to the heart from the abdominal organs collects in the portal vein and travels through the liver before entering the vena cava. Portal hypertension can be caused by a variety of conditions that increase resistance to hepatic blood flow, including prehepatic, posthepatic, and intrahepatic obstructions (with *hepatic* referring to the liver lobules rather than the entire liver).[4] Prehepatic causes of portal hypertension include portal vein thrombosis and external compression due to cancer or enlarged lymph nodes that produce obstruction of the portal vein before it enters the liver.

PORTAL HYPERTENSION

- Venous blood from the gastrointestinal tract empties into the portal vein and travels through the liver before moving into the general venous circulation.
- Obstruction of blood flow in the portal vein produces an increase in the hydrostatic pressure within the peritoneal capillaries, contributing to the development of ascites, splenic engorgement with sequestration and destruction of blood cells and platelets, and shunting of blood to collateral venous channels causing varicosities of the hemorrhoidal and esophageal veins.

Posthepatic obstruction refers to any obstruction to blood flow through the hepatic veins beyond the liver lobules, either within or distal to the liver. It is caused by conditions such as thrombosis of the hepatic veins, veno-occlusive disease, and severe right-sided heart failure that impede the outflow of venous blood from the liver. *Budd–Chiari syndrome* refers to congestive disease of the liver caused by occlusion of the hepatic venules, large portal veins, or the inferior vena cava.[44] The principal cause of the Budd–Chiari syndrome is thrombosis of the hepatic veins, in association with diverse conditions such as polycythemia vera, hypercoagulability states associated with malignant tumours, pregnancy, bacterial infection, metastatic disease of the liver, and trauma. *Hepatic veno-occlusive disease* is a variant of the Budd–Chiari syndrome seen most commonly in persons treated with certain cancer chemotherapeutic drugs, hepatic irradiation, or bone marrow

FIGURE 38.14 • Mechanisms of disturbed liver function related to portal hypertension.

transplantation—possibly due to graft-versus-host disease in the latter instance.[4]

Intrahepatic causes of portal hypertension include conditions that cause obstruction of blood flow within the liver. In alcoholic cirrhosis, which is the major cause of portal hypertension, bands of fibrous tissue and fibrous nodules distort the architecture of the liver and increase the resistance to portal blood flow, which leads to portal hypertension.

Complications of portal hypertension arise from the increased pressure and dilation of the venous channels behind the obstruction (Fig. 38.14). In addition, collateral channels open that connect the portal circulation with the systemic circulation. The major complications of the increased portal vein pressure and the opening of collateral channels are ascites, splenomegaly, and the formation of portosystemic shunts with bleeding from esophageal varices.[3,4]

Ascites. Ascites occurs when the amount of fluid in the peritoneal cavity is increased, and is a late-stage manifestation of cirrhosis and portal hypertension.[45] It is not uncommon for persons with advanced cirrhosis to present with an accumulation of 15 L or more of ascitic fluid. These persons often experience abdominal discomfort, dyspnea, and insomnia. They may also have difficulty walking or caring for themselves.

Although the mechanisms responsible for the development of ascites are not completely understood, several factors seem to contribute to fluid accumulation, including an increase in capillary pressure due to portal hypertension and obstruction of venous flow through the liver, salt and water retention by the kidney, and decreased colloidal osmotic pressure due to impaired synthesis of albumin by the liver. Diminished blood volume (*i.e.*, underfill theory) and excessive blood volume (*i.e.*, overfill theory) have been used to explain the increased salt and water retention by the kidney. According to the underfill theory, a contraction in the effective blood volume constitutes an afferent signal that causes the kidney

to retain salt and water. The effective blood volume may be reduced because of loss of fluid into the peritoneal cavity or because of vasodilation caused by the presence of circulating vasodilating substances. The overfill theory proposes that the initial event in the development of ascites is renal retention of salt and water caused by disturbances in the liver itself. These disturbances include failure of the liver to metabolize aldosterone, causing an increase in salt and water retention by the kidney. Another likely contributing factor in the pathogenesis of ascites is a decreased colloidal osmotic pressure, which limits reabsorption of fluid from the peritoneal cavity (see Chapter 31).

Treatment of ascites usually focuses on dietary restriction of sodium and administration of diuretics. Water intake also may need to be restricted. Because of the many limitations in sodium restriction, the use of diuretics has become the mainstay of treatment for ascites. Two classes of diuretics are used: a diuretic that acts in the distal part of the nephron to inhibit aldosterone-dependent sodium reabsorption, and a loop diuretic such as furosemide (see Chapter 30). Oral potassium supplements often are given to prevent hypokalemia. The upright position is thought to be associated with the activation of the renin–angiotensin–aldosterone system but studies have not shown that bed rest increases the efficacy of diuretics rather it likely leads to more complications such as muscle atrophy and thus bed rest is no longer recommended.[46] Large-volume paracentesis (removal of 5 L or more of ascitic fluid) may be done in persons with massive ascites and pulmonary compromise. Because the removal of fluid produces a decrease in vascular volume along with increased plasma renin activity and aldosterone-mediated sodium and water reabsorption by the kidneys, a volume expander such as albumin usually is administered to maintain the effective circulating volume.[32,45,46] A transjugular intrahepatic portosystemic shunt (TIPS) may be inserted in persons with refractory ascites (to be discussed).[45]

Spontaneous bacterial peritonitis is a complication in persons with both cirrhosis and ascites. The infection is serious and carries a high mortality rate even when treated with antibiotics. Presumably, the peritoneal fluid is seeded with bacteria from the blood or lymph or from passage of gram negative enteric bacteria such as *Escherichia coli* and *Klebsiella pneumonia* through the bowel wall. Symptoms include fever and abdominal pain. Other symptoms include worsening of hepatic encephalopathy, diarrhea, hypothermia, and shock. It is diagnosed by an ascitic fluid neutrophil count of 0.25×10^9/L or higher.[32,49]

Splenomegaly. The spleen enlarges progressively in portal hypertension because of shunting of blood into the splenic vein. The enlarged spleen often gives rise to sequestering of significant numbers of blood elements and development of a syndrome known as *hypersplenism.* Hypersplenism is characterized by a decrease in the life span of all the formed elements of the blood and a subsequent decrease in their numbers, leading to anemia, thrombocytopenia, and leukopenia. The decreased life span of the blood elements is thought to result from an increased rate of removal because of the prolonged transit time through the enlarged spleen.[3]

Portosystemic Shunts. With the gradual obstruction of venous blood flow in the liver, the pressure in the portal vein increases, and large collateral channels develop between the portal and systemic veins that supply the lower rectum, the esophagus, and the umbilical veins of the falciform ligament that attaches to the anterior wall of the abdomen. The collaterals between the inferior and internal iliac veins may give rise to hemorrhoids. In some persons, the fetal umbilical vein is not totally obliterated; it forms a channel on the anterior abdominal wall. Dilated veins around the umbilicus are called *caput medusae.* Portopulmonary shunts also may develop and cause blood to bypass the pulmonary capillaries, interfering with blood oxygenation and producing cyanosis.

Clinically, the most important collateral channels are those connecting the portal and gastric coronary veins that lead to reversal of flow and formation of thin-walled varicosities in the submucosa of the esophagus (Fig. 38.15). These thin-walled *esophageal varices* are subject to rupture, producing massive and sometimes fatal hemorrhage. Impaired hepatic synthesis of coagulation factors and decreased platelet levels (*i.e.,* thrombocytopenia) due to splenomegaly may further complicate the control of esophageal bleeding.[50,51] Esophageal varices develop in approximately 40% of persons with advanced cirrhosis and cause massive hemorrhage and death in approximately half of them.[3]

Treatment of portal hypertension and esophageal varices is directed at prevention of initial hemorrhage, management of acute hemorrhage, and prevention of recurrent hemorrhage. Pharmacologic therapy is used to lower portal venous pressure and prevent initial hemorrhage. β-Adrenergic blocking drugs (*e.g.,* propranolol) commonly are used for this purpose. These agents reduce portal venous pressure by decreasing splanchnic blood flow and thereby decreasing blood flow in collateral channels.[50,51]

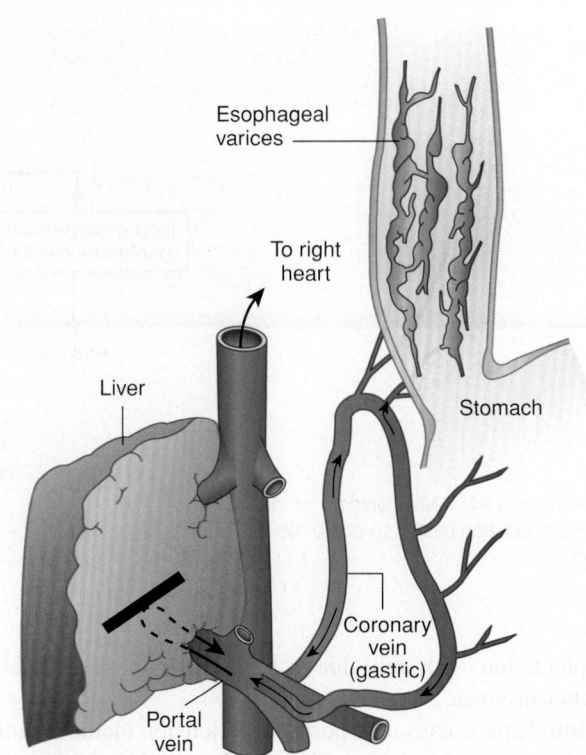

FIGURE 38.15 • Obstruction of blood flow in the portal circulation, with portal hypertension and diversion of blood flow to other venous channels, including the gastric and esophageal veins.

Several methods are used to control acute hemorrhage, including administration of octreotide or vasopressin, balloon tamponade, endoscopic injection sclerotherapy, vessel ligation, or esophageal transection.[50] Octreotide, a long-acting synthetic analog of somatostatin, reduces splanchnic and hepatic blood flow and portal pressures in persons with cirrhosis. Vasopressin, a hormone from the posterior pituitary, is a nonselective vasoconstrictor that also can be used to control variceal bleeding. Because octreotide has fewer side effects and appears to be more effective than vasopressin, it has become the drug of choice for pharmacologic management of acute variceal bleeding. Balloon tamponade provides short-term compression of the varices and is accomplished through the insertion of a tube with inflatable gastric and esophageal balloons. After the tube has been inserted, the balloons are inflated; the esophageal balloon compresses the bleeding esophageal veins, and the gastric balloon helps to maintain the position of the tube. During endoscopic sclerotherapy, the varices are injected with a sclerosing solution that obliterates the vessel lumen. Short-term antibiotics are often added to the management of acute variceal hemorrhages.

Prevention of recurrent hemorrhage focuses on lowering portal venous pressure and diverting blood flow away from the easily ruptured collateral channels. Two procedures may be used for this purpose: the surgical creation of a portosystemic shunt or a TIPS. *Surgical portosystemic shunt* procedures involve the creation of an opening between the portal vein and a systemic vein. These shunts have a considerable complication rate, and TIPS has evolved as the preferred treatment for refractory portal hypertension. The TIPS procedure involves insertion of an expandable metal stent between a branch of the hepatic vein and the portal vein using a catheter inserted through the internal jugular vein. A limitation of the procedure is that stenosis and thrombosis of the stent occurs in most cases over time, with consequent risk of rebleeding. A complication that is associated with the creation of a portosystemic shunt is hepatic encephalopathy, which is thought to result when ammonia and other neurotoxic substances from the gut pass directly into the systemic circulation without going through the liver.

Liver Failure

The most severe clinical consequence of liver disease is hepatic failure. It may result from sudden and massive liver destruction, as in fulminant hepatitis, or be the result of progressive damage to the liver, as occurs in alcoholic cirrhosis. Whatever the cause, 80% to 90% of hepatic functional capacity must be lost before liver failure occurs.[3] In many cases, the progressive decompensating effects of the disease are hastened by intercurrent conditions such as gastrointestinal bleeding, systemic infection, electrolyte disturbances, or superimposed diseases such as heart failure.

Manifestations. The manifestations of liver failure reflect the various synthesis, storage, metabolic, and elimination functions of the liver (Fig. 38.16). *Fetor hepaticus* refers to a characteristic musty, sweetish odour of the breath of patients in advanced liver failure, resulting from the metabolic byproducts of the intestinal bacteria.[3]

Hematologic Disorders. Liver failure can cause anemia, thrombocytopenia, coagulation defects, and leukopenia. Anemia may be caused by blood loss, excessive red blood cell destruction, and impaired formation of red blood cells. A folic acid deficiency may lead to severe megaloblastic anemia. Changes in the lipid composition of the red blood cell membrane increase hemolysis. Because factors V, VII, IX, and X, prothrombin, and fibrinogen are synthesized by the liver, their decline in liver disease contributes to bleeding disorders. Malabsorption of the fat-soluble vitamin K contributes further to the impaired synthesis of these clotting factors. Thrombocytopenia often occurs as the result of splenomegaly. The person with liver failure is subject to purpura, easy bruising, hematuria, and abnormal menstrual bleeding, and is vulnerable to bleeding from the esophagus and other segments of the gastrointestinal tract.

Endocrine Disorders. The liver metabolizes the steroid hormones. Endocrine disorders, particularly disturbances in gonadal (sex hormone) function, are common accompaniments of cirrhosis and liver failure. Women may have menstrual irregularities (usually amenorrhea), loss of libido, and

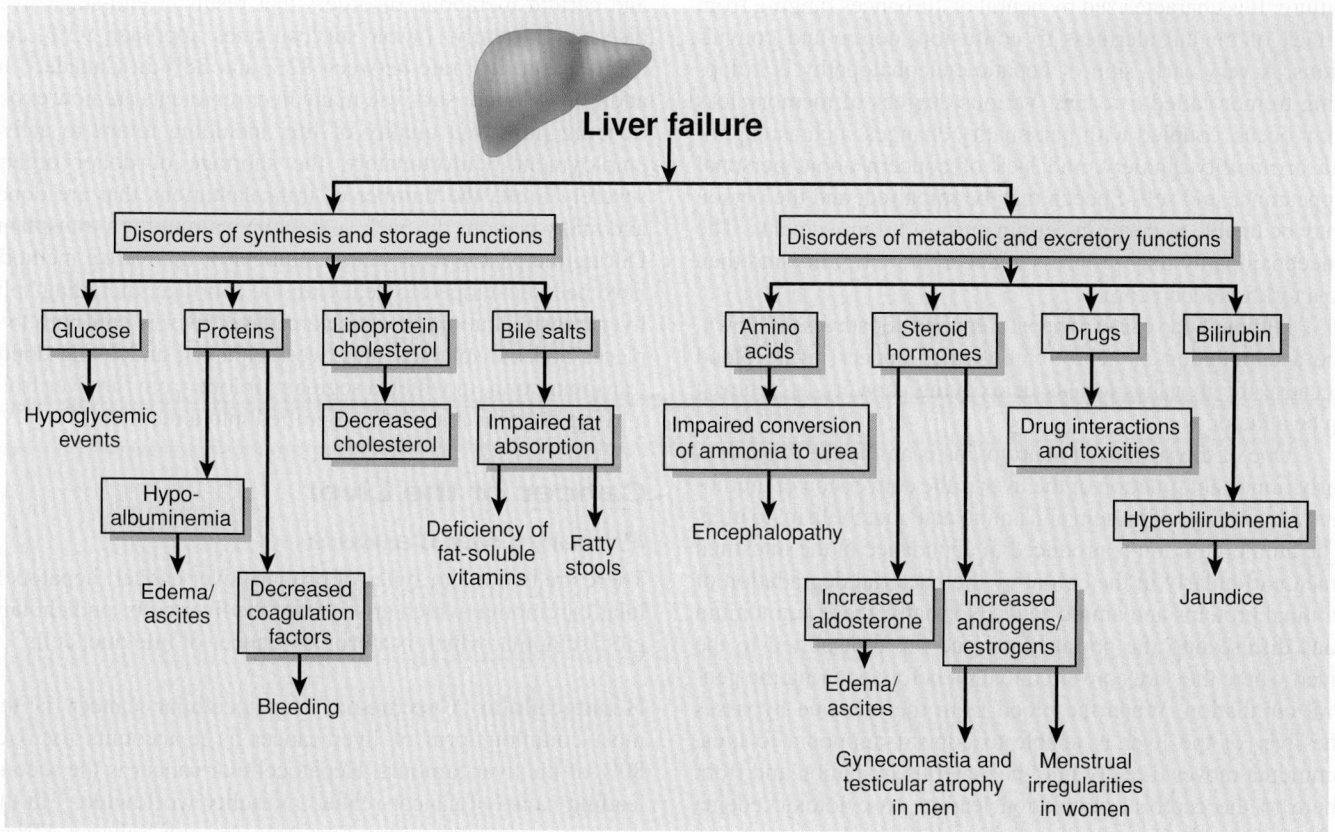

FIGURE 38.16 • Alterations in liver function and manifestations of liver failure.

sterility. In men, testosterone levels usually fall, the testes atrophy, and loss of libido, impotence, and gynecomastia occur. A decrease in aldosterone metabolism may contribute to salt and water retention by the kidney, along with a lowering of serum potassium resulting from increased elimination of potassium.

Skin Disorders. Liver failure brings on numerous skin disorders. These lesions, called by various names such as *vascular spiders, telangiectases, spider angiomas,* and *spider nevi,* are seen most often in the upper half of the body. They consist of a central pulsating arteriole from which smaller vessels radiate. Palmar erythema is redness of the palms, probably caused by increased blood flow from higher cardiac output. Clubbing of the fingers may be seen in persons with cirrhosis. Jaundice usually is a late manifestation of liver failure.[52]

Hepatorenal Syndrome. The hepatorenal syndrome refers to a functional renal failure sometimes seen during the terminal stages of liver failure with ascites.[53] It is characterized by progressive azotemia, increased serum creatinine levels, and oliguria. Although the basic cause is unknown, a decrease in renal blood flow is believed to play a part. Ultimately, when renal failure is superimposed on liver failure, azotemia and elevated levels of blood ammonia occur; this condition is thought to contribute to hepatic encephalopathy and coma.

Hepatic Encephalopathy. Hepatic encephalopathy refers to the totality of central nervous system manifestations of liver failure. It is characterized by neural disturbances ranging from a lack of mental alertness to confusion, coma, and convulsions. A very early sign of hepatic encephalopathy is a flapping tremor called *asterixis.* Various degrees of memory loss may occur, coupled with personality changes such as euphoria, irritability, anxiety, and lack of concern about personal appearance and self. Speech may be impaired, and the person may be unable to perform certain purposeful movements. The encephalopathy may progress to decerebrate rigidity and then to a terminal deep coma.[54]

Although the cause of hepatic encephalopathy is unknown, the accumulation of neurotoxins, which appear in the blood because the liver has lost its detoxifying capacity, is believed to be a factor.

One of the suspected neurotoxins is ammonia. A particularly important function of the liver is the conversion of ammonia, a byproduct of protein and amino acid metabolism, to urea. The ammonium ion is produced in abundance in the intestinal tract, particularly in the colon, by the bacterial degradation of luminal proteins and amino acids. Normally, these ammonium ions diffuse into the portal blood and are transported to the liver, where they are converted to urea before entering the general circulation. When the blood from the intestine bypasses the liver or the liver is unable to convert ammonia to urea, ammonia moves directly into the general circulation and from there to the cerebral circulation leading to cytotoxic edema of astrocytes.[54] Hepatic encephalopathy may become worse after a large protein meal or gastrointestinal tract bleeding.

Narcotics and tranquilizers are poorly metabolized by the liver, and administration of these drugs may cause central nervous system depression and precipitate hepatic encephalopathy.

The minimally absorbable broad spectrum antibiotic, rifaximin is more commonly used compared to the nonabsorbable antibiotic, such as neomycin, but both work to eradicate bacteria from the bowel and thus prevent this cause of ammonia production. Another drug that may be given is lactulose. It is not absorbed from the small intestine but moves directly to the large intestine, where it is catabolized by colonic bacteria to small organic acids that cause production of large, loose stools with a low pH. The low pH favours the conversion of ammonia to ammonium ions, which are not absorbed by the blood. The acid pH also inhibits the intestinal degradation of amino acids, proteins, and blood.[54]

Treatment. The treatment of liver failure is directed toward eliminating alcohol intake when the condition is caused by alcoholic cirrhosis; preventing infections; providing sufficient carbohydrates and calories to prevent protein breakdown; correcting fluid and electrolyte imbalances, particularly hypokalemia; and decreasing ammonia production in the gastrointestinal tract by controlling protein intake.

In many cases, liver transplantation remains the only effective treatment. Liver transplantation rapidly is becoming a realistic form of treatment for many persons with irreversible chronic liver disease, fulminant liver failure, primary biliary cirrhosis, chronic active hepatitis, sclerosing cholangitis, and certain metabolic disorders that result in end-stage liver disease. Currently, 1-year survival rates approach 92%, and a 3-year survival rate between 82% and 88% in Canada.[55] In addition to longer survival, many liver recipients are now experiencing improved quality of life, including return to active employment. Unfortunately, the shortage of donor organs severely limits the number of transplantations that are done, and many persons die each year while waiting for a transplant. During the past several years a number of innovative methods have been developed to deal with the shortage, including split liver transplantation, in which a cadaver liver is split into two pieces and transplanted into two recipients; and living donor transplantation, in which a segment or lobe from the liver from a living donor is resected and grafted into a recipient.[56]

Cancer of the Liver

Primary Liver Cancers

There are two major types of primary liver cancer: hepatocellular carcinoma, which arises from the liver cells, and cholangiocarcinoma, which is a primary cancer of bile duct cells.[57]

Hepatocellular Carcinoma. Hepatocellular cancer is the most common form of liver cancer as it accounts for over 80% of the liver tumours. Hepatocellular cancer is the second leading cause of cancer-related mortality worldwide.[58] In the developing country within East Asia and sub-Saharan Africa, the high incidence of 20 cases per 100,000 is a consequence of increased chronic HCV infections. In Mediterranean countries such as Italy, Spain, and Greece, the incidence rate is approximately 10 to 20 per 100,000. For North and South America, the incidence rate is the lowest with less than 5 cases per 100,000.[58] Although primary tumours of the liver are relatively rare in developed countries of the world, the liver shares with the lung the distinction of being the most common site of metastatic tumours.

Among the factors identified as etiologic agents in liver cancer are chronic viral hepatitis (*i.e.*, HBV, HCV, HDV), cirrhosis, long-term exposure to environmental agents such as aflatoxin, and drinking water contaminated with arsenic.[57] Just how these etiologic agents contribute to the development of liver cancer is still unclear. With HBV and HCV, both of which become integrated into the host DNA, repeated cycles of cell death and regeneration afford the potential for development of cancer-producing mutations. Aflatoxins, produced by food spoilage moulds in certain areas endemic for hepatocellular carcinoma, are particularly potent carcinogenic agents.[3] They are activated by hepatocytes and their products incorporated into the host DNA with the potential for developing cancer-producing mutations. A particularly susceptible site for aflatoxin mutation is the *TP53* tumour suppressor gene[3,59] (see Chapter 8).

The manifestations of hepatocellular cancer often are insidious in onset and masked by those related to cirrhosis or chronic hepatitis. The initial symptoms include weakness, anorexia, weight loss, fatigue, bloating, a sensation of abdominal fullness, and a dull, aching abdominal pain.[59] Ascites, which often obscures weight loss, is common. Jaundice, if present, usually is mild. There may be a rapid increase in liver size and worsening of ascites in persons with pre-existing cirrhosis. Usually, the liver is enlarged when these symptoms appear. Various paraneoplastic syndromes (*e.g.*, disturbances due to ectopic hormone or growth factor production by the tumour [see Chapter 8]) have been associated with hepatocellular cancer, including erythrocytosis (erythropoietin), hypoglycemia (insulin-like growth factor), and hypercalcemia (parathyroid-related protein). Serum α-fetoprotein, which is present during fetal life but barely detectable in the serum after the age of 2 years, is present in 50% to 75% cases of hepatocellular carcinoma. However, the test lacks specificity and is not very useful as a surveillance or diagnostic tool.[3,59] Diagnostic methods include ultrasonography, CT scans, and MRI. Liver biopsy may be used to confirm the diagnosis.

Primary cancers of the liver usually are far advanced at the time of diagnosis. The treatment of choice is subtotal hepatectomy, if conditions permit. Chemotherapy and radiation therapy are largely palliative. Although liver transplantation may be an option for people with well-compensated cirrhosis and small tumours, it often is impractical because of the shortage of donor organs.

Cholangiocarcinoma. Cholangiocarcinoma, with an average incidence of 1 per 100,000 in North America, occurs much less frequently than hepatocellular carcinoma. The etiology, clinical features, and prognosis vary considerably with the part of the biliary tree that is the site of origin. Cholangiocarcinoma is not associated with the same risk factors as hepatocellular carcinoma. Instead, most of the risk factors revolve around long-standing inflammation and injury of the bile duct epithelium. Cholangiocarcinoma often presents with pain, weight loss, anorexia, and abdominal swelling or awareness of a mass in the right hypochondrium. Tumours affecting the central or distal bile ducts may present with jaundice.[3,4,59]

Metastatic Tumours

Metastatic tumours of the liver are much more common than primary tumours. Common sources include colorectal cancer and those spread from breast, lung, or urogenital cancer. In addition, tumours of neuroendocrine origin spread to the liver. It often is difficult to distinguish primary from metastatic tumours with the use of CT scans, MRI, or ultrasonography. Usually the diagnosis is confirmed by biopsy.

IN SUMMARY

The liver is subject to most of the disease processes that affect other body structures, such as vascular disorders, inflammation, metabolic diseases, toxic injury, and neoplasms. As the major drug-metabolizing and detoxifying organ in the body, the liver is subject to potential damage from the enormous array of pharmaceutical and environmental chemicals. Drugs and chemicals can exert their effects by causing hepatocyte injury and death or by cholestatic liver damage due to injury of biliary drainage structures. Drug reactions can be predictable based on the drug's chemical structure and metabolites, or unpredictable (idiosyncratic) based on individual characteristics of the person receiving the drug. Early identification of drug-induced liver disease is important because withdrawal of the drug is curative in most cases.

Hepatitis is characterized by inflammation of the liver. Acute viral hepatitis is caused by hepatitis viruses A, B, C, D, and E. Although all these viruses cause acute hepatitis, they differ in terms of mode of transmission, incubation period, mechanism, degree and chronicity of liver damage, and the ability to evolve to a carrier state. HBV, HCV, and HDV infections have the potential for progression to the carrier state, chronic hepatitis, and hepatocellular carcinoma.

Intrahepatic biliary diseases disrupt the flow of bile through the liver, causing cholestasis and biliary cirrhosis. Among the causes of intrahepatic biliary diseases are primary biliary cirrhosis, primary sclerosing cholangitis, and secondary biliary cirrhosis. Because alcohol competes for use of intracellular cofactors normally needed by the liver for other metabolic processes, it tends to disrupt the metabolic functions of the liver. The spectrum of alcoholic liver disease includes fatty liver disease, alcoholic hepatitis, and cirrhosis.

Cirrhosis represents the end stage of chronic liver disease in which much of the functional liver tissue has been replaced by fibrous tissue. The fibrous tissue replaces normally functioning liver tissue and forms constrictive bands that disrupt flow in the vascular channels and biliary duct systems of the liver. The disruption of vascular channels predisposes to portal hypertension and its complications, loss of liver cells, and eventual liver failure. Portal hypertension is characterized by increased resistance to flow and increased pressure in the portal venous system; the pathologic consequences of the disorder include ascites, the formation of collateral bypass channels (*e.g.*, esophageal varices) from the portosystemic circulation, and splenomegaly. Liver failure represents the end stage of a number of liver diseases and occurs when less than 20% of liver tissue is functional. The manifestations of liver failure reflect the various functions of the liver, including hematologic disorders, disruption of endocrine function, skin disorders, hepatorenal syndrome, and hepatic encephalopathy.

There are two types of primary cancers of the liver: hepatocellular (the most common form, derived from hepatocytes and their precursors) and cholangiocarcinoma (bile duct cancer, arising from biliary epithelium). Hepatocellular carcinoma is associated with HBV and HCV hepatitis, alcoholic cirrhosis, and food contaminants (*e.g.*, aflatoxins). Cholangiocarcinoma occurs primarily in older persons with a history of chronic disorders of the bile ducts. Although primary tumours of the liver are relatively rare in developed countries of the world, the liver shares with the lung the distinction of being the most common site of metastatic tumours.

CONCEPTSin action **ANIMATI◉N**

DISORDERS OF THE GALLBLADDER AND EXOCRINE PANCREAS

After completing this section of the chapter, you should be able to meet the following objectives:

- Explain the function of the gallbladder in regulating the flow of bile into the duodenum and relate to the formation of cholelithiasis (gallstones).
- Describe the clinical manifestations of acute and chronic cholecystitis.
- Characterize the effects of choledocholithiasis and cholangitis on bile flow and the potential for hepatic and pancreatic complications.
- Cite the possible causes and describe the manifestations and treatment of acute and chronic pancreatitis.
- State the reason for the poor prognosis in pancreatic cancer.

Disorders of the Gallbladder and Extrahepatic Bile Ducts

The hepatobiliary system consists of the gallbladder, the left and right hepatic ducts, which come together to form the common hepatic duct, the cystic duct, which extends to the gallbladder, and the common bile duct, which is formed by the union of the common hepatic duct and the cystic duct (Fig. 38.17). The

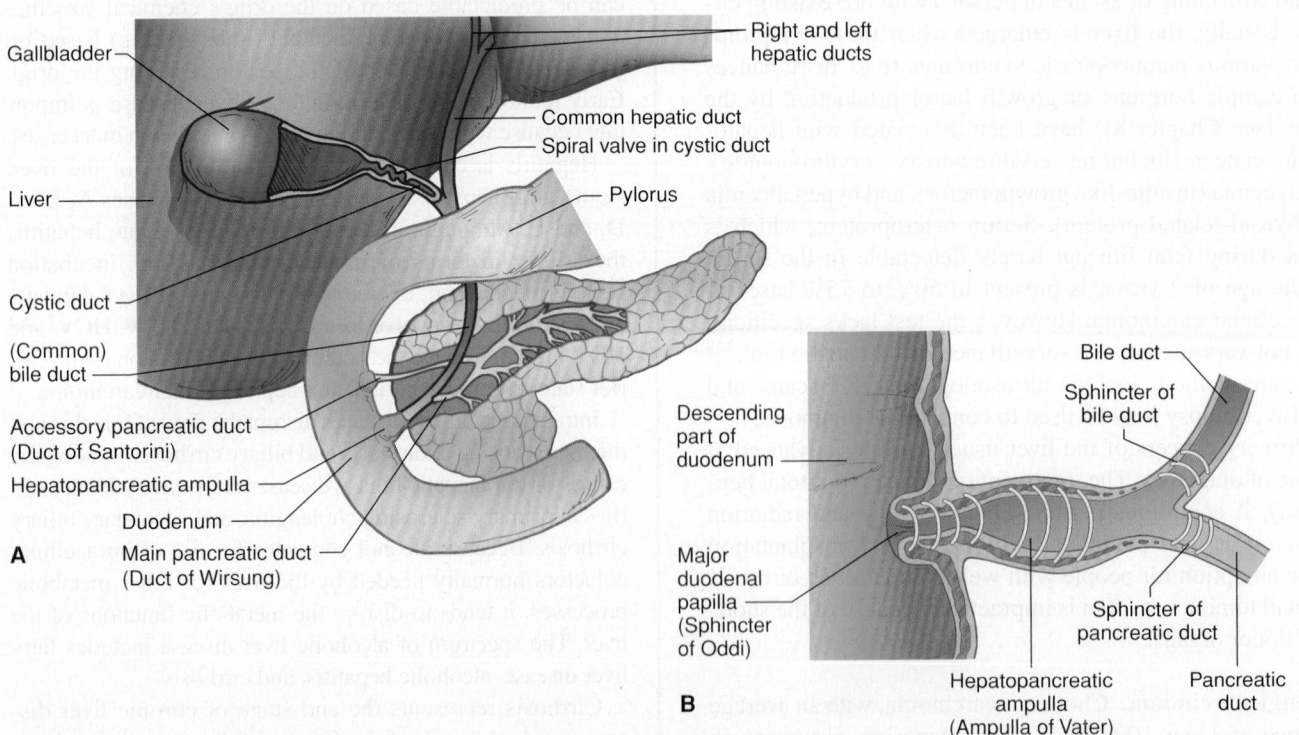

FIGURE 38.17 • **A:** Extrahepatic bile passages, gallbladder, and pancreatic ducts. **B:** Entry of bile duct and pancreatic duct into the hepatopancreatic ampulla, which opens into the duodenum.

common bile duct descends posteriorly to the first part of the duodenum, where it comes in contact with the main pancreatic duct. These ducts unite to form the hepatopancreatic ampulla. The circular muscle around the distal end of the bile duct is thickened to form the sphincter of the bile duct.

The gallbladder is a distensible, pear-shaped muscular sac located on the ventral surface of the liver. It has an outer serous peritoneal layer, a middle smooth muscle layer, and an inner mucosal layer that is continuous with the linings of the bile duct. The function of the gallbladder is to store and concentrate bile. Bile contains bile salts, cholesterol, bilirubin, lecithin, fatty acids, and water and the electrolytes normally found in the plasma. The cholesterol found in bile has no known function; it is assumed to be a byproduct of bile salt formation, and its presence is linked to the excretory function of bile. Normally insoluble in water, cholesterol is rendered soluble by the action of bile salts and lecithin, which combine with it to form micelles. In the gallbladder, water and electrolytes are absorbed from the liver bile, causing the bile to become more concentrated. Because neither lecithin nor bile salts are absorbed in the gallbladder, their concentration increases along with that of cholesterol; in this way, the solubility of cholesterol is maintained.

Entrance of food into the intestine causes the gallbladder to contract and the sphincter of the bile duct to relax, such that bile stored in the gallbladder moves into the duodenum. The stimulus for gallbladder contraction is primarily hormonal. Products of food digestion, particularly lipids, stimulate the release of a gastrointestinal hormone called *cholecystokinin* from the mucosa of the duodenum. Cholecystokinin provides a strong stimulus for gallbladder contraction. The role of other gastrointestinal hormones in bile release is less clearly understood.

Passage of bile into the intestine is regulated largely by the pressure in the common duct. Normally, the gallbladder regulates this pressure. It collects and stores bile as it relaxes and the pressure in the common bile duct decreases, and it empties bile into the intestine as the gallbladder contracts, producing an increase in common duct pressure. After gallbladder surgery, the pressure in the common duct changes, causing the common duct to dilate. The flow of bile then is regulated by the sphincters in the common duct.

Two common disorders of the biliary system are cholelithiasis (*i.e.*, gallstones) and inflammation of the gallbladder (cholecystitis) or common bile duct (cholangitis). At least 10% of adults in developed countries have gallstones but most people remain asymptomatic.[3,4] There is an increased prevalence with age, and approximately twice as many white women as men have gallstones.[3] In both circumstances, hypersecretion of biliary cholesterol appears to play a major role.

Cholelithiasis

Cholelithiasis or gallstones is caused by precipitation of substances contained in bile, mainly cholesterol and bilirubin. Approximately 80% of gallstones are composed primarily of cholesterol; the other 20% are black or brown pigment stones consisting of calcium salts with bilirubin.[3] Many stones have

FIGURE 38.18 • Cholesterol gallstones. The gallbladder has been opened to reveal numerous yellow cholesterol gallstones. (From Rubin R., Strayer D. S. (Eds.). (2012). *Rubin's pathology: Clinicopathologic foundations of medicine* (6th ed., p. 732). Philadelphia, PA: Lippincott Williams & Wilkins.)

a mixed composition. Figure 38.18 shows a gallbladder with numerous cholesterol gallstones.

Two main factors contribute to the formation of gallstones: abnormalities in the composition of bile and the stasis of bile.[3,4,60] The formation of cholesterol stones is associated with increasing age, obesity and occurs more frequently in women, especially women who have had multiple pregnancies or who are taking oral contraceptives.[60] All of these factors cause the liver to excrete more cholesterol into the bile. Estrogen reduces the synthesis of bile acid in women. Gallbladder sludge (thickened gallbladder mucoprotein with tiny trapped cholesterol crystals) is thought to be a precursor of gallstones. Sludge frequently occurs with pregnancy, starvation, and rapid weight loss. Drugs that lower serum cholesterol levels, such as clofibrate, also cause increased cholesterol excretion into the bile. Malabsorption disorders stemming from ileal disease or intestinal bypass surgery, for example, tend to interfere with the absorption of bile salts, which are needed to maintain the solubility of cholesterol. Inflammation of the gallbladder alters the absorptive characteristics of the mucosal layer, allowing excessive absorption of water and bile salts. Cholesterol gallstones are extremely common among northern European descent, Hispanic populations, and Native Americans, which suggests that a genetic component may have a role in gallstone formation.[61] Pigment stones containing bilirubin are seen in persons with hemolytic disease (*e.g.*, sickle cell disease) and hepatic cirrhosis.

Clinical Manifestations. Many persons with gallstones have no symptoms. Gallstones cause symptoms when they obstruct bile flow or cause inflammation.[62] Small stones (*i.e.,* <8 mm in diameter) pass into the common duct, producing symptoms of indigestion and biliary colic. Larger stones are more likely to obstruct flow and cause jaundice. The sharp pain of biliary colic is usually located in the upper right quadrant or epigastric area and may be referred to the upper back, the right shoulder or midscapular region. Typically the pain is abrupt in onset, increases steadily in intensity, persists for 30 minutes to 5 hours, and is followed by soreness in the upper right quadrant.

Acute and Chronic Cholecystitis

Acute cholecystitis is a diffuse inflammation of the gallbladder, usually secondary to obstruction of the gallbladder outlet. Most cases of acute cholecystitis (90%) are associated with the presence of gallstones (calculous cholecystitis).[3,4,62] The remaining cases (acalculous cholecystitis) are associated with sepsis, severe trauma, or infection of the gallbladder. It has been theorized that obstruction of the cystic duct by a gallstone leads to the release of phospholipase from the epithelium of the gallbladder. In turn, this enzyme may hydrolyze lecithin and release lysolecithin, a membrane-active toxin.[3,4] At the same time, disruption of the normally protective mucous lining of the epithelium renders the mucosal cells vulnerable to damage by the detergent action of concentrated bile salts. Acute acalculous cholecystitis is thought to result from ischemia. The cystic artery is an end artery with essentially no collateral circulation.[3] Contributing factors may include dehydration and multiple blood transfusions, leading to increased pigment load; gallbladder stasis, as might occur with hyperalimentation and assisted ventilation; and inflammation and edema of the gallbladder wall. Acute acalculous cholecystitis can rapidly progress to gangrene and perforation because the process appears to involve a transmural infarction, rather than inflammatory changes associated with stones.

Chronic cholecystitis results from repeated episodes of acute cholecystitis or chronic irritation of the gallbladder by stones. It is characterized by varying degrees of chronic inflammation. Gallstones almost always are present. Cholelithiasis with chronic cholecystitis may be associated with acute exacerbations of gallbladder inflammation, common duct stones, pancreatitis, and, rarely, carcinoma of the gallbladder.[62]

Clinical Manifestations. Persons with acute cholecystitis usually experience an acute onset of upper right quadrant or epigastric pain, frequently associated with mild fever, anorexia, nausea, and vomiting. Whereas in biliary colic the cystic duct obstruction is transient, in acute cholecystitis it is persistent. Persons with calculous cholecystitis usually, but not always, have experienced previous episodes of biliary pain. The pain may appear with remarkable suddenness and constitute a surgical emergency. In the absence of medical attention, the attack usually subsides in 7 to 10 days and frequently within 24 hours. In persons who recover, recurrence is common. The onset of acalculous cholecystitis tends to be more insidious because the manifestations are obscured by the underlying conditions precipitating the attack. In the severely ill patient, early recognition is crucial because a delay in treatment can prove life-threatening. Persons with acute cholecystitis usually have an elevated white blood cell count and many have mild elevations in AST, ALT, alkaline phosphatase, and bilirubin.

The manifestations of chronic cholecystitis are more vague than those of acute cholecystitis. There may be intolerance to fatty foods, belching, and other indications of discomfort. Often, there are episodes of colicky pain with obstruction of biliary flow caused by gallstones. The gallbladder, which in chronic cholecystitis usually contains stones, may be enlarged, shrunken, or of normal size.

Diagnosis and Treatment. The methods used to diagnose gallbladder disease include ultrasonography, cholescintigraphy (nuclear scanning), and CT scans.[62] Ultrasonography is widely used in diagnosing gallbladder disease and has largely replaced the oral cholecystogram in most medical centres. It can detect stones as small as 1 to 2 cm, and its overall accuracy in detecting gallbladder disease is high. In addition to stones, ultrasonography can detect wall thickening, which indicates inflammation. It also can rule out other causes of right upper quadrant pain such as tumours. Cholescintigraphy, also called a *gallbladder scan,* relies on the ability of the liver to extract a rapidly injected radionuclide, technetium-99m, bound to one of several iminodiacetic acids, that is excreted into the bile ducts. Serial scanning images are obtained within several minutes of the injection of the tracer and every 10 to 15 minutes during the next hour. The gallbladder scan is highly accurate in detecting acute cholecystitis. Although CT is not as accurate as ultrasonography in detecting gallstones, it can show thickening of the gallbladder wall or pericholecystic fluid associated with acute cholecystitis. MRI can also identify hepatobiliary and/or abdominal pathology but accessibility limits this test.

Gallbladder disease usually is treated by removing the gallbladder. The gallbladder stores and concentrates bile, and its removal usually does not interfere with digestion. Laparoscopic cholecystectomy has become the treatment of choice for symptomatic gallbladder disease.[62] The procedure involves insertion of a laparoscope through a small incision near the umbilicus, and surgical instruments are inserted through several stab wounds in the upper abdomen. Although the procedure requires more time than the older open surgical procedure, most people go home the same day as the surgery. A major advantage of the procedure is that patients are able to return to work between 2 days and 2 weeks, compared with 4 to 6 weeks after an open cholecystectomy.

Choledocholithiasis and Cholangitis

Choledocholithiasis refers to stones in the common duct and *cholangitis* to inflammation of the common duct. Common duct stones usually originate in the gallbladder, but can form spontaneously in the common duct.

Clinical Manifestations. The manifestations of choledocholithiasis are similar to those of gallstones and acute cholecystitis. There is a history of acute biliary colic and right upper abdominal pain, with chills, fever, and jaundice associated with episodes of abdominal pain. Bilirubinuria and an elevated serum bilirubin are present if the common duct is obstructed. Complications include acute suppurative cholangitis when purulent bile fills and distends bile ducts. It is characterized by the presence of an altered sensorium, lethargy, and septic shock.[3] Acute suppurative cholangitis represents an endoscopic or surgical emergency. Common duct stones also can obstruct the outflow of the pancreatic duct, causing a secondary pancreatitis.

Diagnosis and Treatment. Ultrasonography, CT scans, and radionuclide imaging may be used to demonstrate dilation of bile ducts and impaired blood flow. Endoscopic ultrasonography and magnetic resonance cholangiography are used for detecting common duct stones. Both percutaneous transhepatic cholangiography (PTC) and endoscopic retrograde cholangiopancreatography (ERCP) provide a direct means for determining the cause, location, and extent of obstruction. PTC involves the injection of dye directly into the biliary tree. It requires the insertion of a thin, flexible needle through a small incision in the skin with advancement into the biliary tree. ERCP involves the passage of an endoscope into the duodenum and the passage of a catheter into the hepatopancreatic ampulla. ERCP can be used to enlarge the opening of the sphincter of Oddi, which may allow the lodged stone to pass, or an instrument may be inserted into the common duct to remove the stone.

Common duct stones in persons with cholelithiasis usually are treated by stone extraction followed by laparoscopic cholecystectomy. Antibiotic therapy, with an agent that penetrates the bile, is used to treat the infection. Emergency decompression of the common duct, usually by ERCP, may be necessary for persons who are septic or fail to improve with antibiotic treatment.

Cancer of the Gallbladder

Cancer of the gallbladder is slightly more common in women, occurs more often after 60 years of age, and in Canada there is a higher incidence in First Nation populations.[63] The onset of symptoms usually is insidious, and they resemble those of cholecystitis; the diagnosis often is made unexpectedly at the time of gallbladder surgery. About 70% to 80% of persons with gallbladder cancer have cholelithiasis. Because of its ability to produce chronic irritation of the gallbladder mucosa, it is believed that cholelithiasis plays a role in the development of gallbladder cancer. It is seldom resectable at the time of diagnosis, and the mean survival of people with advanced, unresectable cancer is about 2 to 4 months.[63]

Disorders of the Exocrine Pancreas

The pancreas lies transversely in the posterior part of the upper abdomen. The head of the pancreas is at the right of the abdomen; it rests against the curve of the duodenum in the area of the hepatopancreatic ampulla and its entrance into the duodenum. The body of the pancreas lies beneath the stomach.

The tail touches the spleen. The pancreas is virtually hidden because of its posterior position; unlike many other organs, it cannot be palpated. Because of the position of the pancreas and its large functional reserve, symptoms from conditions such as cancer of the pancreas do not usually appear until the disorder is far advanced.

The pancreas is both an endocrine and exocrine organ. Its function as an endocrine organ is discussed in Chapter 42. The exocrine pancreas is made up of lobules that consist of acinar cells, which secrete digestive enzymes into a system of microscopic ducts. For most persons these ducts empty into the main pancreatic duct (Duct of Wirsung), which extends from left to right through the substance of the pancreas. The main pancreatic duct and the bile duct unite to the form hepatopancreatic ampulla, which empties into the duodenum via the major duodenal papilla. The sphincter of the pancreatic duct controls the flow of pancreatic secretions into duodenum (Fig. 38.17). Up to 70% of persons also have an accessory pancreatic duct (Duct of Santorini) which drains part of the head of the pancreas and drains into the duodenum via the minor duodenal papilla.

The pancreatic secretions contain proteolytic enzymes that break down dietary proteins, including trypsin, chymotrypsin, carboxypolypeptidase, ribonuclease, and deoxyribonuclease. The pancreas also secretes pancreatic amylase, which breaks down starch, and lipases, which hydrolyze neutral fats into glycerol and fatty acids. The pancreatic enzymes are secreted in the inactive form and become activated in the intestine. This is important because the enzymes would digest the tissue of the pancreas itself if they were secreted in the active form. The acinar cells secrete a trypsin inhibitor, which prevents trypsin activation. Because trypsin activates other proteolytic enzymes, the trypsin inhibitor prevents subsequent activation of the other enzymes.

Two types of pancreatic disease are discussed in this chapter: acute and chronic pancreatitis and cancer of the pancreas.

Acute Pancreatitis

Acute pancreatitis represents a reversible inflammatory process of the pancreatic acini brought about by premature activation of pancreatic enzymes.[64,65] Although the disease process may be limited to pancreatic tissue, it also can involve peripancreatic tissues or those of more distant organs.

The pathogenesis of acute pancreatitis involves the autodigestion of pancreatic tissue by inappropriately activated pancreatic enzymes. The process is thought to begin with the activation of trypsin. Once activated, trypsin can then activate a variety of digestive enzymes that cause pancreatic injury, resulting in an intense inflammatory response. The acute inflammatory response itself causes substantial tissue damage and may progress beyond the pancreas to produce a systemic inflammatory response syndrome and multiorgan failure (see Chapter 26). Although a number of factors are associated with the development of acute pancreatitis, most cases result from gallstones (stones in the common duct) or alcohol abuse.[64] In the case of biliary tract obstruction due to gallstones, pancreatic duct obstruction or biliary reflux is believed to activate the enzymes in the pancreatic duct system. The precise mechanisms whereby alcohol exerts its action are largely unknown. Alcohol is known to be a potent stimulator of pancreatic secretions, and it also is known to cause partial obstruction of the sphincter of the pancreatic duct. Acute pancreatitis also is associated with hyperlipidemia, hypercalcemia, infections (particularly viral), abdominal and surgical trauma, and drugs such as thiazide diuretics.[64]

Clinical Manifestations. The manifestations of acute pancreatitis can range from mild with minimal organ dysfunction to severe and life-threatening. Overall, about 30% of persons with acute pancreatitis have a severe course with systemic inflammation and organ failure, and 25% to 35% of those with severe pancreatitis die.[64] Abdominal pain is a cardinal manifestation of acute pancreatitis. The pain is usually located in the epigastric or periumbilical region and may radiate to the back, chest, or flank areas. Physical examination findings are variable and include fever, tachycardia, hypotension, severe abdominal tenderness, respiratory distress, and abdominal distension. Recognized markers of severe disease include laboratory values that measure the inflammatory response (*e.g.,* C-reactive protein), scoring systems that assess inflammation or organ failure, and findings on imaging studies. Clinical findings such as thirst, poor urine output, progressive tachycardia, tachypnea, hypoxemia, agitation, confusion, a rising hematocrit level, and lack of improvement in symptoms within the first 48 hours are warning signs of impending severe disease. Complications include the systemic inflammatory response, acute respiratory distress syndrome, acute tubular necrosis, and organ failure. An important disturbance related to acute pancreatitis is the loss of a large volume of fluid into the retroperitoneal and peripancreatic spaces and the abdominal cavity.

Diagnosis and Treatment. Serum amylase and lipase are the laboratory markers most commonly used to establish a diagnosis of acute pancreatitis. The serum lipase may remain elevated slightly longer than amylase. However, the level of elevation of the serum amylase or lipase does not correlate with the severity of the disorder. The white blood cell count may be increased, and hyperglycemia and an elevated serum bilirubin level may be present. Determination of the cause is important in guiding the immediate management and preventing recurrence. Abdominal ultrasonography is usually performed to assess for gallstones. CT scans and dynamic contrast-enhanced CT of the pancreas are used to detect necrosis and fluid accumulation. Recent research has focused on potential biomarkers for predicting the severity and prognosis of pancreatitis. Trypsinogens and pancreatic proteases, enzymes involved in the autodigestive processes, appear promising. Other investigational serologic markers include tumour necrosis factor, C-reactive protein, procalcitonin, phospholipase A$_2$, and other cytokines.

Treatment measures depend on the severity of the disease. Persons who present with persistent or severe pain, vomiting, dehydration, or signs of impending severe acute pancreatitis require hospitalization. Treatment measures are directed at

pain relief, restoration of lost plasma volume, nutrition, and prevention of infection.[64] Intravenous opiates are usually required for pain relief and evidence does not support which specific opiate is best. Intravenous fluids and electrolytes are administered to replace those lost from the circulation and to combat hypotension and shock. Intravenous colloid solutions are given to replace the fluid that has become sequestered in the abdomen and retroperitoneal space. Nutrition has changed over the past decades with the understanding that withholding oral foods and fluids to prevent further stimulation of the secretion of pancreatic enzymes actually undermines the integrity of the intestinal mucosal lining. It is preferred that oral or enteral nutrition be instituted as soon as possible for pancreatic patients to protect the mucosal layer and prevent potential bacterial translocations leading to systemic infections.[64,65]

Complications. Sequelae in persons surviving an episode of severe acute pancreatitis include fluid collections and infection.[64,65] In 30% of persons with acute necrotizing pancreatitis, the necrotic debris becomes infected, usually by gram-negative organisms from the alimentary canal, further complicating the condition. Fluid collections with a high level of pancreatic enzymes are usually associated with pancreatic duct disruptions and may eventually form pseudocysts (a collection of pancreatic fluid enclosed in a layer of inflammatory tissue). A pseudocyst most often is connected to a pancreatic duct, so that it continues to increase in mass. The symptoms depend on its location; for example, jaundice may occur when a cyst develops near the head of the pancreas, close to the common duct. Pseudocysts may resolve or, if they persist, may require surgical intervention.[65]

Chronic Pancreatitis

Chronic pancreatitis is characterized by progressive destruction of the exocrine pancreas, fibrosis, and in the later stages, by destruction of the endocrine pancreas.[66] Most factors that cause acute pancreatitis can also cause chronic pancreatitis. However, the chief distinction between the two conditions is the irreversibility of pancreatic function that is characteristic of chronic pancreatitis. The risk of progression to chronic disease is greatest among people who smoke or have a history of long-term alcohol ingestion. Less common causes are long-standing obstruction of the pancreatic duct by pseudocysts, calculi, or neoplasms; autoimmune chronic pancreatitis, which occurs in association with autoimmune disorders such as Sjögren syndrome, primary sclerosing cholangitis, and inflammatory bowel disease; idiopathic chronic pancreatitis, associated with cystic fibrosis (discussed in Chapter 29); and hereditary pancreatitis, a rare autosomal dominant disorder that is associated with both acute and chronic pancreatitis.

Clinical Manifestations. Chronic pancreatitis is manifested in episodes that are similar to, albeit of lesser severity than, those of acute pancreatitis. Patients have persistent, recurring episodes of epigastric and upper left quadrant pain; the attacks often are precipitated by alcohol abuse or overeating. Anorexia, nausea, vomiting, constipation, and flatulence are common. Eventually the disease progresses to the extent that endocrine and exocrine pancreatic functions become deficient. At this point, signs of diabetes mellitus and the malabsorption syndrome (*e.g.*, weight loss, fatty stools [steatorrhea]) become apparent.

Treatment. Treatment consists of measures to treat coexisting biliary tract disease. A low-fat diet usually is prescribed. The signs of malabsorption may be treated with pancreatic enzymes. When diabetes is present, it is treated with insulin. Alcohol is forbidden because it frequently precipitates attacks. Because of the frequent episodes of pain, narcotic addiction is a potential problem in persons with chronic pancreatitis. Surgical intervention sometimes is needed to relieve the pain and usually focuses on relieving any obstruction that may be present. In advanced cases, a subtotal or total pancreatectomy may be necessary.[32,66]

Cancer of the Pancreas

Pancreatic cancer is now the fourth leading cause of death from cancer in Canada. It is estimated that in 2014, 4,700 will be diagnosed and 4,400 will die from pancreatic cancer. Considered to be one of the most deadly malignancies, locally advanced pancreatic cancer is associated with a 5-year survival rate of only 8%.[67]

The cause of pancreatic cancer is unknown. Age is a major risk factor. Pancreatic cancer rarely occurs in persons younger than 50 years of age, and the risk increases with age. The most significant and reproducible environmental risk factor is cigarette smoking.[67,68] The incidence of pancreatic cancer is twice as high among smokers than nonsmokers. Diabetes and chronic pancreatitis also are associated with pancreatic cancer, although neither the nature nor the sequence of the possible cause-and-effect relation has been established. There has been a recent focus on the molecular genetics of pancreatic cancer as approximately 5% to 10% of persons have a family history of the disease.

Clinical Manifestations. Almost all pancreatic cancers are adenocarcinomas of the ductal epithelium, and symptoms are primarily caused by mass effect rather than disruption of exocrine or endocrine function. The clinical manifestations depend on the size and location of the tumour as well as its metastasis. Pain, jaundice, and weight loss constitute the classic presentation of the disease. The most common pain is a dull epigastric pain often accompanied by back pain, often worse in the supine position, and relieved by sitting forward. Although the tumour can arise anywhere in the pancreas, the most frequent site is the head (60% to 70%), followed by the body (10%), and tail (10% to 15%). The pancreas is diffusely involved in the remaining 15%.[69] Because of the proximity of the pancreas to the common duct and the hepatopancreatic ampulla, cancer of the head of the pancreas tends to obstruct bile flow. Jaundice frequently is the presenting symptom of a person with cancer of the head of the pancreas, and it usually is accompanied by complaints of pain and pruritus. Cancer of the body of the pancreas usually impinges on the celiac ganglion, causing pain. The pain usually worsens with ingestion of food or assumption of the supine position. Cancer of the tail of the pancreas usually has metastasized before symptoms appear.

Migratory thrombophlebitis (deep vein thrombosis) develops in about 10% of persons with pancreatic cancer, particularly when the tumour involves the body or tail of the pancreas.[69] Thrombi develop in multiple veins, including the deep veins of the legs, the subclavian vein, the inferior and superior mesentery veins, and even the vena cava. It is not uncommon for the migratory thrombophlebitis to provide the first evidence of pancreatic cancer, although it may present in other cancers as well. The mechanism responsible for the hypercoagulable state is largely unclear, but may relate to activation of clotting factors by proteases released from the tumour cells.[69]

Diagnosis and Treatment. Patient history, physical examination, and elevated serum bilirubin and alkaline phosphate levels may suggest the presence of pancreatic cancer, but are not diagnostic.[68] The serum cancer antigen (CA) 19–9, a Lewis blood group antigen, may help confirm the diagnosis in symptomatic patients and may help predict prognosis and recurrence after resection. However, CA 19–9 lacks the sensitivity and specificity to screen asymptomatic patients effectively.[68] Ultrasonography and CT scanning are the most frequently used diagnostic methods to confirm the disease. Intravenous and oral contrast–enhanced spiral CT is the preferred method for imaging the pancreas. Percutaneous fine-needle aspiration cytology of the pancreas has been one of the major advances in the diagnosis of pancreatic cancer. Unfortunately, the smaller and more curable tumours are most likely to be missed by this procedure. ERCP may be used for evaluation of persons with suspected pancreatic cancer and obstructive jaundice.

Most cancers of the pancreas have metastasized by the time of diagnosis. Surgical resection of the tumour is done when the tumour is localized, or as a palliative measure. Radiation therapy may be useful when the disease is not resectable but appears to be localized. The use of irradiation and chemotherapy for pancreatic cancer continues to be investigated. Pain control is one of the most important aspects in the management of persons with end-stage pancreatic cancer.[68]

> ### IN SUMMARY
>
> The biliary tract serves as a passageway for the delivery of bile from the liver to the intestine. This tract consists of the bile ducts and gallbladder. The most common causes of biliary tract disease are cholelithiasis and cholecystitis. Three factors contribute to the development of cholelithiasis: abnormalities in the composition of bile, stasis of bile, and inflammation of the gallbladder. Cholelithiasis predisposes to obstruction of bile flow, causing biliary colic and acute or chronic cholecystitis. Cancer of the gallbladder has a poor 5-year survival rate.
>
> The pancreas is an endocrine and exocrine organ. The exocrine pancreas produces digestive enzymes that are secreted in an inactive form and for most persons are transported to

the small intestine through the main pancreatic duct, which usually empties into the hepatopancreatic ampulla and then into the duodenum through the sphincter of the pancreatic duct. The most common diseases of the exocrine pancreas are acute and chronic forms of pancreatitis, and cancer. Acute and chronic pancreatitis are associated with biliary reflux and chronic alcoholism. Acute pancreatitis is an inflammatory condition of the pancreas due to inappropriate activation of pancreatic enzymes, with manifestations that can range from mild to severe and life-threatening. Chronic pancreatitis causes progressive destruction of the endocrine and exocrine pancreas. It is characterized by episodes of pain and epigastric distress that are similar to but less severe than those that occur with acute pancreatitis. Cancer of the pancreas is the fourth leading cause of cancer death in Canada. It usually is far advanced at the time of diagnosis, and the 5-year survival rate is 8%.

REVIEW EXERCISES

1. A 24-year-old woman reports to her healthcare professional with complaints of a yellow discolouration of her skin, loss of appetite, and a feeling of upper gastric discomfort. She denies use of intravenous drugs and has not received blood products. She cannot recall eating uncooked shellfish or drinking water that might have been contaminated. She has a daughter who attends daycare.
    A. *What tests could be done to confirm a diagnosis of hepatitis A?*
    B. *What is the most common mode of transmission for hepatitis A? It is suggested that the source might be the daycare centre that her daughter attends. Explain.*
    C. *What methods could be used to protect other family members from getting the disease?*

2. A 56-year-old man with a history of heavy alcohol consumption and a previous diagnosis of alcoholic cirrhosis and portal hypertension is admitted to the emergency department with acute gastrointestinal bleeding due to a tentative diagnosis of bleeding esophageal varices and signs of circulatory shock.
    A. *Relate the development of esophageal varices to portal hypertension in persons with cirrhosis of the liver.*
    B. *Many persons with esophageal varices have blood coagulation problems. Explain.*
    C. *What are the possible treatment measures for this man, both in terms of controlling the current bleeding episode and preventing further bleeding episodes?*

3. A 40-year-old woman presents in the emergency department with a sudden episode of vomiting and severe right epigastric pain that developed after eating a fatty evening meal. Although there is no evidence of jaundice in her skin, the sclera of her eyes is noted to have a yellowish discolouration. Palpation reveals tenderness of the upper right quadrant with muscle splinting and rebound pain. Right upper quadrant abdominal ultrasonography confirms the presence of gallstones. The woman is treated conservatively with pain and antiemetic medications. She is subsequently scheduled for a laparoscopic cholecystectomy.
    A. *Relate this woman's signs and symptoms to gallstones and their effect on gallbladder function.*
    B. *Explain the initial appearance of jaundice in the eyes as opposed to the skin. Which of the two laboratory tests for bilirubin would you expect to be elevated—direct (conjugated) or indirect (unconjugated or free)?*
    C. *What effect will removal of the gallbladder have on the storage and release of bile into the intestine, particularly as it relates to meals?*

References

1. Hall J. E. (2011). *Textbook of medical physiology* (12th ed.). Philadelphia, PA: W. B. Saunders.
2. Rhoades R. A., Bell D. R. (2013). *Medical physiology: Principles for clinical medicine* (4th ed.). Philadelphia, PA: Lippincott Williams & Wilkins.
3. Crawford J. M., Liu C. (2010). Chapter 18: Liver and biliary tract. In Kumar V., Abbas A. K., Fausto N., et al. (Eds.), *Robbins and cotran pathologic basis of disease* (8th ed.). Philadelphia, PA: Elsevier Saunders.
4. Herrine S. K., Navarro V. J., Rubin R. (2012). Chapter 14: The liver and biliary system. In Rubin R., Strayer D. S. (Eds.), *Rubin's pathology: Clinicopathologic foundations of medicine* (6th ed.). Philadelphia, PA: Lippincott Williams & Wilkins.
5. Gilmore I., Garvey C. J. (2009). Jaundice. *Medicine, 37*(1), 42–46.
6. Barrington K. J., Sankaran K. (2011). Guidelines for detection, management and prevention of hyperbilirubinemia in term and later preterm newborn infants—Updated. Available online at: http://www.cps.ca/documents/position/hyperbilirubinemia-newborn#authors. Accessed July 11, 2014.
7. Pratt D. S., Kaplan M. M. (2012). Chapter 302: Evaluation of liver function. In Longo D., Fauci A., Kasper D. L., et al. (Eds.), *Harrison's principles of internal medicine* (18th ed.). New York: McGraw-Hill.
8. Giannini E. G., Testa R., Savarino V. (2005). Liver enzyme alteration: A guide for clinicians. *Canadian Medical Association Journal, 172*(3), 367–379.
9. Katzung B. G., Masters S. B., Trevor A. J. (2012). *Basic & clinical pharmacology* (12th ed.). New York: McGraw-Hill Companies, Inc.
10. Bunchorntavakul C., Reddy K. R. (2013). Acetaminophen-related hepatotoxicity. *Clinics in Liver Disease, 17*(4), 587–607.
11. Lin J. H., Yamazaki M. (2003). Role of P-glycoprotein in pharmacokinetics: Clinical implications. *Clinical Pharmacokinetics, 42*(1), 59–98.
12. Lewis J. H. (2000). Drug-induced liver disease. *Medical Clinics of North America, 84*(5), 1275–1311.
13. Tujios S., Fontana R. J. (2011). Mechanisms of drug-induced liver injury: From bedside to bench. *Nature Reviews Gastroenterology & Hepatology, 8*(4), 202–211.
14. Feld J. J., Heathcote E. J. (2010). Chapter 81: Hepatitis caused by other viruses. In Feldman M., Friedman L. S., Brandt L. J. (Eds.), *Sleisenger*

and Fordtran's gastrointestinal and liver disease: pathophysiology, diagnosis, management (9th ed.). Philadelphia, PA: Saunders Elsevier.

15. Public Health Agency of Canada. (2012). Hepatitis. Available online at: http://www.phac-aspc.gc.ca/hep/index-eng.php. Accessed July 11, 2014.

16. Bernal W., Auzinger G., Ahawan A., et al. (2010). Acute liver failure. Lancet, 376(9736), 190–201.

17. Dienstag J. L. (2012). Chapter 304: Acute viral hepatitis. In Longo D., Fauci A., Kasper D. L., et al., (Eds.), Harrison's principles of internal medicine (18th ed.). New York: McGraw-Hill.

18. World Health Organization. (2014). Hepatitis B Fact sheet no. 204. Available online at: http://www.who.int/mediacentre/factsheets/fs204/en/. Accessed July 11, 2014.

19. Sjogren M. H., Cheatham J. G. (2010). Chapter 77: Hepatitis A. In Feldman M., Friedman L. S., Brandt L. J. (Eds.), Sleisenger and Fordtran's gastrointestinal and liver disease: pathophysiology, diagnosis, management (9th ed.). Philadelphia, PA: Saunders Elsevier.

20. Public Health Agency of Canada. (2012). Canadian immunization guide: Hepatitis A vaccine. Available online at: http://www.phac-aspc.gc.ca/publicat/cig-gci/p04-hepa-eng.php#post. Accessed July 11, 2014.

21. Public Health Agency of Canada. (2011). Brief report: Hepatitis B infection in Canada. Available online at: http://www.phac-aspc.gc.ca/id-mi/pdf/hepB-eng.pdf. Accessed July 11, 2014.

22. Mast E. E., Weinbaum C. M., Fiore A. E., et al. (2006). A comprehensive immunization strategy to eliminate transmission of hepatitis B virus infection in the United States: Recommendations of the Advisory Committee on Immunization Practices (ACIP) Part II: immunization of adults. Morbidity and Mortality Weekly Report, 55(RR 16), 1–33.

23. Dandri M., Locarnini S. (2012). New insight in the pathobiology of hepatitis B virus infection. Gut, 61(Suppl 1), i6–i17.

24. Public Health Agency of Canada. (2012). Canadian immunization guide: Hepatitis B vaccine. Available online at: http://www.phac-aspc.gc.ca/publicat/cig-gci/p04-hepb-eng.php#a9. Accessed July 11, 2014.

25. Rosen H. R. (2011). Chronic hepatitis C infection. New England Journal Medicine, 364(25), 2429–2438.

26. Wong T., Lee S. S. (2006). Hepatitis C: A review for primary care physicians. Canadian Medical Association Journal, 174(5), 649–659.

27. Bialek S. R., Terrault N. A. (2006). The changing epidemiology and natural history of hepatitis C virus infection. Clinics in Liver Disease, 10(4), 679–715.

28. O'Leary J. G., Davis G. L. (2010). Chapter 79: Hepatitis C. In Feldman M., Friedman L. S., Brandt L. J. (Eds.), Sleisenger and Fordtran's gastrointestinal and liver disease: pathophysiology, diagnosis, management (9th ed.). Philadelphia, PA: Saunders Elsevier.

29. World Health Organization. (2014). Hepatitis C fact sheet no. 164. Available online at: http://www.who.int/mediacentre/factsheets/fs164/en/. Accessed July 11, 2014.

30. World Health Organization. (2014). Hepatitis E fact sheet no. 280. Available online at: http://www.who.int/mediacentre/factsheets/fs280/en/. Accessed July 11, 2014.

31. Kamar N., Bendall R., Abravanel F. L., et al. (2012). Hepatitis E. Lancet, 379(9835), 2477–2488.

32. Friedman L. S. (2014). Chapter 16: Liver, biliary tract, & pancreas disorders. In Papadakis M. A., McPhee S. J., Rabow M. V. (Eds.), Current medical diagnosis and treatment 2014. New York: McGraw-Hill.

33. Crespo G., Marino Z., Navasa M., et al. (2012). Viral hepatitis in liver transplantation. Gastroenterology, 142(6), 1373–1383.

34. Liberal R., Grant C. R., Mieli-Vergani G., Vergani D. (2013). Autoimmune hepatitis: A comprehensive review. Journal of Autoimmunity, 41, 123–139.

35. Czaja A. J. (2010). Chapter 88: Autoimmune hepatitis. In Feldman M., Friedman L. S., Brandt L. J. (Eds.), Sleisenger and Fordtran's gastrointestinal and liver disease: Pathophysiology, diagnosis, management (9th ed.). Philadelphia, PA: Saunders Elsevier.

36. Selmi C., Bowlus C. L., Gershwin M. E., et al. (2011). Primary biliary cirrhosis. Lancet, 377(9777), 9–13.

37. Centre for Addiction and Mental Health (CAMH). (2012). About alcohol. Available online at: http://www.camh.ca/en/hospital/health_information/a_z_mental_health_and_addiction_information/alcohol/Pages/about_alcohol.aspx. Accessed July 11, 2014.

38. Seth D., Haber P. S., Syn W., et al. (2011). Pathogenesis of alcohol-induced liver disease: Classical concepts and recent advances. Journal of Gastroenterology and Hepatology, 26(7), 1089–1105.

39. Zakhari S. (2006). Overview: How is alcohol metabolized by the body? Alcohol Research & Health, 29(4), 245–254.

40. Leiber C. S. (2005). Metabolism of alcohol. Clinics in Liver Disease, 9(1), 1–35.

41. Carithers R. L., McClain C. J. (2010). Chapter 84: Alcoholic liver disease. In Feldman M., Friedman L. S., Brandt L. J. (Eds.), Sleisenger and Fordtran's gastrointestinal and liver disease: pathophysiology, diagnosis, management (9th ed.). Philadelphia, PA: Saunders Elsevier.

42. Rubin E., Lieber C. S. (1968). Alcohol-induced hepatic injury in non-alcoholic volunteers. New England Journal Medicine, 278(16), 869–876.

43. Pinzani M., Rosselli M., Zuckermann M. (2011). Liver cirrhosis. Best Practice & Research Clinical Gastroenterology, 25(2), 281–290.

44. Ferral H., Behrens G., Lopera J. (2012). Budd-Chiari syndrome. American Journal of Roentgenology, 199(4), 737–745.

45. Moore C. M., Thiel D. H. (2013). Cirrhotic ascites review: Pathophysiology, diagnosis and management. World Journal of Hepatology, 5(5), 251–263.

46. Moore K. P., Aithal G. P. (2006). Guidelines on the management of ascites in cirrhosis. Gut, 55(Suppl 6) vi1–vi12.

47. Tuyama A. C., Chang C. Y. (2012). Non-alcoholic fatty liver disease. Journal of Diabetes, 4(3), 266–280.

48. Dureja P., Mellinger J., Agni R., et al. (2011). NAFLD recurrence in liver transplant recipients. Transplantation, 91(6), 684–689.

49. Liou I. W. (2014). Management of end-stage liver disease. Medical Clinics of North America, 98(1), 119–152.

50. Garcia-Tsao G., Bosch J. (2010). Management of varices and variceal hemorrhage in cirrhosis. New England Journal Medicine, 362(9), 823–832.

51. Bari K., Garcia-Tsao G. (2012). Treatment of portal hypertension. World Journal of Gastroenterology, 18(11), 116–1175.

52. Hazin R., Tamimi T. I. A., Abuzetun J. Y., et al. (2009). Recognizing and treating cutaneous signs of liver disease. Cleveland Clinic Journal of Medicine, 76(10), 599–606.

53. Arroyo V., Fernandez J. (2011). Management of hepatorenal syndrome in patients with cirrhosis. Nature Reviews Nephrology, 7(9), 517–526.

54. Felipo V. (2013). Hepatic encephalopathy: Effect of liver failure on brain function. Nature Reviews Neuroscience, 14(12), 851–858.

55. Canadian Institute for Health Information. (2014). Canadian organ replacement register annual report: Treatment of end-stage organ failure in Canada, 2003 to 2012. Available online at: https://secure.cihi.ca/free_products/2014_CORR_Annual_Report_EN.pdf. Accessed July 11, 2014.

56. Martin P., Rosen H. R. (2010). Chapter 95: Liver transplantation. In Feldman M., Friedman L. S., Brandt L. J. (Eds.), Sleisenger and Fordtran's gastrointestinal and liver disease: pathophysiology, diagnosis, management (9th ed.). Philadelphia, PA: Saunders Elsevier.

57. Canadian Cancer Society. (2014). Liver cancer. Available online at: http://www.cancer.ca/en/cancer-information/cancer-type/liver/liver-cancer/?region = bc. Accessed July 11, 2014.

58. Mittal S., El-Serag H. B. (2013). Epidemiology of hepatocellular carcinoma: Consider the population. Journal of Clinical Gastroenterology, 47(Suppl 1), S2–S6.

59. Di Bisceglie A. M., Befeler A. S. (2010). Chapter 94: Tumors and cysts of the liver. In Feldman M., Friedman L. S., Brandt L. J. (Eds.), Sleisenger and Fordtran's gastrointestinal and liver disease: pathophysiology, diagnosis, management (9th ed.). Philadelphia, PA: Saunders Elsevier.

60. Reshetnyak V. I. (2012). Concept of the pathogenesis and treatment of cholelithiasis. World Journal of Hepatology, 4(2), 18–34.

61. Shaffer E. A. (2005). Epidemiology and risk factors for gallstone disease: Has the paradigm changed in the 21st century? Current Gastroenterology Reports, 7(2), 132–140.

62. Knab L. M., Boller A., Mahvi D. M. (2014). Cholecystitis. Surgical Clinics of North America, 94(2), 455–470.

63. Canadian Cancer Society. (2014). Gallbladder cancer. Available online at: http://www.cancer.ca/en/cancer-information/cancer-type/gallbladder/gallbladder-cancer/?region=mb. Accessed July 11, 2014.

64. Schepers N. J., Besselink M. G., van Santvoort H. C., et al. (2013). Early management of acute pancreatitis. *Best Practice & Research Clinical Gastroenterology, 27*(5), 727–743.

65. Wu B. U., Banks P. A. (2013). Clinical management of patients with acute pancreatitis. *Gastroenterology, 144*(6),1272–1281.

66. Forsmark C. E. (2013). Management of chronic pancreatitis. *Gastroenterology, 144*(6), 1282–1291.

67. Canadian Cancer Society. (2014). *Pancreatic cancer.* Available online at: http://www.cancer.ca/en/cancer-information/cancer-type/pancreatic/pancreatic-cancer/?region=nb. Accessed July 11, 2014.

68. Hidalgo M. (2010). Pancreatic cancer. *New England Journal Medicine, 362*(17), 1605–1617.

69. Kilmstra D. S., Stelow E. B. (2012). Chapter 15: The pancreas. In Rubin R., Strayer D. S. (Eds.), *Rubin's pathology: Clinicopathologic foundations of medicine* (6th ed.). Philadelphia, PA: Lippincott Williams & Wilkins.

Visit thePoint **http://thePoint.lww.com for animations, journal articles, and more!**

Alterations in Nutritional Status

39

Nutritional status describes the condition of the body related to the availability and utilization of nutrients. Nutrients are chemicals that are essential for biologic processes. Macronutrients refer to carbohydrates, proteins, and fat, whereas micronutrients include vitamins and minerals. Macronutrients that are digested and absorbed into the body provide the energy needed to perform various body functions. In healthy persons, the stability and composition of body weight over time requires that their energy intake be balanced with energy expenditure. When a person's nutrient intake consistently exceeds expenditure, most of the nutrients are stored and body weight increases; conversely, when energy expenditure exceeds nutrient intake, energy stores are lost and body weight decreases. This chapter discusses the regulation of energy expenditure and storage, nutritional needs, overnutrition and obesity, and undernutrition and eating disorders.

NUTRITIONAL STATUS

After completing this section of the chapter, you should be able to meet the following objectives:

- Define nutritional status.
- Define calorie and state the number of calories derived from the oxidation of 1 g of protein, fat, or carbohydrate.
- Explain the difference between anabolism and catabolism.
- Relate the processes of glycogenolysis and gluconeogenesis to the regulation of blood glucose by the liver.
- Define basal metabolic rate and cite factors that affect it.
- Describe the function of adipose tissue in terms of energy storage and as an endocrine organ.

The nutrients that the body uses to maintain its nutritional status are derived from the digestive tract through the ingestion of foods or, in some cases, through liquid feedings that are delivered directly into the gastrointestinal tract by a synthetic tube (*i.e.*, tube feeding or enteral nutrition). The exception occurs in persons with certain illnesses in which the digestive tract is nonfunctional (*e.g.,* short-bowel syndrome, large-bowel obstruction, etc.). In those instances, the gut is bypassed and nutrients are infused directly into the circulatory system via parenteral nutrition. Once inside the body, nutrients can be used for energy as the building blocks for tissue growth and repair and/or they can act as cofactors that support various metabolic processes. When some nutrients are available in excess, they frequently can be stored for future use. If these required nutrients are unavailable, the body adapts by conserving and using its nutrient stores.

Energy Metabolism

Energy is measured in heat units called *calories.* A calorie, spelled with a small *c* and also called a *gram calorie,* is the amount of heat or energy required to raise the temperature of 1 g of water by 1°C. A *kilocalorie* (kcal), or *large Calorie,* which is equivalent to 1,000 calories, is the amount of energy needed to raise the temperature of 1 kg of water by 1°C.[1] Because a gram calorie is so small, the kilocalorie or large Calorie, spelled with a capital "C," is often used when discussing energy metabolism. The oxidation of proteins provides 4 kcal/g; fats, 9 kcal/g; carbohydrates, 4 kcal/g; and alcohol, 7 kcal/g.

Metabolism is the organized process through which nutrients such as carbohydrates, fats, and proteins are transformed into either smaller or larger substances, or otherwise converted into cellular energy. The process of metabolism is unique in that it enables the continual release of energy, and it couples this energy with physiologic functioning. For example, the energy used for muscle contraction is derived largely from energy sources that are stored in muscle cells and then released as the muscle contracts. Because most of our energy sources come from the nutrients in the food that is ingested, the ability to store energy and control its release is important.

ENERGY METABOLISM

- All body activities require energy, whether they involve a single cell, a single organ, or the entire body.
- Energy, which is measured in calories (cal), is obtained from foods.
- Fats, which are a concentrated water-free energy source, contain 9 kcal/g. They are stored in fat cells as triglycerides, which are the main storage sites for energy.
- Carbohydrates are hydrated fuels, which supply 4 kcal/g. They are stored in limited quantities as glycogen and can be converted to fatty acids and stored in fat cells as triglycerides.
- Proteins are broken down into amino acids that generate 4 kcal/g. Amino acids are used in building body proteins. Amino acids in excess of those needed for protein synthesis can be converted to fatty acids, ketones, or glucose and are stored or used as metabolic fuel.

Anabolism and Catabolism

There are two phases of metabolism: anabolism and catabolism. *Anabolism* is the phase of metabolic storage and synthesis of cell constituents. Anabolism does not provide energy for the body; it requires energy. *Catabolism* involves the breakdown of complex molecules into substances that can be used in the production of energy. The chemical intermediates for anabolism and catabolism are called *metabolites* (*i.e.,* lactic acid is a metabolite formed when glucose is broken down in the absence of oxygen). Both anabolism and catabolism are catalyzed by enzyme systems located in body cells. A *substrate* is a substance on which an enzyme acts. Enzyme systems selectively transform fuel substrates into cellular energy and facilitate the use of energy in the process of assembling molecules to form energy substrates and storage forms of energy.

Body energy cannot be stored as heat, thus the cellular oxidative processes that release energy are low-temperature reactions that convert food component to chemical energy that can be stored or dissipated. The body transforms carbohydrates, fats, and proteins into the intermediary compound, *adenosine triphosphate* (ATP).[1] ATP is called the *energy currency of the cell* because almost all body cells store and use ATP as their energy source (see Chapter 4). The metabolic events involved in ATP formation allow cellular energy to be stored, used, and replenished. However, under some circumstances energy expenditure decreasing metabolic efficiency can increase energy expenditure: an uncoupling of ATP synthesis within the mitochondria results in a loss of energy as released heat. This process may have relevance to obesity (the more energy "wasted" as heat loss, the less weight gain), but is also important in maintaining body warmth in newborns. This is because the increased proportion of brown fat found in neonates is much less efficient at generating ATP than white fat, resulting in increased heat production (see subsequent discussion on brown and white fat).

Energy Expenditure

The expenditure of body energy results from five mechanisms of heat production (*i.e.,* thermogenesis): basal metabolic rate or resting energy expenditure, diet-induced thermogenesis, exercise-induced thermogenesis, nonexercise activity thermogenesis, and thermogenesis in response to changes in environmental conditions. The amount of energy used varies with age, body size, rate of growth, and state of health.

Basal Metabolic Rate

The *basal metabolic rate* (BMR) refers to the chemical reactions occurring when the body is at rest.[1] These reactions are necessary to provide energy for maintenance of normal body temperature, cardiovascular and respiratory function, muscle tone, and other essential activities of tissues and cells in the resting body. The BMR constitutes 50% to 70% of body energy needs.[1] The BMR is measured using an instrument called an *indirect calorimeter* that measures a person's rate of oxygen use. Oxygen consumption is measured under basal conditions:

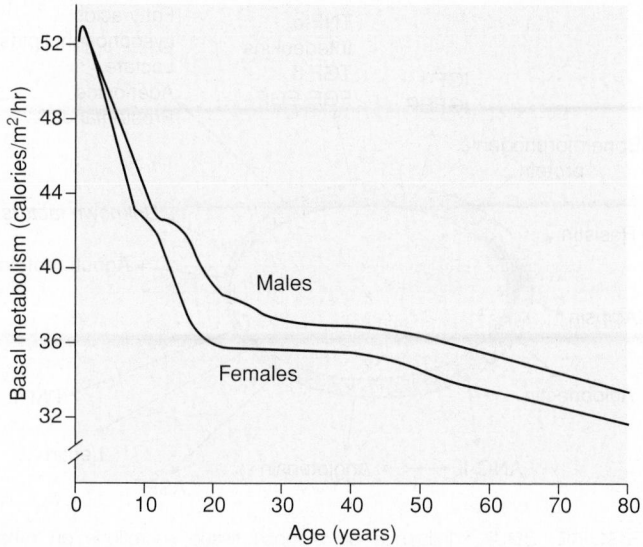

FIGURE 39.1 • Normal basal metabolic rates at different ages for each sex. (From Hall J. E. (2011). *Textbook of medical physiology* (12th ed., p. 864). Philadelphia, PA: W. B. Saunders.)

after a full night's sleep, after at least 12 hours without food, after no strenuous activity for 1 hour, and while the person is awake and at rest in a warm and comfortable room. The BMR is then calculated in terms of calories per hour and normally averages approximately 65 to 70 calories per hour in an average 70-kg man.[1] Women in general have a 5% to 10% lower BMR than men because of their higher percentage of adipose tissue. Although much of the BMR is accounted for by essential activities of the central nervous system, kidneys, and other body organs, the variations in BMR among different individuals are related largely to skeletal muscle mass and body size. Under normal resting conditions, skeletal muscle accounts for 20% to 30% of the BMR.[1] For this reason, the BMR is commonly corrected for body size by expressing it as calories per hour per square metre of body surface area. Factors that affect the BMR are age, sex, physical state, and pregnancy. A progressive decline in the normal BMR occurs with aging and is likely related to the loss of muscle mass and replacement with adipose tissue[1] (Fig. 39.1). The BMR can be used to predict the calorie needs for maintenance of nutrition.

The *resting energy expenditure* (REE) is used for predicting basal energy expenditure. The most accurate way to determine REE is by indirect calorimetry. However, this is expensive and requires trained personnel. Numerous equations that estimate REE based on variables such as weight, height, and age have been published. Examples of such equations include the Harris–Benedict[2], Owen,[3,4] and Mifflin–St Jeor[5] equations. Some illnesses (*e.g.,* severe infection/sepsis, long bone fractures, cancer, trauma, burns, closed head injury) elicit a catabolic state; thus, energy requirements are subsequently higher. To better predict energy expenditure in these conditions, REE is sometimes multiplied by a stress factor ranging from 1.1 to 1.6 depending on the clinical state. In other instances, predictive equation have been developed for specific physical states

such as critical illness.[6] Despite the abundance of predictive equations, their accuracy for use in hospitalized patients is questionable and their use is associated with under- and overestimation of true energy requirements.[7]

Diet- and Exercise-Induced Thermogenesis

Diet-induced thermogenesis, or the thermic effect of food, describes the energy used by the body for the digestion, absorption, and assimilation of food after its ingestion. It is energy expended over and above the caloric value of the food and accounts for approximately 8% of the total calories expended. When food is eaten, the metabolic rate rises and then returns to normal within a few hours.

The type of activity performed, the length of participation, and the person's weight and physical fitness determine the amount of energy expended for physical activity. The most significant increases in metabolic rate come from strenuous activity.

Nonexercise Activity Thermogenesis

Energy expenditure can be increased by increasing voluntary physical activity and/or nonexercise activity thermogenesis. Nonexercise activity thermogenesis includes the energy expended in maintaining posture and in activities such as fidgeting.[8] This can range from 15% of total daily energy in very sedentary individuals to 50% or more in those who are more active.[8] Nonexercise activity thermogenesis may be related to a propensity to gain weight. Individuals with increased nonexercise activity thermogenesis may have less fat gain than those with decreased nonexercise activity thermogenesis.

Energy Storage

Adipose Tissue

More than 90% of body energy is stored in adipose tissue. *Adipocytes,* or fat cells, occur singly or in small groups in loose connective tissue. In many parts of the body, they cushion body organs such as the kidneys. In addition to isolated groups of fat cells, entire regions of fat tissue are committed to fat storage. Collectively, fat cells constitute a large body organ that is metabolically active in the uptake, synthesis, storage, and mobilization of lipids, which are the main source of stored fuel for the body. Some tissues, such as liver cells, are able to store small amounts of lipids, but when these lipids accumulate (so-called ectopic deposition, as occurs in fatty liver), they begin to interfere with normal cell function. Adipose tissue not only serves as a storage site for body fuels, it provides insulation for the body, fills body crevices, and protects body organs.

Studies of adipocytes in the laboratory have shown that fully differentiated cells do not divide. However, such cells have a long life span, and anyone born with large numbers of adipocytes runs the risk of becoming obese. Some immature adipocytes (termed *preadipocytes*) capable of division are present in postnatal life.[1] Fat deposition can result from proliferation of these existing immature adipocytes. Some medications can also have an important effect on fat cell numbers.

The thiazolidinedione class of antidiabetic drugs (*i.e.,* rosiglitazone, pioglitazone) can also stimulate the formation of new fat cells from preadipocytes, allowing increased uptake of glucose into these cells (and storage as fat) and resulting in the desired reduction in serum glucose levels, but with unwanted weight gain. In contrast, some drugs can cause loss of fat cells, resulting in lipodystrophy. This occurs in human immunodeficiency virus (HIV)-associated lipodystrophy in persons treated with highly active antiretroviral therapy (HAART). The mechanism of fat loss is unknown; however, it may be due to increased programmed cell death of the adipocytes (*i.e.,* increased apoptosis).

There are two types of adipose tissue: white fat and brown fat. White fat, which despite its name is cream-coloured or yellow, is the prevalent form of adipose tissue in postnatal life. It constitutes 10% to 20% of body weight in adult men and 15% to 25% in adult women. At body temperature, the lipid content of fat cells exists as an oil. It consists of triglycerides, which are three molecules of fatty acids esterified to a glycerol molecule. Triglycerides, which contain no water, have the highest caloric content of all nutrients and are an efficient form of energy storage. Fat cells synthesize triglycerides, the major fat storage form, from dietary fats and carbohydrates. Insulin is required for transport of glucose into fat cells. When calorie intake is restricted for any reason, fat cell triglycerides are broken down, and the resultant fatty acids and glycerol are released as energy sources.

Brown fat differs from white fat in terms of its thermogenic capacity or ability to produce heat. Brown fat, the site of diet-induced thermogenesis and nonshivering thermogenesis, is found primarily in early neonatal life in humans and in animals that hibernate. This type of fat contains a higher concentration of specialized mitochondria, which enable this process.[1] In humans, brown fat decreases with age but is still detectable in the sixth decade. This small amount of brown fat has a minimal effect on energy expenditure.

Adipose Tissue as an Endocrine Organ

Adipose tissue is now recognized as an endocrine and paracrine organ that secretes a number of important factors.[9] These factors are termed *adipokines,* and include leptin, certain cytokines (*e.g.,* tumour necrosis factor-α [TNF-α], interleukin [IL]-6), adiponectin, and growth factors. Figure 39.2 identifies many of the substances produced by adipose tissue.

Leptin. The discovery of leptin (from the Greek meaning "thin"), a peptide released from adipocytes, has led to renewed interest in adipose tissue and its role in energy homeostasis. Recent studies suggest that leptin acts at the level of the hypothalamus to decrease food intake and increase energy expenditure through an increase in thermogenesis and sympathetic nervous system activity.[10] Leptin is also involved in glucose metabolism and normal sexual maturation and reproduction, and has interactions with the hypothalamic–pituitary–adrenal, thyroid, and growth hormones axes.[11,12]

Leptin acts by binding to and activating specific leptin receptors found in several peripheral tissues and in many areas

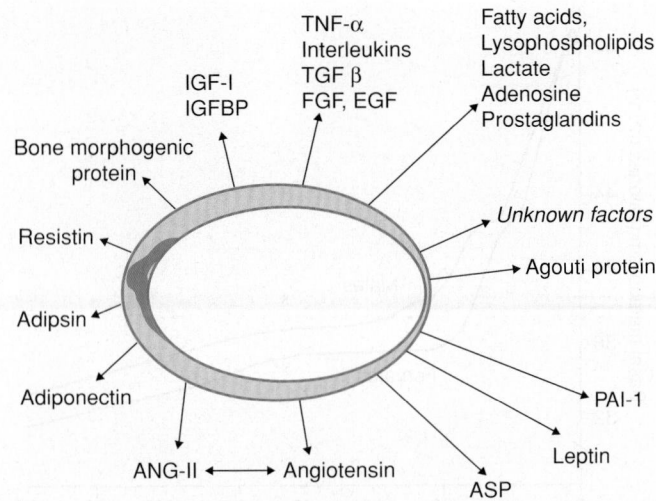

FIGURE 39.2 • Influence on adipose tissue secretions on other organs. Multiple protein and metabolites are secreted by adipose tissue and act locally or at a distance in other organs. They have an impact on food intake, insulin signalling, vascular function, energy expenditure, and other homeostatic processes in the body. ANG-II, angiotensin II; ASP, acetylation-stimulating protein; EGF, epidermal growth factor; FGF, fibroblast growth factor; IGF, insulin-like growth factor; IGFBP, insulin-like growth factor-binding protein; PAI-1, plasminogen activator inhibitor-1; TGF, transforming growth factor; TNF, tumour necrosis factor. (From Rubin R., Strayer D. S. (Eds.). (2012). *Rubin's pathology: Clinicopathologic foundations of medicine* (6th ed., p. 1085). Philadelphia, PA: Lippincott Williams & Wilkins.

of the brain, including specific regions of the hypothalamus.[13] Receptors in these hypothalamic regions are known to be involved in appetite, food intake,[13] sympathetic nervous system activity, temperature regulation, and insulin release by the pancreatic beta cells. Leptin levels tend to rise after food intake and fall during fasting. Adipose tissue signals the brain via leptin that sufficient storage of calories has been achieved, and increased food intake is not necessary. *Leptin resistance* or a failure to respond to the high levels of leptin may result in obesity.[14]

IN SUMMARY

Nutritional status describes the condition of the body related to the availability and use of nutrients. Nutrients provide the energy and materials necessary for performing the activities of daily living and for the growth and repair of body tissues. Metabolism is the organized process whereby nutrients such as carbohydrates, fats, and proteins are broken down, transformed, or otherwise converted to cellular energy. Energy is measured in heat units called kilocalories. Glucose, fats, and amino acids from proteins serve as fuel sources for cellular metabolism. These fuel sources are ingested during meals and stored for future use. Glucose is stored as glycogen or converted to triglycerides in fat cells for storage. Fats are stored in adipose tissue as triglycerides. Fat also functions as an endocrine organ in producing adipokines such as leptin, and cytokines, which affect weight gain. Amino acids are the building blocks of proteins, and most of the stored amino acids are contained in body proteins and as fuel sources for cellular metabolism.

The expenditure of body energy results from heat production (*i.e.,* thermogenesis) associated with the BMR or basal energy equivalent, diet-induced thermogenesis, exercise-induced thermogenesis, nonexercise activity thermogenesis, and thermogenesis in response to changes in environmental conditions.

NUTRITIONAL NEEDS

After completing this section of the chapter, you should be able to meet the following objectives:

* Discuss the different dietary standards that are utilized to formulate uniform diet guidelines for calories, protein, fats, carbohydrates, fibre, vitamins, and minerals.
* Describe methods used for a nutritional assessment.
* State the factors used in determining body mass index and explain its use in evaluating body weight in terms of undernutrition and overnutrition.

Dietary Reference Intakes

The *Dietary Reference Intakes* (DRIs) include a set of nutrient-based reference values: the recommended dietary allowance (RDA), the adequate intake (AI), the estimated average requirement (EAR), the tolerable upper intake level (UL), and the acceptable macronutrient distribution range (AMDR), each of which has specific uses.[15] The DRIs replaced the previously published Recommended Nutrient Intakes (RNIs) in Canada and the Recommended Dietary Allowances (RDAs) in the United States. They are established by Canadian and American scientists through a review process overseen by the National Academy of Sciences and are updated periodically. The DRIs are used to advise persons about the level of nutrient intake they need to prevent nutritional deficiencies and reduce the risk of chronic disease. The current recommended DRIs for selected vitamins and minerals are available on the US Department of Agriculture's (USDA) Food and Nutrition Information Center website at: http://fnic.nal.usda.gov/fnic/interactiveDRI/. This site contains an interactive tool that calculates a person's current nutritional needs based on gender, height, weight, age, and activity levels.[16]

The *recommended dietary allowance* (RDA) defines the intakes that meet the nutrient needs of almost all healthy persons in a specific age and sex group. An *estimated average requirement* (EAR) is the intake that meets the estimated nutrient need of half of the persons in a specific age and sex group. This figure is used as the basis for developing the RDA and is used by nutrition policy makers in the evaluation of the adequacy of a nutrient for a specific group and for planning how much of the nutrient the group should consume. The *adequate intake* (AI) is established when there is not enough scientific evidence to determine an EAR. A nutrient will have either an RDA or an AI. The AI is derived from experimental or observational data that show a mean intake that appears to sustain a desired indicator of health. The *tolerable upper intake* level (UL) is the maximum intake that is judged unlikely to pose a health risk in almost all healthy persons in a specified group. It refers to the total intakes from food, fortified food, and nutrient supplements. As intake increases above the UL, the risk of adverse effects increases. The UL is not intended to be a recommended level of intake and there are no established benefits for persons who consume nutrients beyond the RDA or AI levels.[15]

In Canada, most prepackaged foods are required to have a standardized *Nutrition Facts* table which contains % *Daily Value* (DV) as a benchmark to allow consumers to evaluate the nutrient content of the food quickly and easily. The % DV is based on a 2,000 calorie reference diet and it is mandatory for % DV to be listed for the following nutrients (with the standard reference value following in parentheses): fat (65 g or ~30% of total energy), saturated and trans fat (20 g or ~10% of total energy), carbohydrate (300 g or ~60% of total energy), fibre (25 g), cholesterol (300 mg), sodium (2,400 mg), vitamin A (1,000 RE), vitamin C (60 mg), calcium (1,100 mg), and iron (14 mg).[17] The % DVs are intended to be a general guide for the population and are meant to assist with food choices, by indicating to the consumer what percentage of the DV one serving of a food supplies.

Proteins, fats, carbohydrates, vitamins, and minerals each have their own function in providing the body with what it needs to maintain life and health. Recommended allowances have not been established for every nutrient; some are given as a safe and adequate intake, but others, such as carbohydrates and fats, are expressed as a percentage of the calorie intake.

Nutritional Needs

Calories

Energy requirements are greater during growth periods. A person requires approximately 115 kcal/kg of body weight at birth, 105 kcal/kg at 1 year of age, and 80 kcal/kg from 1 to 10 years of age. During adolescence, boys require 45 kcal/kg of body weight and girls require 38 kcal/kg. During pregnancy, a woman needs an extra 350 and 450 kcal/day above her usual requirement, in the second trimester and third trimesters, respectively. During breast-feeding, a woman requires an additional 350 to 400 additional calories daily, however, this is only an approximation as caloric requirements can vary based on weight loss and milk production.[18]

Proteins

Protein is required for growth and maintenance of body tissues, enzymes and antibody formation, fluid and electrolyte balance, and nutrient transport. Proteins are composed of amino acids, nine of which are essential to the body (*i.e.,* they cannot be synthesized by the body and must be derived from dietary sources). These are leucine, isoleucine, methionine, phenylalanine, threonine, tryptophan, valine, lysine, and histidine. Complete protein foods are those that provide these essential amino acids in adequate amounts. Complete proteins most often are derived from animal sources and include milk, eggs, meat, fish, and poultry. However, there are a few vegetable-derived complete protein sources, including soy and quinoa. Other vegetable proteins, including dried peas and beans, nuts, seeds, and grains, contain all the essential amino acids but in less than adequate proportions. These proteins need to be combined with each other to meet the amino acid requirements for protein synthesis (though combining them at one meal is not necessary). The AMDR recommends protein make up 10% to 35% of daily caloric intake,[15] however these recommendations are controversial and likely underestimate true requirements. Overall protein requirements are dependent on age, weight, and level of physical activity, but it is recommended that at least 1.0 to 1.2 g of protein be kilogram body weight be consumed daily.[19,20] Diets that are inadequate in protein can result in kwashiorkor. If calories and protein are inadequate, protein-calorie malnutrition occurs.

The average protein consists of about 16% nitrogen. About 90% of this is excreted in the urine as urea, uric acid, creatinine, and other, less important nitrogen breakdown products, with the rest being excreted in the feces.[1] Therefore, the rate of protein breakdown can be estimated by measuring the amount of nitrogen in the urine. If the amount of nitrogen taken in as protein is equivalent to the nitrogen excreted, the person is said to be in nitrogen balance. A person is in positive nitrogen balance when the nitrogen consumed through protein is greater than the amount excreted. This occurs during growth, pregnancy, or healing after surgery or injury. A negative nitrogen balance often occurs with fever, illness, infection, trauma, or burns, when more nitrogen is excreted than is consumed[1] and represents a state of lean tissue breakdown.

Fats

Dietary fats are composed primarily of triglycerides (*i.e.,* a mixture of fatty acids and glycerol). The fatty acids are saturated (*i.e.,* no double bonds), monounsaturated (*i.e.,* one double bond), or polyunsaturated (*i.e.,* two or more double bonds). The saturated fatty acids elevate blood cholesterol, whereas the monounsaturated and polyunsaturated fats lower blood cholesterol. Saturated fats usually are from animal sources and remain solid at room temperature. With the exception of coconut and palm oils (which are saturated), unsaturated fats are found in plant oils and usually are liquid at room temperature. *Trans fatty acids* are produced when unsaturated oils are partially hydrogenated and are called *artificial trans fats.* They are found primarily in vegetable shortenings and some margarines and in foods containing either of these. Natural sources of trans fatty acids include dairy products, some meats (*e.g.,* beef and lamb) and other animal-based foods. Trans fatty acids increase low-density lipoprotein (LDL) cholesterol and decrease high-density lipoprotein (HDL) cholesterol.

However, the naturally occurring trans fats may have a beneficial effect. Dietary fats provide energy, function as carriers for the fat-soluble vitamins, serve as precursors of prostaglandins, and are a source of fatty acids.

Polyunsaturated fatty acids, including linoleic acid (an omega-6 fatty acid) and alpha (α) linolenic acid (an omega-3 fatty acid), are examples of essential fatty acids. This means that they are not synthesized in the body and must be included in the diet. An AI has been set for both linoleic and α-linoleic acids.[15] Because certain vegetable oils are rich sources of α-linoleic and linoleic acids, the AI can be met by including two teaspoons per day of vegetable oil in the diet. Deficiency of linoleic acid results in dermatitis and deficiency of α-linolenic acid can result in neurologic abnormalities and poor growth.

Omega-3 and omega-6 fatty acids have been found to contribute to both formation and treatment of many disease states. Gamma linolenic acid, a derivative of linoleic acid may promote inflammation, while α-linolenic acid has been effective in treating some disease states with inflammatory states, but not in others.[1] Much is still unknown about the effects of this group of nutrients. Omega-3 acids are primarily found in cold water fish, walnuts, and flaxseeds. Omega-6 fatty acids are found in seeds and nuts. In general, omega-6 fatty acids promote inflammation, blood clotting, and cell proliferation, while omega-3 fatty acids decrease these functions.

Cholesterol, a waxy lipid produced in the liver, is contained in every body cell. It is necessary for numerous body functions, including hormone production, metabolism of many vitamins, nerve function, and cell permeability. Cholesterol is transmitted throughout the body by lipoproteins; LDL, HDL, and triglycerides. Excess cholesterol in the body can cause significant harm to the cardiovascular system and increase risk of serious cardiac disease. Careful monitoring of blood levels and reduction of dietary intake of cholesterol help to keep cholesterol levels in balance.

In a joint position statement, Dietitians of Canada and the American Dietetic Association released the following recommendations for dietary fat: 20% to 35% of total calories in the diet should come from fats; consumption of saturated fatty acids should be no more than 10% of total energy intake; trans fat intake should be as low as possible; omega-6 polyunsaturated fatty acids comprise 5% to 10% of total energy; and aim for omega-3 polyunsaturated fatty acid intake of 0.5% to 2%.[21] As dietary fat consumption is a primary determinant of serum cholesterol levels, Canada has not set specific recommendations for cholesterol intake, relying instead on limits for total and saturated fat intake and other dietary modifications to achieve healthy blood cholesterol levels.[22]

Carbohydrates

Dietary carbohydrates are composed of simple sugars, complex carbohydrates, and indigestable carbohydrates (*i.e.,* fibre). Because of their vitamin, mineral, and fibre content, it is recommended that the bulk of the carbohydrate content in the diet be in the complex form rather than as simple sugars that contain few nutrients.

There is no specific dietary requirement for carbohydrates. All of the energy requirements of the body can be met by dietary fats and proteins, however, a carbohydrate-deficient diet usually results in the loss of tissue proteins and the development of ketosis. Because protein and fat metabolism increase the production of osmotically active metabolic wastes that must be eliminated through the kidneys, there is a danger of dehydration and electrolyte imbalances in diets deficient in carbohydrates. The amount of carbohydrate needed to prevent tissue wasting and ketosis is 50 to 100 g/day. In practice, most of the daily energy requirement should be supplied by carbohydrate because many protein sources also are high in fat and more expensive. The AMDR indicates that carbohydrate intake should consist of 45% to 65% of the daily calories in the diet.[15] Carbohydrates should be in the form of whole grains, vegetables and fruits, which have higher fibre content compared to refined flour and sugar products.

Fibre

Dietary fibre, the nondigestible carbohydrates found in plants such as fruits, vegetables, beans, nuts, and whole grains; and functional fibre, isolated nondigestible carbohydrates that have beneficial physiologic benefits, together form total fibre. Functional fibres are synthetic or extracted from plant sources and added to food. Examples include psyllium and methylcellulose, and they are commonly found in processed foods. Dietary fibre provides increased bulk, viscosity, and fermentation. Bulking slows gastric emptying, therefore increasing satiety, and increases the rate of transport through the gastrointestinal tract, thereby increasing stool bulk and facilitating normal bowel movements. Viscosity thickens the lining of the intestinal track, helps moderate blood glucose levels, and lowers cholesterol levels. Fermentation contributes to growth of healthy intestinal bacteria and to immune system functioning. Current dietary fibre recommendations for men and women between the ages of 19 to 50 years are 38 and 25 g, respectively, whereas the recommendations for adults older than 50 years are 30 and 21 g, respectively, each day.[15]

Vitamins and Minerals

Vitamins. Vitamins are a group of organic compounds that act as catalysts in various chemical reactions. A compound cannot be classified as a vitamin unless it is shown that a deficiency of it causes disease. Contrary to popular belief, vitamins do not provide energy directly. As catalysts, they are part of the enzyme systems required for the release of energy from protein, fat, and carbohydrates. Vitamins also are necessary for the formation of red blood cells, hormones, genetic materials, and the nervous system. They are essential for normal growth and development.

There are two types of vitamins: fat soluble and water soluble. The four fat-soluble vitamins are vitamins A, D, E, and K. The nine required water-soluble vitamins are thiamine, riboflavin, niacin, pyridoxine (vitamin B_6), pantothenic acid, vitamin B_{12}, folic acid, biotin, and vitamin C. Water-soluble vitamins are excreted in the urine, therefore they are less likely to accumulate in the body to toxic levels; however, the fat-soluble vitamins are stored in the body and they may reach toxic levels. Table 39.1 lists sources and functions of vitamins.

Minerals. Minerals serve many functions. They are involved in acid–base balance and in the maintenance of osmotic pressure in body compartments. Minerals are components of vitamins, hormones, and enzymes. They maintain normal hemoglobin levels, play a role in nervous system function, and are involved in muscle contraction and skeletal development and maintenance. Minerals that are present in relatively large amounts in the body are called *macrominerals*. These include calcium, phosphorus, sodium, chloride, potassium, magnesium, and sulphur. The remainder are classified as *trace minerals;* they include iron, manganese, copper, iodine, zinc, cobalt, fluorine, and selenium. Table 39.2 provides a list of mineral sources and their functions.

Regulation of Food Intake and Energy Storage

Stability of body weight and composition over time requires that energy intake match energy utilization. Environmental, cultural, genetic, and psychological factors all influence food intake and energy expenditure. In addition, body weight is tightly controlled by various physiologic feedback control systems that contribute to the regulation of hunger and food intake.[1]

Hunger, Appetite, and Food Intake

The sensation of *hunger* is associated with several sensory perceptions, such as the rhythmic contractions of the stomach and that "empty feeling" in the stomach that stimulates a person to seek food. A person's *appetite* is the desire for a particular type of food. It is useful in helping the person determine the type of food that is eaten. *Satiety* is the feeling of fullness or decreased desire for food.

Two centres in the brain interact with various hormones and neurotransmitters to help control food intake and energy output. The arcuate nucleus of the hypothalamus has been identified as the centre for hunger and satiety. However, current research indicates other centres in the brainstem also contribute to the mechanisms[23] (Fig. 39.3). These centres receive neural input from the gastrointestinal tract that provides information about stomach filling, chemical signals from nutrients (glucose, amino acids, and fatty acids) in the blood, and input from the cerebral cortex regarding the smell, sight, and taste of the food. Centres in the hypothalamus also control the secretion of several hormones (*i.e.,* thyroid and adrenocortical hormones) that regulate energy balance and metabolism.

The control of food intake is subject to short-term regulation, which is concerned with the amount of food that is consumed at a meal or snack, and intermediate and long-term regulation, which is concerned with the maintenance of energy stores over time.[1]

Neurotransmitters and hormones can influence the short-term regulation of food intake and they are categorized as

TABLE 39.1 SOURCES AND FUNCTIONS OF VITAMINS

VITAMIN	MAJOR FOOD SOURCES	FUNCTIONS
Fat-Soluble Vitamins		
Vitamin A (retinol, provitamin, carotenoids)	Retinol: liver, butter, whole milk, cheese, egg yolk; provitamin A: carrots, green leafy vegetables, sweet potatoes, pumpkin, winter squash, apricots, cantaloupe, fortified margarine	Essential for normal retinal function; plays an essential role in cell growth and differentiation, particularly epithelial cells. Epidemiologic evidence suggests a role in preventing certain cancers
Vitamin D (calciferol)	Fortified dairy products, fortified margarine, fish oils, egg yolk	Increases intestinal absorption of calcium and promotes ossification of bones and teeth
Vitamin E (tocopherol)	Vegetable oil, margarine, shortening, green and leafy vegetables, wheat germ, whole-grain products, egg yolk, butter, liver	Functions as an antioxidant protecting vitamins A and C and fatty acids; prevents cell membrane injury
Water-Soluble Vitamins		
Vitamin C (ascorbic acid)	Broccoli, sweet and hot peppers, collards, brussel sprouts, kale, potatoes, spinach, tomatoes, citrus fruits, strawberries	Potent antioxidant involved in many oxidation–reduction reactions; required for synthesis of collagen; increases absorption of nonheme iron; is involved in wound healing and drug metabolism
Thiamin (vitamin B_1)	Pork, liver, meat, whole grains, fortified grain products, legumes, nuts	Coenzyme required for several important biochemical reactions in carbohydrate metabolism; thought to have an independent role in nerve conduction
Riboflavin (vitamin B_2)	Liver, milk, yogurt, cottage cheese, meat, fortified grain products	Coenzyme that participates in a variety of important oxidation–reduction reactions and an important component of a number of enzymes
Niacin (nicotinamide, nicotinic acid)	Liver, meat, poultry, fish, peanuts, fortified grain products	Essential component of the coenzymes nicotinamide adenine dinucleotide (NAD) and nicotinamide dinucleotide diphosphate (NADP), which are involved in many oxidative–reduction reactions
Folacin (folic acid)	Liver, legumes, green leafy vegetables	Coenzyme in amino acid and nucleoprotein metabolism; promotes red cell formation
Vitamin B_6 (pyridoxine)	Meat, poultry, fish, shellfish, green and leafy vegetables, whole-grain products, legumes	A major coenzyme involved in the metabolism of amino acids; required for synthesis of heme
Vitamin B_{12}	Meat, poultry, fish, shellfish, eggs, dairy products	Coenzyme involved in nucleic acid synthesis; assists in development of red cells and maintenance of nerve function
Biotin	Kidney, liver, milk, egg yolk, most fresh vegetables	Coenzyme in fat synthesis, amino acid metabolism, and glycogen formation
Pantothenic acid	Liver, kidney, meats, milk, egg yolk, whole-grain products, legumes	Coenzyme involved in energy metabolism

orexigenic substances that stimulate feeding or *anorexigenic* substances that inhibit feeding.[1] Also stretch receptors in the gastrointestinal tract monitor gastrointestinal filling and send inhibitory impulses by way of the vagal nerve to the feeding centre to suppress the desire for food. While several genes involved in the regulation of food intake have been identified, researchers continue to develop insights into this complex system.[23,24]

Three main short-term messengers that promote orexigenic effects include ghrelin, produced mainly in the stomach, and neuropeptide Y, and agouti-related protein, both produced in the hypothalamus. Ghrelin, a neuropeptide, is released when the stomach is empty and as the stomach fills and stretches the secretion of ghrelin stops suggesting it may stimulate eating. The gastrointestinal hormones cholecystokinin (CCK) and

glucagon-like peptide-1 (GLP-1) have a strong anorexigenic effect on the hypothalamic feeding centre to signal satiety. Cholecystokinin is released in response to fat in the duodenum, and glucagon-like peptide-1 is released from the lower small bowel in response to nutrients, especially carbohydrates. The presence of food in the stomach increases the release of insulin and glucagon, both of which suppress the neurogenic feeding signals from the brain.[1] The act of tasting, chewing, and swallowing also appears to suppress the feeling of hunger. It seems multiple messengers send messages of satiety that ultimately help decrease food intake.[25]

The intermediate and long-term regulation of food intake is determined by the amount of nutrients that are in the blood and in storage sites. It has long been known that a decrease in blood

TABLE 39.2 SOURCES AND FUNCTIONS OF MINERALS

MINERAL	MAJOR SOURCES	FUNCTIONS
Calcium	Milk and milk products, fish with bones, greens	Bone formation and maintenance; tooth formation, vitamin B absorption, blood clotting, nerve and muscle function
Chloride	Table salt, meats, milk, eggs	Regulates pH of stomach, acid–base balance, osmotic pressure of extracellular fluids
Cobalt	Organ meats, meats	Aids in maturation of red blood cells (as part of B_{12} molecule)
Copper	Cereals, nuts, legumes, liver, shellfish, grapes, meats	Catalyst for hemoglobin formation, formation of elastin and collagen, energy release (cytochrome oxidase and catalase), formation of melanin, formation of phospholipids for myelin sheath of nerves
Fluoride	Fluorinated water	Strengthens bones and teeth
Iodine	Iodized salt, fish (saltwater and anadromous)	Thyroid hormone synthesis and its function in maintenance of metabolic rate
Iron	Meats, heart, liver, clams, oysters, lima beans, spinach, dates, dried nuts, enriched and whole-grain cereals	Hemoglobin synthesis, cellular energy release (cytochrome pathway), killing bacteria (myeloperoxidase)
Magnesium	Milk, green vegetables, nuts, bread, cereals	Catalyst of many intracellular nerve impulses, retention of reactions, particularly those related to intracellular enzyme reactions; low magnesium levels produce an increase in irritability of the nervous system, vasodilation, and cardiac arrhythmias
Phosphorus	Meats, poultry, fish, milk and cheese, cereals, legumes, nuts	Bone formation and maintenance; essential component of nucleic acids and energy exchange forms such as adenosine triphosphate (ATP)
Potassium	Oranges, dried fruits, bananas, meats, potatoes, peanut butter, coffee	Maintenance of intracellular osmolality, acid–base balance, transmission of nerve impulses, catalyst in energy metabolism, formation of proteins, formation of glycogen
Sodium	Table salt, cured meats, meats, milk, olives	Maintenance of osmotic pressure of extracellular fluids, acid–base balance, neuromuscular function; absorption of glucose
Sulphur	Meats, poultry, fish, milk and cheese, eggs, legumes, nuts	Present in sulphur-containing amino acids required for synthesis of essential metabolites
		Functions in oxidation–reduction reactions as part of thiamine and biotin
Zinc	Whole-wheat cereals, eggs, legumes	Integral part of many enzymes, including carbonic anhydrase, which facilitates combination of carbon dioxide with water in red blood cells; component of lactate dehydrogenase, which is important in cellular metabolism; component of many peptidases; important in digestion of proteins in gastrointestinal tract

glucose causes hunger. In contrast, an increase in breakdown products of lipids such as ketoacids produces a decrease in appetite. A ketogenic weight-loss diet (*i.e.*, very low-carbohydrate diets) relies partly on the appetite-suppressant effects of ketones in the blood.

Adipocytes release leptin in proportion to the amount of fat stores. The stimulation of leptin receptors in the hypothalamus produces a decrease in appetite and food intake as well as an increase in metabolic rate and energy consumption. It also produces a decrease in insulin release from the beta cells, which decreases energy storage in fat cells.[23]

Nutritional Assessment

Components of a nutrition assessment include a variety of measures including a review of a person's basic health history to identify any illnesses or gastrointestinal symptoms that might affect food intake, a record of diet intake, a physical assessment, and together linking this information to body measurements and laboratory studies.

Health History

Obtaining a health history facilitates identification of illnesses that may affect a person's nutritional status. For example, some neurologic disorders such as multiple sclerosis, amyotrophic lateral sclerosis, or a cerebral vascular incident (stroke) can cause impaired swallowing which can limit the types and amounts of food ingested thus placing a person at higher nutritional risk. Another example is inflammatory bowel disease (IBD) (*i.e.*, Crohn disease or ulcerative colitis); persons with IBD might experience abdominal pain, cramping, nausea, vomiting, diarrhea, all of which can affect nutrition intake and status. Conditions that are also associated with an acute inflammatory response (*i.e.*, infection/sepsis, burns, major surgery, closed head injury, critical illness) or chronic inflammation (*i.e.*, diabetes, cardiovascular disease, kidney disease etc.) are also associated with increased nutrition risk.[26]

Diet History

Another component of nutritional assessment is an evaluation of a person's usual or typical diet. This can be accomplished

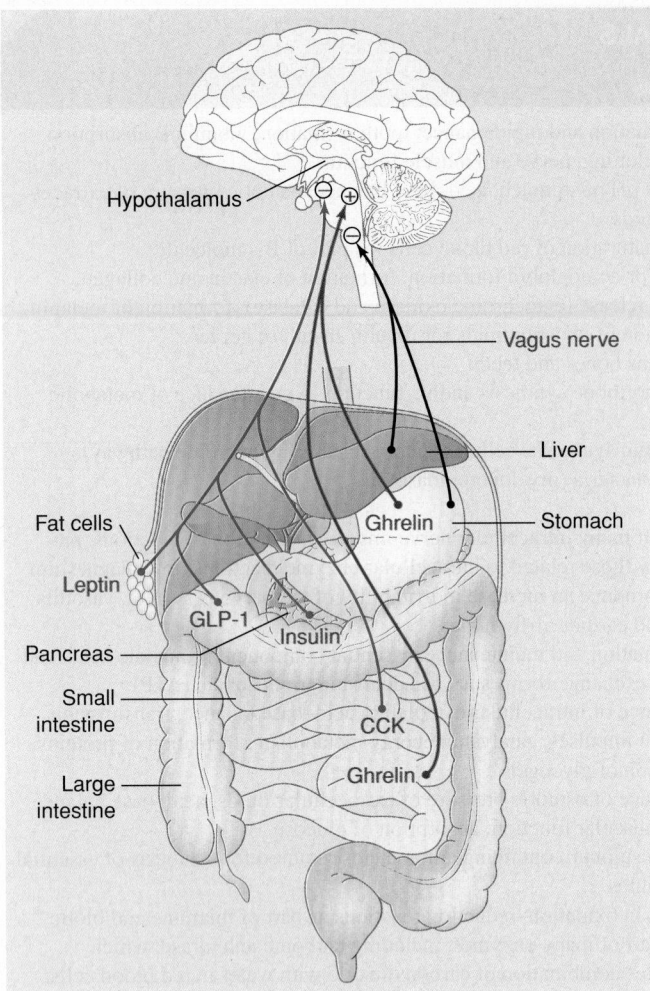

FIGURE 39.3 • Feedback mechanisms for control of food intake. Stretch receptors in the stomach activate sensory afferent pathways in the vagus and inhibit food intake. Glucagon-like peptide-1 (GLP-1), cholecystokinin (CCK), and insulin are gastrointestinal hormones that are released by the ingestion of food and suppress further feeding. Ghrelin is released by the stomach and small intestine, especially during fasting, and stimulates appetite. Leptin is a hormone produced by fat cells as they increase in number and size; it inhibits food intake. (Modified from Hall J. E. (2011). *Textbook of medical physiology.* (12th ed., p. 846). Philadelphia, PA: W. B. Saunders.)

using several different methods including: record of food consumed (*i.e.,* maintaining a food record or diary), the 24-hour recall method, and/or via the administration of a food frequency questionnaire. Each technique has its own shortcomings. For example, persons completing food records have the tendency to underreport food consumption or alter eating habits when it is known that they are being observed or reported.[27]

Physical Examination

A physical examination is a valuable tool in assessing nutritional status. Physical features that may be related to malnutrition include changes in weight, muscle wasting, decreased subcutaneous fat, edema, changes in the quality of the hair or condition of the gums, absence of body hair, and skin

breakdown (*i.e.,* impaired wound healing, development of pressure ulcers), and a decline in physical functioning (*i.e.,* decreased ability to complete activities of daily living).[26] Comparison of a person's current weight with previous weights identifies whether the person's weight is stable, has changed drastically or tends to fluctuate, and whether changes seen have occurred over a short or longer period of time. Rapid weight loss over a short period of time can be a sign of illness (*i.e.,* cancer, hyperthyroidism) or decreased nutritional intake which may be intentional (*i.e.,* self-imposed starvation) or unintentional (*i.e.,* secondary to food insecurity or illness related anorexia). A history of fluctuating weight could be associated with chronic dieting or disordered eating. Regardless of etiology, the effects of malnutrition are broad, affecting every physiologic system in the body.

Anthropometric Assessment

Anthropometry was originally defined as "measurements of the variations of the physical dimensions and the gross composition of the human body at different age levels and degrees of nutrition."[28] Evaluating body composition serves several purposes including determination of growth patterns in children and appropriateness of current weight in adults. Several methods exist to evaluate body composition.

Weight. Body weight is the most frequently used method of assessing nutritional status and measurement of weight over time can help to identify trends in weight changes that may positively or negatively affect health status. For weight measurement, subjects should ideally be in light clothing, without shoes, fasting, and have an empty bladder. Repeat measurements are best made at the same time of the day using the same scale to ensure validity of the measures.

Body Mass Index. Body mass index (BMI) is an index used estimate body fatness and evaluate health risk based on a person's height and weight (Table 39.3). It is calculated by dividing weight in kilograms by height in metres squared (BMI = weight [kg]/height [m^2]). A BMI between 18.5 and 24.9 kg/m^2 is considered normal, whereas a BMI greater than 25 kg/m^2 (classified as overweight or obese) is associated with an increased risk of comorbidities.[29] While BMI is a simple and easy measurement, its use is predominantly as a tool to evaluate the health of a population. Its use in establishing individual health risk is limited. For example, individuals with increased muscle mass may have a higher BMI but not have the associated increase in health risk.

Body weight and BMI evaluate body composition at the whole-body level. They do not describe body composition at the tissue level, for example, they do not quantify the amount of lean or adipose (fat) tissue in the body. However, several methods that can estimate body composition at the tissue level exist, some of which include skinfold and circumference measures, bioelectrical impedance analysis (BIA), air plethysmography, dual-energy x-ray absorptiometry (DEXA), computed

TABLE 39.3 BODY WEIGHT CLASSIFICATION BY BMI AND WAIST CIRCUMFERENCE AND ASSOCIATED HEALTH RISK

	BMI (kg/m²)	RISK OF DEVELOPING HEALTH PROBLEMS[a]	HEALTH RISK CLASSIFICATION USING BOTH BMI AND WC	
			MEN ≤102 cm WOMEN ≤88 cm	MEN >102 cm WOMEN >88 cm
Underweight	<18.5	Increased	—	—
Normal weight	18.5–24.9	Least	Least risk	Increased risk
Overweight	25.0–29.9	Increased	Increased risk	High risk
Obese				
Class I	30.0–34.9	High	High risk	Very high risk
Class II	35.0–39.9	Very high	—[b]	—[b]
Class III	≥40.0	Extremely high	—[b]	—[b]

[a]Health problems include type 2 diabetes, dyslipidemia, hypertension, coronary heart disease, gallbladder disease, obstructive sleep apnea, certain cancers, undernutrition, osteoporosis, infertility, impaired immunocompetence.
[b]For BMIs ≥35.0, WC measurement does not provide additional information regarding level of risk.
BMI, body mass index; WC, waist circumference.

tomography (CT), and magnetic resonance imaging (MRI). When percentage body fat is calculated, it can be compared to existing percent body fat standards for adults as another means to assess health status.[30]

Skinfold and Circumference Measures. Skinfold thickness and body circumference measurements can be utilized to estimate percent body fat and fat-free mass. Skinfold measures provide an estimate of subcutaneous fat and are typically taken at the triceps, biceps, subscapula, and suprailiac sites. These measures are then entered into various regression equations to estimate percentage body fat. Measurements of mid-arm circumference, either alone or combined with triceps skinfold thickness, allows for the estimation of protein stores in the body also through the use of regression equations. Limitations to these measurements are that they are difficult to perform and subject to considerable variation between observers.[31] Another measurement is the *waist circumference* and this has received attention because excess visceral (or intra-abdominal) fat is closely associated with the metabolic syndrome. Studies have indicated that waist circumference at the abdomen (which is a surrogate measure of visceral fat) is highly correlated with insulin resistance, hypertension, dyslipidemia—all hallmark features of the metabolic syndrome (see Chapter 42).

Bioelectrical Impedance Analysis (BIA). *Bioimpedance* is a portable method of assessing body composition that is performed by attaching electrodes at the wrist and ankle that send a harmless current through the body. The flow of the current is affected by the amount of water in the body. Fat-free tissue contains virtually all the water and conducting electrolytes, therefore measurements of the resistance (*i.e.,* impedance) to current flow can be used to estimate the percentage of body fat present.[32]

Radiologic Methods of Assessing Body Composition. Radiologic methods of body composition include the use of DEXA, CT and MRI. DEXA is a radiographic technique based on the differential absorption of x-rays by bone and soft tissues. It enables whole-body estimation of lean soft tissue mass, fat-free mass, fat mass and bone mineral content. CT and MRI allow for in vivo quantification of body composition at the tissue-organ level. Radiologic methods tend to be limited to research settings due to their expense and lack of portability.[33]

Laboratory Studies

Various laboratory tests can aid in evaluating nutritional status. Some of the most commonly performed tests are serum albumin and prealbumin to assess the protein status; total lymphocyte count and delayed hypersensitivity reaction to assess cellular immunity; and creatinine–height index to assess skeletal muscle protein. Vitamin and mineral deficiencies can be determined by measurements of their levels in blood, saliva, and other body tissues or by measuring nutrient-specific chemical reactions. All of these tests are limited by confounding factors and therefore need to be evaluated along with other clinical data.

IN SUMMARY

The body requires more than 40 nutrients on a daily basis. Nutritional status reflects the continued daily intake of nutrients over time and the deposition and use of these nutrients in the body. The DRIs classify the amounts of essential nutrients considered to be adequate to meet the known nutritional needs of healthy persons. The DRIs have 22 age and sex classifications and include recommendations for calories, protein, fat, carbohydrates, vitamins, and minerals. Hunger and satiety are controlled by a complex group of neurohormones, many of which are produced in the gastrointestinal tract. These messengers function to either stimulate hunger or signal satiety to control both short and long-term effects. While much information has been revealed through research in recent years, there is still much to be learned in order to effectively manage the complex process more effectively.

The nutritional status of a person can be assessed by evaluation of a person's health history, diet history, a physical examination, anthropometric measures/body composition and laboratory tests. Methods used for the assessment of body composition may include those that assess whole-body composition (*i.e.,* height, weight and BMI) or body composition at the tissue level (*i.e.,* skinfold and circumference measures, BIA, DEXA, CT scans or MRI scans).

OVERWEIGHT AND OBESITY

After completing this section of the chapter, you should be able to meet the following objectives:

- Define and discuss the causes of obesity and health risks associated with obesity.
- Differentiate upper and lower body obesity and their implications in terms of health risk.
- Discuss the treatment of obesity in terms of diet, behaviour modification, exercise, social support, pharmacotherapy, and surgical methods.
- Explain the use of body mass index in evaluating body weight in terms of overnutrition.

Obesity is defined as having excess body fat accumulation with multiple organ-specific pathologic consequences and an increased number of fat cells. Obesity has become a significant global health problem. In 2008, almost 1.5 billion people were classified as overweight, 500 million of which were obese.[34] Clinically, obesity and overweight have been defined in terms of the BMI. Historically, various world bodies have used different BMI cutoff points to define obesity. In 1997, the World Health Organization (WHO) defined the various classifications of overweight (BMI ≥25) and obesity (BMI ≥30); this classification system is also employed by Health Canada[35,36] (Table 39.3).

In Canada, data from the Canadian Health Measures Survey (2009–2011) showed that almost two of three adults are overweight or obese, with approximately 40% of adults classified as overweight and a further 27% classified as obese.[36] In Canadian aboriginals, the prevalence of obesity is 38%, significantly higher than the nonaboriginal population.[37,38] The prevalence of overweight and obesity is alarming not only because of the number of people affected but because the prevalence continues to increase from previous surveys. In comparing data from the 1978/1979 to the 2009/2011 Canadian Community Health Surveys, the prevalence of obesity

has increased from 13.8% of the population to 27%.[36,39] Perhaps of greater concern is that 32% of Canadian children (5 to 17 years of age) are overweight or obese.[40]

OVERWEIGHT AND OBESITY

- Obesity results from an imbalance between energy intake and energy consumption. Because fat is the main storage form of energy, obesity represents an excess of body fat.
- Overweight and obesity are determined by measurements of body mass index (BMI; weight [kg]/height [m²]) and waist circumference. A BMI of 25 to 29.9 is considered overweight; a BMI of 30 or greater as obese; and a BMI greater than 40 as very or morbidly obese.
- Waist circumference is used to determine the distribution of body fat. Central, or abdominal, obesity is an independent predictor of morbidity and mortality associated with obesity.

Causes of Obesity

The epidemic of obesity results from many causative factors, and research is adding to the body of knowledge almost daily. Many factors contribute to both the development of obesity and the body's response to attempts to control it. Commonly acknowledged contributing causes include diet, genetics, metabolism, behaviour, environment, culture, and socioeconomic status.[41] Medical conditions such as thyroid disorder, Cushing syndrome and polycystic ovarian syndrome can also contribute to weight gain and obesity, as do many medications.

The relationship between genetics and weight gain is complex, and, as yet, not fully understood. The most recent and last update of the human obesity gene map series, completed in 2005, reported 135 candidate genes had been identified that are associated with obesity-related phenotypes.[24,42] Many of these relate to known brain-gut controls of hunger and satiety, metabolism, and the body's storage mechanisms. Researchers theorize this may help to explain differences in obesity levels found in various populations. Identification of these genetic influences may allow for more targeted treatment interventions in the future. It is yet unknown how genes and mutations may directly or indirectly interact with environmental causes of obesity. One description for the complex interaction between environment and genetics is attributed to George Bray, a noted expert on obesity, who stated "the genetic background loads the gun, but the environment pulls the trigger."[43] There is new evidence that behaviour-based interventions may attenuate the genetic influence of obesity.[44]

Though genetic research gives new insight into the genesis of obesity, environmental influence remains the major contributor to this worldwide issue.[45] Obesity rates have reached epidemic proportions in populations with high availability of calorie rich foods and few opportunities for physical activity.[44,45] Influences such as family eating patterns, inactivity because of labour-saving devices and time spent on the computer and watching television, reliance on the automobile for transportation, easy access to food, higher energy density of food, increased consumption of sugar-sweetened beverages, and increasing portion sizes. More recent epidemiologic studies indicate that while decreased physical activity plays a role in increasing rates of overweight and obesity, diet changes due to increased availability of cheap, tasty, highly promoted, obesogenic types of food appears to have caused a much more steep rise in obesity.[45]

Psychological factors are another area of influence on behaviour related to weight gain. Eating may be a way to cope with stress, boredom, or anxiety. However, the relationships of these behaviours to mental health and obesity are complex and poorly understood.[46,47] No specific personality traits characteristic of obese people have been identified.[47] While the causal relationship of psychological behaviours is not clear, binge-eating disorder (BED) behaviours, described as uncontrolled consumption of large quantities of food, have been found in 20% to 30% of obese people seeking weight loss treatment.[47]

Culture and socioeconomic status are also believed to be contributing factors in the increased rates of overweight and obesity. Increased rates of obesity are seen in Canadian Aboriginal populations, African American, and Hispanic groups, particularly in women. Although many theories have been set forth it is not yet clear what impact cultural food choices and accepted cultural behaviours have on these rates. It is clear that interventions will need to be developed to address the needs of different cultures, as well as address the socioeconomic barriers to improved dietary choices.[48] Much discussion and debate will continue related to causative factors, especially as effective means to treat and prevent obesity are sought.

Types of Obesity

Two types of obesity based on distribution of fat have been described: upper body and lower body obesity. *Upper body obesity* is also referred to as *central, abdominal, visceral,* or *male ("android")* obesity. Lower body obesity is also known as *peripheral, gluteal-femoral,* or *female ("gynoid")* obesity. Subjects with upper body obesity are often referred to as being shaped like an "apple," compared with lower body obesity, which is more "pear" shaped (Fig. 39.4). In general, men have more intra-abdominal fat and women more subcutaneous fat. As men age, the proportion of intra-abdominal fat to subcutaneous fat increases. After menopause, women tend to acquire more central fat distribution.

The obesity type is determined by dividing the waist by the hip circumference. A waist-to-hip ratio greater than 1.0 in men and 0.8 in women indicates upper body or central obesity. Central obesity can be further differentiated into intra-abdominal adipose tissue (visceral fat) and subcutaneous abdominal adipose tissue by the use of CT or MRI scans. Waist circumference, which is a measure of central fat distribution, measures both subcutaneous abdominal adipose tissue and intra-abdominal adipose tissue. One of the characteristics

FIGURE 39.4 • Distribution of adipose tissue in (**A**) upper body or central (visceral) obesity and (**B**) lower body or peripheral (subcutaneous) obesity. People with upper body obesity are often described as having an "apple-shaped" body and those with lower body obesity as having a "pear-shaped" body.

of visceral fat is the release of adipokines (such as TNF-α and adiponectin) and fatty acids directly to the liver before entering the systemic circulation, having a potentially greater impact on hepatic function (*i.e.,* the increased fatty acids are deposited in the liver, causing fatty liver, resulting in insulin resistance in the liver). Higher levels of these adipokines and circulating free fatty acids in obese people, particularly those with upper body obesity, are thought to be associated with many of the adverse effects of obesity.[49]

The presence of excess fat in the abdomen out of proportion to total body fat is an independent predictor of risk factors and mortality. Both BMI and waist circumference are positively correlated with total-body adipose tissue, but waist circumference is a better predictor of abdominal or visceral fat content than BMI.[50] A waist circumference greater than 102 cm in men and 88 cm in women is considered high risk for cardiovascular disorders for most Canadians but for some ethnicities (*i.e.,* Asians and south Americans) the cutoff numbers are 90 cm for men and 80 cm for women.[50] Weight loss causes a preferential loss of visceral fat (due to higher turnover of visceral fat cells than subcutaneous) and can result in improvements in metabolic and hormonal abnormalities. Although peripheral obesity is associated with varicose veins in the legs and mechanical problems, it is not as strongly associated with cardiometabolic risk. In terms of weight reduction, some studies have shown that persons with upper body obesity are easier to treat than those with lower body obesity. Other studies have shown no difference in terms of success with weight reduction programs between the two types of obesity.

Weight cycling (the losing and regaining of weight) has been found to have little or no effect on metabolic variables, central obesity, or cardiovascular risk factors or future amount of weight loss. More research is needed to determine its effect on dietary preference for fat, psychological adjustment, disordered eating, and mortality. It is postulated that it is the underlying obesity and not the weight fluctuation that affects life expectancy.[51]

Health Risks Associated With Obesity

The excess body fat associated with obesity often impairs health. It has been predicted that the health effects of obesity will result in a shorter life expectancy for today's youth.[52] Obese people have a 50% to 100% increased risk of premature death from all causes compared to people with a healthy weight.[53] Obesity affects nearly every body system[54] (Fig. 39.5). It is associated with an increased risk of cardiac disease, hypertension, hypertriglyceridemia, and decreased HDL cholesterol. Significant weight gain increases the risk of developing type 2 diabetes, obstructive sleep apnea, gastric reflux, urinary stress incontinence, and gallbladder disease. Limited mobility and increased joint disorders are functional results of increased weight on the body's skeletal system. In women, obesity can contribute to infertility, higher risk pregnancy, gestational diabetes, maternal hypertension and difficulty in labour and delivery. Infants who are born to obese mothers are more likely to be high birth weight, contributing to an increased rate of Caesarean section delivery. Several types of cancer are seen in higher frequency in people who are obese, including endometrial, colon, gallbladder, prostate, kidney and postmenopausal breast cancer. Obesity also causes non alcoholic steatohepatitis and fatty liver disease (see Chapter 38).[54] Because some drugs are lipophilic and exhibit increased distribution in fat tissue, the administration of these drugs, including some anesthetic agents, can be more dangerous in obese persons. If surgery is required, the obese person often heals more slowly than the nonobese person of the same age. Massive obesity, because of its close association with so many health problems, can be regarded as a disease in its own right.

FIGURE 39.5 • Complications of obesity. (From Rubin R., Strayer D. (Eds.). (2012). *Rubin's pathology: Clinicopathologic foundations of medicine* (p. 1085). Philadelphia, PA: Lippincott Williams & Wilkins.)

Labels in figure:
Cerebral atherosclerosis, stroke
Hypertension, left ventricular hypertrophy
Hypoventilation ("Pickwickian" syndrome)
Coronary artery artherosclerosis, myocardial infarction
Gallstones
Diabetes
Osteoarthritis
Hyperlipoproteinemia

In Canada and many other countries, there are many negative stereotypes associated with obesity.[55,56] People, especially women, are expected to be thin, and obesity may be seen as a sign of lack of self-control. Obesity may negatively affect employment and educational opportunities, as well as marital status. Obesity also may play a role in a person's treatment by health professionals. Although nurses, physicians, and other health professionals are aware of the low success rate and difficulty in treating weight problems, they still may place the blame on the obese patient.[55,57]

Prevention and Treatment of Obesity

Prevention

Obesity in epidemic proportions has led to much discussion on methods of prevention, yet few effective approaches have resulted. More research is now being focused on prevention efforts directed at children and adolescents. Most interventions involve modification of lifestyle behaviours to promote healthy food choices and more physical activity. Public debate is also focused on policy methods to regulate availability of less desirable food choices, such as high calorie snacks and sweetened drinks.

Major public education and policy efforts are being undertaken by federal agencies. The Pan-Canadian Healthy Living Strategy is a government endorsed conceptual framework that aspires to a future where the health of Canadians is improved and chronic disease reduced. The targets of this program, to be achieved by 2015, include increasing the proportion of Canadians making healthy food choices, participating in physical activity 30 minutes per day and achieving a BMI within the healthy range (18.5 to 24.9) by 20%.[58] Health Canada has developed *Canada's Food Guide* which translates dietary guidelines into demonstrable eating behaviours. In addition to the traditional print version, *Canada's Food Guide* is also accessible via an interactive websites and applications for electronics that enables individuals to create a personalized food guide and provides tips on maintaining healthy habits (*i.e.,* EATracter.ca).[18] Mass media strategies employed to combat obesity have included the nationwide *ParticipACTION* campaign[59] which brings together partners from the public, private and non-profit sectors to promote physical activity and fitness, and the *Half Your Plate* campaign[60] that aims to increase fruit and vegetable consumption. Ultimately, successful prevention measures will utilize not only governmental agency strategies and regulatory measures, but also private sector initiatives and communication as well.[45,53]

Treatment

The current Canadian recommendations stipulate that weight loss management is indicated in all individuals who have a BMI of 25 or higher or who have a waist circumference above the cutoff point.[61] Treatment should focus on individualized lifestyle modification through a combination of a reduced calorie diet, increased physical activity, and cognitive-behaviour therapy. These three modes of therapy form the basis of all weight management programs. Pharmacotherapy and surgery are available as an adjunct to lifestyle changes in individuals who meet specific criteria.

Before treatment begins, an assessment should be made of the degree of overweight and the overall risk status. This should include assessment of the following risk factors or complications (as well as many other important considerations): coronary heart disease and other atherosclerotic diseases, sleep apnea, gynecologic abnormalities, osteoarthritis, gallstones, stress incontinence, cigarette smoking, depression, eating and/or mood disorders, hypertension, high LDL cholesterol levels, reduced HDL cholesterol levels, high triglyceride levels, prediabetes or type 2 diabetes, family history of premature coronary heart disease, and physical inactivity.[61]

It also is advisable to determine the person's barriers and readiness to lose weight.[61] Several factors can be evaluated to make this assessment. These include reasons and motivations for weight loss, previous history of weight loss attempts, social support, attitude toward physical activity, ability to participate in physical activity, time available for attempting intervention and, understanding the causes of the obesity and its contribution to disease. These help identify the person's emotional, psychological, physical, and social barriers for making changes.

Dietary Therapy. The two major components of all diet therapy are caloric restriction and diet composition. While diet modification and caloric restriction are important components of weight loss therapy, no one method has been shown to be most effective. Therefore, dietary therapy should be individually prescribed based on the person's overweight status and risk profile. The diet should be a personalized plan with realistic goals.

Caloric restriction may vary from low calorie diets to very low calorie diets. Low calorie diets typically restrict caloric intake to 1,200 kcal/day. This results in a variable reduction, depending on the initial dietary intake of the individual. Very low calorie diets restrict calories to approximately 450 kcal/day, primarily made up of protein. This diet has higher risks, including abnormal heart rhythms, and cholelithiasis, and anyone on this diet should be under direct supervision of a medical professional.

A more conservative dietary approach is to reduce the current dietary intake by 500 to 1,000 kcal/day. Total caloric intake should be distributed in four or five meals or snacks throughout the day. Portion control is an effective technique to help achieve calorie reduction. Many overweight people have not practiced or monitored portion size. One strategy is to keep daily diet logs of all food ingested to facilitate awareness of both content and frequency. Meal replacements, such as protein shakes with vitamins and minerals, may also be used as a substitute for solid food meals.

After caloric restriction is determined diet composition should be addressed. There are many methods of altering dietary content, including low fat diets, and low carbohydrate/high protein diets. Low fat diets strive to limit daily calories from fat to 10% to 15% of total calorie intake. This level may be difficult to achieve, and often is less palatable. Low carbohydrate/high

protein diets became popular in the 1960s and 1970s. Although effective for weight loss, especially in the initial stages, they can contribute to health risks. Higher protein diets can increase the risk of kidney stones, and the decrease in fibre can also increase risks of cancer and raise cholesterol levels.

Physical Activity. There is convincing evidence that increased physical activity decreases the risk of overweight and obesity. In addition, it reduces cardiovascular and diabetes risk beyond that achieved by weight loss alone. Physical activity is an important part of weight loss therapy and helps with maintaining weight loss. In addition, it may help reduce abdominal fat, increase cardiorespiratory fitness, and prevent the decrease in muscle mass that often occurs with weight loss. Exercise should be started slowly with the duration and intensity increased independently of each other. The goal should be 60 minutes or more of moderate to vigorous activity on most days of the week to maintain weight, and 60 to 90 minutes when trying to sustain weight loss.[18,58,59] The activity can be performed at one time or intermittently over the day.

Behaviour Therapy. Lifestyle modification is an essential factor in treating weight loss. Strategies include helping participants learn to self-monitor eating habits, including where and when they eat, and identifying situations that trigger eating behaviour. Techniques for changing behaviour include stress management, stimulus control, problem solving, contingency management, cognitive restructuring, social support, and relapse prevention.[62] Another important aspect to behaviour modification is helping the person to set realistic weight loss goals.[62] Weight loss from diet therapy, exercise, and behavioural therapy typically is 10% below the initial baseline.[63] In many cases, this level can lessen health risks, but often falls short of individual expectations.

Pharmacotherapy. Pharmacotherapy can be used as an adjunct to the aforementioned regimen in some patients with a BMI of 30 or more with no other risk factors or diseases, and for patients with a BMI of 27 or more with concomitant risk factors or diseases.[61] Risk factors and diseases defined as warranting pharmacotherapy are coronary heart disease, type 2 diabetes, metabolic syndrome, gynecologic abnormalities, osteoarthritis, gallbladder disease, stress incontinence, and sleep apnea.[61]

In Canada, there are now two prescription drugs that have been approved and are available for long-term weight loss therapy. Orlistat (Xenical) is an oral lipase inhibitor that works by decrease fat absorption in the intestine by approximately 30%.[61] The newest addition is the subcutaneous injection glucagon-like peptide-1 (GLP-1) receptor antagonist called liraglutide (Saxenda). While this same drug is used at lower doses (i.e., Victoza) for diabetes management it has recently been introduced as an adjunct for weight loss. Other agents such as: sibutramine (Meridia) was withdrawn in Canada in 2010 due to health concerns; rimonabant, a cannabinoid type 1 receptor antagonist is used in Europe but has not been approved for use in Canada or the United States; and historically any drugs containing Fen-phen were removed from the market again due to health concerns. A growing area of research and drug utilization includes non-Health Canada approved usage of medications approved for other indications. Examples include antidepressants such as bupropion and fluoxetine, antiepileptic drugs such as topiramate, antidiabetic medications such as metformin, pramlintide, and exenatide. With all such applications, use should be carefully monitored for any untoward side effects, as well as for desired weight loss effects.

Weight Loss (Bariatric) Surgery. In selected patients with acceptable operative risk factors, surgical therapy is currently the most effective treatment of severe obesity with respect to degree and duration of weight reduction achieved.[64] Bariatric surgery, although invasive, does afford significant weight loss, long-term weight loss maintenance, improved quality of life, decreased incidence of associated diseases, and decreased all-cause mortality (including mortality due to cardiovascular disease and cancer). This option is usually limited to persons with a BMI greater than 40; those with a BMI greater than 35 who have comorbid conditions and in whom efforts at medical therapy have failed; and those who have complications of extreme obesity. This weight loss surgery provides medically significant weight loss sustained for 5 years in most people.[61]

There are three types of weight loss surgery: (1) restrictive procedures, which reduce the amount of food that can be taken in (*e.g.*, adjustable gastric band, sleeve gastrectomy), (2) malabsorptive procedures, which bypass sections of the intestine and result in less nutrients being absorbed (*e.g.*, biliopancreatic diversion with duodenal switch), and (3) combined restrictive and malabsorptive procedures (*e.g.*, Roux-en-Y gastric bypass). Each surgery has specific risks and potential complications and requires lifelong nutritional monitoring after surgery. The key to long-term success and maintenance of weight loss after these surgical procedures is participation in a program that provides guidance in nutrition, physical activity, behavioural therapy and social support.

Childhood Obesity

The global prevalence of childhood obesity is rising dramatically over the past three decades with substantially greater increases observed in economically developed regions.[65,66] In 2014, the Canadian adapted World Health Organization (WHO) BMI-for-age growth charts for boys and girls aged 2 to 19 years was released.[67] Other growth charts that are used less frequently in Canada are the U.S. Canter for Disease Control (CDC) charts. Subsequently, the definition for obesity in Canadian children (ages 5 to 19) using the WHO charts is defined as a BMI at or above the sex- and age-specific 97th percentile, whereas a BMI between the 85th and 97th percentiles is defined as being overweight.[67] In North America, childhood obesity has become rampant. Findings from the Canadian Health Measures Survey (CHMS) indicated obesity has increased 2.5 times in the last decades (Fig. 39.6).[38] Childhood obesity prevalence data surveys were further stratified

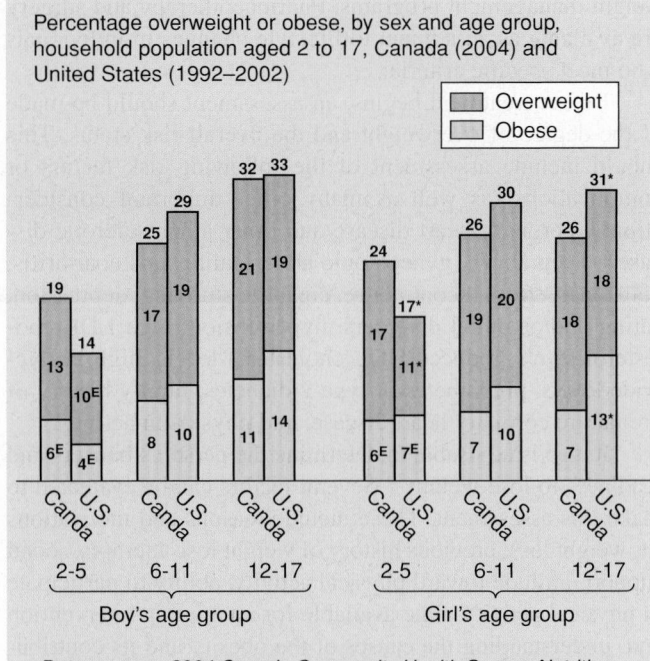

Data sources: 2004 Canada Community Health Survey: Nutrition; 1992-2002. National Health and Nutrition Examination Survey
Note: Because of rounding, detail may not add to totals.
E Coefficient of variation 16.6% to 33.3% (interpret with caution)
*Significantly different from estimate for Canada (p < 0.05)

FIGURE 39.6 • Percentage of overweight or obese children and youth by sex and age groups, comparing Canada (2004) and the United States (1999–2002). (From Minister of Industry. (2012). *Health fact sheet: Body mass index of Canadian children and youth, 2009 to 2011.* Statistics Canada, Catalogue No. 82-625-X.)

by ethnicity and in Canada, the prevalence of obesity amongst young individuals of Aboriginal origin is much greater than the national average.[38] In the United States, obesity prevalence amongst young black, Hispanic, and Mexican Americans was significantly greater than among their Caucasian counterparts.

The major concern of childhood obesity is that obese children will grow up to become obese adults. Pediatricians are now beginning to see hypertension, dyslipidemia, type 2 diabetes, orthopedic complications and psychosocial stigma in obese children and adolescents.[66] In Canada, a study found that 95% of children newly diagnosed with type 2 diabetes were obese.[68] In addition, there is a growing concern that childhood and adolescent obesity may be associated with negative psychosocial consequences, such as low self-esteem and discrimination by adults and peers.[38]

Childhood obesity is determined by a combination of hereditary and environmental factors. It is associated with obese parents, gestational diabetes and excessive weight gain during pregnancy, formula feeding, parenting style, parental eating, energy-dense food choices, erratic eating patterns, ethnicity, and sedentary lifestyle.[38,66] Children with overweight parents are at highest risk. One of the factors leading to childhood obesity is the increase in inactivity, including increased time indoors engaging in sedentary activities such as television viewing and computer usage. Television viewing is associated with consumption of calorie-dense snacks and decreased indoor activity. Studies have shown preschool children watching more than two hours per days of screens (TV or video games) were 34% more likely to be overweight or at risk for becoming overweight compared to children who watch less than two hours per day.[69] Obese children also may have a deficit in recognizing hunger sensations, stemming perhaps from parents who use food as gratification. Increasing perceptions that neighbourhoods are unsafe has resulted in less time spent outside playing and walking. Fast food, increased portion sizes, increased energy density, sugar-sweetened soft drinks, and foods with a high glycemic index are all likely contributing to the increased weights in children and adolescents.

Assessment

Because of the enormity of the problem of overweight and obesity in children, Obesity Canada (a not-for-profit organisation) convened a panel of experts to establish Canadian recommendations for the management of both adult and pediatric obesity.[61] The Canadian guidelines recommend measuring BMI in all children and adolescents aged 2 years and older.[61]

Assessment of the dietary habits of the overweight or obese child is an important component of the overall health assessment. This assessment should include self-efficacy and readiness to change; frequency of eating at restaurants or fast food outlets; frequency of consumption of sweetened beverages, 100% fruit juice, and foods high in energy density; examination of portion sizes in relation to appropriateness for age; frequency and quality of breakfast and snacks; and frequency of vegetable and fruit consumption. Time spent engaging in physical and sedentary activities should also be assessed.

Prevention and Treatment

Because adolescent obesity is predictive of adult obesity, treatment of childhood obesity is desirable.[66-69] The goals of therapy in uncomplicated obesity are directed toward healthy eating and activity behaviours, with the focus on sustainable lifestyle changes rather than weight or food restrictions Families should be taught awareness of current eating habits, activity, and parenting behaviour and how to modify them. For children with complications secondary to the obesity, the goal should be normalization of weight and treatment of the complications. The weight loss interventions should include all family members and caregivers; begin early at a point when the family is ready for change; assist the family to learn to monitor eating and activity patterns and make small and acceptable changes in these patterns; and be designed to encourage and emphasize, not criticize. They should include information about the medical complications of obesity and be directed at permanent changes, not short-term diets or exercise programs aimed at rapid weight loss.

It is recommended that health care providers counsel parents and caregivers of children with a BMI between the 5th and 84th percentiles to limit sugar-sweetened beverages and encourage the recommended amount of vegetables and fruits, limit screen time to no more than 2 hours daily, remove television and computer screens from the child's sleeping area, have the child eat breakfast daily, limit portion size and eating out, especially at fast food restaurants, and encourage family meals where parents and children eat together.[38,61] Primary and secondary schools (grades 1 through 12) are pivotal in the promotion of active living and schools have been encouraged to increase daily physical activity and opportunities for recreation.[61]

Education regarding the prevention of childhood obesity can begin in the prenatal stage. The Canadian obesity guidelines encourage discussions regarding the prevention of childhood obesity with pregnant women. In addition, it is recommended that infants be breast-fed exclusively to 6 months of age and that discussion should ensue with the family encouraging limited intake of energy-dense snacks and foods that are high in fat and sugar.[61]

The first treatment options for overweight or obese children include dietary counselling (with the goal of reducing energy intake) and promotion of regular physical activity. An optimal diet plan to achieve a healthy body weight should be developed by a qualified health practitioner (preferably a Registered Dietitian).[61] Dietary goals should focus on well-balanced, healthy meals with a healthy approach to eating. Specific strategies can include reduction of specific high-calorie foods or an appropriate balance of foods that are low, medium, and high calorie. Commercial diets should be used with caution. Pharmacologic therapy (*i.e.,* orlistat) may be considered in adolescents to aid in weight reduction and/or maintenance when added to a regimen of lifestyle intervention.[66] Due to lack of evidence, pharmacologic therapy is not recommended in prepubertal children. Bariatric surgery in adolescents should be limited to exceptional cases and only be carried out by experienced health care teams.[61]

IN SUMMARY

Obesity is defined as excess body fat accumulation with multiple organ-specific pathologic consequences. Genetic, socioeconomic, cultural, and environmental factors, psychological influences, and activity levels have been implicated as causative factors in the development of obesity. The health risks associated with obesity affect almost every body system. There are two types of obesity—upper body and lower body obesity. Upper body obesity is associated with a higher incidence of complications. The treatment of obesity focuses on nutritionally adequate weight loss diets, behaviour modification, exercise, social support, and, in situations of marked obesity, pharmacotherapy and surgical methods.

Obesity is the most prevalent nutritional disorder affecting the Canadian pediatric populations. Factors that predispose to childhood obesity include erratic eating patterns, calorie-dense food choices, and lack of exercise and sedentary lifestyle. The major concern of childhood obesity is that obese children will grow up to become obese adults. Pediatricians are now beginning to see hypertension, dyslipidemia, type 2 diabetes, orthopedic complications, and psychosocial stigma in obese children and adolescents. Because of the scope of the problem, it is recommended that the weight status of all children be evaluated yearly and that measures to prevent and treat obesity be included in the health care plan for all children.

UNDERNUTRITION AND EATING DISORDERS

After completing this section of the chapter, you should be able to meet the following objectives:

- List the major causes of malnutrition and starvation.
- State the difference between protein-calorie starvation (*i.e.,* marasmus) and protein malnutrition (*i.e.,* kwashiorkor).
- Explain the effect of malnutrition on muscle mass, respiratory function, acid–base balance, wound healing, immune function, bone mineralization, the menstrual cycle, and testicular function.
- State the causes of malnutrition in severely ill or traumatized patients.
- Compare the eating disorders of anorexia and bulimia nervosa and the complications associated with each.

Undernutrition continues to be a major health problem throughout the world. In 2011–2013, 12% of the global population (842 million individuals) was unable to meet their daily energy needs. The majority of the undernourished individuals in the world can be found in Sub-Saharan Africa (25%), Eastern Asia (22%), Caribbean (19%), and Southern Asia (17%).[70] Even in developed nations, malnutrition remains a problem. It is unknown how many Canadian children consume diets that are below the recommended allowances.

Malnutrition and Starvation

Malnutrition and starvation are conditions in which a person does not receive or is unable to use an adequate amount of nutrients for body function. A diet should provide adequate energy in the form of carbohydrates, fats, and proteins; essential amino acids and fatty acids for use as building blocks for synthesis of structural and functional proteins and lipids; and vitamins and minerals, needed to function as coenzymes or hormones in vital metabolic processes, or, as in the case of calcium and phosphate, as important structural components of bone.

Among the many causes of malnutrition are poverty, lack of knowledge, acute and chronic illness, and self-imposed dietary restriction. Homeless persons, older adults, and children of lower socioeconomic status often demonstrate the effects of protein and energy malnutrition, as well as vitamin

and mineral deficiencies. Even the affluent may fail to recognize that infants, adolescents, and pregnant women have increased nutritional needs. Some types of malnutrition are caused by acute and chronic illnesses, such as occurs in persons with Crohn disease who experience impaired nutrient absorption. Anorexia nervosa and less overt eating disorders affect a large population of persons who are concerned about body image or athletic performance.

Protein–Energy Malnutrition

Protein and energy (calorie) malnutrition represents a depletion of the body's lean tissues caused by starvation or a combination of starvation and catabolic stress. The lean tissues are the fat-free, metabolically active tissues of the body, namely, skeletal muscle, viscera, and cells of the blood and immune system. Because lean tissues are the largest body compartment, their rate of loss is the main determinant of total body weight in most cases of protein–energy malnutrition.

Much of the literature on malnutrition and starvation has dealt with infants and children in underdeveloped countries in which food deprivation results in an inadequate intake of protein and calories to meet the body's energy needs. Protein–energy malnutrition in this population commonly is divided into two distinct conditions: marasmus (protein and calorie deficiency) and kwashiorkor (protein deficiency). The pathologic changes for both types of malnutrition include humoral and cellular immunodeficiencies resulting from protein deficiency and lack of immune mediators. There is impaired synthesis of pigments of the hair and skin (*e.g.,* hair colour may change and the skin may become hyperpigmented) because of a lack of substrate (tyrosine) and coenzymes.

There are two functional compartments involved in the distribution of proteins within the body: the somatic compartment, represented by the skeletal muscles, and the visceral compartment, represented by protein stores in body organs, principally the liver.[71] These two compartments are regulated differently, with the somatic compartment being affected more severely in marasmus and the visceral compartment more severely in kwashiorkor.

Marasmus represents a progressive loss of muscle mass and fat stores due to inadequate food intake that is equally deficient in calories and protein.[71,72] It results in a reduction in body weight adjusted for age and size. The child with marasmus has a wasted appearance, with loss of muscle mass, stunted growth, and loss of subcutaneous fat; a protuberant abdomen (from muscular hypotonia); wrinkled skin; sparse, dry, and dull hair; and depressed heart rate, blood pressure, and body temperature. Diarrhea is common. Because immune function is impaired, concurrent infections occur and place additional stress on an already weakened body. An important characteristic of marasmus is growth failure; if sufficient food is not provided, these children will not reach their full potential stature.[72]

Kwashiorkor results from a deficiency in protein in diets relatively high in carbohydrates.[71,72] The term *kwashiorkor* comes from an African word meaning "the disease suffered by the displaced child," because the condition develops soon after a child is displaced from the breast after the arrival of a new infant and placed on a starchy gruel feeding. Kwashiorkor is a more severe form of malnutrition than marasmus. Unlike marasmus, severe protein deficiency is associated with extensive loss of the visceral protein compartment with a resultant hypoalbuminemia that gives rise to generalized or dependent edema. The child with kwashiorkor usually presents with edema, desquamating skin, discoloured hair, anorexia, and extreme apathy (Fig. 39.7). There are "flaky paint" lesions of the skin on the face, extremities, and perineum and the hair becomes a sandy or reddish colour, with linear depigmentation (flag sign).[72] There is generalized growth failure and muscle wasting as in marasmus, but subcutaneous fat is normal because calorie intake is adequate. Other manifestations include skin lesions, hepatomegaly and distended abdomen, cold extremities, and decreased cardiac output and tachycardia.

Marasmus–kwashiorkor is an advanced protein–energy deficit coupled with increased protein requirement or loss. This results in a rapid decrease in anthropometric measurements with obvious edema and wasting and loss of organ mass. One essential aspect of severe protein–energy malnutrition is fatty degeneration of organs such as the heart and liver. This degeneration causes subclinical and overt cardiac dysfunction, especially when malnutrition is accompanied by edema. A second injurious aspect is the loss of subcutaneous fat, which markedly reduces the body's capacity for temperature regulation and water storage. As a consequence, malnourished children become dehydrated and hypothermic more quickly and more severely than normally nourished children.[73] Most children with severe protein–energy malnutrition have asymptomatic infections because their immune systems fail to respond appropriately. A child's immune system is so depressed that he or she is unable to produce the fever that is typical of an acute infection.[73]

Malnutrition in Trauma and Illness

In industrialized societies, protein–energy malnutrition most often occurs secondary to trauma or illness. Kwashiorkor-like secondary protein–energy malnutrition occurs most commonly in association with hypermetabolic acute illnesses, such as trauma, burns, and sepsis.[74] Marasmus-like secondary protein–energy malnutrition typically results from chronic illnesses such as chronic obstructive pulmonary disease, congestive heart failure, cancer, and HIV infection.[74] Approximately half of all persons with cancer experience tissue wasting, in which the tumour induces metabolic changes leading to a loss of adipose tissue and muscle mass.[75]

In healthy adults, body protein homeostasis is maintained by a cycle in which the net loss of protein in the postabsorptive state is matched by a net postprandial gain of protein. In persons with severe injury or illness, net protein breakdown is accelerated and protein rebuilding disrupted. Protein mass is lost from the liver, gastrointestinal tract, kidneys, and heart. As protein is lost from the liver, hepatic synthesis of serum proteins decreases and decreased levels of serum proteins are observed. There is an increased risk of infection due to a decrease in immune cell production and multiple immunologic malfunctions. In addition, wound healing is compromised. The gastrointestinal tract undergoes mucosal atrophy with loss of villi in the small intestine, resulting in malabsorption. The loss of protein from cardiac muscle leads to a decrease in myocardial contractility and cardiac output. The intercostals muscles become weakened when muscle proteins are used as a fuel source, and respiratory function becomes compromised. A reduction in respiratory function has many implications, especially for persons with burns, trauma, infection, or chronic respiratory disease, and for persons who are being mechanically ventilated because of respiratory failure.

In hospitalized patients, malnutrition increases morbidity and mortality rates, incidence of complications, and length of stay. Malnutrition may present at the time of admission or develop during hospitalization. The hospitalized patient often finds eating a healthful diet difficult and commonly has restrictions on food and water intake in preparation for tests and surgery. Pain, medications, special diets, and stress can decrease appetite. Even when the patient is well enough to

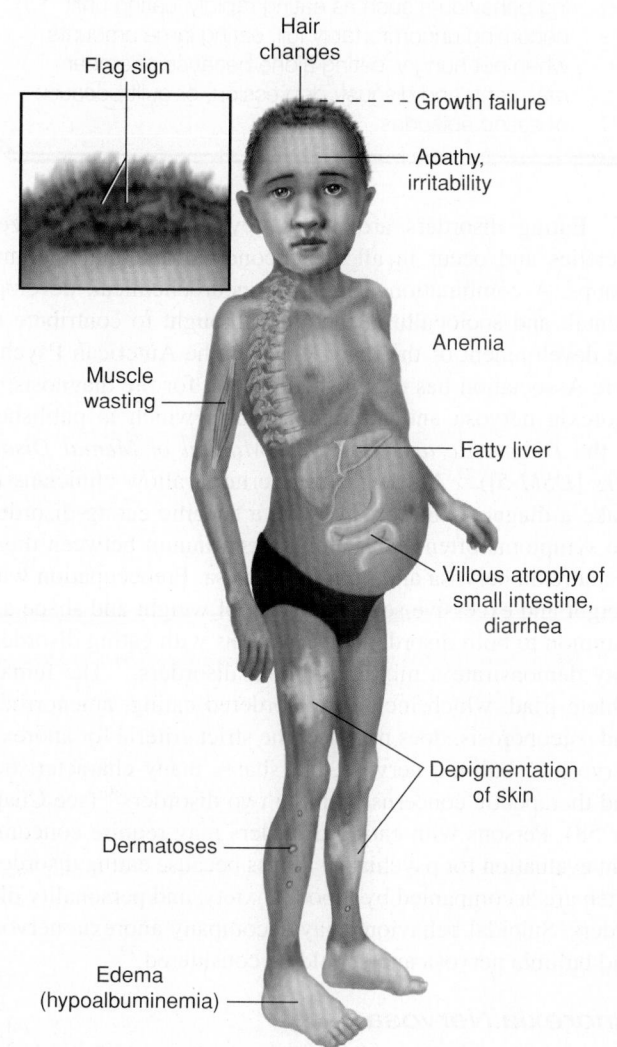

FIGURE 39.7 • Clinical manifestations of kwashiorkor.

eat, being alone in a room where unpleasant treatments may be given is not conducive to eating. Although hospitalized patients may appear to need fewer calories because they are on bed rest, their actual need for caloric intake may be higher because of other energy expenditures. For example, more calories are expended during fever, when the metabolic rate is increased. There also may be an increased need for protein to support tissue repair after trauma or surgery.

Diagnosis and Treatment

No single diagnostic measure is sufficiently accurate to serve as a reliable test for malnutrition. Techniques of nutritional assessment, as previously discussed include completion of medical and dietary intake, physical examination, anthropometric measurements, and laboratory tests.[76] Evaluation of weight is particularly important. Body weight can be assessed in relation to height using the BMI. Evaluation of body composition can be performed by visual assessment or using anthropometric measurements such as skinfold thickness. Serum albumin and prealbumin can be useful in the diagnosis of protein-calorie malnutrition. Albumin, which has historically been used as a determinant of nutrition status, has a relatively large body pool and a half-life of 20 days and is less sensitive to changes in nutrition than prealbumin, which has a shorter half-life and a relatively small body pool.[74]

The treatment of severe protein–energy malnutrition involves the use of measures to correct fluid and electrolyte abnormalities and replenish proteins, calories, and micronutrients.[76] Treatment is started with modest quantities of proteins and calories based on the person's actual weight. Concurrent administration of vitamins and minerals is required and can be given orally, enterally, or parenterally. The treatment should be undertaken slowly to avoid complications. The administration of water and sodium with carbohydrates can overload a heart that has been weakened by malnutrition and result in heart failure and severe electrolyte imbalances (i.e., the refeeding syndrome). Enteral feedings can result in malabsorptive symptoms due to abnormalities in the gastrointestinal tract. Refeeding edema is benign dependent edema that results from renal sodium reabsorption and poor skin and blood vessel integrity. It is treated by elevation of the dependent area and modest sodium restrictions. Diuretics are ineffective and may aggravate electrolyte deficiencies.

Eating Disorders

Eating disorders, which include anorexia nervosa, bulimia nervosa, and binge-eating disorder, incorporate serious disturbances in eating, such as restriction of intake and binging, with an excessive concern over body shape or body weight.[77] Eating disorders manifest in both men and women, typically begin in adolescence or young adulthood and can affect women 10 times more than men. While Canadian prevalence is unclear, the prevalence of anorexia nervosa is estimated to be between 0.3% to 1.0% and potentially three times that for bulimia nervosa.[78]

EATING DISORDERS

- Eating disorders are serious disturbances in eating, such as willful restriction of intake and binge eating, as well as excessive concern over body weight and shape.
- Anorexia nervosa is characterized by a refusal to maintain a minimally normal body weight (e.g., at least 85% of minimal expected weight); an excessive concern over gaining weight and how the body is perceived in terms of size and shape; and amenorrhea (in girls and women after menarche).
- Bulimia nervosa is characterized by recurrent binge eating; inappropriate compensatory behaviours such as self-induced vomiting, fasting, or excessive exercise that follow the binge-eating episode; and extreme concern over body shape and weight.
- Binge eating consists of consuming unusually large quantities of food during a discrete period (e.g., within any 2-hour period) along with lack of control over the binge-eating episode.
- Binge-eating disorders are characterized by eating behaviours such as eating rapidly, eating until becoming uncomfortably full, eating large amounts when not hungry, eating alone because of embarrassment, and disgust, depression, or guilt because of eating episodes.

Eating disorders are more prevalent in industrialized societies and occur in all socioeconomic and major ethnic groups. A combination of genetic, neurochemical, developmental, and sociocultural factors is thought to contribute to the development of the disorders.[78,79] The American Psychiatric Association has established criteria for the diagnosis of anorexia nervosa and bulimia nervosa, which is published in the *Diagnostic and Statistical Manual of Mental Disorders* [*DSM-5*].[77] Although these criteria allow clinicians to make a diagnosis in persons with a specific eating disorder, the symptoms often occur along a continuum between those of anorexia nervosa and bulimia nervosa. Preoccupation with weight and excessive self-evaluation of weight and shape are common to both disorders, and persons with eating disorders may demonstrate a mixture of both disorders.[77] The female athlete triad, which includes disordered eating, amenorrhea, and osteoporosis, does not meet the strict criteria for anorexia nervosa or bulimia nervosa, but shares many characteristics and therapeutic concerns with the two disorders[80] (see Chapter 58). Persons with eating disorders may require concomitant evaluation for psychiatric illness because eating disorders often are accompanied by mood, anxiety, and personality disorders. Suicidal behaviour may accompany anorexia nervosa and bulimia nervosa and should be considered.[77]

Anorexia Nervosa

Anorexia nervosa is an eating disorder that usually begins in adolescence and is characterized by determined dieting, often accompanied by compulsive exercise and, in a subgroup of persons, purging behaviour with or without binge eating, resulting in sustained low weight.[77] Other features include a disturbed body image, a pervasive fear of becoming obese, and obsessions with severely restricted caloric intake and/or excessive physical exercise. Anorexia nervosa is more prevalent among young women than men. The lifetime risk for the full disorder among women is estimated to be 0.3% to 1% (with a greater frequency of subclinical anorexia nervosa); the risk among men is about one tenth of the rate for women.[78]

The causes of anorexia nervosa appear to be multifactorial, with determinants that include genetic influence, personality traits of perfectionism and compulsiveness, anxiety disorders, family history of depression and obesity, and peer, familial, and cultural pressures with respect to appearance.[81] The *DSM-5* diagnostic criteria for anorexia nervosa are (1) restriction of energy intake relative to requirements, leading to a significantly low body weight in the context of age, sex, developmental trajectory and physical health; (2) an intense fear of gaining weight or becoming fat; and (3) a disturbance in the way one's body size, weight, or shape is perceived.[77] Other psychiatric disorders often coexist with anorexia nervosa, including major depression or dysthymia, and obsessive-compulsive disorder (see Chapter 53). Alcohol and substance abuse may also be present, more often among those with binging-purging type of anorexia nervosa.[77]

Many organ systems are affected by the malnutrition that accompanies anorexia nervosa. The severity of the abnormalities tends to be related to the degree of malnutrition and is reversed by reestablishing eating and nutritional intake. The most frequent complication of anorexia is amenorrhea and loss of secondary sex characteristics associated with decreased levels of estrogen, which can eventually lead to osteoporosis. Bone loss can occur and symptomatic compression fractures and kyphosis have been reported. Constipation, cold intolerance and failure to shiver in cold, bradycardia, hypotension, decreased heart size, electrocardiographic changes, blood and electrolyte abnormalities, and increased growth of lanugo (*i.e.,* fine hair) are common. Abnormalities in cognitive function may also occur. The brain loses both white and grey matter during severe weight loss; weight restoration results in return of white matter, but some loss of grey matter persists.[81] As anorexia is a form of starvation it can lead to death if left untreated and the risk appears to increase as weight drops to less than 35% to 40% of ideal weight. It is believed that these deaths are caused by myocardial degeneration and heart failure rather than arrhythmias.

The most exasperating aspect of the treatment of anorexia nervosa is the inability of the person with anorexia to recognize that there is a problem. However, persons with the disorder are usually willing to talk about their preoccupation with weight loss, food refusal and rituals about food, and excessive exercise routines; purging and laxative use; and withdrawal from activities and relationships. A multidisciplinary approach appears to be the most effective method of treating persons with the disorder.[82] The goals of treatment are eating and weight gain, resolution of issues with the family, healing of pain from the past, and efforts to work on psychological, relationship, and emotional issues. Specialized eating disorder treatment programs may include in patient hospitalization, partial hospitalization, or intensive outpatient specialty eating disorder programs, depending on the level of weight loss, medical complications and availability of family support.

However, adults whose weight loss is more than 25% below the expected weight (or with less weight loss if there are coexisting medical or psychiatric conditions, or both), and children or adolescents who are losing weight rapidly, generally require hospitalization to facilitate adequate food intake and limit physical activity.[81]

Bulimia Nervosa

Bulimia nervosa is defined by recurrent binge eating with activities such as vomiting, fasting, excessive exercise, and use of diuretics, laxatives, or enemas to compensate for that behaviour. Binge eating is characterized by the consumption of an unusually large quantity of food during a discrete time (*i.e.,* within a 2-hour period) along with lack of control over the binge-eating episode. Bulimia nervosa usually begins during adolescence, with a peak period of onset around older adolescence and young adulthood. The lifetime prevalence is 3%, and the ratio of women to men is approximately 10:1.[77]

The *DSM-5* criteria for bulimia nervosa are (1) recurrent binge eating, characterized by eating a large amount of food than what most individuals would eat in a discrete period of time and a lack of control during the episode; (2) recurrent inappropriate compensatory behaviours such as self-induced vomiting, abuse of laxatives or diuretics, fasting, or excessive exercise; (3) this binge eating occurs on average at least once per week for three months; (4) self-evaluation that is unduly influenced by body shape and weight; and (5) a determination that the eating disorder does not occur exclusively during episodes of anorexia nervosa.[77] The disorder may be associated with other psychiatric disorders such as anxiety disorder or depression. There is also an association with substance abuse and risky and self-destructive behaviours.[77]

The complications of bulimia nervosa include those resulting from overeating, self-induced vomiting, and cathartic and diuretic abuse.[83] Among the complications of self-induced vomiting are dental disorders, parotitis, and fluid and electrolyte disorders. Dental abnormalities, such as sensitive teeth, increased dental caries, and periodontal disease, occur with frequent vomiting because the high acid content of the vomitus causes tooth enamel to dissolve. Esophagitis, dysphagia, and esophageal strictures are common. With frequent vomiting, there often is reflux of gastric contents into the lower esophagus because of relaxation of the lower esophageal sphincter. Vomiting may lead to aspiration pneumonia, especially in intoxicated or debilitated persons. Potassium, chloride, and hydrogen are lost in the vomitus, and frequent vomiting predisposes to metabolic acidosis with hypokalemia (see Chapter 32). An unexplained physical response to vomiting is the development of benign, painless parotid gland enlargement.

The weights of persons with bulimia nervosa may fluctuate, although not always to the dangerously low levels seen in anorexia nervosa. Their thoughts and feelings range from fear of not being able to stop eating to a concern about gaining too much weight. They may also experience feelings of sadness, anger, guilt, shame, and low self-esteem.

Treatment strategies include psychological and pharmacologic treatments. Cognitive behavioural therapy is the psychosocial therapy predominantly used.[82] This therapy is designed to help the individual become aware of other ways to cope with the feelings that precipitate the desire to purge and to try to correct maladaptive beliefs regarding their self-image. Unlike persons with anorexia nervosa, persons with bulimia nervosa or binge eating are upset by the behaviours practiced and the thoughts and feelings experienced, and they are more willing to accept help. Antidepressants such as serotonin reuptake inhibitors have been found to be useful in treating bulimia and binge-eating disorders and one, fluoxetine, has been clinically indicated for treatment.[82]

Binge-Eating Disorder

Binge-eating disorder (BED) is now recognized as a discrete disorder in the *DSM-5*. It is characterized by: (1) recurrent episodes of binge eating, characterized by eating a large amount of food than what most individuals would eat in a discrete period of time, and a lack of control during the episode; (2) the binge-eating episodes are associated with at least three (or more) of the following: eating rapidly, eating until becoming uncomfortably full, eating large amounts when not hungry, eating alone because of embarrassment, and/or disgust, depression or guilt because of eating episodes; (3) marked distress regarding binge eating; (4) the binge eating occurs at least once a week for 3 months; and (5) the binge eating does not occur exclusively during the course of bulimia nervosa or anorexia nervosa. The great majority of persons with binge-eating disorder are overweight and, in turn, obese persons have a higher prevalence of binge-eating disorder than the nonobese population.[77]

The primary goal of therapy for binge-eating disorder is to establish a regular, healthful eating pattern. Persons with binge-eating disorders who have been successfully treated for their eating disorder have reported that making meal plans, eating a balanced diet at three regular meals a day, avoiding high-sugar foods and other binge foods, recording food intake and binge-eating episodes, exercising regularly, finding alternative activities, and avoiding alcohol and drugs are helpful in maintaining their more healthful eating behaviours after treatment.

IN SUMMARY

Undernutrition can range from a selective deficiency of a single nutrient to starvation, in which there is deprivation of all nutrients. Malnutrition and starvation are among the most widespread causes of morbidity and mortality in the world. Protein–energy malnutrition in this population commonly is divided into two distinct conditions: marasmus (protein and calorie deficiency) and kwashiorkor (protein deficiency). There are two functional compartments involved in the distribution of proteins within the body: the somatic compartment, represented by the skeletal muscles, and the visceral compartment, represented by protein stores in body organs, principally the liver. In marasmus, there is a greater loss of protein from the skeletal muscle compartment, and in kwashiorkor, a greater loss of visceral proteins, particularly those of the liver. Malnutrition is common during illness, recovery from trauma, and hospitalization. The effects of malnutrition and starvation on body function are widespread. They include loss of muscle mass, impaired wound healing, impaired immunologic function, decreased appetite, loss of calcium and phosphate from bone, anovulation and amenorrhea in women, and decreased testicular function in men.

Anorexia nervosa, bulimia nervosa, and binge eating are eating disorders that result in malnutrition. In anorexia nervosa, distorted attitudes about eating lead to determined dieting, significant and inappropriate weight loss, and malnutrition. Bulimia nervosa is characterized by secretive episodes or binges of eating large quantities of easily consumed, high-calorie foods, followed by compensatory behaviours such as fasting, self-induced vomiting, or abuse of laxatives or diuretics. Binge-eating disorder is characterized by characterized by secretive episodes or binges of eating large quantities of food that may be associated with physical discomfort and emotional distress. It is not associated with the inappropriate compensatory behaviours seen in bulimia nervosa.

REVIEW EXERCISES

1. A 25-year-old woman is 165 cm tall and weighs 136 kg. She works as a receptionist in an office, brings her lunch to work with her, spends her evenings watching television, and gets very little exercise. She reports that she has been fat ever since she was a little girl, has tried "every diet under the sun," and when she diets she loses some weight, but gains it all back again.
   A. *Calculate her BMI.*
   B. *How would you classify her obesity?*
   C. *What are her risk factors for obesity?*
   D. *What would be one of the first steps in helping her develop a plan to lose weight?*

2. A 16-year-old high school student is brought into the physician's office by her mother, who is worried because her daughter insists on dieting because she thinks she is too fat. The daughter is 170 cm tall and weighs 44 kg. Her history reveals that she is a straight-A student, plays in the orchestra, and is on the track team. Although she had been having regular menstrual periods, she has not had a period in 4 months. She is given a tentative diagnosis of anorexia nervosa.

A. What are the criteria for a diagnosis of anorexia nervosa?

B. What is the physiologic reason for her amenorrhea?

C. What are some of the physiologic manifestations associated with malnutrition and severe weight loss?

References

1. Hall J. E. (2011). *Textbook of medical physiology* (12th ed.). Philadelphia, PA: W. B. Saunders.

2. Harris J. A., Benedict F. G. (1919). *A biometric study of basal metabolism in man.* Publication No. 279. Washington, DC: Carnegie Institute.

3. Owen O. E., Kavle E., Owen R. S., et al. (1986). A reappraisal of caloric requirements in healthy women. *American Journal of Clinical Nutrition, 44*(1), 1–19.

4. Owen O. E., Holup J. L., D'Alessio D. A., et al. (1987). A reappraisal of caloric requirements in healthy men. *American Journal of Clinical Nutrition, 46*(6), 875–885.

5. Mifflin M. D., St Jeor S. T., Hill L. A., et al. (1990). A new predictive equation for resting energy expenditure in healthy individuals. *American Journal of Clinical Nutrition, 51*(2), 241–247.

6. Kross E. K., Sena M., Schmidt K., et al. (2012). A comparison of predictive equations of energy expenditure and measured energy expenditure in critically ill patients. *Journal of Critical Care, 27*(3), e5–e12.

7. Boullata J., Williams J., Cottrell F., et al. (2007). Accurate determination of energy needs in hospitalized patients. *Journal of the American Dietetic Association, 107*(3),393–401.

8. Levine J. A. (2004). Nonexercise activity thermogenesis (NEAT). *Nutritional Reviews, 62*(Suppl 2), S82–S97.

9. Alvarez-Castro P., Sangiao-Alvarellos S., Brandón-Sandá I., et al. (2011). Endocrine function in obesity. *Endocrinology Nutrition, 58*(8), 422–432.

10. Kershaw E. E., Flier J. S. (2004). Adipose tissue as an endocrine organ. *Journal of Clinical Endocrinology and Metabolism, 89*(6), 2548–2556.

11. Jéquier E. (2002). Leptin signaling, adiposity, and energy balance. *Annals of the New York Academy of Sciences, 967*, 379–388.

12. Robertson S. A., Leinninger G. M., Myers M. G. (2008). Molecular and neural mediators of leptin action. *Physiology and Behavior, 94*(5), 637–642.

13. Sahu A. (2004). Leptin signaling in the hypothalamus: emphasis on energy homeostasis and leptin resistance. *Frontiers in Neuroendocrinology, 24*(4), 225–253.

14. Myers M. G., Cowley M. A., Munzberg H. (2008). Mechanisms of leptin action and leptin resistance. *Annual Review of Physiology, 70*, 537–556.

15. Food and Nutrition Board, Institute of Medicine of the National Academies. (2005). *Dietary reference intakes for energy, carbohydrate, fiber, fat, fatty acids, cholesterol, protein, and amino acids.* Washington, DC: The National Academies Press.

16. United States Department of Agriculture, Food and Nutrition Information Center. (2014). Interactive DRI for Health care professionals. Available online at: http://fnic.nal.usda.gov/interactiveDRI./ Accessed July 23, 2014.

17. Canadian Food Inspection Agency. (2014). *Nutrition labelling.* Available online at: http://www.inspection.gc.ca/food/labelling/food-labelling-for-industry/nutrition-labelling/eng/1386881685057/1386881685870. Accessed July 23, 2014.

18. Health Canada. (2011). *Eating well with Canada's food guide.* Available online at: http://www.hc-sc.gc.ca/fn-an/food-guide-aliment/index-eng.php. Accessed July 23, 2014.

19. Elango R., Humayun M. A., Ball R., et al. (2010). Evidence that protein requirements have been significantly underestimated. *Current Opinion in Clinical Nutrition and Metabolic Care, 13*(1), 52–57.

20. Bauer J., Biolo G., Cederholm T., et al. (2013). Evidence-based recommendations for optimal dietary protein intake in older people: A position paper from the PROT-AGE Study Group. *Journal of the American Medical Directors Association, 14*(8), 542–549.

21. Academy of Nutrition and Dietetics. (2014). Dietary fatty acids for healthy adults. *Journal of the Academy of Nutrition and Dietetics, 114*(1),136–153.

22. McDonald B. E. (2004). The Canadian experience: Why Canada decided against an upper limit for cholesterol. *Journal of the American College of Nutrition, 23*(Suppl 6), 616S–620S.

23. Suzuki K., Simpson K. A., Minnion J. S., et al. (2010). The role of gut hormones and the hypothalamus in appetite regulation. *Endocrine Journal, 57*(5), 359–372.

24. Choquet H., Meyre D. (2011). Genetics of obesity: What have we learned? *Current Genomics, 12*(3), 169–179.

25. Perry B., Wang Y. (2012). Appetite regulation and weight control: the role of gut hormones. *Nutrition and Diabetes, 2*(1), e26.

26. Jensen G. L., Hsiao P. Y., Wheeler D. (2012). Adult nutrition assessment tutorial. *Journal of Parenteral and Enteral Nutrition, 36*(3), 267–274.

27. Bingham S. A. (1991). Limitations of the various methods for collecting dietary intake data. *Annals of Nutrition & Metabolism, 35*(3), 117–127.

28. Jelliffe D. B. (1966). *The assessment of the nutritional status of the community.* WHO Monograph No. 53. Geneva: World Health Organization.

29. World Health Organization. (2000). *Obesity: Preventing and managing the global epidemic. Report of a WHO consultation on obesity.* Geneva: World Health Organization

30. Lobman T. G., Houtkooper L., Going S. B. (1997). Body fat measurement goes high-tech. Not all are created equal. *ACSM's Health & Fitness Journal 1*(1), 30–35.

31. Gibson R. S. (2005). *Principles of nutritionals assessment* (2nd ed.). Oxford: Oxford University Press.

32. Kyle U. G., Bosaeus I., De Lorenzo A. D., et al. (2004). Bioelectrical impedance analysis part I: Review of principles and methods. *Clinical Nutrition, 23*(5):1226–1243.

33. Duren D. L., Sherwood R. J., Czerwinski S. A., et al. (2008). Body composition methods: Comparisons and interpretation. *Journal of Diabetes Science and Technology, 2*(6), 1139–1146.

34. World Health Organization. (2014). *Obesity and overweight fact sheet no. 311.* Available online at: http://www.who.int/mediacentre/factsheets/fs311/en/index.html. Accessed on July 23, 2014.

35. Health Canada. (2003). *Canadian guidelines for body weight classification in adults.* Ottawa: Health Canada Publications.

36. Health Statistics Division. (2012). *Body composition of canadian adults, 2009 to 2011.* Available online at: http://www.statcan.gc.ca/pub/82-625-x/2012001/article/11708-eng.htm. Accessed July 23, 2014.

37. Katzmarzyk P. (2008). Obesity and physical activity among Aboriginal Canadians. *Obesity, 16*(1), 184–190.

38. Public Health Agency of Canada, Canadian Institute for Health Information. (2011). *Obesity in Canada.* Available online at: https://secure.cihi.ca/free_products/Obesity_in_canada_2011_en.pdf. Accessed July 23, 2014.

39. Tjepkema M. (2005). *Adult obesity in Canada: Measured height and weight.* Statistics Canada Catalogue no. 82–620-MWE2005001.

40. Statistics Canada. (2012). *Body mass index of Canadian children and youth, 2009 to 2011.* Available online at: http://www.statcan.gc.ca/pub/82-625-x/2012001/article/11712-eng.htm. Accessed July 23, 2014.

41. Nammi S., Koka S., Chinnala K. M., et al. (2004). Obesity: An overview on its current perspectives and treatment options. *Nutrition Journal, 3*, 3.

42. Rankinen T., Zuberi A., Chagnon Y. C., et al. (2006). The human obesity gene map: The 2005 update. *Obesity, 14*(4), 529–644.

43. Bray G. A. (2004). The epidemic of obesity and changes in food intake: The fluoride hypothesis. *Physiological Behavior, 82*(1), 115–121.

44. Temelkova-Kurktschiev T., Stefanov T. (2012). Lifestyle and genetics in obesity and type 2 diabetes. *Experimental and Clinical Endocrinology and Diabetes, 120*(1), 1–6.

45. Swinburn B. A., Sacks G., Hall K. D., et al. (2011). The global obesity pandemic: Shaped by global drivers and local environments. *Lancet, 378*(9793), 804–814.

46. Koch F. S., Sepa A., Ludvigsson J. (2008). Psychological stress and obesity. *Journal of Pediatrics, 153*(6), 839–844.

47. Talen M. R., Mann M. M. (2009). Obesity and mental health. *Primary Care, 36*(2), 287–305.

48. Calzada P., Anderson-Worts P. (2009). The obesity epidemic: are minority individuals equally affected? *Primary Care: Clinics in Office Practice. 36*, 307–317.

49. Ruderman N. B., Carling D., Prentki M., Cacicedo J. M. (2013). AMPK, insulin resistance, and the metabolic syndrome. *Journal of Clinical Investigation, 123*(7), 2764–2772.

50. Heart & Stroke Foundation. (2010). Healthy waists. Available online at: http://www.heartandstroke.com/site/c.ikIQLcMWJtE/b.3876195./ Accessed July 23, 2014.

51. Montani J., Viecelli A. K., Prevot A., et al. (2006). Weight cycling during growth and beyond as a risk factor of later cardiovascular diseases: The 'repeated overshoot' theory. *International Journal of Obesity, 30*(Suppl 4), S58–S66.

52. Boardley D., Pobocik R. S. (2009). Obesity on the rise. *Primary Care, 36*(2), 243–255.

53. Gortmaker S. L., Swinburn B. A., Levy D., et al. (2011). Changing the future of obesity: Science, policy and action. *Lancet, 378*(9793), 838–847.

54. Malnick S. D., Knobler H. (2006). The medical complications of obesity. *QJM, 99*(9), 565–579.

55. Puhl R. M., Heuer C. A. (2009). The stigma of obesity: a review and update. *Obesity, 17*(5), 941–964.

56. Puhl R. M., Heuer C. A. (2010). Obesity stigma: Important considerations in public health. *American Journal of Public Health, 100*(6), 1019–1028.

57. Teixeira M. E., Budd G. M. (2010). Obesity stigma: A newly recognized barrier to comprehensive and effective type 2 diabetes management. *Journal of the American Academy of Nurse Practitioners, 10*(10), 527–533.

58. The Secretariat for the Intersectoral Healthy Living Network in partnership with the F/P/T Healthy Living Task Group and the F/P/T Advisory Committee on Population Health and Health Security (ACPHHS). (2005). *The integrated Pan-Canadian healthy living strategy.* Health Canada, Catalogue No. HP10–1/2005.

59. ParticipACTION. (2013). Participaction: Let's get moving. Available online at: http://www.participaction.com. Accessed July 23, 2014.

60. Canadian Produce Marketing Association. (2014). Fruits and veggies! Half your plate. Available online at: http://halfyourplate.ca/home. Accessed July 23, 2014.

61. Lau D. C., Douketis J. D., Morrison K. M., et al.; Obesity Canada Clinical Guidelines Expert Panel. (2007). 2006 Canadian clinical practice guidelines on the management and prevention of obesity in adults and children [summary]. *Canadian Medical Association Journal, 176*(Suppl 8), S1–13.

62. Jacob J. J., Isaac R. (2012). Behavioral therapy for management of obesity. *Indian Journal of Endocrinology and Metabolism, 16*(1), 28–32.

63. Wadden T. A., Butryn M. L., Wilson C. (2007). Lifestyle modification for the management of obesity. *Gastroenterology, 132*(6), 2226–2238.

64. Dixon J. B., Zimmet P., Albertit K. G., et al. (2011). Bariatric surgery: An IDF statement for obese type 2 diabetes. *Diabetic Medicine, 28*(6), 628–642.

65. Ng M., Fleming T., Robinson M., et al. (2014). Global, regional and national prevalence of overweight and obesity in children and adults during 1980–2013: A systemic analysis for the Global Burden of Disease Study 2013. *Lancet, 384*(9945):766–781.

66. Han J. C., Lawlor D. A., Kimm S. Y (2010). Childhood obesity. *Lancet* 375(9727), 1737–1748.

67. Dieticians of Canada. (2014). WHO growth charts for Canada: Updated March 2014. Available online at: http://www.dietitians.ca/Secondary-Pages/Public/WHO-Growth-Charts.aspx. Accessed July 23, 2014.

68. Amed S., Dean H. J., Panagiotopoulos C., et al. (2010). Type 2 diabetes, medication-induced diabetes, and monogenic diabetes in Canadian children. *Diabetes Care, 33*(4), 786–791.

69. Steffen L. M., Sinaiko A. R., Zhou X., et al. (2013). Relation of adiposity, television and screen time in offspring to their parents. *BMC Pediatrics, 13*, 133.

70. Food and Agricultural Organization of the United Nations (FAO). (2013). *The state of food insecurity in the world: The multiple dimensions of food security.* Rome: FAO.

71. Kumar V., Abbas A. K., Fausto N., et al. (Eds.). (2010). Chapter 9: Environmental and nutritional diseases. *Robbins and Cotran pathologic basis of disease* (8th ed.). Philadelphia, PA: Elsevier Saunders.

72. Grover Z., Ee L. C. (2009). Protein energy malnutrition. *Pediatric Clinics of North America, 56*(5), 1055–1068.

73. Müller O., Krawinkel M. (2005). Malnutrition and health in developing countries. *Canadian Medical Association Journal, 173*(3), 279–286.

74. Baron R. B. (2014). Chapter 29: Nutritional disorders. In Papadakis M. A., McPhee S. J., Rabow M. V. (Eds.), *Current medical diagnosis and treatment 2014.* New York: McGraw-Hill.

75. Tisdale M. J. (1999). Wasting in cancer. *Journal of Nutrition, 129* (Suppl 1), 43S–46S.

76. Mehanna H. M., Moledina J., Travis J. (2008). Refeeding syndrome: What it is, and how to prevent and treat it. *British Medical Journal, 336*(7659), 1495–1498.

77. American Psychiatric Association. (2013). *Diagnostic and Statistical manual of mental disorders* (5th ed.). Arlington, VA: American Psychiatric Publishing.

78. Langlois K. A., Samokhvalov A. V., Rehm J., et al. (2011). *Health state descriptions for Canadians: Mental illnesses.* Catalogue No. 82–619-MIE2005002. Ottawa: Statistics Canada.

79. Ricanati E. H., Rome E. S. (2005). Eating disorders: Recognizing early to prevent complications. *Cleveland Clinic Journal of Medicine, 72*(10), 895–902.

80. Zach K. N., Smith Machin A. L., Hoch A. Z. (2011). Advances in management of the female athlete triad and eating disorders. *Clinics in Sports Medicine, 30*(3), 551–573.

81. Yager J., Anderson A. E. (2005). Anorexia nervosa. *New England Journal of Medicine, 353*(14), 1481–1488.

82. Brown T. A., Keel P. K. (2012). Current and emerging directions in the treatment of eating disorders. *Substance Abuse: Research and Treatment, 6*, 33–61

83. Judge B. S., Eisenga B. H. (2005). Disorders of fuel metabolism: Medical complications associated with starvation, eating disorders, dietary fads, and supplements. *Emergency Medicine Clinics of North America, 23*(3), 789–813.

Visit the Point **http://thePoint.lww.com for animations, journal articles, and more!**

Unit X

Disorders of Endocrine Function

By the end of the Middle Ages, a great storehouse of anatomic knowledge existed; however, this repository had been culled from a combination of incomplete observations, religious beliefs, extrapolation from animal structures, and philosophical guesswork. Scientists slavishly adhered to these teachings, many of which were the products of the early Greeks (such as Aristotle and Galen), even though personal experience provided them with contradictory evidence.

The endocrine system fell victim to the outdated theories postulated long before. Even when some of its parts were discovered, their importance went unrecognized. For example, the pituitary gland, first noted in 1524 by Jacob Berengar of Carpi, was considered to be necessary to the cooling function of the brain. The brain was thought to secrete *pituita,* phlegm (mucus), and discharge it from the nose as part of its cooling process. The gland received its name from Andreas Vesalius, who referred to it in his text *De Fabrica* (1543) as *glandula pituitam cerebri excipiens,* or the gland that receives the phlegm from the brain. It was not until the late 19th and early 20th centuries that the field of endocrinology had its beginnings. It was then that the importance of the pituitary gland was finally realized, and it was called the master endocrine gland.

Unit X

Disorders of
Endocrine Function

Mechanisms of Endocrine Control

40

THE ENDOCRINE SYSTEM

Hormones
> Paracrine and Autocrine Actions
> Structural Classification
> Synthesis and Release
> Transport
> Metabolism and Elimination
> Mechanisms of Action

Control of Hormone Levels
> Hypothalamic–Pituitary Regulation
> Feedback Regulation

Diagnostic Tests
> Blood Tests
> Urine Tests
> Stimulation and Suppression Tests
> Genetic Tests
> Imaging

The endocrine system is involved in all of the integrative aspects of life, including growth, sex differentiation, metabolism, and adaptation to an ever-changing environment. This chapter focuses on general aspects of endocrine function, organization of the endocrine system, hormone receptors and hormone actions, and regulation of hormone levels.

THE ENDOCRINE SYSTEM

After completing this section of the chapter, you should be able to meet the following objectives:

- Characterize a hormone.
- Describe mechanisms of hormone transport and inactivation.
- State the function of a hormone receptor and the difference between cell surface hormone receptors and intracellular hormone receptors.
- Describe the role of the hypothalamus in regulating pituitary control of endocrine function.
- State the major difference between positive and negative feedback control mechanisms.
- Describe methods used in diagnosis of endocrine disorders.

The endocrine system uses chemical substances called *hormones* as a means of regulating and integrating body functions. The endocrine system participates in the regulation of digestion and the usage and storage of nutrients; growth and development; electrolyte and water metabolism; and reproductive functions. The endocrine network of organs and mediators does not work in isolation. The functions of the endocrine system are closely linked with those of the nervous system (*i.e.,* neuroendocrine, psychoneuroendocrine) and the immune system. For example, neurotransmitters such as epinephrine can act as neurotransmitters or as hormones. The functions of the immune system also are closely linked with those of the endocrine system. The immune system responds to foreign agents by means of chemical messengers (cytokines, such as interleukins, interferons) and complex receptor mechanisms (see Chapter 17). The immune system also is extensively regulated by hormones such as the adrenal corticosteroid hormones.

Hormones

Hormones generally are thought of as chemical messengers that are transported in body fluids. They are highly specialized organic molecules produced by endocrine organs that exert their action on specific target cells. Hormones do not initiate reactions but function as modulators of cellular and systemic responses. Most hormones are present in body fluids at all times, but in greater or lesser amounts depending on the needs of the body.

A characteristic of hormones is that a single hormone can exert various effects in different tissues or, conversely, a single function can be regulated by several different hormones. For example, estradiol, which is produced by the ovary, can act on the ovarian follicles to promote their maturation, on the uterus to stimulate its growth and maintain the cyclic changes in the uterine mucosa, on the mammary gland to stimulate ductal growth, on the hypothalamic–pituitary system to regulate the secretion of gonadotropins and prolactin, on the bone to maintain skeletal integrity, and on general metabolic processes to affect adipose tissue distribution. Lipolysis, which is the release of free fatty acids from adipose tissue, is an example of a single function that is regulated by several hormones, including the catecholamines, insulin, and glucagon, but also by the cytokine, tumour necrosis factor-α. Table 40.1 lists the major actions and sources of body hormones.

Paracrine and Autocrine Actions

Endocrine hormones are typically chemical substances that are released into the bloodstream and transported to distant target sites, where they exerted their action. Although many hormones travel by this mechanism, some hormones and hormone-like substances never enter the bloodstream but instead act locally in the vicinity in which they are released (see Chapter 4, Fig. 4.8). When they act locally on cells other than those that produced the hormone, the action is called *paracrine*. The action of sex steroids on the ovary is a paracrine action.

HORMONES

- Hormones function as chemical messengers, moving through the blood to distant target sites of action, or acting more locally as paracrine or autocrine messengers that incite more local effects.
- Most hormones are present in body fluids at all times, but in greater or lesser amounts depending on the needs of the body.
- Hormones exert their actions by interacting with high-affinity receptors, which in turn are linked to one or more effector systems in the cell. Some hormone receptors are located on the surface of the cell and act through second messenger mechanisms, and others are located in the cell, where they modulate the synthesis of enzymes, transport proteins, or structural proteins.

Hormones also can exert an *autocrine* action on the same cells from which they were produced. For example, the release of insulin from pancreatic beta cells can inhibit its release from the same cells.

Structural Classification

Hormones, which have diverse structures ranging from single amino acids to complex proteins and lipids, are divided into three categories: (1) amines and amino acids; (2) peptides, polypeptides, proteins, and glycoproteins; and (3) steroids (Table 40.2). The first category, the amines, includes norepinephrine and epinephrine, which are derived from a single amino acid (*i.e.*, tyrosine), and the thyroid hormones, which are derived from two iodinated tyrosine amino acid residues. The second category, the peptides, polypeptides, proteins, and glycoproteins, can be as small as thyrotropin-releasing hormone (TRH), which contains 3 amino acids, and as large and complex as growth hormone (GH) and follicle-stimulating hormone (FSH), which have approximately 200 amino acids. Glycoproteins are large peptide hormones associated with a carbohydrate (*e.g.*, FSH). The third category consists of the steroid hormones, which are derivatives of cholesterol.

Synthesis and Release

The mechanisms for hormone synthesis and release vary with hormone structure. Hormones such as the protein and polypeptide hormones are synthesized and stored in vesicles in the cytoplasm of the endocrine cell until secretion is required. These hormones are released by fusion of the vesicle with the cell membrane. Their release may or may not be coupled with the stimulus for synthesis. Other hormones, such as the steroid hormones, are secreted upon synthesis. For these hormones, there typically is no distinction between the stimulus for synthesis and release.

The protein and polypeptide hormones comprise the most prominent class of hormones whose synthesis and release is vesicle mediated. These hormones are synthesized in the rough endoplasmic reticulum of the endocrine cell in a manner similar to the synthesis of other proteins (see Chapter 4). The appropriate amino acid sequence is dictated by messenger ribonucleic acids (mRNAs) from the nucleus. Usually, synthesis involves the production of a precursor hormone, which is modified by the addition of peptides or sugar units. These precursor hormones often contain extra peptide units that ensure proper folding of the molecule and insertion of essential linkages. If extra amino acids are present, as in insulin, the precursor hormone is called a *prohormone*. After synthesis and sequestration in the endoplasmic reticulum, the protein and peptide hormones move into the Golgi complex, where they are packaged in vesicles. It is in the Golgi complex that prohormones are converted into hormones. Stimulation of the endocrine cell causes the vesicles to move to the cell membrane and release their hormones. The vesicle-mediated pathway is also used for secretion of a number of nonpolypeptide hormones and neurotransmitters such as the catecholamines (dopamine, epinephrine, and norepinephrine). However, these small molecules do not pass through the full range of

TABLE 40.1 MAJOR ACTION AND SOURCE OF SELECTED HORMONES

SOURCE	HORMONE	MAJOR ACTION

Hypothalamus	Releasing and inhibiting hormones
	  Corticotropin-releasing hormone (CRH)
	  Thyrotropin-releasing hormone (TRH)
	  Growth hormone–releasing hormone (GHRH)
	  Gonadotropin-releasing hormone (GnRH)
		Control the release of pituitary hormones

	Somatostatin	Inhibits GH and TSH
	Dopamine	Inhibits prolactin release from anterior pituitary
Anterior pituitary	Growth hormone (GH)	Stimulates growth of bone and muscle, promotes protein synthesis and fat metabolism, decreases carbohydrate metabolism
	Adrenocorticotropic hormone (ACTH)	Stimulates synthesis and secretion of adrenal cortical hormones
	Thyroid-stimulating hormone (TSH)	Stimulates synthesis and secretion of thyroid hormone
	Follicle-stimulating hormone (FSH)	Female: stimulates growth of ovarian follicle, ovulation Male: stimulates sperm production
	Luteinizing hormone (LH)	Female: stimulates development of corpus luteum, release of oocyte, production of estrogen and progesterone Male: stimulates secretion of testosterone, development of interstitial tissue of testes
	Prolactin	Prepares female breast for breast-feeding
Posterior pituitary	Antidiuretic hormone (ADH)	Increases water reabsorption by kidney
	Oxytocin	Stimulates contraction of pregnant uterus, milk ejection from breasts after childbirth
Adrenal cortex	Mineralocorticosteroids, mainly aldosterone	Increase sodium absorption, potassium loss by kidney
	Glucocorticoids, mainly cortisol	Affect metabolism of all nutrients; regulates blood glucose levels, affects growth, has anti-inflammatory action, and decreases effects of stress
	Adrenal androgens, mainly dehydroepi-androsterone (DHEA) and androstenedione	Have minimal intrinsic androgenic activity; they are converted to testosterone and dihydrotestosterone in the periphery
Adrenal medulla	Epinephrine Norepinephrine	Serve as neurotransmitters for the sympathetic nervous system
Thyroid (follicular cells)	Thyroid hormones: triiodothyronine (T_3), thyroxine (T_4)	Increase the metabolic rate; increase protein and bone turnover; increase responsiveness to catecholamines; necessary for fetal and infant growth and development
Thyroid C cells	Calcitonin	Lowers blood calcium and phosphate levels
Parathyroid glands	Parathyroid hormone (PTH)	Regulates serum calcium
Pancreatic islet cells	Insulin	Lowers blood glucose by facilitating glucose transport across cell membranes of muscle, liver, and adipose tissue
	Glucagon	Increases blood glucose concentration by stimulation of glycogenolysis and glyconeogenesis
	Somatostatin	Delays intestinal absorption of glucose
Kidney	1,25-Dihydroxyvitamin D	Stimulates calcium absorption from the intestine
Ovaries	Estrogen	Affects development of female sex organs and secondary sex characteristics
	Progesterone	Influences menstrual cycle; stimulates growth of uterine wall; maintains pregnancy
Testes	Androgens, mainly testosterone	Affect development of male sex organs and secondary sex characteristics; aid in sperm production

intracellular mechanisms seen in the synthesis and secretion of the larger protein and polypeptide hormones.

Hormones synthesized by nonvesicle-mediated pathways include the glucocorticoids, androgens, estrogens, and mineralocorticoids—all steroids derived from cholesterol. These hormones are synthesized in the smooth endoplasmic reticulum, and steroid-secreting cells can be identified by their large amounts of smooth endoplasmic reticulum. Certain steroids serve as precursors for the production of other hormones. In the adrenal cortex, for example, progesterone and other steroid intermediates are enzymatically converted into aldosterone, cortisol, or androgens (see Chapter 41). The release

TABLE 40.2 CLASSES OF HORMONES BASED ON STRUCTURE

AMINES AND AMINO ACIDS	PEPTIDES, POLYPEPTIDES, AND PROTEINS	STEROIDS
Dopamine	Corticotropin-releasing hormone (CRH)	Aldosterone
Epinephrine	Growth hormone-releasing hormone (GHRH)	Glucocorticoids
Norepinephrine	Thyrotropin-releasing hormone (TRH)	Estrogens
Thyroid hormone	Adrenocorticotropic hormone (ACTH)	Testosterone
	Follicle-stimulating hormone (FSH)	Progesterone
	Luteinizing hormone (LH)	Androstenedione
	Thyroid-stimulating hormone (TSH)	1,25-Dihydroxyvitamin D
	Growth hormone (GH)	Dihydrotestosterone (DHT)
	Antidiuretic hormone (ADH)	Dehydroepiandrosterone (DHEA)
	Oxytocin	
	Insulin	
	Glucagon	
	Somatostatin	
	Calcitonin	
	Parathyroid hormone (PTH)	
	Prolactin	

of hormones synthesized by nonvesicle-mediated pathways is not fully understood. Historically it was thought to occur by simple diffusion. In recent years, however, specific transporters have been implicated in directing some of these classes of hormones out of the cell. Whether all hormones produced by nonvesicle-mediated pathways depend on transporters for their secretion remains a subject for further investigation.

Transport

Hormones that are released into the bloodstream circulate as either free or unbound molecules, or as hormones attached to transport carriers (Fig. 40.1). Peptide hormones and protein hormones usually circulate unbound in the blood. Steroid hormones and thyroid hormone are carried by specific carrier proteins synthesized in the liver. The extent of carrier binding influences the rate at which hormones leave the blood and enter the cells. The half-life of a hormone—the time it takes for the body to reduce the concentration of the hormone by one half—is positively correlated with its percentage of protein binding. Thyroxine, which is more than 99% protein bound, has a half-life of 6 days. Aldosterone, which is only 15% bound, has a half-life of only 25 minutes. Drugs that compete with a hormone for binding with transport carrier molecules increase hormone action by increasing the availability of the active unbound hormone. For example, aspirin competes with thyroid hormone for binding to transport proteins. When this drug is administered to persons with excessive levels of circulating thyroid hormone, such as during thyroid crisis, serious effects may occur due to the dissociation of free hormone from the binding proteins.

Metabolism and Elimination

Hormones secreted by endocrine cells must be inactivated continuously to prevent their accumulation. Intracellular and extracellular mechanisms participate in the termination

of hormone function. Most peptide hormones and catecholamines are water soluble and circulate freely in the blood. They are usually degraded by enzymes in the blood or tissues and then excreted by the kidneys and liver. For example, the catecholamines are rapidly degraded by catechol-O-methyl transferase (COMT) and monoamine oxidase (MAO). Because of their short half-life, their production can be measured by some of their metabolites. In general, peptide hormones also have a short life span in the circulation. Their major mechanism of degradation is through binding to cell surface receptors,

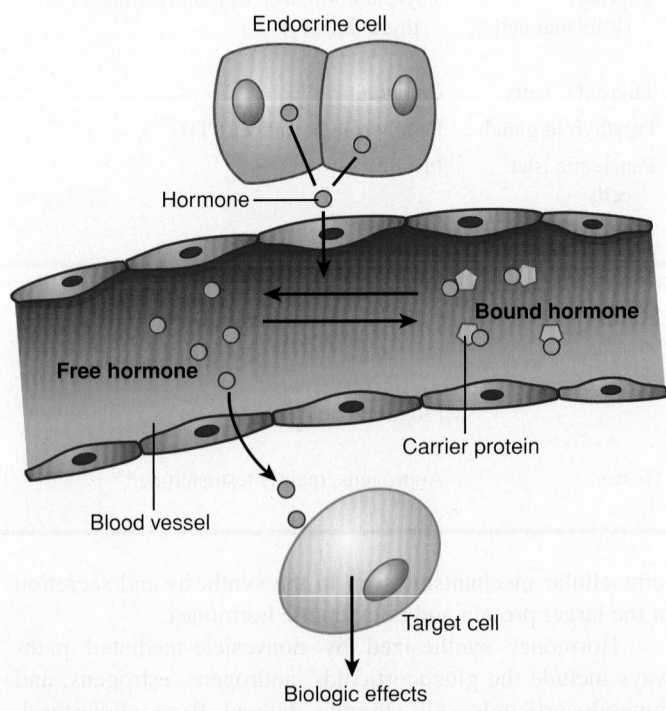

FIGURE 40.1 • Relationship of free and carrier-bound hormones.

with subsequent uptake and degradation by peptide-splitting enzymes in the cell membrane or inside the cell. Steroid hormones are bound to protein carriers for transport and are inactive in the bound state. Their activity depends on the availability of transport carriers. Unbound adrenal and gonadal steroid hormones are conjugated in the liver, which renders them inactive, and then excreted in the bile or urine. Thyroid hormones also are transported by carrier molecules. The free hormone is rendered inactive by the removal of amino acids (*i.e.,* deamination) in the tissues, and the hormone is conjugated in the liver and eliminated in the bile.

Mechanisms of Action

Hormones produce their effects through interaction with high-affinity receptors, which in turn are linked to one or more effector systems within the cell. These mechanisms involve many of the cell's metabolic activities, ranging from ion transport at the cell surface to stimulation of nuclear transcription of complex molecules. The rate at which hormones react depends on their mechanism of action. The neurotransmitters, which control the opening of ion channels, have a reaction time of milliseconds. Thyroid hormone, which functions in the control of cell metabolism and synthesis of intracellular signalling molecules, requires days for its full effect to occur.

Receptors. Hormone receptors are complex molecular structures that are located either on the surface of or inside target cells. The function of these receptors is to recognize a specific hormone and translate the hormonal signal into a cellular response. The structure of these receptors varies in a manner that allows target cells to respond to one hormone and not to others. For example, receptors in the thyroid are specific for thyroid-stimulating hormone, and receptors on the gonads respond to the gonadotropic hormones.

The response of a target cell to a hormone varies with the *number* of receptors present and with the *affinity* of these receptors for hormone binding. A variety of factors influence the number of receptors that are present on target cells and their affinity for hormone binding.

There are approximately 2,000 to 100,000 hormone receptor molecules per cell. The number of hormone receptors on a cell may be altered for any of several reasons. Antibodies may destroy or block the receptor proteins. Increased or decreased hormone levels often induce changes in the activity of the genes that regulate receptor synthesis. For example, decreased hormone levels often produce an increase in receptor numbers by means of a process called *upregulation;* this increases the sensitivity of the body to existing hormone levels. Likewise, sustained levels of excess hormone often bring about a decrease in receptor numbers by *downregulation,* producing a decrease in hormone sensitivity. In some instances, the reverse effect occurs, and an increase in hormone levels appears to recruit its own receptors, thereby increasing the sensitivity of the cell to the hormone. The process of upregulation and downregulation of receptors is regulated largely by inducing or repressing the transcription of receptor genes.

CHART 40.1 HORMONE–RECEPTOR INTERACTIONS

Second Messenger Interactions
Glucagon
Insulin
Epinephrine
Parathyroid hormone (PTH)
Thyroid-stimulating hormone (TSH)
Adrenocorticotropic hormone (ACTH)
Follicle-stimulating hormone (FSH)
Luteinizing hormone (LH)
Antidiuretic hormone (ADH)
Secretin

Intracellular Interactions
Estrogens
Testosterone
Progesterone
Adrenal cortical hormones
Thyroid hormones

Some hormone receptors are located on the surface of the cell and act through second messenger mechanisms, and others are located within the cell, where they modulate the synthesis of enzymes, transport proteins, or structural proteins. The receptors for thyroid hormones, which are found in the nucleus, are thought to be directly associated with controlling the activity of genes located on one or more of the chromosomes. Chart 40.1 lists examples of hormones that act through the two types of receptors.

Cell Surface Receptors. Because of their low solubility in the lipid layer of cell membranes, peptide hormones and catecholamines cannot readily cross the cell membrane. Instead, these hormones interact with surface receptors in a manner that incites the generation of an intracellular signal or message. The intracellular signal system is termed the *second messenger,* and the hormone is considered to be the first messenger. For example, the first messenger, glucagon, binds to surface receptors on liver cells to incite glycogen breakdown by way of the second messenger system.

The most widely distributed second messenger is cyclic adenosine monophosphate (cAMP), which is formed from adenosine triphosphate (ATP) by the enzyme adenylate cyclase, a membrane-bound enzyme that is located on the inner aspect of the cell membrane. Adenylate cyclase is functionally coupled to various cell surface receptors by the regulatory actions of G-proteins. A second messenger similar to cAMP is cyclic guanosine monophosphate (cGMP), derived from guanosine triphosphate (GTP). As a result of binding to specific cell receptors, many peptide hormones incite a series of enzymatic reactions that produce an almost immediate increase in cAMP and target cell response. Some hormones

Understanding Hormone Receptors

Hormones bring about their effects on cell activity by binding to specific cell receptors. There are two general types of receptors: (1) cell surface receptors that exert their actions through cytoplasmic second messenger systems, and (2) intracellular nuclear receptors that modulate gene expression by binding to DNA or promoters of target genes.

1. Cell Surface Receptors

Water-soluble peptide hormones, such as parathyroid hormone and glucagon, which cannot penetrate the lipid layer of the cell plasma membrane, exert their effects through intracellular second messengers. They bind to a portion of a membrane receptor that protrudes through the surface of the cell. This produces a structural change in the receptor molecule itself, causing activation of a hormone-regulated signal system located on the inner aspect of the cell membrane. This system allows the cell to sense extracellular events and pass this information to the intracellular environment. There are several types of cell surface receptors, including G-protein–coupled receptors that mediate the actions of catecholamines, prostaglandins, thyroid-stimulating hormone, and others. Binding of the hormone to the receptor activates a G-protein, which in turn acts on an effector such as adenyl cyclase to generate a second messenger such as cyclic adenosine monophosphate (cAMP). The second messenger, in turn, activates other enzymes that participate in cellular secretion, gene activation, or other target cell responses.

act to decrease cAMP levels and have another or an opposite effect on cell responses.

In some cells, the binding of a hormone or neurotransmitter to a surface receptor acts directly, rather than through a second messenger, to open an ion channel in the cell membrane. The influx of ions then serves as an intracellular signal to convey the hormonal message to the interior of the cell. In many instances, the activation of hormone receptors results in the opening of calcium channels. The increasing cytoplasmic concentration of calcium ions may result in the direct activation of calcium-dependent enzymes or in the formation of calcium–calmodulin complexes with their attendant effects.

Intracellular Receptors. A second type of receptor mechanism is involved in mediating the action of hormones such as the steroid and thyroid hormones. These hormones are lipid soluble and pass freely through the cell membrane. They then attach to intracellular receptors and form a hormone–receptor complex that travels to the cell nucleus. The hormone–messenger complex binds to hormone response elements (HREs) that then activate or suppress intracellular mechanisms such as gene activity, with the subsequent production or inhibition of mRNA and protein synthesis.

Control of Hormone Levels

Hormone secretion varies widely over a 24-hour period. Some hormones, such as GH and adrenocorticotropic hormone (ACTH), have diurnal fluctuations that vary with the sleep–wake cycle. Others, such as the female sex hormones, are secreted in a complicated cyclic manner. The levels of hormones such as insulin and antidiuretic hormone (ADH) are regulated by feedback mechanisms that monitor substances such as glucose (insulin) and water (ADH) in the body. The levels of

2. Nuclear Receptors

Steroid hormones, vitamin D, thyroid hormones, and other lipid-soluble hormones diffuse across the cell membrane into the cytoplasm of the target cell. Once inside, they bind to an intracellular receptor that is activated by the interaction. The activated hormone–receptor complex then moves to the nucleus, where the hormone binds to a hormone response element (HRE) in the promoters on a target gene or to another transcription factor. Attachment to the HRE results in transcription of a specific messenger RNA (mRNA). The mRNA then moves into the cytoplasm, where the "transcribed message" is translated and used by cytoplasmic ribosomes to produce new cellular proteins or changes in the production of existing proteins. These proteins promote a specific cellular response or, in some cases, the synthesis of a structural protein that is exported from the cell.

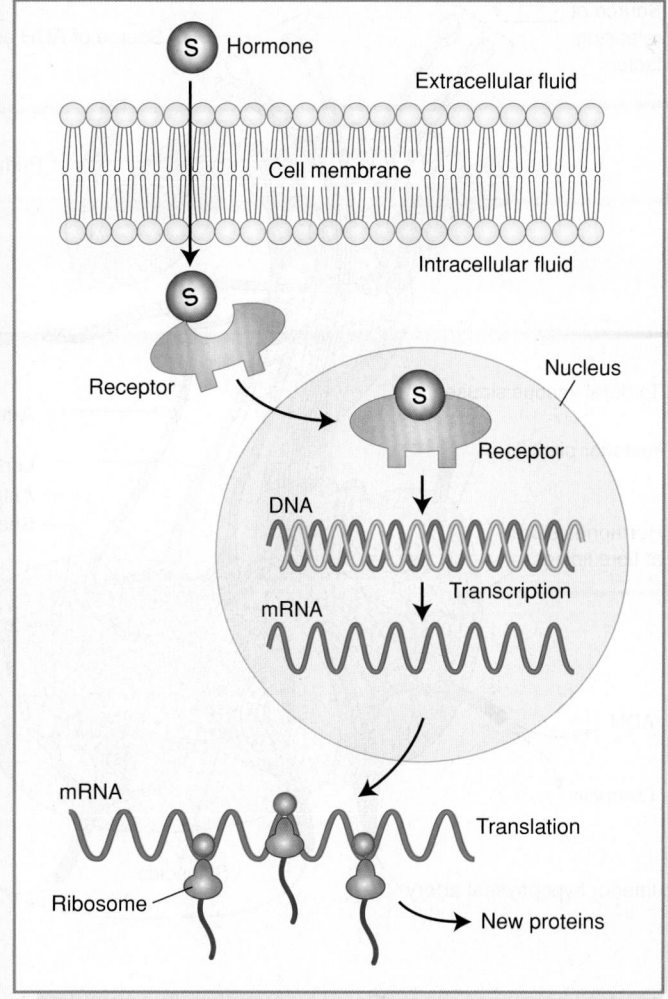

many of the hormones are regulated by feedback mechanisms that involve the hypothalamic–pituitary–target cell system.

Hypothalamic–Pituitary Regulation

The hypothalamus and pituitary (*i.e.,* hypophysis) form a unit that exerts control over many functions of several endocrine glands as well as a wide range of other physiologic functions. These two structures are connected by blood flow in the hypophysial portal system, which begins in the hypothalamus and drains into the anterior pituitary gland, and by the nerve axons that connect the supraoptic and paraventricular nuclei of the hypothalamus with the posterior pituitary gland (Fig. 40.2). The pituitary is enclosed in the bony sella turcica ("Turkish saddle") and is bridged over by the diaphragma sellae. Embryologically, the anterior pituitary gland develops from glandular tissue and the posterior pituitary develops from neural tissue.

Hypothalamic Hormones. The synthesis and release of anterior pituitary hormones are largely regulated by the action of releasing or inhibiting hormones from the hypothalamus, which is the coordinating centre of the brain for endocrine, behavioural, and autonomic nervous system function. It is at the level of the hypothalamus that emotion, pain, body temperature, and other neural input are communicated to the endocrine system (Fig. 40.3). The posterior pituitary hormones, ADH and oxytocin, are synthesized in the cell bodies of neurons in the hypothalamus that have axons that travel to the posterior pituitary. The release and function of ADH are discussed in Chapter 31.

The hypothalamic hormones that regulate the secretion of anterior pituitary hormones include GH-releasing hormone (GHRH), somatostatin, dopamine, TRH, corticotropin-releasing hormone (CRH), and gonadotropin-releasing hormone (GnRH). With the exception of GH and prolactin, most of the

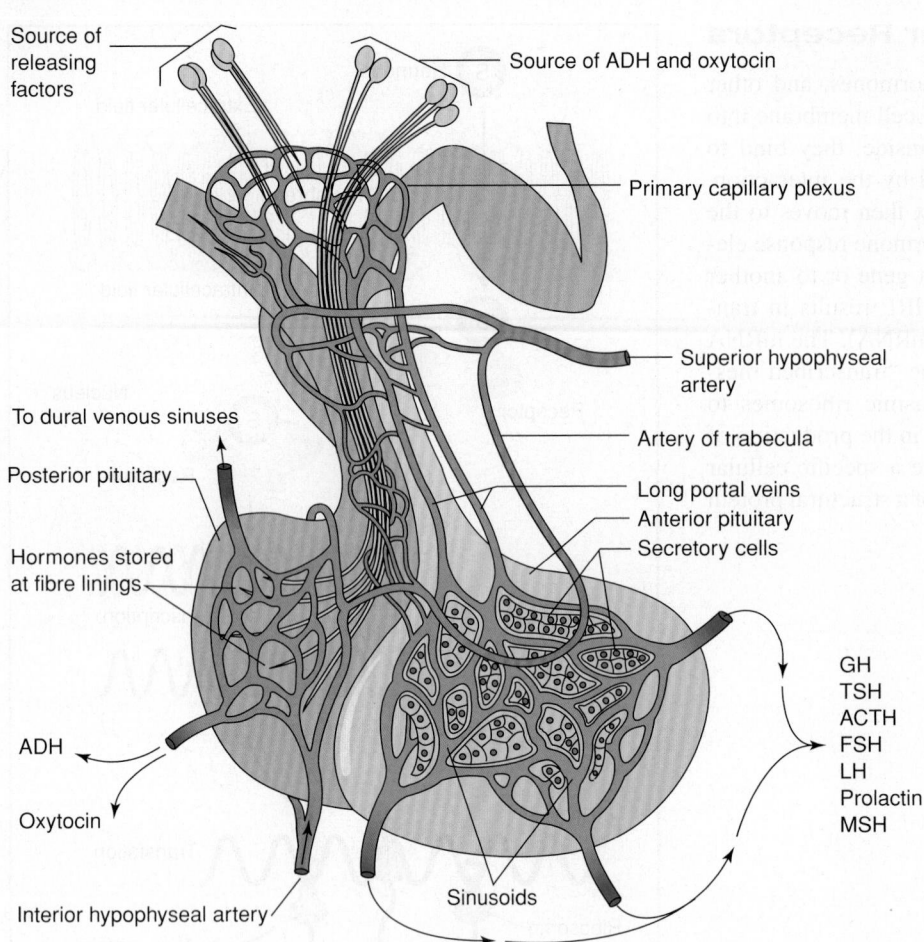

Source of releasing factors

Source of ADH and oxytocin

Primary capillary plexus

Superior hypophyseal artery

Artery of trabecula

To dural venous sinuses

Posterior pituitary

Long portal veins

Anterior pituitary

Secretory cells

Hormones stored at fibre linings

ADH

Oxytocin

Interior hypophyseal artery

Sinusoids

GH
TSH
ACTH
FSH
LH
Prolactin
MSH

FIGURE 40.2 • The hypothalamus and the anterior and posterior pituitary. The hypothalamic releasing or inhibiting hormones are transported to the anterior pituitary through the portal vessels. Antidiuretic hormone and oxytocin are produced by nerve cells in the supraoptic and paraventricular nuclei of the hypothalamus and then transported through the nerve axon to the posterior pituitary, where they are released into the circulation. ACTH, adrenocorticotropic hormone; ADH, antidiuretic hormone; FSH, follicle-stimulating hormone; GH, growth hormone; LH, luteinizing hormone; MSH, melanocyte stimulating hormone; TSH, thyroid-stimulating hormone.

pituitary hormones are regulated by hypothalamic stimulatory hormones. GH secretion is stimulated by GHRH; thyroid-stimulating hormone (TSH) by TRH; ACTH by CRH; and luteinizing hormone (LH) and FSH by GnRH. Somatostatin functions as an inhibitory hormone for GH and TSH. Prolactin secretion is inhibited by dopamine; thus, persons receiving antipsychotic drugs that block dopamine often have increased prolactin levels.

The activity of the hypothalamus is regulated by both hormonally mediated signals (*e.g.*, negative feedback signals) and by neuronal input from a number of sources. Neuronal signals are mediated by neurotransmitters and neuropeptides such as acetylcholine, dopamine, norepinephrine, serotonin, γ-aminobutyric acid (GABA), and opioids. Cytokines that are involved in immune and inflammatory responses, such as the interleukins, also are involved in the regulation of hypothalamic function (see Chapter 17). This is particularly true of the hormones involved in the hypothalamic–pituitary–adrenal axis. Thus, the hypothalamus can be viewed as a bridge by which signals from multiple systems are relayed to the pituitary gland.

Pituitary Hormones. The pituitary gland has been called the *master gland* because its hormones control the functions of many target glands and cells. The anterior pituitary gland contains five cell types: (1) thyrotrophs, which produce

thyrotropin, also called *thyroid-stimulating hormone* (TSH); (2) corticotrophs, which produce corticotrophin, also called *adrenocorticotropic hormone* (ACTH); (3) gonadotrophs, which produce the gonadotropins, *luteinizing hormone* (LH) and *follicle-stimulating hormone* (FSH); (4) somatotrophs, which produce *growth hormone* (GH); and (5) lactotrophs, which produce *prolactin.* Hormones produced by the anterior pituitary control body growth and metabolism (GH), function of the thyroid gland (TSH), glucocorticoid hormone levels (ACTH), function of the gonads (FSH and LH), and breast growth and milk production (prolactin). *Melanocyte-stimulating hormone* (MSH), which is involved in the control of pigmentation of the skin, is produced by the pars intermedia of the pituitary gland. The functions of many of these hormones are discussed in other parts of this book (*e.g.*, thyroid hormone, GH, and the corticosteroids in Chapter 41, the sex hormones in Chapters 44 and 46, and ADH from the posterior pituitary in Chapter 31).

Feedback Regulation

The level of many of the hormones in the body is regulated by negative feedback mechanisms. The function of this type of system is similar to that of the thermostat in a heating system. In the endocrine system, sensors detect a change in the hormone level and adjust hormone secretion so that body levels are maintained within an appropriate range. When the sensors

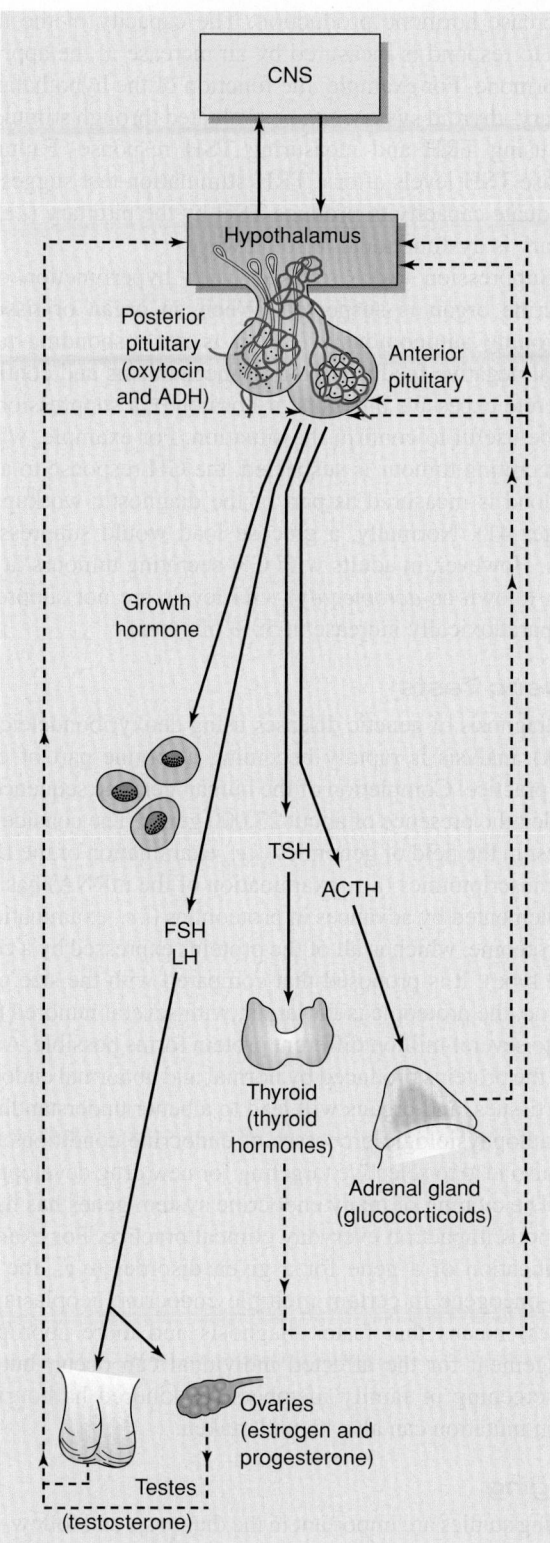

detect a decrease in hormone levels, they initiate changes that cause an increase in hormone production; when hormone levels rise above the set point of the system, the sensors cause hormone production and release to decrease. For example, an increase in thyroid hormone is detected by sensors in the hypothalamus or anterior pituitary gland, and this causes a reduction in the secretion of TSH, with a subsequent decrease in the output of thyroid hormone from the thyroid gland. The feedback loops for the hypothalamic–pituitary feedback mechanisms are illustrated in Figure 40.3.

Exogenous forms of hormones (given as drug preparations) can influence the normal feedback control of hormone production and release. One of the most common examples of this influence occurs with the administration of the corticosteroid hormones, which causes suppression of the hypothalamic–pituitary–target cell system that regulates the production of these hormones.

Although most hormones levels are regulated by negative feedback mechanisms, a small number are under positive feedback control, in which rising levels of a hormone cause another gland to release a hormone that is stimulating to the first. There must, however, be a mechanism for shutting off the release of the first hormone, or its production would continue unabated. An example of such a system is that of the female ovarian hormone estradiol. Increased estradiol production during the follicular stage of the menstrual cycle causes increased gonadotropin (FSH) production by the anterior pituitary gland. This stimulates further increases in estradiol levels until the demise of the follicle, which is the source of estradiol, results in a fall in gonadotropin levels.

In addition to positive and negative feedback mechanisms that monitor changes in hormone levels, some hormones are regulated by the level of the substance they regulate. For example, insulin levels normally are regulated in response to blood glucose levels, and those of aldosterone in response to body levels of sodium and potassium. Other factors such as stress, environmental temperature, and nutritional status can alter feedback regulation of hormone levels.

Diagnostic Tests

Several techniques are available for assessing endocrine function and hormone levels. One technique measures the effect of a hormone on body function. Measurement of blood glucose, for example, is an indirect method of assessing insulin availability. The most common method is to measure hormone levels directly.

Blood Tests

Blood tests for endocrine disorders are vast and compass a wide variety of strategies to assess endocrine function. Blood hormone levels provide information about hormone levels at a specific time. For example, blood insulin levels can be measured along with blood glucose after administration of a challenge dose of glucose to measure the time course of change in blood insulin levels.

FIGURE 40.3 • Control of hormone production by the hypothalamic–pituitary–target cell feedback mechanism. Hormone levels from the target glands regulate the release of hormones from the anterior pituitary through a negative feedback system. The *dashed line* represents feedback control.

Plasma hormone levels can be measured using radio-immunoassay (RIA) methods. This method uses a radiolabelled form of the hormone and a hormone antibody that has been prepared from a purified form of the hormone. The unlabelled hormone in the sample being tested competes with the radio-labelled hormone for attachment to the binding sites of the antibody. Measurement of the radiolabelled hormone–antibody complex then provides a means of arriving at a measure of the hormone level in the sample. Because hormone binding is competitive, the amount of radiolabelled hormone–antibody complex that is formed decreases as the amount of unlabelled hormone in the sample is increased. Limitations for RIA include the lack of specificity due to cross reactivity with more than on hormone, limited shelf life of the radiolabelled hormone, and the cost for the disposal of radioactive waste. Another technique is the immunoradiometric assay (IRMA) which uses the same principle of antibody recognition with two antibodies instead of one. These two antibodies are directed against two different parts of the molecule, and therefore IRMA assays are more specific. Research is looking at the high performance liquid chromatography with tandem mass spectrometry technique as a more precise way to identify and quantitate multiple peptide or steroid compounds from one sample. The increased cost and level of laboratory expertise remain limiting factors.

Other substances that are routinely measured in endocrine disorders include various autoantibodies. For example, anti-thyroid peroxidase (anti-TPO) antibodies are measured during the initial diagnostic work-up and subsequent follow-up of patients with Hashimoto thyroiditis. Other endocrine disorders that use autoantibody testing include type 1 diabetes, Graves disease, autoimmune hypoparathyroidism, and autoimmune Addison disease.

Urine Tests

Measurements of urinary hormone or hormone metabolite excretion often are done on a 24-hour urine sample and provide a better measure of hormone levels during that period compared to hormones measured in an isolated blood sample. The advantages of a urine test include the relative ease of obtaining urine samples and the fact that blood sampling is not required. The disadvantage is that reliably timed urine collections often are difficult to obtain. For example, a person may be unable to urinate at specific timed intervals, and urine samples may be accidentally discarded or inaccurately preserved. Because many urine tests involve the measure of a hormone metabolite rather than the hormone itself, drugs or disease states that alter hormone metabolism may interfere with the test result. Some urinary hormone metabolite measurements include hormones from more than one source and are of little value in measuring hormone secretion from a specific source. For example, urinary 17-ketosteroids are a measure of both adrenal and gonadal androgens.

Stimulation and Suppression Tests

Stimulation tests are used when hypofunction of an endocrine organ is suspected. A tropic or stimulating hormone can be administered to test the capacity of an endocrine organ to increase hormone production. The capacity of the target gland to respond is measured by an increase in the appropriate hormone. For example, the function of the hypothalamic–pituitary–thyroid system can be evaluated through stimulation tests using TRH and measuring TSH response. Failure to increase TSH levels after a TRH stimulation test suggests an inadequate capacity to produce TSH by the pituitary (*i.e.,* the pituitary is dysfunctional in some way).

Suppression tests are used when hyperfunction of an endocrine organ is suspected. When an organ or tissue is functioning autonomously (*i.e.,* it is not responding to the normal negative feedback control mechanisms and continues to secrete excessive amounts of hormone), a suppression test may be useful to confirm the situation. For example, when a GH-secreting tumour is suspected, the GH response to a glucose load is measured as part of the diagnostic workup (see Chapter 41). Normally, a glucose load would suppress GH levels. However, in adults with GH-secreting tumours (a condition known as *acromegaly*), GH levels are not suppressed (and paradoxically increase in 50% of cases).

Genetic Tests

The diagnosis of genetic diseases using deoxyribonucleic acid (DNA) analysis is rapidly becoming a routine part of endocrine practice. Completion of the human genome sequence has revealed the presence of about 23,000 genes. The considerable interest in the field of genomics (*i.e.,* examination of the DNA) and transcriptomics (*i.e.,* examination of the mRNA) has been complemented by advances in proteomics (*i.e.,* examination of the proteome, which is all of the proteins expressed by a cell or tissue type). It is proposed that compared with the size of the genome, the proteome is far larger, with several hundred thousand to several million different protein forms possible. Analysis of the proteins produced by normal and abnormal endocrine cells, tissues, and organs will lead to a better understanding of the pathophysiologic processes of endocrine conditions. This may also lead to selective targeting for new drug development.

The cloning of many endocrine system genes has had an enormous impact on everyday clinical practice. For example, identification of a gene for a given disorder (*e.g.,* the *RET* proto-oncogene in certain multiple endocrine neoplasia syndromes) means that faster diagnosis and more appropriate management for the affected individual can occur, but also that screening of family members for kindred harbouring a known mutation can also be undertaken.

Imaging

Imaging studies are important in the diagnosis and follow-up of endocrine disorders. Imaging modalities related to endocrinology can be divided into isotopic and nonisotopic types. Isotopic imaging includes radioactive scanning of the thyroid (*e.g.,* using radioiodine), parathyroids (*e.g.,* using sestamibi), and adrenals (*e.g.,* using MIBG to detect pheochromocytoma). Nonisotopic imaging includes magnetic resonance imaging (MRI), which is the preferred choice for pituitary and hypothalamic imaging, and computed tomography (CT) scanning, which is preferred

Understanding Feedback Regulation of Hormone Levels

Like many physiologic systems, the endocrine system is regulated by feedback mechanisms that enable the endocrine cells to change their rate of hormone secretion. Feedback can be negative or positive and may involve complex feedback loops involving hypothalamic–pituitary regulation.

1. Negative Feedback

With negative feedback, the most common mechanism of hormone control, some feature of hormone action directly or indirectly inhibits further hormone secretion so that the hormone level returns to an ideal level or set point. In the simple negative feedback loop, the amount of hormone or its effect on a physiologic mechanism regulates the response of the endocrine gland. After a meal, for example, a rise in blood glucose stimulates the pancreas to secrete insulin; insulin acts on target cells to take up the glucose, thus lowering blood glucose. The lowered glucose levels, in turn, suppress insulin release, causing blood glucose to rise.

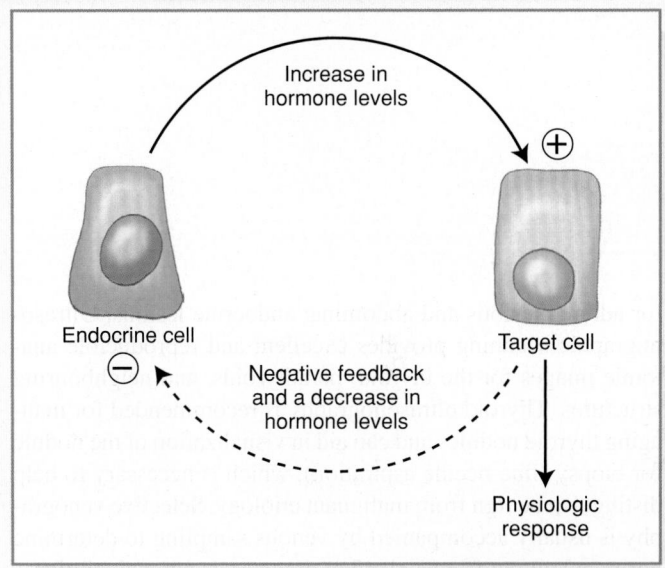

2. Hypothalamic–Pituitary–Target Cell Feedback

Hormones of the thyroid, adrenal cortex, and the gonads are regulated by more complex loops involving the hypothalamus and anterior pituitary gland. The hypothalamus produces a releasing hormone that stimulates the production of a tropic hormone by the anterior pituitary. The tropic hormone then stimulates the peripheral target gland to secrete its hormone, which acts on target cells to produce a physiologic response. A rise in blood levels of the target gland hormone also feeds back to the hypothalamus and anterior pituitary gland, resulting in a decrease in tropic hormone secretion and a subsequent reduction in hormone secretion by the target gland. As a result, blood levels of the hormone vary only within a narrow range.

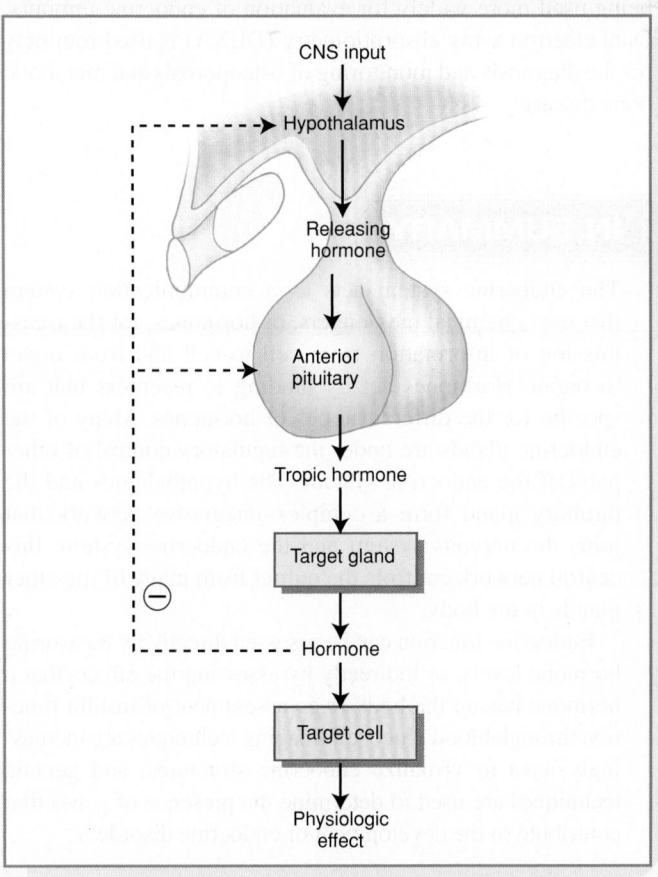

3. Positive Feedback

A small number of hormones are regulated by positive feedback. In this type of regulation, a hormone stimulates continued secretion until appropriate levels are reached. An example of positive feedback is the preovulatory surge in luteinizing hormone (LH) levels that trigger ovulation. At that time, an increase in estrogen levels exerts a positive feedback effect on the anterior pituitary secretion of LH.

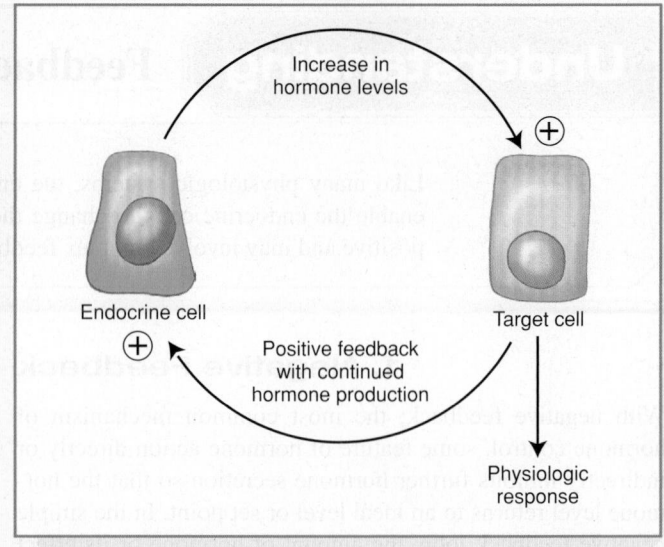

for adrenal lesions and abdominal endocrine lesions. Ultrasonographic scanning provides excellent and reproducible anatomic images for the thyroid, parathyroids, and neighbouring structures. Thyroid ultrasonography is recommended for managing thyroid nodules and can aid in visualization of the nodule for biopsy (fine-needle aspiration), which is necessary to help distinguish benign from malignant etiology. Selective venography is usually accompanied by venous sampling to determine hormonal output from a gland or organ (*e.g.*, adrenal, pituitary, and kidney). Positron emission tomography (PET) scanning is being used more widely for evaluation of endocrine tumours. Dual electron x-ray absorptiometry (DEXA) is used routinely for the diagnosis and monitoring of osteoporosis and metabolic bone diseases.

IN SUMMARY

The endocrine system acts as a communication system that uses chemical messengers, or hormones, for the transmission of information from cell to cell and from organ to organ. Hormones act by binding to receptors that are specific for the different types of hormones. Many of the endocrine glands are under the regulatory control of other parts of the endocrine system. The hypothalamus and the pituitary gland form a complex integrative network that joins the nervous system and the endocrine system; this central network controls the output from many of the other glands in the body.

Endocrine function can be assessed directly by measuring hormone levels, or indirectly by assessing the effects that a hormone has on the body (*e.g.*, assessment of insulin function through blood glucose). Imaging techniques are increasingly used to visualize endocrine structures, and genetic techniques are used to determine the presence of genes that contribute to the development of endocrine disorders.

REVIEW QUESTIONS

1. Thyroid hormones are transported in the serum bound to transport proteins such as thyroid-binding globulin and albumin.
   A. *Explain why free thyroxine (T$_4$) levels are usually used to assess thyroid function rather than total T$_4$ levels.*
2. People who are being treated with exogenous forms of corticosteroid hormones often experience diminished levels of ACTH and exogenously produced cortisol.
   A. *Explain, using information regarding the hypothalamic–pituitary feedback, control of cortisol production by the adrenal cortex.*

Bibliography

Erdelyi D. J., Elliott M., Phillips B. (2011). Urine catecholamines in paediatrics. *Archives of Disease in Childhood Education & Practice Edition, 96*(3), 107–111.

Gardner D. G., Shoback D. (Eds.). (2011). *Greenspan's basic and clinical endocrinology* (9th ed.). New York: Lange Medical Books/McGraw-Hill.

Hall J. E. (2011). *Textbook of medical physiology* (12th ed.). Philadelphia, PA: W. B. Saunders.

Jameson J. L. (Ed.), (2013). *Harrison's endocrinology* (3rd ed.). New York: McGraw-Hill.

Kovacs W. J., Sergio R. O. (2011). *Textbook of endocrine physiology* (6th ed.). New York: Oxford University Press.

Melmed S., Polonsky K. S., Larsen P. R., Kronenberg H. M. (Eds.). (2011). *Williams textbook of endocrinology* (12th ed.). Philadelphia, PA: Elsevier Saunders.

Molina P. E. (2010). *Endocrine physiology* (3rd ed.). New York: Lange Medical Books/McGraw-Hill.

Rhoades R. A., Bell D. R. (2013). *Medical physiology: Principles for clinical medicine* (4th ed.). Philadelphia, PA: Lippincott Williams & Wilkins.

Soldin S. J., Soldin O. P. (2009). Steroid hormone analysis by tandem mass spectrometry. *Clinical Chemistry, 55*(8), 1061–1066.

Visit thePoint **http://thePoint.lww.com for animations, journal articles, and more!**

Disorders of Endocrine Control of Growth and Metabolism

41

The endocrine system affects all aspects of body function, including growth and development, energy metabolism, muscle and adipose tissue distribution, sexual development, fluid and electrolyte balance, and inflammation and immune responses. This chapter focuses on disorders of pituitary function, growth and growth hormone, thyroid function, and adrenal cortical function.

GENERAL ASPECTS OF ALTERED ENDOCRINE FUNCTION

After completing this section of the chapter, you should be able to meet the following objectives:

- Describe the mechanisms of endocrine hypofunction and hyperfunction.
- Differentiate primary, secondary, and tertiary endocrine disorders.

Hypofunction and Hyperfunction

Disturbances of endocrine function usually can be divided into two categories: hypofunction and hyperfunction. Hypofunction of an endocrine gland can occur for a variety of reasons. Congenital defects can result in the absence or impaired development of the gland or the absence of an enzyme needed for hormone synthesis. The gland may be destroyed by a disruption in blood flow, infection, inflammation, autoimmune responses, or neoplastic growth. There may be a decline in function with aging, or the gland may atrophy as the result of drug therapy or for unknown reasons. Some endocrine-deficient states are associated with receptor defects: hormone receptors may be absent, the receptor binding of hormones may be defective, or the cellular responsiveness to the hormone may be impaired. It is suspected that in some cases a gland may produce a biologically inactive hormone or that an active hormone may be destroyed by circulating antibodies before it can exert its action.

Hyperfunction is usually associated with excessive hormone production. This can result from excessive stimulation and hyperplasia of the endocrine gland or from a hormone-producing tumour of the gland. A tumour can produce hormones that are not normally secreted by the tissue from which the tumour is derived (so-called ectopic hormone production); for example, certain bronchogenic tumours produce hormones such as antidiuretic hormone (ADH) and adrenocorticotropic hormone (ACTH).

Primary, Secondary, and Tertiary Disorders

Endocrine disorders in general can be divided into primary, secondary, and tertiary groups. *Primary defects* in endocrine function originate in the target gland responsible for producing the hormone. In *secondary disorders* of endocrine function, the target gland is essentially normal, but its function is altered by defective levels of stimulating hormones or releasing factors from the pituitary system. For example, total thyroidectomy produces a primary deficiency of thyroid hormones. Removal or destruction of the pituitary gland eliminates ACTH stimulation of the adrenal cortex and brings about a secondary deficiency. A *tertiary disorder* results from hypothalamic dysfunction (as may occur with craniopharyngiomas or cerebral irradiation); thus, both the pituitary and target organ are understimulated.

> ## IN SUMMARY
>
> Endocrine disorders are the result of hypofunction or hyperfunction of an endocrine gland. They can occur as a primary defect in hormone production by a target gland or as a secondary or tertiary disorder resulting from a defect in the hypothalamic–pituitary system that controls a target gland's function.

PITUITARY AND GROWTH DISORDERS

After completing this section of the chapter, you should be able to meet the following objectives:

- Discuss the classification of pituitary tumours.
- Describe the clinical features and causes of hypopituitarism.
- Review the effects of a deficiency or excess in growth hormone.
- Differentiate genetic short stature from constitutional short stature.
- List three causes of tall stature.
- Explain why children with isosexual precocious puberty are tall-statured children but short-statured adults.

The pituitary gland, or hypophysis, is a pea-sized gland located at the base of the brain, where it lies in a saddle-shaped depression in the sphenoid bone called the *sella turcica*. A short funnel-shaped stalk, the *infundibulum,* connects the pituitary gland with the hypothalamus (see Chapter 40, Fig. 40.2). The pituitary gland has two components: a posterior lobe (neurohypophysis) or neural component (discussed in Chapter 31) and an anterior lobe (adenohypophysis) or glandular component.

The anterior lobe of the pituitary gland produces ACTH, thyroid-stimulating hormone (TSH), growth hormone (GH), the gonadotrophic hormones (follicle-stimulating hormone [FSH] and luteinizing hormone [LH]), and prolactin (see Chapter 40, Fig. 40.3).[1] Four of these, ACTH, TSH, LH, and FSH, control the secretion of hormones from other endocrine glands. ACTH controls the release of cortisol from the adrenal gland, TSH controls the secretion of thyroid hormone from the thyroid gland, LH regulates sex hormones, and FSH regulates fertility.

Assessment of Hypothalamic–Pituitary Function

The assessment of hypothalamic–pituitary function has been made possible by many newly developed imaging and radio-immunoassay methods. Assessment of the baseline status of the hypothalamic–pituitary target cell hormones involves measuring the following (ideally at 8:00 AM): (1) serum cortisol, (2) serum prolactin, (3) serum thyroxine and TSH, (4) serum testosterone (male)/serum estrogen (female) and serum LH/FSH, (5) serum GH/insulin-like growth factor-1, and (6) plasma osmolality and urine osmolality. Imaging studies (*e.g.,* magnetic resonance imaging [MRI] of the hypothalamus/pituitary) also should be performed as required. When further information regarding pituitary function is required, combined hypothalamic–pituitary function tests are undertaken (although these are performed less often today).[1] These tests consist mainly of hormone stimulation tests (*e.g.,* rapid ACTH stimulation test) or suppression tests (*e.g.,* GH suppression test).

It is often important to test pituitary function, especially if pituitary adenomas are discovered and surgery or radiation treatment is being considered. Diagnostic methods include both static and dynamic testing, and radiologic assessment as required. Any of the systems discussed previously may be affected by either deficiency or excess of the usual hormones secreted.

Pituitary Tumours

Pituitary tumours can be divided into primary or secondary tumours (*i.e.,* metastatic lesions). Tumours of the pituitary can be further divided into functional tumours that secrete pituitary hormones and nonfunctional tumours that do not secrete hormones. They can range in size from small lesions that do not enlarge the gland (microadenomas, <10 mm) to large, expansive tumours (macroadenomas, >10 mm) that erode the sella

TABLE 41.1 FREQUENCY OF ADENOMAS OF THE ANTERIOR PITUITARY

CELL TYPE	HORMONE	FREQUENCY (%)
Lactotrope	Prolactin (PRL)	32
Somatotrope	Growth hormone (GH)	21
Lactotrope/ somatotrope	Mixed PRL/GH	<6
Corticotrope	Adrenocorticotropic hormone (ACTH)	13
Gonadotrope	Follicle-stimulating hormone (FSH)	
	Luteinizing hormone (LH)	<4
Thyrotrope	Thyroid-stimulating hormone (TSH)	
Nonfunctional tumours		25

turcica and impinge on surrounding cranial structures.[1] Small, nonfunctioning tumours are found in up to 20% of adult autopsies. Benign adenomas account for most of the functioning anterior pituitary tumours. Carcinomas of the pituitary are less common. Functional adenomas can be subdivided according to cell type and the type of hormone secreted (Table 41.1).

Hypopituitarism

Hypopituitarism, which is characterized by a decreased secretion of pituitary hormones, is a condition that affects many of the other endocrine systems.[1] Typically, 70% to 90% of the anterior pituitary must be destroyed before hypopituitarism becomes clinically evident. The cause may be congenital or result from a variety of acquired abnormalities (Chart 41.1). The manifestations of hypopituitarism usually occur gradually, but it can present as an acute and life-threatening condition. Patients usually complain of being chronically unfit, with weakness, fatigue, loss of appetite, impairment of sexual function, and cold intolerance. However, ACTH deficiency (secondary adrenal insufficiency) is the most serious endocrine deficiency, leading to weakness, nausea, anorexia, fever, and postural hypotension. Hypopituitarism is associated with increased morbidity and mortality.

Anterior pituitary hormone loss tends to follow a typical sequence, especially with progressive loss of pituitary reserve due to tumours or previous pituitary radiation therapy (which may take 10 to 20 years to produce hypopituitarism). The sequence of loss of pituitary hormones can be remembered by the mnemonic "*G*o *L*ook *F*or *T*he *A*denoma," for *G*H (GH secretion typically is first to be lost), *L*H (results in sex hormone deficiency), *F*SH (causes infertility), *T*SH (leads to secondary hypothyroidism), and *A*CTH (usually the last to become deficient, results in secondary adrenal insufficiency).

Treatment of hypopituitarism includes treating any identified underlying cause. Hormone deficiencies should be treated as dictated by baseline hormone levels, and more

CHART 41.1 CAUSES OF HYPOPITUITARISM

- Tumours and mass lesions—pituitary adenomas, cysts, metastatic cancer, and other lesions
- Pituitary surgery or radiation
- Infiltrative lesions and infections—hemochromatosis, lymphocytic hypophysitis
- Pituitary infarction—infarction of the pituitary gland after substantial blood loss during childbirth (Sheehan syndrome)
- Pituitary apoplexy—sudden hemorrhage into the pituitary gland
- Genetic diseases—rare congenital defects of one or more pituitary hormones
- Empty sella syndrome—an enlarged sella turcica that is not entirely filled with pituitary tissue
- Hypothalamic disorders—tumours and mass lesions (*e.g.,* craniopharyngiomas and metastatic malignancies), hypothalamic radiation, infiltrative lesions (*e.g.,* sarcoidosis), trauma, infections

sophisticated pituitary testing where appropriate (and safe). Cortisol replacement is started when ACTH deficiency is present; thyroid replacement when TSH deficiency is detected; and sex hormone replacement when LH and FSH are deficient. GH replacement is indicated for pediatric GH deficiency, and is being used increasingly to treat GH deficiency in adults.[1,2]

Growth and Growth Hormone Disorders

Several hormones are essential for normal body growth and maturation, including growth hormone (GH), insulin, thyroid hormone, and androgens.[2] In addition to its actions on carbohydrate and fat metabolism, insulin plays an essential role in growth processes. Children with diabetes, particularly those with poor control, often fail to grow normally even though GH levels are normal. When levels of thyroid hormone are lower than normal, bone growth and epiphyseal closure are delayed. Androgens such as testosterone and dihydrotestosterone exert anabolic growth effects through their actions on protein synthesis. Glucocorticoids at excessive levels inhibit growth, apparently because of their antagonistic effect on GH secretion.

Growth Hormone

Growth hormone, also called *somatotropin,* is a 191-amino-acid polypeptide hormone synthesized and secreted by special cells in the anterior pituitary called *somatotropes.*[2] For many years, it was thought that GH was produced primarily during periods of growth. However, this has proved to be incorrect because the rate of GH production in adults is almost as great as in children. GH is necessary for growth and contributes to the regulation of metabolic functions (Fig. 41.1). GH stimulates

GROWTH HORMONE

- Growth hormone (GH), which is produced by somatotropes in the anterior pituitary, is necessary for linear bone growth in children. It also increases the rate at which cells transport amino acids across their cell membranes, and it increases the rate at which they utilize fatty acids and decreases the rate at which they use carbohydrates.
- The effects of GH on linear growth require insulin-like growth factor (IGFs), which are produced mainly by the liver.
- GH (or IGF) deficiency in children interferes with linear bone growth, resulting in short stature or dwarfism.
- In children, GH excess results in increased linear growth or gigantism; in adults it results in overgrowth of the cartilaginous parts of the skeleton, enlargement of the heart and other organs, and metabolic disturbances in fat and carbohydrate metabolism.

all aspects of cartilage growth. One of the most obvious effects of GH is on linear bone growth, resulting from its action on the epiphyseal growth plates of long bones. The width of bone increases because of enhanced periosteal growth. Visceral and endocrine organs, skeletal and cardiac muscle, skin, and connective tissue all undergo increased growth in response to GH. In many instances, the increased growth of visceral and endocrine organs is accompanied by enhanced functional capacity.

For example, increased growth of cardiac muscle is accompanied by an increase in cardiac output.

In addition to its effects on growth, GH facilitates the rate of protein synthesis by all of the cells of the body; it enhances fatty acid mobilization and increases the use of fatty acids for fuel; and it maintains or increases blood glucose levels by decreasing the use of glucose for fuel. GH has an initial effect of increasing insulin levels. However, the predominant effect of prolonged GH excess is to increase glucose levels despite an insulin increase. This is because GH induces a resistance to insulin in the peripheral tissues, inhibiting the uptake of glucose by muscle and adipose tissues.[1]

Many of the effects of GH depend on a family of peptides called *insulin-like growth factors* (IGFs), also called *somatomedins,* which are produced mainly by the liver.[2] GH cannot directly produce bone growth; instead, it acts indirectly by causing the liver to produce IGF. These peptides act on cartilage and bone to promote their growth. At least four IGFs have been identified; of these, IGF-1 (somatomedin C) appears to be the more important in terms of growth, and it is the one that is usually measured in laboratory tests. The IGFs have been sequenced and have structures that are similar to those of proinsulin. This undoubtedly explains the insulin-like activity of the IGFs and the weak action of insulin on growth. IGF levels are themselves influenced by a family of at least six binding factors called *IGF-binding proteins* (IGFBPs).[3]

GH is carried unbound in the plasma and has a half-life of approximately 10 to 20 minutes. The secretion of GH is

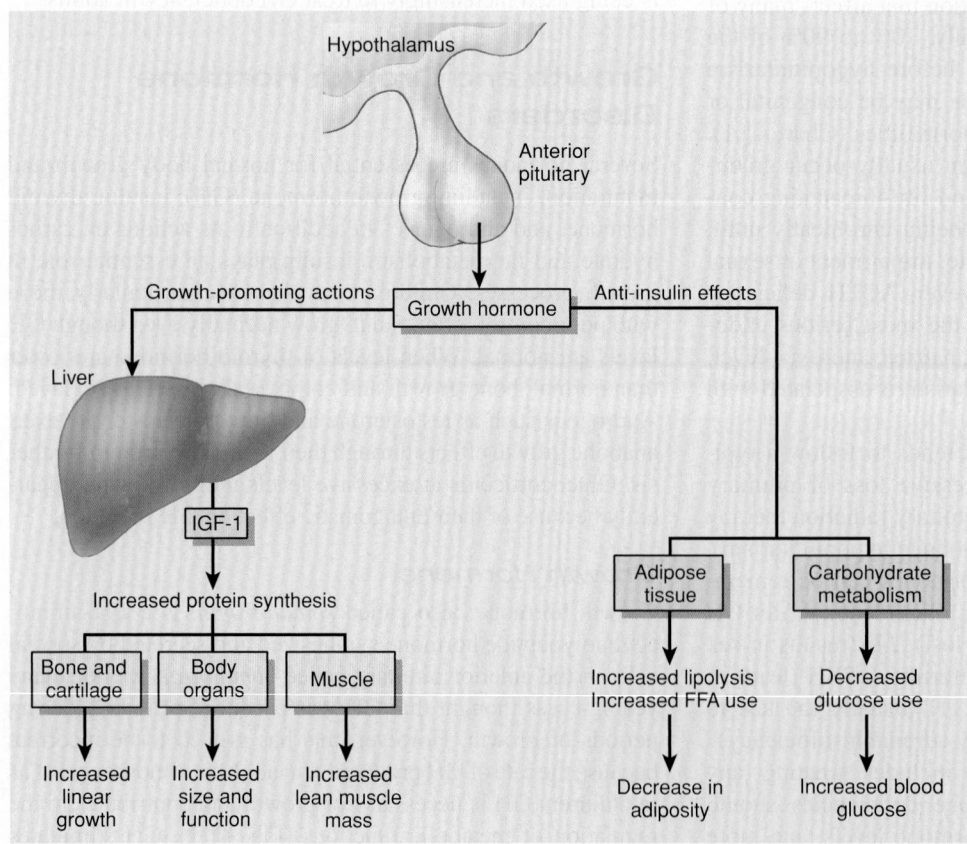

FIGURE 41.1 • Growth-promoting and anti-insulin effects of growth hormone. FFA, free fatty acids; IGF-1, insulin-like growth factor-1.

regulated by two main hypothalamic hormones: GH-releasing hormone (GHRH), which increases GH release, and somatostatin, which inhibits GH release. These hypothalamic influences (*i.e.,* GHRH and somatostatin) are tightly regulated by neural, metabolic, and hormonal factors. The secretion of GH fluctuates over a 24-hour period, with peak levels occurring 1 to 4 hours after onset of sleep (*i.e.,* during sleep stages 3 and 4 [see Chapter 52]). The nocturnal sleep bursts, which account for 70% of daily GH secretion, are greater in children and tend to decrease with age.[1] A third hormone, ghrelin, also may be important. Ghrelin, as well being associated with food intake, seems to act through the GHRH receptor to simulate the GH release but exact role in this regulation is controversial.[4-6]

GH secretion is stimulated by hypoglycemia, fasting, starvation, increased blood levels of amino acids (particularly arginine), and stress conditions such as trauma, excitement, emotional stress, and heavy exercise. GH is inhibited by increased glucose levels, free fatty acid release, cortisol, and obesity. Impairment of secretion, leading to growth retardation, is not uncommon in children with severe emotional deprivation.

Short Stature in Children

Short stature is a condition in which the attained height is well below the third percentile or linear growth is below normal for age and sex. Short stature, or growth retardation, has a variety of causes, including chromosomal abnormalities such as Turner syndrome (see Chapter 7), GH deficiency, hypothyroidism, and panhypopituitarism (*i.e.,* deficiency of *all* pituitary-derived hormones).[2] Other conditions known to cause short stature include protein-calorie malnutrition, chronic diseases such as chronic kidney disease and poorly controlled diabetes mellitus, malabsorption syndromes, and certain therapies such as excessive glucocorticoid administration. Emotional disturbances can lead to functional endocrine disorders, causing psychosocial dwarfism. The causes of short stature are summarized in Chart 41.2.

Accurate measurement of height is an extremely important part of the physical examination of children. Completion of the developmental history and growth charts is essential. Growth curves and growth velocity studies also are needed. Diagnosis of short stature is not made on a single measurement, but is based on sequential height measurements and on velocity of growth and parental height.[5]

The diagnostic procedures for short stature include tests to exclude nonendocrine causes. If the cause is hormonal, extensive hormonal testing procedures are initiated. Usually, GH and IGF-1 levels are determined (IGFBP-3 levels also are useful). Tests can be performed using insulin (to induce hypoglycemia), GHRH, levodopa, and arginine, all of which stimulate GH secretion so that GH reserve can be evaluated.[2,5] Because administration of pharmacologic agents can result in false-negative responses, two or more tests are usually performed. The normal response is a prompt rise in GH. Physiologic tests of GH reserve (*e.g.,* GH response to exercise) also can be performed. Levels of IGF-1 usually reflect those of GH and may be used to indicate GH deficiency. Radiologic films,

---

CHART 41.2 CAUSES OF SHORT STATURE

Variants of Normal
Genetic or "familial" short stature
Constitutional short stature

Low Birth Weight (*e.g.,* intrauterine growth retardation)

Endocrine Disorders
Growth hormone (GH) deficiency
  Primary GH deficiency
    Idiopathic GH deficiency
    Pituitary agenesis
  Secondary GH deficiency (panhypopituitarism)
Biologically inactive GH production
Deficient IGF-1 production in response to normal or
  elevated GH (Laron-type dwarfism)
Hypothyroidism
Diabetes mellitus in poor control
Glucocorticoid excess
  Endogenous (Cushing syndrome)
  Exogenous (glucocorticoid drug treatment)
Abnormal mineral metabolism
  (*e.g.,* pseudohypoparathyroidism)

Chronic Illness and Malnutrition
Chronic organic or systemic disease (*e.g.,* asthma,
  especially when treated with glucocorticoids; heart
  or renal disease)
Nutritional deprivation
Malabsorption syndrome (*e.g.,* celiac sprue)

Functional Endocrine Disorders (Psychosocial Dwarfism)

Chromosomal Disorders (*e.g.,* Turner syndrome)

Skeletal Abnormalities (*e.g.,* achondroplasia)

---

most commonly of the hand-wrist, may reveal delayed bone age or skeletal defects facilitating this diagnosis.[5] MRI of the hypothalamic–pituitary area is recommended if a lesion is clinically suspected. After the cause of short stature has been determined, treatment can be initiated.

Genetic and Constitutional Short Stature. Two forms of short stature, genetic short stature and constitutional short stature, are not disease states but variations from population norms. Genetically short children tend to be well proportioned and to have a height close to the mid-parental height of their parents. The mid-parental height or target height estimate for boys can be calculated by adding 13 cm to the height of the mother, adding the father's height, and dividing the total by two. For girls, 13 cm is subtracted from the father's height, the result is added to the mother's height, and the total is divided by two. Ninety-five percent of children are within 8.5 cm (*i.e.*, ± 2 standard deviations) of the mid-parental height.[5]

Constitutional short stature is a term used to describe children (particularly boys) who have moderately short stature, thin build, delayed skeletal and sexual maturation, and absence of other causes of decreased growth. *Catch-up growth* is a term used to describe an abnormally high growth rate that occurs after the correction of growth-retarding disorders. It can occur after the initiation of therapy for GH deficiency and hypothyroidism and management of chronic diseases. This is usually short lived and as a child approaches normal height for age standard growth is resumed.[2]

Psychosocial Dwarfism. Psychosocial dwarfism involves a functional hypopituitarism and is seen in some emotionally deprived children. These children usually present with poor growth, potbelly, and poor eating and drinking habits. Typically, there is a history of disturbed family relationships in which the child has been severely neglected or disciplined. Often, the neglect is confined to one child in the family. GH function usually returns to normal after the child is removed from the constraining environment. The prognosis depends on improvement in behaviour and catch-up growth. Family therapy is usually indicated, and foster care may be necessary.

Growth Hormone Deficiency in Children

There are several forms of GH deficiency that present in childhood. Children with idiopathic GH deficiency lack the hypothalamic GHRH but have adequate somatotropes, whereas children with pituitary tumours or agenesis of the pituitary lack somatotropes. The term *panhypopituitarism* refers to conditions that cause a deficiency of all of the anterior pituitary hormones. In a rare form of dwarfism called *Laron syndrome*, GH levels are normal or elevated, but there is a hereditary defect in IGF production that can be treated directly with IGF-1 replacement.[3]

Congenital GH deficiency is associated with decreased birth length, followed by a decrease in growth rate that can be identified by careful measurement during the first year and that becomes obvious by 1 to 2 years of age. Persons with classic GH deficiency have normal intelligence, short stature, obesity with immature facial features, and some delay in skeletal maturation (Fig. 41.2). Puberty often is delayed, and males with the disorder have microphallus (abnormally small penis), especially if the condition is accompanied by gonadotropin-releasing hormone (GnRH) deficiency. In the neonate, GH deficiency can lead to hypoglycemia and seizures; if ACTH deficiency also is present, the hypoglycemia often is more severe. Acquired GH deficiency develops in later childhood; it may be caused by a hypothalamic–pituitary tumour, particularly if it is accompanied by other pituitary hormone deficiencies.

When short stature is caused by a GH deficiency, recombinant human GH (rhGH) replacement therapy is the treatment of choice. rhGH is administered by daily subcutaneous injection during the period of active growth, and can be continued into adulthood. With early diagnosis and treatment plus

FIGURE 41.2 • Child with growth hormone deficiency. A 5.5-year-old boy (**left**) with growth hormone deficiency was significantly shorter than his fraternal twin sister (**right**), with discrepancy beginning early in childhood. Notice his chubby, immature appearance compared with his sister. (From Korenman S. G., Molitch M. E. (Eds.). (2000). *Atlas of clinical endocrinology, Volume IV: Neuroendocrinology and pituitary disease* (p. 38). Philadelphia, PA: Current Medicine.)

monitoring and appropriate rhGH titration, most will reach their genetic potential for adult height.[2]

Children with short stature due to Turner syndrome and chronic renal insufficiency also are treated with rhGH. This hormone replacement may be considered for children with short stature but without GH deficiency. Several studies suggest that short-term treatment with GH increases the rate of growth in these children. Although the effect of GH on adult height is not great, it can result in improved psychological well-being. There are concerns about misuse of the drug to produce additional growth in children with normal GH function who are of near-normal height. Guidelines for use of the hormone continue to be established.[2]

Growth Hormone Deficiency in Adults

There are two categories of GH deficiency in adults: (1) GH deficiency that was present in childhood, and (2) GH deficiency that developed during adulthood, mainly as the result of hypopituitarism resulting from a pituitary tumour or its treatment or central nervous system trauma.[6] GH levels also can decline with aging, and there has been interest in the effects of declining GH levels in the elderly (described as the *somatopause*). GH replacement obviously is important in the growing child; however, the role in adults (especially for the somatopause) is being assessed. Some of the differences between childhood and adult-onset GH deficiency are described in Table 41.2.

TABLE 41.2 DIFFERENCES BETWEEN CHILDHOOD AND ADULT-ONSET GROWTH HORMONE DEFICIENCY

CHARACTERISTIC	CHILDHOOD ONSET	ADULT ONSET
Adult height	↓	Normal
Body fat	↑	↑
Lean body mass	↓↓	↓
Bone mineral density	↓	Normal, ↓
Insulin-like growth factor (IGF)-1	↓↓	Normal, ↓
IGF binding protein-3	↓	Normal
Low-density lipoprotein cholesterol	↑	↑
High-density lipoprotein cholesterol	Normal, ↓	↓

Several studies have shown that cardiovascular mortality is increased in GH-deficient adults.[6] A higher prevalence of atherosclerotic plaques and endothelial dysfunction has been reported in both childhood and adult GH deficiency. The GH deficiency syndrome is associated with a cluster of cardiovascular risk factors, including central adiposity (associated with increased visceral fat), insulin resistance, and dyslipidemia. These features also are associated with the *metabolic syndrome* (see Chapter 42). In addition to these so-called traditional cardiovascular risk factors, nontraditional cardiovascular risk factors (*e.g.,* high-sensitivity C-reactive protein [hsCRP], which is a marker of the inflammatory pathway) are also elevated. GH therapy can improve many of these factors.[2,6]

The diagnosis of GH deficiency in adults is made by finding subnormal serum GH responses to provocative stimuli. A low IGF-1 level in the presence of known pituitary disease may also indicate GH deficiency. Measurements of the basal GH levels do not distinguish reliably between normal and subnormal GH secretion in adults. Insulin-induced hypoglycemia is the gold standard test for GH reserve. The arginine plus GHRH test is probably the next best test. Other stimulation tests involve the use of arginine, L-dopa, clonidine (an α-adrenergic agonist), glucagon, or GHRH alone.[6]

GH replacement therapy may lead to increased lean body mass and decreased fat mass, increased bone mineral density, increased glomerular filtration rate, decreased lipid levels, increased exercise capacity, and improved sense of well-being in GH-deficient adults.[6] The most common side effects of GH treatment in adults with hypopituitarism are peripheral edema, arthralgias and myalgias, carpal tunnel syndrome, paresthesias, and decreased glucose tolerance. Side effects appear to be more common in people who are older and heavier, and who are overtreated, as judged by a high serum IGF-1 concentration during therapy. Women seem to tolerate higher doses better than men.[1–3]

Tall Stature in Children

Just as there are children who are short for their age and sex, there also are children who are tall for their age and sex.[2,7]

Tall stature is defined as height above the 97th percentile for age and sex.[8] Normal variants of tall stature include genetic tall stature and constitutional tall stature. Children with exceptionally tall parents tend to be taller than children with shorter parents. The term *constitutional tall stature* is used to describe a child who is taller than his or her peers and is growing at a velocity that is within the normal range for bone age. Other causes of tall stature are genetic or chromosomal disorders such as Marfan syndrome, homocystinuria, or XYY syndrome (see Chapter 7).[7,8] Endocrine causes of tall stature include sexual precocity because of early onset of estrogen and androgen secretion and excessive GH.

Exceptionally tall children (*i.e.,* genetic tall stature and constitutional tall stature) can be treated with sex hormones—estrogens in girls and testosterone in boys—to effect early epiphyseal closure. Such treatment is undertaken only after full consideration of the risks involved. To be effective, such treatment must be instituted 3 to 4 years before expected epiphyseal fusion.[2,7]

Growth Hormone Excess in Children

Growth hormone excess occurring before puberty and the fusion of the epiphyses of the long bones results in *gigantism* (Fig. 41.3). Excessive secretion of GH by somatotrope adenomas causes gigantism in the prepubertal child. It occurs when

FIGURE 41.3 • Primary gigantism. A 22-year-old man with gigantism due to excess growth hormone is shown to the left of his identical twin. (From Gagel R. F., McCutcheon I. E. (1999). Images in clinical medicine. *New England Journal of Medicine, 340,* 524. Copyright © 2003. Massachusetts Medical Society.)

the epiphyses are not fused and high levels of IGF stimulate excessive skeletal growth. Fortunately, the condition is rare because of early recognition and treatment of the adenoma.

Growth Hormone Excess in Adults

When GH excess occurs in adulthood or after the epiphyses of the long bones have fused, the condition is referred to as *acromegaly*. Acromegaly results from excess levels of GH that stimulate the hepatic secretion of IGF-1, which causes most of the clinical manifestations of acromegaly. The annual incidence of acromegaly is 3 to 4 cases per 1 million people, with a mean age at the time of diagnosis of 40 years.[1]

The most common cause (95%) of acromegaly is a somatotrope adenoma. Approximately 75% of persons with acromegaly have a somatotrope macroadenoma at the time of diagnosis, and most of the remainder have microadenomas. The other causes of acromegaly (<5%) are excess secretion of GHRH by hypothalamic tumours, ectopic GHRH secretion by nonendocrine tumours such as carcinoid tumours or small cell lung cancers, and ectopic secretion of GH by nonendocrine tumours.[1,9]

The disorder usually has an insidious onset, and symptoms often are present for a considerable period before a diagnosis is made. When the production of excessive GH occurs after the epiphyses of the long bones have closed, as in the adult, the person cannot grow taller, but the soft tissues continue to grow. Enlargement of the small bones of the hands and feet and of the membranous bones of the face and skull results in a pronounced enlargement of the hands and feet, a broad and bulbous nose, a protruding lower jaw, and a slanting forehead (Fig. 41.4). The teeth become splayed, causing a disturbed bite and difficulty in chewing. The cartilaginous structures in the larynx and respiratory tract also become enlarged, resulting in a deepening of the voice and tendency to develop bronchitis. Vertebral changes often lead to kyphosis, or hunchback. Bone overgrowth often leads to arthralgias and degenerative arthritis of the spine, hips, and knees. Virtually every organ of the body is increased in size. Enlargement of the heart and accelerated atherosclerosis may lead to an early death.[1,9]

The metabolic effects of excess levels of GH include alterations in fat and carbohydrate metabolism. GH causes increased release of free fatty acids from adipose tissue, leading to increased concentration of free fatty acids in body fluids. In addition, GH enhances the formation of ketones and the use of free fatty acids for energy in preference to use of carbohydrates and proteins. GH exerts multiple effects on carbohydrate metabolism, including decreased glucose uptake by tissues such as skeletal muscle and adipose tissue, increased glucose production by the liver, and increased insulin secretion. Each of these changes results in GH-induced insulin resistance (see Chapter 42). This leads to glucose intolerance, which stimulates the beta cells of the pancreas to produce additional insulin. Long-term elevation of GH results in overstimulation of the beta cells, causing them literally to "burn out." Impaired glucose tolerance occurs in as much as 50% to 70% of persons with acromegaly; overt diabetes mellitus subsequently can result.[1]

FIGURE 41.4 • Clinical manifestations of acromegaly.

Labels on figure:
- Somatotropic adenoma of pituitary
- Acromegalic facies
- Goiter
- Cardiomegaly (hypertension)
- Hyperostosis (thoracic vertebrae)
- Barrel chest
- Abnormal glucose tolerance secondary to insulin resistance
- Increased size (hands, feet)
- Male sexual dysfunction (or menstrual disorders in women)
- Degenerative arthritis
- Peripheral neuropathy
- Thickened skin (hypertrophy of sebaceous and sweat glands)

The pituitary gland is located in the pituitary fossa of the sphenoid bone (*i.e.,* sella turcica), which lies directly below the optic nerve. Enlargement of the pituitary gland eventually causes erosion of the surrounding bone, and because of its location, this can lead to headaches, visual field defects resulting from compression of the optic nerve (classically, bitemporal hemianopia), and palsies of cranial nerves III, IV, and VI. Compression of other pituitary structures can cause secondary hypothyroidism, hypogonadism, and adrenal insufficiency. The hypogonadism can result from direct damage to the hypothalamic or pituitary system, or indirectly from hyperprolactinemia due to prevention of the prolactin inhibitory factor (dopamine) from reaching pituitary lactotropes (cells that secrete prolactin) because of damage by the pituitary tumour.

Other manifestations include excessive sweating with an unpleasant odour, oily skin, heat intolerance, moderate weight gain, muscle weakness and fatigue, menstrual irregularities, and decreased libido. Hypertension is relatively common. Sleep apnea syndrome is present in 50% to 70% of patients. The pathogenesis of the sleep apnea syndrome is obstructive in the majority of patients, due to increased pharyngeal soft tissue accumulation. Paresthesias may develop because of nerve entrapment and compression caused by excess soft tissue and accumulation of subcutaneous fluid (especially carpal tunnel syndrome). Acromegaly also is associated with an increased risk of colonic polyps and colorectal cancer. The mortality rate of patients with acromegaly is two to three times the expected rate, mostly from cardiovascular diseases and cancer. The cardiovascular disease results from the combination of cardiomyopathy, hypertension, insulin resistance and hyperinsulinemia, and hyperlipidemia.[1,9]

Acromegaly often develops insidiously, and only a small number of persons seek medical care because of changes in appearance. The diagnosis of acromegaly is facilitated by the typical features of the disorder—enlargement of the hands and feet and coarsening of facial features. Laboratory tests to detect elevated levels of GH not suppressed by a glucose load are used to confirm the diagnosis. MRI scans can detect and localize the pituitary lesions. Because most of the effects of GH are mediated by IGF-1, IGF-1 levels may provide information about disease activity.

The treatment goals for acromegaly focus on the correction of metabolic abnormalities, and include normalization of the GH response to an oral glucose load; normalization of IGF-1 levels to age- and sex-matched control levels; removal or reduction of the tumour mass; relieving the central pressure effects; improvement of adverse clinical features; and normalization of the mortality rate.[9] Pituitary tumours can be removed surgically using the transsphenoidal approach or, if that is not possible, a transfrontal craniotomy. Conventional radiation therapy is rarely used as remission (reduction in GH levels) may not occur for several years after therapy. Radiation therapy also significantly increases the risk of hypopituitarism, leading to hypothyroidism, hypoadrenalism, and hypogonadism. Gamma knife radiosurgery can be used for tumours confined to the sella turcica but currently only 50% to 70% remission rates occur two years after this therapy.[1]

Medical therapy is usually given in an adjunctive role.[1] Somatostatin analogs (especially long-acting formulations of octreotide and lanreotide) produce feedback inhibition of GH, and are effective in the medical management of acromegaly. Dopamine agonists (*e.g.,* cabergoline) reduce GH levels and have been used with some success in the medical management of acromegaly. Growth hormone receptor antagonists (*e.g.,* pegvisomant) are analogs of human GH that have been structurally altered. GH receptor antagonists bind to GH receptors on the cell surfaces, where they block the binding of endogenous GH and thus interfere with GH signal transduction. This results in a decrease in serum IGF-1 levels in more than 90% of patients.[1,10]

Isosexual Precocious Puberty

Isosexual or central precocious puberty is defined as early activation of the hypothalamic–pituitary–gonadal axis, resulting in the development of appropriate sexual characteristics and fertility.[11,12] Precocious puberty is defined as the appearance of secondary sexual development before the age of 7 years in white girls and 6 years in African-American girls. In boys of both races, the lower age limit remains 9 years; however, it is recognized that puberty can develop earlier in boys with obesity (an increasingly common problem).[12] Precocious sexual development may be idiopathic or may be caused by gonadal, adrenal, or hypothalamic disease. Benign and malignant tumours of the central nervous system (CNS) can cause precocious puberty. These tumours are thought to remove the inhibitory influences normally exerted on the hypothalamus during childhood. CNS tumours are found more often in boys with precocious puberty than in girls. In girls, most cases are idiopathic.[12]

Diagnosis of precocious puberty is based on physical findings of early thelarche (*i.e.,* beginning of breast development), adrenarche (*i.e.,* beginning of augmented adrenal androgen production), and menarche (*i.e.,* beginning of menstrual function) in girls. The most common sign in boys is early genital enlargement. Radiologic findings looking at the wrist-hand may indicate advanced bone age. Persons with precocious puberty usually are tall for their age as children but short as adults because of the early closure of the epiphyses. MRI or CT should be used to exclude intracranial lesions.

Depending on the cause of precocious puberty, the treatment may involve surgery, medication, or no treatment. Administration of a long-acting GnRH agonist results in a decrease in pituitary responsiveness to GnRH, leading to decreased secretion of gonadotropic hormones and sex steroids (due to downregulation of GnRH receptors). Parents often need education, support, and anticipatory guidance in dealing with their feelings and the child's physical needs and in relating to a child who appears older than his or her years.[11,12]

IN SUMMARY

Pituitary tumours can result in deficiencies or excesses of pituitary hormones. Hypopituitarism, which is characterized by a decreased secretion of pituitary hormones, is a condition that affects many of the other endocrine systems. Depending on the extent of the disorder, it can result in decreased levels of GH, thyroid hormones, adrenal corticosteroid hormones, and testosterone in the male and estrogens and progesterone in the female.

A number of hormones are essential for normal body growth and maturation, including GH, insulin, thyroid hormone, and androgens. GH exerts its growth effects through IGF-1. GH also exerts an effect on metabolism and is produced in the adult and in the child. Its metabolic effects include a decrease in peripheral use of carbohydrates and an increased mobilization and use of fatty acids.

In children, alterations in growth include short stature, isosexual precocious puberty, and tall stature. Short stature is a condition in which the attained height is well below the third percentile or the linear growth velocity is below normal for a child's age or sex. Short stature can occur as a variant of normal growth (*i.e.,* genetic short stature or constitutional short stature) or as the result of endocrine disorders, chronic illness, malnutrition, emotional disturbances, or chromosomal disorders. Short stature resulting from GH deficiency can be treated with recombinant human GH preparations. In adults, GH deficiency represents a deficiency carried over from childhood or one that develops during adulthood as the result of a pituitary tumour or its treatment. GH levels also can decline with aging, and there has been interest in the effects of declining GH levels in the elderly (described as the somatopause).

Tall stature refers to the condition in which children are tall for their age and sex. It can occur as a variant of normal growth (*i.e.,* genetic tall stature or constitutional tall stature) or as the result of a chromosomal abnormality or GH excess. GH excess in adults results in acromegaly, which involves proliferation of bone, cartilage, and soft tissue along with the metabolic effects of excessive hormone levels. Isosexual precocious puberty defines a condition of early activation of the hypothalamic–pituitary–gonadal axis, resulting in the development of appropriate sexual characteristics and fertility. It causes tall stature during childhood but results in short stature in adulthood because of the early closure of the epiphyses.

THYROID DISORDERS

After completing this section of the chapter, you should be able to meet the following objectives:

* Characterize the synthesis, transport, and regulation of thyroid hormone.
* Diagram the hypothalamic–pituitary–thyroid feedback system.
* Describe tests used in the diagnosis and management of thyroid disorders.
* Relate the functions of thyroid hormone to hypothyroidism and hyperthyroidism.
* Characterize the manifestations and treatment of myxedematous coma and thyroid storm.

Control of Thyroid Function

The thyroid gland is a shield-shaped structure located immediately below the larynx in the anterior middle portion of the neck (Fig. 41.5A). It is composed of a large number of tiny, saclike structures called *follicles* (Fig. 41.5B). These are the functional units of the thyroid. Each follicle is formed by a single layer of epithelial (follicular) cells and is filled with a secretory substance called *colloid,* which consists largely of a glycoprotein–iodine complex called *thyroglobulin.*

The thyroglobulin that fills the thyroid follicles is a large glycoprotein molecule that contains 140 tyrosine amino acids. In the process of thyroid synthesis, iodine is attached to these tyrosine molecules. Both thyroglobulin and iodide are secreted into the colloid of the follicle by the follicular cells.

The thyroid is remarkably efficient in its use of iodide. A daily absorption of 150 to 200 μg or 50 mg per year of dietary iodide is sufficient to form normal quantities of thyroid hormone.[13,14] In the process of removing it from the blood and storing it for future use, iodide is pumped into the follicular cells against a concentration gradient. Iodide (I^-) is transported across the basement membrane of the thyroid cells by an intrinsic membrane protein called the Na^+/I^- *symporter* (NIS).[14] At the apical border, a second I^- transport protein called *pendrin* moves iodine into the colloid, where it is involved in hormonogenesis. The NIS derives its energy from Na^+K^+-ATPase, which drives the process. As a result, the concentration of iodide in the normal thyroid gland is approximately 40 times that in the blood.[13]

The NIS is stimulated by both TSH and the TSH receptor–stimulating antibody found in Graves disease (to be discussed). Pendrin, encoded by the Pendred syndrome gene (*PDS*), is a transporter of chloride and iodide. Mutations in the *PDS* gene have been found in patients with goitre and congenital deafness (Pendred syndrome).[13]

Once inside the follicle, most of the iodide is oxidized by the enzyme thyroid peroxidase (TPO) in a reaction that facilitates combination with a tyrosine molecule to form monoiodotyrosine (MIT) and then diiodotyrosine (DIT). Two diiodotyrosine residues are coupled to form thyroxine (T_4), or a monoiodotyrosine and a diiodotyrosine are coupled to form triiodothyronine (T_3). Only T_4 (90%) and T_3 (10%) are released into the circulation (Fig. 41.5C). There is evidence that T_3 is the more potent form of the hormone and that T_4 is converted to T_3 before it can act physiologically.

Thyroid hormones are bound to thyroxine-binding globulin (TBG) and other plasma proteins for transport in the blood. Only the free hormone enters cells and regulates the pituitary feedback mechanism. Protein-bound thyroid hormone forms a large reservoir that is slowly drawn on as free thyroid hormone is needed. There are three major thyroid-binding proteins: TBG, transthyretin (formerly known as thyroxine-binding prealbumin [TBPA]), and albumin. More than 99% of T_4 and T_3 is carried in the bound form. TBG carries approximately 70% of T_4 and T_3; transthyretin binds approximately 10% of circulating T_4 and lesser amounts of T_3; and albumin binds approximately 15% of circulating T_4 and T_3.[13]

A number of disease conditions and pharmacologic agents can decrease the amount of binding protein in the plasma or influence the binding of hormone. Congenital TBG deficiency is an X-linked trait that occurs in 1 of every 5,000 live births. Glucocorticoid medications and systemic disease conditions such as protein malnutrition, nephrotic syndrome, and cirrhosis decrease TBG concentrations. Medications such as phenytoin,

B

Blood capillary   Follicular cell   Lumen with colloid

A

Iodide transporter

I⁻ → I⁻ → I⁻

Amino acids

TPO

Iodination of thyroglobulin

ER → TG → TG | MIT | DIT

Thyroglobulin in vesicles

Triiodothyronine (T₃)
Thyroxine (T₄)

Pinocytosis

Secretion T₃ ← T₃
T₄   T₄

Proteolysis

Thyroxine (T₄)

HO —⬡— O —⬡— CH_2–CH–$COOH$ with NH_2

C   Triiodothyronine (T₃)

HO —⬡— O —⬡— CH_2–CH–$COOH$ with NH_2

FIGURE 41.5 • **A:** The thyroid gland. **B:** Microscopic structure of thyroid follicles. **C:** Cellular mechanisms for transport of iodide (I⁻), oxidation of I⁻ by thyroperoxidase (TPO), coupling of oxidized I⁻ with thyroglobulin to thyroid hormones, and movement of T₃ and T₄ into the follicular cell by pinocytosis and release into the blood.

salicylates, and diazepam can affect the binding of thyroid hormone to normal concentrations of binding proteins.

The secretion of thyroid hormone is regulated by the hypothalamic–pituitary–thyroid feedback system (Fig. 41.6). In this system, thyrotropin-releasing hormone (TRH), which is produced by the hypothalamus, controls the release of TSH from the anterior pituitary gland. TSH increases the overall activity of the thyroid gland by increasing thyroglobulin breakdown and the release of thyroid hormone from follicles into the bloodstream, activating the iodide pump (by increasing NIS activity), increasing the oxidation of iodide and the coupling of iodide to tyrosine, and increasing the number and the size of the follicle cells. The effect of TSH on the release of thyroid hormones occurs within approximately 30 minutes, but the other effects require days or weeks.[14]

Increased levels of thyroid hormone act in the feedback inhibition of TRH or TSH. High levels of iodide also cause a temporary decrease in thyroid activity that lasts for several weeks, probably through a direct inhibition of TSH on the thyroid. Cold exposure is one of the strongest stimuli for increased thyroid hormone production and probably is mediated through TRH from the hypothalamus. Various emotional reactions also can affect the output of TRH and TSH and therefore indirectly affect secretion of thyroid hormones.

Actions of Thyroid Hormone

All the major organs in the body are affected by altered levels of thyroid hormone. Thyroid hormone has two major functions: it increases metabolism and protein synthesis, and it is necessary for growth and development in children, including mental development and attainment of sexual maturity. These actions are mainly mediated by T₃. In the cell, T₃ binds to a nuclear receptor, resulting in transcription of specific thyroid hormone response genes.[13]

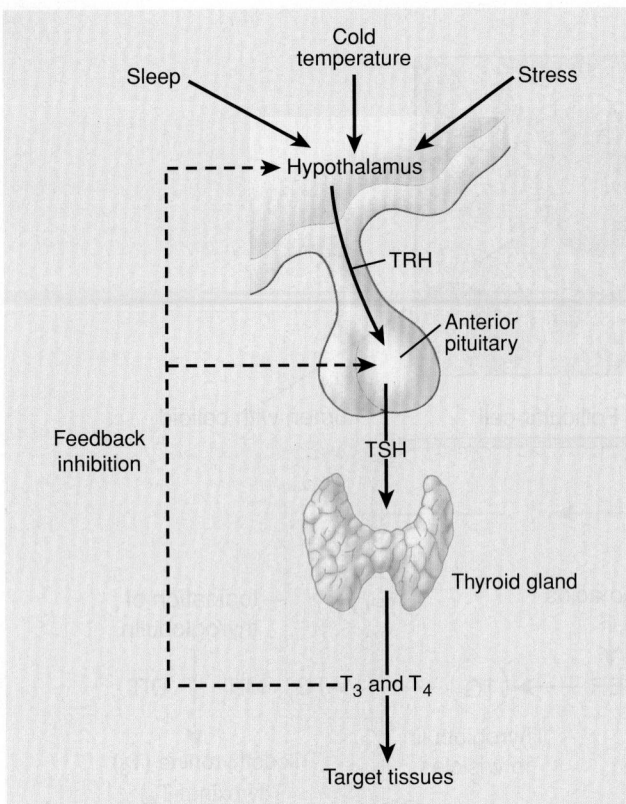

FIGURE 41.6 • The hypothalamic–pituitary–thyroid feedback system, which regulates the body levels of thyroid hormone. TRH, thyrotropin-releasing hormone; TSH, thyroid-stimulating hormone.

Metabolic Rate. Thyroid hormone increases the metabolism of all body tissues except the retina, spleen, testes, and lungs. The basal metabolic rate can increase by 60% to 100% above normal when large amounts of T_4 are present. As a result of this higher metabolism, the rate of glucose, fat, and protein use increases. Lipids are mobilized from adipose tissue, and the catabolism of cholesterol by the liver is increased. Blood

THYROID HORMONE

- Thyroid hormone increases the metabolism and protein synthesis in nearly all of the tissues of the body.
- It also is necessary for growth and brain development in infants and small children. Infants born with decreased or absent thyroid function have impaired mental and physical development.
- When hypothyroidism occurs in older children or adults, it produces a decrease in metabolic rate, an accumulation of a hydrophilic mucopolysaccharide substance (myxedema) in the connective tissues throughout the body, and an elevation in serum cholesterol.
- Hyperthyroidism has an effect opposite that of hypothyroidism. It produces an increase in metabolic rate and oxygen consumption, increased use of metabolic fuels, and increased sympathetic nervous system responsiveness.

levels of cholesterol are decreased in hyperthyroidism and increased in hypothyroidism. Muscle proteins are broken down and used as fuel, probably accounting for some of the muscle fatigue that occurs with hyperthyroidism. The absorption of glucose from the gastrointestinal tract is increased. Because vitamins are essential parts of metabolic enzymes and coenzymes, an increase in metabolic rate "speeds up" the use of vitamins and tends to cause vitamin deficiency.[14]

Cardiovascular Function. Cardiovascular and respiratory functions are strongly affected by thyroid function. With an increase in metabolism, there is a rise in oxygen consumption and production of metabolic end products, with an accompanying increase in vasodilation. Blood flow to the skin, in particular, is augmented as a means of dissipating the body heat that results from the higher metabolism. Blood volume, cardiac output, and ventilation all are increased as a means of maintaining blood flow and oxygen delivery to body tissues. Heart rate and cardiac contractility are enhanced as a means of maintaining the needed cardiac output. On the other hand, blood pressure is likely to change very little because the increase in vasodilation tends to offset the increase in cardiac output.

Gastrointestinal Function. Thyroid hormone enhances gastrointestinal function, causing an increase in motility and production of gastrointestinal secretions that often results in diarrhea. An increase in appetite and food intake accompanies the higher metabolic rate that occurs with increased thyroid hormone levels. At the same time, weight loss occurs because of the increased use of calories.

Neuromuscular Effects. Thyroid hormone has marked effects on neural control of muscle function and tone. Slight elevations in hormone levels cause skeletal muscles to react more vigorously, and a drop in hormone levels causes muscles to react more sluggishly. In the hyperthyroid state, a fine muscle tremor is present. The cause of this tremor is unknown, but it may represent an increased sensitivity of the neural synapses in the spinal cord that control muscle tone. In the infant, thyroid hormone is necessary for normal brain development. The hormone enhances cerebration; in the hyperthyroid state, it causes extreme nervousness, anxiety, and difficulty in sleeping.

Evidence suggests a strong interaction between thyroid hormone and the sympathetic nervous system. Many of the signs and symptoms of hyperthyroidism suggest overactivity of the sympathetic division of the autonomic nervous system, such as tachycardia, palpitations, and sweating. Tremor, restlessness, anxiety, and diarrhea also may reflect autonomic nervous system imbalances. Drugs that block sympathetic activity have proved to be valuable adjuncts in the treatment of hyperthyroidism because of their ability to relieve some of these undesirable symptoms.

Tests of Thyroid Function

Various tests aid in the diagnosis of thyroid disorders.[13–16] Measures of T_3, T_4, and TSH have been made available through immunoassay methods. The free T_4 test measures the unbound

TABLE 41.3 MANIFESTATIONS OF HYPOTHYROID AND HYPERTHYROID STATES

LEVEL OF ORGANIZATION	HYPOTHYROIDISM	HYPERTHYROIDISM
Basal metabolic rate	Decreased	Increased
Sensitivity to catecholamines	Decreased	Increased
General features	Myxedematous features Deep voice Impaired growth (child)	Exophthalmos (in Graves disease) Lid lag Accelerated growth (child)
Blood cholesterol levels	Increased	Decreased
General behaviour	Mental retardation (infant) Mental and physical sluggishness Somnolence	Restlessness, irritability, anxiety Hyperkinesis Wakefulness
Cardiovascular function	Decreased cardiac output Bradycardia	Increased cardiac output Tachycardia, atrial arrhythmias, palpitations
Gastrointestinal function	Constipation Decreased appetite	Diarrhea Increased appetite
Respiratory function	Hypoventilation	Dyspnea
Muscle tone and reflexes	Decreased	Increased, with tremor and twitching
Temperature tolerance	Cold intolerance	Heat intolerance
Skin and hair	Decreased sweating Coarse and dry skin and hair	Increased sweating Thin and silky skin and hair
Weight	Gain	Loss

portion of T_4 that is free to enter cells to produce its effects. TSH levels are used to differentiate between primary and secondary thyroid disorders. T_3, T_4, and free T_4 levels are low in primary hypothyroidism, and the TSH level is elevated. The assessment of thyroid autoantibodies (*e.g.,* anti-TPO antibodies in Hashimoto thyroiditis) is important in the diagnostic workup and consequent follow-up of patients with thyroid disorders.

The radioiodine (^{123}I) uptake test measures the ability of the thyroid gland to remove and concentrate iodine from the blood. Thyroid scans (^{123}I, ^{99m}Tc-pertechnetate) can be used to detect thyroid nodules and determine the functional activity of the thyroid gland. Ultrasonography can be used to differentiate cystic from solid thyroid lesions, and CT and MRI scans are used to demonstrate tracheal compression or impingement on other neighbouring structures. Fine-needle aspiration biopsy of a thyroid nodule has proved to be the best method for differentiation of benign from malignant thyroid disease.[13]

Alterations in Thyroid Function

An alteration in thyroid function can represent a hypofunctional or a hyperfunctional state. The manifestations of these two altered states are summarized in Table 41.3. Disorders of the thyroid may be due to a congenital defect in thyroid development, or they may develop later in life, with a gradual or sudden onset.

Goitre is an increase in the size of the thyroid gland (Fig. 41.7). It can occur in hypothyroid, euthyroid, and hyperthyroid states. Goitres may be diffuse, involving the entire gland without evidence of nodularity, or they may contain

FIGURE 41.7 • Goitre. The thyroid has enlarged to produce a conspicuous neck mass. (From Rubin R., Strayer D. S. (Eds.). (2012). *Rubin's pathology: Clinicopathologic foundations of medicine* (6th ed., p. 1047). Philadelphia, PA: Lippincott Williams & Wilkins.)

nodules. Diffuse goitres usually become nodular. Goitres may be toxic, producing signs of extreme hyperthyroidism, or thyrotoxicosis, or they may be nontoxic. Diffuse nontoxic and multinodular goitres are the result of compensatory hypertrophy and hyperplasia of follicular epithelium from some derangement that impairs thyroid hormone output.

The degree of thyroid enlargement is usually proportional to the extent and duration of thyroid deficiency. Multinodular goitres produce the largest thyroid enlargements. When sufficiently enlarged, they may compress the esophagus and trachea, causing difficulty in swallowing, a choking sensation, and inspiratory stridor. Such lesions also may compress the superior vena cava, producing distension of the veins of the neck and upper extremities, edema of the eyelids and conjunctiva, and syncope with coughing.

Hypothyroidism

Hypothyroidism can occur as a congenital or an acquired defect. Congenital hypothyroidism develops prenatally and is present at birth. Acquired hypothyroidism develops later in life because of primary disease of the thyroid gland or secondary to disorders of hypothalamic or pituitary origin.

Congenital Hypothyroidism

Congenital hypothyroidism is a common cause of preventable mental retardation. It affects approximately 1 of 4,000 infants. Hypothyroidism in the infant may result from a congenital lack of the thyroid gland or from abnormal biosynthesis of thyroid hormone or deficient TSH secretion. With congenital lack of the thyroid gland, the infant usually appears normal and functions normally at birth because hormones have been supplied in utero by the mother.

Thyroid hormone is essential for normal growth and brain development, almost half of which occurs during the first 6 months of life. If untreated, congenital hypothyroidism causes mental retardation and impairs physical growth. The manifestations of untreated congenital hypothyroidism are referred to as *cretinism*. However, the term does not apply to the normally developing infant in whom replacement thyroid hormone therapy was instituted shortly after birth. Fortunately, universal neonatal screening tests have been instituted to detect congenital hypothyroidism during early infancy. Screening is usually done in the hospital nursery. In this test, a drop of blood is taken from the infant's heel and analyzed for T_4 and TSH.

Transient congenital hypothyroidism has been recognized more frequently since the introduction of neonatal screening. It is characterized by high TSH levels and low or normal thyroid hormone levels. The fetal and infant thyroids are sensitive to iodine excess. Iodine crosses the placenta and mammary glands and is readily absorbed by infant skin. Transient hypothyroidism may be caused by maternal or infant exposure to substances such as povidone-iodine used as a disinfectant (*i.e.*, vaginal douche or skin disinfectant in the nursery). Antithyroid drugs such as propylthiouracil and methimazole can cross the placenta and block fetal thyroid function.

Congenital hypothyroidism is treated by hormone replacement. Evidence indicates that it is important to normalize T_4 levels as rapidly as possible because a delay is accompanied by poorer psychomotor and mental development. Dosage levels are adjusted as the child grows. When early and adequate treatment regimens are followed, the risk of mental retardation in infants detected by screening programs essentially is nonexistent.

Acquired Hypothyroidism and Myxedema

Hypothyroidism in older children and adults causes a general slowing down of metabolic processes and myxedema. Myxedema implies the presence of a nonpitting mucous type of edema caused by an accumulation of a hydrophilic mucopolysaccharide substance in the connective tissues throughout the body.[14] The hypothyroid state may be mild, with only a few signs and symptoms, or it may progress to a life-threatening condition called *myxedematous coma*. It can result from destruction or dysfunction of the thyroid gland (*i.e.*, primary hypothyroidism), or it can be a secondary disorder caused by impaired pituitary function or as a tertiary disorder caused by a hypothalamic dysfunction.

Primary hypothyroidism is much more common than secondary (and tertiary) hypothyroidism. It may result from thyroidectomy (*i.e.*, surgical removal) or ablation of the gland with radiation. Certain goitrogenic agents, such as lithium carbonate (used in the treatment of manic-depressive states) and the antithyroid drugs propylthiouracil and methimazole in continuous dosage, can block hormone synthesis and produce hypothyroidism with goitre. Large amounts of iodine (*i.e.*, ingestion of kelp tablets or iodide-containing cough syrups, or administration of iodide-containing radiographic contrast media or the cardiac drug amiodarone, which contains 75 mg of iodine per 200-mg tablet) also can block thyroid hormone production and cause goitre, particularly in persons with autoimmune thyroid disease. Iodine deficiency, which can cause goitre and hypothyroidism, is rare in Canada because of the widespread use of iodized salt and other iodide sources.[15] However, iodine deficiency affects an estimated 100 million people worldwide.

The most common cause of hypothyroidism is Hashimoto thyroiditis, an autoimmune disorder in which the thyroid gland may be totally destroyed by an immunologic process.[17] It is the major cause of goitre and hypothyroidism in children and adults. Hashimoto thyroiditis is predominantly a disease of women. The course of the disease varies. At the onset, only a goitre may be present. In time, hypothyroidism usually becomes evident. Although the disorder usually causes hypothyroidism, a hyperthyroid state may develop midcourse in the disease. The transient hyperthyroid state is caused by leakage of preformed thyroid hormone from damaged cells of the gland. Subacute thyroiditis, which can occur in up to 10% of pregnancies postpartum (postpartum thyroiditis), also can result in hypothyroidism.

Hypothyroidism may affect almost all body functions. The manifestations of the disorder are related largely to two factors: the hypometabolic state resulting from thyroid hormone deficiency, and myxedematous involvement of body

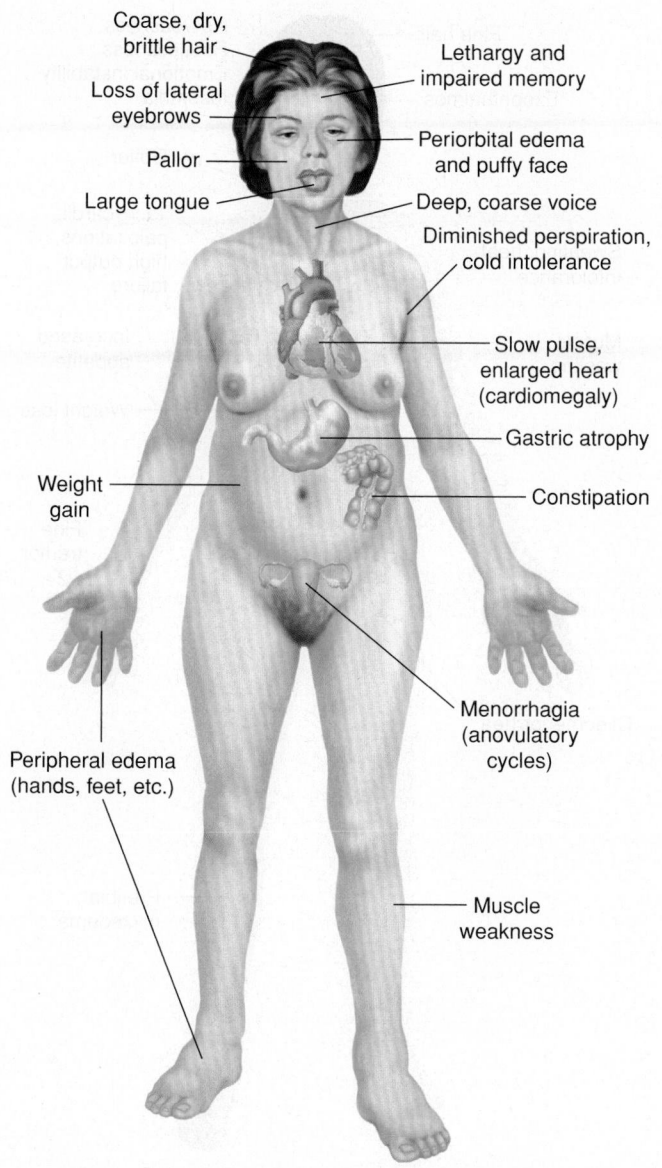

Coarse, dry, brittle hair

Loss of lateral eyebrows

Pallor

Large tongue

Weight gain

Peripheral edema (hands, feet, etc.)

Lethargy and impaired memory

Periorbital edema and puffy face

Deep, coarse voice

Diminished perspiration, cold intolerance

Slow pulse, enlarged heart (cardiomegaly)

Gastric atrophy

Constipation

Menorrhagia (anovulatory cycles)

Muscle weakness

FIGURE 41.8 • Clinical manifestations of hypothyroidism.

tissues. The hypometabolic state associated with hypothyroidism is characterized by a gradual onset of weakness and fatigue, a tendency to gain weight despite a loss of appetite, and cold intolerance (Fig. 41.8). As the condition progresses, the skin becomes dry and rough and acquires a pale yellowish cast, which primarily results from carotene deposition; the hair becomes coarse and brittle; the face becomes puffy with edematous eyelids; and there is thinning of the outer third of the eyebrows. Fluid may collect in almost any serous cavity and in the middle ear, giving rise to conductive deafness. Gastrointestinal motility is decreased, producing constipation, flatulence, and abdominal distension. Delayed relaxation of deep tendon reflexes and bradycardia are sometimes noted. Central nervous system involvement is manifested in mental dullness, lethargy, and impaired memory.[13,15,17]

Although the myxedeous fluid is usually most obvious in the face, it can collect in the interstitial spaces of almost

any body structure and is responsible for many of the manifestations of the severe hypothyroid state. The tongue is often enlarged, and the voice becomes hoarse and husky. Carpal tunnel and other entrapment syndromes are common, as is impairment of muscle function with stiffness, cramps, and pain. Pericardial or pleural effusion may develop. Mucopolysaccharide deposits in the heart cause generalized cardiac dilation, bradycardia, and other signs of altered cardiac function. The signs and symptoms of hypothyroidism are summarized in Table 41.3.

Diagnosis of hypothyroidism is based on history, physical examination, and laboratory tests. A low serum T_4, and elevated TSH levels are characteristic of primary hypothyroidism. The tests for antithyroid antibodies should be done when Hashimoto thyroiditis is suspected (anti-TPO antibody titres is the preferred test).

Hypothyroidism is treated by replacement therapy with synthetic preparations of T_3 or T_4. Most people are treated with T_4. Serum TSH levels are used to estimate the adequacy of T_4 replacement therapy. When the TSH level is normalized, the T_4 dosage is considered satisfactory (for primary hypothyroidism only). A "start-low and go-slow" approach should be considered in the treatment of elderly people with hypothyroidism because of the risk of inducing acute coronary syndromes in the susceptible individual.

Myxedematous Coma

Myxedematous coma is a life-threatening, end-stage expression of hypothyroidism. It is characterized by coma, hypothermia, cardiovascular collapse, hypoventilation, and severe metabolic disorders that include hyponatremia, hypoglycemia, and lactic acidosis. The pathophysiology of myxedema coma involves three major aspects: (1) carbon dioxide retention and hypoxia, (2) fluid and electrolyte imbalance, and (3) hypothermia.[13] It occurs most often in elderly women who have chronic hypothyroidism from a spectrum of causes. The fact that it occurs more frequently in winter months suggests that cold exposure may be a precipitating factor. The severely hypothyroid person is unable to metabolize sedatives, analgesics, and anesthetic drugs, and buildup of these agents may precipitate coma.

Treatment includes aggressive management of precipitating factors; supportive therapy such as management of cardiorespiratory status, hyponatremia, and hypoglycemia; and thyroid replacement therapy. If hypothermia is present (a low-reading thermometer should be used), active rewarming of the body is contraindicated because it may induce vasodilation and vascular collapse. Prevention is preferable to treatment and entails special attention to high-risk populations, such as women with a history of Hashimoto thyroiditis. These persons should be informed about the signs and symptoms of severe hypothyroidism and the need for early medical treatment.

Hyperthyroidism

Thyrotoxicosis is the clinical syndrome that results when tissues are exposed to high levels of circulating thyroid hormone.[13,16] In most instances, thyrotoxicosis is due to hyperactivity of the thyroid gland, or hyperthyroidism.[11,14] The most common cause of hyperthyroidism is Graves disease, which is accompanied by ophthalmopathy (or dermopathy) and diffuse goitre. Other causes of hyperthyroidism are multinodular goitre, adenoma of the thyroid, and thyroiditis. Iodine-containing agents can induce hyperthyroidism as well as hypothyroidism. Thyroid crisis, or storm, is an acutely exaggerated manifestation of the thyrotoxic state.[13,16]

Many of the manifestations of hyperthyroidism are related to the: increase in oxygen consumption; use of metabolic fuels associated with the hypermetabolic state leading to an increase in tissue thermogenesis; and an increase in sympathetic nervous system activity.[13,16] The fact that many of the signs and symptoms of hyperthyroidism resemble those of excessive sympathetic nervous system activity suggests that thyroid hormone may heighten the sensitivity of the body to the catecholamines or that it may act as a pseudo-catecholamine. With the hypermetabolic state, there are frequent complaints of nervousness, irritability, and fatigability (Fig. 41.9). Weight loss is common despite a large appetite. Other manifestations include tachycardia, palpitations, shortness of breath, excessive sweating, muscle cramps, and heat intolerance. The person appears restless and has a fine muscle tremor. Even in persons without exophthalmos (*i.e.,* bulging of the eyeballs seen in ophthalmopathy), there is an abnormal retraction of the eyelids and infrequent blinking such that they appear to be staring. The hair and skin usually are thin and have a silky appearance. The signs and symptoms of hyperthyroidism are summarized in Table 41.3.

The treatment of hyperthyroidism is directed toward reducing the level of thyroid hormone. This can be accomplished with eradication of the thyroid gland with radioactive iodine, through surgical removal of part or all of the gland, or the use of drugs that decrease thyroid function and thereby the effect of thyroid hormone on the peripheral tissues. Eradication of the thyroid with radioactive iodine is used more frequently than surgery. The β-adrenergic blocking drugs (propranolol, metoprolol, atenolol, and nadolol are preferred) are administered to block the effects of the hyperthyroid state on sympathetic nervous system function. They are given in conjunction with antithyroid drugs such as propylthiouracil and methimazole. These drugs prevent the thyroid gland from converting iodine to its organic (hormonal) form and block the conversion of T_4 to T_3 in the tissues (propylthiouracil only).[13,16]

Graves Disease

Graves disease is a state of hyperthyroidism, goitre, and ophthalmopathy (or, less commonly, dermopathy).[13,16] The onset is usually between the ages of 20 and 40 years, and women are ten times more likely to develop the disease than men.[18] Graves disease is an autoimmune disorder characterized by abnormal stimulation of the thyroid gland by thyroid-stimulating antibodies (TSH-receptor antibodies) that act through the normal TSH receptors. It may be associated with other autoimmune disorders such as myasthenia gravis and pernicious anemia.

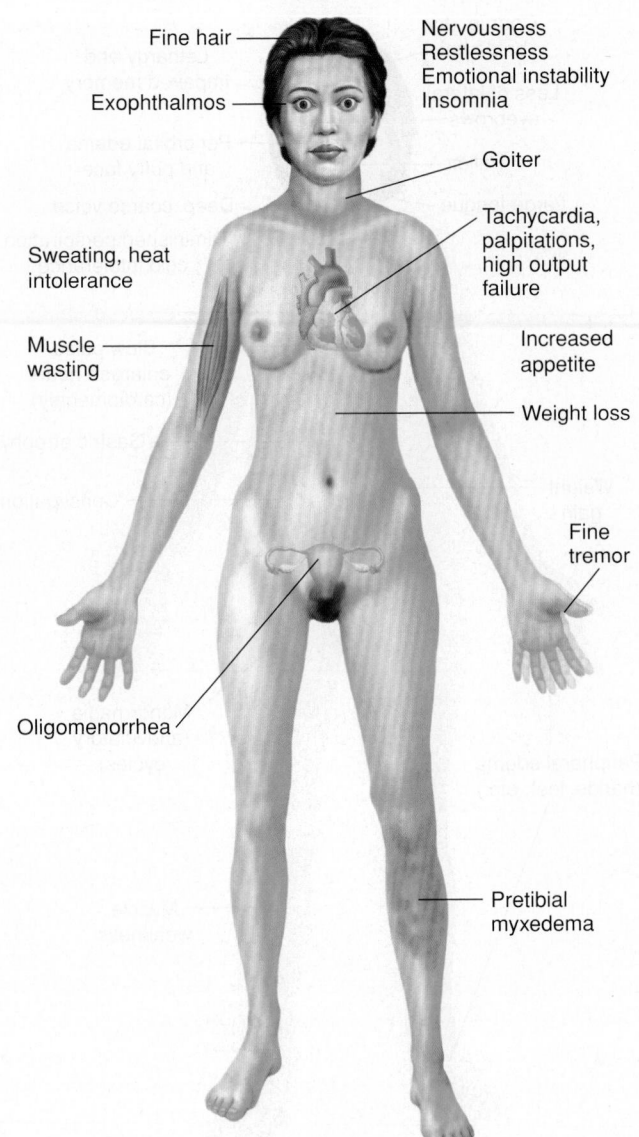

Fine hair

Exophthalmos

Nervousness
Restlessness
Emotional instability
Insomnia

Goiter

Tachycardia,
palpitations,
high output
failure

Sweating, heat
intolerance

Muscle
wasting

Increased
appetite

Weight loss

Fine
tremor

Oligomenorrhea

Pretibial
myxedema

FIGURE 41.9 • Clinical manifestations of hyperthyroidism.

The disease is associated with immune–function genes, human leukocyte antigen (HLA)-DR3 and HLA-B8, and a familial tendency is evident.[18]

The ophthalmopathy, which occurs in up to 25% of persons with Graves disease, is thought to result from a cytokine-mediated activation of fibroblasts in orbital tissue behind the eyeball.[13] Humoral autoimmunity also is important; an ophthalmic immunoglobulin may exacerbate lymphocytic infiltration of the extraocular muscles. The ophthalmopathy of Graves disease can cause severe eye problems, including tethering of the extraocular muscles resulting in diplopia; involvement of the optic nerve, with some visual loss; and corneal ulceration because the lids do not close over the protruding eyeball (due to the exophthalmos). The ophthalmopathy usually tends to stabilize after treatment of the hyperthyroidism. However, ophthalmopathy can worsen acutely after radioiodine treatment. Often glucocorticoids are prescribed for several weeks

FIGURE 41.10 • Graves disease. A young woman with hyperthyroidism presented with a mass in the neck and exophthalmos. (From Rubin R., Strayer D. S. (Eds.). (2012). *Rubin's pathology: Clinicopathologic foundations of medicine* (6th ed., p. 1050). Philadelphia, PA: Lippincott Williams & Wilkins.)

surrounding the radioiodine treatment if the person had signs of ophthalmopathy. Unfortunately, not all of the ocular changes are reversible with treatment. Ophthalmopathy also can be aggravated by smoking, which should be strongly discouraged. Figure 41.10 shows a woman with Graves disease.

Thyroid Storm

Thyroid storm, or thyrotoxic crisis, is an extreme and life-threatening form of thyrotoxicosis, rarely seen today because of improved diagnosis and treatment methods.[13,16,18] When it does occur, it is seen most often in undiagnosed cases or in persons with hyperthyroidism who have not been adequately treated. It often is precipitated by stress such as an infection (usually respiratory), by diabetic ketoacidosis, by physical or emotional trauma, or by manipulation of a hyperactive thyroid gland during thyroidectomy. Thyroid storm is manifested by a very high fever, extreme cardiovascular effects (*i.e.*, tachycardia, congestive failure, and angina), and severe CNS effects (*i.e.*, agitation, restlessness, and delirium). The mortality rate is high.

Thyroid storm requires rapid diagnosis and implementation of treatment. Often this requires admission to an intensive care unit for hemodynamic stabilization. Peripheral cooling is initiated with cold packs and a cooling mattress. For cooling to be effective, the shivering response must be prevented. General supportive measures to replace fluids, glucose, and electrolytes are essential during the hypermetabolic state. A β-adrenergic blocking drug, such as propranolol, is given to block the undesirable effects of T_4 on cardiovascular function. Glucocorticoids are used to correct the relative adrenal insufficiency resulting from the stress imposed by the hyperthyroid state and to inhibit the peripheral conversion of T_4 to T_3. Propylthiouracil or methimazole may be given to block thyroid synthesis. Aspirin increases the level of free thyroid hormones by displacing the hormones from their protein carriers, and should not be used during thyroid storm.[13,16,18]

IN SUMMARY

Thyroid hormones play a role in the metabolic process of almost all body cells and are necessary for normal physical and mental growth in the infant and young child. Key blood tests (TSH, free T_4, T_3 and thyroid autoantibodies) are used to detect alterations in thyroid function that can manifest as a hypothyroid or a hyperthyroid state. Hypothyroidism can occur as a congenital or an acquired defect. Congenital hypothyroidism leads to mental retardation and impaired physical growth unless treatment is initiated during the first months of life. Acquired hypothyroidism, such as Hashimoto thyroiditis, leads to a decrease in metabolic rate and an accumulation of a mucopolysaccharide substance in the intercellular spaces; this substance attracts water and causes a mucous type of edema called myxedema. Hyperthyroidism causes an increase in metabolic rate and alterations in body function similar to those produced by enhanced sympathetic nervous system activity. Graves disease is characterized by the triad of hyperthyroidism, goitre, and ophthalmopathy (or dermopathy), and the life-threatening complication of a thyroid storm can occur if left untreated.

DISORDERS OF ADRENAL CORTICAL FUNCTION

After completing this section of the chapter, you should be able to meet the following objectives:

- Describe the function of the adrenal cortical hormones and their feedback regulation.
- State the underlying cause of congenital adrenal hyperplasia.
- Relate the functions of the adrenal cortical hormones to Addison disease (*i.e.*, adrenal insufficiency) and Cushing syndrome (*i.e.*, glucocorticoid excess).

Control of Adrenal Cortical Function

The adrenal glands are small, bilateral structures that weigh approximately 4 to 5 g each and lie retroperitoneally at the apex of each kidney (Fig. 41.11). The medulla or inner portion of the gland, which constitutes a small part of each adrenal,

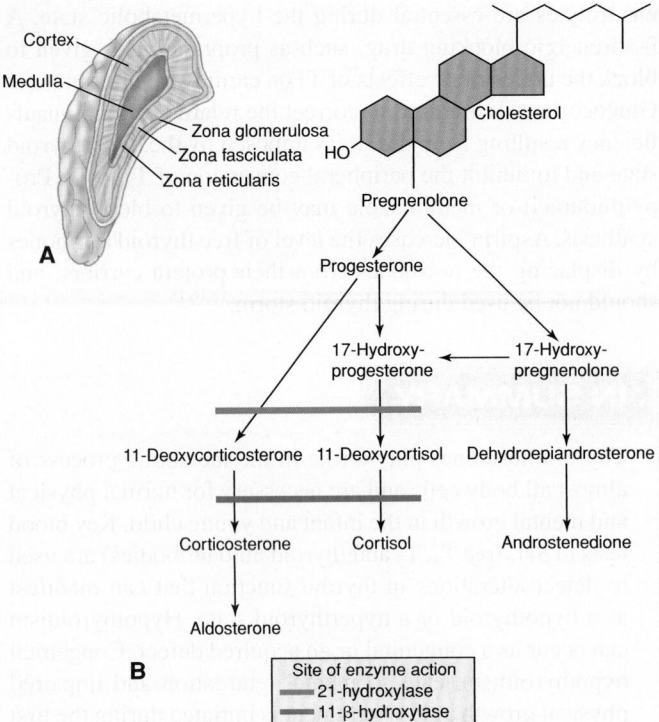

FIGURE 41.11 • A: The adrenal gland, showing the medulla and the three layers of the cortex. The outer layer of the cortex (zona glomerulosa) is primarily responsible for mineralocorticoid production, and the middle layer (zona fasciculata) and the inner layer (zona reticularis) produce the glucocorticoids and the adrenal sex hormones. **B:** Predominant biosynthetic pathways of the adrenal cortex. Critical enzymes in the biosynthetic process include 11-β-hydroxylase and 21-hydroxylase. A deficiency in one of these enzymes blocks the synthesis of hormones dependent on that enzyme and routes the precursors into alternative pathways.

secretes epinephrine and norepinephrine and is part of the sympathetic nervous system. The cortex forms the bulk of the adrenal gland (approximately 80% to 90%) and is responsible for secreting three types of hormones: the glucocorticoids, the mineralocorticoids, and the adrenal androgens.[14,19] Because the sympathetic nervous system also secretes epinephrine and norepinephrine, adrenal medullary function is not essential for life, but adrenal cortical function is. The total loss of adrenal cortical function is fatal in 4 to 14 days if untreated.[14] This section of the chapter describes the synthesis and function of the adrenal cortical hormones and the effects of adrenal cortical insufficiency and excess.

Biosynthesis, Transport, and Metabolism

More than 30 hormones are produced by the adrenal cortex. Of these hormones, aldosterone is the principal mineralocorticoid, cortisol (hydrocortisone) is the major glucocorticoid, and androgens are the chief sex hormones. All of the adrenal cortical hormones have a similar structure in that all are steroids and are synthesized from acetate and cholesterol. Each of the steps involved in the synthesis of the various hormones requires a specific enzyme (Fig. 41.11). The secretion of the

glucocorticoids and the adrenal androgens is controlled by the ACTH secreted by the anterior pituitary gland.

Cortisol, aldosterone, and the adrenal androgens are secreted in an unbound state and bind to plasma proteins for transport in the circulatory system. Cortisol binds largely to corticosteroid-binding globulin and to a lesser extent to albumin. Aldosterone and androgens circulate mostly bound to albumin. It has been suggested that the pool of protein-bound hormones may extend the duration of their action by delaying metabolic clearance.

The main site for metabolism of the adrenal cortical hormones is the liver, where they undergo a number of metabolic conversions before being conjugated and made water soluble. They are then eliminated in either the urine or the bile.

Adrenal Androgens

The adrenal androgens are synthesized primarily by the zona reticularis and the zona fasciculata of the cortex (Fig. 41.11A). These sex hormones probably exert little effect on normal sexual function. There is evidence, however, that the adrenal androgens (the most important of which is dehydroepiandrosterone [DHEA] and its sulphate [DHEA-S]) contribute to the pubertal growth of body hair, particularly pubic and axillary hair in women. They also may play a role in the steroid hormone economy of the pregnant woman and the fetal-placental unit. Because the testes produce these hormones, there is no rationale for requiring DHEA-S replacement in men. The levels of DHEA-S decline to approximately one-sixth the levels of a 20 year old by 60 years of age (the *adrenopause*). The value of routine replacement of DHEA-S in the adrenopause is controversial, but replacement may nominally improve general well-being and sexuality.[20]

Mineralocorticoids

The mineralocorticoids play an essential role in regulating potassium and sodium levels and water balance. They are produced in the zona glomerulosa, the outer layer of cells of the adrenal cortex. Aldosterone secretion is regulated by the renin–angiotensin mechanism and by blood levels of potassium. Increased levels of aldosterone promote sodium retention by the distal tubules of the kidney while increasing urinary losses of potassium. The influence of aldosterone on fluid and electrolyte balance is discussed in Chapter 31.

Glucocorticoids

The glucocorticoid hormones, mainly cortisol, are synthesized in the zona fasciculata and the zona reticularis of the adrenal gland.[14,19] The blood levels of these hormones are regulated by negative feedback mechanisms of the hypothalamic–pituitary–adrenal (HPA) system (Fig. 41.12). Just as other pituitary hormones are controlled by releasing factors from the hypothalamus, corticotropin-releasing hormone (CRH) is important in controlling the release of ACTH. Cortisol levels increase as ACTH levels rise and decrease as ACTH levels fall. There

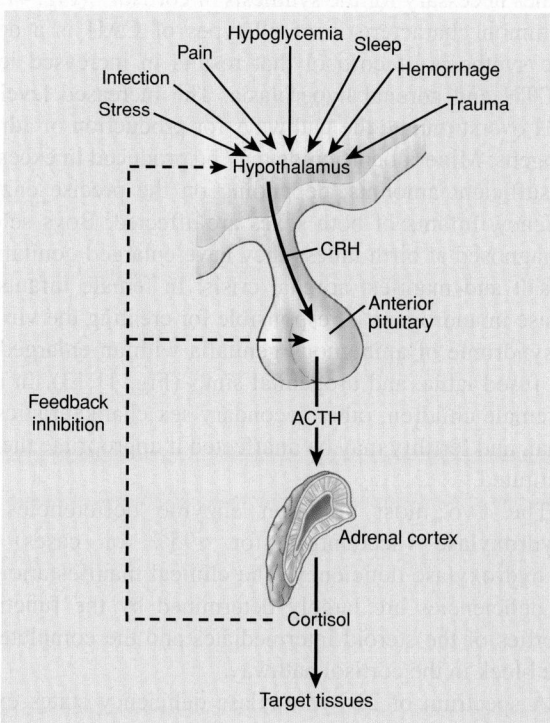

FIGURE 41.12 • The hypothalamic–pituitary–adrenal (HPA) feedback system that regulates glucocorticoid (cortisol) levels. Cortisol release is regulated by adrenocorticotropic hormone (ACTH). Stress exerts its effects on cortisol release through the HPA system and corticotropin-releasing hormone (CRH), which controls the release of ACTH from the anterior pituitary gland. Increased cortisol levels incite a negative feedback inhibition of ACTH release.

TABLE 41.4 ACTIONS OF CORTISOL

MAJOR INFLUENCE	EFFECT ON BODY
Glucose metabolism	Stimulates gluconeogenesis Decreases glucose use by the tissues
Protein metabolism	Increases breakdown of proteins Increases plasma protein levels
Fat metabolism	Increases mobilization of fatty acids Increases use of fatty acids
Anti-inflammatory action (pharmacologic levels)	Stabilizes lysosomal membranes of the inflammatory cells, preventing the release of inflammatory mediators Decreases capillary permeability to prevent inflammatory edema Depresses phagocytosis by white blood cells to reduce the release of inflammatory mediators Suppresses the immune response Causes atrophy of lymphoid tissue Decreases eosinophils Decreases antibody formation Decreases the development of cell-mediated immunity Reduces fever Inhibits fibroblast activity
Psychic effect	May contribute to emotional instability
Permissive effect	Facilitates the response of the tissues to humoral and neural influences, such as that of the catecholamines, during trauma and extreme stress

is considerable diurnal variation in ACTH levels, which reach their peak in the early morning (around 6 to 8 AM) and decline as the day progresses. This appears to be due to rhythmic activity in the CNS, which causes bursts of CRH secretion and, in turn, ACTH secretion. This diurnal pattern is reversed in people who work during the night and sleep during the day. The rhythm also may be changed by physical and psychological stresses, endogenous depression, manic-depressive psychosis, and liver disease or other conditions that affect cortisol metabolism. One of the earliest signs of Cushing syndrome, a disorder of glucocorticoid excess, is the loss of diurnal variation in CRH and ACTH secretion.

The glucocorticoids perform a necessary function in response to stress and are essential for survival. When produced as part of the stress response, these hormones aid in regulating the metabolic functions of the body and in controlling the inflammatory response. The actions of cortisol are summarized in Table 41.4. Many of the anti-inflammatory actions attributed to cortisol result from the administration of pharmacologic levels of the hormone.[14,19]

Metabolic Effects. Cortisol stimulates glucose production by the liver, promotes protein breakdown, and causes mobilization of fatty acids. As body proteins are broken down, amino acids are mobilized and transported to the liver, where they are used in the production of glucose (*i.e.*, gluconeogenesis). Mobilization of fatty acids converts cell metabolism from the use of glucose for energy to the use of fatty acids instead. As glucose production by the liver rises and peripheral glucose use falls, a moderate resistance to insulin develops. In persons with diabetes and those who are diabetes prone, this has the effect of raising the blood glucose level.[14,19]

Psychological Effects. The glucocorticoid hormones appear to be involved directly or indirectly in emotional behaviour. Receptors for these hormones have been identified in brain tissue, which suggests that they play a role in the regulation of behaviour. Persons treated with adrenal cortical hormones have been known to display behaviour ranging from mildly aberrant to psychotic.

Immunologic and Inflammatory Effects. Cortisol influences multiple aspects of immunologic function and inflammatory responsiveness. Large quantities of cortisol are required for an effective anti-inflammatory action. This is achieved by the administration of pharmacologic rather than physiologic doses of synthetic cortisol. The increased cortisol blocks inflammation at an early stage by decreasing capillary permeability and stabilizing the lysosomal membranes so that inflammatory mediators are not released. Cortisol suppresses the immune response by reducing humoral and cell-mediated immunity. With this lessened inflammatory response comes a reduction in fever. During the healing phase, cortisol suppresses fibroblast activity and thereby lessens scar formation. Cortisol also inhibits prostaglandin synthesis, which may account in large part for its anti-inflammatory actions.[14,19]

Pharmacologic Suppression of Adrenal Function

A highly significant aspect of long-term therapy with pharmacologic preparations of the glucocorticoids is adrenal insufficiency on withdrawal of the drugs. The deficiency results from suppression of the HPA system. Chronic suppression causes atrophy of the adrenal gland, and the abrupt withdrawal of drugs can cause acute adrenal insufficiency. Recovery to a state of normal adrenal function may be prolonged, requiring up to 12 months or more.

Tests of Adrenal Function

Several diagnostic tests can be used to evaluate adrenal cortical function and the HPA system.[19] Blood levels of cortisol, aldosterone, and ACTH can be measured using immunoassay methods. A 24-hour urine specimen measuring the excretion of various metabolic end products of the adrenal hormones provides information about alterations in the biosynthesis of the adrenal cortical hormones. The 24-hour urinary free cortisol, late-night (between 11 PM and midnight) serum or salivary cortisol levels, and the overnight 1 mg dexamethasone

suppression test (to be discussed later) are excellent screening tests for Cushing syndrome.[17,19,20]

Suppression and stimulation tests afford a means of assessing the state of the HPA feedback system. For example, a test dose of ACTH can be given to assess the response of the adrenal cortex to stimulation. Similarly, administration of dexamethasone, a synthetic glucocorticoid drug, provides a means of measuring negative feedback suppression of ACTH. Adrenal tumours and ectopic ACTH-producing tumours usually are unresponsive to ACTH suppression by dexamethasone. CRH tests can be used to diagnose a pituitary ACTH-secreting tumour (*i.e.*, Cushing disease), especially when combined with inferior petrosal venous sampling (this allows the blood drainage of the pituitary to be sampled directly). Metyrapone blocks the final step in cortisol synthesis, resulting in the production of 11-dehydroxycortisol, which does not inhibit ACTH. This test measures the ability of the pituitary to release ACTH. The gold standard test for assessing the integrity of HPA axis and its ability to respond to stress is the insulin hypoglycemic stress test.[19]

Congenital Adrenal Hyperplasia

Congenital adrenal hyperplasia (CAH), or the adrenogenital syndrome, describes a congenital disorder caused by an autosomal recessive trait in which a deficiency exists in any of the enzymes necessary for the synthesis of cortisol[21] (Fig. 41.11). A common characteristic of all types of CAH is a defect in the synthesis of cortisol that results in increased levels of ACTH and adrenal hyperplasia. The increased levels of ACTH overstimulate the pathways for production of adrenal androgens. Mineralocorticoids may be produced in excessive or insufficient amounts, depending on the precise enzyme deficiency. Infants of both sexes are affected. Boys seldom are diagnosed at birth unless they have enlarged genitalia or lose salt and manifest adrenal crisis. In female infants, an increase in androgens is responsible for creating the virilization syndrome of ambiguous genitalia with an enlarged clitoris, fused labia, and urogenital sinus (Fig. 41.13). In male and female children, other secondary sex characteristics are normal, and fertility may be unaffected if appropriate therapy is instituted.[21]

The two most common enzyme deficiencies are 21-hydroxylase (accounting for >95% of cases) and 11-β-hydroxylase deficiency. The clinical manifestations of both deficiencies are largely determined by the functional properties of the steroid intermediates and the completeness of the block in the cortisol pathway.[21]

A spectrum of 21-hydroxylase deficiency states exists, ranging from simple virilizing CAH to a complete salt-losing enzyme deficiency.[21,22] Simple virilizing CAH impairs the synthesis of cortisol, and steroid synthesis is shunted to androgen production. Persons with these deficiencies usually produce sufficient aldosterone or aldosterone intermediates to prevent signs and symptoms of mineralocorticoid deficiency. The salt-losing form is accompanied by deficient production

FIGURE 41.13 • A female infant with congenital adrenal hyperplasia demonstrating virilization of the genitalia with hypertrophy of the clitoris and partial fusion of labioscrotal folds. (From Rubin R., Strayer D. S. (Eds.). (2012). *Rubin's pathology: Clinicopathologic foundations of medicine* (6th ed., p. 1067). Philadelphia, PA: Lippincott Williams & Wilkins.)

TABLE 41.5 CLINICAL FINDINGS OF ADRENAL INSUFFICIENCY

FINDING	PRIMARY	SECONDARY/TERTIARY
Anorexia and weight loss	Yes (100%)	Yes (100%)
Fatigue and weakness	Yes (100%)	Yes (100%)
Gastrointestinal symptoms, nausea, diarrhea	Yes (50%)	Yes (50%)
Myalgia, arthralgia, abdominal pain	Yes (10%)	Yes (10%)
Orthostatic hypotension	Yes	Yes
Hyponatremia	Yes (85–90%)	Yes (60%)
Hyperkalemia	Yes (60–65%)	No
Hyperpigmentation	Yes (>90%)	No
Secondary deficiencies of testosterone, growth hormone, thyroxine, antidiuretic hormone	No	Yes
Associated autoimmune conditions	Yes	No

of aldosterone and its intermediates. This results in fluid and electrolyte disorders after the fifth day of life, including hyponatremia, hyperkalemia, vomiting, dehydration, and shock.

The 11-β-hydroxylase deficiency is rare and manifests a spectrum of severity. Affected persons have excessive androgen production and impaired conversion of 11-deoxycorticosterone to corticosterone. The overproduction of 11-deoxycorticosterone, which has mineralocorticoid activity, is responsible for the hypertension that accompanies this deficiency. Diagnosis of CAH depends on the precise biochemical evaluation of metabolites in the cortisol pathway and on clinical signs and symptoms. Genetic testing is also invaluable; however, correlation between the phenotype and genotype is not always straightforward.[21,22]

Medical treatment of CAH includes oral or parenteral glucocorticoid replacement. Fludrocortisone acetate, a mineralocorticoid, also may be given to children who are salt losers. Depending on the degree of virilization, reconstructive surgery during the first 2 years of life is indicated to reduce the size of the clitoris, separate the labia, and exteriorize the vagina. Advances in surgical techniques have led to earlier use of single-stage surgery—between 2 and 6 months of life in girls with 21-hydroxylase deficiency, a time when the tissues are maximally pliable and psychological trauma to the child is minimized.[22] Surgery has provided excellent results and does not usually impair sexual function.

Adrenal Cortical Insufficiency

There are two forms of adrenal insufficiency: primary and secondary[23] (see Table 41.5 for distinguishing features).

Primary adrenal insufficiency, or Addison disease, is caused by destruction of the adrenal gland. Secondary adrenal insufficiency results from a disorder of the HPA system.

Primary Adrenal Cortical Insufficiency

Primary adrenal insufficiency or Addison disease, is a relatively rare disorder in which all the layers of the adrenal cortex are destroyed causing a deficiency in adrenal cortical hormones and ACTH levels are elevated because of lack of feedback inhibition.[19] Autoimmune destruction is the most common cause of Addison disease in Canada. Before 1950, tuberculosis was the major cause of Addison disease in Canada and the United States, and it continues to be a major cause of the disease in countries where it is more prevalent. Rare causes include metastatic carcinoma, fungal infection (particularly histoplasmosis), cytomegalovirus infection, amyloid disease, and hemochromatosis. Bilateral adrenal hemorrhage may occur in persons taking anticoagulants, during open heart surgery, and during birth or major trauma. Adrenal insufficiency can be caused by acquired immunodeficiency syndrome, in which the adrenal gland is destroyed by a variety of opportunistic infectious agents. Drugs that inhibit synthesis or cause excessive breakdown of glucocorticoids can also result in adrenal insufficiency (*e.g.*, ketoconazole).

The adrenal cortex has a large reserve capacity, and the manifestations of adrenal insufficiency usually do not become apparent until approximately 90% of both glands have been destroyed. These manifestations are related primarily to mineralocorticoid deficiency, glucocorticoid deficiency, and hyperpigmentation resulting from elevated ACTH levels. Although lack of the adrenal androgens (*i.e.*, DHEA-S) exerts few effects in men because the testes produce these hormones, women have sparse axillary and pubic hair.[19]

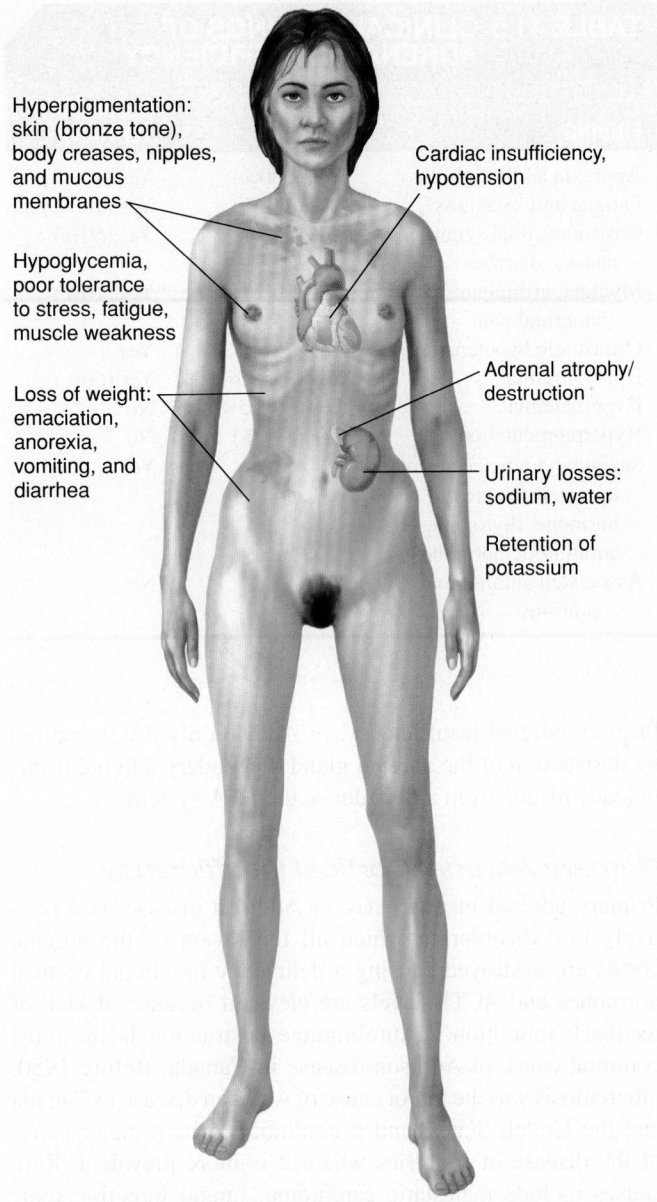

Hyperpigmentation: skin (bronze tone), body creases, nipples, and mucous membranes

Cardiac insufficiency, hypotension

Hypoglycemia, poor tolerance to stress, fatigue, muscle weakness

Loss of weight: emaciation, anorexia, vomiting, and diarrhea

Adrenal atrophy/ destruction

Urinary losses: sodium, water

Retention of potassium

FIGURE 41.14 • Clinical manifestations of primary (Addison disease) and secondary adrenal insufficiency.

Mineralocorticoid deficiency causes increased urinary losses of sodium, chloride, and water, along with decreased excretion of potassium (Fig. 41.14). The result is hyponatremia, loss of extracellular fluid, decreased cardiac output, and hyperkalemia. There may be an abnormal appetite for salt. Orthostatic hypotension is common. Dehydration, weakness, and fatigue are common early symptoms. If loss of sodium and water is extreme, cardiovascular collapse and shock ensue. Because of a lack of glucocorticoids, the person with Addison disease has poor tolerance to stress. This deficiency causes hypoglycemia, lethargy, weakness, fever, and gastrointestinal symptoms such as anorexia, nausea, vomiting, and weight loss.

Hyperpigmentation results from elevated levels of ACTH. The skin looks bronzed or suntanned in exposed and unexposed areas, and the normal creases and pressure points tend to become especially dark. The gums and oral mucous membranes may become bluish-black. The amino acid sequence of ACTH is strikingly similar to that of melanocyte-stimulating hormone; hyperpigmentation occurs in greater than 90% of persons with Addison disease and is helpful in distinguishing the primary and secondary forms of adrenal insufficiency.[19]

Addison disease, like type 1 diabetes mellitus, is a chronic metabolic disorder that requires lifetime hormone replacement therapy. The daily regulation of the chronic phase of Addison disease is usually accomplished with oral replacement therapy, with higher doses being given during periods of stress. The pharmacologic agent that is used should have both glucocorticoid and mineralocorticoid activity. Mineralocorticoids are needed only in primary adrenal insufficiency. Hydrocortisone is usually the drug of choice. In mild cases, hydrocortisone alone may be adequate. Fludrocortisone (a mineralocorticoid) is used for persons who do not obtain a sufficient salt-retaining effect from hydrocortisone. DHEA-S replacement also may be helpful in the female patient.[19]

Because persons with the disorder are likely to have episodes of hyponatremia and hypoglycemia, they need to have a regular schedule for meals and exercise. Persons with Addison disease also have limited ability to respond to infections, trauma, and other stresses. Such situations require immediate medical attention and treatment. All persons with Addison disease should be advised to wear a medical alert bracelet or medallion.

Secondary Adrenal Cortical Insufficiency

Secondary adrenal insufficiency can occur as the result of hypopituitarism or because the pituitary gland has been surgically removed. Tertiary adrenal insufficiency results from a hypothalamic defect. However, a far more common cause than either of these is the rapid withdrawal of glucocorticoids that have been administered therapeutically. These drugs suppress the HPA system, with resulting adrenal cortical atrophy and loss of cortisol production. This suppression continues long after drug therapy has been discontinued and can be critical during periods of stress or when surgery is performed.

Acute Adrenal Crisis

Acute adrenal crisis is a life-threatening situation.[23] If Addison disease is the underlying problem, exposure to even a minor illness or stress can precipitate nausea, vomiting, muscular weakness, hypotension, dehydration, and vascular collapse. The onset of adrenal crisis may be sudden, or it may progress over a period of several days. The symptoms may occur suddenly in children with salt-losing forms of CAH. Massive bilateral adrenal hemorrhage causes an acute fulminating form of adrenal insufficiency. Hemorrhage can be caused by meningococcal septicemia (*i.e.*, Waterhouse–Friderichsen syndrome), adrenal trauma, anticoagulant therapy, adrenal vein thrombosis, or adrenal metastases.

Adrenal insufficiency is treated with hormone replacement therapy that includes a combination of glucocorticoids and mineralocorticoids. For acute adrenal insufficiency, the *five S's* of management should be followed: (1) *S*alt replacement, (2) *S*ugar (dextrose) replacement, (3) *S*teroid replacement, (4) *S*upport of physiologic functioning, and (5) *S*earch for and treat the underlying cause (*e.g.,* infection). Extracellular fluid volume should be restored with several litres of 0.9% saline and 5% dextrose. Glucocorticoid replacement is accomplished through the intravenous administration of either dexamethasone or hydrocortisone. Dexamethasone is preferred acutely for two reasons: it is long acting (12 to 24 hours) and it does not interfere with measurement of serum or urinary steroids during subsequent corticotropin (ACTH) stimulation tests if diagnosis needs to be established. Thereafter, hydrocortisone often is given either intravenously or intramuscularly at 6-hour intervals and then tapered over 1 to 3 days to maintenance levels. Oral hydrocortisone replacement therapy can be resumed once the saline infusion has been discontinued and the person is taking food and fluids by mouth. Mineralocorticoid therapy is not required when large amounts of hydrocortisone are being given, but as the dose is reduced it is usually necessary to add fludrocortisone. Glucocorticoid and mineralocorticoid replacement therapy is monitored using heart rate and blood pressure measurements; serum electrolyte values; and titration of plasma renin activity into the upper-normal range.[19,23]

Glucocorticoid Hormone Excess (Cushing Syndrome)

The term *Cushing syndrome* refers to the manifestations of hypercortisolism from any cause.[19,24] Three important forms of Cushing syndrome result from excess glucocorticoid production by the body. One is a pituitary form, which results from excessive production of ACTH by a tumour of the pituitary gland. This form of the disease was the one originally described by Cushing; therefore, it is called *Cushing disease.* The second form is the adrenal form, caused by a benign or malignant adrenal tumour. The third form is ectopic Cushing syndrome, caused by a nonpituitary ACTH-secreting tumour. Certain extrapituitary malignant tumours such as small cell carcinoma of the lung may secrete ACTH or, rarely, CRH, and produce Cushing syndrome. Cushing syndrome also can result from long-term therapy with one of the potent pharmacologic preparations of glucocorticoids; this form is called *iatrogenic Cushing syndrome.*

The major manifestations of Cushing syndrome represent an exaggeration of the many actions of cortisol (see Table 41.4). Altered fat metabolism causes a peculiar deposition of fat characterized by a protruding abdomen; subclavicular fat pads or "buffalo hump" on the back; and a round, plethoric "moon face" (Figs. 41.15 and 41.16). There is muscle weakness, and the extremities are thin because of protein breakdown and muscle wasting. In advanced cases, the skin over the forearms and legs becomes thin, having the appearance of parchment. Purple striae, or stretch marks, from stretching

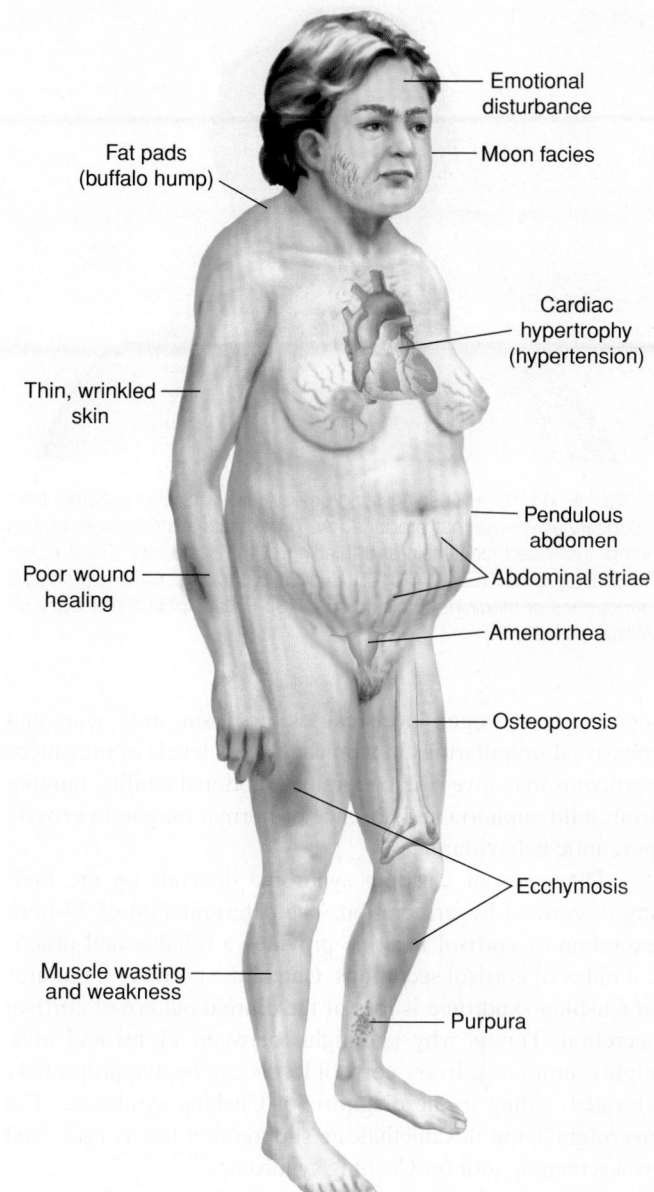

FIGURE 41.15 • Clinical features of Cushing syndrome.

of the catabolically weakened skin and subcutaneous tissues are distributed over the breast, thighs, and abdomen. Osteoporosis may develop because of destruction of bone proteins and alterations in calcium metabolism, resulting in back pain, compression fractures of the vertebrae, and rib fractures. As calcium is mobilized from bone, renal calculi may develop.

Derangements in glucose metabolism are found in approximately 60% of patients, with clinically overt diabetes mellitus occurring in approximately 20%. The glucocorticoids possess mineralocorticoid properties; this causes hypokalemia as a result of excessive potassium excretion and hypertension resulting from sodium retention. Inflammatory and immune responses are inhibited, resulting in increased susceptibility to infection. Cortisol increases gastric acid secretion, which may provoke gastric ulceration and bleeding. An accompanying

FIGURE 41.16 • Cushing syndrome. A woman who suffered from a pituitary adenoma that produced ACTH exhibits a moon face, buffalo hump, increased facial hair, and thinning of the scalp hair. (From Rubin R., Strayer D. S. (Eds.). (2012). *Rubin's pathology: Clinicopathologic foundations of medicine* (6th ed., p. 1073). Philadelphia, PA: Lippincott Williams & Wilkins.)

increase in androgen levels causes hirsutism, mild acne, and menstrual irregularities in women. Excess levels of the glucocorticoids may give rise to extreme emotional lability, ranging from mild euphoria and absence of normal fatigue to grossly psychotic behaviour.

Diagnosis of Cushing syndrome depends on the finding of cortisol hypersecretion. The determination of 24-hour excretion of cortisol in urine provides a reliable and practical index of cortisol secretions. One of the prominent features of Cushing syndrome is loss of the diurnal pattern of cortisol secretion. This is why late-night (between 11 PM and midnight) serum or salivary cortisol levels can be inappropriately elevated, aiding in the diagnosis of Cushing syndrome. The overnight 1 mg dexamethasone suppression test is also used as a screening tool for Cushing syndrome.[19,24]

After the diagnosis of Cushing syndrome has been confirmed further tests to determine the cause for excess cortisol secretion are done such the measurement of plasma ACTH levels.[19,24] ACTH levels should be normal or elevated in ACTH-dependent Cushing syndrome (Cushing disease and ectopic ACTH), and low in non-ACTH–dependent Cushing syndrome (adrenal tumours). Various suppression or stimulation tests of the HPA system are performed to delineate the cause further. MRI or CT scans afford a means for locating adrenal or pituitary tumours.

Untreated, Cushing syndrome produces serious morbidity and even death. The choice of surgery, irradiation, or pharmacologic treatment is determined largely by the cause of the hypercortisolism. The goal of treatment for Cushing syndrome is to remove or correct the source of hypercortisolism without causing permanent pituitary or adrenal damage. Transsphenoidal removal of a pituitary adenoma, or a hemihypophysectomy, is the preferred method of treatment for Cushing disease. This allows removal of only the tumour rather than the entire pituitary gland. After successful removal, the person must receive cortisol replacement therapy for 6 to 12 months or until adrenal function returns. Patients also may receive pituitary radiation therapy, but the full effects of treatment may not be realized for 3 to 12 months. Unilateral or bilateral adrenalectomy may be done in the case of adrenal adenoma. When possible, ectopic ACTH-producing tumours are removed. Pharmacologic agents that block steroid synthesis (*i.e.,* mitotane, ketoconazole, and metyrapone) may be used to treat persons with ectopic tumours or adrenal carcinomas that cannot be resected.[19,24] Many of these patients also require *Pneumocystis jiroveci* (formerly known as *Pneumocystis carinii*) pneumonia prophylaxis because of the profound immunosuppression caused by the excessive glucocorticoid levels.

Incidental Adrenal Mass

An incidentaloma is a mass lesion found unexpectedly in an adrenal gland by an imaging procedure—most commonly CT but also MRI and ultrasonography—done for other reasons. With the increasing use of imaging these incidentalomas have been reported with increasing frequency since the early 1980s. The prevalence of adrenal incidentalomas is approximately 3% to 4%. Incidentalomas also can occur in other organs (*e.g.,* pituitary, thyroid). The two most important questions are (1) is the mass malignant, and (2) is the mass hormonally active (*i.e.,* is it functioning)?[25]

Primary adrenal carcinoma is quite rare, but other cancers, particularly lung cancers, commonly metastasize to the adrenal gland; other cancers include breast, stomach, pancreas, colon, kidney, melanomas, and lymphomas. The size and imaging characteristics of the mass may help determine whether the tumour is benign or malignant. The risk of cancer is high in adrenal masses larger than 4 cm. Many experts recommend surgical removal of masses larger than 4 cm.[19,25] Appropriate screening to exclude a hormonally active lesion includes tests to rule out pheochromocytoma, Cushing syndrome, and Conn syndrome (mineralocorticoid excess).

IN SUMMARY

The adrenal cortex produces three types of hormones: mineralocorticoids, glucocorticoids, and adrenal androgens. The mineralocorticoids, along with the renin–angiotensin mechanism, aid in controlling body levels of sodium and potassium. The glucocorticoids have anti-inflammatory actions and aid in regulating glucose, protein, and fat metabolism during periods of stress. These hormones are under the control of the HPA system. The adrenal androgens exert little effect on daily control of body function, but they probably contribute to the development of body hair in women. CAH describes a genetic defect in the cortisol pathway resulting from a deficiency of one of the enzymes needed for its synthesis. Depending on the enzyme involved, the disorder causes virilization of female infants and, in some instances, fluid and electrolyte disturbances because of impaired mineralocorticoid synthesis.

Chronic adrenal insufficiency can be caused by destruction of the adrenal gland (Addison disease) or by dysfunction of the HPA system. Adrenal insufficiency requires replacement therapy with adrenal cortical hormones. Acute adrenal insufficiency is a life-threatening situation. Cushing syndrome refers to the manifestations of excessive glucocorticoid levels. This syndrome may be a result of pharmacologic doses of glucocorticoids, a pituitary or adrenal tumour, or an ectopic tumour that produces ACTH. The clinical manifestations of Cushing syndrome reflect the very high level of glucocorticoid that is present.

An incidentaloma is a mass lesion found unexpectedly in an adrenal gland (and other glands) by an imaging procedure done for other reasons. They are being recognized with increasing frequency, emphasizing the need for correct diagnosis and treatment.

REVIEW EXERCISES

1. A 59-year-old man was referred to a neurologist for evaluation of headaches. Subsequent MRI studies revealed a large suprasellar mass (2.5×2.4 cm), consistent with a pituitary tumour. His history is positive for hypertension and, on direct inquiry, he says that he believes his hands are slightly larger than before, with increased sweating. Family history is negative, as are weight change, polyuria and polydipsia, visual disturbance, and erectile dysfunction. Subsequent laboratory findings reveal a baseline serum growth hormone (GH) of 8.7 µg/L (normal for males is 0 to 4 µg/L), which is unsuppressed after oral glucose tolerance testing; glucose intolerance; and increased insulin-like growth factor-1 (IGF-1) on two occasions (1,044 and 1,145 µg/L [upper limit of normal is 480 µg/L]). Other indices of pituitary function are within the normal range.
   A. *What diagnosis would this man's clinical features, MRI, and laboratory findings suggest?*
   B. *What is the reason for asking the patient about weight change, polyuria and polydipsia, visual disturbance, and erectile dysfunction?*
   C. *How would you explain his impaired glucose tolerance?*
   D. *What are the possible local effects of a large pituitary tumour?*
2. A 76-year-old woman presents with weight gain, subjective memory loss, dry skin, and cold intolerance. On examination she is found to have a multinodular goitre. Laboratory findings reveal a low serum T_4 and elevated TSH.
   A. *What diagnosis would this woman's history, physical, and laboratory tests suggest?*
   B. *Explain the possible relationship between the diagnosis and her weight gain, dry skin, cold intolerance, and subjective memory loss.*
   C. *What type of treatment would be indicated?*
3. A 45-year-old woman presents with a history of progressive weakness, fatigue, weight loss, nausea, and increased skin pigmentation (especially of creases, pressure areas, and nipples). Her blood pressure is 120/78 mm Hg when supine and 105/52 mm Hg when standing. Laboratory findings reveal a serum sodium of 120 mmol/L (normal is 135 to 145 mmol/L); potassium level of 5.9 mmol/L (normal is 3.5 to 5.0 mmol/L); and low plasma cortisol and high ACTH levels.
   A. *What diagnosis would this woman's clinical features and laboratory findings suggest?*
   B. *Would her diagnosis be classified as a primary or secondary endocrine disorder?*
   C. *What is the significance of her darkened skin?*
   D. *What type of treatment would be indicated?*

References

1. Javorsky B. R., Aron D. C., Findling J. W. (2011). Chapter 4: Hypothalamus and pituitary gland. In Gardner D. G., Shoback D. (Eds.), *Greenspan's basic and clinical endocrinology* (9th ed.). New York: Lange Medical/McGraw-Hill.
2. Styne D. (2011). Chapter 6: Growth. In Gardner D. G., Shoback D. (Eds.), *Greenspan's basic and clinical endocrinology* (9th ed.). New York: Lange Medical Books/McGraw-Hill.
3. Cooke D. W., Divall S. A., Radovick S. (2011). Chapter 24: Normal and aberrant growth. In Melmed S., Polonsky K. S., Larsen P. R., et al. (Eds.), *Williams textbook of endocrinology* (12th ed.). Philadelphia, PA: Elsevier Saunders.
4. Nass R. (2013). Growth hormone axis and aging. *Endocrinology and Metabolism Clinics of North America, 42*(2), 187–199.
5. Rogol A. D., Hayden G. F. (2014). Etiologies and early diagnosis of short stature and growth failure in children and adolescents. *Journal of Pediatrics, 164* (Suppl 1), S1–S14.
6. Kargi A. Y., Merriam G. R. (2013). Diagnosis and treatment of growth hormone deficiency in adults. *Nature Reviews Endocrinology, 9*(6), 335–345.
7. Davies J. H., Cheetham T. (2014). Investigation and management of tall stature. *Archives of Disease in Childhood, 99*(8), 772–777.
8. Kumar S. (2013). Tall stature in children: differential diagnosis and management. *International Journal of Pediatric Endocrinology, 2013*(Suppl 1), P53.
9. Lugo G., Pena L., Cordido F. (2012). Clinical manifestations and diagnosis of acromegaly. *International Journal of Endocrinology, 2012,* 540389.
10. Sherlock M., Woods C., Sheppard M. C. (2011). Medical therapy in acromegaly. *Nature Reviews Endocrinology, 7*(5), 291–300.
11. Synovitz L., Chopak-Foss J. (2013). Precocious puberty: Pathology, related risks, and support strategies. *Journal of Preventive Medicine, 3*(9), 504–509.
12. Styne D. (2011). Chapter 15: Puberty. In Gardner D. G., Shoback D. (Eds.), *Greenspan's basic and clinical endocrinology* (9th ed.). New York: Lange Medical Books/McGraw-Hill.
13. Cooper D. S., Ladenson P. W. (2011). Chapter 7: The thyroid gland. In Gardner D. G., Shoback D. (Eds.), *Greenspan's basic and clinical endocrinology* (9th ed.). New York: Lange Medical Books/McGraw-Hill.

14. Hall J. E. (2011). *Textbook of medical physiology* (12th ed.). Philadelphia, PA: W.B. Saunders.

15. Dubbs S. B., Spangler R. (2014). Hypothyroidism: Causes, killers, and life-saving treatments. *Emergency Medicine Clinics of North America, 32*(2), 303–317.

16. Devereaux D., Tewelde S. Z. (2014). Hyperthyroidism and thyrotoxicosis. *Emergency Medicine Clinics of North America, 32*(2), 277–292.

17. Caturegli P., Remigis A. D., Rose N. R. (2014). Hashimoto thyroiditis: Clinical and diagnostic criteria. *Autoimmunity Reviews, 13*(4–5), 391–397.

18. Merino M. J., Quezado M. (2012). Chapter 21: The endocrine system. In Rubin R., Strayer D. S. (Eds.), *Rubin's pathology: Clinicopathologic foundations of medicine* (6th ed.). Philadelphia, PA: Lippincott Williams & Wilkins.

19. Carroll T. B., Aron D. C., Findling J. W., et al. (2011). Chapter 9: Glucocorticoids and adrenal androgens. In Gardner D. G., Shoback D. (Eds.), *Greenspan's basic and clinical endocrinology* (9th ed.). New York: Lange Medical Books/McGraw-Hill.

20. Chakera A. J., Vaidya B. (2010). Addison disease in adults: Diagnosis and management. *The American Journal of Medicine, 123*(5), 409–413.

21. Simpson H., Hughes I. (2013). Congenital adrenal hyperplasia. *Medicine, 41*(9), 529–531.

22. Speiser P. W., White P. C. (2003). Congenital adrenal hyperplasia. *New England Journal of Medicine, 349*(8), 776–788.

23. Bornstein S. R. (2009). Predisposing factors for adrenal insufficiency. *New England Journal of Medicine, 360*(22), 2328–2339.

24. Guaraldi F., Salvatori R. (2012). Cushing syndrome: Maybe not so uncommon of an endocrine disease. *Journal of the American Board of Family Medicine, 25*(2), 199–208.

25. Willatt J. M., Francis I. R. (2010). Radiologic evaluation of incidentally discovered adrenal masses. *American Family Physician, 81*(11), 1361–1366.

Visit thePoint **http://thePoint.lww.com for animations, journal articles, and more!**

Diabetes Mellitus and the Metabolic Syndrome

42

According to the Canadian Diabetes Association, diabetes mellitus is a chronic health problem affecting 2.4 million people in Canada (approximately 6.8% of the population) and at least 371 million people worldwide. The number of people diagnosed with diabetes is expected to rise to 552 million (1 in 10 adults) worldwide by the year 2030.[1] Canada's Aboriginal peoples (namely First Nation, Inuit and Métis individuals) have an increased prevalence of 3 to 5 times higher than the general Canadian population of developing type 2 diabetes. It has been identified that diabetes and the associated complications are also more prevalent among people with South Asian, Chinese, African, and Latin ancestry.[1]

Diabetes, and the resulting impact of short-term and long-term blood glucose fluctuations, can lead to a variety of complications ranging from acute medical emergencies to disability and death. Diabetes is a significant risk factor in coronary heart disease and stroke, and it is the leading cause of blindness and chronic kidney disease, as well as a major contributor to lower extremity amputations. Optimizing glycemic control, through a variety of interventions, minimizes the complications associated with diabetes.

HORMONAL CONTROL OF GLUCOSE, FAT, AND PROTEIN METABOLISM

After completing this section of the chapter, you should be able to meet the following objectives:

- State the functions of glucose, fats, and proteins in meeting the energy needs of the body.
- Characterize the actions of insulin with reference to glucose, fat, and protein metabolism.
- Explain what is meant by *counter-regulatory hormones,* and describe the actions of glucagon, epinephrine, growth hormone, and the glucocorticoid hormones in regulation of blood glucose levels.

Glucose, Fat, and Protein Metabolism

The body uses glucose, fatty acids, and other substrates as fuel to satisfy its energy needs. Although the respiratory and

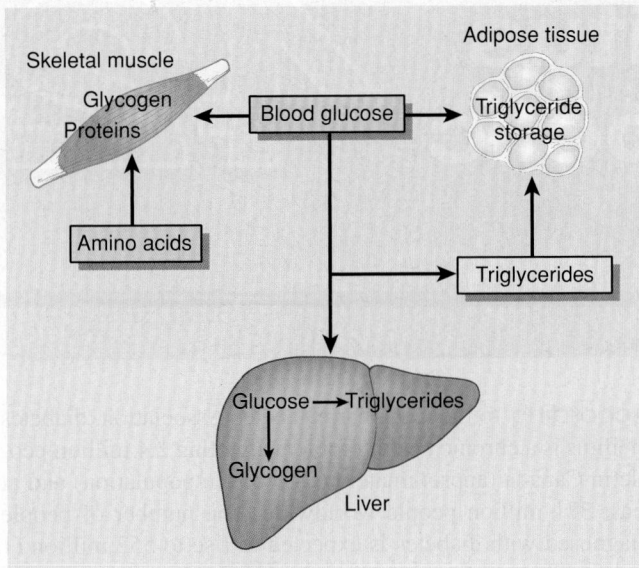

FIGURE 42.1 • Hormonal and hepatic regulation of blood glucose.

circulatory systems combine efforts to furnish the body with the oxygen needed for metabolic purposes, it is the liver, in concert with hormones from the endocrine pancreas, that controls the body's fuel supply (Fig. 42.1).

Glucose Metabolism

Glucose is a six-carbon molecule; it is an efficient fuel that, when metabolized in the presence of oxygen, breaks down to form carbon dioxide and water. Although many tissues and organ systems are able to use other forms of fuel, such as fatty acids and ketones, the brain and nervous system rely almost exclusively on glucose as a fuel source. Because the brain can neither synthesize nor store more than a few minutes' supply of glucose, normal cerebral function requires a continuous supply from the circulation. Severe and prolonged hypoglycemia can cause brain death, and even moderate hypoglycemia can result in substantial brain dysfunction.

Body tissues obtain glucose from the blood. In individuals without diabetes, fasting blood glucose levels are tightly regulated between 4.4 and 5.0 mmol/L. After a meal, blood glucose levels rise and insulin is secreted in response to this rise in glucose. Approximately two thirds of the glucose that is ingested with a meal is removed from the blood and stored in the liver as glycogen. Between meals, the liver releases glucose as a means of maintaining the blood glucose within its normal range.[2]

Glucose that is not needed for energy is removed from the blood and stored as glycogen or converted to fat. When tissues such as those in the liver and skeletal muscle become saturated with glycogen, the additional glucose is converted into fatty acids by the liver and then stored as triglycerides in fat cells. When blood glucose levels fall below normal, as they do between meals, glycogen is broken down by a process called *glycogenolysis,* and glucose is released. Although skeletal muscle has glycogen stores, it lacks the enzyme

glucose-6-phosphatase that allows glucose to be broken down sufficiently to pass through the cell membrane and enter the bloodstream, limiting its usefulness to the muscle cell.

In addition to mobilizing its glycogen stores, the liver synthesizes glucose from amino acids, glycerol, and lactic acid in a process called *gluconeogenesis.* This glucose may be released directly into the circulation or stored as glycogen.

Fat Metabolism

Fat is the most efficient form of fuel storage, providing 9 kcal/g of stored energy, compared with the 4 kcal/g provided by carbohydrates and proteins.[2] Ideally 20% to 35% of the calories in the normal Canadian diet should be obtained from fats, whereas at least 45% should be obtained from carbohydrates and approximately 15% to 20% from proteins.[1] In addition, many of the carbohydrates consumed in the diet are converted to triglycerides for storage in adipose tissue.

A triglyceride contains three fatty acids linked by a glycerol molecule. The mobilization of fatty acids for use as an energy source is facilitated by the action of enzymes (lipases) that break triglycerides into a glycerol molecule and three fatty acids. The glycerol molecule can enter the glycolytic pathway and be used along with glucose to produce energy, or it can be used to produce glucose. The fatty acids are transported to tissues where they are used for energy. Almost all body cells, with the exception of the brain, nervous tissue, and red blood cells, can use fatty acids interchangeably with glucose for energy. Although many cells readily use fatty acids as a fuel source, fatty acids cannot be converted to the glucose needed by the brain for energy.

A large share of the initial degradation of fatty acids occurs in the liver, especially when excessive amounts of fatty acids are being used for energy. The liver uses only a small amount of the fatty acids for its own energy needs; it converts the rest into ketones and releases them into the blood. In situations that favour fat breakdown, such as diabetes mellitus and fasting, large amounts of ketones are released into the bloodstream. Because ketones are organic acids, they cause ketoacidosis when they are present in excessive amounts.

Protein Metabolism

Proteins are essential for the formation of all body structures, including genes, enzymes, contractile structures in muscle, matrix of bone, and the hemoglobin of red blood cells.[2] Amino acids are the building blocks of proteins. Significant quantities of amino acids are present in body proteins. Unlike glucose and fatty acids, there is only a limited capacity for the storage of excess amino acids in the body. Most of the stored amino acids are contained in body proteins. Amino acids in excess of those needed for protein synthesis are converted to fatty acids, ketones, or glucose and then stored or used as metabolic fuel. Because fatty acids cannot be converted to glucose, the body must break down proteins and use the amino acids as a major substrate for gluconeogenesis during periods when metabolic needs exceed food intake.[2]

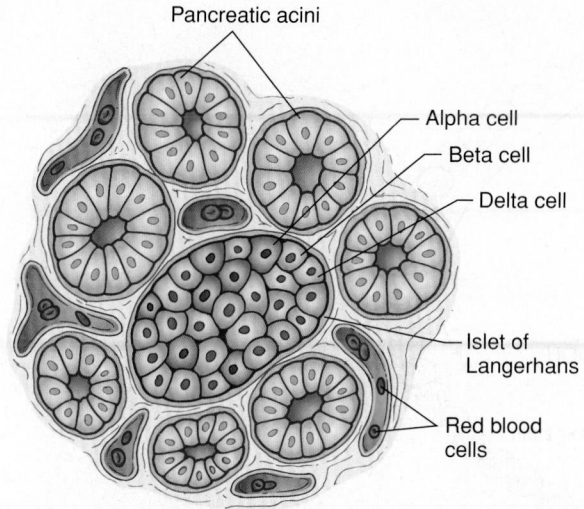

Pancreatic acini

Alpha cell

Beta cell

Delta cell

Islet of Langerhans

Red blood cells

FIGURE 42.2 • Islet of Langerhans in the pancreas.

Glucose-Regulating Hormones

The hormonal control of blood glucose resides largely with the endocrine pancreas. The pancreas is made up of two major tissue types: the acini and the islets of Langerhans (Fig. 42.2). The acini secrete digestive juices into the duodenum, whereas the islets of Langerhans, which account for only about 1% to 2% of volume of the pancreas, secrete hormones into the blood. Each islet is composed of beta cells that secrete insulin and amylin, alpha cells that secrete glucagon, and delta cells that secrete somatostatin. In addition, at least two other types of cell, the PP cell, is present in small numbers in the islets and secretes a hormone of uncertain function called *pancreatic polypeptide,* and the epsilon cell that secrets ghrelin.[2,3] Ghrelin is also secreted from the gastric mucosa and plays a role in gastric emptying and satiety, however the role of islet-derived ghrelin is unclear.[3]

Insulin

Although several hormones are known to increase blood glucose levels, insulin is the only hormone known to have a direct effect in lowering blood glucose levels. The actions of insulin are threefold: (1) it promotes glucose uptake by target cells and provides for glucose storage as glycogen, (2) it prevents fat and glycogen breakdown, and (3) it inhibits gluconeogenesis and increases protein synthesis[2,3] (Table 42.1). Insulin acts to promote fat storage by increasing the transport of glucose into fat cells. It also facilitates triglyceride synthesis from glucose in fat cells and inhibits the intracellular breakdown of stored triglycerides. Insulin also inhibits protein breakdown and increases protein synthesis by increasing the active transport

TABLE 42.1 ACTIONS OF INSULIN AND GLUCAGON ON GLUCOSE, FAT, AND PROTEIN METABOLISM

	INSULIN	GLUCAGON
Glucose		
Glucose transport	Increases glucose transport into skeletal muscle and adipose tissue	
Glycogen synthesis	Increases glycogen synthesis	Promotes glycogen breakdown
Gluconeogenesis	Decreases gluconeogenesis	Increases gluconeogenesis
Fats		
Fatty acid and triglyceride synthesis	Promotes fatty acid and triglyceride synthesis by the liver	
Fat storage in adipose tissue	Increases the transport of fatty acids into adipose cells	
	Increases conversion of fatty acids to triglycerides by increasing the availability of α-glycerol phosphate through increased transport of glucose in adipose cells	
	Maintains fat storage by inhibiting breakdown of stored triglycerides by adipose cell lipase	Activates adipose cell lipase, making increased amounts of fatty acids available to the body for use as energy
Proteins		
Amino acid transport	Increases active transport of amino acids into cells	Increases amino acid uptake by liver cells and their conversion to glucose by gluconeogenesis
Protein synthesis	Increases protein synthesis by increasing transcription of messenger RNA and accelerating protein synthesis by ribosomal RNA	
Protein breakdown	Decreases protein breakdown by enhancing the use of glucose and fatty acids as fuel	

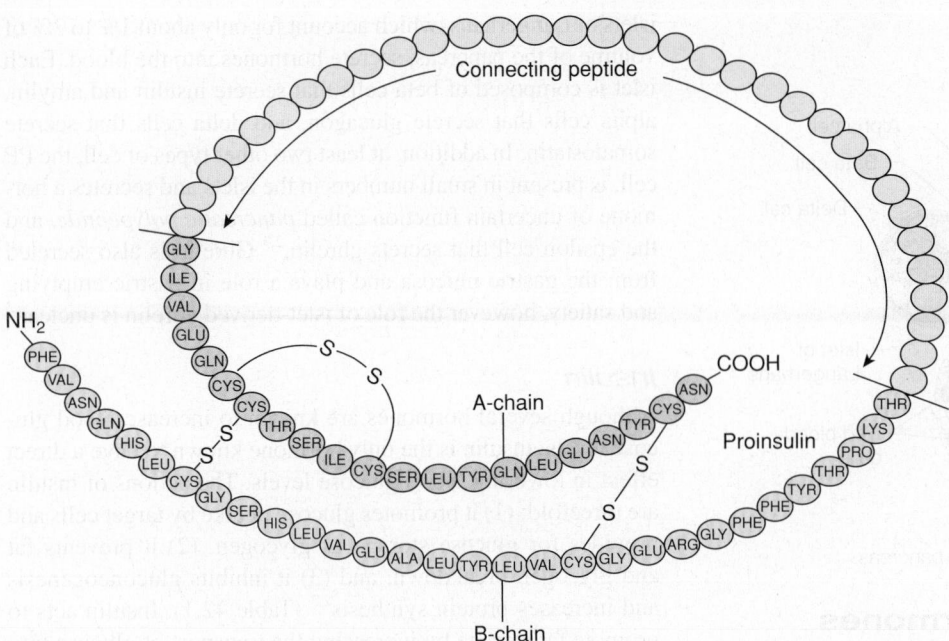

FIGURE 42.3 • Structure of proinsulin. With removal of the connecting peptide (C-peptide), proinsulin is converted to insulin.

of amino acids into body cells; and it inhibits gluconeogenesis, or the building of glucose from new sources, mainly amino acids. When sufficient glucose and insulin are present, protein breakdown is minimal because the body is able to use glucose and fatty acids as a fuel source. In children and adolescents, insulin is needed for normal growth and development.

The active form of insulin is composed of two polypeptide chains—an A chain and a B chain (Fig. 42.3). Active insulin is formed in the beta cells from a larger molecule called *proinsulin.* In converting proinsulin to insulin, enzymes in the beta cell cleave proinsulin at specific sites to form two separate substances: active insulin and a biologically inactive C-peptide (connecting peptide) chain that joined the A and B chains before they were separated. Active insulin and the inactive C-peptide chain are packaged into secretory granules

and released simultaneously from the beta cell. The C-peptide chains can be measured clinically, and this measurement can be used to study beta-cell function. For example, in patients with type 2 diabetes with very little or no remaining beta cell function, the patient will have very low or nonexistent levels of C-peptide in the blood, and thus will likely need insulin replacement for treatment.

The release of insulin from the pancreatic beta cells is regulated by blood glucose levels, increasing as blood glucose levels rise and decreasing when blood glucose levels decline. Blood glucose enters the beta cell by means of the glucose transporter, is phosphorylated by an enzyme called *glucokinase,* and metabolized to form the adenosine triphosphate (ATP) needed to close the potassium channels and depolarize the cell (Fig. 42.4). Depolarization, in turn, results in opening

FIGURE 42.4 • One model of control of release of insulin by the pancreatic beta cells and the action of the sulfonylurea agents. In the resting beta cell with low ATP levels, potassium diffuses through the ATP-gated channels, maintaining the resting membrane potential. As blood glucose rises and is transported into the beta cell by the glucose transporter, ATP rises, causing the potassium channels to close and depolarization to occur. Depolarization results in opening of the voltage-gated calcium channels, which results in insulin secretion. (Modified from Karam J. H. (1992). Type II diabetes and syndrome X. Pathogenesis and glycemic management. *Endocrinology and Metabolism Clinics of North America,* 21(2), 329–350).

FIGURE 42.5 • Biphasic insulin response to a constant glucose stimulus. The peak of the first phase in humans is 3 to 5 minutes; the second phase begins at 2 minutes and continues to increase slowly for at least 60 minutes or until the stimulus stops. (From Ward W. K., Beard J. C., Halter J. B., et al. (1984). Pathology of insulin secretion in non-insulin-dependent diabetes mellitus. *Diabetes Care, 7*(5), 491–502. Used with permission.)

of the calcium channels and insulin secretion.[3] Secretion of insulin occurs in a biphasic, pulsatile fashion. After exposure to glucose, which is a nutrient secretagogue, an initial, rapid first-phase release of stored preformed insulin occurs, followed by a more sustained second-phase release of newly synthesized insulin (Fig. 42.5). Diabetes may result from dysregulation or deficiency in any of the steps involved in this process (*e.g.,* impaired function of the glucose transporters, intracellular metabolic defects, glucokinase deficiency).

Serum insulin levels begin to rise within minutes after a meal, reach a peak in approximately 30 to 45 minutes, and then return to baseline levels within 2 to 3 hours.[3]

Insulin secreted by the beta cells enters the portal circulation and travels directly to the liver, where approximately 50% is used or degraded. Insulin, which is rapidly bound to peripheral tissues or destroyed by the liver or kidneys, has a half-life of approximately 15 minutes once it is released into the general circulation. To initiate its effects on target tissues, insulin binds to a membrane receptor. The insulin receptor is a combination of two subunits—a larger α subunit that extends outside the cell membrane and is involved in insulin binding, and the smaller β subunit that is predominantly inside the cell membrane and contains a kinase enzyme that becomes activated during insulin binding (Fig. 42.6). Activation of the kinase enzyme results in autophosphorylation of the β subunit itself. Phosphorylation of the β subunit in turn activates some enzymes and inactivates others, thereby directing the desired intracellular effect of insulin on glucose, fat, and protein metabolism.[2]

Because cell membranes are impermeable to glucose, they require a special carrier, called a *glucose transporter,* to move glucose from the blood into the cell. These transporters move glucose across the cell membrane at a faster rate than would occur by diffusion alone. Considerable research has revealed a family of glucose transporters termed *GLUT-1, GLUT-2,* and so forth, each with their own tissue distribution.[4] GLUT-4 is the insulin-dependent glucose transporter for skeletal muscle and adipose tissue (Fig. 42.7). It is sequestered inside the membrane of these cells and thus is unable

FIGURE 42.6 • Insulin receptor. Insulin binds to the α subunits of the insulin receptor, which increases glucose and amino acid transport and causes autophosphorylation of the β subunit of the receptor, which induces tyrosine kinase activity. Tyrosine phosphorylation, in turn, activates a cascade of intracellular signalling proteins that mediate the effects of glucose on glucose, fat, and protein metabolism.

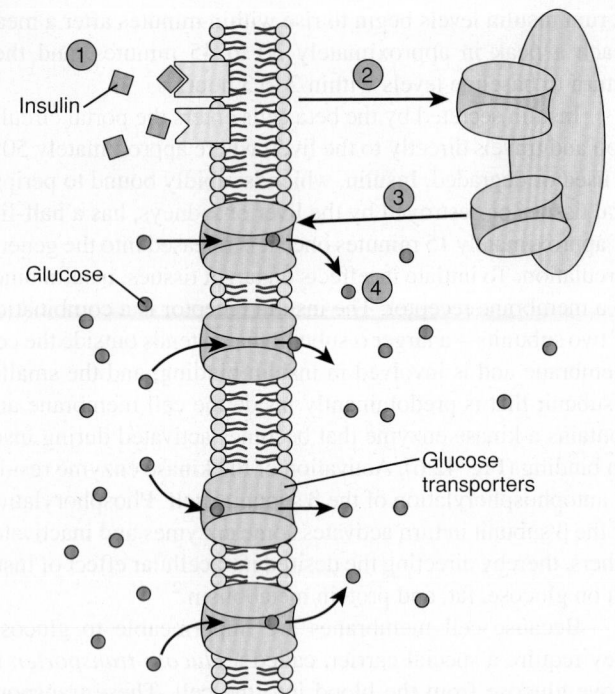

FIGURE 42.7 • Insulin-dependent glucose transporter (GLUT-4). (1) Binding of insulin to insulin receptor on the surface of the cell membrane, (2) generation of intracellular signal, (3) insertion of GLUT-4 receptor from its inactive site into the cell membrane, and (4) transport of glucose across the cell membrane.

to function as a glucose transporter until a signal from insulin causes it to move from its inactive site into the cell membrane, where it facilitates glucose entry. GLUT-2 is the major transporter of glucose into beta cells and liver cells. It has a low affinity for glucose and acts as a transporter only when plasma glucose levels are relatively high, such as after a meal. GLUT-1 is present in all tissues and mediates basal glucose uptake. It does not require the actions of insulin and is important in transport of glucose into cells of the nervous system.

Glucagon

Glucagon, a polypeptide molecule produced by the alpha cells of the islets of Langerhans, maintains blood glucose between meals and during periods of fasting.[2,3] Like insulin, glucagon travels through the portal vein to the liver, where it exerts its main action. In contrast to insulin, glucagon produces an increase in blood glucose (Table 42.1). The most dramatic effect of glucagon is its ability to initiate *glycogenolysis* or the breakdown of liver glycogen as a means of raising blood glucose, usually within a matter of minutes. Glucagon also increases the transport of amino acids into the liver and stimulates their conversion into glucose, a process called *gluconeogenesis*. Because liver glycogen stores are limited, gluconeogenesis is important in maintaining blood glucose levels over time. Other actions of glucagon occur only when the hormone is present in high concentrations, usually well above those normally present in the blood. At high concentrations, glucagon activates adipose cell lipase, making fatty acids available for use as energy.[2] At very

high concentrations, glucagon can increase the strength of the heart, increase blood flow to some tissues, including the kidneys, enhance bile secretion, and inhibit gastric acid secretion.

As with insulin, glucagon secretion is regulated by blood glucose. A decrease in blood glucose concentration to a hypoglycemic level produces an immediate increase in glucagon secretion, and an increase in blood glucose to hyperglycemic levels produces a decrease in glucagon secretion. High concentrations of amino acids, as occur after a protein meal, also can stimulate glucagon secretion.[2] In this way, glucagon increases the conversion of amino acids to glucose as a means of maintaining the body's glucose levels. Glucagon levels also increase during strenuous exercise as a means of preventing a decrease in blood glucose.

Amylin, Somatostatin, and Gut-Derived Hormones

Islet amyloid polypeptide (IAPP), or *amylin,* was originally identified as a major constituent of pancreatic amyloid deposits in persons with type 2 diabetes and subsequently shown to be a polypeptide that is cosecreted with insulin from the beta cells in the pancreas.[3,4] Plasma levels of amylin increase in response to nutritional stimuli to produce inhibition of gastric emptying and glucagon secretion. As with insulin, the active monomeric form, amylin, is derived from a larger proamylin precursor. Although the active monomeric form of amylin is soluble and acts as a hormone, there has been renewed interest in the less soluble oligomeric and insoluble polymeric forms that may contribute to the pathogenesis of overt diabetes.[5]

Somatostatin is a polypeptide hormone containing only 14 amino acids that has an extremely short half-life.[2,3] Somatostatin acts locally in the islets of Langerhans to inhibit the release of insulin and glucagon. It also decreases gastrointestinal activity after ingestion of food. Almost all factors related to ingestion of food stimulate somatostatin secretion. By decreasing gastrointestinal activity, somatostatin is thought to extend the time during which food is absorbed into the blood, and by inhibiting insulin and glucagon, it is thought to extend the use of absorbed nutrients by the tissues.[2]

Several *gut-derived hormones* have been identified as having what is termed an *incretin effect,* meaning that they increase insulin release after an oral nutrient load[2,3,6] (see Chapter 36). This suggests that gut-derived factors can stimulate insulin secretion after a predominantly carbohydrate meal. The two hormones that account for about 90% of the incretin effect are glucagon-like peptide-1, which is released from L cells in the distal small bowel, and glucose-dependent insulinotropic polypeptide (previously known as *gastric inhibitory polypeptide*), which is released by K cells in the upper gut (mainly the jejunum). Currently incretin derived medications have shown benefits of improved glycemic control, improved satiety, delayed gastric emptying, and weight loss.[4]

Counter-Regulatory Hormones

Other hormones that can affect blood glucose include the catecholamines, growth hormone, and the glucocorticoids.

These hormones, along with glucagon, are sometimes called *counter-regulatory hormones* because they counteract the storage functions of insulin in regulating blood glucose levels during periods of fasting, exercise, and other situations that either limit glucose intake or deplete glucose stores.

Epinephrine. *Epinephrine,* one of the catecholamines released from the adrenal medulla, helps to maintain blood glucose levels during periods of stress. Epinephrine has the potent effect of causing glycogenolysis in the liver, thus causing large quantities of glucose to be released into the blood. It also inhibits insulin release from the beta cells and thereby decreases the movement of glucose into muscle cells, while at the same time increasing the breakdown of muscle glycogen stores. The glucose that is released from muscle glycogen cannot be released into the blood; nevertheless, the mobilization of these stores for muscle use conserves blood glucose for use by other tissues such as the brain and the nervous system. Epinephrine also has a direct lipolytic effect on adipose cells, thereby increasing the mobilization of fatty acids for use as an energy source. The blood glucose-elevating effect of epinephrine is an important homeostatic mechanism during periods of hypoglycaemia.

Growth Hormone. Growth hormone has many metabolic effects. It increases protein synthesis in all cells of the body, mobilizes fatty acids from adipose tissue, and antagonizes the effects of insulin. Growth hormone decreases cellular uptake and use of glucose, thereby increasing the level of blood glucose. The increased blood glucose level stimulates further insulin secretion by the beta cells. The secretion of growth hormone normally is inhibited by insulin and increased levels of blood glucose.[6] During periods of fasting, when both blood glucose levels and insulin secretion fall, growth hormone levels increase. Exercise such as running and cycling, and various stresses, including anesthesia, fever, and trauma, increase growth hormone levels.

Chronic hypersecretion of growth hormone, as occurs in acromegaly (see Chapter 41), can lead to glucose intolerance and the development of diabetes mellitus. In people who already have diabetes, moderate elevations in growth hormone levels that occur during periods of stress and periods of growth in children can produce the entire spectrum of metabolic abnormalities associated with poor regulation, despite optimized insulin treatment.[6]

Glucocorticoid Hormones. The glucocorticoid hormones, which are synthesized in the adrenal cortex along with other corticosteroid hormones, are critical to survival during periods of fasting and starvation. They stimulate gluconeogenesis by the liver, sometimes producing a six- to tenfold increase in hepatic glucose production.[2] These hormones also moderately decrease tissue use of glucose. In predisposed persons, the prolonged elevation of glucocorticoid hormones can lead to hyperglycemia and the development of diabetes mellitus. In people with diabetes, even transient increases in cortisol can complicate control.

There are several steroid hormones with glucocorticoid activity; the most important of these is cortisol, which accounts for approximately 95% of all glucocorticoid activity (see Chapter 41). Almost any type of stress, whether physical or emotional, causes an immediate increase in adrenocorticotropic hormone (ACTH) secretion by the anterior pituitary gland, followed within minutes by greatly increased secretion of cortisol by the adrenal gland. Hypoglycemia is a potent stimulus for cortisol secretion. The excess cortisol secreted in persons with Cushing syndrome can also lead to prediabetes and development of diabetes mellitus.

IN SUMMARY

The body uses glucose, fatty acids, and other substrates as fuel to satisfy its energy needs. Body tissues, including the brain, which depends exclusively on glucose for its energy, obtain glucose from the blood. The liver stores excess glucose as glycogen and it uses gluconeogenesis to convert amino acids, lactate, and glycerol into glucose during fasting or when glucose intake does not keep pace with demand. Blood glucose levels reflect the difference between the amount of glucose released into the circulation by the liver and the amount of glucose removed from the blood by body tissues. Fats, which serve as an efficient source of fuel for the body with the exception of the brain, are stored in adipose tissue as triglycerides, which consist of three fatty acids linked to a glycerol molecule. In situations that favour fat breakdown, such as fasting or diabetes mellitus, the triglycerides in adipose tissue are broken down and the fatty acids are used as fuel or transported to the liver, where they are converted to ketones. Proteins, which are made up of amino acids, are essential for the formation of all body structures. Unlike glucose and fatty acids, there is only a limited capacity for storage of excess amino acids in the body. Because fatty acids cannot be converted to glucose, the body must break down proteins and use the amino acids for gluconeogenesis.

Energy metabolism is controlled by a number of hormones, including insulin, glucagon, epinephrine, growth hormone, and the glucocorticoids. Of these hormones, only insulin has the effect of lowering the blood glucose level. Insulin's blood glucose-lowering action results from its ability to increase the transport of glucose into body cells and decrease hepatic production and release of glucose into the bloodstream. Other hormones—glucagon, epinephrine, growth hormone, and the glucocorticoids—maintain or increase blood glucose concentrations and are referred to as counter-regulatory hormones. Glucagon and epinephrine promote glycogenolysis. Glucagon and the glucocorticoids increase gluconeogenesis. Growth hormone decreases the peripheral use of glucose. Epinephrine and glucagon also increase the use of fat for energy by increasing the release of fatty acids from adipose cells.

DIABETES MELLITUS

After completing this section of the chapter, you should be able to meet the following objectives:

- Compare the distinguishing features of type 1 and type 2 diabetes mellitus, list causes of other specific types of diabetes, and cite the criteria for gestational diabetes.
- Describe what is meant by the term *prediabetes*.
- Relate the physiologic functions of insulin to the manifestations of diabetes mellitus.
- Define the metabolic syndrome and describe its associations with the development of type 2 diabetes.
- Discuss the role of diet and exercise in the management of diabetes mellitus.
- Characterize the blood glucose-lowering actions of the hypoglycemic agents used in treatment of type 2 diabetes.
- Name and describe the types (according to duration of action) of insulin.
- Differentiate between the causes and clinical manifestations of diabetic ketoacidosis and the hyperosmolar hyperglycemic state.
- Describe alterations in physiologic function that accompany diabetic peripheral neuropathy, retinopathy, and nephropathy.
- Describe the causes of foot ulcers in people with diabetes mellitus.
- Explain the relation between diabetes mellitus and infection.

The term *diabetes* is derived from a Greek word meaning "going through," and *mellitus* from the Latin word for "honey" or "sweet." Reports of the disorder can be traced back to the first century AD, when Aretaeus the Cappadocian described the disorder as a chronic affliction characterized by intense thirst and voluminous, honey-sweet urine: "the melting down of flesh into urine." It was the discovery of insulin by Banting and Best in 1922 that transformed the once-fatal disease into a manageable chronic health problem.[7]

Diabetes is a disorder of carbohydrate, protein, and fat metabolism resulting from an imbalance between insulin availability and insulin need. It can represent an absolute insulin deficiency, impaired release of insulin by the pancreatic beta cells, inadequate or defective insulin receptors, inadequate or defective insulin postreceptor regulation, or the production of inactive insulin or insulin that is destroyed before it can carry out its action. A person with uncontrolled diabetes is unable to transport glucose into fat and muscle cells; as a result, body cells are starved, and the breakdown of fat and protein is increased to generate alternative fuels.

Classification and Etiology

Although diabetes mellitus clearly is a disorder of insulin availability, it is not a single disease and the Canadian Diabetes Association Clinical Practice Guidelines Expert Committee adopted the American classification system that was updated in 2012[1] (Table 42.2). Type 2 diabetes currently accounts for at least 90% of the cases of diabetes. Included in the classification system are the categories of gestational diabetes mellitus (*i.e.,* diabetes that develops during pregnancy) and other specific types of diabetes, many of which occur secondary to other conditions (*e.g.,* Cushing syndrome, acromegaly, pancreatitis, hemochromatosis).[1]

The revised classification system also includes a system for diagnosing diabetes according to stages of glucose intolerance[1] (Table 42.3). The revised criteria have a category of *impaired glucose tolerance* (IGT), a category of *impaired fasting plasma glucose* (IFG), and a *glycated hemoglobin* (HbA$_{1C}$ or A$_{1C}$). The categories of IFG, IGT, and A$_{1C}$ refer to metabolic stages intermediate between normal glucose homeostasis and diabetes, and are labelled together as *prediabetes*. A fasting plasma glucose (FPG) of less than 6.0 mmol/L or a result of 5.0 to 8.0 mmol/L 2 hours after a meal are considered normal. The Canadian Diabetes Association (CDA) defines prediabetes as an AIC between 6.0% and 6.4% (compared to the American Diabetes Association of 5.7% to 6.4%), and IFG as an elevated FPG concentration of 6.1 to 6.9 mmol/L, noting that the International Diabetes Federation (IDF) identifies 5.6 to 6.9 mmol/L as IFG. IGT reflects abnormal fasting plasma glucose measurements of 6.1 to 6.9 mmol/L and after a 2-hour, 75-g oral glucose tolerance test (OGTT) a result of 7.8 to 11.0 mmol/L.[1] IFG and IGT (*i.e.,* prediabetes) categories are associated with increased risk of atherosclerotic heart disease and increased risk of progression to type 2 diabetes. IFG and IGT have different rates of progression to diabetes because of different pathophysiologic mechanisms; however an IFG and prediabetes A$_{1C}$ value is 100% predictive of progression to type 2 diabetes within a 5-year period.[1] Calorie restriction and weight reduction (even 5% to 10%) are important in overweight people with prediabetes.[8] Persons with an FPG of 7.0 mmol/L or more, or a 2-hour OGTT of 11.1 mmol/L or more after a 75-g glucose load are considered to have *provisional diabetes*.[1] If asymptomatic, a repeat confirmatory test (FPG, A$_{1C}$, or a 2-hour PG in a 75-g OGTT) must be done. If symptomatic, the diagnosis should be made, and begin treatment. The criteria in Chart 42.1 are used to confirm the diagnosis of diabetes in persons with provisional diabetes.

Type 1 Diabetes Mellitus

Type 1 diabetes mellitus or T1DM is characterized by destruction of the pancreatic beta cells.[9] Type 1 diabetes is subdivided into two types: type 1A immune-mediated diabetes, and type 1B idiopathic (nonimmune-related) diabetes. In Canada, United States, and Europe, approximately 90% to 95% of people with type 1 diabetes mellitus have type 1A immune-mediated diabetes, however from a treatment perspective, the types of type 1 diabetes are not differentiated.

TABLE 42.2 ETIOLOGIC CLASSIFICATION OF DIABETES MELLITUS

TYPE	SUBTYPES	ETIOLOGY OF GLUCOSE INTOLERANCE
I. Type 1[a]	Beta cell destruction usually leading to absolute insulin deficiency	
	A. Immune mediated	Autoimmune destruction of beta cells
	B. Idiopathic	Unknown
II. Type 2[a]	May range from predominantly insulin resistance with relative insulin deficiency to a predominantly secretory defect with insulin resistance	
III. Other specific types	A. Genetic defects in beta cell function, *e.g.,* glucokinase	Dysregulation insulin secretion due to a defect in glucokinase generation
	B. Genetic defects in insulin action, *e.g.,* leprechaunism, Rabson–Mendenhall syndrome	Pediatric syndromes that have mutations in insulin receptors
	C. Diseases of exocrine pancreas, *e.g.,* pancreatitis, neoplasms, cystic fibrosis	Loss or destruction of insulin-producing beta cells
	D. Endocrine disorders, *e.g.,* acromegaly, Cushing syndrome	Diabetogenic effects of excess hormone levels
	E. Drug or chemical induced, *e.g.,* Vacor, atypical antipsychotics, glucocorticosteroids, thiazide diuretics, interferon-alfa	Toxic destruction of beta cells Insulin resistance Impaired insulin secretion Production of islet cell antibodies
	F. Infections, *e.g.,* congenital rubella, cytomegalovirus	Beta cell injury followed by autoimmune response
	G. Uncommon forms of immune-mediated diabetes, *e.g.,* "stiff man syndrome"	Autoimmune disorder of central nervous system with immune-mediated beta cell destruction
	H. Other genetic syndromes sometimes associated with diabetes, *e.g.,* Down syndrome, Klinefelter syndrome, Turner syndrome	Disorders of glucose tolerance related to defects associated with chromosomal abnormalities
IV. Gestational diabetes mellitus (GDM)	Any degree of glucose intolerance with onset or first recognition during pregnancy	Combination of insulin resistance and impaired insulin secretion

[a]Patients with any form of diabetes may require insulin treatment at some stage of the disease. Such use of insulin, does not, of itself, classify the patient.
Adapted and updated from American Diabetes Association. (2012). Diagnosis and classification of diabetes mellitus. *Diabetes Care, 35*(Suppl 1), S64–S71.

Type 1A Immune-Mediated Diabetes. Type 1A diabetes, commonly referred to simply as type 1 diabetes, is characterized by immune-mediated destruction of beta cells. This type of diabetes, formerly called *juvenile diabetes,* occurs more commonly in young persons but can occur at any age. The rate of beta cell destruction is quite variable, being rapid in some individuals and slow in others. The rapidly progressive

form commonly is observed in children, but also may occur in adults. The slowly progressive form usually occurs in adults and is sometimes referred to as *latent autoimmune diabetes in adults* (LADA). LADA may account for up to 10% of adults who are currently classified as having type 2 diabetes.[8]

Type 1 diabetes is a catabolic disorder characterized by an absolute lack of insulin, an elevation in blood glucose, and

TABLE 42.3 EXPERT COMMITTEE ON THE DIAGNOSIS AND CLASSIFICATION OF DIABETES MELLITUS CRITERIA FOR CLASSIFICATION OF DIABETES USING FASTING PLASMA GLUCOSE AND ORAL GLUCOSE TOLERANCE TEST

TEST	NORMOGLYCEMIC	PREDIABETES	DIABETES MELLITUS[‡]
FPG[a]	<6.0 mmol/L	6.1–6.9 mmol/L	≥7.0 mmol/L
2-hr OGTT[b]	<8.0 mmol/L	7.8–11.0 mmol/L	≥11.1 mmol/L
A$_{1C}$ (%)	<6.0%	6.0–6.4%	≥6.5%
Other			Symptoms of diabetes mellitus and casual plasma glucose ≥11.1 mmol/L

[a]Fasting is defined as no caloric intake for at least 8 hours.
[b]OGTT with 2-hour measurement of venous plasma or serum glucose after a 75-g carbohydrate load.
FPG, fasting plasma glucose; OGGT, oral glucose tolerance test.
[‡]In the absence of unequivocal hyperglycemia with acute metabolic decompensation, these criteria should be confirmed by repeat testing on a separate day.
Developed from data in Canadian Diabetes Association Clinical Practice Guidelines Expert Committee. (2013). Canadian Diabetes Association 2013 clinical practice guidelines for the prevention and management of diabetes in Canada. *Canadian Journal of Diabetes, 37*(Suppl 1), S8–S11.

a breakdown of body fats and proteins. The absolute lack of insulin in people with type 1 diabetes mellitus means that they are particularly prone to the development of ketoacidosis. One of the actions of insulin is the inhibition of *lipolysis (i.e.,* fat breakdown) and release of free fatty acids (FFA) from fat cells. In the absence of insulin, ketosis develops when these fatty acids are released from fat cells and converted to ketones in the liver. Because of the loss of insulin response, all people with type 1A diabetes require exogenous insulin replacement to reverse the catabolic state, control blood glucose levels, and prevent ketosis.

DIABETES MELLITUS

- Diabetes mellitus is a disorder of carbohydrate, fat, and protein metabolism brought about by impaired beta cell synthesis or release of insulin, or the inability of tissues to use insulin.
- Type 1 diabetes results from loss of beta cell function and an absolute insulin deficiency.
- Type 2 diabetes results from impaired ability of the tissues to use insulin (insulin resistance) accompanied by a relative lack of insulin or impaired release of insulin in relation to blood glucose levels (beta cell dysfunction).

Type 1A diabetes is thought to be an autoimmune disorder resulting from a genetic predisposition (*i.e.,* diabetogenic genes); an environmental triggering event, such as an infection; and a T-lymphocyte–mediated hypersensitivity reaction against some beta cell antigen (see Chapter 19). Much evidence has focused on the inherited major histocompatibility complex (MHC) genes on chromosome 6 that encode human leukocyte antigens HLA-DQ and HLA-DR, especially DR-3 and DR-4.[3] In addition to the MHC susceptibility genes for type 1 diabetes on chromosome 6, an insulin gene regulating beta cell replication and function has been identified on chromosome 11.

Type 1A diabetes-associated autoantibodies may exist for years before the onset of hyperglycemia. There are two major types of autoantibodies: insulin autoantibodies (IAAs), and islet cell autoantibodies and antibodies directed at other islet autoantigens, including glutamic acid decarboxylase (GAD) and the protein tyrosine phosphatase IA-2.[3,9] Testing for antibodies to GAD or IA-2 and for IAAs using sensitive radiobinding assays can identify more than 90% of cases of new type 1 diabetes.[9] The appearance of IAAs may precede that of antibodies to GAD or IA-2, and IAAs may be the only antibodies detected at diagnosis in young children. These people also may have other autoimmune disorders such as Graves disease, rheumatoid arthritis, and Addison disease.

The fact that type 1 diabetes is thought to result from an interaction between genetic and environmental factors has led to research into methods directed at prevention and early control of the disease. These methods include the identification of genetically susceptible persons and early intervention in newly diagnosed persons with type 1 diabetes. After the diagnosis of type 1 diabetes, there often is a short period of beta cell regeneration, during which symptoms of diabetes disappear and insulin injections are reduced or not needed. This is sometimes called the *honeymoon period.* Immune interventions (immunomodulation) designed to interrupt the destruction of beta cells before development of type 1 diabetes are being investigated in various trials. Unfortunately, none of the interventions studied to date has shown real clinical utility. Modulation of environmental influences, such as infant diet and breast-feeding, has also led to conflicting results.[3,9]

Idiopathic Type 1B Diabetes. The term *idiopathic type 1B diabetes* is used to describe those cases of beta cell destruction in which no evidence of autoimmunity is present. Only a small number of people with type 1 diabetes fall into this category; most are of African or Asian descent. Type 1B diabetes is strongly inherited. People with the disorder have episodic ketoacidosis due to varying degrees of insulin deficiency with periods of absolute insulin deficiency that may come and go.

Type 2 Diabetes Mellitus and the Metabolic Syndrome

Type 2 diabetes mellitus accounts for 90% to 95% of cases and is a heterogeneous condition that describes the presence of hyperglycemia in association with *relative* insulin deficiency and not the autoimmune destruction of beta cells. Depending on the level of deficiency, people with type 2 diabetes may eventually require insulin treatment. Although many people with type 2 diabetes are adults and overweight recent trends indicate type 2 diabetes has become a more common occurrence in obese adolescents and children.[10] Due to confusion previous terms such as adult onset diabetes and non-insulin–dependent diabetes are considered obsolete and no longer are used to describe type 2 diabetes

Type 2 diabetes has a strong genetic component.[3] A number of genetic and acquired pathogenic factors have been implicated in the progressive impairment of beta cell function in persons with prediabetes and type 2 diabetes. More than one-third of people who develop type 2 diabetes have at least one parent with diabetes. Monozygotic twins have greater than 90% concordance rates for lifetime development of type 2 diabetes. Despite the strong familial predisposition, the genetics of type 2 diabetes is poorly defined. This is probably because of the heterogeneous nature of the disorder as well as the difficulty in sorting out the contribution of acquired factors affecting insulin action and glycemic control.[3,11]

The metabolic abnormalities that lead to type 2 diabetes include (1) insulin resistance, (2) deranged secretion of insulin by the pancreatic beta cells, and (3) increased glucose production by the liver[12] (Fig. 42.8). In contrast to type 1 diabetes, where *absolute* insulin deficiency is present, persons with type 2 diabetes may have high, normal, or low insulin levels. Insulin resistance initially stimulates an increase in insulin secretion, often to a level of modest hyperinsulinemia, as the beta cells attempt to maintain a normal blood glucose level. In time, the increased demand for insulin secretion leads to beta cell exhaustion and failure. This results in elevated postprandial blood glucose levels and an eventual increase in glucose production by the liver. Because people with type 2 diabetes

do not have an absolute insulin deficiency, they are less prone to ketoacidosis than are people with type 1 diabetes.

Insulin resistance is said to be present when the biologic effects of insulin are less than expected for both glucose disposal in skeletal muscle and suppression of glucose production by the liver.[3,12] In the basal state, hepatic insulin resistance is manifested by overproduction of glucose despite fasting hyperinsulinemia, with the rate of glucose production being the primary determinant of the elevated FPG in persons with type 2 diabetes. Although muscle glucose uptake is increased in absolute terms after a meal, the efficiency with which it is taken up (glucose clearance) is diminished, resulting in an increase in postprandial blood glucose levels. Although the insulin resistance seen in persons with type 2 diabetes can be caused by a number of factors, it is strongly associated with obesity and physical inactivity. A number of circulating hormones, cytokines, and metabolic fuels such as FFAs originate in adipose tissue and modulate insulin action.

Specific causes of beta cell dysfunction are unclear but seem to include an initial decrease in the beta cell mass related to genetic or prenatal factors (*e.g.,* intrauterine growth retardation; see Chapter 2); increased apoptosis or decreased beta cell regeneration; beta cell exhaustion due to long-standing insulin resistance; glucotoxicity (*i.e.,* glucose toxicity-induced beta cell desensitization); lipotoxicity (*i.e.,* toxic effects of lipids on beta cells); and amyloid deposition or other conditions that have the potential to reduce beta cell mass.[12]

Insulin Resistance and the Metabolic Syndrome. There is increasing evidence to suggest that insulin resistance not only contributes to the hyperglycemia in persons with type 2 diabetes, but may play a role in other metabolic abnormalities. These include obesity, high levels of plasma triglycerides

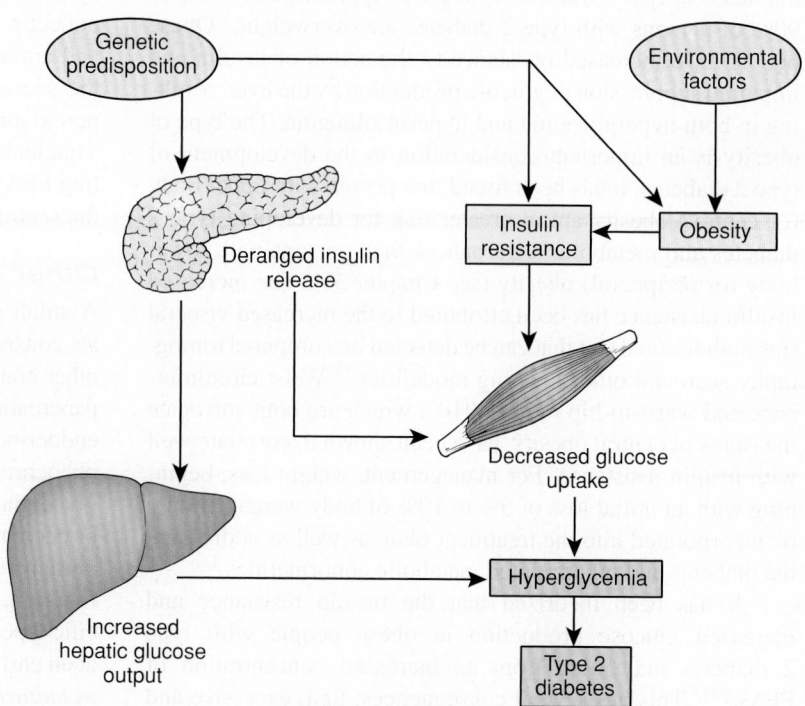

FIGURE 42.8 • Pathogenesis of type 2 diabetes mellitus.

CHART 42.2 **NCEP ATP III CRITERIA FOR A DIAGNOSIS OF METABOLIC SYNDROME**

Three or more of the following:

- Abdominal obesity: waist circumference >88 cm in women or >102 cm in men
- Triglycerides ≥1.7 mmol/L
- High-density lipoproteins (HDL) <1.3 mmol/L in women or <1.0 mmol/L in men
- Blood pressure >130/85 mm Hg
- Fasting plasma glucose 5.7–7.0 mmol/L

Developed from Grundy S. M., Panel Chair. (2001). *Third report of the National Cholesterol Education Program (NCEP) expert panel on detection, evaluation, and treatment of high blood cholesterol in adults (Adult Treatment Panel III)*. NIH publication no. 01–3670. Bethesda, MD: National Institutes of Health.

and low levels of high-density lipoproteins (HDL), hypertension, systemic inflammation (as detected by C-reactive protein [CRP] and other mediators), abnormal fibrinolysis, abnormal function of the vascular endothelium, and macrovascular disease (coronary artery, cerebrovascular, and peripheral arterial disease). This constellation of abnormalities often is referred to as the *insulin resistance syndrome, syndrome X*, or, the preferred term, *metabolic syndrome*.[3,13,14] The clinical signs, laboratory abnormalities, and illnesses associated with this syndrome are described in Chart 42.2. Insulin resistance and increased risk of developing type 2 diabetes are also seen in women with polycystic ovary syndrome[11] (see Chapter 46).

A major factor in persons with the metabolic syndrome that leads to type 2 diabetes is obesity. Approximately 80% to 90% of persons with type 2 diabetes are overweight.[1] Obese people have increased resistance to the action of insulin and impaired suppression of glucose production by the liver, resulting in both hyperglycemia and hyperinsulinemia. The type of obesity is an important consideration in the development of type 2 diabetes. It has been found that people with upper body (or central) obesity are at greater risk for developing type 2 diabetes and metabolic disturbances than persons with lower body (or peripheral) obesity (see Chapter 39). The increased insulin resistance has been attributed to the increased visceral (intra-abdominal) fat that can be detected on computed tomography scan and other imaging modalities.[15] Waist circumference and waist-to-hip ratio (WHR), which are both surrogate measures of central obesity, have been shown to correlate well with insulin resistance. For management, weight loss, beginning with an initial loss of 5% to 10% of body weight, should be incorporated into the treatment plan, as well as addressing the diabetes and other related metabolic abnormalities.[1]

It has been theorized that the insulin resistance and increased glucose production in obese people with type 2 diabetes may stem from an increased concentration of FFAs.[16,17] This has several consequences: first, excessive and chronic elevation of FFAs can cause beta cell dysfunction (lipotoxicity); second, FFAs act at the level of the peripheral tissues to cause insulin resistance and glucose underutilization by inhibiting glucose uptake and glycogen storage; and third, the accumulation of FFAs and triglycerides reduces hepatic insulin sensitivity, leading to increased hepatic glucose production and hyperglycemia, especially in the fasting state. Thus, the increase in FFAs that occurs in obese individuals (especially those with visceral obesity) with a genetic predisposition to type 2 diabetes may eventually lead to beta cell dysfunction, increased insulin resistance, and greater hepatic glucose production. A further consequence is the diversion of excess FFAs to nonadipose tissues, including the liver, skeletal muscle, heart, and pancreatic beta cells.[3,17] In the liver, the uptake of FFAs from the portal blood can lead to hepatic triglyceride accumulation and nonalcoholic fatty liver disease (see Chapter 38).

Adipocytes are the source of a number of important factors (*e.g.*, adiponectin, leptin, FFAs) involved in a wide range of processes related to the features of the metabolic syndrome, including glucose and lipid metabolism, inflammation, and thrombosis.[16–19] In obesity and type 2 diabetes, there is a reduction in the production of some factors that are normally synthesized by adipocytes (*e.g.*, adiponectin), and an accelerated release of other factors such as angiotensinogen, plasminogen activator inhibitor-1, leptin, and proinflammatory cytokines (*e.g.*, tumour necrosis factor-α).[18] Adiponectin, which is secreted by adipocytes and circulates in the blood, is the only known adipocyte-secreted factor that increases tissue sensitivity to insulin.[19] It has been shown that decreased levels of adiponectin coincide with insulin resistance in patients with obesity and type 2 diabetes. In skeletal muscle, adiponectin has been shown to decrease tissue triglyceride content by increasing the use of fatty acids as a fuel source.[19] Adiponectin also appears to have antidiabetic, anti-inflammatory, and antiatherogenic effects. Moreover, there is evidence that the secretion of adiponectin might be partially regulated by peroxisome proliferator-activated receptor gamma (PPAR-γ), a nuclear receptor that leads to the regulation of genes controlling FFA levels and glucose metabolism[18,19] (discussed later in the section on thiazolidinediones [oral antidiabetic agents]).

Other Specific Types of Diabetes

A small percentage of the overall number of cases of diabetes consist of specific types of diabetes associated with certain other conditions and syndromes. Such diabetes can occur with pancreatic disease or the removal of pancreatic tissue and with endocrine diseases, such as acromegaly, Cushing syndrome, or pheochromocytoma.[1] Endocrine disorders that produce hyperglycemia do so by increasing the hepatic production of glucose or decreasing the cellular use of glucose. Several specific types of diabetes are associated with monogenetic defects in beta cell function. These rare autosomal dominant types of inherited specific types of diabetes, which resemble type 2 diabetes but occur at an earlier age (usually before 25 years of age), are referred to as *maturity-onset diabetes of the young* (MODY).[1,3,11]

Several medications commonly used for treatment of other diseases can cause significant alterations in glucose. For example, diuretics especially thiazide and loop diuretics can elevate blood glucose. These diuretics increase potassium loss, which is thought to impair beta cell release of insulin. Other drugs and therapies known to cause hyperglycemia include diazoxide, glucocorticoids, oral contraceptives, antipsychotic agents, and total parenteral nutrition (*i.e.,* hyperalimentation). Drug-related increases in blood glucose usually are reversed after the drug has been discontinued.

Gestational Diabetes

Gestational diabetes mellitus (GDM) refers to any degree of glucose intolerance that is first detected during pregnancy. The prevalence of GDM for Canadians is estimated at 3.7% for non-Aboriginals up to 18% for Aboriginal populations, with an average of approximately 1 in every 10 pregnant women over the age of 30 years developing GDM.[1,20,21] It most frequently affects women with a family history of diabetes; with a history of stillbirth or spontaneous abortion, fetal anomalies in a previous pregnancy, or a previous large- or heavy-for-date infant; and who are obese, of advanced maternal age, or who have had five or more pregnancies.

All pregnant women should undergo risk assessment for diabetes during their first prenatal visit to determine the need for additional screening tests. Women who are younger than 25 years of age, were of normal body weight before pregnancy, have no family history of diabetes or poor obstetric outcome, and are not members of a high-risk ethnic/racial group (*e.g.,* Aboriginal, Hispanic, South Asian, Asian, African) may not need to be screened.[1] Those with significant risk factors should undergo plasma glucose testing as soon as is feasible. If they are found not to have GDM at the initial screening, they should be retested between 24 and 28 weeks. Women with average risk should be tested at 24 to 28 weeks' gestation. Women with an FPG greater than 7.0 mmol/L or casual glucose greater than 11.1 mmol/L meet the threshold for diabetes, if confirmed on a subsequent day, and do not need to undergo oral glucose tolerance testing.[1] Women with high or average GDM risk who do not demonstrate this degree of hyperglycemia on FPG testing should undergo further screening using the OGTT. In Canada, the recommended screening test consists of 50 g of glucose given without regard to the last meal, followed in 1 hour by a venous blood sample for glucose concentration. If the plasma glucose level is greater than 7.8 mmol/L, then a 75-g 2-hour or a 100-g 3-hour OGTT is indicated to establish the diagnosis of GDM.[1]

Diagnosis and careful medical management are essential because women with GDM are at higher risk for complications of pregnancy, mortality, and fetal abnormalities.[3,21] Fetal abnormalities include macrosomia (*i.e.,* large body size), hypoglycemia, hypocalcemia, polycythemia, and hyperbilirubinemia.

Treatment of GDM includes close observation of mother and fetus because even mild hyperglycemia has been shown to be detrimental to the fetus.[1] Maternal fasting and postprandial blood glucose levels should be measured regularly. Fetal surveillance depends on the degree of risk for the fetus. The frequency of growth measurements and determinations of fetal distress depends on available technology and gestational age. All women with GDM require nutritional guidance because nutrition is the cornerstone of therapy. The nutrition plan should provide the necessary nutrients for maternal and fetal health, result in normoglycemia and proper weight gain, and prevent ketosis.[3] If dietary management alone does not achieve a fasting blood glucose level no greater than 6.0 mmol/L or a 2-hour postprandial blood glucose no greater than 8.0 mmol/L, the Canadian Diabetes Association and the Society of Obstetricians and Gynaecologists (SOGC) recommends therapy with insulin.[1,15] Self-monitoring of blood glucose levels is essential.

After 9 years, 20% of women with GDM will develop type 2 diabetes.[22] Predictors of future diabetes or prediabetes include maternal obesity, elevated FBG on OGTT, elevated A_{1C}, and diagnosis of GDM early in gestation. Women in whom GDM is diagnosed should be followed after delivery to detect diabetes early in its course.

Clinical Manifestations of Diabetes

Diabetes mellitus may have a rapid or an insidious onset. In type 1 diabetes, signs and symptoms often arise suddenly. Type 2 diabetes usually develops more insidiously, often over years and its presence may be detected during a routine medical examination or when a patient seeks medical care for other reasons.

The most commonly identified signs and symptoms of diabetes are referred to as the *three polys:* (1) polyuria (*i.e.,* excessive urination), (2) polydipsia (*i.e.,* excessive thirst), and (3) polyphagia (*i.e.,* excessive hunger). These three symptoms are closely related to the hyperglycemia and glycosuria of diabetes. Glucose is a small, osmotically active molecule. When blood glucose levels are sufficiently elevated, the amount of glucose filtered by the glomeruli of the kidney exceeds the amount that can be reabsorbed by the renal tubules; this results in glycosuria accompanied by large losses of water in the urine. Thirst results from the intracellular dehydration that occurs as blood glucose levels rise and water is pulled out of body cells, including those in the hypothalamic thirst centre. This early symptom may be easily overlooked in people with type 2 diabetes, particularly in those who have had a gradual increase in blood glucose levels. Polyphagia usually is not present in people with type 2 diabetes. In type 1 diabetes, it probably results from cellular starvation and the depletion of cellular stores of carbohydrates, fats, and proteins.

Weight loss despite normal or increased appetite is a common occurrence in people with uncontrolled type 1 diabetes. The cause of weight loss is twofold. First, loss of body fluids results from osmotic diuresis. Vomiting may exaggerate the fluid loss in ketoacidosis. Second, body tissue is lost because the lack of insulin forces the body to use its fat stores and cellular proteins as sources of energy. In terms of weight loss, there often is a marked difference between type 2 diabetes and type 1 diabetes. Weight loss is a frequent phenomenon in people with uncontrolled type 1 diabetes, whereas many people with uncomplicated type 2 diabetes often have problems with obesity.

Other signs and symptoms of hyperglycemia include recurrent blurred vision, fatigue, paresthesias, and skin infections.[1] In type 2 diabetes, these often are the symptoms that prompt a person to seek medical treatment. Blurred vision develops as the lens and retina are exposed to hyperosmolar fluids. Lowered plasma volume produces weakness and fatigue. Paresthesias reflect a damage to blood vessels and of the peripheral nerves. Chronic skin infections can occur and are more common in people with type 2 diabetes. Hyperglycemia and glycosuria favour the growth of yeast organisms. Pruritus and vulvovaginitis due to *Candida* infections are common initial complaints in women with diabetes. Balanitis or balanoposthitis secondary to *Candida* infections can occur in men.[23]

Diagnostic Tests

The diagnosis of diabetes mellitus is confirmed through the use of laboratory tests that measure blood glucose levels (see Table 42.3). Screening tests for diabetes should be considered in all individuals 40 years of age and older.[1] Testing should be considered at a younger age in people who are obese, have a first-degree relative with diabetes, are members of a high-risk group, have delivered an infant weighing more than 9 pounds, have been diagnosed with GDM, have hypertension or hyperlipidemia, or have met the criteria for IGT or IFG (*i.e.*, prediabetes) on previous testing.[1]

Blood Tests

Blood glucose measurements are used in both the diagnosis and management of diabetes. Diagnostic tests include the FPG, casual plasma glucose, and the glucose tolerance test. Laboratory and capillary or finger-stick glucose tests are used for glucose management in people with diagnosed diabetes. Glycated hemoglobin (A_{1C}, previously termed HbA_{1C}) can be used as a diagnostic test or to provide information of glucose control over time. Table 42.4 shows the correlation between A_{1C} levels and the average plasma glucose levels reflecting overall glycemic control in persons with diabetes.[1]

TABLE 42.4 CORRELATION BETWEEN HEMOGLOBIN A_{1C} LEVEL AND MEAN PLASMA GLUCOSE LEVELS

HEMOGLOBIN A_{1C} (%)	MEAN PLASMA GLUCOSE (mmol/L)
6	7.0
7	8.6
8	10.2
9	11.8
10	13.4
11	14.9
12	16.5

Adapted from American Diabetes Association (2014). Standards of medical care in diabetes—2014. *Diabetes Care, 37*(Suppl 1), S14–S80.

Fasting Blood Glucose Test. The fasting blood or plasma glucose (FPG) has been suggested as the preferred diagnostic test because of ease of administration, convenience, patient acceptability, and cost.[1] Glucose levels are measured after food has been withheld for at least 8 hours. An FPG level below 6.0 mmol/L is considered normal (see Table 42.3). A level between 6.1 and 6.9 mmol/L is significant and is defined as impaired fasting glucose. If the FPG level is 7.0 mmol/L or more on two occasions, diabetes is diagnosed.[1]

Random Blood Glucose Test. A random plasma glucose is one that is done without regard to the time of the last meal. A casual plasma glucose concentration that is unequivocally elevated (≥ 11.1 mmol/L) in the presence of classic symptoms of diabetes such as polydipsia, polyphagia, polyuria, and blurred vision is diagnostic of diabetes mellitus at any age.

Oral Glucose Tolerance Test. The OGTT is an important screening test for diabetes. The test measures the body's ability to store glucose by removing it from the blood. In men and women, the test measures the plasma glucose response to 75 g of concentrated glucose solution at selected intervals, usually 1 and 2 hours. In pregnant women, the preferred approach is to start with a glucose load of 50 g and proceed to 75 g if applicable. In people with normal glucose tolerance, blood glucose levels return to normal within 2 to 3 hours after ingestion of a glucose load, in which case it can be assumed that sufficient insulin is present to allow glucose to leave the blood and enter body cells. Because a person with diabetes lacks the ability to respond to an increase in blood glucose by releasing adequate insulin to facilitate storage, blood glucose levels rise above those observed in normal people and remain elevated for longer periods (see Table 42.3).

Capillary Blood Glucose Monitoring. Technologic advances have provided the means for monitoring blood glucose levels by using a drop of capillary blood. This procedure has provided health professionals with a rapid means for monitoring blood glucose and has given people with diabetes a way of maintaining near-normal blood glucose levels through self-monitoring of blood glucose. These methods use a drop of capillary blood obtained by lancing the finger or forearm with a special needle or small lancet. Small trigger devices make use of the lancet virtually painless. The drop of capillary blood is placed on or absorbed by a reagent strip, and glucose levels are determined electronically using a glucose meter.

Laboratory tests that use plasma for measurement of blood glucose give results that are 10% to 15% higher than the finger-stick method, which uses whole blood.[3] Most blood glucose monitors approved for home use and test strips calibrate blood glucose readings to plasma values. It is important that people with diabetes know whether their monitors or glucose strips provide whole-blood or plasma test results.

Continuous glucose monitoring systems are becoming available to fine-tune glucose management. The various systems have small catheters that are implanted in the subcutaneous tissue to provide frequent samples. The real time glucose information can transmitted to a display unit or integrated with an insulin pump to optimize glycemic management. The variety and accuracy of these systems is continually improving. However, finger-stick glucose monitoring remains the standard of care.[1]

Glycated Hemoglobin Testing. Glycated hemoglobin, also referred to as glycohemoglobin, glycosylated hemoglobin, HBA$_{1C}$, or A$_{1C}$ (the preferred term), is a term used to describe hemoglobin into which glucose has been incorporated. Hemoglobin normally does not contain glucose when it is released from the bone marrow. During its 120-day life span in the red blood cell, hemoglobin normally becomes glycated to form hemoglobins A$_{1A}$ and A$_{1B}$ (2% to 4%), and A$_{1C}$ (4% to 6%). Because glucose entry into red blood cells is not insulin dependent, the rate at which glucose becomes attached to the hemoglobin molecule depends on blood glucose levels. Glycosylation is essentially irreversible, and the level of A$_{1C}$ present in the blood provides an index of blood glucose levels over the previous 6 to 12 weeks. In uncontrolled diabetes or diabetes with hyperglycemia, there is an increase in the level of A$_{1C}$. The Canadian Diabetes Association (CDA) recommends this test for both screening for diabetes and monitoring the glycemic control of persons with diabetes. The CDA also recommends initiating corrective measures for A$_{1C}$ levels greater than 7%. The goal is to lower the A$_{1C}$ to less than 7.0% for most people. For more intensive glucose control, a target of $\leq$6.5% may be considered for some individuals with type 2 diabetes, and conversely a target of $\leq$8.5% may be more appropriate for other individuals with advanced co-morbidities and concerns about severe hypoglycemic events.[1]

Urine Tests

The ease, accuracy, and convenience of self-administered blood glucose monitoring techniques have made urine testing for glucose obsolete for most people with diabetes. These tests only reflect urine glucose levels and are influenced by such factors as the renal threshold for glucose, fluid intake and urine concentration, urine testing methodologies, and some drugs. It is recommended that all people with diabetes self-monitor their blood glucose. Urine ketone determinations remain an important part of monitoring diabetic control, particularly in people with type 1 diabetes who are at risk for development of ketoacidosis, and in pregnant diabetic women to check the adequacy of nutrition and glycemic control.[1]

Diabetes Management

The desired outcome of glycemic control in both type 1 and type 2 diabetes is normalization of blood glucose as a means of preventing short- and long-term complications. Treatment plans involve medical nutrition therapy, exercise, and medication. People with type 1 diabetes require insulin therapy from the time of diagnosis. Weight loss and dietary management

may be sufficient to control blood glucose levels in people with type 2 diabetes. However, most require follow-up care because insulin secretion from the beta cells may decrease or insulin resistance may persist or worsen, in which case oral antidiabetic agents are prescribed.

Among the methods used to achieve these treatment goals are education in self-management and problem solving. Individual treatment goals should take into account the person's age and other disease conditions, the person's capacity to understand and carry out the treatment regime, and socioeconomic factors that might influence adherence with the treatment plan. Optimal control of both type 1 and type 2 diabetes is associated with prevention or delay of chronic diabetes complications.[1]

Dietary Management

Dietary management usually is prescribed to meet the specific needs of each person with diabetes. The term *medical nutrition therapy*, which was introduced by the American Diabetes Association, is defined as the use of specific nutrition services to treat an illness, injury, or condition and involves both the assessment of the nutrition status and the treatment measure, including nutrition therapy, counselling, and use of specialized nutritional supplements.[24] The diabetic diet has undergone marked changes over the years, particularly in the recommendations for distribution of calories among carbohydrates, proteins, fats, and fibre. There no longer is a specific diabetic or CDA diet but rather an individualized dietary prescription based on nutrition assessment and treatment goals. A coordinated team effort, including the person with diabetes, is needed to individualize the nutrition plan.

Goals and principles of diet therapy differ between type 1 and type 2 diabetes, as well as for lean and obese people. Integral to diabetes management is a prescribed plan for nutrition therapy.[1] Therapy goals include maintenance of near-normal blood glucose levels, achievement of optimal lipid levels, adequate calories to maintain and attain reasonable weights, prevention and treatment of chronic diabetes complications, and improvement of overall health through optimal nutrition. Initial guidelines may include 45% to 60% carbohydrate, 20% to 35% fat and 15% to 20% protein.[1]

For a person with type 1 diabetes, the usual food intake is assessed and used as a basis for adjusting insulin therapy to fit with the person's lifestyle. Eating consistent amounts and types of food at specific and routine times is encouraged. Home blood glucose monitoring provides immediate feedback about nutritional intake, glycemic response, and the influence of physical activity. For those with type 1 diabetes, improvements in insulin regimes and increasing use of insulin pumps allow for more flexibility with meals.[1]

Most people with type 2 diabetes are overweight. Nutrition therapy goals focus on achieving glucose, lipid, and blood pressure goals, and weight loss if indicated. Mild to moderate weight loss (5% to 10% of total body weight) has been shown to improve diabetes control, even if desirable weight is not achieved.[1]

The registered dietitian plays an essential role in the diabetes care team and is able to select from a variety of methods such as carbohydrate counting, food exchanges, healthy food choices, and total available glucose to tailor the meal plan to meet individual needs. The Glycemic Index (GI) is another scale that ranks carbohydrate-rich foods as to how much they raise blood glucose levels. Factors that influence the GI are the types of starch, type of cooking, food processing, fat content, and acid content of the food. The glycemic response is also affected by the speed of the stomach emptying: fats and proteins will slow the rate at which the stomach empties; thus, food will be digested at a slower rate and there will be a decrease in glycemic response. Simpler recommendations have been associated with improved client understanding and dietary adherence. Carbohydrate counting uses product label information that is easily available to people with diabetes.[1] Regardless of food source, total grams of carbohydrate are counted, placing an emphasis on the nutrient that most affects blood glucose control.

Medical nutrition therapy is also important in preventing, or at least slowing, the development of complications. Because diabetes is a risk factor for cardiovascular disease, it is recommended that less than 7% of daily calories should be obtained from saturated fat[1] and that dietary cholesterol be limited to 200 mg or less, and intake of trans fats minimized. Periodic fasting lipid panels may identify concomitant lipid disorders. If lipid disorders are identified, appropriate modifications according to the Canadian Cardiovascular Society (CCS) Guidelines should be followed.[25] For people with diabetic nephropathy, studies suggest lowering the intake of protein to 0.8/kg body weight per day according to the degree of kidney impairment.[1] As other associated conditions of diabetes develop additional nutritional considerations such as sodium intake and other nutrients, may be required to optimize outcomes.

Exercise

The benefits of exercise include cardiovascular fitness and psychological well-being. For many people with type 2 diabetes, the benefits of exercise include a decrease in body fat, better weight control, and improvement in insulin sensitivity.[1] Exercise is so important in diabetes management that a planned program of regular exercise usually is considered an integral part of the therapeutic regimen for every person with diabetes. In general, sporadic exercise has only transient benefits; a regular exercise or training program is the most beneficial. It is better for cardiovascular conditioning and can maintain a muscle–fat ratio that enhances peripheral insulin receptivity.

In people with diabetes, the beneficial effects of exercise are accompanied by an increased risk of hypoglycemia. Although muscle uptake of glucose increases significantly, the ability to maintain blood glucose levels is hampered by failure to suppress the absorption of injected insulin and activate the counter-regulatory mechanisms that maintain blood glucose. Not only is there an inability to suppress insulin levels, but insulin absorption may increase. This increased absorption is more pronounced when insulin is injected into the subcutaneous tissue of the exercised muscle, but it occurs even when insulin is injected into other body areas. Even after exercise ceases, insulin's lowering effect on blood glucose continues. In some people with type 1 diabetes, the symptoms of hypoglycemia occur several hours after cessation of exercise, perhaps because subsequent insulin doses (in people using multiple daily insulin injections) are not adjusted to accommodate the exercise-induced decrease in blood glucose. The cause of hypoglycemia in people who do not administer a subsequent insulin dose is unclear. It may be related to the fact that the liver and skeletal muscles increase their uptake of glucose after exercise as a means of replenishing their glycogen stores, or that the liver and skeletal muscles are more sensitive to insulin during this time. People with diabetes should be aware that delayed hypoglycemia can occur after exercise and that they may need to alter their diabetes medication dose, their carbohydrate intake, or both.

Although of benefit to people with diabetes, exercise must be weighed on the risk–benefit scale. Before beginning an exercise program, persons with diabetes should undergo an appropriate evaluation for macrovascular and microvascular diseases.[1] The goal of exercise is safe participation in activities consistent with an individual's lifestyle. As with nutrition guidelines, exercise recommendations need to be individualized. Considerations include the potential for hypoglycemia, hyperglycemia, ketosis, cardiovascular ischemia and arrhythmias (particularly silent ischemic heart disease), exacerbation of proliferative retinopathy, and lower extremity injury. For those with long standing diabetes, the complications of vigorous exercise can be harmful and cause eye hemorrhage and other problems. For people with type 1 diabetes who exercise during periods of poor control (i.e., when blood glucose is elevated, exogenous insulin levels are low, and ketonemia exists), blood glucose and ketones rise to even higher levels because the stress of exercise is superimposed on pre-existing insulin deficiency and increased counter-regulatory hormone activity.

Oral and Injectable Antidiabetic Agents

The last few years have seen not only new medications for diabetes treatment, but new categories of medications, No longer are the choices oral agents or insulin. Medications to treat diabetes now include new injectable antidiabetic agents (e.g., amylin analogs and glucagon-like peptide-1 [GLP-1] analogs). Because people with type 1 diabetes are deficient in insulin, they are in need of exogenous insulin replacement therapy from the start. People with type 2 diabetes can have increased hepatic glucose production; decreased peripheral utilization of glucose; decreased utilization of ingested carbohydrates; and, over time, impaired insulin secretion and excessive glucagon secretion from the pancreas (Fig. 42.9). The antidiabetic agents used in the treatment of type 2 diabetes attack each one of these areas and sometimes all.[1] If good glycemic control cannot be achieved with one or a combination of antidiabetic agents, insulin can be added or used by itself.

Oral antidiabetic agents fall into six categories: (1) insulin secretagogues (i.e., sulfonylureas, repaglinide, and nateglinide), (2) biguanides, (3) α-glucosidase inhibitors, (4) dipeptidyl

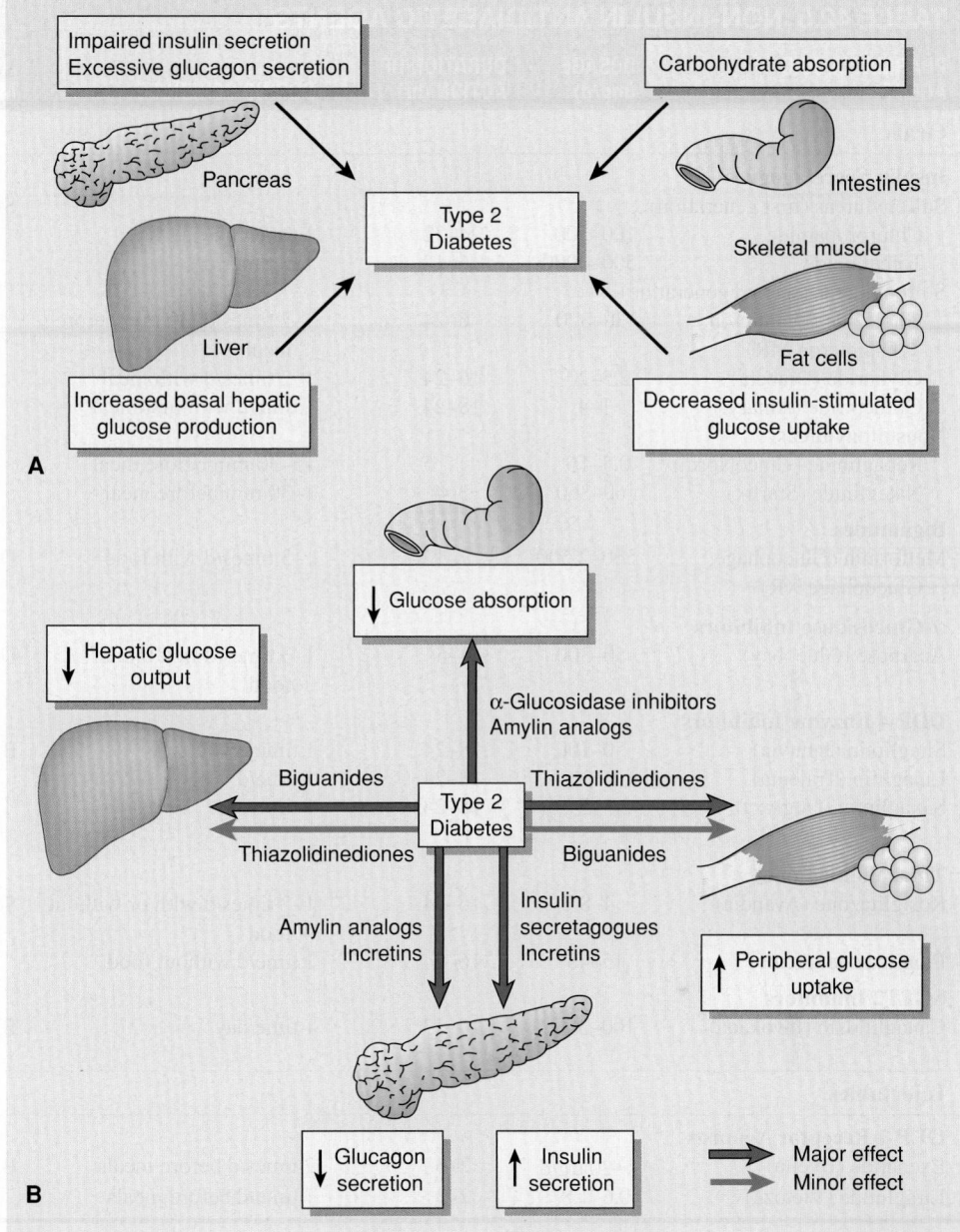

FIGURE 42.9 • **A:** Mechanisms of elevated blood glucose in type 2 diabetes mellitus. **B:** Action sites of hypoglycemic agents and mechanisms of lowering blood glucose in type 2 diabetes. The incretins are the dipeptidyl peptidase-4 (DPP-4) inhibitors and glucagon-like peptide-1 (GLP-1) agonists.

peptidase-4 (DPP-4) enzyme inhibitors, (5) thiazolidinediones (TZDs), and the newest class sodium glucose cotransporter-2 (SGLT2)[1,3,26] (Table 42.5). In addition, injectable formulations of GLP-1 agonists have been introduced in Canada but amylin agonist injections are not available in Canada.

Insulin Secretagogues: Sulfonylureas. The sulfonylureas were discovered accidentally in 1942, when scientists noticed that one of the sulfonamide drugs being developed at the time caused hypoglycemia. These drugs reduce blood glucose by stimulating the release of insulin from beta cells in the pancreas. These agents are effective only when some residual beta cell function remains. The sulfonylureas act by binding to a high-affinity sulfonylurea receptor on the beta cell that is linked to an adenosine triphosphate (ATP)-sensitive potassium

channel (Fig. 42.4). Binding of a sulfonylurea closes the channel, resulting in a coupled reaction that leads to an influx of calcium ions and insulin secretion.

The sulfonylureas are used in the treatment of type 2 diabetes and cannot be substituted for insulin in people with type 1 diabetes, who have an absolute insulin deficiency. Slight modifications in the basic structure of the members of this drug group produce agents that have similar qualitative actions but markedly different potencies. The sulfonylureas traditionally are grouped into first- and second-generation agents (Table 42.5). These agents differ in dosage and duration of action. The second-generation drugs (*e.g.,* glyburide, gliclazide, glimepiride) are considerably more potent than the first-generation drugs and are more widely prescribed than the first-generation agents.

TABLE 42.5 NON-INSULIN ANTIDIABETIC AGENTS[a]

PHARMACOLOGIC AGENT	DOSAGE (mg/d)	DURATION OF ACTION (hr)	DOSING SCHEDULE	MECHANISM OF ACTION
Orals				
Insulin Secretagogues				
Sulfonylureas (first generation)				Stimulates release of insulin from beta cells in the pancreas
Chlorpropamide	100–500	24–72	1 time/d	
Tolbutamide	500–3000	6–12	1–3 times/d	
Sulfonylureas (second generation)				
Gliclazide (Diamicron, Diamicron MR)	30–320	6–24	1–2 times/d, 30 min before meal	
Glyburide (Diabeta)	2.5–20	16–24	1–2 times/d with meal	
Glimepiride (Amaryl)	1–4	18–24	1 time/d with first meal	
Nonsulfonylureas				
Repaglinide (GlucoNorm)	0.5–16	5	15–30 min before meal	
Nateglinide (Starlix)	60–360	3–4	1–30 min before meal	
Biguanides				
Metformin (Glucophage, Glucophage XR)	500–2,500	7–12	1–3 times/d with food	Decreases production and release of glucose by the liver
α-Glucosidase Inhibitors				
Acarbose (Glucobay)	50–300	4–6	1–3 times/d first bite of food	Delays the breakdown and absorption of carbohydrates from the intestine
DDP-4 Enzyme Inhibitors				
Sitagliptin (Januvia)	50–100	18–24	1 time/d	Blocks enzyme DPP-4 (which breaks down GLP-1 and GIP), thereby increasing the release of insulin after blood glucose rises
Linaglitin (Trajenta)	5	18–24	1 time/d	
Saxagliptin (Onglyza)	2.5–5	18–24	1 time/d	
Thiazolidinediones				
Rosiglitazone (Avandia)[b]	4–8	16–24	1–2 times/d with or without food	Sensitizes body cells to the action of insulin
Pioglitazone (Actos)	15–45	16–24	1 time/d without food	
SGLT2 Inhibitors				
Canagliflozin (Invokana)	100–300	10–13	1 time/day	Blocks the resorption of glucose promoting glycosuria
Injectables				
GLP-1 Receptor Agonists				
Exenatide (Byetta)	5–20 µg/d	2–3	2 times/d before meals	Binds to GLP-1 receptor decreasing fasting and postprandial glucose
Liraglutide (Victoza)	0.6–1.8	2–3	1 time/d before meals	

[a]List may not be inclusive.
[b]2007 analysis suggested association with increased risk of myocardial infarction.

Because the sulfonylureas increase insulin levels and the rate at which glucose is removed from the blood, it is important to recognize that they can cause hypoglycemic reactions. This problem is more common in elderly people with impaired hepatic and renal function who are taking the longer-acting sulfonylureas.

Insulin Secretagogues: Repaglinide and Nateglinide. Repaglinide and nateglinide are nonsulfonylurea insulin secretagogues that require the presence of glucose for their main action. These agents exert their action by closing the ATP-dependent potassium channel in the beta cells (Fig. 42.4). Insulin release is glucose dependent and diminishes at low glucose levels. These agents, which are rapidly absorbed from the gas-

trointestinal tract, are taken shortly before meals (repaglinide 15 to 30 minutes and nateglinide 1 to 30 minutes). Both repaglinide and nateglinide can produce hypoglycemia; thus, proper timing of meals in relation to drug administration is essential.

Biguanides. The biguanides are older oral antidiabetic drugs. Phenformin, the earliest biguanide, was used extensively in the 1960s but was removed from the Canadian market in 1977 because of the occurrence of lactic acidosis in some patients treated with it. Unlike its precursor, metformin rarely results in lactic acidosis (0.03 cases per 1,000 patients). Metformin inhibits hepatic glucose production and increases the sensitivity of peripheral tissues to the actions of insulin. Because metformin does not stimulate insulin secretion, it does not produce hypoglycemia as a side effect. Secondary benefits of metformin therapy include weight loss and improved lipid profiles. Whereas the primary action of the sulfonylurea drugs is to increase insulin secretion, metformin exerts its beneficial effects on glycemic control through increased peripheral use of glucose and decreased hepatic glucose production (main effect). To decrease the risk of lactic acidosis, metformin is contraindicated in people with elevated serum creatinine levels (a test of renal function), clinical and laboratory evidence of hepatic disease, and any condition associated with hypoxemia or dehydration.[1]

α-Glucosidase Inhibitors. In patients with type 2 diabetes, sulfonylureas, biguanides, or both may have beneficial effects on FPG levels. However, postprandial hyperglycemia persists in more than 60% of these patients and probably accounts for sustained increases in A_{1C} levels. An alternative approach to the problem of postprandial hyperglycemia is the use of drug acarbose (or miglitol which is not available in Canada); these are inhibitors of α-glucosidase, which is a small intestine brush border enzyme that breaks down complex carbohydrates. By delaying the breakdown of complex carbohydrates, the α-glucosidase inhibitors delay the absorption of carbohydrates from the gut and blunt the postprandial increase in plasma glucose and insulin levels. Although not a problem with monotherapy or combination therapy with a biguanide, hypoglycemia may occur with concurrent sulfonylurea treatment. If hypoglycemia does occur, it should be treated with glucose (dextrose) and not sucrose (table sugar), whose breakdown may be blocked by the action of the α-glucosidase inhibitors.

Thiazolidinediones. The TZDs (or glitazones) are the only class of drugs that directly target insulin resistance, a fundamental defect in the pathophysiology of type 2 diabetes. The TZDs improve glycemic control by increasing insulin sensitivity in the insulin-responsive tissues—liver, skeletal muscle, and fat—allowing the tissues to respond to endogenous insulin more efficiently without increased output from already dysfunctional beta cells.[27] Pioglitazone and rosiglitazone are the most potent insulin sensitizers and were approved by Health Canada in 2000. Another TZD, troglitazone, was approved in 1997, but because of hepatic safety concerns, it is no longer available, having been withdrawn worldwide in March 2000. Pioglitazone and rosiglitazone are both approved for use as monotherapy and in combination therapy. Because of the previous problem with liver toxicity in this class of drugs, liver enzymes should be monitored according to guidelines. In 2007, a published meta-analysis suggested that rosiglitazone may be associated with an increased risk of myocardial infarction.[28] This finding was not seen with pioglitazone. Both agents can cause fluid accumulation and are therefore contraindicated in patients with New York Heart Association stage III and IV heart failure (see Chapter 26, Table 26.2). In addition, an increased risk of bone fractures was recently observed in postmarketing studies of both compounds.

The mechanism of action of the TZDs is complex and not fully understood. The action of the TZDs is associated

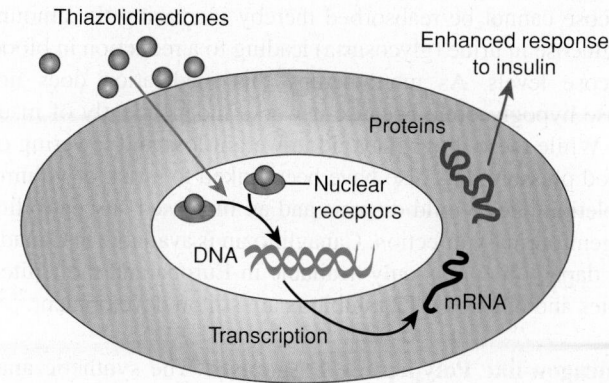

FIGURE 42.10 • Action of the thiazolidinediones on activation of the nuclear peroxisome proliferator. Activated receptor gamma (PPAR-γ) regulates gene transcription of proteins that regulate glucose uptake and reduce fatty acid release. mRNA, messenger ribonucleic acid.

with binding to the PPAR-γ nuclear receptor[29] (Fig. 42.10). Binding of the TZDs to the PPAR-γ receptor begins a cascade of events leading to regulation of genes involved in lipid and glucose metabolism. The result is an increase in the number of GLUT-4 transporters and increased insulin-mediated uptake of glucose in the peripheral tissues. *Adiponectin* which is produced by adipocytes and directly sensitizes the body to the actions of insulin, may be a part of the missing link in explaining insulin resistance in persons with type 2 diabetes.[3] The TZDs are thought to decrease insulin resistance, at least in part, by increasing adipocyte production of adiponectin. Additional effects of TZDs are numerous, and include correction of many of the abnormal metabolic features associated with type 2 diabetes. This includes a decrease in FFA and triglycerides, microalbuminuria, blood pressure, inflammatory mediators (*e.g.*, fibrinogen and CRP), and procoagulation factors.

Dipeptidyl Peptidase-4 Enzyme Inhibitors. Incretins are insulinotropic substances released into the circulation by the gastrointestinal tract after a meal, especially one high in carbohydrates.[30] Incretins act by stimulating insulin secretion by the beta cell. In normal individuals, incretins account for approximately 20% to 60% of insulin secretion after a meal. The main incretins secreted are *GLP-1* and *glucose-dependent insulinotropic polypeptide* (GIP). Both GLP-1 and GIP are rapidly degraded by the enzyme, DPP-4. DPP-4 enzyme inhibitors (*i.e.*, saxagliptin, linagliptin, sitagliptin) work by inhibiting the DPP-4 enzyme and increasing GLP-1 and GIP levels, which then increase insulin release. GLP-1 also helps to suppress glucagon release.

Sodium-Glucose Cotransporter-2 Inhibitors. This is the newest class of oral antidiabetic medications for the treatment of type 2 diabetes. While the 12 known isoforms of SGLT work together to absorb and reabsorb glucose, it is the SGLT2 transporter in the proximal tubule of the nephron that is responsible for reabsorbing 80% to 90% glucose from the renal filtrate. When the SGLT2 transporter is blocked by these medications glucose cannot be reabsorbed thereby increasing the amount of glucose in urine (glycosuria) leading to a reduction in blood glucose levels. As monotherapy this medication does not cause hypoglycemia because it works independently of insulin. While these drugs may aid in weight loss and lowering of blood pressure they also have been linked to a risk of volume depletion due to mild diuresis and an increased susceptibility of genitourinary infection. Canagliflozin is available in Canada but dapagliflozine is only available in Europe and the United States and other SGLT2 inhibitors are still in development.[26,27]

Glucagon-like Polypeptide-1 Agonists. The synthetic analogs of GLP-1, exenatide and liraglutide are available in Canada for the treatment of diabetes. These drugs are an injectable adjunctive therapy for people with type 2 diabetes treated with metformin or sulfonylureas who still have suboptimal glycemic control. These drugs have been shown to have multiple actions such as potentiation of glucose-mediated insulin release, slowed gastric emptying, and a central loss of appetite. Injectable GLP-1 agonists generally produce a tenfold increase in normal blood levels of GLP-1, as opposed to oral DPP-4 enzyme inhibitors, which produce a two- to threefold increase. Exenatide is injected subcutaneously 60 minutes before a meal. When added to pre-existing sulfonylurea therapy, the oral hypoglycemic dosage may need to be lowered to prevent hypoglycemia. Liraglutide is given subcutaneously once a day without regard to meals. The major side effects are nausea and weight loss.[27,30] Another weekly injectable drug in this class, dulaglutide, is only available in the United States.

Amylin Analogs. Pramlintide, is a synthetic analog of amylin, which is an injectable antidiabetic agent that modulates postprandial glucose levels and is approved for use in type 1 and type 2 diabetes in the United States only. Amylin is a 37-amino-acid peptide that is produced, stored, and cosecreted with insulin in response to glucose and other beta cell stimulators.[3] Therefore, in states of diabetes in which the beta cells and insulin secretion are largely depleted or dysfunctional, amylin secretion is also lost or dysfunctional. Pramlintide is injected (in a separate injection from insulin) before meals in those individuals who are unable to achieve their target postprandial blood glucose levels. Pramlintide, which has a rapid onset of action, suppresses glucagon release, slows gastric emptying, and tends to decrease appetite. The major side effects of pramlintide are hypoglycemia and gastrointestinal symptoms such as anorexia, nausea, and vomiting.

Insulin

Type 1 diabetes mellitus *always* requires treatment with insulin, and many people with type 2 diabetes eventually require insulin therapy. Insulin is destroyed in the gastrointestinal tract and must be administered by injection or inhalation. Biosynthetic human insulin is manufactured using recombinant deoxyribonucleic acid (DNA) technology and all exogenous insulins are measured in international units (IU). Most types of insulin are available in U-100 strength (*i.e.*, 100 units of insulin/1 ml). Insulin preparations are categorized according to onset, peak, and duration of action. An inhaled form of insulin (Exubera) was on the market for a short time in the United States only, but was withdrawn for commercial reasons. Other inhaled insulin formulations are in clinical development.

Insulin types are classified by length and peaking of action.[27] There are four principal types of insulin: rapid-acting, short-acting, intermediate-acting, and long-acting (Table 42.6). The rapid-acting insulins (lispro, aspart, and glulisine) are produced by recombinant technology with an amino acid substitution. These insulins have a more rapid onset, peak, and duration of action than short-acting regular insulin, approximately 5 to 15 minutes. The rapid-acting insulins, which are used in combination with intermediate or long-acting insulins, are usually administered immediately before a meal. Due to such a rapid onset they also can be administered during or immediately after meals and can be beneficial for people with unpredictable oral intake such as the pediatric populations. Short-acting insulin (regular) is a soluble crystalline insulin whose effects begin within 30 minutes after subcutaneous injection and generally last for 5 to 8 hours. Intermediate- to long-acting insulins include NPH, glargine, and detemir. These insulins have slower onsets and a longer duration of action. They require several hours to reach therapeutic levels, so their use in type 1 diabetes requires supplementation with rapid- or short-acting insulin. Glargine and detemir have a slower, more prolonged absorption than NPH insulin and provide a relatively constant concentration over 12 to 24 hours. The advantage of these "peakless" insulins is the provision of basal coverage. All forms of insulin have the potential to produce hypoglycemia or "insulin reaction" as a side effect (to be discussed).

Intensive Insulin Treatment Regimens. Two intensive treatment regimens—multiple daily injections and continuous subcutaneous infusion of insulin—closely simulate the normal pattern of insulin secretion by the body. With each method, a basal insulin level is maintained, and bolus doses of short- or rapid-acting insulin are delivered before meals. The choice of management is determined by the person with diabetes in collaboration with the healthcare team.

With *multiple daily injections* (MDI), the basal insulin requirements are met by an intermediate- or long-acting insulin administered once or twice daily. Boluses of rapid- or short-acting insulin are used before meals. The development of convenient injection devices (*e.g.*, pen injectors) has made it easier for people with diabetes to comply with algorithms for these insulins that are administered before meals.

The *continuous subcutaneous insulin infusion* (CSII) method uses an insulin pump. With this method, the basal insulin requirements are met by continuous infusion of subcutaneous insulin, the rate of which can be varied to accommodate variations in lifestyle. The CSII technique involves the insertion of a small needle or plastic catheter into the subcutaneous tissue of the abdomen. Tubing from the catheter is connected to a syringe set into a small infusion pump worn on a belt or in a jacket pocket. The computer-operated pump then delivers one or more set basal amounts of insulin. In addition to the basal

TABLE 42.6 ACTIVITY PROFILES OF INSULIN PREPARATIONS IN CANADA[a]

TYPE (HUMAN INSULIN)	ONSET	PEAK (hr)	DURATION (hr)
Rapid-Acting			
Lispro (Humalog)	5–15 min	1–1.5	3–5
Aspart (NovoRapid)	5–15 min	1–1.5	3–5
Glulisine (Apidra)	5–15 min	1–1.5	3–5
Short-Acting			
Regular Insulin	0.5–1 hr	2–4	5–8
Intermediate-Acting			
Isophane insulin suspension (NPH)	2–4 hrs	4–10	10–18
Long-Acting			
Detemir (Levemir)	2–4 hrs	No peak	6–23
Glargine (Lantus)[b]	2–4 hrs	No peak	20–24
Premixed			
70% NPH/30% regular	0.5–1 hrs	Dual	10–18
50% NPH/50% regular	0.5–1 hrs	Dual	10–18
75% NPL (insulin lispro protamine)/25% lispro (Humalog Mix 25)	5–15 min	Dual	10–18
50% NPL/50% lispro (Humalog Mix 50)	5–15 min	Dual	10–18
70% NPA (insulin aspart protamine)/30% aspart (NovoMix 30)	5–15 min	Dual	10–18

[a]List may not be inclusive.

[b]Lantus insulin should never be mixed with or administered using the same syringe used to administer any other type of insulin.

amount delivered by the pump, a bolus amount of insulin may be delivered when needed (*e.g.,* before a meal) by pushing a button.

Self-monitoring of blood glucose levels is a necessity when using the CSII method of management. Each basal and bolus dose is determined individually and programmed into the infusion pump computer. Although the pump's safety has been proven, strict attention must be paid to signs of hypoglycemia. However, investigations have found CSII therapy to be associated with a marked and sustained reduction in the rate of severe hypoglycemia. Ketotic episodes caused by pump failure, catheter clogging, and infections at the needle site also are possible complications. Candidate selection is crucial to the successful use of the insulin pump. Only people who are highly motivated to do frequent blood glucose tests and make daily insulin adjustments are candidates for this method of treatment. Today's insulin pumps are very sophisticated and can allow multiple setting based on an individual's specific needs. Newer technology is looking at the continuous glucose monitoring to work with the insulin pumps to give real time glucose information and responses improving glycemic control.[31] Other options are to provide a closed-loop insulin pump to sense glucose levels and respond with insulin secretions independently.

Pancreas or Islet Cell Transplantation

Pancreas or islet cell transplantation does not cure type 1 diabetes. It does, however, afford the potential for significantly improving the quality of life through reduction or elimination of insulin injections. Islet cell transplantation is done worldwide according to the Edmonton protocol, which ongoing research continues to determine the most accurate procedure to recover and transplant cells.[1]

Acute Complications

The three major acute complications of diabetes are diabetic ketoacidosis, hyperosmolar hyperglycemic state, and hypoglycemia. All are life-threatening conditions that demand immediate recognition and treatment. These complications account of a significant number of hospitalizations and consumption of healthcare resources.

Diabetic Ketoacidosis

Diabetic ketoacidosis (DKA) most commonly occurs in a person with type 1 diabetes, in whom the lack of insulin leads to mobilization of fatty acids from adipose tissue because of the unsuppressed adipose cell lipase activity that breaks down triglycerides into fatty acids and glycerol. The increase in fatty acid levels leads to ketone production by the liver (Fig. 42.11). It can occur at the onset of the disease, often before the disease has been diagnosed. For example, a mother may bring a child into the clinic or emergency department with reports of lethargy, vomiting, and abdominal pain, unaware that the child

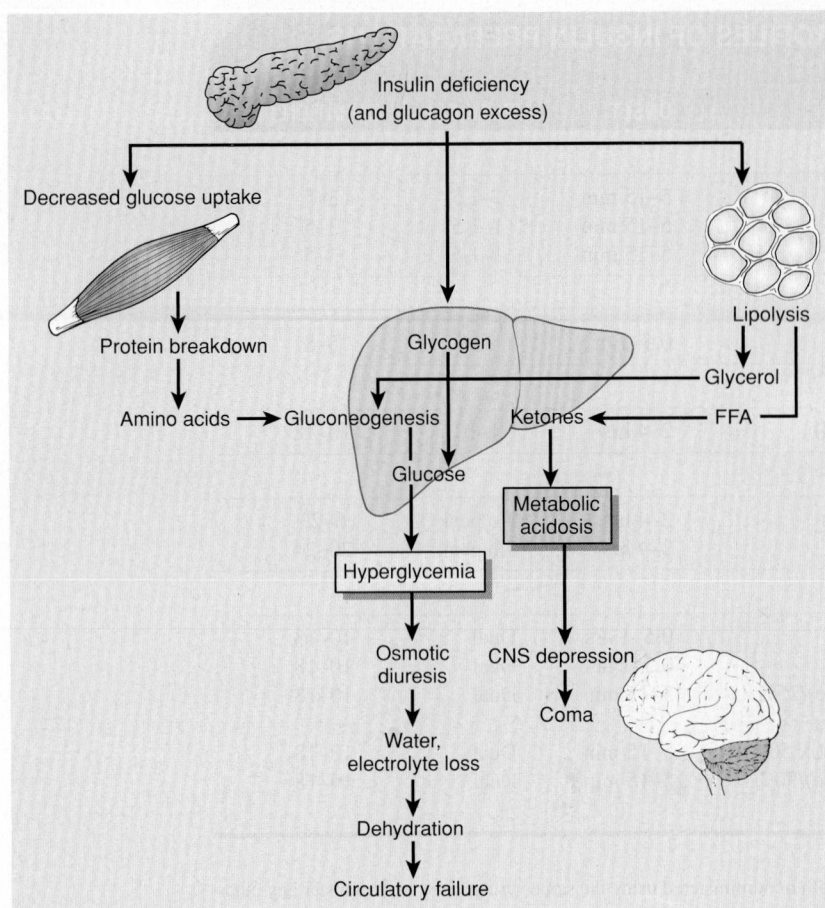

FIGURE 42.11 • Mechanisms of diabetic ketoacidosis. Diabetic ketoacidosis is associated with very low insulin levels and extremely high levels of glucagon, catecholamines, and other counter-regulatory hormones. Increased levels of glucagon and the catecholamines lead to mobilization of substrates for gluconeogenesis and ketogenesis by the liver. Gluconeogenesis in excess of that needed to supply glucose for the brain and other glucose-dependent tissues produces a rise in blood glucose levels. Mobilization of free fatty acids (FFA) from triglyceride stores in adipose tissue leads to accelerated ketone production and ketosis. CNS, central nervous system.

has diabetes. Stress increases the release of gluconeogenic hormones and predisposes the person to the development of ketoacidosis. DKA often is preceded by physical or emotional stress, such as infection, pregnancy, or extreme anxiety. In clinical practice, ketoacidosis also occurs with the omission or inadequate use of insulin.

The three major metabolic derangements in DKA are hyperglycemia, ketosis, and metabolic acidosis. The definitive diagnosis of DKA consists of hyperglycemia (blood glucose levels ≥14.0 mmol/L), low serum bicarbonate (≤15 mmol/L), an anion gap >12 mmol/L, and low pH (≤7.3), with ketonemia (positive at 1:2 dilution) and moderate ketonuria.[1,3,32,33] Hyperglycemia leads to osmotic diuresis, dehydration, and a critical loss of electrolytes. Hyperosmolality of extracellular fluids from hyperglycemia leads to a shift of water and potassium from the intracellular to the extracellular compartment. Extracellular sodium concentration frequently is low or normal despite enteric water losses because of the intracellular–extracellular fluid shift. This dilutional effect is referred to as *pseudohyponatremia*. Serum potassium levels may be normal or elevated, despite total potassium depletion resulting from protracted polyuria and vomiting. Metabolic acidosis is caused by the excess ketoacids that require buffering by bicarbonate ions; this leads to a marked decrease in serum bicarbonate levels.

The appearance of DKA is commonly preceded by a day or more of polyuria, polydipsia, nausea, vomiting, and

marked fatigue, with eventual alterations in cognition that can progress to coma. Abdominal pain and tenderness may be experienced without abdominal disease. The breath has a characteristic fruity smell because of the presence of the volatile ketoacids. Hypotension and tachycardia may be present because of a decrease in blood volume. A number of the signs and symptoms that occur in DKA are related to compensatory mechanisms. The heart rate increases as the body compensates for a decrease in blood volume, and the rate and depth of respiration increase (*i.e.,* Kussmaul respiration) as the body attempts to prevent further decreases in pH. Metabolic acidosis is discussed further in Chapter 32.

The goals in treating DKA are to improve circulatory volume and tissue perfusion, decrease blood glucose, correct the acidosis, and correct electrolyte imbalances. These objectives usually are accomplished through the administration of insulin and intravenous fluid and electrolyte replacement solutions. Because insulin resistance accompanies severe acidosis, low-dose insulin therapy is used. An initial loading dose of regular insulin often is given intravenously, followed by continuous low-dose infusion. Frequent laboratory tests are used to monitor blood glucose and serum electrolyte levels and to guide fluid and electrolyte replacement. It is important to replace fluid and electrolytes and correct pH while bringing the blood glucose concentration to a normal level. Too rapid a drop in blood glucose may cause hypoglycemia. A sudden change in the osmolality of extracellular fluid can also occur when blood glucose levels are lowered too rapidly, and this can cause cerebral edema. Serum potassium levels often fall as acidosis is corrected and potassium moves from the extracellular into the intracellular compartment. Thus, it may be necessary to add potassium to the intravenous infusion. Identification and treatment of the underlying cause, such as infection, also are important. With the better understanding of the pathogenesis of DKA, early recognition, and more uniform agreement on diagnosis and treatment, the mortality rate has been reduced to less than 5%.[1,3,32]

Hyperosmolar Hyperglycemic State

The hyperosmolar hyperglycemic state (HHS) is characterized by hyperglycemia (blood glucose ≥34.0 mmol/L), hyperosmolarity (plasma osmolarity >320 mOsm/L) and dehydration, the absence of ketoacidosis, and depression of the sensorium.[1,33] HHS may occur in various conditions, including type 2 diabetes, acute pancreatitis, severe infection, myocardial infarction, and treatment with oral or parenteral nutrition solutions. It is seen most frequently in people with type 2 diabetes. A partial or relative insulin deficiency may initiate the syndrome by reducing glucose utilization while inducing hyperglucagonemia and increasing hepatic glucose output. With massive glycosuria, obligatory water loss occurs. If the person is unable to maintain adequate fluid intake because of associated acute or chronic illness or has excessive fluid loss, dehydration develops. As the plasma volume contracts, renal insufficiency develops and the resultant limitation of renal glucose losses leads to increasingly higher blood glucose levels and severity of the hyperosmolar state.

In hyperosmolar states, the increased serum osmolarity has the effect of pulling water out of body cells, including brain cells. The condition may be complicated by thromboembolic events arising because of the high serum osmolality. The most prominent manifestations are weakness, dehydration, polyuria, neurologic signs and symptoms, and excessive thirst. Neurologic signs include hemiparesis, seizures, and coma can occur. The onset of HHS often is insidious, and because it occurs most frequently in older people, it may be mistaken for a stroke.

The treatment of HHS requires judicious medical observation and care as water moves back into brain cells, posing a threat of cerebral edema. Extensive potassium losses that also have occurred during the diuretic phase of the disorder require correction. Because of the problems encountered in the treatment and the serious nature of the disease conditions that cause HHS, the prognosis for this disorder is less favourable than that for ketoacidosis.

Hypoglycemia

Hypoglycemia is defined as the development of cognitive impairment or neuroglycopenic symptoms, a low blood glucose level less than 4.0 mmol/L, and symptoms responding after carbohydrates are administered.[1] It occurs most commonly in people treated with insulin injections, but prolonged hypoglycemia also can result from some oral hypoglycemic agents. There are many factors that can precipitate an insulin

reaction in a person with type 1 diabetes, including error in insulin dose, failure to eat, increased exercise, decreased insulin need after removal of a stress situation, medication changes, and a change in insulin injection site. Alcohol decreases liver gluconeogenesis, and people with diabetes need to be cautioned about its potential for causing hypoglycemia, especially if it is consumed in large amounts or on an empty stomach.

Hypoglycemia usually has a rapid onset and progression of symptoms. The signs and symptoms of hypoglycemia can be divided into two categories: (1) those caused by altered cerebral function, and (2) those related to activation of the autonomic nervous system. Because the brain relies on blood glucose as its main energy source, hypoglycemia produces behaviours related to altered cerebral function. Headache, difficulty in problem solving, disturbed or altered behaviour, coma, and seizures may occur. At the onset of the hypoglycemic episode, activation of the parasympathetic nervous system often causes hunger. The initial parasympathetic response is followed by activation of the sympathetic nervous system; this causes anxiety, tachycardia, sweating, and constriction of the skin vessels (*i.e.,* the skin is cool and clammy).

The signs and symptoms of hypoglycemia are highly variable, and not everyone manifests all or even most of the symptoms. The signs and symptoms are particularly variable in children and in older adults. Older adults may not display the typical autonomic responses associated with hypoglycemia but frequently develop signs of impaired function of the central nervous system, including mental confusion. Some people develop hypoglycemic unawareness.[29,34] Unawareness of hypoglycemia should be suspected in people who do not perceive sensations or report symptoms when their blood glucose concentrations are less than 2.8 to 3.3 mmol/L. This occurs most commonly in people who have a longer duration of diabetes and A_{1C} levels within the normal range.[34] Some medications, such as β-adrenergic blocking drugs, interfere with the sympathetic response normally seen in hypoglycemia. If hypoglycemia occurs with α-glucosidase inhibitors, it should be treated with glucose (dextrose) and not sucrose (table sugar), whose breakdown may be blocked by the action of the α-glucosidase inhibitors.

The most effective treatment of an insulin reaction is the immediate administration of 15 to 20 g of glucose in a concentrated carbohydrate source then retesting blood glucose levels 15 minutes later. A further 15 g of glucose can be repeated if necessary (15/15 rule). Monosaccharides such as glucose, which can be absorbed directly into the bloodstream, work best. Complex carbohydrates can be administered after the acute reaction has been controlled to sustain blood glucose levels. It is important not to overtreat hypoglycemia and cause hyperglycemia. Alternative methods for increasing blood glucose may be required when the person having the reaction is unconscious or unable to swallow. Glucagon may be given intramuscularly or subcutaneously. Glucagon acts by hepatic glycogenolysis to raise blood sugar. The liver contains only a limited amount of glycogen (approximately 75 g); glucagon is ineffective in people whose glycogen stores have been depleted. Some people report becoming nauseated after glucagon administration, which also could be in response to the severe hypoglycemia. A small amount of glucose gel (available in most pharmacies) may be inserted into the buccal pouch when glucagon is unavailable. In situations of severe or life-threatening hypoglycemia, it may be necessary to administer glucose (20 to 50 ml of a 50% solution) intravenously.

Counter-Regulatory Mechanisms and the Somogyi Effect and Dawn Phenomenon

The Somogyi effect describes a cycle of insulin-induced post-hypoglycemic episodes. In 1924, Joslin and associates noticed that hypoglycemia was associated with alternate episodes of hyperglycemia. It was not until 1959 that Somogyi presented the results of his 20 years of studies, which confirmed the observation that "hypoglycemia begets hyperglycemia."[35] In people with diabetes, insulin-induced hypoglycemia produces a compensatory increase in blood levels of catecholamines, glucagon, cortisol, and growth hormone. These counter-regulatory hormones cause blood glucose to become elevated and produce some degree of insulin resistance. The cycle begins when the increase in blood glucose and insulin resistance is treated with larger insulin doses.

Clinically, high blood glucose levels in the morning can complicate medical treatment of diabetes if not fully understood to be a counter-regulatory result of hypoglycemia. The hypoglycemic episode often occurs during the night or at a time when it is not recognized, rendering the diagnosis of the phenomenon more difficult. Without proper evaluation an increase in medication can exacerbate the situation. When a Somogyi situation is suspected, people may be asked to test blood sugars in the middle of the night (or use continuous insulin sensors in selected patients) to identify possible hypoglycemic occurrences. Overall measures to prevent hypoglycemia and the subsequent activation of counter-regulatory mechanisms include a redistribution of dietary carbohydrates and an alteration in insulin dose or time of administration.

The dawn phenomenon is characterized by increased levels of fasting blood glucose or insulin requirements, or both, between 5 and 9 AM without antecedent hypoglycemia (as opposed to the Somogyi).[36] It occurs in people with type 1 or type 2 diabetes. It has been suggested that the dawn phenomenon is not fully understood but has been attributed to an increased rate of insulin clearance, decreased insulin sensitivity, or both. Several hormones such as growth hormone, cortisol, and glucagon have been studied in relation to this phenomenon.[37] When the dawn phenomenon occurs alone, it may produce only mild hyperglycemia, but when it is combined with the Somogyi effect, it may produce profound hyperglycemia.

Chronic Complications

The chronic complications of diabetes include disorders of the microvasculature (*i.e.,* neuropathies, nephropathies, and

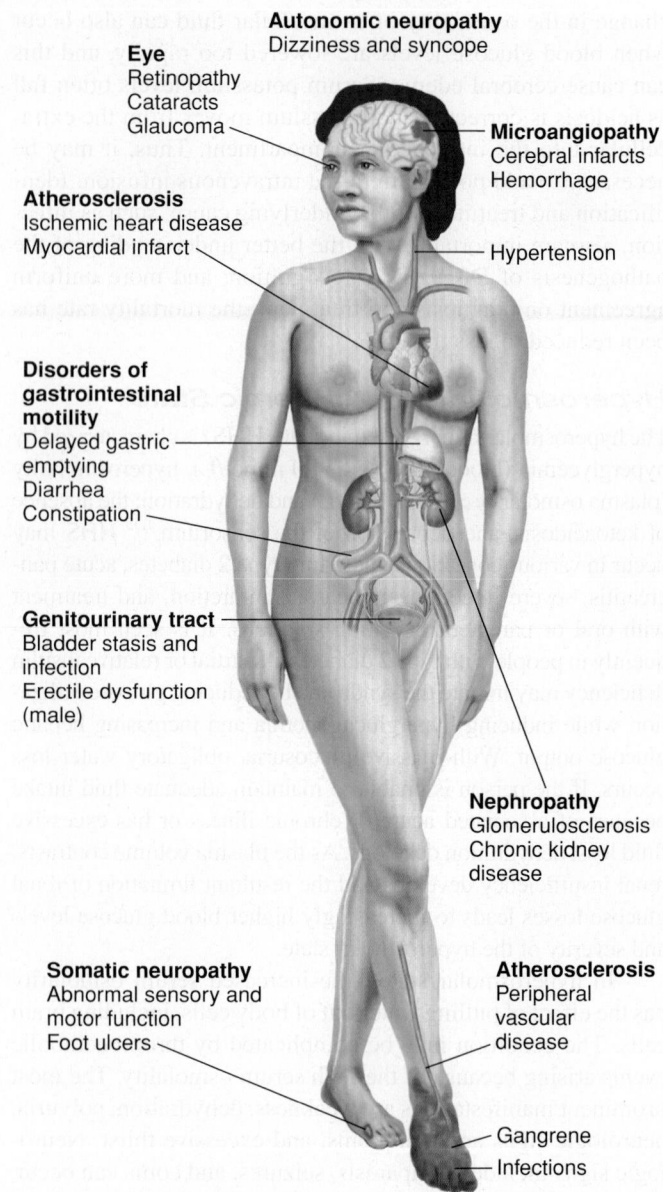

Autonomic neuropathy
Dizziness and syncope

Eye
Retinopathy
Cataracts
Glaucoma

Microangiopathy
Cerebral infarcts
Hemorrhage

Atherosclerosis
Ischemic heart disease
Myocardial infarct

Hypertension

Disorders of gastrointestinal motility
Delayed gastric emptying
Diarrhea
Constipation

Genitourinary tract
Bladder stasis and infection
Erectile dysfunction (male)

Nephropathy
Glomerulosclerosis
Chronic kidney disease

Somatic neuropathy
Abnormal sensory and motor function
Foot ulcers

Atherosclerosis
Peripheral vascular disease

Gangrene
Infections

FIGURE 42.12 • Long-term complications of diabetes mellitus.

retinopathies), macrovascular complications (*i.e.,* coronary artery, cerebral vascular, and peripheral vascular disease), and foot ulcers (Fig. 42.12). The level of chronic hyperglycemia is the best-established concomitant factor associated with diabetic complications. The Diabetes Control and Complications Trial (DCCT), which was conducted with 1,441 patients with type 1 diabetes, demonstrated that the incidence of retinopathy, nephropathy, and neuropathy can be reduced by intensive diabetic treatment.[38] Similar results have been demonstrated by the United Kingdom Prospective Diabetes Study (UKPDS) in 5,000 patients with type 2 diabetes.[39]

Recent studies have also determined the positive benefits of excellent glycemic control during hospitalization, surgery, and acute illness states.[1] All patients with diabetes admitted to acute healthcare facilities need to be identified and have an

CHRONIC COMPLICATIONS OF DIABETES

- The chronic complications of diabetes result from elevated blood glucose levels and associated impairment of lipid and other metabolic pathways.
- Diabetic nephropathy, which is a leading cause of chronic kidney disease, is associated with the increased work demands and microalbuminuria imposed by poorly controlled blood glucose levels.
- Diabetic retinopathy, which is a leading cause of blindness, is closely linked to elevations in blood glucose and hyperlipidemia seen in persons with uncontrolled diabetes.
- Diabetic neuropathies, which can affect the somatic and autonomic nervous systems, result from the demyelinating effect of long-term uncontrolled diabetes.
- Macrovascular disorders such as coronary heart disease, stroke, and peripheral vascular disease reflect the combined effects of unregulated blood glucose levels, elevated blood pressure, and hyperlipidemia.
- The chronic complications of diabetes are best prevented by measures aimed at tight control of blood glucose levels, maintenance of normal lipid levels, and control of hypertension.

order for blood glucose monitoring. Goals for blood glucose control for hospitalized patients are as close to 6.0 mmol/L as possible, and generally less than 8.0 mmol/L for critically ill patients and less than 10.0 mmol/L for noncritically ill patients.

Theories of Pathogenesis

The interest among researchers in explaining the causes and development of chronic lesions in a person with diabetes has led to a number of theories. Several of these theories have been summarized to prepare the reader for understanding specific chronic complications.

Polyol Pathway. The polyol pathway is present in many tissues but is specifically linked to microvascular complications of the retina, kidney, and nerves—all insulin-independent cells (that is they do not require insulin for glucose to enter the cell). When the normal glycolytic pathway becomes saturated due to high levels of intracellular glucose the excess glucose is converted to sorbitol with the enzyme, aldose reductase, in the polyol pathway. In the sorbitol pathway, the sorbitol is further metabolized to fructose using the enzyme, sorbitol dehydrogenase. Although glucose is converted readily to sorbitol, this molecule becomes trapped as it cannot move freely across cell membrane and the rate at which sorbitol can be converted to fructose and then metabolized is limited. Sorbitol is osmotically active, and it has been hypothesized that the presence of excess intracellular amounts may alter cell function in those tissues that use this pathway (e.g., lens, kidneys, nerves, blood vessels). In the lens, for example, the osmotic effects of sorbitol cause swelling and opacity. Increased sorbitol also is

associated with a decrease in myoinositol and reduced adenosine triphosphatase activity. The reduction of these compounds may contribute to the pathogenesis of neuropathies caused by impaired axonal transport and Schwann cell damage. Aldose reductase inhibitors are in development with the aim of reducing complications resulting from this pathway.[40]

Formation of Advanced Glycation End Products. Glycoproteins, or what could be called *glucose proteins,* are normal components of the basement membrane in smaller blood vessels and capillaries. With excessive glucose, a nonenzymatic reaction with these proteins, lipids, or nucleic acids generates intra- and extracellular *advanced glycation end products* (AGEs).[40,41] Increased levels of AGEs can induce oxidative stress and inflammation which can promote further irreversible AGE formation. On the extracellular surface these abnormal glycoproteins are thought to produce structural defects in the basement membrane of the microcirculation and intracellularly the AGEs change properties critical to cellular homeostasis.[41] Some of the altered cellular functions resulting from AGEs are due to binding to specific receptors for AGEs (RAGE).

Protein Kinase C. Diacylglycerol (DAG) and protein kinase C (PKC) are critical intracellular signalling molecules that can regulate many vascular functions, including permeability, vasodilator release, endothelial activation, and growth factor signalling. Levels of DAG and PKC are elevated in diabetes. Activation of PKC in blood vessels of the retina, kidney, and nerves can produce vascular damage.

Oxidative Stress. Ultimately linking each of these theories is the hyperglycemia causing glucose toxicity and inflammation. All of these various abnormalities (i.e., sorbitol, AGEs, PKC, plus other inflammatory cytokines) can ultimately result in increased free reactive oxygen species (i.e., free radicals or ROS) generation and disordered mitochondrial function in response to chronic hyperglycemia.[40–42]

Neuropathies

The risk of neuropathies, along with other chronic complications, has been shown to increase in the presence of long-term hyperglycemia. Ten years after a diagnosis of type 1 or type 2 diabetes 40% to 50% of people will develop detectable sensorimotor polyneuropathy.[1] Although the incidence of neuropathies is high among people with diabetes, it is difficult to document exactly how many people are affected by these disorders because of the diversity in clinical manifestations and because the condition often is far advanced before it is recognized.

Two types of pathologic changes have been observed in connection with diabetic neuropathies. The first is a thickening of the walls of the nutrient vessels that supply the nerve, leading to the assumption that vessel ischemia plays a major role in the development of these neural changes. The second finding is a segmental demyelinization process that affects the Schwann cell. This demyelinization process is accompanied by a slowing of nerve conduction.

Although there are several methods for classifying the diabetic neuropathies, a simplified system divides them into the somatic and autonomic nervous system neuropathies (Chart 42.3).

Somatic Neuropathy. A distal symmetric polyneuropathy, in which loss of function occurs in a stocking–glove pattern, is the most common form of peripheral neuropathy. Somatic sensory involvement usually occurs first and usually is bilateral and symmetric, and associated with diminished perception of vibration, pain, and temperature, particularly in the lower extremities. In addition to the discomforts associated with the loss of sensory or motor function, lesions in the peripheral nervous system predispose a person with diabetes to other complications. As peripheral neuropathy is often associated with the insensate foot the loss of feeling, touch, and position sense increases the risk of falling. Impairment of temperature and pain sensation increases the risk of serious burns and injuries to the feet.[43]

Painful diabetic neuropathy involves the somatosensory neurons that carry pain impulses. This disorder, which causes hypersensitivity to light touch and occasionally severe "burning pain," particularly at night, can become physically and emotionally disabling. Treatment options for this can include pharmacologic (*i.e.*, antidepressants antiepileptics, opioid agonist) or alternative interventions (*i.e.*, acupuncture) to help control the pain as few persons have complete relief.[1,43]

Autonomic Neuropathy. The autonomic neuropathies involve disorders of sympathetic and parasympathetic nervous system function.[1,43] There may be disorders of vasomotor function, decreased cardiac responses, inability to empty the bladder, and sexual dysfunction. Defects in vasomotor reflexes can lead to dizziness and syncope when the person moves from the supine to the standing position (see Chapter 23). Incomplete emptying of the bladder predisposes to urinary stasis and bladder infection and increases the risk of renal complications.

In the male, disruption of sensory and autonomic nervous system function may cause sexual dysfunction (see Chapter 44). Diabetes is the leading physiologic cause of erectile dysfunction, and it occurs in both type 1 and type 2 diabetes. Of Canadian men with diabetes, 34% to 45% have erectile dysfunction. The current treatment, if no contraindications to its use, includes phosphodiesterase type 5 (PDE5) inhibitors to improve erectile function and quality of life.[1]

Disorders of Gastrointestinal Motility. Gastrointestinal motility disorders are common in persons with long-standing diabetes. Although the pathogenesis of these disorders is poorly understood, neuropathy and metabolic abnormalities secondary to hyperglycemia are thought to play an important role.[44] The symptoms vary in severity and include constipation, diarrhea and fecal incontinence, nausea and vomiting, and upper abdominal discomfort referred to as *dyspepsia.*

Gastroparesis (delayed emptying of the stomach) is commonly seen in persons with diabetes.[44] The disorder is characterized by complaints of epigastric discomfort, nausea, postprandial vomiting, bloating, and early satiety. Erratic blood glucose can occur due to delayed food absorption. Diagnostic measures include the use of endoscopy or barium radiography to exclude mechanical obstruction due to peptic ulcer disease or cancer. Management includes the use of prokinetic agents (*e.g.,* metoclopramide, erythromycin) as well as antiemetic agents. Strict control of blood glucose is important because hyperglycemia may slow gastric emptying even in the absence of diabetic neuropathy.

Diarrhea is another common symptom seen mostly in persons with poorly controlled type 1 diabetes and autonomic neuropathy.[44] The pathogenesis is thought to be multifactorial. Diabetic diarrhea is typically intermittent, watery, painless, and nocturnal and may be associated with fecal incontinence. Management includes the use of antidiarrheal agents (loperamide, diphenoxylate). Clonidine (an α_2-adrenergic agonist) and octreotide (a long-acting somatostatin analog) have been used with some success in persons with rapid transit. Antibiotics are used for those with small bowel bacterial overgrowth secondary to slow transit. As with gastroparesis, strict control of blood glucose is important.

Nephropathies

Diabetic nephropathy is the leading cause of chronic kidney disease. In Canada it is estimated that 50% of people with diabetes have chronic kidney disease and this accounts for 34% of all people who seek renal replacement therapy (see Chapter 34).[1,45] The complication affects people with both type 1 and type 2 diabetes. The term *diabetic nephropathy* is used to describe the combination of lesions that often occur concurrently in the diabetic kidney. The most common kidney lesions in people with diabetes are those that affect the glomeruli. Various glomerular changes may occur in people with diabetic nephropathy, including capillary basement membrane thickening, diffuse glomerular sclerosis, and nodular glomerulosclerosis[11] (see Chapter 33). Changes in the capillary basement membrane take the form of thickening of basement membranes along the length of the glomeruli. Diffuse glomerulosclerosis consists of thickening of the basement membrane and the mesangial matrix. Nodular glomerulosclerosis, also called *intercapillary glomerulosclerosis* or *Kimmelstiel–Wilson syndrome,* is a form of glomerulosclerosis that involves the development of nodular lesions in the glomerular capillaries of the kidneys, causing impaired blood flow with progressive loss of kidney function and, eventually, renal failure. Nodular glomerulosclerosis is thought to occur only in people with diabetes. Changes in the basement membrane in diffuse glomerulosclerosis and Kimmelstiel–Wilson syndrome allow plasma proteins to escape in the urine, causing proteinuria and the development of hypoproteinemia, edema, and others signs of impaired kidney function.

Not all people with diabetes develop clinically significant nephropathy; for this reason, attention is focusing on risk factors for the development of this complication. Among the suggested risk factors are genetic and familial predisposition, elevated blood pressure, poor glycemic control, smoking, hyperlipidemia, and microalbuminuria. Diabetic nephropathy occurs in family clusters, suggesting a familial predisposition, although this does not exclude the possibility of environmental factors shared by siblings. The risk for development of kidney disease is greater among Aboriginal, Asian, South Asian, Pacific Island, African/Caribbean, and Hispanic peoples.[46]

Kidney enlargement, nephron hypertrophy, and hyperfiltration occur early in the disease, reflecting the increased work performed by the kidneys in reabsorbing excessive amounts of glucose. One of the first manifestations of diabetic nephropathy is an increase in urinary albumin excretion (*i.e.,* microalbuminuria), which is easily assessed by laboratory methods. Microalbuminuria is defined as a urine protein loss between 30 and 300 mg/day or an albumin-to-creatinine ratio (A/C ratio) between 2.0 and 20.0 mg/mmol (normal <2.0 mg/mmol) from a spot urine collection.[1] It is recommended that the A/C ratio be the preferred screen for microalbuminuria. Once kidney disease is established the stage of nephropathy is determined by the estimated glomerular filtration rate (eGFR).[1] Measures to prevent diabetic nephropathy or its progression in persons with diabetes include achievement of glycemic control; maintenance of blood pressure (<130/80 mm Hg); prevention or reduction in the level of proteinuria (using angiotensin-converting enzyme inhibitors or angiotensin receptor blockers, or protein restriction in selected patients); treatment of hyperlipidemia; and smoking cessation in people who smoke.[1] Both systolic and diastolic hypertension accelerate the progression of diabetic nephropathy. Even moderate lowering of blood pressure can decrease the risk of chronic kidney disease. Smoking increases the risk of chronic kidney disease in both persons with and without diabetes. People with type 2 diabetes who smoke have a greater risk of microalbuminuria, and their rate of progression to chronic kidney disease is approximately twice as rapid as in those who do not smoke.[1]

Retinopathies

Diabetes is the leading cause of acquired blindness and it is estimated that 500,000 Canadians have diabetic retinopathy with higher prevalence rates in the First Nations populations.[1,47] Although people with diabetes are at increased risk for development of cataracts and glaucoma, retinopathy is the most common pattern of eye disease. Diabetic retinopathy is estimated to be the most frequent cause of newly diagnosed blindness under the age 50.[1,47]

Diabetic retinopathy is characterized by abnormal retinal vascular permeability, microaneurysm formation, neovascularization and associated hemorrhage, scarring, and retinal detachment[48] (see Chapter 54). Twenty years after the onset of diabetes, nearly all people with type 1 diabetes and more than 60% of people with type 2 diabetes have some degree of retinopathy.[45] Pregnancy, puberty, and cataract surgery can accelerate these changes. Among the suggested risk factors associated with diabetic retinopathy are poor glycemic control, elevated blood pressure, and hyperlipidemia. The strongest case for control of blood glucose comes from the DCCT and UKPDS studies, which demonstrated a reduction in retinopathy with improved glucose control.[38,39]

Because of the risk of retinopathy, it is important that people with diabetes have regular dilated eye examinations. They should have an initial examination for retinopathy shortly after the diagnosis of diabetes is made. The recommendation for follow-up examinations is based on the type of examination that was done and the findings of that examination. People with persistently elevated glucose levels or proteinuria should be examined yearly.[1] Women who are planning a pregnancy should be counselled on the risk of development or progression of diabetic retinopathy. Women with diabetes who become pregnant should be followed closely throughout pregnancy. This does not apply to women in whom GDM develops because such women are not at risk for development of diabetic retinopathy.

People with macular edema, moderate to severe nonproliferative retinopathy, or any proliferative retinopathy should receive the care of an ophthalmologist who is knowledgeable and experienced in the management and treatment of diabetic retinopathy. Methods used in the treatment of diabetic retinopathy include the destruction and scarring of the proliferative lesions with laser photocoagulation, the use of intraocular injections of antagonists to growth factors (*e.g.,* vascular endothelial growth factor) and vitreoretinal surgery.[1]

Macrovascular Complications

Diabetes mellitus is a major risk factor for coronary artery disease, cerebrovascular disease, and peripheral vascular disease. The prevalence of these macrovascular complications is increased twofold to fourfold in people with diabetes. Approximately 65% to 80% of all people with type 2 diabetes will die of a macrovascular problem.[1]

Multiple risk factors for macrovascular disease, including obesity, hypertension, hyperglycemia, hyperinsulinemia, hyperlipidemia, altered platelet function, endothelial dysfunction, systemic inflammation (as evidenced by increased C-reactive protein), and elevated fibrinogen levels, frequently are found in people with diabetes. There appear to be differences between type 1 and type 2 diabetes in terms of duration of disease and the development of macrovascular disease. In people with type 2 diabetes, macrovascular disease may be present at the time of diagnosis.

Aggressive management of cardiovascular risk factors should include smoking cessation and management of hypertension, plus lipid lowering, diabetes control, and antiplatelet agents (aspirin or clopidogrel) if not contraindicated[1] (see Chapter 22). Lifestyle changes are an integral component to help reduce cardiovascular risk and should include maintenance of health body weight, diet, and exercise.[1]

Diabetic Foot Ulcers

Foot problems are common among people with diabetes and may become severe enough to cause ulceration, infection, and, eventually, the need for amputation. Foot problems have been reported as the most common complication leading to hospitalization among people with diabetes. In people with diabetes, lesions of the feet represent the effects of neuropathy and vascular insufficiency. Approximately 15% of people with diabetes will develop ulceration over their lifetime and this is typically located on the plantar aspect of the foot.

Distal symmetric neuropathy is a major risk factor for foot ulcers. People with sensory neuropathies have impaired pain sensation and often are unaware of the constant trauma to the feet caused by poorly fitting shoes, improper weight bearing, hard objects or pebbles in the shoes, or infections such as athlete's foot. Neuropathy prevents people from detecting pain; they are unable to adjust their gait to avoid walking on an area of the foot where pressure is causing trauma and necrosis. Motor neuropathy with weakness of the intrinsic muscles of the foot may result in foot deformities, which lead to focal areas of high pressure. When the abnormal focus of pressure is coupled with loss of sensation, a foot ulcer can occur. Common sites of trauma are the back of the heel, the plantar metatarsal area, or the great toe, where weight is borne during walking (Fig. 42.13).

All persons with diabetes should receive a full foot examination at least once a year. This examination should include assessment of protective sensation, foot structure and

FIGURE 42.13 Neuropathic ulcers occur on pressure points in areas with diminished sensation in diabetic polyneuropathy. Pain is absent (and therefore the ulcer may go unnoticed). (From Stephen T. C., Skillen D. L., Day R. A., et al. (2010). *Canadian Bates' guide to physical assessment for nurses* (p. 599). Philadelphia, PA: Lippincott Williams & Wilkins.)

biomechanics, vascular status, and skin integrity.[1,3,49] Evaluation of neurologic function should include a somatosensory test using either the Semmes–Weinstein monofilament or vibratory sensation. The Semmes–Weinstein monofilament is a simple, inexpensive device for testing sensory status (Fig. 42.14). The monofilament is held in the hand or attached to a handle at one end. When the unattached or unsupported end of the

FIGURE 42.14 • Use of a monofilament to test for impaired sensation in the foot of a person with diabetes.

monofilament is pressed perpendicularly against the skin until it buckles or bends slightly, it delivers 10 g of pressure at the point of contact. The test has the person being tested report the sensation when touched by the monofilamenton 4 and 10 sites per foot. An incorrect response at even one site indicates increased risk of neuropathy and foot complications.

Because of the constant risk of foot problems, it is important that people with diabetes wear shoes that have been fitted correctly and inspect their feet daily, looking for blisters, open sores, and fungal infection (*e.g.,* athlete's foot) between the toes. If their eyesight is poor, a family member should do this for them. In the event a lesion is detected, prompt medical attention is needed to prevent serious complications. Specially designed shoes have been demonstrated to be effective in preventing relapses in people with previous ulcerations.[1,49] Smoking should be avoided because it causes vasoconstriction and contributes to vascular disease. Because cold produces vasoconstriction, appropriate foot coverings should be used to keep the feet warm and dry. Toenails should be cut straight across to prevent ingrown toenails. The toenails often are thickened and deformed, requiring the services of a podiatrist.

Persons with diabetes mellitus develop more extensive and rapidly progressive peripheral vascular disease than do individuals without diabetes. Cardiovascular risk factors should be addressed in patients with diabetic ulcers and peripheral vascular disease. Advances in the field of chronic wound care have increased treatment options for ulcers that are resistant to standard therapy. Applications of growth factors provide a means by which cells communicate with each other and can have profound effects on cell proliferation, migration, and extracellular matrix synthesis. Use of hyperbaric oxygen therapy, wound care specialty services, and minimally invasive surgeries are often part of the multimodal strategies utilized.[49]

Infections

Although not specifically an acute or a chronic complication, infections are a common concern of people with diabetes as they are considered to be immunocompromised. Certain types of infections occur with increased frequency in people with diabetes: soft tissue infections of the extremities, osteomyelitis, urinary tract infections and pyelonephritis, candidal infections of the skin and mucosal surfaces, dental caries and periodontal disease, and tuberculosis.[1,49,50]

Suboptimal response to infection in a person with diabetes is caused by the presence of chronic complications, such as vascular disease and neuropathies, and by the presence of hyperglycemia and altered neutrophil function. Sensory deficits may cause a person with diabetes to ignore minor trauma and infection, and vascular disease may impair circulation and delivery of blood cells and other substances needed to produce an adequate inflammatory response and effect healing. Pyelonephritis and urinary tract infections are relatively common in persons with diabetes, and it has been suggested that these infections may bear some relation to the presence of a

neurogenic bladder or nephrosclerotic changes in the kidneys. Hyperglycemia and glycosuria may influence the growth of microorganisms and increase the severity of the infection. Diabetes and elevated blood glucose levels also may impair host defences such as the function of neutrophils and immune cells. Polymorphonuclear leukocyte function, particularly adherence, chemotaxis, and phagocytosis, is depressed in persons with diabetes, particularly those with poor glycemic control. In acute illness, increased efforts to control blood sugars for surgical patients and medical conditions cite an impact on infections.[51]

IN SUMMARY

Diabetes mellitus is a disorder of carbohydrate, protein, and fat metabolism resulting from an imbalance between insulin availability and insulin need. The disease can be classified as type 1 diabetes in which there is destruction of beta cells and an absolute insulin deficiency, or type 2 diabetes in which there is a lack of insulin availability or effectiveness. Type 1 diabetes can be further subdivided into type 1A immune-mediated diabetes, which is thought to be caused by autoimmune mechanisms, and type 1B idiopathic diabetes, for which the cause is unknown. GDM develops during pregnancy, and although glucose tolerance often returns to normal after childbirth, it indicates an increased risk for the development of diabetes. The metabolic syndrome represents a constellation of metabolic abnormalities characterized by obesity, insulin resistance, high triglyceride levels and low HDL levels, hypertension, cardiovascular disease, insulin resistance, and increased risk for development of type 2 diabetes.

The most commonly identified symptoms of type 1 diabetes are polyuria, polydipsia, polyphagia, and weight loss despite normal or increased appetite. Although persons with type 2 diabetes may present with one or more of these symptoms, they are often asymptomatic initially. The diagnosis of diabetes mellitus is based on clinical signs of the disease, fasting blood glucose levels, A_{1C} levels, random plasma glucose measurements, and results of the glucose tolerance test. Glycosylation involves the irreversible attachment of glucose to the hemoglobin molecule; the measurement of A_{1C} provides an index of blood glucose levels over the previous 3 months. Self-monitoring provides a means of maintaining near-normal blood glucose levels through frequent testing of blood glucose and adjustment of insulin dosage.

Dietary management focuses on maintaining a well-balanced diet, controlling calories to achieve and maintain an optimum weight, and regulating the distribution of carbohydrates, proteins, and fats. Two types of antidiabetic agents are used in the management of diabetes: injectable insulin and oral/injectable diabetic drugs. Type 1 diabetes, and sometimes type 2, requires treatment with injectable insulin. Antidiabetic drugs now include six categories.

These drugs require a functioning pancreas and may be used in the treatment of type 2 diabetes.

The metabolic disturbances associated with diabetes affect almost every body system. The acute complications of diabetes include diabetic ketoacidosis, hyperglycemic hyperosmolar state, and hypoglycemia in people with insulin-treated diabetes. The chronic complications of diabetes affect the microvascular system (including the retina, kidneys, and peripheral nervous system) and the macrovascular system (coronary, cerebrovascular, and peripheral arteries). The diabetic foot is usually a combination of both microvascular and macrovascular dysfunction. Infection is also a frequent cofactor in the diabetic foot.

REVIEW EXERCISES

1. A 6-year-old boy is admitted to the emergency department with nausea, vomiting, and abdominal pain. He is very lethargic; his skin is warm, dry, and flushed; his pulse is rapid; and he has a sweet smell to his breath. His parents relate that he has been very thirsty during the past several weeks, his appetite has been poor, and he has been urinating frequently. His initial plasma glucose is 23.0 mmol/L, and a urine test for ketones is strongly positive.
   A. *What is the most likely cause of this boy's elevated blood glucose and ketonuria?*
   B. *Explain his presenting signs and symptoms in terms of the elevated blood glucose and metabolic acidosis.*
   C. *What type of treatment will this boy require?*
2. A 53-year-old accountant presents for his routine yearly examination. His history indicates that he was found to have a fasting glucose of 6.7 mmol/L on two prior occasions. Currently, he is asymptomatic. He has no other medical problems and does not use any medications. He neither smokes nor drinks alcohol. His father had type 2 diabetes at age 60 years. His physical examination reveals a blood pressure of 125/80 mm Hg, BMI (body mass index) of 32 kg/m^2, and waist circumference of 114 cm. Laboratory study results are as follows: complete blood count (CBC), thyroid-stimulating hormone (TSH), and alanine aminotransferase (ALT) are within normal limits. The lipid panel shows an HDL of 0.8 mmol/L, low-density lipoprotein (LDL) of 3.5 mmol/L, and triglycerides of 2.3 mmol/L (normal <1.7 mmol/L).
   A. *What is this man's probable diagnosis?*
   B. *Based on this man's blood glucose level and the CDA diabetes classification system, what diabetic status would you place this man in?*

Does he need a 75-g oral glucose tolerance test (OGTT) for further assessment of his IFG?
C. *His OGTT test result reveals a 2-hour glucose value of 9.6 mmol/L. What is the diagnosis? What type of treatment would be appropriate for this man?*

References

1. Canadian Diabetes Association Clinical Practice Guidelines Expert Committee; Booth G., Cheng A. Y. (2013). Canadian Diabetes Association 2013 clinical practice guidelines for the prevention and management of diabetes in Canada. *Canadian Journal of Diabetes, 37*(Suppl 1), S1–S212.
2. Hall J. E. (2011). *Textbook of medical physiology* (12th ed.). Philadelphia, PA: W. B. Saunders.
3. Masharnai U., German M. S. (2011). Chapter 17: Pancreatic hormones and diabetes mellitus. In Gardner D. G., Shobeck D. (Eds.), *Greenspan's basic and clinical endocrinology* (9th ed.). New York: McGraw-Hill.
4. Hayes M. R., Mietlicki-Baase E. G., Kanoski S. E., et al. (2014). Incretins and amylin: Neuroendocrine communication between the gut, pancreas, and brain in control of food intake and blood glucose. *Annual Review of Nutrition, 34*, 207–236.
5. Pillay K., Govender P. (2013). Amylin uncovered: A review on the polypeptide responsible for type II diabetes. *BioMed Research International, 2013*, 826706.
6. Yuen K. C., Chong L. E., Riddle M. C. (2013). Influence of glucocorticoids and growth hormone on insulin sensitivity in humans. *Diabetes Medicine, 30*(6), 651–663.
7. Goldfine I. R., Youngren J. F. (1998). Contributions of the American Journal of Physiology to the discovery of insulin. *American Journal of Physiology: Endocrinology and Metabolism, 274*(2), E207–E209.
8. Roh M. O., Jung C. H., Kim B. Y., et al. (2013). The prevalence and characteristics of latent autoimmune diabetes in adults (LADA). *Acta Diabetologica, 50*(2), 129–134.
9. Atkinson M. A., Eisenbarth G. S., Michels A. W. (2014). Type 1 diabetes. *Lancet, 383*(9911), 69–82.
10. Dabelea D., Mayer-Davis E. J., Saydah S., et al. (2014). Prevalence of type 1 and type 2 diabetes among children and adolescents from 2001 to 2009. *Journal of the American Medical Association, 311*(17), 1778–1786.
11. Williams K. J., Siraj E. S. (2012). Chapter 22: Obesity, diabetes mellitus and the metabolic syndrome. In Rubin R., Strayer D. S. (Eds.), *Rubin's pathology: Clinicopathologic foundations of medicine* (6th ed.). Philadelphia, PA: Lippincott Williams & Wilkins.
12. Kahn S. E., Cooper M. E., Del Prato S. (2014). Pathophysiology and treatment of type 2 diabetes: Perspectives on the past, present, and future. *Lancet, 383*(9922), 1068–1083.
13. Gallagher E. J., LeRoith D., Karnieli E. (2011). The metabolic syndrome: From insulin resistance to obesity and diabetes. *Medical Clinics of North America, 95*(5), 855–873.
14. Kassi E., Pervanidou P., Kaltsas G., et al. (2011). Metabolic syndrome: Definitions and controversies. *BMC Medicine, 9*(48), 1–13.
15. Berger H., Crane J., Farine D. (2002). Screening for gestational diabetes mellitus. *Journal of Obstetrics and Gynaecology Canada, 24*(11), 894–903.
16. Redinger R. N. (2007). The pathophysiology of obesity and its clinical manifestations. *Gastroenterology & Hepatology, 3*(11), 856–863.
17. Shanik M. H., Xu Y., Skrha J., et al. (2008). Insulin resistance and hyperinsulinemia. Is hyperinsulinemia the cart or the horse? *Diabetes Care, 31*(Suppl 2), S262–S268.
18. Makki K., Froguel P., Wolowczuk I. (2013). Adipose tissue in obesity-related inflammation and insulin resistance: Cells, cytokines, and chemokines. *ISRN Inflammation, 2013*, 139239.

19. Turer A. T., Scherer P. E. (2012). Adiponectin: Mechanistic insights and clinical implications. *Diabetologia, 55*(9), 2319–2326.

20. Buresi M. C., Lee J., Gill S., et al. (2010). The prevalence of gestation diabetes mellitus and glucose abnormalities in pregnant women with hepatitis C virus infection in British Columbia. *Journal of Obstetrics and Gynaecology Canada, 32*(10), 935–941.

21. Feig D. S., Hwee J., Shah B. R., et al. (2014). Trends in incidence of diabetes in pregnancy and serious perinatal outcome: A large, population based study in Ontario, Canada, 1996–2010. *Diabetes Care, 37*(6), 1590–1596.

22. Feig D. S., Zinman B., Wang X., et al. (2008). Risk of development of diabetes mellitus after diagnosis of gestational diabetes. *Canadian Medical Association Journal, 179*(3), 229–234.

23. Verma S. B., Wollina U. (2011). Looking through the cracks of diabetic candida balanoposthitis. *International Journal of General Medicine, 4,* 511–513.

24. Pastors J. G., Warshaw H., Daly A., et al. (2002). The evidence for the effectiveness of medical nutrition therapy in diabetes management. *Diabetes Care, 25*(3), 608–613.

25. Anderson T. J., Gregoire J., Hegele R. A., et al. (2013). 2012 update of the Canadian Cardiovascular Society guidelines for the diagnosis and treatment of dyslipidemia for the prevention of cardiovascular disease in the adult. *Canadian Journal of Cardiology, 29*(2), 151–167.

26. Bailey A. V., Day C. (2014). The role of SGLT2 inhibitors in type 2 diabetes. *British Journal of Family Medicine, 2*(4), 29–33.

27. Mansell K., Arnason T. (updated 2014). Endocrine and metabolic disorders: Diabetes mellitus. In Repchinsky C. (Ed.), *e-Therapeutics.* [Online] Ottawa: Canadian Pharmacists Association.

28. Nissen S. E., Wolski K. (2007). Effect of rosiglitazone on the risk of myocardial infarction and death from cardiovascular causes. *New England Journal of Medicine, 356*(24), 2457–2471.

29. Cryer P. E. (2013). Mechanisms of hypoglycemia-associated autonomic failure in diabetes. *New England Journal of Medicine, 369*(4), 362–372.

30. Ahren B. (2013). Incretin therapy for type 2 diabetes: GLP-1 receptor agonists and DPP-4 inhibitors. *European Diabetes Nursing, 10*(1), 31–36.

31. Langendam M., Luijf Y. M., Hooft L., et al. (2012). Continuous glucose monitoring systems for type 1 diabetes mellitus (Review). *Cochrane Database of Systematic Reviews, 2012*(1), CD008101.

32. Westerberg D. P. (2013). Diabetic ketoacidosis: Evaluation and treatment. *American Family Physician, 87*(5), 337–346.

33. Maletkovic J., Drexler A. (2013). Diabetic ketoacidosis and hyperglycemic hyperosmolar state. *Endocrinology and Metabolism Clinics of North America, 42*(4), 677–695.

34. Masharnai U., Gitelman S. E. (2011). Chapter 18: Hypoglycemic disorders. In Gardner D. G., Shobeck D. (Eds.), *Greenspan's basic and clinical endocrinology* (9th ed.). New York: McGraw-Hill.

35. Somogyi M. (1957). Exacerbation of diabetes in excess insulin action. *American Journal of Medicine, 26*(2), 169–191.

36. Porcellati F., Lucidi P., Bolli G. B., Fanelli C. G. (2013). Thirty years of research on the dawn phenomenon: Lessons to optimize blood glucose control in diabetes. *Diabetes Care, 36*(12), 3860–3862.

37. Harmon C., Willoughby D., Floyd C. (2004). A lesson in early morning hyperglycemia. *Nurse Practitioner, 29*(11), 58–63.

38. The Diabetes Control and Complications Trial Research Group. (1993). The effect of intensified treatment of diabetes on the development and progression of long-term complications in insulin-dependent diabetes mellitus. *New England Journal of Medicine, 329*(14), 955–977.

39. Stratton I. M., Adler A. I., Neil H. A., et al. (2000). Association of glycaemia with macrovascular and microvascular complications in type 2 diabetes (UKPDS 35): Prospective observational study. *British Medical Journal, 321*(7258), 405–412.

40. Sytze Van Dam P., Cotter M. A., Bravenboer B., et al. (2013). Pathogenesis of diabetic neuropathy: Focus on neurovascular mechanisms. *European Journal of Pharmacology, 719*(1–3), 180–186.

41. Bodiga V. L., Eda S. R., Bodiga S. (2014). Advanced glycation end products: Role in pathology of diabetic cardiomyopathy. *Heart Failure Reviews, 19*(1), 49–63.

42. Campos C. (2012). Chronic hyperglycemia and glucose toxicity: Pathology and clinical sequelae. *Postgraduate Medicine, 124*(6), 90–97.

43. Vinik A. I., Nevoret M., Casellini C., et al. (2013). Diabetic neuropathy. *Endocrinology and Metabo Clinics of North America, 42*(4), 747–787.

44. Boland B. S., Edelman S. V., Wolosin J. D. (2013). Gastrointestinal complications of diabetes. *Endocrinology and Metabolism Clinics of North America, 42*(4), 809–832.

45. Public Health Agency of Canada. (2011). *Diabetes in Canada: Factors and figures from a public health perspective.* Ottawa: PHAC.

46. Shlipak M. (2011). Diabetic nephropathy: Preventing progression. *American Family Physician, 83*(6), 739–740.

47. CNIB. (2014). Eye connect: Diabetic retinopathy. Available online at: http://www.cnib.ca/en/your-eyes/eye-conditions/eye-connect/DR/Pages/default.aspx. Accessed September 24, 2014.

48. Rosberger D. F. (2013). Diabetic retinopathy: Current concepts and emerging therapy. *Endocrinology and Metabolism Clinics of North America, 42*(4), 721–745.

49. Kim P. J., Steinberg J. S. (2013). Complications of the diabetic foot. *Endocrinology and Metabolism Clinics of North America, 42*(4), 833–847.

50. Casquiero J., Casquiero J., Alves C. (2012). Infections in patient with diabetes mellitus: A review of the pathogenesis. *Indian Journal of Endocrinology and Metabolism, 16*(Suppl 1), S27–S36.

51. Umpeirrez G. E., Smiley D., Jacobs S., et al. (2011). Randomized study of basal-bolus insulin therapy in the impatient management of patients with type 2 diabetes undergoing general surgery. *Diabetes Care, 34*(2), 256–261.

Visit thePoint **http://thePoint.lww.com for animations, journal articles, and more!**

Unit XI

Disorders of Genitourinary and Reproductive Function

There is a long history of misunderstanding and myths about human reproduction, especially the female reproductive system. Early on, the uterus was deemed the most important structure of the female reproductive anatomy. One of the first representations of the uterus appears in ancient Egyptian hieroglyphs (c. 2900 BC). Its importance was a direct result of the understanding that it was from the uterus that a child was born. That a woman was the carrier of the next generation was enough to establish her importance to society. However, society also imposed harsh restrictions on women that made it difficult, if not impossible, for further understanding. Until the Renaissance, custom and manners dictated that a woman's body could not be represented unless it was fully clothed.

To a regrettable extent, the associations made in ancient times that surmised a destiny for women based on the anatomy peculiar to their sex still affect how women are viewed today. The Greek philosopher Plato (approximately 427–347 BC) postulated that the unused womb became "indignant" and wandered around the body, inhibiting the body's "spirits," or life force, and causing disease. The reasonings of Aristotle (384–322 BC) were equally fanciful. It was he, believing as others of the time did that women were irrational and prone to emotional outbursts, who provided the nomenclature for the womb, naming it *hystera* (ustera). Their concept that emotional excitability or instability was the domain of women is confirmed by another word that was coined by the Greeks: hysteria.

Unit XI

Disorders of Genitourinary and Reproductive Function

Structure and Function of the Male Genitourinary System

43

The male genitourinary system is composed of the paired gonads, or testes, genital ducts, accessory organs, and penis (Fig. 43.1). The dual function of the testes is to produce androgens (*i.e.,* male sex hormones), mainly testosterone, and spermatozoa (*i.e.,* male germ cells). The internal accessory organs produce the fluid constituents of semen, and the ductile system aids in the storage and transport of spermatozoa. The penis functions in urine elimination and sexual function. This chapter focuses on the structure of the male reproductive system, spermatogenesis and control of male reproductive function, neural control of sexual function, and changes in function that occur at puberty and as a result of the aging process.

STRUCTURE OF THE MALE REPRODUCTIVE SYSTEM

After completing this section of the chapter, you should be able to meet the following objectives:

- Characterize the embryonic development of the male reproductive organs and genitalia.
- Describe the structure and function of the testes and scrotum, the genital ducts, accessory organs, and penis.

Embryonic Development

The sex of a person is determined at the time of fertilization by the sex chromosomes. In the early stages of embryonic development, the tissues from which the male and female reproductive organs develop are undifferentiated and considered bipotential. Until approximately the seventh week of gestation, it is impossible to determine whether an embryo is male or female unless the chromosomes are studied. Until this time, the male and female genital tracts consist of two wolffian ducts, from which the male genitalia develop, and two müllerian ducts, from which the female genital structures develop. During this period of gestation, the gonads (*i.e.,* ovaries and testes) also are undifferentiated.[1-3]

Between the sixth and eighth weeks of gestation, the testes begin their development under the influence of the Y chromosome. Differentiation of the indifferent gonad into a testis

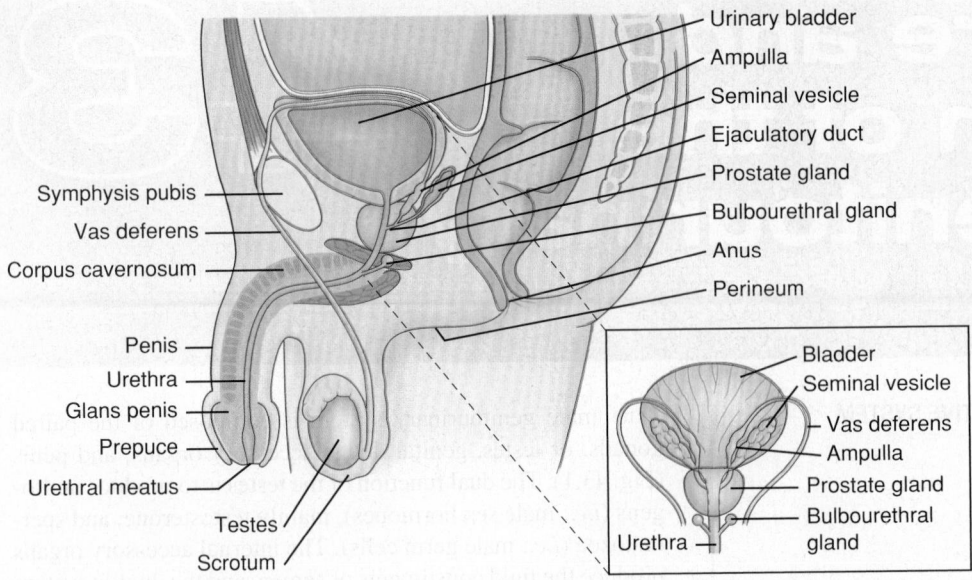

FIGURE 43.1 • The structures of the male reproductive system. (From Stephen T. C., Skillen D. L., Day R. A., et al. (2012). *Canadian Jensen's nursing health assessment: A best practice approach* (p. 756). Philadelphia, PA: Lippincott Williams & Wilkins.)

is initiated by the actions of a single gene on the short arm of the Y chromosome. This gene is called the *sex*-determining *region* of the *Y* chromosome (*SRY*).[1] In the presence of the *SRY* gene, the embryonic gonads develop into testes, and in its absence, the gonads develop into ovaries.

During this time, the testicular cells of the male embryo begin producing an anti-müllerian hormone (AMH) and testosterone. The AMH suppresses the müllerian ducts and prevents development of the uterus and fallopian tubes in the male. In parallel, testosterone stimulates the wolffian ducts to develop into the epididymis, vas deferens, and seminal vesicles.[1] Testosterone also is the precursor of a third hormone, dihydrotestosterone (DHT), which functions in the formation of the male urethra, prostate, and external genitalia. The conversion of testosterone to DHT, predominantly in the peripheral tissues, is performed by the enzyme 5α-reductase. Although testosterone and DHT share the same nuclear androgen receptor, they have marked differences in tissue activity: DHT exerts most of its effects on the external genitalia, including the prostate, but is also subsequently important for the development of facial and body hair, including temporal hair recession. In the absence of testosterone (and DHT), a male embryo with an XY chromosomal pattern develops female external genitalia.[1]

Testes and Scrotum

The testes, or male gonads, are two egg-shaped structures located outside the abdominal cavity in the scrotum. The adult male testes are approximately 15 to 25 ml in volume (>4 ml indicates pubertal onset), with 80% of this volume being cells involved in spermatogenesis and 20% in testosterone production. Embryologically, the testes develop in the abdominal cavity and then descend through the inguinal canal into a pouch of peritoneum (which becomes the tunica vaginalis) in the scrotum. Testicular descent occurs in two stages. The first occurs between 7 and 12 weeks of fetal life, with

AMH being responsible for descent to the inguinal region. The second occurs between 7 and 9 months of fetal life, with testosterone being responsible for descent into the scrotum. As they descend, the testes pull their arteries, veins, lymphatics, nerves, and conducting excretory ducts with them. These structures are encased by the cremaster muscle and layers of fascia that constitute the spermatic cord (Fig. 43.2A). After descent of the testes, the inguinal canal closes almost completely. Failure of this canal to close predisposes to the development of an inguinal hernia later in life (Fig. 43.2B). An inguinal hernia or "rupture" is a protrusion of the parietal peritoneum and part of the intestine through an abnormal opening from the abdominal cavity. A loop of small bowel may become incarcerated in an inguinal hernia (strangulated hernia), in which case its lumen may become obstructed and its vascular supply compromised (see Chapter 37).

The testes are enclosed in a double-layered membrane, the tunica vaginalis, which is derived embryologically from the abdominal peritoneum[2,3] (Fig. 43.2). An outer covering, the tunica albuginea, is a tough, white, fibrous sheath that resembles the sclera of the eye. The tunica albuginea protects the testes and gives them their ovoid shape. The cremaster muscles, which are bands of skeletal muscle arising from the internal oblique muscles of the trunk, elevate the testes. The testes receive their arterial blood supply from the long testicular arteries, which branch from the abdominal artery. The testicular veins, which drain the testes, arise from a venous network called the *pampiniform plexus* that surrounds the testicular artery. The testes are innervated by fibres from both divisions of the autonomic nervous system. Associated sensory nerves transmit pain impulses, resulting in excruciating pain especially when the testes are hit forcibly.

The scrotum, which houses the testes, is made up of a thin outer layer of skin that forms rugae, or folds, and is continuous with the perineum and outer skin of the groin. Under the outer skin lies a thin layer of fascia and smooth muscle

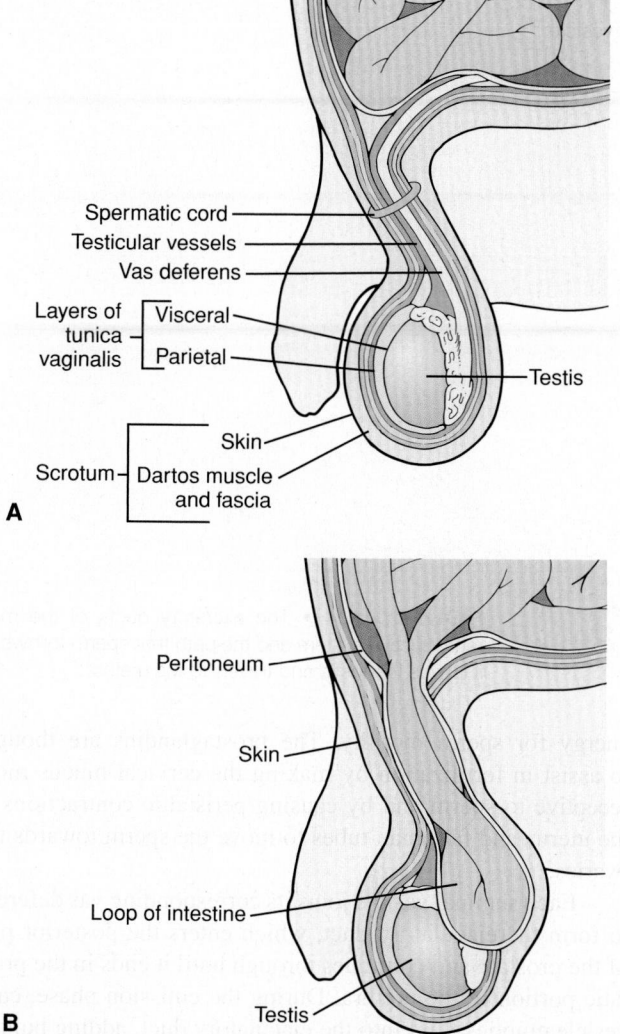

A

B

FIGURE 43.2 • A: Anterior view of the spermatic cord and inguinal canal and coverings of the spermatic cord and testes. **B:** Indirect inguinal hernia. (Adapted from Moore K. L., Agur A. M., Dalley A. F. (2011). *Essential clinical anatomy* (4th ed., p. 129). Philadelphia, PA: Lippincott Williams & Wilkins. Also adapted from Moore K. L., Agur A. M. (2002). *Essentials of clinical anatomy* (2nd ed., p. 138). Philadelphia, PA: Lippincott Williams & Wilkins.)

(*i.e.*, dartos muscle). This layer contains a septum that separates the two testes. The dartos muscle responds to changes in temperature. When it is cold, the muscle contracts, bringing the testes closer to the body, and the scrotum becomes shorter and heavily wrinkled. When it is warmer, the muscle relaxes, allowing the scrotum to fall away from the body.

The location of the testes in the scrotum is important for sperm production, which is optimal at 2°C to 3°C below body temperature.[4] Two systems maintain the temperature of the testes at a level consistent with sperm production. One is the pampiniform plexus of testicular veins that surrounds the testicular artery. This plexus absorbs heat from the arterial blood, cooling it as it enters the testes. The other is the cremaster muscles, which respond to decreases in testicular temperature

by moving the testes closer to the body. Prolonged exposure to elevated temperatures, as a result of hot tubs, sauna, spas, prolonged fever, or the dysfunction of thermoregulatory mechanisms, can impair spermatogenesis. Some tight-fitting undergarments hold the testes against the body and are thought to contribute to a decrease in sperm counts and infertility by interfering with the thermoregulatory function of the scrotum. Cryptorchidism, the failure of the testes to descend into the scrotum, also exposes the testes to the higher temperature of the body (see Chapter 44).

Genital Duct System

Internally, the testes are composed of several hundred compartments or lobules (Fig. 43.3). Each lobule contains one or more coiled seminiferous tubules. These tubules are the site of sperm production. As the tubules lead into the efferent ducts, the seminiferous tubules become the rete testis. From the rete testis, 10,000 to 20,000 efferent ducts emerge to join the epididymis, which is the final site for sperm maturation. Because the spermatozoa are not motile at this stage of development, peristaltic movements of the ductal walls of the epididymis aid in their movement. The spermatozoa continue their migration through the ductus deferens, also called the *vas deferens*. The ampulla of the vas deferens serves as a storage reservoir for sperm. Sperm are stored in the ampulla until they are released through the penis during ejaculation (Fig. 43.4). Spermatozoa can be stored in the genital ducts for as long as 42 days and still maintain their fertility. Surgical disconnection of the vas deferens in the scrotal area (*e.g.*, vasectomy) serves as an effective method of male contraception. Because sperm are stored in the ampulla, men can remain fertile for 4 to 5 weeks after performance of a vasectomy.

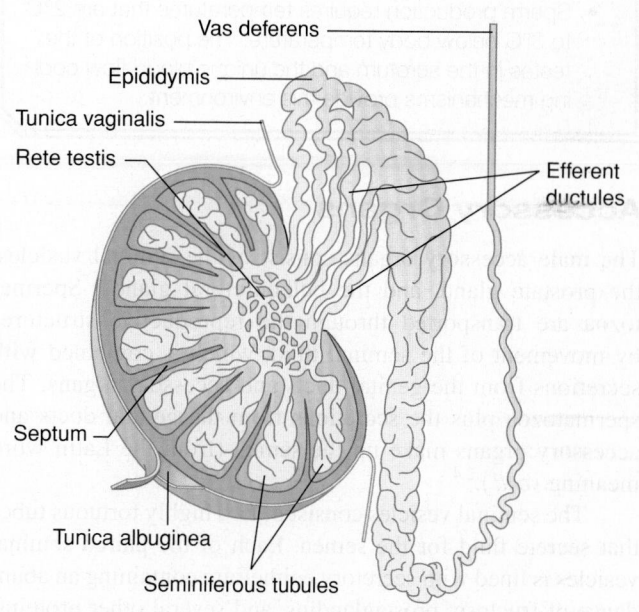

FIGURE 43.3 • The parts of the testes and epididymis.

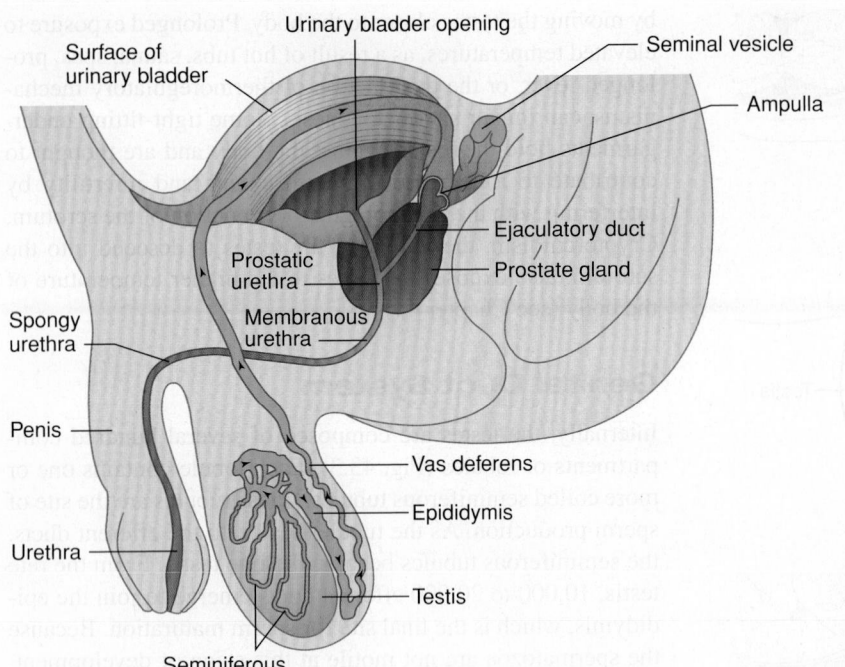

Surface of
urinary bladder

Urinary bladder opening

Seminal vesicle

Ampulla

Ejaculatory duct

Prostatic
urethra

Prostate gland

Membranous
urethra

Spongy
urethra

Penis

Vas deferens

Urethra

Epididymis

Testis

Seminiferous
tubules

FIGURE 43.4 • The excretory ducts of the male reproductive system and the path that sperm follows as it leaves the testis and travels to the urethra.

MALE REPRODUCTIVE SYSTEM

- The male genitourinary system functions in both urine elimination and reproduction.
- The testes function in both production of male germ cells (spermatogenesis) and secretion of the male sex hormone, testosterone.
- The ductile system (epididymides, vas deferens, and ejaculatory ducts) transports and stores sperm, and assists in their maturation; and the accessory glands (seminal vesicles, prostate gland, and bulbourethral glands) prepare the sperm for ejaculation.
- Sperm production requires temperatures that are 2°C to 3°C below body temperature. The position of the testes in the scrotum and the unique blood flow cooling mechanisms provide this environment.

Accessory Organs

The male accessory organs consist of the seminal vesicles, the prostate gland, and the bulbourethral glands. Spermatozoa are transported through the reproductive structures by movement of the seminal fluid, which is combined with secretions from the genital ducts and accessory organs. The spermatozoa plus the secretions from the genital ducts and accessory organs make up the semen (from the Latin word meaning *seed*).[2,4]

The seminal vesicles consist of two highly tortuous tubes that secrete fluid for the semen. Each of the paired seminal vesicles is lined with secretory epithelium containing an abundance of fructose, prostaglandins, and several other proteins. The fructose secreted by the seminal vesicles provides the

energy for sperm motility. The prostaglandins are thought to assist in fertilization by making the cervical mucus more receptive to sperm and by causing peristaltic contractions in the uterus and fallopian tubes to move the sperm towards the ovaries.

Each seminal vesicle joins its corresponding vas deferens to form the ejaculatory duct, which enters the posterior part of the prostate and continues through until it ends in the prostatic portion of the urethra. During the emission phase, each vesicle empties fluid into the ejaculatory duct, adding bulk to the semen. Approximately 70% of the ejaculate originates in the seminal vesicles.

The prostate is a fibromuscular and glandular organ lying just inferior to the bladder. The prostate gland secretes a thin, milky, alkaline fluid containing citric acid, calcium, acid phosphate, a clotting enzyme, and a profibrinolysin. During ejaculation, the capsule of the prostate contracts and the added fluid increases the bulk of the semen. Both vaginal secretions and the fluid from the vas deferens are strongly acidic. Because sperm mobilization occurs at a pH of 6.0 to 6.5, the alkaline nature of the prostatic secretions is essential for successful fertilization of the ovum. The bulbourethral or Cowper glands lie on either side of the membranous urethra and secrete alkaline mucus, which further aids in neutralizing acids from the urine that remain in the urethra.[4]

The prostate gland also functions in the elimination of urine and consists of a thin, fibrous capsule that encloses the circularly oriented smooth muscle fibres and collagenous tissue that surround the urethra where it joins the bladder. The segment of urethra that traverses the prostate gland is called the *prostatic urethra*. It is lined by a thin, longitudinal layer of smooth muscle that is continuous with the bladder wall. The smooth muscle incorporated with the prostate gland is derived primarily from the longitudinal bladder musculature. This smooth muscle represents the true involuntary sphincter of the male prostatic urethra. Because the prostate surrounds the urethra, enlargement of the gland can produce urinary obstruction.

The prostate gland is made up of many secretory glands arranged in three concentric areas surrounding the prostatic urethra, into which they open. The component glands of the prostate include the small mucosal glands associated with the urethral mucosa, the intermediate submucosal glands that lie peripheral to the mucosal glands, and the large main prostatic glands that are situated towards the outside of the gland. It is the overgrowth of the mucosal glands that causes benign prostatic hyperplasia (BPH) in older men (see Chapter 44).

Penis

The penis is the external genital organ through which the urethra passes. Anatomically, the external penis consists of a shaft that ends in a tip called the *glans* (Fig. 43.5). The loose skin of the penis shaft folds to cover the glans, forming the prepuce, or foreskin. The glans of the penis contains many sensory nerves, making this the most sensitive portion of the penile shaft. It is the foreskin that is removed during male circumcision.

The cylindrical body or shaft of the penis is composed of three masses of erectile tissue held together by fibrous strands and covered with a thin layer of skin. The two lateral masses of tissue are called the *corpora cavernosa*. The third, ventral mass is called the *corpus spongiosum*. The corpora cavernosa and corpus spongiosum are cavernous sinuses that normally are relatively empty but become engorged with blood during penile erection.

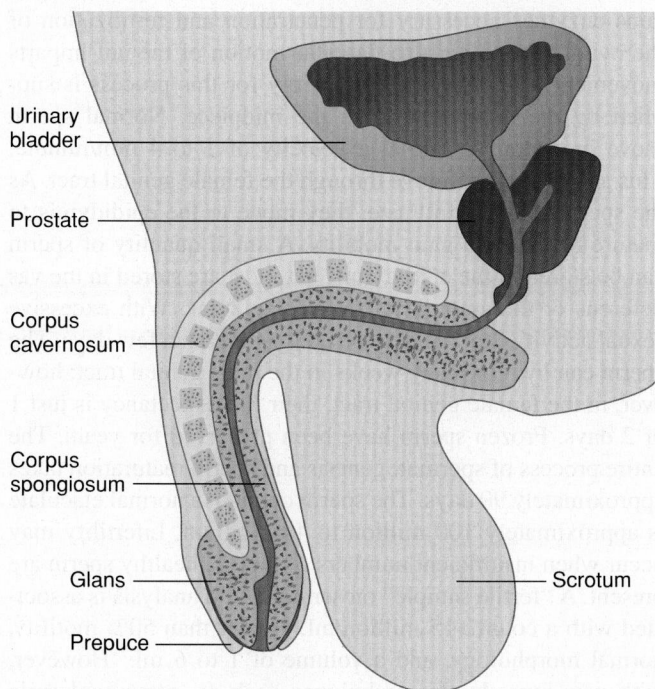

FIGURE 43.5 • Sagittal section of the penis, showing the prepuce, glans, corpus cavernosum, and corpus spongiosum.

Labels on figure: Urinary bladder, Prostate, Corpus cavernosum, Corpus spongiosum, Glans, Prepuce, Scrotum

IN SUMMARY

The male reproductive system consists of a pair of gonads (*i.e.,* testes), a system of excretory ducts (*i.e.,* seminiferous tubules and efferent ducts), the accessory organs (*i.e.,* epididymis, seminal vesicles, prostate, and Cowper glands), and the penis. The sex of a person is determined by the sex chromosomes at the time of fertilization. During the seventh week of gestation, the XY chromosome pattern and the *SRY* gene in the male embryo are responsible for the development of the testes; with the subsequent production of AMH and testosterone, development of the internal and external male genital structures occurs. Before this period of embryonic development, the tissues from which the male and female reproductive structures develop are undifferentiated. In the absence of testosterone production (and its derivative DHT), the male embryo with an XY chromosomal pattern develops female external genitalia.

SPERMATOGENESIS AND HORMONAL CONTROL OF MALE REPRODUCTIVE FUNCTION

After completing this section of the chapter, you should be able to meet the following objectives:

- Describe the process of spermatogenesis.
- State the functions of testosterone.
- Draw a diagram illustrating the secretion, site of action, and feedback control of gonadotropin-releasing hormone, luteinizing hormone, follicle-stimulating hormone, and inhibin.
- Describe the function of follicle-stimulating hormone in terms of spermatogenesis.
- Describe the classification and clinical features of male hypogonadism.

During childhood, the gonads remain essentially quiescent. At puberty, the male gonads and testes begin to mature and to carry out spermatogenesis and hormone production. At approximately 10 or 11 years of age, the adenohypophysis, or anterior pituitary, under the control of the hypothalamus, begins to secrete the gonadotropins that stimulate testicular function and cause the interstitial Leydig cells to begin producing testosterone. At approximately the same time, hormonal stimulation induces mitotic activity of the germ cells that develop into sperm. After cell maturation has begun, the testes begin to enlarge rapidly as the individual tubules grow. Full maturity and spermatogenesis usually are attained by 15 or 16 years of age.

Spermatogenesis

Spermatogenesis refers to the generation of spermatozoa or sperm. It begins at an average age of 13 years and continues throughout the reproductive years of a man's life. Spermatogenesis occurs in the seminiferous tubules of the testes (Fig. 43.3). These tubules, if placed end to end, would measure approximately 250 m. The outer layer of the seminiferous tubules is made up of connective tissue and smooth muscle; the inner lining is composed of Sertoli cells, which are embedded with sperm in various stages of development (Fig. 43.6A). Sertoli cells secrete a special fluid that contains nutrients to bathe and nourish the immature germ cells. They provide digestive enzymes that play a role in spermiation (*i.e.,*

converting the spermatocytes to sperm), and they are thought to play a role in shaping the head and tail of the sperm. Sertoli cells also secrete several hormones, including AMH, which is secreted by the testes during fetal life to inhibit development of fallopian tubes; estradiol, the principal feminizing sex hormone, which seems to be required in the male for spermatogenesis; inhibin, which controls the function of Sertoli cells through feedback inhibition of follicle-stimulating hormone (FSH) from the anterior pituitary gland; and androgen-binding protein, which binds to testosterone and DHT keeping a high intratesticular testosterone concentration required for spermiogenesis.[4–6]

In the first stage of spermatogenesis, small and unspecialized diploid germinal cells located immediately adjacent to the tubular wall, called the *spermatogonia,* undergo rapid mitotic division and provide a continuous source of new germinal cells. As these cells multiply, the more mature spermatogonia divide into two daughter cells, which grow and become the primary spermatocytes—the precursors of sperm. Over several weeks, large primary spermatocytes divide by a process called *meiosis* to form two smaller secondary spermatocytes. Each of the secondary spermatocytes divides to form two spermatids, each containing 23 chromosomes. Meiosis is a unique form of cell division that occurs only in the gonads. It consists of two consecutive nuclear divisions with formation of four daughter cells, each containing a single set of 23 chromosomes rather than a pair of 46 chromosomes, as occurs during mitotic cell division in other body cells (see Chapter 6).

The spermatid elongates into a *spermatozoon,* or mature sperm cell, with a head and tail (Fig. 43.6B). The outside of the anterior two thirds of the head, called the *acrosome,* contains enzymes necessary for penetration and fertilization of the ovum. The to-and-fro flagellar motion of the tail imparts movement to the sperm. The energy for this process is supplied by the mitochondria in the midpiece. Normal sperm move in a straight line at a velocity of 1 to 4 mm/minute. This allows them to move through the female genital tract. As the sperm grow to full size, they move to the epididymis to mature further and gain mobility. A small quantity of sperm can be stored in the epididymis, but most are stored in the vas deferens or the ampulla of the vas deferens. With excessive sexual activity, storage may be no longer than a few days. The sperm can live for many weeks in the male genital tract; however, in the female genital tract, their life expectancy is just 1 or 2 days. Frozen sperm have been preserved for years. The entire process of spermatogenesis and sperm maturation takes approximately 90 days. The sperm count in a normal ejaculate is approximately 100 million to 400 million. Infertility may occur when insufficient numbers of motile, healthy sperm are present. A "fertile sample" on seminal fluid analysis is associated with a count >15 million/ml, greater than 50% motility, normal morphology, and a volume of 1 to 6 ml.[7] However, with new reproductive techniques such as intracytoplasmic sperm injection (ICSI), as few as 20 sperm in the semen may be effective (see Chapter 46).

FIGURE 43.6 • The various stages of spermatogenesis. **A:** Cross-section of seminiferous tubule. **B:** Stages of development of spermatozoa.

Hormonal Control of Male Reproductive Function

Testosterone and Other Male Sex Hormones

The male sex hormones are called *androgens*. The testes secrete several male sex hormones, including *testosterone* (the main testicular hormone), *dihydrotestosterone,* and *androstenedione.* The testes also secrete small quantities of estradiol and estrone. Smaller quantities (<5% of the total male androgens) of androgens are also produced in the adrenal cortex.[4–6]

Testosterone is produced and secreted by the interstitial Leydig cells in the testes. Under the influence of luteinizing hormone (LH), Leydig cells produce approximately 6 mg/day of testosterone (peak at 4 to 8 AM).[5] It is metabolized in the liver and excreted by the kidneys. In the bloodstream, testosterone exists in a free (unbound) or a bound form. The bound form is attached to plasma proteins, including albumin and the sex hormone-binding globulin (SHBG) produced by the liver. Only approximately 2% of circulating testosterone is unbound and therefore able to enter the cell and exert its metabolic effects. Much of the testosterone that becomes fixed to the tissues is converted to DHT by the 5α-reductase enzyme, especially in certain target tissues such as the prostate gland. Some of the actions of testosterone depend on this conversion, whereas others do not. Testosterone also can be aromatized or converted to estradiol in the peripheral tissues.

Testosterone (and DHT) exerts a variety of biologic effects in the male (Chart 43.1). In the male embryo, testosterone is essential for the appropriate differentiation of the internal and external genitalia, and it is necessary for descent of the testes in the fetus. Testosterone is essential to the development of primary and secondary male sex characteristics during puberty and for the maintenance of these characteristics during

adult life.[4,7] It causes growth of pubic, chest, and facial hair; it produces changes in the larynx that result in the male bass voice; and it increases the thickness of the skin and increases the activity of the sebaceous glands, predisposing to acne.

All or almost all of the actions of testosterone and other androgens result from increased protein synthesis in target tissues. Androgens function as anabolic agents in males and females to promote metabolism and musculoskeletal growth. Testosterone and the androgens have a great effect on the development of increasing musculature during puberty, with boys averaging approximately a 50% increase in muscle mass compared with girls.[4]

Action of the Hypothalamic and Anterior Pituitary Hormones

The hypothalamus and the anterior pituitary gland play an essential role in promoting spermatogenic activity in the testes and maintaining the endocrine function of the testes by means of the gonadotropic hormones. The synthesis and release of the gonadotropic hormones from the pituitary gland are regulated by gonadotropin-releasing hormone (GnRH), which is synthesized by the hypothalamus and secreted into the hypothalamic–hypophysial portal circulation (Fig. 43.7).

Two gonadotropic hormones are secreted by the pituitary gland: FSH and LH. The production of testosterone by the interstitial Leydig cells is regulated by LH (Fig. 43.7). FSH

CHART 43.1	MAIN ACTIONS OF TESTOSTERONE

Induces differentiation of the male genital tract during fetal development

Induces development of primary and secondary sex characteristics

    Gonadal function

    External genitalia and accessory organs

    Male voice timbre

    Male skin characteristics

    Male hair distribution

Anabolic effects

    Promotes protein metabolism

    Promotes musculoskeletal growth

    Influences subcutaneous fat distribution

Promotes spermatogenesis (in FSH-primed tubules) and maturation of sperm

Stimulates erythropoiesis

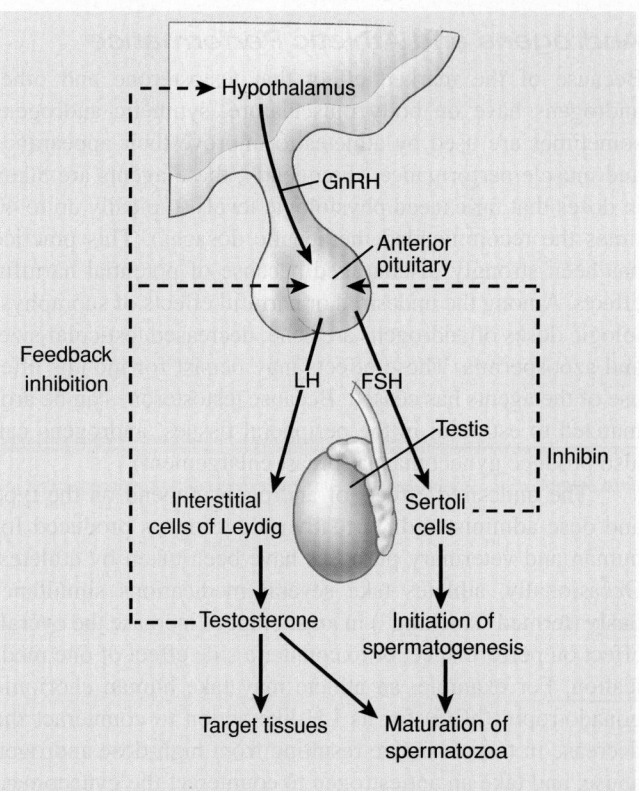

FIGURE 43.7 • Hypothalamic–pituitary feedback control of spermatogenesis and testosterone levels in the male. The *dashed line* represents negative feedback. FSH, follicle-stimulating hormone; GnRH, gonadotropin-releasing hormone; LH, luteinizing hormone.

binds selectively to Sertoli cells surrounding the seminiferous tubules, where it functions in the initiation of spermatogenesis. Under the influence of FSH, Sertoli cells produce androgen-binding protein, plasminogen activator, and inhibin. Androgen-binding protein binds testosterone and serves as a carrier of testosterone in Sertoli cells and as a storage site for testosterone. Although FSH is necessary for the initiation of spermatogenesis, full maturation of the spermatozoa requires testosterone (the intratesticular concentration of testosterone is 100 times greater than serum levels). Androgen-binding protein also serves as a carrier of testosterone from the testes to the epididymis. Plasminogen activator, which converts plasminogen to plasmin, functions in the final detachment of mature spermatozoa from Sertoli cells.

Circulating levels of the gonadotropic hormones are regulated in a negative feedback manner by testosterone. High levels of testosterone suppress LH secretion through a direct action on the pituitary and an inhibitory effect on the hypothalamus. FSH is thought to be inhibited by a substance called *inhibin,* produced by Sertoli cells. Inhibin suppresses FSH release from the pituitary gland. The pituitary gonadotropic hormones and Sertoli cells in the testes form a classic negative feedback loop in which FSH stimulates inhibin and inhibin suppresses FSH.[5,6] Unlike the cyclic hormonal pattern in females, in males, FSH, LH, and testosterone secretion and spermatogenesis occur at relatively unchanging rates during adulthood.

Androgens and Athletic Performance

Because of the marked effect that testosterone and other androgens have on body musculature, synthetic androgens sometimes are used by athletes to improve their appearance and muscle performance.[8] Frequently, these agents are taken in doses that far exceed physiologic levels (typically up to 40 times the recommended therapeutic dosages). This practice has been strongly discouraged because of potential harmful effects. Among the undesired or harmful effects of supraphysiologic doses of androgens are acne, decreased testicular size, and azoospermia. These effects may persist for months after use of the agents has ceased. Because testosterone can be aromatized to estradiol in the peripheral tissues, androgens can also produce gynecomastia (breast enlargement).

The undesired effects of androgens depend on the type and dose administered. Virtually all androgens produced for human and veterinary purposes have been taken by athletes. Occasionally, athletes take several medications simultaneously (termed "stacking") in an attempt to increase the overall effect on performance, or to counter a side effect of one medication. For example, an athlete may take human chorionic gonadotropin (hCG) for its LH-like action to counteract the decrease in testicular size resulting from high-dose androgen abuse, and take an antiestrogen to counteract the gynecomastia from administration of high doses of hCG and androgens.

Attention has also focused on androgen precursors, including oral androstenedione and dehydroepiandrosterone (DHEA) products that are available over the counter and often are marketed as safe natural alternatives to androgens for building muscle.[5] Androstenedione and DHEA exert only weak androgenic activity, but their main purpose is to act as a key precursor for testosterone after peripheral conversion. Whether large doses of these over-the-counter products can produce some of the serious side effects seen with standard anabolic steroids is largely unknown.

Other performance-enhancing agents can be used either alone or in combination with androgens or other agents in an attempt to improve performance. These include stimulants, erythropoietin (EPO), growth hormone, insulin-like growth factor-1 (IGF-1), insulin, and creatine.[8,9]

Hypogonadism

Hypogonadism can be primary (testicular failure due to problem in the testes) or secondary (failure resulting from lack of stimulation by gonadotropins [LH and FSH] from the pituitary). Tertiary hypogonadism also occurs and is caused by lack of stimulation of LH and FSH secretion from the pituitary, due to decreased or absent GnRH secretion from the hypothalamus. In men, primary hypogonadism is characterized by low androgens and sperm count and is due to lack of negative feedback at the hypothalamic–pituitary level, coupled with high levels of gonadotropins (*i.e.,* low testosterone and high LH and FSH). Secondary (and tertiary) hypogonadism, which also is characterized by low androgens and sperm count, is due to lack of secretion of gonadotropins from the hypothalamic–pituitary level, coupled with low levels of gonadotropins (*i.e.,* low testosterone and low LH and FSH). The clinical features of male hypogonadism depend on whether the impairment involves only spermatogenesis (FSH increase reflects Sertoli cell damage) or if testosterone secretion is also impaired (LH increase reflects Leydig cell damage). There are only two clinical manifestations of impaired spermatogenesis: subfertility/infertility and decreased testicular size (80% of testicular size is related to sperm production and 20% to testosterone production). In contrast, there are several possible clinical manifestations of impaired testosterone secretion, which are determined by its time of onset. Onset occurring in the adult is associated with fatigue, depression, decreased sexual desire/activity, erectile dysfunction, loss of secondary sex characteristics, changes in body composition (including loss of muscle mass and increase in fat mass), osteoporosis, and subfertility/infertility.[10]

Diagnosis of hypogonadism includes measurement of total testosterone levels (ideally at 8:00 AM, when the testosterone level is at its peak) in the ambulatory man. If the initial total testosterone level is low, the diagnosis of hypogonadism should be confirmed with either a repeat measure of total testosterone or a measure of free (bioavailable) testosterone. Once the diagnosis of hypogonadism is established, the LH and FSH levels should also be measured. A subsequently high LH and FSH indicates a primary hypogonadism (hypergonadotropic hypogonadism), and low or inappropriately normal LH and FSH indicates a secondary or tertiary hypogonadism (hypogonadotropic hypogonadism).[8] Seminal fluid analysis should be considered in both types of hypogonadism if fertility is a concern. In men with hypogonadotropic hypogonadism, other pituitary hormones should be assessed and a pituitary magnetic resonance imaging (MRI) scan done. In cases of hypergonadotropic hypogonadism, a karyotype (chromosome) analysis may be indicated because Klinefelter syndrome is the most common chromosomal abnormality associated with male hypogonadism (see Chapter 7). The usual karyotype is 47,XXY, although mosaicism or variants can present with a similar phenotype (the normal male is 46,XY and the normal female is 46,XX). Males with Klinefelter syndrome characteristically have small, firm testes (unlike many other cases of hypogonadism, in which the testicular consistency is soft). Other common causes of primary hypogonadism are listed in Chart 43.2.

Testosterone for treatment of androgen deficiency should be administered only to men with confirmed hypogonadism (as evidenced by a distinctly subnormal serum testosterone concentration). The principal goal of testosterone therapy is to restore the serum testosterone concentration to the normal range while balancing the risks and benefits, especially with men diagnosed with or at risk for BPH or prostate cancer.[10]

IN SUMMARY

The function of the male reproductive system is under the negative feedback control of the hypothalamus and the anterior pituitary gonadotropic hormones FSH and LH. Spermatogenesis is initiated by FSH and the production of testosterone is regulated by LH. Testosterone, the major male sex hormone, is produced by the interstitial Leydig

cells in the testes. In addition to its role in the differentiation of the internal and external genitalia in the male embryo, testosterone is essential for the development of secondary male characteristics during puberty, the maintenance of these characteristics during adult life, and spermatozoa maturation.

Because of the marked effect that testosterone and other androgens have on body musculature, synthetic androgens sometimes are used by athletes to improve their appearance and muscle performance. Among the undesired or harmful effects of supraphysiologic doses of androgens are acne, decreased testicular size, azoospermia, and a change in libido (increase/decrease).

Hypogonadism refers to a decrease in testicular function. It can present as a primary hypogonadism originating in the testes; a secondary hypogonadism arising from lack of stimulation from the pituitary gonadotropins (LH and FSH); or as a tertiary hypogonadism due to decreased or absent GnRH secretion from the hypothalamus.

NEURAL CONTROL OF SEXUAL FUNCTION AND AGING CHANGES

After completing this section of the chapter, you should be able to meet the following objectives:

- Describe the autonomic and nonautonomic nervous systems' control of erection, emission, and ejaculation.
- Describe changes in the male reproductive system that occur with aging.
- In the man, the stages of the sexual act involve erection, emission, ejaculation, and detumescence. The physiology of the sexual act involves a complex interaction between spinal cord reflexes, higher neural centres, the vascular system, and the endocrine system.

Neural Control

The most important source of impulse stimulation for initiating the male sexual act is the glans penis, which contains a highly organized sensory system. Afferent impulses from sensory receptors in the glans penis pass through the pudendal nerve to ascending fibres in the spinal cord by way of the sacral plexus. Stimulation of other perineal areas, such as the anal epithelium, the scrotum, and the testes, can transmit signals to higher brain centres, such as the limbic system and cerebral cortex, through the cord, adding to sexual arousal.

The psychic element to sexual stimulation, such as thinking sexual thoughts, can cause erection and ejaculation. Although psychic involvement and higher-centre functions contribute to the sex act, they are not necessary for sexual performance. Genital stimulation can produce erection and

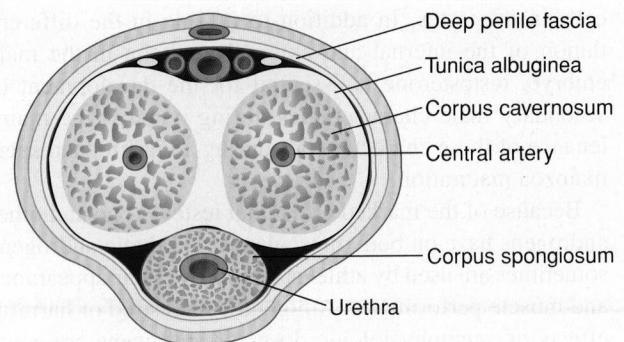

Deep penile fascia
Tunica albuginea
Corpus cavernosum
Central artery
Corpus spongiosum
Urethra

FIGURE 43.8 • Erectile tissue of the penis.

ejaculation in some men with complete transection of the spinal cord (see Chapter 50).

Erection involves the shunting of blood into the corpus cavernosum. It is controlled by the sympathetic, parasympathetic, and nonadrenergic–noncholinergic (NANC) systems. Nitric oxide is the locally released NANC mediator that produces relaxation of vascular smooth muscle. In the flaccid or detumescent state, sympathetic discharge through α-adrenergic receptors maintains contraction of the arteries that supply the penis and vascular sinuses of the corpora cavernosa and corpus spongiosum (Fig. 43.8). Parasympathetic stimulation produces erection by inhibiting sympathetic neurons that cause detumescence and by stimulating the release of nitric oxide to effect a rapid relaxation of the smooth muscle in the sinusoidal spaces of the corpus cavernosum. During sexual stimulation, parasympathetic impulses also cause the urethral and bulbourethral glands to secrete mucus to aid in lubrication. Parasympathetic innervation is effected through the pelvic nerve and sacral segments of the spinal cord. Sympathetic innervation exits the spinal cord at the L1 and L2 levels. Erectile dysfunction can be caused by disease or dysfunction of the brain, spinal cord, cavernous or pudendal nerves, or terminal nerve endings or receptors[11] (see Chapter 44).

Emission and ejaculation, which constitute the culmination of the male sexual act, are a function of the sympathetic nervous system. As with erection, emission and ejaculation are mediated through spinal cord reflexes. With increasing intensity of the sexual stimulus, reflex centres of the spinal cord begin to emit sympathetic impulses that leave the cord at the L1 and L2 levels and pass through the hypogastric plexus to the genital organs to initiate emission, which is the forerunner of ejaculation. Emission causes the sperm to move from the epididymis to the urethra. Efferent impulses from the spinal cord produce contraction of smooth muscle in the vas deferens and ampulla that move sperm forward and close the internal urethral sphincter to prevent retrograde ejaculation into the bladder.

Ejaculation represents the expulsion of the sperm from the urethra. It involves contraction of the seminal vesicles and prostate gland, which add fluid to the ejaculate and propel it forward. Ejaculation is accompanied by contraction of the ischiocavernous and bulbocavernous muscles at the base

of the penis. The filling of the internal urethra elicits signals that are transmitted through the pudendal nerves from the spinal cord, giving the sudden feeling of fullness of the genital organs. Rhythmic increases in pressure in the urethra cause the semen to be propelled to the exterior, resulting in ejaculation. At the same time, rhythmic contractions of the pelvic and trunk muscles produce thrusting movements of the pelvis and penis, which help propel the ejaculate into the vagina.

The period of emission and ejaculation is called *male orgasm*. After ejaculation, erection ceases within 1 to 2 minutes. A man usually ejaculates approximately 2 to 5 ml of semen. The ejaculate may vary with frequency of intercourse. It is less with frequent ejaculation and may increase to 2 to 4 times its normal amount during periods of abstinence. The semen that is ejaculated is 98% fluid and approximately 2% sperm.

Aging Changes

Like other body systems, the male reproductive system undergoes degenerative changes as a result of the aging process; it becomes less efficient with age. The declining physiologic efficiency of male reproductive function occurs gradually and involves the endocrine, circulatory, and neuromuscular systems. Compared with the marked physiologic changes in aging females, the changes in the aging male are more gradual and less drastic. Gonadal and reproductive failure usually are not related directly to age because a man remains fertile into advanced age; 80- and 90-year-old men have been known to father children.

As the male ages, his reproductive system becomes measurably different in structure and function from that of the younger male. Male sex hormone levels, particularly of testosterone, decrease with age, but the rate varies in different individuals and is affected by multiple variables.[12] Beginning at about 25 to 30 years of age in healthy, nonobese men, testosterone levels gradually decrease at approximately 10% per decade. The term *andropause* has been used to describe an ill-defined collection of symptoms in aging men, typically those older than 50 years, who have a relative or absolute hypogonadism associated with aging.[8,11,12] The existence and significance of andropause has important public health implications given the current number of men older than 65 years of age, a number that is expected to double over the next 30 years.

The sex hormones play a part in the structure and function of the reproductive system and other body systems from conception to old age; they affect protein synthesis, salt and water balance, bone growth, and cardiovascular function. Low testosterone levels have an atherogenic effect that may explain the higher incidence of heart disease in androgen-deficient men.[8,11,12] Decreasing levels of testosterone affect sexual energy, muscle strength, and the genital tissues. The testes become smaller and lose their firmness. The seminiferous tubules, which produce spermatozoa, thicken and begin a degenerative process that finally inhibits sperm production, resulting in a decrease in viable spermatozoa. The prostate gland enlarges and its contractions become weaker.

The force of ejaculation decreases because of a reduction in the volume and viscosity of the seminal fluid. The seminal vesicle changes little from childhood to puberty. The pubertal increases in the fluid capacity of the gland remain throughout adulthood and decline after 60 years of age. After 60 years of age, the walls of the seminal vesicles thin, the epithelium shrinks, and the muscle layer is replaced by connective tissue. Age-related changes in the penis consist of fibrotic changes in the trabecula in the corpus spongiosum, with progressive sclerotic changes in arteries and veins. Sclerotic changes also follow in the corpora cavernosa, with the condition becoming generalized in 55- to 60-year-old men.

Erectile dysfunction (see Chapter 44) in the older adult often is directly related to the general physical condition of the person.[13] *Erectile dysfunction* (ED) has largely replaced the term *impotence.* It is defined as the persistent inability to achieve and maintain an erection sufficient to permit satisfactory sexual intercourse. Aging is a major etiologic factor in this condition. However, even among younger men (those in their 40s), 2% to 9% report at least occasional difficulty obtaining or maintaining an erection. The rate increases to 20% to 40% in men aged 60 to 69 years, and the figure approaches 50% to 100% in 70-year-olds.

Diseases that accompany aging can have a direct bearing on male reproductive function. Various cardiovascular, respiratory, hormonal, neurologic, and hematologic disorders can be responsible for secondary impotence. For example, vascular disease affects male potency because it may impair blood flow to the pudendal arteries or their tributaries, resulting in loss of blood volume with subsequent poor distension of the vascular spaces of erectile tissue. Diseases affecting potency include hypertension, diabetes, cardiac disease, and malignancies of the reproductive organs. Common lifestyle factors such as obesity, limited or absence of exercise, smoking, and lower urinary tract symptoms have also been linked with the development of erectile dysfunction.[13] In addition, certain medications can have an effect on sexual function.

One of the greatest inhibitors of sexual functioning in older men is the loss of self-esteem and the development of a negative self-image. The emphasis on youth pervades much of our society. The image of success for a man often involves qualities of masculinity and sexual attractiveness. When queried about success, men often mention such things as work, managing money well, participating in sports or other activities, discussing politics or world events, advising younger persons, and being attractive to women. When a man feels good about himself and expresses self-confidence, sexual attractiveness is communicated, regardless of age. Many older men live in environments that are not conducive to the importance of helping them maintain a positive self-image. Premature cessation of the aforementioned esteem-building activities can contribute to loss of libido and zest for life in the older man.

Testosterone and other synthetic androgens may be used in older men with confirmed low androgen levels to improve muscle strength and vigour. Preliminary studies of androgen replacement in aging men with low androgen levels show an increase in lean body mass and a decrease in bone turnover. Before testosterone replacement therapy is initiated, all men should be screened for prostate cancer.[11] Testosterone is available in several different formulations, including an injectable form (administered every 1 to 3 weeks), transdermal patch, topical gel, or an oral capsule. Side effects of replacement therapy may include acne, gynecomastia, and reduced high-density lipoprotein cholesterol levels. It also may contribute to a worsening of sleep apnea in men who are troubled by this problem.[8,11]

At present, it is not recommended that routine treatment of elderly men with testosterone should be undertaken. A trial of testosterone administration, however, might be warranted in an elderly man whose serum testosterone concentration is less than 10.5 nmol/L (although some believe it should be even lower, *i.e.,* <7.0 nmol/L) and who has manifestations of testosterone deficiency.[8] If treatment is undertaken, the man should be screened before treatment and monitored during therapy for evidence of testosterone-dependent diseases.

IN SUMMARY

The sex act involves erection, emission, ejaculation, and detumescence. The physiology of these functions involves a complex interaction between autonomic-mediated spinal cord reflexes, higher neural centres, and the vascular system. Erection is mediated by the parasympathetic nervous system and emission and ejaculation by the sympathetic nervous system. Like other body systems, the male reproductive system undergoes changes as a result of the aging process. The changes occur gradually and involve parallel changes in endocrine, circulatory, and neuromuscular function. Testosterone levels decrease (andropause), the size and firmness of the testes decrease, sperm production declines, and the prostate gland enlarges. There usually is a decrease in frequency of intercourse, intensity of sensation, speed of attaining erection, and force of ejaculation. However, sexual thought, interest, and activity usually continue into old age.

REVIEW EXERCISES

1. In the absence of the *SRY* gene on the Y chromosome, a developing embryo with an XY genotype will develop female genitalia.
   A. *Explain.*
2. Men who have had a vasectomy often remain fertile for 4 to 5 weeks after the procedure has been done.
   A. *Explain.*
3. A 55-year-old man presents with various vague symptoms (fatigue, depression). On examination, he is noted to have small testes (8 ml bilaterally), marked gynecomastia, and scanty body hair. He

is obese at 122 kg, with a body mass index (BMI) of 34.2. Investigations reveal low testosterone and elevated gonadotropin (LH and FSH) levels.

A. *What endocrine diagnosis is related to this phenotype and these biochemical manifestations?*

References

1. Rey R. A., Grinspon R. P. (2011). Normal male sexual differentiation and aetiology of disorders of sex development. *Best Practice & Research Clinical Endocrinology & Metabolism, 25*(2), 221–238.
2. Tanagho E. A., Nguyen H. T. (2013). Chapter 2: Embryology of the genitourinary system. In McAninch J. W., Lue T. F. (Eds.), *Smith & Tanagho's general urology* (18th ed.). New York: McGraw-Hill Professional.
3. Moore K. L., Persaud T. V. N., Torchia M. G. (2013). *The developing human: Clinical oriented embryology* (9th ed.). Philadelphia, PA: Saunders/Elsevier.
4. Hall J. E. (2011). *Textbook of medical physiology* (12th ed.). Philadelphia, PA: W. B. Saunders.
5. Melmed S., Polonsky K. S., Larsen P. R., et al. (Eds.). (2011). *Williams textbook of endocrinology* (12th ed.). Philadelphia, PA: Saunders/Elsevier.
6. Gardner D. G., Shobeck D. (Eds.). (2011). *Greenspan's basic and clinical endocrinology* (9th ed.). New York: McGraw-Hill.
7. Cooper T. G., Noonan E., von Eckardstein S., et al. (2010). World Health Organization reference values for human semen characteristics. *Human Reproductions Update, 16*(3), 231–245.
8. Basaria S. (2010). Androgen abuse in athletes: Detection and consequences. *Journal of Clinical Endocrinology Metabolism, 95*(4), 1533–1543.
9. Viswanathan V., Eugster E. A. (2009). Etiology and treatment of hypogonadism in adolescents. *Endocrinology & Metabolism Clinics of North America, 38*(4), 719–738.
10. Bhasin S., Cunningham G. R., Hayes F. J., et al; Task Force, Endocrine Society. (2010). Testosterone therapy in men with androgen deficiency syndromes: An Endocrine Society clinical practice guideline. *J Clin Endocrinol Metabol, 95*(6), 2536–2559.
11. Basaria S., Travison T. G., Bhasin S. (2013). Risks and benefits of testosterone therapy in older men. *Nature Reviews Endocrinology, 9*(7), 414–424.
12. Harvey J. H., Berry J. A. (2009). Andropause in the aging male. *Journal for Nurse Practitioners, 5*(3), 207–212.
13. Shamloul R., Ghanem H. (2013). Erectile dysfunction. *Lancet, 381*(9861), 153–165.

Visit the**Point** **http://thePoint.lww.com for animations, journal articles, and more!**

Disorders of the Male Genitourinary System

44

The male genitourinary system is subject to structural defects, inflammation, and neoplasms, all of which can affect urine elimination, sexual function, and fertility. This chapter discusses disorders of the penis, the scrotum and testes, and the prostate.

 DISORDERS OF THE PENIS

After completing this section of the chapter, you should be able to meet the following objectives:

* State the difference between hypospadias and epispadias.
* Cite the significance of phimosis.
* Describe the anatomic changes that occur with Peyronie disease.
* Explain the physiology of penile erection and relate it to erectile dysfunction and priapism.
* Describe the appearance of balanitis xerotica obliterans.
* List the signs of penile cancer.

The penis is the external male genital organ through which the urethra passes to the exterior of the body. It is involved in urinary and sexual function. Disorders of the penis include congenital and acquired defects, inflammatory conditions, and neoplasms.

Congenital and Acquired Disorders

Hypospadias and Epispadias

Hypospadias and epispadias are congenital disorders of the penis resulting from embryologic defects in the development of the urethral groove and penile urethra (Fig. 44.1). In hypospadias, which affects approximately 1 in 250 male infants, the termination of the urethra is on the ventral surface of the penis.[1–3] It is common to categorize hypospadias as glandular (involving the glans penis), midpenile, or posterior (penoscrotal, scrotal, or perineal). The etiology in most cases is unknown. Single-gene defects, chromosomal abnormalities, and maternal progestational drug ingestion in early pregnancy account for only about one fourth of cases. The

Hypospadias

Epispadias

FIGURE 44.1 • Hypospadias and epispadias.

testes are undescended in 10% of boys born with hypospadias and chordee (*i.e.,* ventral bowing of the penis), and inguinal hernia also may accompany the disorder. In the newborn with severe hypospadias and cryptorchidism (undescended testes), the differential diagnosis should consider ambiguous genitalia and masculinization that is seen in females with congenital adrenal hyperplasia (see Chapter 41).

Surgery is the treatment of choice for hypospadias.[1,3,4] Circumcision is avoided because the foreskin is used for surgical repair. Factors that influence the timing of surgical repair include anesthetic risk, penile size, and the psychological effects of the surgery on the child. In mild cases, the surgery is done for cosmetic reasons only. In more severe cases, repair becomes essential for normal sexual functioning and to prevent the psychological sequelae of having malformed genitalia. In contrast to the practices of several decades ago, when surgical repair often was delayed until the child was 2 to 6 years of age, surgical repair is now done between the ages of 6 and 12 months. Judicious use of testosterone supplementation may also be warranted.[4]

Epispadias, in which the opening of the urethra is on the dorsal surface of the penis, is a less common defect. Although epispadias may occur as a separate entity, it often is associated with exstrophy of the bladder, a condition in which the abdominal wall fails to cover the bladder. The treatment depends on the extent of the developmental defect.

Phimosis and Paraphimosis

Phimosis refers to a tightening of the prepuce or penile foreskin that prevents its retraction over the glans. Embryologically, the foreskin begins to develop during the eighth week of gestation as a fold of skin at the distal edge of the penis that eventually grows forward over the base of the glans.[1] By the 16th week of gestation, the prepuce and the glans are adherent. Only a small percentage of newborns have a fully retractable foreskin. With growth, a space develops between

the glans and foreskin, and by 3 years of age, approximately 90% of boys have retractable foreskins.

Because the foreskins of many boys cannot be fully retracted in early childhood, it is important that the area be cleaned thoroughly. There is no need to retract the foreskin forcibly because this could lead to infection, scarring, or paraphimosis. As the child grows, the foreskin becomes retractable, and the glans and foreskin should be cleaned routinely. If symptomatic phimosis occurs after childhood, it can cause difficulty with voiding or sexual activity. Circumcision is then the treatment of choice. Phimosis is also one of the most important predisposing factors for penile cancer.

In a related condition called *paraphimosis,* the foreskin is so tight and constricted that it cannot cover the glans. A tight foreskin can constrict the blood supply to the glans and lead to ischemia and necrosis. Many cases of paraphimosis result from the foreskin being retracted for an extended period, as in the case of catheterized uncircumcised males.

Balanitis and Balanoposthitis

Balanitis is an acute or chronic inflammation of the glans penis. *Balanoposthitis* refers to inflammation of the glans and prepuce. It usually is encountered in men with phimosis or a large, redundant prepuce that interferes with cleanliness and predisposes to bacterial growth in the accumulated secretions and smegma (*i.e.,* debris from the desquamated epithelia). If left untreated, the condition may cause ulcerations of the mucosal surface of the glans; these ulcerations may lead to inflammatory scarring of the prepuce and further aggravate the condition.

Acute superficial balanoposthitis is characterized by erythema of the glans and prepuce. An exudate in the form of malodorous discharge may be present. Extension of the erythema and edema may result in phimosis. The condition may result from infection, trauma, or irritation. Infective balanoposthitis may be caused by a wide variety of organisms. *Chlamydia* and mycoplasmas have been identified as causative organisms in this disease. Gonococcal balanitis may develop as a complication of infection in uncircumcised men. The inflammatory reaction is nonspecific, and correct identification of the specific organism requires microbial smears and cultures.

Balanitis due to candidal infection may be a presenting feature or result from poorly controlled diabetes mellitus. Balanitis also can result from noninfectious causes, such as circinate balanitis, which is seen in reactive arthritis (see Chapter 59). Lesions are superficial, painless ulcers that heal without scarring.

Balanitis xerotica obliterans is a chronic, sclerosing, atrophic process of the glans penis that occurs in uncircumcised men. It is clinically and histologically similar to the lichen sclerosus that is seen in women (see Chapter 46). Typically, the lesions consist of whitish plaques on the surface of the glans penis and the prepuce. The foreskin is thickened and fibrous and is not retractable. Although balanitis xerotica obliterans was once considered a benign condition, it has been associated with several reports of penile cancer and is now recognized as a precancerous state. Treatment measures

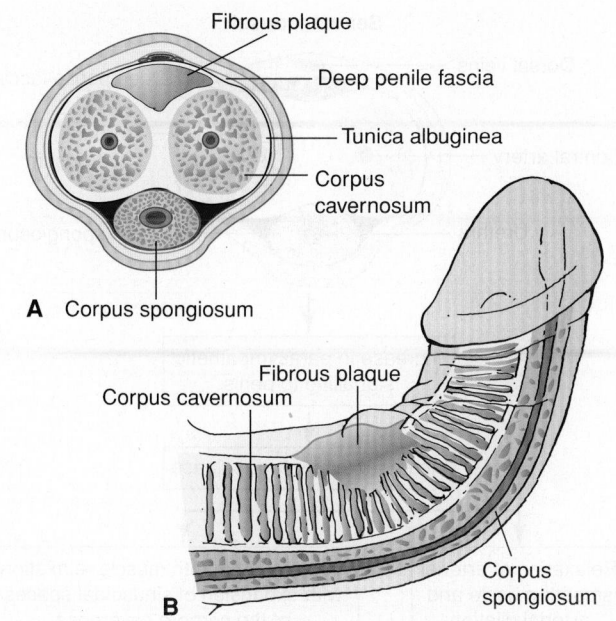

FIGURE 44.2 • Peyronie disease. **A:** Penile cross-section showing plaque between the corpora. **B:** Penile curvature.

include circumcision and topical or intralesional injections of corticosteroids.[5,6]

Peyronie Disease

Peyronie disease involves a localized and progressive fibrosis of unknown origin that affects the tunica albuginea (*i.e.,* the tough, fibrous sheath that surrounds the corpora cavernosa) of the penis.[7,8] The disorder is characterized initially by an inflammatory process that results in dense fibrous plaque formation. The plaque usually is on the dorsal midline of the shaft, causing upward bowing of the shaft during erection (Fig. 44.2). Some men may develop scarring on both the dorsal and ventral aspects of the shaft, causing the penis to be straight but shortened or have a lateral bend.[7,8] The fibrous tissue prevents lengthening of the involved area during erection, making intercourse difficult and painful. The disease usually occurs in men older than 40 years of age.[8,9] Although the cause of the disorder is unknown, many experts agree that Peyronie disease is a result of repetitive trauma to the tissues surrounding the cavernosal bodies.[10] Up to 47% of men with Peyronie disease have another condition associated with fascial tissue fibrosis, such as Dupuytren contracture (fibrosis of the palmar fascia).[7]

The manifestations of Peyronie disease include painful erection, bent erection, and the presence of a hard mass at the site of fibrosis. Approximately two thirds of men complain of pain as a symptom. The pain is thought to be generated by inflammation of the adjacent fascial tissue and usually disappears as the inflammation resolves. During the first year or so after formation of the plaque, while the scar tissue is undergoing the process of remodelling, penile distortion may increase, remain static, or resolve and disappear completely.[7] In some

cases, the scar tissue may progress to calcification and formation of bonelike tissue.

Diagnosis is based on history and physical examination. Doppler ultrasonography may be used to assess causation of the disorder. Although surgical intervention can be used to correct the disorder, it often is delayed because in many cases the disorder is self-limiting, resolving spontaneously within 6 to 18 months.[7] Indications for surgery include penile shortening, persistent pain, severe curvature, and penile narrowing or indentation. Less invasive treatments include the administration of oral agents with antioxidant properties (*e.g.,* colchicine), and intralesional treatments such as corticosteroids or the calcium channel blocker, verapamil. Other therapies include low-dose radiation therapy and various modes of energy transfer, including ultrasound and short-wave diathermy. At present, these methods have been inadequately studied and most have met with variable degrees of success.[7]

Disorders of Erectile Function

Erection is a neurovascular process involving the autonomic nervous system, neurotransmitters and endothelial relaxing factors, the vascular smooth muscle of the arteries and veins supplying the penile tissue, and the trabecular smooth muscle of the sinusoids of the corpora cavernosa (Fig. 44.3). The penis is innervated by both the autonomic and somatic nervous systems. In the pelvis, the sympathetic and parasympathetic components of the autonomic nervous systems merge to form what are called the *cavernous nerves*. Erection is under the control of the parasympathetic nervous system, and ejaculation and detumescence (penile relaxation) are under sympathetic

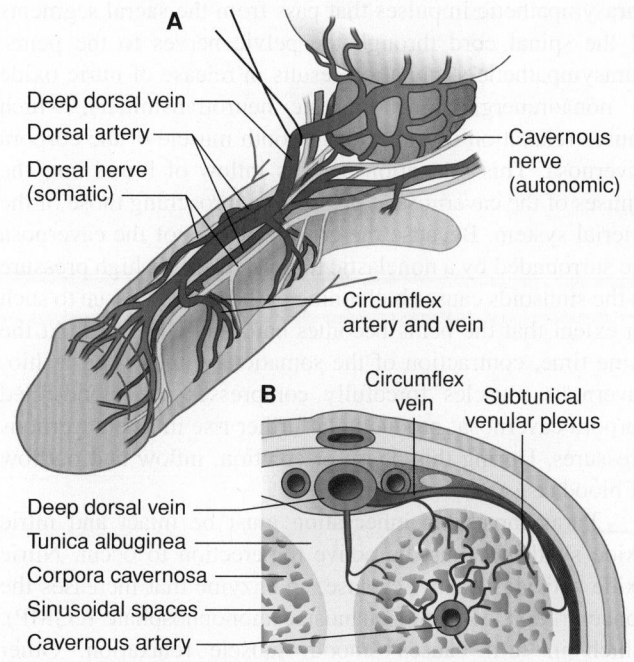

FIGURE 44.3 • Anatomy and mechanism of penile erection. **A:** Innervation and arterial and venous blood supply to the penis. **B:** Cross-section of the sinusoidal system of the corpora cavernosa.

nervous system control. Somatic innervation, which occurs through the pudendal nerve, is responsible for penile sensation and contraction and relaxation of the extracorporeal striated muscles (bulbocavernous and ischiocavernous).

DISORDERS OF PENILE ERECTION

- Erection is a neurovascular process involving the autonomic nervous system, the somatic nervous system by way of the pudendal nerve, the vascular system, and the sinusoidal spaces of the corpora cavernosa.
- Parasympathetic innervation through the pelvic nerves initiates relaxation of the trabecular smooth muscle of the corpora cavernosa through the action of nitric oxide, the inflow of arterial blood, and cessation of venous outflow.
- Erectile failure can result from disorders in one or a combination of the neural, vascular, or chemical mediator aspects of the erectile process.
- Priapism is an abnormal, painful, sustained erection that can lead to ischemic damage of penile structures. It can occur at any age and is one of the possible complications of sickle cell disease.

Penile erection is the first effect of male sexual stimulation, whether psychological or physical (Fig. 44.4). It involves increased inflow of blood into the corpora cavernosa due to relaxation of the trabecular smooth muscle that surrounds the sinusoidal spaces and compression of the veins controlling outflow of blood from the venous plexus. Erection is mediated by parasympathetic impulses that pass from the sacral segments of the spinal cord through the pelvic nerves to the penis. Parasympathetic stimulation results in release of nitric oxide (a nonadrenergic–noncholinergic neurotransmitter), which causes relaxation of trabecular smooth muscle of the corpora cavernosa. This relaxation permits inflow of blood into the sinuses of the cavernosa at pressures approaching those of the arterial system. Because the erectile tissues of the cavernosa are surrounded by a nonelastic fibrous covering, high pressure in the sinusoids causes ballooning of the erectile tissue to such an extent that the penis becomes hard and elongated. At the same time, contraction of the somatically innervated ischiocavernous muscles forcefully compresses the blood-filled corpora cavernosa, producing a further rise in intercavernous pressures. During this phase of erection, inflow and outflow of blood cease.

Parasympathetic innervation must be intact and nitric oxide synthesis must be active for erection to occur. Nitric oxide activates guanyl cyclase, an enzyme that increases the concentration of cyclic guanosine monophosphate (cGMP), which in turn causes smooth muscle relaxation. Other smooth muscle relaxants (*e.g.*, prostaglandin E$_1$ analogs and α-adrenergic antagonists) can independently cause sufficient cavernosal relaxation to result in erection, if present in high

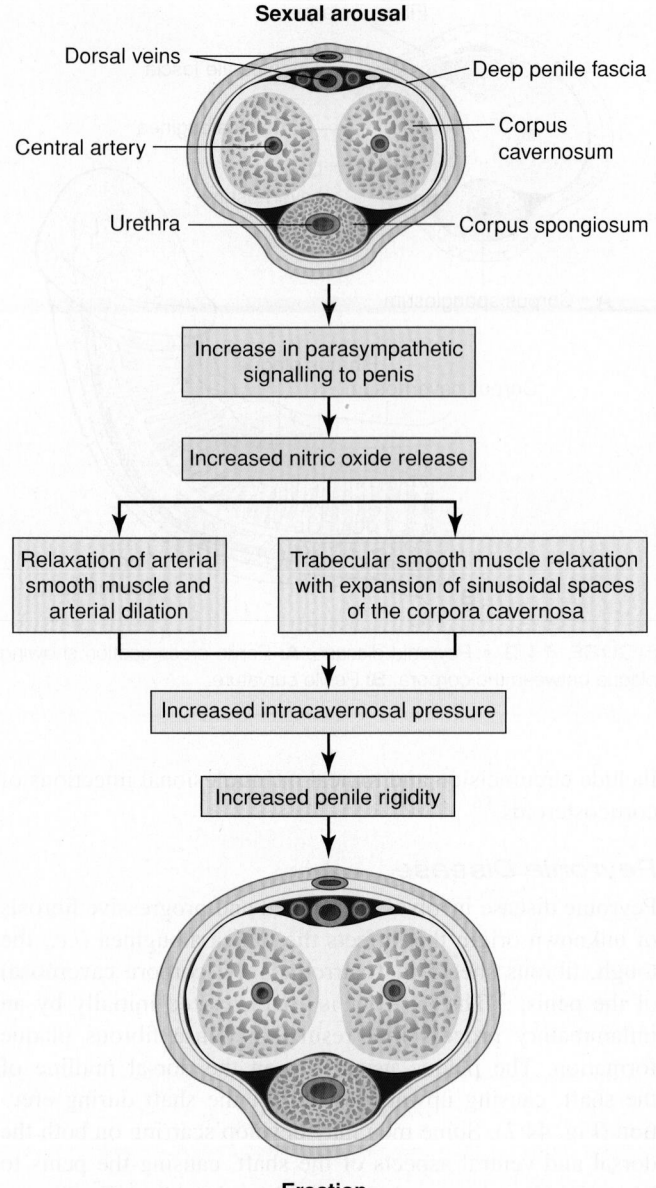

FIGURE 44.4 • Mechanisms of penile erection.

enough concentrations. Many of the drugs that have been developed to treat erectile dysfunction act at the level of these mediators.[11]

Detumescence or penile relaxation is largely a sympathetic nervous system response. It can result from a cessation of neurotransmitter release, the breakdown of second messengers such as cGMP, or sympathetic discharge during ejaculation. Contraction of the trabecular smooth muscle opens the venous channels so that the trapped blood can be expelled and penile flaccidity return.

Erectile Dysfunction

Erectile dysfunction is defined as "the inability to attain and/or maintain an erection sufficient for successful sexual intercourse.[12] It has been estimated that this widespread disorder affects about 150 million men worldwide; this number is expected to reach 322 million by 2025.[12] Erectile dysfunction is commonly classified as psychogenic, organic, or, most commonly, mixed psychogenic and organic.[12–15]

Psychogenic Causes. Psychogenic causes of erectile dysfunction include performance anxiety, a strained relationship with a sexual partner, depression, and overt psychotic disorders such as schizophrenia. Depression is a common cause of erectile dysfunction.[12] Psychogenic factors can be further exacerbated by the side effects of many of the therapies used to treat these disorders, which can themselves cause erectile dysfunction.

Organic Causes. Organic causes of erectile dysfunction span a wide range of pathologic processes. They include neurogenic, hormonal, vascular, drug-induced, and penile-related etiologies.

Neurogenic disorders such as Parkinson disease, stroke, and cerebral trauma often contribute to erectile dysfunction by decreasing libido or preventing the initiation of erection. In spinal cord injury, the extent of neural impairment depends on the level, location, and extent of the lesion. Somatosensory involvement of the genitalia is essential to the reflex mechanisms involved in erection; this becomes important with aging and conditions such as diabetes that impair peripheral nerve function. Extensive pelvis surgery, especially radical prostatectomy (even with the so-called "nerve-sparing" procedures), is a common cause of erectile dysfunction due to both direct and indirect nerve damage.

Hormonal causes of erectile dysfunction include a decrease in androgen levels because of both primary and secondary hypogonadism. Androgen levels may be decreased because of aging (andropause). Hyperprolactinemia from any cause interferes with both reproduction and erectile function. This is because prolactin acts centrally to inhibit the release of the hypothalamic gonadotropin-releasing hormone (GnRH) that controls the release of the pituitary gonadotropic hormones, luteinizing hormone (LH) and follicle-stimulating hormone (FSH). Elevated prolactin levels may also interfere with normal functioning at the level of the gonad.

Common risk factors for generalized penile arterial insufficiency include hypertension, hyperlipidemia, cigarette smoking, diabetes mellitus, and pelvic irradiation.[14] In hypertension, erectile function is impaired not so much by the increased blood pressure as by the associated stenotic arterial lesions. Focal stenosis of the common penile artery most often occurs in men who sustain blunt pelvic or perineal trauma (*e.g.,* from bicycling accidents). Failure of the veins to close completely during an erection (veno-occlusive dysfunction) may occur in men with large venous channels that drain the corpora cavernosa. Other disorders that impair venous occlusion are degenerative changes involving the tunica albuginea, as in Peyronie disease.

Many drugs are reported to cause erectile dysfunction, including antidepressants, antipsychotics, antiandrogens, and antihypertensives.[14] Cigarette smoking can induce vasoconstriction and penile venous leakage because of its effects on cavernous smooth muscle and can double the risk of erectile dysfunction.[13] Alcohol in small amounts may increase libido and improve erection; however, in large amounts it can cause central sedation, decreased libido, and transient erectile dysfunction.

Aging is known to increase the risk of erectile dysfunction[12] (see Chapter 43). Many of the pathologic processes that contribute to erectile dysfunction are more common in older men, including diabetes, hyperlipidemia, vascular disease, and the long-term effects of cigarette smoking. Age-related declines in testosterone may also play a role (andropause). Psychosocial problems such as depression, esteem issues, partner relationships, history of substance abuse, and anxiety and fear of performance failure also may contribute to erectile dysfunction in older men.[12,14]

Diagnosis and Treatment. A diagnosis of erectile dysfunction requires careful history (medical, sexual, and psychosocial), physical examination, and laboratory tests aimed at determining what other tests are needed to rule out organic causes of the disorder. Because many medications, including prescribed, over-the-counter, and illicit drugs, can cause erectile dysfunction, a careful drug history is indicated.

Erectile dysfunction is now recognized as a marker for cardiovascular disease, and is now considered a component of the metabolic syndrome (a collection of cardiovascular risk factors; see Chapter 42).[12] The association between erectile dysfunction and the metabolic syndrome may be related to the underlying endothelial dysfunction seen in both conditions.[12,14] A patient with erectile dysfunction should be thoroughly evaluated for coexisting vascular disease. Any cardiovascular risk factors should be modified or treated (*e.g.,* smoking, diabetes, hypertension, and hyperlipidemia).[12,14]

Any treatment regimens should always take into account the partner's attitude about the problem and the likely response to effective treatment. Erectile dysfunction is a disease of couples.[16] Treatment methods include psychosexual counselling, androgen replacement therapy (when androgen deficiency is confirmed), oral and intracavernous drug therapy, vacuum constriction devices, and surgical treatment (prosthesis and vascular surgery).[11] Among the commonly prescribed drugs are sildenafil, vardenafil, tadalafil, alprostadil, phentolamine and yohimbine. Sildenafil, tadalafil, and vardenafil are selective inhibitors of phosphodiesterase type 5 (PDE-5), the enzyme that inactivates cGMP. This inactivation of cGMP acts by facilitating corporeal smooth muscle relaxation in response to sexual stimulation (Fig. 44.4). The concomitant use of PDE-5 inhibitors and nitrates (which are used, *e.g.,* in ischemic heart disease) is absolutely contraindicated because of the risk of profound hypotension and decreased coronary perfusion.[17] The PDE-5 inhibitors are taken orally. Alprostadil, a prostaglandin E_1 analog, acts by producing relaxation of cavernous smooth muscle. It is either injected directly into the cavernosa (with diffusion into the opposite cavernosa) or placed in the urethra as a minisuppository. Phentolamine (via intracavernous injections) and yohimbine (oral preparations) are α_2-adrenergic receptor antagonists.

Priapism

Priapism is an involuntary, prolonged (>4 hours), abnormal and painful erection that continues beyond, or is unrelated to, sexual stimulation.[18] Priapism is a true urologic emergency because the prolonged erection can result in ischemia and fibrosis of the erectile tissue with significant risk of subsequent impotence. Priapism can occur at any age, in the newborn as well as in other age groups. Sickle cell disease or neoplasms are the most common cause in boys between 5 and 10 years of age.

Priapism is caused by impaired blood flow in the corpora cavernosa of the penis. Priapism is classified as primary (idiopathic) or secondary to a disease or drug effect. Secondary causes include hematologic conditions such as leukemia, sickle cell disease, and thrombocytopenia; neurologic conditions such as stroke, spinal cord injury, and other central nervous system lesions; and renal failure. Between 6% and 42% of males with sickle cell disease are affected at some stage by priapism.[18] The relative deoxygenation and stasis of cavernosal blood during erection is thought to increase sickling. Various medications, such as antihypertensive drugs, anticoagulant drugs, antidepressant drugs, alcohol, and marijuana, can contribute to the development of priapism. Currently, intracavernous injection therapy for erectile dysfunction is one of the more common causes of priapism.

The diagnosis of priapism usually is based on clinical findings. Colour Doppler studies of penile blood flow, penile ultrasonography, and computerized tomography (CT) scans may be used to determine intrapelvic pathology.

Initial treatment measures include analgesics, sedation, and hydration. Urinary retention may necessitate catheterization. Local measures include ice packs and cold saline enemas, aspiration and irrigation of the corpus cavernosum with plain or heparinized saline, or instillation of α-adrenergic drugs. If less aggressive treatment does not produce detumescence, a temporary surgical shunt may be established between the corpus cavernosum and the corpus spongiosum.

The prognosis for whether fibrosis or erectile failure will occur is determined by the severity and duration of blood stasis. Persistent stasis priapism is known to result in impaired erectile function and tissue fibrosis unless resolved within 24 to 48 hours of onset.[18]

Cancer of the Penis

Squamous cell cancer of the penis is most common in men between 45 and 60 years of age. Although relatively rare in developed countries (less than 1% of male genital tumours), it may account for 10% to 20% of all malignant lesions in areas such as Africa and South America.[19,20] When it is diagnosed early, penile cancer is highly curable. The greatest hindrance to early diagnosis is a delay in seeking medical attention.

The cause of penile cancer is unknown. Several risk factors have been suggested, including increasing age, poor hygiene, smoking, human papillomavirus (HPV) infections types 16 and 18, ultraviolet radiation exposure, and immunodeficiency states. There is an association between penile cancer and poor genital hygiene and phimosis. This type of cancer is rare in Jewish and Muslim men, who are circumcised routinely. One theory postulates that smegma accumulation under the phimotic foreskin may produce chronic inflammation, leading to carcinoma. The HPVs have been implicated in the genesis of several genital cancers, including cancer of the penis.[20] Ultraviolet radiation also is thought have a carcinogenic effect on the penis.[21] Men who were treated for psoriasis with ultraviolet A radiation (i.e., PUVA) have had a reported increased incidence of genital squamous cell carcinomas. Immunodeficiency states (e.g., acquired immunodeficiency syndrome) also may play a role in the pathogenesis of penile cancer.[20]

Dermatologic lesions with precancerous potential include balanitis xerotica obliterans and giant condylomata acuminata.[22] Giant condylomata acuminata are cauliflower-like lesions arising from the prepuce or glans that result from HPV infection.

Approximately 95% of penile cancers are squamous cell carcinoma.[22] They are thought to progress from an in situ lesion to an invasive carcinoma. Penile lesions with histologic features of carcinoma in situ require careful follow-up because of their potential to progress to invasive carcinoma.

Invasive carcinoma of the penis begins as a small lump or ulcer. If phimosis is present, there may be painful swelling, purulent drainage, or difficulty urinating. Palpable lymph nodes may be present in the inguinal region. Diagnosis usually is based on physical examination and biopsy results. Cavernosonography, urethroscopy, CT scans, and magnetic resonance imaging (MRI) studies may be used in the diagnostic workup.

Treatment options vary according to stage, size, location, and invasiveness of the tumour. Carcinoma in situ may be treated conservatively with fluorouracil cream application or laser treatment. Conservative treatment requires frequent follow-up examinations.[21] Surgery remains the mainstay of treatment for invasive carcinoma. Superficial primary lesions that are freely movable, do not invade the corpora, and show no evidence of metastatic disease can be treated with sleeve resection. Partial or total penectomy with appropriate lymph node dissection is indicated for invasive lesions.

Cumulative data reveal that men with penile cancer have an overall 5-year survival rate of 66%.[23] The most important prognostic indicator is the lymph node status.[24]

IN SUMMARY

Disorders of the penis can be congenital or acquired. Hypospadias and epispadias are congenital defects in which there is malpositioning of the urethral opening: it is located on the ventral surface in hypospadias and on the dorsal surface in epispadias. Phimosis is the condition in which the opening of the foreskin is too tight to permit retraction over the glans. Balanitis is an acute or chronic inflammation of the glans penis, and balanoposthitis is an inflammation of the glans and prepuce. Peyronie disease is characterized by the growth of a band of fibrous tissue on top of the penile shaft. Erectile dysfunction is defined as the inability to attain and/or maintain an erection sufficient to permit satisfactory sexual intercourse. It can be caused by psychogenic factors, organic disorders, or mixed psychogenic and organic conditions. Priapism is a prolonged, painful erection that can lead to thrombosis with ischemia and necrosis of penile tissue. Cancer of the penis accounts for less than 1% of male genital cancers in developed countries. Although the tumour is slow growing and highly curable when diagnosed early, the greatest hindrance to successful treatment is a delay in seeking medical attention.

DISORDERS OF THE SCROTUM AND TESTES

After completing this section of the chapter, you should be able to meet the following objectives:

- State the physical manifestations and potential risks associated with uncorrected cryptorchidism.
- Compare the cause, appearance, and significance of hydrocele, hematocele, spermatocele, and varicocele.
- State the difference between extravaginal and intravaginal testicular torsion.
- Describe the symptoms of epididymitis.
- State the manifestations and possible complications of mumps orchitis.
- Relate environmental factors to development of scrotal cancer.
- State the cell types involved in seminoma, embryonal carcinoma, teratoma, and choriocarcinoma tumours of the testes.

The scrotum is a skin-covered pouch that contains the testes and their accessory organs. Defects of the scrotum and testes include cryptorchidism, disorders of the scrotal sac, vascular disorders, inflammation of the scrotum and testes, and neoplasms.

Congenital and Acquired Disorders

Cryptorchidism

Cryptorchidism, or undescended testes, occurs when one or both of the testicles fail to move down into the scrotal sac. The condition usually is unilateral, but it may be bilateral in 10% of cases. The testes develop intra-abdominally in the fetus and usually descend into the scrotum through the inguinal canal during the seventh to ninth months of gestation.[1] The undescended testes may remain in the lower abdomen or at a point of descent in the inguinal canal (Fig. 44.5).

FIGURE 44.5 • Possible locations of undescended testes.

The incidence of cryptorchidism is directly related to birth weight and gestational age; infants who are born prematurely or are small for gestational age have the highest incidence of the disorder. Approximately 30% of premature infants and 3% to 5% of full-term infants are born with undescended testicles.[1] The cause of cryptorchidism in full-term infants is poorly understood. Most cases are idiopathic, but some may result from genetic or hormonal factors.

The major manifestation of cryptorchidism is the absence of one or both testes from the scrotum. The testis either is not palpable or can be felt external to the inguinal ring. Spontaneous descent often occurs during the first 3 months of life, and by 6 months of age the incidence decreases to 0.8%. Spontaneous descent rarely occurs after 6 months of age.[1]

In boys with cryptorchidism, histologic abnormalities of the testes reflect intrinsic defects in the testicle or adverse effects of the extrascrotal environment. The undescended testicle is normal at birth, but pathologic changes can be demonstrated at 6 to 12 months.[1] There is a delay in germ cell development, changes in the spermatic tubules, and a reduced number of Leydig cells. These changes are progressive over time if the testes remain undescended.

The consequences of cryptorchidism include infertility, malignancy, testicular torsion (10-fold increased risk), and the possible psychological effects of an empty scrotum. Indirect inguinal hernias usually accompany the undescended testis but rarely are symptomatic. Recognition of the condition and early treatment are important steps in preventing adverse consequences.

The risk of malignancy in the undescended testis is 2 to 4 times higher than in the general population.[1] The increased risk of testicular cancer is not significantly affected by orchiopexy (surgical placement and fixation of the testes in the scrotum), hormonal therapy, or late spontaneous descent after the age of 2 years. Orchiopexy, however, does allow for earlier detection of a testicular malignancy by positioning the testis in a more easily palpable location.

As a group, men with unilateral or bilateral cryptorchidism usually have decreased sperm counts, poorer-quality sperm, and lower fertility rates than men whose testicles descend normally. The likelihood of decreased fertility increases when the condition is bilateral. Unlike the risk of testicular cancer, there seems to be some advantage to early orchiopexy for protection of fertility.[22,26,27]

Diagnosis and Treatment. Diagnosis is based on careful examination of the genitalia in male infants. Undescended testes due to cryptorchidism should be differentiated from retractable testes that retract into the inguinal canal in response to an exaggerated cremaster muscle reflex. Retractable testes usually are palpable at birth but become nonpalpable later. They can be brought down with careful palpation in a warm room. Retractable testes usually assume a scrotal position during puberty. They have none of the complications associated with undescended testes due to cryptorchidism.[1]

Improved techniques for testicular localization include ultrasonography (*i.e.,* visualization of the testes by recording the pulses of ultrasonic waves directed into the tissues), gonadal venography and arteriography (*i.e.,* radiography of the veins and arteries of the testes after the injection of a contrast medium), and laparoscopy (*i.e.,* examination of the interior of the abdomen using a visualization instrument). Adrenal hyperplasia in a genetic female should be considered in a phenotypically male infant with bilateral nonpalpable testes (see Chapter 41).

The treatment goals for boys with cryptorchidism include measures to enhance future fertility potential, placement of the gonad in a favourable place for cancer detection, and improved cosmetic appearance. Regardless of the type of treatment used, it should be carried out between 6 and 15 months of age.[1] Treatment modalities for boys with unilateral or bilateral cryptorchidism include initial hormone therapy with human chorionic gonadotropin (hCG) or pulsatile GnRH, a hypothalamic hormone that stimulates production of the gonadotropic hormones (LH and FSH) by the anterior pituitary gland. For boys who do not respond to hormonal treatment, orchiopexy has proved effective. Approximately 89% of bilateral undescended testicles develop azoospermia if untreated. Those treated with either medical or surgical intervention have 32% to 46% chance of developing azoospermia. Approximately

13% of individuals with a unilateral undescended testicle will develop azoospermia regardless of treatment.[1,27]

Treatment of males with undescended testes should include lifelong follow-up, considering the sequelae of testicular cancer and infertility. Parents need to be aware of the potential issues of infertility and increased risk of testicular cancer. On reaching puberty, boys should be instructed in the necessity of testicular self-examination.

Hydrocele

The testes and epididymis are completely surrounded by the tunica vaginalis, a serous pouch derived from the peritoneum during fetal descent of the testes into the scrotum. The tunica vaginalis has an outer parietal layer and a deeper visceral layer that adheres to the dense fibrous covering of the testes, the tunica albuginea. A space exists between these two layers that typically contains a few millilitres of clear fluid. A hydrocele forms when excess fluid collects between the layers of the tunica vaginalis (Fig. 44.6C). It may be unilateral or bilateral and can develop as a primary congenital defect or as a secondary condition. Acute hydrocele may develop after local injury, testicular torsion, epididymitis or orchitis, gonorrhea, lymph obstruction, or germ cell testicular tumour, or as a side effect of radiation therapy. Chronic hydrocele is more common; fluid collects about the testis and the mass grows gradually.

Most cases of hydrocele in male infants and children are caused by a patent processus vaginalis, which is continuous with the peritoneal cavity. There usually are reports that the mass increases in size during the day and decreases at night if the hydrocele communicates with the peritoneal cavity. In many cases they are associated with an indirect inguinal hernia. Most hydroceles of infancy close spontaneously; therefore, they are not repaired before the age of 1 year. If the hydrocele persists beyond 18 months of age, surgical treatment usually is indicated.[1]

Hydroceles are palpated as cystic masses that may attain massive proportions. If there is enough fluid, the mass may be mistaken for a solid tumour. Transillumination of the scrotum (*i.e.,* shining a light through the scrotum to visualize its internal structures) or ultrasonography can help to determine

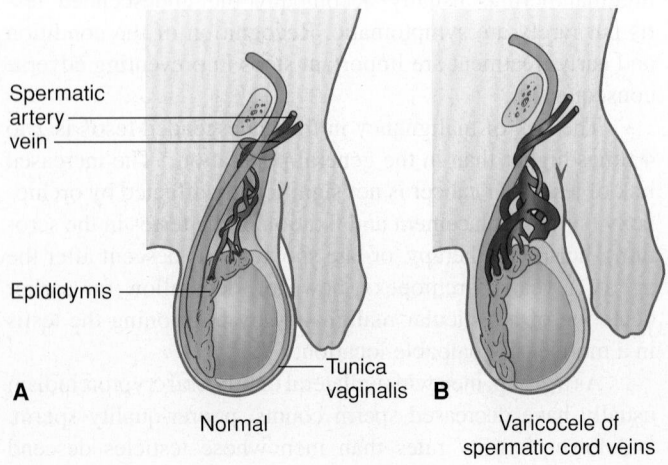

Spermatic
artery
vein

Epididymis

A Normal

Tunica
vaginalis

B Varicocele of
spermatic cord veins

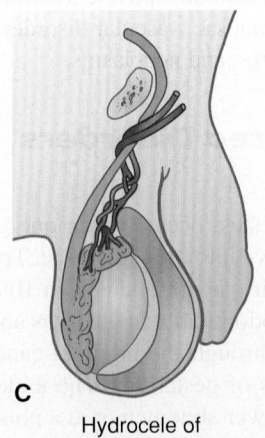

C Hydrocele of
tunica vaginalis

FIGURE 44.6 • (A) Normal testis and appendages, **(B)** varicocele, and **(C)** hydrocele.

whether the mass is solid or cystic and whether the testicle is normal. A dense hydrocele that does not illuminate should be differentiated from a testicular tumour. If a hydrocele develops in a young man without apparent cause, careful evaluation is needed to exclude cancer or infection.

In an adult male, a hydrocele is a relatively benign condition. The condition often is asymptomatic, and no treatment is necessary. When symptoms do occur, the feeling may be that of heaviness in the scrotum or pain in the lower back. In cases of secondary hydrocele, the primary condition is treated. If the hydrocele is painful or cosmetically undesirable, surgical correction is indicated. Surgical repair may be done inguinally or transscrotally.

Hematocele

A hematocele is an accumulation of blood in the tunica vaginalis, which causes the scrotal skin to become dark red or purple. It may develop as a result of an abdominal surgical procedure, scrotal trauma, a bleeding disorder, or a testicular tumour.

Spermatocele

A spermatocele is a painless, sperm-containing cyst that forms at the end of the epididymis. It is located above and posterior to the testis, is attached to the epididymis, and is separate from the testes. Spermatoceles may be solitary or multiple and usually are less than 1 cm in diameter. They are freely movable and should transilluminate. Spermatoceles rarely cause problems, but a large one may become painful and require excision.

Varicocele

A varicocele is characterized by varicosities of the pampiniform plexus, a network of veins supplying the testes (Fig. 44.6B). The left side is more commonly affected because the left internal spermatic vein inserts into the left renal vein at a right angle, whereas the right spermatic vein usually enters the inferior vena cava. Incompetent valves are more common in the left internal spermatic veins, causing a reflux of blood back into the veins of the pampiniform plexus. The force of gravity resulting from the upright position also contributes to venous dilation. If the condition persists, there may be damage to the elastic fibres and hypertrophy of the vein walls, as occurs in formation of varicose veins in the leg. Sperm concentration and motility are decreased in men with varicocele.

Varicoceles rarely are found before puberty. Symptoms of varicocele include an abnormal feeling of heaviness in the left scrotum, although many varicoceles are asymptomatic. Usually, the varicocele is readily diagnosed on physical examination with the patient in the standing and recumbent positions. Typically, the varicocele disappears in the lying position because of venous decompression into the renal vein. Scrotal palpation of a varicocele has been compared to feeling a "bag of worms." Small varicoceles sometimes are difficult to identify. The Valsalva manoeuvre (*i.e.,* forced expiration against a closed glottis) may be used to accentuate small varicosities. If the varicocele is present, retrograde blood flow to the scrotum can be detected by colour Doppler ultrasonography. Other diagnostic aids include radioisotope scanning and spermatic venography.

Treatment options include surgical ligation or sclerosis using a percutaneous transvenous catheter under fluoroscopic guidance. Both can be performed as outpatient procedures. The benefits of the percutaneous technique include a slightly lower recurrence rate and more rapid return to full physical activity. It has been suggested that men with abnormalities in their semen and a varicocele show some degree of improvement in fertility after obliteration of the dilated veins.[28] However, the effectiveness of varicocele treatment in men from subfertile couples is still debated, especially when other assisted reproductive techniques (*e.g.,* intracytoplasmic sperm injection [ICSI]) may be effective with as few as 20 sperm[29] (see Chapter 46). Aside from improving fertility, other reasons for surgery include the relief of the sensation of "heaviness" and cosmetic improvement.

Testicular Torsion

Testicular torsion is a twisting of the spermatic cord that suspends the testis (Fig. 44.7). It is the most common acute scrotal disorder in the pediatric and young adult population.[30] Testicular torsion can be divided into two distinct clinical entities, depending on the level of spermatic cord involvement: extravaginal and intravaginal torsion.[31]

Extravaginal torsion, which occurs almost exclusively in neonates, is the less common form of testicular torsion.[31] It occurs when the testicle and the fascial tunicae that surround it rotate around the spermatic cord at a level well above the tunica vaginalis. The torsion probably occurs during fetal or neonatal descent of the testes before the tunica adheres to the scrotal wall. At birth or shortly thereafter, a firm, smooth, painless scrotal mass is identified. The scrotal skin appears red, and some edema is present. Differential diagnosis is relatively easy because testicular tumours, epididymitis, and orchitis are exceedingly rare in neonates; a hydrocele is softer and can

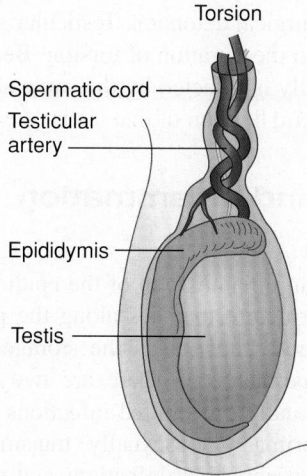

FIGURE 44.7 • Testicular torsion with twisting of the spermatic cord that suspends the testis and the spermatic vessels that supply the testis with blood.

be transilluminated, and physical examination can exclude the presence of hernia. The use of surgical treatment (orchiopexy and orchiectomy or removal of the testicle[s]) is controversial.

Intravaginal torsion is considerably more common than extravaginal torsion. It occurs when the testis rotates on its long axis in the tunica vaginalis. In most cases, congenital abnormalities of the tunica vaginalis or spermatic cord exist. The tunica vaginalis normally surrounds the testis and epididymis, allowing the testicle to rotate freely in the tunica. Although anomalies of suspension vary, the epididymal attachment may be loose enough to permit torsion between the testis and the epididymis. More commonly, the testis rotates about the distal spermatic cord. Because this abnormality is developmental, bilateral anomalies are common.

Intravaginal torsion occurs most frequently between the ages of 8 and 18 years and rarely is seen after 30 years of age. Patients usually present in severe distress within hours of onset and often have nausea, vomiting, and tachycardia. The affected testis is large and tender, with pain radiating to the inguinal area. Extensive cremaster muscle contraction causes a thickening of the spermatic cord.

Testicular torsion must be differentiated from epididymitis, orchitis, and trauma to the testis. On physical examination, the testicle often is high in the scrotum and in an abnormal orientation. These changes are caused by the twisting and shortening of the spermatic cord. The degree of scrotal swelling and redness depends on the duration of symptoms. The testes are firm and tender. The cremasteric reflex, normally elicited by stroking the medial aspect of the thigh and observing testicular retraction, frequently is absent.[1] Colour Doppler ultrasonography is increasingly used in the evaluation of suspected testicular torsion.[32]

Intravaginal testicular torsion is a true surgical emergency, and early recognition and treatment are necessary if the testicle is to be saved. Irreversible damage occurs within 4 to 6 hours; testosterone production is affected with 12 hours of ischemia.[31] Treatment includes surgical detorsion and orchiectomy.[1] Orchiectomy is carried out when the testis is deemed nonviable after surgical detorsion. Testicular salvage rates are directly related to the duration of torsion. Because the opposite testicle usually is affected by the same abnormal attachments, prophylactic fixation of that testis often is performed.[1]

Infection and Inflammation

Epididymitis

Epididymitis is an inflammation of the epididymis, the elongated cordlike structure that lies along the posterior border of the testis, whose function is the storage, transport, and maturation of spermatozoa. There are two major types of epididymitis: sexually transmitted infections associated with urethritis and primary nonsexually transmitted infections associated with urinary tract infections and prostatitis. Most cases of epididymitis are caused by bacterial pathogens.

In primary nonsexual infections, the pressure associated with voiding or physical strain may force pathogen-containing urine from the urethra or prostate up the ejaculatory duct, through the vas deferens and into the epididymis. Infections also may reach the epididymis through the lymphatics of the spermatic cord. In rare cases, organisms from other foci of infection reach the epididymis through the bloodstream. In prepubertal children, the disorder usually is associated with congenital urinary tract abnormalities and infection with gram-negative rods. In postpubertal males, several factors may predispose to development of epididymitis, including sexual activity, heavy physical exertion, and bicycle or motorcycle riding. Sexually transmitted acute epididymitis occurs mainly in young men without underlying genitourinary disease and is most commonly caused by *Chlamydia trachomatis* and *Neisseria gonorrhoeae* (individually or in combination).[33] In men older than 35 years of age, epididymitis often is associated with pathogens such as *Escherichia coli*, *Pseudomonas*, and gram-positive cocci.[34]

Epididymitis is characterized by unilateral pain and swelling, accompanied by erythema and edema of the overlying scrotal skin that develops over a period of 24 to 48 hours. Initially, the swelling and induration are limited to the epididymis. However, the distinction between the testis and epididymis becomes less evident as the inflammation progresses, and the testis and epididymis become one mass. In contrast to patients with testicular torsion, patients with epididymitis usually have a normal cremasteric reflex. There may be tenderness over the groin (spermatic cord) or in the lower abdomen. Fever and complaints of dysuria occur in approximately one half of cases. Whether urethral discharge is present depends on the organism causing the infection; it usually accompanies gonorrheal infections, is common in chlamydial infections, and is less common in infections caused by gram-negative organisms.

Laboratory findings usually reveal an elevated white blood cell count. Urinalysis and urine culture are important in the diagnosis of epididymitis, with bacteriuria and pyuria suggestive of the disorder; however, the urinalysis may be normal. The cause of epididymitis can be differentiated by Gram stain examination or culture of a midstream urine specimen or a urethral specimen. If the diagnosis remains uncertain, colour Doppler ultrasonography may be useful, revealing increased blood flow to the affected testis.

Treatment during the acute phase (which usually lasts for 3 to 4 days) includes bed rest, scrotal elevation and support, and antibiotics.[1] Bed rest with scrotal support improves lymphatic drainage. The choice of antibiotics is determined by age, physical findings, urinalysis, Gram stain results, cultures, and sexual history.[33] Oral analgesics and antipyretics usually are indicated. Sexual activity or physical strain may exacerbate the infection and worsen the symptoms, and should be avoided. If a sexually transmitted disease is suspected as an etiology, it is important to ensure that the sexual partner is screened and treated as necessary (see Chapter 47).

Orchitis

Orchitis is an infection of the testes. It can be precipitated by a primary infection in the genitourinary tract, or the infection can be spread to the testes through the bloodstream or the lymphatics. Epididymitis with subsequent infection of the testis is commonly related to genitourinary tract infections (cystitis, urethritis, genitoprostatitis) that travel to the epididymis and testis through the vas deferens or the lymphatics of the spermatic cord.

Orchitis can develop as a complication of a systemic infection, such as parotitis (*i.e.,* mumps), scarlet fever, or pneumonia. Probably the best known of these complications is orchitis caused by the mumps virus, although this origin is unusual now in Canada because of immunizations.[1,34,35] Mumps orchitis is the most common complication of mumps infection in the postpubertal male, occurring in approximately 20% to 30% of men with mumps. The onset of mumps orchitis is sudden; it usually occurs approximately 3 to 4 days after the onset of the parotitis and is characterized by fever, painful enlargement of the testes, and small hemorrhages into the tunica albuginea. Unlike epididymitis, the urinary symptoms are absent. The symptoms usually run their course in 7 to 10 days. Microscopically, an acute inflammatory response is seen in the seminiferous tubules, with proliferation of neutrophils, lymphocytes, and histiocytes causing distension of the tubules. The residual effects seen after the acute phase include hyalinization of the seminiferous tubules and atrophy of the testes (seen in half of affected men). In less than 30% of cases the orchitis is bilateral. Atrophy of the testes may occur, impacting spermatogenesis, but permanent sterility is rare even with bilateral involvement. Androgenic hormone function is usually maintained in these cases.[1,36]

Neoplasms

Tumours can develop in the scrotum or the testes. Benign scrotal tumours are common and often do not require treatment. Carcinoma of the scrotum is rare and usually is associated with exposure to carcinogenic agents. Almost all solid tumours of the testes are malignant.

Scrotal Cancer

Cancer of the scrotum was the first cancer directly linked to a specific occupation when, in the 1800s, it was associated with chimney sweeps.[37] Studies have linked this cancer to exposure to tar, soot, and oils. Most squamous cell cancers of the scrotum are linked to poor hygiene and chronic inflammation. Exposure to PUVA or HPV also has been associated with the disease. The mean age of presentation with the disease is 60 years, often preceded by 20 to 30 years of chronic irritation.

In the early stages, cancer of the scrotum may appear as a small tumour or wartlike growth that eventually ulcerates. The thin scrotal wall lacks the tissue reactivity needed to block the malignant process; more than one half of the cases seen involve metastasis to the lymph nodes. Because this tumour does not respond well to chemotherapy or irradiation, the treatment includes wide local excision of the tumour with inguinal and femoral node dissection.[38] Prognosis correlates with lymph node involvement.

Testicular Cancer

Testicular cancer accounts for 1% of all male cancers and 3% of male urogenital cancers. Although relatively rare, it is the most common cause of cancer in the 15- to 29-year-old age group.[39] In the past, testicular cancer was a leading cause of death among men entering their most productive years. However, since the late 1970s, advances in therapy have transformed an almost invariably fatal disease into one that is highly curable. With the exception of men with advanced metastatic disease at the time of presentation or those who relapse after primary chemotherapy, most men with these tumours are cured with available therapy (>90% of all newly diagnosed patients will be cured). The prognosis and extent of treatment required for testicular cancer are related to the stage of the disease at the time of presentation.

Although the cause of testicular cancer is unknown, several predisposing influences may be important: cryptorchidism, genetic factors, and disorders of testicular development.[39,40] The strongest association has been with cryptorchid testis. Males with cryptorchidism are at 2 to 4 times the risk of developing malignancy; the higher the location of the undescended testis, the greater the risk.[1] Genetic predisposition also appears to be important. Family clustering of the disorder has been described, although a well-defined pattern of inheritance has not been established. An increased incidence of testicular germ cell tumours, particularly seminomas, has been described in human immunodeficiency virus–infected men. Men with disorders of testicular development, including those with Klinefelter syndrome and testicular feminization, have a higher risk of germ cell tumours.

Approximately 90% of malignant tumours arising in the testis are germ cell tumours.[40] Germ cell tumours can be classified as seminomas and nonseminomas based on their origin in primordial germ cells and their ability to differentiate in vivo. Because these tumours derive from germ cells in the testis, they are multipotential (able to differentiate into different tissue types) and often secrete polypeptide hormones or enzymes representing earlier stages of development.

Seminomas account for approximately 50% of germ cell tumours and are most frequent in the fourth decade of life.[40] They almost never occur before the onset of puberty.[40] Seminomas are thought to arise from the seminiferous epithelium of the testes and are the type of germ cell tumour most likely to produce a uniform population of cells.

The nonseminoma tumours include embryonal carcinoma, teratoma, choriocarcinoma, and yolk cell carcinoma derivatives. Nonseminoma tumours usually contain more than one cell type and are less differentiated than seminomas.[41] Embryonal carcinomas are the least differentiated of the tumours, with the totipotential capacity to differentiate into other nonseminomatous cell types. They occur most commonly in the third decade of life. Choriocarcinoma is a rare and highly malignant form of testicular cancer that is identical to tumours that arise in placental tissue. Yolk sac tumours (also known as endodermal sinus tumours) mimic the embryonic yolk sac histologically. Teratomas are composed of somatic cell types from two or more germ-line layers (ectoderm, mesoderm, or endoderm). They can occur at any age from infancy to old age.[40,41]

Often the first sign of testicular cancer is a slight enlargement of the testicle that may be accompanied by some degree of discomfort. This may be an ache in the abdomen or groin or a sensation of dragging or heaviness in the scrotum. Frank pain may be experienced in the later stages, when the tumour is growing rapidly and hemorrhaging occurs. Testicular cancer can spread when the tumour may be barely palpable. Signs of metastatic spread include swelling of the lower extremities, back pain, neck mass, cough, hemoptysis, or dizziness. Gynecomastia (breast enlargement) may result from hCG-producing tumours and occurs in about 5% of men with germ cell tumours. Regular self-examinations of the testes have not been studied enough to show that the practice lowers the death rate from this cancer.[40,42] However, the Canadian Cancer Society does recommend periodic self-examination for men.[43]

The diagnosis of testicular cancer requires a thorough urologic history and physical examination. A painless testicular mass may be cancer. Conditions that produce an intrascrotal mass similar to testicular cancer include epididymitis, orchitis, hydrocele, or hematocele. The examination for masses should include palpation of the testes and surrounding structures, transillumination of the scrotum, and abdominal palpation. Testicular ultrasonography can be used to differentiate testicular masses. CT scans and MRI are used in assessing metastatic spread.

Tumour markers, assayed by immunoassay methods that measure protein antigens produced by malignant cells, provide information about the existence of a tumour and the type of tumour present. These markers may detect tumours that are too small to be found on physical examination or radiographs. Three tumour markers are useful in evaluating the tumour response to therapy: α-*fetoprotein,* a glycoprotein that normally is present in fetal serum in large amounts; *hCG,* a hormone that normally is produced by the placenta in pregnant women; and *lactate dehydrogenase* (LDH), a cellular enzyme normally found in muscle and the liver, kidneys, and brain.[40,41] During embryonic development, the totipotential germ cells of the testes travel down normal differentiation pathways and produce different protein products. The reappearance of these protein markers in the adult suggests activity of undifferentiated cells in a testicular germ cell tumour.

The clinical staging (TNM classification) for testicular cancer is as follows: stage I, tumour confined to testes, epididymis, or spermatic cord; stage II, tumour spread to retroperitoneal lymph nodes below the diaphragm; and stage III, metastases outside the retroperitoneal nodes or above the diaphragm (see Chapter 8). Staging procedures include CT scans of the chest, abdomen, and pelvis; ultrasonography for detection of bulky inferior nodal metastases; and occasionally lymphangiography.[40–42]

The basic treatment of all testicular cancers includes orchiectomy, which is done at the time of diagnostic exploration. The widely used surgical procedure is the unilateral radical orchiectomy through an inguinal incision. Surgical therapy is advantageous because it enables precise staging of the disease.

Recommendations for further therapy (*e.g.,* retroperitoneal lymph node dissection, chemotherapy, radiation therapy) are based on the pathologic findings from the surgical procedure.

Treatment after orchiectomy depends on the histologic characteristics of the tumour and the clinical stage of the disease. Seminomas are highly radiosensitive; the treatment of stage I or II seminoma is irradiation of the retroperitoneal and homolateral lymph nodes to the level of the diaphragm. Patients with bulky retroperitoneal or distant metastases often are treated with multiagent chemotherapy. Seminoma is probably the most curable of all solid tumours. Men with nonseminomatous tumours usually are managed with observation, chemotherapy, or retroperitoneal lymph node dissection. Rigorous follow-up in all men with testicular cancer is necessary to detect recurrences, most of which occur within 2 years of the end of treatment.[45] Testicular cancer is a disease in which even recurrence is highly treatable. With appropriate treatment, the prognosis for men with testicular cancer is excellent. The 5-year survival rate for patients is 97%.[40] Even patients with more advanced disease have excellent chances for long-term survival. Patients subsequently cured of testicular cancer are also at increased risk for the development of other cancers later in life.[44]

Therapy for testicular cancer can have potentially adverse effects on sexual functioning. Men who have retroperitoneal lymph node dissection may experience retrograde ejaculation or failure to ejaculate because of severing of the sympathetic plexus. Infertility may result from retrograde ejaculation, retroperitoneal lymph node dissection, or the toxic effects of chemotherapy or radiation therapy on the germ cells in the remaining testis. Sperm banking should be considered for men undergoing these treatments.[42]

IN SUMMARY

Disorders of the scrotum and testes include cryptorchidism (*i.e.,* undescended testes), hydrocele, hematocele, spermatocele, varicocele, and testicular torsion. Inflammatory conditions can involve the scrotal sac, epididymis, or testes. Tumours can arise in the scrotum or the testes. Scrotal cancers usually are associated with exposure to petroleum products such as tar, pitch, and soot. Testicular cancers account for 1% of all male cancers. With current treatment methods, a large percentage of men with these tumours can be cured.

DISORDERS OF THE PROSTATE

After completing this section of the chapter, you should be able to meet the following objectives:

- Compare the pathology and symptoms of acute bacterial prostatitis, chronic bacterial prostatitis, and chronic prostatitis/pelvic pain syndrome.

- Describe the urologic manifestations and treatment of benign prostatic hyperplasia.
- List the methods used in the diagnosis and treatment of prostate cancer.

The prostate is a firm, glandular structure that surrounds the urethra. It produces a thin, milky, alkaline secretion that aids sperm motility by helping to maintain an optimum pH. The contraction of the smooth muscle in the gland promotes semen expulsion during ejaculation.

Infection and Inflammation

Prostatitis refers to a variety of inflammatory disorders of the prostate gland, some bacterial and some not. It may occur spontaneously, as a result of catheterization or instrumentation, or secondary to other diseases of the male genitourinary system. The classification system for prostatitis syndromes that is used in Canada is based on the criteria established in 1998 by the American National Institute of Health and reconfirmed in 2002. This includes: acute bacterial prostatitis, chronic bacterial prostatitis, chronic inflammatory and noninflammatory prostatitis/pelvic pain syndrome, and asymptomatic inflammatory prostatitis.[45] Men with asymptomatic inflammatory prostatitis have no subjective symptoms, and are detected incidentally on biopsy or examination of prostatic fluid. It is estimated that up to 50% of men experience prostatitis at some time.[45]

Acute Bacterial Prostatitis

Acute bacterial prostatitis often is considered a subtype of urinary tract infection. The most likely etiology of acute bacterial prostatitis is an ascending urethral infection or reflux of infected urine into the prostatic ducts. The most common organism is *E. coli*. Other gram-negative bacteria (*Proteus, Klebsiella, Pseudomonas,* and *Serratia* species) and enterococci are less frequent pathogens.[46] Anaerobic and gram-positive bacteria are rarely a cause of acute prostatitis. The manifestations of acute bacterial prostatitis include fever and chills, malaise, myalgia, arthralgia, frequent and urgent urination, dysuria, and urethral discharge.[42] Dull, aching pain often is present in the perineum, rectum, or sacrococcygeal region. The urine may be cloudy and malodorous because of urinary tract infection. Rectal examination reveals a firm, swollen, very tender, warm prostate with scattered soft areas. Prostatic massage produces a thick discharge with white blood cells that grows large numbers of pathogens on culture.

Treatment of acute bacterial prostatitis depends on the severity of symptoms. It usually includes antibiotics, minimal activity, adequate hydration, antipyretics, analgesics (preferably nonsteroidal anti-inflammatory drugs) to alleviate pain, and stool softeners. Men who are extremely ill, such as those with sepsis, may require hospitalization. A suprapubic catheter may be indicated if voiding is difficult or painful.

Acute prostatitis usually responds to appropriate antimicrobial therapy chosen in accordance with the sensitivity of the causative agents in the urethral discharge. Depending on the urine culture results, antibiotic therapy usually is continued for at least 4 weeks. Because acute prostatitis often is associated with anatomic abnormalities, a thorough urologic examination usually is performed after treatment is completed.

A persistent fever indicates the need for further investigation for an additional site of infection or a prostatic abscess. CT scans and transrectal ultrasonography of the prostate are useful in the diagnosis of prostatic abscesses. Prostatic abscesses, which are relatively uncommon since the advent of effective antibiotic therapy, are found more commonly in diabetic or immunosuppressed men.

Chronic Bacterial Prostatitis

In contrast to acute bacterial prostatitis, chronic bacterial prostatitis is a subtle disorder that is difficult to treat. Men with the disorder typically have recurrent urinary tract infections with persistence of the same strain of pathogenic bacteria in prostatic fluid and urine. Organisms responsible for chronic bacterial prostatitis usually are the gram-negative enterobacteria (*E. coli, Proteus,* or *Klebsiella*) or *Pseudomonas.*[46] Infected prostatic calculi may develop and contribute to the chronic infection.

The symptoms of chronic prostatitis are variable and include frequent and urgent urination, dysuria, perineal discomfort, and low back pain. Occasionally, myalgia and arthralgia accompany the other symptoms. Secondary epididymitis sometimes is associated with the disorder. Many men experience relapsing lower or upper urinary tract infections because of recurrent invasion of the bladder by the prostatic bacteria. Bacteria may exist in the prostate gland even when the prostatic fluid is sterile. The most accurate method of establishing a diagnosis is by localizing cultures. This four step method is based on sequential collections of the first part of the voided urine (urethral specimen), midstream specimen (bladder specimen), the expressed prostatic secretion (obtained by prostatic massage), and the urine voided after prostatic massage. The last two specimens are considered prostatic urine. A positive expressed prostatic specimen establishes the diagnosis of bacterial prostatitis, excluding nonbacterial prostatitis.[45,46]

Even after an accurate diagnosis has been established, treatment of chronic prostatitis often is difficult and frustrating.[47] Unlike their action in the acutely inflamed prostate, antibacterial drugs penetrate poorly into the chronically inflamed prostate. Long-term therapy (6 to 12 weeks) with an appropriate low-dose oral antimicrobial agent often is used to treat the infection. Adding α_1-adrenergic blocking drugs (*e.g.,* prazosin, doxazosin) to antibacterial drugs may significantly improve symptoms and reduce recurrence.[45]

Chronic Prostatitis/Chronic Pelvic Pain Syndrome

Chronic prostatitis/pelvic pain syndrome is both the most common and least understood of the prostatitis syndromes.[42,45]

The category is divided into two types, inflammatory and non-inflammatory, based on the presence of leukocytes in the prostatic fluid. The inflammatory type was previously referred to as *nonbacterial prostatitis,* and the noninflammatory type as *prostatodynia.*

Inflammatory Prostatitis. A large group of men with prostatitis have pains along the penis, testicles, and scrotum; painful ejaculation; low back pain; rectal pain that spreads to the inner thighs; urinary symptoms; decreased libido; and impotence, but they have no bacteria in the urinary system. Men with nonbacterial prostatitis often have inflammation of the prostate with an elevated leukocyte count and abnormal inflammatory cells in their prostatic secretions. The cause of the disorder is unknown, and efforts to prove the presence of unusual pathogens (*e.g.,* mycoplasmas, *Chlamydia,* trichomonads, viruses) have been largely unsuccessful. It also is thought that nonbacterial prostatitis may be an autoimmune disorder.

Noninflammatory Prostatitis. Men with noninflammatory prostatitis or prostatodynia have symptoms resembling those of nonbacterial prostatitis but have negative urine culture results and no evidence of prostatic inflammation (*i.e.,* normal leukocyte count). The cause of noninflammatory prostatitis is unknown, but because of the absence of inflammation, the search for the cause of symptoms has been directed toward extraprostatic sources. In some cases, there is an apparent functional obstruction of the bladder neck near the external urethral sphincter; during voiding, this results in higher-than-normal pressures in the prostatic urethra that cause intraprostatic urine reflux and chemical irritation of the prostate by urine. In other cases, there is an apparent myalgia (*i.e.,* muscle pain) associated with prolonged tension of the pelvic floor muscles. Emotional stress and depression also may play a role.

Treatment. Treatment methods for chronic prostatitis/pelvic pain syndrome are highly variable and require further study. Antibiotic therapy is used when an occult infection is suspected. Treatment often is directed toward symptom control. Sitz baths and nonsteroidal anti-inflammatory drugs may provide some symptom relief. In men with irritative urination symptoms, anticholinergic agents (*e.g.,* oxybutynin) or α-adrenergic blocking agents may be beneficial. Reassurance can be helpful. It is important that these men know that the condition is neither infectious nor contagious, nor is it known to cause cancer.[42,45]

Hyperplasia and Neoplasms

Benign Prostatic Hyperplasia

Benign prostatic hyperplasia (BPH) is an age-related, non-malignant enlargement of the prostate gland (Fig. 44.8). It is characterized by the formation of large, discrete lesions in the periurethral region of the prostate rather than the peripheral zones, which commonly are affected by prostate cancer (Fig. 44.9). BPH is one of the most common diseases of aging

FIGURE 44.8 • Nodular hyperplasia of the prostate. Cut surface of a prostate enlarged by nodular hyperplasia shows numerous, well-circumscribed nodules of prostatic tissue. The prostatic urethra (paper clip) has been compressed to a narrow slit. (From Rubin R., Strayer D. S. (Eds.). (2012). *Rubin's pathology: Clinicopathologic foundations of medicine* (6th ed., p. 841). Philadelphia, PA: Lippincott Williams & Wilkins.).

Anterior

Prostatic urethra

Posterior

NORMAL PROSTATE

NODULAR PROSTATIC HYPERPLASIA

CARCINOMA OF PROSTATE

FIGURE 44.9 • Normal prostate, nodular benign prostatic hypertrophy, and cancer of the prostate. (From Rubin R., Strayer D. S. (Eds.). (2012). *Rubin's pathology: Clinicopathologic foundations of medicine* (6th ed., p. 840). Philadelphia, PA: Lippincott Williams & Wilkins.).

men. It has been reported that more than 50% of men older than 60 years of age and up to 90% of men over the age of 80 have BPH.[47,48] Between 15% and 30% of these men will develop lower urinary tract symptoms (LUTS).

The exact cause of the BPH is unknown. Potential risk factors include age, family history, race, ethnicity, dietary fat and meat consumption, and hormonal factors. The incidence of BPH increases with advanced age and is highest in African Americans and lowest in native Japanese. Men with a family history of BPH are reported to have had larger prostates than those of control subjects, and higher rates of BPH were found in monozygotic twins than in dizygotic twins.

Both androgens (testosterone and dihydrotestosterone) and estrogens appear to contribute to the development of BPH. The prostate consists of a network of glandular elements embedded in smooth muscle and supporting tissue, with testosterone being the most important factor for prostatic growth. Dihydrotestosterone (DHT), the biologically active metabolite of testosterone, is thought to be the ultimate mediator of prostatic hyperplasia, with estrogen serving to sensitize the prostatic tissue to the growth-producing effects of DHT. Free plasma testosterone enters prostatic cells, where at least 90% is converted into DHT by the action of 5α-reductase. The discovery that DHT is the active factor in BPH is the rationale for the use of 5α-reductase inhibitors (*e.g.*, finasteride, dutasteride) in the treatment of the disorder. Although the exact source of the estrogen is uncertain, small amounts of estrogen are produced in the male. It has been postulated that a relative increase in estrogen levels that occurs with aging may facilitate the action of androgens in the prostate despite a decline in testicular output of testosterone. Other hormonal factors that have been implicated include increased intraprostate levels of insulin-like growth factor-1 (IGF-1).[49]

The anatomic location of the prostate at the bladder neck contributes to the pathophysiology and symptoms of BPH. There are two prostatic components to the obstructive properties of BPH and development of LUTS: dynamic and static.[49] The static component of BPH is related to an increase in prostatic size and gives rise to symptoms such as a weak urinary stream, postvoid dribbling, frequency of urination, and nocturia. The dynamic component of BPH is related to prostatic smooth muscle tone. The α_1-adrenergic receptors are the main receptors for the smooth muscle component of the prostate. The recognition of the role of α_1-adrenergic receptors on neuromuscular function in the prostate is the basis for use of α_1-adrenergic receptor blockers in treating BPH. A third component, detrusor instability and impaired bladder contractility, may contribute to the symptoms of BPH independent of the outlet obstruction created by an enlarged prostate[49] (see Chapter 35). It has been suggested that some of the symptoms of BPH might be related to a decompensating or aging bladder rather than being primarily related to outflow obstruction. An example is the involuntary contraction that results in urgency and an attempt to void that occurs because of small bladder volume.

The clinical significance of BPH resides in its tendency to compress the urethra and cause partial or complete

---

HYPERPLASIA AND CANCER OF THE PROSTATE

- The prostate gland surrounds the urethra and periurethral enlargement causes manifestations of urinary obstruction.
- Benign prostatic hyperplasia is an age-related enlargement of the prostate gland with formation of large, discrete lesions in the periurethral region of the prostate. These lesions compress the urethra and produce symptoms of dysuria or difficulty urinating.
- Prostate cancer begins in the peripheral zones of the prostate gland and usually is asymptomatic until the disease is far advanced and the tumour has eroded the outer prostatic capsule and spread to adjacent pelvic tissues or metastasized.

---

obstruction of urinary outflow. As the obstruction increases, acute retention may occur with overdistension of the bladder. The residual urine in the bladder causes increased frequency of urination and a constant desire to empty the bladder, which becomes worse at night. With marked bladder distension, overflow incontinence may occur with the slightest increase in intra-abdominal pressure.

The resulting obstruction to urinary flow can give rise to urinary tract infection, destructive changes of the bladder wall, hydroureter, and hydronephrosis. Hypertrophy and changes in bladder wall structure develop in stages. Initially, the hypertrophied fibres form trabeculations and then herniations, or sacculations; finally, diverticula develop as the herniations extend through the bladder wall (see Chapter 35, Fig. 35.4). Because urine seldom is completely emptied from them, these diverticula are readily infected. Back-pressure on the ureters and collecting system of the kidneys promotes hydroureter, hydronephrosis, and danger of eventual renal failure.

Diagnosis. It is now thought that the single most important factor in the evaluation and treatment of BPH is the man's own experiences related to the disorder. The International Prostate Symptom Score (IPSS) questionnaire consists of seven questions about symptoms regarding incomplete emptying, frequency, intermittency, urgency, weak stream, straining, and nocturia. Each question is rated with a score of 0 (mild) to 5 (severe). A maximum score of 35 indicates severe symptoms. Total scores below 7 are considered mild; those between 8 and 19, moderate; and scores over 20, severe. A final question relates to quality of life due to urinary problems.

In 2010, the Canadian Urological Association (CUA) published clinical practice guidelines for management of BPH.[50] These guidelines suggest that the initial evaluation of men for a diagnosis of BPH include history, physical examination, digital rectal examination, urinalysis, blood for prostate-specific antigen (PSA), and urine flow rate. Blood for serum creatinine and urine analyses are used as adjuncts to determine BPH complications. Urinalysis is done to detect bacteria, white blood cells, or microscopic hematuria in the presence of infection and inflammation. The serum creatinine test is used as an estimate of the glomerular filtration rate and renal function. The PSA test is used to screen for prostate cancer. These evaluation measures, along with the symptom index, are used to describe the extent of obstruction, determine whether other diagnostic tests are needed, and establish the need for treatment.

The digital rectal examination is used to examine the external surface of the prostate. Enlargement of the prostate due to BPH usually produces a large, palpable prostate with a smooth, rubbery surface. Hardened areas of the prostate gland suggest cancer and should be sampled for biopsy. An enlarged prostate found during a digital rectal examination does not always correlate with the degree of urinary obstruction. Some men can have greatly enlarged prostate glands with no urinary obstruction, but others may have severe symptoms without a palpable enlargement of the prostate.

Residual urine measurement may be made by ultrasonography or postvoiding catheterization for residual urine volume. Residual urines greater than 100 ml are considered high. Uroflowmetry provides an objective measure of urine flow rate. The patient is asked to void with a relatively full bladder (at least 150 ml) into a device that electronically measures the force of the stream and urine flow rate. A urinary flow rate of greater than 15 ml/second is considered normal, and less than 10 ml/second is indicative of obstruction.

Transabdominal or transrectal diagnostic ultrasonography can be used to evaluate the kidneys, ureters, and bladder. Urethrocystoscopy is indicated in men with a history of hematuria, stricture disease, urethral injury, or prior lower urinary tract surgery. It is used to evaluate the length and diameter of the urethra, the size and configuration of the prostate, and bladder capacity. It also detects the presence of trabeculations, bladder stones, and small bladder cancers. CT scans, MRI studies, and radionuclide scans are reserved for rare instances of tumour detection.

Treatment. Treatment of BPH is determined by the degree of symptoms that the condition produces and complications due to obstruction. When a man develops mild symptoms related to BPH, a "watchful waiting" stance often is taken. The condition does not always run a predictable course; it may remain stable or even improve.

Until the 1980s, surgery was the mainstay of treatment to alleviate urinary obstruction due to BPH. Currently, there is an emphasis on less invasive methods of treatment, including use of pharmacologic agents. However, when more severe signs of obstruction develop, surgical treatment is indicated to provide comfort and avoid serious kidney damage.

Pharmacologic management includes the use of 5α-reductase inhibitors and α$_1$-adrenergic blocking drugs.[50] The 5α-reductase inhibitors such as finasteride reduce prostate size by blocking the effect of androgens on the prostate. Finasteride causes atrophy of the prostate glandular epithelial cells; the onset is slow (3 to 6 months), but long-lasting. The

side effects of finasteride are minimal but include erectile dysfunction (4% to 16%) and decreased libido (1% to 10%).[42] The presence of α-adrenergic receptors in prostatic smooth muscle has prompted the use of α$_1$-adrenergic blocking drugs (*e.g.*, prazosin, terazosin) to relieve prostatic obstruction and increase urine flow. All α$_1$-adrenergic blocking drugs in current use have a rapid onset of action (within weeks), and similar effectiveness. Combinations of 5α-reductase inhibitors and α$_1$-adrenergic blocking agents seem to be more effective than either monotherapy.[50]

Herbal therapies have been used for many years by men for the treatment of BPH and LUTS. Several studies have looked at the effects of these agents, including the extract of the saw palmetto berry. Improvements in peak urine flow rates and nocturia can occur compared with placebo, but the durability of these effects is unproven. The long-term toxicity and mechanism of action of these agents remain unclear.[42]

The surgical removal of an enlarged prostate can be accomplished by the transurethral, suprapubic, or perineal approach. Currently transurethral prostatectomy (TURP) is the most commonly used technique in Canada. With this approach, an instrument is introduced through the urethra, and prostate tissue is removed using a resectoscope and electrocautery. Immediate complications of TURP include the inability to urinate, postoperative hemorrhage or clot retention, and urinary tract infection. Late complications of TURP include erectile dysfunction, incontinence, and bladder neck contractures. Retrograde ejaculation is another problem that may occur because of resection of bladder neck tissue.

Many new and experimental techniques have also been used to treat BPH (*e.g.*, transurethral incision of the prostate [TUIP], laser surgery, transurethral vaporization, transurethral microwave therapy, transurethral needle ablation), and each has advantages and disadvantages when considered as an alternative treatment. Other therapies currently not recommended due to lack of evidence include a balloon dilation approach, absolute ethanol injection, and intraprostatic botulinum toxin injection.[50]

For men who have heart or lung disease or a condition that precludes major surgery, a stent may be used to widen and maintain the patency of the urethra. A stent is a device made of tubular mesh that is inserted under local or regional anesthesia. Within several months, the lining of the urethra grows to cover the inside of the stent.

Prostate Cancer

Prostate cancer is the most common nonskin cancer in Canada, and is third to lung cancer and colon/rectal cancer as a cause of cancer-related death in Canadian men.[51] The Canadian Cancer Society estimates that during 2015, approximately 24,000 men in Canada will be diagnosed with prostate cancer, and 4,100 men will die of the disorder.[51] The increase in diagnosed cases is thought to reflect earlier diagnosis because of the widespread use of PSA testing since the early 1990s. The incidence of prostate cancer varies markedly from country to country and varies among races in the same country.[51] Men of African ancestry have the highest reported incidence for prostate cancer at all ages. Prostate cancer also tends to be diagnosed at a later stage in these African men. Men of Asian and Native American ancestry have the lowest rate. Prostate cancer also is a disease of aging. The incidence increases rapidly after 50 years of age.[51]

The precise cause of prostate cancer is unclear. As with other cancers, it appears that the development of prostate cancer is a multistep process involving genes that control cell differentiation and growth. Several risk factors, such as age, race, heredity, and environmental influences (*e.g.*, a high-fat diet), are suspected of playing a role.[51] Male hormone levels also play a role. There is insufficient evidence linking socioeconomic status, infectious agents, smoking, vasectomy, sexual behaviour, or BPH to the pathogenesis of prostate cancer.[51]

The incidence of prostate cancer appears to be higher in relatives of men with prostate cancer. It has been estimated that men who have an affected first-degree relative (*e.g.*, father, brother) and an affected second-degree relative (*e.g.*, grandfather, uncle) have an eightfold increase in risk. It has been suggested that dietary patterns, including increased dietary fats, may alter the production of sex hormones and growth factors and increase the risk of prostate cancer.[51] Supporting the role of dietary fats as a risk factor for prostate cancer has been the observation that the diet of Japanese men, who have a low rate of prostate cancer, is much lower in fat content than that of North American men, who have a much higher incidence.

In terms of hormonal influence, androgens are believed to play a role in the pathogenesis of prostate cancer.[51] Evidence favouring a hormonal influence includes the presence of steroid receptors in the prostate, the requirement of sex hormones for normal growth and development of the prostate, and the fact that prostate cancer almost never develops in men who have been castrated. The response of prostate cancer to estrogen administration or androgen deprivation further supports a correlation between the disease and testosterone levels.

Prostatic adenocarcinomas, which account for 98% of all primary prostate cancers, are commonly multicentric and located in the peripheral zones of the prostate (Fig. 44.8). The high frequency of invasion of the prostatic capsule by adenocarcinoma relates to its subcapsular location. Invasion of the urinary bladder is less frequent and occurs later in the clinical course. Metastasis to the lung reflects lymphatic spread through the thoracic duct and dissemination from the prostatic venous plexus to the inferior vena cava. Bony metastases, particularly to the vertebral column, ribs, and pelvis, produce pain that often presents as a first sign of the disease.

Most men with early-stage prostate cancer are asymptomatic. The presence of symptoms often suggests locally advanced or metastatic disease. Depending on the size and location of prostate cancer at the time of diagnosis, there may be changes associated with the voiding pattern similar to those found in BPH. These include urgency, frequency, nocturia, hesitancy, dysuria, hematuria, or blood in the ejaculate.

On digital rectal examination, the prostate can be nodular and fixed. Bone metastasis often is characterized by low back pain. Pathologic fractures can occur at the site of metastasis. Men with metastatic disease may experience weight loss, anemia, or shortness of breath.

Screening. Because early cancers of the prostate usually are asymptomatic, screening tests are important. The screening tests currently available are digital rectal examination, PSA testing, and transrectal ultrasonography. The controversial PSA test measures a glycoprotein produced and secreted into the cytoplasm of benign and malignant prostatic cells that is not found in other normal tissues or tumours. However, a positive PSA test indicates only the possible presence of prostate cancer. It also can be positive in cases of BPH and prostatitis. It has been reported that one in four men with elevated PSA levels have prostate cancer determined by biopsy, and the remainder do not.[52] Measures to increase the specificity of PSA testing in terms of predicting prostate cancer are being developed and evaluated. For example, because PSA levels increase with age, age-specific ranges have been established.[53] PSA velocity (a change of PSA level over time), PSA density (*i.e.*, PSA level/prostate volume as measured by rectal ultrasonography), kallikreins, and other molecular biomarkers are being studied to ascertain if they will be more effective predictors of indolent versus aggressive prostate cancer.[54]

The Canadian Cancer Society and the Canadian Urological Association (CUA) recommend that men 50 years of age or older should undergo a measurement of PSA and digital rectal examination for early detection of prostate cancer.[52,55] The CUA further suggests that men at higher risk for prostate cancer, such as those with African ancestry and/or those with a strong family history, should undergo annual screening beginning at 40 years of age.[55] However, some controversy regarding the widespread use of PSA for screening remains. In 2014, the Canadian Task Force on Preventive Health Care summarized international screening recommendations and decided to strongly recommend against most PSA testing.[56] Ultimately, informed decision making regarding any screening with PSA is warranted.

A new approach, transrectal ultrasonography, may detect cancers that are too small to be detected by physical examination. This method is not used for first-line detection because of its expense, but it may benefit men who are at high risk for development of prostate cancer.

Diagnosis. The diagnosis of prostate cancer is based on history and physical examination and confirmed through biopsy methods. Transrectal ultrasonography is used to guide a biopsy needle and document the exact location of the sampled tissue. It also is used for providing staging information. Newly developed small probes for transrectal MRI have been shown to be effective in detecting the presence of cancer in the prostate. Radiologic examination of the bones of the skull, ribs, spine, and pelvis can be used to reveal metastases, although radionuclide bone scans are more sensitive.

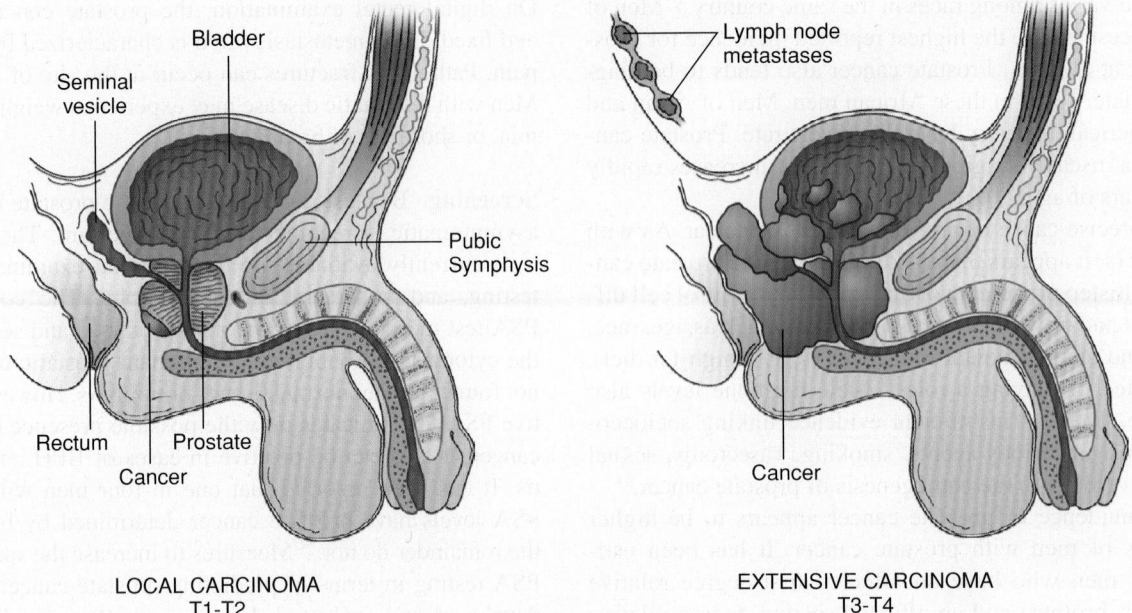

FIGURE 44.10 • TNM staging for prostate cancer. Stage T1 and T2 tumours are localized to the prostate, whereas stage T3 and T4 tumours have spread outside the prostate. (From Rubin R., Strayer D. S. (Eds.). (2012). *Rubin's pathology: Clinicopathologic foundations of medicine* (6th ed., p. 845). Philadelphia, PA: Lippincott Williams & Wilkins.).

Staging. Cancer of the prostate, like other forms of cancer, is graded and staged (see Chapter 8). Prostatic adenocarcinoma commonly is classified using the Gleason grading system.[42,51] Well-differentiated tumours are assigned a grade of 1, and poorly differentiated tumours a grade of 5. The TNM system for staging includes primary-stage tumours (T1) are asymptomatic and discovered on histologic examination of prostatic tissue specimens; T2 tumours are palpable on digital examination but are confined to the prostate gland; T3 tumours have extended beyond the prostate; and T4 tumours have pushed beyond the prostate to involve adjacent structures (Fig. 44.10). Regional lymph node (N) and distant metastases (M) are described as Nx or Mx (cannot be assessed), N0 or M0 (not present), and N1 or M1 (present).[51]

PSA levels are important in the staging and management of prostate cancer. In untreated cases, the level of PSA correlates with the volume and stage of disease. A rising PSA after treatment is consistent with progressive disease, whether it is locally recurring or metastatic. Measurement of PSA is used to detect recurrence after total prostatectomy. Because the prostate is the source of PSA, levels should drop to zero after surgery; a rising PSA indicates recurring disease.

Treatment. Cancer of the prostate is treated by active surveillance, surgery, radiation therapy, and hormonal manipulations.[51] Chemotherapy has shown limited effectiveness in the treatment of prostate cancer. Treatment decisions are based on tumour grade and stage and on the age and health of the man. Expectant therapy (watchful waiting) may be used if the tumour is not producing symptoms, is expected to grow slowly, and is small and contained in one area of the prostate.

This approach is particularly suited for men who are elderly or have other health problems. Most men with an anticipated survival greater than 10 years are considered for surgical or radiation therapy.[42] Radical prostatectomy involves complete removal of the seminal vesicles, prostate, and ampullae of the vas deferens. Refinements in surgical techniques ("nerve-sparing" prostatectomy) have allowed maintenance of continence in most men and erectile function in selected cases. Radiation therapy can be delivered by a variety of techniques, including external-beam radiation therapy and transperineal implantation of radioisotopes (brachytherapy).

Metastatic disease often is treated with androgen deprivation therapy. Androgen deprivation may be induced at several levels along the pituitary-gonadal axis using a variety of methods or agents. Orchiectomy often is effective in reducing symptoms and extending survival as this eliminates most of the male hormones. The GnRH analogs (*e.g.,* leuprolide, triptorelin) block LH (and FSH) release from the pituitary and reduce testosterone levels. When given continuously (as opposed to pulsatile dosing, which is the normal physiologic secretory rhythm) and in therapeutic doses, these drugs desensitize GnRH receptors in the pituitary, thereby preventing the release of LH. However, initially, because these agents are GnRH *agonists,* LH and FSH rise and cause testosterone levels to increase.[51] This can cause a clinical flare that can be especially important in certain circumstances, such as the presence of spinal cord compression due to metastatic disease. This clinical flare can be decreased by pretreatment with antiandrogens. The nonsteroidal antiandrogens (*e.g.,* flutamide, bicalutamide) block the uptake and actions of androgens in the target tissues. Although testosterone is the main circulating androgen, the adrenal gland also secretes androgens. Complete androgen blockade can be achieved by blocking androgens of adrenal origin by combining an antiandrogen with a GnRH agent or orchiectomy. Inhibitors of adrenal androgen synthesis (*i.e.,* ketoconazole, abiraterone, aminoglutethimide [unavailable in Canada]) may also be used for treating men with advanced prostate cancer who present with spinal cord compression, bilateral ureteral obstruction, or disseminated intravascular clotting. This is because these men need rapid decreases in their testosterone levels—ketoconazole, for instance, can produce chemical castration within 24 hours. Palliative care includes adequate pain control and focal irradiation of symptomatic or unstable bone disease. In men with advanced prostate cancer, the bisphosphonates (*e.g.,* pamidronate, zoledronic acid), which act mainly by inhibiting osteoclastic activity (see Chapter 58), have several potential uses in prostate cancer. These include (1) prevention of osteopenia that accompanies the use of androgen deprivation therapy; (2) prevention and delay of skeletal complications (*e.g.,* the need for local radiation treatment, fractures) in patients with metastatic bone involvement; (3) palliation of bone pain; and (4) treatment of hypercalcemia of malignancy.

IN SUMMARY

The prostate is a firm, glandular structure that surrounds the urethra. Inflammation of the prostate occurs as an acute or a chronic process. Chronic prostatitis probably is the most common cause of relapsing urinary tract infections in men. BPH is a common disorder in men older than 50 years of age. Because the prostate encircles the urethra, BPH exerts its effect through obstruction of urinary outflow from the bladder. Advances in the treatment of BPH include laser surgery, prostatic stents, and pharmacologic treatment using 5α-reductase inhibitors such as finasteride, which reduce prostate size by blocking the effects of androgen on the prostate, and α₁-adrenergic receptor blockers, which inhibit contraction of prostatic smooth muscle.

Prostate cancer is the most common nonskin cancer in Canada and is third to lung cancer and colon/rectal cancer as a cause of cancer-related death in men. A recent increase in diagnosed cases is thought to reflect earlier diagnosis because of widespread use of PSA testing. The incidence of prostate cancer increases with age and is greater in men of African ancestry of all ages. Most prostate cancers are asymptomatic and are incidentally discovered on rectal examination. Screening for prostate cancer has become controversial as a method for early identification of prostate cancer. The Canadian Cancer Society and Canadian Urological Association suggest that every man 50 years of age or older should have regular digital rectal examinations and PSA tests. Cancer of the prostate, like other forms of cancer, is graded according to the histologic characteristics of the tumour and staged clinically using the TNM system. Treatment, which is based on the extent of the disease, includes surgery, radiation therapy, and hormonal manipulation.

REVIEW EXERCISES

1. A 64-year-old man presents to his family physician with erectile dysfunction. He is on multiple medications for his "heart disease." An initial physical examination is unremarkable.
   A. *What additional information should be obtained?*
   B. *Given his medical history, what are possible factors contributing to his problem?*

2. A 23-year-old man presents to the emergency department in severe distress. His left testicle is large and tender, and he has pain radiating to the inguinal area.
   A. *What would be a tentative diagnosis for this man?*
   B. *Why would this problem necessitate immediate diagnosis and surgical intervention?*

3. A 72-year-old man had a radical prostatectomy for localized prostate cancer. After surgery, his PSA level was undetectable. He presents 5 years later having been "lost to follow-up." He complains of pain in his hip and lower back. His PSA level is now markedly elevated.
   A. *What initial investigations are warranted?*
   B. *What therapies are available for this complication?*

References

1. Kliegman R. M., Stanton B. F., St. Geme J. W., et al. (Eds.). (2011). *Nelson textbook of pediatrics* (19th ed.). Philadelphia, PA: Elsevier Saunders.
2. Brouwers M. M., van der Zanden L. F., de Gier R. P., et al. (2010). Hypospadias: Risk factor patterns and different phenotypes. *BJU International, 105*(2), 254–262.
3. Springer A., Krois W., Horcher E. (2011). Trends in hypospadias surgery: Results of a worldwide survey. *European Urology, 60*(6), 1184–1189.
4. Steven L., Cherian A., Yankovic F., et al. (2013). Current practice in paediatric hypospadias surgery: A specialist survey. *Journal of Pediatric Urology, 9*(Part B), 1126–1130.
5. Clouston D., Hall A., Lawrentschuk N. (2011). Penile lichen sclerosus (balanitis xerotica obliterans). *BJU International, 108*(2), 14–19.
6. Wilkinson D. J., Lansdale N., Everitt L. H., et al. (2012). Foreskin preputioplasty and intralesional triamcinolone: A valid alternative to circumcision for balanitis xerotica obliterans. *Journal of Pediatric Surgery, 47*(4), 756–759.
7. Ralph D., Gonzalez-Cadavid N., Mirone V., et al. (2010). The management of Peyronie's disease: Evidence-based 2010 guidelines. *Journal of Sexual Medicine, 7*(7), 2359–2374.
8. Almannie R., Carrier S. (2012). Sexual dysfunction after surgical treatment of Peyronie's disease. *Sexologies, 21*(2), 48–54.
9. Tal R., Heck M., Teloken P., et al. (2010). Peyronie's disease following radical prostatectomy: Incidence and predictors. *Journal of Sexual Medicine, 7*(3), 1254–1261.
10. Chung E., Clendinning E., Lessard L., et al. (2011). Five-year follow-up of Peyronie's graft surgery: Outcomes and patient satisfaction. *Journal of Sexual Medicine, 8*(2), 594–600.
11. Eardley I., Donatucci C., Corbin J., et al. (2010). Pharmacotherapy for erectile dysfunction. *Journal of Sexual Medicine, 7*(1), 524–540.

12. Shamloul R., Ghanem H. (2013). Erectile dysfunction. *Lancet, 381*(9861), 153–165.

13. Harte C. B. (2014). Concurrent relations among cigarette smoking status, resting heart rate variability, and erectile response. *Journal of Sexual Medicine, 11*(5), 1230–1239.

14. Araujo A., Travison T., Ganz P., et al. (2009). Erectile dysfunction and mortality. *Journal of Sexual Medicine, 6*(9), 2445–2454.

15. Katz A., Katz A. (2010). Erectile dysfunction. *CMAJ, 182*(4), 381–382.

16. Fisher W., Eardley I., McCabe M., et al. (2009). Erectile dysfunction (ED) is a shared sexual concern of couples part I: Couple conceptions of ED. *Journal of Sexual Medicine, 6*(10), 2746–2760.

17. Chrysant S. (2013). Effectiveness and safety of phosphodiesterase 5 inhibitors in patients with cardiovascular disease and hypertension. *Current Hypertension Reports, 15*(5), 475–483.

18. Broderick G., Kadioglu A., Bivalacqua T., et al. (2010). Priapism: Pathogenesis, epidemiology, and management. *Journal of Sexual Medicine, 7*(1), 476–500.

19. Larke N., Thomas S., Silva I., et al. (2011). Male circumcision and penile cancer: A systematic review and meta-analysis. *Cancer Causes & Control, 22*(8), 1097–1110.

20. Heinlen J., Buethe D., Culkin D. (2012). Advanced penile cancer. *International Urology and Nephrology, 44*(1), 139–148.

21. Bleeker M., Heideman D., Snijders P., et al. (2009). Penile cancer: Epidemiology, pathogenesis and prevention. *World Journal of Urology, 27*(2), 141–150.

22. Muneer A., Kayes O., Ahmed H., et al. (2009). Molecular prognostic factors in penile cancer. *World Journal of Urology, 27*(2), 161–167.

23. Djajadiningrat R. S., Graafland N. M., Werkhoven E., et al. (2014). Contemporary management of regional nodes in penile cancer—Improvement of Survival? *Journal of Urology, 191*(1), 68–73.

24. Guimarães G., Rocha R., Zequi S., et al. (2011). Penile cancer: Epidemiology and treatment. *Current Oncology Reports, 13*(3), 231–239.

25. Callewaert P. R., Rahnama'i M. S., Biallosterski B. T., et al. (2010). Scrotal approach to both palpable and impalpable undescended testes: Should it become our first choice? *Urology, 76*(1), 73–76.

26. Tomiyama H., Sasaki Y., Huynh J., et al. (2005). Testicular descent, cryptorchidism and inguinal hernia: The Melbourne perspective. *Journal of Pediatric Urology, 1*(1), 11–25.

27. Chan E., Wayne C., Nasr A., et al.; FRCSC for Canadian Association of Pediatric Surgeon Evidence-Based Resource. (2014). Ideal timing of orchiopexy: A systematic review. *Pediatric Surgery International, 30*(1), 87–97.

28. Merriman L., Kirsch A. (2012). Varicocele in adolescence: Where are we now? *Current Urology Reports, 13*(4), 311–317.

29. Samplaski M. K., Yu C., Kattan M. W., et al. (2014). Nomograms for predicting changes in semen parameters in infertile men after varicocele repair. *Fertility and Sterility, 102*(1), 68–74.

30. Drlík M., Kočvara R. (2013). Torsion of spermatic cord in children: A review. *Journal of Pediatric Urology, 9*(3), 259–266.

31. Callewaert P. R., Kerrebroeck P. E. (2010). New insights into perinatal testicular torsion. *European Journal of Pediatrics, 169*(6), 705–712.

32. DaJusta D. G., Granberg C. F., Villanueva C., et al. (2013). Contemporary review of testicular torsion: New concepts, emerging technologies and potential therapeutics. *Journal of Pediatric Urology, 9*(6 Pt A), 723–730.

33. Tracy C., Costabile R. (2009). The evaluation and treatment of acute epididymitis in a large university based population: Are CDC guidelines being followed? *World Journal of Urology, 27*(2), 259–263.

34. Trojian T. H., Lishnak T. S., Heiman D. (2009). Epididymitis and orchitis: An overview. *American Family Physician, 79*(7), 583–587.

35. Davis N. F., McGuire B. B., Mahon J. A., et al. (2010). The increasing incidence of mumps orchitis: A comprehensive review. *BJU International, 105*(8), 1060–1065.

36. Lane T. M., Hines J. (2006). The management of mumps orchitis. *BJU International, 97*(1), 1–2.

37. Waldron H. A. (1983). A brief history of scrotal cancer. *British Journal of Industrial Medicine, 40*(4), 390–401.

38. Vandeweyer E., Deraemaecker R. (2000). Basal cell carcinoma of the scrotum. *Journal of Urology, 163*(3), 914.

39. American Society of Clinical Oncology (ASCO). (2014). Testicular cancer overview. Available online at: http://www.cancer.net/cancer-types/testicular-cancer/overview. Accessed December 8, 2014.

40. Canadian Cancer Society. (2014). Testicular cancer. Available online at: https://www.cancer.ca/en/cancer-information/cancer-type/testicular/testicular-cancer/?region=on. Accessed December 8, 2014.

41. Bosl G. J., Feldman D. R., Bajorin D. F., et al. (2011). Chapter 99: Cancer of the testes. In DeVita V. T., Hellman S., Rosenberg S. A. (Eds.), *Cancer: Principles and practice of oncology* (9th ed.). Philadelphia, PA: Lippincott Williams & Wilkins.

42. Goroll A. H., Mulley A. G. (2009). *Primary care medicine* (6th ed.). Philadelphia, PA: Lippincott Williams & Wilkins.

43. Canadian Cancer Society. (2014). Detecting testicular cancer. Available online at: https://www.cancer.ca/en/prevention-and-screening/early-detection-and-screening/finding-cancer-early/detecting-testicular-cancer/?region = on. Accessed December 8, 2014.

44. Abouassaly R., Fossa S. D., Giwercman A., et al. (2011). Sequelae of treatment in long-term survivors of testis cancer. *European Urology, 60*(3), 516–526.

45. Public Health Agency of Canada (PHAC). (2013). Prostatitis. Available online at: http://www.phac-aspc.gc.ca/std-mts/sti-its/cgsti-ldcits/section-4-5-eng.php. Accessed December 8, 2014.

46. Wagenlehner F.M., Pilatz A., Bschleipfer T., et al. (2013). Bacterial prostatitis. *World Journal of Urology, 31*(4), 711–716.

47. Thiruchelvam N. (2014). Benign prostatic hyperplasia. *Surgery (Oxford), 32*(6), 314–322.

48. Ribal M. J. (2013). The link between benign prostatic hyperplasia and inflammation. *European Urology Supplements, 12*(5), 103–109.

49. Sarma A. V., Parsons J. K., McVary K., et al. (2009). Diabetes and benign prostatic hyperplasia/lower urinary tract symptoms: What do we know? *Journal of Urology, 182*(6), S32–S37.

50. Nickel J. C., Méndez-Probst C. E., Whelan T. F., et al. (2010). 2010 Update: Guidelines for the management of benign prostatic hyperplasia. *Canadian Urological Association Journal, 4*(5), 310–316.

51. Canadian Cancer Society. (2014). Prostate cancer. Available online at: http://www.cancer.ca/en/cancer-information/cancer-type/prostate/prostate-cancer/?region=on. Accessed December 8, 2014.

52. Canadian Cancer Society. (2014). Prostate-specific antigen (PSA) test. Available online at: http://www.cancer.ca/en/cancer-information/diagnosis-and-treatment/tests-and-procedures/prostate-specific-antigen-psa/?region=on. Accessed December 8, 2014.

53. Luboldt H. J., Schindler J. F., Rubben H. (2007). Age-specific reference ranges for prostate-specific antigen as a marker for prostate cancer. *EAU-EBU Update Series, 5*(1), 38–48.

54. Artibani W. (2012). Landmarks in prostate cancer diagnosis: The biomarkers. *BJU International, 110*(Suppl 1), 8–13.

55. Izawa J. I., Klotz L., Siemens D. R., et al. (2011). Prostate cancer screening: Canadian Guidelines 2011. *Canadian Urological Association Journal, 5*(4), 235–240.

56. Canadian Task Force on Preventive Health Care. (2014). Recommendations on screening for prostate cancer with the prostate-specific antigen test. *Canadian Medical Association Journal, 186*(16), 1225–1234.

Visit the**Point** **http://thePoint.lww.com for animations, journal articles, and more!**

Structure and Function of the Female Reproductive System

45

The female genitourinary system consists of internal paired ovaries, fallopian or uterine tubes, the uterus, vagina, external mons pubis, labia majora, labia minora, clitoris, urethra, and perineal body. Although the female urinary structures are anatomically separate from the genital structures, their anatomic proximity provides a means for cross-contamination and shared symptomatology between the two systems (Fig. 45.1). This chapter focuses on the internal and external genitalia. It includes a discussion of hormonal and physical changes that occur throughout the life cycle in response to the gonadotropic hormones. The reader is referred to a specialty text for a discussion of pregnancy.

REPRODUCTIVE STRUCTURES

After completing this section of the chapter, you should be able to meet the following objectives:

- Describe the anatomic relationship of the structures of the external genitalia.
- Name the three layers of the uterus and describe their function.
- Cite the location of the ovaries in relation to the uterus, fallopian tubes, broad ligaments, and ovarian ligaments.
- Explain the function of the fallopian tubes.
- State the function of endocervical secretions.

External Genitalia

The external genitalia, also known collectively as the vulva, are located at the base of the pelvis in the perineal area and include the mons pubis, labia majora, labia minora, clitoris, and perineal body. The urethra and anus, although not genital structures, usually are considered in a discussion of the external genitalia (Fig. 45.2).

The *mons pubis* is a rounded, skin-covered fat pad located anterior to the symphysis pubis. Puberty stimulates an increase in the amount of fat and the development of darker and coarser hair over the mons. Normal pubic hair distribution in the female follows an inverted triangle with the base centred

FIGURE 45.1 • Female reproductive system as seen in sagittal section. (Adapted from Stephen T. C., Skillen D. L., Day R. A., et al. (2012). *Canadian Jensen's nursing health assessment: A best practice approach* (p. 791). Philadelphia, PA: Lippincott Williams & Wilkins.)

over the mons. Hair colour and texture varies from person to person and among racial groups. There is an abundance of sebaceous glands in the skin that can become infected owing to normal variations in glandular secretions or poor hygiene. The mons pubis is the most common site of pubic lice infestation in the female. The *labia majora* (singular, labium majus) are analogous to the male scrotum. These structures are the outermost lips of the vulva, beginning anteriorly at the base of the mons pubis and ending posteriorly at the anus. The labia

majora are composed of folds of skin and fat and become covered with hair at the onset of puberty. Before puberty, the labia majora have a skin covering similar to that covering the abdomen. With sufficient hormonal stimulation, the labia of a mature woman close over the urethral and vaginal openings; this can change after childbirth or surgery.

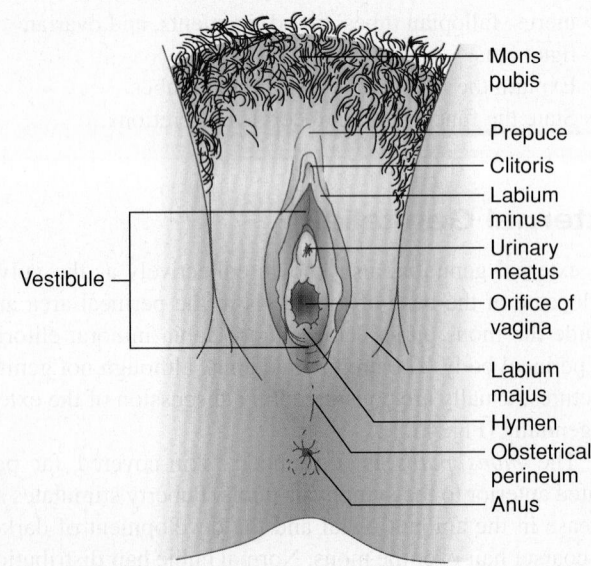

FIGURE 45.2 • External genitalia of the female.

THE FEMALE GENITOURINARY SYSTEM

- The external genitalia (labia majora, labia minora, clitoris, and vestibular glands) surround the openings of the urethra and vagina. Although the female urinary and genital structures are anatomically separate, their close proximity provides a means for cross-contamination and shared symptomatology.

- The internal genitalia of the female reproductive system are specialized to participate in sexual intercourse (the vagina), to produce and maintain the female egg cells (the ovaries), to transport these cells to the site of fertilization (the fallopian tubes), to provide a favourable environment for development of offspring (the uterus), and to produce the female sex hormones (the ovaries).

The *labia minora* (singular, labium minus) are located between the labia majora. These delicate cutaneous structures are smaller than the labia majora and are composed of skin, fat, and some erectile tissue. Unlike the skin of the labia majora, that of the labia minora is hairless and usually light pink.

ood of the clitoris
na. During sexual
d with blood; with
normal size. The
or prepuce, which
minora. The female
ar and nervous sup-
ghly sensitive organ
nulation.
called the *vestibule.*
and vaginal openings
e *urethra,* or urinary
ernal urinary bladder.
clitoris and usually is
clitoris. The urethral
hich have a lubricating
y known as the *introi-*
and internal genitalia.
determined by a con-
men that surrounds the
rcular, or sievelike and
d. Occlusion may occur
partially intact hymen.
hymen does not indicate
tretched without tearing.
At pu...... opening may require sur-
gical intervention to permit discharge of menstrual fluids.

The *perineal body* is that tissue located posterior to the vaginal opening and anterior to the anus. It is composed of fibrous connective tissue and is the site of insertion of several perineal muscles.

Internal Genitalia

Vagina

Connecting the internal and external genitalia is a fibromuscular tube called the *vagina.* The vagina, which is essentially free of sensory nerve fibres, is located behind the urinary bladder and urethra and anterior to the rectum. The uterine cervix projects into the vagina at its upper end, forming recesses called *fornices* (Fig. 45.3). The vagina functions as a route for discharge of menses and other secretions. It also serves as an organ of sexual fulfillment and reproduction.

The membranous vaginal wall forms two longitudinal folds and several transverse folds, or rugae. The vagina is lined with mucus-secreting stratified squamous epithelial cells. Vaginal tissue usually is moist, with a mild acidic pH maintained within the bacteriostatic range of 3.8 to 4.5.

The epithelial cells of the vagina, like other tissues of the reproductive system, respond to changing levels of the ovarian sex hormones. Estrogen stimulates the proliferation and maturation of the vaginal mucosa; this results in a thickening of the vaginal mucosa and an increased glycogen content of the epithelial cells. The glycogen is fermented to lactic acid by the lactobacilli (*i.e.,* Döderlein bacilli) that are part of the normal vaginal flora, accounting for the mildly acid pH of vaginal

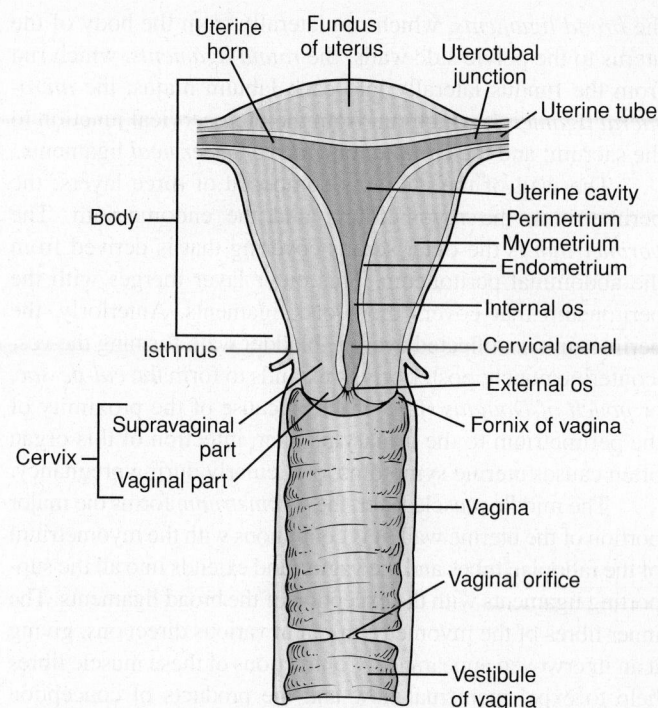

FIGURE 45.3 • Median section of the vagina and uterus. (From Moore K. L., Agur A. M., Dalley A. F. (2011). *Essential clinical anatomy* (4th ed., p. 239). Baltimore, MD: Lippincott Williams & Wilkins.)

fluid. The vaginal ecology can be disrupted at many levels, rendering it susceptible to infection. Pregnancy and the use of oral contraceptive agents increase the amount of estrogen in the system. Diabetes or a prediabetic state may increase the glycogen content of the cells. The use of systemic antibiotics may decrease the number of lactobacilli in the vagina.

Decreased estrogen stimulation after menopause causes the vaginal mucosa to become thin and dry, often resulting in dyspareunia (*i.e.,* painful intercourse), atrophic vaginitis, and occasionally in vaginal bleeding. Estrogen levels can be estimated by means of vaginal scrapings obtained during a routine pelvic examination. The scrapings are used for a test, the *maturation index,* that examines the cellular structure and configuration of the vaginal epithelial cells. The maturation index determines the ratio of parabasal (least mature), intermediate, and superficial (most mature) cells. Typically, this index is 0–40–60 during the reproductive years. With diminished estrogen levels, there is a shift to the left, producing an index of 30–40–30 during the perimenopausal period and an index of 75–25–0 during the postmenopausal period.

Uterus and Cervix

The uterus is a thick-walled, muscular organ. This pear-shaped, hollow structure is located between the bladder and the rectum. The uterus can be divided into three parts: the portion above the insertion of the fallopian tubes, called the *fundus;* the lower, constricted part, called the *cervix;* and the portion between the fundus and the cervix, called the *body of the uterus.* The uterus is supported on both sides by four sets of ligaments:

the *broad ligaments,* which run laterally from the body of the uterus to the pelvic side walls; the *round ligaments,* which run from the fundus laterally into each labium majus; the *utero-sacral ligaments,* which run from the uterocervical junction to the sacrum; and the *cardinal* or *transverse cervical* ligaments.

The wall of the uterus is composed of three layers: the perimetrium, the myometrium, and the endometrium. The *perimetrium* is the outer serous covering that is derived from the abdominal peritoneum. This outer layer merges with the peritoneum that covers the broad ligaments. Anteriorly, the perimetrium is reflected over the bladder wall, forming the vesicouterine pouch; posteriorly, it extends to form the *cul-de-sac,* or *pouch of Douglas* (Fig. 45.1). Because of the proximity of the perimetrium to the urinary bladder, infection of this organ often causes uterine symptoms, particularly during pregnancy.

The middle muscle layer, the *myometrium,* forms the major portion of the uterine wall. It is continuous with the myometrium of the fallopian tubes and the vagina and extends into all the supporting ligaments with the exception of the broad ligaments. The inner fibres of the myometrium run in various directions, giving it an interwoven appearance. Contractions of these muscle fibres help to expel menstrual flow and the products of conception during miscarriage or childbirth. When pain accompanies the contractions associated with menses, it is called *dysmenorrhea.* The myometrium has an amazing ability to change length during pregnancy and labour, increasing the uterine capacity from 70 g to 1,100 g to accommodate gestation.[1]

The *endometrium,* the inner layer of the uterus, is continuous with the lining of the fallopian tubes and vagina. The endometrium is made up of a basal and a superficial layer. The superficial layer is shed during menstruation and regenerated by cells of the basal layer. Ciliated cells promote the movement of tubal/uterine secretions out of the uterine cavity into the vagina.

The round *cervix* is the neck of the uterus that projects into the vagina. The cervix is a firm structure, composed of a connective tissue matrix of glands and muscular tissue elements that become soft and pliable under the influence of hormones produced during pregnancy. Glandular tissue provides a rich supply of protective mucus that changes in character and quantity during the menstrual cycle and during pregnancy. The cervix is richly supplied with blood from the uterine artery and can be a site of significant blood loss during delivery.

The opening of the cervix, the os, forms a pathway between the uterus and the vagina. The vaginal opening is called the *external os* and the uterine opening is called the *internal os* (Fig. 45.3). The space between these two openings is the endocervical canal. Secretions from the columnar epithelium of the endocervix protect the uterus from infection, alter receptivity to sperm, and form a mucoid "plug" during pregnancy. The endocervical canal provides a route for menstrual discharge and sperm entrance.

Fallopian Tubes

The *fallopian,* or uterine, tubes are slender, cylindrical structures attached bilaterally to the uterus and supported by the upper folds of the broad ligament. The end of the fallopian tube nearest the ovary forms a funnel-like opening with fringed, finger-like projections, called *fimbriae,* that pick up the ovum after its release into the peritoneal cavity after ovulation (Fig. 45.4). The fallopian tubes are formed of smooth muscle and lined with a ciliated, mucus-producing epithelial layer. The beating of the cilia, along with contractile movements of the smooth muscle, propels the nonmobile ovum

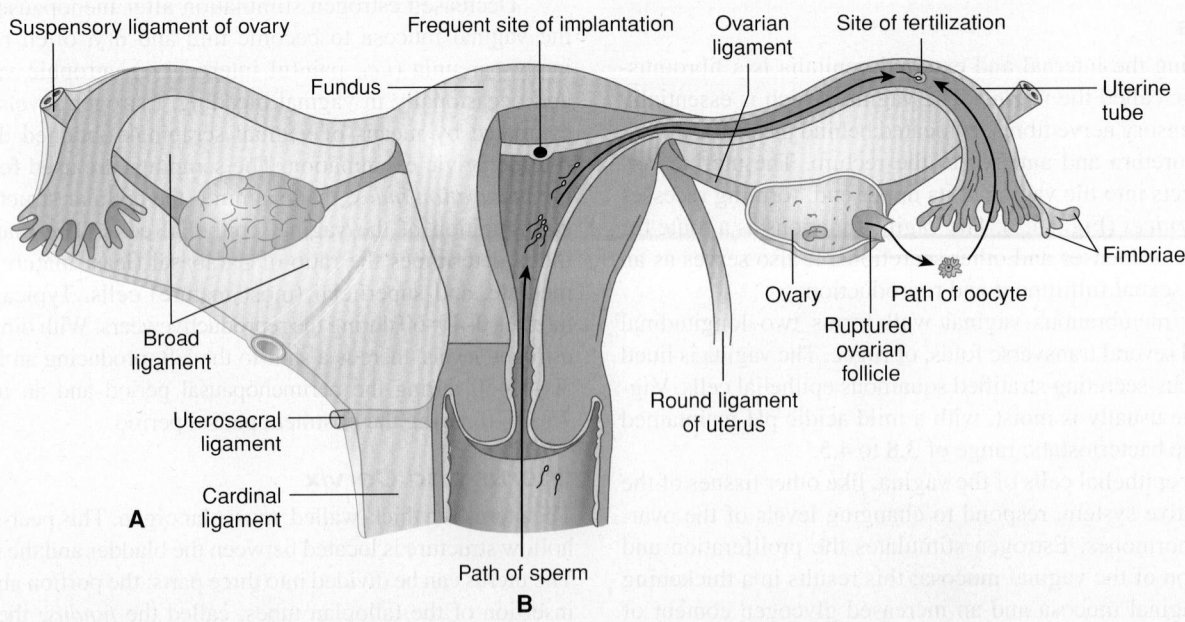

FIGURE 45.4 • Schematic drawing of female reproductive organs, showing (**A**) suspensory ligament of the ovary and the broad, uterosacral, and cardinal ligaments on the left, and (**B**) the path of the oocyte as it moves from the ovary into the fallopian (uterine) tube; the path of sperm is also shown, as is the usual site of fertilization.

towards the uterus. If coitus has occurred recently, fertilization normally occurs in the middle to outer portion of the fallopian tube. Besides providing a passageway for ova and sperm, the fallopian tubes provide for drainage of tubal secretions into the uterus.

Ovaries

By the third month of fetal life, the *ovaries* have fully developed and descended to their permanent pelvic position. Remnants of the primitive genital system provide lateral supporting attachments to the uterus; in the mature female, these supporting structures evolve into the round and suspensory ligaments. Remnants that do not evolve may form cysts, which may become symptomatic later in life.

Oogenesis is the process of generation of ova by mitotic division that begins at the sixth week of fetal life. These primitive germ cells ultimately provide the 1 to 2 million oocytes that are present in the ovaries at birth. At puberty, this number is reduced through *apoptosis* (organized, programmed cell death) or *atresia* (process of cell degeneration) to approximately 200,000, and only 400 to 500 of these oocytes will actually be released during ovulation.[2,3]

The neonate's ovaries are smooth, pale, and elongated. They become shorter, thicker, and heavier before the onset of menarche, which is initiated by pituitary influence. The initial hormonal stimulus for this development is believed to come from ovarian rather than systemic estrogen.

In the reproductive-aged female, the ovaries are flat, almond-shaped structures that are 3 to 5 cm long and weigh 2 to 3 g, but with menopause there is a decrease in function and size of the ovaries. The ovaries are located on either side of the uterus below the fimbriated ends of the two oviducts, or fallopian tubes. The ovaries are attached to the posterior surface of the broad ligament and to the uterus by the ovarian ligament. They are covered with a thin layer of surface epithelium that is continuous with the lining of the peritoneum. The integrity of this covering is periodically broken at the time of ovulation.

The ovaries, like the male testes, have a dual function: they store the female germ cells, or ova, and produce the female sex hormones, estrogen and progesterone. Unlike the male gonads, which produce sperm throughout a man's reproductive life, the female gonads contain a fixed number of ova at birth that diminishes throughout a woman's life.

Structurally, the mature ovary is divided into a highly vascular inner medulla, which contains supporting connective tissue, and an outer cortex of stroma and epithelial follicles (*i.e.,* vesicles), which contain the primary oocytes, or germ cells. After puberty, the pituitary gonadotropic hormones—follicle-stimulating hormone (FSH) and luteinizing hormone (LH)—stimulate the primordial follicles to develop into *mature graafian follicles*. The graafian follicle produces estrogen, which begins to stimulate the development of the endometrium in the uterus. Although several follicles begin to develop during each ovulatory cycle, only one or two complete the entire developmental process and rupture to release a mature ovum. After ovulation, the follicle becomes luteinized; as the corpus luteum, it produces estrogen and progesterone to support the endometrium until conception occurs or the cycle begins again.[1–3]

IN SUMMARY

The female reproductive system consists of internal paired ovaries, fallopian or uterine tubes, uterus, vagina, external mons pubis, labia majora, labia minora, clitoris, urethra, and perineal body. The genitourinary system as a whole serves sexual and reproductive functions throughout the life cycle. The uterus is a thick-walled, muscular organ. The wall of the uterus is composed of three layers: the outer perimetrium; the myometrium or muscle layer, which is continuous with the myometrium of the fallopian tubes and the vagina; and the inner lining or endometrium, which is continuous with the lining of the fallopian tubes and vagina. The gonads, or ovaries, which are internal in the female (unlike the testes in the male), have the dual function of storing the female germ cells, or ova, and producing the female sex hormones. Through the regulation and release of sex hormones, the ovaries influence the development of secondary sexual characteristics, regulation of menstrual cycles, maintenance of pregnancy, and advent of menopause.

MENSTRUAL CYCLE

After completing this section of the chapter, you should be able to meet the following objectives:

- Describe the feedback control of estrogen and progesterone levels by means of gonadotropin-releasing hormone, LH, FSH, and ovarian follicle function.
- List the actions of estrogen and progesterone.
- Describe the four functional compartments of the ovary.
- Relate FSH and LH levels to the stages of follicle development and to estrogen and progesterone production.
- Describe the endometrial changes that occur during the menstrual cycle.
- Describe the composition of normal cervical mucus and the changes that occur during the menstrual cycle.
- Describe the physiology of normal menopause.

Between menarche (*i.e.,* first menstrual bleeding) and menopause (*i.e.,* last menstrual bleeding), the female reproductive system undergoes cyclic changes called the *menstrual cycle.* This includes the maturation and release of oocytes from the ovary during ovulation and periodic vaginal bleeding resulting from the shedding of the endometrial lining. It is not necessary for a woman to ovulate to menstruate. Anovulatory cycles do occur, leading to irregular menses. The menstrual cycle produces changes in the breasts, uterus, skin, and ovaries.

The maintenance of the cycle affects biologic and sociologic aspects of a woman's life, including fertility, reproduction, sexuality, and femaleness.

MENSTRUAL CYCLE

- The menstrual cycle begins at menarche and continues until menopause. It includes the maturation and release of oocytes from the ovary during ovulation and periodic vaginal bleeding resulting from the shedding of the endometrial lining.
- The menstrual cycle is controlled by rhythmic synthesis and release of ovarian hormones (the estrogens and progesterone) under feedback control from the hypothalamic gonadotropin-releasing hormone and the anterior pituitary gonadotropic follicle-stimulating and luteinizing hormones.

Hormonal Control

Normal menstrual function results from interactions among the central nervous system, hypothalamus, anterior pituitary, ovaries, and associated target tissues (Fig. 45.5). Although each part of the system is essential to normal function, the ovaries are primarily responsible for controlling the cyclic changes and the length of the menstrual cycle. In most women in the middle reproductive years, menstrual bleeding occurs every 25 to 35 days, with a median length of 28 days.

The hormonal control of the menstrual cycle is complex. For example, the biosynthesis of estrogens that occurs in adipose tissue may be a significant source of the hormone. There is evidence that a certain minimum body weight (48 kg) and fat content (16% to 22%) are necessary for menarche to occur and for the menstrual cycle to be maintained.[4] This is supported by the observation of amenorrhea in women with anorexia nervosa, chronic disease, and malnutrition and in

FIGURE 45.5 • Hormonal and morphologic changes during the normal menstrual cycle. (From Stephen T. C., Skillen D. L., Day R. A., et al. (2012). *Canadian Jensen's nursing health assessment: A best practice approach* (p. 792). Philadelphia, PA: Lippincott Williams & Wilkins.)

those who are long-distance runners. In women with anorexia nervosa, gonadotropin and estradiol secretion, including LH release and responsiveness to the hypothalamic gonadotropin-releasing hormone (GnRH), can revert to prepubertal levels. With resumption of weight gain and attainment of sufficient body mass, the normal hormonal pattern usually is reinstated. Obesity or significant weight gain also are associated with oligomenorrhea or amenorrhea and infertility, although the mechanism is not well understood.

Hypothalamic and Pituitary Hormones

Growth, prepubertal maturation, the reproductive cycle, and sex hormone secretion in males and females are regulated by FSH and LH from the anterior pituitary gland (Fig. 45.6). Because these hormones promote the growth of cells in the ovaries and testes as a means of stimulating the production of sex hormones, they are called the *gonadotropic hormones*. GnRH from the hypothalamus stimulates the secretion of LH and FSH. In addition to LH and FSH, the anterior pituitary also secretes *prolactin*. The primary function of prolactin is the stimulation of lactation in the postpartum period. During pregnancy, prolactin, along with other hormones such as estrogen, progesterone, insulin, and cortisol, contributes to breast development in preparation for lactation. Although prolactin does not appear to play a physiologic role in ovarian function,

hyperprolactinemia leads to hypogonadism. This may include an initial shortening of the luteal phase with subsequent anovulation, oligomenorrhea or amenorrhea, and infertility. The hypothalamic control of prolactin secretion is primarily inhibitory, and dopamine is the most important inhibitory factor. Hyperprolactinemia may occur as an adverse effect of drug treatment using phenothiazine derivatives (*i.e.,* antipsychotic drugs that block dopamine receptors).

Ovarian Hormones

The ovaries produce estrogens, progesterone, and androgens. Ovarian hormones are secreted in a cyclic pattern as a result of the interaction between the hypothalamic GnRH and the pituitary gonadotropic hormones, FSH and LH. The steroid sex hormones enter cells by passive diffusion, bind to specific receptor proteins in the cytoplasm, and then move to the nucleus, where they bind to specific sites on the chromosomes. These hormones exert their effects through gene–hormone interactions that stimulate the synthesis of specific messenger ribonucleic acid (mRNA). In addition, estrogen appears to have the ability to influence cell activity through other, nongenomic mechanisms. These nongenomic effects take place in cells that have no steroid receptors, possibly mediated by other membrane receptors. This may explain in part some of the nonreproductive effects of estrogen. An example of a nongenomic cardioprotective effect might be the antioxidant activity of estrogen in preventing endothelial injury that can lead to platelet adherence.[5] The number of hormonal receptor sites on a cell is not fixed; evidence suggests that they are constantly being removed and replaced. An increase or a decrease in the number of receptors can serve as a mechanism for regulating hormonal activity. For example, estrogen may induce the development of an increased number of estrogen receptors in some tissues and may stimulate the synthesis of progesterone receptors in others. In contrast, progesterone may cause a reduction in the number of estrogen and progesterone receptors.

There are two types of estrogen receptors that differ in structure (*i.e.,* ERα and ERβ), tissue distribution (*i.e.,* some organs have both types in equal numbers, other organs have only one type, and some organs have both but within different cell types), and expression. The estrogen receptor subtypes and their expression are primary factors that determine tissue specific estrogen responsiveness.[6,7] Likewise, the progesterone receptor has two major forms (A and B), expressed by a single gene, but promoted differently in a complex system of transcription regulation.

Estrogens. Estrogens are a family of structurally related female sex hormones synthesized and secreted by cells in the ovaries and, in small amounts, by cells in the adrenal cortex. Androgens can be converted to estrogens peripherally, especially in fat tissue. Three estrogens occur naturally in humans: estrone (E_1), estradiol (E_2), and estriol (E_3).[7] Of these, estradiol is the most biologically potent and abundantly secreted product of the ovary. Estrogens are secreted throughout the menstrual cycle. Two peaks occur: one before ovulation and one in the middle of the luteal phase. Estrogens are transported

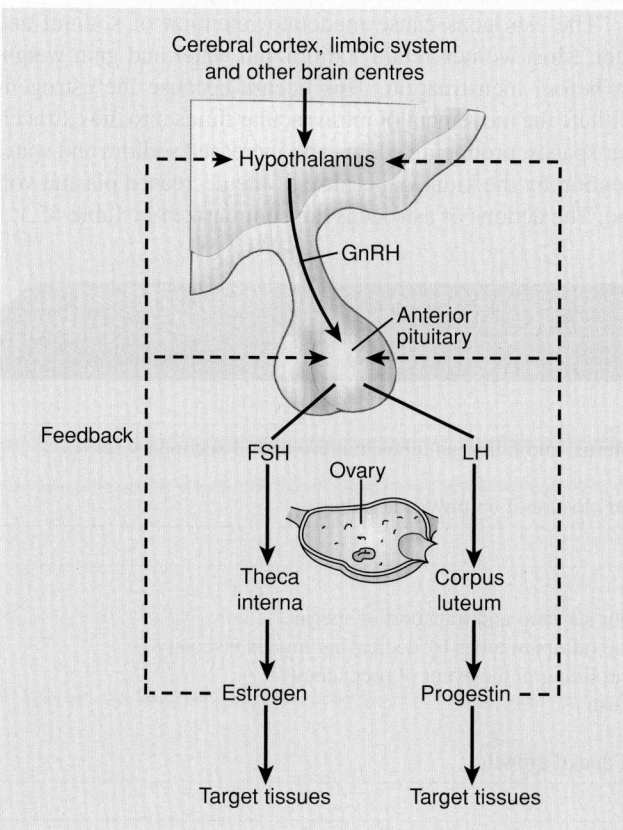

FIGURE 45.6 • Hypothalamic–pituitary feedback control of estrogen and progesterone levels in the female. The *dashed line* represents negative feedback.

in the blood bound to plasma proteins (such as albumin and sex hormone-binding globulin [SHBG] which can also bind testosterone), inactivated and conjugated in the liver, and then excreted in the bile.

Estrogens are necessary for normal female physical maturation. In concert with other hormones, estrogens provide for the reproductive processes of ovulation, implantation of the products of conception, pregnancy, parturition, and lactation by stimulating the development and maintaining the growth of the accessory organs. In the absence of androgens, estrogens stimulate the intrauterine development of the vagina, uterus, and uterine tubes from the embryonic müllerian system. They also stimulate the stromal development and ductal growth of the breasts at puberty, are responsible for the accelerated pubertal skeletal growth phase and for closure of the epiphyses of the long bones, contribute to the growth of axillary and pubic hair, and alter the distribution of body fat to produce the typical female body contours, including the accumulation of body fat around the hips and breasts. Larger quantities of estrogen stimulate pigmentation of the skin in the nipple, areolar, and genital regions.

In addition to their effects on the growth of uterine muscle, estrogens play an important role in the development of the endometrial lining. During anovulatory cycles, continued exposure to estrogens for prolonged periods leads to abnormal hyperplasia of the endometrium and abnormal bleeding patterns. When estrogen production is poorly coordinated during the normal menstrual period, inappropriate bleeding and shedding of the endometrium also can occur (see Chapter 46).

Estrogens have a number of important extragenital metabolic effects. They are responsible for maintaining the normal structure of skin and blood vessels in women. Estrogens decrease the rate of bone resorption by antagonizing the effects of parathyroid hormone on bone; for this reason, osteoporosis is a common problem in estrogen-deficient postmenopausal women. In the liver, estrogens increase the synthesis of transport proteins for thyroxine, estrogen, testosterone, and other hormones. Estrogens also affect the composition of the plasma lipoproteins. They produce an increase in high-density lipoproteins (HDLs), a slight reduction in low-density lipoproteins (LDLs), and a reduction in cholesterol levels (see Chapter 22).

Estrogens have additional cardioprotective actions, including direct atheroprotective effects on the arterial wall (augmentation of vasodilating and antiplatelet aggregation factors such as nitric oxide and prostacyclin), vasodilation through endothelium-independent mechanisms, antioxidant activity, reduction of levels of angiotensin-converting enzyme and renin, reduction of homocysteine levels, improvement of peripheral glucose metabolism with improved insulin sensitivity, and direct effects on cardiac function (*i.e.,* angiogenesis promoting). Estrogens also increase plasma triglyceride levels and they enhance the coagulability of blood by effecting increased circulating levels of plasminogen and factors II, VII, IX, and X.

Estrogens are thought to have both neurotropic and neuroprotective effects on cognitive function and memory, as they affect the neurons. It remains unclear whether estrogens play a role in the prevention of Alzheimer disease through anti-inflammatory mechanisms to prevent vascular injury, increased cerebral blood flow, and altered brain activation. Estrogens promote dendritic branching and enhance presynaptic and postsynaptic signal transmission through increased production of neurotransmitters and receptors.[4]

The estrogens cause moderate retention of sodium and water. Most women retain sodium and water and gain weight just before menstruation. This occurs because the estrogens facilitate the movement of intravascular fluids into the extracellular spaces, producing edema and increased sodium and water retention by the kidneys because of the decreased plasma volume. The actions of estrogens are summarized in Table 45.1.

TABLE 45.1 ACTIONS OF ESTROGENS

GENERAL FUNCTION	SPECIFIC ACTIONS
Growth and Development	
Reproductive organs	Stimulate development of vagina, uterus, and fallopian tubes in utero and of secondary sex characteristics during puberty
Skeleton	Accelerate growth of long bones and closure of epiphyses at puberty
Reproductive Processes	
Ovulation	Promote growth of ovarian follicles
Fertilization	Alter the cervical secretions to favour survival and transport of sperm
	Promote motility of sperm within the fallopian tubes by decreasing mucus viscosity
Implantation	Promote development of endometrial lining in the event of pregnancy
Vagina	Proliferate and cornify vaginal mucosa
Cervix	Increase mucus consistency
Breasts	Stimulate stromal development and ductal growth
General Metabolic Effects	
Bone resorption	Decrease rate of bone resorption
Plasma proteins	Increase production of thyroid and other binding globulins
Lipids	Increase high-density lipoproteins and triglycerides and slightly decrease low-density lipoproteins

Progesterone. Although the word *progesterone* refers to a substance that maintains pregnancy, progesterone is secreted as part of the normal menstrual cycle. The corpus luteum of the ovary secretes large amounts of progesterone after ovulation, and the adrenal cortex secretes small amounts. The hormone circulates in the blood, attached to a specific plasma protein. It is metabolized in the liver and conjugated for excretion in the bile.

The local effects of progesterone on reproductive organs include the glandular development of the lobular and alveolar tissue of the breasts and the cyclic glandular development of the endometrium. Progesterone also can compete with aldosterone at the level of the renal tubule, causing a decrease in sodium reabsorption, with a resultant increase in secretion of aldosterone by the adrenal cortex, as occurs in pregnancy. Although the mechanism is uncertain, progesterone is responsible for the increase in basal body temperature that occurs with ovulation. Smooth muscle relaxation under the influence of progesterone plays an important role in maintaining pregnancy by decreasing uterine contractions, and is responsible for many of the common discomforts of pregnancy, such as edema, nausea, constipation, flatulence, and headaches. The increased progesterone present during pregnancy and the luteal phase of the menstrual cycle enhances the ventilatory response to carbon dioxide, leading to a measurable change in arterial and alveolar carbon dioxide (PCO$_2$) levels.

Androgens. In addition to estrogen and progesterone, the normal female produces androgens such as testosterone, dehydroepiandrosterone (DHEA) and its sulphate (DHEA-S). Approximately 25% of these androgens are secreted from the ovaries, 25% from the adrenal cortex, and 50% from ovarian or adrenal precursors. In the female, androgens contribute to normal hair growth at puberty and may have other important metabolic effects.

Ovarian Follicle Development and Ovulation

The tissues of the adult ovary can be conveniently divided into four compartments, or units: the stroma, or supporting tissue; the interstitial cells; the follicles; and the corpus luteum. The *stroma* is the connective tissue substance of the ovary in which the follicles are distributed. The *interstitial cells* are estrogen-secreting cells that resemble the Leydig cells, or interstitial cells, of the testes.

Beginning at puberty, a cyclic rise in the anterior pituitary hormones FSH and LH stimulates the development of several graafian, or mature, follicles. Follicles at all stages of development can be found in both ovaries, except in menopausal women (Fig. 45.7). Most follicles exist as primary follicles, each of which consists of a round oocyte surrounded by a single layer of flattened, epithelium-derived granulosa cells and a basement membrane. The primary follicles constitute an

FIGURE 45.7 • A: Cross-section of preovulatory follicle. **B:** Schematic diagram of an ovary, showing the sequence of events in the origin, growth, and rupture of an ovarian follicle and the formation and retrogression of a corpus luteum. The atretic follicles are those that show signs of degeneration and death.

inactive pool of follicles from which all the ovulating follicles develop. Under the influence of endocrine stimulation, 6 to 12 primary follicles develop into secondary follicles once every ovulatory cycle. During the development of the secondary follicle, the primary oocyte increases in size, and the granulosa cells proliferate to form a multilayered wall around it. During this time, a membrane called the *zona pellucida* develops and surrounds the oocyte and small pockets of fluid begin to appear between the granulosa cells. Blood vessels, however, do not penetrate the basement membrane; the granulosa cell layer remains avascular until after ovulation has occurred.

As the follicles mature, FSH stimulates the development of the cell layers. Cells from the surrounding stromal tissue align themselves to form a cellular wall called the *theca.* The cells of the theca become differentiated into two layers: an inner theca interna, which lies adjacent to the follicular cells, and an outer theca externa. As the follicle enlarges, a single large cavity, or *antrum,* is formed, and a portion of the granulosa cells and the oocyte are displaced to one side of the follicle by the fluid that accumulates. The secondary oocyte remains surrounded by a crown of granulosa cells, the corona radiata. As the follicle ripens, ovarian estrogen is produced by the granulosa cells. Selection of a dominant follicle occurs with the conversion to an estrogen microenvironment. The lesser follicles, although continuing to produce some estrogen, atrophy or become atretic. The dominant follicle accumulates a greater mass of granulosa cells, and the theca becomes richly vascular, giving the follicle a hyperemic appearance. High levels of estrogen exert a negative feedback effect on FSH, inhibiting multiple follicular development and causing an increase in LH levels. This represents the follicular stage of the menstrual cycle. As estrogen suppresses FSH, the actions of LH predominate, and the mature follicle (measuring approximately 20 mm) bursts; the oocyte, along with the corona radiata, is ejected from the follicle. The ovum normally is then picked up and transported through the fallopian tube towards the uterus.

After ovulation, the follicle collapses, and the luteal stage of the menstrual cycle begins. The granulosa cells are invaded by blood vessels and yellow lipochrome-bearing cells from the theca layer. A rapid accumulation of blood and fluid forms a mass called the *corpus luteum.* Leakage of this blood onto the peritoneal surface that surrounds the ovary is thought to contribute to the *mittelschmerz* ("middle [or intermenstrual] pain") of ovulation. During the luteal stage, progesterone is secreted from the corpus luteum. If fertilization does not take place, the corpus luteum atrophies and is replaced by white scar tissue called the *corpus albicans;* the hormonal support of the endometrium is withdrawn and menstruation occurs. In the event of fertilization, a hormone called *human chorionic gonadotropin* (hCG) is produced by the trophoblastic cells in the blastocyst. This hormone prevents luteal regression. The corpus luteum remains functional for 3 months and provides hormonal support for pregnancy until the placenta is fully functional. Figure 45.5 shows the hormonal changes that occur during the development of the ovarian follicle and ovulation.

Endometrial Changes

The endometrium consists of two distinct layers, or zones, that are responsive to hormonal stimulation: a basal layer and a functional layer. The *basal layer* lies adjacent to the myometrium and is not sloughed off during menstruation. The *functional layer* arises from the basal layer and undergoes proliferative changes and menstrual sloughing. It can be subdivided into two components: a thin, superficial, compact layer and a deeper spongiosa layer that makes up most of the secretory and fully developed endometrium. The endometrial cycle can be divided into three phases: the proliferative, or preovulatory, phase, during which the glands and stroma of the superficial layer grow rapidly under the influence of estrogen; the secretory, or postovulatory, phase, during which progesterone produces glandular dilation and active mucus secretion and the endometrium becomes highly vascular and edematous; and the menstrual phase, during which the superficial layer degenerates and sloughs off (Fig. 45.5).

Cervical Mucus Changes

Cervical mucus is a complex, heterogeneous secretion produced by the glands of the endocervix. It is composed of 92% to 98% water and 1% inorganic salts, mainly sodium chloride. The mucus also contains simple sugars, polysaccharides, proteins, and glycoproteins. Its pH usually is alkaline, ranging from 6.5 to 9.0. Its characteristics are strongly influenced by serum levels of estrogen and progesterone. Estrogen stimulates the production of large amounts of clear, watery mucus through which sperm can penetrate most easily. Progesterone, even in the presence of estrogen, reduces the secretion of mucus. During the luteal phase of the menstrual cycle, mucus is scant, viscous, and cellular.

Two methods are used to examine the properties of cervical mucus and correlate them with hormonal activity. *Spinnbarkeit* is the property that allows cervical mucus to be stretched or drawn into a thread. Spinnbarkeit can be estimated by stretching a sample of cervical mucus between two glass slides and measuring the maximum length of the thread before it breaks. At mid-cycle, spinnbarkeit usually exceeds 10 cm. A second method of estimating hormonal levels is *ferning,* or arborization. Ferning refers to the characteristic microscopic pattern that results from the crystallization of the inorganic salts in the cervical mucus when it is dried. As the estrogen levels increase, the composition of the cervical mucus changes, so that dried mucus begins to demonstrate ferning in the later part of the follicular phase. The absence of ferning can indicate inadequate estrogen stimulation of the endocervical glands or inhibition of the endocervical glands by increased secretion of progesterone. Persistent ferning throughout the menstrual cycle suggests anovulatory cycles or insufficient progesterone secretion.

Menopause

Menopause is the cessation of menstrual cycles. Like menarche, it is more of a process than a single event. Most women typically begin to experience menopausal symptoms between 40 and 58 years of age. *Perimenopause* includes the time period prior to menopause and the first 12 months after cessation of menses. This usually lasts for 2 to 8 years and is characterized by menstrual irregularity and other menopausal symptoms. *Climacteric* is a less common term that refers to the entire transition to the nonreproductive period of life. Premature ovarian failure describes the approximately 1% of women who experience menopause before the age of 40 years. A woman who has not menstruated for a full year or who has a persistently elevated FSH level (>30 IU/L) is considered menopausal.[4,8]

Functional Changes

Menopause results from the gradual cessation of ovarian function and the resultant diminished levels of estrogen. Although estrogens derived from the adrenal cortex continue to circulate in a woman's body, they are insufficient to maintain the secondary sexual characteristics in the same manner as ovarian estrogens. As a result, body hair, skin elasticity, and subcutaneous fat decrease. The breasts become pendulous with a decrease in tissue mass, leaving only the ducts, fat, and connective tissue. The ovaries and uterus diminish in size; and the cervix and vagina become pale and friable. Vaginal pH increases, and levels above 4.5 can be associated with estrogen deficiency.

Problems that can arise as a result of urogenital atrophy include vaginal dryness, urinary stress incontinence, urgency, nocturia, vaginitis, and recurrent urinary tract infections (UTIs). The woman may find intercourse painful and traumatic, although some type of commercially prepared vaginal lubrication may be helpful.

Systemically, a woman may experience significant vasomotor instability secondary to the decrease in estrogens and the relative increase in other hormones, including FSH, LH, GnRH, DHEA, androstenedione, epinephrine, corticotropin, b-endorphin, growth hormone, and calcitonin gene-related peptide. This instability may give rise to "hot flashes," palpitations, dizziness, and headaches as the blood vessels dilate. Despite the association with these biochemical changes, the underlying cause of hot flashes is unknown.[6] Tremendous variation exists in the onset, frequency, severity, and length of time that women experience hot flashes. When they occur at night and are accompanied by significant perspiration, they are referred to as *night sweats*. Insomnia as well as frequent awakening because of vasomotor symptoms can lead to sleep deprivation. A woman may experience irritability, anxiety, and depression as a result of these uncontrollable and unpredictable events.

In addition to changes that closely follow the cessation of ovarian function, there are changes that over many years influence the health and well-being of postmenopausal women. Consequences of long-term estrogen deprivation include osteoporosis due to an imbalance in bone remodelling (*i.e.,* bone resorption occurs at a faster rate than bone formation), and an increased risk for cardiovascular disease (atherosclerosis is accelerated), which is the leading cause of death for women after menopause. Other potential health threats, which reflect both aging and cessation of ovarian function, are loss of vision due to macular degeneration, and cognitive impairment.

Hormone Therapy

Over the past four to five decades, hormone therapy (HT) became increasingly prescribed for postmenopausal women. Initially, HT was used only for symptom management, and later for prevention of osteoporosis. During the 1990s, HT evolved to the status of *replacement* (HRT) for a vital hormone lost due to an endocrine organ failure (menopause). It was routinely offered to all postmenopausal women based on mounting evidence of preventive benefits in numerous areas. During this time, data from observational studies demonstrated a 50% reduction in coronary heart disease (CHD) mortality rates in women using HT.[4,9] Other reported advantages to HT included a reduced risk of neurocognitive loss, decreased risk of colon cancer,[10] increased bone density, and reduced risk of periodontal disease.

The type of HT prescribed was determined by whether or not the woman had an intact uterus. Women with an intact uterus received a combination of estrogen and progesterone (EPT or HRT), and those who had previously had their uterus removed received estrogen (ET or ERT) only. The addition of progesterone to HT was the established protocol for women with an intact uterus because the association between unopposed estrogen and the development of endometrial cancer was noted in the 1970s. Unopposed estrogen can lead to the development of endometrial hyperplasia, which in some cases can increase a woman's risk for endometrial cancer. HT that involves the use of both estrogen and progesterone is not associated with endometrial cancer. When used cyclically (*i.e.,* in continuous sequential estrogen–progesterone therapy [CSEPT]), progesterone is added for 12 to 14 days to mature any endometrium that has developed in response to the estrogen. Progesterone withdrawal results in endometrial shedding (*i.e.,* a cyclic bleeding episode). When used continuously, a small amount of progesterone is added to the daily estrogen regimen. This continuous exposure to progesterone inhibits endometrial development. Eventually, the continuous-combined estrogen–progesterone therapy (CCEPT) results in no bleeding; however, it can be associated with irregular bleeding and spotting until the lining becomes atrophic. Prevention of endometrial hyperplasia either by shedding the endometrial build-up or by preventing its development minimizes the risk of endometrial cancer. This protection must now be considered when weighing the risks and benefits of HT.

Women's Health Initiative and Other Studies. With the current shift to evidence-based medicine, randomized, controlled trials were undertaken to confirm the reported benefits of HT using an experimental model and to demonstrate that the intervention (HT) was in fact responsible for the outcome, and not other variables. Several randomized, controlled trials have now demonstrated that HT does not prevent and can in fact increase the likelihood of a cardiovascular event in women with established heart disease.[11–14] Other studies looking at the effect of HT on cognition and Alzheimer disease have failed to show benefit.[15]

The American Women's Health Initiative (WHI) was planned as an 8- to 10-year nationwide research effort with an observational study component (93,700 women) and a multicentre, prospective, randomized, double-blind, placebo-controlled clinical trial component (68,000 women) to define the risks and benefits of strategies that could reduce the incidence of heart disease, breast and colorectal cancer, and fractures in postmenopausal women. Between 1993 and 1998, the WHI enrolled 161,809 mostly healthy postmenopausal women (50 to 79 years of age) into a set of clinical trials (trials of low-fat diet, calcium and vitamin D supplementation, and two parallel trials of postmenopausal HT).[16]

The two parallel trials of HT were undertaken to determine whether estrogen plus progestin (CCEPT; for women with an intact uterus) or estrogen alone (ET; for women with prior hysterectomy) would reduce the incidence of cardiovascular disease and lead to any change in risk for breast or colorectal cancer in postmenopausal women. A total of 16,608 women with an intact uterus were enrolled in the estrogen plus progestin arm. The study was stopped prematurely in 2002 after 5.2 years of data analysis when it was determined that the risks of HT outweighed its benefits. The study found that the risk of breast cancer crossed the predetermined safety boundary and that incidences of CHD, stroke, and venous thromboembolic disease were all increased. On the positive side, there was a reduction in colorectal cancer and hip fractures among the women using HT.[16] The ET-only clinical trial was also stopped prematurely, after 6.8 years.[17] It demonstrated no increased risk of breast cancer or heart disease, but showed a similar increased risk of stroke and venous thromboembolic disease.

Results from a 3-year follow-up study of women in the CCEPT arm of the WHI trial indicate that the increased cardiovascular risk observed at the time the intervention was stopped were not maintained, but that a greater risk of fatal and nonfatal malignancies occurred (global risk index was 12% higher in women from the CCEPT group as compared with the placebo group).[18] The follow-up study also found that the positive effects of CCEPT, such as decreased risk of colorectal cancer and hip fractures, also stopped when therapy ended.[18]

Cardiovascular Risk. Subsequent critical reassessment and subgroup analyses of the WHI, as well as findings from other studies, have led to a reevaluation of some of the conclusions that were made. A complete review of the literature surrounding HT is beyond the scope of this chapter. However, the following summary statements represent some of the current thinking.

First, the average age (63.7 years) and length of time since menopause (18 years) have been identified as indications that the women in WHI were already potentially predisposed to CHD and that the WHI may, in truth, have been a secondary prevention trial. Analyses of risk by age[19] and time since menopause[20] in the CCEPT trial reveal that the younger women (younger than 60 years of age) and those who started HT within 10 years of menopause demonstrated a trend towards lower rates of CHD. It has been hypothesized that HT, given during a "critical window" after menopause, may continue the cardioprotective actions provided by premenopausal levels of estrogen. However, when HT is started beyond this window period (when women may already have pre-existing subclinical atherosclerosis), it may stimulate inflammatory cytokines that predispose to atherosclerotic plaque rupture and development of symptomatic CHD.[21] The majority (70%) of the women in the WHI were in the age group that could be expected to have subclinical changes at the start of the study and therefore would be less likely to benefit from HT.

Second, data from the American Nurses' Health Study also suggest that women starting HT near the onset of menopause had a significantly reduced risk (30%) of CHD.[21]

Third, a meta-analysis[22] showed a 32% decrease in CHD in younger postmenopausal women. Although there was a reported initial increase in incidence of CHD during the first year in older postmenopausal women (those who started HT after age 60 years), there was a reduced incidence after 2 years. It is still a matter of debate whether the presence of the daily progestin contributed to the higher levels of CHD in the CCEPT group compared with the ET group.

The increased risk of venous thromboembolism does appear to be consistently associated with the use of HT. The absolute risk is low, appears to be greatest in the first 2 years of HT use, and declines thereafter. Women with a history of venous thromboembolism or who have a predisposition to clot formation as a result of coagulation defects such as factor V Leiden are generally advised to avoid the use of HT.

Breast Cancer Risk. The association with breast cancer has long been the other area of concern with HT. In studies reporting estimated risks of breast cancer associated with HT, most of the confidence intervals cross the relative risk of 1 and therefore are not statistically significant.[23] The WHI added to breast cancer concern by reporting a 26% increased risk of invasive breast cancer in the women using CCEPT.[16] Results from a 3-year WHI follow-up study revealed that the breast cancer risk of women who stopped taking CCEPT continued at a rate similar to that observed during the intervention.[18] The use of ET alone did not increase breast cancer risk in the WHI, but it did appear to increase the need for additional follow-up mammograms due to the added density of the breasts in women using estrogen HT.[24]

An update from the Nurses' Health Study showed no increased risk of invasive breast cancer with estrogen HT until 20 years of use.[25] In contrast, another large European study recruited over 1 million women aged 50 to 64 years and analyzed the 80% who were postmenopausal for breast cancer incidence (2.6 years average follow-up) and mortality (4.1 years average follow-up). Approximately half the women had used HT at some time. Results of this observational study revealed increased risk among current users of HT. The largest increase in risk was associated with CCEPT, was slightly less with ET, and declined after discontinuation and returned to baseline within 5 years.[26]

Current thinking postulates that these studies may, in fact, constitute detection studies rather than incidence studies, because it is known that breast cancer cells can be present in the body for 8 to 10 years before the cancer can be detected by any currently available means. Estrogen may accelerate the growth of these cells to a point where the cancer can then be detected, which may explain why some studies show a positive correlation between estrogen and breast cancer and others do not.[7] In this case, the increase in breast cancer detection may in fact be a positive outcome because it can be discovered while the cancer is still curable. At present there is insufficient evidence to support estrogen as the cause (initiator) of breast cancer. Thus, a more reasonable approach may involve identifying predisposing factors for breast cancer and finding better ways for early detection. This would assist women in assessing their own risk–benefit ratio, taking into account their individual circumstances, when making decisions about HT.

Hip Fracture and Other Risks. The release of data from the other two clinical trials within the WHI (low-fat dietary patterns, calcium and vitamin D supplementation) has challenged conventional wisdom in other areas. The use of calcium (1,000 mg/day) plus vitamin D (200 IU/day) was shown to result in a small but significant improvement in hip bone density, but failed to reduce the risk of hip fractures. Women using the supplements did have a slightly increased risk of kidney stones.[27] In addition, following a diet that is low in fat and plentiful in fruits, vegetables, and grains did not make a significant difference in the incidence of breast cancer, colorectal cancer, or heart disease.[28–30] Traditionally, calcium and vitamin D have been discussed with respect to bone health, but newer research is suggesting that there is a difference between calcium dietary intake versus calcium supplementation, with the former lowering CV disease risk and the latter linked to increasing it.[31] Currently the Society of Obstetricians and Gynaecologists of Canada (SOGC) recommends for postmenopausal women a total daily intake of 1,200 mg of elemental calcium from dietary and supplemental sources with 800 to 2,000 IU of vitamin D.[32]

Current Recommendations. Although the average age of menopause has not changed substantially since 1900, life expectancy has increased dramatically. Today, the average woman will live almost one third of her life after menopause. Menopause now represents only the end of reproductive capability. Estrogen's role in many other bodily functions has been well documented, but its replacement after the ovary ceases production has become highly controversial. The Canadian Task Force on Preventive Health Care recommends against the routine use of HT for preventing chronic conditions (*e.g.,* cardiovascular disease, osteoporosis).[33] Statements from the American National Institute of Health State-of-the-Science Conference on Management of Menopausal-related symptoms,[34] the North American Menopause Society (NAMS),[35] the Society of Obstetricians and Gynaecologists of Canada (SOGC),[8] and Health Canada all indicate that estrogen is the most consistently effective therapy for treating menopausal symptoms. Use of HT in younger, recently menopausal women appears less likely to result in the increased risks reported in the WHI and Heart and Estrogen/Progestin Replacement Study (HERS), which studied predominantly older, asymptomatic women who were on average 10 or more years beyond menopause.

Current recommendations for HT, in light of the findings of the WHI and other clinical trials, are to avoid HT for primary or secondary prevention of CHD; develop an individual risk profile for every woman contemplating HT and provide information regarding known risks; use HT only in those women who require relief from menopausal symptoms that affect quality of life; consider lower-than-standard doses and alternative routes of administration; limit the use of HT to the shortest duration consistent with goals, benefits, and risks of treatment for each woman; and because of the potential risks associated with HT products consider alternative therapies if available (i.e., bisphosphonates for osteoporosis prevention) if the woman is not symptomatic.[8,33–35]

Due to the mixed results of the WHI, there has been increased interest in alternative methods for management of postmenopausal symptoms, including the use of bio-identical hormones. Bio-identical HT uses "natural" substances derived from plant oils that are similar in molecular structure to human steroid hormones, and "phytoestrogens," substances occurring in nature with estrogen-like properties such as isoflavones (soy, red clover). Many patients are moving away from traditional pharmaceutical HRT and wanting to use custom-compound hormones, but very little safety data exists for this type of individualized treatment. Many statements released discuss the overall lack of evidence—that "natural" doesn't automatically equate to safer; that benefits and risks likely do not differ for synthetic and bio-identical hormones—but the data is inconclusive. Further, due to the lack of compounding regulations, the consumers might not be fully informed of their risks. Other medications such as selective serotonin reuptake inhibitors (SSRIs), gabapentin, and clonidine have been studied for prevention of hot flashes, showing some improvement over placebos in randomized control trials.[4] Ultimately the use of any botanical and pharmaceuticals for menopausal symptoms remains as options for women and their providers but continued studies are needed to further evaluate efficacy.[36]

Because the risk of osteoporosis remains high, there is a continued search for methods to prevent or decrease the rate of bone loss in postmenopausal women. At present, therapies with demonstrated effectiveness in treating osteoporosis include bisphosphonates, calcitonin, raloxifene (a selective estrogen receptor modulator [SERM] that works only on certain estrogen receptors, but not others), calcium, fluoride, and parathyroid hormone (see Chapter 59).

IN SUMMARY

Between the menarche and menopause, the female reproductive system undergoes cyclic changes called the menstrual cycle. The normal menstrual cycle results from complex interactions among the hypothalamus, which produces GnRH; the anterior pituitary gland, which synthesizes and releases FSH, LH, and prolactin; the ovaries, which synthesize and release estrogens, progesterone, and androgens; and associated target tissues, such as the endometrium and the vaginal mucosa. Although each component of the system is essential for normal functioning, the ovarian hormones are largely responsible for controlling the cyclic changes and length of the menstrual cycle. Estrogens are necessary for normal female physical maturation, for growth of ovarian follicles, for generation of a climate that is favourable to fertilization and implantation of the ovum, and for promoting the development of the endometrium in the event of pregnancy. Estrogens also have a number of extragenital effects, including prevention of bone resorption and regulation of the composition of cholesterol-carrying lipoproteins (HDL and LDL) in the blood. The functions of progesterone include the glandular development of the lobular and alveolar tissue of the breasts, the cyclic glandular development of the endometrium, and maintenance of pregnancy. Androgens contribute to hair distribution in the female and may have important metabolic effects.

Menopause is the cessation of menstrual cycles. Systemically, a woman may experience significant vasomotor instability and "hot flashes" secondary to the decrease in estrogens and the relative increase in other hormones, including FSH, LH, GnRH, dehydroepiandrosterone, and androstenedione. The long-term effects of estrogen deprivation include osteoporosis due to an imbalance in bone remodelling (*i.e.*, bone resorption occurs at a faster rate than bone formation) and an increased risk for cardiovascular disease (atherosclerosis is accelerated), which is the leading cause of death in women after menopause. Hormone replacement therapy for postmenopausal women has come under scrutiny as a result of the WHI, which indicates that CCEPT (continuous-combined estrogen and progestin) may increase the risk for cardiovascular disease and breast cancer. At this time, an analysis of a woman's risks versus benefits should be completed, and for women who are placed on HRT a low dose for the shortest interval in earlier menopause is preferred.

BREASTS

After completing this section of the chapter, you should be able to meet the following objectives:

- Describe the anatomy of the female breast.
- Describe the influence of hormones on breast development.
- Characterize the changes in breast structure that occur with pregnancy and lactation.

Although anatomically separate, the breasts are functionally related to the female genitourinary system in that they respond to the cyclic changes in sex hormones and produce milk for infant nourishment. The breasts also are important for their sexual function and for cosmetic appearance. Breast cancer represents the most common malignancy among women in Canada. The high rate of breast cancer has drawn even greater attention to the importance of the breasts throughout the life span.

Structure and Function

The breasts, or mammary tissues, are located between the third and seventh ribs of the anterior chest wall and are supported by the pectoral muscles and superficial fascia. They are specialized glandular structures that have an abundant shared nervous, vascular, and lymphatic supply (Fig. 45.8). What are commonly called "breasts" are actually two parts of a single anatomic breast. This contiguous nature of breast tissue is important in health and illness. Men and women alike are born with rudimentary breast tissue, with the ducts lined with epithelium. In women, the pituitary release of FSH, LH, and prolactin at puberty stimulates the ovary to produce and release estrogen. This estrogen stimulates the growth and proliferation of the ductile system. With the onset of ovulatory cycles, progesterone is released and this stimulates the growth and development of ductile and alveolar secretory epithelium. By adolescence, the breasts have developed characteristic fat deposition patterns and contours.

Structurally, the breast consists of fat, fibrous connective tissue, and glandular tissue. The superficial fibrous connective tissue is attached to the skin, a fact that is important in the visual observation of skin movement over the breast during breast self-examination. The breast mass is supported by the fascia of the pectoralis major and minor muscles and by the fibrous connective tissue of the breast. Fibrous tissue ligaments, called *Cooper ligaments,* extend from the outer boundaries of the breast to the nipple area in a radial manner, like the spokes on a wheel (Fig. 45.8). These ligaments further support the breast and form septa that divide the breast into 15 to 25 lobes. Each lobe consists of grapelike clusters—alveoli or glands—that are interconnected by ducts. The alveoli are lined with secretory cells capable of producing milk or fluid under the proper hormonal conditions (Fig. 45.9). The route of descent of milk and other breast secretions is from alveoli to duct, to intralobar duct, to lactiferous duct and reservoir, to nipple. Breast milk is produced secondary to complex hormonal changes associated with pregnancy. Fluid is produced and reabsorbed during the menstrual cycle. The breasts respond to the cyclic changes in the menstrual cycle with fullness and discomfort.

The nipple is made up of epithelial, glandular, erectile, and nervous tissue. Areolar tissue surrounds the nipple and is recognized as the darker, smooth skin between the nipple and the breast. The small bumps or projections on the areolar surface known as *Montgomery tubercles* are sebaceous

FIGURE 45.8 • The breasts, showing the shared vascular and lymphatic supply as well as the pectoral muscles.

glands that keep the nipple area soft and elastic. At puberty and during pregnancy, increased levels of estrogen and progesterone cause the areola and nipple to become darker and more prominent and the Montgomery glands to become more active. The erectile tissue of the nipple is responsive to psychological and tactile stimuli, which contributes to the sexual function of the breasts.

There are many individual variations in breast size and shape. The shape and texture vary with hormonal, genetic, nutritional, and endocrine factors and with muscle tone, age, and pregnancy. A well-developed set of pectoralis muscles supports the breast mass higher on the chest wall. Poor posture, significant weight loss, and lack of support may cause the breasts to droop.

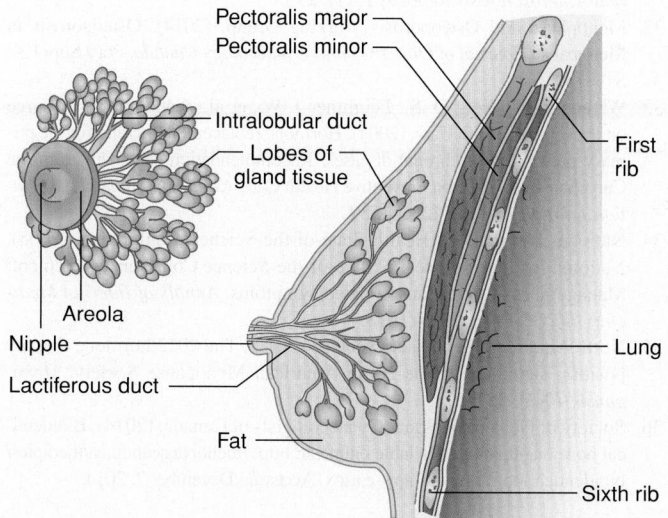

FIGURE 45.9 • The breast, showing the glandular tissue and ducts of the mammary glands.

Pregnancy

During pregnancy, the breasts are significantly altered by increased levels of estrogen and progesterone. Estrogen stimulates increased vascularity of the breasts and the growth and extension of the ductile structures, causing "heaviness" of the breasts. Progesterone causes marked budding and growth of the alveolar structures. The alveolar epithelium assumes a secretory state in preparation for lactation. The progesterone-induced changes that occur during pregnancy may confer some protection against cancer. Cellular changes that occur in the alveolar lining are thought to change the susceptibility of these cells to estrogen-mediated changes later in life.

Lactation

During lactation, milk is secreted by alveolar cells, which are under the influence of the anterior pituitary hormone prolactin. Milk ejection from the ductile system occurs in response to the release of oxytocin from the posterior pituitary. The suckling of the infant also provides the stimulus for milk ejection. Suckling produces feedback to the hypothalamus, stimulating the release of oxytocin from the posterior pituitary. Oxytocin causes contraction of the myoepithelial cells lining the alveoli and ejection of milk into the ductal system. A woman may have breast leakage for 3 months to 1 year after the termination of breast-feeding as breast tissue and hormones regress to the nonlactating state. Overzealous breast stimulation with or without pregnancy can likewise cause breast leakage.

IN SUMMARY

The breast is a complex structure of variable size, consistency, and composition. Although anatomically distinct, the breasts are functionally related to the female genitourinary system in that they respond to cyclic changes in sex hormones and produce milk for infant nourishment.

REVIEW EXERCISES

1. Diabetes mellitus and treatment with broad-spectrum antibiotics increase the risk of vaginal infections.
   A. *Explain how these two conditions change the vaginal ecology, making it more susceptible to infection.*
   B. *Most oral contraceptive agents use low doses of estrogen and progestin to prevent conception.*
2. Use Figure 45.4 and 45.5 to explain how oral contraceptive agents prevent ovulation and pregnancy.

References

1. Cunningham F. G., Leveno K. J., Bloom S. L., et al. (2014). *Williams obstetrics* (24th ed.). New York: McGraw-Hill Education.
2. Rhoades R. A., Bell D. R. (2013). *Medical physiology: Principles for clinical medicine* (4th ed.). Philadelphia, PA: Lippincott Williams & Wilkins.
3. DeCherney A. H., Nathan L., Laufer N., et al. (2013). *Current diagnosis & treatment: Obstetrics & gynecology* (11th ed.). New York: McGraw-Hill Medical.
4. Fritz M. A., Speroff L. (2011). *Clinical gynecological endocrinology and infertility* (8th ed.). Philadelphia, PA: Lippincott Williams & Wilkins.
5. Murphy E. (2011). Estrogen signaling and cardiovascular disease. *Circulation Research, 109*(6), 687–696.
6. Nilsson S., Gustafsson J. A. (2011). Estrogen receptors: Therapies targeted to receptor subtypes. *Clinical Pharmacology and Therapeutics, 89*(1), 44–55.
7. Liang J., Shang Y. (2013). Estrogen and cancer. *Annual Review of Physiology, 75*, 225–240.
8. Menopause and Osteoporosis Working Groups. (2014). Managing menopause. *Journal of Obstetrics and Gynaecology Canada, 36*(9 Suppl 2), S1–S80.
9. Grodstein F., Manson J. E., Colditz G. A., et al. (2000). A prospective, observational study of postmenopausal hormone therapy and primary prevention of cardiovascular disease. *Annals of Internal Medicine, 133*(12), 933–941.
10. Seifer D. B., Kennard E. A. (1999). *Menopause: Endocrinology and management.* Totowa, NJ: Humana Press.
11. Yang X., Reckelhoff J. F. (2011). Estrogen, hormonal replacement therapy and cardiovascular disease. *Current Opinion in Nephrology and Hypertension, 20*(2), 133–138.
12. Kallen A. N., Pal L. (2011). Cardiovascular disease and ovarian function. *Current Opinion in Obstetrics and Gynecology, 23*(4), 258–267.
13. Kass-Wolff J. H., Fisher, J.E. (2011). Menopause and the hormone controversy: Clarification or confusion? *Nurse Practitioner, 36*(7), 22–29.
14. Gurney E. P., Nachtigall M. J., Nachtigall L. E., et al. (2014). The Women's Health Initiative trial and related studies 10 years later: A clinician's view. *Journal of Steroid Biochemistry and Molecular Biology, 142*, 4–11.
15. Henderson V. W. (2014). Alzheimer's disease: Review of hormone therapy trials and implications for treatment and prevention after menopause. *Journal of Steroid Biochemistry and Molecular Biology, 142*, 99–106.
16. Writing Group of the Women's Health Initiative Investigators. (2002). Risks and benefits of estrogen plus progestin in healthy postmenopausal women: Principal results from the Women's Health Initiative randomized controlled trial. *Journal of the American Medical Association, 288*(3), 321–333.
17. Anderson G. L., Limacher M., Assaf A. R., et al.; Women's Health Initiative Steering Committee. (2004). Effects of conjugated equine estrogen in postmenopausal women with hysterectomy: The Women's Health Initiative randomized controlled trial. *Journal of the American Medical Association, 291*(14), 1701–1712.
18. Heiss G., Wallace R., Anderson G. L., et al. (2008). Health risks and benefits 3 years after stopping randomized treatment with estrogen and progestin. *Journal of the American Medical Association, 299*(9), 1036–1045.
19. Hsia J., Langer R. D., Manson J. E., et al.; Women's Health Initiative Investigators. (2006). Conjugated equine estrogens and coronary heart disease: The Women's Health Initiative. *Archives of Internal Medicine, 166*(3), 357–365.
20. Manson J. E., Hsia J., Johnson K. C., et al.; Women's Health Initiative Investigators. (2003). Estrogen plus progestin and the risk of coronary heart disease. *The New England Journal of Medicine, 349*(6), 523–534.
21. Hodis H. N., Mack W. J. (2014). Hormone replacement therapy and the association with coronary heart disease and overall mortality: Clinical application of the timing hypotheses. *Journal of Steroid Biochemistry and Molecular Biology, 142*, 68–75.
22. Salpeter S. R., Walsh J. M., Greyber E., et al. (2006). Coronary heart disease events associated with hormone therapy in younger and older women: A meta-analysis. *Journal of General Internal Medicine, 21*(4), 363–366.
23. Speroff L. (2000). Postmenopausal estrogen-progestin therapy and breast cancer: A clinical response to an epidemiologic report. *Climacteric, 3*(1), 3–12.
24. Stefaniak M. L., Anderson G. L., Margolis K. L., et al.; WHI Investigators. (2006). Effects of conjugated equine estrogens on breast cancer and mammography screening in postmenopausal women with hysterectomy. *Journal of the American Medical Association, 195*(14), 1647–1657.
25. Chen W. Y., Manson J. E., Hankinson S. E., et al. (2006). Unopposed estrogen therapy and the risk of invasive breast cancer. *Archives of Internal Medicine, 166*(9), 1027–1032.
26. Beral V. (2003). Breast cancer and hormone-replacement therapy in the Million Women Study. *Lancet, 362*(9382),419–427.
27. Cauley J. A., Chlebowski R. T., Wende J., et al. (2013). Calcium plus vitamin D supplementation and health outcomes five years after active intervention ended: The Women's Health Initiative. *Journal of Women's Health, 22*(11), 915–929.
28. Prentice R. L., Caan B., Chlebowski R. T., et al. (2006). Low-fat dietary pattern and risk of invasive breast cancer. *Journal of the American Medical Association, 295*(6), 629–642.
29. Beresford S. A., Johnson K. C., Ritenbaugh C., et al. (2006). Low-fat dietary pattern and risk of colorectal cancer. *Journal of the American Medical Association, 295*(6),643–654.
30. Howard B. V., VanHorn L., Hsai J., et al. (2006). Low-fat dietary pattern and risk of cardiovascular disease. *Journal of the American Medical Association, 295*(6), 655–666.
31. Lutsey P. L., Michos E. D. (2013). Vitamin D, calcium, and atherosclerotic risk: Evidence from serum levels and supplementation studies. *Current Atherosclerosis Reports, 15*(1), 293.
32. Menopause and Osteoporosis Working Group. (2014). Osteoporosis in Menopause. *Journal of Obstetrics and Gynaecology Canada, 36*(9 Suppl 3), S1-S15.
33. Wathen C. N., Feig D. S., Feightner J. W., et al.; Canadian Task Force on Preventive Health Care. (2004). Hormone replacement therapy for the primary prevention of chronic diseases: Recommendation statement from the Canadian Task Force on Preventive Health Care. *Canadian Medical Association Journal, 170*(10), 1535–1539.
34. National Institutes of Health State-of-the-Science Conference. (2005). National Institutes of Health State-of-the-Science Conference statement: Management of menopause-related symptoms. *Annals of Internal Medicine, 142*(12 Pt 1), 1003–1013.
35. North American Menopause Society. (2012). The 2012 hormone therapy position statement of the North American Menopause Society. *Menopause, 19*(3), 257–271.
36. Society of Obstetricians and Gynaecologists of Canada. (2014). Bioidentical hormone therapy. Available online at: http://menopauseandu.ca/therapies/bioidentical-hormone-therapy_e.aspx. Accessed December 7, 2014.

Visit thePoint **http://thePoint.lww.com for animations, journal articles, and more!**

Disorders of the Female Reproductive System

46

Disorders of the female genitourinary system have widespread effects on physical and psychological function, including general health status, sexuality, and reproductive potential. The reproductive structures are located close to other pelvic structures, particularly those of the urinary system, and disorders of the reproductive system may affect urinary function. This chapter focuses on infection and inflammation, benign conditions, and neoplasms of the female reproductive structures; disorders of pelvic support and uterine position; alterations in menstruation; and an overview of infertility.

DISORDERS OF THE EXTERNAL GENITALIA AND VAGINA

After completing this section of the chapter, you should be able to meet the following objectives:

- Compare the abnormalities associated with Bartholin gland cyst, nonneoplastic epithelial disorders, vulvodynia, and cancer of the vulva.
- State the role of Lactobacillus in maintaining the normal ecology of the vagina.
- Describe the conditions that predispose to vaginal infections and the methods used to prevent and treat these infections.

Disorders of the External Genitalia

Diseases of the external genitalia are similar to those that affect hair-bearing skin elsewhere in the body. Most skin cysts, nevi, and malignant neoplasms can occur on the skin of the external genitalia as well as on the skin in other parts of the body. The vulva (composed of the mons pubis, labia majora and minora, clitoris, and vaginal vestibule) is particularly prone to skin infections because it is constantly exposed to secretions and moisture. Nonspecific vulvitis is particularly common in women with diabetes, chronic kidney disease, blood dyscrasias, and malnutrition.

Bartholin Gland Cyst and Abscess

A Bartholin gland cyst is a fluid-filled sac that results from occlusion of the duct system in the Bartholin gland (Fig. 46.1). If the cyst becomes infected, an abscess may develop in the gland. Bartholin gland abscesses were formerly associated with gonorrhea, but are now more commonly caused by *Escherichia coli*, staphylococcal, anaerobes, and polymicrobial infections.[1]

Acute symptoms are usually the result of infection and include pain, tenderness, and dyspareunia. The treatment of symptomatic cysts consists of the administration of appropriate antibiotics, local application of moist heat, and incision and drainage. Cysts that frequently are abscessed or are large

FIGURE 46.1 • Bartholin gland cyst. The 4-cm lesion is located to the right of and posterior to the vaginal introitus. (From Rubin R., Strayer D. S. (Eds.). (2012). *Rubin's pathology: Clinicopathologic foundations of medicine* (6th ed., p. 854). Philadelphia, PA: Lippincott Williams & Wilkins.)

enough to cause blockage of the introitus may require surgical intervention. Because the Bartholin glands usually shrink during menopause, a vulvar growth in postmenopausal women should be evaluated for malignancy.

Nonneoplastic Epithelial Disorders

The term *nonneoplastic epithelial disorders* refers to nonmalignant atrophic and hyperplastic changes of the vulvar skin and mucosa that can develop at any age and can progress to malignancy.[2] The condition, commonly referred to as *leukoplakia,* presents as white lesions of the vulva. Itching is the most common symptom, and dyspareunia (painful intercourse) is common. Depending on clinical and histologic characteristics, the lesions can be further categorized as lichen simplex chronicus, lichen sclerosus, or other dermatoses such as psoriasis or chronic dermatitis.

Lichen simplex chronicus, or *chronic dermatitis,* presents as thickened, grey-white plaques with an irregular surface. Presumed to be a response of the genital skin to some type of irritant, this diagnosis is used only when human papillomavirus (HPV) infection, fungal infections, or other known causative conditions have been excluded.[3] Vulvar pruritus is the most common presenting complaint. Scaling is generally present, and excoriations due to recent scratching can often be seen.

Lichen sclerosus is an inflammatory disease of the vulva characterized by plaquelike areas that may progress to parchment-thin epithelium with focal areas of ecchymosis and superficial ulceration secondary to scratching. Atrophy and contracture of the vulvar tissues with eventual stenosis of the introitus are common when this condition becomes chronic. Itching is common and dyspareunia is frequent. The condition develops insidiously and is progressive. There is a high risk associated with developing a vulvar malignancy, and evidence supports that lichen sclerosus has an identical p53 gene mutation as invasive squamous cell carcinoma.

Current treatment measures for lichen sclerosus favour the use of potent topical corticosteroids.[3] Hyperplastic areas respond well to a combination corticosteroid (betamethasone) and antipruritic cream (crotamiton). Lichen sclerosus frequently recurs, and lifetime maintenance therapy may be required. Hyperplastic areas that occur in the field of lichen sclerosus may be sites of malignant change and warrant close follow-up and possible biopsy.

Vulvodynia

Vulvodynia is a syndrome of unexplained vulvar pain, previously referred to as *vulvar pain syndrome* or *burning vulva syndrome.* The International Society for the Study of Vulvovaginal Disorders (ISSVD) defines it as a condition characterized by vulvar pain occurring in the absence of any underlying recognizable disease. Vulvodynia is further classified as localized or generalized, and as to whether it is provoked, unprovoked, or of mixed origin.[4]

Localized vulvodynia or *vestibulodynia,* formerly referred to as *vulvar vestibulitis syndrome,* is characterized by pain at onset of intercourse (*i.e.,* insertional dyspareunia), localized point tenderness near the vaginal opening, and sensitivity to tampon placement, tight-fitting pants, bicycling, or prolonged sitting. It is the leading cause of dyspareunia in women younger than 50 years of age. The pain can be primary (present from first contact) or secondary (developing after a period of comfortable sexual relations). The etiology is unknown, but the problem may evolve from chronic vulvar inflammation or trauma. Nerve fibres that supply the vestibular epithelium may become highly sensitized, causing neurons in the dorsal horn of the spinal cord to respond abnormally, thus transforming the sensation of touch in the vestibule into pain (allodynia).[5] Surgical vestibulectomy may be necessary for symptom relief when medical management fails. A majority of current therapeutic options have been established based on expert opinion, clinical experience and observational studies with no single effective treatment identified. Instead, a multidisciplinary approach should be considered.[4]

Generalized vulvodynia, formerly called *vulvar dysesthesia* or *essential vulvodynia,* involves severe, constant, widespread burning that interferes with daily activities. No abnormalities are found on examination, but there is diffuse and variable hypersensitivity and altered sensation to light touch. The quality of this unprovoked pain shares many of the features of other neuropathic pain disorders, particularly complex regional pain syndrome (see Chapter 49) or pudendal neuralgia. Although the cause of the neuropathic pain is unknown, it has been suggested that it may result from myofascial restrictions affecting the sacral and pelvic floor nerves. Surface electromyography-assisted pelvic floor muscle rehabilitation has been shown to be an effective primary therapy or adjunct to medical or surgical therapy for generalized vulvodynia.[4,5]

There are many proposed triggers for vulvodynia, including chronic recurrent vaginal infections; chemical irritation or drug effects, especially prolonged use of topical steroid creams; the irritating effects of elevated urinary levels of calcium oxalate; and immunoglobulin A deficiency or other disorders of immune regulation.[4,5] Often it is multifactorial in origin.

Careful history taking and physical assessment are essential for differential diagnosis and treatment. *Vulvodynia* is a diagnosis of exclusion after ruling out infections, such as candidiasis and genital herpes; inflammatory conditions, such as lichen simplex chronicus and lichen sclerosus; vulvar cancer; or neurologic disorders, such as herpes neuralgia or spinal nerve compression, as causes for the pain.

Treatment for this chronic, often debilitating problem is aimed at symptom relief, is frequently long term, and often needs to be managed from a multidimensional, chronic pain perspective.[4,5] Regimens can include long-term vaginal or oral antifungal therapy, avoidance of potential irritants, sitz baths with baking soda, emollients such as vitamin E or vegetable oil for lubrication, anesthetic or steroid ointments, capsaicin cream (topical analgesic), physical therapy, and surgery. Oral medications, including tricyclic antidepressants, other antidepressants (*e.g.,* selective serotonin receptor uptake inhibitors [SSRIs]), or gabapentin (an antiepileptic drug), are often used to treat the neuropathic pain associated with vulvodynia. Because this condition can cause strain in sexual, family, and work relationships, psychosocial support often is needed.[4]

Cancer of the Vulva

Carcinoma of the vulva accounts for approximately 5% of all cancers of the female genital tract malignancies. It typically affects older women; the peak age of diagnosis is 75 years.[6] Approximately 90% of vulvar malignancies are squamous cell carcinomas, meaning they begin in squamous cells, the main type of skin cell. Less common forms of vulvar cancer are malignant melanomas, adenocarcinoma, basal cell carcinoma, and sarcoma.[7]

> ## GYNECOLOGIC CANCERS
>
> - Cancers of the vulva, cervix, endometrium, and ovaries represent a spectrum of malignancies.
> - Cancers of the vulva and cervix are mainly squamous cell carcinomas. Certain types of sexually transmitted human papillomaviruses are risk factors for cervical intraepithelial neoplasia, which can be a precursor lesion of invasive carcinoma.
> - Endometrial cancers, which are seen most frequently in women 55 to 65 years of age, are strongly associated with conditions that produce excessive estrogen stimulation and endometrial hyperplasia.
> - Ovarian cancer is the second most common female cancer and the most lethal. The most significant risk factors for ovarian cancer are the length of time that a woman's ovarian cycles are not suppressed by pregnancy, lactation, or oral contraceptive use, and family history.

In terms of etiology, pathogenesis, and clinical presentation, vulvar carcinoma can be divided into two general groups. The first group is associated with vulvar intraepithelial neoplasia (VIN), a precursor lesion of squamous cell carcinoma. One third to one half of VIN cases appear to be caused by the cancer-promoting potential of certain strains (subtypes 16 and 18) of HPV that are sexually transmitted and are associated with the type of vulvar cancer found in younger women (*i.e.,* younger than 40 years of age).[7] VIN lesions may take many forms. They may be singular or multicentric; macular or papular; red or white and plaquelike.[8] Microscopically, VIN presents as a proliferative process, characterized by epithelial cells with atypical nuclei, increased mitosis, and lack of surface differentiation. The risk of progression to invasive cancer increases in older women and in women with suppressed immune function.

The second form of vulvar cancer, which is seen more often in older women, is generally preceded by vulvar non-neoplastic disorders such as chronic vulvar irritation or lichen sclerosus. The etiology of this group of vulvar cancers is unclear, but they are not typically associated with HPV.

Neoplastic changes may arise from lichen sclerosus lesions or hyperplasia, leading directly to malignancy.[7]

The initial lesion of squamous cell vulvar carcinoma may appear as an inconspicuous thickening of the skin, a small raised area or lump, or an ulceration that fails to heal. It may be single or multiple and vary in colour from white to velvety red or black. The lesions may resemble eczema or dermatitis and may produce few symptoms other than pruritus, local discomfort, and exudation. The symptoms frequently are treated with various home remedies before medical treatment is sought. The lesion may become secondarily infected, causing pain and discomfort. The malignant lesion gradually spreads superficially or as a deep furrow involving all of one labial side. Because there are many lymph channels around the vulva, the cancer metastasizes freely to the regional lymph nodes. The most common extension is to the superficial inguinal, deep femoral, and external iliac lymph nodes.[2,7,8]

Early diagnosis is important in the treatment of vulvar carcinoma. Because malignant lesions can vary in appearance and commonly are mistaken for other conditions, biopsy and treatment often are delayed. Treatment is primarily wide surgical excision of the lesion for noninvasive cancer and radical excision or vulvectomy with node resection for invasive cancer. Postoperative groin and pelvic radiation is recommended when groin lymph nodes are involved.

Disorders of the Vagina

The normal vaginal ecology depends on the delicate balance of hormones and bacterial flora. Normal estrogen levels maintain a thick, protective squamous epithelium that contains glycogen. The vaginal flora consists of various bacteria mostly from the *Lactobacillus* species that metabolizes glycogen, and in the process produces the lactic acid that normally maintains the vaginal pH of 3.8 to 4.5.[9,10] Disruptions in these normal environmental conditions predispose to infection.

Vaginitis

Vaginitis represents an inflammation of the vagina that is characterized by vaginal discharge and burning, itching, redness, and swelling of vaginal tissues. Pain often occurs with urination and sexual intercourse. Vaginitis may be caused by chemical irritants, foreign bodies, or infectious agents. The causes of vaginitis differ in various age groups. In premenarchal girls, most vaginal infections have nonspecific causes, such as poor hygiene, intestinal parasites, or the presence of foreign bodies. *Candida albicans, Trichomonas vaginalis,* and bacterial vaginosis are the most common causes of vaginitis in the childbearing years, and some of these organisms can be transmitted sexually[2,3,10] (see Chapter 47).

In postmenopausal women, atrophic vaginitis is the most common form. Atrophic vaginitis is an inflammation of the vagina that occurs after menopause or removal of the ovaries and their estrogen supply. Estrogen deficiency results in a lack of regenerative growth of the vaginal epithelium, rendering these tissues more susceptible to infection and irritation. Since the vaginal bacteria normally gain nutrients from sloughed epithelial cells and glandular secretions, over time the lactobacilli disappear and the vaginal secretions become less acidic. The symptoms of atrophic vaginitis include itching, burning, and painful intercourse. These symptoms usually can be reversed by local application of estrogen.[2,3,9]

Every woman normally experiences vaginal discharge during the menstrual cycle, but it should not cause burning or itching or have an unpleasant odour. These symptoms suggest inflammation or infection. Because these symptoms are common to the different types of vaginitis, precise identification of the organism is essential for proper treatment. A careful history should include information about systemic disease conditions, the use of drugs such as antibiotics that foster the growth of yeast, dietary habits, stress, and other factors that alter the resistance of vaginal tissue to infections. A physical examination usually is done to evaluate the nature of the discharge and its effects on the genital structures. Microscopic examination of a saline or potassium hydroxide (KOH) wet-mount smear (prepared by placing a sample of vaginal mucus in each solution) is the primary means of identifying the organism responsible for the infection.[10] Culture methods may be needed when the organism is not apparent on the wet-mount preparation.[3]

The prevention and treatment of vaginal infections depend on proper health habits and accurate diagnosis and treatment of ongoing infections (see Chapter 47). Measures to prevent infection include keeping the genital area clean and dry, maintaining normal vaginal flora and healthy vaginal mucosa, and avoiding contact with organisms known to cause vaginal infections. Perfumed products, such as feminine deodorant sprays, douches, bath powders, soaps, and even toilet paper, can be irritating and may alter the normal vaginal flora. Tight clothing prevents the dissipation of body heat and evaporation of skin moisture and promotes favourable conditions for irritation and the growth of pathogens. Cotton undergarments that can withstand hot water and bleach (a fungicide) may be preferable for women to prevent such infections. Avoiding sexual contact whenever an infection is known to exist or suspected should limit that route of transmission.

Cancer of the Vagina

Primary cancers of the vagina are extremely rare, accounting for approximately 1% to 2% of all cancers of the female reproductive system.[11,12] Like vulvar carcinoma, carcinoma of the vagina is largely a disease of older women. Most women are 60 years of age or older at the time of diagnosis. The exception to that is the clear cell adenocarcinoma associated with diethylstilbestrol (DES) exposure in utero, which is still seen, although rarely, in offspring of women who were treated with DES. Vaginal cancers may result from local extension of cervical cancer, from exposure to sexually transmitted HPV, or rarely from local irritation such as occurs with prolonged use of a pessary. Smoking and human immunodeficiency virus (HIV) infection also increase the risk of vaginal cancer.[12]

Approximately 80% to 90% of vaginal cancers are squamous cell carcinomas, with other common types being adenocarcinomas (5% to 10%), sarcomas (3% to 4%), and melanomas (3% to 5%).[12] Squamous cell carcinomas begin in the epithelium and progress over many years from precancerous lesions called *vaginal intraepithelial neoplasia* (VAIN), 65% to 80% of which contain HPV deoxyribonucleic acid (DNA).

The most common symptom of vaginal carcinoma is abnormal bleeding. Other signs or symptoms include an abnormal vaginal discharge, a palpable mass, or pain during intercourse. Most women with preinvasive vaginal carcinoma are asymptomatic, with the cancer being discovered during a routine pelvic examination. The anatomic proximity of the vagina to other pelvic structures (urethra, bladder, and rectum) permits early spread to these areas. Pelvic pain, dysuria, and constipation can be associated symptoms.[12]

Since most preinvasive and early invasive cancers are silent, the use of the vaginal cytology (Papanicolaou [Pap] smear) is the most effective way to detect vaginal cancer. Women who have had a hysterectomy performed for reproductive cancer should continue to have vaginal cytologic studies every 3 to 5 years after surgery. Diagnosis requires biopsy of suspect lesions or areas.

Treatment of vaginal cancer must take into consideration the type of cancer, the size, location, and spread of the lesion, and the woman's age. Local excision, laser vaporization, or a loop electrode excision procedure (LEEP) can be considered with stage 0 squamous cell cancers. Radical surgery and radiation therapy are both curative with more advanced cancers. When there is upper vaginal involvement, radical surgery may be required. This includes a total hysterectomy, pelvic lymph node dissection, partial vaginectomy, and placement of a graft from the buttock to the area from which the vagina was excised. Vaginal reconstruction often is possible to allow for sexual intercourse. The ovaries usually are preserved unless they are diseased. Extensive lesions and those located in the middle or lower vaginal area usually are treated by radiation therapy, which can be intracavitary, interstitial, or external beam.

The prognosis depends on the stage of the disease, involvement of lymph nodes, and the degree of mitotic activity of the tumour. With appropriate treatment and follow-up, the 5-year survival rate for squamous cell carcinoma and adenocarcinoma confined to the vagina (stage I) is 84%, whereas it is only 57% for those with extensive spread (stages III and IV).[12]

IN SUMMARY

The surface of the vulva is affected by disorders that affect skin on other parts of the body. Bartholin cysts are the result of occluded ducts in Bartholin glands. They often are painful and can become infected. Nonneoplastic epithelial disorders are characterized by thinning or hyperplastic thickening of vulvar tissues. Vulvodynia is a chronic vulvar pain syndrome with several classifications and variable treatment results. Cancer of the vulva, which accounts for 5% of all female genital tract cancers, is associated with

HPV infections in younger women and lichen sclerosus in older women.

The normal vaginal ecology depends on the delicate balance of hormones and bacterial flora. Disruptions in these normal environmental conditions predispose to vaginal infections. Vaginitis or inflammation of the vagina is characterized by vaginal discharge and burning, itching, redness, and swelling of vaginal tissues. It may be caused by chemical irritants, foreign bodies, or infectious agents. Primary cancers of the vagina are relatively uncommon, accounting for 1% to 2% of all cancers of the female reproductive system. Daughters of women treated with DES to prevent miscarriage are at increased risk for development of adenocarcinoma of the vagina.

DISORDERS OF THE CERVIX AND UTERUS

After completing this section of the chapter, you should be able to meet the following objectives:

- Describe the importance of the cervical transformation zone in the pathogenesis of cervical cancer.
- Compare the lesions associated with nabothian cysts and cervical polyps.
- List the complications of untreated cervicitis.
- Describe the development of cervical cancer from the appearance of atypical cells to the development of invasive cervical cancer and relate to the importance of the Pap smear in early detection of cervical cancer.
- Cite the rationale for describing cervical cancer as a sexually transmitted infection and the rationale for use of the HPV vaccine in prevention of cervical cancer.
- Compare the pathology and manifestations of endometriosis and adenomyosis.
- Cite the major early symptom of endometrial cancer and describe the relationship between unopposed estrogen stimulation of the endometrium and development of endometrial cancer.
- Compare the location and manifestations of intramural and subserosal leiomyomas.

Disorders of the Uterine Cervix

The cervix is composed of two distinct types of tissue. The exocervix, or visible portion, is covered with stratified squamous epithelium, which also lines the vagina. The endocervix is the canal that leads to the endometrial cavity. It is lined with columnar epithelium that contains large, branched mucus-secreting glands. During each menstrual cycle, the cervical glands undergo important functional changes related to the transport of spermatozoa within the cervical canal. The

Columnar
epithelium

Squamous
epithelium

FIGURE 46.2 • Common locations of the squamocolumnar junction (transformation zone) in menarchial (**A**), menstruating (**B**), menopausal (**C**), and postmenopausal women (**D**).

amount and properties of the mucus secreted by the gland cells vary during the menstrual cycle under the influence of the ovarian hormones. Blockage of the mucosal glands results in trapping of mucus in the deeper glands, leading to the formation of dilated cysts in the cervix called *nabothian cysts.* These are benign cysts that require no treatment unless they become so numerous that they cause cervical enlargement.

The junction of the squamous epithelium of the exocervix and mucus-secreting columnar epithelium of the endocervix (*i.e.,* squamocolumnar junction) appears at various locations on the cervix at different points in a woman's life (Fig. 46.2). During periods of high estrogen production, particularly menarche and the first pregnancy, the cervix everts or turns outward, exposing the columnar epithelium to the vaginal environment. The combination of estrogen and low vaginal pH leads to a gradual transformation from columnar to squamous epithelium—a process called *metaplasia* (see Chapter 5). The dynamic area of change where metaplasia takes place is called the *transformation zone.*[2,11]

The transformation zone is a critical area for the development of cervical cancer. During metaplasia, the newly developed squamous epithelial cells are vulnerable to development of dysplasia and genetic change if exposed to cancer-producing agents. *Dysplasia* means disordered growth or development (see Chapter 5). Although initially a reversible cell change, untreated dysplasia can develop into carcinoma. All Pap smear results will comment on the presence or absence of the transformation zone, but the significance of this commentary is under debate. Assuming that the smear sample is satisfactory for evaluation, most Canadian guidelines now state that the absence of the transformation zone is not a reason to rescreen any sooner than the recommended interval.[13] Ideally this zone is the area of the cervix that should be sampled during a Pap smear and is the area most carefully examined during colposcopy. Colposcopy is a vaginal examination using an instrument called a *colposcope* that affords a well-lit and magnified stereoscopic view of the cervix. During colposcopy, the cervical tissue may be stained with an iodine solution (*i.e.,* Schiller test) or acetic acid solution to accentuate topographic or vascular changes that can differentiate normal from abnormal tissue. A biopsy sample may be obtained from suspect areas and examined microscopically.

Cervicitis and Cervical Polyps

Cervicitis is an acute or chronic inflammation of the cervix. Acute cervicitis may result from the direct infection of the cervix or may be secondary to a vaginal or uterine infection. It may be caused by a variety of infective agents, including *C. albicans, T. vaginalis, Neisseria gonorrhoeae, Gardnerella vaginalis, Chlamydia trachomatis, Ureaplasma urealyticum,* and herpes simplex virus. *C. trachomatis* is the organism most commonly associated with mucopurulent cervicitis. With acute cervicitis, the cervix becomes reddened and edematous. Irritation from the infection results in copious mucopurulent drainage and leukorrhea. Depending on the causative agent, acute cervicitis is treated with appropriate antibiotic therapy.

Chronic cervicitis represents a low-grade inflammatory process. It is common in parous women and may be a sequela to minute lacerations that occur during childbirth, instrumentation, or other trauma. The organisms usually are nonspecific—often staphylococcal, streptococcal, or coliform bacteria. The symptoms of chronic cervicitis are less well defined than those of acute cervicitis. The cervix may be ulcerated or normal in appearance; it may contain nabothian cysts; the cervical os may be distorted by old lacerations or everted to expose areas of columnar epithelium; and a mucopurulent drainage may be present.

Untreated cervicitis may extend to include the development of pelvic cellulitis, low back pain, dyspareunia, cervical stenosis, dysmenorrhea, and ascending infection of the uterus or fallopian tubes. Diagnosis of chronic cervicitis is based on vaginal examination, colposcopy, cytologic (Pap) smears, and occasionally biopsy to exclude malignant changes. Treatment usually involves cryosurgery or cauterization, which causes the tissues to slough and leads to eradication of the infection. Colposcopically guided laser vaporization of the abnormal epithelium is the newest but most expensive treatment for cervicitis.

Polyps are the most common lesions of the cervix. They can be found in women of all ages, but their incidence is higher during the reproductive years. Polyps are soft, velvety, red lesions; they usually are pedunculated and often are found protruding through the cervical os. They usually develop as a result of inflammatory hyperplasia of the endocervical mucosa. Polyps typically are asymptomatic but may be associated with postcoital bleeding. Most are benign, but they should be removed and examined by a pathologist to exclude the possibility of malignant change.

Cancer of the Cervix

Cervical cancer is readily detected and, if detected early, is the most easily cured of all the cancers of the female reproductive system. According to Public Health Agency of Canada the incidence rates for cervical cancer have been steadily declining since 1972 and now account for approximately 1% of all female cancer deaths.[15] The Canadian Cancer Society estimates 1,500 cases of invasive cervical cancer will be diagnosed in Canada in 2015 with approximately 380 deaths from cervical cancer during the same period.[16]

Risk Factors and Pathogenesis. A preponderance of evidence identifies a causal link between HPV infection and cervical cancer. Cervical cancer is rare among celibate women. Risk factors for both HPV and cervical cancer include early age at first intercourse, multiple sexual partners, a promiscuous male partner, smoking, a history of sexually transmitted infections (STIs), a weakened immune system (*e.g.*, HIV), DES exposure, or multiple full-term pregnancies. Specific strains of HPV have been associated with cervical cancer versus condylomata or genital warts (see Chapter 47). The strongest link with cervical cancer is with HPV types 16, 18, 31, 33, and 45.[16] Other factors such as smoking, nutrition, and coexisting sexual infections such as *C. trachomatis,* herpes simplex virus type 2, and HIV may play a contributing role in determining whether a woman with HPV infection develops cervical cancer.[2,16]

There are three available vaccines in the defense against HPV infection—a quadrivalent vaccine (Gardasil) to prevent infection with the HPV subtypes 16, 18, 6, and 11, a bivalent vaccine (Cervarix) for subtypes 16 and 18 and the newest Gardasil-9 vaccine with the same subtypes as Gardasil plus HPV 31, 33, 45, 52, and 58.[17] The vaccines target the two strains of HPV (HPV 16 and 18) responsible for 70% of cervical cancer. The quadrivalent also targets the two most common benign strains (HPV 6 and 11), which account for up to 90% of genital warts.[17] Clinical studies have confirmed that the vaccines appear safe and effective in inducing long-term immunity to HPV.[17] Current National Advisory Committee on Immunization (NACI) guidelines have approved the quadrivalent vaccine for use in men and women aged 9 to 26 and women aged 26 to 45. The bivalent vaccine is approved for use in women only. All provinces and territories now have provincially funded access to the quadrivalent vaccine for school-aged girls.[17]

Cervical Intraepithelial Neoplasia (Dysplasia of the Cervix). One of the most important advances in the early diagnosis and treatment of cancer of the cervix was made possible by the observation that this cancer arises from precancerous lesions that begin with the development of atypical cervical cells. Atypical cells differ from normal cervical squamous epithelium. There are changes in the nuclear and cytoplasmic parts of the cell and more variation in cell size and shape (*i.e.,* dysplasia). These precancerous changes represent a continuum of morphologic changes with indistinct boundaries that may gradually progress to cancer in situ and then to invasive cancer, or they may spontaneously regress.[2]

A system of grading devised to describe the dysplastic changes of cancer precursors uses the term *cervical intraepithelial neoplasia* (CIN).[11] This histologic terminology system divides the precursors according to the thickness of cervical epithelial involvement (Table 46.1). Although previously presumed to represent a single progressive disease process, current understanding of the pathogenesis of cervical cancer precursors now suggests two distinct entities: (1) a productive HPV infection that can regress spontaneously (mild dysplasia or CIN 1, now more commonly referred to as atypical squamous cells [ASCs] in Canada); and (2) a true neoplastic process confined to the cervical squamous epithelium (previously called CIN 2 or 3). CIN histologic terminology has been replaced with cytopathologic terms for these two biologic entities: low-grade squamous intraepithelial lesion (LSIL) and high-grade squamous intraepithelial lesion (HSIL).[2]

Studies of the natural history of cervical cancer precursor lesions have yielded variable rates of progression and regression. Generally, only a small percentage of lesions progress to invasive carcinoma. HSIL has a much greater potential for progressing than does LSIL. De novo development of HSIL has also been demonstrated, challenging the concept that LSIL is always a precursor to HSIL. Cancers of the cervix have a long latent period; untreated dysplasia gradually progresses to carcinoma in situ, which may remain static for 7 to 10 years before it becomes invasive. After the preinvasive period, growth may

TABLE 46.1 CLASSIFICATION SYSTEMS FOR PAPANICOLAOU SMEARS

DYSPLASIA/NEOPLASIA	CIN	BETHESDA SYSTEM
Benign	Benign	Negative for intraepithelial lesion or malignancy
Benign with inflammation	Benign with inflammation	Negative for intraepithelial lesion or malignancy, ASC-US
Mild dysplasia	CIN 1	Low-grade SIL or LSIL, ASC-H
Moderate dysplasia	CIN 2	High-grade SIL or HSIL
Severe dysplasia and carcinoma in situ (CIS)	CIN 3	High-grade SIL or HSIL
Invasive cancer	Invasive cancer	Invasive cancer

CIN, cervical intraepithelial neoplasia; SIL, squamous intraepithelial lesion; ASC-US, atypical squamous cells of undetermined significance; LSIL, low-grade squamous intraepithelial lesion; ASC-H, cannot rule out high-grade SIL.

be rapid, and survival rates decline significantly depending on the extent of disease at the time of diagnosis.[2]

The accepted format for reporting cervical and vaginal cytologic diagnoses, called *The Bethesda System* (TBS), was developed during a National Cancer Institute Workshop in 1989 and updated in 1991 and 2001 (Table 46.1). The TBS 2001 terminology includes the following components: specimen type (conventional vs. liquid based); specimen adequacy; general categorization (negative for intraepithelial lesion or malignancy vs. epithelial cell abnormality); and interpretation/result.[18]

The atypical cellular changes that precede frank neoplastic changes consistent with cancer of the cervix can be recognized by a number of direct and microscopic techniques, including the Pap smear, colposcopy, and cervicography. Currently, Pap smears are used for cervical cancer screening. The Canadian Task Force on Preventive Health Care (CTFPHC) revised its screening guidelines in 2013 to include the recommendations to lengthen the interval between screenings in healthy women to 3 years.[19] Although many clinicians, and women themselves, are reluctant to move away from yearly Pap smears, the evidence about the natural progression of cervical cancer supports the position that the updated provincial guidelines present a more cost-effective approach to screening. Each province and territory has evaluated these guidelines and established their own recommendations for clinicians to follow.[14]

It has been estimated that approximately 20% of women with intraepithelial lesions have normal Pap smear results, indicating that care must be taken to obtain an adequate smear from the transformation zone that includes endocervical cells and ensuring that the cytologic examination is done by a competent laboratory. New techniques of specimen collection, slide preparation and processing, and computer-assisted evaluation of Pap smears are being evaluated and offer hope of improved accuracy in diagnosis of precancerous cervical changes. HPV DNA testing is approved by Health Canada, yet the availability is limited within Canada and is not currently available in all provinces and territories. If used, it is most effective for women older than 30 years of age, as well as in the management of women with questionable cytologic results.[20,21] It is not recommended as a screening tool for women younger than 30 years of age because the prevalence of HPV is quite high in this population.

The presence of normal endometrial cells in a cervical cytologic sample during the luteal phase of the menstrual cycle or during the postmenopausal period has been associated with endometrial disease and warrants further evaluation with endometrial biopsy. This demonstrates that shedding of even normal cells at an inappropriate time may indicate disease. Because adenocarcinoma of the cervix is being detected more frequently, especially in women younger than 35 years of age, a Pap smear result of atypical glandular cells warrants further evaluation by endocervical or endometrial curettage, hysteroscopy, or, ultimately, a cone biopsy if the abnormality cannot be located or identified through other means.[2,3]

In 2001, a task force comprising representatives of the Bethesda 2001 group members and the American Society of Colposcopy and Cervical Pathology (ASCCP) provided additional guidance regarding minimally abnormal Pap smear results.[23] Current Canadian guidelines indicate that the management of women with ASCs depends on whether the Pap smear is subcategorized as "of undetermined significance (ASC-US)" or as "cannot exclude HSIL (ASC-H)." With a liquid-based Pap smear, a portion of the fluid can be sent for HPV DNA testing. If HPV testing is negative, the ASC-US is likely related to inflammation, atrophy, or other temporary or reversible processes, and the Pap smear can be repeated in 1 year. Referral for colposcopy or other definitive diagnostic measures is recommended for women with positive HPV DNA test results; ASC-H, LSIL, or HSIL lesions; or if compliance with follow-up observation is uncertain. Colposcopy can also be used if women have suspect findings on examination or are immunocompromised.[21]

Before the availability of colposcopy, many women with abnormal Pap smear results required surgical cone biopsy for further evaluation. Cone biopsy involves the removal of a cone-shaped wedge of cervix, including the entire transformation zone and at least 50% of the endocervical canal. Postoperative hemorrhage, infection, cervical stenosis, infertility, and incompetent cervix are possible sequelae that warrant avoidance of this procedure unless it is truly necessary.

The LEEP or LLETZ (large loop excision of the transformation zone), a refinement of loop diathermy techniques dating back to the 1940s, is quickly becoming the first-line management for SIL. This outpatient procedure allows for the simultaneous diagnosis and treatment of dysplastic lesions found on colposcopy. It uses a thin, rigid, wire loop electrode attached to a generator that blends high-frequency, low-voltage current for cutting and a modulated higher voltage for coagulation. In skilled hands, this wire can remove the entire transformation zone, providing adequate treatment for the lesion while obtaining a specimen for further histologic evaluation.

Diagnosis and Treatment of Cervical Cancer. In its early stages, cervical cancer often manifests as a poorly defined lesion of the endocervix. Frequently, women with cervical cancer present with abnormal vaginal bleeding, spotting, and discharge. Although bleeding may assume any course, it is reported most frequently after intercourse. Women with more advanced disease may present with pelvic or back pain that may radiate down the leg, hematuria, fistulas (rectovaginal or vesicovaginal), or evidence of metastatic disease to supraclavicular or inguinal lymph node areas.

Early treatment of cervical cancer involves removal of the lesion by one of various techniques. Biopsy or local cautery may be therapeutic in and of itself. Electrocautery, cryosurgery, or carbon dioxide laser therapy may be used to treat moderate to severe dysplasia that is limited to the exocervix (*i.e.*, squamocolumnar junction clearly visible). Therapeutic conization becomes necessary if the lesion extends into the endocervical canal and can be done surgically or with LEEP in the physician's office.[3]

Depending on the stage of involvement of the cervix, invasive cancer is treated with radiation therapy, surgery, or both. External-beam irradiation and intracavitary irradiation or *brachytherapy (i.e.,* insertion of radioactive materials into the body) can be used in the treatment of cervical cancer (see Chapter 8). Intracavitary radiation provides direct access to the central lesion and increases the tolerance of the cervix and surrounding tissues, permitting curative levels of radiation to be used. External-beam radiation eliminates metastatic disease in pelvic lymph nodes and other structures, as well as shrinking the cervical lesion to optimize the effects of intracavitary radiation. Surgery can include trachelectomy (*i.e.,* removal of the cervix) in women with early stage cancer desiring fertility, extended hysterectomy (*i.e.,* removal of the uterus, fallopian tubes, ovaries, and upper portion of the vagina) without pelvic lymph node dissection, radical hysterectomy with pelvic lymph node dissection, or pelvic exenteration (*i.e.,* removal of all pelvic organs, including the bladder, rectum, vulva, and vagina). The choice of treatment is influenced by the stage of the disease as well as the woman's age and health.[3]

Disorders of the Uterus

Endometritis

The endometrium and myometrium are relatively resistant to infections, primarily because the endocervix normally forms a barrier to ascending infections. Acute endometritis is uncommon and usually occurs after the cervical barrier is compromised by abortion, delivery, or instrumentation.[11,22] Curettage is diagnostic and often curative because it removes the necrotic tissue that has served as a site of infection.

Chronic inflammation of the endometrium is associated with pelvic inflammatory disease (PID), instrumentation of the uterus (*e.g.,* after endometrial biopsy or implantation of an intrauterine device [IUD]), and retained products of conception after delivery or abortion. The presence of plasma cells (which are not present in the normal endometrium) is required for diagnosis. The clinical picture is variable, but often includes abnormal vaginal bleeding, mild to severe uterine tenderness, fever, malaise, and foul-smelling discharge. Treatment involves oral or intravenous antibiotic therapy, depending on the severity of the condition.

Endometriosis

Endometriosis is the condition in which functional endometrial tissue is found in ectopic sites outside the uterus. It is a progressively inflammatory chronic disease leading to implants, scarring, adhesions, and ovarian cysts called endometriomas. The sites where endometriosis may occur include the ovaries, posterior broad ligaments, uterosacral ligaments, pouch of Douglas (cul-de-sac), pelvis, vagina, vulva, perineum, or intestines (Fig. 46.3). Rarely, endometrial implants have been found in the nostrils, umbilicus, lungs, and limbs.[23]

The cause of endometriosis is unknown. There appears to have been an increase in its incidence in the developed Western countries during the past four to five decades. Approximately 10% of premenopausal women have endometriosis, and up to 50% of women with infertility have some degree of endometriosis.[24]

Several theories attempt to explain the origin of the dispersed endometrial lesions that occur in women with endometriosis.[11] One theory, the *regurgitation/implantation theory* (also known as Sampson theory), suggests that menstrual blood containing fragments of endometrium is forced upward through the fallopian tubes into the peritoneal cavity.[23] Retrograde menstruation is not an uncommon phenomenon, and it is unknown why endometrial cells implant and grow in some women but not in others. A second theory, the *metaplastic theory,* proposes that dormant, immature cellular elements, spread over a wide area during embryonic development, persist into adult life and

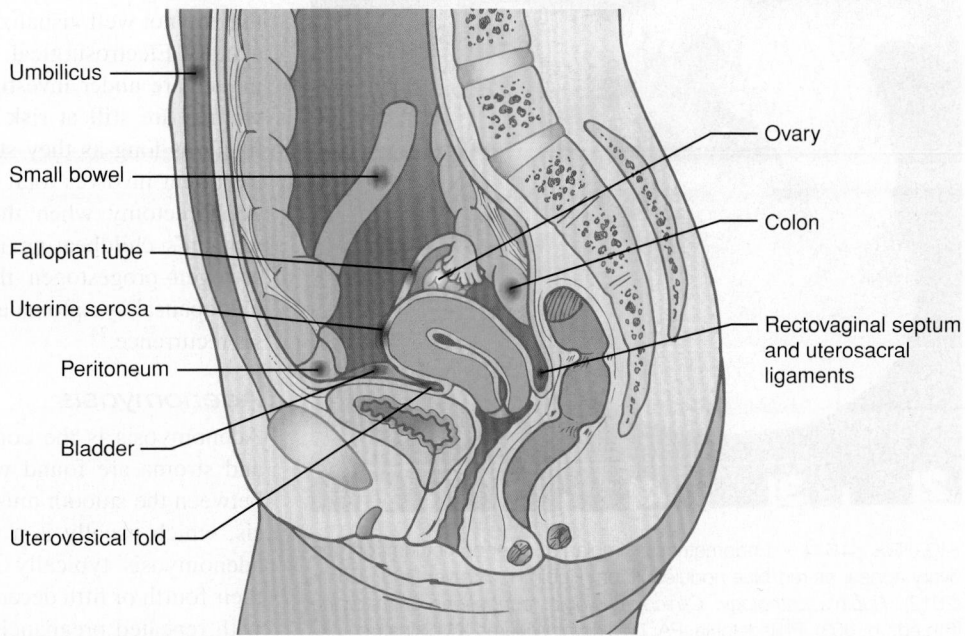

FIGURE 46.3 • Common locations of endometriosis in the pelvis and abdomen.

Umbilicus

Small bowel

Fallopian tube

Uterine serosa

Peritoneum

Bladder

Uterovesical fold

Ovary

Colon

Rectovaginal septum and uterosacral ligaments

then differentiate into endometrial tissue. Another theory, the *vascular* or *lymphatic theory,* suggests that the endometrial tissue may metastasize through the lymphatics or vascular system. Genetic and immune factors also have been studied as contributing factors to the development of endometriosis.[2,3,23]

Endometriosis usually becomes apparent in the reproductive years when the lesions are stimulated by ovarian hormones in the same way as normal endometrium, becoming proliferative, then secretory, and finally undergoing menstrual breakdown. Bleeding into the surrounding structures can cause pain and the development of significant pelvic adhesions. Symptoms tend to be strongest premenstrually, subsiding after cessation of menstruation. Pelvic pain is the most common presenting symptom; other symptoms include back pain, dyspareunia, and pain on defecation and micturition. Endometriosis is associated with infertility because of adhesions that distort the pelvic anatomy and cause impaired ovum release and transport.

The gross pathologic changes that occur in endometriosis differ with location and duration. In the ovary, the endometrial tissue may form cysts (*i.e.,* endometriomas filled with old blood that resembles chocolate syrup [chocolate cysts]). Rupture of these cysts can cause peritonitis and adhesions. Elsewhere in the pelvis, the tissue may take the form of small hemorrhagic lesions that may be black, bluish, red, clear, or opaque (Fig. 46.4). Some may be surrounded by scar tissue.

Endometriosis may be difficult to diagnose because its symptoms mimic those of other pelvic disorders and the severity of the symptoms does not always reflect the extent of the disease. Unfortunately, there are no serum markers or noninvasive tests that screen for endometriosis. Definitive diagnosis can be accomplished only through laparoscopy. This minimally invasive surgery allows direct visualization of pelvic organs to determine the presence and extent of endometrial lesions. Imaging techniques, including ultrasonography and magnetic resonance imaging (MRI), can be useful tools in evaluating endometriomas and deep endometriosis.[24]

Treatment modalities fall into three categories: pain relief, endometrial suppression, and surgery. In young women, simple observation and analgesics (nonsteroidal anti-inflammatory drugs [NSAIDs]) may be sufficient treatment. The use of hormones to induce physiologic amenorrhea is based on the observation that pregnancy and menopause afford pain relief by inducing atrophy of the endometrial tissue. This can be accomplished through administration of oral contraceptive pills, continuous progestogen agents (medroxyprogesterone acetate [oral or depot injection] or the levonorgestrel intrauterine system), or Danazol (a synthetic androgen that is less commonly used now given the increased side effect profile). In women with severe endometriosis, long-acting gonadotropin-releasing hormone (GnRH) analogs that inhibit the pituitary gonadotropins and suppress ovulation may be used.[3,23,24]

Surgery may offer more definitive therapy for women with large or symptomatic endometriomas, or those who have failed medical therapy for endometriosis. The goal of surgical treatment is to restore normal anatomic relationships, remove all visible lesions and slow progression of the disease—all done in a way that minimizes development of pelvic adhesions and avoids injury to normal surrounding structures. Laparoscopy is the preferred surgical approach today and has demonstrated equivalent pain relief with shorter perioperative recovery compared with laparotomy. Laparoscopic treatment options include the use of cautery, laser ablation, and excision techniques.[23,24] Advantages of laser surgery include better hemostasis, more precision in vaporizing lesions with less damage to surrounding tissue, and better access to areas that are not well visualized or would be difficult to reach with cautery. Electrosurgical, thermal, and ultrasonic ablation techniques are under investigation. Even with extensive surgery, women are still at risk for continued symptoms postoperatively as long as they still have menstrual cycles. Definitive treatment involves total hysterectomy and bilateral salpingo-oophorectomy when the symptoms are unbearable or the woman's childbearing is completed. Continuous combined estrogen–progestogen therapy is recommended to manage menopausal symptoms and minimize the risk of endometriosis recurrence.[24]

Adenomyosis

Adenomyosis is the condition in which endometrial glands and stroma are found within the myometrium, interspersed between the smooth muscle fibres. In contrast to endometriosis, which usually is a problem of young, infertile women, adenomyosis typically is found in multiparous women in their fourth or fifth decade. It is thought that events associated with repeated pregnancies, deliveries, and uterine involution

FIGURE 46.4 • Endometriosis. Implants of endometrium on the ovary appear as red-blue nodules. (From Rubin R., Strayer D. S. (Eds.). (2012). *Rubin's pathology: Clinicopathologic foundations of medicine* (6th ed., p. 903). Philadelphia, PA: Lippincott Williams & Wilkins.)

may cause the endometrium to be displaced throughout the myometrium. Adenomyosis frequently coexists with uterine myomas or endometrial hyperplasia. The diagnosis of adenomyosis often occurs as an incidental finding in a uterus removed for symptoms suggestive of myoma or hyperplasia. Heavy, painful periods with clots and painful intercourse are common complaints of women with adenomyosis. Although in the past the diagnosis was made primarily through careful history and the pelvic examination findings of an enlarged, boggy uterus, MRI is now considered an excellent diagnostic tool for confirming this condition. Adenomyosis resolves with menopause. Conservative therapy using oral contraceptives or GnRH agonists is the first choice for treatment. Hysterectomy (with preservation of the ovaries in premenopausal women) is considered when this approach fails.[25]

Endometrial Cancer

Endometrial cancer is the most common cancer found in the female pelvis, occurring more than twice as often as cervical cancer. In 2015, the Canadian Cancer Society estimates that approximately 6,300 women will be diagnosed with endometrial cancer and 1,050 will die of this disorder.[26] Endometrial cancer occurs more frequently in older women (peak ages of 55 to 65 years), with only 8% occurring in women younger than 45 years of age.

Although the proportion of cases of endometrial cancer with a background of familial risk is low, endometrial cancer can develop as part of a hereditary cancer syndrome. Women with a family history of hereditary nonpolyposis colorectal cancer (also known as Lynch syndrome) may have an inherited disorder in DNA mismatch repair genes that predisposes to endometrial and ovarian cancers, as well as colorectal cancer. This autosomal dominant disease carries a 40% to 60% risk of developing cancer of some type for those who inherit the mutation.[27]

Incidence and Pathogenesis. In terms of potential pathogenesis, two general groups of endometrial cancer can be identified. The first develops on a background of prolonged estrogen stimulation and endometrial hyperplasia, whereas the second is less commonly associated with hyperestrogenism and endometrial hyperplasia.

Most endometrial cancers (about 85%) are moderately well-differentiated adenocarcinomas that develop on a background of endometrial hyperplasia. These tumours, also known as *type 1 endometrial cancers,* are typically hormone sensitive, low grade, and have a favourable prognosis. They are associated with long-duration unopposed estrogen stimulation and tend to be well differentiated, mimicking normal endometrial glands in histologic appearance, or display altered differentiation (mucinous, tubal, squamous differentiation).[11,28]

The endometrium undergoes structural modification and cellular changes in response to fluctuations in estrogen and progesterone levels that occur during the menstrual cycle. Prolonged unopposed estrogen stimulation leads to endometrial hyperplasia, which increases the chance of development of atypical hyperplasia and eventually type 1 endometrial cancer. Although the molecular basis for this process is still unknown, anovulatory cycles, disorders of estrogen metabolism, unopposed estrogen therapy, estrogen-secreting granulosa cell tumour, and obesity are all known to increase the risk of endometrial cancer.[2,3,29]

Ovulatory dysfunction that causes infertility at any age or occurs with declining ovarian function in perimenopausal women also can result in unopposed estrogen and increase the risk of endometrial cancer. A sharp rise in endometrial cancer was seen in the 1970s among middle-aged women who had received unopposed estrogen therapy (*i.e.,* estrogen therapy without progesterone) for menopausal symptoms. It was later determined that it was not the estrogen exposure that increased the risk of cancer, but that the hormone was administered without progesterone. It is the presence of progesterone in the second half of the menstrual cycle that matures the endometrium, and the withdrawal of progesterone that ultimately results in endometrial sloughing. Long-term unopposed estrogen exposure without periodic addition of progesterone allows for continued endometrial growth and hyperplasia, which increases the chance of development of atypical cells. Hyperplasia usually regresses after treatment with cyclic progesterone. Sequential oral contraceptives (estrogen alone for 15 days followed by 7 days of combined estrogen and progestin) were withdrawn from the market in the 1970s because of potential risk of endometrial hyperplasia. In contrast, combination oral contraceptives (estrogen and progestin in each pill) effectively prevent hyperplasia and decrease the risk of cancer by 50%.[3] Tamoxifen, a drug that blocks estrogen receptor sites and is used in treatment of breast cancer, exerts a weak estrogenic effect on the endometrium and represents another exogenous risk factor for endometrial cancer.

Diabetes mellitus, hypertension, and polycystic ovary syndrome (PCOS) are conditions that alter estrogen metabolism and elevate estrogen levels. Excessive fat consumption and being overweight are important risk factors for endometrial cancer. In premenopausal women, overweight causes insulin resistance, ovarian androgen excess, anovulation, and chronic progesterone deficiency. In postmenopausal women, estrogens are synthesized in body fats from adrenal and ovarian androgen precursors. Because of its effect on insulin-like growth factor-1 (IGF-1) and its binding protein, obesity can be a risk factor even when circulating levels of estrogen are normal. Estrogen receptor transcriptional activity can be induced by IGF-1 signalling even in the absence of estrogen.

A second subset of endometrial cancers (about 10%) are high-grade tumours with a tendency to recur, even in early stages. These tumours, also known as *type 2 endometrial cancers,* are not estrogen driven, typically occur in women who acquire the disease at a somewhat older age, and are mostly associated with endometrial atrophy rather than hyperplasia.[11,22,28] Overall, this type of endometrial cancer usually has a poorer prognosis than that associated with prolonged estrogen stimulation and endometrial hyperplasia.

Clinical Course. The major symptom of endometrial hyperplasia or overt endometrial cancer is abnormal, painless bleeding. In menstruating women, this takes the form of bleeding between periods or excessive, prolonged menstrual flow. In postmenopausal women, any bleeding is abnormal and warrants investigation. Abnormal bleeding is an early warning sign of the disease, and because endometrial cancer tends to be slow growing in its early stages, the chances of cure are good if prompt medical care is sought. Later signs of uterine cancer may include cramping, pelvic discomfort, postcoital bleeding, lower abdominal pressure, and enlarged lymph nodes.

Although the Pap smear can identify a small percentage of endometrial cancers, it is not a good screening test for this type of gynecologic cancer. Endometrial biopsy (tissue sample obtained in an office procedure by direct aspiration of the endometrial cavity) is far more accurate. Dilation and curettage (D&C), which consists of dilating the cervix and scraping the uterine cavity, is the definitive procedure for diagnosis because it provides a more thorough evaluation. Transvaginal ultrasonography (TVS) used to measure the endometrial thickness is being evaluated as an initial test for postmenopausal bleeding because it is less invasive than endometrial biopsy and less costly than D&C when biopsy is not possible.[29]

The prognosis for endometrial cancer depends on the clinical stage of the disease when it is discovered and its histologic grade and type. Surgery and radiation therapy are the most successful methods of treatment for endometrial cancer. When used alone, radiation therapy has a 20% lower cure rate than surgery for stage I disease. It may be the best option, however, in women who are not good surgical candidates. Total abdominal hysterectomy with bilateral salpingo-oophorectomy plus sampling of regional lymph nodes and peritoneal washings for cytologic evaluation of occult disease is the treatment of choice whenever possible. Postoperative radiation therapy may be added in cases of advanced disease for more complete treatment and to prevent recurrence or metastasis, although the benefits of this as adjuvant therapy are still controversial. The 5-year relative survival rate of early diagnosed endometrial cancers is 96%. The survival rate for all endometrial cancers (those diagnosed early and late stage) is approximately 83%.[30]

Leiomyomas

Uterine leiomyomas (commonly called *fibroids*) are benign neoplasms in premenopausal women of smooth muscle origin. These are the most common form of pelvic tumour and are believed to occur in one of every four or five women older than 35 years of age. They are seen more often and their rate of growth is more rapid in black women than in white women.[31] Leiomyomas usually develop as submucosal, subserosal, or intramural tumours in the corpus of the uterus (Fig. 46.5). Intramural fibroids are embedded in the myometrium. They are the most common type of fibroid, and present as a symmetric enlargement of the nonpregnant uterus. Subserosal tumours are located beneath the perimetrium of the uterus. These tumours are recognized as irregular projections on the

FIGURE 46.5 • A: Submucosal, intramural, and subserosal leiomyomas. **B:** A bisected uterus displays a prominent, sharply circumscribed, fleshy tumour. (From Rubin R., Strayer D. S. (Eds.). (2012). *Rubin's pathology: Clinicopathologic foundations of medicine* (6th ed., pp. 882, 883). Philadelphia, PA: Lippincott Williams & Wilkins.)

uterine surface; they may become pedunculated, displacing or impinging on other genitourinary structures and causing hydroureter or bladder problems. Submucosal fibroids displace endometrial tissue and are more likely to cause bleeding, necrosis, and infection than either of the other types.

Leiomyomas are asymptomatic approximately half of the time and may be discovered during a routine pelvic examination, or they may cause menorrhagia (excessive menstrual bleeding), anemia, urinary frequency, rectal pressure/constipation, abdominal distension, and infrequently pain. Their rate of growth is variable, but they may increase in size during pregnancy or with exogenous estrogen stimulation (*i.e.,* oral contraceptives or menopausal estrogen replacement therapy). Interference with pregnancy is rare unless the tumour is submucosal and interferes with implantation or obstructs the cervical outlet. These tumours may outgrow their blood supply, become infarcted, and undergo degenerative changes.

Leiomyomas should regress with menopause, but if bleeding, pressure on the bladder, pain, or other problems persist, hysterectomy may be required. Myomectomy (removal of just the tumours) can be done to preserve the uterus for future childbearing. Cesarean section may be recommended if the uterine cavity is entered during myomectomy. Hypothalamic GnRH agonists (*e.g.,* leuprolide) may be used to suppress leiomyoma growth before surgery.[32] Uterine artery embolization done by an interventional radiologist is a nonsurgical therapy that has demonstrated short-term advantages but generally higher frequency of reintervention compared to surgery. Additionally, most patients experience acute abdominal pain postembolization with no correlation to the number or size of myoma and with 5% to 10% of women the pain persists for 2 weeks. It is assumed that this pain is due to nonspecific ischemia of the leiomyoma.

IN SUMMARY

Disorders of the cervix and uterus include inflammatory conditions (*i.e.,* cervicitis and endometritis), cancer (*i.e.,* cervical and endometrial cancer), endometriosis, and leiomyomas. Cervicitis is an acute or chronic inflammation of the cervix. Acute cervicitis may result from the direct infection of the cervix or may be secondary to a vaginal or uterine infection. It may be caused by a variety of infectious agents. Chronic cervicitis represents a low-grade inflammatory process resulting from trauma or nonspecific infectious agents. Cervical cancer arises from precursor lesions that can be detected on a Pap smear and if detected early, is the most easily cured of all the cancers of the female reproductive system. Evidence suggests a causal link between HPV infection and cervical cancer. Vaccines against several strains of the HPV are available and show promise for the prevention of cervical cancer.

Endometritis represents an ill-defined inflammation or infection of the endometrium that produces variable symptoms. Endometriosis is the condition in which functional endometrial tissue is found in ectopic sites outside the uterus, particularly in dependent parts of the pelvis and in the ovaries. It causes dysmenorrhea, dyspareunia, and infertility. Adenomyosis is the condition in which endometrial glands and stroma are found in the myometrium, interspersed between the smooth muscle fibres. Endometrial cancer is the most common cancer found in the female pelvis, occurring more than twice as often as cervical cancer. Prolonged estrogen stimulation with hyperplasia of the endometrium has been identified as a major risk factor for endometrial cancer.

Leiomyomas are benign uterine wall neoplasms in premenopausal women of smooth muscle origin. They can develop in the corpus of the uterus and can be submucosal, subserosal, or intramural. Submucosal fibroids displace endometrial tissue and are more likely to cause bleeding, necrosis, and infection than either of the other types.

DISORDERS OF THE FALLOPIAN TUBES AND OVARIES

After completing this section of the chapter, you should be able to meet the following objectives:

- List the common causes and symptoms of pelvic inflammatory disease.
- Describe the risk factors and symptoms of ectopic pregnancy.
- State the underlying cause of ovarian cysts.
- Differentiate benign ovarian cyst from polycystic ovary syndrome.
- List the hormones produced by the three types of functioning ovarian tumours.
- State the reason that ovarian cancer may be difficult to detect in an early stage.

Pelvic Inflammatory Disease

Pelvic inflammatory disease (PID) is a polymicrobial infection of the upper reproductive tract (uterus, fallopian tubes, or ovaries) associated with the sexually transmitted organisms *N. gonorrhoeae* or *C. trachomatis* as well as with endogenous organisms, including anaerobes, *Haemophilus influenzae,* enteric gram-negative rods, and streptococci.[33,34,35,36] The organisms ascend through the endocervical canal to the endometrial cavity, and then to the tubes and ovaries. The endocervical canal is slightly dilated during menstruation, allowing bacteria to gain entrance to the uterus and other pelvic structures. After entering the upper reproductive tract, the organisms multiply rapidly in the favourable environment of the sloughing endometrium and ascend to the fallopian tube (Fig. 46.6).

Factors that predispose women to the development of PID include an age of 16 to 24 years, nulliparity, history of multiple sexual partners, and previous history of PID. Although the use of an IUD has been associated with a three- to fivefold increased risk for development of PID, studies have shown that women with only one sexual partner who are at low risk of acquiring STIs have no significant risk for development of PID from using an IUD.

Clinical Course

The symptoms of PID include lower abdominal pain, which may start just after a menstrual period; dyspareunia; back pain; purulent cervical discharge; and the presence of adnexal tenderness and exquisitely painful cervix on bimanual pelvic examination. Fever (>38°C), increased erythrocyte sedimentation rate, and an elevated white blood cell count (>10 ×10^9/L) commonly are seen, even though the woman may not appear acutely ill. Elevated C-reactive protein levels equate with inflammation and can be used as another diagnostic tool. Laparoscopy, which allows for direct visualization of the ovaries, fallopian tubes, and uterus, is one of the most specific

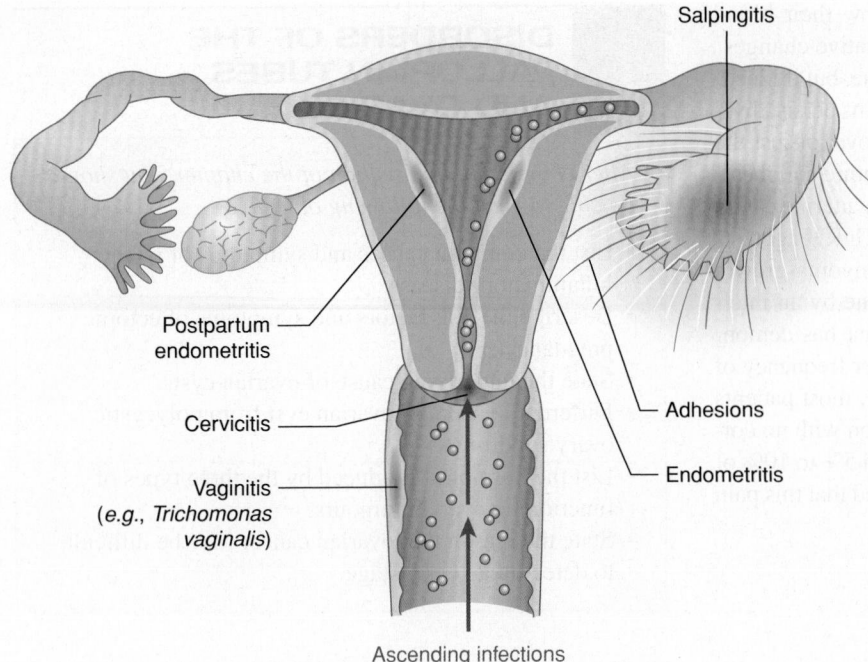

Salpingitis

Postpartum
endometritis

Cervicitis

Vaginitis
(*e.g.*, *Trichomonas
vaginalis*)

Adhesions

Endometritis

Ascending infections
(*e.g.*, *Gonococcus, Staphylococcus*, anaerobes,
Streptococcus, Chlamydia)

FIGURE 46.6 • Pelvic inflammatory disease. Microbial agents enter through the vagina and ascend to involve the uterus, fallopian tubes, and pelvic structures.

procedures for diagnosing PID, but is costly and carries the inherent risks of surgery and anesthesia.[33] Minimal criteria for a presumptive diagnosis of PID require only the presence of lower abdominal pain, adnexal tenderness, and cervical motion tenderness on bimanual examination with no other apparent cause.[33–35]

Outpatient antibiotic therapy is usually sufficient. However, treatment may involve hospitalization with intravenous administration of antibiotics in some cases. Antibiotic regimens should be selected according to STI treatment guidelines, which are published by the Public Health Agency of Canada (PHAC; see Chapter 47).[34] Treatment is aimed at preventing complications, which can include pelvic adhesions, infertility, ectopic pregnancy, chronic abdominal pain, and tubo-ovarian abscesses. Accurate diagnosis and appropriate antibiotic therapy may decrease the severity and frequency of PID sequelae. The PHAC recommends empiric treatment with a presumptive diagnosis of PID, while waiting for confirmation by culture or other definitive test results.[34,35]

Ectopic Pregnancy

Although pregnancy is not discussed in detail in this text, it is reasonable to mention ectopic pregnancy because it represents a true gynecologic emergency and should be considered when a woman of reproductive age presents with the complaint of pelvic pain. Ectopic pregnancy occurs when a fertilized ovum implants outside the uterine cavity, the most common site being the fallopian tube (Fig. 46.7). It accounts for 1% to 2% of spontaneously conceived pregnancies and is consistent across maternal age ranges and ethnic origins.[36,37] Updated estimates for incidence rates are difficult to determine because

many women are now treated on an outpatient basis, so data from hospital discharge records are no longer representative of the scope of the problem. Although ectopic pregnancy is the leading cause of maternal mortality in the first trimester, the death rate has steadily declined as a result of improved diagnostic methods. Earlier detection reduces the risk of tubal

FIGURE 46.7 • Ectopic pregnancy. An enlarged fallopian tube has been opened to disclose a minute fetus. (From Rubin E., Gorstein F., Rubin R., et al. (Eds.). (2004). *Rubin's pathology: Clinicopathologic foundations of medicine* (4th ed., p. 966). Philadelphia, PA: Lippincott Williams & Wilkins.)

rupture, which could result in intra-abdominal hemorrhage, major complications, future infertility, or death.[37]

The cause of ectopic pregnancy is delayed ovum transport, which may result from decreased tubal motility or distorted tubal anatomy (*i.e.,* narrowed lumen, convolutions, or diverticula). Risk factors most strongly associated with ectopic pregnancy include previous tubal surgery, tubal ligation or reversal, previous ectopic pregnancy, and a tubal lesion or abnormality. Smoking, current IUD use, history of PID or therapeutic abortion, and the use of fertility drugs to induce ovulation have also been associated with an increased risk for ectopic pregnancy.[36,37]

Clinical Course

The site of implantation in the tube (*e.g.,* isthmus, ampulla) may determine the onset of symptoms and the timing of diagnosis. As the tubal pregnancy progresses, the surrounding tissue is stretched. The pregnancy eventually outgrows its blood supply, at which point the pregnancy terminates or the tube itself ruptures because it can no longer contain the growing pregnancy.

Symptoms can include lower abdominal discomfort—diffuse or localized to one side—that progresses to severe pain caused by rupture, spotting, syncope, referred shoulder pain from bleeding into the abdominal cavity, and amenorrhea. Physical examination usually reveals adnexal tenderness; an adnexal mass is found in only 50% of cases.[37] Although rarely used today, culdocentesis (needle aspiration from the cul-de-sac) may reveal blood if rupture has occurred.

Diagnostic tests for ectopic pregnancy include a urine pregnancy test, ultrasonography, and β-human chorionic gonadotropin (hCG; a hormone produced by placental cells) levels. Serial hCG tests may detect lower-than-normal hCG production. Transvaginal ultrasonographic studies after 5 weeks' gestation may demonstrate an empty uterine cavity or presence of the gestational sac outside the uterus. In a comparison of various protocols for diagnosing ectopic pregnancy, ultrasonography followed by serial hCG levels was found to yield the best results.[36,37] Definitive diagnosis may require laparoscopy. Differential diagnosis for this type of pelvic pain includes ruptured ovarian cyst, threatened or incomplete abortion, PID, acute appendicitis, and degenerating fibroid.

Treatment is aimed at resolving the problem with minimal morbidity and protecting future fertility where possible. Advances in detection now make it possible to treat early ectopic pregnancies medically or in some cases expectantly. Methotrexate (an antimetabolite used in treatment of chronic inflammatory diseases and cancer) is often used to as primary treatment in cases where the pregnancy is diagnosed early and is unruptured. This folic acid antagonist interferes with DNA and ribonucleic acid (RNA) synthesis, thus inhibiting the growth of trophoblastic cells at the placental implantation site. Close follow-up with serial hCG levels is necessary to ensure that no residual pregnancy tissue remains. Surgical removal of the pregnancy is required when it is unlikely that medical management will be effective (*e.g.,* large ectopic pregnancy,

presence of a fetal heartbeat, noncompliance of the patient), when rupture is imminent or has already occurred, or when the woman is hemodynamically unstable.[37] Laparoscopic treatment of ectopic pregnancy is well tolerated and more cost effective than laparotomy because of shorter convalescence and the reduced need for postoperative analgesia. Laparotomy, which involves an open incision into the abdominopelvic cavity, becomes necessary when there is uncontrolled internal bleeding, when the ectopic site cannot be visualized through the laparoscope, or when the surgeon is not trained in operative laparoscopy.

Cancer of the Fallopian Tube

Although a common site of metastases, primary cancer of the fallopian tube is rare, accounting for less than 1% of all female genital tract cancers. Fewer than 3,000 cases have been reported worldwide. Most primary tubal cancers are papillary adenocarcinomas, and these tumours develop bilaterally in 30% of patients with advanced disease.

Symptoms are uncommon, but intermittent serosanguineous vaginal discharge, abnormal vaginal bleeding, and colicky low abdominal pain have been reported. An adnexal mass may be present; however, the preoperative diagnosis in most cases is leiomyoma or ovarian tumour. Management is similar to that for ovarian cancer and usually includes total hysterectomy, bilateral salpingo-oophorectomy, and pelvic lymph node dissection. More extensive procedures may be warranted, depending on the stage of the disease.[2,38]

Ovarian Cysts and Tumours

The ovaries have a dual function: they produce germ cells, or ova, and they synthesize the female sex hormones. Disorders of the ovaries frequently cause menstrual and fertility problems. Benign conditions of the ovaries can present as primary lesions of the ovarian structures or as secondary disorders related to hypothalamic, pituitary, or adrenal dysfunction.

Ovarian Cysts

Cysts are the most common form of ovarian tumour. Many are benign. A follicular cyst is one that results from occlusion of the duct of the follicle. Each month, several follicles begin to develop and are blighted at various stages of development. These follicles form cavities that fill with fluid, producing a cyst. The dominant follicle normally ruptures to release the egg (*i.e.,* ovulation), but occasionally persists and continues growing. Likewise, a luteal cyst is a persistent cystic enlargement of the corpus luteum that is formed after ovulation and does not regress in the absence of pregnancy. Functional cysts are asymptomatic unless there is substantial enlargement or bleeding into the cyst. This can cause considerable discomfort or a dull, aching sensation on the affected side. These cysts usually regress spontaneously. Occasionally a cyst may become twisted or may rupture into the intra-abdominal cavity (Fig. 46.8).

FIGURE 46.8 • Follicular cyst of the ovary. The rupture of this thin-walled follicular cyst (dowel stick) led to intra-abdominal hemorrhage. (From Rubin R., Strayer D. S. (Eds.). (2012). *Rubin's pathology: Clinicopathologic foundations of medicine* (6th ed., p. 886). Philadelphia, PA: Lippincott Williams & Wilkins.)

Polycystic Ovary Syndrome

Polycystic ovary syndrome (PCOS) is a common endocrine disorder affecting 5% to 10% of women of reproductive age, and is a frequent source of chronic anovulation. The diagnosis of PCOS is made after other endocrine diseases are ruled out and the patient has varying degrees of ovarian dysfunction (*e.g.*, oligomenorrhea [irregular infrequent menses] or amenorrhea [no menses]), biochemical or clinical signs of hyperandrogenism (acne, excess body hair [hirsutism], male-pattern hair loss), and infertility.[39,40] About 50% of women who are diagnosed with PCOS are obese, and most have polycystic ovaries. Hyperinsulinemia and insulin resistance have recently been hypothesized to play a role in the pathogenesis of the disorder.

The precise etiology of this condition is still being debated, but is probably multifactorial. A possible genetic basis has been suggested with an autosomal dominant mode of inheritance and premature balding as the phenotype in males.[42] There is increasing evidence that the disorder may begin before adolescence and that many of the manifestations of PCOS begin to make their appearance at that time. Because many of the symptoms common to PCOS, such as excess hair, acne, and obesity, can be detrimental to a teenage girl's health and self-esteem, early detection and treatment of PCOS in adolescents is essential.[40]

Although this syndrome has been the subject of considerable research, the underlying mechanisms remain unclear. Chronic anovulation is thought to be the underlying cause of the amenorrhea or irregular menses and enlarged, "polycystic" ovaries associated with this condition. Most women with PCOS have elevated luteinizing hormone (LH) levels with normal estrogen and follicle-stimulating hormone (FSH) production. Elevated levels of circulating total testosterone, free testosterone, and dehydroepiandrosterone sulfate (DHEA-S) are not uncommon, and these women occasionally have hyperprolactinemia or hypothyroidism. Persistent anovulation results in an estrogen environment that alters the hypothalamic release of GnRH with a resultant increase in LH secretion and suppression of FSH release by the pituitary gland. This altered LH/FSH ratio often is used as a diagnostic criterion for this condition, but it is not universally present. Although the presence of some FSH allows for new follicular development, full maturation is not attained, and ovulation does not occur. The elevated LH level results in increased androgen production, which in turn prevents normal follicular development and contributes to the vicious cycle of anovulation.[39]

The association between hyperandrogenism and hyperinsulinemia is now well recognized. It has been shown that the cause of hyperinsulinemia is insulin resistance. The frequency and degree of hyperinsulinemia in women with PCOS is often amplified by the presence of obesity. Insulin may cause hyperandrogenism in several ways, although the exact mechanism has not been well defined. It has been shown that the ovary possesses insulin receptors and there is evidence that insulin may act directly on the ovary. Several reports have shown that normal ovulation and sometimes pregnancy have occurred when women with hyperandrogenism were treated with insulin-sensitizing drugs.[39,40]

In addition to its clinical manifestations, long-term health problems including cardiovascular disease and diabetes have been linked to PCOS. There is also concern that women with PCOS who are anovulatory do not produce progesterone. This may, in turn, subject the uterine lining to an unopposed estrogen environment, which is a significant risk factor for development of endometrial cancer.[41] Although there also is a reported association with breast, endometrial, and ovarian cancer, PCOS has not been conclusively shown to be an independent risk factor for any of these malignancies.

The diagnosis PCOS can be suspected from the clinical presentation. Although there is no consensus as to which tests should be used, laboratory evaluations to exclude hyperprolactinemia, late-onset adrenal hyperplasia, and androgen-secreting tumours of the ovary and adrenal gland are commonly done. Although fasting blood glucose, 2-hour oral glucose tolerance test, and insulin levels are often measured to evaluate for hyperinsulinemia, this testing is not required prior to treatment as insulin resistance is almost universal in women with PCOS. Confirmation with ultrasonography or laparoscopic visualization of the ovaries is often done, but not required.[39–41]

The overall goal of treatment should be directed towards symptom relief, prevention of potential malignant endometrial sequelae, protection for potential fertility, and reduction in risk for development of diabetes and cardiovascular disease. The preferred and most effective treatment for PCOS is lifestyle modification. Weight loss may be beneficial in restoring normal ovulation when obesity is present. Although numerous medications and protocols are available, the choice depends on the manifestations that are most bothersome to the woman and her stage in reproductive life. Combined contraceptive agents ameliorate menstrual irregularities and improve hirsutism and acne. The addition of spironolactone, an antimineralocorticoid that inhibits the production of androgens by the adrenal gland, may be beneficial to women with severe hirsutism.[39,42]

Metformin, an insulin-sensitizing drug, used with or without ovulation-inducing medications, is emerging as an important component of PCOS treatment. In addition to expected improvements in insulin sensitivity and glucose metabolism, it has been associated with reductions in androgen and LH levels and is highly effective in restoring normal menstrual regularity and ovulatory cycles.

When fertility is desired, the condition is usually treated with metformin and alternative medications can include the administration of the hypothalamic–pituitary-stimulating drug

clomiphene citrate or injectable gonadotropins to induce ovulation. These drugs must be used carefully because they can induce extreme enlargement of the ovaries.[39–42]

Benign and Functioning Ovarian Tumours

Ovarian tumours are extremely common. Most are benign, but malignant ovarian tumours are the leading cause of death from reproductive cancers. Ovarian tumours can arise from any of the ovarian tissue types—serosal epithelium, germ cell layers, or gonadal stromal tissue[11,22] (Fig. 46.9). Serous and mucinous cystadenomas are the most common benign ovarian neoplasms. Endometriomas are the "chocolate cysts" that develop secondary to ovarian endometriosis. Ovarian fibromas are connective tissue tumours composed of fibrocytes and collagen. They range in size from 6 to 20 cm. Cystic teratomas, or dermoid cysts, are derived from primordial germ cells and are composed of various combinations of well-differentiated ectodermal, mesodermal, and endodermal elements. Not uncommonly, they contain sebaceous material, hair, or teeth.

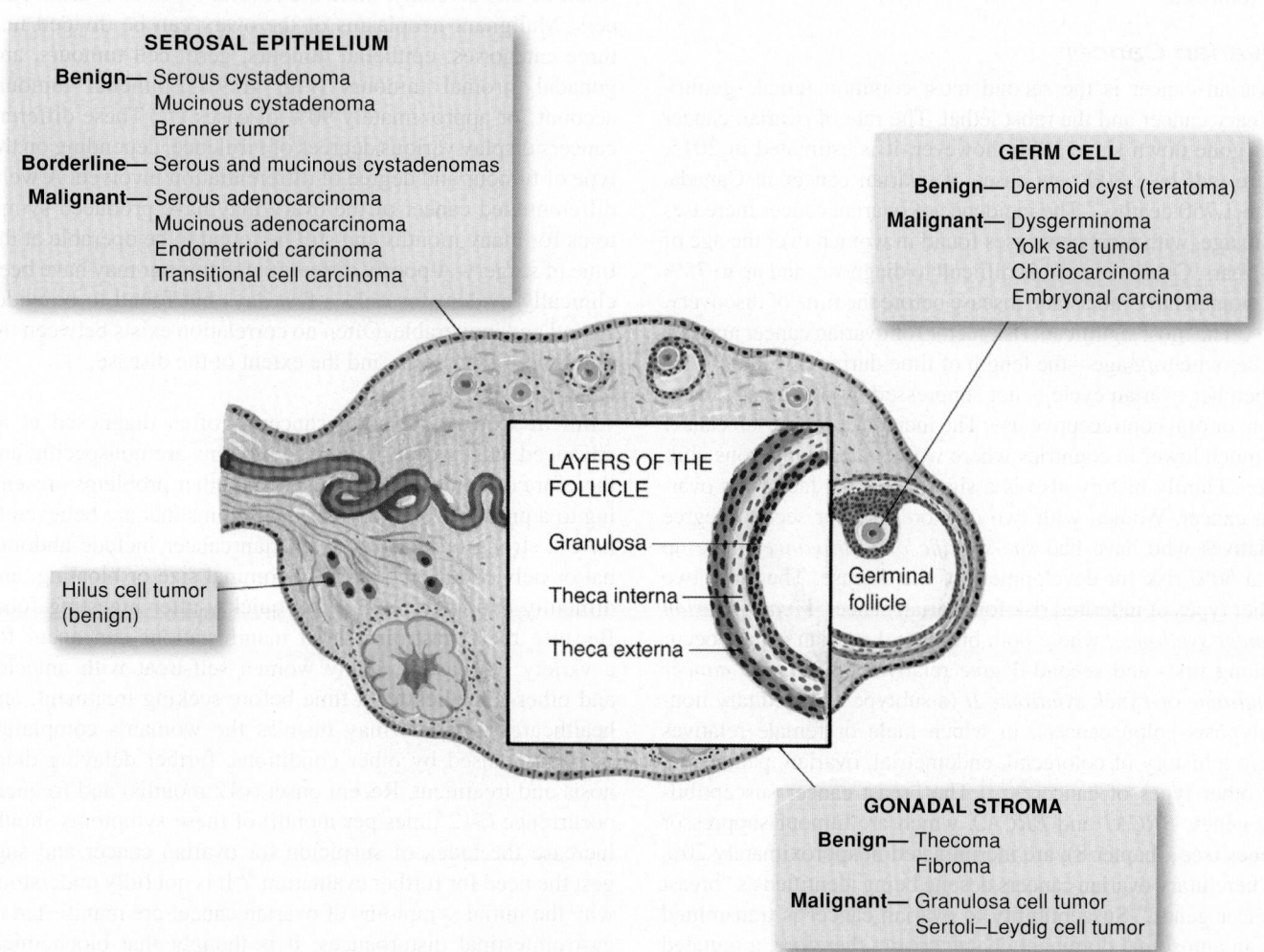

SEROSAL EPITHELIUM

Benign— Serous cystadenoma
Mucinous cystadenoma
Brenner tumor

Borderline— Serous and mucinous cystadenomas

Malignant— Serous adenocarcinoma
Mucinous adenocarcinoma
Endometrioid carcinoma
Transitional cell carcinoma

GERM CELL

Benign— Dermoid cyst (teratoma)

Malignant— Dysgerminoma
Yolk sac tumor
Choriocarcinoma
Embryonal carcinoma

LAYERS OF THE FOLLICLE

Granulosa
Theca interna
Theca externa

Germinal follicle

Hilus cell tumor (benign)

GONADAL STROMA

Benign— Thecoma
Fibroma

Malignant— Granulosa cell tumor
Sertoli–Leydig cell tumor

FIGURE 46.9 • Classification of ovarian neoplasms based on cell type. (From Rubin R., Strayer D. S. (Eds.). (2012). *Rubin's pathology: Clinicopathologic foundations of medicine* (6th ed., p. 888). Philadelphia, PA: Lippincott Williams & Wilkins.)

Although most ovarian tumours are nonfunctional, some are hormonally active.[11] These tumours may be benign or cancerous. One such tumour, the granulosa cell tumour, is associated with excess estrogen production. When it develops during the reproductive period, the persistent and uncontrolled production of estrogen interferes with the normal menstrual cycle, causing irregular and excessive bleeding, endometrial hyperplasia, or amenorrhea and fertility problems. When it develops after menopause, it causes postmenopausal bleeding, stimulation of the glandular tissues of the breast, and other signs of renewed estrogen production. Androgen-secreting tumours (*i.e.,* Sertoli–Leydig cell tumour or androblastoma) inhibit ovulation and estrogen production. They tend to cause hirsutism and development of masculine characteristics, such as baldness, acne, oily skin, breast atrophy, and deepening of the voice.

Treatment for all ovarian tumours is surgical excision. Ovarian tissue that is not affected by the tumour can be left intact if frozen-section analysis does not reveal malignancy. When ovarian tumours are very large, as is frequently the case with serous or mucinous cystadenomas, the entire ovary must be removed.

Ovarian Cancer

Ovarian cancer is the second most common female genitourinary cancer and the most lethal. The rate of ovarian cancer has gone down since 1986; however, it is estimated in 2015, there will be 2,800 new cases of ovarian cancer in Canada, with 1,750 deaths.[43] The incidence of ovarian cancer increases with age, with most new cases found in women over the age of 50 years. Ovarian cancer is difficult to diagnose, and up to 75% of women have metastatic disease before the time of discovery.

The most significant risk factor for ovarian cancer appears to be ovulatory age—the length of time during a woman's life when her ovarian cycle is not suppressed by pregnancy, lactation, or oral contraceptive use. The incidence of ovarian cancer is much lower in countries where women bear numerous children. Family history also is a significant risk factor for ovarian cancer. Women with two or more first- or second-degree relatives who have had *site-specific ovarian cancer* have up to a 50% risk for development of the disease. There are two other types of inherited risk for ovarian cancer: *breast–ovarian cancer syndrome,* where both breast and ovarian cancer occur among first- and second-degree relatives; and *family cancer syndrome* or *Lynch syndrome II* (a subtype of hereditary nonpolyposis colon cancer), in which male or female relatives have a history of colorectal, endometrial, ovarian, pancreatic, or other types of cancer.[2,22,44] The breast cancer susceptibility genes, *BRCA1* and *BRCA2,* which are tumour suppressor genes (see Chapter 8), are incriminated in approximately 20% of hereditary ovarian cancers despite being identified as "breast cancer genes." Susceptibility to ovarian cancer is transmitted as an autosomal dominant characteristic; therefore, a mutated gene from either parent is sufficient to cause the problem.[45] A high-fat Western diet and use of powders containing talc in the genital area are other factors that have been linked to the development of ovarian cancer.[43,44]

Chemoprevention strategies that have been suggested include long-term oral contraceptive use, NSAIDs, acetaminophen, or retinoids (analogs of vitamin A).[46] Each of these agents acts in slightly different ways. The NSAIDs are thought to exert their protective effects through growth inhibition and increased apoptosis (programmed cell death) of ovarian cancer cell lines. The structure of acetaminophen bears a similarity to the sex hormones, suggesting a potential sex steroid-antagonist property. Support for the use of retinoids comes from experimental data in which retinoic acid was shown to induce the differentiation of cultured ovarian cancer cells. Additional clinical trials are needed to support the effectiveness of these chemoprevention agents. Surgical strategies that have reduced the risk of developing ovarian cancer include prophylactic removal of both fallopian tubes and ovaries. These strategies have generally been reserved for women at highest risk, and those who undergo surgical intervention must be counselled that there is still a small risk of developing peritoneal cancer.[44–46]

Cancer of the ovary is a complex neoplasm because of the diversity of tissue types that originate in the ovary. As a result of this diversity, there are several types of ovarian cancers. Malignant neoplasms of the ovary can be divided into three categories: epithelial tumours, germ cell tumours, and gonadal stromal tumours (Fig. 46.9). Epithelial tumours account for approximately 90% of cases.[22,43] These different cancers display various degrees of virulence, depending on the type of tumour and degree of differentiation involved. A well-differentiated cancer of the ovary may have produced symptoms for many months and still be found to be operable at the time of surgery. A poorly differentiated tumour may have been clinically evident for only a few days but found to be widespread and inoperable. Often no correlation exists between the duration of symptoms and the extent of the disease.

Clinical Course. Ovarian cancer is often diagnosed at an advanced stage because many symptoms are nonspecific and therefore difficult to distinguish from other problems presenting to a primary care provider. Symptoms that are believed to have a strong correlation to ovarian cancer include abdominal or pelvic pain, increased abdominal size or bloating, and difficulty eating or feeling full quickly after ingesting food. Because these gastrointestinal manifestations can occur for a variety of reasons, many women self-treat with antacids and other remedies for a time before seeking treatment, and healthcare providers may dismiss the woman's complaints as being caused by other conditions, further delaying diagnosis and treatment. Recent onset (<12 months) and frequent occurrence (>12 times per month) of these symptoms should increase the index of suspicion for ovarian cancer and suggest the need for further evaluation.[47] It is not fully understood why the initial symptoms of ovarian cancer are manifested as gastrointestinal disturbances. It is thought that biochemical changes in the peritoneal fluids may irritate the bowel or that pain originating in the ovary may be referred to the abdomen and be interpreted as a gastrointestinal disturbance. Clinically evident ascites (*i.e.,* fluid in the peritoneal cavity) is seen in approximately one fourth of women with malignant ovarian tumours and is associated with a worse prognosis.

No good screening tests or other early methods of detection exist for ovarian cancer. The serum tumour marker CA-125 is a cell surface antigen; its level is elevated in 80% to 90% of women with stage II to IV nonmucinous ovarian epithelial cancers. The result is negative, however, for as much as 50% of women with stage I disease. In a postmenopausal woman with a pelvic mass, an elevated CA-125 has a positive predictive value of greater than 70% for cancer. It also can be used in monitoring therapy and recurrences when preoperative levels have been elevated. Despite its role in diagnostic evaluation and follow-up, CA-125 is not cancer or tissue specific for ovarian cancer and therefore does not have the sensitivity or specificity required to be a valid single screening test. Levels also are elevated in the presence of endometriosis, uterine fibroids, pregnancy, liver disease, and other benign conditions and with cancers of the endometrium, cervix, fallopian tube, and pancreas.

Transvaginal ultrasonography (TVS) has been used to evaluate ovarian masses for malignant potential. Although TVS has demonstrated high sensitivity and specificity as a screening tool, cost precludes its use as universal screening method. Molecular biologic studies have identified tumour suppressor genes that may play a role in the cause of ovarian cancer. Further evaluation in this area is ongoing and may eventually lead to identification of appropriate screening techniques for ovarian cancer.

When ovarian cancer is suspected, surgical evaluation is required for diagnosis, complete and accurate staging, and cytoreduction and debulking procedures to reduce the size of the tumour. The most common surgery involves removal of the uterus, fallopian tubes, ovaries, and omentum. The liver, diaphragm, retroperitoneal and aortic lymph nodes, and peritoneal surface are examined and biopsies are taken as needed. Cytologic washings are done to test for cancerous cells in the peritoneal fluid. Women with very early cancer who may wish to become pregnant will sometimes have only the affected ovary removed. Recommendations regarding treatment beyond surgery and prognosis depend on the stage of the disease. Women with limited disease (well-differentiated stage Ia or Ib) usually do not require adjuvant treatment; women with intermediate disease (stage Ic or II) or advanced disease (stage III or IV) can benefit from intravenous or intraperitoneal chemotherapy using a combination of a platinum compound (cisplatin or carboplatin) and a taxane (paclitaxel or docetaxel). When this combination therapy fails, salvage chemotherapy with newer drugs may prolong survival. Irradiation rarely plays a major role in treatment of ovarian cancer because of the difficulty in irradiating the entire abdomen without causing life-threatening damage to vital organs.[48]

The lack of accurate screening tools and the resistant nature of ovarian cancers significantly affect the success of treatment and survival. The 5-year survival rate is 94% for women whose ovarian cancer is detected and treated early; however, only 20% of all cases are detected at the localized stage. Overall, the 5-year survival rate is 45%.[43,49]

IN SUMMARY

PID is an inflammation of the upper reproductive tract that involves the uterus (endometritis), fallopian tubes (salpingitis), or ovaries (oophoritis). It is most commonly caused by *N. gonorrhoeae* or *C. trachomatis*. Accurate diagnosis and appropriate antibiotic therapy are aimed at preventing complications such as pelvic adhesions, infertility, ectopic pregnancy, chronic abdominal pain, and tubo-ovarian abscesses.

Ectopic pregnancy occurs when a fertilized ovum implants outside the uterine cavity; the most common site is the fallopian tube. Causes of ectopic pregnancy are delayed ovum transport resulting from complications of PID, therapeutic abortion, tubal ligation or tubal reversal, previous ectopic pregnancy, or other conditions such as use of fertility drugs to induce ovulation. It represents a true gynecologic emergency. Cancer of the fallopian tube is rare; the diagnosis is difficult, and the condition usually is well advanced when diagnosed.

Disorders of the ovaries include benign cysts, functioning ovarian tumours, and cancer of the ovary; they usually are asymptomatic unless there is substantial enlargement or bleeding into the cyst, or the cyst becomes twisted or ruptures. PCOS is characterized by anovulation with varying degrees of menstrual irregularity and infertility; hyperandrogenism with hirsutism, acne, male-pattern of hair loss, and obesity; polycystic ovaries; and hyperinsulinemia with insulin resistance. Benign ovarian tumours consist of endometriomas (chocolate cysts that develop secondary to ovarian endometriosis); ovarian fibromas (connective tissue tumours composed of fibrocytes and collagen); and cystic teratomas or dermoid cysts (germ cell tumours composed of various combinations of ectodermal, mesodermal, and endodermal elements). Functioning ovarian tumours may be benign or malignant and are of three types: estrogen secreting, androgen secreting, and mixed estrogen–androgen secreting. Cancer of the ovary is the second most common female genitourinary cancer and the most lethal. It can be divided into three categories: epithelial tumours, germ cell tumours, and gonadal stromal tumours. There are no effective screening methods for ovarian cancer, and often the disease is well advanced at the time of diagnosis.

DISORDERS OF PELVIC SUPPORT AND UTERINE POSITION

After completing this section of the chapter, you should be able to meet the following objectives:

- Characterize the function of the supporting ligaments and pelvic floor muscles in maintaining the position of the pelvic organs, including the uterus, bladder, and rectum.

- Describe the manifestations of cystocele, rectocele, enterocele, and uterine prolapse.
- Explain how uterine anteflexion, retroflexion, and retroversion differ from normal uterine position.

Disorders of Pelvic Support

The uterus and the pelvic structures are maintained in proper position by the four pairs of ligaments, namely the uterosacral ligaments, the round ligaments, the broad ligaments, and the cardinal ligaments. The two cardinal ligaments maintain the cervix in its normal position (see Chapter 45, Fig. 45.4). The uterosacral ligaments hold the uterus in a forward position and the broad ligaments suspend the uterus, fallopian tubes, and ovaries in the pelvis. The vagina is encased in the semirigid structure of the strong supporting fascia (Fig. 46.10A). The muscular floor of the pelvis is a strong, slinglike structure that supports the uterus, vagina, urinary bladder, and rectum (Fig. 46.11). In the female anatomy, nature is faced with the problems of supporting the pelvic viscera against the force of gravity and increases in intra-abdominal pressure associated

with coughing, sneezing, defecation, and laughing while at the same time allowing for urination, defecation, and normal reproductive tract function, especially the delivery of an infant. Three supporting structures are provided for the abdominal pelvic diaphragm. The bony pelvis provides support and protection for parts of the digestive tract and genitourinary structures, and the peritoneum holds the pelvic viscera in place. The main support for the viscera, however, is the pelvic diaphragm, made up of muscles and connective tissue that stretch across the bones of the pelvic outlet. The openings that must exist for the urethra, rectum, and vagina cause an inherent weakness in the pelvic diaphragm. Congenital or acquired weakness of the pelvic diaphragm results in widening of these openings, particularly the vagina, with the possible herniation of pelvic viscera through the pelvic floor (*i.e.*, prolapse).

Relaxation of the pelvic outlet usually comes about because of overstretching of the perineal supporting tissues during pregnancy and childbirth. Although the tissues are stretched only during these times, there may be no difficulty until later in life, such as in the fifth or sixth decade, when further loss of elasticity and muscle tone occurs. Even in a woman who has not borne children, the combination of aging and postmenopausal changes may give rise to problems related to

Small bowel

Colon

Rectovaginal septum
and uterosacral ligaments

Cervix

Vaginal rectal fascia

Rectum

Intact perineum

Uterus

Bladder

Urethra

Vagina

A

B   **C**   **D**

FIGURE 46.10 • (**A**) Normal support of the uterus and vagina, (**B**) cystocele, (**C**) rectocele, and (**D**) uterine prolapse.

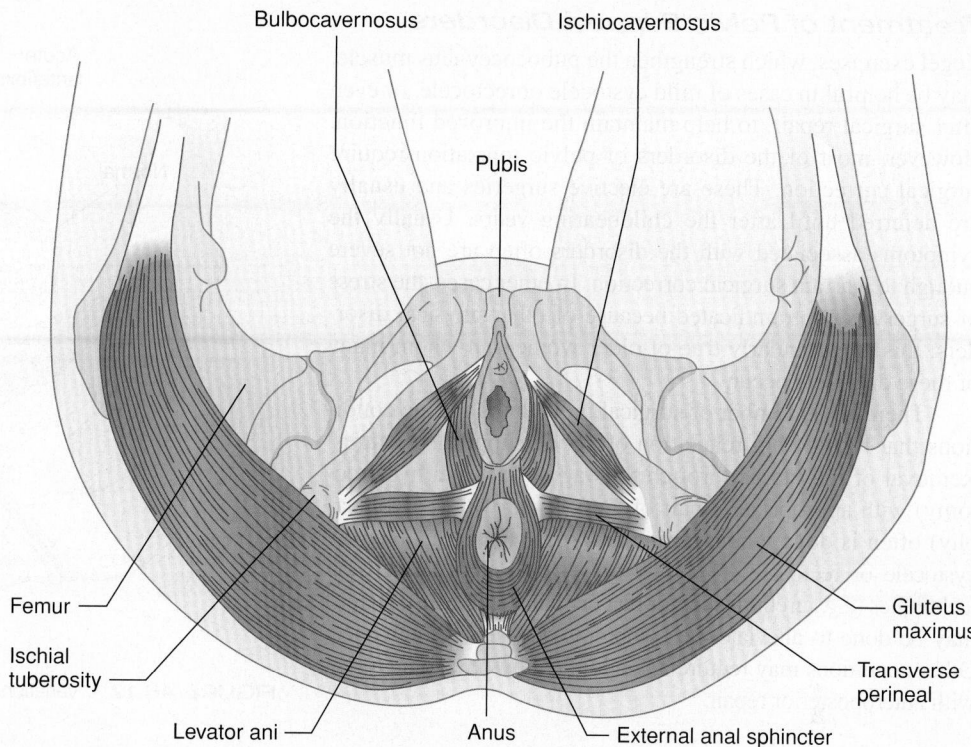

FIGURE 46.11 • Muscles of the pelvic floor (female perineum).

relaxation of the pelvic support structures. The three most common conditions associated with this relaxation are cystocele, rectocele, and uterine prolapse. These may occur separately or together.

Cystocele

Cystocele is a herniation of the bladder into the vagina. It occurs when the normal muscle support for the bladder is weakened, and the bladder sags below the uterus. This causes the anterior vaginal wall to stretch and bulge downward, allowing the bladder to herniate into the vagina due to the force of gravity and pressures from coughing, lifting, or straining at stool (Fig. 46.10B). The symptoms of cystocele include an annoying bearing-down sensation, difficulty in emptying the bladder, frequency and urgency of urination, and cystitis. Stress incontinence may occur at times of increased abdominal pressure, such as during squatting, straining, coughing, sneezing, laughing, or lifting.

Rectocele and Enterocele

Rectocele is the herniation of the rectum into the vagina. It occurs when the posterior vaginal wall and underlying rectum bulge forwards, ultimately protruding through the introitus as the pelvic floor and perineal muscles are weakened. The symptoms include discomfort because of the protrusion of the rectum and difficulty in defecation (Fig. 46.10C). Digital pressure (*i.e.*, splinting) on the bulging posterior wall of the vagina may become necessary for defecation. The area between the uterosacral ligaments just posterior to the cervix may weaken and form a hernial sac into which the small bowel protrudes when the woman is standing. This defect, called an *enterocele*,

may extend into the rectovaginal septum. It may be congenital or acquired through birth trauma. Enterocele can be asymptomatic or cause a dull, dragging sensation and occasionally low backache.

Uterine Prolapse

Uterine prolapse is the bulging of the uterus into the vagina that occurs when the primary supportive ligaments (*i.e.*, cardinal ligaments) are stretched (Fig. 46.10D). Prolapse is ranked as first, second, or third degree, depending on how far the uterus protrudes through the introitus. First-degree prolapse shows some descent, but the cervix has not reached the introitus. In second-degree prolapse, the cervix or part of the uterus has passed through the introitus. The entire uterus protrudes through the vaginal opening in third-degree prolapse (*i.e.*, procidentia).

The symptoms associated with uterine prolapse result from irritation of the exposed mucous membranes of the cervix and vagina and the discomfort of the protruding mass. Prolapse often is accompanied by perineal relaxation, cystocele, or rectocele. Like cystocele, rectocele, and enterocele, it occurs most commonly in multiparous women because childbearing is accompanied by injuries to pelvic structures and uterine ligaments. It also may result from pelvic tumours and neurologic conditions, such as spina bifida and diabetic neuropathy, that interrupt the innervation of pelvic muscles. A pessary may be inserted to hold the uterus in place and may stave off surgical intervention in women who want to have children or in older women for whom the surgery may pose a significant health risk. A newer conservative approach to treatment involves use of a space-occupying device (Colpexin sphere) to elevate the prolapse while performing pelvic floor muscle contractions.[50]

Treatment of Pelvic Support Disorders

Kegel exercises, which strengthen the pubococcygeus muscle, may be helpful in cases of mild cystocele or rectocele, or even after surgical repair, to help maintain the improved function. However, most of the disorders of pelvic relaxation require surgical correction. These are elective surgeries and usually are deferred until after the childbearing years. Usually the symptoms associated with the disorders often are not severe enough to warrant surgical correction. In other cases, the stress of surgery is contraindicated because of other physical disorders; this is particularly true of older women, in whom many of these disorders occur.

There are a number of surgical procedures for the conditions that result from relaxation of pelvic support structures. Removal of the uterus through the vagina (vaginal hysterectomy) with appropriate repair of the vaginal wall (colporrhaphy) often is done when uterine prolapse is accompanied by cystocele or rectocele. A variety of vesicourethral suspension techniques (*e.g.*, urethral sling or bladder sling, colposuspension) may be done to alleviate the symptoms of stress incontinence. Other conditions may require an abdominal hysterectomy along with anteroposterior repair.

Variations in Uterine Position

Variations in the position of the uterus are common. Some variations are innocuous; others, which may be the result of weakness and relaxation of the perineum, give rise to various problems that compromise the structural integrity of the pelvic floor, particularly after childbirth.

The uterus usually is flexed approximately 45 degrees anteriorly, with the cervix positioned posteriorly and downward in the anteverted position. When the woman is standing, the angle of the uterus is such that it lies practically horizontal, resting lightly on the bladder.

Asymptomatic, normal variations in the axis of the uterus in relation to the cervix and physiologic displacements that arise after pregnancy or with pathology of the cul-de-sac include anteflexion, retroflexion, and retroversion (Fig. 46.12). An anteflexed uterus is flexed forward on itself. Retroflexion is flexion backward at the isthmus. Retroversion describes the condition in which the uterus inclines posteriorly while the cervix remains tilted forward. Simple retroversion of the uterus is the most common displacement, found in 30% of normal women. It usually is a congenital condition caused by a short anterior vaginal wall and relaxed uterosacral ligaments; together, these force the uterus to fall back into the cul-de-sac. Retroversion also can follow certain diseases, such as endometriosis and PID, which produce fibrous tissue adherence with retraction of the fundus posteriorly. Large leiomyomas also may cause the uterus to move into a posterior position. Dyspareunia with deep penetration or low back pain with menses can be associated with retroversion. Most symptoms in these women are caused by the associated condition (*e.g.*, adhesions, fibroids) rather than congenital retroversion.

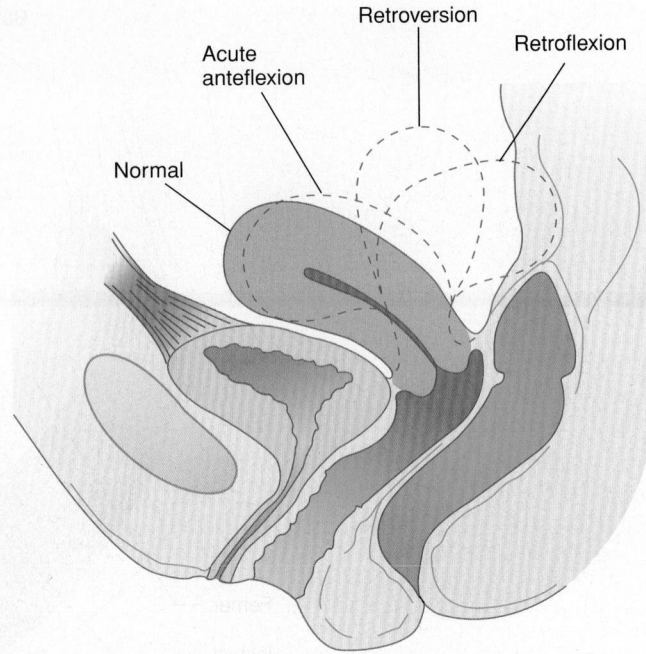

FIGURE 46.12 • Variations in uterine position.

IN SUMMARY

Alterations in pelvic support frequently occur because of weaknesses and relaxation of the pelvic floor and perineum. Cystocele and rectocele involve herniation of the bladder or rectum into the vagina. Uterine prolapse occurs when the uterus bulges into the vagina. Pelvic relaxation disorders typically result from overstretching of the perineal supporting muscles during pregnancy and childbirth. The loss of elasticity in these structures that is a normal accompaniment of aging contributes to these problems. Variations in uterine position include anteflexion, retroflexion, and retroversion. These disorders, which often are innocuous, can be the result of a congenital shortness of the vaginal wall, development of fibrous adhesions secondary to endometriosis or PID, or displacement caused by large uterine leiomyomas.

MENSTRUAL DISORDERS

After completing this section of the chapter, you should be able to meet the following objectives:

- Define the terms amenorrhea, hypomenorrhea, oligomenorrhea, menorrhagia, metrorrhagia, and menometrorrhagia.
- Relate the alteration in estrogen and progesterone levels to the development of dysfunctional menstrual cycles.
- Differentiate between primary dysmenorrhea and secondary dysmenorrhea.
- Characterize the manifestations of the premenstrual syndrome, its possible causes, and the methods of treatment.

Abnormal Uterine Bleeding

Although unexplained uterine bleeding can occur for many reasons, such as pregnancy, abortion, bleeding disorders, and neoplasms, the most frequent cause in the nonpregnant woman is what is commonly called *abnormal menstrual cycle* or *bleeding*. Abnormal cycles may take the form of *amenorrhea* (absence of menstruation), *hypomenorrhea* (scanty menstruation), *oligomenorrhea* (infrequent menstruation, periods more than 35 days apart), *polymenorrhea* (frequent menstruation, periods less than 21 days apart), *menorrhagia* (excessive menstruation), or *metrorrhagia* (bleeding between periods). *Menometrorrhagia* is heavy bleeding during and between menstrual periods.

ABNORMAL UTERINE BLEEDING

- The pattern of menstrual bleeding tends to be fairly consistent in most healthy women with regard to frequency, duration, and amount of flow.
- Abnormal bleeding in postpubertal women can take the form of absent or scanty periods, infrequent periods, excessive and irregular periods, excessive bleeding during periods, and bleeding between periods.
- When the basic pattern of bleeding is changed, it is most often due to a lack of ovulation and disturbances in the pattern of hormone secretion.
- When the basic pattern is undisturbed and there are superimposed episodes of bleeding or spotting, the etiology is more likely to be related to organic lesions or hematologic disorders.

Abnormal uterine bleeding is related to alterations in the hormones that support normal cyclic endometrial changes (see Chapter 45). Estrogen deprivation causes retrogression of a previously built-up endometrium and bleeding. Such bleeding often is irregular in amount and duration, with the flow varying with the time and degree of estrogen stimulation and with the degree of estrogen withdrawal. A lack of progesterone can cause abnormal menstrual bleeding; in its absence, estrogen induces development of a much thicker endometrial layer with a richer blood supply. The absence of progesterone results from the failure of any of the developing ovarian follicles to mature to the point of ovulation, with the subsequent formation of the corpus luteum and production and secretion of progesterone.

Periodic bleeding episodes alternating with amenorrhea are caused by variations in the number of functioning ovarian follicles present. If sufficient follicles are present and active and if new follicles assume functional capacity, high levels of estrogen develop, causing the endometrium to proliferate for weeks or even months. In time, estrogen withdrawal and bleeding develop. This can occur for two reasons: an absolute estrogen deficiency may develop when several follicles simultaneously degenerate, or a relative deficiency may develop as the needs of the enlarged endometrial tissue mass exceed the capabilities of the existing follicles, even though estrogen levels remain constant. Estrogen and progesterone deficiencies are associated with the absence of ovulation, hence the term *anovulatory bleeding*. Because the vasoconstriction and myometrial contractions that normally accompany menstruation are caused by progesterone, anovulatory bleeding seldom is accompanied by cramps, and the flow frequently is heavy. Anovulatory cycles are common among adolescents during the first several years after menarche, when ovarian function is becoming established, among perimenopausal women, whose ovarian function is beginning to decline, and, commonly, in obese women with PCOS.

Abnormal uterine bleeding can originate as a primary disorder of the ovaries or as a secondary defect in ovarian function related to hypothalamic–pituitary stimulation. The latter can be initiated by emotional stress, marked variation in weight (*i.e.,* sudden gain or loss), or nonspecific endocrine or metabolic disturbances. Nonhormonal causes of irregular menstrual bleeding include endometrial polyps, submucosal myoma (*i.e.,* fibroid), bleeding disorder (*e.g.,* von Willebrand disease, platelet dysfunction), infection, endometrial cancer, and pregnancy.

The treatment of abnormal bleeding depends on what is identified as the probable cause. The minimum evaluation should include a detailed history with emphasis on bleeding pattern and a physical examination. Endocrine studies (*e.g.,* FSH/LH ratio, prolactin, testosterone, DHEA-S levels), β-hCG pregnancy test, ultrasonography of the endometrium, endometrial biopsy, D&C with or without hysteroscopy, and progesterone withdrawal tests may be needed for diagnosis. Nonhormonal causes generally require surgical intervention. D&C can be therapeutic as well as diagnostic. Endometrial ablation (thinning or elimination of the basal layer of the endometrium from which the monthly buildup generates) has become a primary treatment strategy for heavy bleeding; it can be accomplished using heat, cold, microwave, chemicals, or radiofrequency energy sources. This procedure is not used for women who wish to preserve their fertility as this treatment leads to endometrial scarring which is considered irreversible.[51] If nonhormonal problems have been excluded and alterations in hormone levels are the primary cause, treatment may include the use of oral contraceptives, cyclic progesterone therapy, or long-acting progesterone via injection or an IUD.

Amenorrhea

There are two types of amenorrhea: primary and secondary. Primary amenorrhea is the failure to menstruate by 15 years of age, or by 13 years of age if failure to menstruate is accompanied by absence of secondary sex characteristics. Secondary amenorrhea is the cessation of menses for at least 6 months in a woman who has established normal menstrual cycles. Primary amenorrhea usually is caused by gonadal dysgenesis, congenital müllerian agenesis, testicular feminization, or a hypothalamic–pituitary–ovarian axis disorder. Causes of secondary amenorrhea include pregnancy; ovarian, pituitary, or hypothalamic dysfunction; intrauterine adhesions; infections (*e.g.*, tuberculosis, syphilis); pituitary tumour; anorexia nervosa; or strenuous physical exercise, which can alter the critical body fat–muscle ratio needed for menses to occur.[52]

Diagnostic evaluation resembles that for dysfunctional uterine bleeding, with the possible addition of a computed tomographic scan or MRI to exclude a pituitary tumour. Treatment is based on correcting the underlying cause and inducing menstruation with cyclic progesterone or combined estrogen–progesterone regimens.

Dysmenorrhea

Dysmenorrhea is pain or discomfort with menstruation. Although not usually a serious medical problem, it causes some degree of monthly disability for a significant number of women. There are two forms of dysmenorrhea: primary and secondary. Primary dysmenorrhea is menstrual pain that is not associated with a physical abnormality or pathologic process.[53] It usually occurs with ovulatory menstruation beginning 6 months to 2 years after menarche. Symptoms may begin 1 to 2 days before menses, peak on the first day of flow, and subside within several hours to several days. Severe dysmenorrhea may be associated with systemic symptoms such as headache, nausea, vomiting, diarrhea, fatigue, irritability, dizziness, and syncope. The pain typically is described as dull, lower abdominal aching or cramping, spasmodic or colicky in nature, often radiating to the lower back, labia majora, or upper thighs.

Secondary dysmenorrhea is menstrual pain caused by specific organic conditions, such as endometriosis, uterine fibroids, adenomyosis, pelvic adhesions, IUDs, or PID. Laparoscopy often is required for diagnosis of secondary dysmenorrhea if medication for primary dysmenorrhea is ineffective.

Treatment for primary dysmenorrhea is directed at symptom control. Although analgesic agents such as aspirin and acetaminophen may relieve minor uterine cramping or low back pain, prostaglandin synthetase inhibitors (*e.g.*, ibuprofen, naproxen, mefenamic acid, indomethacin) are more specific for dysmenorrhea and the treatment of choice if contraception is not desired. Ovulation suppression and symptomatic relief of dysmenorrhea can be instituted simultaneously with the use of oral contraceptives. Relief of secondary dysmenorrhea depends on identifying the cause of the problem. Medical or surgical intervention may be needed to eliminate the problem.

Premenstrual Symptom Disorders

According to surveys, 80% of women experience premenstrual emotional or physical changes, with 20% to 30% of the adult female population indicating these mild to moderate monthly symptoms cause some difficulty; only 3% to 8% report extreme or severe symptoms that have a negative impact on their life.[54–56] It appears there is a spectrum of premenstrual symptom disorders that runs from *premenstrual molimina* on the mild end; through *premenstrual syndrome* (PMS), which is characterized by mild to moderate physical and psychological symptoms limited to 3 to 14 days preceding menstruation and relieved by onset of the menses; to *premenstrual dysphoric disorder* (PMDD), which is the most severe form of premenstrual distress and generally is associated with mood disorders. How many of these women have symptoms that are severe enough to warrant treatment is unknown. The incidence of PMS seems to increase with age. It is less common in women in their teens and twenties, and most of the women seeking help for the problem are in their mid-thirties. The disorder is not culturally distinct, as it affects women from all cultural backgrounds. There is some dispute about whether PMS occurs more frequently in women who have had children or in those who have not.

Physical symptoms of PMS include painful and swollen breasts, bloating, abdominal pain, headache, and backache. Psychologically, there may be depression, anxiety, irritability, and behavioural changes. In some cases, there are puzzling alterations in motor function, such as clumsiness and altered handwriting. Women with PMS may report one or several symptoms, with symptoms varying from woman to woman and from month to month in the same patient. Signs and symptoms associated with this disorder are summarized in Table 46.2. PMS can significantly affect a woman's ability to perform at normal levels.

TABLE 46.2	**SYMPTOMS OF PREMENSTRUAL SYNDROME (PMS) BY SYSTEM**
BODY SYSTEM	**SYMPTOMS**
Cerebral	Irritability, anxiety, nervousness, fatigue, exhaustion, increased physical and mental activity, lability, crying spells, depression, inability to concentrate
Gastrointestinal	Craving for sweets or salt, lower abdominal pain, bloating, nausea, vomiting, diarrhea, constipation
Vascular	Headache, edema, weakness, fainting
Reproductive	Swelling and tenderness of the breasts, pelvic congestion, ovarian pain, altered libido
Neuromuscular	Trembling of the extremities, changes in coordination, clumsiness, backache, leg aches
General	Weight gain, insomnia, dizziness, acne

Although the causes of PMS are poorly documented, they probably are multifactorial. Like dysmenorrhea, it is only recently that PMS has been recognized as a bona fide disorder rather than merely a psychosomatic illness. There has been a tendency to link the disorder with endocrine imbalances such as hyperprolactinemia, estrogen excess, and alteration in the estrogen–progesterone ratio. Prolactin concentration affects sodium and water retention, is higher in the luteal phase than in the follicular phase, and can be increased by estrogens, stress, hypoglycemia, pregnancy, and oral contraceptives. Estrogens stimulate anxiety and nervous tension, and increased progesterone levels may produce depression. The role of hormonal factors in the cause of PMS is supported by two well-established phenomena. First, women who have undergone a hysterectomy but not an oophorectomy may have cyclic symptoms that resemble PMS. Second, PMS symptoms are rare in postmenopausal women. However, there is no research available to confirm these theories.

Other hypotheses suggest that increased aldosterone may contribute to symptoms associated with fluid retention (*e.g.,* headache, bloating, breast tenderness, weight gain); that pyridoxine (vitamin B$_6$) deficiency may lead to estrogen excess or decreased production of the neurotransmitters dopamine and serotonin, which may contribute to PMS symptoms; or that decreased prostaglandin E$_1$ concentrations can lead to abnormal sensitivity to prolactin, with associated fluid retention, irritability, and depression. In addition, increased appetite, binge eating, fatigue, and depression have been associated with altered endorphin activity and subclinical hypoglycemia. Learned beliefs about menstruation may also contribute to the development of PMS or at least affect the woman's response to the symptoms.

The most recent theory to emerge suggests a relationship between normal gonadal fluctuations and central neurotransmitter activity, particularly serotonin. It is unclear whether decreased levels of serotonin are present during the luteal phase, and only susceptible women respond with varying degrees of premenstrual symptoms, or if women with PMDD have a neurotransmitter abnormality.[3,56]

A complete history and physical examination are necessary to exclude other physical causes of the symptoms. Depending on the symptom pattern, blood studies, including thyroid hormones, glucose, and prolactin assays, may be done. Psychosocial evaluation is helpful to exclude emotional illness that is merely exacerbated premenstrually. The diagnosis focuses on identification of symptoms by means of a daily calendar on which the woman records her symptoms for 2 to 3 consecutive months. Although validated tools are available for recording symptoms, any calendar used for this purpose should include information regarding specific symptoms, severity, timing in relation to the menstrual cycle, and baseline level of symptoms in the follicular phase.[3] PMDD is a psychiatric diagnosis that has been developed to distinguish those women whose symptoms are severe enough to interfere significantly with activities of daily living. It requires prospective symptom charting, and a minimum of 5 of the 11 symptom groups as described in the fifth edition of the *Diagnostic and Statistical Manual of*

BOX 46.1 | *DSM-5* CRITERIA FOR PREMENSTRUAL DYSPHORIC DISORDER (PMDD)

PMDD, patient must exhibit five or more symptoms, including at least one core symptom during the premenstrual period, confirmed by prospective charting during at least two consecutive menstrual cycles. Symptoms must cause marked impairment in the woman's ability to carry out her usual activities, must abate within a few days of the onset of menses, and not recur during the week after menses.

Core Symptoms
Affective lability (*i.e.,* mood swings)
Anger, irritability, increased interpersonal conflicts
Depressed mood
Anxiety, tension, edginess, nervousness

Other Symptoms
Fatigue, lethargy
Insomnia, hypersomnia
Difficulty concentrating
Appetite changes or cravings
Diminished interest in usual activities
Feeling overwhelmed or out of control
Physical symptoms (headache, breast tenderness or swelling, bloating, joint and muscle pain)

From American Psychiatric Association. (2013). Premenstrual dysphoric disorder. In *Diagnostic and statistical manual of mental disorders* (5th ed.). Washington, DC: Author.

Mental Disorders (DSM-5)[56], in order to establish a diagnosis of PMDD (Box 46.1). The symptom groups must be present in the week before the onset of menses, improve as menses is initiated, and resolve by the week following. Presence of a single symptom is sufficient for the diagnosis of PMS.[56]

Management of PMS/PMDD has been largely symptomatic and includes education and support directed towards lifestyle changes for women with mild symptoms. Treatment includes diuretics to reduce fluid retention; analgesics for pain, and anxiolytic drugs to treat mood changes. An integrated program of personal assessment by diary, regular exercise, avoidance of caffeine, and a diet low in simple sugars and high in lean proteins is often beneficial. Additional therapeutic regimens that have been used include vitamin or mineral supplements (particularly pyridoxine, vitamin E, and magnesium); evening primrose oil (which contains linoleic acid, a precursor of prostaglandin E$_1$); natural progesterone supplements; low-dose oral monophasic contraceptives; GnRH agonists; bromocriptine for prolactin suppression; danazol (a synthetic androgen); and spironolactone (an aldosterone antagonist and inhibitor of adrenal androgen synthesis).[57] Although a body of knowledge has evolved that offers a variety of therapeutic choices, few treatments have been adequately evaluated in randomized, controlled clinical trials. The SSRI antidepressants, however, have demonstrated significant improvement in overall symptoms compared with placebo, whether used continuously or only in the luteal phase, and are recommended as first-line therapy for severe PMS or PMDD.[3,57]

IN SUMMARY

Menstrual disorders include abnormal uterine bleeding, dysmenorrhea, and PMS. Abnormal uterine bleeding, which involves amenorrhea, oligomenorrhea, metrorrhagia, or menorrhagia, occurs when the hormonal support of the endometrium is altered. Estrogen deprivation causes retrogression of a previously built-up endometrium and bleeding. A lack of progesterone can cause abnormal menstrual bleeding; in its absence, estrogen induces development of a much thicker endometrial layer with a richer blood supply. The absence of progesterone results from the failure of any of the developing ovarian follicles to mature to the point of ovulation, with subsequent formation of the corpus luteum and production of progesterone.

Dysmenorrhea is characterized by pain or discomfort during menses. It can occur as a primary or secondary disorder. Primary dysmenorrhea is not associated with other disorders and begins soon after menarche. Secondary dysmenorrhea is caused by a specific organic condition, such as endometriosis or pelvic adhesions. It occurs in women with previously painless menses.

Premenstrual symptom disorders represent a spectrum from molimina, which is present to some degree in most ovulatory women, to PMS and PMDD. PMS represents a cluster of physical and psychological symptoms that precede menstruation by 1 to 2 weeks. PMDD describes the most severe, disabling form of PMS. The true incidence and nature of PMS has been recognized only recently, and its cause and methods for treatment are still under study.

DISORDERS OF THE BREAST

After completing this section of the chapter, you should be able to meet the following objectives:

- Describe changes in breast function that occur with galactorrhea, mastitis, and ductal ectasia.
- Describe the manifestations of fibrocystic breast changes.
- Describe the methods used in the diagnosis and treatment of breast cancer.

Most breast disease may be described as benign or cancerous. Breast tissue is never static; the breast is constantly responding to changes in hormonal, nutritional, psychological, and environmental stimuli that cause continual cellular changes. Benign breast conditions are nonprogressive; some forms of benign disease, however, increase the risk of malignant disease. In light of this, strict adherence to a dichotomy of benign versus malignant disease may not always be appropriate. This dichotomy, however, is useful for the sake of simplicity and clarity.

Galactorrhea

Galactorrhea is the secretion of breast milk in a nonlactating breast. Galactorrhea may result from vigorous nipple stimulation during lovemaking, exogenous hormones, internal hormonal imbalance, or local chest infection or trauma. A pituitary tumour may produce large amounts of prolactin and cause galactorrhea. Galactorrhea occurs in men and women and usually is benign. Observation may be continued for several months before diagnostic hormonal screening. Spontaneous leaking from the breast (occurring without any type of stimulation) is pathologic and warrants investigation.[58]

Mastitis

Mastitis is inflammation of the breast. It most frequently occurs during lactation but may also result from other conditions. In the lactating woman, inflammation most often results from an ascending infection that travels from the nipple to the ductile structures. The most common bacterial organisms isolated are *Staphylococcus* and *Streptococcus*.[3] The offending organisms originate from the suckling infant's nasopharynx or the mother's hands. During the early weeks of nursing, the breast is particularly vulnerable to bacterial invasion because of minor cracks and fissures that occur with vigorous suckling. Infection and inflammation cause obstruction of the ductile system. The breast area becomes hard, inflamed, and tender if not treated early. Without antibiotic treatment, the area becomes walled off and may abscess, requiring incision and drainage. It is also possible for breastfeeding women to acquire a fungal infection most commonly caused by *C. albicans*. The intense breast and nipple pain is not associated with feeding and can be mistaken for mastitis. It is advisable for the mother to continue breastfeeding during treatment for the infections.

Mastitis is not confined to the postpartum period; it can occur as a result of hormonal fluctuations, tumours, trauma, or skin infection. Cyclic inflammation of the breast occurs most frequently in adolescents, who commonly have fluctuating hormone levels. Tumours may cause mastitis secondary to skin involvement or lymphatic obstruction. Local trauma or infection may develop into mastitis because of ductal blockage of trapped blood, cellular debris, or the extension of superficial inflammation. Treatment for mastitis symptoms includes application of heat or cold, excision, aspiration, mild analgesics, topical agents, antibiotics, and a supportive brassiere or breast binder.

Ductal Disorders

Ductal ectasia manifests in older women as a spontaneous, intermittent, usually unilateral, greyish-green nipple discharge.

Palpation of the breast increases the discharge. Ectasia occurs during or after menopause and is symptomatically associated with burning, itching, pain, and a pulling sensation of the nipple and areola. The disease results in inflammation of the ducts and subsequent thickening. The treatment requires removal of the involved ductal mass.

Intraductal papillomas are benign epithelial tissue tumours that grow within a dilated duct and may range in size from 2 mm to 5 cm. Papillomas usually manifest with a bloody nipple discharge. The tumour may be palpated in the areolar area or incidentally found on mammograms. Because epithelial hyperplasia and apocrine metaplasia are frequently present, most benign papillomas are excised as a precautionary measure.[59]

Fibroadenoma and Fibrocystic Changes

Fibroadenomas are seen in premenopausal women, most commonly in the third and fourth decades. The clinical findings include a firm, rubbery, sharply defined round mass. On palpation, the mass "slides" between the fingers and is easily movable. These masses usually are singular; only 15% are multiple or bilateral. Fibroadenomas are asymptomatic and usually found by accident. They are not thought to be precancerous. Treatment involves simple excision.

Fibrocystic changes is the most frequent lesion of the breast. It is most common in women 20 to 50 years of age and is rare in postmenopausal women not receiving hormone.[58–61] Although the incidence does vary, most studies suggest that fibrocystic breast disease occurs in 50% to 60% of all women.[61] Fibrocystic changes usually present as nodular (*i.e.,* "lumpy bumpy"), granular breast masses that are more prominent and painful during the luteal or progesterone-dominant portion of the menstrual cycle. Discomfort ranges from heaviness to exquisite tenderness, depending on the degree of vascular engorgement and cystic distension.

Fibrocystic changes encompass a wide variety of lesions and breast changes. Microscopically, fibrocystic changes refer to a constellation of morphologic changes manifested by (1) cystic dilation of terminal ducts, often with some apocrine metaplasia, (2) relative increase in fibrous tissue as cysts rupture and release secretory material into the adjacent stroma, and (3) adenosis or variable proliferation of terminal duct epithelial elements.[68] Although fibrocystic changes have been thought to increase the risk of breast cancer, only certain variants in which proliferation of the epithelial components is demonstrated represent a true risk. Presence of large cysts and proliferative epithelial lesions with atypia are more common in women who are at increased risk for development of breast cancer. The nonproliferative form of fibrocystic changes that does not carry an increased risk for development of cancer is more common.

Diagnosis of fibrocystic changes is made by physical examination, mammography, ultrasonography, and biopsy (*i.e.,* aspiration or tissue sample). The use of mammography for diagnosis in high-risk groups younger than 35 years of age on a routine basis remains controversial. Mammography may be helpful in establishing the diagnosis, but increased breast tissue density in women with fibrocystic changes may make an abnormal or cancerous mass difficult to discern among the other structures and often requires an MRI. Ultrasonography is useful in differentiating a cystic from a solid mass. Because a mass caused by fibrocystic changes may be indistinguishable from carcinoma on the basis of clinical findings, suspect lesions should undergo biopsy. Fine-needle aspiration may be used, but if a suspect mass that was nonmalignant on cytologic examination does not resolve over several months, it should be removed surgically. Any discrete mass or lump on the breast should be viewed as possible carcinoma, and cancer should be excluded before instituting the conservative measures used to treat fibrocystic changes.

Treatment for fibrocystic changes is usually symptomatic. Mild analgesics (*e.g.,* aspirin, acetaminophen, or NSAIDs), evening primrose oil, and local application of heat or cold may be used for pain relief. Prominent or persistent cysts may be aspirated and any fluid obtained sent to the laboratory for cytologic analysis. Tamoxifen or danazol, a synthetic androgen, may be used for women with severe pain.[61]

Breast Cancer

Cancer of the breast is the most common female cancer. One in nine women in Canada will have breast cancer in her lifetime. In 2015, it is estimated that breast cancer will be diagnosed in 25,000 Canadian women, and approximately 5,000 deaths will occur in women. In that same time period, 220 men will be diagnosed and 60 will die from breast cancer.[62] Although the breast cancer mortality rate has shown a slight decline, it is second only to lung cancer as a cause of cancer-related deaths in women. Incidence rates for carcinoma in situ have increased dramatically since the mid-1970s because of recommendations regarding mammography screening. Death rates have decreased, particularly in women younger than 50 years of age. The decline in the breast cancer mortality rate is due to earlier diagnosis through screening programs and increased awareness, as well as improvements in cancer treatments.[62]

Risk factors for breast cancer include gender, increasing age, personal or family history of breast cancer (*i.e.,* at highest risk are those with multiple affected first-order relatives), history of benign breast disease (*i.e.,* primary "atypical" hyperplasia), and hormonal influences that promote breast maturation and may increase the chance of cell mutation (*i.e.,* early menarche, late menopause, and no term pregnancies or first child after 30 years of age). Modifiable risk factors include obesity (particularly after menopause), physical inactivity, alcohol intake greater than one drink per day, and long-term use of postmenopausal hormone therapy (especially combined estrogen and progestin).[62] Most women with breast cancer have no identifiable risk factors.

Approximately 5% to 10% of all breast cancers are hereditary, with genetic mutations causing up to 80% of breast cancers in women younger than 50 years of age.[59,60,63] Two breast cancer susceptibility genes—*BRCA1* on chromosome 17 and *BRCA2* on chromosome 13—may account for most inherited forms of breast cancer (see Chapter 8). *BRCA1* is known to be involved in tumour suppression. A woman with known mutations in *BRCA1* has a lifetime risk of 60% to 85% for breast cancer and an increased risk of ovarian cancer. *BRCA2* is another susceptibility gene that carries an elevated cancer risk similar to that with *BRCA1*.[48,63,64] Genetic risk assessments including family history and future recommendations are available through the Canadian Cancer Society.[62] Breast cancer risk reduction options available to known carriers of *BRCA1* and *BRCA2* mutations include surveillance and surgery. Breast evaluation using MRI is generally preferred over standard mammography for these women because of its enhanced sensitivity and lack of radiation exposure, which may be safer for them. Prophylactic surgery, in the form of bilateral mastectomy, bilateral oophorectomy, or both, has been shown to decrease but not negate the risk of developing cancer. These controversial surgeries can have physical and psychological side effects that warrant careful consideration before proceeding. The use of aromatase inhibitors for prevention in these women is controversial because many cancers in these genetically susceptible women are estrogen-receptor negative.[64]

Detection

Cancer of the breast may manifest clinically as a mass, a puckering, nipple retraction, or unusual discharge. Many cancers are found by women themselves—sometimes when only a thickening or subtle change in breast contour is noticed. The variety of symptoms and potential for self-discovery underscore the need for all women to have an awareness of what their normal breast appearance and texture are like. In 2001, the CTFPHC dropped its recommendation that all women perform regular, systematic self-examination; in 2013, it removed the recommendation for clinical breast examination as well. Research has indicated that most women who discover their own cancer do so outside of scheduled breast self-examination (BSE).[65] The Canadian Cancer Society's screening guidelines now place primary emphasis for breast cancer diagnosis on mammography and clinical breast exam, while encouraging women in the area of self-awareness.[62] Premenopausal women who choose to perform BSE should conduct the examination right after menses. This time is most appropriate in relation to cyclic breast changes that occur in response to fluctuations in hormone levels. Postmenopausal women and women who have had a hysterectomy can perform the examination any day of the month. Examination may be done in the shower or bath or at bedtime. The most important aspect of BSE is to devise a systematic, convenient, and consistent method of examination.

Mammography is the only effective screening technique for the early detection of clinically inapparent lesions. Since breast cancer is generally a slow-growing form of cancer, it may be present for 2 to 9 years before it reaches 1 cm, the smallest mass normally detected by palpation. Mammography can disclose lesions as small as 1 mm and the clustering of calcifications that may warrant biopsy to exclude cancer. Mammography has a sensitivity of 80% to 90% for the detection of breast cancer even when performed by the most capable institutions. Therefore, even if the mammogram is negative, a palpable mass requires further evaluation. Approximately 40% of breast cancers can be detected only by palpation and another 40% only by mammography. The most comprehensive approach to screening is a combination of individual self-awareness, clinical breast evaluation by a health professional, and mammography. The Canadian Cancer Society recommends evaluation for women after 50 to 69 years of age every 2 to 3 years. Since healthcare delivery in Canada is under provincial/territorial jurisdiction, the schedule for mammography screening has been developed and implemented independently across the country. Overall, Canadian women between 50 and 69 years of age have access to an organized program that recalls women for their mammography based on their age and previous findings, except for women in Nunavut, who must travel outside their territory for this service.

Diagnosis and Classification

Procedures used in the diagnosis of breast cancer include physical examination, mammography, ultrasonography, percutaneous needle aspiration, stereotactic needle biopsy (*i.e.,* core biopsy), and excisional biopsy. Figure 46.13 illustrates the appearance of breast cancer on mammography. Breast cancer often manifests as a solitary, painless, firm, fixed lesion with poorly defined borders. It can be found anywhere in the breast but is most common in the upper outer quadrant. Because of

FIGURE 46.13 • Carcinoma of the breast. **A:** Mammogram. An irregularly shaped, dense mass (*arrows*) is seen in this otherwise fatty breast. **B:** Mastectomy specimen. The irregular white, firm mass in the centre is surrounded by fatty tissue. (From Rubin R., Strayer D. S. (Eds.). (2012). *Rubin's pathology: Clinicopathologic foundations of medicine* (6th ed., p. 939). Philadelphia, PA: Lippincott Williams & Wilkins.)

the variability in presentation, any suspect change in breast tissue warrants further investigation. The diagnostic use of mammography enables additional definition of the clinically suspect area (*e.g.,* appearance, character, calcification). Placement of a wire marker under radiographic guidance can ensure accurate surgical biopsy of nonpalpable suspect areas. Ultrasonography is useful as a diagnostic adjunct to differentiate cystic from solid tissue in women with nonspecific thickening.

Fine-needle aspiration is a simple in-office procedure that can be performed repeatedly in multiple sites and with minimal discomfort. It can be accomplished by stabilizing a palpable mass between two fingers or in conjunction with handheld sonography to define cystic masses or fibrocystic changes and to provide specimens for cytologic examination. Fine-needle aspiration can identify the presence of malignant cells, but it cannot differentiate in situ from infiltrating cancers. Stereotactic needle biopsy is an outpatient procedure done with the guidance of a mammography machine. After the lesion is localized radiologically, a large-bore needle is mechanically thrust quickly into the area, removing a core of tissue. Discomfort is similar to that with ear piercing, and even when multiple cores are obtained, healing occurs quite rapidly. Cells are available for histologic evaluation with 96% accuracy in detecting cancer. This procedure is less costly than excisional biopsy. Excisional biopsy to remove the entire lump provides the only definitive diagnosis of breast cancer, and often is therapeutic without additional surgery. MRI, positron emission tomography (PET), and computer-based or digital mammography are available as additional diagnostic modalities for breast cancer, and may be recommended to supplement conventional mammography in women with radiographically dense breasts or a strong family history of cancer, or who are known carriers of *BRCA1* or *BRCA2.*[66]

Tumours are classified histologically according to tissue characteristics and staged clinically according to tumour size, nodal involvement, and presence of metastasis. It is recommended that estrogen and progesterone receptor analysis be performed on surgical specimens. Information about the presence or absence of estrogen and progesterone receptors can be used in predicting tumour responsiveness to hormonal manipulation. High levels of both receptors improve the prognosis and increase the likelihood of remission.

Treatment

The treatment methods for breast cancer include surgery, chemotherapy, radiation therapy, and hormonal manipulation. Radical mastectomy (*i.e.,* removal of the entire breast, underlying muscles, and all axillary nodes) rarely is used today as a primary surgical therapy unless breast cancer is advanced at the time of diagnosis. Modified surgical techniques (*i.e.,* mastectomy plus axillary dissection or lumpectomy for breast conservation) accompanied by chemotherapy or radiation therapy have achieved outcomes comparable with those obtained with radical surgical methods and constitute the preferred treatment methods.

The prognosis is related more to the extent of nodal involvement than to the extent of breast involvement. Greater nodal

involvement requires more aggressive postsurgical treatment, and many cancer specialists believe that a diagnosis of breast cancer is not complete until dissection and testing of the axillary lymph nodes has been accomplished. A newer technique for evaluating lymph node involvement is a sentinel lymph node (SLN) biopsy. A radioactive substance or dye is injected into the region of the tumour. In theory, the dye is carried to the first (sentinel) node to receive lymph from the tumour. This would therefore be the node most likely to contain cancer cells if the cancer has spread. If the sentinel node biopsy is positive, more nodes are removed. If it is negative, further lymph node evaluation may not be needed. Successful identification of the SLN occurs 92% to 98% of the time, and when blue dye and isotope are used together, SLN has a positive predictive value approaching 100% and a negative predictive value near 95%.[3]

Systemic therapy refers to the administration of chemotherapy, biologic therapy, or hormonal therapy. Neoadjuvant therapy is given before surgery to shrink the tumour and make surgical removal more effective. Adjuvant therapy is given after surgery to women with and without detectable metastatic disease. The goal of this therapy depends on nodal involvement, menopausal status, and hormone receptor status. Systemic adjuvant therapy has been widely studied and has demonstrated benefits in reducing rates of recurrence and death from breast cancer.[3,67] Biologic therapy with trastuzumab (Herceptin), a drug developed in Canada, is used to stop the growth of breast tumours that express the HER2/neu receptor on their cell surface. The HER2/neu receptor binds an epidermal growth factor that contributes to cancer cell growth. Trastuzumab is a recombinant DNA-derived monoclonal antibody that binds to the HER2/neu receptor, thereby inhibiting proliferation of tumour cells that overexpress the receptor gene.[68]

Hormone therapy is used to block the effects of estrogen on the growth of breast cancer cells. Tamoxifen is a nonsteroidal antiestrogen that binds to estrogen receptors and blocks the effects of estrogens on the growth of malignant cells in the breast. Decreased cancer recurrence, decreased mortality rates, and increased 5-year survival rates have been found in women with estrogen receptor-positive tissue samples who have been treated with the drug. Aromatase inhibitors block the enzyme that converts androstenedione and testosterone to estrogen in the peripheral tissues. This reduces the circulating estrogen levels in postmenopausal women and is becoming the most effective adjuvant therapy for women with early-stage breast cancer.[69] Autologous bone marrow transplantation and peripheral stem cell transplantation are experimental therapies that may be used for treatment of advanced disease or in women at increased risk for recurrence.

The 5-year survival rate for localized cancer is almost 100%; with nodal involvement, it is approximately 86%; and it is approximately 20% with distant metastasis.[62] The overall 5-year survival rates for all stages of breast cancer is 88%.[62]

Paget Disease

Paget disease accounts for 1% of all breast cancers. The disease presents as an eczematoid lesion of the nipple and areola

FIGURE 46.14 • Paget disease of the nipple. (From Rubin, R., Strayer, D.S. (Eds.). (2012). *Rubin's pathology: Clinicopathologic foundations of medicine* (6th ed., p. 937). Philadelphia, PA: Lippincott Williams & Wilkins.)

(Fig. 46.14). Paget disease usually is associated with an infiltrating, intraductal carcinoma. When the lesion is limited to the nipple only, the rate of axillary metastasis is approximately 5%. Complete examination is required and includes a mammogram and biopsy. Treatment depends on the extent of spread.

IN SUMMARY

The breasts are subject to benign and malignant diseases. Mastitis is inflammation of the breast, occurring most frequently during lactation. Galactorrhea is an abnormal secretion of milk that may occur as a symptom of increased prolactin secretion. Ductal ectasia and intraductal papilloma cause abnormal drainage from the nipple. Fibroadenoma and fibrocystic changes are characterized by abnormal masses in the breast that are benign. By far the most important disease of the breast is breast cancer, which is a significant cause of death of women. Mammography and clinical breast examination afford a woman the best protection against breast cancer. They provide the means for early detection of breast cancer and, in many cases, allow early treatment and cure.

INFERTILITY

After completing this section of the chapter, you should be able to meet the following objectives:

* Provide a definition of infertility.
* List male and female factors that contribute to infertility.
* Briefly describe methods used in the treatment of infertility.

Infertility is the inability to conceive a child after 1 year of unprotected intercourse. Primary infertility refers to situations in which there has been no prior conception. Secondary infertility is infertility that occurs after one or more previous pregnancies. Sterility is the inability to father a child or to become pregnant because of congenital anomalies, disease, or surgical intervention. Approximately 11% to 16% of couples in Canada are affected by infertility.[70]

The complexity of the process that must occur to achieve a pregnancy is taken for granted by most couples. For some couples, pregnancy occurs easily, whereas for others, despite many resources, they are unable to bring about this event. Although a full discussion of the diagnosis and treatment of infertility is beyond the scope of this book, an overview of the areas in which problems can occur is presented.

The causes of infertility are almost equally divided between male factors (30% to 40%), female factors (30% to 40%), and combined factors (30% to 40%). In approximately 10% to 25% of infertile couples, the cause remains unknown even after a full workup.

Male Factors

For pregnancy to occur, the man must be able to provide sperm in sufficient quantity, delivered to the upper end of the vagina, with adequate motility to traverse the female reproductive tract. The male contribution to this process is assessed by means of a semen analysis, which evaluates volume of semen (normally 1 to 6 ml), sperm density (>15 million/ml), motility (50% good progressive), viability (50%), morphology (60% normal), and viscosity (full liquefaction within 20 minutes). The specimen is best collected by masturbation into a sterile container after 3 days of abstinence. Because of variability in specimens, abnormal results should lead to a repeat test before the need for treatment is presumed (Fig. 46.15).

Azoospermia is the absence of sperm; *oligospermia* refers to decreased numbers of sperm; and *asthenospermia* refers to poor motility of sperm. Tests of sperm function include cervical mucus penetration tests (*e.g.,* postcoital test), sperm penetration assay (*i.e.,* Hamster Zona Free Ovum test), sperm capacitation, and sperm antibody testing. None of these tests are included in the routine infertility evaluation.[71]

The causes of male infertility include varicocele, ejaculatory dysfunction, hyperprolactinemia, hypogonadotropic

FIGURE 46.15 • Semen analysis identifying normal compared to a variety of abnormal sperm morphology.

hypogonadism, infection, immunologic problems (*i.e.,* anti-sperm antibodies), obstruction, and congenital anomalies. Risk factors for sperm problems include a history of mumps orchitis, cryptorchidism (*i.e.,* undescended testes), testicular torsion, hypospadias, previous urologic surgery, infection, and exposure to known gonadotoxins (see Chapter 44). Treatment depends on the cause and may include surgery, medication, or the use of artificial insemination to deliver a more concentrated specimen directly to the cervical canal or uterine fundus. Artificial insemination with donor sperm can be offered if the man is sterile and if this is an alternative acceptable to the man and woman.

Female Factors

The female contribution to pregnancy is more complex, requiring production and release of a mature ovum capable of being fertilized; production of cervical mucus that assists in sperm transport and maintains sperm viability in the female reproductive tract; patent fallopian tubes with the motility potential to pick up and transfer the ovum to the uterine cavity; development of an endometrium that is suitable for the implantation and nourishment of a fertilized ovum; and a uterine cavity that allows for growth and development of a fetus. Each of these factors is discussed briefly, along with an overview of diagnostic tests and treatment.

Ovulatory Dysfunction

In a normally menstruating woman, ovulatory cycles begin several months to a year after menarche. Release of FSH from the pituitary causes the development of several primordial follicles in the ovary. At some point, a dominant follicle is selected and the remaining follicles undergo atresia. When the dominant follicle has become large enough to contain a mature ovum (16 to 20 mm in diameter) and is producing sufficient estradiol to ensure adequate proliferation of the endometrium, production of LH increases (*i.e.,* the LH surge), and the increased LH level induces release of the ovum from the follicle (*i.e.,* ovulation).

After ovulation, under the influence of LH, the former follicle luteinizes and begins producing progesterone in addition to estradiol. The progesterone stimulates the development of secretory endometrium, which has the capability to nourish a fertilized ovum if one should implant.

The presence of progesterone after ovulation causes a rise in the woman's basal body temperature (BBT). This thermogenic property of progesterone provides the basis for the simplest, most inexpensive beginning test of ovulatory function—the measurement of BBT. Women should be able to detect at least a 0.2°C rise in their BBT (at rest) after ovulation that should be maintained throughout the luteal phase. This biphasic temperature pattern demonstrates that ovulation has taken place, where in the cycle it occurred, and the length of the luteal phase. BBT can be influenced by many other factors, including restless sleep, alcohol intake, drug use, fever due to illness, and change in usual rising time.

Other tests for ovulation can include the LH predictor kits, which can usually be bought at local pharmacies. This test detects LH in urine, which should appear after the LH surge has occurred indicating ovulation. Serum progesterone can be measured after expected ovulation to confirm if ovulation has occurred. A luteal phase defect (LPD) is suggested by an abnormal serum progesterone level 7 days after ovulation. This diagnosis indicates that, although ovulation is occurring, endometrial development is insufficient and implantation may not be possible since pregnancy requires both fertilization and implantation. It can be treated directly with supplemental progesterone after ovulation or with the use of clomiphene citrate to stimulate increased pituitary production of FSH and LH. Finally, an endometrial biopsy can be done to provide histologic evidence of the secretory endometrium and the level of maturation of the lining. This information is compared to the current phase of the woman's cycle and, if a discrepancy of more than 2 days exists, the woman is said to have an LPD. However given the invasiveness of this last test, it is not usually done.

Anovulation (no ovulation) and oligo-ovulation (irregular ovulation) are other forms of ovulatory dysfunction. These problems can be identified by the tests for LPD previously described, but are more often identified and treated based on a history of menstrual irregularity. Ovulatory problems can be primary problems of the ovary or secondary problems related to endocrine dysfunction. When disturbances in ovulation are confirmed, it is reasonable to rule out other endocrine system problems before initiating treatment. If the results of tests for pituitary hormones (*e.g.,* FSH, LH, prolactin), thyroid studies, and tests of adrenal function (*e.g.,* DHEA-S, androstenedione) are normal, ovulatory dysfunction is primary and should respond to treatment. Abnormalities in any of the other endocrine areas should be further evaluated as needed and treated appropriately. Hyperprolactinemia responds well to bromocriptine or cabergoline, but pituitary microadenoma may need to be excluded first. Hypothyroidism requires thyroid replacement, and hyperthyroidism requires suppressive therapy and, sometimes, surgical intervention with thyroid replacement later. Adrenal suppression can be instituted with dexamethasone, a glucocorticoid analog. Normal ovulatory function may resume without further intervention; if not, treatment can be concurrent with management of other endocrine problems.

Cervical Mucus Problems

High preovulatory levels of estradiol stimulate the production of large amounts of clear, stretchy cervical mucus that aids the transport of sperm into the uterine cavity and helps to maintain an environment that keeps the sperm viable for up to 72 hours. Insufficient estrogen production (i.e., inherent or secondary to treatment with clomiphene citrate, an antiestrogen), cervical abnormalities from disease or invasive procedures (e.g., DES exposure, stenosis, conization), and cervical infection (e.g., chlamydial infection, mycoplasmal infection, gonorrhea) can adversely affect the production of healthy cervical mucus.

A postcoital test (Sims–Huhner) involves evaluation of the cervical mucus 1 to 8 hours after intercourse within the 48 hours before ovulation. A sample of cervical mucus is obtained using a special syringe and evaluated grossly for amount, clarity, and stretch (i.e., spinnbarkeit) and microscopically for cellularity, number and quality of motile sperm, and the presence of ferning after the sample has air dried on the slide. To obtain good-quality mucus, it is essential to obtain the sample within the 48 hours before ovulation. Tests may have to be repeated in the same cycle or in subsequent cycles to ensure appropriate timing. This can be a source of stress and frustration, as well as added cost, to the couple. Intrauterine insemination (IUI) with the man's sperm can bypass the cervical mucus, and is often offered empirically as an alternative to postcoital testing.

If inadequate estrogen effect is seen (poor-quality mucus), supplemental oral estrogen can be given in the first 9 days of the next cycle, and the test can be repeated. If the quality of the mucus is good but sperm are inadequate in number or motility, further evaluation of the male may be needed. Both the man and woman can be tested for antisperm antibodies when repeated postcoital tests reveal that the sperm are all dead or agglutinated; however, IUI is the only effective treatment for sperm antibodies and is frequently offered without the need for further testing.

Cervical cultures for gonorrhea, chlamydial infection, and mycoplasmal infection should be obtained and treatment instituted as needed. Prophylactic treatment with antibiotics can be provided before IUI or other procedures that pass through the cervical canal as a more cost-effective alternative to obtaining cervical cultures.

Uterine Cavity Abnormalities

Alterations in the uterine cavity can occur because of DES exposure, submucosal fibroids, cervical polyps, bands of scar tissue, or congenital anomalies (e.g., bicornuate septum, single horn). These defects may be suspected from the patient's history or pelvic examination and require confirmation with a hysterosonography (i.e., ultrasound study injecting sterile saline into the uterine cavity to enlarge it and allow for visualization and measurements), hysterosalpingography (i.e., x-ray study in which dye is placed through the cervix to outline the uterine cavity and demonstrate tubal patency), or hysteroscopy (i.e., study in which a lighted fibreoptic endoscope placed through the cervix under general anesthesia allows direct visualization of the uterine cavity). Treatment is surgical when possible.

Tubal Factors

Tubal patency is required for fertilization and can be disrupted secondary to PID, ectopic pregnancy, large myomas, endometriosis, pelvic adhesions, and previous tubal ligation. Hysterosalpingography can reveal the location and type of any blockage, such as fimbrial, cornual, or hydrosalpinx. Microsurgical repair sometimes is possible.

Even when tubal patency is demonstrated, tubal disease may make ovum pickup impossible. Contrary to popular belief, the ovum is not extruded directly into the fallopian tube. The tube must be free to move to engulf the ovum after release. Pelvic adhesions from previous infection, surgery, or endometriosis can interfere with the tube's mobility. Laparoscopic evaluation of the pelvis is needed for diagnosis. Laser ablation or cautery can be used to lyse adhesions and remove endometriosis through the laparoscope or, if severe, by means of laparotomy.

Assisted Reproductive Technologies

The reported number of assisted reproductive technology (ART) cycles performed annually in Canada has exponentially increased from 7,884 cycles in 2001 to 11,806 in 2010, and now accounts for 1.7% to 4% of all pregnancies.[72,73] In vitro fertilization (IVF) was developed in 1978 for women with significantly damaged or absent tubes to provide them with an opportunity for pregnancy where none normally exists. The ovaries are superstimulated to produce multiple follicles using clomiphene citrate, human menopausal gonadotropins (e.g., Repronex, Menopur) containing FSH and LH, pure FSH (e.g., Gonal F, Bravelle), or a combination of these drugs. Follicular maturation is monitored by means of ultrasonography and assay of serum estradiol levels. When preovulatory criteria are met, an injection of hCG is given to simulate an LH surge; 35 hours later, the follicles are aspirated transvaginally using ultrasound guidance. The follicular fluid is evaluated microscopically for the presence of ova. When found, they are removed and placed into culture media in an incubator.

The ova or eggs are inseminated with sperm from the male that have been prepared by a washing technique that removes the semen, begins the capacitation process, and allows the strongest sperm to be used for fertilization. When very low numbers of normal motile sperm are available, microsurgical techniques can be used to assist with fertilization. Earlier procedures such as *partial zona dissection* (PZD), which involves the creation of a small opening in the layer (*i.e.,* zona pellucida) that surrounds the egg, and subzonal insertion, where several sperm are inserted into the space just beneath the protective layer, are rarely used today. The most definitive form of micromanipulation is a procedure called *intracytoplasmic sperm injection* (ICSI), where a single spermatozoon is injected directly into the cytoplasm of the egg. More than 70% of all IVF procedures performed in 2012 used ICSI for fertilization.[74]

Between 12 and 24 hours after insemination, the ova are evaluated for signs of fertilization. If signs are present, the ova are returned to the incubator, and 2 to 5 days after egg retrieval, the fertilized eggs, now known as zygotes, are placed into the woman's uterus by means of a transcervical catheter. Because many embryos will not advance to the 5 to 6 day blastocyst stage in vitro, this therapy may be limited to those women who have produced a significant number of embryos. In 2012, 41% of embryos were transferred on day 5, compared with 46% transferred on day 3. In all age groups success rates were higher for day 5 transfers. The overall clinical pregnancy rate in 2012 for all forms of ART was 31%, as reported by the Canadian Assisted Reproductive Technology Register (CARTR).[74]

We have been successful in Canada in reducing the number of multiple (twin, triplet, or greater) pregnancies. The Canadian Fertility and Andrology Society reported in 2013 that the rate of multiple pregnancies in ART has decreased from 32% in 2009 to 18.4% in 2012.[75] This is significant, as the costs to the healthcare system from complications of multiple births, such as prematurity and higher risk of maternal complications, has been estimated by the CIHI in 2006 as $295 million.[76] This reduction is in part due to guidelines, published by the Society of Obstetricians and Gynecologist of Canada (SOGC) in 2010, that recommend the elective transfer of only a single embryo in favourable conditions of embryo quality and maternal age.[77]

Hormonal supplementation of the luteal phase is typically used to increase the possibility of implantation. Indications for IVF have been expanded to include male factors (*i.e.,* severe oligospermia or asthenospermia), ovulatory dysfunction, uterine factors, endometriosis, and idiopathic infertility (*i.e.,* infertility of unknown cause). The substantial risk of multiple births with IVF procedures has been reduced with the availability of cryopreservation, which allows freezing of excess embryos and limits the number of fresh embryos transferred. The pregnancy rate in 2012 after frozen embryo transfer was just over 30%.[74]

The use of donor gametes (oocytes, sperm, embryos) provides an alternative for achieving pregnancy for those couples who are unable to use their own gametes and are comfortable raising a child that is not genetically related to them. Donor eggs provide a much higher likelihood of success for women older than 40 years of age, when both egg numbers and egg quality decline. In 2012, there were over 1,100 cycles using donor oocytes in either fresh or frozen transfer cycles, with a 50% pregnancy rate in fresh transfers and over 35% rate in frozen transfers.[74]

Future research for assisted productive technology will focus on understanding and improving the implantation process in an effort to decrease the risk of multiple births while providing an optimal chance for pregnancy.

IN SUMMARY

Infertility is the inability to conceive a child after 1 year of unprotected intercourse. Male factors are related to number and motility of sperm and their ability to penetrate the cervical mucus and the ovum. Causes of male infertility include varicocele, ejaculatory dysfunction, hyperprolactinemia, hypogonadotropic hypogonadism, infection, immunologic problems (*i.e.,* antisperm antibodies), obstruction, and congenital anomalies. Risk factors for sperm disorders include a history of mumps orchitis, cryptorchidism, testicular torsion, hypospadias, previous urologic surgery, infection, and exposure to known gonadotoxins.

The female contribution to pregnancy is more complex, requiring oocyte production and release of a mature ovum capable of being fertilized; production of cervical mucus that assists in sperm transport and maintains sperm viability in the female reproductive tract; patent fallopian tubes with the mobility potential to pick up and transfer the ovum to the uterine cavity; development of an endometrium that is suitable for the implantation and nourishment of a fertilized ovum; and a uterine cavity that allows for growth and development of a fetus.

Evaluation and treatment of infertility can be lengthy and highly stressful for the couple. Options for therapy continue to expand, but newer ART modalities are expensive, and financial resources can be strained while couples seek to fulfill their sometimes elusive dream of having a child.

REVIEW EXERCISES

1. A 32-year-old woman has been told that the report of her annual Pap test revealed the presence of mild dysplasia.
   A. *What questions should this woman ask as a means of becoming informed about the significance of these findings?*
   B. *In obtaining additional information about the results of her Pap test, the woman is informed that dysplastic changes are consistent with a LSIL classification.*
      1. *Does this mean that the woman has cervical cancer?*

2. *Cervical cancer is often referred to as a sexually transmitted infection. Explain.*
3. *What type of follow-up care would be indicated?*

2. A 30-year-old woman consults her gynecologist because of amenorrhea and inability to become pregnant. Physical examination reveals an obese woman with hirsutism. The physician tells the woman that she might have a condition known as polycystic ovary syndrome and that further laboratory tests are indicated.

A. *Among tests ordered were fasting blood glucose, LH, FSH, and DHEA-S levels. What information can these tests provide that would help in establishing a diagnosis of polycystic ovary syndrome?*

B. *What is the probable cause of this woman's amenorrhea, hirsutism, and failure to become pregnant?*

C. *What type of treatment might be used to help this woman become pregnant?*

3. A 45-year-old woman makes an appointment to see her physician because of a painless lump in her breast that she discovered while doing her routine monthly breast self-examination.

A. *What tests should be done to confirm the presence or absence of breast cancer?*

B. *During the removal of breast cancer, a sentinel lymph node biopsy is often done to determine whether the cancer has spread to the lymph nodes. Explain how this procedure is done and its value in determining lymph node spread.*

C. *After surgical removal of breast cancer, tamoxifen may be used as an adjuvant systemic therapy for women without detectable metastatic disease. The presence or absence of estrogen receptors in the cytoplasm of tumour cells is important in determining the selection of an agent for use in adjuvant therapy. Explain.*

References

1. Kessous R., Aricha-Tamir B., Sheizaf B., et al. (2013). Clinical and microbiological characteristics of Bartholin gland abscesses. *Obstetrics & Gynecology, 122*(4), 794–799.
2. Kurman R. J., Ellenson L. H., Ronnett B. M. (2011). *Blaustein's pathology of the female genital tract* (6th ed.). Boston, MA: Springer US.
3. Gibbs R. S, Karlan B. Y., Haney A. F., et al. (2008). *Danforth's obstetrics and gynecology* (10th ed.). Philadelphia, PA: Lippincott Williams & Wilkins.
4. Eppsteiner E., Boardman L., Stockdale C. K. (2014). Vulvodynia. *Best Practice & Research Clinical Obstetrics and Gynaecology, 28*(7), 1000–1012.
5. Cooper A. S., Boardman L. A. (2005). Diagnosing and treating vulvar pain syndromes. *Women's Health Gynecology Edition, 5*(3), 153–162.
6. Alberta Health Services. (2013). Squamous cell carcinoma of the vulva. Available online at: http://www.albertahealthservices.ca/hp/if-hp-cancer-guide-gyne006-vulva.pdf. Accessed December 16, 2014.
7. Canadian Cancer Society. (2014). Vulvar cancer. Available online at: www.cancer.ca. Accessed December 15, 2014.
8. Preti M., Scurry J., Marchitelli C. E., et al. (2014). Vulvar intraepithelial neoplasia. *Best Practice & Research Clinical Obstetrics and Gynaecology, 28*(7), 1051–1062
9. Ma B., Forney L. J., Ravel J. (2012). The vaginal microbiome: Rethinking health and diseases. *Annual Review of Microbiology, 66,* 371–389.
10. Eckert L. O. (2006). Acute vulvovaginitis. *New England Journal of Medicine, 355*(12), 1244–1252.
11. Ellenson L. H., Pirog E. C. (2010). Chapter 22: The female genital tract. In Kumar V., Abbas A. K., Fausto N., et al. (Eds.), *Robbins and Cotran pathologic basis of disease* (8th ed.). Philadelphia, PA: Elsevier Saunders.
12. Canadian Cancer Society. (2014). Vaginal cancer. Available online at: www.cancer.ca. Accessed December 15, 2014.
13. Cancer Care Ontario. (2012). Ontario cervical screening cytology guidelines summary. Available online at: https://cancercare.on.ca/common/pages/UserFile.aspx?fileId=13104. Accessed December 15, 2014.
14. Elumir-Tanner L., Doraty M.; Southern Alberta Primary Care Research Network (SAPCReN). (2013). Management of Papanicolaou test results that lack endocervical cells. *Canadian Medical Association Journal, 183* (5), 563–568.
15. Public Health Agency of Canada. (2014). Cervical cancer. Available online at: http://www.phac-aspc.gc.ca/cd-mc/cancer/cervical_cancer-cancer_du_col_uterus-eng.php. Accessed December 15, 2014.
16. Canadian Cancer Society. (2014). Cervical cancer. Available online at: www.cancer.ca. Accessed December 15, 2014.
17. National Advisory Committee on Immunization. (2012). Update on human Papillomavirus (HPV) vaccines. *Canada Communicable Disease Report Weekly [electronic resource], 38*(ACS-1), 1–62.
18. Solomon D., Davey D., Kurman R., et al. (2002). The 2001 Bethesda System: Terminology for reporting results of cervical cytology. *Journal of American Medicine Association, 287*(16), 2114–2119.
19. Canadian Task Force on Preventive Health Care. (2013). Screening for cervical cancer. Available online at: http://canadiantaskforce.ca/ctfphc-guidelines/2013-cervical-cancer/. Accessed December 15, 2014.
20. Canadian Cancer Society. (2014). HPV testing. Available online at: www.cancer.ca/en/prevention-and-screening. Accessed December 15, 2014
21. Society of Obstetricians and Gynecologists of Canada. (2007). Canadian consensus guidelines on human papillomavirus. *Journal of Obstetrics and Gynecology Canada, 29*(8, Suppl 3), S1–S56.
22. Mutter G. L., Prat J., Schwartz D. A. (2012). Chapter 18: The female reproductive system, the peritoneum and pregnacy. In Rubin R., Strayer D. S. (Eds.), *Rubin's pathology: Clinicopathologic foundations of medicine* (6th ed.). Philadelphia, PA: Lippincott Williams & Wilkins.
23. Harada T. (2014). Endometriosis: Pathogenesis and treatment. Tokyo, Japan: Springer.
24. Giudice L. C. (2010). Clinical practice. Endometriosis. *New England Journal of Medicine, 362*(25), 2389–2398.
25. Garcia L., Isaacson K. (2011). Adenomyosis: Review of the literature. *Journal of Minimally Invasive Gynecology, 18*(4), 428–437.
26. Canadian Cancer Society. (2014). Uterine cancer. Available online at: www.cancer.ca. Accessed December 15, 2014.
27. Canadian Cancer Society. (2014). Lynch syndrome. Available online at: http://www.cancer.ca/en/cancer-information/cancer-101/what-is-a-risk-factor/genetic-risk/lynch-syndrome/?region=on. Accessed December 15, 2014.
28. Sorosky J. I. (2012). Endometrial cancer. *Obstetrics & Gynecology, 120*(2), 383–397.
29. Society of Obstetricians and Gynaecologists of Canada. (2013). Epidemiology and investigations for suspected endometrial cancer, *Journal of Obstetrics and Gynecology Canada, 35*(4), 380–383.
30. American Cancer Society. (2014). Survival by stage of endometrial cancer. Available online at: http://www.cancer.org/cancer/endometrialcancer/detailedguide/endometrial-uterine-cancer-survival-rates. Accessed December 15, 2014.
31. Falcone T., Parker W. H. (2013). Surgical management of leiomyomas for fertility or uterine preservation. *Obstetrics & Gynecology, 121*(4), 856–868.

32. Society of Obstetricians and Gynaecologists of Canada. (2015). The management of uterine leiomyomas: Introduction and medical management. *Journal of Obstetrics and Gynecology Canada, 37*(2), 157–181.

33. Gradison M. (2012). Pelvic inflammatory disease. *American Family Physician, 85*(8), 791–796.

34. Public Health Agency of Canada. (2014). Canadian guidelines on sexually transmitted infections. Available online at: http://www.phac-aspc.gc.ca/std-mts/sti-its/cgsti-ldcits/index-eng.php. Accessed December 16, 2014.

35. Public Health Agency of Canada. (2013). Pelvic inflammatory disease. Available online at: http://www.phac-aspc.gc.ca/std-mts/sti-its/cgsti-ldcits/section-4-4-eng.php. Accessed December 16, 2014.

36. Perry S. E., Hockenberry M. J., Lowdermilk D. L., et al. (2013) *Maternal child nursing care in Canada.* Toronto, Canada: Mosby Elsevier.

37. Sivalingam V. N., Duncan W. C., Kirk E., et al. (2011). Diagnosis and management of ectopic pregnancy. *Journal of Family Planning & Reproductive Health Care, 37*(4), 231–240.

38. Pectasides D., Pectasides E., Economopoulos T. (2006). Fallopian tube carcinoma: A review. *Oncologist, 11*(8), 902–912.

39. Fritz M. A., Speroff L. (2011). *Clinical gynecological endocrinology and infertility* (8th ed.). Philadelphia, PA: Lippincott Williams & Wilkins.

40. Nandi A., Chen Z., Patel R., et al. (2014). Polycystic ovary syndrome. *Endocrinology and Metabolism Clinics of North America, 43*(1), 123–147.

41. Franks S. (2013). Polycystic ovary syndrome. *Medicine, 41*(10), 553–556.

42. Rosen M., Cedars M. I. (2011). Chapter 13: Female reproductive endocrinology and infertility. In Gardner D. G., Shobeck D. (Eds.), *Greenspan's basic and clinical endocrinology* (9th ed.). New York: McGraw-Hill.

43. Canadian Cancer Society. (2014). Ovarian cancer. Available online at: www.cancer.ca. Accessed December 16, 2014.

44. Hunn J., Rodriguez G. C. (2012). Ovarian cancer: Etiology, risk factors, and epidemiology. *Clinical Obstetrics and Gynecology, 55*(1), 3–23.

45. Vaughan S., Coward J. I., Bast R. C., et al. (2011). Rethinking ovarian cancer: Recommendations for improving outcomes. *Nature Reviews Cancer, 11*(10), 719–725.

46. Barnes, M.N., Grizzle, W.E., Grubbs, C.J., et al. (2002). Paradigms for primary prevention of ovarian carcinoma. *CA A Cancer Journal for Clinicians, 52*(4), 216–225.

47. Goff B. A., Mandel L. S., Drescher C. W., et al. (2007). Development of an ovarian cancer symptom index: Possibilities for earlier detection. *Cancer, 109*(2), 221–227.

48. American Cancer Society. (2014). Detailed guide: Ovarian cancer. Available online at: http://www.cancer.org/cancer/ovariancancer/detailedguide/index. Accessed December 22, 2014.

49. American Cancer Society. (2014). Ovarian cancer. Available online at: http://www.cancer.org/cancer/ovariancancer/index. Accessed December 22, 2014.

50. Davila W. G. (2006). Treating genital prolapse. *American Journal for Nurse Practitioners, 10*(5), 49–55.

51. Practice Committee of the American Society for Reproductive Medicine. (2006). Indications and options for endometrial ablation. *Fertility and Sterility, 86*(5 Suppl 1), S6–S10.

52. Klein D. A., Poth M. A. (2013). Amenorrhea: An approach to diagnosis and management. *American Family Physician, 87*(11), 781–788.

53. Goodwin T. M., Montoro M. N., Muderspach L. (2010). *Management of common problems in obstetrics and gynecology* (5th ed.). Hoboken, NJ: Wiley-Blackwell.

54. Dennerstein L., Lehert P., Heinemann K. (2012). Epidemiology of premenstrual symptoms and disorders. *Menopause International, 18*(2), 48–51.

55. Rapkin A. J., Skopains A. L. (2012). Pathophysiology of premenstrual syndrome and premenstrual dysphoric disorder. *Menopausal International, 18*(2), 52–59.

56. American Psychiatric Association. (2013). Premenstrual dysphoric disorder. In *Diagnostic and Statistical Manual of Mental Disorders: DSM-5.* Washington, DC: Author.

57. Panay N. (2012). Treatment of premenstrual syndrome: A decision-making algorithm. *Menopause International, 18*(2), 90–92.

58. Santen R. J., Mansel R. (2005). Benign breast disorders. *New England Journal of Medicine, 353*(3), 275–285.

59. Lester S. C. (2010). Chapter 23: The breast. In Kumar V., Abbas A. K., Fausto, N., et al. (Eds.), *Robbins and Cotran pathologic basis of disease* (8th ed.). Philadelphia, PA: Elsevier Saunders.

60. Mulligan A. M., O'Malley F. P. (2012). Chapter 19: The breast. In Rubin R., Strayer D. S. (Eds.). *Rubin's pathology: Clinicopathologic foundations of medicine* (6th ed.). Philadelphia, PA: Lippincott Williams & Wilkins.

61. Bilodeau C. C., Wise S. S. (2013). Fibrocystic breast disease. In McGarry K. A., Tong I. L. (Eds.), *The 5-minute consult clinical companion to women's health* (2nd ed.). Philadelphia, PA: Wolters Kluwer Health.

62. Canadian Cancer Society. (2014). Breast cancer. Available online at: www.cancer.ca. Accessed December 15, 2014.

63. Njiaju U. O., Olopade O. I. (2012). Genetic determinants of breast cancer risk: A review of current literature and issues pertaining to clinical application. *Breast Journal, 18*(5), 436–442.

64. Hofstatter E. W., Chung G. G., Harris L. N. (2011). Chapter 105: Molecular biology of breast cancer. In DeVita V. T., Hellman S., Rosenberg S. A. (Eds.), *Cancer: Principles and practice of oncology* (9th ed.). Philadelphia, PA: Lippincott Williams & Wilkins.

65. Canadian Task Force on Preventative Health Care. (2011). Recommendations on screening for breast cancer in average-risk women aged 40–74 years. *Canadian Medical Association Journal, 183*(17), 1991–2001.

66. Pisano E. D., Gatsonis C., Hendrick E., et al.; Digital Mammographic Imaging Screening Trial (DMIST) Investigators Group. (2005). Diagnostic performance of digital versus film mammography for breast-cancer screening. *New England Journal of Medicine, 353*(17), 1773–1783.

67. Burstein H. J., Harris J. R., Morrow M. (2011). Chapter 106: Malignant tumors of the breast. In DeVita V. T., Hellman S., Rosenberg S. A. (Eds.), *Cancer: Principles and practice of oncology* (9th ed.). Philadelphia, PA: Lippincott Williams & Wilkins.

68. Piccart-Gebhart M. J., Procter M., Leylan-Jones B., et al.; Herceptin Adjuvant (HERA) Trial Study Team. (2005). Trastuzumab after adjuvant chemotherapy in Her2-positive cancer. *New England Journal of Medicine, 353*(16), 1659–1672.

69. Geller M. L., Chlebowski R. T. (2006). The role of aromatase inhibitors in breast cancer therapy. *Female Patient, 31*(1), 23–32.

70. Bushnik T., Cook J. L., Yuzpe A. A., et al. (2012). Estimating the prevalence of infertility in Canada. *Human Reproduction, 27*(3), 738–746.

71. Vasan S. S. (2011). Semen analysis and sperm function tests: How much to test? *Indian Journal of Urology, 27*(1), 41–48.

72. Canadian Fertility and Andrology Society. (2014). Canadian ART register annual reports. Available online at: http://www.cfas.ca/index.php?option=com_content&view=article&id=1076&Itemid=668. Accessed December 28, 2014.

73. Okun N., Sierra S. (2014). Pregnancy outcomes after assisted human reproduction. *Journal of Obstetrics and Gynaecology Canada, 36*(1), 64–83.

74. Canadian Fertility and Andrology Society. (2012). Assisted productive technologies (ART) in Canada: 2012 results from the Canadian ART register. Available online at: http://www.cfas.ca/images/stories/pdf/CARTR_2012.pdf. Accessed December 28, 2014.

75. Pierson R., Yupze A., Bissonnette F. (2013). Human assisted reproduction 2013 live birth rates for Canada. Available online at: http://www.cfas.ca/index.php?option=com_content&view=article&id=1205%3Alive-birth-rates-2013&catid=929%3Apress-releases&Itemid=460. Accessed December 28, 2014.

76. Canadian Institute for Health Information (2006). Giving birth in Canada: The costs. Available online at: https://secure.cihi.ca/free_products/Costs_Report_06_Eng.pdf. Accessed December 28, 2014.

77. Min J. K., Hughes E., Young D. (2010). Elective single embryo transfer following in vitro fertilization. *Journal of Obstetrics and Gynaecology Canada, 32*(4), 363–377.

Visit thePoint **http://thePoint.lww.com for animations, journal articles, and more!**

Sexually Transmitted Infections

47

Sexually transmitted infections (STIs), previously referred to as sexually transmitted diseases (STDs), encompass a broad range of infectious diseases that are spread by sexual contact. STIs continue to be a significant public health concern in Canada as the number of reported for chlamydia, gonorrhea, and infectious syphilis has been rising since the late 1990s.[1] The actual figures are probably much higher than those reported because many of the STIs are either not reportable or go unreported. The agents of infection can include bacteria, *Chlamydia*, viruses, fungi, protozoa, parasites, and unidentified microorganisms (see Chapter 16). Portals of entry include the mouth, genitalia, urinary meatus, rectum, and skin. The rates of many STIs are highest among adolescents; all STIs are more common in persons who have more than one sexual partner; and it is not uncommon for a person to be concurrently infected with more than one type of STI.

There are many factors that contribute to the increased prevalence and the continued spread of STIs, including the fact that STIs are frequently asymptomatic, which promotes the spread of infection by persons who are unaware that they are carrying the disease. Furthermore, partners of infected persons are often difficult to notify and treat. Condoms could prevent the spread of many STIs, but they often are not used or are used improperly. In addition, there currently are no cures for viral STIs (*e.g.,* human immunodeficiency virus [HIV], herpes simplex virus); although there are drugs available that may help to manage the infections, they do not entirely control the spread. Also, drug-resistant microorganisms are rapidly emerging, making treatment of many STIs more difficult.

This chapter discusses the manifestations of STIs in men and women in terms of infections of the external genitalia, vaginal infections, and infections that have genitourinary as well as systemic manifestations. HIV infection is presented in Chapter 20.

INFECTIONS OF THE EXTERNAL GENITALIA

After completing this section of the chapter, you should be able to meet the following objectives:

- List common portals of entry for STIs.
- Name the organisms responsible for condylomata acuminata, genital herpes, molluscum contagiosum,

- chancroid, granuloma inguinale, and lymphogranuloma venereum.
- State the significance of being infected with high-risk strains of the human papillomavirus.
- Explain the pathogenesis of recurrent genital herpes infections.

STIs can selectively infect the mucocutaneous tissues of the external genitalia, cause vaginitis in women, or produce both genitourinary and systemic effects. Some STIs may be transmitted by an infected mother to a fetus or newborn, causing congenital defects or death of the child. The discussion in this section of the chapter focuses on STIs that affect the mucocutaneous tissues of the oropharynx and external genitalia, and anorectal tissues. These infections include condylomata acuminata, genital herpes, molluscum contagiosum, chancroid, granuloma inguinale, and lymphogranuloma venereum (LGV).

Condylomata Acuminata (Genital Warts)

Condylomata acuminata, or genital warts, are caused by the human papillomavirus (HPV). Although recognized for centuries, HPV-induced genital warts have become one of the fastest growing STIs of the past decade. The Society of Obstetricians and Gynaecologists of Canada (SOGC) estimates HPV affects 550,000 Canadians each year.[1,2] Risk factors for acquiring HPV include young age (<25 years), early age of first intercourse (<16 years), increased numbers of sex partners, and having a male partner with multiple sex partners. HPV infection can occur with any skin-to-skin contact (*i.e.,* penis, scrotum, vagina, vulva, anus) with or without vaginal or anal penetration and is common in men having sex with men and women having sex with women. Oral–genital and manual–genital contact are less likely means of spreading this infection. Most HPV infections are asymptomatic and transient, and resolve without treatment.[1–4] However, in some cases, HPV infection results in genital warts, Papanicolaou (Pap) test abnormalities, or, rarely, cervical cancer.

SEXUALLY TRANSMITTED INFECTIONS

- In general, STIs due to bacterial pathogens can be successfully treated and the pathogen eliminated by antimicrobial therapy. However, many of these pathogens are developing antibiotic resistance.
- STIs due to viral pathogens such as genital herpes simplex virus infections (HSV-1 and HSV-2) are not eliminated by current treatment modalities and persist with risk of recurrence (HSV infections).

HPVs are nonenveloped, double-stranded deoxyribonucleic acid (DNA) viruses that cause proliferative lesions of the squamous epithelium.[3] More than 100 distinct HPV subtypes have been identified, over 40 of which affect the anogenital area.[1–5] These subtypes have been divided into three categories based on their likelihood of inducing dysplasia and carcinoma. HPV types 6 and 11 are considered low risk. They are found in most external genital warts but usually are benign, with only a low potential for dysplasia. Types 31, 33, 35, 39, 45, 51, 52, 56, 58, and 68 are considered to be intermediate risk because they are common causes of intraepithelial neoplasia, but less common causes of squamous cell carcinoma. HPV types 16 and 18 are strongly associated with cervical dysplasia and anogenital cancers and are considered high risk. Only a subset of women infected with HPV go on to develop cervical cancer, however, suggesting that even the most virulent HPV strains may vary in terms of their oncogenic potential. Cofactors that may increase the risk for cancer include smoking, immunosuppression, and exposure to hormonal alteration (*e.g.,* pregnancy, oral contraceptives).[1–5]

HPV infection begins with viral inoculation into a stratified squamous epithelium, where infection stimulates replication of the squamous epithelium, producing the various HPV-proliferative lesions.[5] The incubation period for HPV-induced genital warts ranges from 6 weeks to 8 months. Most individuals with a healthy immune system will be likely to clear or suppress this virus; 10% to 30% will spontaneously clear the virus over 3 months, and approximately 90% will clear the virus naturally within 2 years. However, in another small proportion of patients, the infection will persist, and they will be chronically/latently infected.[3,4,6] Genital warts typically present as soft, raised, fleshy lesions on the external genitalia, including the penis (Fig. 47.1), vulva, scrotum, perineum, and

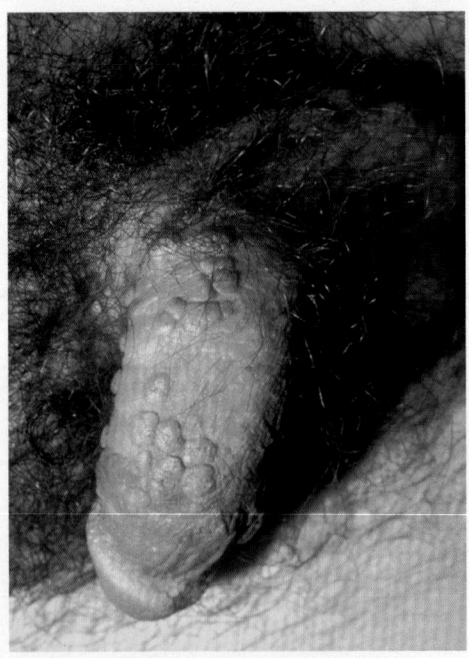

FIGURE 47.1 • Condylomata of the penis. Raised circumscribed lesions are seen on the shaft of the penis. (From Rubin R., Strayer D.S. (Eds.). (2012). *Rubin's pathology: Clinicopathologic foundations of medicine* (6th ed., pp. 825). Philadelphia, PA: Lippincott Williams & Wilkins.)

perianal skin. External warts may appear as small bumps, or they may be flat, rough surfaced, or pedunculated. Less commonly, they can appear as smooth reddish or brown raised papules or as dome-shaped lesions on keratinized skin. Internal warts are cauliflower-shaped lesions that affect the mucous membranes of the vagina, urethra, anus, or mouth. They may cause discomfort, bleeding, or painful intercourse.[3–5]

Subclinical infection occurs more frequently than visible genital warts. Both spontaneous resolution and infection with new HPV types are common. Many women with transient HPV infections develop atypical squamous cells of undetermined significance (ASC-US) or low-grade squamous intraepithelial lesions (LSIL) of the cervix as detected on a Pap test, colposcopy, or biopsy (see Chapter 46). In men, transient HPV infection may be associated with intraepithelial neoplasia of the penis and anus. Development of an effective immune response helps clear the infection, but it is possible for the virus to remain dormant for years and reactivate at a later time. Although reinfection from sexual partners has been considered a reason for the high prevalence of this disease, it is now thought that reinfection with the same HPV type is infrequent.

The association with premalignant and malignant changes has increased the concern regarding the diagnosis and treatment of this viral infection. Lack of regular cervical cancer screening (Pap test) is the primary risk factor for development of invasive cervical cancer.[1–3] There are no approved serologic tests for HPV or routine methods for culturing the virus. Although not available in all provinces or territories, the tests commonly used in Canada are the solution hybridization method or the polymerase chain reaction (PCR) assay to test for 13 high-risk types of HPV DNA.[3,7] The HPV DNA test detects whether one or more of the high-risk types of HPV is present; it does not identify the individual HPV type. HPV DNA testing is warranted with equivocal (ASC-US) Pap test results, and is now recommended to determine which women older than 30 years of age need annual Pap smear screening verses colposcopy (see Chapter 46).

There are three vaccines (Gardasil, Cervarix, and now Gradasil-9) currently available to protect against specific HPV strains. All protect against types 16 and 18, which cause 70% of cervical cancers, and both Gardasil vaccines also protect against types 6 and 11, which are known to lead to genital warts.[8] This vaccine consists of the L1 capsid protein of each of the HPV types. The protein product self-assembles into a noninfectious (as it lacks viral DNA) virus-like particle (VLP) which has the identical shape and size to the natural virus, facilitating the recognition and development of immunity.[8] Currently, however, there is no treatment to eradicate the HPV once a person has become infected. Treatment goals are aimed at elimination of symptomatic warts, surveillance for malignancy and premalignant changes, and education and counselling to decrease psychosocial distress.

Genital condylomata should be considered in any woman who presents with the primary complaint of vulvar pruritus or who has had an abnormal Pap smear result. Microscopic examination of a wet-mount slide preparation and cultures are used to exclude associated vaginitis. Careful inspection of the vulva, with magnification as needed, generally reveals the characteristic lesions, and specimens for biopsy can be taken from questionable areas. Colposcopic examination of the cervix and vagina may be advised as a follow-up measure when there is an abnormal Pap smear result or when HPV lesions are identified on the vulva.

The choice of treatment is based on the number, size, site, and morphology of the lesions, as well the person's preference. Genital warts can resolve spontaneously, so expectant management is acceptable if the person is comfortable with this approach. Evaluation and treatment of sexual partners may be suggested, although this may be difficult considering that warts often do not become clinically apparent for several years after exposure.

The Public Health Agency of Canada (PHAC) identifies several pharmacologic treatments for symptomatic removal of visible genital warts, including patient-applied (podofilox, imiquimod, and sinecatechins [approved in 2013 but not marketed yet in Canada]) and provider-administered (podophyllin and trichloroacetic acid) therapies.[3] Podofilox is a topical antimitotic agent that results in visible necrosis of wart tissue. The safety of podofilox during pregnancy has not been established. Imiquimod cream is a therapeutic agent that stimulates the body's immune system (i.e., production of interferon-α and other cytokines). It is a category B drug and therefore potentially safe for use in pregnancy. Podophyllin, a topical cytotoxic agent, has long been used for treatment of visible external growths. Multiple applications may be required for resolution of lesions. The amount of drug used and the surface area treated should be limited with each treatment session to avoid systemic absorption and toxicity. This treatment is contraindicated in pregnancy for the same reason. An alternative therapy is the topical application of a solution of trichloroacetic acid. This weak destructive agent produces an initial burning in the affected area, followed in several days by a sloughing of the superficial tissue. Several applications at 1- to 2-week intervals may be necessary to eradicate the lesion. Sexual abstinence is suggested during any type of treatment to enhance healing.

Genital warts also may be removed using cryotherapy (i.e., freezing therapy), surgical excision, laser vaporization, or electrocautery. Because it can penetrate deeper than other forms of therapy and can be done as an office-based procedure, cryotherapy often is the treatment of choice for cervical HPV lesions. Surgical options such as laser surgery can be used to remove large or widespread lesions of the cervix, vagina, or vulva, or lesions that have failed to respond to other first-line methods of treatment, but residual scarring may occur.

Genital Herpes

Genital herpes is one of the most common causes of genital ulcers.[9] Because herpesvirus infection is not reportable in all provinces and territories, reliable data on its true incidence (estimated number of new cases every year) and prevalence (estimated number of people currently infected) are lacking. From the late 1970s to early 1990s, genital herpes prevalence increased 30%. Incidence rates have been relatively stable since 1990.[9] Women have a greater mucosal surface area exposed in the genital area and therefore are at greater risk of acquiring the infection.

Herpesviruses are large, encapsulated viruses with a double-stranded genome.[10] There are eight types of herpesviruses, belonging to three groups, that cause infections in humans: (1) neurotropic α-group viruses, which infect epithelial cells and produce latent infections in neurons, including herpes simplex virus type 1 (HSV-1; usually associated with cold sores) and HSV-2 (usually associated with genital herpes); varicella-zoster virus (causes chickenpox and shingles); (2) lymphotropic β-group viruses which infect and produce latent infections in a variety of cell types, including cytomegalovirus, roseolovirus (causes roseola rash); and (3) γ-group viruses, which mainly produce latent infection in lymphoid cells, including Epstein–Barr virus (causes infectious mononucleosis and Burkitt lymphoma) and human herpesvirus type 8 (the apparent cause of Kaposi sarcoma).[10]

HSV-1 and HSV-2 are genetically similar; both cause a similar set of primary and recurrent infections, and both can cause genital lesions.[9,10] These viruses replicate in the skin and mucous membranes at the site of infection (oropharynx or genitalia), where they cause vesicular lesions of the epidermis and infect the neurons that innervate the area. HSV-1 and HSV-2 are *neurotropic* viruses, meaning that they grow in neurons and share the biologic property of latency.[11] Latency refers to the ability to maintain disease potential in the absence of clinical signs and symptoms. In genital herpes, the virus ascends through the peripheral nerves to the sacral dorsal root ganglia. The virus can remain dormant in the dorsal root ganglia, or it can reactivate, in which case the viral particles are transported back down the nerve root to the skin, where they multiply and cause a lesion to develop. During the dormant or latent period, the virus replicates in a different manner so that the immune system or available treatments have no effect on it. It is not known what reactivates the virus. It may be that the body's defence mechanisms are altered. Numerous studies have shown that host responses to infection influence initial development of the disease, severity of infection, development and maintenance of latency, and frequency of HSV recurrences.[11]

HSV is transmitted by contact with infectious lesions or secretions. HSV-1 is transmitted by oral secretions, and infections frequently occur in childhood. HSV-1 may be spread to the genital area by autoinoculation after poor handwashing or through oral–genital contact. It has been estimated that among sexually active adults, new genital HSV-1 infections are almost as common as new HSV-2 infections. HSV-2 usually is transmitted by sexual contact and both HSV-1 and HSV-2 can be passed to an infant during childbirth if the virus is actively being shed from the genital tract. Most cases of HSV-2 infection are subclinical, manifesting as truly asymptomatic or symptomatic but unrecognized infections. These subclinical infections can occur in people who have never had

a symptomatic outbreak or they can occur between recognized clinical recurrences. Genital herpes is spread through asymptomatic shedding by people who do not realize they have the infection.[14] This "unknown" transmission of the virus to sex partners explains why this infection has reached epidemic proportions throughout the world. The incubation period for HSV is 2 to 10 days.

Genital HSV infection may manifest as a first-episode or recurrent infection. There are two types of clinically apparent first-episode eruptions. The first is a true primary infection that occurs in a person who is seronegative for antibodies to HSV-1 or HSV-2. The second is a nonprimary clinical eruption in a person who is seropositive for antibodies to the opposite HSV type (usually genital herpes in someone seropositive to HSV-1). Recurrent infections refer to the second or subsequent outbreak due to the same virus type. First-episode infections have more numerous and scattered vesicles and more systemic manifestations. Viral shedding lasts longer with first-episode infections (10 to 15 days) and new lesions continue to form for about 10 days after the initial infection. Many "severe" presumed primary cases are actually first-recognized recurrences in persons with long-standing infection.

The initial symptoms of primary genital herpes infections include tingling, itching, and pain in the genital area, followed by eruption of small pustules and vesicles. These lesions rupture on approximately the fifth day to form wet ulcers that are excruciatingly painful to touch and can be associated with dysuria, dyspareunia, and urine retention. This period is followed by a 10- to 12-day interval during which the lesions crust over and gradually heal. Involvement of the cervix, vagina, urethra, and inguinal lymph nodes is common in women with primary infections. In men, the infection can cause urethritis and lesions of the penis and scrotum. Rectal and perianal infections are possible with anal contact. Systemic symptoms associated with primary infections include fever, headache, malaise, muscle ache, and lymphadenopathy. Primary infections may be debilitating enough to require hospitalization, particularly in women.

Recurrent HSV episodes are usually milder than the initial episode—there typically are fewer lesions, and viral shedding occurs at a lower concentration and for a shorter duration (about 3 days). However, the prodromal symptoms of itching, burning, and tingling at the lesion site are similar. Except for the greater tendency of HSV-2 to recur, the clinical manifestations of HSV-2 and genital HSV-1 infections are similar. The frequency and severity of recurrence vary from person to person. Numerous factors, including emotional stress, lack of sleep, overexertion, other infections, vigorous or prolonged coitus, and premenstrual or menstrual distress, have been identified as triggering mechanisms.

Diagnosis of genital herpes is based on the symptoms, appearance of the lesions, and identification of the virus from swab tests taken from the lesions for cell culture. The chance of obtaining a positive culture from a crusted lesion is slight, and persons suspected of having genital herpes should be instructed to have a culture within 48 hours of development of new lesions, particularly as the wet-excreting lesions have a higher viral load. PCR testing for HSV DNA is more sensitive than culture (see Chapter 16). This type of testing is more expensive than culture, but even small amounts of the virus will result in a positive test, the results can be obtained more quickly, and the method can distinguish between HSV-1 and HSV-2. In many clinics, PCR testing has become the preferred method of testing when active lesions are present.

Type-specific (HSV-1 and HSV-2) serologic tests are available for determining past infection. Because almost all HSV-2 infections are sexually acquired, the presence of type-specific HSV-2 antibodies usually indicates anogenital infection, whereas the presence of HSV-1 antibodies does not distinguish between anogenital and orolabial infections. The SOGC recommends that type-specific glycoprotein G (gG) assays be requested when serologic testing is performed. This type of testing may prove useful in confirming infection in persons with recurrent genital symptoms and negative HSV cultures, or in establishing a clinical diagnosis of genital herpes without laboratory confirmation or in a partner of a person with genital herpes.[12]

There is no known cure for genital herpes, and the methods of treatment are largely symptomatic. The antiviral drugs acyclovir, valacyclovir, and famciclovir have become the cornerstone for management of genital herpes.[12,13] By interfering with viral DNA replication, these drugs decrease the frequency of recurrences, shorten the duration of active lesions, reduce the number of new lesions formed, and decrease viral shedding with primary infections. Valacyclovir, the active component of acyclovir, and famciclovir have greater bioavailability, which enables improved dosing schedules and increased compliance. Episodic intervention reduces the duration of viral shedding and the healing time for recurrent lesions. Continuous antiviral suppressive therapy may be advised when more than six outbreaks occur within 1 year.[13] These drugs are well tolerated, with few adverse effects. This long-term suppressive therapy does not limit latency, and reactivation of the disease frequently occurs after the drug is discontinued.

Good hygiene is essential during HSV outbreaks to prevent secondary infections. Fastidious handwashing is recommended to avoid hand-to-eye spread of the infection. Sometimes symptomatic relief can be obtained with cool compresses (i.e., Burow soaks), sitz baths, topical anesthetic agents, and oral analgesic drugs. Loose-fitting clothing and cotton undergarments are helpful. To prevent spread of the infection, intimate contact should be avoided until lesions are completely healed.

Current information indicates the risk of neonatal infection is very low when the mother has developed type-specific antibodies, which are then protective to the neonate. Newborns at highest risk are those born to women who shed the virus and have not developed antibodies from previous infections. Disseminated neonatal infection carries high mortality and morbidity rates. Active infection during labour may necessitate cesarean delivery, ideally before membranes rupture. Recommendations from the Canadian Paediatric Society direct care providers to obtain HSV cultures before delivery when a woman has an HSV infection during the pregnancy even if no active lesions are present. Vaginal delivery is acceptable if visible lesions are not present at the onset of labour and women may be counselled to use acyclovir or valacyclovir as suppressive treatment starting at 36 weeks until delivery.[14]

Molluscum Contagiosum

Molluscum contagiosum is a common viral disease of the skin that gives rise to multiple umbilicated papules (Fig 47.2). The infection is mildly contagious; it is transmitted by skin-to-skin contact, fomites, and autoinoculation. Lesions are dome-like and have a dimpled appearance. A curd-like material can be expressed from the centre of the lesion.[15] Necrosis and secondary infection are possible. Diagnosis is based on the appearance of the lesion and microscopic identification of intracytoplasmic molluscum bodies. Molluscum is a benign and self-limited infection.

Spontaneous regression of mature lesions followed by continued emergence of new lesions is common with molluscum, and in the absence of therapy this cycle may persist for 6 months to 5 years. Recurrence is frequent after treatment; therefore, the goal of therapy is to hasten the resolution of individual lesions and reduce the likelihood of further spread.[15] Ablative in office treatments such as curettage, cryotherapy, laser surgery, or even topical chemical destructive agents (e.g., trichloroacetic acid, cantharidin) can cause scarring and pain. Other options are self-applied chemical agents (i.e., retinoic acid, podofilox), immune modulators (i.e., imiquimod), and antiviral medications (i.e., cidofovir), but no single intervention is effective and acceptable to all patients.[15]

Chancroid

Chancroid (i.e., soft chancre) is an infection of the external genitalia and lymph nodes. The causative organism is the gram-negative bacterium *Haemophilus ducreyi,* which causes acute ulcerative lesions with profuse discharge. This disease has become uncommon in Canada with only three reported cases in 1995, no reported cases in 1999, and in 2000 chancroid was removed from the national surveillance database.[16] It typically occurs in discrete outbreaks rather than as an endemic disease. It is more prevalent in Southeast Asia, the West Indies, and North Africa. As a highly infectious disease, chancroid usually is transmitted by sexual intercourse or through skin and mucous membrane abrasions. Autoinoculation may lead to multiple chancres.

Lesions begin as macules, progress to pustules, and then rupture. This painful ulcer has a necrotic base and jagged edges. In contrast, the syphilitic chancre is nontender and indurated. Subsequent discharge can lead to further infection of self or others. On physical examination, lesions and regional lymphadenopathy may be found. Secondary infection may cause significant tissue destruction. Diagnosis usually is made clinically, but may be confirmed through culture. Gram stain rarely is used today because it is insensitive and

FIGURE 47.2 • Typical flesh-coloured, umbilicated, pearly lesions of molluscum contagiosum. (**A**) On the neck, (**B**) Close-up view, (**C**) of vulvar area, and (**D**) with atopic eczema in the antecubital fossae area. (From Hall, B. J., Hall, J. C. (2010). Sauer's manual of skin diseases (10th ed., 236). Philadelphia, PA: Lippincott Williams & Wilkins.)

nonspecific. No useful serology tests exist, and PCR testing methods are not available commercially for definitive identification of *H. ducreyi;* thus, culture is still a primary method of diagnosis in Canada. The PHAC recommends treatment with ciprofloxacin, azithromycin, erythromycin, or ceftriaxone.[17]

Granuloma Inguinale

Granuloma inguinale (*i.e.,* granuloma venereum) is caused by a gram-negative bacillus, *Klebsiella granulomatis* (previously known as *Calymmatobacterium* [*Donovania*] *granulomatis*), which is a tiny, encapsulated intracellular parasite. This disease is almost nonexistent in North America. It is found most frequently in India, Brazil, the West Indies, and parts of Australia, and Africa.[18,19]

Granuloma inguinale causes ulceration of the genitalia, beginning with an innocuous papule. The papule progresses through nodular or vesicular stages until it begins to break down as pink, granulomatous tissue. At this final stage, the tissue becomes thin and friable and bleeds easily. There are complaints of swelling, pain, and itching. Extensive inflammatory scarring may cause late sequelae, such as lymphatic obstruction with the development of enlarged and elephantoid external genitalia. The liver, bladder, bone, joint, lung, and bowel tissue may become involved. Genital complications include

tubo-ovarian abscess, fistula, vaginal stenosis, and occlusion of vaginal or anal orifices. Lesions may become neoplastic.

Diagnosis is made through the identification of Donovan bodies (*i.e.,* large mononuclear cells filled with intracytoplasmic gram-negative rods) in tissue smears, biopsy samples, or culture. A minimum 3-week period of treatment, preferably with doxycycline, or, alternatively, with azithromycin, ciprofloxacin, erythromycin, or trimethoprim-sulfamethoxazole, can be used in treating the disorder.[18]

Lymphogranuloma Venereum

Lymphogranuloma venereum (LGV) is an acute and chronic venereal disease caused by *Chlamydia trachomatis* types L1, L2, and L3. The disease, although found worldwide, has a low incidence outside the tropics. Most cases reported in Canada are in men.[19,20] There appears to be a new variant, L2b, that is causing a resurgence of LGV in Europe, the United States, and Canada, particularly in men who have sex with men.[19]

The lesions of LGV can incubate for a few days to several weeks and thereafter cause small, painless papules or vesicles that may go undetected. An important characteristic of the infection is the early development (within 2 to 6 weeks of the primary lesion) of large, tender, and sometimes fluctuant inguinal lymph nodes called *buboes*. There may be flu-like symptoms with joint pain, rash, weight loss, pneumonitis, tachycardia, splenomegaly, and proctitis. In later stages of the disease, a small percentage of affected persons develop elephantiasis of the external genitalia, caused by lymphatic obstruction or fibrous strictures of the rectum or urethra from inflammation and scarring. Urethral involvement may cause pyuria and dysuria. Cervicitis is a common manifestation of primary LGV, and could extend to perimetritis or salpingitis, which are known to occur in other chlamydial infections. Anorectal structures may be compromised to the point of incontinence. Complications of LGV may be minor or extensive, involving compromise of whole systems or progression to a cancerous state.

Diagnosis usually is accomplished by nucleic acid amplifications tests (NAATs) of urine, urethral, cervical, and/ or vaginal swabs. If the test result is positive for *C. trachomatis,* the samples are then forwarded to specific laboratories for LGV genotyping. Serology is no longer recommended due to the cross-reactions with other *Chlamydia* species and the potential difficulties with interpreting the results. First-line treatment involves 3 weeks of doxycycline; erythromycin or azithromycin can be used as alternative medications.[20] Surgery may be required to correct sequelae such as strictures or fistulas or to drain fluctuant lymph nodes.

IN SUMMARY

STIs that primarily affect the external genitalia include HPV-induced genital warts, genital herpes, molluscum contagiosum, chancroid, granuloma inguinale, and LGV. The lesions of these infections occur on the external genitalia of sexually active males and females. Of concern is the relation between HPV and genital neoplasms. Genital herpes is caused by a neurotropic HSV (HSV-2 and, sometimes, HSV-1) that ascends through the peripheral nerves to reside in the sacral dorsal root ganglia. The herpesvirus can be reactivated, producing recurrent lesions in genital structures that are supplied by the peripheral nerves of the affected ganglia. There is no permanent cure for herpes infections. Molluscum contagiosum is a benign and self-limited infection that is only mildly contagious. Chancroid, granuloma inguinale, and LGV are uncommon in Canada. These infections produce external genital lesions with various degrees of inguinal lymph node involvement.

VAGINAL INFECTIONS

After completing this section of the chapter, you should be able to meet the following objectives:

* State the difference between wet-mount slide and culture methods of diagnosis of STIs.
* Compare the signs and symptoms of infections caused by *Candida albicans, Trichomonas vaginalis,* and bacterial vaginosis.

Candidiasis, trichomoniasis, and bacterial vaginosis are vaginal infections that can be associated with sexual activity. Trichomoniasis is the only form of vaginitis that is known to be sexually transmitted and requires partner treatment. The male partner usually is asymptomatic.

Candidiasis

Also called *yeast infection, thrush,* and *moniliasis, candidiasis* is the second leading cause of vulvovaginitis in Canada. Approximately 75% of women in Canada will experience one episode in their lifetime, 40% to 45% experience two or more infections, and approximately 5% of reproductive-age women will have recurrent symptomatic episodes with four or more per year.[21,22]

Candida albicans is the most commonly identified organism in vaginal yeast infections. However, other *Candida* species, such as *Candida glabrata* and *Candida tropicalis,* may also be present and responsible for complicated candidiasis. These organisms are present in 10% to 20% of healthy women without causing symptoms, and alteration of the host vaginal environment usually is necessary before the organism can cause pathologic effects.[22] Although vulvovaginal candidiasis usually is not transmitted sexually, it is included in the Canadian Guidelines on Sexually Transmitted Infections because it often is diagnosed in women being evaluated for STIs.[21] The possibility of sexual transmission has been recognized for many years; however, candidiasis requires a favourable environment for growth of the organism. The gastrointestinal tract also serves as a reservoir for this organism, and candidiasis can develop through autoinoculation in women who are not sexually active. Although studies have documented the presence of *Candida* on the penis of male partners of women with vulvovaginal candidiasis, few men develop balanoposthitis that requires treatment.[22]

Reported risk factors for the overgrowth of *C. albicans* include recent antibiotic therapy, which suppresses the normal protective bacterial flora; high hormone levels owing to pregnancy or the use of oral contraceptives, which cause an increase in vaginal glycogen stores; and uncontrolled diabetes mellitus or HIV infection, because they compromise the immune system.[21] Women with vulvovaginal candidiasis commonly complain of vulvovaginal pruritus accompanied by irritation, erythema, swelling, dysuria, and dyspareunia. The characteristic discharge, when present, is usually thick, white, and odourless. In obese persons, *Candida* may grow in skin folds underneath the breast tissue, the abdominal flap, and the inguinal folds.

Accurate diagnosis is made by identification of budding yeast filaments (*i.e.,* hyphae) or spores on a wet-mount slide using a saline or potassium hydroxide (KOH) solution (Fig. 47.3). The pH of the discharge, which is checked with litmus paper, typically is less than 4.5. When the wet-mount technique is negative but the clinical manifestations are suggestive of candidiasis, a culture may be necessary.

Antifungal agents such as clotrimazole, miconazole, and terconazole, in various forms, are effective in treating

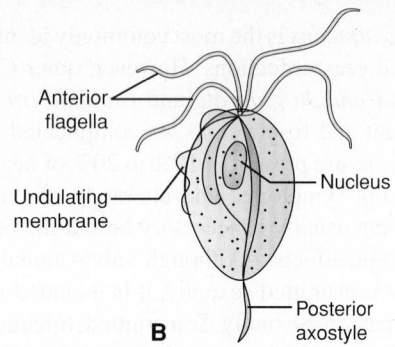

FIGURE 47.3 • Organisms that cause vaginal infections. **A:** *Candida albicans* (blastospores and pseudohyphae). **B:** *Trichomonas vaginalis* (flagella, undulating membrane, and axostyle). (From Centers for Disease Control and Prevention Public Health Image Library. Available online at: http://phil.cdc.gov/phil/details.asp)

candidiasis. These drugs, with the exception of terconazole, are available without prescription for use by women who have had a previously confirmed diagnosis of candidiasis. Oral fluconazole has been shown to be as safe and effective as the standard intravaginal regimens.[21] Chronic vulvovaginal candidiasis, defined as four or more mycologically confirmed episodes within 1 year, can be difficult to manage. Subsequent prophylaxis (maintenance therapy) often is required for long-term management of this problem.[21]

Trichomoniasis

Trichomoniasis is credited with being a far more prevalent STI than either chlamydial infection or gonorrhea. In Canada, the prevalence has not been determined, whereas globally it is estimated that 170 million new cases of trichomoniasis appear annually.[23] Epidemiologically, *T. vaginalis* infections are commonly associated with other STIs and are therefore a marker for high-risk sexual behaviour.

An anaerobic protozoan that can be transmitted sexually, *T. vaginalis* is shaped like a turnip or pear and has four anterior flagella with the fifth flagellum positioned posterior and surrounded by an undulating membrane[23] (Fig. 47.3). Trichomonads can reside in the paraurethral glands of both

FIGURE 47.4 • Strawberry appearance of the cervix due to *Trichomonas vaginalis* infection, or trichomoniasis. The cervical mucosa reveals punctate hemorrhages along with accompanying vesicles and papules. (From the Centers for Disease Control and Prevention Public Health Image Library. Available online at: http://phil.cdc.gov/phil/home.asp)

sexes. Men harbour the organism in the urethra and prostate and are asymptomatic. Although 10% to 50% of women can be asymptomatic, trichomoniasis is a common cause of vaginitis when some imbalance allows the protozoan to proliferate. This extracellular parasite feeds on the vaginal mucosa and ingests bacteria and leukocytes. The infection causes a copious, frothy, malodorous, green or yellow discharge. There commonly is erythema and edema of the affected mucosa, with occasional itching and irritation. Sometimes, small hemorrhagic areas, called *strawberry spots,* appear on the cervix[21,23] (Fig. 47.4).

Trichomoniasis can cause a number of complications.[21–23] It is a risk factor for HIV transmission and infectivity in both men and women. In women, it increases the risk of tubal infertility and atypical pelvic inflammatory disease (PID; see Chapter 46), and it is associated with adverse outcomes such as premature birth in pregnant women. Trichomonads attach easily to mucous membranes. They may serve as vectors for the spread of other organisms, carrying pathogens attached to their surface into the fallopian tubes. In men, it is a common cause of nongonococcal urethritis and is a risk factor for infertility, altering sperm motility and viability. It has also been associated with chronic prostatitis.[21–24]

Diagnosis can be made microscopically by quickly identifying the motile protozoan on a wet-mount slide preparation or with a Gram stain identifying polymorphonuclear leukocytes and trichomonads. The pH of the discharge usually is greater than 4.5. Cultures, including urethral or vaginal swabs, urine, or semen cultures, are more commonly utilized, but results can take seven days for laboratory growth to occur. Newer forms of NAAT are available in some provinces and territories and have the capability of testing for trichomonas, chlamydia, and gonorrhea in a single vaginal or urethral swab.

Because the organism resides in other urogenital structures besides the vagina, systemic treatment is recommended. The treatment of choice is oral metronidazole, which is effective against anaerobic protozoans.[21] Metronidazole is chemically similar to disulfiram (Antabuse), a drug used in the treatment of alcohol addiction that causes nausea, vomiting, flushing of the skin, headache, palpitations, and lowering of the blood pressure when alcohol is ingested. Gastrointestinal disturbances and a metallic taste in the mouth are potential adverse effects of the drug. Metronidazole is considered safe for use during pregnancy. Sexual partners should be treated to avoid reinfection, and abstinence is recommended until the full course of therapy is completed.[21]

Bacterial Vaginosis

Bacterial vaginosis is the most prevalent form of vaginal infection seen by healthcare professionals. It is estimated that 10% to 30% of pregnant women and 10% of family practice patients have this vaginal infection.[21] The disorder is associated with having multiple sex partners, a new sex partner, douching, and a lack of vaginal lactobacilli. Its relation to sexual activity is not clear. Sexual activity is believed to be a catalyst rather than a primary mode of transmission, and endogenous factors may play a role in the development of symptoms.

The pathogenesis of bacterial vaginosis is poorly understood. It is a complex polymicrobial disorder characterized by a shift in the vaginal flora from one dominated by hydrogen peroxide-producing lactobacilli to one with greatly reduced numbers of *Lactobacillus* species and an overgrowth of other organisms, including *Gardnerella vaginalis, Mobiluncus* species, *Mycoplasma hominis,* and numerous anaerobes.[21,22,25] The massive overgrowth of vaginal anaerobes is associated with increased conversion of vaginal peptides to a variety of amines that, in high pH, become volatile and malodorous. The amines are associated with increased vaginal transudation and squamous epithelial cell exfoliation, creating the typical discharge.[27] In conditions of elevated pH, *G. vaginalis* more efficiently adhere to the exfoliating epithelial cells, creating clue cells (squamous epithelial cells covered with masses of coccobacilli, often with large clumps of organisms floating free from the cell). Amines further provide a suitable substrate for *M. hominis* growth.

The predominant symptom of bacterial vaginosis is a thin, greyish-white discharge that has a foul, fishy odour. Burning, itching, and erythema usually are absent because the bacteria have only minimal inflammatory potential. Because of the lack of inflammation, the term *vaginosis* rather than *vaginitis* is used to describe the condition. The organisms associated with bacterial vaginosis may be carried asymptomatically by men and women.

In addition to causing bothersome symptoms, bacterial vaginosis is associated with an increased risk of PID, preterm labour, premature rupture of membranes, chorioamnionitis, and postpartum endometritis linked to the organisms associated with bacterial vaginosis. Postoperative infections, including postabortion PID, posthysterectomy cuff cellulitis, and post-cesarean endometritis, have been shown to be associated with asymptomatic bacterial vaginosis.

The diagnosis of bacterial vaginosis is made when at least three of the following characteristics are present: homogeneous, thin, white discharge; production of a fishy, amine odour when a saline or potassium hydroxide solution is dropped onto the secretions; vaginal pH above 4.5 (usually 5.0 to 6.0); and appearance of characteristic "clue cells" on wet-mount microscopic studies. Because *G. vaginalis* can be a part of the normal vaginal flora, cultures should not be done routinely.

When indicated, treatment is aimed at relieving the vaginal symptoms and signs of infection and reducing the risk of infectious complications after abortion or hysterectomy. All women who have symptomatic disease should be treated. Other potential benefits might include a reduction in the risk of other STIs. The PHAC recommends treatment by oral metronidazole, metronidazole vaginal gel, or clindamycin vaginal cream. The same treatment regimens used for nonpregnant women can be used in pregnancy. Routine screening for bacterial vaginosis is not advocated, but all pregnant women with bacterial vaginosis should be treated, and women at increased risk for preterm labour should be screened during the first trimester.[21,22,25] Treatment of sexual partners is not recommended.[21]

IN SUMMARY

Candidiasis, trichomoniasis, and bacterial vaginosis are common vaginal infections that become symptomatic because of changes in the vaginal ecosystem. Only trichomoniasis is spread through sexual contact. The infection, which is caused by the anaerobic protozoan *T. vaginalis,* incites the production of a copious, frothy, yellow or green, malodorous discharge. It is a risk factor for HIV transmission and infectivity in both men and women. In women, it increases the risk of tubal infertility and atypical PID and it is associated with adverse outcomes such as premature birth in pregnant women. Candidiasis, also called a yeast infection, is a frequent cause of vulvovaginitis. Candida can be present without producing symptoms; usually some host factor, such as altered immune status, contributes to the development of vulvovaginitis. It can be treated with over-the-counter medications. Bacterial vaginosis is the most common cause of vaginal discharge. It is a complex polymicrobial disorder characterized by a shift in the vaginal flora from one dominated by hydrogen peroxide-producing lactobacilli to one with greatly reduced numbers of lactobacilli and an overgrowth of other organisms. The predominant symptom of bacterial vaginosis is a thin, greyish-white discharge that has a foul, fishy odour. Because it does not produce inflammation, it is referred to as vaginosis rather than vaginitis.

VAGINAL–UROGENITAL–SYSTEMIC INFECTIONS

After completing this section of the chapter, you should be able to meet the following objectives:

- Compare the signs and symptoms of gonorrhea in male and female.
- Describe the three stages of syphilis.
- State the genital and nongenital complications that can occur with chlamydial infections, gonorrhea, and syphilis.
- State the treatment for chlamydial urogenital infections, gonorrhea, nonspecific urogenital infections, and syphilis.

Some STIs infect both male and female genital and extragenital structures. Among the infections of this type are chlamydial infections, gonorrhea, and syphilis. Many of these infections also pose a risk to infants born to infected mothers. Some infections, such as syphilis, may be spread to the infant while in utero, whereas others, such as chlamydial and gonorrheal infections, can be spread to the infant during the birth process.

Chlamydial Infections

Chlamydial infection is the most prevalent STI in Canada, with an incidence estimated to be more than twice that of gonorrhea. Mandatory reporting to the local public health authorities is required for all chlamydial infections for all provinces and territories and since 1997 the reported infection rates have continued to increase. The PHAC estimates that chlamydial infections occur at a rate of 100,000 new cases each year, predominantly among individuals younger than 30 years of age. The highest reported rate was among young adults between 20 and 24 years of age, and in 2011 in this age group the rate among females was more than twice as high the rate among males. For older age groups, the gap between female and male chlamydia rates is smaller, and in the 60 years or older age group the rates of reported cases were higher among men.[26,27] The increase in chlamydial infection rates is due in part to an increase in screening programs, improved sensitivity of diagnostic tests, and improved surveillance and reporting systems. Reported rates are higher in women largely because of screening efforts, although with the increasing availability of urine testing, reported infection rates in men have also risen dramatically.[26]

Chlamydia trachomatis is an obligate intracellular bacterial pathogen that is closely related to gram-negative bacteria.[5,10] It resembles a virus in that it requires tissue culture for isolation, but like bacteria, it has ribonucleic acid (RNA) and DNA and is susceptible to some antibiotics. *C. trachomatis* causes a wide variety of genitourinary infections, including nongonococcal urethritis in men and PID in women. The

closely related organisms *Chlamydia pneumoniae* and *Chlamydia psittaci* cause mild and severe pneumonia, respectively. *C. trachomatis* can be serologically subdivided into types A, B, and C, which are associated with trachoma and chronic keratoconjunctivitis; types D through K, which are associated with genital infections and their complications; and types L1, L2, and L3, which are associated with LGV. *C. trachomatis* can cause significant ocular disease in neonates; it is a leading cause of blindness in underdeveloped countries. In these countries, the organism is spread primarily by flies, fomites, and nonsexual personal contact. In industrial countries, the organism is spread almost exclusively by sexual contact and therefore affects primarily the genitourinary structures.

Chlamydiae exist in two forms: elementary bodies, which are the infectious particles capable of entering uninfected cells, and the initiator or reticulate bodies, which multiply by binary fission to produce the inclusions identified in stained cells.[10] The 48-hour growth cycle starts with attachment of the elementary body to the susceptible host cell, after which it is ingested by a process that resembles phagocytosis (Fig. 47.5). Once inside the cell, the elementary body is organized into the reticulate body, the metabolically active form of the organism that is capable of reproduction. The reticulate body is not infectious and cannot survive outside the body. The reticulate bodies divide in the cell for up to 36 hours and then condense to form new elementary bodies, which are released when the infected cell bursts.

The signs and symptoms of chlamydial infection resemble those produced by gonorrhea. The most significant difference between chlamydial and gonococcal salpingitis is that chlamydial infections may be asymptomatic or clinically nonspecific. In women, chlamydial infections may cause dyspareunia, dysuria, and vaginal discharge.[27] The most common symptom is a mucopurulent cervical discharge. The cervix itself frequently hypertrophies and becomes erythematous, edematous, and extremely friable. Seventy-five percent of women and 50% of men with chlamydial infection have no symptoms; therefore, most cases are undiagnosed, unreported, and untreated.[28] This can lead to greater fallopian tube damage and increase the reservoir for further chlamydial infections.

In men, chlamydial infections cause urethritis, including meatal erythema and tenderness, urethral discharge, dysuria, and urethral itching. Prostatitis and epididymitis with subsequent infertility may develop. The most serious complication of untreated chlamydial infection is the development of Reiter syndrome, a reactive arthritis that includes the triad of urethritis, conjunctivitis, and painless mucocutaneous lesions[5] (see Chapter 59). Women can also develop reactive arthritis, but the male-to-female ratio for this complication is 5:1. The arthritis begins 1 to 3 weeks after the onset of chlamydial infection. The joint involvement is asymmetric, with multiple affected joints and a predilection for the lower extremities. The mucocutaneous lesions are papulosquamous eruptions that tend to occur on the palms of the hands and soles of the feet. Annual screening for sexually active adolescents and young adults has been suggested by the PHAC and the Canadian Task Force on

FIGURE 47.5 • Chlamydial growth cycle. EB, elementary body; RB, reticulate body.

Periodic Health Examination (CTFPHE) in an effort to minimize these serious sequelae of asymptomatic infection.[27,29]

Diagnosis of chlamydial infections takes several forms. The identification of polymorphonuclear leukocytes on Gram stain of penile discharge in the man or cervical discharge in the woman provides presumptive evidence. The direct fluorescent antibody test and the enzyme-linked immunosorbent assay that use antibodies against an antigen in the *Chlamydia* cell wall are rapid tests that are highly sensitive and specific. The positive predictive value of these tests is excellent among high-risk groups, but false-positive results occur more often in low-risk groups. The methodologic challenges of culturing this organism have led to the development of non–culture-based tests that amplify and detect *C. trachomatis*-specific DNA and RNA sequences. One of the newest sets of nonculture techniques, NAATs, do not require viable organisms for detection, and can produce a positive signal from as little as a single copy of the target DNA or RNA.[30] The amplification procedures that are now commercially available for chlamydial testing are PCR, transcription-mediated amplification (TMA) of RNA, and strand displacement amplification (SDA). These amplification methods are highly sensitive and, if properly monitored, very specific. Because NAATs can be performed on urine and self-collected swab specimens from the distal vagina as well as on the traditional endocervical and urethral specimens, this easy, convenient means of accurate detection has become the diagnostic method of choice.[30] Detection rates (specificity) for chlamydiae in urine and vaginal samples are nearly identical to those for cervical and urethral samples. Most NAATs in use today detect both *C. trachomatis* and *Neisseria gonorrhoeae* in a single test. However, PCR assays on urine samples are not reliable enough to rule out gonococcal infections in women. Cost often is a factor in determining which type of testing to use.

The PHAC recommends the use of azithromycin or doxycycline in the treatment of chlamydial infection; penicillin is ineffective. Azithromycin is the preferred choice in pregnancy. Simultaneous antibiotic treatment of both sexual partners is recommended. Abstinence from sexual activity is encouraged to facilitate cure.

Gonorrhea

Gonorrhea is a reportable STI caused by the bacterium *N. gonorrhoeae*. It is the second most commonly diagnosed and reported bacterial STI. Since 1997 there has been a gradual and steady increase in cases in Canada.[31] In 2010 there were 11,397 reported cases with the majority of cases reported in people under 30 years of age.[26] Similar to chlamydial infection, gonorrhea is frequently underdiagnosed but improved screening efforts as well as greater use of more sensitive nonculture methods of testing may have contributed to the increased incidence.

The gonococcus is a pyogenic (*i.e.,* pus-forming), gram-negative diplococcus that evokes inflammatory reactions characterized by purulent exudates.[10] Humans are the only natural host for *N. gonorrhoeae*. The organism grows best in warm, mucus-secreting epithelia. The portal of entry can be the genitourinary tract, eyes, oropharynx, anorectum, or skin.

Transmission usually is by heterosexual or homosexual intercourse. Autoinoculation of the organism to the conjunctiva is possible. Neonates born to infected mothers can acquire the infection during passage through the birth canal and are in danger of developing gonorrheal conjunctivitis, with resultant blindness unless treated promptly (Fig. 47.6). An amniotic infection syndrome characterized by premature rupture of the membranes, premature delivery, and increased risk of infant morbidity and mortality has been identified as an additional complication of gonococcal infections in pregnancy. Genital gonorrhea in young children should raise the possibility of sexual abuse.

The infection commonly manifests 2 to 7 days after exposure. It typically begins in the anterior urethra, accessory urethral glands, Bartholin or Skene glands, and the cervix. If

FIGURE 47.6 • Newborn with gonococcal ophthalmia neonatorum caused by maternally transmitted gonococcal infection. (From the Centers for Disease Control and Prevention Public Health Image Library. Available online at: http://phil.cdc.gov/phil/home.asp)

untreated, gonorrhea spreads from its initial sites upward into the genital tract. In males, it spreads to the prostate and epididymis; in females, it commonly moves to the fallopian tubes[5] (Fig. 47.7). Pharyngitis may follow oral–genital contact. The organism also can invade the bloodstream (*i.e.,* disseminated gonococcal infection), causing serious sequelae such as bacteremic involvement of joint spaces, heart valves, meninges, and other body organs and tissues.

Persons with gonorrhea may be asymptomatic and may unwittingly spread the disease to their sexual partners. Men are more likely to be symptomatic than women.[5,31] In men, the initial symptoms include urethral pain and a creamy yellow,

FIGURE 47.7 • Gonorrhea of the fallopian tube. Cross-section of a "pus tube" shows thickening of the wall and lumen swollen with pus. (From Rubin R., Strayer D. S. (Eds.). (2012). *Rubin's pathology: Clinicopathologic foundations of medicine* (6th ed., p. 356). Philadelphia, PA: Lippincott Williams & Wilkins.)

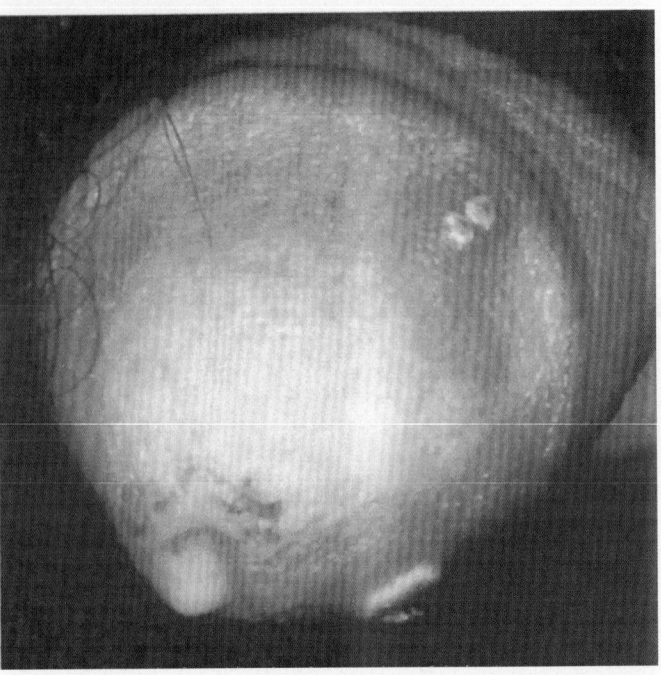

FIGURE 47.8 • Purulent penile discharge due to gonorrhea with overlying pyodermal lesions. (From the Centers for Disease Control and Prevention Public Health Image Library. Available online at: http://phil.cdc.gov/phil/home.asp)

sometimes bloody, discharge (Fig. 47.8). The disorder may become chronic and affect the prostate, epididymis, and periurethral glands. Rectal infections are common in homosexual men. In women, recognizable symptoms include unusual genital or urinary discharge, dysuria, dyspareunia, pelvic pain or tenderness, unusual vaginal bleeding (including bleeding after intercourse), fever, and proctitis. Symptoms may occur or increase during or immediately after menses because the bacterium is an intracellular diplococcus that thrives in menstrual blood but cannot survive long outside the human body. There may be infections of the uterus and development of acute or chronic infection of the fallopian tubes (*i.e.,* salpingitis), with ultimate scarring and sterility.

Diagnosis is based on the history of sexual exposure and symptoms. It is confirmed by identification of the organism on Gram stain or culture. A Gram stain usually is an effective means of diagnosis in symptomatic men (*i.e.,* those with discharge). In women and asymptomatic men, a culture usually is preferred because the Gram stain often is unreliable. Culture has been the gold standard, particularly when the Gram stain is negative. A specimen should be collected from the appropriate site (*i.e.,* endocervix, urethra, anal canal, or oropharynx), inoculated onto a suitable medium, and transported under appropriate conditions. *N. gonorrhoeae* is a fastidious organism with specific nutrient and environmental needs. Detection by NAATs (PCR) is possible using urine and urethral swab specimens[31] (see information about NAATs in the previous section on Chlamydial Infections). Men are often more willing to provide a urine specimen than to have a urethral swab done, and NAAT can be offered to women in locations where pelvic examination is not possible.

Recommendations from the PHAC suggest that clinicians screen all sexually active men and women for gonorrhea who are at increased risk for infection (*i.e.,* younger than 25 years of age, new or multiple sexual partners, inconsistent condom use, sex work, or drug use).[27,31] In Canada, routine testing for STIs, particularly syphilis and chlamydial infection, is suggested but not always included at the time of annual examinations. However, pregnant women are routinely screened at the time of their first prenatal visit; high-risk populations should have repeat cultures during the third trimester. Neonates are routinely treated with various antibacterial agents applied to the conjunctiva within 1 hour of birth to protect against undiagnosed gonorrhea and other diseases.

Penicillin-resistant strains of *N. gonorrhoeae* are prevalent worldwide and strains with other kinds of antibiotic resistance continue to evolve and spread. The current treatment recommendation to combat tetracycline- and penicillin-resistant strains of *N. gonorrhoeae* is ceftriaxone in a single injection and azithromycin in a single oral dose.[26,31] Quinolone-resistant strains are now common in Canada, so the PHAC currently recommends avoiding the use of any quinolones for treatment. More recently there is a concern associated with the increasing treatment failures suggesting that drug-resistant strains of gonorrhea are emerging. All sex partners within 60 days prior to discovery of the infection should be contacted, tested, and treated. Patients are instructed to refrain from intercourse until therapy is completed and symptoms are no longer present, and repeat screening is recommended 6 months post treatment.[31]

Syphilis

Syphilis is a reportable STI caused by a spirochete, *Treponema pallidum.* After declining every year from 1990 to 2000, the rate of primary and secondary syphilis has increased every year since 2001. In 2002, 482 cases of syphilis were reported in Canada (1.5 per 100,000 population), which increased in 2011 to 1,757 cases (5.1 per 100,000), with the highest rates in Quebec and New Brunswick.[26,32] Even though syphilis transmission occurred over a wider geographic area than in the past and there was a significant increase in the rates among whites, it continues disproportionately to affect aboriginal populations.[32]

T. pallidum is spread by direct contact with an infectious moist lesion, usually through sexual intercourse. Bacteria-laden secretions may transfer the organism during kissing or intimate contact. Skin abrasions provide another possible portal of entry. There is rapid transplacental transmission of the organism from the mother to the fetus after 16 weeks' gestation, so that an active infection in the mother during pregnancy can produce congenital syphilis in the fetus. Untreated syphilis can cause prematurity, stillbirth, and congenital defects and active infection in the infant. Because the manifestations of maternal syphilis may be subtle, testing for syphilis is mandatory in all pregnancies. Once treated for syphilis, a pregnant

FIGURE 47.9 • Syphilitic chancre of the penis shaft. (From the Centers for Disease Control and Prevention Public Health Image Library. Available online at: http://phil.cdc.gov/phil/home.asp)

woman usually is followed throughout pregnancy by repeat testing of serum titres.

The clinical disease is divided into three stages: primary, secondary, and tertiary. Primary syphilis is characterized by the appearance of a chancre at the site of exposure, such as on the penis, vulva, anus, or mouth.[10,32] Chancres typically appear within 3 weeks of exposure but may incubate for 3 days to 3 months. The primary chancre begins as a single, indurated, button-like papule up to several centimetres in diameter that erodes to create a clean-based ulcerated lesion on an elevated base. These lesions usually are painless and located at the site of sexual contact. Primary syphilis is readily apparent in men, where the lesion appears on the scrotum or penis (Fig. 47.9). Although chancres can develop on the external genitalia in women, they are more common on the vagina or cervix, and primary syphilis therefore may go untreated since they are not visible without a speculum examination. There usually is an accompanying regional lymphadenopathy.[5] The infection is highly contagious at this stage, but because the symptoms are mild, it frequently goes unnoticed. The chancre usually heals within 3 to 12 weeks, with or without treatment.[5,32]

The timing of the second stage of syphilis varies even more than that of the first, lasting from 2 weeks to 6 months. The symptoms of a rash, (especially on the palms (Fig. 47.10) and soles), fever, sore throat, stomatitis, nausea, loss of appetite, and inflamed eyes may come and go for a year but usually last for 2 to 12 weeks. Secondary manifestations may include alopecia and genital condylomata lata. Condylomata lata are elevated, red-brown lesions that may ulcerate and produce a foul discharge. They are 2 to 3 cm in diameter, contain many spirochetes, and are highly infectious.

FIGURE 47.10 • Secondary syphilis. A maculopapular rash is present on the palm. (From Rubin R., Strayer D. S. (Eds.). (2012). *Rubin's pathology: Clinicopathologic foundations of medicine* (6th ed., p. 376). Philadelphia, PA: Lippincott Williams & Wilkins.)

After the second stage, syphilis frequently enters a latent phase that may last the lifetime of the person or progress to tertiary syphilis at some point. Persons can be infective during the first 1 to 2 years of latency.

Tertiary syphilis is a delayed response to the untreated disease. It can occur decades after the initial infection. Only approximately one third of those with untreated syphilis progress to the tertiary stage of the disease, and symptoms develop in approximately one half of these. When syphilis does progress to the symptomatic tertiary stage, it commonly takes one of three forms: development of localized destructive lesions called *gummas*, development of cardiovascular lesions, or development of central nervous system lesions.[5,32] The syphilitic gumma is a peculiar, rubbery, necrotic lesion that is caused by noninflammatory tissue necrosis. Gummas can occur singly or multiply and vary in size from microscopic lesions to large, tumorous masses. They most commonly are found in the liver, testes, and bone. Central nervous system lesions can produce dementia, blindness, or injury to the spinal cord, with ataxia and sensory loss (*i.e.,* tabes dorsalis). Cardiovascular manifestations usually result from scarring of the medial layer of the thoracic aorta with aneurysm formation. These aneurysms produce enlargement of the aortic valve ring with aortic valve insufficiency.

T. pallidum is difficult to culture and requires special dark field microscopy to adequately detect the organism.

As it evokes a humoral immune response and production of antibodies, this provides the basis for serologic tests. Although PCR tests have been developed for syphilis, serology remains the mainstay for diagnosis.[10,32] Because the disease's incubation period may delay test sensitivity, serologic tests usually are repeated after 6 weeks if the initial test results were negative.

Two types of antibodies—nonspecific and specific—are produced.[10] The nonspecific tests measure antibody to cardiolipin, a phospholipid that is present in both host cells and the *T. pallidum*. These antibodies are detected by flocculation tests such as the Venereal Disease Research Laboratory (VDRL) test or the rapid plasma reagin (RPR) test. Because these tests are nonspecific, positive results can occur for diseases other than syphilis. The tests are easy to perform, rapid, and inexpensive and frequently are used as screening tests for syphilis. Results become positive 4 to 6 weeks after infection or 1 to 3 weeks after the appearance of the primary lesion. Because these tests are quantitative, they can be used to measure the degree of disease activity or treatment effectiveness. The VDRL titre usually is high during the secondary stage of the disease and becomes less so during the tertiary stage. A falling titre during treatment suggests a favourable response. The fluorescent treponemal antibody absorption test or microhemagglutinin test is used to detect specific antibodies to *T. pallidum*. These qualitative tests are used to determine whether a positive result on a nonspecific test such as the VDRL is attributable to syphilis.

The treatment of choice for syphilis is penicillin.[32] Because of the spirochetes' long generation time, effective tissue levels of penicillin must be maintained for several weeks. Long-acting injectable forms of penicillin must be used. Doxycycline or ceftriaxone are used for treatment in persons who are sensitive to penicillin. Pregnant patients should be desensitized and treated with penicillin because erythromycin does not treat fetal infections. Sexual partners should be evaluated and treated prophylactically even though they may show no sign of infection. All treated individuals should be reexamined clinically and serologically at 6 and 12 months after completing therapy; more frequent monitoring (3-month intervals) is suggested for individuals with HIV infection.[32]

IN SUMMARY

The vaginal–urogenital–systemic STIs—chlamydial infections, gonorrhea, and syphilis—can severely involve the genital structures and manifest as systemic infections. Gonorrheal and chlamydial infections can cause a wide variety of genitourinary complications in men and women, and both can cause ocular disease and blindness in neonates born to infected mothers. Syphilis is caused by a spirochete, *T. pallidum*. It can produce widespread systemic effects and is transferred to the fetus of infected mothers through the placenta.

REVIEW EXERCISES

1. A 25-year-old woman has been told that her Pap test indicates infection with HPV type 16.
   A. *What are the possible implications of infection with HPV 16?*
   B. *How might she have acquired this infection?*
   C. *What treatments are currently available for treatment of this infection?*

2. A 35-year-old woman presents with vulvar pruritus, dysuria, dyspareunia, and an odourless, thick, cheesy vaginal discharge. She has diabetes mellitus and has recently recovered from a respiratory tract infection, which required antibiotic treatment.
   A. *Given that these manifestations are consistent with a Candida infection, what tests might be used to confirm the diagnosis?*
   B. *What risk factors does this woman have that predispose to this type of vaginitis?*
   C. *How might this infection be treated?*

References

1. Public Health Agency of Canada (PHAC). (2014). Report on sexually transmitted infections in Canada: 2011. Ottawa: PHAC.

2. Society of Obstetricians and Gynaecologists of Canada (SOCG). (2007). HPV information. Available online at: http://www.hpvinfo.ca. Accessed December 29, 2014.

3. PHAC. (2014). Canadian guidelines on sexually transmitted infections: Human papillomavirus (HPV) infections. Available online at: http://www.phac-aspc.gc.ca/std-mts/sti-its/cgsti-ldcits/section-5-5-eng.php. Accessed December 29, 2014.

4. Steben M., Garland S. M., (2014). Genital warts. *Best Practice & Research Clinical Obstetrics and Gynaecology, 28*(7), 1063–1073.

5. Rubin R., Strayer D. S. (Eds.). (2012). *Rubin's pathology: Clinicopathologic foundations of medicine* (6th ed.). Philadelphia, PA: Lippincott Williams & Wilkins.

6. Center for Disease Control. (2013). Incidence, prevalence, and cost of sexually transmitted infections in the United States. Available online at: http://www.cdc.gov/std/stats/sti-estimates-fact-sheet-feb-2013.pdf. Accessed December 29, 2014.

7. SOGC. (2007). Canadian consensus guidelines on human papillomavirus. *Journal of Obstetrics and Gynaecology Canada, 29*(8, Suppl 3), S1–S56.

8. National Advisory Committee on Immunizations (NACI). (2012). Update on human papillomavirus (HPV) vaccines. *Canada Communicable Disease Report Weekly, 28*(1), 1–62.

9. Aslam M., Kropp K. Y., Jayaraman G., et al. (2012). Genital herpes in Canada: Deciphering the hidden epidemic. *Canadian Journal of Infectious Diseases & Medical Microbiology, 23*(1), e6–e9.

10. Kumar, V., Abbas A. K., Faustos N., et al. (Eds.). (2010). *Robbins and Cotran pathologic basis of disease* (8th ed.). Philadelphia, PA: Elsevier Saunders.

11. Steiner I., Benninger F. (2013). Update on herpes virus infections of the nervous system. *Current Neurology and Neuroscience Reports, 13*(12), 1–7.

12. Money D., Steben M. (2008). Genital Herpes: Gynaecological aspects. *Journal of Obstetrics and Gynaecology Canada, 30*(4), 347–353.

13. PHAC. (2014). Canadian guidelines on sexually transmitted infections: Genital herpes simplex virus (HSV) infections. Available online at: http://www.phac-aspc.gc.ca/std-mts/sti-its/cgsti-ldcits/section-5-4-eng.php. Accessed December 29, 2014.

14. Allen U. D., Robinson J. L.; Canadian Paediatric Society, Infectious Diseases and Immunization Committee. (2014). Prevention and management of neonatal herpes simplex virus infections. *Paediatrics & Child Health, 19*(4), 201–206.

15. Chen X., Anstey A. V., Bugert J. J. (2013). Molluscum contagiosum virus infection. *Lancet Infectious Diseases, 13*(10), 877–888.

16. PHAC. (2006). Notifiable diseases on-line: Chancroid. Available online at: http://dsol-smed.phac-aspc.gc.ca/dsol-smed/ndis/list-eng.php. Accessed October 4, 2015.

17. PHAC. (2014). Canadian guidelines on sexually transmitted infections: Chancroid. Available online at: http://www.phac-aspc.gc.ca/std-mts/sti-its/cgsti-ldcits/section-5-1-eng.php. Accessed December 29, 2014.

18. Centers for Disease Control and Prevention. (2011). Diseases characterized by genital, anal, or perianal ulcers. Available online at: http://www.cdc.gov/std/treatment/2010/genital-ulcers.htm. Accessed December 29, 2014.

19. Basta-Juzbasic A., Cerovic R. (2014). Chancroid, lymphogranuloma venerum, granuloma inguinale, genital herpes simplex infection, and molluscum contagiosum. *Clinics in Dermatology, 32*(2), 290–298.

20. PHAC. (2014). Canadian guidelines on sexually transmitted infections: Lymphogranuloma venereum (LGV) supplementary statement. Available online at: http://www.phac-aspc.gc.ca/std-mts/sti-its/cgsti-ldcits/assets/pdf/appendix-supp-lgv-eng.pdf. Accessed December 29, 2014.

21. PHAC. (2013). Canadian guidelines on sexually transmitted infections: Vaginal discharge. Available online at: http://www.phac-aspc.gc.ca/lab-bio/res/psds-ftss/trichomonas-eng.php. Accessed December 29, 2014.

22. Centers for disease Control and Prevention. (2011). Diseases characterized by vaginal discharge. Available online at: http://www.cdc.gov/std/treatment/2010/vaginal-discharge.htm. Accessed December 29, 2014.

23. PHAC. (2010). Trichomonas vaginalis. Available online at: http://www.phac-aspc.gc.ca/lab-bio/res/psds-ftss/trichomonas-eng.php. Accessed December, 29, 2014.

24. Meites E. (2013). Trichomoniasis. *Infectious Disease Clinics of North America, 27*(4), 755–764.

25. Hay P. (2014). Bacterial vaginosis. *Medicine, 42*(7), 359–363.

26. PHAC. (2014). Report on sexually transmitted infections Canada: 2011. Available online at: http://www.catie.ca/sites/default/files/64–02–14–1200-STI-Report-2011_EN-FINAL.pdf. Accessed December 29, 2014.

27. PHAC. (2013). Canadian guidelines on sexually transmitted infections: Chlamydial infections. Available online at: http://www.phac-aspc.gc.ca/std-mts/sti-its/cgsti-ldcits/section-5-2-eng.php. Accessed December 29, 2014.

28. Grimshaw-Mulcahy L. J. (2008). Now I know my STDs: Part II. *Journal of Nurse Practitioners, 4*(4), 271–281.

29. Canadian Task Force on Preventive Health Care. (2014). CTFPHC Guidelines Overview. Available online at: http://canadiantaskforce.ca/ctfphc-guidelines/overview/. Accessed on December 29, 2014.

30. Centers for Disease Control and Prevention. (2014). Recommendations for the laboratory-based detection of *Chlamydia trachomatis* and *Neisseria gonorrhoeae* – 2014. *Morbidity and Mortality Weekly Report, 63*(2), 1–19.

31. PHAC. (2013). Canadian guidelines on sexually transmitted infections: Gonococcal infections. Available online at: http://www.phac-aspc.gc.ca/std-mts/sti-its/cgsti-ldcits/section-5-6-eng.php. Accessed December 29, 2014.

32. PHAC. (2014). Canadian guidelines on sexually transmitted infections: Syphilis. Available online at: http://www.phac-aspc.gc.ca/std-mts/sti-its/cgsti-ldcits/section-5-10-eng.php. Accessed December 29, 2014.

Visit thePoint **http://thePoint.lww.com for animations, journal articles, and more!**

Unit XII

Disorders of Neural Function

For centuries, the nervous system was ignored or even deemed unimportant. Aristotle (384–322 BC), the great Greek philosopher, decreed that the heart was the seat of the soul, whereas the brain—which he assumed was composed largely of water—simply cooled it. Although Galen (AD 130–200) was able to show that the spinal cord was essential to many sensations and movements, his experiments were conducted only on animals. Not until the 1500s, when the Flemish anatomist Andreas Vesalius (1514–1564) dissected "the heads of executed criminals, still warm," was the overarching importance of the human brain and spinal cord established.

Investigations continued with scientists debating whether the brain should be considered as a whole or as consisting of separate areas, each responsible for specific functions. Progress in brain research took an impressive, if accidental, leap in 1841, when an explosion at a railroad work site in Vermont shot an iron rod into the left cheek of Phineas Gage, through his brain, and out the top of his head. Gage survived the accident, but it became clear to all who knew him that he had changed greatly. Formerly a conscientious, hardworking man, he became fitful, obstinate, foul-mouthed, and capricious. Gage died in 1860, and an autopsy showed destruction of the left lobe of his brain and damage to his right lobe. Scientists concluded that his personality change was the result of the grievous damage to the frontal lobes, an observation that supported the then-emerging concept that different parts of the brain serve different functions.

Organization and Control of Neural Function

48

The nervous system, in coordination with the endocrine system, provides the means by which cell and tissue functions are integrated into a solitary, surviving organism. It controls skeletal muscle movement and helps to regulate cardiac and visceral smooth muscle activity. The nervous system enables the reception, integration, and perception of sensory information; it provides the substratum necessary for intelligence, anticipation, and judgment; and it facilitates adjustment to an ever-changing external environment.

All portions of the nervous system can be divided into two basic components: the central nervous system (CNS) and the peripheral nervous system (PNS). The CNS consists of the brain and spinal cord, which are protected by the skull and vertebral column, whereas the PNS is found outside these structures. Inherent in the basic design of the nervous system is the provision for the concentration of computational and control functions in the CNS. In this design, the PNS functions as an input–output system for relaying information to the CNS and for transmitting output messages that control effector organs, such as muscles and glands.

This chapter is divided into five parts: (1) nervous tissue cells, (2) neurophysiology, (3) developmental organization of the nervous system, (4) the structure and function of the spinal cord, brain, and (5) autonomic nervous system.

NERVOUS TISSUE CELLS

After completing this section of the chapter, you should be able to meet the following objectives:

- Distinguish between the functions of the neurons and neuroglial cells of the nervous system.
- List the three parts of a neuron and describe their structure and function.
- Name the neuroglial cells in the central nervous system and peripheral nervous system and state their functions.
- Describe the energy requirements of nervous tissue.

THE STRUCTURAL ORGANIZATION OF THE NERVOUS SYSTEM

- The nervous system is divided into two parts: the central nervous system (CNS), consisting of the brain and spinal cord, which are located in the skull and spinal column, and the peripheral nervous system (PNS), which is located outside these structures.
- The nervous system contains two major types of cells: neurons, which are functioning cells of the nervous system, and glial cells, which protect the nervous system and supply metabolic support.
- The neurons consist of a cell body with cytoplasm-filled processes, the dendrites, and the axons.
- There are two types of neurons: afferent neurons or sensory neurons, which carry information to the CNS, and efferent neurons or motor neurons, which carry information from the CNS to the effector organs.

Neurons

Neurons, which are the functioning cells of the nervous system, have three distinct parts: the cell body, and its cytoplasm-filled processes, the dendrites and axon. These processes form the functional connections, or synapses, with other nerve cells, with receptor cells, or with effector cells. Axonal processes are particularly designed for rapid communication with other neurons and the many body structures innervated by the nervous system. Afferent (sensory) neurons transmit information to the CNS, whereas efferent (motor) neurons carry information away from the CNS (Fig. 48.1). Interspersed between the afferent and efferent neurons is a network of interconnecting neurons (also called *interneurons* or *internuncial* neurons) that modulate and control the body's response to sensory input from the internal and external environments.

The cell body (soma) of a neuron contains a large, vesicular nucleus with one or more distinct nucleoli and a well-developed rough endoplasmic reticulum. A neuron's nucleus has the same deoxyribonucleic acid (DNA) and genetic code content present in other cells of the body, and its nucleolus, which is composed of portions of several chromosomes, produces ribonucleic acid (RNA) needed for protein synthesis. The cytoplasm contains large masses of ribosomes that are prominent in most neurons. These acidic RNA masses, which are involved in protein synthesis, stain as dark *Nissl bodies* with basic histologic stains (Fig. 48.1).

Dendrites (*i.e.,* "treelike") are multiple, short, branched extensions of the nerve cell body; they conduct information

Nervous tissue contains two types of cells: neurons and neuroglial cells. The neurons are the functional cells of the nervous system. They exhibit membrane excitability and conductivity and secrete neurotransmitters and hormones, such as epinephrine and antidiuretic hormone. The neuroglial or glial cells protect the nervous system and provide metabolic support for the neurons.

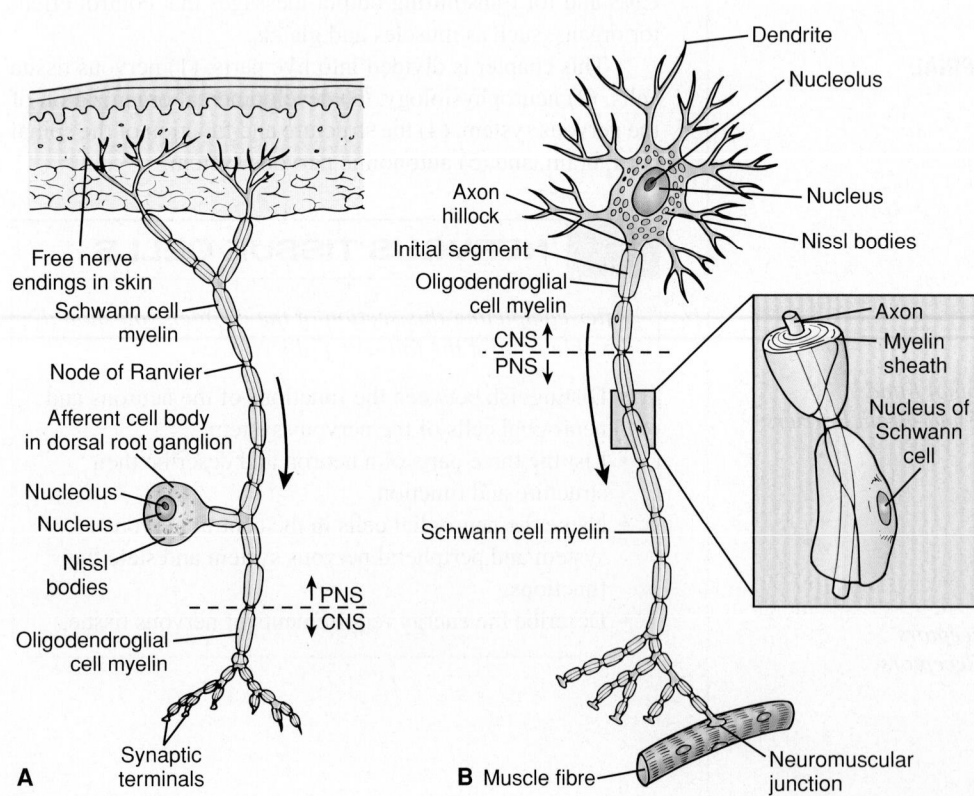

FIGURE 48.1 • Afferent (**A**) and efferent neurons (**B**), showing the soma or cell body, dendrites, and axon. *Arrows* indicate the direction for conduction of action potentials.

toward the cell body and are the main source of information for the neuron. The dendrites and cell body are studded with synaptic terminals that communicate with axons and dendrites of other neurons.

Axons are long efferent processes that project from the cell body. Most neurons have only one axon; however, axons may exhibit multiple branching that results in many axonal terminals. The axon of a neuron conducts nerve impulses from the cell body to its synapse. The axon also provides a physical conduit for the transport of materials between the cell body and the synaptic terminals of the axon. The cell body of the neuron is equipped for a high level of metabolic activity. This is necessary because the cell body must synthesize the cytoplasmic and membrane constituents required to maintain the function of the soma plus the many proteins and other cytoplasmic materials used by the axon and its synaptic terminals. Some of these axons can be very short (0.1 mm); others can extend for a distance of 1 to 1.5 m, and these have a volume that is 200 to 500 times greater than the cell body itself.

A bidirectional axonal transport system exists to carry materials to the nerve terminal (anterograde direction) and back to the cell body (retrograde direction). The anterograde component consists of fast and slow components. Fast anterograde systems transport molecules such as neurosecretory granules via an energy-dependent system at the rate of 200 to 400 mm/day. Another component of the fast anterograde system transports organelles, including mitochondria, at the rate of 50 to 100 mm/day. The antidiuretic hormone and oxytocin use the fast anterograde system to travel from hypothalamic neurons through their axons to the posterior pituitary, where the hormones are released into the blood. The slow anterograde component transports materials such as tubulin and cytoplasmic enzymes at a rate of 0.1 to 6 mm/day. A fast retrograde component of axonal transport carries materials that are shipped back to the cell body for degradation or reuse at the rate of 100 to 200 mm/day. Although much of this material is degraded in lysosomes, retrograde transport is also used to deliver signals to the cell body. The retrograde system does not have a slow component.

Continuous direct observation of axonal transport using video-enhanced light microscopy has revealed that axonal transport depends on microtubules that provide an essentially stationary track on which particles move by means of molecular motors. The microtubule tracks possess inherent polarity and are uniformly oriented with the fast-growing (plus) ends projecting toward the synapse and the slow-growing (minus) ends toward the cell body (Fig. 48.2). Two motor proteins (kinesin and cytoplasmic dynein) are involved in the transport process. Kinesins are generally plus-end-directed motor proteins that transport their cargo anterograde toward the synapse. Cytoplasmic dyneins are minus-end-directed motor proteins that transport their cargo retrograde toward the cell body.

Axonal transport mechanisms are involved in the transport of several pathogens (*e.g.*, herpes simplex, rabies, and polio viruses) and bacterial toxins (*e.g.*, tetanus toxin). After a bite by a rabid animal, rabies viral particles bind to the acetylcholine

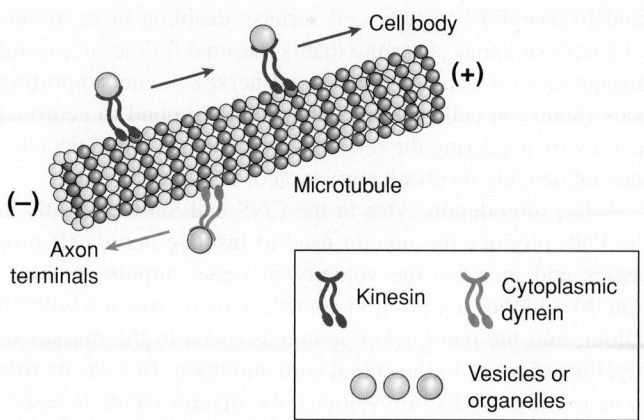

FIGURE 48.2 • The cellular mechanism for axonal transport. Two cellular motor proteins, kinesin and cytoplasmic dynein, are shown transporting vesicles or organelles in the anterograde (kinesin) and retrograde (cytoplasmic dynein) directions. Kinesin transports vesicles toward the rapidly forming (+) end of the microtubule, whereas cytoplasmic dynein transports toward the minus (–) or slower-growing end of the microtubule. (Courtesy of Edward W. Carroll.)

receptors in muscle synapses near the bite and are carried by retrograde transport to the cell bodies of neurons living in the CNS. Affected neurons spread the rabies virus to other neurons throughout the CNS. Affected neurons then transport the virus particles along peripheral nerves by anterograde axonal transport to the salivary glands, where they can be transmitted by another bite. The retrograde axonal transport of the tetanus toxin produced by *Clostridium tetani* bacteria blocks the release of inhibitory substances at synapses, thereby permitting unopposed neural stimulation and sustained contraction of skeletal muscles (tetany). There is also evidence that disorders of axonal transport may be involved in the pathogenesis of neurodegenerative diseases such as Huntington disease and Alzheimer disease.

Neuroglial Cells

The neuroglial or glial cells of the nervous system, including several types of neuroglial cells of the CNS and the Schwann and satellite cells of the PNS, give the neurons protection and metabolic support. These supporting cells segregate the neurons into isolated metabolic compartments, which are required for normal neural function. Some types of supporting cells (astrocytes in the CNS) help to form the blood–brain barrier that prevents toxic materials in the blood from entering the brain. Two types of supporting cells (oligodendrocytes in the CNS and Schwann cells in the PNS) produce the myelin used to insulate nerve cell processes that conduct electrical signals.

Recent research suggests that many supporting cells of the PNS and CNS have functions other than protection and support. For example, evidence suggests that Schwann cells release developmental signals in embryonic nervous tissue that are crucial for survival of neonatal neurons. Postnatally, Schwann cells synthesize and release self-regulating autocrine substances that bind to receptors on their cell surface, enabling them to survive without axons, a feature that is essential for the successful regeneration of damaged peripheral nerves. Some supporting cells (Schwann cells and astrocytes) also respond to neuronal activity by triggering the release of communication molecules, thus influencing feedback regulation of neuronal function.

The oligodendrocytes in the CNS and Schwann cells in the PNS produce the myelin used to insulate nerve cell processes and increase the velocity of nerve impulse conduction. Myelin has a high lipid content, which gives it a whitish colour, and the name *white matter* is given to the masses of myelinated fibres in the spinal cord and brain. Besides its role in increasing conduction velocity, the myelin sheath is essential for the survival of larger neuronal processes, perhaps by the secretion of neurotrophic compounds.

In some pathologic conditions, such as multiple sclerosis in the CNS and Guillain–Barré syndrome in the PNS, the myelin may degenerate or be destroyed. This leaves a section of the axonal process without myelin while leaving the nearby Schwann or oligodendroglial cells intact. Unless remyelination takes place, the axon eventually dies.

Supporting Cells of the Peripheral Nervous System

Schwann cells and satellite cells are the two types of supporting or neuroglial cells in the PNS. Normally, the nerve cell bodies in the PNS are collected into ganglia, such as the dorsal root and autonomic ganglia. Each of the cell bodies and processes of the peripheral nerves is separated from the connective tissue framework of the ganglion by a single layer of flattened capsular cells called *satellite cells*. Satellite cells secrete a basement membrane that protects the cell body from the diffusion of large molecules.

The processes of larger afferent and efferent neurons are surrounded by the cell membrane and cytoplasm of Schwann cells, which are close relatives of the satellite cells. During myelination, the Schwann cell wraps around each nerve process several times in a "jelly roll" fashion (Fig. 48.3). Schwann cells line up along the neuronal process, and each of these cells forms its own discrete myelin segment. The end of each myelin segment attaches to the cell membrane of the axon by means of intercellular junctions. Successive Schwann cells are separated by short extracellular fluid gaps, called the *nodes of Ranvier,* where the myelin is missing and voltage-gated sodium channels are concentrated (Fig. 48.4). The nodes of Ranvier increase nerve conduction by allowing the impulse to jump from node to node through the extracellular fluid in a process called *saltatory conduction* (from the Latin *saltare,* "to jump"). In this way, the impulse can travel more rapidly than it could if it were required to move systematically along the entire nerve process. This increased conduction velocity greatly reduces reaction time, or time between the application of a stimulus and the subsequent motor response. The short reaction time is especially important in peripheral nerves with long distances (sometimes 1 to 1.5 m) for conduction between the CNS and distal effector organs.

FIGURE 48.3 • Section of a peripheral nerve containing both afferent (sensory) and efferent (motor) neurons. Schwann cells form a myelin sheath around the larger nerve fibres in the peripheral nervous system. Successive Schwann cells are separated by short extracellular fluid gaps called the *nodes of Ranvier,* where the myelin is missing and the voltage-gated sodium channels are concentrated.

Each of the Schwann cells, along a peripheral nerve, is encased in a continuous tube of basement membrane, which in turn is surrounded by a multilayered sheath of loose connective tissue known as the *endoneurium* (Fig. 48.3). The endoneurial sheath, which is essential to the regeneration of peripheral nerves, provides a collagenous tube through which a regenerating axon can again reach its former target. The endoneurial sheath does not penetrate the CNS. The absence of the endoneurial sheaths is thought to be a major factor in the limited axonal regeneration of CNS nerves compared with those of the PNS.

The endoneurial sheaths are bundled with blood vessels into small bundles or clusters of nerves called *fascicles.* In the nerve, the fascicles consisting of bundles of nerve fibres are surrounded by another protective covering called the *perineurium.* Usually, several fascicles are further surrounded by the heavy, protective *epineurial sheath* of the peripheral nerve. The protective layers that surround the peripheral nerve processes are continuous with the connective tissue capsule of the sensory nerve endings and the connective tissue that surrounds the effector structures, such as the skeletal muscle cell. Centrally, the connective tissue layers continue along the dorsal and ventral roots of the nerve and fuse with the meninges that surround the spinal cord and brain.

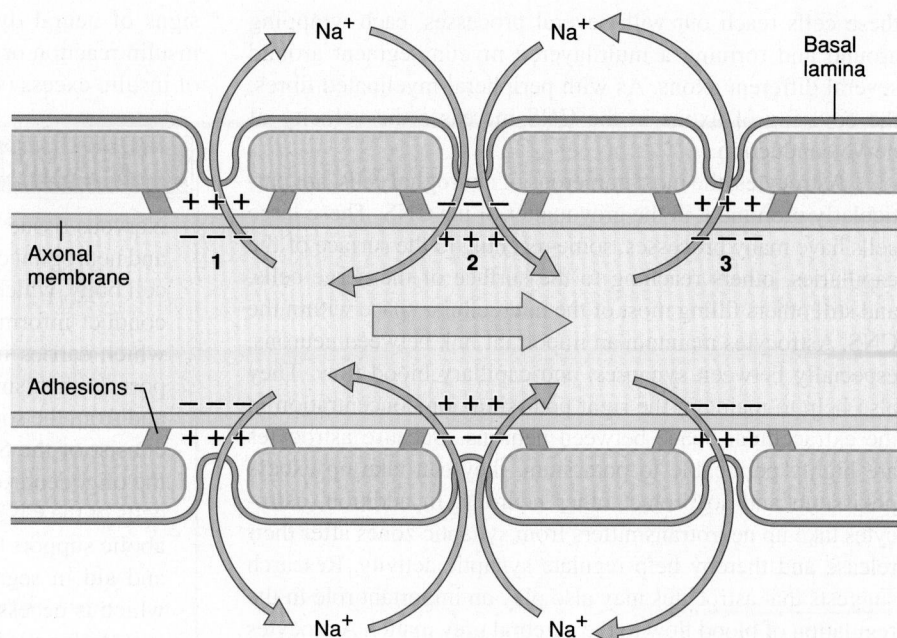

FIGURE 48.4 • Schematic drawing of a longitudinal section of a myelinated axon in the peripheral nervous system. Schwann cells insulate the axon, decreasing flow through the membrane. Action potentials occur at the nodes of Ranvier, which are unmyelinated areas of the basal lamina between the Schwann cells. The impulses jump from node to node in a process called *saltatory conduction,* which greatly increases the velocity of conduction. (*1*) represents the trailing hyperpolarized region behind the action potential, (*2*) the hypopolarized region at the action potential, and (*3*) the leading hyperpolarized area ahead of the action potential. The Schwann cell adhesions (*red*) to the plasma membrane of the axon block the leakage of current under the myelin.

Myelin formation is essentially the same in both the PNS and CNS; both contain myelin basic protein and both involve the winding of plasma membranes around the nerve fibre. During the wrapping of myelin, the cytoplasm between two adjacent inner leaflets of the plasma membrane is expelled. The two adjacent inner leaflets and any remaining cytoplasm appear as a dark line called the *major dense line.* Likewise, during the wrapping of the plasma membranes to form myelin, adjacent outer plasma membrane leaflets become opposed, creating the interperiod or *minor dense line.* Linking proteins,

proteolipid protein (PLP) found only in the CNS and *myelin protein zero* (MPZ) found only in the PNS, help stabilize adjacent plasma membranes of the myelin sheath.

Supporting Cells of the Central Nervous System

Supporting or neuroglial cells of the CNS consist of the oligodendrocytes, astrocytes, microglia, and ependymal cells (Fig. 48.5). The *oligodendrocytes* form the myelin in the CNS. Instead of forming a myelin covering for a single axon,

FIGURE 48.5 • The neuroglial cells of the central nervous system (CNS). Diagrammatic view of relationships between the glial elements (astrocyte, oligodendrocyte, microglial cell, and the ependymal cells), the capillaries, the cerebrospinal fluid, and the cell bodies of CNS neurons.

these cells reach out with several processes, each wrapping around and forming a multilayered myelin segment around several different axons. As with peripheral myelinated fibres, the covering of axons in the CNS increases the velocity of nerve conduction.

Astrocytes, the most numerous of neuroglial cells, are particularly prominent in the grey matter of the CNS. These large cells have many processes, some reaching to the surface of the capillaries, others reaching to the surface of the nerve cells, and still others filling most of the intercellular space within the CNS. Astrocytes maintain an important link between neurons, especially between synapses, and capillary blood flow. They also help to maintain the right potassium ion concentration in the extracellular space between neurons. Because astrocytes are highly permeable to potassium, they can take up excess potassium and so protect other neurons. In addition, astrocytes take up neurotransmitters from synaptic zones after their release and thereby help regulate synaptic activity. Research suggests that astrocytes may also play an important role in the regulation of blood flow to the cerebral grey matter. Astrocytes are also the principal cells responsible for repair and scar formation in the brain. They can fill their cytoplasm with microfibrils (*i.e.*, fibrous astrocytes), and masses of these cells form the special type of scar tissue that develops in the CNS when tissue is destroyed, a process called *gliosis.*

A third type of neuroglial cell, the *microglia,* is a small phagocytic cell that is available for cleaning up debris after cellular damage, infection, or cell death. The fourth type of cell, the *ependymal cell,* forms the lining of the neural tube cavity, the ventricular system. In some areas, these cells combine with a rich vascular network to form the *choroid plexus,* where production of the cerebrospinal fluid (CSF) takes place.

Metabolic Requirements of Nervous Tissue

Nervous tissue has a high rate of metabolism. Although the brain comprises only 2% of the body's weight, it receives approximately 15% of the resting cardiac output and consumes 20% of its oxygen. Despite its substantial energy requirements, the brain cannot store oxygen or effectively engage in anaerobic metabolism. An interruption in the blood or oxygen supply to the brain rapidly leads to clinically observable signs and symptoms. Without oxygen, brain cells continue to function for approximately 10 seconds. Unconsciousness occurs almost simultaneously with cardiac arrest, and the death of brain cells begins within 4 to 6 minutes. Interruption of blood flow also leads to the accumulation of metabolic byproducts that are toxic to neural tissue.

Glucose is the major fuel source for the nervous system, but neurons have no provision for storing glucose. Ketones can provide for limited temporary energy requirements; however, these sources are rapidly depleted. Unlike muscle cells, neurons have no glycogen stores and must rely on glucose from the blood or the glycogen stores of supporting neuroglial cells. Persons receiving insulin for diabetes may experience

signs of neural dysfunction and loss of consciousness (*i.e.*, insulin reaction or shock) when blood glucose drops because of insulin excess (see Chapter 42).

IN SUMMARY

Nervous tissue is composed of two types of cells: neurons and neuroglial cells. Neurons are composed of three parts: a cell body, which controls cell activity; the dendrites, which conduct information toward the cell body; and the axon, which carries impulses from the cell body. Axonal transport mechanisms provide the means to convey materials to and from the soma and axon terminals. The neuroglial cells consist of the Schwann and satellite cells of the PNS and the oligodendrocytes, astrocytes, microglia and ependymal cells of the CNS. Supporting cells protect and provide metabolic support for the neurons, help to regulate blood flow, and aid in segregating them into isolated compartments, which is necessary for normal neuronal function. Nervous system function demands a high proportion of metabolic energy. Glucose is the major fuel for the nervous system. The brain comprises only 2% of body weight but receives 15% of the resting cardiac output.

CONCEPTS in action **ANIMATION**

NEUROPHYSIOLOGY

After completing this section of the chapter, you should be able to meet the following objectives:

- Describe the three phases of an action potential and relate the functional importance of ion channels to the different phases.
- State the difference between electrical and chemical synapses.
- Describe the interaction of the presynaptic and post-synaptic terminals.
- Characterize the role of excitatory and inhibitory postsynaptic potentials as they relate to spatial and temporal summation of membrane potentials.
- Briefly describe how neurotransmitters are synthesized, stored, released, and inactivated.

Neurons are characterized by the ability to communicate with other neurons and body cells through electrical impulses or action potentials. Neurons transfer information from one location to another via the frequency and pattern of action potentials.

Action Potentials

The cell membranes of excitable tissue, including those of nerve and muscle cells, contain ion channels that are responsible for generating action potentials (see Chapter 4, Fig. 4.15). These membrane channels are guarded by voltage-dependent gates that open and close with changes in the membrane potential. Separate voltage-gated channels exist for the sodium, potassium, and calcium ions. Each type of ion channel has a characteristic membrane potential that opens and closes its channels. Also present are ligand-gated channels that respond to chemical messengers such as neurotransmitters, mechanically gated channels that respond to physical changes in the cell membrane, and light-gated channels that respond to fluctuations in light levels.

Nerve signals are transmitted by action potentials, which are abrupt, pulsatile changes in electrical charge of the membrane potential that last a few ten-thousandths to a few thousandths of a second. Action potentials can be divided into three phases: the resting or polarized state, depolarization, and repolarization (Fig. 48.6).

The *resting membrane potential* (typically –70 mV for most neurons to –90 mV for large nerve fibres) is the undisturbed period of the action potential during which the nerve is not transmitting impulses (discussed in Chapter 4). During this period, the membrane is said to be *polarized* because of the large separation of charge (*i.e.*, positive on the outside and negative on the inside). The resting phase of the membrane potential continues until some event causes the membrane to increase its permeability to sodium. A *threshold potential* (approximately –60 mV in large nerve fibres) represents the membrane potential at which neurons or other excitable tissues are stimulated to fire. When the threshold potential is reached, the gatelike structures in the ion channels open.

Below the threshold potential, these gates remain tightly closed. The gates function on an all-or-none basis; they are either fully open or fully closed. Under ordinary circumstances, the threshold stimulus is sufficient to open many ion channels, triggering massive depolarization of the membrane (the action potential).

Depolarization is characterized by the flow of electrically charged ions. During the depolarization phase, the membrane suddenly becomes permeable to sodium ions; the rapid inflow of sodium ions produces local currents that travel through the adjacent cell membrane, causing the sodium channels in this part of the membrane to open. In neurons, sodium ion gates remain open for approximately a quarter of a millisecond. During this phase of the action potential, the inner face of the membrane becomes positive (approximately +30 to +45 mV).

Repolarization is the phase during which the polarity of the resting membrane potential is reestablished. This is accomplished with closure of the sodium channels and opening of the potassium channels. The outflow of positively charged potassium ions across the cell membrane returns the membrane potential to negativity. The sodium–potassium adenosine triphosphatase (Na^+/K^+-ATPase) pump gradually reestablishes the resting ionic concentrations on each side of the membrane. Membranes of excitable cells must be sufficiently repolarized before they can be reexcited. During repolarization, the membrane remains refractory (*i.e.*, is unable to fire) until repolarization is approximately one third complete. This period, which lasts approximately one half a millisecond, is called the *absolute refractory period*. During one portion of the recovery period, the membrane can be excited, although only by a stronger-than-normal stimulus. This period is called *the relative refractory period*.

The excitability of neurons can be affected by conditions that alter the resting membrane potential, moving it either closer to or further from the threshold potential. *Hypopolarization* increases the excitability of the postsynaptic neuron by bringing the membrane potential closer to the threshold potential so that a smaller subsequent stimulus is needed to cause the neuron to fire. *Hyperpolarization* brings the membrane potential further from threshold and has the opposite, inhibitory effect, decreasing the likelihood that an action potential will be generated.

Synaptic Transmission

Neurons communicate with each other through structures known as *synapses*. Two types of synapses are found in the nervous system: electrical and chemical. *Electrical synapses* permit the passage of current-carrying ions through small openings called *gap junctions* that penetrate the cell junction of adjoining cells and allow current to travel in either direction. The gap junctions allow an action potential to pass directly and quickly from one neuron to another. They may link neurons having close functional relationships into circuits.

The most common type of synapse is the *chemical synapse*. Chemical synapses involve special presynaptic and postsynaptic membrane structures, separated by a synaptic

FIGURE 48.6 • Time course of the action potential recorded at one point of an axon with one electrode inside and one on the outside of the plasma membrane. The rising part of the action potential is called the *spike.* The rising phase plus approximately the first half of the repolarization phase is the absolute refractory period (**A**). The portion of the repolarization phase that extends from the threshold to the resting membrane potential represents the relative refractory period (**B**). The remaining portion of the repolarization phase to the resting membrane potential is the negative afterpotential (**C**). The relative refractory period is the period during which the membrane becomes hyperpolarized as the potential drops below the resting membrane potential.

cleft. The presynaptic terminal secretes one and often several chemical transmitter molecules (*i.e.,* neurotransmitters or neuromodulators). The secreted neurotransmitters diffuse into the synaptic cleft and unite with receptors on the postsynaptic membrane. In contrast to an electrical synapse, a chemical synapse serves as a rectifier, permitting only one-way communication. Chemical synapses are divided into two types: excitatory and inhibitory. In excitatory synapses, binding of the neurotransmitter to the receptor produces depolarization of the postsynaptic membrane. Binding of the neurotransmitter to the receptor in an inhibitory synapse reduces the postsynaptic neuron's ability to generate an action potential. Most inhibitory neurotransmitters induce hyperpolarization of the postsynaptic membrane by making the membrane more permeable to potassium or chloride, or both (see Chapter 31).

Chemical synapses are the slowest component in progressive communication through a sequence of neurons, such as in a spinal reflex. In contrast to the conduction of electrical action potentials, each successive event at the chemical synapse—transmitter secretion, diffusion across the synaptic cleft, interaction with postsynaptic receptors, and generation of a subsequent action potential in the postsynaptic neuron—consumes time.

A neuron's cell body and dendrites are covered by thousands of synapses, any or many of which can be active at any moment. Because of the interaction of this rich synaptic input, each neuron resembles a little integrator, in which circuits of many neurons interact with one another. It is the complexity of these interactions and the subtle integrations involved in producing behavioural responses that gives the system its intelligence.

Chemical synapses exhibit several relationships. Axons can synapse with dendrites (axodendritic), with the cell body (axosomatic), or with the axon (axoaxonic). Dendrites can synapse with axons (dendroaxonic), other dendrites (dendrodendritic), or the soma of other neurons (dendrosomatic). Synapses between the nerve cell body and axons (somatoaxonic synapses) also have been observed. Synapses occurring between the soma of neighbouring neurons (somatosomatic) are uncommon, except between some efferent nuclei. The mechanism of communication between the presynaptic and the postsynaptic neuron is similar in all types of synapses; the action potential sweeps into the axonal terminals of the afferent neuron and triggers the rapid release of neurotransmitter molecules from the axonal, or presynaptic, surface.

Excitatory and Inhibitory Postsynaptic Potentials

Many CNS neurons possess thousands of synapses on their dendritic or somatic surfaces, each of which can produce partial excitation or inhibition of the postsynaptic neuron. When the combination of a neurotransmitter with a receptor site causes partial depolarization of the postsynaptic membrane, it is called an *excitatory postsynaptic potential* (EPSP). In other synapses, the combination of a transmitter with a receptor site is inhibitory in the sense that it causes the local nerve membrane to become hyperpolarized and less excitable. This is called an *inhibitory postsynaptic potential* (IPSP).

Action potentials do not begin in the membrane adjacent to the synapse. They begin in the initial segment of the axon, near the *axon hillock* (Fig. 48.1), that lies just before the first myelin segment. The initial segment of the axon is more excitable than the rest of the neuron. The local currents resulting from an EPSP (sometimes called a *generator potential*) are usually insufficient to reach threshold and cause depolarization of the axon's initial segment. However, if several EPSPs occur simultaneously, the area of depolarization can become large enough and the currents at the initial segment can become strong enough to exceed the threshold potential and initiate an action potential. This summation of depolarized areas is called *spatial summation.* EPSPs also can summate and cause an action potential if they occur in rapid succession. This temporal aspect of the occurrence of two or more EPSPs is called *temporal summation.*

IPSPs also can undergo spatial and temporal summation with each other and with EPSPs, reducing the effectiveness of the latter by a roughly algebraic summation. If the sum of EPSPs and IPSPs keeps the depolarization at the initial segment below threshold levels, no action potential occurs.

Spatial and temporal summation during synaptic activity serves as a sensitive and complicated switch that requires the right combination of incoming activity before the cell can elicit an action potential. The occurrence and frequency of action potentials in axons constitute an all-or-none language (*i.e.,* a digital language), which varies only as to the presence or absence of such impulses and their frequency.

Messenger Molecules

The function of the nervous system relies on chemical messengers. These messengers include the neurotransmitters, neuromodulators, and neurotrophic or nerve growth factors.

Neurotransmitters

Neurotransmitters are chemical substances that excite, inhibit, or modify signals between neurons. They are small molecules that incorporate a positively charged nitrogen atom; they include several amino acids, peptides, and monoamines. *Amino acids* are the building blocks of proteins and are present in body fluids. The amino acids glutamine, glycine, and gamma-aminobutyric acid (GABA) serve as neurotransmitters at most CNS synapses. GABA mediates most synaptic inhibition in the CNS. Drugs such as the benzodiazepines (*e.g.,* diazepam) and the barbiturates (*e.g.,* phenobarbital) exert their action by binding to their own distinct receptor on a GABA-operated ion channel. The drugs by themselves do not open the channel, but they change the effect that GABA has when it binds to the channel at the same time as the drug. *Peptides* are low-molecular-weight molecules that are made up of two or more amino acids. They include substance P and the endorphins and enkephalins, which are involved in pain sensation and perception (see Chapter 49). A *monoamine* is an amine molecule containing one amino group (NH_2). Serotonin, dopamine,

Understanding Synaptic Transmission

Neurons communicate with each other through chemical synapses and the use of neurotransmitters. Chemical synapses consist of a presynaptic neuron, a synaptic cleft, and a postsynaptic neuron. The communication process relies on (1) synthesis and release of the neurotransmitter from a presynaptic neuron, (2) binding of the neurotransmitter to receptors in the postsynaptic neuron, and (3) removal of the neurotransmitter from the receptor site.

1. Neurotransmitter Synthesis and Release

Neurotransmitters are synthesized in the presynaptic neuron, and then stored in synaptic vesicles. Communication between the two neurons begins with a nerve impulse that stimulates the presynaptic neuron, followed by movement of the synaptic vesicles to the cell membrane and release of neurotransmitter into the synaptic cleft.

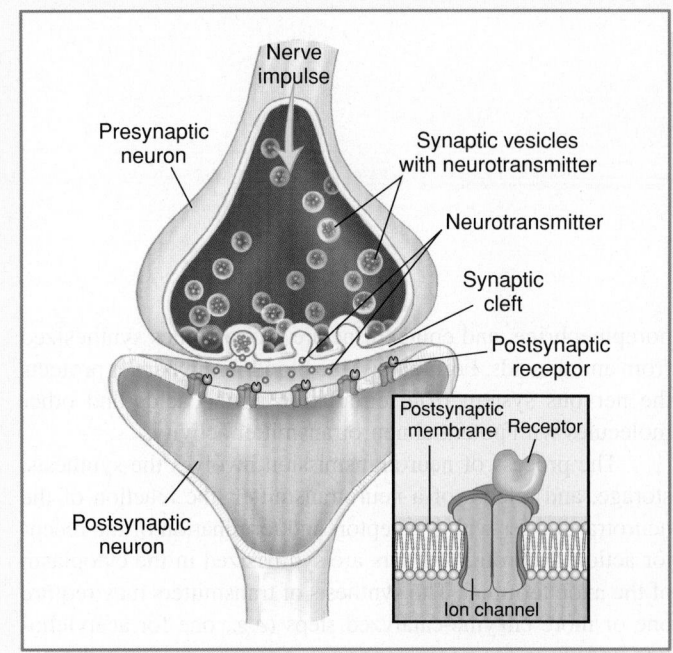

2. Receptor Binding

Once released from the presynaptic neuron, the neurotransmitter moves across the synaptic cleft and binds to receptors on the postsynaptic neuron. The action of a neurotransmitter is determined by the type of receptor (excitatory or inhibitory) to which it binds. Binding of a neurotransmitter to a receptor with an excitatory function often results in the opening of an ion channel, such as the sodium channel. Many presynaptic neurons also have receptors to which a neurotransmitter binds. The presynaptic receptors function in a negative feedback manner to inhibit further release of the neurotransmitter.

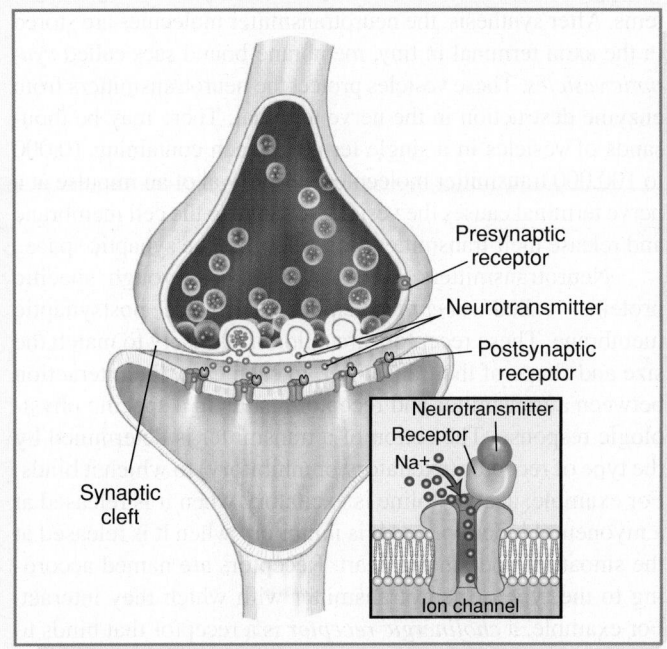

3. Neurotransmitter Removal

Precise control of synaptic function relies on the rapid removal of the neurotransmitter from the receptor site. A released neurotransmitter can (1) be taken back up into the neuron in a process called reuptake, (2) diffuse out of the synaptic cleft, or (3) be broken down by enzymes into inactive substances or metabolites. The action of norepinephrine is largely terminated by the reuptake process, in which the neurotransmitter is taken back into the neuron in an unchanged form and reused. It can also be broken down by enzymes in the synaptic cleft or in the nerve terminals. The neurotransmitter acetylcholine is rapidly broken down by the enzyme acetylcholinesterase.

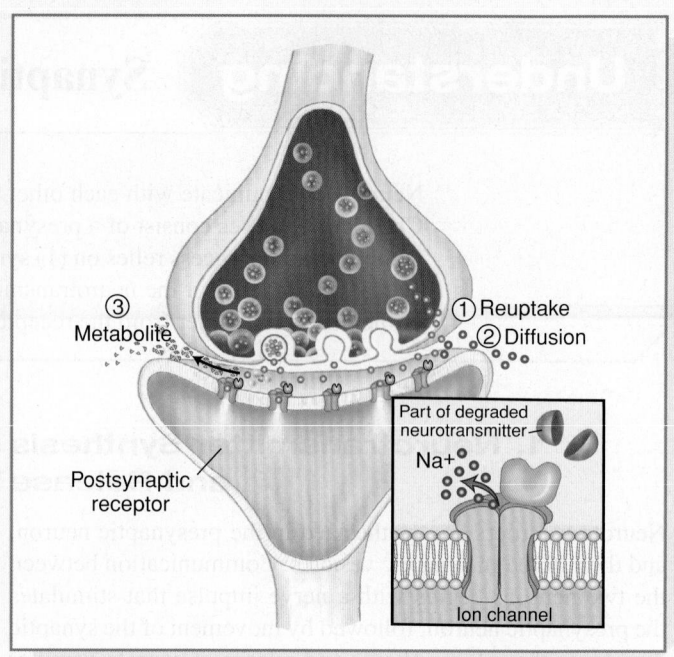

norepinephrine, and epinephrine are monoamines synthesized from amino acids. Fortunately, the blood–brain barrier protects the nervous system from circulating amino acids and other molecules with potential neurotransmitter activity.

The process of neurotransmission involves the synthesis, storage, and release of a neurotransmitter; the reaction of the neurotransmitter with a receptor; and termination of the receptor action. Neurotransmitters are synthesized in the cytoplasm of the axon terminal. The synthesis of transmitters may require one or more enzyme-catalyzed steps (*e.g.,* one for acetylcholine and three for norepinephrine). Neurons are limited as to the type of transmitter they can synthesize by their enzyme systems. After synthesis, the neurotransmitter molecules are stored in the axon terminal in tiny, membrane-bound sacs called *synaptic vesicles*. These vesicles protect the neurotransmitters from enzyme destruction in the nerve terminal. There may be thousands of vesicles in a single terminal, each containing 10,000 to 100,000 transmitter molecules. The arrival of an impulse at a nerve terminal causes the vesicles to move to the cell membrane and release their transmitter molecules into the synaptic space.

Neurotransmitters exert their actions through specific proteins, called *receptors,* embedded in the postsynaptic membrane. These receptors are tailored precisely to match the size and shape of the transmitter. In each case, the interaction between a transmitter and receptor results in a specific physiologic response. The action of a transmitter is determined by the type of receptor (excitatory or inhibitory) to which it binds. For example, acetylcholine is excitatory when it is released at a myoneural junction, and it is inhibitory when it is released at the sinoatrial node in the heart. Receptors are named according to the type of neurotransmitter with which they interact. For example, a *cholinergic receptor* is a receptor that binds to acetylcholine.

Rapid removal of a transmitter, once it has exerted its effects on the postsynaptic membrane, is necessary to maintain precise control of neural transmission. A released transmitter can undergo one of three fates: (1) it can be broken down into inactive substances by enzymes; (2) it can be taken back up into the presynaptic neuron in a process called *reuptake;* or (3) it can diffuse into the intercellular fluid until its concentration is too low to influence postsynaptic excitability. For example, acetylcholine is rapidly broken down by acetylcholinesterase into acetic acid and choline, with the choline being taken back into the presynaptic neuron for reuse in acetylcholine synthesis. The catecholamine norepinephrine is largely taken back into the neuron in an unchanged form for reuse. Norepinephrine also can be degraded by enzymes in the synaptic space or in the nerve terminals.

Neuromodulators

Other classes of messenger molecules, known as *neuromodulators,* also may be released from axon terminals. Neuromodulator molecules react with presynaptic or postsynaptic receptors to alter the release of or response to neurotransmitters. Neuromodulators may act on postsynaptic receptors to produce slower and longer-lasting changes in membrane excitability. This alters the action of the faster-acting neurotransmitter molecules by enhancing or decreasing their effectiveness. By combining with autoreceptors on its own presynaptic membrane, a transmitter can act as a neuromodulator to augment or inhibit further nerve activity. In some nerves, such as the peripheral sympathetic nerves, a messenger molecule can have both transmitter and modulator functions. For example, norepinephrine can activate α_1-adrenergic postsynaptic receptors to produce vasoconstriction or stimulate α_2-adrenergic presynaptic receptors to inhibit further norepinephrine release.

Neurotrophic Factors

Neurotrophic or nerve growth factors are required to maintain the long-term survival of the postsynaptic cell and are secreted by axon terminals independent of action potentials. Examples include neuron-to-neuron trophic factors in the sequential synapses of CNS sensory neurons. Trophic factors from target cells that enter the axon and are necessary for the long-term survival of presynaptic neurons also have been demonstrated. Target cell-to-neuron trophic factors probably have great significance in establishing specific neural connections during normal embryonic development.

IN SUMMARY

Neurons are characterized by the ability to communicate with other neurons and body cells through electrical signals called action potentials. The cell membranes of neurons contain ion channels that are responsible for generating action potentials. These channels are guarded by voltage-dependent gates that open and close with changes in the membrane potential. Action potentials are divided into three parts: the resting membrane potential, during which the membrane is polarized but no electrical activity occurs; the depolarization phase, during which sodium channels open, allowing rapid inflow of the sodium ions that generate the electrical impulse; and the repolarization phase, during which the membrane is permeable to potassium ions, allowing for the efflux of potassium ions and the return to the resting membrane potential.

Synapses are structures that permit communication between neurons. Two types of synapses have been identified: electrical and chemical. Electrical synapses consist of gap junctions between adjacent cells that allow action potentials to move rapidly from one cell to another. Chemical synapses involve special presynaptic and postsynaptic structures, separated by a synaptic cleft. They rely on chemical messengers, released from the presynaptic neuron, that cross the synaptic cleft and then interact with receptors on the postsynaptic neuron.

Neurotransmitters are chemical messengers that control neural function; they selectively cause excitation or inhibition of action potentials. Three major types of neurotransmitters are known: amino acids such as glutamic acid and GABA, peptides such as the endorphins and enkephalins, and monoamines such as epinephrine and norepinephrine. Neurotransmitters interact with cell membrane receptors to produce either excitatory or inhibitory actions. Neuromodulators are chemical messengers that react with membrane receptors to produce slower and longer-acting changes in membrane permeability. Neurotrophic or growth factors, also released from presynaptic terminals, are required to maintain the long-term survival of postsynaptic neurons.

CONCEPTSin action **ANIMATI☉N**

DEVELOPMENTAL ORGANIZATION OF THE NERVOUS SYSTEM

After completing this section of the chapter, you should be able to meet the following objectives:

- Use the segmental approach to explain the development of the nervous system and the organization of the postembryonic nervous system.
- Define the terms afferent, efferent, ganglia, association neuron, cell column, and tract.
- State the origin and destination of nerve fibres contained in the dorsal and ventral roots.
- State the structures innervated by general somatic afferent, special visceral afferent, general visceral afferent, special somatic afferent, general visceral efferent, pharyngeal efferent, and general somatic efferent neurons.

The organization of the nervous system can be described in terms of its development, in which newer functions and greater complexity resulted from the modification and enlargement of more primitive structures. Thus, the rostral or front end of the CNS became specialized, with the more basic organization being retained in the brain stem and spinal cord. The dominance of the front end of the CNS is reflected in what has been termed a *hierarchy of control,* with the forebrain having control over the brain stem and the brain stem having control over the spinal cord. In the developmental process, newer functions were added to the surface of functionally older systems. As newer functions became concentrated at the rostral end of the nervous system, they also became more vulnerable to injury. Nothing exemplifies this principle better than the persistent vegetative state (discussed in Chapter 51) that occurs when severe brain injury causes irreversible damage to higher cortical centres, while lower stem centres such as those that control breathing remain functional.

Somatic and Visceral Development

All body tissues and organs have developed from the three embryonic layers (*i.e.,* endoderm, ectoderm and mesoderm) that were present during the third week of embryonic life. The body is organized into the soma and viscera (see Chapter 4, Fig. 4.16). The *soma,* or body wall, includes all of the structures derived from the embryonic ectoderm, such as the epidermis of the skin and the CNS. Mesodermal connective tissues of the soma include the dermis of the skin, skeletal muscle, bone, and the outer lining of the body cavity (*i.e.,* parietal pleura and peritoneum). The nervous system innervates all somatic structures plus the internal structures making up the viscera. *Viscera* include the great vessels derived from the intermediate mesoderm, the urinary system, and the gonadal structures; it also includes the inner lining of the body cavities, such as the visceral pleura and peritoneum, and the mesodermal tissues that surround the endoderm-lined gut and its derivative organs (*e.g.*, lungs, liver, pancreas).

The nervous system appears very early in embryonic development (week 3). This early development is essential because it influences the development and organization of many other body systems, including the axial skeleton, skeletal muscles, and sensory organs such as the eyes and ears. Throughout life, the organization of the nervous system retains many patterns that were established during embryonic life. It is this early pattern of segmental development in the embryo that is presented as a framework for understanding the nervous system.

THE DEVELOPMENTAL ORGANIZATION OF THE NERVOUS SYSTEM

- Embryologically, the nervous system begins its development as a hollow tube, the cephalic portion of which becomes the brain and the more caudal part the spinal cord.
- In the process of development, the basic organizational pattern is that of a longitudinal series of segments, each repeating the same basic fundamental organizational pattern: a body wall or soma containing the axial skeleton and a neural tube, which develops into the nervous system.
- On cross-section, the embryonic neural tube develops into a central canal surrounded by grey matter or cellular portion (cell columns) and the white matter, or tract system of the central nervous system (CNS).
- As the nervous system develops, it becomes segmented, with a repeating pattern of afferent neuron axons forming the dorsal roots of each succeeding segmental nerve, and the exiting efferent neurons forming the ventral roots of each succeeding segmental nerve.
- The nerve cells in the grey matter are arranged longitudinally in cell columns, with afferent sensory neurons located in the dorsal columns and efferent motor neurons located in the ventral columns.
- The axons of the cell column neurons project out into the white matter of the CNS, forming the longitudinal tract systems.

During the second week of development, embryonic tissue consists of two layers, the endoderm and the ectoderm. At the beginning of week 3, the ectoderm begins to invaginate and migrates between the two layers, forming a third layer called the *mesoderm* (Fig. 48.7). Mesoderm along the entire midline of the embryo forms a specialized rod of embryonic tissue called the *notochord*. The notochord and adjacent

mesoderm provide the necessary induction signal for the overlying ectoderm to differentiate and form a thickened structure called the *neural plate,* the primordium of the nervous system. Within the neural plate an axial groove (*i.e.*, neural groove) develops and sinks into the underlying mesoderm, allowing its walls to fuse across the top and form an ectodermal tube called the *neural tube.* This process, called *closure,* occurs during the later third and fourth weeks of gestation and is vital to the survival of the embryo.

During embryonic development, the neural tube develops into the CNS, while the notochord becomes the foundation around which the vertebral column ultimately develops. The surface ectoderm separates from the neural tube and fuses over the top to become the outer layer of skin. Initial closure of the neural tube begins at the cervical and high thoracic levels and zippers rostrally toward the cephalic end of the embryo and caudally toward the sacrum. Complete closure occurs at the rostral-most end of the brain (*i.e.*, anterior neuropore) around day 25, and about day 27 in the lumbosacral region (*i.e.*, posterior neuropore).

As the neural tube closes, ectodermal cells called *neural crest cells* migrate away from the dorsal surface of the neural tube to become the progenitors of the neurons and supporting cells of the PNS. During this period of embryonic development, neural cell adhesive molecules (N-CAMs) are produced to decrease migration of neural crest cells. In addition, fibronectin molecules are produced to increase the formation of pathways that guide the neural crest cells during their migration. Some of these cells gather into clusters to form the *dorsal root ganglia* at the sides of each spinal cord segment and the *cranial ganglia* that are present in most brain segments. Neurons of these ganglia become the afferent or sensory neurons of the PNS. Other neural crest cells become the pigment cells of the skin or contribute to the formation of the meninges, many structures of the face, and the peripheral ganglion cells of the autonomic nervous system (ANS), including those of the adrenal cortex.

During development, the more rostral portions of the embryonic neural tube—approximately 10 segments—undergo extensive modification and enlargement to form the brain (Fig. 48.8). In the early embryo, three swellings, or primary vesicles, develop, subdividing these 10 segments into the prosencephalon, or forebrain, containing the first two segments; the mesencephalon, or midbrain, which develops from segment 3; and the rhombencephalon, or hindbrain, which develops from segments 4 to 10. The brain stem is formed from modifications of the 10 rostral segments of the wall of the neural tube. In the prosencephalon or forebrain, two pairs of lateral outpouchings develop: the optic cup, which becomes the optic nerve and retina, and the telencephalic vesicles, which become the cerebral hemispheres. Within the prosencephalon, the hollow central canal expands to become enlarged CSF-filled cavities, the first and second (lateral) ventricles. The remaining diencephalic portion of the neural tube develops into the thalamus and hypothalamus. The neurohypophysis (posterior pituitary) grows as a midline ventral

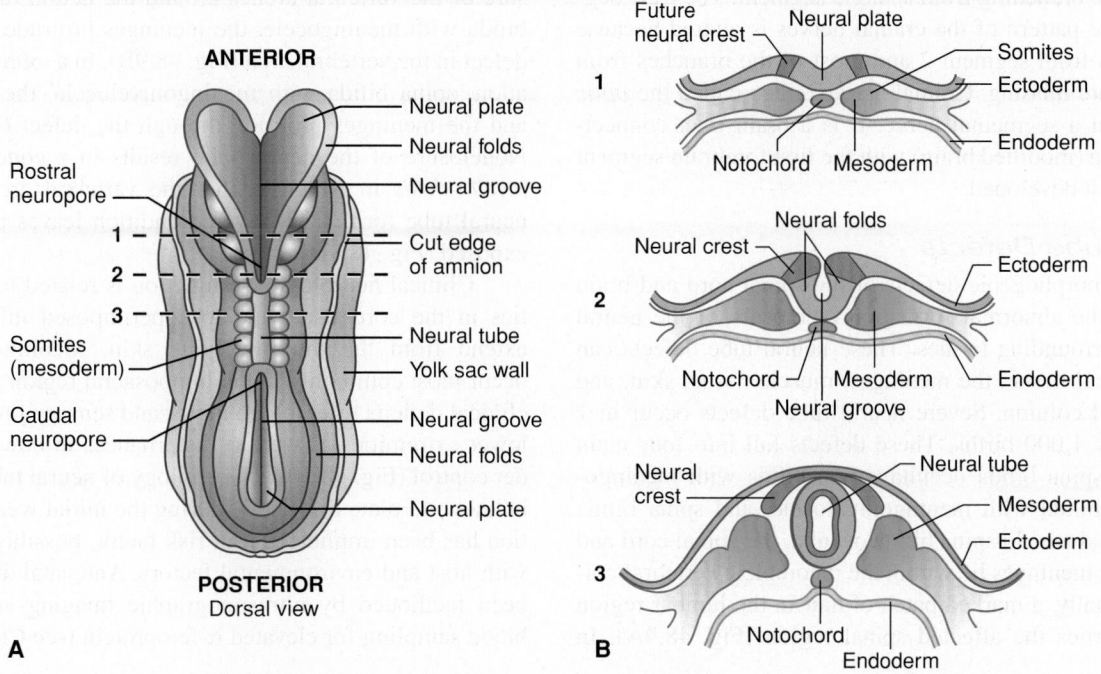

FIGURE 48.7 • Folding of the neural tube. (**A**) Dorsal view of a six-somite embryo (22 to 23 days) showing the neural folds, neural groove, and the fused neural tube. The anterior neuropore closes at about day 25 and the posterior neuropore at about day 27. (**B**) Three cross-sections taken at the levels indicated in **A.** The sections indicate where the neural tube is just beginning to form.

outgrowth at the junctions of segments 1 and 2. A dorsal outgrowth, the pineal body, develops between segments 2 and 3.

All brain segments, except segment 2, retain some portion of the basic segmental organization of the nervous system. Further development of the brain continues with the cranial and upper cervical paired segmental nerves. This reflects the

original pattern of a segmented neural tube, each segment of which has multiple paired branches containing a grouping of component axons. One segment would have paired branches to body muscles and another set to visceral structures, and so on. The classic pattern of spinal nerve organization, which consists of a pair of dorsal and a pair of ventral roots, is a later

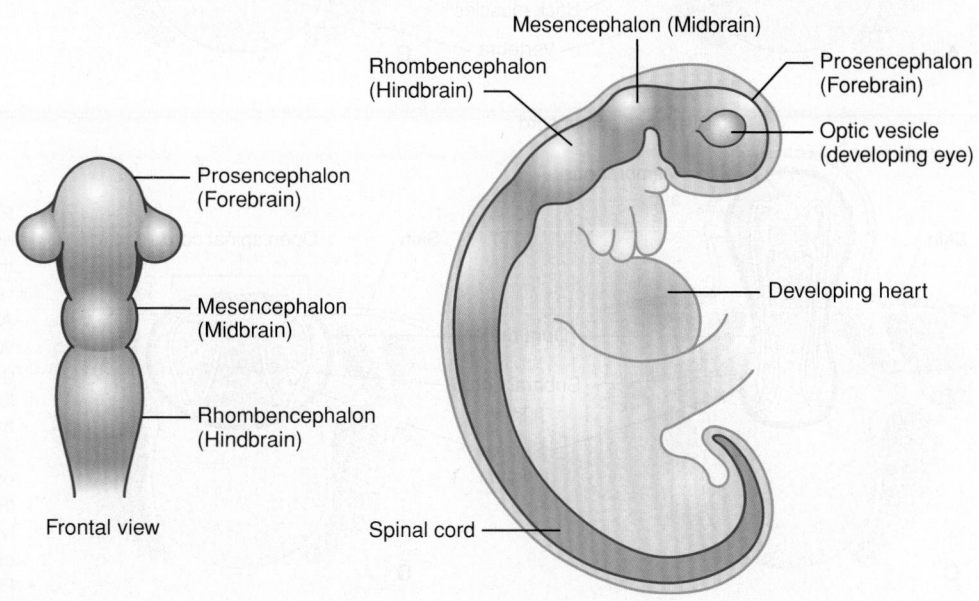

FIGURE 48.8 • Frontal and lateral views of a 5-week-old embryo showing the brain vesicles and three embryonic divisions of the brain and brain stem.

development that has not occurred in the cranial nerves. Consequently, the cranial nerves, which are arbitrarily numbered 1 through 12, retain the ancient pattern, with more than one cranial nerve branching from a single segment. The truly segmental nerve pattern of the cranial nerves is altered because all branches from segment 2 and most of the branches from segment 1 are missing. Cranial nerve 2, also called the *optic nerve,* is not a segmental nerve. It is a brain tract connecting the retina (modified brain) with the first forebrain segment from which it developed.

Neural Tube Defects

The major morphogenic defects of the spinal cord and brain are due to the abnormal formation or closure of the neural tube and surrounding tissues. These neural tube defects can involve neural tissue, the meninges, muscle tissue, skin, and the vertebral column. Severe neural tube defects occur in 1 out of every 1,000 births. These defects fall into four main categories: spina bifida occulta, spina bifida with meningocele, spina bifida with meningomyelocele, and spina bifida with myeloschisis. In spina bifida occulta, the spinal cord and surrounding meninges lie within the incomplete vertebral column. Externally, a marked patch of hair in the lumbar region usually overlies the affected spinal region (Fig. 48.9A). In both spina bifida occulta and spina bifida cystica (spina bifida with meningocele or meningomyelocele), the neural tube has closed but inductive messages fail to promote complete closure of the vertebral arches around the neural tube. In spina bifida with meningocele, the meninges protrude through the defect in the vertebral arch (Fig. 48.9B). In a more severe situation, spina bifida with meningomyelocele, the spinal cord and the meninges protrude through the defect (Fig. 48.9C). Nonclosure of the neural tube results in a condition called *myeloschisis* in which neither the vertebral arches nor the neural tube form. This severe condition leaves neural tissue exposed (Fig. 48.9D).

Clinical neurologic dysfunction is related to abnormalities in the cord itself and to superimposed infections that extend from the thin overlying skin. Meningomyeloceles occur most commonly in the lumbosacral region and produce clinical deficits referable to motor and sensory function in the lower extremities as well as disturbances in bowel and bladder control (Fig. 48.10). The etiology of neural tube defects is unknown. Folate deficiency during the initial weeks of gestation has been implicated as a risk factor, possibly interacting with host and environmental factors. Antenatal diagnosis has been facilitated by ultrasonographic imaging and maternal blood sampling for elevated α-fetoprotein (see Chapter 7).

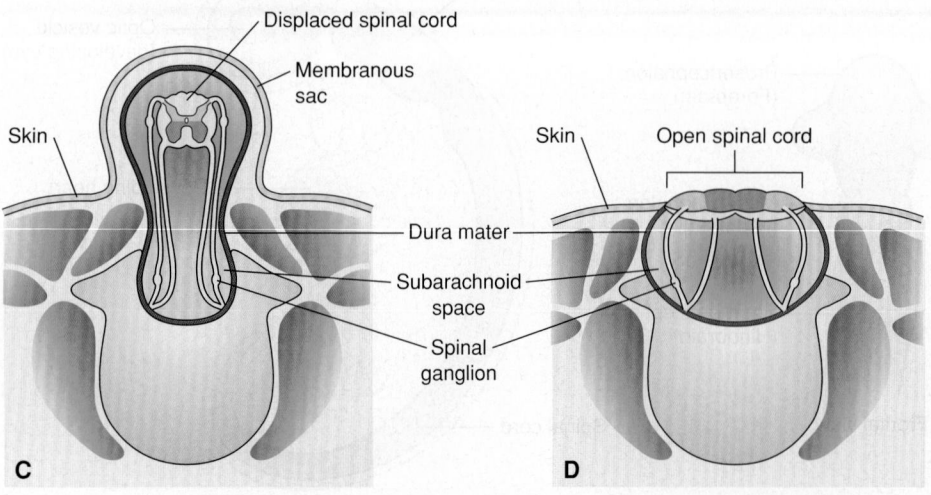

FIGURE 48.9 • Diagrammatic sketches illustrating various types of spina bifida and the commonly associated anomalies of the vertebral arch, spinal cord, and meninges. **A:** Spina bifida occulta. Note the unfused vertebral arch. **B:** Spina bifida with meningocele. **C:** Spina bifida with meningomyelocele. **D:** Spina bifida with myeloschisis. The types illustrated in **B** and **C** are referred to collectively as *spina bifida cystica* because of the cystlike sac associated with them. (From Moore K. L., Persaud T. V. N., Torchia M. G. (2013). *The developing human: Clinically oriented embryology* (9th ed., p. 399). Philadelphia, PA: Saunders Elsevier.)

FIGURE 48.10 • Infant with spina bifida with meningomyelocele in the lumbar region. (From Moore K. L., Persaud T. V. N., Torchia M. G. (2013). *The developing human: Clinically oriented embryology* (9th ed., p. 401). Philadelphia, PA: Saunders Elsevier.)

Segmental Organization

Developmentally, the basic organizational pattern of the body is that of a longitudinal series of segments, each repeating the same fundamental pattern. Although the early muscular, skeletal, vascular, and excretory systems and the nerves that supply the somatic and visceral structures have the same segmental pattern, it is the nervous system that most clearly retains this organization in postnatal life. The CNS and its associated peripheral nerves consist of approximately 41 segments, 31 of which form the spinal cord and spinal nerves, and 10 of which form the brain and its cranial nerves.

Each segment of the CNS is accompanied by bilateral pairs of bundled nerve fibres, or roots, a ventral pair and a dorsal pair (Fig. 48.11). The paired dorsal roots connect a pair

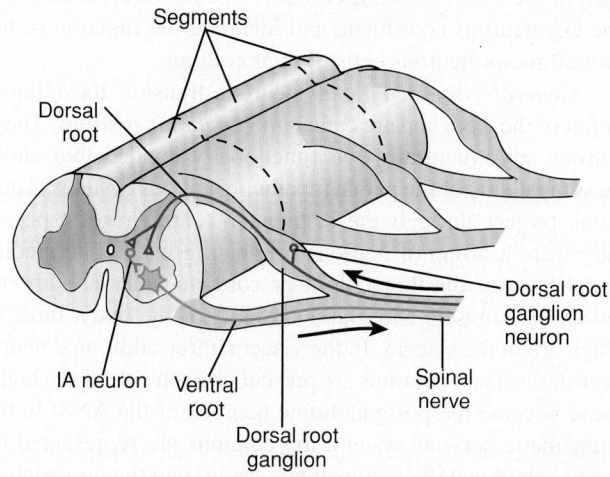

FIGURE 48.11 • In this diagram of three segments of the spinal cord, three dorsal roots enter the dorsal lateral surface of the cord, and three ventral roots exit. The dorsal root ganglion contains dorsal root ganglion cells, whose axons bifurcate: one process enters the spinal cord in the dorsal root, and the other extends peripherally to supply the skin and muscle of the body. The ventral root is formed by axons from motor neurons in the spinal cord. IA, input association.

of dorsal root ganglia and their corresponding CNS segment. The dorsal root ganglia contain many afferent nerve cell bodies, each having two axon-like processes—one that ends in a peripheral receptor and another that enters the central neural segment. These axon-like processes that enter the central neural segment communicate with neurons called *input association* (IA) *neurons*. Somatic afferent (SA) neurons transmit information from the soma to somatic IA (SIA) neurons, and visceral afferent (VA) neurons transmit information from the viscera to visceral IA (VIA) neurons. The paired ventral roots of each segment are bundles of axons that provide efferent output to effector sites such as the muscles and glandular cells of the body segment.

On cross-section, the hollow embryonic neural tube can be divided into a central canal, or ventricle, containing CSF and the wall of the tube. The latter develops into an inner grey cellular portion, which is functionally divided into longitudinal columns of neurons called the *cell columns*. These cell columns contain nerve cell bodies surrounded by a superficial white matter region containing the longitudinal tract systems of the CNS. These tract systems are composed of many nerve cell processes. The dorsal half, or *dorsal horn* of the grey matter, contains afferent neurons. The ventral portion, or *ventral horn,* contains efferent neurons that communicate by way of the ventral roots with effector cells of the body segment. Many CNS neurons develop axons that grow longitudinally as tract systems that communicate between neighbouring and distal segments of the neural tube.

Cell Columns

The organizational structure of the nervous system can be best explained and simplified as a pattern in which functionally specific PNS and CNS neurons are repeated as parallel cell columns running lengthwise along the nervous system. In this organizational pattern, afferent neurons, dorsal horn cells, and ventral horn cells are organized as a bilateral series of 11 cell columns.

The cell columns on each side can be further grouped according to their location in the PNS: four in the dorsal root ganglia that contain sensory neurons; four in the dorsal horn containing sensory IA neurons; and three in the ventral horn that contain motor neurons (Fig. 48.12). Each column of dorsal root ganglia projects to its particular column of IA neurons in the dorsal horn, which then distribute the afferent information to local reflex circuits and to more rostral and elaborate segments of the CNS. The ventral horns contain output association (OA) neurons and lower motor neurons (LMNs). The LMNs provide the final circuitry for organizing efferent nerve activity.

Between the IA neurons and the OA neurons are networks of small internuncial (interneuronal) neurons arranged in complex circuits. Internuncial neurons provide the discreteness, appropriateness, and intelligence of responses to stimuli. Most of the billions of CNS cells in the spinal cord and brain grey matter are internuncial neurons.

FIGURE 48.12 • A: Cell columns of the central nervous system. The cell columns in the dorsal horn contain input association (IA) neurons for the general visceral afferent (GVA), special visceral afferent (SVA), special sensory afferent (SSA), and general somatic afferent (GSA) neurons with cell bodies in the dorsal root ganglion. The cell columns in the ventral horn contain the general visceral efferent (GVE), pharyngeal efferent (PE), and general somite efferent (GSE) neurons and their output association (OA) neurons. **B:** Schematic of the GVE cell column showing both parasympathetic and sympathetic components. The column is not continuous but is interrupted in the brain stem because only the nuclei of cranial nerves III, VII, IX, and X contain preganglionic parasympathetic neurons. The column again is interrupted until levels T-1 to L-1 or L-2, where the preganglionic neurons of the sympathetic portion are found in the lateral horn of the spinal cord. Another gap is evident until the sacral portion of the parasympathetic nervous system.

Dorsal Horn Cell Columns. Four columns of afferent (sensory) neurons in the dorsal root ganglia directly innervate four corresponding columns of IA neurons in the dorsal horn. These columns are categorized as special and general afferents: special somatic afferent, general somatic afferent, special visceral afferent, and general visceral afferent (see Fig. 48.12).

Special somatic afferent fibres are concerned with internal sensory information such as joint and tendon sensation (*i.e.,* proprioception). Neurons in the special SIA column cells relay their information to local reflexes concerned with posture and movement. These neurons also relay information to the cerebellum, contributing to coordination of movement, and to the forebrain, contributing to experience. Afferents innervating the labyrinth and derived auditory end organs of the inner ear also belong to the special somatic afferent category.

General somatic afferents innervate the skin and other somatic structures, and respond to stimuli such as those that produce pressure or pain. General SIA column cells relay the sensory information to protective and other reflex circuits and project the information to the forebrain, where it is perceived as painful, warm, cold, and the like.

Special visceral afferent cells innervate specialized gut-related receptors, such as the taste buds and receptors of the olfactory mucosa. Their central processes communicate with special VIA column neurons that project to reflex circuits producing salivation, chewing, swallowing, and other responses. Forebrain projection fibres from these association cells provide sensations of taste and smell.

General visceral afferent neurons innervate visceral structures such as the gastrointestinal tract, urinary bladder, and heart and great vessels; they project to the general VIA column, which relays information to vital reflex circuits and sends information to the forebrain regarding visceral sensations such as stomach fullness, bladder pressure, and sexual sensation.

Ventral Horn Cell Columns. The ventral horn contains three longitudinal cell columns: general visceral efferent, pharyngeal efferent, and general somatic efferent (Fig. 48.12). Each of these cell columns contains OA and efferent neurons. The OA neurons coordinate and integrate the function of the efferent motor neurons cells of their column.

General visceral efferent neurons transmit the efferent output of the ANS and are called *preganglionic neurons.* These neurons are structurally and functionally divided into either the sympathetic or the parasympathetic nervous systems. Their axons project through the segmental ventral roots (specifically from a group of neurons originating in the intermediolateral horn of the thoracolumbar cord) to innervate smooth and cardiac muscle and glandular cells of the body, most of which are in the viscera. In the viscera, three additional neural crest-derived cell columns are present on each side of the body. These become the postganglionic neurons of the ANS. In the sympathetic nervous system, the columns are represented by paravertebral ganglia (sympathetic chain) and the prevertebral series of ganglia (*e.g.,* celiac ganglia) associated with the dorsal aorta (to be discussed). For the parasympathetic system, these become the enteric plexus in the wall of the gut-derived organs and a series of ganglia in the head. This column is not continuous but is interrupted by the brain stem, because only the nuclei for cranial nerves (CN) III, VII, IX, and X contain preganglionic parasympathetic neurons. The column is again interrupted until thoracic (T) levels T-1 to lumbar (L) levels L-1 or L-2, where the preganglionic neurons of the sympathetic nervous system are found in the lateral horn of the spinal cord. Another gap is evident until the sacral portion of the parasympathetic nervous system.

Pharyngeal efferent neurons innervate the brachial arch skeletal muscles: the muscles of mastication and facial expression, and muscles of the pharynx and larynx. Pharyngeal efferent neurons also innervate muscles responsible for moving the head.

The *general somatic efferent* neurons supply somite-derived muscles of the body and head, which include the skeletal muscles of the body and limbs, the tongue, and extrinsic eye muscles. These efferent neurons transmit the commands of the CNS to peripheral effectors, the skeletal muscles. They are the "final common pathway neurons" in the sequence leading to motor activity. They are often called LMNs because they are under the control of higher levels of the CNS, including precise control by upper motor neurons (UMNs).

Peripheral Nerves. With rare exceptions, peripheral nerves, including the cranial nerves, contain afferent and efferent

processes of more than one of the four afferent and three efferent cell columns. This provides the basis for assessing the function of any peripheral nerve. The functional components of each of the cranial nerves and spinal nerve roots are presented in Table 48.1.

Longitudinal Tracts

The grey matter of the cell columns in the CNS is surrounded by bundles of myelinated axons (*i.e.,* white matter) and unmyelinated axons that travel longitudinally along the length of the neural axis. This white matter can be divided into three layers: an inner, middle, and outer layer (Fig. 48.13). The inner layer, or *archilayer,* contains short fibres that project for a maximum of approximately five segments before reentering the grey matter. The middle layer, or *paleolayer,* projects to six or more segments. Archilayer and paleolayer fibres have many branches, or collaterals, that enter the grey matter of intervening segments. In the outer layer, or *neolayer,* are found large-diameter axons that can travel the entire length of the nervous system (Table 48.2). *Suprasegmental* is a term that refers to higher levels of the CNS, such as the brain stem and cerebrum and structures above a given CNS segment. Paleolayer and neolayer fibres have suprasegmental projections.

TABLE 48.1 THE SEGMENTAL NERVES AND THEIR COMPONENTS

SEGMENT AND NERVE	COMPONENT	INNERVATION	FUNCTION
1. Forebrain			
I. Olfactory	SVA	Receptors in olfactory mucosa	Reflexes, olfaction (smell)
2. II. Optic nerve		Optic nerve and retina (part of brain system, not a peripheral nerve)	
3. Midbrain			
V. Trigeminal (V$_1$) ophthalmic division	SSA	Muscles: upper face, forehead, upper lid	Facial expression, proprioception
	GSA	Skin, subcutaneous tissue, conjunctiva, frontal/ethmoid sinuses	Somesthesia Reflexes (blink)
III. Oculomotor	GVE	Iris sphincter Ciliary muscle	Pupillary constriction Accommodation
	GSE	Extrinsic eye muscles	Eye movement, lid movement
4. Pons			
V. Trigeminal (V$_2$) maxillary division	SSA	Muscles: facial expression	Proprioception Reflexes (sneeze), somesthesia
	GSA	Skin, oral mucosa, upper teeth, hard palate, maxillary sinus	
V. Trigeminal (V$_3$) mandibular division	SSA	Lower jaw, muscles: mastication	Proprioception, jaw jerk
	GSA	Skin, mucosa, teeth, anterior ⅔ of tongue	Reflexes, somesthesia
	PE	Muscles: mastication tensor tympani tensor veli palatini	Mastication: speech Protects ear from loud sounds Tenses soft palate
IV. Trochlear	GSE	Extrinsic eye muscle	Moves eye down and in
5. Caudal Pons			
VIII. Vestibular, cochlear (vestibulocochlear)	SSA	Vestibular end organs	Reflexes, sense of head position
		Organ of Corti	Reflexes, hearing

(continued)

TABLE 48.1 THE SEGMENTAL NERVES AND THEIR COMPONENTS (*continued*)

SEGMENT AND NERVE	COMPONENT	INNERVATION	FUNCTION
VII. Facial nerve, intermedius portion	GSA	External auditory meatus	Somesthesia
	GVA	Nasopharynx	Gag reflex: sensation
	SVA	Taste buds of anterior ⅔ of tongue	Reflexes: gustation (taste)
	GVE	Nasopharynx	Mucus secretion, reflexes
		Lacrimal, sublingual, submandibular glands	Lacrimation, salivation
Facial nerve	PE	Muscles: facial expression, stapedius	Facial expression
			Protects ear from loud sounds
VI. Abducens	GSE	Extrinsic eye muscle	Lateral eye deviation
6. Middle Medulla			
IX. Glossopharyngeal	SSA	Stylopharyngeus muscle	Proprioception
	GSA	Posterior external ear	Somesthesia
	SVA	Taste buds of posterior ⅓ of tongue	Gustation (taste)
	GVA	Oral pharynx	Gag reflex: sensation
	GVE	Parotid gland; pharyngeal mucosa	Salivary reflex: mucus secretion
	PE	Stylopharyngeus muscle	Assists swallowing
7, 8, 9, 10. Caudal Medulla			
X. Vagus	SSA	Muscles: pharynx, larynx	Proprioception
	GSA	Posterior external ear	Somesthesia
	SVA	Taste buds, pharynx, larynx	Reflexes, gustation
	GVA	Visceral organs (esophagus to midtransverse colon, liver, pancreas, heart, lungs)	Reflexes, sensation
	GVE	Visceral organs as above	Parasympathetic efferent
	PE	Muscles: pharynx, larynx	Swallowing, phonation, emesis
XIII. Hypoglossal	GSE	Muscles of tongue	Tongue movement, reflexes
Spinal Segments			
C-1–C-4 Upper Cervical	PE	Muscles: sternocleidomastoid, trapezius	Head, shoulder movement
XI. Spinal accessory nerve			
Spinal nerves	SSA	Muscles of neck	Proprioception, DTRs
	GSA	Neck, back of head	Somesthesia
	GSE	Neck muscles	Head, shoulder movement
C-5–C-8 Lower Cervical	SSA	Upper limb muscles	Proprioception, DTRs
	GSA	Upper limbs	Reflexes, somesthesia
	GSE	Upper limb muscles	Movement, posture
T-1–L-2 Thoracic, Upper Lumbar	SSA	Muscles: trunk, abdominal wall	Proprioception
	GSA	Trunk, abdominal wall	Reflexes, somesthesia
	GVA	All of viscera	Reflexes and sensation
	GVE	All of viscera	Sympathetic reflexes, vasomotor control, sweating, piloerection
	GSE	Muscles: trunk, abdominal wall, back	Movement, posture, respiration
L-2–S-1 Lower Lumbar, Upper Sacral	SSA	Lower limb muscles	Proprioception, DTRs
	GSA	Lower trunk, limbs, back	Reflexes, somesthesia
	GSE	Muscles: trunk, lower limbs, back	Movement, posture
S-2–S-4 Lower Sacral	SSA	Muscles: pelvis, perineum	Proprioception
	GSA	Pelvis, genitalia	Reflexes, somesthesia
	GVA	Hindgut, bladder, uterus	Reflexes, sensation
	GVE	Hindgut, visceral organs	Visceral reflexes, defecation, urination, erection
S-5–Co-2 Lower Sacral, Coccygeal	SSA	Perineal muscles	Proprioception
	GSA	Lower sacrum, anus	Reflexes, somesthesia
	GSE	Perineal muscles	Reflexes, posture

Afferent (sensory) components: SSA, special somatic afferent; GSA, general somatic afferent; SVA, special visceral afferent; GVA, general visceral afferent.
Efferent (motor) components: GVE, general visceral efferent (autonomic nervous system); PE, pharyngeal efferent; GSE, general somatic efferent; DTRs, deep tendon reflexes.

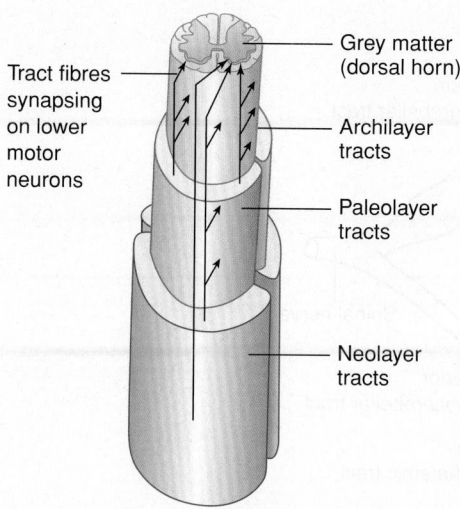

Tract fibres
synapsing
on lower
motor
neurons

Grey matter
(dorsal horn)

Archilayer
tracts

Paleolayer
tracts

Neolayer
tracts

FIGURE 48.13 • The three concentric subdivisions of the tract systems of the white matter. Migration of neurons into the archilayer converts it into the reticular formation of the white matter.

The longitudinal layers are arranged in bundles, or fibre tracts, that contain axons that have the same destination, origin, and function (Fig. 48.14). These longitudinal tracts are named systematically to reflect their origin and destination; the origin is named first, and the destination is named second. For example, the spinothalamic tract originates in the spinal cord and terminates in the thalamus. The corticospinal tract originates in the cerebral cortex and ends in the spinal cord.

The Inner Layer. Lying next to the superficial grey matter, the inner layer of white matter contains the axons of neurons that connect neighbouring segments of the nervous system. Axons of this layer permit motor neurons of several segments to work together as a functional unit. They also allow the afferent neurons of one segment to trigger reflexes that activate motor units in neighbouring segments as well as in the same one. It is the first of the longitudinal layers to become functional and can be referred to as the *archilayer*, with its circuitry limited to reflex types of movements, including reflex movements of the fetus (*i.e.*, quickening) that begin during the fifth month of intrauterine life.

The inner layer of the white matter differs from the other two layers in one important aspect. Many neurons in the embryonic grey matter migrate out into this layer, resulting in a rich mixture of neurons and local fibres called the *reticular formation*. The circuitry of most reflexes is contained in the reticular formation. In the brain stem, the reticular formation becomes quite large and contains major portions of vital reflexes, such as those controlling respiration, cardiovascular function, swallowing, and vomiting. A functional system called the *reticular activating system* (RAS) operates in the lateral portions of the reticular formation of the medulla, pons, and especially the midbrain. Information derived from all sensory modalities, including those of the somesthetic, auditory, visual, and visceral afferent nerves, bombards the neurons of this system.

The RAS has descending and ascending portions. The descending portion communicates with all spinal segmental levels through paleolevel reticulospinal tracts and serves to facilitate many cord-level reflexes. For example, it speeds reaction time and stabilizes postural reflexes. The ascending portion accelerates brain activity, particularly thalamic and cortical activity. This is reflected by the appearance of awake-type patterns of brain wave activity. Sudden stimuli result in protective and attentive postures and increased awareness.

The Middle Layer. The middle layer of the white matter contains most of the major fibre tract systems required for sensation and movement, including the ascending spinoreticular and spinothalamic tracts. This layer consists of larger-diameter and longer suprasegmental fibres, which ascend to the brain stem and are largely functional at birth. These tracts are sometimes called the *paleolayer*. It facilitates many primitive functions, such as the auditory startle reflex, which occurs in response to loud noises. This reflex consists of turning the head and body toward the sound, dilation of the pupils of the eyes, catching of the breath, and quickening of the pulse.

The Outer Layer. The outer layer of the tract systems is sometimes called the *neolayer*. It becomes functional during approximately the second year of life, and it includes the pathways needed for bladder training. Myelination of these suprasegmental tracts, which include many pathways required for delicate and highly coordinated skills, is not complete until approximately the fifth year of life. This includes the development of tracts needed for fine manipulative skills, such as the finger–thumb coordination required for using tools and the toe movements needed for acrobatics. Neolayer tracts are situated more superficially on the brain and spinal cord and

CHARACTERISTICS	ARCHILAYER TRACTS	PALEOLAYER TRACTS	NEOLAYER TRACTS
Segmental span	Intersegmental (<5 segments)	Suprasegmental (≥5 segments)	Suprasegmental
Number of synapses	Multisynaptic	Multisynaptic but fewer than archilayer tracts	Monosynaptic with target structures
Conduction velocity	Very slow	Fast	Fastest
Examples of functional systems	Flexor withdrawal reflex circuitry	Spinothalamic tracts	Corticospinal tracts

TABLE 48.2 CHARACTERISTICS OF THE CONCENTRIC SUBDIVISIONS OF THE LONGITUDINAL TRACTS IN THE WHITE MATTER OF THE CENTRAL NERVOUS SYSTEM

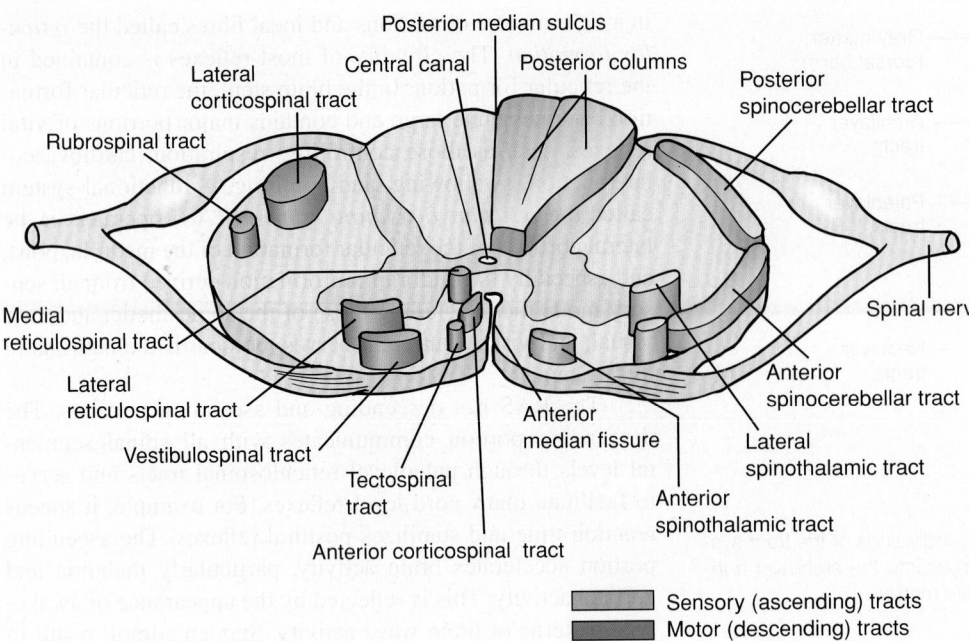

FIGURE 48.14 • Transverse section of the spinal cord showing selected sensory and motor tracts. The tracts are bilateral but are indicated only on one half of the cord.

Posterior median sulcus
Central canal
Lateral corticospinal tract
Posterior columns
Posterior spinocerebellar tract
Rubrospinal tract
Medial reticulospinal tract
Spinal nerve
Lateral reticulospinal tract
Vestibulospinal tract
Tectospinal tract
Anterior median fissure
Anterior corticospinal tract
Anterior spinocerebellar tract
Lateral spinothalamic tract
Anterior spinothalamic tract

☐ Sensory (ascending) tracts
☐ Motor (descending) tracts

are the most vulnerable to injury. When neolayer tracts are damaged, the paleolayer and archilayer tracts often remain functional, and rehabilitation methods can result in effective use of the older systems. Delicacy and refinement may be lost, but basic function remains. For example, when the corticospinal system, an important neolayer system that permits the fine manipulative control required for writing, is damaged, the remaining paleolayer systems, if intact, permit the grasping and holding of objects. The hand can still be used to perform basic functions, but the fine manipulative functions of the fingers are lost.

Collateral Communication Pathways. Axons in the archilayer and paleolayer characteristically possess many collateral branches that move into the grey cell columns or synapse with fibres of the reticular formation as the axon passes each succeeding CNS segment. Should a major axon be destroyed at some point along its course, these collaterals provide multisynaptic alternative pathways that bypass the local damage. Neolayer tracts do not possess these collaterals but instead project mainly to the target neurons with which they communicate. Because of this, damage to the neolayer tracts causes permanent loss of function. Damage to the archilayer or paleolayer systems is usually followed by a slow return of function, presumably through the collateral connections.

IN SUMMARY

The CNS develops from the ectoderm of the early embryo by formation of a hollow tube that closes along its longitudinal axis and sinks below the surface. This hollow tube forms the ventricles of the brain and spinal canal, and the side wall develops to form the brain stem and spinal cord.

Development of the CNS requires the coordinated production of many embryonic inductive factors. The brain stem and spinal cord are subdivided into the dorsal horn, which contains neurons that receive and process incoming or afferent information, and the ventral horn, which contains efferent motor neurons that handle the final stages of output processing. The PNS develops from ectodermal cells called neural crest cells that migrate away from the dorsal surface of the forming neural tube.

Throughout life, the organization of the nervous system retains many patterns established during early embryonic life. This segmental pattern of early embryonic development is retained in the fully developed nervous system. Each of the 43 or more body segments is connected to corresponding CNS or neural tube segments by segmental afferent and efferent neurons. Afferent neuronal processes enter the CNS through the dorsal root ganglia and the dorsal roots. Afferent neurons of the dorsal root ganglia are of four types: general somatic afferent, special somatic afferent, general visceral afferent, and special visceral afferent. Each of these afferent neurons synapses with its appropriate IA neurons in the cell columns of the dorsal horn (*e.g.*, general somatic afferents synapse with neurons in the general somatic afferent IA cell column). Efferent fibres from motor neurons in the ventral horn exit the CNS in the ventral roots. General somatic efferent neurons are LMNs that innervate somite-derived skeletal muscles, and general visceral efferent neurons are preganglionic fibres that synapse with postganglionic fibres that innervate visceral structures. This pattern of afferent and efferent neurons, which is usually repeated in each segment of the body, forms parallel cell columns running lengthwise through the CNS and PNS.

Longitudinal communication between CNS segments is provided by neurons that send the axons into nearby segments by means of the innermost layer of the white matter, the archilayer system of fibres. These cells provide coordination between neighbouring segments. Neurons have invaded this layer, and the mix of these cells and axons is called the reticular formation. The reticular formation is the location of many important reflex circuits of the spinal cord and brain stem. Paleolayer tracts, located outside the archilayer, provide the longitudinal communication between more distant segments of the nervous system; this layer includes most of the important ascending and descending tracts. The neolayer systems, which become functional during infancy and childhood, travel outside the white matter and provide the means for very delicate and discriminative function. The outer position of the neolayer tracts and their lack of collateral and redundant pathways make them the most vulnerable to injury.

STRUCTURE AND FUNCTION OF THE SPINAL CORD AND BRAIN

After completing this section of the chapter, you should be able to meet the following objectives:

- Describe the longitudinal and transverse structures of the spinal cord.
- Trace an afferent and efferent neuron from its site in the periphery through its entrance into or exit from the spinal cord.
- Explain the innervation and function of spinal cord reflexes.
- List the structures of the hindbrain, midbrain, and forebrain and describe their functions.
- Name the cranial nerves and cite their location and function.
- Describe the characteristics of the CSF and trace its passage through the ventricular system.
- Contrast and compare the blood–brain and CSF–brain barriers.

Spinal Cord

In the adult, the spinal cord is found in the upper two thirds of the spinal canal of the vertebral column (Fig. 48.15). It extends from the foramen magnum at the base of the skull to a cone-shaped termination, the conus medullaris, usually at the level of the first or second lumbar vertebra (L-1 or L-2) in the adult. Consequently, the dorsal and ventral roots of the more caudal portions of the cord elongate during development and angle downward from the cord, forming what is called the *cauda equina* (from the Latin for "horse's tail"). The filum terminale, which is composed of nonneural tissues and the pia mater, continues caudally and attaches to the second sacral vertebra (S-2).

The spinal cord is somewhat oval on transverse section. Internally, the grey matter has the appearance of a butterfly or the letter "H" on cross-section (see Fig. 48.15). Some neurons that make up the grey matter of the cord have processes or axons that leave the cord, enter the peripheral nerves, and supply tissues such as autonomic ganglia or skeletal muscles. The white matter of the cord that surrounds the grey matter contains nerve fibre tracts or descending axons that transmit information between segments of the cord or from higher levels of the CNS, such as the brain stem or cerebrum.

Internally, the extensions of the grey matter that form the letter "H" are called the *horns.* Those that extend posteriorly are called the *dorsal horns,* and those that extend anteriorly are called the *ventral horns.* Dorsal horns contain IA neurons that receive afferent impulses through the dorsal roots and other connecting neurons. Ventral horns contain OA neurons and the efferent LMNs that leave the cord through the ventral roots. The central portion of the cord, which connects the dorsal and ventral horns, is called the *intermediate grey matter.* The intermediate grey matter surrounds the central canal. In the thoracic area, the small, slender projections that emerge from the intermediate grey matter are called the *intermediolateral columns* of the horns. These columns contain the visceral OA neurons and the efferent neurons of the sympathetic nervous system.

The amount of grey matter is proportional to how much tissue is innervated by a given segment of the cord (see Fig. 48.15). Larger amounts of grey matter are present in the lower lumbar and upper sacral segments, which supply the lower extremities, and in the fifth cervical segment to the first thoracic segment, which supply the upper limbs. The white matter in the spinal cord also increases progressively toward the brain because ever more ascending fibres are added and the number of descending axons is greater.

The spinal cord and the dorsal and ventral roots are covered by a connective tissue sheath, the pia mater, which also contains the blood vessels that supply the white and grey matter of the cord (Fig. 48.16). On the lateral sides of the spinal cord, extensions of the pia mater, the denticulate ligaments, attach the sides of the spinal cord to the bony walls of the spinal canal. Thus, the cord is suspended by both the denticulate ligaments and the segmental nerves. A fat- and vessel-filled epidural space intervenes between the spinal dura mater and the inner wall of the spinal canal.

The spinal cord and nerves and their supporting structures are protected by the vertebral column. The vertebral body is the anterior, more massive part of the bone that gives strength to the vertebral column and supports body weight. Each vertebral body has two pedicles that extend posteriorly and support the laterally oriented transverse processes of the laminae, which arch medially and fuse to continue as the spinal processes. The vertebral arch and posterior surface of the vertebral body form the wall of the vertebral foramen. The succession of vertebral foramina in the articulated spinal column forms the vertebral canal (spinal canal), which contains

Posterior view

First cervical nerve

First cervical vertebrae

Cervical plexus
(C-1–C-5)

Brachial plexus
(C-5–T-1)

Lumbar plexus
(L-1–L-4)

Sacral plexus
(L-4–S-5)

Sciatic nerve

C-1

C-8
T-1

T-12
L-1

L-5

S-1

S-5

Cervical
nerves
(8 pairs)

Thoracic
nerves
(12 pairs)

Lumbar
nerves
(5 pairs)

Sacral
nerves
(5 pairs)

Coccygeal nerves
(1 pair)

A

Dorsal horn
of grey matter

Ventral horn
of grey matter

Cervical

White matter

Intermediolateral
horn of grey matter

Thoracic

Lumbar

B

FIGURE 48.15 • **A:** Posterior view of the spinal cord, including portions of the major spinal nerves and some of the components of the major nerve plexuses. **B:** Cross-sectional views of the spinal cord, showing regional variations in grey matter and increasing white matter as the cord ascends.

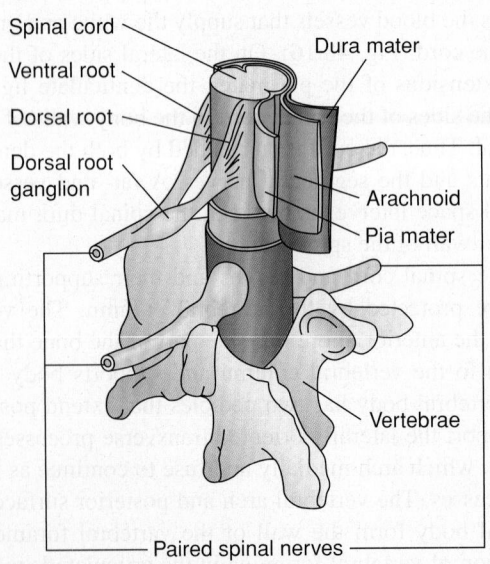

Spinal cord

Ventral root

Dorsal root

Dorsal root
ganglion

Dura mater

Arachnoid

Pia mater

Vertebrae

Paired spinal nerves

FIGURE 48.16 • Spinal cord and meninges.

the spinal cord, meninges, fat, and spinal nerve roots. The spaces between the vertebral bodies are filled with fibrocartilaginous disks and stabilized with tough ligaments. A gap, the intervertebral foramen, occurs between each two succeeding pedicles, allowing for the exit of the segmental nerves and passage of blood vessels. Supporting structures of the spinal cord are discussed further in Chapter 50.

Early in fetal life, the spinal cord extends the entire length of the vertebral column and the spinal nerves exit through the intervertebral foramina (openings) near their level of origin. Because the vertebral column and spinal dura grow faster than the spinal cord, a disparity develops between each succeeding cord segment and the exit of its dorsal and ventral nerve roots through the corresponding intervertebral foramina. In the newborn, the cord terminates at vertebral level L-2 or L-3, whereas the adult cord usually terminates at the inferior border of L-1. In addition, the arachnoid and its enclosed subarachnoid space, which is filled with CSF, do not close down on the filum terminale until they reach the second sacral vertebra. This results in the formation of a pocket of CSF, the *dural cisterna spinalis,* which extends from approximately L-2 to S-2. Because this area contains an abundant supply of CSF and the spinal cord does not extend this far, the area is often used for sampling the CSF. A procedure called a *spinal tap,* or *lumbar puncture,* can be done by inserting a special needle into the dural sac at L-3 or L-4. The spinal roots, which are covered with pia mater, are in little danger of trauma from the needle used for this purpose.

Spinal Nerves

The peripheral nerves that carry information to and from the spinal cord are called *spinal nerves.* Usually, 31 or more pairs of spinal nerves are present (*i.e.,* 8 cervical, 12 thoracic, 5 lumbar, 5 sacral, and 1 or more coccygeal); each pair is named for the segment of the spinal cord from which it exits. Because the first cervical spinal nerve exits the spinal cord just above the first cervical vertebra (C-1), the nerve is given the number of the bony vertebra just below it. The numbering is changed for all lower levels, however. Cervical nerve 8 (C-8), exits above the T-1 vertebra, and each subsequent nerve is numbered for the vertebra just above its point of exit (Fig. 48.15).

Each spinal cord segment communicates with its corresponding body segment through the paired segmental spinal nerves (Fig. 48.11). Each spinal nerve, accompanied by the blood vessels supplying the spinal cord, enters the spinal canal through an intervertebral foramen, where it divides into two branches, or roots. One branch enters the dorsolateral surface of the cord (*i.e.,* dorsal root), carrying the axons of afferent neurons into the CNS. The other branch leaves the ventrolateral surface of the cord (*i.e.,* ventral root), carrying the axons of efferent neurons into the periphery. These two branches or roots fuse at the intervertebral foramen, forming the mixed spinal nerve—"mixed" because it has both afferent and efferent axons.

After emerging from the vertebral column, the spinal nerve divides into two branches or *rami* (singular, *ramus*): a small dorsal primary ramus and a larger ventral primary ramus (Fig. 48.17). Thoracic and upper lumbar spinal nerves also produce a third branch, the ramus communicans, which contains sympathetic axons supplying the blood vessels, the genitourinary system, and the gastrointestinal system. The dorsal primary ramus contains sensory fibres from the skin and motor fibres to muscles of the back. The ventral primary ramus contains motor fibres that innervate the skeletal muscles of the anterior body wall and the legs and arms.

Spinal nerves do not go directly to skin and muscle fibres; instead, they form complicated nerve networks called *plexuses* (Fig. 48.15). A plexus is a site of intermixing nerve branches. Many spinal nerves enter a plexus and connect with other spinal nerves before exiting from the plexus. Nerves emerging from a plexus form progressively smaller branches that supply the skin and muscles of the various parts of the body. The PNS contains four major plexuses: the cervical plexus, the brachial plexus, the lumbar plexus, and the sacral plexus.

Dorsal
- Pia mater
- Subarachnoid space
- Dorsal root
- Arachnoid
- Dura mater
- Meningeal branch
- Dorsal primary ramus
- Ventral primary ramus
- Rami communicans
- Denticulate ligament
- Ventral root
- Third thoracic vertebra

Ventral

FIGURE 48.17 • Cross-section of vertebral column at the level of the third thoracic vertebra, showing the meninges, the spinal cord, and the origin of a spinal nerve and its branches or rami.

Spinal Reflexes

A *reflex* is a highly predictable relationship between a stimulus and an elicited motor response. Its anatomic basis consists of an afferent (sensory) neuron, the connection or synapse with CNS interneurons that communicate with the effector (motor) neuron, and the effector (motor) neuron that innervates a muscle or organ. Reflexes are essentially "wired in" to the CNS in that normally they are always ready to function; with training, most reflexes can be modulated to become parts of more complicated movements. A reflex may involve neurons in a single cord segment (*i.e.,* segmental reflexes), several or many segments (*i.e.,* intersegmental reflexes), or structures in the brain (*i.e.,* suprasegmental reflexes). Two important types of spinal motor reflexes are the withdrawal reflex and myotatic reflex.

The withdrawal reflex is stimulated by a painful (nociceptive) stimulus and quickly moves the body part away from the offending stimulus, usually by flexing a limb part (Fig. 48.18). The withdrawal reflex is a powerful reflex, taking precedence over other reflexes associated with locomotion. Any of the major joints may be involved, depending on the site of afferent stimulation. All the joints of an extremity (*e.g.,* finger, wrist, elbow, shoulder) typically are involved. This complex, protective, polysynaptic reflex also shifts postural support to the opposite side of the body with a crossed extensor reflex and simultaneously alerts the forebrain to the offending stimulus event. The withdrawal reflex also can produce contraction of muscles other than the extremities. For example, irritation of the abdominal viscera may cause contraction of the abdominal muscles.

The myotatic or stretch reflex controls muscle tone and helps maintain posture. Specialized sensory nerve terminals in skeletal muscles and tendons relay information on muscle stretch and joint tension to the CNS (see Chapter 50). This information, which drives postural reflex mechanisms, also is

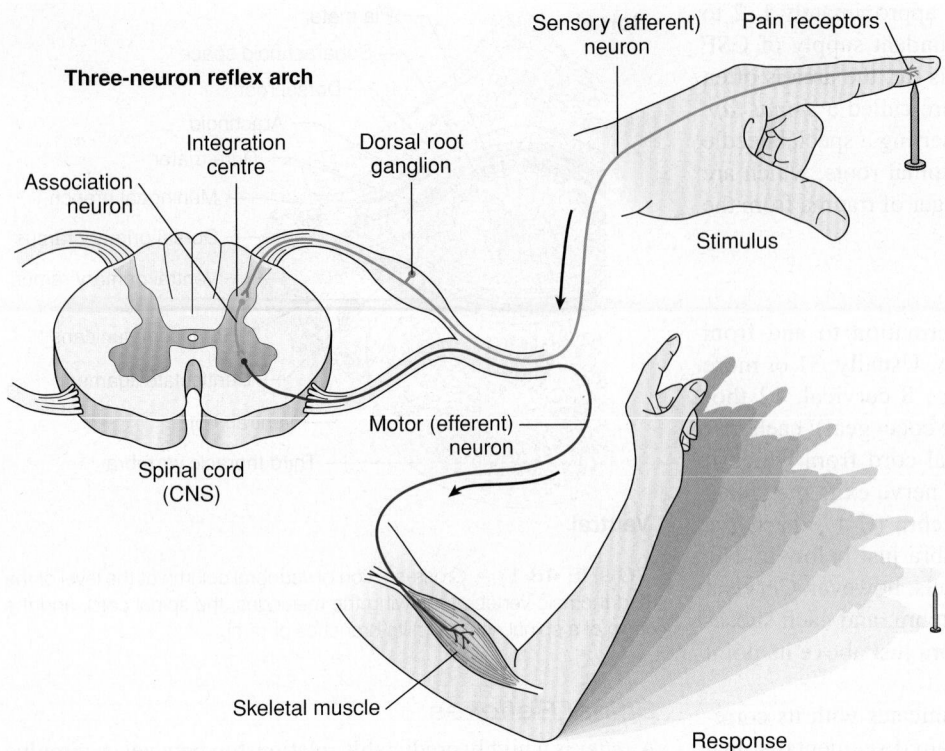

Three-neuron reflex arch

Association neuron

Integration centre

Dorsal root ganglion

Sensory (afferent) neuron

Pain receptors

Stimulus

Spinal cord (CNS)

Motor (efferent) neuron

Skeletal muscle

Response

FIGURE 48.18 • Diagram of withdrawal reflex, showing the essential elements in a spinal reflex arc–a receptor in a sensory neuron, an integration centre with an association neuron, and an effector (skeletal muscle).

relayed to the thalamus and the sensory cortex and is experienced as *proprioception,* the sense of body movement and position. To provide this information, the muscles and their tendons are supplied with two types of sensory receptors: muscle spindle receptors and Golgi tendon organs. *Muscle spindles* are stretch receptors distributed throughout the belly of a muscle that transmit information about muscle length and rate of stretch. The *Golgi tendon organs* are found in muscle tendons and transmit information about muscle tension or force of contraction at the junction of the muscle and the tendon that attaches to bone. A likely role of the tendon organs is to equalize the contractile forces of the separate muscle groups, spreading the load over all the fibres to prevent the local muscle damage that might occur when small numbers of fibres are overloaded.

The Brain

Based on its embryonic development, the brain is divided into three regions: the hindbrain, the midbrain, and the forebrain (Fig. 48.8). The hindbrain includes the medulla oblongata, the pons, and its dorsal outgrowth, the cerebellum. Midbrain structures include two pairs of dorsal enlargements, the superior and inferior colliculi. The forebrain, which consists of two hemispheres and is covered by the cerebral cortex, contains central masses of grey matter, the basal ganglia, and the rostral end of the neural tube, the diencephalon, with its adult derivatives—the thalamus and hypothalamus.

An important concept is that the more rostral, recently developed parts of the neural tube gain dominance or control over regions and functions at lower levels. They do not replace

the circuitry but merely dominate it. After damage to the more vulnerable parts of the forebrain, as occurs with brain injury, a brain stem-controlled organism remains that is capable of breathing and may survive if the environmental temperature is regulated and nutrition and other aspects of care are provided. However, all aspects of intellectual function, experience, perception, and memory are usually permanently lost. The organization of content in this section moves from the circuitry of the hindbrain to the more dominant structures of the forebrain.

Hindbrain

The hindbrain consists of the myelencephalon (medulla oblongata) and the metencephalon (pons and cerebellum), which together support vital bodily functions. This area of the brain assists in managing motor activity, posture, conduction of sensory information, and controlling basic autonomic functions (*e.g.,* breathing, heart rate, digestion).

Brain Stem. The term *brain stem* is often used to include the medulla, pons, and midbrain (Fig. 48.19B). These regions of the neural tube have the organization of spinal cord segments, except that more of the longitudinal cell columns are present, reflecting the increased complexity of the cranial segmental nerves. In the brain stem, the structure and function of the reticular formation have been greatly expanded. In the pons and medulla, the reticular formation contains networks controlling basic breathing, eating, and locomotion functions. Higher-level integration of these functions occurs in the midbrain. The reticular formation is surrounded on the outside by the long tract systems that connect the forebrain with lower parts of the CNS.

FIGURE 48.19 • **A:** Mid-sagittal section of the brain, showing the structures of the forebrain, midbrain, and hindbrain. **B:** Diencephalon, brain stem, and the cerebral aqueduct connecting the third and fourth ventricles. **C:** Lateral view of the cerebral hemispheres.

Medulla. The *medulla oblongata* represents the caudal five segments of the brain part of the neural tube; the cranial nerve branches entering and leaving it have functions similar to the spinal segmental nerves. Although the ventral horn areas in the medulla are quite small, the dorsal horn areas are enlarged, processing a large amount of the information pouring through the cranial nerves. The segmental peripheral nerve components of the medulla can be divided into those leaving the neural tube ventromedially (*i.e.*, hypoglossal and abducens cranial nerves) or dorsolaterally (*i.e.*, vagus, spinal accessory, glossopharyngeal, and vestibulocochlear cranial nerves). Because pathologic signs and symptoms reflect the spatial segregation of brain stem components, neurologic syndromes resulting from trauma, tumours, aneurysms, and cerebrovascular accidents are often classified as ventral or dorsolateral syndromes.

The general somatic efferent LMNs of the lower segments of the medulla supply the extrinsic and intrinsic muscles of the tongue by means of the *hypoglossal nerve* (CN XII). Damage to the hypoglossal nerve results in weakness or paralysis of tongue muscles. When the tongue is protruded, it deviates toward the damaged and therefore weaker side because of the greater protrusion strength on the normal side. Axons of the hypoglossal nerve exit the medulla adjacent to two long, longitudinal ridges along the medial undersurface of the medulla. These ridges, called the *pyramids*, contain the corticospinal fibres, most of which cross to descend in the lateral column to the opposite side of the spinal cord. Lesions of the ventral surface of the caudal medulla result in the syndrome of

alternating hypoglossal hemiplegia. These lesions are characterized by signs of ipsilateral (*i.e.*, same side) denervation of the tongue and contralateral (*i.e.*, opposite side) weakness or paralysis of both the upper and lower extremities.

The *vagus nerve* (CN X) has several afferent (sensory) and efferent (motor) components. General somatic afferent neurons innervate the external ear, whereas special visceral afferent neurons innervate the pharyngeal taste buds. Sensory and motor components of the nerve innervate the pharynx, the gastrointestinal tract (from the laryngeal pharynx to the mid-transverse colon), the heart, the spleen, and the lungs. Initiation of many essential reflexes and normal functions depends on intact vagal innervation. For example, 80% of the fibres of the vagus are afferents, some of which are involved in vomiting and hiccup reflexes and in ongoing feedback during swallowing and speech. The unilateral loss of vagal function can result in slowed gastrointestinal motility, a permanently husky voice, and deviation of the uvula away from the damaged side. Bilateral loss of vagal function can seriously damage reflex maintenance of cardiovascular and respiratory reflexes. Swallowing may become difficult and, occasionally, paralysis of laryngeal structures causes life-threatening airway obstruction.

The sternocleidomastoid, a powerful head-turning muscle, and the trapezius muscle, which elevates the shoulders, are innervated by the *spinal accessory nerve* (CN XI), with LMNs in the upper four cervical spinal segments. Intermediate rootlets from these segmental levels combine and enter the cranial cavity through the foramen magnum and exit the jugular foramen with CNs IX and X. Loss of spinal accessory nerve function results in drooping of the shoulder on the damaged side and weakness when turning the head to the opposite side.

The dorsolateral *glossopharyngeal nerve* (CN IX) contains the same components as the vagus nerve but for a more rostral segment of the gastrointestinal tract and the pharynx. This nerve provides the special visceral sensory innervation of the taste buds of the oral pharynx and the back of the tongue; the afferent innervation of the oral pharynx and the baroreceptors of the carotid sinus; the efferent innervation of the otic ganglion, which controls the salivary function of the parotid gland; and the efferent innervation of the stylopharyngeus muscles of the pharynx. This cranial nerve is seldom damaged, but when it is, anesthesia of the ipsilateral oral pharynx develops along with dry mouth resulting from reduced salivation.

The special sensory afferent *vestibulocochlear nerve* (CN VIII), also called the *auditory or acoustic nerve,* is attached laterally at the junction of the medulla oblongata and the pons, often called the *caudal pons.* It consists of two distinct fibre divisions, the cochlear and vestibular divisions, both of which are sensory. Cell bodies in the cochlea of the inner ear produce fibres of the cochlear division. These fibres transmit impulses related to the sense of hearing. The vestibular division arises from two ganglia that innervate cell bodies in the utricle, saccule, and semicircular canals and transmit impulses related to head position and movement of the body through space. Irritation of the cochlear division results in tinnitus (*i.e.,* ringing of the ears); destruction of the nerve results in nerve deafness. Injury to the vestibular division leads to vertigo, nystagmus, and some postural instability (see Chapter 55).

The *facial nerve* (CN VII) and its intermediate component (the intermedius) is a mixed nerve that has both afferent and efferent components. It emerges from the junction of the pons and medulla. The nervus intermedius, containing the general somatic afferent, special visceral afferent, general visceral afferent, and general visceral efferent neurons, innervates the nasopharynx and taste buds of the palate. It also innervates the anterior two thirds of the tongue, the submandibular and sublingual salivary glands, the lacrimal glands, and the mucous membranes of the nose and roof of the mouth. Loss of this branch of the facial nerve can lead to eye dryness with risk of corneal scarring and blindness. The pharyngeal efferent LMNs of the facial nerve proper innervate muscles that control facial expression, such as wrinkling of the brow and smiling. Unilateral loss of facial nerve function results in flaccid paralysis of the muscles of half the face, a condition called *Bell's palsy.*

Pons. The pons (from the Latin for "bridge") develops from the fifth neural tube segment. Internally, the central canal of the spinal cord, which is enlarged in the pons and rostral medulla, forms the fourth ventricle (Fig. 48.19B). An enlarged area on the ventral surface of the pons contains the pontine nuclei, which receive information from all parts of the cerebral cortex. Axons of these neurons form a massive bundle that swings around the lateral side of the fourth ventricle to enter the cerebellum. In the pons, the reticular formation is large and contains the circuitry for masticating food and manipulating the jaws during speech.

The *abducens nerve* (CN VI), which arises from the caudal pons, sends LMNs out ventrally on either side of the pyramids and then forward into the orbit to innervate the lateral rectus muscle of the eye. As the name suggests, the abducens nerve abducts the eye (lateral or outward rotation); peripheral damage to this nerve results in medial strabismus, which is a weakness or loss of eye abduction (see Chapter 54).

The *trigeminal nerve* (CN V), which has both sensory and motor subdivisions, exits the brain stem laterally on the forward surface of the pons. The trigeminal is the main sensory nerve conveying the modalities of pain, temperature, touch, and proprioception to the superficial and deep regions of the face. Regions innervated include the skin of the anterior scalp and face, the conjunctiva and orbit, the meninges, the paranasal sinuses, and the mouth, including the teeth and the anterior two thirds of the tongue. LMNs of the trigeminal nerve innervate skeletal muscles involved with mastication and contribute to swallowing and speech, movements of the soft palate, and tension of the tympanic membrane through the tensor tympani muscle. The tensor tympani muscle has a protective reflex function, dampening movement of the middle ear ossicles during high-intensity sound.

Cerebellum. The *cerebellum* is located in the posterior fossa of the cranium superior to the pons (Fig. 48.17A). It is separated from the cerebral hemispheres by a fold of dura mater, the tentorium cerebelli. The cerebellum consists of a small unpaired median portion, called the *vermis,* and two large lateral masses, the *cerebellar hemispheres.* In contrast to the brain stem with its external white matter and internal grey nuclei, the cerebellum, like the cerebrum, has an outer cortex of grey matter overlying the white matter. Next to the fourth ventricle, several masses of grey matter, called the *deep cerebellar nuclei,* border the roof of the fourth ventricle. Cells of the cerebellar cortex and deep nuclei interact, and axons from the latter send information to many regions, particularly to the motor cortex, by means of a thalamic relay. Synergistic functions of the cerebellum (*i.e.,* temporal and spatial smoothing) contribute to all movements of the limbs, trunk, head, larynx, and eyes, whether the movement is part of a voluntary movement or of a highly learned semiautomatic or automatic movement. During highly skilled movements, the motor cortex sends signals to the cerebellum, informing it about the movement that is to be performed. The cerebellum makes continuous adjustments, resulting in smoothness of movement, particularly during delicate maneuvres. Highly skillful movement requires extensive motor training, and considerable evidence suggests many of these learned movement patterns involve cerebellar circuits.

The cerebellum receives proprioceptor input from the vestibular system; feedback from the muscles, tendons, and joints; and indirect signals from the somesthetic, visual, and auditory systems that provide background information for ongoing movement. Sensory and motor information from a given area of the body is sent to the same area in the cerebellum. In this way, the cerebellum can assess continuously the status of each body part—position, rate of movement, and forces such as gravity that are opposing movement. The cerebellum compares what is actually happening with what is intended to happen. It then transmits the appropriate corrective signals back to the motor system, instructing it to increase or decrease the activity of the participating muscle groups so that smooth and accurate movements can be performed.

Another function of the cerebellum is the dampening of muscle movement. All body movements are essentially pendular (*i.e.*, swinging back and forth). As movement begins, momentum develops and must be overcome before the movement can be stopped. This momentum would cause movements to overshoot if they were not dampened. In the intact cerebellum, automatic signals stop movement precisely at the intended point. The cerebellum analyzes proprioceptive information to predict the future position of moving parts, their rapidity of movement, and the projected time course of the movement. This allows the cerebellum to inhibit agonist muscles and excite antagonist muscles when movement approaches the intended target.

Midbrain

The midbrain or mesencephalon develops from the fourth segment of the neural tube, and its organization is similar to that of a spinal segment. Internally, the central canal is reestablished as the cerebral aqueduct, connecting the fourth ventricle with the third ventricle (Fig. 48.19B). Two general somatic efferent cranial nerves, the oculomotor nerve (CN III) and the trochlear nerve (CN IV), exit the midbrain.

Two prominent bundles of nerve fibres, the *cerebral peduncles,* pass along the ventral surface of the midbrain. These fibres include the corticospinal tracts and are the main motor pathways between the forebrain and the pons. On the dorsal surface, four "little hills," the *superior* and *inferior colliculi,* are areas of cortical formation. The inferior colliculi are involved in directional turning and, to some extent, in experiencing the direction of sound sources, whereas the superior colliculi are essential to the reflex mechanisms that control conjugate eye movements when the visual environment is surveyed.

The ventral central grey matter (*i.e.*, ventral horn) of the midbrain contains the LMNs that innervate most of the skeletal muscles that move the optic globe and raise the eyelids. These axons leave the midbrain through the oculomotor nerve (CN III). This nerve also contains the parasympathetic LMNs that control pupillary constriction and ciliary muscle focusing of the lens (see Table 48.1). Damage to the ventrally exiting CN III and to the adjacent cerebral peduncle, which contains the corticospinal axon system on one side, results in paralysis of eye movement combined with contralateral hemiplegia.

A small group of cells in the ventral part of the caudal central grey matter contains the trochlear nerve (CN IV),

which innervates the superior oblique eye muscle. This muscle moves the upper part of the eye downward and toward the nose when the eye is adducted, or turned inward. The trochlear nerve exits the dorsal surface of the midbrain and decussates (crosses over) before exiting the brain stem. Lesions of the trochlear nerve affect downward gaze on the side opposite the denervated muscle, producing diplopia, or double vision. Walking downstairs becomes particularly difficult. Because the superior oblique muscle has inward rotation of the optic globe as its major function, persons with trochlear nerve damage usually carry their heads tilted to the side of damage.

Forebrain

The most rostral part of the brain, the forebrain consists of the telencephalon, or "end brain," and the diencephalon, or "between brain." The diencephalon forms the core of the forebrain, and the telencephalon forms the cerebral hemispheres.

Diencephalon. Three of the most forward brain segments form an enlarged dorsal horn and ventral horn with a narrow, deep, enlarged central canal—the third ventricle—separating the two sides. This region is called the *diencephalon.* The dorsal horn part of the diencephalon is the thalamus and subthalamus, and the ventral horn part is the hypothalamus (Fig. 48.20). The optic nerve (CN II) and retina are outgrowths of the diencephalon. The structure and function of the optic nerve are presented in Chapter 54.

The *thalamus* consists of two large, egg-shaped masses, one on either side of the third ventricle. It is divided into several major parts, and each part is divided into distinct nuclei, which are the major relay stations for information going to and from the cerebral cortex. All sensory pathways have direct projections to thalamic nuclei, which convey the information to restricted areas of the sensory cortex. Coordination and integration of peripheral sensory stimuli occur in the thalamus, along with some crude interpretation of highly emotion-laden auditory experiences that not only occurs but can be remembered. For example, a person can recover from a deep coma in which cerebral cortex activity is minimal and remember some of what was said at the bedside.

The thalamus also plays a role in relaying critical information regarding motor activities to and from selected areas of the motor cortex. Two neuronal circuits are significant in this regard. One is the pathway from the cerebral cortex to the pons and cerebellum and then, by way of the thalamus, back to the motor cortex. The second is the feedback circuit that travels from the cortex to the basal ganglia, then to the thalamus, and from the thalamus back to the cortex. The subthalamus also contains movement control systems related to the basal ganglia.

Through its connections with the ascending RAS, the thalamus processes neural influences that are basic to cortical excitatory rhythms (*i.e.*, those recorded on the electroencephalogram), to essential sleep–wakefulness cycles, and to the process of attending to stimuli. Besides their cortical connections, the thalamic nuclei have connections with each other

FIGURE 48.20 • Frontal section of the brain passing through the third ventricle, showing the thalamus, subthalamus, hypothalamus, internal capsule, corpus callosum, basal ganglia (caudate nucleus, lentiform nucleus), amygdaloid complex, insula, and parietal cortex.

and with neighbouring nonthalamic brain structures such as the limbic system. Through their connections with the limbic system, some thalamic nuclei are involved in the relation between stimuli and the emotional responses they evoke.

Inferior to the thalamus and representing the ventral horn portion of the diencephalon is the *hypothalamus*. It also borders the third ventricle and includes a ventral extension, the neurohypophysis (*i.e.*, posterior pituitary). The hypothalamus is the area of master-level integration of homeostatic control of the body's internal environment. Maintenance of blood gas concentrations, water balance, food consumption, and major aspects of endocrine and ANS control require hypothalamic function.

The internal capsule is a broad band of projection fibres that lies between the thalamus medially and the basal ganglia laterally (Fig. 48.20). It contains all of the fibres that connect the cerebral cortex with deeper structures, including the basal ganglia, thalamus, midbrain, pons, medulla, and spinal cord.

Telencephalon. This is the largest division of the brain and consists of the cerebral cortex with the two cerebral hemispheres, and the several subcortical structures and connections such as the corpus callosum, basal ganglia, and components of the limbic system.

Corpus Callosum. A massive commissure, or bridge, of myelinated axons called the *corpus callosum* connects the cerebral cortex of the two sides of the brain, allowing the transfer of information between both hemispheres (Fig. 48.20). Two smaller commissures, the anterior and posterior commissures, connect the two sides of the more specialized regions of the cerebrum and diencephalon.

Basal Ganglia. A section through the cerebral hemispheres reveals the surface of the cerebral cortex, a subcortical layer

of white matter made up of masses of myelinated axons, and deep masses of grey matter: the basal ganglia that border the lateral ventricle. The basal ganglia lie on either side of the internal capsule, just lateral to the thalamus. The basal ganglia consist of the comma-shaped *caudate* (tailed) *nucleus,* the shield-shaped *putamen,* and the *globus pallidus* ("pale globe"). The term *striatum* ("striped body") refers to the caudate plus the putamen. Together, the globus pallidus and putamen make up the *lentiform* (lens-shaped) *nucleus.*

The basal ganglia supply axial and proximal unlearned and learned postures and movements, which enhance and add gracefulness to UMN-controlled manipulative movements. These background movement functions are called *associated movements*. Intact and functional basal ganglia provide arm swinging during walking and running. Basal ganglia also are involved in follow-through movements that accompany throwing a ball or swinging a club. As with the motor cortex, the nuclei on the left side control movement on the right side of the body, and vice versa. Circuits connecting the premotor cortex and supplementary motor cortex, the basal ganglia, and parts of the thalamus provide associated movements that accompany highly skilled behaviours. Parkinson disease, Huntington chorea, and some forms of cerebral palsy, among other dysfunctions involving the basal ganglia, result in a frequent or continuous release of abnormal postural or axial and proximal movement patterns. If damage to the basal ganglia is localized to one side, the movements occur on the opposite side of the body. These automatic movement patterns stop only in sleep, but in some conditions, the movements are so violent that falling asleep becomes difficult.

Limbic System. The medial aspect of the cerebrum is organized into concentric bands of cortex, the *limbic system* (from the Latin for "border"), which surrounds the connection between the lateral and third ventricles. The innermost band

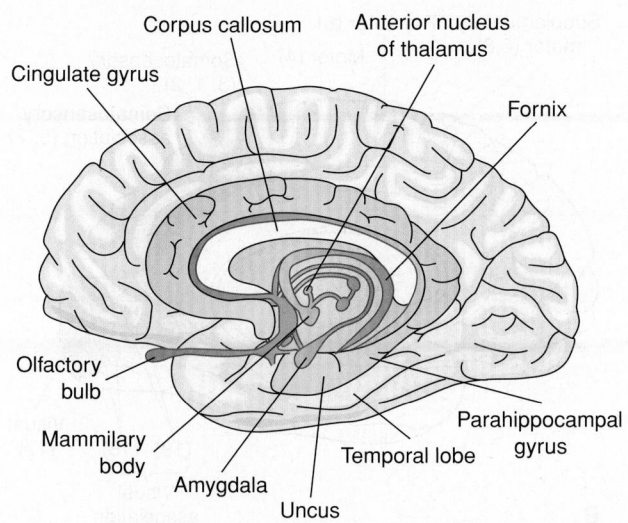

FIGURE 48.21 • The limbic system includes the limbic cortex (cingulate gyrus, parahippocampal gyrus, uncus) and associated subcortical structures (thalamus, hypothalamus, amygdala).

just above and below the cut surface of the corpus callosum is folded out of sight but is a three-layered cortex ending as the hippocampus in the temporal lobe. Just outside the folded area is a band of transitional cortex, which includes the cingulate and the parahippocampal gyri (Fig. 48.21). The limbic lobe has reciprocal connections with the medial and the intralaminar nuclei of the thalamus, with the deep nuclei of the cerebrum (*e.g.*, amygdaloid nuclei, septal nuclei), and with the hypothalamus. Overall, this region of the brain is involved in emotional experience and in the control of emotion-related behaviour. Stimulation of specific areas in this system can lead to feelings of dread, high anxiety, or exquisite pleasure. It also can result in violent behaviours, including attack, defence, or explosive and emotional speech.

Cerebral Hemispheres

The two cerebral hemispheres are lateral outgrowths of the diencephalon. Internally, the cerebral hemispheres contain the lateral ventricles (*i.e.*, ventricles I and II), which are connected to the third ventricle of the diencephalon by a small opening called the *interventricular foramen* (Fig. 48.19A). Axons of the olfactory nerve (CN I) terminate in the most ancient portion of the cerebrum, the olfactory bulb, where initial processing of olfactory information occurs. Projection axons from the olfactory bulb relay information through the olfactory tracts to the thalamus and to other parts of the cerebral cortex (*i.e.*, orbital cortex), where olfactory-related reflexes and olfactory experience occur.

The surfaces of the hemispheres are lateral (side), medial (area between the two sides of the brain), and basal (ventral). Many ridges and grooves are present on the surface of the hemispheres. A *gyrus* is the ridge between two grooves, and the groove is called a *sulcus* or *fissure*. The cerebral cortex is arbitrarily divided into lobes named after the bones that cover them: the frontal, parietal, temporal, and occipital lobes

(Fig. 48.19C). Early in the 20th century Korbinian Brodmann, a German neurologist, generated a map of about 50 distinct areas of the cerebral cortex; this cytoarchitecture was originally numbered according to histology and function. Today these Brodmann's areas are used by neurophysiologists and neurologists to refer by number to many of the different functional areas of the cortex (*e.g.*, area 4 constitutes primary motor cortex).

Frontal Lobe. The frontal lobe extends from the frontal pole to the central sulcus (*i.e.*, fissure) and is separated from the temporal lobe by the lateral sulcus. Each frontal lobe can be subdivided rostrally into the frontal pole and laterally into the superior, middle, and inferior gyri, which continue on the undersurface over the eyes as the orbital cortex. These areas are associated with the medial thalamic nuclei, which also are related to the limbic system. Functionally, the prefrontal cortex is thought to be involved in anticipation and prediction of consequences of behaviour.

The precentral gyrus (area 4), next to the central sulcus, is the *primary motor cortex* (Fig. 48.22). This area of the cortex provides precise movement control for distal flexor muscles of the hands and feet and of the phonation apparatus required for speech. Just rostral to the precentral gyrus is a region of the frontal cortex called the *premotor* or *motor association cortex*. This region (area 8 and rostral area 6) is involved in the planning of complex learned movement patterns, and damage to these areas results in dyspraxia or apraxia. Such people can manipulate a screwdriver, for instance, but cannot use it to loosen a screw. The primary motor cortex and the association motor cortex are connected with lateral thalamic nuclei, through which they receive feedback information from the basal ganglia and cerebellum. On the medial surface of the hemisphere, the premotor area includes a *supplementary motor cortex* involved in the control of bilateral movement patterns requiring great dexterity.

Parietal Lobe. The parietal lobe of the cerebrum lies behind the central sulcus (*i.e.*, postcentral gyrus) and above the lateral sulcus. A strip of cortex bordering the central sulcus is called the *primary somatosensory cortex* (areas 3, 1, and 2) because it receives very discrete sensory information from the lateral nuclei of the thalamus. Just behind the primary sensory cortex is the *somesthetic association cortex* (areas 5 and 7), which is connected with the thalamic nuclei and with the primary sensory cortex (Fig. 48.22). This region is necessary for somesthetic perception (*i.e.*, appreciation of the meaningfulness of integrated sensory information from various sensory systems), especially concerning perception of "where" the stimulus is in space and in relation to body parts. Localized lesions of this region can result in the inability to recognize the meaningfulness of an object (a condition called *agnosia*). With the eyes closed, a person can feel a screwdriver and describe its shape and texture. Nevertheless, the person cannot integrate the sensory information required to identify it as a screwdriver.

FIGURE 48.22 • Motor and sensory areas of the cerebral cortex. **A:** Left lateral view of the cerebral cortex. **B:** This diagram represents the areas in a brain that has been sectioned in the median plane.

Temporal Lobe. The temporal lobe lies below the lateral sulcus and merges with the parietal and occipital lobes. It includes the temporal pole and three primary gyri, the superior, middle, and inferior gyri. The primary auditory cortex (area 41) involves the part of the superior temporal gyrus that extends into the lateral sulcus (Fig. 48.22). This area is particularly important in discrimination of sounds entering opposite ears. It receives auditory input projections through the inferior colliculus of the midbrain and a ventrolateral thalamic nucleus. The more exposed part of the superior temporal gyrus involves the auditory association or perception area (area 22). The aspects of hearing that attach meaning to certain sound patterns require that this area function properly. The remaining portions of the temporal cortex are less well defined, but apparently are important in long-term memory recall. This is particularly true with respect to perception and memory of complex sensory patterns such as geometric figures and faces (*i.e.,* recognition of "what" or "who" the stimulus is).

Occipital Lobe. The occipital lobe lies posterior to the temporal and parietal lobes and is arbitrarily separated from them. The medial surface of the occipital lobe contains a deep sulcus extending from the limbic lobe to the occipital pole, the *calcarine sulcus,* which is surrounded by the primary visual cortex (area 17). Just superior and inferior and extending onto the lateral side of the occipital pole is the *visual association cortex* (areas 18 and 19). This area is closely connected with the primary visual cortex and with complex nuclei of the thalamus. Integrity of the association cortex is required for gnostic visual function, by which the meaningfulness of visual experience, including experiences of colour, motion, depth perception, pattern, form, and location in space, takes place.

The neocortical areas of the parietal lobe, between the somesthetic and the visual cortices, have a function in relating the texture, or "feel," and location of an object with its visual image. Between the auditory and visual association areas, the *parieto-occipital region* is necessary for relating the meaningfulness of a sound and image to an object or person.

Meninges

Inside the skull and vertebral column, the brain and spinal cord are loosely suspended and protected by several connective tissue sheaths called the *meninges* (Fig. 48.23). All surfaces of the spinal cord, brain, and segmental nerves are covered with a delicate connective tissue layer called the *pia mater* (Latin for "delicate mother"). Surface blood vessels and those that penetrate the brain and spinal cord are encased in this protective tissue layer. A second, very delicate, nonvascular,

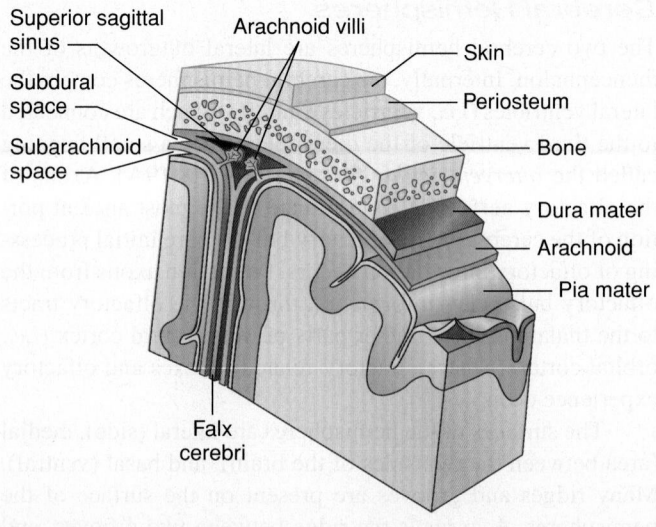

FIGURE 48.23 • The cranial meninges. Arachnoid villi, shown within the superior sagittal sinus, are one site of cerebrospinal fluid absorption into the blood.

FIGURE 48.24 • Schematic diagram of the three connective tissue membranes (pia, arachnoid, and dura) constituting the meninges of the central nervous system. Cerebrospinal fluid is resorbed (*arrows*) through the arachnoid villi projecting into the dural sinuses. (From Cormack D. H. (1987). *Ham's histology* (9th ed., p. 367). Philadelphia, PA: J. B. Lippincott.)

and waterproof layer, called the *arachnoid,* encloses the entire CNS (Fig. 48.24). The arachnoid layer is named for its spider-web appearance. The CSF is contained in the subarachnoid space. Immediately outside the arachnoid is a continuous sheath of strong connective tissue, the *dura mater* ("tough mother"), which provides the major protection for the brain and spinal cord. The cranial dura often splits into two layers, with the outer layer serving as the periosteum of the inner surface of the skull.

The inner layer of the dura forms two major infoldings—a longitudinal infolding called the *falx cerebri* and a transverse infolding called the *tentorium cerebelli*—that anchor the brain to the skull (Fig. 48.25). The falx cerebri (from the Latin *falx,* "sickle-shaped") lies in the longitudinal fissure and separates the two cerebral hemispheres. It attaches to the crista of the ethmoid bone anteriorly and ends by becoming continuous with the tentorium cerebelli. The tentorium cerebelli is a wide crescentic septum that acts as a hammock, supporting the occipital lobes above the cerebellum. The falx cerebri attaches to the tentorium cerebri and holds it up, giving it a tentlike appearance. The tentorium attaches to the petrous portion of the temporal bone and the dorsum sellae of the cranial floor,

with a semicircular gap, or incisura, formed at the midline to permit the midbrain to pass forward from the posterior fossa. It also forms a tough septum, separating the anterior and middle cranial fossae, which contain the cerebral hemispheres, from the posterior fossa, found interiorly and containing the brain stem and cerebellum. This compartmentalization is the basis for the commonly used terms *supratentorial* (*i.e.,* above the tentorium) and *infratentorial* (*i.e.,* below the tentorium). The cerebral hemispheres and the diencephalon are supratentorial structures, and the pons, cerebellum, and medulla are infratentorial structures.

The tentorium and falx cerebri normally support and protect the brain, which floats in CSF within the enclosed space. During extreme trauma, however, the sharp edges of these folds can damage the brain. Space-occupying lesions such as enlarging tumours or hematomas can squeeze the brain against these edges or through the incisura of the tentorium (*i.e.,* herniation). As a result, brain tissue can be compressed, contused, or destroyed, often causing permanent deficits (see Chapter 52).

Ventricular System and Cerebrospinal Fluid

The ventricular system is a series of CSF-filled cavities in the brain (Fig. 48.26). The CSF provides a supporting and protective fluid in which the brain and spinal cord float. CSF helps maintain a constant ionic environment that serves as a medium for diffusion of nutrients, electrolytes, and metabolic end products into the extracellular fluid surrounding CNS neurons and neuroglia. Filling the ventricles, the CSF supports the mass of the brain. Because it fills the subarachnoid space surrounding the CNS, a physical force delivered to either the skull or spine is to some extent diffused and cushioned.

The ventricles and central canal of the spinal cord are lined by a thin membrane of neuroglial cells collectively termed the *ependyma.* There is a tremendous expansion of the ependyma in the roof of the lateral, third, and fourth ventricles. The CSF is produced by tiny reddish masses of specialized ependymal cells and capillaries, called the *choroid plexus,* that project into the ventricles. CSF is an ultrafiltrate of blood plasma, composed of 99% water with other constituents, making it close

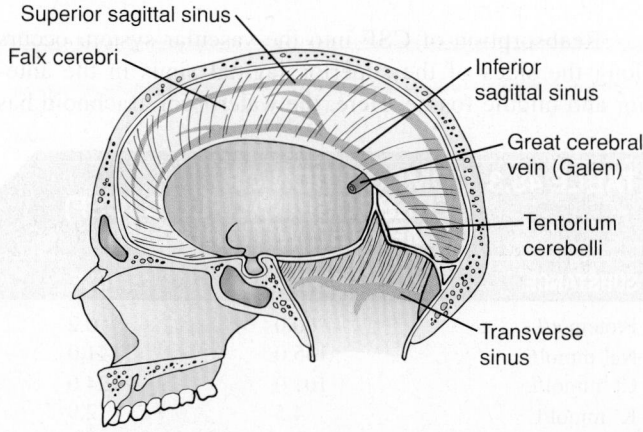

FIGURE 48.25 • Cranial dura mater. The skull is open to show the falx cerebri and the right and left portions of the tentorium cerebelli, as well as some of the cranial venous sinuses.

FIGURE 48.26 • A: The flow of cerebrospinal fluid (CSF) from the time of its formation from blood in the choroid plexuses until its return to the blood in the superior sagittal sinus. Plexuses in the lateral ventricles are not illustrated. **B:** CSF is a blood filtrate produced by the choroids plexus epithelium that is found in each brain ventricle. CSF flows from the lateral ventricles through the interventricular foramen (Monroe) into the third ventricle. From the third ventricle, CSF is conveyed to the fourth ventricle via the cerebral aqueduct (Sylvius). Three openings, a midline foramen of Magendie and two lateral foramina (Luschka), pass the CSF into the subarachnoid space, where it is returned to the venous circulation through the arachnoid villi.

to the composition of the brain extracellular fluid (Table 48.3). Humans secrete approximately 500 ml of CSF each day. However, only approximately 150 ml is in the ventricular system at any one time, meaning that the CSF is continuously being absorbed.

The CSF produced in the ventricles must flow through the interventricular foramen, the third ventricle, the cerebral aqueduct, and the fourth ventricle to exit from the ventricular system. Three openings, or foramina, allow the CSF to pass into the subarachnoid space. Two of these, the foramina of Luschka, are located at the lateral corners of the fourth ventricle. The third, the medial foramen of Magendie, is in the midline at the caudal end of the fourth ventricle (Fig. 48.26). Approximately 30% of the CSF passes down into the subarachnoid space that surrounds the spinal cord, mainly on its dorsal surface, and moves back up to the cranial cavity along its ventral surface.

Reabsorption of CSF into the vascular system occurs along the sides of the superior sagittal sinus in the anterior and middle fossae. Here, the waterproof arachnoid has

TABLE 48.3 COMPOSITION OF CEREBROSPINAL FLUID (CSF) COMPARED WITH PLASMA

SUBSTANCE	PLASMA	CSF
Protein g/L	60.0	0.2
Na^+ mmol/L	145.0	141.0
Cl^- mmol/L	101.0	124.0
K^+ mmol/L	4.5	2.9
HCO_3^- mmol/L	25.0	24.0
pH	7.4	7.32
Glucose mmol/L	5.1	3.4

protuberances, the *arachnoid villi*, that penetrate the inner dura and walls of the superior sagittal sinus (Fig. 48.24). Reabsorption of CSF into the vascular system occurs along a pressure gradient. The normal CSF pressure is approximately 130 mm H_2O (10 mm Hg) in the lateral recumbent position, although it may range from as low as 65 mm H_2O to as high as 195 mm H_2O, even in healthy persons. The microstructure of the arachnoid villi are such that if the CSF pressure falls below approximately 50 mm H_2O, the passageways collapse and reverse flow is blocked. Thus, the arachnoid villi function as one-way valves, permitting CSF outflow into the venous blood of the sagittal sinus but not allowing blood to pass into the arachnoid spaces.

Blood–Brain and Cerebrospinal Fluid–Brain Barriers

Maintenance of a chemically stable environment is essential to the function of the brain. In most regions of the body, extracellular fluid undergoes small fluctuations in pH and concentrations of hormones, amino acids, and potassium ions during routine daily activities such as eating and exercising. If the brain were to undergo such fluctuations, the result would be uncontrolled neural activity because some substances such as amino acids act as neurotransmitters, and ions such as potassium influence the threshold for neural firing. Two barriers, the blood–brain barrier and the CSF–brain barrier, provide the means for maintaining the stable chemical environment of the brain. Only water, carbon dioxide, and oxygen enter the brain with relative ease; the transport of other substances between the brain and the blood is slower and more controlled.

The blood–brain barrier depends on the unique characteristics of the brain capillaries. Endothelial cells of brain capillaries are joined by continuous tight junctions. In addition, most brain capillaries are surrounded by a basement membrane and by the processes of the CNS neuroglial cells, called *astrocytes* (Fig. 48.27). The blood–brain barrier permits passage of essential substances while excluding unwanted materials. Reverse transport systems remove materials from the brain. Large molecules, such as proteins and peptides, are largely excluded from crossing the blood–brain barrier. Acute cerebral lesions, such as trauma and infection, increase the permeability of the blood–brain barrier and alter brain concentrations of proteins, water, and electrolytes.

The blood–brain barrier prevents many drugs from entering the brain. Most highly water-soluble compounds are excluded from the brain, especially molecules with high ionic charge such as many of the catecholamines. In contrast, many lipid-soluble molecules cross the lipid layers of the blood–brain barrier with ease. Some drugs, such as the antibiotic chloramphenicol, are highly lipid soluble and therefore enter the brain readily. Other medications have a low solubility in lipids and enter the brain slowly or not at all. Alcohol, nicotine, and heroin are very lipid soluble and rapidly enter the brain. Some substances that enter the capillary endothelium are converted by metabolic processes to a chemical form incapable of moving into the brain.

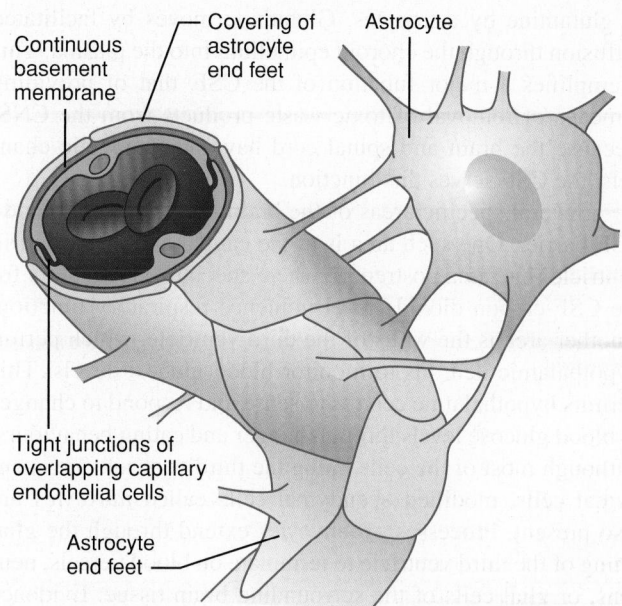

FIGURE 48.27 • The three components of the blood–brain barrier: the astrocyte and astrocyte end feet that encircle the capillary, the capillary basement membrane, and the tight junctions that join the overlapping capillary endothelial cells.

The cerebral capillaries are much more permeable at birth than in adulthood, and the blood–brain barrier develops during the early years of life. In severely jaundiced infants, bilirubin can cross the immature blood–brain barrier, producing kernicterus and brain damage (see Chapter 15). In adults, the mature blood–brain barrier prevents bilirubin from entering the brain, and the nervous system is not affected.

The ependymal cells covering the choroid plexus are linked together by tight junctions, forming a blood–CSF barrier to diffusion of many molecules from the blood plasma of choroid plexus capillaries to the CSF. Water is transported through the choroid epithelial cells by osmosis. Oxygen and carbon dioxide move into the CSF by diffusion, resulting in partial pressures roughly equal to those of plasma. The high sodium and low potassium contents of the CSF are actively regulated and kept relatively constant. Lipids and nonpeptide hormones diffuse through the barrier rather easily, but most large molecules, such as proteins, peptides, many antibiotics, and other medications, do not normally get through. The choroid epithelium uses energy in the form of adenosine triphosphate (ATP) to actively secrete many components into the CSF, including proteins, sodium ions, and several micronutrients such as vitamins C, B_6 (pyridoxine), and folate. Because the resultant CSF has a relatively high sodium content, the negatively charged chloride and bicarbonate diffuse into the CSF along an ionic gradient. The choroid cells also generate bicarbonate from carbon dioxide in the blood. This bicarbonate is important to the regulation of the pH of the CSF.

Mechanisms exist that facilitate the transport of other molecules such as glucose without energy expenditure. Ammonia, a toxic metabolite of neuronal activity, is converted to glutamine by astrocytes. Glutamine moves by facilitated diffusion through the choroid epithelium into the plasma. This exemplifies a major function of the CSF, that of providing a means of removal of toxic waste products from the CNS. Because the brain and spinal cord have no lymphatic channels, the CSF serves this function.

Several specific areas of the brain do not have a blood–CSF barrier. One such area is at the caudal end of the fourth ventricle (*i.e.,* area postrema), where specialized receptors for the CSF carbon dioxide level influence respiratory function. Another area is the walls of the third ventricle, which permit hypothalamic neurons to monitor blood glucose levels. This permits hypothalamic centres to sense and respond to changes in blood glucose levels through hunger and eating behaviours. Although most of the cells lining the third ventricle are ependymal cells, modified ependymal cells called *tanycytes* are also present. Processes of tanycytes extend through the glial lining of the third ventricle to terminate on blood vessels, neurons, or glial cells of the surrounding brain tissue. Evidence suggests that tanycytes may have important neuroendocrine functions besides their function as barrier cells. For example, tanycytes express high levels of the enzyme needed to convert thyroxine (T_4) into the more potent triiodothyronine (T_3) form.

IN SUMMARY

In the adult, the spinal cord is in the upper two thirds of the spinal canal of the vertebral column. On transverse section, the spinal cord has an oval shape. Internally, the grey matter has the appearance of a butterfly or letter "H." The dorsal horns contain the IA neurons and receive afferent information from dorsal root and other connecting neurons. The ventral horns contain the OA neurons and efferent LMNs that leave the cord by the ventral roots.

Thirty-one pairs of spinal nerves (*i.e.,* 8 cervical, 12 thoracic, 5 lumbar, 5 sacral, and 1 or more coccygeal) are present. Each pair communicates with its corresponding body segments. The spinal nerves and the blood vessels that supply the spinal cord enter the spinal canal through an intervertebral foramen. After entering the foramen, they divide into two branches, or roots, one of which enters the dorsolateral surface of the cord (*i.e.,* dorsal root), carrying the axons of afferent neurons into the CNS. The other root leaves the ventrolateral surface of the cord (*i.e.,* ventral root), carrying the axons of efferent neurons into the periphery. These two roots fuse at the intervertebral foramen, forming the mixed spinal nerve.

A reflex provides a highly reliable relation between a stimulus and a motor response. Its anatomic basis consists of an afferent neuron, the connection or synapse with CNS neurons that communicate with the effector neuron, and the effector neuron that innervates a muscle or organ. Reflexes are essentially "wired in" to the CNS in that normally they are always ready to function; with training, most reflexes

can be modulated to become parts of more complicated movements.

The brain can be divided into three parts: the hindbrain, midbrain, and forebrain. The hindbrain, consisting of the medulla oblongata, pons, and cerebellum, contains the neuronal circuits for the eating, breathing, and locomotive functions required for survival. Cranial nerves XII, XI, X, IX, VIII, VII, VI, and V are located in the hindbrain, and CNs III and IV arise from the midbrain. The forebrain is the most rostral part of the brain; it consists of the diencephalon and the telencephalon. The dorsal horn part of the diencephalon comprises the thalamus and subthalamus, and the ventral horn part is the hypothalamus. The telencephalon consists of the cerebrum, including the corpus callosum and subcortical structures such as the basal ganglia and components of the limbic system. The limbic system, which is involved in emotional experience and release of emotional behaviours, is located in the medial aspect of the cerebrum. These cortical areas are reciprocally connected with underlying thalamic nuclei through the internal capsule. Thalamic involvement is essential for normal forebrain function. The cerebral hemispheres are lateral outgrowths of the diencephalon.

The cerebral hemispheres are arbitrarily divided into lobes—the frontal, parietal, temporal, and occipital lobes—named after the bones of the skull that cover them. Contained in the frontal lobe are the prefrontal premotor area and primary motor cortex; the primary sensory cortex and somesthetic association area are in the parietal cortex; the primary auditory cortex and the auditory association area are in the temporal lobe; and the primary visual cortex and association visual cortex are in the occipital lobe.

The brain is enclosed and protected by the pia mater, arachnoid, and dura mater. The protective CSF in which the brain and spinal cord float isolates them from minor and moderate trauma. CSF is secreted into the ventricles by the ependymal cells of the choroid plexus, circulates through the ventricular system, and is reabsorbed into the venous system through the arachnoid villi. The CSF–brain barrier, the arachnoid–CSF barrier, and the blood–brain barrier protect the brain from substances in the blood that would disrupt brain function.

THE AUTONOMIC NERVOUS SYSTEM

After completing this section of the chapter, you should be able to meet the following objectives:

- Compare the sensory and motor components of the autonomic nervous system with those of the CNS.
- Compare the anatomic location and functions of the sympathetic and parasympathetic nervous systems.
- Describe neurotransmitter synthesis, release, degradation, and receptor function in the sympathetic and parasympathetic nervous systems.

The ability to maintain homeostasis and perform the activities of daily living in an ever-changing physical environment is largely vested in the ANS. This portion of the nervous system functions at the subconscious level and is involved in regulating, adjusting, and coordinating vital visceral functions such as blood pressure and blood flow, body temperature, respiration, digestion, metabolism, and elimination. The ANS is strongly affected by emotional influences and is involved in many of the expressive aspects of behaviour. Blushing, pallor, palpitations of the heart, clammy hands, and dry mouth are several emotional expressions mediated through the ANS. Biofeedback and relaxation exercises have been used for modifying the subconscious functions of the ANS.

THE AUTONOMIC NERVOUS SYSTEM (ANS)

- The ANS functions at the subconscious level and is responsible for maintaining homeostatic functions of the body.
- The ANS has two divisions: the sympathetic and parasympathetic systems. Although the two divisions function in concert, they are generally viewed as having opposite and antagonistic actions.
- The sympathetic division functions in maintaining vital functions and responding when there is a critical threat to the integrity of the individual—the "fight-or-flight" response.
- The parasympathetic nervous system is concerned with conservation of energy, resource replenishment, and maintenance of organ function during periods of minimal activity—the "rest-and-digest" response.
- The outflow of both divisions of the ANS consists of a two-neuron pathway: a preganglionic and a postganglionic neuron. Acetylcholine is the neurotransmitter for the preganglionic neurons for both ANS divisions, as well as the postganglionic neurons of the parasympathetic nervous system. Norepinephrine and epinephrine are the neurotransmitters for most sympathetic postganglionic neurons.

As with the somatic nervous system, the ANS is represented in both the CNS and the PNS. Traditionally, the ANS has been defined as a general efferent system innervating visceral organs. The efferent outflow from the ANS has two divisions: the sympathetic nervous system and the parasympathetic nervous system. Afferent inputs to the ANS are provided by visceral afferent neurons and are not usually considered a part of the ANS.

The functions of the sympathetic nervous system include maintaining body temperature and adjusting blood flow and blood pressure to meet the changing needs of the body. These adjustments occur in response to changes in routine activities of daily living, such as moving from the supine to the standing position. The sympathoadrenal system also can discharge as a unit when there is a critical threat to the integrity

of the individual—the so-called *fight-or-flight* response. During a stress situation, the heart rate accelerates; blood pressure rises; blood flow shifts from the skin and gastrointestinal tract to the skeletal muscles and brain; blood sugar increases; the bronchioles and pupils dilate; the sphincters of the stomach and intestine and the internal sphincter of the urethra constrict; and the rate of secretion of exocrine glands involved in digestion diminishes. Emergency situations often require vasoconstriction and shunting of blood away from the skin and into the muscles and brain, a mechanism that, should a wound occur, provides for a reduction in blood flow and preservation of vital functions needed for survival. Sympathetic function is often summarized as "catabolic" in that its actions predominate during periods of pronounced energy expenditure, such as when survival is threatened.

In contrast to the sympathetic nervous system, the functions of the parasympathetic nervous system are concerned with conservation of energy, resource replenishment and storage, and maintenance of organ function during periods of minimal activity—the *rest-and-digest* response. The parasympathetic nervous system slows heart rate, stimulates gastrointestinal function and related glandular secretion, promotes bowel and bladder elimination, and contracts the pupil, protecting the retina from excessive light during periods when visual function is not vital to survival. The two divisions of the ANS are usually viewed as having opposite and antagonistic actions (*i.e.*, if one activates, the other inhibits a function). Exceptions are functions, such as sweating and regulation of arteriolar blood vessel diameter, that are controlled by a single division of the ANS, in this case the sympathetic nervous system.

The sympathetic and parasympathetic nervous systems are continually active. The effect of this continual or basal (baseline) activity is referred to as *tone*. The tone of an effector organ or system can be increased or decreased and is usually regulated by a single division of the ANS. For example, vascular smooth muscle tone is controlled by the sympathetic nervous system. Increased sympathetic activity produces local vasoconstriction from increased vascular smooth muscle tone, and decreased activity results in vasodilation due to decreased tone. In structures such as the sinoatrial node and atrioventricular node of the heart, which are innervated by both divisions of the ANS, one division predominates in controlling tone. In this case, the tonically active parasympathetic nervous system exerts a constraining or braking effect on heart rate, and when parasympathetic outflow is withdrawn, similar to releasing a brake, the heart rate increases. The increase in heart rate that occurs with vagal withdrawal can be further augmented by sympathetic stimulation. Table 48.4 describes the responses of effector organs to sympathetic and parasympathetic impulses.

Autonomic Efferent Pathways

The outflow of both divisions of the ANS follows a two-neuron pathway. The first motor neuron, called the *preganglionic neuron,* lies in the intermediolateral cell column of the spinal cord or its equivalent location in the brain stem. The

TABLE 48.4 CHARACTERISTICS OF THE SYMPATHETIC AND PARASYMPATHETIC NERVOUS SYSTEMS

CHARACTERISTIC	SYMPATHETIC OUTFLOW	PARASYMPATHETIC OUTFLOW
Location of preganglionic cell bodies	T-1–T-12, L-1 and L-2	Cranial nerves: III, VII (intermedius), IX, and X; sacral segments 2, 3, and 4
Relative length of preganglionic fibres	Short—to paravertebral chain of ganglia or to aortic prevertebral of ganglia	Long—to ganglion cells near or in the innervated organ
General function	Catabolic—mobilizes resources in anticipation of challenge for survival (preparation for "fight-or-flight" response)	Anabolic—concerned with conservation, renewal, and storage of resources
Nature of peripheral response	Generalized	Localized
Transmitter between preganglionic terminals and postganglionic neurons	ACh	ACh
Transmitter of postganglionic neuron	ACh (sweat glands and skeletal muscle vasodilator fibres); norepinephrine (most synapses); norepinephrine and epinephrine (secreted by adrenal gland)	ACh

ACh, acetylcholine.

second motor neuron, called the *postganglionic neuron,* synapses with a preganglionic neuron in an autonomic ganglion in the PNS. The two divisions of the ANS differ as to location of their preganglionic cell bodies, the relative length of their preganglionic fibres, the nature of their peripheral responses, and their preganglionic and postganglionic neurotransmitters (see Table 48.4). This two-neuron pathway and the interneurons in the autonomic ganglia that add further modulation to ANS function are distinctly different from arrangements in the somatic nervous system.

Most visceral organs are innervated by both sympathetic and parasympathetic fibres. Exceptions include structures such as blood vessels and sweat glands that have input from only one division of the ANS. The fibres of the sympathetic nervous system are distributed to effectors throughout the body and, as a result, sympathetic actions tend to be more diffuse than those of the parasympathetic nervous system, in which there is a more localized distribution of fibres. The preganglionic fibres of the sympathetic nervous system may traverse a considerable distance and pass through several ganglia before synapsing with postganglionic neurons, and their terminals contact many postganglionic fibres. In some ganglia, the ratio of preganglionic to postganglionic cells may be 1:20; because of this, the effects of sympathetic stimulation are diffuse. Considerable overlap exists, and one ganglion cell may be supplied by several preganglionic fibres. In contrast to the sympathetic nervous system, the parasympathetic nervous system has its postganglionic neurons located very near or in the organ of innervation. Because the ratio of preganglionic to postganglionic communication is often 1:1, the effects of the parasympathetic nervous system are much more circumscribed.

Sympathetic Nervous System

The neurons of the sympathetic nervous system are located primarily in the intermediolateral cell column of the thoracic and upper lumbar segments (T-1 to L-2) of the spinal cord;

hence, the sympathetic nervous system is often called the *thoracolumbar division* of the ANS. These preganglionic neurons have axons that are largely myelinated and relatively short. Postganglionic neurons of the sympathetic nervous system are located in the paravertebral ganglia of the sympathetic chain of ganglia that lie on either side of the vertebral column, or in prevertebral sympathetic ganglia such as the celiac ganglia (Fig. 48.28). Besides postganglionic efferent neurons, the sympathetic ganglia contain neurons of the internuncial, short-axon type, similar to those associated with complex circuitry in the brain and spinal cord. Many of these inhibit and others modulate preganglionic-to-postganglionic transmission.

The axons of the preganglionic neurons leave the spinal cord through the ventral roots of the spinal nerves (T-1 to L-2), enter the ventral primary rami, and leave the spinal nerve through white rami of the rami communicantes to reach the paravertebral ganglionic chain (Fig. 48.29). In the sympathetic chain of ganglia, preganglionic fibres may synapse with neurons of the ganglion they enter, pass up or down the chain and synapse with one or more ganglia, or pass through the chain and move outward through a splanchnic nerve to terminate in prevertebral ganglia (*i.e.,* celiac, superior mesenteric, or inferior mesenteric) scattered along the dorsal aorta and its branches.

Preganglionic fibres from the thoracic segments of the cord pass upward to form the cervical chain connecting the inferior, middle, and superior cervical sympathetic ganglia with the rest of the sympathetic chain at lower levels (Fig. 48.28). Postganglionic sympathetic axons of the cervical and lower lumbosacral chain ganglia spread further through nerve plexuses along continuations of the great arteries. Cranial structures, particularly blood vessels, are innervated by the spread of postganglionic axons along the external and internal carotid arteries into the face and the cranial cavity. The sympathetic fibres from T-1 usually continue up the sympathetic chain into the head; those from T-2 pass into the neck; those from T-1 to T-5 travel to the heart: those from T-3, T-4, T-5,

Sympathetic

A = Superior cervical ganglion
B = Middle cervical ganglion
C = Inferior cervical ganglion

To skin and skeletomuscular system

A
B
C

Greater splanchnic nerve

Lesser splanchnic nerve

1
2
3

1 = Celiac ganglion
2 = Superior mesenteric ganglion
3 = Inferior mesenteric ganglion

Parasympathetic

Ciliary ganglion
Eye
Pterygopalatine ganglion
Lacrimal gland
Submandibular and sublingual glands
Submandibular ganglion
Parotid gland
Otic ganglion
Heart
Trachea
Lung
Liver
Gallbladder
Stomach
Small intestine
Adrenal gland
Kidney
Large intestine
Bladder
Genitalia

III
VII
IX
X
Midbrain
Medulla
Cervical
Thoracic
Lumbar
Sacral

FIGURE 48.28 • The autonomic nervous system. The involuntary organs are depicted with their parasympathetic innervation (craniosacral) indicated on the right and sympathetic innervation (thoracolumbar) on the left. Preganglionic fibres are *solid lines;* postganglionic fibres are *dashed lines.* For purposes of illustration, the sympathetic outflow to the skin and skeletomuscular system is shown separately (to the far left); effectors include sweat glands, pilomotor muscles and blood vessels of the skin, and blood vessels of the skeletal muscles and bones. (Modified from Hemer L. (1983). *The human brain and spinal cord: Functional neuroanatomy and dissection guide.* New York: Springer-Verlag.)

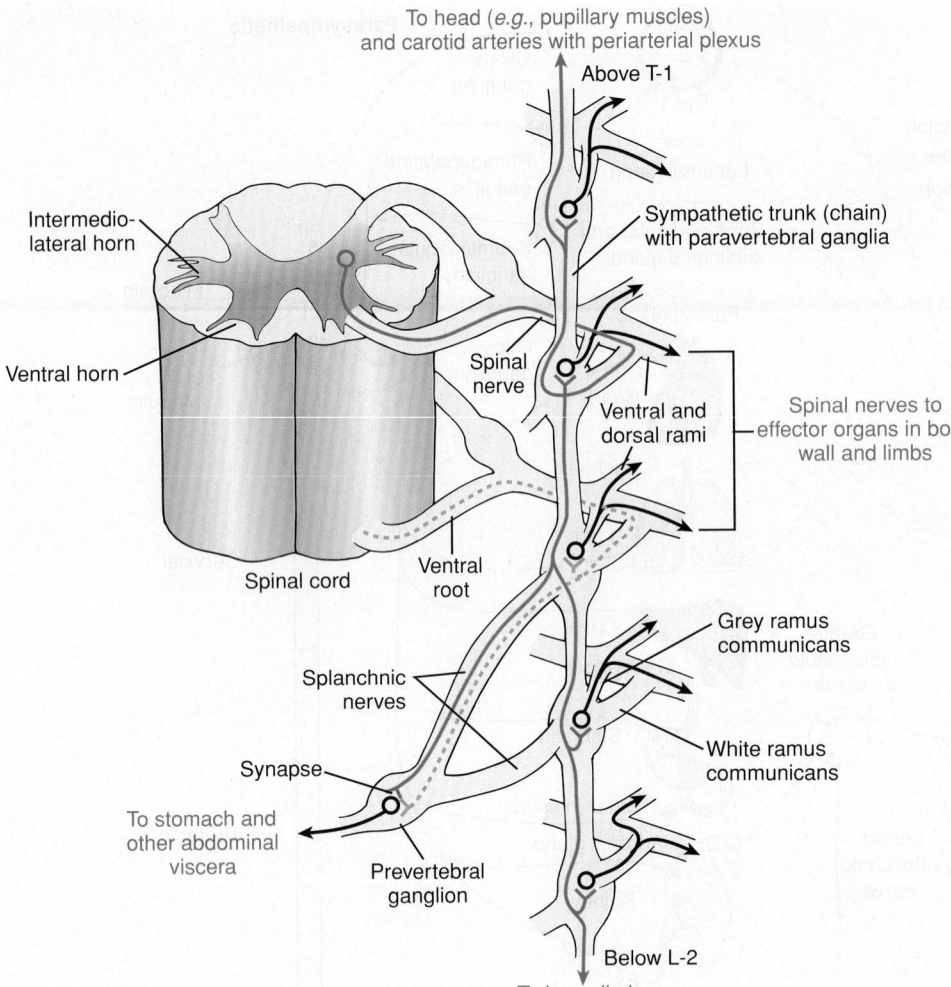

To head (*e.g.*, pupillary muscles)
and carotid arteries with periarterial plexus

Above T-1

Sympathetic trunk (chain)
with paravertebral ganglia

Intermedio-
lateral horn

Ventral horn

Spinal
nerve

Ventral and
dorsal rami

Spinal nerves to
effector organs in body
wall and limbs

Spinal cord

Ventral
root

Grey ramus
communicans

Splanchnic
nerves

White ramus
communicans

Synapse

To stomach and
other abdominal
viscera

Prevertebral
ganglion

Below L-2

To lower limbs

FIGURE 48.29 • Sympathetic pathways. Sympathetic preganglionic fibres (*blue*) leave the spinal cord by way of the ventral root of the spinal nerves, enter the ventral primary rami, and pass through the white rami to the prevertebral or paravertebral ganglia of the sympathetic chain, where they synapse with postganglionic neurons (*black*). Other preganglionic neurons (*red dotted lines*) travel directly to their destination in the various effector organs.

and T-6 proceed to the thoracic viscera; those from T-7, T-8, T-9, T-10, and T-11 pass to the abdominal viscera; and those from T-12, L-1, L-2, and L-3 pass to the kidneys and pelvic organs. Many preganglionic fibres from the fifth to the last thoracolumbar segments pass through the paravertebral ganglia to continue as the splanchnic nerves. Most of these fibres do not synapse until they reach the celiac or superior mesenteric ganglion; others pass to the adrenal medulla.

The adrenal medulla, which is part of the sympathetic nervous system, contains postganglionic sympathetic neurons that secrete sympathetic neurotransmitters directly into the bloodstream. Some postganglionic fibres, all of which are unmyelinated, exit the paravertebral ganglionic chain and reenter the segmental nerve through unmyelinated branches, called *grey rami*. These segmental nerves are then distributed to all parts of the body wall in the spinal nerve branches. These fibres innervate the sweat glands, piloerector muscles of the hair follicles, all blood vessels of the skin and skeletal muscles, and the CNS itself.

Parasympathetic Nervous System

The preganglionic fibres of the parasympathetic nervous system, also called the *craniosacral division* of the ANS,

originate in some segments of the brain stem and the sacral segments of the spinal cord (Fig. 48.28). The central regions of origin are the midbrain, pons, medulla oblongata, and the sacral spinal cord. The midbrain outflow passes through the oculomotor nerve (CN III) to the ciliary ganglion that lies in the orbit behind the eye; it supplies the pupillary sphincter muscle of each eye and the ciliary muscles that control lens thickness for accommodation. From the caudal pontine outflow originate the preganglionic fibres of the intermedius component of the facial nerve (CN VII) complex. This outflow synapses in the submandibular ganglion, which sends postganglionic fibres to supply the submandibular and sublingual glands. In addition, preganglionic fibres are distributed to the pterygopalatine ganglia to synapse on postganglionic neurons that supply the lacrimal and nasal glands. Fibres in the glossopharyngeal nerve (CN IX) synapse in the otic ganglia, which supply the parotid salivary glands. Approximately 75% of parasympathetic efferent fibres are carried in the vagus nerve (CN X). The vagus nerve provides parasympathetic innervation for the heart, trachea, lungs, esophagus, stomach, small intestine, proximal half of the colon, liver, gallbladder, pancreas, kidneys, and upper portions of the ureters. The gastrointestinal tract has its own intrinsic network of ganglionic cells located between the smooth muscle layers, called the *enteric nervous system,* which controls local peristaltic and secretory functions (see Chapter 38). The action of the enteric nervous system can be modified by the activity of the ANS.

Sacral preganglionic axons leave the S-2 to S-4 segmental nerves by gathering into the pelvic nerves, also called the *nervi erigentes.* The pelvic nerves leave the sacral plexus on each side of the cord and distribute their peripheral fibres to the bladder, uterus, urethra, prostate, distal portion of the transverse colon, descending colon, and rectum. Sacral parasympathetic fibres also supply the venous outflow from the external genitalia to facilitate erectile function.

Except for CNs III, VII, and IX, which synapse in discrete ganglia, the long parasympathetic preganglionic fibres pass uninterrupted to short postganglionic fibres in the organ walls. In the walls of these organs, postganglionic neurons send axons to smooth muscle and glandular cells that modulate their functions.

Central Integrative Pathways

General visceral afferent fibres accompany the sympathetic and parasympathetic outflow into the spinal and cranial nerves, bringing chemoreceptor, pressure, organ capsule stretch, and nociceptive information from organs of the viscera to the brain stem, thoracolumbar cord, and sacral cord. Local reflex circuits relating visceral afferent and autonomic efferent activity are integrated into a hierarchic control system in the spinal cord and brain stem. Progressively greater complexity in the responses and greater precision in their control occur at each higher level of the nervous system. Most visceral reflexes contain contributions from the LMNs that innervate skeletal muscles as part of their response patterns. The distinction between purely visceral and somatic reflex hierarchies becomes less and less meaningful at the higher levels of hierarchic control and behavioural integration.

For most autonomically mediated functions, the hypothalamus serves as the major control centre. The hypothalamus, with connections to the cerebral cortex, the limbic system, and the pituitary gland, is in a prime position to receive, integrate, and transmit information to other areas of the nervous system. Signals from the hypothalamus can affect almost all the brain stem control centres. For example, stimulation of certain areas, mainly in the posterior hypothalamus, can cause the cardiovascular control centres to increase the arterial blood pressure to more than twice normal. Likewise, other hypothalamic centres control body temperature and increase salivation and gastrointestinal activity.

Reflex adjustments of cardiovascular and respiratory function occur at the level of the brain stem. A prominent example is the carotid sinus baroreflex. Increased blood pressure in the carotid sinus results in increased discharge from afferent fibres that travel by way of CN IX to cardiovascular centres in the brain stem. These centres increase the activity of descending efferent vagal fibres that slow heart rate, while inhibiting sympathetic fibres that increase heart rate and

blood vessel tone. Striking features of the ANS are the rapidity and intensity with which it can change visceral function. Within 3 to 5 seconds, it can increase the heart rate to approximately twice its resting level. Bronchial smooth muscle tone is largely controlled by parasympathetic fibres carried in the vagus nerve. These nerves produce mild to moderate constriction of the bronchioles.

Other important ANS reflexes are located at the level of the spinal cord. As with other spinal reflexes, these reflexes are modulated by input from higher centres. When there is a loss of communication between the higher centres and the spinal reflexes, as occurs in spinal cord injury, these reflexes function in an unregulated manner (see Chapter 50). This results in uncontrolled sweating, vasomotor instability, and reflex bowel and bladder function.

Autonomic Neurotransmission

The generation and transmission of impulses in the ANS occur in the same manner as in other neurons. There are self-propagating action potentials with transmission of impulses across synapses and other tissue junctions by neurohumoral transmitters. However, the somatic motor neurons that innervate skeletal muscles divide into many branches, with each branch innervating a single muscle fibre; in contrast, the distribution of postganglionic fibres of the ANS forms a diffuse neural plexus at the site of innervation. The membranes of the cells of many smooth muscle fibres are connected by conductive protoplasmic bridges, called *gap junctions,* that permit rapid conduction of impulses through whole sheets of smooth muscle, often in repeating waves of contraction. Autonomic neurotransmitters released near a limited portion of these fibres provide a modulating function extending to many effector cells. Smooth muscle layers of the gut and of the bladder wall are examples. Sometimes, isolated smooth muscle cells are individually innervated by the ANS, such as the piloerector cells that elevate the hair on the skin during cold exposure.

The main neurotransmitters of the ANS are acetylcholine and the catecholamines, epinephrine and norepinephrine (Fig. 48.30). Acetylcholine is released at all preganglionic synapses in the autonomic ganglia of both sympathetic and parasympathetic nerve fibres and from postganglionic synapses of all parasympathetic nerve endings. It also is released at sympathetic nerve endings that innervate the sweat glands and cholinergic vasodilator fibres found in skeletal muscle. Norepinephrine is released at most sympathetic nerve endings. The adrenal medulla, which is a modified prevertebral sympathetic ganglion, produces epinephrine along with small amounts of norepinephrine. Dopamine, which is an intermediate compound in the synthesis of norepinephrine, also acts as a neurotransmitter. It is the principal inhibitory transmitter of internuncial neurons in the sympathetic ganglia. It also has vasodilator effects on renal, splanchnic, and coronary blood vessels when given intravenously and is sometimes used in the treatment of shock (see Chapter 26).

FIGURE 48.30 • Comparison of neurotransmission in the somatic and autonomic nervous systems. In the somatic nervous system, all lower motor neurons release acetylcholine (ACh) as their neurotransmitter. In the autonomic nervous system, both sympathetic and parasympathetic preganglionic neurons release ACh as their neurotransmitter. Parasympathetic postganglionic neurons release ACh at the site of organ innervation. Most postganglionic neurons of the sympathetic nervous system release norepinephrine (NE) at the site of organ innervation. The principal neurotransmitter released by the adrenal gland is epinephrine (Epi), which travels to the site of organ innervation through the bloodstream. The postganglionic neurons innervating the sweat gland are sympathetic fibres that use ACh as their neurotransmitter.

Acetylcholine and Cholinergic Receptors

Acetylcholine (ACh) is synthesized in the cholinergic neurons from choline and acetyl coenzyme A (acetyl CoA; Fig. 48.31). After acetylcholine is secreted by the cholinergic nerve endings, it is rapidly broken down by the enzyme acetylcholinesterase (AChE). The choline molecule is transported back into the nerve ending, where it is used again in the synthesis of acetylcholine.

Receptors that respond to acetylcholine are called *cholinergic receptors*. Two types of cholinergic receptors are known: muscarinic and nicotinic. Muscarinic receptors are present on the innervational targets of postganglionic fibres of the parasympathetic nervous system and the sweat glands, which are innervated by the sympathetic nervous system. Nicotinic receptors are found in autonomic ganglia and the end plates of skeletal muscle. Acetylcholine is excitatory to most muscarinic and nicotinic receptors, except those in the heart and lower esophagus, where it has an inhibitory effect. The drug atropine is an antimuscarinic or muscarinic cholinergic blocking drug that prevents the action of acetylcholine at excitatory and inhibitory muscarinic receptor sites. Because it is a muscarinic blocking drug, it exerts little effect at nicotinic receptor sites.

Catecholamines and Adrenergic Receptors

The catecholamines, which include norepinephrine, epinephrine, and dopamine, are synthesized in the axoplasm of sympathetic nerve terminal endings from the amino acid tyrosine (Fig. 48.31). During catecholamine synthesis, tyrosine is hydroxylated (*i.e.,* has a hydroxyl group added) to form DOPA, and DOPA is decarboxylated (*i.e.,* has a carboxyl group removed) to form dopamine. Dopamine in turn is hydroxylated to form norepinephrine. In the adrenal gland, an additional step occurs during which norepinephrine is methylated (*i.e.,* a methyl group is added) to form epinephrine.

Each step in sympathetic neurotransmitter synthesis requires a different enzyme, and the type of neurotransmitter produced depends on the types of enzymes that are available in a nerve terminal. For example, the postganglionic sympathetic neurons that supply blood vessels synthesize norepinephrine, but postganglionic neurons in the adrenal medulla produce epinephrine or norepinephrine. Epinephrine accounts for approximately 80% of the catecholamines released from the adrenal gland. The synthesis of epinephrine by the adrenal medulla is influenced by glucocorticoid secretion from the adrenal cortex. These hormones are transported through an intra-adrenal vascular network from the adrenal cortex to the adrenal medulla, where they cause the sympathetic neurons to increase their production of epinephrine through increased enzyme activity. Thus, any situation sufficiently stressful to evoke increased levels of glucocorticoids also increases epinephrine levels. As the catecholamines are synthesized, they are stored in vesicles. The final step of norepinephrine synthesis occurs in these vesicles. When an action potential reaches an axon terminal, the neurotransmitter molecules are released from the storage vesicles. The storage vesicles provide a means for concentrated storage of the catecholamines and protect the neurotransmitters from the cytoplasmic enzymes that degrade them.

Besides neuronal synthesis, a second major mechanism exists for the replenishment of norepinephrine in sympathetic nerve terminals. This mechanism consists of the active recapture or reuptake of the released neurotransmitter into the nerve terminal. Between 50% and 80% of the norepinephrine released during an action potential is removed from the synaptic area by an active reuptake process. This process stops the action of the neurotransmitter and allows it to be reused by the neuron. The

FIGURE 48.31 • Schematic illustration of cholinergic parasympathetic (**A**) and noradrenergic sympathetic (**B**) neurotransmitter synthesis, release, receptor binding, neurotransmitter degradation, and metabolite transport back into the presynaptic neuron (acetylcholine) and reuptake (norepinephrine). COMT, catechol-*O*-methyltransferase.

remainder of the released catecholamines diffuses into the surrounding tissue fluids or is degraded by two special enzymes: catechol-*O*-methyltransferase, which is diffusely present in all tissues, and monoamine oxidase (MAO), which is found in the nerve endings. Some drugs, such as the tricyclic antidepressants, are thought to increase the level of catecholamines at the site of nerve endings in the brain by blocking the reuptake process. Others, such as the MAO inhibitors, increase the levels of neurotransmitters by decreasing their enzymatic degradation.

Catecholamines can cause excitation or inhibition of smooth muscle contraction, depending on the site, dose, and type of receptor present. Norepinephrine has potent excitatory activity and low inhibitory activity. Epinephrine is potent as both an excitatory and an inhibitory agent. The excitatory or inhibitory responses of organs to sympathetic neurotransmitters are mediated by interaction with special structures in the cell membrane called *adrenergic receptors*. In 1948, Ahlquist proposed the designations α and β for the receptor sites where catecholamines produce their excitatory (α) and inhibitory (β) effects.

In vascular smooth muscle, excitation of α receptors causes vasoconstriction, and excitation of β receptors causes vasodilation. Endogenously and exogenously administered norepinephrine produces marked vasoconstriction of the blood vessels in the skin, kidneys, and splanchnic circulation that are supplied with α receptors. The β receptors are most prevalent in the heart, the blood vessels of skeletal muscle, and the bronchioles. Blood vessels in skeletal muscle have α and β receptors. In these vessels, high levels of norepinephrine produce vasoconstriction; low levels produce vasodilation. The low levels are thought to have a diluting effect on norepinephrine levels in the arteries of these blood vessels so that the β effect predominates. With respect to vessels having few α receptors, such as those that supply the lungs, brain, and heart, norepinephrine has little effect.

α-Adrenergic receptors have been further subdivided into α_1 and α_2 receptors, and β-adrenergic receptors into β_1, β_2, and β_3 receptors. β_1-Adrenergic receptors are found primarily in the heart and can be selectively blocked by β_1 receptor blocking drugs. β_2-Adrenergic receptors are found in the bronchioles and in other sites that have β-mediated functions whereas β_3 adrenergic receptors are found in adipose tissue and impact energy metabolism. α_1-Adrenergic receptors are found primarily in postsynaptic effector sites; they mediate responses in vascular smooth muscle. α_2-Adrenergic receptors are mainly located presynaptically and can inhibit the release of norepinephrine from sympathetic nerve terminals. α_2-Adrenergic receptors are abundant in the CNS and are thought to influence the central control of blood pressure.

The various classes of adrenergic receptors provide a mechanism by which the same adrenergic neurotransmitter can have many selective effects on different effector cells. This mechanism also permits neurotransmitters carried in the bloodstream, whether from neuroendocrine secretion by the adrenal gland or from subcutaneously or intravenously administered drugs, to produce the same effects. The catecholamines produced and released from sympathetic nerve endings are called *endogenous neuromediators*. Sympathetic nerve endings also can be activated by exogenous forms of these neuromediators, which reach the nerve endings through the bloodstream after being injected into the body or administered orally. These drugs mimic the action of the neuromediators and are said to have a *sympathomimetic action*. Other drugs can selectively block the receptor sites on the neurons and temporarily prevent the neurotransmitter from exerting its action.

IN SUMMARY

The ANS regulates, adjusts, and coordinates the visceral functions of the body. The ANS, which is divided into the sympathetic and parasympathetic systems, is an efferent system. It receives its afferent input from visceral afferent neurons. The ANS has CNS and PNS components. The outflow of the sympathetic and parasympathetic nervous systems follows a two-neuron pathway, which consists of a preganglionic neuron in the CNS and a postganglionic neuron located outside the CNS. Sympathetic fibres leave the CNS at the thoracolumbar level, and the parasympathetic fibres leave at the cranial and sacral levels. Usually, the sympathetic and parasympathetic nervous systems have opposing effects on visceral function—if one excites, the other inhibits. The hypothalamus serves as the major control centre for most ANS functions; local reflex circuits relating visceral afferent and autonomic efferent activity are integrated in a hierarchic control system in the spinal cord and brain stem.

The main neurotransmitters for the ANS are acetylcholine and the catecholamines, epinephrine and norepinephrine. Acetylcholine is the transmitter for all preganglionic neurons, for postganglionic parasympathetic neurons, and for selected postganglionic sympathetic neurons. The catecholamines are the neurotransmitters for most postganglionic sympathetic neurons. Neurotransmitters exert their target action through specialized cell surface receptors—cholinergic receptors that bind acetylcholine and adrenergic receptors that bind the catecholamines. The cholinergic receptors are divided into nicotinic and muscarinic receptors, and adrenergic receptors are divided into α and β receptors. Different receptors for the same transmitter at various sites in the same tissue or in other tissues result in differences in tissue responses to the same transmitter. This arrangement also permits the use of pharmacologic agents that act at specific receptor types.

REVIEW EXERCISES

1. Herpes zoster or shingles is a painful vesicular skin eruption involving the dermatomal distribution of a general somatic afferent nerve that is caused by reactivation of the chickenpox virus (varicella-zoster virus) that has remained dormant in the dorsal root ganglion since a childhood infection.
   A. *Explain.*
2. An event such as cardiac arrest, which produces global ischemia of the brain, can produce a selective loss of recent memory and cognitive skills, while the more vegetative and life-sustaining functions such as breathing are preserved.
   A. *Use principles related to the development of the nervous system and hierarchy of control to explain why.*
3. Usually spinal cord injury or disease produces both sensory and motor deficits. An exception is infection by the poliomyelitis virus, which produces weakness and paralysis without loss of sensation in the affected extremities.
   A. *Explain, using information on the cell column organization of the spinal cord.*
4. The functions of the sympathetic nervous system are often described in relation to the "fight-or-flight" response. Using this description, explain the physiologic advantage for the following distribution of sympathetic nervous system receptors:
   A. *The presence of β_2 receptors on the blood vessels that provide blood flow to the skeletal muscles during "fight or flight," and the presence of α_1 receptors on the resistance vessels that control blood pressure.*
   B. *The presence of acetylcholine receptors on the sweat glands that allow for evaporative loss of body heat during "fight or flight," and the presence of α_1 receptors that constrict the skin vessels that control blood flow to the skin.*
   C. *The presence of β_2 receptors that produce relaxation in the detrusor muscle of the bladder during "fight or flight," and the presence of α_1 receptors that produce contraction of the smooth muscle in the internal sphincter of the bladder.*

Bibliography

Albert B., Johnson A., Lewis J., et al. (2015). *Molecular biology of the cell* (6th ed.). New York: Garland Science.

Bear M. F., Connors B. W., Paradiso M. A. (2016). *Neuroscience: Exploring the brain* (4th ed.). Philadelphia, PA: Lippincott Williams & Wilkins.

Boron W. F., Boulpaep E. L. (2009). *Medical physiology* (2nd ed.). Philadelphia, PA: Saunders.

Carlson B. M. (2014). *Human embryology and developmental biology* (5th ed.). Philadelphia, PA: Elsevier Saunders.

Cochard L. R. (2012). *Netter's atlas of human embryology* (Updated ed.). Philadelphia, PA: Elsevier Saunders.

Filosa J. A., Bonev A. D., Straub S. V., et al. (2006). Local potassium signaling couples neuronal activity to vasodilation in the brain. *Nature Neuroscience, 9*, 1397–1403.

Hall J. E. (2011). *Textbook of medical physiology* (12th ed.). Philadelphia, PA: W. B. Saunders.

Hickey J. V. (2014). *The clinical practice of neurological and neurosurgical nursing* (7th ed.). Philadelphia, PA: Lippincott Williams & Wilkins.

Melmed S., Polonsky K. S., Larsen P. R., et al. (2011). *Williams textbook of endocrinology* (12th ed.). Philadelphia: Elsevier Saunders.

Moore K. L., Dalley A. F., Agur A. M. R. (2014). *Clinically oriented anatomy* (7th ed.). Philadelphia, PA: Lippincott Williams & Wilkins.

Moore K. L., Persaud T. V. N., Torchia M. G. (2013). *The developing human: Clinically oriented embryology* (9th ed.). Philadelphia, PA: Saunders Elsevier.

Rhoades R. A., Bell D. R. (2013). *Medical physiology: Principles for clinical medicine* (4th ed.). Philadelphia, PA: Lippincott Williams & Wilkins.

Roberts S. A., Lloyd A. C. (2012). Aspects of cell growth control illustrated by the Schwann cell. *Current Opinion in Cell Biology, 24*(6), 852–857.

Snell R. S. (2010). *Clinical neuroanatomy* (7th ed.). Philadelphia, PA: Lippincott Williams & Wilkins.

Squire L. R., Berg D., Bloom F. E., et al. (2013). *Fundamental neuroscience* (4th ed.). Boston, MA: Academic Press.

Tortora G. J., Derrickson B. (2014). *Principles of anatomy and physiology* (14th ed.). Hoboken, NJ: John Wiley & Sons.

Visit thePoint, **http://thePoint.lww.com for animations, journal articles, and more!**

Somatosensory Function, Pain, and Headache

49

Sensory mechanisms provide individuals with a continuous stream of information about their bodies, the outside world, and the interactions between the two. The somatosensory component of the nervous system provides an awareness of body sensations such as touch, temperature, limb position, and pain. Other sensory components of the nervous system include the special senses of vision, hearing, smell, and taste, which are discussed in other chapters. The sensory receptors for somatosensory function consist of discrete nerve endings in the skin and other body tissues. Between 2 and 3 million sensory neurons deliver a steady stream of encoded information. Only a small proportion of this information reaches awareness; most provides input essential for a myriad of reflex and automatic mechanisms that keep us alive and manage our functioning.

This chapter is organized into two distinct parts. The first part describes the organization and control of somatosensory function, and the second focuses on pain as a somatosensory modality.

ORGANIZATION AND CONTROL OF SOMATOSENSORY FUNCTION

After completing this section of the chapter, you should be able to meet the following objectives:

- Describe the four major classes of somatosensory modalities.
- Describe the organization of the somatosensory system in terms of first-, second-, and third-order neurons.

- Characterize the structure and function of the dorsal root ganglion neurons in terms of sensory receptors, conduction velocities, and spinal cord projections.
- Compare the discriminative pathway with the anterolateral pathway, and explain the clinical usefulness of this distinction.
- Compare the tactile, thermal, and position sense modalities in terms of receptors, adequate stimuli, ascending pathways, and central integrative mechanisms.
- Describe the role of clinical examination in assessing somatosensory function.

The somatosensory system is designed to provide the central nervous system (CNS) with information related to deep and superficial body structures as compared with the special senses such as sight and hearing. Sensory neurons can be divided into three types that vary in distribution and the type of sensation detected: general somatic, special somatic, and general visceral. *General somatic afferent neurons* have branches with widespread distribution throughout the body and with many distinct types of receptors that result in sensations such as pain, touch, and temperature. *Special somatic afferent neurons* have receptors located primarily in muscles, tendons, and joints. These receptors sense position and movement of the body. *General visceral afferent neurons* have receptors on various visceral structures that sense fullness and discomfort.

Sensory Systems

Sensory systems can be conceptualized as a serial succession of neurons consisting of first-order, second-order, and third-order neurons. *First-order neurons* transmit pain, temperature, and light touch (sensory information) from the periphery to the CNS. *Second-order neurons* within the spinothalamic tract convey pain and temperature sensation through the spinal cord directly to the thalamus. *Third-order neurons* relay information from the thalamus to the cerebral cortex (Fig. 49.1).

This organizing framework corresponds with the three primary levels of neural integration in the somatosensory system: the sensory units, which contain the sensory receptors; the ascending pathways; and the central processing centres in the thalamus and cerebral cortex. Sensory information usually is relayed and processed in a cephalad (toward the head) direction by the three orders of neurons. Many interneurons process and modify the sensory information at the level of the second- and third-order neurons, and many more participate before coordinated and appropriate learned-movement responses occur. The number of participating neurons increases exponentially from the primary through the secondary and the secondary through the tertiary levels.

The Sensory Unit

The somatosensory experience arises from information provided by a variety of receptors distributed throughout the

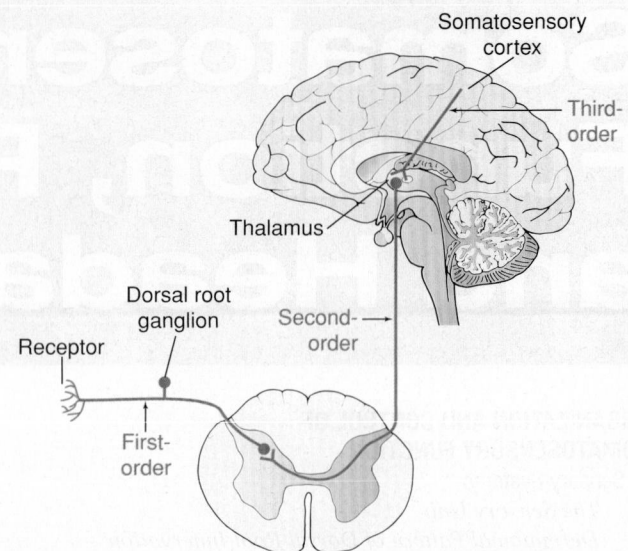

FIGURE 49.1 • Arrangement of first-order, second-order, and third-order neurons of the somatosensory system.

body. These receptors monitor four major types or modalities of sensation: discriminative touch, which is required to identify the size and shape of objects and their movement across the skin; temperature sensation; sense of movement of the limbs and joints of the body; and nociception, or pain.

Each of the somatosensory modalities is mediated by a distinct system of receptors and pathways to the brain; however, all somatosensory information from the limbs and trunk shares a common class of sensory neurons called *dorsal root ganglion neurons*. Somatosensory information from the face and cranial structures is transmitted by the trigeminal sensory neurons, which function in the same manner as the dorsal root ganglion neurons. The cell body of the dorsal root ganglion neuron, its peripheral branch (which innervates a small area of periphery), and its central axon (which projects to the CNS) form what is called a *sensory unit*.

THE SOMATOSENSORY SYSTEM

- The somatosensory system relays information about four major modalities: touch, temperature, pain, and body position.
- The system is organized segmentally into dermatomes, with each segment supplied by a single dorsal root ganglion that contains the neuronal cell bodies for the sensory units of the segment.
- Somatosensory information is sequentially transmitted over three types of neurons: first-order neurons, which transmit information from sensory receptors to dorsal horn neurons; second-order CNS association neurons, which communicate with various reflex circuits and transmit information to the thalamus; and third-order neurons, which forward the information from the thalamus to the sensory cortex.

FIGURE 49.2 • Cutaneous distribution of spinal nerves (dermatomes) based on the studies of Foerster (1933). (From Barr M. (1993). *The human nervous system*. New York: Harper & Row.)

The fibres of different dorsal root ganglion neurons conduct impulses at varying rates, ranging from 0.5 to 120 m/sec. This rate depends on the diameter of the nerve fibre. There are three types of nerve fibres that transmit somatosensory information: types A, B, and C. Type A fibres, which are myelinated, have the fastest rate of conduction.[1,2] Type A fibres convey cutaneous pressure and touch sensation, cold sensation, mechanical pain, and heat pain. Type B fibres, which also are myelinated, transmit information from cutaneous and subcutaneous mechanoreceptors. The unmyelinated type C fibres have the smallest diameter and the slowest rate of conduction. They convey warm–hot, mechanical and chemical sensation, as well as heat- and cold-induced pain sensation.

Dermatomal Pattern of Dorsal Root Innervation

The somatosensory innervation of the body, including the head, retains a basic segmental organizational pattern that was established during embryonic development. Thirty-three paired spinal (*i.e.,* segmental) nerves provide sensory and motor innervation of the body wall, the limbs, and the viscera (see Chapter 48). Sensory input to each spinal cord segment is provided by sensory neurons with cell bodies in the dorsal root ganglia.

The region of the body wall that is supplied by a single pair of dorsal root ganglia is called a *dermatome*. These dorsal root ganglion-innervated strips occur in a regular sequence moving upward from the second coccygeal segment through the cervical segments, reflecting the basic segmental organization of the body and the nervous system (Fig. 49.2). The cranial nerves that innervate the head send their axons to equivalent nuclei in the brain stem. Neighbouring dermatomes overlap one another sufficiently so that a loss of one dorsal root or root ganglion results in reduced but not total loss of sensory innervation of a dermatome (Fig. 49.3). Dermatome maps are helpful in interpreting the level and extent of sensory deficits that are the result of segmental nerve and spinal cord damage.

Spinal Circuitry and Ascending Neural Pathways

On entry into the spinal cord, the central axons of the somatosensory neurons branch extensively and project to neurons in the spinal cord grey matter. Some branches become involved in local spinal cord reflexes and directly initiate motor reflexes (*e.g.,* flexor-withdrawal reflex). Two parallel pathways, the *discriminative pathway* and the *anterolateral pathway,* carry the information from the spinal cord to the thalamic level of sensation, each taking a different route through the CNS. The

Central
processes

Dorsal
root ganglia

Peripheral
processes

Dermatomes

FIGURE 49.3 • The dermatomes formed by the peripheral processes of adjacent spinal nerves overlap on the body surface. The central processes of these fibres also overlap in their spinal distribution.

discriminative pathway crosses at the base of the medulla and the anterolateral pathway crosses within the first few segments of entering the spinal cord. These pathways relay information to the brain for three purposes: perception, arousal, and motor control. Having a two-pathway system has several advantages. It adds richness to the sensory input by allowing

sensory information to be handled in two different ways, and it ensures that if one pathway is damaged, the other still can provide input.

The Discriminative Pathway. The discriminative pathway, also known as the dorsal column-medial lemniscal pathway, is used for the rapid transmission of sensory information such as discriminative touch. It contains branches of primary afferent axons that travel up the ipsilateral (*i.e.,* same side) dorsal columns of the spinal cord white matter and synapse with highly evolved somatosensory input association neurons in the medulla. The discriminative pathway uses only three neurons to transmit information from a sensory receptor to the somatosensory strip of the parietal cerebral cortex of the opposite side of the brain: (1) the primary dorsal root ganglion neuron, which projects its central axon to the dorsal column nuclei; (2) the dorsal column neuron, which sends its axon through a rapid conducting tract, called the *medial lemniscus,* that crosses at the base of the medulla and travels to the thalamus on the opposite side of the brain, where basic sensation begins; and (3) the thalamic neuron, which projects its axons through the somatosensory radiation to the primary sensory cortex[1] (Fig. 49.4A). The medial lemniscus is joined by fibres

Primary
somatosensory
cortex

Thalamus

Medulla

Dorsal root
ganglion

Dorsal
column

A

Spinal cord

Somatosensory
and other areas
of cerebral cortex

Reticular formation

Paleospinothalamic tract
Neospinothalamic tract

Dorsal horn

B

Spinal cord

FIGURE 49.4 • **A:** Rapid-transmitting discriminative (dorsal column–medial lemniscal) pathway carrying axons mediating tactile sensation and proprioception. **B:** Neospinothalamic and paleospinothalamic subdivisions of the anterolateral sensory pathway. The neurons of anterolateral pathways cross within the same segment as the cell body and ascend in the contralateral side of the spinal cord. The neospinothalamic tract travels mainly to thalamic nuclei that have third-order fibres projecting to the somatosensory cortex. The paleospinothalamic tract sends collaterals to the reticular formation and other structures, from which further fibres project to the thalamus.

from the sensory nucleus of the trigeminal nerve (cranial nerve V) that supplies the face. Sensory information arriving at the sensory cortex by this route can be discretely localized and discriminated in terms of intensity.

One of the distinct features of the discriminative pathway is that it relays precise information regarding spatial orientation. This is the only pathway taken by the sensations of muscle and joint movement, vibration, and delicate discriminative touch, which is required to differentiate correctly the location of touch on the skin at two neighbouring points (*i.e.,* two-point discrimination). One of the important functions of the discriminative pathway is to integrate the input from multiple receptors. Recognition of the sense of shape and size of an object in the absence of visualization, called *stereognosis,* is based on precise afferent information from muscle, tendon, and joint receptors. For example, a screwdriver is perceived as being different from a knife in terms of its texture (tactile sensibility) and shape based on the relative position of the fingers as they move over the object. This complex interpretive perception requires that both the discriminative system and the higher-order parietal association cortex are functioning properly. If the discriminative somatosensory pathway is functional but the parietal association cortex has become discretely damaged, the person can correctly describe the object but does not recognize that it is a screwdriver. This deficit is called *astereognosis.*

The Anterolateral Pathway. The anterolateral pathways (anterior and lateral spinothalamic pathways) consist of bilateral, multisynaptic, slow-conducting tracts (see Chapter 48, Fig. 48.14). These pathways provide for transmission of sensory information such as pain, thermal sensations, crude touch, and pressure that does not require discrete localization of signal source or fine discrimination of intensity. The fibres of the anterolateral pathway originate in the dorsal horns at the level of the segmental nerve, where the dorsal root neurons enter the spinal cord. They cross in the anterior commissure, within a few segments of origin, to the opposite anterolateral pathway, where they ascend upward toward the brain. The spinothalamic tract fibres synapse with several nuclei in the thalamus, but en route they give off numerous branches that travel to the reticular activating system of the brain stem. These projections provide the basis for increased wakefulness or awareness after strong somatosensory stimulation and for the generalized startle reaction that occurs with sudden and intense stimuli. They also stimulate autonomic nervous system responses, such as a rise in heart rate and blood pressure, dilation of the pupils, and the pale, moist skin that results from constriction of the cutaneous blood vessels and activation of the sweat glands.

There are two subdivisions in the anterolateral pathway: the *neospinothalamic tract* and the *paleospinothalamic tract*[1] (Fig. 49.4B). The neospinothalamic tract consists of a sequence of at least three neurons with long axons. It provides for relatively fast transmission of localized, acute and sharp pain sensations to the thalamus. The paleospinothalamic

pathway consists of bilateral, multisynaptic, slow-conducting tracts that transit sensory signals such as diffuse aching and throbbing sensations that do not require discrete localization or discrimination of fine gradations in intensity. This slower-conducting pathway also projects into the intralaminar nuclei of the thalamus, which have close connections with the limbic cortical systems. This circuitry gives touch its affective or emotional aspects, such as the particular unpleasantness of heavy pressure and the peculiar pleasantness of the tickling and gentle rubbing of the skin.

Central Processing of Somatosensory Information

Perception, or the final processing of somatosensory information, involves awareness of the stimuli, localization and discrimination of their characteristics, and interpretation of their meaning. As sensory information reaches the thalamus, it begins to enter the level of consciousness. In the thalamus, the sensory information is roughly localized and perceived as a crude sense. The full localization, discrimination of the intensity, and interpretation of the meaning of the stimuli require processing by the somatosensory cortex.

The somatosensory cortex is located in the parietal lobe, which lies behind the central sulcus and above the lateral sulcus (Fig. 49.5). The strip of parietal cortex that borders the central sulcus is called the *primary somatosensory cortex* because it receives primary sensory information by direct projections from the thalamus. A distorted map of the body and head surface, called the *sensory homunculus,* reflects the density of cortical neurons devoted to sensory input from afferents in corresponding peripheral areas. As depicted in Figure 49.6, most of the cortical surface is devoted to areas

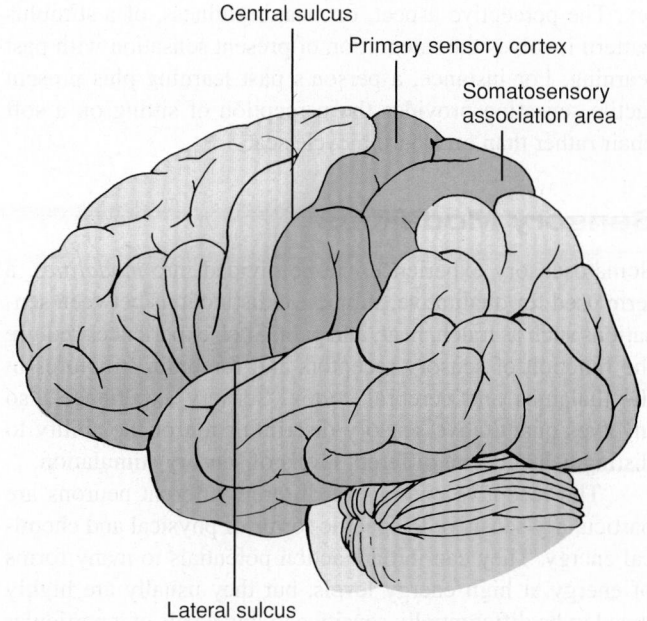

FIGURE 49.5 • Primary somatosensory cortex and somatosensory association area.

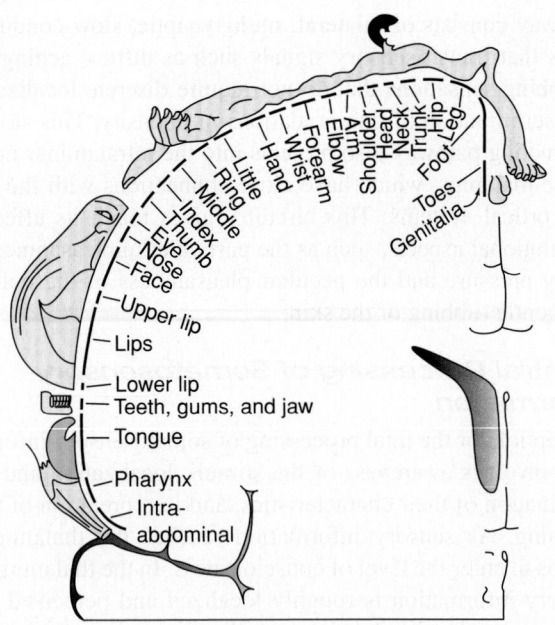

FIGURE 49.6 • Homunculus, as determined by stimulation studies on the human cortex during surgery. (From Penfield E., Rasmussen T. (1955). *The cerebral cortex of man.* New York: Macmillan. Copyright © by Macmillan Publishing Co., Inc., renewed 1978 by Theodore Rasmussen.)

of the body such as the thumb, forefinger, lips, and tongue, where fine touch and pressure discrimination are essential for normal function.

Parallel to and just behind the primary somatosensory cortex (*i.e.,* toward the occipital cortex) lie the somatosensory association areas, which are required to transform the raw material of sensation into meaningful learned perception. Most of the perceptive aspects of body sensation, or somesthesia, require the function of this parietal association cortex. The perceptive aspect, or meaningfulness, of a stimulus pattern involves the integration of present sensation with past learning. For instance, a person's past learning plus present tactile sensation provides the perception of sitting on a soft chair rather than on a hard bicycle seat.

Sensory Modalities

Somatosensory experience can be divided into *modalities,* a term used for qualitative, subjective distinctions between sensations such as touch, heat, and pain. Such experiences require the function of sensory receptors and forebrain structures in the thalamus and cerebral cortex. Sensory experience also involves quantitative sensory discrimination or the ability to distinguish between different levels of sensory stimulation.

The receptive endings of different afferent neurons are particularly sensitive to specific forms of physical and chemical energy. They can initiate action potentials to many forms of energy at high energy levels, but they usually are highly tuned to be differentially sensitive to low levels of a particular energy type. For instance, a receptive ending may be particularly sensitive to a small increase in local skin temperature.

Stimulating the ending with electric current or strong pressure also can result in action potentials. The amount of energy required, however, is much greater than it is for a change in temperature. Other afferent sensory terminals are most sensitive to slight indentations of the skin, and their signals are subjectively interpreted as touch. Cool versus warm, sharp versus dull pain, and delicate touch versus deep pressure are all based on different populations of afferent neurons or on central integration of simultaneous input from several differently tuned afferents.

When information from different primary afferents reaches the forebrain, where subjective experience occurs, the qualitative differences between warmth and touch are called *sensory modalities.* Although the receptor-detected information is relayed to the thalamus and cortex over separate pathways, the experience of a modality, such as cold versus warm, is uniquely subjective.

Stimulus Discrimination

The ability to discriminate the location of a somesthetic stimulus is called *acuity* and is based on the sensory field in a dermatome innervated by an afferent neuron. High acuity (*i.e.,* the ability to make fine discriminations of location) requires a high density of innervation by afferent neurons. For example, acuity is higher on the lips and cheek but lower on the arm or back. High acuity also requires a projection system through the CNS to the forebrain that preserves distinctions between levels of activity in neighbouring sensory fields. Receptors or receptive endings of primary afferent neurons differ as to the intensity at which they begin to fire. For instance, it is possible to assess two-point discrimination by using an open paperclip with its ends bent together to 5 mm apart. When placed on the lips or cheek, the person will readily detect two points of contact. On the back or arm, the ends of the paperclip must be moved progressively farther apart before two points of contact can be detected.

Tactile Sensation

The tactile system, which relays sensory information regarding touch, pressure, and vibration, is considered the basic somatosensory system. Loss of temperature or pain sensitivity leaves the person with no awareness of deficiency. If the tactile system is lost, however, total anesthesia (*i.e.,* numbness) of the involved body part results.

Touch sensation results from stimulation of tactile receptors in the skin and in tissues immediately beneath the skin, pressure from deformation of deeper tissues, and vibration from rapidly repetitive sensory signals. There are at least six types of specialized tactile receptors in the skin and deeper structures: free nerve endings,[1,2] Meissner corpuscles, Merkel disks, pacinian corpuscles, hair follicle end-organs, and Ruffini end-organs (Fig. 49.7).

Free nerve endings are found in skin and many other tissues, including the cornea. They detect touch and pressure. *Meissner corpuscles* are elongated, encapsulated nerve endings present in nonhairy parts of the skin. They are particularly

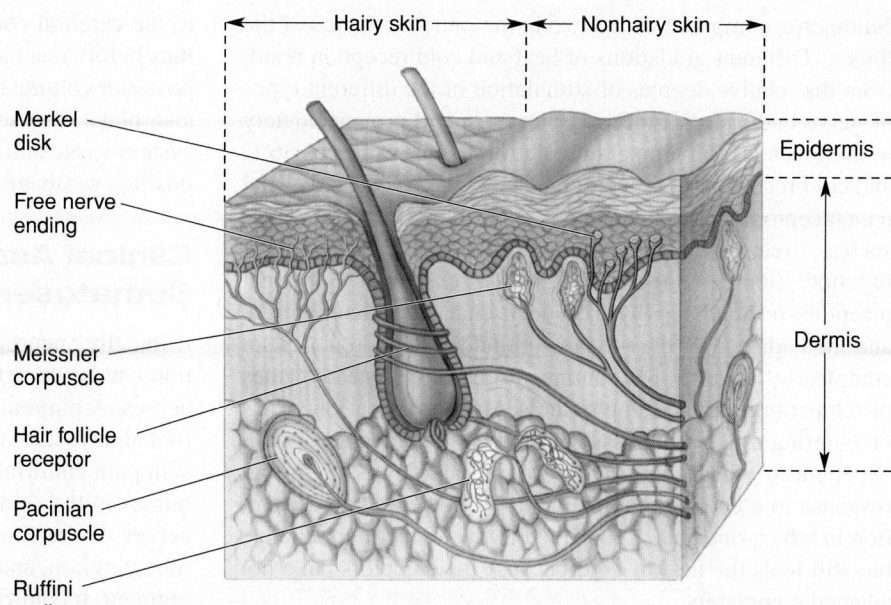

FIGURE 49.7 • Somatic sensory receptors in the skin. Hairy and nonhairy skin have a variety of sensory receptors within the skin. (Adapted from Bear M. F., Connors B. W., Paradiso M. A. (2016). *Neuroscience: Exploring the brain* (4th ed., p. 417). Philadelphia, PA: Lippincott Williams & Wilkins.)

abundant in the fingertips, lips, and other areas where the sense of touch is highly developed. *Merkel disks* are dome-shaped receptors found in nonhairy areas and in hairy parts of the skin. In contrast to Meissner corpuscles, which adapt within a fraction of a second, Merkel disks transmit an initial strong signal that diminishes in strength but is slow in adapting. For this reason, Meissner corpuscles are particularly sensitive to the movement of very light objects over the surface of the skin and to low-frequency vibration. Merkel disks are responsible for giving steady-state signals that allow for continuous determination of touch against the skin.

The *pacinian corpuscles* are located immediately beneath the skin and deep in the fascial tissues of the body. Receptors of this type, which are stimulated by rapid movement of the tissues and adapt within a few hundredth of a second, are important in detecting tissue vibration. The *hair follicle end-organ* consists of afferent unmyelinated fibres entwined around most of the length of the hair follicle. These receptors, which are rapidly adapting, detect movement on the surface of the body. *Ruffini end-organs* are found in the skin and deeper structures, including the joint capsules. These receptors, which have multibranched encapsulated endings, have very little adaptive capacity and are important for signalling continuous states of deformation, such as heavy and continuous touch and pressure.

Almost all the specialized touch receptors, such as Merkel disks, Meissner corpuscles, hair follicle end-organs, pacinian corpuscles, and Ruffini end-organs, transmit their signals in large myelinated nerve fibres (*i.e.,* types Aα, Aβ) that have transmission velocities ranging from 30 to 70 m/sec. Most free nerve endings transmit signals by way of small myelinated fibres (*i.e.,* type Aδ) with conduction velocities of 5 to 30 m/sec.[1]

The sensory information for tactile sensation enters the spinal cord through the dorsal roots of the spinal nerves. All tactile sensation that requires rapid transmission is transmitted through the discriminative pathway to the thalamus by way of the medial lemniscus. This includes touch sensation requiring a high degree of localization or fine gradations of intensity, vibratory sensation, and sensation that signals movement against the skin. In addition to the ascending discriminative pathway, tactile sensation uses the more primitive and crude anterolateral pathway. The afferent axons that carry tactile information up the dorsal columns have many branches or collaterals, and some of these synapse in the dorsal horn near the level of dorsal root entry. After several synapses, axons are projected up both sides of the anterolateral aspect of the spinal cord to the thalamus. Few fibres travel all the way to the thalamus. Most synapse on reticular formation neurons that then send their axons on toward the thalamus. The lateral nuclei of the thalamus are capable of modulating a crude, poorly localized sensation from the opposite side of the body. From the thalamus, some projections travel to the somatosensory cortex, especially to the side opposite the stimulus.

Because of these multiple routes, total destruction of the anterolateral pathway seldom occurs. The only time this crude alternative system becomes essential is when the discriminative pathway is damaged. Then, despite projection of the anterolateral system information to the somatosensory cortex, only a poorly localized, high-threshold sense of touch remains. Such persons lose all sense of joint and muscle movement, body position, and two-point discrimination.

Thermal Sensation

Thermal sensation is discriminated by three types of receptors: cold, warmth, and pain. The cold and warmth receptors are located immediately under the skin at discrete but separate points, each serving an area of approximately 1 mm². In some areas, there are more cold receptors than warmth receptors. For example, the lips have 15 to 25 cold receptors per square centimetre, compared with 3 to 5 in the same-sized area of the finger.[1] Different gradations of heat and cold reception result from the relative degrees of stimulation of the different types of nerve endings. Warmth receptors respond proportionally to increases in skin temperature above resting values of 36°C and cold receptors to temperatures below 32°C.[2] The thermal pain receptors are stimulated only by extremes of temperature such as "freezing cold" (temperatures below 10°C) and "burning hot" (temperatures above 45°C) sensations.[2] Thermal receptors respond rapidly to sudden changes in temperature and then adapt over the next few minutes. They do not adapt completely, however, but continue to respond to steady states of temperature. For example, the sensation of heat one feels on entering a tub of hot water or the extreme degree of cold experienced when going outside on a cold day is the initial response to a change in temperature, followed by an adaptation in which one gets accustomed to the temperature change but still feels the heat or cold because the receptors have not adapted completely.

Thermal afferents, with receptive thermal endings in the skin, send their central axons into the segmental dorsal horn of the spinal cord. On entering the dorsal horn, thermal signals are processed by second-order input association neurons. These association neurons activate projection neurons whose axons then cross to the opposite side of the cord and ascend in the multisynaptic, slow-conducting anterolateral system to the opposite side of the brain. Thalamic and cortical somatosensory regions for temperature are mixed with those for tactile sensibility.

Conduction of thermal information through peripheral nerves is quite slow compared with the rapid tactile afferents that travel through the discriminative system. If a person places a foot in a tub of hot water, the tactile sensation occurs well in advance of the burning sensation. The foot has been removed from the hot water by the local withdrawal reflex well before the excessive heat is perceived by the forebrain. Local anesthetic agents block the small-diameter afferents that carry thermal sensory information before they block the large-diameter axons that carry discriminative touch information.

Position Sensation

Position sense refers to the sense of limb and body movement and position without using vision. It is mediated by input from proprioceptive receptors (muscle spindle receptors and Golgi tendon organs) found primarily in muscles, tendons, and joint capsules (see Chapter 50). There are two submodalities of proprioception: the stationary or static component (limb position sense) and the dynamic aspects of position sense (kinesthesia). Both of these depend on constant transmission of information to the CNS regarding the degree of angulation of all joints and the rate of change in angulation. In addition, stretch-sensitive receptors in the skin (Ruffini end-organs, pacinian corpuscles, and Merkel cells) also signal postural information. Signals from these receptors are processed through the dorsal column–medial lemniscus pathway. In addition to the transmission of signals from the periphery

to the cerebral cortex, the signals are processed in the thalamus before reaching the cerebral cortex. Lesions affecting the posterior column impair position sense. The vestibular system also plays an essential role in position sense. The vestibular system's role and the diseases affecting it and thus impairing position sense are discussed in Chapter 55.

Clinical Assessment of Somatosensory Function

Clinically, neurologic assessment of somatosensory function can be done by testing the integrity of spinal segmental nerves. A pinpoint pressed against the skin of the sole of the foot that results in a withdrawal reflex and a complaint of skin pain confirms the functional integrity of the afferent terminals in the skin, the entire pathway through the peripheral nerves of the foot, leg, and thigh to the sacral (S-1) dorsal root ganglion, and through the dorsal root into the spinal cord segment. It confirms that the somatosensory input association cells receiving this information are functioning and that the reflex circuitry of the cord segments (L-5 to S-2) is functioning. In addition, the lower motor neurons of the L-4 to S-1 ventral horn can be considered operational, and their axons through the ventral roots, the mixed peripheral nerve, and the motor neuron to the muscles producing the withdrawal response can be considered intact and functional. If the communication between the lower motor neuron and the muscle cells is functional, then these muscles have normal responsiveness and strength.

Testing is done at each segmental level, or dermatome, moving upward along the body and neck from coccygeal segments through the high cervical levels to test the functional integrity of all the spinal nerves. Similar dermatomes cover the face and scalp, and these, although innervated by cranial segmental nerves, are tested in the same manner.

Observation of a normal withdrawal reflex rules out peripheral nerve disease, disorders of the dorsal root and ganglion, diseases of the myoneural junction, and severe muscle diseases. Normal reflex function also indicates that many major descending CNS tracts are functioning within normal limits. If the person is able to report the pinprick sensation and accurately identify its location, many ascending systems through much of the spinal cord and brain also are functioning normally, as are basic intellect and speech mechanisms.

The integrity of the discriminative dorsal column–medial lemniscus pathway compared with the anterolateral tactile pathways is tested, with the person's eyes closed, by gently brushing the skin with a wisp of cotton, touching an area with one or two sharp points, touching corresponding parts of the body on each side simultaneously or in random sequence, and passively bending the person's finger one way and then another in random order. If only the anterolateral pathway is functional, the tactile threshold is markedly elevated, two-point discrimination and proprioception are missing, and the patient has difficulty discriminating which side of the body received stimulation.

The somatosensory component of the nervous system provides an awareness of body sensations such as touch, temperature, position sense, and pain. There are three primary levels of neural integration in the somatosensory system: the sensory units containing the sensory receptors, the ascending pathways, and the central processing centres in the thalamus and cerebral cortex. A sensory unit consists of a single dorsal root ganglion neuron, its receptors, and its central axon that terminates in the dorsal horn of the spinal cord or medulla. The part of the body innervated by the somatosensory afferent neurons of one set of dorsal root ganglia is called a dermatome. Ascending pathways include the discriminative pathway, which crosses at the base of the medulla, and the anterolateral pathway, which crosses within the first few segments of entering the spinal cord. Perception, or the final processing of somatosensory information, involves centres in the thalamus and somatosensory cortex. In the thalamus, the sensory information is crudely localized and perceived. The full localization, discrimination of the intensity, and interpretation of the meaning of the stimuli require processing by the somatosensory cortex. A distorted map of the body and head surface, called the sensory homunculus, reflects the density of cortical neurons devoted to sensory input from afferents in corresponding peripheral areas.

The tactile system relays the sensations of touch, pressure, and vibration. It uses two anatomically separate pathways to relay touch information to the opposite side of the forebrain: the dorsal column discriminative pathway and the anterolateral pathway. Delicate touch, vibration, position, and movement sensations use the discriminative pathway to reach the thalamus, where third-order relay occurs to the primary somatosensory strip of the parietal cortex. Crude tactile sensation is carried by the bilateral slow-conducting anterolateral pathway. Temperature sensations of warm–hot and cool–cold are the result of stimulation to thermal receptors of sensory units projecting to the thalamus and cortex through the anterolateral system on the opposite side of the body. Proprioception is the sense of limb and body movement and position without using vision. Proprioceptive information is processed through the rapid-transmitting dorsal column–medial lemniscus pathway. Testing of the ipsilateral dorsal column (discriminative touch) system or the contralateral temperature projection system permits diagnostic analysis of the level and extent of damage in the somatosensory pathways.

PAIN

After completing this section of the chapter, you should be able to meet the following objectives:

- Differentiate among the specificity, pattern, gate control, and neuromatrix theories of pain.
- Characterize the response of nociceptors to stimuli that produce pain.
- State the difference between the Aδ- and C-fibre neurons in the transmission of pain information.
- Trace the transmission of pain signals with reference to the neospinothalamic, paleospinothalamic, and reticulospinal pathways, including the role of chemical mediators and factors that modulate pain transmission.
- Describe the function of endogenous analgesic mechanisms as they relate to transmission of pain information.
- Compare pain threshold and pain tolerance.
- Differentiate acute pain from chronic pain in terms of mechanisms, manifestations, and treatment.
- Describe the mechanisms of referred pain, and list the common sites of referral for cardiac and other types of visceral pain.
- Describe three methods for assessing pain.
- State the proposed mechanisms of pain relief associated with the use of heat, cold, transcutaneous electrical nerve stimulation, and acupuncture and acupressure.
- Cite the mechanisms whereby nonnarcotic and narcotic analgesics, tricyclic antidepressants, and antiseizure drugs relieve pain.

Pain is an "unpleasant sensory and emotional experience associated with actual and potential tissue damage, or described in terms of such damage."[3] The early work by Sir Charles Sherrington[4] introduced the important concept that pain perception and reaction to pain can be separated. This is particularly important for clinical pain because suffering is more heavily influenced by the reaction to pain than by actual pain intensity. Attention, motivation, past experience, and the meaning of the situation influence the individual's perception and reaction to pain. Thus, pain involves anatomic structures and physiologic behaviours, as well as psychological, social, cultural, and cognitive factors.

Pain is a common symptom that varies widely in intensity and spares no age group. When pain is extremely severe, it disrupts a person's customary behaviour and can consume all of a person's attention. It can be equally devastating for infants and children, young and middle-aged adults, as well as adults over 65 years of age. Both acute pain and chronic pain can be major health problems. Pain is the most common symptom for which patients seek medical attention. Acute pain often results from injury, surgery, or invasive medical procedures. It also can be a presenting symptom for some infections (*e.g.,* pharyngitis, appendicitis, otitis media). Chronic pain can be symptomatic of a wide range of health problems (*e.g.,* arthritis, back injury, trauma, cancer). It is estimated that 19% of Canadians suffer from chronic, noncancer pain, with an increased frequency in women and the older age groups; 31% suffer from severe chronic pain; and

1 in 5 Canadians have chronic pain that interferes with their quality of life and productivity.[5,6]

The experience of pain depends on both sensory stimulation and perception. The perception of pain can be heavily influenced by the endogenous analgesia system that modulates the sensation of pain. This is perhaps most dramatically illustrated by the phenomenon of soldiers injured in battle or athletes injured during a game who do not perceive major injuries as painful until they leave the battlefield or the game.

Pain can be either nociceptive or neuropathic in origin. When nociceptors (pain receptors) are activated in response to actual or impending tissue injury, *nociceptive pain* is the consequence. *Neuropathic pain,* on the other hand, arises from direct injury or dysfunction of the sensory axons of peripheral or central nerves. Tissue and nerve injury can result in a wide range of symptoms. These include pain from noninjurious stimuli to the skin (*allodynia*), extreme sensitivity to pain (*hyperalgesia*), and the absence of pain from stimuli that normally would be painful (*analgesia*). The latter, although not painful, can be extremely serious (*e.g.,* in diabetic persons with peripheral neuropathy) because the normally protective early warning system for the presence of tissue injury is absent.

Pain Theories

Traditionally, two theories have been offered to explain the physiologic basis for the pain experience. The first, *specificity theory,* regards pain as a separate sensory modality evoked by the activity of specific receptors that transmit information to pain centres or regions in the forebrain where pain is experienced.[7] The second theory includes a group of theories collectively referred to as *pattern theory*. It proposes that pain receptors share endings or pathways with other sensory modalities, but that different patterns of activity (*i.e.,* spatial or temporal) of the same neurons can be used to signal painful and nonpainful stimuli.[7] For example, light touch applied to the skin would produce the sensation of touch through low-frequency firing of the receptor; intense pressure would produce pain through high-frequency firing of the same receptor. Both theories focus on the neurophysiologic basis of pain, and both probably apply. Specific nociceptive afferents have been identified; however, almost all afferent stimuli, if driven at a very high frequency, can be experienced as painful.

Gate control theory, a modification of specificity theory, was proposed by Melzack and Wall in 1965 to meet the challenges presented by the pattern theories. This theory postulated the presence of neural gating mechanisms at the segmental spinal cord level to account for interactions between pain and other sensory modalities.[8] The original gate control theory proposed a spinal cord-level network of transmission or projection cells and internuncial neurons that inhibits the transmission cells, forming a segmental-level gating mechanism that could block projection of pain information to the brain.

According to the gate control theory, the internuncial neurons involved in the gating mechanism are activated by large-diameter, faster-propagating fibres that carry tactile information.

The simultaneous firing of the large-diameter touch fibres has the potential for blocking the transmission of impulses from the small-diameter myelinated and unmyelinated pain fibres. Pain therapists have long known that pain intensity can be temporarily reduced during active tactile stimulation. For example, repeated sweeping of a soft-bristled brush on the skin (*i.e.,* brushing) over or near a painful area may result in pain reduction for several minutes to several hours.

Pain modulation is now known to be a much more complex phenomenon than that proposed by the original gate control theory. Tactile information is transmitted by small- and large-diameter fibres. Major interactions between sensory modalities, including the so-called gating phenomenon, occur at several levels of the CNS rostral to the input segment. Perhaps the most puzzling aspect of locally applied stimuli, such as brushing, that can block the experience of pain is the relatively long-lasting effect (minutes to hours) of such treatments. This prolonged effect has been difficult to explain on the basis of specificity theories, including the gate control theory. Other important factors include the effect of endogenous opioids and their receptors at the segmental and brain stem level, descending feedback modulation, altered sensitivity, learning, and culture. Despite this complexity, the Melzack and Wall theory served a useful purpose. It sparked interest in pain and stimulated research and clinical activity related to the pain-modulating systems, and provided recognition for the complexity and diversity of pain assessment tools and pain intervention strategies.

Melzack developed the *neuromatrix theory* to address further the brain's role in pain as well as the multiple dimensions and determinants of pain.[9] This theory is particularly useful in understanding chronic pain and phantom limb pain, in which there is not a simple one-to-one relationship between tissue injury and pain experience. The neuromatrix theory proposes that the brain contains a widely distributed neural network, called the *body–self neuromatrix,* that contains somatosensory, limbic, and thalamocortical components. Genetic and sensory influences determine the synaptic architecture of an individual's neuromatrix that integrates multiple sources of input and yields the neurosignature pattern that evokes the sensory, affective, and cognitive dimensions of pain experience and behaviour. These multiple sources include somatosensory inputs; other sensory inputs affecting interpretation of the situation; phasic and tonic inputs from the brain addressing such things as attention, expectation, culture, and personality; intrinsic neural inhibitory modulation; and various components of stress regulation systems. This theory may open entire new areas of research, such as an understanding of the role that cortisol plays in chronic pain, the effect estrogen has on pain mediated through the release of peripheral cytokines, and the reported increase in chronic pain that occurs with age.

Pain Mechanisms and Pathways

Pain usually is viewed in the context of tissue injury. The term *nociception,* which means "pain sense," comes from the

Latin word *nocere,* "to injure." Nociceptive stimuli are objectively defined as stimuli of such intensity that they cause or are close to causing tissue damage. Researchers often use the withdrawal reflex (*e.g.,* the reflexive withdrawal of a body part from a tissue-damaging stimulus) to determine when a stimulus is nociceptive. Stimuli used include pressure from a sharp object, strong electric current to the skin, or application of heat or cold of approximately 10°C above or below normal skin temperature. At low levels of intensity these noxious stimuli do activate nociceptors (pain receptors), but typically are perceived as painful only when the intensity reaches a level where tissue damage occurs or is imminent.

The mechanisms of pain are many and complex. As with other forms of somatosensation, the pathways are composed of first-, second-, and third-order neurons (Fig. 49.8). The first-order neurons and their receptive endings detect stimuli that threaten the integrity of innervated tissues. Second-order neurons are located in the spinal cord and process nociceptive information. Third-order neurons project pain information to the brain. The thalamus and somatosensory cortex integrate

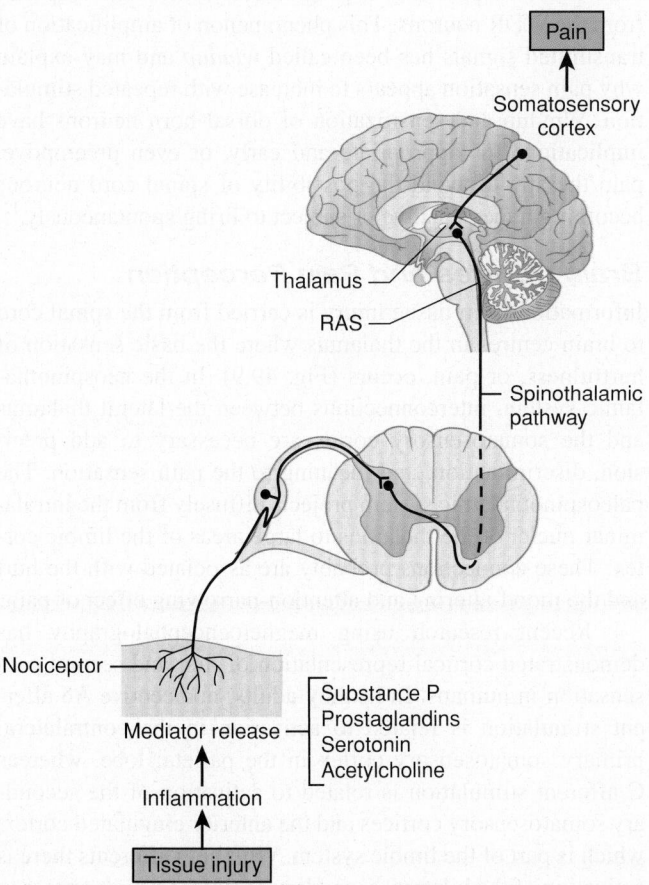

FIGURE 49.8 • Mechanism of acute pain. Tissue injury leads to release of inflammatory mediators with subsequent nociceptor stimulation. Pain impulses are then transmitted to the dorsal horn of the spinal cord, where they make contact with second-order neurons that cross to the opposite side of the cord and ascend by the spinothalamic tract to the reticular activating system (RAS) and thalamus. The localization and meaning of pain occur at the level of the somatosensory cortex.

and modulate pain as well as the person's subjective reaction to the pain experience.

Pain Receptors and Mediators

Nociceptors, or pain receptors, are sensory receptors that are activated by noxious insults to peripheral tissues. Structurally, the receptive endings of the peripheral pain fibres are free nerve endings. These receptive endings, which are widely distributed in the skin, dental pulp, periosteum, meninges, and some internal organs, translate the noxious stimuli into action potentials that are transmitted by a dorsal root ganglion to the dorsal horn of the spinal cord.

Nociceptive action potentials are transmitted through two types of afferent nerve fibres: myelinated Aδ fibres and unmyelinated C fibres.[1,2] The larger Aδ fibres have considerably greater conduction velocities, transmitting impulses at a rate of 6 to 30 m/sec. The C fibres are the smallest of all peripheral nerve fibres; they transmit impulses at the rate of 0.5 to 2.0 m/sec.[1] Pain conducted by Aδ fibres traditionally is called *fast pain* or first pain and typically is elicited by mechanical or thermal stimuli. C-fibre pain often is described as *slow-wave pain* or second pain because it is slower in onset and longer in duration. It typically is incited by chemical stimuli or by persistent mechanical or thermal stimuli. The slow postexcitatory potentials generated in C fibres are now believed to be responsible for central sensitization to chronic pain.

Stimulation of Nociceptors. Unlike other sensory receptors, nociceptors respond to several forms of stimulation, including mechanical, thermal, and chemical. Some receptors respond to a single type of stimuli (mechanical or thermal) and others, called *polymodal receptors,* respond to all three types of stimuli (mechanical, thermal, and chemical).[10] Mechanical stimuli can arise from intense pressure applied to skin or from the violent contraction or extreme stretch of a muscle. Both extremes of heat and cold can stimulate nociceptors. Chemical stimuli arise from a number of sources, including tissue trauma, ischemia, and inflammation. A wide range of chemical mediators are released from injured and inflamed tissues, including hydrogen and potassium ions, prostaglandins, leukotrienes, histamine, bradykinin, acetylcholine, and serotonin. These chemical mediators produce their effects by directly stimulating nociceptors or sensitizing them to the effects of nociceptive stimuli; perpetuating the inflammatory responses that lead to the release of chemical agents that act as nociceptive stimuli; or inciting neurogenic reflexes that increase the response to nociceptive stimuli. For example, bradykinin, histamine, serotonin, and potassium activate and also sensitize nociceptors.[1] Adenosine triphosphate, acetylcholine, and platelets act alone or in concert to sensitize nociceptors through other chemical agents such as prostaglandins. Aspirin and other nonsteroidal anti-inflammatory drugs (NSAIDs) are effective in controlling pain because they block the enzyme needed for prostaglandin synthesis.

Nociceptive stimulation that activates C fibres can cause a response known as *neurogenic inflammation* that produces vasodilation and an increased release of chemical mediators to which nociceptors respond.[11] This mechanism is thought to be mediated by a dorsal root neuron reflex that produces retrograde transport and release of chemical mediators, which in turn causes increasing inflammation of peripheral tissues. This reflex can set up a vicious cycle, which has implications for persistent pain and hyperalgesia.

Mediators in the Spinal Cord. In the spinal cord, the transmission of impulses between the nociceptive neurons and the dorsal horn neurons is mediated by chemical neurotransmitters released from central nerve endings of the nociceptive neurons. Some of these neurotransmitters are amino acids (*e.g.,* glutamate), others are amino acid derivatives (*e.g.,* norepinephrine), and still others are low-molecular-weight peptides composed of two or more amino acids. The amino acid glutamate is a major excitatory neurotransmitter released from the central nerve endings of the nociceptive neurons. Substance P, a neuropeptide, also is released in the dorsal horn by C fibres in response to nociceptive stimulation. Substance P elicits slow excitatory potentials in dorsal horn neurons. Unlike glutamate, which confines its action to the immediate area of the synaptic terminal, some neuropeptides released in the dorsal horn can diffuse some distance because they are not inactivated by reuptake mechanisms. In persistent pain, this may help to explain the excitability and unlocalized nature of many painful conditions. Neuropeptides such as substance P also appear to prolong and enhance the action of glutamate. If these neurotransmitters are released in large quantities or over extended periods, they can lead to secondary hyperalgesia, a condition in which the second-order neurons are overly sensitive to low levels of noxious stimulation. Understanding how chemical mediators function in nociception is an active area of research that has implications for the development of new treatments for pain.

Spinal Cord Circuitry and Pathways

On entering the spinal cord through the dorsal roots, the pain fibres bifurcate and ascend or descend one or two segments before synapsing with association neurons in the dorsal horn. From the dorsal horn, the axons of association projection neurons cross through the anterior commissure to the opposite side and then ascend upward in the previously described neospinothalamic and paleospinothalamic pathways.

The faster-conducting fibres in the neospinothalamic tract (Fig. 49.9) are associated mainly with the transmission of sharp–fast pain information to the thalamus. In the thalamus, synapses are made and the pathway continues to the contralateral parietal somatosensory area to provide the precise location of the pain. Typically, the pain is experienced as bright, sharp, or stabbing in nature.

The paleospinothalamic tract is a slower-conducting, multisynaptic tract concerned with the diffuse, dull, aching, and unpleasant sensations that commonly are associated with chronic and visceral pain. This information travels through the small, unmyelinated C fibres. Fibres of this system also project up the contralateral (*i.e.,* opposite) anterolateral pathway to terminate in several thalamic regions, including the intralateral nuclei, which project to the limbic system. It is associated with the emotional or affective–motivational aspects of pain. Spinoreticular fibres from this pathway project bilaterally to the reticular formation of the brain stem. This component of the paleospinothalamic system facilitates avoidance reflexes at all levels. It also contributes to an increase in the electroencephalographic activity associated with alertness and indirectly influences hypothalamic functions associated with sudden alertness, such as increased heart rate and blood pressure. This may explain the tremendous arousal effects of certain pain stimuli.

Dorsal horn (second-order) neurons are divided primarily into two types: wide-dynamic-range (WDR) neurons that respond to different low-intensity stimuli, and nociceptive-specific neurons that respond only to noxious or nociceptive stimuli. When stimuli are increased to a noxious level, the WDR neurons respond more intensely. After more severe damage to peripheral sensory afferents, Aδ and C fibres respond more intensely as they are increasingly stimulated. When C fibres are repetitively stimulated at a rate of once per second, each stimulus produces a progressively increased response from the WDR neurons. This phenomenon of amplification of transmitted signals has been called *windup* and may explain why pain sensation appears to increase with repeated stimulation. Windup and sensitization of dorsal horn neurons have implications for appropriate and early, or even preemptive, pain therapy to avoid the possibility of spinal cord neurons becoming hypersensitive or subject to firing spontaneously.[12]

Brain Centres and Pain Perception

Information from tissue injury is carried from the spinal cord to brain centres in the thalamus where the basic sensation of hurtfulness, or pain, occurs (Fig. 49.9). In the neospinothalamic system, interconnections between the lateral thalamus and the somatosensory cortex are necessary to add precision, discrimination, and meaning to the pain sensation. The paleospinothalamic system projects diffusely from the intralaminar nuclei of the thalamus to large areas of the limbic cortex. These connections probably are associated with the hurt and the mood-altering and attention-narrowing effect of pain.

Recent research using magnetoencephalography has demonstrated cortical representation of first and second pain sensation in humans. In healthy adults, nociceptive Aδ afferent stimulation is related to activation in the contralateral primary somatosensory cortex in the parietal lobe, whereas C afferent stimulation is related to activation of the secondary somatosensory cortices and the anterior cingulated cortex, which is part of the limbic system. With both afferents there is activation of the bilateral secondary somatosensory cortices in the posterior parietal lobes.[13]

Central Pathways for Pain Modulation

A major advance in understanding pain was the discovery of neuroanatomic pathways that arise in the midbrain and brain stem, descend to the spinal cord, and modulate ascending pain

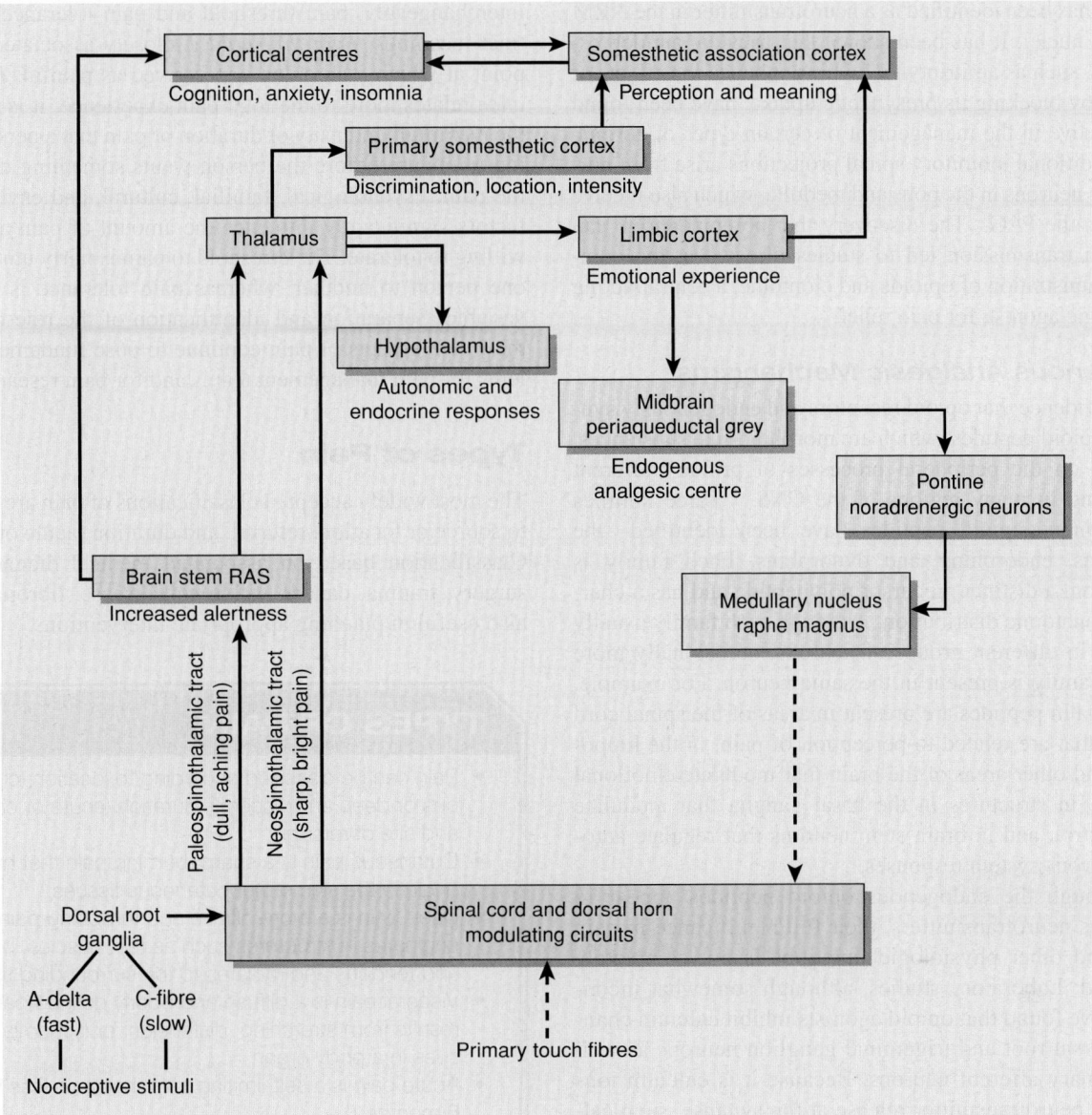

FIGURE 49.9 • Primary pain pathways. The transmission of incoming nociceptive impulses is modulated by dorsal horn circuitry that receives input from primary touch receptors and from descending pathways that involve the limbic cortical systems (orbital frontal cortex, amygdala, and hypothalamus), the periaqueductal endogenous analgesic centre in the midbrain, pontine noradrenergic neurons, and the nucleus raphe magnus (NRM) in the medulla. *Dashed lines* indicate inhibition or modulation of pain transmission by dorsal horn projection neurons. (RAS, reticular activating system)

impulses. One such pathway begins in an area of the midbrain called the *periaqueductal grey* (PAG) region. Research studies demonstrated that electrical stimulation of the midbrain PAG regions produced a state of analgesia that lasted for many hours.[2] This stimulation-induced analgesia was found to be remarkably specific and was not associated with changes in either the levels of consciousness or the reactions to auditory and visual stimuli. Subsequently, opioid receptors were found to be highly concentrated in this and other regions of the CNS where electrical stimulation produced analgesia. Because of these findings, the PAG area of the midbrain often is referred to as the *endogenous analgesia centre.*[1]

The PAG area receives input from widespread areas of the CNS, including the cerebral cortex, hypothalamus, brain stem reticular formation, and spinal cord by way of the paleospinothalamic and neospinothalamic tracts. This region is intimately connected to the limbic system, which is associated with emotional experience. The neurons of the PAG have axons that descend into an area in the rostral medulla called the *nucleus raphe magnus* (NRM). The axons of these NRM neurons project to the dorsal horn of the spinal cord, where they terminate in the same layers as the entering primary pain fibres (Fig. 49.9). In the spinal cord these descending pathways inhibit pain transmission by dorsal horn projection neurons.[2]

Serotonin has been identified as a neurotransmitter in the NRM medullary nuclei. It has been shown that tricyclic antidepressant drugs, such as amitriptyline, which enhance the effects of serotonin by blocking its presynaptic uptake, have been found to be effective in the management of certain types of chronic pain.[14] Additional inhibitory spinal projections arise from noradrenergic neurons in the pons and medulla, which also receive input from the PAG.[2] The discovery that norepinephrine can block pain transmission led to studies directed at the combined administration of opioids and clonidine, a central-acting α-adrenergic agonist, for pain relief.

Endogenous Analgesic Mechanisms

There is evidence that opioid receptors and endogenously synthesized opioid peptides, which are morphine-like substances, are found on the peripheral processes of primary afferent neurons and in many regions of the CNS.[15] Three families of endogenous opioid peptides have been identified—the enkephalins, endorphins, and dynorphins. Each family is derived from a distinct precursor polypeptide and has a characteristic anatomic distribution. Although each family usually is located in different groups of neurons, occasionally more than one family is present in the same neuron. For example, proenkephalin peptides are present in areas of the spinal cord and PAG that are related to perception of pain, in the hippocampus and other areas of the brain that modulate emotional behaviour, in structures in the basal ganglia that modulate motor control, and in brain stem neurons that regulate autonomic nervous system responses.

Although the endogenous opioid peptides appear to function as neurotransmitters, their full significance in pain control and other physiologic functions is not completely understood. Laboratory studies, although somewhat inconsistent, have found that opioid agonists inhibit calcium channels in dorsal root and trigeminal ganglion neurons as well as on primary afferent neurons. Because it is calcium ions that cause neurotransmitter release at the synapse, such calcium blockage would inhibit synaptic transmission of pain impulses. Other studies are focusing on the effect of opioids on sodium and potassium channels that influence the transmission of pain impulses.[15]

Probably of greater importance in understanding mechanisms of pain control has been the characterization of receptors that bind the endogenous opioid peptides (to be discussed). The identification of these receptors has facilitated a more thorough understanding of the actions of available opioid drugs, such as morphine, and it also has facilitated ongoing research into the development of newer preparations—for example, if one could develop an opioid that acted exclusively on the peripheral opioid receptors of sensory neurons, then centrally mediated side effects should not occur.[15]

Pain Threshold and Tolerance

Pain threshold and tolerance affect an individual's response to a painful stimulus. Although the terms often are used interchangeably, pain threshold and pain tolerance have distinct meanings. *Pain threshold* is closely associated with the point at which a stimulus is perceived as painful. *Pain tolerance* relates more to the total pain experience; it is defined as the maximum intensity or duration of pain that a person is willing to endure before the person wants something done about the pain. Psychological, familial, cultural, and environmental factors significantly influence the amount of pain a person is willing to tolerate. The threshold to pain is fairly uniform from one person to another, whereas pain tolerance is extremely variable. Separation and identification of the role of each of these two aspects of pain continue to pose fundamental problems for pain management teams and for pain researchers.

Types of Pain

The most widely accepted classifications of pain are according to source or location, referral, and duration (acute or chronic). Classification based on associated medical diagnosis (*e.g.,* surgery, trauma, cancer, sickle cell disease, fibromyalgia) is also useful in planning appropriate interventions.

TYPES OF PAIN

- Pain can be classified according to location (cutaneous or deep and visceral), duration (acute or chronic), and site of referral.
- Cutaneous pain is a sharp, burning pain that has its origin in the skin or subcutaneous tissues.
- Deep pain is a more diffuse and throbbing pain that originates in structures such as the muscles, bones, and tendons and radiates to the surrounding tissues.
- Visceral pain is a diffuse and poorly defined pain that results from stretching, distension, or ischemia of tissues in a body organ.
- Acute pain is a self-limiting pain that lasts less than 6 months.
- Chronic pain is persistent pain that lasts longer than 6 months, lacks the autonomic and somatic responses associated with acute pain, and is accompanied by loss of appetite, sleep disturbances, depression, and other debilitating responses.
- Referred pain is pain that originates at a visceral site but is perceived as originating in the part of the body wall that is innervated by neurons entering the same segment of the nervous system.

Cutaneous and Deep Somatic Pain

Cutaneous pain arises from superficial structures, such as the skin and subcutaneous tissues. A paper cut on the finger is an example of easily localized superficial, or cutaneous, pain. It is a sharp pain with a burning quality and may be abrupt or slow in onset. It can be localized accurately and may be distributed along the dermatomes. Because there is an overlap of nerve fibre distribution between the dermatomes, the boundaries of pain frequently are not as clear-cut as dermatome diagrams indicate.

Deep somatic pain originates in deep body structures, such as the periosteum, muscles, tendons, joints, and blood vessels. This pain is more diffuse than cutaneous pain. Various stimuli, such as strong pressure exerted on bone, ischemia to a muscle, and tissue damage, can produce deep somatic pain. This is the type of pain a person experiences from a sprained ankle. Radiation of pain from the original site of injury can occur. For example, damage to a nerve root can cause a person to experience pain radiating along its fibre distribution.

Visceral Pain

Visceral, or splanchnic, pain has its origin in the visceral organs and is one of the most common pains produced by disease. While similar to somatic pain in many ways, both the neurologic mechanisms and the perception of visceral pain differ from somatic pain. One of the most important differences between surface pain and visceral pain is the type of damage that causes pain.[16] For example, a surgeon can cut the bowel entirely in two in a patient who is awake without causing significant pain.[1] In contrast, strong contractions, distension, or ischemia affecting the walls of the viscera can induce severe pain. Also, visceral pain is not evoked from all viscera (*e.g.*, the liver, lung parenchyma). Another difference is the diffuse and poorly localized nature of visceral pain, its tendency to be referred to other locations and to be accompanied by symptoms associated with autonomic reflexes (*e.g.*, nausea).[17] There are several explanations for this. There is a low density of nociceptors in the viscera compared with the skin. There is functional divergence of visceral input within the CNS, which occurs when many second-order neurons respond to a stimulus from a single visceral afferent. There is also convergence between somatic and visceral afferents in the spinal cord and in the supraspinal centres and possibly also between visceral afferents (*e.g.*, bladder, uterus, cervix, and vagina).[17]

Visceral afferents are predominantly small, unmyelinated pain fibres that terminate in the dorsal horn of the spinal cord and express peptide neurotransmitters such as substance P. There are thought to be two classes of nociceptive receptors that innervate the viscera: high-threshold and intensity-coding receptors.[16,17] High-threshold receptors have a high threshold for stimulation and respond only to stimuli within the noxious range. Intensity-coding receptors have a lower threshold for stimulation and an encoding function that incorporates the intensity of the stimulus into the magnitude of their discharge. Acute visceral pain, such as pain produced by intense contraction of a hollow organ, is thought to be triggered initially by high-threshold receptors. More extended forms of visceral stimulation, such as that caused by hypoxia and inflammation, often result in sensitization of the receptors. Once sensitized, these receptors begin to respond to otherwise innocuous stimuli (*e.g.*, motility and secretory activity) that normally occur in the viscera. This sensitization may resolve more slowly than the initial injury and thus visceral pain may persist longer than expected based on the initial injury.[16]

Visceral nociceptive afferents from the thorax and abdomen travel along the cranial and spinal nerve pathways of the autonomic nervous system. For many years it was believed that the spinothalamic and spinoreticular tracts carried visceral nociceptive information. More recently, additional pathways have been identified: the dorsal column pathway, the spino(trigemino)-parabrachio-amygdaloid pathway, and the spinohypothalamic pathway. Identification of new pathways can be quite useful clinically. For example, knowledge of the dorsal column pathway has led to new surgical approaches to visceral pain due to pelvic cancer, such as midline myelotomy.[17]

Referred Pain

Referred pain is pain that is perceived at a site different from its point of origin but innervated by the same spinal segment. It is hypothesized that visceral and somatic afferent neurons converge on the same dorsal horn projection neurons (Fig. 49.10). For this reason, it can be difficult for the brain to correctly identify the original source of pain. Pain that originates in the abdominal or thoracic viscera is diffuse and poorly localized and often perceived at a site far removed from the affected area. For example, the pain associated with myocardial infarction commonly is referred to the left arm, neck, and chest, which may delay diagnosis and treatment of a potentially life-threatening condition.

Referred pain may arise alone or concurrent with pain located at the origin of the noxious stimuli. This lack of correspondence between the location of the pain and the location of the painful stimuli can make diagnosis difficult. Although the term *referred* usually is applied to pain that originates in the viscera and is experienced as if originating from the body wall, it also may be applied to pain that arises from somatic structures. For example, pain referred to the chest wall could be caused by nociceptive stimulation of the peripheral portion of the diaphragm, which receives somatosensory innervation from the intercostal nerves. An understanding of pain referral is of great value in diagnosing illness. The typical pattern of pain referral can be derived from our understanding that the afferent neurons from visceral or

FIGURE 49.10 • Convergence of cutaneous and visceral inputs onto the same second-order projection neuron in the dorsal horn of the spinal cord. Although virtually all visceral inputs converge with cutaneous inputs, most cutaneous inputs do not converge with other sensory inputs.

Skin in which pain is perceived

Intestine: site of injury

Anterolateral column axon

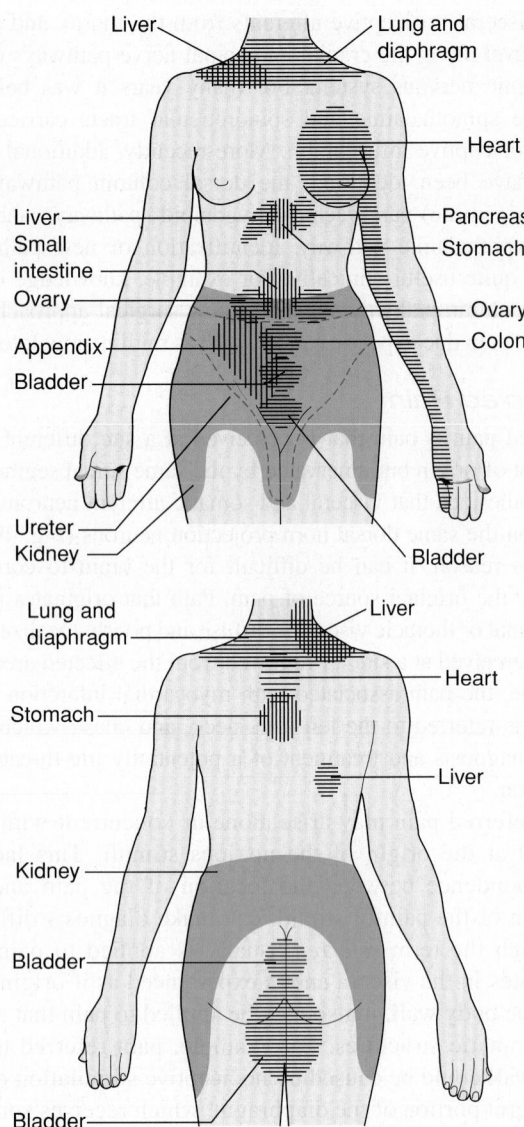

FIGURE 49.11 • Areas of referred pain. **Top:** Anterior view. **Bottom:** Posterior view.

deep somatic tissue enter the spinal cord at the same level as the afferent neurons from the cutaneous areas to which the pain is referred (Fig. 49.11).

The sites of referred pain are determined embryologically with the development of visceral and somatic structures that share the same site for entry of sensory information into the CNS and then move to more distant locations. For example, a person with peritonitis may complain of pain in the shoulder. Internally, there is inflammation of the peritoneum that lines the central part of the diaphragm. In the embryo, the diaphragm originates in the neck, and its central portion is innervated by the phrenic nerve, which enters the cord at the level of the third to fifth segments (C-3 to C-5). As the fetus develops, the diaphragm descends to its adult position between the thoracic and abdominal cavities, while maintaining its embryonic pattern of innervation. Thus, fibres that enter the spinal cord at the C-3 to C-5 levels carry information from both the neck area and the diaphragm, and the diaphragmatic pain is interpreted by the forebrain as originating in the shoulder or neck area.

Although the visceral pleura, pericardium, and peritoneum are said to be relatively free of pain fibres, the parietal pleura, pericardium, and peritoneum do react to nociceptive stimuli. Visceral inflammation can involve parietal and somatic structures, and this may give rise to diffuse local or referred pain. For example, irritation of the parietal peritoneum resulting from appendicitis typically gives rise to pain directly over the inflamed area in the lower right quadrant. Such stimuli can evoke pain referred to the umbilical area.

Muscle spasm, or *guarding,* occurs when somatic structures are involved. Guarding is a protective reflex rigidity; its purpose is to protect the affected body parts (*e.g.,* an abscessed appendix or a sprained muscle). This protective guarding may cause blood vessel compression and give rise to the pain of muscle ischemia, causing local and referred pain.

Acute and Chronic Pain

It is common to classify pain according to its duration. Pain research of the past three decades has emphasized the importance of differentiating acute pain from chronic pain. The diagnosis and therapy for each is distinctive because they differ in cause, function, mechanisms, and psychological sequelae (Table 49.1).

Traditionally, the distinction between acute and chronic pain has relied on a single continuum of time with some interval (*e.g.,* 6 months) since the onset of pain used to designate the onset of acute pain or the transition when acute pain became chronic.[18] A more recent conceptualization includes both time and pathophysiologic dimensions.[18,19] Some conditions such as osteoarthritis exhibit dimensions of both acute and chronic pain.

Acute Pain. Acute pain is pain that is elicited by injury to body tissues and activation of nociceptive stimuli at the site of local tissue damage.[20] It is generally of short duration and remits when the underlying pathologic process has resolved.[18] The purpose of acute pain is to serve as a warning system. Besides alerting the person to the existence of actual or impending tissue damage, it prompts a search for professional help. The pain's location, radiation, intensity, and duration, as well as those factors that aggravate or relieve it, provide essential diagnostic clues.

Acute pain can lead to anxiety and secondary reflex musculoskeletal spasms, which in turn tend to worsen the pain.[21] Interventions that alleviate the pain usually relieve the anxiety and musculoskeletal spasms as well. Inadequately treated pain can provoke physiologic responses that alter circulation and tissue metabolism and produce physical manifestations, such as tachycardia, reflective of increased sympathetic activity. Inadequately treated acute pain tends to decrease mobility and respiratory movements such as deep breathing and coughing to the extent that it may complicate or delay recovery.

TABLE 49.1 CHARACTERISTICS OF ACUTE AND CHRONIC PAIN

CHARACTERISTIC	ACUTE PAIN	CHRONIC PAIN
Onset	Recent	Continuous or intermittent
Duration	Short (<6 months)	6 months or more
Autonomic responses	Consistent with sympathetic fight-or-flight response[a] Increased heart rate Increased stroke volume Increased blood pressure Increased pupillary dilation Increased muscle tension Decreased gut motility Decreased salivary flow (dry mouth)	Absence of autonomic responses
Psychological component	Associated anxiety	Increased irritability Associated depression Somatic preoccupation Withdrawal from outside interests Decreased strength of relationships
Other types of response		Decreased sleep Decreased libido Appetite changes

[a]Responses are approximately proportional to intensity of the stimulus.

Chronic Pain. Chronic pain is pain that persists longer than might be reasonably expected after an inciting event and is sustained by factors that are both pathologically and physically remote from the originating cause. Chronic pain continues for long periods and generally represents low levels of an underlying pathologic process that do not explain the presence or extent of the pain.[18] Chronic pain can be quite variable. It may be unrelenting and extremely severe, as in metastatic bone pain. It can be relatively continuous with or without periods of escalation, as with some forms of back pain. Some conditions with recurring episodes of acute pain are particularly problematic because they have characteristics of both acute and chronic pain. These include the pain associated with sickle cell crisis or migraine headaches.

Chronic pain is a leading cause of disability. Unlike acute pain, persistent chronic pain usually serves no useful function. To the contrary, it imposes physiologic, psychological, familial, and economic stresses and may exhaust a person's resources. In contrast to acute pain, psychological and environmental influences may play an important role in the development of behaviours associated with chronic pain.

The biologic factors that contribute to chronic pain include peripheral mechanisms, peripheral–central mechanisms, and central mechanisms.[19] Peripheral mechanisms result from persistent stimulation of nociceptors. They contribute to the pain associated with chronic musculoskeletal, visceral, and vascular disorders. Peripheral–central mechanisms involve abnormal function of the peripheral and central portions of the somatosensory system. These disorders include conditions such as those resulting from partial or complete loss of descending inhibitory pathways or spontaneous firing of regenerated nerve fibres. They include conditions such as causalgia, phantom limb pain, and postherpetic neuralgia. Central pain mechanisms are associated with disease or injury of the CNS. Central pain is characterized by burning, aching, hyperalgesia, dysesthesia, and other abnormal sensations. Central pain is associated with conditions such as thalamic lesions (thalamic pain), spinal cord injury, surgical interruption of pain pathways, and multiple sclerosis.

Persons with chronic pain may not exhibit the somatic, autonomic, or affective behaviours often associated with acute pain. As painful conditions become prolonged and continuous, autonomic nervous system responses tend to decrease. In addition, chronic pain often is associated with loss of appetite, sleep disturbances, and depression. Amazingly, depression commonly is relieved once the pain is removed. The link between depression and decreased pain tolerance may be explained by the similar manner in which both respond to changes in the biologic pathways of serotonergic and noradrenergic systems. Tricyclic antidepressants and other medications with serotonergic and noradrenergic effects have been shown to relieve a variety of chronic pain syndromes, lending credence to the theory that chronic pain and depression share a common biologic pathway.[22]

Assessment of Pain

Careful assessment of pain assists clinicians in diagnosing, managing, and relieving the patient's pain. Assessment includes such things as the nature, severity, location, and radiation of the pain. As with other disease states, eliminating the cause of the pain is preferable to simply treating the symptom. A careful history often provides information about the triggering factors (*i.e.*, injury, infection, or disease) and the site of nociceptive stimuli (*i.e.*, peripheral receptor or visceral organ). Clinical Practice Guideline No. 1, *Acute Pain Management: Operative and Medical Procedures and Trauma* (released in 1992 by the Agency for Health Care Policy and Research [AHCPR], currently the Agency for Healthcare Research and Quality, Public Health Service, in the United States) emphasizes that "the single most reliable indicator of the existence and intensity of acute pain—and any resultant affective discomfort or distress—is the patient's self report."[23] A comprehensive pain history should include pain onset; description, localization, radiation, intensity, quality, and pattern of the pain; anything that relieves or exacerbates it; and the individual's personal reaction to the pain.

Unlike many other bodily responses, such as temperature and blood pressure, the nature, severity, and distress of pain cannot be measured objectively. To overcome this problem, various methods have been developed for quantifying a person's pain based on the patient's report. They include numeric pain intensity, visual analogue, and verbal descriptor scales. Most pain questionnaires assess a single aspect of pain such as pain intensity. For example, a *numeric pain intensity* scale would have patients select which number best represents the intensity of their pain, where 0 represents no pain and 10 represents the most intense pain imaginable. A *visual analog* scale also can be used; it is a straight line, often 10 cm in length, with a word description (*e.g.*, "no pain" and "the most intense pain imaginable") at each of the ends of the line representing the continuum of pain intensity. Patients are asked to choose a point on the continuum that represents the intensity of their pain. The response can be quantified by measuring the line to determine the distance of the mark, measured in millimetres, from the "no pain" end of the line. *Verbal descriptor* scales consist of several numerically ranked choices of words such as none = 0, slight = 1, mild = 2, moderate = 3, and severe = 4. The word chosen is used to determine the numeric representation of pain severity on an ordinal scale.

Some pain questionnaires are multidimensional (*e.g.*, the McGill Pain Questionnaire) in that they include several sections or sets of questions that are scored into subscales that quantify various aspects of pain. The McGill Pain Questionnaire[24] is divided into four parts. The first part uses a drawing of the body on which the person indicates the location of pain. The second part uses a list of 20 words to describe the sensory, affective, evaluative, and other qualities of pain, with the selected words being given a numeric score (*e.g.*, words implying the least pain are assigned a value of 1, moderate pain a value of 2, and so on). The third part asks the person to select words such as *brief, momentary,* and *constant* to describe the pattern of pain. The fourth part of the instrument evaluates the present pain intensity on a scale with scores from 0 to 5. The Memorial Pain Assessment Card, another multidimensional instrument, can be used to determine the intensity of pain, mood, and effectiveness of analgesia.[23]

Scales developed for use in children rely on behavioural and physiologic signs for assessment of pain in preverbal children. The Objective Pain Scale was developed for use in children 6 months to 3 years of age, evaluating blood pressure, crying, movement, and agitation.[25] The CRIES scale was developed for use in neonates and infants up to 6 months of age, evaluating crying, need for oxygen to maintain saturation, vital signs, expression, and sleeplessness.[26] Scales also exist for pain assessment in older adults, mentally challenged, and non-verbal populations. Many organizations have developed pain guidelines. Implementation of the guidelines has resulted in improved patient satisfaction, a reduction in pain scores, and decreased nursing frustration.

Management of Pain

The therapeutic approaches to acute and chronic pain differ markedly. In acute pain, therapy is directed at providing pain relief by interrupting the nociceptive stimulus. Because the pain is self-limited, in that it resolves as the injured tissues heal, long-term therapy usually is not needed. Chronic pain management is much more complex and is based on multiple considerations, including life expectancy.

Acute Pain

Acute pain should be aggressively managed and pain medication provided before the pain becomes severe. This allows the person to be more comfortable and active and to assume a greater role in directing his or her own care. Part of the reluctance of healthcare workers to provide adequate relief for acute pain has been fear of addiction. However, addiction to opioid medications is thought to be virtually nonexistent when these drugs are prescribed for acute pain. Usually, less medication is needed when the drug is given before the pain becomes severe and the pain pathways become sensitized.

The AHCPR guideline, which addresses pain from surgery, medical procedures, and trauma, emphasizes the need for (1) a collaborative, interdisciplinary approach to pain control, which includes members of the healthcare team and input from the patient and the patient's family when appropriate; (2) an individualized, proactive pain control plan developed before surgery (if possible) by patients and providers; (3) the assessment and frequent reassessment of the patient's pain, facilitated by a pain management log or flow sheet; (4) the use of drug and nondrug therapies to control or prevent pain; and (5) a formal, institutional approach to management of acute pain with clear lines of responsibility.[23]

Chronic Pain

Management of chronic pain requires early attempts to prevent pain and adequate therapy for acute bouts of pain. Specific treatment depends on the cause of the pain, the natural history of the underlying health problem, as well as the life expectancy of the individual. If the organic illness causing the pain cannot be cured, then noncurative methods of pain control become the cornerstone of treatment. Treatment methods for chronic pain can include neural blockade, electrical modalities (*e.g.*, transcutaneous electrical nerve stimulation), physical therapy, cognitive-behavioural interventions, and nonnarcotic and narcotic medications. Nonnarcotic medications such as tricyclic antidepressants, antiseizure medications, and NSAIDs serve as useful adjuncts to opioids for the treatment of different types of chronic pain. Chronic pain is best handled by a multidisciplinary team that includes specialists in areas such as anesthesiology, nursing, physical therapy, social services, and surgery.[19]

Cancer is a common cause of chronic pain. The goal of chronic cancer pain management should be pain alleviation and prevention. Preemptive therapy tends to reduce sensitization of pain pathways and provides for more effective pain control. In 1994, the AHCPR published Clinical Practice Guideline No. 9, *Management of Cancer Pain.*[27] Although dated, this guideline remains a standard and highlights the fact that pain control remains a significant problem despite the advances in understanding and management of pain. The report emphasizes that pain control merits high priority because pain diminishes activity, appetite, and sleep and can further weaken a person already debilitated by cancer. It also emphasizes that pain interferes with productive employment, enjoying recreation, and taking an active part in family life. Like the AHCPR acute pain guideline, the cancer pain guideline emphasizes the need for a collaborative multidisciplinary approach to cancer pain management. Clinically useful interventions are described in the guideline. Some of these (*e.g.*, analgesics, adjuvant drugs, cognitive or behavioural strategies, physical modalities, and nerve blocks) are used for many forms of chronic pain. Depending on the form and stage of the cancer, other treatments such as palliative radiation, antineoplastic therapies, and palliative surgery may help to control the pain. The AHCPR guideline also stresses that written patient education materials at an appropriate reading level should be provided. The basic World Health Organization analgesic ladder for cancer pain is still relevant, although a newer version for general pain (acute, chronic noncancer, and cancer pain) also includes a fourth step of neurosurgical procedures (brain stimulators) and invasive techniques (nerve blocks).[28]

Nonpharmacologic Treatment

A number of nonpharmacologic methods of pain control often are used in pain management. These include cognitive-behavioural interventions, physical agents such as heat and cold, and electroanalgesia. Often these methods are used in addition to analgesics rather than as the only form of pain management.

Cognitive-Behavioural Interventions. Cognitive-behavioural interventions, which often are helpful for individuals experiencing acute as well as chronic pain, include relaxation, distraction, cognitive reappraisal, imagery, meditation, and biofeedback. If the person is having surgery or a painful procedure, it is ideal to teach these techniques before the pain begins (*e.g.*, before surgery). If the person is already in severe pain, the use of cognitive-behavioural interventions should be based on the person's ability to master the technique as well as his or her response to the intervention. For example, it may be a more appropriate adjunct to analgesics for a terminally ill

person in severe pain to use self-selected relaxing music rather than trying to teach that person an intervention requiring more attention (*e.g.*, meditation or cognitive reappraisal).

Relaxation is one of the best-evaluated cognitive-behavioural approaches to pain relief. The relaxation method need not be complex. Relatively simple strategies, such as slow, rhythmic breathing and brief jaw relaxation procedures, have been successful in decreasing self-reported pain and analgesic use.

Distraction (*i.e.*, focusing a person's attention on stimuli other than painful stimuli or negative emotions) does not eliminate pain, but it can make pain more tolerable. It may serve as a type of sensory shielding whereby attention to pain is sacrificed in order to pay attention to other stimuli that are easily perceived. Examples of distraction include counting, repeating phrases or poems, and engaging in activities that require concentration, such as projects, activities, work, conversation, or describing pictures. Television, adventure movies, music, and humour also can provide distraction. *Cognitive reappraisal* is a form of self-distraction or cognitive control in which individuals focus their attention on the positive aspects of the experience and away from their pain. Individuals using distraction may not appear to be in severe pain. Nonetheless, it is inappropriate to assume that a person who copes with pain by using distraction does not have pain. Prescribed analgesics should not be denied to patients simply because they appear to be coping with their pain without medication. Appropriate assessment is needed to determine the patient's level of pain and what other interventions for pain may be needed.

Imagery consists of using one's imagination to develop a mental picture. In pain management, therapeutic guided imagery (*i.e.*, goal-directed imaging) is used. It can be used alone or in conjunction with other cognitive behavioural interventions (*e.g.*, relaxation or biofeedback) to develop sensory images that may decrease the perceived intensity of pain. It also can be used to lessen anxiety and reduce muscle tension. *Meditation* also can be used, but it requires practice and the ability to concentrate to be effective.

Biofeedback is used to provide feedback to a person concerning the current status of some body function (*e.g.*, finger temperature, temporal artery pulsation, blood pressure, or muscle tension). It involves a process of learning designed to make the person aware of certain of his or her own body functions for the purpose of modifying these functions at a conscious level. Interest in biofeedback has increased with the possibility of its use in the management of migraine and tension headaches or for other pain that has a muscle tension component.

Physical Agents. Heat and cold are physical agents that are used to provide pain relief. The choice of physical agent depends on the type of pain being treated and, in many cases, personal preference.

Heat has long been used to relieve pain. Heat dilates blood vessels and increases local blood flow; it also can influence the transmission of pain impulses and increase collagen extensibility. An increase in local circulation can reduce the level of nociceptive stimulation by reducing local ischemia caused by muscle spasm or tension, increase the removal of metabolites and inflammatory mediators that act as nociceptive stimuli, and help to reduce swelling and relieve pressure on local nociceptive endings. The heat sensation is carried to the posterior horn of the spinal cord and may exert its effect by modulating projection of pain transmission. It also may trigger the release of endogenous opioids. Heat alters the viscosity of collagen fibres in ligaments, tendons, and joint structures so that they are more easily extended and can be stretched further before the nociceptive endings are stimulated. Thus, heat often is applied before therapy aimed at stretching joint structures and increasing range of motion. Care must be taken not to use excessive heat. When excessive heat is used, the heat itself becomes a noxious stimulus, which results in actual or impending tissue damage and pain. In certain conditions, the use of heat is controversial, and in some conditions (*e.g.*, peripheral vascular disease) where increased blood flow or metabolism would be detrimental, the use of heat is contraindicated.

Like heat, the application of *cold* may produce a dramatic reduction in pain. Cold exerts its effect on pain through circulatory and neural mechanisms. The initial response to local application of cold is sudden local vasoconstriction. This initial vasoconstriction is followed by alternating periods of vasodilation and vasoconstriction during which the body "hunts" for its normal level of blood flow to prevent local tissue damage. This gives rise to the so-called *hunting reflex*, whereby the circulation to the cooled area causes alternating periods of pallor due to ischemia and flushing due to hyperemia.[29] The vasoconstriction is caused by local stimulation of sympathetic fibres and direct cooling of blood vessels, and the hyperemia by local autoregulatory mechanisms. In situations of acute injury, cold is used to produce vasoconstriction and prevent extravasation of blood into the tissues; pain relief results from decreased swelling and decreased stimulation of nociceptive endings. The vasodilation that follows can be useful in removing substances that stimulate nociceptive endings.

Cold also can have a marked and dramatic effect on pain that results from the spasm-induced accumulation of metabolites in muscle. In terms of pain modulation, cold may reduce afferent activity reaching the posterior horn of the spinal cord by modulating sensory input. The application of cold is a noxious stimulus and may influence the release of endogenous opioids from the PAG area. Cold packs should be flexible to conform to body parts easily, adequately wrapped to protect the skin, and applied for no more than 10 to 20 minutes at a time. Cold should be used only with great caution in anyone whose circulation is compromised.

Stimulus-Induced Analgesia. Stimulus-induced analgesia is one of the oldest known methods of pain relief. Historical references to the use of electricity to decrease or control pain date back to 46 AD, when a Roman physician, Scribonius Largus, described how the stimulus from an electric eel was able to provide pain relief for headache and gout.[30] Electrical stimulation methods of pain relief include transcutaneous electrical nerve stimulation (TENS), electrical acupuncture, and neurostimulation. TENS refers to the transmission of electrical energy across the surface of the skin to the peripheral nerve fibres. TENS units have been developed that are convenient, easily transported, and relatively economical to use. Most are approximately the size of a deck of cards. These battery-operated units deliver an electrical current to a target site.

The system usually consists of three parts: a pair of electrodes, lead wires, and a stimulator. The electrical stimulation is delivered in a pulsed waveform that can be varied in terms of pulse amplitude, width, and rate. The type of stimulation used varies with the type of pain being treated. Electrode placement is determined by the physiologic pathways and an understanding of the pain mechanisms involved. They may be placed on either side of a painful area, over an affected dermatome, over an affected peripheral nerve where it is most superficial, or over a nerve trunk. For example, the electrodes commonly are placed medial and lateral to the incision when treating postoperative pain.

There probably is no single explanation for the physiologic effects of TENS. Each specific type of stimulator may have different sites of action and may be explained by more than one theory. The gate control theory was proposed as one possible mechanism. According to this theory, pain information is transmitted by small-diameter Aδ and C fibres. Large-diameter afferent A fibres and small-diameter fibres carry tactile information mediating touch, pressure, and kinesthesia. TENS may function on the basis of differential firing of impulses in the large fibres that carry nonpainful information. Accordingly, increased activity in these larger fibres purportedly modulates transmission of painful information to the forebrain. A second possible explanation is that the high-frequency stimulation (50 to 60 Hz) produced by some units simply acts as a counterirritant.[31] A third possible explanation is that stimulators that produce strong rhythmic contractions may act through the release of endogenous analgesics such as the endorphins and enkephalins that suppress or modulate pain transmission. A fourth, and probably the best, explanation for quick analgesia with brief, intense stimulation is that it acts as a conduction block.[31,32] TENS has the advantage that it is noninvasive, easily regulated by the patient or health professional, and effective in some forms of acute and chronic pain. Its use can be taught before surgery, affording a reduction in postoperative analgesic medication and, possibly, preventing the development of persistent pain.

Acupuncture. The practice of acupuncture involves introducing needles into specific points on the surface of the body. Charts are available that describe the points of needle placement that are used to relieve pain at certain anatomic sites. In addition to needles, sometimes palpation is used. The practice of acupuncture dates back thousands of years to ancient China, when the stimulation was achieved by using needles made of bone, stone, or bamboo. Each year Canadians use acupuncture to relieve pain. Acupuncture is widely available in pain clinics with accumulating evidence now showing the effectiveness of acupuncture for various pain conditions.[33] Different theories of how acupuncture achieves analgesia have been proposed, including the gate control theory and the neurohumoral theory, involving the cascade of endorphins and monoamines.[34]

Neurostimulation. Neurostimulation delivers low-voltage electrical stimulation to the spinal cord or targeted peripheral nerve to block the sensation of pain. Melzack and Wall (gate theory) proposed that neurostimulation activates the body's pain-inhibiting system.[8] The neurostimulation system implanted in the epidural space stimulates pain-inhibiting nerve fibres in the dorsal horn of the spinal cord, masking the sensation of pain with a tingling sensation (paresthesia).[35]

There are two types of neurostimulation systems: one that is completely internal (surgically implanted) and one that has both internal and external components.[32,35] For a totally implantable system, the power source (battery) and lead(s) are surgically implanted. In the other type of system, the radiofrequency receiver and leads are implanted and the power source with an antenna is worn externally. The latter type of system may be used as a precursor to an implantable system.

Pharmacologic Treatment

Analgesics have been used for many years to relieve pain of short duration, enabling the person to achieve mobility after surgery, for example, voluntary coughing is used as an exercise to expand the lungs and prevent atelectasis. The use of analgesics is only one aspect of a comprehensive pain management program with acute pain, and even more so with chronic pain. An analgesic is a medication that acts on the nervous system to decrease or eliminate pain without inducing loss of consciousness. Analgesic drugs do not cure the underlying cause of the pain, but their appropriate use may prevent acute pain from progressing to chronic pain. The AHCPR cancer pain guideline classifies pain medications into three categories: aspirin, other NSAIDs, and acetaminophen; opioid analgesics; and adjuvant analgesics.[27]

The ideal analgesic would be effective, nonaddictive, and inexpensive. In addition, it would produce minimal adverse effects and not affect the person's level of consciousness. Although long-term treatment with opioids can result in opioid tolerance (*i.e.,* more drug being needed to achieve the same effect) and physical dependence, this should not be confused with addiction. Long-term drug-seeking behaviour is rare in persons who are treated with opioids only during the time that they require pain relief. The unique needs and circumstances presented by each person in pain must be addressed to achieve satisfactory pain management.

Nonnarcotic Analgesics. Common nonnarcotic oral analgesic medications include aspirin, other NSAIDs, and acetaminophen. Aspirin, or acetylsalicylic acid, acts centrally and peripherally to block the transmission of pain impulses. It also has antipyretic and anti-inflammatory properties. The action of aspirin and other NSAIDs is through the inhibition of the

cyclooxygenase (COX) enzymes, which mediate the biosynthesis of prostaglandins. Prostaglandins (particularly, prostaglandin E_2) exert their effect through peripheral sensitization of nociceptors to chemical mediators such as bradykinin and histamine.[36] The NSAIDs also decrease the sensitivity of blood vessels to bradykinin and histamine, affect cytokine production by T lymphocytes, reverse vasodilation, and decrease the release of inflammatory mediators from granulocytes, mast cells, and basophils. Acetaminophen is an alternative to the NSAIDs. Although usually considered equivalent to aspirin as an analgesic and antipyretic agent, it lacks anti-inflammatory properties.

Opioid Analgesics. The term *opioid* or *narcotic* is used to refer to a group of medications, natural or synthetic, with morphine-like actions.[36] The older term *opiate* was used to designate drugs derived from opium—morphine, codeine, and many other semisynthetic congeners of morphine. Opioids are used for relief of short-term pain and for more long-term use in conditions such as cancer pain. When given for temporary relief of severe pain, such as that occurring after surgery, there is much evidence that opioids given routinely before the pain starts (preemptive analgesia) or becomes extreme are far more effective than those administered in a sporadic manner. Persons who are treated in this manner seem to require fewer doses and are able to resume regular activities sooner.

Opioids also are used for persons with limited life expectancy. Too often, because of undue concern about the possibility of addiction, many chronic pain sufferers with a short life expectancy receive inadequate pain relief. Most pain experts agree that it is appropriate to provide the level of opioid necessary to relieve the severe, intractable pain of persons whose life expectancy is limited. Addiction is not considered a problem in patients with cancer.[37,38] In persons with chronic cancer pain, morphine remains the most useful strong opioid. The World Health Organization has recommended that oral morphine be part of the essential medication list and be made available throughout the world as the medication of choice for cancer pain.[27,39] Oral forms of morphine are well absorbed from the gastrointestinal tract and have a half-life of approximately 2.5 hours and a duration of action of 4 to 6 hours. Liquid forms of the medication usually are given at 4-hour intervals to maintain an adequate blood level for analgesia, while minimizing the potential for toxic side effects. Controlled-release forms of the drug also are available, lasting 8 to 20 hours.

Although the analgesic and psychopharmacologic properties of morphine have been known for centuries, the fact that the brain contains its own endogenous opioid-like chemicals, the endorphins (enkephalins, endorphins, and dynorphins), has become known only within the last 40 to 50 years. It has been hypothesized that part of the pain-relieving properties of exogenous opioids such as morphine involves the release of these endogenous opioid peptides.[36]

The opioid analgesics are characterized by their interaction with three types of opioid receptors, designated mu (μ, for "morphine"), delta (δ), and kappa (κ).[36,40] Each receptor type has been cloned and subtypes have been identified using receptor binding and molecular studies. Morphine and most opioids that are used clinically exert their effects through the mu receptor. Kappa receptor opioids are effective analgesics, but their side effects have proven troublesome, and the clinical impact of delta receptor opioids has been negligible.

It is well documented that the mu receptors modulate both the therapeutic effect of analgesia, as well as the side effects of respiratory depression, miosis, reduced gastrointestinal motility (causing constipation), feelings of well-being or euphoria, and physical dependence. The mu receptors are found at presynaptic and postsynaptic sites in the spinal dorsal horn, and in the ascending pathways of the brain stem, thalamus, and cortex, as well as the descending inhibitory system that modulates pain at the spinal cord. Their spinal location has been used clinically by direct application of opioid analgesics to the spinal cord by injection, infusion, or implantable intrathecal device (pump), which provides regional anesthesia while minimizing the unwanted respiratory depression, nausea and vomiting, and sedation that occur with systemically administered drugs that act at the brain level. Mu receptors are also found in peripheral sensory neurons after inflammation. This location supports the exploration and eventual clinical use of locally applied opioids (*e.g.*, intra-articular instillation of opioids after knee surgery).

As more information becomes available regarding the opioids and their receptors, it seems likely that pain medications can be developed that act selectively at certain receptor sites, providing more effective pain control while producing fewer adverse effects and affording less danger of addiction. For example, it might be possible to develop opioid drugs that produce effective analgesia but not undesirable adverse effects, such as respiratory depression and the most common complication, constipation.[41]

One of the problems with the need for long-term use of opioids, as in relief of cancer pain, is the development of tolerance or the need for larger and larger doses to achieve the same level of pain relief. Clinicians have long noted two important phenomena that suggest the possibility of multiple mu opioid receptor subtypes and support the importance of research in this area.[38] First, there are often noteworthy differences in patient responses to mu opioids. Patient-specific responses to these drugs include both the extent of relief obtained and the side effect profiles observed. Second, patients who become tolerant to one mu opioid are often far less tolerant to another mu opioid. The difference in tolerance across mu opioids is called *incomplete cross-tolerance.*[40]

Some clinicians use opioid rotation to improve analgesia once opioid tolerance becomes problematic. It is important to note that the standard equianalgesic conversion tables are based primarily on single-dose studies and as such do not account for incomplete cross-tolerance. When opioid rotation is used with patients demonstrating a tolerance to opioids, it is recommended that the new opioid be started at a fraction of the dosage that is predicted to be equivalent to the current opioid dosage.[40]

Adjuvant Analgesics. Adjuvant analgesics include medications such as tricyclic antidepressants, antiseizure medications, and neuroleptic anxiolytic agents. The fact that the pain suppression system has nonendorphin synapses raises the possibility that potent, centrally acting, nonopiate medications may be useful in relieving pain. Serotonin has been shown to play an important role in producing analgesia. The tricyclic antidepressant medications (*i.e.,* imipramine, amitriptyline, and doxepin) that block the removal of serotonin from the synaptic cleft have been shown to produce pain relief in some persons. These medications are particularly useful in some chronic painful conditions, such as postherpetic neuralgia, but their safety profile may limit their usefulness.

Certain antiseizure medications, such as carbamazepine, pregabalin, and gabapentin, have analgesic effects in some pain conditions. These medications, which suppress spontaneous neuronal firing, are particularly useful in the management of pain that occurs after nerve injury (neuropathic pain), including diabetic neuropathy and chronic regional pain syndrome. Other agents, such as the corticosteroids, may be used to decrease inflammation and the nociceptive stimuli responsible for pain.

Surgical Intervention

If surgery removes the problem causing the pain, such as a tumour pressing on a nerve or an inflamed appendix, it can be curative. In other instances, surgery is used for symptom management rather than for cure. However, with rare exceptions, noninvasive analgesic approaches should precede invasive palliative approaches.[20] Surgery for severe, intractable pain of peripheral or central origin has met with some success. It can be used to remove the cause or block the transmission of intractable pain from phantom limb pain, severe neuralgia, inoperable cancer of certain types, and causalgia.

IN SUMMARY

Pain is an elusive and complex phenomenon; it is a symptom common to many illnesses. It is a highly individualized experience that is shaped by a person's culture and previous life experiences, and it is difficult to measure. Traditionally, there have been two principal theories of pain: the specificity and pattern theories. Scientifically, pain is viewed within the context of nociception. Nociceptors are receptive nerve endings that respond to noxious stimuli. Pain receptors respond to mechanical, thermal, and chemical stimuli. Nociceptive neurons transmit impulses to the dorsal horn neurons using chemical neurotransmitters. The neospinothalamic and the paleospinothalamic pathways are used to transmit pain information to the brain. Several neuroanatomic pathways as well as endogenous opioid peptides modulate pain in the CNS.

Pain can be classified according to location, referral, and duration as well as associated medical diagnoses. Pain can arise from cutaneous, deep somatic, or visceral locations.

Referred pain is pain perceived at a site different from its origin. Acute pain is self-limiting pain that ends when the injured tissue heals, whereas chronic pain is pain that lasts much longer than the anticipated healing time for the underlying cause of the pain. Pain threshold, pain tolerance, age, sex, and other factors affect an individual's reaction to pain.

Treatment modalities for pain include the use of physiologic, cognitive, and behavioural measures; heat and cold; stimulation-induced analgesic methods; and pharmacologic agents singly or in combination. It is becoming apparent that even with chronic pain, the most effective approach is early treatment or even prevention. After pain is present, the greatest success in pain assessment and management is achieved with the use of an interdisciplinary approach.

ALTERATIONS IN PAIN SENSITIVITY AND SPECIAL TYPES OF PAIN

After completing this section of the chapter, you should be able to meet the following objectives:

- Define allodynia, hypoesthesia, hyperesthesia, paresthesias, hyperpathia, analgesia, and hypoalgesia and hyperalgesia.
- Describe the cause, characteristics and treatment of neuropathic pain, trigeminal neuralgia, postherpetic neuralgia, and complex regional pain syndrome.
- Cite possible mechanisms of phantom limb pain.

Alterations in Pain Sensitivity

Sensitivity to and perception of pain vary among persons and in the same person under different conditions and in different parts of the body. Irritation, mild hypoxia, and mild compression of a peripheral nerve often result in hyperexcitability of the sensory nerve fibres or cell bodies. This is experienced as unpleasant hypersensitivity (*i.e., hyperesthesia*) or increased painfulness (*i.e., hyperalgesia*). Primary hyperalgesia describes pain sensitivity that occurs directly in damaged tissues. Secondary hyperalgesia occurs in the surrounding uninjured tissue. Possible causes of hyperalgesia include increased sensitivity to noxious stimuli, a decrease in the threshold of nociceptors, an increase in pain produced by suprathreshold stimuli, and the windup phenomenon. Hyperalgesia can also be induced by mediators released by immune cells during an inflammatory or allergic response that act directly on nociceptors or indirectly through the release of other mediators, such as the prostaglandins.[42]

Hyperpathia is a syndrome in which the sensory threshold is raised, but when it is reached, continued stimulation, especially if repetitive, results in a prolonged and unpleasant experience. This pain can be explosive and radiates through a peripheral nerve distribution. It is associated with pathologic changes in peripheral nerves, such as localized ischemia.

Spontaneous, unpleasant sensations called *paresthesias* occur with more severe irritation (*e.g.,* the pins-and-needles sensation that follows temporary compression of a peripheral nerve). The general term *dysesthesia* is given to distortions (usually unpleasant) of somesthetic sensation that typically accompany partial loss of sensory innervation.

More severe pathologic processes can result in reduced or lost tactile (*e.g., hypoesthesia, anesthesia*), temperature (*e.g., hypothermia, athermia*), and pain sensation (*i.e., hypoalgesia*). *Analgesia* is the absence of pain on noxious stimulation or the relief of pain without loss of consciousness. The inability to sense pain may result in trauma, infection, and even loss of a body part or parts. Inherited insensitivity to pain may take the form of congenital indifference or congenital insensitivity to pain. Congenital indifference occurs when the transmission of nerve impulses appears normal but appreciation of painful stimuli at higher levels appears to be absent. Congenital insensitivity occurs when a peripheral nerve defect apparently exists such that transmission of painful nerve impulses does not result in perception of pain. Whatever the cause, persons who lack the ability to perceive pain are at constant risk of tissue damage because pain is not serving its protective function.

Allodynia (Greek *allo*, "other," and *odynia*, "painful") is the term used for the puzzling phenomenon of pain that follows a nonnoxious stimulus to apparently normal skin. Non-noxious stimuli may include wind, touching sheets, and showering. This term is intended to refer to instances in which otherwise normal tissues may be abnormally innervated or may be referral sites for other loci that give rise to pain with nonnoxious stimuli. It can result from increased responsiveness within the spinal cord (central sensitization) or a reduction in the threshold for nociceptor activation (peripheral sensitization). With central sensitization, activity in non-nociceptive nerve fibres can produce pain. With peripheral sensitization, tissue damage and inflammation (referred to as the "inflammatory soup") may cause the area to become hypersensitive, in which case a normally subthreshold stimulus is sufficient to trigger the sensation of pain.

One type of allodynia involves *trigger points*, which are highly localized points on the skin or mucous membrane that can produce immediate intense pain at that site or elsewhere when stimulated by light tactile stimulation. Myofascial trigger points are foci of exquisite tenderness found in many muscles and can be responsible for pain projected to sites remote from the points of tenderness. Trigger points are widely distributed in the back of the head and neck and in the lumbar and thoracic regions. These trigger points cause reproducible myofascial pain syndromes in specific muscles. These pain syndromes are the major source of pain in clients at chronic pain treatment centres.

Special Types of Pain

Neuropathic Pain

Neuropathic pain refers to pain that is initiated or caused by pathology of the nervous system. It can affect up to 4% to 8%

of the population in the developed world, suggesting that up to two million Canadians have this condition.[43] When peripheral nerves are affected by injury or disease, it can lead to unusual and sometimes intractable sensory disturbances. The notable features that point to neuropathic processes as a cause of pain include widespread pain that is not otherwise explainable, evidence of sensory deficit (*e.g.*, numbness, paresthesias), burning pain, pain that occurs with light stroking of the skin, and attacks of pain that occur without seeming provocation.[43] Depending on the cause, few or many axons could be damaged and the condition could be unilateral or bilateral. Neuropathic pain is distinguished from other pain conditions where the pain stimulus begins in nonneuronal tissues.

Causes of neuropathic pain can be categorized according to the extent of peripheral nerve involvement. Conditions that can lead to pain by causing damage to peripheral nerves in a single area include nerve entrapment, nerve compression from a tumour mass, and various neuralgias (*e.g.*, trigeminal, postherpetic, and post-traumatic). Conditions that can lead to pain by causing damage to peripheral nerves in a wide area include diabetes mellitus, long-term alcohol use, hypothyroidism, renal insufficiency, and drug treatment with neurotoxic agents.[44] Diabetes often causes a length-dependent neuropathy (meaning that the longest axons in a peripheral nerve are most vulnerable). Injury to a nerve also can lead to a multisymptom, multisystem syndrome called *complex regional pain syndrome*. Nerve damage associated with amputation is believed to be a cause of phantom limb pain.

Neuropathic pain can vary with the extent and location of disease or injury. There may be allodynia or pain that is stabbing, jabbing, burning, or shooting. The pain may be persistent or intermittent. The diagnosis depends on the mode of onset, the distribution of abnormal sensations, the quality of the pain, and other relevant medical conditions (*e.g.*, diabetes, hypothyroidism, alcohol use, rash, or trauma). Injury to peripheral nerves sometimes results in pain that persists beyond the time required for the tissues to heal. Peripheral pathologic processes (*e.g.*, neural degeneration, neuroma formation, and generation of abnormal spontaneous neural discharges from the injured sensory neuron) and neural plasticity (*i.e.*, changes in CNS function) are the primary working hypotheses to explain persistent neuropathic pain.

Treatment methods include measures aimed at restoring nerve function or preventing further nerve damage (*e.g.*, surgical resection of a tumour causing nerve compression, improving glycemic control for diabetic patients with painful neuropathies), and interventions for the palliation of pain. Although many adjuvant analgesics are used for neuropathic pain, pain control often is difficult. The Canadian Pain Society's initial approach in seeking adequate pain control is to try these drugs in sequence and then in combination as outlined in the 2014 revised Consensus Statement.[43] The first-line analgesics are antidepressants (tricyclics [TCAs] or serotonin noradrenaline reuptake inhibitors [SNRIs]) and anticonvulsant medications; second-line includes tramadol and opioids analgesics; third-line suggests cannabinoids; and fourth-line

consists of selective serotonin reuptake inhibitors (SSRIs), Lamotrigine (a novel anticonvulsant agent), methadone, topical lidocaine, and miscellaneous agents such as tapentadol, topical capsaicin or botulinum toxin.[43] The adjuvant analgesics can be further divided into three general classes according to the pain they are used to treat: burning, tingling, or aching pain; stabbing or shooting pain; and neurogenic pain. For pain that is burning, tingling or aching, tricyclic antidepressants and the α_2-adrenergic agonist clonidine frequently are used. For the stabbing or shooting pain of neuralgias, anticonvulsant medications or baclofen, a drug used in treatment of spasticity, may be used.[44]

Poor pain control or unacceptable side effects may lead to a trial with other medications. If there has been a poor response to the adjuvant analgesics, opioids also can be used. However, concerns about side effects and the remote possibility of addiction must be considered. When opioids are used, the use of long-acting opioids with a plan for breakthrough pain is desirable because it addresses the typically continuous nature of neuropathic pain. Nonpharmacologic therapies also are used for neurogenic pain. Electrical stimulation of the peripheral nerve or spinal cord can be used for radiculopathies and neuralgias. As a last resort, neurolysis or neurosurgical blockade sometimes is used.

Neuralgia

Neuralgia is characterized by severe, brief, often repetitive attacks of lightning-like or throbbing pain. It occurs along the distribution of a spinal or cranial nerve and usually is precipitated by stimulation of the cutaneous region supplied by that nerve.

Trigeminal Neuralgia. Trigeminal neuralgia, or *tic douloureux,* is one of the most common and severe neuralgias. It is manifested by facial tics or spasms and characterized by paroxysmal attacks of stabbing pain that usually are limited to the unilateral sensory distribution of one or more branches of the trigeminal nerve, most often the maxillary or mandibular divisions.[44,45] Although intermittent, the pain often is excruciating and may be triggered by light touch, movement, drafts, and eating.[45] Considerable controversy remains regarding the pathophysiology of trigeminal neuralgia. One theory suggests that peripheral injury or disease of the trigeminal nerve increases afferent firing in the nerve. Failure of central inhibitory mechanisms may be involved as well.[45]

Treatment of trigeminal neuralgia includes pharmacologic and surgical modalities. Other interventions include avoidance of precipitating factors (*e.g.*, stimulation of trigger spots) and eye injury due to irritation; provision for adequate nutrition; and avoidance of social isolation. Carbamazepine, an anticonvulsant drug, is recognized as a first-line agent for treatment of trigeminal neuralgia.[45] Surgical release of vessels, dural structures, or scar tissue surrounding the semilunar ganglion or root in the middle cranial fossa often eliminates the symptoms. If not, percutaneous blocking or partial destruction of peripheral branches of the trigeminal nerve with heat, glycerol, or balloon compression may be used.[45] Gamma knife radiosurgery, a form of stereotactic radiosurgery, is one of the newest and least invasive neurosurgical techniques for trigeminal neuralgia.[45] The procedure uses a stereotactic head frame, stereotactic imaging of the trigeminal nerve root entry zone, and radiation of the trigeminal nerve. There has also been recent interest in the use of botulinum toxin as a treatment modality.[45]

Postherpetic Neuralgia. Herpes zoster (also called *shingles*) is caused by the same herpesvirus (varicella-zoster virus) that causes chickenpox and is thought to represent a localized recurrent infection by the varicella-zoster virus that has remained latent in the dorsal root ganglia since the initial attack of chickenpox[46,47] (see Chapter 61). Reactivation of viral replication is associated with a decline in cellular immunity, such as occurs with aging. Thus, the probability of developing herpes zoster increases strikingly with aging, and most cases occur in older adults.[47] Impaired cellular immunity also increases the risk of herpes zoster.

During the acute attack of herpes zoster, the reactivated virus travels from the affected sensory ganglia and peripheral nerve to the skin of the corresponding dermatomes, causing a unilateral localized vesicular eruption and hyperpathia (*i.e.,* abnormally exaggerated subjective response to pain). In the acute infection, proportionately more of the large nerve fibres are destroyed. Regenerated fibres appear to have smaller diameters. Because there is a relative loss of large fibres with age, older adults are particularly prone to suffering because of the shift in the proportion of large- to small-diameter nerve fibres.

Most recent definitions of postherpetic neuralgia describe the presence of pain more than 90 to 120 days after the onset of the herpes rash, which eliminates pain from acute inflammation and ensures that the person has true chronic neuropathic pain.[46] Persons with postherpetic neuralgia may suffer from constant pain ("burning, aching, throbbing"), intermittent pain ("stabbing, shooting"), and stimulus-evoked pain (allodynia). Persons with allodynia often suffer from excruciating pain after the slightest touch to affected skin by such things as cold wind or clothing.[46] These subtypes of pain may interfere with sleep and basic activities of living, causing chronic fatigue, depression, anorexia, weight loss, and social isolation.

Early treatment of shingles with antiviral drugs such as acyclovir or valacyclovir that inhibit herpesvirus deoxyribonucleic acid (DNA) replication may reduce the severity of herpes zoster. Initially, postherpetic neuralgia can be treated with a topical anesthetic agent, lidocaine-prilocaine cream or 5% lidocaine gel. Another topical agent used is capsaicin; however, it can cause intense burning and many users experience a worsening of burning pain while waiting for relief to start. New to the American market but currently unavailable in Canada is a capsaicin patch (Qutenza) that seems to provide longer relief. A tricyclic antidepressant medication, such as amitriptyline or desipramine, may be used for pain relief. Regional nerve blockade (*i.e.,* stellate ganglion, epidural, local infiltration, or peripheral nerve block) has been used with limited success.

A recent trial investigating a new live attenuated herpes zoster vaccine among adults 60 years of age and older, designed to boost their cell-mediated immunity to the varicella-zoster virus, demonstrated dramatic decreases in the incidence of herpes zoster and postherpetic neuralgia.[48] In 2008, the vaccine was approved by Health Canada for the prevention of herpes zoster in persons 50 years of age and older. It is not indicated for treatment of herpes zoster or postherpetic neuralgia.

Complex Regional Pain Syndrome

The complex regional pain syndrome (CRPS), formerly known as *reflex sympathetic dystrophy* (RSD), is a rare disorder of the extremities characterized by autonomic and vasomotor instability.[49–51] There are two forms of CRPS: CRPS I (equivalent of RSD) and CRPS II, also known as *causalgia.* The preferred Budapest criteria for diagnosis of CRPS is based on continuing pain and the grouping of signs and symptoms into four distinct categories: *sensory* with allodynia (perception of pain from a nonpainful stimulus) and/or hyperalgesia (disproportionate to the inciting event); *vasomotor* with temperature asymmetry, skin colour changes, and/or skin colour symmetry; *sudomotor/edema* with edema, sweating changes, and/or sweating symmetry; and *motor/trophic* with decreased range of motion, motor dysfunction (weakness, tremor, dystonia) and/or tropic changes (hair, skin, nails). The diagnosis is excluded by the existence of any condition that would otherwise account for the degree of pain and dysfunction.[49,50]

Traditionally, CRPS II (*i.e.,* causalgia) was diagnosed as the presence of continuing pain, allodynia, or hyperalgesia after a nerve injury, not necessarily limited to the distribution of the injured nerve, with evidence at some time of edema, changes in skin blood flow, or abnormal sensorimotor activity in the region of pain.[51] The diagnosis is excluded by the existence of any condition that would otherwise account for the degree of pain and dysfunction. However, the signs and symptoms of the two subtypes are similar, and there is no evidence that they differ in terms of pathophysiologic mechanisms or treatment responsiveness.[51]

The hallmark of CRPS is pain and mobility problems more severe than the injury warrants. Characteristically, the pain is severe and burning with or without deep aching. Usually, the pain can be elicited with the slightest movement or touch to the affected area, it increases with repetitive stimulation, and it lasts even after the stimulation has stopped. The pain can be exacerbated by emotional upsets or any increased peripheral sympathetic nerve stimulation. All the variations of CRPS include sympathetic components. These are characterized by vascular and trophic (*e.g.,* dystrophic or atrophic) changes to the skin, soft tissue, and bone, and can include rubor or pallor, sweating or dryness, edema (often sharply demarcated), and, with time, patchy osteoporosis.

The pathophysiologic process of CRPS remains obscure. In 1916, Leriche proposed that increased local sympathetic outflow in response to heightened afferent activity was the cause of symptoms such as pain, redness, heat, and edema.

Although abnormalities in sympathetic activity are observed, recent experimental data suggest sensitization of small-diameter, polymodal C and Aδ fibres to noxious stimuli may be the basis for hyperalgia to heat and nociceptive stimuli.[52] There is also evidence that central mechanisms may play a role in sensitization of central neurons (the previously described dorsal horn WDR neurons) that occurs after intense peripheral mechanical stimuli or continuous activity in nociceptors. The role of the α₁-adrenergic receptors in sympathetic efferent or afferent coupling, either directly or indirectly through prostaglandin or α₁-adrenergic receptor activity, is considered to contribute to the excitation and sensitization of the nociceptive afferents. Other proposed mechanisms include neurogenic inflammation caused by the activation of neuromediators, such as substance P, calcitonin gene-related peptide, and histamine, which also mediates inflammation and vasodilation of microvessels.[49] Recent research demonstrated the presence of autoantibodies against autonomic nervous system structures in patients with CRPS, suggesting that the disorder may result from dysfunction of the autonomic nervous system caused by an autoimmune attack.[49]

Early mobilization after injury or surgery reduces the likelihood of developing the syndrome.[52] In addition to addressing the underlying disorder, treatment is directed at restoration of function. Physical therapy is a cornerstone of therapy. Pain management involves the use of standard pharmacologic agents used in the management of neuropathic pain, namely antidepressants (*e.g.,* amitriptyline) and anticonvulsant drugs (*e.g.,* gabapentin). Short-term corticosteroid (prednisone) treatment may be used in resistant cases. If these do not lead to improvement, treatment by sympathetic blockade (lumbar sympathetic block or stellate ganglion block) may provide relief from pain, as well as helping to determine the extent to which the pain is sympathetically maintained. The latter mechanism, when present, might respond to the use of an α₁-adrenergic receptor antagonist (*e.g.,* terazosin, phenoxybenzamine). Electrical neurostimulation of the spinal cord may also be considered. Neurostimulation may provide analgesia and, in addition, may reduce the burning dysesthesia of which many patients complain. It may also improve circulation in the affected extremity by blocking the sympathetic efferent pathways.[52,53]

Phantom Limb Pain

Phantom limb pain, a type of neurologic pain, follows amputation of a limb or part of a limb. As many as 50% to 85% of amputees experience phantom limb pain.[54] The pain often begins as sensations of tingling, heat and cold, or heaviness, followed by burning, cramping, or shooting pain. It may disappear spontaneously or persist for many years. One of the more troublesome aspects of phantom pain is that the person may experience painful sensations that were present before the amputation, such as that of a painful ulcer or bunion.

Several theories have been proposed as to the causes of phantom limb pain.[54] One theory is that the end of a regenerating nerve becomes trapped in the scar tissue of the amputation site. It is known that when a peripheral nerve is cut, the scar tissue that forms becomes a barrier to regenerating outgrowth of the axon. The growing axon often becomes trapped in the scar tissue, forming a tangled growth (*i.e.,* neuroma) of small-diameter axons, including primary nociceptive afferents and sympathetic efferents. It has been proposed that these afferents show increased sensitivity to innocuous mechanical stimuli and to sympathetic activity and circulating catecholamines. A related theory moves the source of phantom limb pain to the spinal cord, suggesting that the pain is due to the spontaneous firing of spinal cord neurons that have lost their normal sensory input from the body. In this case, a closed self-exciting neuronal loop in the posterior horn of the spinal cord is postulated to send impulses to the brain, resulting in pain. Even the slightest irritation to the amputated limb area can initiate this cycle. Other theories propose that the phantom limb pain may arise in the brain itself. In one hypothesis, the pain is caused by changes in the flow of signals through somatosensory areas of the brain. In other words, there appears to be plasticity even in the adult CNS. Treatment of phantom limb pain has been accomplished by the use of sympathetic blocks, TENS of the large myelinated afferents innervating the area, hypnosis, relaxation training, and the new mirror therapy. This promising therapy utilizes a mirror image of the normal body limb to help reorganize and integrate the mismatch between motor intention, proprioception, and visual system.[54]

IN SUMMARY

Pain may occur with or without an adequate stimulus, or it may be absent in the presence of an adequate stimulus—either of which describes a pain disorder. There may be analgesia (absence of pain), hyperalgesia (increased sensitivity to pain), hypoalgesia (a decreased sensitivity to painful stimuli), hyperpathia (an unpleasant and prolonged response to pain), hyperesthesia (an abnormal increase in sensitivity to sensation), hypoesthesia (an abnormal decrease in sensitivity to sensations), paresthesia (abnormal touch sensation such as tingling or "pins and needles" in the absence of external stimuli), or allodynia (pain produced by stimuli that do not normally cause pain).

Neuropathic pain may be due to trauma to or disease of neurons in a focal area or in a more global distribution (*e.g.,* from endocrine disease or neurotoxic medications). Neuralgia is characterized by severe, brief, often repetitive attacks of lightning-like or throbbing pain that occur along the distribution of a spinal or cranial nerve and usually are precipitated by stimulation of the cutaneous region supplied by that nerve. Trigeminal neuralgia, or tic douloureux, is one of the most common and severe neuralgias. It is manifested by facial tics or spasms. Postherpetic neuralgia is a chronic pain that can occur after shingles, an infection of the dorsal root ganglia and corresponding areas of innervation by the varicella-zoster virus. CRPS is a severe pain syndrome characterized by severe pain and sensory, vasomotor, sudomotor/edema, and/or motor/tropic changes. Phantom limb pain, a neurologic pain, can occur after amputation of a limb or part of a limb.

HEADACHE AND ASSOCIATED PAIN

After completing this section of the chapter, you should be able to meet the following objectives:

- State the importance of distinguishing between primary and secondary types of headache.
- Differentiate between the periodicity of occurrence and manifestations of migraine headache, cluster headache, tension-type headache, and headache due to temporomandibular joint syndrome.
- Characterize the nonpharmacologic and pharmacologic methods used in treatment of headache.
- Cite the most common cause of temporomandibular joint pain.

Headache

Headache is a very common health problem, with over 90% of adults reporting having had a headache at least once. Seventy-six percent of women and 57% of men report at least one headache a month.[55] Twenty-five percent of adults report having recurrent severe headaches and 4% report having daily or near-daily headaches.[56] Although head and facial pain have characteristics that distinguish them from other pain disorders, they also share many of the same features.

Headache is caused by a number of conditions. Some headaches represent primary disorders and others occur secondary to other disease conditions in which head pain is a symptom. The most common types of primary or chronic headaches are migraine headache, tension-type headache, cluster headache, and chronic daily headache. Individuals can also experience problems with headaches post-concussion or after a mild traumatic brain injury. Although most causes of secondary headache are benign, some are indications of serious disorders such as meningitis, brain tumour, or cerebral aneurysm. The sudden onset of a severe, intractable headache in an otherwise healthy person is more likely related to a serious intracranial disorder, such as subarachnoid hemorrhage or meningitis, than to a chronic headache disorder. Headaches that disturb sleep, exertional headaches (*e.g.,* triggered by physical or sexual activity or a Valsalva maneuver), and headaches accompanied by neurologic symptoms such as drowsiness, visual or limb disturbances, or altered mental status also are suggestive of underlying intracranial lesions or other pathologic processes. Other red flags for secondary headache disorder include a fundamental change or progression in headache pattern or a new headache in individuals younger than 5

or older than 50 years of age, or in individuals with cancer, immunosuppression, or who are pregnant.[56]

The diagnosis and classification of headaches often is difficult. It requires a comprehensive history and physical examination to exclude secondary causes. The history should include factors that precipitate headache, such as foods and food additives, missed meals, and association with the menstrual period. A careful medication history is essential because many medications can provoke or aggravate headaches. Alcohol also can cause or aggravate headache. A headache diary in which the person records his or her headaches and concurrent or antecedent events may be helpful in identifying factors that contribute to headache onset. Appropriate laboratory and imaging studies of the brain may be done to rule out secondary headaches.

In 2013, the International Headache Society (IHS) published the third edition of *The International Classification of Headache Disorders* (ICHD-3 beta). The classification system is divided into three sections: (1) primary headaches, (2) headaches secondary to other medical conditions, and (3) cranial neuropathies, other facial pain, and other headaches.[57,58] Primary headaches include migraine, tension-type headache, cluster headache, and other trigeminal autonomic cephalalgias.

Migraine Headache

Migraine headaches affect approximately 3.0 million persons in Canada and are a common disability worldwide. Lifetime prevalence is estimated at 24% in women and 9% in men; women consistently are almost three times more likely to suffer migraines than men.[59] Migraine headaches tend to run in families and are thought to be inherited as an autosomal dominant trait with incomplete penetrance. It is noteworthy that the genetic influence is stronger for migraine with aura than for migraine without aura.[60]

The ICHD-3 classifies migraine headaches into six major categories, the two most important of which are migraine without aura, which accounts for approximately 85% of migraines, and migraine with aura, which accounts for most of the remaining migraines.[58] Migraine without aura is a pulsatile, throbbing, unilateral headache that typically lasts 1 to 2 days and is aggravated by routine physical activity. The headache is accompanied by nausea and vomiting, which often is disabling, and sensitivity to light and sound. Visual disturbances occur quite commonly and consist of visual hallucinations such as stars, sparks, and flashes of light. Migraine with aura has similar symptoms, but with the addition of reversible visual symptoms, including positive features (*e.g.,* flickering lights, spots, or lines) or negative features (loss of vision); fully reversible sensory symptoms, including positive features (feeling of pins or needles) or negative features (numbness); and fully reversible speech disturbances or neurologic symptoms that precede the headache.[58] The aura usually develops over a period of 5 to 20 minutes and lasts from 5 minutes to an hour. Although only a small percentage of persons with migraine experience an aura before an attack, many persons without aura have prodromal symptoms, such as fatigue and irritability that precede the attack by hours or even days.

The other ICHD-3 migraine headache subcategories include retinal migraine, complications of migraine (*e.g.,* chronic migraine, migrainous infarction, and migraine-triggered seizures), and childhood periodic syndromes that are commonly precursors of migraine. Retinal migraines are a rare form of migraine characterized by recurrent attacks of fully reversible scintillations (visual sensation of sparks or flashes of light), scotomata (visual blind spots), or blindness affecting one eye, followed within an hour by migrainous headache. The ICHD-3 classifies chronic migraine when a headache meeting the criteria for migraine is present on 15 or more days per month for 3 months or more, in the absence of medication overuse. Migrainous infarction is an uncommon occurrence in which one or more otherwise typical aura symptoms persists beyond 1 hour and neuroimaging confirms ischemic infarction. Strictly applied, these criteria distinguish this disorder from stroke, which must be excluded.[58] Migraine headache also can present as a mixed headache, including symptoms typically associated with tension-type headache, sinus headache, or chronic daily headache. These are called *transformed migraine* and are difficult to classify. Although nasal symptoms are not one of the diagnostic criteria for migraine, they frequently accompany migraine and are probably due to cranial parasympathetic activation. Pain in the sinus area may indicate either inflammation or migraine. In a recent study, 96% of those self-diagnosed with sinus headache in fact met the IHS criteria for migraine or migrainous headache.[61]

Migraine headaches occur in children as well as adults.[57,62,63] Before puberty, migraine headaches are equally distributed between the sexes. The essential diagnostic criterion for migraine in children is the presence of recurrent headaches separated by pain-free periods. Diagnosis is based on at least three of the following symptoms or associated findings: abdominal pain, nausea or vomiting, throbbing headache, unilateral location, associated aura (visual, sensory, motor), relief during sleep, and a positive family history.[63] Symptoms vary widely among children, from those that interrupt activities and cause the child to seek relief in a dark environment to those detectable only by direct questioning. A common feature of migraine in children is intense nausea and vomiting. The vomiting may be associated with abdominal pain and fever; thus, migraine may be confused with other conditions such as appendicitis. Because headaches in children can be a symptom of other, more serious disorders, including intracranial lesions, it is important that other causes of headache that require immediate treatment be ruled out.

The pathophysiologic mechanisms of the pain associated with migraine headaches remain poorly understood. Although many alternative theories exist, it is well established that during a migraine the trigeminal nerve becomes activated.[60,64] Activation of the trigeminal sensory fibres may lead to the release of neuropeptides, causing painful neurogenic inflammation within the meningeal vasculature characterized by plasma protein extravasation, vasodilation, and mast cell degranulation.[65] Another possible mechanism implicates neurogenic vasodilation of meningeal blood vessels as a key component of the inflammatory processes that occur during migraine. Activation of trigeminal sensory fibres evokes a neurogenic dural vasodilation mediated by calcitonin gene-related peptide. It also has been observed that the calcitonin gene-related peptide level is elevated during migraine and is normalized after successful treatment with sumatriptan.[64] Supporting the neurogenic basis for migraine is the frequent presence of premonitory symptoms before the headache begins; the presence of focal neurologic disturbances, which cannot be explained in terms of cerebral blood flow; and the numerous accompanying symptoms, including autonomic and constitutional dysfunction.

Hormonal variations, particularly in estrogen levels, play a role in the pattern of migraine attacks. For many women, migraine headaches coincide with their menstrual periods. The greater predominance of migraine headaches in women is thought to be related to the aggravating effect of estrogen on the migraine mechanism. Dietary substances, such as monosodium glutamate, aged cheese, and chocolate, also may precipitate migraine headaches. The actual triggers for migraine are the chemicals in the food, not allergens.

Treatment. The treatment of migraine headaches includes preventive and abortive nonpharmacologic and pharmacologic treatment.[65] In 2012, the Canadian Headache Society produced a set of evidence-based guidelines for the nonpharmacologic and pharmacologic management and prevention of migraine headaches in primary care settings for adults.[59]

Nonpharmacologic treatment includes the avoidance of migraine triggers, such as foods, that precipitate an attack. Many persons with migraines benefit from maintaining regular eating and sleeping habits. Measures to control stress, which also can precipitate an attack, also are important. During an attack, many persons find it helpful to retire to a quiet, darkened room until symptoms subside.

Pharmacologic treatment involves both abortive therapy for acute attacks and preventive therapy. A wide range of medications is used to treat the acute symptoms of migraine headache. Based on clinical trials, first-line agents include acetylsalicylic acid; combinations of acetaminophen, acetylsalicylic acid, and caffeine; NSAIDs (*e.g.,* naproxen sodium, ibuprofen); serotonin ($5-HT_1$) receptor agonists (*e.g.,* sumatriptan, naratriptan, rizatriptan, zolmitriptan); ergotamine derivatives (*e.g.,* dihydroergotamine); and antiemetic medications (*e.g.,* ondansetron, metoclopramide). Nonoral routes of administration may be preferred in individuals who develop severe pain rapidly or on awakening, or in those with severe nausea and vomiting. Both sumatriptan and dihydroergotamine have been approved for intranasal administration. Intranasal lidocaine has also shown promise as an abortive agent. For intractable migraine headache, dihydroergotamine may be administered parenterally with an antiemetic or opioid analgesic (transnasal butorphanol).[66] Frequent use of abortive headache medications may cause rebound headache.

Preventive pharmacologic treatment may be necessary if migraine headaches become disabling, if they occur more than two or three times a month, if abortive treatment is being used more than two times a week, or if the individual has hemiplegic migraine, migraine with prolonged aura, or migrainous infarction. In most cases, preventative treatment must be taken daily for months to years. First-line agents include β-adrenergic blocking medications (*e.g.,* propranolol, atenolol), antidepressants (amitriptyline), and anticonvulsant medications (divalproex sodium, valproate).[64,67] When a decision to discontinue preventive therapy is made, the medications should be gradually withdrawn to prevent exacerbation of headaches.

Other effective medications are available, but they can have serious side effects in some individuals. For example, because of the risk of coronary vasospasm, the 5-HT$_1$ receptor agonists should not be given to persons with coronary artery disease. Ergotamine preparations can cause uterine contractions and should not be given to pregnant women. They also can cause vasospasm, and should be used with caution in persons with peripheral arterial disease.

Cluster Headache

Cluster headaches are relatively uncommon headaches that occur in about 1 in 1,000 individuals, affecting men (80% to 85%) more frequently than women and typically beginning in the third decade of life and rarely beginning beyond the age of 70.[68] These headaches tend to occur in clusters over weeks or months, followed by a long, headache-free remission period. Cluster headache is a type of primary neurovascular headache that typically includes severe, unrelenting, unilateral pain located, in order of decreasing frequency, in the orbital, retro-orbital, temporal, supraorbital, and infraorbital regions.[68–70] The pain is of rapid onset and builds to a peak in approximately 10 to 15 minutes, lasting for 15 to 180 minutes. The pain behind the eye radiates to the ipsilateral trigeminal nerve (*e.g.,* temple, cheek, gum). The headache frequently is associated with one or more symptoms such as restlessness or agitation, conjunctival redness, lacrimation, nasal congestion, rhinorrhea, forehead and facial sweating, miosis, ptosis, and eyelid edema. Because of their location and associated symptoms, cluster headaches are often mistaken for sinus infections or dental problems.

The underlying pathophysiologic mechanisms of cluster headaches are not completely known, although recently it has been noted that heredity, through an autosomal dominant gene, plays some role in the pathogenesis of cluster headache. The most likely pathophysiologic mechanisms include the interplay of vascular, neurogenic, metabolic, and humoral factors. Activation of the trigemino-vascular system and the cranial autonomic parasympathetic reflexes is thought to explain the pain and autonomic symptoms. The hypothalamus is believed to play a key role. The possible role of the regulating centres in the anterior hypothalamus is implicated from observations of circadian biologic changes and neuroendocrine disturbances (*e.g.,* changes in cortisol, prolactin, and testosterone) that occur in both active periods and during clinical remission. The hypothalamic grey matter also has been implicated. Positron emission tomography (PET) scanning has demonstrated

increased blood flow as well as structural changes in the hypothalamic grey area on the painful side during an attack.[68–70] Magnetic resonance imaging has demonstrated dilated intracranial arteries on the painful side. Loss of vascular tone is believed to result from a defect in the sympathetic perivascular innervation.

Treatment. Because of the relatively short duration and self-limited nature of cluster headaches, oral preparations typically take too long to reach therapeutic levels. The most effective treatments are those that act quickly (*e.g.,* oxygen inhalation and subcutaneous sumatriptan). Intranasal lidocaine also may be effective.[69,70] Oxygen inhalation may be indicated for home use. Many prophylactic medications for cluster headaches are available such as ergotamine, verapamil, topiramate, methysergide, lithium carbonate, corticosteroids, valproate, etc. Deep-brain surgical neurostimulation is an experimental approach beginning to show promise in the elimination of cluster headaches.[69]

Tension-Type Headache

The most common type of headache is tension-type headache. Unlike migraine and cluster headaches, tension-type headache usually is not sufficiently severe that it interferes with daily activities. Tension-type headaches frequently are described as dull, aching, diffuse, nondescript headaches, occurring in a hatband distribution around the head, and not associated with nausea or vomiting or worsened by activity. They can be infrequent, episodic, or chronic.

The exact mechanisms of tension-type headache are not known and the hypotheses of causation are contradictory. One popular theory is that tension-type headache results from sustained tension of the muscles of the scalp and neck; however, research has found no correlation between muscle contraction and tension-type headache. Many authorities now believe that tension-type headaches are forms of migraine headache.[71] It is thought that migraine headache may be transformed gradually into chronic tension-type headache. Tension-type headaches also may be caused by oromandibular dysfunction, psychogenic stress, anxiety, depression, and muscular stress. They also may result from overuse of analgesics or caffeine. Daily use of caffeine, whether in beverages or medications, can produce addiction, and a headache can develop in such persons who go without caffeine for several hours.[72]

Treatment. Tension-type headaches often are more responsive to nonpharmacologic techniques, such as biofeedback, massage, acupuncture, relaxation, imagery, and physical therapy, than other types of headache. For persons with poor posture, a combination of range-of-motion exercises, relaxation, and posture improvement may be helpful.

The medications of choice for acute treatment of tension-type headaches are analgesics, including acetylsalicylic acid, acetaminophen, and NSAIDs.[72] Persons with infrequent tension-type headache usually self-medicate using over-the-counter analgesics to treat the acute pain, and do not require prophylactic medication. These agents should be used cautiously because rebound headaches can develop when the medications are taken regularly.

Because the "dividing lines" between tension-type headache, migraine, and chronic daily headache often are vague, addition of medications as well as the entire range of migraine medications may be tried in refractory cases. Other medications used concomitantly with analgesics include sedating antihistamines (*e.g.,* promethazine and diphenhydramine), antiemetics (*e.g.,* metoclopramide and prochlorperazine), or sedatives (*e.g.,* butalbital). Prophylactic treatment for chronic tension-type headaches can include antidepressants (*e.g.,* amitriptyline) and selective serotonin reuptake inhibitors (SSRIs; *e.g.,* paroxetine, venlafaxine, and fluoxetine).[72]

Chronic Daily Headache

The term *chronic daily headache* (CDH) is used to refer to headaches that occur 15 days or more a month, including those due to medication overuse.[73–75] Little is known about the prevalence and incidence of CDH. Diagnostic criteria is now provided in the IHS Classification System (new daily persistent headache). The cause of CDH is unknown, although there are several hypotheses. They include transformed migraine headache, evolved tension-type headache, new daily persistent headache, and post-traumatic headache. In many persons, CDH retains certain characteristics of migraine, whereas in others it resembles chronic tension-type headache. CDH may be associated with chronic and episodic tension-type headache. New daily persistent headache may have a fairly rapidly onset, with no history of migraine, tension-type headache, trauma, or psychological stress. Although overuse of symptomatic medications (*e.g.,* analgesics, ergotamine) has been related to CDH, there is a group of patients in whom CDH is unrelated to excessive use of medications.

Treatment. For patients with CDH, a combination of pharmacologic and behavioural interventions may be necessary. As with tension-type headaches, nonpharmacologic techniques, such as biofeedback, massage, acupuncture, relaxation, imagery, and physical therapy, may be helpful. Measures to reduce or eliminate the overuse of medications, including caffeine, may be helpful. If the patient is abusing medications, the overuse must be managed before prophylactic agents will be effective.[74] Most of the medications used for prevention of CDH have not been examined in well-designed, double-blind studies.

Temporomandibular Joint Pain

A common cause of headache is temporomandibular joint (TMJ) syndrome. It usually is caused by an imbalance in joint movement because of poor bite, bruxism (*i.e.,* teeth grinding), or joint problems such as inflammation, trauma, and degenerative changes.[76] The pain almost always is referred

and commonly presents as facial muscle pain, headache, neck ache, or earache. Referred pain is aggravated by jaw function. Headache associated with this syndrome is common in adults and children and can cause chronic pain problems.

Treatment of TMJ pain is aimed at correcting the problem, and in some cases this may be difficult. The initial therapy for TMJ should be directed toward relief of pain and improvement in function. Pain relief often can be achieved with use of the NSAIDs. Muscle relaxants may be used when muscle spasm is a problem. In some cases, the selected application of heat or cold, or both, may provide relief. Referral to a dentist who is associated with a team of therapists, such as a psychologist, physical therapist, or pain specialist, may be indicated.[76]

IN SUMMARY

Head pain is a common disorder that is caused by a number of conditions. Some headaches represent primary disorders and others occur secondary to another disease state in which head pain is a symptom. Primary headache disorders include migraine headache, tension-type headache, cluster headache, and chronic daily headache. Although most causes of secondary headache are benign, some are indications of serious disorders such as meningitis, brain tumour, or cerebral aneurysm. TMJ syndrome is one of the major causes of headaches. It usually is caused by an imbalance in joint movement because of poor bite, teeth grinding, or joint problems such as inflammation, trauma, and degenerative changes.

PAIN IN CHILDREN AND OLDER ADULTS

After completing this section of the chapter, you should be able to meet the following objectives:

- State how the pain response may differ in children and older adults.
- Explain how pain assessment may differ in children and older adults.
- Explain how pain treatment may differ in children and older adults.

Pain frequently is underrecognized and undertreated in both children and older adults. In addition to the common obstacles to adequate pain management, such as concern about the effects of analgesia on respiratory status and the potential for addiction to opioids, there are additional deterrents to adequate pain management in children and older adults. With regard to both children and older adults, there are stereotypic beliefs that they feel less pain than other patients.[77–80] These beliefs may affect a clinician's opinion about the need for pain control. In very young children and confused elderly, there are several additional factors. These include the extreme difficulty of assessing the location and intensity of pain in individuals who are cognitively immature or cognitively impaired, and the argument that even if they feel pain, they do not remember it. Research during the past few decades has added a great deal to the body of knowledge about pain in children and older adults.

Pain in Children

Human responsiveness to painful stimuli begins in the neonatal period and continues through the life span. Although the specific and localized behavioural reactions are less marked in the younger neonate or the more cognitively impaired individual, protective or withdrawal reflexes in response to nociceptive stimuli are clearly demonstrated. Pain pathways, cortical and subcortical centres, and neurochemical responses associated with pain transmission are developed and functional by the last trimester of pregnancy.[78] Neonates clearly perceive pain, as demonstrated by their integrated physiologic response to nociceptive stimuli. In fact, pain may be accentuated because descending inhibitory pathways to the dorsal horn are not as well developed at birth.[81] Furthermore, dorsal horn neurons in neonates have a wider receptive field and lower excitatory threshold than those in older children.

As infants and children mature, their responses to pain become more complex and reflective of their maturing cognitive and developmental processes. Children do feel pain and have been shown to reliably and accurately report pain at as young as 3 years of age.[82] They also remember pain, as evidenced in studies of children with cancer, whose distress during painful procedures increases over time without intervention, and in neonates in intensive care units, who demonstrate protective withdrawal responses to a heel stick after repeated episodes.

Pain Assessment

To treat pain adequately, ongoing assessment of the presence of pain and response to treatment is essential.[78,79] Self-report is usually regarded as the most reliable estimate of pain. With children 8 years of age or older, numeric scales (*i.e.,* 1 to 10) and word graphic scales (*i.e.,* "none," "a little," "most I have ever experienced") can be used. With children 3 to 8 years of age, scales with faces of actual children or cartoon faces can be used to obtain a report of pain. Another supplementary strategy for assessing a child's pain is to use a body outline and ask the child to indicate where the hurt is located. Particular care must be taken in assessing children's reports of pain because their reports may be influenced by a variety of factors, including age, anxiety and fear levels, and parental presence. In very young children, infants, and neonates as well as in children with disabilities that impair cognition or communication, clinicians must rely on physiologic parameters or age/development-appropriate behavioural pain scales.[78] Some physiologic measures, such as heart rate, are convenient to measure and respond rapidly to brief nociceptive stimuli,

but they are nonspecific. Relying on indicators of sympathetic nervous system activity and behaviours can also be problematic because they can be caused by things other than pain (*e.g.,* anxiety and activity) and they do not always accompany pain, particularly chronic pain.

Pain Management

The management of children's pain basically falls into two categories: pharmacologic and nonpharmacologic. In terms of pharmacologic interventions, many of the analgesics used in adults can be used safely and effectively in children and adolescents. However, it is critical when using specific medications to determine that the medication has been approved for use with children and that it is dosed appropriately according to the child's weight and level of physiologic development. Age-related differences in physiologic functioning, notably in neonates, will affect drug action. Neonates have decreased fat and muscle and increased water, which increases the duration of action for some water-soluble drugs; neonates also have decreased concentration of plasma proteins (albumin and α_1-glycoprotein), which increases the unbound concentration of protein-binding drugs.[81] Neonates and infants have decreased levels of the hepatic enzymes needed for metabolism of many analgesics. The levels of these hepatic enzymes quickly increase to adult levels in the first few months of life. Drug clearance in the 2- to 6-year-old age group is actually higher than adult levels because of the larger hepatic mass relative to body weight.[81,83] The renal excretion of drugs depends on renal blood flow, glomerular filtration rate, and tubular secretion, all of which are decreased in neonates, particularly premature neonates. Renal function reaches adult levels by 1 year of age.[81,83]

As with any person in pain, the type of analgesic used should be matched to the type and intensity of pain; and whether the patient is a child or adult, the management of chronic pain may require a multidisciplinary team.[83] The overriding principle in all pediatric pain management is to treat each child's pain on an individual basis and to match the analgesic agent with the cause and the level of pain. A second principle involves maintaining the balance between the level of side effects and pain relief such that pain relief is obtained with as little opioid and sedation as possible. One strategy toward this end is to time the administration of analgesia so that a steady blood level is achieved and, as much as possible, pain is prevented. This requires that the child receive analgesia on a regular dosing schedule, not "as needed." Also, most drugs are packaged primarily for adult use, and dose calculations and serial dilutions may predispose to medication errors. Common errors include milligram–microgram errors, decimal point errors, confusion between daily dose and fractional dose (*e.g.,* 100 mg/kg per day divided by 6 hours versus 100 mg/kg per dose every 6 hours), and dilution errors.[83]

Nonpharmacologic strategies can be very effective in reducing the overall amount of pain and amount of analgesia used. In addition, some nonpharmacologic strategies can reduce anxiety and increase the child's level of self-control during pain. In full-term infants, ingesting 2 ml of a sucrose solution has been found to relieve the pain from a heel stick.[84] Children as young as 4 years of age can use TENS,[85] and they can be taught to use simple distraction and relaxation and other techniques such as application of heat and cold.[86] Other nonpharmacologic techniques can be taught to the child to provide psychological preparation for a painful procedure or surgery. These include positive self-talk, imagery, play therapy, modelling, and rehearsal. The nonpharmacologic interventions must be developmentally appropriate and, if possible, the child and parent should be taught these techniques when the child is not in pain (*e.g.*, before surgery or a painful procedure) so that it is easier to practice the technique.

Pain in Older Adults

Among adults, the prevalence of pain in the general population increases with age, with a higher prevalence in women compared to men. Among the elderly the most common self-attributed causes of pain are getting older (88%) and arthritis (69%). In long-term care facilities, it has been estimated that 85% of individuals experience pain on a regular basis.[80] Research is inconsistent about whether there are age-related changes in pain perception. Some apparent age-related differences in pain may be due to differences in willingness to report the pain rather than actual differences in pain. The older adult may be reluctant to report pain so as not to be a burden or out of fear of the diagnoses, tests, medications, or costs that may result from an attempt to diagnose or treat their pain.

Pain Assessment

The assessment of pain in the elderly can range from relatively simple in a well-informed, alert, cognitively intact individual with pain from a single source and no comorbidities, to extraordinarily difficult in a frail individual with severe dementia and many concurrent health problems.[80,87,88] When possible, a patient's report of pain is the gold standard, but behavioural signs of pain should be considered as well. Accurately diagnosing pain when the individual has many health problems or some decline in cognitive function can be particularly challenging. In recent years, there has been increased awareness of the need to address issues of pain in individuals with dementia. The Assessment for Discomfort in Dementia Protocol is one example of the efforts to improve assessment and pain management in these individuals. It includes behavioural criteria for assessing pain and recommended interventions for pain. Its use has been shown to improve pain management.[80,87,88]

Pain Management

When prescribing pharmacologic and nonpharmacologic methods of pain management for the older population, care must be taken to consider the cause of the pain, the patient's health status, the concurrent therapies, and the patient's mental status. In the older population, where the risk of adverse events is higher, the nonpharmacologic options are usually less costly and cause fewer side effects.

Common nonpharmacologic interventions include application of cold (which suppresses the release of products from tissue damage) and heat (which promotes the release of endogenous endorphins).[80] The role of mental focus and anxiety is important, and relaxation techniques, massage, and biofeedback may be useful. Physical therapy and occupational therapy bring a variety of modalities, including the use of braces or splints, changes in biomechanics, and exercise, all of which have been shown to promote pain relief.

Although efficacy is important when considering the use of pharmacologic agents for pain relief in the older adult population, cost and safety must also be considered. Safety issues that must be considered among older adults include changes in drug metabolism, other disease comorbidity, and polypharmacy. The elderly may have physiologic changes that affect the pharmacokinetics of medications prescribed for pain management. These changes include decreased blood flow to organs, delayed gastric motility, reduced kidney function, and decreased albumin related to poor nutrition.[36] Older adults also often have many coexisting health problems, leading to polypharmacy. On the average, a 70-year-old takes seven different medications.[80] The addition of analgesics to a complex medication regimen is even more likely to cause drug interactions and complicate compliance in older adults. However, these considerations should not preclude the appropriate use of analgesic drugs to achieve pain relief. Nonopioids are generally the first line of therapy for mild to moderate pain, and acetaminophen is usually the first choice because it is relatively safe for older adults.[80] Opioids are used for more severe pain and for palliative care. As with younger persons, adjuvant analgesics are effectively used for treatment of pain in older adults. The use of some assessment tool to evaluate the level of pain and effectiveness of treatment is essential. Monitoring for side effects is also critical.

IN SUMMARY

Children experience and remember pain, and even fairly young children are able to accurately and reliably report their pain. Recognition of this has changed the clinical practice of health professionals involved in the assessment of children's pain. Pharmacologic (including opioids) and nonpharmacologic pain management interventions have been shown to be effective in children. Nonpharmacologic techniques must be based on the developmental level of the child and should be taught to both children and parents.

Pain is a common symptom in older adults. Assessment, diagnosis, and treatment of pain in older adults can be complicated. Older adults may be reluctant or cognitively unable to report their pain. Diagnosis and treatment can be complicated by comorbidities and age-related changes in cognitive and physiologic function.

REVIEW EXERCISES

1. A 25-year-old man is admitted to the emergency department with acute abdominal pain that began in the epigastric area and has now shifted to the lower right quadrant of the abdomen. There is localized tenderness and guarding or spasm of the muscle over the area. His heart rate and blood pressure are elevated, and his skin is moist and cool from perspiring. He is given a tentative diagnosis of appendicitis and referred for surgical consultation.

   A. *Describe the origin of the pain stimuli and the neural pathways involved in the pain that this man is experiencing.*

   B. *Explain the neural mechanisms involved in the spasm of the overlying abdominal muscles.*

   C. *What is the significance of his cool, moist skin and increased heart rate and blood pressure?*

2. A 65-year-old woman with breast cancer is receiving hospice care in her home. She is currently receiving a long-acting opioid analgesic supplemented with a short-acting combination opioid and nonnarcotic medication for breakthrough pain.

   A. *Explain the difference between the mechanisms and treatment of acute and chronic pain.*

   B. *Describe the action of opioid drugs in the treatment of pain.*

   C. *Define the term tolerance and cross-tolerance as they refer to the use of opioids for treatment of pain.*

   D. *Describe the common side effects associated with the use of opioid drugs to relieve pain in persons with cancer.*

3. A 42-year-old woman presents with sudden, stabbing-type facial pain that arises near the right side of her mouth and then shoots toward the right ear, eye, and nostril. She is holding her hand to protect her face because the pain is "triggered by touch, movement, and drafts." Her initial diagnosis is trigeminal neuralgia.

   A. *Explain the distribution and mechanisms of the pain, particularly the triggering of the pain by stimuli applied to the skin.*

   B. *What are possible treatment methods for this woman?*

4. A 21-year-old woman presents to the student health centre with complaints of a throbbing pain on the left side of her head, nausea and vomiting, and extreme sensitivity to light, noise, and head movement. She also tells you she had a similar headache 3 months ago that lasted for 2 days and states that she thinks she is developing migraine headaches like her mother. She is concerned because she has been unable to attend classes and has exams next week.

   A. *Are this woman's history and symptoms consistent with migraine headaches? Explain.*

   B. *Use the distribution of the trigeminal nerve and the concept of neurogenic inflammation to explain this woman's symptoms.*

5. A 72-year-old man presents to the emergency department after a fall with a complaint of the "worst headache ever experienced." He is able to answer your questions with increasing difficulty.

   A. *Differentiate primary headache from secondary headache.*

   B. *Given the information that you have, what type of headache do you suspect, and why?*

References

1. Hall J. E. (2011). *Textbook of medical physiology* (12th ed.). Philadelphia, PA: W. B. Saunders.
2. Kandel E. R., Schwartz J. H., Jessell T. M., et al. (2013). *Principles of neural science* (5th ed.). New York: McGraw-Hill Medical.
3. Merskey H., Bogduk N. (1994). *Classification of chronic pain: Description of chronic pain and definitions of pain terms* (2nd ed.). Seattle, WA: IASP Publications.
4. Sherrington C. (1947). *The integrative action of the nervous system.* New Haven, CT: Yale University Press.
5. Schopflocher D., Taenzer P., Jovey R. (2011). The prevalence of chronic pain in Canada. *Pain Research & Management, 16*(6), 445–450.
6. Pain Resource Centre. (2014). Pain in Canada fact sheet. Available online at: http://prc.canadianpaincoalition.ca/en/canadian_pain_fact_sheet.html. Accessed June 15, 2015.
7. Bonica J. J. (1991). History of pain concepts and pain theory. *Mount Sinai Journal of Medicine, 58,* 191–202.
8. Melzack R., Wall P. D. (1965). Pain mechanisms: A new theory. *Science, 150,* 971–979.
9. Melzack R. (1999). From the gate to the neuromatrix. *Pain, 6*(Suppl), S121–S126.
10. Reichling D. B., Green P. G., Levine J. D. (2013). The fundamental unit of pain is the cell. *Pain, 154,* S2–S9.
11. Chiu I. M., von Hehn C. A., Woolf C. J. (2012). Neurogenic inflammation and the peripheral nervous system in host defense and immunopathology. *Nature Neuroscience, 15*(8), 1063–1067.
12. Vase L., Svensson P., Nikoljsen L., et al. (2013). The effects of menthol on cold allodynia and wind-up-like pain in upper limb amputees with different levels of phantom limb pain. *Neuroscience Letters, 534,* 52–57.
13. Ploner M., Gross J., Timmerman L., et al. (2002). Cortical representation of first and second pain sensation in humans. *Proceedings of the National Academy of Sciences of the United States of America, 99,* 12444–12448.
14. McMahon S. B., Koltzenburg M., Tracey I., et al. (2013). *Wall & Melzack's textbook of pain* (6th ed.). Philadelphia, PA: Elsevier Saunders.
15. Stein C. (2003). Opioid receptors on peripheral sensory neurons. In Machelska, H., Stein C. (Eds.), *Immune mechanisms of pain and analgesia* (pp. 69–76). New York: Kluwer Academic/Plenum.
16. Sikandar S., Dickenson A. H. (2012). Visceral pain: The ins and outs, the ups and downs. *Current Opinion in Supportive and Palliative Care, 6*(1), 17–26.
17. Al-Chaer E. D., Traub R. J. (2002). Biological basis of visceral pain: Recent developments. *Pain, 96,* 221–225.

18. Turk D. C., Okifuji A. (2010). Chapter 2: Pain terms and taxonomies of pain. In Fishman S. M., Ballantyne J. C., Rathmell J. P. (Ed.), *Bonica's management of pain* (4th ed.). Philadelphia, PA: Lippincott Williams & Wilkins.

19. Turk D. C., Robinson J. P. (2010). Chapter 23: Multidisciplinary assessment to patients with chronic pain. In Fishman S. M., Ballantyne J. C., Rathmell J. P. (Ed.), *Bonica's management of pain* (4th ed.). Philadelphia, PA: Lippincott Williams & Wilkins.

20. Fink W. A. Jr. (2005). The pathophysiology of acute pain. *Emergency Medicine Clinics of North America, 23*, 277–284.

21. Reichling D. B., Levine J. D. (2009). Critical role of nociceptor plasticity in chronic pain. *Trends in Neurosciences, 32*(12), 611–918.

22. Maizels M., McCarberg B. (2005). Antidepressant and antiepileptic drugs for chronic non-cancer pain. *American Family Physician, 71*, 483–490.

23. Acute Pain Management Guideline Panel. (1992). *Clinical practice guideline no. 1. Acute pain management: Operative or medical procedures and trauma.* AHCPR publication no. 92–0032. Rockville, MD: Agency for Health Care Policy and Research, Public Health Service, U.S. Department of Health and Human Services.

24. Melzack R. (1975). The McGill pain questionnaire: Major properties and scoring methods. *Pain, 1*, 277–299.

25. Norden J., Hanallah R. (1991). Reliability of an objective pain scale in children. *Journal of Pain and Symptom Management, 6*, 196.

26. Krechel S. W., Bilder J. (1995). CRIES: A new neonatal postoperative pain management score: Initial testing of validity. *Pediatric Anesthesia, 5*(1), 53–61.

27. Jacox A., Carr D. B., Payne R., et al. (1994). *Clinical practice guideline no. 9. Management of cancer pain.* AHCPR publication no. 94–0592. Rockville, MD: Agency for Health Care Policy and Research, Public Health Service, U.S. Department of Health and Human Services.

28. Vargas-Schaffer G. (2010). Is the WHO analgesic ladder still valid? Twenty-four years of experience. *Canadian Family Physician, 56*, 514–517.

29. Mohr W. J., Jenabzadeh K., Ahrenholz D. H. (2009). Cold injury. *Hand Clinics, 25*(4), 481–496.

30. Hymes A. (1984). A review of the historical area of electricity. In Mannheimer J. S., Lampe G. N. (Eds.), *Clinical Transcutaneous Electrical Stimulation* (pp. 1–5). Philadelphia, PA: F.A. Davis.

31. Jones I., Johnson M. I. (2009). Transcutaneous electrical nerve stimulation. *Continuing Education in Anaesthesia, Critical Care & Pain, 9*(4), 130–135.

32. Dorsi M. J., Belzerg A. J. (2010). Chapter 94: Peripheral nerve stimulation. In Fishman S. M., Ballantyne J. C., Rathmell J. P. (Ed.), *Bonica's management of pain* (4th ed.). Philadelphia, PA: Lippincott Williams & Wilkins.

33. Kelly R. B. (2009). Acupuncture for pain. *American Family Physician, 80*(5), 481–484.

34. Ezzo J., Berman B., Hadhazy A., et al. (2000). Is acupuncture effective for the treatment of chronic pain? A systematic review. *Pain, 86*, 217–225.

35. Shealey C. N., Mortimer J. T., Reswick J. B. (2007). Electrical inhibition of pain by stimulation of the dorsal columns: Preliminary clinical report. *Anesthesia and Analgesia, 46*, 489–491.

36. Katzung B. G., Trevor A. J. (2015). *Basic and clinical pharmacology* (13th ed.). New York: Lange Medical Books/McGraw-Hill.

37. Inturrisi C. E. (2002). Clinical pharmacology of opioids for pain. *Clinical Journal of Pain, 18*(4 Suppl), S3-S13.

38. Melzack R. (1990). The tragedy of needless pain. *Scientific American, 262*(2), 2–8.

39. Kurz A., Sessler D. (2003). Opioid-induced bowel dysfunction: Pathophysiology and potential new therapies. *Drugs, 63*, 649–671.

40. Pasternak G. W. (2011). *The Opiate receptors* (2nd ed.). Totowa, NJ: Humana Press.

41. Swerdlow M., Stjerward J. (1982). Cancer pain relief: An urgent problem. *World Health Forum, 3*, 325–330.

42. Marchand F., Perretti D., McMahon S. B. (2005). Role of the immune system in chronic pain. *Nature Reviews Neuroscience, 6*, 521–532.

43. Moulin D. E., Boulanger A., Clark A. J., et al. (2014). Pharmacological management of chronic neuropathic pain: Revised consensus statement from the Canadian Pain Society. *Pain Research & Management, 19*(6), 328–335.

44. Rozen T. D. (2004). Trigeminal neuralgia and glossopharyngeal neuralgia. *Neurologic Clinics, 22*, 185–206.

45. Liu J. K., Apfelbaum R. I. (2004). Treatment of trigeminal neuralgia. *Neurosurgical Clinics of North America, 15*, 319–334.

46. Philip A., Thakur R. (2011). Postherpetic neuralgia. *Journal of Palliative Medicine, 14*(6), 765–773.

47. Schmader K. (2007). Herpes zoster and postherpetic neuralgia in older adults. *Clinics in Geriatric Medicine, 23*, 615–632.

48. Kimberlin D. W., Whitley R. J. (2007). Varicella-zoster vaccine for the prevention of herpes zoster. *New England Journal of Medicine, 356*, 1338–1343.

49. Marinus J., Moseley G. L., Birklein F., et al. (2011). Clinical features and pathophysiology of complex regional pain syndrome. *Lancet Neurology, 10*(7), 637–648.

50. Harden R. N., Bruehl S., Stanton-Hicks M., et al. (2007). Proposed new diagnostic criteria for complex regional pain syndrome. *Pain Medicine, 8*(4),326–31.

51. Bruehl S. (2010). An update on the pathophysiology of complex regional pain syndrome. *Anesthesiology, 113*(3), 713–725.

52. Stanton-Hicks M. (2003). Complex regional pain syndrome. *Anesthesia Clinics of North America, 21*, 733–744.

53. Tram D. Q., Duong S., Bertini P., et al. (2010). Treatment of complex regional pain syndrome: A review of the evidence. *Canadian Journal of Anesthesia, 57*(2), 149–166.

54. Weeks S. R., Anderson-Barnes V. C., Tsao J. W. (2010). Phantom limb pain: Theories and therapies. *The Neurologist, 16*(5), 277–286.

55. Robbins M. S., Lipton R. B. (2010). The epidemiology of primary headache disorders. *Seminars in Neurology, 30*(2), 107–119.

56. Kaniecki R. (2003). Headache assessment and management. *Journal of American Medical Association, 289*, 1430–1433.

57. Headache Classification Subcommittee of the International Headache Committee. (2013). The International Classification of headache disorders, 3rd edition (beta version). *Cephalalgia, 33*(9), 629–808.

58. Lipton R. B., Biglal M. E., Stiener T. J., et al. (2004). Classification of primary headaches. *Neurology, 63*, 427–435.

59. Pringsheim T., Davenport W., Mackie G., et al. (2012). Canadian headache society guidelines for migraine prophylaxis. *Canadian Journal of Neurological Sciences, 39*(Suppl 2), S1–S61.

60. Pietrobon D., Moskowitz M. A. (2013). Pathophysiology of migraine. *Annual Review of Physiology, 75*, 365–391.

61. Cady R., Schreiber C. (2003). Sinus headache or migraine? Considerations in making a differential diagnosis. *Headache, 43*, 305.

62. Babineau S. E., Green M. W. (2012). Headaches in children. *Continuum, 18*(4), 853–868.

63. Hershey A. D.. (2011). Chapter 588: Headaches. In Kliegman R. M., Stanton B. F., St. Geme J. W., et al. (Eds.), *Nelson textbook of pediatrics* (19th ed.). Philadelphia, PA: Saunders Elsevier.

64. Williamson D. H., Hargreaves R. J. (2001). Neurogenic inflammation in the context on migraine. *Microscopy Research and Technique 53*, 167–178.

65. Gilmore B., Michael M. (2011). Treatment of acute migraine headache. *American Family Physician, 83*(3), 271–280.

66. Silberstein S. D. (2000). Practice parameter: Evidence-based guidelines for migraine headache. *Neurology 55*, 754–763.

67. Silberstein S. D. (2009). Preventive migraine treatment. *Neurologic Clinics, 27*(2), 429–443.

68. Ekbom K., Hardebo J. E. (2002). Cluster headache aetiology, diagnosis and management. *Drugs, 62*, 61–69.

69. May A. (2005). Cluster headache: Pathogenesis, diagnosis, and management. *Lancet, 366*, 843–855.

70. Beck E., Sieber W. J., Trejo R. (2005). Management of cluster headache. *American Family Physician, 71*, 717–728.

71. Gladstein J. (2006). Headache. *Medical Clinics of North America, 90*, 275–290.

72. Millea P. J., Brodie J. J. (2002). Tension-type headache. *American Family Physician, 66,* 797–804.

73. Biondi D. M. (2005). Chronic daily headache. *Clinics in Family Practice, 7,* 463–491.

74. Maizels M. (2004). The patient with daily headaches. *American Family Physician, 70,* 2299–2306, 2313–2314.

75. Lake A., Saper J. (2002). Chronic headache: New advances in treatment strategies. *Neurology, 59*(5 Suppl 2), S8–S13.

76. Cairns B. E. (2010). Pathophysiology of TMD pain: Basic mechanisms and their implications for pharmacotherapy. *Journal of Oral Rehabilitation, 37*(6), 391–410.

77. Palmermo T. M. (2009). Assessment of chronic pain in children: Current status and emerging topics. *Journal of the Canadian Pain Society, 14*(1), 21–26.

78. Howard R. F. (2003). Current status of pain management in children. *Journal of American Medical Association, 290,* 2464–2469.

79. Committee on Psychological Aspects of Child and Family Health. (2001). The assessment and management of acute pain in infants, children, and adolescents. *Pediatrics, 108*(3), 793–797.

80. Abdulla A., Adams N., Bone M., et al. (2013). Guidance on the management of pain in older people. *Age and Ageing, 42* (Suppl 1), 1–57.

81. Brislin R. P., Rose J. B. (2005). Pediatric acute pain management. *Anesthesia Clinics of North America, 23,* 789–814.

82. Zeltzer L. K, Krane E. J. (2011). Chapter 71: Pediatric pain management. In Kliegman R. M., Stanton B. F., St. Geme J. W., et al. (Eds.), *Nelson textbook of pediatrics* (19th ed.). Philadelphia, PA: Saunders Elsevier.

83. Berde C. B., Sethna N. F. (2002). Analgesics for the treatment of pain in children. *New England Journal of Medicine, 347,* 1094–1103.

84. Haouari N., Wood C., Griffiths G., et al. (1995). The analgesic effect of sucrose in full term infants: A randomized controlled trial. *BMJ, 310,* 1498–1500.

85. Merkel S. I., Gutstein H. B., Malviya S. (1999). Use of transcutaneous electrical nerve stimulation in a young child with pain from open perineal lesions. *Journal of Pain and Symptom Management, 18,* 376–381.

86. Gold J., Kim S. H., Kant A. J., et al. (2006). Effectiveness of virtual reality for pediatric pain distraction during IV placement. *CyberPsychology & Behavior, 9,* 207–212.

87. Achterberg W. P., Pieper M. J., van Dalen-Kok A. H., et al. (2013). Pain management in patients with dementia. *Clinical Interventions in Aging, 8,* 1471–1482.

88. Barkin. R. L., Barkin S. J., Barkin D.S. (2005). Perception, assessment, treatment, and management of pain in the elderly. *Clinics in Geriatric Medicine, 21,* 465–490.

Visit thePoint **http://thePoint.lww.com for animations, journal articles, and more!**

Disorders of Motor Function

Just as our perceptual skills reflect the ability of our sensory systems to detect, analyze, and estimate the significance of our physical environment, the ability to carry out skilled movements requires skeletal muscles that contract and neural pathways that plan, coordinate, and execute these contractions in a manner that provides for smooth and coordinated movement. In some cases, purposeless and disruptive movements can be almost as disabling as relative or complete absence of movement. This chapter provides an introduction to the organization and control of motor function, followed by a discussion of disorders of skeletal muscle, peripheral nerve, the basal ganglia and cerebellum, and upper motor neurons (UMNs).

ORGANIZATION AND CONTROL OF MOTOR FUNCTION

After completing this section of the chapter, you should be able to meet the following objectives:

- Understand the hierarchy of motor function and its relationship to performing a complicated movement such as writing your name or throwing a ball.
- Define motor unit and describe its mechanism of controlling skeletal muscle movement.
- Describe the distribution of upper and lower motor neurons within the central nervous system.
- Differentiate between the functions of the primary, premotor, and supplemental motor cortices.
- Compare the effect of upper and lower motor neuron lesions on the spinal cord stretch reflex and on muscle strength, bulk, and tone.

Motor function, whether it involves walking, running, or precise finger movements, requires movement and maintenance of posture. Posture can be described as the relative position of various parts of the body with respect to one another (limb extension, flexion) or to the environment (standing, supine).[1] Posture also can be described as the active muscular resistance to the displacement of the body by gravity or acceleration. The structures that control posture and movement are located throughout the neuromuscular system. The system consists of the motor unit (motor neuron and the muscle fibres it innervates); the spinal cord, which contains the basic reflex circuitry for posture and movement; and the descending pathways from brain stem, the cerebellum, basal ganglia, and the motor cortex.

MOTOR SYSTEMS

- Motor systems require upper motor neurons (UMNs) that project from the motor cortex to the brain stem or spinal cord, where they directly or indirectly innervate the lower motor neurons (LMNs) of the contracting muscles; sensory feedback from the involved muscles that is continuously relayed to the cerebellum, basal ganglia, and sensory cortex; and a functioning neuromuscular junction that links nervous system activity with muscle contraction.
- The pyramidal motor system originating in the motor cortex provides control of delicate muscle movement, and the extrapyramidal system originating in the basal ganglia provides the background for the more crude, supportive movement patterns.
- The efficiency of the movement by the motor system depends on a background of muscle tone provided by the stretch reflex and vestibular system input to maintain stable postural support.

Organization of Movement

As with other parts of the nervous system, the motor systems are organized in a functional hierarchy, each concerned with increased levels of complexity.[2] (Fig. 50.1). The lowest level of the hierarchy occurs at the spinal cord, which contains the basic reflex circuitry needed to coordinate the function of the motor units involved in the planned movement. Above the spinal cord is the brain stem, and above the brain stem are the cerebellum and basal ganglia, structures that modulate the actions of the brain stem. Overseeing these supraspinal structures are the motor centres in the cerebral cortex. The highest level of function, which occurs at the level of the frontal cortex, is concerned with the purpose and planning of the motor movement. The efficiency of movement depends on input from sensory systems that operate in parallel with the motor systems.

The Spinal Cord

The spinal cord contains the neuronal circuits that mediate a variety of reflexes and automatic rhythmic movements. Similar circuits governing reflex movements of the face and mouth are located in the brain stem. The simplest circuits are monosynaptic, containing only a primary motor neuron. However, most reflexes are more complex or polysynaptic, involving one or more interposed interneurons. Interneurons and motor neurons receive input from axons descending from higher centres. These supraspinal signals can modify reflex responses to peripheral stimuli by facilitating or inhibiting different populations of interneurons. They also coordinate movements through these interneurons.

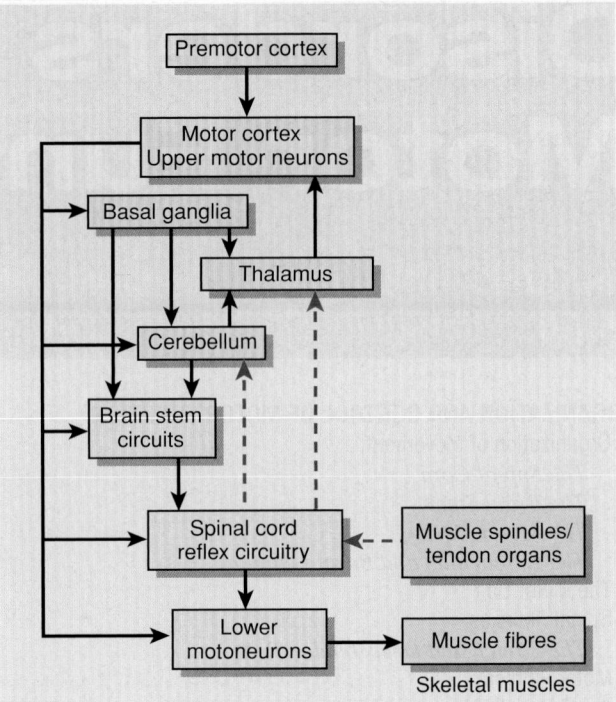

FIGURE 50.1 • The motor control system. The final common pathway transmits all central nervous system commands to the skeletal muscles. This path is influenced by sensory input from the muscle spindles and tendon organs (*dashed lines*) and descending signals from the cerebral cortex and brain stem. The cerebellum and basal ganglia influence the motor function indirectly, using brain stem and cortical pathways.

The Brain Stem

The brain stem contains, in addition to the facial nerves, many groups of neurons that project from the spinal grey matter. These projections are grouped into two main systems: the medial and lateral brain stem pathways.[2] The medial pathways provide for the basic postural control systems that the cortical motor areas use to organize highly differentiated movement. They consist of tracts that descend in the ipsilateral ventral columns of the spinal cord and terminate in the interneurons that influence motor neurons of axial and proximal muscles that are responsible for postural reflexes, such as those needed for pacing of steps during walking or running and recovery of posture when balance is disrupted. The lateral brain stem pathways are more concerned with goal-directed movements. They terminate on the interneurons in the dorsolateral part of the spinal grey matter and thus influence the motor neurons that control distal muscles of the limbs. These descending pathways modify the activity of extensor and flexor motor neurons to produce more complex motor movements such as walking and running.

The Motor Cortex

The cortex represents the highest level of motor function. Precise, skillful, and intentional movements of the distal and especially flexor muscles of the limbs and speech apparatus are initiated and controlled by the primary, premotor, and

FIGURE 50.2 • Primary motor cortex. (**Top**) The location of the primary, premotor, and supplementary cortex on the medial surface of the brain. (**Bottom**) The location of the primary and premotor cortex on the lateral surface of the brain. (Courtesy of Carole Russell Hilmer, CMI.)

complex "patterns" of movement than the discrete patterns generated by the primary motor cortex. For example, the movement patterns of throwing a ball or picking up a fork are programmed by the prefrontal association cortex and associated thalamic nuclei.

The supplementary motor cortex, which contains representations of all parts of the body, is located on the medial surface of the hemisphere in the premotor region (areas 6 and 8). It is involved in the performance of complex, skillful movements involving both sides of the body.

The Cerebellum and Basal Ganglia

In addition to the brain stem and cerebral cortex, two other parts of the brain assist in the planning and execution of motor movements. The cerebellum and the basal ganglia provide feedback circuits that regulate cortical and brain stem motor areas.[2] They receive inputs from various areas of the cortex and project to the motor cortex through the thalamus. The cerebellum and basal ganglia do not send significant output directly to the spinal cord, but act directly on motor neurons in the brain stem.

The cerebellum and the basal ganglia are both needed for smooth movement and posture. The basal ganglia lend gracefulness to the performance, and provide the supportive posture for highly skilled movements. As will be discussed, degenerative diseases of the basal ganglia such as Parkinson disease produce involuntary movements and posture. In this disease, cerebellar circuits are involved with the timing and coordination of movements in progress, and with learning of motor skills. Damage to the cerebellum by vascular lesions of certain familial degenerative disorders produces cerebellar ataxia, a characteristic loss of coordination and accuracy of limb movement.

The Motor Unit

The neurons that control motor function are referred to as *motor neurons* or sometimes as *alpha motor neurons*.[3,5] The motor neuron and the group of muscle fibres it innervates in a muscle are called a *motor unit*. When the motor neuron develops an action potential, all of the muscle fibres in the motor unit it innervates develop action potentials, causing them to contract simultaneously. Thus, a motor neuron and the muscle fibres it innervates function as a single unit—the basic unit of motor control.

Each motor neuron undergoes multiple branchings, making it possible for a single motor neuron to innervate a few to thousands of muscle fibres. In general, large muscles—those containing hundreds or thousands of muscle fibres and providing gross motor movement—have large motor units. In contrast, those that control the hand, tongue, and eye movements have small motor units that permit very precise control.

The motor neurons supplying a motor unit are located in the ventral horn of the spinal cord and are called *lower motor neurons* (LMNs). *UMNs,* which exert control over LMNs, are contained entirely within the central nervous system and

supplementary motor cortices located in the posterior part of the frontal lobe.[1,3] (Fig. 50.2). These motor areas receive information directly from the thalamus and somatosensory cortex and, indirectly, from the cerebellum and basal ganglia.

The primary motor cortex (area 4 if using Brodmann classification of the brain cortical areas), also called the *motor strip,* is located on the rostral surface and adjacent portions of the central sulcus.[3] The primary motor cortex controls specific muscle movement sequences and is the first level of descending control for precise motor movements. The neurons in the primary motor cortex are arranged in a somatotopic array or distorted map of the body called the *motor homunculus*[4] (Fig. 50.3). The parts of the body that require the greatest dexterity have the largest cortical areas devoted to them. More than half of the primary motor cortex is concerned with controlling the muscles of the hands and face, including facial expression and vocalization.

The premotor cortex (areas 6 and 8), located anterior to the primary motor cortex, sends some fibres into the corticospinal tract but mainly innervates the primary motor strip. Nerve signals generated by the premotor cortex produce more

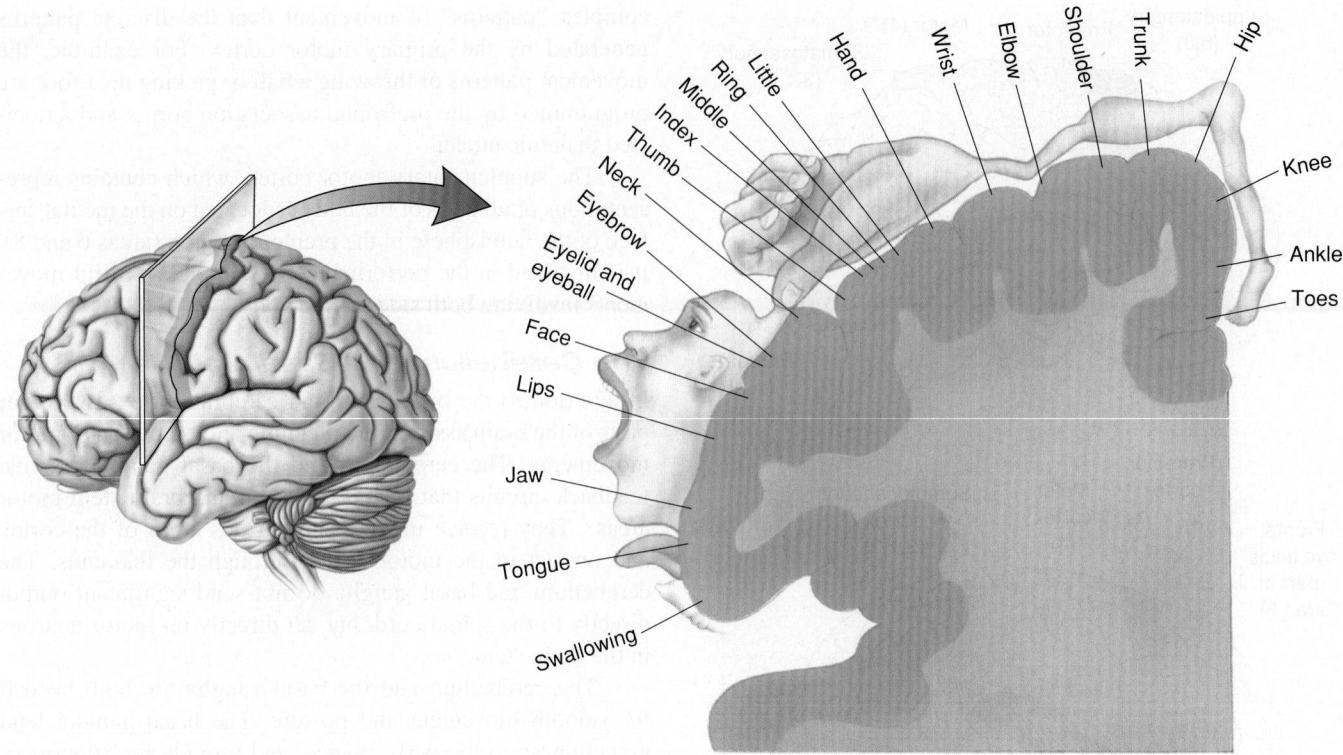

FIGURE 50.3 • The motor homunculus. This is a representation of the relative extent of motor cortical area 4 devoted to muscles of the various body regions. Medial surface is at the right, lateral fissure is at the left, with pharyngeal and laryngeal muscle representation extending toward the insula. (From Stephen T. C., Skillen D. L., Day R. A., et al. (2012). *Canadian Jensen's nursing health assessment: A best practice approach.* (p. 699) Philadelphia, PA: Lippincott Williams & Wilkins.)

project from the motor strip in the cerebral cortex to the ventral horn of the spinal cord (Fig. 50.4).

Spinal Reflexes

Reflexes are coordinated, involuntary motor responses initiated by a stimuli applied to peripheral receptors.[3,6] Some reflexes, such as the flexor withdrawal reflex, initiate movements to avoid hazardous situations, whereas others, such as the stretch reflex or crossed extensor reflex, serve to integrate motor movements so that they function in a coordinated manner. The anatomic basis of a reflex consists of an afferent neuron that synapses either directly with an effector neuron innervating a muscle, or with an interneuron that synapses with an effector neuron. Reflexes are essentially "wired into" the CNS so they are always ready to function. With training, most reflexes can be modulated to become parts of more complicated movements. A reflex may involve neurons in a single cord segment (*i.e.,* segmental reflexes), several or many segments (*i.e.,* intersegmental reflexes), or structures in the brain (*i.e.,* suprasegmental reflexes).

In many cases, reflex activities go on without our conscious awareness. There is a significant amount of reflex circuitry in the spinal cord for the coordinated control of movements, particularly stereotyped movements concerned with locomotion. Many of these reflexes work equally well in decerebrate animals (those in which the brain has been destroyed) as long as the spinal cord is intact. Other spinal reflexes require the activity of the brain for their successful completion. More specifically, the brain is advised of many types of spinal cord reflex activities and can either inhibit or facilitate them.

The Stretch and Deep Tendon Reflexes

If the skeletal muscle is to perform normally, the brain must be continually informed of the current state of the muscles; and the muscles must exhibit healthy tone (resistance to active and passive stretch at rest). The first requirement depends on the transmission of information regarding the sense of body position, movement, and muscle tone to the CNS. Information from these sensory afferents is relayed to the cerebellum and cerebral cortex and is experienced as *proprioception* or the sense of body movement and position, independent of vision. To provide this information, the muscles and their tendons are supplied with two types of receptors: muscle spindle receptors and Golgi tendon organs. The muscle spindles, which are distributed throughout the belly of a muscle, relay information about muscle length and rate of stretch. The *Golgi tendon organs* are found in muscle tendons and transmit information about muscle tension or force of contraction at the junction of the muscle and the tendon that attaches to bone. Healthy muscle tone depends on stretch reflexes initiated by the muscle spindles, which monitor changes in muscle length.

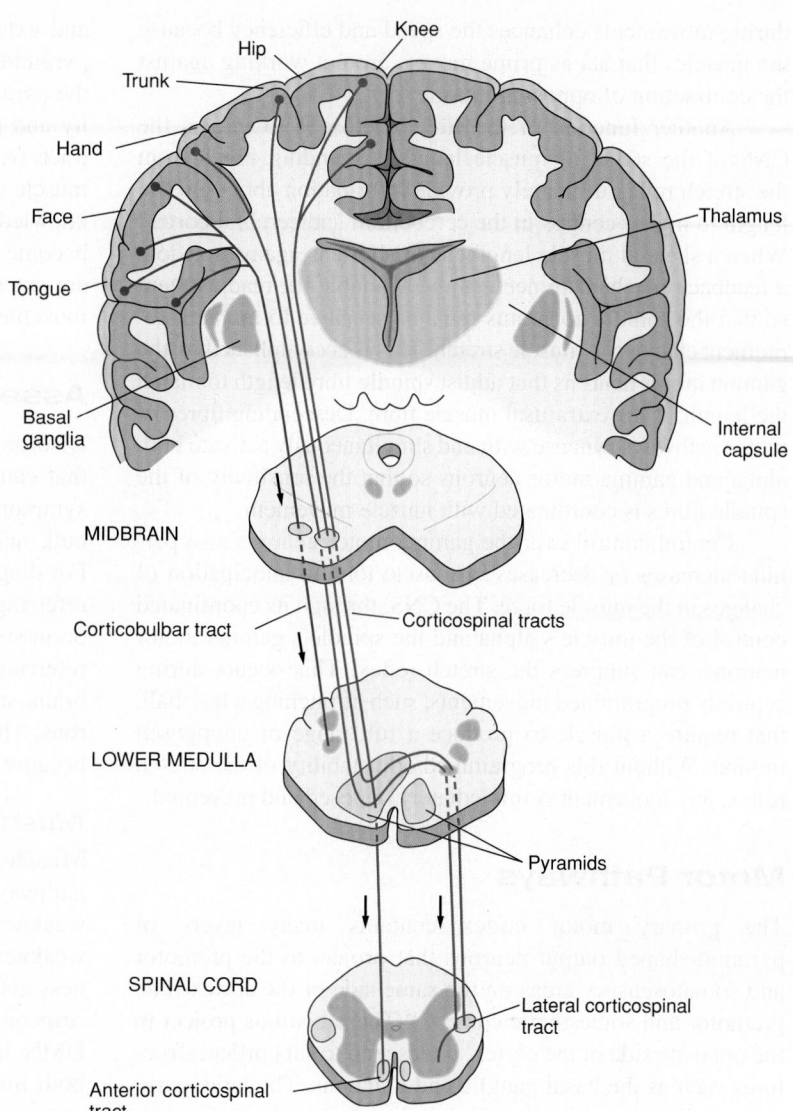

FIGURE 50.4 • Motor pathways: corticospinal and corticobulbar tracts carrying information from the cortex to cranial and peripheral nerves. (From Stephen T. C., Skillen D. L., Day R. A., et al. (2012). *Canadian Jensen's nursing health assessment: A best practice approach.* (p. 704) Philadelphia, PA: Lippincott Williams & Wilkins.)

The stretch reflex, a contraction of muscle fibres that occurs when a muscle is stretched, is essential to the control of muscle tone and maintenance of posture (see Understanding the Stretch Reflex and Muscle Tone). Stretch reflexes can be evoked in many muscles throughout the body and are tested (*e.g.,* knee-jerk reflex) during clinical examination. Stretch reflexes tend to be hypoactive or absent in cases of peripheral nerve damage or ventral horn injury involving the test area. However, they are hyperactive when lesions of the corticospinal tract (*e.g.,* stroke or spinal cord injury [SCI]) reduce or disrupt the inhibitory effect of the brain on the spinal cord.

The muscle spindles consist of a group of specialized miniature skeletal muscle fibres called *intrafusal fibres* that are encased in a connective tissue capsule and attached to the extrafusal fibres of a skeletal muscle. In the centre of the receptor area, a large sensory neuron spirals around the intrafusal fibre, forming the so-called *primary* or *annulospiral ending.* The intrafusal muscle fibres function as stretch receptors. When a skeletal muscle is stretched, the spindle and its

intrafusal fibres are stretched, resulting in increased firing of their afferent nerve fibres. Axons of these afferent neurons enter the spinal cord through several branches of the dorsal root. Some branches end in the segment of entry; others ascend to adjacent segments, influencing intersegmental reflex function; and still others ascend in the dorsal column of the cord to the medulla of the brain stem. Segmental branches make connections, along with other branches, that pass directly to the anterior grey matter of the spinal cord and establish monosynaptic contact with each of the LMNs that have motor units in the muscle containing the spindle receptor. This produces an opposing muscle contraction. Another segmental branch of the same afferent neuron innervates an internuncial neuron that is inhibitory to motor units of antagonistic muscle groups. This disynaptic inhibitory pathway is the basis for the reciprocal activity of agonist and antagonist muscles (*i.e.,* when an agonist muscle is stretched, the antagonists relax). Reciprocal innervation is useful not only for the stretch reflex, but for voluntary movements. Relaxation of the antagonist muscle during movements enhances the speed and efficiency because the muscles that act as prime movers are not working against the contraction of opposing muscle.[1]

Another function of the stretch reflex is to inform the CNS of the status of muscle length. Ascending fibres from the stretch reflex ultimately provide information about muscle length to higher centres in the cerebellum and cerebral cortex. When a skeletal muscle lengthens or shortens against tension, a feedback mechanism needs to be available for readjustment so that the spindle apparatus remains sensitive to moment-to-moment changes in muscle stretch. This is accomplished by the gamma motor neurons that adjust spindle fibre length to match the length of the extrafusal muscle fibre. Descending fibres of motor pathways synapse with and simultaneously activate both alpha and gamma motor neurons so that the sensitivity of the spindle fibres is coordinated with muscle movement.

Central control over the gamma motor neurons also permits increases or decreases in muscle tone in anticipation of changes in the muscle force. The CNS, through its coordinated control of the muscle's alpha and the spindle's gamma motor neurons, can suppress the stretch reflex. This occurs during centrally programmed movements, such as pitching a baseball, that require a muscle to produce a full range of unopposed motion. Without this programmed adjustability of the stretch reflex, any movement is immediately opposed and prevented.

Motor Pathways

The primary motor cortex contains many layers of pyramid-shaped output neurons that project to the premotor and somatosensory areas on the same side of the cortex (*i.e.,* premotor and somesthetic cortices). These neurons project to the opposite side of the cortex, or descend to subcortical structures such as the basal ganglia and thalamus. The large pyramidal cells located in the fifth layer project to the brain stem and spinal cord. The axons of these UMNs project through the subcortical white matter and internal capsule to the deep surface of the brain stem, through the ventral bulge of the pons, and to the ventral surface of the medulla, where they form a ridge or pyramid (Fig. 50.4). About 80% to 90% of the corticospinal UMNs cross the midline in the pyramidal decussation at the junction of the medulla and cervical spinal cord to form the lateral corticospinal tract in the lateral white matter of the spinal cord.[7] Most of the remaining uncrossed fibres travel down the ventral column of the cord, mainly to cervical levels, where they cross and innervate contralateral LMNs.

Traditionally, motor tracts have been classified as belonging to one of two motor systems: the pyramidal and extrapyramidal systems. According to this classification system, the pyramidal system consists of the motor pathways originating in the motor cortex and terminating in the corticobulbar fibres in the brain stem and the corticospinal fibres in the spinal cord. Other fibres from the cortex and basal ganglia project to the brain stem reticular formation and reticulospinal systems, following an alternative pathway to LMNs of proximal

and extensor muscles. These fibres do not decussate in the pyramids, hence the name *extrapyramidal system*. Disorders of the pyramidal tracts (*e.g.,* stroke) are characterized by spasticity and paralysis, whereas those affecting the extrapyramidal tracts (*e.g.,* Parkinson disease) result in involuntary movements, muscle rigidity, and immobility without paralysis. As increased knowledge regarding motor pathways has emerged, it has become evident that the extrapyramidal and pyramidal systems are extensively interconnected and cooperate in the control of movement.[1]

Assessment of Motor Function

Disorders of the motor system produce signs and symptoms that can be used in localizing the disorder. These signs and symptoms include changes in muscle characteristics (strength, bulk, and tone), spinal reflex activity, and motor coordination.[8] For diagnostic purposes, clinicians often use the terms *LMN,* referring to neurons that are located in the spinal cord and brain stem and directly innervate skeletal muscle, and *UMN,* referring to neurons that originate in higher regions of the brain, such as the motor cortex, and synapse with motor neurons. The distinction between LMNs and UMNs is important because each class of neurons produces distinctive symptoms.

Muscle Strength, Bulk, and Tone

Muscle Strength. Abnormalities in any part of the motor pathway can impair muscle strength and result in muscle weakness. *Paralysis* refers to loss of movement, and *paresis,* to weakness or incomplete loss of strength. The pattern of weakness may be helpful in the localization of the lesion. *Monoparesis* or *monoplegia* results from the destruction of pyramidal UMN innervation of one limb; *hemiparesis* or *hemiplegia,* both limbs on one side; *diparesis* or *diplegia* or *paraparesis* or *paraplegia,* both upper or lower limbs; and *tetraparesis* or *tetraplegia,* also called *quadriparesis* or *quadriplegia,* all four limbs (Fig. 50.5).

Paresis or paralysis can be further designated as of UMN or LMN origin. UMN lesions of the motor cortex or corticospinal tract typically affect the extensors in the upper extremities more than the flexors, whereas in the lower extremities, the flexors are more affected. In LMN or peripheral nerve disorders, the weakness is predominantly in the distal limb, whereas in muscle disorders, such as muscular dystrophy, proximal limb function may be affected earlier than distal limb function.

Muscle Bulk. The size of muscle (whether muscles are normal sized, enlarged, or atrophied) also helps localize the lesion, and sometimes provides helpful hints to the pathologic process. Muscular atrophy, or loss of muscle bulk, usually results from LMN lesions as well as diseases of the muscles themselves. Hypertrophy refers to an increase in muscle bulk with a proportionate increase in strength. Pseudohypertrophy, as occurs with Duchenne muscular dystrophy (DMD), refers

Understanding The Stretch Reflex and Muscle Tone

Muscle tone is controlled by the stretch reflex, which monitors changes in muscle length. The activity of the stretch reflex can be divided into three steps: (1) activation of the stretch receptors, (2) integration of the reflex in the spinal cord, and (3) regulation of reflex sensitivity by higher centres in the brain. Testing the (4) knee-jerk reflex provides a means of assessing that reflex.

1. Stretch Reflex Receptors

Skeletal muscle is composed of two types of muscle fibres: a large number of extrafusal fibres, which control muscle movement, and a smaller number of intrafusal fibres, which control muscle tone. The intrafusal fibres are encapsulated in sheaths, forming a muscle spindle that runs parallel to the extrafusal fibres. Each intrafusal fibre is innervated by a large Ia sensory nerve fibre, which encircles the central noncontractile portion of the fibre to form the so-called *annulospiral ending*. Because the spindles are oriented parallel to the extrafusal muscle fibres, stretching of the extrafusal fibres also stretches the spindle fibres and stimulates the receptive endings of the Ia afferent neuron.

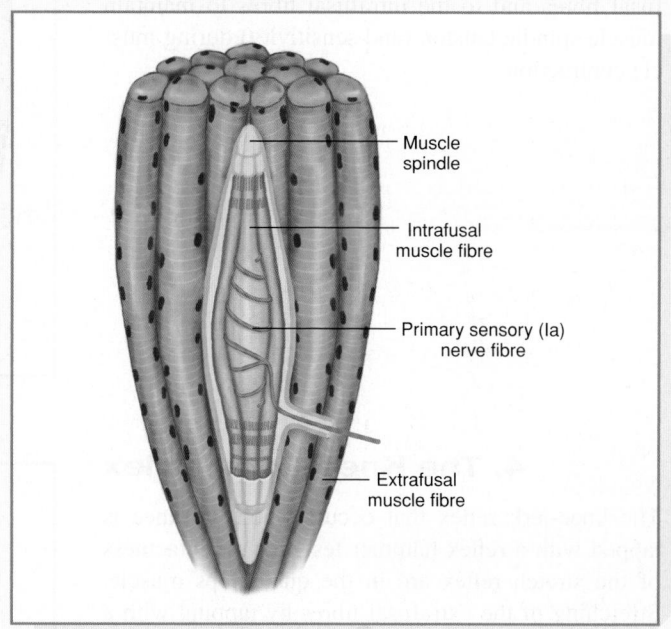

2. Spinal Reflex Centres

Afferent impulses from the Ia sensory fibre of the muscle spindle are transmitted to the spinal cord, where they synapse with alpha motor neurons of the stretched muscle to form a monosynaptic reflex arc—"monosynaptic" because only one synapse separates the primary sensory input from the motor neuron output. The reflex muscle contraction that follows resists further stretching of the muscle. As this spinal reflex activity is occurring, impulses providing information on muscle length are transmitted to higher centres in the brain. It is the coordinated activity of all the monosynaptic reflexes supplying the extrafusal fibres in a skeletal muscle that provides the muscle tone needed for organized movement.

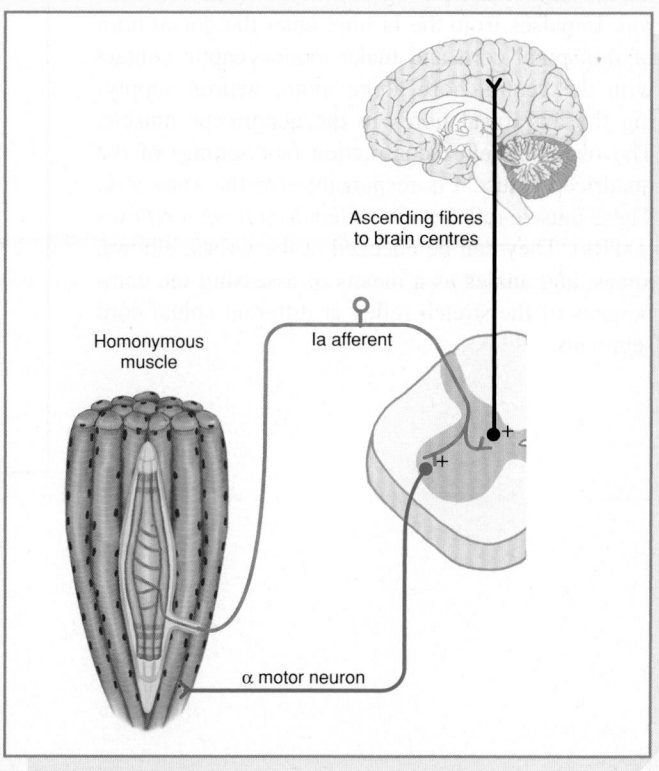

3. Brain Centre Connections

Although a spinal reflex can function independently, its sensitivity is adjusted by higher centres in the brain. Both types of muscle fibres are supplied with motor neurons—the extrafusal fibres with large alpha motor neurons, which produce muscle contraction; and the intrafusal fibres with smaller gamma motor neurons, which control the sensitivity of the stretch reflex. Descending fibres of motor pathways synapse with both alpha and gamma motor neurons, and the impulses are sent simultaneously to the large extrafusal fibres and to the intrafusal fibres to maintain muscle spindle tension (and sensitivity) during muscle contraction.

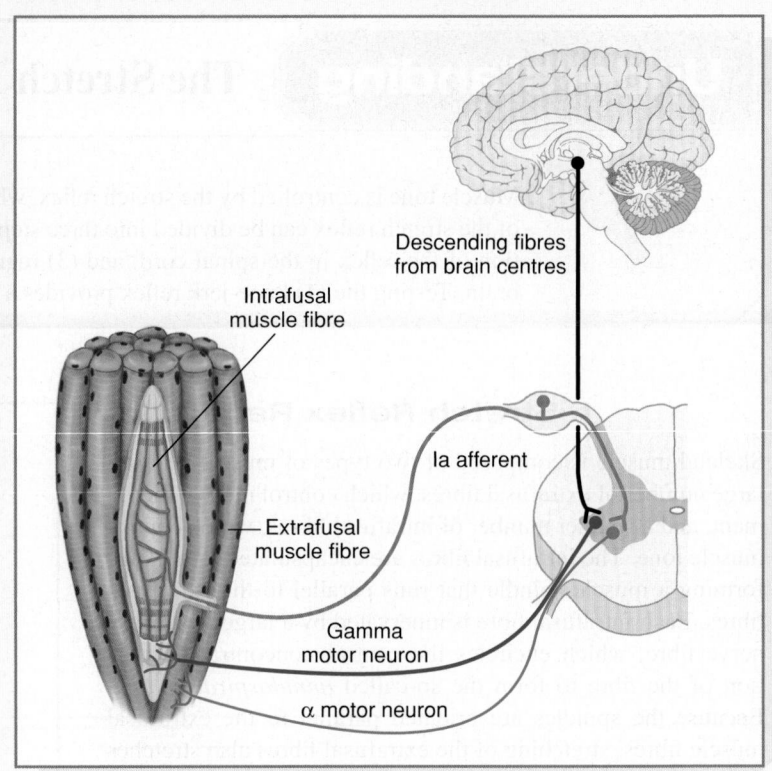

4. The Knee-Jerk Reflex

The knee-jerk reflex that occurs when the knee is tapped with a reflex hammer tests for the intactness of the stretch reflex arc in the quadriceps muscle. Stretching of the extrafusal fibres by tapping with a reflex hammer leads to lengthening of the intrafusal fibres and increased firing of the type Ia afferent neuron. Impulses from the Ia fibre enter the dorsal horn of the spinal cord and make monosynaptic contact with the ventral horn alpha motor neuron supplying the extrafusal fibres in the quadriceps muscle. The resultant reflex contraction (shortening) of the quadriceps muscle is responsible for the knee jerk. These muscle reflexes are called *deep tendon reflexes* (DTRs). They can be checked at the wrists, elbows, knees, and ankles as a means of assessing the components of the stretch reflex at different spinal cord segments.

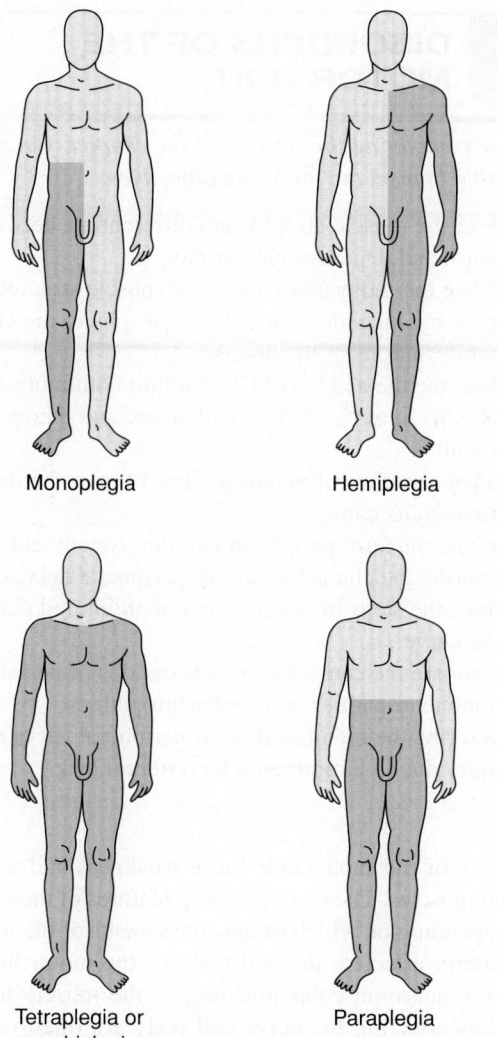

Monoplegia

Hemiplegia

Tetraplegia or quadriplegia

Paraplegia

FIGURE 50.5 • Areas of the body affected by monoplegia, hemiplegia, tetraplegia or quadriplegia, and paraplegia. The *shaded area* shows the extent of motor and sensory loss. (Adapted from Hickey J. V. (2014). *The clinical practice of neurological and neurosurgical nursing* (7th ed.). Philadelphia, PA: Lippincott Williams & Wilkins.)

to an increase in bulk without an accompanying increase in strength.

Fasciculations are visible twitching movements of muscle fibres that can be seen as flickers under the skin. They are caused by spontaneous contractions of all the muscle fibres in a motor unit due to irritation and hyperexcitability of the cell body and its motor neuron, and suggest LMN disease.

Muscle Tone. Muscle tone is the normal state of muscle tension. It is assessed by palpating the muscle while at rest and during passive stretching. With the person at rest, the joints are moved through the normal range of motion (flexion and extension) by the examiner. Disorders of skeletal muscle tone are characteristic of many nervous system lesions. Any interruption of the myotatic or stretch reflex circuitry by peripheral

nerve injury, alterations at the neuromuscular junction, injury to the spinal cord, or damage to the corticospinal system can result in disturbances of muscle tone.

Abnormalities of muscle tone may be described as hypotonia (less than normal) or flaccidity (absent), or hypertonia, rigidity, spasticity, or tetany (all indicating higher-than-normal tone). Typically, UMN lesions produce increased tone, whereas LMN lesions produce decreased tone. Increased resistance that varies and becomes worse at the extremes of range of motion (ROM) is called *spasticity*. Resistance that becomes worse throughout the range and in both directions is called *lead-pipe rigidity*. Decreased resistance suggests disease of the LMNs or the acute stages of SCI. Marked floppiness indicates hypotonic or flaccid muscles.

Spinal Reflex Activity

Testing of deep tendon reflexes (DTRs; see Understanding the Stretch Reflex and Muscle Tone) can provide important information about the CNS and its ability to control muscle function. Hyperactive reflexes are suggestive of an UMN disorder. *Clonus* is the rhythmic contraction and alternate relaxation of a limb that is caused by suddenly stretching a muscle and gently maintaining it in the stretched position. It is seen in the hypertonia of spasticity associated with UMN lesions, such as SCI. *Hyporeflexia* or *areflexia* suggests the presence of an LMN lesion. The distribution of abnormality in the reflexes is also helpful in determining the location of the lesion. For example, hyperreflexia in both lower extremities would suggest a lesion in the spinal cord, whereas hyperreflexia on one side of the body would suggest a lesion in the UMN along the motor pathway (*e.g.,* in the motor cortex or internal capsule).

Coordination of Movement

Coordination of muscle movement requires that four areas of the nervous system function in an integrated manner—the motor system for muscle strength, the cerebellar system for rhythmic movement and steady posture, the vestibular system for posture and balance, and the sensory system for position sense.

In cerebellar disease, one movement cannot be followed quickly by its opposite movement and movements are slow, irregular, clumsy, unsteady, and inappropriately varying in their speed, force, and direction. *Dysdiadochokinesia* is the failure to accurately perform rapid alternating movements. *Ataxia* is a term used to describe a wide-based, unsteady gait. *Dysmetria* describes inaccuracies of movement leading to a failure to reach a specified target. This can be tested by having the person touch the examiner's finger and then alternately touch his or her finger. These movements are normally smooth and accurate. Asking the person to touch the examiner's finger with an outstretched arm and finger, first with the eyes open and then closed, provides a test for position sense. Repetitive and consistent deviation to one side (referred to as past pointing), which is worse with the eyes closed, suggests cerebellar or vestibular disease.

Chorea (abnormal writhing movements), *dystonia* (abnormal simultaneous contractions of agonist and antagonist muscles, leading to abnormal postures), *tremor* (rhythmic movements of a particular body part), *bradykinesia* (slowness of movements), and *myoclonus* (involuntary jerking movement) indicate abnormalities in the basal ganglia, although the exact localization may be difficult to determine.

IN SUMMARY

Motor function, whether it involves walking, running, or precise finger movements, requires movement and maintenance of posture. The system consists of the LMNs, which are located in the ventral horn of the spinal cord and the group of muscle fibres it innervates in the muscle; the spinal cord circuitry and reflexes; and the descending UMNs that project from the motor cortex to the opposite side of the medulla, where they form a pyramid before crossing the midline to form the lateral corticospinal tract in the spinal cord. Voluntary control of motor function is directed by the motor cortex, which consists of the primary, premotor, and supplementary motor cortex. The primary motor cortex is responsible for execution of a movement, the premotor cortex for generating a plan of movement, and the supplemental motor cortex for rehearsing the motor sequences of a movement, including those involving both sides of the body. As with other parts of the nervous system, the motor systems are organized in a functional hierarchy consisting of spinal cord, brain stem, and motor cortex, each with circuits that contribute to the organization and regulation of complex motor responses.

Proper control of muscle function requires not only excitation of the muscle by the LMNs located in the spinal cord, but the function of reflex circuitry that monitors the functional status of the muscle fibres on a moment-by-moment basis. The muscle spindles of the stretch reflex monitor and correct for changes in muscle length when extrafusal fibres are either shortened (by contraction) or lengthened (by stretch).

Assessments of muscle strength and muscle bulk, muscle tone and motor reflexes, and patterns of motor movement and posture provide the means for determining the location of disorders of motor function. Paresis (weakness) and paralysis (loss of muscle movement) reflect a loss of muscle strength. UMN lesions tend to produce spastic paralysis and LMN lesions flaccid paralysis. Changes in muscle bulk are characterized by a loss of muscle mass (atrophy) or an increase in muscle mass (hypertrophy). Muscle tone is maintained through the combined function of the spinal cord stretch reflex, and the higher centres that monitor and buffer UMN innervation of LMNs. Hypotonia is a condition of less-than-normal muscle tone, and hypertonia or spasticity is a condition of excessive tone. Abnormal and uncoordinated movements and postures are suggestive of a cerebellar or basal ganglia pathologic process.

DISORDERS OF THE MOTOR UNIT

After completing this section of the chapter, you should be able to meet the following objectives:

- Describe muscle atrophy and differentiate between disuse and degenerative atrophy.
- Relate the molecular changes in muscle structure that occur in Duchenne muscular dystrophy to the clinical manifestations of the disease.
- Describe the actions of Clostridium botulinum neurotoxins in terms of their pathologic and therapeutic potential.
- Relate the clinical manifestations of myasthenia gravis to its cause.
- Define the term peripheral nervous system and describe the characteristics of peripheral nerves.
- Trace the steps in regeneration of an injured peripheral nerve.
- Compare the cause and manifestations of peripheral mononeuropathies with polyneuropathies.
- Describe the manifestation of peripheral nerve root injury due to a ruptured intervertebral disk.

Disorders of the motor unit cause weakness and wasting of skeletal muscles. The distinguishing features of these diseases vary depending on which of the components of the motor unit is primarily affected: the cell body of the motor neuron, its axon, the neuromuscular junction, or the muscle fibres.[5,9,10] Disorders affecting the nerve cell body are often referred to as *LMN disorders;* those affecting the nerve axon as *peripheral neuropathies;* and primary disorders affecting the muscle fibres as *myopathies.*

Skeletal Muscle Disorders

Muscle Atrophy

Maintenance of muscle strength requires relatively frequent movements against resistance. Reduced use results in muscle atrophy, which is characterized by a reduction in the diameter of the muscle fibres because of a loss of protein filaments.[10] When a normally innervated muscle is not used for long periods, the muscle cells shrink in diameter, and although the muscle cells do not die, they lose much of their contractile proteins and become weakened. This is called *disuse atrophy,* and it occurs with conditions such as immobilization and chronic illness.

The most extreme examples of muscle atrophy are found in persons with disorders that deprive muscles of their innervation. This is called *denervation atrophy.* During early embryonic development, outgrowing skeletal nerves innervate partially mature muscle cells. If the developing muscle cells are not innervated, they do not mature and eventually die. In the process of innervation, randomly contracting muscle cells become enslaved by the innervating neurons, and from then on, the muscle cell contracts only when stimulated by that particular neuron. If the LMN dies or its axon is destroyed, the skeletal muscle cell is again free of neural domination. When this happens, it begins to have temporary spontaneous contractions, called *fibrillations.* In contrast to previously described fasciculations, fibrillations are not visible clinically and can be detected only by electromyography (EMG).[5] The muscle also begins to lose its contractile proteins and, after several months, if not reinnervated, it is replaced by fibrous connective tissue, which makes a person's rehabilitation difficult. Atrophy of denervation can often be delayed by electrically stimulating the muscle periodically while waiting to determine if the damaged nerve fibre regenerates.

Muscular Dystrophy

Muscular dystrophy is a term applied to a group of genetic disorders that produce progressive deterioration of skeletal muscles because of mixed muscle cell hypertrophy, atrophy, and necrosis. Dystrophies are primary diseases of muscle tissue and probably do not involve the nervous system. As the muscle undergoes necrosis, fat and connective tissue replace the muscle fibres, which increases muscle size and results in muscle weakness. The increase in muscle size resulting from connective tissue infiltration is called *pseudohypertrophy.* The muscle weakness is insidious in onset but continually progressive, varying with the type of disorder.

The most common form of the disease is *Duchenne muscular dystrophy* (DMD) affecting one in every 3,500 live male births worldwide.[10-12] DMD is inherited as a recessive single-gene defect on the X chromosome and is transmitted from the mother to her male offspring. A spontaneous (mutation) form may occur in girls. Another form of dystrophy, *Becker muscular dystrophy,* is similarly X-linked but manifests later in childhood or adolescence and has a slower course of progression.

DMD is caused by mutations in a gene located on the short arm of the X chromosome that codes for a protein called *dystrophin.* Dystrophin is a large cytoplasmic protein located on the inner surface of the sarcolemma or muscle fibre membrane. The dystrophin molecules are concentrated over the Z-bands of the muscle, where they form a strong link between the actin filaments of the intracellular contractile apparatus and the extracellular connective tissue matrix[9,10] (see Chapter 4, Fig. 4. 21). It is thought that abnormalities in the dystrophin-associated protein complex compromise sarcolemma integrity, particularly with sustained contractions. This disruption in integrity may be responsible for the observed increased fragility of dystrophic muscle, excessive influx of calcium ions, and release of soluble muscle enzymes such as creatine kinase into the serum.

The degenerative process in DMD consists of a relentless necrosis of muscle fibres, accompanied by a continuous process of repair and regeneration, and progressive fibrosis. The degenerative process eventually outpaces the regenerative capacity of the muscle, causing a gradual replacement of muscle fibres by fibrofatty connective tissue. The end stage is characterized

FIGURE 50.6 • A boy with Duchenne muscular dystrophy demonstrating pseudohypertrophy of his calves and climbing from a sitting position because of proximal muscle weakness. (From Bird T., Sumi S. (2002). *Atlas of clinical neurology.* Edited by Roger N. Rosenberg. © Current Medicine, Inc.)

by almost complete loss of skeletal muscle fibres, with relative sparing of intrafusal fibres of the muscle spindles.[10]

Clinical Course. Children with DMD are usually asymptomatic at birth and during infancy.[14] Early gross movements such as rolling, sitting, and standing are usually achieved at the proper ages. The postural muscles of the hips and shoulders are usually the first to be affected. Pseudohypertropy of the calf muscles eventually develops (Fig. 50.6). Signs of muscle weakness usually become evident beginning at 2 to 3 years, when frequent falling begins to occur. Imbalances between agonist and antagonist muscles lead to abnormal postures and the development of contractures and joint immobility. Scoliosis is common. Wheelchairs usually are needed at approximately 7 to 12 years of age.[14] Function of the distal muscles usually is preserved well enough that the child can continue to use eating utensils and a computer keyboard. Function of the extraocular muscles also is well preserved, as is the function of the smooth muscle controlling bladder and bowel activity. Incontinence is an uncommon and late event. Respiratory muscle involvement results in weak and ineffective cough, frequent respiratory infections, and decreasing respiratory reserve. DMD also affects cardiac muscle, and cardiomyopathy is a common feature of the disease. The severity of cardiac involvement, however, does not necessarily correlate with skeletal muscle weakness. Some patients die at an early age from severe cardiomyopathy, whereas others maintain adequate cardiac function until the terminal stages of the disease. Death from respiratory and cardiac muscle involvement usually occurs in young adulthood.

Observation of the child's voluntary movements and a complete family history provide important diagnostic data for the disease. Serum levels of the enzyme creatine kinase, which leaks from damaged muscle fibres, can be used to assist the diagnosis. Muscle biopsy showing a mixture of muscle cell degeneration and regeneration and reveals fat and scar tissue replacement is diagnostic of the disorder. Echocardiography, electrocardiography, and chest radiography are used to assess cardiac function. A specific molecular genetic diagnosis is possible by demonstrating defective dystrophin through the use of immunohistochemical staining of sections of muscle biopsy tissue or by polymerase chain reaction (PCR) analysis of genomic deoxyribonucleic acid (DNA) derived from leukocytes in a blood sample. The same methods of DNA analysis may be used on blood samples to establish carrier status in female relatives at risk, such as sisters and cousins. Prenatal diagnosis is possible as early as 12 weeks' gestation by sampling chorionic villi for DNA analysis[1] (see Chapter 7).

As this is a genetic disease, the management is directed toward maintaining ambulation and preventing deformities. Passive stretching, correct or counter posturing, and splints help to prevent deformities. Use of specific types of steroids such as Deflazacort may enable walking for a bit longer time, although side effects may be significant. Precautions should be taken to avoid respiratory infections. Recently Canadian researchers identified a mutation in unique muscle fibres that results in regrowth of the dystrophin protein. Since this is the missing protein for DMD, the hope is for a drug therapy to be developed for the treatment of DMD.[13] Even with these advances, however, currently there is no known cure.

Disorders of the Neuromuscular Junction

The neuromuscular junction serves as a synapse between a motor neuron and a skeletal muscle fibre. It consists of the axon terminals of a motor neuron and a specialized region of the muscle membrane called the *motor endplate*. The transmission of impulses at the neuromuscular junction is mediated by the release of the neurotransmitter *acetylcholine* from the axon terminals. Acetylcholine binds to specific receptors in the endplate region of the muscle fibre surface to cause muscle contraction (Fig. 50.7). Acetylcholine is active in the neuromuscular junction only for the brief period it takes to generate an action potential in the innervated muscle cell. In the synaptic space are large quantities of the enzyme *acetylcholinesterase*, which destroys acetylcholine a few milliseconds after it has been released. The rapid inactivation of acetylcholine allows repeated muscle contractions and gradations of contractile force.

Drug- and Toxin-Induced Disorders

A number of drugs and agents can alter neuromuscular function by changing the release, inactivation, or receptor binding of acetylcholine. Curare-type drugs act on the postjunctional membrane of the motor endplate to prevent the depolarizing effect of the neurotransmitter. Blocking of neuromuscular transmission by curare-type drugs is used during many types of surgical procedures to facilitate relaxation of involved musculature. Drugs such as physostigmine and neostigmine inhibit the action of acetylcholinesterase and allow acetylcholine released from the motor neuron to accumulate and prolong its action. These drugs are used in the treatment of myasthenia gravis.[15]

Neurotoxins from the botulism organism (*Clostridium botulinum*) produce paralysis by blocking acetylcholine release.[10,16] Clostridia are anaerobic, gram-positive, spore-forming bacilli found worldwide in soils, marine and fresh water sediments, and the intestines of many animals. Classic food-borne botulism occurs through ingestion of soil-grown foods that are not properly cooked or preserved.[17] Spores can be dormant, are resistant to heat, and germinate in low-acidity and low-nitrate environments. Canned vegetables, items preserved in garlic oil, and soups are usually the cause of sporadic outbreaks. Ingestion of the spores leads to toxin synthesis and absorption of the toxins from the intestinal tract. Wound botulism occurs through colonization of wounds with *C. botulinum*. Although postsurgical cases were initially the cause of wound botulism, almost all recent adult cases have involved intravenously injected heroin users.[17]

Infant botulism, now the most commonly reported form of the disease, occurs through infant ingestion of *C. botulinum* spores.[18] An infant's immature gastrointestinal tract allows the spores to germinate and elaborate the botulinum toxins. Infant botulism is rare in Canada with 42 cases reported since 1979.[19] It can affect healthy children who are less than 1 year of age. Usually these infants develop botulism by ingesting

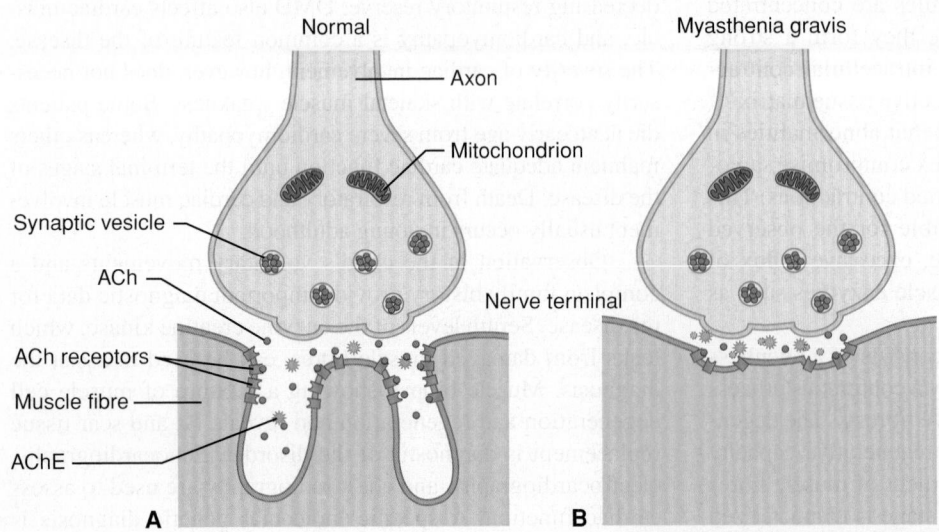

FIGURE 50.7 • Neuromuscular junction. **A:** Acetylcholine (ACh) released from the motor neurons in the myoneural junction crosses the synaptic space to reach receptors that are concentrated in the folds of the endplate of the muscle fibre. Once released, ACh is rapidly broken down by the enzyme acetylcholinesterase (AChE). **B:** Decrease in ACh receptors in myasthenia gravis.

C. botulinum spores, which are found in the soil or in honey products. According to microbiologic studies, 25% of honey products have been found to contain spores.[17] Therefore, it is recommended that honey not be given to infants younger than 1 year of age. The classic clinical features include constipation, cranial nerve abnormalities (loss of head control, loss of facial expression, weak cry), hypotonia, hyperreflexia, and respiratory distress. Constipation may be present in affected infants for a variable time and precede weakness by several weeks.

Pharmacologic preparations of the botulinum toxin (botulinum type A toxin [Botox] and botulinum type B toxin [Myobloc]) have become available for use in treating eyelid and eye movement disorders such as blepharospasm and strabismus.[10,15] It also is used for treatment of spasmodic torticollis, spasmodic dysphonias (laryngeal dystonia), and other dystonias. The drug is injected into the target muscle using the electrical activity recorded from the tip of a special electromyographic injection needle to guide the injection. The treatment is not permanent and usually needs to be repeated approximately every 3 months.

The aminoglycoside antibiotics (*e.g.*, gentamicin) may produce a clinical disturbance similar to botulism by preventing the release of acetylcholine from nerve endings. The symptoms usually subside rapidly once the drug is eliminated from the body. These drugs are particularly dangerous in persons with pre-existing disturbances of neuromuscular transmission, such as myasthenia gravis.

The organophosphates that are used in some insecticides bind acetylcholinesterase to prevent the breakdown of acetylcholine. They produce excessive and prolonged acetylcholine action with a depolarization block of cholinergic receptors, including those of the neuromuscular junction.[15] The organophosphates are well absorbed from the skin, lungs, gut, and conjunctiva of the eye, making them particularly effective as insecticides but also potentially dangerous to humans. Malathion and certain other organophosphates are rapidly metabolized to inactive products in humans and are considered safe for sale to the general public. The sale of other insecticides, such as parathion, which is not effectively metabolized to inactive products, has been banned. Other organophosphate compounds were developed as "nerve gases" with military potential; if absorbed in high enough concentrations, they have lethal effects from depolarization block and loss of respiratory muscle function.

Myasthenia Gravis

Myasthenia gravis is a disorder of transmission at the neuromuscular junction that affects communication between the motor neuron and the innervated muscle cell. The disease may occur at any age, but the peak incidence occurs between 20 and 30 years of age, and the disease is approximately three times more common in women than men. A smaller, second peak occurs in later life and affects men more often than women.[20] The Lambert–Eaton myasthenic syndrome is a special type of myasthenic syndrome that develops in association with neoplasms, particularly small cell carcinoma of the lung (see Chapter 8).

This autoimmune disease is caused by an antibody-mediated loss of acetylcholine receptors in the neuromuscular junction.[20–22] (Fig. 50.7). Although the exact mechanism that triggers the autoimmune response is unclear, it is thought to be caused by sensitized helper T cells and an antibody-directed attack on the acetylcholine receptor in the neuromuscular junction. The antibody attack leads to a shedding of the acetylcholine receptor-rich terminal portions of the folds in the endplate of the muscle fibre, a decreased number of receptors, and a widened synaptic space that impairs signal transmission.[11] Approximately 75% of persons with myasthenia gravis also have thymic abnormalities, such as a thymoma (*i.e.*, thymus tumour) or thymic hyperplasia (*i.e.*, increased thymus weight from an increased number of thymus cells).[20] Transient neonatal myasthenia gravis, caused by placental transfer of the acetylcholine receptor antibody, occurs in about 10% to 15% of infants born to mothers with the disease. Spontaneous resolution of symptoms usually occurs within a few months of birth. Myasthenia gravis in juveniles is uncommon.

In persons with myasthenia gravis who have a reduced postsynaptic membrane area and fewer acetylcholine receptors, each release of acetylcholine from the presynaptic membrane results in a lower-amplitude endplate potential. This results in both muscle weakness and fatigability with sustained effort. Most commonly affected are the eye and periorbital muscles, with ptosis due to eyelid weakness or diplopia due to weakness of the extraocular muscles as an initial symptom. The disease may progress from ocular muscle weakness to generalized weakness, including respiratory muscle weakness. Chewing and swallowing may be difficult. Weakness in limb movement usually is more pronounced in proximal than in distal parts of the extremity, so that climbing stairs and lifting objects are difficult. As the disease progresses, the muscles of the lower face are affected, causing speech impairment. In most persons, symptoms are least evident when arising in the morning, but grow worse with effort and as the day proceeds.

Persons with myasthenia gravis may experience a sudden exacerbation of symptoms and weakness known as *myasthenic crisis*. Myasthenic crisis occurs when muscle weakness becomes severe enough to compromise ventilation to the extent that ventilatory support and airway protection are needed. This usually occurs during a period of stress, such as infection, emotional upset, pregnancy, alcohol ingestion, extreme exposure to cold or heat, or surgery. It also can result from inadequate or excessive doses of the anticholinesterase drugs used in treatment of the disorder.

Diagnosis and Treatment. The diagnosis of myasthenia gravis is based on history and physical examination, the anticholinesterase test, nerve stimulation studies, and an assay for acetylcholine receptor antibodies. The anticholinesterase test uses a drug that inhibits acetylcholinesterase, the enzyme that breaks down acetylcholine. Edrophonium (Tensilon), a short-acting acetylcholinesterase inhibitor, is commonly used for the test. When this drug is administered intravenously, it decreases the breakdown of acetylcholine in the neuromuscular junction.

When weakness is caused by myasthenia gravis, a dramatic transitory improvement in muscle function occurs. Electrophysiologic studies can be done to demonstrate a decremental muscle response to repetitive 2- or 3-Hz stimulation of motor nerves. An advance in diagnostic methods for myasthenia gravis is single-fibre EMG, which is available in many medical centres. Single-fibre EMG detects delayed or failed neuromuscular transmission in muscle fibres supplied by a single nerve fibre.[20–22] An immunoassay test can be used to detect the presence of antiacetylcholine receptor antibodies circulating in the blood. A chest computed tomography (CT) or magnetic resonance imaging (MRI) is done on all patients with confirmed myasthenia gravis to exclude the presence of a thymoma.

Treatment methods include the use of pharmacologic agents; immunosuppressive therapy, including corticosteroid drugs; management of myasthenic crisis; thymectomy; and plasmapheresis or intravenous immunoglobulin.[20–22] Treatment is individualized and depends on the person's severity of illness, muscle weakness, age, and presence of other comorbidities. Medications that may exacerbate myasthenia gravis, such as the aminoglycoside antibiotics, should be avoided. Pharmacologic treatment with reversible anticholinesterase drugs inhibits the breakdown of acetylcholine at the neuromuscular junction by acetylcholinesterase, thereby enhancing communication across the junction. Pyridostigmine and neostigmine are the drugs of choice. Immunosuppressant drugs (e.g., azathioprine, cyclosporine) may also be used. In cases of crisis or a poor response to anticholinesterase drugs and thymectomy, corticosteroid drugs (e.g., prednisone), which suppress the immune response, are used.[20]

In combination with pharmacologic measures and/or surgery, plasmapheresis may be an effective short-term solution. Plasmapheresis removes antibodies from the circulation and provides short-term clinical improvement. It is used primarily to stabilize the condition of persons in myasthenic crisis or for short-term treatment in persons undergoing thymectomy or other surgery. Intravenous immunoglobulin also produces improvement in persons with myasthenia gravis. Although the effect is temporary, it may last for weeks to months. The indications for its use are similar to those for plasmapheresis. The mechanism of action of intravenous immunoglobulin is unknown. Thymectomy, or surgical removal of the thymus, may be used as a treatment for myasthenia gravis. The mechanism whereby this surgery has an effect is not completely understood. Thymectomy is performed in persons with thymoma, regardless of age, and in persons between puberty and 55 years of age with generalized myasthenia gravis.[20–22]

Lower Motor Neuron Disorders

Lower motor neuron diseases are progressive neurologic illnesses that selectively affect the anterior horn cells of the spinal cord and cranial nerve motor neurons.[9,23] An example of a disorder that involves purely LMNs is a distinctive group of degenerative disorders that begin in childhood or adolescence called *spinal muscular atrophy* (SMA). Weakness and muscle atrophy are prominent findings in all forms of the disorder.

This condition is likely to be inherited, usually in an autosomal recessive fashion, and is caused by the deletion of the survival motor neuron-1 gene (*SMN1*). Some forms of SMA result from degeneration of the anterior horn cells but are not caused by deletion of the *SMN1* gene. The most severe form may be symptomatic at birth or in the first months of life. In addition to hypotonia in the infant, patients frequently die from respiratory failure. More indolent forms may become symptomatic later in life, from infancy to as late as adolescence.[23]

Peripheral Nerve Disorders

The peripheral nervous system consists of the motor and sensory branches of the cranial and spinal nerves, the peripheral parts of the autonomic nervous system, and the peripheral ganglia. A peripheral neuropathy is any primary disorder of the peripheral nerves. The result usually is muscle weakness, with or without atrophy and sensory changes.

Unlike nerves in the CNS, peripheral nerves are fairly strong and resilient. They contain a series of connective tissue sheaths that enclose their nerve fibres. An outer fibrous sheath called the *epineurium* surrounds the medium-sized to large nerves; inside, a sheath called the *perineurium* invests each bundle of nerve fibres; and within each bundle, a delicate sheath of connective tissue known as the *endoneurium* surrounds each nerve fibre (see Chapter 48, Fig. 48.3). Inside the endoneurial sheath are the Schwann cells that produce the myelin sheath that surrounds the peripheral nerves. Each Schwann cell can myelinate only one segment of a single axon—the one that it covers—so that myelination of an entire axon requires the participation of a long line of these cells.

Peripheral Nerve Injury and Repair

There are two main types of peripheral nerve injury, depending on the area of insult: segmental demyelination involving the Schwann cell and axonal degeneration involving the neuronal cell body or its axon.[9,10] The peripheral nerve disorders can affect a spinal nerve or nerve root, a nerve plexus, or a peripheral nerve trunk (mononeuropathies), or multiple peripheral nerves (polyneuropathies).

Segmental Demyelination. Segmental demyelination occurs when there is a disorder of the Schwann cell (as in Guillain–Barré syndrome) or damage to the myelin sheath (e.g., sensory neuropathies), without a primary abnormality of the axon. It typically affects some Schwann cells while sparing others. The denuded axon provides a stimulus for remyelination, and the population of cells in the endoneurium has the capacity to replace the injured Schwann cells. These cells proliferate and encircle the axon, and in time remyelinate the denuded portion. However, the new myelin sheath is thin in proportion to the axon, and over time, many chronic demyelinating neuropathies give way to axonal injury.

Axonal Degeneration. Axonal degeneration is caused by primary injury to a neuronal cell body or its axon. Damage to the axon may be due either to a focal event occurring at some point along the length of the nerve (*e.g.,* trauma or ischemia) or to a more generalized abnormality affecting the neuronal cell body (neuropathy).

Damage to a peripheral nerve axon, whether due to injury or neuropathy, results in degenerative changes, followed by breakdown of the myelin sheath and Schwann cells. In distal axonal degeneration, the proximal axon and neuronal cell body, which synthesizes the material required for nourishing and maintaining the axon, remain intact. In neuropathies and crushing injuries in which the endoneurial tube remains intact, the outgrowing fibre will grow down this tube to the structure that was originally innervated by the neuron (Fig. 50.8). However, it can take weeks or months for the regrowing fibre to reach its target organ and for communicative function to be reestablished. More time is required for the Schwann cells to form new myelin segments and for the axon to recover its original diameter and conduction velocity.

The successful regeneration of a nerve fibre in the peripheral nervous system depends on many factors. If a nerve fibre is destroyed relatively close to the neuronal cell body, the chances are that the nerve cell will die, and if it does, it will not be replaced. If a crushing type of injury has occurred, partial or often full recovery of function occurs. Cutting-type trauma to a nerve is an entirely different matter. Connective scar tissue forms rapidly at the wound site, and when it does, only the most rapidly regenerating axonal branches are able to get through to the intact distal endoneurial tubes. A number of scar-inhibiting agents have been used in an effort to reduce this hazard, but have met with only moderate success. In another attempt to improve nerve regeneration, various types of tubular implants have been placed to fill longer gaps in the endoneurial tube.

Neuropathies involving the neuronal cell body are much less common than those affecting the axons. In these cases, there is little potential for recovery of function because death of the neuronal cells precludes axonal regeneration.

Mononeuropathies

Mononeuropathies usually are caused by localized conditions such as trauma, compression, or infection that affect a single spinal nerve, plexus, or peripheral nerve trunk. Fractured bones may lacerate or compress nerves; excessively tight tourniquets may injure nerves directly or produce ischemic injury; and infections such as herpes zoster may affect a single segmental afferent nerve distribution. Recovery of nerve function usually is complete after compression lesions and incomplete or faulty after nerve transection.

Carpal Tunnel Syndrome. Carpal tunnel syndrome is a relatively common compression-type mononeuropathy.[7,24,25] It is caused by compression of the median nerve as it travels with the flexor tendons through a canal made by the carpal bones and transverse carpal ligament (Fig. 50.9). The condition can be caused by a variety of conditions that produce a reduction in the capacity of the carpal tunnel (*i.e.,* bony or ligamentous changes) or an increase in the volume of the tunnel contents (*i.e.,* inflammation of the tendons, synovial swelling, or tumours). Carpal tunnel syndrome may be a feature of a number of systemic diseases, such as rheumatoid arthritis, hypothyroidism, acromegaly, and diabetes mellitus.[25] Most cases, however, are due to repetitive use of the wrist (*i.e.,* flexion–extension movements and stress associated with pinching and gripping motions, or use of vibratory tools).

Carpal tunnel syndrome is characterized by pain, paresthesia, and numbness of the thumb and first two and one half digits of the hand; pain in the wrist and hand, which worsens at night; atrophy of the abductor pollicis muscle; and weakness in precision grip. All of these abnormalities may contribute to clumsiness of fine motor activity.

Early diagnosis and treatment are important to avoid permanent damage to the median nerve. Diagnosis usually is based on sensory disturbances confined to median nerve distribution and a positive Tinel or Phalen sign.[25] The *Tinel sign* is the development of a tingling sensation radiating into the palm of the hand that is elicited by light percussion over the median nerve at the wrist. The *Phalen maneuver* is performed

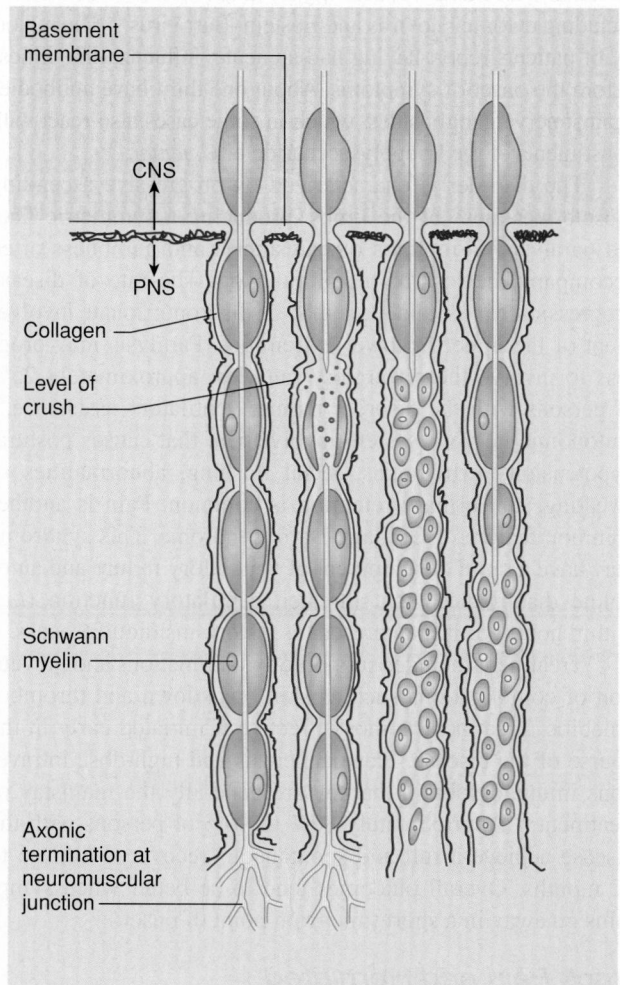

Basement membrane

CNS

PNS

Collagen

Level of crush

Schwann myelin

Axonic termination at neuromuscular junction

FIGURE 50.8 • Sequential stages in efferent axon degeneration and regeneration within its endoneurial tube, after peripheral nerve crush injury. CNS, central nervous system; PNS, peripheral nervous system.

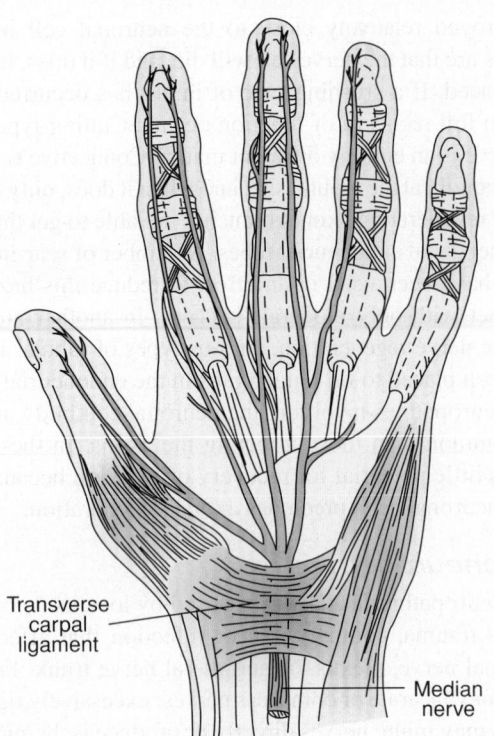

Transverse carpal ligament

Median nerve

FIGURE 50.9 • Carpal tunnel syndrome: compression of the median nerve by the transverse carpal ligament. (Courtesy Carole Russell Hilmer, CMI.)

by having the person hold the wrist in complete flexion for approximately a minute; if numbness and paresthesia along the median nerve are reproduced or exaggerated, the test result is considered to be positive. EMG and nerve conduction studies are often done to confirm the diagnosis and exclude other causes of the disorder.

Treatment falls under two categories: conservative and surgical. Conservative measures include the avoidance of movements that cause nerve compression, splinting, and anti-inflammatory medications. Identifying and decreasing any causative repetitive movements should be initiated. Splints may be confined to nighttime use. When splinting is ineffective, corticosteroids may be injected into the carpal tunnel to reduce inflammation and swelling. Measures to treat a systemic disease, if this is the cause, are important prior to surgical intervention. Surgery consists of operative division of the volar carpal ligaments as a means of relieving pressure on the median nerve.[25]

Polyneuropathies

Polyneuropathies involve demyelination or axonal degeneration of multiple peripheral nerves that leads to symmetric sensory, motor, or mixed sensorimotor deficits. Typically, the longest axons are involved first, with symptoms beginning in the distal part of the extremities. If the autonomic nervous system is involved, there may be postural hypotension, constipation, and impotence. Polyneuropathies can result from immune mechanisms (*e.g.,* Guillain–Barré syndrome), toxic agents (*e.g.,* arsenic polyneuropathy, lead polyneuropathy,

alcoholic polyneuropathy), and metabolic diseases (*e.g.,* diabetes mellitus, uremia). Different causes tend to affect axons of different diameters and to affect sensory, motor, or autonomic neurons to different degrees.

Guillain–Barré Syndrome. Guillain–Barré syndrome is an acute immune-mediated polyneuropathy.[26] The syndrome defines a clinical entity that is characterized by rapidly progressive limb weakness and loss of tendon reflexes. It has been described as the most common cause of acute, flaccid paralysis in developed countries, now that poliomyelitis has been eliminated. As a syndrome, there are several subtypes of the disorder, including pure motor axonal degeneration, axonal degeneration of both motor and sensory nerves, and a variant characterized by ophthalmoplegia, ataxia, and areflexia.[26]

The disorder is manifested by infiltration of mononuclear cells, consisting mainly of T cell and macrophages, around the capillaries of the peripheral neurons, edema of the endoneurial compartment, and demyelination of ventral spinal roots. The cause of the Guillain–Barré syndrome probably has an immune component. Controlled epidemiologic studies have linked it to infection with *Campylobacter jejuni* in addition to other viruses, including cytomegalovirus and Epstein–Barr virus.[26] The majority of patients report having had an acute, influenza-like illness before the onset of symptoms. About one third have antibodies against nerve gangliosides, which in some cases also react with constituents of the lipopolysaccharide of *C. jejuni*.[26]

The disorder is characterized by progressive ascending muscle weakness of the limbs, producing a symmetric flaccid paralysis. Symptoms of paresthesia and numbness often accompany the loss of motor function. The rate of disease progression varies, and there may be disproportionate involvement of the upper or lower extremities. Paralysis may progress to involve the respiratory muscles; approximately 25% of persons with the disorder require ventilatory assistance.[26] Autonomic nervous system involvement that causes postural hypotension, arrhythmias, facial flushing, abnormalities of sweating, and urinary retention is common. Pain is another common feature of Guillain–Barré syndrome. This syndrome may have a rapid development of ventilatory failure and autonomic disturbances that threaten circulatory function (*i.e.,* within hours) or it may present as a slow, insidious process.

Treatment includes support of vital functions and prevention of complications such as skin breakdown and thrombophlebitis. Treatment is most effective if initiated early in the course of the disease. Plasmapheresis and high-dose intravenous immunoglobulin therapy are generally the mainstay of treatment.[26] Approximately 80% to 90% of persons with the disease achieve a full and spontaneous recovery within 6 to 12 months. Overall outcomes tend to be better when symptoms go away in a short time from point of onset.

Back Pain and Herniated Intervertebral Disk

Back problems are among the most common chronic conditions in Canada. The lifetime prevalence is reported to be as high as 84%, with 11% to 12% of the population being disabled by low back pain.[27] It affects men and women equally, with onset most often between the ages of 30 and 50 years.[28] Risk factors include heavy lifting, twisting, bodily vibration, obesity, and poor conditioning, but low back pain is common even in persons without these risk factors. Other risks include psychological factors such as depression and chronic stress. Although acute low back pain resolves within 3 to 6 weeks in most persons, recurrences are common.[28]

Back pain can result from a number of interrelated problems involving spinal structures, including facet joints, the vertebral periosteum, ligaments, paravertebral musculature and fascia, and spinal nerve roots. Perhaps the most common are musculoligamentous injuries and age-related degenerative changes in the intervertebral disks and facet joints. Other causes include disk herniation (to be discussed) and spinal stenosis. Spinal stenosis is characterized by narrowing of the central canal, typically from hypertrophic degenerative changes.[28]

The diagnostic measures used in the evaluation of back pain include history and physical examination, including a thorough neurologic examination. Other diagnostic methods include radiographs of the back and MRI. MRI or radiography is not generally recommended early in the course of low back pain. The diagnostic challenge is to identify those persons who require further evaluation for more serious problems.

Treatment of back pain usually is conservative and consists of analgesic medications, skeletal muscle relaxants, superficial heat, and instruction in the correct mechanics for lifting and methods of protecting the back.[27–29] Pain relief is usually provided using nonsteroidal anti-inflammatory drugs (NSAIDS). Muscle relaxants may be used on a short-term basis, but should be used with caution because of CNS adverse effects. Bed rest does not increase the speed of recovery, rather sometimes delays recovery.[27]

Herniated Intervertebral Disk. The intervertebral disk is considered the most critical component of the load-bearing structures of the spinal column. The intervertebral disk consists of a soft, gelatinous centre called the *nucleus pulposus,* which is encircled by a strong, ring-like collar of fibrocartilage called the *annulus fibrosus.*[3,30] The structural components of the disk make it capable of absorbing shock and changing shape while allowing movement. With dysfunction, the nucleus pulposus can be squeezed out of place and herniate through the annulus fibrosus, a condition referred to as a *herniated* or *slipped disk* (Fig. 50.10A, B).

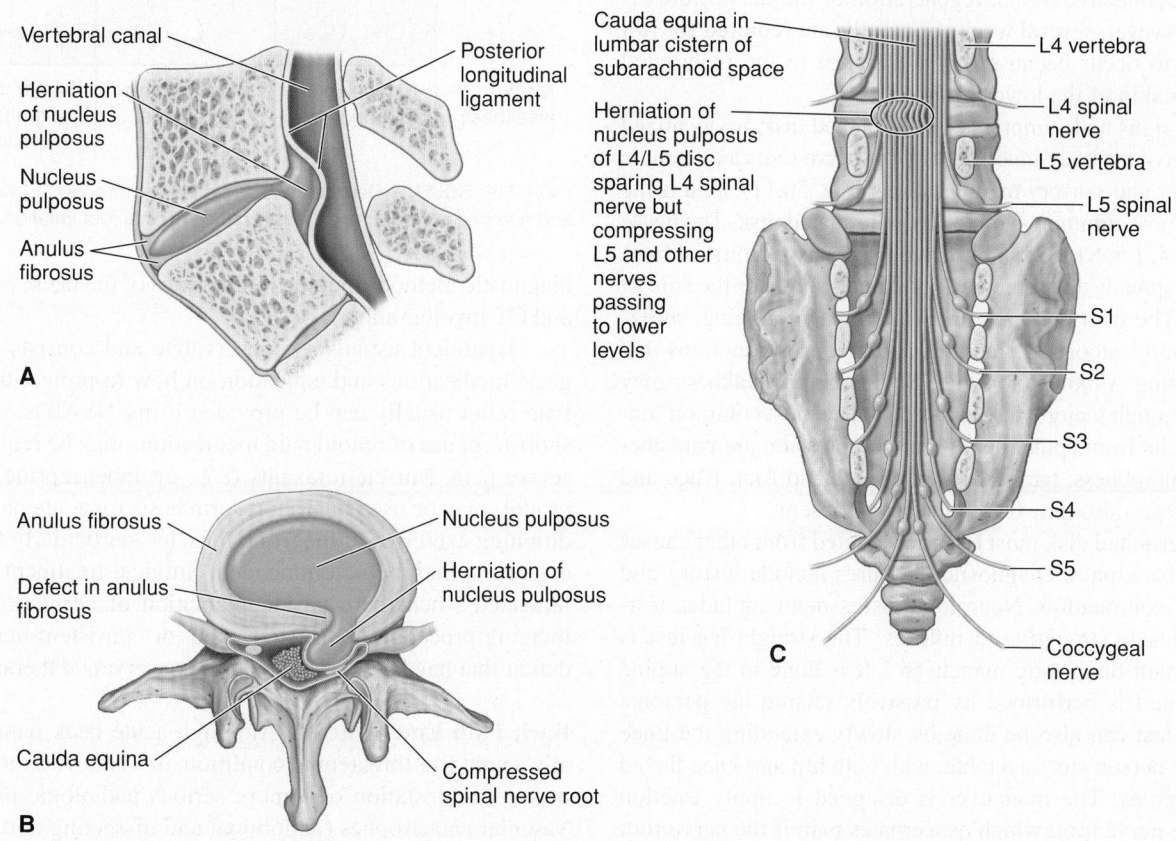

FIGURE 50.10 • Herniated intervertebral disk. **A:** Longitudinal section. **B:** Cross-section. **C:** Location of L4–L5 and S1–S5 spinal nerves, with site of L4/L5 herniation of nucleus pulposus indicated. (Modified from Moore K. L., Dalley A. F., Agur A. M. R. (2014). *Clinical oriented anatomy* (7th ed., p. 475). Philadelphia, PA: Lippincott Williams & Wilkins.)

The intervertebral disk can become dysfunctional because of trauma, the effects of aging, or degenerative disorders of the spine. Trauma results from activities such as lifting while in the flexed position, slipping, falling on the buttocks or back, or suppressing a sneeze. With aging, the gelatinous centre of the disk dries out and loses much of its elasticity, causing it to fray and tear. Degenerative processes such as osteoarthritis or ankylosing spondylitis predispose to malalignment of the vertebral column.

The cervical and lumbar regions are the most flexible areas of the spine and are most often involved in disk herniations. Usually, herniation occurs at the lower levels of the lumbar spine, where the mass being supported and the bending of the vertebral column are greatest. The majority of lumbar herniations occur in the L4 or L5 to S1 regions. With herniations of the cervical spine, the most frequently involved levels are C6 to C7 and C5 to C6. Protrusion of the nucleus pulposus usually occurs posteriorly and toward the intervertebral foramen and its contained spinal nerve root, where the annulus fibrosus is relatively thin and poorly supported by either the posterior or anterior ligaments (Fig. 50.10A).

The level at which a herniated disk occurs is important (Fig. 50.10C). When the injury occurs in the lumbar area, only the nerve fibres of the cauda equina are involved. Because these elongated dorsal and ventral roots contain endoneurial tubes of connective tissue, regeneration of the nerve fibres is likely. However, several weeks or months are required for full recovery to occur because of the distance to the innervated muscle or skin of the lower limbs.

The signs and symptoms of a herniated disk are localized to the area of the body innervated by the nerve roots and include both motor and sensory manifestations (Fig. 50.11). Pain is the first and most common symptom of a herniated disk. The nerve roots of L4, L5, S1, S2, and S3 give rise to a syndrome of back pain that spreads down the back of the leg and over the sole of the foot. The pain is usually intensified with coughing, sneezing, straining, stooping, standing, and the jarring motions that occur during walking or riding. Slight motor weakness may occur, although major weakness is rare. The most common sensory deficits from spinal nerve root compression are paresthesias and numbness, particularly of the leg and foot. Knee and ankle reflexes also may be diminished or absent.

A herniated disk must be differentiated from other causes of acute back pain. Diagnostic measures include history and physical examination. Neurologic assessment includes testing of muscle strength and reflexes. The straight-leg test is an important diagnostic maneuver.[28] It is done in the supine position and is performed by passively raising the person's leg. The test can also be done by slowly extending the knee while the person sits on a table, with both hip and knee flexed at 90 degrees. The maneuver is designed to apply traction along the nerve root, which exacerbates pain if the nerve root is acutely inflamed. Normally, it is possible to raise the leg approximately 90 degrees without causing discomfort of the hamstring muscles. The test result is positive if pain is produced when the leg is raised to 60 degrees or less.[28] Other

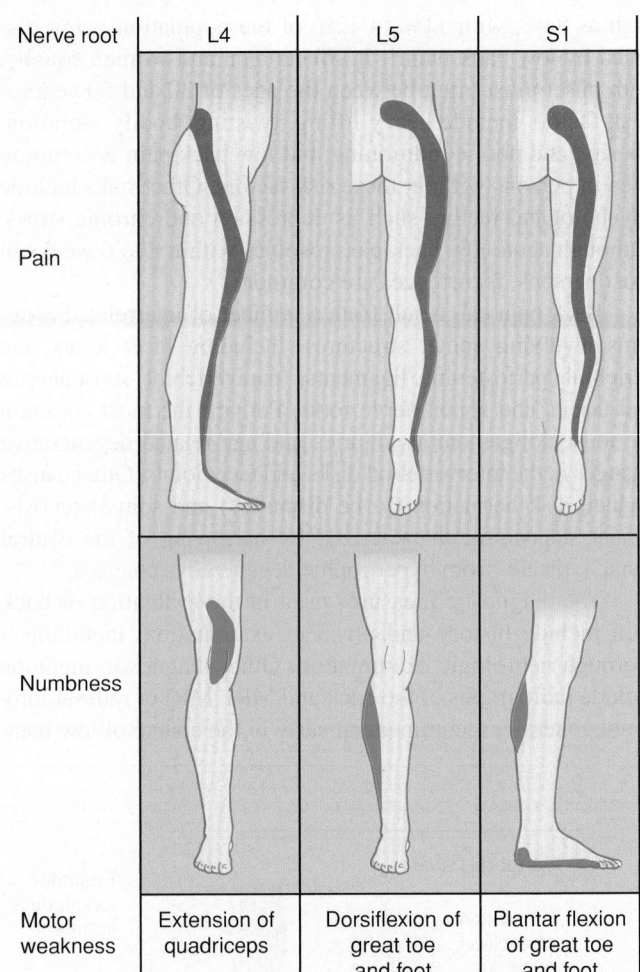

Nerve root	L4	L5	S1
Pain			
Numbness			
Motor weakness	Extension of quadriceps	Dorsiflexion of great toe and foot	Plantar flexion of great toe and foot

FIGURE 50.11 • Dermatomes of the leg (L1 through S5) where pain and numbness would be experienced with spinal root irritation.

diagnostic methods include radiographs of the back, MRI, CT, and CT myelography.

Treatment usually is conservative and consists of analgesic medications and education on how to protect the back. Pain relief usually can be provided using NSAIDs, although short-term use of opioid pain medications may be required for severe pain. Muscle relaxants (*e.g.*, cyclobenzaprine, carisoprodol) may be used on a short-term basis for acute pain. Conditioning exercises of the trunk muscles, particularly the back extensors, may be recommended. Surgical treatment may be indicated when there is documentation of herniation by an imaging procedure, consistent pain, or consistent neurologic deficit that has failed to respond to conservative therapy.

Back Pain Emergencies. Although acute back pain is usually a non–life-threatening condition, in 5% to 10% of persons it is a manifestation of a more serious pathologic process.[31] Vascular catastrophes (abdominal and dissecting aortic aneurysms), malignancy, spinal cord compression syndromes, and infectious processes may all present as acute back pain.

Clinical findings or *red flags* indicate the possibility of more serious disease. These include gradual onset of pain; age younger than 20 years or older than 50 years; thoracic back pain; history of trauma, fever, chills, night sweats, immunosuppression or malignancy; unintentional weight loss; recent procedure known to cause bacteremia; and history of intravenous drug use.[28,31] The gradual onset of pain may be indicative of malignancy or infection. Back pain that begins before 20 years of age suggests congenital or developmental disorders, and new-onset pain in persons 50 years of age or older is more likely to be a manifestation of serious conditions such as an aortic aneurysm, malignancy, or compression fracture. Pain that is aggravated by lying down is a red flag for malignancy or infection; and pain that improves with sitting or slight flexion of the spine suggests the presence of spinal stenosis. Reports of neurologic symptoms such as paresthesia, motor weakness, urinary or fecal incontinence, or gait abnormalities require additional diagnostic tests to rule out spinal cord compression.

IN SUMMARY

The motor unit consists of the LMN, the neuromuscular junction, and the skeletal muscle that the nerve innervates. Disorders of the neuromuscular unit include muscular dystrophy and myasthenia gravis. Muscular dystrophy is a term used to describe a number of disorders that produce progressive deterioration of skeletal muscle. Muscle necrosis is followed by replacement with fat and connective tissue. One form, DMD, is inherited as an X-linked trait and transmitted by the mother to her male offspring. Myasthenia gravis is a disorder of the neuromuscular junction resulting from a deficiency of functional acetylcholine receptors, which causes weakness of the skeletal muscles. Because the disease affects the neuromuscular junction, there is no loss of sensory function. The most common manifestations are weakness of the eye muscles, with ptosis and diplopia.

Peripheral nerve disorders involve motor and sensory neurons outside the CNS. There are two main types of peripheral nerve injury based on the target of the insult: segmental demyelination involving the Schwann cell, and axonal degeneration involving the nerve axon or cell body. Peripheral nerve disorders include mononeuropathies, involving a single spinal nerve, plexus, or peripheral nerve; and polyneuropathies that involve demyelination or axonal degeneration of multiple peripheral nerves that leads to symmetric sensory, motor, or mixed sensorimotor deficits. Carpal tunnel syndrome, a mononeuropathy, is caused by compression of the median nerve that passes through the carpal tunnel in the wrist. Guillain–Barré syndrome is a subacute polyneuropathy, probably caused by immune mechanisms, that causes progressive ascending motor, sensory, and autonomic nervous system manifestations. Respiratory involvement may occur and necessitate mechanical ventilation.

Acute back pain is most commonly the result of conditions such as muscle strain; treatment focuses on measures to improve activity tolerance. A herniated intervertebral disk is characterized by protrusion of the nucleus pulposus into the spinal canal with irritation or compression of the nerve root. Usually, herniation occurs at the lower levels of the lumbar and sacral (L4 or L5 to S1) and cervical (C6 to C7 and C5 to C6) regions of the spine. The signs and symptoms of a herniated disk are localized to the area of the body innervated by the affected nerve roots and include pain and both motor and sensory manifestations.

DISORDERS OF THE CEREBELLUM AND BASAL GANGLIA

After completing this section of the chapter, you should be able to meet the following objectives:

- Relate the functions of the cerebellum to production of vestibulocerebellar ataxia, decomposition of movement, and cerebellar tremor.
- Describe the functional organization of the basal ganglia and communication pathways with the thalamus and cerebral cortex.
- State the possible mechanisms responsible for the development of Parkinson disease and characterize the manifestations and treatment of the disorder.

Disorders of the Cerebellum

The cerebellum is a cauliflower-shaped structure located in the posterior fossa and attached to the pons, medulla, and midbrain by the three paired cerebellar peduncles[3,32] (see Chapter 48). It has sometimes been referred to as the *silent area* of the brain because electrical stimulation does not produce any conscious sensation and rarely causes any motor movements.[3] However, removal or damage to the cerebellum causes movements to become highly abnormal. The cerebellum is especially vital during rapid muscular activities such as running, typing, and even talking. Loss of cerebellar function can result in total incoordination of these functions even though paralysis does not ensue.

The functions of the cerebellum are integrated into many connected afferent and efferent pathways throughout the brain. An extensive and important afferent pathway is the *corticopontocerebellar* pathway, which originates in the cerebral motor and premotor cortices as well as the somatosensory cortex. Other important afferent pathways link the cerebellum to input from the basal ganglia, muscle and joint tension information from the stretch receptors, visual input from the eyes, and balance and equilibrium sensation from the vestibular system in the inner ear. There are three general efferent pathways leading out of the cerebellum: the *vestibulocerebellar pathway* that functions in close association with the brain stem vestibular nuclei to maintain equilibrium and posture; the *spinocerebellar pathway* that provides the circuitry for coordinating the movements of the distal portions of the limbs, especially the hands and fingers; and the *cerebrocerebellar pathway* that transmits output information in the upward direction to the brain, functioning in a feedback manner with the motor and somatosensory systems to coordinate sequential body and limb movements.

Cerebellum-Associated Movement Disorders

The signs of cerebellar dysfunction can be grouped into three classes: vestibulocerebellar disorders, cerebellar ataxia or decomposition of movement, and cerebellar tremor. These disorders occur on the side of cerebellar damage, whether because of congenital defect, vascular accident, or growing tumour. Visual monitoring of movement cannot compensate for cerebellar defects, and the movement abnormalities occur whether the eyes are open or closed.

Damage to the part of the cerebellum associated with the vestibular system leads to difficulty or inability to maintain a steady posture of the trunk, which normally requires constant readjusting movements. This is seen as an unsteadiness of the trunk, called *truncal ataxia,* and can be so severe that standing is not possible. The ability to fix the eyes on a target also can be affected. Constant conjugate readjustment of eye position, called *nystagmus,* results and makes reading extremely difficult, especially when the eyes are deviated toward the side of cerebellar damage.

Cerebellar ataxia and tremor are different aspects of defects in the smooth, continuously correcting functions. Cerebellar dystaxia or, if severe, ataxia is characterized by a decomposition of movement, with each succeeding component of a complex movement occurring separately instead of being blended into a smoothly proceeding action. Because ethanol specifically affects cerebellar function, persons who are inebriated often walk with a staggering and unsteady gait. Rapid alternating movements such as supination–pronation–supination of the hands are jerky and performed slowly. Reaching to touch a target breaks down into small sequential components, each going too far, followed by overcorrection. The finger moves jerkily toward the target, misses, corrects in the other direction, and misses again, until the target is finally reached. This is called *over- and underreaching* or *dysmetria.*

Cerebellar tremor is a rhythmic back-and-forth movement of a finger or toe that worsens as the target is approached. The tremor results from the inability of the damaged cerebellar system to maintain ongoing fixation of a body part and to make smooth, continuous corrections in the trajectory of the movement; overcorrection occurs, first in one direction and then the other. Often, the tremor of an arm or leg can be detected during the beginning of an intended movement. The common term for cerebellar tremor is *intention tremor.* Cerebellar function, as it relates to tremor, can be assessed by asking a person to touch one heel to the opposite knee and move it down the leg, to gently move the toes along the back of the opposite shin, or to touch the nose with a finger.

Cerebellar function also can affect the motor skills of chewing and swallowing (dysphagia) and of speech (dysarthria). Normal speech requires smooth control of respiratory muscles and highly coordinated control of the laryngeal, lip, and tongue muscles. Cerebellar dysarthria is characterized by slow, slurred speech of continuously varying loudness. Rehabilitative efforts directed by speech therapists include learning strategies to slow the rate of speech and to compensate as much as possible through the use of less-affected muscles.

Disorders of the Basal Ganglia

The basal ganglia are a group of deep, interrelated subcortical nuclei that play an essential role in control of movement. They function in the organization of inherited and highly learned and rather automatic movement programs, especially those affecting the trunk and proximal limbs. The basal ganglia are thought to be particularly important in starting, stopping, and monitoring movements ordered and executed by the cortex, especially those that are relatively slow and sustained, or stereotyped, such as arm swinging during walking. They also help to regulate the intensity of these movements, and they act to inhibit antagonistic or unnecessary movements. The function of the basal ganglia is not limited to motor functions; they also are involved in cognitive and perceptual functions.

The structural components of the basal ganglia include the caudate nucleus, putamen, and globus pallidus.[3,33] They are located lateral and caudal to the thalamus, occupying a large portion of the interior of both cerebral hemispheres. The caudate and putamen are collectively referred to as the *striatum,* and the putamen and the globus pallidus form a wedge-shaped region called the *lentiform nucleus.* Two other structures, the *substantia nigra* of the midbrain and *subthalamic nucleus* of the diencephalon, are considered part of the basal ganglia (Fig. 50.12). The dorsal part of the substantia nigra contains cells that use dopamine as a neurotransmitter and are rich in a black pigment called *melanin.* The high concentration of melanin gives the structure a black colour, hence the name *substantia nigra.* The axons of the substantia nigra form the *nigrostriatal pathway,* which supplies dopamine to the striatum. The subthalamic nucleus lies just below the thalamus and above the anterior portion of the substantia nigra. The glutaminergic cells of this nucleus are the only excitatory projections to the basal ganglia.

Associated with the basal ganglia are several thalamic nuclei. For the motor and premotor cartices, these nuclei are the ventral lateral (VL) and the ventral anterior (VA) nuclei. Each region of the cerebral cortex is interconnected with a corresponding region of the ventral row of thalamic nuclei. The cortex-to-thalamus and thalamus-to-cortex feedback circuitries are excitatory and, if unmodulated, would produce hyperactivity of the cortical area, causing stiffness and rigidity of the face, body, and limbs, and, if alternating, a continuous tremor (*i.e.,* tremor at rest). For many semiautomatic stereotyped movements, thalamic excitability is modulated through inhibition by the basal ganglia. The basal ganglia form a

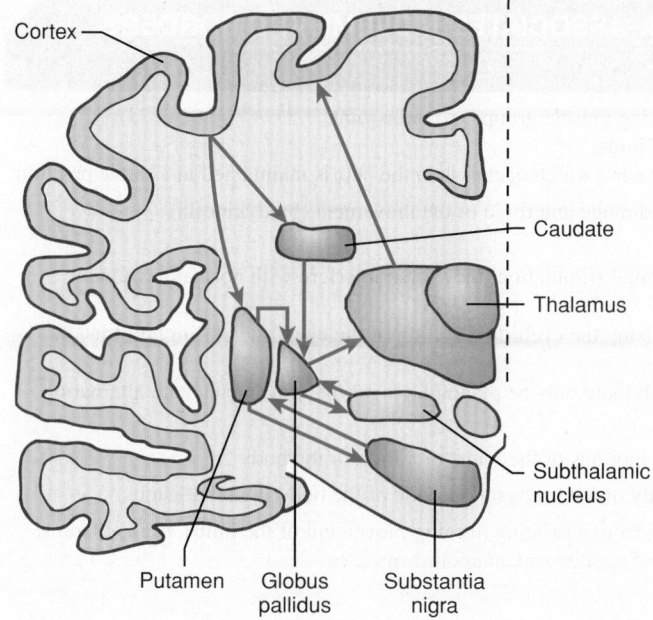

FIGURE 50.12 • Structures and basal neural circuitry of the basal ganglia.

major component of an inhibitory loop from each specific cortical region. Discrete inhibitory cortex-to-basal ganglia and thalamus-to-cortex loops modulate the function of all cerebral cortex regions.

The basal ganglia have input structures that receive afferent information from outside structures, internal circuits that connect the various structures of the basal ganglia, and output structures that deliver information to other brain centres. The striatum represents the major input structure for the basal ganglia. Virtually all principal pathways for executing learned patterns of movement pass through the striatum. Other basal ganglia structures such as the substantia nigra and subthalamic nuclei are interconnected with one another or with the input and output nuclei, and are considered to be components of the internal structures.

The output functions of the basal ganglia are mainly inhibitory. Looping circuits from specific cortical centres pass through the basal ganglia to modulate the excitability of certain thalamic nuclei and thus influence the cortical control of highly learned, automatic, and stereotyped motor functions. The two output nuclei of the basal ganglia, the globus pallidus and the substantia nigra, tonically inhibit their target nuclei in the thalamus. This inhibitory output is thought to be mediated by two parallel pathways that project from the striatum to the two output nuclei: one direct and one indirect.[33] These efferent pathways have opposing effects on the basal ganglia nuclei and thus on the targets of these nuclei. Activation of the direct pathway disinhibits the thalamus, thereby increasing thalamocortical activity, whereas activation of the indirect pathway further inhibits the thalamocortical neurons. As a result, activation of the direct pathway facilitates movement, and activation of the indirect pathway inhibits movement.

The basal ganglia also have a cognitive function in that they monitor sensory information coming into the brain and apply it to information stored in memory as a means of planning and sequencing motor movements.[3] The cognitive control of motor activities determines, subconsciously and within seconds, which patterns of movement will be needed to achieve a goal. The caudate nucleus, which receives large amounts of input from the association areas of the brain, plays a major role in the cognitive control of motor activity.

Multiple pathways provide excitatory signals that balance the large number of inhibitory signals transmitted by GABA (γ-aminobutyric acid) and dopaminergic neurons. One of these circuits involves a *neostriatal inhibitory projection* on the substantia nigra. The substantia nigra projects dopaminergic axons back on the striatum. A deficiency in the dopaminergic projection of this modulating circuit is implicated in parkinsonism. The function of the striatum also involves local cholinergic interneurons, and their destruction is thought to be related to the choreiform movements of Huntington disease, another basal ganglia–related syndrome (see Chapter 53).

Basal Ganglia–Associated Movement Disorders

Disorders of the basal ganglia comprise a complex group of motor disturbances characterized by tremor and other involuntary movements, changes in posture and muscle tone, and poverty and slowness of movement. They include tremors and tics, hypokinetic disorders, and hyperkinetic disorders[1] (Table 50.1).

Unlike disorders of the motor cortex and corticospinal (pyramidal) tract, lesions of the basal ganglia disrupt movement but do not cause paralysis. The various types of involuntary movements often occur in combination and appear to have a common underlying cause. Recent studies indicate that hypokinetic and hyperkinetic disorders can be explained as specific disturbances in the indirect and direct pathways that link the basal ganglia with the thalamocortical motor circuit.[33] Accordingly, overactivity of the indirect pathway would result in *hypokinetic* disorders such as Parkinson disease, and underactivity of the indirect pathway would result in *hyperkinetic* disorders such as chorea and ballismus.

Parkinson Disease

Parkinson disease is a degenerative disorder of basal ganglia function that results in variable combinations of tremor, rigidity, and bradykinesia. The disorder is characterized by progressive destruction of the nigrostriatal pathway, with subsequent reduction in striatal concentrations of dopamine. The prevalence of Parkinson disease in Canada is estimated at 0.2% of the general population.[34] It is estimated that approximately 55,000 Canadians have Parkinson disease. The average age at which people experience symptoms is 64 years, and the incidence increases with age.[34,50]

The clinical syndrome arising from the degenerative changes in basal ganglia function often is referred to as *parkinsonism*. Parkinson disease, the most common form of parkinsonism, is named after James Parkinson, a British physician who

TABLE 50.1 CHARACTERISTICS OF BASAL GANGLIA–ASSOCIATED MOVEMENT DISORDERS

MOVEMENT DISORDER	CHARACTERISTICS
Tremor	Involuntary, oscillating contractions of opposing muscle groups around a joint Usually fairly uniform in frequency and amplitude Can occur as resting tremors and postural tremors, which occur when the part is maintained in a stable position
Hypokinetic disorders	Slowness in initiating movement, and reduced range and force of the movement (bradykinesia)
Chorea	Irregular wriggling and writhing movements Accentuated by movement and by environmental stimulation; they often interfere with normal movement patterns May be grimacing movements of the face, raising the eyebrows, rolling of the eyes, and curling, protrusion, withdrawal of the tongue In the limbs, the movements largely are distal; there may be piano playing–type movements with alternating extension and flexion of the fingers
Athetosis	Continuous, worm-like, twisting and turning motions of the joints of a limb or the body
Ballismus	Violent, sweeping, flinging motions, especially of the limbs on one side of the body (hemiballismus)
Dystonia	Abnormal maintenance of a posture resulting from a twisting, turning movement of the limbs, neck, or trunk Often the result of simultaneous contraction of agonist and antagonist muscles Can result in grotesque and twisted postures
Dyskinesias	Bizarre wriggling and writhing movements Frequently involve the face, mouth, jaw, and tongue, causing grimacing, pursing of the lips, or protrusion of the tongue Limbs affected less often Tardive dyskinesia is an untoward reaction that can develop with long-term use of some antipsychotic medications

first described the disease in a paper he published in 1817 on the "shaking palsy."[35] In Parkinson disease, also known as *idiopathic parkinsonism,* dopamine depletion results from degeneration of the dopamine nigrostriatal system. Parkinsonism can also develop as a postencephalitic syndrome, as a side effect of therapy with antipsychotic drugs that block dopamine receptors, as a toxic reaction to a chemical agent, or as an outcome of severe carbon monoxide poisoning. Drug-induced parkinsonism can follow the administration of antipsychotic drugs in high doses (*e.g.,* phenothiazines, butyrophenones). These drugs block dopamine receptors and dopamine output by the cells of the substantia nigra. Symptoms of parkinsonism also may accompany conditions such as cerebral vascular disease, brain tumours, repeated head trauma, or degenerative neurologic diseases that structurally damage the nigrostriatal pathway.

The primary brain abnormality found in all persons with Parkinson disease is degeneration of the nigrostriatal dopamine neurons.[36–38] Other brain areas are affected to a lesser extent. On microscopic examination, there is loss of pigmented substantia nigra neurons. Some residual nerve cells are atrophic, and few contain *Lewy bodies,* which are visualized as spherical, eosinophilic cytoplasmic inclusions.

Although the cause of Parkinson disease is still unknown, it is widely believed that most cases are caused by an interaction of environmental and genetic factors. Over the past several decades, several pathologic processes (*e.g.,* oxidative stress, apoptosis, and mitochondrial disorders) that might lead to degeneration have been identified. Evidence suggests that welders exposed to manganese may have an occupational hazard of

developing Parkinson disease more often compared to people not exposed.[28,39] Certainly there are multiple other toxins in the environment that, similar to manganese, trigger manifestations of neurotoxicity that may lead to parkinsonism. Multiple genes have been identified that illustrate there are different types of Parkinson disease depending on whether the person inherits a dominant or recessive gene.[39] In fact, it has been found that the recessive form causes a milder set of symptoms than the dominant form, which resembles the more complex and severe form of Parkinson disease with Lewy bodies.[39]

The first genetic mutation associated with Parkinson disease was found in the gene encoding α-synuclein, a member of a small family of proteins that are expressed preferentially in the substantia nigra.[36,37] Although mutations in this gene cause a very rare, autosomal dominant form of the disease, the mutation has received considerable attention because α-synuclein is one of the major components of the Lewy bodies that are found in brain tissue of persons with Parkinson disease.[36–40] Mutations in a second gene coding the protein *parkin* is associated with an autosomal recessive, early-onset form of Parkinson disease. The parkin protein acts as an enzyme (*i.e.,* ubiquitin ligase) in the ubiquitin-conjugating system that targets defective and abnormally folded proteins for destruction (see Chapter 5). Loss of normal parkin function is postulated to cause abnormal proteins to aggregate and cause neurodegenerative changes. Thus, the genetics of Parkinson disease are beginning to provide molecular clues that help explain the etiology of parkinsonism, just as epidemiologic studies have delineated multiple environmental risks, which can now be explored in the context of gene expression.

Clinical Manifestations. The cardinal manifestations of Parkinson disease are tremor, rigidity, and bradykinesia or slowness of movement.[35–39] Tremor is the most visible manifestation of the disorder. The tremor affects the distal segments of the limbs, mainly the hands and feet; head, neck, face, lips, and tongue; or jaw. It is characterized by rhythmic, alternating flexion and contraction movements (4 to 6 beats per minute) that resemble the motion of rolling a pill between the thumb and forefinger. The tremor usually is unilateral, occurs when the limb is supported and at rest, and disappears with movement and sleep. The tremor eventually progresses to involve both sides of the body.

Rigidity is defined as resistance to movement of both flexors and extensors throughout the full range of motion. It is most evident during passive joint movement, and involves jerky, cogwheel-type or ratchet-like movements that require considerable energy to perform. Flexion contractions may develop as a result of the rigidity. As with tremor, rigidity usually begins unilaterally but progresses to involve both sides of the body.

Bradykinesia is characterized by slowness in initiating and performing movements and difficulty with sudden, unexpected stopping of voluntary movements. Unconscious associative movements occur in a series of disconnected steps rather than in a smooth, coordinated manner. This is the most disabling of the symptoms of Parkinson disease. Persons with the disease have difficulty initiating walking and difficulty turning. While walking, they may freeze in place and feel as if their feet are glued to the floor, especially when moving through a doorway or preparing to turn. When they walk, they lean forward to maintain their centre of gravity and take small, shuffling steps without swinging their arms, and they have difficulty changing their stride (Fig. 50.13).

Manifestations of advanced-stage parkinsonism include falls, fluctuations in motor function, neuropsychiatric disorders, and sleep disorders. Loss of postural reflexes predisposes the affected person to falling, often backward. Emotional and voluntary facial movements become limited and slow as the disease progresses, and facial expression becomes stiff and mask-like. There is loss of the blinking reflex and a failure to express emotion. The tongue, palate, and throat muscles become rigid; the person may drool because of difficulty in moving the saliva to the back of the mouth and swallowing it. The speech becomes slow and monotonous, without modulation, and poorly articulated.

Because the basal ganglia also influence the autonomic nervous system, persons with Parkinson disease often have excessive and uncontrolled sweating, sebaceous gland secretion, and salivation. Autonomic symptoms, such as lacrimation, dysphagia, orthostatic hypotension, thermal regulation, constipation, impotence, and urinary incontinence, may be present, especially late in the disease.

Cognitive dysfunction may also be an important feature associated with Parkinson disease. It occurs in approximately 20% of persons with the disease. Deficits in visuospatial discrimination, frontal lobe executive function, and memory retrieval (compared with formation of new memories, as seen in

FIGURE 50.13 • The clinical features of Parkinson disease. (From Timby B. K., Smith N. E. (2013). *Introductory medical-surgical nursing* (11th ed.). Philadelphia, PA: Lippincott Williams & Wilkins.)

Alzheimer disease) are more typical of the cognitive dysfunction seen in persons with Parkinson disease than in other forms of dementia. Deficits in executive functioning may be among the earliest signs of cognitive decline, as evidenced by difficulty in planning, starting, and carrying out tasks. Dementia, when it does occur, is usually a late manifestation of the disease, and the rate of decline is slow compared with Alzheimer disease.

Treatment. The approach to treatment of Parkinson disease must be highly individualized and is focused on the management of symptoms. It includes nonpharmacologic, pharmacologic, and, when indicated, surgical methods.[38] Nonpharmacologic interventions offer group support, education, daily exercise, and adequate nutrition. Botulinum toxin injections may be used in the treatment of dystonias such as eyelid spasm and limb dystonias that frequently are associated with Parkinson disease. Persons with parkinsonism other than idiopathic Parkinson disease usually do not respond significantly to medications developed for Parkinson disease.

Pharmacologic treatment usually is determined by the severity of symptoms, with the aim to restore balance of acetylcholine and dopamine. Antiparkinson drugs act by increasing the functional ability of the underactive dopaminergic system, or by reducing the excessive influence of excitatory cholinergic neurons. Drugs that improve the function of the dopaminergic system include those that increase dopamine levels (levodopa), stimulate dopamine receptors (dopamine receptor agonists), or retard the breakdown of dopamine (monoamine oxidase inhibitors). Because dopamine transmission is disrupted in Parkinson disease, there is a preponderance of cholinergic activity, which may be treated with anticholinergic drugs.

Dopamine does not cross the blood–brain barrier. Administration of levodopa, a precursor of dopamine that does cross the blood–brain barrier, has yielded significant improvement in clinical symptoms of Parkinson disease and remains the most effective drug for treatment. The evidence of decreased dopamine levels in the striatum in Parkinson disease led to the administration of large doses of the synthetic compound levodopa, which is absorbed from the intestinal tract, crosses the blood–brain barrier, and is converted to dopamine by centrally acting dopa decarboxylase. Unfortunately, only a small fraction of administered levodopa enters the brain unaltered; the remainder is metabolized outside the brain, predominantly by decarboxylation to dopamine, which cannot cross the blood–brain barrier.[17] However, when levodopa (a decarboxylase inhibitor) is given in combination with carbidopa, the peripheral metabolism of levodopa is reduced, plasma levels of levodopa are increased and its half-life is longer, more levodopa is available for entry into the brain, and a smaller dose is needed. A later adverse effect of levodopa treatment is the so-called *on–off phenomenon,* in which frequent, abrupt, and unpredictable fluctuations in motor performance occur during the day. These fluctuations include "on" periods without dyskinesia, "on" periods with dyskinesia, and periods of bradykinesia (the "off" response). Some fluctuations reflect the timing of drug administration, in which case the "on" response coincides with peak drug levels and the "off" response with low drug levels.

Bromocriptine, pramipexole, and ropinirole are dopamine agonists that act directly to stimulate dopamine receptors.[15,38] Rotigotine is a dopamine agonist that is supplied in a transdermal system. Apomorphine is another dopamine agonist that can be given intravenously. Bromocriptine, pramipexole, and ropinirole can be used as initial or adjunctive therapy in Parkinson disease. They can be given in combination with carbidopa/levodopa.

Amantadine was introduced as an antiviral agent for prophylaxis of A_2 influenza and was unexpectedly found to cause symptomatic improvement in persons with Parkinson disease with dyskinesias. Although the exact mechanism of action remains to be elucidated, it may augment release of dopamine from the remaining intact dopaminergic terminals in the nigrostriatal pathway of persons with Parkinson disease.[41]

Selegiline and rasagiline are monoamine oxidase type B inhibitors that inhibit the metabolic breakdown of dopamine. Selegiline and most recently rasagiline may be used as adjunctive treatment to reduce mild on–off fluctuations in the responsiveness of persons who are receiving levodopa.

Anticholinergic drugs (*e.g.,* trihexyphenidyl, benztropine) are thought to restore a "balance" between reduced dopamine and uninhibited cholinergic neurons in the striatum. They are more useful in alleviating tremor and rigidity than bradykinesia. The anticholinergic drugs lessen the tremors and rigidity and afford some improvement of function. However, their potency seems to decrease over time, and increasing the dosage merely increases side effects such as blurred vision, dry mouth, bowel and bladder problems, cognitive dysfunction, and hallucinations.

Before the advent of deep brain stimulation, surgical treatment for Parkinson disease was limited to thalamotomy and pallidotomy performed using stereotactic surgery. With these procedures, part of the thalamus or globus pallidus in the basal ganglia is destroyed using an electrical stimulator or the supercooled tip of a metal probe (cryothalamotomy). Brain mapping is done during the surgery to identify and prevent injury to sensory and motor tracts. Thalamotomy and pallidotomy are generally confined to one side of the brain because of adverse effects associated with bilateral lesioning procedures. Surgical transplantation of adrenal medullary tissue or fetal substantia nigra tissue was studied in clinical trials, but neither was proven to be helpful.

In the last few years, deep brain stimulation, which involves the implantation of electrodes into the subthalamic nuclei or the pars interna of the globus pallidus, is performed for treatment of Parkinson disease.[42] The electrodes are connected to a surgically implanted impulse generator that delivers electrical simulation to block the abnormal nerve activity that causes tremor and abnormal motor activity in Parkinson disease. The deep brain stimulation system allows the stimulation to be programmed to control the individual patient's symptoms, and the stimulating parameters can be changed over time as the disease progresses. Deep brain stimulation is used for persons with Parkinson disease who respond to levodopa but experience side effects associated with it (*e.g.,* motor fluctuation or dyskinesia). It is not a cure but serves to increase the duration of the "on" periods, allows for a reduction in medication dosages (in subthalamic nuclei stimulation), and improves function. Depending on use, stimulators may last 3 to 5 years. Of note, other movement disorders can be treated by placing electrodes in different target sites (*e.g.,* thalamus for tremor and globus pallidus internus for dystonia).

IN SUMMARY

Alterations in coordination of muscle movements and abnormal muscle movements result from disorders of the cerebellum and basal ganglia. The functions of the cerebellum, which are especially vital during rapid muscular movements, use afferent input from various sources, including the stretch receptors, proprioceptors, tactile receptors in the skin, visual input, and the vestibular system. Cerebellar disorders include vestibulocerebellar dysfunction, cerebellar ataxia, and cerebellar tremor.

The basal ganglia organize basic movement patterns into more complex patterns and release them when commanded by the motor cortex, contributing gracefulness to cortically initiated and controlled skilled movements. Disorders of the basal ganglia are characterized by involuntary movements, alterations in muscle tone, and disturbances in posture. These disorders include tremor, tics, hemiballismus, chorea, athetosis, dystonias, and dyskinesias.

Parkinsonism, a disorder of the basal ganglia, is characterized by destruction of the nigrostriatal pathway, with a subsequent reduction in striatal concentrations of dopamine. This results in an imbalance between the inhibitory effects of dopaminergic basal ganglia functions and an increase in the excitatory cholinergic functions. The disorder is manifested by resting tremor, increased muscle tonus and rigidity, slowness of movement (*i.e.,* bradykinesia), gait disturbances, and impaired autonomic postural responses. The disease usually is slowly progressive over several decades. The tremor often begins in one or both hands and then becomes generalized. Postural changes and gait disturbances continue to become more pronounced, resulting in significant disability.

UPPER MOTOR NEURON DISORDERS

After completing this section of the chapter, you should be able to meet the following objectives:

- Relate the pathologic UMN and LMN changes that occur in amyotrophic lateral sclerosis to the manifestations of the disease.
- Explain the significance of demyelination and plaque formation in multiple sclerosis.
- Describe the manifestations of multiple sclerosis.
- Relate the structures of the vertebral column to mechanisms of spinal cord injury.
- Explain how loss of UMN function contributes to the muscle spasms that occur after recovery from spinal cord injury.
- State the effects of spinal cord injury on ventilation and communication, the autonomic nervous system, cardiovascular function, sensorimotor function, and bowel, bladder, and sexual function.

UMN disorders involve neurons that are fully contained within the CNS. They include the motor neurons arising in the motor areas of the cortex and their fibres as they project through the brain and descend in the spinal cord. Disorders that affect UMNs include multiple sclerosis (MS) and SCI. Stroke, which is a common cause of UMN damage, is

discussed in Chapter 51. Amyotrophic lateral sclerosis is a mixed UMN and LMN disorder.

Amyotrophic Lateral Sclerosis

Amyotrophic lateral sclerosis (ALS), also known as *Lou Gehrig disease* after the famous New York Yankees baseball player, is a devastating neurologic disorder that selectively affects motor function. ALS has an annual incidence of 1 to 2 per 100,000.[43] ALS is primarily a disorder of middle to late adulthood, affecting persons between 55 and 60 years of age, with men developing the disease nearly twice as often as women. The disease typically follows a progressive course, with a mean survival period of 2 to 5 years from the onset of symptoms.

ALS affects motor neurons in three locations: the anterior horn cells of the spinal cord; the motor nuclei of the brain stem, particularly the hypoglossal nuclei; and the UMNs of the cerebral cortex.[36,37,43] The fact that the disease is more extensive in the distal parts of the affected tracts in the lower spinal cord rather than the proximal parts suggests that affected neurons first undergo degeneration at their distal terminals and that the disease proceeds in a centripetal direction until ultimately the parent nerve cell dies. A remarkable feature of the disease is that the entire sensory system, the regulatory mechanisms of control and coordination of movement, and the intellect remain intact. The neurons for ocular motility and the parasympathetic neurons in the sacral spinal cord also are spared.

The death of LMNs leads to denervation, with subsequent shrinkage of musculature and muscle fibre atrophy. It is this fibre atrophy, called *amyotrophy,* which appears in the name of the disease. The loss of nerve fibres in lateral columns of the white matter of the spinal cord, along with fibrillary gliosis, imparts a firmness or sclerosis to this CNS tissue; the term *lateral sclerosis* designates these changes.

The cause of LMN and UMN destruction in ALS is uncertain. Five percent to 10% of cases are familial; the others are believed to be sporadic, with no family history of the disease.[44] The gene for a subset of familial ALS has been mapped to superoxide dismutase 1 (*SOD1*) on chromosome 21. The mutation accounts for 20% of familial ALS, with the remaining 80% being caused by mutations in other genes.[44] Five percent of persons with sporadic ALS also have *SOD1* mutations. Possible targets of *SOD1*-induced toxicity include the neurofilament proteins, which function in the axonal transport of molecules necessary for the maintenance of axons[44] (see Chapter 48, Fig. 48.2). Other genetic loci for ALS have been mapped but not yet cloned. Another suggested mechanism of pathogenesis in ALS is exotoxic injury through activation of glutamate-gated ion channels, which are distinguished by their sensitivity to *N*-methyl-D-aspartic acid (see Chapter 51). The possibility of glutamate excitotoxicity has also been implicated in the pathogenesis of ALS. Although autoimmunity has been suggested as a cause of ALS, the disease does not respond to the immunosuppressant agents that normally are used in treatment of autoimmune disorders.

The symptoms of ALS may be linked to UMN or LMN involvement. Manifestations of UMN lesions include weakness, spasticity or stiffness, and impaired fine motor control.[36] Dysphagia (difficulty swallowing), dysarthria (impaired articulation of speech), and dysphonia (difficulty making the sounds of speech) may result from brain stem LMN involvement or from dysfunction of UMNs descending to the brain stem. Manifestations of LMN destruction include fasciculations, weakness, muscle atrophy, and hyporeflexia. Muscle cramps involving the distal legs often are an early symptom. The most common clinical presentation is slowly progressive weakness and atrophy in distal muscles of one upper extremity. This is followed by regional spread of clinical weakness, reflecting involvement of neighbouring areas of the spinal cord. Eventually, UMNs and LMNs involving multiple limbs and the head are affected. In the more advanced stages, muscles of the palate, pharynx, tongue, neck, and shoulders become involved, causing impairment of chewing, swallowing, and speech. Dysphagia with recurrent aspiration and weakness of the respiratory muscles produces the most significant acute complications of the disease. Death usually results from involvement of cranial nerves and respiratory musculature.

Currently, there is no cure for ALS. The treatment of persons with ALS, which requires management of medical problems, progressive disability, and psychosocial problems, is best provided by a multidisciplinary team.[43–45] Measures to assist persons with the disorder to manage their symptoms (*e.g.,* weakness and muscle spasms, dysphagia, communication difficulty, excessive watery saliva, and emotional lability), nutritional needs, and respiratory muscle weakness allow people with the disorder to survive longer than would otherwise have been the case. An antiglutamate drug, riluzole, is the only drug approved by the FDA and Health Canada for treatment of ALS.[43] The drug is designed to decrease the release of glutamate and reduce damage to motor neurons, thereby slowing the progression of the disease.

Demyelinating Disorders of the Central Nervous System

Multiple Sclerosis

As with other demyelinating disorders, multiple sclerosis (MS) is characterized by inflammation and selective destruction of CNS myelin.[36,37,46] The peripheral nervous system is spared and there is usually no evidence of an associated systemic disease. Prevalent rates range from 1 to 2 per 1,000 people across Canada. Canada is known as a high-risk area, similar to other countries that are further away from the equator.[47] The age of onset is typically between 15 and 40 years in Western societies, MS is second only to trauma as a cause of neurologic disability in early and young adulthood. As such, MS results in significant functional and often work-related disability in persons who are in the prime of their productivity.

Epidemiology and Genetics. MS occurs more commonly in individuals of European ancestry and is uncommon in certain ethnic groups such as Inuit, Native Americans, and Africans. The highest known prevalence of MS occurs in the Orkney Islands, located north of Scotland, and similarly high rates are found throughout northern Europe, the northern United States, and Canada.[48] The prevalence is low in Japan, in other parts of Asia, in equatorial Africa, and in the Middle East. It has been observed that the disease is more common in northern latitudes, perhaps related to the vitamin D deficiency during winter months.[47–49]

The risk for developing MS is 15-fold higher when the disease is present in a first-degree relative, and is even greater in monozygotic twins.[37] People with the human leukocyte antigen HLA-DR2 haplotype (see Chapter 17) are particularly susceptible. The molecular basis for the influence of this particular haplotype is unknown.

Pathogenesis. MS is believed to be an immune-mediated disorder that occurs in genetically susceptible people. Although the target antigen has not been identified, the data suggest an immune response to a protein in the CNS.

The lesions of MS consist of hard, sharp-edged, demyelinated or sclerotic patches that are macroscopically visible throughout the white matter of the CNS.[36,37,46] These lesions, which represent the end result of acute myelin breakdown, are called *plaques.* The lesions have a predilection for the optic nerves, periventricular white matter, brain stem, cerebellum, and spinal cord white matter. In an active plaque, there is evidence of ongoing myelin breakdown. The sequence of myelin breakdown is not well understood, although it is known that the lesions contain small amounts of myelin basic proteins and increased amounts of proteolytic enzymes, macrophages, lymphocytes, and plasma cells. Oligodendrocytes are decreased in number and may be absent, especially in older lesions. Acute, subacute, and chronic lesions often are seen at multiple sites throughout the CNS.

MRI has shown that the lesions of MS may occur in two stages: a first stage that involves the sequential development of small inflammatory lesions, and a second stage during which the lesions extend and consolidate and in which demyelination and gliosis (scar formation) occur. It is not known whether the inflammatory process, present during the first stage, is directed against myelin or against the oligodendrocytes that produce myelin. Remyelination of the nervous system was considered to be impossible until the late 1990s. Evidence now suggests that remyelination can occur in the CNS if the process that initiated the demyelination is halted before the oligodendrocyte dies.[50]

Manifestations and Clinical Course. The pathophysiology of MS involves the demyelination of nerve fibres in the white matter of the brain, spinal cord, and optic nerve. In the CNS, myelin is formed by the oligodendrocytes, chiefly those lying among the nerve fibres in the white matter. This function of the oligodendrocytes is equivalent to that of the Schwann cells in the peripheral nervous system (see Chapter 48). The properties of the myelin sheath—high electrical resistance and low capacitance—permit it to function as an electrical insulator. Demyelinated nerve fibres display a variety of conduction abnormalities, ranging from decreased conduction velocity to conduction blocks. The interruption of neural conduction in the demyelinated nerves is manifested by a variety of symptoms, depending on the location and extent of the lesion. Areas commonly affected by MS are the optic nerve (visual field), corticobulbar tracts (speech and swallowing), corticospinal tracts (muscle strength), cerebellar tracts (gait and coordination), spinocerebellar tracts (balance), medial longitudinal fasciculus (conjugate gaze function of the extraocular eye muscles), and posterior cell columns of the spinal cord (position and vibratory sensation). Typically, an otherwise healthy person presents with an acute or subacute episode of paresthesias, optic neuritis (*i.e.,* visual clouding or loss of vision in part of the visual field with pain on movement of the globe), diplopia, or specific types of gaze paralysis.

Paresthesias are evidenced as numbness, tingling, burning sensations, or pressure on the face or involved extremities, with symptoms ranging from annoying to severe.[51] The *Lhermitte sign* is an electric shock-like tingling down the back and onto the legs that is produced by flexion of the neck occurs at some point in the disease for up to one third of people with MS. Pain from spasticity also may be a factor that can be alleviated by appropriate stretching exercises. Other common symptoms are abnormal gait, bladder and sexual dysfunction, vertigo, nystagmus, fatigue, and speech disturbance. These symptoms usually last for several days to weeks, and then completely or partially resolve. After a period of normal or relatively normal function, new symptoms appear. Psychological manifestations, such as mood swings, may represent an emotional reaction to the nature of the disease or, more likely, involvement of the white matter of the cerebral cortex. Depression, euphoria, inattentiveness, apathy, forgetfulness, and loss of memory may occur.[51]

Fatigue is one of the most common problems for persons with MS. Fatigue often is described as a generalized low-energy feeling not related to depression and different from weakness. Fatigue has a harmful impact on activities of daily living and sustained physical activity. Interventions such as spacing activities with rest periods and setting priorities are often helpful.

The course of the disease may fall into one of four categories: relapsing-remitting, secondary progressive, primary progressive, or progressive relapsing.[51] The *relapsing-remitting* form of the disease is the most common and is characterized by episodes of acute worsening with recovery and a stable course between relapses. *Secondary progressive disease* involves a gradual neurologic deterioration with or without superimposed acute relapses in a person with previous relapsing-remitting disease. *Primary progressive disease* is characterized by slow, but continuous neurologic deterioration from onset of symptoms. The *progressive relapsing* category of disease is relatively rare and involves steady neurologic deterioration from the onset of symptoms but with subsequent superimposed relapses.[51]

Diagnosis. The diagnosis of MS is based on established clinical and, when necessary, laboratory criteria. Advances in cerebrospinal fluid analysis and MRI have greatly simplified the procedure. A definite diagnosis of MS requires evidence of one of the following patterns: two or more episodes of exacerbation separated by 1 month or more and lasting more than 24 hours, with subsequent recovery; a clinical history of clearly defined exacerbations and remissions, with or without complete recovery, followed by progression of symptoms over a period of at least 6 months; or slow and stepwise progression of signs and symptoms over a period of at least 6 months.[51] Primary progressive MS may be suggested by a progressive course that lasts longer than 6 months. A person who has not had a relapse or progression of symptoms is described as having stable MS.

MRI can be used as an adjunct to clinical diagnosis. MRI studies can detect lesions even when CT scans appear normal. A computer-assisted method of MRI can measure lesion size. Many new areas of myelin abnormality are asymptomatic. Serial MRI studies can be done to detect asymptomatic lesions, monitor the progress of existing lesions, and evaluate the effectiveness of treatment. Although MRI can be used to provide evidence of disseminated lesions in persons with the disease, normal findings do not exclude the diagnosis. Electrophysiologic evaluations (*e.g.,* evoked potential studies) and CT scans may assist in the identification and documentation of lesions.

Although no laboratory test can be used to diagnose MS, examination of the cerebrospinal fluid is helpful. A large percentage of patients with MS have elevated immunoglobulin G (IgG) levels, and some have oligoclonal patterns (*i.e.,* discrete electrophoretic bands) even with normal IgG levels. Total protein or lymphocyte levels may be mildly elevated in the cerebrospinal fluid. These test results can be altered in a variety of inflammatory neurologic disorders and are not specific for MS.

Treatment. Most treatment measures for MS are directed at modifying the course and managing the primary symptoms of the disease. The variability in symptoms, unpredictable course, and lack of specific diagnostic methods has made the evaluation and treatment of MS difficult. Persons who are minimally affected by the disorder require no specific treatment. The person should be encouraged to maintain as healthy a lifestyle as possible, including good nutrition and adequate rest and relaxation. Physical therapy may help maintain muscle tone. Every effort should be made to avoid excessive fatigue, physical deterioration, emotional stress, viral infections, and extremes of environmental temperature, including whirlpool and hot showers, which may precipitate an exacerbation of the disease.

The pharmacologic agents used in the treatment of MS fall into three categories: those used to (1) treat acute attacks or initial demyelinating episodes, (2) modify the course of the disease, and (3) treat symptoms of the disorder.[51] Corticosteroids are the mainstay of treatment for acute attacks of MS. These agents are thought to reduce inflammation, improve nerve conduction, and have important immunologic effects. Long-term administration does not, however, appear to alter the course of the disease and can have harmful side effects. Adrenocorticotropic hormone (ACTH) also may be used in treatment of MS. Plasmapheresis has also proved beneficial in some cases.

The agents used to modify the course of the disease include interferon-beta, glatiramer acetate, and mitoxantrone.[51] These agents have shown some benefit in reducing exacerbations in persons with relapsing-remitting MS. Interferon-beta is a cytokine that acts as an immune enhancer. Two forms of recombinant interferon have been approved for treatment of MS—interferon-beta-1a (Avonex, Rebif) and interferon-beta-1b (Betaseron, Extavia). Both types of interferon are administered by injection, and both are usually well tolerated. The most common side effects are flu-like symptoms for 24 to 48 hours after each injection, and these usually subside after 2 to 3 months of treatment. Glatiramer acetate (copaxone) is a synthetic polypeptide that simulates parts of the myelin basic protein. Although the exact mechanism of action is unknown, the drug seems to block myelin-damaging T cells by acting as a myelin decoy. The drug is given daily by subcutaneous injection.

Mitoxantrone is an antineoplastic agent developed in the 1970s. It prevents the ligation of DNA strands and thus delays the cell-cycle progression. It also has immunomodulatory properties, inhibiting proliferation of macrophages and B and T lymphocytes.[51,52] Acute side effects of the drug include nausea and alopecia. In Canada, other immunomodulating agents such as azathioprine, fingolimod, teriflunomide, methotrexate, and sirolimus have been suggested to delay progression of relapsing-remitting and secondary progressive MS.[51,52] Natalizumab and alemtuzmab, now approved for relapsing-remitting MS, are monoclonal antibodies. Natalizumab works against leukocyte α4 integrins, and its primary mechanism of action is suppression of leukocyte entry into the CNS, whereas alemtuzumab targets an antigen (CD52) that is present at high levels mature lymphocytes.[51]

Among the medications used to manage the chronic problems associated with MS are dantrolene, baclofen, zanaflex, or diazepam for spasticity; cholinergic drugs for bladder problems; and antidepressant drugs for depression.

Vertebral and Spinal Cord Injury

Spinal cord injury (SCI) represents damage to the neural elements of the spinal cord. SCI is primarily a disorder of young people, with most injuries occurring in the 16- to 30-year age group.[53] The most common cause of SCI is motor vehicle collisions, followed by falls, violence (*e.g.,* gunshot wounds), and recreational sporting activities.[53] Life expectancy for persons with SCI continues to increase, but is somewhat below life expectancy for those without SCI. Mortality rates are significantly higher during the first year after injury than during subsequent years, particularly for severely injured persons.[53]

Most SCIs involve damage to the vertebral column or supporting ligaments as well as the spinal cord. Because of extensive tract systems that connect sensory afferent neurons and LMNs with high brain centres, SCIs commonly involve both sensory and motor function. Although the discussion in this section of the chapter focuses on traumatic SCI, much of the content is applicable to SCI caused by other disorders, such as congenital deformities (*e.g.,* spina bifida), tumours, ischemia and infarction, and bone disease with pathologic fractures of the vertebrae.

Injury to the Vertebral Column

Injuries to the vertebral column include fractures, dislocations, and subluxations. A fracture can occur at any part of the bony vertebrae, causing fragmentation of the bone. It most often involves the pedicle, lamina, or processes (*e.g.,* facets). Dislocation or subluxation (partial dislocation) injury causes the vertebral bodies to become displaced, with one overriding another and preventing correct alignment of the vertebral column. Damage to the ligaments or bony vertebrae may make the spine unstable. In an unstable spine, further unguarded movement of the spinal column can impinge on the spinal canal, causing compression or overstretching of neural tissue.

Most injuries result from some combination of compressive force or bending movements.[7] Flexion injuries occur when forward bending of the spinal column exceeds the limits of normal movement. Typical flexion injuries result, for example, when the head is struck from behind, as in a fall with the back of the head as the point of impact. Extension injuries occur with excessive forced bending (*i.e.,* hyperextension) of the spine backward. A typical extension injury involves a fall in which the chin or face is the point of impact, causing hyperextension of the neck. Injuries of flexion and extension occur more commonly in the cervical spine (C4 to C6) than in any other area. Limitations imposed by the ribs, spinous processes, and joint capsules in the thoracic and lumbar spine make this area less flexible and less susceptible to flexion and extension injuries than the cervical spine.

A compression injury, causing the vertebral bones to shatter, squash, or even burst, occurs when there is spinal loading from a high-velocity blow to the top of the head or when landing forcefully on the feet or buttocks[7] (Fig. 50.14A). This typically occurs at the cervical level (*e.g.,* diving injuries) or in the thoracolumbar area (*e.g.,* falling from a distance and landing on the buttocks). Compression injuries may occur when the vertebrae are weakened by conditions such as osteoporosis and cancer with bone metastasis. Axial rotation injuries can produce highly unstable injuries. Maximal axial rotation occurs in the cervical region, especially between C1 and C2, and at the lumbosacral joint[7] (Fig. 50.14B). Coupling of vertebral motions is common in injury when two or more individual motions occur (*e.g.,* lateral bending and axial rotation).

Acute Spinal Cord Injury

SCI involves damage to the neural elements of the spinal cord. The damage may result from direct trauma to the cord from penetrating wounds or indirect injury resulting from vertebral fractures, fracture dislocations, or subluxations of the spine. The spinal cord may be contused, not only at the site of injury

FIGURE 50.14 • **A:** Compression vertebral fracture secondary to axial loading as occurs when a person falls from a height and lands on the buttocks. **B:** Rotational injury, in which there is concurrent fracture and tearing of the posterior ligamentous complex, is caused by extreme lateral flexion or twisting of the head or neck. (Modified from Hickey J.V. (2003). *The clinical practice of neurological and neurosurgical nursing* (5th ed., pp. 411–412). Philadelphia, PA: Lippincott Williams & Wilkins.)

but above and below the trauma site.[7] Traumatic injury may be complicated by the loss of blood flow to the cord or significant edema around the injury site, with resulting infarction.

Sudden, complete transection of the spinal cord results in complete loss of motor, sensory, reflex, and autonomic function below the level of injury. The immediate response to SCI is often referred to as *spinal cord shock*. It is characterized by flaccid paralysis with loss of tendon reflexes below the level of injury, absence of somatic and visceral sensations below the level of injury, and loss of bowel and bladder function. Loss of systemic sympathetic vasomotor tone may result in vasodilation, increased venous capacity, and hypotension. These manifestations occur regardless of whether the level of the lesion eventually will produce spastic (UMN) or flaccid (LMN) paralysis. The basic mechanisms accounting for transient spinal shock are unknown. Spinal shock may last for hours, days, or weeks. Usually, if reflex function returns by the time the person reaches the hospital, the neuromuscular changes are reversible. This type of reversible spinal shock may occur in football-type injuries, in which jarring of the spinal cord produces a concussion-like syndrome with loss of movement and reflexes, followed by full recovery within days. In persons in whom the loss of reflexes persists, hypotension and bradycardia may become critical but manageable problems. In general, the higher the level of injury, the greater is the effect.

Pathophysiology. The pathophysiology of acute SCI can be divided into two types: primary and secondary.[7,54] The *primary neurologic injury* occurs at the time of mechanical injury and is irreversible. It is characterized by small hemorrhages in the grey matter of the cord, followed by edematous changes in the white matter that lead to necrosis of neural tissue. This type of injury results from the forces of compression, stretch,

and shear associated with fracture or compression of the spinal vertebrae, dislocation of vertebrae (*e.g.*, flexion, extension, subluxation), and contusions due to jarring of the cord in the spinal canal. Penetrating injuries produce lacerations and direct trauma to the cord and may occur with or without spinal column damage. Lacerations occur when there is cutting or tearing of the spinal cord, which injures nerve tissue and causes bleeding and edema.

Secondary injuries follow the primary injury and promote the spread of injury. Although there is considerable debate about the pathogenesis of secondary injuries, the tissue destruction that occurs ends in progressive neurologic damage. After SCI, several pathologic mechanisms come into play, including vascular damage, neuronal injury that leads to loss of reflexes below the level of injury, and release of vasoactive agents and cellular enzymes. Vascular lesions (*i.e.*, vessel trauma and hemorrhage) can lead to ischemia, increased vascular permeability, and edema. Blood flow to the spinal cord may be further compromised by spinal shock that results from a loss of vasomotor tone and neural reflexes below the level of injury. The release of vasoactive substances (*i.e.*, norepinephrine, serotonin, dopamine, and histamine) from the wound tissue causes vasospasm and impedes blood flow in the microcirculation, producing further necrosis of blood vessels and neurons. The release of proteolytic and lipolytic enzymes from injured cells causes delayed swelling, demyelination, and necrosis in the neural tissue in the spinal cord.

Management. The goal of management of acute SCI is to reduce the neurologic deficit and prevent any additional loss of neurologic function. SCI may require emergency resuscitation at the trauma site or in the emergency department, depending on the urgency of the situation.[7] Most traumatic injuries to the spinal column render it unstable, mandating measures such as immobilization with hard collars and backboards and limiting the movement of persons at risk for or with known SCI. Every person with multiple trauma or head injury, including victims of traffic or sport injuries, should be suspected of having sustained an acute SCI until this is ruled out with imaging.[7]

The nature of the injury determines further methods of stabilization and treatment.[55] In unstable injuries of the cervical spine, cervical traction improves or restores spinal alignment, decompresses neural structures, and facilitates recovery. Fractures and dislocations of the thoracic and lumbar vertebrae may be initially stabilized by restricting the person to bed rest and turning him or her in a log-rolling manner to keep the spine rigid. Gunshot or stab wounds of the spinal column may not produce structural instability and may not require immobilization.

The goal of early surgical intervention for an unstable spine is to provide internal skeletal stabilization so that early mobilization and rehabilitation can occur. One of the more important aspects of early SCI care is the prevention and treatment of spinal or systemic shock and the hypoxia associated with compromised respiration. Correcting hypotension or hypoxia is essential to maintaining circulation to the injured cord.

A short-acting corticosteroid such as methylprednisolone has been used extensively in the treatment of inflammatory and allergic disorders. In acute SCI, it is thought to stabilize cell membranes, enhance impulse generation, improve blood flow, and inhibit free radical formation. However, evidence supporting the use of methylprednisolone treatment as a standard of care remains insufficient, and so it is considered a treatment option.[56] Treatment with high-dose methylprednisolone is associated with complications such as increased frequency of gastric bleeding, wound infection, venous thrombosis, and steroid myopathy.[15] Other neuroprotective agents, including monosialoganglioside sodium (GM-1 ganglioside), naloxone, and tirilazad, have been tested in multicentre clinical trials, but primary end points have not been achieved.[55,57]

Types and Classification of Spinal Cord Injury

Alterations in body function that result from SCI depend on the level of injury and the amount of cord involvement. *Tetraplegia,* sometimes referred to as *quadriplegia,* is the impairment or loss of motor or sensory function (or both) after damage to neural structures in the cervical segments of the spinal cord.[7,58] It results in impairment of function in the arms, trunk, legs, and pelvic organs (Fig. 50.5). *Paraplegia* refers to impairment or loss of motor or sensory function (or both) in the thoracic, lumbar, or sacral (but not cervical) segments of the spinal cord from damage of neural elements in the spinal canal. With paraplegia, arm functioning is spared, but depending on the level of injury, functioning of the trunk, legs, and pelvic organs may be impaired.[58] Paraplegia includes conus medullaris and cauda equina injuries (discussed later).

The American Spinal Injury Association (ASIA) impairment scale is used in Canada to describe the extent of neurologic damage as *complete* or *incomplete*[58] (Chart 50.1).

CHART 50.1 **THE STANDARD AMERICAN SPINAL INJURY ASSOCIATION (ASIA) IMPAIRMENT SCALE**

A = Complete: No motor or sensory function is preserved in sacral segments S4–S5.

B = Incomplete: Sensory but not motor function is preserved below the neurologic level and includes sacral segments S4–S5.

C = Incomplete: Motor function is preserved below the neurologic level, and more than half of the key muscles below the neurologic level have a muscle grade less than 3.

D = Incomplete: Motor function is preserved below the neurologic level, and at least half of the key muscles below the level of injury have a muscle grade of 3 or more.

E = Normal: Motor and sensory functions are normal.

Muscle grading: (0) total paralysis; (2) active movement, full range of motion, gravity eliminated; (3) active movement, full range of motion, against gravity; (4) active movement, full range of motion, against gravity and provides some resistance; (5) active movement, full range of motion, against gravity and provides normal resistance.
Developed from the American Spinal Injury Association. (2011). *International standards for neurological classification of SCI, revised 2011.* Chicago: American Spinal Cord Injury Association.

Complete cord injuries can result from severance of the cord, disruption of nerve fibres although they remain intact, or interruption of blood supply to that segment, resulting in complete destruction of neural tissue and UMN or LMN paralysis. With complete injuries, no motor or sensory function is preserved in sacral segments S4 to S6. Incomplete SCI implies there is some residual motor or sensory function below the level of injury. The prognosis for return of function is better in an incomplete injury because of preservation of axonal function. Incomplete injuries may manifest in a variety of patterns, but can be organized into certain patterns or "syndromes" that occur more frequently and reflect the predominant area of the cord that is involved. Types of incomplete lesions include the central cord syndrome, anterior cord syndrome, Brown-Séquard syndrome, and conus medullaris syndrome.

Central Cord Syndrome. A condition called *central cord syndrome* occurs when injury is predominantly in the central grey or white matter of the cord[27] (Fig. 50.15). Because the corticospinal tract fibres are organized with those controlling the arms located more centrally and those controlling the legs located more laterally, some external axonal transmission may remain intact. Motor function of the upper extremities is affected, but the lower extremities may not be affected or may be affected to a lesser degree, with some sparing of sacral sensation. Bowel, bladder, and sexual functions usually are affected to various degrees, and this may parallel the degree of lower extremity involvement. This syndrome occurs almost

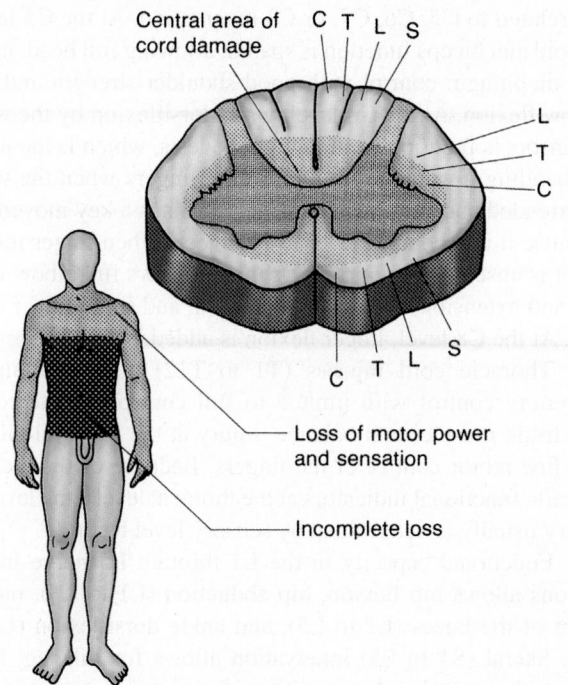

FIGURE 50.15 • Central cord syndrome. A cross-section of the cord shows central damage and the associated motor and sensory loss. C, cervical; T, thoracic; L, lumbar; S, sacral. (From Hickey J. V. (2014). *The clinical practice of neurological and neurosurgical nursing* (7th ed., p. 400). Philadelphia, PA: Lippincott Williams & Wilkins.)

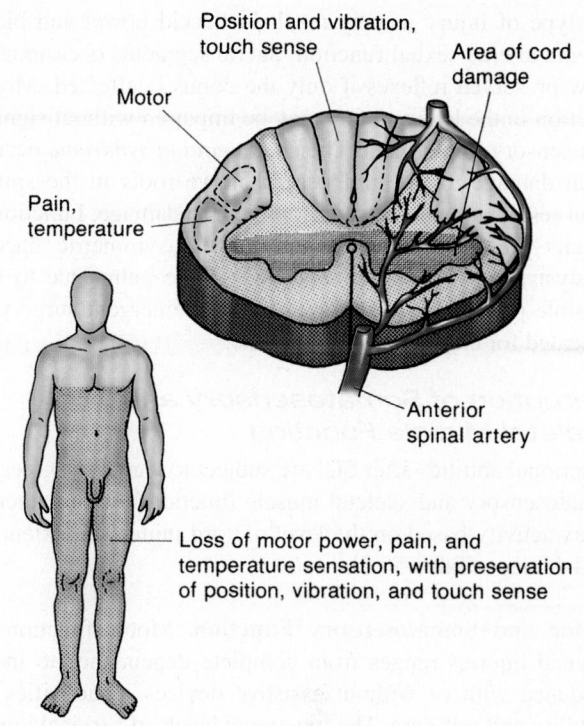

FIGURE 50.16 • Anterior cord syndrome. Cord damage and associated motor and sensory loss are illustrated. (From Hickey J. V. (2014). *The clinical practice of neurological and neurosurgical nursing* (7th ed., p. 400). Philadelphia, PA: Lippincott Williams & Wilkins.)

exclusively in the cervical cord, rendering the lesion a UMN lesion with spastic paralysis. Central cord damage is more frequent in elderly persons with narrowing or stenotic changes in the spinal canal that are related to arthritis. Damage also may occur in persons with congenital stenosis.

Anterior Cord Syndrome. Anterior cord syndrome usually is caused by damage from infarction of the anterior spinal artery, resulting in damage to the anterior two thirds of the cord[7] (Fig. 50.16). The deficits include loss of motor function provided by the corticospinal tracts and loss of pain and temperature sensation from damage to the lateral spinothalamic tracts. The posterior one third of the cord is relatively unaffected, preserving the dorsal column axons that convey position, vibration, and touch sensation.

Brown-Séquard Syndrome. A condition called *Brown-Séquard syndrome* results from damage to a hemisection of the anterior and posterior cord.[7] (Fig. 50.17). The effect is a loss of voluntary motor function from the corticospinal tract, proprioception loss from the ipsilateral side of the body, and contralateral loss of pain and temperature sensation from the lateral spinothalamic tracts for all levels below the lesion.

Conus Medullaris and Cauda Equina Syndromes. The conus medullaris syndrome involves damage to the conus medullaris or the sacral cord (*i.e.,* conus) and lumbar nerve roots in the neural canal. Functional deficits resulting from

FIGURE 50.17 • Brown-Séquard syndrome. Cord damage and associated motor and sensory loss are illustrated. (From Hickey J. V. (2014). *The clinical practice of neurological and neurosurgical nursing* (7th ed., p. 400). Philadelphia, PA: Lippincott Williams & Wilkins.)

this type of injury usually result in flaccid bowel and bladder and altered sexual function. Sacral segments occasionally show preserved reflexes if only the conus is affected. Motor function in the legs and feet may be impaired without significant sensory impairment. The *cauda equina syndrome* occurs when damage to the lumbosacral nerve roots in the spinal canal results in LMN and sensory neuron damage. Functional deficits present as various patterns of asymmetric flaccid paralysis, sensory impairment, and severe pain. Due to the possible permanent neurologic damage, emergent surgery is indicated for cauda equina syndrome.[7]

Disruption of Somatosensory and Skeletal Muscle Function

Functional abilities after SCI are subject to various degrees of somatosensory and skeletal muscle function loss and altered reflex activity based on the level of cord injury and extent of cord damage (Table 50.2).

Motor and Somatosensory Function. Motor function in cervical injuries ranges from complete dependence to independence with or without assistive devices in activities of mobility and self-care. The functional levels of cervical injury

are related to C5, C6, C7, or C8 innervation. At the C5 level, deltoid and biceps function is spared, allowing full head, neck, and diaphragm control with good shoulder strength and full elbow flexion. At the C6 level, wrist dorsiflexion by the wrist extensors is functional, allowing tenodesis, which is the natural bending inward and flexion of the fingers when the wrist is extended and bent backward. Tenodesis is a key movement because it can be used to pick up objects when finger movement is absent. A functional C7 injury allows full elbow flexion and extension, wrist plantar flexion, and some finger control. At the C8 level, finger flexion is added.

Thoracic cord injuries (T1 to T12) allow full upper extremity control with limited to full control of intercostal and trunk muscles and balance. Injury at the T1 level allows full fine motor control of the fingers. Because of the lack of specific functional indicators at the thoracic levels, the level of injury usually is determined by sensory level testing.

Functional capacity in the L1 through L5 nerve innervations allows hip flexion, hip abduction (L1 to L3), movement of the knees (L2 to L5), and ankle dorsiflexion (L4 to L5). Sacral (S1 to S5) innervation allows for full leg, foot, and ankle control and innervation of perineal musculature for bowel, bladder, and sexual function.

TABLE 50.2 FUNCTIONAL ABILITIES BY LEVEL OF CORD INJURY

INJURY LEVEL	SEGMENTAL SENSORIMOTOR FUNCTION	DRESSING, EATING	ELIMINATION	MOBILITY[a]
C1	Little or no sensation or control of head and neck; no diaphragm control; requires continuous ventilation	Dependent	Dependent	Limited. Voice-controlled or sip-n-puff electric wheelchair
C2–C3	Head and neck sensation; some neck control. Independent of mechanical ventilation for short periods	Dependent	Dependent	Same as for C1
C4	Good head and neck sensation and motor control; some shoulder elevation; diaphragm movement	Dependent; may be able to eat with adaptive sling	Dependent	Limited to voice-, mouth-, head-, chin-, or shoulder-controlled electric wheelchair
C5	Full head and neck control; shoulder strength; elbow flexion	Independent with assistance	Maximal assistance	Electric or modified manual wheelchair, needs transfer assistance
C6	Fully innervated shoulder; wrist extension or dorsiflexion	Independent or with minimal assistance	Independent or with minimal assistance	Independent in transfers and wheelchair
C7–C8	Full elbow extension; wrist plantar flexion; some finger control	Independent	Independent	Independent; manual wheelchair
T1–T5	Full hand and finger control; use of intercostal and thoracic muscles	Independent	Independent	Independent; manual wheelchair
T6–T10	Abdominal muscle control, partial to good balance with trunk muscles	Independent	Independent	Independent; manual wheelchair
T11–L5	Hip flexors, hip abductors (L1–3); knee extension (L2–4); knee flexion and ankle dorsiflexion (L4–5)	Independent	Independent	Short distance to full ambulation with assistance
S1–S5	Full leg, foot, and ankle control; innervation of perineal muscles for bowel, bladder, and sexual function (S2–4)	Independent	Normal to impaired bowel and bladder function	Ambulate independently with or without assistance

[a]Assistance refers to adaptive equipment, setup, or physical assistance.

Reflex Activity. Spinal cord reflexes are fully integrated in the spinal cord and can function independent of input from higher centres. Altered spinal reflex activity after SCI is essentially determined by the level of injury and whether UMNs or LMNs are affected. With UMN injuries at T12 and above, the cord reflexes remain intact, whereas communication pathways with higher centres are interrupted. This results in spasticity of involved skeletal muscle groups and of smooth and skeletal muscles that control bowel, bladder, and sexual function. In LMN injuries at T12 or below, the reflex circuitry itself has been damaged at the level of the spinal cord or spinal nerve, resulting in a decrease or absence of reflex function. The LMN injuries cause flaccid paralysis of involved skeletal muscle groups and the smooth and skeletal muscles that control bowel, bladder, and sexual function. However, injuries near the T12 level may result in mixed UMN and LMN deficits (*e.g.,* spastic paralysis of the bowel and bladder with flaccid muscle tone).

After the period of spinal shock in a UMN injury, isolated spinal reflex activity and muscle tone that is not under the control of higher centres return. This may result in hypertonia and spasticity of skeletal muscles below the level of injury.[7] These spastic movements are involuntary instead of voluntary, a distinction that needs to be explained to persons with SCI and their families. The antigravity muscles, the flexors of the arms and extensors of the legs, are predominantly affected.

The stimuli for reflex muscle spasm arise from somatic and visceral afferent pathways that enter the cord below the level of injury. The most common of these stimuli are muscle stretching, bladder infections or stones, fistulas, bowel distension or impaction, pressure areas or irritation of the skin, and infections. Because the stimuli that precipitate spasms vary from person to person, careful assessment is necessary to identify the factors that precipitate spasm in each individual. Passive range-of-motion exercises to stretch the spastic muscles help to prevent spasm induced by muscle stretching, such as occurs with a change in body position.

Spasticity in itself is not detrimental and may even facilitate maintenance of muscle tone to prevent muscle wasting, improve venous return, and aid in mobility. Spasms become detrimental when they impair safety; they also reduce the ability to make functional gains in mobility and activities of daily living. Spasms also may cause trauma to bones and tissues, leading to joint contractures and skin breakdown.

Respiratory Muscle Function. Ventilation requires movement of the expiratory and inspiratory muscles, all of which receive innervation from the spinal cord.[7] The main muscle of ventilation, the diaphragm, is innervated by segments C3 to C5 through the phrenic nerves. The intercostal muscles, which function in elevating the rib cage and are needed for coughing and deep breathing, are innervated by spinal segments T1 through T7. The major muscles of expiration are the abdominal muscles, which receive their innervation from levels T6 to T12.

Although the ability to inhale and exhale may be preserved at various levels of SCI, functional deficits in ventilation are most apparent in the quality of the breathing cycle and the ability to oxygenate tissues, eliminate carbon dioxide, and mobilize secretions. Cord injuries involving C1 to C3 result in a lack of respiratory effort, and affected patients require mechanical ventilation. Although a C3 to C5 injury allows partial or full diaphragmatic function, ventilation is diminished because of the loss of intercostal muscle function, resulting in shallow breaths and a weak cough. Below the C5 level, as less intercostal and abdominal musculature is affected, the ability to take a deep breath and cough is less impaired. Maintenance therapy consists of muscle training to strengthen existing muscles for endurance and mobilization of secretions. The ability to speak is compromised with assisted ventilation, whether continuous or intermittent. Thus, ensuring adequate communication of needs is also essential.

Disruption of Autonomic Nervous System Function

In addition to its effects on skeletal muscle function, SCI interrupts autonomic nervous system function below the site of injury.[59] This includes sympathetic outflow from the thoracic and lumbar cord and parasympathetic outflow from the sacral cord. Because of their sites of exit from the CNS, the cranial nerves, such as the vagus, are unaffected. Depending on the level of injury, the spinal reflexes that control autonomic nervous system function are largely isolated from the rest of the CNS. Afferent sensory input that enters the spinal cord is unaffected, as is the efferent motor output from the cord. This results in a situation in which the autonomic reflexes below the level of injury are uncontrolled, whereas those above the level of injury function in a relatively controlled manner.

Sympathetic nervous system regulation of circulatory function and body temperature (*i.e.,* thermoregulation) presents some of the most severe problems in SCI. The higher the level of injury and the greater the surface area affected, the more profound are the effects on circulation and thermoregulation. Persons with injury at the T6 level or above experience problems in regulating vasomotor tone; those with injuries below the T6 level usually have sufficient sympathetic function to maintain adequate vasomotor function. The level of injury and its corresponding problems may vary among persons, and some dysfunctional effects may be seen at levels below T6. With lower lumbar and sacral injuries, sympathetic function remains essentially unaltered.

Vasovagal Response. The vagus nerve (cranial nerve X), which is unaffected in SCI, normally exerts a continuous inhibitory effect on heart rate. Vagal stimulation that causes a marked bradycardia is called the *vasovagal response.* Visceral afferent input to the vagal centres in the brain stem of persons with tetraplegia or high-level paraplegia can produce marked bradycardia when unchecked by a dysfunctional sympathetic nervous system. Severe bradycardia and even asystole can result when the vasovagal response is elicited by deep endotracheal suctioning or rapid position change. Preventive measures, such as hyperoxygenation before, during, and after suctioning, are advised. Rapid position changes should be avoided or anticipated, and anticholinergic drugs should be immediately available to counteract severe episodes of bradycardia.

Autonomic Dysreflexia. Autonomic dysreflexia, also known as *autonomic hyperreflexia,* represents an acute episode of exaggerated sympathetic reflex responses that occur in persons with injuries at T6 and above, in which CNS control of spinal reflexes is lost[60] (Fig. 50.18). It does not occur until spinal shock has resolved and autonomic reflexes return, most often within the first 6 months after injury. It is most unpredictable during the first year after injury, but can occur throughout the person's lifetime.

Autonomic dysreflexia is characterized by vasospasm, hypertension ranging from mild (20 mm Hg above baseline) to severe (systolic can reach 300 mm Hg), skin pallor, and "goosebumps" associated with the piloerector response.[61]

Because baroreceptor function and parasympathetic control of heart rate travel by way of the cranial nerves, these responses remain intact. Continued hypertension produces a baroreflex-mediated vagal slowing of the heart rate to bradycardic levels. There is an accompanying baroreflex-mediated vasodilation, with flushed skin and profuse sweating above the level of injury, headache ranging from dull to severe and pounding, nasal stuffiness, and feelings of anxiety. A person may experience one, several, or all of the symptoms with each episode.

The stimuli initiating the dysreflexic response include visceral distension, such as a full bladder or rectum; stimulation of pain receptors, as occurs with pressure ulcers, ingrown toenails, dressing changes, and diagnostic or operative procedures; and visceral contractions, such as ejaculation, bladder spasms, or uterine contractions. In many cases, the dysreflexic response results from a full bladder.

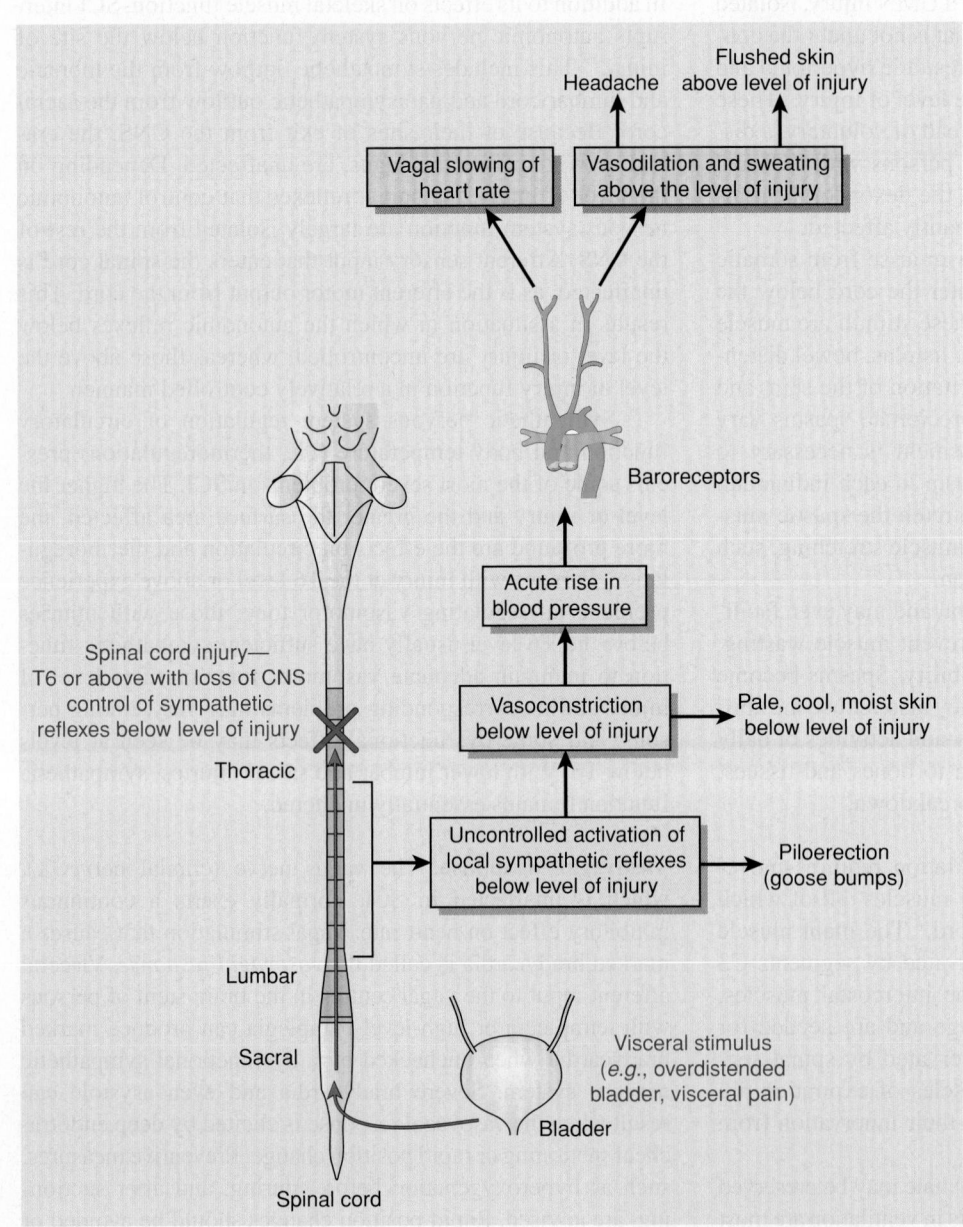

FIGURE 50.18 • Mechanisms of autonomic dysreflexia.

Autonomic dysreflexia is a clinical emergency.[60] Without prompt and adequate treatment, convulsions, loss of consciousness, and even death can occur. The major components of treatment include monitoring blood pressure while removing or correcting the initiating cause or stimulus. The person should be placed in an upright position, and all support hose or binders should be removed to promote venous pooling of blood and reduce venous return, thereby decreasing blood pressure. If the stimuli are removed or the stimuli cannot be identified and the upright position is established but the blood pressure remains elevated, drugs that block autonomic function are administered. Prevention of the type of stimuli that trigger the dysreflexic event is advocated.[61]

Postural Hypotension. Postural, or orthostatic, hypotension usually occurs in persons with injuries at T4 to T6 and above and is related to the interruption of descending control of sympathetic outflow to blood vessels in the extremities and abdomen. Pooling of blood, along with gravitational forces, impairs venous return to the heart, and there is a subsequent decrease in cardiac output when the person is placed in an upright position. The signs of orthostatic hypotension include dizziness, pallor, excessive sweating above the level of the lesion, complaints of blurred vision, and possibly fainting. Postural hypotension usually is prevented by slow changes in position and measures to promote venous return.

Disruption of Bladder, Bowel, and Sexual Function

Among the most devastating consequences of SCI is the loss of bowel, bladder, and sexual function.[7] Loss of bladder function results from disruption of neural pathways between the bladder and the reflex voiding centre at the S2 to S4 level (*i.e.,* an LMN lesion) or between the reflex voiding centre and higher brain centres for communication and coordinated sphincter control (*i.e.,* a UMN lesion). Persons with UMN lesions or spastic bladders lack awareness of bladder filling (*i.e.,* storage) and voluntary control of voiding (*i.e.,* evacuation). In LMN lesions or flaccid bladder dysfunction, lack of awareness of bladder filling and lack of bladder tone render the person unable to void voluntarily or involuntarily (see Chapter 35).

Bowel elimination is a coordinated function involving the enteric nervous system, the autonomic nervous system, and the CNS. Persons with SCI above S2 to S4 develop spastic functioning of the defecation reflex and loss of voluntary control of the external anal sphincter. Damage to the cord at the S2 to S4 level causes flaccid functioning of the defecation reflex and loss of anal sphincter tone. Even though the enteric nervous system innervation of the bowel remains intact, without the defecation reflex, peristaltic movements are ineffective in evacuating stool.

Sexual function, like bladder and bowel control, is mediated by the S2 to S4 segments of the spinal cord. The genital sexual response in SCI, which is manifested by an erection in men and vaginal lubrication in women, may be initiated by mental or touch stimuli, depending on the level of injury. The T11 to L2 cord segments have been identified as the mental stimulus, or psychogenic, sexual response area, where autonomic nerve pathways in communication with the forebrain leave the cord and innervate the genitalia. The S2 to S4 cord segments have been identified as the sexual-touch reflex centre. In T10 or higher injuries, reflex sexual response to genital touch may occur freely. However, a sexual response to mental stimuli (T11 to L2) does not occur because of the spinal lesion blocking the communication pathway. In an injury at T12 or below, the sexual reflex centre may be damaged, and there may be no response to touch.

In men, the lack of erectile ability or inability to experience penile sensations or orgasm is not a reliable indicator of fertility, which should be evaluated by an expert. In women, fertility is parallel to menses; usually, it is delayed for 3 months to 5 months after injury. There are hazards to pregnancy, labour, and use of birth control devices relative to SCI that require the input of knowledgeable healthcare providers.

Disruption of Other Functions

Temperature Regulation. The central mechanisms for thermoregulation are located in the hypothalamus (see Chapter 10). In response to cold, the hypothalamus stimulates vasoconstrictor responses in peripheral blood vessels, particularly those of the skin. This results in decreased loss of body heat. Heat production results from increased metabolism, voluntary activity, or shivering. To reduce heat, hypothalamus-stimulated mechanisms produce vasodilation of skin blood vessels to dissipate heat, and sweating to increase evaporative heat losses.

After SCI, the communication between the thermoregulatory centres in the hypothalamus and the sympathetic effector responses below the level of injury is disrupted; the ability to control blood vessel responses that conserve or dissipate heat is lost, as are the abilities to sweat and shiver. Higher levels of injury tend to produce greater disturbances in thermoregulation. In tetraplegia and high paraplegia, there are few defences against changes in the environmental temperature, and body temperature tends to assume the temperature of the external environment, a condition known as *poikilothermy.* Persons with lower-level injuries have various degrees of thermoregulation. Disturbances in thermoregulation are chronic and may cause continual loss of body heat. Treatment consists of education in the adjustment of clothing and awareness of how environmental temperatures affect the person's ability to accommodate to these changes.

Deep Vein Thrombosis and Edema. Persons with SCI are at an extremely high risk for development of deep vein thrombosis (DVT) and pulmonary embolism, particularly during the first month after injury.[7,62] Fatal pulmonary embolism has been reported in 9.7% of all persons with SCI within the first year of injury.[7] The high risk for DVT in patients with acute SCI is due to immobility, decreased vasomotor tone below the level of injury, and hypercoagulability and stasis of blood flow. Prevention strategies include the use of low-molecular-weight heparin, graduated compression stockings, sequential compression boots, and early mobilization.[7] Electrical stimulation applied to the lower limbs has been reported to provide some benefit by achieving muscular contraction and improving venous flow. Local pain, a common symptom of DVT, is often absent because of sensory deficits. Thus, a regular schedule of visual inspection for local signs of DVT (*e.g.,* swelling) is important. Testing of persons at high risk for DVT includes plethysmography and duplex ultrasonography.

Edema is also a common problem in persons with SCI. The development of edema is related to decreased peripheral vascular resistance, decreased muscle tone in the paralyzed limbs, and immobility that causes increased venous pressure and abnormal pooling of blood in the abdomen, lower limbs, and upper extremities. Edema in the dependent body parts usually is relieved by positioning to minimize gravitational forces or by using compression devices (*e.g.,* support stockings, binders) that encourage venous return.

Skin Integrity. The entire surface of the skin is innervated by cranial or spinal nerves organized into dermatomes that show cutaneous distribution. The CNS and autonomic nervous system also play a vital role in skin function. The sympathetic nervous system, through control of vasomotor and sweat gland activity, influences the health of the skin by providing adequate circulation, excretion of body fluids, and temperature regulation. The lack of sensory warning mechanisms and voluntary motor ability below the level of injury, coupled with circulatory changes, place the spinal cord-injured person at major risk for disruption of skin integrity (see Chapter 61). Significant factors associated with disruption of skin integrity are pressure, shearing forces, and localized trauma and irritation. Relieving pressure, allowing adequate circulation to the skin, and skin inspection are primary ways of maintaining skin integrity. Of all the complications after SCI, skin breakdown is the most preventable.

Future Directions in Repair of the Injured Spinal Cord

There is a continued effort to determine new and innovative strategies for repairing the injured spinal cord.[62] At present, these strategies focus on promoting the regrowth of interrupted nerve fibre tracts, using nerve growth-stimulating factors or molecules that suppress inhibitors of neuronal extension; bridging spinal cord lesions with scaffolds that are impregnated with nerve growth factors, which promote axon growth and reduce the barriers caused by scar tissue; repairing damaged myelin and restoring nerve fibre conductivity in the lesion area; and enhancing CNS plasticity by promoting compensatory growth of spared, intact nerve fibres above and below the level of injury. Although these strategies may not allow for complete repair of the spinal cord so as to recreate what was present before the injury, even small successes may be useful for someone with SCI. Much of the newer research is focusing on the potential of stem cell transplants. For a person with an injury in the cervical region, "a return of function over even one spinal segment would improve the quality of life, while return to function over three or four segments would transform it."[63]

IN SUMMARY

UMN lesions are those involving neurons completely contained in the CNS. Amyotrophic lateral sclerosis is a progressive and devastating neurologic disorder that selectively affects motor function. It affects LMNs in the spinal cord as well as UMNs in the brain stem and cerebral cortex. MS is a slowly progressive demyelinating disease of the CNS. The most common symptoms are paresthesias, optic neuritis, and motor weakness. The disease is usually characterized by exacerbations and remissions. Initially, near-normal function returns between exacerbations.

SCI is a disabling neurologic condition most commonly caused by motor vehicle collisions, falls, and sports injuries. Dysfunctions of the nervous system after SCI comprise various degrees of sensorimotor loss and altered reflex activity based on the level of injury and extent of cord damage. Depending on the level of injury, the physical problems of SCI include spinal shock; ventilation and communication problems; autonomic nervous system dysfunction that predisposes to the vasovagal response, autonomic hyperreflexia, impaired body temperature regulation, and postural hypotension; impaired muscle pump and venous innervation leading to edema of dependent areas of the body and risk for deep vein thrombosis; altered sensorimotor integrity that contributes to uncontrolled muscle spasms, altered pain responses, and threats to skin integrity; alterations in bowel and bladder elimination; and impaired sexual function.

REVIEW EXERCISES

1. A 32-year-old woman presents with complaints of drooping eyelids, difficulty chewing and swallowing, and weakness of her arms and legs that is less severe in the morning but becomes worse as the day progresses. She complains that climbing stairs and lifting objects are becoming increasingly difficult. Clinical examination confirms weakness of the eyelid and jaw muscles. She is told that she may have myasthenia gravis and is scheduled for a test using the short-acting acetylcholinesterase inhibitor edrophonium (Tensilon).

   A. *Explain the pathogenesis of this woman's symptoms as it relates to myasthenia gravis.*

   B. *Explain how information from the administration of the acetylcholinesterase inhibitor edrophonium can be used to assist in the diagnosis of the disorder.*

   C. *Explain the rationale for avoiding the use the aminoglycoside antibiotics for treatment of infections in this woman.*

2. A 16-year-old boy has approached you for assistance in preparing a poster for the science fair at

his high school. He is interested in baseball and wants to focus his presentation on the neurophysiology of the pitching and catching of a baseball.

   A. *How would you go about helping him to outline the role of the cerebellum and basal ganglia in performing the motor movements associated with these maneuvers?*

3. A 20-year-old man suffered a spinal cord injury at the C2 to C3 level as the result of a motorcycle accident.

   A. *Explain the effects of this man's injury on ventilation and communication; sensorimotor function; autonomic nervous system function; bowel, bladder, and sexual function; and temperature regulation.*

   B. *Autonomic dysreflexia, which is a threat to persons with spinal cord injury at T6 or above, is manifested by hypertension, often to extreme levels, and bradycardia; constriction of skin vessels below the level of injury; and severe headache and nasal stuffiness. Explain the origin of the elevated blood pressure and bradycardia.*

   C. *Autonomic dysreflexia does not occur until after shock has resolved, and usually occurs only in persons with injuries at T6 and above. Explain.*

References

1. Macpherson J. M., Horak F. B. (2013). Chapter 41: Posture. In Kandel E. R., Jessell T. M., Schwartz J. H., et al. (Eds.), *Principles of neural science* (5th ed.). New York, NY: McGraw-Hill Medical.
2. Wolpert D. M., Pearson K. G., Ghez C. P. (2013). Chapter 33: The organization and planning of movement. In Kandel E. R., Jessell T. M., Schwartz J. H., et al. (Eds.), *Principles of neural science* (5th ed.). New York, NY: McGraw-Hill Medical.
3. Hall J. E. (2011). *Textbook of medical physiology* (12th ed.). Philadelphia, PA: W. B. Saunders.
4. Penfield W., Rasmussen T. (1950). *The cerebral cortex of man.* New York, NY: Macmillan.
5. Brown R. H., Cannon S. C., Rowland L. P. (2013). Chapter 14: Diseases of the motor unit. In Kandel E. R., Jessell T. M., Schwartz J. H., et al. (Eds.), *Principles of neural science* (5th ed.). New York, NY: McGraw-Hill Medical.
6. Pearson K., Gordon J. (2013). Chapter 35: Spinal reflexes. In Kandel E. R., Jessell T. M., Schwartz J. H., et al. (Eds.), *Principles of neural science* (5th ed.). New York, NY: McGraw-Hill Medical.
7. Hickey J. V. (2014). *The clinical practice of neurological and neurosurgical nursing* (7th ed.). Philadelphia, PA: Lippincott Williams & Wilkins.
8. Stephen T. C., Skillen D. L., Day R. A., et al. (2010). *Canadian Bates' guide to physical assessment for nurses* Philadelphia, PA: Lippincott Williams & Wilkins.
9. Anthony D. P., Frosch M. P., De Girolami U. (2010). Chapter 27: Peripheral nerve and skeletal muscle. In Kumar V., Abbas A. K., Fausto N., et al. (Eds.), *Robbins and Cotran pathologic basis of disease* (8th ed.). Philadelphia, PA: Elsevier Saunders.
10. Kenyon L. C. (2012). Chapter 27: Skeletal muscle. In Rubin R., Strayer D. S. (Eds.). *Rubin's pathology: Clinicopathologic foundations of medicine* (6th ed.). Philadelphia, PA: Lippincott Williams & Wilkins.
11. Deconinck N., Dan B. (2007). Pathophysiology of Duchenne muscular dystrophy: Current hypothesis. *Pediatric Neurology, 36*(1), 1–7.
12. Canadian Institute of Health Research. (2013). Success story in muscle, treating a devastating disease: The case of Duchenne muscular dystrophy. Available online at: http://www.cihr-irsc.gc.ca/e/47129.html. Accessed May 11, 2015.
13. Echigoya Y., Lee J., Rodrigues M. et al. (2013). Mutation types and aging differently affect revertant fiber expansion in dystrophic Mdx and Mdx52 mice. *Plos ONE, 8*(7), e69194.
14. Sarnat H. B. (2011). Chapter 601: Muscular dystrophies. In Kliegman R. M., Stanton B. F., St. Geme J. W., et al. (Eds.), *Nelson textbook of pediatrics* (19th ed.). Philadelphia, PA: Saunders Elsevier.
15. Katzung B. G., Masters S. B., Trevor A. J. (Eds.). *Basic & clinical pharmacology* (12th ed.). Norwalk, CT: Appleton & Lange.
16. Rhoades R. A., Bell D. R. (2013). *Medical physiology: Principles for clinical medicine* (4th ed.). Philadelphia, PA: Lippincott Williams & Wilkins.
17. Horowitz B. Z. (2005). Botulinum toxin. *Critical Care Clinics, 21,* 825–839.
18. Famularo C. A. (2009). Infantile botulism: Clinical manifestations, treatment, and the role of the nurse practitioner. *Journal for Nurse Practitioners, 5*(5), 335–343.
19. Government of Canada. (2013). Infant botulism. Available online at: http://www.healthycanadians.gc.ca/eating-nutrition/safety-salubrite/vulnerable-populations/infant-botulism-botulisme-eng.php. Accessed May 11, 2015.
20. Meriggioli M. N., Sanders D. B. (2009). Autoimmune myasthenia gravis: Emerging clinical and biological heterogeneity. *The Lancet Neurology, 8*(5), 475–90.
21. Drachman D. B. (2012). Chapter 381: Myasthenia gravis and other diseases of the neuromuscular junction. In Longo D., Fauci A., Kasper D. L., et al. (Eds.), *Harrison's principles of internal medicine* (18th ed.). New York, NY: McGraw-Hill.
22. Kothari M. J. (2004). Myasthenia gravis. *Journal of the American Osteopathic Association, 104,* 377–384.
23. Russman B. S. (2007). Spinal muscular atrophy: Clinical classification and disease heterogeneity. *Journal of Child Neurology, 22,* 946–951.
24. Viera A. J. (2003). Management of carpal tunnel syndrome. *American Family Physician, 68,* 265–272.
25. Ibrahim I., Khan W. S., Goddard N., et al. (2012). Carpal tunnel syndrome: A review of the recent literature. *The Open Orthopaedics Journal, 6*(Suppl 1), 69–76.
26. Yuki N., Hartung H. (2012). Guillain-Barré syndrome. *New England Journal of Medicine, 366*(24), 2294–2304.
27. Balague F., Mannion A. F., Pellise F., et al. (2012). Non-specific low back pain. *Lancet, 379*(9814), 482–491.
28. Dunphy L. M., Windland-Brown J. E., Porter B. O., et al. (2011). *Primary care: The art and science of advance practice nursing* (3rd ed.). Philadelphia, PA: FA Davis.
29. McCarberg B. H. (2010). Acute back pain: Benefits and risks of current treatments. *Current Medical Research and Opinion, 26*(1), 179–190.
30. Moore K. L., Dalley A. F., Agur A. M. R. (2014). *Clinical oriented anatomy* (7th ed.). Philadelphia, PA: Lippincott Williams & Wilkins.
31. Winters M. E., Kluetz P., Ziberstein J. (2006). Back pain emergencies. *Medical Clinics of North America, 90,* 505–523.
32. Lisberger S. G., Thach W. T. (2013). Chapter 42: The cerebellum. In Kandel E.R., Jessell T. M., Schwartz J. H., et al. (Eds.), *Principles of neural science* (5th ed.). New York, NY: McGraw-Hill Medical.
33. Wichmann T., DeLong M. R. (2013). Chapter 43: The basal ganglia. In Kandel E. R., Jessell T. M., Schwartz J. H., et al. (Eds.), *Principles of neural science* (5th ed.). New York, NY: McGraw-Hill Medical.
34. Wong S. L., Gilmour H., Ramage-Morin P. L. (2014). Parkinson's disease: Prevalence, diagnosis and impact. *Health Reports, 25*(11), 10–14.
35. Parkinson J. (1817). *An essay on the shaking palsy.* London: Sherwood, Nelley & Jones.
36. Fuller G. N., Goodman J. C., Bouldin T. W. (2012). Chapter 28: The nervous system. In Rubin, R., Strayer, D.S. (Eds.). *Rubin's pathology: Clinicopathologic foundations of medicine* (6th ed.). Philadelphia, PA: Lippincott Williams & Wilkins.

37. Frosch M. P., Anthony D. C., De Girolami U. (2010). Chapter 28: The central nervous system. In Kumar V., Abbas A. K., Fausto N., et al. (Eds.), *Robbins and Cotran pathologic basis of disease* (8th ed.). Philadelphia, PA: Elsevier Saunders.

38. Gazewood J. D., Richards D. R., Clebak K. (2013). Parkinson disease: An update. *American Family Physician, 87*(4), 267–273.

39. Wu Y., Le W., Jankovic J. (2011). Preclinical markers of Parkinson disease. *Archives of Neurology, 68*(1), 22–30.

40. Meissner W. G., Frasier M., Basser T., et al. (2011). Priorities in Parkinson's disease research. *Nature Reviews Drug Discovery, 10*(5), 377–393.

41. Fernandex H. H. (2012). Updates in the medical management of Parkinson disease. *Cleveland Clinic Journal of Medicine, 79*(1), 28–35.

42. Okun M. S. (2012). Deep-brain stimulation for Parkinson's disease. *New England Journal of Medicine, 367*(16), 1529–1538.

43. Shoesmith C. L., Strong M. J. (2006). Amyotrophic lateral sclerosis. *Canadian Family Physician, 52*, 1563–1569.

44. Kiernan M. C., Vucic S., Cheah B. C., et al. (2011). Amyotrophic lateral sclerosis. *Lancet, 377*(9769), 942–955.

45. Malik R., Lui A., Lomen-Hoerth C. (2014). Amyotrophic lateral sclerosis. *Seminars in Neurology, 34*(5), 534–541.

46. Lassmann H., van Horssen J., Mahad D. (2012). Progressive multiple sclerosis: Pathology and pathogenesis. *Nature Reviews Neurology, 8*(11), 647–656.

47. Poppe A. Y., Wolfson C., Zhu B. (2008). Prevalence of multiple sclerosis in Canada: A systematic review. *Canadian Journal of Neurological Sciences, 35*(5), 593–601.

48. Hauser S. L., Goodin D. S. (2012). Chapter 458: Multiple sclerosis and other demyelinating diseases. In Longo D., Fauci A., Kasper D. L., et al. (Eds.), *Harrison's principles of internal medicine* (18th ed.). New York, NY: McGraw-Hill.

49. Kantarci O., Wingerchuk D. (2006). Epidemiology and natural history of multiple sclerosis: New insights. *Current Opinion in Neurology, 19*(3), 248–254.

50. Calabresi P. A. (2004). Diagnosis and management of multiple sclerosis. *American Family Physician, 70*, 1935–1944.

51. Goodin D. S. (Ed) (2014). Multiple sclerosis and related disorders. *Handbook of Clinical Neurology, 122*, 2–715.

52. Multiple Sclerosis Society of Canada. (2015). Treatment. Available online at: https://beta.mssociety.ca/about-ms/treatments. Accessed May 11, 2015.

53. National Spinal Cord Injury Statistical Center. (2014). Spinal cord injury: Facts and figures at a glance. Available online at: https://www.nscisc.uab.edu/PublicDocuments/fact_figures_docs/Facts%202014.pdf. Accessed May 11, 2015.

54. Oyinbo C. A. (2011). Secondary injury mechanism in traumatic spinal cord injury: A nugget of the multiply cascade. *Acta Neurobiology Experiments, 71*(2), 281–299.

55. Cadotte D. W., Fehlings M. G. (2011). Spinal cord injury: A systematic review of current treatment options. *Clinical Orthopaedics and Related Research, 469*(3), 732–741.

56. Canadian Association of Emergency Physicians (2013). Steroids in acute spinal cord injury. Position statement. Available online at: http://caep.ca/resources/position-statements-and-guidelines/steroids-acute-spinal-cord-injury. Accessed May 11, 2015.

57. Sipski M., Pearse D. D. (2006). Methylprednisolone and other confounders to spinal cord injury trials. *Nature Clinical Practice Neurology, 2*, 402–403.

58. Kirshblum S. C., Burns S. P., Biering-Sorensen F., et al. (2011). International standards for neurological classification of spinal cord injury. *Journal of Spinal Cord Medicine, 34*(6), 535–546.

59. Garstang S. V., Miller-Smith S. A. (2007). Autonomic nervous system dysfunction after spinal cord injury. *Physical Medicine and Rehabilitation Clinics of North America, 18*, 275–296.

60. Cragg J., Krassioukov A. (2012). Autonomic dysreflexia. *Canadian Medical Association Journal, 184*(1), 66.

61. Krassioukov A., Balckmer J., Teasell R. W., et al. (2014). Autonomic dysreflexia following spinal cord injury. *Spinal Cord Injury Rehabilitation,* Version 5.0, 1–35.

62. Malhotra M., Bhatoe H. S., Sudambrekar S. M. (2010). Spinal cord injuries. *Medical Journal, Armed Forces India, 66*(4), 325–328.

63. Fawcett J. (2002). Repair of spinal cord injuries: Where are we, where are we going? *Spinal Cord, 40*(12), 615–623.

Visit the Point **http://thePoint.lww.com for animations, journal articles, and more!**

Disorders of Brain Function

51

MANIFESTATIONS AND MECHANISMS OF BRAIN INJURY

The brain is the most complex structure in the body. It controls our ability to think and be aware of things around us, and our interactions with the outside world. Brain functions are diverse and highly localized within the brain. Therefore, unlike other organs that have a global function, the brain is much more vulnerable to focal lesions. For example, an isolated renal infarct would not be expected to have a significant effect on kidney function, whereas an infarct of comparable size in the brain could have a serious impact on brain function, such as complete paralysis on one side of the body.

MANIFESTATIONS AND MECHANISMS OF BRAIN INJURY

After completing this section of the chapter, you should be able to meet the following objectives:

- Define consciousness and trace the rostral-to-caudal progression of consciousness in terms of pupillary changes, respiration, and motor function as the effects of brain dysfunction progress to involve structures in the diencephalon, midbrain, pons, and medulla.
- State two criteria for the diagnosis of brain death.
- Differentiate cerebral hypoxia from cerebral ischemia and focal from global ischemia.
- Characterize the role of excitatory amino acids as a common pathway for neurologic disorders.
- State the determinants of intracranial pressure and describe compensatory mechanisms used to prevent large changes in intracranial pressure when there are changes in brain, blood, and cerebrospinal fluid volumes.
- Explain the causes of tentorial herniation of the brain and its consequences.
- Compare the causes of communicating and noncommunicating hydrocephalus.
- Compare cytotoxic, vasogenic, and interstitial cerebral edema.
- Differentiate primary and secondary brain injuries due to head trauma.

- Describe the mechanism of brain damage in coup–contrecoup injuries.
- List the constellation of symptoms involved in the postconcussion syndrome.
- Differentiate among the location, manifestations, and morbidity of epidural, subdural, and intracerebral hematoma.

The brain is protected from external forces by the rigid confines of the skull and the cushioning provided by the cerebrospinal fluid (CSF). The metabolic stability required by its electrically active cells is maintained by a number of regulatory mechanisms, including the blood–brain barrier and autoregulatory mechanisms that ensure its blood supply. Nonetheless, the brain remains remarkably vulnerable to injury by ischemia, trauma, tumours, degenerative processes, and metabolic derangements.

Manifestations of Brain Injury

Brain injury, whether due to head trauma, stroke, or other pathologic processes, is manifested by alterations in sensory, motor, and cognitive function and by changes in the level of consciousness. In contrast to focal injury, which causes focal neurologic deficits without altered consciousness, global injury nearly always results in altered levels of consciousness, ranging from inattention to stupor or coma. Severe injury that seriously compromises brain function may result in brain death.

The cerebral hemispheres are the most susceptible to damage, and the most frequent sign of brain dysfunction is an altered level of consciousness and change in behaviour. As the brain structures in the diencephalon, midbrain, pons, and medulla are sequentially affected, additional signs related to pupillary and eye movement reflexes, motor function, and respiration become evident (Table 51.1). Hemodynamic and respiratory instability are the last signs to occur because their regulatory centres are located low in the medulla.

With progressive brain deterioration, the person's neurologic capabilities appear to deteriorate in stepwise fashion.

Similarly, if neurologic function returns, there appears to be stepwise progress to higher levels of consciousness. Deterioration of brain function from supratentorial lesions tends to follow a rostral-to-caudal stepwise progression, which is observed as the brain initially compensates for injury and subsequently decompensates with loss of autoregulation and cerebral perfusion. Infratentorial (brain stem) lesions may lead to an early, sometimes abrupt disturbance in consciousness without any orderly rostrocaudal progression of neurologic signs.

BRAIN INJURY AND LEVELS OF CONSCIOUSNESS

- Consciousness is a global function that depends on a diffuse neural network that includes activity of the reticular activating system (RAS) and both cerebral hemispheres.
- Impaired consciousness implies diffuse brain injury to the RAS at any level (medulla through thalamus) or both cerebral hemispheres simultaneously.
- In contrast, local brain injury causes focal neurologic deficit but does not disrupt consciousness.

Altered Levels of Consciousness

All forms of brain injury and disease can lead to altered levels of consciousness. Consciousness is the state of awareness of self and the environment and of being able to orient to new stimuli. It has traditionally been divided into two components: (1) arousal and wakefulness, and (2) content and cognition.[1–3] The content and cognition aspects of consciousness are determined by a functioning cerebral cortex. Arousal and wakefulness require the concurrent functioning of both cerebral hemispheres and an intact reticular activation system (RAS) in the brain stem.

Anatomic and Physiologic Basis of Consciousness. The reticular formation is a diffuse, primitive system of interlacing nerve cells and fibres in the brain stem that receive input from multiple sensory pathways (Fig. 51.1). Anatomically, the reticular formation constitutes the central core of the brain stem,

TABLE 51.1	KEY SIGNS IN ROSTRAL-TO-CAUDAL PROGRESSION OF BRAIN LESIONS
LEVEL OF BRAIN INJURY	**KEY CLINICAL SIGNS**
Diencephalon	Impaired consciousness; small, reactive pupils; intact oculocephalic reflex; decorticate posturing; Cheyne–Stokes respirations
Midbrain	Coma; fixed, midsize pupils; impaired oculocephalic reflex; neurogenic hyperventilation; decerebrate posturing
Pons	Coma; fixed, irregular pupils; dysconjugate gaze; impaired cold caloric stimulation; loss of corneal reflex; hemiparesis/quadriparesis; decerebrate posturing; apneustic respirations
Medulla	Coma; fixed pupils; flaccidity; loss of gag and cough reflexes; ataxic/apneic respirations

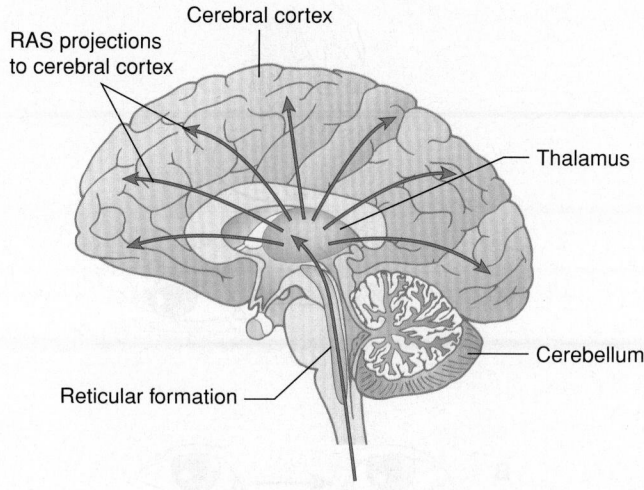

Cerebral cortex

RAS projections to cerebral cortex

Thalamus

Cerebellum

Reticular formation

FIGURE 51.1 • The brain stem reticular formation and reticular activating system (RAS). Ascending sensory tracts send axon collateral fibres to the reticular formation. These give rise to fibres synapsing in the nonspecific nuclei of the thalamus. From there, the nonspecific thalamic projections influence widespread areas of the cerebral cortex and limbic system.

extending from the medulla through the pons to the midbrain, which is continuous caudally with the spinal cord and rostrally with the subthalamus, the hypothalamus, and the thalamus.[4] Fibres from the reticular activating system (RAS) also project to the autonomic nervous system and motor systems. The hypothalamus plays a predominant role in maintaining homeostasis through integration of somatic, visceral, and endocrine functions. Inputs from the reticular formation, vestibulospinal projections, and other motor systems are integrated to provide a continuously adapting background of muscle tone and posture to facilitate voluntary motor actions. Reticular formation neurons that function in regulation of cardiovascular, respiratory, and other visceral functions are intermingled with those that maintain other reticular formation functions.

Ascending fibres of the reticular formation, known as the ascending RAS, transmit activating information to all parts of the cerebral cortex. The flow of information in the ascending RAS activates the hypothalamic and limbic structures that regulate emotional and behavioural responses such as those that occur in response to pain and loud noises, and they exert facilitatory effects on cortical neurons. Without cortical activation, a person is less reactive to environmental stimuli, and the level of consciousness is reduced.

The pathways for the ascending RAS travel from the medulla through the midbrain, such that lesions of the brain stem can interrupt RAS activity, leading to altered levels of consciousness and coma. Any deficit in level of consciousness, from mild confusion to stupor or coma, indicates either direct injury to the RAS or to both cerebral hemispheres concurrently. For example, consciousness may decline owing to severe systemic metabolic derangements that affect both hemispheres, or from head trauma causing shear injuries to white matter of both the RAS and the cerebral hemispheres. Brain injuries that affect a hemisphere unilaterally and also spare the RAS, such as cerebral infarction, usually do not cause impaired consciousness.

Levels of Consciousness. Levels of consciousness reflect awareness of and response to the environment. A fully conscious person is totally aware of her or his surroundings and able to react to stimuli in the environment.[2,5] Levels of consciousness exist on a continuum that includes consciousness, confusion, delirium, obtundation, stupor, and coma (Table 51.2).

The earliest signs of diminution in level of consciousness are inattention, mild confusion, disorientation, and blunted responsiveness. With further deterioration, the delirious person becomes markedly inattentive and variably lethargic or agitated. The person may progress to become obtunded and may respond only to vigorous or noxious stimuli.

Because of its simplicity of application, the Glasgow Coma Scale has gained universal acceptance as a method for assessing the level of arousal in persons with brain injury[2] (Table 51.3). Numbered scores are given to responses of eye opening, verbal utterances, and motor responses. The total score is the sum of the best response in each category. Lower scores are representative of a poor state of arousal.

TABLE 51.2 DESCENDING LEVELS OF CONSCIOUSNESS AND THEIR CHARACTERISTICS

LEVEL OF CONSCIOUSNESS	CHARACTERISTICS
Confusion	Disturbance of consciousness characterized by impaired ability to think clearly, and to perceive, respond to, and remember current stimuli; also disorientation
Delirium	State of disturbed consciousness with motor restlessness, transient hallucinations, disorientation, and sometimes delusions
Obtundation	Disorder of decreased alertness with associated psychomotor retardation
Stupor	A state in which the person is not unconscious but exhibits little or no spontaneous activity
Coma	A state of being unarousable and unresponsive to external stimuli or internal needs; often determined by the Glasgow Coma Scale

TABLE 51.3 THE GLASGOW COMA SCALE

TEST	SCORE[a]
Eye Opening Response (E)	
Spontaneous	4
To verbal command	3
To pain	2
None	1
Motor Response (M)	
Obeys commands	6
Localizes pain	5
Normal flexion (withdrawal)	4
Abnormal flexion (decorticate posturing)	3
Extension (decerebrate posturing)	2
None (flaccid)	1
Verbal Response (V)	
Oriented	5
Confused conversation	4
Inappropriate words	3
Incomprehensible sounds	2
None	1

[a]GSC Score = E + M + V. Best possible score = 15; worst possible score = 3.

Other Manifestations of Deteriorating Brain Function

Additional elements in the initial neurologic evaluation of a person with brain injury include checking for abnormalities in the size of the pupils and their reaction to light, evidence of decorticate or decerebrate posturing, and altered patterns of respiration.

Pupillary Reflexes and Eye Movements. Although the pupils may initially respond briskly to light, they become unreactive and dilated as brain function deteriorates. A bilateral loss of the pupillary light response is indicative of lesions of the brain stem. A unilateral loss of the pupillary light response may be due to a lesion of the optic or oculomotor pathways. The oculocephalic reflex (doll's-head eye movement) can be used to determine whether the brain stem centres for eye movement are intact (Fig. 51.2). If the oculocephalic reflex is inconclusive, and if there are no contraindications, the oculovestibular test (*i.e.,* cold caloric test, in which cold water is instilled into the ear canal) may be used to elicit nystagmus (see Chapter 55).

Decorticate and Decerebrate Posturing. With the early onset of unconsciousness, there is some combative and purposeful movement in response to pain. As coma progresses, noxious stimuli can initiate rigidity and abnormal postures if the motor tracts are interrupted at specific levels. These abnormal postures are classified as decorticate and decerebrate posturing, and may be referred to as flexor and extensor respectively.[2] Decorticate (flexor) posturing is characterized by flexion of the arms, wrists, and fingers, with abduction of the upper extremities, internal rotation, and plantar flexion of the

FIGURE 51.2 • Doll's-head response. The *doll's-head eye response* demonstrates the always-present vestibular static reflexes without forebrain interference or suppression. Severe damage to the forebrain or to the brain stem rostral to the pons often results in loss of rostral control of these static vestibular reflexes. If the person's head is moved from side to side or up and down, the eyes will move in conjugate gaze to the opposite side (**A**), much like those of a doll with counterweighted eyes. If the doll's-head phenomenon is observed, brain stem function at the level of the pons is considered intact (in a comatose person). In the unconscious person without intact brain stem function and vestibular static reflexes, the eyes stay in mid-position (fixed) or turn in the same direction (**B**) as the head is turned.

lower extremities (Fig. 51.3A). This type of posturing results from lesions of the cerebral hemisphere or internal capsule. Decerebrate (extensor) posturing results from increased muscle excitability (Fig. 51.3B). It is characterized by rigidity of the arms with palms of the hands turned away from the body and with stiffly extended legs and plantar flexion of the feet. This response occurs with rostral-to-caudal deterioration, when lesions of the diencephalon extend to involve the midbrain and upper brain stem. Both types of posturing are poor prognostic signs.

Respiratory Responses. As brain function deteriorates, early respiratory changes include yawning and sighing, with progression to Cheyne–Stokes breathing. With progression of injury continuing to the midbrain, respirations change to neurogenic hyperventilation, in which the frequency of respirations may exceed 40 breaths per minute because of uninhibited stimulation of inspiratory and expiratory centres. With medullary involvement, respirations become ataxic (*i.e.,* totally uncoordinated and irregular). Apnea may occur because of a lack of responsiveness to carbon dioxide stimulation. Complete ventilatory assistance is often required at this point.

Brain Death

Brain death or neurologically determined death has specific clinical criteria. It has been described as the irreversible loss of function of the brain, including the brain stem.[6,7] Irreversibility implies that brain death cannot be reversed. Some

FIGURE 51.3 • Abnormal posturing. **A:** Decorticate rigidity. In decorticate rigidity, one or both of the upper arms are held at the sides with elbows, wrists, and fingers flexed. The legs are extended and internally rotated. The feet are plantar flexed. **B:** Decerebrate rigidity. In decerebrate rigidity, the jaws are clenched and neck extended. The arms are adducted and stiffly extended at the elbows with the forearms pronated and the wrists and fingers flexed. (From Hickey J. V. (2014). The clinical practice of neurological and neurosurgical nursing (7th ed., p. 173). Philadelphia, PA: Lippincott Williams & Wilkins.)

A *Flexor or decorticate posturing response*

B *Extensor or decerebrate posturing*

conditions such as drug and metabolic intoxication can cause cessation of brain functions that is completely reversible, even when they produce clinical cessation of brain functions and electroencephalographic (EEG) silence. This needs to be excluded before declaring a person brain dead.

With advances in scientific knowledge and technology that have provided the means for artificially maintaining ventilatory and circulatory function, the definition of brain death has been continually reexamined. In 2003, a large Canadian forum of healthcare professionals collaborated to initiate the development of standards for neurologically determined death. According to these recommendations, the following minimal criteria were recommended: (1) irreversible brain death with established etiology capable of causing neurologic death; (2) deep, unresponsive coma with absent motor responses, excluding spinal reflexes; (3) absent brain stem reflexes (gag, cough) and absence of corneal responses, pupillary responses with pupils at mid-size or greater and vestibulo-ocular responses; (4) absent respiratory effort based on apnea test (disconnection of the ventilator after pre-oxygenation, and observation for spontaneous breathing); and finally, (5) absent confounding factors (*e.g.,* unresuscitated shock, hypothermia, drug intoxications, neuromuscular blockade).[7] Key clinical considerations have been defined for each of these criteria. Ancillary tests such as cerebral angiography may also be performed to support clinical findings of brain death. National consensus for brain death requires further discussion.

Persistent Vegetative State

Advances in the care of brain-injured persons during the past several decades have resulted in survival of many persons who previously would have died. Unfortunately, most persons in prolonged coma who survive evolve to what is called the *persistent vegetative state.* In this state, the brainstem is mostly spared, although the grey and white matter in both hemispheres are severely damaged. There is loss of all cognitive functions and unawareness of self and surroundings. Reflex and vegetative functions remain, including sleep–wake cycles.[8] These individuals have spontaneous eye opening without concurrent awareness, often leading to confusion and concern in hopeful families. Persons in the vegetative state require enteral feeding and full nursing care.

The criteria for diagnosis of vegetative state include absence of awareness of self and environment and an inability to interact with others; absence of sustained or reproducible voluntary behavioural responses; lack of language comprehension; sufficiently preserved hypothalamic and brain stem function to maintain life; bowel and bladder incontinence; and variably preserved cranial nerve (*e.g.,* pupillary, gag) and spinal cord reflexes.[8] The diagnosis of persistent vegetative state requires that the condition has continued for at least 1 month. The minimally conscious state has been more recently defined as a state of arousal similar to persistent vegetative state, but with the distinction of the objective presence of some awareness on the part of the patient.[9]

Mechanisms of Injury

Injury to brain tissue can result from a number of conditions, including trauma, tumours, stroke, metabolic derangements, and degenerative disorders. Brain damage resulting from these disorders involves several common pathways, including the effects of ischemia, excitatory amino acid injury, cerebral edema, and injury due to increased intracranial pressure (ICP). In many cases, the mechanisms of injury are interrelated.

Hypoxic and Ischemic Injury

The energy requirements of the brain are provided mainly by adenosine triphosphate (ATP); the ability of the cerebral circulation to deliver oxygen in sufficiently high concentrations to facilitate metabolism of glucose and generate ATP is essential to brain function. Although the brain makes up only 2% of the body's weight, it receives 15% of the resting cardiac output and accounts for 20% of the oxygen consumption.[2,5] Thus, deprivation of oxygen or blood flow can have a deleterious effect on brain structures.

By definition, hypoxia denotes a deprivation of oxygen to brain tissue and cells while maintaining adequate blood flow (perfusion), whereas ischemia is a situation of greatly reduced or interrupted blood flow. The brain tends to have different sensitivities to the two conditions. Whereas hypoxia interferes with the delivery of oxygen, ischemia interferes with delivery of oxygen and glucose as well as the removal of metabolic wastes. Hypoxia usually is seen in conditions such as exposure to reduced atmospheric pressure, carbon monoxide poisoning, severe anemia, and hypoxemia or failure to oxygenate the blood. Because hypoxia indicates decreased oxygen levels in all brain tissue, it produces a generalized depressant effect on the brain. Contrary to belief, neurons are capable of substantial anaerobic metabolism and are fairly tolerant of pure hypoxia, which commonly produces euphoria, listlessness, drowsiness, and impaired problem solving. Unconsciousness and seizure activity may occur when hypoxia is sudden, severe, or prolonged.

Cerebral ischemia can be focal, as in stroke, or global, as in cardiac arrest. In global ischemia, the blood flow to the entire brain is compromised. In contrast, during focal ischemia only a region of the brain is not adequately perfused. An ischemic stroke is an example of focal ischemia. Collateral circulation provides blood flow to uninvolved brain areas during focal ischemia. The collateral perfusion may even provide sufficient substrates to the borders of the focal ischemic region to maintain a low level of metabolic activity, thereby preserving membrane integrity. At the same time, interruption in delivery of glucose under these anaerobic conditions may result in additional lactic acid production and depletion of ATP stores.[5]

Global Ischemia. Global ischemia occurs when blood flow is inadequate to meet the metabolic needs of the entire brain. The result is a spectrum of neurologic disorders reflecting global brain dysfunction. Unconsciousness occurs within seconds of severe global ischemia, such as that resulting from complete cessation of blood flow, as in cardiac arrest, or from a marked decrease in blood flow, as in serious cardiac arrhythmias. If cerebral circulation is restored immediately, consciousness is regained quickly. However, if blood flow is not promptly restored, severe pathologic changes take place. Energy sources (*i.e.,* glucose and glycogen), are exhausted in 2 to 4 minutes, and cellular ATP stores are depleted in 4 to 5 minutes. Approximately 50% to 75% of the total energy requirement of neuronal tissue is spent on mechanisms for maintenance of ionic gradients across the cell membrane (*e.g.,* sodium-potassium pump), resulting in fluxes of sodium, potassium, and calcium ions (Table 51.4). Excessive influx of sodium results in neuronal and interstitial edema. The influx of calcium initiates a cascade of events, including release of intracellular and nuclear enzymes that cause cell destruction (see section on Excitotoxic Injury). When ischemia is sufficiently severe or prolonged, infarction or death of all the cellular elements of the brain occurs. Even if blood flow is restored, if the ischemic thresholds for injury were exceeded, then permanent cell death ensues. Furthermore, reperfusion of injured tissues can lead to secondary brain injury through the delivery of inflammatory cells and toxic byproducts, including

TABLE 51.4 PATHOPHYSIOLOGIC CONSEQUENCES OF IMPAIRED CEREBRAL PERFUSION

CONSEQUENCES	TIMING
Depletion of oxygen	10 sec
Depletion of glucose	2–4 min
Conversion to anaerobic metabolism	2–4 min
Exhaustion of cellular ATP	4–5 min
Consequences	
Efflux of potassium	
Influx of sodium	
Influx of calcium	

excitatory amino acids. Such reperfusion injury compounds the initial ischemic damage.

The pattern of global ischemia reflects the anatomic arrangement of the cerebral vessels and the sensitivity of various brain tissues to oxygen deprivation.[9] Selective neuronal sensitivity to a lack of oxygen is most apparent in the Purkinje cells of the cerebellum and neurons in the Sommer sector of the hippocampus, where cell death occurs earliest after global ischemia. The anatomic arrangement of the cerebral blood vessels predisposes to two types of injury: watershed infarcts and laminar necrosis.

Watershed infarcts are concentrated in anatomically vulnerable border zones between the overlapping territories supplied by the major cerebral arteries, notably the middle, anterior, and posterior cerebral arteries. The overlapping territory at the distal ends of these vessels forms extremely vulnerable areas in terms of global ischemia, called *watershed zones*. During events such as severe hypotension, these distal territories undergo a profound lowering of blood flow, predisposing to focal ischemia and infarction of brain tissues. Therefore, global ischemia can result in focal infarcts that occur in the border zones between major vascular territories. This is in contrast to primarily focal ischemia in which the pattern of infarction is within a vascular territory. Laminar necrosis refers to short, serpiginous segments of necrosis that occur within and parallel to the cerebral cortex, in areas supplied by the penetrating arteries. The grey matter of the cerebral cortex receives its major blood supply through short penetrating arteries that emerge at right angles from larger vessels in the pia mater and then form a cascade as they repeatedly branch, forming a rich capillary network. An abrupt loss of arterial blood pressure markedly diminishes flow through these capillary channels. Because the third cortical layer is most sensitive to ischemia, the necrosis that develops is laminar and is most severe in this deep layer of the cortex.

The neurologic deficits that result from global ischemic injury vary widely. If the period of nonflow or low flow is minimal, the neurologic damage is usually minimal to nonexistent. When the period is extensive or resuscitation is lengthy, the early neurologic clinical picture is that of fixed and dilated pupils, abnormal motor posturing, and coma. If the victim survives, there may be gradual improvement in neurologic status, although permanent cognitive and focal deficits usually persist and can prevent a return to preischemic levels of functioning.

An exception to this time frame is the circumstance of cold-water drowning in which the person, especially a child, is submerged in cold water for longer than 10 minutes.[10] Hypothermia develops and reduces the cerebral metabolic requirements for oxygen, minimizes intracellular acidosis, and lessens the effects of excitotoxic byproducts. In this case, recovery can be rapid and remarkable, and resuscitation efforts should not be discontinued precipitously.

Treatment of global cerebral ischemia varies with the underlying cause (*e.g.,* cardiac arrest, asthma attack). General goals common to all causes are aimed at providing oxygen to the troubled brain and decreasing the metabolic needs of brain tissue during the nonflow state. Hemodynamic support aimed at restoring systemic and cerebral perfusion is required. Respiratory support including mechanical ventilation and supplemental oxygen may be indicated. Methods that decrease brain temperature as a means of decreasing brain metabolism are effective in certain patients after cardiac arrest.[11] Normovolemic hemodilution may be used to overcome sludging of cerebral blood flow during reperfusion. Because both hypoglycemia and hyperglycemia adversely affect the outcome in persons with global ischemia, control of blood glucose within a range of 4.0 to 7.0 mmol/L is appropriate, and even narrower targets have been advocated in acute stroke.[10,12] Recent interest has focused on other neuroprotective therapies and pharmacologic agents that could minimize injury (from free radicals, excitatory amino acids such as glutamate, and other forms of secondary injury) and salvage brain tissue.

Excitotoxic Brain Injury

In many neurologic disorders, injury to neurons may be caused by various mediators, including excitatory amino acids, catecholamines, nitric oxide, free radicals, inflammatory cells, apoptosis, and intracellular proteases.[12] The earliest and most studied of these is the overstimulation of receptors for specific amino acids, such as glutamate and aspartate, that act as excitatory neurotransmitters. The neurologic conditions involved in excitotoxic injury range from acute insults such as stroke, hypoglycemic injury, and trauma to chronic degenerative disorders such as Huntington disease and possibly Alzheimer disease. The term *excitotoxicity* has been coined for the final common pathway for neuronal cell injury and death triggered by excessive activity of the excitatory neurotransmitters and their receptor-mediated effects.

Glutamate is the principal excitatory neurotransmitter in the brain, and its interaction with specific receptors is responsible for many higher-order functions, including memory, cognition, movement, and sensation.[2,12] Many of the actions of glutamate are coupled with receptor-operated ion channels. One subtype in particular, the glutamate *N*-methyl-D-aspartate (NMDA) receptor, has been implicated in causing central nervous system (CNS) injury.[2,12] This subtype of

glutamate receptor opens a large-diameter calcium channel that permits calcium and sodium ions to enter the cell and allows potassium ions to exit, resulting in prolonged (seconds) action potentials. The intracellular concentration of glutamate is approximately 16 times that of the extracellular concentration. Normally, extracellular concentrations of glutamate are tightly regulated, with excess amounts removed and actively transported into astrocytes and neurons.

During prolonged ischemia, the glutamate transport mechanisms become immobilized, causing extracellular glutamate to accumulate. In addition, intracellular glutamate is released from the damaged cells. This glutamate excess then drives the uncontrolled opening of NMDA receptor-operated channels, producing an increase in intracellular calcium. Excess intracellular calcium leads to a series of calcium-mediated processes called the *calcium cascade* (Fig. 51.4), including the release of intracellular enzymes that cause protein breakdown, free radical formation, lipid peroxidation, fragmentation of deoxyribonucleic acid (DNA), mitochondrial injury, nuclear breakdown, and eventually brain cell death.

The effects of acute glutamate toxicity may be reversible if the excess glutamate can be removed or if its effects can be blocked before the full cascade of events progresses. Current research continues to explore the efficacy of *neuroprotectants* in reducing brain cell injury by interfering with the calcium cascade.[13] These pharmacologic strategies may protect viable

FIGURE 51.4 • The role of the glutamate-NMDA receptor in brain cell injury.

brain cells from irreversible damage in the setting of excitotoxicity. Pharmacologic strategies being explored include those that inhibit the synthesis or release of excitatory amino acid transmitters; block the NMDA receptors; stabilize the membrane potential to prevent initiation of the calcium cascade using lidocaine and certain barbiturates; and specifically block certain intracellular proteases, endonucleases, and lipases that are known to be cytotoxic.[13] The drug riluzole, which acts presynaptically to inhibit glutamate release, is currently used in the treatment of amyotrophic lateral sclerosis (see Chapter 50). In the setting of ischemic stroke, multiple mechanisms of pharmacologic action, including NMDA receptor blockade, nitric oxide manipulation, inflammatory suppression, and potassium channel opening, are being studied.[13,14]

CNS neurons can be divided into two major categories: macroneurons and microneurons. Macroneurons are large cells with long axons that leave the local network of intercommunicating neurons to send action potentials to other regions of the nervous system at distances of centimetres to metres (e.g., upper motor neurons originating in the motor cortex that communicate with lower motor neurons of the spinal cord that control leg movement). Macroneurons number in the thousands. Microneurons are very small cells intimately involved in local circuitry, and count in the billions. Their axons transmit action potentials to other members of the same local network. It is the microneuron network that provides the analytic, integrative, and learning circuitry that is the basis for the higher-order function of the CNS. Many macroneurons use glutamate as a neurotransmitter in their excitatory communication with microneurons. The microneurons of the cerebral cortex and hippocampus are particularly vulnerable to excessive stimulation of the glutamate NMDA receptors and the neurotoxic effects of increased intracellular calcium levels. Because of their increased vulnerability, many of the small interneurons that make up essential parts of the complex control and memory functions of the brain are selectively damaged, even if the remainder of the brain survives the insult. This pattern may account for the long-term effects of brain insult, which frequently include subtle reductions in cognitive and memory functions.

Increased Intracranial Volume and Pressure

The adult brain is enclosed within a nonexpandable rigid skull or cranium, making it particularly susceptible to increases in intracranial pressure (ICP). Increased ICP is a common pathway for brain injury from different types of insults and agents. Excessive ICP can obstruct cerebral blood flow, destroy brain cells, displace brain tissue (as in herniation), and otherwise damage delicate brain structures.

The cranial cavity within the skull contains blood (approximately 10%), brain tissue (approximately 80%), and cerebral spinal fluid (CSF) (approximately 10%).[2] Each of these three volumes contributes to the ICP, which normally is maintained within a range of 0 to 15 mm Hg when measured in the lateral ventricles. The volumes of each of these components can vary slightly without causing marked changes in ICP. This is because small increases in the volume of one component can be compensated for by a decrease in the volume of one or both of the other two components. This association is called the *Monro–Kellie hypothesis*.[2] Normal fluctuations in ICP occur with respiratory movements and activities of daily living such as straining, coughing, and sneezing.

Abnormal variation in intracranial volume with subsequent changes in ICP can be caused by a volume change in any of the three intracranial components. For example, an increase in tissue volume can result from a brain tumour, cerebral edema, or bleeding into brain tissue. An increase in blood volume develops when there is vasodilation of cerebral vessels or obstruction of venous outflow. Excess production, decreased absorption, or obstructed circulation of CSF may increase the CSF component. When the change in volume is caused by a brain tumour, it tends to occur slowly and is usually localized to the immediate area, whereas the increase resulting from head injury or vascular disruption usually develops rapidly.

According to the modified Monro–Kellie hypothesis, reciprocal compensation occurs among the three intracranial compartments. Of the three intracranial volumes, tissue volume is relatively restricted in its ability to undergo change; CSF and blood volume are best able to compensate for changes in ICP. Initial increases in ICP are buffered by a translocation of CSF to the spinal subarachnoid space and increased reabsorption of CSF. The compensatory ability of the blood compartment is limited by the small amount of blood that is in the cerebral circulation. The cerebral blood vessels contain less than 10% of the intracranial volume, most of which is contained in the low-pressure venous system. As the volume-buffering capacity of this compartment becomes exhausted, venous pressure increases, and cerebral blood volume and ICP rise. Also, cerebral blood flow is highly controlled by autoregulatory mechanisms, which affect its compensatory capacity. Conditions such as ischemia and an elevated partial pressure of carbon dioxide (PCO_2) in the blood produce a compensatory vasodilation of the cerebral blood vessels. A decrease in PCO_2 has the opposite effect; for this reason, hyperventilation, which results in a decrease in PCO_2 levels, is sometimes used to decrease a significant increase in ICP.

The impact of increases in blood, brain tissue, or CSF volumes on ICP varies among individuals and depends on the amount of increase, the effectiveness of compensatory mechanisms, and the compliance of brain tissue. Compliance represents the ratio of change in volume to the resulting change in pressure (compliance = change in volume/change in pressure).[2] In the case of intracranial volumes and pressure, an increase in intracranial volume will have little, or no, effect on ICP as long as compliance is high. Factors that influence compliance include the amount of volume increase, the time frame for accommodation, and the size of the intracranial compartments. For example, small volume increments over long periods of time can be accommodated more easily than a comparable amount introduced over a short time.

The cerebral perfusion pressure (CPP), which represents the difference between the mean arterial blood pressure (MAP)

Understanding ▸ Intracranial Pressure

The intracranial pressure (ICP) is the pressure within the intracranial cavity. It is determined by (1) the pressure–volume relationships among the brain tissue, cerebrospinal fluid (CSF), and blood in the intracranial cavity; (2) the Monro–Kellie hypothesis, which relates to reciprocal changes among the intracranial volumes; and (3) the compliance of the brain and its ability to buffer changes in intracranial volume.

1. Intracranial Volumes and Pressure

The ICP represents the pressure exerted by the essentially incompressible tissue and fluid volumes of the three compartments contained within the rigid confines of the skull—the brain tissue and interstitial fluid (80%), the blood (10%), and the CSF (10%).

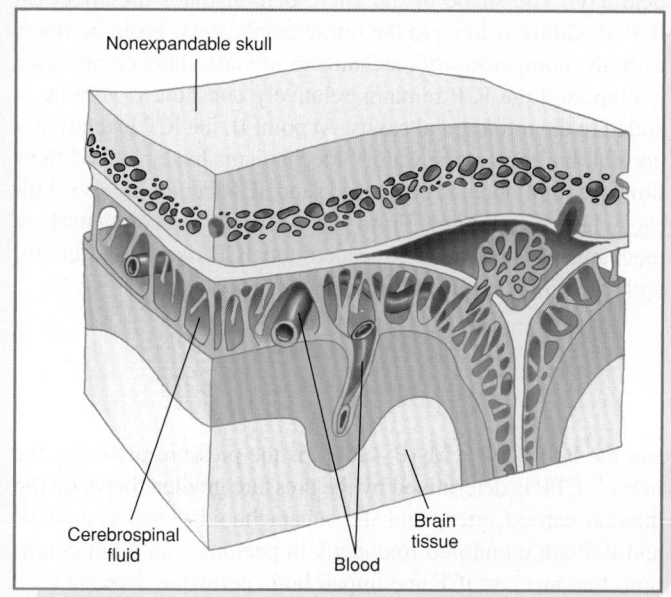

Nonexpandable skull

Cerebrospinal fluid

Blood

Brain tissue

2. Monro–Kellie Hypothesis

Normally, a reciprocal relationship exists among the three intracranial volumes such that the ICP is maintained within normal limits. Because these volumes are practically incompressible, a change in one component must be balanced by an almost equal and opposite effect in one or both of the remaining components. This is known as the *Monro–Kellie hypothesis.*

Of the three intracranial volumes, the fluid in the CSF compartment is the most easily displaced. The CSF (A) can be displaced from the ventricles and cerebral subarachnoid space to the spinal subarachnoid space, and it can also undergo increased absorption or decreased production. Because most of the blood in the cranial cavity is contained in the low-pressure venous system, venous compression (B) serves as a means of displacing blood volume.

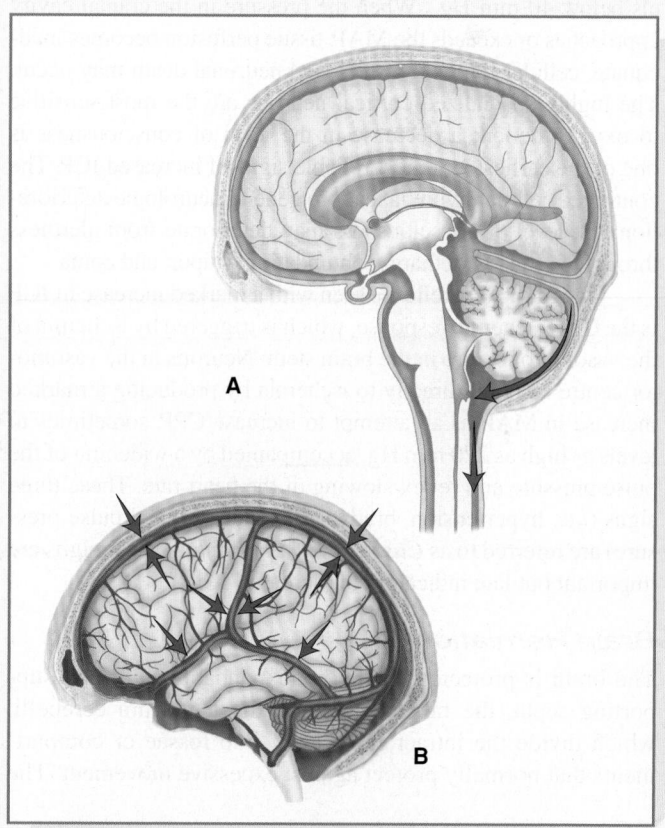

A

B

3. Compliance and the Volume–Pressure Curve

Compliance, which refers to the ease with which a substance can be compressed or deformed, is a measure of the brain's ability to maintain its ICP during changes in intracranial volume. Compliance (C) represents the ratio of change (Δ) in volume (V) to change in pressure (P): $C = \Delta V / \Delta P$.

The dynamic effects of changes in intracranial volume and compliance on ICP can be illustrated on a graph with the volume represented on the horizontal axis and ICP on the vertical axis. The shape of the curve demonstrates the effect on ICP of adding volume to the intracranial cavity. From points A to B, the compensatory mechanisms are adequate, compliance is high, and the ICP remains relatively constant as volume is added to the intracranial cavity. At point B, the ICP is relatively normal, but the compensatory mechanisms have reached their limits, compliance is decreased, and ICP begins to rise with each change in volume. From points C to D, the compensatory mechanisms have been exceeded and ICP rises significantly with each increase in volume as compliance is lost.

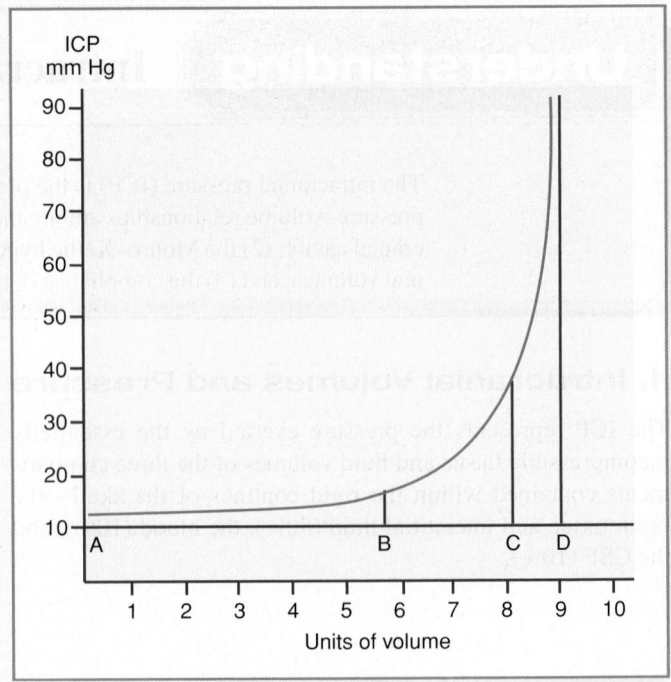

and the ICP (CPP = MAP – ICP), is the pressure perfusing the brain.[15] CPP is determined by the pressure gradient between the internal carotid artery and the subarachnoid veins. The MAP and ICP are monitored frequently in persons with brain conditions that increase ICP and impair brain perfusion. Normal CPP ranges from 70 to 100 mm Hg. Brain ischemia develops at levels below 40 mm Hg.[2] When the pressure in the cranial cavity approaches or exceeds the MAP, tissue perfusion becomes inadequate, cellular hypoxia results, and neuronal death may occur. The highly specialized cortical neurons are the most sensitive to oxygen deficit; a decrease in the level of consciousness is one of the earliest and most reliable signs of increased ICP. The continued cellular hypoxia leads to general neurologic deterioration; the level of consciousness may deteriorate from alertness through confusion, lethargy, obtundation, stupor, and coma.

One of the late reflexes seen with a marked increase in ICP is the CNS ischemic response, which is triggered by ischemia of the vasomotor centre in the brain stem. Neurons in the vasomotor centre respond directly to ischemia by producing a marked increase in MAP as an attempt to increase CPP, sometimes to levels as high as 270 mm Hg, accompanied by a widening of the pulse pressure and reflex slowing of the heart rate. These three signs (*i.e.,* hypertension, bradycardia, and widened pulse pressure) are referred to as *Cushing's triad or reflex*. These signs are important but late indicators of increased ICP.[16]

Brain Herniation

The brain is protected by the nonexpandable skull and supporting septa, the falx cerebri and the tentorium cerebelli, which divide the intracranial cavity into fossae or compartments that normally protect against excessive movement. The

falx cerebri is a sickle-shaped septum that separates the two hemispheres. The tentorium cerebelli divides the cranial cavity into anterior and posterior fossae (Fig. 51.5A). This inflexible dural sheath extends posteriorly from the bony petrous ridges and anterior to the clinoid process, sloping downward and outward from its medial edge to attach laterally to the occipital bone. Extending posteriorly into the centre of the tentorium is a large semicircular opening called the *incisura* or *tentorial notch*. The temporal lobe rests on the tentorial incisura, and the midbrain occupies the anterior portion of the tentorial notch. The cerebellum is closely opposed to the dorsum of the midbrain and fills the posterior part of the notch. Other important anatomic associations exist among the anterior cerebral, internal carotid, posterior communicating, and posterior and superior cerebellar arteries and the incisura (Fig. 51.5B). The oculomotor nerve (cranial nerve III) emerges from the mediolateral surface of each peduncle just caudal to the tentorium.

Brain herniation represents a displacement of brain tissue under the falx cerebri or through the tentorial notch or incisura of the tentorium cerebelli. It occurs when an elevated ICP in one brain compartment causes displacement of the cerebral tissue toward an area of lower ICP. The different types of herniation syndromes are based on the area of the brain that has herniated and the structure under which it has been pushed (Fig. 51.5). They commonly are divided into two broad categories, supratentorial and infratentorial, based on whether they are located above or below the tentorium.

Supratentorial Herniations. Three major patterns of supratentorial herniation were described by Plum and Posner in their classic work: cingulate, central transtentorial, and uncal

FIGURE 51.5 • Supporting septa of the brain and patterns of herniation. **A:** The falx cerebri [1], tentorium cerebelli [2], foramen magnum [3]. **B:** The location of the incisura or tentorial notch in relation to the cerebral arteries and oculomotor nerve. **C:** Herniation of the cingulate gyrus under the falx cerebri [1], central or transtentorial herniation [2], uncal herniation of the temporal lobe into the tentorial notch [3], and infratentorial herniation of the cerebellar tonsils [4]. (Courtesy of Carole Hilmer, CMI.)

transtentorial.[17] Table 51.5 describes the key structures and clinical signs of these three types of herniations. Of the three, cingulate herniation poses the least serious threat in terms of clinical outcomes.[2] Transtentorial herniations result in two distinct syndromes: an uncal syndrome and a central syndrome. Clinically, they display distinct patterns early in their course, but both merge in a similar pattern once they begin to involve the midbrain level and below (brain stem structures). In addition, alterations of consciousness vary depending on the herniation pattern.[18]

Cingulate herniation involves displacement of the cingulate gyrus and hemisphere beneath the sharp edges of the falx cerebri to the opposite side of the brain. Displacement of the falx can compress the local brain tissue and blood supply from the anterior cerebral artery, causing ischemia and edema, which further increase ICP levels. Unilateral or bilateral leg weakness is an early sign of impending cingulate herniation.

Central transtentorial herniations involve the downward displacement of the cerebral hemispheres, basal ganglia, diencephalon, and midbrain through the tentorial incisura. The diencephalon may be compressed tightly against the midbrain with such force that edema and hemorrhage result. It may or may not be associated with uncal or lateral herniation. In the early diencephalic stage, there is clouding of consciousness, bilaterally small pupils (approximately 2 mm in diameter) with a full range of constriction, and motor responses to pain that are purposeful or semipurposeful (localizing) and often asymmetric. The change in consciousness, which is often a first sign of central herniations, is caused by pressure on the reticular activating system (RAS) in the upper midbrain, which is responsible for wakefulness. As the herniation progresses to the late diencephalic stage, painful stimulation results in decorticate posturing, which may be asymmetric (Fig. 51.3A), and there is waxing and waning of respirations with periods of apnea (Cheyne–Stokes respirations). With midbrain involvement, the pupils are fixed and midsize (approximately 5 mm in diameter), and reflex adduction of the eyes is impaired; pain elicits cerebrate posturing (Fig. 51.3B); and respirations

TABLE 51.5 KEY STRUCTURES AND CLINICAL SIGNS OF CINGULATE, CENTRAL, AND UNCAL HERNIATIONS

HERNIATION SYNDROME	KEY STRUCTURES INVOLVED	KEY CLINICAL SIGNS
Cingulate	Anterior cerebral artery	Leg weakness
Central transtentorial	Reticular activating system	Altered level of consciousness
	Corticospinal tract	Decorticate posturing
		Rostral–caudal deterioration
Uncal	Cerebral peduncle	Hemiparesis
	Oculomotor nerve	Ipsilateral pupil dilation
	Posterior cerebral artery	Visual field loss
	Cerebellar tonsil	
	Respiratory centre	Respiratory arrest

change from Cheyne–Stokes to neurogenic hyperventilation, in which the frequency may exceed 40 breaths per minute because of uninhibited stimulation of the inspiratory and expiratory centres. Progression of brain herniation involving the lower pons and upper medulla produces fixed, midpoint (3- to 5-mm) pupils with loss of reflex abduction and adduction of the eyes, and absence of motor responses or only leg flexion on painful stimuli. Once the area of herniation has progressed beyond the diencephalon and into the midbrain and brain stem, the process is generally irreversible and the prognosis is extremely poor.[2]

Uncal herniation occurs when a lateral mass pushes the brain tissue centrally and forces the medial aspect of the temporal lobe, which contains the uncus and hippocampal gyrus, under the edge of the tentorial incisura and into the posterior fossa. As a result, the diencephalon and midbrain are compressed and displaced laterally to the opposite side of the tentorium. Cranial nerve III (oculomotor nerve) and the posterior cerebral artery frequently are caught between the uncus and the tentorium. The oculomotor nerve controls pupillary constriction; entrapment of this nerve results in ipsilateral pupillary dilation, which usually is an early sign of uncal herniation. Consciousness may be unimpaired because the RAS has not yet been affected. However, after any signs of herniation or brain stem compression appear, deterioration may proceed rapidly, making it important to recognize the distinguishing early features of uncal herniations.

As uncal herniations progress, the descending motor pathways become compressed, causing changes in motor strength and coordination of voluntary movements. It is not unusual for initial changes in motor function to occur ipsilateral to the side of the brain damage because of compression of the contralateral cerebral peduncles. This may result in a false localizing sign of hemiparesis on the same side as cranial nerve III, rather than on the opposite side, which would be the case if a singular lesion in the midbrain were the cause. As the condition progresses, bilateral positive Babinski responses and respiratory changes (*e.g.,* Cheyne–Stokes respirations, ataxic patterns) occur. Decorticate and decerebrate posturing may develop, followed by dilated, fixed pupils, flaccidity, and respiratory arrest.

Infratentorial Herniation. Infratentorial herniation results from increased pressure in the infratentorial compartment. It often progresses rapidly and can cause death because it is likely to involve the lower brain stem centres that control vital cardiopulmonary functions. Herniation may occur superiorly (upward) through the tentorial incisura or inferiorly (downward) through the foramen magnum.

Upward displacement of brain tissue can cause blockage of the aqueduct of Sylvius and lead to hydrocephalus and coma. Downward displacement of the midbrain through the tentorial notch or of the cerebellar tonsils through the foramen magnum can interfere with medullary functioning and cause cardiac or respiratory arrest. In cases of pre-existing ICP elevations, herniation may occur when the pressure is released from below, such as in a lumbar puncture. If the CSF pathway is blocked and fluid cannot leave the ventricles, the volume expands, and fluid is displaced downward through the tentorial notch. The expanding volume causes all function at a given level to cease as destruction progresses in a rostral-to-caudal direction. The result of this displacement is brain stem ischemia and hemorrhage extending from the diencephalon to the pons. If the lesion expands rapidly, displacement and obstruction occur quickly, leading to irreversible infarction and hemorrhage.

Cerebral Edema

Cerebral edema, or brain swelling, is an increase in tissue volume secondary to abnormal fluid accumulation. There are two types of cerebral edema: vasogenic and cytotoxic.[5] Vasogenic edema occurs when integrity of the blood–brain barrier is disrupted, allowing fluid to escape into the extracellular fluid that surrounds brain cells. Cytotoxic edema involves the actual swelling of brain cells themselves. Cerebral edema may or may not increase ICP. The impact of cerebral edema depends on the brain's compensatory mechanisms and the extent of the swelling.

Vasogenic Edema. Vasogenic edema occurs with conditions that impair the function of the blood–brain barrier and allow transfer of water and protein from the vascular into the interstitial space. It occurs in conditions such as tumours, prolonged ischemia, hemorrhage, brain injury, and infectious processes (*e.g.,* meningitis). Vasogenic edema occurs primarily in the white matter of the brain, possibly because the white matter is more compliant than the grey matter. Vasogenic edema can displace a cerebral hemisphere and can be responsible for various types of herniation. The functional manifestations of vasogenic edema include focal neurologic deficits, disturbances in consciousness, and severe intracranial hypertension.

Cytotoxic Edema. Cytotoxic edema involves an increase in intracellular fluid. It can result from hypoosmotic states such as water intoxication or severe ischemia that impair the function of the sodium–potassium membrane pump. Ischemia also results in the inadequate removal of anaerobic metabolic end products such as lactic acid, producing extracellular acidosis. If blood flow is reduced to low levels for extended periods or to extremely low levels for a few minutes, cellular edema can cause the cell membrane to rupture, allowing the escape of intracellular contents into the surrounding extracellular fluid. This leads to damage of neighbouring cells. The altered osmotic conditions result in water entry and cell swelling. Major changes in cerebral function, such as stupor and coma, occur with cytotoxic edema. The edema associated with ischemia may be severe enough to produce cerebral infarction with necrosis of brain tissue.

Treatment. Although cerebral edema is viewed as a pathologic process, it does not necessarily disrupt brain function unless it increases the ICP. The localized edema surrounding a brain tumour often responds to corticosteroid therapy (*e.g.*, dexamethasone), but use of these drugs for generalized edema is controversial. The mechanism of action of the corticosteroid drugs in the treatment of cerebral edema is unknown, but in therapeutic doses, they seem to stabilize cell membranes and scavenge free radicals. Osmotic diuretics (*e.g.*, mannitol) may be useful in the acute phase of vasogenic and cytotoxic edema when hypo-osmolarity is present.

Hydrocephalus

Enlargement of the CSF compartment occurs with hydrocephalus, which is defined as an abnormal increase in CSF volume in any part or all of the ventricular system. The two causes of hydrocephalus are decreased absorption of CSF and overproduction of CSF. There are two types of hydrocephalus: noncommunicating and communicating.

Noncommunicating or obstructive hydrocephalus occurs when obstruction in the ventricular system prevents the CSF from reaching the arachnoid villi. CSF flow can be obstructed by congenital malformations, from tumours encroaching on the ventricular system, and by inflammation or hemorrhage. The ependyma (*i.e.*, lining of ventricles and CSF-filled spaces) is especially sensitive to viral infections, particularly during embryonic development; ependymitis is believed to be the cause of congenital aqueductal stenosis.[9]

Communicating hydrocephalus is caused by impaired reabsorption of CSF from the arachnoid villi into the venous system. Decreased absorption can result from a block in the CSF pathway to the arachnoid villi or a failure of the villi to transfer the CSF to the venous system. It can occur if too few villi are formed, if postinfective (meningitis) scarring occludes them, or if the villi become obstructed with fragments of blood or infectious debris. Adenomas of the choroid plexus can cause an overproduction of CSF. This form of hydrocephalus is much less common than that resulting from decreased absorption of CSF.

Similar pathologic patterns occur with noncommunicating and communicating types of hydrocephalus. The cerebral hemispheres become enlarged, and the ventricular system beyond the point of obstruction is dilated. The sulci on the surface of the brain become effaced and shallow, and the white matter is reduced in volume. The presence and extent of the ICP is determined by fluid accumulation and the type of hydrocephalus, the age at onset, and the rapidity and extent of pressure rise. Computed tomographic (CT) and magnetic resonance imaging (MRI) scans are used to diagnose all types of hydrocephalus. The usual treatment is a shunting procedure, which provides an alternative route for return of CSF to the circulation.

Signs and symptoms of hydrocephalus vary greatly, depending on the rapidity of onset. When hydrocephalus develops in utero or before the cranial sutures have fused in infancy, the ventricles expand beyond the point of obstruction, the cranial sutures separate, the head expands, and there is bulging of the fontanels. Because the skull is able to expand, signs of increased ICP may be absent, and intelligence spared.

However, seizures are not uncommon, and in severe cases, optic nerve atrophy leads to blindness. Weakness and uncoordinated movement are common. Surgical placement of a shunt allows for diversion of excess CSF fluid, preventing extreme enlargement of the head and neurologic deficits.

In adults, head enlargement does not occur because the cranial sutures are fully fused. Thus, signs and symptoms are likely to occur earlier. Slowly developing hydrocephalus is unlikely to produce an increase in ICP, but it may still produce deficits such as progressive dementia and gait changes, as in normal-pressure hydrocephalus ("pseudotumour cerebri") in older adults. In contrast, acute-onset hydrocephalus in adults usually is marked by symptoms of increased ICP, including headache, vomiting, and papilledema, or lateral rectus palsy from pressure effects on the cranial nerves. If the obstruction is not relieved, progression to herniation ensues (see previous discussion of herniation). Treatment includes surgical decompression and shunting.

Traumatic Head Injury

The brain is enclosed in the protective confines of the rigid bony skull. Although the skull generally affords protection to the soft tissues of the CNS from external forces, it also imposes risks as a source of injury from internal forces. The bony structures of the internal surface of the skull can induce traumatic and ischemic brain injuries when intracranial tissues increase in volume (swelling or bleeding) or shift (swelling or mechanical trauma). Furthermore, fractures of the skull can compress sections of the nervous system and cause penetrating wounds.

The term *head injury* is used to describe all structural damage to the head and has become synonymous with *traumatic brain injury.*[19] In Canada, the impact of head injury is most prevalent in the young (birth to 19) and older (above 60) age groups.[20] Interestingly, Canada has seen a 35% decline in hospitalizations due to traumatic head injuries in the last 10 years. In the young (birth to 19 years of age), hospital admissions rates have fallen 53%.[20]

Head injuries can involve both closed injuries and open wounds. Skull fractures can be divided into three groups: simple, depressed, and basilar. A simple or linear skull fracture is a break in the continuity of bone. A comminuted skull fracture refers to a splintered or multiple fracture line. When bone fragments are embedded into the brain tissue, the fracture is said to be depressed. A fracture of the bones that form the base of the skull is called a basilar skull fracture.

Radiologic examination usually is needed to confirm the presence and extent of a skull fracture. This evaluation is important because of the possible damage to the underlying tissues. The ethmoid cribriform plate, through which the olfactory fibres enter the skull, represents the most fragile portion of the neurocranium and is shattered in basal skull fractures. A frequent complication of basilar skull fractures is leakage of CSF from the nose (rhinorrhea) or ear (otorrhea); this occurs because of the proximity of the base of the skull to the nose and ears. This break in protection of the brain becomes a probable source of infection of the meninges or of brain substance. There may be lacerations to the vessels of the dura, with resultant intracranial bleeding. Skull fractures can damage the cranial nerves (I, II, III, VII, and VIII) as they exit the cranial vault.

Types of Brain Injuries

The effects of traumatic head injuries can be divided into two categories: primary or direct injuries, in which damage is caused by impact; and secondary injuries, in which damage results from the subsequent brain swelling, infection, or cerebral hypoxia.[19] The direct brain injuries include diffuse axonal injury and the focal lesions of laceration, contusion, and hemorrhage. Secondary brain injuries are often diffuse or multifocal, including concussion, infection, and hypoxic brain injury. Although the skull and CSF provide protection for the brain, they can also contribute to trauma. When the mechanical forces inducing head injury cause bouncing of the brain in the closed confines of the rigid skull, a coup–contrecoup injury occurs. Because the brain floats freely in the CSF, blunt force to the head accelerates the brain within the skull, and then the brain decelerates abruptly on hitting the inner skull surfaces. The direct contusion of the brain at the site of external force is referred to as a *coup* injury, whereas the rebound injury on the opposite side of the brain is the *contrecoup* injury. As the brain strikes the rough surface of the cranial vault, brain tissue, blood vessels, nerve tracts, and other structures are bruised and torn, resulting in contusions and hematomas.

Ischemia is considered the most common cause of secondary brain injury. It can result from the hypoxia and hypotension that occur during the resuscitation process or from the impairment of regulatory mechanisms by which cerebrovascular responses maintain an adequate blood flow and oxygen supply.[19,21] Insults that occur immediately after injury or in the course of resuscitation efforts are important determinants of the outcome from severe brain injury. More than 25% of patients with severe head injury sustain one or more secondary insults in the time between injury and resuscitation, indicating the need for improved airway management and circulatory status. The significance of secondary injuries depends in part upon the extent of damage caused by the primary injury. Certain secondary injuries have been discussed, including increased ICP, cerebral edema, and brain herniation.

In mild head injury, there may be momentary loss of consciousness without demonstrable neurologic symptoms or residual damage, except for possible residual amnesia. Microscopic neuroinflammatory changes usually can be detected in the neurons and glia within hours of injury, but brain imaging is negative.[21] Concussion refers to "a complex pathophysiologic process affecting the brain, induced by traumatic biomechanical forces."[19] Although recovery usually takes place within 24 hours, about 10% to 15% of persons with a mild head injury experience symptoms, such as headache, irritability, insomnia, and poor concentration and memory, that persist after 1 year. This is known as the *postconcussion syndrome*.[19]

The memory loss usually includes an interval of time preceding the injury (retrograde amnesia) and after the injury (anterograde amnesia). The duration of retrograde amnesia correlates with the severity of the brain injury. Because these cognitive complaints are vague and subjective, they sometimes are regarded as being of psychological origin. Postconcussion syndrome can have a significant effect on interpersonal relationships, activities of daily living and return to employment. Persons with postconcussion syndrome may need cognitive retraining, medications, and/or psychological support. Additional concussions, such as might occur with contact sports, increase the risk of altered function and symptoms.

In moderate head injury, many small hemorrhages and some swelling of brain tissue occur. These contusions often are distributed along the rough, irregular inner surface of the brain and are more likely to occur in the frontal or temporal lobes, resulting in cognitive and motor deficits. Moderate head injury is characterized by a period of unconsciousness and may be associated with focal manifestations such as hemiparesis, aphasia, and cranial nerve palsy. In this type of injury, the contusions often can be visualized on CT scan.

Severe head injury involves deficits to arousal, usually coma, and extensive mechanical and secondary damage to brain structures. In severe head injury, contusions and intracerebral, subdural, epidural, and subarachnoid hemorrhages are often evident on CT scan. The mechanical damage is instantaneous and irreversible, resulting from shearing and pressure forces that cause diffuse axonal injury, disruption of blood vessels, and tissue damage. Often, there are severe neurologic deficits such as coma, hemiplegia, and all the other signs of elevated ICP (see earlier). Severe head injuries do not usually occur in isolation. Often there is injury to other parts of the body such as extremities, chest, and abdomen, which often limits the examiner's ability to carefully assess neurologic deficits.

Hematomas

Hematomas result from vascular injury and bleeding. Depending on the anatomic position of the ruptured vessel, bleeding can occur in any of several compartments, including the epidural, subdural, and subarachnoid spaces or into the brain itself (intracerebral hematoma).

Epidural Hematoma. Epidural hematomas usually are caused by head injury in which the skull is fractured. An epidural (extradural) hematoma is one that develops between the inner table of the bones of the skull and the dura (Fig. 51.6). It usually results from a tear in an artery, most often the middle meningeal, usually in association with a skull fracture.[5] Because bleeding is arterial in origin, rapid expansion of the hematoma compresses the brain. Anatomically, injury to the temporal lobe has a significantly high risk for epidural hematomas. Epidural hematoma more commonly occurs in a young person because the dura is less firmly attached to the skull surface than in an older person; as a consequence, the dura can be easily separated from the inner surface of the skull, allowing the hematoma to grow.

Anterior

Epidural
hematoma

Subdural
hematoma

Intracerebral
hematoma

Posterior

FIGURE 51.6 • Location of epidural, subdural, and intracerebral hematomas.

Typically, a person with an epidural hematoma presents with a history of head injury and a brief period of unconsciousness followed by a lucid period in which consciousness is regained, followed by rapid progression to unconsciousness. The lucid interval does not always occur or may be missed as it is brief, but when observed, it is of great diagnostic value. With rapidly developing unconsciousness, there are focal symptoms related to the area of the brain involved. These symptoms can include ipsilateral (same side) pupil dilation and contralateral (opposite side) hemiparesis from uncal herniation. If the hematoma is not removed, the condition progresses, with increased ICP, tentorial herniation, and death. However, prognosis is excellent if the hematoma is removed before loss of consciousness occurs.

Subdural Hematoma. A subdural hematoma develops in the area between the dura and the arachnoid (subdural space) and usually is the result of a tear in the small bridging veins that connect veins on the surface of the cortex to dural sinuses (Fig. 51.6). The bridging veins pass from the pial vessels through the CSF-filled subarachnoid space, penetrate the arachnoid and the dura, and empty into the intradural sinuses.[9] These veins are readily snapped in head injury when the brain moves suddenly in relation to the cranium. Bleeding can occur between the dura and arachnoid (*i.e.,* subdural hematoma) or into the CSF-filled subarachnoid space (*i.e.,* subarachnoid hematoma).

The venous source of bleeding in a subdural hematoma develops more slowly than the arterial bleeding in an epidural hematoma. Subdural hematomas are classified as acute, subacute, or chronic. This classification system is based on the approximate time before the appearance of symptoms. Symptoms of acute hematoma are seen within 24 hours of the injury, whereas subacute hematoma does not produce symptoms until 2 to 10 days after injury. Symptoms of chronic subdural hematoma may not arise until several weeks after the injury, particularly in older adults.

Acute subdural hematomas progress rapidly and have a high mortality rate because of the severe secondary injuries related to edema and increased ICP. The high mortality rate has been associated with uncontrolled ICP increase, loss of consciousness, decerebrate posturing, and delay in surgical removal of the hematoma. The clinical picture is similar to that of epidural hematoma, except that there usually is no lucid interval. Morbidity and mortality rates are higher with acute subdural hematoma than with epidural and intracerebral hematoma. By contrast, in subacute hematoma, there may be a period of improvement in the level of consciousness and neurologic symptoms, only to be followed by deterioration if the hematoma is not removed.

Symptoms of chronic subdural hematoma develop weeks after a head injury, so much later that the person may not remember having had a head injury. Chronic subdural hematoma is more common in older persons because brain atrophy causes the brain to shrink away from the dura and stretch fragile bridging veins. These veins rupture, causing slow seepage of blood into the subdural space. Fibroblastic activity causes the hematoma to become encapsulated. The sanguineous fluid in this encapsulated area has high osmotic pressure and draws in fluid from the surrounding subarachnoid space; the mass expands, exerting pressure on the cranial contents. In some instances, the clinical picture is less defined, with the most prominent symptom being a decreasing level of consciousness indicated by drowsiness, confusion, headache, and apathy.

Traumatic Intracerebral Hematomas. Traumatic intracerebral hematomas may be single or multiple. They can occur in any lobe of the brain but are most common in the frontal or temporal lobes, related to the bony prominences on the inner skull surface (Fig. 51.7). They may occur in association with the severe motion that the brain undergoes during head injury, or a contusion can coalesce into a hematoma. Intracerebral hematomas occur more frequently in older persons and alcoholics, whose cerebral vessels are more friable.

The signs and symptoms produced by an intracerebral hematoma depend on its size and location in the brain. Signs of increased ICP can be manifested if the hematoma is large and encroaching on vital structures. A hematoma in the temporal lobe can be dangerous because of the potential for lateral herniation.

Treatment of an intracerebral hematoma can be medical or surgical depending on the size and impact of the hematoma. For a large hematoma with a rapidly deteriorating neurologic

Epidural hematoma

Cerebral contusions

Subarachnoid hemorrhage

FIGURE 51.7 • Computed tomography scan of brain in traumatic brain injury, showing hemorrhagic cerebral contusions in right temporal and bifrontal lobes, subarachnoid hemorrhage, and epidural hematoma.

condition, surgery to evacuate the clot usually is indicated. Surgery may not be needed in someone who is neurologically stable despite neurologic deficits; in this case, the hematoma may resolve spontaneously much like a contusion.

IN SUMMARY

Many of the agents that cause brain damage do so through common pathways, including hypoxia or ischemia, accumulation of excitatory neurotransmitters, increased ICP, and cerebral edema. Deprivation of oxygen (*i.e.,* hypoxia) or blood flow (*i.e.,* ischemia) can have deleterious effects on the brain structures. Focal ischemia causes localized brain injury, as in stroke. Global ischemia, as in cardiac arrest, occurs when blood flow to the entire brain is inadequate, causing global deficits such as altered mental status.

The term head injury is used to describe all structural damage to the head and has become synonymous with brain injury. The effects of traumatic head injuries can be divided into two categories: primary and secondary injuries. Primary injuries result from direct impact, resulting in skull fracture, concussion, or contusion. In secondary injuries, damage results from the subsequent brain swelling; epidural, subdural, or intracerebral hematoma formation; infection; cerebral hypoxia; and ischemia. Even if there is no break in the skull, a blow to the head can cause severe and diffuse brain damage. Such closed injuries vary in severity and can be classified as focal or diffuse. Diffuse injuries include concussion and diffuse axonal injury. Focal injuries include contusion, laceration, and hemorrhage.

Brain injury is manifested by alterations in sensory and motor function and by changes in the level of consciousness. Consciousness is a state of awareness of self and environment. It exists on a continuum from normal wakefulness and sleep to the pathologic states of stupor and coma. In progressive brain injury, the onset of coma may follow a rostral-to-caudal progression with characteristic changes in levels of consciousness, respiratory activity, pupillary and oculovestibular reflexes, and muscle tone occurring as the diencephalon through the medulla are affected.

Brain death is defined as the irreversible loss of function of the brain, including that of the brain stem. Clinical examination must disclose at least the absence of responsiveness, brain stem reflexes, and respiratory effort. The vegetative state is characterized by loss of all cognitive functions and the unawareness of self and surroundings, whereas reflex and vegetative functions remain intact.

CEREBROVASCULAR DISEASE

After completing this section of the chapter, you should be able to meet the following objectives:

- List the major vessels in the cerebral circulation and state the contribution of the internal carotid arteries, the vertebral arteries, and the circle of Willis to the cerebral circulation.
- Describe the autoregulation of cerebral blood flow.
- Explain the substitution of "brain attack" for stroke in terms of making a case for early diagnosis and treatment.
- Differentiate the pathologies of ischemic and hemorrhagic stroke.
- Explain the significance of transient ischemic attacks, the ischemic penumbra, and watershed zones of infarction and how these conditions relate to ischemic stroke.
- Cite the most common cause of subarachnoid hemorrhage and state the complications associated with subarachnoid hemorrhage.
- Describe the alterations in cerebral vasculature that occur with arteriovenous malformations.
- Describe the patterns of motor deficits and typical problems with speech and language that occur as a result of stroke.

Cerebrovascular disease encompasses a number of disorders involving vessels in the cerebral circulation. These disorders include stroke and transient ischemic attacks (TIAs), aneurysmal subarachnoid hemorrhage, and arteriovenous malformations.

Cerebral Circulation

Cerebral Blood Vessels

The blood flow to the brain is supplied by the two internal carotid arteries anteriorly and the vertebral arteries posteriorly (Fig. 51.8A). The internal carotid artery, a terminal branch of the common carotid artery, branches into several arteries: ophthalmic, posterior communicating, anterior choroidal, anterior cerebral, and middle cerebral (Fig. 51.8B). Most of the arterial blood in the internal carotid arteries is distributed through the anterior and middle cerebral arteries. The anterior cerebral arteries supply the medial surface of the frontal and parietal lobes and the anterior half of the thalamus, the corpus striatum, part of the corpus callosum, and the anterior limb of the internal capsule. The genu and posterior limb of the internal capsule and medial globus pallidus are fed by the anterior choroidal branch of the internal carotid artery. The middle cerebral

artery passes laterally, supplying the lateral basal ganglia and the insula, and then emerges on the lateral cortical surface, supplying the inferior frontal gyrus, the motor and premotor frontal cortex concerned with delicate face and hand control. It is the major vascular source for the language cortices (frontal and superior temporal), the primary and association auditory cortex (superior temporal gyrus), and the primary and association somesthetic cortex for the face and hand (postcentral gyrus, parietal). The middle cerebral artery is functionally a continuation of the internal carotid; emboli of the internal carotid most frequently become lodged in branches of the middle cerebral artery. The consequences of ischemia of these areas may be the most devastating, resulting in damage to the fine manipulative skills of the face and upper limbs and to receptive and expressive communication functions (*e.g.,* aphasia).

The two vertebral arteries arise from the subclavian artery, enter the foramina in the transverse spinal processes at

FIGURE 51.8 • Cerebral circulation. **A:** Branches of the right external carotid artery. The internal carotid artery ascends to the base of the brain. The right vertebral artery is also shown as it ascends through the transverse foramen of the cervical vertebrae. **B:** The cerebral arterial circle (circle of Willis).

the level of the sixth cervical vertebra, and continue upward through the foramina of the upper six vertebrae; they wind behind the atlas, enter the skull through the foramen magnum, and unite to form the basilar artery, which then diverges to terminate in the posterior cerebral arteries. Branches of the basilar and vertebral arteries supply the medulla, pons, cerebellum, midbrain, and caudal part of the diencephalon. The posterior cerebral arteries supply the remaining occipital and inferior regions of the temporal lobes and the thalamus.

The distal branches of the internal carotid and vertebral arteries communicate at the base of the brain through the circle of Willis; this anastomosis of arteries can provide continued circulation if blood flow through one of the main vessels is disrupted (Fig. 51.8B). For instance, occlusion of one middle cerebral artery may have limited consequences if the anterior and posterior communicating arteries are patent, allowing collateral flow from the ipsilateral posterior cerebral and opposite carotid arteries. Without collateral input, cessation of blood flow in cerebral arteries results in ischemic neural damage as metabolic needs of electrically active cells exceed nutrient supply.

The cerebral circulation is drained by two sets of veins that empty into the dural venous sinuses: the deep (great) cerebral venous system and the superficial venous system. In contrast to the superficial cerebral veins that travel through the pia mater on the surface of the cerebral cortex, the deep system is well protected. These vessels connect directly to the sagittal sinuses in the falx cerebri by bridging veins. They travel through the CSF-filled subarachnoid space and penetrate the arachnoid and then the dura to reach the dural venous sinuses. This system of sinuses returns blood to the heart primarily through the internal jugular veins. Alternate routes for venous flow also exist; for example, venous blood may exit through the emissary veins that pass through the skull and through veins that traverse various foramina to empty into extracranial veins.

The intracranial venous system has no valves. The direction of flow depends on gravity or the relative pressure in the venous sinuses compared with that of the extracranial veins. Increases in intrathoracic pressure, as can occur with coughing or performance of the Valsalva maneuvre (*i.e.,* exhaling against a closed glottis), produce a rise in central venous pressure that is reflected back into the internal jugular veins and to the dural sinuses. This briefly raises the ICP.

Regulation of Cerebral Blood Flow

The blood flow to the brain is maintained at approximately 750 ml/min or one sixth of the resting cardiac output.[16] The regulation of blood flow to the brain is controlled largely by autoregulatory or local mechanisms that respond to the metabolic needs of the brain. Cerebral autoregulation has been classically defined as the ability of the brain to maintain constant cerebral blood flow despite changes in systemic arterial pressure. This allows the cerebral cortex to adjust cerebral blood flow locally to satisfy its metabolic needs. The autoregulation of cerebral blood flow is maintained within a MAP range of approximately 60 to 140 mm Hg.[16] Although total cerebral blood flow remains relatively stable throughout marked

changes in cardiac output and arterial blood pressure, regional blood flow may vary markedly in response to local changes in metabolism. If mean arterial blood pressure falls below 60 mm Hg, cerebral blood flow becomes severely compromised, and if it rises above the upper limit of autoregulation, blood flow increases rapidly and overstretches the cerebral vessels. In persons with hypertension, this autoregulatory range shifts to higher MAP levels.

At least three metabolic factors affect cerebral blood flow: carbon dioxide, and hydrogen ion and oxygen concentration. Increased carbon dioxide provides a potent stimulus for vasodilation—a doubling of the PCO_2 in the blood results in a doubling of cerebral blood flow. Increased hydrogen ion concentrations also increase cerebral blood flow, serving to wash away the neurally depressive acidic materials.[16] Profound extracellular acidosis induces vasomotor paralysis, in which case cerebral blood flow may depend entirely on the systemic arterial blood pressure. Decreased oxygen concentration also increases cerebral blood flow.

The deep cerebral blood vessels appear to be completely controlled by autoregulation. However, the superficial and major cerebral blood vessels are innervated by the sympathetic nervous system. Under normal physiologic conditions, local regulatory and autoregulatory mechanisms override the effects of sympathetic stimulation. However, when local mechanisms fail, sympathetic control of cerebral blood pressure becomes important.[16] For example, when the arterial pressure rises to very high levels during strenuous exercise or in other conditions, the sympathetic nervous system constricts the large and intermediate-sized superficial blood vessels as a means of protecting the smaller, more easily damaged vessels. Sympathetic reflexes are believed to cause vasospasm in the intermediate and large arteries in some types of brain damage, such as that caused by rupture of a cerebral aneurysm.

Stroke (Brain Attack)

Stroke is the syndrome of acute focal neurologic deficit from a vascular disorder that injures brain tissue. Stroke is the number one cause of adult disability in Canada and the third leading cause of death.[22–27] Each year, approximately 50,000 Canadians (one every 10 minutes) have a stroke and about 315,000 are living in the community with the effects of a stroke, which can include a range of disabilities. Although mortality rates from strokes have greatly decreased over the past 10 years, there has been an increase in strokes in younger people; strokes have risen 24% among people in their 50s.[23] More women than men die from stroke. In addition, ethnic populations such as African, South Asian, First Nations, Inuit and Métis, who are more at risk for hypertension and diabetes, are at a greater risk for stroke.[24] The term *brain attack* has been promoted to raise awareness that time-dependent tissue damage occurs and that rapid emergency treatment is necessary, similar to that with heart attack.

There are two main types of strokes: ischemic and hemorrhagic. Ischemic strokes are caused by an interruption of

BOX 51.1	STROKE RISK FACTORS

Unmodifiable Factors	Modifiable Factors
• Age	• Hypertension
• Sex	• Hyperlipidemia
• Race	• Smoking
• Heredity	• Diabetes
	• Heart disease
	Atrial fibrillation
	Wall motion defects
	• Carotid disease
	• Coagulation disorders
	• Obesity/inactivity
	• Heavy alcohol use
	• llicit drug use

STROKE/BRAIN ATTACK

- Stroke is an acute focal neurologic deficit due to a disturbance in the blood vessels supplying the brain. It can be due to ischemia caused by thrombi or emboli that interrupt blood flow or rupture of a blood vessel with bleeding into brain tissue.
- The term *brain attack* as a description for stroke is intended to alert people to the need for immediate treatment at the first sign of a stroke.
- During the evolution of an ischemic stroke, there usually is a central core of dead or dying cells surrounded by an ischemic band of minimally perfused cells called a *penumbra*. Whether the cells of the penumbra continue to survive depends on the successful timely return of adequate circulation.
- The realization that there is a window of opportunity during which ischemic but viable brain tissue can be salvaged has led to the use of fibrinolytic agents in the early treatment of ischemic stroke.

blood flow in a cerebral vessel and are the most common type of stroke, accounting for 80% of all strokes.[22] The less common hemorrhagic strokes are caused by bleeding into brain tissue. This type of stroke usually is from a blood vessel rupture caused by hypertension, aneurysm, arteriovenous malformation, head injury, or blood dyscrasias and has a much higher fatality rate than ischemic strokes.

Risk Factors

Among the major risk factors for stroke are age, sex, race, family history, hypertension, smoking, diabetes mellitus, asymptomatic carotid stenosis, sickle cell disease, hyperlipidemia, and atrial fibrillation[23] (Box 51.1). The incidence of stroke increases with age, with men's stroke incidence rates being greater than women's at younger ages, but not at older ages. Because women live longer than men, more women die of stroke each year. Blood pressure is a powerful determinant of stroke risk. Persons with a blood pressure less than 120/80 mm Hg have about half the lifetime risk of stroke compared with persons with hypertension.[23] Atrial fibrillation and other conditions that predispose to clot formation on the wall of the heart or valve leaflets, or to paradoxical embolism through right-to-left shunting, predisposes to cardioembolic stroke. Polycythemia, sickle cell disease (during sickle cell crisis), and blood disorders predispose to clot formation in the cerebral vessels.

Other, modifiable risk factors include obesity, physical inactivity, alcohol and drug abuse, hypercoagulability disorders, hormone replacement therapy, and oral contraceptive use.[22–24] Clinical trial data indicate that estrogen plus progestin, as well as estrogen alone, increase stroke risk for generally healthy postmenopausal women, and provide no protection for women with established heart disease.[24] Although extensively used in the past, the use of hormone therapy for protection is no longer recommended (see Chapter 45). Light to moderate alcohol consumption is associated with reduced risk of stroke, but heavier or excessive consumption increases risk for stroke. Illicit drug usage (*i.e.*, cocaine, amphetamines) causes both

ischemic and hemorrhagic strokes by inducing vasospasm, enhanced platelet activity, and increased blood pressure, heart rate, body temperature, and metabolic rate.[28] Cocaine stroke victims range in age from newborn (*i.e.*, from maternal cocaine use) to older adult.

Elimination or control of risk factors for cerebrovascular disease (*e.g.*, use of tobacco, control of blood lipids and blood sugar, reduction of hypertension, anticoagulants with atrial fibrillation) offers the best opportunity to prevent cerebral ischemia from cerebral atherosclerosis. Primary prevention of stroke by early detection and treatment of modifiable risk factors offers significant advantages over waiting until a serious event has occurred.

Ischemic Stroke

Ischemic strokes are caused by cerebrovascular obstruction by thrombosis or emboli (Fig. 51.9). Various methods have been used to classify ischemic cerebrovascular disease. A common classification system identifies the five main mechanisms of stroke as stroke subtypes and their frequency: 20% large artery atherosclerotic disease (both thrombosis and arterial emboli); 25% small vessel or penetrating artery disease (so-called lacunar stroke); 20% cardiogenic embolism; 30% cryptogenic stroke (undetermined cause); and 5% other, unusual causes[2] (*i.e.*, migraine, vessel dissection, coagulopathy).

Ischemic Penumbra in Evolving Stroke. During the evolution of a stroke, there usually is a central core of dead or dying cells, surrounded by an ischemic band or area of minimally perfused cells called the *penumbra* ("halo"). Brain cells of the penumbra receive marginal blood flow, and their metabolic activities are impaired; although the area undergoes an "electrical failure," the structural integrity of the brain cells is maintained.[29] Whether the cells of the penumbra continue to

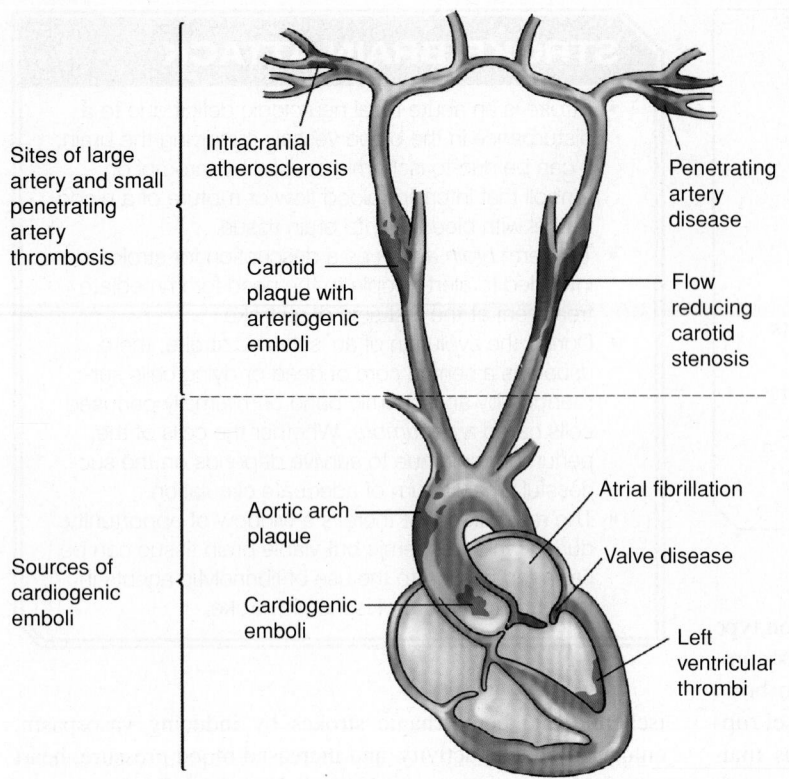

Sites of large artery and small penetrating artery thrombosis

Intracranial atherosclerosis

Penetrating artery disease

Carotid plaque with arteriogenic emboli

Flow reducing carotid stenosis

Sources of cardiogenic emboli

Aortic arch plaque

Atrial fibrillation

Valve disease

Cardiogenic emboli

Left ventricular thrombi

FIGURE 51.9 • The most frequent sites of arterial and cardiac abnormalities causing ischemic stroke. (From Hickey J. V. (2014). The clinical practice of neurological and neurosurgical nursing (7th ed., p. 531). Philadelphia, PA: Lippincott Williams & Wilkins.)

survive depends on the successful timely return of adequate circulation, the volume of toxic products released by the neighbouring dying cells, the degree of cerebral edema, and alterations in local blood flow. If the toxic products result in additional death of cells in the penumbra, the core of dead or dying tissue enlarges, and the volume of surrounding ischemic tissue increases.

Transient Ischemic Attacks. Transient ischemic attack (TIA) is a transient episode of neurologic dysfunction caused by focal brain, spinal cord, or retina ischemia without acute infarction.[30] A TIA or "ministroke" is equivalent to "brain angina" and reflects a temporary disturbance in focal cerebral blood flow, which reverses before infarction occurs, analogous to angina in relation to heart attack.[2,30] The causes of TIAs are the same as those of ischemic stroke and include atherosclerotic disease of cerebral vessels and emboli. TIAs are important because they may provide warning of impending stroke. Approximately 11% of patients after a TIA will experience a disabling stroke within 3 months and of those 50% will do so within the first 48 hours following the TIA.[30] Diagnosis of TIA before a stroke may permit surgical or medical intervention that prevents an eventual stroke and the associated neurologic deficits.

Thrombotic (Large Vessel) Stroke. Thrombi are the most common cause of ischemic strokes, usually occurring in atherosclerotic blood vessels. In the cerebral circulation, atherosclerotic plaques are found most commonly at arterial bifurcations. Common sites of plaque formation include larger

vessels of the brain, notably the origins of the internal carotid and vertebral arteries, and junctions of the basilar and vertebral arteries. Cerebral infarction can result from an acute local thrombosis and occlusion at the site of chronic atherosclerosis, with or without embolization of the plaque material distally, or from critical perfusion failure distal to a stenosis (watershed). These infarcts often affect the cortex, causing aphasia or neglect, visual field defects, or transient monocular blindness (amaurosis fugax). In most cases of stroke, a single cerebral artery and its territories are affected. Usually, thrombotic strokes are seen in older persons and frequently are accompanied by evidence of atherosclerotic heart or peripheral arterial disease. The thrombotic stroke is not associated with activity and may occur in a person at rest.

Small Vessel Stroke (Lacunar Infarct). Lacunar infarcts are small (1.5- to 2-cm) to very small (3- to 4-mm) infarcts located in the deeper, noncortical parts of the brain or in the brain stem. They are found in the territory of single deep penetrating arteries supplying the internal capsule, basal ganglia, or brain stem. They result from occlusion of the smaller penetrating branches of large cerebral arteries, commonly the middle cerebral and posterior cerebral arteries. In the process of healing, lacunar infarcts leave behind small cavities, or *lacunae* ("lakes"). They are thought to result from arteriolar lipohyalinosis or microatheroma, commonly in the settings of chronic hypertension or diabetes. Six basic causes of lacunar infarcts have been proposed: embolism, hypertension, small vessel occlusive disease, hematologic abnormalities, small intracerebral hemorrhages, and vasospasm. Because of their size and location, lacunar infarcts usually do not cause cortical deficits like aphasia or apraxia. Instead, they produce classic recognizable "lacunar syndromes" such as pure motor hemiplegia, pure sensory hemiplegia, and dysarthria with the clumsy hand syndrome. Because CT scans are not sensitive enough to detect these tiny infarcts, diagnosis used to depend on clinical features alone. The use of MRI has allowed frequent visualization of small vessel infarcts and is obligatory to confirm such a lesion.

Cardiogenic Embolic Stroke. An embolic stroke is caused by a moving blood clot that travels from its origin to the brain. It usually affects the larger proximal cerebral vessels, often lodging at bifurcations. The most frequent site of embolic strokes is the middle cerebral artery, reflecting the large territory of this vessel and its position as the terminus of the carotid artery. Although most cerebral emboli originate from a thrombus in the left heart, they also may originate in an atherosclerotic plaque in the carotid arteries. The embolus travels quickly to the brain and becomes lodged in a smaller artery through which it cannot pass. Embolic stroke usually has a sudden onset with immediate maximum deficit.

Various cardiac conditions predispose to formation of emboli that produce embolic stroke, including rheumatic heart disease, atrial fibrillation, recent myocardial infarction, ventricular aneurysm, mobile aortic arch atheroma, and bacterial endocarditis. More recently, the use of transesophageal echocardiography, which better images the interatrial septum, has implicated a patent foramen ovale as a source for paradoxical venous emboli to the arterial system. Advances in the diagnosis and treatment of heart disease can be expected to alter favourably the incidence of embolic stroke.

Hemorrhagic Stroke

The most frequently fatal stroke is a spontaneous hemorrhage into the brain substance resulting in an intracerebral hemorrhage.[2,5,9] With rupture of a blood vessel, hemorrhage into the brain tissue occurs, resulting in a focal hematoma and sometimes intraventricular hemorrhage, edema, compression of the brain contents, or spasm of the adjacent blood vessels. The most common predisposing factors are advancing age and hypertension. Other causes of hemorrhage are trauma, erosion of the vessels by tumours, blood coagulation disorders, vasculitis, and drugs. Aneurysms and arteriovenous malformations are structural abnormalities that can also cause sudden hemorrhage. A cerebral hemorrhage occurs suddenly, usually when the person is active. Vomiting commonly occurs at the onset, and headache often occurs. Focal symptoms depend on which vessel is involved. In the most common situation, hemorrhage into the basal ganglia results in contralateral hemiplegia, with initial flaccidity progressing to spasticity. The hemorrhage and resultant edema exert great pressure on the brain substance, and the clinical course progresses rapidly to coma and frequently to death.

Manifestations of Acute Stroke or TIA

The specific manifestations of stroke or TIA are determined by the cerebral artery that is affected, by the area of brain tissue that is supplied by that vessel, and by the adequacy of the collateral circulation. Symptoms of stroke/TIA always are sudden in onset and focal, and usually are one-sided. The most common symptom is weakness of the face and arm, sometimes also of the leg. Other frequent stroke symptoms are unilateral numbness, vision loss in one eye (amaurosis fugax) or to one side (hemianopia), language disturbance (aphasia), slurred speech (dysarthria), and sudden, unexplained imbalance or ataxia. In the event of TIA, symptoms rapidly resolve spontaneously, usually within minutes, although the underlying mechanisms are the same as for stroke. The specific stroke signs depend on the specific vascular territory compromised (Table 51.6). As a generalization, carotid ischemia causes monocular visual loss or aphasia (dominant hemisphere) or hemineglect (nondominant hemisphere), contralateral sensory or motor loss, or other discrete cortical signs such as apraxia and agnosia. Vertebrobasilar ischemia induces ataxia, diplopia, hemianopia, vertigo, cranial nerve deficits, contralateral hemiplegia, sensory deficits (either contralateral or crossed, *i.e.,* contralateral body and ipsilateral face), and arousal defects. Discrete subsets of these vascular syndromes usually occur, depending on which branches of the involved artery are blocked.

Stroke-Related Motor Deficits. Motor deficits are most common, followed by deficits of language, sensation, and cognition. After a stroke affecting the corticospinal tract such as the motor cortex, posterior limb of the internal capsule, basis pontis, or medullary pyramids, there is profound weakness on the contralateral side (hemiparesis; see Chapter 50, Fig. 50.5). Involvement at the level of the motor cortex is most often in the territory of the middle cerebral artery, usually with a sparing of the leg, which is supplied by the anterior cerebral artery. Subcortical lesions of the corticospinal tracts cause equal weakness of the face, arm, and leg. Within 6 to 8 weeks, the initial weakness and flaccidity is replaced by hyperreflexia and spasticity. Spasticity involves an increase in the tone of affected muscles and usually an element of weakness. The flexor muscles usually are more strongly affected in the upper extremities and the extensor muscles more strongly affected in the lower extremities. There is a tendency toward foot drop; outward rotation and circumduction of the leg with gait; flexion at the wrist, elbow, and fingers; lower facial paresis; slurred speech; an upgoing toe to plantar stimulation (Babinski sign); and dependent edema in the affected extremities. A slight corticospinal lesion may be indicated only by clumsiness in carrying out fine coordinated movements rather than by obvious weakness. Passive range-of-motion exercises help to maintain joint function and to prevent edema, shoulder subluxation (*i.e.,* incomplete dislocation), and muscle atrophy, and may help to reestablish motor patterns. If no voluntary movement or movement on command appears within a few months, significant function usually will not return to that extremity.

Stroke-Related Dysarthria and Aphasia. Two key aspects of verbal communication are speech and language. Speech involves the mechanical act of articulating language, the

TABLE 51.6 SIGNS AND SYMPTOMS OF STROKE BY INVOLVED CEREBRAL ARTERY

CEREBRAL ARTERY	BRAIN AREA INVOLVED	SIGNS AND SYMPTOMS[a]
Anterior cerebral	Infarction of the medial aspect of one frontal lobe if lesion is distal to communicating artery; bilateral frontal infarction if flow in other anterior cerebral artery is inadequate	Paralysis of contralateral foot or leg; impaired gait; paresis of contralateral arm; contralateral sensory loss over toes, foot, and leg; problems making decisions or performing acts voluntarily; lack of spontaneity, easily distracted; slowness of thought; aphasia depends on the hemisphere involved; urinary incontinence; cognitive and affective disorders
Middle cerebral	Massive infarction of most of lateral hemisphere and deeper structures of the frontal, parietal, and temporal lobes; internal capsule; basal ganglia	Contralateral hemiplegia (face and arm); contralateral sensory impairment; aphasia; homonymous hemianopia; altered consciousness (confusion to coma); inability to turn eyes toward paralyzed side; denial of paralyzed side or limb (hemiattention); possible acalculia, alexia, finger agnosia, and left–right confusion; vasomotor paresis and instability
Posterior cerebral	Occipital lobe; anterior and medial portion of temporal lobe	Homonymous hemianopia and other visual defects such as colour blindness, loss of central vision, and visual hallucinations; memory deficits; perseveration (repeated performance of same verbal or motor response)
	Thalamus involvement	Loss of all sensory modalities; spontaneous pain; intentional tremor; mild hemiparesis; aphasia
	Cerebral peduncle involvement	Oculomotor nerve palsy with contralateral hemiplegia
Basilar and vertebral	Cerebellum and brain stem	Visual disturbance such as diplopia, dystaxia, vertigo, dysphagia, dysphonia

[a]Depend on hemisphere involved and adequacy of collaterals.

"motor act" of verbal expression, whereas language involves the written or spoken use of symbolic formulations, such as words or numbers. *Dysarthria* is a disorder of speech, manifest as the imperfect articulation of speech sounds or changes in voice pitch or quality. It results from a stroke affecting the muscles of the pharynx, palate, tongue, lips, or mouth and does not relate to the content of speech. A person with dysarthria may demonstrate slurred speech while still retaining language ability, or may have a concurrent language problem as well. *Aphasia* is a general term that encompasses varying degrees of inability to comprehend, integrate, or express language. Aphasia may be localized to the dominant cerebral cortex or thalamus, usually the left side in 95% of people who are right handed and 70% of people who are left handed. In children, language dominance can readily shift to the unaffected hemisphere, resulting in more transient language deficits after stroke. A stroke in the territory of the middle cerebral artery is the most common aphasia-producing stroke.

Aphasia can be categorized as receptive or expressive, or as fluent or nonfluent. Fluency relates to the ease and spontaneity of conversational speech and is more strictly defined by the rate of speech, with "fluent" denoting many words, and "nonfluent," few words. Expressive or nonfluent aphasia is characterized by an inability to easily communicate spontaneously or translate thoughts or ideas into meaningful speech or writing. Speech production is limited, effortful, and halting and often may be poorly articulated because of a concurrent dysarthria. The person may be able, with difficulty, to utter or write two or three words, especially those with an emotional overlay.

Comprehension is normal, and the person seems to be fully aware of his or her deficits but is unable to correct them. This often leads to frustration, anger, or depression. Expressive, nonfluent aphasia is associated with lesions of the Broca area at the dominant inferior frontal lobe cortex (areas 44 and 45).

Fluent speech requires little or no effort, is articulate, and is of increased quantity. The term *fluent* refers only to the ease and rate of verbal output, and does not relate to the content of speech or the ability of the person to comprehend what is being said. Verbal utterances are often paraphrasic, meaning that letters, syllables, or whole words are substituted for the target words. There are three categories of fluent aphasia: Wernicke, anomic, and conductive aphasia. Wernicke aphasia is characterized by an inability to comprehend the speech of others or to comprehend written material. Lesions of the posterior superior temporal or lower parietal lobe (areas 22 and 39) are associated with receptive, fluent aphasia. Anomic aphasia is speech that is nearly normal except for a difficulty with finding singular words. Conductive aphasia is manifest as impaired repetition and speech riddled with letter substitutions, despite good comprehension and fluency. Conductive aphasia (*i.e.,* disconnection syndrome) results from destruction of the fibre system under the insula that connects the Wernicke and Broca areas.

Stroke-Related Cognitive and Other Deficits. Stroke can also cause cognitive, sensory, visual, and behavioural deficits. One distinct cognitive syndrome is that of hemineglect or hemi-inattention. Usually caused by strokes affecting the nondominant (right) hemisphere, hemineglect is the inability to attend to and react to stimuli coming from the contralateral (left) side of space. Patients may not visually track, orient, or reach to the neglected side. They may neglect to use the limbs on that side, despite normal motor function, and may not shave, wash, or comb that side. Such persons are unaware of this deficit, which is another form of their neglect (*anosognosia*). Other cognitive deficits include apraxia (impaired ability to carry out previously learned motor activities despite normal sensory and motor function), agnosia (impaired recognition with normal sensory function), memory loss, behavioural syndromes, and depression. Sensory deficits affect the body contralateral to the lesion and can manifest as numbness, tingling paresthesias, or distorted sensations such as dysesthesia and neuropathic pain. Visual disturbances from stroke are diverse, but most common are hemianopia from a lesion of the optic radiations between the lateral geniculate body and the temporal or occipital lobes, or monocular blindness from occlusion of the ipsilateral central retinal artery, a branch of the internal carotid.

Diagnosis and Treatment

Diagnosis. Accurate diagnosis of acute stroke is based on a complete history and thorough physical and neurologic examination. A careful history, including documentation of previous TIAs, the time of onset and pattern and rapidity of system progression, the specific focal symptoms (to determine the likely vascular territory), and any coexisting diseases, can help to determine the type of stroke that is involved. The diagnostic evaluation should aim to determine the presence of hemorrhage or ischemia, identify the stroke or TIA mechanism (*i.e.*, large vessel or small vessel atherothrombotic, cardioembolic, hemorrhagic, other or cryptogenic), characterize the severity of clinical deficits, and unmask the presence of risk factors.

Brain imaging studies document the brain infarction, whereas vascular imaging reveals the anatomy and pathologic processes of the related blood vessels. CT scans and MRI have become essential brain imaging tools in diagnosing stroke, differentiating cerebral hemorrhage from ischemia and excluding intracranial lesions that mimic stroke clinically. CT scans are a necessary screening tool in the acute setting for rapid identification of hemorrhage, but are insensitive to ischemia within 24 hours and to any brain stem or small infarcts. MRI is superior for imaging ischemic lesions in all territories, and for differentiating other nonstroke pathologic processes (*e.g.*, tumours, contusion, infection). MRI techniques such as perfusion- and diffusion-weighted imaging (DWI) can reveal cerebral ischemia immediately after onset and identify areas of potentially reversible damage (*i.e.*, penumbra). MR DWI is used in settings of emergency stroke evaluation to rapidly identify the area and volume of ischemia, identifying candidates for emergency treatments.

Vascular imaging is accomplished with CT angiography (CTA), magnetic resonance angiography (MRA), catheter-based "conventional" arteriography, and ultrasonography. All except ultrasonography can demonstrate the site of vascular abnormality (intracranial and extracranial) and afford visualization of most intracranial vascular areas. However, each modality has relative strengths and weaknesses. MRA is noninvasive and most widely available, but less sensitive and specific than CTA or catheter angiography. CTA is exquisitely detailed for a noninvasive technique, but is limited in availability and requires iodinated contrast, which is nephrotoxic. Catheter angiography remains the gold standard in sensitivity, and allows visualization of dynamic patterns of collateral flow, but is invasive and requires significant contrast doses. CTA and MRA have largely replaced angiography as a screening tool for vascular lesions. Ultrasonographic techniques allow quick bedside assessment of the carotid bifurcation (duplex ultrasonography) or of flow velocities in the cerebral circulation (transcranial Doppler).

Treatment. Treatment of acute ischemic stroke has changed markedly since the early 1990s, with an emphasis on salvaging brain tissue, preventing secondary stroke, and minimizing long-term disability. The care of patients with stroke has shifted away from the "nearest hospital" to *stroke centres*.[31] Stroke centres can manage stroke patients with appropriate care throughout the continuum, from emergency treatments, through the inpatient stay, and into the rehabilitation phase. With this advancement, the medical and lay communities together acknowledge that care of the patient with stroke requires specialized personnel and resources to minimize the devastating costs to society from stroke, the leading cause of adult disability in Canada and North America overall.

Stroke care begins with emergency treatments aimed at reversing the evolving ischemic brain injury. Although the results of emergent treatment of hemorrhagic stroke have been less dramatic, continued efforts to reduce disability have been promising. The realization that there is a window of opportunity during which ischemic but viable brain tissue can be salvaged has led to the use of reperfusion techniques and neuroprotective strategies in the early treatment of ischemic stroke. Reperfusion techniques include fibrinolytic drugs (administered either intravenously or intra-arterially), catheter-directed mechanical clot disruption, and augmentation of CPP during acute stroke. The use of fibrinolytic agents for treatment of stroke was first investigated in the late 1960s, but it was quickly abandoned because of hemorrhagic complications resulting from treatment many hours beyond the time window of penumbral cell viability and because exclusion of persons with hemorrhagic stroke was difficult before CT scanning was available. The renewed interest in fibrinolytic therapy has come about because of the development of new fibrinolytic agents and the availability of rapid diagnostic scanning methods that are able to differentiate between ischemic and hemorrhagic stroke.

Fibrinolytic agents include streptokinase, urokinase, and recombinant tissue-type plasminogen activator (tPA) (see Chapter 13), although only tPA is approved for treatment of acute ischemic stroke.[14,32] The Canadian Stroke Consortium, a national network of neurologists, has developed guidelines for the use of tPA for acute stroke.[33] These guidelines recommend that in persons with suspected stroke, the diagnosis of hemorrhagic stroke be excluded through the use of CT scanning before administration of fibrinolytic therapy, which must be administered within 4.5 hours of onset of symptoms.[33] The major risk of treatment with fibrinolytic agents is intracranial hemorrhage of the infarcted brain. A number of conditions, including therapeutic levels of oral anticoagulant medications, a history of gastrointestinal or urinary tract bleeding in the previous 21 days, prior stroke or head injury within 3 months, major surgery within the past 14 days, and a blood pressure greater than 185/110 mm Hg, are considered contraindications to intravenous fibrinolytic therapy.[32,33]

Emerging experimental treatments for ischemic stroke are being increasingly used as alternative methods of reperfusion beyond intravenous thrombolysis. New catheter-based methods allow recanalization of a directly visualized cerebral clot with intra-arterial techniques.[34] The interventional specialist might mechanically disrupt the clot, deliver fibrinolytic drug intra-arterially at the clot surface, or urgently stent intracranial vessels to restore flow. Generally, although patient selection is more stringent for these invasive methods, patients can be treated past the 4.5-hour time window for intravenous tPA. However, these methods require an experienced interventional angiography team and extensive institutional infrastructure, and thus remain limited to tertiary care centres.[33] Other experimental treatments include neuroprotection with drugs that limit the calcium cascade (Fig. 51.6) and treatments like hypothermia that decrease brain metabolic demands in the setting of ischemia.

Poststroke treatment is aimed at preventing recurrent stroke and medical complications, while promoting the fullest possible recovery of function. The risk of stroke recurrence is highest in the first week after stroke or TIA, so the early implementation of antiplatelet agents in most cases, or warfarin (an anticoagulant) in cardioembolic stroke, is imperative. Long-term stroke recurrence is most effectively prevented with aggressive reduction of risk factors, primarily hypertension, diabetes, smoking, and hyperlipidemia. In cases of carotid territory stroke with carotid stenosis, revascularization with surgery or stenting should be considered. Early hospital care also requires careful prevention of aspiration, deep vein thrombosis, and falls. Recovery is maximized with early and aggressive rehabilitation efforts that include all members of the rehabilitation team—physician, nurse, speech therapist, physical therapist, and occupational therapist—and the family. Much research is ongoing into the determinants and mechanisms of stroke recovery.

The successful treatment of stroke depends on education of the public, paramedics, and healthcare professionals about the need for both early diagnosis and treatment and for risk factor reduction and prevention. As with heart attack, the message should be that prevention is the key, and to treat stroke symptoms as an emergency "brain attack." Effective medical and surgical procedures may preserve brain function and prevent disability.

FIGURE 51.10 • Berry aneurysm. A saccular aneurysm (*arrow*) arises from the posterior cerebral artery. The dark color is a result of subarachnoid blood from this aneurysm that ruptured. (From Rubin R., Strayer D. S. (Eds.), *Rubin's pathology: Clinicopathologic foundations of medicine* (6th ed., p. 1316). Philadelphia, PA: Lippincott Williams & Wilkins.)

Aneurysmal Subarachnoid Hemorrhage

Aneurysmal subarachnoid hemorrhage represents bleeding into the subarachnoid space caused by a ruptured cerebral aneurysm. Bleeding into the subarachnoid space can extend well beyond the site of origin, flooding the basal cistern, ventricles, and spinal subarachnoid space.[5,9,34] An aneurysm is a bulge at the site of a localized weakness in the muscular wall of an arterial vessel. Most cerebral aneurysms are small saccular aneurysms called *berry aneurysms* (Fig. 51.10). They usually occur in the anterior circulation and are found at bifurcations and other junctions of vessels such as those in the circle of Willis (Fig. 51.11). They are thought to arise from a congenital defect in the media of the involved vessels. Their incidence is higher in persons with certain disorders, including polycystic kidney disease, fibromuscular dysplasia, coarctation of the aorta, and arteriovenous malformations of the brain.[5,9] Other causes of cerebral aneurysms are atherosclerosis, hypertension, and bacterial infections.

Rupture of a cerebral aneurysm results in subarachnoid hemorrhage. The probability of rupture increases with the size of the aneurysm; most ruptured aneurysms tend to be less than

FIGURE 51.11 • Pathophysiology of saccular aneurysm. **A:** Common sites of saccular and berry aneurysms, which preferentially involve the proximal carotid tributaries, are shown. **B:** The lesion evolves as a result of blood under pressure acting on an early embryonic defect of the vascular wall at bifurcations. (From Strayer D. S., Rubin E., Saffitz J. E., et al. (Eds.), *Rubin's pathology: Clinicopathologic foundations of medicine* (7th ed., p. 1433). Philadelphia, PA: Lippincott Williams & Wilkins.)

7 mm.[34] Rupture often occurs with acute increases in ICP. Of the various environmental factors that may predispose to aneurysmal subarachnoid hemorrhage, cigarette smoking, hypertension, and excessive alcohol intake appear to constitute the greatest threat.[34,35] Intracranial aneurysms are rare in children, and the mean age for subarachnoid hemorrhage is approximately 50 years. The mortality and morbidity rates with aneurysmal subarachnoid hemorrhage are high, with only one third of persons recovering without major disability.[35]

The signs and symptoms of cerebral aneurysms can be divided into two phases: those presenting before rupture and bleeding and those presenting after rupture and bleeding. Most small aneurysms are asymptomatic and intact aneurysms frequently are found at autopsy as an incidental finding.[5] Large aneurysms may cause chronic headache, neurologic deficits, or both. Approximately 50% of persons with subarachnoid hemorrhage have a history of atypical headaches occurring days to weeks before the onset of hemorrhage, suggesting the presence of a small leak. These headaches are characterized by sudden onset and often are accompanied by nausea, vomiting, and dizziness. Persons with these symptoms may be mistakenly diagnosed as having tension or migraine headaches.

The onset of subarachnoid aneurysmal rupture often is heralded by a sudden and severe headache, described as "the worst headache of my life."[35,36] If the bleeding is severe, the headache may be accompanied by collapse and loss of consciousness. Vomiting may accompany the presenting symptoms. Other manifestations include signs of meningeal irritation such as nuchal rigidity (neck stiffness) and photophobia (light intolerance); cranial nerve deficits, especially cranial nerve II, and sometimes III and IV (diplopia and blurred vision); stroke syndromes (focal motor and sensory deficits); cerebral edema and increased ICP; and pituitary dysfunction (diabetes insipidus and hyponatremia). Hypertension, a frequent finding, and cardiac arrhythmias result from massive release of catecholamines triggered by the subarachnoid hemorrhage.

The diagnosis of subarachnoid hemorrhage and intracranial aneurysms is made by clinical presentation, CT scan, lumbar puncture, and angiography.[2,35] Lumbar puncture may reveal the presence of blood in the CSF, whereas CT may demonstrate the location and extent of subarachnoid blood. To identify the aneurysm at the source of bleeding, conventional angiography, MRA, and helical (spiral) CTA are used. Conventional catheter angiography is the definitive diagnostic tool for detecting the aneurysm. MRA is noninvasive and does not require the intravascular administration of contrast, but is less sensitive. Helical CTA does require intravenous contrast, but can be used in persons after aneurysmal clipping, when the use of MRI may be contraindicated.

The course of treatment after aneurysm rupture depends on the extent of neurologic deficit. The best outcomes are achieved when the aneurysm can be secured early and prevention of complications initiated.[35] Persons with mild to no neurologic deficits may undergo cerebral arteriography and early surgery, usually within 24 to 72 hours. Surgery involves craniotomy and inserting a specially designed silver clip that is tightened around the neck of the aneurysm. This procedure offers protection from rebleeding and may permit removal of the hematoma. The use of endovascular techniques such as balloon embolization and platinum coil electrothrombosis is an alternative to surgery, particularly in surgically inaccessible aneurysms or poor surgical candidates. Some persons with subarachnoid hemorrhage are managed medically for 10 days or more in an attempt to improve their clinical status before surgery.

The complications of aneurysmal rupture include rebleeding, vasospasm with cerebral ischemia, hydrocephalus, hypothalamic dysfunction, and seizure activity. Rebleeding and vasospasm are the most serious and most difficult to treat. Rebleeding, which has its highest incidence on the first day after the initial rupture, results in further and usually catastrophic neurologic deficits.

Vasospasm is a common complication of aneurysmal rupture. The condition is difficult to treat and is associated with a high incidence of morbidity and mortality. Although the description of aneurysm-associated vasospasm is relatively uniform, its proposed mechanisms are controversial. Usually, the condition develops within 3 to 10 days (peak, 7 days) after aneurysm rupture and involves a focal narrowing of the cerebral artery or arteries that can be visualized by arteriography or by transcranial Doppler. The neurologic status gradually deteriorates as blood supply to the brain in the region of the spasm is decreased; this usually can be differentiated from the rapid deterioration seen in rebleeding. Vasospasm is treated by attempting to maintain adequate CPP through the use of vasoactive drugs or administration of large amounts of intravenous fluids to increase intravascular volume and produce hemodilution. There is risk for rebleeding from this therapy. Early surgery may provide some protection from vasospasm. Endovascular techniques, including balloon dilation, have been developed to treat spasmodic arterial segments mechanically. Nimodipine is a vasodilatory drug that blocks calcium channels and selectively acts on cerebral blood vessels. It is used to prevent or treat vasospasm and initially persons should be monitored for systemic hypotension.

Another complication of aneurysm rupture is the development of hydrocephalus. It is caused by plugging of the arachnoid villi with products from lysis of blood in the subarachnoid space. Hydrocephalus is diagnosed by serial CT scans showing increasing size of the ventricles and by the clinical signs of increased ICP. Hydrocephalus may respond to osmotic diuretics, but if neurologic deterioration is significant, surgical placement of a shunt is indicated.

Arteriovenous Malformations

Arteriovenous malformation (AVM) is a complex tangle of abnormal arteries and veins linked by one or more fistulas.[2] These vascular networks lack a capillary bed, and the small arteries have a deficient muscularis layer. Arteriovenous malformations are thought to arise from failure in development of the capillary network in the embryonic brain. As the child's brain grows, the malformation acquires additional arterial contributions that enlarge to form a tangled collection of thin-walled vessels that shunt blood directly from the arterial to the venous circulation. Arteriovenous malformations typically present before 40 years of age and affect men and women equally. Rupture of vessels in the malformation causing hemorrhagic stroke accounts for approximately 2% of all strokes.[37]

The hemodynamic effects of arteriovenous malformations are twofold. First, blood is shunted from the high-pressure arterial system to the low-pressure venous system without the buffering advantage of the capillary network. The draining venous channels are exposed to high levels of pressure, predisposing them to rupture and hemorrhage. Second, the elevated arterial and venous pressures divert blood away from the surrounding tissue, impairing tissue perfusion. Clinically, this is evidenced by slowly progressive neurologic deficits. The major clinical manifestations of arteriovenous malformations are intracerebral and subarachnoid hemorrhage, seizures, headache, and progressive neurologic deficits. Headaches often are severe, and persons with the disorder may describe them as throbbing and synchronous with their heartbeat. Other, focal symptoms depend on the location of the lesion and include visual symptoms (i.e., diplopia and hemianopia), hemiparesis, mental deterioration, and speech deficits.

Definitive diagnosis often is obtained through cerebral angiography. Treatment methods include surgical excision, endovascular occlusion, and radiation therapy.[2,37] Because of the nature of the malformation, each of these methods is accompanied by some risk for complications. If the arteriovenous malformation is accessible, surgical excision usually is the treatment of choice. Endovascular treatment involves the insertion of microcatheters into the cerebral circulation for delivery of embolic materials (e.g., microballoons, sclerosing agents, microcoils, or quick-drying glue) into the arteriovenous malformation vessels.[37,38] Radiation therapy (also known as *radiosurgery*) may involve the use of a gamma knife, proton beam, or linear accelerator.

IN SUMMARY

A stroke, or "brain attack," is an acute focal neurologic deficit caused by a vascular disorder that injures brain tissue. It is the third leading cause of death in Canada and a major cause of disability. There are two main types of stroke: ischemic and hemorrhagic. Ischemic stroke, which is the most common type, is caused by cerebrovascular obstruction by a thrombus or emboli. Hemorrhagic stroke, which is associated with greater morbidity and mortality, is caused by the rupture of a blood vessel and bleeding into the brain. The acute manifestations of stroke depend on the location of the blood vessel that is involved and can include motor, sensory, language, speech, and cognitive disorders. Early diagnosis and treatment with fibrinolytic agents can prevent disabling brain injury from ischemic stroke. Treatment of long-term neurologic deficits from stroke is primarily symptomatic, involving the combined efforts of the healthcare team, the patient, and the family.

A subarachnoid hemorrhage involves bleeding into the subarachnoid space. Most subarachnoid hemorrhages are the result of a ruptured cerebral aneurysm. Presenting symptoms include headache, nuchal rigidity, photophobia, and nausea. Complications include rebleeding, vasospasm, and hydrocephalus.

Arteriovenous malformations are congenital abnormal communications between arterial and venous channels that result from failure in development of the capillary network in the embryonic brain. The vessels in the arteriovenous malformations may enlarge to form a space-occupying lesion, become weak and predispose to bleeding, and divert blood away from other parts of the brain; they can cause brain hemorrhage, seizures, headache, and other neurologic deficits.

INFECTIONS AND NEOPLASMS

After completing this section of the chapter, you should be able to meet the following objectives:

- List the sequence of events that occur with meningitis.
- Describe the symptoms of encephalitis.
- List the major categories of brain tumours and interpret the meaning of benign and malignant as related to brain tumours.
- Describe the general manifestations of brain tumours.
- List the methods used in diagnosis and treatment of brain tumours.

Infections

Infections of the CNS may be classified according to the structure involved: the meninges, meningitis; the brain parenchyma, encephalitis; the spinal cord, myelitis; and the brain and spinal cord, encephalomyelitis. They also may be classified by the type of invading organism: bacterial, viral, or other. In general, the pathogens enter the CNS through the bloodstream by crossing the blood–brain barrier or by direct invasion through skull fracture or a bullet hole, or, rarely, by contamination during surgery or lumbar puncture.

Meningitis

Meningitis is an inflammation of the pia mater, the arachnoid, and the CSF-filled subarachnoid space. Inflammation spreads rapidly because of CSF circulation around the brain and spinal cord. The inflammation usually is caused by an infection, but chemical meningitis can occur. There are two types of acute infectious meningitis: acute purulent meningitis (usually bacterial) and acute lymphocytic (usually viral) meningitis.[5]

Factors responsible for the severity of meningitis include virulence factors of the pathogen, host factors, cerebral edema, and the presence of permanent neurologic sequelae.

Bacterial Meningitis. Most cases of bacterial meningitis are caused by *Streptococcus pneumoniae* (the pneumococcus) or *Neisseria meningitidis* (the meningococcus), except in neonates (infected most by group B streptococci).[39–41] The incidence of *Haemophilus influenzae* and *S. pneumoniae* meningitis have both declined dramatically during recent years because of vaccination. Other pathogens in adults are gram-negative bacilli and *Listeria monocytogenes*. The very young and the very old are at highest risk for pneumococcal meningitis. Risk factors associated with contracting meningitis include head trauma with basilar skull fractures, otitis media, sinusitis or mastoiditis, neurosurgery, dermal sinus tracts, systemic sepsis, or immunocompromise. Despite the use of antibiotics, morbidity and mortality rates remain high for bacterial meningitis. For adults, the overall mortality rate is 34% for *S. pneumoniae* and 10% for *N. meningitidis* with long-term complications affecting up to 50% of survivors.[40]

In the pathophysiologic process of bacterial meningitis, the bacterial organisms replicate and undergo lysis in the CSF, releasing endotoxins or cell wall fragments. These substances initiate the release of inflammatory mediators, which set off a complex sequence of events permitting pathogens, neutrophils, and albumin to move across the capillary wall into the CSF. As the pathogens enter the subarachnoid space, they cause inflammation, characterized by a cloudy, purulent exudate (Fig. 51.12). Thrombophlebitis of the bridging veins and dural sinuses or obliteration of arterioles by inflammation may develop, causing vascular congestion and infarction in the surrounding tissues. Ultimately, the meninges thicken and

FIGURE 51.12 • Purulent meningitis. A creamy exudate opacifies the leptomeninges in bacterial meningitis. The superficial veins are engorged and may develop thrombosis, and the arteries on the surface of the brain may also develop thrombosis, leading to infarcts. (From Strayer D. S., Rubin E., Saffitz J. E., et al. (Eds.), *Rubin's pathology: Clinicopathologic foundations of medicine* (7th ed., p. 1436). Philadelphia, PA: Lippincott Williams & Wilkins.)

adhesions form. These adhesions may impinge on the cranial nerves, giving rise to cranial nerve palsies, or may impair the outflow of CSF, causing hydrocephalus.

The most common symptoms of acute bacterial meningitis are fever and chills; headache; stiff neck; back, abdominal, and extremity pains; and nausea and vomiting.[2,5,41] Other signs include seizures, cranial nerve palsies, and focal cerebral signs. Meningococcal meningitis causes a petechial rash with palpable purpura in most people. These petechiae vary in size from pinhead to large ecchymoses or even areas of skin gangrene that slough if the person survives. Other types of meningitis also may produce a petechial rash. Persons infected with *H. influenzae* or *S. pneumoniae* may present with difficulty in arousal and seizures, whereas those with *N. meningitidis* infection may present with delirium or coma. The development of cerebral edema, hydrocephalus, or increased cerebral blood flow can increase ICP.

Meningeal signs (*e.g.*, photophobia and nuchal rigidity), such as those seen in subarachnoid hemorrhage, also may be present. Two assessment techniques can help determine whether meningeal irritation is present. The Kernig sign is resistance to extension of the knee while the person is lying with the hip flexed at a right angle. The Brudzinski sign is elicited when flexion of the neck induces flexion of the hip and knee. These postures reflect resistance to the painful stretching of the inflamed meninges from the lumbar level to the head. Cranial nerve damage (especially the eighth nerve, with resulting deafness) and hydrocephalus may occur as complications of pyogenic meningitis.

Diagnosis of bacterial meningitis is based on the history and physical examination, along with laboratory data. Lumbar puncture findings, which are necessary for accurate diagnosis, include a cloudy and purulent CSF under increased pressure. The CSF typically contains large numbers of polymorphonuclear neutrophils (up to 90×10^9/L), increased protein content, and reduced sugar content. Bacteria can be seen on smears and can easily be cultured with appropriate media. Occasionally, previous antibiotic use limits culture sensitivities, in which case latex agglutination can be used, or polymerase chain reaction (PCR) testing for *N. meningitidis*, *H. influenzae*, and *Listeria* species. Because complications associated with lumbar puncture include life-threatening cerebral herniation, at-risk patients (*i.e.*, those who are immunocompromised, have had a seizure within a week, have papilledema, or have specific neurologic abnormalities) should have a CT scan before undergoing the procedure.

Treatment includes urgent antibiotics while diagnostic testing ensues.[39] Delay in initiation of antimicrobial therapy, most frequently because of performance of medical imaging before performance of lumbar puncture or transfer to another medical facility, can result in poor outcomes.[41] Initial choice of antibiotics includes broad-spectrum coverage with a third-generation cephalosporin, vancomycin, and sometimes ampicillin. Further adjustment of antibiotics is driven by results of CSF cultures. Effective antibiotics produce rapid lysis of the pathogen, which produces inflammatory mediators that have the potential for exacerbating the abnormalities of the blood–brain barrier. To suppress this pathologic inflammation, adjunctive corticosteroid therapy is increasingly administered with or just before the first dose of antibiotics in patients of all ages.[41]

Persons who have been exposed to someone with meningococcal meningitis should be treated prophylactically with antibiotics. Effective polysaccharide vaccines are available to protect against meningococcal groups. Current vaccines in Canada include a monovalent (Group C), quadrivalent (Groups A, C, Y, and W-135), and the latest multicomponent vaccine (Group B).[42] These vaccines are recommended for military recruits, college students, and travellers, who are at increased risk for invasive meningococcal disease.

Viral Meningitis. Viral meningitis manifests in much the same way as bacterial meningitis, but the course is less severe and the CSF findings are markedly different. There are lymphocytes in the fluid rather than polymorphonuclear cells, the protein content is only moderately elevated, and the sugar content usually is normal. The acute viral meningitides are self-limiting and usually require only symptomatic treatment, except for herpes simplex virus (HSV) type 2, which responds to intravenous acyclovir. Viral meningitis can be caused by many different viruses, most often enteroviruses, including coxsackievirus, poliovirus, and echovirus. Others include Epstein–Barr virus, mumps virus, HSV, and West Nile virus. Although often the virus cannot be identified, newer assays are allowing in some circumstances for rapid identification of viral ribonucleic acid (RNA) in CSF.

Encephalitis

Encephalitis represents a generalized infection of the parenchyma of the brain or spinal cord. It usually is caused by a virus, but it also may be caused by bacteria, fungi, and other organisms. The nervous system is subject to invasion by many viruses, such as arbovirus, poliovirus, and rabies virus. The mode of transmission may be the bite of a mosquito (arbovirus), a rabid animal (rabies virus), or ingestion (poliovirus). Common causes of encephalitis are HSV and West Nile virus. Less frequent causes of encephalitis are toxic substances such as ingested lead and vaccines for measles and mumps. Encephalitis caused by human immunodeficiency virus (HIV) infection is discussed in Chapter 20.

The pathologic picture of encephalitis includes local necrotizing hemorrhage, which ultimately becomes generalized, with prominent edema. There is progressive degeneration of nerve cell bodies. The histologic picture, although rather general, may demonstrate some specific characteristics. For example, the poliovirus selectively destroys the cells of the anterior horn of the spinal cord.

Like meningitis, encephalitis is characterized by fever, headache, and nuchal rigidity, but more often patients also experience neurologic disturbances, such as lethargy, disorientation, seizures, focal paralysis, delirium, and coma. Diagnosis of encephalitis is made by clinical history and presenting symptoms, in addition to traditional CSF studies.

Brain Tumours

Primary brain tumours account for 2% of all cancer deaths. The Canadian Cancer Society estimated that there will be 3,000 new cases and more than 2,100 deaths from brain and spinal cord cancers in 2015.[25] It is estimated that 20% to 40% of intracranial tumours are metastatic, coming from other sites such as lung and breast. The incidence of brain and spinal tumours increases with age and a majority of these tumours are found in people between the ages of 50 and 70. In Canada, brain tumours in children and adolescents are the second most common neoplasm.[25]

Types of Tumours

The term *brain tumour* refers to a collection of intracranial neoplasms, each with its own histology, site of origin, prognosis, and treatment. For most neoplasms, the term *malignant* is used to describe the tumour's lack of cell differentiation, its invasive nature, and its ability to metastasize. However, the terms *benign* and *malignant* do not apply to brain tumours in the same sense as they do to tumours in other parts of the body. In the brain, even a well-differentiated and histologically benign tumour may grow and cause death because of its location. Also, tumours in the brain are rarely benign because surgery rarely cures.[25] Most histologically benign tumours infiltrate the normal brain tissue, preventing total resection and allowing for tumour recurrence. Furthermore, brain tumours seldom metastasize, except within the CNS itself. Because of difficulty with pathologic discrimination and absence of metastasis, the clinical staging systems used for other cancers are not used for describing brain tumours. Instead, the terms *low-grade tumours* and *high-grade tumours* are often used.[25]

Brain tumours can be divided into three basic types: primary intracranial tumours of neuroepithelial tissue (*e.g.,* neurons, neuroglia), primary intracranial tumours that originate in the skull cavity but are not derived from the brain tissue itself (*e.g.,* meninges, pituitary gland, pineal gland, primary CNS lymphoma), and metastatic tumours.[9] Collectively, neoplasms of astrocytic origin are the most common type of primary brain tumour in adults, followed by primary CNS lymphoma.

Glial Tumours. Glial tumours are divided into two main categories: astrocytic and oligodendroglial. For purposes of classification, astrocytic tumours can be subdivided into fibrillary (infiltrating) astrocytic tumours and pilocytic astrocytomas.

Fibrillary or diffuse astrocytomas account for 70% of adult primary brain tumours.[25] They are most common in middle age, with the anaplastic astrocytomas having a peak incidence in the sixth decade. Although they usually are found in the cerebral hemispheres, they also can occur in the cerebellum, brain stem, or spinal cord. Astrocytomas of the cerebral hemispheres commonly are divided into three grades of increasing pathologic anaplasia and rapidity of progression: well-differentiated lesions, designated *astrocytomas;* intermediate-grade tumours, termed *anaplastic astrocytomas;* and the least differentiated and most aggressive, designated *glioblastoma multiforme.*

Clinically, infiltrating astrocytic tumours present with symptoms of increased ICP (*e.g.,* headache) or focal abnormalities related to their position (*e.g.,* seizures).

Pilocytic astrocytomas are distinguished from other astrocytomas by their cellular appearance and their benign behaviour. Typically, they occur in children and young adults and usually are located in the cerebellum, but they also can be found in the floor and walls of the third ventricle, in the optic chiasm and nerves, and occasionally in the cerebral hemispheres. The prognosis of persons with pilocytic astrocytomas is influenced primarily by their location. The prognosis is usually better for persons with surgically resectable tumours, such as those located in the cerebellar cortex, than for persons with less accessible tumours, such as those involving the hypothalamus or brain stem.

Oligodendrogliomas are tumours of the oligodendrocytes or their precursors, or with histologic features representing both oligodendrocytes and astrocytes. They represent approximately 5% to 18% of glial tumours and are most common in middle life.[25] The prognosis of persons with oligodendrogliomas is less predictable than for persons with infiltrating astrocytomas. It depends on the histologic grade of the tumour, its location, and, more recently, recognition of molecular features that can be linked to chemosensitivity. The oligodendroglial tumours are prone to spontaneous hemorrhage owing to their delicate vasculature.

Ependymomas. Ependymomas are derived from the single layer of epithelium that lines the ventricles and spinal canal. Although they can occur at any age, they are most likely to occur under the age of 5 and most frequently affect the fourth ventricle; they constitute 5% to 10% of brain tumours in this age group.[27] The spinal cord is the most common site for ependymomas occurring in middle age. The clinical features depend on the location of the neoplasm. Intracranial tumours are often associated with hydrocephalus and evidence of increased ICP.

Meningiomas. Meningiomas develop from the meningothelial cells of the arachnoid and are outside the brain. They usually have their onset in the middle or later years of life and constitute approximately 20% of primary brain tumours in this age group. Meningiomas are slow growing, well circumscribed, and often highly vascular tumours. They usually are benign, and complete removal is possible if the tumour does not involve vital structures.

Primary Central Nervous System Lymphomas. Primary CNS lymphomas are deep, periventricular, and diffuse tumours especially common in immunocompromised patients and are associated with the Epstein–Barr virus and derived from large B cells. This type of lymphoma accounts for approximately 3% of all CNS tumours with most being malignant, and recurrence is common despite treatment.[43] Behavioural and cognitive changes, which are the most common presenting symptoms, occur in about 65% of patients; hemiparesis, aphasia, and visual field deficits in about 50%; and seizures in 15% to 20%.[44]

Etiology

The etiology of brain tumours is largely unknown. Although a large number of studies have examined the relationship between environmental and occupational factors, only two have shown a relationship to brain cancer: ionizing radiation and immunosuppression.[26] High-dose irradiation given to treat intracranial and extracranial cancers, including prophylactic irradiation for leukemia, increases the incidence of gliomas, meningiomas, and nerve sheath tumours. Immunosuppression, either congenital or acquired (*e.g.,* immunosuppression to prevent organ rejection, HIV infection), increases the risk of primary CNS lymphomas. There may also be a hereditary factor. A few inherited disorders predispose to the development of brain tumours. For example, neurofibromatosis (see Chapter 7) is associated with primary brain tumours. Some childhood tumours, such as medulloblastoma, are considered to be of embryonic origin.

Manifestations

Intracranial tumours give rise to focal disturbances in brain function and increased ICP. Focal disturbances occur because of brain compression, tumour infiltration, disturbances in blood flow, and cerebral edema.

Tumours may be located intra-axially (*i.e.,* within brain tissue) or extra-axially (*i.e.,* outside brain tissue, but within the cranium). Disturbances in brain function usually are greatest with fast-growing, infiltrative, intra-axial tumours because of compression, infiltration, and necrosis of brain tissue. Extra-axial tumours, such as meningiomas, may reach a large size without producing signs and symptoms. Cysts may form in tumours and contribute to brain compression. The clinical manifestations of brain tumours depend on the size and location of the tumour. General signs and symptoms include headache, nausea, vomiting, mental changes, papilledema, visual disturbances (*e.g.,* diplopia), alterations in sensory and motor function, and seizures. Because the volume of the intracranial cavity is fixed, brain tumours cause a generalized increase in ICP when they reach sufficient size or produce edema. Cerebral edema usually is of the vasogenic type, which develops around the tumours and is characterized by increased brain water and expanded extracellular fluid. The edema is thought to result from increased permeability of tumour capillary endothelial cells. Tumours can also obstruct the flow of CSF in the ventricular cavities and produce hydrocephalic dilation of the proximal ventricles and atrophy of the cerebral hemispheres. With very slow-growing tumours, complete compensation of ventricular volumes can occur, but with rapidly growing tumours, increased ICP is an early sign. Depending on the location of the tumour, brain displacement and herniation of the uncus or cerebellum may occur.

The brain itself is insensitive to pain. The headache that accompanies brain tumours results from compression or distortion of pain-sensitive dural or vascular structures. It may be felt on the same side of the head as the tumour, but more commonly is diffuse. In the early stages, the headache is mild and occurs in the morning on awakening and improves with head elevation. The headache becomes more constant as the tumour enlarges and often is worsened by coughing, bending, or sudden movements of the head.

Vomiting occurs with or without nausea, may be projectile, and is a common symptom of increased ICP and brain stem compression. Direct stimulation of the vomiting centre, which is located in the medulla, may contribute to the vomiting that occurs with brain tumours. The vomiting is often associated with headache. Papilledema (edema of the optic disk) results from increased ICP and obstruction of the CSF pathways. It is associated with decreased visual acuity, diplopia, and deficits in the visual fields. Visual defects associated with papilledema often are the reason that persons with brain tumour seek medical care.

Personality and mental changes are common with brain tumours. They may demonstrate irritability initially and later become quiet and apathetic. They may become forgetful, seem preoccupied, and appear to be psychologically depressed. Because of these changes, a psychiatric consultation may be sought before a diagnosis of brain tumour is made.

Focal signs and symptoms are determined by the location of the tumour. Tumours arising in the frontal lobe may grow to large size, increase the ICP, and cause signs of generalized brain dysfunction before focal signs are recognized. Tumours that impinge on the visual system cause visual loss or visual field defects long before generalized signs develop. Certain areas of the brain have a relatively low threshold for seizure activity. Temporal lobe tumours often produce seizures as their first symptom. Hallucinations of smell or hearing and déjà vu phenomena are common focal manifestations of temporal lobe tumours. Brain stem tumours commonly produce upper and lower motor neuron signs, such as weakness of facial muscles and ocular palsies that occur with or without involvement of sensory or long motor tracts. Cerebellar tumours often cause ataxia of gait.

Diagnosis and Treatment

The diagnosis of brain tumours in the modern era rests mainly on MRI. Gadolinium-enhanced MRI is the test of choice for identifying and localizing the presence and extent of tumour involvement. CT scans may fail to reveal certain mass lesions such as low-grade tumours or posterior fossa masses. Diagnostic maneuvres that suggest a possible tumour and indicate the need for MRI include physical and neurologic examinations, visual field and funduscopic examination, and sometimes EEG. Approximately 75% of persons with a brain tumour have an abnormal EEG, which can indicate an underlying structural lesion warranting MRI. Cerebral angiography can be used to visualize the tumour's vascular supply, information that is important when planning surgery. MRI may be supplemented with positron emission tomography (PET) scan to better characterize the metabolic properties of the tumour, useful in planning treatment.[26] MRA and CTA can be used to distinguish vascular masses from tumours.

The three general methods for treatment of brain tumours are surgery, irradiation, and medications. Surgery is part of the initial management of virtually all brain tumours; it establishes the diagnosis and achieves tumour removal in many cases. The development of microsurgical neuroanatomy, the operating microscope, and advanced stereotactic and ultrasonographic technology; the fusion of imaging systems with resection techniques; and the intraoperative monitoring of evoked potentials or the EEG have improved the effectiveness of surgical resection. However, the degree of removal may be limited by the location of the tumour and its invasiveness. Stereotactic surgery uses three-dimensional coordinates and CT and MRI to localize a brain lesion precisely. Ultrasonographic technology has been used for localizing and removing tumours. The ultrasonic aspirator, which combines a vibrating head with suction, permits atraumatic removal of tumours from cranial nerves and important cortical areas. Intraoperative monitoring of evoked potentials is an important adjunct to some types of surgery. For example, evoked potentials can be used to monitor auditory, visual, speech or motor responses during surgery done under local anesthesia.

Most malignant brain tumours respond to external irradiation. Irradiation can increase longevity and sometimes can allay symptoms when tumours recur. The treatment dose depends on the tumour's histologic type, radioresponsiveness, and anatomic site and on the level of tolerance of the surrounding tissue. The technique called *gamma knife* combines stereotactic localization of tumour with radiosurgery, allowing delivery of high-dose radiation to deep tumours while sparing surrounding brain. Radiation therapy is avoided in children younger than 2 years of age because of the long-term effects, which include developmental delay, panhypopituitarism, and secondary tumours.

The use of medications, including chemotherapy, and biologic therapies (*e.g.,* bevacizumab) for brain tumours is somewhat limited by the blood–brain barrier. Chemotherapeutic agents can be administered intravenously, intra-arterially, intrathecally (*i.e.,* into the spinal canal), as wafers impregnated with a drug and implanted into the tumour at the time of surgery, or intraventricularly. Future agents being developed will target specific genetic features and molecular profiles of a tumour.

IN SUMMARY

Infections of the CNS may be classified according to the structures involved (*e.g.,* meningitis, encephalitis) or the type of organism causing the infection. The damage caused by infection may predispose to hydrocephalus, seizures, or other neurologic defects.

Brain tumours account for 2% of all cancer deaths and are the second most common type of cancer in children. Brain tumours can arise primarily from intracranial structures, and tumours from other parts of the body often metastasize to the brain. Primary brain tumours can arise from any structure in the cranial cavity. Most begin in brain tissue, but the pituitary, the pineal region, and the meninges also are sites of tumour development. Brain tumours cause focal disturbances in brain function and increased ICP. Focal disturbances result from brain compression, tumour infiltration, disturbances in blood flow, and cerebral edema. The clinical manifestations of brain tumour depend on the size and location of the tumour. General signs and symptoms include headache, nausea, vomiting, mental changes, papilledema, visual disturbances, alterations in motor and sensory function, and seizures. Diagnostic tests include physical examination, visual field testing and funduscopic examination, CT scans, MRI studies, EEG, and cerebral angiography. Treatment includes surgery, irradiation, and medications.

SEIZURE DISORDERS

After completing this section of the chapter, you should be able to meet the following objectives:

- Explain the difference between a seizure and epilepsy.
- State four or more causes of seizures other than epilepsy.
- Differentiate between the origin of seizure activity in focal and generalized forms of epilepsy and compare the manifestations of each.
- Characterize status epilepticus.

A seizure represents the abnormal behaviour caused by an electrical discharge from neurons in the cerebral cortex. A seizure is a discrete clinical event with associated signs and symptoms that vary according to the site of neuronal discharge in the brain. Manifestations of seizure generally include sensory, motor, autonomic, or psychic phenomena. A convulsion refers to the specific seizure type of a motor seizure involving the entire body, and this affects approximately 0.6% of the Canadian population.[45] Seizure activity is the most common disorder encountered in pediatric neurology, and among adults its incidence is exceeded only by cerebrovascular disorders. In most persons, the first seizure episode occurs before 20 years of age. After 20 years of age, a seizure is caused most often by a structural change, trauma, tumour, or stroke.[45,46]

A seizure is not a disease but a symptom of underlying CNS dysfunction. Seizures may occur during almost all serious illnesses or injuries affecting the brain, including metabolic derangements, infections, tumours, drug abuse, vascular lesions, congenital deformities, and brain injury. A seizure represents the clinical manifestations of an abnormal, uncontrolled electrical discharge from a group of neurons. Seizures are one feature of epileptic syndromes. Epilepsy refers to the syndromes of associated seizure types, EEG patterns, examination findings, hereditary patterns, and precipitating factors.

SEIZURES

- Seizures are paroxysmal motor, sensory, or cognitive manifestations of spontaneous, abnormally synchronous electrical discharges from collections of neurons in the cerebral cortex.
- The site of seizure generation and the extent to which the abnormal neural activity is conducted to other areas of the brain determine the type and manifestations of the seizure activity.
- Focal seizures originate in a small group of neurons localized to one hemisphere. There are two major groups for focal seizures: without impairment of consciousness and with impaired consciousness.
- Generalized seizures show simultaneous disruption of normal brain activity in both hemispheres from the onset. They include unconsciousness and varying bilateral degrees of symmetric motor responses without evidence of localization to one hemisphere. These types of seizure include tonic–clonic, absence, myoclonic, clonic, tonic, and atonic.

Patients with an epileptic syndrome may have several seizure types. The newest classification system endorsed by the International League Against Epilepsy categorizes both seizure type (generalized or focal), and epilepsy syndromes.

Etiology: Provoked and Unprovoked Seizures

Many theories have been proposed to explain the cause of the abnormal brain electrical activity that occurs with seizures. Seizures may be caused by alterations in cell membrane permeability or distribution of ions across the neuronal cell membranes. Another cause may be decreased inhibition of cortical or thalamic neuronal activity or structural changes that alter the excitability of neurons. Neurotransmitter imbalances such as an acetylcholine excess or γ-aminobutyric acid (GABA, an inhibitory neurotransmitter) deficiency have been proposed as causes. Certain epilepsy syndromes have been linked to specific genetic mutations causing ion channel defects.[47]

Clinically, seizures may be categorized as unprovoked (primary or idiopathic) or provoked (secondary or acute symptomatic). Unprovoked or idiopathic seizures are those for which no identifiable cause can be determined, and are thought to be genetic. Most unprovoked seizures occur in the setting of an epileptic syndrome. These patients usually require chronic administration of antiepileptic medications to limit seizure recurrences. Provoked or symptomatic seizures include febrile seizures, seizures precipitated by systemic metabolic conditions, and those that follow a primary insult to the CNS. Most provoked seizures are best prevented by treatment of the underlying cause. For example, the most common subgroup is that of febrile seizures in children.[48] In susceptible children, a high fever, usually over 40°C, may provoke a generalized seizure.

Treatment includes aggressive use of antipyretics to prevent seizures during a febrile illness. Transient systemic metabolic disturbances may precipitate seizures. Examples include electrolyte imbalances, hypoglycemia, hypoxia, hypocalcemia, uremia, alkalosis, and rapid withdrawal of sedative drugs. Specific CNS injuries such as toxemia of pregnancy, water intoxication, meningoencephalitis, trauma, cerebral hemorrhage and stroke, and brain tumours may precipitate a seizure. In all cases of provoked seizures, treatment of the immediate underlying cause often results in their resolution.

Classification

The International Classification of Epileptic Seizures determines seizure type by clinical symptoms and EEG activity and has developed an organization of epilepsy syndromes. The classification was revised and published in 2010.[46] It divides seizures into categories depending on whether the seizure begins in a specific or focal area of one cerebral hemisphere or begins simultaneously in both cerebral hemispheres[46,47] (Chart 51.1). Further classification of epileptic syndromes characterizes the underlying diseases that cause the seizures, and divides seizures into genetic (previously referred to as

CHART 51.1 REVISED CLASSIFICATION OF SEIZURES AND EPILEPSIES

Focal Seizures
Without impairment of consciousness or awareness
With impairment of consciousness or awareness
Evolving to bilateral, convulsive seizure with tonic and/or clonic components

Generalized Seizures
Tonic–clonic (in any combination)
Absence seizures
  Typical absence
  Atypical absence
  Absence with special features
    Myoclonic absence
    Eyelid myoclonia
Myoclonic
  Myoclonic
  Myoclonic atonic
  Myoclonic tonic
Clonic
Tonic
Atonic

Unknown
Epileptic spasms
Febrile seizures

Source: Berg A. T., Berkovic S. F., Brodie M. J. (2010). Revised terminology and concepts for organization of seizures and epilepsies: Report of the ILAE Commission on Classification and Terminology, 2005–2009. *Epilepsia, 51,* 676–685.

idiopathic), structural/metabolic (resulting from some CNS injury, previously *symptomatic*), and unknown (presumed to be symptomatic of some unidentified cause, previously *cryptogenic*).[46,47] The system also has categories for unknown seizures of undetermined origin such as neonatal seizures and epileptic spasms.

Focal Seizures

Focal seizures are the most common type of seizure among newly diagnosed cases in all groups older than 10 years of age. Focal seizures are categorized as *focal seizure with alteration in consciousness or awareness* (formerly known as *simple partial seizure*), *focal seizure without alteration in consciousness or awareness* (formerly known as *complex partial seizure*), or *evolving, bilateral, convulsive seizure*. Although the terms have changed, evaluation of patients must still consider descriptors of impairment in consciousness/awareness or other dyscognitive features, localization, and progression of ictal events, which previously differentiated simple and complex partial seizures.

Focal Seizures WITHOUT Impairment of Consciousness or Awareness.

Focal seizures usually involve only one hemisphere and are not accompanied by loss of consciousness or responsiveness. These seizures also have previously been referred to as elementary partial seizures, partial seizures with elementary symptoms, or focal seizures.

The observed clinical signs and symptoms depend on the area of the brain where the abnormal neuronal discharge is taking place. If the motor area of the brain is involved, the earliest symptom is motor movement corresponding to the location of onset on the contralateral side of the body. The motor movement may remain localized or may spread to other cortical areas. If the sensory portion of the brain is involved, there may be no observable clinical manifestations. Sensory symptoms correlating with the location of seizure activity on the contralateral side of the brain may involve somatic sensory disturbance (*e.g.,* tingling and crawling sensations) or special sensory disturbance (*i.e.,* visual, auditory, gustatory, or olfactory phenomena). When abnormal cortical discharge stimulates the autonomic nervous system, flushing, tachycardia, diaphoresis, hypotension or hypertension, or pupillary changes may be evident.[46,47]

The term *prodrome* or *aura* traditionally has meant a stereotyped warning sign of impending seizure activity described by the affected person. The aura actually represents a simple partial seizure, reflecting only a small area of abnormal electrical activity in the brain. Simple partial seizures may progress to complex partial seizures or generalized tonic–clonic seizures that result in unconsciousness. Most patients perceive the aura as a warning sign of impending complex partial seizures or other generalized seizures.

Focal Seizures WITH Impairment of Consciousness or Awareness.

These types of seizures involve impairment of consciousness and often arise from the temporal lobe. The seizure begins in a localized area of the brain but may progress rapidly to involve both hemispheres. These seizures were sometimes referred to as *psychomotor seizures,* reflecting their typical manifestations.[46,47]

These types of seizures often are accompanied by automatisms. Automatisms are repetitive, nonpurposeful activities such as lip smacking, grimacing, patting, or rubbing clothing. Confusion during the postictal state (after a seizure), or dyscognition, is common. Hallucinations and illusional experiences such as déjà vu (familiarity with unfamiliar events or environments) or jamais vu (unfamiliarity with a known environment) have been reported. There may be overwhelming fear, uncontrolled forced thinking or a flood of ideas, and feelings of detachment and depersonalization. A person with a complex partial seizure disorder sometimes is misdiagnosed as having a psychiatric disorder.

Evolving Convulsive Seizures.

These seizures are focal at onset but then become generalized as the ictal neuronal discharge spreads, involving deeper structures of the brain, such as the thalamus or the reticular formation.[47] Discharges spread to both hemispheres, resulting in progression to tonic–clonic seizure activity. These seizures may start as focal seizures and may be preceded by an aura. The aura, often a stereotyped peculiar sensation that precedes the seizure, is the result of partial seizure activity. A history of an aura is clinically useful to identify the seizure as partial and not generalized in onset. However, absence of an aura does not reliably exclude a focal onset because many evolving convulsive seizures generalize too rapidly to generate an aura.

Generalized-Onset Seizures

Generalized-onset seizures are the most common type in young children. These seizures are classified as generalized as clinical signs, symptoms, and supporting EEG changes indicate involvement of both hemispheres at onset. The clinical symptoms include unconsciousness and involve varying bilateral degrees of symmetric motor responses without evidence of localization to one hemisphere. These seizures include tonic–clonic, absence (typical, atypical, and with special features), myoclonic, clonic, tonic, and atonic types.[46,47]

Tonic–Clonic Seizures.

Tonic–clonic seizures, formerly called grand mal seizures, are the most common major motor seizure. Frequently, a person has a vague warning (possibly a focal seizure) and experiences a sharp tonic contraction of the muscles with extension of the extremities and immediate loss of consciousness. Incontinence of bladder and bowel is common. Cyanosis may occur from contraction of airway and respiratory muscles. The tonic phase is followed by the clonic phase, which involves rhythmic bilateral contraction and relaxation of the extremities. At the end of the clonic phase, the person remains unconscious until the RAS begins to function again. This is called the *postictal phase*. The tonic–clonic phases last approximately 60 to 90 seconds.

Absence Seizures.

Absence seizures are generalized, nonconvulsive epileptic events and are expressed mainly as disturbances in consciousness. Formerly referred to as *petit mal seizures,* absence seizures typically occur in children and cease in adulthood or evolve to generalized motor seizures. Children may present with a history of school failure that predates the first evidence of seizure episodes. Although typical absence seizures have been characterized as a blank stare, motionlessness, and unresponsiveness, motion occurs in many cases of absence seizures. This motion takes the form of automatisms such as lip smacking, mild clonic motion (usually in the eyelids), increased or decreased postural tone, and autonomic phenomena. There often is a brief loss of contact with the environment. The seizure usually lasts only a few seconds, and then the person is able to resume normal activity immediately. The manifestations often are so subtle that they may pass unnoticed. Because automatisms and unresponsiveness are common to focal seizures, the latter often are mistakenly labelled as absence seizures.

Atypical absence seizures are similar to typical absence seizures except for greater alterations in muscle tone and less abrupt onset and cessation. In practice, it is difficult to distinguish typical from atypical absence seizures without the benefit of supporting EEG findings. However, it is important to distinguish between focal and absence seizures because the drugs of choice for treatment are different. Medications that are effective for partial seizures may increase the frequency of absence seizures.

Myoclonic Seizures. Myoclonic seizures involve sudden brief involuntary muscle contractions induced by stimuli of cerebral origin. A myoclonic seizure involves bilateral jerking of muscles, generalized or confined to the face, trunk, or one or more extremities.

Clonic Seizures. Clonic seizures begin with a loss of consciousness and sudden hypotonia. This is followed by limb jerking that may or may not be symmetrical. The jerking consists of repeated contractions and relaxations of the same muscle groups.

Tonic Seizures. Tonic seizures are characterized by a rigid, violent contraction of the muscles, fixing the limbs in a strained position. This sustained contraction can last for a few seconds to minutes.

Atonic Seizures. In akinetic or atonic seizures, there is a sudden, split-second loss of muscle tone leading to slackening of the jaw, drooping of the limbs, or falling to the ground. These seizures also are known as *drop attacks.*

Unknown Seizures

Unclassified seizures are those that cannot be placed in one of the previous categories. These seizures are observed in the neonatal and infancy periods. Determination of whether the seizure is focal or generalized is not possible. Unclassified seizures are difficult to control with medication. In this new unknown category, epileptic spasms or infantile spasms, are more commonly seen in infants but can also be persist in adults. When presenting with unique seizure like rhythmic movements but does not fit into any of the previously mentioned categories, this is now referred to as an epileptic spasms.[46,47]

Diagnosis and Treatment

The diagnosis of seizure disorders is based on a thorough history and neurologic examination, including a full description of the seizure. The physical examination and laboratory studies help exclude any metabolic disease or alteration (*e.g.,* hyponatremia) that could precipitate seizures. MRI scans are used to identify structural defects such as temporal lobe sclerosis or underlying congenital malformations causing the seizure. One of the most useful diagnostic tests is the EEG, which is used to record changes in the brain's electrical activity. It is used to support the clinical diagnosis of epilepsy, to provide a guide for prognosis, and to assist in classifying the seizure disorder.

The first rules of treatment are to protect the person from injury during a seizure, preserve brain function by aborting or preventing seizure activity, and treat any underlying disease. Persons with epilepsy should be advised to avoid situations that could be dangerous or life-threatening if seizures occur. Treatment of the underlying disorder may reduce the frequency of seizures.

After the underlying disease is treated, the aim of treatment is to bring the seizures under control with the least possible disruption in lifestyle and minimum side effects from medication. Since the late 1970s, the therapy for epilepsy has changed drastically because of an improved classification system, the ability to measure serum anticonvulsant levels, and the availability of potent new anticonvulsant drugs. With proper drug management, 60% to 80% of persons with epilepsy can obtain good seizure control.

Anticonvulsant Medications

Multiple drugs are now available for the treatment of epilepsy. Until 1990, the available antiseizure drugs included carbamazepine, phenytoin, ethosuximide, valproic acid, phenobarbital, primidone, and clonazepam.[14,49] Newer antiepileptic drugs that have been marketed since 1996 include gabapentin, lamotrigine, felbamate, topiramate, levetiracetam, tiagabine, oxcarbazepine, and vigabatrin.[14]

The choice of drugs used as first-line therapy for seizure disorders has changed since the newer drugs were introduced because they have much better side-effect profiles.[14,49] In selecting the appropriate antiepileptic drug, the following principles should be kept in mind: seizure type, mechanism of seizure action, side effects, interactions with other medications, length of time for onset of drug, and cost. This pharmacologic decision-making in treating seizures is complex and requires an individualized patient approach as seizure activity will vary. Generally, complete seizure control can be attained in 50% of patients with another 25% improving significantly.[49]

Women of childbearing age on antiseizure medications require special consideration concerning fertility, contraception, and pregnancy. Many of the drugs interact with oral contraceptives; some affect hormone function or decrease fertility. All such women should be advised to take folic acid supplementation. For women with epilepsy who become pregnant, antiseizure drugs increase the risk for congenital abnormalities and other perinatal complications. Carbamazepine, phenytoin, phenobarbital, primidone, and valproic acid can interfere with vitamin D metabolism and predispose to osteoporosis.[14]

Whenever possible, a single drug should be used in epilepsy therapy. Monotherapy eliminates drug interactions and additive side effects. Determining the proper dose of the anticonvulsant drug is often a long and tedious process, which can be very frustrating for the person with epilepsy. Consistency in taking the medication is essential. Anticonvulsant drugs never should be discontinued abruptly; the dose should be decreased slowly to prevent seizure recurrence. The most frequent cause of recurrent seizures is patient noncompliance with drug regimens. Ongoing education and support are extremely important in the management of seizures. The psychosocial implications of a diagnosis of epilepsy continue to have a large impact on those affected with the disorder.

The neurologist and primary care provider must work together when a person on anticonvulsant medication becomes ill and must take additional medications. Some drugs act synergistically, and others interfere with the actions of anticonvulsant medications. This situation needs to be carefully monitored to avoid overmedication or interference with successful seizure control.

Surgical Therapy

Surgical treatment may be an option for persons with epilepsy that is refractory to drug treatment.[50] With the use of modern neuroimaging and surgical techniques, a single epileptogenic lesion can be identified and removed without leaving a neurologic deficit. The most common surgery consists of removal of the amygdala and an anterior part of the hippocampus and entorhinal cortex, as well as a small part of the temporal pole, leaving the lateral temporal neocortex intact. Another surgical procedure involves partial removal of the corpus callosum to prevent spread of a unilateral seizure to a generalized seizure. Some refractory patients benefit from an implantable electrical stimulator of the vagus nerve. Modern epilepsy surgery requires a multidisciplinary team of highly skilled surgeons and specialists working together in an epilepsy centre. Most procedures require only a few hours in the operating room and a few days' stay in the hospital after surgery. Epilepsy surgery is increasingly considered a treatment modality for persons with medically intractable epilepsy.

Status Epilepticus

Seizures that do not stop spontaneously or occur in succession without recovery are called *status epilepticus*. There are as many types of status epilepticus as there are types of seizures. Tonic–clonic or convulsive status epilepticus is a medical emergency and, if not promptly treated, may lead to respiratory failure and death.

The disorder occurs most frequently in the young children and in the elderly. Morbidity and mortality rates are highest in older adults and persons with acute symptomatic seizures, such as those related to anoxia or cerebral infarction.[51] Approximately one third of patients have no history of a seizure disorder, and in another one third, status epilepticus occurs as an initial manifestation of epilepsy.[51] If status epilepticus is caused by neurologic or systemic disease, the cause needs to be identified and treated immediately because the seizures probably will not respond until the underlying cause has been corrected.

Treatment consists of appropriate life support measures. Medications are given to control seizure activity. Intravenously administered diazepam or lorazepam is considered first-line therapy for the condition. The prognosis is related to the underlying cause as well as the duration of the seizures themselves.

IN SUMMARY

Seizures are caused by spontaneous, uncontrolled, paroxysmal, transitory discharges from cortical centres in the brain. Seizures may occur as a reversible symptom of another disease condition or as a recurrent condition called "epilepsy." Epileptic seizures are classified as generalized, focal, or unknown. Generalized seizures involve both hemispheres from the start and include unconsciousness and rapidly occurring, widespread, bilateral symmetric motor responses. Focal seizures have evidence of local onset, beginning in one hemisphere. Control of seizures is the primary goal of treatment and is accomplished with anticonvulsant medications. Anticonvulsant medications interact with each other and need to be monitored closely when more than one drug is used.

REVIEW EXERCISES

1. A 20-year-man is an unbelted driver involved in a motor vehicle collision and presents in coma.
   A. *What are the clinical signs of coma?*
   B. *Where does the source of coma localize in the brain?*
   C. *Which complications of traumatic head injury might lead to coma?*
   D. *What are the key treatment options to manage elevated intracranial pressure?*
2. A 65-year-old woman presents with a 1-hour history of right-sided weakness and aphasia. An immediate CT scan of the brain is negative.
   A. *Where in the brain is the pathologic process?*
   B. *What are the indications to administer intravenous tissue plasminogen activator?*

C. *What are the possible causes of this stroke, and what diagnostic tests would reveal the cause?*

3. A child is taken to the emergency department with lethargy, fever, and a stiff neck on examination.

A. *What findings on initial lumbar puncture indicate bacterial versus viral meningitis?*

B. *In the case of bacterial meningitis, what are the most likely organisms?*

4. A 60-year-old man develops involuntary shaking of his right arm, which spreads to the face; then he collapses with whole-body shaking and loss of consciousness. After 1 minute, the shaking stops, and he is confused and disoriented.

A. *What type of seizure is suggested by the clinical manifestations?*

B. *Assuming this is his first seizure, what diagnostic tests should be performed to identify a cause for the seizure?*

C. *If he has a long history of similar recurrent seizures, what treatments should be instituted? What treatments should be considered if he has failed multiple adequate trials of anticonvulsant medications?*

References

1. Gosseries O., Vanhaudenhuyse A., Bruno M., et al. (2011). Chapter 2: Disorders of consciousness: Coma, vegetative, and minimally conscious states. In Cvetkovic D., Cosic I. (Eds.), *States of consciousness*. Berlin: Springer-Verlag.

2. Hickey J. V. (2014). *The clinical practice of neurological and neurosurgical nursing* (7th ed.). Philadelphia, PA: Lippincott Williams & Wilkins.

3. Giacino J. T., Fins J. J., Lauareys S., Schiff N. D. (2014). Disorders of consciousness after acquired brain injury: The state of the science. *Nature Reviews Neurology, 10*(2), 99–114.

4. Rhoades R. A., Bell D. R. (2013). *Medical physiology: Principles for clinical medicine* (4th ed.). Philadelphia, PA: Lippincott Williams & Wilkins.

5. Frosch M. P., Anthony D., De Girofami U. (2010). Chapter 28: The central nervous system. In Kumar V., Abbas A. K., Fausto N., et al. (Eds.), *Robbins and Cotran pathologic basis of disease* (8th ed.). Philadelphia, PA: Elsevier Saunders.

6. Wijdicks E. F., Varelas P. N., Gronseth G. S., Greer D. M.; American Academy of Neurology. (2010). Evidence-based guideline update: Determining brain death in adults: Report of the Quality Standards Subcommittee of the American Academy of Neurology. *Neurology, 74*(23), 1911–1918.

7. Shemie S. D., Doig C., Dickens B., et al.; Pediatric Reference Group; Neonatal Reference Group. (2006). Severe brain injury to neurological determination of death: Canadian forum recommendations. *Canadian Medical Association Journal, 174*(6), S1–S12.

8. Quality Standards Subcommittee of American Academy of Neurology. (1995). Practice parameters for determining brain death in adults. *Neurology, 45*(5), 1012–1014.

9. Fuller G. N., Goodman J. C., Bouldin T. W. (2012). Chapter 28: The nervous system. In Rubin R., Strayer D. S. (Eds.). *Rubin's pathology: Clinicopathologic foundations of medicine* (6th ed.). Philadelphia, PA: Lippincott Williams & Wilkins.

10. Hopkins R. O. (2008). Does near drowning in ice water prevent anoxic induced brain injury? *Journal of the International Neuropsychological Society, 14*(4), 656–659.

11. Peberdy M. A., Callaway C. W., Neumar R. W., et al.; American Heart Association. (2010). Part 9: Post-cardiac arrest care: 2010 American Heart Association Guidelines for Cardiopulmonary Resuscitation and Emergency Cardiovascular Care. *Circulation, 122*(18 Suppl 3), S768–S786.

12. Cornelius C., Crupi R., Calabrese V., et al. (2013). Traumatic brain injury: Oxidative stress and neuroprotection. *Antioxidants & Redox Signaling, 19*(8), 836–853.

13. De Keyser J., Uyttenboogaart, M., Koch M. W., et al. (2005). Neuroprotection in acute ischemic stroke. *Acta Neurologica Belgica, 105*(3), 144–148.

14. Katzung B. G., Masters S. B., Trevor A. J. (Eds.), *Basic & clinical pharmacology* (12th ed.). Norwalk, CT: Appleton & Lange.

15. Silver J. M., McAllister T. W., Yudofsky S. C. (2011). *Textbook of traumatic brain injury* (2nd ed.). Arlington, TX: American Psychiatric Publishing.

16. Hall J. E. (2011). *Textbook of medical physiology* (12th ed.). Philadelphia, PA: W. B. Saunders.

17. Plum F., Posner J. B. (1980). *The diagnosis of stupor and coma* (3rd ed.). Philadelphia, PA: F. A. Davis.

18. Young G. B. (2011). Impaired consciousness and herniation syndromes. *Neurologic Clinics, 29*(4), 765–772.

19. Blennow K., Hardy J., Zetterberg H. (2012). The neuropathology and neurobiology of traumatic brain injury. *Neuron, 76*(5), 886–899.

20. Canadian Institute for Health Information (CIHI). (2006). Head injuries in Canada: A decade of change. Available online at: https://secure.cihi.ca/free_products/ntr_head_injuries_2006_e.pdf. Accessed May 18, 2015.

21. Rathbone A. T., Tharmaradinam S., Jiang S., et al. (2015). A review of the neuro- and systemic inflammatory responses in post-concussion symptoms: Introduction of the "post inflammatory brain syndrome" PIBS. *Brain, Behavior, and Immunity, 46*, 1–16.

22. Heart & Stroke Foundation. (2015). Statistics. Available online at: http://www.heartandstroke.on.ca/site/c.pvI3IeNWJwE/b.3581729/k.359A/Statistics.htm#stroke. Accessed May 18, 2015.

23. Heart & Stroke Foundation. (2014). 2014 Stroke report. Available online at: http://www.heartandstroke.com/atf/cf/%7B99452D8B-E7F1-4BD6-A57D-B136CE6C95BF%7D/HSF_SMReport2014E_Final.pdf. Accessed May 18, 2015.

24. Heart and Stroke Foundation. (2011). First Nations, Inuit & Métis resources. Available online at: http://www.heartandstroke.on.ca/site/c.pvI3IeNWJwE/b.3581613/k.16/First_Nations_Inuit__M233tis_Resources.htm. Accessed May 18, 2015.

25. Canadian Cancer Society. (2015). Brain and spinal tumours. Available online at: https://www.cancer.ca/en/cancer-information/cancer-type/brain-spinal/brain-and-spinal-tumours/?region=on. Accessed October 23, 2015.

26. Mehta M., Vogelbaum M. A., Chang S., et al. (2011). Chapter 121: Neoplasms of the central nervous system. In DeVita V. T., Hellman S., Rosenberg S. A. (Eds.), *Cancer: Principles and practice of oncology* (9th ed.). Philadelphia, PA: Lippincott Williams & Wilkins.

27. Canadian Cancer Society. (2015). Childhood brain and spinal tumours. Available online at: https://www.cancer.ca/en/cancer-information/cancer-type/brain-spinal-childhood/childhood-brain-and-spinal-tumours/?region = on. Accessed May 18, 2015.

28. Fonseca A. C., Ferro J. M. (2013). Drug abuse and stroke. *Current Neurology and Neuroscience Reports, 13*(2), 325.

29. Fisher M., Bastan B. (2012). Identifying and utilizing the ischemic penumbra. *Neurology, 79*(13, Suppl 1), S79–S85.

30. Siket M. S., Edlow J. A. (2012). Transient ischemic attack: Reviewing the evolution of the definition, diagnosis, risk stratification, and management for the emergency physician. *Emergency Medicine Clinics of North America, 30*(3), 745–770.

31. Heart & Stroke Foundation. (2015). Canadian stroke best practice recommendations. Available online at: http://www.strokebestpractices.ca/. Accessed May 18, 2015.

32. Phillips S. J., Gubitz G. (updated 2014). Cardiovascular disorders: Acute stroke. In Repchinsky C. (Ed.), *e-Therapeutics*. Ottawa, ON: Canadian Pharmacists Association.

33. Canadian Best Practices Recommendations for Stroke Care Group. (2013). Taking action towards optimal stroke care. Available online at: http://www. strokebestpractices.ca/wp-content/uploads/2013/05/CSBP-Taking-Action-Resource-OVERVIEW_EN_22May13F.pdf. Accessed May 18, 2015.

34. Goyal M., Demchuk A. M., Menon B. K., et al.; ESCAPE Trial Investigators. (2015). Randomized assessment of rapid endovascular treatment of ischemic stroke. *New England Journal of Medicine, 372*(11), 1019–1030.

35. Bederson J. B., Connolly S., Batjer H. H.; ESCAPE Trial Investigators. (2009). Guidelines for the management of aneurysmal subarachnoid hemorrhage. *Stroke, 40*(3), 994–1025.

36. Chalouhi N., Hoh B. L., Hasan D. (2013). Review of cerebral aneurysm formation, growth, and rupture. *Stroke, 44*(12), 3613–3622.

37. Friedlander R. M. (2007). Arteriovenous malformations of the brain. *New England Journal of Medicine, 356*, 2704–2712.

38. Ogilvy C. S., Stieg P. E., Awad I., et al.; Special Writing Group of the Stroke Council, American Heart Association. (2001). Recommendations for management of intracranial arteriovenous malformations. *Stroke, 32*, 1458–1471.

39. Brouwer M. C., Tunkel A. R., van de Beek D. (2010). Epidemiology, diagnosis, and antimicrobial treatment of acute bacterial meningitis. *Clinical Microbiology Reviews, 23*(3), 467–492.

40. Koedel U., Klein M., Pfister H. (2010). New understanding on the pathophysiology of bacterial meningitis. *Current Opinion in Infectious Diseases, 23*(3), 217–223.

41. Le Saux N. (2014). Guidelines for the management of suspected and confirmed bacterial meningitis in Canadian children older than one month of age. *Paediatrics & Child Health, 19*(3), 141–146.

42. Public Health Agency of Canada. (2014). Canadian immunization guide: Part 4, active vaccines, meningococcal vaccine. Available online at: http://www. phac-aspc.gc.ca/publicat/cig-gci/p04-eng.php. Accessed May 11, 2015.

43. Norden A. D., Reardon D. A., Wen P. C. (2011). *Primary central nervous system tumors.* New York: Springer Science.

44. DeAngelis L. M. (2001). Brain tumors. *New England Journal of Medicine, 344*, 114–123.

45. Epilepsy Canada. (2005). Epilepsy facts. Available online at: http://www. epilepsy.ca/en-CA/Facts/Epilepsy-Facts.html. Accessed May 18, 2015.

46. Berg A. T., Berkovic S. F., Brodie M. J., et al. (2010). Revised terminology and concepts for the organization of seizures and epilepsies: Report of the ILAE Commission on classification and terminology, 2005–2009. *Epilepsia, 51*(4), 676–685.

47. Berg A. T., Millichap J. J. (2013). The 2010 revised classification of seizure and epilepsy. *Continuum (Minneap Minn), 19*(3), 571–597.

48. Mikati M. A. (2011). Chapter 586: Seizures in childhood. In Kliegman R. M., Stanton B. F., St. Geme J. W., et al. (Eds.), *Nelson textbook of pediatrics* (19th ed.). Philadelphia, PA: Saunders Elsevier.

49. Goldenberg M. M. (2010). Overview of drugs used for epilepsy and seizures: Etiology, diagnosis, and treatment. *Pharmacy and Therapeutics, 35*(7), 392–415.

50. Perry M. S., Duchowny M. (2013). Surgical versus medical treatment for refractory epilepsy: Outcomes beyond seizure control. *Epilepsia, 54*(12), 2060–2070.

51. Huff J. S., Fountain N. B. (2011). Pathophysiology and definitions of seizures and status epilepticus. *Emergency Medicine Clinics of North America, 29*(1), 1–13.

Visit thePoint **http://thePoint.lww.com for animations, journal articles, and more!**

Sleep and Sleep Disorders

52

As humans, we spend approximately a third of our lives asleep. We all know what sleep feels like. Yet defining sleep, describing what happens when we sleep, and explaining why we sleep are more difficult. Of equal concern is an understanding of factors that interfere with sleep. For many people, the inability to engage in appropriate periods of normal, restful sleep seriously impairs their functioning. The content in this chapter is divided into three parts: (1) the neurobiology of sleep, (2) sleep disorders, and (3) sleep and sleep disorders in children and older adults.

NEUROBIOLOGY OF SLEEP

After completing this section of the chapter, you should be able to meet the following objectives:

- Cite the major brain structures that are involved in sleep.
- Describe the different stages of sleep in terms of the electroencephalogram tracing, eye movements, motor movements, heart rate, blood pressure, and cerebral activity.
- Characterize the circadian rhythm as it relates to sleep and wakefulness.
- Describe the possible role of melatonin in regulation of sleep.

Sleep is part of what is called the *sleep–wake cycle.* In contrast to wakefulness, which is a time of mental activity and energy expenditure, sleep is a period of inactivity and restoration of mental and physical function. It has been suggested that sleep provides time for entering information that has been acquired during periods of wakefulness into memory and for reestablishing communication between various parts of the brain. Sleep also is a time when other body systems restore their energy and repair their tissues. Muscle activity and digestion decrease and sympathetic nervous system activity is diminished. Many hormones, such as growth hormone, are produced in a cyclic manner correlating with the sleep–wake cycle, suggesting that growth and tissue repair may occur during sleep.

FIGURE 52.1 • A: Brain structures involved in sleep. **B:** Location of the suprachiasmatic nucleus (biologic clock) with input from the retina and its association with the pineal gland and melatonin production.

Neural Structures and Pathways

Anatomically, the sleep–wake cycle involves structures in the thalamus, associated areas of the cerebral cortex, and interneurons in the reticular formation of the midbrain, the pons, and the brain stem (Fig. 52.1). The reticular formation of the midbrain, pons, and brain stem monitors and modulates the activity of various circuits controlling wakefulness. The thalamus and the cerebral cortex function in tandem, with all sensory information being relayed to the thalamus and from there to the cerebral cortex. For example, visual impulses from the retina go to the thalamus and are then relayed to the visual cortex. The pathways between each sensory area of the thalamus and the cortex form two-way communication loops called *thalamocortical loops.*[1] Communication between each sensory area of the thalamus and its companion area in the cortex is kept orderly by several neuronal control systems, including the midbrain reticular formation that controls the level of background activity so that external stimuli can be processed.

The Sleep–Wake Cycle

The sleep–wake cycle normally consists of a synchronous pattern of wakefulness and sleep. Wakefulness is a state of being aware of the environment—of receiving and responding to information arriving from all the senses, placing that information into memory, and recalling and integrating present experiences with previously stored memories. During wakefulness,

both the thalamocortical loop and brain stem centres are active. A full repertoire of motor movements are made possible by corticospinal circuits that travel through the brain stem. Sleep represents a period of diminished consciousness from which a person can be aroused by sensory or other stimuli. It occurs in stages during which the brain remains active but does not effectively process sensory information. However, during sleep, a person does have inward conscious experiences such as dreams.

Brain Waves

Many of the advances in understanding the sleep–wake cycle have come about because of the ability to record brain waves through the use of the electroencephalogram (EEG). In 1928 the German psychiatrist Hans Berger first successfully recorded continuous electrical activity from the scalp of human subjects.[1] The source of the brain waves is the alternating excitatory and inhibitory nerve activity in postsynaptic neurons.[2] During the recording of an EEG, the postsynaptic potentials are averaged and filtered to improve the quality of the signal. As such, the EEG does not measure the activity of a single neuron, but rather the combined activity and "cross-talk" among many hundreds of neurons responding to a given stimulus.

The normal EEG consists of brain waves of various frequencies (measured in cycles per second, or hertz [Hz]) and amplitude (measured in microvolts [μV]; Fig. 52.2). Four types of EEG rhythms are used to describe brain activity during the sleep–wake cycle: alpha, beta, delta, and theta rhythms.[2–4] The

FIGURE 52.2 • The amplitude and frequency characteristics of an EEG tracing.

alpha rhythm, which has a frequency of 8 to 14 Hz, occurs when a person is awake with eyes closed. When the eyes are open, the EEG becomes desynchronized and the dominant frequency changes to the low-amplitude *beta* rhythm with a frequency greater than 14 Hz. The increased frequency of the beta waves is thought to reflect a higher level of brain activity produced by firing of a large number of neurons, and the low amplitude a lack of synchronization resulting from nerve activity occurring in many different brain sites at the same time. The *delta* (0.5 to 4 Hz) and *theta* (4 to 7 Hz) rhythms are observed during sleep. The low-frequency, higher-amplitude waves that occur during sleep indicate that fewer neurons are firing and that those that are active are more highly synchronized and less affected by sensory stimulation.

Sleep Stages

There are two types of sleep: rapid eye movement (REM) and nonREM sleep.[2,4,5] These two types of sleep alternate with each other and are characterized by differences in eye movements, muscle tone and body movements, heart rate and blood pressure, breathing patterns, brain wave activity, and

dreaming (Table 52.1). A complete sleep cycle takes about 90 to 110 minutes.

Nonrapid Eye Movement Sleep. Nonrapid Eye Movement (nonREM) sleep is a quiet type of sleep characterized by a relatively inactive, yet fully regulating brain, and a fully movable body.[5] The brain stem coordinates activity between the spinal cord and various reflexes such as swallowing and chewing. NonREM sleep normally is encountered when the person first becomes drowsy. It is divided into four stages that reflect an increasing depth of sleep (Fig. 52.3). *Stage 1* consists of low-voltage, mixed-frequency EEG activity. It occurs at sleep onset and is a brief (1 to 7 minutes) transitional stage between wakefulness and true sleep. During this stage, persons can be easily aroused simply by touching them, calling their name, or quietly closing a door. People may experience sudden muscle twitches called hypnic (hypnagogic) jerks, brief contractions of the body that occur at sleep onset. Often these movements are associated with a sensation of falling. In addition to its role at sleep onset, stage 1 serves as a transitional stage for repeated sleep cycles throughout the night. A common sign

TABLE 52.1 ELECTROENCEPHALOGRAM, EYE AND MOTOR MOVEMENTS, VITAL FUNCTIONS, AND CEREBRAL ACTIVITY DURING SLEEP

SLEEP STAGE	ELECTRO-ENCEPHALOGRAM	EYE MOVEMENTS	MOTOR MOVEMENTS	HEART RATE, BLOOD PRESSURE, RESPIRATIONS	CEREBRAL ACTIVITY
Stage 1	Low voltage, mixed frequency	Slow, rolling movements	Moderate activity	Slows	Decreases
Stage 2	Low voltage, 12- to 14-Hz spindles	Slow, rolling movements	Moderate activity	Slows	Decreases
Stages 3 and 4 (deep sleep)	Delta (0.5–4 Hz) waves (slow-wave sleep)	Slow, rolling movements	Moderate activity	Slows	Decreases
REM sleep	Low voltage, mixed frequency	Clusters of rapid eye movements	Suppressed with loss of muscle tone	Increases, variable	Increases

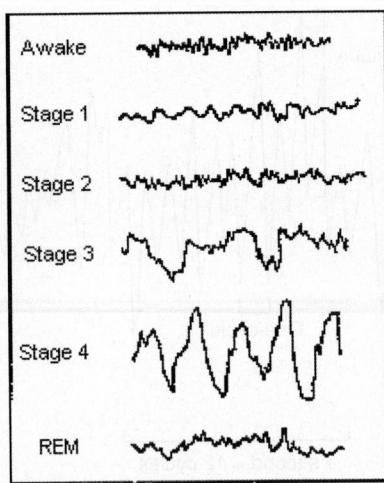

FIGURE 52.3 • Brain waves during wakefulness; nonREM stages 1, 2, 3, and 4; and REM sleep.

of severely disrupted sleep is an increase or decrease in stage 1 sleep. *Stage 2,* which lasts approximately 10 to 25 minutes, is a deeper sleep during which EEG activity is interrupted by sleep spindles consisting of bursts of high-frequency (12 to 14 Hz) waves. *Stages 3* and *4* represent deep sleep and are dominated by high-voltage, low-frequency (0.5 to 4 Hz) waves. Stage 3 usually lasts only a few minutes and is transitional to

stage 4, which lasts for approximately 20 to 40 minutes. During deep sleep, the muscles of the body relax and posture is adjusted intermittently. The heart rate and blood pressure decrease and gastrointestinal activity is slowed. An incrementally larger stimulus is required for arousal from slow-wave sleep.

Rapid Eye Movement Sleep. Rapid eye movement (REM) sleep is associated with rapid eye movements, loss of muscle movements, and vivid dreaming.[5,6] External sensory input is inhibited, whereas internal sensory circuits such as those of the auditory and visual systems are aroused. During this time, the brain can replay previous memories but cannot acquire new sensory information (Fig. 52.4). At the same time, motor systems that control body movements are inhibited. There is a loss of muscle movement and muscle tone. The result is an extraordinary set of paradoxes, in which people see things in their dreams, but cannot move. They imagine being engaged in activities such as running, flying, or dancing but are paralyzed.

There also are changes in autonomic nervous system–controlled functions during REM sleep—blood pressure, heart rate, and respirations increase and fluctuate and temperature regulation is lost. Cerebral blood flow and metabolic rate decrease. Sleep-related penile erection occurs during this stage of sleep.

Visual input is blocked

Movement is blocked

FIGURE 52.4 • Dreaming during REM sleep when sensory and motor activity are blocked.

It has been shown that adequate amounts of REM sleep are necessary for normal daytime functioning. Deprivation of REM sleep is associated with anxiety, irritability, inability to concentrate, and, if deprivation is severe enough, disturbed behaviour.

Moving Between Sleep Stages. There is a rather predictable pattern of shifting between one nonREM stage and another during a typical night's sleep.[4] At sleep onset, there is a stepwise descent from lighter stage 1 sleep to deeper stage 4 sleep, followed by an abrupt ascent back toward stage 1. However, in place of stage 1, the first REM episode usually occurs. REM sleep is comparatively short (1 to 5 minutes) during the first sleep cycle, but gradually becomes longer across the night. Stages 3 and 4 occupy less time in the second and subsequent sleep cycles and disappear altogether in later cycles.

Breathing During Sleep

Breathing normally changes during sleep. Stages 1 and 2 of nonREM sleep are characterized by a cyclic waning and waxing of the tidal volume and respiratory rate, which may include brief periods (5 to 15 seconds) of apnea. After sleep has stabilized during stages 3 and 4 of nonREM sleep, breathing becomes more regular. Ventilation usually is 1 to 2 L/min less than during quiet wakefulness; the arterial carbon dioxide partial pressure (PCO_2) is 2 to 4 mm Hg greater, and the arterial oxygen partial pressure (PO_2) is 3 to 9 mm Hg less.[7] Involuntary respiratory control mechanisms, such as responses to hypercapnia, hypoxia, and lung inflation, are intact during nonREM sleep and critically important to maintaining ventilation.

During REM sleep, respirations become irregular, but not periodic, and may include short periods of apnea. Breathing during REM sleep has many features of the voluntary control that integrates breathing with acts such as walking, talking, and swallowing. However, their influence on breathing is diminished.

Dreaming

Dreams are recollections of mental activity that occurred during sleep. They occur during all stages of sleep, but are more frequent during REM sleep. Approximately 80% of dreams occur during REM and sleep onset (stages 1 and 2).[8] Dreams that occur during REM sleep tend to be bizarre with colourful, storybook-like detail.[1] Most nightmares occur during REM sleep. Dreams that occur during stages 1 and 2 of sleep tend to be shorter, have fewer associations, and lack the colour and emotion of those that occur during REM sleep.

The purpose of dreaming is unclear. Evidence suggests that dreaming, like other physiologic functions, is important to learning and memory processing.[8] It has been suggested that dreaming may be the result of reprogramming of the central nervous system (CNS; *i.e.,* rearranging previous experiences) in preparation for the next day's conscious experiences.

Circadian Rhythms

Normally, sleep and wakefulness occur in a cyclic manner, integrated into the 24-hour light–dark solar day. The term *circadian,* from the Latin *circa* ("about") and *dies* ("day"), is used to describe these 24-hour diurnal rhythms. The function of the circadian time system is to provide a temporal organization for physiologic processes and behaviours as a means of promoting effective adaptation to the environment. At the behavioural level, this is expressed in regular cycles of sleep and waking and body functions such as temperature regulation and hormone secretion based on changes in the 24-hour light–dark solar day.

The daily rhythm of the sleep–wake cycle is part of a timekeeping system created by an internal pacemaker or clock.[9,10] Time isolation experiments, in which people were placed in an environment without time cues, showed that the cycle length of the human internal clock is in general from 23.5 to 26.5 hours.[8] Because the intrinsic cycle tends to be longer than 24 hours, a daily resetting of the circadian clock is necessary to synchronize with the environmental day. This process is called *entrainment* and normally is accomplished by exposure to the light–dark changes of the solar day.

The circadian clock appears to be controlled by a small group of hypothalamic cells, called the *suprachiasmatic nucleus* (SCN), located just above the optic chiasm and lateral to the third ventricle[9–11] (Fig. 52.1). The SCN, which receives light–dark input from the retina, exhibits a rhythm of neuronal firing that is high during the day and low during the night. Although light serves as the primary stimulus for resetting the circadian clock, other stimuli such as locomotion and activity contribute to its regulation. The major projections from the SCN are to the anterior pituitary, with lesser ones to the basal forebrain and midline thalamus. Projections to the anterior pituitary provide for diurnal regulation of growth hormone and cortisol secretion; those to hypothalamic centres, for changes in metabolism and body temperature; and those to the brain stem reticular formation, for changes in autonomic nervous system-regulated functions such as heart rate and blood pressure (Fig. 52.5).

Melatonin

Melatonin, a hormone produced by the pineal gland, is thought to help regulate the sleep–wake cycle and, possibly, circadian rhythm.[12–14] The pineal gland synthesizes and releases melatonin at night, a rhythm that is under direct control of the SCN (Fig. 52.1). Large numbers of melatonin receptors are present in the SCN, suggesting a feedback loop between the SCN and the pineal gland. Administration of melatonin produces phase-shifting changes in the circadian rhythm, similar to those caused by light. There has been recent interest in the use of melatonin in treatment of various sleep disorders, particularly those related to a shift in the circadian rhythm. Although synthetic preparations are available without prescription in health food stores and pharmacies, their potency, purity, safety, and effectiveness cannot be ensured. There also is a lack of clinical trial evidence about appropriate dosage, adverse effects,

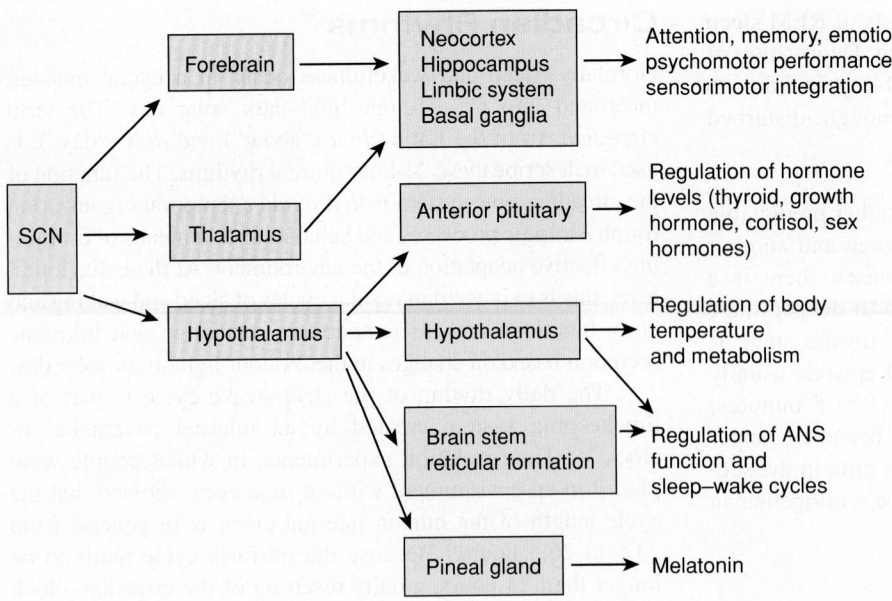

FIGURE 52.5 • Projections from the suprachiasmatic nucleus (SCN) to the forebrain, thalamus, and hypothalamus. ANS, autonomic nervous system.

drug interactions, and the effects of melatonin on various disease states.[13] A pharmacologic melatonin-receptor agonist (Ramelteon) is available as an American prescription drug but is not available in Canada.[12]

IN SUMMARY

Sleep is part of what is called the sleep–wake cycle. In contrast to wakefulness, which is a time of mental activity and energy expenditure, sleep is a period of inactivity and restoration of mental and physical function. There are two types of sleep: REM and nonREM sleep. REM sleep is associated with rapid eye movements, loss of muscle movements, and vivid dreaming. External sensory input is inhibited, whereas internal sensory circuits such as those of the auditory and visual systems are aroused. NonREM sleep is a quiet type of sleep characterized by a relatively inactive, yet fully regulating brain, and a fully movable body. It is divided into four stages that reflect an increasing depth of sleep. Stage 1 is a brief transitional stage that occurs at the onset of sleep, during which a person is easily aroused. Stage 2 is a deeper sleep, lasting approximately 10 to 25 minutes, during which EEG activity is interrupted by sleep spindles consisting of bursts of high-frequency waves. Stages 3 and 4 represent deep sleep, during which the muscles of the body relax, the heart rate and blood pressure decrease, and gastrointestinal activity is slowed.

Normally, sleep and wakefulness occur in a cyclic manner, called the circadian rhythm, that is integrated into the 24-hour light–dark solar day. The circadian clock is thought to be controlled by the SCN in the hypothalamus. The SCN, which receives light–dark input from the retina, exhibits a rhythm of neuronal firing that is high during the day and low during the night. Melatonin, a hormone produced by the pineal gland, is thought to help regulate the sleep–wake cycle.

SLEEP DISORDERS

After completing this section of the chapter, you should be able to meet the following objectives:

- List the four categories of sleep disorders included in the *International Classification of Sleep Disorders*.
- Describe the methods used in diagnosis of sleep disorders, including the sleep history, sleep diary, polysomnography, and wrist actigraphy.
- Characterize the non-24-hour sleep–wake syndrome experienced by visually impaired individuals, sleep disorders associated with acute shifts in the sleep–wake cycle due to intercontinental travel and shift work, and advanced sleep phase and delayed sleep phase circadian rhythm sleep disorders.
- Describe the causes, manifestations, diagnosis, and treatment of acute and chronic insomnia.
- Differentiate periodic limb movement disorder and restless legs syndrome in terms of manifestations and treatment.
- Explain the physiologic mechanisms, contributing factors, and manifestations of obstructive sleep apnea and describe the methods used in diagnosis and treatment of the disorder.
- Define the term *parasomnias* and relate it to the manifestations of nightmare, sleep terrors, and sleep walking.

Sleep disorders cover a broad spectrum of symptoms including the inability to fall asleep and stay asleep, circadian rhythm and sleep–wake transition disorders, sleep-related breathing and movement disorders, and excessive sleepiness. While sleep disorders have existed for centuries, it is only

CHART 52.1 **INTERNATIONAL CLASSIFICATION OF SLEEP DISORDERS**

- Insomnia
- Sleep-related breathing disorders
- Hypersomnia of central origin not due to circadian rhythm disorder or other cause of disturbed nocturnal sleep
- Circadian rhythm sleep disorders
- Parasomnias
- Sleep-related movement disorders
- Isolated symptoms, apparently related to normal variants and unresolved issues
- Other sleep disorders

Adapted from American Academy of Sleep Medicine. (2005). *International classification of sleep disorders: Diagnostic and coding manual* (2nd ed.). Westchester, IL: Author.

within the last 3 to 4 decades that attention has focused on their diagnosis and classification. The development of the *Diagnostic Classification of Sleep and Arousal Disorders* by the Association of Sleep Disorders in 1979 heralded the emergence of the discipline of sleep medicine. This was followed by the *International Classification of Sleep Disorders* (ICSD), which was produced by the American Academy of Sleep Medicine, in association with the European Sleep Research Society, the Japanese Society of Sleep Research, and the Latin American Sleep Society. First produced in 1990, the ICSD was revised in 1997 and again in 2005 as ICSD-2.[15,16] ICSD-2 classifies sleep disorders into eight major categories (Chart 52.1).

Diagnostic Methods

The diagnosis of sleep disorders usually is based on an adequate sleep history and physical examination. A sleep diary or sleep log often is helpful in describing sleep problems and arriving at a diagnosis.[17] In some cases, sleep laboratory studies may be needed to arrive at an accurate diagnosis.

Sleep History

A sleep history is fundamental to the process of identifying the nature of a sleep disorder.[17] The history should include the person's perception of the sleep problem, sleep schedule (*e.g.,* times of retiring and arising), problems with falling asleep and maintaining sleep, quality of sleep, daytime sleepiness and impact of the sleep disorder on daytime functioning, general emotional and physical problems, sleep hygiene (*e.g.,* eating and drinking before retiring), and sleep environment (*e.g.,* bed comfort, room temperature, noise, light). Because drugs such as over-the-counter medications, herbal preparations, and prescription medications can influence sleep, a careful drug history is important. It also is important to obtain information about the use of alcohol, caffeine, tobacco, and illegal substances.

Sleep Log/Diary

A sleep log/diary is a person's written account of his or her sleep experience. It usually is recommended that the diary be kept for at least 2 weeks. The diary should record the person's account of their bedtime, wakeup time, total sleep time, time of sleep onset, time needed to prepare for bed and to fall asleep, use of sleep medications, number of awakenings, subjective assessment of sleep quality, time out of bed in the morning, and daytime naps and symptoms. A number of sample forms are available to healthcare professionals for distribution to their clients.

SLEEP DISORDERS

- Circadian rhythm sleep disorders represent a misalignment between a person's sleep pattern and societal norms.
- Hypersomnia (*e.g.,* narcolepsy) is characterized by excessive daytime sleepiness not related to disturbed nocturnal sleep or circadian rhythm disorders.
- The insomnias represent a repeated difficulty with sleep initiation, duration, and quality of sleep.
- The sleep-related breathing disorders are characterized by disordered respirations during sleep (sleep apnea) and sleep-related movement by disturbing limb movements (periodic limb movement and restless legs syndrome).
- The parasomnias, which are undesirable physical phenomena that occur almost exclusively during sleep or are exaggerated by sleep, include nightmares, sleepwalking, and sleep terrors.

Actigraphy and Polysomnography

Actigraphy. Actigraphy measures muscle motion and is used to obtain objective measurements of sleep duration and efficiency outside the sleep laboratory.[18] The actigraph is a compact device that is worn on the wrist or ankle to measure body movement, which is an indirect indicator of wakefulness and sleep. Depending on the type of unit that is used, actigraphs can collect up to several weeks' worth of information.

Polysomnography. A typical sleep study, or *polysomnography,* involves use of the EEG, electro-oculogram (EOG), electromyogram (EMG), electrocardiogram (ECG), breathing movements, and pulse oximetry.[4] The EOG records eye movements. Because the eye is like a small battery with the retina negative to the cornea, an electrode placed on the skin near the eye records changes in voltage as the eye rotates in its socket. The EMG records the electrical activity from muscle movement. It is recorded from the surface of the skin, typically from under the chin because muscles in this area of the body show very dramatic changes associated with the sleep cycle. The ECG is used to measure the heart rate and detect cardiac arrhythmias. The pulse oximeter (placed on the ear or finger) estimates arterial oxygen saturation.

The multiple sleep latency test (MSLT) is used to evaluate daytime sleepiness. This test usually is completed the morning after a diagnostic sleep study. An average adult requires 10 or more minutes to fall asleep. An MSLT result of less than 8 minutes is considered abnormal. Polysomnographic recordings are made during three to five naps spaced 2 hours apart during the day. Special attention is paid to how much time elapses from when the lights go out to the first evidence of sleep. This interval is called *sleep latency.*

Circadian Rhythm Disorders

Circadian sleep disorders are characterized by a disturbance between an "individual's sleep pattern and that which is desired or considered to be within the societal norm."[19] Sleep problems due to alterations in circadian rhythm tend to fall into three categories: non-24-hour sleep–wake syndrome (disorders of visual input and SCN function); acute shifts in the sleep–wake cycle (jet lag and shift work); and changes in sleep phase disorders (advanced and delayed sleep phase disorders).[10,20–22]

Non-24-hour Sleep–Wake Syndrome

The non-24-hour sleep–wake syndrome consists of a lack of synchronization between the internal sleep–wake rhythm and the external 24-hour day. Most persons with the disorder are blind or have brain lesions that affect the SCN. Studies have shown that 50% or more of blind persons have chronic sleep–wake complaints.[20]

The non-24-hour sleep–wake syndrome often goes unrecognized. In sighted persons, a neurologic examination, including magnetic resonance imaging to detect possible SNC lesions, often is indicated. The disorder usually is unresponsive to sedative and stimulant medications. Some blind people seem to respond to a schedule of strict light–dark 24-hour cues as the circadian visual pathways remain intact for some blind people. Bright light exposure and melatonin administration has been shown to be effective for both sighted and blind persons.[20]

Acute Shifts in the Sleep–Wake Cycle

The normal diurnal clock is set for a 24-hour day and resists changes in its pattern of as little as 1 to 2 hours per day. This means that there is a limited range of day lengths to which humans can synchronize. Imposed sleep–wake schedules of less than 23 hours or more than approximately 26 hours, such as those that occur with intercontinental jet travel and switches in the work shift, produce increasing sleep difficulties.

Time Zone Change (Jet Lag) Syndrome. *Jet lag,* a popular term for symptoms of sleep disturbance that occur with air travel that crosses several time zones, is caused by the sudden loss of synchrony between a traveller's intrinsic circadian clock and the local time of the flight's destination. The severity and duration of symptoms vary depending on the number of times zones crossed, direction of travel (eastward versus westward), takeoff and arrival times, and age. Most people who cross three or four time zones experience some sleep disturbance, usually lasting two to four nights.

Circadian rhythms take longer to resynchronize to local time after eastward flights than westward flights, presumably because of the longer-than-24-hour intrinsic circadian period in most people. There is a natural tendency for the circadian clock to move later each day, making it more difficult to phase advance than to phase delay. Eastward travel requires a phase advance, so bedtime arrives before the person's' internal clock is ready for sleep.[21,22] Because the human time system seems to be less flexible in adjusting to sudden time changes after 35 years of age, age also affects adjustment to time zone changes.

Manifestations of jet lag syndrome include insomnia, daytime sleepiness, and decreased alertness and performance. Other symptoms, such as eye and nasal irritation, headache, abdominal distension, dependent edema, and intermittent dizziness, result from cabin conditions and usually remit sooner than symptoms of jet lag. Frequent travellers, such as airline personnel and business travellers, may develop chronic sleep disturbances accompanied by malaise, irritability, and performance impairment. Jet lag usually is milder in infrequent travellers, but may reduce the enjoyment of a vacation or effectiveness of business transactions. Persons with preexisting sleep disorders such as sleep apnea often experience a worsening of symptoms with jet travel.

Management of jet lag focuses on efforts either to maintain the home time schedule or to adapt to the new time zone schedule. For persons crossing four or fewer time zones for only a few days, trying to maintain a schedule that is nearer to the home time schedule may be helpful, especially with westward travel. For longer stays, adapting to the new time schedule as quickly as possible is probably a better strategy. Use of artificial light may enhance the adjustment to the time shift. Getting outdoors and engaging in local social events enhances resynchronization by providing social cues and increasing exposure to the new light–dark environment.[21]

Shift Work Sleep Disorder. The sleep disruption of night-shift work can be attributed to a clash between shift demands for wakefulness as part of the work environment and the sleep setting of the worker's intrinsic circadian clock.[24] Shift work usually creates an environment in which some circadian clock-setting cues (*e.g.,* artificial light and rest–activity) are shifted, whereas others (*e.g.,* natural light–dark schedule, family and social routines) are not. This situation almost never allows for a complete shift of the circadian system. To complicate the situation, most night-shift workers revert to a nighttime sleeping schedule on days off. The effect of abruptly attempting to sleep at normal hours after working nights and sleeping days is biologically equivalent to a 6- to 10-hour eastbound jet flight.

Manifestations of sleep disorders of night-shift workers include shortened and interrupted daytime sleep after the night shift, somnolence and napping at work, sleepiness while commuting home, and insomnia on the nights off from work. The abrupt transitions required of workers and interruptions that occur from sleeping during the day hours results in a degree of sleep deprivation.[23] Permanent night workers report averaging 6 hours of sleep on work days, approximately an hour less than evening and day workers.[24]

Arriving at a sleep schedule that is most supportive of the worker's intrinsic circadian rhythm often is difficult for night-shift workers. Beginning sleep at noon rather than earlier in the morning may produce a more normal sleep period in relation to shift onset, but exacerbate insomnia on nights off. Sleeping in absolute darkness during daytime by using blackout shades or eye masks may benefit the night worker's sleep.

Change in Sleep Phase Disorders

Change in sleep phase disorders include delayed sleep phase syndrome and advanced sleep phase syndrome. The disorders may arise because of developmental changes in the sleep–wake cycle or because of poor sleep habits.

The main symptoms of *delayed sleep phase syndrome* (DSPS) are extreme difficulty falling asleep at a conventional hour of the night and awakening on time in the morning for school, work, or other responsibilities. Although most chronically sleep-deprived persons are sleepy in the late afternoon or evening, persons with DSPS report greatest alertness at these times of the day.[21]

The disorder is more common in adolescents and in persons older than 50 years of age.[21] In adults, there is evidence of association between some psychopathological disorders and DSPS. Most cases are adolescents whose frustrated parents cannot wake them up in time for school and have trouble getting them to go to bed at night. Staying up late is fairly common among teenagers, who are strongly influenced by peer pressure, defiance of parental rules, and other factors. It has been suggested that social pressure may contribute to, but may not be the only reason for, changes in a teenager's sleep pattern. Rather, puberty may be accompanied by a lengthening of the intrinsic circadian rhythm, with a corresponding increase in evening wakefulness, which in turn leads to later sleep onset and arising.

Diagnosis of DSPS usually can be made from information in a sleep history and confirmed with a 2-week sleep log or diary. The presence of concurrent psychopathological disorders or chronic sedative or alcohol use should be considered. There are no quick remedies for DSPS. In adolescents, common-sense remedies such as setting earlier bedtimes and using multiple alarm clocks for waking up have been used, but with minimal success. The use of bright light may be helpful in maintaining morning wakefulness. For some people, engagement in a regular morning exercise program, such as taking a daily 20- to 30-minute walk outdoors as soon as possible after arising each morning, may prove beneficial. In persons with psychopathological disorders or sedative abuse, treatment of the underlying disorder is indicated.[21,22]

Advanced sleep phase syndrome (ASPS) basically is the mirror image of DSPS—early sleep onset and early arising. People with ASPS have trouble staying awake in the evening and have to curtail evening activities to avoid falling asleep. Unlike persons with depression, who awaken early with feelings of hopelessness and sadness, the person with ASPS obtains a normal amount of consolidated sleep and wakes up feeling refreshed.[21] The pathophysiologic basis of ASPS is presumed to be a partial defect in phase delay capability, with the possibility that persons with the disorder have an inherently fast circadian timing system. This disorder often is found in the elderly. Time isolation studies in middle-aged and older subjects suggest that the circadian timing system shortens with aging, usually beginning sometime in the sixth decade of life.[21] Diagnosis of ASPS is based on history and information from a sleep log. Other pathologic causes, such as sleep apnea and depression, should be ruled out. The need for treatment depends on how disruptive a person perceives the problem to be. Current treatment methods, which focus largely on sleep schedule changes, are somewhat limited.

Insomnia

Insomnia has been defined as three or more of the following: difficulty initiating sleep, difficulty maintaining sleep, waking up too early with the inability to return to sleep, or sleep that is chronically nonrestorative or poor in quality.[25–29] To be classified as insomnia, these symptoms must be accompanied by at least one of the following forms of daytime impairment: fatigue or daytime sleepiness, impairment of attention, concentration, or memory; poor social, occupational, or academic performance; mood disturbance or irritability; proneness to errors or accidents at work or while driving; tension headaches or gastrointestinal distress due to sleep loss; or worries about sleep. Primary insomnia is sleep difficulty in which other causes of sleep disruption have been ruled out or treated, whereas secondary insomnia can be associated with medical conditions (*e.g.,* chronic pain), psychiatric disorders (*e.g.,* anxiety, depression, bipolar disorder), neurologic disorders (*e.g.,* Parkinson disease), primary sleep disorders (*e.g.,* sleep apnea, restless legs syndrome), and drugs.[17,25–29]

Estimates of the prevalence of insomnia vary depending on the method used in the diagnosis and monitoring of the condition. According to the fifth edition of the *Diagnostic and Statistical Manual of Mental Disorders,* one third of adults report insomnia symptoms.[27] An estimated 3.3 million Canadians, or anywhere from 10% to 15% of adults have chronic insomnia.[25–27] Chronic insomnia is more common in women, especially in the postmenopausal years; in older people, perhaps as a consequence of declining health and institutionalization; and in persons with psychological and other disease conditions. Insomnia was independently associated with painful chronic conditions, activity limitations, mood and anxiety disorders, life stress, frequent use of alcohol or cannabis, obesity, and low education.[25]

Adjustment or Acute Insomnia

Adjustment or acute insomnia is characterized by short periods (days or weeks) of sleep difficulty that is expected to resolve with either adaptation or resolution of the stressor.[27,28] Acute insomnia often is caused by emotional and physical discomfort. Some common examples include an unfamiliar or nonconducive sleep environment, stress-related events, and sleep schedule problems. Probably one of the most common causes of acute insomnia is an unfamiliar sleep environment, such as that encountered when travelling.

Factors that contribute to a nonconducive sleep environment include excessive noise, extremes of temperature, an uncomfortable sleep surface, or being forced to sleep in an uncomfortable position. Hospital intensive care units with their noise, intensive lighting, and frequent interruptions for monitoring vital signs and providing treatments are excellent examples of nonconducive sleep environments. Common stress-related causes of insomnia are expected occurrences such as being on call or stressful life events. Sleep schedule changes include jet lag and sleep disruption due to shift work.

Chronic Insomnia

Chronic insomnia should be distinguished from acute insomnia yet there is no clear definition. It may be defined in terms of severity (mild, moderate, severe), frequency (once a week, 3 to 4 times per week, etc.), or duration (less than a month, more than a month, greater than 6 months).[25] Persons with chronic insomnia lasting longer than a month frequently complain of fatigue; mood changes, such as irritability and depression; difficulty concentrating; and impaired performance.

Chronic insomnia often is related to medical or psychiatric disorders. Factors such as pain, immobility, and hormonal changes associated with pregnancy or menopause also can cause insomnia. Interrupted sleep can accompany other sleep disorders such as restless legs syndrome and sleep apnea. Many health problems worsen during the night. Heart failure, respiratory disease, and gastroesophageal reflux can cause frequent awakening during the night. Mood and anxiety disorders are the most frequent cause of insomnia in persons with psychiatric diagnoses.

A number of drugs can lead to poor-quality sleep. Drugs commonly related to insomnia are caffeine, nicotine, stimulating antidepressants, alcohol, and recreational drugs. Although alcohol initially may induce sleep, it often causes disrupted and fragmented sleep. Sleep also is disrupted in persons undergoing alcohol or sleep medication withdrawal.

Diagnosis and Treatment

The diagnosis of insomnia is aided by a sleep history. Questions should address both sleep and daytime functioning. If the person has a bed partner, it is important to ask if the person snores, has unusual movement during sleep, or is excessively drowsy during the day.[29] Because sleep needs vary from person to person, a 1- to 2-week sleep diary can be useful in diagnosing the sleep problem and in serving as a baseline for treatment effects.[17,25] Other factors that need to be explored are the use of drugs such as caffeine, tobacco, and alcohol, as well as prescription and over-the-counter drugs that affect the sleep–wake cycle. Identification of physical and psychological factors that interfere with sleep also is important. Actigraphy or polysomnography may be used as diagnostic tools. Polysomnography

is the most sensitive tool to evaluate sleep and wakefulness. However, it is expensive and because of the numerous monitoring electrodes can actually disrupt sleep. Its use as a diagnostic tool for insomnia is usually limited to cases in which other sleep disorders, such as sleep apnea, are suspected.[25]

Treatment of insomnia includes education and counselling regarding better sleep habits (sleep hygiene), behavioural therapy aimed at changing maladaptive sleep habits, and the judicious use of pharmacologic interventions. The cause and duration of insomnia are particularly important in deciding on a treatment strategy. With transient insomnia, treatment stresses the development of good sleep hygiene and judicious short-term use of sedatives or hypnotics. Long-term and chronic insomnia require careful assessment to determine the cause of the disorder. Depending on the findings, treatment options include behavioural strategies such as relaxation therapy, sleep restriction therapy, stimulus control therapy, and cognitive therapy. Sedatives and hypnotics, which tend to become less effective with time and may cause dependence, are used with caution.

Sleep hygiene refers to a set of rules and information about personal and environmental activities that affect sleep. These rules include establishing a regular wakeup time to help set the circadian clock and regularity of sleep onset; maintaining a practice of sleeping only as long as needed to feel refreshed; providing a quiet sleep environment that is neither too hot nor too cold; and avoiding the use of alcohol and caffeine (coffee, colas, tea, chocolate) before retiring for sleep.

Behavioural therapies include relaxation therapy, sleep restriction therapy, stimulus control therapy, and cognitive therapy.[25–31] Relaxation therapy is based on the premise that persons with insomnia tend to display high levels of physiologic, cognitive, and emotional arousal during both the day and the night. Sleep restriction therapy consists of curtailing the amount of time spent in bed in an effort to increase the sleep efficiency (time asleep/time in bed). People with insomnia often increase their time in bed in the misguided belief that it will provide more opportunity to sleep. Stimulus control therapy focuses on reassociating the bed and bedroom with sleep rather than sleeplessness. It is important that the bed and bedroom be identified with sleep and not with reading, watching television, or working. Persons who cannot fall asleep should be instructed to turn on the light and do something else outside the bed, preferably in another room. Cognitive therapy involves the identification of dysfunctional beliefs and attitudes about sleep and replacing them with more adaptive substitutes.

Pharmacologic treatment usually is reserved for short-term management of insomnia—either as the sole treatment or as adjunctive therapy until the underlying problem can be addressed. The most common type of agents used to promote sleep are the benzodiazepine receptor agonists and a new class of nonbenzodiazepine hypnotics with only zolpidem and zopiclone available in Canada (eszopiclone, ramelteon, and zaleplon are not available in Canada). The nonbenzodiazepine is often preferred because of its rapid onset and shorter duration of action. In Canada, there are four benzodiazepines indicated for the treatment of insomnia—flurazepam, nitrazepam, temazepam, and triazolam. Each of these have hypnotic and sedative properties and must be used with caution in older adults.[31]

Sedating antidepressants also may be prescribed, particularly when insomnia is due to depression. Antihistamines have sedative effects and may be used to induce sleep. The most commonly used agents are diphenhydramine and doxylamine. Most over-the-counter sleep medications include an antihistamine. Adverse effects of antihistamines include daytime sleepiness, cognitive impairments, and anticholinergic effects. Falls and fractures are more frequent in persons using hypnotic or other psychotherapeutic agents. Melatonin, available in both natural and synthetic forms, is one of the most popular over-the-counter sleep aids. The pharmacokinetics of melatonin have not been established because of differences in dosing, large variations in absorption, and diversity of study subjects.[27,31]

Narcolepsy

Narcolepsy is a syndrome characterized by abnormal sleep tendencies, including excessive daytime sleepiness, disturbed nocturnal sleep, and manifestations related to REM sleep such as cataplexy (brief periods of muscle weakness), hypnagogic hallucinations, and sleep paralysis.[32–36] Daytime sleepiness is the most common initial symptom of narcolepsy. It is most apparent in boring, sedentary situations and often is relieved by movement. Although the sleepiness that occurs with narcolepsy is similar to that experienced after sleep deprivation, it is different in that no amount of nighttime sleep produces full alertness. The periods of daytime sleep usually are brief, lasting 30 minutes or less, and often are accompanied by brief interruptions of speech or irrelevant words, lapses in memory, and nonsensical activities. Cataplexy is characterized by brief periods of muscle weakness brought about by emotional reactions such as laughter, anger, or fear. Sleep paralysis is a terrifying experience that occurs on falling asleep or on awakening, during which persons find themselves unable to move, speak, or even breathe deeply.

Hypnagogic hallucinations are vivid hallucinations that occur at the onset of sleep. Similar hallucinations may occur on awakening (*i.e.,* hypnopompic hallucinations). Visual hallucinations, either simple or bizarre and fantastic, are the rule, although auditory and tactile components may occur.[34] The exact boundary between hypnagogic/hypnopompic hallucinations and dreams is not a clear one. Although the symptoms of narcolepsy generally begin in puberty, they have been reported in children and in adults up to 68 years of age. The impact of sleepiness is often underappreciated because persons with the disorder may be reluctant to report problems that may adversely affect their ability to work, drive, or obtain insurance.[36]

The mechanisms underlying the manifestations of narcolepsy appear to be linked to an abnormality in REM sleep regulation. The occurrence of REM sleep at sleep onset or within 10 to 15 minutes of sleep onset is the most characteristic and striking manifestation of the disorder. Periods of sleep-onset REM are thought to indicate impaired sleep–wake regulation rather than increased need for REM sleep. The sleep paralysis, dreamlike hallucinations, and the loss of muscle tone that occur during cataplexy are similar to behaviours that occur during REM sleep.

Although the cause of narcolepsy is unknown, there are indications that the disorder may have a genetic component. Persons with narcolepsy have been shown to have an unusually high rate of a specific human leukocyte antigen (HLA) subtype (HLA DQB1–0602).[34,35] This association is seen in approximately 85% of cases with cataplexy.[35] Importantly, this association is substantially lower in persons who have received the diagnosis of narcolepsy, but do not have cataplexy.[34,35] The strong association between HLA type and cataplexy raises the possibility that narcolepsy is an autoimmune disease.

Recent research has suggested a link between a newly identified group of neurotransmitters called *hypocretins* and narcolepsy. The hypocretins (hypocretin 1 and hypocretin 2) are secreted by cells in the area of the hypothalamus that is related to wakefulness.[33–36] The results of several studies suggest that narcolepsy with cataplexy is caused by a loss of hypocretin-producing neurons. Narcolepsy may also be caused by neurologic insults that affects levels of hypocretin, such as hypothalamic lesions, vascular disruptions, inflammatory mediators, or brain trauma.[37]

Usually, sleep laboratory studies are required for accurate diagnosis of narcolepsy. Both daytime and nighttime studies usually are done.[36] Nighttime studies usually are performed after the person has been on a regular sleep schedule for 10 days or more to determine the presence and severity of sleep apnea, limb movement disorders, and nocturnal sleep disturbance. A daytime MSLT usually is done the next day. People with narcolepsy are observed to have a short period of sleep latency (less than 5 minutes) during daytime studies, along with a rapid onset of REM sleep (usually within 10 minutes). A mean sleep latency of less than 8 minutes and two or more periods of sleep-onset REM during the repeated nap opportunities is considered diagnostic of narcolepsy.[34]

The treatment of narcolepsy focuses on the use of stimulant medications, such as methylphenidate, amphetamines, and modafinil, to counteract daytime sleepiness.[34,36,38] Modafinil, a nonamphetamine stimulant, has been studied and approved for use in treatment of narcolepsy. The mechanism of action of modafinil is unknown, although animal studies indicate the drug acts in areas of the brain involved in the sleep–wake cycle. Sodium oxybate, a central nervous system depressant, can be used to decrease the number of cataplexy attacks; however this medication has a very short half-life (requiring two doses per night) and number of serious side effects.[38] Tricyclic antidepressants may also be used to treat the cataleptic attacks.[36] Nonpharmacologic treatments include prevention of sleep deprivation, regular sleep and wake times, a stimulating work environment, and avoidance of shift work. Scheduled short naps may be effective in reducing daytime sleepiness.

Sleep-Related Movement Disorders

A variety of spontaneous limb movements occur during normal sleep. Many of these movements demonstrate characteristic rates and patterns during certain stages of sleep, with movements being minimal during nonREM sleep and maximal during REM sleep. Many movement disorders occur during stage 2 nonREM sleep. Some occur during normal sleep in all persons at one time or another. Others are not part of normal sleep patterns and can be disruptive of sleep. Among the abnormal motor disorders are periodic limb movement disorder (PLMD) and restless legs syndrome (RLS).[38–42]

Periodic Limb Movement Disorder

PLMD is characterized by episodes of repetitive movement of the large toe with flexion of the ankle, knee, and hip during sleep.[38–42] It can occur simultaneously in both legs, alternate between legs, or occur unilaterally. The condition occurs most frequently during light (stages 1 and 2 nonREM) sleep compared with deep (stages 3 and 4 nonREM) sleep and REM sleep.

The incidence of the disorder, which occurs equally in men and women, increases with age. It may occur in as much as 29% of persons older than 50 years of age.[42] The disorder frequently accompanies RLS. It has been reported that approximately 80% of persons with RLS exhibit evidence of PLMD during polysomnographic studies.[40–42] Persons with PLMD are often unaware of periodic limb movements, but their bed partners may report the symptoms.

The cause of PLMD is largely unknown. It has been observed that the movements mimic the Babinski reflex, suggesting removal of an excitatory influence over a subcortical inhibitory system allowing for facilitation of abnormal movements during sleep.[40] Diagnosis of PLMD is facilitated with use of EMG recordings from both tibialis anterior muscles.[38,40] Four or more consecutive muscle contractions, each lasting 5 to 90 seconds (typically 20 to 40 seconds) and recurring at intervals of 5 to 90 seconds, is indicative of PLMD.

Restless Legs Syndrome

The NIH Consensus Panel recently characterized RLS as (1) an urge to move the limbs with or without sensations, (2) worsening at rest, (3) improving with activity, and (4) worsening in the evening or night.[43] The prevalence of the condition peaks in middle age and reportedly occurs in 2% to 15% of the elderly population. Although the prevalence increases with age, it has a variable age of onset and can even occur in children.

The disorder, which is thought to have its origin in the CNS, can occur as a primary or secondary disorder. There is a high familial incidence of primary RLS, suggesting a genetic disorder. Secondary causes of RLS include iron deficiency, neurologic disorders such as spinal cord and peripheral nerve lesions, pregnancy, uremia, and medications. Although the neurologic basis of RLS has not been determined, recent research suggests that it may involve homeostatic mechanisms that regulate the influx and efflux of iron from cells of the CNS that regulate motor movements.[42] Cerebrospinal fluid ferritin (the main iron storage molecules in the CNS) levels are lower in persons with RLS. Of interest is the role of iron in dopaminergic transmission in the CNS. Iron is an important cofactor for tyrosine hydroxylase, the rate-limiting enzyme in dopamine synthesis, and also plays a major role in the functioning of postsynaptic dopamine receptors.[38,42]

Diagnosis of RLS is based on a history of (1) a compelling urge to move the legs, usually associated with paresthesias; (2) motor restlessness, as seen by activities such as pacing, tossing and turning in bed, or rubbing the legs; (3) symptoms that become worse at rest and are relieved by activity; and (4) symptoms that are worse in the evening or at night.[43] Laboratory tests to determine secondary causes of RLS usually are done. Because RLS may be a symptom of iron deficiency, serum ferritin and iron saturation should be assessed. This is important because iron deficiency is frequently present in the absence of anemia. Sleep studies usually are not required because the condition can be diagnosed on the basis of history and clinical findings.

Treatment of RLS varies depending on the severity of symptoms. Dopaminergic agents are the first-line drugs for most persons with RLS.[38–42] The treatment of choice are the dopamine agonists (pergolide, pramipexole, ropinirole). Other alternative agents include precursors of dopamine (carbidopa-levodopa), facilitating agents (selegiline), antiseizure agents (gabapentin), benzodiazepines (*e.g.,* clonazepam, temazepam), and opioids (*e.g.,* codeine) or opioid agonists (*e.g.,* tramadol).[38–42] Supplementation with folic acid, and magnesium continue to be investigated for RLS.[41] Although pharmacologic treatment is helpful for many persons with RLS, those with mild symptoms may not require medications. For many persons, deliberate manipulation of the muscles through ambulation, kicking movements, stretching, or massage may provide relief. Good sleep habits are important. Because a high prevalence of iron deficiency has been found among persons with RLS, treatment of the deficiency may improve or resolve symptoms.

Sleep Apnea

Sleep apnea is sleep-disordered breathing, accompanied by daytime symptoms, most often excessive sleepiness. There are two types of sleep apnea: central and obstructive.[44,45] *Central sleep apnea,* which is caused by disorders affecting the respiratory centre in the brain, is rare. It is characterized by a cessation or decrease in ventilatory effort during sleep and is usually associated with oxygen desaturation. *Obstructive sleep apnea,* which is caused by upper airway obstruction and characterized by snoring, disrupted sleep, and excessive daytime sleepiness, is the much more common type. Although airflow ceases, respiratory muscles continue to function. This is one of the features that distinguishes central from obstructive sleep apnea.

Obstructive Sleep Apnea

Apnea is defined as cessation of airflow through the nose and mouth for 10 seconds or longer.[44,45] The apneic periods typically last for 15 to 120 seconds, and some persons may have as many as 100 apneic periods per night. An accompanying reduction in tidal volume due to a decrease in the depth and rate of respiration (called *hypopnea*) is associated with a decrease in arterial oxygen saturation. The average number of apnea–hypopnea periods per hour is called the *apnea–hypopnea index* (AHI).[46,47] An adult may experience up to five events an hour without symptoms. As the AHI increases, so does the severity of symptoms. An AHI of five or greater in combination with reports of excessive daytime sleepiness is indicative of sleep apnea.[45,48]

A critical pathophysiologic feature of obstructive sleep apnea is sleep-related collapse of the upper airway at the level of the pharynx.[46,49] All skeletal muscles except the diaphragm undergo a decrease in tone during sleep. This loss of muscle tone is most pronounced during REM sleep. The loss of muscle tone in the upper airways predisposes to airway obstruction as the negative airway pressure produced by contraction of the diaphragm brings the vocal cords together, collapses the pharyngeal wall, and sucks the tongue back into the throat (Fig. 52.6). Airway collapse is accentuated in persons with conditions that cause narrowing of the upper airway or weakness of the throat muscles.

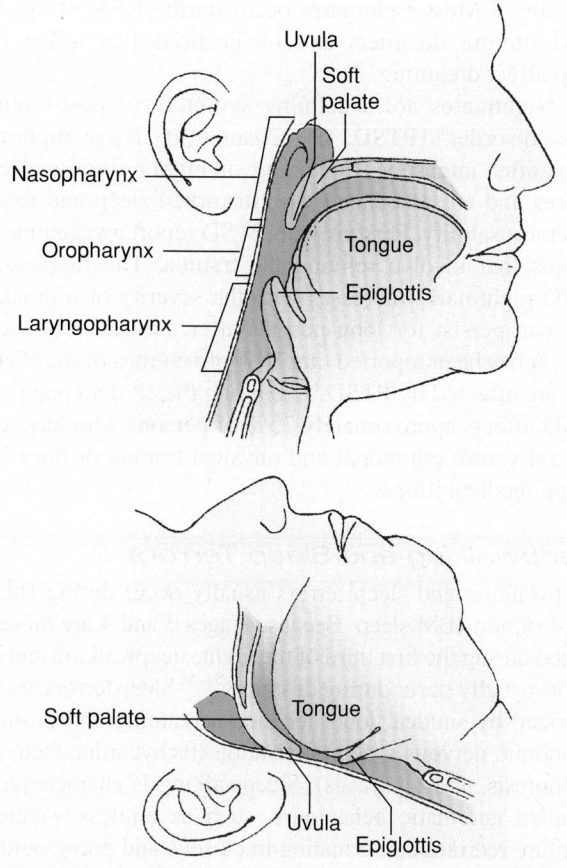

FIGURE 52.6 • Principal mechanism of obstructive sleep apnea. When the person is awake (**top**), the airway is kept open by the activity of the pharyngeal musculature. During sleep (**bottom**), this activity is decreased, causing airway obstruction, most commonly in the area behind the uvula, soft palate, and posterior tongue.

Conditions that predispose to sleep apnea include male sex, increasing age, positive family history, and obesity. Alcohol and other drugs that depress the CNS tend to increase the severity of obstructive episodes. Most persons who develop sleep apnea are obese. Large neck girth in both male and female snorers is highly predictive of sleep apnea. Neck circumference greater than 40 cm is correlated with obstructive sleep apnea, even more so than body mass index (BMI). The Pickwickian syndrome, named after the markedly obese boy in Charles Dickens' *The Posthumous Papers of the Pickwick Club,* published in 1837, is characterized by obesity, hypersomnolence, periodic breathing, hypoxemia, and right-sided heart failure.[50] Men have a higher risk for obstructive sleep apnea than women. The reason for this is not entirely clear, but gonadal hormones may play a role.[44] Postmenopausal women are at higher risk than premenopausal women. Individuals with specific endocrine disorders, namely acromegaly, Cushing syndrome, hypothyroidism, and diabetes mellitus, are at higher risk for obstructive sleep apnea. In each of these disorders, hormonal imbalances lead to structural distortion of the airways that leads to obstruction.[45]

Obstructive sleep apnea is characterized by loud snoring interrupted by periods of silence. Abnormal gross motor movements during sleep are common. In many cases, the snoring precedes by many years the onset of other signs of sleep apnea. Persons with sleep apnea often complain of persistent daytime sleepiness, morning headache, memory and judgment problems, irritability, difficulty concentrating, and depression. They also are more likely to fall asleep at inappropriate times and have higher rates of automobile and work-related accidents. Nocturia may also be a symptom of obstructive sleep apnea, although this can be mistaken for benign prostatic hypertrophy or an overactive bladder. Men may complain of impotence. In children, a decline in school performance may be the only indication of the problem.

Sleep apnea also is associated with sleep-related cardiac arrhythmias and hypertension. Usually bradycardia is observed, but ventricular tachycardia may occur in situations of severe hypoxemia. Frequent apneic periods may result in increased systemic and pulmonary blood pressures. The morning blood pressure has been shown to increase almost linearly with increasing apnea episodes. In severe cases, pulmonary hypertension, polycythemia, and cor pulmonale may develop. Signs and symptoms of obstructive sleep apnea are summarized in (Chart 52.2).

Diagnosis and Treatment. Obstructive sleep apnea usually is suspected from a history of snoring, disturbed sleep, and daytime sleepiness. A definitive diagnosis is accomplished with sleep studies done in a sleep laboratory using polysomnography.[48,51] Currently, this procedure requires an overnight stay in a sleep laboratory. The procedure consists of EEG and EOG to determine the sleep stages; monitoring of the airflow; an ECG to detect arrhythmias; methods to measure ventilatory effort; and pulse oximetry to detect changes in oxygen saturation. An MSLT may be done to rule out narcolepsy in persons who exhibit excessive daytime sleepiness. Home evaluation

CHART 52.2	SIGNS AND SYMPTOMS OF SLEEP APNEA

- Excessive daytime sleepiness
- Noisy snoring
- Insomnia
- Abnormal movements during sleep
- Morning headaches
- Cognitive and personality changes
- Sexual impotence
- Systemic hypertension
- Pulmonary hypertension, cor pulmonale
- Polycythemia
- Nocturia

using pulse oximetry and portable monitors may be used to screen for sleep apnea. This method is less expensive than laboratory sleep tests but often is less accurate.[48] It is most useful in persons with severe sleep apnea, in whom the results clearly are positive.

The treatment of obstructive sleep apnea is determined by the severity of the condition.[48,51] Behavioural measures may be the only treatment needed for persons with mild sleep apnea. These include weight loss, eliminating evening alcohol and sedatives, and proper bed positioning. Weight loss often is beneficial for persons with obstructive apnea. In many instances, the disordered breathing events are confined to the supine sleeping position, so that training the person to sleep in the lateral position may help to alleviate the problem.

Oral or dental appliances that displace the tongue forward and move the mandible to a more anterior and forward position may be an option for persons with mild to moderate sleep apnea. Persons who snore but do not have sleep apnea also may use these devices. They should be fitted by a dentist or orthodontist experienced in their use. Side effects of the devices include excessive salivation and temporomandibular joint discomfort.

The application of nasal continuous positive airway pressure (NCPAP) at night has proven helpful in treating obstructive sleep apnea. This method uses an occlusive nasal mask or a device that fits into the nares, an expiratory valve and tubing, and a blower system to generate positive pressure. The main difficulty with NCPAP is that many persons find it unacceptable. Common complaints include dryness of the mouth, claustrophobia, and noise.

Several surgical procedures have been used to correct airway obstruction, including nasal septoplasty (*i.e.,* repair of the nasal septum) and uvulopalatopharyngoplasty (*i.e.,* excision of excess soft tissue on the palate, uvula, and posterior pharyngeal wall). Both of these procedures have met with limited success. Severe cases of sleep apnea may require a tracheostomy (*i.e.,* surgical placement of a tube into the trachea for the purpose of maintaining an open airway). The tracheostomy tube remains occluded during the day and is opened during the night.

Parasomnias

The parasomnias are undesirable physical phenomena that occur almost exclusively during sleep or are exaggerated by sleep.[52–54] They include nightmares, sleepwalking (somnambulism) and sleep terrors, teeth grinding, and bed-wetting (enuresis). Sleepwalking, sleep terrors, and bed-wetting often are seen in children and may be considered normal to some degree at a certain age. They are less common in adults and may be indicative of other pathologic processes. For example, sleepwalking and sleep terrors may occur in persons with poorly controlled cardiac insufficiency after myocardial infarction. In rare cases, sleepwalking and sleep terrors may be the first sign of a slowly evolving brain tumour. Finally, sleepwalking and sleep terrors may be triggered by disorders interacting with the sleep–wake cycle. Particularly in older adults, health problems such as a febrile illness may enhance nonREM sleep nightmares, sleep terrors, and sleepwalking.

Nightmares

Nightmares are vivid and terrifying nocturnal episodes in which the dreamer is abruptly awakened from sleep. Usually there is difficulty returning to sleep. Nightmares affect 20% to 39% of children between 5 and 12 years of age and 5% to 8% of adults.[53] Most nightmares occur during REM sleep. Most REM-altering disorders and medications that affect REM sleep affect dreaming.

Nightmares are a defining symptom of post-traumatic stress disorder[8] (PTSD; see Chapter 9). These nightmares occur after intensely frightening or highly emotional experiences and are associated with disturbed sleep and daytime hyperarousability. Persons with PTSD report awakening from dreams that involve reliving the trauma. The frequency of PTSD nightmares increases with the severity of trauma, and they can persist for long periods after the traumatic experience. It has been reported that 30% of veterans of the Vietnam War are affected by PTSD.[8,53] Among the civilian population, PTSD affects approximately 25% of persons who have experienced severe emotional and physical trauma or have had a severe medical illness.

Sleepwalking and Sleep Terrors

Sleepwalking and sleep terrors usually occur during stages 3 and 4 of nonREM sleep. Because stages 3 and 4 are more prolonged during the first third of the night, sleepwalking and sleep terrors usually occur during this time.[53–55] Sleep terrors are characterized by sudden, loud, terrified screaming and prominent autonomic nervous system activation (tachycardia, tachypnea, diaphoresis, and mydriasis). Sleepwalking is characterized by complex automatic behaviours, such as aimless wandering, furniture rearranging, urinating in closets, and going outdoors. During a typical episode, the sleepwalker appears dazed and relatively unresponsive to the communication efforts of others. On awakening, there may be a brief period of confusion or disorientation. The sleepwalker usually has no memory or only a vague awareness of what has happened.

Sleep terrors are more common in children and are discussed later in the chapter. In children, sleepwalking usually is a benign and self-limited disorder. In adults, sleepwalking occurs almost three times more often per year and persists for a longer period than in children. It often is associated with stress or major life events.[55] New-onset sleepwalking in older adults is uncommon and usually is a manifestation of another disorder such as delirium, drug toxicity, or seizure disorders.[55] Although rare, sleepwalking can occur during complex partial seizures.

Diagnosis and treatment of sleepwalking and sleep terrors depend on age. Because most children eventually outgrow the disorders, parents may simply need to be reassured and instructed in safety measures. Insufficient sleep may precipitate episodes of sleepwalking, so parents should make certain that the child goes to bed on time and gets enough sleep. In adults, a thorough medical, psychiatric, and sleep history should be done to eliminate other causes of the disorder. Because sleepwalking can be dangerous, it is important that the environment be safe. Dangerous objects should be removed and bolts should be placed on doors and windows. No attempt should be made to interrupt the sleepwalking event because such efforts may be frightening.

Pharmacologic treatment includes the selective use of the benzodiazepines (particularly diazepam and clonazepam) or the tricyclic antidepressant imipramine.[55] In older adults, treatment focuses on reversing the underlying causes of delirium. Because medications are a frequent cause of delirium in older adults, a complete drug history should be done with the intent of eliminating medications that might be causing the disorder.

IN SUMMARY

Sleep disorders include the circadian rhythm sleep disorders, insomnias, narcolepsy, sleep-related movement disorders, sleep apnea, and the parasomnias. Sleep problems due to alterations in circadian rhythm tend to fall into three categories: non-24-hour sleep–wake syndrome (disorders of visual input and SCN function); acute shifts in the sleep–wake cycle (jet lag and shift work); and changes in sleep phase disorders (advanced and delayed sleep phase disorders). Insomnia represents a subjective problem of insufficient or nonrestorative sleep despite an adequate opportunity to sleep. It includes transient and chronic problems in falling asleep and maintaining sleep, waking up too early, or nonrefreshing sleep.

Narcolepsy is a disorder of daytime sleep attacks, cataplexy, hallucinations occurring at the onset of sleep, and sleep paralysis. Among the movement disorders that occur during sleep are PLMD and RLS. PLMD is characterized by episodes of repetitive movement of the large toe with flexion of the ankle, knee, and hip during sleep, usually involving both legs. RLS is a neurologic disorder characterized by an irresistible urge to move the legs, usually owing to a "creeping," "crawling," or uncomfortable

sensation. It usually is worse during periods of inactivity and often interferes with sleep.

Obstructive sleep apnea is a serious, potentially life-threatening disorder characterized by brief periods of apnea or breathing cessation during sleep, loud snoring interrupted by periods of silence, and abnormal gross motor movements. It is accompanied by complaints of persistent daytime sleepiness, morning headache, memory and judgment problems, irritability, difficulty concentrating, and depression. Sleep apnea also is associated with sleep-related cardiac arrhythmias and hypertension. The parasomnias are undesirable physical phenomena that occur almost exclusively during sleep or are exaggerated by sleep. They include nightmares, sleepwalking and sleep terrors, teeth grinding, and bed-wetting (enuresis).

SLEEP AND SLEEP DISORDERS IN CHILDREN AND OLDER ADULTS

After completing this section of the chapter, you should be able to meet the following objectives:

- Characterize normal sleep patterns of the infant and small child and relate them to the development of sleep disorders.
- Describe the normal changes in sleep stages that occur with aging and relate them to sleep problems in older adults.

It has been said that "sleep is of the brain, by the brain, and for the brain."[1] Thus, sleep changes as the brain develops in the fetus and neonate, matures during adolescence and early adulthood, and begins to decline with aging.

Sleep and Sleep Disorders in Children

Sleep Patterns in Children

A child's circadian rhythms and sleep patterns are established early in life. There is evidence that many of the sleep patterns in the newborn are present at birth.[1] The first behavioural manifestations of sleep patterns occur between 28 and 30 weeks of gestation, when movement of the fetus is interrupted by periods of quiet.[56] At 32 weeks, periods of quiescence begin to occur at regular intervals, suggesting the beginnings of a sleep–wake cycle.

An infant born at full term sleeps approximately 16 to 17 hours a day, half of which is spent in REM sleep. The other half of the infant's sleep resembles adult nonREM sleep.[1,57] Not only does the infant spend more time in REM sleep than adults, but the behavioural manifestations of REM sleep are more exaggerated. This probably is because inhibitory systems in the infant's brain are relatively immature. Thus, an infant's sleep behaviour includes a wide range of physical behaviours such as changes in facial expression, cooing sounds, and movement and stretching of the extremities.

Although infants have some capacity to concentrate sleep in one part of the day, this capacity must be developed in the weeks after birth. As development progresses, the infant is able to concentrate sleep during the night and remain awake for longer periods during the day. By 5 to 6 months, the infant may sleep through the night and may nap at predictable times during the day. As the cyclic structure of the sleep–wake cycle progresses, the amount of time spent in REM sleep decreases. By the time the child is 8 months of age, the duration of sleep has decreased to approximately 13 hours and REM sleep occupies only approximately one third of that time. At 12 to 15 years of age, sleep has decreased to approximately 8 hours, with one fourth being spent in REM sleep.

Sleep Disorders in Children

Although sleep complaints are common among adults, children usually do not complain about sleep problems, although their parents might. The usual concerns of parents include irregular sleep habits, insufficient or too much sleep, nightmares, sleep terrors, sleepwalking, and bed-wetting. Complaints of excessive daytime sleepiness or sleep attacks not accounted for by an inadequate amount of sleep may be due to a more serious health or sleep problem (*e.g.,* narcolepsy), in which case a careful sleep history, physical examination, and other diagnostic tests may be needed. Three of the more common sleep problems of children are discussed in this section of the chapter: sleep terrors, confusional arousals, and sleepwalking.

Sleep Terrors. Sleep terrors are marked by repeated episodes of awakening from sleep. They usually occur during the first half of sleep in the first interval of nonREM sleep.[57–59] The age of onset usually is between 2 and 4 years of age.[59] The course is variable, usually occurring at intervals of days or weeks. The disorder gradually resolves in children and usually disappears during adolescence. In a typical episode, the child sits up abruptly in bed, appears frightened, and demonstrates signs of extreme anxiety, including dilated pupils, excessive perspiration, rapid breathing, and tachycardia. Until the agitation and confusion subside, efforts to comfort or help the child are futile. There usually is no memory of the episode. Occasionally, the child recounts a sense of terror on being aroused during a night terror, but there is only fragmentary recall of dreamlike images. Treatment consists primarily of educating and reassuring the family. The child should be assisted in settling down without awakening. The child must be protected if he or she gets up and walks about during the episodes.

Confusional Arousals. Confusional arousals are common in infants and toddlers.[58] They usually occur during the first third of the night when the brain is partially asleep while remaining partially awake. During these events, children present with marked confusion, slow and inappropriate responses to questions, and nonpurposeful activities. They do not express fear, terror, or panic. Children spontaneously return to sleep and have no recollection of the event in the morning. Recovery from sleep deprivation tends to increase the incidence of confusional arousals.

Sleepwalking. Sleepwalking involves repeated episodes of complex motor movements that lead to leaving the bed and walking without the child being conscious of the episode or remembering that it occurred. As with sleep terrors, it normally occurs in nonREM sleep stages 3 and 4 during the first third of the sleep period.

A sleepwalking episode typically lasts for a few minutes to half an hour, during which time the child sits up; makes purposeful movements such as picking at the bed coverings; then proceeds to semipurposeful movements such as getting out of bed, walking around, opening doors, dressing, or going to the bathroom. Often they end up in the parent's bedroom. Commonly, they are unresponsive to the efforts of others to communicate with them. Confusion and disorientation are typical of the events, and on awakening there is no memory of the event. There may be manifestations of extreme autonomic nervous system activity such as tachycardia, rapid breathing, perspiration, and urination.

Approximately 10% to 15% of children have had isolated sleepwalking events.[55] It occurs more commonly in boys than in girls and is more frequent in children in whom there is a family history of sleepwalking. The onset usually is between 4 and 8 years of age, and it lasts several years. Usually symptoms resolve by the end of the teens or in the early twenties. The primary concern is injury during an episode. Children may bump into things, fall down stairs, or even leave their home during an episode. Therefore, gates should be placed across stairs and windows and doors should be locked so the child cannot leave the house.

Sleep and Sleep Disorders in Older Adults

Complaints of difficulty sleeping occur in over 50% of older adults, and approximately 40% in those over 65 years of age experience chronic insomnia.[60] However, this increased prevalence should not be expected as a phenomenon of aging. Instead, the difficulties with sleeping are often the result of medical and psychosocial comorbidities.[62] The consequences of chronic sleep problems in older adults can be considerable. Left uncorrected, a sleep disorder affects the quality of life. Loss of sleep and use of sedating medications may lead to falls and accidents. Sleep-related disorders of breathing may have serious cardiovascular, pulmonary, and CNS effects.

There are a number of changes that occur in the sleep–wake cycle as a person ages. Older adults have more fragmented sleep and shorter duration of stages 3 and 4 sleep. Although REM sleep tends to be preserved, the deepest stages of nonREM sleep frequently are reduced or nonexistent.[61–63]

Compared with younger persons, adults in their 70s need 30 to 60 minutes less sleep than adults in their 20s.[64] They often take longer to fall asleep, they awaken earlier, and they have more nighttime arousals. Environmental influences, particularly auditory stimuli, often are more disruptive in older adults. With an increase in nighttime wakefulness, there is an increase in daytime fatigue and daytime napping. An often overlooked cause of nocturnal awakenings in the older adult population is nocturia or need to urinate during the night.[61]

The causes of sleep disorders in older adults include age-related changes in sleep architecture, secondary sleep disturbances, primary sleep disorders, lack of exercise, and poor sleep habits. Factors that predispose to secondary sleep disturbances include physical and mental illness, medication effects, and emotional stress. A variety of medical illnesses contribute to sleep disorders in older adults, including arthritic pain, respiratory problems and cardiac disease, and neurologic disorders. Nightmares and nighttime fears are common in older adults with Parkinson disease, particularly those who are receiving levodopa. Psychiatric illness, such as depression, is a common cause of disturbed sleep in this age group. Primary sleep disorders such as sleep apnea, RLS, and PLMD also increase in old age. Many medications have stimulating effects and interfere with sleep. These include some of the antidepressants, decongestants, bronchodilators, corticosteroids, and some antihypertensives. Certain over-the-counter medications can cause or exacerbate sleep disturbances.[62] Alcohol use also may serve as a deterrent to sleep in older adults. Sleep–wake problems may be compounded further by inappropriate interventions initiated by the older person, his or her family, or healthcare providers.

Sleep also is disturbed in disorders characterized by dementia. Episodes of nocturnal wandering, confusion, and delirium can occur despite normal daytime functioning. Persons with Alzheimer disease often have increased periods of nighttime awakening and daytime napping.

Diagnosis of sleep disorders in older adults requires a comprehensive sleep history, inquiries about pain and anxiety or depression, review of current sleep hygiene practices, drug use history, spousal or bed partner reports, a comprehensive physical examination, and appropriate laboratory tests.[64] Treatment of a medical disorder and changes in medication regimes and timing of medication doses can often improve sleep. Avoidance of alcohol and stimulants before bedtime and improving sleep hygiene are other measures that can be used to improve sleep. Although hypnotics can be used to treat transient insomnia, they often fail to provide long-term relief of chronic sleep disturbances.

IN SUMMARY

Circadian rhythms and sleep patterns are established early in life. In the newborn, REM sleep occurs at sleep onset, and periods of sleep and awakening are distributed throughout the day. As the cyclic structure of the sleep–wake cycle progresses, the amount of time spent in REM sleep decreases.

By the time the child is 8 months of age, the duration of sleep has decreased to approximately 13 hours and REM sleep occupies only approximately one third of that time. At 12 to 15 years of age, sleep has decreased to approximately 8 hours, with one fourth being spent in REM sleep. Although sleep complaints are common among adults, children usually do not complain about sleep problems, although their parents might. The usual concerns of parents include irregular sleep habits, insufficient or too much sleep, nightmares, sleep terrors, sleepwalking, and bed-wetting.

Complaints of sleep disorders are common in older adults. The sleep–wake cycle changes that occur with aging are evidenced by more fragmented sleep, shorter duration of stage 3 and 4 sleep, and reduced REM sleep. Older adults also have more health problems that interrupt sleep, they are apt to be on medications that interfere with sleep, and they are more likely to have sleep disorders such as insomnia, RLS, and sleep apnea. Left uncorrected, sleep disorders in older adults affect the quality of life. Loss of sleep and use of sedating medications may lead to falls and accidents.

REVIEW EXERCISES

1. A frustrated mother complains that her teenage son stays up at night and then has trouble waking up and getting to school on time.
   A. *Is there a developmental explanation for these behaviours?*
   B. *What suggestions would you make to this mother?*

2. A 30-year-old woman presents with complaints of fatigue, irritability, and difficulty concentrating. She relates that for the past 3 months or more, she has had difficulty falling asleep and staying asleep despite remaining in bed and focusing on measures to help her sleep. She laughingly tells you she has even tried counting sheep.
   A. *What type of diagnostic measure would prove useful in determining whether this woman's problem is related to insomnia?*
   B. *If the woman is diagnosed with insomnia, what type of treatment would be indicated?*

3. A 50-year-old man presents with hypertension, daytime sleepiness and difficulty concentrating, and injuries sustained from an automobile collision that occurred when he fell asleep at the wheel. He weighs 113 kg (250 lb), is 175 cm (69 in) tall, and leads a sedentary lifestyle. He states that his wife has moved into the guest bedroom because his snoring disturbs her sleep.
   A. *What is the possible cause of this man's problems?*
   B. *What diagnostic tests could be used to confirm the diagnosis?*
   C. *What type of lifestyle changes and other treatments might be used?*

References

1. Hobson J. A. (1989). *Sleep.* New York: Scientific American Library.
2. McCarley R. W. (2008). Chapter 27: Sleep, dreams, and states of consciousness. In Conn P. M. (Ed.), *Neuroscience in medicine* (3rd ed.). Totowa, NJ: Humana Press.
3. Carskadon M. A., Dement W. C. (2011). Chapter 2: Normal human sleep: An overview. In Kryger M. H., Roth T., Dement W. C. (Eds.), *Principles and practice of sleep medicine* (5th ed.). Philadelphia, PA: Elsevier Saunders.
4. Keenan S., Hirshkowitz M. (2011). Chapter 141: Monitoring and staging human sleep. In Kryger M. H., Roth T., Dement W. C. (Eds.), *Principles and practice of sleep medicine* (5th ed.). Philadelphia, PA: Elsevier Saunders.
5. Siegel J. M. (2011). Chapter 8: REM sleep. In Kryger M. H., Roth T., Dement W. C. (Eds.), *Principles and practice of sleep medicine* (5th ed.). Philadelphia, PA: Elsevier Saunders.
6. National Institute of Neurological Disorders and Stroke. (2014). Brain basics: Understanding sleep. Available online at: http://www.ninds.nih.gov/disorders/brain_basics/understanding_sleep.htm. Accessed June 1, 2015.
7. Douglas N. J. (2005). Chapter 22: Respiratory physiology: Understanding the control of ventilation. In Kryger M. H., Roth T., Dement W. C. (Eds.), *Principles and practice of sleep medicine* (5th ed.). Philadelphia, PA: Elsevier Saunders.
8. Pagel J. F. (2000). Nightmares and disorders of dreaming. *American Family Physician, 61,* 2037–2042, 2044.
9. Moore M. C., Czeisler C. A., Richardson G. S. (1983). Circadian timekeeping in health and disease. Part 1. Basic properties of circadian pacemakers. *The New England Journal of Medicine, 309,* 469–473.
10. Moore R. Y. (1997). Circadian rhythms: Basic neurobiology and clinical applications. *Annual Review of Medicine, 48,* 253–266.
11. Czeisler C. A., Buxton O. M. (2011). Chapter 35: The human circadian timing system and sleep–wake regulation. In Kryger M. H., Roth T., Dement W. C. (Eds.), *Principles and practice of sleep medicine* (5th ed.). Philadelphia, PA: Elsevier Saunders.
12. McMillan J. M., Aitken E., Holroyd-Leduc J. M. (2013). Management of insomnia and long-term use of sedative-hypnotic drugs in older patients. *Canadian Medical Association Journal, 185*(17), 1499–1505.
13. Ahrendt J. (2000). Melatonin, circadian rhythms, and sleep. *The New England Journal of Medicine, 343,* 1114–1115.
14. Guardiola-Lemaitre B., Quera-Salva M. A. (2011). Chapter 36: Melatonin in the regulation of sleep and circadian rhythms. In Kryger M. H., Roth T., Dement W. C. (Eds.), *Principles and practice of sleep medicine* (5th ed.). Philadelphia, PA: Elsevier Saunders.
15. American Academy of Sleep Medicine. (2005). *International classification of sleep disorders: Diagnostic and coding manual* (2nd ed.). Westchester, IL: Author.
16. Thorpy M. J. (2012). Classification of sleep disorders. *Neurotherapeutics, 9*(4), 687–701.
17. Morin C. M., Benca R. (2012). Chronic insomnia. *Lancet, 379*(9821), 1129–1141.
18. Stone K. L., Ancoli-Israel S. (2011). Chapter 147: Actigraphy. In Kryger M. H., Roth T., Dement W. C. (Eds.), *Principles and practice of sleep medicine* (5th ed.). Philadelphia, PA: Elsevier Saunders.
19. Lu Brandon S., Zee P. S. (2006). Circadian rhythm sleep disorders. *Chest, 130*(6), 1915–1923.
20. Zhu L., Zee P. C. (2012). Circadian rhythm sleep disorders. *Neurological Clinics, 30*(4), 1167–1191.
21. Fahey C. D., Zee P. C. (2006). Circadian rhythm sleep disorders and phototherapy. *Psychiatric Clinics of North America, 29*(4), 989–1007.
22. Eastman C. I., Burgess H. J. (2009). How to travel the world without jet lag. *Sleep Medicine Clinics, 4*(2), 241–255.
23. Morris C. J., Aeschbach D., Scheer F. A. (2012). Circadian system, sleep and endocrinology. *Molecular and Cellular Endocrinology, 349*(1), 91–104.
24. Pilcher J. J., Lambert B. J., Huffcutt A. I. (2000). Differential effects of permanent and rotating shifts on self-report sleep length: A meta-analytic view. *Sleep, 23,* 155–163.
25. Tjepkema M. (2005). Insomnia. *Health Reports, 17*(1), 9–25.
26. Morin C. M., LeBlanc M., Belanger L., et al. (2011). Prevalence of insomnia and its treatment in Canada. *Canadian Journal of Psychiatry, 56*(9), 540–548.
27. American Psychiatric Association. (2013). Sleep-wake disorders. In *Diagnostic and statistical manual of mental disorders: DSM-5.* Washington, DC: Author.
28. Budur K., Rodriguez C., Foldvary-Schaefer N. (2007). Advances in treating insomnia. *Cleveland Clinic Journal of Medicine, 74,* 251–266.
29. Silber M. H. (2005). Clinical practice. Chronic insomnia. *The New England Journal of Medicine, 353,* 803–810.
30. Sateia M. J., Nowell P. D. (2004). Insomnia. *Lancet, 364,* 1959–1973.
31. Fleming A. E. (updated 2015). Psychiatric disorders: Insomnia. In Repchinsky, C. (Ed.): *e-Therapeutics.* Ottawa, ON: Canadian Pharmacists Association.
32. Ahmed I., Thorpy M. (2010). Clinical features, diagnosis, and treatment of narcolepsy. *Clinics in chest medicine, 31,* 371–381.
33. Mignot E. (2005). Chapter 84: Narcolepsy: pathophysiology and genetics predisposition. In Kryger M. H., Roth T., Dement W. C. (Eds.), *Principles and practice of sleep medicine* (5th ed.). Philadelphia, PA: Elsevier Saunders.
34. Guilleminault C., Cao M. T. (2011). Chapter 85: Narcolepsy: Diagnosis and management. In Kryger M. H., Roth T., Dement W. C. (Eds.), *Principles and practice of sleep medicine* (5th ed.). Philadelphia, PA: Elsevier Saunders.
35. Singh A. K., Mahlios J., Mignot E. (2013). Genetic association, seasonal infections and autoimmune basis of narcolepsy. *Journal of Autoimmunity, 43,* 26–31
36. Dyken M. E., Yamada T. (2005). Narcolepsy and disorders of excessive somnolence. *Primary Care Clinics in Office Practice, 32,* 389–413.
37. Akintomide S. G., Rickards H. (2011). Narcolepsy: A review. *Neuropsychiatric Disease and Treatment, 7,* 507–518.
38. Ramar K., Olson E. J. (2013). Management of common sleep disorders. *American Family Physician, 88*(4), 231–238.
39. Montplaisir J., Allen R. P., Walters A. S., et al. (2011). Chapter 90: Restless legs syndrome and periodic limb movements during sleep. In Kryger M. H., Roth T., Dement W. C. (Eds.), *Principles and practice of sleep medicine* (5th ed.). Philadelphia, PA: Elsevier Saunders.
40. Trenkwalder C., Paulus W., Walters A. S. (2005). The restless legs syndrome. *Lancet Neurology, 4,* 465–474.
41. Yeh P., Walters A. S., Tsuang J. W. (2012). Restless legs syndrome: A comprehensive overview on its epidemiology, risk factors, and treatment. *Sleep and Breathing, 16*(4), 987–1007.
42. Ondo W. G. (2005). Restless legs syndrome. *Neurology Clinics, 23,* 1165–1185.
43. National Center on Sleep Disorders Research. (2000). *Restless legs syndrome: Detection and management in primary care.* NIH publication no. 00–3788. Bethesda, MD: National Institutes of Health.
44. Guilleminault C., Stoohs R., Quera-Salva M. (1992). Sleep-related obstructive and nonobstructive apneas and neurologic disorders. *Neurology, 42*(Suppl 6), 53–60.
45. Pashayan A. G., Passannante A. N., Rock P. (2005). Pathophysiology of obstructive sleep apnea. *Anesthesiology Clinics of North America, 23,* 431–443.
46. White D. P., Younes M. K. (2012). Obstructive sleep apnea. *Comprehensive Physiology, 2*(4), 2541–2594.
47. Caples S. M., Gami A. S., Somers V. K. (2005). Obstructive sleep apnea. *Annals of Internal Medicine, 142,* 187–197.
48. Flemons W. W. (2002). Obstructive sleep apnea. *The New England Journal of Medicine, 347,* 498–504.
49. Ryan C. M., Bradley T. D. (2005). Pathogenesis of obstructive sleep apnea. *Journal of Applied Physiology, 99,* 2240–2450.
50. Burwell C. S., Robin E. D., Whaley R. D., et al. (1956). Extreme obesity associated with alveolar hypoventilation: A Pickwickian syndrome. *American Journal of Medicine, 21,* 811–818.
51. Baldwin C. M., Quan S. F. (2002). Sleep disordered breathing. *Nursing Clinics of North America, 37,* 633–654.

52. Howell M. J. (2012). Parasomnias: An updated review. *Neurotherapeutics, 9*(4), 753–775.

53. Plante D. T., Winkleman J. W. (2006). Parasomnias. *Psychiatric Clinics of North America, 29,* 969–987.

54. Mahowald M. W. (2004). Parasomnias. *Medical Clinics of North America, 88,* 660–678.

55. Masand R., Popli A. P. (1995). Sleepwalking. *American Family Physician, 51,* 649–653.

56. Graven S. (2006). Sleep and brain development. *Clinical Perinatology, 33,* 693–706.

57. Ferber R. (1996). Childhood sleep disorders. *Neurologic Clinics, 14,* 493–451.

58. Ward T., Mason T. B. (2002). Sleep disorders in children. *Nursing Clinics of North America, 37,* 693–706.

59. Sheldon S. H. (2004). Parasomnias in childhood. *Pediatric Clinics of North America, 51,* 69–88.

60. Crowley K. (2011). Sleep and sleep disorders in older adults. *Neuropsychology Review, 21*(1), 41–53.

61. Bliwise D. L. (2011). Chapter 3: Normal aging. In Kryger M. H., Roth T., Dement W. C. (Eds.), *Principles and practice of sleep medicine* (5th ed.). Philadelphia, PA: Elsevier Saunders.

62. Bloom H. G., Ahmend I., Alessi C. A., et al. (2009). Evidence-based recommendations for the assessment and management of sleep disorders in older persons. *Journal of the American Geriatrics Society, 57*(5), 761–789.

63. Avidan A. (2005). Sleep disorders in the older patient. *Primary Care Clinics in Office Practice, 32,* 563–586.

64. Townsend-Roccichelli J., Sanford J. T., VandeWaa E. (2010). Managing sleep disorders in the elderly. *Nurse Practitioner, 35*(5), 30–37.

Visit thePoint **http://thePoint.lww.com for animations, journal articles, and more!**

Disorders of Thought, Mood, and Memory

Psychiatric disorders are characterized by changes in a person's thoughts, mood, or behaviours that preclude ordinary functioning in one or more spheres of life. Throughout the course of history, persons in the healing professions have tried to uncover the causes of and find effective treatments for diseases that alter the way in which people experience the world and behave in it. Over the centuries, the pendulum has swung between those practitioners who espouse the view that mental disease arises from inadequate interpersonal relationships and those who espouse the view that mental disease arises from alterations in brain structure or activity. In the late 20th century, and now in the early years of the 21st, the conversation between these two apparently divergent philosophies continues, perhaps to conclude with a new synthesis of nurture versus nature and therefore new and effective therapies for those with mental illness.

The purpose of this chapter is to review the understanding of the pathogenesis and treatment of mental illness, and to relate the anatomy of the brain and its integrated regional functions to the causes, manifestations, and treatment of selected thought, mood, anxiety, and cognitive disorders.

EVOLUTION IN UNDERSTANDING OF MENTAL ILLNESS

After completing this section of the chapter, you should be able to meet the following objectives:

- Define the terms *biologic psychiatry* and *psychosocial psychiatry* and compare them in terms of their definitions of the origins of mental disease.
- Describe the changes in the treatment of mental illness over the past three centuries.
- Explain the role that heredity plays in the epidemiology and development of mental illness.

Historical Perspectives

Psychiatry was not an organized specialty before the end of the 18th century, but mental disorders are as old as the human race. Even early artefacts and cave drawings indicate that what we now call psychotic disorders were known back then. Over the ages, the explanations of mental disorders have ranged from possession by gods and demons, to the breaking of taboos, to the idea that a harmful substance had entered the body. Persons with psychiatric disorders were treated with prayers, magic, and exorcisms. In some communities, people with mental illness were viewed with fear and often turned out of their homes, villages, and towns. In other communities, families took care of those with mental illness, but often these people were neglected or locked up in barns or cellars.[1]

The history of our understanding of psychiatric illnesses reveals a tension between two schools of thought as to the origin of mental disease. The pendulum has swung between these two apparently opposite viewpoints across the centuries. One view of psychiatric illness is that mental disorders are due to anatomic, developmental, and functional disorders of the brain, and is called *biologic psychiatry.* Another view is that mental disorders are due to impaired psychological development, a consequence of poor child rearing or environmental stress, and is called *psychosocial psychiatry.*[1] These differences of emphasis in terms of the pathogenesis of mental illness are important because the prevailing theory about the origins of mental disease influences which therapies for psychiatric illness predominate.

Early biologic psychiatry in the late 1800s to early 1900s emphasized the correlation of neurologic symptoms with postmortem microscopic study of anatomic changes in the brain. Although this research was of immense importance in terms of regional localization of brain functions (*e.g.,* Wernicke aphasia), it provided little help to the clinical psychiatrists of the time. Emil Kraepelin, a German psychiatrist, was the first to begin to classify psychiatric disorders by systematically studying the natural history of the disease. The intent was to be able to predict outcomes. In the sixth edition of his textbook, *Psychiatrie* (1899), Kraepelin laid the groundwork for the *Diagnostic and Statistical Manual of Mental Disorders* (*DSM;* the current fifth edition is titled *DSM-5* and was released in 2013) of the American Psychiatric Association, which is used in Canada.[2] He divided all mental disorders into 13 groups, including psychoses, which he divided into two distinct groups: those with an affective component, which he called *manic–depressive psychosis,* and those without, which he called *dementia praecox.*[1]

In the mid-20th century, the psychoanalytic view of mental disorders took hold, reaching its zenith in the 1950s and 1960s. Psychiatric illness was explained as the result of unconscious conflicts over events in an individual's past. Alterations in nurture, not nature, became the underlying cause of psychiatric illness.

In the last half of the 20th century, biologic psychiatry became important once again. During the 1970s, techniques of neuroimaging became available that allowed the neuroscientist to visualize brain structures and function.[1] The results of genetic studies examining the correlation between family relationships and incidence of psychiatric illness, in particular the studies of monozygotic and dizygotic twins, suggested that depression and schizophrenia had a strong genetic component. The introduction of chlorpromazine, a first-generation phenothiazine antipsychotic, as a treatment for schizophrenia revolutionized psychiatry because although it did not cure psychosis, it did control the symptoms of the disease, increasing the potential for more traditional therapies to work and allowing previously institutionalized individuals to lead much more normal lives. It also suggested strongly that mental illness had a biologic foundation. Chlorpromazine soon was followed by other drugs for psychosis and depression.

This move to biologic psychiatry, however, has not excluded the healing value of the therapist–client relationship. It appears that pharmacotherapy in conjunction with psychotherapy is of greater healing power than either alone. Perhaps this effort is most clearly reflected in the most recent efforts to categorize diagnoses and treatment in the newest version of the Diagnostic and Statistical Manual. One of the primary distinctions in the current *DSM-5* edition is the clustering of disorders into factors which are "internalized" (*i.e.,* somatic, anxiety, depressive symptoms) and those which are "externalized" (*i.e.,* disruptive behaviours, impulsive actions and symptoms of addiction).

As an expansion of diagnostic criteria, the use of nonaxial descriptors, based on careful history with inclusions of culturally diverse responses and socially deviant behaviours associated with developmental processes in clinically significant disturbances, become more focused. These shifts demonstrate an effort to account for genetic and genomic vulnerability, familial influences, environmental exposures, and individual neurocircuitry in a means allowing for organization of information and clearer specificity while enhancing treatment options and decisions.[3]

These expansions are an effort to consider the disorder process with a broadened view to pattern development and treatment interventions. These shifts in diagnostic criteria are intended to be more expanded, with increased flexibility, and it would be a misunderstanding of the intent to not maintain the historic definitions and descriptors for various disorders of thought and mood, insofar as those historical definitions are based in scientific evidence. Perhaps, the best view of *DSM-5* is to consider this update as a means of visualizing what is known about disorders, providing a more global means of discussing the criteria, and developing a practice view toward interventions and treatment. Further, there are issues of increased use of medication and the abnormalization of normal behaviours that must be considered in the clinical decision-making process regarding diagnostics and treatment.

Perhaps we are beginning to realize the distinction drawn between biologic and psychosocial disease is arbitrary. Current research in mindfulness and awareness/noticing techniques in psychotherapy shows promise for nonpharmacologic interventions which impact the interface between mind and body;

as well as treating the nonverbal or limited-verbal patient.[4] While none of these are included in the *DSM-5* as alternative treatment choices to medication the evidence from research overwhelmingly supports the inclusion of these modalities as part of a more psychosocial approach to healing. Research has also documented through findings in neuroplasticity that the brain changes itself for health or illness through a process of feedback and reexperiencing.[5] Indeed, experiments indicate that learning and sensory stimulation or deprivation can in fact weaken or strengthen synaptic connections, which in turn could change brain function and thus behaviour.[6]

Treatment of Mental Illness

Asylums have existed since the Middle Ages, but until the end of the 18th century, their only function was custodial. One of the oldest asylums was the Priory of St. Mary of Bethlehem, founded in London in the 13th century. Its name was eventually shortened to *Bedlam,* a term that has become synonymous with madness. The asylum as a therapeutic establishment did not become an important concept until the end of the 18th century.[1]

At this time, madness was viewed as an excessive irritation of the nerves, so establishing a calming environment was crucial. These asylums often had a very rigid schedule of daily activities meant to focus the patient and afford mental rest. It was also during this time that practitioners attempted to systematize the techniques known to establish a therapeutic relationship between the doctor and the patient.

In the 1800s, the number of patients in asylums was, at the most, in the hundreds. By the mid-1900s, the numbers were in the thousands. Unfortunately, by the early 1900s, asylums had become little more than warehouses for those living with chronic mental illness.[7] Whether this was due to the failure of asylums as a therapeutic environment or to the increased number of persons housed in them, overwhelming the available resources, remains a matter of debate. The reason for the increased numbers of persons in asylums in the 19th century also is debated. Was there an increased incidence of mental illness, or did society become increasingly intolerant of deviant behaviour?

This debate exploded in the 1960s, during which time several writers suggested that there was no such thing as mental illness but rather that there had been a medicalizing of deviance, and that psychiatric institutions were evil. Schizophrenia in this view was a gifted and creative state of consciousness, not an illness. This antipsychiatry attitude, coupled with the advent of psychopharmacology, laid the foundations for the deinstitutionalization of the mentally ill and the move to community psychiatry. Unfortunately, deinstitutionalization was neither carefully planned nor adequately funded, leaving many mentally ill homeless and without proper care (Fig. 53.1).[1]

The Role of Heredity in Mental Illness

Who we are and how we express ourselves through behaviour depends on the complex influences of genetic and environmental factors on neural development and function. Since the early 1990s, the scientific knowledge base in genetics has grown exponentially and has created new tools to study the role of genetic inheritance in the development of mental illness. Research into the complexities of the regulation of gene expression can only deepen our understanding of the etiology of mental disorders, increase our ability to treat the disorders with more precisely targeted psychotherapeutic drugs, and ultimately lead to the discovery of ways to prevent the development of psychiatric illness.

Epidemiologic studies of twins, of adopted children, and of family histories or pedigrees have shed light on the debate over the relative influence of nurture versus nature in the development of mental illness. Twin studies compared the incidence of mental illness among monozygotic (identical) twins, dizygotic (fraternal) twins, and their siblings. If a disease were at all genetically determined, higher rates of coexistence of the disorder (concordance) would be expected among monozygotic twins compared with dizygotic twins, nontwin siblings, or the general population. Adoption studies questioned whether children with a genetic history of mental illness, adopted by parents with no history of psychiatric illness, had a greater risk of developing mental illness than children with no genetic history of mental illness who were adopted by parents with a psychiatric illness. Also, if a mental illness has a genetic component, it would be expected that higher numbers of persons in a family would have the disorder than would be found in the general population.[8] The overwhelming conclusions of these studies have been that both genetic vulnerability and environmental influences play significant roles in the development of mental illness.

For example, studies of twins have shown a 45% concordance for schizophrenia among monozygotic twins, compared with 15% for dizygotic twins or other siblings. With bipolar depression, there is an 80% concordance in monozygotic twins, compared with 10% for siblings. In monozygotic twins living apart, the concordance rate for affective disorders is 40% to 60%.[9] Even the concordance rates among siblings for these two disorders is suggestive of a genetic influence, because schizophrenia has approximately a 1% incidence and depression a 5% incidence among the general population.[9] The rate of occurrence of either disorder also is higher in the biologic families of adopted children than in the adoptive families. The incidence of suicide is six times higher among biologic relatives of adoptees with depressive illness than among the biologic relatives of adoptees without depression.

Although the evidence for a genetic basis for mental illness is compelling, the fact that the concordance among monozygotic twins is not 100% indicates that other factors may be involved in the development of a mental illness. It certainly is highly likely that mental illnesses are polygenic and multifactorial rather than simply inherited through transmission of a classic disordered dominant or recessive mendelian trait

FIGURE 53.1 • **A:** Canada's first hospital for the mentally ill opening in 1835 in Saint John, New Brunswick (From Austin W., Body M. A. (2010). *Psychiatric & mental health nursing for Canadian Practice* (2nd ed., p. 6). Philadelphia, PA: Lippincott Williams & Wilkins and from Provincial Archives of New Brunswick, Saint John Stereographs, P86–67.) **B–D:** Earlsworth Asylum, Redhill, England (T. S. Crowther; courtesy of the National Library of Medicine, National Institutes of Health.)

(see Chapter 6). In addition, mental disorders exhibit variable expressivity. It is possible that a person with the disease genotype needs to have the right environmental stressors (*e.g.,* viral illness, physical or emotional abuse, substance abuse) to express the disease phenotype, or that there are gene–gene interactions that influence the extent to which a mental illness is manifested.[10,11]

Recent research in epigenetics is shifting the way we view the psychiatric process of disorder development and genetics. The current view of genetic implications in psychiatric disorders does not require the change of DNA but rather shifts in the epigenetics and methylation process of the histones which allows for activation or silencing of the genes. This in part, may answer such questions as the difference between expression of genes in twins where one is exhibiting psychiatric disorders and the other is not, while giving insight into the processes in the portion of the population developing disorders. It may also point the way for

research leading to interventions allowing for the switching to be reversed.[10,11]

IN SUMMARY

Psychiatric disorders are characterized by alterations in thought, mood, or behaviour that may interfere with a person's ability to engage in ordinary social interactions and may in some instances require temporary or long-term institutionalization. Our understanding of the pathogeneses of mental disease is still in its infancy, and the historical debate over the relative importance of nurture and nature in the development of mental illness continues. It is likely that the cause of mental illness is multifactorial and includes a dynamic interplay among genetic predisposition, alterations in early neurodevelopment, and dysfunctional social interactions in a family.

ANATOMIC AND NEUROCHEMICAL BASIS OF BEHAVIOUR

After completing this section of the chapter, you should be able to meet the following objectives:

- Name the cerebral cortical structures and structures of the primitive brain involved in thought and emotion.
- Describe the major functions of each brain structure in terms of thought processes, learning, and emotion.
- Describe the cortical pathways by which learning and the development of memory occur.
- Define the terms *synapse, synaptic transmission,* and *neuromediators.*
- Name the major neuromediators in the brain, their major location and source, and possible involvement of each in the manifestations of mental illness.

Behavioural Anatomy of the Brain

There is scientific evidence that anatomic and biochemical alterations in the brain play a critical role in the behaviours observed in mental illness. The brain is extraordinarily complex, divided into several distinct groups of functional neurons that are highly interconnected and thus able to influence each other's activity.[12] Information processing occurs within nanoseconds. However, for persons with brain injury or degenerative changes, information processing and cognitive function may be impaired.

Cerebral Cortical Structures

The cerebral cortex covers the outermost part of the brain. The cortex, which contains the centres for elaboration of thought, voluntary motor and sensory function, speech, and memory patterns, has extensive connections with deeper parts of the brain. The thalamus, in particular, forms important connections with the cerebral cortex. Thalamic excitation is necessary for almost all cortical activity. Thus, the loss of function is much greater when the thalamus is damaged along with the cerebral cortex than when damage is limited to the cortex. Table 53.1 summarizes the cerebral cortical structures and their functions.

Prefrontal Cortex. The frontal lobe is the largest lobe and often is referred to as the "chief administrator" of the brain (Fig. 53.2). It is responsible for planning, problem solving, intellectual insight, judgment, and expression of emotion. It is the function of the prefrontal areas to keep track of many bits of information simultaneously and then to recall this information as it is needed for subsequent intellectual tasks. Before the discovery of modern drugs to treat psychiatric conditions, some patients were treated surgically with a procedure called *prefrontal lobotomy* that severed the connections between the prefrontal areas of the brain and the remainder of the brain. Subsequent studies of these patients revealed a lack of ability to solve complex problems, link sequential tasks together, and learn to do parallel tasks at the same time. Their social responses were also inappropriate, and their levels of aggression were decreased to the point where they lost all ambition. They were, however, still able to perform at their previous level of motor function, talk, and comprehend language, but they were unable to carry through with any long-term trains of thought.

Temporal Lobe. The temporal lobe integrates and interprets somatic, visual, and auditory information that is critical for recognition of the familiar, as well as appropriate interpretation of and response to social contexts. The temporal lobe also contains the area of the brain (*Wernicke area*) that is responsible for language comprehension. It is one of the more important areas of the brain in terms of intellect because almost all intellectual functions depend on language.

Part of an appropriate social response is the accurate interpretation of emotions and the ability to respond with

TABLE 53.1 SELECTED FUNCTIONS OF SEVERAL BRAIN REGIONS

FRONTAL LOBE	TEMPORAL LOBE	PARIETAL LOBE	OCCIPITAL LOBE
Abstract vs. concrete reasoning	Visual–spatial recognition	Sensory integration and spatial relations	Vision
Motivation–volition	Attention	Bodily awareness	Possible information holding area
Concentration	Motivation	Filtration of background stimuli	
Decision making	Emotional modulation and interpretation	Personality factors and symptom denial	
Purposeful behaviour	Impulse and aggression control	Memory and nonverbal memory	
Memory and historical sense of self	Interpretation and meaning of social context	Concept formation	
Sequencing	Aspects of sexual action and meaning		
Making meaning of language			
Speech organization			
Speech production (Broca area)			
Aspects of emotional response—blunting			

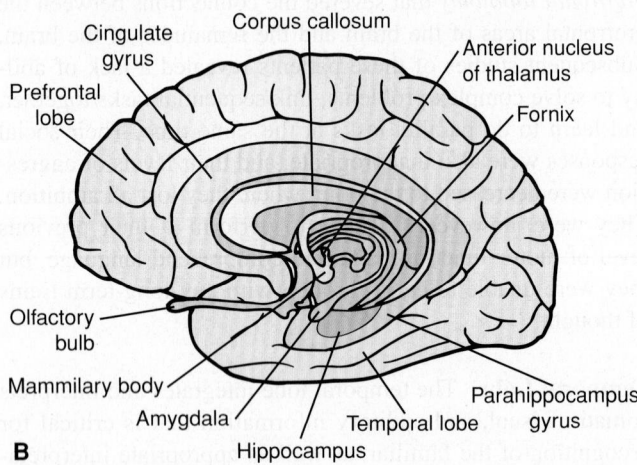

FIGURE 53.2 • **A:** Lateral aspects of the cerebral hemispheres, including the frontal, temporal, parietal, and occipital lobes. **B:** The structure of the limbic cortex, which includes the limbic cortex (cingulate gyrus, parahippocampal gyrus, hippocampus) and associated subcortical structures (thalamus, hypothalamus, amygdala).

the socially appropriate level of emotionality and language. Impulse control, the management of aggression and sexual expression, including the culturally determined stereotypy of what it means to be male or female in a given society, also are temporal lobe functions. Emotion originates in the amygdala of the limbic system (discussed later), but the modulation and "fine-tuning" of that emotion to an appropriate level of intensity occur in the temporal lobe.

Parietal Lobe. The parietal lobe is essential in the integration and processing of sensory (visual, tactile, and auditory) input. It is in the parietal lobe that sensory experiences first begin to coalesce into the cognitions we experience as thinking in the frontal lobes. The coordination of spatial awareness occurs in the parietal lobe and involves not only visual content, but the ability to experience, claim, and care for all of one's body. Another important parietal lobe function is to filter out extraneous information. The ability to filter out background

and extraneous noise and sensations is critical to normal daily functioning.

Occipital Lobe. The occipital lobe is the most posterior of the lobes and is responsible for receiving visual information from the eyes. The visual association cortex of the occipital lobe is important for the interpretation of visual experiences, including depth perception and location in space.

Association Areas. A large part of the cerebral cortex forms association areas that add perception and meaning to incoming sensory information. The most important of these are the parieto-occipitotemporal association area, the prefrontal association area, and the limbic association area (Fig. 53.3).

The *parieto-occipitotemporal association area* lies in the large parietal–occipital cortical space bounded by the somatosensory cortex, the visual cortex, and the auditory cortex (see Chapter 48). This association area computes the coordinates of incoming visual, auditory, and somatosensory information, providing information about the location of body parts and their relationship to the environment. It also contains the major area for comprehending language, processing visual language (reading), and naming objects.

The *prefrontal association area* functions in close connection with the motor cortex to plan and execute complex motor movements. This area uses input from sensory receptors in muscles and joints, as well as sensory input from the skin and vestibular system. The prefrontal association area is also important in carrying out thought processes that involve input from multiple sensory modalities. It is often described as being the area for short-term "working memories" that are used to analyze each new thought as it is entering the brain. A special area of the frontal cortex,

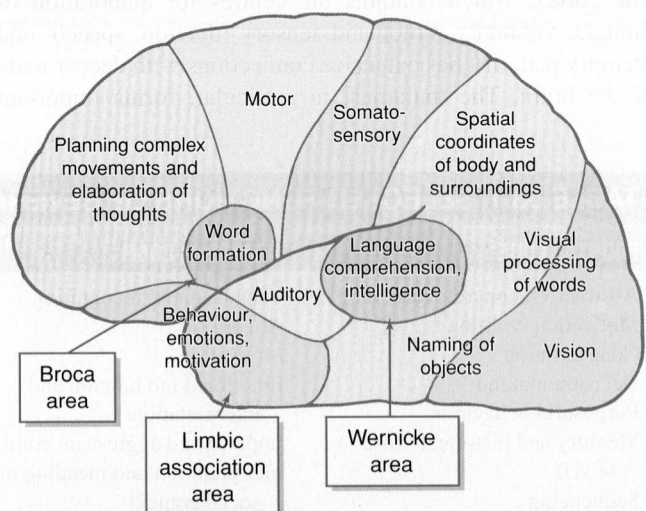

FIGURE 53.3 • Map of specific functional areas in the cerebral cortex, showing especially the Wernicke and Broca areas of language comprehension and speech production, which in 95% of all people are located in the left hemisphere. (Adapted from Hall J. E. (2011). *Textbook of medical physiology* (12th ed., p. 703). Philadelphia, PA: W. B. Saunders.)

called the *Broca area,* provides the neural circuitry for word formation.

The *limbic association area* is found in the anterior pole of the temporal lobe and in the cingulate gyrus on the medial aspect of the brain. It is concerned primarily with behaviour, emotions, and motivation.

The Limbic System

The limbic system is a complex group of neurons that regulate our emotional behaviour. It comprises several discrete structures in the deep part of the brain, including the hippocampus, parahippocampal gyrus, cingulate gyrus, amygdala, and a bridgelike structure called the *fornix,* which is a bundle of nerve fibres connecting the hippocampus with the hypothalamus (Fig. 53.2). Higher and lower brain centres communicate with the limbic system to link thoughts and autonomic nervous system responses to emotions. The hippocampus, along with its adjacent temporal and parietal lobe structures, has numerous indirect connections with many portions of the cerebral cortex as well as other parts of the limbic system. The hippocampus plays a major role in the encoding, consolidation, and retrieval of memories. Almost all types of sensory information activate some part of the hippocampus. In turn, the hippocampus distributes information to the anterior thalamus, hypothalamus, and other parts of the limbic system. The hippocampus also groups and schematizes input in preparation for memory encoding. It plays a significant role in converting short-term memory to long-term memory. Hippocampal atrophy has been noted in diseases in which memory problems play an important role, such as Alzheimer disease.

The amygdala is located deep in the medial temporal lobe. It receives neuronal signals from the temporal and occipital lobes of the cortex and has many bidirectional connections with the hypothalamus, as well as other parts of the limbic system. Through these connections, the amygdala helps a person relate to the surrounding environment and then pattern appropriate behaviour. Because of the many connections, the amygdala has been called the "window" through which a person sees the world. The amygdala is important in emotional function and regulation and modulation of affective responses in social settings. Sexual arousal, aggression, and fear also are functions of the amygdala.

The hypothalamus, although not strictly an anatomic part of the limbic system, plays a critical role in it because of the extensive connections it has with the limbic system. The hypothalamus has a multitude of regulatory functions related to basic survival needs of the body, such as regulation of body temperature, sleep–rest patterns, hunger, sexual drive, and hormonal secretion.

Physiology of Perception, Thought, and Memory

Perception is the final stage of information processing. It is the conscious awareness of sensory stimuli and results in behavioural responses to that sensation. Information from the senses

is received by the thalamus and then projected to the somatosensory cortex and prefrontal association area. The prefrontal association area keeps track of where information has been put in long-term memory and is responsible for retrieving and then integrating memories with sensory input for decision making.

Learning and Memory

Behaviour is altered by environmental cues that are processed through learning and memory. Learning is the process of acquiring knowledge, whereas memory is the process of storing and retrieving what has been learned. There are two forms of memory: implicit memory, which is involved in learning reflexive motor and perceptual skills, and explicit memory, which is involved with processing the factual knowledge of persons, places, and things and their meanings.[6] Psychiatric patients and brain-injured persons not only experience specific cortical dysfunctions, but may experience difficulty in the proposed pathways for learning and memory. These difficulties are likely to influence their behaviour and may have an impact on the design of effective interventions.

Thought processes probably involve a pattern of stimuli from many parts of the nervous system at the same time and in a definite sequence. Each thought requires simultaneous input from portions of the cerebral cortex, the thalamus, the limbic system, and the reticular formation in the brain stem. The prefrontal association cortex processes information from many areas of the brain and is necessary to achieve thinking. It has the ability to keep track of bits of information and recall them simultaneously from working memory. This allows us to plan, set goals, and solve problems. Thoughts are expressed in the form of language through the functions of the Broca area for word formation and the Wernicke area for language comprehension.

Physiologically, thought and memories are the result of synaptic transmission between neurons. During the process, new or reactivated pathways transmit neural circuits, sometimes called *memory traces,* through the brain.[13] Although we often think of memories as being positive recollections of past experiences, the greatest share of memories are probably negative encounters that the brain disregards as adverse or unimportant information. It is the basal regions of the limbic system that determine whether information is important and whether to store the thought as a memory trace or to suppress it. This aspect of memory selection is vital to the brain. Without it, the constant inundation of sensory information would exceed the capacity of the brain within minutes.

Memories can last minutes, hours, months, or years. For the purpose of classification, memory can be classified as short term, intermediate term, or long term. Short-term memory is typically confined to the remembering of information for a period of several seconds to minutes (*e.g.,* 7 to 10 digits of a telephone number). It is thought that these memories involve nerve signals that travel around and around a temporary memory trace.[6] Intermediate-term memory involves the remembering of information for a period of many minutes to weeks. These memories become lost unless memory traces are established. Long-term memory, which lasts for years, is generally thought to result from actual structural changes in the synapses. For example, there might be an increase in the number of presynaptic structures responsible for neurotransmitter synthesis or release.

Disorders of Perception

Two disorders of information processing, hallucinations and delusional thoughts, are common symptoms of many psychiatric disorders. These symptoms may also occasionally occur in healthy persons, they may accompany other health problems, or they may be a side effect of drugs.

Hallucinations

Perception consists of the input of sensory information from the outside world and the processing of this information into meaning. All sensory information from the external world is transmitted to the thalamus; from there it is relayed to various parts of the brain and then transformed into meaningful experience. For example, visual stimuli from the retina are transmitted to centres in the thalamus through the optic nerve; from there, they are relayed to the primary visual cortex in the occipital lobe and then to the visual association cortex, where they gain meaning (see Chapter 54).

Hallucinations are described as "sensory perceptions with a compelling sense of reality."[12] Hallucinations should be differentiated from illusions, which are misinterpreted sensory perceptions that are stimulated by actual external stimuli. The pathophysiologic process of hallucinations can occur at several levels. The disorder may originate at the end organ, occur during sensory transmission, or be based on abnormal cortical reception, perception, or interpretation.

Hallucinations can be classified in several ways, such as by the structure or function involved, the etiology, or the affected sense perception. One functional method categorizes hallucinations as *release hallucinations* and *ictal hallucinations*. Release hallucinations occur when a normal sensory input is blocked and, as a replacement, stored images are experienced, whereas ictal hallucinations are produced by abnormal neuronal discharges. Visual ictal hallucinations tend to be of brief duration, stereotyped in content, and geometric in design. These are the types of hallucinations that occur during the aura in people with epilepsy. Hallucinations that are classified according to etiology may occur as the result of disorders of brain structure or function (brain tumours, epilepsy, metabolic disorders), drug reactions, sensory deprivation, sleep deprivation, or psychotic disorders. The type and content of hallucinations often provide insight into their etiology.

The most commonly used classification of hallucinations is based on the sensory perception involved (*e.g.*, visual, auditory, olfactory, tactile). Within this system, hallucinatory experiences involving the visual system are the most clearly categorized. Several types of visual hallucinations are normal life experiences (*e.g.*, images seen in a dream). Several ophthalmologic stimuli also are accompanied by visual hallucinations. Ocular phosphenes, which are produced by vigorous rubbing

of the eye, are a form of visual hallucination. The Charles Bonnet syndrome is an organic disorder occurring in the elderly that is characterized by complex visual hallucinations. It is associated with loss of vision and is seen in older adults with preserved intellectual function.[14] While the prevalence varies, it is estimated that approximately 10% of persons (mean age of 75 years) with severe visual disability experienced visual hallucinations. These persons retained insight into the problem and needed only reassurance that their hallucinations did not represent mental illness. Visual hallucinations associated with psychiatric disorders tend to be complex, may be enhanced by auditory hallucinations, and often lead to delusional beliefs.

Auditory hallucinations include misperceptions of sounds such as ringing and buzzing noises, music, and voices. Although they commonly occur in psychiatric disorders, particularly schizophrenia, they also occur in other disorders. Musical hallucinations featuring the perception of music without an external stimulus can be seen in disorders ranging from hearing impairment, especially in depressed elderly women, to temporal lobe lesions.[15] When associated with brain pathology, the lesion is usually on the right side of the brain. Auditory hallucinations are commonly reported as part of the aura of epilepsy. Tinnitus, the perception of ringing, buzzing, or whistling sounds, is often the result of disorders of the inner ear (see Chapter 55). Withdrawal states, particularly from alcohol, are known to cause auditory hallucinations.

A variety of psychiatric disorders are accompanied by auditory hallucinations, such as the sound of voices. Often the source of the sound, which is sensed as occurring within the head, is difficult to localize. The voice often comments on the person's behaviour and echoes his or her thoughts. Voices are rarely described as supportive; they are most often described as critical and negative in tone. Strategies of distraction used by persons hearing voices include listening to music, especially through headphones, or snapping rubber bands on their wrists. In addition, keeping a record helps to identify hallucinatory precipitants and thus helps individuals avoid those situations that act as precipitants.[16]

Hallucinations involving smell and taste are often the result of damage to the olfactory bulb. Tumours at the base of the brain that extend into the olfactory cortex can produce olfactory hallucinations. Persons with migraine headaches may also experience an aura consisting of olfactory or gustatory hallucinations. Somatosensory hallucinations, such as phantom limb pain, are discussed in Chapter 49.

Delusions

Delusions are characterized by a false belief and the persistent, unshakable acceptance of the false belief. In contrast to hallucinations, which are abnormalities of perception, delusions are abnormalities of thought. Delusions are formed from and coloured by an individual's background, including personal, family, and social experiences; educational background; and cultural (including religious) influences. Delusional thinking may include, among others, delusions of persecution (*e.g.*, believing one's self or property is being threatened), influence (*e.g.,* believing thoughts can move through radio or atomic rays), ill health, grandeur (*e.g.,* believing oneself to be a great person, such as the King of England), poverty, and possession (*e.g.,* believing one's body is possessed by God or some great power).

The causes or mechanisms underlying delusional thinking are unclear. It has been suggested that delusional thinking is the product of repeated stress, rather than a disorder based on a single, acute situational problem. Interestingly, delusions have been associated with conditions that produce sensory deprivation, such as hearing loss. In one study that used a case-control method, elderly persons with late-life psychoses that included paranoid symptomatology were four times more likely to have hearing impairments than control subjects.[17]

Role of Neuromediators

Many of the new advances in the understanding and treatment of mental illness are derived from an increased understanding of how nerve cells in the brain communicate with one another. Nerve cells of discrete brain regions communicate with each other rapidly and over long distances by electrochemical signals that are propagated along the length of each neuron. The point at which two neurons meet is called a *synapse,* and the process by which the signal from one neuron to another is communicated is called *synaptic transmission* or *neurotransmission* (see Chapter 48). Chemical substances called *neurotransmitters* or *neuromediators* are released from the axonal terminal of one neuron (presynaptic cell), cross the synapse, bind to receptors on the postsynaptic cells, and cause excitatory or inhibitory actions.[6]

Neurotransmission involves several discrete steps: (1) the synthesis of a transmitter substance, (2) the storage and release of the transmitter, (3) binding of the transmitter to receptors on the postsynaptic membrane, and (4) removal of the transmitter from the synaptic cleft. The classic neurotransmitters include small-molecule transmitters and neuroactive peptides. These molecules typically are stored in vesicles in the presynaptic axonal terminal and released by the process of exocytosis[6] (see Chapter 48, section on Understanding Synaptic Transmission).

The substances generally agreed on to be neurotransmitters and that are implicated in mental illness include acetylcholine, the biogenic amines (dopamine, epinephrine, norepinephrine, and serotonin), and amino acids (gamma-aminobutyric acid [GABA], glutamate, glycine, and aspartate). Table 53.2 summarizes the major source and effect of each neurotransmitter.

Emergence of Psychotropic Medications

The treatment of many psychiatric disorders is based on pharmacologic interventions that alter neurotransmitter or receptor properties of the brain. In the 1950s, a French neurosurgeon, Henri Laborit, was searching for a drug that would reduce the affects of preoperative anxiety-induced histamine release in his patients. Through trial and error, he found chlorpromazine to be the most effective calming agent and recommended the drug to his psychiatric colleagues. It was subsequently found that high doses of chlorpromazine were efficacious in calming agitated persons with schizophrenia and bipolar disorders. It eventually became clear that chlorpromazine was not simply a tranquilizer but also had some specific antipsychotic effects. Chlorpromazine and

TABLE 53.2 THE SOURCE AND EFFECT OF BRAIN NEUROMEDIATORS

NEUROMEDIATOR	MAJOR SOURCE IN THE BRAIN	EFFECT AND IMPLICATIONS FOR MENTAL ILLNESS
Acetylcholine (ACh)	Formed in many synapses of the brain; in high concentration in basal ganglia and motor cortex Derived from choline	Can be excitatory or inhibitory, depending on the area of the brain Underactivity implicated in Alzheimer disease
Dopamine (DA)	Substantia nigra and ventral segmental area in the midbrain Derived from tyrosine	Usually excitatory Involved in motivation, thought, and emotional regulation Overactivity thought to be involved in schizophrenia and other psychotic disorders
Norepinephrine (NE) and epinephrine (E)	Locus ceruleus in brain stem Derived from dopamine	Can be excitatory or inhibitory, depending on the area of the brain Noradrenergic pathways to cerebral cortex, limbic system, and brain stem Underactivity thought to be involved in some depressions
Serotonin (5-HT)	Raphe nucleus in the brain stem Derived from tryptophan	Involved in the regulation of attention and complex cognitive functions Pathways to cerebral cortex, limbic system, and brain stem Underactivity thought to be involved in some depressions and obsessive-compulsive disorder
γ-Aminobutyric acid (GABA), glutamate, aspartate, and glycine	No single major source	GABA and glycine usually are inhibitory; glutamate is excitatory Implicated in anxiety disorders

related drugs in the phenothiazine class attenuated or abolished delusions, hallucinations, and disordered thinking.

There are now four major groups of antipsychotic agents used to treat schizophrenia, divided into two major categories: the typical and the atypical antipsychotics. The typical antipsychotics include the phenothiazines (*e.g.,* chlorpromazine), butyrophenones (*e.g.,* haloperidol), and thioxanthenes (*e.g.,* chlorprothixene). The atypical antipsychotics (*e.g.,* clozapine, risperidone, olanzapine) are more effective in treating the negative symptoms of schizophrenia (to be discussed) and produce fewer extrapyramidal effects. Both categories of drugs exert their effect by blocking dopamine receptors, although the atypical antipsychotics have a more refined blockade action. The atypical antipsychotics also exert some of their effects through blockade of serotonin (5-hydroxytryptamine [HT]) receptors.

Psychopharmacology has been particularly productive in developing highly effective treatments for affective disorders. Antidepressants alleviate depressive symptoms by increasing the activity of norepinephrine and serotonin at postsynaptic membrane receptors. The most widely used antidepressants can be divided into four major categories: the monoamine oxidase (MAO) inhibitors, the tricyclic compounds, the serotonin reuptake inhibitors (SRIs), and the novel, or dual action, antidepressants.[18]

The MAO inhibitors (*e.g.,* phenelzine, tranylcypromine) increase the concentration of serotonin and norepinephrine by reducing the degradation of these neurotransmitters by MAO. The tricyclic antidepressants (TCAs; *e.g.,* amitriptyline, imipramine, nortriptyline) block the reuptake of serotonin and norepinephrine by the presynaptic membrane, whereas the SRIs inhibit the reuptake of serotonin.

The formulations of the SRIs vary and target different neurotransmitters. These include the selective SRIs (SSRIs; *e.g.,* fluoxetine, fluvoxamine, paroxetine, citalopram, sertraline), the serotonin antagonist and reuptake inhibitors (SARIs; *e.g.,* nefazodone, discontinued in Canada in 2003), and the serotonin and norepinephrine reuptake inhibitors (SNRIs; *e.g.,* venlafaxine, duloxetine). Other novel or dual action antidepressants include bupropion (inhibits norepinephrine and dopamine reuptake), trazodone (a serotonin receptor antagonist with some SRI), and mirtazapine (increases serotonergic and noradrenergic neurotransmission).[18]

The therapeutic effect of the antipsychotic and antidepressant drugs probably is not entirely due to increasing or decreasing the neural levels of one or more neurotransmitters. For example, the clinical effect of the antidepressants typically is slow (weeks), even though the drugs rapidly block receptors. This suggests that the real mechanism of these drugs may be due to their effects on expression of receptors at the cellular membrane or on other intracellular pathways that regulate protein synthesis.[18]

Neuroimaging

Abnormalities in brain structure and function can contribute to the manifestations of mental illness. Since the early 1970s,

FIGURE 53.4 • Positron emission tomography (PET) scan showing differences in frontal lobe activity of a pair of twins, one with schizophrenia, and one who does not have the disorder. (From Austin W., Boyd M. A. (2010). *Psychiatric & mental health nursing in Canadian practice* (2nd ed., p. 145). Philadelphia, PA: Lippincott Williams & Wilkins. Courtesy of Drs. K. F. Berman and D. R. Weinberger, Clinical Brain Disorders Branch, National Institutes of Health.)

imaging techniques have been developed that allow practitioners and researchers to map brain anatomy in exquisite detail and to estimate brain activity by measuring brain blood flow and metabolic rate. These imaging studies have suggested intriguing correlations between brain lesions and psychiatric manifestations that provide clues to the pathogenesis of mental disorders. Brain imaging techniques, however, remain research tools and have not yet been applied clinically, which means that imaging cannot be used to make a diagnosis of mental illness. The techniques include computed tomography (CT) scans, magnetic resonance imaging (MRI), magnetoencephalography (MEG), positron emission tomography (PET), and single-photon emission computed tomography (SPECT; Fig. 53.4).

A CT scan of the brain provides a three-dimensional view of brain structures that can differentiate fine densities. Abnormalities in a CT scan are not diagnostic of any particular mental illness; however, they suggest a brain-based problem. Structural abnormalities of the brain have been measured in people with schizophrenia, mood disorders, and dementias. MRI is used primarily for diagnosis of structural changes in the brain, although newer techniques are able to measure brain function as well. Unlike CT, MRI is able to distinguish between grey and white matter. MEG detects the minute magnetic fluctuations of regional brain activity.[19] The basis of PET is the variable brain tissue uptake of an infused radioactive substance. The tissue uptake of the substance depends on tissue type and metabolic activity. Labelled drugs can be infused to study neurotransmitter receptor activity or concentration in the brain. SPECT is similar to PET but is less expensive and uses more stable substances and different detectors to visualize blood flow patterns. This is useful for diagnosis of cerebrovascular accidents and brain tumours.[19]

IN SUMMARY

The symptoms of mental illness arise from alterations in neural functioning or from destruction of neurons in the brain. Because the brain integrates the processes of learning, memory, and emotions, the manifestations of mental disease may be primarily cognitive impairment, emotional impairment, or a combination of both. Psychiatric patients and brain-injured persons not only experience specific cortical dysfunctions but may experience difficulty in the proposed pathways for learning and memory. These difficulties are likely to influence behaviour and may have an impact on the design of effective interventions.

Many of the new advances in the understanding and treatment of mental illness and symptoms such as hallucinations, mood disruptions, and cognitive dysfunction are derived from an increased understanding of how nerve cells in the brain communicate with one another. Neurotransmission involves several discrete steps: (1) the synthesis of a transmitter substance, (2) the storage and release of the transmitter, (3) the binding of the transmitter to receptors on the postsynaptic membrane, and (4) the removal of the transmitter from the synaptic cleft. The substances generally agreed to be neurotransmitters and that are implicated in mental illness include acetylcholine, the biogenic amines, and amino acids.

New diagnostic tools, such as increasingly sophisticated neuroimaging techniques, may help in the development of more precise correlations between behaviour, thought, and mood disorders and microscopic alterations in brain structure and neuron function. In addition, an increased understanding of the complex interactions among the different parts of the brain will assist in the development of more effective psychotherapies and more efficacious psychotropic drugs.

DISORDERS OF THOUGHT AND VOLITION

After completing this section of the chapter, you should be able to meet the following objectives:

- Define the term *schizophrenia*.
- Describe the epidemiology of schizophrenia.
- Describe the manifestations of schizophrenia, both positive and negative symptoms, and their underlying neuropathophysiology.
- Cite the diagnostic criteria for schizophrenia according to the *DSM-5* classification.
- Describe the treatment for the positive and negative manifestations of schizophrenia.

Schizophrenia

Schizophrenia is a chronic debilitating psychotic disorder that involves the disconnection between thought and language. It affects a person's thoughts, feelings, perceptions, and overall behaviours while interfering with filtering of stimuli from the environment.[20] Although the word *schizophrenia* means "splitting of the mind," it should not be confused with "split personality." The onset of the disorder typically occurs between 17 and 25 years of age. The peak age of onset for males is between 10 and 25 years of age, and for females between 25 and 35 years of age.[20] Ninety percent of those in treatment are between 15 and 55 years of age. Onset before 10 or after 60 years of age is rare. Schizophrenia affects 1% of the Canadian population and men and women seem to be affected equally.[21] Risk factors for schizophrenia include having a close relative with schizotypal personality disorder or schizophrenia (first-degree relatives of a person with schizophrenia have a 10-fold greater prevalence of the illness than the population at large), winter/spring birth date, second-trimester prenatal influenza infection, and early history of attentional deficits.[20]

Manifestations

Recent research and data concerning schizophrenia present a complex image of brain dysfunction with alterations in anatomic structures, biochemical variations, and functional disturbances.[12,20] The psychopathology of schizophrenia can be organized in various ways, but all such systems consider the positive and negative symptoms of the disease. *Positive* or *psychotic symptoms* reflect the presence of abnormal behaviours and include incomprehensible speech; delusions (*e.g.*, that one is being controlled by an outside force); hallucinations (hearing voices is the most common); and grossly disorganized or catatonic behaviour. Alterations in speech patterns can include using invented words (neologisms), derailment (loose associations), tangentiality (inability to stick to the original point), incoherence (loss of logical connections), or word salad (groups of disconnected words; Fig. 53.5). Frequently, persons with schizophrenia lose the ability to sort and interpret incoming stimuli, which impairs

SCHIZOPHRENIA

- Schizophrenia is a psychotic disorder of thought and language that is characterized by disorganized speech, delusions, visual and auditory hallucinations, and possible catatonic behaviour.
- The positive symptoms of schizophrenia include delusions, or fixed false beliefs, and hallucinations, or abnormal sensory perceptions, that occur without external visual or auditory input.
- The negative symptoms of schizophrenia reflect the absence of normal social and interpersonal relationships such as lack of motivation, apathy, and flattening of emotional expression.

FIGURE 53.5 • A sample of noncommunicative writing by a patient with chronic paranoid schizophrenia. This letter, written to the patient's psychiatrist, illustrates lack of control over the writing process with repeated meaningless words or phrases (verbigeration) with some nonsensical and unrecognizable words that only have meaning to the writer (neologisms). (From Sadock B. J., Sadock V. A., Ruiz P. (2015). *Kaplan & Sadock's synopsis of psychiatry: Behavioral sciences/clinical psychiatry* (11th ed., p. 314). Philadelphia, PA: Lippincott Williams & Wilkins.)

the ability to respond appropriately to the environment. An enhancement or a blunting of the senses is very common in the early stages of schizophrenia. Sounds may be experienced as louder and more intrusive; colours may be brighter and sharper. In addition, the person with schizophrenia often experiences sensory overload owing to a loss of the ability to screen external sensory stimuli.[19,22,23]

Delusions and hallucinations may be related to the inability of the person with schizophrenia to filter, interpret, and respond appropriately to stimuli. Delusions are fixed, false ideas believed by the affected person that cannot be corrected by reason. They range from simply believing that people are watching them to beliefs that they are being controlled and manipulated by others. Delusions may be characterized according to the type of false beliefs. The most common type is persecutory delusions or the belief that one will be harmed by an individual, organization, or group. Grandiose delusions of being a historical figure (*e.g.,* Jesus Christ or the Queen of England) or having exceptional abilities also are common. Other delusions may include: a belief that the affected person is able to control others with his or her thoughts (control); falsely believing that another individual is in love with him or her (erotomanic); a belief that an impending major catastrophic event will occur (nihilistic); and beliefs that are focused on a bodily sensation, defective functional components, or medical condition (somatic).[2,23]

Hallucinations are very common in schizophrenia, especially the auditory type. In these cases, the individual sees and hears things that are not in the external world but nevertheless are very real phenomena to the person experiencing them. Hallucinations may represent the end of the spectrum of increasing intensity of sensual stimuli. Auditory hallucinations range from simple repetitive sounds to many voices speaking at once. Sometimes the voices are pleasant, but often they accuse and curse. When visual hallucinations occur, they usually are in conjunction with auditory hallucinations.[19–23]

The *negative symptoms* of schizophrenia reflect the absence of normal social and interpersonal behaviours and include alogia (tendency to speak very little), avolition (lack of motivation for goal-oriented activity), apathy, affective flattening (lack of emotional expression), inappropriate affect, and anhedonia (an inability to experience pleasure in things that ordinarily are pleasurable). Some persons with schizophrenia have a blunted response to pain. Negative symptoms are the most difficult to treat, and often are severe and persistent between acute episodes of illness.[12]

Another component of schizophrenia concerns what is referred to alternatively as the *disorganized dimension, cognitive symptoms,* or *disorganization symptom cluster.*[12,24] It involves thought disorders and overlaps the categories of positive and negative symptoms. This component involves the disorganized speech and behaviour described previously, and the incongruent mood and affect that interfere with relating to the environment.

These three dimensions of behaviour—positive or psychotic symptoms, negative symptoms, and disorganization—are used in evaluating the neurocognitive impairment that occurs with schizophrenia. Studies have found less cognitive impairment when psychotic symptoms predominate, such as in paranoid schizophrenia. Conversely, there is more cognitive impairment related to negative and disorganized symptoms.[24]

Neurophysiology of Symptoms

The exact pathogenesis of schizophrenia is unknown. No single lesion in the brain appears to be specific to schizophrenia or to the brains of all persons with schizophrenia.[25] With the advent of neuroimaging techniques of the 1960s, it became possible to document what had long been suspected: that schizophrenia was associated with brain abnormalities. These abnormalities are present at the first episode and in unmedicated persons. This suggests that the anatomic changes are not the result of progressive brain deterioration or the effects of psychiatric medications, but are caused by abnormalities in neurodevelopment that occur in prenatal or early postnatal life. There is an enlargement of the lateral and third ventricles; a reduction in frontal lobe, temporal lobe, and whole-brain volumes; and diminished neuronal content in both the thalamus and hippocampus.[25] Schizophrenia also is characterized by reduced metabolic activity in the frontal cortex on PET scan, although marked decreases in activity can be seen in almost every area of the brain, depending on the individual and the particular symptoms being experienced at the time of the scan[26] (Fig. 53.4).

It is not known at what age these differences might be visible with imaging because children usually are not subjected to imaging techniques without a specific event indicating a clinical need for the procedure. Adolescents and young adults who are at high risk for development of schizophrenia because of a strong family history also have enlarged ventricles and smaller medial temporal lobes.[27] Studies have also found other brain abnormalities in nonpsychotic first-degree relatives of persons with schizophrenia. These were most pronounced in the hippocampus.[27]

An additional anatomic finding is an increased density of dopamine (D_2) receptor sites, particularly in the basal ganglia. With the finding that effective antipsychotic drugs are dopamine antagonists and that dopamine-releasing agents such as amphetamine can cause psychosis, the "dopamine hypothesis" was developed; it proposes that the symptoms of schizophrenia are due to dopaminergic overactivity. This hypothesis, however, cannot explain types of schizophrenia in which negative symptoms predominate, or the residual symptoms of an acute psychotic episode. In addition, it is possible that the increased density of dopamine receptors found in some studies is related to the effects of antipsychotic drugs. Other neurotransmitter changes implicated in the development of schizophrenia include a decreased activity of serotonin

(through the $5\text{-}HT_{2A}$ receptor) and a decreased activity of glutamate through dysfunction of its N-methyl-D-aspartate receptor (see Chapter 51). Norepinephrine and GABA have also been implicated in the pathophysiology of schizophrenia.

Diagnostic Criteria

According to the *DSM-5* classification system, a diagnosis of schizophrenia requires that two or more of the following symptoms be present for a significant portion of 1 month: delusions, hallucinations, disorganized speech, grossly disorganized or catatonic behaviour, or negative symptoms such as changes in affective lability, volition, or amount of speech.[2] In addition, one or more areas of functioning must be significantly impaired compared with premorbid abilities, and continuous signs of the disturbance must persist for at least 6 months.[2] Previous editions of the DSM had subtypes of schizophrenia (paranoid, disorganized, catatonic, undifferentiated, and residual types) that have been eliminated in the *DSM-5* because of difficulties with reliability, validity, and stability of diagnosis.

Treatment

The goals of treatment for schizophrenia are to induce a remission, prevent a recurrence, and improve behavioural, cognitive, and psychosocial functions. Schizophrenia is a chronic illness, and for the person living with schizophrenia, the goal is *recovery.* The Canadian Mental Health Association (CMHA) reiterates that with the use of proper, improved medications, community support, and psychotherapy, many people with schizophrenia are able to function in the community—including living and working independently.[28] The implications and reality are that outcomes from this illness are varied, and some individuals function at a much higher level than originally thought. One example is the Nobel Prize winner John Forbes Nash Jr., who struggles with schizophrenia. Hospitalization may be indicated if the patient is a danger to self or others, is unable to provide basic care for self, or refuses to eat or drink.[28]

Pharmacotherapy and psychosocial interventions, the latter of which include patient and family education, housing support, vocational rehabilitation, and case management, are components in the treatment of persons with schizophrenia. The positive symptoms of schizophrenia (delusions, hallucinations, agitation, thought broadcasting, loose associations, suspiciousness, and poor hygiene and dress) are most likely to respond to drug therapy. Both typical and atypical antipsychotic drugs address these positive symptoms. The negative symptoms of schizophrenia respond more favourably to the atypical antipsychotic drugs (*e.g.,* olanzapine, ziprasidone). Often antipsychotics are combined with benzodiazepines or antiparkinson agents during the acute phase of treatment to reduce the risk of extrapyramidal effects from large doses of antipsychotic agents.

Psychosocial interventions are important to help patients learn about and live successfully with their illness. Assistance with housing, employment or disability benefits, socialization, and cooccurring illnesses may be indicated and may require the involvement of a case manager. Family members may need assistance in learning about the illness and the best ways to support each other and their family member with schizophrenia. Maintenance of pharmacotherapy may be difficult for a variety of reasons, including side effects of medications, cost of medications, and beliefs that they are no longer necessary. Social support and nursing interventions aimed at identifying and assisting with noncompliance issues can lead to improved compliance and reminding patients and families that recovery is possible.

IN SUMMARY

Schizophrenia is a chronic psychotic disorder of thought and volition in which thought and language become disconnected. It is characterized by both positive symptoms, negative symptoms, and disorganized thinking. Positive symptoms are abnormal behaviours (*e.g.,* incomprehensible speech), delusions, and auditory or visual hallucinations. Negative symptoms are the lack of normal social and interpersonal behaviours (*e.g.,* lack of emotional expression) and an inability to experience pleasure. The onset of the disorder typically occurs between the ages of 17 and 25 years, with an equal incidence in men and women. Risk factors for schizophrenia include having a close relative with schizotypal personality disorder or schizophrenia. The pathogenesis of schizophrenia is unknown, although neuroimaging studies reveal anatomic and functional changes in regions of the brain, including enlargement of the ventricles and diminished volumes in several areas of the brain, including the hippocampus and temporal cortex. Abnormalities in neurotransmission have been implicated, including changes in concentration and activity of the neurotransmitters dopamine, serotonin, norepinephrine, GABA, and glutamate. Treatment includes both psychosocial interventions and psychotropic medications.

DISORDERS OF MOOD

After completing this section of the chapter, you should be able to meet the following objectives:

- Define the terms *depression* and *mania*.
- Describe the epidemiology and manifestations of major depression.
- Describe the manifestations of bipolar and related disorders.
- Cite the diagnostic criteria for depression according to the *DSM-5* classification.
- Describe the treatment modalities for depression.

Mood disorders are disorders of emotion (mania and depression) rather than disturbances of thought. Although relatively common, with estimates that 10% of Canadians are affected, they are highly underdiagnosed and undertreated illnesses.[28]

Mood disorders previously combined major depression and bipolar (manic–depressive) disorders. However, the *DSM-5* has split these two categories into a category for each. Therefore, there is a category for depression with its own diagnostic criteria and one for bipolar disorder with its own criteria. Depression is among the leading causes of disability worldwide with approximately 8% of adults experiencing major depressive episodes at some time in their lives.[21] The prevalence of major depression among women is double that in men. The prevalence of bipolar disorder is approximately 1% in the population at large, approximately equally distributed between men and women.[2,21]

Depressive Disorders

Depressive disorders in the *DSM-5* now include the major depressive disorder (MDD), persistent depressive disorder as well as disruptive mood dysregulation, premenstrual dysphoric disorder (PMDD), substance/medication-induced depression, and other unspecified causes of depression.[2] Prevalence of depression is higher in individuals from families with a history of depressive disorders than in the population at large, indicating a genetic component to the etiology. Depression can vary in intensity and often is recurrent. The average age of onset of is in the mid-30s, although this has been decreasing. The earlier and more frequent the onset of symptoms, the more likely it is that the affected individual will require medications for symptom relief. Depression in older adults often appears with an element of confusion and often is left untreated. A first episode of depression that occurs after 65 years of age can be a precursor to dementia and should precipitate both assessment and treatment of the depression, as well as a thorough evaluation for dementia. Early intervention often greatly retards the progression of dementia, maintaining the individual's independence and quality of life. Mood disorders are thought to occur with equal prevalence among races, although it is more frequently misdiagnosed as schizophrenia among nonwhite populations.[29] Depression rates are also higher among individuals living in or near poverty.

MOOD DISORDERS

- Mood disorders, which include a range of depressive disorders and bipolar and related disorders, represent a disturbance in emotion rather than thought.
- Major depression is characterized by feelings of worthlessness and guilt, decreased concentration, alterations in sleep and appetite, and possible suicidal ideation.
- Bipolar disorders are characterized by periods of mania, during which there is a decreased need for food and sleep, racing thoughts, irritability, and high distractibility. These episodes may be followed by hypomanic or even major depressive episodes.

As with schizophrenia, genetic factors appear to play an important role in the development of mood disorders. Several studies have identified genetic loci that might contribute to the vulnerability to depression in families and individuals. However, the expression of affective disorders is not 100% in vulnerable families, and additional factors, such as environment, life history, development, and biologic challenges, and epigenetic changes likely interact to cause mood disorders.[6]

Depression can vary in intensity and often is recurrent. The earlier and more frequent the onset of symptoms, the more likely it is that the affected individual will require medications for symptom relief. Depression in the elderly often appears with an element of confusion and often is left untreated. A first episode of depression that occurs after 65 years of age can be a precursor to dementia and should precipitate both assessment and treatment of the depression, as well as a thorough evaluation for dementia. Early intervention often greatly retards the progression of dementia, maintaining the individual's independence and quality of life.

Major Depressive Disorder

A *major depressive disorder (MDD)* may first appear at any age and is characterized by the either a depressed mood or a loss of interest or pleasure. Features may include anhedonia (inability to experience pleasure), feelings of worthlessness or excessive guilt, decreased concentration, psychomotor agitation or retardation, insomnia or hypersomnia, decreased libido, change in weight or appetite, and thoughts of death or suicidal ideation.

The *DSM-5* diagnostic criteria for a major depressive episode include the simultaneous presence of five or more of the aforementioned symptoms during a 2-week period, and these must represent a change from previous functioning.[2] Depression must be differentiated from grief reactions, medication side effects, and sequelae of medical illnesses. It should be noted, however, that depression often coexists with physical illnesses, notably myocardial infarction. It is estimated that 50% of hospitalized patients with coronary artery disease have some depressive symptoms, with up to 20% developing major depression.[30] Depression impairs prognosis, affecting both behavioural and physiologic aspects of recovery, and increases the risk of death.[30]

MDD may also have various subclassifications distinguished by symptom patterns. Depression with *melancholic features* is characterized by depression that is worse in the morning, insomnia with early morning awakening, anorexia with significant weight loss, psychomotor retardation or agitation, excessive or inappropriate guilt, loss of interest in activity, inability to respond to pleasurable stimuli, and a complete loss of capacity for joy. The symptoms of *atypical* depression are opposite those of melancholic depression; it is characterized by a depression that becomes worse as the day progresses, overeating, and hypersomnia (excessive sleep). Depression with *psychotic features* involves the presence of delusions or hallucinations that may or may not be mood congruent. The classification of depression with *catatonic features* is applied when symptoms include excessive mobility or motoric immobility, extreme negativism, repetitive speech, and peculiar voluntary movements. The *chronic* specifier is applied if symptoms of major depression persist for 2 or more years.

A *postpartum* specifier is included if the onset is within 6 weeks of childbirth. Many women experience some mild letdown of mood in the postpartum period. For some, the symptoms are more severe and similar to those seen in serious depression, with increased emphasis related to the infant (obsessive thoughts about harming it or an inability to care for it). When psychotic symptoms occur, there is frequently associated sleep deprivation, volatility of behaviour, and manic-like symptoms. Biologic vulnerability with hormonal changes and psychological stressors all play a role.[2]

Persistent Depressive Disorder (Dysthymia)

Dysthymia is characterized by the same symptoms as major depression, but in a milder form.[2] These include low self-esteem, sleep and energy problems, and appetite disturbances. The insidious and chronic nature of this disorder often makes it difficult for the person dealing with this illness to separate it from the usual manner of functioning and to recognize the symptoms as part of an illness. Persons with dysthymia are at risk for development of major depression and other psychiatric disorders, including substance abuse disorders.[6,23]

Disruptive Mood Dysregulation Disorder

Disruptive Mood Dysregulation Disorder (DMDD) is associated with chronic, severe persistent irritability and is common among children presenting to mental health clinics. Symptoms begin before the age of 10, but children are not diagnosed with this before the age of 6 or after the age of 18 year of age. This type of mood disorder goes far beyond temper tantrums, and these outbursts are severe, recurrent, and grossly out of proportion in intensity or duration to the situation. These usually occur three or more time per week and persist over a year. Also for children with DMDD, the child's mood is persistently negative between these frequent, severe explosions of temper.[2]

Premenstrual Dysphoric Disorder

Prior to menses, a woman with *premenstrual dysphoric disorder (PMDD)* experiences severe symptoms of depression and anxiety, causing disruption to her functioning ability. It is estimated between 2% to 8% of menstruating women may experience this disorder. Symptoms usually begin 7 to 10 days prior to menses (late luteal phase) and subside shortly after menstruation begins. PMDD is not the same as premenstrual syndrome (PMS); rather PMDD is a debilitating condition causing extreme mood shifts.[2]

Other Depressive Disorders

Within the *DSM-5* there are other causes for depressive symptoms. *Substance/medication-induced depressive disorder* occurs when a substance or medication (*e.g.*, cocaine, alcohol, dexamethasone) causes depression. This is associated with depressive symptoms that develop during or soon after exposure to the substance and persist past the expected length of the substance's effect. *Depressive disorder due to another medical condition* may be evident when depression is directly related to physiological effects of another medical condition. These might include: neuroanatomical conditions (*e.g.,* traumatic brain injury, Huntington disease, Parkinson disease); neuroendocrine conditions (*e.g.,* Cushing disease, hypothyroidism), and other causal conditions (*e.g.,* multiple sclerosis). There are other specified and unspecified categories for any other presentations that do not meet the full criteria of other depressive disorders yet still cause clinically significant impairment.[2]

Bipolar and Related Disorders

In the *DSM-5* the bipolar disorder category includes an emphasis on changes in activity and energy as well as mood, while separating it from the category of MDD. Bipolar disorder is diagnosed on the basis of the pattern of occurrence of manic, hypomanic, and depressed episodes over time that are not due to medications or other therapies. The frequency, duration, and severity of the manic or depressive periods are unique to each individual. Mania, particularly in its severe delusional forms, also needs to be differentiated from schizophrenia or drug-induced states.

The bipolar disorder category also has multiple sub-classifications, all of which are characterized by episodes of elation and irritability (mania) with or without episodes of depression.[2,31] The spectrum of bipolar disorders include bipolar I disorder (at least one manic episode), bipolar II disorder (hypomania with major depression), cyclothymic disorder (periods of hypomanic symptoms and depressive symptoms), substance/medication-induced bipolar and related disorder (elevated, expansive mood occurs with exposure to a substance and persists), plus other specific and unspecified conditions not meeting the previous criteria. Although mania without associated depression (previously called unipolar mania) can occur, it is rare. Mania, in persons with bipolar disorder, can be precipitated by antidepressant medications and the somatic therapies used to treat depression, such as electroconvulsive therapy (ECT).

The manifestations of mania include decreased need for food and sleep, labile mood, irritability, racing thoughts, high distractibility, rapid and pressured speech, inflated self-esteem, and excessive involvement with pleasurable activities, some of which may be high risk. In its minor forms, the subjective experience of mania can be quite pleasurable to the individual, with a heightened sense of well-being and increased alertness. The severity of manic symptoms runs the gamut from a condition called *cyclothymia,* in which mood fluctuates between mild elation and depression, to severe delusional mania. Mania may begin abruptly within hours or days, or develop over a few weeks. Bipolar episodes, left untreated, become more severe with age. Rapid cycling is said to occur when an individual has four or more shifts in mood from normal within a 1-year period. Women are more likely than men to be rapid cyclers.[23]

Kindling is a hypothesized phenomenon in which a stressor creates an electrophysiologic vulnerability to future stressful events by causing long-lasting changes in neuronal function. This may be the basis for the phenomenon of rapid cycling in bipolar depression. The more frequently a person has a shift in mood, cycling into either mania or depression, the easier it becomes to have another episode. There now is evidence that many psychiatric disorders, not just bipolar disorder, are subject to this phenomenon. The better the control of the illness and the fewer cycles an individual has, the better his or her quality of life is likely to be.[23]

Neurophysiology of Symptoms

In some cases of familial MDD and bipolar disorder, PET and MRI studies have demonstrated a reduction in the volume of grey matter in the prefrontal cortex, with an associated decrease in activity in the region. Structural imaging studies have consistently found abnormalities in the subgenual prefrontal cortex in patients with familial bipolar disorder, a region related to responses to emotional experiences.[32] Clinical studies have suggested that this area of the brain is important for mood states and has extensive connections with the limbic system. Physiologically, there is evidence of decreased functioning in the frontal and temporal lobes, although it is not known if this is a cause or an effect of depression because the activity returns to normal with the resolution of the symptoms[15,32] (Fig. 53.6). The amygdala tends to have increased blood flow and oxygen consumption during depression. Unlike

FIGURE 53.6 • Acute effects of antidepressant medications in patients with affective disorder showing widespread effects on the cortex that vary dramatically with the medication used. Positron emission tomography (PET) is useful in revealing specific patterns of metabolic change in the brain and in providing clues to the mechanisms of antidepressant response. (Courtesy of Monte S. Buchsbaum, MD. The Mount Sinai Medical Center and School of Medicine, New York.)

those areas where function returns to normal with the resolution of depression, the amygdala continues to be excessively active for 12 to 24 months after the resolution of depression. It is hypothesized that relapse into depression is more likely to occur if medications are decreased or stopped before the amygdala returns to normal functioning. Other studies suggest abnormal neurodevelopment of the amygdala.[32] Neurologic disorders of the limbic system and basal ganglia are also involved in the development of mood disorders.[27]

A number of neurotransmitters, serotonin and norepinephrine in particular, are implicated in depression.[15,23] The biogenic amine hypothesis suggests that decreased levels of these neurotransmitters in the synaptic cleft, due either to decreased presynaptic release or decreased postsynaptic sensitivity, is the underlying pathologic process in depression. The hypothesis is derived from the fact that drugs that deplete brain serotonin and norepinephrine cause depression, and drugs that increase brain levels of norepinephrine and serotonin decrease depression. Dopamine activity has also been implicated in mood disorders, with decreased dopamine activity found in depression, and increased dopamine activity in mania.[15,33] It has become increasingly clear, however, that a simple decrease in the concentration of amines in neuronal synapses cannot entirely explain the complexities of depression. Neuromodulatory systems in the brain interact with each other in complex ways. For example, cholinergic and GABA-ergic pathways also may play a role in the development of depression because both of these pathways influence the activity of brain norepinephrine neurons.[32,33]

Disturbances in the function of the hypothalamic–pituitary–adrenal (HPA) axis also may play a critical role in depression. In the general population, cortisol levels usually are flat from late in the afternoon until a few hours before dawn, when they begin to rise. In persons with depression, cortisol levels spike erratically over the 24 hours of the day. Cortisol levels return to the normal pattern as depression resolves. In 40% of those diagnosed with depression, hypersecretion of cortisol is resistant to feedback inhibition by dexamethasone, indicating a dysfunction of the HPA axis.[15,33] About 5% to 10% of persons with depression have a decrease in thyroid function, in which case the person is less likely to have a vigorous response to medical intervention.

Alteration in the sleep–wake cycle is common in many mental illnesses and often is one of the prodromal signs of relapse. Researchers have found that the normal sleep cycle is reversed in depression. Persons with depression often have what is called *dream pressure sleep*. The depressed individual falls into light and dream-state sleep early in the sleep cycle and reaches deep stage 4 sleep only late in the sleep cycle. This finding helps explain why many inpatients report they did not sleep all night and the staff reports that the patient was asleep all night. Although the sleep cycle usually reverts to normal after the resolution of the depression, it may not be completely normal for weeks to months. Decreasing or halting medications before the sleep disturbances resolve may lead to a relapse of depressive symptoms. Fatigue and hypersomnia

are common among individuals with depressive disorder, and individuals who complain of chronic fatigue are at risk for development of MDD.[34]

Circadian rhythms also are an area of serious research interest. A specific type of depression known as *seasonal affective disorder* (SAD) is triggered for some persons in the winter by the shortening of daylight hours as fall commences, with symptoms of depression usually resolving in the spring when daylight hours again lengthen. Circadian rhythm considerations are also critical in symptom management for persons with bipolar depression. One of the fastest ways to precipitate a manic episode is for the individual to stay up all night. It is not unusual for a first manic episode to occur when someone "pulls an all-nighter" studying for final examinations. Persons with bipolar disorder should have a fairly rigid schedule for sleeping and awakening if cycling is to be minimized. Although exercise is important, the person with bipolar disorder should exercise before mid-afternoon to prevent the normal increase in metabolic rate from disrupting the sleep cycle.

Treatment

Effective treatments exist for the range of depressive and bipolar disorders, including antidepressant drugs, ECT, phototherapy, lithium, anticonvulsants, and psychotherapy.[6,18] The antidepressants most often used are SSRIs, which inhibit the reuptake of serotonin; MAO inhibitors, which block the degradation of norepinephrine and serotonin; TCAs, which block the reuptake of norepinephrine and serotonin; and novel or dual action antidepressants.[18] ECT, a procedure that electrically stimulates a generalized seizure, is a highly effective treatment for depression, with 70% to 90% of clients showing a good response.[35] Because the motor component of the seizure does not contribute to the therapeutic effects of the treatment, modern ECT is always given under general anesthesia with complete muscle relaxation. On an average, six to eight treatments are given at 2-day intervals over a period of 2 to 4 weeks.

Phototherapy, or light therapy, uses artificial light to influence the production of melatonin and the function of the catecholamine systems. It is often a first-line treatment for depression associated with seasonal changes, such as SAD.[36]

Lithium and several anticonvulsant agents are used in the treatment of bipolar depression. Lithium's exact mechanism of action is unknown. It is known to inhibit the accumulation of cyclic adenosine monophosphate (cAMP), and may down-regulate second-messenger systems that are associated with cAMP-linked receptors.[37] Anticonvulsant agents, especially carbamazepine and valproate, have also proved to be effective agents for treatment of bipolar depression. However, the mechanism by which these drugs act is not completely understood. One theory for the mechanism of action proposes blocked effects of the excitatory amino acid glutamate.[37]

Newer therapies, such as vagal nerve stimulation and transcranial magnetic stimulation, are being considered as treatment for depression that does not respond to pharmacologic interventions. The effectiveness of these treatments is still unclear.[38]

Psychotherapy is an important component of therapy for persons and families with MDDs. Individuals and families can learn how to deal with stressful life events and heal disrupted interpersonal relationships. Unfortunately, many people with bipolar disorder do not believe they need treatment, particularly during the manic phase of the illness, and tend to self-medicate with alcohol or recreational drugs. It is not unusual for people with bipolar depression to be diagnosed with substance abuse. When in the manic phase, they often feel exceptionally creative and talented. When helping people make the decision to enter treatment, it is important that they understand the treatment will not stop their creativity.

IN SUMMARY

Mood disorders are disorders of emotion rather than disturbances of thought. Mood disorders include major depressive disorder (characterized by a persistent unpleasant mood), dysthymia (characterized by chronic mild depressive symptoms), and bipolar disorder (characterized by alternating periods of depression and mania). Depression is characterized by an inability to experience pleasure, feelings of worthlessness and excessive guilt, alterations in sleeping patterns and appetite, and thoughts of death or suicidal ideation. Mania is characterized by elation, irritability, high distractibility, and, often, engagement in high-risk pleasurable activities. As with schizophrenia, genetic factors appear to play an important role in the development of mood disorders. Neuroimaging techniques have revealed several anatomic and functional abnormalities in different regions of the brain. Abnormalities in neurotransmission also have been implicated in the development and maintenance of depression, including changes in concentration and activity of the neurotransmitters norepinephrine, serotonin, acetylcholine, and GABA. Treatment of depressive disorders includes the use of antidepressant medications, ECT, phototherapy, and psychotherapy. Bipolar disorders are usually treated with lithium or an anticonvulsant agent that has been shown to be effective in treating the disorder.

ANXIETY DISORDERS

After completing this section of the chapter, you should be able to meet the following objectives:

- Define the terms panic disorder, generalized anxiety disorder, social phobia, and obsessive-compulsive disorder.
- Describe the manifestations of panic disorder, generalized anxiety disorder, social phobia, and obsessive-compulsive disorder and the underlying neuropathophysiology of each.

- Cite the diagnostic criteria for panic disorder, generalized anxiety disorder, social phobia, and obsessive-compulsive disorder according to the *DSM-5* classification.
- Describe the treatment for panic disorder, generalized anxiety disorder, social phobia, and obsessive-compulsive disorder.

Anxiety disorders are characterized by intense fearfulness that occurs without a precipitating potentially dangerous event, accompanied by subjective as well as objective manifestations. Just as grief is a normal response to personal loss, anxiety is a normal response to threatening situations. Anxiety disorders are the most prevalent of the psychiatric disorders. Anxiety disorders affect approximately 10% to 12% of Canadians, women more often than men.[28] Anxiety disorders have a higher rate of occurrence among family members, but there is not yet any clearly delineated genetic link.

A key component of anxiety disorders is increased fear accompanied by subjective as well as objective manifestations. The subjective manifestations range from heightened awareness to deep fear of impending disaster or death. The objective manifestations, which occur with activation of the sympathetic cascade through the HPA axis, include restlessness, sweating, palpitations, an increase in heart rate and blood pressure, dry mouth, and a desire to run and escape. According to the new *DSM-5* classification system, anxiety has been restructured into three distinct groups: (1) anxiety; (2) obsessive-compulsive and other related disorders; and (3) trauma- and stressor-related disorders. The anxiety component is subdivided into various types, depending on clinical characteristics and response to pharmacologic agents, such as panic disorder, generalized anxiety disorder, and social phobia. The new *DSM-5* separates obsessive-compulsive disorder (OCD) into its own diagnostic category, but it will be discussed here. The *DSM-5* also places posttraumatic stress disorder (PTSD) in a separate diagnostic category

ANXIETY DISORDERS

- Anxiety disorders constitute a group of disorders that are characterized by intense episodes of fearfulness with symptoms related to activation of the sympathetic nervous system through the hypothalamic–pituitary–adrenal axis.
- Panic disorder is characterized by an experience of intense fear with neurologic, cardiac, respiratory, and psychological symptoms.
- Generalized anxiety disorder is characterized by excessive, uncontrollable worry.
- Social phobia is an intense fear reaction to social interaction.
- Obsessive-compulsive disorder is characterized by repetitive thoughts and actions.

of trauma- and stressor-related disorders; PTSD is discussed in Chapter 9. However, the sequential order of these sections in *DSM-5* reflects the close relationships among these topics.[2]

Panic Disorder

Panic disorder is a disabling condition commonly seen in patients in the primary care setting.[15,39] The disorder has been reported to occur in 3% to 8% of persons seen by primary care physicians and may effect up to 2 million Canadians.[28] The disorder is twice as common in women as men, and there appears to be a bimodal distribution in age of onset, with one peak in late adolescence and a second peak in the mid-thirties.[39] The diagnosis of panic disorder may be made more difficult by the presence of symptoms such as chest pain and shortness of breath that also are associated with potentially more serious conditions.

Persons with panic disorder typically have attacks characterized by neurologic symptoms (dizziness or lightheadedness, paresthesias, fainting), cardiac symptoms (tachycardia, chest pain, palpitations), respiratory symptoms (shortness of breath, feeling of smothering or choking), sweating, nausea or abdominal distress, and psychological symptoms (feelings of impending doom, fear of dying, and a sense of unreality). Panic attacks, which are unexpected and not related to external events, usually last 15 to 30 minutes, but sometimes continue for an hour. Depression may coexist in 40% to 80% of persons with panic disorder, and substance abuse disorders are not uncommon.[27]

Both biologic and environmental factors appear to be involved in the causation of panic attacks.[15] Monozygotic twins have a significantly higher concordance of the disorder than dizygotic twins. First-degree relatives of persons with panic disorder have a 3- to 21-fold higher risk of developing panic disorder than unrelated persons. Approximately 80% of persons with panic disorder report major life stressors during the previous 12 months. Persons with a history of sexual or physical abuse have a higher risk for panic disorder than those without such history.[15]

Neurophysiologic studies suggest that the attacks may result from an abnormally sensitive "fear network" that is centred in the amygdala and involves interactions with the hippocampus and prefrontal cortex.[27] Projections from the amygdala to hypothalamic and brain stem sites account for many of the observed signs (*e.g.*, sweating, increased heart rate, respiratory responses) of the fear response. Responses to medications indicate that multiple mechanisms and neurotransmitters are involved in initiating the panic attack. Norepinephrine, serotonin, and GABA are the three neurotransmitters most associated with this disorder.[27] Persons experiencing panic attacks have been found to have somewhat lower levels of serotonin than do persons with no known mental illness, but the mechanism for that decrease is not known.

Treatment includes the use of behavioural, psychological, and drug therapies. All antidepressants, except bupropion, are effective in the treatment of panic disorders. There is

growing evidence in the greater effectiveness of SSRIs in the treatment of panic, but full response to medication can take 12 or more weeks.[15,18] Many individuals may require the use of more than one class of medication for the management of panic attacks. However, treatment is most effective when psychotherapy focused on cognitive and behavioural changes is included as part of a comprehensive program. If inadequately treated, persons with panic disorder frequently develop phobias, particularly agoraphobia, which can be so debilitating that the person cannot leave his or her home.

Generalized Anxiety Disorder

In 1980, generalized anxiety disorder was first recognized as a separate entity from panic disorder in the *DSM-III*. Since then, the diagnostic criteria have been sharpened in an attempt to improve the ability of practitioners to discriminate the disorder. The central characteristic of generalized anxiety disorder is prolonged (>6 months), excessive worry that is not easily controlled by the person and causes significant distress or impairment. The characteristics of the disorder include muscle tension, autonomic hyperactivity, sleep disturbances, and vigilance and scanning (exaggerated startle response, inability to concentrate).[2]

While a definitive pathophysiologic mechanism has not yet been determined, neurotransmitter dysregulation is thought to underlie all anxiety disorders. Disruptions of the neurotransmitter GABA system and its receptors are associated with symptoms of anxiety, particularly as many persons respond to treatment with benzodiazepines.[40] The benzodiazepine medications (*e.g.*, chlordiazepoxide, diazepam) are particularly effective drugs in treating anxiety as these drugs increase the activity of the $GABA_A$ receptor, which increases the flow of chloride ions across the cell membrane, hyperpolarizing the membrane and thus inhibiting firing of target cells.[27] Other considerations include the serotonergic and noradrenergic neurotransmitter systems with underactivation of the serotonergic and overactivation of the noradrenergic systems leading to anxiety presentations. The glutamatergic hypothesis suggests that an elevated level of excitatory glutamate signalling contributes to panicogenicity particularly in the amygdala area that processes emotional responses to stressful conditions.[41]

Buspirone is another effective medication for treating generalized anxiety disorder, but may take up to 2 weeks to show antianxiety effects, and up to 6 weeks for maximum benefits. SSRIs are also used in the treatment of generalized anxiety disorder, and it is thought that they result in limbic, paralimbic, and frontal hyperactivity normalization. Other medications used in the treatment of generalized anxiety disorder include other antidepressants (tricyclic and atypical antidepressants) and β-adrenergic blockers, the latter of which block the symptoms of anxiety rather than treating the anxiety disorder itself.

Social Phobia

Social phobia, also called *social anxiety disorder*, is a generalized or specific, intense, irrational, and persistent fear of being scrutinized or negatively evaluated by others. Diagnostic criteria include the development of symptoms of anxiety when the person is exposed to the feared social situation, recognition by the person that the fear is irrational, avoidance by the person of the social situation, and interference of the anxiety or avoidance behaviour with the person's normal routine. The fear must not be related to any physiologic effects of a substance and must be present for at least 6 months.[2]

Social phobia is a fairly common disorder with a lifetime prevalence of 12% and a slight tendency to occur more often in women than in men.[42] Typically, the onset occurs between 11 and 19 years of age. The major adverse effects of social phobia are felt in employment and school, causing a loss of earning power and socioeconomic status. In addition, approximately one half of persons with social phobia also have a drug or alcohol problem. Several drugs have proved efficacious for the treatment of social phobia, including SSRIs, benzodiazepines, and MAO inhibitors. β-Adrenergic blockers are useful in specific social performance situations. Social phobia also has been particularly responsive to behavioural and cognitive therapies.

Obsessive-Compulsive and Related Disorders

In the *DSM-5* the OSDs have been renamed and includes additional related disorders including body dysmorphic disorder, hoarding disorder, trichotillomania (hair-pulling disorder), excoriation (skin-picking) disorder, substance/medication-induced obsessive-compulsive and related disorder, and obsessive-compulsive and related disorder due to another medical condition. As a stress disorder, OCD is characterized by recurrent *obsessions* (repeated thoughts) and *compulsions* (repeated acts).[2,43]

To be defined as compulsive, the behaviour (activities such as handwashing, ordering, or checking, or mental activities such as praying, counting, or repeating words) must be repeated excessively and the repetition must not be related to any environmental condition. These behaviours are time consuming or distressing to the individual. Usually, the person experiencing the symptoms recognizes that the rituals are unreasonable. For instance, the person may have to recheck the stove many times before she is able to leave for work or may have to check the stairwells at work repeatedly for debris to ensure that no one is injured. Between 2% and 3% of the world's population has OCD, and OCD is the 10th most disabling disease worldwide.[43] This disorder is found with equal frequency among men and women, and there is a higher prevalence among family members. The average age of onset is approximately 20 years, although the disorder also may occur in children and, if undiagnosed, may appear as behaviour problems and angry outbursts that can seem impulsive and may be confused with attention deficit or hyperactivity disorders.[44]

Although the neurophysiology of OCD remains under investigation, the general anatomic model suggests dysfunction of the prefrontal cortex and structures of the basal ganglia, particularly the caudate nucleus and globus pallidus.[41] Studies have also suggested increased activity in the thalamus and the putamen of the basal ganglia, as well as a decrease in serotonin activity. Several other neurologic syndromes that involve the basal ganglia, such as tic disorders, Sydenham chorea, postencephalitic Parkinson disease, and Huntington disease, often are associated with a component of OCD.[45]

Diagnosis of OCD is based on the history and clinical observation. Treatment methods for OCD include behavioural therapy (involving exposure to feared situations and the prevention of compulsive behaviour), cognitive therapy (in which maladaptive thoughts are challenged), and specific medications. About 50% to 60% of persons with OCD respond to SSRIs, but often require a higher dose than that prescribed for treatment of depression. The TCA clomipramine is sometimes prescribed if there is a poor response to SSRIs, and an atypical antipsychotic may be added in severe cases. This disorder is particularly amenable to cognitive-behavioural therapy, and for most persons with OCD, combining cognitive-behavioural therapy with medication is the best approach.[43]

IN SUMMARY

Anxiety disorders include panic disorder, generalized anxiety disorder, and social phobia. A common characteristic of the disorders is an intense fear that occurs in the absence of a precipitating dangerous event. The symptoms of anxiety disorders suggest an inappropriate and intense activation of the sympathetic nervous system. Panic disorder is characterized by neurologic, cardiac, respiratory, and psychological symptoms. The central characteristic of generalized anxiety disorder is excessive worry not easily controlled by the person and lasting more than 6 months. Social phobia is a generalized or specific, intense, irrational, and persistent fear of being scrutinized or negatively evaluated by others. OCD (now a separate category) is characterized by recurrent obsessions (repeated thoughts) and compulsions (repeated acts).

SUBSTANCE-RELATED AND ADDICTIVE DISORDERS

After completing this section of the chapter, you should be able to meet the following objectives:

- Define substance dependence.
- Describe the epidemiology of addiction disorders.
- Describe the neurophysiologic alterations associated with substance dependence.
- Cite the actions of medications used in the treatment of substance dependence.

The *DSM-5* uses the term *substance use disorders* to include substance abuse and substance dependence.[2] *Substance abuse* refers to repeated use of alcohol or other drugs, resulting in functional problems.[46] *Dependence* refers to the behaviours exhibited when an individual is unable to control the use of drugs or alcohol and continues to use them in spite of negative consequences. In the *DSM-5* these two descriptors are combined and accompanied by criteria for 10 separate classes of drug intoxication, withdrawal, and unspecified substance-induced disorders, where relevant.[2] *Addiction* is a difficult term to define; there is no clear consensus on a definition, nor is it defined in the *DSM-5*. Addiction usually describes a combination of craving, compulsive use, and high risk of relapse after withdrawal. The *DSM-5* has expanded criteria to include cannabis and caffeine withdrawal as well as alcohol, hallucinogens, inhalants, tobacco, opioids, sedatives, stimulants, and others. Within this section gambling is now included as a behavioural addiction.

Problems related to alcohol and drug abuse exact a large toll on individuals and families, including financial, social, and physical. In 2012, it was estimated that 21.6% (approximately 6 million) of Canadians met the criteria for a substance use disorder during their lifetime. Approximately 3.2% of Canadians were dependent on alcohol, 1.3% were dependent on cannabis, and 0.7% were dependent on illicit drugs.[47] Although substance abuse is not a new problem—people have been abusing drugs and alcohol for thousands of years—our understanding of abuse and addiction as diseases is more recent. Although early understandings of these disorders attributed them to poor character and moral weakness, current and ongoing research has pointed to a neurophysiologic basis to addiction disorders, leading to a better understanding of the ongoing risk of relapse, even after a lengthy period of abstinence.

The vulnerability of certain individuals to substance abuse disorders and dependence appears to be multifactorial, involving a genetic disposition, environmental factors, and physiologic mechanisms resulting from repeated drug use. It has been suggested that self-medication of symptoms associated with psychiatric disorders provides another source for the initiation of drug abuse. Substance abuse disorders are more common among individuals with mood and anxiety disorders, and schizophrenia, all populations with altered levels of the neurotransmitter dopamine.[47,48] Epidemiologic data indicate that there is a high comorbidity between drug dependence and depression. Approximately 40% of those with alcohol abuse or dependence also meet the criteria for MDD, and people who abuse substances are 20 times more likely to commit suicide than the general population.[27] Research has also indicated that there is a high comorbidity between depression, posttraumatic stress, and cannabis use.[49]

Habitual use of drugs, including alcohol, is thought to induce adaptations in brain systems that alter the normal dopamine pathways and increase dopamine transmission. A neural pathway called the *mesolimbic dopamine system* is thought to gate signals that regulate biologic drives and motivation. These neurons send their axons to the nucleus accumbens, the striatum of the basal ganglia, and the frontal cortex. Drugs that facilitate dopamine transmission enhance the processes whereby otherwise neutral stimuli acquire incentive and reinforcing properties and facilitate drug-seeking behaviour.[50] Some drugs, such as cocaine and amphetamines, raise the level of dopamine in the nucleus accumbens by blocking the dopamine transporter, thereby prolonging the time that dopamine remains in the synaptic cleft. Although many drugs of abuse alter dopamine levels, not all of them act by way of the dopamine transporter. Nicotine, perhaps the most addictive of all drugs, enhances the release of dopamine by acting on presynaptic cholinergic receptors.

The rewarding effect of drug abuse results not only from the release of dopamine; as addiction develops, behaviour also is influenced by a glutamatergic pathway. Glutamine is the major excitatory transmitter in the brain and spinal cord. Animal studies focusing on stimuli for relapse have found that exposure to a cue associated with substance use (*i.e.,* stress, or a single dose of the substance) results in activation of glutamatergic projections from areas of the brain that stimulate dopamine release from the nucleus accumbens.[15,50] In addition, there is a reported increase in GABA (a neurotransmitter that activates inhibitory receptors) levels during alcohol intoxication and opiate use.[15,50] Opioid agonists appear to be rewarding because they inhibit GABA-ergic neurons that normally suppress dopaminergic neurons.

Treatment of addiction requires an understanding of physiologic alterations in brain function that can cause relapse, even after years of abstinence. Precipitants for relapse include stress, environmental cues, and exposure to the substance. Relapses are not uncommon and should not be considered as failures in treatment, but rather as a reflection of the nature of the illness. Because there is a high comorbidity between depression and drug dependence, professional treatment of pre-existing psychiatric problems may also decrease the use of illicit substances and help prevent relapse.[46,49]

Treatments are varied and include biologic, behavioural, and psychosocial interventions. Biologic interventions are used in the maintenance of recovery from alcohol and opiates, such as heroin. Methadone, used in opiate addictions, has the narcotic properties of addiction and sedation, but lacks the euphoric effects of heroin and other opiates. Buprenorphine is a recently approved analgesic for treatment of opioid addictions with less euphoric and sedative properties than methadone. Naltrexone is used in treatment of alcohol and opiate addictions, and works by blocking the opioid receptors and euphoric effects. It does not, however, eliminate cravings. These medications work best in conjunction with other therapies, such as self-help groups (Alcoholics Anonymous), individual therapy, family therapy, behavioural contracting, and social skills training.

IN SUMMARY

Substance abuse refers to repeated use of alcohol or other drugs, resulting in functional problems; dependence refers to the behaviours exhibited when an individual is unable to control the use of drugs or alcohol; and addiction to a combination of craving, compulsive use, and high risk of relapse after withdrawal. Substance abuse disorders are more common among individuals with mood and anxiety disorders or schizophrenia, all populations with altered levels of the neurotransmitter dopamine. The vulnerability of certain individuals to substance abuse disorders appears to be multifactorial, related to genetic disposition, environmental factors, and physiologic adaptations to repeated drug use. Habitual use of drugs, including alcohol, is thought to induce adaptations in brain systems that alter the normal dopamine pathways and increase dopamine transmission. Treatments are varied and include biologic, behavioural, and psychosocial interventions.

NEUROCOGNITIVE DISORDERS

After completing this section of the chapter, you should be able to meet the following objectives:

- State the criteria for a diagnosis of dementia.
- Compare the causes associated with Alzheimer disease, vascular dementia, frontotemporal dementia, Creutzfeldt–Jakob disease, Wernicke–Korsakoff syndrome, and Huntington disease.
- Describe the changes in brain tissue that occur with Alzheimer disease.
- Use the three stages of Alzheimer disease to describe its progress.
- Cite the difference between Wernicke disease and the Korsakoff component of the Wernicke–Korsakoff syndrome.

In the shift to the *DSM-5* this category was redefined from delirium, dementia, and amnestic and other cognitive disorders to the current neurocognitive disorders. Primarily, this shift covers delirium, dementia, and the subtypes of dementia, and also includes personality disorders. While the criteria for the disorders have not changed from the DSM-IV-TR, there is an effort to provide an alternative approach to the diagnosis of personality disorders.[2,51]

Cognition refers to all the processes by which the sensory input is transformed, reduced, elaborated, stored, recovered, and used. It involves the perception of sensory input and the ability to learn and manipulate new information, recognize familiar objects and recollect past experiences, solve problems, think abstractly, and make judgments. Dementia is a syndrome of deterioration in cognitive function severe enough to interfere with occupational or social performance.[52,53] It is a common and disabling disorder in older adults and is becoming a growing public health problem because of rapidly increasing numbers of older adults in the developed countries of the world.

Normal Cognitive Aging

Memory shows a slow, progressive impairment over the life span, and it is important to differentiate what can be termed "normal cognitive aging" from disorders of memory and cognition. Many older adults remain intellectually intact, and some make outstanding contributions later in life.

Short-term memory typically is well preserved during normal cognitive aging unless there is a high demand placed on processing resources.[53] However, older adults may have greater difficulty than younger people in manipulating the information that is held in short-term memory. With regard to long-term memory, age-related impairments in free recall of stories and word lists are evident by age 50 years. However, when structure is provided by the use of recognition cues, the age differences diminish, which suggests greater impairment of retrieval processes than of encoding and retrieval.[53]

Memory problems associated with normal aging tend to reflect a generalized decrease in the efficiency with which information is processed and retrieved. Memory of a past event can be based on retrieval that is accompanied by recollection of specific details or on the feeling that the event is old or new, based on its familiarity.[53] There is evidence that recollection is more dependent on the hippocampus, whereas familiarity is more dependent on the entorhinal cortex, and that healthy aging has greater effects on recollection than on familiarity.[53]

Evidence suggest that knowledge is first acquired through processing in one of the three polymodal association cortices (the prefrontal, limbic, and parieto–occipital–temporal cortices) that synthesize visual, auditory, and somatic sensory information[6] (Fig. 53.7). From there the information is conveyed to a series of parahippocampal and perirhinal cortices, then to the entorhinal cortex, dentate gyrus, hippocampus, and subiculum, and finally back to the entorhinal cortex. From the entorhinal cortex, the information is sent back to the parahippocampal cortices and finally back to the polymodal association areas of the neocortex.[6] Thus, in processing information for explicit memory storage, the entorhinal cortex has dual functions. It is the main input to the hippocampus and it is the major output to the hippocampus. With aging, there appears to be a reduced connectivity in the network that connects the hippocampus and association cortices but increased connectivity in the network that connects the entorhinal and association cortices.[53] This suggests that older adults may compensate for hippocampal deficits by relying more on the entorhinal cortex.

Originally, it was believed that the laying down and retrieval of memories was due primarily to action of a single neurotransmitter, acetylcholine. This led to the development of acetylcholinesterase inhibitors to treat cognitive impairment. The further recognition of the role of the glutamate *N*-methyl-D-aspartate receptor led to the development of memantine (discussed in the section on Alzheimer disease). More recently, it was recognized that several neuropeptides (*i.e.,* neuropeptide Y, orexin A, and the endogenous opioid peptides) also play an important role in memory.[53] Although

FIGURE 53.7 • **A:** Key structures of the medial temporal lobe important for memory storage. **B:** Input and output pathways for the hippocampal formation. (Adapted from Kandel E. R., Schwartz J. H., Jessel T. M. (2000). *Principles of neural science* (4th ed., p. 1232). New York: McGraw-Hill.)

these peptides have the potential for enhancing memory at low levels, they can inhibit memory at high levels. There is also emerging evidence that several gastrointestinal hormones may contribute to memory, as evidenced by the observation that tasks learned before a meal is ingested are recalled better at a later time.[53] This is thought to be related to the release of the gastrointestinal hormone cholecystokinin, which, through its stimulation of the vagus nerve, eventually leads to activation of neurons in the hippocampus.[13] Another hormone, ghrelin, which is produced in the fundus of the stomach, has receptors in the hippocampus and is also thought to enhance memory.

Dementia

Dementia or nonnormative cognitive decline can be caused by any disorder that permanently damages large association areas of the cerebral hemispheres or subcortical areas subserving memory and learning. Based on criteria in the *DSM-5*, for a major or minor neurocognitive disorder the essential feature of the cognitive decline is impairment of short- and long-term memory, which is associated with deficits in abstract thinking, impaired judgment and other higher cortical functions, or personality change. For a major neurocognitive disorder the disturbance should be sufficiently severe as to interfere significantly with work or social activities.[2] Common causes of dementia are Alzheimer disease, vascular dementia, frontotemporal dementia (FTD), Creutzfeldt–Jakob disease (CJD), Wernicke–Korsakoff syndrome, and Huntington chorea.

The diagnosis of dementia is based on assessment of the presenting problem; history about the person that is provided by an informant (someone who has known the person over time, usually a family member); complete physical and

neurologic examination; evaluation of cognitive, behavioural, and functional status; and laboratory and imaging studies. In 2012, the Fourth Canadian Consensus Conference on the Diagnosis and Treatment of Dementia recommended structural neuroimaging (which may include CT or MRI) only for individuals with specific clinical features and screening of all for depression, anemia, electrolyte imbalances, diabetes, vitamin B_{12} deficiency, folic acid deficiency, hypothyroidism, and routine urinalysis.[54,55] Depression is the most common treatable illness that may masquerade as dementia, and it must be excluded when a diagnosis of dementia is considered (see Chapter 3). This is important because cognitive functioning usually returns to baseline levels after depression is treated. Screening evaluations for subdural hematoma, cerebral infarcts, cerebral tumours, and normal-pressure hydrocephalus (discussed in Chapter 51) are also recommended. These and other reversible forms of dementia that should be ruled out can be remembered by the mnemonic DEMENTIA: *D*rugs (drugs with anticholinergic activity), *E*motional (depression), *M*etabolic (hypothyroidism), *E*yes and ears (declining vision and hearing), *N*ormal-pressure hydrocephalus, *T*umour or other space-occupying lesions, *I*nfection (human immunodeficiency virus infection or syphilis), *A*nemia (vitamin B_{12} or folate deficiency).[53]

Alzheimer Disease

Dementia of the Alzheimer type occurs in middle or late life and accounts for 64% of all cases of dementia. The disorder affects more than 500,000 Canadians and is expected to increase to 1.1 million cases by the year 2038 unless a cure or prevention is developed.[55] The risk for development of Alzheimer disease increases with age, and it is estimated

Normal brains   Alzheimer's brains

A

B

FIGURE 53.8 • Gross examination (**A**) and coronal slices (**B**) show the extensive shrinkage of the brain from Alzheimer disease. (From Higgins E. S., George M. S. (2013). *Neuroscience of clinical psychiatry: The pathophysiology of behavior and mental illness* (2nd ed., p. 289). Philadelphia, PA: Lippincott Williams & Wilkins.)

that almost 50% of individuals 85 years of age and older live with this illness, which affects almost twice as many women as men.[56]

Pathophysiology. The pathophysiologic aspects of Alzheimer disease involve neuropathologic and neurotransmitter changes. Alzheimer disease is characterized by cortical atrophy and loss of neurons, particularly in the parietal and temporal lobes.[44,57,58] With significant atrophy, there is ventricular enlargement (*i.e.,* hydrocephalus) from the loss of brain tissue (Fig. 53.8).

The major microscopic features of Alzheimer disease are the presence of neuritic (senile) plaques, neurofibrillary tangles, and amyloid angiopathy.[57,58] The *neuritic plaques* are patches or flat areas composed of clusters of degenerating nerve terminals arranged around a central amyloid core.[44] The dominant component of the amyloid core is amyloid beta ($A\beta$), a peptide derived from the proteolysis of a larger membrane-spanning amyloid precursor protein (APP). There is increasing evidence that $A\beta$ is the critical molecule in the pathogenesis of Alzheimer disease. Full-length APP has an intracellular region, a membrane-spanning sequence, and an extracellular region. The normal degradation of APP involves cleavage in the middle of the $A\beta$ domain by a proteolytic α-secretase enzyme, with the release of two soluble nonamyloidogenic pieces. However, APP can also be cleaved at either end of the $A\beta$ domain, leading to the release of intact and highly amyloidogenic $A\beta$ that accumulates in senile plaques as amyloid fibrils. There are at least three distinct forms of secretase enzymes: α-, β-, and γ-secretase. Evidence suggests that cleavage by the β- and γ-secretase leads to the generation of $A\beta$.[44]

The *neurofibrillary tangles,* found in the cytoplasm of abnormal neurons, consist of fibrous proteins that are wound around each other in a helical fashion. These tangles are resistant to chemical or enzymatic breakdown, and they persist in brain tissue long after the neuron in which they arose has died and disappeared. A major component of the paired helical filaments is an abnormally hyperphosphorylated form of the protein *tau,* an axonal microtubule-associated protein that enhances microtubule assembly.[44,57,58]

Some plaques and tangles can be found in the brains of older persons who do not show cognitive impairment. The number and distribution of the plaques and tangles appear to contribute to the intellectual deterioration that occurs with Alzheimer disease. In persons with Alzheimer disease, the plaques and tangles and associated neuronal loss and glial reaction are evident earliest in the entorhinal cortex, then spread through the hippocampal formation and isocortex, and then extend to the neocortex.[44] Neurochemically, Alzheimer disease has been associated with a decrease in the level of choline acetyltransferase activity in the cortex and hippocampus. This enzyme is required for the synthesis of acetylcholine, a neurotransmitter that is associated with memory. The reduction in choline acetyltransferase is quantitatively related to the numbers of neuritic plaques and the severity of dementia.

It is likely that Alzheimer disease is caused by several factors that interact differently in different persons. Progress on the genetics of inherited early-onset Alzheimer disease shows mutations in at least three genes—the *APP* gene on chromosome 21; presenilin-1 (*PS1*), a gene on chromosome 14; and presenilin-2 (*PS2*), a gene on chromosome 1—can cause Alzheimer disease in certain families.[52] The *APP* gene is associated with an autosomal dominant form of early-onset Alzheimer disease, and can be tested clinically. Persons with Down syndrome (trisomy 21) develop the pathologic changes of Alzheimer disease and a comparable decline in cognitive functioning at a relatively young age, usually in their 40s. Virtually all persons with Down syndrome exhibit the pathologic features of Alzheimer disease as they age. PS1 and PS2, both intracellular proteins, are components of γ-secretase and possibly part of a multiprotein complex containing the proteolytic site for breakdown of $A\beta$. A fourth gene, an allele (ϵ4) of the apolipoprotein E (ApoE) gene found on chromosome 19, increases the risk of Alzheimer disease and lowers the age of onset. ApoE can bind $A\beta$ and is present in plaques, but how this allele increases the risk of Alzheimer disease has not been established.[44]

Although age is the greatest risk, additional factors have been identified as adding to the risks for development of Alzheimer disease. These include head trauma, inflammatory factors, and oxidative stress. Education has been identified as a protective factor, with suggestions that education can increase synaptic density.[59] Other studies have looked at exercise as a possible protective factor in maintaining hippocampal health and increasing hippocampal size.[60]

Manifestations. Alzheimer-type dementia follows an insidious and progressive course, with an average survival of 8 to 10 years after diagnosis.[27] The hallmark symptoms are loss of short-term memory and denial of such memory loss, with eventual disorientation, impaired abstract thinking, apraxias, and changes in personality and affect. Three stages of the disease have been recognized, as identified by the Consensus statement and the Alzheimer Association. All are characterized by progressive degenerative changes.[61] The initial change is subtle, characterized by short-term memory loss that often is difficult to differentiate from the normal forgetfulness that occurs in the elderly, and usually is reported by caregivers and denied by the patient. Although most older adults have trouble retrieving from memory incidental information and proper names, persons with Alzheimer disease randomly forget important and unimportant details. They forget where things are placed, get lost easily, and have trouble remembering appointments and performing novel tasks. Mild changes in personality, such as lack of spontaneity, social withdrawal, and loss of a previous sense of humour, occur during this stage.

As the disease progresses, the person with Alzheimer disease enters the moderate stage. This stage may last several years and is marked by a more global impairment of cognitive functioning. During this stage, there are changes in higher cortical functioning needed for language, spatial relationships, and problem solving. Depression may occur in persons who are aware of their deficits. There is extreme confusion, disorientation, lack of insight, and inability to carry out the activities of daily living. Personal hygiene is neglected, and language becomes impaired because of difficulty in remembering and retrieving words. Behavioural changes can include agitation, sleep problems, restlessness and wandering, aggression, and suspiciousness. Some persons may become hostile and abusive toward family members. Persons who enter this stage become unable to live alone and should be assisted in making decisions about supervised placement with family members or friends or in a community-based facility.

Severe Alzheimer disease is the last stage of the disease. It is characterized by a loss of ability to respond to the environment. Individuals in this stage require total care, and spend most of their time bedridden. Death can occur as a result of complications related to chronic debilitation.

Diagnosis and Treatment. Alzheimer disease is essentially a diagnosis of exclusion. There are no peripheral biochemical markers or tests for the disease. The diagnosis can be confirmed only by microscopic examination of tissue obtained from a cerebral biopsy or at autopsy. The diagnosis is based on clinical findings.

The diagnostic procedures for Alzheimer disease involve numerous steps, and a differential diagnosis in Alzheimer Algorithm has been developed.[61] A diagnosis of Alzheimer disease requires the presence of dementia established by clinical examination and documented by results of a Mini-Mental State Examination, Blessed Dementia Test, or similar mental status test; no disturbance in consciousness; onset between 40 and 90 years of age, most often after 65 years of age; and absence of systemic or brain disorders that could account for the memory or cognitive deficits. Brain imaging, CT scan, or MRI is done to exclude other brain disease. Metabolic screening should be done for known reversible causes of dementia such as vitamin B_{12} deficiency, thyroid dysfunction, and electrolyte imbalance.

There is no curative treatment for Alzheimer dementia. Drugs are used primarily to slow the progression and to control depression, agitation, or sleep disorders. Two major goals of care are maintaining the person's socialization and providing support for the family. Self-help groups that provide support for family and friends have become available, with support from the Alzheimer Society of Canada. Day care and respite centres are available in many areas to provide relief for caregivers and appropriate stimulation for the patient.

Although there is no current drug therapy that is curative for Alzheimer disease, some show promise in terms of slowing the progress of the disease. Cholinesterase inhibitors have been shown to be effective in slowing the progression of the disease by potentiating the action of available acetylcholine.[62,63] These drugs—donepezil, rivastigmine, and galantamine—inhibit acetylcholinesterase, preventing the metabolism of endogenous acetylcholine, and are used in the early stages of the disease for mild cognitive impairment. Thus far, such therapy has not halted disease progression, but it can slow the disease progression by approximately 6 to 12 months. The therapeutic effects cease when the medication is discontinued.

Memantine, an *N*-methyl-D-aspartate antagonist, was approved by Health Canada for treatment of moderate to severe Alzheimer disease.[62,63] This medication may act by interfering with the glutamatergic excitotoxicity (see Chapter 51, Fig. 51.4) caused by the ischemia and amyloid deposits associated with the disease, or it may provide symptomatic improvement through effects on the function of hippocampal neurons. This medication, like the cholinesterase inhibitors, does not reverse the disease, but does provide a modest delay in functional loss.

Other treatments for Alzheimer disease include agents that are thought to have a neuroprotective effect. Aβ seems to exert its neurotoxic effects through a variety of secondary mechanisms, including oxidative injury and lipid peroxidation of cell membranes, and inflammation. Several strategies have involved the use of anti-inflammatory agents and antioxidants (omega-3 polyunsaturated fatty acids, vitamin E, and *Ginkgo biloba*).[52,63] Several, but not all, epidemiologic studies provide evidence supporting the concept that vitamin E and vitamin C have a role in delaying the onset of Alzheimer disease. In some, but not all, trials, *G. biloba* had small but statistically significant effects compared with placebo in persons with Alzheimer disease.

Psychotropic medications, such as antipsychotics and mood stabilizers, may be used to assist in the behavioural management of the disease. Interventions also include environmental adjustments, behavioural intervention, and education and support for caregivers. Caregiver support is essential because they are responsible for supervising persons who live in the community and continue to visit and provide support after the person has been institutionalized. They are also responsible for administering medications, implementing nonpharmacologic treatments, and promoting the person's general health and well-being.

Current research efforts are focusing on aspects of amyloid production, which initiates neuronal dysfunction. The enzymes responsible for liberating Aβ from APP are the β- and γ-secretases.[63] Inhibitors of these enzymes are under current study. Strategies aimed at reducing the aggregation of Aβ offer another therapeutic avenue to be explored. The metabolism of cholesterol is intimately involved in the generation of Aβ, and preliminary evidence suggests that the statin drugs may be beneficial in reducing the accumulation of Aβ.[63] A program to vaccinate humans was implemented after the observation that immunization with Aβ reduces pathologic signs of Alzheimer disease in transgenic mice with APP mutations. This clinical trial was terminated when encephalitis developed in 6% of the patients. It has been suggested that passive immunization (*i.e.,* administration of Aβ antibodies) represents an alternative and perhaps safer vaccination strategy.[63]

Vascular Dementia

Vascular dementia is caused by brain injury resulting from ischemic or hemorrhagic damage. Up to 20% of dementias in persons over the age of 65 are vascular in origin, making it the second most common cause of dementia.[64,65] The incidence is closely associated with hypertension, but also with arrhythmias, myocardial infarction, peripheral vascular disease, lipid abnormalities, diabetes mellitus, autoimmune and infectious vasculitis, and smoking.[52,58] The usual onset is between the ages of 55 and 70 years, and more men are affected than women.[52]

Vascular dementia differs from Alzheimer disease in its presentation and tissue abnormalities. Slowness in psychomotor functioning is a main clinical feature of this dementia, and symptoms of depression are often present.[58] The onset may be gradual or abrupt, the course usually is a stepwise progression, and there are focal neurologic symptoms related to local areas of infarction.

Frontotemporal Dementia

Frontotemporal dementia (FTD) refers to a group of disorders associated with atrophy of the frontal and anterior temporal lobes of the brain.[66] Originally known as *Pick disease,* FTD now refers to a syndrome that includes primary progressive aphasia, corticobasal degeneration, progressive supranuclear palsy, and semantic dementias.[6,52] The disease occurs with the same frequency in men and women, with onset between 35 and 75 years of age.[52] The median age of onset for FTD is about 58 years, with 22% of persons with the disorder having onset after 65 years of age.

There are two distinct clinical presentations that reflect the symptoms of FTD: behaviour and language. The former is more common, with behavioural presentations of disinhibited and impulsive actions or apathy, with inappropriate social behaviour. The behavioural abnormalities can be quite extreme, and can be misdiagnosed as schizophrenia or psychotic depression. The second type of FTD involves disturbances in understanding or expressing language.[2]

Diagnosis is based on evidence of cognitive impairment and exclusion of other illnesses that cause cognitive and behavioural deficits. Neuroimaging can be helpful in distinguishing FTD from other types of cognitive disorders. Typically, structural imaging shows anterior temporal and frontal lobe atrophy.[2] The course of the disease is relentless, with death ensuing within 2 to 10 years. The immediate cause of death usually is infection.

Creutzfeldt–Jakob Disease

Creutzfeldt–Jakob disease (CJD) is included in the major or mild neurocognitive disorder due to prion disease classification. CJD is an extremely rare, rapidly degenerative form of dementia thought to be caused by an infective protein agent called a *prion*[85] (see Chapter 16). There are four subtypes of CJD: sporadic, hereditary, acquired, and variant. Sporadic, in which the disease occurs without known risk factors, is the most common form, accounting for up to 85% of the cases. Familial or hereditary CJD represents 10% to 15% of cases, whereas the other subtypes of CJD are rare, representing less than 1% of cases. Variants of the disease occur in animals, including scrapie in sheep and goats and bovine spongiform encephalopathy (BSE; mad cow disease) in cattle.[67]

CJD causes degeneration of the pyramidal and extrapyramidal systems and is distinguished most readily by its rapid course. Affected persons usually are demented within 6 months of onset. The disease is uniformly fatal, with death often occurring within months, although a few persons may survive for several years.[52] The early symptoms consist of abnormalities in personality and visual-spatial coordination, and impaired memory and judgment. Extreme dementia, insomnia, and ataxia follow as the disease progresses.[67] There is no medical treatment for the disease.

Wernicke–Korsakoff Syndrome

Wernicke–Korsakoff syndrome most commonly results from chronic alcoholism. Wernicke disease is characterized by acute weakness and paralysis of the extraocular muscles, nystagmus, ataxia, and confusion.[68] The affected person also may have signs of peripheral neuropathy. The person has an unsteady gait and complains of diplopia. There may be signs attributable to alcohol withdrawal such as delirium, confusion, and hallucinations. This disorder is caused by a deficiency of thiamine (vitamin B_{12}), which directly interferes with production of glucose, the brain's main nutrient. Many of the symptoms are reversed when thiamine is administered parenterally and overall nutrition is improved.[68]

The Korsakoff component of the syndrome involves the chronic phase with severe impairment of recent memory. There often is difficulty in dealing with abstractions, and the person's capacity to learn is defective. Confabulation (*i.e.,* recitation of imaginary experiences to fill in gaps in memory) probably is the most distinctive feature of the disease. Polyneuritis also is common. Unlike Wernicke disease, Korsakoff psychosis does not improve significantly with treatment.

Huntington Disease

Huntington disease is a hereditary neurodegenerative disorder characterized by chronic progressive chorea, psychological changes, and dementia. Although the disease is inherited as an autosomal dominant disorder, the age of onset most commonly is in the fourth and fifth decades. By the time the disease has been diagnosed, the person often has passed the gene on to his or her children. Approximately 10% of Huntington cases involve juvenile onset.[52,69] Children with the disease rarely live to adulthood.

Huntington disease is caused by a single genetic mutation on chromosome 4 (4p16:3) that encodes the information for the huntingtin protein. The cellular functions of this large protein are not completely understood, but without its protection it leads to localized death of brain cells.[69,70] The first and most severely affected neurons are of the caudate nucleus and putamen of the basal ganglia. The neurochemical changes that occur with the disease are complex. The neurotransmitter GABA is an inhibitory neurotransmitter in the basal ganglia. Postmortem studies have shown a decrease of GABA and GABA receptors in the basal ganglia of persons with Huntington disease. Likewise, the levels of acetylcholine, an excitatory neurotransmitter in the basal ganglia, are reduced in persons with Huntington disease. The dopaminergic pathway of the nigrostriatal system, which is affected in Parkinson disease, is preserved in Huntington disease, suggesting that an imbalance in dopamine and acetylcholine may contribute to manifestations of the disease.

Depression and personality changes are the most common early psychological manifestations; memory loss often is accompanied by impulsive behaviour, moodiness, antisocial behaviour, and a tendency toward emotional outbursts.[52] An estimated 30% of persons with Huntington disease experience MDD or dysthymic disorder, with about 6% of deaths attributed to suicide.[52] Other early signs of the disease are lack of initiative, loss of spontaneity, and inability to concentrate. Fidgeting or restlessness may represent early signs of dyskinesia, followed by choreiform and some dystonic posturing. Eventually, progressive rigidity and akinesia (rather than chorea) develop in association with dementia. Symptoms of juvenile onset of Huntington disease include Parkinson-like dystonias and seizures.

There is no cure for Huntington disease. The treatment is largely symptomatic. Drugs may be used to treat the dyskinesias and behavioural disturbances. It is hoped that with further genetic information about the huntingtin protein other biomarkers might be found to help promote disease-modifying therapeutics for delaying and slowing the progression.[69]

IN SUMMARY

Cognition refers to all the processes by which sensory input is transformed, reduced, elaborated, stored, recovered, and used. It is important to differentiate what can be termed "normal cognitive aging" from disorders of memory and cognition. Memory problems that are associated with normal aging tend to reflect a generalized decrease in the efficiency with which information is processed and retrieved. Memory of a past event can be based on retrieval that is accompanied by recollection of specific details, or on the feeling that the event is old or new based on its familiarity. There is evidence that recollection is more dependent on the hippocampus, whereas familiarity is more dependent on the entorhinal cortex, and that healthy aging has greater effects on recollection than on familiarity.

Dementia represents a syndrome of deterioration in cognitive function severe enough to interfere with occupational or social performance. The diagnosis of dementia is based on history; complete physical and neurologic examination; evaluation of cognitive, behavioural, and functional status; and laboratory (particularly electrolytes, thyroid hormone and vitamin B_{12}) and neuroimaging studies. There are several potentially reversible causes of dementia that can be remembered by the mnemonic DEMENTIA: *D*rug (any drug with anticholinergic activity), *E*motional (depression), *M*etabolic (thyroid function), *E*yes and ears declining, *N*ormal-pressure hydrocephalus, *T*umour or other space-occupying lesion, *I*nfection (HIV or syphilis), *A*nemia (vitamin B_{12} or folate deficiency).

The major syndromes of progressive dementia include Alzheimer disease, vascular dementia, FTD, CJD, Wernicke–Korsakoff syndrome, and Huntington disease. By far the most common cause of dementia is Alzheimer disease. The condition is a major health problem among older adults. It is characterized by cortical atrophy and loss of neurons, and the presence of neuritic plaques, granulovacuolar degeneration, and cerebrovascular deposits of amyloid. The disease follows an insidious and progressive course that begins with memory impairment and terminates in an inability to recognize family or friends and the loss of control over bodily functions. Ischemic or hemorrhagic damage is associated with vascular dementia, and FTD with atrophy of the frontal and temporal lobes. CJD is a rare, rapidly progressive form of dementia. Wernicke–Korsakoff syndrome most often results from chronic alcoholism. Huntington disease is a hereditary disorder characterized by chronic and progressive chorea, psychological changes, and dementia.

REVIEW EXERCISES

1. A 45-year-old woman was brought to the emergency department after being picked up by the police. She was wandering in and out of traffic saying someone was after her and was recognized as a homeless person. Her appearance is dirty and dishevelled and she is wearing several layers of clothing, although it is summer. She smacks her lips and at times does not seem to understand

questions. Periodically she laughs for no apparent reason and often repeats the words of her questioner. She has a 20-year history of schizophrenia with multiple admissions.

    A. *List the positive and negative signs she exhibits.*

    B. *What are the brain areas and transmitters responsible for these signs?*

    C. *What are the DSM-5 criteria that would have led to her diagnosis?*

2. A 35-year-old woman was recently admitted with suicidal tendencies shortly after a diagnosis of major depression. She had lost 18 kg in the last 6 months. She appears tired and supplies only short answers to questions. She complains of dizziness and informs the nurse that it is not her business to discuss her suicidal thoughts. Her husband says she relies heavily on alcohol.

    A. *Describe some of her manifestations. Why is she using alcohol?*

    B. *Provide an explanation for her tiredness.*

    C. *What areas of the brain and neurotransmitters are involved in depression? How is it different from mania?*

    D. *What are the possible roles of thyroid and adrenal hormones?*

3. A 40-year-old woman is seen in the emergency department in a state of severe panic. She has had panic attacks for several months and had not sought treatment until her husband came home and found her sitting in the bedroom unable to move. She had been there all day and had soiled her clothing. In the emergency department she appeared frightened and paced in one area. She had difficulty understanding questions and cooperated only as long as she could pace. The husband relates that his wife had been under a lot of stress in her job and had recently lost some important clients.

    A. *What are some manifestations of her panic?*

    B. *What is the biologic cause of anxiety disorders (the brain structures and neurotransmitters)?*

    C. *Describe the physiologic manifestations of a panic attack.*

References

1. Shorter E. (1997). *A history of psychiatry: From the era of the asylum to the age of Prozac.* New York: John Wiley & Sons.
2. American Psychiatric Association. (2013). *Diagnostic and Statistical Manual of Mental Disorders: DSM-5.* Washington, DC, Author.
3. Shin L, Liberzon I. (2010). The neurocircuitry of fear, stress, and anxiety disorders. *Neuropsychopharmacology, 35*(1), 169–191.
4. Quinn K. (2015). *Mandala Art: Inter-professional Mindfulness Education Techniques for Self-awareness and Self-Transformation.* Springfield, MO: American Association of Integrative Medicine.
5. Hanson R. (2009). Mind changing brain changing mind. *Insight Journal, 32,* 9–15.
6. Kandel E. R., Schwartz J. H., Jessell T. M., et al. (2013). *Principles of neural science* (5th ed.). New York: McGraw-Hill Medical.
7. Grob G. N. (1994). *The mad among us: A history of the care of America's mentally ill.* New York: Macmillan.
8. Gelernter J. (2015). Genetics of complex traits in psychiatry. *Biological Psychiatry, 77*(1), 36–42.
9. Hall L. L. (Ed.) (1996). *Genetics and mental illness: Evolving issues for research and society.* New York: Plenum Press.
10. Stahl S. (2009). Epigenetics and methylomics in psychiatry. *Journal of Clinical Psychiatry, 70*(9), 1204–1205.
11. Abdolmaleky H., Smith C., Zhou J., et al. (2008). Chapter 9: Epigenetic alterations of the dopaminergic system in major psychiatric disorders. In Yan Q. (Ed). *Pharmacogenomics in Drug Discovery and Development.* New York: Humana Press.
12. Austin W., Boyd M. A. (2010). *Psychiatric & mental health nursing for Canadian practice* (2nd ed.). Philadelphia, PA: Lippincott Williams & Wilkins.
13. Hall J. E. (2011). *Textbook of medical physiology* (12th ed.). Philadelphia, PA: W. B. Saunders.
14. Schadlu A. P., Schadlu R., Shepherd J. B. (2009). Charles Bonnet syndrome: A review. *Current Opinion in Ophthalmology, 20*(3), 219–222.
15. Yudofsky S. C., Hales R. E. (2004). *Essentials of neuropsychiatry and clinical neurosciences.* Washington, DC: American Psychiatric Publishing.
16. National Empowerment Center. (2013). Hearing voices that are distressing: Self-help resources. Available online at: http://www.power2u.org/articles/selfhelp/voices.html. Accessed June 9, 2015.
17. Hariri A. G., Ozer G., Ceylan M. E. (2009). Acquired hearing loss and psychiatric symptoms. *Archives of Neuropsychiatry, 46*(4), 149–156.
18. Kennedy S. H., Parikh S.V., Grigoriadis S. (updated 2015). Psychiatric disorders: Depression. In Repchinsky C. (Ed.), *e-Therapeutics.* Ottawa, ON: Canadian Pharmacists Association.
19. Yudofsky S. C., Hales R. E. (2010). *Essentials of neuropsychiatry and behavioral neurosciences* (2nd ed.). Washington, DC: American Psychiatric Publishing.
20. Torrey E. F. (2006). *Surviving schizophrenia: A manual for families, patients, and providers.* New York: Harper & Row.
21. Canadian Mental Health Association. (2015). Fast facts: Mental health/mental illness. Available online at: http://www.cmha.ca/media/fast-facts-about-mental-illness/#.VXflmvlVhHw. Accessed June 9, 2015.
22. Cannon C., Clarke M. C. (2005). Risk for schizophrenia: Broadening the concepts, pushing back the boundaries. *Schizophrenia Research, 79,* 5–13.
23. Varcarolis E. M., Carson V. B., Shoemaker N. C. (2006). *Foundations of psychiatric mental health nursing: A clinical approach* (5th ed.). St. Louis, MO: Elsevier Saunders.
24. Flashman L. A., Green M. F. (2004). Review of cognition and brain structure in schizophrenia: Profiles, longitudinal course, and effects of treatment. *Psychiatric Clinics of North America, 27,* 1–18.
25. Shepherd A. M., Laurens K. R., Matheson S. L., et al. (2012). Systematic meta-review and quality assessment of the structural brain alterations in schizophrenia. *Neuroscience and Biobehavioral Reviews, 36*(4), 1342–1356.
26. Boos H. B., Aleman A., Cahn W., et al. (2007). Brain volumes in relatives of patients with schizophrenia. *Archives of General Psychiatry, 64,* 297–304.
27. Sadock B. J., Sadock V. A., Ruiz P. (2009). *Kaplan & Sadock's comprehensive textbook of psychiatry* (9th ed.). Philadelphia, PA: Lippincott Williams & Wilkins.
28. Canadian Mental Health Association. (2009). Understanding mental illness. Available online at: http://www.cmha.ca/mental-health/understanding-mental-illness. Accessed June 9, 2015.
29. Read J. (2010). Can poverty drive you mad? 'Schizophrenia', socio-economic status and the case for primary prevention. *New Zealand Journal of Psychology, 39*(2), 7–19.
30. Agency for Healthcare Research and Quality. (2005). Post-myocardial infarction depression. Available online at: http://archive.ahrq.gov/clinic/tp/mideptp.htm. Accessed June 9, 2015.

31. Lojko D., Suwalska A., Rybakowski J. (2014). Bipolar and related disorders and depressive disorders in DSM-5. *Psychiatria Polska, 48*(2), 245–260.

32. Hajek T., Carrey N., Alda M. (2005). Neuroanatomical abnormalities as risk factors for bipolar disorder. *Bipolar Disorders, 7*, 393–403.

33. Brunswick D. J., Amsredam J. D., Mozley P. D., et al. (2003). Greater availability of brain dopamine transporters in major depression shown by [99mTc] TRODAT-1 SPECT imaging. *American Journal of Psychiatry, 160*, 1836–1841.

34. Baldwin D. S., Papakostas G. I. (2006). Symptoms of fatigue and sleepiness in major depressive disorder. *Journal of Clinical Psychiatry, 67*(6), 9–15.

35. Trevino K., McClintock S. M., Husain M. M. (2010). A review of continuation electroconvulsive therapy: Application, safety, and efficacy. *The Journal of ECT, 26*(3), 186–195.

36. Kurlanski S. L., Ibay A. D. (2013). Seasonal affective disorder. *American Family Physician, 86*(11), 1037–1041.

37. Beimaker R. H. (2004). Bipolar disorders. *The New England Journal of Medicine, 351*(5), 476–486.

38. Shuchman M. (2007). Approving the vagus-nerve stimulator for depression. *The New England Journal of Medicine, 356*, 1604–1607.

39. Katon W. J. (2006). Panic disorder. *The New England Journal of Medicine, 354*, 2360–2367.

40. Mohler H. (2012). The GABA system in anxiety and depression and its therapeutic potential. *Neuropharmacology, 62*(1), 42–53.

41. Bermudo-Soriano C. R., Perez-Rodriguez M. M., Vaquero-Lorenzo C., Baca-Garcia E. (2012). New perspectives in glutamate and anxiety. *Pharmacology, Biochemistry and Behavior, 100*(4), 752–774.

42. Greene J. A. (2006). Chapter 18: The client with an anxiety disorder. In Mohr W. K. *Johnson's psychiatric-mental health nursing* (6th ed.). Philadelphia, PA: Lippincott Williams & Wilkins.

43. Jenike M. A. (2004). Obsessive-compulsive disorder. *The New England Journal of Medicine, 350*, 259–265.

44. Kumar V., Abbas A. K., Faustos N., et al. (Eds.). (2010). *Robbins and Cotran pathologic basis of disease* (8th ed.). Philadelphia, PA: Elsevier Saunders.

45. Anderson K. E., Savage C. R. (2004). Cognitive and neurobiological findings in obsessive-compulsive disorder. *Psychiatric Clinics of North America, 27*, 37–47.

46. Tjepkema M. (2004). Alcohol and illicit drug dependence. *Health Reports, 15*(Suppl), 9–19

47. Pearson C., Janz T., Ali J. (2013). *Health at a Glance: Mental and substance use disorders in Canada*, No. 82–624-X. Minister of Industry: Statistics Canada.

48. Green A. I., Drake R. E., Brunette M. F., et al. (2007). Schizophrenia and co-occurring substance use disorder. *American Journal of Psychiatry, 163*, 402–408.

49. Bruinjnzeel A. W., Repetto M., Gold M. (2004). Neurobiological mechanisms of addiction and psychiatric disorders. *Psychiatric Clinics of North America, 27*, 661–674.

50. Kalivas P. W., Volkow N. D. (2005). The neural basis of addiction: A pathology of motivation and choice. *American Journal of Psychiatry, 162*, 1403–1413.

51. Simpson J. R. (2014). DSM-5 and neurocognitive disorders. *Journal of the American Academy of Psychiatry and the Law, 42*(2), 159–164.

52. Millsap P. (2007). Neurological system. In Linton A. D., Lach H. W. *Matteson & McConnell's gerontological nursing: Concepts and practice* (3rd ed.). St. Louis, MO: Elsevier Saunders.

53. Josshi S., Morley J. E. (2006). Cognitive impairment. *Medical Clinics of North America, 90*, 769–787.

54. Gauthier S., Patterson C., Chertkow H., et al. (2012). Recommendations for the 4th Canadian consensus conference on the diagnosis and treatment of dementia. *Canadian Geriatrics Journal, 15*(4), 120–126.

55. Moore A., Patterson C., Lee L., et al; Canadian Consensus Conference on the Diagnosis and Treatment of Dementia. (2014). Fourth Canadian consensus conference on the diagnosis and treatment of dementia. *Canadian Family Physician, 60*, 433–438.

56. Alzheimer Association. (2015). 2015 Alzheimer's disease facts and figures. *Alzheimers & Dementia, 11*(3), 332–384.

57. Holtzman D. M., Morris J. C., Goate A. M. (2011). Alzheimer's disease: The challenge of the second century. *Science Translational Medicine, 3*(77), 77sr1.

58. Rubin R., Strayer D. S. (Eds.). (2012). *Rubin's pathology: Clinicopathologic foundations of medicine* (6th ed.). Philadelphia, PA: Lippincott Williams & Wilkins.

59. National Institute of Aging. (2015). About Alzheimer's disease: Alzheimer's basics. Available online at: https://www.nia.nih.gov/alzheimers/topics/alzheimers-basics. Accessed June 10, 2015.

60. Erickson K. I., Voss M. W., Prakash R. S., et al. (2011). Exercise training increases size of hippocampus and improves memory. *Proceedings of the National Academy of Science of USA, 108*(7), 3017–3022.

61. Alzheimer's Association. (2015). Diagnostic procedures. Available online at: http://www.alz.org/professionals_and_researchers_diagnostic_procedures.asp. Accessed June 10, 2015.

62. Rockwood K., Bosma M. (updated 2015). Psychiatric disorders: Dementia. In Repchinsky C., (Ed.), *e-Therapeutics*. Ottawa, ON: Canadian Pharmacists Association.

63. Mangialasche F., Solomon A., Winblad B., et al. (2010). Alzheimer's disease: Clinical trials and drug development. *The Lancet Neurology, 9*(7), 702–716.

64. Black S. E. (2011). Vascular cognitive impairment: Epidemiology, subtypes, diagnosis and management. *Journal of the Royal College of Physicians of Edinburgh, 41*(1), 49–56.

65. Iadecola C. (2013). The pathobiology of vascular dementia. *Neuron, 80*(4), 844–866.

66. Hornberger M., Piguet O. (2012). Episodic memory in frontotemporal dementia: A critical review. *Brain, 135*(3), 678–692.

67. Gencer A., Pelin Z., Kucukali C. I., et al. (2011). Creutzfeldt-Jakob disease. *Psychogeriatrics, 11*(2), 119–124.

68. Isenberg-Grzeda E., Kutner H. E., Nicolson S. E. (2012). Wernicke-Korsakoff-syndrome: Under-recognized and under-treated. *Psychosomatics, 53*(6), 507–516.

69. Ross C. A., Aylward E. H., Wild E. J., et al. (2014). Huntington disease: Natural history, biomarkers and prospects for therapeutics. *Nature Reviews Neurology, 10*(4), 204–216.

70. Ross C. A., Tabrizi S. J. (2011). Huntington's disease: From molecular pathogenesis to clinical treatment. *The Lancet Neurology, 10*(1), 83–98.

Visit thePoint **http://thePoint.lww.com for animations, journal articles, and more!**

Unit XIII

Disorders of Special Sensory Function

Of all the ancient civilizations, it was the Greeks who led the way in understanding the body and its workings. One of the earliest Greek anatomists was Alcmaeon of Croton (c. 500 BC). Through his animal dissections, Alcmaeon came to recognize many structures and was the first to mention the eye in his writings. He described the optic nerve and decided that three things were necessary for vision—external light, the "fire" in the eye (he assumed there must be fire in the eye because a blow to the eye produces sparks, or stars), and the liquid in the eyeball.

The Greeks also developed early surgical procedures, among them techniques for the removal of cataracts. However, it was the Roman encyclopedist, Aulus Cornelius Celsus (1st century AD), whose most important surviving works are concerned with medicine, who provided a vivid description of the procedure:

The needle is to be sharp enough to penetrate, yet not too fine; and this is to be inserted straight through...at a spot between the pupil of the eye and the angle adjacent to the temple, away from the middle of the cataract, in such a way that no vein is wounded. The needle, however, should not be inserted timidly. When the spot is reached, the needle is to be sloped against the coloured area [lens] itself and rotated gently, guiding it little by little below the pupil; when the cataract has passed below the pupil, it is pressed upon more firmly in order that it may settle below.

Disorders of Visual Function

54

There are 285 million people worldwide who are visually impaired—39 million are blind and 246 million have partial vision loss that cannot be corrected, a visual impairment known as *low vision*. Without intervention, the number of people with impaired vision could double by 2020. The prevalence of vision impairment increases with age.[1] An estimated 500,000 Canadians are living with significant vision loss that impacts their quality of life.[2]

Alterations in vision can result from disorders of the eyelids and optic globe (conjunctiva, cornea, and uvea), intraocular pressure (glaucoma), lens (cataract), vitreous humour and retina (retinopathy and macular degeneration), optic pathways and visual cortex, and extraocular muscles and eye movement (Fig. 54.1).

DISORDERS OF THE ACCESSORY STRUCTURES OF THE EYE

After completing this section of the chapter, you should be able to meet the following objectives:

- State the cause of eyelid weakness.
- Define the terms *entropion* and *ectropion*.

FIGURE 54.1 • A scene as it might be viewed by a person with (**A**) normal vision, (**B**) age-related macular degeneration, (**C**) cataract, and (**D**) glaucoma. (From National Eye Institute, National Institutes of Health. Available online at: www.nei.nih.gov/photo.)

- Explain the differences between marginal blepharitis, a hordeolum, and a chalazion as to causes and manifestations.
- State the causes and treatment of dry eye.

The optic globe, commonly called the *eyeball,* is a remarkably mobile, nearly spherical structure contained in a pyramid-shaped cavity of the skull called the *orbit.* Only the anterior one fifth of the orbit is occupied by the eyeball; the remainder is filled with muscles, nerves, the lacrimal gland, and adipose tissue that support the normal position of the optic globe (Fig. 54.2). Exposed surfaces of the eyes are protected by the eyelids, which are mucous membrane-lined skin flaps that provide a means for shutting out most light, and protecting the globe. Tears bathe the anterior surface of the eye; they prevent friction between it and the lid, maintain hydration of the cornea, and protect the eye from infection and irritation by foreign objects.

Three distinct layers form the wall of the eyeball: the sclera or outer supporting layer, the choroid or middle vascular layer, and the retina, which is composed of the neuronal retinal layer and the outer pigmented layer (Fig. 54.2). The outer layer of the eyeball consists of a tough, opaque, white, fibrous layer called the *sclera.* It is strong yet elastic,

VISION

- Vision is a special sensory function that incorporates the visual receptor activities of the eyeball, the optic nerve, and optic pathways that carry and distribute sensory information from the optic globe to the central nervous system, and the primary and visual association cortices that translate the sensory signals into visual images.
- The eyeball is a hollow spherical structure that functions in the reception of the light rays that provide the stimuli for vision. The refractive surface of the cornea and accommodative properties of the lens serve to focus the light signals from near and far objects on the photoreceptors in the retina.
- Visual information is carried to the brain by axons of the retinal cells that form the optic nerve. The two optic nerves fuse in the optic chiasm, where axons of the nasal retina of each eye cross to the contralateral side and travel with axons of the ipsilateral temporal retina to form the fibres of the optic radiations that travel to the visual cortex.
- Binocular vision depends on the coordination of three pairs of extraocular nerves that provide for the conjugate eye movements, with optical axes of the two eyes maintained parallel with one another as the eyes rotate in their sockets.

FIGURE 54.2 • The eye and its appendages: lateral view.

and maintains the shape of the globe. The sclera is continuous with the cornea anteriorly and with the cranial dural sheath that surrounds and protects the optic nerve posteriorly. The choroid predominantly provides vascular support of the retina, whereas the retina is the neurosensory tissue that provides the sensory input for sight.

Disorders of the Eyelids

The upper and lower eyelids, the *palpebrae,* are modified folds of skin with associated muscle and cartilaginous plates that protect the eyeball. The palpebral fissure is the oval opening between the upper and lower eyelids. At the corners of the eye,

where the upper and lower lids meet, is an angle called the *canthus;* the lateral canthus is the outer, or temporal, angle, and the medial canthus is the inner, or nasal, angle. In each lid, a tarsus, or plate of dense connective tissue, gives the lid its shape (Fig. 54.3). Each tarsus contains modified sebaceous glands, called *meibomian glands,* the ducts of which open onto the eyelid margins. Sebaceous secretions of the meibomian glands enable airtight closure of the lids and prevent rapid evaporation of tears.

Three striated muscles, the levator palpebrae superioris, Müller muscle, and the orbicularis oculi, provide for movement of the eyelids. The main elevator, the levator palpebrae superioris, innervated by the oculomotor nerve (cranial nerve

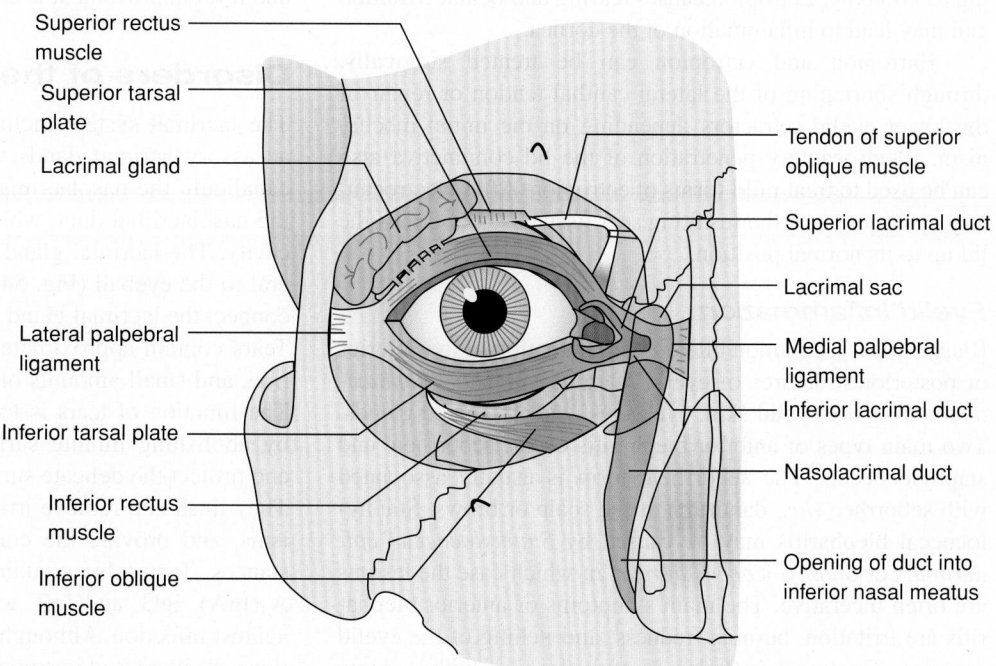

FIGURE 54.3 • The eye and its appendages: anterior view.

[CN] III), serves to raise the upper lid, along with the sympathetically innervated Müller muscle. Encircling the eye is the orbicularis oculi muscle, which is supplied by the facial nerve (CN VII). When this muscle contracts, it closes the eyelids. Between the nose and medial angle of the eye is the medial palpebral ligament, which connects to the medial margin of the orbit (Fig. 54.3). A similar palpebral ligament attaches to the lateral margin of the orbit. The orbicularis oculi nerve inserts into the medial palpebral ligament that passes through each eyelid and inserts into the lateral palpebral junction. The four recti and two oblique muscles provide for movement of the eyeball (discussed under disorders of eye movement).

Eyelid Weakness

Drooping of the eyelid is called *ptosis*. It can result from weakness of the levator muscle that elevates the upper lid in conjunction with the unopposed action of the orbicularis oculi that forcefully closes the eyelids. Weakness of the orbicularis oculi causes an open eyelid, a condition called lagophthalmos, but not ptosis. Neurologic causes of eyelid weakness include damage to the innervating cranial nerves or to the nerves' central nuclei in the midbrain and the caudal pons, as well as damage to the sympathetic nerves innervating Müller muscle.

Normally, the edges of the eyelids, or lid margins, are in such a position that the palpebral conjunctiva that lines the eyelids are not exposed and the eyelashes do not rub against the cornea. Turning in of the lid margin is called *entropion*. It is usually caused by degeneration of the fascial attachments to the lower lid that occurs with aging, which leads to lid laxity, or disinsertion of the eyelid retractors. Corneal irritation may occur as the eyelashes turn inward. *Ectropion* refers to eversion of the lower lid margin. The condition is usually bilateral and caused by relaxation of the orbicularis oculi muscle because of CN VII weakness or the aging process, again leading to lid laxity. Ectropion causes tearing and ocular irritation and may lead to inflammation of the cornea.

Entropion and ectropion can be treated surgically, through shortening of the lateral canthal tendon or repair of the lower eyelid retractors depending on the initial mechanism. Electrocautery penetration of the lid conjunctiva also can be used to treat mild forms of ectropion. After electrocautery, contraction of the resulting scar tissue usually draws the lid up to its normal position.

Eyelid Inflammation

Blepharitis is a common bilateral inflammation of the anterior or posterior structures of eyelid margins. *Anterior blepharitis* involves the eyelid skin, eyelashes, and associated glands. Two main types of anterior blepharitis occur: seborrheic and staphylococcal.[3] The seborrheic form is usually associated with seborrhea (*i.e.,* dandruff) of the scalp or brows. Staphylococcal blepharitis may be caused by *Staphylococcus epidermidis* or *Staphylococcus aureus,* in which case the lesions are often ulcerative. The main symptoms of anterior blepharitis are irritation, burning, redness, and itching of the eyelid margins. Treatment includes careful cleaning with a damp applicator to remove the scales. When the disorder is associated with a microbial infection, an antibiotic ointment or drops are prescribed.

Posterior blepharitis is inflammation of the eyelids that involves the meibomian glands. It may result from a bacterial infection, particularly with staphylococci, or dysfunction of the meibomian glands, in which there is a strong association with acne rosacea[3] (see Chapter 61). The meibomian glands and their orifices are inflamed, with dilation of the glands, plugging of the orifices, and abnormal secretions. The tears may be frothy and abnormally greasy from the meibomian secretions. Treatment of posterior blepharitis is determined by associated conjunctival and corneal changes. Initial therapies can include warm compression of the lids, daily judicious use of topical lubricating drops, and use of flaxseed or fish oil tablets to provide omega-3 fatty acid benefits to meibomian oil secretions. Long-term, low-dose systemic antibiotic therapy guided by results of bacterial cultures along with short-term topical steroids may also be needed.

A *hordeolum,* or *stye,* is caused by infection of the sebaceous glands of the eyelid and can be internal (meibomian gland) or external (glands of Zeis or Moll). The main symptoms are pain, redness, and swelling. The treatment is similar to that for abscesses in other parts of the body. Heat such as a warm compress is applied, and short-term treatment with systemic antibiotics (*e.g.,* doxycycline) may be used to reduce or eliminate the infection. Incision or expression of the infectious contents of the abscess may be necessary.

A *chalazion* is a chronic inflammatory granuloma of a meibomian gland that may follow an internal hordeolum. It is characterized by a small, nontender nodule on the upper or lower lid. The conjunctiva around the chalazion is red and elevated. If the chalazion is large enough, it may press on the eyeball and distort vision. Treatment consists initially of topical steroids, and if no improvement is observed, incision and curettage.

Disorders of the Lacrimal System

The lacrimal system includes the major lacrimal gland and accessory lacrimal glands, which produce the tears, the puncta, canaliculi, the nasolacrimal sac, which collect the tears, and the nasolacrimal duct, which empties the tears into the nasal cavity. The lacrimal gland lies in the orbit, superior and lateral to the eyeball (Fig. 54.3). Approximately 12 small ducts connect the lacrimal gland to the superior conjunctival fornix. Tears contain approximately 98% water, 1.5% sodium chloride, and small amounts of potassium, albumin, and glucose. The function of tears is to provide a smooth optical surface by abolishing minute surface irregularities. Tears also wet and protect the delicate surface of the cornea and conjunctiva. They flush and remove irritating substances and microorganisms, and provide the cornea with necessary nutrient substances. Tears also contain lysozymes and immunoglobulin A (IgA), IgG, and IgE, which synergistically act to protect against infection. Although IgA predominates, IgE concentrations are increased in some allergic responses.

Dry Eyes

The thin film of tears that covers the cornea is essential in preventing drying and damage of the outer layer of the cornea. This tear film is composed of three layers: (1) a superficial lipid layer, which is derived from the meibomian glands and thought to retard evaporation; (2) an aqueous layer, secreted by the lacrimal glands; and (3) a mucinous layer, which overlies the cornea and epithelial cells. Because the epithelial cell membranes are hydrophobic and cannot be wetted by aqueous solutions alone, the mucinous layer plays an essential role in wetting these surfaces. Periodic blinking of the eyes is needed to maintain a continuous tear film over the ocular surface.

Several conditions reduce the functioning of the lacrimal glands. With aging, the lacrimal glands diminish their secretion, and as a result, some older persons awaken from a night's sleep with highly irritated eyes. Dry eyes also can result from loss of reflex lacrimal gland secretion because of congenital defects, infection, irradiation, damage to the parasympathetic innervation of the gland, and medications such as antihistamines and drugs with anticholinergic action. Wearing contact lenses can contribute to an interruption of the normal tear film. *Sjögren syndrome* is a systemic disorder in which lymphocytes and plasma cells infiltrate the lacrimal and parotid glands. The disorder is associated with diminished salivary and lacrimal secretions, resulting in keratoconjunctivitis sicca (*i.e.,* dry eye syndrome) and xerostomia (*i.e.,* dry mouth). The syndrome occurs mainly in women near menopause and is often associated with connective tissue disorders such as rheumatoid arthritis.

Persons with dry eyes complain of a dry or gritty sensation in the eye, burning and itching, inability to produce tears, photosensitivity, redness, pain, and difficulty in moving the eyelids. Some persons experience excess tearing as the eyes attempt to react to dry symptoms, but these tears are mainly composed of an aqueous component that quickly evaporates, repeating the cycle. Dry eyes and the absence of tears can cause keratinization of the cornea and conjunctival epithelium. In severe cases, corneal ulcerations can occur.

The treatment of dry eyes includes frequent instillation of artificial tear solutions into the conjunctival sac.[3] More prolonged duration of action can be obtained from topical preparations containing methylcellulose or polyvinyl alcohol. An ointment is useful for prolonged lubrication. Overall, these artificial tear preparations are safe and without side effects. However, the preservatives necessary to maintain their sterility can be irritating to the cornea.[3] Further treatment can include occlusion of the lacrimal puncta with silicone plugs, use of therapeutic topical drugs to increase natural tear volume, topical anti-inflammatories, immunosuppressants such as cyclosporine, and oral doxycycline.[4] Increased intake of omega-3 fatty acids has also been shown to provide improvement in dry eye symptoms.

Dacryocystitis

Dacryocystitis is an infection of the nasolacrimal sac. It occurs most often in infants or in persons older than 50 years of age with an increased incidence noted for postmenopausal women.[3–6] It is usually unilateral and most often occurs secondary to obstruction of the nasolacrimal duct. Often the cause of the obstruction is unknown, although there may be a history of severe trauma to the midface. The symptoms include tearing and discharge, pain, swelling, and tenderness. The treatment includes application of warm compresses and antibiotic therapy. In chronic forms of the disorder, surgical repair of the tear duct may be necessary.

In infants, dacryocystitis is usually caused by failure of the nasolacrimal ducts to open spontaneously before birth. When a duct fails to open, a secondary dacryocystitis may develop. These infants are usually treated with gentle massage of the tear sac, instillation of antibiotic drops into the conjunctival sac, and, if that fails, surgical probing is done to open the tear duct. The majority resolve without surgery by the age of 1 year.

IN SUMMARY

The eyelids serve to protect the eye. Ptosis refers to drooping of the upper lid, which is caused by injury to CN III. Entropion, which refers to turning in the upper eyelid and eyelashes, is discomforting and causes corneal irritation. Ectropion, or eversion of the lower eyelid, causes tearing and may lead to corneal inflammation. Marginal blepharitis is the most common disorder of the eyelids. It commonly is caused by a staphylococcal infection or seborrhea (*i.e.,* dandruff).

The lacrimal system includes the major lacrimal gland, which produces the tears, the puncta and tear sac, which collect the tears, and the nasolacrimal duct, which empties the tears into the nasal cavity. Tears protect the cornea from drying and irritation. Impaired tear production or conditions that prevent blinking and the spread of tears produce drying of the eyes and predispose them to corneal irritation and injury. Dacryocystitis is an infection of the lacrimal sac.

DISORDERS OF THE CONJUNCTIVA, CORNEA, AND UVEAL TRACT

After completing this section of the chapter, you should be able to meet the following objectives:

- Compare symptoms associated with red eye caused by conjunctivitis, corneal irritation, and acute glaucoma.
- Describe the appearance of corneal edema.
- Characterize the manifestations, treatment, and possible complications of bacterial, *Acanthamoeba*, and herpes keratitis.
- Describe the structures of the uveal tract.
- Describe tests used in assessing the pupillary reflex and cite the possible causes of abnormal pupillary reflexes.

Disorders of the Conjunctiva

The conjunctiva is a delicate mucous membrane that lines the anterior surface of both eyelids as the *palpebral conjunctiva* and folds back over the anterior surface of the optic globe as the *bulbar* or *ocular conjunctiva*[5,7,8] (Fig. 54.2). The bulbar conjunctiva covers only the sclera or white portion of the optic globe, not the cornea. When both eyes are closed, the conjunctiva lines the closed conjunctival sac. Although the conjunctiva protects the eye, its main function is the production of a lubricating mucus from goblet cells that bathes the eye and keeps it moist.

Conjunctivitis, or inflammation of the conjunctiva (*i.e.,* red or pink eye), is one of the most common forms of eye disease.[7,8] It may result from bacterial or viral infection, allergens, chemical agents, physical irritants, or radiant energy. Depending on the cause, conjunctivitis can vary in severity from a mild hyperemia (redness) with tearing to severe conjunctivitis with purulent drainage. The conjunctiva is extremely sensitive to irritation and inflammation. Symptoms of conjunctivitis are a foreign body sensation, a scratching or burning sensation, itching, and photophobia. Severe pain suggests the presence of corneal rather than conjunctival disease. A discharge, or exudate, may be present. It is usually watery when the conjunctivitis is caused by allergy, a foreign body, or viral infection, and mucopurulent in the presence of bacterial or fungal infection. A characteristic of many forms of conjunctivitis is papillary hypertrophy. This occurs because the palpebral conjunctiva is bound to the tarsus by fine fibrils. As a result, inflammation that develops between the fibrils causes the conjunctiva to be elevated in mounds called *papillae*. When the papillae are small, the conjunctiva has a smooth, velvety appearance. Red papillary conjunctivitis suggests bacterial or chlamydial conjunctivitis. In allergic conjunctivitis, the papillae often become flat-topped, polygonal, and milky in colour and have a cobblestone appearance.

The diagnosis of conjunctivitis is based on history, physical examination, and microscopic and culture studies to identify the cause. Because a red eye may be the sign of several eye conditions, it is important to differentiate between redness caused by conjunctivitis and that caused by more serious eye disorders, such as corneal lesions and acute glaucoma. In contrast to corneal lesions and acute glaucoma, conjunctivitis produces injection (*i.e.,* enlargement and redness) of the peripheral conjunctival blood vessels rather than those radiating around the corneal limbus (Fig. 54.4). Conjunctivitis also produces only mild discomfort compared with the moderate to severe discomfort associated with corneal lesions or the severe and deep pain associated with acute glaucoma. Infectious forms of conjunctivitis are usually bilateral and may involve other family members and associates. Unilateral disease suggests sources of irritation such as foreign bodies or chemical irritation.

Allergic Conjunctivitis

Allergic conjunctivitis encompasses a spectrum of conjunctival conditions usually characterized by itching. The most

FIGURE 54.4 • Gonococcal conjunctivitis of right eye. Note injection of the peripheral conjunctival blood vessels. (From the Centers for Disease Control and Prevention Public Health Image Library. Available online at: http://phil.cdc.gov/phil/home.asp.)

common of these is seasonal allergic rhinoconjunctivitis, or hay fever. Seasonal allergic conjunctivitis is an IgE-mediated hypersensitivity reaction precipitated by small airborne allergens such as pollens.[9] It typically causes bilateral tearing, itching, and redness of the eyes.

The treatment of seasonal allergic rhinoconjunctivitis includes allergen avoidance and the use of cold compresses and eye washes with tear substitute. Allergic conjunctivitis also has been successfully treated with topical mast cell stabilizers, histamine type 1 (H_1) receptor antagonists, and topical nonsteroidal anti-inflammatory drugs.[9] Systemic antihistamines may be useful in prolonged allergic conjunctivitis. In severe cases, a short course of topical corticosteroids may be required to afford symptomatic relief.

Infectious Conjunctivitis

The agents of infectious conjunctivitis include bacteria, viruses, and chlamydiae. Infections may spread from areas adjacent to the conjunctiva or may be bloodborne, as in measles or chickenpox. Newborns can contract conjunctivitis during the birth process.

Bacterial Conjunctivitis. Bacterial conjunctivitis may present as a hyperacute, acute, or chronic infection. *Hyperacute conjunctivitis* is a severe, sight-threatening ocular infection. The infection has an abrupt onset and is characterized by a copious amount of yellow-green drainage. The symptoms, which typically are progressive, include conjunctival redness, chemosis (swelling around the cornea), lid swelling, and tender, swollen preauricular lymph nodes. The most common causes of hyperacute purulent conjunctivitis are *Neisseria gonorrhoeae* and *Neisseria meningitidis,* with *N. gonorrhoeae* being the most common.[8] Gonococcal ocular infections left untreated result in corneal ulceration, ultimately leading to perforation and sometimes permanent loss of vision. Diagnostic methods include immediate Gram staining of ocular specimens and special cultures for *Neisseria* species. Treatment includes systemic antibiotics supplemented with ocular antibiotics and treatment to cover concurrent *Chlamydia* infection. Because of the increasing prevalence of penicillin-resistant *N. gonorrhoeae,* antibiotic choice should be determined by current information regarding antibiotic sensitivity.

Acute bacterial conjunctivitis typically presents with burning, tearing, and mucopurulent or purulent discharge. Common agents of bacterial conjunctivitis are *S. aureus, Streptococcus pneumoniae, Haemophilus influenzae,* and in children also *Moraxella catarrhalis.*[8] The eyelids are sticky, with possible excoriation of the lid margins. Treatment may include local application of antibiotics. The disorder is usually self-limited, lasting approximately 10 to 14 days if untreated. Scrupulous handwashing plus prompt treatment of infected persons and their contacts are essential.[8]

Chronic bacterial conjunctivitis most commonly is caused by *Staphylococcus* species, although other bacteria may be involved. It is often associated with blepharitis and bacterial colonization of eyelid margins. The symptoms of chronic bacterial conjunctivitis vary and can include itching, burning, foreign body sensation, and morning eyelash crusting. Other symptoms include flaky debris and erythema along the lid margins, eyelash loss, and eye redness. Some people with chronic bacterial conjunctivitis also have recurrent styes and chalazia of the lid margins. Treatment includes good eyelid hygiene and application of topical antibiotics.

Viral Conjunctivitis. Etiologic agents of viral conjunctivitis include adenoviruses, herpesviruses, and enteroviruses. Viruses cause up to 80% of all cases of acute conjunctivitis.[8] The infection, which causes generalized conjunctival hyperemia, copious tearing, and minimal exudate, is usually accompanied by pharyngitis, fever, and malaise. Children are affected more often than adults. Swimming pools contaminated because of inadequate chlorination are common sources of infection.

Viral epidemic keratoconjunctivitis is caused by adenoviruses types 8, 19, 29, and 37.[7] It presents with marked discomfort and is highly contagious, with rapid spread from person to person. The disease lasts for at least 2 weeks and may be complicated by visual symptoms due to epithelial and subepithelial involvement. Topical antibiotics are ineffective in controlling the inciting viral agent, but may be used to prevent secondary bacterial infection. For severe cases, an ophthalmologist referral may be required and topical corticosteroids may be prescribed. The most important aspect of treatment is education regarding the highly transmissible nature of the infection. Instructions should include the need for scrupulous handwashing and avoiding the shared use of eyedroppers, eye makeup, goggles, and towels. Persons who use contact lenses should avoid them and wear their prescription glasses instead.

Chlamydial Conjunctivitis. Chlamydial conjunctivitis is usually a benign suppurative conjunctivitis transmitted by the type of *Chlamydia trachomatis* (serotypes D through K) that causes venereal infections[10] (see Chapter 47). It is spread by contaminated genital secretions and occurs in newborns of mothers with *C. trachomatis* infections of the birth canal. It also can be contracted through swimming in unchlorinated pools. The incubation period varies from 5 to 12 days, and the disease may last for several months if untreated. The infection is usually treated with appropriate oral antibiotics.

A more serious form of infection is caused by a different strain of *C. trachomatis* (serotypes A, B, and C).[10] This form of chlamydial infection affects the conjunctiva and causes ulceration and scarring of the cornea. It is the leading cause of preventable blindness in the world. Although the agent is widespread, it is seen mostly in developing countries, particularly those of Africa, Asia, and the Middle East.[7,10] It is transmitted by direct human contact, contaminated objects (fomites), and flies.

Ophthalmia Neonatorum

Ophthalmia neonatorum is a form of conjunctivitis that occurs in newborns younger than 1 month of age and is usually contracted during or soon after vaginal delivery. Many causes are known, including *N. gonorrhoeae, Pseudomonas,* and *C. trachomatis.*[7,11] Epidemiologically, these infections reflect those sexually transmitted infections most common in a particular area. Once the most common form of conjunctivitis in the newborn, gonococcal ophthalmia neonatorum now has an estimated incidence of 0.5 per 100,000 live births, or less than 1% of all reported cases in Canada.[12,13] In comparison, *C. trachomatis* has an incidence of 6 per 100,000 live births, or up to 40% of all cases with ophthalmia neonatorum.[12,13] The primary prevention for all neonates for the prevention of gonococcal ophthalmia is to apply 0.5% erythromycin ointment drops immediately after birth, as 1% silver nitrate, or 1% tetracycline hydrochloride drops are no longer used or available in Canada.[13]

Signs of ophthalmia neonatorum include redness and swelling of the conjunctiva, swelling of the eyelids, and discharge, which may be purulent. The conjunctivitis caused by silver nitrate occurs within 6 to 12 hours of birth and clears within 24 to 48 hours.[12] The incubation period for *N. gonorrhoeae* is 2 to 5 days and for *C. trachomatis,* 5 to 14 days. Infection should be suspected when conjunctivitis develops 48 hours after birth. Ophthalmia neonatorum is a potentially blinding condition, and it can cause serious and potentially systemic manifestations. It requires immediate diagnosis and treatment.

Disorders of the Cornea

At the anterior part of the eyeball, the outer covering of the eye is modified to form the transparent cornea, which bulges anteriorly from its junction with the sclera (Fig. 54.5). The major part of the refraction (*i.e.,* bending) of light rays and focusing of vision occurs in the cornea, responsible for focusing 70% of the light rays. Three layers of tissue form the cornea: an extremely thin outer epithelial layer, which is continuous with the bulbar conjunctiva; a middle layer called the *substantia propria*

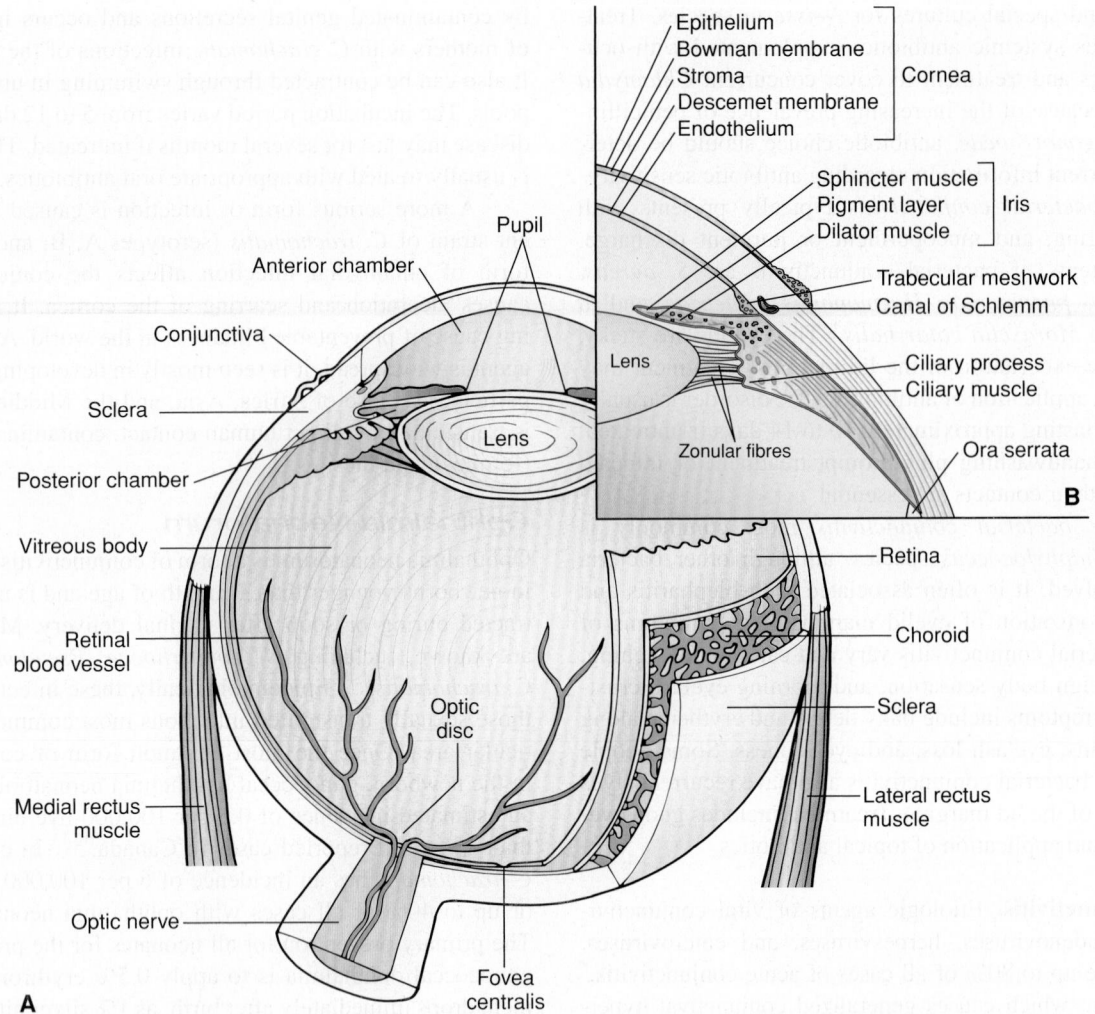

FIGURE 54.5 • A: Transverse section of the eyeball. **B:** Enlargement of the anterior and posterior chambers of the eye, showing the layers of the cornea, the structures of the iris, and aqueous drainage system (trabecular meshwork, Schlemm canal), and the ciliary process and ciliary muscle.

or *stroma;* and an inner endothelial layer, which lies next to the aqueous humour of the anterior chamber.[5,10] The substantia propria is composed of regularly arranged collagen bundles embedded in a mucopolysaccharide matrix. This organization of the collagen fibres, which makes the substantia propria transparent, is necessary for light transmission. Hydration within a limited range is necessary to maintain the spacing of the collagen fibres and transparency. Three layers of the cornea are separated by two important basement membranes: Bowman and Descemet membranes. *Bowman membrane,* which is not a true basement membrane, lies between the corneal epithelium and stroma, acts as a barrier to infection. It does not regenerate and if damaged, an opaque scar forms that can impair vision. *Descemet membrane,* which lies between the corneal endothelium and stroma, has a felt-like appearance and consists of interwoven fibres and pores. Unlike Bowman membrane, it regenerates readily after injury as long as the endothelium is intact.

The cornea is avascular and obtains its nutrient and oxygen supply by diffusion from blood vessels of the adjacent sclera, from the aqueous humour at its deep surface, and from

tears.[10] The corneal epithelium is heavily innervated by sensory neurons (trigeminal nerve [CN V], ophthalmic division [CN V_1]). Epithelial damage causes discomfort that ranges from a foreign body sensation and burning of the eyes to severe, incapacitating pain. Reflex lacrimation is common.

Disorders of the cornea include trauma, inflammation and infection, abnormal corneal deposits, and degenerative processes such as arcus senilis. Diagnosis of corneal disorders is based on history of trauma, medication use, and signs and symptoms associated with corneal irritation and disease.[14] Because of the discomfort involved, examination of the eye is often eased by instillation of a local anesthetic agent. Fluorescein staining can be used to outline an ulcerated area. The biomicroscope (slit lamp) is used for proper examination of the cornea. In cases of an infectious etiology, scrapings from the ulcer are obtained for staining and culture studies.

Corneal Trauma

The integrity of the epithelium and the endothelium is necessary to maintain hydration of the cornea within a limited range. Damage to either structure leads to edema and loss of transparency. Among the causes of corneal edema is the prolonged wearing of contact lenses, which can deprive the epithelium of oxygen, disrupting its integrity. Corneal edema also occurs after a sudden rise in intraocular pressure. With corneal edema, the cornea appears dull, uneven, and hazy; visual acuity decreases, and iridescent vision (*i.e.,* rainbows around lights) occurs.

Trauma that causes abrasions of the cornea can be extremely painful, but if minor, the abrasions usually heal in a few days. The epithelial layer can regenerate, and small defects heal without scarring. If the stroma is damaged, healing occurs more slowly, and the danger of infection is increased. Injuries to the Bowman membrane and the stromal layer heal with scar formation that impairs the transmission of light.

Keratitis

Keratitis refers to inflammation of the cornea. It can be caused by infections, misuse of contact lenses, hypersensitivity reactions, ischemia, trauma, defects in tearing, and interruption in sensory innervation, as occurs with local anesthesia. Scar tissue formation due to keratitis is the leading cause of blindness and impaired vision throughout the world. Most of this vision loss is preventable if the condition is diagnosed early and appropriate treatment is begun.

Keratitis can be divided into two types: nonulcerative, in which all the layers of the epithelium are affected but the epithelium remains intact, and ulcerative, in which parts of the epithelium, stroma, or both are destroyed. Nonulcerative or interstitial keratitis is associated with many diseases, including syphilis, tuberculosis, and lupus erythematosus. It also may result from a viral infection entering through a small defect in the cornea. Treatment usually consists of topical antibiotics and possibly anti-inflammatory agents.

Causes of ulcerative keratitis include infectious agents such as those causing conjunctivitis (*e.g., Staphylococcus, S. pneumoniae, Chlamydia*), exposure trauma, and use of extended-wear contact lenses. Bacterial keratitis is aggressive and demands immediate care. Exposure trauma may result from deformities of the lid, paralysis of the lid muscles, or severe exophthalmos. Mooren ulcer is a chronic, painful, indolent ulcer that occurs in the absence of infection. It is usually seen in older persons and may affect both eyes. Although the cause is unknown, an autoimmune origin is suspected.

Herpes Simplex Keratitis. Herpes simplex virus (HSV) keratitis with stromal scarring is the most common cause of corneal ulceration and blindness in the Western world.[14] Most cases are caused by HSV type 1, the cause of oral infections. However, in neonatal infections acquired during passage through the birth canal, approximately 80% are caused by HSV type 2 (the cause of genital herpes). The disease can occur as a primary or recurrent infection.[14] Primary epithelial infections are the optical counterpart of labial herpes with similar immunologic and pathologic features as well as a similar time course. During childhood, mild primary HSV

infection may go unnoticed. After the initial primary infection, the virus may persist in a quiescent or latent state in the trigeminal ganglion and possibly in the cornea without causing signs of infection.

Recurrent infection may be precipitated by various poorly understood, stress-related factors that reactivate the virus. Involvement is usually unilateral. The first symptoms are irritation, photophobia, and tearing. Some reduction in vision may occur when the lesion affects the central part of the cornea. Because corneal anesthesia occurs early in the disease, the symptoms may be minimal, and the person may delay seeking medical care. A history of fever blisters or other herpetic infection is often noted, but corneal lesions may be the only sign of recurrent herpes infection. Most typically, the corneal lesion involves the epithelium and has a typical branching pattern. These epithelial lesions heal without scarring. Herpetic lesions that involve the stromal layer of the cornea produce increasingly severe corneal opacities. Although previously thought to be a purely immunologic response to viral particles or virally induced cellular changes, there is increasing evidence that infection due to active viral particles can occur in stromal and possibly endothelial cells, as well as other tissues in the anterior segment such as the iris and trabecular endothelium.

The treatment of HSV keratitis focuses on eliminating viral replication in the cornea while minimizing the damaging effects of the inflammatory process. It involves the use of epithelial debridement and drug therapy. Debridement is used to remove the virus from the corneal epithelium. Topical antiviral agents, such as trifluridine or idoxuridine drops, are used to promote healing.[14] Oral antiviral agents (*e.g.,* acyclovir) may be helpful for treatment of severe keratitis and as prophylaxis against recurrence, particularly in persons with compromised immune function. Although corticosteroids may control the damaging inflammatory responses, they do so at the expense of facilitating viral replication. With a few exceptions, their use is contraindicated.

Varicella Zoster Ophthalmicus. Herpes zoster or shingles is a relatively common infection caused by herpesvirus type 3, the same virus that causes varicella (chickenpox).[14] It occurs when the varicella virus, which has remained dormant in the neurosensory ganglia since the primary infection, is reactivated. Herpes ophthalmicus, which represents 10% to 20% of all cases of herpes zoster, occurs when reactivation of the latent virus occurs in the ganglia of the ophthalmic division of the trigeminal nerve.[15] Immunocompromised persons, particularly those with human immunodeficiency virus (HIV) infection, are at higher risk for developing herpes zoster ophthalmicus than those with a normally functioning immune system.

Herpes zoster ophthalmicus usually presents with malaise, fever, headache, and burning and itching of the periorbital area. These symptoms commonly precede the ocular eruption by a day or two. The rash, which is initially vesicular, becomes pustular and then crusting (see Chapter 61). Involvement of the tip of the nose and lid margins indicates a high likelihood of ocular involvement (*i.e.,* Hutchinson sign). Ocular signs include conjunctivitis, keratitis, episcleritis, and anterior uveitis, often with elevated intraocular pressure. Persons with corneal disease present with varying degrees of decreased vision, pain, and sensitivity to light. Persons who are immunocompromised are at a high risk for retinal necrosis, requiring immediate treatment.

Treatment includes the use of high-dose oral antiviral drugs (*i.e.,* acyclovir, famciclovir, valacyclovir). Initiation of treatment within the first 72 hours after the appearance of the rash reduces the incidence of ocular complications and subsequent risk of postherpetic neuralgia (see Chapter 49).

Acanthamoeba **Keratitis.** *Acanthamoeba* is a free-living protozoan that thrives in contaminated water.[10] *Acanthamoeba* keratitis is a rare but serious and sight-threatening complication of wearing soft contact lenses, particularly when they are worn overnight beyond doctor-recommended periods or when poor disinfection techniques are used. It also may occur in noncontact lens wearers after exposure to contaminated water or soil. It is characterized by pain that is disproportionate to the clinical manifestations, redness of the eye, and photophobia. The disorder commonly is misdiagnosed as herpes keratitis. Diagnosis is confirmed by scrapings and culture with specially prepared medium. In the early stages of infection, epithelial debridement may be beneficial. Treatment includes a combination of antibacterial, antifungal, and antiparasitic agents. However, the organism may encyst within the corneal stroma, making treatment more difficult. Keratoplasty may be necessary in advanced disease to arrest the progression of the infection.

Abnormal Corneal Deposits

The cornea frequently is the site for deposition of abnormal metabolic products. In hypercalcemia, calcium salts can precipitate in the cornea, producing a cloudy band keratopathy. Cystine crystals are deposited in cystinosis, cholesterol esters in hypercholesterolemia, and a golden ring of copper (*i.e.,* Kayser–Fleischer ring) in hepatolenticular degeneration due to Wilson disease. Pharmacologic agents, such as chloroquine, can result in crystal deposits in the cornea.

Arcus senilis is an extremely common, bilateral, benign corneal degeneration that may occur at any age, but is more common in the elderly. It consists of a greyish-white infiltrate, approximately 2 mm wide, that occurs at the periphery of the cornea. It represents an extracellular lipid infiltration and commonly is associated with hyperlipidemia. Arcus senilis does not produce visual symptoms, and there is no treatment for the disorder.

Corneal Transplantation

Advances in ophthalmologic surgery permit corneal transplantation using a cadaver cornea. Unlike kidney or heart transplantation procedures, which are associated with considerable risk of rejection of the transplanted organ (see Chapter 19), the use of cadaver corneas entails minimal danger of rejection.

The low rejection rate is due to several factors: the cornea is avascular, including lymphatics, thereby limiting perfusion by immune elements; major histocompatibility complexes (class II) are virtually absent in the cornea; antigen-presenting cells are not present in great numbers; the cornea secretes immunosuppressive factors; and corneal cells secrete substances (*e.g.,* Fas ligand) that protect against apoptosis, thereby minimizing inflammation.[16]

Disorders of the Uveal Tract

The middle vascular layer, or uveal tract, is an incomplete ball with gaps at the pupil and the optic nerve. The pigmented uveal tract has three distinct regions: the choroid, ciliary body, and the iris. The *choroid* is a highly vascular, dark brown membrane that forms the posterior five sixths of the uveal tract. Its blood vessels provide nourishment for the other layers of the eyeball. Its brown pigment, produced by melanocytes, absorbs light within the eyeball and light that penetrates the retina. The light absorptive function prevents the scattering of light and is important for visual acuity, particularly with high background illumination levels. The *ciliary body* is a thickened ring of tissue that encircles the lens. It has smooth muscle and secretory functions. Its smooth muscle function contributes to changes in lens shape and its secretory function to the production of aqueous humour.

The *iris* is an adjustable diaphragm that permits changes in pupil size and in the light entering the eye. The posterior surface of the iris is formed by a two-layer epithelium continuous with those layers covering the ciliary body. The anterior layer contains the dilator or radial muscles of the iris. Just anterior to these muscles is a layer of highly vascular connective tissue. Embedded in this layer are concentric rings of smooth muscle that compose the sphincter muscle of the pupil. The anterior layer of the iris forms an irregular anterior surface, containing many fibroblasts and melanocytes. Eye colour differences result from the density of the pigment. The amount of pigment decreases from that found in dark brown eyes through shades of brown and green to that found in blue eyes.

Several mutations affect the pigment of the uveal tract, including albinism. *Albinism* is a genetic (autosomal recessive trait) deficiency of tyrosinase, the enzyme needed for the synthesis of melanin by the melanocytes. Tyrosinase-negative albinism, also called *classic albinism,* is characterized by an absence of tyrosinase; affected persons have white hair, pink skin, and light blue eyes. In these persons, excessive light penetrates the unpigmented iris and choroid, and, to some extent, the anterior sclera. Their photoreceptors are flooded with excess light, and visual acuity is markedly reduced, often leading to abnormal jerking movements of the eyes. Excess stimulation of the photoreceptors at normal or high illumination levels is experienced as painful photophobia.

Uveitis

Inflammation of the entire uveal tract, which supports the lens and neural components of the eye, is called *uveitis.* It is one of several inflammatory disorders of ocular tissue with clinical features in common and an immunologically based cause.[17] Uveitis can be divided into anterior uveitis, (also known as iritis), intermediate uveitis, posterior uveitis, or panuveitis. Careful history and clinical evaluation must be performed to determine if there is an infectious agent (viral, bacterial, fungal, or parasitic) or inflammatory agent (autoimmune, malignant, or idiopathic) causing the disease. A serious consequence of uveitis can be the involvement of the underlying retina. Parasitic invasion of the choroid can result in local atrophic changes that usually involve the retina; examples include toxoplasmosis and histoplasmosis. Once infection is ruled out, treatment can include topical steroids, oral steroids, and even oral disease modifying agents like methotrexate, or biologics.

The Pupil and Pupillary Reflexes

Changes in pupil size are controlled by contraction or relaxation of the sphincter and radial muscles of the iris. The pupillary reflex, which controls the size of the pupillary opening, is controlled by the autonomic nervous system, with the parasympathetic nervous system producing pupillary constriction or *miosis* and the sympathetic nervous system producing pupillary dilation or *mydriasis*. The sphincter muscle that produces pupillary constriction is innervated by postganglionic parasympathetic neurons of the ciliary ganglion and other scattered ganglion cells between the scleral and choroid layers. Part of the oculomotor (CN III) nucleus is called the *Edinger–Westphal nucleus*.[18] This autonomic nucleus, found in the midbrain, provides the preganglionic innervation for these parasympathetic axons. Pupillary dilation by the radial muscles is provided by sympathetic innervation under excitatory descending control from the hypothalamus. Innervation is derived from preganglionic neurons in the upper thoracic cord, which send axons along the sympathetic chain to synapse with postganglionic neurons in the superior ciliary ganglion (see Chapter 48, Fig. 48.28). Postganglionic fibres travel along the surfaces of the internal carotid artery and smaller arteries to reach the eye.

The pupillary reflex is controlled by a region in the midbrain called the *pretectum*. Pretectal areas on each side of the brain are connected, explaining the binocular aspect of the light reflex. The afferent stimuli for pupillary constriction arise in the ganglionic cells of the retina and are transmitted to the *pretectal nuclei* at the junction of the thalamus and the midbrain, and from there to preganglionic neurons in the oculomotor (CN III) nuclei (Fig. 54.6).

Normal function of the pupillary reflex mechanism can be tested by shining a penlight into one eye of the person being tested. To avoid a change in pupil size due to accommodation, the person is asked to stare into the distance. A rapid constriction of the pupil exposed to light should occur; this is called the *direct pupillary light reflex*. Because the reflex is normally bilateral, the contralateral pupil also should constrict, a reaction called the *consensual pupillary light reflex*. The circuitry of the light reflex is partially separated from

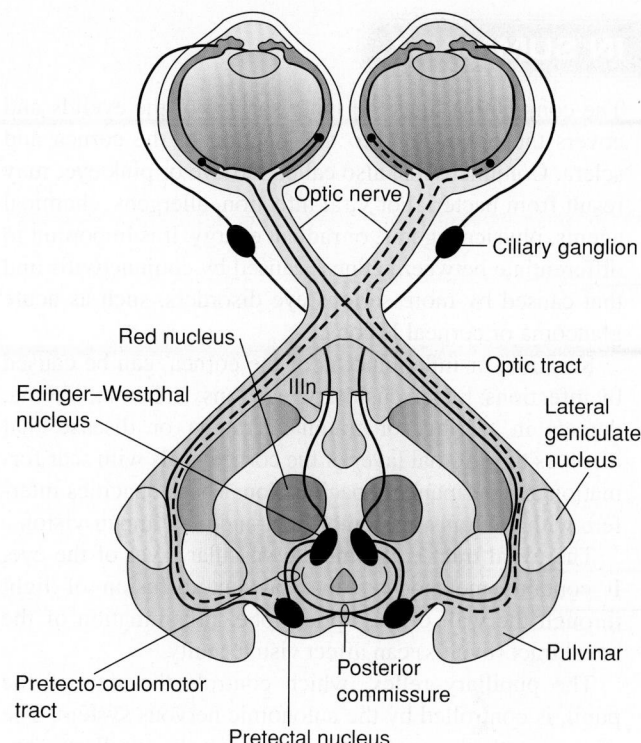

FIGURE 54.6 • Diagram of the path of the pupillary light reflex. (Reproduced with permission from Walsh F. B., Hoyt W. F. (1969). *Clinical neuro-ophthalmology* (3rd ed., Vol. 1). Baltimore: Williams & Wilkins.)

the main optic pathway. This is illustrated by the fact that the pupillary reflex remains unaffected when lesions to the optic radiations or the visual cortex occur.

Integrity of the dual autonomic control of pupillary diameter is vulnerable to trauma, tumour enlargement, or vascular disease. With diffuse damage to the forebrain involving the thalamus and hypothalamus, the pupils are typically small but respond to light. Damage to the CN III nucleus results in permanent pupillary dilation in the affected eye. Lesions affecting the cervical spinal cord or the ascending sympathetic ganglionic chain in the neck or internal carotid artery (*e.g.,* Horner syndrome) can interrupt the sympathetic control of the iris dilator muscle, resulting in permanent pupillary constriction. Tumours of the orbit that compress structures behind the eye can eliminate all pupillary reflexes, usually before destroying the optic nerve.

Pupillary size can also be differentially affected by pharmacologic agents. Bilateral pupillary constriction is characteristic of opiate usage. Pupillary dilation results when topical parasympathetic blocking agents such as atropine are applied and sympathetic pupillodilatory function is left unopposed. Dilation can be enhanced by sympathomimetic agents. These medications are used by ophthalmologists and optometrists to facilitate the examination of the transparent media and fundus of the eye. Miotic drugs (*e.g.,* pilocarpine), which are used in the treatment of angle-closure glaucoma (to be discussed), produce pupil constriction and in that manner facilitate aqueous humour circulation.

IN SUMMARY

The conjunctiva lines the inner surface of the eyelids and covers the optic globe to the junction of the cornea and sclera. Conjunctivitis, also called red eye or pink eye, may result from bacterial or viral infection, allergens, chemical agents, physical agents, or radiant energy. It is important to differentiate between redness caused by conjunctivitis and that caused by more serious eye disorders, such as acute glaucoma or corneal lesions.

Keratitis, or inflammation of the cornea, can be caused by infections, hypersensitivity reactions, ischemia, trauma, defects in tearing, or trauma. Trauma or disease that involves the stromal layer of the cornea heals with scar formation and permanent opacification. These opacities interfere with the transmission of light and may impair vision.

The uveal tract is the middle vascular layer of the eye. It contains melanocytes that prevent diffusion of light through the wall of the optic globe. Inflammation of the uveal tract (uveitis) can affect visual acuity.

The pupillary reflex, which controls the size of the pupil, is controlled by the autonomic nervous system. The parasympathetic nervous system controls pupillary constriction, and the sympathetic nervous system controls pupillary dilation.

INTRAOCULAR PRESSURE AND GLAUCOMA

After completing this section of the chapter, you should be able to meet the following objectives:

- Describe the formation and outflow of aqueous humour from the eye and relate to the development of glaucoma.
- Compare open-angle and angle-closure glaucoma in terms of pathology, symptomatology, and diagnosis and treatment.
- Explain why glaucoma leads to blindness.

Glaucoma comprises a group of diseases defined by characteristic progressive optic nerve degeneration with the development of distinctive patterns of visual dysfunction, leading to irreversible blindness if untreated. While elevated intraocular pressure is a primary risk factor and often associated with glaucoma, its absence or presence does not have a role in the definition of the disease. It is one of the leading causes of blindness worldwide, and is second only to age-related macular degeneration as the leading cause of blindness in North America.[2,19] The condition is often asymptomatic, and a significant loss of peripheral vision may occur before medical attention is sought (Fig. 54.1D).

Control of Intraocular Pressure

The intraocular pressure is largely regulated by the aqueous humour, which fills the anterior chamber of the eye. The aqueous humour is produced by the ciliary body and passes from the posterior chamber through the pupil into the anterior chamber[20] (Fig. 54.7A). Aqueous humour leaves through the iridocorneal angle between the anterior surface of the iris and the sclera. Here it filters through the trabecular meshwork and enters the canal of Schlemm for return to the venous circulation. The canal of Schlemm is actually a thin-walled vein that extends circumferentially around the iris of the eye. Its endothelial membrane is so porous that even large protein molecules up to the size of a red blood cell can pass from the posterior chamber into the canal of Schlemm.

The pressure of the aqueous humour results from a balance of several factors, including the rate of aqueous secretion, the resistance to flow between the iris and the ciliary body, and the resistance to resorption at the trabeculated region of the sclera at the iridocorneal angle. Normally, the rate of aqueous production is equal to the rate of aqueous outflow, and the intraocular pressure is maintained within a normal range of 9 to 21 mm Hg.[21]

Tonometry is the measurement of intraocular pressure. The most widely used instrument is the Goldmann applanation tonometer, which is attached to a slit lamp and measures the force required to flatten a fixed area on the cornea. Central corneal thickness, which can be measured by either optical or ultrasonic methods, is thought to influence the accuracy of measurement, with intraocular pressure being overestimated in eyes with a thick cornea and underestimated in eyes with a thin cornea.[20] Another type of tonometer, the noncontact ("airpuff") tonometer, which uses the rebound force of a small puff of air blown against the cornea to estimate the intraocular pressure, is not as accurate as the applanation tonometer. However, this method does not require anesthetic drops because no instrument touches the eye. It is therefore more easily used by technicians and is useful in screening programs.[20]

Glaucoma

Glaucoma usually results from congenital or acquired lesions of the anterior segment of the eye that mechanically obstruct aqueous outflow.[10,20] Glaucoma is commonly classified as open-angle (*i.e.*, wide-angle) or angle-closure (*i.e.*, narrowangle) glaucoma, depending on the location of the compromised outflow, and may occur as a primary or secondary disorder. Primary glaucoma occurs without evidence of preexisting ocular or systemic disease. Secondary glaucoma can result from inflammatory processes that affect the eye, from tumours, or from blood cells of trauma-produced hemorrhage that obstruct the outflow of aqueous humour.

In persons with glaucoma, temporary or permanent impairment of vision results from degenerative changes in the retina and optic nerve and from corneal edema and opacification. Damage to optic nerve axons in the region of the optic

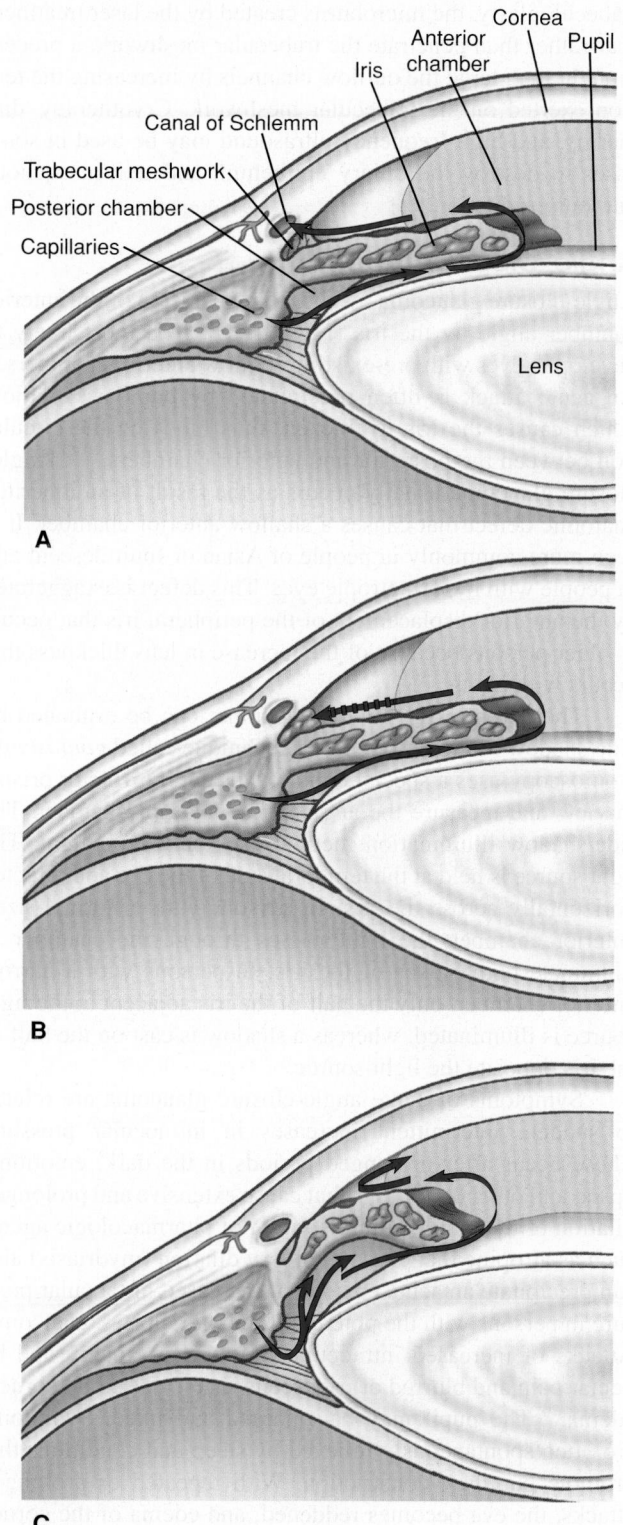

A

B

C

FIGURE 54.7 • A: Normally, aqueous humour, which is secreted in the posterior chamber, gains access to the anterior chamber by flowing through the pupil. In the angle of the anterior chamber, it passes through the canal of Schlemm into the venous system. **B:** In open-angle glaucoma, the outflow of aqueous humour is obstructed at the trabecular meshwork. **C:** In angle-closure glaucoma, the aqueous humour encounters resistance to flow through the pupil. Increased pressure in the posterior chamber produces a forward bowing of the peripheral iris, so that the iris blocks the trabecular meshwork.

nerve can be recognized on ophthalmoscopic examination. The normal optic disc has a central depression called the *optic cup.* With progressive atrophy of axons caused by increased intraocular pressure, pallor of the optic disc develops, and the size and depth of the optic cup increase.[19] Because changes in the optic cup precede visual field loss, regular ophthalmoscopic examinations are important for detecting eye changes that occur with increased intraocular pressure. Many attempts have been made to quantify the optic disc changes in people with glaucoma using various photographic techniques and, more recently, scanning laser imaging systems and optical coherence tomography.

Advances in computer technology allow detection and quantification of visual changes due to glaucoma. These tests of vision include white-on-white and blue-on-yellow visual field testing, testing of contrast sensitivity, and dark adaptation. Scanning laser technology and optical coherence tomography tests can detect damage to retinal ganglion axons before visual field loss occurs.

Open-Angle Glaucoma

Primary open-angle glaucoma is the most common form of glaucoma.[20,22,23] The condition is characterized by an abnormal increase in intraocular pressure that occurs without obstruction at the iridocorneal angle, hence the name *open-angle glaucoma.* Instead, it usually occurs because of an abnormality of the trabecular meshwork that controls the flow of aqueous humour into the canal of Schlemm[10,20] (Fig. 54.7B). Secondary open-angle glaucoma occurs as a result of other conditions, including the formation of red cell fragments after trauma and iris pigment epithelial granules that may clog the trabecular meshwork.

The condition is usually asymptomatic and chronic, causing progressive damage to the optic nerve and visual field loss unless it is appropriately treated. Elevated intraocular pressure is a primary factor for open-angle glaucoma, but it is not the only diagnostic factor. Some people maintain a higher intraocular pressure without evidence of optic nerve damage or visual field loss, demonstrating a condition described as *glaucoma suspect* or *ocular hypertension.*[20] It is questionable whether damage to the optic nerve results from excessive intraocular pressure, decreased blood flow to the optic nerve, or both factors.

The etiology of primary open-angle glaucoma remains unclear. Major risk factors for this disorder include an age of 40 years and older, black race, a positive first-degree family history, myopia, and increased intraocular pressure.[22] Other risk factors with moderate to fair epidemiologic evidence include hypertension, type 2 diabetes, hyperthyroidism, migraine headaches, and sleep apnea. In some persons, the use of moderate amounts of topical or inhaled corticosteroid medications can cause an increase in intraocular pressure. Sensitive persons also may sustain an increase in intraocular pressure with the use of systemic corticosteroid drugs. There is emerging evidence that central corneal thickness is also an important predictor for the development of primary open-angle glaucoma, and it may be a relevant predictor of both glaucoma progression and response to intraocular pressure-lowering drugs.[22]

Diagnostic methods include applanation tonometry, ophthalmoscopic visualization of the optic nerve, and central visual field testing. Measurement of intraocular pressures provides a means of assessing glaucoma risk. Because the condition is usually asymptomatic, persons at risk for open-angle glaucoma should have regular direct ophthalmoscopic examinations, on both eyes, concentrating on the optic disc. Optic disc changes frequently are noted before visual field defects become apparent. Periodic stereoscopic assessment of the optic disc by an eye care provider trained in the detection of glaucoma is strongly recommended for at-risk patients.

The elevation in intraocular pressure in persons with open-angle glaucoma is usually treated pharmacologically or, in cases where pharmacologic treatment fails, by increasing aqueous outflow through a surgically created pathway. Drugs used in the long-term management of glaucoma fall into five classes: β-adrenergic antagonists, prostaglandin analogs, adrenergic agonists, carbonic anhydrase inhibitors, and cholinergic agonists.[20] Most glaucoma drugs are applied topically. However, systemic side effects may occur. When treatment with one drug does not reduce the intraocular pressure to the target level, a drug from a different class may be used or a second medication may be added as adjunctive therapy.

Topical β-adrenergic antagonists are usually the drugs of first choice for lowering intraocular pressure. The β-adrenergic antagonists are thought to lower intraocular pressure by decreasing aqueous humour production in the ciliary body. Systemic absorption of these eye drops can cause bradycardia and bronchospasm in persons with asthma. Carbonic anhydrase inhibitors reduce the secretion of aqueous humour by the ciliary epithelium. The topical carbonic anhydrase inhibitors (dorzolamide and brinzolamide) are often used as adjunctive therapy, but rarely as initial therapy. Selective α_2-adrenergic agonists (*i.e.,* brimonidine and apraclonidine) increase aqueous outflow in addition to decreasing aqueous production. They are effective as an adjunctive, or occasionally as a primary treatment agent. Local ocular allergy often limits the usefulness of apraclonidine.

Several classes of drugs increase aqueous outflow. Prostaglandins are locally acting substances found in most tissues. At low concentrations, prostaglandin $F_2\alpha$ increases the outflow of aqueous humour through the iris root and ciliary body, either by decreasing the extracellular matrix or by relaxing the ciliary musculature. Latanoprost, a topical prostaglandin analog, is now one of the most frequently prescribed glaucoma drugs. Acetylcholine is the postganglionic neuromediator for the parasympathetic nervous system; it increases aqueous outflow through contraction of the ciliary muscle and pupillary constriction (miosis). Pilocarpine, a parasympathomimetic miotic and once the mainstay of treatment, has largely been replaced by newer and more effective drugs.

When a reduction in intraocular pressure cannot be maintained through pharmacologic methods, laser or surgical trabeculoplasty may become necessary. With laser trabeculoplasty, the microburns created by the laser treatment scar rather than penetrate the trabecular meshwork, a process thought to enlarge the outflow channels by increasing the tension exerted on the trabecular meshwork. Cryotherapy, diathermy, and high-frequency ultrasound may be used in some cases to destroy the ciliary epithelium and reduce aqueous humour production.

Angle-Closure Glaucoma

Angle-closure glaucoma results from occlusion of the anterior chamber angle by the iris (Fig. 54.7C). It is most likely to develop in eyes with pre-existing shallow anterior chambers.[23] An acute attack is often precipitated by pupillary dilation, which causes the iris to thicken, thus blocking the circulation between the posterior and anterior chambers.[10,20] Angle-closure glaucoma usually occurs as the result of an inherited anatomic defect that causes a shallow anterior chamber. It is seen more commonly in people of Asian or Inuit descent and in people with hypermetropic eyes. This defect is exaggerated by the anterior displacement of the peripheral iris that occurs in older persons because of the increase in lens thickness that occurs with aging.

The depth of the anterior chamber can be evaluated by side/shadow illumination or by a technique called *gonioscopy*. Gonioscopy uses a special contact lens and mirrors or prisms to view and measure the angle of the anterior chamber. The side/shadow illumination method uses only a penlight. The light source is held at the temporal side of the eye and directed horizontally across the iris. In persons with a normal-sized anterior chamber, the light passes through the chamber to illuminate both halves of the iris. In persons with a narrow anterior chamber, only the half of the iris adjacent to the light source is illuminated, whereas a shadow is cast on the half of the iris opposite the light source.

Symptoms of acute angle-closure glaucoma are related to sudden, intermittent increases in intraocular pressure. These occur after prolonged periods in the dark, emotional upset, and other conditions that cause extensive and prolonged dilation of the pupil. Administration of pharmacologic agents such as atropine that cause pupillary dilation (mydriasis) also can precipitate an acute episode of increased intraocular pressure in persons with the potential for angle-closure glaucoma. Attacks of increased intraocular pressure are manifested by ocular pain and blurred or iridescent vision caused by corneal edema.[20] The pupil may be enlarged and fixed. Symptoms are often spontaneously relieved by sleep and conditions that promote pupillary constriction. With repeated or prolonged attacks, the eye becomes reddened, and edema of the cornea may develop, giving the cornea a hazy appearance. A unilateral, often excruciating, headache is common. Nausea and vomiting may occur, causing the headache to be confused with migraine.

Some persons with congenitally narrow anterior chambers never develop symptoms, and others develop symptoms only in older age. Because of the dangers of vision loss, those with narrow anterior chambers should be warned about the significance of blurred vision, halos, and ocular pain. Sometimes, decreased visual acuity and an unreactive pupil may be the only clues to angle-closure glaucoma in older adults.

Acute angle-closure glaucoma is an ophthalmic emergency. Treatment is initially directed at reducing the intraocular pressure, usually with pharmacologic agents, including oral, topical, and intravenous medications. Once the intraocular pressure is under control, a laser peripheral iridotomy is performed to create a permanent opening between the anterior and posterior chambers, allowing the aqueous humour to bypass the pupillary block. The anatomic abnormalities responsible for angle-closure glaucoma are usually bilateral, and prophylactic surgery is often performed on the other eye.[23]

Congenital and Infantile Glaucoma

There are several types of childhood glaucoma, including congenital glaucoma, which is present at birth, and infantile glaucoma, which develops during the first 2 to 3 years of life. As with glaucoma in adults, childhood glaucoma can occur as a primary or secondary disorder.

Congenital glaucoma is caused by a disorder in which the anterior chamber retains its fetal configuration, with aberrant trabecular meshwork extending to the root of the iris, or is covered by a membrane. In general it has a much poorer prognosis than infantile glaucoma. Primary infantile glaucoma occurs in approximately 1 in 10,000 live births.[20] It is bilateral in 65% to 80% of cases, and occurs more commonly in boys than girls. About 10% of cases have a familial origin, and the rest are either sporadic or possibly multifactorial with reduced penetrance. The familial cases are usually transmitted as an autosomal dominant trait with potentially high penetrance. Recent studies suggest a mutation in chromosome 2 (2p21-p22 regions). This gene is expressed in the tissues of the anterior chamber of the eye and its protein product plays an important role in the metabolism of molecules that are used in signalling pathways during the terminal stages of anterior chamber development.[24]

The earliest symptoms of congenital or infantile glaucoma are excessive lacrimation and photophobia. Affected infants tend to be fussy, have poor eating habits, and rub their eyes frequently. Diffuse edema of the cornea usually occurs, giving the eye a greyish-white appearance. Chronic elevation of the intraocular pressure before the age of 3 years causes enlargement of the entire optic globe. Early surgical treatment is necessary to prevent blindness.

IN SUMMARY

Glaucoma is a leading cause of blindness worldwide. It is characterized by conditions that cause an increase in intraocular pressure and that, if untreated, can lead to atrophy of the optic disc and progressive blindness. The aqueous humour is formed by the ciliary epithelium in the posterior chamber and flows through the pupil to the angle formed by the cornea and the iris. Here, it filters through the trabecular meshwork and enters the canal of Schlemm for return to the venous circulation. Glaucoma results from overproduction or impeded outflow of aqueous humour from the anterior chamber of the eye.

There are two types of glaucoma: open-angle and angle-closure. Open-angle glaucoma is caused by microscopic obstruction of the trabecular meshwork. Open-angle glaucoma is usually asymptomatic, and considerable loss of the visual field often occurs before medical treatment is sought. Routine screening by applanation tonometry provides one of the best means for early detection of glaucoma before vision loss has occurred. Angle-closure glaucoma is caused by a narrow anterior chamber and blockage of the outflow channels at the angle formed by the iris and the cornea. This occurs when the iris becomes thickened during pupillary dilation. Congenital glaucoma is caused by a disorder in which the anterior chamber retains its fetal configuration, with aberrant trabecular meshwork extending to the root of the iris or covered by a membrane. Early surgical treatment is necessary to prevent blindness.

DISORDERS OF THE LENS AND LENS FUNCTION

After completing this section of the chapter, you should be able to meet the following objectives:

- Describe changes in eye structure that occur with nearsighted and farsighted vision.
- Describe the changes in lens structure that occur with cataract.
- Cite risk factors and visual changes associated with cataract.
- Describe the treatment of persons with cataracts.

The function of the eye is to transform light energy into nerve signals that can be transmitted to the cerebral cortex for interpretation. Optically, the eye is similar to a camera. It contains a lens system that focuses an inverted image, an aperture (*i.e.,* the pupil) for controlling light exposure, and a retina that corresponds to the film and records the image.

Disorders of Refraction and Accommodation

The lens is an avascular, transparent, biconvex body, the posterior side of which is more convex than the anterior side. A thin, highly elastic lens capsule is attached to the surrounding ciliary body by delicate suspensory radial ligaments called *zonules,* which hold the lens in place (Fig. 54.5). The tough elastic sclera, in providing for a change in lens shape, acts as a bow, and the zonule and the lens capsule act as the bowstring. The suspensory ligaments and lens capsule are normally under tension, causing the lens to have a flattened shape for distant vision. Contraction of the muscle fibres of the ciliary body narrows the diameter of the ciliary body, relaxes the fibres of the suspensory ligaments, and allows the lens to relax to a more convex shape for near vision.

When light passes from one medium to another, its velocity is decreased or increased, and the direction of light transmission is changed. This change in direction of light rays is called *refraction*. When light rays pass through the centre of a lens, their direction is not changed; however, other rays passing peripherally through a lens are bent (Fig. 54.8). The refractive power of a lens is usually described as the distance (in metres) from its surface to the point at which the rays come into focus (*i.e.*, focal length). Usually, this is reported as the reciprocal of this distance (*i.e.*, diopters).[21] For example, a lens that brings an object into focus at 0.5 m has a refractive power of 2 diopters (1/0.5 = 2). With a fixed power lens, the closer an object is to the lens, the further behind the lens is

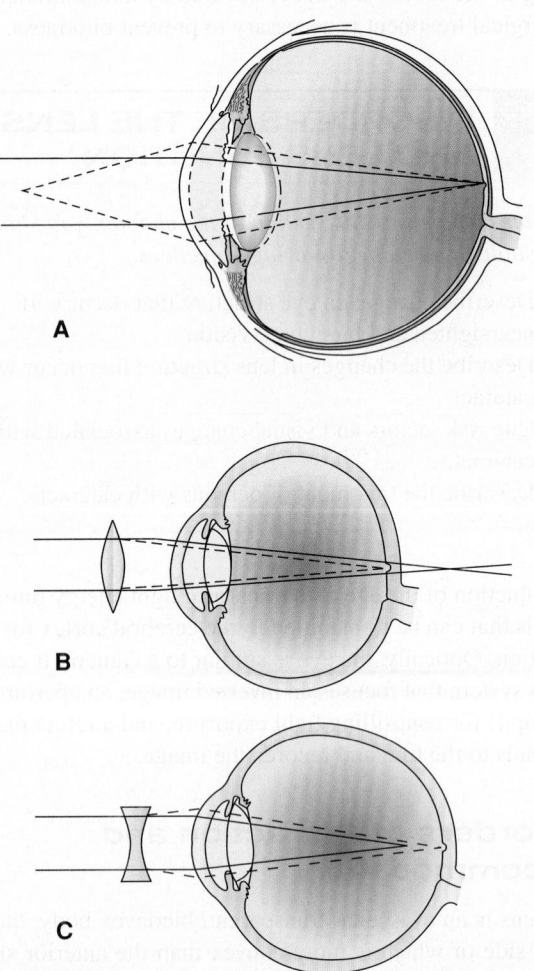

FIGURE 54.8 • A: Accommodation. The *solid lines* represent rays of light from a distant object, and the *dotted lines* represent rays from a near object. The lens is flatter for the former and more convex for the latter. In each case, the rays of light are brought to a focus on the retina. **B:** Hyperopia corrected by a biconvex lens, shown by the *dotted lines.* **C:** Myopia corrected by a biconcave lens, shown by the *dotted lines.*

its focus point. The closer the object, the stronger and more precise the focusing system must be.

In the eye, the major refraction of light begins at the convex corneal surface. Further refraction occurs as light moves from the posterior corneal surface to the aqueous humour, from the aqueous humour to the anterior lens surface, from the anterior lens surface to the posterior lens surface, and from the posterior lens surface to the vitreous humour.

Disorders of Refraction

A perfectly shaped optic globe and cornea result in optimal visual acuity, producing a sharp image in focus at all points on the retinal surface in the posterior part, or fundus, of the eye. Unfortunately, individual differences in formation and growth of the eyeball and cornea frequently result in inappropriate focal image formation. If the anterior–posterior dimension of the eyeball is too short, the image is theoretically focused posterior to (behind) the retina. This is called *hyperopia* or *farsightedness* (Fig. 54.8B). In such cases, the accommodative changes of the lens can bring distant images into focus, but near images become blurred. Hyperopia is corrected by appropriate convex-surface lenses. If the anterior–posterior dimension of the eyeball is too long, the focus point for an infinitely distant target is anterior to the retina. This condition is called *myopia* or *nearsightedness* (Fig. 54.8C). Persons with myopia can see close objects without problems because accommodative changes in their lens bring near objects into focus, but distant objects are blurred. Myopia can be corrected with an appropriate concave-surface lens. Refractive corneal surgeries such as laser in situ keratomileusis (LASIK) and photorefractive keratectomy can be performed to correct the corneal curvature to create accurate optical focus.[14,25]

Refractive defects of the corneal surface do not permit the formation of a sharp image. Nonuniform curvature of the refractive medium with regard to the horizontal and vertical planes is called *astigmatism*. Astigmatism is usually the result of an asymmetric bowing of the cornea, but it can result from defects in the cornea, the lens, or the retina. Lens correction is available to sharpen focus in case of such refractive error.

Disorders of Accommodation

Because the retina is at a fixed distance from the lens, adjustability in the refractive power of the lens is needed so that a clear image is maintained as gaze is shifted from a far to a near object. The process by which the refractive power of the lens is increased, and the diverging light rays are bent more sharply, is called *accommodation*. Accommodation is neurologically associated with convergence of the eyes and pupillary constriction, and results from thickening of the lens through contraction of the ciliary muscle. Contraction of the ciliary muscles is controlled mainly by the parasympathetic fibres of the oculomotor cranial nerve (CN III). In near vision, pupillary constriction (*i.e.*, miosis) improves the clarity of the retinal image. This must be balanced against the resultant decrease in light intensity reaching the retina. During changes from near to far vision, pupillary dilation partially compensates for the reduced size of the retinal image by increasing the light entering the pupil. A third component of accommodation involves the reflex narrowing of the palpebral opening during near vision and widening during far vision.

Paralysis of the ciliary muscle, with loss of accommodation, is called *cycloplegia*. Pharmacologic cycloplegia is sometimes necessary to aid refractive examination of the eye, especially in small children who are unable to hold a steady degree of accommodation during the examination. Lens shape is totally controlled by the pretectal region and the parasympathetic pathways through the oculomotor nerve to the ciliary muscle. Accommodation is lost with destruction of this pathway.

The term *presbyopia* refers to a decrease in accommodation that occurs because of aging. The lens consists of transparent fibres arranged in concentric layers, of which the external layers are the newest and softest. No loss of lens fibres occurs with aging; instead, additional fibres are added to the outermost portion of the lens. As the lens ages, it thickens, and its fibres become less elastic, so that the range of focus or accommodation is diminished to the point where reading glasses become necessary for near vision.

Cataracts

A cataract is a lens opacity that interferes with the transmission of light to the retina. Cataracts are the most common cause of age-related visual loss in the world; they are found in approximately 50% of those between 65 and 74 years of age, and in 70% of those older than 75 years.[1,26] Cataract surgery is the most common surgical procedure in Canada, with more than 250,000 procedures performed annually in Canada and over 1.5 million cataract surgeries in North America. More than 95% of persons undergoing cataract surgery experience visual improvement if there is no ocular comorbidity.[2]

Causes and Types of Cataracts

The cause of cataract development is thought to be multifactorial, with different factors being associated with different types of opacities.[26] The pathogenesis of cataracts is not completely understood. Several risk factors have been proposed, including the effects of aging, genetic influences, environmental and metabolic influences, drugs, and injury. Metabolically induced cataracts are caused by disorders of carbohydrate metabolism (diabetes) or inborn errors of metabolism.[26] Long-term exposure to sunlight (ultraviolet B radiation) and heavy smoking have been associated with increased risk of cataract formation. Occasionally, cataracts occur as a developmental defect (*i.e.,* congenital cataracts) or secondary to trauma or diseases.

Cataracts can result from several drugs. Corticosteroids drugs have been implicated as causative agents in cataract formation. Both systemic and inhaled corticosteroids have been cited as risk factors.[27] Other drugs associated with cataracts include the phenothiazines, amiodarone, and strong miotic ophthalmic drugs such as phospholine iodine. Frequent examination of lens transparency should accompany the use of these and any other medications with potential cataract-forming effects.

Traumatic Cataract. Traumatic cataracts are usually caused by foreign body injury to the lens or blunt trauma to the eye. Foreign body injury that interrupts the lens capsule allows aqueous and vitreous humour to enter the lens and initiate cataract formation. Other causes of traumatic cataract are overexposure to heat (*e.g.,* glassblower cataract) or to ionizing radiation. The radiation dose necessary to cause a cataract varies with the amount and type of energy; younger lenses are most vulnerable.

Congenital Cataract. A congenital cataract is one that is present at birth. Among the causes of congenital cataracts are genetic defects, toxic environmental agents, and viruses such as rubella.[11] Cataracts and other developmental defects of the ocular apparatus depend on the total dose of the agent and the embryonic stage at the time of exposure. During the last trimester of fetal life, genetically or environmentally influenced malformation of the superficial lens fibres can occur. Congenital lens opacities may occur in children of diabetic mothers.

Most congenital cataracts are not progressive and are not dense enough to cause significant visual impairment. However, if the unilateral cataract is visually significant, it should be removed by 6 weeks, and if the cataracts are bilateral and the opacity is significant, lens extraction should be done on one eye by the age of 10 weeks to permit the development of vision (see later section on amblyopia). If the surgery is successful, the contralateral lens should be removed within 2 weeks postsurgery.

Senile Cataract. Cataracts are the most common cause of age-related vision loss in the world.[28] With normal aging, the nucleus and the cortex of the lens enlarge as new fibres are formed in the cortical zones of the lens. In the nucleus, the old fibres become more compressed and dehydrated. Metabolic changes occur and lens proteins become more insoluble, and concentrations of calcium, sodium, potassium, and phosphate increase. During the early stages of cataract formation, a yellow pigment and vacuoles accumulate in the lens fibres. The unfolding of protein molecules, cross-linking of sulfhydryl groups, and conversion of soluble to insoluble proteins lead to the loss of lens transparency. The onset is gradual, and the only symptoms are increasingly blurred vision and visual distortion.

Manifestations

The manifestations of cataract depend on the extent of opacity and whether the defect is bilateral or unilateral. With the exception of traumatic or congenital cataract, most cataracts are bilateral. Age-related cataracts, which are the most common type, are characterized by increasingly blurred vision and visual distortion (Fig. 54.1C). Visual acuity for far and near objects decreases. Dilation of the pupil in dim light improves vision. With nuclear cataracts (those involving the lens nucleus), the refractive power of the anterior segment often increases to produce an acquired myopia. Persons with hyperopia may experience a "second sight" or improved reading acuity until increasing opacity reduces acuity. Central lens opacities may divide the visual axis and cause an optical defect in which two or more blurred images are seen. Posterior subcapsular cataracts are located in the posterior cortical layer and usually involve the central visual axis. In addition to decreased visual acuity, cataracts tend to cause light entering the eye to be scattered, thereby producing glare or the abnormal presence of light in the visual field.

Diagnosis and Treatment

Diagnosis of cataract is based on ophthalmoscopic examination and the degree of visual impairment on the Snellen vision test. On ophthalmoscopic examination, cataracts may appear as a gross opacity filling the pupillary aperture or as an opacity silhouetted against the red background of the fundus. A Snellen test acuity of 20/50 is a common requirement for drivers of motor vehicles so tests of potential vision (*i.e.*, the ability to see well after surgery) may be done to ensure that the visual loss can be corrected to necessary functional levels if the cataract were removed.

There is no effective medical treatment for cataract. Strong bifocals, magnification, appropriate lighting, and visual aids may be used as the cataract progresses. Surgery is the only treatment for correcting cataract-related vision loss. Surgery usually involves lens extraction and intraocular lens implantation. It is commonly performed on an outpatient basis with the use of local anesthesia. The use of extracapsular surgery, which leaves the posterior capsule of the lens intact, has significantly improved the outcomes of cataract surgery. The cataract lens is usually removed using phacoemulsification techniques.[28] Phacoemulsification involves ultrasonic fragmentation of the lens into fine pieces, which then are aspirated from the eye.

One of the greatest advances in cataract surgery has been the development of reliable intraocular implants. Monofocal intraocular lenses that correct for distance vision are available, and eyeglasses may be needed for near vision, although in some cases this can be aided by the use of multifocal intraocular lenses.[26]

IN SUMMARY

The lens is a biconvex, avascular, colourless, and almost transparent structure suspended behind the iris. The shape of the lens is controlled by the ciliary muscle, which contracts and relaxes the zonule fibres, thus changing the tension on the lens capsule and altering the focus of the lens. Refraction, which refers to the ability to focus an object on the retina, depends on the size and shape of the eyeball and the cornea and on the focusing ability of the lens. Errors in refraction occur when the visual image is not focused on the retina because of individual differences in the size or shape of the eyeball or cornea. In hyperopia,

or farsightedness, the image theoretically falls behind the retina. In myopia, or nearsightedness, the image falls in front of the retina. Accommodation is the process by which a clear image is maintained as the gaze is shifted from a far to a near object. It is associated with convergence of the eyes and pupillary constriction, and thickening of the lens results from contraction of the ciliary muscle. Presbyopia is a change in the lens that occurs because of aging such that the lens becomes thicker and less able to change shape and accommodate for near vision.

A cataract develops when the lens becomes opaque. It can occur as the result of congenital influences, metabolic disturbances, infection, injury, and aging. The most common type of cataract is the senile cataract that occurs with aging. The treatment for a totally opaque or mature cataract is surgical extraction. An intraocular lens implant may be inserted during the surgical procedure to replace the removed lens; otherwise, thick convex lenses or contact lenses are used to compensate for the loss of lens function.

DISORDERS OF THE VITREOUS AND RETINA

After completing this section of the chapter, you should be able to meet the following objectives:

- Relate the phagocytic function of the retinal pigment epithelium to the development of retinitis pigmentosa.
- Cite the manifestations and long-term visual effects of papilledema.
- Describe the pathogenesis of background and proliferative diabetic retinopathies and their mechanisms of visual impairment.
- Relate the role of posterior vitreous detachment to the development of retinal tears and detachment.
- Explain the pathology and visual changes associated with macular degeneration.

The posterior segment, comprising five sixths of the eyeball, contains the transparent vitreous humour, the retina, and the choroid. The innermost layer of the eyeball, the fundus, is visualized through the pupil with an ophthalmoscope.

Disorders of the Vitreous

Vitreous humour (*i.e.*, vitreous body) is a colourless, amorphous biologic gel that fills the posterior cavity of the eye (Fig. 54.5). It consists of approximately 99% water, some salts, glycoproteins, proteoglycans, and dispersed collagen fibrils. The vitreous is attached to the peripheral retina in the region of the ora serrata and to the periphery of the optic disc, as well as the macular and retinal vessels.

Disease, aging, and injury can disturb the factors that maintain the water of the vitreous humour in suspension, causing liquefaction of the gel to occur. With the loss of gel structure, fine fibres, membranes, and cellular debris develop. When this occurs, floaters (images) can often be noticed as these substances move within the vitreous cavity during head movement. In disease, blood vessels may grow from the surface of the retina or optic disc onto the posterior surface of the vitreous, and blood may fill the vitreous cavity.

In a procedure called a *vitrectomy,* the removal and replacement of the vitreous with a balanced saline solution can restore sight in some persons with vitreous opacities resulting from hemorrhage or vitreoretinal membrane formations that cause legal blindness. Using this procedure, a small probe with a cutting tip is used to remove the opaque vitreous and membranes. The procedure is difficult and requires complex instrumentation. It is of no value if the retina is not functional.

Disorders of the Retina

The function of the retina is to receive visual images, partially analyze them, and transmit this modified information to the brain.[18] It is composed of two layers: the inner neural retina that contains the photoreceptors and an outer melanin-containing layer that it rests on (called the retinal pigmented epithelium or RPE), and is firmly attached to, the choriocapillaris, the capillary layer of the choroid. A non–light-sensitive portion of the retina, along with the RPE, continues anteriorly to form the posterior surface of the iris. A wavy border called the *ora serrata* exists at the junction between the light-sensitive and the non–light-sensitive retinas. Separating the vascular portion of the choroid from pigmented cells of the retina is a thin layer of elastic tissue, the *Bruch membrane,* which contains collagen fibrils in its superficial and deep portions. Cells of the pigmented layer receive their nourishment by diffusion from the choriocapillaris.

Disorders of the retina and its function include derangements of the RPE (*e.g.,* retinitis pigmentosa); ischemic conditions caused by disorders of the retinal blood supply; disorders of the retinal vessels such as retinopathies that cause hemorrhage and the development of opacities; separation of the pigment and sensory layers of the retina (*i.e.,* retinal detachment); abnormalities of the Bruch membrane and choroid (*e.g.,* macular degeneration); and malignant tumours of the nuclear layer of the retina (*i.e.,* retinoblastoma). Because the retina has no pain fibres, most diseases of the retina are painless and do not cause redness of the eye.

The Neural Retina

The neural retina is composed of three layers of neurons: a posterior layer of photoreceptors, a middle layer of bipolar cells, and an inner layer of ganglion cells that communicate with the photoreceptors (Fig. 54.9). A pattern of light on the retina falls on a massive array of photoreceptors. These photoreceptors synapse with bipolar and other interneurons before action potentials in ganglion cells relay the message to specific regions of the brain and the brain stem associated with vision. For rods, this microcircuitry involves the convergence of signals from many rods on a single ganglion cell. This arrangement maximizes spatial summation and the detection of stimulated (light versus dark) receptors. The interneurons, composed of horizontal and amacrine cells, have cell bodies in the bipolar layer, and they play an important role in modulating retinal function. A superficial marginal layer contains the axons of the ganglion cells as they collect and leave the eye through the optic nerve. These fibres lie beside the vitreous

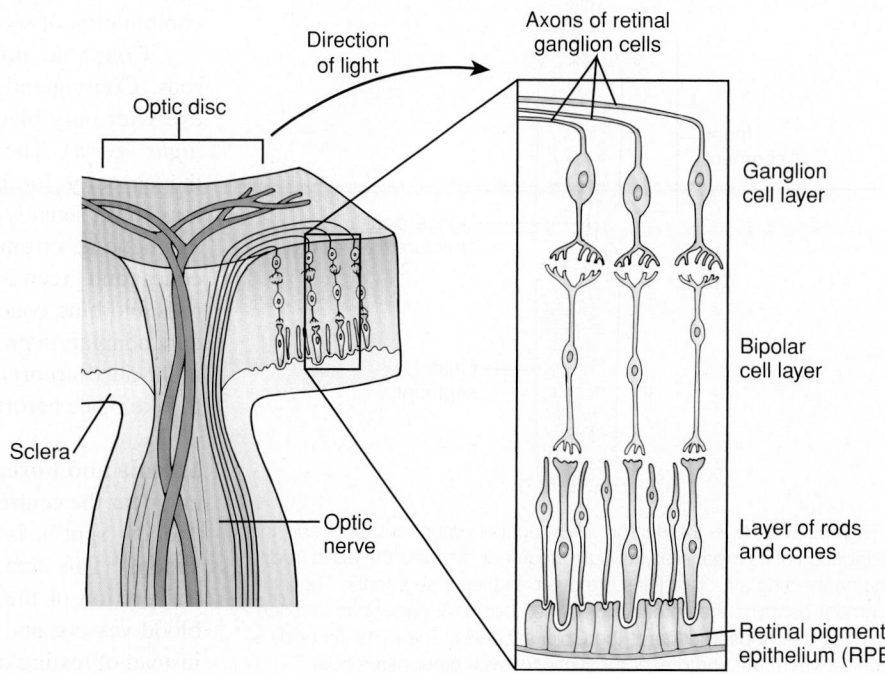

FIGURE 54.9 • Organization of the human retina. The optic pathway begins with photoreceptors (rods and cones) in the retina. The responses of the photoreceptors are transmitted by the bipolar cells to the ganglion cell layer of the retina.

humour. Light must pass through the transparent inner layers of the sensory retina before it reaches the photoreceptors.

Photoreceptors

Two types of photoreceptors are present in the retina: rods, capable of black–white discrimination, and cones, capable of colour discrimination.[18] Both types of photoreceptors are thin, elongated, mitochondria-filled cells with a single, highly modified cilium (Fig. 54.10). The cilium has a short base, or inner segment, and a highly modified outer segment. The plasma membrane of the outer segment is tightly folded to form membranous discs (rods) or conical shapes (cones) containing visual pigment. These discs are continuously synthesized at the base of the outer segment and shed at the distal end. Discarded membranes are phagocytized by the retinal pigment cells. If this phagocytosis is disrupted, as in retinitis pigmentosa, the sensory retina degenerates.

Rods. Photoreception involves the transduction of light energy into an altered ionic membrane potential of the rod cell. Light passing through the eye penetrates the nearly transparent neural elements to produce decomposition of the photochemical substance (visual pigment) called *rhodopsin* in the outer segment of the rod. Light that is not trapped by a rhodopsin molecule is absorbed by the retinal pigment melanin or deeper choroid melanin. Rhodopsin consists of a protein

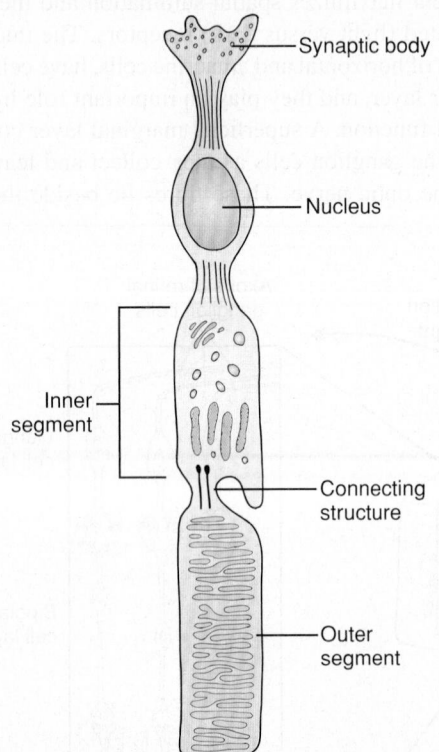

FIGURE 54.10 • Retinal rod, showing its component parts and the distribution of its organelles. Its outer segment contains the discs (rods). The connecting structure joins the outer and inner segments. The inner segment contains the mitochondria, the ribosomal endoplasmic reticulum, the free ribosomes, and the Golgi saccules. The synaptic body is the site where the photoreceptor synapses with other nerve cells.

called *opsin* and a vitamin A-derived pigment called *retinal.* During light stimulation, rhodopsin is broken down into its component parts, opsin and retinal; retinal subsequently is converted into vitamin A. The reconstitution of rhodopsin occurs during total darkness; vitamin A is transformed into retinal, and then opsin and retinal combine to form rhodopsin. Considerable stores of vitamin A are present in the retinal pigment cells and in the liver; therefore, a vitamin A deficiency must be present for weeks or months to affect the photoreceptive process. Reduced sensitivity to light, a symptom of vitamin A deficiency, initially affects night vision; however, this is quickly reversed by injection or ingestion of the vitamin.

Rod-based vision is particularly sensitive to detecting light, especially moving light stimuli, at the expense of clear pattern discrimination. Rod vision is particularly adapted for night and low-level illumination. Dark adaptation is the process by which rod sensitivity increases to the optimum level. This requires approximately 4 hours in total or near-total darkness and is referred to as scotopic vision (night vision). During daylight or high-intensity bombardment, the concentration of vitamin A increases, whereas the concentration of the photopigment retinal decreases. During dark adaptation, an increase in synthesis of retinal from vitamin A results in a higher concentration of rhodopsin available to capture light energy.

Cones and Colour Sensitivity. Cone receptors that are selectively sensitive to different wavelengths of light provide the basis for colour vision. Three types of cones, or cone-colour systems, respond to the blue, green, and red portions of the visible electromagnetic spectrum. This selectivity reflects the presence of one of three colour-sensitive molecules to which the photochemical substance (visual pigment) is bound. The decomposition and reconstitution processes of the cone visual pigments are believed to be similar to that of the rods. The colour a person perceives depends on which set of cones or combination of sets of cones is stimulated in a given image.

Cones do not have the dark adaptation capability of rods. Consequently, the dark-adapted eye is a rod receptor eye with only black–grey–white discrimination (*scotopic* or *night vision*). The light-adapted eye (*photopic vision*) adds the capacity for colour discrimination. Rhodopsin has its maximum sensitivity in the blue-green region of the electromagnetic spectrum. If red lenses are worn in daylight, the red cones (and green cones to some extent) are in use, whereas the rods and blue cones are essentially in the dark, and therefore dark adaptation proceeds. This method is used by military and night-duty airport control tower personnel to allow adaptation to take place before they go on duty in the dark.

Macula and Fovea. An area approximately 1.5 mm in diameter near the centre of the retina, called the *macula lutea* (i.e., "yellow spot"), is especially adapted for acute and detailed vision.[18] This area is composed entirely of cones. In the central portion of the macula, the *fovea centralis* (foveola), the blood vessels, and innermost layers are displaced to one side instead of resting on top of the cones (Fig. 54.11). This allows

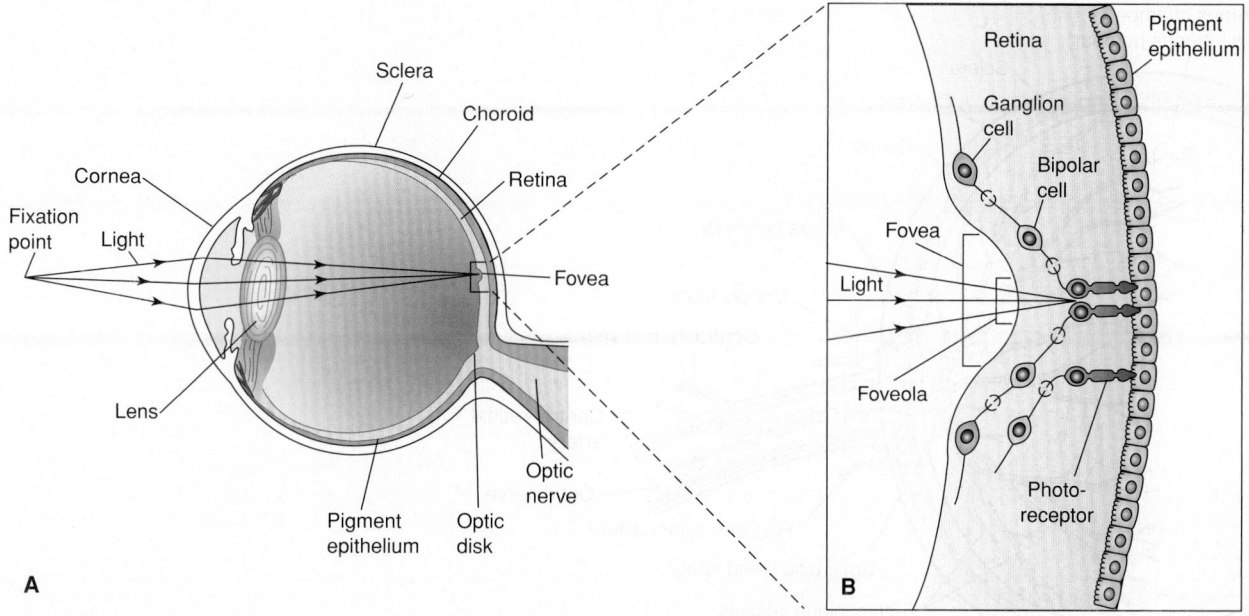

FIGURE 54.11 • Reflection of light onto the retina (**A**), focusing of light in the fovea (**B**). (From Kandel, E. R., Schwartz, J. H., Jessel, T. M. (1991). *Principles of neural science* (3rd ed., New York: Elsevier.)

light to pass unimpeded to the cones without passing through several layers of the retina. Of the approximately 6.4 million cones in the retina, 200,000 are located in the fovea. The density of cones drops off rapidly away from the fovea. Rods are not present in the fovea, but their numbers increase as the cones decrease in density toward the periphery of the retina.

Colour Blindness. "Colour blindness" is a misnomer for a condition in which persons appear to confuse or mismatch colours, or experience reduced acuity for colour discrimination. Such persons are often unaware of their defect until they attempt to discriminate between red and green traffic lights or experience difficulty matching colours. Colour blindness is inherited as an X-linked deficiency of a specific type of retinal photoreceptor. The most common abnormality is red-green colour blindness. The deficiency is usually partial but can be complete. Rarely are two of the colour mechanisms missing; when this occurs, usually red and green are missing. Complete lack of colour discrimination is rare; for such people, the world is experienced entirely as black, grey, and white.

The genetically colour-blind person has never experienced the full range of normal colour vision and is unaware of what he or she is missing. Colour discrimination is necessary for everyday living, and colour-blind persons, knowingly or unknowingly, make colour discriminations based on other criteria, such as brightness or position. For example, the red light of a traffic signal is always the upper light, and the green is the lower light. Colour-blind persons experience difficulties when brightness differences are small and discrimination must be based on hue and saturation qualities.

Retinitis Pigmentosa. Retinitis pigmentosa represents a group of hereditary diseases that cause slow degenerative changes in the retinal photoreceptors. The disease can be inherited as an autosomal dominant (20% to 40% of cases), autosomal recessive (50% to 60%), sex-linked (5% to 15%) trait, or sporadic mutations (up to 50%). With advances in genetics technology, there are now 100 known or predicted retinitis pigmentosa mutation genes.[29] The group of genes most commonly mutated encodes proteins in the visual cascade of the photoreceptor outer segment. Although retinitis pigmentosa is a disease usually confined to the eye, approximately 20% to 30% of persons have associated nonocular disease. Usher syndrome, in which retinitis pigmentosa is associated with hearing impairment, is the most frequent of these combined syndromes.[30] The hearing loss can be either profound, present at birth, and associated with vestibular ataxia, or moderate to mild and nonprogressive.

In typical cases, known as *rod–cone retinitis pigmentosa,* the rods are the predominantly affected photoreceptor cells. This generally produces a number of characteristic clinical symptoms, including night blindness, which is usually an early symptom, and bilateral symmetric loss of midperipheral fields. Although there is relative preservation of macular vision, the visual field defects gradually increase both centrally and peripherally. With progression, cone photoreceptor cells are also affected and day vision and central visual acuity are compromised. The rate of visual failure is variable. Some people are severely visually handicapped before the age of 20 years, whereas others experience few symptomatic visual deficits even after 60 years of age.[30]

Disorders of Retinal Blood Supply

The blood supply for the retina is derived from two sources: the choriocapillaris (*i.e.,* the capillary layer of the choroid) and branches of the central retinal artery (Fig. 54.12). Oxygen and other nutritional substances needed by the retina and its component parts (pigment cells, rods, and cones) are supplied by diffusion from blood vessels in the choroid. Because the choriocapillaris provides the only blood supply for the fovea centralis

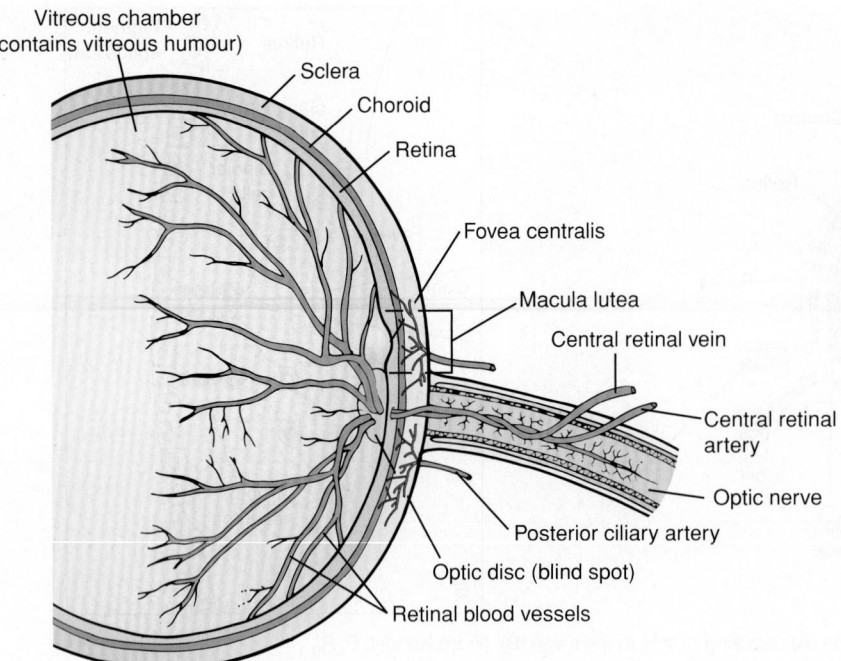

FIGURE 54.12 • Retinal circulation.

(*i.e.*, foveola), detachment of this part of the sensory retina from the pigment epithelium causes irreparable visual loss.

DISORDERS OF THE RETINAL BLOOD SUPPLY

- The blood supply for the retina is derived from the central retinal artery, which supplies blood flow for the entire inside of the retina, and from vessels in the choroid, which supply the rods and cones.
- The retinopathies, which are disorders of the retinal vessels, interrupt blood flow to the visual receptors, leading to visual impairment.
- Retinal detachment separates the visual receptors from the choroid, which provides their major blood supply.

The bipolar, horizontal, amacrine, and ganglion cells, and the ganglion cell axons that gather at the optic disc, are supplied by branches of the retinal artery.[28] The central artery of the retina is a branch of the ophthalmic artery. It enters the globe through the optic disc. Branches of this artery radiate over the entire retina, except the central fovea, which is surrounded by, but is not crossed by, arterial branches. The central artery of the retina is an end artery, meaning that it does not anastomose with other arteries. This is critical because an infarct in this artery will totally deprive distal structures of their vascular supply. Retinal veins follow a distribution parallel to the arterial branches and carry venous blood to the central vein of the retina, which exits the back of the eye through the optic disc.

Funduscopic examination of the eye with an ophthalmoscope provides an opportunity to examine the retinal blood vessels and other aspects of the retina (Fig. 54.13). Because the retina is an embryonic outgrowth of the brain and the blood vessels are to a considerable extent representative of brain blood vessels, the ophthalmoscopic examination of the fundus of the eye permits the study and diagnosis of metabolic and vascular diseases of the brain as well as pathologic processes that are specific to the retina.

Functioning of the retina, like that of other cellular portions of the central nervous system (CNS), depends on an

FIGURE 54.13 • Funduscopic image of normal retina. Retinal venules (wider) and retinal arterioles (narrower) radiate from the centre of the oval optic disc. The dark area lateral to the disc is the macula. Branches of retinal vessels extend toward this area, but do not reach its centre, the fovea centralis—the area of most acute vision. (From Moore K. L., Dalley A. F., Agur A.M. (2014). *Clinical oriented anatomy* (7th ed., p. 897). Philadelphia, PA: Lippincott Williams & Wilkins.)

oxygen supply from the vascular system. One of the earliest signs of decreased perfusion pressure in the head region is a greying-out or blackout of vision, which usually precedes loss of consciousness. This can occur during large increases in intrathoracic pressure, which interfere with the return of venous blood to the heart, as occurs with the Valsalva maneuver; with systemic hypotension; and during sudden postural changes (*e.g.,* postural hypotension).

Ischemia of the retina occurs during general circulatory collapse. If a person survives cardiopulmonary arrest, for instance, permanently decreased visual acuity can occur as a result of edema and the ischemic death of retinal neurons. This is followed by primary optic nerve atrophy proportional to the extent of ganglionic cell death. The ophthalmic artery, the source of the central artery of the retina, takes its origin from the internal carotid artery.[28] Intermittent retinal ischemia can accompany internal carotid or common carotid stenosis. *Amaurosis fugax* is characterized by transient episodes of monocular visual loss lasting 5 to 10 minutes.[28] Persons with the disorder often describe a curtain coming down from above or across their vision, usually with complete return of vision within seconds or minutes. Besides the vision loss, contralateral hemiplegia or sensory deficits may accompany the episodes. The condition, commonly due to emboli, is most often the result of carotid artery disease.[28]

Papilledema. The central retinal artery enters the eye through the optic papilla in the centre of the optic nerve. An accompanying vein exits the eye along the same path. The entrance and exit of the central retinal artery and vein through the tough scleral tissue at the optic papilla can be compromised by any condition causing persistent increased intracranial pressure. The most common of these conditions are cerebral tumours, subdural hematomas, hydrocephalus, idiopathic intracranial hypertension, and malignant hypertension. Papilledema is bilateral optic disc swelling.

Usually, the thin-walled, low-pressure veins are the first to collapse, with the consequent backup and slowing of arterial blood flow. Under these conditions, capillary permeability increases and leakage of fluid results in edema of the optic papilla, called *papilledema.* The interior surface of the papilla is normally cup-shaped and can be evaluated for cupping with an ophthalmoscope. With papilledema, sometimes called *choked disc,* the optic cup is distorted by protrusion into the interior of the eye (Fig. 54.14). Because this sign does not occur until the intracranial pressure is significantly elevated, compression damage to the optic nerve fibres passing through the lamina cribrosa may have begun. As a warning sign, papilledema occurs quite late. Unresolved papilledema results in the destruction of the optic nerve axons and blindness. Pseudopapilledema can result from infiltration or optic disc drusen (calcified deposits in the optic papilla).

Retinopathies

Disorders of the retinal vessels can result in microaneurysms, neovascularization, hemorrhage, and formation of retinal

FIGURE 54.14 • Chronic papilledema. The optic nerve head is congested and protrudes anteriorly toward the interior of the eye. It has blurred margins, and vessels within it are poorly seen. (From Rubin R., Strayer D. S. (Eds.). (2012). *Rubin's pathology: Clinicopathologic foundations of medicine* (6th ed., p. 1408). Philadelphia, PA: Lippincott Williams & Wilkins.)

opacities. *Microaneurysms* are outpouchings of the retinal vasculature. On ophthalmoscopic examination, they appear as minute, unchanging red dots associated with blood vessels. These microaneurysms tend to leak plasma, resulting in localized edema that gives the retina a hazy appearance. Microaneurysms can be identified with certainty using fluorescein angiography; the fluorescein dye is injected intravenously, and the retinal vessels subsequently are photographed using a special ophthalmoscope and fundus camera. The microaneurysms may bleed, but areas of hemorrhage and edema tend to clear spontaneously. However, they reduce visual acuity if they encroach on the macula and cause degeneration before they are absorbed.

Neovascularization involves the formation of new blood vessels. They can develop from the choriocapillaris, extending between the pigment layer and the sensory layer, or from the retinal veins, extending between the sensory retina and the vitreous cavity and sometimes into the vitreous. These new blood vessels are fragile, leak protein, and are likely to bleed. Neovascularization occurs in many conditions that impair retinal blood flow, including stasis because of hyperviscosity of blood or decreased flow, vascular occlusion, sickle cell disease, sarcoidosis, diabetes mellitus, and retinopathy of prematurity, as well as following ischemia. Although the cause of neovascularization is uncertain, research links the process with a vascular endothelial growth factor (VEGF) produced by the lining of blood vessels.[31,32] Hypoxia is a key regulator of VEGF-induced retinal neovascularization. Another factor, pigment epithelium-derived factor (PEDF), synthesized elsewhere in the eye and throughout the body, is thought to inhibit neovascularization. It is likely that other growth factors and signalling systems are also involved.

Hemorrhage can be preretinal, intraretinal, or subretinal. *Preretinal hemorrhages* occur between the retina and the vitreous. These hemorrhages are usually large because the blood vessels are only loosely restricted; they may be associated with a subarachnoid or subdural hemorrhage and are usually regarded as a serious manifestation of the disorder. They usually reabsorb without complications unless they penetrate into the vitreous. *Intraretinal hemorrhages* occur because of abnormalities of the retinal vessels, diseases of the blood, increased pressure in the retinal vessels, or vitreous traction on the vessels. Systemic causes include diabetes mellitus, hypertension, and blood dyscrasias. *Subretinal hemorrhages* are those that develop between the choroid and pigment layer of the retina. A common cause of subretinal hemorrhage is neovascularization. Microaneurysms and neovascularization can be treated with photocoagulation and, more recently, with the use of intravitreal-injected anti-VEGF agents such as bevacizumab and ranibizumab.

Light normally passes through the transparent inner portions of the sensory retina before reaching the photoreceptors. *Opacities* such as hemorrhages, exudate, cotton-wool spots, edema, and tissue proliferation can produce a localized loss of transparency observable with an ophthalmoscope. Exudates are opacities resulting from inflammatory processes. The development of exudates often results in the destruction of the underlying retinal pigment and choroid layer. Deposits are localized opacities consisting of lipid-laden macrophages or accumulated cellular debris. Cotton-wool spots are retinal opacities with hazy, irregular outlines. They occur in the nerve fibre layer and contain cell organelles. Cotton-wool patches are associated with retinal trauma, severe anemia, papilledema, and diabetic retinopathy.

Diabetic Retinopathy. Diabetic retinopathy is the third leading cause of blindness for all ages in the industrialized countries of the world. It ranks first as the cause of newly reported cases of blindness in persons between the ages of 20 and 74 years. Advances in treatment have greatly reduced the risk of blindness from diabetes, but because diabetes is so common, retinopathy remains an important cause of visual impairment.

Diabetic retinopathy can be divided into two types: *nonproliferative* (*i.e.,* background) and *proliferative*.[32,33] Background or nonproliferative retinopathy is confined to the retina. It involves engorgement of the retinal veins, thickening of the capillary endothelial basement membrane, and development of capillary microaneurysms (Fig. 54.15A,B). Small intraretinal hemorrhages may develop and microinfarcts may cause cotton-wool spots and leakage of exudates. A sensation of glare (because of the scattering of light) is a common complaint. The most common cause of decreased vision in persons with background retinopathy is macular edema. The edema is caused primarily by the breakdown of the inner blood–retina barrier at the level of the capillary endothelium, allowing leakage of fluid and plasma constituents into the surrounding retina.

Proliferative diabetic retinopathy represents a more severe retinal change than background retinopathy (Fig. 54.15C,D).

It is characterized by formation of new, fragile blood vessels (*i.e.,* neovascularization) at the disc and elsewhere in the retina. These vessels grow in front of the retina along the posterior surface of the vitreous or into the vitreous. They threaten vision in two ways. First, because they are abnormal, they often bleed easily, leaking blood into the vitreous cavity and decreasing visual acuity. Second, the blood vessels attach firmly to the retinal surface and posterior surface of the vitreous, such that normal movement of the vitreous may exert a pull on the retina, causing retinal detachment and progressive blindness. Because early proliferative diabetic retinopathy is likely to be asymptomatic, it must be identified early, before bleeding occurs and obscures the view of the fundus or leads to fibrosis and retinal detachment.

The cause of diabetic retinopathy is uncertain. Several biochemical mechanisms have been proposed as explanations for the development and progression of diabetic retinopathy and have led to exploration of possible treatments.[32] However, except for the demonstration that chronically elevated levels of blood glucose contribute to the development and progression of retinopathy and other complications of diabetes, no mechanism can be regarded as established. The increased expression of VEGF has become a focus of current research on the pathogenesis of diabetic retinopathy as well as other retinal and choroidal vascular disorders. Hypertension is also thought to increase the risk for the development and progression of diabetic retinopathy. Recent evidence suggests that the renin–angiotensin system is activated by chronically elevated levels of blood glucose. Angiotensin II increases vascular permeability and promotes angiogenesis, and it has been suggested that a relationship may exist between angiotensin II and VEGF in ocular tissues.[34] Accordingly, angiotensin-converting enzyme inhibitors or receptor blockers may be useful agents for preventing the progression of diabetic retinopathy. In addition to chronic hyperglycemia and hypertension, several studies have indicated the association of diabetic exudative retinopathy with hypercholesteremia and combined inflammatory mediators on the retinal microvasculature.[34]

Preventing diabetic retinopathy from developing or progressing is considered the best approach to preserving vision. Growing evidence suggests that careful control of blood glucose levels in persons with diabetes mellitus may retard the onset and progression of retinopathy. The ACCORD study demonstrated that intensive management of persons with type 1 diabetes to maintain blood glucose at near-normal levels limited the risk of developing retinopathy. There also is a need for intensive management of hypertension and hyperlipidemia, both of which have been shown to increase the risk of diabetic retinopathy in persons with diabetes.[35]

Regular dilated eye examinations are an effective approach to detecting and treating vision-threatening diabetic retinopathy. Current guidelines recommend that persons with diabetes have eye examinations every 1 to 2 years, although deviations from this guideline are appropriate in certain low-risk groups.[35] For persons with moderate to severe nonproliferative retinopathy, more frequent examinations are often

FIGURE 54.15 • **A:** Nonproliferative (background) retinopathy showing microaneurysms. **B:** Ocular fundus of a patient with background diabetic retinopathy. Several yellowish "hard" exudates (which are rich in lipids) and several relatively small retinal hemorrhages are present. **C:** Proliferative retinopathy. **D:** Ocular fundus in a patient with proliferative retinopathy. A vascular frond (branching pattern of preretinal neovascularization) has extended anterior to the retina. (**B** and **D** from Rubin R., Strayer D. S. (Eds.). (2012). *Rubin's pathology: Clinicopathologic foundations of medicine* (6th ed., p. 1403). Philadelphia, PA: Lippincott Williams & Wilkins.)

necessary to determine when to initiate treatment. Persons with any levels of macular edema, severe nonproliferative diabetic retinopathy, or any proliferative retinopathy require the prompt care of an ophthalmologist who is knowledgeable and experienced in the management and treatment of diabetic retinopathy.[36] Women with pre-existing diabetes who plan to become pregnant should have a comprehensive eye examination and be counselled about the risk for initiation or progression of diabetic retinopathy. Women with diabetes who become pregnant should have a comprehensive eye examination in the first trimester and close follow-up throughout pregnancy.[35]

Photocoagulation using an argon laser provides the major direct treatment modality for diabetic retinopathy.[31,32] Treatment strategies include laser photocoagulation applied directly to leaking microaneurysms and grid photocoagulation with a checkerboard pattern of laser burns applied to diffuse areas of leakage and thickening.[31] Because laser photocoagulation destroys the proliferating vessels and the ischemic retina, it reduces the stimulus for further neovascularization. However, photocoagulation of neovascularization near the disc is not recommended.[31] Vitrectomy has proved effective in removing vitreous hemorrhage and severing vitreoretinal membranes that develop.

Because of the limitations of current treatment measures, new pharmacologic therapies that target the underlying biochemical mechanisms that cause diabetic retinopathy are being investigated. Recent interest has focused on intravitreal corticosteroid or VEGF inhibitor injections (discussed in the section on Macular Degeneration).

Hypertensive Retinopathy. As with other blood vessels in the body, the retinal vessels undergo changes in response to chronically elevated blood pressure. In the initial, vasoconstrictor stage, there is vasospasm and an increase in retinal arterial tone because of local autoregulatory mechanisms. On ophthalmoscopy, this stage is represented by a general narrowing of the retinal arterioles. Persistently elevated blood pressure results in the compensatory thickening of arteriolar walls, which effectively reduces capillary perfusion pressure.[37] With severe, uncontrolled hypertension, there is disruption of the blood–retina barrier, necrosis of smooth muscle and endothelial cells, exudation of blood and lipids, and retinal ischemia. These changes are manifested in the retina by microaneurysms, intraretinal hemorrhages, hard exudates, and cotton-wool spots. Swelling of the optic disc may occur at this stage and usually indicates severely elevated blood pressure (malignant hypertension). Older adults often have more rigid vessels that are unable to respond to the same degree as those of younger individuals.

Studies have shown that signs of hypertensive retinopathy regress with control of blood pressure.[37] There is also evidence that advanced signs of hypertensive retinopathy (*e.g.,* retinal hemorrhages, microaneurysms, and cotton-wool spots) predict stroke and death from stroke independent of elevated blood pressure and other risk factors.[37] Persons with these signs may benefit from close monitoring of cerebrovascular risk and intensive measures to reduce the risk.

Retinal Detachment

Retinal detachment involves the separation of the neurosensory retina from the pigment epithelium (Fig. 54.16). It occurs when traction on the inner sensory layer or a tear in this layer allows fluid, usually vitreous, to accumulate between the two layers.[31,38] There are three types of retinal detachments: exudative, traction, and rhegmatogenous.[31]

Exudative (or serous) *retinal detachment* results from the accumulation of serous or hemorrhagic fluid in the subretinal space due to severe hypertension, inflammation, or neoplastic effusions. It usually resolves with successful treatment of the underlying disease and without visual impairment. *Traction retinal attachment* occurs with mechanical forces on the retina, usually mediated by fibrotic tissue, resulting from previous hemorrhage (*e.g.,* from diabetic retinopathy), injury, infection, or inflammation. Intraocular surgery such as cataract extraction may produce traction on the peripheral retina that causes eventual detachment months or even years after surgery. Correction of traction retinal detachment requires disengaging scar tissue from the retinal surface, and vision outcomes are often poor.

Rhegmatogenous detachment (*rhegma* is the Greek for "rent" or "hole") is the most common type of retinal detachment. The vitreous is a hydrated gel whose structure is maintained by a collagenous and mucopolysaccharide matrix. As persons age, this macromolecular network begins to liquefy and collapse. As this occurs, the vitreous shrinks and partly separates from the retinal surface, a condition known as *posterior vitreous detachment* (Fig. 54.16). Rhegmatogenous detachment occurs when the liquid vitreous enters the subretinal space through the retinal tear. Detachment of the neural retina from the retinal pigment layer separates the receptors from their major blood supply, the choroid. If retinal detachment continues for some time, permanent destruction and blindness of that part of the retina occur.

Risk factors for retinal detachment include advancing age and myopia. Development of a posterior vitreous detachment occurs in less than 10% of persons younger than

FIGURE 54.16 • Pathogenesis of rhegmatogenous retinal detachment. (**A**) Changes in the vitreous structure cause it to shrink and separate from the retina, causing posterior vitreous detachment; (**B**) sustained fluid collection and tractional forces cause the retina to tear (rhegmatogenous retinal detachment). **C:** Ophthalmoscopic photograph of retinal detachment (*arrows,* wrinkles in detached retina). (**C** from Moore K. L., Dalley A. F., Agur A.M. (2014). *Clinical oriented anatomy* (7th ed., p. 910). Philadelphia, PA: Lippincott Williams & Wilkins.)

60 years, but in 27% between the ages of 60 and 69 years and in 63% older than 70 years.[38] In about 11% to 15% of these persons, a retinal tear or hole forms as the vitreous pulls away from the retina, especially in the periphery where the retina is thinner.[38] Persons with high grades of myopia may have abnormalities in the peripheral retina that predispose to sudden detachment. In moderate to severe myopia or nearsightedness, the axial (anteroposterior) length of the eye is increased, resulting in an egg-shaped globe. As a result, there is greater vitreoretinal traction, and posterior vitreous detachment may occur at a younger age than in persons without myopia. Also, the retina tends to be thinner and more prone to formation of a hole or tear. Other, less common risk factors include a family history of retinal detachment, a history of congenital eye disease (glaucoma, cataracts), and hereditary vitreopathies with abnormal vitreous gel.

The primary symptom of retinal detachment consists of painless changes in vision. Commonly, flashing lights or sparks, followed by small floaters or spots in the field of vision, occur as the vitreous pulls away from the posterior pole of the eye. As detachment progresses, the person perceives a shadow or dark curtain progressing across the visual field. Because the process begins in the periphery and spreads circumferentially and posteriorly, initial visual disturbances may involve only one quadrant of the visual field. Large peripheral detachments may occur without involvement of the macula, so that visual acuity remains unaffected.

Diagnosis is based on a history of visual disturbances (*e.g.,* presence of floaters, luminous rays or light flashes) and the ophthalmoscopic appearance of the retina. The direct (hand-held) ophthalmoscope is useful in detecting an altered red reflex sometimes associated with retinal detachment. However, because the view is narrow, a negative examination with direct ophthalmoscopy cannot exclude the diagnosis of retinal detachment. Ophthalmologists and optometrists use indirect examination techniques that greatly enhance visualization of the peripheral retina.[31]

Because there is a variable interval between a retinal break and retinal detachment, treatment methods focus on early detection and prevention of further vitreous detachment and retinal tear formation. Symptomatic retinal breaks are usually treated with laser or cryotherapy to seal the retinal tears so that the vitreous can no longer leak into the subretinal space. The treatment is more than 95% effective in preventing progression of a retinal tear and preventing retinal detachment.[31] The primary treatment of traction retinal detachment is vitreoretinal surgery and may involve vitrectomy, membrane removal, scleral buckling, or pneumatic retinopexy. Scleral buckling is the primary surgical procedure performed to reattach the retina.[31,38] With scleral buckling, a piece of silicone (*i.e.,* the buckle) is sutured and infolded into the sclera, physically indenting the sclera so it contacts the separated pigment and retinal layers. A less invasive procedure, pneumatic retinopexy, involves the intraocular injection of an expandable gas to bring the retina and choroid into contact.[38]

Macular Degeneration

Macular degeneration is characterized by degenerative changes in the central portion of the retina (the macula) that result primarily in loss of central vision (Fig. 54.1B). Age-related macular degeneration is the most common cause of reduced vision in the older adult population in the Western world.[39] The causes of age-related macular degeneration are poorly understood. In addition to older age, identifiable risk factors include female sex, white race, hypertension, obesity, and cigarette smoking. Increasing evidence suggests that genetic factors may also play a role.[39] Careful attention should be paid to cardiovascular risk factors, which appear to be more common in patients with age-related macular degeneration.

There are two types of age-related macular degeneration: an atrophic nonexudative or "dry" form and an exudative or "wet" form. Although both types are progressive, they differ in terms of manifestations, prognosis, and management. Although most people with age-related macular degeneration manifest nonproliferative changes only, those who experience severe vision loss do so from the development of the exudative form of the disease.[31,39]

Nonexudative age-related macular degeneration is characterized by various degrees of atrophy and degeneration of the outer retina, Bruch membrane, and the choriocapillaris. It does not involve leakage of blood or serum; hence it is called *dry age-related macular degeneration* (Fig. 54.17). On ophthalmoscopic examination, there are visible changes in the retinal pigmentary epithelium and pale yellow spots, called *drusen,* that may occur individually or in groups throughout the macula. Histopathologically, most drusen contain remnants of materials representative of focal detachment of the pigment epithelium. With time, the drusen enlarge, coalesce, and increase in number. The level of associated visual impairment is variable and may be minimal. Most people with macular drusen do not experience significant loss of central vision, and the atrophic changes may stabilize or progress slowly. However, people with the nonexudative form of age-related macular degeneration need to be followed closely because the exudative stage may develop suddenly, at any time. Careful monitoring for metamorphopsia, or distorted vision of straight lines, can aid in the early detection of retinal damage.

The exudative or "wet form" of macular degeneration is characterized by the formation of a choroidal neovascular membrane that separates the pigmented epithelium from the neuroretina. These new blood vessels have weaker walls than normal and are prone to leakage. The leakage of serous or hemorrhagic fluid into the subretinal space causes separation of the pigmented epithelium from the neurosensory retina. Over time, the subretinal hemorrhages organize to form scar tissue, causing death of the underlying retinal tissue and loss of all visual function in the corresponding macular area (Fig. 54.17). The early stages of subretinal neovascularization may be difficult to detect with an ophthalmoscope. Therefore, there is a need to be alert for recent or sudden changes in central vision, blurred vision, or scotomata in persons with evidence of age-related macular degeneration.

FIGURE 54.17 • Funduscopic view of different stages of age-related macular degeneration (AMD). (**A**) Early intermediate AMD (*white arrow*), (**B**) intermediate AMD, (**C**) advanced AMD with fibrosis. (From the National Eye Institute, National Institutes of Health.)

Although some subretinal neovascular membranes may regress spontaneously, the natural course of exudative macular degeneration is toward irreversible loss of central vision. Persons with late-stage disease often find it difficult to see at long distances (*e.g.,* in driving), do close work (*e.g.,* reading), see faces clearly, or distinguish colours. However, they may not be severely incapacitated because the peripheral retinal function usually remains intact. With the use of low-vision aids, many of them are able to continue many of their normal activities.

Effective therapies for exudative or wet-type macular degeneration include thermal laser photocoagulation, photodynamic therapy, intravitreal injections of VEGF inhibitors, and intravitreal and periocular corticosteroid injections.[39] The decision about specific therapies must take into account the likelihood of visual recovery, which is greater with smaller, more recent lesions, as well as the risks of the various therapies. Currently there is no established effective treatment for the dry form of macular degeneration, and most current therapies and new investigational treatments are directed at choroidal (or subretinal) neovascularization.

Photodynamic laser therapy, which involves the intravenous injection of a dye that is subsequently activated by retinal laser irradiation to produce selective vascular damage, is indicated when the neovascular membrane is well defined.[31] Conventional photocoagulation of subfoveal neovascular membranes is associated with an inevitable immediate reduction in vision because of associated retinal damage and thus is indicated only for extrafoveal membranes. Various surgical procedures to excise subfoveal neovascular membranes or position the macula away from them continue to be investigated.

The VEGF inhibitors that are administered by intravitreal injection include pegaptanib, ranibizumab, and bevacizumab.[39] Pegaptanib is a VEGF inhibitor used for the treatment of slow vision loss in eyes affected by all subtypes of age-related macular degeneration. In Canada, ranibizumab and bevacizumab are recombinant humanized monoclonal antibodies with specificity for VEGF for the treatment of the wet form of age-related macular degeneration. The corticosteroids have an angiostatic activity that appears to be independent of their hormone activity. The intravitreal injection of these agents bypasses the blood–ocular barrier, achieving therapeutic levels in the eye while avoiding systemic side effects. Further research is looking into intravitreal injections with aflibercept, an engineered protein that has greater binding to VEGF receptors preventing angiogenesis formation, as another treatment for age-related macular degeneration.[39]

In addition to currently used and forthcoming treatments, there is interest in the preventative category of treatments. Tobacco smoking is consistently identified as a preventable age-related macular degeneration risk; thus, its elimination should be one the first therapeutic recommendations. Preventative recommendations also include dietary supplementation with antioxidants and minerals such as vitamin E (α-tocopherol), vitamin C (ascorbic acid), zinc, and β-carotene for persons at risk for developing macular degeneration and for slowing the progression of age-related macular degeneration in persons with the disease according to the AREDS study.[36]

Retinoblastoma

Retinoblastoma is the most common intraocular malignant neoplasm of children, affecting approximately 1 in 15,000

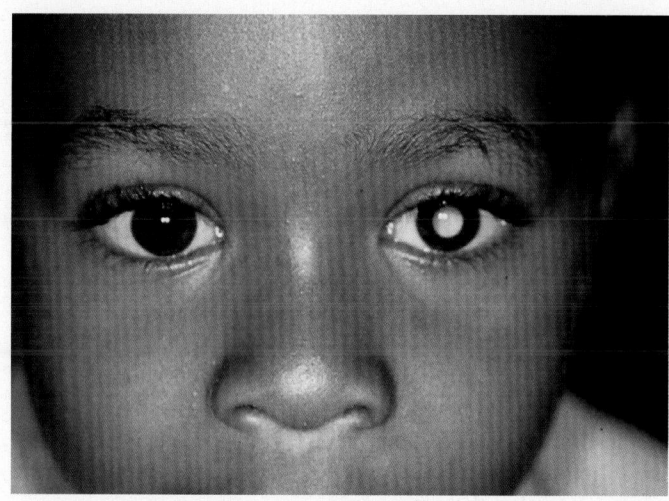

FIGURE 54.18 • The white pupil reflex (leukokoria) in the left eye of a child with retinoblastoma. (From Rubin R., Strayer D. S. (Eds.). (2012). *Rubin's pathology: Clinicopathologic foundations of medicine* (6th ed., p. 1413). Philadelphia, PA: Lippincott Williams & Wilkins.)

worldwide.[10,40] The tumour occurs most frequently in children younger than 3 years of age and may even be found at birth. Retinoblastomas are related inherited or acquired mutations in the retinoblastoma (*Rb*) tumour suppressor gene, located on the long arm of chromosome 13 (13q14; see Chapter 8). If untreated, almost all children die of intracranial extension and disseminated disease. However, new diagnostic and treatment methods allow for a high rate of cure (96% to 98% survival in Canada).[41,42]

Leukokoria (*i.e.*, cat's-eye reflex, white reflex, or white pupil) is the most common presenting sign and is often noticed by the family; light entering the eye commonly reflects a yellowish-white colour similar to that of the membranous covering of a cat's eye (Fig. 54.18). Strabismus (*i.e.*, crossed eye, lazy eye) is the second most common sign.[10] Red, tearing, and painful eyes are a late sign of the disorder. Limited or poor vision is also a late sign. Most retinoblastomas occur sporadically and are unilateral. Up to 25% of sporadic retinoblastomas and most inherited forms of the disorder are bilateral.

Diagnostic measures for detection of retinoblastoma are usually prompted by abnormal results of an eye examination in the hospital nursery or healthcare provider's office. All children with a family history of retinoblastoma should be screened soon after birth. Screening should be repeated every 4 to 6 weeks until 1 year of age, and then every 2 to 3 months until 3 years of age.[42] Congenital cataracts are an important cause of childhood leukokoria and should be ruled out. A definitive diagnosis usually requires ophthalmoscopic examination under general anesthesia by an ophthalmologist to obtain complete visualization of both eyes, which facilitates photographing and mapping of the tumours. CT or MRI scans are used to evaluate the extent of the intraocular disease and extraocular spread.

The treatment of retinoblastoma has changed dramatically in recent years owing to the evolution of treatment options. The goals of treatment are primarily to save the child's life and secondarily to save the eye. Treatment options include laser thermotherapy, radioactive plaque therapy, cryotherapy, chemotherapy, external beam radiation, and enucleation (removal of the eye).[40,42,43] The choice of treatment is determined by the size of the tumour and its location and extension, as well as the visual potential and age of the child. Up to 45% of children treated with eye-preserving therapy may need subsequent therapy for recurrence of tumour, and up to 10% of children with unilateral tumours will develop a tumour in the contralateral eye.[43]

IN SUMMARY

The neural retina covers the inner aspect of the posterior two thirds of the eyeball and is continuous with the optic nerve. It contains the neural receptors for vision, and it is here that light energy of different frequencies and intensities is converted to graded local potentials, which then are converted to action potentials and transmitted to visual centres in the brain. The photoreceptors normally shed portions of their outer segments. These segments are phagocytized by cells in the pigment epithelium. Failure of phagocytosis, as occurs in one form of retinitis pigmentosa, results in degeneration of the pigment layer and blindness.

The retina receives its blood from two sources: the choriocapillaris, which supplies the pigment layer and the outer portion of the sensory retina adjacent to the choroid, and the branches of the retinal artery, which supply the inner half of the retina. Retinal blood vessels are normally apparent through the ophthalmoscope. Neovascularization involves the formation of new, fragile blood vessels that leak protein, and are likely to bleed. Although the cause of neovascularization is uncertain, research links the process with a VEGF produced by the lining of blood vessels. Hypoxia is a key regulator of VEGF-induced retinal neovascularization.

Disorders of retinal vessels can result from many local and systemic disorders, including diabetes mellitus and hypertension. They cause vision loss through changes that result in hemorrhage, production of opacities, and separation of the pigment epithelium and sensory retina. Retinal detachment involves separation of the sensory receptors from their blood supply; it causes blindness unless reattachment is accomplished promptly. Macular degeneration is characterized by loss of central vision due to destructive changes of the macula of the retina. There are two types of age-related macular degeneration: a nonexudative "dry form" that causes atrophy and degeneration of the outer retina and an exudative "wet form" that results in formation of a choroidal neovascular membrane with vessels that leak blood and serum and predispose to separation of the pigmented epithelium from the neuroretina. Although there are currently no effective therapies for the dry form of age-related macular degeneration, effective forms of treatment for the wet form include photodynamic therapy, laser photocoagulation, and intravitreal injection of corticosteroids and VEGF inhibitors.

Retinoblastoma is an intraocular malignant neoplasm of children (most often those younger than 2 years of age) that is caused by inherited or acquired mutations in the retinoblastoma (*Rb*) tumour suppressor gene. The most common presenting sign is leukokoria (white reflex or white pupil), with strabismus being the second most common sign. With new diagnostic and treatment methods, retinoblastomas in Canada can be cured.

DISORDERS OF NEURAL PATHWAYS AND CORTICAL CENTRES

After completing this section of the chapter, you should be able to meet the following objectives:

- Characterize what is meant by a *visual field defect.*
- Explain the use of perimetry in the diagnosis of a visual field defect.
- Define the terms *hemianopia, quadrantanopia, heteronymous hemianopia,* and *homonymous hemianopia* and relate them to disorders of the optic pathways.
- Describe visual defects associated with disorders of the visual cortex and visual association areas.

Full visual function requires the normally developed brain-related functions of photoreception and the pupillary reflex. These functions depend on the integrity of all optic pathways,

including retinal circuitry and the pathway from the optic nerve to the visual cortex and other visual regions of the brain and brain stem.

Optic Pathways

Visual information is carried to the brain by axons of the retinal ganglion cells, which form the optic nerve. Surrounded by pia mater, cerebrospinal fluid, arachnoid, and the dura mater, the optic nerve represents an outgrowth of the brain rather than a peripheral nerve. The optic nerve extends from the back of the optic globe through the orbit and the optic foramen, into the middle cranial fossa, and on to the optic chiasm at the base of the brain[18] (Fig. 54.19). Axons from the nasal portion of the retina remain medial, and those from the temporal retina remain lateral in the optic nerve.

The two optic nerves meet and fuse in the optic chiasm, beyond which they are continued as the optic tracts. In the optic chiasm, axons from the nasal retina of each eye cross to the opposite side and join with the axons of the temporal retina of the contralateral eye to form the optic tracts. Thus, one optic tract contains fibres from both eyes that transmit information from the same visual hemifield (half-field).

Visual Cortex

The primary visual cortex (area 17) surrounds the calcarine fissure, which lies in the occipital lobe. It is at this level that visual sensation is first experienced (Fig. 54.20). Immediately surrounding area 17 are the visual association cortices (areas 18 and 19) and several other association cortices.[18] These association cortices, with their thalamic nuclei, must be functional to add meaningfulness to visual perception.

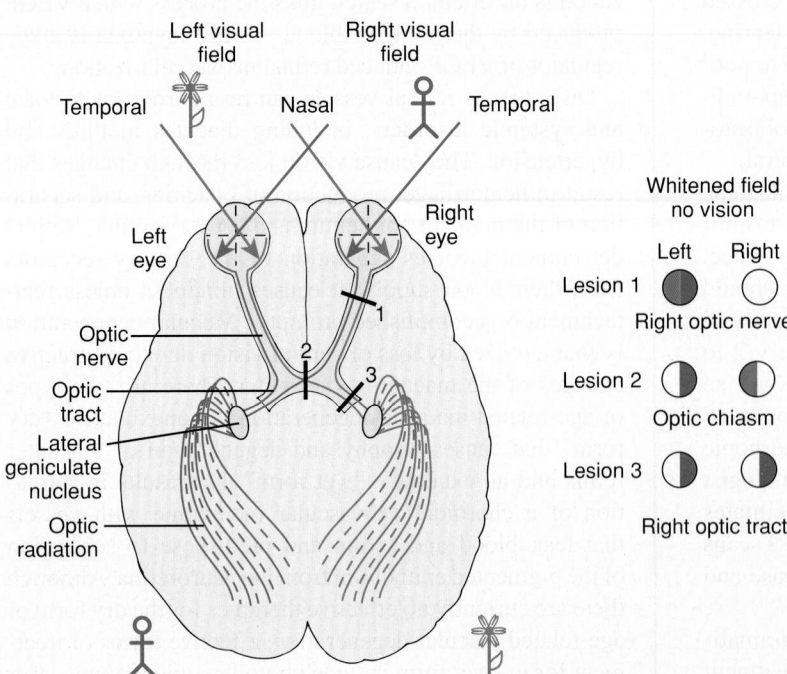

FIGURE 54.19 • Diagram of optic pathways. The *red lines* indicate the right visual field and the *blue lines* the left visual field. Note the crossing of fibres from the medial half of each retina at the optic chiasm. Lesion 1 (right optic nerve) produces unilateral blindness. Lesion 2 (optic chiasm) may involve only those fibres that originate in the nasal half of each retina and cross to the opposite side in the optic chiasm; visual loss involves the temporal half of each field (bitemporal hemianopia). Lesion 3 (right optic tract) interrupts fibres (and vision) originating on the same side of both eyes (homonymous) with loss of vision from half of each field (hemianopia).

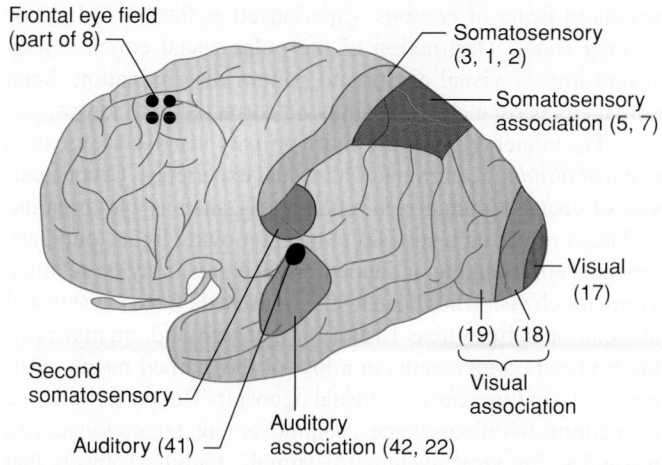

FIGURE 54.20 • Lateral view of the cortex illustrating the location of the visual, visual association, auditory, and auditory association areas.

Visual Fields

The *visual field* refers to the area that is visible during fixation of vision in one direction. Because visual system deficits are often expressed as visual field deficits rather than as direct measures of neural function, the terminology for normal and abnormal visual characteristics usually is based on visual field orientation.

Most of the visual field is *binocular,* or seen by both eyes. This binocular field is subdivided into central and peripheral portions. Central portions of the retina provide high visual acuity and correspond to the field focused on the central fovea; the peripheral and surrounding portion provides the capacity to detect objects, particularly moving objects. Beyond the visual field shared by both eyes, the left lateral periphery of the visual field is seen exclusively by the left nasal retina, and the right peripheral field is seen by the right nasal retina.

As with a camera, the simple lens system of the eye inverts the image of the external world on each retina. In addition, the right and left sides of the visual field also are reversed. The right binocular visual field is seen by the left retinal halves of each eye—the nasal half of the right eye and the temporal half of the left eye.

Once the level of the retina is reached, the nervous system plays a consistent role. The upper half of the visual field is received by the lower half of the retinas of both eyes.

Representations of this upper half of the field are carried in the lower half of each optic nerve: they synapse in the lower half of the lateral geniculate nucleus (LGN) of each side of the brain (Fig. 54.19). Neurons in this part of the LGN send their axons through the inferior half of the optic radiation, looping into the temporal lobe to terminate in the lower half of the primary visual cortex on each side of the brain.

Because of the lateral separation of the two eyes, each eye contributes a different image of the world to the visual field. This is called *binocular disparity.* Disparity between the laterally displaced images seen by the two eyes provides a powerful source of three-dimensional depth perception for objects within a distance of 30 m. Beyond that distance, binocular disparity becomes insignificant: depth perception is based on other cues (*e.g.,* the superimposition of the image of near objects over that of far objects, and the faster movement of near objects than of far objects).

Visual Field Defects

Visual field defects result from damage to the retina, optic pathways, or the visual cortex. Perimetry or visual field testing, in which the limits of the visual field of each eye are measured and plotted in an arc, is used to identify defects and determine the location of lesions.

Retinal Defects. All of us possess a hole, or *scotoma,* in our visual field, of which we are unaware. Because the optic disc, where the optic nerve fibres exit the retina, does not contain photoreceptors, the corresponding location in the visual field constitutes a blind spot approximately 15 degrees temporal to fixation of each eye. Local retinal damage caused by small vascular lesions and other localized pathologic processes can produce additional blind spots. As with the normal blind spot, persons are usually not aware of the existence of scotomata in their visual field unless they encounter problems seeing objects in certain restricted parts of the visual field.

Absences near or in the centre of the bilateral visual field can be annoying and even disastrous. Although the hole is not recognized as such, the person finds that a part of a printed page appears or disappears, depending on where the fixation point is held. Most persons learn to position their eyes to use the remaining central foveal vision for high-acuity tasks. Defects in the peripheral visual field, including the monocular peripheral fields, are less annoying but potentially more dangerous. Persons who are unaware of the defect, when walking or driving an automobile, do not see cars or bicyclists until their image reaches the functional visual field—sometimes too late to avert an accident. Once these persons become aware of the defect, they can learn to shift their gaze constantly to obtain visual coverage of important parts of the visual field. If the damage is at the retinal or optic nerve level, only the monocular field of the damaged eye becomes a problem. A lesion affecting the central foveal vision of one eye can result in complaints of eyestrain during reading and other close work because only one eye is being used.

Disorders of the Optic Pathways

Localized damage to the optic tracts, LGN, optic radiation, or primary visual cortex affects corresponding parts of the visual fields of both eyes (Fig. 54.19). Examination of visual system function is of particular importance because lesions at various points along the pathway have characteristic symptoms that assist in the localization of the lesion.

Among the disorders that can interrupt the optic pathway are vascular lesions, trauma, and tumours. For example, normal visual system function depends on adequate perfusion of the ophthalmic artery and its branches; the central artery of the retina; the anterior and middle cerebral arteries, which supply the intracranial optic nerve, chiasm, and optic tracts; and the posterior cerebral artery, which supplies the LGN, optic radiation, and visual cortex. The adequacy of posterior cerebral artery function depends on that of the vertebral and basilar arteries that supply the brain stem. Vascular insufficiency in any one of these arterial systems can seriously affect vision.

Visual field defects of each eye and of the two eyes together are useful in localizing lesions affecting the system. Blindness in one eye is called *anopia.* If half of the visual field for one eye is lost, the defect is called *hemianopia,* and if a quarter of the field is lost, it is called *quadrantanopia.* Enlarging pituitary tumours can produce longitudinal damage through the optic chiasm with loss of the medial fibres of the optic nerve representing both nasal retinas and both temporal visual half-fields. The loss of different half-fields in the two eyes is called a *heteronymous loss,* and the abnormality is called *heteronymous hemianopia.* Destruction of one or both lateral halves of the chiasm is common with multiple aneurysms of the circle of Willis (see Chapter 50). In this condition, the function of one or both temporal retinas is lost, and the nasal fields of one or both eyes are lost. The loss of the temporal fields (nasal retina) of both eyes is called *bitemporal heteronymous hemianopia.* With both eyes open, the person with bilateral defects still has the full binocular visual field.

Loss of the optic tract, LGN, full optic radiation, or complete visual cortex on one side results in loss of the corresponding visual half-fields in each eye. *Homonymous* means "the same" for both eyes. In left-side lesions, the right visual field is lost for each eye and is called *complete right homonymous hemianopia.* Partial injury to the left optic tract, LGN, or optic radiation can result in the loss of a quarter of the visual field in both eyes. This is called *homonymous quadrantanopia,* and depending on the lesion, it can involve the upper (superior) or lower (inferior) fields. Because the optic radiation fibres for the superior quarter of the visual field traverse the temporal lobe, superior quadrantanopia is more common.

Disorders of the Visual Cortex

Discrete damage to the binocular portion of the primary visual cortex also can result in scotomata in the corresponding visual fields. The central high-acuity portion of the visual field is located at the occipital pole. If the visual loss is in the central high-acuity part of the field, severe loss of visual acuity and pattern discrimination occurs. Mechanical trauma to the cortex results in firing of neurons, experienced as flashes of light or "seeing stars." Destruction of the polar visual cortex causes severe loss of visual acuity and pattern discrimination. Such damage is permanent and cannot be corrected with lenses.

The bilateral loss of the entire primary visual cortex, called *cortical blindness,* eliminates all visual experience. Crude analysis of visual stimulation at reflex levels, such as eye-orienting and head-orienting responses to bright moving lights, pupillary reflexes, and blinking at sudden bright lights, may be retained even though vision has been lost. Extensive damage to the visual association cortex (areas 18 and 19) that surrounds an intact primary visual cortex results in a loss of the learned meaningfulness of visual images (*i.e.,* visual agnosia). The person can see the patterns of colour, shapes, and movement, but no longer can recognize formerly meaningful stimuli. Familiar objects can be described but not named or reacted to meaningfully. However, if other sensory modalities, such as hearing and touch, can be applied, full recognition occurs. This disorder represents a problem of recognition rather than intellect.

Testing of Visual Fields

Crude testing of the binocular visual field and the visual field of each individual eye (*i.e.,* monocular vision) can be accomplished without specialized equipment. In the confrontation method, the examiner stands or sits in front of the person to be tested and instructs the person to focus with one eye closed on the examiner's nose while random presentations of finger quantities are presented roughly 1 m from the observer in each of the four major field quadrants to assess for the awareness of the finger quantities. In a kinetic assessment of the expansiveness of the gross visual field, an object such as a penlight is moved from the centre toward the periphery of the person's visual field and from the periphery toward the centre, and the person is instructed to report the presence or absence of the object. By moving the object through the vertical, horizontal, and oblique aspects of the visual field, a crude estimate can be made of the visual field. Large field defects can be estimated by the confrontation method, and it may be the only way for testing young children and uncooperative adults.

Accurate determination of the presence, size, and shape of smaller holes, or scotomata, in the visual field of a particular eye can be demonstrated only by perimetry. This is done by having the person look with one eye toward a central spot directly in front of the eye while the head is stabilized by a chin rest or bite board. A small dot of light or a coloured object is moved back and forth in all areas of the visual field. The person reports whether the stimulus is visible and, if a coloured stimulus is used, what the perceived colour is. A hemispheric support is used to control and standardize the movement of the test object, and a plot of radial coordinates of the visual field is made. Automated perimetry uses static dots of varying intensity and colour, as well as flicker frequency stimuli, to assess higher levels of retinal cell function. Perimetry provides a means of determining alterations from normal and, with repeated testing, a way of following the progress of the condition causing the visual field defect or its treatment.

IN SUMMARY

Visual information is carried to the brain by axons of the retinal ganglion cells that form the optic nerve. The two optic nerves meet and fuse in the optic chiasm. The axons of each nasal retina cross in the chiasm and join the uncrossed fibres of the temporal retina of the opposite eye in the optic tract to form the optic tracts. The fibres of each optic tract then synapse in the LGN, and from there, travel by way of the optic radiations to the primary visual cortex in the calcarine area of the occipital lobe. Damage to the visual association cortex can result in the phenomenon of seeing an object without the ability to recognize it (*i.e.,* visual agnosia). Optic pathway or visual cortex damage leads to visual field defects that can be identified through visual field testing. Perimetry, which maps the sensitivity contours of the visual field, can be used to determine the presence, size, and shape of smaller holes, or scotomata, in the visual field of an eye.

DISORDERS OF EYE MOVEMENT

After completing this section of the chapter, you should be able to meet the following objectives:

- Describe the function and innervation of the extraocular muscles.
- Recognize the use of smooth pursuit, saccadic, and vergence conjugate gaze movements in self or others.
- Explain the difference between paralytic and nonparalytic strabismus.
- Define *amblyopia* and explain its pathogenesis.
- Explain the need for early diagnosis and treatment of eye movement disorders in children.

For complete visual function, it is necessary that the two eyes focus on the same fixation point, that the image of the object falls simultaneously on the fovea of each eye, and that the retinal and CNS visual mechanisms are functional. It is through these mechanisms that an object is simultaneously imaged on the fovea of both eyes and perceived as a single image. Strabismus and amblyopia are two disorders that affect this highly integrated system.

Extraocular Eye Muscles and Their Innervation

Each eyeball can rotate around its vertical axis (lateral or medial rotation in which the pupil moves away from or toward the nose), its horizontal left-to-right axis (vertical elevation or depression, in which the pupil moves up or down), and torsional rotations on the longitudinal horizontal axis (in which the top of the pupil moves toward or away from the nose).

Three pairs of extraocular muscles—the superior and inferior recti, the medial and lateral recti, and the superior and inferior obliques—control the movement of each eye (Fig. 54.21). The four rectus muscles are named according to where they insert into the sclera on the medial, lateral, inferior, and superior surfaces of each eye. The two oblique muscles insert on the lateral posterior quadrant of the eyeball—the superior oblique on the upper surface and the inferior oblique on the lower. Each of the three sets of muscles in each eye is reciprocally innervated so that one muscle relaxes when the other contracts. Reciprocal contraction of the medial and lateral recti moves the eye from side to side (adduction and abduction); the superior and inferior recti move the eye up and down (elevation and depression). The oblique muscles rotate (intorsion and extorsion) the eye around its optic axis and have a role in elevation and depression. A seventh muscle, the levator palpebrae superioris, elevates the upper lid.

The extraocular muscles are innervated by three cranial nerves. The abducens nerve (CN VI) innervates the lateral rectus,

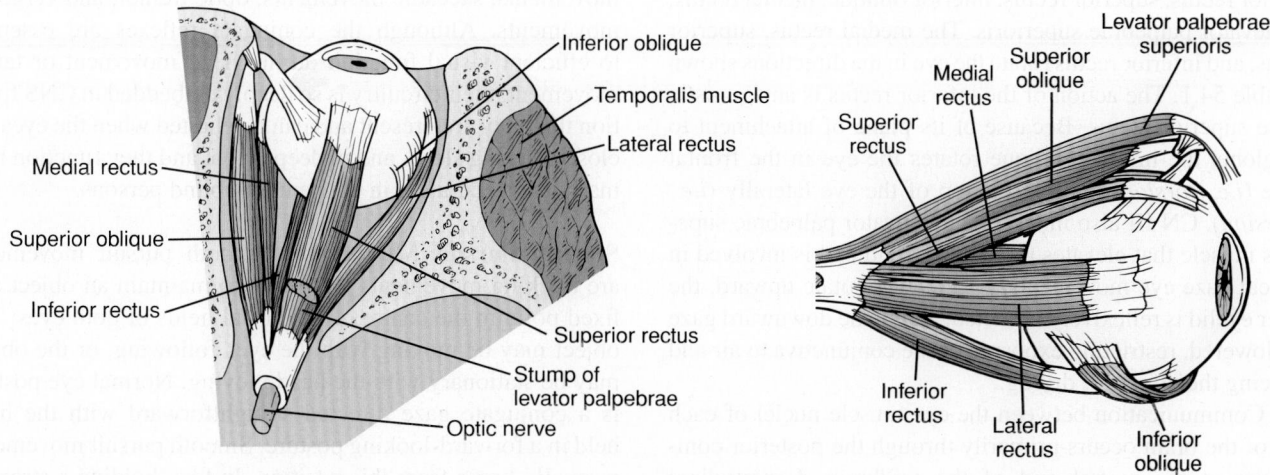

FIGURE 54.21 • Extraocular muscles of the right eye.

III–SR   IO–III   III–IO   SR–III

VI–LR   ○   MR III   MR III   ○   LR–VI

III–IR   SO–IV   IV–SO   IR–III

TABLE 54.1 EYE IN PRIMARY POSITION: EXTRINSIC OCULAR MUSCLE ACTIONS

MUSCLE[a]	INNERVATION	PRIMARY	SECONDARY	TERTIARY
MR: medial rectus	III	Adduction		
LR: lateral rectus	VI	Abduction		
SR: superior rectus	III	Elevation	Intorsion	Adduction
IR: inferior rectus	III	Depression	Extorsion	Adduction
SO: superior oblique	IV	Intorsion	Depression	Abduction
IO: inferior oblique	III	Extorsion	Elevation	Abduction

[a]In the schema of the functional roles of the six extraocular muscles, the major directional force applied by each muscle is indicated on the top. These muscles are arranged in functionally opposing pairs per eye and in parallel opposing pairs for conjugate movements of the two eyes. The numbers associated with each muscle indicate the cranial nerve innervation: 3, oculomotor (III) cranial nerve; 4, trochlear (IV) cranial nerve; 6, abducens (VI) cranial nerve.

the trochlear nerve (CN IV) innervates the superior oblique, and the oculomotor nerve (CN III) innervates the remaining four muscles (Table 54.1). The CN VI (abducens) nucleus, in the caudal pons, innervates the lateral rectus muscle, which rotates the ipsilateral (same-side) eye laterally (abduction). Partial or complete damage to this nerve results in weakness or complete paralysis of the muscle. Medial gaze is normal, but the affected eye fails to rotate laterally with an attempted gaze toward the affected side, giving the appearance of an esotropia. The CN IV (trochlear) nucleus, at the junction of the pons and midbrain, innervates the contralateral or opposite-side superior oblique muscle, which rotates the top of the globe inward toward the nose, a movement called *intorsion*. In combination with other muscles, it also contributes strength to movement of the innervated eye downward and inward.

The CN III (oculomotor) nucleus, which extends through a considerable part of the midbrain, contains clusters of lower motor neurons for each of the five eye muscles it innervates: inferior rectus, superior rectus, inferior oblique, medial rectus, and levator palpebrae superioris. The medial rectus, superior rectus, and inferior rectus rotate the eye in the directions shown in Table 54.1. The action of the inferior rectus is antagonistic to the superior rectus. Because of its plane of attachment to the globe, the inferior oblique rotates the eye in the frontal plane (*i.e.*, torsion), pulling the top of the eye laterally (*i.e.*, extorsion). CN III also innervates the levator palpebrae superioris muscle that elevates the upper eyelid and is involved in vertical gaze eye movements. As the eyes rotate upward, the upper eyelid is reflexively retracted, and in the downward gaze it is lowered, restricting exposure of the conjunctiva to air and reducing the effects of drying.

Communication between the eye muscle nuclei of each side of the brain occurs primarily through the posterior commissure at the rostral end of the midbrain. Longitudinal communication among the three nuclei occurs along a fibre tract called the *medial longitudinal fasciculus* (MLF), which extends from the midbrain to the upper part of the spinal cord. Each pair of eye muscles is reciprocally innervated, by the MLF or other associated pathways, so that as one muscle contracts, the other relaxes. These MLF-linked communication paths are vulnerable to damage in the caudal midbrain and pons. Damage to the pontine MLF on one side of the brain results in loss of this linkage, so that lateral deviation of the ipsilateral eye is no longer linked to adduction on the contralateral side. If the MLF is damaged bilaterally, the linkage is lost for lateral gaze in either direction. This can occur in patients with multiple sclerosis or ischemic damage.

Eye Movements and Gaze

Conjugate movements are those in which the optical axes of the two eyes are kept parallel, sharing the same visual field. *Gaze* refers to the act of looking steadily in one direction. Eye movements can be categorized into smooth pursuit movements, saccadic movements, optic tremor, and vergence movements. Although the conjugate reflexes are essential to efficient visual function during head movement or target movement, their circuitry is so deeply embedded in CNS function that they are present and can be elicited when the eyes are closed, during sleep, and in deep coma, and they function normally and accurately in congenitally blind persons.

Smooth Pursuit Movements. Smooth pursuit movements are tracking movements that serve to maintain an object at a fixed point in the centre of the visual fields of both eyes. The object may be moving with the eyes following, or the object may be stationary with the head moving. Normal eye posture is a conjugate gaze directed straightforward with the head held in a forward-looking posture. Smooth pursuit movements normally begin from this position. In fact, holding a strongly deviated gaze becomes tiring after about 30 seconds, and most people will make head and body rotation adjustments to bring the eyes to a central position within that time.

Voluntary pursuit movements are tested by asking the person to follow a finger or another object as it is moved slowly through the visual field. Successful conjugate following requires a functional optic system communicating to the superior colliculus and with the primary visual cortex.

Saccadic Eye Movements. Saccadic eye movements are sudden, jerky conjugate movements that quickly change the fixation point. During reading, the fixation pattern involves a focus on a word or short series of words and then a sudden jump of the eyes to a new fixation point on the next word or phrase. During the saccade, a person does not experience the blur of the rapidly moving visual field. Saccadic movements are automatic reflex movements that, in most situations, operate at the brain stem level. Saccadic shifts of a gaze toward the source of a sudden, unexpected visual, auditory, tactile, or painful stimulus are a component of the startle pattern. This is functionally a visual grasping reflex, redirecting conjugate gaze in the direction of the startle stimulus.

The frontal eye fields of the premotor cortex are important for voluntary saccadic movements such as reading. If this frontal premotor area is not functional, a person can describe objects in the visual field but cannot voluntarily search the visual environment.

Eye Tremor. An eye tremor refers to involuntary, rhythmic, oscillatory eye movements, occurring approximately 10 times per second. Small-range optical tremors are a normal and useful independent function of each eye. One function of the fine optic tremor is to constantly move a bright image onto a new bank of cones, permitting previously stimulated receptors to quickly recover from adaptation.

Vergence Eye Movements. Vergence eye movements are those that move the eyes in opposite directions to keep the image of an object precisely positioned on the fovea of each eye. Convergence and divergence, which assist in maintaining a binocularly fixed image in near vision, have a major role in accurate depth perception. The vergence system is driven by retinal disparity (*i.e.,* differential placement of an object's image on each retina). A nearby target (<10 m) moving in the same dimension as the optical axis elicits a reflex mechanism that provides redirection of the optical axes of each eye away from parallel (*i.e.,* in opposite directions) in the horizontal plane. This process permits a continued binocular focus on the near target. Perception of depth is a higher-order function of the cortical visual system and is based on one or more of several classes of stimuli, such as superimposition and relative movement.

Strabismus

Strabismus, also referred to as "squint" or "crossed eye," refers to any abnormality of eye coordination or alignment that results in loss of binocular vision.[44] When images from the same spots in visual space do not fall on corresponding points of the two retinas, diplopia, or double vision, occurs. Strabismus affects approximately 4% of children younger than 6 years of age.[44] Because 30% to 50% of these children sustain permanent secondary loss of vision, or amblyopia, if the condition is left untreated, early diagnosis and treatment are essential.

In standard terminology, the disorders of eye movement are described according to the direction of movement. *Esotropia* refers to medial (inward) deviation, *exotropia* to lateral (outward) deviation, *hypertropia* to upward deviation, *hypotropia* to downward deviation, and *cyclotropia* to torsional deviation. The term *concomitance* refers to equal deviation in all directions of gaze. A nonconcomitant strabismus is one that varies with the direction of gaze. Strabismus may be divided into nonparalytic (concomitant) forms, in which there is no primary muscle impairment, and paralytic (nonconcomitant) forms, in which there is weakness or paralysis of one or more of the extraocular muscles. Strabismus is called *intermittent,* or *periodic,* when there are periods in which the eyes are parallel. It is monocular when the same eye always deviates and the opposite eye fixates. Figure 54.22 illustrates abnormalities in eye movement associated with esotropia and exotropia.

Nonparalytic Strabismus

Nonparalytic esotropia is the most common type of strabismus. The individual ocular muscles have no obvious defect and the amount of deviation is constant, or relatively constant in the various directions of gaze. With persistent deviation, secondary abnormalities may develop because of overactivity or underactivity of the extraocular muscles in some fields of gaze.

The disorder may be nonaccommodative, accommodative, or a combination of the two. Infantile esotropia is the most common cause of nonaccommodative strabismus. It occurs in the first 6 months of life, with large-angle deviations, in an otherwise developmentally and neurologically normal infant. Eye movements are full, and the child often uses each eye independently to alter fixation (cross-fixation). The cause of the disorder is unclear. Research suggests that idiopathic strabismus may have a genetic basis; siblings often present with similar disorders.

Accommodative strabismus is caused by disorders such as uncorrected hyperopia of a significant degree, in which the esotropia occurs with accommodation that is undertaken to focus clearly. Onset of this type of esotropia characteristically occurs between 18 months and 4 years of age because accommodation is not well developed until that time. The disorder most often is monocular but may be alternating.

Paralytic Strabismus

Paralytic strabismus results from paresis (*i.e.,* weakness) or plegia (*i.e.,* paralysis) of one or more of the extraocular muscles. When the normal eye fixates, the affected eye is in the position of primary deviation. In the case of esotropia, there is weakness of one of the lateral rectus muscles, usually due to a disorder of the abducens nerve (CN VI). When the affected eye

A Primary position: right esotropia

B Left gaze: no deviation

C Right gaze: left esotropia

D Right hypertropia

E Right exotropia

FIGURE 54.22 • A–C: Paralytic strabismus associated with paralysis of the right lateral rectus muscle: (**A**) primary position of the eyes (looking straight ahead); (**B**) left gaze with no deviation; and (**C**) right gaze with left esotropia. **D:** Primary position of the eyes with weakness of the right inferior rectus and right hypertropia. **E:** Primary position of the eyes with weakness of the right medial rectus and right exotropia.

fixates, the unaffected eye is in a position of secondary deviation. The secondary deviation of the unaffected eye is greater than the primary deviation of the affected eye. This is because the affected eye requires an excess of innervational impulse to maintain fixation; the excess impulses also are distributed to the unaffected eye, causing overaction of its muscles.[44]

Paralytic strabismus is uncommon in children but accounts for nearly all cases of adult strabismus; it can be caused by infiltrative processes (*e.g.,* Graves disease; see Chapter 41), myasthenia gravis, stroke, and direct optical trauma. The pathway of the oculomotor, trochlear, and abducens nerves through the cavernous sinus and the back of the orbit make them vulnerable to basal skull fracture and tumours of the cavernous sinus or orbit. In infants, paralytic strabismus can be caused by birth injuries affecting the extraocular muscles or the cranial nerves supplying these muscles. In general, paralytic strabismus in an older child or adult does not produce amblyopia, and binocular vision can be maintained when the strabismus is corrected. Most adult strabismus represents deterioration of childhood strabismus, which can occur even decades after good ocular alignment.

Treatment

Treatment of strabismus is directed toward the development of normal visual acuity, correction of the deviation, and superimposition of the retinal images to provide binocular vision.

Early and adequate treatment is crucial because a delay in or lack of treatment can lead to amblyopia and permanent loss of vision. In addition to its effects on visual function, strabismus can have an adverse impact on interpersonal relationships, self-image, schoolwork, and participation in extracurricular activities. Children begin to develop negative attitudes toward classmates with strabismus as early as 6 years of age.

Treatment includes both surgical and nonsurgical methods. Infantile esotropia is usually treated surgically by weakening the medial rectus muscle on each eye while the infant is under general anesthesia. Surgery in children with esotropia should be done as early as possible to preserve stereoptic acuity. Early surgical treatment also appears to result in better outcomes than later intervention. Recurrent strabismus is common with infantile esotropia, and multiple surgeries are often required.

Nonsurgical treatment includes glasses, occlusive patching, and eye exercises (*i.e.,* pleoptics). Glasses are often used in the treatment of accommodative esotropia that occurs with hypermetropia (farsightedness). Because accommodation is linked with convergence, focusing drives the eyes inward, producing esotropia. Intermittent exotropia is commonly treated with patching, use of overminus glasses, and eye exercises. Although no appreciable deviation is present when the child with intermittent strabismus sees near objects, the deviation becomes obvious when the child views distant objects or is fatigued. Patching for 1 to 2 hours daily for several months works by preventing, rather than treating, suppression of an eye. Patching is most effective in infants, and the efficacy is limited once the child passes the age of 10. The use of over-minus glasses stimulates accommodative convergences, which contracts the exotropic drift. Vision therapy involves exercises to stimulate convergence (*e.g.,* focusing on reading-distance targets up to 30 minutes several times a day) and techniques to train the visual system to recognize the suppressed images. Surgical treatment of intermittent exotropia is indicated when conservative methods fail to correct the deviation. Early treatment of children with intermittent exotropia is not as crucial as it is for those with constant deviations because stereopsis can still develop.

A relatively new form of treatment involves the injection of botulinum toxin type A (Botox) into the extraocular muscle to produce a dose-dependent paralysis of that extraocular muscle. Paralysis of the muscle shifts the eye into the field of action of the antagonist muscle. During the time the eye is deviated the paralyzed muscle is stretched, whereas the antagonistic muscle is contracted. Usually two or more injections of the drug are necessary to obtain a lasting effect.

Amblyopia

Amblyopia, sometimes called *lazy eye,* describes a decrease in visual acuity resulting from abnormal visual development in infancy or early childhood.[44] The vision loss ranges from mild (worse than 20/25) to severe (legal blindness, 20/200 or worse). It is the leading cause of visual impairment, affecting 1% to 4% of the population. With early detection and treatment, most cases of amblyopia are reversible and the most severe forms of the condition can be prevented.

Normal development of the thalamic and cortical circuitry necessary for binocular visual perception requires simultaneous binocular use of each fovea during a critical period early in life (0 to 5 years). Amblyopia can result from visual deprivation (*e.g.,* cataracts, ptosis) or abnormal binocular interactions (*e.g.,* strabismus, anisometropia) during visual immaturity. In infants with unilateral cataracts that are dense, central, and larger than 2 mm in diameter, this time is before 2 months of age.[44] In conditions causing abnormal binocular interactions, one image is suppressed to provide clearer vision. In esotropia, vision of the deviated eye is suppressed to prevent diplopia. A similar situation exists in anisometropia, in which the refractive indexes of the two eyes are different. Although the eyes are correctly aligned, they are unable to focus together, and the image of one eye is suppressed.

The reversibility of amblyopia depends on the maturity of the visual system at the time of onset and the duration of the abnormal experience. Occasionally in strabismus, some persons alternate eye fixation and do not experience deep amblyopia or diplopia. With late adolescent or adult onset, this habit pattern must be unlearned after correction. Amblyopia is remarkably responsive to treatment if the treatment is initiated early in life; thus, all infants and young children should be evaluated for visual conditions that could lead to amblyopia (see the section on Eye Examination in Infants and Children).

The treatment of children with the potential for development of amblyopia must be instituted well before the age of 6 years to avoid the suppression phenomenon. Surgery for congenital cataracts and ptosis should be done early. Severe refractive errors should be corrected. In children with strabismus, the alternate blocking of the vision in one eye and then the other forces the child to use both eyes for form discrimination. The duration of occlusion of vision in the good eye must be short (2 to 5 hours per day) and closely monitored, or deprivation amblyopia can develop in the good eye as well. Although amblyopia is not likely to occur after 8 or 9 years of age, some plasticity in central circuitry is evident even in adulthood. For example, after refractive correction for long-standing astigmatism in adults, visual acuity improves slowly, requiring several months to reach normal levels.

Eye Examination in Infants and Children

Early detection and prompt treatment of ocular disorders in children are important to prevent amblyopia and lifelong visual impairment.[45] The Canadian Paediatric Society in association with the Canadian Ophthalmologic Society recommends that all newborn infants be examined in the nursery for structural abnormalities and have a red reflex test performed to check for abnormalities in the back of the eye (posterior segment) and opacities in the visual axis, such as cataracts or corneal opacity.[45] An infant with an abnormal red reflex requires immediate referral to an eye care specialist. Visual examinations should then be performed on all well-child visits. These should include age-appropriate evaluation of visual acuity, ocular alignment, and ocular media clarity (cataracts, tumours).

Visual assessment of infants and children younger than 3 years of age is accomplished by determining whether each eye can fixate on an object, maintain fixation, and then follow the object in various gaze positions. Failure to perform these maneuvers indicates significant visual impairment. The assessment should be done binocularly and monocularly. If poor fixation is noted binocularly after 3 months of age, a significant bilateral eye or brain abnormality should be suspected and the child should be referred for further evaluation. Emphasis should be placed on screening for visual acuity as soon as the child is cooperative enough to complete the examination. Decreased vision in one eye requires evaluation for ocular deviation or other ocular abnormalities, which may be difficult to discern on screening examination.[11,45] Strabismus deviations of only a few degrees, too small to be detected by gross inspection, can lead to amblyopia and vision loss.

Every effort should be made to ensure that eye examinations are performed by properly prepared examiners, using appropriate testing conditions, instruments, and techniques (the reader is referred to an appropriate reference source for a detailed description of the various methods that are used).[45,46] The provincial and territorial healthcare plans offer yearly screening for potential eye and vision problems as a complement to the eye screening provided in a pediatric well-care visit up to the age of 18 years.

The results of vision assessments and visual acuity measurements, along with instructions for follow-up care, should be clearly communicated to the parents. Parents' observations are also important. Questions about whether the child's eyes seem straight or seem to cross or drift, or appear lazy; whether the child's eyelids droop or one eyelid tends to close; and, in older children, whether the child seems to see well or tends to hold objects close to his or her face when trying to focus, can provide helpful information.[43–46]

IN SUMMARY

Binocular vision depends on the extraocular muscles and their innervating cranial nerves to move the eye up and down and rotate it around its optical axis. For full visual function, it is necessary that the two eyes point toward the same fixation point and the two images become fused. Binocular fusion is controlled by ocular reflex mechanisms that adjust the orientation of each eye to produce a single image. The term conjugate gaze refers to the use of both eyes to look steadily in one direction. During conjugate eye movements, the optical axes of the two eyes are maintained parallel to each other as the eyes rotate upward, downward, or from side to side in their sockets.

Strabismus refers to abnormalities in the coordination of eye movements, with loss of binocular eye alignment. This inability to focus a visual image on corresponding parts of the two retinas results in diplopia. Esotropia refers to medial deviation, exotropia to lateral deviation, hypertropia to upward deviation, hypotropia to downward deviation, and cyclotropia to torsional deviation. Paralytic strabismus is caused by weakness or paralysis of the extraocular muscles, whereas nonparalytic strabismus results from the inappropriate length or insertion of the extraocular muscles or from accommodation disorders.

Amblyopia (*i.e.*, lazy eye) is a decrease in visual acuity resulting from abnormal visual development in infancy and early childhood. It results from inadequately developed CNS circuitry because of visual deprivation (*e.g.*, cataracts) or abnormal binocular interactions (*e.g.*, strabismus) during visual immaturity.

REVIEW EXERCISES

1. The mother of a 3-year-old boy notices that his left eye is red and watering when she picks him up from day care. He keeps rubbing his eye as if it itches. The next morning, however, she notices that both eyes are red, swollen, and watering. Being concerned, she takes him to the family physician in the morning and is told that he has "pink eye." She is told that the infection should go away by itself.
   A. *What part of the eye is involved?*
   B. *What type of conjunctivitis do you think this child has: bacterial, viral, or allergic?*
   C. *Why didn't the pediatrician order an antibiotic?*
   D. *Is the condition contagious? What measures should she take to prevent its spread?*

2. During a routine eye examination to get new glasses because she had been having difficulty with her distant vision, a 75-year-old woman is told that she is developing cataracts.
   A. *What type of visual changes occurs as the result of a cataract?*
   B. *What can the woman do to prevent the cataracts from getting worse?*
   C. *What treatment may she eventually need?*

3. A 50-year-old woman is told by her "eye doctor" that her intraocular pressure is slightly elevated and that although there is no evidence of damage to her eyes at this time, she is at risk for developing glaucoma and should have regular eye examinations.
   A. *Describe the physiologic mechanisms involved in the regulation of intraocular pressure.*
   B. *What are the risk factors for developing glaucoma?*
   C. *Explain how an increase in intraocular pressure produces its damaging effects.*

4. The parents of a newborn infant have been told that their son has congenital cataracts in both eyes and will require cataract surgery to prevent loss of sight.
   A. *Explain why the infant is at risk for losing his sight if the cataracts are not removed.*
   B. *When should this procedure be done to prevent loss of vision?*

References

1. WHO. (2012). Global data on visual impairment 2010. Available online at: http://www.who.int/entity/blindness/GLOBALDATAFINALforweb.pdf?ua=1. Access May 18, 2015.
2. CNIB. (2015). Fast facts about vision loss. Available online at: http://www.cnib.ca/en/about/media/vision-loss/Pages/default.aspx. Accessed May 18, 2015.
3. Vagefi M. R., Sullivan J. H., Correa Z. M., et al. (2011). Chapter 4: Lids, lacrimal apparatus and tears. In Riordan-Eva P., Cunningham E. T. (Eds.), *Vaughan & Ashbury's general ophthalmology* (18th ed.). New York: Lange Medical Books.
4. Dogru M., Tsubota K. (2011). Pharmacotherapy of dry eye. *Expert Opinion on Pharmacotherapy, 12*(3), 325–334.
5. Riordan-Eva P. (2011). Chapter 1: Anatomy and embryology of the eye. In Riordan-Eva P., Cunningham E. T. (Eds.), *Vaughan & Ashbury's general ophthalmology* (18th ed.). New York: Lange Medical Books.

6. Pinar-Sueiro S., Sota M., Lerchundi T., et al. (2012). Dacryocystitis: Systematic approach to diagnosis and therapy. *Current Infectious Disease Reports, 14*(2), 137–146.

7. Nijm L. M., Garcia-Ferrier F., Schwab J. R., et al. (2011). Chapter 5: Conjunctivita and tears. In Riordan-Eva P., Cunningham E. T. (Eds.), *Vaughan & Ashbury's general ophthalmology* (18th ed.). New York: Lange Medical Books.

8. Azari A. A., Barney N. P. (2013). Conjunctivitis: A systemic review of diagnosis and treatment. *Journal of the American Medical Association, 310*(16), 1721–1729.

9. La Rosa M., Lionetti E., Reibaldi M., et al. (2013). Allergic conjunctivitis: A comprehensive review of the literature. *Italian Journal of Pediatrics, 39*(18).

10. Kumar V., Abbas A. K., Faustos N., et al. (Eds.). (2010). *Robbins and Cotran pathologic basis of disease* (8th ed.). Philadelphia, PA: Elsevier Saunders.

11. Olitsky S. E., Hug D., Plummer L. S., et al. (2011). Part XXIX: Disorders of the eye. In Kliegman R. M., Stanton B. F., St. Geme J. W., et al. (Eds.), *Nelson textbook of pediatrics* (19th ed.). Philadelphia, PA: Saunders Elsevier.

12. Matejcek A., Goldman R. D. (2013). Treatment and prevention of ophthalmia neonatorum. *Canadian Family Physician, 59*(11), 1187–1190.

13. Moore D. L., MacDonald N. E. (2015). Preventing ophthalmia neonatorum. *Paediatrics & Child Health, 20*(2), 93–96.

14. Biswell R. (2011). Chapter 6: Cornea. In Riordan-Eva P., Cunningham E. T. (Eds.), *Vaughan & Ashbury's general ophthalmology* (18th ed.). New York: Lange Medical Books.

15. Sampathkumar P., Drage L. A., Martin D. P. (2009). Herpes zoster (shingles) and postherpetic neuralgia. *Mayo Clinic Proceedings, 84*(3), 274–280.

16. Keirszenbaum A. L., Tres L. L. (2012). *Histology and cell biology: An introduction to pathology* (3rd ed.). Philadelphia: Elsevier.

17. Cunningham E. T., Augsburger J. J., Correa Z. A., et al. (2011). Chapter 7: Uveal tract and sclera. In Riordan-Eva P., Cunningham E. T. (Eds.), *Vaughan & Ashbury's general ophthalmology* (18th ed.). New York: Lange Medical Books.

18. Kandel E. R., Schwartz J. H., Jessell T. M. (2013). *Principles of neural science* (5th ed.). New York: McGraw-Hill Medical.

19. Almasieh M., Wilson A. M., Morquette B., et al. (2012). The molecular basis or retinal ganglion cell death in glaucoma. *Progress in Retinal and Eye Research, 31*(2), 152–181.

20. Salmon J. F. (2011). Chapter 11: Glaucoma. In Riordan-Eva P., Cunningham E. T. (Eds.), *Vaughan & Ashbury's general ophthalmology* (18th ed.). New York: Lange Medical Books.

21. Hall J. E. (2011). *Textbook of medical physiology* (12th ed.). Philadelphia, PA: W. B. Saunders.

22. Kwon Y. H., Fingert J. H., Kuehn M. H., Alward W. L. (2009). Primary open-angle glaucoma. *The New England Journal of Medicine, 360*(11), 1113–1124.

23. Patel K., Patel S. (2014). Angle-closure glaucoma. *Disease-a-Month, 60*(6), 254–262.

24. Fan B. J., Wiggs J. L. (2010). Glaucoma: Genes, phenotypes, and new directions for therapy. *Journal of Clinical Investigation, 120*(9), 3064–3072.

25. Messmer J. J. (2010). LASIK: A primer for family physicians. *American Family Physician, 81*(1), 42–48.

26. Harper R. A., Shock J. P. (2011). Chapter 8: Lens. In Riordan-Eva P., Cunningham E. T. (Eds.), *Vaughan & Ashbury's general ophthalmology* (18th ed.). New York: Lange Medical Books.

27. Wang J. J., Rochtchina E., Tan A. G., et al. (2009). Use of inhaled and oral corticosteroids and the long-term risk of cataract. *Ophthalmology, 116*(4), 652–657.

28. Pringle E., Graham E. M. (2011). Chapter 15: Ocular disorders associated with systemic diseases. In Riordan-Eva P., Cunningham E. T. (Eds.), *Vaughan & Ashbury's general ophthalmology* (18th ed.). New York: Lange Medical Books.

29. National Human Genome Research institute. (2013). Learning about retinitis pigmentosa. Available online at: https://www.genome.gov/13514348. Accessed May 18, 2015.

30. Harton D. T., Berson E. L., Dryja T. P. (2006). Retinitis pigmentosa. *Lancet, 368*, 1795–1809.

31. Fletcher E. C., Chong N. V., Augsburger J. J., et al. (2011). Chapter 10: Retina. In Riordan-Eva P., Cunningham E. T. (Eds.), *Vaughan & Ashbury's general ophthalmology* (18th ed.). New York: Lange Medical Books.

32. Fante R. J., Durairaj V. D., Oliver S. C. (2010). Diabetic retinopathy: An update on treatment. *American Journal of Medicine, 123*(3), 213–216.

33. ACCORD A Study Group and ACCORD Eye Study Group. (2010). Effects of medical therapies on retinopathy progression in type 2 diabetes. *The New England Journal of Medicine, 363*(3), 233–244.

34. Cuspidi C., Negri F., Giudici V., Sala C. (2009). Retinal changes and cardiac remodelling in systemic hypertension. *Therapeutic Advances in Cardiovascular Disease, 3*(3), 205–214.

35. Hooper P., Boucher M. C., Cruess A., et al. (2012). Canadian Ophthalmological Society evidence-based clinical practice guidelines for the management of diabetic retinopathy. *Canadian Journal of Ophthalmology, 47*(Suppl 1), S1–S30.

36. The Age-Related Eye Disease Study 2 (ARED2) Research Group. (2013). Lutein + zeaxanthin and omega-3 fatty acids for age-related macular degeneration. *Journal of the American Medical Association, 309*(19), 2005–2015.

37. Wong T. Y., Mitchell P. (2004). Hypertensive retinopathy. *The New England Journal of Medicine, 351*, 2310–2317.

38. D'Amico D. J. (2008). Primary retinal detachment. *The New England Journal of Medicine, 359*(22), 2346–2354.

39. Laurence S. L., Mitchell P., Seddon J. M., et al. (2012). Age-related macular degeneration. *Lancet, 379*(9827), 1728–1738.

40. Dimaras H., Kimani K., Dimba E. A., et al. (2012). Retinoblastoma. *Lancet, 379*(9824), 1436–1446.

41. Canadian Cancer Society. (2015). Retinoblastoma. Available online at: https://www.cancer.ca/en/cancer-information/cancer-type/retinoblastoma/retinoblastoma/?region=on. Accessed May 18, 2015.

42. Canadain Retinoblasotma Society. (2009). National retinoblastoma strategy Canadian guidelines for Care. *Canadian Journal of Ophthalmology, 44*(Suppl 2), S1–S88.

43. Melamud A., Palekar R., Singh A. (2006). Retinoblastoma. *American Family Physician, 73*, 1039–1044.

44. Motley W. W., Asbury T. (2011). Chapter 12: Strabismus. In Riordan-Eva P., Cunningham E. T. (Eds.), *Vaughan & Ashbury's general ophthalmology* (18th ed.). New York: Lange Medical Books.

45. Bell A. L., Rodes M. E., Kellar L. C. (2013). Childhood eye examination. *American Family Physician, 88*(4), 241–248.

46. Amit M., Canadian Paediatric Society. (2014). Vision screening in infants, children and youth. *Paediatrics & Child Health, 14*(4), 246–248.

Visit thePoint **http://thePoint.lww.com for animations, journal articles, and more!**

Disorders of Hearing and Vestibular Function

55

The ears are paired organs consisting of an external and middle ear, which function in capturing, transmitting, and amplifying sound, and an inner ear that contains the receptive organs that are stimulated by sound waves (*i.e.,* hearing) or head position and movement (*i.e.,* vestibular function). Acute otitis media, or inflammation of the middle ear, is a leading cause of primary care visits and the number one reason for antimicrobial prescriptions for children. Hearing loss is a very common disability experienced by people in Canada, particularly among older adults. It is also a cause of impaired language development in children. Vertigo, a disorder of vestibular function, is also a common cause of disability among older adults. This chapter is divided into two parts: the first focuses on disorders of the ear and auditory function, and the second on disorders of the inner ear and vestibular function.

DISORDERS OF THE AUDITORY SYSTEM

After completing this section of the chapter, you should be able to meet the following objectives:

- List the structures of the external, middle, and inner ear and cite their function.
- Describe two common disorders of the outer ear.
- Relate the functions of the eustachian tube to the development of middle ear problems, including acute otitis media and otitis media with effusion.
- Describe anatomic variations as well as risk factors that make infants and young children more prone to develop acute otitis media.
- List three common symptoms of acute otitis media.
- Describe the disease process associated with otosclerosis and relate it to the progressive conductive hearing loss that occurs.
- Characterize tinnitus.
- Differentiate between conductive, sensorineural, and mixed hearing loss and cite the more common causes of each.

- Describe methods used in the diagnosis and treatment of hearing loss.
- Characterize the causes of hearing loss in infants and children and describe the need for early diagnosis and treatment.

Disorders of the External Ear

The external ear consists of the auricle, which collects sound, and the external acoustic meatus or ear canal, which conducts the sound to the tympanic membrane[1,2] (Fig. 55.1). The auricle, or pinna, is composed of an irregularly shaped plate of elastic cartilage that is covered by thin skin. Its rim is somewhat thicker, and its fleshy earlobe lacks surrounding cartilage. The funnel shape of the auricle concentrates high-frequency sound entering from the lateral-forward direction into the ear canal. This shape also helps to prevent front-to-back confusion of sound sources.

The external acoustic meatus, or ear canal, is S-shaped and spans 2 to 3 cm in adults. In infants and young children, the canal is relatively shorter so that extra care must be taken when inspecting it with an otoscope. A thin layer of skin containing fine hairs, sebaceous glands, and ceruminous glands lines the ear canal. These glands produce cerumen, or earwax, which has certain antimicrobial properties and is thought to serve a protective function.

The anterior portion of the auricle and external part of the ear canal are innervated by branches of the trigeminal nerve (cranial nerve [CN] V). The posterior portions of the auricle and the wall of the ear canal are innervated by auricular branches of the facial (CN VII), glossopharyngeal (CN IX), and vagus (CN X) nerves. Because of the vagal innervation, the insertion of a speculum or an otoscope into the external ear canal can stimulate coughing or vomiting reflexes, particularly in young children.

The tympanic membrane, approximately 1 cm in diameter, is a thin, transparent membrane that separates the external ear from the middle ear. The tympanic membrane is covered with thin skin externally and the mucous membrane of the middle ear internally. The tympanic membrane is attached in a manner that allows it to vibrate freely when audible sound waves enter the external auditory canal. Movements of the membrane are transmitted through the middle ear to the inner ear.

When viewed through an otoscope, the tympanic membrane appears as a shallow, oval cone pointing inward toward its apex, the umbo (Fig. 55.2). Light usually is reflected from the pars tensa at approximately the 4 o'clock position, and is referred to as the *cone of light*. Landmarks include the lightened stripe over the handle of the malleus; the umbo at the end of the handle; the pars tensa (tense part), which constitutes most of the drum; and a thinner membrane, the pars flaccida (flaccid part), the small area above the malleus attachment. A bright light reflected from the otoscope's illuminator, called the cone of light, radiates anteroinferiorly from the umbo. The tympanic membrane is semitransparent, and a small, whitish cord, which traverses the middle ear from back to front, can be seen just under its upper edge. This is the *chorda tympani*, a branch of the intermedius component of the facial nerve (CN VII).

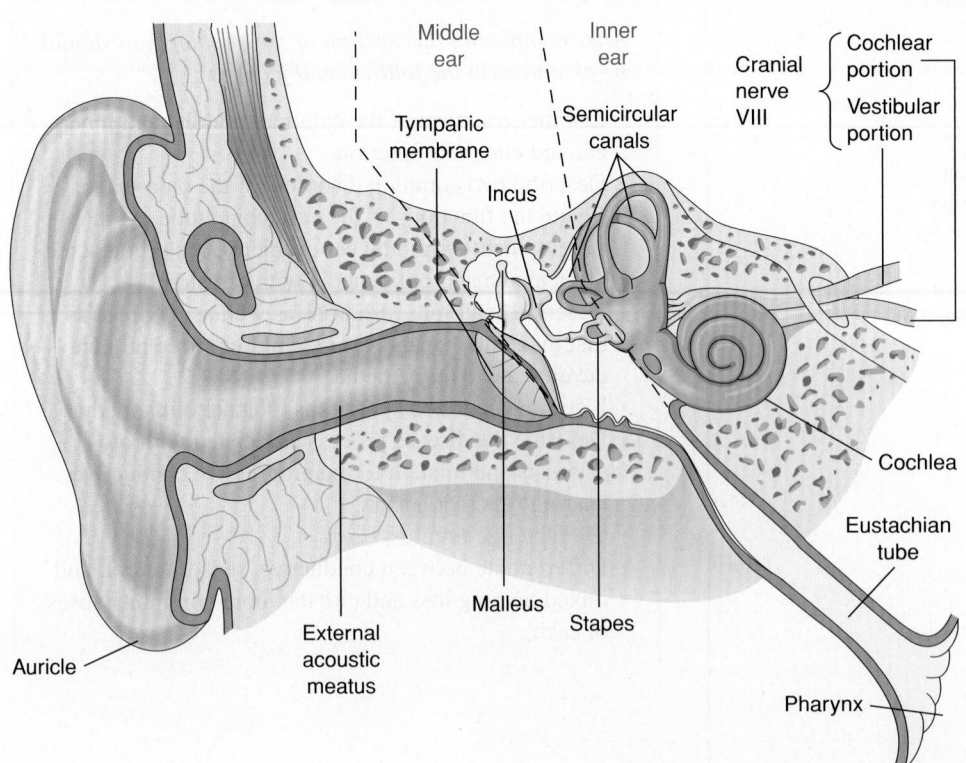

FIGURE 55.1 • External, middle, and internal subdivisions of the ear.

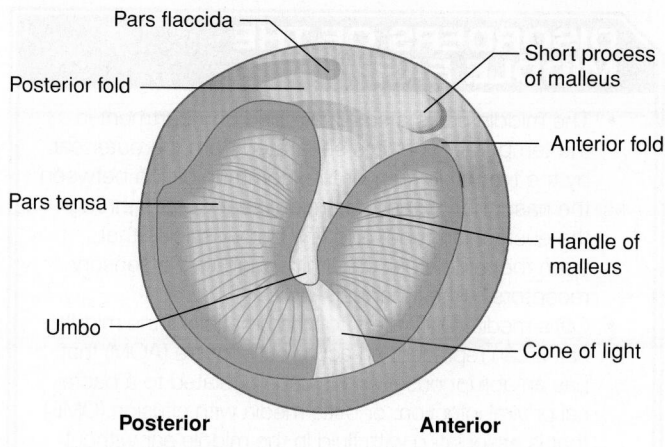

FIGURE 55.2 • Right eardrum.

(figure labels:) Pars flaccida, Posterior fold, Pars tensa, Umbo, Posterior, Short process of malleus, Anterior fold, Handle of malleus, Cone of light, Anterior

The function of the external ear is disturbed when sound transmission is obstructed by impacted cerumen, inflammation (*i.e.*, otitis externa), or drainage from the external ear (otorrhea).

Impacted Cerumen

Cerumen, or earwax, is a protective secretion produced by the sebaceous and ceruminous glands of the skin that lines the ear canal. Although the ear normally is self-cleaning, the cerumen can accumulate and narrow the canal, causing reversible hearing loss.[3,4]

Impacted cerumen usually produces no symptoms unless it hardens and touches the tympanic membrane, or the canal becomes irritated by a buildup of hardened cerumen. Clinical symptoms may include pain, itching, and a sensation of fullness. As the canal becomes completely occluded, a person may experience a feeling of fullness, a conductive hearing loss, and tinnitus (*i.e.*, ringing in the ears). Because the external auditory canal is innervated by the auricular branch of the vagus nerve, coughing or even cardiac deceleration can result from stimulation of the canal by cerumen impaction or removal attempts.[3]

In most cases, cerumen can be removed by irrigation using a bulb syringe and warm tap water. Warm water is used to avoid inducing a feeling of disequilibrium due to the vestibular caloric response. The ear canal should be dried thoroughly after irrigation to avoid introducing an infection. Irrigation should be avoided in an only-hearing ear or one that is postsurgical, prone to infection, or suspect for perforation of the tympanic membrane. Alternatively, healthcare professionals may remove cerumen using an otoscope and a metal curette.

Cerumen that has become hardened or impacted can be softened by instillation of a few drops of a commercially available ceruminolytic agent or a mineral oil and acetic acid combination. Typically, these agents are instilled in the affected ear one or two times daily for up to 7 days before irrigation. Overuse should be avoided because this may make the condition worse. Ceruminolytic agents should not be used in ears that may have a perforated tympanic membrane.

Otitis Externa

Otitis externa is an inflammation of the external ear that can vary in severity from mild allergic dermatitis to severe cellulitis. It can be caused by infectious agents, irritation (*e.g.*, wearing hearing aids or earphones), or allergic reactions. Predisposing factors include frequent exposure to moisture in the ear canal (*i.e.*, swimmer's ear), trauma to the canal caused by cleaning or scratching, and allergies or skin conditions such as psoriasis. The most common pathogens are bacterial (such as *Pseudomonas aeruginosa* and *Staphylococcus aureus*) and fungi such as *Aspergillus* and *Candida* that grow in the presence of excess moisture.[5,6] Otitis externa commonly occurs in the summer and is manifested by itching, redness, tenderness, and narrowing of the ear canal because of edema. Inflammation of the pinna or canal makes movement of the ear painful. There may be watery or purulent drainage and intermittent hearing loss.

Treatment usually includes the use of ear drops containing an appropriate antimicrobial or antifungal agent. For bacterial infections, a corticosteroid may be combined with an antimicrobial to reduce inflammation. Systemic oral agents are rarely needed. Protection of the ear from additional moisture (*i.e.*, use of ear plugs) and avoidance of trauma from scratching with cotton-tipped applicators and other devices are important. Preventing recurrences is important, particularly in persons who swim frequently. Instillation of a dilute alcohol, acetic acid, or Burow otic solution (available in over-the-counter ear drops) immediately after contact with water is an effective prophylaxis.

Disorders of the Middle Ear and Eustachian Tube

The middle ear, or tympanic cavity, is a small, mucosa-lined cavity in the petrous portion of the temporal bone[1,7] (Fig. 55.3A). It is bounded laterally by the tympanic membrane and medially by a bony wall with two openings, the superior oval (vestibular) window and the round (cochlear) window. It is connected anteriorly with the nasopharynx by the *eustachian tube*, also called the *pharyngotympanic tube*. Posteriorly, it is connected with small air pockets in the temporal bone called *mastoid air spaces* or *cells*.

Three tiny bones, the auditory ossicles, are suspended from the roof of the middle ear cavity and connect the tympanic membrane with the oval window. They are connected by synovial joints and are covered with the epithelial lining of the cavity.[1,2] The *malleus* ("hammer") has its handle firmly fixed to the upper portion of the tympanic membrane. The head of the malleus articulates with the *incus* ("anvil"), which articulates with the *stapes* ("stirrup"), which is inserted and sealed into the oval window by an annular ligament. Arrangement of the ear ossicles is such that their lever movements transmit vibrations from the tympanic membrane to the oval window and from there to the fluid in the inner ear. Two tissue-covered openings in the medial wall, the oval and the round windows, provide for the transmission of sound waves between the air-filled middle ear and the fluid-filled inner ear. It is the piston-like action of the stapes footplate that sets up compression waves in the inner ear fluid.

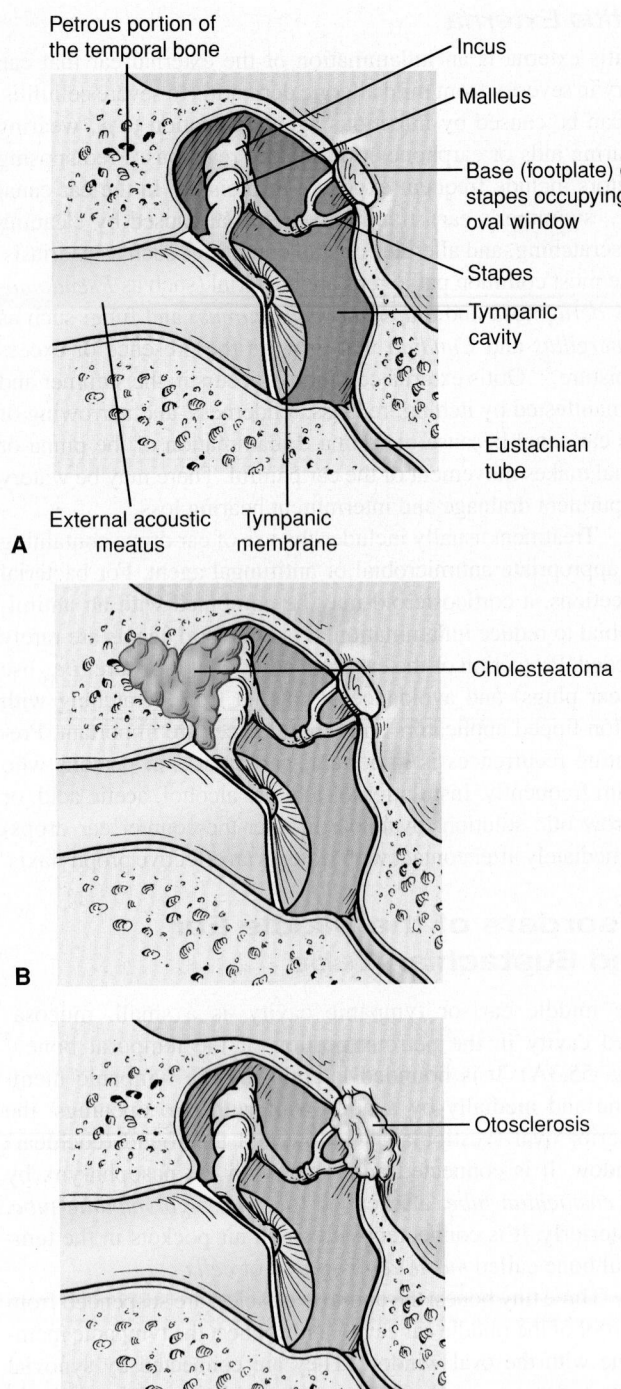

Petrous portion of
the temporal bone

Incus

Malleus

Base (footplate) of
stapes occupying
oval window

Stapes

Tympanic
cavity

Eustachian
tube

External acoustic   Tympanic
meatus   membrane

A

Cholesteatoma

B

Otosclerosis

C

FIGURE 55.3 • Disorders of the middle ear. **A:** Otitis media. Otitis involves inflammation of the tympanic cavity. Infection often enters through the eustachian tube. **B:** Cholesteatoma, a cystlike mass of the middle ear that often extends to involve the temporal bone. **C:** Otosclerosis involving formation of new, spongy bone around the stapes and oval window.

Eustachian Tube Dysfunction

The eustachian tube, which connects the nasopharynx with the middle ear, is located in a gap in the bone between the anterior and medial walls of the middle ear (Fig. 55.1). The eustachian tube serves three basic functions: (1) ventilation

---

DISORDERS OF THE MIDDLE EAR

- The middle ear is a small, air-filled compartment in the temporal bone. It is separated from the outer ear by the tympanic membrane; communication between the nasopharynx and the middle ear occurs through the eustachian tube; and tiny bony ossicles that span the middle ear transmit sound to the sensory receptors in the inner ear.
- Otitis media (OM) refers to inflammation of the middle ear. It can represent an acute otitis media (AOM) that has an abrupt onset and is usually related to a bacterial or viral infection, or otitis media with effusion (OME) that is associated with fluid in the middle ear without the manifestations of infection and which does not usually require treatment with antimicrobial agents.
- The function of the middle ear is to conduct sound waves from the external to the inner ear. Impaired conduction of sound waves and hearing loss occur when the tympanic membrane has been perforated; air in the middle ear has been replaced with fluid (OME); or the function of the bony ossicles has been impaired (otosclerosis).

of the middle ear, along with equalization of middle ear and ambient pressures; (2) protection of the middle ear from unwanted nasopharyngeal sound waves and secretions; and (3) drainage of middle ear secretions into the nasopharynx.[2,7] The nasopharyngeal entrance to the eustachian tube, which usually is closed, is opened by the action of the trigeminal (CN V)-innervated *tensor veli palatini muscle.* Opening of the eustachian tube, which normally occurs with swallowing and yawning reflexes, provides the mechanism for equalizing the pressure of the middle ear with that of the atmosphere. This equalization ensures that the pressures on both sides of the tympanic membrane are the same, so that sound transmission is not reduced and rupture does not result from sudden changes in external pressure, as occurs during plane travel.

The eustachian tube is lined with a mucous membrane that is continuous with the pharynx and the mastoid air cells. Infections from the nasopharynx can travel from the nasopharynx along the mucous membrane of the eustachian tube to the middle ear, causing acute otitis media. Toward the nasopharynx, the eustachian tube becomes lined by columnar epithelium with mucus-secreting cells. Hypertrophy of the mucus-secreting cells is thought to contribute to the mucoid secretions that develop during certain types of otitis media.

Abnormalities in eustachian tube function are important factors in the pathogenesis of middle ear infections. There are two important types of eustachian tube dysfunction: abnormal patency and obstruction (Fig. 55.4). The *abnormally patent tube* does not close or does not close completely. In infants and children with an abnormally patent tube, air and secretions often are pumped into the eustachian tube during crying and nose blowing.

FIGURE 55.4 • Pathophysiology of the eustachian tube. TVP, tensor veli palatini. (Developed from Bluestone C. D. (1981). Recent advances in the pathogenesis, diagnosis, and management of otitis media. *Pediatric Clinics of North America, 28,* 737. With permission from Elsevier Science.)

Obstruction can be functional or mechanical. *Functional obstruction* results from the persistent collapse of the eustachian tube due to a lack of tubal stiffness or poor function of the tensor veli palatini muscle that controls the opening of the eustachian tube. It is common in infants and young children because the amount and stiffness of the cartilage supporting the eustachian tube is less than in older children and adults. Changes in the craniofacial base also render the tensor muscle less efficient for opening the eustachian tube in this age group. In addition, craniofacial disorders, such as a cleft palate, alter the attachment of the tensor muscle, producing functional obstruction of the eustachian tube.

Mechanical obstruction results from internal obstruction or external compression of the eustachian tube. Ethnic differences in the structure of the palate may increase the likelihood of obstruction. The most common internal obstruction is caused by swelling and secretions resulting from allergy and viral respiratory infections. External compression by prominent or enlarged adenoidal tissue surrounding the opening of the eustachian tube may make drainage less effective. Tumours also may obstruct drainage. With obstruction, air in the middle ear is absorbed, causing a negative pressure and the transudation of serous capillary fluid into the middle ear.

Barotrauma

Barotrauma represents injury resulting from the inability to equalize middle ear with ambient pressure during air travel or, less commonly, underwater diving. It occurs most often during air travel, when there is a sudden change in atmospheric pressure. The pressure in the middle ear parallels atmospheric pressure; it decreases at high altitudes and increases at lower altitudes. The problem occurs during rapid airplane descent, when the negative pressure in the middle ear tends to cause the eustachian tube to collapse. If air cannot pass back through the eustachian tube, hearing loss and discomfort develop.

Barotrauma most often occurs in persons who travel while suffering from an upper respiratory tract infection. Autoinflation measures such as yawning, swallowing, and chewing gum facilitate opening of the eustachian tube, which equalizes air pressure in the middle ear. Intranasal or systemic decongestants may be used to prevent symptoms. Acute negative middle ear pressure that persists on the ground is treated with decongestants and attempts at autoinflation. More severe hearing loss or discomfort may require that the person consult an otolaryngologist. Myringotomy (*i.e.,* surgical incision in the tympanic membrane) provides immediate relief and may be used in cases of acute otalgia and hearing loss. Placement of ventilation tubes may be considered for persons with repeated episodes of barotrauma related to frequent air travel.

Otitis Media

Otitis media (OM) refers to inflammation of the middle ear without reference to etiology or pathogenesis (Fig. 55.3A). Acute OM is the most common infection for which antimicrobial agents are prescribed for children in Canada, with 75% of children having at least one episode by the age of 1 year.[8] As such, the diagnosis and management of OM has a significant impact on the health of children, cost of providing care, and overall use of antimicrobial agents.[8]

Several terms are important in reference to OM. *Acute otitis media* (AOM) refers to an acute middle ear infection.[6,9] It usually has an abrupt onset of signs and symptoms related to middle ear inflammation and effusion. *Otitis media with effusion* (OME) refers to the presence of fluid in the middle ear without signs and symptoms of acute ear infection.[6] OME is more common than AOM.[9] It can develop spontaneously because of poor eustachian tube function, accompany a viral upper respiratory tract infection, or occur as a prelude or a sequela to AOM.[6,8,9] Because OME does not usually require treatment with antimicrobial agents, it is important to differentiate OME from AOM to avoid unnecessary use of antimicrobial agents.

Risk Factors. Although AOM may occur in any age group, it is the most frequent primary diagnosis in preschool-age children.[8] Infants and young children between the ages of 3 months and 3 years are at highest risk for AOM, with the peak incidence between 6 and 11 months.[10] There is a second peak incidence at about 5 years of age that is believed to be associated with entrance into school.[10] Risk factors include premature birth, male gender, ethnicity (Native American, Inuit, Métis, First Nation), family history of recurrent otitis media, presence of siblings in the household, genetic syndromes, and low socioeconomic status.[6,8,11] AOM is more frequent in children with orofacial abnormalities such as cleft lip and palate.

The most important factor that contributes to AOM is believed to be a dysfunction of the eustachian tube that allows reflux of fluid and bacteria into the middle ear space from the nasopharynx. There are two reasons for the increased risk of AOM in infants and young children: the eustachian tube is shorter, more horizontal, and wider in this age group than in older children and adults; and infection can spread more easily through the eustachian canal of infants who spend most of their day in the supine position.[8-11] Bottle-fed infants have a higher incidence of AOM than breast-fed infants, probably because they are held in a more horizontal position during feeding, and swallowing while in the horizontal position facilitates the reflux of milk into the middle ear. Breast-feeding also provides for the transfer of protective maternal antibodies to the infant.

Measures to reduce the risk for development of AOM during the first 6 months of life include breast-feeding and reduction or elimination of pacifier use.[8,9] Other ways to reduce the risk of developing AOM include minimal exposure to group settings and the avoidance or elimination of bottle-propping as well as exposure to passive tobacco smoke.[8,9] Efficacy in prevention of OM during the respiratory illness season has been demonstrated by immunoprophylaxis with killed and live-attenuated intranasal influenza vaccines.[9] The recommendation by the National Advisory Committee on Immunization (NACI) to immunize children older than 6 months of age with influenza virus eliminates the specific need for using the vaccine in the prevention of OM. Immunization with pneumococcal 10 or 13-valent conjugate vaccine (Synflorix, Prevnar-13) has also been shown to reduce the incidence of OM caused by vaccine-serotype *Pneumococcus*, but the overall effect has been small.[9,12]

Etiology. Acute OM may be of either bacterial or viral origin. The mucosal lining of the middle ear is continuous with the eustachian tube and nasopharynx, and most middle ear infections enter through the eustachian tube (Fig. 55.1). Bacteria may replicate in fluid of the middle ear to cause bacterial OM; respiratory viruses may infect the middle ear mucosa, either alone, leading to viral OM, or in combination with bacteria. Most cases of AOM follow an uncomplicated upper respiratory tract infection that has been present for several days. Respiratory syncytial virus is the most common viral pathogen in middle ear fluid from children with AOM, although other viruses (*e.g.,* rhinovirus, parainfluenza virus, adenovirus) have been isolated.[10] The most common bacteria in AOM are *Streptococcus pneumoniae, Haemophilus influenzae,* and *Moraxella catarrhalis.*[6,10,13] Respiratory viruses (or virus-derived ribonucleic acid [RNA]) may also be found in the middle ear exudates of children with AOM, either alone or, more commonly, in association with pathogenic bacteria. Emergence of a multiple-drug–resistant strain of *S. pneumoniae* has led to increased numbers of treatment failures.[14] There is also evidence that the formation of bacterial biofilms may play a role in the pathogenesis of recurrent AOM that does not respond to antimicrobial therapy.[15] Biofilms consist of aggregated

bacteria, usually adherent to a surface and surrounded by an extracellular matrix covering that isolates and protects them from antimicrobial agents (see Chapter 16).

Clinical Manifestations. Acute OM is characterized by acute onset of otalgia (or pulling of the ears in an infant), fever (up to 40°C), and hearing loss. Children older than 3 years of age may have rhinorrhea or running nose, vomiting, and diarrhea. In contrast, younger children often have nonspecific signs and symptoms that manifest as ear tugging, irritability, nighttime awakening, and poor feeding. Key diagnostic criteria include distinct otalgia (earache that interferes with activity or sleep) or tympanic membrane erythema, and middle ear effusion.[6,9] Ear pain usually increases as the effusion accumulates behind the tympanic membrane. Perforation of the tympanic membrane may occur acutely, allowing purulent material from the eustachian tube to drain into the external auditory canal. This may prevent spread of the infection into the temporal bone or intracranial cavity. Healing of the tympanic membrane usually follows resolution of the middle ear infection.

OME is a condition in which the tympanic membrane is intact and there is an accumulation of fluid in the middle ear without signs or symptoms of infection. The duration of the effusion may range from less than 3 weeks to more than 3 months. The similarity between OME and AOM is that hearing loss may be present in both conditions. Many cases of OME resolve spontaneously, but some can last longer than a year and some patients can experience recurrent OME. Persistent middle ear fluid from OME results in decreased motility of the tympanic membrane and serves as a barrier to sound conduction.

Diagnosis. Distinguishing between AOM and OME on clinical grounds is often straightforward, but because each condition may evolve into the other without any clearly differentiating physical findings, any system for distinguishing between them is somewhat arbitrary. Because of the increasing antimicrobial resistance, distinguishing between AOM and OME has become increasingly important.

Both AOM without otorrhea (drainage from the ear) and OME are accompanied by otoscopic signs of middle ear effusion, namely, the presence of at least two of three tympanic membrane abnormalities: white, yellow, amber (or occasionally blue) discolouration; opacification other than scarring; and decreased or absent motility. With OME the tympanic membrane is often cloudy with distinct impairment of mobility, and an air–fluid level or bubble may be visible in the middle ear.

A definitive diagnosis of AOM requires the following: history of acute onset of signs and symptoms, the presence of middle ear effusion, and signs and symptoms of middle ear inflammation.[8-11] Signs of middle ear inflammation include fullness or bulging of the tympanic membrane with or without erythema, limited or absent mobility of the tympanic membrane, a purulent (pus-containing) effusion, and ear pain that interferes with normal activity. Unless intense, erythema alone is insufficient to support a diagnosis of AOM because erythema without other abnormalities may result from crying or vascular flushing. The malleus may be obscured and the tympanic membrane may resemble a bagel without a hole, but with a central indentation.[11]

The diagnosis of AOM should be confirmed with pneumatic otoscopy and can be supplemented with tympanometry and acoustic reflectometry. The use of the pneumatic otoscope permits the introduction of air into the ear canal for the purpose of determining tympanic membrane flexibility. The movement of the tympanic membrane is decreased in some cases of AOM and absent in chronic middle ear infection. The diagnosis of AOM can also be confirmed using tympanometry or acoustic reflectometry. *Tympanometry* is helpful in detecting effusion in the middle ear or high negative middle ear pressure.[9,16] Portable tympanometers (resembling an otoscope) and desktop instruments are available. A tympanogram is obtained by using a small probe that is placed snugly into the external ear canal. A sound stimulus generator then transmits acoustic energy into the canal, while a vacuum pump introduces positive and negative pressures into the ear canal. A microphone in the instrument detects returning sound energy. The tympanogram provides a determination of the degree of negative pressure present in the middle ear. It detects disease when present but is less reliable when disease is absent. *Acoustic reflectometry* detects reflected sound waves from the middle ear and provides information on whether an effusion is absent or present. Increased reflected sound correlates with an increased likelihood of effusion. This technique is most useful in children older than 3 months, and its success depends on user technique.

Tympanocentesis (puncture of the tympanic membrane with a needle) may be done to relieve pain from an effusion or to obtain a specimen of middle ear fluid for culture and sensitivity testing. The procedure involves the insertion of a needle through the inferior part of the tympanic membrane. Because of the cost, effort, and lack of availability, it is not routinely used in management of AOM.[10] In selected cases of refractory or recurrent middle ear disease, tympanocentesis can help improve diagnostic accuracy, guide treatment, and avoid unnecessary medical or surgical interventions. In instances where the tympanic membrane has perforated with resultant drainage into the external ear, a specimen can be obtained and microbiologic studies can be done to identify the organism and the antimicrobial sensitivities.

Treatment. The treatment of OM focuses on symptom control and management of the underlying pathologic process. A number of options for pain management are available, including the local application of heat and use of analgesic drugs such as acetaminophen, ibuprofen, and naproxen. Myringotomy (incision of the tympanic membrane) can be used for relief of pressure in the child who is in severe pain, providing almost immediate relief.[9]

The extensive use of antimicrobial agents contributes to the development of bacterial resistance, and evidence exists for the efficacy and safety of two alternative approaches to routine antibiotic prescription: delayed prescription and watchful waiting.[8,9] Observation without antimicrobial agents is an option in a child over 6 months of age with uncomplicated AOM. These approaches involve waiting for 24 hours to 72 hours (greater than 6 months of age) to see if symptoms improve before institution of antibiotic therapy. Factors to consider when deciding whether to defer treatment include the child's age, severity of illness, comorbidities, and certainty of the diagnosis. If observation is recommended, it is essential that the parent or caregiver have ready access to communication, follow-up, and a mechanism for obtaining medication if needed.[8,13]

Most cases of OME resolve spontaneously within a 3-month period.[17] The management options for this duration include observation only, antibiotic therapy, or combination antibiotic and corticosteroid therapy. Topical and systemic decongestants usually are of little value in clearing middle ear effusion.[6] Referral to an otolaryngologist is indicated if the effusion persists for 4 months or longer. Because there is concern over hearing loss and its effect on learning and speech, a hearing evaluation is recommended when OME persists for 3 months or longer or at any time that language delay, learning problems, or a significant hearing loss are suspected.[17] Children with recurrent OM should be evaluated to rule out any anatomic variations (*e.g.,* enlarged adenoids), allergies, and immunologic abnormalities. Children with immunoglobulin G subclass deficiencies (see Chapter 19) and poor responses to polysaccharide vaccines are more likely to develop recurrent OM.

Surgical treatment (*e.g.,* tympanostomy tubes, adenoidectomy) may be indicated if the effusion has persisted for 4 months or longer and is accompanied by persistent hearing loss and other manifestations; if recurrent or persistent effusion occurs in children at risk regardless of hearing status; or if there is structural damage to the tympanic membrane or middle ear.[6,9,17] Tympanostomy tube insertion is the preferred initial procedure and does not typically include the removal of adenoids unless the child has additional indications, such as postnasal obstruction from enlarged adenoids. The tubes usually are inserted under general anesthesia. The ears of children with tubes must be kept out of water. The adverse effects of tube placement include recurrent otorrhea; persistent perforation, scarring, and atrophy of the tympanic membrane; and cholesteatoma. Adenoidectomy plus myringotomy (without tube insertion) has been shown to have comparable efficacy in older children. Recent research indicates that prompt insertion of tympanostomy tubes for persistent OME in otherwise healthy children who were younger than 3 years of age did not improve developmental outcomes (*e.g.,* literacy, attention, social skills, and academic achievement) as compared with delayed insertion in children in whom effusion continued unremittingly.[18]

Complications of Otitis Media. The complications of OM include hearing loss, adhesive OM, cholesteatoma, mastoiditis, and intracranial complications such as otologic meningitis.

Hearing loss, which is a common complication of OM, usually is conductive and temporary based on the duration of the effusion. Hearing loss that is associated with fluid collection usually resolves when the effusion clears. Permanent hearing loss may occur as the result of damage to the tympanic membrane or other middle ear structures. Cases of sensorineural hearing loss are rare. Persistent and episodic conductive hearing loss in children may impair their cognitive, linguistic, and emotional development.[6,9,17] Children younger than 3 years of age with recurrent OME are at increased risk of impaired language development. Additional studies indicate that before 3 years of age, time spent with middle ear effusion correlates with decreased cognitive development as measured by standardized inventories. However, the degree and duration of hearing loss required to produce such effects are unknown.

Adhesive OM involves an abnormal healing reaction in an inflamed middle ear.[11] It produces irreversible thickening of the mucous membranes and may cause impaired movement of the ossicles and possibly conductive hearing loss. Tympanosclerosis involves the formation of whitish plaques and nodular deposits on the submucosal surface of the tympanic membrane, with possible adherence of the ossicles and conductive hearing loss.

Cholesteatomas are cystlike lesions of the middle ear, usually associated with chronic otitis media[11] (Fig. 55.3B). Measuring 1 to 4 cm in diameter, they are lined with keratinizing squamous epithelium or metaplastic mucus-secreting epithelium and filled with amorphous debris (derived largely from desquamated epithelium).[11,19] Although precise mechanisms involved in their development are unclear, it is proposed that chronic inflammation and perforation of the eardrum with ingrowth of squamous epithelium or metaplasia of the secretory epithelium of the middle are contributing factors. Sometimes the cyst ruptures, enhancing the inflammatory reaction. These lesions, by progressive enlargement, can erode the ossicles, the labyrinth, the adjacent mastoid bone, and the surrounding soft tissues. Although often thought of as a complication of otitis media, a cholesteatoma may also occur as a congenital condition. Symptoms commonly include painless drainage from the ear and hearing loss. Treatment involves microsurgical techniques to remove the cholesteatomatous material.[19]

The mastoid antrum and air cells constitute a portion of the temporal bone and may become inflamed as an extension of acute or chronic OM.[11] The disorder causes necrosis of the mastoid process and destruction of the bony intercellular matrix, which are visible by radiologic examination. Mastoid tenderness and drainage of exudate through a perforated tympanic membrane can occur. Chronic mastoiditis can develop as the result of chronic middle ear infection. The usefulness of antimicrobial agents for this condition is limited. Mastoid or middle ear surgery, along with other medical treatment, may be indicated. The incidence of mastoiditis has markedly decreased compared with the preantimicrobial era.

Intracranial complications are uncommon since the advent of antimicrobial therapy. Although rare, these complications can develop when the infection spreads through vascular channels, by direct extension, or through preformed pathways such as the round window.[11] These complications are seen more often with chronic suppurative OM and mastoiditis. They include otogenic meningitis, brain abscess, lateral sinus thrombophlebitis or thrombosis, labyrinthitis, and facial nerve paralysis. Any child who develops persistent headache, tinnitus, stiff neck, or visual or other neurologic symptoms should be investigated for possible intracranial complications.

Otosclerosis

Otosclerosis refers to the formation of new spongy bone around the stapes and oval window, which results in progressive deafness[20] (Fig. 55.3C). In most cases, the condition is familial and follows an autosomal dominant pattern with variable penetrance. Otosclerosis may begin at any time in life but usually does not appear until after puberty, most frequently between the ages of 20 and 30 years. White, middle-aged women are most at risk, and this disease process accelerates during pregnancy.

Otosclerosis begins with resorption of bone in one or more foci. During active bone resorption, the bone structure appears spongy and softer than normal (i.e., osteospongiosis). The resorbed bone is replaced by an overgrowth of new, hard, sclerotic bone.[20] The process is slowly progressive, involving more areas of the temporal bone, especially in front of and posterior to the stapes footplate. As it invades the footplate, the pathologic bone increasingly immobilizes the stapes, reducing the transmission of sound. Pressure of otosclerotic bone on middle ear structures or the vestibulocochlear nerve (CN VIII) may contribute to the development of tinnitus, sensorineural hearing loss, and vertigo.

The symptoms of otosclerosis involve an insidious hearing loss. Initially, the affected person is unable to hear a whisper or someone speaking at a distance. In the earliest stages, the bone conduction by which the person's own voice is heard remains relatively unaffected. At this point, the person's own voice sounds unusually loud, and the sound of chewing becomes intensified. Because of bone conduction, most of these persons can hear fairly well on the telephone, which provides an amplified signal. Many are able to hear better in a noisy environment, probably because the masking effect of background noise causes other persons to speak louder.

The treatment of otosclerosis can be medical or surgical. A carefully selected, well-fitting hearing aid may allow a person with conductive deafness to lead a normal life. Sodium fluoride has been used with some success in the medical treatment of osteospongiosis.[20] Because much of the conductive hearing loss associated with otosclerosis is caused by stapedial fixation, surgical treatment involves stapedectomy with stapedial reconstruction using the patient's own stapes or a stapedial prosthesis. The argon laser may be used in the surgical procedure.

Disorders of the Inner Ear

The inner ear contains a labyrinth or system of intercommunicating channels and the receptors for hearing and position sense.[1,2,21,22] Structurally, it consists of an outer bony labyrinth located in the otic capsule of the petrous part of the temporal bone and an inner membranous labyrinth (Fig. 55.5). The membranous labyrinth lies in the bony labyrinth and consists of a complex system of sacs and ducts (i.e., semicircular ducts). The bony labyrinth, which occupies a space with a

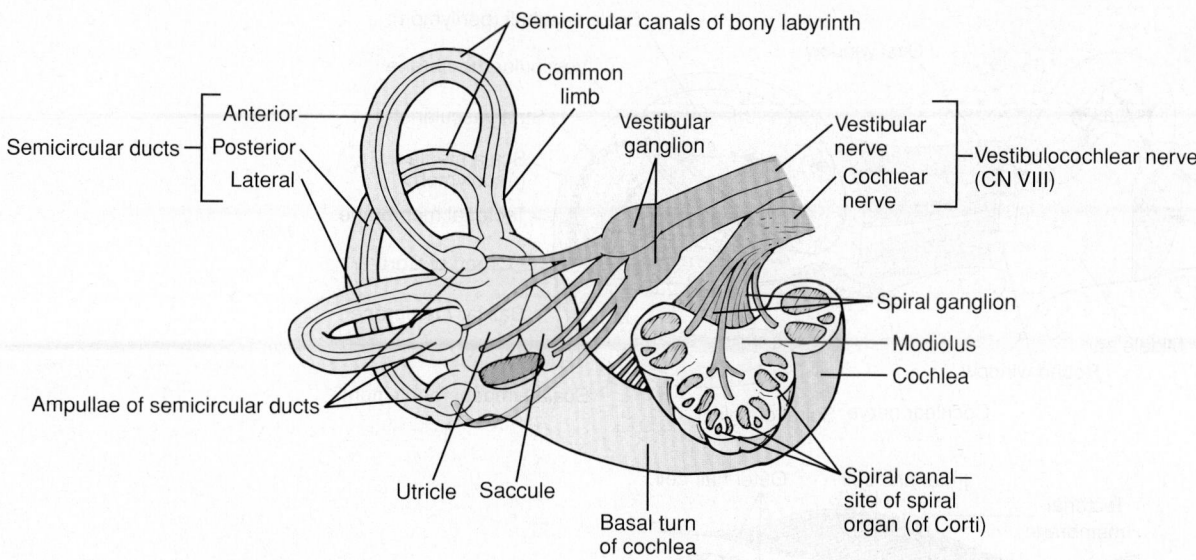

FIGURE 55.5 • Schematic lateral view of the bony canals of the vestibular system showing the membranous labyrinth in a closed system of ducts and chambers filled with endolymph and bathed in perilymph with the bony labyrinth. Observe the parts of the membranous labyrinth: the semicircular ducts and the saccule and utricle within the vestibule. (Adapted from Moore K. L., Dalley A. F. (1999). *Clinically oriented anatomy* (4th ed., p. 1102). Philadelphia, PA: Lippincott Williams & Wilkins.)

diameter less than 1.5 cm, is a series of cavities (the cochlea, vestibule, and semicircular canals). The receptors for hearing are contained in the cochlea and those for head position sense are contained in the semicircular ducts, the utricle, and the saccule. The vestibule is the central egg-shaped cavity of the bony labyrinth that lies posterior to the cochlea and anterior to the semicircular canals. It contains the utricle and saccule and parts of the balancing apparatus (vestibular labyrinth). The vestibule features the oval window on its lateral wall, occupied by the base of the stapes.

The cochlea is the shell-shaped part of the bony labyrinth that contains the inner membranous cochlear duct, the part of the inner ear concerned with hearing. The spiral canal of the cochlea, which is shaped like a snail shell, begins at the vestibule and winds around a central core of spongy bone called the *modiolus* (Fig. 55.5). The modiolus contains canals for blood vessels and for distribution of the cochlear nerve. The cochlea consists of three tubes coiled side by side: (1) the *scala vestibuli,* (2) the *scala media,* and (3) the *scala tympani* (Fig. 55.6). The scala vestibuli and scala media are separated from each other by the vestibular membrane, also known as *Reissner membrane,* and the scala tympani is separated from the scala media by the basilar membrane. On the surface of the basilar membrane lies the spiral organ of Corti, which contains a series of electromechanically sensitive cells, the *hair cells.* They are the receptive organs that generate nerve impulses in response to sound vibrations.

Two separate fluids are found in the cochlea of the inner ear: the endolymph and perilymph. The scala vestibuli and scala tympani communicate directly with the subarachnoid space around the brain, so the perilymph is similar to cerebrospinal fluid.[21] The endolymph that fills the scala media is an entirely different fluid that is secreted by the stria vascularis on the outer wall of the scala media (Fig. 55.6A). The perilymph that fills the scala vestibuli and scala tympani has a high sodium (Na^+) concentration, whereas the endolymph that fills the scala media has a high potassium (K^+) content. A direct-current resting membrane potential of about +80 mV exists between the endolymph and perilymph, with positivity inside the scala media and negativity outside. This current, which is called the *endolymphatic potential,* is generated by the continual secretion of K^+ ions into the scala media by Na^+/K^+-adenosine triphosphatase (ATPase) pumps in the stria vascularis. This current is believed to sensitize the hair cells of the organ of Corti, increasing their ability to respond to the slightest sound. Degeneration of the stria vascularis, which has been called the "battery of the cochlea," and the resultant decline in the endolymphatic potential, is thought to be one of the causes of hearing loss that occurs with aging.[23]

Unlike light, which can be transmitted through a vacuum such as outer space, sound is a pressure disturbance originating from a vibrating object and propagated by the molecules of an elastic medium. Sound waves, which are delivered by the stapes footplate to the perilymph, travel throughout the fluid of the inner ear, including up the scala vestibuli, to the apex of the cochlea (Fig. 55.6A). Because of the thinness of the vestibular membrane, sound vibrations from the scala vestibuli are readily transmitted into the scala media. Therefore, as far as sound conduction is concerned, the scala media and scala vestibuli function as a single chamber.

As the pressure wave descends through the endolymph of the scala media it sets the entire basilar membrane vibrating. The basilar membrane, which becomes progressively more massive from its base to its distal apex, resonates at higher frequencies

A

B

FIGURE 55.6 • **A:** Path taken by sound waves reaching the inner ear. **B:** Spiral organ of Corti has been removed from the cochlear duct and greatly enlarged to show the inner and outer hair cells, the basilar membrane, and cochlear nerve fibres.

near the base and at lower frequencies toward its apex as the fluid pressure wave travels up the cochlear spiral. This "tuned" aspect of the basilar membrane results in increased amplitude of displacement at the resonant locations, responding to a particular sound frequency and greater firing of cochlear neurons innervating this region. This mechanism provides the major basis for the discrimination of sound frequency.

Perched on the basilar membrane and extending along its entire length is an elaborate arrangement of columnar epithelium called the *spiral organ of Corti* (Fig. 55.6B). Continuous rows of hair cells separated into inner and outer rows can be found in the columnar arrangement of the spiral organ. The cells have hairlike cilia that protrude through openings in an overlying supporting reticular membrane into the endolymph of the cochlear duct. A gelatinous mass, the tectorial membrane, extends from the medial side of the duct to enclose the cilia of the outer hair cells. The hair cells in the organ of Corti are programmed to respond to deformation of the cochlear duct induced by compression waves moving through the perilymph, which ascend and descend in the surrounding scala vestibule and scala tympani. Selective destruction of hair cells in a particular segment of the cochlea can lead to hearing loss of particular tones.

Neural Pathways

Information flows from the hair cells in the organ of Corti to neurons that have their cell bodies in the cochlear ganglion, which follows a spiral course in the bony modiolus of the cochlear spiral. Afferent fibres from the spiral ganglion (*i.e.,*

vestibulocochlear, auditory, or acoustic nerve [CN VIII]) travel to the cochlear nuclei in the caudal pons (Fig. 55.5). Many secondary nerve fibres from the cochlear nuclei pass to the opposite side of the pons. These secondary fibres may project to such cell groups as the trapezoid or the superior olivary nucleus, or rostrally toward the inferior colliculus of the midbrain. Ipsilateral projections and interconnections between the nuclei of the two sides occur throughout the central auditory system. Consequently, impulses from either ear are transmitted through the auditory pathways to both sides of the brain stem.

From the inferior colliculus, the auditory pathway passes to the medial geniculate nucleus of the thalamus, where all the fibres synapse. From the medial geniculate nuclei, the auditory tract spreads through the auditory radiation to the primary auditory cortex (area 41), located mainly in the superior temporal gyrus and insula (see Chapter 48, Fig. 48.22). This area and its corresponding higher-order thalamic nuclei are required for high-acuity loudness discrimination and precise discrimination of pitch. The auditory association cortex (areas 42 and 22) borders the primary cortex on the superior temporal gyrus. This area and its associated higher-order thalamic nuclei are necessary for auditory gnosis, or the meaningfulness of sound, to occur. Experience and the precise analysis of momentary auditory information are integrated during this process.

Tinnitus

Tinnitus (from the Latin *tinniere,* meaning ."to ring") is the perception of abnormal ear or head noises, not produced by an external stimulus.[24–26] Although it often is described as "ringing of the ears," it may also assume a hissing, roaring, buzzing, or humming sound. Tinnitus may be constant, intermittent, and unilateral or bilateral. The prevalence is estimated to be 10% to 15% of the general population, but 1% to 2% of persons find that these noises seriously impair their quality of life.[24] The condition affects males more often than female, is most prevalent between 40 and 70 years of age, and occasionally affects children.[26]

Although tinnitus is subjective, for clinical purposes it is subdivided into objective and subjective tinnitus.[24–26] *Objective tinnitus* refers to those rare cases in which the sound is detected or potentially detectable by another observer. Typical causes of objective tinnitus include vascular abnormalities or neuromuscular disorders. In some vascular disorders, for example, sounds generated by turbulent blood flow (*e.g.,* arterial bruits or venous hums) are conducted to the auditory system. Vascular disorders typically produce a pulsatile form of tinnitus.

Subjective tinnitus refers to noise perception when there is no noise stimulation of the cochlea. A number of causes and conditions have been associated with subjective tinnitus. Intermittent periods of mild, high-pitched tinnitus lasting for several minutes are common in normal-hearing persons. Impacted cerumen is a benign cause of tinnitus, which resolves after the earwax is removed. Medications such as aspirin and stimulants such as nicotine and caffeine can cause transient tinnitus. Conditions associated with more persistent tinnitus include noise-induced hearing loss, presbycusis (sensorineural hearing loss that occurs with aging), hypertension, atherosclerosis, head injury, and cochlear or labyrinthine infection or inflammation.

The physiologic mechanism underlying subjective tinnitus is largely unknown. It seems likely that there are several mechanisms, including abnormal firing of auditory receptors, dysfunction of cochlear neurotransmitter function or ionic balance, damage to the auditory nerve, or alterations in central processing of the signal.

Because tinnitus is a symptom, the diagnosis relies heavily on the person's description of the problem, including onset, frequency, description, and location of the tinnitus; perceived cause; and the extent to which the person is bothered by the problem.[24] A history of medication or stimulant use and dietary factors that may cause tinnitus should be obtained. Tinnitus often accompanies hearing disorders, and tests of auditory function usually are done. Causes of objective tinnitus, such as serious vascular abnormalities, should be ruled out.

Treatment measures are designed to treat the symptoms rather than effect a cure.[24,26] They include elimination of ototoxic drugs, such as aminoglycosides, NSAIDs, furosemide, and some chemotherapy drugs, and a review of other medications for potential tinnitus side effects. The use of an externally produced sound (*e.g.,* noise generators or tinnitus-masking devices) may be used to mask or inhibit the tinnitus. Medications, including antihistamines, anticonvulsant drugs, calcium channel blockers, benzodiazepines, and antidepressants, have been used for tinnitus alleviation, but most are not

effective, and many produce undesirable side effects. For persistent tinnitus, psychological interventions may be needed to help the person deal with the stress and distraction associated with the condition. Tinnitus retraining therapy, which includes directive counselling and extended use of low-noise generators to facilitate auditory adaptation to the tinnitus, has met with considerable success. Surgical intervention (*i.e.,* cochlear nerve section, vascular decompression) is a last resort for persons for whom all other interventions have failed and in whom the disorder is disabling.

Disorders of the Central Auditory Pathways

The auditory pathways in the brain involve communication between the two sides of the brain at many levels. As a result, strokes, tumours, abscesses, and other focal abnormalities seldom produce more than a mild reduction in auditory acuity on the side opposite the lesion. For intelligibility of auditory language, lateral dominance becomes important. On the dominant side, usually the left side, the more medial and dorsal portion of the auditory association cortex is of crucial importance. This area is called the *Wernicke area,* and damage to it is associated with auditory receptive aphasia. Persons with damage to this area of the brain can speak intelligibly and read normally but are unable to understand the meaning of major aspects of audible speech.

Irritative foci that affect the auditory radiation or the primary auditory cortex can produce roaring or clicking sounds, which appear to come from the auditory environment of the opposite side (*i.e.,* auditory hallucinations). Focal seizures that originate in or near the auditory cortex often are immediately preceded by the perception of ringing or other sounds

---

HEARING LOSS

- Hearing is a special sensory function that incorporates the sound-transmitting properties of the external ear canal, the eardrum that separates the external and middle ear, the bony ossicles of the middle ear, the sensory receptors of the cochlea in the inner ear, the neural pathways of the vestibulocochlear or auditory nerve, and the primary auditory and auditory association cortices.
- Hearing loss represents impairment of the ability to detect and perceive sound.
- It can range from mild, affecting sounds of different tones and intensities, to moderate or profound.
- Hearing loss can be caused by conductive disorders, in which auditory stimuli are not transmitted through the structures of the outer and middle ears to the sensory receptors in the inner ear; by sensorineural disorders that affect the inner ear, auditory nerve, or auditory pathways; or by a combination of conductive and sensorineural disorders.

preceded by a prodrome (*i.e.*, aura). Damage to the auditory association cortex, especially if bilateral, results in deficiencies of sound recognition and memory (*i.e.*, auditory agnosia). If the damage is in the dominant hemisphere, speech recognition can be affected (*i.e.*, sensory or receptive aphasia).

Hearing Loss

The Canadian Association of the Deaf estimates that there are 3.15 million Canadians who are hard of hearing, with approximately 350,000 profoundly deaf or deafened Canadians; however, they note that there has never been a full census for people with hearing loss in Canada.[27] It affects persons of all age groups. It is estimated that 6 of every 1,000 children in Canada have some form of hearing loss, and of these 6, 9 out of 10 children who are born deaf are born to parents who can hear.[28] The prevalence increases dramatically with age; hearing loss affects approximately 37% of people ages 61 to 70 years, 60% ages 71 to 80 years, and more than 80% of those 85 years of age and older.[29]

Hearing is a specialized sense that provides the ability to perceive vibration of sound waves. Functions of the ear include receiving sound waves, distinguishing their frequency, translating this information into nerve impulses, and transmitting these impulses to the central nervous system (CNS). The compression waves that produce sound have frequency and intensity. *Frequency* indicates the number of waves per unit time (reported in cycles per second [cps] or hertz [Hz]). The human ear is most sensitive to waves in the frequency range of 1,000 to 3,000 Hz. Most persons cannot hear compression waves that have a frequency higher than 20,000 Hz. Waves of higher frequency are called *ultrasonic waves,* meaning that they are above the audible range. In the audible frequency range, the subjective experience correlated with sonic frequency is the pitch of a sound. Waves below 20 to 30 Hz are experienced as a rattle or drum beat rather than a tone.

Wave intensity is represented by amplitude or units of sound pressure. By convention, the intensity (in power units or ergs per square centimetre) of a sound is expressed as the ratio of intensities between the sound and a reference value. A 10-fold increase in sound pressure is called a *bel,* after Alexander Graham Bell. Because this representation is too crude to be of use, the decibel (dB), or 1/10 of a bel, is used. For purposes of hearing evaluation, the threshold for perception of sound at a given frequency in persons with normal hearing is set at 0 dB.

Hearing loss is classified as mild (21 to 40 dB), moderate (41 to 55 dB), moderately severe (56 to 70 dB), severe (71 to 90 dB), or profound (91 dB or greater). The term "hard of hearing" is sometime used for people who have slight difficulty hearing and is defined as hearing loss greater than 20 to 25 dB in adults and greater than 15 dB in children.

There are many causes of hearing loss or deafness. Most fit into the categories of conductive, sensorineural, or mixed deficiencies that involve a combination of conductive and sensorineural function deficiencies of the same ear.[29–31] Hearing

---

CHART 55.1 | **COMMON CAUSES OF CONDUCTIVE AND SENSORINEURAL HEARING LOSS**

Conductive Hearing Loss
- External ear conditions
  - Impacted earwax or foreign body
  - Otitis externa
- Middle ear conditions
  - Trauma
  - Otitis media (acute and with effusion)
  - Otosclerosis
  - Tumours

Sensorineural Hearing Loss
- Trauma
  - Head injury
  - Noise
- Central nervous system infections (*e.g.*, meningitis)
- Degenerative conditions
  - Presbycusis
- Vascular
  - Atherosclerosis
  - Sudden deafness
- Ototoxic drugs (*e.g.*, aminoglycosides, salicylates, loop diuretics)
- Tumours
  - Vestibular schwannoma (acoustic neuroma)
  - Meningioma
  - Metastatic tumours
- Idiopathic
  - Ménière disease

Mixed Conductive and Sensorineural Hearing Loss
- Middle ear conditions
  - Barotrauma
  - Cholesteatoma
  - Otosclerosis
- Temporal bone fractures

---

loss may be hereditary or acquired, sudden or progressive, unilateral or bilateral, partial or complete, reversible or irreversible. Age and suddenness of onset provide important clues as to the cause of hearing loss. Chart 55.1 summarizes common causes of conductive and sensorineural hearing loss.

Conductive Hearing Loss

Conductive hearing loss occurs when auditory stimuli are not adequately transmitted through the auditory canal, tympanic membrane, middle ear, or ossicle chain to the inner ear. Temporary hearing loss can occur as the result of impacted cerumen in the outer ear or fluid in the middle ear. Foreign bodies, including pieces of cotton and insects, may impair hearing. More permanent causes of hearing loss are thickening or damage of the tympanic membrane or involvement of the bony structures (ossicles and oval window) of the middle ear due to otosclerosis or Paget disease.

Sensorineural Hearing Loss

Sensorineural, or perceptive, hearing loss occurs with disorders that affect the inner ear, auditory nerve, or auditory pathways of the brain.[29] With this type of deafness, sound waves are conducted to the inner ear, but abnormalities of the cochlear apparatus or auditory nerve decrease or distort the transfer of information to the brain. Tinnitus often accompanies cochlear nerve irritation. Abnormal function resulting from damage or malformation of the central auditory pathways and circuitry is included in this category.

Sensorineural hearing loss is usually irreversible and occurs most commonly in the higher frequencies. Sensorineural hearing loss may have a genetic cause or may result from intrauterine infections such as maternal rubella, or developmental malformations of the inner ear. Genetic hearing loss may result from mutation in a single gene (monogenetic) or from a combination of mutations in different genes and environmental factors (multifactorial). It has been estimated that 60% to 70% of all inherited cases of profound deafness in children have a monogenetic basis.[32] The inheritance pattern for monogenetic hearing loss is autosomal recessive in approximately 75% to 80% of cases.[32] Hearing loss may begin before development of speech (prelingual) or after speech development (postlingual). Most prelingual forms are present at birth. Hereditary forms of hearing loss also can be classified as being part of a syndrome in which other abnormalities are present, or as nonsyndromic, in which deafness is the only abnormality.

Sensorineural hearing loss also can result from trauma to the inner ear, tumours that encroach on the inner ear or sensory neurons, vascular disorders with hemorrhage, or thrombosis of vessels that supply the inner ear. Other causes of sensorineural deafness are infections and drugs. Sudden sensorineural hearing loss represents an abrupt loss of hearing that occurs instantaneously or on awakening. It most commonly is caused by viral infections, circulatory disorders, or rupture of the labyrinth membrane that can occur during tympanotomy.

Environmentally induced deafness can occur through direct exposure to excessively intense sound, as in the workplace or at a concert. This is a particular problem in older adults who were working in noisy environments before the mid-1960s, when there were no laws mandating use of devices to protect hearing. Sustained or repeated exposure to noise pollution at sound intensities greater than 100 to 120 dB can cause corresponding mechanical damage to the organ of Corti. If the damage is severe, permanent sensorineural deafness to the corresponding sound frequencies occurs. Wearing earplugs or ear protection is important in many industrial settings and for musicians and music listeners exposed to high sound amplification.

A number of infections can cause hearing loss. Deafness or some degree of hearing impairment is the most common serious complication of bacterial meningitis in infants and children.

The mechanism causing hearing impairment seems to be a suppurative labyrinthitis or neuritis resulting in the loss of hair cells and damage to the auditory nerve. Untreated suppurative otitis media also can extend into the inner ear and cause sensorineural hearing loss through the same mechanisms.

Among the neoplasms that impair hearing are *acoustic neuromas*. Acoustic neuromas are benign Schwann cell tumours affecting CN VIII. These tumours usually are unilateral and cause hearing loss by compressing the cochlear nerve or interfering with blood supply to the nerve and cochlea. Other neoplasms that can affect hearing include meningiomas and metastatic brain tumours. The temporal bone is a common site of metastases. Breast cancer may metastasize to the middle ear and invade the cochlea.

Drugs that damage inner ear structures are labelled *ototoxic*. Vestibular symptoms of ototoxicity include lightheadedness, giddiness, and dizziness; if toxicity is severe, cochlear symptoms consisting of tinnitus or hearing loss occur. Hearing loss is sensorineural and may be bilateral or unilateral, transient or permanent. Several classes of drugs have been identified as having ototoxic potential, including the aminoglycosides and some other basic antimicrobial agents, antimalarial drugs, some chemotherapeutic drugs, loop diuretics, and salicylates (*e.g.,* aspirin).[29,33] The symptoms of drug-induced hearing loss may be transient, as often is the case with salicylates and diuretics, or they may be permanent. The risk of ototoxicity depends on the total dose of the drug and its concentration in the bloodstream. It is increased in persons with impaired kidney function and in those previously or currently treated with another potentially ototoxic drug.

Diagnosis and Treatment

Diagnosis. Diagnosis of hearing loss is aided by careful history of associated otologic factors such as otalgia, otorrhea, tinnitus, and self-described hearing difficulties; physical examination to detect the presence of conditions such as otorrhea, impacted cerumen, or injury to the tympanic membrane; and hearing tests.[29,31] A history of occupational and noise exposure is important, as is the use of medications with ototoxic potential. Testing for hearing loss includes a number of methods, including a person's reported ability to hear an observer's voice, use of a tuning fork to test air and bone conduction, audioscopes, and auditory brain stem-evoked responses (ABRs).

Tuning forks are used to differentiate conductive and sensorineural hearing loss. A 512-Hz or higher-frequency tuning fork is used because frequencies below this level elicit a tactile response. The Weber test evaluates conductive hearing loss by lateralization of sound. It is done by placing the lightly vibrating tuning fork on the forehead or vertex of the head. In persons with conductive losses, the sound is louder on the side with the hearing loss, but in persons with sensorineural loss, it radiates to the side with the better hearing. The Rinne test compares air and bone conduction. The test is done by placing the tuning fork alternately on the mastoid bone and in front of the ear canal. In conductive losses, bone conduction exceeds air conduction; in sensorineural losses, the opposite occurs.

An audioscope is a rechargeable battery-powered, hand-held instrument that combines a pure-tone screening audiometer and otoscope into a single unit. It produces pure sounds at 500, 1,000, 2,000, and 4,000 Hz, at loudness levels of 20, 25, and 40 dB. If a person cannot hear pure tones at 1,000 to 2,000 Hz (usual speech frequencies), referral for a full audiogram is indicated. The audiogram is an important method of analyzing a person's hearing, and is generally considered the gold standard for diagnosis of hearing loss. It is done by an audiologist and requires highly specialized sound production and control equipment. Pure tones of controlled intensity are delivered, usually to one ear at a time, and the minimum intensity needed for hearing to be experienced is plotted as a function of frequency.

The ABR is a noninvasive method that permits functional evaluation of certain defined parts of the central auditory pathways. Electroencephalographic (EEG) electrodes and high-gain amplifiers are required to produce a record of the electrical wave activity elicited during repeated acoustic stimulations of either or both ears. ABR recording involves subjecting the ear to loud clicks and using a computer to pick up nerve impulses as they are processed in the midbrain. With this method, certain of the early waves that come from discrete portions of the pons and midbrain auditory pathways can be correlated with specific sensorineural abnormalities. Imaging studies such as computed tomography (CT) scans and magnetic resonance imaging (MRI) may be done to determine the site of a lesion and the extent of damage.

Treatment. Hearing loss can have many consequences. It produces a loss of the important communicative function of auditory language. Social isolation and depressive disorders are common in hearing-impaired older adults. Safety issues and functional decline, both in and out of the home, may become significant.

Treatment of hearing loss can range from simple removal of impacted cerumen in the external auditory canal to surgical procedures such as those used to reconstruct the tympanic membrane. For other people, hearing aids and cochlear implants are option. Although many assistive devices are available to persons with hearing loss, understanding on the part of family and friends is perhaps the most important. The interpretation of speech involves both visual and auditory clues. It is important that people speaking to persons with hearing impairment face the person and articulate so that lip reading cues can be used. Adequate lighting is important. Distractions such as background noise can make communication difficult and should be avoided when possible.

Hearing aids remain the mainstay of treatment for many persons with conductive and sensorineural hearing loss. With the advent of microcircuitry, hearing aids are now designed with computer chips that allow multiple programs to be placed in a single hearing aid. The various programs allow the user to select a specific setting for different listening situations. The development of microcircuitry has also made it possible for hearing aids to be miniaturized to the point that,

in many cases, they can be placed deep in the ear, where they take advantage of the normal shape of the external ear and ear canal. Although modern hearing aids have improved greatly, they cannot replicate the hearing person's ability to hear both soft and loud noises. They also fail to consistently filter out distorted or background noise. Many persons who are fitted with hearing aids use them inconsistently, often because of social embarrassment, increase in background noise, or the sound of their own voice being transmitted through the hearing aid.[34] Other aids for the hearing impaired include alert and signal devices, assisted-listening devices from telephone companies, and dogs trained to respond to various sounds.

Surgically implantable cochlear prostheses for the profoundly deaf have been successfully used in adults and children 8 months of age or older. Small studies are now looking into cochlear implant surgeries for children younger than 6 months.[35] These prostheses are inserted into the scala tympani of the cochlea and work by providing direct stimulation to the auditory nerve, bypassing the stimulation that typically is provided by transducer cells but that is absent or nonfunctional in a deaf cochlea. For the implant to work, the auditory nerve must be functional. Although early implants used a single electrode, current implants use multielectrode placement, enhancing speech perception. Much of the progress in implant performance has been achieved through improvements in the speech processors that convert sound into electrical stimuli. Advances in the development of the multichannel implant have improved performance such that cochlear implants have been established as an effective option for adults and children with profound hearing impairment.[35] Most persons who are deafened after learning speech derive substantial benefit when cochlear implants are used in conjunction with lip reading; some are able to understand some speech without lip reading; and some are able to communicate by telephone.

Hearing Loss in Infants and Children

Even mild or unilateral hearing loss can have a detrimental effect on the language development and hearing-associated learning of the young child.[11,36] Although estimates vary depending on the group surveyed and testing methods used, from 1 to 2 per 1,000 newborns have moderate (30 to 50 dB), severe (50 to 70 dB), or profound (≥70 dB) sensorineural hearing loss.[11] An additional 1 to 2 per 1,000 may have milder or unilateral impairments. When considering less severe or transient conductive hearing loss that is commonly associated with middle ear disease in young children, the numbers are even greater.

The cause of hearing impairment in children may be conductive or sensorineural. Most conductive hearing loss is caused by middle ear infections. Causes of sensorineural hearing impairment include genetic, infectious, traumatic, and ototoxic factors. Genetic causes are probably responsible for as much as 50% of sensorineural hearing loss in children.

The most common infectious cause of congenital sensorineural hearing loss is cytomegalovirus (CMV), which infects 0.3% to 2.2% of all live births in Canada.[37] Most newborns with a symptomatic congenital CMV infection (*i.e.*, with significant clinical illness) will go on to have neurologic sequelae, including sensorineural hearing loss. Of particular concern are the newborns who are asymptomatic at birth; approximately 13.5% will have neurodevelopmental abnormalities including sensorineural hearing loss that appear in infancy or later in childhood.[37]

Postnatal causes of sensorineural hearing loss include β-hemolytic streptococcal sepsis in the newborn and bacterial meningitis. *S. pneumoniae* is the most common cause of bacterial meningitis that results in sensorineural hearing loss after the neonatal period. This cause may become less frequent with the routine administration of the conjugate pneumococcal vaccine. Other causes of sensorineural hearing loss are toxins and trauma. Early in pregnancy, the embryo is particularly sensitive to toxic substances, including ototoxic drugs such as the aminoglycosides and loop diuretics. Trauma, particularly head trauma, may cause sensorineural hearing loss.

Hearing impairment can have a major impact on the development of a child; therefore, early identification through screening programs is strongly advocated. The Canadian Paediatric Society advocates for universal screening of all newborns by physiologic measurements before 12 weeks of age, with proper intervention no later than 6 months of age.[49] Most Canadian provinces and territories have now enacted legislation resulting in newborn hearing screening programs in nurseries. The currently recommended screening techniques are either the transient evoked otoacoustic emissions (TEOAE) or the ABR. Both methodologies are noninvasive, relatively quick (<5 minutes), and easy to perform. The TEOAE measures sound waves generated in the inner ear (cochlea) in response to clicks or tone bursts emitted and recorded by a minute microphone placed in the external ear canals of the infant. The ABR uses three electrodes pasted to the infant's scalp to measure the EEG waves generated by clicks. Because many children become hearing impaired after the neonatal period and are not identified by neonatal screening programs, the recommendations that all infants with risk factors for delayed onset of progressive hearing loss receive ongoing audiologic and medical monitoring and at appropriate intervals thereafter.

Once hearing loss has been identified, a full developmental and speech and language evaluation is needed. Parental involvement and counselling are essential. Children with sensorineural hearing loss should be evaluated for possible hearing aid use by a pediatric audiologist. Hearing aids may be fitted for infants as young as 2 months of age. The use of surgically implanted cochlear prostheses in children with profound hearing loss has been approved for children 8 months of age and older.[38] One limitation with implantation in children over 1 year of age is that the critical period of auditory input for the acquisition of oral language has passed; however, with surgical advances, earlier ages are now being considered.[35] Because of the increased risk of pneumococcal meningitis, children who receive implants should receive age-appropriate immunization against pneumococcal disease.[11] At present, the best educational approach to children with significant hearing loss is open to controversy. Some members of the hearing-impaired community have objected to the use of cochlear implants in children, maintaining that the child can develop adequate communication skills using more conventional strategies such as sign language and lip reading.

Hearing Loss in Older Adults

The term *presbycusis* is used to describe degenerative hearing loss that occurs with advancing age.[21] Hearing loss is a prevalent chronic condition in older Canadians. Between 25% and 40% of the population aged 65 years and older is hearing impaired.[39] Because of its high prevalence, presbycusis is a common social and health problem. People with the disorder have difficulty proportional to the degree of hearing impairment in conversation, music appreciation, orientation to alarms, and participation in social activities.

The hearing loss associated with presbycusis is typically gradual, bilateral, and characterized by high-frequency hearing loss. It is further characterized by reduced hearing sensitivity and speech understanding in noisy environments, slowed central processing of acoustic information, and impaired localization of sound sources. The disorder first reduces the ability to understand speech and, later, the ability to detect, identify, and localize sounds. The most common complaint of persons with presbycusis is not that they cannot hear, but rather that they cannot understand what is being said. For example, they often confuse words like *mash* with *math, map* with *mat,* and *Sunday* with *some day.* High-frequency warning sounds, such as beepers, turn signals, and escaping steam, are not heard and localized, with potentially dangerous results.

Although the degeneration with aging of the sensory cells in the cochlea, supporting cells, and cochlear nerve are well described, the cause of presbycusis is largely unknown. Because of the age at which the problems occur varies widely, it seems likely that the disorder results from a mixture of acquired auditory stresses, trauma, and otologic diseases superimposed on an intrinsic, genetically controlled aging process.[40]

Given the high prevalence of presbycusis in people of retirement age and the adverse effects of hearing loss on well-being, screening for hearing loss should be performed at annual healthcare visits. The single question "do you have a hearing problem?" is usually an effective method of screening. The 10-item Hearing Handicap Inventory for the Elderly—Screening Version (HHIE-S) is also a widely used screening tool.[29] Clinical measures for hearing loss such as whispered voice tests and finger friction tests are reportedly imprecise and are not reliable methods for screening. Screening audiometry administered by someone trained in its use is a practical and cost-effective method for detecting significant hearing loss. The equipment needed for screening audiometry is lightweight, low cost, and well accepted by persons being tested.

Several otologic abnormalities can be identified and treated. Cerumen impaction may result in substantial hearing loss and can be found in up to 30% of older adults with hearing loss.[3] Many older adults are on multiple medications, some of which may possess ototoxic potential. A frequently overlooked ototoxic agent is aspirin. Little is known about what level of dosage causes ototoxicity, but it is generally believed that 81 mg of aspirin on a daily basis is safe. Fortunately, in most cases, the resulting tinnitus and hearing loss are temporary and reversible with cessation of the drug.

The majority of hearing loss in older adults is sensorineural. In mild to severe loss, the most effective treatment is hearing amplification with hearing aids, speech reading, and assistive-listening devices (*e.g.*, hearing aids with the telephone, captioning on televised programs, flashing alarms). Cochlear implants are indicated at any age for people with bilateral hearing losses not materially helped by hearing aids.

IN SUMMARY

Hearing is a specialized sense whose external stimulus is the vibration of sound waves. Our ears receive sound waves, distinguish their frequencies, translate this information into nerve impulses, and transmit them to the CNS. Anatomically, the auditory system consists of the outer ear, middle ear, and inner ear, the auditory pathways, and the auditory cortex. The middle ear is a tiny, air-filled cavity in the temporal bone. A connection exists between the middle ear and the nasopharynx. This connection, called the eustachian tube, allows equalization of pressure between the middle ear and the atmosphere. The inner ear contains the receptors for hearing.

Disorders of the auditory system include infections of the external and middle ear, otosclerosis, and conductive and sensorineural deafness. Otitis externa is an inflammatory process of the external ear. Otitis media is an inflammation of the middle ear without reference to etiology or pathogenesis. Acute OM, which refers to an acute middle ear infection, is one of the most common illnesses in children. It usually follows an upper respiratory tract infection, has an abrupt onset, and is characterized by otalgia, fever, and hearing loss. OM with effusion refers to the presence of fluid in the inner ear without signs and symptoms of acute ear infection. The effusion that accompanies OM can persist for weeks or months, interfering with hearing and impairing speech development. It is important to differentiate OME from AOM to avoid unnecessary antimicrobial use. Otosclerosis is a familial disorder of the otic capsule. It causes bone resorption followed by excessive replacement with sclerotic bone. The disorder eventually causes immobilization of the stapes and conduction deafness.

Deafness, or hearing loss, can develop as the result of a number of auditory disorders. It can be conductive, sensorineural, or mixed. Conductive deafness occurs when transmission of sound waves from the external to the inner ear is impaired. Sensorineural deafness can involve cochlear structures of the inner ear or the neural pathways that transmit auditory stimuli. Sensorineural hearing loss can result from genetic or congenital disorders, trauma, infections, vascular disorders, tumours, or ototoxic drugs. Hearing

loss in infants and young children impairs language and speech development. In older adults, hearing loss is a common condition resulting in significant loss of social well-being. Treatment of hearing loss includes the use of hearing aids and, in some cases of profound deafness, implantation of a cochlear prosthesis.

CONCEPTS in action **ANIMATI** **N**

DISORDERS OF VESTIBULAR FUNCTION

After completing this section of the chapter, you should be able to meet the following objectives:

- Explain the function of the vestibular system with respect to postural reflexes and maintaining a stable visual field despite marked changes in head position.
- Relate the function of the vestibular system to nystagmus and vertigo.
- Differentiate the structures of peripheral and central vestibular function.
- Characterize the physiologic cause of motion sickness.
- Compare the manifestations and pathologic processes associated with benign paroxysmal positional vertigo and Ménière disease.
- Differentiate the manifestations of peripheral and central vestibular disorders.

The Vestibular System and Vestibular Reflexes

The vestibular receptive organs, which are located in the inner ear, and their connections to the CNS contribute to the reflex activity necessary for effective posture and movement in a physical world governed by momentum and a gravitational field.[21] Because the vestibular apparatus is part of the inner ear and located in the head, it is head position and acceleration that is sensed. The vestibular system serves two general and related functions. It maintains and assists recovery of stable body and head position through control of postural reflexes, and it maintains a stable visual field despite marked changes in head position.

Peripheral Vestibular Apparatus

The peripheral apparatus of the vestibular system is contained in the bony labyrinth of the inner ear next to and continuous with the cochlea of the auditory system. Like the cochlea, it consists of two fluid-filled compartments—an outer bony labyrinth that is filled with perilymph and an inner membranous labyrinth that is filled with endolymph[21,41,42] (Fig. 55.7A). The bony labyrinth is divided into three semicircular canals and a central vestibule or egg-shaped cavity that lies posterior to the cochlea and anterior to the semicircular canals. Suspended in

DISORDERS OF THE VESTIBULAR SYSTEM

- The receptors concerned with the sense of balance and position in space are located in fluid (endolymph)-filled semicircular canals of the vestibular system of the inner ear.
- The vestibular system has extensive interconnections with neural pathways controlling vision, hearing, and autonomic nervous system function. Disorders of the vestibular system are characterized by vertigo, nystagmus, tinnitus, nausea and vomiting, and autonomic nervous system manifestations.
- Disorders of vestibular function can result from repeated stimulation of the vestibular system such as during car, air, and boat travel (motion sickness); acute infection of the vestibular pathways (acute vestibular neuritis); dislodgement of otoliths that participate in the receptor function of the vestibular system (benign paroxysmal positional vertigo); or distension of the endolymphatic compartment of the inner ear (Ménière disease).

the perilymph and united by a duct are two membranous labyrinth sacs, the saccule and utricle. The smaller saccule is continuous with the membranous labyrinth extending anteriorly into the cochlea through the ductus reuniens, which connects with the cochlear duct; whereas the utricle is continuous with the ducts extending into the semicircular canals posteriorly. The receptors of the vestibular system consist of small patches of hair cells located in membranous ampullae of three semicircular ducts and the maculae of the saccule and utricle.

The cavities of the three semicircular canals, the lateral, anterior, and posterior canals, are oriented in one of three planes of space.[42] The lateral (horizontal) canals are in the same plane, whereas the anterior (superior) canal of one side is parallel with the posterior (inferior) canal on the other side, and the two function as a pair. Located in each semicircular canal is a corresponding semicircular duct, which communicates with the utricle. Each of these ducts has an enlarged swelling at one end called an *ampulla* (Fig. 55.7A). The ampulla of each of the semicircular canals contains a ridge that is covered by a sensory epithelium with hair cells that are raised into a crest, called the crista ampullaris, which lies at a right angle to the duct (Fig. 55.7B). These hair cells are innervated by the primary afferents of the vestibular nerve, which is a subdivision of the eighth cranial nerve. The hair cells of the crista ampullaris extend into a flexible gelatinous mass, called the *cupula,* which essentially closes off fluid flow through the semicircular ducts (Fig. 55.7C).

When the head begins to rotate around the axis of a semicircular canal (*i.e.,* undergoes angular acceleration), the momentum of the endolymph causes an increase in pressure on one side of the cupula. This is similar to the lagging behind of the water in a glass that is suddenly rotated, except that the endolymph cannot flow past the cupula. Instead, the endolymph applies a differential pressure to the two sides of the cupula, bending the hair bundles. Because all the hair cells in each semicircular canal share a common orientation, angular acceleration in one direction depolarizes hair cells and

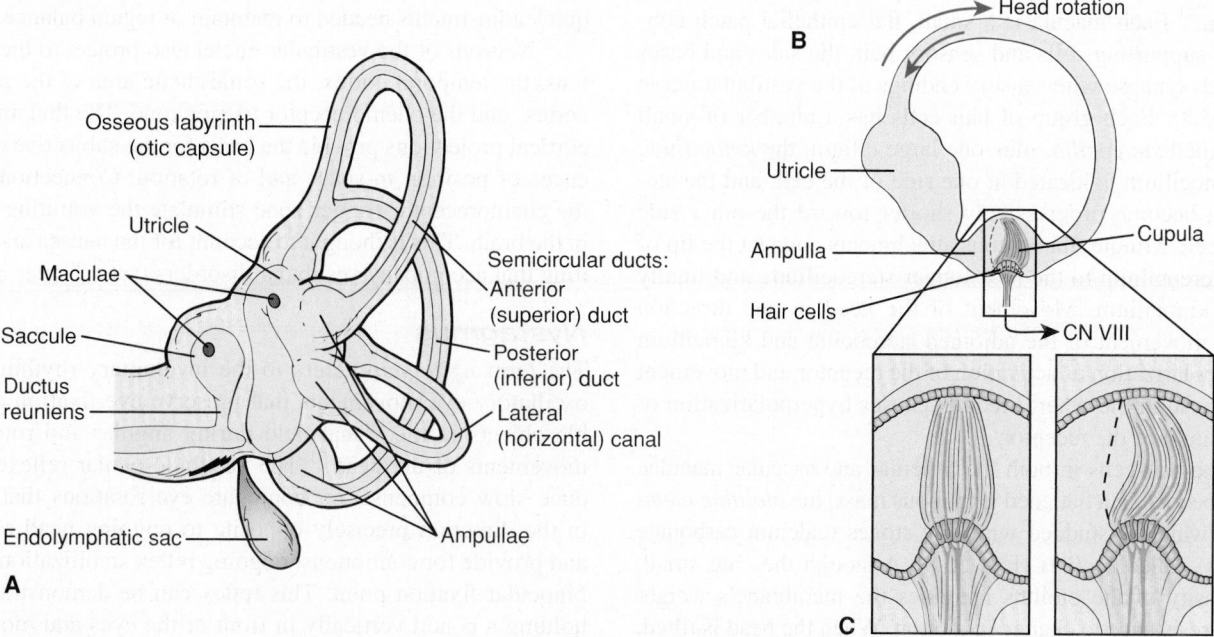

FIGURE 55.7 • A: The osseous and membranous labyrinth of the left ear showing the utricle and saccule with their maculae and three semicircular canals and their ampullae. **B:** Location of the crista ampullaris and its connection to the vestibular branch of CN VIII. **C:** The location of the cupula and movement of hair cells of the crista ampullaris with head movement.

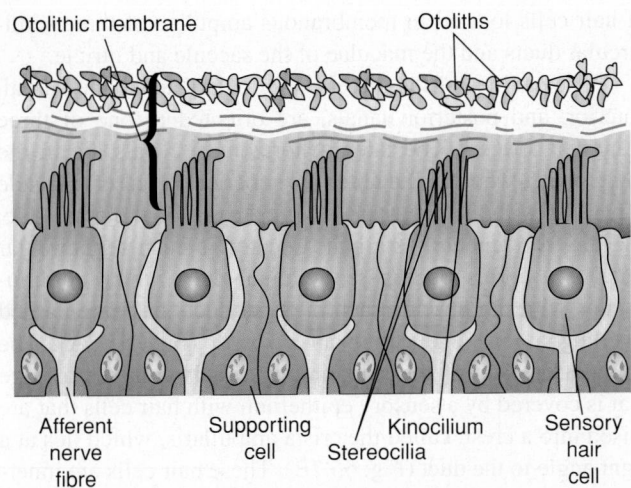

FIGURE 55.8 • The relation of the otoliths to the sensory cells in the maculae of the utricle and saccule. (From Ross M. H., Pawlina W. (2011). *Histology: A text and atlas* (6th ed., p. 938). Philadelphia, PA: Lippincott Williams & Wilkins.)

increases afferent neurons, whereas acceleration in the opposite direction hyperpolarizes the receptor cells and diminishes nerve activity. Impulses from the semicircular ducts are particularly important in reflex movement of the eyes. Vestibular nystagmus (to be discussed) is a complex phenomenon that occurs during and immediately after rotational motion. As you rotate your head, your eyes slowly drift in the opposite direction and then jump rapidly back toward the direction of rotation to establish a new fixation point.

The saccule and utricle house equilibrium receptors called *maculae* that respond to the pull of gravity and head position.[42] Each macula is a small, flat epithelial patch containing supporting cells and sensory hair, the sides and bases of which synapse with sensory endings of the vestibular nerve (Fig. 55.8). Each group of hair cells has a number of small cilia called *stereocilia,* plus one large cilium, the *kinocilium.* The kinocilium is located at one side of the cell, and the stereocilia become progressively shorter toward the other side of the cell. Minute filamentous attachments connect the tip of each stereocilium to the next longer stereocilium, and finally to the kinocilium. Movement of the head in one direction causes movement of the adjoined stereocilia and kinocilium and depolarization or activation of the receptor and movement of the head in the other direction causes hyperpolarization or inactivation of the receptor.

The hair cells in both the utricular and saccular maculae are embedded in a flattened gelatinous mass, the *otolithic membrane,* which is studded with tiny stones (calcium carbonate crystals) called *otoliths* (Fig. 55.8). Although they are small, the density of the otoliths increases the membrane's weight and its resistance to change in motion. When the head is tilted, the gelatinous mass shifts its position because of the pull of the gravitational field, bending the stereocilia of the macular hair cells. Although each hair cell becomes more or less excitable depending on the direction in which the cilia are bending,

the hair cells are oriented in all directions, making these sense organs sensitive to static or changing head position in relation to the gravitational field. In a condition called *benign paroxysmal positional vertigo* (BPPV, sensation of whirling or spinning motion), the otoliths become dislodged from their gelatinous base, causing a vertigo that is precipitated by changes in the recumbent head position (to be discussed).

Neural Pathways

The response to body imbalance, such as stumbling, must be fast and reflexive. Hence, information from the vestibular system goes directly to reflex centres in the brain stem, rather than to the cerebral cortex. Ganglionic cells, homologous with dorsal root ganglion cells, form afferent ganglia: the superior and inferior vestibular ganglia that innervate the hair cells of the peripheral vestibular apparatus (Fig. 55.5). The central axons of these ganglion cells become the superior and inferior vestibular nerves, which become part of the vestibulocochlear nerve (CN VIII).

Impulses from the vestibular nerves initially pass to one of two destinations: the vestibular nuclear complex in the brain stem, or the cerebellum. The vestibular nuclei, which form the main integrative centre for balance, also receive input from visual and somatic receptors, particularly from proprioceptors in the neck muscles that report the angle or inclination of the head. The vestibular nuclei integrate this information and then send impulses to the brain stem centres that control the extrinsic eye movements (CN III, IV, and VI) and reflex movements of the neck, limb, and trunk muscles (through the vestibulospinal tracts). These reflexes include the vestibulo-ocular reflexes that keep the eyes still as the head moves and the vestibulospinal reflexes that enable the musculoskeletal system to make the quick adjustments needed to maintain or regain balance.

Neurons of the vestibular nuclei also project to the thalamus, the temporal cortex, the somesthetic area of the parietal cortex, and the chemoreceptor trigger zone. The thalamic and cortical projections provide the basis for the subjective experiences of position in space and of rotation. Connections with the chemoreceptor trigger zone stimulate the vomiting centre in the brain. This is thought to account for the nausea and vomiting that accompany vestibular disorders (see Chapter 36).

Nystagmus

The term *nystagmus* refers to the involuntary rhythmic and oscillatory eye movements that preserve eye fixation on stable objects in the visual field during angular and rotational movements of the head.[21] The vestibulo-ocular reflexes produce slow compensatory conjugate eye rotations that occur in the direction precisely opposite to ongoing head rotation and provide for continuous, ongoing reflex stabilization of the binocular fixation point. This reflex can be demonstrated by holding a pencil vertically in front of the eyes and moving it from side to side through a 10-degree arc at a rate of approximately five times per second. At this rate of motion, the pencil appears blurred because a different and more complex reflex, smooth pursuit, cannot compensate quickly enough. However,

	Direction of spin
Horizontal canals	
Left ear Right ear	Direction of endolymph movement
	Hair displacement
	Nerve discharge
Slow Slow Fast Fast	Nystagmus

FIGURE 55.9 • Effect of spinning a subject clockwise. On acceleration, the endolymph in the horizontal canals will lag behind with respect to movement of the canal wall. The hairs of cristae will be displaced to the left. In the left semicircular canal, hair displacement is away from the kinocilium, leading to decreased nerve discharges below the resting level. On the right, hair displacement is toward the kinocilium, leading to an increase in nerve discharge above the resting level. (From Sekurt F. E. (1982). *Basic physiology for the health professions* (2nd ed., p. 140). Boston, MA: Little, Brown.)

if the pencil is maintained in a stable position and the head is moved back and forth at the same rate, the image of the pencil is clearly defined. The eye movements are the same in both cases. The reason that the pencil image remains clear in the second situation is because the vestibulo-ocular reflexes keep the image of the pencil on the retinal fovea. When compensatory vestibulo-ocular reflexes carry the conjugate eye rotations to their physical limit, a very rapid conjugate movement moves the eyes in the direction of head rotation to a new fixation point, followed by a slow vestibulo-ocular reflex as the head continues to rotate past the new fixation point. This pattern of slow–fast–slow movements is called *nystagmus* (Fig. 55.9). Clinically, the direction of nystagmus is named for the fast phase of nystagmus.

Nystagmus can be classified according to the direction of eye movement: horizontal, vertical, rotary (torsional), or mixed. If head rotation is continued, friction between endolymph and semicircular duct walls results in endolymph rotating at the same velocity as the head, and nystagmus adapts to a stable eye posture. If rotation is suddenly stopped, vestibular nystagmus reappears in the direction precisely opposite to the angular accelerating nystagmus. This results because the inertia of the endolymph is again bending ampullary hair cells of a now stationary ampulla.

Spontaneous nystagmus that occurs without head movement or visual stimuli is always pathologic. It seems to appear more readily and more severely with fatigue and to some extent can be influenced by psychological factors. Nystagmus due to a CNS pathologic process, in contrast to vestibular end-organ or vestibulocochlear nerve sources, seldom is accompanied by vertigo. If present, the vertigo is mild. Nystagmus eye movements can be tested by caloric stimulation or rotation (to be discussed).

Vertigo

Disorders of vestibular function are characterized by a condition called *vertigo,* in which an illusion of motion occurs. With vertigo, the person may be stationary and the environment in motion (*i.e.,* objective vertigo) or the person may be in motion and the environment stationary (*i.e.,* subjective vertigo). Persons with vertigo frequently describe a sensation of spinning, "to-and-fro" motion, or falling.

Vertigo should be differentiated from lightheadedness, faintness, unsteadiness, or syncope[43] (loss of consciousness; Table 55.1). Presyncope, which is characterized by a feeling

TABLE 55.1 DIFFERENCES IN PATHOLOGY AND MANIFESTATIONS OF DIZZINESS ASSOCIATED WITH BENIGN PAROXYSMAL POSITIONAL VERTIGO, PRESYNCOPE, AND DISEQUILIBRIUM STATE

TYPE OF DISORDER	PATHOLOGY	SYMPTOMS
Benign paroxysmal positional vertigo (BPPV)	Disorder of otoliths	Vertigo initiated by a change in head position, usually lasts less than a minute
Presyncope	Orthostatic hypotension	Lightheadedness and feeling faint on assumption of standing position
Disequilibrium	Sensory (*e.g.,* vision, proprioception) deficits	Dizziness and unsteadiness when walking, especially when turning; relieved by additional proprioceptive stimulation such as touching wall or table

of lightheadedness or "blacking out," is commonly caused by postural hypotension (see Chapter 23) or a stenotic lesion in the cerebral circulation that limits blood flow. An inability to maintain normal gait may be described as dizziness despite the absence of objective vertigo. The unstable gait may be caused by disorders of sensory input (*e.g.,* proprioception), peripheral neuropathy, gait problems, or disorders other than vestibular function and usually is corrected by touching a stationary object such as a wall or table.

Vertigo or dizziness can result from central or peripheral vestibular disorders. Approximately 85% of persons with vertigo have a peripheral vestibular disorder, whereas only 15% have a central disorder.[44] Vertigo due to peripheral vestibular disorders tends to be severe in intensity and episodic or brief in duration. In contrast, vertigo due to central vestibular causes tends to be mild and constant and chronic in duration.

Motion Sickness

Motion sickness is a form of normal physiologic vertigo. It is caused by repeated rhythmic stimulation of the vestibular system, such as that encountered in car, air, or boat travel. Vertigo, malaise, nausea, and vomiting are the principal symptoms. Autonomic signs, including lowered blood pressure, tachycardia, and excessive sweating, may occur. Hyperventilation, which commonly accompanies motion sickness, produces changes in blood volume and pooling of blood in the lower extremities, leading to postural hypotension and sometimes to syncope. Some persons experience a variant of motion sickness, complaining of sensing the rocking motion of the boat after returning to ground. This usually resolves after the vestibular system becomes accustomed to the stationary influence of being back on land.

Motion sickness can usually be suppressed by supplying visual signals that more closely match the motion signals being supplied to the vestibular system. For example, looking out the window and watching the environment move when experiencing motion sickness associated with car travel provides the vestibular system with the visual sensation of motion, but reading a book provides the vestibular system with the miscue that the environment is stable. Motion sickness usually decreases in severity with repeated exposure. Antimotion sickness drugs also may be used to reduce or ameliorate the symptoms. These drugs work by suppressing the activity of the vestibular system.

Disorders of Peripheral Vestibular Function

Disorders of peripheral vestibular function occur when signals from the peripheral vestibular apparatus are distorted, as in BPPV, or are unbalanced by unilateral involvement of one of the vestibular organs, as in Ménière disease. The inner ear is vulnerable to injury caused by fracture of the petrous portion of the temporal bones; by infection of nearby structures,

including the middle ear and meninges; and by blood-borne toxins and infections. Damage to the vestibular system can occur as an adverse effect of certain drugs or from allergic reactions to foods. The aminoglycosides (*e.g.,* streptomycin, gentamicin) have a specific toxic affinity for the vestibular portion of the inner ear. Alcohol can cause transient episodes of vertigo. The cause of peripheral vertigo remains unknown in approximately half of the cases.

Severe irritation or damage of the vestibular end organs or nerves results in severe balance disorders reflected by instability of posture, ataxia, and falling accompanied by vertigo. With irritation, falling is away from the affected side; with destruction, it is toward the affected side. Adaptation to asymmetric stimulation occurs within a few days, after which the signs and symptoms diminish and eventually are lost. After recovery, there usually is a slightly reduced acuity for tilt, and the person walks with a somewhat broadened base to improve postural stability. The neurologic basis for this adaptation to unilateral loss of vestibular input is not understood. After adaptation to the loss of vestibular input from one side, the loss of function of the opposite vestibular apparatus produces signs and symptoms identical to those resulting from unilateral rather than bilateral loss. Within weeks, adaptation is again sufficient for locomotion and even for driving a car. Such a person relies heavily on visual and proprioceptive input from muscle and joint sensors and has severe orientation difficulty in the dark, particularly when traversing uneven terrain.

Benign Paroxysmal Positional Vertigo

Benign paroxysmal positional vertigo (BPPV) is the most common cause of pathologic vertigo, it is more common in women, and prevalence in the older adult population may approach 9%.[45] It is characterized by brief periods of vertigo, usually lasting less than 1 minute, that are precipitated by a change in head position. The most prominent symptom of BPPV is vertigo that occurs in bed when the person rolls into a lateral position. It also commonly occurs when the person is getting in and out of bed, bending over and straightening up, or extending the head to look up. It also can be triggered by amusement rides that feature turns and twists.

BPPV is thought to result from damage to the delicate sensory organs of the inner ear, the semicircular ducts, and otoliths (Fig. 55.9). In persons with BPPV, the calcium carbonate particles (otoliths, also called otoconia) from the utricle become dislodged and become free-floating debris within the endolymph of a semicircular canal, most commonly the posterior canal, which is the most dependent part of the inner ear.[45] Movement of the free-floating debris causes this portion of the vestibular system to become more sensitive, such that any movement of the head in the plane parallel to the posterior duct may cause vertigo and nystagmus. There usually is a several-second delay between head movement and onset of vertigo, representing the time it takes to generate the exaggerated endolymph activity. Symptoms usually subside with continued movement, probably because the movement causes the debris to be redistributed throughout the endolymph system and away from the posterior semicircular canal.

Diagnosis is based on tests that involve the use of a change in head position to elicit vertigo and nystagmus, such as the Dix–Hallpike manoeuvres.[45] BPPV often is successfully treated with drug therapy to control vertigo-induced nausea. Nondrug therapies using habituation exercises and canalith repositioning are successful in many people. Canalith repositioning involves a series of manoeuvres in which the head is moved to different positions in an effort to reposition the free-floating debris in the endolymph of the semicircular canals.[45]

Acute Vestibular Neuronitis

Acute vestibular neuronitis represents the unilateral inflammation of the vestibular nerve and is characterized by an acute onset (usually hours) of vertigo, nausea, and vomiting lasting several days and not associated with auditory or other neurologic manifestations. Most persons experience gradual improvement over 1 to 2 weeks, but some develop recurrent episodes. A large percentage report an upper respiratory tract illness 1 to 2 weeks before onset of symptoms, suggesting a viral origin. The condition also can occur in persons with herpes zoster oticus. In some persons, attacks of acute vestibulopathy recur over months or years. There is no way to determine whether a person who experiences a first attack will have repeated attacks.

Ménière Disease

Ménière disease is a disorder of the inner ear linked to distension of the endolymphatic compartment of the inner ear, causing a triad of hearing loss, vertigo, and tinnitus.[46,47] It has been associated with a primary lesion in the endolymphatic sac, which is thought to be responsible for endolymph filtration and excretion. A number of pathogenetic mechanisms have been hypothesized, including an increased production of endolymph, decreased production of perilymph accompanied by a compensatory increase in volume of the endolymphatic sac, and decreased absorption of endolymph caused by malfunction of the endolymphatic sac or blockage of endolymphatic pathways. Newer research is focusing on the immunologic function of the endolymphatic sac and inflammatory responses involved.[46]

Ménière disease is characterized by fluctuating episodes of tinnitus, feelings of ear fullness, and violent rotary vertigo that often renders the person unable to sit or walk. There is a need to lie quietly with the head fixed in a comfortable position, avoiding all head movements that aggravate the vertigo.[47] Symptoms referable to the autonomic nervous system, including pallor, sweating, nausea, and vomiting, usually are present. The more severe the attack, the more prominent are the autonomic manifestations. A fluctuating hearing loss occurs with a return to normal after the episode subsides. Initially the symptoms tend to be unilateral, resulting in rotary nystagmus caused by an imbalance in vestibular control of eye movements. Because initial involvement usually is unilateral and because the sense of hearing is bilateral, many persons with the disorder are not aware of the full extent of their hearing loss. However, as the disease progresses, the hearing loss stops fluctuating and progressively worsens, with both ears tending to be affected so that the prime disability becomes one of deafness. The episodes of vertigo diminish and then disappear, although the person may be unsteady, especially in the dark.

The cause of Ménière disease is unknown. A number of conditions, such as trauma, infection (*e.g.,* syphilis), and immunologic, endocrine (*i.e.,* adrenal–pituitary insufficiency and hypothyroidism), and vascular disorders have been proposed as possible causes of Ménière disease.[46] The most common form of the disease is an idiopathic form thought to be caused by a single viral injury to the fluid transport system of the inner ear. One area of investigation has been the relation between autoimmune disorders and Ménière disease.

Methods used in the diagnosis of Ménière disease include audiograms, vestibular testing by electronystagmography (ENG), electrocochleography, and CT or MRI. The administration of hyperosmolar substances, such as glycerin and urea, often produces acute temporary hearing improvement in persons with Ménière disease and sometimes is used as a diagnostic measure of endolymphatic hydrops. The diuretic furosemide also may be used for this purpose.

The management of Ménière disease focuses on attempts to reduce the distension of the endolymphatic space, and can be medical or surgical. Pharmacologic management consists of suppressant drugs (*e.g.,* prochlorperazine, promethazine, diazepam), which act centrally to decrease the activity of the vestibular system. Diuretics are used to reduce endolymph fluid volume. A low-sodium diet is recommended in addition to these medications.[47] Intratympanic gentamicin therapy has been used for ablation of the vestibular system. Persons who are candidates for intratympanic gentamicin infusion include those who have frequent attacks of Ménière disease, disease that involves one ear, good contralateral vestibular function, or normal or near-normal balance between episodes. This treatment is mainly effective in controlling vertigo and does not alter the underlying pathologic process. Newer treatment is using intratympanic steroids with success.[46–48]

Surgical methods include the creation of an endolymphatic shunt in which excess endolymph from the inner ear is diverted into the subarachnoid space or the mastoid (endolymphatic sac surgery), and vestibular nerve section. Advances in vestibular nerve section have facilitated the monitoring of CN VII and CN VIII potentials. These methods are used to prevent hearing damage. In unilateral cases, vestibular nerve section has a high success rate and provides relief of vertigo 2 years after surgery. The surgery, however, involves an intracranial procedure with possible postoperative morbidity.

Disorders of Central Vestibular Function

Abnormal nystagmus and vertigo can occur as a result of CNS lesions involving the cerebellum and lower brain stem. Central causes of vertigo include brain stem ischemia, tumours, and multiple sclerosis. When brain stem ischemia is the cause of vertigo, it usually is associated with other brain stem signs such as diplopia, ataxia, dysarthria, or facial weakness. Compression of the vestibular nuclei by cerebellar tumours invading the fourth ventricle results in progressively severe signs and symptoms. In addition to abnormal nystagmus and vertigo, vomiting and a broad-based and dystaxic gait become progressively more evident. The central demyelinating effects of multiple sclerosis can present with vertigo up to 10% of the time, and up to one third of persons with multiple sclerosis experience vertigo and nystagmus at some time in the course of the disease.[49]

Centrally derived nystagmus usually has equal excursion in both directions (*i.e.,* pendular). In contrast to peripherally generated nystagmus, CNS-derived nystagmus is relatively constant rather than episodic, can occur in any direction rather than being primarily in the horizontal or torsional (rotatory) dimensions, often changes direction through time, and cannot be suppressed by visual fixation. Repeated induction of nystagmus results in rapid diminution or "fatigue" of the reflex with peripheral abnormalities, but fatigue is not characteristic of central lesions. Abnormal nystagmus can make reading and other tasks that require precise eye positional control difficult.

Diagnosis and Treatment of Vestibular Disorders

Diagnostic Tests

Diagnosis of vestibular disorders is based on a description of the symptoms, a history of trauma or exposure to agents that are destructive to vestibular structures, and physical examination. Physical examination methods include use of the Romberg test, evaluation of gait, and observation for the presence of nystagmus.[50] Tests for hearing function can include: audiometry to monitor hearing over time: electrocochleography, which measures how sounds move from the tympanic membrane to the auditory nerve and can identify elevated endolymphatic fluid levels; and vestibular-evoked myogenic potential, a neurophysiologic assessment to determine the integrity of the saccule and utricle. Other tests of vestibular function include ENG and the caloric stimulation test.[51,52]

In peripheral lesions, nystagmus is usually horizontal and with a rotary component; the fast beat usually beats away from the disease side (Fig. 55.9). Several types of manoeuvres can be used to provoke vertigo and observe for nystagmus. The Dix–Hallpike test usually involves the person sitting upright on an examining table with the head turned toward the side being examined, and the eyes open and focused on the examiner's finger.[45,51] The person is then properly supported and lowered rapidly to the supine position with the head extending over the upper end of the examining table and placed about 30 degrees lower than the body. The person is observed for nystagmus for about 30 to 45 seconds while in that position. The test can be performed with the head turned to either side or with the person looking straight ahead.

Vertigo arising from central lesions tends to develop gradually, and nystagmus is not always present, can occur in any direction, and can be dissociated in the two eyes. The associated nystagmus is often nonfatigable, vertical rather than horizontal, and not suppressed by visual fixation.[51] ENG is often useful in documenting these characteristics. Further evaluation of central vertigo usually requires MRI.

Romberg Test. The Romberg test is used to demonstrate disorders of static vestibular function. The person being tested is requested to stand with feet together and arms at their sides, observing for the degree of sway and positional stability. The person then is asked to close his or her eyes. When visual clues are removed, postural stability is based on proprioceptive sensation from the joints, muscles, and tendons and from static vestibular reception. Deficiency in vestibular static input is indicated by greatly increased sway. The *pronator drift,* with the person extending their arms forward and palms facing up, can be added to monitor any drifting of the arms toward the side of deficiency. This is also done initially with the eyes open and then with the eyes closed.

If vestibular input is severely deficient, the subject falls toward the deficient side. Care must be taken because defects of proprioceptive projection to the forebrain also result in some arm drift and postural instability toward the deficient side. Only if two-point discrimination and vibratory sensation from the lower and upper limbs are bilaterally normal can the deficiency be attributed to the vestibular system.

Electronystagmography. Electronystagmography (ENG) is an examination that records eye movements in response to vestibular, visual, cervical (vertigo triggered by somatosensory input from head and neck movements), rotational, and positional stimulation. Electrodes are placed lateral to the outer canthus of each eye and above and below each eye. A ground electrode is placed on the forehead. With ENG, the velocity, frequency, and amplitude of spontaneous or induced nystagmus and the changes in these measurements brought by a loss of fixation, with the eyes open or closed, can be quantified. Alternatively, eye movements can be recorded by videonystagmography (VNG) when the patient wears an infrared camera mounted inside goggles. The advantages of ENG and VNG are that they are easily administered, are noninvasive, do not interfere with vision, and do not require head restraint.[52]

Caloric Stimulation. Caloric testing involves elevating the head 30 degrees and irrigating each external auditory canal separately with 30 to 50 ml of cold or even ice water. The resulting changes in temperature, which are conducted through the petrous portion of the temporal bone, set up convection currents in the endolymph that mimic the effects of angular acceleration. In a conscious person, this produces an immediate severe vertigo and in an unconscious person with a functional brain stem and intact oculovestibular reflexes, the eyes exhibit a jerk nystagmus lasting 2 to 3 minutes, with the slow component toward the irrigated ear followed by rapid movement away from the ear (see Chapter 51, Fig. 51.2). With impairment of brain stem function, the response becomes blunted and eventually disappears. An advantage of the caloric stimulation method is the ability to test the vestibular apparatus on one side at a time. The test is never done on persons who do not have an intact eardrum or who have blood or fluid collected behind the eardrum.

Treatment

Pharmacologic Methods. Depending on the cause, vertigo may be treated pharmacologically.[53,54] The drugs used to suppress the illusion of motion include antihistamines (*e.g.,* meclizine, dimenhydrinate, promethazine, betahistine) and anticholinergic drugs (*e.g.,* scopolamine, atropine) that suppress the vestibular system. Although the antihistamines have long been used in treating vertigo, little is known about their mechanism of action. Antidopaminergic drugs (*e.g.,* phenothiazines) and benzodiazepines commonly are used to relieve the nausea and vomiting that can accompany the condition. Steroids have been advocated for treatment of Ménière disease and vestibular neuritis to help with vertigo and the inflammatory process.[54]

Vestibular Rehabilitation Exercises. Vestibular rehabilitation has been shown to be helpful as a treatment modality for peripheral vestibular disorders.[45,55] It commonly is done by physical therapists and uses a home exercise program that incorporates habituation exercises, balance retraining exercises, and a general conditioning program.[55] The habituation exercises take advantage of physiologic fatigue of the neurovegetative response to repetitive movement or positional stimulation and are done to decrease motion-provoked vertigo, lightheadedness, and unsteadiness. The exercises are selected to provoke the vestibular symptoms. The person moves quickly into the position that causes symptoms, holds the position until the symptoms subside (*i.e.,* fatigue of the neurovegetative response), relaxes, and then repeats the exercise for a prescribed number of times. The exercises usually are repeated twice daily. The habituation effect is characterized by decreased sensitivity and duration of symptoms. It may occur in as little as 2 weeks or take as long as 6 months.

Balance-retraining exercises consist of activities directed toward improving individual components of balance that may be abnormal. General conditioning exercises, a vital part of the rehabilitation process, are individualized to the person's preferences and lifestyle.[55] They should consist of motion-oriented activity that the person is interested in and should be done on a regular basis, usually about five times per week.

IN SUMMARY

The vestibular system plays an essential role in the equilibrium sense, which is closely integrated with the visual and proprioceptive (position) senses. Receptors in the semicircular canals, utricle, and saccule of the vestibular system, located in the inner ear, respond to changes in linear and angular acceleration of the head. The vestibular nerve fibres travel in CN VIII to the vestibular nuclei at the junction of the medulla and pons; some fibres pass through the nuclei to the cerebellum. Cerebellar connections are necessary for temporally smooth, coordinated movements during ongoing head movements, tilt, and angular acceleration. The vestibular nuclei also connect with nuclei of the oculomotor (CN III), trochlear (CN IV), and abducens (CN VI) nerves that control eye movement. Nystagmus is a term used to describe vestibular-controlled eye movements that occur in response to angular and rotational movements of the head. The vestibulospinal tract, which provides for the control of muscle tone in the axial muscles, including those of the back, provides the support for maintaining balance. Neurons of the vestibular nuclei also project to the thalamus, to the temporal cortex, and to the somesthetic area of the parietal cortex. The thalamic and cortical projections provide the basis for the subjective experiences of position in space and of rotation and vertigo.

Vertigo, an illusory sensation of motion either of oneself or of one's surroundings, tinnitus, and hearing loss are common manifestations of vestibular dysfunction, as are autonomic manifestations such as perspiration, nausea, and vomiting. Common disorders of the vestibular system include motion sickness, BPPV, and Ménière disease.

BPPV is a condition believed to be caused by free-floating particles in the posterior semicircular canal. It presents as a sudden onset of dizziness or vertigo that is provoked by certain changes in head position. Ménière disease is characterized by severe, disabling episodes of tinnitus; feelings of ear fullness; and violent rotary vertigo. The diagnosis of vestibular disorders is based on a description of the symptoms, a history of trauma or exposure to agents destructive to vestibular structures, and tests of eye movements (*i.e.,* nystagmus) and muscle control of balance and equilibrium. Among the methods used in treatment of the vertigo that accompanies vestibular disorders are habituation exercises and antivertigo drugs. These drugs act by diminishing the excitability of neurons in the vestibular nucleus.

REVIEW EXERCISES

1. A mother notices that her 13-month-old child is fussy and tugging at his ear, and he refuses to eat his breakfast. When she takes his temperature, it is 37.8°C. Although the child attends daycare, the mother has kept him home and made an appointment with the child's pediatrician. In the physician's office, his temperature is 37.9°C, he is somewhat irritable, and he has a clear nasal drainage. His left tympanic membrane shows normal landmarks and motility on pneumatic otoscopy. His right tympanic membrane is erythematous and there is decreased motility on pneumatic otoscopy.
   A. *What risk factors are present that predispose this child to the development of acute otitis media?*

B. *Are his signs and symptoms typical of otitis media in a child this age?*

C. *What are the most likely pathogens? What treatment would be indicated?*

D. *Later in the week, the mother notices that the child does not seem to hear as well as he did before developing the infection. Is this a common occurrence and should the mother be concerned about transient hearing loss in a child of this age?*

2. A granddaughter is worried that her grandfather is "losing his hearing." Lately, he has been staying away from social gatherings that he always enjoyed, saying everybody mumbles. He is defiant in maintaining that there is nothing wrong with his hearing. However, he does complain that his ears have been ringing a lot lately.

A. *What are common manifestations of hearing loss in older adults?*

B. *What type of evaluation would be appropriate for determining if this man has a hearing loss and the extent of his hearing loss?*

C. *What are some things that the granddaughter might do so that her grandfather could hear her better when she is talking to him?*

3. A 70-year-old man complains that he gets this terrible feeling "like the room is moving around" and becomes nauseated when he rolls over in bed or bends over suddenly. It usually goes away once he has been up for a while. He has been told that his symptoms are consistent with benign paroxysmal positional vertigo.

A. *What is the pathophysiology associated with this man's vertigo?*

B. *Why do the symptoms subside once he has been up for a while?*

C. *What methods are available for treatment of the disorder?*

References

1. Moore K. L., Dalley A. F., Agur A. M. (2014). *Clinical oriented anatomy* (7th ed.). Philadelphia, PA: Lippincott Williams & Wilkins.
2. Rhoades R. A., Bell D. R. (2013). *Medical physiology: Principles for clinical medicine* (4th ed.). Philadelphia, PA: Lippincott Williams & Wilkins.
3. McCarter D. F., Courtney A. U., Pollart S. M. (2007). Cerumen impaction. *American Family Physician, 75*(10), 1523–1530.
4. Bagai A., Thavendiranathan P., Detsky A. S. (2006). Does this patient have hearing impairment? *Journal of the American Medical Association, 295*(4), 416–428.
5. Rosenfeild R. M., Schwartz S. R., Cannon C. R., et al. (2014). Clinical practice guideline: Acute otitis externa. *Otolaryngology Head and Neck Surgery, 150*(Suppl 1), S1–S24.
6. Lee H., Kim J., Nguyen V. (2013). Ear infections: Otitis externa and otitis media. *Primary Care, 40*(3), 671–686.
7. Seibert J. W., Danner C. J. (2006). Eustachian tube function and the middle ear. *Otolaryngologic Clinics of North America, 39*(6), 1221–1235.
8. Forgie S., Zhanel G., Robinson J.. (2009). Management of acute otitis media. *Paediatrics & Child Health, 14*(7), 457–460.
9. Lieberthal A. S., Carroll A. E., Chonmaitree T., et al. (2013). The diagnosis and management of acute otitis media. *Pediatrics, 131*(3), e964–e999.
10. Bhetwal N., McConaghy J. R. (2007). The evaluation and treatment of children with acute otitis media. *Primary Care Clinics in Office Practice, 34*(1), 59–70.
11. Haddad J., Kerschner J. E. (2011). Part 30: The ear. In Kliegman R. M., Stanton B. F., St. Geme J. W., et al. (Eds.), *Nelson textbook of pediatrics* (19th ed.). Philadelphia, PA: Saunders Elsevier.
12. Public Health Agency of Canada. (2015). Canadian Immunization Guide: Part 4, active vaccines. Available online at: http://www.phac-aspc.gc.ca/publicat/cig-gci/p04-eng.php. Accessed May 4, 2015.
13. Anti-infective Review Panel. (2013). *Anti-infective guidelines for community-acquired infections.* Toronto: MUMS Guideline Clearinghouse.
14. Pelton S. I. (2005). Otitis media: Re-evaluation of diagnosis and treatment in the era of antimicrobial resistance, pneumococcal conjugate vaccine, and evolving morbidity. *Pediatric Clinics of North America, 52*(3), 711–728.
15. Saylam G., Tatar E. C., Tatar I., et al. (2010). Association of adenoid surface biofilm formation and chronic otitis media with effusion. *Archives of Otolaryngology Head and Neck Surgery, 136*(6), 550–555.
16. Hunter L. L., Sanford C. A. (2014). Chapter 9: Tympanometry and wideband acoustic immittance. In Katz J., Chasin M., English K., et al. (Eds.), *Handbook of clinical audiology* (7th ed.). Philadelphia, PA: Lippincott Williams & Wilkins.
17. Morris P. S., Leach A. J. (2009). Acute and chronic otitis media. *Pediatric Clinics of North America, 56*(6), 1383–1399.
18. Paradise J. L., Feldman H. M., Campbell T. F., et al. (2007). Tympanostomy tubes and developmental outcomes at 9 to 11 years of age. *The NewEngland Journal of Medicine, 356*(3), 248–261.
19. Narayan S. R. (2014). Cholesteatoma: The silent killer. *Asian Journal of Pharmaceutical and Clinical Research, 7*(Suppl 1), 157–161.
20. Thomas J. P., Minovi A., Dazert S. (2011). Current aspects of etiology, diagnosis and therapy of otosclerosis. *Otolaryngologia Polska, 65*(3), 162–170.
21. Hall J. E. (2011). *Textbook of medical physiology* (12th ed.). Philadelphia, PA: W. B. Saunders.
22. Kandel E. R., Schwartz J. H., Jessell T. M., et al. (2013). *Principles of neural science* (5th ed.). New York: McGraw-Hill.
23. Terao K., Cureoglu S., Schachern P. A., et al. (2011). Cochlear changes in presbycusis with tinnitus. *American Journal of Otolaryngology, 32*(3), 215–220.
24. Langguth B., Kreuzer P. M., Kleinjung T., et al. (2013). Tinnitus: Causes and clinical management. *Lancet Neurology, 12*(9), 920–930.
25. Canadian Academy of Audiology. (2015). Tinnitus. Available online at: https://canadianaudiology.ca/consumer/tinnitus.html. Accessed May 11, 2015.
26. American Tinnitus Association. (2015). Understanding the facts. Available online at: https://www.ata.org/understanding-facts. Accessed May 11, 2015.
27. Canadian Association of the Deaf. (2007). Statistics on deaf Canadians. Available online at: http://www.cad.ca/statistics_on_deaf_canadians.php. Accessed May 11, 2015.
28. Canadian Hard of Hearing Association. (2008). Frequently asked questions about hearing loss. Available online at: http://www.chha.ca/chha/publications-booklets.php. Accessed May 11, 2015.
29. Walling A. D., Dickson G. M. (2012). Hearing loss in older adults. *American Family Physician, 85*(12), 1150–1156.
30. American Speech-Language-Hearing Association. (2011). Type, degree, and configuration of hearing loss. Available online at: http://www.asha.org/public/hearing/disorders/types.htm. Accessed May 11, 2015.
31. Uy J., Forciea M. A. (2013). Hearing loss. *Annals of Internal Medicine, 158*(7), ITC4-1; quiz ITC4-16.

32. Mahboubi H., Dwabe S., Fradkin M., et al. (2012). Genetic of hearing loss: Where are we standing now? *European Archives of Otorhinolaryngology, 269*(7), 1733–1745.

33. Cannizzaro E., Cannizzaro C., Plescia F., et al. (2014). Exposure to ototoxic agents and hearing loss: A review of current knowledge. *Hearing, Balance and Communication, 12*(4), 166–175.

34. Palmer C. V., Ortmann A. (2005). Hearing loss and hearing aids. *Neurologic Clinics, 23*(3), 901–918.

35. Colletti L., Mandala M., Colletti V. (2012). Cochlear implant in children younger than 6 months. *Otolaryngology Head and Neck Surgery, 147*(1), 139–146.

36. Papsin B. C., Gordon K. A. (2007). Cochlear implants for children with severe-to-profound hearing loss. *The New England Journal of Medicine, 357*(23), 2380–2387.

37. Vaudry W., Lee B. E., Rosychuk R. J. (2014). Congenital cytomegalovirus infection in Canada: Active surveillance for cases diagnosed by paediatricians. *Paediatrics & Child Health, 19*(1), e1–e5.

38. Patel H., Feldman M. (2011, Reaffirmed 2014). Universal newborn hearing screening. *Paediatrics & Child Health, 16*(5), 301–305.

39. Bance M. (2007). Hearing and aging. *Canadian Medical Association Journal, 176*(7), 925–927.

40. Gates G. A. (2012). Presbycusis: A brain disorder? The ears listen, the brain hears. *Seminars in Hearing, 33*(3), 225–230.

41. Ross M. H., Pawlina W. (2011). *Histology: A text and atlas* (6th ed.). Philadelphia, PA: Lippincott Williams & Wilkins.

42. Holstein G. R. (2012). Chapter 35: The vestibular system. In Mai J. K., Paxinos, G. *The human nervous system* (3rd ed.). San Diego: Elsevier Inc.

43. Hogue J. D. (2015). Office evaluation of dizziness. *Primary Care Clinics in Office Practice, 42*(2), 249–258.

44. Chawla N., Olshaker J. S. (2006). Diagnosis and management of dizziness and vertigo. *Medical Clinics of North America, 90*(2), 291–304.

45. Gold D. R., Morris L., Kheradmand A., Schubert M. C. (2014). Repositioning maneuvers for benign paroxysmal positional vertigo. *Current Treatment Options in Neurology, 16*(8), 307.

46. Berlinger N. T. (2011). Meniere's disease. *Minnesota Medicine, 94*(11), 33–36.

47. Semaan M. T., Megerian C. A. (2011). Meniere's disease: A challenging and relentless disorder. *Otolaryngologic Clinics of North America, 44*(2), 383–403.

48. McCall A. A., Swan E. E., Borenstein J. T., et al. (2010). Drug delivery for treatment of inner ear disease: Current state of knowledge. *Ear and Hearing, 31*(2), 156–165.

49. Baloh R. W. (2003). Vestibular neuritis. *The New England Journal of Medicine, 348*(11), 1027–1032.

50. Valente L. M. (2011). Assessment technique for vestibular evaluation in pediatric patients. *Otolaryngologic Clinics of North America, 44*(2), 273–290.

51. Labuguen R. H. (2006). Initial evaluation of vertigo. *American Family Physician, 73*(2), 244–254.

52. Lang E. E., Walsh R. M. (2010). Vestibular function testing. *Irish Journal of Medical Science, 179*(2), 173–178.

53. Hain T. C., Yacovino D. (2005). Pharmacologic treatment of persons with vertigo. *Neurologic Clinics, 23*(3), 831–853.

54. Bisht M., Bist S. S. (2010). An update on pharmacotherapy of vertigo. *Journal of Chemical and Pharmaceutical Research, 2*(3), 381–386.

55. Herdman S. J. (2013). Vestibular rehabilitation. *Current Opinion in Neurology, 26*(1), 96–101.

Visit thePoint **http://thePoint.lww.com for animations, journal articles, and more!**

Unit XIV

Disorders of Musculoskeletal Function

Some of the most significant investigations of the skeleton and muscles took place during the Renaissance—a time that celebrated the human body and lifted the knowledge of the body and its workings out of medieval murkiness.

The first comprehensive description of musculature was presented by Andreas Vesalius (1514–1564), a professor of anatomy and surgery at Padua. The product of his scrupulous dissections was the masterwork *De Humani Corporis Fabrica* (On the Structure of the Human Body), the second volume of which dealt with muscles and their structure. The work was beautifully illustrated with elegantly poised cadavers set against backgrounds of medieval Italy. Vesalius' effort successfully challenged many of the long-held pronouncements of Galen. The studies of artist Leonardo da Vinci (1452–1519) sought not to dispute or confirm previous teachings but to learn of the "divine form" so that it could be better rendered. A physician of the time wrote that "in order that he might be able to paint the various joints and muscles as they bend and extend according to the laws of nature, he [Leonardo] dissected in medical schools the corpses of criminals, indifferent to this inhuman and nauseating work." Although da Vinci was primarily a painter studying anatomy for the sake of art, there is little doubt that had his anatomic drawings been published during his lifetime or shortly after, science would have been advanced by years.

Unit XIV

Disorders of Musculoskeletal Function

Structure and Function of the Musculoskeletal System

The bones of the skeletal system serve as a framework for the attachment of muscles, tendons, and ligaments. The skeletal system protects and maintains soft tissues in their proper position, provides stability for the body, and maintains the body's shape. The bones act as a storage reservoir for calcium, and the central cavity of some bones contains the hematopoietic connective tissue in which blood cells are formed. Coordinated movement of the skeleton is made possible by the tendons and ligaments that join bones at joints.

For our purposes, the skeletal system is considered to include the bones and cartilage of the skeletal system, as well as the connective tissue structures (*i.e.,* ligaments and tendons) that connect the bones and join muscles to bone.

BONY STRUCTURES OF THE SKELETAL SYSTEM

After completing this section of the chapter, you should be able to meet the following objectives:

- Describe locations and characteristics of compact and cancellous bone.
- Describe the structure of a long bone.
- Cite the characteristics and name at least one location of elastic cartilage, hyaline cartilage, and fibrocartilage.
- Name and characterize the function of the four types of bone cells.
- State the function of parathyroid hormone, calcitonin, and vitamin D in terms of bone formation and metabolism.

The skeletal system consists of the axial and appendicular skeleton. The *axial skeleton,* which is composed of the bones of the skull, thorax, and vertebral column, forms the axis of the body. The *appendicular skeleton* consists of the bones of the upper and lower extremities, including the shoulder and hip. The skeletal system contains both bone and cartilage tissue. Bones provide protection for internal organs and rigid support for the extremities, whereas cartilage provides for flexibility and cushioning of bony structures and for skeletal development in both prenatal and postnatal life.

THE SKELETAL SYSTEM

- Two types of connective tissue are found in the skeletal system: (1) cartilage, a semirigid and slightly flexible structure that plays an essential role in prenatal and childhood development of the skeleton and as a surface for the articulating ends of skeletal joints; and (2) bone, which provides for the firm structure of the skeleton and serves as a reservoir for calcium and phosphate storage.
- Both bone and cartilage tissue are composed of living cells and a nonliving intercellular matrix that is secreted by the living cells.
- Bone matrix is maintained by four types of cells: osteoblasts, which synthesize and secrete the constituents of bone; osteoclasts, which resorb surplus bone and are required for bone remodelling; osteocytes, which make up the osteoid tissue of bone; and osteoprogenitor cells, which are the source of all bone cells, except osteoclasts.

Bone Structures

There are two types of mature bones, compact and cancellous bone (Fig. 56.1). Cancellous (spongy) bone is found in the interior of bones and is composed of *trabeculae,* or *spicules,* of bone that form a lattice-like pattern. These lattice-like structures are lined with osteogenic cells and filled with red or yellow bone marrow. Cancellous bone is relatively light, but its structure is such that it has considerable tensile strength and weight-bearing properties. Compact (cortical) bone, which forms the outer shell of a bone, has a densely packed, calcified intercellular matrix that makes it more rigid than cancellous bone. Although bones contain both cancellous and compact elements, their proportions vary in different bones throughout the body and in different parts of the same bone, depending on the relative needs for strength and lightness. Compact bone is the major component of tubular bones. It is also found along the lines of stress on long bones and forms an outer protective shell on other bones.

Types of Bones

Bones are classified by shape as long, short, flat, and irregular. Long bones are found in the upper and lower extremities. Short bones are irregularly shaped bones located in the ankle and the wrist. Except for their surface, which is compact bone, these bones are spongy throughout. Flat bones are composed of a layer of cancellous bone between two layers of compact bone. They are found in areas such as the skull and rib cage, where extensive protection of underlying structures is needed, or, as in the scapula, where a broad surface for muscle attachment must be provided. Irregular bones, because of their shapes, cannot be classified in any of the previous groups. This group includes bones such as the vertebrae and the bones of the jaw.

A typical long bone has a shaft, or *diaphysis,* and two ends, called *epiphyses* (Fig. 56.2). Long bones usually are narrow in the mid-portion and broad at the ends so that the weight they bear can be distributed over a wider surface. The shaft of a long bone is formed mainly of compact bone roughly hollowed out to form a marrow-filled medullary canal. The ends of long bones are covered with articular cartilage.

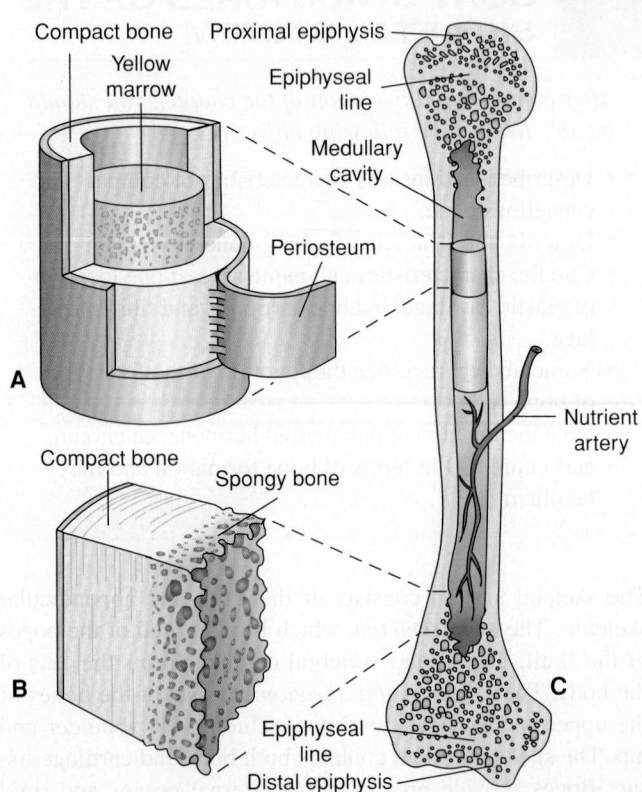

FIGURE 56.1 • A long bone shown in longitudinal section. **A:** Periosteum and bone marrow, **B:** compact and cancellous bone, **C:** epiphysis and source of blood supply from epiphysial and nutrient arteries.

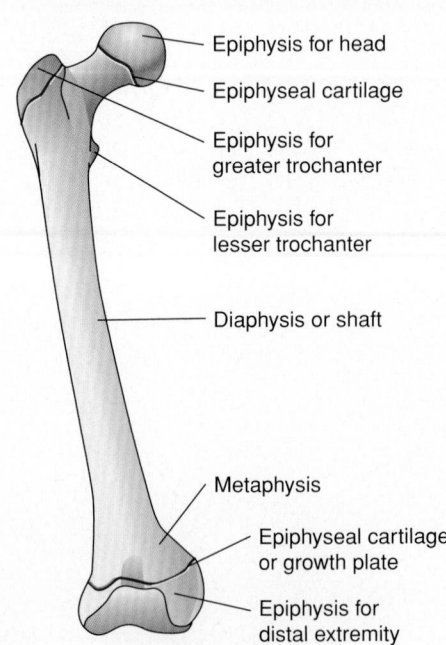

FIGURE 56.2 • A femur, showing epiphyseal cartilages for the head, metaphysis, trochanters, and distal end of the bone.

In growing bones, the part of the bone shaft that funnels out as it approaches the epiphysis is called the *metaphysis*. It is composed of bony trabeculae that have cores of cartilage. In the child, the epiphysis is separated from the metaphysis by the cartilaginous growth plate. After puberty, the metaphysis and epiphysis merge, and the growth plate is obliterated.

Periosteum and Endosteum

Bones are covered, except at their articular ends, by a membrane called the *periosteum* (Fig. 56.1). The periosteum has an outer fibrous layer and an inner layer that contains the osteoprogenitor cells needed for bone growth and development. The periosteum contains blood vessels and acts as an anchorage point for vessels as they enter and leave the bone. The endosteum is the membrane that lines the spaces of spongy bone, the marrow cavities, and the haversian canals of compact bone. It is composed mainly of osteoprogenitor cells, which contribute to the growth and remodelling of bone and are necessary for bone repair.

Bone Marrow

Bone marrow occupies the medullary cavities of the long bones throughout the skeleton and the cavities of cancellous bone in the vertebrae, ribs, sternum, and flat bones of the pelvis. The cellular composition of the bone marrow varies with age and skeletal location. Red bone marrow contains developing red blood cells and is the site of blood cell formation. Yellow bone marrow is composed largely of adipose cells. At birth, nearly all of the marrow is red and hematopoietically active. As the need for red blood cell production decreases during postnatal life, red marrow is gradually replaced with yellow bone marrow in most of the bones. In the adult, red marrow persists in the vertebrae, ribs, sternum, and ilia.

Blood Supply

The compact bone of long tubular bones is provided with blood supply from two sources, nutrient arteries and perforating arteries. The nutrient arteries enter the bone through a nutrient foramen and supply the marrow space and the internal one half of the cortex. The perforating arteries are small arteries that extend inward from the periosteal arteries on the external surface of the periosteum and anastomose in the cortex with branches of the nutrient arteries coming from the bone marrow. The distribution of blood in the cortex occurs through the haversian and Volkmann canals (Fig. 56.3). Haversian canals are spaces in the bone of the cortex that run

Osteocyte
Canaliculi
Lacuna
Haversian canal

Inner circumferential lamellae
Spongy bone

Compact bone

Outer circumferential lamellae

Haversian system

Periosteum

Blood vessel into marrow

Volkmann canal
Haversian canal
Vessel of haversian canal

FIGURE 56.3 • Haversian systems as seen in a wedge of compact bone tissue. The periosteum has been peeled back to show a blood vessel entering a Volkmann canal. (**Top**) Osteocytes lying within lacunae; canaliculi permit interstitial fluid to reach each lacuna.

parallel through the long axis of the bone for a short distance and then branch and communicate with other, similar canals. Each canal carries one or two blood vessels, lymphatics, and some nerve fibres. Volkmann canals, which also contain blood vessels, are spaces in the cortex that run perpendicular to the long axis of the cortex to connect adjacent haversian canals.

Cancellous bone is usually not penetrated by blood vessels. Instead, the bone cells of cancellous bone are nourished by diffusion from the endosteal surface through canaliculi, which interconnect their surrounding fluid-filled lacunae and extend to the bone surface.

Bone Tissue

Bone is connective tissue in which the intercellular matrix has been impregnated with inorganic calcium salts so that it has great tensile and compressive strength but is light enough to be moved by coordinated muscle contractions. The intercellular matrix is composed of two types of substances—organic matter and inorganic salts. The organic matter, including bone cells, blood vessels, and nerves, constitutes approximately one third of the dry weight of bone; the inorganic salts make up the other two thirds.

The organic matter consists primarily of collagen fibres embedded in an amorphous ground substance of other proteins, lipids, and glycosaminoglycans. The inorganic matter consists of hydroxyapatite, an insoluble macrocrystalline structure of calcium phosphate salts, and small amounts of calcium carbonate and calcium fluoride. Bone may also take up lead and other heavy metals, thereby removing these toxic substances from the circulation. This can be viewed as a protective mechanism. The antibiotic tetracycline is readily bound to calcium deposited in newly formed bones and teeth. When tetracycline is given during pregnancy, it can be deposited in the teeth of the fetus, causing discolouration and deformity. Similar changes can occur if the drug is given for long periods to children younger than 6 years of age.

Lamellar and Woven Bone

There are two types of bone tissue: lamellar bone and woven bone. Both forms of bone can be mineralized or unmineralized,

the latter being referred to as *osteoid. Lamellar bone* is a strong, mature form of bone that is formed slowly and is highly organized. It is the mature bone found in the adult skeleton; anything other than lamellar bone in an adult skeleton is abnormal. Lamellar bone is composed largely of cylindrical units called *osteons* or *haversian systems.* The osteons consist of concentric lamellae of bone matrix, surrounding a central canal, called the *haversian canal,* that contains the blood vessels and nerve supply for the osteon (Fig. 56.3). In compact bone, the central haversian canal runs essentially parallel to the long axis of the bone. Between the osteons are remnants of previous concentric lamellae, called the *interstitial lamella.* Circumferential lamellae follow the entire inner and outer shaft of a long bone, appearing much like the growth rings of a tree. Cancellous bone is also composed of lamellae, but, as mentioned previously, its trabeculae usually are not penetrated by blood vessels.

Woven bone is deposited more rapidly than lamellar bone. It is of low tensile strength, serving as temporary scaffolding for support. It is found in the developing fetus, in areas surrounding tumours and infections, and as part of a healing fracture.

Bone Cells

Four types of bone cells participate in the formation and maintenance of bone tissue: osteoprogenitor cells, osteoblasts, osteocytes, and osteoclasts (Table 56.1).

Osteoprogenitor Cells. The undifferentiated osteoprogenitor cells are found in the periosteum, endosteum, and epiphyseal plate of growing bone. These cells differentiate into osteoblasts and are active during normal growth; they may also be activated in adult life during healing of fractures and other injuries. Osteoprogenitor cells also participate in the continual replacement of worn-out bone tissue.

Osteoblasts. The osteoblasts, or bone-building cells, are responsible for the formation of the bone matrix. Bone formation occurs in two stages: ossification and calcification. Ossification involves the formation of osteoid, or prebone. Calcification of bone involves the deposition of calcium salts

TABLE 56.1 FUNCTION OF BONE CELLS

TYPE OF BONE CELL	FUNCTION
Osteoprogenitor cells	Undifferentiated cells that differentiate into osteoblasts. They are found in the periosteum, endosteum, and epiphyseal growth plate of growing bones.
Osteoblasts	Bone-building cells that synthesize and secrete the organic matrix of bone. Osteoblasts also participate in the calcification of the organic matrix.
Osteocytes	Mature bone cells that function in the maintenance of bone matrix. Osteocytes also play an active role in releasing calcium into the blood.
Osteoclasts	Bone cells responsible for the resorption of bone matrix and the release of calcium and phosphate from bone.

in the osteoid tissue. The osteoblasts synthesize collagen and other proteins that make up osteoid tissue. They also participate in the calcification process of the osteoid tissue, probably by controlling the availability of calcium and phosphate. Osteoblasts secrete the enzyme *alkaline phosphatase,* which is thought to act locally in bone tissue to raise calcium and phosphate levels to the point at which precipitation occurs. The activity of the osteoblasts undoubtedly contributes to the increase in serum levels of alkaline phosphatase that follows bone injury and fractures. In addition, the osteoblasts can secrete many growth factors and tumour necrosis factor, which are needed for bone growth regulation.

Osteocytes. The osteocytes are mature bone cells that are actively involved in maintaining the bony matrix. Death of the osteocytes results in the resorption of this matrix. The osteocytes lie in a small lake filled with extracellular fluid, called a *lacuna,* and are surrounded by a calcified intercellular matrix (Fig. 56.3). Extracellular fluid-filled passageways permeate the calcified matrix and connect with the lacunae of adjacent osteocytes. These passageways are called *canaliculi.* Because diffusion does not occur through the calcified matrix of bone, the canaliculi serve as communicating channels for the exchange of nutrients and metabolites between the osteocytes and the blood vessels on the surface of the bone layer.

Osteoclasts. Osteoclasts are "bone-chewing" cells that function in the resorption of bone, removing the mineral content and the organic matrix. They are large phagocytic cells of monocyte/macrophage lineage. Although the mechanism of osteoclast formation and activation remains elusive, it is known that parathyroid hormone (PTH) increases the number and resorptive function of the osteoclasts. Calcitonin is thought to reduce the number and resorptive function of the osteoclasts. Estrogen also reduces the number and function of the osteoclasts; thus, the decrease in estrogen levels that occurs at menopause results in increased resorption of bone. The mechanism whereby osteoclasts exert their resorptive effect on bone is unclear. These cells may secrete an acid that removes calcium from the bone matrix, releasing the collagenic fibres for digestion by osteoclasts or mononuclear cells. Osteoclasts, by virtue of their phagocytic lineage, also imbibe minute particles of bone matrix and crystals, eventually dissolving and releasing them into the blood.

Cartilage

Cartilage is an essential part of the skeletal system. It constitutes the articular cartilage of joints; it is found in the tendinous and ligamentous insertions, menisci, the symphysis pubis, and insertions of joint capsules. It is also essential for growth before and after birth. In the embryo, most of the axial and appendicular skeleton is formed first as a cartilage model and then replaced by bone. In postnatal life, cartilage continues to play an essential role in the growth of long bones and persists as articular cartilage in the adult.

As a tissue, cartilage both resembles and differs from bone. Both of these connective tissue types consist of living cells, nonliving intercellular fibres, and an amorphous (shapeless) ground substance. The tissue cells are responsible for secreting and maintaining the intercellular substances in which they are housed. However, cartilage consists of more extracellular substance than bone, and its fibres are embedded in a firm gel rather than a calcified cement-like substance. Hence, cartilage has the flexibility of a firm plastic material rather than the rigid characteristics of bone.

There are three types of cartilage: elastic cartilage, hyaline cartilage, and fibrocartilage. *Elastic cartilage* contains some elastin in its intercellular substance. It is found in areas, such as the ear, where some flexibility is important. Pure cartilage is called *hyaline cartilage* (from a Greek word meaning "glass") and is pearly white. It is the type of cartilage seen on the articulating ends of fresh soup bones found in the supermarket. *Fibrocartilage* has characteristics that are intermediate between dense connective tissue and hyaline cartilage. It is found in the intervertebral disks, in areas where tendons are connected to bone, and in the symphysis pubis.

Hyaline cartilage is the most abundant type of cartilage. It forms much of the cartilage of the fetal skeleton. In the adult, hyaline cartilage forms the costal cartilages that join the ribs to the sternum and vertebrae, many of the cartilages of the respiratory tract, the articular cartilages, and the epiphyseal plates.

Cartilage cells, which are called *chondrocytes,* are located in lacunae. The lacunae are surrounded by an uncalcified, gel-like intercellular matrix of collagen fibres and ground substance. Cartilage is devoid of blood vessels and nerves. The free surfaces of most hyaline cartilage, with the exception of articular cartilage, are covered by a layer of fibrous connective tissue called the *perichondrium.*

It has been estimated that approximately 80% of the wet weight of cartilage is water held in its gel structure. Because cartilage has no blood vessels, this tissue fluid allows the diffusion of gases, nutrients, and wastes between the chondrocytes and blood vessels outside the cartilage. Diffusion cannot take place if the cartilage matrix becomes impregnated with calcium salts, and cartilage dies if it becomes calcified.

Hormonal Control of Bone Formation and Metabolism

The process of bone formation and mineral metabolism is complex. It involves the interplay among the actions of PTH, calcitonin, and vitamin D. Other hormones, such as cortisol, growth hormone, thyroid hormone, and the sex hormones, also influence bone formation directly or indirectly (Table 56.2).

Parathyroid Hormone

PTH is one of the important regulators of calcium and phosphate levels in the blood. PTH prevents serum calcium levels from falling below and serum phosphate levels from rising above normal physiologic concentrations (see Chapter 41). The secretion of PTH is regulated by negative feedback;

TABLE 56.2 ACTIONS OF PARATHYROID HORMONE, CALCITONIN, AND VITAMIN D

ACTIONS	PARATHYROID HORMONE	CALCITONIN	VITAMIN D
Intestinal absorption of calcium	Increases indirectly through increased activation of vitamin D	Probably not affected	Increases
Intestinal absorption of phosphate	Increases	Probably not affected	Increases
Renal excretion of calcium	Decreases	Increases	Probably increases, but less effect than PTH
Renal excretion of phosphate	Increases	Increases	Increases
Bone resorption	Increases	Decreases	$1,25\text{-}(OH)_2D_3$ increases
Bone formation	Decreases	Uncertain	$24,25\text{-}(OH)_2D_3$ increases (?)
Serum calcium levels	Produces a prompt increase	Decreases with pharmacologic doses	No effect
Serum phosphate levels	Prevents an increase	Decreases with pharmacologic doses	No effect

increased serum levels of ionized calcium inhibit PTH release. PTH maintains serum calcium levels by initiation of calcium release from bone, by conservation of calcium by the kidney, by enhanced intestinal absorption of calcium through activation of vitamin D, and by reduction of serum phosphate levels (Fig. 56.4). PTH also increases the movement of calcium and phosphate from bone into the extracellular fluid. Calcium is immediately released from the canaliculi and bone cells; a more prolonged release of calcium and phosphate is mediated by increased osteoclast activity. In the kidney, PTH stimulates tubular reabsorption of calcium while reducing the reabsorption of phosphate. The latter effect ensures that

increased release of phosphate from bone during mobilization of calcium does not produce an elevation in serum phosphate levels. This is important because an increase in calcium and phosphate levels could lead to crystallization in soft tissues. PTH increases intestinal absorption of calcium because of its ability to stimulate activation of vitamin D by the kidney.

Calcitonin

Whereas PTH increases blood calcium levels, the hormone calcitonin lowers blood calcium levels. Calcitonin, sometimes called *thyrocalcitonin,* is secreted by the parafollicular, or C, cells of the thyroid gland. Calcitonin inhibits the release of calcium from bone into the extracellular fluid. It is thought to act by causing calcium to become sequestered in bone cells and by inhibiting osteoclast activity. Calcitonin also reduces the renal tubular reabsorption of calcium and phosphate; the decrease in serum calcium level that follows administration of pharmacologic doses of calcitonin may be related to this action.

The major stimulus for calcitonin synthesis and release is an increase in serum calcium. The role of calcitonin in overall mineral homeostasis is uncertain. There are no clearly definable syndromes of calcitonin deficiency or excess, which suggests that calcitonin does not directly alter calcium metabolism. It has been suggested that the physiologic actions of calcitonin are related to the postprandial handling and processing of dietary calcium. This theory proposes that after meals, calcitonin maintains PTH secretion at a time when it normally would be reduced by calcium entering the blood from the digestive tract. Although excess or deficiency states associated with alterations in physiologic levels of calcitonin have not been observed, it has been shown that pharmacologic doses of the hormone reduce osteoclastic activity. Because of this action, calcitonin has proved effective in the treatment of Paget disease (see Chapter 59). The hormone is also used to reduce serum calcium levels during hypercalcemic crises.

Parathyroid glands

Kidney
Reabsorption of calcium

Bone
Release of calcium and phosphate

Calcium concentration in extracellular fluid

Urinary excretion of phosphate

Activation of vitamin D

Intestine
Reabsorption of calcium via activated vitamin D

FIGURE 56.4 • Regulation and actions of parathyroid hormone.

Vitamin D

Vitamin D and its metabolites are not true vitamins but steroid hormones. There are two forms of vitamin D: vitamin D_2 (ergocalciferol) and vitamin D_3 (cholecalciferol). The two forms differ by the presence or absence of a double bond, but they have identical biologic activity. The term *vitamin D* is used to indicate both forms. Vitamin D is a valuable hormone involved in immune system modulation, bone mineralization, and even suppression of malignant cells.

Vitamin D has little or no physiologic activity until it has been converted to its active form by metabolic pathways that mediate its activity. Figure 56.5 depicts sources of vitamin D and pathways for activation. The first step of the activation process occurs in the liver, where vitamin D is hydroxylated to form the metabolite 25-hydroxyvitamin D_3 [25-(OH)D_3]. From the liver, 25-(OH)D_3 is transported to the kidneys, where it undergoes conversion to 1,25-dihydroxyvitamin D_3 [1,25-(OH)$_2D_3$] or 24,25-dihydroxyvitamin D_3 [24,25-(OH)$_2D_3$]. Other metabolites of vitamin D have been and still are being discovered.

There are two sources of vitamin D: intestinal absorption and skin production. Intestinal absorption occurs mainly in the jejunum and includes vitamin D_2 and vitamin D_3. The most important dietary sources of vitamin D are fish, liver, and irradiated milk. Because vitamin D is fat soluble, its absorption is mediated by bile salts and occurs by means of the lymphatic vessels. In the skin, ultraviolet radiation from sunlight spontaneously converts 7-dehydrocholesterol D_3 to vitamin D_3. A circulating vitamin D-binding protein provides a mechanism to remove vitamin D from the skin and make it available to the rest of the body.

With adequate exposure to sunlight, the amount of vitamin D that can be produced by the skin is usually sufficient to meet physiologic requirements. The importance of sunlight exposure is evidenced by population studies that report lower vitamin D levels in northern countries, such as Canada and England, which have less sunlight than the southern United States, especially in the fall and winter months. Older adults who are housebound or institutionalized frequently have low vitamin D levels. The deficiency often goes undetected until there are problems such as pseudofractures or electrolyte imbalances. Seasonal variations in vitamin D levels probably reflect changes in sunlight exposure.

The most potent of the vitamin D metabolites is 1,25-(OH)$_2D_3$. This metabolite increases intestinal absorption of calcium and promotes the actions of PTH on resorption of calcium and phosphate from bone. Bone resorption by the osteoclasts is increased, and bone formation by the osteoblasts is decreased; there is also an increase in acid phosphatase and a decrease in alkaline phosphatase. Intestinal absorption and bone resorption increase the amount of calcium and phosphorus available to the mineralizing surface of the bone. The role of 24,25-(OH)$_2D_3$ is less clear. There is evidence that 24,25-(OH)$_2D_3$, in conjunction with 1,25-(OH)$_2D_3$, may be involved in normal bone mineralization.

The regulation of vitamin D activity is influenced by several hormones. PTH and prolactin stimulate 1,25-(OH)$_2D_3$ production by the kidney. States of hyperparathyroidism are associated with increased levels of 1,25-(OH)$_2D_3$, and hypoparathyroidism leads to lowered levels of this metabolite. Prolactin may have an ancillary role in regulating vitamin D metabolism during pregnancy and lactation. Calcitonin inhibits 1,25-(OH)$_2D_3$ production by the kidney. In addition to hormonal influences, changes in the concentration of ions such as calcium, phosphate, hydrogen, and potassium exert an effect on 1,25-(OH)$_2D_3$ and 24,25-(OH)$_2D_3$ production. Under conditions of phosphate and calcium deprivation, 1,25-(OH)$_2D_3$ levels are increased, whereas hyperphosphatemia and hypercalcemia decrease the levels of metabolite.

FIGURE 56.5 • Sources and pathways for activation of vitamin D.

IN SUMMARY

Skeletal tissue consists of the bones and cartilage that form the appendicular and axial skeleton. There are two types of bone: compact bone, which forms the outer shell of a bone, and cancellous or spongy bone that forms the interior. The endosteum is the membrane that lines the spaces of spongy bone, the marrow cavities, and the haversian canals of compact bone. The periosteum, the membrane that covers bones, contains blood vessels and acts as an anchorage point for vessels as they enter and leave the bone. Mature bone is largely made up of cylindrical units called osteons, formed from concentric layers or lamellae of bone matrix and surrounding a central haversian canal. The haversian canals contain the blood vessels and nerve supply for the osteon. There are four types of bone cells: osteocytes, or mature bone cells; osteoblasts, or bone-building cells; osteoclasts, which function in bone resorption; and osteoprogenitor cells, which differentiate into osteoblasts.

Cartilage is a firm, flexible type of skeletal tissue that is essential for growth before and after birth. There are three types of cartilage: elastic, hyaline, and fibrocartilage. Hyaline cartilage, which is the most abundant type, forms the costal cartilages that join the ribs to the sternum and vertebrae, many of the cartilages of the respiratory tract, and the articular cartilages. The process of bone formation and mineral metabolism involves the interplay among the actions of PTH, calcitonin, and vitamin D. PTH acts to maintain serum levels of ionized calcium; it increases the release of calcium and phosphate from bone, the conservation of calcium and elimination of phosphate by the kidney, and the intestinal reabsorption of calcium through vitamin D. Calcitonin inhibits the release of calcium from bone and increases renal elimination of calcium and phosphate, thereby serving to lower serum calcium levels. Vitamin D functions as a hormone in regulating body calcium. It increases absorption of calcium from the intestine and promotes the actions of PTH on bone.

dense connective tissue found in tendons and ligaments has a limited blood supply and is composed largely of intercellular bundles of collagen fibres arranged in the same direction and plane. Collagen is an inelastic and insoluble fibrous protein. Because of its molecular configuration, collagen has great tensile strength; the breaking point of collagenous fibres found in human tendons is reached with a force of several hundred kilograms per square centimetre. Fresh collagen is colourless, and tissues that contain large numbers of collagenous fibres generally appear white.

SKELETAL JOINTS

- Articulations, or joints, are sites where two or more bones meet to hold the skeleton together and give it mobility.
- There are two types of joints: synarthroses, which are immovable joints, and synovial joints, which are freely movable joints.
- All limb joints are synovial (diarthroidal) joints, which are enclosed in a joint cavity containing synovial fluid.
- The articulating surfaces of synovial joints are covered with a layer of avascular cartilage that relies on oxygen and nutrients contained in the synovial fluid.
- Regeneration of articular cartilage of synovial joints is slow, and healing of injuries often is slow and unsatisfactory.

ARTICULATIONS AND JOINTS

After completing this section of the chapter, you should be able to meet the following objectives:

- State the characteristics of tendons and ligaments.
- State the difference between synarthroses and synovial joints.
- Describe the source of blood supply to a synovial joint.
- Explain why pain is often experienced in all the joints of an extremity when only a single joint is affected by a disease process.
- Describe the structure and function of a bursa.
- Explain the pathology associated with a torn meniscus of the knee.

Articulations, or joints, are areas where two or more bones meet. The term *arthro* is the prefix used to designate a joint; for example, *arthrology* is the study of joints, and *arthroplasty* is the repair of a joint.

Tendons and Ligaments

In the skeletal system, tendons and ligaments are dense connective tissue structures that connect muscles and bones. The

Tendons, which attach skeletal muscles to bone, are relatively inextensible because of their richness in collagen fibres. The collagen bundles of tendons aggregate into bundles that are enveloped by loose connective tissue, blood vessels, and nerves. Tendons that may rub against bone or other friction-generating surfaces are enclosed in double-layered sheaths. An outer connective tissue tube is attached to the structures surrounding the tendon, and an inner sheath encloses the tendon and is attached to it. The space between the inner and outer sheath is filled with a fluid similar to synovial fluid. Overuse can result in *tendonitis* or inflammation of the tendon.

Ligaments are fibrous thickenings of the articular capsule that join one bone to its articulating mate. They vary in size and shape depending on their specific role. Although most ligaments are considered inelastic, they are pliable enough to permit movement at the joints. However, ligaments tear rather than stretch when exposed to excess stress. Torn ligaments are extremely painful and accompanied by local swelling.

Types of Joints

Joints exhibit a variety of movements. Some joints have no movement; others allow only slight movement; and some are freely moveable, such as the shoulder joint. There are two classes of joints based on their movement and the presence or absence of a joint cavity: synarthroses and synovial joints.

Synarthroses

Synarthroses are joints that lack a joint cavity and move little or not at all. There are three types of synarthroses: synostoses, synchondroses, and syndesmoses. *Synostoses* are nonmovable joints in which the surfaces of the bones are joined by dense connective tissue or bone. The bones of the skull are joined by synostoses; they are joined by dense connective tissue in children and young adults and by bone in older persons. *Synchondroses* are joints in which bones are connected by hyaline cartilage and have limited motion. The ribs are attached to the sternum by this type of joint. *Syndesmoses* permit a certain amount of movement; they are separated by a fibrous disk and joined by interosseous ligaments. The symphysis pubis of the pelvis and the vertebral bodies joined by intervertebral disks are examples of syndesmoses.

Synovial (Diathrodial) Joints

Synovial or diarthrodial joints are freely movable joints. Most joints in the body are of this type. Although they are classified as freely movable, their movement ranges from almost none (*e.g.*, sacroiliac joint), to simple hinge movement (*e.g.*, interphalangeal joint), to movement in many planes (*e.g.*, shoulder or hip joint). The bony surfaces of these joints are covered with thin layers of articular cartilage, and the cartilaginous surfaces of these joints slide past each other during movement. As discussed in Chapter 59, diarthrodial joints are the joints most frequently affected by rheumatic disorders.

In a diarthrodial joint, the articulating ends of the bones are not connected directly but are indirectly linked by a strong fibrous capsule (*i.e.*, joint capsule) that surrounds the joint and is continuous with the periosteum (Fig. 56.6). This capsule supports the joint and helps to hold the bones in place. Additional support may be provided by ligaments that extend between the bones of the joint.

The joint capsule consists of two layers: an outer fibrous layer and an inner membrane, the synovium. The synovium

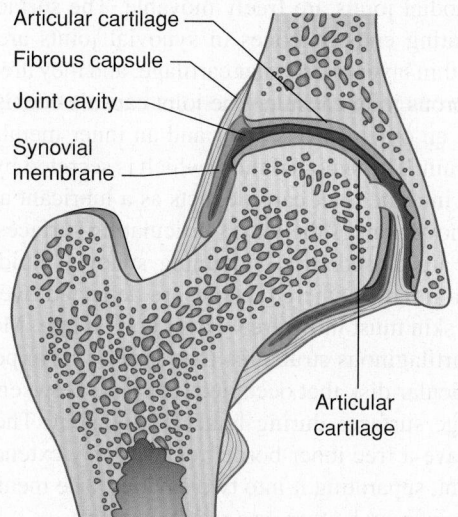

FIGURE 56.6 • Synovial (diathroidal) joint, showing the articular cartilage, fibrous joint capsule, joint cavity, and synovial membrane.

surrounds the tendons that pass through the joints and the free margins of other intra-articular structures such as ligaments and menisci. The synovium forms folds that surround the margins of articulations but do not cover the weight-bearing articular cartilage. These folds permit stretching of the synovium so that movement can occur without tissue damage.

The synovium secretes a slippery fluid with the consistency of egg white called *synovial fluid*. This fluid acts as a lubricant and facilitates the movement of the articulating surfaces of the joint. Normal synovial fluid is clear or pale yellow, and viscous. It is made up of the large charged molecule, hyaluronate, which has a high affinity for water, plus other glycoproteins, proteinases, and collagenases. It does not clot, and it contains fewer than 0.1×10^9/L white blood cells. The cells are predominantly mononuclear cells derived from the synovium. The composition of the synovial fluid is altered in many inflammatory and pathologic joint disorders. Aspiration and examination of the synovial fluid play an important role in the diagnosis of joint diseases.

The articular cartilage is an example of hyaline cartilage and is unique in that its free surface is not covered with perichondrium. It has only a peripheral rim of perichondrium, and calcification of the portion of cartilage abutting the bone may limit or preclude diffusion from blood vessels supplying the subchondral bone. Articular cartilage is apparently nourished by the diffusion of substances contained in the synovial fluid bathing the cartilage. Regeneration of most cartilage is slow; it is accomplished primarily by growth that requires the activity of perichondrium cells. In articular cartilage, which has no perichondrium, superficial injuries heal slowly.

Blood Supply and Innervation

All the tissues of synovial joints, except the articulating surfaces of the articulating cartilage, receive nourishment either directly or indirectly from blood vessels. The articulating areas are nourished indirectly by the synovial fluid that is distributed over the surface of the articular cartilage.

The blood supply to a joint arises from blood vessels that enter the subchondral bone at or near the attachment of the joint capsule and form an arterial circle around the joint. The synovial membrane has a rich blood supply, and constituents of plasma diffuse rapidly between these vessels and the joint cavity. Because many of the capillaries are near the surface of the synovium, blood may escape into the synovial fluid after relatively minor injuries. Healing and repair of the synovial membrane usually are rapid and complete. This is important because synovial tissue is injured in many surgical procedures that involve the joint.

The nerve supply to joints is provided by the same nerve trunks that supply the muscles that move the joints. These nerve trunks also supply the skin over the joints. As a rule, each joint of an extremity is innervated by all the peripheral nerves that cross the articulation; this accounts for the referral of pain from one joint to another. For example, hip pain may be perceived as pain in the knee.

The synovial membrane is innervated only by autonomic fibres that control blood flow. It is relatively free of pain fibres,

Suprapatellar bursa

Femur

Synovial
membrane

Prepatellar
bursa

Patella

Patellar ligament

Tibia

Anterior cruciate
ligament

FIGURE 56.7 • Sagittal section of knee joint, showing prepatellar and suprapatellar bursae.

as evidenced by the fact that surgical procedures on the joint are often done under local anesthesia. The joint capsule and the ligaments have pain receptors; these receptors are more easily stimulated by stretching and twisting than are other joint structures. Pain arising from the capsule tends to be diffuse and poorly localized.

The tendons and ligaments of the joint capsule are sensitive to position and movement, particularly stretching and twisting. These structures are supplied by the large sensory nerve fibres that form proprioceptor endings (see Chapter 48). The proprioceptors function reflexively to adjust the tension of the muscles that support the joint and are particularly important in maintaining muscular support for the joint. For example, when a weight is lifted, there is a proprioceptor-mediated reflex contraction and relaxation of appropriate muscle groups to support the joint and protect the joint capsule and other joint structures. Loss of proprioception and reflex control of muscular support leads to destructive changes in the joint.

Bursae

In some diarthrotic joints, the synovial membrane forms closed sacs that are not part of the joint. These sacs, called *bursae,* contain synovial fluid. Their purpose is to prevent friction on a tendon. Bursae occur in areas where pressure is exerted because of close approximation of joint structures (Fig. 56.7). Such conditions occur when tendons are deflected over bone or where skin must move freely over bony tissue. Bursae may become injured or inflamed, causing discomfort, swelling, and limitation in movement of the involved area. A bunion is an inflamed bursa of the metatarsophalangeal joint of the great toe.

Intra-articular Menisci

Intra-articular menisci are fibrocartilage structures that develop from portions of the articular disk that occupied the space between articular cartilage surfaces during fetal development. Menisci may extend partway through the joint and have a free

inner border, as at the lateral and medial articular surfaces of the knee, or they may extend through the joint, separating it into two separate cavities, as in the sternoclavicular joint. The menisci of the knee joint may be torn as the result of an injury (see Chapter 57).

IN SUMMARY

Articulations or joints are areas where two or more bones meet. Tendons and ligaments are dense connective tissue structures that connect muscles and bones. Tendons connect muscles to bones and ligaments connect the movable bones of joints.

Synarthroses are joints in which bones are joined together by fibrous tissue, cartilage, or bone; they lack a joint cavity and have little or no movement. Synovial or diarthrodial joints are freely movable. The surfaces of the articulating ends of bones in synovial joints are covered with a thin layer of articular cartilage, and they are enclosed in a fibrous joint capsule. The joint capsule consists of two layers: an outer fibrous layer and an inner membrane, the synovium. The synovial fluid, which is secreted by the synovium into the joint capsule, acts as a lubricant and facilitates movement of the joint's articulating surfaces. Bursae, which are closed sacs containing synovial fluid, prevent friction in areas where tendons are deflected over bone or where skin must move freely over bony tissue. Menisci are fibrocartilaginous structures that develop from portions of the articular disk that occupied the space between articular cartilage surfaces during fetal development. The menisci may have a free inner border, or they may extend through the joint, separating it into two cavities. The menisci in the knee joint may be torn as a result of injury.

CONCEPTS in action **ANIMATI**◌◌**N**

REVIEW EXERCISES

1. Often pain from injury to the knee is experienced as pain in the hip.
   A. *Explain why this might occur.*
2. Persons with end-stage kidney disease have a deficiency of activated vitamin D.
   A. *Explain why this occurs and what effect it would have on the person's bones.*
3. Recent studies have revealed that estrogen deficiency as well as normal aging may produce a decrease in osteoblast activity.
   A. *Explain how this would contribute to the development of osteoporosis.*

Bibliography

Christakos S., Hewison M., Gardner D. G., et al. (2013). Vitamin D: beyond the bone. *Annals of the New York Academy of Sciences, 1287*(1), 45–58.

Garcia R. A., Klein M. J., Schiller A. L. (2012). Chapter 26: Bones and joints. In Rubin R., Strayer D. S. (Eds.), *Rubin's pathology: Clinicopathologic foundations of medicine* (6th ed.). Philadelphia, PA: Lippincott Williams & Wilkins.

Hall J. E. (2011). *Textbook of medical physiology* (12th ed.). Philadelphia, PA: W. B. Saunders.

Hossein-Nezhad A., Holick M. F. (2013). Vitamin D for health: A global perspective. *Mayo Clinic Proceedings, 88*(7), 720–755.

Moore K. L., Dalley A. F., Agur A. M. (2014). *Clinical oriented anatomy* (7th ed.). Philadelphia, PA: Lippincott Williams & Wilkins.

Rhoades R. A., Bell D. R. (2013). *Medical physiology: Principles for clinical medicine* (4th ed.). Philadelphia, PA: Lippincott Williams & Wilkins.

Rosenberg A. E. (2010). Chapter 26: Bones, joints, and soft tissue tumors. In Kumar V., Abbas A. K., Fausto N., et al. (Eds.), *Robbins and Cotran Pathologic Basis of Disease* (8th ed.). Philadelphia, PA: Elsevier Saunders.

Ross M. H., Pawlina W. (2011). *Histology: A text and atlas* (6th ed.). Philadelphia, PA: Lippincott Williams & Wilkins.

Schwalfenberg G. (2007). Not enough vitamin D: Health consequences for Canadians. *Canadian Family Physician, 53*(5), 841–854.

Visit thePoint **http://thePoint.lww.com for animations, journal articles, and more!**

57

Disorders of Musculoskeletal Function: Trauma, Infection, and Neoplasms

The musculoskeletal system includes the bones, joints, and muscles of the body together with associated structures such as ligaments and tendons. This system, which constitutes more than 70% of the body's mass, is subject to a large number of disorders. These disorders affect persons in all age groups and walks of life, causing pain and disability. The discussion in this chapter focuses on the effects of trauma, infections, ischemia, and neoplasms on musculoskeletal structures of the body.

INJURY AND TRAUMA OF MUSCULOSKELETAL STRUCTURES

After completing this section of the chapter, you should be able to meet the following objectives:

- Describe the physical agents responsible for soft tissue trauma.
- Differentiate among the three types of soft tissue injuries.
- Compare muscle strains and ligamentous sprains.
- Describe the healing process of soft tissue injuries.
- Differentiate open from closed fractures.
- List the signs and symptoms of a fracture.
- Explain the measures used in treatment of fractures.
- Describe the fracture healing process.
- Differentiate the early complications of fractures from later complications of fracture healing.

A broad spectrum of musculoskeletal injuries result from numerous physical forces, including blunt tissue trauma, disruption of tendons and ligaments, and fractures of bony structures. Many of the forces that cause injury to the musculoskeletal system are typical for a particular environmental setting, activity, or age group. The majority of the injuries that occur are classified as unintentional rather than accidental, which indicates and reinforces the importance of prevention aspects.

In Canada, the leading cause of death for the 15- to 24-year age group is motor vehicle injuries, with most involving high speeds.[1] Motorcycle injuries are especially common in young men, resulting in fractures of the distal tibia, midshaft femur, and radius occurring most often. In Canada, as well as other parts of the world, unintentional falls such as falling on playgrounds and bicycle-related injuries are the leading cause of hospitalized injuries for children and youth.[2] In addition, many children older than 5 years of age are treated each year in hospital emergency departments for sports injuries. About two thirds of all team sport injuries occur in hockey, soccer, and basketball.[2] Most injuries are strains and sprains. Teenage athletes are injured at about the same rate as professionals. Unfortunately, this is due in part to the increasing level of competition.[3]

Falls are the most common cause of injury in people 65 years of age and older. Current statistics indicate that one out of three of persons in this age group experience at least one fall each year.[4] Impaired vision and hearing, dizziness, unsteadiness of gait, and medications contribute to falls in the older person. Among older adults, the majority of fractures are caused by falls.[4] Falls can be compounded by osteoporosis, or bone atrophy, which makes fractures more likely. Fractures of the vertebrae, distal radius, and hip are particularly common in this age group. These injuries reduce mobility and independence and increase the risk for premature death.[5]

Athletic Injuries

Athletic injuries are either acute injuries or overuse injuries. Acute injuries are caused by sudden trauma and include injuries to soft tissues (contusion, strains, and sprains) and to bone (fractures). Overuse injuries have been described as chronic injuries, including stress fractures that result from constant high levels of physiologic stress without sufficient recovery time.[6] They commonly occur in the elbow ("Little League elbow" or "tennis elbow") and in tissue where tendons attach to the bone, such as the heel, knee, and shoulder. Contact sports pose a greater threat for injury to the neck, spine, and growth plates in children and adolescents, who have not yet reached maturity. Injuries can be prevented by proper training, use of safety equipment, and limiting the level of competition according to skill and size rather than chronologic age. Adequate warm-up time, hydration, and proper nutrition are also key factors in injury prevention.[3]

Soft Tissue Injuries

Most skeletal injuries are accompanied by soft tissue (muscle, tendon, or ligament) injuries. These injuries include contusions, hematomas, and lacerations. They are discussed here because of their association with musculoskeletal injuries.

A *contusion* is an injury to soft tissue that results from direct trauma and is usually caused by striking a body part against a hard object. With a contusion, the skin overlying the injury remains intact. Initially, the area becomes ecchymotic (*i.e.,* black and blue) because of local hemorrhage; later, the discolouration gradually changes to brown and then to yellow as the blood is reabsorbed. A large area of local hemorrhage is called a *hematoma*. Hematomas cause pain as blood accumulates and exerts pressure on nerve endings. The pain

> ## JOINT INJURIES
>
> - Joints are the weakest part of the skeletal system and common sites for injury due to mechanical overloading or forcible twisting or stretching.
> - Injury can include damage to the tendons, which connect muscle to bone; ligaments, which hold bones together; or the cartilage that covers the articular surface.
> - Healing of the dense connective tissue involved in joint injuries requires time to restore the structures so that they are strong enough to withstand the forces imposed on the joint. Ligamentous injuries may require surgical intervention with approximation of many fibrous strands to facilitate healing.
> - Injuries involving the articular cartilage may predispose to later joint disease.

increases with movement or when pressure is applied to the area. The pain and swelling of a hematoma take longer to subside than that accompanying a contusion. Unlike a contusion, which does not drain, a hematoma may eventually split the skin because of increased pressures and produce drainage or occasionally may need to be aspirated.

Treatment of a contusion and a hematoma consists of elevating the affected part and applying cold for the first 24 hours to reduce the bleeding into the area. A hematoma may need to be aspirated. After the first 24 hours, heat or cold should be applied intermittently for 10–20 minutes at a time.

A *laceration* is an injury in which the skin is torn or its continuity is disrupted. The seriousness of a laceration depends on the size and depth of the wound and on whether there is contamination from the object that caused the injury. Puncture wounds from nails or rusted material provide the setting for growth of anaerobic bacteria such as those that cause tetanus and gas gangrene.

Lacerations are usually treated by wound closure, which is done after the area is sufficiently cleaned; the closed wound is covered with a sterile dressing. It is important to minimize contamination of the wound and to control bleeding. Contaminated wounds and open fractures are copiously irrigated and debrided, and the skin usually is left open to heal to prevent the development of an anaerobic infection or a sinus tract. Antimicrobial agents are selectively used based on the suspected nature of the contaminants.

Joint (Musculotendinous) Injuries

Joints, or articulations, are sites where two or more bones meet. Joints (*i.e.,* diarthrodial joints) are supported by tough bundles of collagenous fibres called *ligaments* that attach to the joint capsule and bind the articular ends of bones together, and by *tendons* that join muscles to the periosteum of the articulating bones (see Chapter 56). Joint injuries involve mechanical overloading or forcible twisting or stretching.

Strains and Sprains

Strains. A *strain* is a stretching injury to a muscle or a musculotendinous unit caused by mechanical overloading. This type of injury may result from an unusual muscle contraction or an excessive forcible stretch. Although there usually is no external evidence of a specific injury, pain, stiffness, and swelling exist. The most common sites for muscle strains are the lower back and the cervical region of the spine. The elbow and the shoulder are also supported by musculotendinous units that are subject to strains. Foot strain is associated with the weight-bearing stresses of the feet; it may be caused by inadequate muscular and ligamentous support, overweight, or excessive exercise such as standing, walking, or running.

In the lumbar and cervical spine regions, muscle strains are more common than sprains. Mechanical low back pain is becoming increasingly common in the adolescent athlete. Overuse, especially hyperextension of the lumbar spine in such sports as track, wrestling, gymnastics, and diving, can tear the muscles, fascia, and ligaments. Careful diagnosis is necessary because chronic low back pain may indicate a stress fracture. Fractures near the top and bottom surface of the vertebrae can occur when the growing lumbar spine is overstressed, causing the disks to push into the spinal nerve roots. Early detection and treatment are important to prevent complications and disability. Treatment of back strains consists of a short period of rest and anti-inflammatory analgesics followed by a gradual return to activities. Cold should be used during the first 24 hours to reduce pain and swelling of the affected area. Exercises, correct posture, and good body mechanics help to reduce the risk for reinjury.

Sprains. A *sprain,* which involves the ligamentous structures (strong bands of connective tissue) surrounding the joint, resembles a strain, but the pain and swelling subside more slowly. It usually is caused by abnormal or excessive movement of the joint. With a sprain, the ligaments may be incompletely torn or, as in a severe sprain, completely torn or ruptured (Fig. 57.1). Occasionally, a chip of bone is evident when the entire ligament, including part of its bony attachment, has been ruptured or torn from the bone. The signs of sprain are pain, rapid swelling, heat, disability, discolouration, and limitation of function.

Any joint may be sprained, but the ankle joint is most commonly involved, especially in fast-moving injuries in which an ankle or knee can be suddenly twisted. Most ankle sprains occur in the lateral ankle when the foot is turned inward under a person, forcing the ankle into inversion beyond the structural limits. Other common sites of sprain are the knee (the collateral ligament and anterior cruciate ligament) and elbow (the ulnar side). As with a strain, the soft tissue injury that occurs with a sprain is not evident on the radiograph. Wrist sprains most often occur with a fall on an outstretched hand.

Healing. If properly treated, musculotendinous injuries usually heal with restoration of the original tensile strength. Repair is accomplished by fibroblasts from the inner tendon

FIGURE 57.1 • Degrees of sprain on the medial side of the right knee: grade 1, mild sprain of the medial collateral ligament; grade 2, moderate sprain with hematoma formation; grade 3, severe sprain with total disruption of the ligament; and grade 4, severe sprain with avulsion of the medial femoral condyle at the insertion of the medial collateral ligament.

sheath or, if the tendon has no sheath, from the loose connective tissue that surrounds the tendon. Capillaries infiltrate the injured area during the initial healing process and supply the fibroblasts with the materials they need to produce large amounts of collagen. Formation of the long collagen bundles occurs within the first 2 weeks, and although tensile strength increases steadily thereafter, it is not sufficient to permit strong tendon pulls for 6 to 8 weeks.[7] During the healing process, there is a danger that muscle contraction will pull the injured ends apart, causing the tendon to heal in the lengthened position. There is also a danger that adhesions will develop in areas where tendons pass through fibrous channels, such as in the distal palm of the hands, rendering the tendon useless.

Treatment. The treatment of muscle strains and ligamentous sprains is similar in several ways. For an injured extremity, elevation of the part followed by local application of cold may be sufficient. Compression, accomplished through the use of adhesive wraps or a removable splint, helps reduce swelling and provides support. A cast is applied for severe sprains, especially those severe enough to warrant surgical repair. Immobilization for a muscle strain is continued until the pain and swelling have subsided. In a sprain, the affected joint is immobilized for several weeks. Immobilization may be followed by graded active exercises. Early diagnosis, treatment, and rehabilitation are essential in preventing chronic ligamentous instability.

Dislocations

A *dislocation* involves the displacement or separation of the bone ends of a joint with loss of articulation. It usually follows a severe trauma that disrupts the holding ligaments. Dislocations are seen most often in the shoulder and acromioclavicular joints. A *subluxation* is a partial dislocation in which the bone ends in the joint are still in partial contact with each other.

Dislocations can be congenital, traumatic, or pathologic. Congenital dislocations occur in the hip and knee. Traumatic dislocations occur after falls, blows, or rotational injuries. For example, car accidents often cause dislocations of the hip and accompanying acetabular fractures because of the direction of impact. This is true both of persons wearing seat belts and those who are unrestrained. In the shoulder and patella, dislocations may become recurrent, especially in athletes. They recur with the same motion but require less and less force each time.

Pathologic dislocation in the hip is a late complication of infection, rheumatoid arthritis, paralysis, and neuromuscular diseases. Dislocations of the phalangeal joints are not serious and are usually reduced by manipulation. Less common sites of dislocation, seen mainly in young adults, are the wrist and midtarsal region. They usually are the result of direct force, such as a fall on an outstretched hand.

Diagnosis of a dislocation is based on history, physical examination, and radiologic findings. The symptoms are pain, deformity, and limited movement. With recurrent dislocations, the person often experiences apprehension during tests of joint rotation, fearing that the joint will slip out of place.

The treatment depends on the site, mechanism of injury, and associated injuries such as fractures. Dislocations that do not reduce spontaneously usually require manipulation or surgical repair. Various surgical procedures also can be used to prevent redislocation of the patella, shoulder, or acromioclavicular joints. Immobilization is necessary for several weeks after reduction of a dislocation to allow healing of the joint structures. In dislocations affecting the knee, alternatives to surgery are isometric quadriceps-strengthening exercises and a temporary brace.

Loose Bodies

Loose bodies are small pieces of bone or cartilage within a joint space. These can result from trauma to the joint or may occur when cartilage has worn away from the articular surface, causing a necrotic piece of bone to separate and become free floating. The symptoms are painful catching and locking of the joint. Loose bodies are commonly seen in the knee, elbow, hip, and ankle. The loose body repeatedly gets caught in the crevice of a joint, pinching the underlying healthy cartilage; unless the loose body is removed, it may cause osteoarthritis and restricted movement. The treatment consists of removal using operative arthroscopy.

Shoulder and Rotator Cuff Injuries

The shoulder is a complex series of joints that produce extraordinary range of motion. The extreme mobility is accomplished at the expense of relative instability. This instability, combined with its relatively exposed position, makes the shoulder extremely vulnerable to injuries such as sprains and dislocations and degenerative processes such as rotator cuff disorders.

The shoulder is composed of three bones: the scapula, the clavicle, and the humerus. The scapula is a thin bone that articulates widely and closely with the chest wall.[8] It also articulates with the humerus by way of the glenoid cavity and with the clavicle at the acromion process. Clavicle fractures are among the most common fractures of childhood.[9] The typical mechanism of fracture is a fall on the point of the shoulder.

Three articulations form the shoulder joint—the acromioclavicular joint that joins the clavicle to the acromion of the scapula, the sternoclavicular joint that joins the sternum to the clavicle, and the glenohumeral joint that connects the head of the humerus to the relatively shallow glenoid cavity in the scapula. The stability of these joints is provided by a series of muscles and tendons. Sprains of the acromioclavicular joint usually occur as a result of a blow to the top of the shoulder but are known to occur with a fall to the lateral or posterior aspects of the shoulder.[9] The most common site of shoulder dislocation is the glenohumeral joint.[9,10] Most acute dislocations involve anterior displacement of the humeral head with respect to the glenoid cavity, the result of the shoulder being abducted and forcefully extended and rotated. Other mechanisms include a fall on an outstretched arm or a blow to the posterior shoulder.

Motion of the arm involves the coordinated movement of muscles of the rotator cuff (supraspinous, infraspinatus, teres minor, subscapularis) and their musculotendinous attachments. These muscles are separated from the overlying coracoacromial arch by two bursae, the subdeltoid and subcoracoid. These two bursae, sometimes referred to as the *subacromial bursae,* often communicate and are affected by lesions of the rotator cuff.

The rotator cuff is not unlike other muscle groups of the body in that its risk for injury increases when it is required to perform a high-stress function in an unconditioned state. Rotator cuff injuries and impingement disorders can result from a number of causes, including excessive use, a direct blow, or stretch injury, usually involving throwing or swinging, as with baseball pitchers or tennis players. Complete tears or rupture of the rotator cuff usually occur in young persons after severe trauma (Fig. 57.2).

Overuse and degenerative disorders have a slower onset and are seen in older persons with minor or no trauma. The tendons of the rotator cuff fuse together near their insertions into the tuberosities of the humerus to form the musculotendinous cuff. Degeneration of these tendons can result from a number of factors, including repetitive microtrauma, impairment of vascularity as a result of aging, or shoulder instability with secondary overload of the cuff. Degeneration is most severe near the tendon insertion, with the supraspinous being affected most often. Chronic irritation of the musculotendinous unit can lead to tendinitis with scarring and thickening

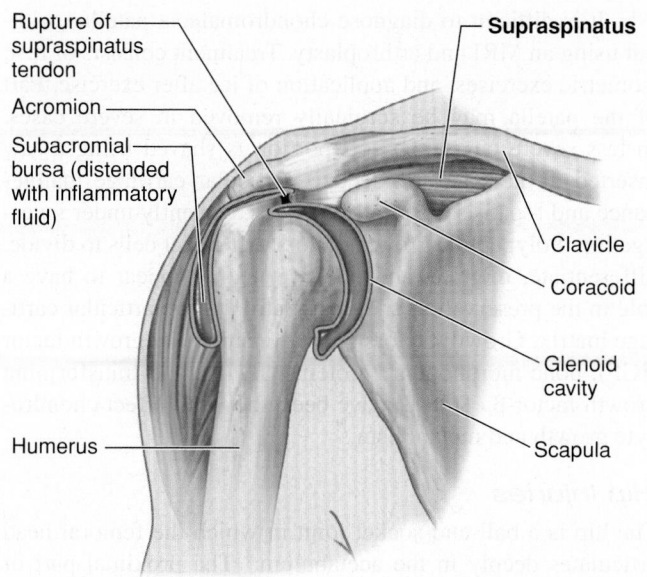

FIGURE 57.2 • Structures of the glenohumeral shoulder joint, showing the location of common rotator cuff injuries. The supraspinatus muscle is the most commonly injured part of the rotator cuff. (Adapted from Moore K. L., Dalley A. F., Agur, A. M. R. (2014). *Clinical oriented anatomy* (7th ed., p. 712). Philadelphia, PA: Lippincott Williams & Wilkins.)

of the tendon and secondary inflammation of the overlying bursae.[8] Thickening of these tissues decreases the distance between the cuff and the overlying coracoacromial arch. Pain and impingement may be noted when motions of the arm squeeze and pinch these tissues between the humerus and the overlying arch. Severe tendinitis also can cause either a partial or complete rotator cuff tear.

Several physical examination manoeuvres are used to define shoulder pathologic processes.[11] The history and mechanism of injury are important. In addition to standard radiographs, arthrography, computed tomography (CT), or magnetic resonance imaging (MRI) may be used. Arthroscopic examination under anesthesia may be used for diagnostic purposes, and operative arthroscopy may be done to repair severe tears. Conservative treatment with anti-inflammatory agents, corticosteroid injections, and physical therapy often is undertaken. A period of rest is followed by a customized exercise and rehabilitation program to improve strength, flexibility, and endurance.

Knee Injuries

The knee is a common site of injury, particularly sport-related injuries in which the knee is subjected to abnormal twisting and compression forces. These forces can result in injury to the menisci, patellar subluxation and dislocation, and chondromalacia. Knee injuries in young adulthood and both knee and hip injuries in middle age substantially increase the risk for osteoarthritis in the same joint later in life.

Meniscus Injuries. The menisci are C-shaped plates of fibrocartilage that are superimposed between the condyles

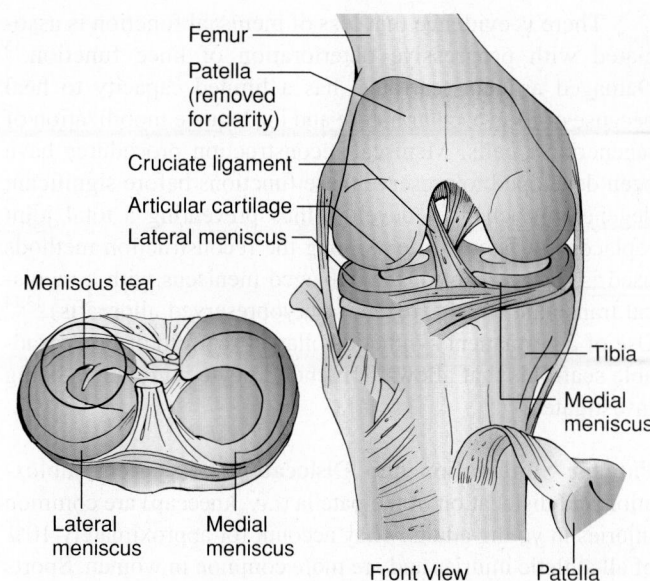

FIGURE 57.3 • The knee, showing the lateral and medial meniscus (with the patella removed for clarity). *Inset* (*lower left*) shows meniscus tear.

of the femur and tibia. There are two menisci in each knee, a lateral and medial meniscus (Fig. 57.3). The menisci are thicker at their external margins and taper to thin, unattached edges at their interior margin. They are firmly attached at their ends to the intercondylar area of the tibia and are supported by the coronary and transverse ligaments of the knee. The menisci play a major role in load bearing and shock absorption. They also help to stabilize the knee by deepening the tibial socket and maintaining the femur and tibia in proper position. In addition, the meniscus assists in joint lubrication and serves as source of nutrition for articular cartilage in the knee.

Meniscus injury commonly occurs as the result of a rotational injury from a sudden or sharp pivot or a direct blow to the knee, as in hockey, basketball, or football. It is often associated with other injuries, such as a torn anterior cruciate ligament (ACL).[12] The type and location of the meniscal tear are determined by the magnitude and direction of the force that acts on the knee and the position of the knee at the time of injury. Meniscus tears can be described by their appearance (*e.g.,* parrot-beak, bucket handle) or their location (*e.g.,* posterior horn, anterior horn). The injured knee is edematous and painful, especially with hyperflexion and hyperextension. A loose fragment may cause knee instability and locking.

Diagnosis is made by examination and confirmed by MRI. A regular radiograph may be needed to rule out osteoarthritis.[12] Initial treatment of meniscal injuries may be conservative. The knee may be placed in a removable knee immobilizer. Isometric quadriceps exercises may be prescribed. Activity usually is restricted until complete motion is recovered. Arthroscopic meniscectomy may be performed when there is recurrent or persistent locking, recurrent effusion, or disabling pain.

There is evidence that loss of meniscal function is associated with progressive deterioration of knee function.[13] Damaged articular cartilage has a limited capacity to heal because of its avascular nature and inadequate mobilization of regenerative cells. Meniscal reconstruction procedures have been developed to preserve these functions before significant degenerative changes develop, thus preventing a total joint replacement later in life. Among the reconstruction methods used is replacement of the damaged meniscus with a meniscal transplant (fresh, frozen, or cryopreserved allografts).[13,14] Use of a permanent synthetic collagen scaffold or biodegradable scaffolds that allows fibrochondrocyte ingrowth is being investigated.[13]

Patellar Subluxation and Dislocations. Recurrent subluxation and dislocation of the patella (*i.e.,* kneecap) are common injuries in young adults. They account for approximately 10% of all athletic injuries and are more common in women. Sports such as skiing or tennis may cause stress on the patella. These sports involve external rotation of the foot and lower leg with knee flexion, a position that exerts rotational stresses on the knee. Congenital knee variations are also a predisposing factor.

There is often a sensation of the patella "popping out" when the dislocation occurs.[8] Other complaints include the knee giving out, swelling, crepitus, stiffness, and loss of range of motion. Treatment can be difficult, but nonsurgical methods are used first. They include immobilization with the knee extended, bracing, administration of anti-inflammatory agents, and isometric quadriceps-strengthening exercises. Surgical intervention often is necessary.

Chondromalacia. Chondromalacia, or softening of the articular cartilage, is seen most commonly on the undersurface of the patella and occurs most frequently in young adults.[8] It can be the result of recurrent subluxation of the patella or overuse in strenuous athletic activities. Persons with this disorder typically complain of pain, particularly when climbing stairs or sitting with the knees bent. Occasionally, the person experiences weakness of the knee.

It is difficult to diagnose chondromalacia patellae without using an MRI and arthroplasty. Treatment consists of rest, isometric exercises, and application of ice after exercise. Part of the patella may be surgically removed in severe cases. In less severe cases, the soft portion is shaved using a saw inserted through an arthroscope. Articular cartilage maintenance and repair is a complex process, currently under investigation. Polypeptide growth factors that direct cells to divide, differentiate, migrate, and produce matrix appear to have a role in the preservation and degradation of the articular cartilage matrix. Growth factors such as insulin-like growth factor (IGF), bone morphogenic proteins (BMP), and transforming growth factor-β (TGF-β) have been shown to affect chondrocyte growth and metabolism.[15]

Hip Injuries

The hip is a ball-and-socket joint in which the femoral head articulates deeply in the acetabulum.[4] The proximal part of the femur consists of a head, neck, and greater trochanter. The vascular anatomy of the femoral head is of critical importance in any disorder of the hip. The main sources of blood supply are the intramedullary vessels and the retinacular arteries arising from the circumflex femoral arteries, both of which course from the intertrochanteric region proximally to nourish the femoral head (Fig. 57.4). Disease or injuries that compromise the circulation may damage the viability of the femoral head and lead to avascular necrosis or osteonecrosis (to be discussed). Disorders of the hip include dislocations and fractures of the hip. Congenital dysplasia of the hip, Legg–Calvé–Perthes disease, and slipped capital femoral epiphysis are discussed in Chapter 58.

Dislocations of the Hip. Dislocations of the hip are the result of severe trauma and are usually posterior in direction.[8] They commonly result from the knee being struck while the hip and knee are in a flexed position. This force drives the femoral head out of the acetabulum posteriorly. Anterior dislocations are less common and usually result from a force on the knee with the thigh abducted.

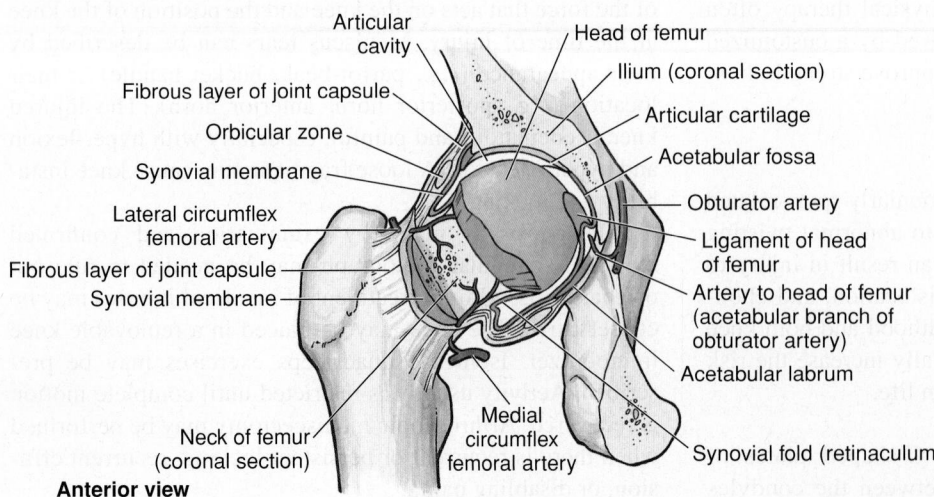

Articular cavity
Fibrous layer of joint capsule
Orbicular zone
Synovial membrane
Lateral circumflex femoral artery
Fibrous layer of joint capsule
Synovial membrane
Neck of femur (coronal section)
Medial circumflex femoral artery

Head of femur
Ilium (coronal section)
Articular cartilage
Acetabular fossa
Obturator artery
Ligament of head of femur
Artery to head of femur (acetabular branch of obturator artery)
Acetabular labrum
Synovial fold (retinaculum)

Anterior view

FIGURE 57.4 • Blood supply of the head and neck of the femur (anterior view). A section of the bone has been removed from the femoral neck. (From Moore K. L., Agur A. M. R., Dalley A. F. (2011). *Essential clinical anatomy* (4th ed., p. 380). Philadelphia, PA: Lippincott Williams & Wilkins.)

Hip dislocation is an emergency.[8] In the dislocated position, great tension is placed on the blood supply to the femoral head and avascular necrosis may result. To prevent this complication, early reduction is indicated. Weight bearing is usually limited after reduction to prevent dislocation from reoccurring and allow healing to occur.

Fractures of the Hip. Hip fracture is a major public health problem in the Western world, particularly among older adults. It results in hospitalization, disability, and loss of independence. The incidence of hip fractures increases with age, doubling for each decade after 50 years of age, and is two to three times higher in women than men.[16,17] The incidence is also higher in white women compared with nonwhite women. Risk factors for hip fracture include excessive consumption of alcohol and caffeine, physical inactivity, low body weight, tall stature, use of certain psychotropic drugs, residence in an institution, visual impairment, and dementia.[17] Osteoporosis is an important contributing factor.

Most hip fractures result from falls. Occasionally, the person may actually fracture the hip before falling, the fracture being caused by twisting or excessive force on a femur that has been weakened by osteoporosis or neoplasms. The characteristics of the fall (the direction, site of impact, and protective response) and environmental factors are important factors influencing the risk of hip fracture from a fall.

A hip fracture is generally a fracture of the proximal femur. Such fractures are commonly categorized according to the anatomic site in which they occur.[16,17] Femoral neck fractures are located in the area distal to the femoral head but proximal to the greater and lesser trochanters and are considered intracapsular because they are located within the capsule of the hip joint. Intertrochanteric fractures occur in the metaphyseal region between the greater and lesser trochanter. Subtrochanteric fractures are those that occur just below the greater trochanter. Femoral neck and intertrochanteric fractures account for over 90% of hip fractures, occurring in approximately equal proportions.[17]

The location of a hip fracture is important in terms of blood flow to the femoral head, which receives its blood supply from vessels that course proximally up the femoral neck (Fig. 57.4). Subtrochanteric and intertrochanteric fractures that occur distal to these vessels do not usually disturb the blood supply to the femoral head, whereas femoral neck fractures, particularly those involving marked displacement, often disrupt the blood supply to the femoral head and are therefore associated with increased incidence of complications (nonunion and avascular necrosis).

Most hip fractures are diagnosed based on clinical findings and standard radiographs. A bone scan or MRI may be done when the radiograph is negative but the clinical findings support the diagnosis of hip fracture.

The primary goal of treatment is a return to preinjury level of function as soon as possible.[8] Undisplaced or impacted fractures have a better prognosis in terms of healing and are often treated nonoperatively or by simple internal fixation to provide

stability. Displaced intracapsular fractures in older adults are usually best treated by surgical hip replacement and early mobilization. Young, healthy people are treated by reduction of the fracture (if needed) and internal fixation. This method allows for preservation of the femoral head, which in this age group is desirable because the long-term results are better than with prosthetic replacement.[17] Intertrochanteric fractures are usually treated with open reduction and internal fixation. This allows for early ambulation by eliminating pain at the fracture site.[17] Nonunion in this type of fracture is much less common than with intracapsular fractures. Weight bearing, however, is usually restricted for 3 months, until union of the fracture has occurred.

Fractures

Fracture, or discontinuity of the bone, is the most common type of bone lesion. Normal bone can withstand considerable compression and shearing forces and, to a lesser extent, tension forces. A fracture occurs when more stress is placed on the bone than it is able to absorb. Grouped according to cause, fractures can be divided into three major categories: fractures caused by sudden injury, fatigue or stress fractures, and pathologic fractures. The most common fractures are those resulting from sudden injury. The force causing the fracture may be direct, such as a fall or blow, or indirect, such as a massive muscle contraction or trauma transmitted along the bone. For example, the head of the radius or clavicle can be fractured by the indirect forces that result from falling on an outstretched hand. A fatigue fracture results from repeated wear on a bone. Pain associated with overuse injuries of the lower extremities, especially posterior medial tibial pain, is one of the most common symptoms that physically active persons, such as runners, experience. Stress fractures in the tibia may be confused with "shin splints," a nonspecific term for pain in the lower leg from overuse in walking and running, because they frequently do not appear on x-ray films until 2 weeks after the onset of symptoms.

A pathologic fracture occurs in bones that already are weakened by disease or tumours. Fractures of this type may occur spontaneously with little or no stress. The underlying disease state can be local, as with infections, cysts, or tumours, or generalized, as in osteoporosis, Paget disease, or cancer metastasis.

Classification

Fractures usually are classified according to location, type, and direction or pattern of the fracture line[8] (Fig. 57.5). A long bone is divided into three parts: proximal, midshaft, and distal. A fracture of the long bone is described in relation to its position in the bone. Other descriptions are used when the fracture affects the head or neck of a bone, involves a joint, or is near a prominence such as a condyle or malleolus.

The type of fracture is determined by its communication with the external environment, the degree of break in continuity of the bone, and the character of the fracture pieces. A fracture can be classified as open or closed. When the bone fragments have broken through the skin, the fracture is called an *open* or

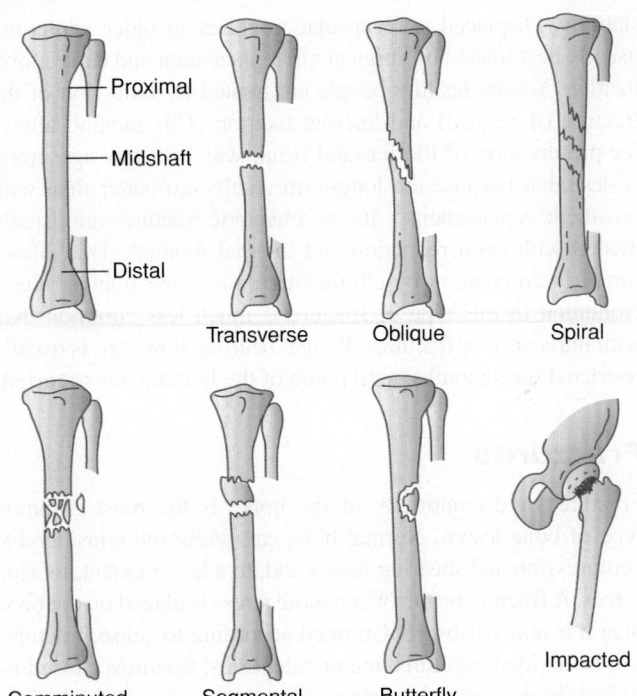

Proximal

Midshaft

Distal

Transverse   Oblique   Spiral

Comminuted   Segmental   Butterfly   Impacted

FIGURE 57.5 • Classification of fractures. Fractures are classified according to location (proximal, midshaft, or distal), the direction of fracture line (transverse, oblique, spiral), and type (comminuted, segmental, butterfly, or impacted).

compound fracture.[8] Open fractures often are complicated by infection, osteomyelitis, delayed union, or nonunion. In a closed fracture, there is no communication with the outside skin.

The degree of a fracture is described in terms of a partial or complete break in the continuity of bone. A *greenstick fracture,* which is seen in children, is an example of a partial break in bone continuity and resembles that seen when a young sapling is broken. This kind of break occurs because children's bones, especially until approximately 10 years of age, are more resilient than the bones of adults.

The character of a fracture is determined by its pieces. A *comminuted fracture* has more than two pieces. A *compression fracture,* as occurs in the vertebral body, involves two bones that are crushed or squeezed together. A fracture is called *impacted* when the fracture fragments are wedged together. This type usually occurs in the humerus, often is less serious, and usually is treated without surgery.

The direction of the trauma or mechanism of injury produces a certain configuration or pattern of fracture. The pattern of a fracture indicates the nature of the trauma and provides information about the easiest method for reduction. *Reduction* is the restoration of a fractured bone to its normal anatomic position. *Transverse fractures* are caused by simple angular forces. A *spiral fracture* results from a twisting motion, or torque. A transverse fracture is not likely to become displaced or lose its position after it is reduced. On the other hand, spiral, oblique, and comminuted fractures often are unstable and may change position after reduction.

Manifestations

The signs and symptoms of a fracture include pain, tenderness at the site of bone disruption, swelling, loss of function, deformity of the affected part, and abnormal mobility. The deformity varies according to the type of force applied, the area of the bone involved, the type of fracture produced, and the strength and balance of the surrounding muscles.

In long bones, three types of deformities—angulation, shortening, and rotation—are seen. Severely angulated fracture fragments may be felt at the fracture site and often push up against the soft tissue to cause a tenting effect on the skin. Bending forces and unequal muscle pulls cause angulation. Shortening of the extremity occurs as the bone fragments slide and override each other because of the pull of the muscles on the long axis of the extremity (Fig. 57.6).

Rotational deformity occurs when the fracture fragments rotate out of their normal longitudinal axis; this can result from rotational strain produced by the fracture or unequal pull by the muscles that are attached to the fracture fragments. A crepitus or grating may be felt as the bone fragments rub against each other. In the case of an open fracture, there is bleeding from the wound where the bone protrudes. Blood loss from a pelvic fracture or multiple long bone fractures can cause hypovolemic shock in a trauma victim.

Shortly after the fracture has occurred, nerve function at the fracture site may be temporarily lost. The area may become numb, and the surrounding muscles may become flaccid. This condition has been called *local shock.* During this period, which may last for a few minutes to half an hour, fractured bones may be reduced with little or no pain. After this brief period, the pain returns and, with it, muscle spasms and contractions occur in the surrounding muscles.

The early complications of fractures are associated with loss of skeletal continuity, injury from bone fragments, pressure from swelling and hemorrhage, involvement of nerve fibres, or development of fat emboli. The extent of early complications depends on the severity of the fracture and the area of the body that is involved. For example, bone fragments from a skull fracture may cause injury to brain tissue, and multiple rib fractures may lead to a flail chest and respiratory insufficiency. With flail chest, the chest wall on the fractured side becomes so unstable that it may move in the opposite direction as the person breathes (*i.e.,* in during inspiration and out during expiration).

Diagnosis

Diagnosis is the first step in the care of fractures and is based on history and physical manifestations. X-ray examination is

FIGURE 57.6 • Displacement and overriding of fracture fragments of a long bone (femur) caused by severe muscle spasm.

TABLE 57.1	OESTERN AND TSCHERNE CLASSIFICATION OF CLOSED FRACTURES	
GRADE	**SOFT TISSUE INJURY**	**BONY INJURY**
Grade 0	Minimal soft tissue damage Indirect injury to limb	Simple fracture pattern
Grade 1	Superficial abrasion/contusion	Mild fracture pattern
Grade 2	Deep abrasion with skin or muscle contusion Direct trauma to limb	Severe fracture pattern
Grade 3	Extensive skin contusion or crush Severe damage to underlying muscle Subcutaneous avulsion Compartmental syndrome may be present	Severe fracture pattern

Court-Brown C. M., Heckman J. D., McQueen M. M., et al. (2014). *Rockwood and Green's fractures in adults* (8th ed., p. 49). Philadelphia, PA: Lippincott Williams & Wilkins.

used to confirm the diagnosis and direct the treatment. The ease of diagnosis varies with the location and severity of the fracture. In the trauma patient, the presence of other, more serious injuries may make diagnosis more difficult. A thorough history includes the mechanism, time, and place of the injury; first recognition of symptoms; and any treatment initiated. A complete history is important because a delay in seeking treatment or a period of weight bearing on a fracture may cause further injury or displacement of the fracture. When a fracture is suspected, the injured part always should be splinted before it is moved.[8] This is essential for preventing further injury.

Determination of the severity of injury to soft tissue is an important component of assessment and management of closed fractures. The response of the soft tissue to blunt injury involves microvascular and inflammatory responses that produce localized tissue hypoxia and acidosis.[18] Incisions placed through such compromised tissue can lead to wound breakdown and infections. Therefore, recognizing the signs of soft tissue injury is the foundation for successful management of closed fractures. The classification of Oestern and Tscherne can be used to characterize the severity of closed fractures[18,19] (Table 57.1). This system remains the only published classification system for the soft tissue injury associated with closed fractures. Fractures are assigned one of four grades, from 0 to 3. The presence of deep skin abrasions, muscle contusion, fracture blisters, and massive soft tissue swelling suggest the need to use external fixation methods to limit further soft tissue injury and facilitate rapid recovery before surgical intervention.

Treatment

There are three objectives for treatment of fractures: reduction of the fracture, immobilization, and preservation and restoration of the function of the injured part.

Reduction and Internal Fixation. Reduction is directed at alignment of the bones in the angular and rotational planes, restoration of proper length, and restoration of apposition of the bone ends.[8] This can be accomplished by closed manipulation or surgical (open) reduction. Closed manipulation uses methods such as manual pressure and traction. Fractures are held in reduction by external or internal fixation devices. The benefits of internal fixation must be balanced against its associated risks. The advantages are precise restoration of the osseous anatomy and early mobilization with at least partial weight bearing. The principal disadvantages are the increased risk of infection and the fact that healing may be impaired if a technique is not used properly. Patients are usually more comfortable after internal fixation than with a cast or external fixation device.[20] Surgical reduction involves the use of various types of hardware to accomplish internal fixation of the fracture fragments (Fig. 57.7).

Immobilization and External Fixation. Immobilization prevents movement of the injured parts and is the single most important element in obtaining union of the fracture fragments. Immobilization can be accomplished through the use of external devices, such as splints, casts, traction, or external fixation devices; or by internal fixation devices inserted during surgical reduction of the fracture.

Splints are made from many different materials. Metal splints or air splints may be used during transport to a healthcare facility as a temporary measure until the fracture has been reduced and another form of immobilization instituted. Plaster of Paris splints, which are moulded to fit the extremity, work well. Splinting should be done if there is any suspicion of a fracture because motion of the fracture site can cause pain, bleeding, more soft tissue damage, and nerve or blood vessel compression. If the fracture has sharp fragments, movement can cause perforation of the skin and conversion of a closed fracture into an open one. When a splint is applied to an extremity, it should extend from the joint above the fracture site to the joint below it.

Casts, which are made of plaster or synthetic material such as fibreglass, are commonly used to immobilize fractures of the extremities. They often are applied with a joint in partial flexion to prevent rotation of the fracture fragments. Without this flexion, the extremity, which is essentially a cylinder, tends to rotate within the cylindrical structure of the cast. A brace may be used after a cast is removed or instead of a cast, as with a tibial stress

FIGURE 57.7 • **A:** A simple tibia and fibula spiral fracture by indirect trauma that required reduction and internal fixation. **B:** Surgical management with a screw and protection plate inserted to stabilize bone. **C:** Healing occurs without callus formation at the 1-year follow-up. (From Court-Brown C. M., Heckman J. D., McQueen M. M., et al. (2014). *Rockwood and Green's fractures in adults* (8th ed., p. 198). Philadelphia, PA: Lippincott Williams & Wilkins.)

fracture. The application of a cast carries the risk for impaired circulation to the extremity because of blood vessel compression. A cast applied shortly after a fracture may not be large enough to accommodate the swelling that inevitably occurs in the hours that follow. After a cast is applied, the peripheral circulation must be observed carefully until this danger has passed. If the circulation becomes inadequate, the parts that are exposed at the distal end of the cast (*i.e.,* the toes with a leg cast and the fingers with an arm cast) usually become cold and cyanotic or pale. An increase in pain may occur initially, followed by paresthesia (*i.e.,* tingling or abnormal sensation) or anesthesia as the sensory neurons that supply the area are affected. There is a decrease in the amplitude or absence of the pulse in areas where the arteries can be palpated. Capillary refill time, which is assessed by applying pressure to the fingernail and observing the rate of blood return, is prolonged to longer than 3 seconds. Signs of impaired circulation demand immediate measures, such as splitting the cast, to restore the circulation and prevent permanent damage to the extremity. A casted extremity should be elevated above the level of the heart for the first 24 hours to minimize swelling.

Traction is another method for achieving immobility, maintaining alignment of the bone ends, and maintaining the reduction, particularly if the fracture is unstable or comminuted. Traction is a pulling force applied to an extremity or part of the body while a counterforce, or countertraction, pulls in the opposite direction. The five goals of traction therapy are to correct and maintain the skeletal alignment of entire bones or joints; reduce pressure on a joint surface; correct, lessen, or prevent deformities such as contractures and dislocations;

decrease muscle spasm; and immobilize the fracture site to promote healing. Traction may be used as a temporary measure before surgery or as a primary treatment method. There are three types of traction: manual traction, skin traction, and skeletal traction. *Manual traction* consists of a steady, firm pull that is exerted by the hands. It is a temporary measure used to manipulate a fracture during closed reduction, for support of a neck injury during transport when a cervical spine fracture is suspected, or for reduction of a dislocated joint. *Skin traction* is a pulling force applied to the skin and soft tissue. It is accomplished by strips of adhesive flannel or foam secured to the injured part. *Skeletal traction* is a pulling force applied directly to the bone. Pins, wires, or tongs are inserted through the skin and subcutaneous tissue into the bone distal to the fracture site. Skeletal traction provides an excellent pull and can be used for long periods with large amounts of weight. It is commonly used for fractures of the femur, the humerus, and the cervical spine (*e.g.,* Crutchfield tongs applied to the skull).

With *external fixation devices,* pins or screws are inserted directly into the bone above and below the fracture site. They are secured to a metal frame and adjusted to align the fracture. This method of treatment is used primarily for open fractures, infections such as osteomyelitis and septic joints, unstable closed fractures, and limb lengthening.

Limb-Lengthening Systems. Limb-lengthening systems, such as the Ilizarov external fixator (Fig. 57.8), are used to lengthen or widen bones, correct angular or rotational defects, or immobilize fractures.[21] The apparatus is applied with a

FIGURE 57.8 • Ilizarov device used to treat a tibial fracture with anterolateral bow and medullary sclerosis: before (**A**), with Ilizarov device in place (**B**), and 3-year follow-up lateral roentgenograph (**C**). (From Paley D., Catagni M., Argnani F., et al. (1992). Treatment of congenital pseudoarthrosis of the tibia using Ilizarov technique. *Clinical Orthopaedics and Related Research, 280*, 84.)

surgical technique called a *corticotomy,* which is a percutaneous osteotomy that preserves the periosteal and endosteal tissues. A circular external apparatus is attached to bone by tensioned Kirschner wires. The corticotomy site is gradually distracted or pulled apart by approximately 1 mm/day until the desired length is achieved. The continuous distraction activates regeneration of bone, soft tissue, nerves, and blood vessels. New bone forms in the distraction gap. This newly formed bone can fill posttraumatic defects or those formed after resection for osteomyelitis, consolidate nonunions, regenerate bone in limb lengthening, correct deformities, and eliminate the need for bone grafting. The apparatus is left on until the desired length is achieved and consolidation is complete.

Preservation and Restoration of Function. During the period of immobilization required for fracture healing, muscles tend to atrophy because of lack of use. Joints stiffen as muscles and tendons contract and shorten. The degree of muscle atrophy and joint stiffness depends on several factors. In adults, the degree of atrophy and muscle stiffness is directly related to the length of immobilization, with longer periods of immobility resulting in greater stiffness. Children have a natural tendency to move on their own, and this movement maintains muscle and joint function. They usually have less atrophy and recover sooner after the source of immobilization has been removed. Associated soft tissue injury, infection, and pre-existing joint disease increase the risk for stiffness. Although limbs are immobilized in a functional position, casts

are removed as soon as fracture healing has taken place so that joint stiffness does not occur.

Exercises designed to preserve function, maintain muscle strength, and reduce joint stiffness in the unaffected and affected extremities should be started early. Active range of motion, in which the person moves the extremity, is done on unaffected extremities, and isometric, or muscle tensing, exercises are done on the affected extremities. In some instances, an electrical muscle stimulator is applied directly to the skin to stimulate isometric muscle contraction as a means of preventing disuse atrophy. After the fracture has healed, a program of physical therapy may be necessary. However, the most important factor in restoring function is the person's own active exercises.

Bone Healing

Bone healing occurs in a manner similar to soft tissue healing. It is, however, a more complex process and takes longer. Although the exact mechanisms of bone healing are open to controversy, four stages of the healing process have been identified: hematoma formation with cellular proliferation, callus formation, ossification, and remodelling.[22–24] The degree of response during each of these stages is in direct proportion to the extent of trauma.

Hematoma formation occurs during the first 1 to 2 days after fracture. It develops from torn blood vessels in the periosteum and adjacent muscles and soft tissue. Disruption of blood vessels also leads to death of bone cells at the fracture site. In 2 to 5 days, the hemorrhage forms a large blood clot. Neovascularization begins peripheral to the blood clot. By the end of the first week, most of the clot is organized by invasion of blood vessels and early fibrosis. Hematoma formation is thought to be necessary for the initiation of the cellular events essential to bone healing.[24] As the result of hematoma formation, clotting factors remain in the injured area to initiate the formation of a fibrin meshwork, which serves as a framework for the ingrowth of fibroblasts and new capillary buds. At the same time, degranulated platelets and migrating inflammatory cells release growth factors, which stimulate osteoclast and osteoblast proliferation.[22,24]

The next event in fracture healing is formation of granulation tissue or soft tissue (fibrocartilaginous) callus. During this stage of bone healing, fibroblasts and osteoblasts migrate into the fracture site from the nearby periosteal and endosteal membranes and begin reconstruction of bone. Some fibroblasts produce collagen that spans the break and connects the broken bone ends, whereas others differentiate into chondrocytes that secrete the collagen matrix. At about the same time, osteoblasts begin depositing bone into this matrix. After a few days, a fibrocartilage "collar" becomes evident around the fracture site. The collar edges on either side of the fracture eventually unite to form a bridge, which connects the bone fragments. The earliest bone, in the form of woven bone, begins its formation sometime after the first week. In an uncomplicated fracture, the repair tissue reaches its maximum girth at the end of the second to third week, which helps stabilize the fracture, but is not yet strong enough for weight bearing.

Ossification and formation of bony callus represent the deposition of mineral salts into the callus. This stage usually occurs during the third to fourth week of fracture healing and is prominent 2 to 3 months after the injury. Continued migration and multiplying of osteoblasts and osteocytes turns the fibrocartilaginous callus into bony callus. The fracture site feels firm and immovable and appears united on the radiograph. At this point, it is safe to remove the cast and allow increased weight bearing.

Remodelling is the final stage of bone healing. It involves resorption of the excess bony callus that develops in the marrow space and encircles the external aspect of the fracture site. Dead bone is removed by the osteoclasts. Compact bone replaces spongy bone around the fracture to reconstruct the shaft. The medullary cavity of the bone is also restored. The remodelling process is directed by mechanical stress and direction of weight bearing. It continues according to the Wolff law—bone responds to mechanical stress by becoming thicker and stronger in relation to its function.

Healing Time. Healing time depends on the site of the fracture, the condition of the fracture fragments, hematoma formation, and other local and host factors. In general, fractures of long bones, displaced fractures, and fractures with less surface area heal more slowly. Function usually returns within 6 months after union is complete. However, return to complete function may take longer. Stress fractures usually require less

time to heal, usually 2 to 4 weeks, during which time a reduction in activity and protection of the area are needed.

Factors that influence bone healing are specific to the person, the type of injury sustained, and local factors that disrupt healing. Individual factors that may delay bone healing are the patient's age; current medications; debilitating diseases, such as diabetes and rheumatoid arthritis; level of immunocompetency; local stress around the fracture site; circulatory problems and coagulation disorders; and poor nutrition.

Impaired Healing

Union of a fracture has occurred when the fracture is solid enough to withstand normal stresses and it is clinically and radiologically safe to remove the external fixation. In children, fractures usually heal within 4 to 6 weeks; in adolescents, they heal within 6 to 8 weeks; and in adults, they heal within 10 to 18 weeks.[25] The increased rate of healing among children compared with adults may be related to the increased cellularity and vascularity of the child's periosteum. A number of factors can contribute to impaired bone healing, including the nature and extent of the injury, the health of the person with the fracture and his or her responses to injury, the adequacy of initial treatment, and pharmacologic factors. For large bone defects caused by trauma or a tumour, bone regeneration may need enhancement. Various growth factors, such as BMP, are thought to induce bone formation and repair bone defects.[26]

Malunion is healing with deformity, angulation, or rotation that is visible on x-ray films. Early, aggressive treatment, especially of the hand, can prevent malunion and result in earlier alignment and return of function. Malunion is caused by inadequate reduction or alignment of the fracture. *Delayed union* is the failure of a fracture to unite within the normal period (e.g., 20 weeks for a fracture of the tibia or femur in an adult). Intraarticular fractures (i.e., those through a joint) may heal more slowly and may eventually produce arthritis. *Nonunion* is failure to produce union and cessation of the processes of bone repair. It is seen most often in the tibia, especially with open fractures or crushing injuries. It is characterized by mobility of the fracture site and pain on weight bearing. Muscle atrophy and loss of range of motion may occur. Nonunion usually is established 6 to 12 months after the time of the fracture. The complications of fracture healing are summarized in Table 57.2.

Treatment methods for impaired bone healing encompass surgical interventions, including bone grafts, bracing, external fixation, or electrical stimulation of the bone ends. The treatment for delayed union consists of determining and correcting the cause of the delay. Electrical stimulation is thought to stimulate the osteoblasts to lay down a network of bone. Three types of commercial bone growth stimulators are available: a noninvasive model, which is placed outside the cast; a seminoninvasive model, in which pins are inserted around the fracture site; and a totally implantable type, in which a cathode coil is wound around the bone at the fracture site and operated by a battery pack implanted under the skin. The Ilizarov method of circular external fixation is used to treat nonunions, especially those that are infected.

TABLE 57.2 COMPLICATIONS OF FRACTURE HEALING

COMPLICATION	MANIFESTATIONS	CONTRIBUTING FACTORS
Delayed union	Failure of fracture to heal within predicted time as determined by x-ray	Large displaced fracture Inadequate immobilization Large hematoma Infection at fracture site Excessive loss of bone Inadequate circulation
Malunion	Deformity at fracture site Deformity or angulation on x-ray	Inadequate reduction Malalignment of fracture at time of immobilization
Nonunion	Failure of bone to heal before the process of bone repair stops Evidence on x-ray Motion at fracture site Pain on weight bearing	Inadequate reduction Mobility at fracture site Severe trauma Bone fragment separation Soft tissue between bone fragments Infection Extensive loss of bone Inadequate circulation Malignancy Bone necrosis Noncompliance with restrictions

Complications of Fractures and Other Musculoskeletal Injuries

The complications of fractures and other orthopedic injuries are associated with loss of skeletal continuity, injury from bone fragments, pressure from swelling and hemorrhage (*e.g.,* fracture blisters, compartment syndrome), involvement of nerve fibres (*e.g.,* complex regional pain syndrome [CRPS]), or development of venous thromboembolism and fat embolism syndrome (FES).

Fracture Blisters

Fracture blisters are skin bullae and blisters representing areas of epidermal necrosis with separation of epidermis from the underlying dermis by edema fluid. They occur when the intra-compartmental pressure is too high to be relieved by normal means. They are seen with more severe, twisting types of injuries (*e.g.,* motor vehicle collisions and falls from heights), but can also occur after excessive joint manipulation, dependent positioning, and heat application, or from peripheral vascular disease. They can be solitary, multiple, or massive depending on the extent of injury. Most fracture blisters occur in the ankle, elbow, foot, knee, or areas where there is little soft tissue between the bone and the skin. The development of fracture blisters reportedly is reduced by early surgical intervention in persons requiring operative repair.[27] This probably reflects the early operative release of the fracture hematoma, reapproximation of the disrupted soft tissues, ligation of bleeding vessels, and fixation of bleeding fracture surfaces. Prevention of fracture blisters is important because they pose an additional risk for infection. They also constitute a warning sign of compartment syndrome.

Compartment Syndrome

The compartment syndrome has been described as a condition of increased pressure within a limited space (*e.g.,* abdominal and limb compartments) that compromises the circulation and function of the tissues in the space. The abdominal compartment syndrome alters cardiovascular hemodynamics, respiratory mechanics, and renal function. The discussion in this chapter is limited to a discussion of the limb compartment syndromes.

The muscles and nerves of an extremity are enclosed in a tough, inelastic fascial envelope called a *muscle compartment*[28–30] (Fig. 57.9). If the pressure in the compartment is

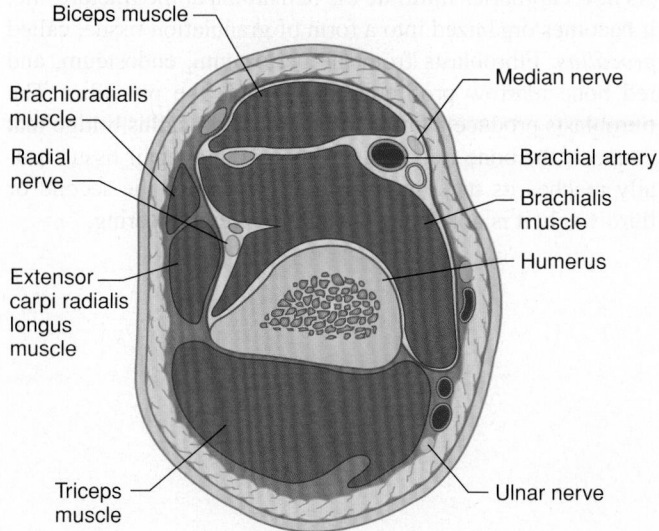

FIGURE 57.9 • The proximal muscle compartment of the arm, showing the location of fascia, muscles, nerves, and blood vessels.

Understanding | Fracture Healing

A fracture, which is any break in a bone, undergoes a healing process to reestablish bone continuity and strength. The repair of simple fractures is commonly divided into four phases: (1) hematoma formation, (2) fibrocartilaginous callus formation, (3) bony callus formation, and (4) remodelling.

1. Hematoma Formation

When a bone breaks, blood vessels in the bone and surrounding tissues are torn and bleed into and around the fragments of the fractured bone, forming a blood clot, or hematoma. The hematoma facilitates the formation of the fibrin meshwork that seals off the fracture site and serves as a framework for the influx of inflammatory cells, the ingrowth of fibroblasts, and the development of new capillary buds (vessels). It is also the source of signalling molecules that initiate the cellular events that are critical to the healing process.

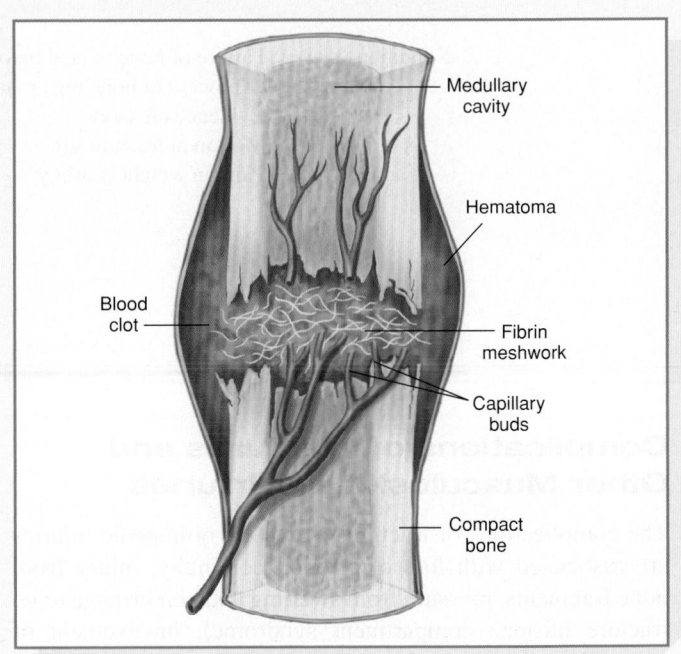

2. Fibrocartilaginous Callus Formation

As new capillaries infiltrate the hematoma at the fracture site, it becomes organized into a form of granulation tissue, called *procallus*. Fibroblasts from the periosteum, endosteum, and red bone marrow proliferate and invade the procallus. The fibroblasts produce a fibrocartilaginous soft callus bridge that connects the bone fragments. Although this repair tissue usually reaches its maximum girth at the end of the second or third week, it is not strong enough for weight bearing.

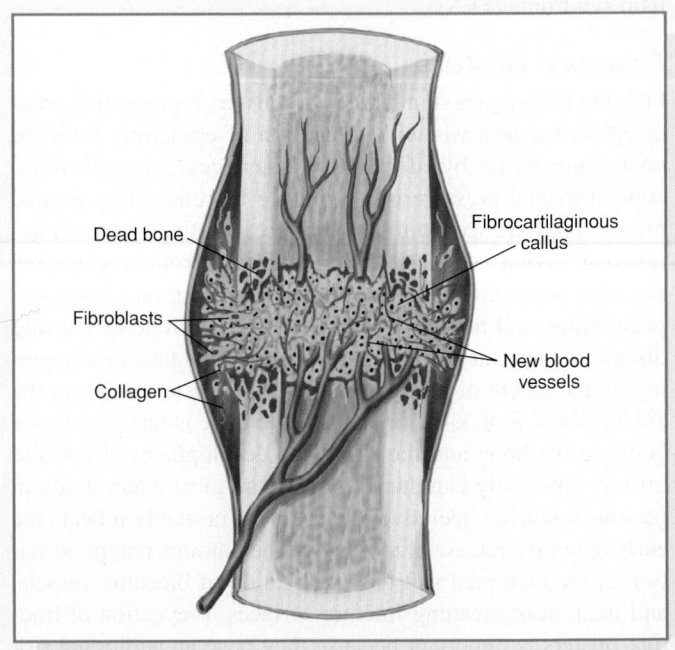

3. Bony Callus Formation

Ossification represents the conversion of the fibrocartilaginous cartilage to bony callus. In areas close to well-vascularized bone tissue, osteogenic cells develop into osteoblasts, or bone-building cells, which produce spongy bone trabeculae. The newly formed osteoblasts first deposit bone on the outer surface of the bone some distance from the fracture site. The formation of bone progresses toward the fracture site until a new bony sheath covers the fibrocartilaginous callus. In time, the fibrocartilage is converted to spongy bone, and the callus is then referred to as bony callus. Gradually, the bony callus calcifies and is replaced by mature bone. Bony callus formation begins 3 to 4 weeks after injury and continues until a firm bony union is formed months later.

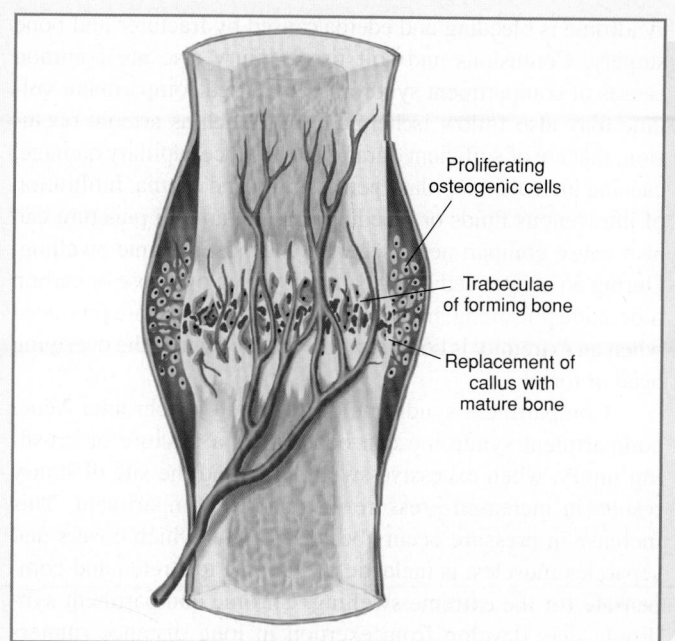

Proliferating osteogenic cells

Trabeculae of forming bone

Replacement of callus with mature bone

4. Remodelling

During remodelling of the bony callus, dead portions of the bone are gradually removed by osteoclasts. Compact bone replaces spongy bone around the periphery of the fracture, and there is reorganization of mineralized bone along the lines of mechanical stress. During this period, the excess material on the outside of the bone shaft and within the medullary cavity is removed and compact bone is laid down to reconstruct the shaft. The final structure of the remodelled area resembles that of the original unbroken bone; however, a thickened area on the surface of the bone may remain as evidence of a healed fracture.

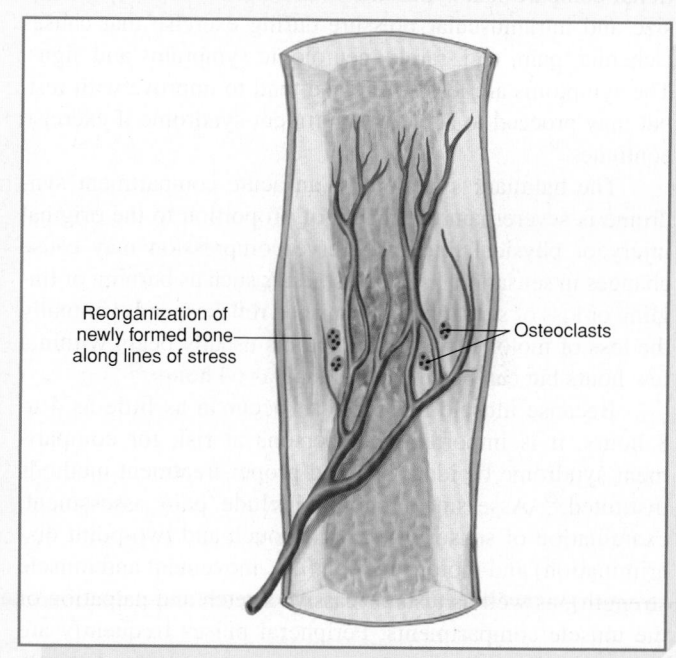

Reorganization of newly formed bone along lines of stress

Osteoclasts

sufficiently high, tissue circulation is compromised, causing death of nerve and muscle cells. Permanent loss of function may occur. The amount of pressure required to produce a compartment syndrome depends on many factors, including the duration of the pressure elevation, the metabolic rate of the tissues, vascular tone, and local blood pressure. Less tissue pressure is required to stop circulation when hypotension or vasoconstriction is present. Intracompartmental pressures greater than 30 mm Hg (normal is approximately 0 to 8 mm Hg) are considered sufficient to impair capillary blood flow.[28]

Compartment syndrome can result from a decrease in compartment size, an increase in the volume of its contents, or a combination of the two factors. Among the causes of decreased compartment size are constrictive dressings and casts, closure of fascial defects, and burns. In persons with circumferential third-degree burns, the inelastic and constricting eschar decreases the size of the underlying compartments (see Chapter 61).

An increase in compartment volume can be caused by trauma, swelling, vascular injury and bleeding, and venous obstruction. One of the most important causes of compartment syndrome is bleeding and edema caused by fractures and bone surgery. Contusions and soft tissue injury also are common causes of compartment syndrome. Increased compartment volume may also follow ischemic events, such as arterial occlusion, that are of sufficient duration to produce capillary damage, causing increased capillary permeability and edema. Infiltration of intravenous fluids or bleeding from an arterial puncture can also cause compartment ischemia and postischemic swelling. During an unattended coma caused by drug overdose or carbon monoxide poisoning, high compartment pressures are produced when an extremity is compressed by the weight of the overlying head or torso.

Compartment syndrome can be acute or chronic. Acute compartment syndrome can occur after a fracture or crushing injury, when excessive swelling around the site of injury results in increased pressure in a closed compartment. This increase in pressure occurs because fascia, which covers and separates muscles, is inelastic and unable to stretch and compensate for the extreme swelling. Chronic compartment syndrome may develop from exertion in long distance runners and others involved in a major change in activity level. Exertional compartment syndrome is an increase in compartment size and intramuscular pressure during exercise that causes ischemia, pain, and, rarely, neurologic symptoms and signs. The symptoms are less severe and tend to improve with rest, but may proceed to acute compartment syndrome if exercise continues.[31]

The hallmark symptom of an acute compartment syndrome is severe pain that is out of proportion to the original injury or physical findings. Nerve compression may cause changes in sensation (*e.g.*, paresthesias such as burning or tingling or loss of sensation), diminished reflexes, and eventually the loss of motor function. Symptoms usually begin within a few hours but can be delayed as long as 64 hours.[29]

Because muscle necrosis can occur in as little as 4 to 8 hours, it is important that persons at risk for compartment syndrome be identified and proper treatment methods instituted.[29] Assessment should include pain assessment, examination of sensory (*i.e.*, light touch and two-point discrimination) and motor function (*i.e.*, movement and muscle strength), as well as tests of passive stretch and palpation of the muscle compartments. Peripheral pulses frequently are normal in the presence of compartment syndrome because the major arteries are located outside the muscle compartments. Although edema may make it difficult to palpate the pulse, the increased compartment pressure seldom is sufficient to occlude flow in a major artery. Doppler methods usually confirm the existence of a pulse. Direct measurements of tissue pressure can be obtained using a needle or wick catheter inserted into the muscle compartment. This method is particularly useful in persons who are unresponsive and in those with nerve deficits.

Treatment consists of reducing compartmental pressures. This entails cast splitting or removal of restrictive dressings. These procedures often are sufficient to relieve most of the underlying pressure and symptoms. Elevating the extremity on pillows can help to reduce edema. However, excessive elevation should be avoided because the effects of gravity can lower the arterial pressure in the limb; thereby decreasing compartment perfusion. When compartment syndrome cannot be relieved by conservative measures, a fasciotomy may become necessary.[28–30] During this procedure, the fascia is incised longitudinally and separated so that the compartment volume can expand and blood flow can be reestablished. Because of potential problems with wound infection and closure, this procedure is usually performed as a last resort.

Complex Regional Pain Syndrome

The complex regional pain syndrome (CRPS), also referred to as *reflex sympathetic dystrophy (RSD) syndrome* and *causalgia* (discussed in Chapter 49), represents soft tissue complications of musculoskeletal injuries that cause pain out of proportion to the injury, and autonomic nervous system dysfunction manifested by hyperhidrosis (increased sweating) and vasomotor instability (either flushed and warm or cold and pale).[27,32]

Pain, which is the prominent symptom of the disorder, is described as severe, aching, or burning. It usually increases in intensity with movement and with noxious and nonnoxious stimuli. The pathophysiologic cause of the pain is unclear, but it is thought to have a sympathetic nervous system component. Muscle wasting, thin and shiny skin, and abnormalities of the nails and bone can occur. Decreased muscle strength and disuse can lead to contractures and osteoporosis. Alleviation of the pain and discomfort is challenging, and treatment focuses on pain management (*i.e.*, physical therapy, sympathetic nerve blocks, emotional support) (see Chapter 49).

Thromboemboli

Because of inactivity and restrictions in weight bearing, the persons with a lower extremity fracture are at risk for the development of venous thromboembolic disorders, which include pulmonary embolism and deep vein thrombosis (see Chapter 22). Expert consensus guidelines recommend thromboprophylaxis medication be given for a minimum of 10 days after surgery.[33] The incidence of venous thromboemboli associated with hip fracture and surgery can be as high as 40% to 60%.[34] It is estimated that the occurrence rate of fatal pulmonary embolism is 7.5% within 3 months of hip fracture surgery.[33] Anticoagulant prophylaxis with unfractionated heparin or low–molecular-weight heparin is effective and safe for individuals with fracture or trauma.[34,35] For high-risk patients, such as those on bed rest, the use of graduated compression stockings or intermittent pneumatic compression devices is the best practice.[34]

The majority of symptomatic venous thromboemboli associated with hospital admissions occur at least 2 months after hospital discharge.[34] Venous Doppler ultrasonography is the accepted test for the diagnosis of lower extremity deep vein thrombosis. A lung scan may be used in the diagnosis of a pulmonary embolus, but it may not differentiate between a thrombus and a fat embolus, especially in an individual with a long bone fracture.

Fat Embolism Syndrome

The fat embolism syndrome (FES) refers to a constellation of clinical manifestations resulting from the presence of fat droplets in the small blood vessels of the lung or other organs after a long bone fracture or other major trauma.[36–39] The fat emboli are thought to be released from the bone marrow or adipose tissue at the fracture site into the venous system through torn veins.

The pathophysiologic process of FES is unclear. Note that *fat embolization* and the *fat embolism syndrome* are not synonymous.[36] Fat embolization involves the presence of fat emboli in the circulation and FES is an identifiable clinical pattern of organ dysfunction associated with fat emboli in the circulation. One suggestion is that, when a bone is fractured, disruption of the venous sinusoids and fat cells allows fat globules to gain access to the venous circulation. The larger particles then become lodged in and block small pulmonary capillaries, whereas the smaller particles may pass through the lung capillaries and enter the systemic circulation. Although fat embolization occurs in many persons with fractures or operative fixation of fractures, FES occurs in only a small percentage of cases, supporting the hypothesis that factors other than fat embolization may be necessary for the development of FES.[36]

The main clinical features of FES are respiratory failure, cerebral dysfunction, and skin and mucosal petechiae. Cerebral manifestations include encephalopathy, seizures, and focal neurologic deficits unrelated to head injury. Initial symptoms of FES begin to develop within a few hours to 3 to 4 days after injury and do not appear beyond 1 week after the injury. The first symptoms include a subtle change in behaviour and signs of disorientation resulting from emboli in the cerebral circulation, combined with respiratory depression. There may be complaints of substernal chest pain and dyspnea accompanied by tachycardia and a low-grade fever. Diaphoresis, pallor, and cyanosis become evident as respiratory function deteriorates. A petechial rash that does not blanch with pressure often occurs 2 to 3 days after the injury. This rash usually is found on the anterior chest, axillae, neck, and shoulders. It also may appear on the soft palate and conjunctiva. The rash is thought to be related to embolization of the skin capillaries or thrombocytopenia.

An important part of the treatment of FES is early diagnosis. Arterial blood gases should be obtained and analyzed immediately after recognition of clinical manifestations. Treatment is directed toward correcting hypoxemia with supplemental oxygen and maintaining adequate fluid balance. Mechanical ventilation may be required. Corticosteroid drugs are administered to decrease the inflammatory response of lung tissues, decrease the edema, stabilize the lipid membranes to reduce lipolysis, and combat bronchospasm. Corticosteroids are also given prophylactically to high-risk persons. The only preventive approach to FES is early stabilization of the fracture.

IN SUMMARY

Many external physical agents can cause trauma to the musculoskeletal system. Particular factors, such as environment, activity, or age, can place a person at greater risk for injury. Some soft tissue injuries, such as contusions, hematomas, and lacerations, are relatively minor and easily treated. Muscle strains and ligamentous sprains are caused by mechanical overload on the connective tissue. They heal more slowly than the minor soft tissue injuries and require some degree of immobilization. Healing of soft tissue begins within 4 to 5 days of the injury and is primarily the function of fibroblasts, which produce collagen. Joint dislocation is caused by trauma to the supporting structures. Repeated trauma to the joint can cause articular softening (*i.e.*, chondromalacia) or the separation of small pieces of bone or cartilage, called loose bodies, in the joint.

Fractures occur when more stress is placed on a bone than the bone can absorb. The nature of the stress determines the type of fracture and the character of the resulting bone fragments. Healing of fractures is a complex process that takes place in five stages: hematoma formation, cellular proliferation, callus formation, ossification, and remodelling. For satisfactory healing to take place, the affected bone has to be reduced and immobilized. Immobilization is accomplished with the use of external devices, such as splints, casts, traction, or an external fixation apparatus, or with a surgically implanted internal fixation device. The complications associated with fractures can occur early because of soft tissue and nerve damage, or later when the healing process of the fracture is interrupted. The early complications of fractures and other orthopedic injuries are associated with swelling and hemorrhage (fracture blisters and compartment syndrome), involvement of nerve fibres (RSD and causalgia), and development of fat emboli. Impaired healing of a fracture can cause malunion with deformity, angulation, or rotation; delayed union, in which the healing process is prolonged; or nonunion, in which the fracture fails to heal.

BONE INFECTIONS

After completing this section of the chapter, you should be able to meet the following objectives:

- Explain the implications of bone infection.
- Differentiate among osteomyelitis due to spread from a contaminated wound, hematogenous osteomyelitis, and osteomyelitis due to vascular insufficiency in terms of etiologies, manifestations, and treatment.
- Cite the characteristics of chronic osteomyelitis.
- Describe the most common sites of tuberculosis of the bone.

Bone infections, including acute and chronic osteomyelitis, are known for their ability to cause pain, disability, and deformity. Despite the common use of antibiotics, they remain difficult to treat and eradicate. A resurgence of tubercular bone infections are occurring in industrialized parts of the world, attributed in part to immigration from developing countries and greater numbers of immunocompromised people.

BONE INFECTIONS

- Bone infections may be caused by a wide variety of microorganisms introduced during injury, during operative procedures, or from the bloodstream.
- Once localized in bone, the microorganisms proliferate, produce cell death, and spread within the bone shaft, inciting a chronic inflammatory response with further destruction of bone.
- Bone infections are difficult to treat and eradicate. Measures to prevent infection include careful cleaning and debridement of skeletal injuries and strict aseptic operating room protocols.

Osteomyelitis

Osteomyelitis represents an acute or chronic infection of the bone. *Osteo* refers to bone, and *myelo* refers to the marrow cavity, both of which are involved in this disease. The infection can be caused by direct penetration or contamination of an open fracture or wound (exogenous origin); seeding through the bloodstream (hematogenous spread); extension from a contiguous site; or skin infections in persons with vascular insufficiency. Osteomyelitis can occur as an acute, subacute, or chronic condition. All types of organisms, including viruses, parasites, fungi, and bacteria, can produce osteomyelitis, but infections caused by certain pyogenic bacteria and mycobacteria are the most common.

The specific agents isolated in pyogenic bacterial osteomyelitis are often associated with the age of the person or the inciting condition (*e.g.,* trauma or surgery). *Staphylococcus aureus* is the most common cause, but organisms such as *Escherichia coli, Neisseria gonorrhoeae, Haemophilus influenzae,* and *Salmonella* species are also seen.[22,24,40-42] *S. aureus* has two characteristics that favour its ability to produce osteomyelitis: (1) it has the ability to produce a collagen-binding adhesion molecule that allows it to adhere to the connective tissue elements of bone; and (2) it has the ability to be internalized and survive in osteoblasts, making the microorganism more resistant to antimicrobial (*e.g.,* antibiotic) therapy.[40]

Hematogenous Osteomyelitis

Hematogenous osteomyelitis originates with infectious organisms that reach the bone through the bloodstream. Acute hematogenous osteomyelitis occurs predominantly in children.[40-42] In adults, it is seen most commonly in debilitated persons and in those with a history of chronic skin infections, chronic urinary tract infections, and intravenous drug use and in those who are immunologically suppressed. Intravenous drug users are at risk for infections with *Streptococcus* and *Pseudomonas*.

Pathogenesis. The pathogenesis of hematogenous osteomyelitis differs in children and adults. In children, the infection usually affects the long bones of the appendicular skeleton. It starts in the metaphyseal region close to the growth plate, where termination of nutrient blood vessels and sluggish blood flow favour the attachment of blood-borne bacteria (Fig. 57.10). With advancement of the infection, purulent exudate collects in the rigidly enclosed bony tissue. Because of the bone's rigid structure, there is little room for swelling and the purulent exudate finds its way beneath the periosteum, shearing off the perforating arteries that supply the cortex with blood, thereby leading to necrosis of cortical bone. The necrotic bone that is formed may separate from the viable

FIGURE 57.10 • Hematogenous osteomyelitis. **A:** Infectious organisms reach the metaphysis through a nutrient blood vessel. **B:** Bacterial growth results in bone destruction and abscess formation. From the abscess cavity, the infection spreads between the trabeculae into the medullary cavity of compact bone and then through the cortex to the outside. **C:** The purulent exudate finds its way beneath the periosteum, shearing off the perforating arteries that supply the cortex with blood, thereby leading to necrosis of cortical bone and formation of devascularized fragments, called *sequestra*.

surrounding bone to form devascularized fragments, called *sequestra*.[22] Eventually, the purulent drainage may penetrate the periosteum and skin to form a draining sinus. In children 1 year of age and younger, the adjacent joint is often involved because the periosteum is not firmly attached to the cortex.[22] From 1 year of age to puberty, subperiosteal abscesses are more common. As the process continues, periosteal new bone formation and reactive bone formation in the marrow tend to wall in the infection. *Involucrum* refers to a lesion in which bone formation forms a sheath around the necrotic sequestrum. It is seen most commonly in cases of chronic osteomyelitis (discussed later).

In adults, the long bone microvasculature no longer favours seeding, and hematogenous infection rarely affects the appendicular skeleton. Instead, vertebrae, sternoclavicular and sacroiliac joints, and the symphysis pubis are involved. Infection typically first involves subchondral bone, then spreads to the joint space.[43] With vertebral osteomyelitis, this causes sequential destruction of the endplate, adjoining disk, and contiguous vertebral body. Infection less commonly begins in the joint and spreads to the adjacent bone.

Manifestations. The signs and symptoms of acute hematogenous osteomyelitis are those of bacteremia accompanied by symptoms referable to the site of the bone lesion. Bacteremia is characterized by chills, fever, and malaise. There often is pain on movement of the affected extremity, loss of movement, and local tenderness followed by redness and swelling. X-ray studies may appear normal initially, but they show evidence of periosteal elevation and increased osteoclast activity after an abscess has formed. Changes are evident on a bone scan 10 to 14 days before any changes are seen on x-ray films.[42]

Treatment. The treatment of hematogenous osteomyelitis begins with identification of the causative organism through blood and bone aspiration cultures.[42] Antimicrobial agents are given first parenterally and then orally. The length of time the affected limb needs to be rested and pain control measures used are based on the person's symptoms. Debridement and surgical drainage also may be necessary.

Direct Penetration and Contiguous Spread Osteomyelitis

Direct penetration or extension of bacteria from an outside (exogenous) source is now the most common cause of osteomyelitis.[22] Bacteria may be introduced directly into the bone by a penetrating wound, an open fracture, or surgery. Inadequate irrigation or debridement, introduction of foreign material into the wound, and extensive tissue injury increase the bone's susceptibility to infection.

Iatrogenic bone infections are those inadvertently brought about by surgery or other treatments. These complications include pin tract infection in skeletal traction, septic (infected) joints in joint replacement surgery, and wound infections after surgery. Staphylococci and streptococci are still commonly implicated, but in 25% of postoperative infections, gram-negative organisms are detected.[22] Measures to prevent these infections include preparation of the skin to reduce bacterial growth before surgery or insertion of traction devices or wires; strict operating room protocols; prophylactic use of antibiotics immediately before and for 24 hours after surgery and as a topical wound irrigation; and maintenance of sterile techniques after surgery when working with drainage tubes and dressing changes.

Pathogenesis. The pathogenesis of osteomyelitis resulting from direct penetration or contiguous spread differs from hematogenous infection in that virtually any traumatized bone may be involved. Although healthy bone is highly resistant to infection, injury from local inflammation and trauma may devitalize bone and surrounding tissue, providing an inert matrix on which microorganisms introduced during trauma thrive.

Manifestations. Osteomyelitis after trauma or bone surgery usually is associated with persistent or recurrent fever, increased pain at the operative or trauma site, and poor incisional healing, which often is accompanied by continued wound drainage and wound separation. Prosthetic joint infections often present with joint pain, fever, and cutaneous drainage.

Diagnosis and Treatment. Diagnosis requires both confirming the infection and identifying the offending microorganism with culture and sensitivity studies. The diagnosis of skeletal infection entails use of various imaging strategies, including conventional radiology, nuclear imaging studies, CT scans, and MRI.[42] Bone biopsy may be used to identify the causative microorganisms.

Treatment includes the use of antibiotics and selective use of surgical interventions. Antimicrobial agents are usually used prophylactically in persons undergoing bone surgery. However, prolonged use of prophylactic antimicrobial agents is associated with emergence of resistant bacterial strains.[44] For persons with osteomyelitis, early antimicrobial treatment, before there is extensive destruction of bone, produces the best results. The choice of agents and method of administration depend on the microorganisms causing the infection. Antimicrobial beads (*e.g.*, vancomycin, tobramycin, or other broad-spectrum antibiotics) can be embedded into the cement as part of the procedure for an infected hip arthroplasty or for a wound infection after spinal cord injury.[45] In acute osteomyelitis that does not respond to antibiotic therapy, surgical decompression is used to release intramedullary pressure and remove drainage from the periosteal area. Prosthesis removal may be necessary in cases of an infected prosthetic joint. The joint is left out while a 2- to 6-week course of therapy is given, after which another joint is implanted.[41]

Chronic Osteomyelitis

Chronic osteomyelitis usually occurs in adults. Generally, these infections occur secondary to an open wound, most often to the bone or surrounding tissue. Chronic osteomyelitis has long been recognized as a disease. However, the incidence has decreased in the past century because of improvements in surgical techniques and the advent of broad-spectrum antibiotic therapy. Chronic osteomyelitis includes all inflammatory processes of bone, excluding those in rheumatic diseases that are caused by microorganisms. It may be the result of delayed or inadequate treatment of acute hematogenous osteomyelitis or osteomyelitis caused by direct contamination of bone by exogenous organisms. Chronic osteomyelitis can persist for years; it may appear spontaneously, after a minor trauma, or when resistance is lowered.

The hallmark feature of chronic osteomyelitis is the presence of infected dead bone, a *sequestrum,* that has separated from the living bone.[22,24,41] A sheath of new bone, called the *involucrum,* forms around the dead bone. Radiologic techniques such as x-ray films, bone scans, and sinograms are used to identify the infected site. Chronic osteomyelitis or infection around a total joint prosthesis can be difficult to diagnose because the classic signs of infection are not apparent and the blood leukocyte count may not be elevated. A subclinical infection may exist for years. Bone scans are used with bone biopsy for a definitive diagnosis.

The treatment of chronic bone infections begins with wound cultures to identify the microorganism and its sensitivity to antibiotic therapy. The goal in selecting antimicrobial treatment for osteomyelitis is to use the drug with the highest bactericidal activity and least toxicity, and at the lowest cost. Intravenous therapy is usually needed for up to 6 weeks.[41] Initial antibiotic therapy is followed by surgery to remove foreign bodies (*e.g.,* metal plates, screws) or sequestra and by long-term antibiotic therapy. Immobilization of the affected part usually is necessary, with restriction of weight bearing on a lower extremity. External fixation devices are sometimes used.

Osteomyelitis With Vascular Insufficiency

In persons with vascular insufficiency, osteomyelitis may develop from a skin lesion. It is most commonly associated with chronic or ischemic foot ulcers in persons with long-standing diabetes. Neuropathy causes a loss of protective reflexes, and impaired arterial circulation and repetitive trauma are the major contributors to skin fissure and ulcer formation.

Persons with vascular insufficiency osteomyelitis often present with seemingly unrelated problems such as ingrown toenails, cellulitis, or a perforating foot ulcer, making diagnosis difficult. Furthermore, pain is often muted by peripheral neuropathy. Osteomyelitis is confirmed when bone is exposed in the ulcer bed or after debridement. Radiologic evidence is a late sign.

Treatment depends on the oxygen tension of the involved tissues. Debridement and antibiotic therapy may benefit persons who have good oxygen tension in the infected site. Hyperbaric oxygen therapy may be used as an adjunctive treatment. Amputation may be indicated when oxygen tension is inadequate.[43]

Tuberculosis of the Bone or Joint

A resurgence of tubercular osteomyelitis is occurring in industrialized countries, attributed to the influx of immigrants from developing countries and the greater numbers of immunocompromised people. In developing countries, affected individuals are usually adolescents or young adults, whereas in the nonimmigrant population of developed countries, the victims tend to be older, except for those who are immunocompromised.

Tuberculosis can spread from one part of the body, such as the lungs or the lymph nodes, to the musculoskeletal system. Any bone, joint, or bursa may be affected, but the spine is the most common site, followed by the knees and hips.[24,46,47] Tubercular osteomyelitis tends to be more destructive and difficult to control than pyogenic osteomyelitis. The infection spreads through large areas of the medullary cavity and causes extensive necrosis. In tuberculosis of the spine, also known as *Pott disease* or *tuberculous spondylitis,* the infection spreads through the intervertebral disks to involve multiple vertebrae and extends into the soft tissue, forming abscesses.

Local symptoms include pain, immobility, and muscle atrophy; joint swelling, mild fever, and leukocytosis also may occur. The most feared complication of spinal tuberculosis is neurologic compromise due to spinal deformity and epidural abscess formation. Because there are no specific radiographic findings in tubercular osteomyelitis, the diagnosis is usually made by tissue biopsy or culture findings. In spinal tuberculosis, a CT-guided biopsy is often used. The mainstay of treatment for tubercular osteomyelitis remains the appropriate three- or four-drug antimicrobial therapy based on current guidelines.[46,47] Conservative treatment is usually as effective as surgery, especially for earlier and milder cases.

> ## IN SUMMARY
>
> Bone infections occur because of the direct or indirect invasion of the musculoskeletal system by microorganisms, most commonly *S. aureus.* Osteomyelitis, or infection of the bone and marrow, can be an acute or chronic disease. Acute osteomyelitis is seen most often as a result of the direct contamination of bone by a foreign object. Chronic osteomyelitis represents an infection that continues beyond 6 to 8 weeks and may persist for years. The incidence of all types of bone infection has been dramatically reduced since the advent of antibiotic therapy. Iatrogenic infections are those inadvertently brought about by surgery or other treatments. Tuberculosis of the bone, which is characterized by bone destruction and abscess formation, is caused by spread of the infection from the lungs or lymph nodes.

OSTEONECROSIS

After completing this section of the chapter, you should be able to meet the following objectives:

- Define osteonecrosis.
- Cite four major causes of osteonecrosis.
- Characterize the blood supply of bone and relate it to the pathologic features of the condition.
- Describe the methods used in diagnosis and treatment of the condition.

Osteonecrosis, or death of a segment of bone, is a condition caused by the interruption of blood supply to the marrow, medullary bone, or cortex[22,24,47–50] (Fig. 57.11). It is a relatively common disorder and can occur in the medullary cavity of the metaphysis and the subchondral region of the epiphysis, especially in the proximal femur, distal femur, and proximal humerus. It is a common complicating disorder of Legg–Calvé–Perthes disease, slipped capital femoral epiphysis, sickle cell disease, steroid therapy, alcohol abuse, and hip trauma, fracture, or surgery. Persons treated with corticosteroids and/or bisphosphonates are more vulnerable to developing osteonecrosis. Approximately 2.5% of the joint replacements performed annually in Canada are for treatment of osteonecrosis.[48]

Although bone necrosis results from ischemia, the mechanisms producing the ischemia are varied and include mechanical vascular interruption such as occurs with trauma or a fracture; thrombosis and embolism (*e.g.,* sickle cell disease, nitrogen

FIGURE 57.11 • Osteonecrosis of the head of the femur. A coronal section shows a circumscribed area of subchondral infarction with partial detachment of the overlying articular cartilage and subarticular bone. (From Rubin R., Strayer D. S. (Eds.). (2012). *Rubin's pathology: Clinicopathologic foundations of medicine* (6th ed., p. 1217). Philadelphia, PA: Lippincott Williams & Wilkins.)

CHART 57.1 CAUSES OF OSTEONECROSIS

Mechanical disruption of blood vessels
    Fractures
    Legg–Calvé–Perthes disease
    Blount disease
Thrombosis and embolism
    Sickle cell disease
    Nitrogen bubbles in decompression sickness
Vessel injury
    Vasculitis
    Connective tissue disease
        Systemic lupus erythematosus
        Rheumatoid arthritis
    Radiation therapy
    Gaucher disease
Corticosteroid therapy

bubbles caused by inadequate decompression during deep sea diving); and vessel injury (*e.g.,* vasculitis, radiation therapy). In many cases, the cause of the necrosis is uncertain. Other than fracture, the most common causes of bone necrosis are idiopathic (*i.e.,* those of unknown cause) and prior steroid therapy. Chart 57.1 lists disorders associated with osteonecrosis.

Bone has a rich blood supply that varies from site to site.[47] The flow in the medullary portion of bone originates in nutrient vessels from an interconnecting plexus that supplies the marrow, trabecular bone, and endosteal half of the cortex. The outer cortex receives its blood supply from periosteal, muscular, metaphyseal, and epiphyseal vessels that surround the bone. Some bony sites, such as the head of the femur, have only limited collateral circulation, so that interruption of the flow, such as with a hip fracture, can cause necrosis of a substantial portion of medullary and cortical bone and irreversible damage.

One of the most frequent causes of osteonecrosis is that associated with administration of corticosteroids.[16,20,47] Despite numerous studies, the mechanism of steroid-induced osteonecrosis remains unclear. The condition may develop after the administration of very high, short-term doses; during long-term treatment; or even from intra-articular injection. Although the risk increases with the dose and duration of treatment, it is difficult to predict who will be affected. The interval between corticosteroid administration and onset of symptoms rarely is less than 6 months and may be more than 3 years. There is no satisfactory method for preventing progression of the disease. Osteonecrosis of the jaw has been reported after long-term use of bisphosphonates.[51] The complication has mainly been reported in patients receiving the drugs intravenously for multiple myeloma and bone metastases from breast cancer.

The pathologic features of bone necrosis are the same, regardless of cause. The site of the lesion is related to the vessels involved. There is necrosis of cancellous bone and marrow. The cortex usually is not involved because of collateral blood flow. In subchondral infarcts (*i.e.,* ischemia below the cartilage), a triangular or wedge-shaped segment of tissue that has the subchondral bone plate as its base and the centre of the epiphysis as its apex, undergoes necrosis. When medullary infarcts occur in fatty bone marrow, the death of bone cells causes calcium release and necrosis of fat cells, with the formation of free fatty acids. Released calcium forms an insoluble "soap" with free fatty acids. Because bone lacks mechanisms for resolving the infarct, the lesions remain for life.

The symptoms associated with osteonecrosis are varied and depend on the extent of infarction. Typically, subchondral infarcts cause chronic pain that is initially associated with activity but that gradually becomes more progressive until it is experienced at rest. Subchondral infarcts often collapse and predispose the patient to severe secondary osteoarthritis.

Diagnosis of osteonecrosis is based on history, physical findings, radiographic findings, and results of special imaging studies, including CT scans and technetium-99m bone scans. Treatment of osteonecrosis depends on the underlying pathologic process. In some cases, only short-term immobilization, nonsteroidal anti-inflammatory drugs, exercises, and limitation in weight bearing are used. Osteonecrosis of the hip is particularly difficult to treat. In persons with early disease, limitation of weight bearing through the use of crutches may allow the condition to stabilize. Although several surgical approaches have been used, the most definitive treatment of advanced osteonecrosis of the knee or hip is total joint replacement. Treatment with hyperbaric oxygenation can also be effective.[52]

IN SUMMARY

Osteonecrosis is a common condition that has long been recognized but is not fully understood. Death of bone is caused by disruption of the blood supply from intravascular or extravascular processes. Sites with poor collateral circulation, such as the femoral head, are most seriously affected. Causative factors include corticosteroid therapy. Symptoms include pain that varies in severity, depending on the extent of infarction. Total joint replacement is the most frequently used treatment for advanced osteonecrosis.

NEOPLASMS

After completing this section of the chapter, you should be able to meet the following objectives:

- Differentiate between the properties of benign and malignant bone tumours.
- Contrast osteogenic sarcoma, Ewing sarcoma, and chondrosarcoma in terms of the most common age groups and anatomic sites that are affected.
- List the primary sites of tumours that frequently metastasize to the bone.
- State the three primary goals for treatment of metastatic bone disease.

TABLE 57.3 CLASSIFICATION OF PRIMARY BONE NEOPLASMS

TISSUE TYPE	BENIGN NEOPLASM	MALIGNANT NEOPLASM
Bone	Osteoid osteoma Benign osteoblastoma	Osteosarcoma Parosteal osteogenic sarcoma
Cartilage	Osteochondroma Chondroma Chrondroblastoma Chondromyxoid fibroma	Chondrosarcoma
Lipid	Lipoma	Liposarcoma
Fibrous and fibro-osseous tissue	Fibrous dysplasia	Fibrosarcoma
Miscellaneous	Giant cell tumour	Malignant fibrous histiocytoma Malignant giant cell Ewing sarcoma
Bone marrow		Multiple myeloma Reticulum cell sarcoma

Neoplasms in the skeletal system are referred to as *bone tumours*. Primary malignant tumours of the bone are uncommon, constituting less than 0.2% of all cancers.[53,54] Metastatic disease of the bone, however, is relatively common. Primary bone tumours may arise from any of the skeletal components, including osseous bone tissue, cartilage, and bone marrow. The discussion in this section focuses on primary benign and malignant bone tumours of osseous or cartilaginous origin and metastatic bone disease. Tumours of bone marrow origin (*i.e.,* leukemia and multiple myeloma) are discussed in Chapter 15.

Like other types of neoplasms, bone tumours may be benign or malignant. Benign tumours far outnumber malignant tumours. The benign types, such as osteochondromas, tend to grow rather slowly and usually do not destroy the supporting or surrounding tissue or spread to other parts of the body. Malignant tumours, such as osteosarcoma, grow rapidly and can spread to other parts of the body through the bloodstream or lymphatics. The two major forms of bone cancer in children and young adults are osteosarcoma and Ewing sarcoma. Both tumour types occur more frequently in the second decade of life.[24] Chondrosarcomas tend to occur during middle to late adulthood.[24] The classification of benign and malignant bone tumours is described in Table 57.3.

Characteristics of Bone Tumours

There are three major manifestations of bone tumours: pain, presence of a mass, and impairment of function. Pain is a feature common to almost all malignant tumours, but may or may not occur with benign tumours. For example, a benign bone cyst usually is asymptomatic until a fracture occurs. Pain that persists at night and is not relieved by rest suggests malignancy. A mass or hard lump may be the first sign of a bone tumour. A malignant tumour is suspected when a painful mass exists that is enlarging or eroding the cortex of the bone. The ease of discovery of a mass depends on the location of the tumour; a small lump arising on the surface of the tibia is easy to detect, whereas a tumour that is deep in the medial portion of the thigh may grow to a considerable size before it is noticed. Benign and malignant tumours may cause the bone to erode to the point at which it cannot withstand the strain of ordinary use. In such cases, even a small amount of bone stress or trauma precipitates a pathologic fracture. A tumour may produce pressure on a peripheral nerve, causing decreased sensation, numbness, a limp, or limitation of movement.

Benign Neoplasms

Benign bone tumours usually are limited to the confines of the bone, have well-demarcated edges, and are surrounded by a thin rim of sclerotic bone. The four most common types of benign bone tumours are osteoma, chondroma, osteochondroma, and giant cell tumour.[22,24] An *osteoma* is a small bony tumour found on the surface of a long bone, flat bone, or the skull. It usually is composed of hard, compact (ivory osteoma), or spongy (cancellous) bone. It may be excised or left alone.

BONE NEOPLASMS

- Neoplasms of the skeletal system can affect bone tissue, cartilage, or bone marrow.
- Benign tumours tend to grow slowly, do not spread to other parts of the body, and exert their effects through the space-occupying nature of the tumour and their ability to weaken bone structures.
- Malignant bone tumours are rare before 10 years of age, have their peak incidence in the teenage years, tend to grow rapidly, and have a high mortality rate.

A *chondroma* is a tumour composed of hyaline cartilage. It may arise on the surface of the bone (*i.e.,* ecchondroma) or in the medullary cavity (*i.e.,* endochondroma). These tumours may become large and are especially common in the hands and feet. A chondroma may persist for many years and then take on the attributes of a malignant chondrosarcoma. A chondroma usually is not treated unless it becomes unsightly or uncomfortable.

An *osteochondroma* is the most common form of benign tumour in the skeletal system, representing 50% of all benign bone tumours and approximately 15% of all primary skeletal lesions. It grows only during periods of skeletal growth, originating in the epiphyseal cartilage plate and growing out of the bone like a mushroom. An osteochondroma is composed of cartilage and bone and usually occurs singly, but may affect several bones in a condition called *multiple exostoses*. Malignant changes are rare, and excision of the tumour is done only when necessary.

A *giant cell tumour,* or *osteoclastoma,* is an aggressive tumour of multinucleated cells that often behaves like a malignant tumour, metastasizing through the bloodstream and recurring locally after excision. It arises most often in people in their 20s to 40s and is found most commonly in the knee, wrist, or shoulder. The tumour begins in the metaphyseal region, grows into the epiphysis, and may extend into the joint surface. Pathologic fractures are common because the tumour destroys the bone substance. Clinically, pain may occur at the tumour site, with gradually increasing swelling. X-ray films show destruction of the bone with expansion of the cortex.

The treatment of giant cell tumours depends on their location. If the affected bone can be eliminated without loss of function, such as the clavicle or fibula, the entire bone or part of it may be removed. When the tumour is near a major joint, such as the knee or shoulder, a local excision is done. Irradiation may be used to prevent recurrence of the tumour.

Malignant Bone Tumours

In contrast to benign tumours, primary malignant tumours tend to be ill defined, lack sharp borders, and extend beyond the confines of the bone. Primary bone tumours occur in all age groups and may arise in any part of the body. However, certain types of tumours tend to target certain age groups and anatomic sites (Fig. 57.12). For example, most osteogenic sarcomas occur in adolescents and are particularly common around the knee joint. Also, people with certain conditions such as Paget disease are at increased risk for development of bone cancer.

The diagnosis of bone tumours includes radiologic staging and biopsy.[51] Radiographs give the most general diagnostic information, such as malignant versus benign and primary versus metastatic status. The radiograph demonstrates the region of bone involvement, extent of destruction, and amount of reactive bone formed. Radioisotope scans are used to estimate the local intramedullary extent of the tumour and screen for other skeletal areas of involvement. CT scans further aid diagnosis and anatomic localization and can identify small pulmonary metastases not seen by conventional radiographs. MRI is the most accurate method of evaluating the intramedullary extent of bone tumour and can demarcate the soft structures in relation to neurovascular structures without the use of contrast media. It is best used in conjunction with a CT scan. Radionuclide bone scans are used to assess for metastasis. A biopsy also is done because the definitive treatment of most bone tumours is based on pathologic interpretation of the biopsy specimen.

Osteosarcoma

Osteosarcoma is an aggressive and highly malignant bone tumour. It is the most common primary malignant bone tumour, representing one fifth of all bone tumours.[22] Osteosarcoma is the most common bone tumour in children and the third most common cancer in children and adolescents.[22,24,54–56] Although osteosarcomas can develop in any bone, they most

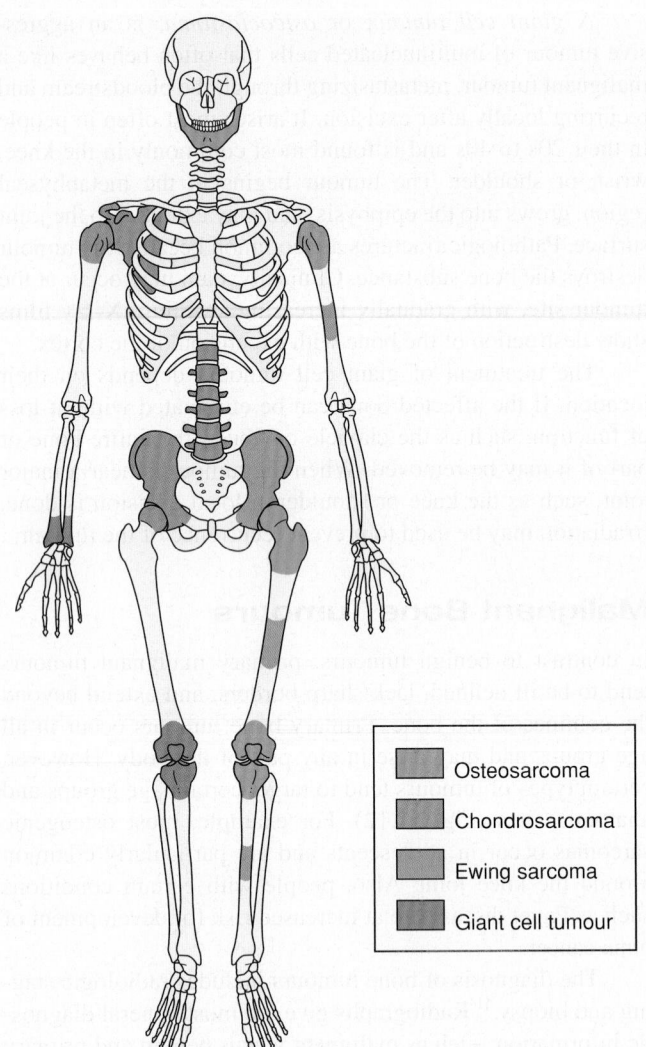

Osteosarcoma

Chondrosarcoma

Ewing sarcoma

Giant cell tumour

FIGURE 57.12 • Common sites of primary malignant bone tumours (chondrosarcoma, osteosarcoma, and Ewing sarcoma) and giant cell tumour, a locally aggressive benign tumour.

commonly arise in the vicinity of the knee (*e.g.,* lower femur or upper tibia or fibula). The proximal humerus is the second most common site. The hands, feet, skull, and jaw are less frequent sites for the disease, being affected most frequently in persons older than 25 years of age.[22]

The cause of osteosarcoma is unknown. The tumour has a bimodal distribution, with 75% occurring in persons younger than 20 years of age. A second peak occurs in the elderly with predisposing factors such as Paget disease, bone infarcts, or prior irradiation.[24] The correlation of age and location of most of the tumours with the period of maximum growth suggests some relation to increased osteoblastic activity. In younger persons, the primary tumour most often is located at the anatomic sites associated with maximum growth velocity—the distal femur, proximal tibia, and proximal humerus. Bone tumours in the elderly are more common in the humerus, pelvis, and proximal femur. Paget disease, which is linked to osteosarcoma in adults, also is associated with increased

osteoblastic activity. Irradiation from an internal source, such as the radioactive pharmaceutical technetium used in bone scans, or an external source, such as x-ray films, also has been associated with osteosarcoma. There are known genetic factors associated with osteosarcoma. Mutations in two genes are reported to increase the susceptibility to the development of osteosarcoma: the retinoblastoma (*RB*) gene and the *TP53* tumour suppressor gene[22] (see Chapter 8).

Osteosarcomas are aggressive tumours that grow rapidly in a circular, ball-like mass in the bone tissue. They often are eccentrically placed in the bone and move from the metaphysis of the bone out into the periosteal surface, with subsequent spread to adjacent soft tissues (Fig. 57.13). The tumour infrequently metastasizes to the lymph nodes because the cells are unable to grow in the node. Nodal metastases usually occur only in the late course of disseminated disease. Most often, the tumour cells exit the primary tumour through the venous end of the capillary, and early metastasis to the lung is common. Lung metastases, even if massive, usually are relatively asymptomatic. The prognosis for a person with osteosarcoma depends on the aggressiveness of the disease, presence or absence of pathologic fractures, size of the tumour, and rapidity of tumour growth. Long-term survival is better in younger people with effective chemotherapy regimens and no metastases.[57] Despite advances in surgery and chemotherapy, the 5-year survival rate has remained unchanged at 54%.[54]

FIGURE 57.13 • Osteosarcoma. The distal femur contains a dense osteoblastic malignant tumour that extends through the centre in the soft tissue and epiphysis. (From Rubin R., Strayer D. S. (Eds.). (2012). *Rubin's pathology: Clinicopathologic foundations of medicine* (6th ed., p. 1244). Philadelphia, PA: Lippincott Williams & Wilkins.)

The primary clinical feature of osteosarcoma is deep, localized pain with nighttime awakening and swelling in the affected bone. Because the pain is often of sudden onset, patients and their families often associate the symptoms with recent trauma.[55] The skin overlying the tumour may be warm, shiny, and stretched, with prominent superficial veins. The range of motion of the adjacent joint may be restricted.

History, physical examination, and radiographic studies are all part of the evaluation of a patient with osteosarcoma. Plain films of the primary site and of the chest are first obtained. MRI, CT scan, and full-body scan are required to evaluate the extent of the local disease and to determine the extent of metastasis if present. Radionuclide bone scans are done to evaluate for lung and bone metastasis. An open biopsy is required to confirm the diagnosis and to determine the histologic features and cell type of the tumour.

Osteosarcoma is treated by surgery in combination with multiagent chemotherapy used both before and after surgery.[53–56] In the past, treatment usually entailed amputation above the level of the tumour. Limb salvage surgical procedures, using a metal prosthesis or cadaver allograft, are now a standard alternative. Studies have shown that limb salvage surgery has no adverse effects on the long-term survival of persons with osteosarcoma. The success of limb salvage appears to depend on the use of a wide surgical margin, improved radiographic imaging studies, multiagent chemotherapy, and more refined surgical reconstructive techniques. Advanced imaging techniques, including serum thallium scans and the use of angiography, assist the surgeon in determining the best type of treatment. Chemotherapy using various drug combinations is the most effective treatment for metastatic osteosarcoma.[58,59] A preoperative regimen of intra-arterial cisplatin and infusional doxorubicin is being used in combination with limb-sparing procedures.[56,58,60]

Amputation is another surgical option. It involves either the removal of expendable bones such as the fibula, ribs, toes, or ulna, or the complete removal of the tumour and the affected limb. The primary objective of overall treatment of patients with osteosarcoma is long-term disease-free survival or cure. Preserving limb function is a secondary objective. In cases in which adequate limb salvage surgery cannot be achieved, limb amputation may be necessary.

Ewing Sarcoma

Ewing sarcoma is a member of a group of small round cell, undifferentiated tumours thought to be of neural crest origin[16,24,55] (see Chapter 48). The family of tumours includes Ewing sarcoma of the bone and soft tissue and peripheral primitive neuroectodermal tumour (PPNET). Of the tumours in this family, Ewing sarcoma accounts for most cases. Ewing sarcoma and osteosarcoma occur in the same sex and age groups, but they can usually be distinguished radiographically and histologically. It can occur at any age, but is seen most commonly in patients 10 to 20 years of age. Males are affected slightly more frequently than females. There is a striking predilection for Caucasians, whereas children with African or Asian ancestry are rarely affected.[24]

The most frequent site of Ewing sarcoma is the femur, usually in the diaphysis. The pelvis represents the second most common site; other sites include the pubis, sacrum, humerus, vertebrae, ribs, skull, and other flat bones. The characteristic pathologic findings of Ewing sarcoma include densely packed, regularly shaped, small cells with round or oval nuclei. A specific reciprocal translocation of chromosomes 11 and 22, or a variant thereof, is found in most of the Ewing sarcoma family of tumours.[22,55] Detection of the translocation by routine cytogenetic or polymerase chain reaction analysis can be helpful in confirming the diagnosis in highly undifferentiated tumours.[55]

Manifestations of Ewing tumour include bone pain, limitation of movement, and tenderness over the involved bone or soft tissue.[55] It often is accompanied by systemic manifestations such as fever or weight loss, which may serve to confuse the diagnosis. There may be a delay in diagnosis when the pain and swelling associated with the tumour are attributed to a sports injury or when the tumour is located in the pelvis and the pain is not localized and the mass is not apparent. Pathologic fractures are common because of bone destruction. The most common sites of metastasis are the lungs, bone marrow, and other bones.

Because Ewing sarcoma is a difficult diagnosis to establish, the diagnostic biopsy is very important. Clinical evaluations include MRI and CT scans of the primary tumour, chest radiographs, CT of the chest, bone scan, bilateral bone marrow aspiration, and biopsy of the primary tumour site.[55] The extent of disease at diagnosis is the most important prognostic factor. The presence of metastatic disease at diagnosis is a poor prognostic factor regardless of the site of the primary lesion.

Treatment methods incorporate a combination of multiagent chemotherapy, surgery, and radiation therapy. Chemotherapy is important because it can shrink the tumour and improve overall survival rates from 10% to 70%.[55] It is generally given before local control measures are initiated. Ewing sarcoma is considered to be a radiosensitive tumour, and local control may be achieved through radiation or surgery. Patients with small, nonmetastatic, distally located tumours generally have the best prognosis. Such patients have up to a 50% to 75% cure rate.[53,54] The presence of metastases at the time of diagnosis decreases the 3-year survival rate to 30% to 60%.[55]

Chondrosarcoma

Chondrosarcoma, a malignant tumour of cartilage that can develop in the medullary cavity or peripherally, is the second most common form of malignant bone tumour. It occurs primarily in middle or later life and slightly more often in men. The tumour arises from points of muscle attachment to bone, particularly the knee, shoulder, hip, and pelvis. Chondrosarcomas can arise from underlying benign lesions such as osteochondroma, chondroblastoma, or fibrous dysplasia.[24]

Chondrosarcomas are slow growing and metastasize late, and often are painless. They can remain hidden in an area such as the pelvis for a long time. This type of tumour, like many primary malignancies, tends to destroy bone and extend into the soft tissues beyond the confines of the bone of origin. Chondrosarcomas mainly affect the bones of the trunk, pelvis, or proximal femur and rarely develop in the distal portion of a bone. Irregular flecks and ringlets of calcification often are prominent radiographic findings.

Early diagnosis is important because chondrosarcoma responds well to early radical surgical excision. It usually is resistant to radiation therapy and available chemotherapeutic agents. Not infrequently, these tumours transform into a highly malignant tumour, mesenchymal chondrosarcoma, which requires a more aggressive treatment, including combination chemotherapy.

Metastatic Bone Disease

Skeletal metastases are the most common malignancy of osseous tissue.[61,62] Approximately half of all people with cancer have bone metastasis at some point in their disease. Metastatic lesions are seen most often in the spine, femur, pelvis, ribs, sternum, proximal humerus, and skull, and are less common in anatomic sites more distant from the trunk of the body. Tumours that frequently spread to the skeletal system are those of the breast, lung, prostate, kidney, and thyroid, although any cancer can ultimately involve the skeleton. More than 85% of bone metastases result from primary lesions in the breast, lung, or prostate.[61] The incidence of metastatic bone disease is highest in persons older than 40 years of age.

The major symptom of bone metastasis is pain with evidence of an impending pathologic fracture.[61,62] It usually develops gradually, over weeks, and is more severe at night. Pain is caused by stretching of the periosteum of the involved bone or by nerve entrapment, as when the nerve roots of the spinal cord are compressed by the vertebral body. Pathologic fractures occur in approximately 10% to 15% of persons with metastatic bone disease. The affected bone appears to be eaten away on x-ray images; in severe cases, it crumbles on impact, much like dried toast. Many pathologic fractures occur in the femur, humerus, and vertebrae.

Radiographic examinations are used along with CT or bone scans to detect, diagnose, and localize metastatic bone lesions. Approximately one third of persons with skeletal metastases have positive bone scans without radiologic findings. This is because 50% of the trabecular bone must be destroyed before a lesion is visible on plain radiographs.[62] Arteriography using radiopaque contrast media may be helpful in outlining the tumour margins. A bone biopsy usually is done when there is a question regarding the diagnosis or treatment. A closed-needle biopsy with CT localization is particularly useful with spine lesions. Serum levels of alkaline phosphatase and calcium often are elevated in persons with metastatic bone disease.

The primary goals in treatment of metastatic bone disease are to prevent pathologic fractures and promote survival with maximum functioning, allowing the person to maintain as much mobility and pain control as possible. Standard treatment methods include chemotherapy, irradiation, and surgical stabilization. Radiation therapy is primarily used as a palliative treatment to alleviate pain and prevent pathologic fractures. After a pathologic fracture has occurred, bracing, intramedullary nailing of the femur, or spine stabilization may be done. Because adequate fixation often is difficult in diseased bone, cement (i.e., methylmethacrylate) often is used with internal fixation devices to stabilize the bone.

Recent research has focused on the role of osteoclastic and osteoblastic activity in the pathogenesis of metastatic bone disease and on the use of the bisphosphonates (e.g., pamidronate disodium, zoledronic acid) for its treatment.[63,64] Bone tissue contains a rich environment of growth factors and cells of various embryonic origins, including hematopoietic, stromal, endothelial, and other cell types. The osteoclasts and osteoblasts, in particular, appear to play a dominant role in the pathogenesis of bone metastasis. Osteoclasts are involved in osteolytic or destructive bone lesions and osteoblasts in the excessive production of new and poor-quality bone.[61] The bisphosphonates, which are now well-established agents for the prevention and treatment of osteoporosis, have recently been shown to decrease symptoms associated with bone metastasis secondary to breast and prostate cancer. These agents bind preferentially to bone at sites of active bone metabolism, are released from the bone matrix during bone resorption, and potentially inhibit osteoclast activity and survival, thereby reducing osteoclast-mediated bone resorption. Recent studies suggest that besides their strong antiosteoclastic activity, these agents may also have some direct antitumour effects.[64]

IN SUMMARY

Bone tumours, like any other type of neoplasm, may be benign or malignant. Benign bone tumours grow slowly and usually do not destroy the surrounding tissues. Malignant tumours can be primary or metastatic. Primary bone tumours are rare, grow rapidly, metastasize to the lungs and other parts of the body through the bloodstream, and have a high mortality rate. Metastatic bone tumours usually are multiple, originating primarily from cancers of the breast, lung, and prostate. The incidence of metastatic bone disease probably is increasing because improved treatment methods enable persons with cancer to live longer. Advances in chemotherapy, radiation therapy, and surgical procedures have substantially increased the survival and cure rates for many types of bone cancers. A primary goal in metastatic bone disease is the prevention of pathologic fractures.

REVIEW EXERCISES

1. A 39-year-old man is in intensive care after a motorcycle crash in which he skidded across the pavement on his right side. He has fractures of his right femur, pelvis, and several ribs on the right side. His leg was crushed beneath the

motorcycle. He is beginning to lose movement in his leg.

A. *What are the priorities in treating his orthopedic injuries? What are the options for stabilizing his leg?*

B. *What risk factors for complications of fractures are present?*

C. *What are the symptoms of compartment syndrome, and how is it treated?*

2. A 73-year-old woman sustained a comminuted fracture in the mid-diaphysis of her left humerus when her husband lifted her up in bed. She has multiple lucent lesions scattered throughout her proximal humerus, radius, and ulna. She was recently hospitalized for confusion and was found to have diffuse bone metastases. Her bone marrow biopsy showed adenocarcinoma. She has a history of breast cancer 30 years ago, but her most recent mammogram was negative.

A. *What would you consider to be the most likely cause of her fracture?*

B. *What are the most common sites for bone metastasis?*

C. *Explain the treatment goals for persons with pathologic fractures.*

3. A 14-year-old boy has complained of recent pain and swelling of his knee, with some restriction in movement. Although he thinks he may have injured his knee playing football, his mother insists that he be seen by an orthopedic specialist, who raises the possibility that the boy may have an osteosarcoma.

A. *Use the theory that osteosarcoma has its origin in sites of maximal growth velocity to explain the site of this boy's possible tumour.*

B. *What diagnostic tests could be used to establish a diagnosis of osteosarcoma?*

C. *The boy and his family are concerned that he will require radical surgery with amputation of the leg. How would you explain possible treatment options to him?*

References

1. Public Health Agency of Canada (PHAC). (2012). Injury in Review, 2012 edition. Available online at: http://www.parachutecanada.org/downloads/research/reports/InjuryInReview2012_EN.pdf. Accessed May 26, 2015.

2. Canadian Hospital Injury Reporting and Prevention Program. (2012). Injury reports. Available online at: http://www.phac-aspc.gc.ca/injury-bles/chirpp/injrep-rapbles/index-eng.php. Accessed May 26, 2015.

3. American Academy of Orthopaedic Surgeons. (2012). High school sports injuries. Available online at: http://orthoinfo.aaos.org/topic.cfm?topic=A00056. Accessed May 26, 2015.

4. American Academy of Orthopedic Surgeons. (2012). Guidelines for preventing falls. Available online at: http://orthoinfo.aaos.org/topic.cfm?topic=A00135. Accessed May 26, 2015.

5. Gourlay M., Richy F., Reginstar J. Y. (2003). Strategies for the prevention of hip fracture. *American Journal of Medicine, 115*, 309–317.

6. Hogan K. A., Gross R. H. (2003). Overuse injuries in pediatric athletes. *Orthopedic Clinics of North America, 34*, 405–415.

7. Weintraub W. (2003). *Tendons and ligament healing.* Brookline, MA: Paradigm Publications.

8. Mercier L. R. (2008). *Practical orthopedics* (6th ed.). St. Louis, MO: Mosby.

9. Gomez J. E. (2002). Upper extremity injuries in youth sports. *Pediatric Clinics of North America, 49*, 593–626.

10. Landry G. L. (2011). Chapters 678–684: Sports medicine. In Kliegman R. M., Stanton B. F., St. Geme J. W., et al. (Eds.), *Nelson textbook of pediatrics* (19th ed.). Philadelphia, PA: Saunders Elsevier.

11. Fongemie A. E., Buss D. D., Rolnick S. J. (2001). Management of shoulder impingement syndrome and rotator cuff tears. *American Family Physician, 57*, 667–679.

12. American Association of Orthopedic Surgeons. (2014). Meniscal tears. Available online at: http://orthoinfo.aaos.org/topic.cfm?topic=a00358. Accessed May 26, 2015.

13. Maitra R. S., Miller M. D., Johnson D. L. (1999). Meniscal reconstruction: I. Indications, techniques, and graft considerations. *American Journal of Orthopedics, 28*, 213–218.

14. Maitra R. S., Miller M. D., Johnson D. L. (1999). Meniscal reconstruction: II. Indications, techniques, and graft considerations. *American Journal of Orthopedics, 28*, 280–286.

15. Falah M., Nierenberg G., Soudry M., et al. (2010). Treatment of articular cartilage lesion of the knee. *International Orthopaedics, 34*(5), 621–630.

16. Brunner L., Eshilian-Oats L. (2003). Hip fractures in adults. *American Family Physician, 67*, 537–542.

17. Zuckerman J. D. (1996). Hip fracture. *New England Journal of Medicine, 334*, 1519–1525.

18. Court-Brown C. M., Heckman J. D., McQueen M. M., et al. (2015). *Rockwood & Green's fractures in adults* (8th ed.). Philadelphia, PA: Lippincott Williams & Wilkins.

19. Tull F., Borrelli J. Jr. (2003). Soft-tissue injury associated with closed fractures: Evaluation and management. *Journal of the American Academy of Orthopedic Surgeons, 11*, 431–438.

20. Schutz M., Ruedi T. P. (2015). Chapter 7: Principles of internal fixation. In Court-Brown C. M., Heckman J. D., McQueen M. M., et al. (Eds.), *Rockwood & Green's fractures in adults* (8th ed.). Philadelphia, PA: Lippincott Williams & Wilkins.

21. Paley D., Catagni M., Argnani F., et al. (1992). Treatment of congenital pseudoarthrosis of the tibia using Ilizarov technique. *Clinical Orthopaedics and Related Research, 280*, 81.

22. Garcia R. A., Klein M. J., Achiller A. L. (2012). Chapter 26: Bones and joints. In Rubin, R., Strayer, D.S. (Eds.), *Rubin's pathology: Clinicopathologic foundations of medicine* (6th ed.). Philadelphia, PA: Lippincott Williams & Wilkins.

23. Einhorn T. A. (1998). The cell and molecular biology of fracture healing. *Clinical Orthopaedics and Related Research, 355*(Suppl), S7–S21.

24. Rosenberg A. E. (2010). Chapter 26: Bones, joints, and soft tissue tumors. In Kumar V., Abbas A. K., Fausto N., et al. (Eds.), *Robbins and Cotran pathologic basis of disease* (8th ed.). Philadelphia, PA: Elsevier Saunders.

25. Hayda R. A., Brighton C. T., Esterhai J. L. (1998). Pathophysiology of delayed healing. *Clinical Orthopaedics and Related Research, 355*(Suppl), S31–S40.

26. Peng H., Wright V., Usas A., et al. (2002). Synergistic enhancement of bone formation and healing of stem cell-expressed VECF and bone morphogenetic protein-4. *Journal of Clinical Investigation, 110*, 751–759.

27. Hoover T. J., Siefert J. A. (2000). Soft tissue complications of orthopedic emergencies. *Emergency Medicine Clinics of North America, 18*, 115–139.

28. Edwards S. (2004). Acute compartment syndrome. *Emergency Nursing, 12*(3), 32–38.

29. Kostler W., Strom P. C., Sudkamp N. P. (2004). Acute compartment syndrome of the limb. *Injury, 35*, 1221–1227.

30. McQueen M. M. (2006). Chapter 29: Acute compartment syndrome. Court-Brown C. M., Heckman J. D., McQueen M. M., et al. (Eds.), *Rockwood & Green's fractures in adults* (8th ed.). Philadelphia, PA: Lippincott Williams & Wilkins.

31. Mohler L. R., Styf J. R., Pedowitz R., et al. (1997). Intramuscular deoxygenation during exercise in patients who have chronic anterior compartment syndrome of the leg. *Journal of Bone and Joint Surgery (American Volume), 79*, 844–849.

32. Schwartzman R. (2000). New treatments for reflex sympathetic dystrophy. *New England Journal of Medicine, 343*, 654–656.

33. Rahme E., Dasgupta K., Burman M., et al. (2008). Postdischarge thromboprophylaxis and mortality risk after hip- or knee-replacement surgery. *CMAJ, 178*(12), 1545–1554.

34. Geerts W. H., Pineo G. F., Bergqvist D., et al. (2004). Prevention of venous thromboembolism: The seventh ACCP conference on antithrombotic and thrombolytic therapy. *Chest, 126*, 338S–400S.

35. Dentali F., Douketis J. D., Gianni M., et al. (2007). Meta-analysis: Anticoagulant prophylaxis to prevent symptomatic venous thromboembolism in hospitalized medical patients. *Annals of Internal Medicine, 146*, 278–288.

36. Parisi D. M., Koval K., Egot K. (2002). Fat embolism syndrome. *American Journal of Orthopedics, 31*, 507–512.

37. Richards R. R. (1997). Fat emboli syndrome. *Canadian Journal of Surgery, 40*, 334–339.

38. Mellor A., Soni M. (2001). Fat embolism. *Anaesthesia, 56*, 145–154.

39. Arai F., Kia T., Nakai T., et al. (2007). Histopathologic features of fat embolism in fulminant fat embolism syndrome. *Anesthesiology, 107*, 509–511.

40. Green N. E., Nania J. J. (2005). Chapter 6: Bone and joint infections in children. In Weinstein S. L., Buckwalter J. A. (Eds.), *Turek's orthopedics: Principles and their application* (6th ed.). Philadelphia, PA: Lippincott Williams & Wilkins.

41. Lew D. P., Waldvogel F. A. (2004). Osteomyelitis. *Lancet, 364*, 369–379.

42. Carek P. J., Dickerson L. M., Sack J. L. (2001). Diagnosis and management of osteomyelitis. *American Family Physician, 63*, 2413–2420.

43. Calhoun J. J., Manring M. M. (2005). Adult osteomyelitis. *Infectious Disease Clinics, 19*, 765–786.

44. Bratzle D. W., Houck P. M. (2005). Antimicrobial prophylaxis for surgery: An advisory statement from the National Surgical Infection Prevention Project. *American Journal of Surgery, 189*, 395–404.

45. Taggart T., Kerry R. M., Norman P., et al. (2002). The use of vancomycin-impregnated cement beads in the management of infection in prosthetic joints. *Journal of Bone and Joint Surgery (British Volume), 84*, 70–72.

46. Fisher D., Elwood D. (2014). Chapter 7: Nonrespiratory tuberculosis. In PHAC. *Canadian tuberculosis standards* (7th ed.). Ottawa.

47. Assouline-Dayan Y., Chang C., Greenspan A., et al. (2002). Pathogenesis and history of osteonecrosis. *Seminars in Arthritis and Rheumatism, 32*, 94–124.

48. Canadian Institute for Health Information. (2014). *Hip and knee replacements in Canada: Canadian Joint Replacement Registry (CJRR) 2014 annual report*. Ottawa: CIHI.

49. Childs S. G. (2005). Osteonecrosis: Death of bone cells. *Orthopedic Nursing, 24*, 295–301.

50. Johnson E. O., Soultanis K., Soucacos P. N. (2004). Vascular anatomy and microcirculation of skeletal zones vulnerable to osteonecrosis: Vascularization of the femoral head. *Orthopedic Clinics of North America, 35*, 285–291.

51. Migliorati C. A., Siegel M. A., Elting L. S. (2006). Bisphosphonate-associated osteonecrosis: A long-term complication of bisphosphonate treatment. *Lancet Oncology, 7*, 508–514.

52. Reis N. O., Schwartz D., Miltianu D., et al. (2003). Hyperbaric oxygen therapy as a treatment for stage I avascular necrosis of the femoral head. *Journal of Bone and Joint Surgery (British Volume), 85*, 371–375.

53. American Cancer Society. (2015). Bone cancer. Available online at: http://www.cancer.org/cancer/bonecancer/index. Accessed May 26, 2015.

54. Canadian Cancer Society. (2015). Bone cancer. Available online at: http://www.cancer.ca/en/cancer-information/cancer-type/bone/bone-cancer/?region=on. Accessed May 26, 2015.

55. Arndt C. A. (2011). Chapter 495: Neoplasms of bone. In Kliegman R. M., Stanton B. F., St. Geme J. W., et al. (Eds.), *Nelson textbook of pediatrics* (19th ed.). Philadelphia, PA: Saunders Elsevier.

56. Hayden J. B., Hoang B. H. (2006). Osteosarcoma: Basic science and implications. *Orthopedic Clinics of North America, 37*, 1–7.

57. Mankin H. J., Hornicek F. J., Rosenberg A. E., et al. (2004). Survival data for 648 patients with osteosarcoma treated at one institution. *Clinical Orthopaedics and Related Research, 429*, 286–291.

58. Matthews E., Snell K., Coats H. (2006). Intra-arterial chemotherapy for limb preservation in patients with osteosarcoma: Nursing implications. *Clinical Journal of Oncology Nursing, 10*, 581–589.

59. Longhi A., Setola E., Versari M., et al. (2005). The role of chemotherapy in the treatment of bone and soft tissue sarcomas. *Current Orthopaedics, 19*, 119–126.

60. Grimer R. J., Taminiau A. M., Cannon S. R. (2002). Surgical outcomes in osteosarcoma. *Journal of Bone and Joint Surgery (British Volume), 84*, 395–400.

61. Roodman G. D. (2004). Mechanisms of bone metastasis. *The New England Journal of Medicine, 350*, 1655–1664.

62. O'Keefe R. J., Schwartz E. M., Boyce B. F. (2000). Bone metastasis: An update on bone resorption and therapeutic strategies. *Current Opinion in Orthopedics, 11*, 353–359.

63. Juan J., Pollock C. B., Kelly K. (2005). Mechanisms of cancer metastasis to the bone. *Cell Research, 15*, 57–62.

64. Hershey M. S. (2004). Toward new horizons: The future of bisphosphonate therapy. *The Oncologist, 9*(Suppl 4), 38–47.

Visit the Point₊ **http://thePoint.lww.com for animations, journal articles, and more!**

Disorders of Musculoskeletal Function: Developmental and Metabolic Disorders

58

The development of skeletal structures begins in utero and continues to change throughout life. During childhood, skeletal structures grow in length and diameter and sustain a large increase in bone mass. The term modelling refers to the formation of the macroscopic skeleton, which ceases at maturity, usually between 18 and 20 years of age. Once skeletal growth has attained its adult size, the process of bone remodelling is responsible for skeletal maintenance. It involves bone resorption and formation and is responsible for skeletal maintenance at sites that require replacement or repair. With aging, bone resorption and formation are no longer perfectly coupled, and there is loss of bone.

Skeletal disorders may develop as a result of abnormal growth and developmental processes that are due to hereditary or congenital influences. Other skeletal disorders can occur later in life as a result of nutritional deficiencies, metabolic disorders, hormonal influences, or the aging process. This chapter is divided into two parts: the first part focuses on alterations in skeletal growth and development, and the second on metabolic bone disorders.

ALTERATIONS IN SKELETAL GROWTH AND DEVELOPMENT

After completing this section of the chapter, you should be able to meet the following objectives:

- Describe the function of the epiphyseal growth plate in skeletal growth.
- Describe common torsional deformities that occur in infants and small children, proposed mechanisms of development, diagnostic methods, and treatment.
- Define genu varum and genu valgum.
- List the problems that occur because of defective tissue synthesis in osteogenesis imperfecta.
- Characterize the abnormalities associated with developmental dysplasia of the hip and methods of diagnosis and treatment.
- Describe the treatment for a newborn with clubfoot.
- Define the term *osteochondroses* and describe the pathology and symptomatology of Legg–Calvé–Perthes disease and Osgood–Schlatter disease.

- Describe the pathology associated with a slipped capital femoral epiphysis and explain why early treatment is important.
- Differentiate between congenital, idiopathic, and neuromuscular scoliosis.

Bone Growth and Remodelling

Embryonic and Fetal Development

The skeletal system develops from the mesodermal and neural crest cells of the developing embryo[1] (see Chapter 48). Development of the vertebrae of the axial skeleton begins at approximately the fourth week in the embryo; during the ninth week, ossification begins with the appearance of ossification centres in the lower thoracic and upper lumbar vertebrae. The paddle-shaped limb buds of the lower extremities make their appearance late in the fourth week of development; the hand pads are developed by days 33 to 36; and the finger rays are evident on days 41 to 43.[1]

Abnormalities originating from the embryonic stage of development are relatively uncommon. When they do occur, they are usually limited to defined embryonic structures (*e.g.*, congenital absence of a phalanx; formation of extra bones [supernumerary digits], or fusion of adjacent digits [syndactylism]). The more common problems are caused by in utero positioning during fetal development. In the newborn, the imprint of in utero positioning may be evident and confused with an abnormality (to be discussed). The effects of in utero positioning are usually physiologic in origin, rather than anatomic. A child may be 3 to 4 years of age before the effects of in utero positioning resolve.

Bone Growth in Childhood

During the first two decades of life, the skeleton undergoes general overall growth. The long bones of the skeleton, which grow at a relatively rapid rate, are provided with a specialized structure called the *epiphyseal growth plate*. As long bones grow in length, the deeper layers of cartilage cells in the growth plate multiply and enlarge, pushing the articular cartilage farther away from the metaphysis and diaphysis of the bone.[2–4] As this occurs, the mature and enlarged cartilage cells at the metaphyseal end of the plate become metabolically inactive and are replaced by bone cells (Fig. 58.1). This process allows bone growth to proceed without changing the shape of the bone or causing disruption of the articular cartilage. The cells in the growth plate stop dividing at puberty, at which time the epiphysis and metaphysis fuse.

Several factors can influence the growth of cells in the epiphyseal growth plate. Epiphyseal separation can occur in children as the result of trauma. The separation usually occurs

FIGURE 58.1 • Anatomy of long bone. **A:** Diagram of femur illustrating the various compartments. **B:** Coronal section of the proximal femur illustrates the various anatomic parts of a long bone. The epiphysis of the femoral head and the apophysis of the greater trochanter are separated from the metaphysis by their respective growth plates. The cortex and medullary cavity are well visualized. The medullary cavity contains cancellous bone until the metaphysis narrows into the diaphysis (shaft) of the bone, at which point the medullary cavity is completely devoid of bone and filled with marrow. **C:** A section of the epiphysis with a zone of proliferating cartilage cells. Beneath this zone, the hypertrophic cartilage cells are arranged in columns. At the bottom, the calcifying matrix is invaded by blood vessels. E, epiphysis; PC, proliferative cartilage; HC, hypertrophic cartilage; V, vascular invasion; CC, calcified cartilage. (From Rubin R., Strayer D. S. (Eds.) (2012). *Rubin's pathology: Clinicopathologic foundations of medicine* (6th ed., p. 1202). Philadelphia, PA: Lippincott Williams & Wilkins.)

in the zone of the mature enlarged cartilage cells, which is the weakest part of the growth plate. The blood vessels that nourish the epiphysis pass through the growth plate. These vessels are ruptured when the growth plate separates. This can cause cessation of growth and a shortened extremity. The growth plate also is sensitive to nutritional and metabolic changes. Scurvy (*i.e.,* vitamin C deficiency) impairs the formation of the organic matrix of bone, causing slowing of growth at the epiphyseal plate and cessation of diaphyseal growth. In rickets (*i.e.,* vitamin D deficiency), calcification of the newly developed bone on the metaphyseal side of the growth plate is impaired. Thyroid and growth hormones are required for normal growth. Alterations in these and other hormones can also affect growth (see Chapter 41). A few years after reaching puberty, the epiphyseal plates in the long bones become increasingly less responsive and eventually totally unresponsive to the hormones.[3] Generally, young adults reach the end of bone growth by the age of 20 as the epiphyseal plate closes. However, some bones remain responsive to hormones and continue to grow, such as skull, finger, feet, and jaw.[3]

Growth in the diameter of bones occurs as new bone is added to the outer surface of existing bone along with an accompanying resorption of bone on the endosteal or inner surface. Such oppositional growth allows for widening of the marrow cavity while preventing the cortex from becoming too thick and heavy. In this way, the shape of the bone is maintained. As a bone grows in diameter, concentric rings are added to the bone surface, much as rings are added to a tree trunk; these rings form the lamellar structure of mature bone. Osteocytes, which develop from osteoblasts, become buried in the rings. Haversian channels form as periosteal vessels running along the long axis become surrounded by bone (see Chapter 56, Fig. 56.3).

Alterations During Normal Growth Periods

Infants and children undergo changes in muscle tone and joint motion during growth and development. Toeing-in, toeing-out, bowlegs, and knock-knees occur frequently in infancy and childhood.[5] They usually cause few problems and are corrected during normal growth processes. The normal folded position of the fetus in utero causes physiologic flexion contractures of the hips and an inward rotation of the lower extremities[6] (Fig. 58.2). The hips are externally rotated and the patellae point outward, whereas the feet appear to point forward because of the internal pulling force of the tibiae. During the first year of life, the lower extremities begin to straighten out in preparation for walking. Internal and external rotations become equal, and the hips extend.

Musculoskeletal assessment of the newborn is important to identify abnormalities that require early intervention, facilitate treatment, establish baselines for future reference, and educate and counsel parents.[6–9] There are many clinical deviations that are easily correctable in a newborn. Many others correct spontaneously as the child grows.

FIGURE 58.2 • Position of fetus in utero, with tibial bowing and legs folded. (From Dunne K. B., Clarren S. K. (1986). The origin of prenatal and postnatal deformities. *Pediatric Clinics of North America, 33,* 1282; with permission from Elsevier Science.)

Torsional Deformities

All infants and toddlers have lax ligaments that become tighter with age and assumption of the weight-bearing posture. The hypermobility that accompanies joint laxity, coupled with the torsional (*i.e.,* rotational) forces exerted on the limbs during growth, is responsible for a number of variants seen in young children. Torsional forces caused by intrauterine positions or sleeping and sitting patterns twist the growing bones and can produce the deformities as a child grows and develops.

In infants, the femur normally is rotated to an anteverted position, with the femoral head and neck rotated anteriorly with respect to the femoral condyles. Femoral anteversion (*i.e.,* medial rotation) decreases from approximately 40 degrees at birth to approximately 15 degrees at maturity (Fig. 58.3). The normal tibia is externally rotated approximately 5 degrees at

DEVELOPMENTAL SKELETAL DISORDERS

- Many disorders of early infancy are caused by intrauterine positions and resolve as the child grows.
- All infants and toddlers have lax ligaments that predispose them to skeletal disorders caused by twisting or torsional forces.
- Bone growth in infants and children occurs at the epiphysis. Separation of the epiphyseal growth plate ruptures the blood vessels that nourish the epiphysis, causing cessation of growth and shortened extremity length.
- Nutritional and metabolic disorders can impair the formation of the organic matrix of bone, causing slowing of growth at the epiphyseal plate.

FIGURE 58.3 • Femoral anteversion and internal tibial rotation. Femoral anteversion normally decreases from about 40 degrees at birth to 15 degrees at maturity, and internal tibial rotation from 5 degrees at birth to 15 degrees at maturity.

birth and 15 degrees at maturity. Torsional abnormalities frequently demonstrate a familial tendency.

Toeing-in and Toeing-out. The foot progression angle describes the angle between the axis of the foot and the line of progression. It is determined by watching the child walking and running, although it is usually less noticeable when the child is running or barefoot. Figure 58.4 illustrates the position of the foot in toeing-in and toeing-out, and the line of progression, when a child is walking.

Toeing-in (*i.e.,* metatarsus adductus) is the most common congenital foot deformity, with an incidence of approximately 1 to 2 per 1,000, and it affects boys and girls equally.[7,8] The forefoot commonly is adducted and gives the foot a kidney-shaped appearance, whereas the hindfoot is normal[6–9] (Fig. 58.5). It can be caused by torsion in the foot, lower leg, or entire leg. Toeing-in due to adduction of the forefoot (*i.e.,* congenital metatarsus adductus) usually is the result of the fetal position maintained in utero. It may occur in one foot or both feet. Diagnostic methods include examination of the plantar aspect of the foot, noting the overall shape of the foot and the presence or absence of an arch. The presence of a skin crease indicates a congenital deformity (Fig. 58.5). Metatarsus adductus is graded based on the foot's flexibility while applying pressure to the medial forefoot. The defect is defined as grade I, grade II, or grade III. Grade I is a supple deformity that can be passively manipulated into a straight position and

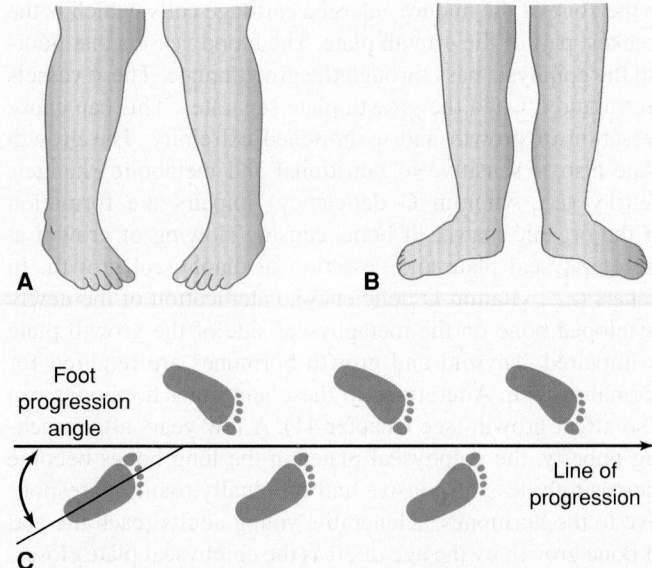

FIGURE 58.4 • **A:** Toeing-in. **B:** Toeing-out. **C:** Toeing-in and toeing-out can be determined by watching a child walk and comparing the long axis of the foot with the direction in which the child is walking. If the foot is directed inward, the angle is negative and indicative of toeing-in; if it is positive, it is indicative of toeing-out.

requires no treatment. A grade II deformity corrects only to a straight lateral border, and a grade III deformity is more rigid and may require further treatment.[6] Treatment consisting of serial long leg casting or a brace that pushes the metatarsals (not the hindfoot) into abduction usually is required in a fixed (rigid) deformity (*i.e.,* one in which the forefoot cannot be passively manipulated into a straight position).

Toeing-out is a common problem in children and is caused by external femoral torsion. This occurs when the femur can be externally rotated to approximately 90 degrees but internally rotated only to a neutral position or slightly beyond. Because the femoral torsion persists when a child habitually sleeps in the prone position, an external tibial torsion also may develop. If external tibial torsion is present, the feet point lateral to the midline of the medial plane. External tibial torsion rarely causes toeing-out; it only intensifies the condition. Toeing-out usually corrects itself as the child becomes proficient in walking. Occasionally, a night splint is used.

FIGURE 58.5 • Shape of foot. The left foot is normal, whereas the right foot has metatarsus adductus.

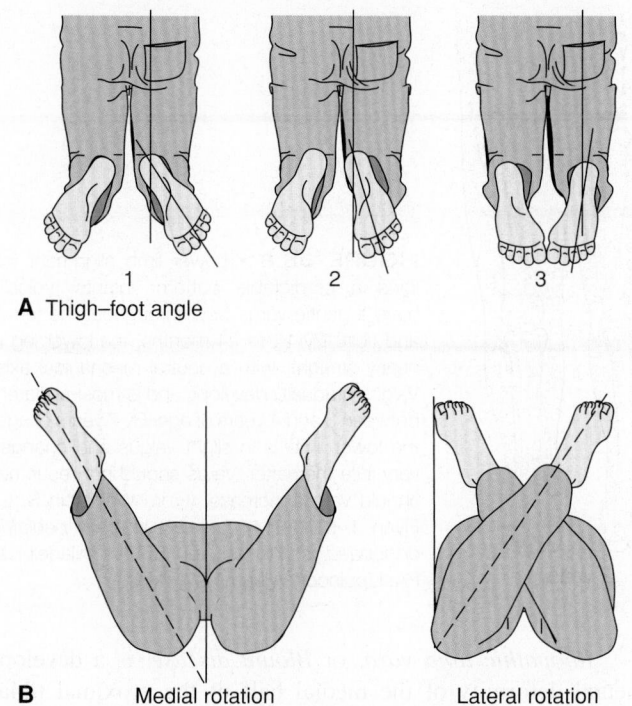

A Thigh–foot angle

B   Medial rotation   Lateral rotation

FIGURE 58.6 • **A:** Assessment for tibial torsion using thigh–foot angle. When the child is in the prone position with the knee flexed, with normal alignment there is slight external rotation (2); internal tibial torsion produces inward rotation (3); external tibial torsion produces outward rotation (1). **B:** Hip rotation is measured with the child prone and knees flexed at a 90-degree angle. On outward rotation the leg produces internal (medial) hip and femoral rotation; on inward rotation the leg produces external hip and femoral rotation. (Adapted from Staheli L. T. (1986). Torsional deformity. *Pediatric Clinics of North America, 33,* 1378; and Kliegman R. M., Greenbaum L. A., Lye P. S. (Eds.). (2004). *Practical strategies in pediatric diagnosis and therapy* (2nd ed.). Philadelphia, PA: W.B. Saunders.)

Tibial Torsion. Tibial torsion is determined by measuring the thigh–foot angle, which is done with the ankle and knee positioned at 90 degrees (Fig. 58.6). In this position, the foot normally rotates outward. *Internal tibial torsion (i.e.,* bowing of the tibia) is a rotation of the tibia that makes the feet appear to turn inward (Fig. 58.3). It is the most common cause of toeing-in in children younger than 2 years of age.[6] It is present at birth and may fail to correct itself if children sleep on their knees with the feet turned in, or sit on in-turned feet. It is thought to be caused by genetic factors and intrauterine compression, such as an unstretched uterus during a first pregnancy or intrauterine crowding with twins or multiple fetuses. Tibial torsion improves naturally with growth, but this may take years.[7]

External tibial torsion, a much less common disorder, is associated with calcaneovalgus foot and is caused by a normal variation of intrauterine positioning or a neuromuscular disorder. It is characterized by an abnormally positive thigh–foot angle of 30 to 50 degrees.[6] The condition corrects itself naturally, and treatment is observational. Significant improvement begins during the first year with the onset of ambulation, and usually is complete by 2 to 3 years of age.[6] The normal adult exhibits about 20 degrees of tibial torsion.

Femoral Torsion. *Femoral torsion* refers to abnormal variations in hip rotation. Hip rotation is measured at the pelvic level with the child in the prone position and the knees flexed at a 90-degree angle. In this position, the hip is in a neutral position. Rotating the lower leg outward produces internal or medial femoral rotation; rotating it inward produces external or lateral rotation. During measurement of hip rotation, the legs are allowed to fall to full internal rotation by gravity alone; lateral rotation is measured by allowing the legs to fall inward and cross. Hip rotation in flexion and extension also can be measured with computed tomography (CT). By 1 year of age, there is normally approximately 45 degrees of internal rotation and 45 degrees of external rotation.[6]

Internal femoral torsion, also called *femoral anteversion* (Fig. 58.3), is a normal variant commonly seen during the first 6 years of life, especially in 3- and 4-year-old girls.[5] Characteristically, there is 80 to 90 degrees of internal rotation of the hip in the prone position.[7] The condition is thought to be related to increased laxity of the anterior capsule of the hip such that it does not provide the stable pressure needed to correct the anteversion that is present at birth. Children are most comfortable sitting in the "W" position, with their hips between their knees (Fig. 58.7). It is believed that this position allows the lower leg to act as a lever, producing torsional changes in the femur. When the child stands, the knees turn in and the feet appear to point straight ahead; when the child walks, the knees and toes point in. Children with this problem are encouraged to sit cross-legged or in the so-called *tailor position.* If left untreated, the tibiae compensate by becoming externally rotated, so that by 8 to 12 years of age, the knees may turn in but the feet no longer do so. This can result in patellofemoral malalignment with patellar subluxation or dislocation and pain.[10] A derotational osteotomy may be done in severe cases or if there is functional disability.

FIGURE 58.7 • Typical sitting position of child with femoral anteversion. (Adapted from Staheli L. T. (1986). Torsional deformity. *Pediatric Clinics of North America, 33,* 1382.)

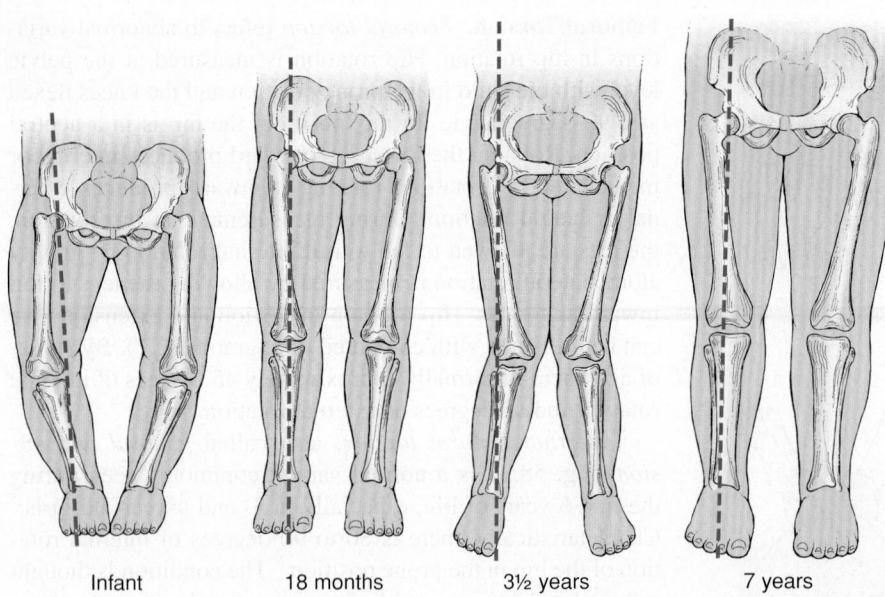

Infant   18 months   3½ years   7 years

FIGURE 58.8 • Lower limb alignment follows a predictable pattern. Infants typically have a gentle varus bow throughout the femur and tibia. By 18 to 24 months, the lower leg is nearly straight, with a neutral mechanical axis. Valgus gradually develops and is most apparent between 3 and 4 years of age. By 7 years of age, the lower limb is in slight valgus and changes very little thereafter. Varus should not recur, nor should valgus increase. (From Weinstein S. L., Flynn J. M. (2014). *Lovell & Winter's pediatric orthopaedics* (7th ed., p. 1277). Philadelphia, PA: Lippincott Williams & Wilkins.)

External femoral torsion is an uncommon disorder characterized by excessive external rotation of the hip. Bilateral external torsion is usually a benign condition, and treatment is observational. When the disorder is unilateral, slipped capital femoral epiphysis should be excluded, particularly if the condition occurs in an obese child or young adolescent[6] (discussed later).

Genu Varum and Genu Valgum

Genu varum, or *bowlegs,* is an outward bowing of the knees greater than 1 inch when the medial malleoli of the ankles are touching. As children grow, lower limb alignment usually follows a predicable pattern (Fig. 58.8). Most infants and toddlers have some bowing of their legs up to 18 months of age. If there is a large separation between the knees (>15 degrees) after 2 years of age, the child may require bracing. The child also should be evaluated for diseases such as rickets or tibia vara (*i.e.,* Blount disease).[10]

Genu valgum, or *"knock-knees,"* is a deformity in which there is decreased space between the knees. The medial malleoli in the ankles cannot be brought in contact with each other when the knees are touching. Valgus gradually develops after age 24 months and is most apparent between 3 and 4 years of age (Fig. 58.8). The condition usually is the result of lax medial collateral ligaments of the knee and may be exacerbated by sitting in the "W" position and by obesity. By 7 years of age, the lower limb is in slight valgus and changes very little thereafter. Genu valgum can be ignored up to 7 years of age, unless it is more than 15 degrees, unilateral, or associated with short stature. It usually resolves spontaneously and rarely requires treatment. If genu varum or genu valgum persists and is uncorrected, osteoarthritis may develop in adulthood as a result of abnormal intra-articular stress. Genu varum can cause gait awkwardness and increased risk for sprains and fractures. Uncorrected genu valgum may cause subluxation and recurrent dislocation of the patella, with a predisposition to chondromalacia and joint pain and fatigue.

Idiopathic tibia vara, or *Blount disease,* is a developmental deformity of the medial half of the proximal tibial epiphysis that results in a progressive varus angulation below the knee[7,10,11] (Fig. 58.9). Onset can occur early in infancy, or later, during adolescence.[10,11] Untreated infantile tibia vera is almost always progressive, with evidence of outward angulation, flexion, internal rotation, and abnormal lateral knee laxity. There is radiographic evidence of progressive depression of the medial metaphysis, the growth plate, and the epiphysis. Fusion of the metaphysis to the epiphysis may occur in severe cases. Night-brace treatment is used for mild early-onset disease. Valgus rotational osteotomy of the tibia is usually indicated if angulation persists beyond 3 years of age. Persistent tibia vara leads to early degenerative changes of the knee.

FIGURE 58.9 • Rotational deformity of the proximal tibia, especially when unilateral, suggests tibia vera (Blount disease).

Adolescent Blount disease occurs in the second decade of life, is seen in persons who are above the 95th percentile in height and weight, and is usually unilateral.[7] It is the most common cause of pathologic genu varum and is seen in obese boys.[10] Radiography shows medial femoral and tibial bowing. Bracing is not practical in obese adolescents. Treatment includes osteotomy to realign the limb or lateral growth plate closure to allow growth to "catch up" medially.

Flatfoot

Flatfoot (*i.e.,* pes planus) is a deformity characterized by the absence of the longitudinal arch of the foot. Infants normally have a wider and fatter foot than adults. The fat pads that normally are accentuated by pliable muscles create an illusion of fullness often mistaken for a flatfoot. Until the longitudinal arch develops at 2 to 3 years of age, all children have flat feet. The true criterion for flatfoot is that the head of the talus points medially and downward, so that the heel is everted and the forefoot must be inverted (toed-in) for the metatarsal heads to be planted equally on the ground. Weight bearing may cause pain in the longitudinal arch and up the leg.

There are two types of flatfoot—flexible and rigid. Most children with flexible (or supple) flatfoot have loose ligaments, allowing the feet to sag when they gain weight. In supple flatfoot, the arch disappears only with weight bearing. No special treatment is needed for flexible flatfoot.[6] People with flexible flatfoot are less prone to pain and injury than those with normal or high arches. The rigid flatfoot is fixed with no apparent arch in any position. It is seen in conjunction with congenitally tight heel cords, neuromuscular diseases such as cerebral palsy, or juvenile rheumatoid arthritis.[6]

In the adult, treatment of flatfoot is conservative and aimed at relieving fatigue, pain, and tenderness. Supportive, well-fitting shoes with arch supports may be helpful and prevent ligaments from becoming overstretched. Women may complain of pain in the forefoot when wearing poorly fitting high heels. Surgery may be done in cases of severe and persistent symptoms.

Hereditary and Congenital Deformities

Congenital deformities are abnormalities that are present at birth. They range in severity from mild limb deformities, which are relatively common, to major limb malformations, which are relatively rare. However, there was an epidemic of limb deformities that occurred from 1957 to 1962 as a result of maternal ingestion of thalidomide. The most common anomaly of the toes or fingers is *polydactyly* or the presence of an extra digit on the hand or foot. Macrodactyly occurs when one or more toes or fingers are hypertrophied and are significantly larger than the surrounding toes or fingers.

There may also be a simple webbing of the fingers or toes (syndactyly), or the absence of a bone such as the phalanx, rib, or clavicle. Joint contractures and dislocations produce more severe deformity, as does the absence of entire bones, joints, or limbs. Surgery is done to relieve functional symptoms, such as pain or difficulty in fitting shoes. The cosmetic goal is to alter the grotesque appearance of the hand or foot and to achieve a similar size to the opposite extremity.

Congenital deformities are caused by many factors, some unknown. These factors include hereditary influences, external agents that injure the fetus (*e.g.,* radiation, alcohol, drugs, viruses), and intrauterine environmental factors. Many of the organic bone matrix components have been identified only recently, and their interactions were found to be more complex than originally thought. Hereditary disorders associated with abnormalities in bone matrix include those with deficient collagen synthesis and decreased bone mass.

Osteogenesis Imperfecta

Osteogenesis imperfecta is a hereditary disease characterized by defective synthesis of or interaction with type I collagen.[4,12–14] It is one of the most common hereditary bone diseases, with an occurrence rate of approximately 1 case in 15,000 to 20,000 births.[12] Although it usually is transmitted as an autosomal dominant trait, a distinct form of the disorder with multiple lethal defects is thought to be inherited as an autosomal recessive trait.[14] Mutations in the genes connected with type I collagen, which impacts the development of bones, joints, ears, ligaments, teeth, sclerae, and skin, cause the problems. Specifically, mutations in *COL1A1* and *COL1A2* genes, which encode for the structure, modification, folding and/or quantity of type I procollagen, cause different structural changes in the types of OI.[12] In some cases, the defect is caused by a spontaneous mutation.

The clinical manifestations of osteogenesis imperfecta include a spectrum of disorders marked by extreme skeletal fragility. While nine subtypes have now been identified, the four more common major subtypes are outlined in Table 58.1[4,12–14] The disorder is characterized by thin and poorly developed bones that are prone to multiple fractures. These children have short limbs and a soft, thin cranium with bifrontal prominences that give a triangular appearance to the face. Other problems associated with defective connective tissue synthesis include thin skin, blue or grey sclera, abnormal tooth development, hypotonic muscles, loose-jointedness, and scoliosis. Hearing loss due to otosclerosis of the tiny bones in the middle ear is common in affected adults.

The most serious defects occur when the disorder is inherited as a recessive trait (type II). Severely affected fetuses have multiple intrauterine fractures and bowing and shortening of the extremities. Many of these infants are stillborn or die during infancy. Less severe forms occur when the disorder is inherited as a dominant trait. The skeletal system is not as weakened, and fractures often do not appear until the child becomes active and starts to walk, or even later in childhood. These fractures heal rapidly, although with a poor-quality callus. In some cases, parents may be suspected of child abuse when the child is admitted to the healthcare facility with multiple fractures. There also is an increased incidence of complications such as hernias and congenital heart abnormalities.

There is no definitive treatment for correction of the defective collagen synthesis that is characteristic of osteogenesis

TABLE 58.1 TYPES OF OSTEOGENESIS IMPERFECTA

TYPE	SUBTYPE	INHERITANCE	MAJOR FEATURES
I	Postnatal fractures, blue sclera	Autosomal dominant	Normal stature, skeletal fragility, hearing impairment, joint laxity, blue sclera
II	Perinatal, lethal	Autosomal recessive	Death in utero, or in days after birth. Skeletal deformity with excessive fragility, multiple fractures, blue sclera
III	Progressive deformity	Autosomal dominant (75%) Autosomal recessive (25%)	Growth retardation, multiple fractures, progressive kyphoscoliosis, hearing impairment, blue sclera at birth
IV	Postnatal fractures, normal sclera	Autosomal dominant	Moderate skeletal fragility, short stature

Developed from Kumar V., Abbas A. K., Faustos N., et al. (Eds). (2010). *Robbins and Cotran pathologic basis of disease* (8th ed., 1212). Philadelphia, PA: Elsevier Saunders.

imperfecta. However, the bisphosphonates (*e.g.*, pamidronate) have been shown to produce an increase in cortical bone width and cancellous bone volume, as well as increased bone strength and mineral content.[12,13,15] Prevention and treatment of fractures are important. Precise alignment is necessary to prevent deformities. Nonunion is common, especially with repeated fractures. Surgical intervention often is needed to stabilize fractures and correct deformities (*e.g.*, internal fixation of long bones may be done with an intramedullary rod that "grows" with the child).

Developmental Dysplasia of the Hip

Developmental dysplasia of the hip (DDH), formerly known as *congenital dislocation of the hip,* is an abnormality in hip development that leads to a wide spectrum of hip problems in infants and children, including hips that are unstable, malformed, subluxated, or dislocated.[6,16–18] In less severe cases, the hip joint may be unstable, with excessive laxity of the joint capsule, or subluxated, so that the joint surfaces are separated and there is a partial dislocation (Fig. 58.10). With dislocated hips, the head of the femur is located outside of the acetabulum.

Specific information is not available for Canada with regard to the incidence of hip instability, dislocation, or dysplasia in newborns.[16] It is generally known that the left hip is involved more frequently than the right hip because of the left occipital

intrauterine positioning of most infants.[10,16] The disorder occurs most frequently in first-born children and is six times more common in female than in male infants.[6] The cause of DDH is multifactorial, with heredity, environmental, and mechanical factors playing a role. A positive family history and generalized laxity of the ligaments are related. The increased frequency in girls is thought to result from their susceptibility to maternal estrogens and other hormones associated with pelvic relaxation. Dislocation also may result from environmental factors such as fetal position, a tight uterus that prevents fetal movement, and breech delivery. Approximately 16% to 25% of children with DDH have a history of breech presentation.[6] The presence of other congenital abnormalities is associated with an increased incidence of DDH. Thus, the hips of children presenting with congenital abnormalities should be examined carefully.

Early diagnosis of DDH is important because treatment is easiest and most effective if begun during the first 6 months of life. Also, repeated dislocations cause damage to the femoral head and the acetabulum. There is no uniformly accepted method for diagnosis of DDH during the newborn period, although clinical examination of the hips is recommended at birth and every several months during the first year of life; additional screening may be done for females born in the breech position or infants with a family history.[16–18] Follow-up clinical examinations should be done in the presence of abnormality. In infants, signs of DDH include asymmetry of the hip or gluteal folds, shortening of the thigh so that one knee (on the affected side) is higher than the other hip, and limited abduction of the affected hip (Fig. 58.11). The asymmetry of gluteal folds is not definitive but indicates the need for further evaluation. The Preventive Health Care update concluded that serial clinical examination for all infants should be done but the evidence was insufficient to recommend additional screening of asymptomatic infants as a means of preventing adverse outcomes.[18]

Several examination techniques can be used to screen for a dislocatable hip.[16] Two specific manoeuvres for assessing hip stability in the newborn are the Ortolani manoeuvre (for reducible dislocation) and the Barlow manoeuvre (for the dislocatable hip)[10,16–18] (Fig. 58.12). The Barlow manoeuvre involves a

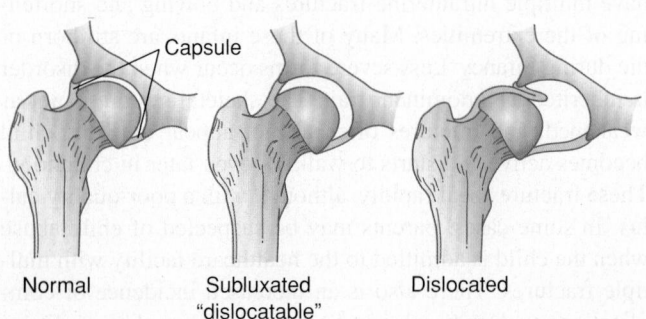

FIGURE 58.10 • Normal (**left**) and abnormal relationships of hip joint structure in subluxation (**middle**) and dislocation (**right**).

Capsule

Normal   Subluxated   Dislocated
                "dislocatable"

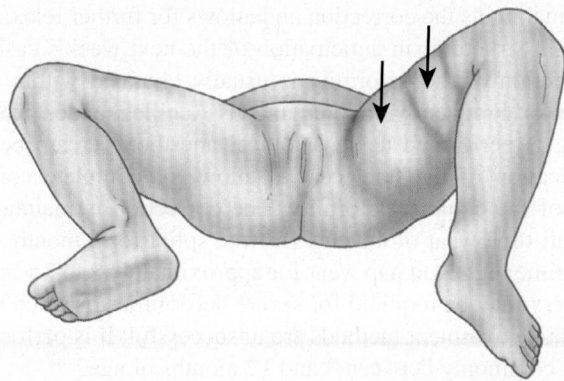

FIGURE 58.11 • Congenital dysplasia of the left hip with shortening of the femur, as indicated by legs in abduction and asymmetric gluteal and thigh folds (*arrows*).

manual attempt to dislocate and reduce the abnormal hip while the infant is in the supine position with both knees flexed. With gentle downward pressure being applied to the knees, the knee and thigh are manually abducted as an upward and medial pressure is applied to the proximal thigh. In infants with the

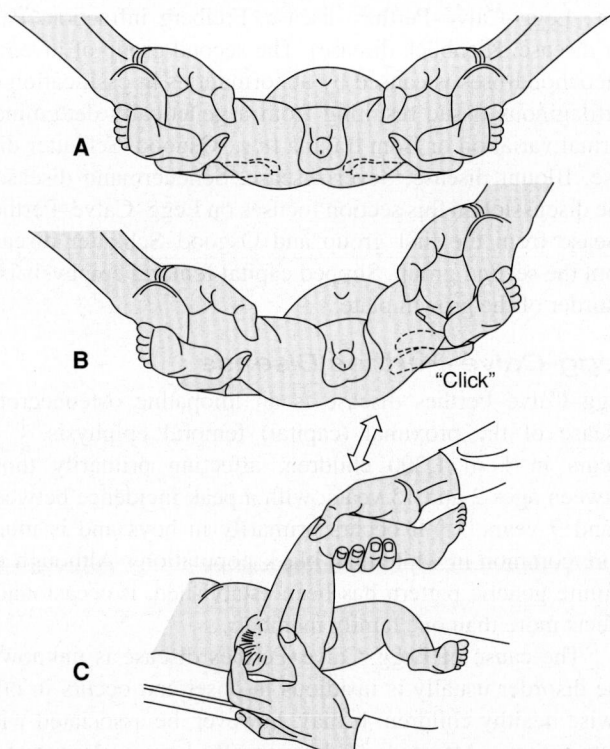

FIGURE 58.12 • Manoeuvres for assessing hip stability in the newborn. **A:** In the newborn, both hips can be equally flexed, abducted and externally rotated without producing a "click." **B:** In the Barlow manoeuvre, which assesses for dislocation of a nondisplaced hip, the examiner adducts and gently pushes the thigh posteriorly in an attempt to dislocate the femoral head. In a positive test the hip will be felt to slide out of the acetabulum. **C:** In the Ortolani manoeuvre for the dislocated hip, the examiner holds the infant's thigh and gently abducts the hip while lifting the greater trochanter with two fingers. When the test is positive, the dislocated hip will fall back into the acetabulum with a "click" as the hip is abducted.

disorder, the initial downward pressure on the knee produces a dislocation of the hip, a positive Barlow sign. This is followed by a palpable or audible click (*i.e.,* Ortolani sign) as the hip is reduced and moves back into the acetabulum. The sensitivity of these tests is improved significantly with the use of trained and experienced examiners. The Galeazzi test is a measurement of the length of the femurs that is done by comparing the height at the knees while they are flexed at 90 degrees. An inequality in the height of the knees is a positive Galeazzi sign and is usually caused by hip dislocation or congenital femoral shortening. This test is not useful in detecting bilateral DDH because both leg lengths will be equal. In an older child, instability of the hip may produce a delay in standing or walking and eventually cause a characteristic waddling gait. When the thumbs are placed over the anterior iliac crest and the hands are placed over the lateral pelvis in examination, the levels of the thumbs are not even; the child is unable to elevate the opposite side of the pelvis (positive Trendelenburg test).

Diagnosis of DDH is confirmed by ultrasonography or radiography. Ultrasonography is used in infants with high risk factors (*e.g.,* female infants born in the breech position) or any abnormal result on examination.[10,16,17] Radiographs of newborns with suspected DDH are of limited value because the femoral heads do not ossify until 4 to 6 months of age. After 6 months of age, the increasing ossification of the femur renders ultrasonography less reliable, and radiographs are preferred.

Treatment of a DDH should be individualized and depends on whether the hip is subluxated or dislocated. Subluxation of the hip at birth often resolves without treatment and should be observed for 2 weeks. When subluxation persists beyond this time, treatment may be indicated and referral is recommended. The best results are obtained if the treatment is begun before changes in the hip structure (*e.g.,* 2 to 3 months) prevent it from being reduced by gentle manipulation or abduction devices. The Pavlik harness is used on newborns (up to 6 months) to maintain the femoral head in the acetabulum.[10,16] The harness allows the child more mobility as the leg is slowly and gently brought into abduction. Infants with dislocated hips caused by anatomic changes and toddlers who lack development of the acetabular socket require more aggressive treatment, such as open reduction and joint reconstruction. Treatment at any age includes reduction of the dislocation and immobilization of the legs in an abducted position. The most serious complication of any treatment is avascular necrosis of the femoral head as a result of the forced abduction.[16] This most often occurs as a complication of a closed or open reduction in an older child. In addition, hyperflexion has the potential to cause femoral nerve palsies. With children younger than 3 years of age, skin traction is used when reduction cannot be easily obtained. This treatment is followed by several months of immobilization in a hip spica cast, plaster splints, or an abduction splint such as an Ilfeld splint. Older children or adults with an unreduced dislocatable hip may require hip surgery because of damage to the articulating surface of the joint. These persons have considerable problems after surgery because of soft tissue contractures.

Congenital Clubfoot

Clubfoot, or talipes, is one of the most common pediatric orthopedic conditions. It has an incidence of approximately 1 to 4 cases per 1,000 live births, is bilateral in about 50% of cases, and affects boys more often than girls.[6,19–22] Like congenital dislocation of the hip, its occurrence follows a multifactorial inheritance pattern. Clubfoot may be associated with chromosomal abnormalities or congenital syndromes that are transmitted by mendelian inheritance patterns. However, it is most commonly idiopathic and found in normal infants in whom no genetic or chromosomal abnormality or other extrinsic cause can be found.

In forefoot adduction, which accounts for approximately 95% of idiopathic cases, the foot is plantar flexed and inverted. This is the so-called *equinovarus type* in which the foot resembles a horse's hoof (Fig. 58.13). The other 5% of cases are of the calcaneovalgus type, or reverse clubfoot, in which the foot is dorsiflexed and everted. The reverse clubfoot can occur as an isolated condition or in association with multiple congenital defects. At birth, the feet of many infants assume one of these two positions, but they can be passively overcorrected or brought back into the opposite position. If the foot cannot be overcorrected, some type of correction may be necessary.

Treatment of clubfoot is begun as soon as the diagnosis is made. When treatment is initiated during the first few weeks of life, a nonoperative procedure may be effective. Serial manipulations and casting are used gently to correct each component of the deformity. One method, called the *Ponseti method*, involves weekly gentle stretching and manipulation of the misaligned bones followed by application of a well-molded long leg plaster cast with the knee held at a right angle.[20] The

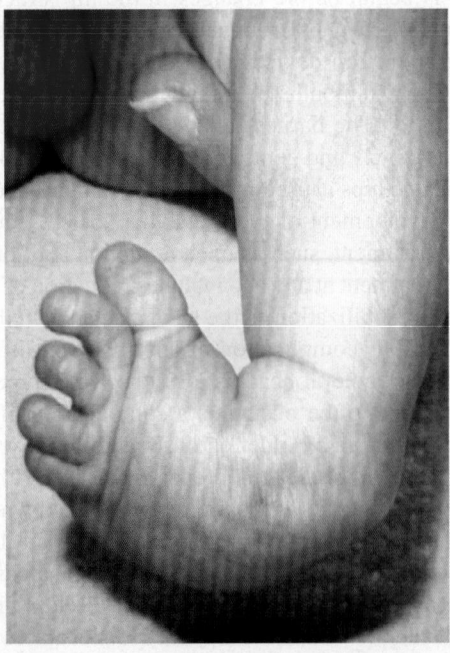

FIGURE 58.13 • Newborn with clubbing of the left foot. (Public Images Library, Centers for Disease Control and Prevention. ID#: 2632. Available at http://phil.cdc.gov/phil/detail.asp.)

cast maintains the correction and allows for further relaxation of tight structures in anticipation of the next week's casting. Correction of the deformity is usually obtained within 6 to 8 weeks. Frequently, a percutaneous Achilles tendon lengthening is performed using a topical anesthetic cream before application of the final cast to allow for complete correction of the equinus deformity. The correction is maintained by full-time wear of a Denis Browne splint for 3 months and part-time night and nap wear for approximately 2 to 3 years.[21] Surgery may be required for severe deformities or when nonoperative treatment methods are unsuccessful. It is performed most commonly between 3 and 12 months of age.[6,10]

Juvenile Osteochondroses

The term *juvenile osteochondroses* is used to describe a group of children's diseases in which one or more growth ossification centres undergoes a period of degeneration, necrosis, or inactivity that is followed by regeneration and usually deformity. The osteochondroses are separated into two groups according to their causes. The first group consists of the true osteonecrotic osteochondroses, so called because the diseases are caused by localized osteonecrosis of an apophyseal or epiphyseal centre (*e.g.,* Legg–Calvé–Perthes disease, Freiberg infraction, Panner disease, Kienböck disease). The second group of juvenile osteochondroses is caused by abnormalities in ossification of cartilaginous tissue resulting from a genetically determined normal variation or from trauma (*e.g.,* Osgood–Schlatter disease, Blount disease, Sever disease, Scheuermann disease). The discussion in this section focuses on Legg–Calvé–Perthes disease from the first group and Osgood–Schlatter disease from the second group. Slipped capital femoral epiphysis is a disorder of the growth plate.

Legg–Calvé–Perthes Disease

Legg–Calvé–Perthes disease is an idiopathic osteonecrotic disease of the proximal (capital) femoral epiphysis.[6,10] It occurs in 1 in 1,200 children, affecting primarily those between ages 2 and 13 years, with a peak incidence between 3 and 9 years.[10,23] It occurs primarily in boys and is much more common in white than black populations. Although no definite genetic pattern has been established, it occasionally affects more than one family member.

The cause of Legg–Calvé–Perthes disease is unknown. The disorder usually is insidious in onset and occurs in otherwise healthy children. It may, however, be associated with acute trauma. Affected children usually have a shorter stature. Undernutrition has been suggested as a causative factor. When girls are affected, they usually have a poorer prognosis than boys because they are skeletally more mature and have a shorter period for growth and remodelling than boys of the same age. In most cases, only one leg is affected, but 10% to 12% of affected children have the condition in both legs.[24,25]

The primary pathologic feature of Legg–Calvé–Perthes disease is an avascular necrosis of the bone and marrow involving the epiphyseal growth centre in the femoral head.

The disorder may be confined to part of the epiphysis, or it may involve the entire epiphysis. In severe cases, there is a disturbance in the growth pattern that leads to a broad, short femoral neck. The necrosis is followed by slow absorption of the dead bone over 2 to 3 years. Although the necrotic trabeculae eventually are replaced by healthy new bone, the epiphysis rarely regains its normal shape. The process occurs in four predictable stages.[25] The *first stage,* which lasts for 6 to 12 months, is the avascular stage, during which the femoral head appears smaller and gradually increases in density. The ossification centre becomes necrotic. Damage to the femoral head is determined by the degree of necrosis that occurs during this stage. The *second stage* is the regenerative or revascularization stage, during which resorption of the necrotic bone takes place. This stage usually lasts 1 to 3 years, during which the necrotic bone is gradually replaced by new immature bone cells and the contour of the bone is remodelled. The *third stage* is the reossification stage, during which radiolucent areas begin to ossify and become dense, while the shape of the femoral head improves. The *fourth stage,* which is the healed or residual stage, involves the formation and replacement of immature bone cells by normal bone cells and the resulting final shape of the femoral head.

The main symptoms of Legg–Calvé–Perthes disease are pain in the groin, thigh, or knee and difficulty in walking. The child may have a painless limp with limited abduction and internal rotation and a flexion contracture of the affected hip. The age of onset is important because young children have a greater capability for remodelling of the femoral head and acetabulum, and thus less flattening of the femoral head occurs. Early diagnosis is important and is based on correlating physical symptoms with radiographic findings that are related to the stage of the disease.

The goal of treatment is to reduce deformity and preserve the integrity of the femoral head. Conservative and surgical interventions are used in the treatment of Legg–Calvé–Perthes disease. Children younger than 4 years of age with little or no involvement of the femoral head may require only periodic observation. In all other children, some intervention is needed to relieve the force of weight bearing, muscular tension, and subluxation of the femoral head. It is important to maintain the femur in a well-seated position in the concave acetabulum to prevent deformity. This is done by keeping the hip in abduction and mild internal rotation. Treatment involves periods of rest, use of assistive devices for walking, non–weight-bearing activities, and abduction braces to keep the legs separated in abduction with mild internal rotation. The Atlanta Scottish Rite brace, which does not extend below the knee, is the most widely used orthosis because it provides containment while allowing free knee motion and ambulation without crutches or external support[6,10] (Fig. 58.14). Surgery may be done to contain the femoral head in the acetabulum. This treatment usually is reserved for children older than 6 years of age who at the time of diagnosis have more serious involvement of the femoral head. The best surgical results are obtained when surgery is done early, before the epiphysis becomes necrotic.

FIGURE 58.14 • Scottish Rite brace for Legg–Calvé–Perthes disease produces containment for abduction and allows free knee motion. (From Crocetti M., Barone M. A. (2004). *Oski's essential pediatrics* (2nd ed., p. 679). Philadelphia, PA: Lippincott, Williams & Wilkins.)

Osgood–Schlatter Disease

Osgood–Schlatter disease involves microfractures in the area where the patellar tendon inserts into the tibial tubercle, which is an extension of the proximal tibial epiphysis.[6] This area is particularly vulnerable to injury caused by sudden or continued strain from the patellar tendon during periods of growth, particularly in athletic individuals. It occurs most frequently in boys between the ages of 10 and 15 years and in girls between 8 and 13 years.

The disorder is characterized by pain in the front of the knee that is associated with inflammation and thickening of the patellar tendon. The pain usually is associated with specific activities such as kneeling, running, bicycle riding, or stair climbing. There is swelling, tenderness, and increased prominence of the tibial tubercle. The symptoms usually are self-limiting. They may recur during growth periods, but usually resolve after closure of the tibial growth plate. In some cases, limitations on activity, tibial bands, or braces to immobilize the knee; anti-inflammatory agents; and application of cold are necessary to relieve the pain. The objective of treatment is to release tension on the quadriceps to permit revascularization and reossification of the tibial tubercle. Complete resolution of symptoms through healing (physical closure) of the tibial tubercle usually requires 12 to 24 months.[6] Occasionally, minor symptoms or an increased prominence of the tibial tubercle may continue into adulthood. In some cases, a high-riding patella can cause dislocation with chondromalacia of the patella and result in degenerative arthritis.

Slipped Capital Femoral Epiphysis

Slipped capital femoral epiphysis, or coxa vara, is a disorder of the growth plate that occurs near the age of skeletal maturity. It involves a three-dimensional displacement of the epiphysis (posteriorly, medially, inferiorly), meaning that the femur is rotated externally from under the epiphysis. The condition is rare, with an estimated frequency of 1 to 10 in 100,000.[6]

The cause of slipped capital femoral epiphysis is obscure, but it may be related to the child's susceptibility to stress on the femoral neck as a result of genetics or structural abnormalities. Boys are affected twice as often as girls, and in approximately half of cases the condition is bilateral. Affected children often are overweight with poorly developed secondary sex characteristics, or, in some instances, are extremely tall and thin. In many cases, there is a history of rapid skeletal growth preceding displacement of the epiphysis. The condition also may be affected by nutritional deficiencies or endocrine disorders such as hypothyroidism, hypopituitarism, and hypogonadism. Rapid growth after administration of growth hormone has been associated with displacement of the epiphysis.

Children with the condition often complain of referred knee pain accompanied by difficulty in walking, fatigue, and stiffness. The diagnosis is confirmed by radiographic studies in which the degree of slipping is determined and graded according to severity (mild, <33%; moderate, 33% to 50%; and severe, >50%).[10] Early treatment is imperative to prevent lifelong crippling. Avoidance of weight bearing on the femur and bed rest are essential parts of the treatment. Traction or gentle manipulation under anesthesia is used to reduce the slip. Surgical insertion of pins to keep the femoral neck and head of the femur aligned is a common method of treatment for children with moderate or severe slips. Crutches are used for several months after surgical correction to prevent full weight bearing until the growth plate closes.

Children with the disorder must be followed closely until the epiphyseal plate closes. Long-term prognosis depends on the amount of displacement that occurs. Complications include avascular necrosis, leg shortening, malunion, and problems with the internal fixation. Degenerative arthritis may develop, requiring joint replacement later in life.

Scoliosis

Scoliosis is a lateral deviation of the spinal column that may or may not include rotation or deformity of the vertebrae. It is a three-dimensional deformity of the spine that often affects the entire skeletal torso. The majority of scoliotic deformities are idiopathic. Others can be congenital, associated with neuromuscular disorders or intraspinal deformities, or are caused by compensation for leg-length discrepancy.[6] The estimated prevalence of scoliosis in the adolescent population is approximately 2%, using a definition of a spinal curve of greater than 10 degrees.[26] The prevalence of curves greater than 30 degrees is 0.1% to 0.3%.[6,27]

Scoliosis is classified as postural or structural. With postural scoliosis, there is a small curve that corrects with bending. It can be corrected with passive and active exercises. Structural scoliosis does not correct with bending. It is a fixed deformity classified according to the cause: congenital, neuromuscular, or idiopathic.

Congenital Scoliosis

Congenital scoliosis is caused by disturbances in vertebral development during the sixth to eighth weeks of embryologic development.[6,27,28] Congenital scoliosis may be divided into failures of formation and failures of segmentation. Failures of formation indicate the absence of a portion of the vertebra, such as hemivertebra (absence of a whole side of the vertebra) and wedge vertebra (missing only a portion of the vertebra). Failure of segmentation is the absence of the normal separation between the vertebrae.[6] The child may have other anomalies and neurologic complications if the spine is involved. Early diagnosis and treatment of progressive curves are essential for children with congenital scoliosis. Surgical intervention is the treatment of choice for progressive congenital scoliosis.[6]

Neuromuscular Scoliosis

Neuromuscular scoliosis develops from neuropathic or myopathic diseases. It is seen with cerebral palsy, myelodysplasia, and poliomyelitis. There is often a long, C-shaped curve from the cervical to the sacral region. In children with cerebral palsy, severe deformity may make treatment difficult. Myopathic neuromuscular scoliosis develops with Duchenne muscular dystrophy and usually is not severe.

Idiopathic Scoliosis

Idiopathic scoliosis, a structural spinal curvature for which no cause has been established, accounts for approximately 80% of scoliosis cases. It occurs in healthy, neurologically normal children. Although the incidence is only slightly greater in girls than boys, it is more likely to progress and require treatment in girls.[6,27] The cause is most likely complex and multifactorial. It seems likely that heredity is involved because mother–daughter pairings are common, but identical twins are not uniformly affected. The magnitude of the curvature in an affected individual is not related to magnitude of curvature in relatives. So far, no single genetic mutation has been linked to idiopathic scoliosis, though a number of candidate genes have been implicated for this multigenic, complex pathogenesis.[29]

Idiopathic scoliosis can be divided into three groups on the basis of age at onset: infantile (birth to 3 years), juvenile (3 to 10 years), and adolescent (11 years and older).[6,27] The infantile form is rare in the United States. It is seen primarily in the United Kingdom and Europe; the incidence is unreported for Canada. It affects boys more often than girls, and the curvature usually is convex and to the left rather than to the right, as in other forms of scoliosis. Although most forms of juvenile scoliosis regress spontaneously, some progress and are difficult to treat effectively. Juvenile idiopathic scoliosis is uncommon. However, in many children with the diagnosis of adolescent scoliosis, the onset may have occurred when they were juveniles but was not diagnosed until later. Adolescent scoliosis is the most common type, accounts for approximately 80% of cases, and is seen more commonly in girls. An increase in joint laxity, which causes excessive joint motion and is found commonly in girls, has been associated with the development of idiopathic scoliosis. Delayed puberty and menarche are other risk factors for the development of adolescent scoliosis.[30]

Although a scoliotic curve may be present in any area of the spine, the most common curve is a right thoracic curve, which produces a rib prominence on the convex side and hypokyphosis from rotation of the vertebral column around its long axis as the spine begins to curve. A spinal curvature of less than 10 degrees is considered a normal variant, not scoliosis.[6,27] Curves greater than 40 degrees usually are considered severe.

Manifestations. Scoliosis usually is first noticed because of the deformity it causes. A high shoulder, prominent hip, or projecting scapula may be noticed by a parent or in a school-based screening program (Fig. 58.15). In girls, difficulty in hemming or fitting a dress may call attention to the deformity. Idiopathic scoliosis usually is a painless process, although pain may be present in severe cases, usually in the lumbar region. The pain may be caused by pressure on the ribs or on the crest of the ilium. There may be shortness of breath as a result of diminished chest expansion and gastrointestinal disturbances from crowding of the abdominal organs. Adults with less severe deformity may experience mild backache. If scoliosis is left untreated, the curve may progress to an extent that compromises cardiopulmonary function and creates a risk for neurologic complications.

Diagnosis and Treatment. Early diagnosis of scoliosis can be important in the prevention of severe spinal deformity. The cardinal signs of scoliosis are uneven shoulders or iliac crest, prominent scapula on the convex side of the curve, malalignment of spinous processes, asymmetry of the flanks, asymmetry of the thoracic cage, and rib hump or paraspinal muscle prominence when bending forward (Fig. 58.15). A complete physical examination is necessary for children with scoliosis because the defect may be indicative of other, underlying pathologic processes.

Diagnosis of scoliosis is made by physical examination and confirmed by radiography. A scoliometer should be used at the apex of the curvature to quantify a prominence; a scoliometer reading of greater than 10 degrees requires referral to orthopedics. The curve is measured by determining the amount of lateral deviation present on radiographs and is labelled "right" or "left" for the convex portion of the curve. Other radiographic procedures may be done, including CT scanning, magnetic resonance imaging (MRI), and myelography.

Screening for scoliosis in schools remains a controversial issue. In Canada in the 1970s, school screening for scoliosis was implemented but by 1979 these provincial programs were stopped as they were not found to be cost effective. The Canadian Task Force on Periodic Health Examination (1994) recommended against the routine screening of asymptomatic adolescents for idiopathic scoliosis.[31] Internationally Australia, Great Britain, and the U.S. Preventive Services Task Force have not found sufficient evidence to support the school screening for scoliosis.[32] Thus, healthcare professionals should be prepared to evaluate idiopathic scoliosis when it is discovered incidentally or when the adolescent or parent expresses concern about scoliosis.[32]

The treatment of scoliosis depends on the severity of the deformity and the likelihood of progression. Larger curves are more likely to progress. Age of presentation also is important. Curves that are detected before menarche are more likely to progress than those detected after menarche. For persons with lesser degrees of curvature (10 to 20 degrees), the trend has been away from aggressive treatment and toward a "wait and see" approach, taking advantage of the more sophisticated diagnostic methods that now are available. Treatment is considered for physically immature patients with curves between 20 and 30 degrees. Curves between 30 and 40 degrees usually are considered for correction with braces, and those greater than 40 to 45 degrees are considered for surgery.

A brace may be used to control the progression of the curvature during growth and can provide some correction. A commonly used brace is the Milwaukee brace, which was developed by Blount and Schmitt in the 1940s. This was the first brace to provide some degree of active correction. It involves a pelvic mold, various pads, and two metal upright supports around the throat. It is cumbersome, and compliance with wearing the brace has been shown to be poor. In an effort to improve compliance, a number of new bracing techniques have been developed. They include underarm or thoracolumbosacral orthoses. These orthoses consist of easily concealed, prefabricated forms that are modified to suit the patient.

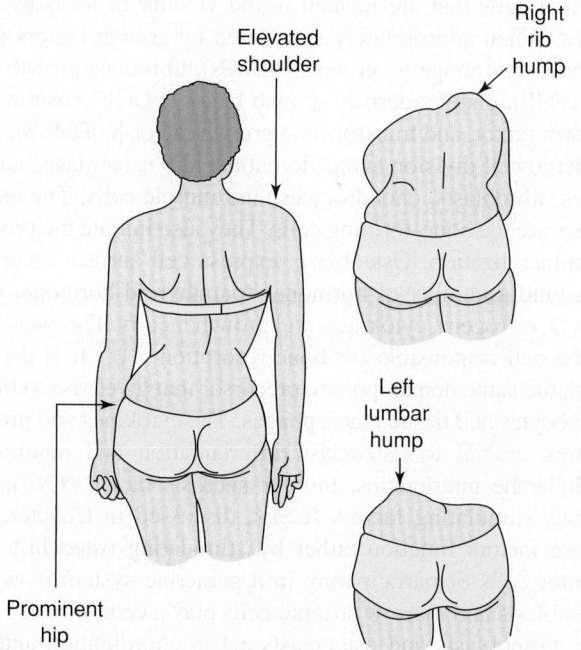

FIGURE 58.15 • Scoliosis: abnormalities to be determined at initial screening examination. (From Gore D. R., Passehl R., Sepic S., et al. (1981). Scoliosis screening: Results of a community project. *Pediatrics,* *67,* 196–200. Copyright 1981 by the American Academy of Pediatrics.)

Elevated shoulder

Right rib hump

Left lumbar hump

Prominent hip

Surgical intervention with instrumentation and spinal fusion is done in severe cases—when the curvature has progressed to 40 degrees or more at the time of diagnosis or when curves of a lesser degree are compounded with imbalance or rotation of the vertebrae. Unlike bracing, which is intended to halt progression of the curvature, surgical intervention is used to decrease the curve. Instrumentation helps correct the curve and balance, and spinal fusion maintains the spine in the corrected position.[6,27,28] Several methods of instrumentation (*i.e.,* rods that attach to the vertebral column and posterior fusion) are used. Combined anterior and posterior surgery is used for more severe curvatures. The newer systems provide better sagittal control and more stable fixation, which allow earlier mobility. Despite great advances in spinal surgery, no one method seems to be the best for all cases. There is recent interest in growth modulation approaches using minimally invasive techniques, which will result in curve correction while maintaining spinal motion and disk and motion segment integrity.[33]

IN SUMMARY

Skeletal disorders can result from congenital or hereditary influences or from factors that occur during normal periods of skeletal growth and development. Newborn infants undergo normal changes in muscle tone and joint motion, causing torsional conditions of the femur or tibia. Many of these conditions are corrected as skeletal growth and development take place. Osteogenesis imperfecta is a rare autosomal hereditary disorder characterized by defective synthesis of connective tissue, including bone matrix. It results in poorly developed bones that fracture easily. DDH includes a range of structural abnormalities. Dislocated hips are always treated to prevent changes in the anatomic structure. Other childhood skeletal disorders, such as the osteochondroses, slipped capital femoral epiphysis, and scoliosis, are not corrected by the growth process. These disorders are progressive, can cause permanent disability, and require treatment. Disorders such as DDH and congenital clubfoot are present at birth and both of these disorders are best treated during infancy. Regular examinations during the first year of life are recommended as a means of achieving early diagnosis of such disorders.

Scoliosis is a lateral deviation of the spinal column that may or may not include rotation or deformity of the vertebrae. Scoliosis is classified as postural, which corrects with bending, or structural, which does not. Structural scoliosis is a fixed deformity classified according to the cause: congenital, which results from defects in vertebral development; neuromuscular, which is caused by diseases such as cerebral palsy; and idiopathic, which is the most common form. Curves between 30 and 40 degrees usually are considered for correction with braces, and those greater than 40 to 45 degrees are considered for surgery.

METABOLIC BONE DISEASE

After completing this section of the chapter, you should be able to meet the following objectives:

- Cite the origin of osteoclasts and osteoblasts and describe their functions in bone remodelling.
- Describe the function of the RANK ligand/RANK receptor, and the osteoprotegerin-blocking molecule in the regulation of bone remodelling.
- Describe risk factors that contribute to the development of osteoporosis and relate them to the prevention of the disorder.
- Describe the primary features of osteoporotic bone.
- Explain the methods used in the diagnosis of osteoporosis.
- Describe the actions of medications used in the treatment of osteoporosis.
- Compare the pathogenesis and manifestations of osteomalacia and rickets.
- Characterize the cause and manifestations of Paget disease.

Bone is an admixture of inorganic elements and organic matrix that is in a constant state of bone resorption and bone formation. The inorganic elements include the calcium and phosphorus that mineralize bone, and the organic matrix includes bone cells and matrix proteins. The bone cells include the osteoprogenitor cells, the osteoblasts, and the osteoclasts[6,34-36] (see Chapter 56). The osteoprogenitor cells are pluripotent mesenchymal cells that are located in the vicinity of all bony surfaces. When appropriately stimulated by growth factors such as bone morphogenic proteins (BMPs), fibroblast growth factor (FGF), platelet-derived growth factor (PDGF), insulin-like growth factor, and transforming growth factor-β (TGF-β), they undergo cell division and differentiate into osteoblasts, adipocytes, fibroblasts, chondrocytes, and muscle cells. The osteoblasts are the bone-forming cells. They also initiate the process of mineralization. Osteoblasts express cell surface receptors that bind a number of hormones (parathyroid hormone, vitamin D, estrogen), cytokines, and growth factors. The osteoclast is the cell responsible for bone resorption.[6,34-36] It is derived from the same hematopoietic precursor that gives rise to blood monocytes and tissue macrophages. The cytokines and growth factors crucial to osteoclast differentiation and maturation include the interleukins, tumour necrosis factor (TNF), and colony-stimulating factors (CSFs; discussed in Chapter 12). These factors function either by stimulating osteoclast progenitor cells or participating in a paracrine system in which osteoblasts and marrow stromal cells play a central role.

Osteoblasts and osteoclasts act in coordination and are considered the functional unit of bone, known as the *basic multicellular unit*. The processes of bone formation and resorption are tightly coupled, and their balance determines skeletal mass at any time. As the skeleton grows and enlarges during childhood, a process called *bone modelling* predominates. It results in a bone having adult form and shape. Peak bone mass is achieved during early adulthood after cessation of modelling. It is determined by a number of factors, including the type of vitamin D receptor inherited, nutrition, level of physical activity, age, and hormonal status. Once skeletal growth has attained its adult size, the breakdown and renewal of bone that is responsible for skeletal maintenance is initiated at sites that require replacement or repair. This process is called *bone remodelling.*

The sequence of bone resorption and bone formation begins with osteoclastic resorption of existing bone, during which the organic (protein matrix) and the inorganic (mineral) components are removed. The sequence proceeds to the formation of new bone by osteoblasts. In the adult, the length of one sequence (*i.e.,* bone resorption and formation) is approximately 4 months. Ideally, the replaced bone should equal the absorbed bone. If it does not, there is a net loss of bone. In older adults, for example, bone resorption and formation no longer are perfectly coupled, and bone mass is lost.

It is only recently that significant progress has been made in understanding the phenomenon of bone remodelling as it relates to the coupling of bone resorption with bone formation. The pivotal paracrine pathway linking these two processes consists of three factors: the *r*eceptor *a*ctivator of *n*uclear factor κB *l*igand (RANKL); its receptor RANK; and a soluble inhibitor receptor for RANKL, osteoprotegerin (OPG).[6,34–37] RANK and RANKL are the factors that express bone resorption, and OPG is a bone resorption inhibitor. RANKL is a member of the TNF superfamily, and both RANK and OPG are members of the TNF receptor family. RANKL is expressed by osteoblasts and their immature precursors and is necessary for osteoclast differentiation and function. RANKL activates its receptor, RANK, which is expressed on osteoclasts and their precursors, thus promoting osteoclast differentiation and activation and prolonging osteoclast survival by suppressing apoptosis. The term *osteoprotegerin* was coined because of its protective effects against bone loss. The effects of RANKL are blocked by OPG, a soluble receptor protein, which acts as a decoy receptor that binds RANKL and prevents it from binding with RANK on osteoclasts.

It is now believed that dysregulation of the RANKL/RANK/OPG pathway plays a prominent role in the pathogenesis of bone diseases such as neoplasia and bone lesions as well as osteoporosis.[35] For example, it has been shown that postmenopausal women express higher levels of RANKL on their marrow stromal cells and lymphocytes than premenopausal women or postmenopausal women taking estrogen. It has also been shown that estrogens and the selective estrogen receptor modulator (SERM), raloxifene, stimulate OPG production in osteoblasts. Glucocorticoid exposure, which can contribute to steroid osteoporosis, enhances RANKL expression and suppresses OPG levels, thus elevating the RANKL-to-OPG ratio. There is also evidence linking the pathogenesis of inflammatory conditions such as rheumatoid arthritis to dysregulation of the RANKL/OPG system. Based

on immunologic and inflammatory conditions such as rheumatoid arthritis or myeloma bone diseases, various hormones and cytokines differentially regulate RANKL and OPG, producing an enhanced RANKL-to-OPG ratio that favours skeletal damage. There is also evidence that RANKL is expressed on T cells, and in vitro studies have shown that activated T cells can regulate the development and activation of osteoclasts through RANKL.[37]

METABOLIC BONE DISORDERS

- Metabolic bone disorders have their origin in the bone remodelling process that involves an orderly sequence of osteoclastic bone reabsorption, the formation of new bone by the osteoblasts, and mineralization of the newly formed osteoid tissue.
- Osteoporosis represents an increased loss of total bone mass due to an imbalance between bone absorption and bone formation, most often related to the aging process and decreased estrogen levels in postmenopausal women.
- Osteomalacia and rickets represent a softening of bone due to inadequate mineralization of the bone matrix caused by a deficiency of calcium or phosphate.
- Paget disease is a disorder involving excessive bone destruction and repair, resulting in structural deformities of the long bones, spine, pelvis, and cranium.

Osteopenia

Osteopenia is a condition that is common to all metabolic bone diseases. It is characterized by a reduction in bone mass greater than expected for age, race, or sex that occurs because of a decrease in bone formation, inadequate bone mineralization, or excessive bone deossification. *Osteopenia* is not a diagnosis but a term used to describe an apparent lack of bone seen on x-ray studies. The major causes of osteopenia are osteoporosis, osteomalacia, malignancies such as multiple myeloma, and endocrine disorders such as hyperparathyroidism and hyperthyroidism.

Osteoporosis

Osteoporosis is a metabolic bone disease characterized by a loss of mineralized bone mass causing increased porosity of the skeleton and susceptibility to fractures.[37–41] The World Health Organization has defined osteoporosis as a bone mineral density (BMD) value greater than 2.5 standard deviations below the mean for normal young white women. The exact number is difficult to determine because bone loss varies in the different parts of the skeleton where bone mass is measured, and definitions of osteoporosis have not been developed for all subpopulations. Although osteoporosis can occur as the result of a number of disorders, it most often is associated with the aging process. With Canada's aging population, the prevalence of osteoporosis and osteopenia is expected to increase. Based upon fracture information, it is estimated that one in three women and one in five men in Canada have osteoporosis.[41] Fractures result in a significant individual and societal burden due to the loss of income, pain, and healthcare costs. It is estimated that the overall yearly cost to the Canadian healthcare system of treating osteoporosis and the associated fractures was over $2.3 billion as of 2010.[41]

Pathogenesis

The pathogenesis of osteoporosis is unclear, but most data suggest an imbalance between bone resorption and formation such that bone resorption exceeds bone formation. Although both of these factors play a role in most cases of osteoporosis, their relative contribution to bone loss may vary depending on age, gender, genetic predisposition, activity level, and nutritional status. Exercise may prevent or delay the onset of osteoporosis by increasing peak BMD during periods of growth. Poor nutrition or an age-related decrease in intestinal absorption of calcium because of deficient activation of vitamin D may contribute to the development of osteoporosis, particularly in older adults.

Under normal conditions, bone mass increases steadily during childhood, reaching a peak in the young adult years. The peak bone mass, or BMD, is an important determinant of the subsequent risk for osteoporosis. It is determined in part by genetic factors, hormone (estrogen) levels, exercise, calcium intake and absorption, and environmental factors. Genetic factors are linked, in largest part, to the maximal amount of bone in a given person, referred to as *peak bone mass*. Race is a key determinant of BMD and the risk of fractures. Incidence rates obtained from studies among racial and ethnic groups demonstrate that although women have higher fracture rates compared with men overall, these differences vary by race and age. White and Asian women had higher rates for all age groups older than 50 years.[38] The highest BMD values and lowest fracture rates have been reported for black women.[38] Body size is another factor affecting the risk of osteoporosis and risk of fractures. Women with smaller body builds are at increased risk of hip fracture because of lower hip BMD.

Hormonal factors play a significant role in the development of osteoporosis, particularly in postmenopausal women.[42,43] Postmenopausal osteoporosis, which is caused by an estrogen deficiency, is manifested by a loss of cancellous bone and a predisposition to fractures of the vertebrae and distal radius. The loss of bone mass is greatest during early menopause, when estrogen levels are withdrawing. Several factors appear to influence the increased loss of bone mass associated with an estrogen deficiency. Decreased estrogen levels are associated with an increase in cytokines (*e.g.,* interleukin-1, interleukin-6, and TNF) that stimulate the production of osteoclast precursors. Estrogen deficiency also influences osteoclast differentiation through the RANK receptor pathways.[14] Estrogen stimulates the production of OPG and thus inhibits the formation of osteoclasts; it also

blunts the responsiveness of osteoclast precursors to RANKL. With menopause and its accompanying estrogen deficiency, this inhibition of osteoclast production is lost.[14] Compensatory osteoblastic activity and new bone formation occurs, but it does not keep pace with the bone that is lost.

Sex hormone deficiency may contribute to bone loss in men with senile osteoporosis, although the effect is not of the same magnitude as that caused by estrogen deficiency. Unlike women, men do not have a midlife loss of sex hormone production.[44] Another factor that provides relative protection for men is the fact that they achieve 8% to 10% more peak bone mass than women. Although androgens have long been assumed to be critical for growth and maintenance of the male skeleton, the estrogens obtained from peripheral conversion of testicular and adrenal hormone precursors may be even more important than androgens in the maintenance of bone mass in men.

Age-related changes in bone density occur in all individuals and contribute to the development of osteoporosis in both sexes. After peak bone mass is attained at about 30 years of age, the rate of bone loss for both sexes is approximately 0.7% per year, and it increases to approximately 2% per year or more in menopausal women.[14,41] Age-related changes in bone cells and matrix have a strong impact on bone metabolism. Osteoblasts from older adults have reduced replicative and biosynthetic potential compared with those of younger persons. Growth factors that stimulate osteoblastic activity also lose their potential over time. The end result is a skeleton that has decreased ability to make bone. Reduced physical activity increases the rate of bone loss because mechanical forces are important stimuli for normal bone remodelling. Thus, the decreased physical activity that often accompanies aging may also contribute to the loss of bone mass in older adults.

Secondary osteoporosis is associated with many conditions, including endocrine disorders, malabsorption disorders, malignancies, alcoholism, and certain medications.[45] Persons with endocrine disorders such as hyperthyroidism, hyperparathyroidism, Cushing syndrome, or diabetes mellitus are at high risk for development of osteoporosis. Hyperthyroidism causes an acceleration of bone turnover. Some malignancies (*e.g.,* multiple myeloma) secrete osteoclast-activating factor, causing significant bone loss. Alcohol is a direct inhibitor of osteoblasts and may also inhibit calcium absorption. Corticosteroid use is the most common cause of drug-related osteoporosis, and long-term corticosteroid use in the treatment of disorders such as rheumatoid arthritis and chronic obstructive lung disease is associated with a high rate of fractures. With the increased use of prednisone and other drugs that act like cortisol for the treatment of many inflammatory and autoimmune diseases, this form of bone loss has become a major clinical concern. The prolonged use of medications that increase calcium excretion, such as aluminum-containing antacids, corticosteroids, and anticonvulsants, also is associated with bone loss. Persons with human immunodeficiency virus (HIV) infection or acquired immunodeficiency syndrome (AIDS) who are being treated with antiretroviral therapy may develop a lower bone density and signs of osteopenia and osteoporosis.[45]

Understanding   Bone Remodelling

Bone remodelling constitutes a process of skeletal maintenance once skeletal growth is complete. It takes place in the (1) osteons of mature bone and consists of a cycle of (2) bone resorption by osteoclasts, (3) followed by bone formation by osteoblasts. Bone remodelling is (4) controlled by cytokines and growth factors that interact with a paracrine system consisting of the RANK ligand (RANKL), the RANK receptor, and osteoprotegerin.

1. Bone Remodelling Cycle

Mature bone is made up of osteons or units of concentric lamellae (bone layers) and the haversian canal they surround. Bone remodelling consists of a sequence of bone resorption within an osteon by osteoclasts, followed by new bone formation by osteoblasts. In the adult, the length of one sequence (*i.e.,* bone resorption and formation) is approximately 4 months. Ideally, the replaced bone should equal the resorbed bone. If it does not, there is net loss of bone. In the elderly, for example, bone resorption and formation no longer are perfectly coupled, and bone mass is lost.

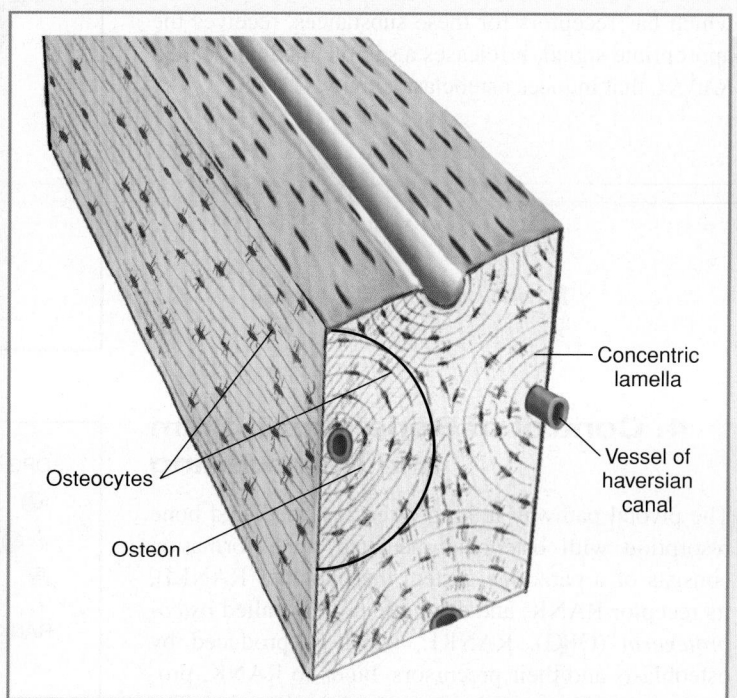

Concentric lamella

Vessel of haversian canal

Osteocytes

Osteon

2. Bone Resorption

The osteoclasts, which are bone-resorbing cells derived from monocyte/macrophage precursors, are the cells involved in the initiation of bone remodelling. The sequence of bone resorption and bone formation is activated by many stimuli, including the action of parathyroid hormone and calcitonin. It begins with osteoclastic resorption of existing bone, during which the organic (protein matrix) and inorganic (mineral) components are removed, creating a tunnel-like space in the osteon. Soluble factors released during resorption aid in the recruitment of osteoblasts to the site, thereby linking bone resorption to bone formation.

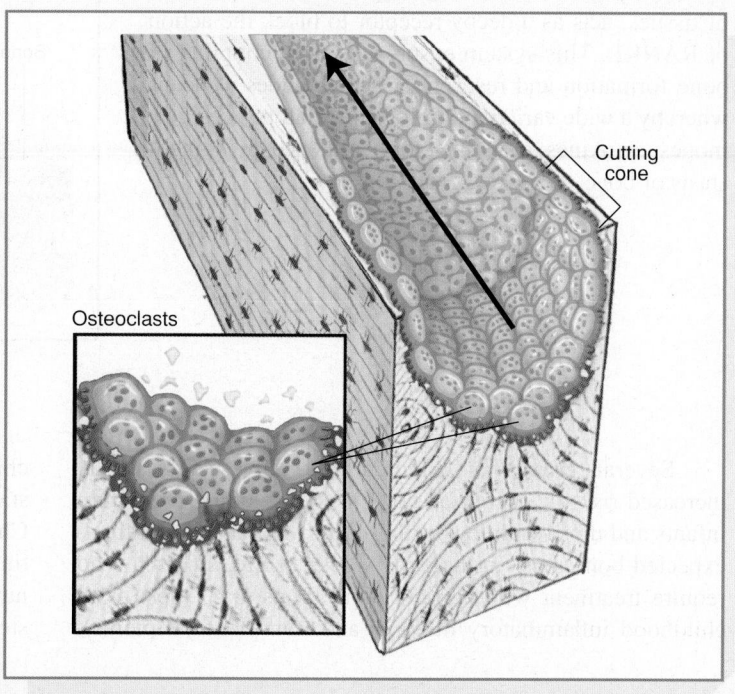

Cutting cone

Osteoclasts

3. Bone Formation

After osteoclastic activity has ceased, osteoblasts begin to deposit the organic matrix (osteoid) on the wall of the osteon canal. As successive lamellae of bone are deposited, the canal ultimately attains the relative proportions of the original osteon. In the formation and maintenance of bone, osteoblasts provide much of the local control because not only do they produce new bone matrix, they play an essential role in mediating osteoclast activity. Many of the primary stimulators of bone resorption, such as parathyroid hormone, have minimal or no direct effects on osteoclasts. Once the osteoblast, which has receptors for these substances, receives the appropriate signal, it releases a soluble mediator called *RANKL* that induces osteoclast activity.

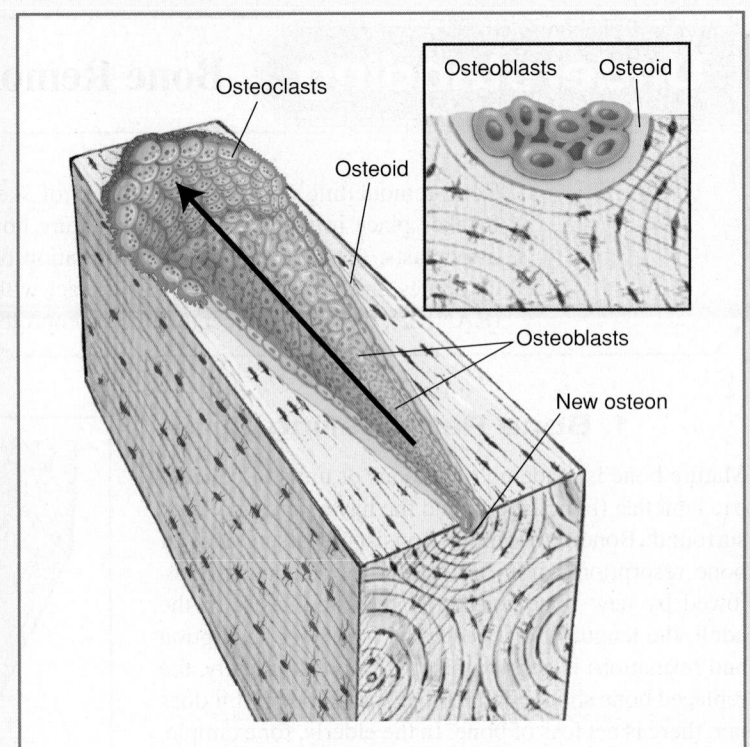

4. Control of Bone Metabolism and Remodelling

The pivotal pathway linking osteoclast-mediated bone resorption with osteoblast-mediated bone formation consists of a paracrine system that includes RANKL, its receptor RANK, and a soluble protein called *osteoprotegerin* (OPG). RANKL, which is produced by osteoblasts and their precursors, binds to RANK, promoting osteoclast differentiation and proliferation. The soluble OPG molecule, which is produced by a number of tissues, acts as a decoy receptor to block the action of RANKL. This system ensures the tight coupling of bone formation and resorption, and provides a means whereby a wide variety of biologic mediators (*e.g.*, hormones, cytokines, growth factors) influence the homeostasis of bone.

Several groups of children and adolescents are at increased risk for decreased bone mass, including premature infants and those with low birth weight who have lower-than-expected bone mass in the early weeks of life, children who require treatment with corticosteroid drugs (*e.g.*, those with childhood inflammatory diseases and transplant recipients), children with cystic fibrosis, and those with hypogonadal states (*e.g.*, anorexia nervosa and the female athlete triad).[40] Children with cystic fibrosis often have impaired gastrointestinal function that reduces the absorption of calcium and other nutrients, and many also require the frequent use of corticosteroid drugs.

Premature osteoporosis is increasingly being seen in female athletes owing to an increased prevalence of eating disorders and amenorrhea.[46–48] It most frequently affects women engaged in endurance sports, such as running and swimming; in activities where appearance is important, such as figure skating, diving, and gymnastics; or in sports with weight categories, such as horse racing, martial arts, and rowing. The *female athlete triad* refers to a pattern of disordered eating that leads to amenorrhea and eventually osteoporosis. Poor nutrition, combined with intense training, can decrease the critical body fat-to-muscle ratio needed for normal menses and estrogen production by the ovary. The decreased levels of estrogen combined with the lack of calcium and vitamin D from dietary deficiencies result in a loss of bone density and increased risk for fractures. There is a concern that athletes with low BMD will be at increased risk for fractures during their competitive years. It is unclear whether osteoporosis induced by amenorrhea is reversible. Data are emerging that even having only one or two elements of the triad greatly increases the risk of these women for long-term morbidity.[46]

Manifestations

Osteoporotic changes occur in the diaphysis and metaphysis of bone. In severe osteoporosis, the bones begin to resemble the fragile structure of a fine porcelain vase. There is loss of trabeculae from cancellous bone and thinning of the cortex to such an extent that minimal stress causes fractures. The changes that occur with osteoporosis have been explained by two distinct disease processes: postmenopausal and senile osteoporosis. In postmenopausal women, the increase in osteoclastic activity affects mainly bones or portions of bone that have increased surface area, such as the cancellous compartment of the vertebral bodies. The osteoporotic trabeculae become thinned and lose their interconnections, leading to microfractures and eventual vertebral collapse. In senile osteoporosis, the osteoporotic cortex is thinned by subperiosteal and endosteal resorption and the haversian systems are widened. In severe cases, the haversian systems are so enlarged that the cortex resembles cancellous bone (Fig. 58.16). Hip fractures, which are seen later in life, are more commonly associated with senile osteoporosis.

Osteoporosis is usually a silent disorder. Often, the first manifestations of the disorder are those that accompany a skeletal fracture—a vertebral compression fracture or fractures of the hip, pelvis, humerus, or any other bone (Fig. 58.17). Typically, the fractures occur with less force than usual, such as a minor fall with daily activities (*e.g.,* on stairs, while walking) or in a gymnast performing a common jump. Women who present with fractures are much more likely to sustain another fracture than are women of the same age without osteoporosis. Wedging and collapse of vertebrae cause a loss of height in the vertebral column and kyphosis, a condition commonly referred to as *dowager hump.* Usually, there is no generalized bone tenderness. When pain occurs, it is related to fractures. Systemic symptoms such as weakness and weight loss suggest that the osteoporosis may be caused by underlying disease.

FIGURE 58.16 • Osteoporosis. Femoral head of an 82-year-old woman with osteoporosis and femoral neck fracture (**right**), compared with a normal control bone cut to the same thickness (**left**). (From Rubin R., Strayer D. S. (Eds.). (2012). *Rubin's pathology: Clinicopathologic foundations of medicine* (6th ed., p. 1226). Philadelphia, PA: Lippincott Williams & Wilkins.)

FIGURE 58.17 • Clinical manifestations of osteoporosis.

Diagnosis and Treatment

An important advance in diagnostic methods used for the identification of osteoporosis has been the use of BMD assessment. The clinical method of choice for BMD studies is dual-energy x-ray absorptiometry (DEXA) of the spine and hip.[49–52] Current practice is to perform DEXA on the total hip, the femoral neck, and the anterior lumbar spine (L1 to L4).[51] The site with the lowest score should be used to make a diagnosis. Measurement of BMD has become increasingly common for early detection and fracture prevention. Measurement of serial heights in older adults is another simple way to screen for osteoporosis. A further advance in the diagnosis of osteoporosis is the refinement of risk factors, permitting better analysis of risk pertaining to particular persons. Testing for BMD should be performed based on the individual person's risk. The Osteoporosis Society of Canada and the Society of Obstetricians and Gynaecologists have recommended that all adults should be assessed for risk factors for osteoporosis and both men and women should have a measurement of BMD at 65 years of age.[51] Risk factors that may indicate a need for testing women at a younger age include fragility fracture after the age of 40 (other than skull, facial bone, ankle, finger, or toe), family history (especially maternal hip fracture), systemic glucocorticoid longer than 3 months (even low doses), early menopause (before the age of 45), low body weight (<57 kg), current smoker, and weight loss with greater than 10% at age of 25.[51]

Prevention and early detection of osteoporosis are essential to the prevention of associated deformities and fractures. Most clinicians now use the Canadian Association of Radiologists and Osteoporosis Canada risk assessment tool (CAROC) or the WHO fracture risk assessment algorithm (FRAX) to predict future 10-year hip fracture risk or the probability of having a major osteoporotic fracture. These tools help categorize patients into low, moderate, and high-risk groups and guide treatment decisions.[51,52] It is important to identify persons in high-risk groups so that treatment can begin early (Chart 58.1). Regular exercise and adequate calcium intake are important factors in preventing osteoporosis. Weight-bearing exercises such as walking, jogging, rowing, and weight lifting are important in the maintenance of bone mass. The recommended total daily intake of elemental calcium (through diet and supplements) for individuals over 50 years of age should be 1,200 mg/day.[51] Most Canadian women do not consume a sufficient quantity of dairy products to meet their calcium needs; thus, calcium supplementation is recommended. Calcium tablets vary in content of elemental calcium. Calcium carbonate contains 40% elemental calcium but requires normal stomach acidity to be absorbed. Calcium citrate is 21% elemental calcium but can be absorbed in the absence of acidity. Vitamin D deficiency may be an important factor in the impaired intestinal absorption of calcium in older adults. On the basis of this evidence, 1,25-dihydroxyvitamin D_3 is being studied as a treatment for osteoporosis. Vitamin D optimizes calcium absorption and inhibits parathyroid secretion, which stimulates calcium resorption from bone. Due to seasonal variations most Canadians have inadequate levels of vitamin D

CHART 58.1 **RISK FACTORS ASSOCIATED WITH OSTEOPOROSIS**

Personal Characteristics
Advanced age
Female
White (fair, thin skin)
Small bone structure
Postmenopausal
Family history

Lifestyle
Sedentary
Calcium deficiency (long-term)
High-protein diet
Excessive alcohol intake
Excessive caffeine intake
Smoking

Drug and Disease Related
Aluminum-containing antacids
Anticonvulsants
Heparin
Corticosteroids or Cushing disease
Gastrectomy
Diabetes mellitus
Chronic obstructive lung disease
Malignancy
Hyperthyroidism
Hyperparathyroidism
Rheumatoid arthritis

at some time during the winter or spring and now the discussion is to change from the daily intake of 400 to 1,000 IU and increase this to 2,000 IU of vitamin D.[51,53]

Pharmacologic treatment of osteoporosis uses two main classes of drugs: antiresorptive agents (drugs that block bone resorption by osteoclasts) and anabolic agents (agents that stimulate bone formation by osteoblasts).[51]

There are three main types of antiresorptive agents: estrogens and SERMs, bisphosphonates, and calcitonin. Estrogen is one of the most effective interventions for reducing the incidence and progression of osteoporosis in postmenopausal women. However, since release of data from the Women's Health Initiative, use of hormone replacement therapy (HRT) is not universally recommended, but instead individually tailored to women's potential health risks and benefits.[54] Raloxifene, a SERM that acts only on specific estrogen receptors, has been approved in Canada for the prevention and treatment of osteoporosis in postmenopausal women. However, it may increase mortality in the event of stroke.[51] The use of phytoestrogens, naturally occurring plant compounds, has gained popularity as an alternative to estrogens; however, information regarding their effect on bone health is conflicting and incomplete.[55]

Bisphosphonates are effective inhibitors of bone resorption and the most effective agents for prevention and treatment of osteoporosis. The bisphosphonates (*e.g.,* alendronate, etidronate, ibandronate, risedronate) are analogues of endogenous inorganic pyrophosphate that the body cannot break down. In bone, they bind to hydroxyapatite and prevent bone resorption by inhibiting osteoclast activity. Bisphosphonates have been shown to be effective in reducing the risk of hip, vertebral, and nonvertebral fractures. Bisphosphonates also have adverse effects such as causing hip fractures although very rarely.[43,51] The most dramatic impact has been in the reduction of multiple spine fractures, showing that treatment can decrease progression of the disease.

Denosumab (Prolia) is a monoclonal antibody that inhibits osteoclast formation by preventing the RANKL–RANK interaction. This subcutaneous medication is given twice a year to treat osteoporosis, often after other therapies have been tried. Side effects are similar to bisphosphonates.[56]

Calcitonin is an endogenous peptide that partially inhibits osteoclastic activity. Nasal calcitonin and subcutaneous calcitonin have been approved for the treatment of postmenopausal osteoporosis. Teriparatide is an analogue of parathyroid hormone approved in Canada for the treatment of osteoporosis; it may also help decrease pain associated with vertebral fractures.[51] Unlike the antiresorptive drugs, parathyroid hormone stimulates bone remodelling by increasing osteoblast-mediated bone formation. While testosterone appears to play an important role in bone homeostasis by stimulating osteoblasts and inhibiting osteoclasts, it is no longer recommended for the treatment of osteoporosis in men.[51]

Persons with osteoporosis have many special needs. Walking and swimming are encouraged. Unsafe conditions that predispose persons to falls and fractures should be corrected or avoided. In treating fractures, it is important to minimize immobility. Surgical intervention is done for stable fracture fixation that allows early restoration of mobility and function; for fractures of the lower extremities, this means early weight bearing. Vertebral fractures are treated symptomatically. Conservative treatment with bracing is most often seen, especially in fractures of the thoracic vertebra.[57] Vertebroplasty and kyphoplasty are minimally invasive spinal procedures that use bone cement to restore vertebral height and relieve pain (Fig. 58.18). Bone cement is instilled directly into the fractured vertebral body to restore height and shape. The procedure for kyphoplasty involves the use of a device called a balloon tamp to create a void for the cement. Kyphoplasty seems to be associated with less cement extravasation and better restoration of vertebral height than vertebroplasty.[58]

Osteomalacia and Rickets

In contrast to osteoporosis, which causes a loss of total bone mass and results in brittle bones, osteomalacia and rickets produce a softening of the bones but do not involve a loss of bone matrix. Approximately 60% of bone is mineral content, approximately 30% is organic matrix, and the remainder is

FIGURE 58.18 • Kyphoplasty. (**A**) Insertion of balloon tamp; (**B**) inflation of balloon tamp with collapsed vertebral bone being restored to normal height; (**C**) bone cavity being filled with cement; (**D**) cavity completely filled with cement. (Adapted from American Academy of Orthopedic Surgeons. Kyphoplasty. Available online at: http://orthoinfo.aaos.org/fact/thr_report.cfm?Thread_ID=470&topcategory.)

living bone cells. The organic matrix and the inorganic mineral salts are needed for normal bone consistency. The term *rickets* refers to the disorder in children in which changes in bone growth produce characteristic skeletal abnormalities, and the term *osteomalacia* is used in adults because the bone that forms during the remodelling process is undermineralized.[59]

Osteomalacia

Osteomalacia is a generalized bone condition in which there is inadequate mineralization of bone. There are two main causes of osteomalacia: (1) insufficient calcium absorption from the intestine because of a lack of dietary calcium or a deficiency of or resistance to the action of vitamin D; and (2) phosphate deficiency caused by increased renal losses or decreased intestinal absorption. Vitamin D deficiency is caused most commonly by lack of production due to low sunlight exposure, or decreased absorption as a result of biliary tract or intestinal diseases that impair fat and fat-soluble vitamin absorption. Vitamin D in the diet has previously been presumed to be sufficient in Canada and the United States because many foods are fortified with the vitamin. However, recent evidence supports supplementation at higher amounts.[53] Anticonvulsant medications, such as phenobarbital and phenytoin, induce hepatic hydroxylases that accelerate breakdown of the active forms of vitamin D.

The incidence of osteomalacia is high among older adults because of diets deficient in calcium and vitamin D, a problem often compounded by the intestinal malabsorption that accompanies aging. Osteomalacia often is seen in countries in which vitamin D is not added to dietary items, such as in northern China, Japan, and northern India. Women in these areas have a higher incidence of the disorder than men because of the combined effects of pregnancy, lactation, and more indoor confinement. Osteomalacia occasionally is seen in strict vegetarians, persons who have had a gastrectomy, and those on long-term anticonvulsant, tranquilizer, sedative, muscle relaxant, or diuretic drugs. There also is a greater incidence of osteomalacia in the colder regions of the world, particularly during the winter months, probably because of lessened exposure to sunlight.

A form of osteomalacia called *renal rickets* occurs in persons with chronic renal failure. It is caused by the inability of the kidney to activate vitamin D and excrete phosphate and is accompanied by hyperparathyroidism, increased bone turnover, and increased bone resorption (see Chapter 34). Another form of osteomalacia results from renal tubular defects that cause excessive phosphate losses. This form of osteomalacia is commonly referred to as *vitamin D–resistant rickets,* and often is a familial disorder.[14] It is inherited as an X-linked dominant gene passed by mothers to one half of their children and by fathers to their daughters only. This form of osteomalacia affects boys more severely than girls. Long-standing primary hyperparathyroidism causes increased calcium resorption from bone and hypophosphatemia, which can lead to rickets in children and osteomalacia in adults.

The clinical manifestations of osteomalacia are bone pain, tenderness, and fractures as the disease progresses. In severe cases, muscle weakness often is an early sign. The cause of muscle weakness is unclear. Osteomalacia predisposes a person to pathologic fractures in the weakened areas, especially in the distal radius and proximal femur. In contrast to osteoporosis, it is not a significant cause of hip fractures. There may be delayed healing and poor retention of internal fixation devices. Osteomalacia usually is accompanied by a compensatory or secondary hyperparathyroidism stimulated by low serum calcium levels. Parathyroid hormone reduces renal reabsorption of phosphate and removes calcium from the bone. Serum calcium levels are only slightly reduced in osteomalacia.

Diagnostic measures are directed toward identifying osteomalacia and establishing its cause. Diagnostic methods include x-ray studies, laboratory tests, bone scan, and bone biopsy. X-ray findings typical of osteomalacia are the development of transverse lines or pseudofractures called *Looser zones.* These apparently are caused by stress fractures that are inadequately healed, or by the mechanical inadequacy of penetrating nutrient vessels.[4] A bone biopsy may be done to confirm the diagnosis of osteomalacia in a person with nonspecific osteopenia who shows no improvement after treatment with exercise, vitamin D, and calcium.

The treatment of osteomalacia is directed at the underlying cause. If the problem is nutritional, restoring adequate amounts of calcium and vitamin D to the diet may be sufficient. Older adults with intestinal malabsorption also may benefit from vitamin D. The least expensive and most effective long-term treatment is a diet rich in vitamin D (*i.e.,* fish, dairy products, and margarine) along with careful exposure to the midday sun. Vitamin D is specific for adult osteomalacia and vitamin D–resistant rickets, but large doses usually are needed to overcome the resistance to calcium absorption action and to prevent renal loss of phosphate. The biologically active forms of vitamin D, 25-OH vitamin D (calciferol) or 1,25-(OH)$_2$ vitamin D (calcitriol), are available for use in the treatment of osteomalacia resistant to vitamin D (*i.e.,* osteomalacia resulting from chronic liver disease and kidney failure). If osteomalacia is caused by malabsorption, the treatment is directed toward correcting the primary disease. For example, adequate replacement of pancreatic enzymes is of paramount importance in pancreatic insufficiency. In renal tubular disorders, the treatment is directed at the altered renal physiology.

Rickets

Rickets is a metabolic bone disorder characterized by a failure or delay in calcification of the cartilaginous growth plate in children whose epiphyses have not yet fused.[4,14,59–61] It is also manifested by widening and deformation of the metaphyseal regions of long bones, and a delay in the mineralization of trabecular, endosteal, and periosteal bone surfaces. There are several forms of rickets, including nutritional rickets, vitamin D–dependent rickets, and vitamin D–resistant rickets. As with osteomalacia in the adult, rickets can result from kidney failure; malabsorptive syndromes such as celiac disease and cystic fibrosis; and medications such as anticonvulsants, which cause target organ resistance to vitamin D, and aluminum-containing antacids, which bind phosphorus and prevent its absorption.

Nutritional rickets results from inadequate sunlight exposure or inadequate intake of vitamin D, calcium, or phosphate. Nutritional rickets occurs primarily in underdeveloped areas of the world and among immigrants to developed countries. The causes are inadequate exposure to sunlight (*e.g.,* children are often kept clothed and indoors) and prolonged breast-feeding without vitamin D supplementation. Although the vitamin D content of human milk is low, the combination of breast milk and sunlight exposure usually provides sufficient vitamin D to prevent rickets. Another cause of rickets is the use of commercial alternative milks (*e.g.,* soy or rice beverages) that are not fortified with vitamin D. Vitamin D–dependent rickets can result from abnormalities in the gene coding for the enzyme that converts inactive vitamin D to the active form of vitamin D, or from an autosomal disorder caused by mutations in the vitamin D receptor.[60] Vitamin D–resistant rickets involves hypophosphatemia or a decrease in serum phosphate levels, the most common form being caused by mutations of the phosphate-regulating gene on the X chromosome.[60] The gene mutation causes renal wasting of phosphate at the proximal tubular level of the kidney.

Rickets is characterized by changes in the growing bones of children with overgrowth of the epiphyseal cartilage due to inadequate provisional calcification and failure of the cartilage cells to disintegrate. Bones become deformed; ossification at the epiphyseal plates is delayed and disordered, resulting in widening of the epiphyseal cartilage plate. Any new bone that does grow is unmineralized. The conformation of the gross skeletal changes depends on the severity and duration of the rachitic process, and in particular on the stresses to which the individual bones are subjected.[4,14] During the nonmobile stage of infancy, the head and chest undergo the greatest stresses. The skull is enlarged and soft, and closure of the fontanels is delayed. Teeth are slow to develop, and the child may have difficulty standing. When an ambulating child develops rickets, deformities are likely to affect the spine, pelvis, and long bones (*i.e.,* tibia), causing, most notably, lumbar lordosis and bowing of the legs. The ends of long bones and ribs are enlarged. The thorax may be abnormally shaped, with prominent rib cartilage (*i.e.,* rachitic rosary). The child usually has stunted growth, with a height sometimes far below the normal range. Weight often is not affected, so that the children, many of whom present with a protruding abdomen (*i.e.,* rachitic potbelly), have been described as presenting a Buddha-like appearance when sitting.

Nutritional rickets is treated with a balanced diet sufficient in calcium, phosphorus, and vitamin D. Exposure to sunlight also is important, especially for premature infants and those on artificial milk feedings. Supplemental vitamin D in excess of normal requirements is given for several months. Maintenance of good posture, positioning, and bracing in older children are used to prevent deformities. After the disease is controlled, deformities may have to be surgically corrected as the child grows.

Children with vitamin D-dependent and vitamin D-independent rickets require special treatment measures. Children with vitamin D-dependent rickets caused by lack of the enzyme needed to convert vitamin D to its active form are treated with calcitriol, the active form of vitamin D.[60] Vitamin D-resistant forms of rickets are treated with oral phosphorus or oral phosphorus and calcitriol.

Paget Disease

Paget disease (*i.e.,* osteitis deformans) is the second most common bone disease after osteoporosis.[4,14,62,63] The disease, which has been described as a "collage of matrix madness" is characterized by focal areas of excessive bone turnover and disorganized osteoid formation.[14] The disease usually begins during mid-adulthood and becomes progressively more common with increasing age. The disease is more common in older people and those of Northern European heritage. Men are about twice as likely as women to have the disease.[63]

Paget disease is a focal process with considerable variation in its stage of development in separate sites. At the onset, the disease is marked by regions of furious osteoclastic bone resorption, followed by a period of hectic bone formation with increased numbers of osteoblasts rapidly depositing bone in a chaotic fashion such that the newly formed bone is of poor quality and is disorganized rather than lamellar. The poor quality of bone accounts for the bowing and fractures that occur in bones affected by the disease. The bone marrow adjacent to the bone-forming surface is replaced by loose connective tissue that contains osteoprogenitor cells and numerous blood vessels, which transport blood to and from these metabolically active sites. The lesions of Paget disease may be solitary or may occur in multiple sites. They tend to localize to the bones of the axial skeleton, including the spine, skull, and pelvis. The proximal femur and tibia may be involved in more widespread forms of the disease. Histologically, Paget lesions show increased vascularity and bone marrow fibrosis with intense cellular activity. The bone has a somewhat mosaic-like pattern caused by areas of density outlined by heavy blue lines, called *cement lines* (Fig. 58.19).

Although the cause of Paget disease remains unclear, there is evidence of both genetic and environmental influences. It has been reported that 15% to 40% of persons with the disease have a first-degree relative with Paget disease, and numerous studies have described extended family members with the disease.[63] It is likely that factors other than genetics

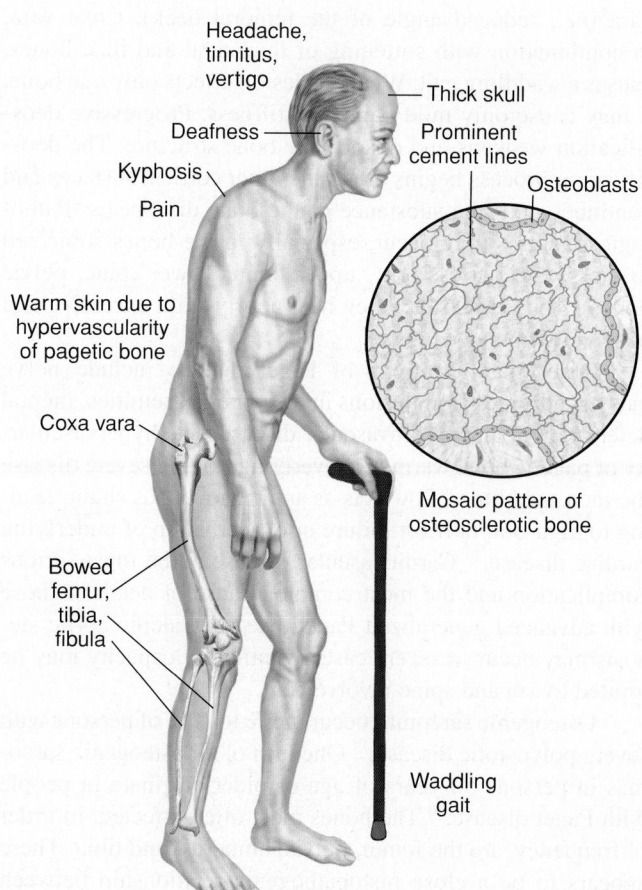

Headache, tinnitus, vertigo

Thick skull

Deafness

Prominent cement lines

Kyphosis

Osteoblasts

Pain

Warm skin due to hypervascularity of pagetic bone

Coxa vara

Mosaic pattern of osteosclerotic bone

Bowed femur, tibia, fibula

Waddling gait

FIGURE 58.19 • Clinical manifestations of Paget disease.

are also involved in the pathogenesis of the disease. Conflicting evidence suggests a probable association with a virus, possibly a paramyxovirus.[14,63,64] This has been supported by the observation of viral particles resembling the paramyxovirus nucleocapsid in the cytoplasm of osteoclasts in persons with Paget disease.

In children, hyperostosis corticalis deformans juvenilis (a rare autosomal recessive disorder), hyperphosphatemia, and diseases that cause diaphyseal stenosis may mimic Paget disease and sometimes are referred to as *juvenile Paget disease*.[65] The disorder presents in infancy or early childhood with pain from debilitating fractures and deformities due to a markedly accelerated rate of bone remodelling throughout the skeleton.

Manifestations

The disease varies in severity from a simple lesion to involvement of many bones. It may be present long before it is detected clinically. The clinical manifestations of Paget disease depend on the specific area involved (Fig. 58.19). Approximately 70% of persons with the disorder are totally asymptomatic, and the disease is discovered accidentally.[62] Involvement of the skull causes headaches, intermittent tinnitus, vertigo, and eventual hearing loss. In the spine, collapse of the anterior vertebrae causes kyphosis of the thoracic spine. The femur and tibia become bowed. Softening of the femoral neck can cause coxa vara (*i.e.,* reduced angle of the femoral neck). Coxa vara, in combination with softening of the sacral and iliac bones, causes a waddling gait. When the lesion affects only one bone, it may cause only mild pain and stiffness. Progressive deossification weakens and distorts the bone structure. The deossification process begins along the inner cortical surfaces and continues until the substance of the bone disappears. Pathologic fractures may occur, especially in the bones subjected to the greatest stress (*e.g.,* upper femur, lower spine, pelvic bones). These fractures often heal poorly, with excessive and poorly distributed callus.

Other manifestations of Paget disease include nerve palsy syndromes from lesions in the upper extremities, mental deterioration, and cardiovascular disease. The hypervascularity of pagetic bone warms the overlying skin; in severe disease the increased blood flow acts as an arteriovenous shunt, leading to high-output heart failure or exacerbation of underlying cardiac disease.[14] Cardiovascular disease is the most serious complication and the most common cause of death in those with advanced generalized Paget disease. Calcific aortic stenosis may occur in severe cases. Ventilatory capacity may be limited by rib and spine involvement.

Osteogenic sarcomas occur in 5% to 10% of persons with severe polyostotic disease.[14] One fifth of all osteogenic sarcomas in persons 50 years of age or older originate in people with Paget disease.[66] The bones most often affected, in order of frequency, are the femur, pelvis, humerus, and tibia. There appears to be a close histopathogenic relationship between Paget disease and the associated sarcoma.[66]

Diagnosis and Treatment

Diagnosis of Paget disease is based on characteristic bone deformities and x-ray changes. Elevated levels of serum alkaline phosphatase and urinary hydroxyproline support the diagnosis, and continued surveillance of these levels may be used to monitor the effectiveness of treatment. Bone scans are used to detect the rapid bone turnover indicative of active disease and to monitor the response to treatment. The scan cannot identify bone activity resulting from malignant lesions. Bone biopsy may be done to differentiate the lesion from osteomyelitis or a primary or metastatic bone tumour.

The treatment of Paget disease is based on the degree of pain and the extent of the disease. Pain can be reduced with nonsteroidal or other anti-inflammatory agents. Suppressive agents such as the bisphosphonates and calcitonin are used to manage pain and prevent further spread of the disease and neurologic defects. Bisphosphonate therapy is the most effective way to control Paget disease.[64] These drugs act by binding directly to bone minerals, inhibiting bone loss by rapidly decreasing bone resorption, followed by a secondary, slower decrease in the rate of bone formation.[62,64] Treatment usually is continued for 3 to 6 months, although recent studies are evaluating shorter courses of treatment. Parenteral bisphosphonates are particularly useful in persons who cannot tolerate oral preparations. Calcitonin also inhibits bone resorption. It is available in injectable and nasal spray forms, but only the injectable form is approved for treatment of Paget disease. Nasal-spray calcitonin, which is approved for other uses, is being studied for use in Paget disease. Persons with Paget disease should receive adequate doses of calcium and vitamin D. A recombinant form of osteoprotegerin is also being used to inhibit osteoclastogenesis in children, slowing the osteoclast activity. Juvenile Paget disease is being described as an osteoprotegerin deficiency.[65]

IN SUMMARY

In addition to its structural function, the skeleton is a homeostatic organ. Metabolic bone diseases such as osteoporosis, osteomalacia, rickets, and Paget disease are the result of a disruption in the equilibrium of bone formation and resorption. Osteoporosis, which is the most common of the metabolic bone diseases, occurs when the rate of bone resorption is greater than that of bone formation. It is seen frequently in postmenopausal women and is the major cause of fractures in persons older than 45 years of age. Osteomalacia and rickets are caused by inadequate mineralization of bone matrix, primarily because of a deficiency of vitamin D. Paget disease results from excessive osteoclastic activity and is characterized by the formation of poor-quality bone. The success rate of the various drugs and hormones that are used to treat metabolic bone diseases varies. Further research is needed to clarify the cause, pathologic process, and treatment of these diseases.

REVIEW EXERCISES

1. A newborn girl was found to have developmental dysplasia of the hip (DDH) during a routine screening examination.
   A. Describe the anatomic abnormalities that are present in the disorder.
   B. Explain the need for early treatment of DDH.

2. A 12-year-old girl was noted to have asymmetry of the shoulders, scapular height, and pelvic height during routine physical examination. On x-ray examination, she is found to have a 30-degree curvature of the spine.
   A. What possible treatments are available for this girl?
   B. Describe the physical problems associated with progressive scoliosis.

3. A 60-year-old postmenopausal woman presents with a compression fracture of the vertebrae. She has also noticed increased backache and loss of height over the past few years.
   A. Explain how the lack of estrogen and aging contribute to the development of osteoporosis.
   B. What other factors should be considered when assessing the risk for development of osteoporosis?
   C. What is the best way to measure bone density?
   D. Name the two most important factors in preventing osteoporosis.
   E. What medications might be used to treat this woman's condition?

References

1. Moore K. L., Persaud T. V. N., Torchia M. G. (2013). *The developing human: Clinically oriented embryology* (9th ed.). Philadelphia, PA: Saunders Elsevier.
2. Ross M. H., Pawlina W. (2011). *Histology: A text and atlas* (6th ed.). Philadelphia, PA: Lippincott Williams & Wilkins.
3. Rhoades R. A., Bell D. R. (2013). *Medical physiology: Principles for clinical medicine* (4th ed.). Philadelphia, PA: Lippincott Williams & Wilkins.
4. Garcia R. A., Klein M. J., Schiller A. L. (2012). Chapter 26: Bones and joints. In Rubin R., Strayer D. S. (Eds.), *Rubin's pathology: Clinicopathologic foundations of medicine* (6th ed.). Philadelphia, PA: Lippincott Williams & Wilkins.
5. Schoeneker P. L., Rich M. M., Gordon J. E. (2014). Chapter 27: The lower extremity. In Weinstein S. L., Flynn J. M. (Eds.), *Lovell & Winter's pediatric orthopaedics* (7th ed.). Philadelphia, PA: Lippincott Williams & Wilkins.
6. Wells L., Sehgal K., Dormans J. P., et al. (2011). Part 32: Bone and joint disorders. In Kliegman R. M., Stanton B. F., St. Geme J. W., et al. (Eds.), *Nelson textbook of pediatrics* (19th ed.). Philadelphia, PA: Saunders Elsevier.
7. Sass P., Hassan G. (2003). Lower extremity abnormalities in children. *American Family Physician, 68*(3), 461–468.
8. Williams C. M., James A. M., Tran T. (2013). Metatarsus adductus: Development of a non-surgical treatment pathway. *Journal of Paediatrics and Child Health, 49*(9), E428–E433.

9. Wall E. J. (2000). Practical primary pediatric orthopedics. *The Nursing Clinics of North America, 35*(1), 95–113.
10. Crocetti M., Barone M. A. (2004). *Oski's essential pediatrics* (2nd ed.). Philadelphia, PA: Lippincott Williams & Wilkins.
11. Kim H. W., Park H. W. (2005). Chapter 18: The pediatric leg and knee. In Weinstein S. L., Buckwalter J. A. (Eds.), *Turek's orthopaedics: Principles and their application* (6th ed.). Philadelphia, PA: Lippincott Williams & Wilkins.
12. Forlino A., Cabral W. A., Barnes A. M., et al. (2011). New perspectives on osteogenesis imperfecta. *Nature Reviews Endocrinology, 7*(9), 540–557.
13. Marini J. C. (2011). Chapter 692: Osteogenesis imperfecta. In Kliegman R. M., Stanton B. F., St. Geme J. W., et al. (Eds.), *Nelson textbook of pediatrics* (19th ed.). Philadelphia, PA: Saunders Elsevier.
14. Rosenberg A. E. (2010). Chapter 26: Bones, joints, and soft tissue tumors. In Kumar V., Abbas A. K., Fausto N., et al. (Eds.), *Robbins and Cotran Pathologic Basis of Disease* (8th ed.). Philadelphia, PA: Elsevier Saunders.
15. Russell R. G. (2011). Bisphosphonates: The first 40 years. *Bone, 49*(1), 2–19.
16. Storer S., Skaggs D. L. (2001). Developmental dysplasia of the hip. *American Family Physician, 74*, 1310–1316.
17. American Academy of Orthopaedic Surgeons. (2014). Detection and non-operative management of paediatric developmental dysplasia of the hip in infants up to six months of age. Available online at: http://www.aaos.org/research/guidelines/DDHGuidelineFINAL.pdf. Accessed June 1, 2015.
18. Patel H.; Canadian Task Force on Preventive Health Care. (2001). Preventive health care, 2001 update: Screening and management of developmental dysplasia of the hip in newborns. *Canadian Medical Association Journal, 164*(12), 1669–1677.
19. Weinstein S. L. (2005). Chapter 20: The pediatric foot. In Weinstein S. L., Buckwalter J. A. (Eds.), *Turek's orthopaedics: Principles and their application* (6th ed.). Philadelphia, PA: Lippincott Williams & Wilkins.
20. Hennessey T. A. (2012). Congenital clubfoot and the Ponseti method: A review of recent literature. *Current Orthopaedic Practice, 23*(5), 442–447.
21. Faulks S. (2005). Changing paradigm for treatment of clubfeet. *Orthopedic Nursing, 26*(1), 25–30.
22. Carroll N. C. (2012). Clubfoot in the twentieth century: Where we were and where we may be going in the twenty-first century. *Journal of Paediatric Orthopaedics Part B, 21*(1), 1–6.
23. Alexander M. (2002). Congenital and developmental disorders. In Maher A. B., Salmond S. W., Pellino T. A. (Eds.), *Orthopaedic nursing* (3rd ed., pp. 567–570). Philadelphia, PA: W.B. Saunders.
24. Gill K. G. (2013). Pediatric hip: Pearls and pitfalls. *Seminars in Musculoskeletal Radiology, 17*(3), 328–338.
25. Kim H. K. W., Herring J. A. (2014). Chapter 17: Legg-Calvé-Perthes disease. In Herring A. J. (Ed.), *Tachdjian's pediatric orthopaedics* (5th ed.). Philadelphia, PA: W.B. Saunders.
26. Yawn B. P., Yawn R. A., Hodge D., et al. (1999). A population-based study of school scoliosis screening. *Journal of the American Medical Association, 282*, 1427–1432.
27. Reamy B. V., Slakey J. B. (2001). Adolescent scoliosis: Review and current comments. *American Family Physician, 64*, 111–116.
28. Weinstein S. (2005). Chapter 16: The thoracolumbar spine. In Weinstein S. L., Buckwalter J. A. (Eds.), *Turek's orthopaedics: Principles and their application* (6th ed.). Philadelphia, PA: Lippincott Williams & Wilkins.
29. Paria N., Wise C. A. (2015). Genetic of adolescent idiopathic scoliosis. *Seminars in Spine Surgery, 27*(1), 9–15.
30. Omey M. L., Micheli L. J., Gerbino P. G. 2nd. (2000). Idiopathic scoliosis and spondylolysis in the female athlete: Tips for treatment. *Clinical Orthopaedics and Related Research, 372*, 74–84.
31. Greig A., Constantin E., Carsley S., et al. (2010). Preventive health care visits for children and adolescents aged 6 to 17 years: The Greig Health Record, technical report. *Paediatrics & Child Health, 15*(3), 157–159.
32. Beausejour M., Goulet L., Parent S., et al.; Members of the Quebec Scoliosis Society and of the Canadian Paediatric Spinal Deformities Study Group. (2013). The effectiveness of scoliosis screening programs:

Methods for systematic review and expert panel recommendations formulation. *Scoliosis, 8*, 12.

33. Lonner B. S. (2007). Emerging minimally invasive technologies for management of scoliosis. *Orthopedic Clinics of North America, 38*, 431–440.

34. Cohen S. (2006). Role of RANK ligand in normal and pathologic bone remodeling and therapeutic potential of novel inhibitory molecules in musculoskeletal disease. *Arthritis and Rheumatism, 55*, 15–18.

35. Hofbauer L. C., Schoppet M. (2004). Clinical implications of osteoprotegerin/RANKL/RANK system for bone and vascular disease. *The Journal of American Medical Association, 292*, 490–495.

36. Rogers A., Eastell R. (2005). Review: Circulating osteoprotegerin and receptor activator for nuclear factor κB ligand: Clinical utility in metabolic bone disease assessment. *Journal of Clinical Endocrinology and Metabolism, 90*, 6323–6331.

37. Rachner T. D., Khosla S., Hofbauer L. C. (2011). Osteoporosis: Now and the future. *Lancet, 377*(9773), 1276–1287.

38. Lane N. E. (2006). Epidemiology, etiology, and diagnosis of osteoporosis. *American Journal of Obstetrics and Gynecology, 194*, S3–S11.

39. Gass M., Dawson-Hughes B. (2006). Preventing osteoporosis-related fractures: An overview. *American Journal of Medicine, 119*, S3–S11.

40. Rodan G. A., Reska H. A. (2003). Osteoporosis and bisphosphonates. *Journal of Bone and Joint Surgery (American Volume), 85*(Suppl 3), 8–12.

41. Osteoporosis Canada. (2015). Osteoporosis facts and statistics. Available online at: http://www.osteoporosis.ca/osteoporosis-and-you/osteoporosis-facts-and-statistics/. Accessed June 1, 2015.

42. Steinweg K. K. (2002). Menopause, bone physiology, and osteoporosis prevention. *Clinics in Family Practice, 4*, 89–111.

43. Rosen C. J. (2005). Postmenopausal osteoporosis. *The New England Journal of Medicine, 353*, 595–603.

44. Mosekilde L., Vestergaard P., Rejnmark L. (2013). The pathogenesis, treatment and prevention of osteoporosis in men. *Drugs, 73*(1), 15–29.

45. Walker-Bone K. (2012). Recognizing and treating secondary osteoporosis. *Nature Reviews Rheumatology, 8*(8), 480–492.

46. Beals K. A., Meyer N. L. (2007). Female athlete triad update. *Clinics in Sports Medicine, 26*, 69–80.

47. Deimel J. F., Dunlap B. J. (2012). The female athlete triad. *Clinics in Sports Medicine, 31*, 247–254.

48. Kazis K., Iglesias E. (2003). Female athlete triad. *Adolescent Medicine, 14*, 87–95.

49. Raisz L. C. (2005). Screening for osteoporosis. *The New England Journal of Medicine, 353*(2), 164–171.

50. Armstrong C. (2006). NAMS updates recommendations on diagnosis and management of osteoporosis in postmenopausal women. *American Family Physician, 74*, 1631–1639.

51. Papaioannou A., Morin S., Cheung A. M., et al.; Scientific Advisory Council of Osteoporosis Canada. (2010). 2010 clinical practice guidelines for the diagnosis and management of osteoporosis in Canada: Summary. *Canadian Medical Association Journal, 182*(17). 1864–1873.

52. Osteoporosis Canada. (2010) Quick reference guide. Available online at: http://www.osteoporosis.ca/multimedia/pdf/Quick_Reference_Guide_October_2010.pdf. Accessed June 1, 2015.

53. Schwalfenberg G. (2007). Not enough vitamin D: Health consequences for Canadians. *Canadian Family Physician, 53*(5), 841–854.

54. Cauley J. A., Robbins J., Chen Z., et al. (2003). Effects of estrogen plus progestin on risk of fracture and bone mineral density: The Women's Health Initiative randomized trial. *Journal of the American Medical Association, 290*, 1729–1738.

55. Sirotkin A. V., Harrath A. H. (2014). Phytoestrogens and their effects. *European Journal of Pharmacology, 741*, 230–236.

56. Hanley D. A. (updated 2013). Musculoskeletal disorders: Osteoporosis. In Repchinsky C. (Ed.), *e-Therapeutics*. Ottawa, ON: Canadian Pharmacists Association.

57. Lavelle W., Lavelle E. D., Khaleel M. A. (2007). Vertebroplasty and kyphoplasty. *Medical Clinics of North America, 91*, 299–314.

58. Pateder D. B., Khanna A. J., Lieberman I. H. (2007). Vertebroplasty and kyphoplasty for the management of osteoporotic vertebral compression fractures. *Orthopedic Clinics of North America, 38*, 409–418.

59. Berg E. E. (2004). Rickets. *Orthopaedic Nursing, 23*(1), 53–55.

60. Nield L. S., Mahajan P., Joshi A., et al. (2006). Rickets: Not a disease of the past. *American Family Physician, 74*, 619–630.

61. Pttifor J. M. (2005). Rickets and vitamin D deficiency in children and adolescents. *Endocrinology and Metabolism Clinics of North America, 34*, 537–553.

62. Schneider D., Hofmann M. T. (2002). Diagnosis and treatment of Paget's disease of bone. *American Family Physician, 65*, 2069–2072.

63. Roodman G. D., Windle J. J. (2005). Paget disease of bone. *Journal of Clinical Investigation, 115*, 200–208.

64. Ralston S. H. (2013). Paget's disease of bone. *New England Journal of Medicine, 368*(7), 644–650.

65. Cundy T., Davidson J., Rutland M. D., et al. (2005). Recombinant osteoprotegerin for juvenile Paget disease. *New England Journal of Medicine, 353*, 918–923.

66. Drake W. M., Kendler D. L., Brown J. P. (2001). Consensus statement on the modern therapy of Paget's disease of bone from a Western Alliance Symposium. Biannual Foothills Meeting on Osteoporosis, Calgary, Alberta, Canada, September 9–10, 2000. *Clinical Therapeutics, 23*(4), 620–626.

Visit thePoint **http://thePoint.lww.com for animations, journal articles, and more!**

Disorders of Musculoskeletal Function: Rheumatic Disorders

59

Arthritis is a descriptive term applied to more than 100 rheumatic diseases, ranging from localized, self-limiting conditions to those that are systemic autoimmune processes. Arthritis affects persons in all age groups.[1] It is estimated that over 4.6 million Canadians older than 15 years of age (approximately 16% of the population) are affected by arthritic and rheumatic diseases, with a higher proportion of the Aboriginal population affected (1.3 to 1.6 times higher when adjusted for the Canadian population composition).[2] Estimates for the year 2036 indicate that this will climb to over 7.5 million Canadians over the age of 15 years (1 in 5) who will be afflicted with arthritic conditions.[2,3] Although arthritis cannot be cured, much can be done to control its progress.

The common use of the term *arthritis* oversimplifies the nature of the varied disease processes, the difficulty in differentiating one form of arthritis or rheumatic disease from another, and the complexity of treatment of these usually chronic conditions. These diverse conditions share inflammation of the joint as a prominent or accompanying symptom. In the systemic rheumatic diseases—those affecting body systems in addition to the musculoskeletal system—the inflammation is primary, resulting from an immune response. In rheumatic conditions limited to a single or few synovial or diarthrodial joints, the inflammation is secondary, resulting from a degenerative process and the resulting joint irregularities that occur as the bone attempts to remodel itself.

This chapter focuses on systemic autoimmune rheumatic diseases, arthritis associated with spondylitis, osteoarthritis syndrome, metabolic diseases associated with arthritis, and rheumatic disease in children and older adults. A review of normal joint structures is presented in Chapter 56.

SYSTEMIC AUTOIMMUNE RHEUMATIC DISEASES

After completing this section of the chapter, you should be able to meet the following objectives:

- Characterize the common characteristics of the different systemic autoimmune rheumatic disorders.
- Describe the pathologic changes that may be found in the joint of a person with rheumatoid arthritis.

- List the extra-articular manifestations of rheumatoid arthritis.
- Describe the immunologic process that occurs in systemic lupus erythematosus.
- List four major organ systems that may be involved in systemic lupus erythematosus.
- Describe the manifestations of systemic sclerosis.

Systemic autoimmune rheumatic diseases are a group of chronic disorders characterized by diffuse inflammatory lesions and degenerative changes in connective tissue. These disorders share similar clinical features and may affect many of the same organs. Rheumatoid arthritis (RA), systemic lupus erythematosus (SLE), polymyalgia rheumatica, temporal arteritis, and juvenile arthritis and dermatomyositis, which share an autoimmune systemic pathogenesis, are discussed in this section.

Rheumatoid Arthritis

Rheumatoid arthritis (RA) is a systemic inflammatory disease that affects approximately 300,000 Canadians, with women affected three times more frequently than men.[3] Although the disease can occur in all age groups, its prevalence increases with age and most often appears between 25 and 50 years of age.[3]

Etiology and Pathogenesis

Although the cause of RA remains uncertain, evidence points to a genetic predisposition and the development of joint inflammation that is immunologically mediated. It has been suggested that the disease is initiated in a genetically predisposed individual by the activation of a T-cell–mediated response to an immunologic trigger, such as a microbial agent (Fig. 59.1). The importance of genetic factors in the pathogenesis of RA is supported by the increased frequency of the disease among first-degree relatives and monozygotic twins.[4] In addition, it is generally agreed that certain major histocompatibility complex (MHC) genes are expressed in a nonrandom manner in persons with RA. An important genetic locus that predisposes to RA is present on the human leukocyte antigen (HLA) II loci on the MHC class II molecules, with a specific set of HLA DR alleles (DR4, DR1, DR14) being consistently increased in

FIGURE 59.1 • Disease process in rheumatoid arthritis.

persons with RA.[4] These alleles are thought to form a shared epitope in the hypervariable segment of the HLA-DRB1 gene, which forms a rheumatoid pocket on the HLA molecule (see Chapter 17). It seems likely that the binding properties of this pocket influence the types of peptides that can be bound by the RA-associated HLA-DR molecules, thereby affecting the immune response.[4]

The pathogenesis of RA can be viewed as an aberrant immune response that leads to synovial inflammation and destruction of the joint architecture. It has been suggested that the disease is initiated by the activation of helper T cells, release of cytokines (*e.g.,* tumour necrosis factor [TNF], interleukin [IL]-1), and antibody formation. Approximately 70% to 80% of persons with the disease have a substance called the *rheumatoid factor* (RF), which is an autologous (self-produced) antibody (Ig RF) that reacts with a fragment of immunoglobulin G (IgG) to form immune complexes.[4,5] Immune complexes (Ig RF ± IgG) and complement components are found in the synovium, synovial fluid, and extra-articular lesions of persons with RA. Although persons with RA may be seronegative (do not have Ig RF in their serum), the presence of a high RF titre is frequently associated with severe and unremitting disease, with mainly systemic complications. Evidence suggests that identification of anticyclic citrullinated peptide antibodies (anti-CCP antibodies) is a more specific diagnostic marker for predicting RA than the RF test.[4]

RHEUMATOID ARTHRITIS

- Rheumatoid arthritis is a chronic systemic inflammatory disease with bilateral involvement of synovial or diarthrodial joints.
- The initial joint changes involve the synovial cells lining the joint. Inflammatory cells accumulate, and angiogenesis and formation of pannus, which proceed to cover the articular cartilage and isolate it from its nutritional synovial fluid, take place.

The role of the autoimmune process in the joint destruction of RA remains obscure. At the cellular level, neutrophils, macrophages, and lymphocytes are attracted to the area. The neutrophils and macrophages phagocytize the immune complexes and, in the process, release lysosomal enzymes capable of causing destructive changes in the joint cartilage (Fig. 59.1). The inflammatory response that follows attracts additional inflammatory cells, setting into motion a chain of events that perpetuates the condition. As the inflammatory process progresses, the synovial cells and subsynovial tissues undergo reactive hyperplasia. Vasodilation and increased blood flow cause warmth and redness. The joint swelling that occurs is the result of the increased capillary permeability that accompanies the inflammatory process.

Characteristic of RA is the development of an extensive network of new blood vessels in the synovial membrane that contributes to the advancement of the rheumatoid synovitis. This destructive vascular granulation tissue, which is called *pannus,* extends from the synovium to involve the "bare area," a region of unprotected bone at the junction between cartilage and subchondral bone. Pannus is a feature of RA that differentiates it from other forms of inflammatory arthritis[6] (Fig. 59.2B). The inflammatory cells found in the pannus have a destructive effect on the adjacent cartilage and bone. Eventually, pannus develops between the joint margins, leading to reduced joint motion and the possibility of eventual ankylosis. With progression of the disease, joint inflammation and the resulting structural changes lead to joint instability, muscle atrophy from disuse, stretching of the ligaments, and involvement of the tendons and muscles. The effect of the pathologic changes on joint structure and function is related to the degree of disease activity, which can change at any time. Unfortunately, the destructive changes are irreversible.

Clinical Manifestations

RA often is associated with extra-articular as well as articular manifestations (Fig. 59.2). It usually has an insidious onset marked by systemic manifestations such as fatigue, anorexia, weight loss, and generalized aching and stiffness. The disease, which is characterized by exacerbations and remissions, may involve only a few joints for brief durations, or it may become relentlessly progressive and debilitating.

Joint Manifestations. Joint involvement usually is symmetric and polyarticular. Any synovial (diarthrodial) joint can be involved. The person may complain of joint pain and stiffness that lasts for 30 minutes and frequently for several hours. The limitation of joint motion that occurs early in the disease usually is because of pain; later, it is because of fibrosis. The most frequently affected joints initially are the fingers, hands, wrists, knees, and feet. Later, other diarthrodial joints may become involved. Spinal involvement usually is limited to the cervical region. In the hands, there usually is bilateral and symmetric involvement of the proximal interphalangeal (PIP) and metacarpophalangeal (MCP) joints in the early stages of RA; the distal interphalangeal (DIP) joints rarely are affected.

The fingers often take on a spindle-shaped appearance because of inflammation of the PIP joints.

Progressive joint destruction may lead to subluxation (*i.e.,* dislocation of the joint resulting in misalignment of the bone ends) and instability of the joint and limitation of movement. Swelling and thickening of the synovium can result in stretching of the joint capsule and ligaments. When this occurs, muscle and tendon imbalances develop, and mechanical forces applied to the joints through daily activities produce joint deformities. In the MCP joints, the extensor tendons can slip to the ulnar side of the metacarpal head, causing ulnar deviation of the fingers (Fig. 59.2A). Subluxation of the MCP joints may develop when this deformity is present. Hyperextension of the PIP joint and partial flexion of the DIP joint is called a *swan neck deformity.* After this condition becomes fixed, severe loss of function occurs because the person can no longer make a fist. Flexion of the PIP joint with hyperextension of the DIP joint is called a *boutonnière deformity.*

The knee is one of the most commonly affected joints and is responsible for much of the disability associated with the disease.[1] Active synovitis may be apparent as visible swelling that obliterates the normal contour over the medial and lateral aspects of the patella. The *bulge sign,* which involves milking fluid from the lateral to the medial side of the patella, may be used to determine the presence of excess fluid when it is not visible. Joint contractures, instability, and genu valgus (knock-knee) deformity are other possible manifestations. Severe quadriceps atrophy can contribute to the disability. A *Baker cyst* may develop in the popliteal area behind the knee. This is caused by enlargement of the bursa but does not usually cause symptoms unless the cyst ruptures, in which case symptoms mimicking thrombophlebitis appear.

Ankle involvement can limit flexion and extension, which can create difficulty in walking. Involvement of the metatarsophalangeal joints can cause subluxation, hallux valgus, and hammer toe deformities. Neck discomfort is common. In rare cases, long-standing disease can lead to neurologic complications such as occipital headaches, muscle weakness, and numbness and tingling in the upper extremities.

Extra-articular Manifestations. Although characteristically a joint disease, RA can affect a number of other tissues. Extra-articular manifestations probably occur with a fair degree of frequency but usually are mild enough to cause few problems. They are most likely to occur in persons who have the RF.

Because RA is a systemic disease, it may be accompanied by complaints of fatigue, weakness, anorexia, weight loss, and low-grade fever when the disease is active. The C-reactive protein (CRP), which commonly is elevated during inflammatory processes, has been found to be more sensitive to the amount of disease activity compared with the erythrocyte sedimentation rate (ESR).[7] Anemia associated with a low serum iron level or low iron-binding capacity is common.[1] This anemia usually is resistant to iron therapy.

Rheumatoid nodules are granulomatous lesions that develop around small blood vessels. The nodules may be

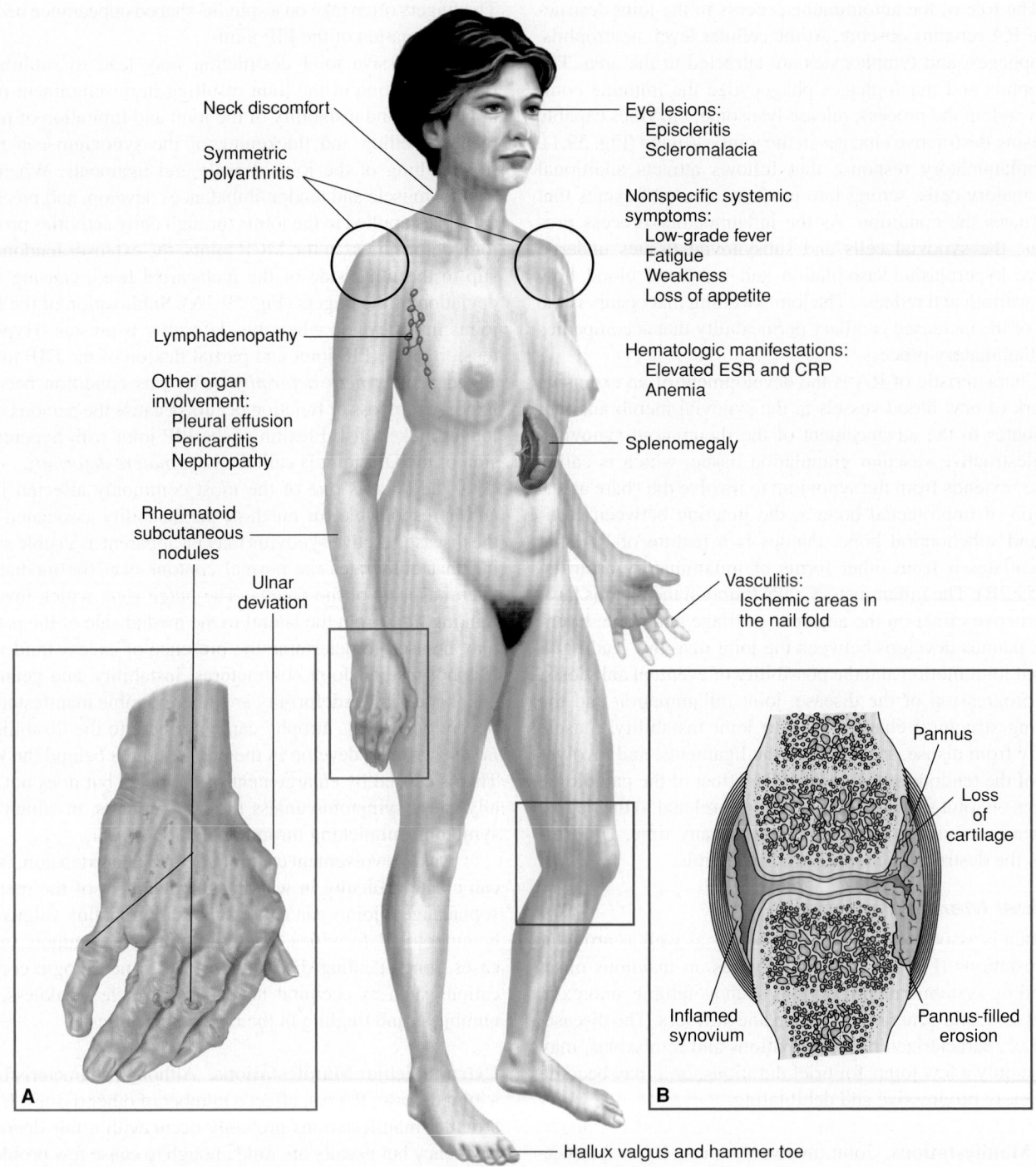

Neck discomfort

Symmetric polyarthritis

Lymphadenopathy

Other organ involvement:
Pleural effusion
Pericarditis
Nephropathy

Rheumatoid subcutaneous nodules

Ulnar deviation

Eye lesions:
Episcleritis
Scleromalacia

Nonspecific systemic symptoms:
Low-grade fever
Fatigue
Weakness
Loss of appetite

Hematologic manifestations:
Elevated ESR and CRP
Anemia

Splenomegaly

Vasculitis:
Ischemic areas in the nail fold

Pannus

Loss of cartilage

Inflamed synovium

Pannus-filled erosion

A

B

Hallux valgus and hammer toe

FIGURE 59.2 • Clinical manifestations of rheumatoid arthritis featuring (**A**) hand and finger manifestations and (**B**) destructive joint changes. ESR, erythrocyte sedimentation rate; CRP, C-reactive protein.

tender or nontender, movable or immovable, and small or large. Typically, they are found over pressure points such as the extensor surfaces of the ulna. The nodules may remain unless surgically removed, or they may resolve spontaneously.

Vasculitis, or inflammation of small and medium-sized arteries, is an uncommon manifestation of RA in persons with a long history of active arthritis and high titres of RF (see Chapter 22). Manifestations include ischemic areas in the nail

fold and digital pulp that appear as brown spots. Ulcerations may occur in the lower extremities, particularly around the malleolar areas. In some cases, neuropathy may be the only symptom of vasculitis. The visceral organs, such as the heart, lungs, and gastrointestinal tract, also may be affected.

Other extra-articular manifestations include eye lesions such as episcleritis, and scleromalacia, which is due to scleral nodules and is capable of causing retinal detachment, and pulmonary and cardiac complications (pleuritis and pericarditis). A small number of persons have splenomegaly and lymph node enlargement.

Diagnosis and Treatment

The diagnosis of RA is based on findings of the history, physical examination, and laboratory tests. Information should be elicited regarding the duration of symptoms, systemic manifestations, stiffness, and family history. The criteria for establishing an RA diagnosis that is used in Canada was developed by the American College of Rheumatology and the European League against Rheumatism (EULAR).[8] A score-based algorithm is used to look at four areas of classification (joint involvement, serology, acute phase reactants, and duration) to identify newly presenting patients and facilitate early treatment.

In the early stages, the disease often is difficult to diagnose. On physical examination, the affected joints show signs of inflammation, swelling, tenderness, and possibly warmth and reduced motion. The joints have a soft, spongy feeling because of the synovial thickening and inflammation. Body movements may be guarded to prevent pain. Changes in joint structure usually are not visible early in the disease.

The RF test results are not diagnostic for RA, but they can be of value in differentiating RA from other forms of arthritis. Between 1% and 5% of healthy persons have the factor, and its presence seems to be more common with advancing age.[9] Also, a person can have RA without the presence of RF. Disease severity and activity tend to correlate with RF levels; patients with high RF levels tend to have a significantly higher frequency of extra-articular involvement (*e.g.,* rheumatoid nodules, vasculitis, neuropathy).[9] The detection of anti-cyclic citrullinated peptide (CCP) antibodies is more useful for diagnosing RA because of its higher specificity. Citrulline is an unusual amino acid that is generated by the enzymatic digestion of arginine. Recent research suggests that citrulline-containing proteins may serve as specific targets for the IgG antibody response in RA.[10,11] Anti-CPP antibodies, which have been detected very early in RA, appear to be a good prognostic marker for the disease and discriminate between erosive and nonerosive forms of the disease.[12]

Radiologic findings also are not diagnostic in RA because joint erosions often are not seen on radiographic images in the early stages of the disorder. Synovial fluid analysis can be helpful in the diagnostic process. The synovial fluid has a cloudy appearance, the white blood cell count is elevated as a result of inflammation, and the complement components are decreased.

The treatment goals for a person with RA are to reduce pain, minimize stiffness and swelling, maintain mobility, and possibly halt the pathologic process. The treatment plan includes education about the disease and its treatment, rest, therapeutic exercises, and medications. Because of the chronicity of the disease and the need for continuous, long-term adherence to the prescribed treatment modalities, it is important that the treatment be integrated with the person's lifestyle.

Strategies to aid in symptom control also involve regulating activity by pacing, establishing priorities, and setting realistic goals. Support groups and group education programs may be beneficial. The home and work environments should be assessed, and interventions should be incorporated as the situation warrants.

Both physical rest and emotional rest are important aspects of care.[1] Physical rest reduces joint stress. Rest of specific joints is recommended to relieve pain. For example, sitting reduces the weight on an inflamed knee, and the use of lightweight splints reduces undue movement of the hand or wrist. Emotional rest decreases outflow from the sympathetic nervous system and helps muscles relax and is often useful for persons who find that emotional stress increases discomfort. Although rest is essential, therapeutic exercises also are important in maintaining joint motion and muscle strength. Range-of-motion exercises involve the active and passive movement of joints. Isometric (muscle-tensing) exercises may be used to strengthen muscles. These exercises are usually taught by a physical therapist and performed daily at home. The difference between normal activity and therapeutic exercise should be emphasized. Aerobic exercise and muscle strengthening exercises can be an important component of the treatment regimen of selected patients. Studies have shown that although persons with RA may have low levels of physical fitness, they can benefit from individualized exercise programs without experiencing joint damage or flare-ups of the disease.[13]

Instruction in the safe use of heat and cold modalities to relieve discomfort and in the use of relaxation techniques also is important. Proper posture, positioning, and body mechanics and the use of supportive shoes can provide further comfort. There often is a need for information about the principles of joint protection and work simplification. Some persons may need assistive devices to reduce pain and improve their ability to perform activities of daily living.

The goals of pharmacologic therapy for RA are to reduce pain, decrease inflammation, maintain or restore joint function, and prevent bone and cartilage destruction. Medications used to achieve these goals are classified as those that provide relief of arthritis symptoms and those that have the potential for modifying the course of the disease. The trend in RA management is toward a more aggressive pharmacologic approach at an earlier stage in the disease. Ideally, disease-modifying antirheumatic drug therapy should be used when the diagnosis of RA is established and before erosive changes appear on radiography.[1] Early treatment is based on the theory that T-cell–dependent pathways, which manifest early in the inflammatory process, are more responsive to treatment than later in the process, when disease progression is controlled by activated fibroblasts and macrophages, and the disease may be more resistant to treatment.

Nonsteroidal anti-inflammatory drugs (NSAIDs) usually are used early in the treatment of RA. The NSAIDs inhibit cyclooxygenase (COX)-mediated synthesis of prostaglandins, which have a damaging effect on joint structures. NSAIDs, including salicylates (*e.g.,* aspirin), provide analgesic and anti-inflammatory effects. Effectiveness, side effects, cost, and dosing schedules are considered when selecting an NSAID.

There is a wide range of responses to the various NSAIDs, and the particular NSAID that works best for any one individual is not always predictable. The incidence of adverse reactions to the NSAIDs (*e.g.*, gastric irritation and bleeding, fluid retention, kidney damage) tends to increase with age and long-term use. The selective COX-2 inhibitors (*e.g.*, celecoxib) were developed with the goal of decreasing the gastrointestinal adverse effects seen with the traditional NSAIDs.[14] There are two COX isomers—COX-1 and COX-2. COX-1 is continuously expressed in many cells and is responsible for the general effects of prostaglandins, including protection of the gastric mucosa, whereas COX-2 is induced by cytokines and mainly expressed in inflammatory tissues.

Early treatment also includes the disease-modifying antirheumatic drugs (DMARDs).[15] DMARDs include gold salts, hydroxychloroquine, sulfasalazine, methotrexate, and azathioprine. Methotrexate has become the drug of choice because of its potency, and it is relatively fast acting (*i.e.*, improvement is seen in 1 month) compared with the slower-acting DMARDs, which can take 3 to 4 months to work. Methotrexate is thought to interfere with purine metabolism, leading to the release of adenosine, a potent anti-inflammatory compound. All of the DMARDs can be toxic and require close monitoring for adverse effects, especially those related to bone marrow suppression.

Corticosteroid drugs may be used to reduce discomfort. These agents interrupt the inflammatory and immune cascade at several levels, such as interfering with inflammatory cell adhesion and migration, impairing prostaglandin synthesis, and inhibiting neutrophil superoxide production. To avoid long-term side effects, they are used only in specific situations for short-term therapy at a low-dose level. They may be used for unremitting disease with extra-articular manifestations. The corticosteroids do not modify the disease and are unable to prevent joint destruction. Intra-articular corticosteroid injections can provide rapid relief of acute or subacute inflammatory synovitis (after infection is excluded) in a few joints. They should not be repeated more than a few times each year.

Second-line antirheumatic drugs include biologic and synthetic DMARDs such as etanercept, infliximab, and adalimumab.[15-17] Infliximab, etanercept, and adalimumab are biologic response-modifying agents that block TNF-α, one of the key proinflammatory cytokines in RA.[17] The anti–TNF-α agents have shown significant efficacy and favourable safety profiles. These agents have also been shown to inhibit radiologic disease progression and improve functional outcomes.

Another approach to RA treatment is combination DMARD therapy.[16,17] This approach is a generally accepted one, and has been shown to be effective in several studies. Individual drugs with different mechanisms of action are given simultaneously to control the disease. The individual drugs are then tapered as symptoms subside and clinical remission is achieved.

Newer biologic response modifiers, abatacept and rituximab, are available for treatment of persons with RA who have had an inadequate response to one or more of the DMARDs. Abatacept, a T-cell modulator, binds to CD80/CD86 on antigen-presenting cells, preventing the costimulatory signal that results in full T-cell activation.[18] Rituximab is a chimeric antibody that binds to the antigen CD20 on pre-B and mature B lymphocytes, causing their destruction. B-cell depletion is associated with reduction of markers of inflammation, including IL-6, C-reactive protein, anti-CCP, and RF.[18]

Surgery also may be a part of the treatment of RA.[1] Synovectomy may be indicated to reduce pain and joint damage when synovitis does not respond to medical treatment. The most common soft tissue surgery is tenosynovectomy (*i.e.*, repair of damaged tendons) of the hand to release nerve entrapments. Total joint replacements (*i.e.*, arthroplasty) may be indicated to reduce pain and increase motion. Arthrodesis (*i.e.*, joint fusion) is indicated only in extreme cases when there is so much soft tissue damage and scarring or infection that a replacement is impossible. Although the course of RA is unpredictable and effective treatments continue to be developed, the goal is to identify and treat this disease as early as possible for the best prognosis.

Systemic Lupus Erythematosus

Systemic lupus erythematosus (SLE) is a chronic inflammatory disease that can affect virtually any organ system, including the musculoskeletal system. It is a major rheumatic disease, with a prevalence of approximately 1 case per 2,000 persons. Approximately 17,000 Canadians and 5 million people worldwide have this disease.[3] There is a female predominance of 10 to 1, and this ratio is closer to 30 to 1 during the childbearing years. SLE is more common in African, Hispanic, and Asian populations compared to Caucasians and within Canada it is more common and severe among Aboriginal people.[19]

Etiology and Pathogenesis

The cause of SLE is unknown. It is characterized by the formation of autoantibodies and immune complexes. Persons with SLE appear to have B-cell hyperreactivity and increased production of antibodies against self (*i.e.*, autoantibodies) and nonself antigens. These B cells are polyclonal, each producing a different type of antibody. The autoantibodies can directly damage tissues or combine with corresponding antigens to form tissue-damaging immune complexes. Antibodies have been identified against an array of nuclear and cytoplasmic cell components (*e.g.*, microtubules, ribosomes, RNA). Some autoantibodies that have been identified in SLE are antinuclear antibodies (ANAs), including antideoxyribonucleic acid (anti-DNA) antibodies, antiphospholipid antibodies, and anti-Smith (Sm) antibodies. In addition to ANAs, persons with lupus have a host of other self-antigens including those directed against elements of the blood (red cells, platelets, lymphocytes) and plasma proteins (clotting and complement factors).

The development of autoantibodies can result from a combination of factors, including genetic, hormonal, immunologic, and environmental factors.[20] Genetic predisposition is evidenced by the occurrence of familial cases of SLE, especially among identical twins. The increased incidence among blacks and Canadian Aboriginals compared with whites also suggests genetic factors.[19] As many as four genes may be involved in the expression of SLE in humans. Genes linked to the HLA-DR and HLA-DQ loci in the MHC class II molecules show strong support for a genetic link in the development of SLE.[21] Studies also suggest that an imbalance in sex hormone levels may play a role in the development of the disease, especially because the disease is so prevalent among women. Androgens appear to protect against the development of SLE, whereas estrogens seem to favour its development. It has been suggested that an imbalance in sex hormone levels may lead to heightened helper T-cell and weakened suppressor T-cell immune responses that could in turn lead to the development of autoantibodies.[1]

Possible environmental triggers include ultraviolet (UV) light, chemicals (*e.g.,* drugs, hair dyes), some foods, and infectious agents.[20] UV light, specifically UVB associated with exposure to the sun or unshielded fluorescent bulbs, may trigger exacerbations. Photosensitivity occurs in approximately one third of patients with SLE. Certain drugs may also provoke a lupus-like disorder in susceptible persons, particularly in older adults. The most common of these drugs are hydralazine and procainamide. Other drugs, such as quinidine, chlorpromazine, methyldopa, isoniazid, minocycline, and phenytoin, also have been known to produce this syndrome. The disease usually recedes when the drug is discontinued.[1]

Clinical Manifestations

SLE can manifest in a variety of ways. The disease has been called the *great imitator* because it has the capacity for affecting many different body systems, including the musculoskeletal system, the skin, the cardiovascular system, the lungs, the kidneys, the central nervous system (CNS), and the red blood cells and platelets (Fig. 59.3). The onset may be acute or insidious, and the course of the disease is characterized by exacerbations and remissions.

CLINICAL MANIFESTATIONS OF SYSTEMIC LUPUS ERYTHEMATOSUS

- SLE is a chronic autoimmune disorder characterized by production of a wide array of autoantibodies against nuclear and cytoplasmic cell components.
- SLE is often described as the great imitator because it can affect almost any organ system, including the joints of the musculoskeletal system, the skin, kidneys, lungs, nervous system, and the heart.

Arthralgias and arthritis are among the most commonly occurring early symptoms of SLE; approximately 90% of all persons with the disease complain of joint pain at some point during the course of their disease.[20] The polyarthritis of SLE initially can be confused with other forms of arthritis, especially RA, because of the symmetric arthropathy. However, on

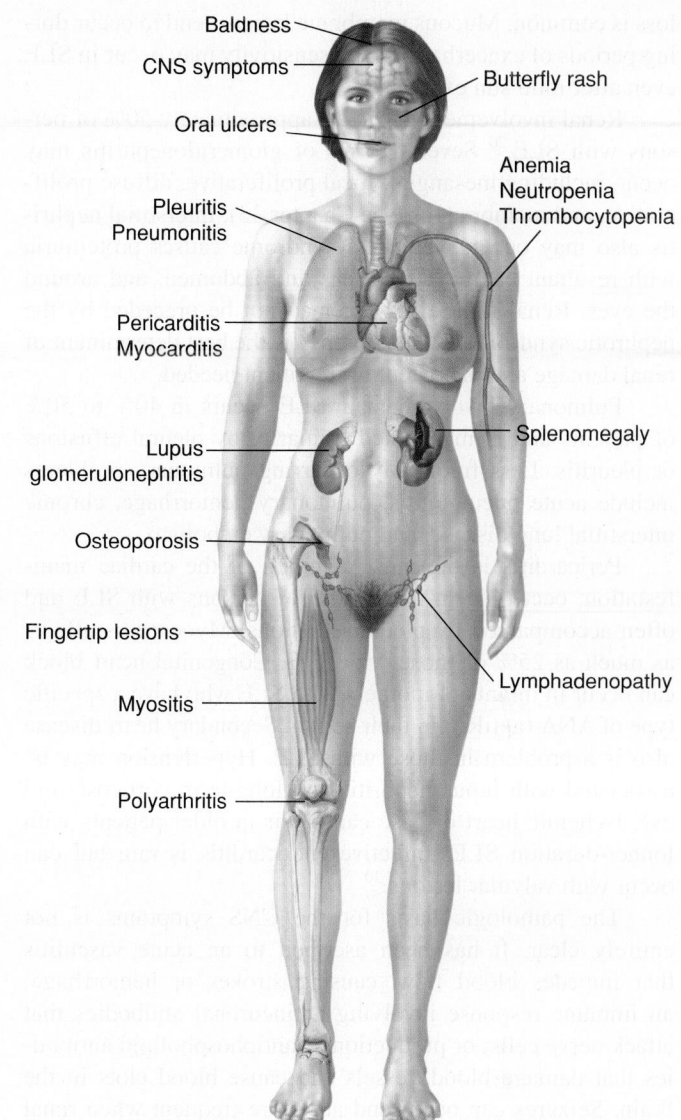

FIGURE 59.3 • Clinical manifestations of systemic lupus erythematosus.

radiologic examination, articular destruction rarely is found. Ligaments, tendons, and the joint capsule may be involved, causing varied deformities in persons with the disease. Flexion contractures, hyperextension of the interphalangeal joints, and subluxation of the carpometacarpal joints contribute to the deformity and subsequent loss of function in the hands. Other musculoskeletal manifestations of SLE include tenosynovitis, rupture of the intrapatellar and Achilles tendons, and avascular necrosis, frequently of the femoral head.

Skin manifestations can vary greatly and may be classified as acute, subacute, or chronic. The acute skin lesions include the classic malar or "butterfly" rash on the nose and cheeks (Fig. 59.3). This rash is seen in SLE but may be associated with other skin lesions, such as hives or livedo reticularis (*i.e.,* reticular cyanotic discolouration of the skin, often precipitated by cold) and fingertip lesions, such as periungual erythema, nail fold infarcts, and splinter hemorrhages. Hair loss is common. Mucous membrane lesions tend to occur during periods of exacerbation. Sun sensitivity may occur in SLE even after mild sun exposure.

Renal involvement occurs in approximately 50% of persons with SLE.[20] Several forms of glomerulonephritis may occur, including mesangial, focal proliferative, diffuse proliferative, and membranous (see Chapter 33). Interstitial nephritis also may occur. Nephrotic syndrome causes proteinuria with resultant edema in the legs and abdomen, and around the eyes. Renal failure may or may not be preceded by the nephrotic syndrome. Kidney biopsy is the best determinant of renal damage and the extent of treatment needed.

Pulmonary involvement in SLE occurs in 40% to 50% of patients and is manifested primarily by pleural effusions or pleuritis. Less frequently occurring pulmonary problems include acute pneumonitis, pulmonary hemorrhage, chronic interstitial lung disease, and pulmonary embolism.

Pericarditis is the most common of the cardiac manifestation, occurring in up to 50% of persons with SLE and often accompanied by pleural effusions. Myocarditis affects as much as 25% of those with SLE. Congenital heart block can occur in infants of mothers with SLE who have a specific type of ANA (antiRo) in their serum. Secondary heart disease also is a problem in those with SLE. Hypertension may be associated with lupus nephritis and long-term corticosteroid use. Ischemic heart disease can occur in older patients with longer-duration SLE. Infective endocarditis is rare but can occur with valvular lesions.[20]

The pathologic basis for the CNS symptoms is not entirely clear. It has been ascribed to an acute vasculitis that impedes blood flow, causing strokes or hemorrhage; an immune response involving antineuronal antibodies that attack nerve cells; or production of antiphospholipid antibodies that damage blood vessels and cause blood clots in the brain. Seizures can occur and are more frequent when renal failure is present. Psychotic symptoms, including depression and unnatural euphoria, as well as decreased cognitive functioning, confusion, and altered levels of consciousness, may develop. More research is being done on the role of psychological factors in triggering the onset of SLE.

Hematologic disorders may manifest as hemolytic anemia, leukopenia, lymphopenia, or thrombocytopenia. Lymphadenopathy also may occur in many patients with SLE.[20] Discoid SLE (*i.e.,* chronic cutaneous lupus) involves plaquelike lesions on the head, scalp, and neck. These lesions first appear as red, swollen patches of skin, and later there can be scarring, depigmentation, and plugging of hair follicles. Most patients with discoid lupus have disease that involves only the skin.

Subacute cutaneous lupus erythematosus (SCLE) is a less severe form of lupus. The skin lesions in this condition may resemble psoriasis. These lesions are found in sun-exposed areas such as the face, chest, upper back, and arms. Patients with SCLE may have mild systemic problems, which usually are limited to joint and muscle pains. There is a low incidence of lupus nephritis among those with SCLE.

Diagnosis and Treatment

The diagnosis of SLE can be complicated and difficult. Diagnosis of SLE in Canada requires that four of the 11 criteria identified by the American College of Rheumatology be present. These criteria include butterfly (malar) rash on the cheeks of the face, patchy redness on the skin (discoid skin rash), photosensitivity, mouth ulcers, arthritis in two or more extremity joints, serositis, renal disorder, neurologic disorder, immunologic disorder, blood count abnormalities, and/or antinuclear antibodies.[22] Diagnosis is based on a complete history, physical examination, and analysis of blood work, as no single test can diagnose SLE in all persons.

The most common laboratory test performed is the immunofluorescence test for ANA. Ninety-five percent of persons with untreated SLE have high ANA levels. The ANA test is not specific for SLE, and positive ANA results may be found in healthy persons or may be associated with other disorders. The anti-DNA antibody test is more specific for the diagnosis of SLE. Other serum tests may reveal moderate to severe anemia, thrombocytopenia, and leukocytosis or leukopenia. Additional immunologic tests may be done to give support to the diagnosis or to differentiate SLE from other connective tissue diseases.

Treatment of SLE focuses on managing the acute and chronic symptoms of the disease. Communication and trust between healthcare providers and the person with SLE are the basis for long-term disease management. The goals of treatment include preventing progressive loss of organ function, reducing the possibility of exacerbations, minimizing disability from the disease process, and preventing complications from medication therapy. Treatment with medications may be as simple as a drug to reduce inflammation, such as an NSAID. NSAIDs can control fever, arthritis, and mild pleuritis. An antimalarial drug (*e.g.,* hydroxychloroquine) may be the next medication considered to treat cutaneous and musculoskeletal manifestations of SLE. Corticosteroids are used to treat more significant symptoms of SLE, such as renal and CNS disorders. High-dose corticosteroid treatment is used for acute symptoms, and the drug is tapered to the lowest therapeutic dose as soon as possible to minimize the adverse effects. Immunosuppressive drugs (*e.g.,* azathioprine, cyclophosphamide,) are used in cases of severe disease. Newer drugs targeting the hyperactive B lymphocytes (*e.g.,* rituximab, belimumab) are showing promising effects.[23]

Systemic Sclerosis/Scleroderma

Systemic sclerosis, sometimes called *scleroderma,* is an autoimmune disease of connective tissue characterized by excessive collagen deposition in the skin and internal organs such as the lungs, gastrointestinal tract, heart, and kidneys. In this disorder, the skin is thickened through fibrosis, with an accompanying fixation of subdermal structures, including the sheaths or fascia covering tendons and muscles.[24,25] Systemic sclerosis affects women up to five times more often than men, with a peak incidence in the 30- to 50-year-old age group.[3] The cause of this rare disorder is poorly understood. There is evidence of both humoral and cellular immune system abnormalities.

Scleroderma presents as two distinct clinical entities: (1) the limited, or CREST, variant or (2) the diffuse or generalized form of the disease. The CREST syndrome is manifested by *calcinosis* (*i.e.,* calcium deposits in the subcutaneous tissue that erupt through the skin), *R*aynaud phenomenon, *e*sophageal dysmotility, *s*clerodactyly (localized scleroderma of the fingers), and *t*elangiectasia.[24] In this syndrome, hardening of the skin (scleroderma) is limited to the hands and face, whereas the skin changes in diffuse scleroderma also involve the trunk and proximal extremities. Almost all persons with scleroderma develop polyarthritis and Raynaud phenomenon, a vascular disorder characterized by reversible vasospasm of the arteries supplying the fingers (see Chapter 22).

Diffuse scleroderma is characterized by severe and progressive disease of the skin and the early onset of organ involvement. The typical person has a "stone facies" due to tightening of the facial skin with restricted motion of the mouth. Involvement of the esophagus leads to hypomotility and difficulty swallowing. Malabsorption may develop if the submucosal and muscular atrophy affect the intestine. Pulmonary involvement leads to dyspnea and eventually respiratory failure. Vascular involvement of the kidneys is responsible for malignant hypertension and progressive renal insufficiency. Cardiac problems include pericarditis, heart block, and myocardial fibrosis.

Treatment of systemic sclerosis is largely symptomatic and supportive. Depending on the presenting clinical features, treatments must be adapted for each person.[26] Studies have indicated that if heart, lung, or kidney involvement is to become severe, it tends to do so early in the disease and is a predictor of shortened survival. Advances in treatment, primarily the use of angiotensin-converting enzyme (ACE) inhibitors in renal involvement, have led to a substantial decrease in the mortality from hypertensive renal disease.[25] Cardiopulmonary manifestations of scleroderma, specifically pulmonary hypertension, can be treated with prostanoids (epoprostenol), phosphodiesterase-5 inhibitors (sildenafil), or endothelial receptor antagonists (Bosentan). Bosentan has been shown to improve survival in patients with scleroderma and pulmonary arterial hypertension.[27]

Polymyositis and Dermatomyositis

Polymyositis and dermatomyositis are chronic inflammatory myopathies. The pathogenesis is multifactorial and includes cellular and humoral immune mechanisms. Systemic manifestations are common, and cardiac and pulmonary complications often adversely affect the outcome. These conditions are characterized by symmetric proximal muscle weakness and occasional muscle pain and tenderness. Sometimes symptoms of these myopathies are confused with chronic muscle weakness due to neuromuscular diseases or genetic disorders such as muscular dystrophies. Treatment for the inflammatory myopathies should seek to control inflammation and prevent long-term damage to muscles, joints, and internal organs. Corticosteroids are the mainstay of treatment for these conditions.

IN SUMMARY

Rheumatoid arthritis is a systemic inflammatory disorder that affects 1% to 2% of the population. Women are affected more frequently than men. This form of arthritis, the cause of which is unknown, has a chronic course and usually is characterized by remissions and exacerbations. Joint involvement is symmetric and begins with inflammatory changes in the synovial membrane. As joint inflammation progresses, structural changes can occur, leading to joint instability and eventual deformity. Systemic manifestations include weakness, anorexia, weight loss, and low-grade fever. Some extra-articular features include rheumatoid nodules and vasculitis. The treatment goals include reducing pain, stiffness, and swelling; and maintaining mobility.

SLE is a chronic autoimmune disorder that affects multiple body systems. There is no known cause of SLE, but the disease may result from an immunoregulatory disturbance brought about by a combination of genetic, hormonal, and environmental factors. Some drugs have been shown to induce SLE, especially in older adults. There is an exaggerated production of autoantibodies, which interact with antigens to produce an immune complex. These immune complexes produce an inflammatory response in affected tissues. Treatment focuses on preventing loss of organ function, controlling inflammation, and minimizing complications of medication therapy.

Systemic sclerosis, often prefixed by the term progressive, is sometimes called scleroderma. In this disorder, the skin is thickened through fibrosis with an accompanying fixation to the subdermal structures, including the sheaths or fascia covering tendons and muscles. Polymyositis and dermatomyositis are chronic inflammatory myopathies. Its pathogenesis is multifactorial and includes cellular and humoral immune mechanisms.

SERONEGATIVE SPONDYLOARTHROPATHIES

After completing this section of the chapter, you should be able to meet the following objectives:

- Cite a definition of the seronegative spondyloarthropathies.
- Cite the primary features of ankylosing spondylitis.
- Describe how the site of inflammation differs in spondyloarthropathies from that in rheumatoid arthritis.
- Contrast and compare ankylosing spondylitis, reactive arthritis, and psoriatic arthritis in terms of cause, pathogenesis, and clinical manifestations.

The *spondyloarthropathies* are an interrelated group of multisystem inflammatory disorders that primarily affect the axial skeleton, particularly the spine. Typically, the inflammation begins at sites where tendon and ligament insert into bone rather than in the synovium. Sacroiliitis is a pathologic hallmark of the disorders. Persons with the spondyloarthropathies may also have inflammation and involvement of the peripheral joints, in which case the signs and symptoms overlap with other inflammatory types of arthritis. Because there is an absence of the RF, these disorders often are referred to as *seronegative spondyloarthropathies* and are recognized as specific disease entities.

The seronegative spondyloarthropathies include ankylosing spondylitis, reactive arthritis, and psoriatic arthritis. Although they differ in terms of factors such as age and type of onset and extent of joint involvement, there is clinical evidence of overlap between the various seronegative spondyloarthropathies. In none of these disorders is the cause or pathogenesis well understood. There is a striking association with the HLA-B27 antigen, but the presence of the HLA-B27 antigen by itself is neither necessary nor sufficient for the development of any of the diseases.[6,28]

Ankylosing Spondylitis

Ankylosing spondylitis is a chronic, systemic inflammatory disease of the joints of the axial skeleton manifested by pain and progressive stiffening of the spine. The disease is more common than once was believed, affecting approximately 150,000 to 300,000 Canadians, with men developing this three times more often than women.[3] Clinical manifestations of ankylosing spondylitis usually begin between 15 and 30 years of age and the disease usually evolves more slowly and is less severe in women.[3]

> ### SERONEGATIVE SPONDYLOARTHROPATHIES
>
> - The seronegative spondyloarthropathies represent a group of related multisystem disorders that lack the RF.
> - The inflammatory process associated with the disorders commonly affects the axial skeleton, involving areas where ligaments and tendons attach to bone.
> - Although the cause of the disorders is unknown, there is a striking association between the HLA-B27 antigen and development of the spondyloarthropathies.

Ankylosing spondylitis produces an inflammatory erosion of the sites where tendons and ligaments attach to bone.[29] Typically, the disease process begins with bilateral involvement of the sacroiliac joints and then moves to the smaller joints of the posterior elements of the spine. The result is ultimate destruction of these joints with ankylosis or posterior fusion of the spine. The vertebrae take on a squared appearance and bone bridges fuse one vertebral body to the next across the intervertebral disks. Progressive spinal changes usually follow an ascending pattern beginning with the sacroiliac area and then moving up the spine to involve the costovertebral

joints and cervical spine. Occasionally, large synovial joints (*i.e.*, hips, knees, and shoulders) may be involved. The small peripheral joints usually are not affected. The disease spectrum ranges from an asymptomatic sacroiliitis to a progressive disease that can affect many body systems.

Etiology and Pathogenesis

Although the pathogenesis of ankylosing spondylitis has not been established, the presence of mononuclear cells in the acutely involved tissue suggests an immune response. Epidemiologic findings indicate that genetic and environmental factors play a role in the pathogenesis of the disease. The HLA-B27 antigen remains one of the best known examples of an association between a disease and a hereditary marker.[28] Although approximately 90% of those with ankylosing spondylitis possess the HLA-B27 antigen and nearly 100% of those who also have uveitis or aortitis have the marker, the HLA-B27 antigen also is present in approximately 8% of the normal population. Several theories have been advanced to account for the association between the HLA-B27 antigen and ankylosing spondylitis. One possibility is that the gene that determines the HLA-B27 antigen may be linked to other genes that determine the pathologic autoimmune phenomena or that lead to increased susceptibility to infections or environmental agents. A second theory postulates molecular mimicry; an autoimmune reaction to an antigenic determinant site in the host's tissues may occur as a consequence of an immunologic response to an identical or closely related antigen of a foreign agent, usually an infectious agent[29] (see Chapter 19).

Clinical Manifestations

The person with ankylosing spondylitis typically complains of low back pain, which may be persistent or intermittent. The pain, which becomes worse when resting, particularly when lying in bed, initially may be blamed on muscle strain or spasm from physical activity. Lumbosacral pain also may be present, with discomfort in the buttocks and hip areas. Sometimes, pain can radiate to the thigh in a manner similar to that of sciatic pain. Prolonged stiffness is present in the morning and after periods of rest. Mild physical activity or a hot shower helps reduce pain and stiffness. Sleep patterns frequently are interrupted because of these manifestations. Walking or exercise may be needed to provide the comfort needed to return to sleep. Muscle spasm also may contribute to discomfort.[29]

Loss of motion in the spinal column is characteristic of the disease (Fig. 59.4). The severity and duration of disease activity influence the degree of mobility. Loss of lumbar lordosis occurs as the disease progresses, and this is followed by kyphosis of the thoracic spine and extension of the neck. A spine fused in the flexed position is the end result in severe ankylosing spondylitis. A kyphotic spine makes it difficult for the patient to look ahead and to maintain balance while walking. The image is one of a person bent over looking at the floor and unable to straighten up. X-ray films show a rigid, bamboo-like spine. The heart and lungs are constricted in the chest cavity. Abnormal weight bearing can lead to degeneration and destruction of the hips,

Kyphosis and extension of the neck

Eyes: Uveitis

Enthesitis (inflammation and tendency for fibrosis and calcification at sites of muscle insertion) at shoulders, hips, knees, and heels

Enthesitis of costovertebral and costosternal junctions with flexion contraction of the diaphragm

Spinal column fused by ossification of disks, joints, and ligaments

FIGURE 59.4 • Clinical manifestations of ankylosing spondylitis.

necessitating joint replacement procedures. Peripheral arthritis is more common in the hips and shoulders. The incidence of hip joint involvement varies from 17% to 36% and potentially is more crippling than involvement in any other joint.[1]

The most common extraskeletal involvement is acute anterior uveitis, which occurs in 25% to 30% of patients at some time in the course of their disease.[1] Systemic features of weight loss, fever, and fatigue may be apparent. Sometimes, the fatigue is a greater problem than pain or stiffness. Osteoporosis can occur, especially in the spine, which contributes to the risk of spinal fracture. Fusion of the costovertebral joints can lead to reduced lung volume.

The disease process varies considerably among individuals. Exacerbations and remissions are common; their unpredictability can create uncertainty in planning daily activities and in setting goals. Fortunately, most of those affected are able to lead productive lives. The prognosis for ankylosing spondylitis in general is good. The first decade of the disease predicts the remainder. Severe disease usually occurs early and is marked by peripheral arthritis, especially of the hip.

Diagnosis and Treatment

The diagnosis of ankylosing spondylitis is based on history, physical examination, and x-ray examination. The early and precise diagnosis of ankylosing spondylitis is closely related to a favourable prognosis. Early recognition allows for implementation of a conservative and usually effective treatment program on a lifelong basis.

Several methods are available to assess mobility and detect sacroiliitis. These methods include pressure on the sacroiliac joints with the person in a forward-bending position to elicit pain and muscle spasm, measurement of the distance between the tips of the fingers and the floor in a bent-over position with straight knees, and a modified Schober test that measures lumbar vertebral column movement. Although these measures alone do not provide a diagnosis of ankylosing spondylitis or other spondyloarthropathies, they can provide useful measurements for monitoring the disease status. Measurement of chest expansion may be used as an indirect indicator of thoracic involvement, which usually occurs late in the disease course.

Laboratory findings frequently include an elevated ESR. The person also may have a mild normocytic normochromic anemia. HLA typing is not diagnostic of the disease and should not be used as a routine screening procedure. Radiologic evaluations help differentiate ankylosing spondylitis from sacroiliitis due to other diseases. However, x-ray images may be negative in early disease. Vertebrae normally are concave on the anterior border. In ankylosing spondylitis, the vertebrae take on a squared appearance (Fig. 59.4).

Treatment of ankylosing spondylitis is directed at controlling pain and maintaining mobility by suppressing inflammation. Proper posture and positioning are important. This includes sleeping in a supine position on a firm mattress and using one small pillow or no pillow. A bed board may be used to supply additional firmness. Therapeutic exercises are important to assist in maintaining motion in peripheral joints and in the spine. Muscle-strengthening exercises for extensor muscle groups also are prescribed. Heat applications or a shower or bath may be beneficial before exercise to improve ease of movement. Swimming is an excellent general conditioning exercise that avoids joint stress and enhances muscle tone. Immobilizing joints is not recommended. Maintaining ideal weight reduces the stress on weight-bearing joints. Smoking should be discouraged because it can exacerbate respiratory problems. Occupational counselling or job evaluation may be warranted because of postural abnormalities.

Pharmacologic treatment includes the use of NSAIDs to reduce inflammation, relieve pain, and reduce muscle spasm. DMARDs are potential second-line therapies, but their efficacy in ankylosing spondylitis is unproven. Sulfasalazine and methotrexate have not shown benefit for spondylitis-associated back pain, but have shown efficacy for the peripheral joint involvement. Anti–TNF-α agents, including etanercept, infliximab, and adalimumab, have demonstrated rapid effectiveness in reducing both the axial and peripheral symptoms of ankylosing spondylitis, as well as improving quality of life.[30]

Reactive Arthropathies

The reactive arthropathies may be defined as sterile inflammatory joint disorders that are distant in time and place from the initial inciting infective process. The infecting agents cannot be cultured, and are not viable once having reached the joints. The list of triggering agents is continuously increasing and may be divided into urogenic, enterogenic, and respiratory tract associated, and the idiopathic arthritides. In some cases, the identity of the causative agent is unknown.[31,32]

The disease develops in a genetically susceptible host after a bacterial infection due to *Chlamydia trachomatis* in the genitourinary tract or *Salmonella, Shigella, Yersinia,* or *Campylobacter* in the gastrointestinal tract.[31] Reactive arthritis also has been observed in persons with acquired immunodeficiency syndrome (AIDS). Spondyloarthropathies such as Reiter syndrome and psoriatic arthritis are more frequent and severe in human immunodeficiency virus (HIV)-infected patients than in the general population. It is thought that the immune response to HIV infection is selective and largely spares the natural killer cells, which may be critical in the pathogenesis of these conditions. This is in contrast to RA and SLE, which dramatically improve as immunodeficiency develops. Reactive arthritis may also result from the presence of a foreign substance in the joint tissue, as in silicone implants in the small joints of the hands or feet or after exposure to industrial gases and oils. However, there is no evidence of antigenicity as the causative substance.

In the strictest sense, the definition of reactive arthritis includes a possibility of immunologic sensitization before arthritic development.[31] Similarities exist between reactive arthritis and bacterial arthritis. Several bacteria cause both diseases. When cultured bacteria are isolated from the synovial fluid, the diagnosis is bacterial arthritis. When they cannot be isolated, even though there has been a preceding infection, the diagnosis of reactive arthritis is made.

Reactive arthritis may follow a self-limited course; it may involve recurrent episodes of arthritis; or, in a small number of cases, it may follow a continuous and unremitting course. The treatment is largely symptomatic. NSAIDs are used in treating the arthritic symptoms. Vigorous treatment of possible triggering infections is thought to prevent relapses of reactive arthritis, but in many cases the triggering infection passes unnoticed or is mild, and the patient contacts a physician only with the onset of definite arthritis. Short antibiotic courses at this time are not effective.

Enteropathic Arthritis

Arthritis that is associated with an inflammatory bowel disease usually is considered an enteropathic arthritis because the intestinal disease is directly involved in the pathogenesis. Most cases of enteropathic arthritis are classified among the spondyloarthropathies. These include cases in which the arthritis is associated with inflammatory bowel disease (*i.e.*, ulcerative colitis and Crohn disease), the reactive arthritides triggered by enterogenic bacteria, some of the undifferentiated spondyloarthropathies, Whipple disease, and reactions after intestinal bypass surgery.[1] There is no direct relation between the activity of the bowel disease and the degree of arthritis activity.

Psoriatic Arthritis

Psoriatic arthritis is a seronegative inflammatory arthropathy that occurs in up to 30% of people with psoriasis.[3] It is a heterogeneous disease with features of the spondyloarthropathies in some persons, RA in others, and features of both coexisting in yet others.

The etiology of psoriasis and psoriatic arthritis is unknown. Genetic, environmental, and immunologic factors appear to affect susceptibility and play a role in expression of both the psoriatic skin disease and the arthritis. Environmental factors that may play a role in the pathogenesis of the disorder include infectious agents and physical trauma. T-cell–mediated immune responses seem to play an important role in the skin and joint manifestations of the disease, as indicated by the observation that there is improvement in disease status after treatment with immunosuppressant agents such as cyclosporine.

Although the arthritis can antedate detectable skin rash, the definitive diagnosis of psoriatic arthritis cannot be made without evidence of skin or nail changes typical of psoriasis. Psoriatic arthritis falls into five subgroups: oligoarticular or asymmetric; spondyloarthropathy; polyarticular, or symmetric; distal interphalangeal; and mutilans.[33] This heterogeneous clinical presentation suggests more than one disease is associated with psoriasis, or that there are various clinical responses to a common cause. Some of those with psoriatic arthritis have an elevated serum level of uric acid. The abnormally elevated serum uric acid level is caused by the rapid skin turnover of psoriasis and the subsequent breakdown of nucleic acid followed by its metabolism to uric acid. This finding may lead to a misdiagnosis of gout. Psoriatic arthritis tends to be slowly progressive, but has a more favourable prognosis than RA.

Basic management is similar to the treatment of RA. Suppression of the skin disease may be important in helping control the arthritis. Often, affected joints are surprisingly functional and only minimally symptomatic. The biologic response modifiers, specifically the TNF-α inhibitors (*e.g.*, etanercept, infliximab, and adalimumab), have been found to be beneficial in controlling the arthritis as well as the psoriasis in patients with psoriatic arthritis.[33]

IN SUMMARY

The seronegative arthropathies are a group of rheumatic disorders that lack the RF. The seronegative spondyloarthropathies affect the axial skeleton, particularly the spine. Inflammation develops at sites where tendons and ligaments insert into bone. They include ankylosing spondylitis, reactive arthritis, and psoriatic arthritis. Ankylosing spondylitis is considered a prototype of this classification category. Bilateral sacroiliitis is the primary feature of ankylosing spondylitis. The disease spectrum ranges from asymptomatic sacroiliitis to a progressive disorder affecting many body systems. The cause remains unknown; however, a strong association between the HLA-B27 antigen and ankylosing spondylitis has been identified. Loss of motion in the spinal column is characteristic of the disease. Peripheral arthritis may occur in some persons. Another form of spondyloarthritis is reactive arthritis. Although there are overlapping features for each of the spondyloarthropathies, identifying etiologic differences and clinical manifestations is important for determining treatment.

Psoriatic arthritis is a seronegative arthropathy that occurs in up to 30% of people with psoriasis. It is a heterogeneous disease with features of the spondyloarthropathies in some persons, RA in others, and features of both coexisting in yet others.

OSTEOARTHRITIS SYNDROME

After completing this section of the chapter, you should be able to meet the following objectives:

- Compare rheumatoid arthritis and osteoarthritis in terms of joint involvement, level of inflammation, and local and systemic manifestations.
- Describe the pathologic joint changes associated with osteoarthritis.
- Characterize the treatment of osteoarthritis.

Osteoarthritis (OA), formerly called *degenerative joint disease,* is the most prevalent form of arthritis affecting more than 3 million Canadians and is a leading cause of disability and pain in older adults.[3] OA is more of a disease process than a specific entity and is considered to have an inflammatory component along with the degenerative aspect. The term encompasses a heterogeneous collection of syndromes, including OA of the hand, knee, hip, foot, and spine. It can occur as a primary idiopathic disorder or as a secondary disorder, although this distinction is not always clear. Idiopathic or primary variants of OA occur as localized or generalized (*i.e.,* involvement of more than three joints) syndromes.[35] Secondary OA has a known underlying cause such as congenital or acquired defects of joint structures, trauma, metabolic disorders, or inflammatory diseases (Chart 59.1).

The joint changes associated with OA, which include a progressive loss of articular cartilage and synovitis, results from the inflammation caused when cartilage attempts to repair itself, creating osteophytes or spurs. These changes are accompanied by joint pain, stiffness, and limitation of motion,

OSTEOARTHRITIS

- Often referred to as "wear-and-tear" arthritis, osteoarthritis is a slowly destructive disorder of the articular cartilage.
- It can present as a primary disease of unknown etiology or as a secondary disorder related to congenital or acquired defects that affect the distribution of joint stress.
- The pathogenesis of osteoarthritis includes the progressive disruption of the smooth surface of the articular cartilage with development of surface cracks that deepen to involve the subchondral bone, followed by complete erosion of the articular cartilage with exposure of ivory-like polished subchondral bone, dislodgment of fragments of free-floating osteocartilaginous bodies, development of bone cysts, and formation of abnormal bony spurs at the joint margins.

and in some cases by joint instability and deformity. Fortunately, changes in the traditional conservative management of this underemphasized condition are occurring. Attitudes regarding the inevitability of the limitations imposed by this condition are changing on the part of healthcare providers and persons with the disease.

CHART 59.1   CAUSES OF OSTEOARTHRITIS

Postinflammatory disorders
  Rheumatoid arthritis
  Septic joint
Posttraumatic disorders
  Acute fracture
  Ligament or meniscal injury
  Cumulative occupational or recreational trauma
Anatomic or bony disorders
  Hip dysplasia
  Avascular necrosis
  Paget disease
  Slipped capital femoral epiphysis
  Legg–Calvé–Perthes disease
Metabolic disorders
  Calcium crystal deposition
  Hemochromatosis
  Acromegaly
  Wilson disease
  Ochronosis
Neuropathic arthritis
  Charcot joint
Hereditary disorders of collagen
Idiopathic or primary variants

Epidemiology and Risk Factors

Age, gender, and race interact to influence the time of onset and the pattern of joint involvement in OA. Men are affected more commonly at a younger age than women, but the rate of women affected exceeds that of men by middle age.[34] Heredity influences the occurrence of hand OA in the DIP joint. Hand OA is more likely to affect white women, whereas knee OA is more common in black women. The incidence of hip OA is lower among the Chinese than Europeans, perhaps representing the influence of other factors such as occupation, obesity, or heredity. Bone mass may also influence the risk of developing OA. In theory, thinner subchondral bone mass may provide a greater shock-absorbing function than denser bone, allowing less direct trauma to the cartilage.

Obesity is a particular risk factor for OA of the knee in women and a contributory biomechanical factor in the pathogenesis of the disease. Excess fat due to adipokines may have a direct metabolic effect on cartilage beyond the effects of excess joint stress.[34] Weight loss reduces the risk of developing symptomatic arthritis of the knee. Although the radiographic incidence of knee OA increases with advancing age, the incidence of symptomatic OA of the knee decreases.

Pathogenesis

The pathogenesis of OA resides in the homeostatic mechanisms that maintain the articular cartilage. Articular cartilage plays two essential mechanical roles in joint physiology. First, it serves as a remarkably smooth weight-bearing surface. In combination with synovial fluid, the articular cartilage provides extremely low friction during movement of the joint. Second, the cartilage transmits the load down to the bone, dissipating the mechanical stress.[36] Thus, the subchondral bone protects the overlying articular cartilage, providing it with a pliable bed and absorbing the energy of the force (Fig. 59.5).

Cartilage is a specialized type of connective tissue. As with other types of tissue, it consists of cells (*i.e.*, chondrocytes)

FIGURE 59.5 • A: A joint normally undergoes deformation of the articular cartilage and the subchondral bone when carrying a load. This maximizes the contact area and spreads the force of the load. **B:** If the joint does not deform with a load, the stresses are concentrated and the joint breaks down.

nested in an extracellular matrix. In articular cartilage, the extracellular matrix is composed of water, proteoglycans, collagen, and ground substance. The proteoglycans, which are large macromolecules made up of disaccharides and amino acids, afford elasticity and stiffness, permitting articular cartilage to resist compression. The ground substance constitutes a highly hydrated, semisolid gel. Collagen molecules consist of polypeptide chains that form long, fibrous strands. They provide form and tensile strength. The primary function of the collagen fibres is to provide a rigid scaffold to support the chondrocytes and ground substance of cartilage. The hydrated proteoglycan molecules, because of their size and charge, are trapped in the collagen meshwork of the extracellular matrix and prevented from expanding to their maximum size. This confers the high interstitial osmotic pressure and fluid volume that is needed for lubrication of the joint.[36] As in the case of adult bone, articular cartilage is not static; it undergoes turnover and its "worn-out" matrix components are continually degraded and replaced. This turnover is maintained by the chondrocytes, which not only synthesize the matrix but secrete matrix-degrading enzymes. Thus, the health of the chondrocytes determines joint integrity. In OA, this integrity can be disturbed by a number of influences.

Popularly known as *wear-and-tear* arthritis, OA is characterized by significant changes in both the composition and mechanical properties of cartilage. Early in the course of the disease, the cartilage contains increased water and decreased concentrations of proteoglycans compared with healthy cartilage. In addition, there appears to be a weakening of the collagen network, presumably caused by a decrease in the local synthesis of new collagen and an increase in the breakdown of existing collagen. The articular cartilage injury that occurs in OA is thought to result from the release of cytokines and growth factors[34,36] (Fig. 59.6). These chemical messengers stimulate production and release of proteases (enzymes) that are destructive to joint structures.[36] The resulting damage predisposes the chondrocytes to more injury and impairs their ability to repair the damage by producing new collagen and proteoglycans. The combined effects of inadequate repair mechanisms and imbalances between the proteases and their inhibitors contribute further to disease progression.

The earliest structural changes in OA include enlargement and reorganization of the chondrocytes in the superficial part of the articular cartilage. This is accompanied by edematous changes in the cartilaginous matrix, principally the intermediate layer. The cartilage loses its smooth aspect and surface cracks or microfractures occur, allowing synovial fluid to enter and widen the crack. As the crack deepens, vertical clefts form and eventually extend through the full thickness of the articular surface and into the subchondral bone.[36] Portions of the articular cartilage eventually become completely eroded and the exposed surface of the subchondral bone becomes thickened and polished to an ivory-like consistency (eburnation). Fragments of cartilage and bone often become dislodged, creating free-floating osteocartilaginous bodies ("joint mice") that enter the joint cavity. Synovial fluid may

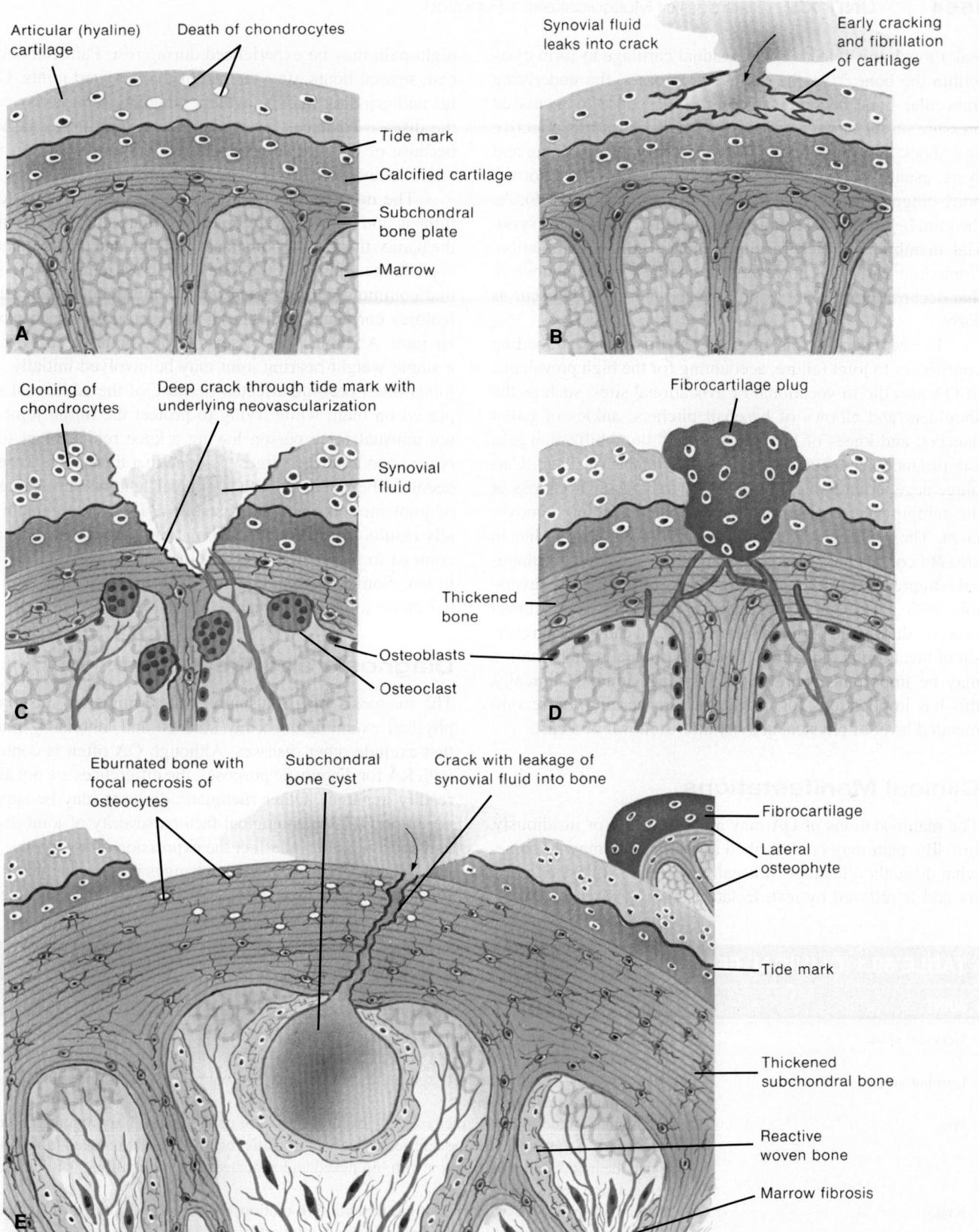

FIGURE 59.6 • Disease process in osteoarthritis. **A, B:** The death of chondrocytes leads to a crack in the articular cartilage that is followed by an influx of synovial fluid and further loss of cartilage. **C:** As a result of this process, cartilage is gradually worn away. Below the tidemark, new vessels grow in from the epiphysis. **D:** Fibrocartilage is deposited. **E:** The fibrocartilage plug is not mechanically sufficient and may be worn away, thus exposing the subchondral bone plate, which becomes thickened. If there is a crack in this region, synovial fluid leaks into the marrow space and produces a subchondral bone cyst. Focal regrowth of the articular surface leads to the formation of osteophytes. (From Rubin R., Strayer D. S. (Eds.). (2012). *Rubin's pathology: Clinicopathologic foundations of medicine* (6th ed., p. 1253). Philadelphia, PA: Lippincott Williams & Wilkins.)

leak though the defects in the residual cartilage to form cysts within the bone.[36] As the disease progresses, the underlying trabecular bone becomes sclerotic in response to increased pressure on the surface of the joint, rendering it less effective as a shock absorber. Sclerosis, or formation of new bone and cysts, usually occurs at the joint margins, forming abnormal bony outgrowths called *osteophytes,* or *spurs* (Fig. 59.6). As the joint begins to lose its integrity, there is trauma to the synovial membrane, which results in nonspecific inflammation. Compared with RA, however, the changes in the synovium that occur in OA are not as pronounced, nor do they occur as early.

In secondary forms of OA, repetitive impact loading contributes to joint failure, accounting for the high prevalence of OA specific to vocational or avocational sites, such as the shoulders and elbows of baseball pitchers, ankles of ballet dancers, and knees of hockey players.[36] Immobilization also can produce degenerative changes in articular cartilage. Cartilage degeneration due to immobility may result from loss of the pumping action of lubrication that occurs with joint movement. These changes are more marked and appear earlier in areas of contact but occur also in areas not subject to mechanical compression. Although cartilage atrophy is rapidly reversible with activity after a period of immobilization, impact exercise during the period of remobilization can prevent reversal of the atrophy. Therefore, slow and gradual remobilization may be important in preventing cartilage injury. Clinically, this has implications for instructions concerning the recommended level of physical activity after removal of a cast.

Clinical Manifestations

The manifestations of OA may arise suddenly or insidiously. Initially, pain may be described as aching and may be somewhat difficult to localize. It usually worsens with use or activity and is relieved by rest. In later stages of disease activity,

night pain may be experienced during rest. Pain can occur at rest, several hours after the use of the involved joints. Crepitus and grinding may be evident when the joint is moved. As the disease advances, even minimal activity may cause pain because of the limited range of motion resulting from intra-articular and periarticular structural damage.

The most frequently affected joints are the hips, knees, lumbar and cervical vertebrae, proximal and distal joints of the hands, the first carpometacarpal joint, and the first metatarsophalangeal joints of the feet. Table 59.1 identifies the joints that commonly are affected by OA and the common clinical features correlated with the disease activity of each particular joint. A single joint or several may be affected. Although a single weight-bearing joint may be involved initially, other joints often become affected because of the additional stress placed on them while trying to protect the initial joint. It is not unusual for a person having a knee replacement to discover soon after the surgery is done that the second knee also needs to be replaced. Other clinical features are limitations of joint motion and joint instability. Joint enlargement usually results from new bone formation; the joint feels hard, in contrast to the soft, spongy feeling characteristic of the joint in RA. Sometimes, mild synovitis or increased synovial fluid can cause joint enlargement.

Diagnosis and Treatment

The diagnosis of OA usually is determined by history and physical examination, x-ray studies, and laboratory findings that exclude other diseases. Although OA often is contrasted with RA for diagnostic purposes, the differences are not always readily apparent. Other rheumatic diseases may be superimposed on OA. Psychological factors, severity of joint disease, and educational level affect the expression of symptoms.[35]

Characteristic radiologic changes initially include medial joint space narrowing, followed by subchondral bony sclerosis,

TABLE 59.1 CLINICAL FEATURES OF OSTEOARTHRITIS

JOINT	CLINICAL FEATURES
Cervical spine	Localized stiffness; radicular or nonradicular pain; posterior osteophyte formation may cause vascular compression
Lumbar spine	Low back pain and stiffness; muscle spasm; decreased back motion; nerve root compression causing radicular pain; spinal stenosis
Hip	Most common in older men; characterized by insidious onset of pain, localized to groin region or inner aspect of the thigh; may be referred to buttocks, sciatic region, or knee; reduced hip motion; leg may be held in external rotation with hip flexed and adducted; limp or shuffling gait; difficulty getting in and out of chairs
Knee	Localized discomfort with pain on motion; limitation of motion; crepitus; quadriceps atrophy due to lack of use; joint instability; genu varus or valgus; joint effusion
First carpometacarpal joint	Tenderness at base of thumb; squared appearance to joint
Proximal interphalangeal joint—Bouchard nodes	Same as for distal interphalangeal joint disease
Distal interphalangeal joint—Heberden nodes	Occurs more frequently in women; usually involves multiple DIPs, lateral flexor deviation of joint, spur formation at joint margins, pain and discomfort after joint use
First metatarsophalangeal joint	Insidious onset; irregular joint contour; pain and swelling aggravated by tight shoes

formation of spikes on the tibial eminence, and osteophytes. The results of laboratory studies usually are normal because the disorder is not a systemic disease. The ESR may be slightly elevated in generalized OA or erosive inflammatory variations of the disease. If inflammation is present, there may be a slight increase in the white blood cell count. The synovial fluid usually is normal.

Because there is no cure, the treatment of OA is symptomatic and includes physical rehabilitative, pharmacologic, and surgical measures. Physical measures are aimed at improving the supporting structures of the joint and strengthening opposing muscle groups involved in cushioning weight-bearing forces. This includes a balance of rest and exercise, use of splints to protect and rest the joint, use of heat and cold to relieve pain and muscle spasm, and adjusting the activities of daily living. Weight reduction is fundamental when the knee is involved. The involved joint should not be further abused, and steps should be taken to protect and rest it. These include weight reduction (when weight-bearing surfaces are involved) and the use of a cane or walker if the hips and knees are involved. Muscle-strengthening exercises may help protect the joint and decrease pain.

Oral medications are aimed at reducing inflammation or providing analgesia. Popular medications used in the treatment of OA are the NSAIDs (oral or topical), many of which are available without a prescription. Ongoing research may confirm that some NSAIDs impede the repair mechanisms in early cartilage lesions. However, studies have shown that the pain of OA may arise from factors other than an inflamed synovium. These factors include stretching of the joint capsule, ligaments, or nerve endings in the periosteum over osteophytes; nontrabecular microfractures; intraosseous hypertension; bursitis or tendinitis; and muscle spasm. In such cases, the pain may be relieved by an NSAID through the analgesic effect of the drug rather than its anti-inflammatory effect.[1] For many persons, acetaminophen may be as effective and less toxic than NSAIDs. Acetaminophen is recommended as the initial systemic treatment for OA in Canada.[37]

Intra-articular corticosteroid injections may be used when other treatment measures have been unsuccessful in adequately relieving symptoms. They are especially helpful in persons who have an effusion of the joint. Injections usually are limited to a total of four and not more than three within 1 year, because their use is thought to accelerate joint destruction.

Viscosupplementation is a newer concept in treatment and is based on the hypothesis that joint lubrication is abnormal in OA. Hyaluronate is injected into the joint weekly for 3 to 5 weeks. Despite numerous studies and meta-analyses, the efficacy of this treatment remains debated and inconclusive.[38] Speculation that other agents (*i.e.,* glucosamine and chondroitin sulphate) may be chondroprotective has prompted other studies, some of which have demonstrated greater pain relief with treatment with either compound than with placebo, and others finding little or no difference.[39] A recent multicentre trial funded by the National Institutes of Health in the United States found that glucosamine hydrochloride was no more efficacious than placebo. It is interesting to note, however, that some studies that used glucosamine sulphate rather than glucosamine hydrochloride reported greater pain relief in their treatment group compared with their placebo group.[39] Other compounds with collagenase-inhibiting properties are being developed and investigated as structure- or disease-modifying agents for OA.[41]

Surgery is considered when the person is having severe pain and joint function is severely reduced. A Cochrane review of surgical lavage and debridement for OA of the knee showed no benefit for both short-term and long-term outcomes.[40] Other procedures include bunion resections, osteotomies to change alignment of the knee and hip joints, and decompression of the spinal roots in osteoarthritic vertebral stenosis. Total hip replacements have provided effective relief of symptoms and improved range of motion for many persons, as have total knee replacements.[34] Joint replacement is available for the first carpometacarpal joint. Arthrodesis (surgical stiffening of a joint) is used in advanced disease to reduce pain; however, this results in loss of motion.

Future management of OA lies in the development of techniques to identify and monitor cartilage lesions at an earlier stage. Potential approaches include bone scanning, magnetic resonance imaging, and arthroscopy.

IN SUMMARY

OA, the most common form of arthritis, is a localized condition affecting primarily the weight-bearing joints. Risk factors for OA progression include older age, OA in multiple joints, neuropathy, and, for knees, obesity. The disorder is characterized by degeneration of the articular cartilage and subchondral bone. It has been suggested that the cellular events responsible for the development of OA begin with some type of abnormal mechanical insult or stimulus, including hormones and growth factors, drugs, mechanical stresses, and the extracellular environment. Studies also implicate immunologic factors in the perpetuation and acceleration of the osteoarthritic change. As cartilage ages, biochemical events such as collagen fatigue and fracture occur with less stress. Attempts at repair by increased matrix synthesis and cellular proliferation maintain the integrity of the cartilage until failure of reparative processes allows the degenerative changes to progress. Joint enlargement usually results from new bone formation, which causes the joint to feel hard. Pain and stiffness are primary features of the disease. Inflammatory mediators (*e.g.,* prostaglandins) may increase the inflammatory and degenerative response.

Treatment is directed toward the relief of pain and maintenance of mobility while preserving the articular cartilage. Although there is no known cure for OA, appropriate treatment can reduce pain, maintain or improve joint mobility, and limit functional disability.

CRYSTAL-INDUCED ARTHROPATHIES

After completing this section of the chapter, you should be able to meet the following objectives:

- Relate the metabolism and elimination of uric acid to the pathogenesis of crystal-induced arthropathy.
- State why asymptomatic hyperuricemia is a laboratory finding and not a disease.
- Describe the clinical manifestations, diagnostic measures, and methods used in the treatment of gouty arthritis.

Metabolic bone and joint disorders result from biochemical and metabolic disorders that affect the joints. Metabolic and endocrine diseases associated with joint symptoms include amyloidosis, osteogenesis imperfecta, diabetes mellitus, hyperparathyroidism, thyroid disease, AIDS, and hypermobility syndromes. The discussion in this chapter is limited to the crystal-induced arthropathy caused by monosodium urate deposition, or gout.

Crystal deposition in joints produces arthritis. In gout, monosodium urate or uric acid crystals are found in the joint cavity. Another condition in which calcium pyrophosphate dihydrate crystals are found in the joints sometimes is referred to as *pseudogout* or *chondrocalcinosis*. A brief discussion of pseudogout is found in the section on rheumatic diseases in older adults.

Gout

Gout is actually a group of diseases known as the *gout syndrome*.[42] It includes acute gouty arthritis with recurrent attacks of severe articular and periarticular inflammation; tophi or the accumulation of crystalline deposits in articular surfaces, bones, soft tissue, and cartilage; gouty nephropathy or renal impairment; and uric acid kidney stones.

The term *primary gout* is used to designate cases in which the cause of the disorder is unknown or an inborn error in metabolism and is characterized primarily by hyperuricemia and gout. Primary gout is predominantly a disease of men, with a peak incidence in the fourth to sixth decade.[1] In secondary gout, the cause of the hyperuricemia is known but the gout is not the main disorder. Asymptomatic hyperuricemia is a laboratory finding and not a disease. Most persons with hyperuricemia do not develop gout.

Pathogenesis

The pathogenesis of gout resides in an elevation of serum uric acid levels. Uric acid is the end product of purine (adenine and guanine from DNA and RNA) metabolism.[43] Two pathways are involved in purine synthesis: (1) a de novo pathway, in which purines are synthesized from nonpurine precursors; and (2) the salvage pathway, in which purine bases are recaptured

from the breakdown of nucleic acids derived from exogenous (dietary) or endogenous sources.[4] The elevation of uric acid and the subsequent development of gout can result from overproduction of purines, decreased salvage of free purine bases, augmented breakdown of nucleic acids as a result of increased cell turnover, or decreased urinary excretion of uric acid. Primary gout, which constitutes 90% of cases, may be a consequence of enzyme defects that result in an overproduction of uric acid; inadequate elimination of uric acid by the kidney; or a combination of the two.[4,36,43] In most cases, the reason is unknown. In secondary gout, the hyperuricemia may be caused by the increased breakdown of nucleic acids, as occurs with rapid tumour cell lysis during treatment for lymphoma or leukemia. Other cases of secondary gout result from chronic renal disease. Some of the diuretics, including the thiazides, can interfere with the excretion of uric acid.

An attack of gout occurs when monosodium urate crystals precipitate in the joint and initiate an inflammatory response. Synovial fluid is a poorer solvent for uric acid than plasma, and uric acid crystals are even less soluble at temperatures below 37°C. Crystal deposition usually occurs in peripheral areas of the body, such as the great toe, where the temperatures are cooler than other parts of the body. With prolonged hyperuricemia, crystals and microtophi (*i.e.,* small, hard nodules with irregular surfaces that contain crystalline deposits of monosodium urate) accumulate in the synovial lining cells and in the joint cartilage. The released crystals are chemotactic to leukocytes and also activate complement. Phagocytosis of urate crystals by polymorphonuclear leukocytes occurs and leads to polymorphonuclear cell death with the release of lysosomal enzymes. As this process continues, the inflammation causes destruction of the cartilage and subchondral bone.

Repeated attacks of acute arthritis eventually lead to chronic arthritis and the formation of the large, hard nodules called *tophi*[42] (Fig. 59.7). They are found most commonly in the synovium, olecranon bursa, Achilles tendon, subchondral bone, and extensor surface of the forearm and may be mistaken for rheumatoid nodules. Tophi usually do not appear until 10 years or more after the first gout attack. This stage of gout, called *chronic tophaceous gout,* is characterized by more frequent and prolonged attacks, which often are polyarticular.

Clinical Manifestations

The typical acute attack of gout is monoarticular and usually affects the first metatarsophalangeal joint. The tarsal joints, insteps, ankles, heels, knees, wrists, fingers, and elbows also may be initial sites of involvement. Acute gout often begins at night and may be precipitated by excessive exercise, certain medications or foods, alcohol, or dieting. The onset of pain typically is abrupt, and redness and swelling are observed. The attack may last for days or weeks. Pain may be severe enough to be aggravated even by the weight of a bed sheet covering the affected area.

In the early stages of gout, after the initial attack has subsided, the person is asymptomatic, and joint abnormalities are not evident. This is referred to as *intercritical gout*. After the

FIGURE 59.7 • Gout. **A:** Gouty tophi of the hands appear as multiple rubbery nodules, one of which is ulcerated. **B:** A cross-section of a digit demonstrates a tophaceous collection of toothpaste-like urate crystals. (From Rubin R., Strayer D. S. (Eds.). (2012). *Rubin's pathology: Clinicopathologic foundations of medicine* (6th ed., p. 1262). Philadelphia, PA: Lippincott Williams & Wilkins.)

first attack, it may be months or years before another attack. As attacks recur with increased frequency, joint changes occur and become permanent.

Diagnosis and Treatment

Although hyperuricemia is the biochemical hallmark of gout, the presence of hyperuricemia cannot be equated with gout because many persons with this condition never develop gout. A definitive diagnosis of gout can be made only when monosodium urate crystals are in the synovial fluid or in tissue sections of tophaceous deposits. Synovial fluid analysis is useful in excluding other conditions, such as septic arthritis, pseudogout, and RA. Diagnostic methods also include measures to determine if the disorder is related to overproduction or to underexcretion of uric acid; the latter form is far more common (90% vs. 10%). This is done through measurement of serum uric acid levels and collection of a 24-hour urine sample for determination of urate excretion in the urine.[43]

The objectives for treatment of gout include the termination and prevention of the acute attacks of gouty arthritis and the correction of hyperuricemia, with consequent inhibition of further precipitation of sodium urate and absorption of urate crystal deposits already in the tissues.

Pharmacologic management of acute gout is directed toward reducing joint inflammation. Hyperuricemia and related problems of tophi, joint destruction, and renal problems are treated after the acute inflammatory process has subsided. NSAIDs, particularly indomethacin and ibuprofen, are used as first-line drugs for the treatment of acute gouty arthritis. Alternative therapies include colchicine and intra-articular deposition of corticosteroids. Treatment with colchicine is used early in the acute stage. Colchicine produces its antiinflammatory effects by inhibition of leukocyte migration and phagocytosis. The acute symptoms of gout usually subside within 48 hours after treatment with oral colchicine has been instituted and within 12 hours after intravenous administration of the drug. The NSAIDs are also effective during the acute stage when used at their maximum dosage and usually are preferred to colchicine because they have fewer toxic side effects. The corticosteroid drugs can be given orally, intravenously, intramuscularly, and intra-articularly and are commonly used in patients who cannot be treated with other first-line medications. Corticosteroids often are preferred for polyarticular gout and for patients with chronic renal disease as this a common comorbidity in older adults with gout.[44]

After the acute attack has been relieved, the hyperuricemia is treated. Treatment of hyperuricemia is aimed at maintaining normal uric acid levels and is lifelong. One method is to reduce hyperuricemia through the use of allopurinol or a uricosuric agent. Allopurinol and febuxostat inhibit xanthine oxidase, an enzyme needed for the conversion of hypoxanthine to xanthine and xanthine to uric acid. The uricosuric drugs (*e.g.*, probenecid or sulfinpyrazone, a phenylbutazone derivative) prevent the tubular reabsorption of urate and increase its excretion in the urine. The serum urate concentrations are monitored to determine efficacy and dosage. Prophylactic NSAIDs or colchicine may be used between gout attacks.

Although gout can often be effectively controlled by nonpharmacologic methods, many persons with gout have a limited understanding of the disease and therefore a poor compliance with treatment. Thus, education about the disease and its management is fundamental to the treatment and management of gout. Some changes in lifestyle may be needed, such as maintenance of ideal weight, moderation in alcohol consumption, and avoidance of purine-rich foods (*e.g.*, liver, kidney, sardines, anchovies, and sweetbreads), particularly by patients with excessive tophaceous deposits.[42]

IN SUMMARY

Crystal-induced arthropathy is characterized by crystal deposition in the joint. Gout is the prototype of this group. Acute attacks of arthritis occur with gout and are characterized by the presence of monosodium urate crystals in the joint. The disorder is accompanied by hyperuricemia, which results from overproduction of uric acid or from the reduced ability of the kidney to rid the body of excess uric acid. Management of acute gout is directed first toward the reduction of joint inflammation, after which the hyperuricemia is treated. Hyperuricemia is treated with uricosuric agents, which prevent the tubular reabsorption of urate, or with medication that inhibits the production of uric acid. Although gout is chronic, most people can control it with appropriate lifestyle changes.

RHEUMATIC DISEASES IN CHILDREN AND OLDER ADULTS

After completing this section of the chapter, you should be able to meet the following objectives:

- List three types of juvenile arthritis and differentiate among their major characteristics.
- Name one rheumatic disease that affects only the older adult population.

Rheumatic Diseases in Children

Children can be affected with almost all of the rheumatic diseases. In addition to disease-specific differences, these conditions affect not only the child but the family. Growth and development require special attention. Adherence to the treatment program requires intervention with the child and parents. School issues also must be addressed.

Juvenile Idiopathic Arthritis

Juvenile idiopathic arthritis (JIA) is not a single disease. Instead the term encompasses all forms of arthritis that begin before the age of 16 years, persist longer than 6 weeks, and are of unknown origin.[45,46] It is characterized by synovitis and can influence epiphyseal growth by stimulating growth of the affected side. Generalized stunted growth also may occur. JIA can be regarded not as a single disease, but as a category of diseases with three principal types of onset: (1) systemic-onset disease, (2) oligoarticular arthritis, and (3) polyarticular disease.

Systemic-onset disease affects approximately 5% to 10% of children with JIA.[45] The symptoms of systemic JIA include a daily intermittent high fever, which usually is accompanied by a rash, generalized lymphadenopathy, hepatosplenomegaly, leukocytosis, and anemia. Most of these children also have joint involvement, which develops concurrently with fever and rash. Systemic symptoms usually subside in 6 to 12 months. This form of JIA also can make an initial appearance in adulthood. Infections, heart disease, and adrenal insufficiency may cause death.

A second subgroup of JIA, oligoarticular arthritis, affects no more than four joints. This disease affects approximately 50% of children with JIA.[1,45] Oligoarticular arthritis affects two distinct groups. The first group generally consists of girls younger than 6 years of age with chronic uveitis. The results of ANA testing in this group usually are positive. The second group, characterized by late-onset arthritis, is made up mostly of boys. The HLA-B27 test results are positive in more than one half of this group. They are affected by sacroiliitis, and the arthritis usually occurs in the lower extremities.

The third subgroup, accounting for approximately 30% of the total cases of JIA, is polyarticular disease.[1,45] It affects five or more joints, often symmetrically, during the first 6 months of the disease. This form of arthritis more closely resembles the adult form of the disease than the other two subgroups. RF sometimes is present and may indicate a more active disease process. Systemic features include a low-grade fever, weight loss, malaise, anemia, stunted growth, slight organomegaly (*e.g.*, hepatosplenomegaly), and adenopathy.[1]

The prognosis for most children with JIA is good. Occupational and physical therapy are integral in the nonpharmacologic management of JIA.[45] NSAIDs are the first-line drugs used in treating JIA. Second-line agents are low-dose methotrexate and, less often, sulfasalazine. Finally, biologic response modifiers and TNF-α inhibitors are also used to treat JIA depending on the symptoms and classifications but a concern remains with potential long-term implications.[45] Other aspects of treatment of children with JIA require careful attention to growth and development and nutritional issues. Children are encouraged to lead as normal a life as possible.

Systemic Lupus Erythematosus

The features of SLE in children are similar to those in adults. The incidence in children is 10 times lower, estimated at 0.3 to 0.9 per 100,000 children.[47] The occurrence in the sexes is almost equal until puberty, after which it approaches the sex ratio seen in adults, which is predominantly female. The clinical manifestations of SLE in children reflect the extent and severity of systemic involvement. The best prognostic indicator in children is the extent of renal involvement, which is more common and more severe in children than in adults with SLE. Infectious complications are the most common cause of death in children with SLE.[47]

Children with SLE may present with constitutional symptoms, including fever, malaise, anorexia, and weight loss. Symptoms of the integumentary, musculoskeletal, central nervous, cardiac, pulmonary, and hematopoietic systems are similar to those of adults. Endocrine abnormalities include Cushing syndrome from long-term corticosteroid use and autoimmune thyroiditis. Adolescents often experience menstrual disturbances, which tend to resolve with disease remission.[1]

Treatment of SLE in children is similar to that in adults. The use of NSAIDs, corticosteroids, antimalarial drugs, and immunosuppressive agents depends on the symptoms. Corticosteroids may cause stunting of growth and necrosis of femoral heads and other joints. Immunization schedules should be maintained using attenuated rather than live vaccines. Rest periods should be balanced with exercise; children should be encouraged to maintain as normal a schedule as possible. The diversity of the clinical manifestations of SLE in the young requires the establishment of a comprehensive treatment or management program.

Juvenile Dermatomyositis

Juvenile dermatomyositis (JDMS) is a rare inflammatory myopathy primarily involving skin and muscle and associated with a characteristic rash. JDMS can affect children of all ages, with a mean age at onset of 8 years. There is an increased incidence among girls. The cause is unknown. Symmetric proximal muscle weakness, elevated muscle enzymes, evidence of vasculitis, and electromyographic changes confirming an inflammatory myopathy are diagnostic for JDMS. Generalized vasculitis is not seen in the adult form of the disease. The rash may precede or follow the onset of proximal muscle weakness. Periorbital edema, erythema, and eyelid telangiectasia are common.

Calcifications can occur in 30% to 50% of children with JDMS and are by far the most debilitating symptom. The calcifications appear at pressure points or sites of previous trauma. JDMS is treated primarily with corticosteroids to reduce inflammation. Occasionally, immunosuppressives are used in cases of refractory disease.[1] Adjunct therapies include using sunblock with a sun protection factor (SPF) greater than 30, a calcium-sufficient diet, and vitamin D therapy.

Juvenile Spondyloarthropathies

Ankylosing spondylitis, reactive arthritis, psoriatic arthritis, and spondyloarthropathies associated with ulcerative colitis and regional enteritis can affect children as well as adults. In children, spondyloarthropathy manifests in peripheral joints first, mimicking pauciarticular JIA, with no evidence of sacroiliac or spine involvement for months to years after onset. The spondyloarthropathies are more common in boys and commonly occur in children who have a positive family history. HLA-B27 typing is helpful in diagnosing children because of the unusual presentation of the disease.

Management of the disease involves physical therapy, education, and attention to school and growth and development issues. Medication includes the use of salicylates or other NSAIDs such as indomethacin. More severe disease or symptoms may require systemic corticosteroids or biologic disease modifiers.[1] Etanercept and infliximab produce more dramatic improvement of disease activity; however, their long-term effects and toxicity are not yet known.[47]

Rheumatic Diseases in Older Adults

Arthritis is the most common complaint of older adults. The pain, stiffness, and muscle weakness affect daily life, often threatening independence and quality of life. Symptoms of the rheumatic diseases can also have an indirect effect on and even threaten the duration of life for older adults. The weakness and gait disturbance that often accompany the rheumatic diseases can contribute to the likelihood of falls and fracture, causing suffering, increased healthcare costs, further loss of independence, and the potential for a decreased life span.

Older adults have more trouble coping with mild to moderately severe disease that in younger people is less likely to lead to serious disability for the same degree of impairment. Unfortunately, older adults and often their healthcare providers think the problems associated with arthritis are an inevitable consequence of aging and fail to take advantage of measures that can improve the quality of life.

Because arthritis is the leading cause of change in the functional status of older adults, a functional approach to the problems of the age group is appropriate. Inactivity is a societal expectation of older adults. Usually any activity there is tends to be low impact (e.g., leisurely walking), and deconditioning results.

Older patients often have multiple problems complicating diagnosis and management. The diagnosis of an older patient with a musculoskeletal problem must consider a wide variety of disorders that usually are regarded as outside the range of typical rheumatic disease. Among these are metastatic malignancy, multiple myeloma, musculoskeletal disorders accompanying endocrine or metabolic disorders, orthopedic conditions, and neurologic disease. The diagnosis may be missed if the assumption is that musculoskeletal problems in the older person are caused by OA.

There is an increased incidence of false-positive test results for RF and ANA in the older adult population with or without rheumatic disease because older persons are better producers of autoantibodies than younger persons. There are differences in the manifestations, diagnosis, and treatment of some of the rheumatic diseases in older adults. The usual presentation of these conditions was discussed earlier in this chapter. One form of rheumatic disease that has a predilection for older adults is polymyalgia rheumatica.

Rheumatoid Arthritis

The prevalence of RA increases with advancing age, possibly due to the decrease in T lymphocyte generation. Seropositive patients are more likely to have had an acute onset with systemic features and higher disease activity. Patients with seronegative, elderly onset RA have a disease that usually follows a mild course. The close resemblance of the manifestations of seronegative RA in older adults to those of polymyalgia rheumatica has led to speculation concerning the relationship of these syndromes. It may be that RA in older adults is a broad disorder that includes a number of distinct subsets with characteristic manifestations, courses, and outcomes.

Systemic Lupus Erythematosus

SLE is another condition with different manifestations in older adults. The disease is accompanied less frequently by renal involvement. However, pleurisy, pericarditis, arthritis, and symptoms closely resembling polymyalgia rheumatica are more common than in younger patients. The characteristics of SLE in older adults closely resemble those of drug-induced SLE, leading to speculation that the syndrome may result from one of the multiple drugs that are taken by many older patients.[48]

Osteoarthritis

Osteoarthritis is by far the most common form of arthritis among older adults. It is the greatest cause of disability and limitation of activity in older populations. It has been suggested that OA begins at a very young age, expressing itself in older adults only after a long period of latency. Too often, it is accepted by the patient or expected by the physician. OA presents a major management problem, but there is much that can be done. Self-control by maintaining a positive attitude and sense of self-esteem is a frequent coping strategy.[49]

Crystal-Induced Arthropathies

Gout. The incidence of clinical gout increases with advancing age, in part because of the increased involvement of joints after years of continued hyperuricemia. High serum urate levels rarely occur in women before menopause; initial attacks of clinical gout occur around the age of 70 years, or 20 years after menopause.[42] Gouty attacks in older women may be precipitated by the use of diuretics. The treatment of gout is often more difficult in the older adult. Although colchicine may be effective in controlling the symptoms of chronic gout, it may cause diarrhea in some patients, limiting its effectiveness in maintenance therapy.

Pseudogout. As part of the tissue aging process, OA develops with associated cartilage degeneration and the shedding of calcium pyrophosphate crystals into the joint cavity. These crystals may produce a low-grade chronic inflammation—the chronic pseudogout syndrome. The accumulation of calcium pyrophosphate and related crystalline deposits in articular cartilage is common in older adults. There are no medications that can remove the crystals from the joints. Although it may be asymptomatic, presence of the crystals may contribute to more rapid cartilage deterioration. This condition may coexist with severe OA. Calcium pyrophosphate deposition disease may also present with proximal muscle pain mimicking polymyalgia rheumatica.[50]

Polymyalgia Rheumatica

Polymyalgia rheumatica is an inflammatory condition of unknown origin characterized by aching and morning stiffness in the cervical regions and shoulder and pelvic girdle areas.[51] Of the forms of arthritis affecting older adults, it is one of the more difficult to diagnose and one of the most important to identify. Older women are especially at risk. Polymyalgia rheumatica is a common syndrome of older patients, rarely occurring before 50 years and usually after 60 years of age. The onset can be abrupt, with the patient going to bed feeling well and awakening with pain and stiffness in the neck, shoulders, and hips.

Diagnosis is based on the pain and stiffness persisting for at least 1 month and an elevated ESR or CRP. The diagnosis is confirmed when the symptoms respond dramatically to a small dose of prednisone, a corticosteroid. Biopsies have shown that the muscles are normal, despite the name, but that a nonspecific inflammation affecting the synovial tissue is present. It is possible that a number of patients are erroneously diagnosed as having RA or OA. For patients with an elevated ESR (>40 mm/hr), the diagnosis usually is based on a 3-day trial of prednisone treatment.[52] Patients with polymyalgia rheumatica typically exhibit striking clinical improvement approximately the second day. Patients with RA also show improvement, although usually days later.

Treatment with NSAIDs provides relief for some patients, but most require continuing therapy with prednisone, with gradual reduction of the dose over the course of 1.5 to 2 years, using the patient's symptoms as the primary guide. Patients need close monitoring during the maintenance phase with prednisone therapy. Because their symptoms are relieved, they often quit taking the prednisone and their symptoms recur, or doses are missed and the decreased dosage leads to an increase in symptoms. Unless careful assessment reveals the frequency of missed doses, the healthcare provider may be misled into increasing the dosage when it is not needed. Because of the side effects of the corticosteroids, the goal is to use the lowest dose of the drug necessary to control the symptoms. Weaning patients off low-dose prednisone therapy after this length of time can be a difficult and extended process.

A certain percentage of patients with polymyalgia rheumatica also develop giant cell arteritis (*i.e.,* temporal arteritis) with involvement of the ophthalmic arteries. The two conditions are considered to represent different manifestations of the same disease. Giant cell arteritis, a form of systemic vasculitis, is a systemic inflammatory disease of large and medium-sized arteries. The inflammatory response seems to be a T-cell response to an antigen.

Clinical manifestations of giant cell arteritis usually begin insidiously and may exist for some time before being recognized.[51] It is potentially dangerous if missed or mistreated, especially if the temporal artery or other vessels supplying the eye are involved, in which case blindness can ensue quickly without treatment. The condition is responsive to appropriate therapy. For those patients at risk, adherence to the medication program is critical, with preservation of sight being the goal. Because this complication can occur so quickly and is relatively asymptomatic, it is vital that the patient understand the importance of taking the correct dose regularly as prescribed. Initial treatment consists of large doses of prednisone. This dosage is continued for 4 to 6 weeks and then decreased gradually.

Management of Rheumatic Diseases in Older Adults

In addition to diagnosis-specific treatment, older adults require special considerations. Management techniques that rely on modalities other than drugs are particularly important for older adults. These include splints, walking aids, muscle-building exercise, and local heat. Muscle-strengthening and stretching exercises are particularly effective in the older person with age-related losses in muscle function and should be instituted early. Rest, the cornerstone of conservative therapy, is hazardous in older adult, who can rapidly lose muscle strength.

In terms of medications, the selection of drugs used in the treatment of arthritic disorders and their dosages may need to be considered when prescribing for this age group. For example, the NSAIDs may be less well tolerated by older adults, and their side effects are more likely to be serious. In addition to bleeding from the gastrointestinal tract and renal insufficiency, there may be cognitive dysfunction manifested by forgetfulness, inability to concentrate, sleeplessness, paranoid ideation, and depression.

Joint arthroplasty can also be used for pain relief and increased function. Chronologic age is not a contraindication to surgical treatment of arthritis. In appropriately selected candidates, survival and functional outcome after surgery are equivalent to those in younger age groups. The more sedentary activity level of older adults makes them even better candidates for joint replacement because they put less stress and demand on the new joint.

IN SUMMARY

Rheumatic diseases that affect children can be similar to the adult diseases, but there also are manifestations unique to the younger population. Children with chronic diseases also have to be approached with different priorities than adults. Managing rheumatic diseases in children requires a team approach to address issues of the family, school, growth and development, and coping strategies and requires a comprehensive disease management program.

Arthritis is the most common complaint of the older adult population. The pain, stiffness, and muscle weakness affect daily life, often threatening independence and quality of life. There is a difference in the manifestations, diagnosis, and treatment of some of the rheumatic diseases in older adults compared with those in the younger population. Osteoarthritis is the most common form of arthritis among older adults. The prevalence of RA and gout increases with advancing age. One form of rheumatic disease that has a predilection for older adults is polymyalgia rheumatica. A certain percentage of patients with polymyalgia rheumatica also have giant cell arteritis, frequently with involvement of the ophthalmic arteries. If this condition is untreated, it carries a serious threat of blindness.

REVIEW EXERCISES

1. A 30-year-old woman, recently diagnosed with rheumatoid arthritis (RA), complains of general fatigue and weight loss along with symmetric joint swelling, stiffness, and pain. The stiffness is more prominent in the morning and subsides during the day. Laboratory measures reveal a rheumatoid factor (RF) of 120 IU/ml (normal <15 IU/ml) and an anti-CPP antibody test of 65 U/L (normal <20 U/L).
   A. Describe the immunopathogenesis of the joint changes that occur with RA.
   B. How do these changes relate to this woman's symptoms?
   C. What is the significance of her test results?
   D. How do her complaints of general fatigue and weight loss relate to the RA disease process?

2. A 65-year-old obese woman with a diagnosis of osteoarthritis (OA) has been having increasing pain in her right knee that is made worse with movement and weight bearing and is relieved by rest. Physical examination reveals an enlarged joint with a varus deformity; coarse crepitus is felt over the joint on passive movement.
   A. Compare the pathogenesis and articular structures involved in OA with those of RA.
   B. What is the origin of the enlargement of the affected joint, the varus deformity, and the crepitus that is felt on movement of the affected knee?
   C. Explain the predilection for involvement of the knee in persons such as this woman.
   D. What types of treatment are available for this woman?

3. A 75-year-old woman is seen by her healthcare provider because of complaints of fever, malaise, and weight loss. She is having trouble combing her hair, putting on a coat, and getting out of chairs because of the stiffness and pain in her shoulders, hip, and lower back. Because of her age and symptoms, the healthcare provider suspects the woman has polymyalgia rheumatica.
   A. What laboratory test can be used to substantiate the diagnosis?
   B. What other diagnostic strategies are used to confirm the diagnosis?
   C. How is the disease treated?

References

1. Klippel J. H., Stone J. H., Crawford L. T., et al. (2008). *Primer on the rheumatic diseases* (13th ed.). New York: Springer New York.
2. Public Health Agency of Canada. (2010). *Life with Arthritis in Canada. A personal and public health challenge.* Ottawa, ON: Health Canada.
3. The Arthritis Society. (2015). Types of arthritis. Available online at: http://www.arthritis.ca/aboutarthritis. Accessed June 25, 2015.
4. Garcia R. A., Klein M. J., Schiller A. L. (2012). Chapter 26: Bones and joints. In Rubin R., Strayer D. S. (Eds.). *Rubin's pathology: Clinicopathologic foundations of medicine* (6th ed.). Philadelphia, PA: Lippincott Williams & Wilkins.
5. McInnes I. B., Schett G. (2011). The pathogenesis of rheumatoid arthritis. *New England Journal of Medicine, 365*(23), 2205–2219.
6. Firestein G. S., Budd R. C., Gabriel S. E., et al. (Eds.), *Kelley's textbook of rheumatology* (9th ed.). Philadelphia, PA: Elsevier Saunders.

7. British Columbia. (2012). Rheumatoid arthritis: Diagnosis, management and monitoring. Available online at: http://www2.gov.bc.ca/assets/gov/health/practitioner-pro/bc-guidelines/rheumatoid_arthritis.pdf. Accessed June 25, 2015.

8. Aletaha D., Neogi T., Silman A. J., et al. (2010). 2010 Rheumatoid Arthritis Classification Criteria. *Annals of the Rheumatic Diseases, 69*(9), 1580–1588.

9. Rindfleisch J. A. (2005). Diagnosis and management of rheumatoid arthritis. *American Family Physician, 72*, 1037–1047.

10. Turkiewicz A. M., Moreland L. W. (2006). Rheumatoid arthritis. In Bartlett S. J., Bingham C. O., Maricic M. J., et al. (Eds.), *Clinical care in the rheumatic diseases* (3rd ed.). Atlanta: Association of Rheumatology Health Professionals.

11. Dollah R., Yaacob A., Ismail A. H., et al. (2011). Anti-CPP antibodies: A better diagnostic tool for rheumatoid arthritis. *International Medical Journal, 18*(1), 53–57.

12. Peoples C., Valiyil R., Davis R. B., et al. (2013). Clinical use of anti-cyclic citrullinated peptide antibody testing. *Journal of Clinical Rheumatology, 19*(6), 351–352.

13. Munnek M., deJong Z., Zwinderman A. H., et al. (2005). Effect of a high intensity weight-bearing exercise program on radiologic damage progression of the large joints in subgroups of patients with rheumatoid arthritis. *Arthritis Care and Research, 53*, 410–417.

14. Singh G., Fort J. G., Goldstein J. L., et al.; SUCCESS-I Investigators. (2006). Celecoxib versus naproxen and diclofenac in osteoarthritis patients: SUCCESS-1 Study. *American Journal of Medicine, 119*, 255–266.

15. Bykerk V. P., Akhavan P., Hazlewood G. S., et al.; Canadian Rheumatology Association. (2012). Canadian rheumatology association recommendations for pharmacological management of rheumatoid arthritis with traditional and biologic disease-modifying anti rheumatic drugs. *Journal of Rheumatology, 39*(8), 1559–1582.

16. Smolen J. S., Landewe R., Breedveld F. C., et al. (2014). EULAR recommendations for the management of rheumatoid arthritis with synthetic and biological disease-modifying antirheumatic drugs: 2013 update. *Annals of the Rheumatic Diseases, 73*(3), 492–509.

17. Hazlewood G., Bykerk V. P. (updated 2015). Musculoskeletal disorders: Rheumatoid arthritis. In Repchinsky C. (Ed.). *e-Therapeutics*. Ottawa, ON: Canadian Pharmacists Association.

18. Calabrese L. H., Cohen M. D. (2006). *Targeting B cells in rheumatoid arthritis: Rationale and results*. Cleveland, OH: Cleveland Clinic Foundation for Continuing Education.

19. Murphy K. A., Spence S. T., McIntosh C. N., et. al. (2006). *Health state descriptions for Canadians: Musculoskeletal diseases* (Catalogue No. 82–619-MIE2006003). Ottawa, ON: Statistics Canada.

20. Dall'Era M., Wofsy D. (2013). Chapter 80: Clinical features of systemic lupus erythematosus. In Firestein G. S., Budd R. C., Gabriel S. E., et al. (Eds.), *Kelley's textbook of rheumatology* (9th ed.). Philadelphia, PA: Elsevier Saunders.

21. James J. A., Dedeke A. B. (2007). How to diagnose and treat systemic lupus erythematosus. *Arthritis Practitioner, 3*(1), 16–20.

22. Yu C., Gershwin E., Chang C. (2014). Diagnostic criteria for systemic lupus erythematosus: A critical review. *Journal of Autoimmunity, 48*, 10–13.

23. Hahn B. H. (2013). Belimumab for systemic lupus erythematosus. *New England Journal of Medicine, 368*(16), 1528–1535.

24. Gabrielli A., Avvedimento E. V., Krieg T. (2009). Scleroderma. *New England Journal of Medicine, 360*(19), 1989–2003.

25. Shanmugam V. K., Steen V. D. (2012). Reanl disease in scleroderma: An update on evaluation, risk stratification, pathogenesis and management. *Current Opinion in Rheumatology, 24*(6), 669–676.

26. Balbir-Gurman A., Braun-Moscovici Y. (2012). Scleroderma: New aspects in pathogenesis and treatment. *Best Practice & Research Clinical Rheumatology, 26*(1), 13–24.

27. Highland K. B. (2014). Recent advances in scleroderma-associate pulmonary hypertension. *Current Opinion in Rheumatology, 26*(6), 637–645.

28. Kuon W., Sieper J. (2003). Identification of HLA-B27 restricted peptides in reactive arthritis and other spondyloarthropathies. *Rheumatic Disease Clinics of North America, 29*, 595–611.

29. Elyan M., Khan M. A. (2006). Diagnosing ankylosing spondylitis. *Journal of Rheumatology, 33*(Suppl 78), 12–23.

30. Clegg D. O. (2006). Treatment of ankylosing spondylitis. *Journal of Rheumatology, 33*(Suppl 78), 24–31.

31. Carter J. D. (2010). Treating reactive arthritis: Insights for the clinician. *Therapeutic Advances in Musculoskeletal Disease, 2*(1), 45–54.

32. Kim P. S., Klausmeier T. L., Orr D. P. (2009). Reactive arthritis: A review. *Journal of Adolescent Health, 44*(4), 309–315.

33. Fitzgerald O. (2013). Chapter 77: Psoriatic arthritis. In Firestein G. S., Budd R. C., Gabriel S. E., et al. (Eds.), *Kelley's textbook of rheumatology* (9th ed.). Philadelphia, PA: Elsevier Saunders.

34. Bijlsma J. W., Berenbaum F., Lafeber F. P. (2011). Osteoarthritis: An update with relevance for clinical practice. *Lancet, 377*(9783), 2115–2126.

35. Lozada C. J., Altman R. D. (2003). Osteoarthritis. In Koopman W., Boulware D., Heudebert G. R. (Eds.), *Clinical primer of rheumatology*. Philadelphia, PA: Lippincott Williams & Wilkins.

36. Rosenberg A. E. (2010). Chapter 26: Bones, joints, and soft tissue tumors. In Kumar V., Abbas A. K., Fausto N., et al. (Eds.), *Robbins and Cotran pathologic basis of disease* (8th ed.). Philadelphia, PA: Elsevier Saunders.

37. Kean W. F., Kean C. A., Hogan M. G. (updated 2015). Musculoskeletal disorders: Osteoarthritis. In Repchinsky C. (Ed.), *e-Therapeutics*. Ottawa, ON: Canadian Pharmacists Association.

38. Hunter D. J. (2015). Viscosupplementation for osteoarthritis of the knee. *New England Journal of Medicine, 372*(11), 1040–1047.

39. Gregory P. J., Fellner C. (2014). Dietary supplements as disease-modifying treatments in osteoarthritis: A critical appraisal. *Pharmacy and Therapeutics, 39*(6), 436–452.

40. Laupattarakasem W., Laipaiboon M., Laupattarakasem P., et al. (2008). Arthroscopic debridement of knee osteoarthritis. *Cochrane Database of Systematic Reviews*, (1):CD005118.

41. Ling S. M., Rudolph K. (2006). Osteoarthritis. In Bartlett S. J., Bingham C. O., Maricic M. J., et al. (Eds.), *Clinical care in the rheumatic diseases* (3rd ed.). Atlanta: Association of Rheumatology Health Professionals.

42. Keenan R. T., Nawatzky J., Pillinger M. H. (2013). Chapter 94: Etiology and pthogeneis of hyperuricemia and gout. In Firestein G. S., Budd R. C., Gabriel S. E., et al. (Eds.), *Kelley's textbook of rheumatology* (9th ed.). Philadelphia, PA: Elsevier Saunders.

43. Rock K. L., Kataoka H., Lai J. (2013). Uric acid as a danger signal in gout and its comorbidities. *Nature Reviews Rheumatology, 9*(1), 13–23.

44. Schlesinger N. (2014). Treatment of acute gout. *Rheumatic Diseases Clinics of North America, 40*(2), 329–341.

45. Gowdie P. J., Tse S. M. (2012). Juvenile idiopathic arthritis. *Pediatric Clinics of North America, 59*(2), 301–327.

46. Prakken B., Albani S., Marini A. (2011). Juvenile idiopathic arthritis. *Lancet, 377*(9783), 2138–2149.

47. Levy D. M., Kamphuis S. (2012). Systemic lupus erythematosus in children and adolescents. *Pediatric Clinics of North America, 59*(2), 345–364.

48. Tomic-Lucic A., Petrovic R., Radak-Perovic M., et al. (2013). Late-onset systemic lupus erythematosus: Clinical features, course, and prognosis. *Clinical Rheumatology, 32*(7), 1053–1058.

49. Rapp S. R., Rejeski W. J., Miller M. E. (2000). Physical function among older adults with knee pain: The role of coping skills. *Arthritis Care and Research, 13*, 270–279.

50. Pego-Reigosa J. M., Rodriguez-Rodriguez M., Hurtado-Hernandez Z., et al. (2005). Calcium pyrophosphate deposition disease mimicking polymyalgia rheumatica: A prospective follow-up study of predictive factors for this condition in patients presenting with polymyalgia symptoms. *Arthritis Care and Research, 53*, 931–938.

51. Weyand C. M., Goronzy J. J. (2003). Giant-cell arteritis and polymyalgia rheumatica. *Annals of Internal Medicine, 139*, 505–515.

52. Frearson R., Cassidy T., Newton J. (2003). Polymyalgia rheumatica and temporal arteritis: Evidence and guidelines for diagnosis and management in older people. *Age and Ageing, 32*, 370–374.

Visit the**Point** **http://thePoint.lww.com for animations, journal articles, and more!**

Unit XV

Disorders of Integumentary Function

The recorded dawn of dermatology—the study of skin, hair, and nails and considered a subspecialty of medicine since ancient times—can be traced to the *Ebers Papyrus,* a work of the Ancient Egyptians dating from the 16th century BC. The papyrus revealed a collection of medical information about visible changes in skin appearance from multiple sources, including skin diseases, cosmetic problems, and therapies. Later in a pivotal 700-page French book, *Tractatus de Morbis Cutaneis* (Lorry, 1777), the skin was described as a living organ working with other organs. Prior to Lorry's book the skin was regarded merely as an enclosure for the body.

Two diseases in particular contributed to the expansion and interest in dermatology; leprosy and syphilis. Around the 15th century in Europe, leprosy became pandemic and syphilis became rampant, both associated with infected, and seemingly incurable, sailors returning home. At this time, dermatology started to detail cutaneous manifestations of these skin disorders.

Ferdinand Ritter von Hebra, a founder of the new Vienna school of dermatology, provided many of the names of numerous skin diseases and clearly described them according to their clinical presentations. His work became the basis for modern dermatology today.

Structure and Function of the Skin

60

The skin, also called the *integumentum,* is the largest and one of the most versatile organs of the body. It has a surface area of 1.5 to 2 m², weighs approximately 4 kg to 5 kg in the average adult, accounts for roughly 16% of the body's weight, and can range in thickness from 0.5 mm (eyelids) to 4.0 mm (heels) with an average of thickness of 1 to 2 mm over most of the body. The skin forms the major interface between the internal organs and the external environment. As the body's first line of defence, the skin is continuously subjected to potentially harmful environmental agents, including solid matter, liquids, gases, sunlight, and microorganisms. Although it may become bruised, lacerated, burned, or infected, it has remarkable properties that allow for a continuous cycle of shedding, healing, and regenerating.

As the outer covering of the body, the skin may demonstrate outwardly what occurs inside the body. A number of systemic diseases are manifested by skin disorders (*e.g.,* rash associated with systemic lupus erythematosus; jaundice due to liver disease). Thus, it is important to recognize that although skin eruptions are frequently caused by primary disorders of the skin, they may also represent manifestations of systemic disease.

STRUCTURE AND FUNCTION OF THE SKIN

After completing this section of the chapter, you should be able to meet the following objectives:

* Describe the protective functions of skin.
* Characterize the changes in a keratinocyte from its inception in the basal lamina to its arrival on the outer surface of the skin.
* List the four specialized cells of the epidermis and describe their functions.
* Describe the structure and function of the dermis and subcutaneous layers of skin.
* Describe the following skin appendages and their functions: sebaceous gland, eccrine gland, apocrine gland, nails, and hair.
* Characterize the skin in terms of sensory and immune functions.

Functions of the Skin

The skin and its derivatives constitute a complex organ with many cell types. The diversity of cell types and their ability to work together provide a number of ways of protecting a person from the elements in the external environment. As a barrier, microorganisms find it almost impossible to penetrate the skin from the outside, and water loss is limited from the inside. The skin surface is covered with a thin lipid film containing bactericidal fatty acids that protect against the entry of harmful microorganisms, and it harbours a constant flora of relatively harmless strains of microorganisms that protect against other, more virulent strains. The skin also plays an important role in immune regulation through skin-associated lymphoid tissues, including Langerhans cells, mast cells, and lymphocytes (see Chapter 17). Langerhans cells, the antigen-presenting cells of the skin, not only protect against harmful pathogens but also play an important role in the development of allergic skin conditions.

FUNCTIONS OF THE SKIN

- The skin is the largest organ of the body.
- As an interface between the internal and external environments, the skin prevents body fluids from leaving the body, protects the body from potentially damaging environmental agents, and serves as an area for heat exchange; in addition, cells of the skin immune system provide protection against invading microorganisms.
- Receptors in the skin relay touch, pressure, temperature, and pain sensation to the central nervous system for localization and discrimination.

The skin serves several other vital functions, including somatosensory function, temperature regulation, and vitamin D synthesis. The skin is richly innervated with pain, temperature, and touch receptors. Skin receptors relay the numerous qualities of touch, such as pressure, sharpness, dullness, and pleasure, to the central nervous system for localization and fine discrimination (see Chapter 49). Most of the heat produced in the body is generated by deep organs, such as the liver, heart, and skeletal muscles, and then transferred to the skin, where it is lost to the surrounding environment. The rate at which heat is dissipated from the body is determined by constriction or dilation of the arterioles that supply blood to the skin and through evaporation of moisture and sweat from the skin surface (see Chapter 10). The skin also functions as an endocrine organ, in which 7-dehydrocholesterol, a substance normally found in epidermal cells, is converted to cholecalciferol (an inactive form of vitamin D) by ultraviolet rays from the sun (discussed further in Chapter 56).

Although broken down into its constituent parts in this chapter, the skin is increasingly being understood as a complex and dynamic system involving neuroendocrine, immunologic, and cutaneous interactions.

Skin Structures

There are great variations in skin structure on different parts of the body; therefore, "normal skin" on any one surface of the body is difficult to describe. Variations are found in the properties of the skin, such as the thickness of skin layers, the distribution of sweat glands, and the number and size of hair follicles. For example, the epidermis is thicker on the palms of the hands and soles of the feet than elsewhere on the body. The dermis, on the other hand, is thickest on the back, whereas the subcutaneous fat layer is thickest on the abdomen and buttocks. Hair follicles are densely distributed on the scalp, axillae, and genitalia, but they are sparse on the inner arms and abdomen. The apocrine sweat glands are confined to the axillae and the anogenital area.

Nevertheless, certain structural properties are common to all skin on all areas of the body. The skin is composed of three layers: the epidermis (outer layer), the dermis (inner layer), and the subcutaneous fat layer. The basement membrane divides the first two layers. The subcutaneous tissue, a layer of loose connective and fatty tissues, binds the dermis to the underlying tissues of the body (Fig. 60.1).

Epidermis

The functions of the skin depend on the properties of its outermost layer, the epidermis. The epidermis covers the body, and it is specialized in areas to form the various skin appendages: hair, nails, and glandular structures. The keratinocytes of the epidermis produce a fibrous protein called *keratin,* which is essential to the protective function of skin. In addition to the keratinocytes, the epidermis has three other types of cells that arise from its basal layer: melanocytes that produce a pigment called *melanin,* which is responsible for skin colour, tanning,

---

ORGANIZATION OF SKIN STRUCTURES

- The skin has two layers, an outer epidermis and an inner dermis, separated by a basement membrane.
- The epidermis, which is avascular, is composed of four to five layers of stratified squamous keratinized epithelial cells that are formed in the deepest layer of the epidermis and migrate to the skin surface to replace cells that are lost during normal skin shedding.
- The basement membrane is a thin adhesive layer that cements the epidermis to the dermis. This is the layer involved in blister formation.
- The dermis is a connective tissue layer that separates the epidermis from the underlying subcutaneous fat layer. It contains the blood vessels and nerve fibres that supply the epidermis.

FIGURE 60.1 • Three-dimensional view of the skin.

and protecting against ultraviolet radiation; Merkel cells that provide sensory information; and Langerhans cells that link the epidermis to the immune system. The epidermis contains openings for two types of glands: sweat glands, which produce watery secretions, and sebaceous glands, which produce an oily secretion called *sebum*.

Keratinocytes

The *keratinocyte* is the major cell of the epidermis, comprising 95% of the cells of this layer. The epidermis is composed of stratified squamous keratinized epithelium, which, when viewed under the microscope, is seen to consist of five distinct layers, or strata, that represent a progressive differentiation or maturation of the keratinocytes: the stratum germinativum, or basal layer; the stratum spinosum; the stratum granulosum; the stratum lucidum; and the stratum corneum.

The deepest layer, the *stratum germinativum* or *stratum basale,* consists of a single layer of basal cells that are attached to the basal lamina. The basal cells, which are columnar, undergo mitosis to produce new keratinocytes that move

toward the skin surface to replace cells lost during normal skin shedding. Unlike the other layers of the epidermis, the basal cells do not migrate toward the skin surface, but remain stationary in the stratum germinativum.

The next layer, the *stratum spinosum,* is formed as the progeny of the basal cell layer move outward toward the skin surface. The stratum spinosum is two to four layers thick, and its cells become differentiated as they migrate outward. Because they develop a spiny appearance where their cell borders interconnect, the cells of this layer are commonly referred to as *prickle cells.*

The *stratum granulosum* is only a few cells thick; it consists of granular cells that are the most differentiated cells of the living skin. The cells in this layer are unique in that two opposing functions are occurring simultaneously: while some cells are losing cytoplasm and nuclear structures, others continue to synthesize keratin.

The *stratum lucidum,* which lies just superficial to the stratum granulosum, is a thin, transparent layer found primarily on the palms of the hands and soles of the feet. It consists

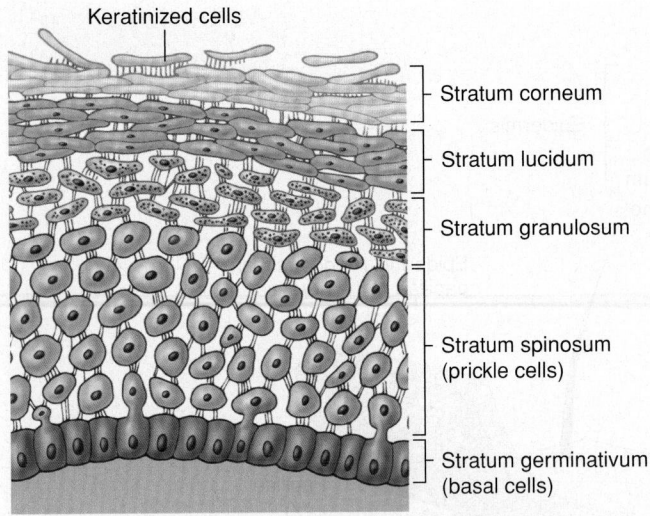

Keratinized cells

Stratum corneum

Stratum lucidum

Stratum granulosum

Stratum spinosum
(prickle cells)

Stratum germinativum
(basal cells)

FIGURE 60.2 • Epidermal cells. The basal cells undergo mitosis, producing keratinocytes that change their size and shape as they move upward, replacing cells that are lost during normal cell shedding.

of transitional cells that retain some of the functions of living skin cells from the layers below but otherwise resemble the cells of the stratum corneum.

The top or surface layer, the *stratum corneum*, consists of dead, keratinized cells. This layer contains the most cell layers and the largest cells of the epidermis. It ranges from 15 layers thick in areas such as the face to 25 layers or more on the arm. Specialized areas, such as the palms of the hands or soles of the feet, have 100 or more layers.

The keratinocytes that originate in the basal layer change morphologically as they are pushed toward the outer layer of the epidermis. For example, in the basal layer, the keratinocyte is round. As it is pushed into the stratum spinosum, the keratinocyte becomes multisided. It becomes flatter in the granular layer and is flattened and elongated in the stratum corneum (Fig. 60.2). Keratinocytes also change cytoplasmic structure and composition as they are pushed outward. This transformation from viable cells to the dead cells of the stratum corneum is called *keratinization*. The migration time of a keratinocyte from the basal layer to the stratum corneum is 20 to 30 days. The rate of production of new keratinocytes needs to be consistent with the rate of shedding old keratinocytes. When the rates are not in balance, skin anomalies occur.

The movement of the keratinocytes to the surface of the skin is best described as random or nonsynchronized. Keratinocytes pass other keratinocytes, melanocytes, and Langerhans cells as they migrate in a seemingly random fashion. However, the cells are connected by minute points of attachment called *desmosomes*. Desmosomes are localized patches or plaques that hold two cells tightly together. They are terminal end points on the cell walls of keratinocytes, made up of fibrous material that is bound into bundles, called *tonofilaments*. Desmosomes keep the cells from detaching and provide some structure to the skin while it is in perpetual motion. The

basal layer provides the underlying structure and stability for the epidermis.

Besides desmosomes, there are three other types of cellular junctions that bind keratinocytes: adherens junctions, gap junctions, and tight junctions (see Chapter 4). *Adherens junctions* are specialized structures that provide strong mechanical connections between cells. They are responsible for adhesion between cells, communicate about the presence of neighbouring cells, and anchor the skin cells. *Gap junctions* are cylindrical channels that permit ions and small molecules to pass between cells. They are composed of proteins called *connexins*.

Keratinocytes produce keratin, a complex protein that forms the surface of the skin and is also the structural protein of the hair and nails. Once believed to be passive cells passing through time while changing morphologically, keratinocytes are now known to be active secretory cells that play an important role in the immunobiology of the skin by communicating with and regulating cells of the immune response and secreting cytokines and inflammatory mediators.

Melanocytes

Melanocytes are pigment-synthesizing cells that are located at or in the basal layer. They function to produce pigment granules called *melanin*, the substance that gives skin its colour. There are two major forms of melanin: *eumelanin* and *pheomelanin*. The two forms of eumelanin are brown and black; pheomelanin is yellow to red. The type of melanin produced depends on the stimulation of specific hormones or proteins and the binding of these substances to receptors on the melanocyte. Eumelanin is the most abundant in humans. Exposure to the sun's ultraviolet rays increases the production of eumelanin, causing tanning to occur. The primary function of such melanin is to protect the skin by absorbing and scattering harmful ultraviolet rays, which are implicated in skin cancers. Localized concentrations of eumelanin are also responsible for the formation of freckles and moles.

Pheomelanin, the yellow to red pigment, is found in all humans. It is particularly concentrated in the lips, nipples, glans penis, and vagina. Besides the skin, it is found in hair, particularly red hair. It has been suggested that the reason fair-haired individuals are more susceptible to skin cancers may be due to the enhanced photoreactivity of pheomelanin, as compared with eumelanin.

The ability to synthesize melanin depends on the ability of the melanocytes to produce an enzyme called *tyrosinase*, which converts the amino acid tyrosine to a precursor of melanin. A genetic lack of this enzyme results in a clinical condition called *albinism*. Persons with this disorder lack pigmentation in the skin, hair, and iris of the eye. Tyrosinase is synthesized in the rough endoplasmic reticulum of the melanocytes and then routed to membranous vesicles in the Golgi complex called *melanosomes*. Melanin is subsequently synthesized in the melanosomes. Melanocytes have long, cytoplasm-filled dendritic processes that contain accumulated melanosomes and extend between the keratinocytes. Although the melanocytes remain in the basal layer, the melanosomes

FIGURE 60.3 • The melanocytes, which are located in the basal layer of the skin, produce melanin pigment granules that give skin its colour. The melanocytes have threadlike, cytoplasm-filled extensions that are used in passing the pigment granules to the keratinocytes.

are transferred to the keratinocytes through their dendritic processes. The dendrite tip containing the melanosome is engulfed by a nearby keratinocyte, and the melanin is transferred (Fig. 60.3).

The amount of melanin in the keratinocytes determines a person's skin colour. Dark-skinned and light-skinned people have approximately the same number of melanocytes, but the production and packaging of pigment is different. In dark-skinned people, *larger* melanin-containing melanosomes are produced and transferred individually to the keratinocyte, whereas in light-skinned people, *smaller* melanosomes are produced and then packaged together in a membrane before being transferred to the keratinocyte. All people, regardless of skin colour, have relatively few or no melanocytes in the epidermis of the palms of the hands or soles of the feet. In light-skinned people, the number of melanocytes decreases with age; the skin becomes lighter and is more susceptible to skin cancer when exposed to ultraviolet light.

Merkel Cells

Merkel cells are clear cells found in the stratum basale of the epidermis; they are connected to other skin cells by desmosomes. Each Merkel cell is connected to an afferent nerve terminal, forming a structure known as a *Merkel disk*. They are the sparsest cells of the epidermis and are found over the entire body, but are most plentiful in the basal layer of the fingers, toes, lips, and oral cavity, and in the outermost sheath of hair follicles (*i.e.,* the touch areas). The exact function of Merkel cells is unclear, but they are believed to be neuroendocrine cells (*i.e.,* they release hormones into the blood in response to neural stimuli) and function as specific, slowly adapting sensory touch receptors. Merkel cells may also be involved in the metabolic support of their associated neurons,

neuron development and regeneration after injury, and neurotransmission for autonomic nerves, blood vessels, and inflammatory cells.

Langerhans Cells

Langerhans cells are scattered in the suprabasal layers of the epidermis among the keratinocytes. They are less numerous (3% to 5% of epidermal cells) than the keratinocytes. They are derived from precursor cells originating in the bone marrow, and continuously repopulate the epidermis. Like melanocytes, they have a dendritic shape and clear cytoplasm. *Birbeck granules* that often resemble tennis racquets are their most distinguishing characteristic microscopically.

Langerhans cells are the immunologic cells responsible for recognizing foreign antigens harmful to the body (Fig. 60.4). As such, Langerhans cells play an important role in defending the body against foreign antigens. Langerhans cells bind antigen to their surface and process it, and, bearing the processed antigen, migrate from the epidermis into lymphatic vessels and

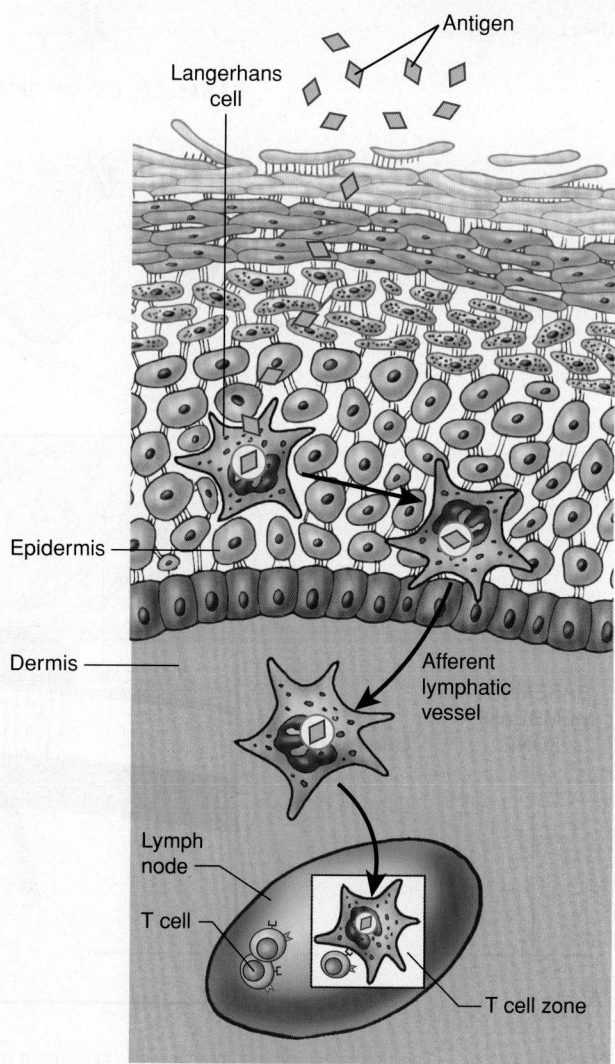

FIGURE 60.4 • Langerhans cells.

then into regional lymph nodes, where they are known as *dendritic cells*. During their migration in the lymph system, the Langerhans cells become potent antigen-presenting cells (see Chapter 17). Langerhans cells are innervated by sympathetic nerve fibres, which may explain why the skin's immune system is altered under stress. An example of this is the exacerbations of acne seen in persons under stress. Langerhans cells and the keratinocytes produce a number of cytokines that stimulate maturation of skin-localizing T lymphocytes.

Basement Membrane

The terms *basement membrane* and *basal lamina* are often used interchangeably. Technically, however, the basal lamina is a component of the basement membrane. The basement membrane is a layer of intercellular and extracellular matrices

that serves as an interface between the dermis and the epidermis (Fig. 60.5). It separates epithelium from the underlying connective tissue, it anchors the epithelium to the loose connective tissue underneath, and it serves as a selective filter for molecules moving between the two layers. It is also a major site of immunoglobulin and complement deposition in skin disease. The basement membrane is involved in skin disorders that cause bullae or blister formation.

The basement membrane consists of three distinct zones or layers—lamina lucida, lamina densa, and lamina fibroreticularis—all of which contribute to the adhesion of the two skin layers. The *lamina lucida* is an electron-lucent layer where adherence proteins are located. It consists of fine anchoring filaments and a cell adhesion glycoprotein, called *laminin*, that plays a role in the organization of the macromolecules in the basement membrane zone and promotes attachment of cells

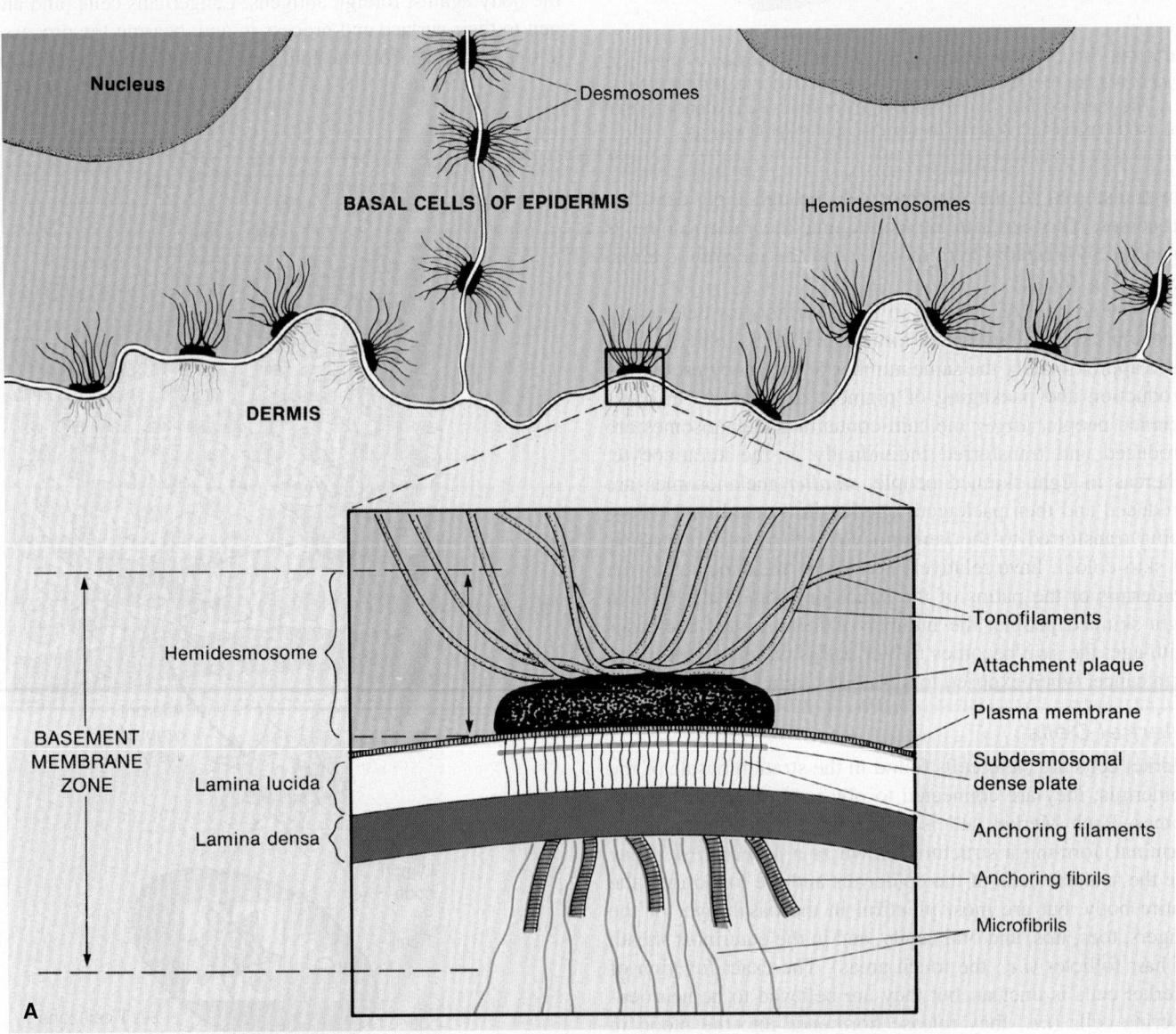

FIGURE 60.5 • The dermal–epidermal interface and basement membrane layers. (From Rubin R., Strayer D. S., (Eds.). (2012). *Rubin's pathology: Clinicopathologic foundations of medicine* (6th ed., p. 1117). Philadelphia, PA: Lippincott Williams & Wilkins.)

to the extracellular matrix. The *lamina densa* contains an adhesive called *type IV collagen* as well as laminin. It is important in dermal–epidermal attachment. Combined, the lamina lucida and the lamina densa comprise what is known as the *basal lamina*. The *lamina fibroreticularis* then completes the basement membrane. This layer contains many anchoring microfibrils. These are short, curved structures that insert into the lamina densa and the upper part of the dermis (superficial dermis), where they are known as *anchoring fibrils*. Type VII collagen, another adherent substance, has been found in the anchoring fibrils and plaques. Another component of the lamina fibroreticularis are elastic fibre bundles that extend to the dermis.

Hemidesmosomes are like half-desmosomes in both structure and function. They lie immediately at the basal plasma membrane and form the site or source of tonofilaments, which attach the dermis and epidermis (Fig. 60.5). Because they form a continuous link between the intracellular keratin filament network and the extracellular basement membrane, they are also involved in relaying signals between the skin systems.

Dermis

The dermis is the connective tissue layer that separates the epidermis from the subcutaneous fat layer (Fig. 60.1). It supports the epidermis and serves as its primary source of nutrition. The two layers of the dermis, the papillary dermis and the reticular dermis, are composed of cells, fibres, ground substances, nerves, and blood vessels. The main component of the dermis is collagen, a group of fibrous proteins. The collagen is enmeshed in a ground substance called hyaluronic acid. Collagen fibres are loosely arranged in the papillary dermis, but are tightly bundled in the reticular dermis.

The pilar (hair) and glandular structures are embedded in this layer and continue through the epidermis. In general, a dark dermis is more compact than the white dermis, and consequently darker-skinned people show less wrinkling.

Papillary Dermis

The *papillary dermis* (pars papillaris) is a thin, superficial layer that lies adjacent to the epidermis. It consists of collagen fibres and ground substance. This layer is densely covered with conical projections called *dermal papillae* (Fig. 60.1). The basal cells of the epidermis project into the papillary dermis, forming *rete ridges*. Microscopically, the junction between the epidermis and the dermis appears like undulating ridges and valleys. It is believed that the dense structure of the dermal papillae serves to minimize the separation of the dermis and the epidermis. Dermal papillae contain capillaries, end arterioles, and venules that nourish the epidermal layers of the skin. This layer of the dermis is richly vascularized. Lymph vessels and nerve tissue also are found in this layer.

Reticular Dermis

The *reticular dermis* (pars reticularis) is the thicker area of the dermis and forms the bulk of the dermal layer. This is the tough layer in animal hides from which leather is made. The reticular dermis is characterized by a complex meshwork of three-dimensional collagen bundles interconnected with large elastic fibres and ground substance, a viscid gel that is rich in mucopolysaccharides. The collagen fibres are oriented parallel to the body's surface in any given area. Collagen bundles may be organized lengthwise, as on the abdomen, or in round clusters, as on the heel. The direction of surgical incisions is often determined by this organizational pattern.

Immune Cells. Over time, the reticular dermis has undergone much study. Once thought to be composed primarily of fibroblasts, it is now believed that the main cells of this layer are dendritic cells, called *dermal dendrocytes*. Dermal dendrocytes are spindle-shaped cells that have both phagocytic and dendritic properties. They are believed to possess antigen-presenting functions and play an important part in the immunobiology of the dermis. In addition, it is possible that dermal dendrocytes may be able either to initiate or respond to immunologic events in the epidermis. Dermal dendrocytes also are thought to be involved in processes such as wound healing, blood clotting, and inflammation.

Immune cells found in the dermis include macrophages, T cells, mast cells, and fibroblasts. Dermal macrophages may present antigen to T cells in the dermis. Most of these T cells are previously activated or memory T cells. T-cell responses to macrophage- or endothelium-associated antigens in the dermis are probably more important in generating an immune response to antigen challenge in previously exposed persons than in initiating a response to a new antigen. The major type of T-cell–mediated immune response in the skin is delayed-type hypersensitivity (see Chapter 19).

Mast cells, which have a prominent role in immunoglobulin E-mediated immediate hypersensitivity, also are present in the dermis. These cells are strategically located at body interfaces such as the skin and mucous membranes and are thought to interact with antigens that come in contact with the skin.

Blood Vessels. The arterial vessels that nourish the skin form two plexuses (*i.e.,* collections of blood vessels), one located between the dermis and the subcutaneous tissue and the other between the papillary and reticular layers of the dermis. The pink colour of light skin results primarily from blood in the vessels of this latter plexus. Capillary flow that arises from vessels in this plexus also extends up and nourishes the overlaying epidermis by diffusion. Blood leaves the skin through small veins that accompany the subcutaneous arteries. The lymphatic system of the skin, which aids in combating certain skin infections, also is limited to the dermis.

The skin is richly supplied with arteriovenous anastomoses in which blood flows directly between an artery and a vein, bypassing the capillary circulation. These anastomoses are important for temperature regulation. They can open up, letting blood flow through the skin vessels when there is a need to dissipate body heat, and close off, conserving body heat if the environmental temperature is cold.

Innervation. The innervation of the skin is complex. The skin, with its accessory structures, serves as an organ for receiving sensory information from the environment. The dermis is well supplied with sensory neurons as well as nerves that supply the blood vessels, sweat glands, and arrector pili muscles.

The receptors for touch, pressure, heat, cold, and pain are widely distributed in the dermis (see Chapter 49). The papillary layer of the dermis is supplied with free nerve endings that serve as nociceptors (*i.e.*, pain receptors) and thermoreceptors. The dermis also contains encapsulated pressure-sensitive receptors that detect pressure and touch. The largest of these are the *pacinian corpuscles,* which are widely distributed in the dermis and subcutaneous tissue. The afferent nerve endings of the pacinian corpuscle are surrounded by concentric layers of modified Schwann cells such that they resemble an onion when sectioned. Pacinian corpuscles are responsible for detecting gross pressure changes and vibrations. Pressure causes the pacinian corpuscle to change its shape, thereby triggering nerve impulses. Pacinian corpuscles are adaptive and respond more to changes than to steady pressure or vibration.

Flat, encapsulated nerve endings found on the palmar surfaces of the fingers and hands and plantar surfaces of the feet are called *Meissner corpuscles.* They are concentrated on the fingertips, palms, soles, lips, tongue, face, and genitalia. They are thick, laminated, ovoid capsules each containing up to six nerve endings. When the corpuscle is deformed by pressure, the nerve endings are stimulated, signalling the somatosensory portion of the cerebral cortex and informing the person about the location and strength of the stimulus. They are rapidly adapting and do not react to constant, steady stimulation.

The deep dermis is supplied with small, oval mechanoreceptors called *Ruffini corpuscles.* Ruffini corpuscles are located in the subcutaneous tissue of hairy and glabrous skin. Several expanded nerve endings branch from a single, myelinated afferent fibre. They are slowly adapting receptors, responding to heavy pressure and joint movement. They are also believed to detect cold.

The skin is also supplied by *Krause end bulbs,* nerve endings contained in a cylindrical or oval capsule. They are found most frequently in the oral cavity, conjunctiva, and genitalia. Although their function is uncertain, they are thought to function as thermoreceptors sensitive to cold.

Most of the skin's blood vessels are under sympathetic nervous system control. The sweat glands are innervated by cholinergic fibres but controlled by the sympathetic nervous system. Likewise, the sympathetic nervous system controls the arrector pili (pilomotor) muscles that cause elevation of hairs on the skin. Contraction of these muscles tends to cause the skin to dimple, producing "goose bumps."

Subcutaneous Tissue

The subcutaneous tissue layer consists primarily of fat and connective tissues that lend support to the vascular and neural structures supplying the outer layers of the skin. There is controversy about whether the subcutaneous tissue should be considered an actual layer of the skin. Because the eccrine glands and deep hair follicles extend to this layer and several skin diseases involve the subcutaneous tissue, the subcutaneous tissue may be considered part of the skin.

Skin Appendages

The skin houses a variety of appendages, including hair, nails, and sebaceous and sweat glands. The distribution and functions of the appendages vary.

Sweat Glands

There are two types of sweat glands: eccrine and apocrine. *Eccrine sweat glands* are simple tubular structures that originate in the dermis and open directly to the skin surface. They are numerous (several million), vary in density, and are located over the entire body surface except the lips and part of the external genitalia. Their purpose is to transport sweat to the outer skin surface to regulate body temperature. *Apocrine sweat glands* are less numerous than eccrine sweat glands. They are larger and located deep in the dermal layer. They open through a hair follicle, even though a hair may not be present, and are found primarily in the axillae and groin. The major difference between these glands and the eccrine glands is that apocrine glands secrete an oily substance. In animals, apocrine secretions give rise to distinctive odours that enable animals to recognize the presence of others. In humans, apocrine secretions are sterile until mixed with the bacteria on the skin surface; they then produce what is commonly known as "body odour."

Sebaceous Glands

The sebaceous glands are located over the entire skin surface except for the palms, soles, and sides of the feet. They are part of the *pilosebaceous unit.* They secrete a mixture of lipids, including triglycerides, cholesterol, and wax. This mixture is called *sebum;* it lubricates hair and skin. Sebum is not the same as the surface lipid film. Sebum prevents undue evaporation of moisture from the stratum corneum during cold weather and helps to conserve body heat. Sebum production is under the control of genetic and hormonal influences. Sebaceous glands are relatively small and inactive until individuals approach adolescence. The glands then enlarge, stimulated by the rise in sex hormones. Gland size directly influences the amount of sebum produced, and the level of androgens influences gland size. The sebaceous glands are the structures that become inflamed in acne (see Chapter 61).

Hair

Hair is a structure that originates from hair follicles in the dermis. Most hair follicles are associated with sebaceous glands, and these structures combine to form the pilosebaceous unit. The entire hair structure consists of the hair follicle, sebaceous gland, hair muscle (arrector pili), and, in some instances, the apocrine gland (Fig. 60.6). Hair is a keratinized structure that is pushed upward from the hair follicle. Growth of the hair is centred in the bulb (*i.e.*, base) of the hair follicle, and the hair

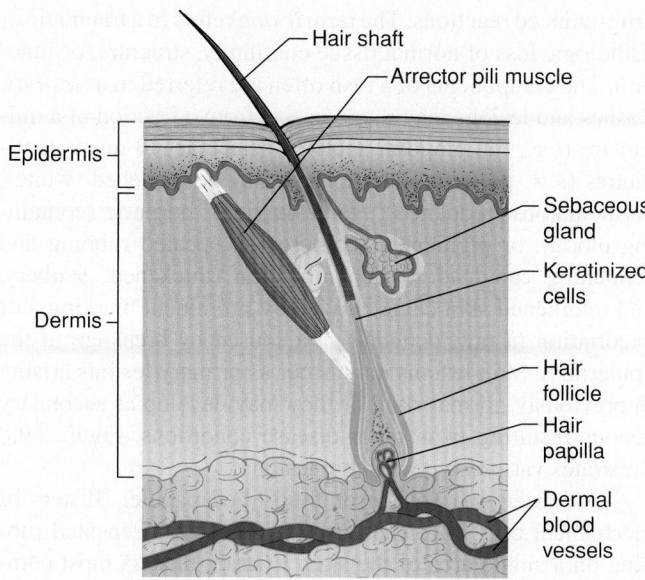

FIGURE 60.6 • Parts of a hair follicle.

Labels: Hair shaft; Arrector pili muscle; Epidermis; Dermis; Sebaceous gland; Keratinized cells; Hair follicle; Hair papilla; Dermal blood vessels

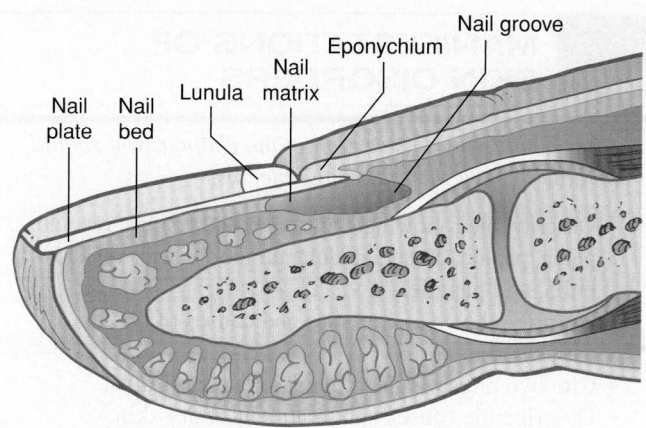

FIGURE 60.7 • Parts of a fingernail.

Labels: Nail plate; Nail bed; Lunula; Nail matrix; Eponychium; Nail groove

undergoes changes as it is pushed outward. Hair goes through three cyclic phases identified as anagen (the growth phase), catagen (the atrophy phase), and telogen (the resting phase, or no growth). Like most animals, human beings shed hair cyclically. However, human hair follicles work independently and therefore, unlike most animals, human beings shed hair asynchronously.

A vascular network at the site of the follicular bulb nourishes and maintains the hair follicle. Melanocytes in the bulb transfer melanosomes to the cells of the bulb matrix in much the same way as in the skin and are therefore responsible for the colour of the hair. Similar to the skin, large melanosomes are found in the hair of darker-skinned persons; aggregated and encapsulated melanosomes are found in persons with light skin. Red hair has spherical melanosomes, whereas grey hair is the result of a decreased number of melanosome-producing melanocytes. The arrector pili muscle, located under the sebaceous gland, provides a thermoregulatory function by contracting to cause goose bumps, thereby reducing the skin surface area that is available for the dissipation of body heat.

Nails

The nails are hardened keratinized plates, called *fingernails* and *toenails*, that protect the fingers and toes and enhance dexterity. The nails grow out from a curved transverse groove called the *nail groove*. The floor of this groove, called the *nail matrix,* is the germinal region of the nail plate (Fig. 60.7). The underlying epidermis, attached to the nail plate, is called the *nail bed.* Like hair, nails are the end product of dead matrix cells that are pushed outward from the nail matrix. Unlike hair, nails grow continuously rather than cyclically, unless permanently damaged or diseased. The epithelium of the fold of skin that surrounds the nail consists of the usual layers of skin. The stratum corneum forms the *eponychium* or cuticle. The nearly transparent nail plate provides a useful window for

viewing the amount of oxygen in the blood, providing a view of the colour of the blood in the dermal vessels. Changes or abnormalities of the nail can also serve to help diagnose skin or systemic diseases.

IN SUMMARY

The skin is primarily an organ of protection. It is the largest organ of the body and forms the major barrier between the internal organs and the external environment. The skin is richly innervated with pain, temperature, and touch receptors; it synthesizes vitamin D and plays an essential role in fluid and electrolyte balance. It contributes to glucose metabolism through its glycogen stores.

The skin is composed of two layers, the epidermis and the dermis, separated by a basement membrane. A layer of subcutaneous tissue binds the dermis to the underlying organs and tissues of the body. The epidermis, the outermost layer of the skin, contains four to five layers, or strata. The major cells of the epidermis are the keratinocytes, melanocytes, Langerhans cells, and Merkel cells. The stratum germinativum, or basal layer, is the source of the cells in all five layers of the epidermis. The keratinocytes, which are the major cells of the epidermis, are transformed from viable keratinocytes to dead keratin as they move from the innermost layer of the epidermis (*i.e.,* stratum germinativum) to the outermost layer (*i.e.,* stratum corneum). The melanocytes are pigment-synthesizing cells that give skin its colour. The dermis provides the epidermis with support and nutrition and is the source of blood vessels, nerves, and skin appendages (*i.e.,* hair follicles, sebaceous glands, nails, and sweat glands). Sensory receptors for touch, pressure, heat, cold, and pain are widely distributed in the dermis. The skin serves as a first line of defence against microorganisms and other harmful agents. The epidermis contains Langerhans cells, which process foreign antigens for presentation to T cells, and the dermis contains macrophages, T cells, mast cells, and fibroblasts, all contributing to the body's immune defences.

MANIFESTATIONS OF SKIN DISORDERS

After completing this section of the chapter, you should be able to meet the following objectives:

- Describe the following skin rashes and lesions: macule, patch, papule, plaque, nodule, tumour, wheal, vesicle, bulla, and pustule.
- Describe the characteristics and causes of blisters, calluses, and corns.
- Cite two physiologic explanations for pruritus.
- Describe the causes and treatment of dry skin.
- State common variations found in dark skin.

No two skin disorders look exactly alike, nor are they necessarily caused by the same agents. The appearance of many skin disorders may be further influenced by excessive itching, infection, or the effects of self-treatment. Skin colour also may influence the appearance. Nevertheless, most skin disorders have some common characteristics that can be used to describe them. This section of the chapter covers lesions and rashes, dry skin, pruritus, skin disorders due to mechanical forces, and variations in dark skin.

Lesions and Rashes

Rashes are temporary eruptions of the skin, such as those associated with childhood diseases, heat, diaper irritation, or drug-induced reactions. The term *lesion* refers to a traumatic or pathologic loss of normal tissue continuity, structure, or function. The components of a rash often are referred to as *lesions.* Rashes and lesions may range in size from a fraction of a millimetre (*e.g.,* the pinpoint spots of petechiae) to many centimetres (*e.g.,* pressure ulcer). They may be blanched (white), erythematous (reddened), hemorrhagic or purpuric (containing blood), or pigmented (coloured). Repeated rubbing and scratching can lead to lichenification (thickened, leathery, and roughened skin characterized by prominent markings) or excoriation (a raw, denuded area caused by breakage of the epidermis). Skin lesions may occur as primary lesions arising in previously normal skin, or they may develop as secondary lesions resulting from other disease conditions. Figure 60.8 illustrates various types of skin lesions.

A *blister* is a vesicle or fluid-filled papule. Blisters of mechanical origin are caused by friction from repeated rubbing on a single area of the skin. Friction blisters most commonly occur on the palmar and plantar surfaces of the hands and feet where the skin is constantly exposed to mechanical trauma, such as from shoes and household tools and appliances. Blisters also develop in bullous skin disorders and from burns. Histologically, there is degeneration of the epidermal cells and a disruption of the intercellular junctions, causing the layers of the skin to separate. As a result, fluid accumulates and a noticeable bleb forms on the skin surface. Friction blisters can be protected by adhesive bandages and gauze to prevent further irritation and rubbing. Breaking the skin of a blister to remove the fluid is inadvisable because of the risk of secondary infection.

Circumscribed, flat, nonpalpable changes in skin colour	Palpable elevated solid masses	Circumscribed superficial elevations of the skin formed by free fluid in a cavity within the skin layers

Macule—Small, up to 1 cm.
  Example: freckle, petechia
Patch—Larger than 1 cm.
  Example: vitiligo
	Papule—Up to 1 cm.
	  Example: elevated nevus
	Plaque—A flat, elevated surface larger than 1 cm, often formed by the coalescence of papules
	Nodule—0.5 cm to 1–2 cm; often deeper and firmer than a papule
	Tumour—Larger than 1–2 cm
	Wheal—A somewhat irregular, relatively transient, superficial area of localized skin edema.
	  Example: mosquito bite, hive
		Vesicle—Up to 1 cm; filled with serous fluid.
		  Example: herpes simplex
		Bulla—Greater than 1 cm; filled with serous fluid.
		  Example: second-degree burn
		Pustule—Filled with pus.
		  Examples: acne, impetigo

FIGURE 60.8 • Primary lesions may arise from previously normal skin. Authorities vary somewhat in their definitions of skin lesions by size. (From Bates B. B. (1995). *A guide to physical examination and history taking* (6th ed.). Philadelphia, PA: J.B. Lippincott.)

A *callus* is a hyperkeratotic plaque of skin due to chronic pressure or friction. It represents hyperplasia of the dead, keratinized cells that make up the cornified or horny layer of the skin. Increased cohesion between cells results in hyperkeratosis and decreased skin shedding. A callus may be filed down but is likely to recur if pressure continues in the localized area.

Corns (helomas) are small, well-circumscribed, conical, keratinous thickenings of the skin. They usually appear on the toes from rubbing or ill-fitting shoes. The corn may be either hard (heloma durum) with a central hard, horny core, or soft (heloma molle), as commonly seen between the toes. They may appear on the hands as an occupational hazard. The hard tissue at the centre of the corn looks like a funnel with a broad top and a pointed bottom, hence the name, "corn." Corns on the feet often are painful, whereas corns on the hands may be asymptomatic. Corns may be abraded or surgically removed, but they recur if the causative agent is not removed.

Pruritus

Pruritus, or the sensation of itch, is a common symptom of skin disorders. Symptoms of pruritus range from mild to severe. In some persons, the condition may be so severe that it interrupts sleep and the general quality of life. Although itching commonly occurs with skin disorders, it can also provide a valuable clue to internal disorders, such as chronic renal disease, diabetes, or biliary disease.

Despite the fact that almost all skin diseases manifest in pruritus, very little is known about it. It is generally agreed that itch is a sensation that originates in free nerve endings in the skin, is carried by small myelinated type C nerve fibres to the dorsal horn of the spinal cord, and is then transmitted to the somatosensory cortex through the spinothalamic tract (see Chapter 49). Until recently, it was believed that pain and itch travelled along the same nerve pathways and that itch was a low-level pain response. It has now been demonstrated through micrographic recordings that there are itch-specific neuronal pathways in the spinothalamic tract and central nervous system that process peripheral itch stimuli. Evidence over the years has supported this finding; for example, it has been shown that itch and pain are antagonistic—pain and peripheral inflammation suppress itch, whereas opioids often provoke itch. Further, itch induces scratching, whereas pain induces withdrawal, and itch and pain can be simultaneously perceived. Finally, the belief in polymodal pain–itch receptors may be discounted by the knowledge that massaging or rubbing the skin, which are sensations conducted by non-itch fibres, often results in the sensation of itch. In other words, although rubbing a painful area tends to decrease pain sensations, it increases itch sensations.

Specific afferent type C fibres, distinct from the polymodal nociceptors that are responsible for pain, may transmit itch sensations. These specific itch neurons are believed to be sensitive to temperature, which explains why itch worsens in warm environments, including warm sleeping environments.

Given these new findings, it has been postulated that itch exists both locally and centrally, that in addition to localized itch, an "itch centre" exists in the somatosensory cortex. For example, a mosquito bite on most people itches momentarily then subsides. However, central itch may be similar to central pain: that is, it is perceived by the brain but does not exist locally. This may explain the presence of localized itch when no skin alterations are observable.

Advances have also been made in understanding peripheral mediators (*i.e.*, substances that cause itch) other than histamine. Mast cell tryptase may be an important itch mediator because it activates a specific receptor in the sensory nerves. Opioids operate centrally and peripherally in producing itch, whereas neuropeptides, such as substance P, induce itch by their effect on mast cells. Substances such as bradykinin and bile salts act locally to stimulate the itch sensation. Prostaglandins are modulators of the itch response, lowering the threshold for other mediators.

Scratching, the well-known response to an itch, is a spinal reflex response that to varying degrees can be controlled by the individual. Many types of itch are not easily localized or relieved by scratching. Excoriations and thickened papular areas develop at the site of repeated scratching or rubbing, and in some skin conditions, such as dry skin, scratching further activates itch sensations. Chronic forms of pruritus can severely affect the quality of a person's life.

Most treatment measures for pruritus are nonspecific. Measures such as using the entire hand to rub over large areas and keeping the fingernails trimmed often can relieve itch and prevent skin damage. Self-limited or seasonal cases of pruritus may respond to treatment measures such as moisturizing lotions, bath oils, and the use of humidifiers. Because vasodilation tends to increase itching, cold applications may provide relief. Cool showers before bed, light sleepwear, and cool home temperatures also may be helpful. Topical corticosteroids may be helpful in some cases, such as itch related to allergy-mediated urticaria. However, unlike for some other skin problems, there is no armamentarium of effective antipruritic drugs available.

Mild cutaneous disorders, such as bug bites, are mediated by histamine; therefore, nonsedating antihistamines tend to be the treatment of choice. However, because most cases of pruritus are not histamine related, their management should be directed at the underlying cause. For example, systemic antihistamines and corticosteroids may be indicated for persons with severe pruritus or atopic dermatitis. Topical capsaicin cream and topical aspirin have been used for localized chronic pruritic disorders. Opioid antagonists may be used for pruritus caused by opioid medications such as morphine. Other modalities that have been used for all cases of pruritus with varying degrees of success are phototherapy, acupuncture, vagus nerve stimulation, antidepressant medications, behaviour modification, and alternative therapies (herbal, nutritional, and reflex therapies). In persons with pruritus due to a systemic cause, itching gradually recedes as the primary condition improves.

Given the recent advances in the science of pruritus, it is anticipated that healthcare professionals will have available in the near future new, effective, and disease-specific antipruritic drugs. Classification schemes for pruritus may also be forthcoming. Similar to pain scales, visual analog scales may be developed and used in the diagnosis and treatment of pruritus.

Dry Skin

Dry skin, also called *xerosis,* may be a natural occurrence, as in the drying of skin associated with aging, or it may be symptomatic of an underlying systemic disease or skin disorder such as contact dermatitis or psoriasis. Most cases of dry skin are caused by dehydration of the stratum corneum. The effects of aging on skin dryness include a change in the composition of sebaceous gland secretions and a decrease in the secretion of moisture from the sweat glands. Aging is also accompanied by a decrease in skin capillaries as well as a flattening of the dermal rete ridges, resulting in less surface area for exchange of fluids between the dermis, epidermis, and skin surface.

Persons with dry skin often experience severe pruritus and discomfort, most commonly of the extremities. Other commonly involved areas include the back, abdomen, and waist. Dry skin appears rough and scaly; there may be increased wrinkles or lines. Skin drying also predisposes the skin to scratching, resulting in cracking, fissuring, and a number of other skin maladies.

Moisturizing agents are the cornerstone of treatment for dry skin. These agents exert their effects by repairing the skin barrier, increasing the water content of the skin, reducing transepidermal water loss, and restoring the lipid barrier's ability to attract, hold, and redistribute water. Moisturizing agents can be classified as emollients, humectants, and occlusives. *Emollients* are fatty acid-containing lotions that replenish the oils on the skin surface, but usually do not leave a residue on the skin. They have a short duration of action and need to be applied frequently. *Humectants* are the additives in lotions, such as alpha-hydroxy acids and urea, that draw out water from the deeper skin layers and hold it on the skin surface. However, the water that is drawn to the skin is transepidermal water, not atmospheric water; thus, continued evaporation from the skin can actually exacerbate dryness. Alpha-hydroxy acids are derived from fruits, hence the abundance of fruit additives in shampoos and lotions in over-the-counter preparations. Urea is a nitrogenous substance that has been quite effective in reducing xerosis when combined with lotions. It is a humectant at lower concentrations (10%), but in higher concentrations (20% to 30%) it is mildly keratolytic. *Occlusives* are thick creams that contain petroleum or some other moisture-proof material. They prevent water loss from the skin. They are the most effective agents for relieving skin dryness, but because of their greasiness and lack of cosmetic appeal, some people do not wish to use them.

Lotion or cream additives include corticosteroids or mild anesthetics, such as camphor, menthol, lidocaine, or benzocaine. These agents work by suppressing itching while moisturizing the skin. Using room humidifiers and keeping room temperatures as low as possible to prevent water loss from the skin also may be helpful. Soaps with moisturizers may be helpful. Glycerine soaps, although popular and visually appealing, are drying and can exacerbate the symptoms.

Variations in Dark-Skinned People

Some skin disorders common to people of African, Hispanic, or East Indian descent are not commonly found in those of European descent. Similarly, some skin disorders, such as skin cancers, affect light-skinned persons more commonly than dark-skinned persons. Because of these differences, serious skin disorders may be overlooked, and normal variations in darker skin may be mistaken for anomalies.

Skin colour is determined by the melanin produced by the melanocytes. Although the number of melanosomes in dark and white skin is the same, black skin produces more melanin, and more quickly, than white skin. Because of their skin colour, dark-skinned persons are better protected against skin cancer, premature wrinkling, and aging of the skin that occurs with sun exposure.

A condition common in people with dark skin is too much or too little colour. Areas of the skin may darken after injury, such as a cut or scrape, or after disease conditions such as acne.

TABLE 60.1 COMMON NORMAL VARIATIONS IN DARK SKIN

VARIATION	APPEARANCE
Epidermal layer	Same thickness of stratum corneum for all races, but there are more layers in black skin
Follicular prominence	Pronounced hair follicle patterns; common in young children
Futcher (Voigt) line	Demarcation between darkly pigmented and lightly pigmented skin in upper arm; follows spinal nerve distribution; common in black and Japanese populations
Midline hypo-pigmentation	Line or band of hypopigmentation over the sternum, dark or faint, lessens with age; common in the Latino and black populations
Nail pigmentation	Linear dark bands down nails or diffuse nail pigmentation, brown, blue, or blue-black
Oral pigmentation	Blue to blue-grey pigmentation of oral mucosa; gingivae also affected
Palmar changes	Hyperpigmented creases, small hyperkeratotic papules, and tiny pits in creases
Plantar changes	Hyperpigmented macules, can be multiple with patchy distribution, irregular borders, and variance in colour

Developed from information in Burns T., Breathnach S., Cox N., et al. (2010). *Rook's textbook of dermatology.* (8th ed., Vol. 1). Malden, MA: Wiley-Blackwell.

These darkened areas may take many months or years to fade. Dry or "ashy" skin also can be a problem for people with dark skin. It often is uncomfortable, and it also is easily noticed because it gives the skin an ashen or greyish appearance. Although using a moisturizer may help relieve the discomfort, it may cause a worsening of acne in predisposed persons.

Normal variations in skin structure and skin tones often make evaluation of dark skin difficult. The darker pigmentation can make skin pallor, cyanosis, and erythema more difficult to observe. Therefore, verbal histories must be relied on to assess skin changes. The verbal history should include the client's description of her or his normal skin tones. Changes in skin colour, in particular hypopigmentation and hyperpigmentation, often accompany disorders of dark skin and are very important signs to observe when diagnosing skin conditions. Common variations in dark skin and nails are described in Table 60.1.

IN SUMMARY

Skin lesions and rashes are the most common manifestations of skin disorders. Rashes are temporary skin eruptions. Lesions result from traumatic or pathologic loss of the normal continuity, structure, or function of the skin. Lesions may be vascular in origin; they may occur as primary lesions in previously normal skin; or they may develop as secondary lesions resulting from primary lesions. Blisters, calluses, and corns result from rubbing, pressure, and frictional forces applied to the skin. Pruritus and dry skin are symptoms common to many skin disorders. Scratching because of pruritus can lead to excoriation, infection, and other complications. Normal variations in dark skin often make evaluation difficult and result in some disorders being overlooked. Changes in colour, especially hypopigmentation or hyperpigmentation, often accompany the skin disorders of dark-skinned people.

REVIEW EXERCISES

1. Bullous pemphigoid is an autoimmune blistering disease caused by autoantibodies to constituents of the dermal–epidermal junction.
   A. *Explain how antibodies, which attack glycoproteins in the lamina lucida and their attachment to the hemidesmosomes, can cause blisters to form (hint: see Fig. 60.5).*
2. "Allergy tests" involve the application of an antigen to the skin, either through a small scratch or intradermal injection.
   A. *Explain how the body's immune system is able to detect and react to these antigens.*

Bibliography

Arda O., Goksugur N., Tuzun Y. (2014). Basic histological structure and functions of facial skin. *Clinics in Dermatology, 32*(1), 3–13.

Bolognia J., Jorizzo J. L., Schaffer J. V. (2012). *Dermatology* (3rd ed.). Philadelphia, PA: Elsevier Saunders.

Buchness M. R. (2006). A practical approach to basic skin care. *Women's Health in Primary Care, 9*(8), 11–15.

Burns T., Breathnach S., Cox N., et al. (2010). *Rook's textbook of dermatology: Volume I* (8th ed.). Malden, MA: Wiley-Blackwell.

Hood A. F., Kwan T. H., Mihm M. C., et al. (2002). *Primer of dermatopathology* (3rd ed.). Philadelphia, PA: Lippincott Williams & Wilkins.

LaMotte R. H., Dong X., Ringkamp M. (2014). Sensory neurons and circuits mediating itch. *Nature Reviews Neuroscience, 15*(1), 19–31.

Storm C. A., Elder D. E. (2012). Chapter 24: The skin. In Rubin R., Strayer D. S. (Eds.). *Rubin's pathology: Clinicopathologic foundations of medicine* (6th ed.). Philadelphia, PA: Lippincott Williams & Wilkins.

Weisshaar E., Szepietowski J. C., Darsow U., et al. (2012). European guideline on chronic pruritus. *Acta Dermato-Venereologica, 92*(5), 563–581.

Visit thePoint **http://thePoint.lww.com for animations, journal articles, and more!**

Disorders of Skin Integrity and Function

61

The skin is a unique organ in that numerous signs of disease or injury are immediately observable on the skin. The skin serves as the interface between the body's internal organs and the external environment. Therefore, skin disorders represent the culmination of environmental forces and the internal functioning of the body. Sunlight, insects, other arthropods, infectious organisms, chemicals, and physical agents all play a role in the pathogenesis of skin diseases. Although most disorders are intrinsic to skin, many are external manifestations of systemic disease. Thus, skin provides a valuable window for the recognition of many systemic disorders.

The skin also has an elusive property that reflects emotional states. It is through the skin that warmth and other responses are given and received. The skin conveys a sense of health, beauty, integrity, and emotion. Human beings emphasize the body and, in particular, the skin to the degree that even slight imperfections may evoke a wide variety of responses.

PRIMARY DISORDERS OF THE SKIN

After completing this section of the chapter, you should be able to meet the following objectives:

- Describe common pigmentary disorders of the skin.
- Relate the behaviour of fungi to the production of superficial skin lesions associated with tinea or ringworm.
- State the cause and describe the appearance of impetigo and ecthyma.
- Compare the viral causes, manifestations, and treatments of verrucae, herpes simplex, and herpes zoster lesions.
- Compare acne vulgaris, acne conglobata, and rosacea in terms of appearance and location of lesions.

- Describe the pathogenesis of acne vulgaris and relate it to measures used in treating the disorder.
- Differentiate allergic and contact dermatitis and atopic and nummular eczema.
- Describe the differences and similarities between erythema multiforme minor, Stevens–Johnson syndrome, and toxic epidermal necrolysis.
- Define the term *papulosquamous* and use the term to describe the lesions associated with psoriasis, pityriasis rosea, and lichen planus.
- Relate the life cycle of *Sarcoptes scabiei* to the skin lesions seen in scabies.
- Use knowledge of the life cycles of *Pediculus humanus corporis* and *Pediculus humanus capitis* to explain the lesions associated with body, head, and pubic lice.

FIGURE 61.1 • Vitiligo of the forearm of a black person. (Neutrogena Skin Care Institute.) (From Hall B. J., Hall J. C. (2010). *Sauer's manual of skin diseases* (10th ed., p. 381). Philadelphia, PA: Lippincott Williams & Wilkins.)

Primary skin disorders are those originating in the skin. They include pigmentary skin disorders, infectious processes, acne, rosacea, papulosquamous dermatoses, allergic disorders and drug reactions, and arthropod infestations. Although most of these disorders are not life-threatening, they can affect the quality of life.

PRIMARY SKIN DISORDERS

- Primary skin disorders originate in the skin.
- Pigmentary skin disorders involve increased, decreased, or absent melanocyte function.
- Infectious skin disorders are caused by viruses, bacteria, and fungi that invade the skin, incite inflammatory responses, and otherwise cause rashes and lesions that disrupt the skin surface.
- Acne involves occlusion of the pilosebaceous unit with noninflammatory and inflammatory lesions resulting from occlusion, inflammation due to the irritating effects of sebum, and infection caused by the *Propionibacterium acnes* organism.
- Allergic and hypersensitivity responses are caused by antigen–antibody responses resulting from sensitization to topical or systemic antigens.
- The papulosquamous dermatoses constitute a group of disorders characterized by scaling papules and plaques that result from uncontrolled keratinocyte proliferation.
- Scabies and lice are arthropod skin infestations that are transmitted from person to person and from animals to humans.

Pigmentary Skin Disorders

Pigmentary skin disorders involve the melanocytes. In some cases, there is an absence of melanin production, as in vitiligo or albinism. In other cases, there is an increase in melanin

or some other pigment, as in mongolian spots or melasma. In either case, the emotional impact can cause much worry and anxiety. Because pigmentary changes can result in social ostracism, it is also important to treat the physiologic, emotional, and social components of these skin disorders.

Vitiligo

Vitiligo is a pigmentary problem of concern to darkly pigmented persons of all races. It also affects white-skinned persons, but not as often, and the effects usually are not as socially problematic. The classic sign of vitiligo is the sudden appearance of white patches on the skin. The lesion is a depigmented macule with definite smooth borders on the face, axillae, neck, or extremities (Fig. 61.1). The patches vary in size from small macules to ones involving large skin surfaces. The large macular type is more common. Depigmented areas appear white, pale-coloured, or sometimes greyish-blue. Histologically, the depigmented areas may contain no melanocytes, greatly altered or decreased amounts of melanocytes, or, in some cases, melanocytes that no longer produce melanin. These areas sunburn easily and they enlarge over time. Vitiligo often is asymptomatic, although pruritus may occur.

Vitiligo appears at any age; roughly half of cases begin before the age of 20 years. Worldwide, it affects people of all races regardless of sex, with an incidence rate of 1% to 2%.[1–3] The cause is unknown, although several hypotheses have been postulated, including (1) a hereditary predisposition—up to 20% of people with vitiligo report a family history; (2) an autoimmune process in which there is immunologic destruction of the melanocytes—the disorder often accompanies other autoimmune diseases, such as diabetes mellitus and thyroid disease; (3) neural mechanisms in which the melanocytes are destroyed by a cytotoxic chemical secreted by nearby nerve endings; (4) a self-destruct phenomenon in which the melanocytes are preprogrammed for self-destruction; (5) a lack of melanocyte growth factors; or (6) a combination of factors in which multiple causes are involved and vary among individuals. In some cases, vitiligo has been reportedly precipitated by emotional stress or physical trauma, such as sunburn.[2,3]

Although there are many treatment regimens for vitiligo, the two goals remain to stop further depigmentation and to induce repigmentation. Self-tanning lotions, skin stains, and cosmetics are used for camouflage. Self-tanning compounds that contain a chemical such as *dihydroxyacetone* do not need melanocytes to colour the skin. Corticosteroids administered topically, intralesionally, and orally have also been used successfully. Narrow-band (focused) ultraviolet B (UVB) irradiation has also been used successfully in the treatment of vitiligo. The combination of psoralen and UVA (PUVA) treatment has also been successful in some people with large areas of skin involvement.[1]

A variety of skin grafting techniques have been used in persons unresponsive to other therapies. Successful skin grafting techniques vary from minigrafting (2-mm full-thickness punch grafts transplanted to involved areas) to grafting melanocytes into involved areas. Micropigmentation (tattooing) has been done on smaller, recalcitrant areas, but it is often risky to attain a correct colour match.[4]

If extensive skin surfaces are involved, the treatment may be reversed and the pigmented areas bleached to match the remainder of the skin colour. A melanocytotoxic agent is used to remove remaining melanocytes from skin areas. This process, which is called *depigmentation,* is permanent and irreversible; patients need to be apprised of this and their need to avoid the sun and use sunscreens for the remainder of their lives.

Albinism

Albinism, a genetic disorder in which there is complete or partial congenital absence of pigment in the skin, hair, and eyes, is found in all races. The prevalence is estimated at 1 in 20,000 people worldwide, and 1 in 17,000 in North America and Europe.[5] Although there are multiple types of albinism, the most common type is recessively inherited oculocutaneous albinism, in which there is a normal number of melanocytes but gene mutations limit tyrosinase, the enzyme needed for synthesis of melanin, or its receptors. It affects the skin, hair, and eyes. Individuals have pale or pink skin, white or yellow hair, and light-coloured or sometimes pink eyes. Persons with albinism have ocular problems, such as extreme sensitivity to light, refractive errors, lack of stereopsis, macular hypoplasia, and nystagmus. There is no cure for albinism. Treatment efforts for people with albinism are aimed at reducing their risk for cancer through protection from solar radiation and screening for malignant skin changes. Efforts to reduce the visual impact are important, such as glasses, preferential seating in classrooms, and large-print books.[6]

Melasma

Melasma is a disorder characterized by darkened facial macules. It is common in all skin types, but most prominent in brown-skinned people from Asia, India, and South America. It occurs in men but is more common in women, particularly during pregnancy or while using oral contraceptives. It may or may not resolve after giving birth or discontinuing hormonal birth control. Melasma is exacerbated by sun exposure. Treatment measures are palliative, mostly consisting of limiting exposure to the sun and using sunscreens. Bleaching agents, containing 2% to 4% hydroquinone, are standard treatments. Tretinoin cream and azelaic acid have been useful in treating severe cases. Depending on the person's ability to tolerate topical treatments, triple combinations (hydroquinone, tretinoin, and fluocinolone acetonide) or double combinations (hydroquinone and tretinoin) have been highly successful, sometimes combined with glycolic acid.[7,8]

Infectious Processes

The skin is subject to invasion by a number of microorganisms, including fungi, bacteria, and viruses. Normally, the skin flora, sebum, immune responses, and other protective mechanisms guard the skin against infection. Depending on the virulence of the infecting agent and the competence of the host's resistance, infections may result.

Superficial Fungal Infections

Fungi are free-living, saprophytic plant-like organisms, certain strains of which are considered part of the normal skin flora (see Chapter 16). There are two types of fungi, yeasts and moulds. Yeasts, such as *Candida albicans,* grow as single cells and reproduce asexually. Moulds grow in long filaments, called *hyphae.* There are thousands of known species of yeasts and moulds, but only about 100 of them cause disease in humans and animals. Fungal or mycotic infections of the skin are traditionally classified as superficial or deep. The superficial mycoses, more commonly known as *tinea* or *ringworm,* invade only the superficial keratinized tissue (skin, hair, and nails). Deep fungal infections involve the epidermis, dermis, and subcutis. Infections that typically are superficial may exhibit deep involvement in immunosuppressed individuals.

Most of the superficial mycoses (or *dermatophytoses*) are caused by the dermatophytes, a group of closely related fungi classified into three genera: *Microsporum* (*M. audouinii, M. canis, M. gypseum*), *Epidermophyton* (*E. floccosum*), and *Trichophyton* (*T. schoenleinii, T. violaceum, T. tonsurans*). Another way of classifying the dermatophytes is according to their ecologic origin—human, animal, or soil. Anthropophilic species (*M. audouinii, M. tonsurans, T. violaceum*) are parasitic on humans and are spread by other infected humans. Zoophilic species (*M. canis* and *T. mentagrophytes*) cause parasitic infections in animals, some of which can be spread to humans. Geophilic species originate in the soil, but may infect animals, which in turn serve to infect humans.

The fungi that cause superficial mycoses live on the dead keratinized cells of the epidermis. They emit an enzyme that enables them to digest keratin, which results in superficial skin scaling, nail disintegration, or hair breakage, depending on the location of the infection. An exception to this is the invading fungus of tinea versicolour, which does not produce a keratolytic enzyme. Deeper reactions involving vesicles, erythema, and infiltration are caused by the inflammation that results from exotoxins liberated by the fungus. Fungi also are capable of producing an allergic or immune response. Superficial fungal infections affect various parts of the body, with the lesions varying according to site and fungal species. Tinea can affect the body (tinea corporis), face and neck (tinea faciale), scalp (tinea capitis), hands (tinea manus), feet (tinea pedis), nails (tinea unguium), or genitalia (tinea cruris).[1,9]

Diagnosis of superficial fungal infections is primarily done by microscopic examination of skin scrapings for fungal spores, the reproducing bodies of fungi. Potassium hydroxide (KOH) preparations are used to prepare slides of skin scrapings. KOH disintegrates human tissue and leaves behind the thread-like filaments, or hyphae, that grow from the fungal spores. Cultures also may be done using a dermatophyte test medium or a microculture slide that produces colour changes and allows for direct microscopic identification. The Wood light (UV light) is another method that can assist with the diagnosis of tinea. Some types of fungi (*e.g.,* *M. canis* and *M. audouinii*) fluoresce yellow-green when the light is directed onto the affected area.[1,2]

Superficial fungal infections may be treated with topical or systemic antifungal agents. Treatment usually follows diagnosis confirmed by KOH preparation or culture, particularly if a systemic agent is to be used. Topical agents, both prescription and over-the-counter, are commonly used in the treatment of tinea infections; however, success often is limited because of the lengthy duration of treatment, poor compliance, and high rates of relapse at specific body sites.

The oral systemic antifungal agents include griseofulvin, the azoles, and the allylamines. Griseofulvin, a fungicidal agent that is no longer available in Canada, was derived from a species of *Penicillium* that is used only in the treatment of dermatophytoses. The azoles are a group of synthetic antifungal drugs that act by inhibiting the fungal enzymes needed for the synthesis of ergosterol, which is an essential part of fungal cell membranes. The azoles are classified as either imidazoles or triazoles. The imidazoles consist of ketoconazole, miconazole, and clotrimazole. The latter two drugs are used only in topical therapy. The triazoles include itraconazole and fluconazole, both of which are used for the systemic treatment of fungal infections. Terbinafine, a synthetic allylamine, acts by interrupting ergosterol synthesis, causing the accumulation of a metabolite that is toxic to the fungus. These synthetic agents are fungicidal. Some of the oral agents can produce serious side effects, such as hepatic toxicity, or interact adversely with other medications. A number of the synthetic fungicides (*e.g.,* ketoconazole, miconazole, clotrimazole, and terbinafine) are available as topical preparations that produce less severe side effects. Topical corticosteroids may be used in conjunction with antifungal agents to relieve itching and erythema secondary to inflammation.

Tinea of the Body or Face. *Tinea corporis* (ringworm of the body) can be caused by any of the fungi but is most frequently caused by *M. canis* in North America and by *T. rubrum* worldwide. There has been an increase in *T. tonsurans* as the

FIGURE 61.2 • Tinea corporis (ringworm) of the arm due to *Trichophyton mentagrophytes.* (Centers for Disease Control and Prevention Public Health Image Library. Available online at: http://phil.cdc.gov/Phil/home.asp)

causative agent of tinea corporis as well. Although tinea corporis affects all ages, children seem most prone to infection. Transmission is most commonly from kittens, puppies, and other children who have infections.[9]

The lesions vary, depending on the fungal agent. The most common types of lesions are oval or circular patches on exposed skin surfaces and the trunk, back, or buttocks (Fig. 61.2). Less common are foot and groin infections. The lesion begins as a red papule and enlarges, often with a central clearing. Patches have raised red borders consisting of vesicles, papules, or pustules. The borders are sharply defined, but lesions may coalesce. Pruritus, a mild burning sensation, and erythema frequently accompany the skin lesion.

Tinea faciale, or ringworm of the face (Fig. 61.3), is an infection caused by *T. mentagrophytes* or *T. rubrum.* Tinea

FIGURE 61.3 • Child with ringworm (tinea faciale) on the left side of his face and ear. Tinea faciale does not include the bearded areas (called *tinea barbae*). Tinea faciale infections are uncommon, and are often initially misdiagnosed. (Centers for Disease Control and Prevention Public Health Image Library. Available online at: http://phil.cdc.gov/Phil/home.asp)

faciale may mimic the annular, erythematous, scaling, pruritic lesions characteristic of tinea corporis. It also may appear as flat erythematous patches. Topical antifungal agents usually are effective in treating tinea corporis and tinea faciale. Oral antifungal agents may be used in resistant cases.

Tinea of the Scalp. There are two common types of *tinea capitis* (ringworm of the scalp): primary (noninflammatory) and secondary (inflammatory). In North America and the United Kingdom, over 95% of the cases of noninflammatory tinea capitis are caused by *T. tonsurans;* however, forms commonly found in Africa and West Asia have been isolated.[9] *T. tonsurans* does not fluoresce green with a Wood lamp. Urban children between the ages of 3 and 9 years are primarily affected, with a higher incidence of tinea capitis among people of African descent.[9] Although there is a lower incidence among adults attributed to the higher content of fatty acids in the sebum after puberty, increasing numbers of adults are being diagnosed.[1,2] The infection is spread most often among household members who share combs and brushes on which the spores are shed and remain viable for long periods. Depending on the invading fungus, the lesions of the noninflammatory type can vary from greyish, round, hairless patches to balding spots, with or without black dots on the head. The lesions vary in size and are most commonly seen on the back of the head (Fig. 61.4). Mild erythema, crust, or scale may be present. The individual usually is asymptomatic, although pruritus may exist.

The inflammatory type of tinea capitis is caused by virulent strains of *T. mentagrophytes, T. verrucosum,* and *M. gypseum.* The onset is rapid, and inflamed lesions usually are localized to one area of the head. The inflammation is believed to be a delayed hypersensitivity reaction to the invading fungus. The initial lesion consists of a pustular, scaly, round patch with broken hairs. A secondary bacterial infection is common and may lead to a painful, circumscribed, boggy, and indurated lesion called a *kerion.*

FIGURE 61.4 • Child with tinea capitis (ringworm of the scalp) caused by a *Microsporum* species. (Centers for Disease Control and Prevention Public Health Image Library. Available online at: http://phil.cdc.gov/Phil/home.asp)

FIGURE 61.5 • Chronic tinea of the sole caused by *Trichophyton rubrum.* (Schering Corp.) (From Hall B. J., Hall J. C. (2010). *Sauer's manual of skin diseases* (10th ed., p. 249). Philadelphia, PA: Lippincott Williams & Wilkins.)

The treatment for both noninflammatory and inflammatory forms of tinea capitis is oral antifungals. Terbinafine is the primary treatment and has been shown to be safe in children.[1,2] Topical ointments or shampoos are occasionally indicated in addition to oral medications, both to decrease the spore population and protect household members. Wet packs, medicated shampoos, steroids, and antibiotics may be prescribed for secondary infections that occur.

Tinea of the Foot and Hand. *Tinea pedis* (athlete's foot) is the most common fungal dermatosis, primarily affecting the spaces between the toes, the soles, or the sides of the feet (Fig. 61.5). It is caused by *T. mentagrophytes* and *T. rubrum.* The lesions vary from a mildly scaling lesion to a painful, exudative, erosive, inflamed lesion with fissuring. Lesions often are accompanied by pruritus, pain, and foul odour. Some persons are prone to chronic tinea pedis. Mild forms are more common during dry environmental conditions. Exacerbations occur as a result of hot weather, sweating, and exercise or when the feet are exposed to moisture, occlusive shoes, and communal swimming.

Tinea manus usually is a secondary infection with tinea pedis as the primary infection. In contrast to other skin disorders, such as contact dermatitis and psoriasis, which affect both hands, tinea manus usually occurs only on one hand. The characteristic lesion is a blister on the palm or finger surrounded by erythema. Chronic lesions are scaly and dry. Cracking and fissuring may occur. The lesions may spread to the plantar surfaces of the hand. If chronic, tinea manus may lead to tinea of the fingernails. Simple forms of tinea pedis and tinea manus are treated with topical applications of antifungals.[9]

Tinea of the Nail. *Tinea unguium* is a dermatophyte infection of the nails. It is a subset of *onychomycosis,* which includes dermatophyte, nondermatophyte, and candidal infections of the nails. There is an increased incidence of fungal nail

FIGURE 61.6 • Tinea of the fingernail caused by *Trichophyton rubrum*. (Duke Laboratories, Inc.) (From Hall B. J., Hall J. C. (2010). *Sauer's manual of skin diseases* (10th ed., p. 253). Philadelphia, PA: Lippincott Williams & Wilkins.)

infections in recent years, probably reflecting better diagnostics, increased numbers of immunocompromised patients who have greater susceptibility, increased use of immunosuppressive drugs, increasing numbers of elderly people, worldwide travel, and increased use of communal bathing facilities.

Distal and lateral subungual onychomycosis, the most common form of tinea unguium, usually is caused by *T. rubrum* or *T. mentagrophytes*. Toenails are involved more commonly than fingernails because fingernails are more exposed to air. The infection often begins at the tip of the nail, where the fungus digests the nail keratin. In some cases, the infection may begin from a crushing injury to a toenail or from the spread of tinea pedis. Initially, the nail appears opaque, white, or silver (Fig. 61.6). The nail then turns yellow or brown. The condition often remains unchanged for years. During this time it may involve only one or two nails and may produce little or no discomfort. Gradually, the nail thickens and cracks as the infection spreads and includes the nail plate. Permanent discoloration and distortion result as the nail plate separates from the nail bed. Less common forms of tinea unguium are superficial white onychomycosis, in which areas of the nails become powdery white and erode, and proximal subungual onychomycosis, in which there is rapid invasion of the nail, leaving it white with no additional thickening of the nail. Although it is one of the less common forms of tinea unguium, proximal subungual onychomycosis has increased among people with human immunodeficiency virus (HIV) infection.

Treatment of tinea unguium usually requires oral antifungal therapy. Toenail infections are usually treated with itraconazole and terbinafine. Fluconazole has been effective, particularly if *Candida* is involved. Itraconazole and terbinafine can be administered in pulses (intermittent weeks with 1 week of therapy repeated every month for 4 to 12 months).[2,10] Fingernail

infections are more easily treated, in part because the fingernails are more exposed to air. Itraconazole and terbinafine have been effective in treating fingernail infections. All of the oral agents require careful monitoring for side effects. A nail lacquer containing the antifungal agent ciclopirox is available for use in the topical management of mild to moderate infections of the fingernails and toenails caused by *T. rubrum*. A new nail may require 3 to 12 months to grow. Thus, people being treated with antifungal agents need to be reminded that the resolution of the infection requires 4 to 6 months for fingernails and longer for toenails.

Although there has been an increase in the cure rate of toenail fungal infections, primarily because of the synthetic antifungals, recalcitrant cases remain. Some authorities recommend removal of the infected toenails. Many cases of tinea unguium would be prevented if primary infections of tinea pedis were diagnosed and treated promptly.

Tinea Versicolour. Tinea versicolour is a fungal infection involving the upper chest, the back, and sometimes the arms, and can cause hypo- or hyperpigmented areas. The causative agent belongs to the *Malassezia* yeast genus, of which a variety of species are found as normal flora on the human body. The characteristic lesion is a yellow, pink, or brown sheet of scaling skin. The name *versicolour* is derived from the multicoloured variations of the lesion. The depigmented patches do not tan when exposed to UV light. These cosmetic defects often bring the patient to the healthcare provider in the summer months. It is believed that the fungus filters the UV light, preventing tanning. In darker-skinned persons, the depigmented areas are more apparent.

Selenium sulphide, found in several shampoo preparations, has been an effective fungistatic treatment measure. Miconazole or ketoconazole creams or shampoos, because of their fungicidal properties, have become the drugs of choice. Oral antifungals are used for extensive cases. The infection may recur after drug therapy.[11]

Tinea Incognito. Tinea incognito is a form of dermatophyte infection that developed with the widespread use of topical corticosteroids. It often is seen in cases where tinea infections are misdiagnosed as eczema and treated with corticosteroids. Because corticosteroids suppress inflammation, scaling and erythema may not be present or it may not resemble a fungal infection at all after several rounds of cortisone therapy. There has been an increased incidence of tinea incognito in persons with HIV infection. Persons with the disorder often present with thickened plaques with lichenification, papules, pustules, and nodules. Telangiectases, atrophy, and striae may be present. Tinea incognito is seen most often on the groin, the palms, or the dorsal aspect of the hand.

Treatment measures include discontinuing topical corticosteroids. Topical or oral antifungal agents are used, depending on the severity of the infection.

Dermatophytid Reaction. A secondary skin eruption may occur in persons allergic to the fungus responsible for the

FIGURE 61.7 • Dermatophytid reaction on the fingers due to a tinea infection. An immunologic reaction, also known as *autoeczematization,* is an itchy, vesicular rash produced in response to an intense inflammatory process that can be located in another region of the body. (Centers for Disease Control and Prevention Public Health Image Library. Available online at: http://phil.cdc.gov/Phil/home.asp)

dermatophytosis. This dermatophytid or allergic reaction may occur during an acute episode of a fungal infection. The most common reaction occurs on the hands in response to tinea pedis. The lesions are vesicles with erythema extending over the palms and fingers, sometimes extending to other areas (Fig. 61.7). Less commonly, a more generalized reaction occurs in which papules or vesicles erupt on the trunk or extremities. These eruptions may resemble tinea corporis. Lesions may become excoriated and infected with bacteria. Treatment is directed at the primary site of infection. The intradermal reaction resolves in most cases without intervention if the primary site is cleared.[2]

Candidal Infections. Candidiasis (moniliasis) is a fungal infection caused by *C. albicans* and occasionally by a few other *Candida* species. This yeast-like fungus is a normal inhabitant of the gastrointestinal tract, mouth, and vagina (see Chapter 47). The skin problems result from the release of irritating toxins on the skin surface. *C. albicans* is found almost always on the surface of the skin; it rarely penetrates to the deeper layers of the skin. Some persons are predisposed to candidal infections by conditions such as diabetes mellitus, antibiotic therapy, pregnancy, oral contraceptive use, poor nutrition, and immunosuppressive diseases. Oral candidiasis may be the first sign of infection with HIV.

C. albicans thrives on warm, moist, intertriginous areas of the body. The rash is red with well-defined borders. Patches erode the epidermis, and there is scaling. Mild to severe itching and burning often accompany the infection. Severe forms of infection may involve pustules or vesiculopustules. In addition to microscopy, a candidal infection often can be differentiated from a tinea infection by the presence of satellite lesions. These satellite lesions are maculopapular and are found outside the clearly demarcated borders of the candidal infection. Satellite lesions often are diagnostic of diaper rash

complicated by *Candida.* The appearance of candidal infections varies according to the site (see Chapter 47 for a discussion of vaginal candidiasis).

Diagnosis usually is based on microscopic examination of skin or mucous membrane scrapings placed in a KOH solution. Treatment measures vary according to the location. Preventive measures such as wearing rubber gloves are encouraged for persons with infections of the hands. Intertriginous areas often are separated with clean cotton cloth and allowed to air dry as a means of decreasing the macerating effects of heat and moisture. Topical and oral antifungal agents, such as clotrimazole, ketoconazole, and miconazole, are used in treatment depending on the site and extent of involvement.

Bacterial Infections

Bacteria are considered normal flora of the skin. Most bacteria are not pathogenic, but when pathogenic bacteria invade the skin, superficial or systemic infections may develop. Bacterial skin infections are commonly classified as primary or secondary infections. Primary infections are superficial skin infections such as impetigo or ecthyma. Secondary infections consist of deeper cutaneous infections, such as infected ulcers. Diagnosis usually is based on cultures taken from the infected site. Treatment measures include antibiotic therapy and measures to promote comfort and prevent the spread of infection.

Impetigo. Impetigo is a common, superficial bacterial infection caused by staphylococci or group A beta-hemolytic streptococci, or both. Impetigo is common among infants and young children, although older children and adults occasionally contract the disease. Its occurrence is highest during warm summer months or in warm, moist climates. Although overcrowded housing and poor hygiene contribute to its incidence, they are not causative. It is highly communicable in the younger population.[12]

Impetigo initially appears as a small vesicle or pustule or as a large bulla on the face or elsewhere on the body. As the primary lesion ruptures, it leaves a denuded area that discharges a honey-coloured serous liquid that hardens on the skin surface and dries as a honey-coloured crust with a "stuck-on" appearance (Fig. 61.8). New vesicles erupt within hours. Pruritus often accompanies the lesions, and skin excoriations that result from scratching multiply the infection sites. Although a very low risk, a possible complication of untreated streptococcal impetigo is poststreptococcal glomerulonephritis (see Chapter 33). Topical mupirocin (Bactroban), which has few side effects, may be effective for limited infections. If the area is large or if there is concern about complications, systemic antibiotics are used.

Another form of impetigo exists, *bullous impetigo,* which is caused by *Staphylococcus aureus.* Bullous impetigo is common among children. Thin bullae erupt that appear clear to cloudy and coalesce. The bullae open, leaving the original bullous rim with central thin, flat, brownish or honey-coloured crusts, or in some cases denuded areas. Bullous impetigo is typically found on the trunk, axilla, extremities,

FIGURE 61.8 • Impetigo of the face. The lesions vary from small vesicles to large bullae that rupture and discharge a honey-coloured serous liquid that hardens on the skin surface and dries as a honey-coloured crust. (Abner Kurten, Folia Dermatologica. No. 2. Geigy Pharmaceuticals.) (From Hall B. J., Hall J. C. (2010). *Sauer's manual of skin diseases* (10th ed., p. 203). Philadelphia, PA: Lippincott Williams & Wilkins.)

and intertriginous (diaper) areas but may occur anywhere on the body. The treatment measures are the same as for nonbullous impetigo.[12]

Ecthyma is an ulcerative form of impetigo, usually secondary to minor trauma. It is caused by group A beta-hemolytic streptococci, *S. aureus,* or *Pseudomonas* species. It frequently occurs on the buttocks and thighs of children (Fig. 61.9). The lesions are similar to those of impetigo. A vesicle or pustule

FIGURE 61.9 • Ecthyma on the buttocks of a 13-year-old boy. (Glaxo-Wellcome Co.) (From Hall B. J., Hall J. C. (2010). *Sauer's manual of skin diseases* (10th ed., p. 204). Philadelphia, PA: Lippincott Williams & Wilkins.)

FIGURE 61.10 • Staphylococcal scalded skin syndrome. (From Fitzpatrick T. B., Johnson R. A., Polona M. K., et al. (1992). Color atlas and synopsis of clinical dermatology (2nd ed., p. 297). New York: McGraw Hill.

ruptures, leaving a skin erosion or ulcer that weeps and dries to a crusted patch, often resulting in scar formation.[1,2] With extensive ecthyma, there is a low-grade fever and extension of the infection to other organs. Treatment usually involves the use of systemic antibiotics.

A less common form of *S. aureus* infection, called *Ritter disease,* manifests with a diffuse, scarlet fever-like rash, followed by skin separation and sloughing (Fig. 61.10). It is also called *staphylococcal scalded skin syndrome* because the skin looks scalded. Ritter disease usually affects children younger than 5 years of age; immunosuppressed adults also are at risk. The disorder, which is considered a deeper skin infection because the superficial layers of the epidermis are separated and shed in sheets, is caused by the hematologic spread of toxins from a focal infection, such as the nasopharynx or a superficial skin abrasion. The onset of the rash may be preceded by malaise, fever, irritability, and extreme tenderness over the skin. The conjunctiva often is inflamed, with purulent drainage. Although the fluid in the unbroken bullae is sterile, cultures usually are obtained from suspected sites of local infection and from the blood. Systemic antibiotics, either oral or parenteral, are used to treat the disorder. Healing usually occurs in 10 to 14 days without scarring.

Cellulitis is a deeper infection affecting the dermis and subcutaneous tissues. It is usually caused by group A beta-hemolytic streptococci or *S. aureus,* but can be caused by bacteria associated with specific activities (*e.g.,* fish handling, swimming in fresh water, or swimming in salt water) or from animal bites or scratches. Pre-existing wounds (*e.g.,* ulcers, erosions) and tinea pedis are often portals of entry. Legs are the most common sites, followed by the hands and pinnae of the

FIGURE 61.11 • Cellulitis on leg infected with *Staphylococcus aureus* and *Pseudomonas*.

ears, but cellulitis may be seen on many body parts. The lesion consists of an expanding red, swollen, tender plaque with an indefinite border, covering a small to wide area (Fig. 61.11). Cellulitis is frequently accompanied by fever, erythema, heat, edema, and pain. Cellulitis often involves the lymph system and, once compromised, repeat infections may impair lymphatic drainage, leading to chronically swollen legs, and eventually dermal fibrosis and lymphedema. Incorrectly treated, it may result in septicemia, nephritis, or death. Treatment measures (oral and intravenous antibiotics) are aimed at the invasive organisms and the extent of the infection.

Viral Infections

Viruses are intracellular pathogens that rely on live cells of the host for reproduction. They have no organized cell structure but consist of a deoxyribonucleic acid (DNA) or ribonucleic acid (RNA) core surrounded by a protein coat. The viruses seen in skin lesion disorders tend to be DNA-containing viruses. Viruses invade the keratinocyte, begin to reproduce, and cause cellular proliferation or cellular death. The rapid increase in viral skin diseases has been attributed to the use of corticosteroid drugs, which have immunosuppressive qualities, and the use of antibiotics, which alter the bacterial flora of the skin. As the number of bacterial infections has decreased, there has been a proportional rise in viral skin diseases.

Verrucae. Verrucae, or warts, are common benign papillomas caused by the DNA-containing human papillomavirus (HPV). Transmission of HPV infection is largely by direct contact between individuals or by autoinoculation. As benign papillomas, warts represent an exaggeration of the normal skin structures. There is an irregular thickening of the stratum spinosum and greatly increased thickening of the stratum corneum. The classification of warts is based largely on morphology and location.

Although warts vary in appearance depending on their location, it is now recognized that the clinically distinct types of warts result not simply because of the anatomic sites in which they arise, but also because of the distinct types of HPV. There are more than 100 types of HPV affecting humans that cause several different kinds of warts, including skin warts and genital warts.[1,13] Many of the HPV types that cause genital warts are sexually transmitted, some of which (types 6, 11, 16, and 18) may increase the risk of cervical cancer (discussed in Chapter 47).

Nongenital warts often occur on the hands and feet. They are commonly caused by HPV types 1, 2, 3, 4, 27, and 57, and are not considered precancerous lesions. They are classified as common warts, flat warts, and plantar or palmar warts. Common warts, or verrucae vulgaris, are the most common type. The lesions can occur anywhere, but most frequently occur on dorsal surfaces of hands, especially the periungual area, where they appear as small, greyish-white to tan, flat to convex papules with a rough, pebble-like surface (Fig. 61.12). Verrucae plana, or flat warts, are common on the face or dorsal surfaces of the hands. The warts are slightly elevated, flat, smooth, tan papules that are slightly larger than verrucae vulgaris. Verrucae plantaris and verrucae palmaris (*i.e.,* plantar and palmar warts, respectively) occur on the soles of the feet and palms of the hands, respectively. They appear as rough, scaly lesions that may reach 1 to 2 cm in diameter, coalesce, and be confused with ordinary calluses. HPV transmission usually occurs through breaks in skin integrity. For example, plantar warts, which occur on the soles of the feet, frequently are transmitted to the abraded, softened heels of children in swimming areas.

Treatment is usually directed at inducing a "wart-free" period without producing scarring. Warts resolve spontaneously when immunity to the virus develops. The immune response, however, may be delayed for years. Because of their appearance or discomfort, people usually desire their removal, rather than waiting for immunity to develop. Removal is usually

FIGURE 61.12 • Common and periungual warts. (From Stephen T. C., Skillen D. L., Day R. A., et al. (2012). *Canadian Jensen's nursing health assessment: A best practice approach* (p. 311). Philadelphia, PA: Lippincott Williams & Wilkins.)

done by applying a keratolytic agent, such as salicylic acid gel or plaster that breaks down the wart tissue, or by freezing with liquid nitrogen. Salicylic acid works by dissolving intercellular cement and producing desquamation of the horny layer of skin without affecting normal epidermal cells. Intralesional bleomycin injections have been effective for recalcitrant warts. Various types of laser surgery, electrosurgery, cryotherapy, immunotherapy, imiquimod, and antiviral therapy (*e.g.,* cidofovir) also have been successful in wart eradication.[14]

Occluding warts with duct tape may be another treatment that is painless and inexpensive.[14] Duct tape is applied on warts for 61/2 days, every 7 days, then repeated for up to 2 months. The mechanism of action for duct tape is unknown, but resolution of other untreated warts on the same person suggests that occluding the wart stimulates the immune response. Another possibility is that the tape debrides the skin surface while also removing the virus attached to it.

Herpes Simplex. Herpes simplex virus (HSV) infections of the skin and mucous membrane (*i.e.,* cold sore or fever blister) are common. Two types of HSV infect humans: type 1 and type 2. HSV-1 is usually associated with oropharynx infections, and the organism is spread by respiratory droplets or by direct contact with infected saliva. HSV-1 may also be transmitted to other parts of the body through occupational hazards, such as skin contact athletics, dentistry, and medicine. Genital herpes usually is caused by HSV-2 (see Chapter 47). HSV-1 genital infections and HSV-2 oral infections are becoming more common, perhaps because of oral–genital sex.

Infection with HSV-1 may present as a primary or recurrent infection. Primary HSV-1 symptoms include fever, sore throat, painful vesicles, and ulcers of the tongue, palate, gingiva, buccal mucosa, and lips. Primary infection results in the production of antibodies to the virus so that recurrent infections are more localized and less severe. After an initial infection, the herpesvirus persists in the trigeminal and other dorsal root ganglia in the latent state, periodically reactivating in recurrent infections. It also may be that reactivation of a herpes infection occurs both in the dorsal root ganglion and locally, where it has been found to exist in the epidermis and other organs. The symptoms of a primary HSV-1 infection most often occur in young children (1 to 5 years of age). It is likely that many adults were exposed to HSV-1 during childhood and therefore have antibodies to the virus.

The recurrent lesions of HSV-1 usually begin with a burning or tingling sensation. Umbilicated vesicles and erythema follow and progress to pustules, ulcers, and crusts before healing (Fig. 61.13). Lesions are most common on the lips, face, mouth, nasal septum, and nose. When a lesion is active, HSV-1 is shed and there is risk of transmitting the virus to others. Pain is common, and healing takes place within 10 to 14 days. Precipitating factors may be stress, menses, or injury. In particular, UVB exposure seems to be a frequent trigger for recurrence.

There is no cure for oropharyngeal herpes; most treatment measures are palliative. Penciclovir cream or docosanol

FIGURE 61.13 • Recurrent herpes simplex of the face. (Dermik Laboratories, Inc.) (From Hall B. J., Hall J. C. (2010). *Sauer's manual of skin diseases* (10th ed., p. 231). Philadelphia, PA: Lippincott Williams & Wilkins.)

cream, topical antiviral agents, applied at the first symptom and then several times daily, reduces the duration of an attack. Application of over-the-counter topical preparations containing antihistamines, antipruritics, and anesthetic agents along with aspirin or acetaminophen may be used to relieve pain. Oral antiviral drugs (*e.g.,* acyclovir, famciclovir, valacyclovir) inhibit herpesvirus replication and may be used prophylactically to prevent recurrences.

Herpes Zoster. Herpes zoster (shingles) is an acute, localized vesicular eruption distributed over a dermatomal segment of the skin. It is caused by the same herpesvirus, varicellazoster, that causes chickenpox. It is believed to be the result of reactivation of a latent varicella-zoster virus infection that has been dormant in the sensory dorsal root ganglia since a primary childhood infection. During an episode of herpes zoster, the reactivated virus travels from the ganglia to the skin of the corresponding dermatome. Although herpes zoster is not as contagious as chickenpox, the reactivated virus can be transmitted to nonimmune contacts.

The lifetime risk of developing varicella is over 95%, whereas the lifetime risk of at least one episode of herpes zoster is estimated to be 30%. More than half of the people who contract the disease are older than 50 years of age and this percentage increases with age.[15] An age-related decline in varicella-zoster T-cell–mediated immunity is thought to account for the increased viral activation in this age group. Other persons at risk because of impaired T-cell–mediated immunity are those with conditions such as HIV infection and certain malignancies, chronic corticosteroid users, and those undergoing chemotherapy and radiation therapy.

The lesions of herpes zoster typically are preceded by a prodrome consisting of a burning pain, a tingling sensation, extreme sensitivity of the skin to touch, and pruritus along the affected dermatome (see Chapter 49). Among the dermatomes, the most frequently involved are the thoracic (53%),

FIGURE 61.14 • **A:** Dermatomal distribution of herpes zoster rash due to varicella-zoster virus in a child with a history of leukemia. (Centers for Disease Control and Prevention Public Health Image Library. Available online at: http://phil.cdc.gov/Phil/home.asp) **B:** Dermatomal distribution due to herpes zoster virus. (From Stephen T. C., Skillen D. L., Day R. A., et al. (2012). *Canadian Jensen's nursing health assessment: A best practice approach* (p. 308). Philadelphia, PA: Lippincott Williams & Wilkins.)

the cervical (20%), the trigeminal (15%), and the lumbosacral (11%).[1] Prodromal symptoms may be present for 1 to 3 days or longer before the appearance of the rash. During this time, the pain may be mistaken for a number of other conditions, such as heart disease, pleurisy, musculoskeletal disorders, or gastrointestinal disorders.

The lesions appear as an eruption of vesicles with erythematous bases that are restricted to skin areas supplied by sensory neurons of a single or associated group of dorsal root ganglia (Fig. 61.14). In immunosuppressed persons, the lesions may extend beyond the dermatome. Eruptions usually are unilateral in the thoracic region, trunk, or face. New crops of vesicles erupt for 3 to 5 days along the nerve pathway. The vesicles dry, form crusts, and eventually fall off. The lesions usually clear in 2 to 3 weeks, although they can persist up to 6 weeks in some elderly persons.

Serious complications can accompany eruptions. Eye involvement can result in permanent blindness and occurs in a large percentage of cases involving the ophthalmic division of the trigeminal nerve (see Chapter 54). *Postherpetic neuralgia,* which is pain that persists longer than 1 to 3 months after the resolution of the rash, is an important complication of herpes zoster (discussed in Chapter 49). It is seen most commonly in persons older than 50 years of age, increasing age being the greatest risk factor. Given the aging population in Canada, the incidence of herpes zoster is expected to increase over the next two decades. Affected persons complain of sharp, burning pain that often occurs in response to nonnoxious stimuli. Even the slightest pressure of clothing and bed sheets may elicit pain. It usually is a self-limited condition that persists for months, with symptoms abating over time.

The treatment of choice for herpes zoster is the administration of an antiviral agent (*e.g.,* acyclovir, valacyclovir, famciclovir). The treatment is most effective when started within 72 hours of rash development. When given in the acute vesicular stage, the antiviral drugs have been shown to decrease the amount of lesion development and pain. Narcotic analgesics, tricyclic antidepressants, gabapentin, anticonvulsant drugs, and nerve blocks have been used for management of postherpetic neuralgia. Local application of capsaicin cream or lidocaine patches may be used in selected cases. Palliative treatments, such as heat and gentle pressure, may also be helpful. In 2008, a live, attenuated vaccine for herpes zoster was approved by Health Canada (Zostavax) and is recommended for use in people older than 50 years of age. When introduced in other countries, the vaccine has been found to reduce (1) the incidence of herpes zoster by 51.3%, and (2) the incidence of postherpetic neuralgia by 66.5%.[16]

Acne and Rosacea

Acne is a disorder of the pilosebaceous unit (hair follicle and sebaceous gland).[17,18] The hair follicle is a tubular invagination of the epidermis in which hair is produced (see Chapter 60, Fig. 60.6). The sebaceous glands empty into the hair follicle, and the pilosebaceous unit opens to the skin surface through a widely dilated opening called a *pore.* The sebaceous glands produce a complex lipid mixture called *sebum,* from the Latin word meaning "tallow" or "grease." Sebum consists of a mixture of free fatty acids, triglycerides, diglycerides, monoglycerides, sterol esters, wax esters, and squalene. Sebum production occurs through what is called a *holocrine process,* in which the sebaceous gland cells that produce the sebum are completely broken down and their lipid contents emptied through the sebaceous duct into the hair follicle. The amount of sebum produced depends on two factors: the size of the sebaceous gland and the rate of sebaceous cell proliferation. The sebaceous glands are largest on the scalp, face, and upper torso, but are present in all areas of the skin except for the soles and palms. Sebaceous cell proliferation and sebum production are uniquely responsive to direct hormonal stimulation by androgens. In men, testicular androgens are the main stimulus for sebaceous activity; in women, adrenal and ovarian androgens maintain sebaceous activity.

The spectrum of acne lesions ranges from noninflammatory to inflammatory lesions.[18] Noninflammatory lesions consist of *comedones* (whiteheads and blackheads). *Blackheads* are plugs of material that accumulate in sebaceous glands that open to the skin surface. The colour of blackheads results from melanin that has moved into the sebaceous glands from adjoining epidermal cells. *Whiteheads* are pale, slightly elevated papules with no visible orifice. Inflammatory lesions consist of papules, pustules, nodules, and, in severe cases, cysts, which can lead to scarring. *Papules* are raised areas less than 5 mm in diameter. *Pustules* have a central core of purulent material. *Nodules* are larger than 5 mm in diameter and may become suppurative or hemorrhagic. Suppurative nodules often are referred to as *cysts* because of their resemblance to inflamed epidermal cysts. The inflammatory lesions are believed to develop from the escape of sebum into the dermis and the irritating effects of the fatty acids contained in the sebum.

Two types of acne occur during different stages of the life cycle: acne vulgaris, which is the most common form among adolescents and young adults, and acne conglobata, which develops later in life. Other types of acne occur in association with various etiologic agents such as drugs (*e.g.,* steroids, iodides), occupational compounds, cosmetics, and other irritating agents. Treatment measures for these acnes depend on the precipitating agent and the extent of the lesions.

Acne Vulgaris

Acne vulgaris is a chronic inflammatory disease of the pilosebaceous unit, affecting almost all persons aged 15 to 17 years and becoming moderate to severe in approximately 15% to 20% of that group. While this is perceived as a teenage disease, it often persists into adulthood.[17] In women, acne may begin earlier and persist longer; overall, however, the incidence and severity are greater in men. Acne vulgaris lesions form primarily on the face and neck and, to a lesser extent, on the back, chest, and shoulders (Fig. 61.15). The lesions may consist of comedones (whiteheads and blackheads) or inflammatory lesions (pustules, nodules, and cysts).

The cause of acne vulgaris remains unknown. There is a hereditary factor; multiple generations of family members often experience it. Several factors are believed to contribute to acne, including (1) increased sebum production, (2) increased proliferation of the keratinizing epidermal cells that form the sebaceous cells, (3) the colonization and proliferation of *Propionibacterium acnes,* and (4) inflammation.[17,18] These factors are probably interrelated. Increased androgen production results in increased sebaceous cell activity, with resultant plugging of the pilosebaceous ducts. The excessive sebum provides a medium for the growth of *P. acnes.* The *P. acnes* organism contains lipases that break down the free fatty acids that produce the acne inflammation. In addition, there have been new findings regarding the physiology of acne. One example is that *P. acnes* forms a biofilm (an extracellular polysaccharide lining in which the bacteria are encased). The biofilm acts as a protective exoskeleton and as a physical barrier to antibiotic treatment, explaining why prolonged antibiotic treatments are necessary.[17]

Over the years, several factors, such as poor hygiene, acne as an infectious process, diets high in fatty content, and certain foods (*e.g.,* chocolate, fried foods) have been studied

FIGURE 61.15 • (**A**) Acne of the face and (**B**) acne of the chest. (From Hall B. J., Hall J. C. (2010). *Sauer's manual of skin diseases* (10th ed., p. 152). Philadelphia, PA: Lippincott Williams & Wilkins.)

empirically and rejected as causal factors in the development of acne. Although general hygienic measures are important, obsessive scrubbing can traumatize the skin and worsen the condition. Instead, it is recommended that the affected areas are washed gently and patted dry.[17]

Diagnosis. The diagnosis of acne is based on history and physical examination. The severity of the acne is generally assessed by the type and number of lesions.[18] *Mild acne* is usually characterized by the presence of a small number (generally <10) of open and closed comedones, with a few inflammatory papules; *moderate acne* by the presence of a moderate number (10 to 40) of erythematous papules and pustules, usually limited to the face; and moderately severe acne by the presence of numerous papules and pustules (40 to 100) and occasionally larger, deeper, nodular inflamed lesions involving the face, chest, and back. Acne conglobata (to be discussed) is a severe chronic form of acne.

Treatment. Treatment of acne focuses on clearing up existing lesions, preventing new lesions, and limiting scar formation. Depending on the extent of involvement and the types of lesions, treatment of acne may involve the use of topical or systemic agents.[17,18] Long-term treatment usually is required. Significant improvement may not be apparent for 4 to 8 weeks after initiation of treatment, and maximum effects may not be apparent for months.[17] An important treatment measure is sensitivity to the client's emotional needs.

A number of topical agents are available for the treatment of acne, including retinoids, benzoyl peroxide, azelaic acid, and antibiotics. Topical retinoids, benzoyl peroxide, and azelaic acid are effective treatments for mild acne. Moderate to severe acne often requires combination therapy with a topical agent and systemic antibiotics. The type of vehicle (cream, gel, or lotion) may be an important consideration in the selection of an agent. Persons with drier skin may benefit from creams, whereas persons with oily skin may have better results using a gel or lotion. Many acne creams and lotions containing keratolytic agents such as sulphur, salicylic acid, phenol, and resorcinol are available as over-the-counter preparations. These agents act chemically to break down keratin, loosen comedones, and exert a peeling effect on the skin.

Benzoyl peroxide is a topical agent that has both antibacterial and comedolytic properties. It is the topical agent most effective in reducing the *P. acnes* population. Bacterial proteins are oxidized by the oxygen-free radicals released from the metabolism of benzoyl peroxide on the skin. Because of its mechanism of action, bacterial resistance does not develop to benzoyl peroxide. The irritant effect of the drug also causes vasodilation and increased blood flow, which may hasten resolution of the inflammatory lesions. *Azelaic acid,* derived from wheat, rye, and barley, has actions similar to benzoyl peroxide. It decreases the proliferation of keratinocytes and has antibacterial actions against *P. acnes.* Azelaic cream is moisturizing and causes only minimal skin irritation.

Topical tretinoin (Retin-A), an acid derivative of vitamin A, acts locally to decrease the cohesiveness of epidermal cells and increase epidermal cell turnover. This is thought to result in an increased extrusion of open comedones and a transformation of closed comedones into open ones. Tretinoin is inactivated by UV light and oxidized to benzoyl peroxide, and should be applied only at night and not with benzoyl peroxide. All tretinoin formulations are irritating to the skin, an effect that is increased with sun exposure. Another form of tretinoin, Retin-A Micro, works by entrapping the drug in microspheres that move into the follicle and serve as reservoirs for drug release. Other retinoid drugs, such as adapalene and tazarotene, have actions similar to tretinoin. Adapalene appears to be as effective as tretinoin, but may be less irritating to the skin.

Topical antibiotics also are effective in treating mild to moderate acne. Topical tetracycline, erythromycin, and clindamycin are used most commonly. They do not affect existing lesions but prevent future lesions by decreasing the amount of *P. acnes* on the skin, thereby reducing subsequent inflammation formed by the presence of sebaceous fatty acid metabolites. Treatment failure can result from development of antibiotic resistance. Combination drugs such as benzoyl peroxide and erythromycin or clindamycin also have been effective.

Oral antibiotics are indicated for moderate to severe disease, and for the treatment of acne on the chest, back, or shoulders. Low-dose tetracycline has been used effectively for many years. Tetracycline has no effect on sebum production, but it decreases bacterial growth and the amount of free fatty acids produced. Tetracycline requires a sufficient treatment period to establish effective blood levels. Side effects are minimal, which is why the drug has remained so useful. However, it does have teratogenic effects on skeletal and tooth development and should not be given to those who are pregnant or lactating, or to children. The more expensive tetracycline derivatives, minocycline and doxycycline, are better tolerated than tetracycline. Doxycycline may cause photosensitivity reactions. Erythromycin and trimethoprim/sulfamethoxazole are also effective in acne treatment, especially when tetracycline and its derivatives cannot be used.

Isotretinoin (Accutane), an orally administered synthetic retinoid or acid form of vitamin A, revolutionized the treatment of recalcitrant cases of acne and cystic acnes. In carefully planned doses, oral isotretinoin has cleared major cases of acne and initiated long-term remissions of the disease. It is administered for 3- to 6-month treatment periods. Although the exact mode of action is unknown, it decreases sebaceous gland activity, prevents new comedones from forming, reduces the *P. acnes* count through sebum reduction, and has an anti-inflammatory effect. Because of its many side effects, it is used only in persons with severe acne or when other treatment is ineffective. Side effects include dryness of the mouth and other mucous membranes, conjunctivitis, and musculoskeletal system abnormalities. Although not confirmed by population-based studies, there have been case reports of depression and suicide attempts, even 6 months after cessation of treatment.[17] Careful clinical and laboratory monitoring is necessary because the drug can produce elevated serum lipid levels, abnormal liver enzyme test results, and hematologic disorders. Isotretinoin is a well-documented and potent teratogen that causes brain, heart, and ear malformations. Baseline and monthly pregnancy tests are also recommended for women taking isotretinoin. In conjunction with the medication, women are encouraged to take oral contraceptives or remain abstinent during therapy.

Estrogens reduce the size and secretion of the sebaceous gland, but because of the high dosages required, they are contraindicated in men. In women, oral contraceptive agents that combine estrogen with a progestin that has low androgenic activity may be used.

Other treatment measures for acne include surgery, UV irradiation, cryotherapy (*e.g.,* freezing with carbon dioxide slushes, liquid nitrogen), laser and light therapy, and intralesional corticosteroid injection. Acne surgery involves the aspiration of comedones with small-bore needles or devices designed to extract comedonal contents. Intralesional injection of corticosteroids using a syringe or needleless injector is limited to severe nodulocystic forms of acne. It has been effective in promoting cyst healing, but usually has to be repeated frequently.[2,17,18]

Acne Conglobata

Acne conglobata occurs later in life and is a chronic form of acne. Comedones, papules, pustules, nodules, abscesses, cysts, and scars occur on the back, buttocks, and chest. Lesions occur to a lesser extent on the abdomen, shoulders, neck, face, upper arms, and thighs. The comedones or cysts have multiple openings, large abscesses, and interconnecting sinuses. Inflammatory nodules are not uncommon. Their discharge is odoriferous, serous or mucoid, and purulent. Healing often leaves deep keloidal lesions. Affected persons have anemia with elevated white blood cell counts, erythrocyte sedimentation rates, and neutrophil counts. When persons with acne conglobata have a sudden onset of a fever and arthralgia with their leukocytosis, plus tender, ulcerating acne lesions, this type of rare, severe acne is diagnosed as *acne fulminans.*[19] For both, the treatment is difficult and stringent. It often includes debridement, systemic corticosteroid therapy, oral retinoids, and systemic antibiotics.

Rosacea

Rosacea is a chronic inflammatory process that occurs in middle-aged and older adults and typically presents between ages 30 to 50.[20] Rosacea is two to three times more prevalent in women, almost exclusively affects the central facial skin, and is estimated to affect over two million Canadians. It is easily confused with acne and may coexist with it. Rosacea is more common in fair-skinned persons. An early characteristic and diagnostic sign is seen in persons who "flush and blush."

The cause of rosacea is unknown; however, it is believed to be an inflammatory process accompanied by vascular instability with leakage of fluid and inflammatory mediators into the dermis. *Demodex folliculorum* mites have been proposed as a pathogenic factor. These tiny mites, as part of the normal flora, live in or near hair follicles and are commonly local to the face. The link to rosacea is poorly understood with theories suggesting increased numbers may be associated with certain subtypes of rosacea or these mites might trigger an immune response.[20,21] In addition to microorganisms, other causes postulated have been genetic, environmental, and vascular.

Rosacea has now been classified into four types: (1) erythematotelangiectatic (flushing and persistent central facial erythema); (2) papulopustular (inflammatory); (3) phymatous (thickening of the skin with irregular surface nodularities and enlargement); and (4) ocular (involving the eyes).[20] In the early stage of rosacea development, there are repeated episodes of blushing. The blush eventually becomes a permanent dark red erythema on the nose and cheeks that sometimes extends to the forehead and chin. This stage often occurs before 20 years of age. Ocular problems occur in at least 50% of persons with rosacea, which may lead to visual losses. Prominent symptoms include eyes that are itchy, burning, or dry; a gritty or foreign body sensation; and erythema and swelling of the eyelid.[20] As the person ages, the erythema persists, and telangiectases with or without acne components (*e.g.,* comedones, papules, pustules, nodules, erythema, edema) develop. After years of affliction, acne rosacea may develop into an

FIGURE 61.16 • Chronic rosacea with rhinophyma. (Hoechst Marion Roussel Pharmaceuticals, Inc.) (From Hall B. J., Hall J. C. (2010). *Sauer's manual of skin diseases* (10th ed., p. 158). Philadelphia, PA: Lippincott Williams & Wilkins.)

irregular bullous hyperplasia (thickening of the skin) of the nose, known as *rhinophyma* (Fig. 61.16). The sebaceous follicles and openings of the nose enlarge, and the skin colour changes to a purple-red, resulting in hypertrophy of the nose and impaired breathing. Although rosacea is more common in women, rhinophyma is more common in men.

Persons with rosacea are heat sensitive. They are instructed to avoid vascular stimulating agents such as heat, sunlight, hot liquids, foods, and alcohol. Treatment measures are similar to those used for acne vulgaris. Topical metronidazole, azelaic acid, and brimonidine have been effective. Topical antibiotics (*e.g.,* clindamycin, erythromycin) have been useful, as well as systemic antibiotics (*e.g.,* tetracycline and its derivatives). Light therapies, such as laser, have been recommended. Rhinophyma can be treated by a number of surgical methods, including electrosurgery, laser ablation, dermabrasion, cryosurgery, and excision.[22]

Allergic and Hypersensitivity Dermatoses

Allergic and hypersensitivity dermatoses involve the inflammatory response to multiple exogenous and endogenous agents. The disorders, which are usually characterized by epidermal edema with separation of epidermal cells, include irritant contact dermatitis, allergy contact dermatitis, atopic and nummular eczema, urticaria, and drug-induced skin eruptions.

Contact and Allergic Dermatitis

Contact dermatitis is a common inflammation of the skin. There are two types of contact dermatitis: allergic and irritant contact dermatitis. *Allergic contact dermatitis* results from a cell-mediated, type IV hypersensitivity response brought about

FIGURE 61.17 • A: Contact dermatitis from shoe material. (Glaxo-Wellcome Co.) (From Hall B. J., Hall J. C. (2010). *Sauer's manual of skin diseases* (10th ed., p. 79). Philadelphia, PA: Lippincott Williams & Wilkins.) **B:** Arm with a blistering oak rash. Note the linear pattern of the lesions. (Centers for Disease Control and Prevention Public Health Image Library. Available online at: http://phil.cdc.gov/Phil/home.asp)

by sensitization to an allergen (see Chapter 19). More than 2,000 allergens have been identified as capable of producing an inflammatory skin response. Crude forms of many naturally occurring substances are in general less allergenic than alloys and synthetic products. Additives such as dyes and perfumes account for the major sources of known allergens. Some of the common topical agents causing allergic rashes are antimicrobial agents (especially neomycin), antihistamines, local anesthetic agents (benzocaine), preservatives (*e.g.*, parabens), and adhesive tape. Additional examples are poison ivy, poison oak, and metal alloys found in jewellery. Also of concern is the increased incidence of contact dermatitis from the heavy use of synthetic latex products, specifically latex gloves and condoms used to prevent communicable diseases. The top 10 causes of allergic contact dermatitis in order of frequency are nickel, gold (jewellery), balsam of Peru (perfume fragrance), thimerosal (preservative in cosmetics), neomycin sulphate, fragrance mix (eight fragrances used for testing fragrance allergies), formaldehyde (preservative in paper, paint, medications, fabrics), cobalt chloride (metal in medical products, hair dye, antiperspirants), bacitracin, and quaternium-15 (preservative in skin products similar to formaldehyde).[23]

The lesions of allergic contact dermatitis range from a mild erythema with edema to vesicles or large bullae (Fig. 61.17). Secondary lesions from bacterial infection may occur. Lesions can occur almost anywhere on the body and the many variations of eczema are often classified according to their location (*e.g.*, ear eczema, hand eczema). The location and pattern often help in identifying causative agents. For example, the typical poison ivy (or oak) lesion consists of vesicles or bullae in a linear pattern (from swiping the plant) on exposed areas. The vesicles and bullae break and weep, leaving an excoriated area.

Irritant contact dermatitis is caused by chemicals (soaps, detergents, organic solvents) that irritate the skin. It can occur from mechanical means such as rubbing (*e.g.*, wool, fibreglass), chemical irritants (*e.g.*, household cleaning products),

or environmental irritants (*e.g.*, plants, urine). In contrast to allergic contact dermatitis, no allergens can be identified. A history of atopic dermatitis, either in the past or concurrent, is a major risk for the development of irritant contact dermatitis. The spectrum of irritant contact dermatitis includes subjective, acute, and chronic cases. Subjective cases have no clinical manifestation, but the person reports burning or stinging sensations when exposed to the irritant, and the effect can be reproduced. Acute episodes are often due to single exposures to the irritant. There may be dryness and erythema or edema, inflammation, and vesicles. Chronic irritant dermatitis results from continued exposure to the irritant; even when the irritant is removed, the reaction may continue for several years. In addition to dryness and erythema, there may be scales, fissures, and vesicles.[24]

With both allergic and irritant contact dermatitis, the location of the lesions is of great benefit in diagnosing the causative agent. Patch testing, in which a small amount of the suspected antigen is applied to the skin, is used to identify the allergens.

Treatment measures for both types of contact dermatitis are aimed at removing the source of the irritant or allergen. This may mean that the person needs to modify his or her behaviour. This may be particularly difficult for the person with hand eczema because it may mean changing employment to avoid contact with the irritant or allergen. Minor cases are treated by washing the affected areas to remove further contamination by the irritant or allergen, applying antipruritic creams or lotions, and bandaging the exposed areas. Topical corticosteroids may be helpful in these cases. Systemic treatment regimens differ according to the type of irritant or allergen and the severity of the reaction. Moderate to extreme cases are treated with wet dressings, oral antihistamines, and systemic corticosteroids.

Atopic Dermatitis and Nummular Eczema

Atopic Dermatitis. Atopic dermatitis (atopic eczema) is an itchy, inflammatory skin disorder that is characterized by poorly defined erythema with edema, vesicles, and weeping at the acute stage and skin thickening (lichenification) in the chronic stage.[25–27] Although often described as an immunoglobulin E (IgE)-mediated hypersensitivity (atopic) disease, allergic causation is difficult to document, and the disorder is increasingly viewed as a skin disease that predisposes to allergies. Greater than 50% of children with atopic dermatitis develop asthma and allergies, typically by the third birthday, and this can persist into adolescence and adulthood.[25]

Atopic dermatitis presents differently at different ages (infantile and adult) and in people of different races. Approximately 70% of cases of atopic allergy start in children younger than 5 years of age.[26] The infantile form of atopic dermatitis is characterized by vesicle formation, oozing, and crusting with excoriations. It usually begins on the cheeks and may progress to involve the scalp, arms, trunk, and legs (Fig. 61.18). The skin of the cheeks may be paler, with extra creases under the eyes, called *Dennie–Morgan folds*. The infantile form may become milder as the child ages, often disappearing by the age of 15 years. However, many individuals have resultant eczematous disorders and rhinitis symptoms throughout life.

Adolescents and adults usually have dry, red patches affecting the face, neck, and upper trunk, but without the thickening and discrete demarcation associated with psoriasis. The bends of the elbows and knees are usually involved. In chronic cases, the skin is dry, leathery, and lichenified. Persons with dark skin may have a papular eruption, and poorly demarcated

FIGURE 61.18 • Atopic eczema on an infant's face and wrist. (Dome Chemicals.) (From Hall B. J., Hall J. C. (2010). *Sauer's manual of skin diseases* (10th ed., p. 85). Philadelphia, PA: Lippincott Williams & Wilkins.)

hypopigmentation patches on the cheeks and extremities. In persons with black skin, pigmentation may be lost from lichenified skin. Acute flares may present with red patches that are weepy, shiny, or lichenified (*i.e.*, thickened, with more prominent markings), and with plaques and papules. Itching may be severe and prolonged with both childhood and adult forms of atopic dermatitis. Secondary infections are common.

Treatment of atopic eczema is designed to target the underlying abnormalities: dryness, pruritus, infection, and inflammation. The guidelines derived consensually from and endorsed by North American and European expert teams include a stepwise approach for the management of atopic dermatitis based on the intensity of the disease process. Underlying all treatment measures is a comprehensive education program regarding the cause of the disorder, treatment measures, and avoidance of temperature changes and stress to minimize vascular and sweat responses. Basic therapy begins with optimal skin care, addressing the skin barrier defect with continuous use of emollients and skin hydration, along with avoiding exposure to environmental irritants and foods that cause exacerbation of the symptoms. Contact with water should be minimized; the person should bathe with warm (not hot) water and mild soap. For moderate to severe cases, adding a minute amount of bleach to the bathwater can decrease microbial activity on the skin surface, limiting secondary infections. Bathing dries the skin, yet it is important to maintain a low level of microorganisms to prevent infection. Although there is no evidence that emollients improve atopic dermatitis directly, they are widely used to relieve the problem of dry skin and pruritus. A key feature of atopic dermatitis is severe dryness of the skin caused by dysfunction of the skin barrier with transepidermal water loss. This is accompanied by intense pruritus and inflammation.[27]

Topical corticosteroids remain an important treatment for acute flare-ups but can cause local and systemic side effects. Potency of topical corticosteroids is classified by the potential for vasoconstriction. In general, only preparations that have weak or moderate potency are used on the face and genital areas, whereas those that have moderate or high potency are used on other areas of the body.[27] Lower-potency corticosteroids may be sufficient on all areas of the body in younger children. One of the main concerns of topical corticosteroid use is skin thinning. Another concern is secondary adrenal suppression and the suppression of growth in children resulting from systemic absorption.[27]

Topical immune modulators (*e.g.*, tacrolimus, pimecrolimus) are demonstrating positive outcomes in atopic dermatitis without the side effect of cortisone therapy (dermal atrophy).[27] Immune modulators are immunosuppressive agents that have been used systemically for the prevention of organ rejection. Tacrolimus is believed to control atopic dermatitis by inhibiting activation of cells involved in atopic dermatitis: T lymphocytes, dendritic cells, mast cells, and keratinocytes. In 2005, a warning was issued to healthcare professionals concerning a potential link between topical tacrolimus and pimecrolimus and cancer (mainly lymphoma and skin cancer) based on animal studies, case reports, and knowledge of how these drugs work. To date these drugs have demonstrated a good safety profile when used as recommended, but continued assessment is needed.[27]

Wet-wrap therapy, in which a wet dressing is applied over emollients in combination with topical antiseptics (*e.g.,* triclosan, chlorhexidine) or topical corticosteroids, has been shown to be beneficial in some cases of severe atopic dermatitis.[27] Secondary infection with *S. aureus* is common and usually treated with short courses of antibiotics.[27] Short-term corticosteroids are also used during acute flare-ups with adult patients. Cyclosporine and azathioprine, both immunosuppressive agents, may also be used, keeping in mind their potentially harmful effects.[28] Topical antihistamines may be used for short-term management of the pruritic components but are not recommended as first-line treatment due to potential systemic toxicity when the skin barrier is broken, and the risk of traumatic effects on local skin, with burning, stinging, or even allergic contact dermatitis resulting. Oral antihistamines are useful for their sedative effects, and may be helpful during severe pruritic episodes.[27] Phototherapy alone or in combination with corticosteroids during acute flares is often practised, with beneficial results.[28]

Less studied is the use of *probiotics,* foods containing live microorganisms, such as *Lactobacillus acidophilus* or *Bifidobacterium bifidum.* These foods include hydrolyzed cow's milk formula (predigested peptides of whey and casein), whey formulas, and yogurts. Probiotics are believed to reduce IgE-mediated reactions.[29]

Nummular Eczema. The lesions of nummular eczema are coin-shaped (hence its other name, *discoid eczema*), papulovesicular patches mainly involving the arms and legs (Fig. 61.19). Lichenification and secondary bacterial infections are common. It is not unusual for the initial lesions seemingly to heal, followed by a secondary outbreak of mirror-image lesions on the opposite side of the body. Nummular eczema is mostly chronic, with weeks to years between exacerbations. Exacerbations are more frequent in the cold winter months. The exact cause of nummular eczema is unknown, although many people have a history of atopy (allergy-related disorders), and there is heavy colonization of lesions with staphylococci. Ingestion of iodides and bromides usually aggravates the condition and should be avoided. Treatment is similar to that for other types of dermatitis. Frequent bathing and stress should be reduced, whereas environmental humidity should be increased. Topical emollients, corticosteroids, coal tar preparations, and UV light treatments may be prescribed as necessary.

Urticaria

Urticaria, or hives, is a common skin disorder characterized by the development of edematous wheals accompanied by intense itching.[30] The lesions typically appear as raised pink or red areas surrounded by a paler halo. They blanch with pressure and vary in size from a few millimetres to centimetres. Angioneuroedema, also referred to as *angioedema,* which can occur alone or with urticaria, is characterized by nonpitting, nonpruritic,

FIGURE 61.19 • Nummular eczema on the legs. (From Hall B. J., Hall J. C. (2010). *Sauer's manual of skin diseases* (10th ed., p. 92). Philadelphia, PA: Lippincott Williams & Wilkins.)

well-defined edematous swelling that involves subcutaneous tissues.[30] It may occur in face, hands, feet, groin, genitals, tongue, or upper airway. Although rare, it may result in airway obstruction. It has been associated with heredity causes, plus responses to drugs including nonsteroidal anti-inflammatory drugs and angiotensin-converting enzyme inhibitors.

Urticaria can be acute or chronic and due to known or unknown causes. Numerous factors, both immunologic and nonimmunologic, can be involved in its pathogenesis. The urticarial wheal results from liberation of histamine from mast cells and basophils. Histamine causes hyperpermeability of the microvessels of the skin and surrounding tissue, allowing fluid to leak into the tissues, causing edema and wheal formation.

Acute immunologic urticaria is commonly the result of an IgE-mediated immune reaction. Most attacks of acute urticaria are thought to be idiopathic (30% to 50%), but other triggers may include foods or drinks, medications (*e.g.,* penicillins), insect stings, viral infections, dust mites, and exposure to pollens or chemicals.[31] Although nonsteroidal anti-inflammatory drugs, including aspirin, do not normally cause urticaria, they may exacerbate the pre-existing disease.

Chronic urticaria affects primarily adults and is more common in women than in men. Usually its cause cannot be determined despite extensive laboratory tests.[30,32] It appears to be an autoimmune disorder in a substantial number of persons. Approximately 30% to 40% of persons with chronic urticaria have circulating IgG antibodies to a subunit of the IgE receptor or to the IgE molecule. These antibodies activate basophils and mast cells to release histamine.[32] In rare cases, urticaria

FIGURE 61.20 • Dermographism on flexor wrist. (From Hall B. J., Hall J. C. (2010). *Sauer's manual of skin diseases* (10th ed., p. 131). Philadelphia, PA: Lippincott Williams & Wilkins.)

is a manifestation of underlying disease, such as certain cancers, collagen diseases, and hepatitis. There is an association between chronic urticaria and autoimmune thyroid disease. Additionally, a hereditary deficiency of a C1 (complement 1) inhibitor also can cause urticaria and angioedema.[30,32]

The physical urticarias constitute another form of chronic urticaria.[38] Physical urticarias are intermittent, usually last less than 2 hours, are produced by appropriate stimuli, have distinctive appearances and locations, and are seen most frequently in young adults. Dermographism, or skin writing, is one form of physical urticaria in which wheals appear in response to simple rubbing of the skin (Fig. 61.20). The wheals follow the pattern of the scratch or rubbing, appearing within 10 minutes and dissolving completely within 20 minutes. Other types of physical urticaria are induced by exercise (cholinergic), cold, delayed pressure, sunlight (solar), water (aquagenic), vibration, and heat (external localized). Appropriate challenge tests (*e.g.,* application of an ice cube to the skin to initiate development of cold urticaria) are used to differentiate physical urticaria from chronic urticaria due to other causes.[30,33]

Most types of urticaria are treated with antihistamines: drugs that block histamine type 1 (H_1) receptors and, less frequently, H_1 receptor blockers in combination with H_2 receptor blockers.[30–33] They control urticaria by inhibiting vasodilation and the escape of fluid into the surrounding tissues. Usually nonsedating antihistamines that alleviate pruritus and decrease the incidence of hives, without producing drowsiness, are used. Leukotriene antagonists (zafirlukast and montelukast) may also be used.[30] Starch or colloid-type (*e.g.,* Aveeno) baths may be used as comfort measures. Persons who experience angioedema of the larynx and pharynx can be counselled to carry a prescription of epinephrine in an autoinjectable instrument (*e.g.,* EpiPen). Oral corticosteroids may be used in the treatment of refractory urticaria.[30]

Drug-Induced Skin Eruptions

Most drugs can cause a localized or generalized skin eruption. Topical drugs are usually responsible for localized contact dermatitis types of rashes, whereas systemic drugs cause generalized skin lesions. Although many drug-induced skin eruptions are morbilliform (*i.e.,* measles-like) or exanthematous, they may mimic most of the skin disorders described in this chapter. Because the lesions vary greatly, the diagnosis depends almost entirely on an accurate patient report, including a full drug history. Management of mild cases is aimed at eliminating the offending drug while treating the symptoms. Severe cases require prompt medical attention and treatment with systemic corticosteroids and antihistamines.

Some drug reactions result in epidermal skin detachment and formation of bullous lesions. Three types of drug reactions that result in bullous skin lesions are *erythema multiforme minor, Stevens–Johnson syndrome,* and *toxic epidermal necrolysis.* Erythema multiforme minor is usually self-limiting. Cases involving less than 10% of the body surface area are called *Stevens–Johnson syndrome,* and detachment of more than 30% of the epidermis is labelled *toxic epidermal necrolysis,* with a 10% to 30% overlap of Stevens–Johnson syndrome and toxic epidermal necrolysis.[34]

Although the cause of erythema multiforme minor may be drug induced or unknown, it frequently occurs after infections, especially HSV infection. It is self-limiting, with a small amount of skin detachment at the lesion sites. Stevens–Johnson syndrome and toxic epidermal necrolysis are caused by hypersensitivity reaction to drugs, the most common being sulfonamides, anticonvulsants, nonsteroidal anti-inflammatory drugs, antimalarials, and allopurinol. Although rare, Stevens–Johnson syndrome and toxic epidermal necrolysis have an annual incidence of 0.4 to 7 per 1 million people and a high mortality rate.[35] Recovery is based on the severity and on quick, aggressive treatment.

The skin detachment seen with bullous skin lesions is different from the desquamation (*i.e.,* peeling) that occurs with other skin disorders. For example, with scarlet fever there is peeling of the dead keratinized layer of the stratum corneum. In the bullous disorders, there is full-thickness detachment of the entire epidermis from the dermis. This leaves the person vulnerable to multiple problems, including loss of body fluids and electrolytes, impaired body temperature control, and a greatly increased risk of infection.

The lesions of erythema multiforme minor and Stevens–Johnson syndrome are similar. The primary lesion of both is a round, erythematous papule, resembling an insect bite. Within hours to days, these lesions change into several different patterns. The individual lesions may enlarge and coalesce, producing small plaques, or they may change to concentric zones of colour appearing as "target" or "iris" lesions (Fig. 61.21). The outermost rings of the target lesions usually are erythematous; the central portion usually is opaque white, yellow, or grey (dusky). In the centre, small blisters on the dusky purpuric macules may form, giving them their characteristic target-like appearance. Although there is wide distribution of lesions over the body surface area, there is a propensity for them to occur on the face and trunk.

Toxic epidermal necrolysis is the most serious drug reaction, with mortality rates of 30% to 50%.[35] The person

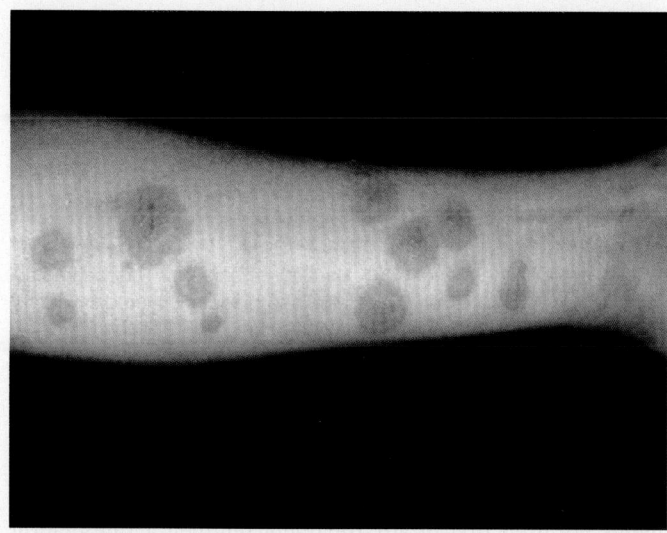

FIGURE 61.21 • Erythema-multiforme–like eruption on the patient's arm. Note the dusky, target-like appearance. (Dermik Laboratories, Inc.) (From Hall B. J., Hall J. C. (2010). *Sauer's manual of skin diseases* (10th ed., p. 133). Philadelphia, PA: Lippincott Williams & Wilkins.)

experiences a prodromal period of malaise, low-grade fever, and sore throat. Within a few days, widespread erythema and large, flaccid bullae appear, followed by the loss of the epidermis, leaving a denuded and painful dermis. The skin surrounding the large denuded areas may have the typical target-like lesions seen with Stevens–Johnson syndrome. Lateral pressure causes the surrounding skin to separate easily from the dermis (*Nikolsky sign*). Usually, the epithelium of mucosal surfaces, especially the mouth and eyes, is also involved and may lead to blindness.

Treatment of erythema multiforme minor and less severe cases of Stevens–Johnson syndrome includes relief of symptoms using compresses, antipruritic drugs, and topical anesthetics. Recurrent cases of erythema multiforme have been prevented with continuous acyclovir therapy. Corticosteroid therapy may be indicated in moderate cases, although its use is controversial. For severe cases of Stevens–Johnson syndrome and toxic epidermal necrolysis, hospitalization is required for fluid replacement, respiratory care, administration of antibiotics and analgesics, and application of moist dressings. When large areas of skin are detached, the care is similar to that of thermal burn patients. Intravenous immunoglobulin may hasten the healing response of the skin. Generally, healing is a slow process, taking 6 weeks or more to regenerate skin.[34,35] The mucous membranes heal slowly and follow-up treatment is often needed for ophthalmologic and mucous membrane sequelae. Avoidance of the responsible drug and chemically related compounds is essential.

Papulosquamous Dermatoses

Papulosquamous dermatoses are a group of skin disorders characterized by scaling papules and plaques. Among the major papulosquamous diseases are psoriasis, pityriasis rosea,

and lichen planus, which are discussed in this section of the chapter.

Psoriasis

Psoriasis is a common, chronic inflammatory skin disease characterized by circumscribed, red, thickened plaques with an overlying silvery-white scale. Psoriasis occurs worldwide, although the incidence is lower in warmer, sunnier climates. In Canada, the United States, and England, it affects 1% to 2.6% of the population.[36] The onset of the disease can occur at any age, but two peaks of onset are noted: an early peak between 16 and 22 years and a later one at 57 to 60 years.[1,2,36] Evidence supports an important genetic component. The early onset of the disease is more strongly associated with a family history than psoriasis occurring in adults older than 30 years of age. The disease, which can persist throughout life and become exacerbated at unpredictable times, is classified as a chronic ailment. A few cases, however, have been known to clear and not recur. There appears to be an association between psoriasis and arthritis as many as one third of patients with psoriasis develop arthritis. Psoriatic arthritis can account for a considerable amount of joint damage[36] (see Chapter 59).

The primary cause of psoriasis is uncertain. The unintended, yet dramatic, clearing of severe, disabling psoriasis with cyclosporine provides strong evidence that psoriasis has a T-cell–mediated autoimmune response to an unidentified antigen.[1,36] It is thought that activated T lymphocytes (T-helper cells—T_h1 and T_h17) produce chemical messengers that stimulate abnormal growth of keratinocytes and dermal blood vessels. Accompanying inflammatory changes are caused by infiltration of neutrophils and monocytes. Skin trauma (*i.e.,* prepsoriasis) is a common precipitating factor in people predisposed to the disease. The reaction of the skin to an original trauma of any type is called the *Köbner reaction*. Stress, infections, trauma, cigarette smoking, xerosis, and use of medications such as angiotensin-converting enzyme inhibitors, beta-adrenergic blocking drugs, lithium, and the antimalarial agent hydroxychloroquine (Plaquenil), may precipitate or exacerbate the condition.

Histologically, psoriasis is characterized by increased epidermal cell turnover with marked epidermal thickening, a process called *hyperkeratosis*. The granular layer (stratum granulosum) of the epidermis is thinned or absent, and neutrophils are found in the stratum corneum. There also is an accompanying thinning of the epidermal cell layer that overlies the tips of the dermal papillae (suprapapillary plate), and the blood vessels in the dermal papillae become tortuous and dilated. These capillary beds show permanent damage even when the disease is in remission or resolved. The close proximity of the vessels in the dermal papillae to the hyperkeratotic scale accounts for multiple, minute bleeding points that are seen when the scale is lifted.

There are several variants or types of psoriasis, including plaque-type psoriasis, guttate psoriasis, pustular psoriasis (localized and generalized), and erythrodermic psoriasis.[44] *Plaque-type psoriasis (psoriasis vulgaris)*, which is the most

FIGURE 61.22 • Psoriasis. This characterized by well-defined plaques covered by silvery scales. (From Stephen T. C., Skillen D. L., Day R. A., et al. (2012). *Canadian Jensen's nursing health assessment: A best practice approach* (p. 303, 896). Philadelphia, PA: Lippincott Williams & Wilkins.)

common type, accounting for approximately 90% of patients, is a chronic stationary form of psoriasis.[36] The lesions may occur anywhere on the skin, but most often involve the elbows, knees, and scalp (Fig. 61.22). The primary lesions are sharply demarcated, thick, red plaques with a silvery scale that vary in size and shape. In darker-skinned persons, the plaques may appear purple. There may be excoriation, thickening, or oozing from the lesions. A differential diagnostic finding is that the plaques bleed from minute points when removed, which is known as the *Auspitz sign.*

Guttate psoriasis is characterized by teardrop-shaped, pink to salmon-coloured scaly lesions, and occurs in children and young adults. Its lesions are usually limited to the upper trunk and extremities. This form of psoriasis usually is brought on by a streptococcal infection. It generally responds to treatments such as UVB phototherapy, only to return with recurrent streptococcal infections.

Pustular psoriasis is characterized by papules or plaques studded with pustules. Localized pustular psoriasis usually is limited to the palms of the hands and soles of the feet. Generalized pustular psoriasis is characterized by more general involvement and may be associated with systemic symptoms such as fever, malaise, and diarrhea. The person may or may not have had pre-existing psoriasis.

Erythrodermic psoriasis is a rare form of psoriasis affecting all body surfaces, including the hands, feet, nails, trunk, and extremities. It is characterized by a process in which the lesions scale and become confluent, leaving much of the body surface bright red, with continuous skin shedding. Severe itching and pain often accompany it. Severe complications may develop related to loss of body fluids, proteins, and electrolytes and disturbances in temperature regulation. Without treatment, death from sepsis is a well-known complication of erythrodermic psoriasis.[36]

Treatment. There is no cure for psoriasis. The goal of treatment is to suppress the signs and symptoms of the disease: hyperkeratosis, epidermal inflammation, and abnormal keratinocyte differentiation. Treatment depends on the severity of the disease, as well as the person's age, sex, treatment history, and level of treatment compliance. Treatment measures are divided into topical and systemic approaches. Usually, topical agents are used first in any treatment regimen. Combination therapies tailored to the needs of the client are most effective. Also, rotating various therapies may decrease the side effects of any one therapy.

Topical agents include emollients, keratolytic agents, coal tar products, anthralin, corticosteroids, and calcipotriene.[36] Emollients hydrate and soften the psoriatic plaques. Petroleum-based products are more effective than water-based, but they are often less acceptable cosmetically to persons with psoriasis. Keratolytic agents are peeling agents. Salicylic acid is the most widely used. It softens and removes plaques. It has been used alone or in conjunction with other topical agents. Coal tar, the by-product of the processing of coke and gas from coal, is one of the oldest yet most effective forms of treatment. The skin is covered with a film of coal tar for up to several weeks. The exact mechanism of action of tar products is unknown, but side effects of the treatment are few.

Anthralin, a synthesized product of Goa powder from Brazilian araroba tree bark, has remained a topical treatment of choice. It has been effective in resolving lesions in approximately 2 weeks. A disadvantage to anthralin is that it stains the uninvolved skin and clothes brown or purple. A treatment variation, called the *Ingram method,* involves coal tar applications and UVB radiation, followed by anthralin paste application.

Topical corticosteroids are widely used and relatively effective. They are generally more acceptable because they do not stain and are easy to use. Topical corticosteroids are available as low-, medium-, and high-potency preparations. Treatment usually is started with a medium-potency agent. Low-potency drugs usually are used on the face and areas of the body, such as the groin and axillary areas, where the skin tends to be thinner. High-potency preparations are reserved for treatment of thick chronic plaques that do not respond to less potent preparations. Although the corticosteroids are rapidly effective in the treatment of psoriasis, they are associated with flare-ups after discontinuation and they have many potential side effects. Their effectiveness is increased when used under occlusive dressings, but there is an increase in side effects. *Calcipotriene,* a topical vitamin D derivative, has been effective for the treatment of psoriasis. It inhibits epidermal cell proliferation and enhances cell differentiation. *Tazarotene,* a synthetic retinoid, also has been effective, but it is teratogenic and should be avoided in women of childbearing age.

Systemic treatments include phototherapy, photochemotherapy, methotrexate, retinoids, corticosteroids, and cyclosporine. The positive effects of sunlight have long been established. Phototherapy with UVB is a widely used treatment, with the narrow-band UVB radiation reportedly more effective than broad-band UVB.[36] Photochemotherapy involves using a light-activated form of the drug methoxsalen. Methoxsalen, a psoralen, exerts its actions when exposed to UVA radiation in 320- to 400-nm wavelengths. The combination treatment regimen of psoralen and UVA is known by the acronym *PUVA*. Methoxsalen is given orally before UVA exposure. Activated by the UVA energy, methoxsalen inhibits DNA synthesis, thereby preventing cell mitosis and decreasing the hyperkeratosis that occurs with psoriasis. Although viewed as one of the safest therapies since its introduction in the 1970s, PUVA increases the risk for squamous cell carcinoma, and it may increase the risk for development of melanoma.

Systemic corticosteroids have been effective in treating severe or pustular psoriasis. However, they cause severe side effects, including Cushing syndrome. Intralesional injection of triamcinolone has proved effective in resistant lesions. The retinoids are another class of systemic psoriasis therapy. These drugs, which are derivatives of vitamin A, are only moderately effective as a monotherapy and are associated with numerous mucocutaneous side effects such as hair loss, cheilitis, and thinning of the nails. However, when used over the short term in combination with UVB phototherapy or PUVA, low-dose acitretin has been shown to be effective, allowing substantial clearing of lesions with fewer physician visits and fewer mucocutaneous side effects.[36] Teratogenicity limits use of retinoids in women of childbearing potential.

Methotrexate, which is used for cancer treatment, is an antimetabolite that inhibits DNA synthesis and prevents cell mitosis. Oral methotrexate has been effective in treating psoriasis when other approaches have failed. The drug has many side effects, including nausea, malaise, leukopenia, thrombocytopenia, and liver function abnormalities. Cyclosporine is a potent immunosuppressive drug used to prevent rejection of organ transplants. It suppresses inflammation and the proliferation of T cells in persons with psoriasis. Its use is limited to severe psoriasis because of serious side effects, including nephrotoxicity, hypertension, and increased risk of cancers. Intralesional cyclosporine also has been effective. Biologic agents that target the activity of: T lymphocytes on the cell surface (*e.g.,* alefacept); cytokines such as TNFα (*e.g.,* adalimumab, etanercept, infliximab); or specific interleukins (*e.g.,* ustekinumab), are effective in modifying and limiting the inflammatory nature of psoriasis, not only with the skin lesions, but in halting the effects of the associated arthritis of psoriasis.[36]

Pityriasis Rosea

Pityriasis rosea is a rash that primarily affects children and young adults. The origin of the rash is unknown, but is thought

FIGURE 61.23 • Pityriasis rosea. Note oval herald patch (*arrow*) on the abdomen as well as a more generalized rash. (Centers for Disease Control and Prevention Public Health Image Library. Available online at: http://phil.cdc.gov/Phil/home.asp)

to be caused by an infective agent. Numerous viruses have been investigated, thus far with no conclusive evidence. Cases occur in clusters and among persons who are in close contact, indicating an infectious spread. However, there are no data to support communicability. It may be an immune response to any number of agents.

The characteristic lesion is an oval macule or papule with surrounding erythema (Fig. 61.23). The lesion spreads with central clearing, much like tinea corporis. This initial lesion is a solitary lesion called the *herald patch* and is usually on the trunk or neck. As the lesion enlarges and begins to fade (2 to 10 days), successive crops of lesions appear on the trunk and neck. The lesions on the back have a characteristic "Christmas tree" pattern. The extremities, face, and scalp may be involved. Mild to severe pruritus may occur. The disease is self-limited and usually disappears within 6 to 8 weeks. Treatment measures are palliative and include topical steroids, antihistamines, and colloid baths. Systemic corticosteroids may be indicated in severe cases.[2]

Lichen Planus

Lichen planus is a skin disorder characterized by small (2 to 10 mm), flat-topped papules with irregular, angulated borders (Fig. 61.24). Lichen planus is a relatively common chronic pruritic disease. It involves inflammation and papular eruption of the skin and mucous membranes. There are variations in the pattern of lesions (*e.g.,* annular, linear) and differences in the sites (*e.g.,* mucous membranes, genitalia, nails, scalp). The characteristic lesion is a purple, polygonal papule covered with a shiny, white, lace-like pattern. The lesions appear on the wrist, ankles, and trunk of the body. Most persons who have skin lesions also have oral lesions, appearing as milky white lacework on the buccal mucosa or tongue. Other mucosal surfaces, such as the genital, nasal, laryngeal, otic, gastric, and anal areas may also be affected. As with psoriasis, lichen planus lesions can develop on scratches or skin injuries (Köbner phenomenon; see Fig. 61.24A).

FIGURE 61.24 • **A:** Lichen planus of the dorsum of the hand. Note the colour of the plaques and the linear Köbner phenomenon. (E.R. Squibb.) (From Hall B. J., Hall J. C. (2010). *Sauer's manual of skin diseases* (10th ed., p. 169). Philadelphia, PA: Lippincott Williams & Wilkins.) **B:** Lichen planus affecting both wrists. (Centers for Disease Control and Prevention Public Health Image Library. Available online at: http://phil.cdc.gov/Phil/home.asp.)

The etiology of lichen planus is unknown, but it is believed to be an abnormal immune response in which epithelial cells are recognized as foreign. The disorder involves the epidermal–dermal junction with damage to the basal cell layer. Some cases of lichen planus have been linked to hepatitis C virus infections or medication use.

Diagnosis is based on the clinical appearance of the lesions and the histopathologic findings from a punch biopsy. For most persons, lichen planus is a self-limited disease. Treatment measures include a review of all medications, followed by treatment with topical corticosteroids and occlusive dressings. Occlusion may be used to enhance the effect of topical medications. Antipruritic agents are helpful in reducing itch. Systemic corticosteroids may be indicated in severe cases. Intralesional corticosteroid injections also may be used. Topical or systemic retinoid agents also may be effective. Because retinoids are teratogenic, they should be avoided in women of childbearing age. Cyclosporine, tacrolimus, other immunosuppressive agents, and phototherapy have been helpful.[2,37]

Lichen Simplex Chronicus

Lichen simplex chronicus is a localized lichenoid pruritic dermatitis resulting from repeated rubbing and scratching. The term *lichen simplex* denotes the absence of a known predisposing skin disorder in the affected person. It is characterized by the occurrence of itchy, reddened, thickened, and scaly patches of dry skin (Fig. 61.25). Persons with the condition may have a single or, less frequently, multiple lesions. The lesions are seen most commonly at the nape of the neck, wrists, ankles, or anal area. The condition usually begins as a

FIGURE 61.25 • Localized lichen simplex chronicus of the leg. (Duke Laboratories, Inc.) (From Hall B. J., Hall J. C. (2010). *Sauer's manual of skin diseases* (10th ed., p. 126). Philadelphia, PA: Lippincott Williams & Wilkins.)

small pruritic patch, which after a repetitive cycle of itching and scratching develops into a chronic dermatosis. Because of the chronic itching and scratching, excoriations and lichenification with thickening of the skin develops, often giving the appearance of tree bark. Treatment consists of measures to decrease scratching of the area. A moderate-potency corticosteroid is often prescribed to decrease the itching and subsequent inflammatory process.

Arthropod Infestations

The skin is susceptible to a variety of disorders as a result of an invasion or infestation by arthropods, including mites and lice. The type of rash or sometimes singular lesion depends on the causative agent.

Scabies

A mite, *S. scabiei,* which burrows into the epidermis, causes scabies. After a female mite is impregnated, she burrows into the skin and lays two to three eggs each day for 4 or 5 weeks. The eggs hatch after 2 to 3 days, and the larvae migrate to the skin surface. At this point, they burrow into the skin only for food or protection. The larvae moult and become nymphs; they moult once more to become adults. After the new adult females are impregnated, the cycle is repeated.[38]

The characteristic lesion is a small burrow (*e.g.*, 2 mm) that may be red to reddish-brown. Small vesicles may cover the burrows. The areas most commonly affected are the interdigital web of the finger, flexor surface of the wrist, inner surface of the elbow, axilla, female nipple, penis, belt line, and gluteal crease (Fig. 61.26). Pruritus is common and may result from the burrows, the fecal material of the mite, or both. Excoriations may develop from scratching, leaving the host vulnerable to secondary bacterial infections and severe skin lesions if left untreated. In immunocompromised patients, a severe form of scabies that involves millions of mites is called *Norwegian* or *crusted scabies;* it differs from common scabies in the large number of mites living on the host and a crusting over of the infested region.[2,38]

Scabies is transmitted by person-to-person contact, including sexual contact. It also is transmitted by contact with mite-infested sheets in hospitals and nursing homes because the mite can live up to 2 days on sheets or clothing.

Diagnosis is done by skin scrapings. A positive diagnosis relies on the presence of mites, ova, or feces. The treatment is simple and curative. After bathing, permethrin, pyrethrins, or other effective mite-killing agents are applied over the entire skin surface for 12 hours. Repeated applications may be recommended in certain cases, but one treatment usually is sufficient. Care must be taken to ensure that close contacts are treated. Clothes and towels are disinfected with hot water and detergent, or they can be isolated for 2 weeks. If symptoms persist after treatment, the patient should be advised not to retreat the condition without consulting a healthcare provider. Oral ivermectin, a broad-spectrum antiparasitic agent, has been used for treatment-resistant scabies.[2,38]

FIGURE 61.26 • (**A**) Pimple-like irritations, burrows, and rash of the skin due to infestation with (**B**) *Sarcoptes scabiei* var. *hominis*, or "itch mite." (Centers for Disease Control and Prevention Public Health Image Library. Available online at: http://phil.cdc.gov/Phil/home.asp)

Pediculosis

Pediculosis is the term for infestation with lice (genus *Pediculus*). Lice are grey, grey-brown, or red-brown, oval, wingless insects that live off the blood of humans and animals (Fig. 61.27A). Lice are host-specific; lice that live on animals do not transfer to humans, and vice versa. Lice also are host-dependent; they cannot live apart from the host beyond a few hours.

Three types of lice affect humans: *Pediculus humanus corporis* (body lice), *Phthirus pubis* (pubic lice), and *Pediculus humanus capitis* (head lice). Although these three types differ biologically, they have similar life cycles. The life cycle of a louse consists of a "nit" or unhatched egg (Fig. 61.27B), three moult stages, an adult reproductive stage, and death. Before adulthood, lice live off the host and are incapable of reproduction. After fertilization, the female louse lays her eggs along hair shafts. The nits appear pearl-grey to brown. Depending on the site, a female louse can lay between 150 and 300 nits in her life. The life span of a feeding louse is 30 to 50 days. Lice are equipped with stylets that pierce the skin. Their saliva contains an anticoagulant that prevents the host's blood from clotting while the louse is feeding. A louse takes up to 1 ml of blood during a feeding.

FIGURE 61.27 • A: Female body louse, *Pediculus humanus corporis,* as it is obtaining a blood meal from a human host. **B:** Unhatched nit of the head louse, *Pediculus humanus capitis,* attached to a human hair. **C:** Pediculosis capitis (head lice) infestation. Unhatched nits are visible on hair shafts. (From Stephen T. C., Skillen D. L., Day R. A., et al. (2012). *Canadian Jensen's nursing health assessment: A best practice approach* (p. 894). Philadelphia, PA: Lippincott Williams & Wilkins.)

Pediculosis Corporis. Pediculosis corporis is infestation with *P. humanus corporis,* or body lice. The lice are transferred chiefly through contact with an infested person, clothing, or bedding. The lice live in clothes fibres, coming out only to feed, usually at night, causing nocturnal pruritus. Unlike pubic and head lice, the body louse can survive 10 to 14 days without the host.

The typical lesion is a macule at the site of the bite. Papules and wheals may develop. The infestation is pruritic and evokes scratching that brings about a characteristic linear excoriation. Eczematous patches are found frequently. Secondary lesions may become scaly and hyperpigmented and leave scars. Areas typically affected are the shoulders, trunk, and buttocks. The presence of nits in the seams of clothes confirms a diagnosis of body lice.

Treatment measures consist of eradicating the louse and nits on the body and on clothing. Dry-cleaning, washing in hot water, or steam pressing clothes are recommended methods. Special attention is given to the seams. Merely storing clothing in plastic bags for 2 weeks also rids clothes of lice. Many healthcare providers prefer not to treat the body unless nits are in evidence on hair shafts. If treatment is indicated, shampoos or topical preparations containing pyrethrins or other pediculicides are recommended. Care must be taken to ensure that close contacts are treated.

Pediculosis Pubis. Pediculosis pubis, the infestation known as crabs or pubic lice, is a nuisance disease that is spread by intimate contact with someone harbouring *P. pubis.* The lice and nits are usually found in the pubic area of men and women, where their bites produce itching and erythematous lesions (Fig. 61.27C). Occasionally, they may be found in sites of secondary sex characteristics, such as the beard in men or the axillae in both sexes. Symptoms include intense itching and irritation of the skin. Diagnosis is made on the basis of symptoms and microscopic examination. The treatment is the same as for head lice.

Pediculosis Capitis. Pediculosis capitis, or infestation with head lice, primarily affects white-skinned persons; it is relatively unknown in darker-skinned persons. The incidence is higher among girls, although hair length has not been indicated as a contributing factor. Infestations of head lice usually are confined to the nape of the neck and behind the ears. Less frequently, head lice are found on the beard, pubic areas, eyebrows, and body hairs. Although head lice can be transmitted by sharing combs and hats, they usually are spread from hair shaft to hair shaft through close personal contact. A positive diagnosis depends on the presence of firmly attached nits or live adult lice on hair shafts. Pruritus and scratching of the head are the primary indicators that head lice may be present. The scalp may appear red and excoriated from scratching. In severe cases, the hair becomes matted together in a crusty, foul-smelling "cap." An occasional morbilliform rash, which may be misdiagnosed as rubella, may occur with lymphadenopathy.

Head lice are treated with permethrin or pyrethrins shampoos or rinses. Repeated treatments may be needed to eliminate the hatching nits. Dead nits may be removed with a fine-toothed comb or over-the-counter nit removal hair rinses. Over the years, permethrin- and pyrethrin-resistant lice have evolved.

The "no-nit" policies that had been adopted over the past several years have been rescinded. The Canadian Paediatric

Society, the American Academy of Pediatrics and the Public Health Medicine Environmental Group in the United Kingdom all recommend not excluding children from school because of residual nits. The primary goal is to control outbreaks and infestations; interventions beyond this are out of proportion to the medical significance of lice.[39]

Bed Bugs

The common *bed bug,* or *Cimex lectularius,* is a parasitic insect that prefers to feed on human blood. These bugs are generally nocturnal and are attracted to carbon dioxide and warmth. They are visible as a tiny reddish-brown, flattened, oval-shaped insect and can usually be found in cracks and crevices in mattresses, furniture, or even walls.[2,40]

As the bed bug feeds, the insect injects saliva that contains various protein fractions to promote anticoagulation and provide an anesthetic property. While some people will not react to the saliva, others may get an intense allergic response. For most individuals the bite reaction occurs within 1 to 9 days as papular urticaria that is seen on exposed skin, often in clusters of three to five bites that may be in a linear or zigzag pattern. Individuals often see some oozing at the bite site or small flecks of blood on bed sheets. Typically these skin lesions will last 4 to 6 weeks after the infestation is eliminated.[2,40]

Treatment is symptomatic with oral or topical antihistamines or topical corticosteroids to control the itch. In severe cases, systemic corticosteroids may be required. All affected furniture should be removed and fumigated.[40]

IN SUMMARY

Primary disorders of the skin include pigmentary skin disorders, infectious processes, inflammatory conditions, immune disorders, allergic reactions, and arthropod infestations. Pigmentary skin disorders include vitiligo, albinism, and melasma. Although the causes of the disorders vary, all involve changes in the amount of melanin produced by the melanocytes. These disorders appear in people of every skin type; however, the manifestations of the disorders vary among light-skinned and dark-skinned persons.

Superficial fungal infections are called dermatophytoses and are commonly known as tinea or ringworm. Tinea can affect the whole body (tinea corporis), face and neck (tinea faciale), scalp (tinea capitis), hands (tinea manus), feet (tinea pedis), or nails (tinea unguium). The deep fungal infections invade the skin more deeply and go into living tissue, and are also capable of involving other organs. Impetigo, which is caused by staphylococci or beta-hemolytic streptococci, is the most common superficial bacterial infection. Viruses are responsible for verrucae (warts), herpes simplex type 1 lesions (cold sores or fever blisters), and herpes zoster (shingles).

Noninfectious inflammatory skin conditions, such as acne, lichen planus, psoriasis, and pityriasis rosea, are of unknown origin. They usually are localized to the skin and are rarely associated with a specific internal disease.

Allergic skin responses involve the body's immune system and are caused by hypersensitivity reactions to allergens such as environmental agents, drugs, and other substances. They include contact dermatitis, atopic dermatitis, and drug-induced skin eruptions (erythema multiforme, Stevens–Johnson syndrome, and toxic epidermal necrolysis).

The skin is also subject to invasion or infestation by a number of arthropod species, including scabies, which is caused by a mite (*S. scabiei*), pediculosis, which is caused by lice, and bed bugs (*C. lectularius*).

ULTRAVIOLET RADIATION, THERMAL, AND PRESSURE INJURY

After completing this section of the chapter, you should be able to meet the following objectives:

- Describe the three types of ultraviolet radiation and relate them to sunburn, aging skin changes, and the development of skin cancer.
- Describe the manifestations, treatment, and prevention of sunburn.
- Compare the tissue involvement in first-degree, second-degree full thickness, and third-degree burns.
- Review the methods to determine body surface area involved in a burn and burn severity classifications.
- Describe the systemic complications of burns.
- Describe the major considerations in treatment of burn injury.
- Cite two causes of pressure ulcers.
- Explain how shearing forces contribute to ischemic skin damage.
- List four measures that contribute to the prevention of pressure ulcers.

Skin Damage Caused by Ultraviolet Radiation

The skin is the protective shield against harmful UV rays from the sun. Skin cancers and other skin disorders such as early wrinkling and aging of the skin have been attributed to the damaging effects of sunlight.

Sunlight is measured in wavelengths of nanometres (nm; one billionth of a metre) ranging from approximately 290 nm in the UV region up to approximately 2,500 nm in the infrared region. UV radiation (UVR) is divided into three types: UVC, UVB, and UVA. UVC rays are short (100 to 290 nm) and do not pass through Earth's atmosphere. However, they can be produced artificially and are damaging to the eyes. UVB rays are 290 to 320 nm. Commonly referred to as *sunburn rays,* they are responsible for nearly all the skin effects of sunlight, including *photoaging*—the wrinkles, pigmentary changes, dryness, and loss of skin tone that occur with and are enhanced by exposure to sunlight. UVA rays are 320 to 400 nm, and can pass through window glass. They are further divided into UVA2 (320 to 339 nm) and UVA1 (340 to 400 nm) because the effects of UVA2 are now believed to be similar to UVB rays.[2,41] In general, it takes approximately 1,000 times more UVA to match the untoward effects of UVB. Nonetheless, UVA, particularly UVA2, contributes greatly to skin alterations. Artificial sources of UVA, such as tanning salons and therapeutic solar interventions (PUVA) for certain skin conditions, also produce the same effects as UVB radiation.

ULTRAVIOLET RADIATION, THERMAL, AND PRESSURE INJURY

- Because the skin covers the body, it is exposed to a number of potentially damaging agents in the external environment.
- The ultraviolet rays of sunlight have the potential for directly damaging skin cells, accelerating the effect of aging on the skin, and predisposing to the development of skin cancer.
- Prolonged pressure can interrupt blood flow, causing pressure ulcers.
- Thermal injury can damage skin and subcutaneous tissue and destroy the barrier function of the skin in terms of preventing the loss of body fluids and protecting against the entry of infectious organisms.

The acute effects of UVA and UVB are short-lived and reversible. They include erythema, pigmentation, and injury to Langerhans cells and keratinocytes in the epidermis. These reactions differ depending on whether the inciting agent is UVA or UVB. For example, UVA-induced erythema occurs immediately, fades within 2 hours, and is believed to be due to the "heat load." UVB-induced erythema has a delayed response, peaking within 6 to 24 hours after exposure to sunlight and fading over 1 or 2 days. Pigmentation or tanning induced by UVA and UVB is due to a delayed increase in the number of melanocytes, elongation and extension of the dendritic processes, and transfer of melanin to keratinocytes (see Chapter 60, Fig. 60.3). For tanning to occur, there must be UVB-induced erythema. Small doses of UVA produce oxidation of melanin with transient, immediate darkening of the skin that fades within 2 hours, whereas higher doses of UVA can produce pigmentary changes lasting for several hours to days.[41] Tanning induced by UVB is protective against subsequent exposures, whereas tanning induced by UVA provides limited protection.

Skin damage induced by UVB is believed to be caused by the generation of reactive oxygen species and by damage to melanin. Cellular proteins and DNA are primarily damaged because of their abundance and ability to absorb UVR. Both UVA and UVB also deplete Langerhans cells and immune cells. It is believed that these effects prevent immune cells

from detecting and removing sun-damaged cells with malignant potential. Both UVA and UVB are now considered causes of cancer. UVA may actually be more carcinogenic than UVB. Although it causes less sunburn, UVA is present during all daylight hours, year-round. UVB, on the other hand, varies by season, location, and time of day. UVA penetrates deeply and causes greater damage in the keratinocytes, where most skin cancers arise.

Drug-Induced Photosensitivity

Some drugs are classified as photosensitive drugs because they produce an exaggerated response to UVR when the drug is taken in combination with sun exposure. Examples include some of the anti-infective agents (sulfonamides, tetracyclines, nalidixic acid), antihistamines (cyproheptadine, diphenhydramine), antipsychotic agents (phenothiazines, haloperidol), diuretics (thiazides, acetazolamide, amiloride), hypoglycemic agents (sulfonylureas), and nonsteroidal anti-inflammatory drugs (phenylbutazone, ketoprofen, naproxen).

Drug-induced photosensitivity, such as UVA photosensitivity induced by the psoralens, may be used in treating skin conditions, such as psoriasis, that respond well to UVR exposure. Because an increased incidence of cancerous lesions has been reported in people who have been treated with these agents, their use requires caution and careful surveillance.

Sunburn

Sunburn is caused by excessive exposure of the epidermal and dermal layers of the skin to UVR, resulting in an erythematous inflammatory reaction. Sunburn ranges from mild to severe. Mild sunburn consists of various degrees of skin redness. The burn continues to develop for 1 to 3 days, occasionally followed by peeling skin in 3 to 8 days. Some peeling and itching may continue for several weeks. Inflammation, blistering, weakness, chills, fever, malaise, and pain often accompany severe forms of sunburn. Scaling and peeling follow any overexposure to sunlight. Dark skin also burns and may appear greyish or grey-black. Severe sunburns are those that cover large portions of the body with blisters or are accompanied by a high fever or intense pain.

Mild to moderate sunburns are treated with anti-inflammatory medications, such as aspirin or ibuprofen, until redness and pain subside. Cold compresses or cool baths, and application of a moisturizing cream, such as aloe, to affected skin help treat the symptoms. Steroid and nonsteroidal agents are used depending on the severity of the burn.[1,2] Blisters should not be broken to preserve the protective layer of the skin, hasten the healing process, and decrease the risk of infection. Extensive second- and third-degree burns may require hospitalization and specialized burn care techniques, as described in the section on Thermal Injury.

Sunscreens and Other Protective Measures

The UV rays of sunlight or other sources can be completely or partially blocked from the skin by sunscreens. There are three primary types of sunscreens available on the market that reduce or prevent UV erythema chemically, physically, or biologically. Chemical agents absorb UVR, physical agents reflect UVR, and biologic agents reduce inflammation by either blocking the inflammatory response or by enhancing biologic repair.[1] Sunscreen agents no longer contain para-aminobenzoic acid (PABA), a chemical blocking agent that protects against UVB, because of its allergenic and staining properties. However, PABA derivatives are used widely, but protect only against UVB. Broad-spectrum suntan lotions protect against both UVA and UVB. These products contain a benzophenone, such as oxybenzone, dioxybenzone, or avobenzone. Newer agents, such as micronized titanium dioxide and microfine zinc, act by reflecting as well as absorbing sunlight. They protect against most of the UV spectrum. Anthelios SX (Mexoryl SX), a sunscreen that is photo-stable and protects against both UVB and UVA, is also used in Canada.

Sunscreens are available as lotions, creams, oils, gels, and sprays. They also are incorporated into cosmetics and lip balms. Sunscreens should be used diligently and according to the person's tendency to burn rather than tan (Table 61.1). Because many skin cancers are correlated with childhood sunburns, children younger than 18 years of age should use broad-spectrum (blocks UVA and UVB) sunscreens that have a Sun Protection Factor (SPF) of at least 30. Health Canada requires an SPF rating on all commercial suntan preparations based on their ability to obstruct UVR absorption.

Sunless suntan creams, such as dihydroxyacetone, produce a tan without exposure to the sun. They come in various tones, with emollients or humectants added for moisturizing or gel or alcohol-based products for drying. Vitamins, herbal extracts, antioxidants, and alpha-hydroxy acids may be added as enhancers. It is important to avoid products that use the sun to create tans; they may exacerbate sun damage. Tanning pills contain the pigment, canthaxanthin, found in carrots and are especially dangerous because of their association with hepatitis and urticaria.

Sunscreens should be considered only one component of an overall program to reduce UVR exposure. Health Canada recommends the following sun-protection behaviours: (a) wear a wide-brimmed hat; (b) cover up in the sun; (c) seek shade; (d) wear wrap-around sunglasses; and (e) avoid the sun during the hours of 10 AM to 4 PM, while using a broad-spectrum sunscreen with an SPF of 15 or higher.[42] It is also important to avoid tanning booths, perform a self-assessment of the skin every month, and obtain a professional skin examination every year. The *Global Solar UV Index* was developed by the WHO and adopted by Environment Canada in 2004 to predict the risk of overexposure to UVR. It helps people determine the degree to which they should take caution when outdoors. The index is based on a scale of 0 to 11+, with 0 being low risk and 11+ extreme risk. It is calculated daily and is based on skin types of people who sunburn easily. For example, a UV Index value (*i.e.*, high) of 5 or 6 means there is a good possibility of UV overexposure.[43]

Thermal Injury

Burn injures may be due to thermal (flame, scald, contact), electrical or chemical causes. Although house fires are the main cause of burn-related deaths, more than half (56%) of hospitalizations are for children with scald burns.[44] The effects and complications of burns fully illustrate the essential function that the skin performs as it protects the body from the many damaging elements in the environment while serving to maintain the constancy of the body's internal environment. The massive loss of skin tissue not only predisposes to penetration of microorganisms that are present in the environment, it allows for the massive loss of body fluids and their contents, it interferes with temperature regulation, it challenges the immune system, and it imposes excessive demands on the metabolic and reparative processes that are needed to restore the body's interface with the environment.

Burns are caused by a number of sources. Flame burns occur because of exposure to direct fire. Scald burns result from hot liquids spilled or poured on the skin surface. In a child, a scald burn may be indicative of child abuse. Chemical burns occur from industrial agents used in occupational sites. Electrical burns occur from contact with live electrical wires in fields or in the home. Electrical burns are usually more extensive because of internal tissue injury and the presence of entrance and exit wounds (see Chapter 5, Fig. 5.5). Lightning, electromagnetic radiation, and ionizing radiation also can cause skin burns.

Classification of Burns

Burns are typically classified according to the depth of involvement as first-degree, second-degree, and third-degree burns.[1,2,45-47] The depth of a burn is largely influenced by the duration of exposure to the heat source and the temperature of the heating agent. *First-degree burns* (superficial

TABLE 61.1 SKIN PHOTOTYPES

SKIN PHOTOTYPE	SUNTAN AND SUNBURN HISTORY
I	Very fair; always burns, never tans, sensitive to sun exposure Eyes blue or green; hair blond or red
II	Fair; burns easily, tans minimally Eyes blue, hazel, or brown; hair blond, red, or brown
III	Medium; burns moderately, tans gradually to light brown
IV	Olive; burns minimally, always tans well to moderately brown
V	Brown; rarely burns, tans profusely to dark
VI	Black; never burns, deeply pigmented, least sensitive

Adapted from Skin Cancer Foundation. (2007). Skin types and at-risk groups. Available online at: www.skincancer.org.

partial-thickness burns) involve only the outer layers of the epidermis. They are red or pink, dry, and painful. There usually is no blister formation. A mild sunburn is an example. The skin maintains its ability to function as a water vapour and bacterial barrier and heals in 3 to 10 days. First-degree burns usually require only palliative treatment, such as pain relief measures and adequate fluid intake. Extensive first-degree burns on infants, the elderly, and persons who receive radiation therapy for cancer may require more care.

Second-degree burns involve both the epidermis and dermis. *Second-degree partial-thickness burns* involve the epidermis and various degrees of the dermis. They are painful, moist, red, and blistered. Underneath the blisters is weeping, bright pink or red skin that is sensitive to temperature changes, air exposure, and touch. When intact, the blisters prevent the loss of body water and superficial dermal cells. Excluding excision of large burn areas, it is important to maintain intact blisters after injury because they serve as protection and may promote wound healing. These burns heal in approximately 1 to 2 weeks.

Second-degree full-thickness burns involve the entire epidermis and dermis. Structures that originate in the subcutaneous layer, such as hair follicles and sweat glands, remain intact. These burns can be very painful because the pain sensors remain intact. Tactile sensation may be absent or greatly diminished in the areas of deepest destruction. These burns appear as mottled pink, red, or waxy white areas with blisters and edema. The blisters resemble flat, dry tissue paper, rather than the bullous blisters seen with superficial partial-thickness injury. After healing, in approximately 1 month, these burns maintain their softness and elasticity, but there may be the loss of some sensation. Scar formation is usual. These burns heal with supportive medical care aimed at preventing further tissue damage, providing adequate hydration, and ensuring that the granular bed is adequate to support reepithelialization.

Third-degree full-thickness burns extend into the subcutaneous tissue and may involve muscle and bone. Thrombosed vessels can be seen under the burned skin, indicating that the underlying vasculature is involved. Third-degree burns vary in colour from waxy white or yellow to tan, brown, deep red, or black. These burns are hard, dry, and leathery. Edema is extensive in the burn area and surrounding tissues. There is no pain because the nerve sensors have been destroyed. However, there is no such thing as a "pure" third-degree burn. Third-degree burns are almost always surrounded by second-degree burns, which are surrounded by an area of first-degree burns. The injury sometimes has an almost target-like appearance because of the various degrees of burn. Full-thickness burns wider than 4 cm usually require skin grafts because all the regenerative (*i.e.,* dermal) elements have been destroyed. Smaller injuries usually heal from the margins inward toward the centre, the dermal elements regenerating from the healthier margins. However, regeneration may take many weeks and leave a permanent scar, even in smaller burns.

In addition to the depth of the wound, the extent of the burn also is important. Extent is measured by estimating the amount of total body surface area (TBSA) involved. Several tools exist for estimating the TBSA (Fig. 61.28). For example, the *rule of nines* counts anatomic body parts as multiples of 9% (the head is 9%, each arm 9%, each leg 18%, anterior trunk 18%, posterior trunk 18%), with the perineum counting as 1%. The Lund and Browder chart includes a body diagram table that estimates the TBSA by age and anatomic part.[46,47] Children are more accurately assessed using this method because it takes into account the difference in relative size of body parts. The estimates of TBSA are then converted to the American Burn Association Classification of Extent of Injury (Table 61.2).

Other factors, such as age, location, other injuries, and pre-existing conditions, are taken into consideration for a full assessment of burn injury.[45–48] These factors can increase the

TABLE 61.2 AMERICAN BURN ASSOCIATION GRADING SYSTEM FOR BURN SEVERITY AND DISPOSITION

	TYPE OF BURN		
	MINOR	**MODERATE**	**MAJOR**
Criteria	<10% TBSA in adult	10–20% TBSA in adult	>20% TBSA in adult
	<5% TBSA in young (<10 years) or old (>50 years)	5–10% TBSA in young or old	>10% TBSA in young or old
	<2% Full-thickness burn	2–5% Full-thickness burn	>5% Full-thickness burn
		High-voltage injury	High-voltage burn
		Suspected inhalation injury	Known inhalation injury
		Circumferential burn	Any significant burn to face, eyes, ears, genitalia, hands, feet, or major joints
		Concomitant medical problem predisposing to infection (*e.g.,* diabetes, sickle cell disease)	Significant associated injuries (*e.g.,* major trauma)
Disposition	Outpatient management	Hospital admission	Referral to burn center

TBSA, total body surface area.
From American Burn Association. (1990). Hospital and prehospital resources for optimal care of patients with burn injury: Guidelines for development and operation of burn centers. *Journal of Burn Care and Rehabilitation, 11,* 98–104.

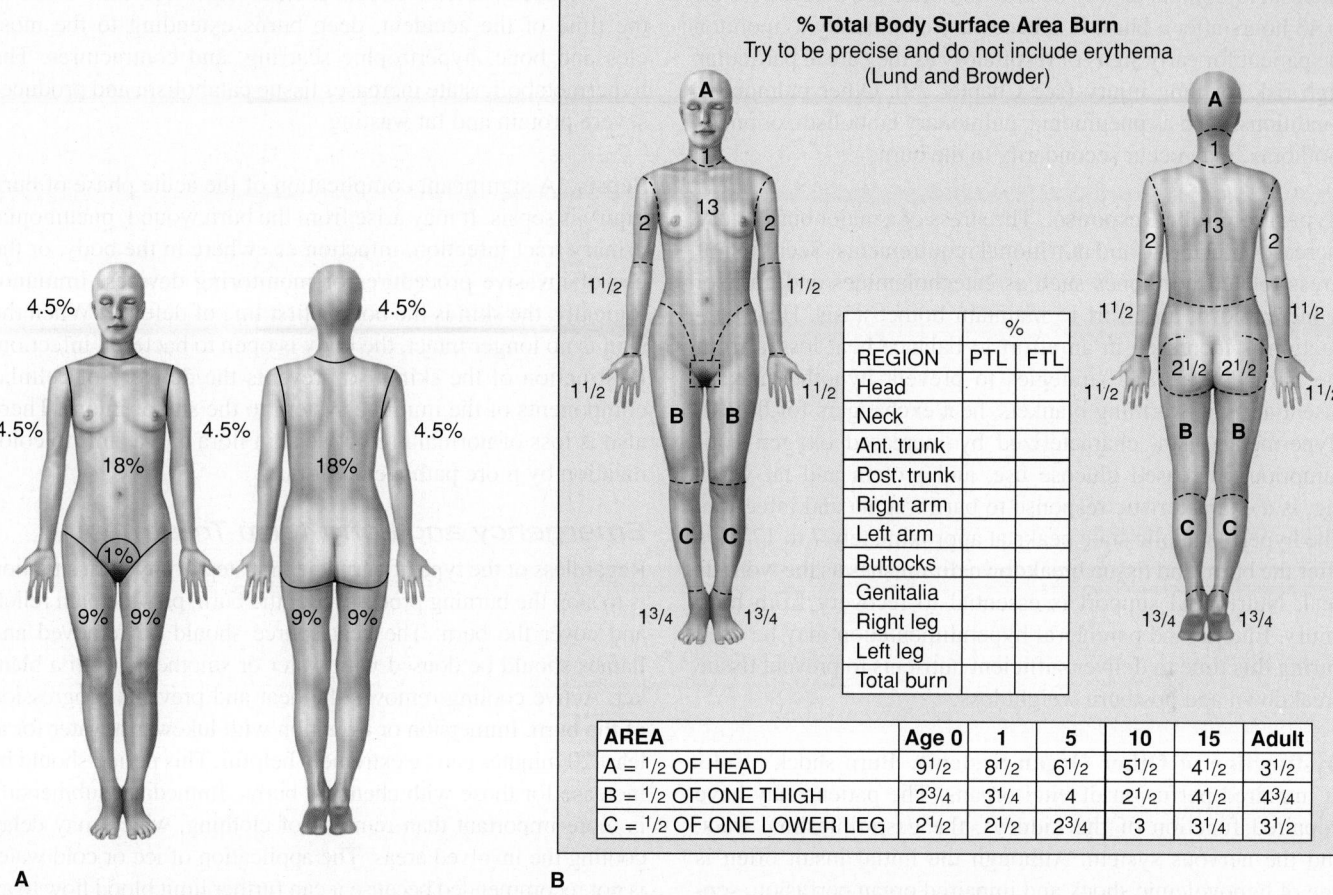

FIGURE 61.28 • Classification of burns. **A:** The rule of nines. **B:** The Lund and Browder chart. (From Lund C. C., Browder N. C. (1944). The estimation of areas of burns. *Surgical Gynecology and Obstetrics, 79,* p. 352.)

assessed severity of the burn and the length of treatment. For example, a first-degree burn is reclassified as a more severe burn if other factors are present, such as burns to the hands, face, and feet; inhalation injury; electrical burns; other trauma; or existence of psychosocial problems. Genital burns almost always require hospitalization because edema may cause difficulty with urination and the location complicates maintenance of a bacteria-free environment.

Systemic Complications

Burn victims often experience multiple life-threatening complications, such as hemodynamic instability, impaired respiratory function, and a hypermetabolic response. They are at high risk for multiple organ dysfunction, infection, or sepsis.[46–49] The magnitude of the response is proportional to the extent of injury, usually reaching a plateau when approximately 60% of the body is burned. In addition to loss of skin, burn victims often have associated injuries or illnesses. The treatment challenge is to provide immediate resuscitation efforts and long-term maintenance of physiologic function. Pain and emotional problems are additional challenges faced by persons with burns.

Hemodynamic Instability. Hemodynamic instability begins almost immediately with injury to capillaries in the burned

area and surrounding tissue. Fluid is lost from the vascular, interstitial, and cellular compartments. Because of a loss of vascular volume, major burn victims often present in the emergency department in a form of hypovolemic shock (Chapter 26) known as *burn shock*. The patient has a decrease in cardiac output, increased peripheral vascular resistance, and impaired perfusion of vital organs. Electrical injuries that cause burns can produce cardiac arrhythmias that require immediate attention.

Respiratory System Dysfunction. Another injury that may occur with burns is smoke inhalation and subsequent acute lung injury. Victims who are trapped in a burning structure may inhale significant amounts of smoke, carbon monoxide, or other toxic fumes. Water-soluble gases, such as ammonia, sulphur dioxide, and chlorine that are found in smoke from burning plastics and rubber, react with mucous membranes to form strong acids and alkalis that induce ulceration of the mucous membrane, bronchospasm, and edema. Lipid-soluble gases, such as nitrous oxide and hydrogen chloride, are transported to the lower airways, where they damage lung tissue. There also may be thermal injury to the respiratory passages. Manifestations of inhalation injury include hoarseness, drooling, an inability to handle secretions, hacking cough, and laboured and shallow breathing. Serial blood gases show a fall in the partial pressure of arterial oxygen (PO_2). Signs of mucosal injury and airway obstruction often are delayed for 24 to 48 hours after a burn. It is necessary continually to monitor the patient for early signs of respiratory as they are at particular high risk for lung injury (see Chapter 29). Other pulmonary conditions, such as pneumonia, pulmonary embolism, or pneumothorax, may occur secondarily to the burn.

Hypermetabolic Response. The stress of a major burn injury increases metabolic and nutritional requirements. Secretion of stress-related hormones such as catecholamines and cortisol is increased in an effort to maintain homeostasis. Heat production is increased in an effort to balance heat losses from the burned area, and strategies to prevent hypothermia are essential (*e.g.*, warming blankets, heat exchangers for fluids). Hypermetabolism, characterized by increased oxygen consumption, increased glucose use, and protein and fat wasting, is a characteristic response to burn trauma and infection. The hypermetabolic state peaks at approximately 7 to 17 days after the burn, and tissue breakdown diminishes as the wounds heal. Nutritional support is essential to recovery from burn injury. Enteral and parenteral hyperalimentation may be used during this time to deliver sufficient nutrients to prevent tissue breakdown and postburn weight loss.

Dysfunction of Other Organ Systems. Burn shock results in impaired perfusion of vital organs. The patient may have impaired function of the kidneys, the gastrointestinal tract, and the nervous system. Although the initial insult often is one of hypovolemic shock and impaired organ perfusion, sepsis may contribute to impaired organ function after the initial resuscitation period.

Renal insufficiency can occur in burn patients as a result of the hypovolemic state, damage to the kidneys at the time of the burn, or from drugs that are administered. Immediately after the burn, a person goes into a short period of relative anuria, followed by a phase of hypermetabolism characterized by increased urine output and nitrogen loss.

The effects of burn injury on the gastrointestinal tract include gastric dilation and decreased peristalsis. These effects are compounded by immobility and narcotic analgesics. Burn victims are observed carefully for vomiting and fecal impaction. Acute ulceration of the stomach and duodenum (called *Curling ulcer*) is a potential complication in burn victims and is thought to be the result of stress and gastric ischemia. It is largely controlled by the prophylactic administration of proton pump inhibitors. Enteral feeding tubes are inserted almost immediately. Tube feeding is intended to mitigate ulcer formation, maintain the integrity of the intestinal mucosa, and provide sufficient calories and protein for the hypermetabolic state.

Neurologic changes can occur from periods of hypoxia. Neurologic damage may result from head injuries, drug or alcohol abuse, carbon monoxide poisoning, fluid volume deficits, and hypovolemia. With an electrical burn, the brain or spine can be directly injured. The responses to neurologic damage may include confusion, memory loss, insomnia, lethargy, and combativeness.

Musculoskeletal effects include fractures that occur at the time of the accident, deep burns extending to the muscles and bone, hypertrophic scarring, and contractures. The hypermetabolic state increases tissue catabolism and produces severe protein and fat wasting.

Sepsis. A significant complication of the acute phase of burn injury is sepsis. It may arise from the burn wound, pneumonia, urinary tract infection, infection elsewhere in the body, or the use of invasive procedures or monitoring devices. Immunologically, the skin is the body's first line of defence. When the skin is no longer intact, the body is open to bacterial infection. Destruction of the skin also prevents the delivery of cellular components of the immune system to the site of injury. There also is loss of normal protective skin flora and a shift to colonization by more pathogenic flora.

Emergency and Long-term Treatment

Regardless of the type of burn, the first step in any burn situation is to stop the burning process, cool the burn, provide pain relief, and cover the burn. The heat source should be removed and flames should be doused with water or smothered with a blanket. Active cooling removes the heat and prevents progression of the burn. Immersion or irrigation with lukewarm water for at least 20 minutes can be extremely helpful. This period should be increase for those with chemical burns. Immediate submersion is more important than removal of clothing, which may delay cooling the involved areas. The application of ice or cold water is not recommended because it can further limit blood flow to an area, turning a partial-thickness into a full-thickness burn.

Medical treatment is determined by the depth and extent of the burn. Emergency care consists of resuscitation and stabilization with intravenous fluids while maintaining cardiac and respiratory function. Frequent evaluation of electrolytes, complete blood count (CBC), coagulation, electrolytes, and lactate levels should be performed.[46–50] Once hospitalized, the immediate treatment regimen focuses on continued maintenance of cardiorespiratory function, pain alleviation, wound care, and emotional support. Intermediate and long-term treatments depend on the extent of injury.

After hemodynamic and pulmonary stability have been established, treatment is directed toward initial care of the wound. Treatment of the burn wound focuses on protection from desiccation and further injury of those burn areas that reepithelialize in 7 to 10 days (superficial second-degree burns). "Nature's own blister" is the best protection for these burns. Topical antimicrobial preparations (*e.g.*, silver sulfadiazine) and dressings are used to cover the wound when the blister has been broken. Wounds that will not heal spontaneously in 7 to 10 days (deep second-degree and third-degree burns) are usually treated by excision and skin grafts. The sloughed tissue, or *eschar*, produced by the burn is excised as soon as possible. This decreases the chance of infection and allows the skin to regenerate faster.

Burns that encircle the entire surface of the body or a body part (*e.g.*, arms, legs, torso) act like tourniquets and can cause major tissue damage to the muscles, tendons, and vasculature under the area of the leathery eschar skin. These burns are called *circumferential burns*. The eschar is incised longitudinally (escharotomy), and sometimes a fasciotomy (surgical incision through the fascia of the muscle) is performed. The timing of these incisions is important. Incision is done after the patient's circulatory condition stabilizes to some degree, thereby limiting some of the massive fluid loss. However, the incisions must be done before eschar formation can cause hypoxia and necrosis of the underlying tissues and organs. This is extremely important when torso burns occur because the pressure placed on the chest can result in inability to breathe and decreased blood return to the heart.

Systemic infection remains a leading cause of morbidity among persons with extensive burns. Continuous microbiologic surveillance is necessary; protective isolation measures are often instituted. There is an increasing trend toward use of prophylactic antibiotic treatment in persons with major burns.

Skin grafts are surgically implanted as soon as possible, often at the same time the burn tissue is excised, to promote new skin growth, limit fluid loss, and act as a dressing. Skin grafts can be permanent or temporary, and either split-thickness or full-thickness. Permanent skin grafts are used over newly excised tissue. Temporary skin grafts are used to cover a burned area until the tissue underneath it has healed.

Various sources of skin grafts exist: *autograft* (skin obtained from the person's own body), *homograft* (skin obtained from another human being, alive or recently dead), and *heterograft* (skin obtained from another species, such as pigs). The best choice is autografting when there is enough uninterrupted skin on the person's body. The thickness of these grafts depends on the donor site and the needs of the burn patient. A *split-thickness skin graft* is one that includes the epidermis and part of the dermis. A split-thickness skin graft can be sent through a skin mesher that cuts tiny slits into the skin, allowing it to expand up to nine times its original size. These grafts are used frequently because they can cover large surface areas and there is less autorejection. *Full-thickness skin grafts* include the entire thickness of the dermal layer. They are used primarily for reconstructive surgery or for deep, small areas. The donor site of a full-thickness skin graft requires a split-thickness skin graft to help it heal.

Synthetic skin grafts generally are composed of a layer of silicone, mimicking the properties of the epidermis, and a layer or matrix of fibres. Skin cells attach to the fibres, enabling dermal skin growth. Once the dermal skin has regenerated, the silicone layer is removed and a thin epidermal skin graft is applied, thus requiring less skin grafting overall.

Other treatment measures include positioning, splinting, and physical therapy to prevent contractures and maintain muscle tone. Because the normal body response to disuse is flexion, the contractures that occur with a burn are disfiguring and cause loss of limb or appendage use. Once the wounds have healed sufficiently, elastic pressure garments, sometimes for the full body, often are used to prevent hypertrophic scarring.

Pressure Ulcers

Pressure ulcers are costly in terms of human suffering, financial expense, and allocation of healthcare resources.[51] The national prevalence of pressure ulcers in Canada estimates that 25% occur in acute care facilities, 30% in nonacute care settings (long-term care, nursing homes, etc.), 22% in mixed healthcare settings, and 15% occur within the community, all require medical intervention.[52,53]

Pressure ulcers are ischemic lesions of the skin and underlying structures caused by unrelieved pressure that impairs the flow of blood and lymph. Pressure ulcers often are referred to as *decubitus ulcers* or *bedsores*. Pressure ulcers are most likely to develop over a bony prominence, but they may occur on any part of the body that is subjected to external pressure, friction, or shearing forces. Several subpopulations are at particular risk, including persons with quadriplegia, older adults with restricted activity and hip fractures, and critically ill persons.

Mechanisms of Development

Many factors contribute to the development of pressure ulcers, including primary extrinsic factors (*i.e.*, undue and prolonged pressure, shearing forces, friction, moisture, impaired mobility) and secondary intrinsic factors (*i.e.*, decreased sensations, nutrition, anemia, medications, cardiovascular changes, smoking).[54] When external pressure between a bony prominence and a support surface exceeds the normal capillary filling pressure, capillary flow essentially is obstructed. If this pressure is applied constantly for 2 hours, oxygen deprivation coupled with an accumulation of metabolic end products leads to irreversible tissue damage. Although 32 mm Hg has been traditionally accepted as the amount of pressure necessary to compress capillaries and interrupt blood flow, this is highly variable among individuals.[54] Persons with impaired circulation require less pressure to interrupt circulation. The same amount of pressure causes more damage when it is distributed over a small area than over a larger area.

Whether a person is sitting or lying down, the weight of the body is borne by tissues covering the bony prominences. A majority of pressure ulcers are located on the lower part of the body, most often over the sacrum, the coccygeal area, the ischial tuberosities, and the greater trochanters. Pressure over a bony area is transmitted from the surface to the underlying dense bone, compressing all of the intervening tissue. As a result, the greatest pressure occurs at the surface of the bone and dissipates outward in a cone-like manner toward the surface of the skin (Fig. 61.29). Thus, extensive underlying tissue damage can be present when a small superficial skin lesion is first noticed.

Altering the distribution of pressure from one skin area to another prevents tissue injury. Pressure ulcers most commonly occur in persons with conditions such as spinal cord injury in which normal sensation and movement to effect redistribution of body weight are impaired. Normally, persons unconsciously shift their weight to redistribute pressure

Skin { Epidermis — Dermis —
Subcutaneous fat
Deep fascia —
Muscle
Periosteum —
Bone —
Pressure

FIGURE 61.29 • Pressure over a bony prominence compresses all intervening soft tissue, with a resulting wide, three-dimensional pressure gradient that causes various degrees of tissue damage. (From Shea J. D. (1975). Pressure sores: Classification and management. *Clinical Orthopedics and Related Research, 112,* 90.)

on the skin and underlying tissues. For example, during the night, people turn in their sleep, preventing ischemic injury of tissues that overlie the bony prominences that support the weight of the body; the same is true for sitting for any length of time. The movements needed to shift the body weight are made unconsciously, and only when movement is restricted do people become aware of discomfort.

Shearing forces are caused by the sliding of one tissue layer over another with stretching and angulation of blood vessels, causing injury and thrombosis. Shear occurs when the skeleton moves, but the skin remains fixed to an external surface, such as occurs with transfer from a stretcher to a bed or pulling a person up in bed. The same thing happens when the head of the bed is elevated, causing the torso to move toward the foot of the bed while friction and moisture cause the skin to remain fixed to the bed linens. *Friction* contributes to pressure ulceration by damaging the skin at the epidermal–dermal interface. It occurs as persons who are bedridden use their elbows and heels to aid in movement. *Moisture* contributes to pressure ulcer formation by weakening the cell wall of individual skin cells and by changing the protective pH of the skin. This makes the skin more susceptible to pressure, shear, and friction injury.

Prevention

The prevention of pressure ulcers is preferable to their treatment. The Canadian Association of Wound Care Advisory Panel developed clinical recommendations for the prevention and treatment of pressure ulcers.[53] The panel recommended many goals, such as identifying at-risk persons who need preventative measures and the specific factors placing them at risk; maintaining and improving tissue tolerance to prevent injury; protecting against the adverse effects of external mechanical forces (*i.e.,* pressure, friction, and shear); maximizing nutritional status; utilizing an interdisciplinary team to stage, assess, and treat the wound and other patient requirements (*e.g.,* pain, psychosocial, etc.); and reducing the incidence of pressure ulcers through educational programs. These recommendations included details for assessment of the person with pressure ulcers, management of tissue load, ulcer care, managing bacterial colonization and infection, operative repair, and education and quality control.[53]

Risk factors identified as contributing to the development of pressure ulcers were those related to sensory perception (*i.e.,* ability to respond meaningfully to pressure-related discomfort), level of skin moisture, urine and fecal continence, nutrition and hydration status, mobility, circulatory status, and presence of shear and friction forces.[53]

Methods for preventing pressure ulcers include frequent position change, meticulous skin care, and frequent and careful observation to detect early signs of skin breakdown. Moisture macerates and injures skin. Sources of moisture include sweat, wound drainage, urine and feces. Both urinary and fecal incontinence increase the risk of pressure ulcers. Food crumbs, intravenous tubing, and other debris in the bed can greatly increase local skin pressure points. The prevention of dehydration improves the circulation. It also decreases the concentration of urine, thereby minimizing skin irritation in persons who are incontinent, and it reduces urinary problems that contribute to incontinence. Maintenance of adequate nutrition is important. Anemia and malnutrition contribute to tissue breakdown and delay healing after tissue injury has occurred.[53]

Staging and Treatment

Pressure ulcers can be staged using four categories. *Stage I ulcers* are characterized by a defined area of persistent redness in lightly pigmented skin or an area of persistent redness with blue or purple hues in darker skin. *Stage II ulcers* represent a partial-thickness loss of skin involving the epidermis or dermis, or both. The ulcer is superficial and presents clinically as an abrasion, a blister, or a shallow crater. *Stage III ulcers* represent a full-thickness skin loss involving damage and necrosis of subcutaneous tissue that may extend down to but not through underlying fascia. The ulcer manifests as a deep crater with or without undermining of adjacent tissue. *Stage IV ulcers* involve full-thickness skin loss and necrosis with extensive destruction or damage to the underlying subcutaneous tissues that may extend to involve muscle, bone, and supporting structures (*e.g.,* tendon or joint capsule).[54]

After skin breakdown has occurred, special treatment measures are needed to prevent further ischemic damage, reduce bacterial contamination and infection, and promote healing. Treatment methods are selected based on the stage of the ulcer.[53,55,56] Stage I ulcers usually are treated with frequent turning and measures to remove pressure. Stage II or III ulcers with little exudate are treated with semipermeable or occlusive dressings. Occlusive dressings are credited with preventing the loss of wound fluid and maintaining a moist environment that is necessary for epithelial cell migration. Wound fluid is thought to contain a variety of growth factors that enhance wound healing. Occlusive dressings may also relieve wound pain and prevent bacterial contamination. There are several types of occlusive dressings available, including polymer films, hydrogels, hydrocolloids, biomembranes, and absorbing granules. The available products differ in their permeability to water vapour and wound protection, and each has advantages and disadvantages.

Necrotic debris increases the possibility of bacterial infection and delays wound healing. Stage III ulcers with exudate and necrotic debris and stage IV ulcers usually require debridement (*i.e.,* removal of necrotic tissue and eschar). This can be done surgically, with wet-to-dry dressings, or through the use of proteolytic enzymes. Stage IV wounds often require packing to obliterate dead space and are covered with nonadherent dressings. Stage IV ulcers may require surgical interventions, such as skin grafts or myocutaneous flaps.

IN SUMMARY

Repeated exposure to the UV rays of the sun predisposes to sunburn, premature aging of the skin (wrinkling, solar elastosis, and irregularities in pigmentation), and skin cancer. Solar and artificial sources of UVR, such as from a tanning parlour, contribute to the amount of radiation to which human beings are exposed. Sunburn, which is caused by excessive exposure to UVR, is an erythematous inflammatory reaction, ranging from mild to severe. Photosensitive drugs can also produce an exaggerated response to UVR when they are taken in combination with sun exposure. Sunscreens are protective agents that work by either reflecting sunlight or preventing its absorption.

Burns cause damage to skin structures, ranging from first-degree burns, which damage the epidermis, to third-degree full-thickness burns, which extend into the subcutaneous tissue and may involve muscle and bone. The extent of injury is determined by the thickness of the burn and the total body surface area involved. In addition to skin involvement, burn injury can cause hemodynamic instability with hypovolemic shock, inhalation injury with respiratory involvement, a hypermetabolic state, organ dysfunction, immune suppression and sepsis, pain, and emotional trauma. Treatment methods vary with the severity of injury and include immediate resuscitation and maintenance of physiologic function, wound cleaning and debridement, application of antimicrobial agents and dressings, and skin grafting. Efforts are directed toward preventing or limiting disfigurement and disability.

Pressure ulcers are caused by ischemia of the skin and underlying tissues. They result from external pressure, which disrupts blood flow, or shearing forces, which cause stretching and injury to blood vessels. Pressure ulcers are divided into four stages, according to the depth of tissue involvement. The prevention of pressure ulcers is preferable to their treatment. The goals of prevention should include identifying at-risk persons who need prevention along with the specific factors placing them at risk; maintaining and improving tissue tolerance to pressure to prevent injury; and protecting against the adverse effects of external mechanical forces (*i.e.,* pressure, friction, and shear).

NEVI AND SKIN CANCERS

After completing this section of the chapter, you should be able to meet the following objectives:

- Describe the origin of nevi and state their relationship to skin cancers.
- Compare the appearance and outcome of basal cell carcinoma, squamous cell carcinoma, and malignant melanoma.

Nevi

Nevi, or moles, are common congenital or acquired tumours of the skin that are benign. Almost all adults have nevi, some in greater numbers than others. Nevi can be pigmented or nonpigmented, flat or elevated, and hairy or nonhairy.

Nevocellular nevi are pigmented skin lesions resulting from proliferation of melanocytes in the epidermis or dermis. Nevocellular nevi are tan to deep brown, uniformly pigmented, small papules with well-defined, rounded borders (Fig. 61.30A). They are formed initially by melanocytes with their long dendritic extensions that are normally interspersed among the basal keratinocytes (see Chapter 60, Fig. 60.2). The melanocytes are transformed into round or oval melanin-containing cells that grow in nests or clusters along the dermal–epidermal junction. Because of their location, these lesions are called *junctional nevi* (Fig. 61.30B). Eventually, most junctional nevi grow into the surrounding dermis as nests or cords of cells. *Compound nevi* contain epidermal and dermal components. In older lesions, the epidermal nests may disappear entirely, leaving a *dermal nevus.* Compound and dermal nevi usually are more elevated than junctional nevi.

Another form of nevus, the *dysplastic nevus,* is important because of its capacity to transform into malignant melanoma. Although the association between nevocellular nevi and malignant melanoma was made over 175 years ago, it was not until 1978 that the role of dysplastic nevi as precursors to malignant melanoma was described in detail. Dysplastic nevi are usually larger than other nevi (often >5 mm in diameter). Their appearance is a flat, slightly raised plaque with a pebbly surface, or a target-like lesion with a darker, raised centre and irregular border (Fig. 61.31). They vary in shade from brown

FIGURE 61.30 • **A:** Normal mole, with no different shades of brown, black, or tan. (Centers for Disease Control and Prevention Public Health Image Library. Available online at: http://phil.cdc.gov/Phil/home.asp) **B:** Junctional nevi on the back of a 16-year-old patient. (Owen Laboratories, Inc.) (From Hall B. J., Hall J. C. (2010). *Sauer's manual of skin diseases* (10th ed., p. 434). Philadelphia, PA: Lippincott Williams & Wilkins.)

and red to flesh tones. A person may have hundreds of these lesions. Unlike other moles or nevi, they occur on both sun-exposed and covered areas of the body. Dysplastic nevi have been documented in multiple members of families prone to development of malignant melanoma.

Because of the possibility of malignant transformation, any mole that undergoes a change warrants immediate medical attention. The changes to observe and report are changes in size, thickness, colour, itching, and bleeding.

Skin Cancer

There has been an alarming increase in skin cancers over the past several decades. The worldwide incidence of malignant melanoma, the most serious form of skin cancer, has continued to increase over the past four decades among white populations.[57] It is estimated in 2015, there will be approximately 6,800 new cases and 1,150 deaths from melanoma in Canada. There will be also approximately 78,300 cases per year of highly curable nonmelanoma (basal cell and squamous cell) cancers.[58]

The rising incidence of skin cancer has been attributed to increased sun exposure associated with social and lifestyle. The thinning of the ozone layer in the earth's stratosphere is thought to be another factor in this increased incidence. Society's emphasis on suntanning also is implicated. People tend to have more leisure time and spend increasing amounts of time in the sun with uncovered skin.

FIGURE 61.31 • Dysplastic nevi. Lesion has a dark brown "pebbly" elevated surface against a lighter tan, macular background. The irregular, indistinct margin helps to distinguish it from the small congenital-pattern nevus, which some dysplastic nevi closely resemble. Its distinct morphology, rather than its size (6 × 6 mm), identifies it as a dysplastic nevus. (National Cancer Institute Visuals. Available online at: http://visualsonline. cancer.gov/browseaction.cfm?topicid=g11.)

SKIN CANCERS

- Increased and unprotected exposure to the ultraviolet rays of sunlight produces sunburn and increases the risk for development of skin cancer.
- The melanocytes, which protect against sunburn through increased production of melanin and suntanning, are particularly vulnerable to the adverse effects of unprotected exposure to ultraviolet light. Malignant melanoma, which is a malignant tumour of melanocytes, is a rapidly progressive and metastatic form of skin cancer.
- Basal cell carcinoma and squamous cell carcinoma, which also reflect the effects of increased sun exposure, are less aggressive forms of skin cancer and are more easily cured.

Although the factors linking sun exposure to skin cancer are not completely understood, both total cumulative exposure and altered patterns of exposure are strongly implicated. Basal cell and squamous cell carcinomas are often associated with total cumulative exposure to UVR. Thus, basal cell and squamous cell carcinomas occur more commonly on maximally sun-exposed parts of the body, such as the face and backs of the hands and forearms. Melanomas occur most commonly on areas of the body that are exposed to the sun intermittently, such as the back in men and the lower legs in women.

Malignant Melanoma

Malignant melanoma is a malignant tumour of the melanocytes. It is a rapidly progressing, metastatic form of cancer. The dramatic increase in the incidence of malignant melanoma over the past several decades has been credited to increased UVR exposure, including tanning salons. Fortunately, the global mortality rates have remained relatively stable since the 1980s.[57] Public health screening measures, early diagnosis, increased knowledge of precursor lesions, and greater public knowledge of the disease may account for earlier intervention.

The risk is greatest in fair-skinned people, particularly those with blond or red hair who sunburn and freckle easily (see Table 61.1). Other risk factors include a family history of malignant melanoma, presence of marked freckling on the upper back, history of three or more blistering sunburns before 20 years of age, and presence of actinic keratoses. Still other significant risk factors for melanoma are atypical mole/dysplastic nevus syndrome, immunosuppression, and prior PUVA therapy.[59]

Severe, blistering sunburns in early childhood and intermittent intense sun exposures (trips to sunny climates) contribute to increased susceptibility to melanoma in young and middle-aged adults. Roughly 90% of malignant melanomas in whites occur on sun-exposed skin. However, in darker-skinned people melanomas often occur on non–sun-exposed areas, such as the mucous membranes and subungual, palmar, and plantar surfaces.

Malignant melanomas differ in size and shape. Usually, they are slightly raised and black or brown. Borders are irregular and surfaces are uneven. Most seem to arise from pre-existing nevi or new mole-like growths (Fig. 61.32). There may be surrounding erythema, inflammation, and tenderness. Periodically, melanomas ulcerate and bleed. Dark melanomas are often mottled with shades of red, blue, and white. These three colours represent three concurrent processes: melanoma growth (blue), inflammation and the body's attempt to localize and destroy the tumour (red), and scar tissue formation (white).

Four types of melanomas have been identified: superficial spreading, nodular, lentigo maligna, and acral lentiginous.[2,59] *Superficial spreading melanoma* is characterized by a raised-edged nevus with lateral growth. It has a disorderly appearance in colour and outline. This lesion tends to have biphasic growth, horizontally and vertically. It typically ulcerates and bleeds with growth. This type of lesion accounts for 70% of all melanomas and is most prevalent in persons who sunburn easily and have intermittent sun exposure. *Nodular melanomas,* which account for 15% of melanomas, are raised, dome-shaped lesions that can occur anywhere on the body. They are commonly a uniform blue-black colour and tend to look

FIGURE 61.32 • Melanoma lesions, demonstrating the ABCDE rule: A (asymmetry), B (irregular borders), C (different colours), D (diameter change in size), and E (elevations/evolving). (National Cancer Institute Visuals and Larry Meyer (photographer). Available online at: http://visualsonline.cancer.gov/browseaction.cfm?topicid=g11.)

like blood blisters. Nodular melanomas tend to rapidly invade the dermis from the start, with no apparent horizontal growth phase. *Lentigo maligna melanomas,* which account for 5% of all melanomas, are slow-growing, flat nevi that occur primarily on sun-exposed areas of older adults. Untreated lentigo maligna tends to exhibit horizontal and radial growth for many years before it invades the dermis to become lentigo maligna melanoma. *Acral lentiginous melanoma,* which accounts for 10% of melanomas, occurs primarily on the palms, soles, nail beds, and mucous membranes. While this type is rare, it is usually aggressive, with rapid changes from radial to vertical growth. It has the appearance of lentigo maligna.[2,59]

Early detection is critical with malignant melanoma. Regular self-examination of the total skin surface in front of a well-lighted mirror provides a method for early detection. It requires that a person undress completely and examine all areas of the body using a full mirror, handheld mirror, and handheld hair dryer (to examine the scalp). An *ABCDE* rule has been developed to aid in early diagnosis and timely treatment of malignant melanoma. The acronym stands for *a*symmetry, *b*order irregularity, *c*olour variegation, *d*iameter greater than 6 mm (pencil eraser size), and *e*levation/*e*volving.[59] People should be taught to watch for these changes in existing nevi or the development of new nevi, as well as other alterations such as bleeding, crusting, or itching. Because of the existence of small-diameter melanomas (*i.e.,* ≤6 mm in diameter), it has been suggested that people routinely screen their skin for all possible manifestations of skin cancer.[59]

Diagnosis of melanoma is based on biopsy findings from a lesion. Consistent with other cancerous tumours, melanoma is commonly staged using the TNM (tumour, lymph node, and metastasis) staging system (see Chapter 8) using the International Union Against Cancer (UICC) or conversely the American Joint Committee on Cancer (AJCC) Staging System for Cutaneous Melanoma, in which the tumour is rated 0 to 4, may be used with further subclassifications depending on numerous factors, including extent of tumour invasion, ulceration, and metastasis.[59,60] Ulceration and invasion of the tumour into the deeper skin tissue result in a poorer prognosis. Although survival rates may vary with individual circumstances, the current 5-year survival rate for stage 0 melanoma is 99%; stage I melanoma, 91% to 95%; stage II melanoma, 45% to 79%; stage III melanoma, 24% to 70%; and stage IV melanoma, 10% to 19%.[59] Early diagnosis and treatment are of extreme importance.

Treatment is usually surgical excision, the extent of which is determined by the thickness of the lesion, invasion into the deeper skin layers, and spread to the regional lymph nodes. When diagnosed in a premetastatic phase, melanoma is now treated in ambulatory settings, lessening the cost and inconvenience of care. Current capability allows for mapping lymph flow to a regional lymph node that receives lymphatic drainage from tumour sites on the skin. This lymph node, which is called the *sentinel lymph node,* is then sampled for biopsy. If tumour cells have spread from the primary tumour to the regional lymph nodes, the sentinel node will be the first node in which tumour cells appear. Therefore, sentinel node biopsy can be used to test for the presence of melanoma cells and determine if radical lymph node dissection is necessary. When nodes are positive, consideration is also given to systemic adjuvant therapy.

FIGURE 61.33 • Basal cell carcinoma on the nose. Note the central crust, ulceration, rolled borders, and telangiectasia. (From Goodheart H. P. (2009). *Goodheart's photoguide to common skin disorders: Diagnosis and management* (3rd ed., p. 409) Philadelphia, PA: Lippincott Williams and Wilkins.)

Routine cancer treatment, such as chemotherapy, is indicated when the disease becomes systemic. Despite many interventions used over the years, efforts to cure melanoma in its later stages have been disappointing. Areas of active research in melanoma therapy include vaccine development, more specific immunotherapy, and alternative treatments such as electrochemotherapy. Vaccines are targeted to treat or prevent the recurrence of melanoma, especially in stages II and III.

Basal Cell Carcinoma

Basal cell carcinoma, which is a neoplasm of the nonkeratinizing cells of the basal layer of the epidermis, is the most common skin cancer in light-skinned people (Fig. 61.33). Like other skin cancers, basal cell carcinoma has increased in incidence over the past several decades. Fair-skinned persons with a history of significant long-term sun exposure are more susceptible. Black- and brown-skinned persons are affected occasionally. Basal cell carcinoma usually occurs in persons who were exposed to great amounts of sunlight. Of the nonmelanoma skin cancers diagnosed each year, 75% are basal cell carcinomas.[61,62] Basal cell carcinoma occurs more frequently in women under the age of 52, but over the age of 52 it occurs more frequently in men.[61]

Basal cell carcinoma usually is a nonmetastasizing tumour that extends wide and deep if left untreated. These tumours are most frequently seen on the head and neck, most often occurring on skin that has hair. They also occur on skin surfaces unexposed to the sun, although less frequently.[61,62] Although there are several histologic types of basal cell carcinoma, nodular ulcerative and superficial basal cell carcinomas are the two most frequently occurring types. *Nodular ulcerative basal cell carcinoma* is the most common, accounting for half of all basal cell carcinomas.[62] It has a nodulocystic structure that begins as a small, flesh-coloured or pink, smooth, translucent nodule that enlarges over time. Telangiectatic vessels frequently are seen beneath the surface. Over the years, a central depression forms that progresses to an ulcer surrounded by the original shiny, waxy border. Basal cell carcinoma in darker-skinned persons usually is darkly pigmented and frequently misdiagnosed as other skin diseases, including melanoma.

The second most common form is *superficial basal cell carcinoma,* which is seen most often on the chest or back. It begins as a flat, nonpalpable, erythematous plaque. The red, scaly areas slowly enlarge, with nodular borders and telangiectatic bases. This type of skin cancer is difficult to diagnose because it mimics other dermatologic problems.[61,62]

Biopsies are obtained from all suspected basal cell carcinomas for diagnosis. It is highly curable if detected and treated early. The treatment depends on the site and extent of the lesion. The most important treatment goal is complete elimination of the lesion. Also important is the maintenance of function and optimal cosmetic effect. Curettage with electrodesiccation, surgical excision, irradiation, laser, cryosurgery, and chemosurgery are effective in removing all cancerous cells. Immune therapy, gene therapy, and photodynamic therapy are emerging treatments. Patients should be checked at regular intervals for recurrences.[61,62]

Squamous Cell Carcinoma

Squamous cell carcinomas are the second most common malignant tumours of the outer epidermis and account for approximately 20% of all skin cancers.[61] The increase in the incidence of squamous cell carcinomas is consistent with increased UVR exposure. Occupational hazards are linked to the development of squamous cell carcinoma; persons exposed to arsenic (*i.e.,* Bowen disease), industrial tars, coal, and paraffin have an increased likelihood of contracting squamous cell carcinoma. HPV has also been implicated in the development of this type of cancer in both immunocompromised and immunocompetent individuals.[62] Men are twice as likely as women to have squamous cell carcinoma. Dark-skinned people are rarely affected.

There are two types of squamous cell carcinoma: intraepidermal and invasive. *Intraepidermal squamous cell carcinoma* remains confined to the epidermis for a long time. However, at some unpredictable time, it penetrates the basement membrane to the dermis and metastasizes to the regional lymph nodes. It then converts to *invasive squamous cell carcinoma.* The invasive type can develop from intraepidermal carcinoma or from a premalignant lesion (*e.g.,* actinic keratoses). It may be slow growing or fast growing with metastasis.[62]

Squamous cell carcinoma is a red-scaling, keratotic, slightly elevated lesion with an irregular border, usually with a shallow chronic ulcer (Fig. 61.34). The lesions usually lack the pearly rolled border and superficial telangiectases found on basal cell carcinomas. Later, lesions grow outward, show large ulcerations, and have persistent crusts and raised erythematous borders. The lesions occur on sun-exposed areas of the skin, particularly the nose, forehead, helix of the ear, lower lip, and back of the hand. In dark-skinned black persons, the

FIGURE 61.34 • Squamous cell carcinoma. Generally found on sun-exposed surfaces. (From Stephen T. C., Skillen D. L., Day R. A., et al. (2012). *Canadian Jensen's nursing health assessment: A best practice approach* (p. 317). Philadelphia, PA: Lippincott Williams & Wilkins.)

lesions may appear as hyperpigmented nodules and occur more frequently on non–sun-exposed areas. Metastasis is more common with squamous cell carcinoma than with basal cell carcinoma.[62]

Treatment measures are aimed at the removal of all cancerous tissue using methods such as cryotherapy, topical chemotherapy and immune modifiers, electrosurgery, excision surgery, chemosurgery, or radiation therapy. After treatment, the person is observed for the remainder of his or her life for signs of recurrence.

IN SUMMARY

Nevi or moles usually are benign. Because they may undergo cancerous transformation, any mole that undergoes a change warrants immediate medical attention. There has been an alarming increase in skin cancers over the past few decades. Repeated exposure to the UV rays of the sun has been implicated as the principal cause of skin cancer. Neoplasms of the skin include malignant melanoma, basal cell carcinoma, and squamous cell carcinoma.

Malignant melanoma is a malignant tumour of the melanocytes. It is a rapidly progressing, metastatic form of cancer. Clinically, malignant melanoma of the skin usually is asymptomatic. The most important clinical sign is the change in size, shape, and colour of pigmented skin lesions, such as moles. As the result of increased public awareness, melanomas are being diagnosed earlier, when they can be cured surgically. Squamous cell carcinoma and basal cell carcinoma are of epidermal origin.

Basal cell carcinomas are the most common form of skin cancer among whites. They are slow-growing tumours that rarely metastasize. The two types of squamous cell carcinoma are intraepidermal and invasive. Intraepidermal squamous cell carcinoma remains confined to the epidermis for a long time. Invasive squamous cell carcinoma can develop from intraepidermal carcinoma or from premalignant lesions such as actinic keratoses.

AGE-RELATED SKIN MANIFESTATIONS

After completing this section of the chapter, you should be able to meet the following objectives:

* Differentiate a hemangioma of infancy from a port-wine stain in terms of appearance and outcome.
* Describe the manifestations and probable causes of diaper dermatitis, prickly heat, and cradle cap.
* Describe the distinguishing features of rashes associated with the following infectious childhood diseases: roseola infantum, rubeola, rubella, and varicella.
* Characterize the physiologic changes of aging skin.
* Describe the appearance of skin tags, keratoses, lentigines, and vascular lesions that are commonly seen in the elderly.

Many skin problems occur more commonly in certain age groups. Because of aging changes, infants, children, and older adults tend to have different skin problems.

Skin Manifestations of Infancy and Childhood

Skin Disorders of Infancy

Infancy connotes the image of perfect, unblemished skin. For the most part, this is true. However, several congenital skin lesions, such as mongolian spots, hemangiomas, and nevi, are associated with the early neonatal period. There are also several acquired skin conditions, including diaper dermatitis, prickly heat, and cradle cap, that are relatively common in infants.

Pigmented and Vascular Birthmarks. Pigmented and vascular lesions comprise most birthmarks. Pigmented birthmarks represent abnormal migration or proliferation of melanocytes. For example, *mongolian spots* are caused by selective pigmentation. They usually occur on the buttocks or sacral area and are seen commonly in Asian and black persons. *Nevi* or moles are small, tan to brown, uniformly pigmented solid macules. *Nevocellular nevi* are formed initially from aggregates of melanocytes and keratinocytes along the dermal–epidermal border. *Congenital melanocytic nevi* are collections of melanocytes that are present at birth or develop within the first year of life. They present as macular, papular, or plaque-like pigmented lesions of various shades of brown, with a black or blue focus. The texture of the lesions varies and they may be with or without hair. They usually are found on the hands, shoulders, buttocks, entire arm, or trunk of the body. Some involve large areas of the body in garment-like fashion. They usually grow proportionally with the child. Congenital melanocytic nevi are clinically significant because of their association with malignant melanoma.

Vascular birthmarks are cutaneous anomalies of angiogenesis and vascular development. Two types of vascular birthmarks commonly are seen in infants and small children: bright red, raised hemangiomas of infancy and flat, reddish-purple port-wine stains.

Hemangiomas of infancy (formerly called *strawberry hemangiomas*) are small, red lesions that are noticed shortly after birth. Infantile hemangiomas are generally benign vascular tumours produced by proliferation of endothelial cells. A small portion of these lesions are present at birth, and the remainder develop within a few weeks after birth. They are seen in approximately 10% of children in the first year of life, with about 60% located on the head and neck.[63] Girls are three times more likely to have hemangiomas than boys, and there is an increased incidence in premature infants (20%).[63,64] They also occur more frequently in white infants born to mothers of advanced maternal age or to mothers with multiple gestations.[65]

Hemangiomas of infancy typically undergo an early period of a proliferation during which they enlarge, followed by a period of slow involution where the growth is reversed until complete resolution. Hemangiomas of infancy can occur anywhere on the body; however, when they occur in the airway, they can be life-threatening. Ulceration, the most frequent complication, can be painful and carries the risk of infection, hemorrhage, and scarring. A small percentage of hemangiomas of infancy develop complications, such as infection or ulceration. Some hemangiomas of infancy are located in anatomic regions associated with other anomalies requiring careful monitoring and early intervention. Most hemangiomas of infancy disappear before 10 years of age without leaving an appreciable scar.

Port-wine stains are pink or red patches that can occur anywhere on the body and are very noticeable (Fig. 61.35). They represent slow-growing capillary malformations that

FIGURE 61.35 • Port-wine stain on the arm and hand. (From Hall B. J., Hall J. C. (2010). *Sauer's manual of skin diseases* (10th ed., p. 429). Philadelphia, PA: Lippincott Williams & Wilkins.)

grow proportionately with the child and persist throughout life. There is progressive dilation of the dermal capillaries, which initially is confined to the immediate epidermis, with gradual involvement of deeper dermal blood vessels, although the greater number is always in the upper dermis. Distribution of lesions on the face roughly corresponds to the sensory branches of the trigeminal nerve. The development of a port-wine stain may follow trauma. Port-wine stains usually are confined to the skin, but may be associated with vascular malformations of the eye, resulting primarily in glaucoma and other neurologic deficits (Sturge–Weber syndrome). Laser surgery has revolutionized the treatment of port-wine stains.

Diaper Dermatitis. Irritant diaper dermatitis, or *diaper rash,* is a form of contact dermatitis caused by the interaction of several factors, including prolonged contact of the skin with a mixture of urine and feces.[66] The wearing of diapers causes an increase in skin wetness and pH because of ammonia from urine. Prolonged wetness leads to softening and maceration of the skin, making it more susceptible to damage by friction from the surface of the diaper and local irritants. The contents of soiled diapers, if not changed frequently, can lead to contact dermatitis, bacterial infections, or other skin conditions. The proteases and lipases contained in feces are particularly irritating.

The appearance of diaper rash ranges from simple (*i.e.,* widely distributed macules on the buttocks and anogenital areas) to severe (*i.e.,* beefy, red, excoriated skin surfaces in the diaper area). Secondary infections with bacteria and yeasts are common; discomfort may be marked because of intense inflammation. Such conditions as contact dermatitis, seborrheic dermatitis, candidiasis, and atopic dermatitis should be considered when the eruption is persistent and recalcitrant to simple therapeutic measures.

Diaper dermatitis often responds to simple measures, including frequent diaper changes with careful cleansing of the irritated area to remove all waste products. Exposing the irritated area to air is helpful. It has been shown that application of a barrier ointment after each diaper change is a valuable component of therapy. Topical corticosteroid therapy is usually effective, but should be used cautiously because infants absorb proportionately greater quantities through their skin than adults.[67] Antifungal therapy should not be used routinely; it should be used only when *Candida* infection is established or suspected. Antibacterial agents should not be used because it is known that bacterial infections are usually not involved in diaper dermatitis, and the normal microflora should be preserved.

Selection of a barrier preparation is important. It is now clear that the barrier function of the skin is provided by the stratum corneum, whose main function is to minimize water loss and prevent inward penetration of toxic substances and microorganisms. Ideally, a barrier should mimic the skin's natural function by forming a long-lasting barrier to increase protection against irritants and microorganisms and to maintain optimum moisture levels. Products containing nonessential ingredients such as perfumes can cause allergic contact

FIGURE 61.36 • Candidal intertrigo after a course of oral antibiotics in a 1-year-old child. (Owen Laboratories, Inc.) (From Hall B. J., Hall J. C. (2010). *Sauer's manual of skin diseases* (10th ed., p. 433). Philadelphia, PA: Lippincott Williams & Wilkins.)

dermatitis and should be avoided. Inclusion of an antiseptic is not necessary or desirable. Ideally, the safety and effectiveness of a barrier product should be clinically proven.

There is controversy regarding the effects of cloth versus disposable diapers in preventing diaper rash. In the early days of disposable diapers, infants who wore cloth diapers without plastic pants had fewer diaper rashes than those who wore disposable diapers. It has been suggested that this may not be true with the newer disposable diapers that use absorbent gelling material.[68] These superabsorbent diapers have the smallest increase in skin wetness compared with conventional disposable diapers and cloth diapers. When cloth diapers are used, they should be washed in gentle detergent and thoroughly rinsed to remove all traces of waste products. Plastic pants should be discouraged.

Intractable and severe cases of diaper dermatitis should be seen by a healthcare provider for treatment of any secondary infections. Secondary candidal (*i.e.,* yeast; Fig. 61.36) or other skin manifestations discussed in this chapter may occur in the diaper area. It is important to differentiate between normal diaper dermatitis and more serious skin problems.

Prickly Heat. Prickly heat (heat rash) results from constant maceration of the skin because of prolonged exposure to a warm, humid environment. Maceration leads to midepidermal obstruction and rupture of the sweat glands. Although commonly seen during infancy, prickly heat may occur at any age. The treatment includes removing excessive clothing, cooling the skin with warm water baths, drying the skin with powders, and avoiding hot, humid environments.

Cradle Cap. Cradle cap is a greasy crust or scale formation on the scalp. It usually is attributed to infrequent and inadequate washing of the scalp. Cradle cap is treated using mild shampoo and gentle combing to remove the scales. Sometimes oil can be left on the head for minutes to several hours, softening the scales before scrubbing. Other emulsifying ointments or creams may be helpful in difficult cases. The scalp may need to be rubbed firmly to remove the buildup of keratinized cells. Recalcitrant cases need to be seen by a healthcare practitioner; serious or chronic forms of seborrheic dermatitis may exist.

Skin Manifestations of Common Infectious Diseases

Infectious childhood diseases that produce rashes include exanthem subitum, rubella, rubeola, varicella, and scarlet fever. Although these diseases are seen less frequently because of successful immunization programs and the use of antibiotics, outbreaks still occur.

Roseola Infantum. Roseola infantum (exanthem subitum or sixth disease) is a contagious disease caused by human herpesvirus type 6 (HHV-6). Because HHV-6 is the etiologic agent, the condition is often referred to as *sixth disease*. Primary HHV-6 infection occurs early in life. More than 95% of roseola cases occur in children younger than 3 years of age, with a peak age of acquisition of 9 months of age.[69] Transplacental antibodies likely protect most infants until 6 months of age. Roseola produces a characteristic maculopapular rash covering the trunk and spreading to the appendages. The rash is preceded by an abrupt onset of high fever (≤40°C), inflamed tympanic membranes, and cold-like symptoms usually lasting 3 to 4 days. These symptoms improve at approximately the same time the rash appears. Because infants with roseola exhibit a unique constellation of symptoms over a short time, the infection may be confused with other childhood exanthems. Blood antibody titres may be taken to determine the actual diagnosis. In most cases, there are no long-term effects from this disease. Infants who spike high temperatures should be seen by their healthcare providers.

Rubella. Rubella (*i.e.,* 3-day measles or German measles) is a childhood disease caused by the rubella virus (a togavirus). It is characterized by a diffuse, punctate, macular rash that begins on the trunk and spreads to the arms and legs (Fig. 61.37). Mild febrile states occur (usually <38°C). Postauricular, suboccipital, and cervical lymph node adenopathy is common. Cold-like symptoms usually accompany the disease in the form of cough, congestion, and coryza (*i.e.,* nasal discharge).

Rubella usually has no long-lasting sequelae; however, the transmission of the disease to pregnant women early in their gestation periods may result in congenital rubella syndrome. Among the clinical signs of congenital rubella syndrome are cataracts, microcephaly, mental retardation, deafness, patent ductus arteriosus, glaucoma, purpura, and bone defects. Canada requires immunization to prevent transmission of rubella. Immunization is accomplished by live-virus injection. Rubella vaccination has close to a 100% immunity response in treated children.[70] Immunization includes a second preschool or later dose of rubella vaccine to increase immunity. Cases and outbreaks of rubella occur in Canada and the United States, especially among foreign-born unvaccinated adults.

FIGURE 61.37 • Rash of rubella on a child's back. Distribution is similar to measles (rubeola), but not as intense. (Centers for Disease Control and Prevention Public Health Image Library. Available online at: http://phil.cdc.gov/Phil/home.asp)

Rubeola. Rubeola (measles, red measles, 7-day measles) is an acute, highly communicable viral disease caused by a morbillivirus. The characteristic rash is macular and blotchy; sometimes the macules become confluent (Fig. 61.38). The rubeola rash usually begins on the face and spreads to the appendages. There are several accompanying symptoms: a fever of 38°C or greater, *Koplik spots* (*i.e.,* small, irregular red spots with a bluish-white speck in the centre) on the buccal mucosa, and mild to severe photosensitivity. The patient commonly has cold-like symptoms, general malaise, and myalgia. In severe cases, the macules may hemorrhage into the skin tissue or onto the outer body surface. This form is called *hemorrhagic measles*. The course of measles is more severe in infants, adults, and malnourished children. The World Health Organization recommends vitamin A treatment for measles in developing countries to reduce morbidity and mortality. There may be severe complications, including blindness, otitis media, pneumonia, and encephalitis. Antibody titres are determined for a conclusive diagnosis of rubeola.

Measles is a disease preventable by vaccine, and immunization is accomplished by the injection of a live-virus vaccine. Measles vaccination produces close to 100% immunity.[70] Outbreaks continue to occur in Canada and the United States because of the high infectivity of measles and the decreasing number of people completing the required immunizations. Ideally, at least 95% of the population needs to be immunized

FIGURE 61.38 • A: Child with measles (rubeola) showing the characteristic conjunctivitis, coryza, and red, blotchy rash that appear around day 3 of illness, first on the face and then becoming more generalized. **B:** Koplik spots (irregularly shaped, bright red spots often with a bluish-white central dot), indicative of the beginning onset of rubeola. (Centers for Disease Control and Prevention Public Health Image Library. Available online at: http://phil.cdc.gov/Phil/home.asp)

to develop herd or community immunity, which can provide some protection for infants, pregnant women, or immunocompromised individuals. The concern is if Canadians decline the measles vaccines, outbreak numbers will continue to increase.

Varicella. Varicella (chickenpox) is a common communicable childhood disease. It is caused by the varicella-zoster virus, which also is the agent in herpes zoster (shingles). The characteristic skin lesion occurs in three stages: macule, vesicle, and granular scab. The macular stage is characterized by development within hours of macules over the trunk, spreading to the limbs, buccal mucosa, scalp, axillae, upper respiratory tract, and conjunctiva (Fig. 61.39). During the second stage, the macules form vesicles with depressed centres. The vesicles break open and a scab forms during the third stage. Crops of lesions occur successively, so that all three forms of the lesion usually are visible by the third day of the illness.

Mild to extreme pruritus accompanies the lesions, which can lead to scratching and subsequent development of secondary bacterial infections. Chickenpox also is accompanied by cold-like symptoms, including cough, coryza, and sometimes photosensitivity. Mild febrile states usually occur, typically beginning 24 hours before lesion outbreak. Side effects, such as pneumonia, septic complications, and encephalitis, are rare.

Varicella in adults may be more severe, with a prolonged recovery rate and greater chances for development of varicella pneumonitis or encephalitis. Immunocompromised persons may experience a chronic, painful form of the infection.

In Canada, two doses of the live attenuated varicella vaccine are recommended to prevent the disease.[70] Outbreaks of mild cases of varicella, called *breakthrough varicella,* have occurred in vaccinated populations. The breakthrough infection is difficult to diagnose because the maculopapular rash does not have the classic sign of vesicles.

Skin Manifestations and Disorders in Older Adults

Older adults experience a variety of age-related skin disorders and exacerbations of earlier skin problems. Aging skin is

FIGURE 61.39 • Blister-like rash on the back of a person with varicella-zoster (*i.e.,* chickenpox). (Centers for Disease Control and Prevention Public Health Image Library. Available online at: http://phil.cdc.gov/Phil/home.asp)

believed to involve a complex process of actinic (solar) damage, normal aging, and hormonal influences. Actinic changes primarily involve increased occurrence of lesions on sun-exposed surfaces of the body.

Normal Age-Related Changes

Normal skin changes associated with aging are seen on areas of the body that have not been exposed to the sun. They include thinning of the dermis and the epidermis, diminution in subcutaneous tissue, a decrease and thickening of blood vessels, and a decrease in the number of melanocytes, Langerhans cells, and Merkel cells. The keratinocytes shrink, but the number of dead keratinized cells at the surface increases. This results in less padding and thinner skin, with colour and elasticity changes. The skin also loses its resistance to environmental and mechanical trauma. Tissue repair takes longer.

With aging, there is also less hair and nail growth, and there is permanent hair pigment loss. Hormonally, there is less sebaceous gland activity, although the glands in the facial skin may increase in size. Hair growth reduction also may be hormonally influenced. Although the reason is poorly understood, the skin in most older adults becomes dry, rough, scaly, and itchy. When there is no underlying pathologic process, it is called *senile pruritus*. Itching and dryness become worse during the winter, when the need for home heating lowers the humidity.

The aging of skin, however, is not just a manifestation of age itself. Most skin changes associated with older adults are the result of cumulative actinic or environmental damage. For example, the wrinkled, leathery look of aged skin, as well as odd scars and ecchymotic spots, are due to solar elastotic degenerative change.

Skin Lesions Common Among Older Adults

The most common skin lesions in older adults are skin tags, keratoses, lentigines, and vascular lesions. Most are actinic manifestations; they occur as a result of exposure to sun and weather over the years.

Skin Tags. Skin tags are soft, brown or flesh-coloured papules. They occur on any skin surface, but most frequently the neck, axilla, and intertriginous areas. They range in size from a pinhead to the size of a pea. Skin tags have the normal texture of the skin. They are benign and can be removed with scissors or electrodesiccation for cosmetic purposes.

Keratoses. A *keratosis* is a horny growth or an abnormal growth of the keratinocytes. A *seborrheic keratosis* (i.e., seborrheic wart) is a benign, sharply circumscribed, wart-like lesion that has a stuck-on appearance (Fig. 61.40). They vary in size up to several centimetres. They are usually round or oval, tan, brown, or black lesions. Less pigmented ones may appear yellow or pink. Keratoses can be found on the face or trunk, as a solitary lesion or sometimes by the hundreds. Seborrheic keratoses are benign, but they must be watched for changes in colour, texture, or size, which may indicate malignant transformation.

Actinic keratoses are the most common premalignant skin lesions that develop on sun-exposed areas. The lesions usually

FIGURE 61.40 • Large seborrheic keratoses on the hand of an 84-year-old woman. (From Hall B. J., Hall J. C. (2010). *Sauer's manual of skin diseases* (10th ed., p. 447). Philadelphia, PA: Lippincott Williams & Wilkins.)

are less than 1 cm in diameter and appear as dry, brown, scaly areas, often with a reddish tinge. Actinic keratoses often are multiple and more easily felt than seen (Fig. 61.41). They often are indistinguishable from squamous cell carcinoma without biopsy. Actinic keratoses may accumulate dense scale on the surface of the skin and become hyperkeratotic (*i.e.,* developing cutaneous growths of fingernail-type tissue that grow into horn-like appendages). This form is more prominent and palpable. Often, there is a weathered appearance to the surrounding skin. Slight changes, such as enlargement or ulceration, may indicate malignant transformation. There is controversy regarding the classification of actinic keratoses. Some believe them to be capable of converting to cancerous growths, some

FIGURE 61.41 • Multiple actinic keratoses of the face of an 80-year-old man. (Dermik Laboratories, Inc.) (From Hall B. J., Hall J. C. (2010). *Sauer's manual of skin diseases* (10th ed., p. 289). Philadelphia, PA: Lippincott Williams & Wilkins.)

believe them to be on a continuum of cancerous growth, and still others believe that actinic keratoses do not convert or progress to cancerous cells, but that they are actual early malignancies.[71] Actinic keratoses are removed with cryosurgery, electrodesiccation, or lasers. When surgery is not indicated they are treated with topical chemotherapy agents, like 5-fluorouracil or imiquimod creams, which erode the lesions.

Lentigines. A *lentigo* is a well-bordered, brown to black macule, usually less than 1 cm in diameter. *Solar lentigines* are tan to brown, benign spots on sun-exposed areas. Commonly referred to as *liver spots,* these lesions are considered risks for the development of skin cancers. Lentigines can be removed surgically (cryotherapy, laser therapy, liquid nitrogen). Topical creams and lotions containing adapalene or tretinoin have been used. Successful treatment depends on avoiding sun exposure and consistently using sunscreens.

Lentigo maligna (i.e., Hutchinson freckle) is a slowly progressive (≤20 years) preoplastic disorder of melanocytes. It occurs on sun-exposed areas, particularly the face. The lesion is a pigmented macule with a well-defined border and grows to 5 cm or sometimes larger. As it grows over the years, it may become slightly raised and wart-like. If untreated, a true malignant melanoma often develops. Surgery, curettage, and cryotherapy have been effective at removing the lentigines. Careful monitoring for conversion to melanoma is important.

Vascular Lesions. Vascular lesions include angiomas, telangiectases, and venous lakes. *Cherry angiomas* are smooth, cherry-red or purple, dome-shaped papules that occur in nearly all people older than 30 years of age. They usually are found on the trunk and are generally benign unless there is a sudden appearance of many cherry angiomas. *Telangiectases* are single dilated blood vessels, capillaries, or terminal arteries that appear on areas exposed to sun or harsh weather, such as the cheeks and the nose. They occur individually or in clusters, measure 1 cm or less, are nonpalpable, and easily blanch. They can become large and disfiguring. Pulsed dye lasers have been effective in removing them. *Venous lakes* are small, dark blue, slightly raised papules that have a lake-like appearance. They occur on exposed body parts, particularly the backs of the hands, ears, and lips. They are smooth and compressible. Venous lakes can be removed by electrosurgery, laser therapy, or surgical excision if a person desires.

IN SUMMARY

Some skin problems occur in specific age groups. Common in infants are diaper rash, prickly heat, and cradle cap. Infectious childhood diseases that are characterized by rashes include roseola infantum, rubella, rubeola, and varicella. Vaccines are available to protect against rubella, rubeola, and varicella.

With aging, there is thinning of the dermis and the epidermis, diminution in subcutaneous tissue, loss and thickening of

blood vessels, and slowing of hair and nail growth. Dry skin is common among older adults, becoming worse during the winter months. Among the skin lesions seen in older adults are skin tags, keratoses, lentigines, and vascular lesions.

REVIEW EXERCISES

1. The mother of a 7-year-old boy notices that he is scratching his head frequently. On close examination she notices a greyish, round, and roughened area, where the hair has broken off. Examination by the child's pediatrician produces a diagnosis of tinea capitis.
   A. *Explain the cause of the infection and propose possible mechanisms for spread of this infection in school-age children, particularly during winter months.*
   B. *Referring to Chapter 16, explain the preference of the superficial mycoses (dermatophytoses) for the skin-covered areas of the body.*
   C. *What methods are commonly used in the diagnosis of superficial fungal infections?*

2. A 75-year-old woman presents with severe burning pain and a vesicular rash covering a strip over the rib cage on one side of the chest. She is diagnosed with herpes zoster or shingles.
   A. *What is the source of this woman's rash and pain?*
   B. *Explain the dermatomal distribution of the lesions.*

3. Psoriasis is a chronically recurring papulosquamous skin disorder, characterized by circumscribed red, thickened plaques with an overlying silvery-white scale.
   A. *Explain the development of the plaques in terms of epidermal cell turnover.*
   B. *Persons with psoriasis are instructed to refrain from rubbing or scratching the lesions. Explain the rationale for these instructions.*
   C. *Among the methods used in the treatment of psoriasis are the use of topical keratolytic agents and corticosteroid skin preparations. Explain how these two different types of agents exert their effect on the plaque lesions.*

4. During the past several decades there has been an alarming increase in the incidence of skin cancers, including malignant melanoma, that has been attributed to increased sun exposure.
   A. *Explain the possible mechanisms whereby ultraviolet radiation promotes the development of malignant skin lesions.*
   B. *Cite two important clinical signs that aid in distinguishing a dysplastic nevus from a malignant melanoma.*

References

1. Burns T., Breathnach S., Cox N., et al. (2010). *Rook's textbook of dermatology: Volumes 1–4.* (8th ed.). Hoboken, NJ: Wiley-Blackwell.

2. Hall B. J., Hall J. C. (2010). *Sauer's manual of skin diseases.* (10th ed.). Philadelphia, PA: Lippincott Williams & Wilkins.

3. Alikhan A., Felsten L. M., Daly M., et al. (2011). Vitiligo: A comprehensive overview Part I. Introduction, epidemiology, quality of life, diagnosis, differential diagnosis, associations, histopathology, etiology, and work-up. *Journal of the American Academy of Dermatology, 65*(3), 473–491.

4. Anbar T. S., Hegazy R. A., Picardo M., Taieb A. (2014). Beyond vitiligo guidelines: Combined stratified/personalized approaches for the vitiligo patient. *Experimental Dermatology, 23*(4), 219–223.

5. Montoliu L., Gronskov K., Wei A. H., et al. (2014). Increasing the complexity: New genes and new types of albinism. *Pigment Cell & Melanoma Research, 27*(1), 11–18.

6. Levin A. V., Stroh E. (2011). Albinism for the busy clinician. *Journal of AAPOS, 15*(1), 59–66.

7. Sheth V. M., Pandya A. G. (2011). Melasma: A comprehensive update: Part I. *Journal of the American Academy of Dermatology, 65*(4), 689–697.

8. Sheth V. M., Pandya A. G. (2011). Melasma: A comprehensive update: Part II. *Journal of the American Academy of Dermatology, 65*(4), 699–714.

9. Kelly B. P. (2012). Superficial fungal infections. *Pediatrics in Review, 33*(4), e22–e37.

10. Moriarty B., Hay R., Morris-Jones R. (2012). The diagnosis and management of tinea. *British Medical Journal, 345*, e4390.

11. Nevas J. (2012). Tinea versicolor: Understanding effective treatment options. *Nurse Practitioner, 37*(1), 11–13.

12. Hartman-Adams H., Banvard C., Junkett G. (2014). Impetigo: diagnosis and treatment. *American Family Physician, 90*(4), 229–235.

13. Chan P. K., Picconi M. A., Cheung T. H., et al. (2012). Laboratory and clinical aspects of human papillomavirus testing. *Critical Reviews in Clinical Laboratory Sciences, 49*(4), 117–136.

14. Lynch M. D., Cliffe J., Morris-Jones R. (2014). Management of cutaneous viral warts. *British Medical Journal, 348*, e3339.

15. Yawn B. P., Gilden D. (2013). The global epidemiology of herpes zoster. *Neurology, 81*(10), 928–930.

16. Public Health Agency of Canada. (2014). Herpes Zoster (shingles) vaccine. Available online at: http://www.phac-aspc.gc.ca/publicat/cig-gci/p04-herp-zona-eng.php. Accessed March 11, 2015.

17. Williams H. C., Dellavalle R. P., Garner S. (2012). Acne vulgaris. *Lancet, 379*(9813), 361–372.

18. Titus S., Hodge J. (2012). Diagnosis and treatment of acne. *American Family Physician, 86*(8), 734–740.

19. Zaba R., Schwartz R. A., Jarmuda S., et al. (2010). Acne fulminans: Explosive systemic form of acne. *Journal of the European Academy of Dermatology and Venereology, 25*(5), 501–507.

20. Leyden J. L. (2013). Rosacea update: Advances from basic and clinical research. *Journal of the American Academy of Dermatology, 69*(Suppl 1), S1–S66.

21. Rather P. A., Hassan I. (2014). Human Demodex mite: The versatile mite of dermatological importance. *Indian Journal of Dermatology, 59*(1), 60–66.

22. Maddin W. S. (updated 2015). Skin Disorders: Rosacea. In Repchinsky C. (Ed.). *e-Therapeutics.* Ottawa, ON: Canadian Pharmacists Association.

23. Davis M. (2007). Top 10 causes of allergic contact dermatitis. *Allergy & Asthma Today, 5*(1), 44.

24. Rustemeyer T., van Hoogstraten I. M., von Blomberg B. M., et al. (2011). Mechanisms of irritant and allergic contact dermatitis. In Johansen J. D., Froasch P. J., Lepoittevin J. P. (Eds.). *Contact dermatitis* (5th ed.). Berlin: Springer.

25. Boguniewicz M., Leung D. Y. (2011). Atopic dermatitis: A disease of altered skin barrier and immune dysregulation. *Immunological Reviews, 242*(1), 233–246.

26. Williams H. C. (2005). Atopic dermatitis. *New England Journal of Medicine, 352*(22), 2314–2324.

27. Eichenfield L. F., Tom W. L., Berger T. G., et al. (2014). Guidelines of care for the management of atopic dermatitis: Section 2 Management and treatment with topical therapies. *Journal of the American Academy of Dermatology, 71*(1), 116–132.

28. Sidbury R., Davis D. M., Cohen D. E., et al; American Academy of Dermatology. (2014). Guidelines of care for the management of atopic dermatitis: Section 3 Management and treatment with phototherapy and systemic agents. *Journal of the American Academy of Dermatology, 71*(2), 327–349.

29. Schuerman G., Vezeau T. (2007) All bugs aren't bad: Probiotics in the treatment of pediatric atopic dermatitis. *American Journal for Nurse Practitioners, 11*(4), 28–36.

30. Sanchez-Borges M., Asero R., Ansotegui I. J., et al; WAO Scientific and Clinical Issues Council. (2012). Diagnosis and treatment of urticarial and angioedema: A worldwide perspective. *World Allergy Organization Journal, 5*(11), 125–147.

31. Sabroe R. A. (2014). Acute urticaria. *Immunology and Allergy Clinics of North America, 34*(1), 11–21.

32. Saini S. (2014). Chronic spontaneous urticaria. *Immunology and Allergy Clinics of North America, 34*(1), 33–52.

33. Abajian M., Schoepke N., Altrichter S., et al. (2014). Physical urticarias and cholinergic urticaria. *Immunology and Allergy Clinics of North America, 34*(1), 73–88.

34. Samim F., Zed C., Williams P. M. (2013). Erythema multiforme. *Dental Clinics of North America, 57*(4), 583–596.

35. Gerull R., Nelle M., Schaible T. (2011). Toxic epidermal necrolysis and Stevens-Johnson syndrome: A review. *Critical Care Medicine, 39*(6), 1521–1532.

36. Canadian Psoriasis Guidelines Committee. (2009). Canadian guidelines for the management of plaque psoriasis (1st ed.). Available online at: http://www.dermatology.ca/wp-content/uploads/2012/01/cdnpsoriasis-guidelines.pdf. Accessed March 11, 2015.

37. LeCleach L., Chosidow O. (2012). Lichen planus. *New England Journal Medicine, 366*(8), 723–732.

38. Golant A. K., Levitt J. O. (2012). Scabies: A review of diagnosis and management based on mite biology. *Pediatrics in Review, 33*(1), e1–e12.

39. Canadian Paediatric Society. (2014). Head lice infestations: A clinical update. Available online at: http://www.cps.ca/documents/position/head-lice. Accessed March 11, 2015.

40. Doggett S. L., Dwyer D. E., Penas P. F., et al. (2012). Bed bugs: Clinical relevance and control options. *Clinical Microbiology Reviews, 25*(1), 164–192.

41. Balk S. J. (2011). Technical report: Ultraviolet radiation, a hazard to children and adolescents. *Pediatrics, 127*(3), e791–e817.

42. Government of Canada. (2014). Sun safety basics. Available online at: http://healthycanadians.gc.ca/healthy-living-vie-saine/environment-environnement/sun-soleil/safety-protection-eng.php. Accessed March 11, 2015.

43. Environment Canada. (2015). Sun protection messages. Available online at: https://ec.gc.ca/uv/default.asp?lang=En&n=DCF1C20A-1. Accessed March 11, 2015.

44. Safe Kids Canada. (2006). Child & youth unintentional injury: 10 years in review. Available online at: http://www.mhp.gov.on.ca/en/prevention/injury-prevention/skc_injuries.pdf. Accessed March 11, 2015.

45. Lloyd E. C., Rodgers B. C., Michener M., Williams M. S. (2012). Outpatient burns: Prevention and care. *American Family Physician, 85*(1), 25–32.

46. Rex S. (2012). Burn injuries. *Current Opinion in Critical Care, 18*(6), 671–676.

47. Purdue G. F., Arnoldo B. D., Hunt J. L. (2011). Acute assessment and management of burn injuries. *Physical Medicine and Rehabilitation Clinics of North America, 22*(2), 201–212.

48. Kowalske K. J. (2011). Burn wound care. *Physical Medicine and Rehabilitation Clinics of North America, 22*(2), 213–227.

49. Latenser B. A. (2009). Critical care of the burn patient: The first 48 hours. *Critical Care Medicine, 37*(10), 2819–2826.

50. Dunne J. A., Rawlins J. M. (2014). Management of burns. *Surgery, 32*(9), 477–484.

51. Gillespie B. M., Chaboyer W. P., McInnes E., et al. (2012). Repositioning for pressure ulcer prevention in adults. *Cochrane Database of Systematic Reviews, 7*, Art No. CD009958.

52. Woodbury M. G., Houghton P. (2004). Prevalence of pressure ulcers in Canadian healthcare settings. *Ostomy Wound Management, 50*(10), 22–38.

53. Keast D. H., Pawslow N., Houghton P. E., et al. (2006). Best practice recommendations for the prevention and treatment of pressure ulcers: Update 2006. *Wound Care Canada, 4*(1), 31–43.

54. Agrawal K., Chauhan N. (2012). Pressure ulcers: Back to the basics. *Indian Journal of Plastic Surgery, 45*(2), 244–254.

55. Qaseem A., Humphrey L. L., Forciea M. A., et al; Clinical Guidelines Committee of the American College of Physicians. (2015). Treatment of pressure ulcers: A clinical practice guideline from the American College of Physicians. *Annals of Internal Medicine, 162*(5), 370–379.

56. Sibbald R. G., Goodman L., Norton L., et al. (2012). Prevention and treatment of pressure ulcers. *Skin Therapy Letter, 17*(8), 4–7.

57. Nicholaou V., Stratigos A. J. (2014). Emerging trend in the epidemiology of melanoma. *British Journal of Dermatology, 170*(1), 11–19.

58. Canadian Cancer Society's Advisory Committee (2014). *Canadian Cancer Statistics, 2014.* Toronto, ON: Canadian Cancer Society.

59. Canadian Cancer Society. (2015). Non-melanoma skin cancer. Available online at: https://www.cancer.ca/en/cancer-information/cancer-type/skin-non-melanoma/non-melanoma-skin-cancer/?region=on. Accessed March 11, 2015.

60. Balch C. M., Gershenwald J. E., Soong S. J., et al. (2009). Final version of 2009 AJCC melanoma staging and classification. *Journal of Clinical Oncology, 27*(36), 6199–6206.

61. Canadian Cancer Society. (2015). Melanoma. Available online at: https://www.cancer.ca/en/cancer-information/cancer-type/skin-melanoma/melanoma/?region=on. Accessed March 11, 2015.

62. Rigel D. S., Robinson J. K., Ross M., et al. (2011). *Cancer of the skin* (2nd ed.). New York, NY: Elsevier Saunders.

63. Macarthur C. J. (2006). Head and neck hemangiomas of infancy. *Current Opinion in Otolaryngology & Head and Neck Surgery, 14*(6), 397–405.

64. Morelli J. G. (2011). Chapter 642: Vascular disorders. In Kliegman R. M., Stanton B. F., St. Geme J. W., et al. (Eds.), *Nelson textbook of pediatrics* (19th ed.). Philadelphia, PA: Saunders Elsevier.

65. Chen T. S., Eichenfield L. F., Friedlander S. F. (2013). Infantile hemangiomas: An update on pathogenesis and therapy. *Pediatrics, 131*(1), 99–108.

66. Coughlin C. C., Eichenfield L. F., Frieden I. J. (2014). Diaper dermatitis: Clinical characteristics and differential diagnosis. *Pediatric Dermatology, 31*(Suppl 1), 19–24.

67. Klunk C., Domingues E., Wiss K. (2014). An update on diaper dermatitis. *Clinics in Dermatology, 32*(4), 477–487.

68. Clark-Greuel J. N., Helmes C. T., Laurence A., et al. (2014). Setting the record straight on diaper rash and disposable diapers. *Clinical Pediatrics (Phila), 53*(9), S23–S26.

69. Stone R. C., Micali G. A., Schwartz R. A. (2014). Roseola infantum and its causal human herpesviruses. *International Journal of Dermatology, 53*(4), 397–403.

70. Public Health Agency of Canada. (2015). Canadian Immunization Guide: Part 4, active vaccines. Available online at: http://www.phac-aspc.gc.ca/publicat/cig-gci/p04-eng.php. Accessed March 11, 2015.

71. Rosen T., Lebwohl M. G. (2013). Prevalence and awareness of actinic keratosis: Barriers and opportunities. *Journal of the American Academy of Dermatology, 68*(Suppl 1), S2–S9.

Visit thePoint **http://thePoint.lww.com for animations, journal articles, and more!**

Appendix A
Lab Values

TABLE A.1 PREFIXES DENOTING DECIMAL FACTORS

PREFIX	SYMBOL	FACTOR
mega	M	10^6
kilo	k	10^3
hecto	h	10^2
deci	d	10^{-1}
centi	c	10^{-2}
milli	m	10^{-3}
micro	μ	10^{-6}
nano	n	10^{-9}
pico	p	10^{-12}
femto	f	10^{-15}

TABLE A.2 HEMATOLOGY

TEST	SI UNITS (USED IN CANADA)	CONVENTIONAL UNITS (USED IN UNITED STATES)
Erythrocyte count (RBC count)	M. $4.2–5.4 \times 10^{12}$/L F. $3.6–5.0 \times 10^{12}$/L	M. $4.2–5.4 \times 10^6$/μL F. $3.6–5.0 \times 10^6$/μL
Hematocrit (Hct)	M. 0.40–0.50 F. 0.37–0.47	M. 40–50% F. 37–47%
Hemoglobin (Hb)	M. 140–165 g/L F. 120–150 g/L	M. 14.0–16.5 g/dL F. 12.0–15.0 g/dL
Mean corpuscular hemoglobin (MCH)	27–34 pg/cell	
Mean corpuscular hemoglobin concentration (MCHC)	310–350 g/L	31–35 g/dL
Mean corpuscular volume (MCV)	80–100 fL/cell	
Reticulocyte count	1.0–1.5% total RBC	
Platelet count	$150–400 \times 10^9$/L	$150–400 \times 10^3$/μL
Leukocyte count (WBC count)	$4.8–10.8 \times 10^9$/L	$4.8–10.8 \times 10^3$/μL
Basophils	0–2%	
Eosinophils	0–3%	
Lymphocytes	24–40%	
Monocytes	4–9%	
Neutrophils (segmented [Segs])	47–63%	
Neutrophils (bands)	0–4%	

TABLE A.3 BLOOD CHEMISTRY[a]

TEST	SI UNITS (USED IN CANADA)	CONVENTIONAL UNITS (USED IN UNITED STATES)
Alanine aminotransferase (ALT, SGPT)	7–56 units/L[b]	
Alkaline phosphatase	41–133 units/L[b,c]	
Ammonia	11–35 µmol/L	18–60 µg/dL
Amylase	20–110 units/L[b]	
Aspartase aminotransferase (AST, SGOT)	0–35 units/L[b]	
Bicarbonate	22–26 mmol/L	22–26 mEq/L
Bilirubin (total)	17.1–21 µmol/L	0.1–1.2 mg/dL
Direct	<8 µmol/L	0.1–0.5 mg/dL
Indirect	<12 µmol/L	0.1–0.7 mg/dL
Blood urea nitrogen (BUN)	2.9–7.1 mmol/L	8–20 mg/dL
Calcium (Ca^{2+})	2.1–2.6 mmol/L	8.5–10.5 mg/dL
Chloride	98–106 mmol/L	98–106 mEq/L
Creatine kinase (CK, CPK)	32–267 units/L[b]	
Creatine kinase (MB)	<16 IU/L[b] or 4% of total CK	
Creatinine (serum)	53–106 µmol/L[c]	0.6–1.2 mg/dL[c]
Gamma-glutamyl-transpeptidase (GGT)	9–85 units/L[b]	
Glucose (plasma, fasting)	<6.0 mmol/L	<100 mg/dL
Glycosylated hemoglobin (HbA_{1c})	0.039–0.069	3.9–6.9%
Lactate dehydrogenase (LDH)	88–230 units/L[b]	
Lipids		
LDL cholesterol (Primary prevention)	≤5.0 mmol/L (low risk)	<130 mg/dL
	≤3.5 mmol/L (moderate risk)	
	<2.0 mmol/L (high risk)	
Total cholesterol : HDL ratio	≤6.0 mmol/L (low risk)	
(secondary prevention)	≤5.0 mmol/L (moderate risk)	
	<4.0 mmol/L (high risk)	
HDL cholesterol	>1.0 mmol/L	Male: 35–65 mg/dL
	>1.3 mmol/L	Female: 35–80 mg/dL
Triglycerides	≤1.7 mmol/L (fasting)	<150 mg/dL
Lipase	0–160 units/L[b]	
Magnesium	0.70–1.25 mmol/L	1.8–3.0 mg/dL
Osmolality	275–295 mmol/kg	275–295 mOsm/kg
pH (arterial)	7.35–7.45	
Phosphorus (inorganic)	0.80–1.45 mmol/L	2.5–4.5 mg/dL
Potassium	3.5–5.0 mmol/L	3.5–5.0 mEq/L
Prostate specific antigen (PSA)	0–4 µg/L	0–4 ng/mL
Protein total	60–80 g/L	6.0–8.0 g/L
Albumin	34–47 g/L	3.4–4.7 g/L
Globulin	23–35 g/L	2.3–3.5 g/L
A/G ratio	1.0–2.2	1.0–2.2
Thyroid tests		
Thyroxine (T_4) total	64–142 nmol/L	5.0–11.0 µg/dL
Thyroxine, free (FT_4)	9–24 pmol/L[b]	
Triiodothyronine (T_3) total	1.5–2.9 nmol/L	95–190 ng/dL
Thyroid-stimulating hormone (TSH)	0.4–4.2 mU/L	0.4–4.2 µU/mL
Thyroglobin	3–42 µg/L	3–42 ng/mL
Sodium	135–145 mmol/L	135–145 mEq/L
Uric acid	Male: 140–440 µmol/L	Male: 2.4–7.4 mg/dL
	Female: 80–350 µmol/L	Female: 1.4–5.8 mg/dL

[a]Values may vary with laboratory. The values supplied by the laboratory performing the test should always be used since the ranges may be method specific.

[b]Laboratory and/or method specific.

[c]Varies with age and muscle mass.

Values obtained from Tierney L. M., McPhee S. J., Papadakis M. A. (2007). *Current medical diagnosis and treatment* (46th ed., pp. 1769–1777). Stamford, CT: Appleton & Lange; Fischbach F. (2004). *A manual of laboratory and diagnostic tests* (7th ed.). Philadelphia: Lippincott Williams & Wilkins; and other sources.

Internet Sites

LRC Hamilton and Hamilton Regional Laboratory Medicine Program (HRLMP) http://www.lrc.hrlmp.ca/AttachedFiles/LRC_All_Tests.pdf

Labquest: Biochemistry Unit Conversion (site has calculator and conversion table for common laboratory tests) http://www.vin.com/calculators/ChemConvCalc.htm

Glossary

Abduction The act of abducting (moving or spreading away from a position near the midline of the body or the axial line of a limb) or the state of being abducted.

Abrasion The wearing or scraping away of a substance or structure, such as the skin, through an unusual or abnormal mechanical process.

Abscess A collection of pus that is restricted to a specific area in tissues, organs, or confined spaces.

Accommodation The adjustment of the lens (eye) to variations in distance.

Acromion The lateral extension of the spine of the scapula, forming the highest point of the shoulder. (Adjective: acromial)

Acuity The clearness or sharpness of perception, especially of vision.

Adaptation The adjustment of an organism to its environment, physical or psychological, through changes and responses to stress of any kind.

Adduction The act of adducting (moving or drawing toward a position near the midline of the body or the axial line of a limb) or the state of being adducted.

Adhesin The molecular components of the bacterial cell wall that are involved in adhesion processes.

Adrenergic Activated by or characteristic of the sympathetic nervous system or its neurotransmitters (*i.e.,* epinephrine and norepinephrine).

Aerobic Growing, living, or occurring only in the presence of air or oxygen.

Afferent Bearing or conducting inward or toward a centre, as an afferent neuron.

Agglutination The clumping together of particles, microorganisms, or blood cells in response to an antigen–antibody reaction.

Agonist A muscle whose action is opposed by another muscle (antagonist) with which it is paired; or a drug or other chemical substance that has affinity for or stimulates a predictable physiologic function.

Akinesia An abnormal state in which there is an absence or poverty of movement.

Allele One of two or more different forms of a gene that can occupy a particular locus on a chromosome.

Alveolus A small saclike structure, as in the alveolus of the lung.

Amblyopia A condition of vision impairment without a detectable organic lesion of the eye.

Amine An organic compound containing nitrogen.

Amorphous Without a definite form; shapeless.

Amphoteric Capable of reacting chemically as an acid or a base.

Ampulla A saclike dilation of a duct, canal, or any other tubular structure.

Anabolism A constructive metabolic process characterized by the conversion of simple substances into larger, complex molecules.

Anaerobic Growing, living, or occurring only in the absence of air or oxygen.

Analog A part, organ, or chemical having the same function or appearance but differing in respect to a certain component, such as origin or development.

Anaplasia A change in the structure of cells and in their orientation to each other that is characterized by a loss of cell differentiation, as in cancerous cell growth.

Anastomosis The connection or joining between two vessels; or an opening created by surgical, traumatic, or pathologic means.

Androgen Any substance, such as a male sex hormone, that increases male characteristics.

Anergy A state of absent or diminished reaction to an antigen or group of antigens.

Aneuploidy A variation in the number of chromosomes within a cell involving one or more missing chromosomes rather than entire sets.

Aneurysm An outpouching or dilation in the wall of a blood vessel or the heart.

Ankylosis Stiffness or fixation of separate bones of a joint, resulting from disease, injury, or surgical procedure. (Verb: to ankylose)

Anorexia Lack or loss of appetite for food. (Adjective: anorexic)

Anoxia An abnormal condition characterized by the total lack of oxygen.

Antagonist A muscle whose action directly opposes that of another muscle (agonist) with which it is paired; or a drug or other chemical substance that can diminish or nullify the action of a neuromediator or body function.

Anterior Pertaining to a surface or part that is situated near or toward the front.

Antigen A substance that generates an immune response by causing the formation of an antibody or reacting with antibodies or T-cell receptors.

Apex The uppermost point, the narrowed or pointed end, or the highest point of a structure, such as an organ.

Aphagia A condition characterized by the refusal or the loss of ability to swallow.

Aplasia The absence of an organ or tissue due to a developmental failure.

Apnea The absence of spontaneous respiration.

Apoptosis A mechanism of programmed cell death, marked by shrinkage of the cell, condensation of chromatin, formation of cytoplasmic blebs, and fragmentation of the cell into membrane-bound bodies eliminated by phagocytosis.

Apraxia Loss of the ability to carry out familiar, purposeful acts or to manipulate objects in the absence of paralysis or other motor or sensory impairment.

Articulation The place of connection or junction between two or more bones of a skeletal joint.

Ascites An abnormal accumulation of serous fluid in the peritoneal cavity.

Asepsis The condition of being free of or freed from pathogenic microorganisms.

Astereognosis A neurologic disorder characterized by an inability to identify objects by touch.

Asterixis A motor disturbance characterized by a hand-flapping tremor, which results when the prolonged contraction of groups of muscles lapses intermittently.

Ataxia An abnormal condition characterized by an inability to coordinate voluntary muscular movement.

Athetosis A neuromuscular condition characterized by the continuous occurrence of slow, sinuous, writhing movements that are performed involuntarily. (Adjective: athetoid)

Atopy Genetic predisposition toward the development of a hypersensitivity or an allergic reaction to common environmental allergens.

Atresia The absence or closure of a normal body orifice or tubular organ, such as the esophagus.

Atrophy A wasting or diminution of size, often accompanied by a decrease in function, of a cell, tissue, or organ.

Autocrine A mode of hormone action in which a chemical messenger acts on the same cell that secretes it.

Autophagy Segregation of part of the cell's own damaged cytoplasmic material within a vacuole and its disposal.

Autosome Any chromosome other than a sex chromosome.

Axillary Of or pertaining to the axilla, or armpit.

Bacteremia The presence of bacteria in the blood.

Bactericide An agent that destroys bacteria. (Adjective: bactericidal)

Bacteriostat An agent that inhibits bacterial growth. (Adjective: bacteriostatic)

Ballismus An abnormal condition characterized by violent flailing motions of the arms and, occasionally, the head, resulting from injury to or destruction of the subthalamic nucleus or its fibre connections.

Baroreceptor A type of sensory nerve ending such as those found in the aorta and the carotid sinus that is stimulated by changes in pressure.

Basal Pertaining to, situated at, or forming the base; or the fundamental or the basic.

Benign Not malignant; or of the character that does not threaten health or life.

Bipolar neuron A nerve cell that has a process at each end—an afferent process and an efferent process.

Bolus A rounded mass of food ready to swallow or such a mass passing through the gastrointestinal tract; or a concentrated mass of medicinal material or other pharmaceutical preparation injected all at once intravenously for diagnostic purposes.

Borborygmus The rumbling, gurgling, or tinkling noise produced by the propulsion of gas through the intestine.

Bruit A sound or murmur heard while auscultating an organ or blood vessel, especially an abnormal one.

Buccal Pertaining to or directed toward the inside of the cheek.

Buffer A substance or group of substances that prevents change in the concentration of another chemical substance.

Bulla A thin-walled blister of the skin or mucous membranes greater than 5 mm in diameter containing serous or seropurulent fluid.

Bursa A fluid-filled sac or saclike cavity situated in places in the tissues at which friction would otherwise develop, such as between certain tendons and the bones beneath them.

Cachexia A condition of general ill health and malnutrition, marked by weakness and emaciation.

Calculus A stony mass formed within body tissues, usually composed of mineral salts.

Capsid The protein shell that envelops and protects the nucleic acid of a virus.

Carcinogen Any substance or agent that causes the development or increases the incidence of cancer.

Carpal Of or pertaining to the carpus, or wrist.

Caseation A form of tissue necrosis in which the tissue is changed into a dry, amorphous mass resembling crumbly cheese.

Catabolism A metabolic process through which living organisms break down complex substances to simple compounds, liberating energy for use in work, energy storage, or heat production.

Catalyst A substance that increases the velocity of a chemical reaction without being consumed by the process.

Catecholamines Any one of a group of biogenic amines having a sympathomimetic action and composed of a catechol molecule and the aliphatic portion of an amine.

Caudal Signifying an inferior position, toward the distal end of the spine.

Cellulitis An acute, diffuse, spreading, edematous inflammation of the deep subcutaneous tissues and sometimes muscle, characterized most commonly by an area of heat, redness, pain, and swelling, and occasionally by fever, malaise, chills, and headache.

Cephalic Of or pertaining to the head, or to the head end of the body.

Cerumen The waxlike secretion produced by vestigial apocrine sweat glands in the external ear canal.

Cheilosis A noninflammatory disorder of the lips and mouth characterized by chapping and fissuring.

Chelate A chemical compound composed of a central metal ion and an organic molecule with multiple bonds, arranged in ring formation, used especially in treatment of metal poisoning.

Chemoreceptor A sensory nerve cell activated by chemical stimuli, as a chemoreceptor in the carotid artery that is sensitive to changes in the oxygen content in the blood and reflexly increases or decreases respiration and blood pressure.

Chemotaxis A response involving cell orientation or cell movement that is either toward (positive chemotaxis) or away from (negative chemotaxis) a chemical stimulus.

Chimeric Relating to, derived from, or being an individual possessing one's own immunologic characteristics and that of another individual; a phenomenon that can occur as the result of procedures such as a bone marrow graft.

Chondrocyte Any one of the mature polymorphic cells that form the cartilage of the body.

Chromatid One of the paired threadlike chromosome filaments, joined at the centromere, that make up a metaphase chromosome.

Chromosome Any one of the structures in the nucleus of a cell containing a linear thread of DNA, which functions in the transmission of genetic information.

Chyme The creamy, viscous, semifluid material produced during digestion of a meal that is expelled by the stomach into the duodenum.

Cilia A minute, hairlike process projecting from a cell, composed of nine microtubules arrayed around a single pair. Cilia beat rhythmically to move the cell around in its environment or they move mucus or fluids over the surface.

Circadian Being, having, pertaining to, or occurring in a period or cycle of approximately 24 hours.

Circumduction The active or passive circular movement of a limb or of the eye.

Cisterna An enclosed space, such as a cavity, that serves as a reservoir for lymph or other body fluids.

Clone One or a group of genetically identical cells or organisms derived from a single parent.

Coagulation The process of transforming a liquid into a semisolid mass, especially of blood clot formation.

Coarctation A condition of stricture or contraction of the walls of a vessel.

Cofactor A substance that must unite with another substance in order to function.

Colic Sharp, intermittent abdominal pain localized in a hollow or tubular organ, resulting from torsion, obstruction, or smooth muscle spasm. (Adjective: colicky)

Collagen The protein substance of the white, glistening, inelastic fibres of the skin, tendons, bone, cartilage, and all other connective tissue.

Collateral Secondary or accessory rather than direct or immediate; or a small branch, as of a blood vessel or nerve.

Complement Any one of the complex, enzymatic serum proteins that are involved in physiologic reactions, including antigen–antibody reaction and anaphylaxis.

Confluent Flowing or coming together; not discrete.

Congenital Present at, and usually before, birth.

Conjugate To pair and fuse in conjugation; or a form of sexual reproduction seen in unicellular organisms in which genetic material is exchanged during the temporary fusion of two cells.

Contiguous In contact or nearly so in an unbroken sequence along a boundary or at a point.

Contralateral Affecting, pertaining to, or originating in the opposite side of a point or reference.

Contusion An injury of a part without a break in the skin, characterized by swelling, discolouration, and pain.

Convolution An elevation or tortuous winding, such as one of the irregular ridges on the surface of the brain, formed by a structure being infolded upon itself.

Corpuscle Any small mass, cell, or body, such as a red or white blood cell.

Costal Pertaining to a rib or ribs.

Crepitus A sound or sensation that resembles a crackling or grating noise.

Cutaneous Pertaining to the skin.

Cyanosis A bluish discolouration, especially of the skin and mucous membranes, caused by an excess of deoxygenated hemoglobin in the blood.

Cytokine Any of a class of polypeptide immunoregulatory substances that are secreted by cells, usually of the immune system, that affect other cells.

Cytology The study of cells, including their origin, structure, function, and pathology.

Cytosol Cytoplasm exclusive of membranous components (*e.g.,* mitochondria, endoplasmic reticulum) and nonmembranous insoluble components.

Decibel A unit for expressing the relative power intensity of electric or acoustic signal power that is equal to one tenth of a bel.

Defecation The evacuation of feces from the digestive tract through the rectum.

Deformation The process of adapting in form or shape; also the product of such alteration.

Degeneration The deterioration of a normal cell, tissue, or organ to a less functionally active form. (Adjective: degenerative)

Deglutition The act or process of swallowing.

Degradation The reduction of a chemical compound to a compound less complex, usually by splitting off one or more groups.

Dehydration The condition that results from excessive loss of water from the body tissues.

Delirium An acute, reversible organic mental syndrome characterized by confusion, disorientation, restlessness, incoherence, fear, and often illusions.

Dendrite One of the branching processes that extends and transmits impulses toward a cell body of a neuron. (Adjective: dendritic)

Depolarization The reduction of a cell membrane potential to a less negative value than that of the potential outside the cell.

Dermatome The area of the skin supplied with afferent nerve fibres of a single dorsal root of a spinal nerve.

Desmosome A small, circular, dense area within the intercellular bridge that forms the site of adhesion between intermediate filaments and cell membranes.

Desquamation A normal process in which the cornified layer of the epidermis is shed in fine scales or sheets.

Dialysis The process of separating colloids and crystalline substances in solution, which involves the two distinct physical processes of diffusion and ultrafiltration; or a medical procedure for the removal of urea and other elements from the blood or lymph.

Diapedesis The outward passage of red or white blood corpuscles through the intact walls of the vessels.

Diaphoresis Perspiration, especially the profuse perspiration associated with an elevated body temperature, physical exertion, exposure to heat, and mental or emotional stress.

Diarthrosis A specialized articulation that permits, to some extent, free joint movement. (Adjective: diarthrodial)

Diastole The dilation of the heart; or the period of dilation, which is the interval between the second and the first heart sound and is the time during which blood enters the relaxed chambers of the heart from the systemic circulation and the lungs.

Differentiation The act or process of development in which unspecialized cells or tissues acquire more specialized characteristics, including those of physical form, physiologic function, and chemical properties.

Diffusion The process of becoming widely spread, as in the spontaneous movement of molecules or other particles in solution from an area of higher concentration to an area of lower concentration, resulting in an even distribution of the particles in the fluid.

Dimer A compound or unit formed by the combination of two identical molecules or radicals of a simpler compound. (Adjective: dimeric)

Diopter A unit of measurement of the refractive power of lenses equal to the reciprocal of the focal length in metres.

Diploid Pertaining to an individual, organism, strain, or cell that has two full sets of homologous chromosomes.

Disseminate To scatter or distribute over a considerable area.

Distal Away from or being the farthest from a point of reference.

Diurnal Of, relating to, or occurring in the daytime.

Diverticulum A pouch or sac of variable size occurring naturally or through herniation of the muscular wall of a tubular organ.

Dorsum The back or posterior. (Adjective: dorsal)

Dysgenesis Defective or abnormal development of an organ or part, typically occurring during embryonic development. (Also called dysgenesia.)

Dyslexia A disturbance in the ability to read, spell, and write words.

Dyspepsia The impairment of the power or function of digestion, especially epigastric discomfort following eating.

Dysphagia A difficulty in swallowing.

Dysphonia Any impairment of the voice that is experienced as a difficulty in speaking.

Dysplasia The alteration in size, shape, and organization of adult cell types.

Eburnation The conversion of bone or cartilage, through thinning or loss, into a hard and dense mass with a worn, polished, ivory-like surface.

Ecchymosis A small hemorrhagic spot, larger than a petechia, in the skin or mucous membrane caused by the extravasation of blood into the subcutaneous tissues.

Ectoderm The outermost of the three primary germ layers of the embryo, and from which the epidermis and epidermal tissues, such as nails, hair, and glands of the skin, develop.

Ectopic Relating to or characterized by an object or organ being situated in an unusual place, away from its normal location.

Edema The presence of an abnormal accumulation of fluid in interstitial spaces of tissues. (Adjective: edematous)

Efferent Conveyed or directed away from a centre.

Effusion The escape of fluid from blood vessels into a part or tissue, as an exudation or a transudation.

Embolus A mass of clotted blood or other formed elements, such as bubbles of air, calcium fragments, or a bit of tissue or tumour, that circulates in the bloodstream until it becomes lodged in a vessel, obstructing the circulation. (Plural: emboli)

Empyema An accumulation of pus in a cavity of the body, especially the pleural space.

Emulsify To disperse one liquid throughout the body of another liquid, making a colloidal suspension, or emulsion.

Endocytosis The uptake or incorporation of substances into a cell by invagination of its plasma membrane, as in the processes of phagocytosis and pinocytosis.

Endoderm The innermost of the three primary germ layers of the embryo, and from which epithelium arises.

Endogenous Growing within the body; or developing or originating from within the body; or produced by internal causes.

Endoscopy The visualization of any cavity of the body with an endoscope.

Enteropathic Relating to any disease of the intestinal tract.

Enzyme A protein molecule produced by living cells that catalyzes chemical reactions of other organic substances without itself being destroyed or altered.

Epiphysis The expanded articular end of a long bone (head) that is separated from the shaft of the bone by the epiphyseal plate until the bone stops growing, the plate is obliterated, and the shaft and the head become united.

Epithelium The covering of the internal and the external surfaces of the body, including the lining of vessels and other small cavities.

Epitope The simplest form of an antigenic determinant that combines with an antibody or a T-cell receptor to cause a specific reaction by an immunoglobulin.

Erectile Capable of being erected or raised to an erect position.

Erythema The redness or inflammation of the skin or mucous membranes produced by the congestion of superficial capillaries. (Adjective: erythematous)

Etiology The study or theory of all factors that may be involved in the development of a disease, including susceptibility of an individual, the nature of the disease agent, and the way in which an individual's body is invaded by the agent; or the cause of a disease.

Eukaryotic Pertaining to an organism with cells having a true nucleus; that is, a highly complex, organized nucleus surrounded by a nuclear membrane containing organelles and exhibiting mitosis.

Euploid Pertaining to an individual, organism, strain, or cell with a balanced set or sets of chromosomes, in any number, that is an exact multiple of the normal, basic haploid number characteristic of the species; or such an individual, organism, strain, or cell.

Evisceration The removal of the viscera from the abdominal cavity, or disembowelment; or the extrusion of an internal organ through a wound or surgical incision.

Exacerbation An increase in the severity of a disease as marked by greater intensity in any of its signs and symptoms.

Exfoliation Peeling and sloughing off of tissue cells in scales or layers. (Adjective: exfoliative)

Exocytosis The discharge of cell particles, which are packaged in membrane-bound vesicles, by fusion of the vesicular membrane with the plasma membrane and subsequent release of the particles to the exterior of the cell.

Exogenous Developed or originating outside the body, as a disease caused by a bacterial or viral agent foreign to the body.

Exophthalmos A marked or abnormal protrusion of the eyeball.

Extension A movement that allows the two elements of any jointed part to be drawn apart, increasing the angle between them, as extending the leg increases the angle between the femur and the tibia.

Extrapyramidal Pertaining to motor systems supplied by fibres outside the corticospinal or pyramidal tracts.

Extravasation A discharge or escape, usually of blood, serum, or lymph, from a vessel into the tissues.

Extubation The process of withdrawing a previously inserted tube from an orifice or cavity of the body.

Exudate Fluid, cells, or other substances that have been slowly exuded or have escaped from blood vessels and have been deposited in tissues or on tissue surfaces.

Fascia A sheet or band of fibrous connective tissue that may be separated from other specifically organized structures, as the tendons, the aponeuroses, and the ligaments.

Febrile Pertaining to or characterized by an elevated body temperature, or fever.

Fibrillation A small, local, involuntary contraction of muscle, resulting from spontaneous activation of a single muscle fibre or of an isolated bundle of nerve fibres.

Fibrin A stringy, insoluble protein formed by the action of thrombin on fibrinogen during the clotting process.

Fibrosis The formation of fibrous connective tissue, as in the repair or replacement of parenchymatous elements.

Filtration The process of passing a liquid through or as if through a filter, which is accomplished by gravity, pressure, or vacuum.

Fimbria Any structure that forms a fringe, border, or edge or the processes that resemble such a structure.

Fissure A cleft or a groove, normal or otherwise, on the surface of an organ or a bony structure.

Fistula An abnormal passage or communication from an internal organ to the body surface or between two internal organs.

Flaccid Weak, soft, and lax; lacking normal muscle tone.

Flatus Air or gas in the intestinal tract that is expelled through the anus. (Adjective: flatulent)

Flexion A movement that allows the two elements of any jointed part to be brought together, decreasing the angle between them, as bending the elbow.

Flora The microorganisms, such as bacteria and fungi, both normally occurring and pathologic, found in or on an organ.

Focal Relating to, having, or occupying a focus.

Follicle A sac or pouchlike depression or cavity.

Fontanelle A membrane-covered opening in bones or between bones, such as the soft spot covered by tough membranes between the bones of an infant's incompletely ossified skull.

Foramen A natural opening or aperture in a membranous structure or bone.

Fossa A hollow or depressed area, especially on the surface of the end of a bone.

Fovea A small pit or depression in the surface of a structure or an organ.

Fundus The base or bottom of an organ or the portion farthest from the mouth of an organ.

Ganglion One of the nerve cell bodies, chiefly collected in groups outside the central nervous system. (Plural: ganglia)

Genotype The entire genetic constitution of an individual, as determined by the particular combination and location of the genes on the chromosomes; or the alleles present at one or more sites on homologous chromosomes.

Glia The neuroglia, or supporting structure of nervous tissue.

Globulin One of a broad group of proteins classified by solubility, electrophoretic mobility, and size.

Gluconeogenesis The formation of glucose from any of the substances of glycolysis other than carbohydrates.

Glycolysis A series of enzymatically catalyzed reactions, occurring within cells, by which glucose is converted to adenosine triphosphate (ATP) and pyruvic acid during aerobic metabolism.

Gonad A gamete-producing gland, as an ovary or a testis.

Gradient The rate of increase or decrease of a measurable phenomenon expressed as a function of a second; or the visual representation of such a change.

Granuloma A small mass of nodular granulation tissue resulting from chronic inflammation, injury, or infection. (Adjective: granulomatous)

Hapten A small, nonproteinaceous substance that is not antigenic by itself but that can act as an antigen when combined with a larger molecule.

Haustrum A structure resembling a recess or sacculation. (Plural: haustra)

Hematoma A localized collection of extravasated blood trapped in an organ, space, or tissue, resulting from a break in the wall of a blood vessel.

Hematopoiesis The normal formation and development of blood cells.

Hemianopia Defective vision or blindness in half of the visual field of one or both eyes.

Heterogeneous Consisting of or composed of dissimilar elements or parts; or not having a uniform quality throughout. (Noun: heterogeneity)

Heterophagy The taking into the cell of an exogenous substance by phagocytosis or pinocytosis and the subsequent digestion of the newly formed vacuole by a lysosome.

Heterozygous Having two different alleles at corresponding loci on homologous chromosomes.

Histology The branch of anatomy that deals with the minute (microscopic) structure, composition, and function of cells and tissue. (Adjective: histologic)

Homolog Any organ or part corresponding in function, position, origin, and structure to another organ or part,

as the flippers of a seal that correspond to human hands. (Adjective: homologous)

Homozygous Having two identical alleles at corresponding loci on homologous chromosomes.

Humoral Relating to elements dissolved in the blood or body fluids.

Hybridoma A tumour of hybrid cells produced by fusion of normal lymphocytes and tumour cells.

Hydrolysis The chemical alteration or decomposition of a compound into fragments by the addition of water.

Hypercapnia Excess amounts of carbon dioxide in the blood.

Hyperemia An excess or engorgement of blood in a part of the body.

Hyperesthesia An unusual or pathologic increase in sensitivity of a part, especially the skin, or of a particular sense.

Hyperplasia An abnormal multiplication or increase in the number of normal cells of a body part.

Hypertonic A solution having a greater concentration of solute than another solution with which it is compared, hence exerting more osmotic pressure than that solution.

Hypertrophy The enlargement or overgrowth of an organ due to an increase in the size of its cells rather than the number of its cells.

Hypesthesia An abnormal decrease of sensation in response to stimulation of the sensory nerves. (Also called hypoesthesia.)

Hypocapnia A deficiency of carbon dioxide in the blood.

Hypotonic A solution having a lesser concentration of solute than another solution with which it is compared, hence exerting less osmotic pressure than that solution.

Hypoxemia An inadequate level of oxygen (PO_2) in the blood.

Hypoxia An inadequate amount of oxygen within the cells or tissues, which may result from either ischemia or hypoxemia.

Iatrogenic Induced inadvertently through the activity of a physician or by medical treatment or diagnostic procedures.

Idiopathic Arising spontaneously or from an unknown cause.

Idiosyncrasy A physical or behavioural characteristic or manner that is unique to an individual or to a group. (Adjective: idiosyncratic)

Incidence The rate at which a certain event occurs (*e.g.*, the number of new cases of a specific disease during a particular period of time in a population at risk).

Inclusion The act of enclosing or the condition of being enclosed; or anything that is enclosed.

Indigenous Native, or natural, to the particular country or region where found.

Infarction Necrosis or death of tissues due to local ischemia resulting from obstruction of blood flow.

Inotropic Influencing the force or energy of muscular contractions.

In situ In the natural or normal place; or something, such as cancer, that is confined to its place of origin and has not invaded neighbouring tissues.

Interferon Any one of a group of small glycoproteins (cytokines) produced in response to viral infection and which inhibit viral replication.

Interleukin Any of several multifunctional cytokines produced by a variety of lymphoid and nonlymphoid cells, including immune cells, that stimulate or otherwise affect the function of lympopoietic and other cells and systems in the body.

Interstitial Relating to or situated between parts or in the interspaces of a tissue.

Intramural Situated or occurring within the wall of an organ.

Intrinsic Pertaining exclusively to a part or situated entirely within an organ or tissue.

In vitro A biologic reaction occurring in an artificial environment, such as a test tube.

In vivo A biologic reaction occurring within the living body.

Involution The act or instance of enfolding, entangling, or turning inward.

Ionize To separate or change into ions.

Ipsilateral Situated on, pertaining to, or affecting the same side of the body.

Ischemia Decreased blood supply to a body organ or part, usually due to functional constriction or actual obstruction of a blood vessel.

Juxta-articular Situated near a joint or in the region of a joint.

Juxtaglomerular Near to or adjoining a glomerulus of the kidney.

Karyotype The total chromosomal characteristics of a cell; or the micrograph of chromosomes arranged in pairs in descending order of size.

Keratin A fibrous, sulphur-containing protein that is the primary component of the epidermis, hair, and horny tissues. (Adjective: keratinous)

Keratosis Any skin condition in which there is overgrowth and thickening of the cornified epithelium.

Ketosis A condition characterized by the abnormal accumulation of ketones (organic compounds with a carboxyl group attached to two carbon atoms) in the body tissues and fluid.

Kinesthesia The sense of movement, weight, tension, and position of body parts mediated by input from joint and muscle receptors and hair cells. (Adjective: kinesthetic)

Kyphosis An abnormal condition of the vertebral column, characterized by increased convexity in the curvature of the thoracic spine as viewed from the side.

Lacuna A small pit or cavity within a structure, especially bony tissue; or a defect or gap, as in the field of vision.

Lateral A position farther from the median plane or midline of the body or a structure; or situated on, coming from, or directed towards the side.

Lesion Any wound, injury, or pathologic change in body tissue.

Lethargy The lowered level of consciousness characterized by listlessness, drowsiness, and apathy; or a state of indifference.

Ligament One of many predominantly white, shiny, flexible bands of fibrous tissue that binds joints together and connects bones or cartilages.

Ligand A group, ion, or molecule that binds to the central atom or molecule in a chemical complex.

Lipid Any of the group of fats and fatlike substances characterized by being insoluble in water and soluble in nonpolar organic solvents, such as chloroform and ether.

Lipoprotein Any one of the conjugated proteins that is a complex of protein and lipid.

Lobule A small lobe.

Lordosis The anterior concavity in the curvature of the lumbar and cervical spine as observed from the side.

Lumen A cavity or the channel within a tube or tubular organ of the body.

Luteal Of or pertaining to or having the properties of the corpus luteum.

Lysis Destruction or dissolution of a cell or molecule through the action of a specific agent.

Maceration Softening of tissue by soaking, especially in acidic solutions.

Macroscopic Large enough to be visible with the unaided eye or without a microscope.

Macula A small, flat blemish, thickening, or discolouration that is flush with the skin surface. (Adjective: macular)

Malaise A vague feeling of bodily fatigue and discomfort.

Manometry The measurement of tension or pressure of a liquid or gas using a device called a manometer.

Marasmus A condition of extreme protein-calorie malnutrition that is characterized by growth retardation and progressive wasting of subcutaneous tissue and muscle and occurs chiefly during the first year of life.

Matrix The intracellular substance of a tissue or the basic substance from which a specific organ or kind of tissue develops.

Meatus An opening or passage through any body part.

Medial Pertaining to the middle; or situated or oriented toward the midline of the body.

Mediastinum The mass of tissues and organs in the middle of the thorax, separating the pleural sacs containing the two lungs.

Meiosis The division of a sex cell as it matures, so that each daughter nucleus receives one half of the number of chromosomes characteristic of the somatic cells of the species.

Mesoderm The middle layer of the three primary germ layers of the developing embryo, lying between the ectoderm and the endoderm.

Metabolism The sum of all the physical and chemical processes by which living organisms are produced and maintained, and also the transformation by which energy is provided for vital processes and activities.

Metaplasia Change in type of adult cells in a tissue to a form that is not normal for that tissue.

Metastasis The transfer of disease (*e.g.,* cancer) from one organ or part to another not directly connected with it. (Adjective: metastatic)

Miosis Contraction of the pupil of the eye.

Mitosis A type of indirect cell division that occurs in somatic cells and results in the formation of two daughter nuclei containing the identical complements of the number of chromosomes characteristic of the somatic cells of the species.

Molecule The smallest mass of matter that exhibits the properties of an element or compound.

Morbidity A diseased condition or state; the relative incidence of a disease or of all diseases in a population.

Morphology The study of the physical form and structure of an organism; or the form and structure of a particular organism. (Adjective: morphologic)

Mosaicism In genetics, the presence in an individual or in an organism of cell cultures having two or more cell lines that differ in genetic constitution but are derived from a single zygote.

Mutagen Any chemical or physical agent that induces a genetic mutation (an unusual change in form, quality, or some other characteristic) or increases the mutation rate by causing changes in DNA.

Mydriasis Physiologic dilation of the pupil of the eye.

Myoclonus A spasm of a portion of a muscle, an entire muscle, or a group of muscles.

Myoglobin The oxygen-transporting pigment of muscle consisting of one heme molecule containing one iron molecule attached to a single globin chain.

Myopathy Any disease or abnormal condition of skeletal muscle, usually characterized by muscle weakness, wasting, and histologic changes within muscle tissue.

Myotome The muscle plate or portion of an embryonic somite that develops into a voluntary muscle; or a group of muscles innervated by a single spinal segment.

Necrosis Localized tissue death that occurs in groups of cells or part of a structure or an organ in response to disease or injury.

Neutropenia An abnormal decrease in the number of neutrophilic leukocytes in the blood.

Nidus The point where a morbid process originates, develops, or is located.

Nociception The reception of painful stimuli from the physical or mechanical injury to body tissues by nociceptors (receptors usually found in either the skin or the walls of the viscera).

Nosocomial Pertaining to or originating in a hospital, such as a nosocomial infection; an infection acquired during hospitalization.

Nystagmus Involuntary, rapid, rhythmic movements of the eyeball.

Oncogene A gene that is capable of causing the initial and continuing conversion of normal cells into cancer cells.

Oncotic Relating to, caused by, or marked by edema or any swelling.

Oocyte A primordial or incompletely developed ovum.

Oogenesis The process of the growth and maturation of the female gametes, or ova.

Opsonization The process of making cells, such as bacteria, more susceptible to the action of phagocytes.

Organelle Any one of the various membrane-bound particles of distinctive morphology and function present within most cells, as the mitochondria, the Golgi complex, and the lysosomes.

Orthopnea An abnormal condition in which a person must be in an upright position in order to breathe deeply or comfortably.

Orthosis An external orthopedic appliance or apparatus, as a brace or splint, used to support, align, prevent or correct deformities, or to improve the function of movable parts of the body.

Osmolality The concentration of osmotically active particles in solution expressed in osmols or milliosmols per kilogram of solvent.

Osmolarity The concentration of osmotically active particles in solution expressed in osmols or milliosmols per litre of solution.

Osmosis The movement or passage of a pure solvent, such as water, through a semipermeable membrane from a solution that has a lower solute concentration to one that has a higher solute concentration.

Osteophyte A bony project or outgrowth.

Palpable Perceptible by touch.

Papilla A small nipple-shaped projection, elevation, or structure, as the conoid papillae of the tongue.

Papule A small, circumscribed, solid elevation of the skin less than one centimetre in diameter. (Adjective: papular)

Paracrine A mode of hormone action in which a chemical messenger that is synthesized and released from a cell acts on nearby cells of a different type and affects their function.

Paralysis An abnormal condition characterized by the impairment or loss of motor function due to a lesion of the neural or muscular mechanism.

Paraneoplastic Relating to alterations produced in tissue remote from a tumour or its metastases.

Parenchyma The basic tissue or elements of an organ as distinguished from supporting or connective tissue or elements. (Adjective: parenchymal)

Paresis Slight or partial paralysis.

Paresthesia Any abnormal touch sensation, which can be experienced as numbness, tingling, or a "pins and needles" feeling, often in the absence of external stimuli.

Parietal Pertaining to the outer wall of a cavity or organ; or pertaining to the parietal bone of the skull or the parietal lobe of the brain.

Parous Having borne one or more viable offspring.

Pathogen Any microorganism capable of producing disease.

Pedigree A systematic presentation, such as in a table, chart, or list, of an individual's ancestors that is used in human genetics in the analysis of inheritance.

Peptide Any of a class of molecular chain compounds composed of two or more amino acids joined by peptide bonds.

Perfusion The process or act of pouring over or through, especially the passage of a fluid through a specific organ or an area of the body.

Peripheral Pertaining to the outside, surface, or surrounding area of an organ or other structure; or located away from a centre or central structure.

Permeable A condition of being pervious, or permitting passage, so that fluids and certain other substances can pass through, as a permeable membrane.

Pervasive Pertaining to something that becomes diffused throughout every part.

Petechia A tiny, perfectly round, purplish red spot that appears on the skin as a result of minute intradermal or submucous hemorrhage. (Plural: petechiae)

Phagocytosis The process by which certain cells engulf and consume foreign material and cell debris.

Phalanx Any one of the bones composing the fingers of each hand and the toes of each foot.

Phenotype The complete physical, biochemical, and physiologic makeup of an individual, as determined by the interaction of both genetic makeup and environmental factors.

Pheresis A procedure in which blood is withdrawn from a donor, a portion (plasma, leukocytes, etc.) is separated and retained, and the remainder is reperfused into the donor. It includes plasmapheresis and leukopheresis.

Pili Hair; or in microbiology, the minute filamentous appendages of certain bacteria. (Singular: pilus)

Plethoric Relating to an excess of any of the body fluids, especially blood; the term used to describe the beefy red coloration of a newborn.

Plexus A network of intersecting nerves, blood vessels, or lymphatic vessels.

Polygene Any of a group of nonallelic genes that interact to influence the same character in the same way so that the effect is cumulative, usually of a quantitative nature, as size, weight, or skin pigmentation. (Adjective: polygenic)

Polymorph One of several, or many, forms of an organism or cell. (Adjective: polymorphic)

Polyp A small, tumour-like growth that protrudes from a mucous membrane surface.

Polypeptide A molecular chain of more than two amino acids joined by peptide bonds.

Presbyopia A visual condition (farsightedness) that commonly develops with advancing years or old age in which the lens loses elasticity causing defective accommodation and inability to focus sharply for near vision.

Prevalence The number of new and old cases of a disease that are present in a population at a given time or occurrences of an event during a particular period of time.

Prodrome An early symptom indicating the onset of a condition or disease. (Adjective: prodromal)

Prokaryotic Pertaining to an organism, such as bacterium, with cells lacking a true nucleus and nuclear membrane that reproduces through simple fission.

Prolapse The falling down, sinking, or sliding of an organ from its normal position or location in the body.

Proliferation The reproduction or multiplication of similar forms, especially cells.

Pronation Assumption of a position in which the ventral, or front, surface of the body or part of the body faces downward. (Adjective: prone)

Propagation The act or action of reproduction.

Proprioception The reception of stimuli originating from within the body regarding body position and muscular activity by proprioceptors (sensory nerve endings found in muscles, tendons, joints).

Prosthesis An artificial replacement for a missing body part; or a device designed and applied to improve function, such as a hearing aid.

Proteoglycans Any one of a group of polysaccharide-protein conjugates occurring primarily in the matrix of connective tissue and cartilage.

Proto-oncogene A normal cellular gene that with alteration, such as by mutation, becomes an active oncogene.

Proximal Closer to a point of reference, usually the trunk of the body, than other parts of the body.

Pruritus The symptom of itching, an uncomfortable sensation leading to the urge to rub or scratch the skin to obtain relief. (Adjective: pruritic)

Purpura A small hemorrhage, up to about 1 cm in diameter, in the skin, mucous membrane, or serosal surface; or any of several bleeding disorders characterized by the presence of purpuric lesions.

Purulent Producing or containing pus.

Quiescent Quiet, causing no disturbance, activity, or symptoms.

Reflux An abnormal backward or return flow of a fluid, such as stomach contents, blood, or urine.

Regurgitation A flow of material that is in the opposite direction from normal, as in the return of swallowed food into the mouth or the backward flow of blood through a defective heart valve.

Remission The partial or complete disappearance of the symptoms of a chronic or malignant disease; or the period of time during which the abatement of symptoms occurs.

Resorption The loss of substance or bone by physiologic or pathologic means, for example, the loss of dentin and cementum of a tooth.

Retrograde Moving backward or against the usual direction of flow; reverting to an earlier state or worse condition (degenerating); catabolic.

Retroversion A condition in which an entire organ is tipped backward or in a posterior direction, usually without flexion or other distortion.

Rhabdomyolysis Destruction or degeneration of muscle, associated with myoglobinuria (excretion of myoglobin in the urine).

Rostral Situated near a beak (oral or nasal region).

Sacroiliitis Inflammation in the sacroiliac joint.

Sclerosis A condition characterized by induration or hardening of tissue resulting from any of several causes, including inflammation, diseases of the interstitial substance, and increased formation of connective tissues.

Scotopic vision Describes vision, especially night vision, when the eye is dark adapted.

Semipermeable Partially but not wholly permeable, especially a membrane that permits the passage of some (usually small) molecules but not of other (usually larger) particles.

Senescence The process or condition of aging or growing old.

Sepsis The presence in the blood or other tissues of pathogenic microorganisms or their toxins; or the condition resulting from the spread of microorganisms or their products. (Adjective: septic)

Serous Relating to or resembling serum; or containing or producing serum, such as a serous gland.

Shunt To divert or bypass bodily fluid from one channel, path, or part to another; a passage or anastomosis between two natural channels, especially between blood vessels, established by surgery or occurring as an abnormality.

Soma The body of an organism as distinguished from the mind; all of an organism, excluding germ cells; the body of a cell.

Spasticity The condition characterized by spasms or other uncontrolled contractions of the skeletal muscles. (Adjective: spastic)

Spatial Relating to, having the character of, or occupying space.

Sphincter A ringlike band of muscle fibres that constricts a passage or closes a natural orifice of the body.

Stenosis An abnormal condition characterized by the narrowing or stricture of a duct or canal.

Stochastic Involving a random process.

Stria A streak or a linear scarlike lesion that often results from rapidly developing tension in the skin; or a narrow bandlike structure, especially the longitudinal collections of nerve fibres in the brain.

Stricture An abnormal temporary or permanent narrowing of the lumen of a duct, canal, or other passage, such as the esophagus, because of inflammation, external pressure, or scarring.

Stroma The supporting tissue or the matrix of an organ as distinguished from its functional element, or parenchyma.

Stupor A lowered level of consciousness characterized by lethargy and unresponsiveness in which a person seems unaware of his or her surroundings.

Subchondral Beneath a cartilage.

Subcutaneous Beneath the skin.

Subluxation An incomplete or partial dislocation in which the relationship between joint surfaces is altered, but contact remains.

Sulcus A shallow groove, depression, or furrow on the surface of an organ, such as a sulcus on the surface of the brain, separating the gyri.

Supination Assuming the position of lying horizontally on the back, or with the face upward. (Adjective: supine)

Suppuration The formation of pus, or purulent matter.

Symbiosis Mode of living characterized by close association between organisms of different species, usually in a mutually beneficial relationship.

Sympathomimetic An agent or substance that produces stimulating effects on organs and structures similar to those produced by the sympathetic nervous system.

Syncope A brief lapse of consciousness due to generalized cerebral ischemia.

Syncytium A multinucleate mass of protoplasm produced by the merging of a group of cells.

Syndrome A complex of signs and symptoms that occur together to present a clinical picture of a disease or inherited abnormality.

Synergist An organ, agent, or substance that aids or cooperates with another organ, agent, or substance.

Synthesis An integration or combination of various parts or elements to create a unified whole.

Systemic Pertaining to the whole body rather than to a localized area or regional portion of the body.

Systole The contraction, or period of contraction, of the heart that drives the blood onward into the aorta and pulmonary arteries.

Tamponade Stoppage of the flow of blood to an organ or a part of the body by pathologic compression, such as the compression of the heart by an accumulation of pericardial fluid.

Teratogen Any agent or factor that induces or increases the incidence of developmental abnormalities in the fetus.

Thrombus A stationary mass of clotted blood or other formed elements that remains attached to its place of origin along the wall of a blood vessel, frequently obstructing the circulation. (Plural: thrombi)

Tinnitus A tinkling, buzzing, or ringing noise heard in one or both ears.

Tophus A chalky deposit containing sodium urate that most often develops in periarticular fibrous tissue, typically in individuals with gout. (Plural: tophi)

Torsion The act or process of twisting in either a positive (clockwise) or negative (counterclockwise) direction.

Trabecula A supporting or anchoring stand of connective tissue, such as the delicate fibrous threads connecting the inner surface of the arachnoid to the pia mater.

Transmural Situated or occurring through the wall of an organ.

Transudate A fluid substance passed through a membrane or extruded from the blood.

Tremor Involuntary quivering or trembling movements caused by the alternating contraction and relaxation of opposing groups of skeletal muscles.

Trigone A triangular-shaped area.

Ubiquitous The condition or state of existing or being everywhere at the same time.

Ulcer A circumscribed excavation of the surface of an organ or tissue, which results from necrosis that ac-companies some inflammatory, infectious, or malignant processes. (Adjective: ulcerative)

Urticaria A pruritic skin eruption of the upper dermis, usually transient, characterized by wheals (hives) of various shapes and sizes.

Uveitis An inflammation of all or part of the uveal tract of the eye.

Vector An invertebrate animal (*e.g.,* tick, mite, mosquito) that serves as a carrier, transferring an infective agent from one vertebrate host to another.

Ventral Pertaining to a position toward the belly of the body; or situated or oriented toward the front or anterior of the body.

Vertigo An illusory sensation that the environment or one's own body is revolving.

Vesicle A small bladder or sac, as a small, thin-walled, raised skin lesion, containing liquid.

Visceral Pertaining to the viscera, or internal organs of the body.

Viscosity Pertaining to the physical property of fluids, caused by the adhesion of adjacent molecules, that determines the internal resistance to shear forces.

Zoonosis A disease of animals that may be transmitted to humans from its primary animal host under natural conditions.

Index

Note: Page numbers followed by the letter f refer to figures; those followed by the letter t refer to tables; those followed by the letter b refer to boxes; and those followed by the letter c refer to charts.

A

ABCDE rule, for malignant melanoma, 1623f, 1624
Abciximab, 271
Abdominal aortic aneurysms, 513
Abdominal obesity, hypertension risk, 532–533
Abducens nerve, 1232
Ablation therapy, for arrhythmias, 621
Abnormal corneal deposits, 1424
Abnormal nystagmus, 1475–1476
ABO blood groups, 303t, 304
Abscess, 347, 400
  Bartholin gland, 1154
  formation of, 400, 401f
  lung, 724
  prostatic, 1129
Absence seizures, 1357–1358
Absolute refractory period
  cardiac conduction system and, 607–608, 608f
  in neurophysiology, 1213
Absorption, 933. *See also* Gastrointestinal (GI) tract
Abuse
  child, 30, 39
  disorders, 1402–1404
  physical, 30
  sexual, 30
  substance, 35, 1403
Acalculous cholecystitis, 1000
Acanthamoeba keratitis, 1424
Acanthosis nigricans, 187, 187t
Acceptable macronutrient distribution range (AMDR), 1011
Accessory muscles of inspiration, 670
Accessory organs
  gastrointestinal tract, 917, 918 (*see also* Gastrointestinal (GI) tract)
  male, 1108–1109
    bulbourethral glands, 1108
    prostate gland, 1108–1109
    seminal vesicles, 1108
Accommodation, 1430
  disorders of, 1430–1431, 1430f
Accutane. *See* Isotretinoin
ACE inhibitors. *See* Angiotensin-converting enzyme (ACE) inhibitors
Acetaminophen
  in fever, 228
  and liver necrosis, 109
  in osteoarthritis treatment, 1565
  overdose, 982
Acetylcholine (ACh), 428, 492, 931, 1216, 1245, 1246, 1247f, 1298
  and drug- and toxin-induced disorders, 607
  and heart rate, 607
  hypermagnesemia and, 824
  in myasthenia gravis, 1299–1300
  in neuromuscular junction disorders, 1298, 1298f
  as neurotransmitter for parasympathetic neurons, 492
  for urinary incontinence, 910
Acetylcholinesterase, 1298

Acetylcholinesterase inhibitors, in dementia, 54
Acetyl-coenzyme A (acetyl-CoA), 79, 977–978, 977f
N-acetylcysteine, 982
Achalasia, 940
Achilles tendons, 1555
Achlorhydria, 47
Achondroplasia, 128, 143t
Acid–base balance, 827–828
  acid–base chemistry, 828
    acid, 828
    base, 828
    dissociation constant, 828
    pH, 828
  disorders of, 836
    chronic kidney disease and, 885–886
    compensatory mechanisms, 836–837
    metabolic acidosis, 837–841, 838c, 838t
    metabolic alkalosis, 841–843, 841t, 842f
    metabolic *versus* respiratory, 836, 837t
    respiratory acidosis, 843–844, 844t
    respiratory alkalosis, 844–845, 844t
    single *versus* mixed, 836–837, 837t
  laboratory tests for, 834–835, 835f, 835t
    anion gap, 835, 835f
    base excess or deficit, 835
    carbon dioxide and bicarbonate levels, 835
  metabolic acid and bicarbonate production, 828–829, 828f
    carbon dioxide and bicarbonate production, 829
    fixed or nonvolatile acids and bases production, 829
    nonvolatile acids, 828–829
  pH
    calculation of, 829
    regulation of, 829–834
  volatile acid, 828
Acid-fast stain, bacteria classification, 340
Acidosis, 836
  metabolic, 837–841, 838c, 838t
  respiratory, 843–844, 844t
Acne, 1599–1600
  conglobata, 1600, 1602
  mild, 1600
  moderate, 1600
  vulgaris, 1600–1601, 1600f
    diagnosis of, 1600
    treatment of, 1600–1601
Acoustic nerve, 1232
Acoustic neuromas, 1467
Acquired conditions, 4
Acquired immunodeficiency syndrome (AIDS), 338, 443, 1538, 1560
  clinical course, 449–454
  diagnostic methods, 455–456
  emergence of, 444
  epidemiology, 443–444, 444t
  management of, 457
  pathophysiology, 446–449
  prevention, 455
  psychosocial issues, 459
  transmission of HIV infection, 444–445
  treatment, 457–459, 458t

Acral lentiginous melanomas, 1624
Acromegaly, 1042, 1052–1053
  causes of, 1052
  clinical manifestations of, 1052–1053, 1052f
  diagnosis of, 1053
  incidence of, 1052
  and sleep apnea syndrome, 1053
  treatment goals for, 1053
Acromioclavicular joint, 1498
ACS. *See* Acute coronary syndrome (ACS)
Action potentials, 84–86, 1212–1213, 1213f
  absolute refractory period, 1213
  depolarization, 1213
  hyperpolarization, 1213
  hypopolarization, 1213
  polarized state, 1213
  relative refractory period, 1213
  repolarization, 1213
  resting membrane potential, 1213
  threshold potential, 1213
Active immunity, 384
Active synovitis, 1551. *See also* Rheumatoid arthritis (RA)
Active transport system, 80f, 81, 81f
  primary, 81
  secondary, 81
Activities of daily living (ADLs), 41, 49
Activity. *See* Exercise
Activity tolerance, assessment of, 243
Acuity, 1256
Acute anterior uveitis, 1559. *See also* Ankylosing spondylitis
Acute bacterial conjunctivitis, 1421
Acute chest syndrome, 296
Acute coronary syndrome (ACS), 560–569, 561f, 563f, 566f–568f
  cardiac rehabilitation programs, 568–569
  clinical presentation of, 563–564
  complications of, 567–568
  electrocardiographic changes with, 560–561, 561f
  management of, 564–567
    coronary artery bypass grafting, 566–567, 566f
    fibrinolytic therapy, 565–566
    percutaneous coronary intervention, 566, 566f
    reperfusion strategies, 565
  non–ST-segment elevation myocardial infarction (NSTEMI), 560, 562
  postinfarction recovery period, 567–568, 567f, 568f
  serum biomarkers for, 561–562
  ST-segment elevation myocardial infarction (STEMI), 560, 562–563, 563f
  unstable angina, 560, 562
Acute disorder, 6
Acute gouty arthritis, 1566. *See also* Gout
Acute heart failure syndromes (AHFSs), 635
Acute lung injury, shock and, 650
Acute lymphocytic (lymphoblastic) leukemia (ALL), 324–326. *See also* Leukemias
Acute myelogenous (myeloblastic) leukemia (AML), 324–326. *See also* Leukemias

PREFIXES

a-, an- without, lack of
apnea (without breath)
anemia (lack of blood)

ab- separation, away from
abductor (leading away from)
aberrant (away from the usual course)

ad- to, toward, near to
adductor (leading toward)
adrenal (near the kidney)

ana- up, again, excessive
anapnea (to breathe again)
anasarca (severe edema)

ante- before, in front of
antecubital (in front of the elbow)
antenatal (occurring before birth)

anti- against, counter
anticoagulant (opposing coagulation)
antisepsis (against infection)

ap-, apo- separation, derivation from
apocrine (type of glandular secretion that contains cast-off parts of the secretory cell)

aut-, auto- self
autoimmune (immunity to self)
autologous (pertaining to self graft or blood transfusion)

bi- two, twice, double
biarticulate (pertaining to two joints)
bifurcation (two branches)

brady- slow
bradyesthesia (slowness or dullness of perception)

cata- down, under, lower, negative, against
catabolism (breaking down)
catalepsy (diminished movement)

circum- around, about
circumflex (winding around)
circumference (surrounding)

contra- against, counter
contraindicated (not indicated)
contralateral (opposite side)

de- away from, down from, remove
dehydrate (remove water)
deaminate (remove an amino group)

dia- through, apart, across, completely
diapedesis (ooze through)
diagnosis (complete knowledge)

dis- apart, reversal, separation
discrete (made up of separated parts)
disruptive (bursting apart)

dys- difficulty, faulty, painful
dysmenorrhea (painful menstruation)
dyspnea (difficulty breathing)

e-, ex- out from, out of
enucleate (remove from)
exostosis (outgrowth of bone)

ec- out from
eccentric (away from center)
ectopic (out of place)

ecto- outside, situated on
ectoderm (outer skin)
ectoretina (outer layer of retina)

em-, en- in, on
empyema (pus in)
encephalon (in the brain)

endo- within, inside
endocardium (within heart)
endometrium (within uterus)

epi- upon, after, in addition
epidermis (on skin)
epidural (upon dura)

eu- well, easily, good
eupnea (easy or normal respiration)
euthyroid (normal thyroid function)

exo- outside
exocolitis (inflammation of outer coat of colon)
exogenous (originating outside)

extra- outside of, beyond
extracellular (outside cell)
extrapleural (outside pleura)

hemi- half
hemialgia (pain affecting only one side of the body)
hemilingual (affecting one side of the tongue)

hyper- extreme, above, beyond
hyperemia (excessive blood)
hypertrophy (overgrowth)

hypo- under, below
hypotension (low blood pressure)
hypothyroidism (underfunction of thyroid)

im-, in- in, into, on
immersion (act of dipping in)
injection (act of forcing fluid into)

im-, in- not
immature (not mature)
inability (not able)

infra- beneath
infraclavicular (below the clavicle)
infraorbital (below the eye)

inter- among, between
intercostal (between the ribs)
intervene (come between)

intra- within, inside
intraocular (within the eye)
intraventricular (within the ventricles)

intro- into, within
introversion (turning inward)
introduce (lead into)

iso- equal, same
isotonia (equal tone, tension, or activity)
isotypical (of the same type)

juxta- near, close by
juxtaglomerular (near an adjoining glomerulus in the kidney)
juxtaspinal (near the spinal column)

macro- large, long, excess
macrocephaly (excessive head size)
macrodystrophia (overgrowth of a part)

mal- bad, abnormal
maldevelopment (abnormal growth or development)
malfunction (to function imperfectly or badly)

mega- large, enlarged, abnormally large size
megaprosopous (having a large face)
megasoma (great size and stature)

meso- middle, intermediate, moderate
mesoderm (middle germ layer of embryo)
mesocephalic (pertaining to a skull with an average breadth–length index)

meta- beyond, after, accompanying
metacarpal (beyond the wrist)
metamorphosis (change of form)

micro- small size or amount
microbe (a minute living organism)
microtiter (a titer of minute quantity)

neo- new, young, recent
neoformation (a new growth)
neonate (newborn)

oligo- few, scanty, less than normal
oligogenic (produced by a few genes)
oligospermia (abnormally low number of spermatozoa in the semen)

para- beside, beyond
paracardiac (beside the heart)
paraurethral (near the urethra)

per- through
perforate (bore through)
permeate (pass through)

peri- around
peribronchia (around the bronchus)
periosteum (around bone)

poly- many, much
polyphagia (excessive eating)
polytrauma (occurrence of multiple injuries)

post- after, behind in time or place
postoperative (after operation)
postpartum (after childbirth)

pre-, pro- in front of, before in time or place
premaxillary (in front of the maxilla)
prognosis (foreknowledge)

pseud-, pseudo- false, spurious
pseudocartilaginous (made up of a substance resembling cartilage)
pseudopregnancy (false pregnancy)

retro- backward, located behind
retrocervical (located behind cervix)
retrograde (going backward)